362 .1 LIPUB)

369 0290918

D1428997

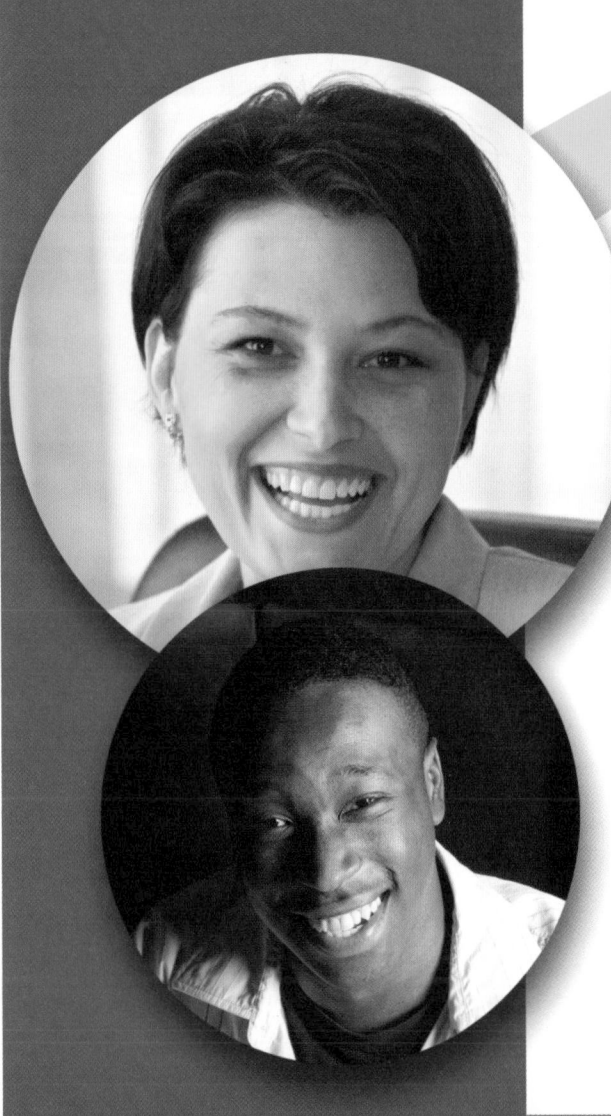

thePoint

Provides flexible learning solutions and resources for students and faculty using

Lippincott Manual of Nursing Practice, Tenth Edition

- **Get the Full text and an online image bank**
- Access medication tips and a dosage calculator
- Prepare for the NCLEX with drug-related NCLEX®-style questions
- Stay current with new clinical studies and the latest FDA updates

Log on today!

Visit **http://thepoint.lww.com/activate** to learn more about **thePoint™** and the resources available. Use the code provided below to access the student

http://thepoint.lww.com/activate

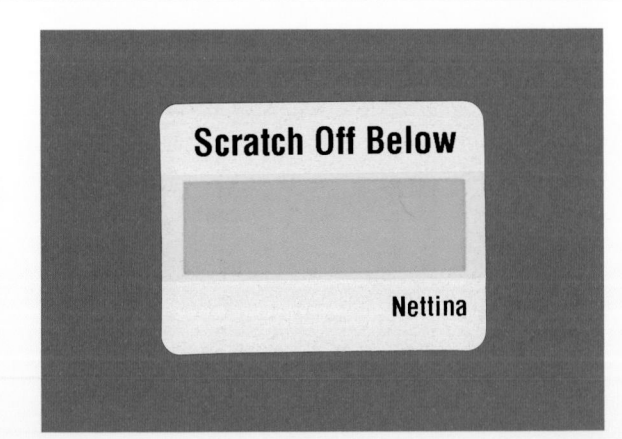

Scratch Off Below

Nettina

Note: Book cannot be returned once panel is scratched off.

The faculty resources are restricted to adopters of the text. Adopters have to be approved before accessing the faculty resources.

 Wolters Kluwer | Lippincott
Health | Williams & Wilkins

Health Improvement Library
Law House
Airdrie Road
Carluke
M18 5ER

LIPPINCOTT
MANUAL OF
NURSING PRACTICE

Tenth Edition

DATE DUE

			PRINTED IN U.S.A.

Health Improvement Library
Law House
Airdrie Road
Carluke
ML8 5ER

LIPPINCOTT
MANUAL OF NURSING PRACTICE

Tenth Edition

SANDRA M. NETTINA, MSN, ANP-BC
Nurse Practitioner
Columbia Medical Practice
Columbia, Maryland
Clinical Preceptor
Johns Hopkins University
School of Nursing
Baltimore, Maryland

Wolters Kluwer | Lippincott Williams & Wilkins
Health

Philadelphia • Baltimore • New York • London
Buenos Aires • Hong Kong • Sydney • Tokyo

Senior Acquistions Editor: Shannon W. Magee
Senior Book Designer: Joan Wendt
Production Project Manager: David Orzechowski
Developmental Editor: Lisa Marshall
Product Manager: Ashley Fischer
Copy Editor: Laura Patchkofsky
Illustrators: Judy Newhouse, Betty Winnberg
Senior Manufacturing Coordinator: Beth J. Welsh
Editorial Assistant: Marsha Gilbert
Compositor: SPi Global

Copyright © 2014 Wolters Kluwer Health | Lippincott Williams & Wilkins.

The clinical treatments described and recommended in this publication are based on research and consultation with nursing, medical, and legal authorities. To the best of our knowledge, these procedures reflect currently accepted practice. Nevertheless, they can't be considered absolute and universal recommendations. For individual applications, all recommendations must be considered in light of the patient's clinical condition and, before administration of new or infrequently used drugs, in light of the latest package insert information. The authors and publisher disclaim any responsibility for any adverse effects resulting from the suggested procedures, from any undetected errors, or from the reader's misunderstanding of the text.
© 2010 by Wolters Kluwer Health | Lippincott Williams & Wilkins.
© 2006, 2001 by Lippincott Williams & Wilkins.
© 1996 by Lippincott-Raven Publishers.
© 1991, 1986, 1982, 1978, 1974 by J. B. Lippincott Company.

All rights reserved. This book is protected by copyright. No part of it may be reproduced, stored in a retrieval system, or transmitted, in any form or by any means — electronic, mechanical, photocopy, recording, or otherwise — without prior written permission of the publisher, except for brief quotations embodied in critical articles and reviews and testing and evaluation materials provided by the publisher to instructors whose schools have adopted its accompanying textbook. Printed in China. For information, write Lippincott Williams & Wilkins, 323 Norristown Road, Suite 200, Ambler, PA 19002-2756.

LMNP9E010509

9 8 7 6 5 4 3 2 1

Not authorised for sale in the United States, Canada, Australia, New Zealand, Puerto Rico, and United States Virgin Islands.

Library of Congress Cataloging-in-Publication Data
Lippincott manual of nursing practice. — 10th ed. / [edited by] Sandra M. Nettina.
    p. ; cm.
  Manual of nursing practice
  Includes bibliographical references and index.
  ISBN 978-1-4511-7354-3
 I. Nettina, Sandra M. II. Title: Manual of nursing practice.
  [DNLM: 1. Nursing Care—Handbooks. WY 49]
  610.73—dc23

    2012045183

To purchase additional copies of this book, call our customer service department at (800) 638-3030 or fax orders to (301) 223-2320. International customers should call (301) 223-2300.

Visit Lippincott Williams & Wilkins on the Internet: http://www.lww.com. Lippincott Williams & Wilkins customer service representatives are available from 8:30 am to 6:00 pm, EST.

Dedicated to the nurses who teach, educate, mentor, precept, and support new and future nurses. Whether you are a paid educator, or a natural role model who assists with clinical training in addition to all your other duties, you are needed and appreciated. The art of nursing must be experienced and nurtured within students and recent graduates. Quality care is not gleaned from science alone. Our profession depends on all those who have followed in the footsteps of the Lady with the lamp…

to improve the health of individuals and the quality of health care.

CONTENTS

PART FIVE
PSYCHIATRIC NURSING

APPENDICES

CONTRIBUTORS
AND REVIEWERS

CONTRIBUTORS

CHAPTER 1   Nursing Practice and the Nursing Process
Sandra M. Nettina, MSN, ANP-BC
Nurse Practitioner
Columbia, Maryland
Clinical Preceptor
Johns Hopkins University School of Nursing
Baltimore, Maryland

CHAPTER 2   Standards of Care and Ethical and Legal Issues
Julia Olijnyk Selah, MSN, RN, ANP-C
Legal Nurse Consultant
Herndon, Virginia
Nurse Practitioner
Clinical Monitoring Research Program
SAIC-Frederick, Inc.
Frederick, Maryland

CHAPTER 3   Health Promotion and Preventive Care
Sandra M. Nettina, MSN, ANP-BC
Nurse Practitioner
Columbia, Maryland
Clinical Preceptor
Johns Hopkins University School of Nursing
Baltimore, Maryland

CHAPTER 4   Genetics and Health Applications
Yvette P. Conley, PhD
Associate Professor of Nursing and Human Genetics
University of Pittsburgh
Pittsburgh, Pennsylvania

CHAPTER 5   Adult Physical Assessment
Sandra M. Nettina, MSN, ANP-BC
Nurse Practitioner
Columbia, Maryland
Clinical Preceptor
Johns Hopkins University School of Nursing
Baltimore, Maryland

CHAPTER 6   Intravenous Therapy
Sandy Hamilton, BSN, MEd, RN, CRNI
Hospice Manager
Horizon Home Health and Hospice
Meridian, Idaho

CHAPTER 7   Perioperative Nursing
Claudia G. King, BSN, CNOR, RNFA
Clinical Mentor/Educator, Surgical Services
Carroll Hospital Center
Westminster, Maryland

CHAPTER 8   Cancer Nursing
Carol DeClue Riley, MSN, CRNP
Nurse Practitioner
Johns Hopkins Kimmel Cancer Center
Baltimore, Maryland

CHAPTER 9   Care of the Older or Disabled Adult
Elizabeth Galik, PhD, CRNP
Assistant Professor

Barbara Resnick, PhD, CRNP, FAAN, FAANP
Professor, Sonya Gershwitz Chair in Gerontology
University of Maryland School of Nursing
Baltimore, Maryland

Ann A. Scheve, MS, RN
Clinical Faculty, College of Nursing
Villanova University
Villanova, Pennsylvania

CHAPTER 10   Respiratory Function and Therapy
Brenda Windemuth, DNP, CRNP
Assistant Professor
University of Maryland School of Nursing
Baltimore, Maryland

CHAPTER 11   Respiratory Disorders
Chris Garvey, MSN, MPA, FNP, FAACVPR
Manager, Pulmonary and Cardiac Rehabilitation
Seton Medical Center
Daly City, California
Nurse Practitioner
Sleep Disorders Center
University of California at San Francisco
San Francisco, California

CHAPTER 12   Cardiovascular Function and Therapy

CHAPTER 13   Cardiac Disorders
Ann Marie Cullen, MSN, CCRN
Nurse Clinician III

Dzifa Dordunoo, MSN, CCRN
Nurse Clinician I

Joy A. Malanyaon, RN, BSN, CCRN
Nurse Clinician II

Mary Grace Nayden, RN, BSN
Nurse Clinician III, Discharge Planner
Johns Hopkins Hospital
Baltimore, Maryland

Alicia Williams, MS, CCRN, CCNS, CRNP
Nurse Practitioner, Cardiac Surgery
University of Maryland Medical Center
Baltimore, Maryland

CHAPTER 14   Vascular Disorders
Theresa E. DeVeaux, MS, ACNP, CCRN
Nurse Practitioner
Maryland Vascular Center at Baltimore Washington Medical Center
Glen Burnie, Maryland

Melody S. Heffline, MSN, ACNS, ACNP
Nurse Practitioner
Southern Surgical Group, Lexington Medical Center
West Columbia, South Carolina

Debra Kohlman-Trigoboff, ACNP-BC, CVN
Nurse Practitioner, Heart and Vascular
Duke University Medical Center
Durham, North Carolina

Marge Lovell, RN, CCRC, MEd
Clinical Trials Nurse, Vascular Surgery
London Health Sciences Center
London, Ontario, Canada

Leslie Beth Sossoman, MSN, ACNP, CPHQ, CVN
Nurse Practitioner, Cardiovascular Institute
Presbyterian Hospital
Charlotte, North Carolina

CHAPTER 15   Neurologic Disorders
Denise Miller Niklasch, DNP, ANP, CNRN
Neuro-critical Care Nurse Practitioner
Medical College of Wisconsin
Milwaukee, Wisconsin

Angela Starkweather, PhD, ACNP-BC, CNRN
Assistant Professor, School of Nursing
Virginia Commonwealth University
Richmond, Virginia

CHAPTER 16   Eye Disorders
Agueda Lara-Smalling, BSN, MPH
Nurse Reviewer-Research
Michael E. DeBakey VA Medical Center
Houston, Texas

CHAPTER 17   Ear, Nose, and Throat Disorders
Doreen Frances Gagné, MS, CRNP, CORLN
Otolaryngology Nurse Practitioner
Summit ENT and Hearing Services
Chambersburg, Pennsylvania

Carol Sailese Maragos, MSN, CRNP, CORLN
Otolaryngology Nurse Practitioner
Johns Hopkins Hospital
Baltimore, Maryland

CHAPTER 18   Gastrointestinal Disorders
Dawn L. Piercy, MS, NP, CCRC
Senior Nurse Practitioner and Clinical Trials Manager
Duke University Medical Center
Durham, North Carolina

CHAPTER 19   Hepatic, Biliary, and Pancreatic Disorders
JoAnn Coleman, DNP, ANP, ACNP, AOCN
Clinical Program Coordinator, Geriatric Surgery
Sinai Hospital
Baltimore, Maryland

Cynthia Cohen, DNP, ACNP, ANP
Nurse Practitioner
Johns Hopkins Comprehensive Transplant Center
Baltimore, Maryland
Assistant Professor of Nursing
University of Maryland
Baltimore, Maryland

CHAPTER 20   Nutritional Problems
Karen Flanders, MSN, NP-C, APRN, BC, CBN
Bariatric Coordinator, Nurse Practitioner
Winchester Hospital
Winchester, Massachusetts

CHAPTER 39   Complications of the Childbearing Experience
Keiko L. Tordersen, MS, RNC
CNO, Perinatal University
Adjunct Faculty for University of Alaska and
    University of Phoenix

Carol A. Curran, MS, RNC, OGNP
Perinatal Clinical Nurse Specialist, Educator
    and Consultant
Clinical Specialists Consulting, Inc. & Perinatal University
Virginia Beach, Virginia

CHAPTER 40   Pediatric Growth and Development

CHAPTER 41   Pediatric Physical Assessment
Laurie Scudder, DNP, PNP-C
President, Nurse Practitioner Alternatives
Editor, Medscape Pediatrics
Columbia, Maryland

CHAPTER 42   Pediatric Primary Care
Chritine Nelson-Tuttle, DNS, PNP-BC
Associate Professor
St. John Fisher College
Rochester, New York

CHAPTER 43   Care of the Sick or Hospitalized Child
Jocelyn Gmerek, MSN, PNP-C
Mary Kate Klarich, MSN, PNP-C
Pediatric Nurse Practitioners, General Surgery
Children's Hospital of Philadelphia
Philadelphia, Pennsylvania

CHAPTER 44   Pediatric Respiratory Disorders
Suzan E. Smallman, MSc, RGN, RSCN, LLBHons, NDNCert
Head of Division, Child Health (retired)
Birmingham City University
Edgbaston, Birmingham, England

CHAPTER 45   Pediatric Cardiovascular Disorders
Debbie Fraser Askin, MN, RNC-NIC
Associate Professor, Faculty of Health Disciplines
Athabascau University
Athabascau, Alberta, Canada

CHAPTER 46   Pediatric Neurologic Disorders
Maria Zak, MN, NP-Paediatrics
Nurse Practitioner-Pediatrics, Division of Neurology

Valerie W. Chan, BScN, RN, CNN
Neurology Clinic Nurse
The Hospital for Sick Children
Toronto, Ontario, Canada

CHAPTER 47   Pediatric Eye and Ear Problems
Zoe Strough O'Brien, MS, PNP-C
Pediatric Nurse Practitioner
Children's Pediatricians and Associates
Gaithersburg, Maryland

CHAPTER 48   Pediatric Gastrointestinal and Nutritional Disorders
Ellen Thomen Clore, MSN, CPNP-AC

Erin Garth, MSN, PNP-BC
Pediatric Nurse Practitioners
Children's National Medical Center
Washington, District of Columbia

CHAPTER 49   Pediatric Renal and Genitourinary Disorders
Catherine Daniels, MS, NP-Paediatrics
Nurse Practitioners, Urology

Anagaile Soriano, MN, NP-Paediatrics
Jill O'Hare, MN, NP-Paediatrics
Nurse Practitioners, Nephrology
The Hospital for Sick Children
Toronto, Ontario, Canada

CHAPTER 50   Pediatric Metabolic and Endocrine Disorders
Chritine Nelson-Tuttle, DNS, PNP-BC
Associate Professor
St. John Fisher College
Rochester, New York

CHAPTER 51   Pediatric Oncology

CHAPTER 52   Pediatric Hematologic Disorders
Katherine E. Heinze, RN, BSN, CPHON
PhD Student
Johns Hopkins University
Baltimore, Maryland

CHAPTER 53   Pediatric Immunologic Disorders
Georgina MacDougall, RN
HIV Clinic Nurse Coordinator

Audrey Bell-Peter, RN, MN
Rheumatology Nurse Coordinator

Holly Convery, BScN, NP-Primary Care
Clinic Nurse, Division of Rheumatology

Brenda Reid, RN, MN
Clinical Nurse Specialist, Immunology/Allergy
The Hospital for Sick Children
Toronto, Ontario, Canada

CHAPTER 54   Pediatric Orthopedic Problems
Catherine M. Haut, DNP, CPNP-AC, CPNP-PC, CCRN
Pediatric NP Program Director
University of Maryland
Pediatric Nurse Practitioner
Children's Hospital at Sinai
Baltimore, Maryland

CHAPTER 55   Pediatric Integumentary Disorders
Tonya L. Appleby, MSN, CCRN, CEN, ACNP-BC, GNP-BC
Acute and Geriatric Nurse Practitioner
Good Samaritan Hospital
Baltimore, Maryland

Pamela K. Fletcher, DNP, FNP-BC, DCNP
Dermatology Nurse Practitioner
UC Health Dermatology
Southgate, Kentucky
Nurse Educator
Northern Kentucky University
Highland Heights, Kentucky

Theodore D. Scott, MSN, FNP-C, DCNP
Nurse Practitioner, Dermatology
Kaiser-Permanente Medical Offices
San Marcus, California

CHAPTER 56   Developmental Disabilities
Chritine Nelson-Tuttle, DNS, PNP-BC
Associate Professor
St. John Fisher College
Rochester, New York

CHAPTER 57   Problems of Mental Health
Matthew R. Sorenson, PhD, RN
Director, Masters Entry to Practice Program
DePaul University
Chicago, Illinois

REVIEWERS

Barbara J. Brown, RN, DNC
Registered Nurse 4
Vanderbilt University Medical Center
Nashville, Tennessee

Carol George, RN, BSN, CRNO
Nurse Manager, Ophthalmology
University of Michigan Health System/Kellogg
   Eye Center
Ann Arbor, Michigan

Barbara Bulik Gottschalk, MSN, CRNP
Nurse Practitioner
The Listening Center at Johns Hopkins
Baltimore, Maryland

Alice Hillenbrand, MSN, RN, CNN, CURN
Renal Urology Education Specialist
Holy Name Medical Center
Teaneck, New Jersey

Betty McGinty, RN, BSHA, CGRN, MS HAS
Director of Gastroenterology Services
Northside Hospital
Atlanta, Georgia

Victoria Ruffing, RN, CCRP
Program Manager
Johns Hopkins Arthritis Center
Baltimore, Maryland

Elizabeth Turcotte, RN-BC, ONC
Nurse Manager
Orthopedic Institute of Central Maine at Maine Medical Center
Lewiston, Maine

PREFACE

I have been involved in direct patient care, clinical education and training, and heath policy leadership for over 35 years. I have been paid to care for patients inside and outside of the hospital, in medical offices, in long-term care facilities, and in homes. I have volunteered to mentor nursing students, provide health care for the homeless, and work at state and national levels to change nursing regulations and statutes. My experiences have been fulfilling, rewarding, exciting at times, and exhausting much of the time. It has been worth every minute, knowing the number of patients I have helped improve their health. It is also gratifying knowing that I played a part in training many nurses who are providing excellent care in many settings.

I now present the 10th edition of the *Lippincott Manual of Nursing Practice* with a challenge. This manual is meant to guide students and nurses in every setting and specialty to provide excellent patient care. I also present this book as a way for nurses to use best practices to help train and mentor other nurses.

ORGANIZATION

This new edition continues to follow a basic outline format for easy readability and access of information. The subheadings continue to follow a medical model—Pathophysiology and Etiology, Clinical Manifestations, Diagnostic Evaluation, Management, and Complications—and a nursing process model—Nursing Assessment, Nursing Diagnoses, Nursing Interventions, Community and Home Care Considerations, Patient Education and Health Maintenance, and Evaluation: Expected Outcomes. Medical model information is presented because nurses need to understand the medical disorder, diagnostic workup, and treatment that are the basis for nursing care. The nursing process section provides a practical overview of step-by-step nursing care for almost any patient scenario.

This edition is divided into five parts to present a comprehensive reference for all types of nursing care. Part One discusses the role of the nurse in the health care delivery system. It comprises chapters on Nursing Practice and the Nursing Process, Standards of Care and Ethical and Legal Issues, Health Promotion and Preventative Care, and Genetics and Health Applications.

Part Two encompasses medical-surgical nursing. General topics are presented in Unit I, including Adult Physical Assessment, Intravenous Therapy, Perioperative Nursing, Cancer Nursing, and Care of the Older or Disabled Adult. Units II through XII deal with body system function and dysfunction and the various disorders seen in adult medical and surgical nursing.

Part Three covers Maternity and Neonatal Nursing. Chapters include Maternal and Fetal Health, Nursing Management during Labor and Delivery, Care of the Mother and Newborn during the Postpartum Period, and Complications of the Childbearing Experience. Chapters reflect the routine childbearing experience as well as frequently encountered high-risk situations and problems that may arise for the mother as well as the infant.

Part Four focuses on Pediatric Nursing. Chapters are divided into two units. One unit covers General Practice Considerations, comprising Pediatric Growth and Development, Pediatric Physical Assessment, Pediatric Primary Care, and Care of the Sick or Hospitalized Child. The other unit contains chapters based on body systems to describe the various disorders and corresponding nursing care seen in pediatric nursing.

Part Five discusses Psychiatric Nursing. Entries follow the *Diagnostic and Statistical Manual of Mental Disorders*, Fourth Edition, Text Revision (DSM-IV-TR) classification of mental illness. Treatments and nursing management for each are discussed.

Sandra M. Nettina, MSN, ANP-BC

NEW TO THIS EDITION

New and Expanded Material

Information has been added to or extensively updated throughout chapters in these areas:

Chapter 1—cultural competency, changing health care systems, patient safety

Chapter 3—updated U.S. Preventive Services Task Force screening guidelines, dietary and exercise guidelines

Chapter 7—perioperative safety, World Health Organization Perioperative Checklist

Chapter 8—chemotherapy administration safety

Chapter 9—updated recommendations for older adult primary and secondary prevention

Chapter 10—extensive updating

Chapter 11—extensive updating

Chapter 12—extensive updating

Chapter 13—extensive updating

Chapter 14—new anticoagulant therapy, new hypertension drugs

Chapter 15—diagnostic imaging, management of many disorders

Chapter 16—drugs that elevate intraocular pressure

Chapter 17—instillation of ear drops

Chapter 20—MyPlate instead of the Food Pyramid, new bariatric surgeries

Chapter 22—new pelvic exam and cervical cancer screening guidelines, STD prevention counseling

Chapter 23—magnetic resonance imaging screening, hormonal treatment

Chapter 25—American Diabetic Association updates

Chapter 26—dietary iron sources

Chapter 27—updated blood and bone marrow stem cell transplantation

Chapter 28—latex safety for patients and health care workers, asthma drug update

Chapter 29—antiretroviral therapy update

Chapter 31—updated infection control guidelines

Chapter 35—characteristics of sepsis, alcohol withdrawal protocol

Chapter 42—lead update

Chapter 45—common pediatric cardiac drugs

Chapter 46—new seizure medications

Chapter 47—risk factors for eustachian tube dysfunction

Chapter 53—pediatric immunodeficiency, treatment of juvenile idiopathic arthritis

Chapter 56—fetal alcohol syndrome

Headings have been changed, eliminated, and made more uniform throughout the book. You will also find updated information on diagnostic tests and medical care for almost every entry. Nursing care has also been extensively updated to reflect new treatments and best practice information.

Evidence Base

Expanded in this edition is the inclusion of references within the text that reflect the evidence base for much of medical and nursing care. While the *Lippincott Manual* has always been prepared based on a combination of research review, extensive literature search, and expert clinical review, many nurses and students wanted to see a more direct line of evidence to the information. We have used a variety of evidence sources, including accepted guidelines and position statements, large research studies and meta-analyses, specialty texts, and review articles from authoritative sources. Based on this evidence base, information has been updated and procedure guidelines have been altered. Evidence has come from accepted sources worldwide.

Graphics

Many new figures, boxes, and tables have been added. A number of diagrams outlining the pathophysiology of important illnesses have been developed. A new and recurring logo, Key Decision Points, has been added to many Procedure Guidelines to highlight step-by-step information that may be necessary to follow during a procedure. All of these features will make it easier to access information in the busy clinical setting and translate that information to patient care.

It has been my pleasure preparing the 10th edition of the *Lippincott Manual of Nursing Practice* for you. I hope that it will serve you well in providing patient care and transferring your nursing expertise to other nurses.

Sandra M. Nettina, MSN, ANP-BC

ACKNOWLEDGMENTS

I would like to thank past and present reviewers and contributors and the entire Lippincott Williams & Wilkins team for their contribution to the *Lippincott Manual of Nursing Practice*, 10th edition. Lisa Marshall, project manager has been invaluable in guiding and supporting me in this project. Bruce Hobart kept the chapters, and all of us involved, moving through production. Christine Nelson-Tuttle provided additional review for all the pediatric chapters. Everyone involved has come to respect the enormity of the task and how each step affects the next. I am proud of our accomplishment.

Nursing Practice and
the Nursing Process

PART ONE

NURSING PROCESS AND PRACTICE

1
Nursing Practice and the Nursing Process

NURSING PRACTICE

Basic Concepts in Nursing Practice

Since Florence Nightingale developed the first model for nursing education in 1873, the role of the professional nurse and nursing scope of practice has evolved. Emphasis now is focused on evidence-based nursing care and preventive health practices. Understanding basic concepts in nursing practice, such as roles of nursing, theories of nursing, licensing, and legal issues, helps enhance performance.

Definition of Nursing

1. Nursing is an art and a science.
2. Earlier emphasis focused on care of the sick patient; now, the promotion of health is stressed.
3. American Nurses Association (ANA) definition, 1980: Nursing is the diagnosis and treatment of the human response to actual and potential health problems.

Roles of Nursing

Whether in a hospital-based or community health care setting, nurses assume three basic roles:

1. Practitioner—involves actions that directly meet the health care and nursing needs of patients, families, and significant others; includes staff nurses at all rungs of the clinical ladder, advanced practice nurses, and community-based nurses.
2. Leader—involves actions, such as deciding, relating, influencing, and facilitating, that affect the actions of others and are directed toward goal determination and achievement; may be a formal nursing leadership role or an informal role periodically assumed by the nurse.
3. Researcher—involves actions taken to implement studies to determine the actual effects of nursing care to further the scientific base of nursing; may include all nurses, not just academicians, nurse scientists, and graduate nursing students.

Theories of Nursing

1. Nursing theories help define nursing as a scientific discipline of its own.
2. The elements of nursing theories are uniform: nursing, patient, environment, and health—also known as the *paradigm* or *model* of nursing.
3. Nightingale was the first nursing theorist; she believed the purpose of nursing was to put the patient in the best condition for nature to restore or preserve health.
4. Theories range from broad to limited in scope.
   a. Grand nursing theories are the broadest and most abstract; they pertain to all nursing situations but are limited in directing or explaining nursing care.
   b. Middle-range nursing theories bridge grand theory with nursing practice; they can generate theoretical research and nursing practice strategies.
   c. Nursing practice theories (micro-range) are limited in scope; they provide framework for nursing interventions and predicted outcomes in specific nursing situations.
5. More recent nursing theorists include:
   a. Levine—nursing supports a patient's adaptation to change due to internal and external environmental stimuli.
   b. Orem—nurses assist the patient to meet universal, developmental, and health deviation self-care requisites.
   c. Roy—nurses manipulate stimuli to promote adaptation in four modes: physiologic, self-concept, role function, and interdependence relations.

d. Leninger—model of transcultural nursing; nurses should provide culturally specific care

e. Pender—nurses promote healthy behavior through a preventive model of health care

f. Rogers—nurses promote harmonious interaction between the patient and environment to maximize health; both are four-dimensional energy fields.

Nursing in the Health Care Delivery System

1. Technology, education, society values, demographics, and health care financing all have an impact on where and how nursing is practiced.

   a. As the population ages, chronic disease rates rise and health care utilization increases.

   b. Almost 50% of the U.S. population has one or more chronic conditions. According to the Center for Medicare and Medicaid Services, 75% of Medicare spending is on individuals with five or more chronic diseases. The cost of health care in the United States was over $2.5 trillion in 2009, or 17.6% of the gross domestic product (GDP).

   c. The World Economic Forum estimates that the global cost of treating the five most common noninfectious diseases (cancer, diabetes, heart disease, lung disease, and mental illness) at $47 trillion between 2011 and 2030, or 75% of the current global GDP.

   d. Health promotion and prevention strategies such as immunizations, health education, and screening tests aimed at reducing the incidence of infectious disease, injuries, and chronic illness save health care dollars and improve well-being. Nurses are well prepared for implementing health promotion strategies.

2. Unsuccessful cost-containing measures and a growing uninsured population led to the passage of the Patient Protection and Affordable Care Act of 2010, also known as health care reform in the United States. Emphasis is on preventive health care and coordination of care. Specific provisions phased in through 2015 ensure more options for people with pre-existing conditions that previously caused exclusion from coverage; allowing young people to stay on parent or family insurance policies until age 26; eliminating lifetime limits on coverage; providing small-business tax credits to provide coverage to employees; providing rebates on Medicare prescription costs; providing funding to states to expand Medicaid coverage; state insurance exchanges to offer more coverage for all citizens; preventive health services offered without extra cost; and linking payments to quality outcomes. For more information, go to *www.healthcare.gov.*

3. More patients are expected to enter the health care system, particularly in primary care, requiring more health care providers, more nurses, and more health care facilities.

   a. A nursing faculty shortage may challenge the ability of nursing to meet the needs of the expanded patient population. According to the American Association of Colleges of Nursing, nursing schools turned away a reported 11,000 qualified applicants in the United States in 2010.

   b. Advanced practice nurses may be utilized as primary care and acute care providers due to a shortage of physicians.

The Institute of Medicine 2010 report "The Future of Nursing" called for removal of regulatory barriers so nurses could practice to the full extent of their education and scope of practice.

Advanced Practice Nursing

1. Registered professional nurses with advanced training, education, and certification are allowed to practice in expanded scope.

2. This includes nurse practitioners, nurse-midwives, nurse-anesthetists, and clinical nurse specialists.

3. Scope of practice and legislation vary by state.

   a. Clinical nurse specialists are included in advanced practice nurse (APN) legislation in at least 25 states (some of these include only psychiatric/mental health clinical nurse specialists).

   b. Nurse practitioners have some type of prescriptive authority in all 50 states and the District of Columbia.

   c. In most cases, nurse practitioners are now eligible for Medicare reimbursement across the United States at 85% of the physician fee schedule and are eligible for Medicaid reimbursement in many states.

   d. Many states give authority to APNs through the Board of Nursing with no requirement for physician oversight or collaboration required.

4. Master's degree preparation is the current requirement for most APN roles; however, many certificate programs have trained APNs in the past 40 years. In addition, doctoral programs are becoming increasingly available, with emphasis on the practice role of APNs.

5. In Canada and other countries, the growth of the number of APNs in practice has been slower than in the United States, except for midwives in many cases.

Licensing, Certification, and Continuing Education

1. Every professional registered nurse must be licensed through the state board of nursing in the United States to practice in that state or the College of Nursing to practice in a Canadian province.

2. Although the state primarily regulates and restricts practice, the framework for scope of practice actually depends on a four-tier hierarchy: (1) the ANA Scope and Standards for Nursing Practice; (2) the particular state Nurse Practice Act; (3) the facility policies and procedures where the nurse is practicing; and (4) the nurse with her or his individual self-determination and competencies. Indeed, it is the nurse's responsibility to maintain competency and practice within the appropriate scope.

3. Continuing education requirements vary depending on state laws, facility policies, and area of specialty practice and certification. Continuing education units can be obtained through a variety of professional nursing organizations and commercial educational services.

4. Many professional nursing organizations exist to provide education, certification, support, and communication among nurses; for more information, contact your state nurses'

association, state board of nursing, or the ANA, 8515 Georgia Avenue, Suite 400, Silver Spring, MD 20910, 800-274-4ANA, *www.nursingworld.org*.

5. The Doctor of Nursing Practice (DNP) was introduced in 2005 to ensure that nursing can meet the demands of the changing health care system with the highest level of scientific knowledge and practice expertise.

   a. The American Association of Colleges of Nursing has proposed that the DNP replace the master's degree as preparation for advanced practice nursing by 2015; however, this is still up for debate.

   b. There are more than 150 DNP programs in the United States and many more are in development.

6. Nursing curriculum and the nursing role has expanded to meet the demands of an aging, chronically ill population; advanced technology in the acute care setting; and expanding preventive strategies and community-based care to promote a healthier population. A wide variety of certifications offered through the American Nurses Credentialing Center (*www.nursecredentialing.org*) acknowledge advanced preparation of nurse practitioners, clinical nurse specialists, home health nurses, case management nurses, and many other specialties.

7. A recent addition to the certification arena is that of the clinical nurse leader, which has a master's degree requirement. It is defined as a nursing generalist whose role is to improve the quality of nursing care. The clinical nurse leader provides direction at the point of care, collaborates with the health care team, provides risk assessment, and implements quality improvement strategies based on evidence-based practice.

Safe Nursing Care

Patient Safety

1. Adequate nursing staffing is essential to reduce nurses' dissatisfaction, burnout, and high turnover rates, as well as reduce patient mortality. Studies have linked inadequate staffing to increased patient mortality.

   a. A recent retrospective observation study at a Magnet hospital identified an average patient exposed to three nursing shifts with below staffing resulted in 6% higher risk of mortality than patients with no below-target mortality.

Evidence Base Needleman, J., Buerhaus, P., Pankratz, V. S., et al. (2011). Nursing staffing and inpatient hospital mortality. *New England Journal of Medicine*, 364(11), 1032–1045.

   b. The American Nursing Association campaign, "Safe Nursing Saves Lives," advocates that hospitals set staffing levels on each unit based on patient acuity, number of patient, nursing skills, support staff, and technology (*www.safestaffingsaveslives.org*).

2. The Institute of Medicine (IOM) of the National Academies has focused on deficient health care systems as the cause of medical errors that are preventable and result in about 50% of adverse events and patient deaths. The IOM offers recommendations for improving systems and processes in

---

> **BOX 1-1** **National Patient Safety Goals—Hospital Program***
>
> Use at least two patient identifiers when providing care, treatment, and services.
>
> Eliminate transfusion errors related to patient misidentification.
>
> Report critical results of tests and diagnostic procedures on a timely basis.
>
> Label all medications, medication containers, and other solutions on and off the sterile field in perioperative and other procedural settings.
>
> Reduce the likelihood of patient harm associated with the use of anticoagulant therapy.
>
> Maintain and communicate accurate patient medication information.
>
> Comply with either the current Centers for Disease Control and Prevention (CDC) hand hygiene guidelines or the current World Health Organization (WHO) hand hygiene guidelines.
>
> Implement evidence-based practices to prevent health care–associated infections due to multidrug-resistant organisms in acute care hospitals.
>
> Implement evidence-based practices to prevent central line–associated bloodstream infections.
>
> Implement evidence-based practices for preventing surgical site infections.
>
> Implement evidence-based practices to prevent indwelling catheter-associated urinary tract infections (CAUTI).
>
> Identify patients at risk for suicide.
>
> Conduct a preprocedure verification process.
>
> Mark the procedure site.
>
> A time-out is performed before the procedure.
>
> ---
>
> *See www.jointcommission.org/assets/1/6/NPSG_EPs_Scoring_HAP_20110706.pdf for elements of performance. http://www.jointcommission.org/hap_2013_npsg/

---

health care organizations to ultimately improve patient safety. For more information, refer to the website *www.iom.edu*.

3. The Agency for Healthcare Research and Quality has compiled a wide array of patient safety literature as a resource for all types of health care providers and settings, available at *http://psnet.ahrq.gov/default.aspx*.

4. The Joint Commission is also committed to improving safety for patients in health care organizations. The National Patient Safety Goals were implemented in 2003 to help address specific concerns for patient safety by health care setting, including ambulatory care, long-term care, behavioral health care, home care, hospital, laboratory services, and office-based surgery. New goals are introduced yearly with suggested performance measures to meet the goals. These are available at *www.jointcommission.org/standards_information/npsgs.aspx*. See Box 1-1 for selected National Patient Safety Goals.

Personal Safety

1. Nurses may be at risk for personal harm in the workplace. The ANA has sponsored initiatives to improve nurses' personal safety. The Position Statement: Risk and Responsibility in Providing Nursing Care acknowledges that there may be

limits to the personal risk a nurse can assume in providing care in any clinical setting.

2. The Centers for Disease Control and Prevention estimates that 380,000 health care workers are injured by needles and other sharps each year, increasing the risk of hepatitis B, hepatitis C, and human immunodeficiency virus. Nurses sustain the largest percentage of these injuries. The ANA's "Safe Needles, Save Lives" (*www.needlestick.org*) campaign was key in promoting the use of safety devices. Nurses and other health care workers are protected by the Needlestick Safety and Prevention Act (P.L. 106-430), which requires health care organizations to use needleless or shielded-needle devices, obtain input from clinical staff in the evaluation and selection of devices, educate staff on the use of safety devices, and have an exposure control plan.

3. The physical work environment, which includes patient handling tasks such as manual lifting, transferring, and repositioning patients, can also place nurses at risk for musculoskeletal disorders such as back injuries and shoulder strains. The ANA's "Handle with Care" campaign (*www.nursingworld.org/handlewithcare*) aims to prevent such injuries and to promote safe patient handling through the use of technology and assistive patient-handling equipment and devices.

Culturally Competent Care

 Evidence Base Expert Panel on Global Nursing and Health. (2010). Standards of practice for culturally competent nursing care executive summary. Available: *www.tcns.org/TCNStandardsofPractice.html*.

The changing demographics of the United States, Canada, the United Kingdom, and other countries bring a diverse array of individuals with varying cultures and beliefs into nursing practice. Nurses must provide culturally competent care by expanding their knowledge about different cultures. Cultural competence involves learning a new set of attitudes, behaviors, and skills to help the nurse provide care effectively in cross-cultural situations. See Box 1-2, Standards of Practice for Culturally Competent Nursing Care. The Transcultural Nursing Society (TCNS) was founded in 1975 by Madaliene Leninger with a focus on human caring. Culturally congruent and competent care results in improved health and well-being for people worldwide. TCNS offers a peer-reviewed evidence-based journal, educational courses, and many other resources to provide information about the values, beliefs, and traditions of various cultures (*www.tcns.org*). However, the nurse must always use caution and avoid generalizing and stereotyping

---

BOX 1-2   Transcultural Nursing Standards of Practice

1. **Social Justice:** Professional nurses shall promote social justice for all. The applied principles of social justice guide decisions of nurses related to the patient, family, community, and other health care professionals. Nurses will develop leadership skills to advocate for socially just policies.

2. **Critical Reflection:** Nurses shall engage in critical reflection of their own values, beliefs, and cultural heritage in order to have an awareness of how these qualities and issues can impact culturally congruent nursing care.

3. **Transcultural Nursing Knowledge:** Nurses shall gain an understanding of the perspectives, traditions, values, practices, and family systems of culturally diverse individuals, families, communities, and populations for whom they care, as well as knowledge of the complex variables that affect the achievement of health and well-being.

4. **Cross-Cultural Practice:** Nurses shall use cross-cultural knowledge and culturally sensitive skills in implementing culturally congruent nursing care.

5. **Health Care Systems and Organizations:** Health care organizations should provide the structure and resources necessary to evaluate and meet the cultural and language needs of their diverse clients.

6. **Patient Advocacy and Empowerment:** Nurses shall recognize the effect of health care policies, delivery systems, and resources on their patient populations, and shall empower and advocate for their patients as indicated. Nurses shall advocate for the inclusion of their patient's cultural beliefs and practices in all dimensions of their health care when possible.

7. **Multicultural Workforce:** Nurses shall actively engage in the effort to ensure a multicultural workforce in health care settings. One measure to achieve a multicultural workforce is through strengthening of recruitment and retention effort in the hospital and academic setting.

8. **Education and Training:** Nurses shall be educationally prepared to promote and provide culturally congruent health care. Knowledge and skills necessary for ensuring that nursing care is culturally congruent shall be included in global health care agendas that mandate formal education and clinical training, as well as required ongoing, continuing education for all practicing nurses.

9. **Cross-Cultural Communication:** Nurses shall use culturally competent verbal and nonverbal communication skills to identify client's values, beliefs, practices, perceptions, and unique health care needs.

10. **Cross-Cultural Leadership:** Nurses shall have the ability to influence individuals, groups, and systems to achieve positive outcomes of culturally competent care for diverse populations.

11. **Policy Development:** Nurses shall have the knowledge and skills to work with public and private organizations, professional associations, and communities to establish policies and standards for comprehensive implementation and evaluation of culturally competent care.

12. **Evidence-Based Practice and Research:** Nurses shall base their practice on interventions that have been systematically tested and shown to be the most effective for the culturally diverse populations that they serve. In areas where there is a lack of evidence of efficacy, nurse researchers shall investigate and test interventions that may be the most effective in reducing the disparities in health outcomes.

Adapted with permission from the Society of Transcultural Nursing.

patients. Culturally competent care begins with an individualized patient assessment, including the patient's own definition of health and expectations for care. Based on this assessment and application of a set of standards, the nurse can develop an individualized care plan.

THE NURSING PROCESS

The nursing process is a deliberate, problem-solving approach to meeting the health care and nursing needs of patients. It involves assessment (data collection), nursing diagnosis, planning, implementation, and evaluation, with subsequent modifications used as feedback mechanisms to promote the resolution of the nursing diagnoses. The process as a whole is cyclical, with the steps being interrelated, interdependent, and recurrent.

Steps in the Nursing Process

Assessment—systematic collection of data to determine the patient's health status and to identify any actual or potential health problems. (Analysis of data is included as part of the assessment. For those who wish to emphasize its importance, analysis may be identified as a separate step of the nursing process.)

Nursing diagnosis—identification of actual or potential health problems that are amenable to resolution by nursing actions.

Planning—development of goals and a care plan designed to assist the patient in resolving the nursing diagnoses.

Implementation—actualization of the care plan through nursing interventions or supervision of others to do the same.

Evaluation—determination of the patient's responses to the nursing interventions and of the extent to which the goals have been achieved.

Assessment

1. The nursing history.
   a. Subjective data obtained by interviewing the patient, family members, or significant other and reviewing past medical records.
   b. Provides the opportunity to convey interest, support, and understanding to the patient and to establish a rapport based on trust.
2. The physical examination.
   a. Objective data obtained to determine the patient's physical status, limitations, and assets.
   b. Should be done in a private, comfortable environment with efficiency and respect.

Nursing Diagnosis

 Evidence Base NANDA International. (2012). *NANDA Nursing Diagnoses: Definitions and classifications, 2012–2014.* DeMoines, IA: Wiley Blackwell.

1. The process of making a clinical judgment about experiences or responses to health problems or life processes; based on an individual, family, or community and done through patient assessment rather than picked from a list of medical diagnoses.

BOX 1-3	NANDA International Domains of Nursing

Health Promotion
Nutrition
Elimination and Exchange
Activity/Rest
Perception/Cognition
Self-Perception
Role Relationships
Sexuality
Coping/Stress Tolerance
Life Principles
Safety/Protection
Comfort
Growth/Development

2. Used to determine the appropriate plan of care (ie, to select nursing interventions that will achieve desired outcomes).
3. Nursing diagnoses are based on the NANDA International taxonomy, which is a standardized nursing language that includes evidence-based definitions, defining characteristics, and etiologic factors.
   a. Nursing diagnoses continue to be developed and refined by NANDA International and the University of Iowa Center for Nursing Classification and Clinical Effectiveness.
   b. There are currently 206 nursing diagnoses grouped in 13 domains (see Box 1-3). Nursing diagnoses are listed throughout this book associated with medical diagnoses and other health conditions, but in reality, nursing diagnoses are formulated through individualized patient assessment.

Planning

See Nursing Care Plan 1-1.

 Evidence Base University of Iowa College of Nursing, Center for Nursing Classification and Clinical Effectiveness. (2013). *CNC-Overview: Nursing Outcomes Classification (NOC).* Available: *www.nursing.uiowa. edu/cncce/nursing-outcomes-classification-overview.*

1. Assign priorities to the nursing diagnoses. Highest priority is given to problems that are the most urgent and critical.
2. Establish goals or expected outcomes derived from the nursing diagnoses.
   a. Specify short-term, intermediate, and long-term goals as established by nurse and patient together.
   b. Goals should be specific, measurable, and patient-focused and should include a time frame.
   c. The Nursing Outcomes Classification developed by the University of Iowa College of Nursing Center is a comprehensive, standardized nursing language of outcomes used to evaluate the effects of nursing interventions. Each of the approximately 490 outcomes includes a list of indicators and is linked to NANDA I nursing diagnoses.

NURSING CARE PLAN 1-1

Example of a Nursing Care Plan

Mr. John Preston, a 52-year-old businessperson, was admitted with chest pain; rule out myocardial infarction. He had experienced substernal chest pain and weakness in his arms after having lunch with a business associate. The pain had lessened by the time he arrived at the hospital. The nursing history revealed that he had been hospitalized 5 months previously with the same complaints and had been told by his physician to go to the emergency department if the pain ever recurred. He had been placed on a low-fat diet and had stopped smoking. Physical examination revealed that Mr. Preston's vital signs were within normal limits. He stated that he had feared he was having a "heart attack" until his pain subsided and until he was told that his electrocardiogram was normal. He verbalized that he wanted to find out how he could prevent the attacks of pain in the future. The physician's orders on admission included activity as tolerated, low-cholesterol diet, and nitroglycerin 0.4 mg (1/500 gr) sublingually as needed.

NURSING DIAGNOSIS

Acute Pain related to angina pectoris/rule out myocardial ischemia

GOAL

Short-term: Relief of pain.
Intermediate: Inclusion of healthy lifestyle measures that decrease myocardial ischemia.
Long-term: Compliance with therapeutic regimen.

Expected Outcomes	Nursing Intervention	Critical Time*	Actual Outcomes (Evaluation)
• Blood pressure (BP), pulse (P), and respiration (R) will remain within normal limits.	Monitor BP, P, R q4h.	24 h	• BP: stable at 116 to 122/72 to 84 • P: stable at 68 to 82 • R: stable at 16 to 20
• Patient will remain free from chest pain.	Assess frequency of chest pain and precipitating events.	24 h	• Denies chest pain; able to walk length of hall, eat meals, and visit with family and friends without chest. discomfort.
• Will tolerate dietary regimen. • Will not experience chest pain after meals. • Will maintain normal bowel elimination. • Will have intake of 1,500 to 2,000 mL fluid/day.	Encourage food and fluid intake that promotes healthy nutrition, digestion, and elimination and that does not precipitate chest pain: light, regular meals; foods low in cholesterol; 1,500 to 2,000 mL fluid/day.	24 h	• Denies chest pain after meals; no constipation or diarrhea; fluid intake 1,700 to 2,100 mL/day.
• Will identify foods low in cholesterol and those foods that are to be avoided. • Will select well-balanced diet within prescribed restrictions.	Request consultation with dietitian. Reinforce diet teaching.	48 h	• Dietitian reviewed diet restrictions with patient and wife; wife counseled in meal planning. Patient selects and eats a balanced diet consisting of foods low in cholesterol.
• Will identify activities and exercises that could precipitate chest pain: those that require sudden bursts of activity and heavy effort. • Will identify emotionally stressful situations; will explain the necessity for alternating periods of activity with periods of rest.	Encourage alterations in activities and exercise that are necessary to prevent episodes of anginal pain.	48 h	• Patient and wife have identified activities and situations that should be avoided; patient and wife have studied their usual daily routine and have made plans to alter the routine to allow for rest periods; teenage son has volunteered to assist with strenuous home-maintenance chores.
• Will describe action, use, and correct administration of nitroglycerin.	Teach about nitroglycerin regimen.	24 h	• Patient has accurately stated action, use, and dosage of nitroglycerin; demonstrated correct administration.

*These times have not been standardized, but are individualized according to the patient's needs.

3. Identify nursing interventions as appropriate for goal attainment.
   a. An intervention is defined as any treatment, based on clinical judgment and knowledge, that a nurse performs to enhance patient/client outcomes.
   b. Include independent nursing actions as well as collaborative interventions based on medical orders.
   c. Should be detailed to provide continuity of care.
   d. Nursing Interventions Classification (NIC) is a standardized language describing treatments performed by nurses in all settings and specialties. More than 550 NIC interventions have been developed through the University of Iowa College of Nursing. NIC is organized into 30 classifications and 7 domains and includes physiologic and psychosocial interventions as well as interventions for illness prevention and treatment. NIC interventions serve a role in documentation, possibly coding, and reimbursement for nursing care in the future.
4. Formulate the nursing care plan. The nursing care plan may be a component of the interdisciplinary/collaborative care plan for the patient.
   a. Include nursing diagnoses, expected outcomes, interventions, and a space for evaluation.
   b. May use a standardized care plan—check off appropriate data and fill in target dates for expected outcomes and frequency and other specifics of interventions.
   c. May use a protocol that gives specific sequential instructions for treating patients with a particular problem, including who is responsible and what specific actions should be taken in terms of assessment, planning, interventions, teaching, recognition of complications, evaluation, and documentation.
   d. May use a care path or clinical pathway (also called *care map* or *critical pathway*) in which the nurse as case manager is responsible for outcomes, length of stay, and use of equipment during the patient's illness; includes the patient's medical diagnosis, length of stay allowed by diagnostic related group (DRG), expected outcomes, and key events that must occur for the patient to be discharged by that date. Key events are not as specific as nursing interventions, but are categorized by day of stay and who is responsible (nurse, physician, other health team member, patient, family).
   e. May also use a computerized care plan that is based on assessment data and allows for the selection of nursing interventions and establishment of expected outcomes.

Implementation

1. Coordinate activities of patient, family, significant others, nursing team members, and other health team members.
2. Delegate specific nursing interventions to other members of the nursing team as appropriate.
   a. Consider the capabilities and limitations of the members of the nursing team.
   b. Supervise the performance of nursing interventions.
3. Record the patient's responses to nursing interventions precisely and concisely.

Evaluation

Determines the success of nursing care and the need to alter the care plan.

1. Collect assessment data.
2. Compare patient's actual outcomes to expected outcomes to determine to what extent goals have been achieved.
3. Include the patient, family, or significant other; nursing team members; and other health team members in the evaluation.
4. Identify alterations that need to be made in the goals and the nursing care plan.

Continuation of the Nursing Process

1. Continue all steps of the nursing process: assessment, nursing diagnosis, planning, implementation, and evaluation.
2. Continuous evaluation provides the means for maintaining the viability of the entire nursing process and for demonstrating accountability for the quality of nursing care rendered.

COMMUNITY AND HOME CARE NURSING

Home Health Concepts

The home care nurse functions in the home and community, outside the walls of health care facilities. The role is more independent and the basic concepts of home health are different from hospital or outpatient nursing.

Roles and Duties of the Home Care Nurse

1. The home care nurse maintains a comprehensive knowledge base of the health of the patient.
2. The home care nurse performs an extensive evaluation of the patient's medical history, physical condition, psychosocial well-being, living environment, and support systems.
3. The home care nurse functions independently, recommending to the primary or specialty health care provider what services are needed in the home.
4. The home care nurse coordinates the services of other disciplines, such as physical therapy, occupational therapy, nutrition, and social work.
5. The home care nurse oversees the entire treatment plan and keeps the health care provider apprised of the patient's progress or lack of progress toward goals.
6. The home care nurse acts as a liaison between patient, family, caregivers, and the primary health care provider and other members of the health care team.
7. The home care nurse may function as supervisor of home health aides who provide direct daily care for the patient.
8. The home care nurse must honor the same patient rights as a health care facility.

Skills for Home Care Nursing

1. Good rapport building—to engage the patient, family, and caregivers in goal attainment.

2. Clear communication—to provide effective teaching to family and caregivers, to relate assessment information about the patient to the health care provider, and to share information with the home care team.
3. Cultural competence—knowledge and appreciation of the cultural norms being practiced in the home. Cultural practices may affect family structure, communication, and decision making in the home; health beliefs, nutrition, and alternative health practices; and spirituality and religious beliefs.
4. Accurate documentation—record keeping in home care is used for reimbursement of nursing services, accreditation and regulatory review, and communication among the home care team.

Reimbursement Issues

1. Home health care services are reimbursed by Medicare, Medicaid, and a variety of commercial insurances and managed care plans.
2. Some patients are willing to pay out of pocket for additional services not covered by insurance because of the well-established value of home care services compared with more expensive hospital and nursing home services.
3. Services are reimbursed by Medicare if they meet the following criteria:
   a. Services are ordered by a physician (current law does not recognize nurse practitioners).
   b. Services are intermittent or needed on a part-time basis.
   c. The patient is homebound.
   d. The services required are skilled (need to be provided by a licensed nurse, physical therapist, or speech therapist; or by an occupational therapist, social worker, or home health aide along with the service of a nurse).
   e. The services requested are reasonable and medically necessary.
4. The home health nurse must evaluate the case and ensure that these criteria apply. This information must be documented so reimbursement won't be denied.

Home Health Practice

The nursing process is carried out in home care as it is in other nursing settings. Patient interactions are structured differently than in the hospital because the nurse will interact with the patient intermittently and in the intimate home environment. Many procedures and nursing interventions are implemented in a similar manner as other nursing settings, as outlined in the rest of this book. Major concerns of the home care nurse are patient teaching, infection control, and safety maintenance.

The Home Care Visit

1. The initial home care visit should be preceded by information gathering and an introductory phone call to the patient.
2. Extensive assessment is carried out at the first visit, including complete medical and psychosocial history, physical examination, home environment assessment, nutritional assessment, medication review, and current treatment plan review.

3. Once assessment (gathered from multiple sources) is complete, nursing diagnoses are formed. The plan of care must be adaptable to the specific home dynamics.
4. Outcome planning (goal setting) is done with the patient, family, and caregivers involved.
5. The plan is implemented over a prescribed time period (the certified period of service). Interventions may be:
   a. Cognitive—involves patient teaching.
   b. Psychosocial—reinforces coping mechanisms, supports caregivers, reduces stress.
   c. Technical—entails procedures, such as wound care and catheter insertion.
6. Evaluation is ongoing at every visit and by follow-up phone calls to adjust and refine the care plan and frequency of service.
7. Recertification for continued service, discharge, or transfer (to a hospital or nursing home) ultimately occurs.

Patient Teaching

1. Patient teaching is directed toward the patient, family, caregivers, and involved significant others.
2. Patient teaching is usually considered skilled and is therefore reimbursable. Topics may include:
   a. Disease process, pathophysiology, and signs and symptoms to monitor treatment.
   b. Administration of injectable medication or complex regimen of oral medications.
   c. Diabetic management for a patient newly diagnosed with diabetes.
   d. Wound or ostomy care.
   e. Catheterization.
   f. Gastrostomy and enteral feedings.
   g. Management of peripheral or central intravenous catheters.
   h. Use of adaptive devices for carrying out activities of daily living and ambulation.
   i. Transfer techniques and body alignment.
   j. Preparation and maintenance of therapeutic diet.
3. Barriers to learning should be evaluated and removed or compensated for.
   a. Environmental barriers, such as noise, poor lighting, and distractions.
   b. Personal barriers, such as sensory deficits, poor reading skills, and drowsiness.
4. The teaching plan should include the three domains of learning:
   a. Cognitive—sharing of facts and information.
   b. Affective—addressing the patient's feelings about the disease and treatment.
   c. Psychomotor—discussing performance of desired behavior or steps in a procedure.
5. Documentation of patient teaching should be specific and include the degree of patient competence of the procedure.
6. Patient teaching plans may include review of teaching started in the hospital and may take several sessions to implement successfully.

Infection Control

1. Nosocomial infection rates are much lower in home care, but patients are still at risk for infection due to weakened immune systems and the variability of a clean or sterile environment at home.
2. The nurse should assess and maintain a clean environment.
   a. Make sure that clean or sterile supplies are readily available when needed.
   b. Make sure that contaminated supplies are disposed of promptly and properly.
      i. Needles should be disposed of in a safe and secure container (usually kept in the home [until full]), which can be disposed of through the home health agency or the patient's pharmacy.
      ii. Supplies, such as dressings, gloves, and catheters, should be securely bagged and disposed of in small amounts through the regular trash collection at the patient's home. However, biohazardous waste disposal may be necessary in some cases.
3. The nurse should be aware of all methods of transmission of infection and implement and teach preventive practices.

 NURSING ALERT Above all else, model and teach good hand-washing practice to everyone in the home.

4. The nurse must perform ongoing assessment for signs and symptoms of infection and teach the patient, family, and caregivers what to look for.
5. The nurse should be aware of community-acquired infections that may be prevalent in certain populations, such as tuberculosis, human immunodeficiency virus infection, hepatitis, and sexually transmitted diseases.
   a. Teach preventive practices.
   b. Encourage and institute screening programs.
   c. Report infections according to the local public health department policy.
6. Encourage and provide vaccination for the patient and household contacts for influenza, pneumococcal pneumonia, hepatitis B, and others as appropriate.

Ensuring Safety

1. Continually assess safety in the home, particularly if the patient is very ill and the care plan is complex.
2. Assess for environmental safety issues—cluttered spaces, stairs, throw rugs, slippery floors, poor lighting.
3. Assess for the patient's personal safety issues—sensory deficits, weakness, problems with eating or swallowing.
4. Assess safety in the bathroom—handrails, bath mat, raised toilet seat, water temperature.
5. Assess safety in the kitchen—proper refrigeration of food, ability to shop for and cook meals, oven safety.
6. Be alert for abuse and neglect, especially of children, dependent elders, and women.
7. Check equipment for electrical and fire safety and that it is being used properly.
8. Be continually cognizant of your own safety—get directions, travel during daylight hours, wear seat belts, do not enter suspicious areas without an escort, be alert to your surroundings.

SELECTED REFERENCES

American Association of Colleges of Nursing. (2011, August). The Doctor of Nursing Practice fact sheet. Available: *www.aacn.nche.edu/media/factsheets/dnp.htm.*

American Association of Colleges of Nursing. (2011, April 22). Nursing faculty shortage fact sheet. Available: *www.aacn.nche.edu/Media/Factsheets/facultyshortage.htm.*

American Association of Colleges of Nursing. (2011). Annual state of the schools. Available: *www.aacn.nche.edu/aacn-publications/annual-reports/AR2011.pdf.*

American Nurses Association. (2006). *Position statement: Risk and responsibility in providing nursing care.* Silver Spring, MD: Author.

American Nurses Association. (2011). ANA's handle with care. Available: *www.nursingworld.org/handlewithcare.htm.*

American Nurses Credentialing Center. (2011). Certification and renewals. Available: *www.nursecredentialing.org/cert/index.htm.*

Andrew, M. A., & Boyle, J. S. (2011). *Transcultural concepts in nursing care* (6th ed.). Philadelphia: Lippincott Williams & Wilkins.

Bloom, D. E., Cafiero, E. T., Jané-Llopis, E., et al. (2011). The global economic burden of non-communicable diseases. Geneva: World Economic Forum. Available: *www.weforum.org.*

Bulechek, G., Butcher, H., Dochterman, J., et al. (Eds.). (2013). *Nursing interventions classification (NIC)* (6th ed.). St. Louis, MO: Elsevier.

Canadian Nurses Association. (2010). Position statement: Promoting cultural competence in Nursing. Available: *www.cna-aiic.ca/CNA/documents/pdf/publications/PS114_Cultural_Competence_2010_e.pdf.*

Carpenito-Moyet, L. J. (2009). *Handbook of nursing diagnosis* (13th ed.). Philadelphia: Lippincott Williams & Wilkins.

Carpenito-Moyet, L. J. (2009). *Nursing diagnosis: Applications to clinical practice* (13th ed.). Philadelphia: Lippincott Williams & Wilkins.

Centers for Medicare and Medicaid Services. (2010). National health expenditure projections 2010–2020. Baltimore: Office of the Actuary, National Health Statistics Group. Available: *www.cms.hhs.gov/nationalhealthexpenddata/.*

Department of Health and Human Services. (2010). The health care law and you: What's changing and when. Available: *www.healthcare.gov/law/timeline/index.html.*

Douglas, M. K., Pierce, J. U., Rosenkoetter, M., et al. (2009). Standards of practice for culturally competent nursing care: A request for comments. *Journal of Transcultural Nursing, 20*(3), 257–269.

Expert Panel on Global Nursing and Health. (2010). Standards of practice for culturally competent nursing care executive summary. Available: *www.tcns.org/TCNStandardsofPractice.html.*

Institute of Medicine. (2006). Preventing medication errors. Available: *www.iom.edu.*

Institute of Medicine. (2010). Future directions for the National Healthcare Quality and Disparities Reports, April 14, 2010. Available: *www.iom.edu/Reports/2010/Future-Directions-for-the-National-Healthcare-Quality-and-Disparities-Reports.aspx.*

Institute of Medicine. (2010, October). The future of nursing: Leading change, advancing health. Available: *www.iom.edu/Reports/2010/The-Future-of-Nursing-Leading-Change-Advancing-Health.aspx.*

The Joint Commission (2012). Hospital 2013 national patient safety goals. Available: *www.jointcommission.org/hap_2013_npsg/.*

Kaiser Family Foundation, (2009). Trends in health care costs and spending, March 2009 (Publication No. 7692-02). Available: *www.kff.org.*

Leininger, M. M., & McFarland, M. R. (2002). *Transcultural nursing: Concepts, theories, research, and practice* (3rd ed.). New York: McGraw-Hill.

Moorhead, S., Johnson, M., Maas, M., et al. (Eds.). (2013). *Nursing outcomes classification (NOC)* (5th ed.). St. Louis, MO: Elsevier.

NANDA International. (2011). Nursing diagnosis frequently asked questions. Available: *www.nanda.org/nursingdiagnosisFAQ.aspx.*

NANDA International. (2012). NANDA nursing diagnoses: Definitions and classifications, 2012–2014. DeMoines, IA: Wiley Blackwell.

National Quality Forum. (2010). *Safe practices for better healthcare: 2010 update.* Washington, DC: Author.

Ray, M. (2010). *Transcultural caring dynamics in nursing and health care.* Philadelphia: Davis.

Sammer, C. E., & James, B. R. (2012). Patient safety culture: The nursing unit leader's role. *OJIN: The Online Journal of Issues in Nursing, 16*(3). Available: *http://www.nursingworld.org/MainMenuCategories/ANAMarketplace/ANAPeriodicals/OJIN/TableofContents/Vol-16-2011/No3-Sept-2011/Patient-Safety-Culture-and-Nursing-Unit-Leader.html.*

Spath, P. L. (Ed.). (2011). *Error reduction in healthcare: A systems approach to improving patient safety* (2nd ed.). San Francisco: Jossey-Bass.

Tzeng, H. M., Hu, H. M., Yin, C. Y. (2011). The relationship of the hospital-acquired injurious fall rate with the quality profile of a hospital's care delivery and nursing staff patterns. *Nursing Economics, 29*(6):299–306.

U.S. Department of Health and Human Services. (2007). Office of Minority Health. Culturally competent nursing care: A cornerstone of caring. Available: *https://ccnm.thinkculturalhealth.hhs.gov.*

University of Iowa College of Nursing. (2013). CNC-Overview: Nursing Interventions Classification (NIC). Available: *www.nursing.iowa.edu/cncce/nursing-interventions-classification-overview.*

University of Iowa College of Nursing. (2013). CNC—Overview: Nursing Outcomes Classification (NOC). Available: *www.nursing.uiowa.edu/cncce/nursing-outcomes-classification-overview.*

Vigorito, M. C., McNicoll, L., Adams, L., et al. (2011). Improving safety culture results in Rhode Island ICUs: Lessons learned from the development of action oriented plans. *Quality Patient Safety, 37*, 509–514.

Young, J. Q., Ranji, S. R., Wachter, R. M., et al. (2011). "July Effect": Impact of the academic year-end changeover on patient outcomes. A systematic review. *Annals of Internal Medicine, 155*, 309–315.

2

Standards of Care and Ethical and Legal Issues

INTRODUCTION

Professional nurses occupy the frontlines of the health care arena. So it is no surprise that they are the part of the health care team patients trust most with their health and welfare. Along with this privilege, nurses carry equal duties of responsibility and accountability to follow ethical principles and standards of care integral to the profession. Greater efforts must be made from within the profession to apply evidence-based research data to daily practice systematically and deliberately, thereby increasing patient safety, improving outcomes, and reducing risk and adverse events. Transformation of the professional culture within the health care system itself would give nurses at the bedside the incentive to join in these efforts as full partners with leaders in health care. Additional measures might include protocol implementation, preceptor performance review, peer review, continuing education, patient satisfaction surveys, and the implementation of risk management techniques. However, in certain instances, either despite or in the absence of such internal mechanisms, claims are made for an alleged injury or alleged malpractice liability. Although the vast majority of claims may be without merit, many professional nurses will have to deal with the unfamiliar legal system. A system of ethical principles and standards of care will be beneficial in such situations. Therefore, it is preferable for the nursing profession to incorporate certain ethical and legal principles and protocols into practice to make sure that the patient receives only safe and appropriate care.

ETHICAL CORE CONCEPTS

Clinical ethics literature identifies four principles and values that are integral to the professional nurse's practice: the nurse's ethical duty to respect the patient's autonomy and to act with beneficence, nonmaleficence, and justice.

Respect for the Individual and Autonomy

1. Respect for the individual's autonomy incorporates principles of freedom of choice, self-determination, and privacy.
2. The professional nurse's duty is to view and treat each individual as an autonomous, self-determining person with the freedom to act in accordance with self-chosen, informed goals, as long as the action does not interfere or infringe on the autonomous action of another.
3. Numerous institutions and health care organizations have developed patient rights statements and policies that impact nursing care.
   a. The National League of Nursing (NLN) has developed an Education Competencies Model for all educational levels of nursing, which names the core values as caring, diversity, ethics, excellence, holism, integrity, and patient centeredness.
   b. The American Nurses Association (ANA) has developed and updated a Code of Ethics for Nurses, which states,

"the nurse in all professional relationships practices with compassion with respect for the inherent dignity, worth, and uniqueness of every individual, unrestricted by considerations of social or economic status, personal attributes, or the nature of health problems.

 Evidence Base National League of Nursing. (2010). *The NLN Education Competencies Model.* New York: Author.
American Nurses Association. (2001). *Code of Ethics for Nurses with Interpretive Statements (Code for Nurses).* Silver Spring, MD: Author.

Beneficence

The principle of beneficence affirms the inherent professional aspiration and duty to help promote the well-being of others and, often, is the primary motivating factor for those who choose a career in the health care profession. Health care professionals aspire to help people achieve a better life through an improved state of health.

Nonmaleficence

1. The principle of nonmaleficence complements beneficence and obligates the professional nurse not to harm the patient directly or with intent.
2. In the health care profession, this principle is actualized only with the complementary principle of beneficence because it is common for the nurse to cause pain or expose the patient to risk of harm when such actions are justified by the benefits of the procedures or treatments.
3. It is best to seek to promote a balance of potential risk-induced harms with benefits, with the basic guideline being to strive to maximize expected benefits and minimize possible harms. Therefore, nonmaleficence should be balanced with beneficence.

Justice

1. Justice, or fairness, relates to the distribution of services and resources.
2. As the health care dollar becomes increasingly scarce, justice seeks to allocate resources fairly and treat patients equally.
3. Dilemmas arise when resources are scarce and insufficient to meet the needs of everyone. How do we decide fairly who gets what in such situations?
4. One might consider whether it is just or fair for many people not to have funding or access to the most basic preventive care, whereas others have insurance coverage for expensive and long-term hospitalizations.
5. Along with respect for people and their autonomy, the complex principle of justice is a culturally comfortable principle in countries such as the United States. Nonetheless, the application of justice is complex and often challenging.

ETHICAL DILEMMAS
Conflicting Ethical Principles

1. Ethical dilemmas arise when two or more ethical principles are in conflict.
2. Such dilemmas can best be addressed by applying principles on a case-by-case basis once all available data are gathered and analyzed.
3. Clinicians should network with their colleagues and consider establishing multidisciplinary ethics committees to provide guidance.

Ethics Committees

1. Ethics committees identify, examine, and promote resolution of ethical issues and dilemmas by:
   a. Protecting the patient's rights.
   b. Protecting the staff and the organization.
   c. Reviewing decisions regarding clinical practice and standards of practice.
   d. Improving the quality of care and services.
   e. Serving as educational resources to staff.
   f. Building a consensus on ethical issues with other professional organizations.
2. Addressing and resolving ethical dilemmas is usually a challenging decision shared with the clinical staff.

Examples of Ethical Dilemmas and Possible Responses
Unsafe Nurse-to-Patient Ratio

1. A pattern of unsafe nurse-to-patient ratio can be caused by temporary or long-term staffing problems.
2. A series of actions to best resolve the problem includes:
   a. Address this unsafe situation verbally and in writing to the unit charge nurse with copies to the nursing supervisor and director of nursing.
   b. This will likely prompt action by the facility, such as creating an as-needed pool of nurses to call for such situations, hiring more staff, or, in the interim, securing contracts with outside nursing agencies and utilizing agency nursing personnel.
3. Tolerance by staff nurses employed under such circumstances will preclude appropriate resolution and will leave the nurse open to unsafe practice and unmet patient needs, potentially increasing the risk of liability.
4. Although the employer is liable for the acts of the employee performed within the scope of employment, the nurse will not be exonerated should a patient's care be compromised in a setting of an unsafe nurse-to-patient ratio.

Nonresponse by Physician

1. A patient arrives to the rehabilitation unit at 9 PM with numerous positive criteria for falling, including poor short-term memory, daily use of a diuretic, daily use of a sleep aid, a history of a fall within the preceding 2 months, and known vision impairment.

a. Patient is oriented to time, place, and person, his new room, facility bed, and call light use.

b. The nurse instructs patient to summon her if he needs to void or otherwise get out of bed, at least until he becomes familiar with his new environment.

c. Upon returning to patient's room 10 minutes later, the nurse finds patient out of bed, arranging his clothes in his closet, standing in a pool of urine on the floor.

d. The nurse weighs the risks and benefits of restraint use and determines whether alternatives are available. She calls the physician for a restraint order if patient continues to jeopardize his safety. The nurse intends to ask the physician for an order with clear specification of the least restrictive method of restraint, the duration, circumstances, frequency of monitoring, and reevaluation if it differs from facility policy. However, the physician does not return her calls. The nurse documents her initial assessment of the patient, her nursing diagnoses, the orientation to room and equipment provided to the patient, the circumstances wherein she found the patient out of bed, and her repeated messages for the physician and the lack of a return telephone call.

2. Again, a series of actions may resolve the problem or at least prevent injury to the patient. Address this situation with intermediate measures while waiting for the physician's return call:

a. Raise side rails on the patient's bed.

b. Move patient to a room close to the nurse's station.

c. Place a sign on patient's room door and above the bed identifying him as being at risk for falling.

d. Place a sign above the bed instructing personnel to raise the bed's side rails fully before leaving patient's room.

e. Check on the patient frequently during the first 24 hours, reminding him of the call light, its use, and the need to call the nurse before getting out of bed.

3. Call the patient's family, advising them of your concern about the patient's safety, and discuss the issue of restraints with them. Discuss the risk for falling and prevention of fall-induced injury versus the restriction of the patient's freedom of movement about the room.

4. Document ongoing assessments of potential problems, calls to the physician, and discussions with family members.

5. Apply restraints according to the policy of the rehabilitation unit until an order is secured from the physician.

a. Consult facility policy on restraint use.

b. Secure an order from the physician for restraints to be used as needed, including specific criteria outlined in step 1d.

6. Reassess the patient's need for diuretic and sleep aid or sedative use. Discuss discontinuation of any unnecessary medications that increase the patient's degree of confusion or risk for falling, if possible.

Inappropriate Orders

1. A 65-year-old patient with a diagnosis of uncontrolled heart failure is presently in the intensive care unit for treatment and hemodynamic monitoring. He is becoming increasingly anxious during your shift, but vital signs are stable and respiratory distress is absent. A house officer is summoned to evaluate this change in clinical status.

a. The house officer, unfamiliar with the patient, spends 2 minutes reviewing the chart, examines the patient for 2 minutes, and orders a sedative to be administered stat and, as needed, every 4 hours.

b. You tell the house officer that you heard decreased breath sounds in the left, lower lung and ask him to order some diagnostic tests, such as a chest x-ray and arterial blood gas analysis, and share your concern that administering a sedative to the patient may mask the underlying cause of the anxiety, lead to respiratory compromise, and delay diagnosis and treatment of the underlying clinical problem. Nevertheless, he leaves the unit.

c. You decide not to give the sedative ordered by the house officer.

2. Although you cannot automatically follow an order you think is unsafe, you cannot just ignore a medical order either.

a. Document the scenario described above in the patient's chart, contact the resident on call, and notify your supervising nurse.

b. If assessment by the resident on call agrees with the house officer, call the attending physician, discuss your concerns with him, obtain appropriate stat orders, and notify the house officer and resident of the attending physician's orders and the actions you took.

c. Notify all involved medical and nursing personnel of the patient's status.

d. Document clearly, succinctly, and in a timely fashion.

3. Your actions reflect concern about the best interest of the patient and, although they may yield negative behaviors by the house officer or resident, it is more important to prevent potential injury to the patient.

LEGAL ASPECTS OF PROFESSIONAL NURSING PRACTICE

Accountability

1. Integral to the practice of any profession is the inherent need to be responsible for actions taken and for omissions.

2. The professional nurse must be proactive and take all appropriate measures to ensure that her own practice is not lacking, remiss, or deficient in any area or way.

3. Useful proactive measures include:

a. Maintaining familiarity of relevant, current facility policies, procedures, and regulations as they apply to the nurse's practice and specialty area.

b. Providing for self-audit.

c. Providing for peer review to assess reasonableness of care in a particular setting for a particular problem.

d. Working with local nursing organizations to make certain that local standards of practice are met.

   e. Examining the quality (accuracy and completeness) of documentation.
   f. Establishing open working relationships with colleagues wherein honest constructive criticism is welcomed for the greater goal of quality patient care.
4. Local standards of practice normally coordinate with those of nationally accepted standards.

Advocacy

The professional nurse has the duty to:
1. Promote what is best for the patient.
2. Ensure that the patient's needs are met.
3. Protect the patient's rights.

Confidentiality

1. The patient's privacy is consistent with the Hippocratic Oath and with the law as part of the constitutional right to privacy.
2. Although the professional nurse should assure the patient of confidentiality, limits on this standard must be clarified and discussed with the patient at the earliest opportunity.
3. It is imperative to clearly understand the process of informed consent and the legal standard for disclosure of confidential patient information to others.
4. The Medical Record Confidentiality Act of 1995, a federal statute, is the primary federal law governing the use of health treatment and payment records. Several practical guidelines include:
   a. Respecting the individual's right to privacy when requesting or responding to a request for a patient's medical records.
   b. Always requiring a signed medical authorization and consent form to release medical records and information to protect and respect patient–provider privilege statutes.
   c. Discussing confidentiality issues with the patient and establishing consent. Addressing concerns or special requests for information not to be disclosed.
5. Based on the Health Insurance Portability and Accountability Act (HIPAA), the Department of Health and Human Services issued guidelines in 2000 to protect the confidentiality of individually identifiable health information. The rule:
   a. Limits the use and disclosure of certain individually identifiable health information.
   b. Gives patients the right to access their medical records.
   c. Restricts most disclosure of health information to the minimum needed for the intended purpose.
   d. Establishes safeguards and restrictions regarding the use and disclosure of records for certain public responsibilities, such as public health, law enforcement, and research.
   e. Provides for criminal or civil sanctions for improper uses or disclosures.
6. The exceptions or limits to confidentiality include situations in which society has judged that the need for information outweighs the principle of confidentiality. However, legal counsel should be consulted because these decisions are made on a case-by-case basis and broad generalizations cannot be assumed.
7. It may be appropriate to breach confidentiality on a limited basis in situations such as the following:
   a. If a patient reveals intent to harm him- or herself or another individual, it is imperative to protect the patient and third parties from such harm.
   b. A clinician employed by a company, school, military unit, or court has split allegiances, and the patient should be so advised at the appropriate time.
   c. Court orders, subpoenas, and summonses in some states may require the clinician to release records for review or testify in court. However, legal counsel should be consulted first to ensure that complying with these orders does not violate HIPAA.
   d. Most insurance companies, health maintenance organizations, and governmental payers require participants to sign a release of their records to the payers.
   e. When a patient places his or her medical condition at issue, such as in personal injury cases, worker's compensation, or in various other cases of patients claiming injuries for which they are seeking compensation from any entity or organization.
   f. Many states have laws requiring clinicians to report the incidence of certain diseases, deaths, and other vital statistics.
   g. Criminal codes in many states require reporting gunshot wounds, incidents of rape, and incidents of child, spousal, or elder abuse if they have reasonable cause to suspect abuse.

Informed Consent

1. The doctrine of informed consent has become a fundamentally accepted principle governing the relationship between professional nurses and all other health care providers and patients.
2. Informed consent relates to the patient's right to accept or reject treatment by a nurse or any other health care provider and is a right of all legally competent adults or emancipated minors.
3. In the majority of circumstances, informed consent is obtained for medical or surgical procedures to be performed by physicians. Therefore, it is the duty of the physician to inform the patient of alternative treatments, the nature of the procedure, and benefits and potential risks. Oftentimes, especially when the patient is hospitalized, the nurse is required to witness the patient's signature before the procedure. It is prudent for the nurse to note witness to signature directly next to the patient's signature.
4. Emancipated minors are individuals who are under age 18 and married, parents of their own children, or are self-sufficiently living away from the family domicile with parental consent.
5. In the case of a minor, informed consent would be obtained from the legal guardian.
6. In the case of individuals incapable of understanding medical treatment issues, informed consent must be obtained through a responsible person such as a guardian.

7. The nurse has the duty to verify that the physician or other health care provider has explained each treatment or procedure in a language the patient (or the responsible person) can comprehend; has warned the patient of any material risks, dangers, or harms inherent in or collateral to the treatment; and has advised the patient of available alternatives. This enables the patient to make an intelligent and informed decision and choice about whether to undergo treatment.

8. The informed consent should be obtained before rendering the treatment or performance of the procedure. For more information on informed consent for patient's surgery, see Chapter 7, page 105.

9. The nurse must document that the informed consent was obtained and that the patient understood the information.

10. A witness signature is desirable and may be required by some health care institutions.

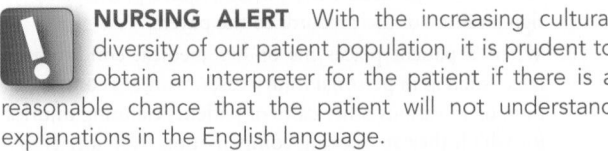 **NURSING ALERT** With the increasing cultural diversity of our patient population, it is prudent to obtain an interpreter for the patient if there is a reasonable chance that the patient will not understand explanations in the English language.

Scope of Practice, Licensure, and Certification

1. The professional nurse's scope of practice is defined and outlined by the State Board of Nursing that governs practice. The National Council of State Boards of Nursing and the NLN have developed standards that guide each State Board in the development of their licensure requirements and scope of practice rules.

2. Licensure is granted by an agency of state government and permits individuals accountable for the practice of professional nursing to engage in the practice of that profession, while prohibiting all others from doing so legally.

3. Certification is provided by a nongovernmental association or agency and certifies that a person licensed to practice as a professional nurse has met certain predetermined standards described by that profession for specialty practice, thereby assuring the patient that a person has mastered a body of knowledge and acquired the skills in a particular specialty.

4. The mechanisms for achieving certification and maintaining a specialty certification vary by association and certifying body, such as a specified number of hours of clinical practice, continuing education, peer review, periodic self-assessment examination, or reexamination.

5. The American Nurses Credentialing Center is one certifying body that provides specialty certification (*www.nursecredentialing.org* or 800-284-2378). Credentialing protects the public by recognizing professional nurses who have successfully completed an approved course of study and achieved a level of specialized knowledge and skill to hold specialized positions.

Standards of Practice
General Principles

1. The practice of professional nursing has standards of practice setting minimum levels of acceptable performance for which its practitioners are accountable.
   a. The authority for the practice of nursing is based on a social contract that acknowledges rights and responsibilities, along with mechanisms for public accountability.
   b. These standards provide patients with a means of measuring the quality of care they receive.

2. Standards of practice were developed by the ANA and have been updated regularly to include 2,800 pages of general standards as well as standards for each nursing specialty. A copy can be purchased from the ANA publications office (*www.nursesbooks.org* or 800-637-0323).
   a. These standards describe what nursing is, what nurses do, and the responsibilities for which nurses are accountable.
   b. Professional nurses are to be guided by the generic standards applicable to all nurses in all areas of practice as well as by specialty area standards.

3. Various specialty groups have developed their own additional standards, but addressing these exceeds the scope of this chapter. The professional nurse needs to be familiar with all standards applicable to her or his own practice areas.

4. Standards and parameters also provide a source of legal protection for the practicing nurse.
   a. Standards and parameters typically consist of a simple, realistic series of steps that would be applicable given the same or similar clinical scenario.
   b. Standards and parameters should outline the minimum requirements for safe care and need to be updated as scientific knowledge changes.

5. A deviation from the protocol should be documented in the patient's chart with clear, concise statements of the nurse's decisions, actions, and reasons for the care provided, including any apparent deviation. This should be done at the time the care is rendered because passage of time may lead to a less than accurate recollection of the specific events.

6. Informal or volunteer practice must be consistent with the applicable standard of care. Documentation that the care rendered was the standard of practice within a community or state may afford the practitioner a degree of protection. Informal or volunteer care still needs to comply with the applicable standard of care.

Common Departures from the Standards of Nursing Care

Legal claims most commonly made against professional nurses include the following departures from appropriate care: failure to assess the patient properly or in a timely fashion, follow physician orders, follow appropriate nursing measures, communicate information about the patient, adhere to facility policy or procedure, document appropriate information in the medical record, administer medications as ordered, and follow physician's orders

BOX 2-1	Common Legal Claims for Departure from Standards of Care

- Failure to monitor or observe a patient's clinical status adequately
- Failure to monitor or observe a change in a patient's clinical status
- Failure to communicate or document a significant change in a patient's condition to appropriate professional
- Failure to obtain a complete nursing history
- Failure to formulate or follow the nursing care plan
- Failure to perform a nursing treatment or procedure properly
- Failure to provide a safe environment and to protect the patient from avoidable injury
- Failure to implement a physician's, advanced practice nurse's, or physician assistant's order properly or in a timely fashion
- Failure to administer medications properly and in a timely fashion or to report and administer omitted doses appropriately
- Failure to observe a medication's action or adverse effect
- Failure to prevent infection
- Failure to obtain help for a patient not receiving proper care from a physician or other health care provider

- Failure to report that a patient is not receiving proper care from a physician or other health care provider
- Failure to use equipment properly
- Failure to evaluate or identify a patient at high risk for falling or to plan and implement a fall prevention program appropriate to the individual patient
- Failure to apply restraints when indicated and ordered
- Failure to apply restraints in a proper manner
- Using equipment that is known to be defective
- Failure to make prompt, accurate entries in a patient's medical record
- Altering a medical record without noting it as a correction with signature, date, and time of change
- Failure to adhere to facility policy or procedural guidelines
- Following medical orders that should not have been followed such as medication dosage errors
- Failure to act as a patient advocate, such as not questioning illegible or incomplete medical orders or not questioning discharge when a patient's clinical status warrants

that should have been questioned or not followed, such as orders containing medication dosage errors (see Box 2-1).

Quality Assurance and Adverse Event Reduction

1. A quality assurance program creates and implements a systematic, deliberate, and ongoing mechanism for the evaluation and monitoring of professional nursing practice aimed at performance improvement and adverse event reduction. Many facilities follow the National Database of Nursing Quality Indicators program, implemented by the ANA. It is a database that is updated regularly to track progress in providing quality care in certain areas, including pressure ulcers, falls, hospital-acquired infections, and restraint prevalence.

2. In 2007, the U.S. Centers for Medicare and Medicaid Services announced that Medicare would be ending payments to facilities for the increased costs attributable to preventable, facility-acquired conditions, including pressure ulcers, catheter-associated urinary tract infections, vascular catheter-associated infections, coronary artery bypass graft–related mediastinitis, and a number of injuries, including dislocations, fractures, intracranial injuries, and burns. More than ever before, nurses delivering care at the frontlines are critical partners in promoting quality care, preventing adverse events, and saving avoidable expenditure of health care dollars.

3. Integral to the creation of such a proactive program are the following key factors:
   a. Create an atmosphere of collegiality.
   b. Develop and implement the consistent application of new policies and procedures for quick, easy, and, if possible, anonymous error reporting, with protection from disciplinary action.

   c. Support employees involved in serious errors, adopting a nonpunitive attitude.
   d. Acknowledge the need for system-wide improvement and for centralization of information. Doing so ensures maximal benefit to the patients of health care and to all disciplines involved in the delivery of care.
   e. Introduce scientifically valid quality and safety solutions universally throughout the health care system, allowing for sharing of successful strategies and measures and reward systems.

      These actions would promote the delivery of high-quality care, a sense of responsibility and accountability, as well as ongoing self- and peer-auditing, thus yielding greater trending, analysis, problem-solving, and system-wide refinements.

4. Consequently, the use of a quality assurance program effectively reduces the professional nurse's exposure to liability, identifies educational needs, and improves the documentation of the care provided.

5. The components of quality assurance include:
   a. Structure—focuses on the organization of patient care.
   b. Process—focuses on tests ordered and procedures performed.
   c. Outcome—focuses on the outcome, such as improvement, absence of complications, timely discharge, patient satisfaction, or death.

6. Mechanisms to incorporate in quality assurance programs may include:
   a. Patient satisfaction surveys to assess nurse interactions and maintain open lines of communication between the provider and the patient.
   b. Peer review to recognize and reward care delivered, lead to higher standards of practice within a community, and discourage practice beyond the scope of legal authority.

c. Audit of clinical records to determine how well-established criteria were met by the care rendered.

d. Utilization review to evaluate the extent to which services or resources were used as measured against a standard.

Management of Liability

1. The sources of legal risk in a professional nurse's practice include patient care, procedures performed, and quality of documentation.

2. Liability can be minimized by the application of risk management systems and activities, which are designed to recognize and intervene to reduce the risk of injury to patients and subsequent claims against professional nurses.

3. Risk management systems and activities are based on the premise that many injuries to patients are preventable.

Malpractice

1. Nursing malpractice refers to a negligent act of a professional nurse engaged in the practice of that profession.

2. Although negligence embraces all negligent acts, malpractice is a specific term referring to negligent conduct in the rendering of professional services.

3. There is no guaranteed way to avoid a medical malpractice suit short of avoiding practicing as a professional nurse. Even the best nurses have been named as defendants.

4. A diligent and reflective nurse can reduce the risks of malpractice by consistently incorporating the following four elements into her or his practice:

a. Excellent communication skills, with consistent efforts to elicit and address the expectations and requests of the patient.

b. Sincere compassion for each patient.

c. Competent practice.

d. Accurate and complete charting with notations of any deviations from the applicable standard of care with the specific reasons (eg, the patient refused chest radiograph due to time constraint) and the patient's noncompliance.

5. Generally, the professional nurse has the duty to:

a. Exercise a degree of diligence and skill that is ordinarily exercised by other professional nurses in the same state and specialty of practice.

b. Apply such knowledge with reasonable care.

c. Keep informed of approved standards of care in general use.

d. Exercise her own best judgment in rendering care to the patient.

6. Some states apply a geographic standard, referred to as a locality rule, which asserts that providers in remote rural areas may have less access to continuing education and various equipment than their colleagues in urban areas. However, because communication and transportation continue to improve rapidly, the locality rule is becoming obsolete.

Burden of Proof for Malpractice

The plaintiff has the burden of proving four elements of malpractice, usually by means of expert testimony.

Duty

1. The plaintiff has a burden to prove that a nurse–patient relationship did, in fact, exist and, by virtue of that relationship, the nurse had the duty to exercise reasonable care when undertaking and providing treatment to the patient.

2. Limits and obligations of duty include:

a. This duty exists only when there is a nurse–patient relationship.

b. The professional nurse is not obligated to enter into a nurse–patient relationship with any individual.

c. Professional nurses generally have the right to decide to whom they will provide professional services and may request to be reassigned to another patient if the nurse–patient relationship is strained, difficult, or otherwise not comfortable.

d. Nurses have limits on their rights to decide, however; they cannot refuse to treat a patient who has relied reasonably on the nurse's apparent willingness to treat all in need (eg, the emergency department in a general facility that advertises its emergency services) and may not abandon an established patient.

e. If a professional nurse wishes to terminate an established relationship with a patient, an alternative with an equivalent level of nursing services must be made available to the patient in a timely fashion.

 NURSING ALERT The professional nurse must use caution when offering telephone advice for which there is no charge; there have been reported cases of patients successfully suing providers because they reasonably relied on the telephone advice of a nurse that caused them to delay seeking care and sustained permanent injuries as a result.

Breach of Duty

1. The plaintiff has the burden to establish that the professional nurse violated the applicable standard of care in treating the patient's condition.

2. The plaintiff must establish by way of expert professional nurse testimony that the "negligent" nurse failed to conform to the applicable standard of care or provided nursing care that fell below the level of care that would have been provided by a prudent and diligent nurse under the same circumstances.

Proximate Cause

1. The plaintiff has the burden of establishing a causal relationship between the breach in the standard of care and the patient's injuries.

2. If a breach in standard of care did not cause the alleged injuries, there is no proximate cause.

Damages

The plaintiff has the burden of establishing the existence of damages to the patient as a result of malpractice.

Malpractice Insurance

1. Malpractice insurance will not protect the professional nurse from charges of practicing outside the scope of practice

if he or she is practicing outside the legal scope of practice permitted within the state.

2. It is critical that the nurse know the exact scope of practice permitted in his or her jurisdiction.

3. It is universally recommended that all professional nurses carry their own liability insurance coverage. This affords one's own legal representation and an attorney who will be looking out solely for the nurse's best interests. Such coverage is recommended over and above the legal coverage and representation afforded by the employer's coverage.

4. Coverage should be by occurrence, rather than claims-made terms. Occurrence policies cover the nurse whenever the occurrence of the care took place, even if the nurse is no longer employed at that location or the policy is not active at the time the claim is made.

Telephone Triage, Advice, and Counseling

1. The use of telephone triage, advice, and counseling has become increasingly prevalent as health care providers have attempted to meet and satisfy the health care needs of their patients, increase access to care, and improve continuity of care, while limiting scheduled appointments to those truly requiring a patient–physician or other health care provider interaction.

2. Health care professionals who provide telephone services must keep in mind that they are legally accountable for gathering an accurate and complete history, application of appropriate protocols for diagnostic impressions, appropriate consultation with other health care providers, advice and counseling given, and facilitation of timely and appropriate access to treatment facilities or referral to specialists to those in need.

3. Internet and other means of electronic communication are becoming acceptable but present concerns for privacy.

4. A number of legal concepts of relevance to telephone triage are outlined in the next section.

Confidentiality

Just as in face-to-face interactions, all information exchanged during a telephone interaction is privileged and is to be used only in the context of the advice being sought, with the sole purpose of providing the most appropriate and timely care needed by the patient.

Implied Relationships

Even if the professional nurse providing telephone advice has never had face-to-face interaction with the patient, the telephone interaction itself will establish a formal and legally binding nurse–patient relationship, for which the practitioner will be accountable legally.

Information Retrieval

1. The professional nurse has the duty to provide advice and counsel in the context of all medical data available to the practice from within the patient's medical record.

2. Therefore, a rapid method for the retrieval of medical record data should be established and integrated into the telephone component of all practices.

3. Telephone advice must not be provided in a vacuum of knowledge about the patient's past history.

4. Because limited time will usually preclude the gathering of all data available in the medical record, advice rendered without the benefit of all known medical history is more subject to error.

Respondeat Superior

1. Employers are held accountable, legally responsible, and liable for all inappropriate advice provided by their employees and all damages that may result.

2. Therefore, employers must be responsible for educating and training employees and updating protocols.

Vicarious Liability

1. Although similar to the concept of respondeat superior, vicarious liability is a broader concept in that a professional nurse providing telephone advice or counseling may be viewed as a representative of the facility physician, practice group, or facility, thereby binding them legally for all acts of omission or commission and damages that result.

2. Thus, if telephone advice and counsel are rendered by an LPN, RN, or unlicensed personnel, the nurse, health care facility, or physicians in the practice may be viewed by a court as vicariously liable for inappropriate advice provided and all resulting damages to the patient.

3. This underscores the reasons for limiting this practice to well-trained nurses, physicians, and other health care providers and following carefully devised office protocols and standards.

4. The professional nurse must be encouraged to consult briefly with the in-office physician or other health care providers to reduce the possibility of advice that is not appropriate or is in error.

Negligent Supervisor

1. This concept relates to the failure of a supervising physician or other health care provider to provide the needed guidance and direction to the telephone advice nurse, despite a prevailing understanding, practice, or policy obligating this supervision.

2. This scenario usually overlaps with respondeat superior or vicarious liability.

Negligence

1. Any telephone assessment and advice rendered must be in accordance with the generally accepted standards and protocols.

2. Violation of the applicable standards of practice or care is considered to be negligent.

3. Evidence of standards of care is established by:
   a. Publications on the topic.
   b. Community practices.
   c. Generally accepted guidelines or treatises on the topic.

Abandonment

1. This concept becomes operational when a patient calls or comes in to report symptoms, seek advice, or request an on-site evaluation or treatment, and this communication is documented or otherwise established as fact, but the telephone advice nurse fails to follow through with the professional component of the interaction (advice).

BOX 2-2	Components of Successful Telephone Practice

- Apply standardized protocols and guidelines for the most frequently reported chief complaints.
- Train nurses in proper history taking, protocol or guideline utilization, and documentation.
- Apply a computer-based approach to manage the telephone encounters to complement existing protocols and guidelines to improve the process and documentation of the encounter.
- Implement a quality assurance system to ensure a regular review of telephone logs.
- Discuss problem cases with telephone advice nurses and perform outcome surveys.
- Maintain a constant availability of physicians and other health care providers to provide consultative assistance to the telephone advice nurse as needed.
- Ensure an ongoing review and revision of protocols and policies to eliminate or improve on problematic policies and protocols.

- Schedule patients with serious problems as soon as possible.
- Ask and confirm that the patient understands and feels comfortable with the plan at the end of the telephone interaction.
- Invite the patient for an after-hours visit if he or she is uncomfortable with receiving home care instructions or with waiting until the next day to see the physician or other health care provider.
- Encourage patients to call back if their condition worsens or if they have additional questions.
- Advise patients to contact their health care provider the next day if the problem has not improved.
- Document succinctly the components of the telephone interaction, including the chief complaint, history of present illness, past medical history, allergies, home care or other instructions given, confirmation of the patient's understanding and comfort with the advice given, emergency precautions provided, and follow-up plans.

2. However, unless an undesirable outcome with serious and permanent damages occurs due to the absence of follow-through by the telephone practitioner, it is doubtful that a legal claim could be brought successfully against the practitioner.

Successful Telephone Practice

1. Policies aimed at minimizing the risk of an untoward outcome resulting from telephone advice, triage, and counseling should be established in every practice.
2. Policies should include protocol use, telephone practitioner training and education, use of an established patient database, communication with a physician or other health care provider, and appropriate documentation of interaction.
3. See Box 2-2 for components of a successful telephone advice practice.
4. The telephone advice nurse must gather and document certain fundamental information from the patient seeking health care advice or treatment. Although the following list is presented, it is not intended to limit inquiry or imply that the list is exhaustive. The inquiry and documentation must minimally include:
   a. Date and time of the call.
   b. Caller information including the name of the patient, relationship to the patient, telephone number with area code, when and where the caller may be reached for return calls, and alternative telephone numbers with area code for backup.
   c. Chief complaint.
   d. History of present illness, with brief description of onset, symptoms, treatment used to date, effectiveness or lack thereof of measures attempted, and aggravating or alleviating factors.
   e. Whether the patient has had this problem before and, if so, when, diagnosis, and method of resolution.
   f. If female, last menstrual period, method of birth control, and follow-up to rule out pregnancy.
   g. Past medical history and other medical problems.
   h. Allergies.
   i. Likely differential diagnosis based on the established protocols and guidelines being utilized by the organization or facility.
   j. Impact of the problem on the caller or patient.
   k. Accessibility of alternative sources of health care.
   l. Nurse's perception of the patient's vulnerability.
   m. Nurse's perception of the patient's understanding and comfort with the plan of care and follow-up plans.

SELECTED REFERENCES

American Nurses Association. (2001). *Code of Ethics for Nurses with Interpretive Statements (Code for Nurses).* Silver Spring, MD: Author.

American Nurses Association. (2010). *Nursing scope and standards of practice* (2nd ed.). Silver Spring, MD: Author.

Buppert, C. (2011). Three frequently asked questions about malpractice insurance. *Journal for Nurse Practitioners, 7*(1), 16–17.

Dunton, N. (2011, March 24). Understanding NDNQI: What it is and why it is important. Presentation for the 58th AORN Congress, Philadelphia. Available: *www.nursingquality.org/Documents/Public/AORN_2011.pdf.*

Fernbach, A. (2011). Parental rights and decision making regarding vaccinations: Ethical dilemmas for the primary care provider. *Journal of the American Academy of Nurse Practitioners, 23*(7), 336–345.

Howie, W. O., Howie, B. A., & McMullen, P. C. (2012). To assist or not assist: good Samaritan considerations for nurse practitioners. *Journal for Nurse Practitioners, 8*(9): 688–693.

Institute of Medicine. (2011). *Health IT and patient safety: Building safer systems for better care.* Washington, DC: Author.

Miller, K. (2012). The national practitioner data bank history and data. *Journal for Nurse Practitioners 8*(9): 698–701.

Murray, T. L., Calhoun, M., & Philipsen, N. C. (2011). Privacy, confidentiality, HIPAA, and HITECH: Implications for the health care practitioner. *Journal for Nurse Practitioners, 7*(9), 747–752.

National Council of State Boards of Nursing. (2010). *National Council of State Boards of Nursing Policy Position Statement: Advancement of nursing education.* Chicago: Author.

National League of Nursing. (2010). *The NLN Education Competencies Model.* New York: Author.

Philipsen, N. (2011). The criminalization of mistakes in nursing. *Journal for Nurse Practitioners, 7*(9), 719–726.

3
Health Promotion and Preventive Care

CONCEPTS IN PROMOTION AND PREVENTION

Principles of Health Promotion

Health promotion is defined as the actions taken to develop a high level of wellness and is accomplished by influencing individual behavior and the environment in which people live.

Levels of Prevention

1. Disease prevention is aimed at avoiding problems or minimizing problems once they occur.
   a. Primary prevention is the total prevention of a condition.
   b. Secondary prevention is the early recognition of a condition and the measures taken to speed recovery.
   c. Tertiary prevention is the care given to minimize the effects of the condition and prevent long-term complications.
2. Preventive care should involve assessment for people at risk for specific disorders.

Healthy People 2020

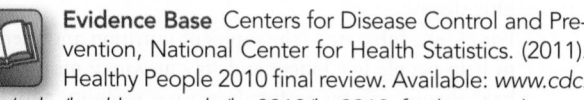 **Evidence Base** Centers for Disease Control and Prevention, National Center for Health Statistics. (2011). Healthy People 2010 final review. Available: *www.cdc. gov/nchs/healthy_people/hp2010/hp2010_final_review.htm*.
Centers for Disease Control and Prevention, National Center for Health Statistics. (2009.) Healthy People 2020. Available: *www.cdc.gov/nchs/healthy_people/hp2020.htm*.

1. Health promotion goes beyond prevention to help people manage their health and live longer and feel better.
2. Health promotion has become a priority since the U.S. Department of Health and Human Services (DHHS) initiated its Healthy People 2000 campaign in 1990.
3. For the Healthy People 2010 campaign, launched in 2000, 23% of the campaign's stated objectives were reached or exceeded, whereas 48% of the stated objectives were approached. The two major goals of Healthy People 2010 were to enhance life expectancy while improving quality of life and to reduce health disparities due to gender, race and ethnicity, income and education, disabilities, and other factors.
4. Healthy People 2020 consists of four overreaching goals with 42 topic areas (see Box 3-1, page 22):
   a. Attain high-quality, longer lives free of preventable disease, disability, injury, and premature death.
   b. Achieve health equity and eliminate disparities.
   c. Create social and physical environments that promote good health for all.
   d. Promote quality of life, healthy development, and healthy behaviors across all life stages.
5. For more information, see *www.healthypeople.gov*.

Millennium Development Goals

1. The Millennium Development Goals (MDGs) were approved by the United Nations in 2000 to address the most pressing needs of the poor worldwide, including some health needs.

BOX 3-1	Healthy People 2020 Topic Areas

- Access to quality health services
- Adolescent health
- Arthritis, osteoporosis, and chronic back conditions
- Blood disorders and blood safety
- Cancer
- Chronic kidney disease
- Dementias, including Alzheimer's disease
- Diabetes
- Disability and secondary conditions
- Early and middle childhood
- Educational and community-based programs
- Environmental health
- Family planning
- Food safety
- Genomics
- Global health
- Health communication
- Health care–associated infections
- Health-related quality of life and well-being
- Hearing and other sensory or communication disorders
- Heart disease and stroke
- Human immunodeficiency virus
- Immunization and infectious disease
- Injury and violence prevention
- Lesbian, gay, bisexual, and transgender health
- Maternal, infant, and child health
- Medical product safety
- Mental health and mental disorders
- Nutrition and weight control
- Occupational safety and health
- Older adults
- Oral health
- Physical activity and fitness
- Preparedness
- Public health infrastructure
- Respiratory disorders
- Sexually transmitted diseases
- Sleep health
- Social determinants of health
- Substance abuse
- Tobacco use
- Vision

2. Goals to be achieved by 2015 focus on the following areas:
   a. Eradicating extreme hunger and poverty.
   b. Achieving universal primary education.
   c. Promoting gender equality.
   d. Reducing child mortality.
   e. Improving maternal health.

f. Combating human immunodeficiency virus (HIV)/acquired immunodeficiency syndrome, malaria, and other diseases.
   g. Ensuring environmental sustainability.
   h. Developing a global partnership for development.
3. Nurses are at the forefront of health care throughout the world and can make tremendous strides in reaching these goals by caring for families and communities and advocating for vulnerable populations.
4. Review progress of the MDGs at *www.un.org/millenniumgoals*.

Nursing Role in Health Promotion

1. Nurses have played key roles in prevention in such areas as prenatal care, immunization programs, occupational health and safety, cardiac rehabilitation and education, and public health care and early intervention.
2. Nurses in all settings can meet health promotion needs of patients, whether their practice is in a hospital, clinic, patient's home, health maintenance organization, private office, or community setting.
3. Health promotion is primarily accomplished through patient education, an independent function of nursing.
4. Health promotion should occur through the life cycle, with topics focused on infancy, childhood, adolescence, adulthood, and older adults. Specific preventive services are evidence-based and recommended by the United States Preventive Services Task Force (*www.ahrq.gov/clinic/prevenix.htm*), the Canadian Task Force on Preventive Health Care (*www.canadiantaskforce.ca/index.html*), the National Institute for Health and Clinical Excellence (*www.nice.org.uk*) in the United Kingdom, as well as other agencies (see Table 3-1).
   a. For infancy, teach parents about the importance of prenatal care, basic care of infants, breastfeeding, nutrition, and infant safety (see Chapter 42).
   b. For childhood, stress the importance of immunizations; proper nutrition to enhance growth and development; and safety practices, such as use of car seats and seat belts, fire prevention, and poison-proofing the home (see Chapter 42).
   c. For adolescence, focus on motor vehicle safety; avoidance of drug, alcohol, and tobacco use; sexual decision making and contraception; and prevention of suicide.
   d. For adulthood, teach patients about nutrition, exercise, and stress management to help them feel better; also teach cancer-screening techniques, such as breast and testicular self-examination; and risk factor reduction for the leading causes of death—heart disease, stroke, cancer, and chronic lung disease.
   e. For older adults, stress the topics of nutrition and exercise to help people live longer and stay fit, safety measures to help them compensate for decreasing mobility and sensory function, and ways to stay active and independent (see Chapter 9).

Theories of Behavior Change

Lifestyle changes that promote wellness and reduce or prevent illness are often difficult to accomplish. Although education and support by nurses are key, lifestyle changes are ultimately up to

Table 3-1 Preventive Services Recommended by the USPSTF

The U.S. Preventive Services Task Force (USPSTF) recommends that clinicians discuss these preventive services with eligible patients and offer them as a priority. All these services have received an "A" (strongly recommended) or "B" (recommended) grade from the Task Force.

RECOMMENDATION	MEN	WOMEN	PREGNANT WOMEN	CHILDREN
Abdominal Aortic Aneurysm, Screening (1)	✓			
Alcohol Misuse Screening and Behavioral Counseling Interventions	✓	✓	✓	
Aspirin for the Primary Prevention of Cardiovascular Events (2)	✓	✓		
Asymptomatic Bacteriuria in Adults, Screening (3)			✓	
Breast Cancer, Screening (4)		✓		
Breast and Ovarian Cancer Susceptibility, Genetic Risk Assessment and BRCA Mutation Testing (5)		✓		
Breast-feeding, Primary Care Interventions to Promote (6)		✓	✓	
Cervical Cancer, Screening (7)		✓		
Chlamydial Infection, Screening (8)		✓	✓	
Colorectal Cancer, Screening (9)	✓	✓		
Congenital Hypothyroidism, Screening (10)				✓
Depression (Adults), Screening (11)	✓	✓		
Folic Acid Supplementation (12)		✓		
Gonorrhea, Screening (13)		✓		
Gonorrhea, Prophylactic Medication (14)				✓
Hearing Loss in Newborns, Screening (15)				✓
Hepatitis B Virus Infection, Screening (16)			✓	
High Blood Pressure, Screening	✓	✓		
Human Immunodeficiency Virus (HIV), Screening (17)	✓	✓	✓	✓
Iron-Deficiency Anemia, Prevention (18)				✓
Iron-Deficiency Anemia, Screening (19)			✓	
Lipid Disorders in Adults, Screening (20)	✓	✓		
Major Depressive Disorder in Children and Adolescents, Screening (21)				✓
Obesity in Adults, Screening (22)	✓	✓		
Obesity in Children and Adolescents, Screening (23)				✓
Osteoporosis, Screening (24)		✓		
Phenylketonuria, Screening (25)				✓
Rh(D) Incompatibility, Screening (26)			✓	
Sexually Transmitted Infections, Counseling (27)	✓	✓		✓

(continued)

Table 3-1	Preventive Services Recommended by the USPSTF (continued)				
RECOMMENDATION		MEN	WOMEN	PREGNANT WOMEN	CHILDREN
Sickle Cell Disease, Screening (28)					✓
Syphilis Infection, Screening (29)		✓	✓	✓	
Tobacco Use and Tobacco-Caused Disease, Counseling and Interventions (30)		✓	✓	✓	
Type 2 Diabetes Mellitus in Adults, Screening (31)		✓	✓		
Visual Impairment in Children Younger Than 5 Years, Screening (32)					✓

1. One-time screening by ultrasonography in men ages 65 to 75 who have ever smoked.
2. When the potential harm of an increase in gastrointestinal hemorrhage is outweighed by a potential benefit of a reduction in myocardial infarctions (men age 45 to 79 years) or in ischemic strokes (women age 55 to 79 years).
3. Pregnant women at 12 to 16 weeks' gestation or at first prenatal visit, if later.
4. Biennial screening mammography for women age 50 to 74 years; (2002 recommendations: age 40 and older, every 1–2 years).
5. Refer women whose family history is associated with an increased risk for deleterious mutations in BRCA1 or BRCA2 genes for genetic counseling and evaluation for BRCA testing.
6. Interventions during pregnancy and after birth to promote and support breastfeeding.
7. Cytology every 3 years (age 21 to 65) or cotest (cytology/HPV testing) every 5 years (age 30–65).
8. Sexually active women age 24 and younger and other asymptomatic women at increased risk for infection. Asymptomatic pregnant women age 24 and younger and others at increased risk.
9. Adults age 50 to 75 using fecal occult blood testing, sigmoidoscopy, or colonoscopy.
10. Newborns.
11. When staff-assisted depression care supports are in place to ensure accurate diagnoses, effective treatment, and follow-up.
12. All women planning or capable of pregnancy take a daily supplement containing 0.4 to 0.8 mg (400 to 800 mcg) of folic acid.
13. Sexually active women, including pregnant women age 25 and younger, or at increased risk for infection.
14. Prophylactic ocular topical medication for all newborns against gonococcal ophthalmia neonatorium.
15. Newborns.
16. Pregnant women at first prenatal visit.
17. All adolescents and adults at increased risk for HIV infection and all pregnant women.
18. Routine iron supplementation for asymptomatic children age 6 to 12 months who are at increased risk for iron-deficiency anemia.
19. Routine screening in asymptomatic pregnant women.
20. Men age 25 to 35 and older and women over age 20 who are at risk for coronary disease; all men age 35 and older.
21. Adolescents (age 12 to 18) when systems are in place to ensure accurate diagnosis, psychotherapy, and follow-up.
22. Intensive counseling and behavioral interventions to promote sustained weight loss for obese adults.
23. Screen children age 6 years and older for obesity and offer them or refer them to comprehensive, intensive behavioral interventions to promote improvement in weight status.
24. Women age 65 and older and women under age 65 at increased risk for osteoporotic fractures.
25. Newborns.
26. Blood type and antibody testing at first pregnancy-related visit. Repeated antibody testing for unsensitized Rh(D)-negative women at 24 to 28 weeks' gestation unless biological father is known to be Rh(D) negative.
27. All sexually active adolescents and adults at increased risk for STIs
28. Newborns.
29. Persons at increased risk and all pregnant women.
30. Ask all adults about tobacco use and provide tobacco cessation interventions for those who use tobacco; provide augmented, pregnancy-tailored counseling to pregnant women who smoke.
31. Asymptomatic adults with sustained blood pressure greater than 135/80 mm Hg.
32. To detect amblyopia, strabismus, and defects in visual acuity; screen children ages 3–5 years.

Guide to Clinical Preventive Services, 2012: Recommendations of the U.S. Preventive Services Task Force. AHRQ Publication No. 12-05154, October 2012. Agency for Healthcare Research and Quality, Rockville, MD. http://www.ahrq.gov/clinic/pocketgd2012/

the patient. Nurses should understand the concepts and processes related to behavior change in order to help direct interventions for successful outcomes in individual patients or groups.

Health Belief Model

The health belief model identifies perceptions that influence an individual's behavior. Nurses can inquire about a patient's perceptions in three areas in order to individualize education and interventions.

1. The first perception is susceptibility to and seriousness of disease or threat of illness. This most directly influences whether a person will take action.
2. The perceived benefit of taking action also affects behavior change.

3. Any perceived barriers to change may prevent or impede action.

Transtheoretical Model

The transtheoretical model of behavior change developed by Prochaska and DiClemente identifies six predictable stages of change. The stages may cycle back and forth several times before change is complete. Education and interventions can be aimed at moving the patient onto the next stage or back into the cycle if a lapse occurs.

1. Precontemplation—no intention to change, may deny that there is a problem, may blame others for any problems.
2. Contemplation—acknowledgment that there is a problem, willing to change but may be ambivalent or anxious about change.
3. Preparation—explores options, actively plans to change, may go public with intent.
4. Action—overtly making a change, substituting desired behavior for old behavior.
5. Maintenance—continuing the change, may devalue old behavior, lapse may occur.
6. *Termination*—takes on a new self-image, old behavior is no longer a threat.

Patient Teaching and Health Education

Health education is included in the American Nurses Association Standards of Care and is defined as an essential component of nursing care. It is directed toward promotion, maintenance, and restoration of health and toward adaptation to the residual effects of illness.

Learning Readiness

1. Assist the patient in physical readiness to learn by trying to alleviate physical distress that may distract the patient's attention and prevent effective learning.
2. Assess and promote the patient's emotional readiness to learn.
   a. Motivation to learn depends on acceptance of the illness or that illness is a threat, recognition of the need to learn, values related to social and cultural background, and a therapeutic regimen compatible with the patient's lifestyle.
   b. Promote motivation to learn by creating a warm, accepting, positive atmosphere; encouraging the patient to participate in the establishment of acceptable, realistic, and attainable learning goals; and providing constructive feedback about progress.
3. Assess and promote the patient's experiential readiness to learn.
   a. Determine what experiences the patient has had with health and illness, what success or failure the patient has had with learning, and what basic knowledge the patient has on related topics.
   b. Provide the patient with prerequisite knowledge necessary to begin the learning process.

Teaching Strategies

1. Patient education can occur at any time and in any setting; however, you must consider how conducive the environment is to learning, how much time you are able to schedule, and what other family members can attend the teaching session.
2. Use a variety of techniques that are appropriate to meet the needs of each individual.
   a. Lecture or explanation should include discussion or a question-and-answer session.
   b. Group discussion is effective for individuals with similar needs; participants commonly gain support, assistance, and encouragement from other members.
   c. Demonstration and practice should be used when skills need to be learned; ample time should be allowed for practice and return demonstration.
   d. Teaching aids include books, pamphlets, pictures, slides, videos, tapes, and models and should serve as supplements to verbal teaching. These can be obtained from government agencies, such as the Department of Health and Human Services, the Centers for Disease Control and Prevention, and the National Institutes of Health; nonprofit groups, such as the American Heart Association or the March of Dimes; various Internet health websites; or pharmaceutical and insurance companies.
   e. Reinforcement and follow-up sessions offer time for evaluation and additional teaching, if necessary, and can greatly increase the effectiveness of teaching.
3. Document patient teaching, including what was taught and how the patient responded; use standardized patient teaching checklists if available.

Health Literacy

1. Health literacy is the ability to read, understand, and act on health information.
2. Health literacy goes beyond ability to read; it encompasses the following processes:
   a. Being able to follow instructions on prescription bottles.
   b. Understanding follow-up and referral appointment information.
   c. Understanding consent forms.
   d. Reading and understanding informational brochures and other instructions.
   e. Being able to negotiate the complex health care system.
3. According to the Institute of Medicine's report "A Prescription to End Confusion," poor health literacy is a stronger predictor of a person's health than age, income, employment status, education level, and race.
4. Vulnerable groups include people over 65 years of age, minorities and immigrants, low-income populations, and people with chronic mental and physical conditions.
5. The majority of Americans read at an eighth-grade level and 20% read at a fifth-grade level or below. Most health-related materials are written at a 10th-grade reading level.
6. Clear communication between patients and health care professionals is critical. Nurses can assess patient literacy skills, use level-appropriate language and written materials, and help patients ask the right questions. The Ask Me 3 program, designed by the Partnership for Clear Health

Communication, encourages patients to ask and understand the answers to the following questions:

a. What is my main problem?

b. What do I need to do?

c. Why is it important for me to do this?

Selected Areas of Health Promotion

Counsel patients about proper nutrition, smoking cessation, physical activity, relaxation, and sexual health to promote well-being.

Nutrition and Diet

 Evidence Base U.S. Department of Health and Human Services and U.S. Department of Agriculture. (2011). Dietary Guidelines for Americans 2010. Executive summary. Available: www.cnpp.usda.gov/Publications/DietaryGuidelines/2010/DGAC/Report/A-ExecSummary.pdf.

1. Poor diet and sedentary lifestyle are linked to cardiovascular disease, type 2 diabetes, hypertension, osteoporosis, and some cancers.

2. The U.S. DHHS and the U.S. Department of Agriculture recommend and update dietary guidelines every 5 years. These guidelines, combined with physical activity, should enhance the health of most individuals. For more information on these guidelines, see *www.dietaryguidelines.gov*.

3. The 2010 guidelines recommend two major interrelated concepts:

   a. Calorie balance over time to achieve or sustain a healthy weight—consume only enough calories to meet the needs expended by physical activity.

   b. Consumption of nutrient-dense foods and beverages—such as vegetables, fruits, whole grains, fat-free to low-fat milk products, seafood, lean meat, poultry, eggs, beans, and nuts.

4. Key recommendations of the 2010 Guidelines include:

   a. Prevent or reduce overweight and obesity through improved eating and increased physical activity.

   b. Control total calorie intake to manage or achieve weight.

   c. Increase physical activity and reduce sedentary activity time.

   d. Maintain appropriate calorie balance during each stage of life.

   e. Reduce sodium intake to less than 2,300 mg daily, or 1,500 mg daily if older than 50 years or if there is a history of hypertension, diabetes, or chronic kidney disease.

   f. Consume less than 10% of calories from saturated fats and use a minimum of trans fats by limiting partially hydrogenated oils and other solid fats.

   g. Consume less than 300 mg cholesterol daily.

   h. Reduce the intake of calories from solid fats and refined sugars.

   i. Limit refined grains, especially those containing solid fats, added sugars, and sodium.

   j. Consume alcohol in moderation—no more than one drink daily for women, two drinks for men.

   k. Increase vegetable and fruit intake; eat a variety, especially dark-green and red and orange vegetables, beans, and peas.

   l. Increase whole-grain intake by replacing refined grains.

   m. Increase fat-free and low-fat milk and milk products or soy beverages.

   n. Choose a variety of protein foods (including eggs, beans, peas, soy, unsalted nuts and seeds).

   o. Use oils to replace solid fats.

   p. Increase foods with potassium, fiber, calcium, vitamin D by increasing vegetables, fruits, whole grains, and milk products.

5. Educate patients about the five basic food groups, optimum weight, calorie requirements, and ways to increase fiber and decrease fat in the diet.

6. Teach patients to add fiber to the diet by choosing whole-grain breads and cereals; raw or minimally cooked fruits and vegetables (especially citrus fruits, squash, cabbage, lettuce and other greens, beans); and any nuts, skins, and seeds. Fiber can also be increased by adding several teaspoons of whole bran to meals each day or taking an over-the-counter fiber supplement, such as psyllium, as directed.

 NURSING ALERT Encourage all patients to follow up closely with their health care providers if they are following high-fat, restricted-carbohydrate diets. Any diet that is unbalanced may require vitamin supplementation and alter biochemical processes such as cholesterol metabolism and fluid balance.

7. Encourage patients to keep food diaries and review them periodically to determine if other adjustments should be made.

8. If weight loss is desired, have the patient weigh in monthly, and review the diet and give praise or corrective advice at this visit. Many people, especially women, respond to group therapy that focuses on education, support, and expression of feelings related to overeating.

Smoking Prevention and Cessation

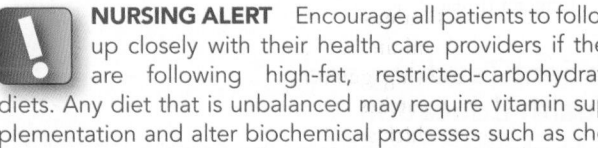 **Evidence Base** National Cancer Institute. (2012, last modified October 23, 2012). Cigarette smoking: Health risks and how to quit (PDQ). Available: http://www.cancer.gov/cancertopics/pdq/prevention/control-of-tobacco-use/HealthProfessional.

1. According to the National Cancer Institute, a smoker's risk of cancer is 2 to 10 times greater than a nonsmoker's risk, depending on how much a person has smoked, and lung cancer is the leading cause of cancer deaths for both men and women.

2. The number of first-time smokers has increased in the United States to approximately 2.4 million first-time smokers each year (6,500 each day), up from about 2 million in 2002.

3. Smoking is a risk factor for hypertension; heart disease; peripheral vascular disease; chronic obstructive pulmonary disease (COPD); and cancer of the lung, colon, larynx, oral cavity, esophagus, bladder, pancreas, and kidney. It also

worsens such conditions as respiratory infections, peptic ulcers, hiatal hernia, and gastroesophageal reflux.

4. Not smoking promotes health by increasing exercise tolerance; enhancing taste bud function; and avoiding facial wrinkles and bad breath.

5. Smoking prevention education should begin during childhood and stressed during adolescence, a time when peer modeling and confusion over self-image may lead to smoking.

6. Smoking cessation can be accomplished through an individualized, multidimensional program that includes:

   a. Information on the short- and long-term health effects of smoking.

   b. Practical behavior-modification techniques to help break the habit—gum chewing, snacking on carrot and celery sticks, sucking on mints and hard candy to provide oral stimulation; working modeling clay, knitting, or other ways to provide tactile stimulation; avoiding coffee shops, bars, or other situations that smokers frequent; delaying each cigarette and recording each cigarette in a log before it is smoked; and incentive plans such as saving money for each cigarette not smoked and rewarding oneself when a goal is reached.

   c. Use of medications designed to reduce physical dependence and minimize withdrawal symptoms, such as nicotine chewing gum, nasal spray, inhaler system, or transdermal patches as well as oral medication such as bupropion, which acts on neurotransmitters in the central nervous system, and varenicline, a selective nicotinic acetylcholine receptor partial agonist.

   d. Use of support groups, frequent reinforcement, and follow-up. Encourage additional attempts if relapse occurs.

Exercise and Fitness

1. Regular exercise as part of a fitness program helps achieve optimal weight, control blood pressure (BP), increase high-density lipoprotein, lower risk of coronary artery disease, increase endurance, and improve the sense of well-being.

2. Long-term goals of regular exercise include decreased absenteeism from work, improved balance and reduced disability among older adults, decreased osteoporosis and fracture risk, and reduced health care costs.

3. Most health benefits occur with at least 150 minutes of physical activity a week, or 30 minutes of moderate-intensity physical activity (in addition to usual activity) most days of the week. Greater benefits can be obtained by increasing intensity and duration of activity.

   a. Children and adolescents should do 60 minutes of physical activity daily that is age appropriate and includes aerobic, muscle-strengthening, and bone-strengthening activities.

   b. For additional health benefits such as managing or losing weight, adults should increase their aerobic activity to 300 minutes (5 hours) of moderate-intensity or 150 minutes (2.5 hours) of vigorous-intensity aerobic activity weekly.

   c. Muscle-strengthening activities that involve all major muscle groups two or more days a week provide additional benefits.

   d. Older adults and those with disabilities should engage in physical activities as their conditions allow. Generally the benefits of physical activity outweigh potential risks.

 Evidence Base U.S. Department of Health and Human Services (2012). The Physical Activity Guidelines for Americans Midcourse Report: Strategies for Increasing Physical Activity Among Youth Available: *http://www.health.gov/paguidelines/midcourse/PAG_Midcourse_Report.pdf.*

4. Suggest walking, jogging, bicycling, swimming, water aerobics, and low-impact aerobic dancing as good low- to moderate-intensity exercise, performed three to five times per week for 45 minutes. Walking can be done safely and comfortably by most patients if the pace is adjusted to the individual's physical condition. Use of weights is important for muscle strengthening throughout the life span.

   a. Exercise programs should include 5- to 10-minute warm-up and cool-down periods with stretching activities to prevent injuries.

   b. Full intensity and duration of exercise should be increased gradually over a period of several weeks to months.

 GERONTOLOGIC ALERT Older adults who are at risk for falling should do exercise that maintains or improves balance.

5. Advise patients to stop if pain, shortness of breath, dizziness, palpitations, or excessive sweating is experienced.

6. Advise patients with cardiovascular, respiratory, and musculoskeletal disorders to check with their health care provider about specific guidelines or limitations for exercise.

 NURSING ALERT Severe cases of COPD, osteoarthritis, and coronary disease are contraindications for unsupervised exercise; check with the patient's health care provider to see if a physical therapy or occupational therapy referral would be helpful.

Relaxation and Stress Management

1. *Stress* is a change in the environment that is perceived as a threat, challenge, or harm to the person's dynamic equilibrium. In times of stress, the sympathetic nervous system is activated to produce immediate changes of increased heart rate, peripheral vasoconstriction, and increased BP. This response is prolonged by adrenal stimulation and secretion of epinephrine and norepinephrine, and is known as the "fight-or-flight" reaction.

2. A limited amount of stress can be a positive motivator to take action; however, excessive or prolonged stress can cause emotional discomfort, anxiety, possible panic, and illness.

3. Prolonged sympathetic–adrenal stimulation may lead to high BP, arteriosclerotic changes, and cardiovascular disease; stress has also been implicated in acute asthma attack, peptic ulcer disease, irritable bowel syndrome, migraine headaches, and other illnesses.

4. Stress management can help patients control illnesses, improve self-esteem, gain control, and enjoy life more fully.

5. Stress management involves the identification of physiologic and psychosocial stressors through assessment of the patient's education, finances, job, family, habits, activities, personal and family health history, and responsibilities. Positive and negative coping methods should also be identified.

6. Relaxation therapy is one of the first steps in stress management; it can be used to reduce anxiety brought on by stress. Relaxation techniques include:
   a. Relaxation breathing—the simplest technique that can be performed at any time. The patient breathes slowly and deeply until relaxation is achieved; however, it can lead to hyperventilation if done incorrectly.
   b. Progressive muscle relaxation—relieves muscle tension related to stress. The patient alternately tenses, then relaxes muscle groups until the entire body feels relaxed.
   c. Autogenic training—can help relieve pain and induce sleep. The patient replaces painful or unpleasant sensations with pleasant ones through self-suggestions; may require extensive coaching at first.
   d. Imagery—uses imagination and concentration to take a "mental vacation." The patient imagines a peaceful, pleasant scene involving multiple senses. It can last as long as the patient decides.
   e. Distraction—uses the patient's own interests and activities to divert attention from pain or anxiety and includes listening to music, watching television, reading a book, singing, knitting, doing crafts or projects, or physical activities.

7. To assist patients with relaxation therapy, follow these steps:
   a. Review the techniques and encourage a trial with several techniques of the patient's choice.
   b. Teach the chosen technique and coach the patient until effective use of the technique is demonstrated.
   c. Suggest that the patient practice relaxation techniques for 20 minutes per day to feel more relaxed and to be prepared to use them confidently when stress increases.
   d. Encourage the patient to combine techniques such as relaxation breathing before and after imagery or progressive muscle relaxation along with autogenic training to achieve better results.

8. Additional steps in stress management include dealing with the stressors or problem areas and increasing coping behaviors.
   a. Help the patient to recognize specific stressors and determine if they can be altered. Then develop a plan for managing that stressor, such as changing jobs, postponing taking an extra class, hiring a babysitter once per week, talking to the neighbor about a problem, or getting up 1 hour earlier to exercise.
   b. Teach the patient to avoid negative coping behaviors, such as smoking, drinking, using drugs, overeating, cursing, and using abusive behavior toward others. Teach positive coping mechanisms, such as continued use of relaxation techniques and fostering of support systems—family, friends, church groups, social groups, or professional support groups.

Sexual Health

1. Because sexuality is inherent to every person and sexual functioning is a basic physiologic need of human beings, nurses can help patients gain knowledge, validate normalcy, prepare for changes in sexuality throughout the life cycle, and prevent harm gained through sexual activity.

2. Education about sexuality should begin with school-age children, increase during adolescence, and continue through adulthood.

3. Topics to cover include:
   a. Relationships, responsibilities, communication.
   b. Normal reproduction—the menstrual cycle, ovulation, fertilization, sperm production.
   c. Prevention of unwanted pregnancy (approximately 1 million teen pregnancies occur in the United States each year) and sexually transmitted diseases (STDs).

4. The Centers for Disease Control and Prevention estimates that there are approximately 19 million new STD infections each year, which cost the U.S. health care system $16.4 billion annually and cost individuals even more in terms of acute and long-term health consequences.
   a. The number of cases of gonorrhea is declining and the number of cases of chlamydia is increasing (probably due to increased screening), but still only about half of people at risk for STDs are screened.
   b. Chlamydia, gonorrhea, and syphilis are reportable to state and local health departments; however, other STDs such as human papilloma virus (HPV) and herpes simplex virus are prevalent and cause chronic effects. Complications of STDs include pelvic inflammatory disease, infertility, serious vital organ damage in the case of tertiary syphilis, cervical cancer in the case of HPV, and increased risk of contracting HIV.
   c. Nurses are in a key position to teach prevention through abstinence and barrier protection, identify cases through screening for earlier treatment, and reduce the burden of these serious and often chronic diseases.

5. Use and refer patients to such resources as the American Social Health Association (*www.ashastd.org*) and Centers for Disease Control and Prevention Health Topics A to Z: (*www.cdc.gov/health/default.htm*).

PATIENT TEACHING AIDS

Copy and distribute the patient teaching aids on pages 29 to 32 to enhance your counseling and promote health.

PATIENT EDUCATION GUIDELINES 3-1

Exercise Guidelines

Aerobic exercise provides a wide range of benefits including weight loss, muscle toning, endurance building, improved circulation, increased high-density lipoprotein (the "good" cholesterol), lowered risk of a heart attack, better controlled BP, and a sense of reduced tension and overall wellness. Aerobic exercise refers to any type of activity that uses oxygen to produce energy. The cardiovascular system is stimulated and fat is burned. Most people can do aerobic exercise of some kind, adjusting the intensity as necessary. Follow these guidelines to develop your own exercise program.

- Choose an activity that you enjoy, is convenient, and you are capable of; consider walking, bicycle riding, jogging, swimming, aerobics or step aerobics, sporting activities, or use of fitness equipment such as a rowing machine, stair stepper, or cross-country ski machine.
- Start out exercising 15 to 20 minutes at a time for the first week or two, then gradually increase the intensity and length of exercise time over several weeks to months.
- Include a 5- to 10-minute warm-up and cool-down period with each exercise session, doing stretching of major muscles, deep breathing, and light calisthenics.
- Exercise most days or a total of at least 150 minutes per week, but remember that some exercise is better than none.
- Exercise at 50% to 70% of your maximum heart rate for moderate intensity or 70% to 90% for high intensity, as tolerated.

CALCULATING TARGET HEART RATE

To get the most out of exercise, calculate your heart rate. First, subtract your age from 220. This is your maximum heart rate; do not exceed this rate while exercising to avoid strain on your heart.

If you are age 40, your maximum heart rate is 220 minus 40, or 180. Your target heart rate is 40% to 50% of maximum for low-intensity exercise, 50% to 70% of maximum for moderate-intensity exercise, or 70% to 90% of maximum for high-intensity exercise. So, if you want to exercise at moderate intensity, 60% of 180 is 108 (180 × 0.6). Your target heart rate is 108. By taking your pulse several times during exercise, you can adjust your pace to stay close to your target heart rate and exercise optimally but safely.

TAKING YOUR PULSE

First take your resting pulse before you begin exercise, counting for 30 seconds and multiplying by 2.

To take your pulse during exercise, slow down and find the carotid pulse point in your neck. Place two or three fingers on your trachea (windpipe) near the base of your neck and then move them over to the left or right about 2 to 3 inches until you feel the beating of your pulse. Press lightly so you do not cause an irregular heartbeat or interrupt circulation to your brain. Use a watch with a second hand to count the number of beats in 6 seconds. Now, multiply by 10 to get an estimate of your true 60-second pulse.

If you counted 10 beats in 6 seconds, your working heart rate is 100 (10 × 10). As you continue to exercise, you can work a little harder to reach your target rate. If your working heart rate is 10 beats or more greater than your target rate, slow down your pace and check your pulse again in 5 to 10 minutes.

When you complete your exercise, your pulse should be no more than 15 beats above your resting pulse; if it is, continue your cool-down activity.

WHEN TO STOP

You should usually never stop exercising abruptly; you must allow the heart to slow down and the blood to redistribute appropriately.

You should slow down if you experience muscle cramps, shortness of breath, or fatigue. You should stop, however, if you experience chest pain, a cold sweat, dizziness, nausea or vomiting, heart palpitations, or fainting. Seek help and notify your health care provider immediately.

For more information, go to *www.healthfinder.gov*.

PATIENT EDUCATION GUIDELINES 3-2

Stress Management

Stress is a common phenomenon among most individuals today and can be related to job, relationship, financial, and other pressures. Known as the "fight-or-flight" reaction, the physiologic and emotional response to stress can lead to tension, anxiety, and a variety of health threats. Stress can be minimized by better coping with it and adapting to its causes. Follow this guide to better manage stress.

RECOGNIZE STRESS

- First, identify signs that you may be under stress (eg, irritability, tension, fatigue, insomnia, loss of interest in activities, feeling overwhelmed, or fighting with spouse and others).
- Next, try to identify the true cause of stress. For example, you may snap at your children for playing the stereo too loudly, but what is the underlying cause of your irritability?
- Examine areas of your job, family life, financial stability, and other roles and responsibilities that may be demanding or problematic.

DO SOMETHING ABOUT IT

- Try to manage stressful areas better—be assertive, negotiate, and say no if necessary. For example, confront the person with whom you are at odds and work out a mutual agreement, put the plan in writing, and try to stick to it.
- Make more time for yourself and important relationships. Say no to responsibilities that you do not have time for and get help from a family member or friend, or hire a babysitter when necessary.

RELAX

When you enter a stressful situation or you feel tension rising, practice the following relaxation techniques; you will be able to think more clearly and function more effectively.

Relaxation Breathing

Concentrate on breathing slowly and deeply with eyes closed (if possible) for several minutes when you need a quick tension reducer or before beginning one of the other methods.

- Breathe in through your nose and mouth with face relaxed for a count of 1 and 2 and 3 and 4.
- Hold your breath for 4 seconds, without straining.
- Breathe out through your nose and pursed lips for a count of 6.
- Repeat two or three times, breathe naturally for about 30 seconds, then repeat one or more sequences.
- If you feel dizzy or tingling in your fingertips, you may be hyperventilating; slow down your breathing and do not breathe out so forcefully.

Progressive Muscle Relaxation

Because stress may cause you to subconsciously contract your muscles, in this exercise you will alternately tense and relax your muscle groups one by one, until your entire body is in a state of relaxation.

- Assume a comfortable position, either sitting or reclining, and close your eyes.
- Start with your forehead and tense the muscles so you feel tightness or strain; hold this position for 5 to 10 seconds.
- Next, relax your forehead, noting the relief; concentrate on this for 10 to 15 seconds.
- Progress from head to toe with each muscle group, including your jaw, shoulders, arms, hands, abdomen, buttocks, legs, and feet (you can do both sides simultaneously).
- Note the feeling of total relaxation in your body once you have relieved tension from all your muscles.
- Complete the exercise by opening your eyes, taking a few deep breaths, stretching, and arising slowly.

Imagery

Imagery allows you to take a mental vacation by using your imagination and diverting your attention from stressful thoughts.

- Assume a comfortable position, breathe deeply, and close your eyes.
- Count backward from 5 and begin to imagine a pleasant place such as a beach or garden.
- Put yourself in that place by imagining it with all your senses (eg, hear the sound of waves washing up on the beach, feel the warm sun saturating your skin, or taste a tangy drink of lemonade).
- Stay in that place for about 5 minutes, imagining different images.
- Slowly let the images fade, breathe deeply, and count to 5 before opening your eyes.

Distraction

You can use many methods of distraction to block your concentration from anxiety and stressful matters. Using your senses to listen to music, petting your dog, or reading can be relaxing.

- Choose activities that you enjoy—reading, watching television, listening to music, taking a walk, playing an instrument, knitting, doing a craft, or drawing or painting.
- Adjust the distraction method to your mood—if you are extremely tense, do not attempt a complex project or listen to loud, lively music. Rather, listen to quiet, soothing music or sketch a free-form design.
- Use a variety of methods—some reserved for longer periods of time and others that can be used on the spot when needed (eg, a portable tape player with headphones and your favorite music or a book of poetry).

If relaxation methods don't help and you are having difficulty coping with stress, contact a health care provider.

PATIENT EDUCATION GUIDELINES 3-3

Eating Healthier

Most American diets include too little whole grains, vegetables, fruits, dairy products, seafood, fiber, and important nutrients; and too much saturated fat, sodium, refined grains, and calories from solid fats and added sugars. There is no one ideal diet, but to help maintain optimal weight, feel better, and reduce the risk of heart disease, cancer, and a variety of health problems, follow these Dietary Guidelines.

BUILD A HEALTHY PLATE

- Before you eat, think about the type of food and how much of it should go on your plate. Make half your plate fruits or vegetables—include red, orange, and dark green vegetables in your main and side dishes.
- Make one quarter of your plate whole grains—choose whole grain breads, rice, crackers, and pasta, as well as 100% whole-grain cereals
- Vary your proteins for the final quarter of your plate—try seafood twice a week, beans, eggs, nuts, seeds, soy products, as well as small, lean portions of meat and poultry. Snack on fruits, vegetables, or unsalted nuts, rather than processed grains such as crackers and chips and foods with added sugar and fat.

CUT BACK

- Cut back on foods with added sugar and salt.
  Drink water and other zero-calorie beverages instead of sugary drinks.
  Choose fruit for dessert. Save sugary desserts for a special occasion.
  Choose 100% fruit juice instead of fruit-flavored drinks.
  Read labels to compare sodium in soup, canned foods, and frozen meals.

Add spices or herbs other than salt to season food.
- Eat fewer foods that are high in solid fats.
  Select lean cuts of meat and poultry.
  Buy fat-free or low-fat milk, yogurt, and cheese.
- Switch from solid fat to oils when preparing food. Solid fats contain more saturated fat, which increases the risk of having a heart attack. So limit solid fats, which come from:
  Meat and poultry
  Butter, cream, and milk fat
  Coconut, palm, and palm kernel oil
  Hydrogenated and partially hydrogenated oils
  Shortening and stick margarine
- When fat is needed in preparing food, use the following oils: canola, corn, cottonseed, olive, peanut, safflower, sunflower; or use tub margarine.

PAY ATTENTION TO CALORIES

- Eat the right amount of calories for you.
  Think before you eat—do I need the calories?
  Avoid oversized portions, use a smaller plate or bowl.
  Cook more often at home, where you are in control of what is in your food.
  When eating out, choose lower-calorie menu options, order a smaller portion, or share.
  Stop eating when you are satisfied, not full.
  Write down what you eat to keep track of how much you eat.
- Use food labels to make better choices.

For more information, go to *www.dietaryguidelines.gov* or *www.choosemyplate.gov*.

PATIENT EDUCATION GUIDELINES 3-4

Smoking Cessation

Cigarette smoking is the single most preventable cause of death and disability today. Smoking is related to about 30% of all cancer deaths, is the leading risk factor for coronary artery disease and emphysema, and has many other effects on health and hygiene. People who smoke tend to have more dental problems, premature aging of the skin, increased acid in the stomach, decreased exercise tolerance, loss of taste bud function, problems with pregnancy and fetal growth, more frequent respiratory infections, and bad breath.

Smoking cessation, however, will reverse most of these risks and allow you to breathe more easily and feel better.

PLAN TO QUIT

- Make a list of all the positive things and all the negative things about smoking; consider the short- and long-term health risks on your list.
- Talk to your health care provider about the use of nicotine chewing gum, nasal spray, or skin patch to aid your stop-smoking program by reducing withdrawal symptoms and cravings for a cigarette. Oral medications that do not contain nicotine are also available by prescription.
- Talk to family and friends and form a support network of people who have quit smoking.
- Set a date to quit and don't make excuses.
- Stock up on low-calorie treats, such as raw vegetables, sugarless gum, popcorn, and sugar-free soft drinks, to enjoy when the urge to smoke hits.

- Remove ashtrays, cigarettes, matches, and lighters from your home, car, and office.

STICK WITH IT

- Avoid smoky environments, such as bars and coffee shops and the smoking section of restaurants.
- Restructure your routine to eliminate times you previously enjoyed a cigarette.
- Anticipate feeling irritable for several days to several weeks while quitting, and avoid stressful situations.
- Increase exercise, such as walking, biking, or sporting activities, to relieve tension, fill free time, and concentrate on healthy activity.
- Occupy your hands with modeling clay, knitting, doodling, or a craft project.
- Brush your teeth often to enjoy fresher breath.
- Reward yourself for not smoking.

TRY, TRY AGAIN

- If you start smoking again, do not be discouraged; many people are successful the second time around.
- Review and revise your plan and pick a new quit date.

For more information on smoking-cessation, go to *www.healthfinder.gov*.

SELECTED REFERENCES

Agency for Healthcare Research and Quality. (2012). The guide to clinical preventive services, 2012. *http://www.ahrq.gov/clinic/pocketgd2012/gcp12s1.htm*.

Centers for Disease Control and Prevention, National Center for Health Statistics. (2009). Healthy People 2020. Available: *www.cdc.gov/nchs/healthy_people/hp2020.htm*.

Centers for Disease Control and Prevention, National Center for Health Statistics. (2011). Healthy People 2010 final review. Available: *www.cdc.gov/nchs/healthy_people/hp2010/hp2010_final_review.htm*.

Committee on Health Literacy. (2004). *Health literacy: A prescription to end confusion*. Washington, DC: National Academies Press.

Fildes, E. E., Wilson, M. A., Crawford, B. J., et al. (2012). Tobacco quitlines in the United States. *Nursing Clinics of North America*, 47(1): 97–107.

National Cancer Institute. (2012, last modified 10/23/12). *http://www.cancer.gov/cancertopics/pdq/prevention/control-of-tobacco-use/HealthProfessional*

National Patient Safety Foundation. Ask Me 3. (2012). Available: *www.npsf.org/for-healthcare-professionals/programs/ask-me-3*.

National Patient Safety Foundation. (2012). Health literacy: Statistics-at-a-glance. Available: *www.npsf.org/wp-content/uploads/2011/12/AskMe3_Stats_English.pdf*.

Substance Abuse and Mental Health Services Administration. (2011). Results from the 2010 National Survey on Drug Use and Health: Mental health findings (Office of Applied Studies, NSDUH Series H-41, DHHS Publication No. SMA 11-4658). Available: *http://store.samhsa.gov/home*.

United Nations. (2011). Millennium development goals report 2011. Available: *www.un.org/millenniumgoals*.

U.S. Department of Health and Human Services. (2008). 2008 physical activity guidelines for Americans. Summary. Available: *www.health.gov/paguidelines/guidelines/summary.aspx*.

U.S. Department of Health and Human Services (2012). The Physical Activity Guidelines for Americans Midcourse Report: Strategies for Increasing Physical Activity Among Youth. Available: *http://www.health.gov/paguidelines/midcourse/PAG_Mid-course_Report.pdf*.

U.S. Department of Health and Human Services, Centers for Disease Control and Prevention. (2009). STD surveillance 2010. Available: *www.cdc.gov/std/stats10/default.htm*.

4
Genetics and Health Applications

HUMAN GENETICS

Human genetics, as it pertains to health care, is the study of the etiology, pathogenesis, and natural history of human conditions that are influenced by genetic factors. Genetic factors extend beyond the limited view of solely distinct genetic syndromes to encompass influences on health, the occurrence of complex disorders, individual biologic responses to illness, potential treatment and medical management approaches, and strategies for prevention or cure.

This tremendous realization is apparent through the accomplishments of the Human Genome Project. This 15-year international collaborative effort was completed in 2003. One significant goal of the Human Genome Project was to identify the approximately 25,000 human genes. These advances and the associated knowledge will continue to affect the delivery of health care and nursing practice significantly. Genetic evaluations, screening, testing, guided treatment, family counseling, and related legal, ethical, and psychosocial issues are becoming daily practice for many nurses.

The impact of genetics on nursing is significant. In 1997, the American Nurses Association (ANA) officially recognized genetics as a nursing specialty. This effort was spearheaded by the International Society of Nurses in Genetics (ISONG), which also initiated credentialing for the Advanced Practice Nurse in Genetics and the Genetics Clinical Nurse. ANA and ISONG have collaborated in the establishment of a scope and standards of practice for nurses in genetics practice. Essential Nursing Competencies and Curricula Guidelines for Genetics and Genomics were finalized in 2006 with Outcome Indicators established in 2008. They reflect the minimal genetic and genomic competencies for every nurse regardless of academic preparation, practice setting, role, or specialty. A copy of these competencies is available through the ANA or the National Human Genome Research Institute websites (*www.genome.gov/17517146*).

The purpose of this chapter is to provide the nurse with practical information, resources, representative examples, and professional considerations critical to integration of genetics knowledge into nursing practice.

Underlying Principles

Readers are encouraged to use the Talking Glossary of Genetic Terms available through the National Human Genome Research Institute to supplement the terms provided here. This glossary can be found at *www.genome.gov/glossary*.

Cell: The Basic Unit of Biology

1. Cytoplasm—contains functional structures important to cellular functioning, including mitochondria, which contain extranuclear deoxyribonucleic acid (DNA) important to mitochondrial functioning.
2. Nucleus—contains 46 chromosomes in each somatic (body) cell, or 23 chromosomes in each germ cell (egg or sperm) (see Figure 4-1, page 34).

Chromosomes

1. Each somatic cell with a nucleus has 22 pairs of autosomes (the same in both sexes) and 1 pair of sex chromosomes.
2. Females have two X sex chromosomes; males have one Y sex chromosome and one X sex chromosome.
3. Normally, at conception, each individual receives one copy of each chromosome from the maternal egg cell (1 genome) and one copy of each chromosome from the paternal sperm cell (1 genome), for a total of 46 chromosomes (2 genomes).
4. *Karyotype* is the term used to define the chromosomal complement of an individual (eg, 46, XY), as is determined by laboratory chromosome analysis.
5. Each chromosome contains a different number of genes, ranging from approximately 380 to 3,000 genes.

33

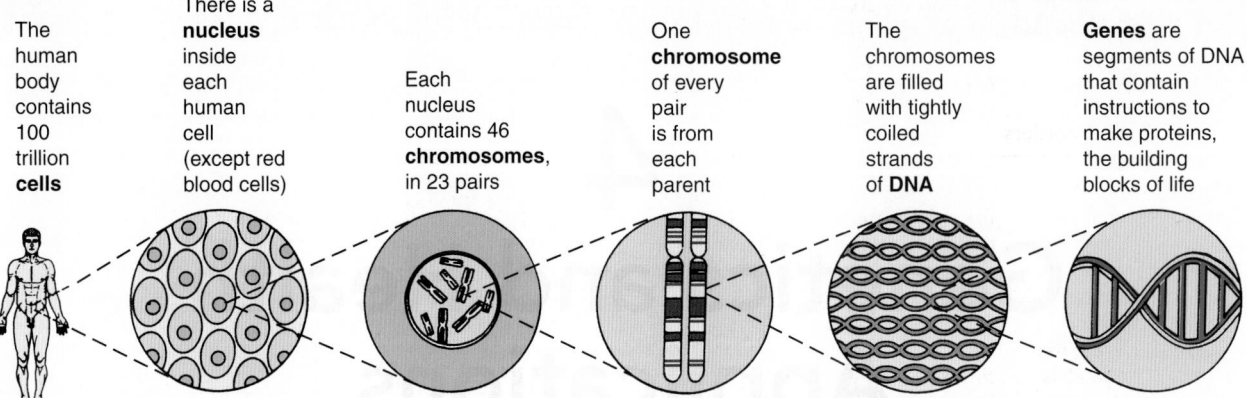

The human body contains 100 trillion **cells**

There is a **nucleus** inside each human cell (except red blood cells)

Each nucleus contains 46 **chromosomes**, in 23 pairs

One **chromosome** of every pair is from each parent

The chromosomes are filled with tightly coiled strands of **DNA**

Genes are segments of DNA that contain instructions to make proteins, the building blocks of life

Figure 4-1. Cells, chromosomes, DNA, and genes.

Genes

1. The basic unit of inherited information.
2. Each copy of the human genome in the nucleus has about 25,000 genes. Cells also have some non-nuclear genes located within the mitochondria within the cytoplasm.
3. Alternate forms of a gene are termed *alleles.*
4. For each gene, an individual receives one allele from each parent, and thus has two alleles for each gene on the autosomes and also on the X chromosomes in females.
5. Males have only one X chromosome and, therefore, have only one allele for all genes on the X chromosome; they are hemizygous for all X-linked genes.
6. At any autosomal locus, or gene site, an individual can have two identical alleles (homozygous) for that locus or can have two different alleles (heterozygous) at a particular locus.
7. *Genotype* refers to the constitution of the genetic material of an individual; for practical purposes, it is commonly used to refer to a particular base or bases in the DNA. For example, the gene for sickle cell disease, the gene for cystic fibrosis, or the gene for familial polyposis.
8. *Phenotype* refers to the physical or biochemical characteristics an individual manifests regarding expression of the presence of a particular feature, or set of features, associated with a particular gene.
9. Each gene is composed of a unique sequence of DNA bases.

DNA: Nuclear and Mitochondrial

1. Human DNA is a double-stranded helical structure comprised of four different bases, the sequence of which codes for the assembly of amino acids to make a protein—for example, an enzyme. These proteins are important for the following reasons:
   a. For body characteristics such as eye color.
   b. For biochemical processes such as the gene for the enzyme that digests phenylalanine.
   c. For body structure such as a collagen gene important to connective tissue and bone formation.
   d. For cellular functioning such as genes associated with the cell cycle.

2. The four DNA bases are adenine, guanine, cytosine, and thymine (A, G, C, and T).
3. A change, or mutation, in the coding sequence, such as a duplicated or deleted region, or even a change in only one base, can alter the production or functioning of the gene or gene product, thus affecting cellular processes, growth, and development.
4. DNA analysis can be done on almost any body tissue (blood, muscle, skin) using molecular techniques (not visible under a microscope) for mutation analysis of a specific gene with a known sequence or for DNA linkage of genetic markers associated with a particular gene.

Normal Cell Division

1. Mitosis occurs in all somatic cells, which, under normal circumstances, results in the formation of cells identical to the original cell with the same 46 chromosomes.
2. Meiosis, or reduction division, occurs in the germ cell line, resulting in gametes (egg and sperm cells) with only 23 chromosomes, one representative of each chromosome pair.
3. During the process of meiosis, parental homologous chromosomes (from the same pair) pair and undergo exchanges of genetic material, resulting in recombinations of alleles on a chromosome and thus variation in individuals from generation to generation.

CLINICAL APPLICATION
Genetic Disorders

Presentations warranting genetic consideration include mental retardation, birth defects, biochemical or metabolic disorders, structural abnormalities, multiple miscarriages, and family history of the same or related disorder.

Examples of disorders that result from abnormalities of chromosomes or genes or that are, at least in part, influenced by genetic factors are described in Table 4-1.

Classification of Genetic Alterations

Chromosomal

1. The entire chromosome or only part can be affected. This is usually associated with birth defects and mental retardation

(Text continues on page 40)

Table 4-1 Selected Genetic Disorders

DISORDER AND INCIDENCE	CHARACTERISTICS	ETIOLOGY AND RECURRENCE RISKS	CONSIDERATIONS AND COMMENTS
Chromosomal Disorders			
Autosomal			
Down syndrome (Trisomy 21) 1 in 700 neonates; incidence increases with advanced maternal age (eg, risk at maternal age 25 is 1 in 1,350; at age 35, 1 in 384; at age 45, 1 in 28)	Brachycephaly: oblique palpebral fissures; epicanthal folds; Brushfield spots; flat nasal bridge; protruding tongue; small, low-set ears; clinodactyly; simian crease; congenital heart defects; hypotonia; mental retardation; growth retardation; dry, scaly skin; increased risk for childhood leukemia and early-onset Alzheimer's disease	• Extra copy of number 21 chromosome (total of three copies). • 94% of cases are trisomy (karyotype 47, +21) for three distinct number 21 chromosomes due to nondisjunction (failure of chromosomal separation during meiosis); recurrence risk 1%, plus maternal age–related risk if older than age 35. • 4% of cases have a translocation—the extra number 21 is attached to another chromosome, usually a number 13 or number 14; half of these translocations are new occurrences, the other half are inherited from a parent. • 2% of cases are mosaic—affected individual has two different cell lines, one with the normal number of chromosomes and the other cell line trisomic for the number 21 chromosome; due to a postconception error in chromosomal division during mitosis.	• Recurrence risk for parents of affected are dependent on one or more of the following: chromosomal type of disorder, maternal age, parental karyotype, family history, and sex of transmitting parent and other chromosome involved (if translocation). • May demonstrate nuccal thickening prenatally on ultrasound examination. • Associated with moderate mental retardation. • No phenotypic differences between trisomy Down syndrome and translocation Down syndrome. • Chromosome analysis should be performed on all persons with Down syndrome. • Prenatal maternal serum screening can adjust risk for the pregnancy.
Trisomy 13 (Patau syndrome) 1 in 5,000 live births	Holoprosencephaly; cleft lip or palate, or both; abnormal helices; cardiac defects; rocker-bottom feet; overlapping positioning of fingers; seizures; severe mental retardation	• Extra number 13 chromosome (total of three copies): Either trisomy form, due to nondisjunction, with less than a 1% recurrence risk; or translocation form, with recurrence risk less than that of translocation Down syndrome and dependent on other factors, including chromosomes involved.	• 44% die within the first month; 18% survive first year of life.
Trisomy 18 (Edwards syndrome) 1 in 6,000 live births	Small for gestational age (may be detected prenatally); feeble fetal activity; weak cry; prominent occiput; low-set, malformed ears; short palpebral fissures; small oral opening; overlapping positioning of fingers (fifth digit over fourth, index over third); nail hypoplasia, short hallux; cardiac defects; inguinal or umbilical hernia; cryptorchidism in males; severe mental retardation	• Extra number 18 chromosome (total of three copies): Majority due to trisomy with less than 1% recurrence risk.	• Most trisomy 18 conceptions miscarry; 90% die within first year of life.

(continued)

Table 4-1   Selected Genetic Disorders (continued)

DISORDER AND INCIDENCE	CHARACTERISTICS	ETIOLOGY AND RECURRENCE RISKS	CONSIDERATIONS AND COMMENTS
Chromosomal Disorders (continued)			
Sex Chromosome			
Klinefelter syndrome 1 in 700 males; 47, XXY abnormality in 90%; other 10% have more than two X chromosomes in addition to the Y chromosome or have mosaicism (about 20%)	Body habitus may be tall, slim, and underweight; long limbs; gynecomastia; small testes; inadequate virilization; azoospermia or low sperm count; cognitive defects; behavioral problems	• Due to nondisjunction during meiosis, except for cases of mosaicism, which are due to mitotic nondisjunction.	• No distinguishing features prenatally. • Diagnosis may not be suspected or pursued before puberty. • Diagnosis in childhood is beneficial in planning for testosterone replacement therapy, in addition to accurate understanding of learning or behavioral problems. • Tend to be delayed in onset of speech, have difficulty in expressive language; may be relatively immature; may have history of recurrent respiratory infections.
Turner syndrome (45, X) 1 in 2,500 female births	Webbing of neck and short stature; lymphedema of hands and feet as neonate; congenital cardiac defects (especially coarctation of the aorta); low posterior hairline; cubitus valgus; widely spaced nipples; underdeveloped breasts; immature internal genitalia (eg, streak ovaries); primary amenorrhea; learning disabilities	• About 50% due to a nondisjunctional error during meiosis (karyotype 45, X); 20% are mosaic due to nondisjunction during mitosis; 30% have two X chromosomes but one is functionally inadequate (eg, due to presence of abnormal gene); generally a sporadic occurrence.	• Webbing of neck and short stature may be detected prenatally by ultrasound. • Early diagnosis enhances optimal health care management (eg, planning for administration of growth hormone therapy, estrogen replacement). • Psychosocial implications associated with short stature, delayed onset of puberty. • Infertility associated with ovarian dysgenesis; oocyte donation and adoption are generally the only options for having children.
Microdeletion/Microduplication			
Fragile X 1 in 1,200 males; 1 in 2,500 females	Motor delays; hypotonia; speech delay and language difficulty; hyperactivity; classic features including long face, prominent ears, and macroorchidism manifest around puberty; autism (about 7% of males); mental retardation in most males; learning disabilities in most affected females	• Mutation in the fragile X mental retardation gene (FMR-1), represented as a large DNA expansion of a normally present trinucleotide. • Carrier mother of an affected male has a 50% risk for future affected males and 50% chance of transmitting the FMR-1 X chromosome to a daughter who would be a carrier, may be unaffected, or manifest features associated with the fragile X syndrome and has a 50% chance of transmitting that gene to future offspring.	• Both cytogenetic testing for expression of the fragile X site and DNA analysis to characterize the size of the DNA expansion are available, but the latter is superior. Testing for methylation status of the DNA increases sensitivity. • Phenotypic expression of this gene in males and females is variable; genetic mechanisms determining expression of this gene are very complicated. • Fragile X should be considered in the differential diagnosis of any male with mental retardation who is undiagnosed; it is the most common mental retardation in males.

Table 4-1   Selected Genetic Disorders (continued)

DISORDER AND INCIDENCE	CHARACTERISTICS	ETIOLOGY AND RECURRENCE RISKS	CONSIDERATIONS AND COMMENTS
Chromosomal Disorders (continued)			
Microdeletion/Microduplication			
Prader-Willi syndrome Estimated incidence 1 in 25,000	Hypotonia and poor sucking ability in infancy; almond-shaped palpebral fissures; small stature; small, slow growth of hands or feet; small penis, cryptorchidism; insatiable appetite, behavioral problems developing in childhood; below-normal intelligence or mental retardation	• Cytogenetic microdeletion in chromosome 15q11 to 13 identified in 50% to 70% of cases; deletion associated with paternally inherited number 15 chromosome. • Generally sporadic occurrence; empiric recurrence risk 1.6%.	• Consider diagnosis in infants presenting with hypotonia and sucking problems where etiology is unknown. • Associated with lack of a functioning paternal gene at this locus; presents clinical evidence for the necessity of two functioning genes, both a maternal and paternal contribution. • Another distinct entity, termed *Angelman syndrome*, is associated with a deletion of the maternal contribution in this same cytogenetic region; it is also associated with mental deficiency, but with a different phenotypic presentation.
Mendelian Disorders—Single Gene			
Autosomal Dominant			
Achondroplasia 1 in 10,000 live births Increased incidence associated with advanced paternal age (>40)	Megalocephaly; small foramen magnum and short cranial base with early spheno-occipital closure; prominent forehead; low nasal bridge; midfacial hypoplasia; small stature; short extremities; lumbar lordosis; short tubular bones; incomplete extension at the elbow; normal intelligence	• Autosomal dominant inheritance; 80% to 90% are due to a new mutation and neither parent is affected. • An affected parent has a 50% risk to transmit the gene to each child.	• Hydrocephalus can be a complication of achondroplasia and may be masked by megalocephaly. • Risk for apnea secondary to cervical spinal cord and lower brain stem compression due to alterations in shape of cervical vertebral bodies; respiratory problems are also a risk because of the small chest and upper airway obstruction. • Can be diagnosed prenatally by ultrasound.
Osteogenesis imperfecta (Type 1) 1 in 15,000 live births	Blue sclerae; fractures (variable number); deafness may occur	• Defect in the procollagen gene associated with decreased synthesis of a constituent chain important to collagen structure. • Can occur as a new mutation in that gene or can be inherited from a parent who has a 50% recurrence risk to transmit the gene; most severe cases represent a sporadic occurrence within a family.	• There are at least four general classifications of osteogenesis imperfecta, each with varying clinical severity, presentation, and pattern of genetic transmission. • Treatment with calcitonin and fluoride may be beneficial in reducing the number of fractures.
Breast and breast/ ovarian cancer syndrome Accounts for 5% to 10% of breast cancer	Breast cancer (usually, but not exclusively, early-age onset, premenopausal); ovarian cancer	• Mutation in the BRCA-1 or BRCA-2 gene; poses increased susceptibility (not certainty) for breast (31% to 78%) and/or ovarian (3% to 54%) cancer.	• Studies have also noted increased risk for prostate cancer, colon cancer in some families; also an association between male breast cancer and BRCA-2 mutations. • Individuals from Ashkenazi Jewish ancestry are at increased risk for mutations in BRCA-1 and BRCA-2.

(continued)

Table 4-1   Selected Genetic Disorders (continued)

DISORDER AND INCIDENCE	CHARACTERISTICS	ETIOLOGY AND RECURRENCE RISKS	CONSIDERATIONS AND COMMENTS
Mendelian Disorders—Single Gene (continued)			
Autosomal Dominant			
Familial adenomatous polyposis (FAP) Accounts for about 1% of colon cancer	Associated with multiple adenomatous colorectal polyps (classic: > 100; atypical: < 100), desmoid tumors, other GI polyps, jaw cysts; family history of polyps or colorectal cancer; polyps progress to cancer; polyps can be present in childhood	• Mutations in the APC gene (a tumor suppressor gene). The majority of mutations result in a truncated protein.	• Genetic testing (protein truncation testing is available). If mutation is identified in affected person, relatives can be tested for the same finding. Relatives at risk, whether by family history or by genetic testing, should start cancer screening by age 18, if not earlier, if there are symptoms or as a baseline. Screening includes colonoscopy, ophthalmologic examination.
Autosomal Recessive			
Sickle cell disease 1 in 400 live births of African Americans	Physically normal in appearance at birth; hemolytic anemia and the occurrence of acute exacerbations (crises), resulting in increased susceptibility to infection and vascular occlusive episodes	• Point mutation in the beta globin gene resulting in an altered gene product; red blood cells susceptible to sickling at times of low oxygen tension. • Parents of an affected individual are both unaffected carriers of one abnormal copy of the beta globin gene (sickle cell trait); together have a 25% risk for recurrence in any offspring.	• 1 in 10 African Americans is a carrier of the beta globin gene mutation; population screening is indicated for these individuals. • Unaffected siblings of an affected individual have a two-thirds, or 67%, risk to have the sickle cell trait and should be screened. • See page 1704 for nursing care. • Prenatal testing is available through DNA analysis from specimen obtained during chorionic villus sampling or amniocentesis.
Cystic fibrosis (CF) 1 in 2,000 live births (predominantly white)	Phenotypically normal at birth; may present with meconium ileus (10%) as neonate or later with persistent cough, recurrent respiratory problems, gastrointestinal complaints, malnutrition, abdominal pain, or infertility	• Mutation in the CF transmembrane conduction regulator gene on chromosome 7 results in an abnormality of a protein integral to the cell membrane. • Parents of an affected individual are both considered obligate carriers of one copy of the abnormal CF gene; thus, together they have a 25% recurrence risk with each conception.	• 1 in 20 individuals from Northern European ancestry is a carrier of a CF gene mutation. • Many different mutations have been identified within the CF gene, the most common of which is Delta-F508, which accounts for about 70% of CF mutations. CF screening can identify about 85% of all CF mutations (95% in Jewish population). • "General population" screening is recommended by the American College of Obstetrics and Gynecology. • DNA analysis of the CF gene is advised for affected individuals and relatives of persons with CF. • See page 1514 for nursing care.

Table 4-1   Selected Genetic Disorders *(continued)*

DISORDER AND INCIDENCE	CHARACTERISTICS	ETIOLOGY AND RECURRENCE RISKS	CONSIDERATIONS AND COMMENTS
Mendelian Disorders—Single Gene *(continued)*			
Autosomal Recessive			
Tay-Sachs disease 1 in 3,600 Ashkenazi Jews	Normal at birth; progressive neurodegenerative manifestations, including loss of developmental milestones and lack of central nervous system maturation; cherry-red spot on macula	• Mutation in the gene for hexosaminidase A, an enzyme important to cellular metabolic processes, results in accumulation of metabolic by-products within the cell (especially brain), impairing functioning and causing the neurodegenerative effects. • Parents of an affected individual are both considered unaffected obligate carriers of one copy of the Tay-Sachs disease gene; together they have a 25% risk of recurrence in their offspring.	• About 1 in 25 Ashkenazi Jews is a carrier of the Tay-Sachs gene; about 1 in 17 French Canadians is a carrier of an abnormal Tay-Sachs gene (different mutation from that of the Jewish ancestry); persons of these ancestries should be screened. • No treatment available; results in death in childhood. • Prenatal and preimplantation testing are available.
X-Linked Recessive			
Duchenne muscular dystrophy (DMD) 1 in 3,500 males	Phenotypically normal at birth; dramatically elevated creatinine kinase level (detectable as early as age 2 days); hypertrophy of the calves; history of tendency to trip and fall (at about age 3); Gowers' sign (tendency to push off oneself when getting up from a sitting position)	• DNA mutation, generally a deletion, detectable in 70% of affected males. • Carrier females have a 25% risk, with each pregnancy, to have an affected male, a 25% risk to have a carrier female, a 25% chance to have a healthy male, and a 25% chance to have a healthy noncarrier female.	• 1 in 1,750 females is a carrier of the DMD gene. • In the case of an isolated affected male, the mother has a two thirds statistical risk that she is a carrier of the DMD gene and a one third chance that her affected son developed as the result of a new mutation in that gene (she is not a carrier). • DNA testing is recommended for affected males; once type of gene mutation is known in that family, prenatal diagnosis and evaluation of potential female carriers can be carried out. • DNA analysis may provide clues as to expected clinical severity.
Hemophilia A 1 in 7,000 males	Phenotypically normal at birth; bleeding tendency (ranging from frequent spontaneous bleeds associated with the severe form to bleeding only after trauma associated with the mild form)	• Deficiency of Factor VIII (antihemophilic factor) due to abnormality in this gene located on the X chromosome. • Carrier females have a 25% risk, with each pregnancy, to have an affected son, a 25% risk to have a carrier daughter, and a 25% chance each to have a healthy unaffected daughter or son. • Mates of affected males should be tested for carrier status. If the female is not a carrier, the affected male will not have any affected children.	• Frequency of carrier females is about 1 in 3,500. • The severe form occurs in about 48% of cases. • Moderate cases account for 31%. • The mild form accounts for 21% of cases. • See page 1712 for nursing care.

(continued)

Table 4-1	Selected Genetic Disorders (continued)		
DISORDER AND INCIDENCE	**CHARACTERISTICS**	**ETIOLOGY AND RECURRENCE RISKS**	**CONSIDERATIONS AND COMMENTS**
Mendelian Disorders—Single Gene (continued)			
X-Linked Recessive			
Glucose 6-phosphate dehydrogenase (G6PD) 10% to 14% of male live births of African American origin	Phenotypically normal at birth; many remain asymptomatic throughout life; may manifest acute hemolysis associated with exposure to outside factors (eg, certain medications)	• Abnormality of the G6PD gene on the X chromosome. • Carrier females have a 25% risk, with each pregnancy, to have an affected male and 25% risk to have a carrier female.	• Be aware of drugs, such as antimalarial drugs or sulfonamides, or chemicals, such as phenylhydrazine (used in silvering mirrors, photography, soldering), associated with hemolysis in G6PD-deficient individuals.
Multifactorial Disorders			
Neural tube defects 1 in 1,000 live births	Abnormalities of neural tube closure, ranging from anencephaly to myelomeningocele to spina bifida occulta	• Probably several genetic factors may predispose certain individuals or families to susceptibility, but certain environmental (eg, prolonged hyperthermia or folate deficiency) and other unknown factors play an additive rule in surpassing an arbitrary threshold, placing the developing fetus at risk. • Recurrence risk for isolated neural tube defects range between 1% and 5%.	• Recurrence risk for isolated neural tube defects is dependent on the severity of the defect (ie, a defect in the neurulation [the cranial end of the neural tube] versus cannulation [the development of the caudal end]) and if there is a positive family history. • Maternal screening can be performed prenatally (after 14 weeks' gestation) through alpha-fetoprotein levels in maternal serum. • Can be associated with chromosomal or genetic disorders.
Cleft lip and/or cleft palate 1 in 1,000 live births	Unilateral or bilateral; cleft lip and cleft palate may occur together or in isolation	• Failure of migration and fusion of the maxillary processes during embryogenesis. • Recurrence risk for first-degree relatives of a person with an isolated cleft lip or cleft palate ranges between 2% and 6%.	• Clefting can occur as an isolated congenital abnormality or be one component of a syndrome, genetic defect, or chromosome abnormality, the latter three of which are associated with a recurrence risk specific to that disorder. • Recurrence for isolated cleft lip or palate is dependent on the type of cleft, the sex of the affected individual, and the family history.

because there are extra or missing copies of all genes associated with the involved chromosome.

  a. Numerical—abnormal number of chromosomes due to nondisjunction (error in chromosomal separation during cell division). Examples are Down and Klinefelter syndromes.

  b. Structural—abnormality involving deletions, additions, or translocations (rearrangements) of parts of chromosomes. Examples are Prader-Willi and Angelman syndromes.

  c. Fragile sites—regions susceptible to chromosomal breakage such as in fragile X syndrome.

2. May involve autosomes or sex chromosomes.

Single Gene or Pair of Genes

1. Manifestations are specific to cells, organs, or body systems affected by that gene.

2. Autosomal dominant—presence of a single copy of an abnormal gene results in phenotypic expression.

  a. These genes may involve proteins of a structural nature such as collagen. Affected individuals are usually of normal intelligence.

  b. Can be inherited from one parent, whose physical manifestations can vary, depending on the specific disorder and the gene's penetrance and expressivity (eg, neurofibromatosis).

  c. Can arise as a result of a new mutation in that gene in the affected individual.

  d. An individual with an autosomal dominant gene has a 50% chance of transmitting that gene to all offspring.

3. Autosomal recessive—requires that both alleles at a gene locus be abnormal for an individual to be affected.

a. These genes are frequently important to biochemical functions, such as the breakdown of phenylalanine. Depending on the gene and the nature of the mutation, affected individuals may be of normal intelligence or have mental retardation.

b. Generally, two healthy parents of an affected child are considered obligate carriers (unaffected) of one copy of the abnormal gene.

c. Such a carrier couple has a 25% chance, with each pregnancy, to have an affected child, a 50% chance for the child to be an unaffected carrier, and a 25% chance for the child to be an unaffected noncarrier.

4. X-linked recessive—due to one or more abnormal genes on the X chromosome.

a. These genes may be important to structure or biochemical function. Depending on the gene and the nature of the mutation, affected individuals may be of normal intelligence or have mental retardation.

b. Recessively inherited, in most cases, meaning that two abnormal genes are required to be affected. However, only one abnormal gene needs to be present for a male to be affected because males are hemizygous for all X-linked genes, as in Duchenne muscular dystrophy.

c. Females are typically only carriers of X-linked recessive disorders because the presence of a corresponding normal gene on the other X chromosome in a female produces enough gene product for normal functioning. Carrier females can be affected to varying degrees in certain circumstances. Incidence of females affected with X-linked recessive conditions is possible and usually have an affected father and a carrier mother.

d. A carrier female has a 25% chance, with each pregnancy, to have an affected son, a 25% chance to have a carrier daughter, a 25% chance to have an unaffected son, and a 25% chance to have an unaffected noncarrier daughter.

e. A male with an abnormal X-linked gene who has children with a noncarrier female will transmit that gene to all of his daughters, who will be carriers of that gene (usually unaffected); none of his sons will inherit his abnormal X-linked gene because they receive his Y chromosome.

5. X-linked dominant—relatively rare.

a. Mutations in these genes are usually lethal to male conceptions, as in Rett syndrome.

b. Depending on the gene and the nature of the mutation, affected females may be of normal intelligence or have mental retardation. An example is incontinentia pigmenti.

6. Mitochondrial—genes whose DNA is within the mitochondria, which are located in the cytoplasm, not in the nucleus, and therefore do not follow Mendelian laws of inheritance.

a. Many of these genes are associated with respiratory functions within mitochondria and thus affect energy capacity of cells. Disorders may be manifested by diminished strength in the involved tissue, or myopathy.

b. Essentially are maternally inherited because the egg cell contains the cytoplasmic material that is involved in the zygote; the sperm cell contributes mainly only nuclear DNA.

c. Varying phenotypes, depending on the number and distribution of abnormal mitochondrial genes.

d. Males and females can have mitochondrial conditions, but males transmit few, if any, mitochondrial genes to their offspring.

Multifactorial

1. Caused by multiple genetic factors in addition to other nongenetic influences (eg, environmental).

2. Because of the genetic components, affected individuals or close relatives are at an increased risk, compared with the general population, to have an affected child or develop the condition themselves.

3. Elimination of known nongenetic risk factors or proactive treatment regimen in some conditions can reduce risk for occurrence (eg, diet modification to manage hypercholesterolemia, cessation of smoking to reduce risk of cancer, or weight control and exercise to prevent type 2 diabetes in susceptible individuals).

Genetic Counseling

Genetic counseling is a communication process that deals with human problems associated with the occurrence or recurrence of a genetic disorder in a family or individual at increased risk for a condition that has a genetic component due to factors such as ancestral background or the results of screening tests. For these individuals or families, specific concern exists about risk associated with a certain problem or because of the relationship to someone who is affected (the proband). Several steps occur in the genetic evaluation, including obtaining and reviewing the medical history and records of the affected; eliciting the family history with special attention to factors pertinent to the diagnosis in the proband; evaluating and examining the affected (if available and indicated); ordering appropriate tests and interpreting results; and then meeting with the person seeking the consultation and/or the proband.

Goals of Genetic Counseling

Assist the patient and proband to:

1. Comprehend the medical facts, including the diagnosis, the possible course of the disorder, and the available management.

2. Understand the inheritance of the disorder, susceptibility to a condition, and the risk of recurrence in specified relatives.

3. Understand the options for dealing with the risk of recurrence.

4. Choose a course of action that seems appropriate to the individuals involved; consider their risk, family goals, and religious beliefs, and act in accordance with that decision.

5. Make the best possible adjustment to the disorder.

6. Understand the individual risks and the types of testing available and assist with interpretation and follow-up of test results.

Identify People in Need of Genetic Assessment and Counseling

1. Parents of a child with a birth defect, mental retardation, or known or possible genetic disorder.

2. Any individual with a genetic or potentially genetic disorder.

3. People with a family history of mental retardation, birth defects, genetic disorder, or condition that tends to run in the family.

4. Pregnant women who will be age 35 or older at the time of delivery.

5. Couples of ethnic origin known to be at an increased risk for a specific genetic disorder.

6. Couples who have experienced two or more miscarriages.

7. Pregnant women who have an elevated or low maternal serum screening test result such as alpha-fetoprotein (AFP).

8. Women who have been exposed to drugs or infections during pregnancy.

9. Couples who are related to each other.

10. Couples who are identified as carriers of autosomal recessive conditions through screening.

11. People who are concerned about the risk for a genetic disorder.

Genetic Screening, Testing, and Research

Screening

1. Screening is the level of testing offered to large populations (eg, neonate) or to high-risk segments of the population at increased risk of being carriers (such as individuals from African ancestry, Ashkenazi Jewish ancestry, and Mediterranean ancestry) to identify individuals with a genetic disorder, increased risk for abnormality, or carriers of a genetic disorder.

2. Criteria include that the test itself must be reliable, appropriate to the designated population, and cost-effective and that the condition being tested must be treatable or that early identification will enhance quality of life.

3. Neonate screening varies among facilities and states; however, all states and facilities test for a minimum of 21 conditions including phenylketonuria, hypothyroidism, sickle cell disease, and galactosemia, with most states testing for up to 50 or more conditions.

 Evidence Base National Newborn Screening and Genetic Resource Center. (2012). Resources on newborn screening including the national newborn screening status reports. Available: *http://genes-r-us.uthscsa .edu/*.

4. Prenatal screening includes multiple-marker screening that uses maternal serum to test AFP level alone or the triple screen (includes measurement of maternal serum AFP, beta-human chorionic gonadotropin, and estriol). A fourth protein, inhibin-A, measured by some laboratories, is called the quadruple screen. These tests are typically conducted after 14 weeks' gestation and can identify pregnancies at increased risk for neural tube defects (NTD), Down syndrome, trisomy 13 (Patau syndrome), and trisomy 18 (Edwards syndrome).

Testing

1. Biochemical testing is done on body tissue or fluid to measure enzyme levels and activity.

2. DNA testing is done on blood or tissue samples to look for a gene mutation or to study DNA linkage.

3. Chromosomal testing is done on nucleated cells (usually white blood cells) or other tissue for detection of various conditions, such as extra, missing, deleted, duplicated, or rearranged chromosomes.

Prenatal Testing

1. Chorionic villus sampling—for chromosomal and DNA testing; done at 9 to 12 weeks' gestation.

2. Amniocentesis—for chromosomal, biochemical, and DNA testing at 13 weeks' gestation (early amniocentesis); AFP can be done at 14 to 18 weeks' gestation.

3. Ultrasound—for dating pregnancy and assessing fetal structures, placenta, and amniotic fluid; done throughout pregnancy, but fetal structures are best visualized after 12 weeks.

4. Acetylcholinesterase—for testing amniotic fluid for suspected NTD.

5. Fetoscopy—for obtaining fetal blood samples or visualizing details of fetal structures; done during the second trimester.

6. Percutaneous umbilical blood sampling—for obtaining fetal blood; done during second trimester.

Preimplantation Diagnosis

1. Requires *in vitro* fertilization so that embryos can form in the laboratory. One or two cells are removed from the embryo and sent for genetic testing. Only embryos lacking the genetic composition for disease are placed into the womb for further development.

2. Useful if the embryo is at an increased risk for a specific genetic condition, for example, an autosomal/X-linked recessive, autosomal/X-linked dominant, or chromosomal condition.

Research

1. Testing is performed to further understand the genetics of a disorder, biochemical process, or individual response to therapies.

2. Genetic research is *not* clinical testing and may have no clinical value to the patient's case.

3. There is ongoing and extensive research on cancer susceptibility genes, genetic abnormalities present in different cancer types, and genes related to therapeutic response to medications.

Additional Genetic Testing Consideration

DNA banking—extraction and storage of one's DNA from blood through a qualified genetics laboratory; requires informed consent, proper collection, and prompt handling.

Nursing Roles and Responsibilities

1. Recognize or suspect genetic disorders by their physical characteristics and clinical manifestations.

2. Demonstrate an understanding of the relationship of genetics and genomics to health, prevention, screening, diagnostics, prognostics, selection of treatment, and monitoring of treatment effectiveness.

3. Create a genetic pedigree (diagram of the family history), including cause of death and any genetically linked ailments (see Figure 4-2).

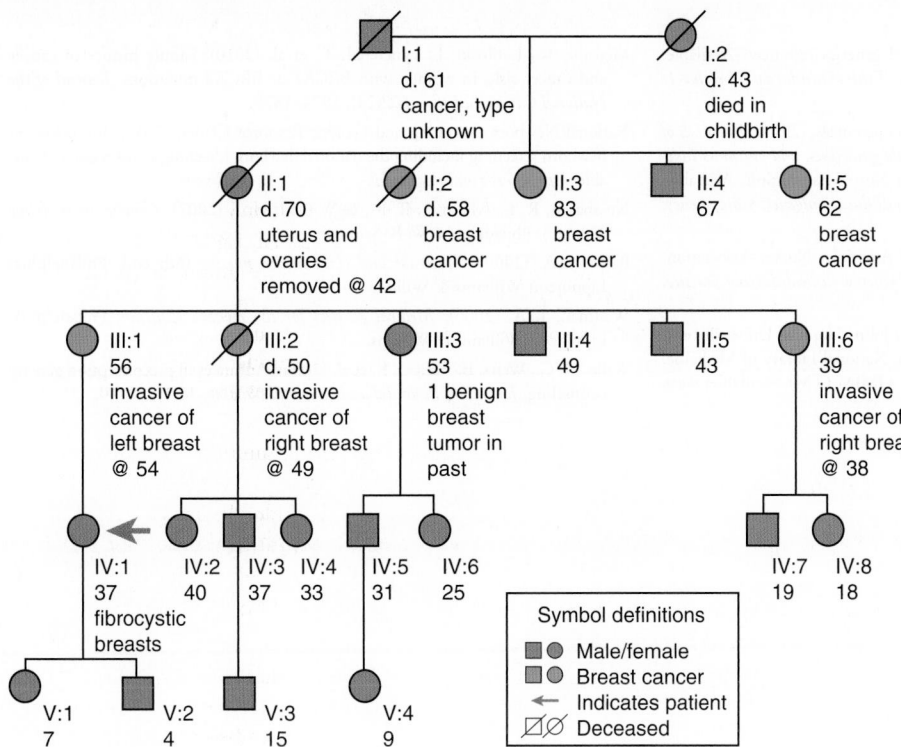

Figure 4-2. Genetic pedigree of a patient with breast cancer. Maternal side only is shown; however, both maternal and paternal sides are assessed. Genetic risk may run through either side.

4. Explain those aspects of diagnosis, prognosis, and treatment that affect the patient and his family. Relate information that parents, affected or at-risk individuals, and caregivers need to know to plan for the care of the patient.

5. Clear up misconceptions and allay feelings of guilt.

6. Assist with the diagnostic process by exploring medical and family history information, using physical assessment skills, procuring samples for testing, and developing a plan of care that incorporates genetic and genomic assessment information.

7. Enhance and reinforce self-image and self-worth of parents, child, or the individual at risk for or presenting with a genetic condition.

8. Advocate for clients' access to genetic/genomic services and resources, including support groups.

9. Refer and prepare family for genetic counseling.

   a. Inform that prenatal testing does not mean termination of pregnancy (eg, it may confirm that the fetus is not affected, thus eliminating worry throughout pregnancy, although the determination of an abnormality is also a possibility).

   b. Encourage parents and patient to allow adequate time to deliberate on a course of action (eg, they should not rush into a test without full knowledge of what the results can and can't tell, nor should they rush to make future reproductive decisions such as tubal ligation because in a few years they may want more children).

   c. Remain nonjudgmental.

10. Check with the state (eg, state health department) or with the Centers for Disease Control and Prevention (*www.cdc.gov*) for information and resources regarding neonatal testing required, state regulations on genetic testing and research.

11. Recognize that there are many ethical, legal, psychosocial, and professional issues associated with obtaining, using, and storing genetic information.

   a. Be aware of associated professional responsibilities, including informed consent, documentation in medical records, medical releases, and individual privacy of information.

   b. Refer to federal legislation (Genetic Information Nondiscrimination Act of 2008 and Health Insurance Portability and Accountability Act, 1997) that deals with protection from genetic discrimination in medical insurance; individual state legislation; genetics professional societies (see below); and the World Health Organization document on ethical considerations in genetic testing and services.

12. Refer for further information and support to:
   - March of Dimes: *www.modimes.org*
   - International Society of Nurses in Genetics: *www.isong.org*
   - Genetic Alliance: *www.geneticalliance.org*
   - Oncology Nursing Society, Genetics Special Interest Group: *www.ons.org*
   - National Society of Genetic Counselors: *www.nsgc.org*
   - CDC Public Health Genomics: *www.cdc.gov/genomics*

SELECTED REFERENCES

American Nurses Association. (2012). Educational genetics resources. Available: *http://nursingworld.org/MainMenuCategories/EthicsStandards/Genetics-1/ Resources.*

Concensus Panel on Genetic/Genomic Nursing Competencies. (2009). *Essentials of genetic and genomic nursing competencies, curricula guidelines, and outcomes indicators* (2nd ed.). Silver Spring, MD: American Nurses Association. Available: *www.genome.gov/Pages/Careers/HealthProfessionalEducation/geneticscompetency. pdf.*

International Society of Nurses in Genetics and American Nurses Association. (2007). *Statement on the scope and standards of genetics clinical nursing practice.* Washington, DC: American Nurses Publishing.

McKusick-Nathans Institute for Genetic Medicine, Johns Hopkins University and National Center for Biotechnology Information, National Library of Medicine. (2012). Online Mendelian Inheritance in Man, OMIM (TM). Available: *www .ncbi.nlm.nih.gov/omim.*

Metcalfe, K., Lubinski, J., Lynch, H. T., et al. (2010). Family history of cancer and cancer risks in women with BRCA1 or BRCA2 mutations. *Journal of the National Cancer Institute, 102*(24), 1874–1878.

National Newborn Screening and Genetic Resource Center. (2012). Resources on newborn screening including the national newborn screening status reports. Available: *http://genes-r-us.uthscsa.edu/.*

Nussbaum, R. L., McInnes, R. R., & Willard, H. F. (2007). *Genetics in medicine* (7th ed.). Philadelphia: W. B. Saunders.

Pillitteri, A. (2009). *Maternal and child health nursing* (6th ed.). Philadelphia: Lippincott Williams & Wilkins.

Westman, J. A. (2006). *Medical genetics for the modern clinician.* Philadelphia: Lippincott Williams & Wilkins.

Wille, M. C., Weitz, B., Kerper, P., et al. (2004). Advances in preconception genetic counseling. *Journal of Perinatal and Neonatal Nursing, 18*(1), 28–40.

PART TWO

MEDICAL-SURGICAL NURSING

5
Adult Physical Assessment

THE PATIENT HISTORY
General Principles

1. The first step in caring for a patient and in soliciting active cooperation is to gather a careful and complete history.
   a. In all patient concerns and problems, an accurate history is the foundation on which data collection and the process of assessment are based.
   b. The comprehensiveness of the history elicited depends on the information available in the patient's record and the reliability of the patient.
2. Time spent early in the nurse–patient relationship gathering detailed information about what the patient knows, thinks, and feels about the problems prevents time-consuming errors and misunderstandings later.
3. Skill in interviewing affects both the accuracy of information elicited and the quality of the relationship established with the patient. This point cannot be overemphasized; the reader is encouraged to consult other sources for detailed discussion of techniques of health interviewing.

4. The purpose of the interview is to encourage an exchange of information between the patient and the nurse and to establish rapport and understanding.

Interviewing Techniques

1. Provide privacy in as quiet a place as possible and see that the patient is comfortable.
2. Begin the interview with a courteous greeting and an introduction. Address the patient as *Mr.*, *Mrs.*, or *Ms.* and shake hands if appropriate. Explain who you are and the reason for your presence.
3. Make sure that facial expressions, body movements, and tone of voice are pleasant, unhurried, and nonjudgmental, and that they convey the attitude of a sensitive listener so the patient will feel free to express thoughts and feelings.
4. Avoid reassuring the patient prematurely (before you have adequate information about the problem). This only cuts off discussion; the patient may then be unwilling to bring up a problem causing concern.

5. At times, a patient gives cues or suggests information, but does not tell enough. It may be necessary to probe for more information to obtain a thorough history.

6. Guide the interview so the necessary information is obtained without cutting off discussion. Controlling a rambling patient is often difficult but, with practice, it can be done without jeopardizing the quality of the information gained.

Components

Identifying Information

1. Date and time.
2. Patient's name, address, telephone number, race, ethnicity, religion, birth date, and age.
3. Name of referring practitioner.
4. Insurance data.
5. Name of informant—the patient may be the person giving the history; if not, record the name, address, telephone number, and relationship to the patient of the person giving the history. (The patient's facility or clinical record may also be a valuable resource.)
6. Accuracy and reliability of informant—this is a judgment based on the consistency of responses to questions and on a comparison of information in the history with your own observations in the physical examination.
7. Explain the reasons why the information is needed to help put the patient at ease.

Chief Complaint

1. A brief statement of the patient's primary problem or concern in the patient's own words, including the duration of the complaint. Example: "hacking cough × 3 weeks."
2. Purpose is to allow the patient to describe his or her own problems and expectations with little or no direction from the interviewer and to identify the overriding problem for which the patient is seeking help (there may be numerous complaints).
3. To obtain information, ask the patient a direct question, such as "For what reason have you come to the facility?" or "What seems to be bothering you most at this time?"
   a. Avoid confusing questions, such as "What brings you here?" ("The bus.") or "Why are you here?" ("That's what I came to find out.")
   b. Ask how long the concern or problem has been present, for example, whether it has been hours, days, or weeks. If necessary, establish the time of onset precisely by offering such clues as "Did you feel this way a month (6 months or 2 years) ago?"
4. Write down what the patient says using quotation marks to identify patient's words.

History of Present Illness

1. A detailed chronological picture, beginning with the time the patient was last well (or, in the case of a problem with an acute onset, the patient's condition just before the onset of the problem) and ending with a description of the patient's current condition.

2. If there is more than one important problem, each is described in a separate, chronologically organized paragraph in the written history of present illness.

3. Investigate the chief complaint by eliciting more information through the use of the pneumonic "OLD CARTS":
   a. **O**nset (setting, circumstances, rapidity, or manner in which it began).
   b. **L**ocation (exact place where the symptom is felt, radiation pattern).
   c. **D**uration (how long; if intermittent, the frequency and duration of each episode).
   d. **C**haracter/course (nature or quality of the symptom, such as sharp pain, interference with activity, how it has changed or evolved over time; ask to describe a typical episode).
   e. **A**ggravating/associated factors (medications, rest, activity, diet; associated nausea, fever, and other symptoms).
   f. **R**elieving factors (lying down, having bowel movement).
   g. **T**reatments tried (pharmacologic and nonpharmacologic methods attempted and their outcomes).
   h. **S**everity (the quantity of the symptom; eg, how severe on scale of 1 to 10).
4. Alternately, use the pneumonic PQRST: **p**rovocative/palliative factors, **q**uality/quantity, **r**egion/radiation, **s**everity, **t**iming.
5. Obtain OLD CARTS data for all the major problems associated with the present illness, as applicable.
6. Clarify the chronology of the illness by asking questions and summarizing the history of present illness for the patient to comment on.

Past Medical History

1. To determine the background health status of the patient, including present status, recent health conditions, and past health conditions, that will serve as a basis for nursing care planning for holistic patient care.
2. General health and lifestyle patterns—sleeping pattern; diet; stability of weight; usual exercise and activities; use of tobacco, alcohol, illicit drugs.
3. Childhood illnesses, such as infectious diseases (if applicable).
4. Immunization—polio, diphtheria, pertussis, tetanus, measles, mumps, rubella, *haemophilus influenza* type b, hepatitis B, hepatitis A, pneumococcal, influenza, varicella, meningitis, human papilloma virus, herpes zoster, last purified protein derivative or other skin test, abnormal or unusual reactions (give date when possible).
5. Operation—indications, diagnosis, dates, facility, surgeon, complications.
6. Previous hospitalizations—physician, facility data (year), diagnosis, treatment.
7. Injuries—type, treatment, outcome.
8. Major acute and chronic illnesses (any serious or prolonged illnesses not requiring hospitalization)—dates, symptoms, course, treatment.
9. Medications—prescription drugs from all providers (including ophthalmologist and dentist); nonprescription drugs including vitamins, supplements, and herbal products; include dosage, length of use, and adherence.

10. Allergies—environmental allergies, food allergies, drug reactions; give type of reaction (hives, rhinitis, local reaction, angioedema, anaphylaxis).
11. Obstetric history (may appear in review of systems).
    a. Pregnancies, miscarriages, abortions.
    b. Describe course of pregnancy, labor, and delivery; date, place of delivery.
12. Psychiatric history (may appear in review of systems)—treatment by a mental health provider, diagnosis, date, place, medications.

Family History

1. Purpose is to present a picture of the patient's family health, including that of grandparents, parents, brothers, sisters, aunts, and uncles because some diseases show a familial tendency or are hereditary.
2. Include age and health status (or age at and cause of death) of maternal and paternal grandparents, parents, siblings.
3. History, in immediate and close relatives, of heart disease, hypertension, stroke, diabetes, gout, kidney disease or stones, thyroid disease, pulmonary disease, blood problems, cancer (types), epilepsy, mental illness, arthritis, alcoholism, obesity.
4. Genetic disorders, such as hemophilia or sickle cell disease.
5. Age and health status of spouse and children.

Review of Systems

1. Purpose is to obtain detailed information about the current state of the patient and any past symptoms, or lack of symptoms, patient may have experienced related to a particular body system.
2. May give clues to diagnosis of multisystem disorders or progression of a disorder to other areas.
3. Include subjective information about what the patient feels or sees with regard to the major systems of the body.
    a. General constitutional symptoms—fever, chills, night sweats, malaise, fatigability, recent weight loss or gain.
    b. Skin—rash, itching, change in pigmentation or texture, sweating, hair growth and distribution, condition of nails, skin care habits, protection from sun.
    c. Skeletal—stiffness of joints, pain, deformity, restriction of motion, swelling, redness, heat. (If there are problems, ask the patient to specify any activities of daily life that are difficult or impossible to perform.)
    d. Head—headaches, dizziness, syncope, head injuries.
    e. Eyes—vision, pain, diplopia, photophobia, blind spots, itching, burning, discharge, recent change in appearance or vision, glaucoma, cataracts, glasses or contact lenses worn, date of last refraction, infection.
    f. Ears—hearing acuity, earache, discharge, tinnitus, vertigo, history of tubes or infection.
    g. Nose—sense of smell, frequency of colds, obstruction, epistaxis, postnasal discharge, sinus pain or therapy, use of nose drops or sprays (type and frequency).
    h. Teeth—pain; bleeding, swollen or receding gums; recent abscesses, extractions; dentures; dental hygiene practices, last dental examination.
    i. Mouth and tongue—soreness of tongue or buccal mucosa, ulcers, swelling.
    j. Throat—sore throat, tonsillitis, hoarseness, dysphagia.
    k. Neck—pain, stiffness, swelling, enlarged glands or lymph nodes.
    l. Endocrine—goiter, thyroid tenderness, tremors, weakness, tolerance to heat and cold, changes in hat or glove size, changes in skin pigmentation, libido, easy bruising, muscle cramps, polyuria, polydipsia, polyphagia, hormone therapy, unexplained weight change.
    m. Respiratory—pain in the chest with breathing, dyspnea, wheezing, cough, sputum (character, quantity), hemoptysis, last tuberculin test or chest x-ray and result (indicate where obtained), exposure to tuberculosis.
    n. Cardiovascular—pain (aggravating and alleviating factors), palpitations, dyspnea, orthopnea (note number of pillows required for sleeping), history of heart murmur, edema, cyanosis, claudication, varicose veins, exercise tolerance, blood pressure (if known), last electrocardiogram and results (indicate where obtained).
    o. Hematologic—anemia (if so, treatment received), tendency to bruise or bleed, thromboses, thrombophlebitis, any known abnormalities of blood cells.
    p. Lymph nodes—enlargement, tenderness, suppuration, duration and progress of abnormality.
    q. Gastrointestinal—appetite and digestion, intolerance to foods, belching, regurgitation, heartburn, nausea, vomiting, hematemesis, bowel habits, diarrhea, constipation, flatulence, stool characteristics, hemorrhoids, jaundice, use of laxatives or antacids, history of ulcer or other conditions, previous diagnostic tests such as colonoscopy.
    r. Urinary—dysuria, pain, urgency, frequency, hematuria, nocturia, polydipsia, polyuria, oliguria, edema of the face, hesitancy, dribbling, loss in size or force of stream, passage of stones, stress incontinence.
    s. Male reproductive—puberty onset, sexual activity, use of condoms, libido, sexual dysfunction, history of sexually transmitted diseases (STDs).
    t. Female reproductive—pattern and characteristics of menses, libido, sexual activity, satisfaction with sexual relations, pregnancies, methods of contraception, STD protection.
    u. Breasts—pain, tenderness, discharge, lumps, mammograms, breast self-examination.
    v. Neurologic—history of loss of consciousness, seizures, confusion, memory, cognitive function, incoordination, weakness, numbness, paresthesia, tremors, muscle cramps.
    w. Psychiatric—how patient views self, mood changes, difficulty concentrating, sadness, nervousness, tension, irritability, change in social interaction, obsessive thoughts, compulsions, manic episodes, suicidal or homicidal thoughts, hallucinations.

Personal and Social History

1. To develop a plan of care that "fits" the patient. Here the interviewer finds out the many personal and family resources an individual has to aid in coping with the situation and determines what health promotion activities may be necessary.

2. Determine personal status—birthplace, education, armed service affiliation, position in the family, education level, satisfaction with life situations (home and job), personal concerns.

3. Identify habits and lifestyle patterns.
   a. Sleeping pattern, number of hours of sleep, difficulty sleeping.
   b. Exercise, activities, recreation, hobbies.
   c. Nutrition and eating habits (diet recall for a typical day).
   d. Alcohol—frequency, amount, type; CAGE questionnaire for problem drinking:
      i. Have you ever thought you should **C**ut down on your drinking?
      ii. Have you ever been **A**nnoyed by criticism of your drinking?
      iii. Have you ever felt **G**uilty about your drinking?
      iv. Do you drink in the morning (ie, an **E**ye-opener)?
   e. Caffeine—type and amount per day.
   f. Illicit drugs (illegal or improperly used prescription or over-the-counter medications).
   g. Tobacco—past and present use, type (cigarettes, cigars, chewing, snuff), pack, years.
   h. Sexual habits (can be part of genitourinary history)—relationships, frequency, satisfaction, number of partners in past year and lifetime, STD and pregnancy prevention.

4. Home conditions.
   a. Marital status, nature of family relationships.
   b. Economic conditions—source of income; health insurance, Medicare, Medicaid.
   c. Living arrangements and housing (owning or renting, heating, sewage, pets).
   d. Involvement with agencies (name, caseworker).
   e. History of physical or sexual abuse.

5. Occupation—past and present employment and working conditions, including exposure to stress and tension, noise, chemicals, pollution.

6. Cultural beliefs, religion or faith—its importance in coping and health practices.

Ending the History

When you have completed the history, it is often helpful to say, "Is there anything else you would like to tell me?" or "What additional concerns do you have?" This allows the patient to end the history by saying what is on his or her mind and what concerns the patient most.

PHYSICAL EXAMINATION

General Principles

1. A complete or partial physical examination is conducted following a careful comprehensive or problem-related history.

2. It is conducted in a quiet, well-lit room with consideration for patient privacy and comfort.

Approaching the Patient

1. When possible, begin with the patient in a sitting position so both the front and back can be examined.

2. Completely expose the part to be examined but drape the rest of the body appropriately.

3. Conduct the examination systematically from head to foot so as not to miss observing any system or body part.

4. While examining each region, consider the underlying anatomic structures, their function, and possible abnormalities.

5. Because the body is bilaterally symmetric for the most part, compare findings on one side with those on the other.

6. Explain all procedures to the patient while the examination is being conducted to avoid alarming or worrying the patient and to encourage cooperation.

Techniques of Examination and Assessment

Use the following techniques of examination, as appropriate, for eliciting findings.

Inspection

1. Begins with the first encounter with the patient and is the most important of all the techniques.

2. It is an organized scrutiny of the patient's behavior and body.

3. With knowledge and experience, the examiner can become highly sensitive to visual clues.

4. The examiner begins each phase of the examination by inspecting the particular part with the eyes.

Palpation

1. Involves touching the region or body part just observed and noting whether these are tender to touch and what the various structures feel like.

2. With experience comes the ability to distinguish variations of normal from abnormal.

3. It is performed in an organized manner from region to region.

Percussion

1. By setting underlying tissues in motion, percussion helps in determining the density of the underlying tissue and whether it is air-filled, fluid-filled, or solid.

2. Audible sounds and palpable vibrations are produced, which can be distinguished by the examiner. The five basic notes produced by percussion can be distinguished by differences in the qualities of sound, pitch, duration, and intensity (see Table 5-1, page 50).

3. The technique for percussion may be described as follows:
   a. Hyperextend the middle finger of your left hand, pressing the distal portion and joint firmly against the surface to be percussed.
      i. Other fingers touching the surface will damp the sound.
      ii. Be consistent in the degree of firmness exerted by the hyperextended finger as you move it from area to area or the sound will vary.

Table 5-1	Five Basic Notes Produced by Percussion			
	RELATIVE INTENSITY	**RELATIVE PITCH**	**RELATIVE DURATION**	**EXAMPLE LOCATION**
Flatness	Soft	High	Short	Thigh
Dullness	Medium	Medium	Medium	Liver
Resonance	Loud	Low	Long	Normal lung
Hyperresonance	Very loud	Lower	Longer	Emphysematous lung
Tymphany	Loud	High*	*	Gastric air bubble or puffed

*Distinguished mainly by its musical timbre.
Adapted from Bickley, L. S. (2008). *Bates' guide to physical examination and history taking* (10th ed.). Philadelphia: Lippincott Williams & Wilkins.

b. Cock the right hand at the wrist, flex the middle finger upward, and place the forearm close to the surface to be percussed. The right hand and forearm should be as relaxed as possible.

c. With a quick, sharp, relaxed wrist motion, strike the extended left middle finger with the flexed right middle finger, using the tip of the finger, not the pad. Aim at the end of the extended left middle finger (just behind the nailbed) where the greatest pressure is exerted on the surface to be percussed.

d. Lift the right middle finger rapidly to avoid damping the vibrations.

e. The movement is at the wrist, not at the finger, elbow, or shoulder; the examiner should use the lightest touch capable of producing a clear sound.

Auscultation

1. This method uses the stethoscope to augment the sense of hearing.

2. The stethoscope must be constructed well and must fit the user. Earpieces should be comfortable, the length of the tubing should be 10 to 15 inches (25 to 38 cm), and the head should have a diaphragm and a bell.

a. The bell is used for low-pitched sounds such as certain heart murmurs.

b. The diaphragm screens out low-pitched sounds and is good for hearing high-frequency sounds such as breath sounds.

c. Extraneous sounds can be produced by clothing, hair, and movement of the head of the stethoscope.

Adult Physical Assessment

EQUIPMENT

- Cotton applicator stick
- Flashlight
- Oto-ophthalmoscope
- Reflex hammer
- Safety pin

- Sphygmomanometer
- Stethoscope
- Thermometer
- Tongue blade
- Tuning fork

- Additional items may include disposable gloves and lubricant for rectal examination and a speculum for examination of female pelvis.

Technique	Findings
VITAL SIGNS	
Importance—Many major therapeutic decisions are based on the vital signs; therefore, accuracy is essential.	
Temperature	
Routinely, where accuracy is not crucial, an oral or ear temperature will suffice.	Temperature—may vary with the time of day. Oral: 98.6° F (37° C) is considered normal.
A rectal temperature is the most accurate, but may be contraindicated with some rectal problems and cardiac arrhythmias.	May vary from 96.4–99.1° F (35.8–37.3° C). Rectal: Higher than oral by 0.7–0.9° F (0.4°–0.5° C).
Pulse	
Palpate the radial pulse and count for at least 30 seconds.	Pulse—Normal adult pulse is 60–80 beats/minute; regular in rhythm. Elasticity of the arterial walls, blood volume, and mechanical action of the heart muscle are some of the factors that affect the strength of the pulse wave, which normally is full and strong.
If the pulse is irregular, count for a full minute and note the number of irregular beats per minute.	
Note whether the beat of the pulse against your finger is strong or weak, bounding or thready.	
Respiration	
Count the number of respirations taken in 15 seconds and multiply that by 4.	Respiration—Normally 16–20 respirations per minute.
Note rhythm and depth of breathing.	
Blood pressure	
Measure the blood pressure (BP) in both arms. Document the patient's position.	Normal BP is < 120/80 mm Hg.
Palpate the systolic pressure before using the stethoscope in order to detect an auscultatory gap.*	A difference of 5–10 mm Hg between arms is common.
Apply the cuff firmly; if it is too loose, it will give a falsely high reading.	Systolic pressure in lower extremities is usually 10 mm Hg higher than reading in upper extremities.
Use an appropriate-sized cuff: a pediatric cuff for children; a large cuff or a leg cuff for obese people.	Going from a recumbent to a standing position can cause the systolic pressure to fall 10–15 mm Hg and the diastolic pressure to rise slightly (by 5 mm Hg).
The cuff should be approximately 1 inch (2.5 cm) above the antecubital fossa.	
HEIGHT, WEIGHT, AND WAIST CIRCUMFERENCE	
Determine the patient's height and weight. Use a measuring stick or tape rather than asking the patient for recent measurements.	Height and weight can be used to determine body mass index.
Determine waist circumference by using tape measure just above the umbilicus at the narrowest point.	Waist circumference is an independent risk factor for cardiovascular disease. Normal is ≤ 40 inches (102 cm) for men and ≤ 35 inches (88 cm) for women.
GENERAL APPEARANCE	
Begin observation on first contact with the patient (in the waiting room or while the patient is in bed); continue throughout the interview systematically.	

*Auscultatory gap:
1. The first sound of blood in the artery is usually followed by continuous sound until nothing is audible with the stethoscope.
2. Occasionally the sound is not continuous and there is a gap after the first sound, after which the sound of blood in the vessel is heard again.
3. If one uses only the auscultatory method and pumps the cuff up until the sound is no longer heard, it is possible, when there is a gap in the sound or when the sound is not continuous, to get a falsely low systolic reading.

(continued)

Adult Physical Assessment *(continued)*

Technique	Findings

GENERAL APPEARANCE *(continued)*

Inspection

Observe for: race, sex, general physical development, nutritional state, mental alertness, affect, evidence of pain, restlessness, body position, clothes, apparent age, hygiene, grooming. Use smell and hearing as well as sight.

Careful observation of the general state of the individual provides many clues about a person's body image, how he or she behaves, and also some idea of how well or ill he or she is.

SKIN

1. Examination of the skin is correlated with the information obtained in the history and other parts of the physical examination.
2. Examine the skin as you proceed through each body system.

Inspection

Observe for: skin color, pigmentation, lesions (distribution, type, configuration, size), jaundice, cyanosis, scars, superficial vascularity, hydration, edema, color of mucous membranes, hair distribution, nails.

"Normal" varies considerably depending on racial or ethnic background, exposure to sun, complexion, pigmentation tendencies (such as freckles).

Palpation

Examine skin for temperature, texture, elasticity, turgor.

The skin is normally warm, slightly moist, and smooth and returns quickly to its original shape when picked up between two fingers and released. There is a characteristic hair distribution over the body associated with gender and normal physiologic function. Nails are present and smooth and cared for in some way.

HEAD

Inspection

Observe for: symmetry of face, configuration of skull, hair color and distribution, scalp.

Normally, the skull and face are symmetric, with distribution of hair varying from person to person. (However, determine by history if there has been any change.)

Palpation

Examine: hair texture, masses, swelling or tenderness of scalp, configuration of skull.

The scalp should be free of flaking, with no signs of nits (small, white louse eggs), lesions, deformities, or tenderness.

EYES AND VISION

Equipment

- Ophthalmoscope
- Snellen chart for visual acuity (see page 573)

Anatomic landmarks

Globes
Palpebral fissures
Lid margins
Conjunctivae
Sclerae
Pupils
Iris

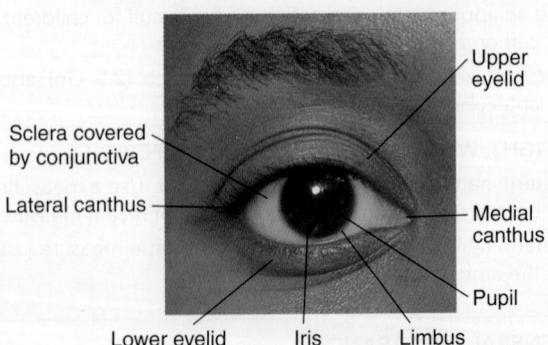

Upper eyelid
Sclera covered by conjunctiva
Lateral canthus
Medial canthus
Pupil
Lower eyelid   Iris   Limbus

Inspection

1. Globes—for protrusion.
2. Palpebral fissures (oval opening between the upper and lower eyelids)—for width and symmetry.

2. Palpebral fissures—appear equal in size when the eyes are open.

   Upper lid—covers a small portion of the iris and cornea.
   Lower lid—margin is just below the junction of the cornea and sclera (limbus).
   Ptosis—drooping of eyelids.

Adult Physical Assessment *(continued)*

Technique	Findings

EYES AND VISION *(continued)*
Inspection *(continued)*

3. Lid margins—for scaling, secretions, erythema, position of lashes.

3. Lid margins—are clear; the lacrimal duct openings (puncta) are evident at the nasal ends of the upper and lower lids.

   Eyelashes—normally are evenly distributed and turn outward.

4. Bulbar and palpebral conjunctivae—for congestion and color. Bulbar conjunctiva—membranous covering of the sclera (contains blood vessels). Palpebral conjunctiva—membranous covering of the inside of the upper and lower lids (contains blood vessels).

4. Bulbar conjunctiva (cover of sclera)—consists of transparent red blood vessels, which may become dilated and produce the characteristic "bloodshot" eye.

   Palpebral conjunctivae—are pink and clear.

   Conjunctivitis—inflammation of the conjunctival surfaces.

5. Sclerae and iris—for color.

5. Sclerae—should be white and clear.

6. Pupils—for size, shape, symmetry, reaction to light and accommodation (ability of the lens to adjust to objects at varying distances).

6. Pupils—normally constrict with increasing light and accommodation. Pupils are normally round and can range in size from very small ("pinpoint") to large (occupying the entire space of the iris).

7. Eye movement—extraocular movements, nystagmus, convergence. (Nystagmus: rapid, lateral, horizontal, or rotary movement of the eye; convergence: ability of the eye to turn in and focus on a very close object.) (See neurologic system, page 75.)

7. Extraocular movement—movement of the eyes in conjugate fashion. (Six muscles control the movement of the eye.) Eyes normally move in conjugate fashion, except when converging on an object that is moving closer.

   Nystagmus—may be seen briefly on lateral movement as a result of eye fatigue; however, vertical nystagmus or prolonged nystagmus should be evaluated.

   Convergence—fails when double vision occurs, usually 4–6 inches (10–15 cm) from the nose.

8. Gross visual fields—by confrontation. (See neurologic system, page 75.)

8. Peripheral vision—is full (medially and laterally, superiorly and inferiorly) in both eyes.

9. Visual acuity—check with a Snellen chart (with and without glasses).

9. Normal vision—20/20.

   Myopia—nearsightedness.

   Hyperopia—farsightedness.

Palpation

1. Determine the strength of the upper lids by attempting to open closed lids against resistance.

1. The examiner should not be able to open the lids when the patient is squeezing them shut.

2. Palpate globes through closed lids for tenderness and tension.

2. Globes normally are not tender when palpated.

Funduscopic examination

1. Red retinal reflex—check the transparency of the anterior and posterior chambers.

1. Red retinal reflex—can be spotted by the examiner while standing 1 foot (30 cm) from the eye.

2. Cornea—check for transparency.

2. Cornea—should be transparent, with the light directed at the pupil.

3. Lens—check for transparency.

3. Lens—should be transparent (retina can be seen).

4. Retina—check for color, pigmentation, hemorrhages, and exudates.

4. Retina—color varies according to the amount of pigment present. There should be no hemorrhages or exudates.

(continued)

Adult Physical Assessment *(continued)*

Technique	Findings

EYES AND VISION *(continued)*

Funduscopic examination *(continued)*

5. Optic disc—check for color, distinction of margins, pigmentation, degree of elevation, cupping.

5. Optic disc—is circular and has a yellowish pink color. Although disc appearance may vary, the margins are normally distinct and regular, with varying amounts of pigment.

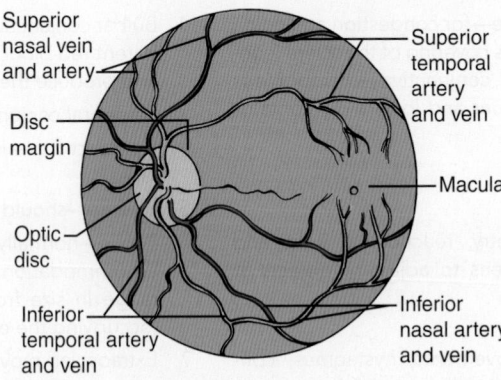

Superior nasal vein and artery — Disc margin — Optic disc — Inferior temporal artery and vein — Superior temporal artery and vein — Macula — Inferior nasal artery and vein

6. Macula—check for color. (Lies at a distance of 2 optic disc diameters laterally from the optic disc.)

6. Macula—because it is free of blood vessels, it is lighter in color than the rest of the retina.

7. Blood vessels—check for diameter, arteriovenous ratio; origin and course; venous–arterial crossings. (Both arteries and veins are present and move outward from the disc nasally and temporally.) Use of the ophthalmoscope.

7. Retinal arteries and veins—arteries are approximately $4/5$ the size of the veins and lighter in color. Where arteries and veins cross, there is usually no disturbance in the course of either. Pulsations may occur in the vein near the optic disc.

Use of the ophthalmoscope

1. Hold the instrument in your right hand and use your right eye to examine the patient's right eye.
   a. Reverse the procedure to examine the patient's left eye.
   b. This approach allows you to get close to the patient without bumping noses.

2. Hold the instrument so your last two fingers are straight, rather than curved around the handle. You can place these fingers against the patient's cheek to steady the instrument and to avoid hitting the patient with it.

3. Begin the funduscopic examination standing about 1 foot (30 cm) away from, and on the same level as, the patient. The room should be darkened.

4. Turn the dial on the head of the ophthalmoscope to 0 diopters.

5. Turn on the ophthalmoscope light and place the eyepiece up to your eye. If you wear glasses or contact lenses, it is best to wear them during the examination so you do not have to accommodate for your vision by turning the dial on the ophthalmoscope.

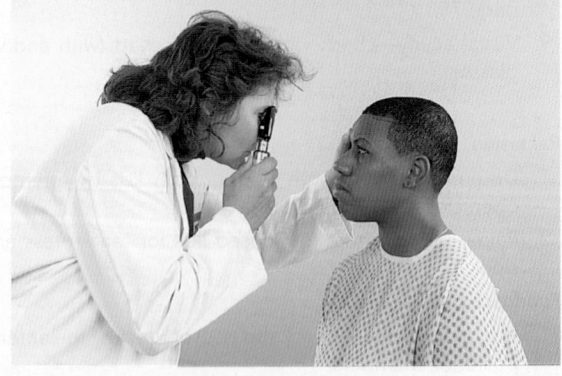

Adult Physical Assessment *(continued)*

Technique	Findings

EYES AND VISION *(continued)*

Use of the ophthalmoscope (continued)

6. Aim the light at the pupil of the eye. You should see the red reflex immediately.

7. Slowly move in toward the patient, continuing to look through the eyepiece and keeping the light directed at the pupil, beyond which is the fundus.

8. With the index finger of the hand holding the ophthalmoscope, turn the dial counterclockwise (to the minus diopters) to focus if the patient is nearsighted, or clockwise (toward the plus diopters) to focus if the patient is farsighted.

   a. This allows you to focus on the various chambers of the eye.

   b. A way to find the eye and pupil is to put your hand on top of the patient's head and your thumb at the outer corner of the eye. If you lose the fundus, you can return to your thumb and get your bearings by moving medially from the thumb nail.

9. Once your hand is resting on the patient's cheek, continue to turn the dial until you can focus on the retina and the blood vessels and the optic disc appear sharp.

10. Once you are focused on the optic disc, it is possible to follow the blood vessels out from the disc inferiorly and superiorly, medially and laterally.

Findings:

6. Absence of the red reflex suggests opacity of the lens (cataract), detached retina, or retinoblastoma (rarely).

10. Abnormal findings include hemorrhages, exudates, and papilledema.

EARS AND HEARING

Equipment

- Tuning fork
- Otoscope

To examine with otoscope

1. Hold the helix of the ear and gently pull the pinna upward and back toward the occiput to straighten the external canal.

2. Gently insert the lighted otoscope, using an earpiece that is a comfortable size for the patient.

3. Once the otoscope is in place, put your eye up to the eyepiece and examine the external canal.

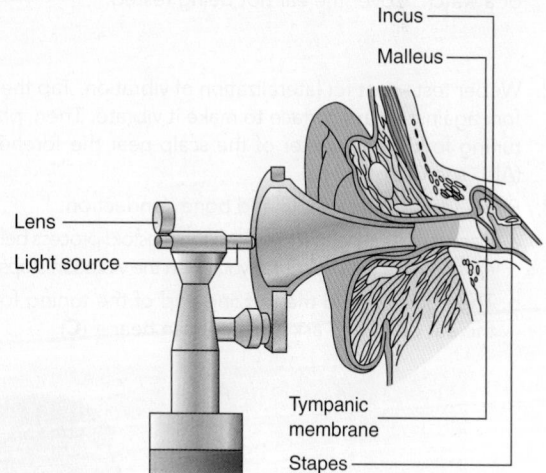

Inspection

1. Pinna—examine for size, shape, color, symmetry, placement on the head, lesions, and masses.

2. External canal—examine with the otoscope for discharge, impacted cerumen, inflammation, masses, or foreign bodies.

Findings:

2. External canal—is normally clear with perhaps minimal cerumen.

(continued)

Adult Physical Assessment *(continued)*

Technique	Findings

EARS AND HEARING *(continued)*

Inspection *(continued)*

3. Tympanic membrane—examine for color, luster, shape, position, transparency, integrity, and scarring.
4. Landmarks—note cone of light, umbo, handle and short process of the malleus, pars flaccida, and pars tensa. Gently move the otoscope to observe the entire drum. (Cerumen may obscure visualization of the drum.)

Palpation

Pinna—examine for tenderness, consistency of cartilage, swelling.

3. Tympanic membrane and landmarks.

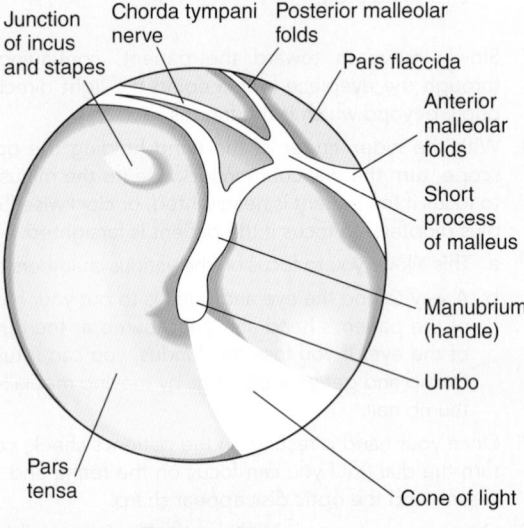

Junction of incus and stapes · Chorda tympani nerve · Posterior malleolar folds · Pars flaccida · Anterior malleolar folds · Short process of malleus · Manubrium (handle) · Umbo · Pars tensa · Cone of light

Right ear drum

Mechanical tests

1. Test each ear for gross hearing acuity using a whispered word or a watch. Cover the ear not being tested.

2. Weber test—test for lateralization of vibration. Tap the tuning fork against a hard surface to make it vibrate. Then, place the tuning fork in the center of the scalp near the forehead (**A**). (Also see Chapter 17.)
3. Rinne test—compares air and bone conduction.
   a. Place the vibrating tuning fork on the mastoid process behind the ear and have the patient tell you when the vibration stops (**B**).
   b. Then quickly hold the buzzing end of the tuning fork near the ear canal and ask if patient can hear it (**C**).

1. A person with normal hearing can hear a whispered word from approximately 15 feet (4.5 m) and a watch from 1 foot (30 cm). The patient should hear the sound equally well in both ears; that is, there is no lateralization.

2. Sound should be heard equally in both ears.

3. Sound should be heard after vibration can no longer be felt; that is, air conduction is greater than bone conduction. Lateralization and conduction findings are altered by damage to the cranial nerve VIII and damage to the ossicles in the middle ear.

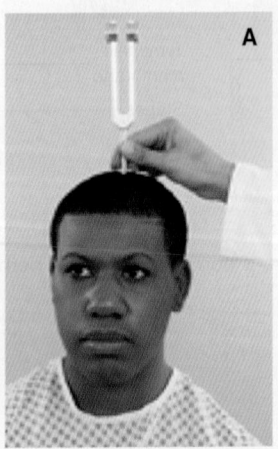
A

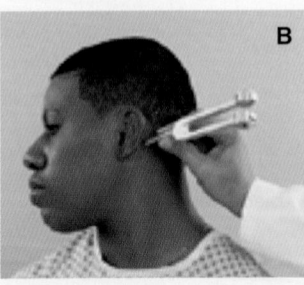
B

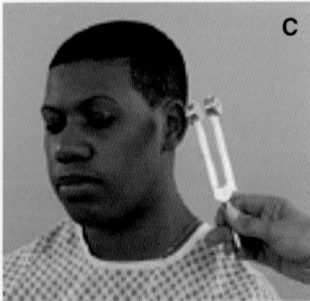
C

Adult Physical Assessment (continued)

Technique	Findings

NOSE AND SINUSES

Equipment
- Otoscope
- Nasal speculum

Inspection
1. Observe for general deformity.
2. With nasal speculum (otoscope, if speculum is unavailable) examine for:
   a. Nasal septum (position and perforation)
   b. Discharge (anteriorly and posteriorly)
   c. Nasal obstruction and airway patency
   d. Mucous membranes for color
   e. Turbinates for color and swelling

Nasal septum—is normally straight and not perforated.

Discharge—none should be present.

Airways—are patent.

Mucous membranes—are normally pink.

Turbinates—three bony projections on each lateral wall of the nasal cavity covered with well-vascularized, mucous-secreting membranes. They warm the air going into the lungs and may become swollen and pale with colds and allergies.

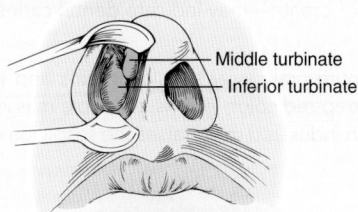

Middle turbinate
Inferior turbinate

Palpation

Sinuses (frontal and maxillary)—for tenderness.

Frontal—direct manual pressure upward toward the wall of the sinus. Avoid pressure on eyes.

Maxillary—with thumbs, direct pressure upward over lower edge of maxillary bones.

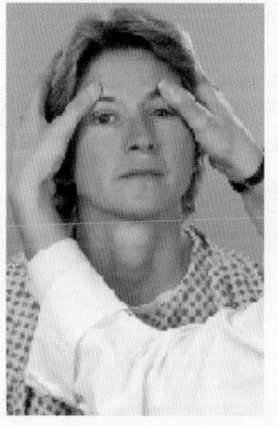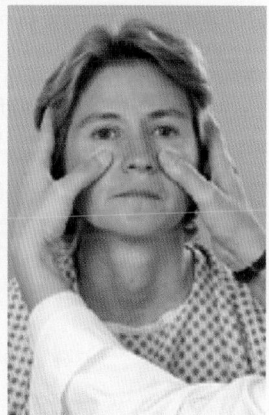

Tenderness of sinuses may indicate sinusitis.

MOUTH

Equipment
- Flashlight
- Tongue blade
- Gloves
- Gauze sponges

Inspection
1. Observe lips for color, moisture, pigment, masses, ulcerations, fissures.

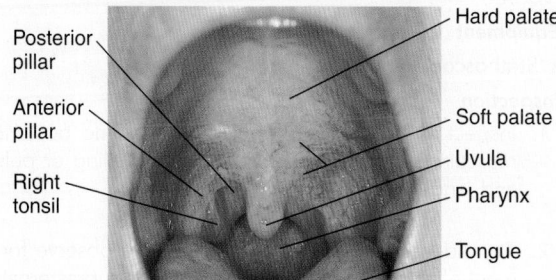

Posterior pillar
Anterior pillar
Right tonsil
Hard palate
Soft palate
Uvula
Pharynx
Tongue

2. Use tongue blade and penlight to examine:
   a. Teeth—number, arrangement, general condition.
   b. Gums—for color, texture, discharge, swelling, retraction.

Teeth—an adult normally has 32 teeth.

Gums—commonly recede in adults. Bleeding is fairly common and may result from trauma, gingival disease, or systemic problems (less common).

(continued)

Adult Physical Assessment *(continued)*

Technique	Findings

MOUTH *(continued)*

Inspection *(continued)*

c. Buccal mucosa—for discoloration, vesicles, ulcers, masses.

d. Pharynx—for inflammation, exudate, masses.

e. Tongue (protruded)—for size, color, thickness, lesions, moisture, symmetry, deviations from midline, fasciculations.

f. Salivary glands—for patency.
   i. Parotid glands
   ii. Sublingual and submaxillary glands

g. Uvula—for symmetry when patient says "ah."

h. Tonsils—for size, ulceration, exudates, inflammation.

i. Breath—for odor.

j. Voice—for hoarseness.

Tongue—is normally midline and covered with papillae, which vary in size from the tip of the tongue to the back. (The circumvallate papillae are large and posterior.)

Parotid glands—open in the buccal pouch at the level of the upper teeth halfway back.

Sublingual and submaxillary glands—open underneath the tongue.

Uvula—should be midline.

Lingual tonsils—can often be seen on the posterior portion of the tongue.

Odor of breath—may indicate dental caries.

Palpation

1. Examine the oral cavity with a gloved hand for masses and ulceration. Palpate beneath the tongue and laterally explore the floor of the mouth.

2. Grasp the tongue with a gauze sponge to retract it; inspect the sides and undersurface of the tongue and the floor of the mouth.

1. Entire oral cavity should be pink and without ulcers, deep-red color, lesions, palpable masses, or swelling. An indurated mass raises the suspicion of malignancy.

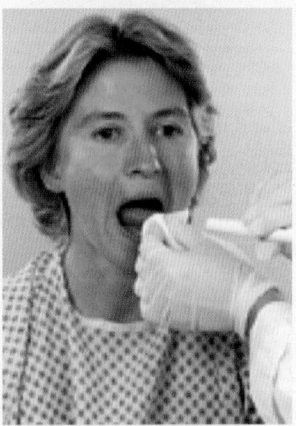

NECK

Equipment

• Stethoscope

Inspection

1. Inspect all areas of the neck anteriorly and posteriorly for muscular symmetry, masses, unusual swelling or pulsations, and range of motion.

2. Thyroid—ask the patient to swallow and observe for movement of an enlarged thyroid gland at the suprasternal notch.

3. Muscular strength.
   a. Cervical muscles—have the patient turn his chin forcefully against your hand.
   b. Trapezius muscles—exert pressure on the patient's shoulders while he shrugs his shoulders.

1. Range of motion—normally, the chin can touch the anterior chest, the head can be extended at least 45 degrees from the vertical position and can be rotated 90 degrees from midline to side.

2. Thyroid—is not usually visible, except in extremely thin people.

3. Strength—see "Findings, cranial nerve XI," page 78.

Adult Physical Assessment (continued)

Technique	Findings

NECK (continued)

Palpation

1. Palpate the 10 areas for cervical lymph nodes as shown here.

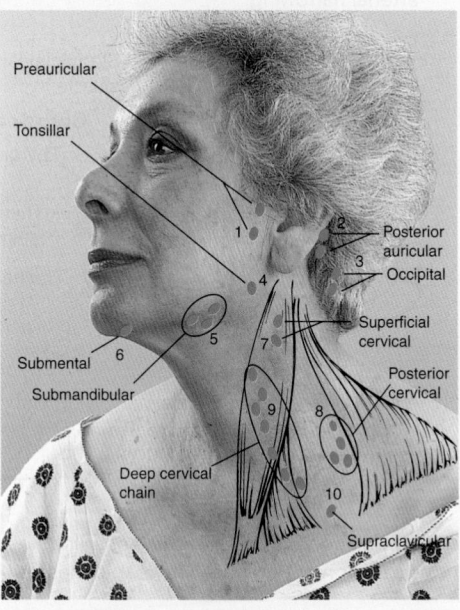

2. Trachea—palpate at the sternal notch. Place one finger along the side of the trachea and note the space between it and the sternomastoid. Compare to the other side.

3. Thyroid

   a. Stand behind the patient and have him flex the neck slightly to relax the muscles.

   b. Place the fingertips of both hands on either side of the trachea just below the cricoid cartilage. Have the patient swallow and feel for any glandular tissue rising under your fingertips.

   c. Palpate the area over the trachea for the isthmus and laterally for the right and left lobes.

   d. Note any enlargement, nodules, masses, consistency.

1. Cervical nodes—in the adult, the cervical lymph nodes are not normally palpable unless the patient is very thin, in which case the nodes are felt as small, freely movable masses. Tender nodes suggest inflammation; hard, fixed nodes suggest malignancy.

2. Trachea—should be midline. Spaces measured by fingers should be symmetrical. Tracheal deviation may be caused by neck mass or problems within the chest.

3. If the thyroid is palpable, it is normally smooth, without nodules, masses, or irregularities.

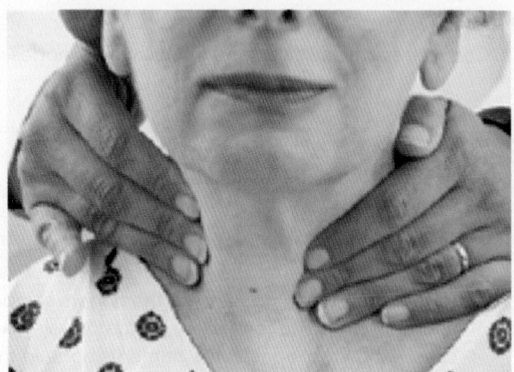

(continued)

Adult Physical Assessment *(continued)*

Technique	Findings

NECK *(continued)*

Palpation *(continued)*

4. Carotid arteries
   a. Palpate the carotids one side at a time.
   b. The carotids lie anterolaterally in the neck—avoid palpating the carotid sinuses at the level of the thyroid cartilage just below the angle of the jaw because this may cause slowing of heart rate.
   c. Note the symmetry of pulsations, strength, and amplitude, as well as any abnormal thrill.

4. A thrill (humming-like vibration) usually indicates arterial narrowing.

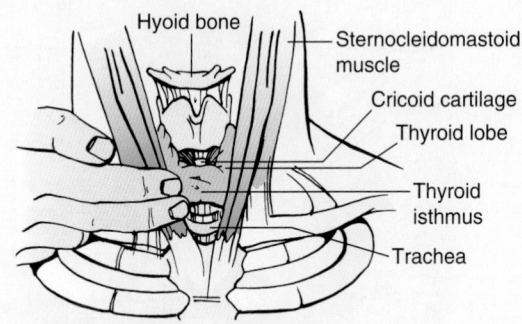

Auscultation

1. Use the diaphragm of the stethoscope to listen for bruits (murmur-like sound) over the carotid arteries.

1. A bruit may indicate arterial narrowing with turbulent blood flow. A cardiac murmur may also be referred to the carotid arteries.

LYMPH NODES

1. It is important at some point in the examination to palpate all areas where lymphadenopathy might appear.
2. Typically, this is done as each region of the body is examined; for example, the cervical nodes are studied when the neck is examined and inguinal nodes are inspected when the abdomen is examined.

1. Lymph nodes are normally nonpalpable or felt as small, nontender, freely moveable masses.

Inspection

Note size, shape, mobility, consistency, tenderness, and inflammation.

Palpation

1. Cervical, supraclavicular, and infraclavicular nodes.

1. Supraclavicular and infraclavicular nodes—not normally palpable. Enlargement may indicate a thoracic problem.

2. Axillary nodes (usually done during breast exam).
   a. Examine the patient while patient is sitting.
   b. Place the patient's arm at his side and examine the apex of the patient's axilla. (Use the fingers of your right hand to examine the left axilla and vice versa.)
   c. Rotate the examining hand so the fingers can palpate the anterior and posterior axillary fossae pressing against the chest wall. Press against the humerus bone in the axilla to examine the lateral fossa for nodes. Conclude the axillary examination by moving the fingers from the apex of the axilla downward in the midline along the chest wall.

2. Axillary nodes—normally nonpalpable. Enlargement may occur with a breast or arm problem.

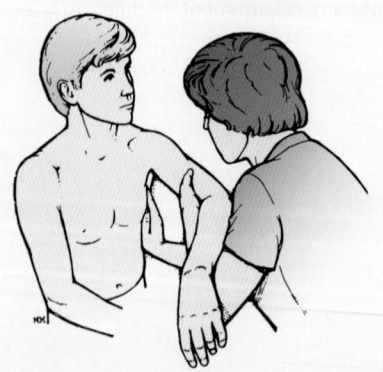

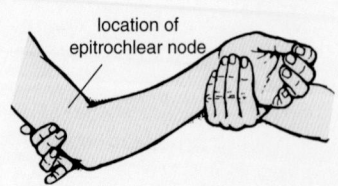

location of epitrochlear node

Adult Physical Assessment *(continued)*

Technique	Findings

LYMPH NODES *(continued)*

Palpation *(continued)*

3. Inguinal nodes—are located in the groin and are usually examined when the abdomen is examined.

4. Epitrochlear nodes—are palpated just above the medial epicondyle, between the biceps and triceps muscles.

3. Inguinal nodes—a few may be felt. Enlargement and acute tenderness may indicate a genital or lower extremity problem.

4. Epitrochlear nodes—not normally palpable. Enlargement may indicate an arm or systemic problem.

BREASTS (MALE AND FEMALE)

Female breast

Inspection

(With the patient sitting, arms relaxed at sides.)

1. Inspect the areolae and nipples for position, pigmentation, inversion, discharge, crusting, and masses. Extra, or supernumerary, nipples may occur normally, most commonly in the anterior axillary region or just below the normal breasts.

2. Examine the breast tissue for size, shape, color, symmetry, surface, contour, skin characteristics, and level of breasts. Note any retraction or dimpling of the skin.

3. Ask the patient to elevate her hands over her head; repeat the observation.

4. Have the patient press her hands to her hips; repeat the observation.

1. The *nipples* should be at the same level and protrude slightly. An *inverted nipple* (one that turns inward), if present since puberty, may be normal.

   A *supernumerary nipple* usually consists of a nipple and a small areola and may be mistaken for a mole.

2. Breast size—in the female it is not uncommon to find a difference in the size of the two breasts. Normal asymmetry has usually been present since puberty and is not a recent phenomenon.

3. If there is a mass attached to the pectoral muscles, contracting the muscles will cause retraction of the breast tissue.

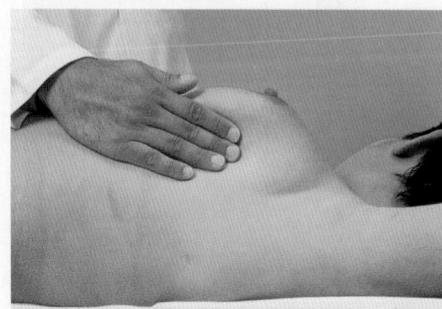

Palpation

(This is best done with the patient in a recumbent position.)

1. The patient with pendulous breasts should be given a pillow to place under the ipsilateral scapula of the breast being palpated so the tissue is distributed more evenly over the chest wall.

2. The arm on the side of the breast being palpated should be raised above the patient's head.

3. Palpate one breast at a time, beginning with the "asymptomatic" breast if the patient complains of symptoms.

4. To palpate, use the palmar aspects of the fingers in a rotating motion, compressing the breast tissue against the chest wall. Don't forget to include the "tail" of the breast tissue, which extends into the axillary region in the upper outer quadrant of the breast.

5. Note skin texture, moisture, temperature, or masses.

6. Gently squeeze the nipple and note any expressible discharge.

7. Repeat the examination on the opposite breast and compare findings.

3. This allows the examiner to palpate the "normal" breast first and then compare the "symptomatic" breast to it.

4. Breast texture—varies according to the amount of subcutaneous tissue present.

   a. In young females, tissue is fairly soft and homogeneous; in postmenopausal women, tissue may feel nodular or stringy.

   b. Consistency also varies with menstrual cycle, being more nodular and edematous just prior to menstruation.

5. Masses—If a mass is palpated, its location, size, shape, consistency, mobility, and associated tenderness are reported.

6. Discharge—In the normal nonpregnant or nonlactating female, there is usually no nipple discharge.

(continued)

Adult Physical Assessment *(continued)*

Technique	Findings

BREASTS (MALE AND FEMALE) *(continued)*

Male breast

Examination of the male breast can be brief but may be important.

1. Observe the nipple and areola for ulceration, nodules, swelling, or discharge.

2. Palpate the areola for nodules and tenderness.

3. Palpate axillary lymph nodes (see page 60).

1. There should be no discharge.

2. Enlargement of glandular tissue is gynecomastia, related to hormone imbalance.

THORAX AND LUNGS

1. Methodical inspection of the thorax requires reference to established "landmarks" to locate specific structures and to report significant findings.

2. The same structural landmarks are used in examining both the lung and the heart.

3. It is important to visualize the underlying structures and organs when examining the thorax.

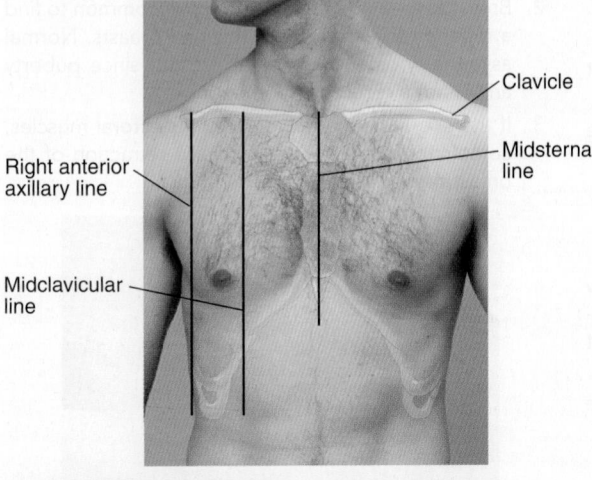

Right anterior axillary line

Midclavicular line

Clavicle

Midsternal line

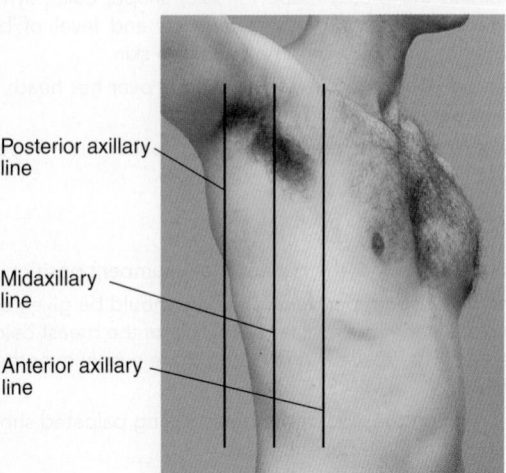

Posterior axillary line

Midaxillary line

Anterior axillary line

Posterior thorax and lungs

Begin the examination with the patient seated; examine posterior chest and lungs.

Inspection

1. Inspect the spine for mobility and any structural deformity.

2. Observe the symmetry of the posterior chest and the posture and mobility of the thorax on respiration. Note any bulges or retractions of the costal interspaces on respiration or any impairment of respiratory movement.

3. Note the anteroposterior diameter in relation to the lateral diameter of the chest.

2. The thorax is normally symmetric; it moves easily and without impairment on respiration. There are no bulges or retractions of the intercostal spaces.

3. The anteroposterior diameter of the thorax in relation to the lateral diameter is approximately 1:2.

Adult Physical Assessment (continued)

Technique	Findings

THORAX AND LUNGS (continued)

Posterior thorax and lungs (continued)

Palpation

1. Palpate the posterior chest with the patient sitting; identify areas of tenderness, masses, inflammation.
2. Palpate the ribs and costal margins for symmetry, mobility, and tenderness and the spine for tenderness and vertebral position.
3. To assess respiratory expansion, place thumbs at the level of the 10th vertebra. With hands held parallel to the 10th ribs as they grasp the lateral rib cage, ask the patient to inhale deeply. Observe the movement of the thumbs while feeling the range and observe the symmetry of the hands.

2. On palpation, there should be no tenderness; chest movement should be symmetric and without lag or impairment. Tenderness may indicate musculoskeletal strain, fracture, or other problems.

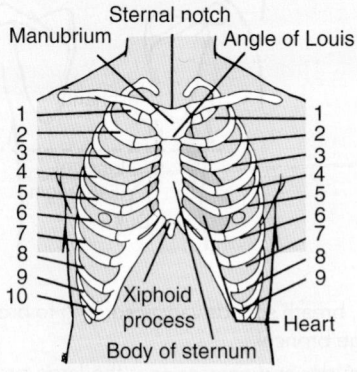
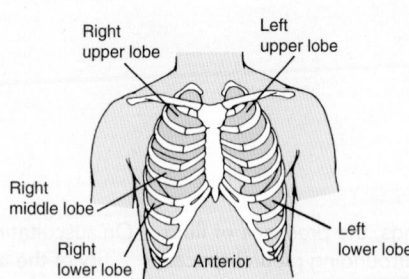
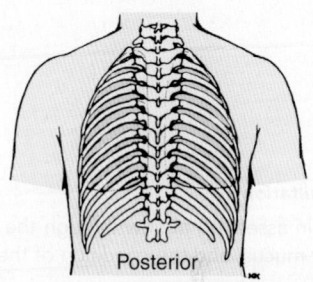

Sternal notch
Manubrium — Angle of Louis
1 2 3 4 5 6 7 8 9 10
Xiphoid process
Body of sternum
Heart

Right upper lobe
Left upper lobe
Right middle lobe
Right lower lobe
Anterior
Left lower lobe

Posterior

4. To elicit vocal and tactile *fremitus* (palpable vibrations transmitted through the bronchopulmonary system on speaking).
   a. Ask the patient to say "99"; palpate and compare symmetric areas of the lungs with the ball of one hand. Begin at the upper lobes and move downward.
   b. Note any areas of increased or decreased fremitus.
   c. If fremitus is faint, ask the patient to speak louder and in a deeper voice.

4. Posteriorly, fremitus is generally equal throughout the lung fields. It may be increased near the large bronchi due to consolidation of tissue resulting from pneumonia. It may be decreased or absent anteriorly and posteriorly when vocal loudness is decreased, when posture is not erect, or when excessive tissue or underlying structures are present, or in cases of pneumothorax and other pathology.

Percussion

As with palpation, the posterior chest is optimally percussed with the patient sitting.

1. Percuss symmetric areas, comparing sides.

1. Percussion normally reveals resonance over symmetric areas of the lung. Percussion sound may be altered by poor posture or the presence of excessive tissue.

2. Begin across the top of each shoulder and proceed down between the scapulae and then under the scapulae, both medially and laterally in the axillary lines.
3. Note and localize any abnormal percussion sound.

3. Dullness may indicate mass or consolidation due to pneumonia.

4. For diaphragmatic excursion, percuss by placing the pleximeter (stationary) finger parallel to the approximate level of the diaphragm below the right scapula. (See diagram on next page.)

4. The lower border of the lungs is approximately at the level of the 10th thoracic spinous process on normal respiration. Unilateral abnormality of decreased excursion may indicate pleural effusion, atelectasis, or paralysis of one side of the diaphragm.

(continued)

Adult Physical Assessment (continued)

Technique	Findings

THORAX AND LUNGS (continued)

Posterior thorax and lungs (continued)

Percussion (continued)

a. Ask the patient to inhale deeply and hold his breath; percuss downward to the point of dullness. Mark this point.

b. Let the patient breathe normally and then ask patient to exhale deeply; percuss upward from the mark to the point of resonance.

c. Mark this point and measure between the two marks—normally 2–2½ inches (5–6 cm).

d. Repeat this procedure on the opposite side of the chest.

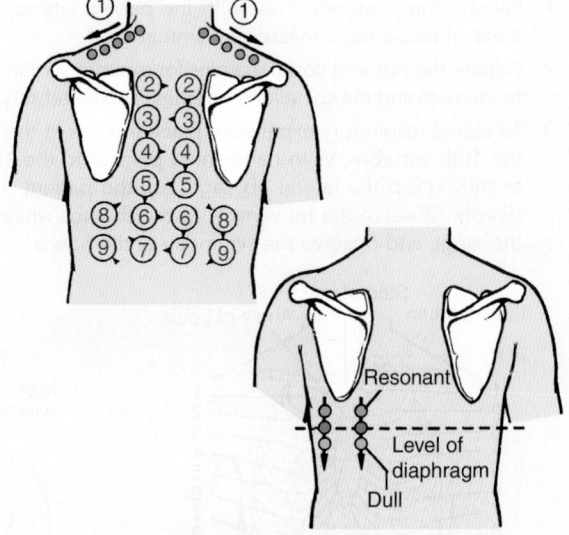

Auscultation

Aids in assessing airflow through the lungs, the presence of fluid or mucus, and the condition of the surrounding pleural space.

1. Have the patient sit erect.*

2. With a stethoscope, listen to the lungs as the patient breathes more deeply than normally with the mouth open. (Let the patient pause, as needed, to avoid hyperventilation.)

3. Place the stethoscope in the same areas on the chest wall as those percussed, and listen to a complete inspiration and expiration in each area.

4. Compare symmetric areas methodically from the apex to the lung bases.

5. It should be possible to distinguish three types of normal breath sounds as indicated in the following table.

On auscultation, breath sounds vary according to proximity of the large bronchi.

– They are louder and coarser near the large bronchi and over the anterior.

– They are softer and much finer (vesicular) at the periphery over the alveolae.

Breath sounds also vary in duration with inspiration and expiration.

Sounds may normally decrease in obese individuals.

5. Pathology will alter the normal bronchial, bronchovesicular, and vesicular breath sounds. Adventitious sounds may indicate crackles, wheezes, and rhonchi.

Breath Sounds	Duration of Inspiration and Expiration	Pitch of Expiration	Intensity of Expiration	Normal Location
Vesicular	Inspiration > Expiration	Low	Soft	Most of lungs
Bronchovesicular	Inspiration = Expiration	Medium	Medium	Near the main stem bronchi (below the clavicles and between the scapulae, especially on the right)
Bronchial or tubular	Expiration > Inspiration	High	Usually loud	Over the trachea

Adapted from Bickley, L. S. (2008). Bates' guide to physical examination and history taking (10th ed.). Philadelphia: Lippincott Williams & Wilkins.

*Note: If the patient is unable to sit without assistance for examination of the posterior chest and lungs, position him or her first on one side and then on the other as you examine the lung fields.

Adult Physical Assessment *(continued)*

Technique	Findings

THORAX AND LUNGS *(continued)*

Anterior thorax and lungs

The patient should be recumbent with his or her arms at sides and slightly abducted.

Inspection

1. Inspect the chest for any structural deformity.
2. Note the width of the costal angle.

2. The angle at the tip of the sternum is determined by the right and left rib margins at the xiphoid process. Normally, the angle is less than 90 degrees.

3. Observe the rate and rhythm of breathing, any bulging or retraction of intercostal spaces on respiration, and use of accessory muscles of respiration (sternocleidomastoid and trapezius on inspiration and abdominal muscles on expiration).

3. There are no bulges or retractions of the intercostal spaces.

4. Note any asymmetry of chest wall movement on respiration.

4. The thorax is normally symmetric and moves easily without impairment on respiration.

Palpation

1. To assess expansion, place your hands along the costal margins and note symmetry and degree of expansion as the patient inhales deeply.
2. Palpate for fremitus with the ball of the hand anteriorly and laterally. (Underlying structures [heart, liver] may damp, or decrease, fremitus.)
3. Compare symmetric areas.
4. If necessary, displace the female breast gently.

Percussion

1. With patient's arms resting comfortably at sides, percuss the anterior and lateral chest. Begin just below the clavicles and percuss downward from one interspace to the next, comparing the sound from the interspace on one side with that of the contralateral interspace.
2. Displace the female breast so breast tissue does not damp the vibration. Continue downward, noting the intercostal space where hepatic dullness is percussed on the right and cardiac dullness on the left.
3. Note the effect of underlying structures.

2. A tympanic sound is produced over the gastric air bubble on the left somewhat lower than the point of liver dullness on the right.

3. Percussion over heart will produce a dull sound. The upper border of the liver will be percussed on the right side, producing a dull note.

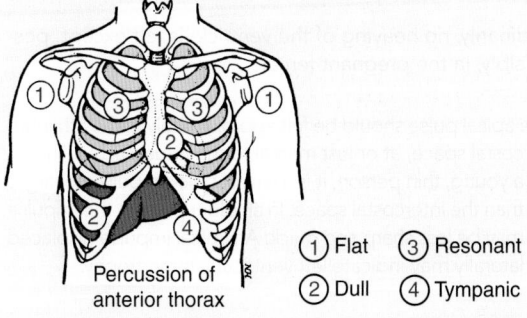

Percussion of anterior thorax

① Flat   ③ Resonant
② Dull   ④ Tympanic

Auscultation

Listen to the chest anteriorly and laterally for the distribution of resonance and any abnormal or adventitious sounds.

(continued)

Adult Physical Assessment *(continued)*

Technique	Findings

HEART
General approach

1. The examiner must visualize the position of the heart under the sternum and the ribs and know certain landmarks for identification of specific structures and significant findings.

2. It is also important to identify those "areas" on the chest wall that will yield the most information initially about the function of the heart and its valves.

   a. In locating the intercostal spaces, begin by identifying the angle of Louis, which is felt as a slight ridge approximately 1 inch (2.5 cm) below the sternal notch, where the manubrium and the body of the sternum are joined.

   b. The 2nd ribs extend to the right and left of this angle.

   c. Once the 2nd rib is located, palpate downward and obliquely away from the sternum to identify the remaining ribs and intercostal spaces.

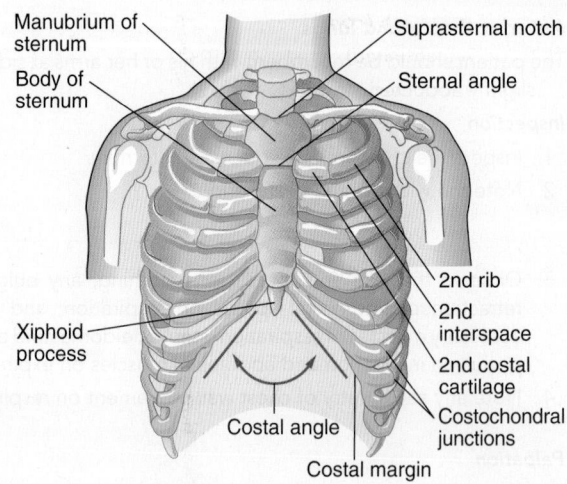

Manubrium of sternum — Suprasternal notch — Body of sternum — Sternal angle — 2nd rib — 2nd interspace — Xiphoid process — 2nd costal cartilage — Costochondral junctions — Costal angle — Costal margin

Inspection

1. Inspect the precordium for any bulging, heaving, or thrusting.

2. Look for the apical impulse in the 5th or 6th intercostal space at or just medial to the midclavicular line.

3. Note any other pulsations. Tangential lighting is most helpful in detecting pulsations.

1. Normally there are no bulges or heaves; these indicate pathology.

2. An apical impulse may or may not be observable.

3. There should be no other pulsations.

Palpation

1. Use the ball of the hand to detect vibrations, or "thrills," which may be caused by murmurs. (Use the fingertips or palmar surface to detect pulsations.)

2. Proceed methodically through the examination so no area is omitted. Palpate for thrills and pulsations in each area (aortic, pulmonic, tricuspid, mitral).

   a. Begin in the aortic area (2nd right intercostal space, close to the sternum) and proceed to the pulmonic area (2nd left intercostal space), and then downward to the apex of the heart. (The mitral area is considered the apex of the heart.)

   b. In the tricuspid area, use the palm of the hand to detect any heaving or thrusting of the precordium (tricuspid area—5th intercostal space next to the sternum).

   c. In the mitral area (5th intercostal space, at or just medial to the midclavicular line), palpate for the apical beat; identify the point of maximal impulse (PMI) and note its size and force.

1. There should be no thrills or other pulsations. (Thrills are vibrations caused by turbulence of blood moving through valves that are transmitted through the skin, which feels similar to a purring cat.)

Ordinarily, no heaving of the ventricle is felt except, possibly, in the pregnant female.

The apical pulse should be felt approximately in the 5th intercostal space, at or just medial to the midclavicular line. In a young, thin person, it is a sharp, quick impulse no larger than the intercostal space. In an older person, the impulse may be less sharp and quick. An apical impulse displaced laterally may indicate left ventricular hypertrophy.

Percussion

1. Outline the heart border or area of cardiac dullness.

   a. The left border generally does not extend beyond 4, 7, and 10 cm left of the midsternal line in the 4th, 5th, and 6th intercostal spaces, respectively.

   b. The right border usually lies under the sternum.

Adult Physical Assessment (continued)

Technique	Findings

HEART (continued)
General approach (continued)
Percussion (continued)

2. Percuss outward from the sternum with the stationary finger parallel to the intercostal space until dullness is no longer heard. Measure the distance from the midsternal line in centimeters.

Auscultation

1. Place the stethoscope in the pulmonic or aortic area.
2. Begin by identifying the first (S₁) and second (S₂) heart sounds.
   a. S_1 is caused by the closing of the tricuspid and mitral valves.
   b. S_2 results from the closing of the aortic and pulmonic valves.

2. The two sounds are separated by a short systolic interval; each pair of sounds is separated from the next pair by a longer, diastolic interval. Normally, two sounds are heard—"lub, dub."
   - In the aortic and pulmonic areas, S_2 is usually louder than S_1. In this way, each of the paired sounds can be distinguished from the other.
   - In the tricuspid area, S_1 and S_2 are of almost equal intensity and, in the mitral area, S_1 is often slightly louder than S_2.

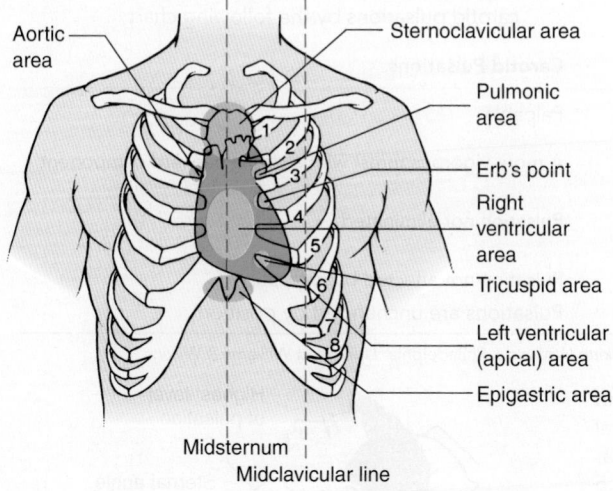

Aortic area — Sternoclavicular area — Pulmonic area — Erb's point — Right ventricular area — Tricuspid area — Left ventricular (apical) area — Epigastric area

Midsternum | Midclavicular line

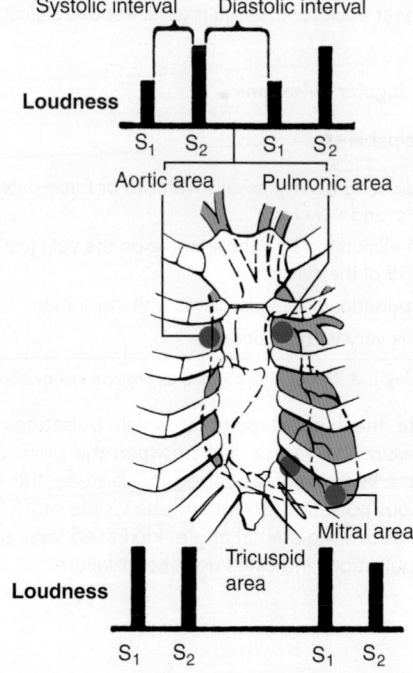

Systolic interval   Diastolic interval

Loudness

S₁ S₂   S₁ S₂

Aortic area   Pulmonic area

Mitral area

Tricuspid area

Loudness

S₁ S₂   S₁ S₂

3. Once the heart sounds are identified, count the rate and note the rhythm as discussed under vital signs. If there is an irregularity, try to determine if there is any pattern to the irregularity in relation to the intervals, heart sounds, or respirations.

3. Normally, the heart sounds are regular, with a rate of 60–80 beats/minute (in the adult). In the athlete or jogger, the resting pulse may be between 40 and 60 beats/minute.

(continued)

Adult Physical Assessment *(continued)*

Technique	Findings

HEART *(continued)*

General approach *(continued)*

Auscultation (continued)

4. Once rate and rhythm are determined, listen in each of the four areas and at Erb's point (3rd left interspace, close to the sternum) systematically, first with the diaphragm (detects higher-pitched sounds) and then with the bell (detects lower-pitched sounds). In each area, listen to S_1 and then to S_2 for intensity and splitting.

4. An extra "woosh" sound between S_1 and S_2 indicates systolic murmur; between S_2 and S_1 indicates a diastolic murmur. Note the area of its greatest intensity (aortic, pulmonic, mitral, tricuspid). An extra sound of short duration usually indicates an S_3 or S_4 gallop.

    Occasionally, there may be a splitting of S_2 in the pulmonic area. This is normal. Splitting of S_2 (two contiguous sounds are heard instead of one) is best heard at the end of inspiration, when right ventricular stroke volume is sufficiently increased to delay closure of the pulmonic valve *slightly* behind closure of the aortic valve.

PERIPHERAL CIRCULATION

Jugular veins

Evaluation of jugular venous distention is most useful in patients with suspected compromise of cardiac function.

Inspection

1. Inspect neck for internal jugular venous pulsations.

1. Jugular venous pulsations can be distinguished from carotid pulsations by the following chart:

Internal Jugular Pulsations	Carotid Pulsations
Rarely palpable	Palpable
Soft, undulating quality, usually with two or three outward components (a, c, and v waves)	A more vigorous thrust with a single outward component
Pulsation eliminated by light pressure on the vein just above the sternal end of the clavicle	Pulsation not eliminated
Level of pulsation barely descends with inspiration	Pulsation not affected by inspiration
Pulsations vary with position	Pulsations are unchanged by position

From Bickley, L. S. (2008). *Bates' guide to physical examination and history taking* (10th ed.). Philadelphia: Lippincott Williams & Wilkins.

2. Note the highest point at which pulsations are seen and measure the vertical line between the point and the sternal angle. With the head raised 30 degrees, the internal jugular venous pulsations should not be visible more than 1 inch (2.5 cm) above the sternal angle. Increased level of internal jugular pulsations indicates right heart failure.

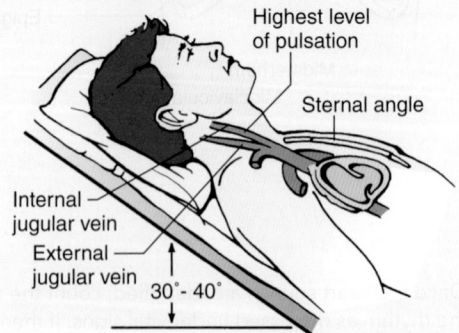

Extremities

Inspection

1. Observe skin over extremities for color, hair distribution, pallor, rubor, and swelling.

1. Extremities should be symmetrically even in color, warmth, and moisture, without swelling. Swelling of feet may occur after prolonged standing or sitting, but will disappear readily when extremity is elevated (dependent edema).

2. Inspect for any superficial vessels.

Adult Physical Assessment *(continued)*

Technique	Findings

PERIPHERAL CIRCULATION *(continued)*

Extremities *(continued)*

Palpation

1. Note the temperature of the skin over extremities, comparing one side to the other.

2. Palpate pulses (radial, femoral, posterior tibial, dorsalis pedis), comparing symmetry from side to side.

   2. Absence of peripheral pulses indicates peripheral vascular disease.

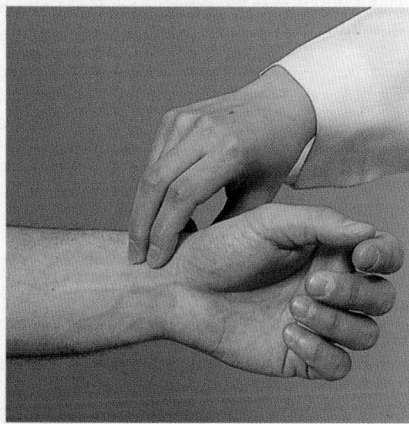 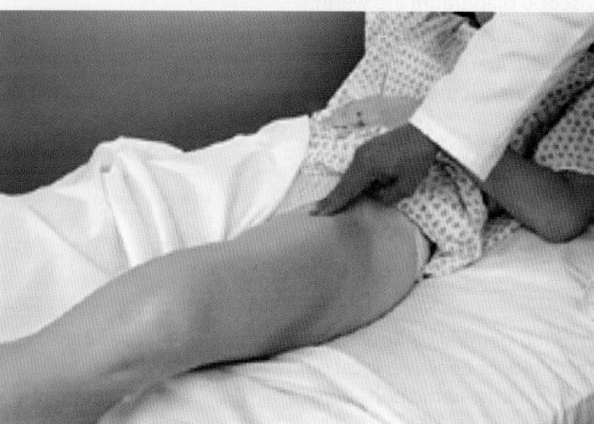

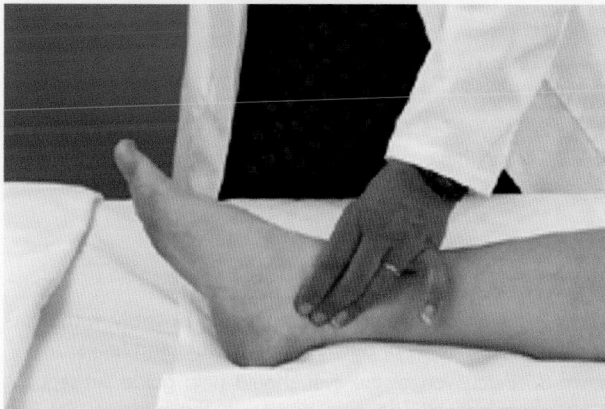 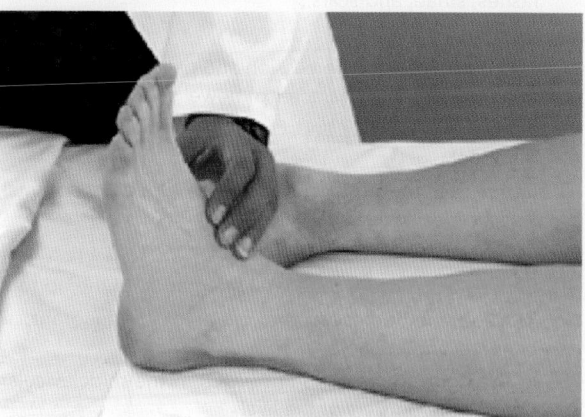

3. Palpate the skin over the tibia for edema by squeezing the skin for 30–60 seconds. Run the pads of your fingers over the area pressed and note indentation. If indentation is noted, repeat the procedure, moving up the extremity, and note the point at which no more swelling is present.

   3. Edema is usually graded from trace to 3+ or 4+ pitting. Trace is a slight indentation that disappears in a short time. Grade 3+ or 4+ is deep pitting that does not disappear readily. At best, these are subjective measurements, which are tried and confirmed through practice and comparison of findings with associates.

(continued)

Adult Physical Assessment *(continued)*

Technique	Findings

ABDOMEN

General approach

1. Make sure the patient has an empty bladder.
2. The patient should be lying comfortably with his or her arms at sides. Bending the knees slightly will help to relax the abdominal muscles and make palpation easier.
3. Expose the abdomen fully. Make sure your hands and the stethoscope diaphragm are warm.
4. Be methodical in visualizing the underlying organs as you inspect, auscultate, percuss, and palpate each quadrant or region of the abdomen.

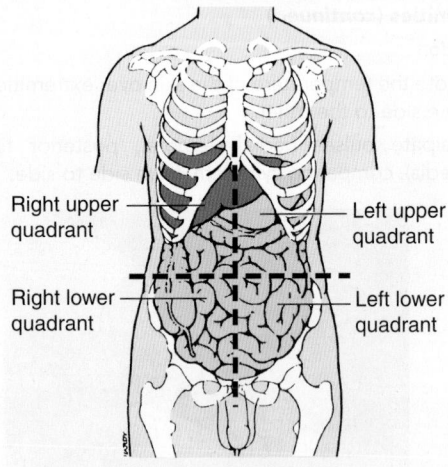

Right upper quadrant · Left upper quadrant

Right lower quadrant · Left lower quadrant

Inspection

1. Observe the general contour of the abdomen (flat, protuberant, scaphoid, or concave; local bulges). Also note symmetry, visible peristalsis, aortic pulsations.
2. Check the umbilicus for contour or hernia and the skin for rashes, striae, and scars.

1. The abdomen may or may not have any scars and should be flat or slightly rounded in the nonobese person.

Auscultation

1. This is done before percussion and palpation because palpation may alter the character of bowel sounds.
2. Note the frequency and character of bowel sounds (pitch, duration).
3. Listen over the aorta, renal arteries (upper quadrants), and iliac arteries (lower quadrants) for bruits.

2. Anywhere from 5 to 35 bowel sounds per minute. May have familiar sound of "growling."
3. Bruits indicate arterial narrowing.

Percussion

1. Percussion provides a general orientation to the abdomen.
2. Proceed methodically from quadrant to quadrant, noting tympany and dullness.
3. In the right upper quadrant (RUQ) in the midclavicular line, percuss the borders of the liver.
   a. Begin at a point of tympany in the midclavicular line of the right lower quadrant (RLQ) and percuss upward to the point of dullness (the lower liver border); mark the point.
   b. Percuss downward from the point of lung resonance above the RUQ to the point of dullness (the upper border of the liver); mark the point.
   c. Measure in centimeters the distance between the two marks in the midclavicular line (the liver span).
   d. Tympany of the gastric air bubble can be percussed in the left upper quadrant over the anterior lower border of the rib cage.

2. Tympany usually predominates, possibly with scattered areas of dullness due to fluid and feces.
3. Percussion of the liver should help guide subsequent palpation. The liver border in the midclavicular line should normally range from 2½ to 4½ inches (6 to 11 cm).

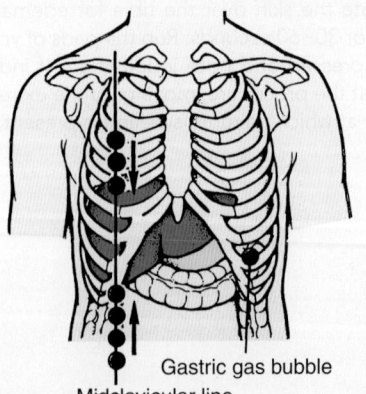

Gastric gas bubble
Midclavicular line

Adult Physical Assessment (continued)

Technique	Findings

ABDOMEN (continued)

General approach (continued)

Percussion (continued)

4. Assess for an enlarged spleen by percussing the lowest interspace of the right anterior axillary line (should be tympanic). Ask the patient to take a deep breath and repeat (should still be tympanic).

4. Change in percussion note to dullness on inspiration indicates an enlarged spleen.

Palpation

1. Perform light palpation in an organized manner to detect any muscular resistance (guarding), tenderness, or superficial organs or masses.

1. Tenderness and involuntary guarding indicate peritoneal inflammation.

2. Perform deep palpation to determine location, size, shape, consistency, tenderness, pulsations, and mobility of underlying organs and masses.

2. Rebound tenderness (pain on quick withdrawal of the fingers following palpation) suggests peritoneal irritation, as in acute appendicitis.

3. Move slowly and gently from one quadrant to the next to relax and reassure the patient.

3. Palpate painful areas last.

4. Use two hands if the abdomen is obese or muscular, with one hand on top of the other. The upper hand exerts pressure downward while the lower hand feels the abdomen.

Liver

1. Palpate the liver by placing the left hand under the patient's lower right rib cage and the right hand on the abdomen below the level of liver dullness. Press gently inward and upward with your fingertips while the patient takes a deep breath.

1. A normal liver edge may be palpable as a smooth, sharp, regular surface. An enlarged liver will be palpable and may be tender, hard, or irregular.

Spleen

1. Place your left hand around and under the patient's left lower rib cage and press your right hand below the left costal margin inward toward the spleen while the patient takes a deep breath.

1. A normal spleen is usually not palpable. Be sure to start low enough so as not to miss the border of an enlarged spleen.

Kidney

1. Next palpate for the left and right kidneys.

1. The kidney is usually felt only in people with very relaxed abdominal muscles (the very young, the aged, and multiparous women). The right kidney is slightly lower than the left. The kidney is felt as a solid, firm, smooth elastic mass.

2. Place the left hand under the patient's back between the rib cage and the iliac crest.

3. Support the patient while you palpate the abdomen with the right palmar surface of the fingers facing the left side of the body.

4. Palpate by bringing the left and right hands together as much as possible slightly below the level of the umbilicus on the right and left.

5. If the kidney is felt, describe its size and shape and note any tenderness.

6. Costal vertebral angle tenderness is palpated with the patient sitting, usually during the examination of the posterior chest. Locate the costal vertebral angle in the flank region and strike firmly with the ulnar surface of your hand. Note any tenderness over the area.

6. There should be no costal vertebral angle tenderness.

(continued)

Adult Physical Assessment *(continued)*

Technique	Findings

ABDOMEN *(continued)*

General approach *(continued)*

Aorta

1. Palpate for the aorta with the thumb and index finger.
2. Press deeply in the epigastric region (roughly in the midline) and feel with the fingers for pulsations, as well as for the contour of the aorta.

1. The aorta is soft and pulsatile.

Other Findings

1. Palpation of the RLQ may reveal the part of the bowel called the *cecum*.
2. The sigmoid colon may be palpated in the lower left quadrant.
3. The inguinal and femoral areas should be palpated bilaterally for lymph nodes.

1. The cecum will be soft.

2. The sigmoid colon is ropelike and vertical and, if filled with feces, may be quite firm.

3. Often small inguinal nodes are present; they are nontender, freely movable, and firm.

MALE GENITALIA AND HERNIAS

This part of the examination, especially for hernias, is best done with the patient standing. (A hernia is the protrusion of a portion of the intestine through an abnormal opening.)

1. Drape the patient's chest and abdomen.
2. Expose the groin and genitalia.

Inspection

1. Inspect the pubic hair distribution and the skin of the penis.
2. Retract the foreskin, if present.

3. Observe the glans penis and the urethral meatus. Note any ulcers, masses, or scars.
4. Note the location of the urethral meatus and any discharge.

5. Observe the skin of the scrotum for ulcers, masses, redness, or swelling. Note size, contour, and symmetry. Lift the scrotum to inspect the posterior surface.
6. Inspect the inguinal areas and groin for bulges (with and without the patient bearing down, as though having a bowel movement).

2. The foreskin of the penis, if present, should be easily retractable.

3. The skin of the glans penis is smooth, without ulceration.

4. The urethral meatus normally is located ventrally on the end of the penis. Normally, there is no discharge from the urethra.

5. The scrotum descends approximately 1½ inches (4 cm) in the adult; the left side is often larger than the right side.

Palpation

Wear gloves.

1. Palpate any lesions, nodules, or masses, noting tenderness, contour, size, and induration. Palpate the shaft of the penis for any induration (firmness in relation to surrounding tissues).
2. Palpate each testis and epididymis separately between the thumb and first two fingers, noting size, shape, consistency, and undue tenderness (pressure on the testis normally produces pain).
3. Palpate the spermatic cord, including the vas deferens within the cord, from the testis to the inguinal ring. Note any nodules or tenderness.

2. The testes are usually rubbery and of approximately equal size. The epididymis is located posterolaterally on each testis and is most easily palpable on the superior portion of the testis.

Adult Physical Assessment *(continued)*

Technique	Findings

MALE GENITALIA AND HERNIAS *(continued)*
Palpation *(continued)*

4. Palpate for inguinal hernias, using the left hand to examine the patient's left side and the right hand to examine the patient's right side.
   a. Insert the right index finger laterally, invaginating the scrotal sac to the external inguinal ring.
   b. If the external ring is large enough, insert the finger along the inguinal canal toward the internal ring and ask the patient to strain down, noting any mass that touches the finger.

4. Normally, there is no palpable herniating mass in the inguinal area.

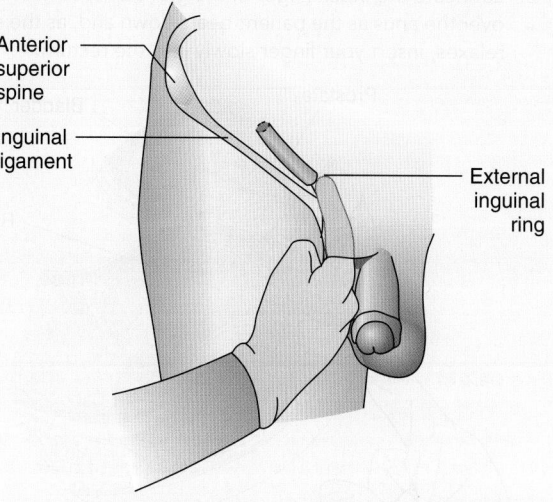

Anterior superior spine
Inguinal ligament
External inguinal ring

5. Palpate the anterior thigh for a herniating mass in the femoral canal. Ask the patient to strain down. (The femoral canal is not palpable; it is a potential opening in the anterior thigh, medial to the femoral artery below the inguinal ligament.)

5. Ordinarily, there is no palpable mass in the femoral area.

FEMALE GENITALIA
See Procedure Guidelines 22-1, page 835.

RECTUM
Equipment
- Glove
- Lubricant

Techniques of examination: Male
General approach

1. If the patient is ambulatory, have him stand and bend over the edge of the table with his toes pointed inward.
2. It is also possible to examine the anus and rectum with the patient lying on the left side, knees drawn up and buttocks close to the edge of the table.
3. The patient should be draped so only the buttocks are exposed.

Inspection

Spread the buttocks and inspect the anus, perianal region, and sacral region for inflammation, nodules, scars, lesions, ulcerations, or rashes. Ask the patient to bear down; note any bulges.

In males and females, the perianal and sacrococcygeal areas are dry, with varying amounts of hair covering them. Anal and perianal lesions include hemorrhoids, abscesses, skin tags, and sexually transmitted genital lesions.

(continued)

Adult Physical Assessment *(continued)*

Technique	Findings

RECTUM *(continued)*
Techniques of examination: Male *(continued)*
Palpation

1. Palpate any abnormal area noted on inspection.
2. Lubricate the index finger of the gloved hand. Rest the finger over the anus as the patient bears down and, as the sphincter relaxes, insert your finger slowly into the rectum.

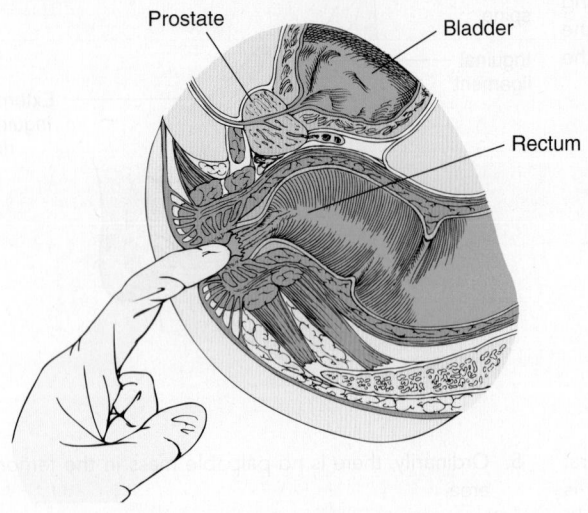

Prostate — Bladder

Rectum

3. Note sphincter tone, any nodules or masses, or tenderness.

    3. The anal canal is approximately 1 inch (2.5 cm) long; it is bordered by the external and internal anal sphincters, which are normally firm and smooth.

4. Insert the finger further and palpate the walls of the rectum laterally and posteriorly while rotating your index finger. Note irregularities, masses, nodules, tenderness.

    4. The wall of the rectum in males and females is smooth and moist.

5. Anteriorly, palpate the two lateral lobes of the prostate gland and its median sulcus for irregularities, nodules, swelling, or tenderness.

    5. The male prostate gland is approximately 1 inch (2.5 cm) long, smooth, regular, nonmovable, nontender, and rubbery.

6. If possible, palpate the superior portion of the lateral lobe, where the seminal vesicles are located. Note induration, swelling, or tenderness.

    6. The seminal vesicles are generally not palpable unless swollen.

7. Just above the prostate anteriorly, the rectum lies adjacent to the peritoneal cavity. If possible, palpate this region for peritoneal masses and tenderness.
8. Continue to insert the finger as far as possible and have the patient bear down so more of the bowel can be palpated.
9. Gently withdraw your finger. Any fecal material on the glove should be tested for occult blood.

    9. There is normally no occult blood in the stools.

Techniques of examination: Female
General approach

1. The examination is usually performed following the pelvic examination with the patient still in the lithotomy position. Gloves are changed to prevent cross-contamination.

Adult Physical Assessment *(continued)*

Technique	Findings

RECTUM *(continued)*
Techniques of examination: Female *(continued)*
General approach (continued)

2. If only the rectal examination is done, the patient may be positioned laterally, as for examination of the male. The lateral position permits better visualization of the sacral region.
3. The technique is basically the same for the female as for the male.
4. Anteriorly, the cervix, and perhaps a retroverted uterus, may be felt.

4. Anteriorly, the cervix is round and smooth.

MUSCULOSKELETAL SYSTEM
General approach

1. Examine the muscles and joints, keeping in mind the structure and functions of each.
2. Observe and palpate joints and muscles for symmetry and examine each joint individually as indicated.
3. The examination is performed with the joints both at rest and in motion, moving through a full range of motion; joints and supporting muscles and tissues are noted.

3. Joints should move freely without resistance or pain.

Inspection

1. Inspect the upper and lower extremities for size, symmetry, deformity, and muscle mass.
2. Inspect the joints for range of motion (in degrees), enlargement, redness.
3. Note gait and posture; observe the spine for range of motion, lateral curvature, or any abnormal curvature.
4. Observe the patient for signs of pain during the examination.

Palpation

1. Palpate the joints of the upper and lower extremities and the neck and back for tenderness, swelling, warmth, any bony overgrowth or deformity, and range of motion.
2. Hold the palm of your hand over the joint as it moves, or move the joint through the fullest range of motion and note any crepitation (crackling feeling within the joint).
3. Palpate the muscles for size, tone, strength, any contractures, and tenderness.
4. Palpate the spine for bony deformities and crepitation. Gently tap the spine with the ulnar surface of your fist from the cervical to the lumbar region and note any pain or tenderness.

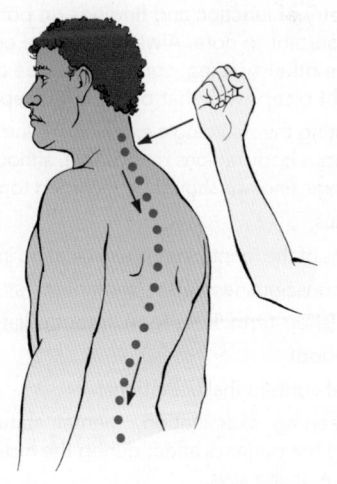

NEUROLOGIC SYSTEM
Equipment

- Safety pin
- Cotton
- Tuning fork
- Reflex hammer
- Flashlight
- Tongue blade
- Ophthalmoscope
- Vision screener
- Cloves, coffee, or other scented items

(continued)

Adult Physical Assessment (continued)

Technique	Findings

NEUROLOGIC SYSTEM (continued)
General information (continued)
Equipment (continued)

1. The examination described in this section is a screening neurologic examination. It is performed on individuals without specific neurologic complaints.
2. The examination is performed with the patient in either the sitting or supine position.
3. Much of the neurologic examination can be performed as different regions of the body are being examined. This facilitates the flow of the entire examination.

Components of the neurologic examination
There are six components of the neurologic examination:

1. Mental status (cerebral function)
2. Cranial nerve function
3. Cerebellar function
4. Motor function
5. Sensory function
6. Deep tendon reflexes

The screening neurologic examination involves testing all of these components at least superficially. Learning these components in order will help in organizing the examination and in avoiding the omission of any part.

Basic principles

1. Symmetry of function and findings on both sides of the body are important to note. Always compare one side of the body with the other side (eg, compare degree of motor strength of the right biceps with that of the left biceps).
2. Integrating the neurologic examination into the examination of the various body regions is advisable, although the results of the neurologic findings should be recorded together as an entity.

Mental status
Components of the mental status examination include the following:

- State of consciousness (alert, somnolent, stuporous, comatose)
- Memory (short term, long term, intermediate)
- Affect (mood)
- Ideational content (hallucinations)

In a screening examination, mental status is evaluated by observing the patient's affect during the history and the content of what he or she says.

1. While recording the history, ask the patient for identifying information (how to spell his or her name, where he or she lives), and ask what the date is. This tests orientation.

2. The patient's ability to remember is also evaluated as the history is taken; ask for his or her past medical history (long-term memory) and dietary habits: "What did you eat for breakfast?" (intermediate memory).

3. Cognition and ideational content are evaluated throughout the history by what the patient says and by his or her articulateness, consistency, and reliability in reporting events.

1. Normally, the individual is alert, knows who he or she is and where he or she lives, and can tell you the date.

2. The patient remembers recent and past events consistently, and willingly admits forgetting something. Older adults often have much better long-term memory than recent memory.

Adult Physical Assessment (continued)

Technique	Findings

NEUROLOGIC SYSTEM (continued)
General information (continued)
Mental status (continued)

4. Affect or mood is evaluated by observing the patient's verbal and nonverbal behavior in response to questions asked, sudden noises, and interruptions. For example, does the patient laugh or smile when talking about normally sad events; is he or she easily startled by unexpected noises?

4. Mood should be appropriate to the content of the conversation.

Cranial nerve function
First (olfactory) nerve

The olfactory nerve is not usually tested unless the patient complains of a disturbance in sense of smell.

1. The airway must be patent.
2. Occlude one nostril; ask the patient to close eyes and then present various substances to smell (coffee, common spices). Occlude the other nostril and repeat.

2. The patient should be able to identify common smells such as cinnamon and coffee.

Second (optic) nerve

Includes tests of visual acuity and of gross visual fields and examination of the optic disc with a funduscope.

Visual acuity

Visual acuity is tested with the use of a Snellen chart (patient uses glasses if required).

1. Have the patient cover one eye at a time and read the smallest print possible on the chart from a distance of 20 feet (6 m).

1. Normal vision and corrected vision should be 20/20.

Visual fields

1. Have the patient cover right eye with the right hand. (You cover your left eye with your left hand.)
2. Stand approximately 2 feet (60 cm) from the patient and have him or her fix gaze on your nose.
3. Bring two wagging fingers in from the periphery (in a plane equidistant from the patient and you) in all quadrants of the visual field and ask the patient to tell you when he or she sees your wagging fingers.

3. Assuming your visual fields are grossly normal, the patient and you should see the wagging fingers approximately simultaneously. (The patient's peripheral vision should approximate the examiner's, assuming that it is normal.)

Optic disc

The optic disc is visualized as part of the funduscopic examination (see page 54.)

Third (oculomotor), fourth (trochlear), and sixth (abducens) nerves

These nerves are tested together. They control the movements of the extraocular muscles of the eye—the superior and inferior oblique and the medial and lateral rectus muscles. The oculomotor nerve also controls pupillary constriction.

1. Hold your index finger approximately 1 foot (30 cm) from the patient's nose. Ask the patient to hold head steady.
2. Ask the patient to follow your finger with his or her eyes.
3. Move your finger to the right as far as the patient's eye moves. Before bringing your finger back to the center, move it up and then down, so that the patient glances up and peripherally and then down and peripherally.
4. Repeat the test, moving your finger to the left.

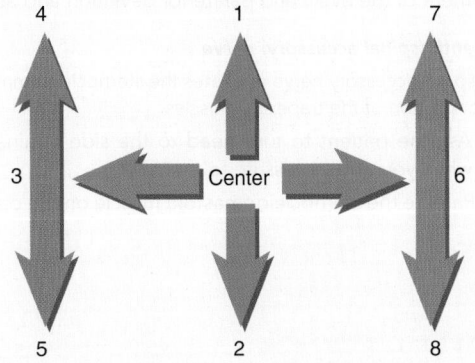

(continued)

Adult Physical Assessment *(continued)*	
Technique	**Findings**

NEUROLOGIC SYSTEM *(continued)*

Cranial nerve function *(continued)*

Fifth (trigeminal) nerve

The trigeminal nerve controls muscles of mastication and has a sensory component that controls sensations of the face.

Motor

1. Have the patient clench teeth while palpating the temporal and masseter muscles of the jaws with both hands.

    1. Muscle strength in the face should be present and should be symmetric.

Sensory

Sensation to light touch.

1. Have the patient close eyes.

    1. Sensation should be present and symmetrical. Always demonstrate to the patient how and with what you are testing sensation—to avoid startling the patient and to encourage cooperation.

2. Touch first one side of the patient's face and then the other (forehead, cheek, and chin), asking the patient if the sensation is present and feels the same on both sides.
3. Sensation to pain (pinprick) is tested similarly.

Seventh (facial) nerve

Motor function is tested by observing facial expression and symmetry of facial movement.

Ask the patient to frown, close eyes, and smile.

    The facial muscles should look symmetric when the patient frowns, closes eyes, and smiles. Notice particularly the symmetry of the nasolabial folds.

Eighth (acoustic) nerve

The acoustic nerve has two branches.

Cochlear (mediates hearing). (See ear examination, page 55.)

Vestibular (helps control equilibrium).

Romberg test: Have the patient stand erect with eyes closed and feet close together.

    Slight swaying may occur, but the patient should not fall. (Stand close to the patient so you can assist if he or she begins to fall.)

Ninth (glossopharyngeal) and tenth (vagus) nerves

These nerves are tested together because they both have a motor portion innervating the pharynx.

1. *Ninth:* Test the presence of the gag reflex.

    1. The gag reflex should be present, and there should be no difficulty in swallowing.

2. *Tenth:* Ask the patient to say "ah" and observe the movement of the uvula and palate for deviation and asymmetry.

    2. The palate and uvula should move symmetrically without deviation.

Eleventh (spinal accessory) nerve

The spinal accessory nerve mediates the sternocleidomastoid and upper portion of the trapezius muscles.

1. Ask the patient to turn head to the side against resistance while you apply pressure to the jaw.
2. Palpate the sternocleidomastoid muscle on the opposite side.

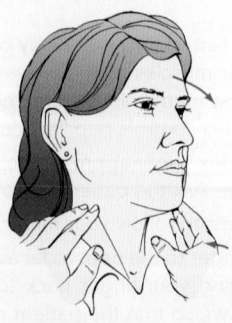

3. Have the patient shrug shoulders while you place your hands on his or her shoulders and apply slight pressure.

    3. Neck and shoulder muscle strength should be symmetric.

Adult Physical Assessment (continued)

Technique	Findings
NEUROLOGIC SYSTEM (*continued*)	

Cranial nerve function (*continued*)

Twelfth (hypoglossal) nerve

Technique	Findings
This nerve innervates muscles of the tongue. It is tested by noting articulation and by having the patient stick out the tongue, noting any deviation or asymmetry.	The tongue should be symmetric and should not deviate.

Cerebellar function

Purpose: to screen for coordination.

Technique	Findings
1. Observe posture and gait.	
2. Ask the patient to walk forward (and then backward) in a straight line.	2. The patient should be able to perform all the tests described with smooth, even movement and without losing balance.
3. To test for muscle coordination in the lower extremities, have the patient run the right heel down the left shin and vice versa.	
4. To test coordination in upper extremities, have the patient close eyes and touch the nose with the index finger (starting position: arms outstretched) first left, then right, in rapid succession.	4. The normal person can do this with rapid, smooth movements without undershooting or overshooting the target.

Motor function

Tested in conjunction with the skeletal system because any bony deformity will affect motor function. Evaluate muscle mass, tone, strength, and any abnormal movements (tics, fasciculations, twitching).

Technique	Findings
1. To assess muscle mass, note symmetry between sides of the body and distribution distally and proximally.	1. Muscle mass is usually considered in relation to sex and body build and to use of various muscle groups.
2. Test muscle tone by noting the resistance the muscle offers to movement on passive motion.	2. Generally there is slight resistance to passive movement of muscles as opposed to flaccidity (no resistance) or rigidity (increased muscle tone).
3. Have the patient do deep knee bends; walk on toes and then heels; hop on one foot and then the other.	3. Strength will vary from person to person but should be equal bilaterally.
4. Have the patient squeeze your fingers with both hands; compare sides of the body. Also, apply resistance to the patient's outstretched arms and when the patient flexes the wrist and elbow; compare sides.	
5. Unusual muscle movements, if present, are noted both when muscle is at rest and when it is moving.	5. Normally, tremors, tics, or fasciculations are not present either at rest or with movement.

Sensory function

Should test sensitivity to light touch (cotton), pain (pinprick), vibration (tuning fork), and position. Compare both sides of the body.

Technique	Findings
1. Ask the patient to close eyes. Brush the skin with a piece of cotton (on the back of hands, forearms, upper arms, dorsal portion of foot laterally and medially, and along the tibia and thigh laterally and medially). Ask the patient to indicate when he or she feels the cotton and to compare the sensation bilaterally.	1. Patient should feel light touch bilaterally.
2. Use a safety pin; touch the skin as lightly as possible to elicit a sharp sensation.	2. Pain should be felt bilaterally.

(continued)

Adult Physical Assessment *(continued)*

Technique	Findings

NEUROLOGIC SYSTEM *(continued)*
Sensory function *(continued)*

3. Test vibration sense by placing a vibrating tuning fork on a bony prominence (wrist, medial and lateral malleoli). Ask the patient to tell you when he or she no longer feels the vibration. Stop the vibration with your hand.

3. The patient should normally feel no vibration within a very short time.

4. Test position sense by having the patient close eyes.
   - Move the patient's digit (finger, great toe) up or down and ask the patient to say in what direction the finger or toe is pointing.
   - Place your thumb and index finger on either side of the digit being moved so the patient will not sense any pressure from your finger in the direction in which you are moving the digit.

4. Normally the patient can tell you without hesitation in what direction his or her digit is pointing.

Deep tendon reflexes

1. Have the patient relax; provide support for the extremity being tested.
2. Compare reflex amplitude of the same tendons on either side of the body.

2. Amplitude of the reflex may vary for different tendons but is equal bilaterally.

Upper extremities
Biceps

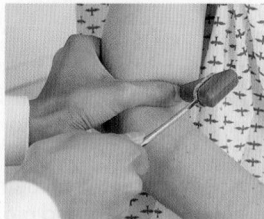

1. Place your right thumb on the patient's right biceps tendon (located in the antecubital fossa) with the patient's arm slightly flexed.
2. Strike your thumb with the pointed end of the hammer head. Hold the hammer loosely so it pivots in your hand when it is moved with a wrist action.
3. Strike your thumb with the least amount of pressure needed to elicit the reflex.

3. The forearm may move, and your thumb should feel the tendon jerk.

Triceps tendon

1. Have the patient hang arm freely while you support it with your nondominant hand or rest the slightly flexed arm in the patient's lap.

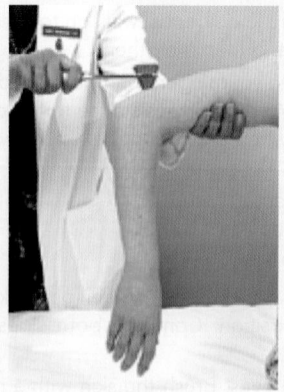
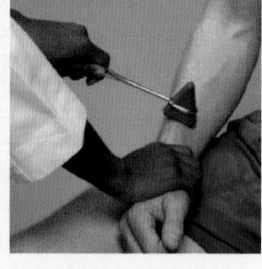

2. With the elbow flexed, strike the tendon directly, using the pointed end of the hammer.

2. The forearm should move slightly.

NURSING ALERT If the reflexes are diminished symmetrically, have the patient grasp hands and contract arm muscles to relax the lower extremities, or tap feet on the floor to relax the upper extremities.

Adult Physical Assessment *(continued)*

Technique	Findings

NEUROLOGIC SYSTEM *(continued)*
Deep tendon reflexes (*continued*)
Upper extremities (continued)
Brachioradialis tendon

1. Strike the forearm with the hammer about 1 inch (2.5 cm) above the wrist over the radius.
2. Be sure the forearm is supported and relaxed.

1. The thumb may be observed moving downward.

Lower extremities
Quadriceps reflex

1. Have the patient sit with legs hanging over the edge of the table or lay down while you support the legs at the knee (slightly bent).
2. Strike the tendon just below the patella.

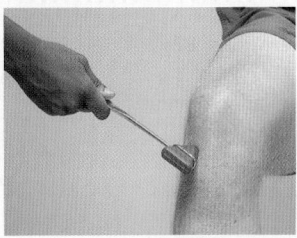

Achilles reflex

1. Support the foot in dorsiflexed position.
2. Tap the Achilles tendon with the hammer.

2. The foot should move downward into your hand.

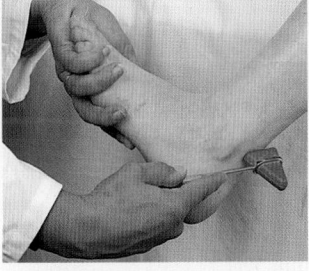

Plantar reflex

1. Stroke the sole of the patient's foot with a flat object such as a tongue blade.

1. Toes normally flex. Dorsiflexion of the great toe and fanning of the other toes is known as a positive Babinski response and indicates a central nervous system problem.

SELECTED REFERENCES

Bickley, L. S. (2012). *Bates' guide to physical examination and history taking* (11th ed.). Philadelphia: Lippincott Williams & Wilkins.

Ewing, J. A. (1984). Detecting alcoholism: The CAGE questionnaire. *Journal of the American Medical Association, 252*(14), 1905–1907.

Jensen, S. (2010). *Nursing health assessment: A best practices approach.* Philadelphia: Lippincott Williams & Wilkins.

Lippincott Williams & Wilkins. (2010). *Professional guide to signs and symptoms* (6th ed.). Philadelphia: Author.

Lippincott Williams & Wilkins. (2012). *Assessment made incredibly easy* (5th ed.). Philadelphia: Author.

6
Intravenous Therapy

GENERAL CONSIDERATIONS

Goals

The goals of intravenous (IV) therapy are to:

1. Maintain or replace body stores of water, electrolytes, vitamins, proteins, fats, and calories in the patient who cannot maintain an adequate intake by mouth.
2. Restore acid-base balance.
3. Restore the volume of blood components.
4. Administer safe and effective infusions of medications by using the appropriate vascular access.
5. Monitor central venous pressure (CVP).
6. Provide nutrition while resting the GI tract.

Physiologic Assimilation of Infusion Solutions

Principles

1. Tissue cells (such as epithelial cells) are surrounded by a semipermeable membrane.
2. Osmotic pressure is the "pulling" pressure demonstrated when water moves through the semipermeable membrane of tissue cells from an area of weaker concentration to stronger concentration of solute (eg, sodium ions and blood glucose). The end result is dilution and equilibration between the intracellular and extracellular compartments.
3. Extracellular compartment fluids primarily include plasma and interstitial fluid.

Types of Fluids

Isotonic

A solution that exerts the same osmotic pressure as that found in plasma.

1. 0.9% sodium chloride solution (normal saline).
2. Lactated Ringer's solution.
3. Blood components.
    a. Albumin 5%.
    b. Plasma.
4. Dextrose 5% in water (D_5W).

Hypotonic

A solution that exerts less osmotic pressure than that of blood plasma. Administration of this fluid generally causes dilution of plasma solute concentration and forces water to move into cells to reestablish intracellular and extracellular equilibrium; cells will then expand or swell.

1. 0.45% sodium chloride solution (half normal saline)
2. 0.33% sodium chloride solution (one third normal saline)

Hypertonic

A solution that exerts a higher osmotic pressure than that of blood plasma. Administration of this fluid increases the solute concentration of plasma, drawing water out of the cells and into the extracellular compartment to restore osmotic equilibrium; cells will then shrink.

1. D_5W in normal saline solution.
2. D_5W in half normal saline solution (only slightly hypertonic because dextrose is rapidly metabolized and renders only temporary osmotic pressure).

3. Dextrose 10% in water.
4. Dextrose 20% in water.
5. 3% or 5% sodium chloride solution.
6. Hyperalimentation solutions.
7. D₅W in lactated Ringer's solution.
8. Albumin 25%.

Composition of Fluids

See Table 6-1.
1. Saline solutions—water and electrolytes (Na^+, Cl^-).
2. Dextrose solutions—water or saline and calories.
3. Lactated Ringer's solution—water and electrolytes (Na^+, K^+, Cl^-, Ca^{++}, lactate).
4. Balanced isotonic solution—varies; water, some calories, electrolytes (Na^+, K^+, Mg^{++}, Cl^-, HCO_3^-, gluconate).
5. Whole blood and blood components.
6. Plasma expanders—albumin, mannitol, dextran, plasma protein fraction 5%, hetastarch; exert increased oncotic pressure, pulling fluid from interstitium into the circulation and temporarily increasing blood volume.
7. Parenteral hyperalimentation—fluid, electrolytes, amino acids, and calories.

Uses and Precautions with Common Types of Infusions

See Table 6-2, page 84, for signs and symptoms of water excess or deficit, and Table 6-3, page 84, for signs and symptoms of isotonic fluid excess or deficit.
1. D₅W
   a. Used to replace water (hypotonic fluid) losses, supply some caloric intake, or administer as carrying solution for numerous medications.
   b. Should be used cautiously in patients with water intoxication (hyponatremia, syndrome of inappropriate antidiuretic hormone release). Should not be used as concurrent solution infusion with blood or blood components.
2. Normal saline solution
   a. Used to replace saline (isotonic fluid) losses, administer with blood components, or treat patients in hemodynamic shock.
   b. Should be used cautiously in patients with isotonic volume excess (heart failure, renal failure).
3. Lactated Ringer's solution
   a. Used to replace isotonic fluid losses, replenish specific electrolyte losses, and moderate metabolic acidosis. Use cautiously in patients with liver failure.

Table 6-1 Composition of Selected IV Solutions

SOLUTION	TONICITY	Na⁺ (mEq/L)	K⁺ (mEq/L)	Cl⁻ (mEq/L)	Ca⁺⁺ (mEq/L)	pH	mOsm/L	CALORIES
5% DW	Isotonic	—	—	—	—	5.0	253	170
10% DW	Hypertonic	—	—	—	—	4.6	561	340
0.9% NS	Isotonic	154	—	154	—	5.7	308	—
0.45% NS	Hypotonic	77	—	7	—	5.3	154	—
5% D and 0.9% NS	Hypertonic	154	—	154	—	4.2	561	170
5% D and 0.45% NS*	Slightly hypertonic	77	—	77	—	4.2	407	170
5% D and 0.2% NS	Isotonic	34	—	34	—	4.2	290	170
Lactated Ringer's solution†	Isotonic	148	4	156	4.5	6.7	309	9
5% DW and lactated Ringer's solution	Slightly hypertonic	130	4	109	3.0	5.1	527	170
Normosol-R	Isotonic	140	5	96	—	6.4	295	—
Sodium lactate	Slightly hypertonic	167	—	—	—	6.9	333	55
1/6 molar								
6% Dextran 75 and 0.9% NS	Isotonic	154	—	154	—	4.3	309	—

DW, dextrose in water; NS, normal saline.
*5% dextrose metabolizes rapidly in the blood and, in reality, produces minimal osmotic effects.
†Lactate converts to bicarbonate in the liver.

Table 6-2	Signs and Symptoms of Water Excess or Deficit	
SITE	**HYPONATREMIA (WATER EXCESS)**	**HYPERNATREMIA (WATER DEFICIT)**
Central nervous system	• Muscle twitching • Hyperactive tendon reflexes • Convulsions • Increased intracranial pressure, coma	• Restlessness • Weakness • Delirium • Coma
Cardiovascular	• Increased blood pressure and pulse (if severe)	• Tachycardia • Hypotension (if severe)
Tissues	• Increased salivation, tears • Watery diarrhea • Fingerprinting of skin	• Decreased saliva and tears • Dry, sticky mucous membranes • Red, swollen tongue • Flushed skin
Other	• None	• Fever

Table 6-3	Signs and Symptoms of Isotonic Fluid Excess or Deficit	
SITE	**EXCESS**	**DEFICIT**
Central nervous system	• Confusion (if severe)	• Fatigue, apathy • Anorexia • Stupor, coma
Cardiovascular	• Elevated venous pressure • Distended neck veins • Increased cardiac output • Heart gallops • Pulmonary edema	• Orthostatic hypotension • Flat neck veins • Fast, thready pulse • Hypotension • Cool, clammy skin
Gastrointestinal	• Anorexia, nausea and vomiting • Edema of stomach, colon, and mesentery	• Anorexia • Thirst • Silent ileus
Tissues	• Pitting edema • Moist pulmonary crackles	• Soft, small tongue with longitudinal wrinkling • Sunken eyes • Decreased skin turgor
Metabolism	• None	• Mild increase in temperature

TYPES OF INTRAVENOUS ADMINISTRATION

IV "Push"

IV "push" (or *IV bolus*) refers to the administration of a medication from a syringe directly into an ongoing IV infusion. It may also be given directly into a vein by way of an intermittent access device (saline or heparin lock).

Indications

1. For emergency administration of cardiopulmonary resuscitative procedures, allowing rapid concentration of a medication in the patient's bloodstream.
2. When quicker response to the medication is required (eg, furosemide or digoxin).
3. To administer "loading" doses of a drug that will be continued by way of infusion (eg, heparin).
4. To reduce patient discomfort by limiting the need for intramuscular injections.
5. To avoid incompatibility problems that may occur when several medications are mixed in one bottle.
6. To deliver drugs to patients unable to take them orally (eg, coma) or intramuscularly (eg, coagulation disorder).
7. Cost-effective method—no need for extra tubing or syringe pump.

Precautions and Recommendations

1. Before medication administration:
   a. Review order and patient allergies.
   b. Dilute the drug as indicated by pharmacy references. Many medications are irritating to veins and require sufficient dilution.
   c. Determine the correct (safest) rate of administration. Consult the pharmacy or pharmaceutical text. Most medications are given slowly (rarely over less than 1 minute); sometimes as long as 30 minutes is required. Too rapid administration may result in serious adverse effects.
   d. If IV push is to be given with an ongoing IV infusion or to follow another IV push medication, check pharmacy for possible incompatibility. It is always wise to flush the IV tubing or cannula with saline before and after administration of a drug.
   e. Assess the patient's condition and ability to tolerate the drug.
   f. Assess patency of the IV line by the presence of blood return.
      i. Lower-running IV bottle.
      ii. Withdraw with syringe before injecting medication.
      iii. Pinch IV tubing gently.
   g. Ascertain the dwell time of the catheter. For infusion of vesicants (some chemotherapy agents), a catheter placement of 24 hours or less is advisable.

2. Watch the patient's reaction to the drug during and after administration.
   a. Be alert for major adverse effects, such as anaphylaxis, respiratory distress, tachycardia, bradycardia, or seizures. Stop the medication. Notify the health care provider and institute emergency procedures as necessary.
   b. Assess for minor adverse effects, such as nausea, flushing, skin rash, or confusion. Stop medication and consult the health care provider.
3. Administer vesicants only through the side port of a running IV infusion.
4. Be familiar with facility policies and guidelines regarding how, where, and by whom IV push medications can be given.

 NURSING ALERT Unusual dosages or unfamiliar drugs should always be confirmed with the health care provider and pharmacist before administration. The nurse is ultimately accountable for the drug administered.

Continuous or Intermittent Infusion Using Infusion Control Devices

Continuous or intermittent IV infusions may be given through traditionally hung bags of solution and tubing, with or without flow rate regulators. IV, intra-arterial, and intrathecal (spinal) infusion may be accomplished through the use of special external or implantable pumps. See Procedure Guidelines 6-1, pages 86 to 88.

General Considerations

1. Advantages
   a. Ability to infuse large and small volumes of fluid with accuracy.
   b. An alarm warns of problems, such as air in line, high pressure required to infuse, or, ultimately, occlusion.
   c. Reduces nursing time in constantly readjusting flow rates.
2. Disadvantages
   a. Usually requires special tubing.
   b. There may be added cost to therapy.
   c. Infusion pumps will continue to infuse despite the presence of infiltration (pump alarms for mechanical problems, not physiological problems).
3. Nursing responsibilities
   a. Remember that a mechanical infusion regulator is only as effective as the nurse operating it.
   b. Continue to check the patient regularly for complications, such as infiltration or infection.
   c. Follow the manufacturer's instructions carefully when inserting the tubing.
   d. Double-check the flow rate.
   e. Be sure to flush all air out of the tubing before connecting it to the patient's IV catheter.
   f. Explain the purpose of the device and the alarm system. Added machines in the room can evoke greater anxiety in the patient and family.

Types

1. Electronic flow rate regulators
   a. These devices deliver a prescribed fluid volume per hour.
   b. Often, pressure gradients may be adjusted so that high pressures are not used to deliver peripheral therapies.
   c. Use of an electronic flow-rate regulator is indicated for continuous infusions of:
      i. Chemotherapy.
      ii. Infant and pediatric therapies.
      iii. Hyperalimentation.
      iv. Fluid and electrolytes on patients at risk for fluid overload.
      v. Most medications.
2. Battery-powered ambulatory infusion pumps
   a. Example: CADD PRISM™ pump (Pharmacia Deltec, Inc.).
   b. These pumps deliver continuous or intermittent medications by way of IV, subcutaneous, or spinal routes.
   c. If used for pain control, patient may deliver a "bolus" injection if relief is not obtained from continuous, prescribed dose.
3. Freon-controlled spring pump (implanted)
   a. Example: Infusaid™ (Neuromed).
   b. Placed subcutaneously, usually in the left lower quadrant of the abdomen.
   c. Will deliver continuous pain medication or chemotherapy by way of an artery, vein, or the spinal canal.
4. Computer-programmable pump (implanted)
   a. Example: SynchroMed pump™ (Medtronic).
   b. Same actions as above.

Intermittent Infusions

Intermittent IV infusions may be given through an intermittent access device (saline lock), "piggybacked" to a continuous IV infusion, or for long-term therapy through a venous access device. See Procedure Guidelines 6-2, 6-3, and 6-4, pages 89 to 92.

Intermittent Access Device (Saline Lock)

1. This intermittent infusion device permits the administration of periodic IV medications and solution without continuous fluid administration.
2. Many facilities do not use heparin solutions to keep short peripheral catheters open. A saline flush (2 mL) is administered and a clamp is tightened or the needle is withdrawn while injecting to create positive pressure and keep the vein open.

"Piggyback" IV Administration

1. Means of administering medication by way of the fluid pathway of an established primary infusion line.
2. Drugs may be given on an intermittent basis through a primary infusion.

(Text continues on page 92)

PROCEDURE GUIDELINES 6-1

Venipuncture Using Needle or Catheter

EQUIPMENT

- Tourniquet (nonlatex preferred)
- Disposable gloves (nonlatex)
- Antiseptic swab (chlorhexidine, alcohol, iodine, povidone-iodine)

If continuous infusion:
- IV solution
- IV tubing

If intermittent access device:
- Extension set or PRN adapter
- Heparin or normal saline solution (1 to 2 mL) in sterile syringe
- Tape
- Transparent IV dressing or other dressing supplies

- Covered armboard (if necessary)
- Desired cannula
  - Catheter (Teflon, Silastic polyurethane, or polyvinyl chloride) in chosen bore size (gauges 14–25)
  - Winged ("butterfly") needle

Note: Thorough handwashing is required before handling sterile supplies and initiating venipuncture.

PROCEDURE

Nursing Action	Rationale
Preparatory phase	
1. Explain the procedure to the patient. Ascertain whether the patient is left- or right-handed.	1. Helps alleviate anxiety about the procedure. Start the infusion in the opposite arm, if possible.
2. Prime all IV and winged-needle tubing (clear the tubing of air with fluid from infusion tubing by attaching a needle, or by irrigating the needle with saline in a sterile syringe).	2. Prevents infusion of air and potential air embolus.
3. Put on gloves.	3. Complies with CDC requirements to minimize passing of blood-borne pathogens between the patient and nurse.
4. Select a site for insertion. (See the discussion on site selection, page 95.)	
5. Apply a tourniquet 2–6 inches (5–15 cm) above the desired insertion site and ascertain satisfactory distention of the vein. Distal pulses should remain palpable.	5. The vein must be visible or palpable before venipuncture is attempted. The tourniquet should not be applied too tightly so it does not interfere with arterial blood flow.
6. Have the patient open and close fist several times.	6. Increases blood supply in the area. Further techniques to aid in vein distention are discussed on page 95. A tourniquet may not be necessary on greatly distended veins.
7. Remove the tourniquet.	7. Prevents trauma to the arm from extended application of the tourniquet. It can be reapplied later.
8. Clip the hair if site is obscured and clean as follows:	8. Reduce the number of skin microorganisms and minimizes risk of infection.
a. Cleanse the skin with a chlorhexidine solution	a. Chlorhexidine is the preferred solution.
b. If preferred over chlorhexidine, clean skin with alcohol first, using the swab in a circular motion outward from the site for at least 30 seconds; then povidone-iodine swab for 1 minute, working from the center of the proposed site to the periphery until a circle of 2–4 inches (5–10 cm) has been disinfected.	b. Alcohol should be used as part of a two-step process, but may be used alone if the patient is allergic to iodine. If a 1%–2% iodine solution is used, it should be used before alcohol for 30–60 seconds and allowed to dry.
c. Allow the area to air-dry.	c. Drying allows for additional disinfection.
9. Reapply a tourniquet.	9. Facilitates catheter insertion.
Performance phase: Catheter insertion	
1. Remove the needle guard.	
2. Hold the patient's arm so your thumb is positioned approximately 2 inches (5 cm) from the site. Exert traction on the skin in the direction of your hand.	2. Stabilizes the vein and facilitates successful cannulation.
3. Insert the needle, bevel up, through the skin at an angle. Use a slow, continuous motion.	3. Bevel-up position allows for the smallest and sharpest point of the needle to enter the vein first.

PROCEDURE GUIDELINES 6-1 *(continued)*

Venipuncture Using Needle or Catheter

PROCEDURE *(continued)*

Nursing Action	Rationale
4. If the vessel rolls, it may be necessary to penetrate the skin first at a 20-degree angle and then apply a second thrust parallel to the skin.	4. Satisfactory penetration is evidenced by a sudden decrease in resistance and by the appearance of blood coming back into catheter.
5. When the vein is entered, lower the catheter to skin level.	5. Prevents puncturing the vessel wall.
6. When inserting, always hold the catheter by the clear plastic flashback chamber and not by the colored hub.	
7. Advance the catheter approximately ¼ to ½ inch (0.5 to 1.5 cm) into the vein.	7. Ensures entry into the vein.
8. Pull back on needle to separate needle from catheter about ¼ inch and advance the catheter into the vein.	8. Pulling back on the needle prevents inadvertent puncture of the vein and provides stability of catheter for insertion.

 Key Decision Point

If resistance is met while attempting to thread the catheter, do not force it. Resistance is a sign the catheter is not positioned well within the lumen of the vein, and attempts to advance the catheter further against resistance may cause vein damage. If the catheter does not freely advance, you may attach IV tubing or a heparin lock and flush, attempting to float the catheter into the vein. If resistance is still met, release the tourniquet and carefully remove the needle and the catheter.

 NURSING ALERT   Never reinsert a stylet back into a catheter once it has been removed. You may puncture or sever the catheter.

9. Once the catheter is positioned within the vein, apply pressure on the vein beyond the catheter tip with your little finger (see illustration); release the tourniquet and slowly remove the needle while holding the catheter hub in place.	9. Reduces blood leakage while removing the needle and connecting tubing to the infusion set.

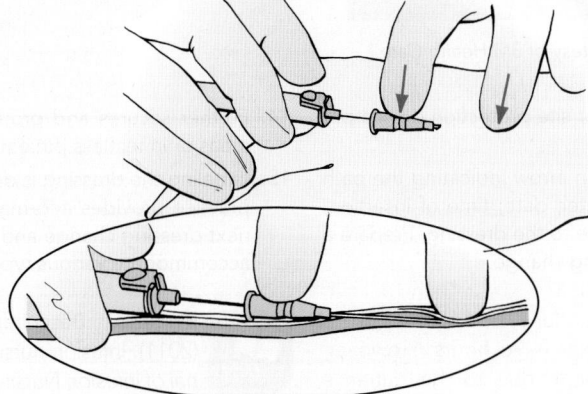

Finger palpation of dorsal venous arch, applying pressure above cannula.

PROCEDURE GUIDELINES 6-1 *(continued)*

Venipuncture Using Needle or Catheter

PROCEDURE *(continued)*

Nursing Action	Rationale
10. If a continuous infusion, attach the primed administration set to the hub of the catheter and adjust the infusion flow at the prescribed rate.	
11. If an intermittent access device, attach lock cap and extension set, taking care to maintain sterility of the set. Flush with 0.5 mL heparin or normal saline solution.	
12. Apply transparent dressing to the site or use dressing according to facility protocol (see illustration).	12. Transparent dressing secures the IV catheter and prevents infection.
13. Loop tubing and tape to dressing or arm.	13. Prevents tension on the IV catheter itself.

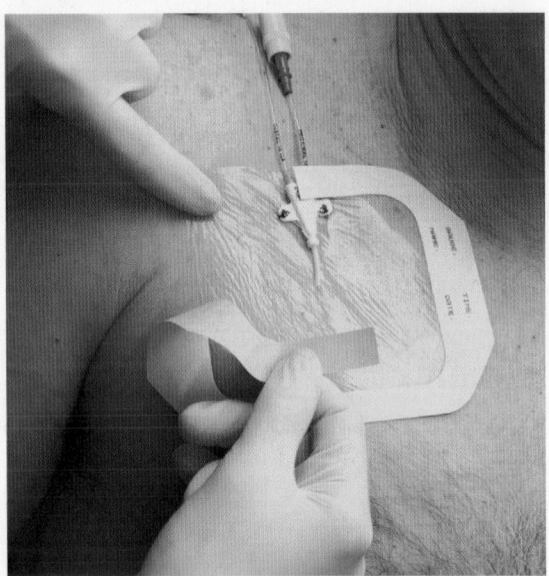

Transparent IV dressing. (Courtesy of 3M Health Care.)

14. Apply a stabilization device or site protection device per facility policy.	14. Further secures and protects site placement in difficult areas or in restless patients.
15. Label the strip of tape with an arrow indicating the path of the catheter, size of catheter, date, time of insertion, and your initials. Affix the tape to the dressing. Prepare a similar label with each dressing change.	15. Labeling the dressing is dictated by facility policy. Such a practice provides information useful in determining the next dressing change and the capability of the needle to accommodate various types of infusion.

NURSING ALERT Standard dwell time for a short peripheral catheter is 96 hours. However, exceptions may be made due to the patient's venous access, type of solution, and catheter material. A facility with a higher than average phlebitis rate should review their policies and procedures regarding dwell time.

 Evidence Base Infusion Nurses Society (INS). (2011). Infusion nursing standards of practice. *Journal of Infusion Nursing, 34*(1S), Standards 37 and 38.

PROCEDURE GUIDELINES 6-2

Intermittent Access Device (Saline Lock)

A saline lock is an intermittent infusion reservoir that permits administration of periodic IV medications and solution without continuous fluid administration and aspiration of blood samples for laboratory analysis. The reservoir indicated here includes the extension set, access valve, and catheter.

EQUIPMENT

- Antiseptic swabs (usually alcohol)
- Syringe with normal saline solution
- Preflushed extension set with 2 mL sterile normal saline solution if converting IV line to existing cannula in vein
- Tape
- Unsterile gloves
- Optional: Syringe containing 1–2 mL flush solution of heparin 10 units/mL

PROCEDURE

Nursing Action	Rationale
Preparatory phase	
1. Wash hands.	1. Minimizes possibility of infection.
2. Explain the procedure to the patient.	2. Minimizes patient anxiety.
3. Put on gloves.	3. Complies with CDC requirements.
Performance phase	
1. Clean the port of the saline lock with alcohol. Insert a normal saline syringe needle into the port and aspirate slightly.	1. Use either a protected needle or a blunt-end syringe to access the port. This equipment avoids accidental needlesticks. If a small-gauge catheter does not show a positive blood return, monitor the site carefully.
2. Inject normal saline solution slowly to flush the reservoir of saline or heparin solution and blood.	2. Not all facilities use heparin to maintain peripheral locks.
3. Check with the patient to ensure he or she has no pain on flushing.	3. May indicate a clot or infiltration.
4. Check for swelling at the needle site when flushing.	4. May indicate a clot or infiltration.
5. Insert medication tubing, administer the drug, and infuse at the prescribed rate.	
6. After drug or solution administration, insert the saline syringe and flush the reservoir slowly. Remove the syringe while still pushing the plunger of the syringe to ensure positive pressure.	6. Prevents blood clotting in the IV cannula. Central venous catheters require more than 2.5 mL of solution to be effective. (INS suggests two times the volume of the catheter and any add-on devices.)
7. *Optional:* If using a heparin lock, insert heparin solution into the reservoir after saline.	
Follow-up phase	
1. Maintain patency of saline lock by flushing it every 8 to 12 hours, regardless of use.	1. If resistance is met, the device should not be flushed. Attempt to remove the occlusion via aspiration. If unable to restore patency, remove the IV device.
2. IV administration set for intermittent therapy should be changed according to facility policy. The tubing should only be used for the same medication.	2. It is recommended that the tubing be changed every 24 hours because the tubing is not maintained as a closed system and therefore poses a risk for infection.

Evidence Base Infusion Nurses Society (INS). (2011). Infusion nursing standards of practice. *Journal of Infusion Nursing, 34*(1S), Standards 37 and 38.

PROCEDURE GUIDELINES 6-3

Setting Up an Automatic IV "Piggyback"

EQUIPMENT

- Sterile infusion set (primary)
- Sterile infusion set (secondary)
- *Optional:* Syringe containing 1–2 mL heparin for a solution of 10 units/mL

PROCEDURE

Follow the procedure of the manufacturer of the "piggyback" infusion set being used. In general, most procedures are similar to the following:

Nursing Action	Rationale
Preparatory phase	
1. Wash hands thoroughly.	1. Minimizes the possibility of infection.
2. Set up the primary infusion set; this may have a check-valve (see **A** in illustration).	2. The primary set should be functioning effectively before the secondary (piggyback) set can be attached.
3. Lower the primary flask on the IV pole; usually, an extension hook accompanies the set.	3. Permits the check-valve to function.
Performance phase	
1. Use an alcohol swab to carefully clean the injection site.	1. Usually, this is a Y-connection on the primary site.
2. Attach secondary tubing to primary tubing—preferably with a needle-free adapter—at entry port.	
3. Lower secondary solution, open clamp, and allow infusate from primary solution to prime secondary tubing. Close clamp.	3. Clears the secondary tubing of air and prevents any loss of medication from the secondary line.

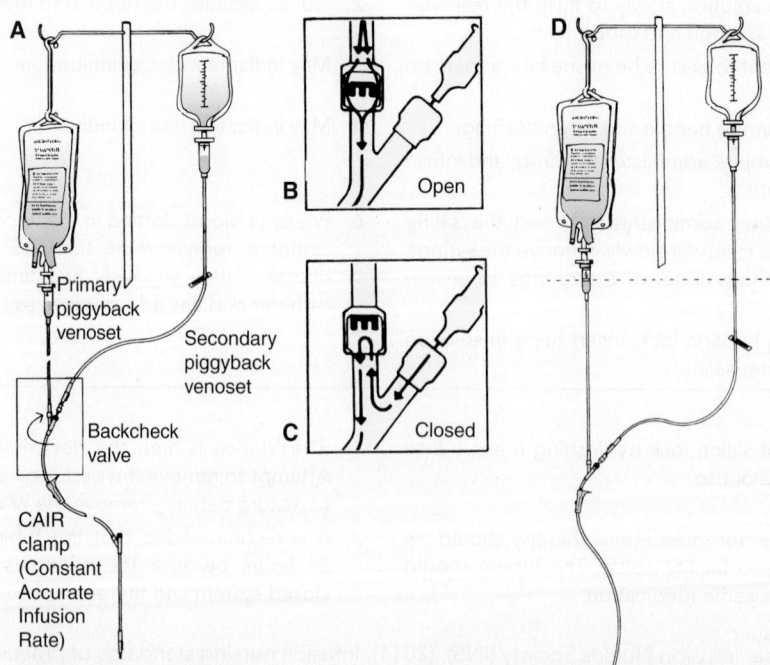

*"Piggyback" IV. (**A**) On the left is the primary infusion flask. Note the use of an extension hook (hanging from the IV pole) to suspend the primary flask. The back check-valve is seen more clearly in B and C. The secondary "piggyback" source is seen on the right. (**B**) Open check-valve. Fluid from primary source flows down on either side of movable disc. Fluid from secondary source is closed off with clamp (not visible). (**C**) Closed check-valve. Note that the fluid source from the secondary flask (where pressure is greater because the flask source is higher) is forcing the movable disc upward, thereby closing off fluid from the primary source. (**D**) When the last of the fluid from the secondary source reaches the level of the fluid in the primary set drip chamber (as indicated by a broken line), hydrostatic pressure between both sets will equalize. This releases the check-valve; flow will shift from the secondary to the primary source. (Adapted from Abbott Laboratories.)*

PROCEDURE GUIDELINES 6-3 (continued)

Setting Up an Automatic IV "Piggyback"

PROCEDURE (continued)

Nursing Action	Rationale
4. Hang secondary solution higher than primary solution. Open roller clamp (see **D** in illustration).	
5. Program pump or controller for rate of infusion for secondary medication.	5. Ensures medication administration over the appropriate time period.

Follow-up phase

Nursing Action	Rationale
1. Change IV administration tubing according to your facility's guidelines.	1. Minimizes risk of infection.
2. If possible, do not detach the secondary tubing from the primary tubing after the infusion regimen has started.	2. If using more than one secondary medication, the same tubing may be used. Back-flush the tubing into old secondary bag or bottle. Dispose of bag or bottle. Hang new secondary medication to same tubing.

 Evidence Base Infusion Nurses Society (INS). (2011). Infusion nursing standards of practice. *Journal of Infusion Nursing, 34*(1S), Standard 43.2.

PROCEDURE GUIDELINES 6-4

Accessing an Implanted Port

Implanted ports are becoming increasingly popular for patients with diseases such as cancer, sickle cell anemia, or cystic fibrosis to administer medications and continuous or intermittent IV fluids.

EQUIPMENT

- Two 10-mL syringes filled with normal saline solution
- Noncoring Huber needle
- Heparin flush solution 100 units/mL
- Alcohol prep pads or swab sticks
- Three povidone-iodine swab sticks
- Chlorhexidine scrub stick (optional)
- Sterile gloves

PROCEDURE

Nursing Action	Rationale
Preparatory phase	
1. Wash hands thoroughly.	1. Minimizes risk of infection.
2. Explain the procedure to the patient.	2. Minimizes anxiety and facilitates learning.
Performance phase	
1. Palpate the port—feel the septum.	1. Ensures placement and patency.
2. Select the appropriate Huber needle—gauge and length.	
3. Flush Huber needle and extension with normal saline solution, leaving one of the 10-mL syringes attached, being careful not to touch the needle with unsterile gloves or fingers.	3. Priming of the needle is essential to prevent infusion of air and ensure patency.
4. Put on sterile gloves and clean site by scrubbing with a chlorhexidine* scrub or alcohol and three povidone-iodine swabs. Allow to dry.	4. Prevents the introduction of organisms into the central line. *If chlorhexidine is used, follow manufacturer's instructions.

(continued)

PROCEDURE GUIDELINES 6-4 *(continued)*

Accessing an Implanted Port

PROCEDURE *(continued)*

Nursing Action	Rationale
Performance phase (continued)	
5. Hold the Huber needle with one hand and stabilize the port with the other hand—again locating septum.	
6. With a firm, steady motion, insert the needle into the port.	
7. Aspirate. If unable to aspirate, flush the port with saline solution and try to aspirate blood again.	7. By aspirating first, you withdraw saline solution that has been in the port.
8. After aspirating blood, flush with 10 mL normal saline solution.	8. The presence of blood confirms correct needle placement in the port.
9. If still no blood return, repeat port access or report findings to the health care provider.	9. May order a radiologic study or urokinase declotting procedure.
10. When placement of the needle is confirmed, attach the IV line or "heparin-lock" the port.	
Follow-up phase	
1. Maintain patency by flushing according to your facility's guidelines. Change the needle every 7 days, or per facility policy.	1–2. Maintains potency and prevents infection.
2. Instruct the patient to have the port flushed monthly when not in use and notify the health care provider of any problems.	

 Evidence Base Infusion Nurses Society (INS). (2011). Infusion nursing standards of practice. *Journal of Infusion Nursing*, *34*(1S), Standard 45.

3. When a check valve is present on the primary tubing, it:
   a. Permits the primary infusion to flow after the medication has been administered.
   b. Prevents air from entering the system.
   c. Prevents secondary fluid from "running dry."
   d. Permits less mixing of primary fluid with secondary solution.
4. Use of an infusion pump or controller will permit rate changes between primary and secondary infusates.

Central Venous Access Devices

Indications
1. Long-term therapy—weeks, months, or years.
2. Chemotherapy, medication, or blood product infusion; blood specimen collection.
3. IV fluids in the home.
4. Limited peripheral venous access due to extensive previous IV therapy, surgery, or previous tissue damage.

Types
See Figure 6-1.
1. Central catheter—nontunneled; commonly called *percutaneous*.
   a. Has one to four lumens.
   b. Dwell time usually less than 1 month.
   c. May be inserted in femoral, jugular, or subclavian veins.

 NURSING ALERT An x-ray to determine placement of central catheter is necessary for all devices that deliver fluid into the subclavian vein or superior vena cava.

2. Central catheter—tunneled.
   a. A tunneled catheter is inserted into a central vein (usually the subclavian, then the superior vena cava) and subcutaneously tunneled to an exit site approximately 4 inches (10 cm) from the insertion site.
   b. A Dacron cuff is located approximately ¾ to 1 inch (2 to 3 cm) from the exit site, providing a barrier against microorganisms.

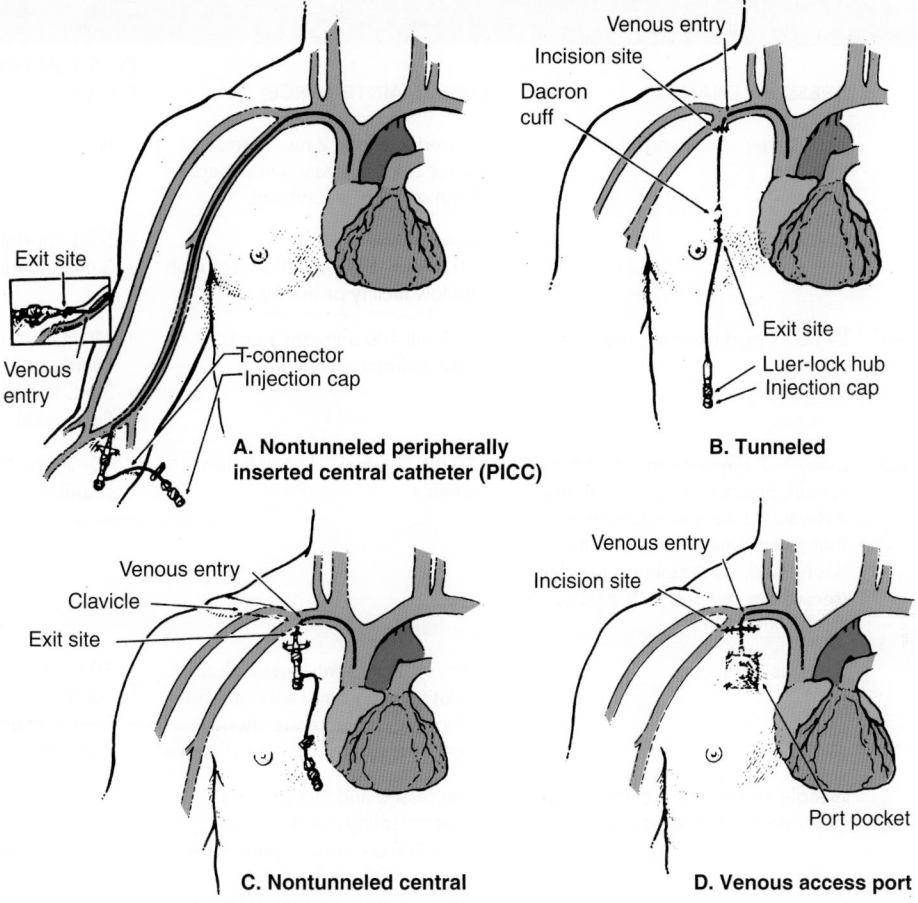

Figure 6-1. Common sites for long-term venous access devices. (Courtesy of American Cancer Society.)

Labels in figure:

A. Nontunneled peripherally inserted central catheter (PICC)
- Exit site
- Venous entry
- T-connector
- Injection cap

B. Tunneled
- Venous entry
- Incision site
- Dacron cuff
- Exit site
- Luer-lock hub
- Injection cap

C. Nontunneled central
- Venous entry
- Clavicle
- Exit site

D. Venous access port
- Venous entry
- Incision site
- Port pocket

c. Examples of the tunneled catheters in current use are Hickman™, Broviac™, and Groshong™.

3. Central implanted device.

   a. A subcutaneous pocket is formed and a reservoir is placed; a catheter is attached to the reservoir and tunneled subcutaneously and inserted into a central vein (usually the catheter tip is in the superior vena cava). This device cannot be seen exteriorly.

   b. Examples of implanted devices in current use include the Port-A-Cath™, Medi-Port™, Infuse-A-Port™, Bard Port systems, and Groshong Port™.

4. Peripheral central—nontunneled.

   a. Peripherally inserted central catheter (PICC); used in patients in acute, long-term, and home care settings.

      i. Inserted in basilic, median cubital, or cephalic veins.

      ii. May be inserted by nurses with special training or interventional radiologists.

      iii. PICC tip placement must be located in superior vena cava (verified by x-ray). Tip placement in subclavian

or innominate vein contraindicated for hyperosmolar solutions (hyperalimentation).

      iv. PICC insertion site and hub should be covered by a transparent dressing.

      v. Extension tubing must be clamped when no solution is being infused. Tape it securely to the patient's arm.

      vi. Positive pressure flushing will keep PICC from clotting (see Table 6-4, page 94).

      vii. PICCs placed in the median cubital vein tend to follow the cephalic vein to central placement. Observe carefully for pain and tenderness because the cephalic vein is smaller than the basilic.

   b. PAS Port™.

      i. Inserted in basilic vein.

      ii. Connected to a subcutaneously implanted port in the forearm.

      iii. Delivers fluid centrally into superior vena cava.

Table 6-4   IV Catheter Maintenance Guidelines

CATHETER	DRESSING CHANGE	FLUSH (MAINTENANCE)	FLUSH (AFTER BLOOD DRAW)
Short peripheral	3 days after site changed	• If used as a lock, 2 mL *normal saline solution every shift or heparin flush solution; 10 units/mL	• N/A
Midline	Every 3–5 days	• 3 mL of 100 units/mL or 10 units/mL heparin flush solution (follow facility protocol)	• 5 mL *normal saline solution • 3 mL heparin flush solution
Peripherally inserted central catheter	24 hours postinsertion, then weekly	• 2–3 mL 100 units/mL heparin flush solution every day	• 10 mL *normal saline solution • 3 mL 100 units/mL heparin flush solution
Groshong (tunneled)	Every 1–2 days postinsertion for 1 week postoperative, then every 3 days until the site is fully healed, then every week; when the site has healed, no dressing is needed (secure the catheter to the patient's chest with tape)	• 10 mL *normal saline solution weekly	• 10–20 mL *normal saline solution
Hickman/Broviac	Same as Groshong	• 3 mL 100 units/mL heparin flush solution every day if accessed every 8 hours or more frequently, no need for heparin between infusions	• 10 mL *normal saline solution • 3 mL 100 units/mL heparin flush solution
Implanted ports (including PAS port)	Needle and dressing change every week when accessed	• If accessed and locked: 5 mL *normal saline solution and 5 mL 100 units/mL heparin flush solution after each infusion • Terminal flush: 5–7 mL 100 units/mL heparin flush solution and every 4 weeks thereafter	• 10 mL *normal saline solution • 5 mL 100 units/mL heparin flush solution
Percutaneous catheters (triple/double lumen)	Every 2–3 days	• 3 mL *normal saline solution • 2 mL 10 units/mL heparin flush solution twice per day or after each infusion	• 3 mL *normal saline solution • 3 mL 10 units/mL heparin flush solution
Quinton/Perm-A catheter (blue lumen, use only with order)	Every 2–3 days	• 2 mL 1,000 units/mL heparin flush solution every 2–3 days (always withdraw heparin first when using catheter)	• 10 mL *normal saline solution • 2 mL 1,000 units/mL heparin flush solution

*Normal saline should be preservative-free 0.9% sodium chloride (USP) when possible. Bacteriostatic 0.9% sodium chloride contains benzyl alcohol as a preservative and, if used, should not exceed 30 mL in a 24-hour period.

 Evidence Base *Infusion Nurses Society (INS). (2011). Infusion nursing standards of practice. Journal of Infusion Nursing, 34(IS), Standard 45.*

 NURSING ALERT If central catheters are placed too deeply and extend into the right atrium, an irregular heartbeat may result. Monitor heart rhythm and notify the health care provider immediately.

5. Midline catheters.
   a. These catheters are inserted into the basilic, cephalic, or median cubital vein and extend 3 to 8 inches (7.5 to 20 cm) up the arm with the proximal tip resting in the upper arm just distal to the axillary arch.
   b. They are inserted by specially trained nurses.
   c. Dwell time—for intermediate therapy of 2 to 6 weeks.
   d. They are considered deep peripheral and not appropriate for hyperosmolar solutions, such as hyperalimentation, and some antibiotics, such as erythromycin and nafcillin.

NURSING ROLE IN INTRAVENOUS THERAPY

Initiating an IV LINE

Nurses must be familiar with the procedure as well as the equipment involved in initiating an IV to provide effective therapy and prevent complications. See Standards of Care Guidelines 6-1.

Selecting a Vein

1. First verify the order for IV therapy unless it is an emergency situation.
2. Explain the procedure to the patient.
3. Select a vein suitable for venipuncture.
   a. Back of hand—metacarpal vein (see Figure 6-2A, page 96). Avoid digital veins, if possible.
      i. The advantage of this site is that it permits arm movement.
      ii. If a vein problem develops later at this site, another vein higher up the arm may be used.
   b. Forearm—basilic or cephalic vein (see Figure 6-2B, page 96).
   c. Inner aspect of elbow, antecubital fossa—median basilic and median cephalic for relatively short-term infusion. However, use of these veins prevents bending of arm.

 NURSING ALERT The median basilic and cephalic veins are not recommended for chemotherapy administration due to the potential for extravasation and poor healing, resulting in impaired joint movement. In addition, these veins may be needed for intermediate or long-term indwelling catheters.

   d. Lower extremities.
      i. Foot—venous plexus of dorsum, dorsal venous arch, medial marginal vein.
      ii. Ankle—great saphenous vein.

 NURSING ALERT Use lower extremities as a last resort. A patient with diabetes or peripheral vascular disease is not a suitable candidate. Obtain an order from the health care provider for the IV site and monitor lower extremity closely for signs of phlebitis, thrombosis, and infection.

4. Central veins are used:
   a. When medications and infusions are hypertonic or highly irritating, requiring rapid, high-volume dilution to prevent systemic reactions and local venous damage (eg, chemotherapy and hyperalimentation).
   b. When peripheral blood flow is diminished (eg, shock) or when peripheral vessels are not accessible (eg, obese patients).
   c. When CVP monitoring is desired.
   d. When moderate or long-term fluid therapy is expected.

Methods of Distending a Vein

1. Apply manual compression above the site where the cannula is to be inserted.
2. Have the patient periodically clench fist if the arm is used.
3. Massage the area in the direction of venous flow.
4. Apply a tourniquet (soft nonlatex) at least 2 to 6 inches (5 to 15 cm) above the planned insertion site, fastening it with a slipknot or hemostat.
5. An alternative is to apply a blood pressure cuff (keep pressure just below systolic pressure).
6. Lightly tap the vein site; this is to be done gently so the vein is not injured.
7. Allow the extremity to be dependent (below heart level) for a few minutes.
8. Apply heat to a possible needle site by using a moist, warm towel.

Selecting Needle or Catheter

1. Use the smallest-gauge catheter suitable for the type and location of the infusion.
2. If a blood transfusion is to be given, use a larger-bore catheter, preferably 20G or larger.
3. For very small veins and an infusion rate below 75 mL/hour, a 24G catheter may be appropriate.
4. Consider local anesthesia.

STANDARDS OF CARE GUIDELINES 6-1
IV Therapy

To prevent adverse effects of IV therapy, perform the following assessments and procedures:

- Before starting IV therapy, consider duration of therapy, type of infusion, condition of veins, and medical condition of the patient to assist in choosing IV site and type of catheter.

- Ensure that you are competent in initiating the type of IV therapy decided on and are familiar with facility policy and procedure before initiating therapy.

- After initiation of IV therapy, monitor the patient frequently for:
  - Signs of infiltration or sluggish flow.
  - Signs of phlebitis or infection.
  - Correct solution, medication, volume, and rate.
  - Dwell time of catheter and need to be replaced.
  - Condition of catheter dressing and frequency of change.
  - Fluid and electrolyte balance.
  - Signs of fluid overload or dehydration.
  - Patient satisfaction with mode of therapy.

This information should serve as a general guideline only. Each patient situation presents a unique set of clinical factors and requires nursing judgment to guide care, which may include additional or alternative measures and approaches.

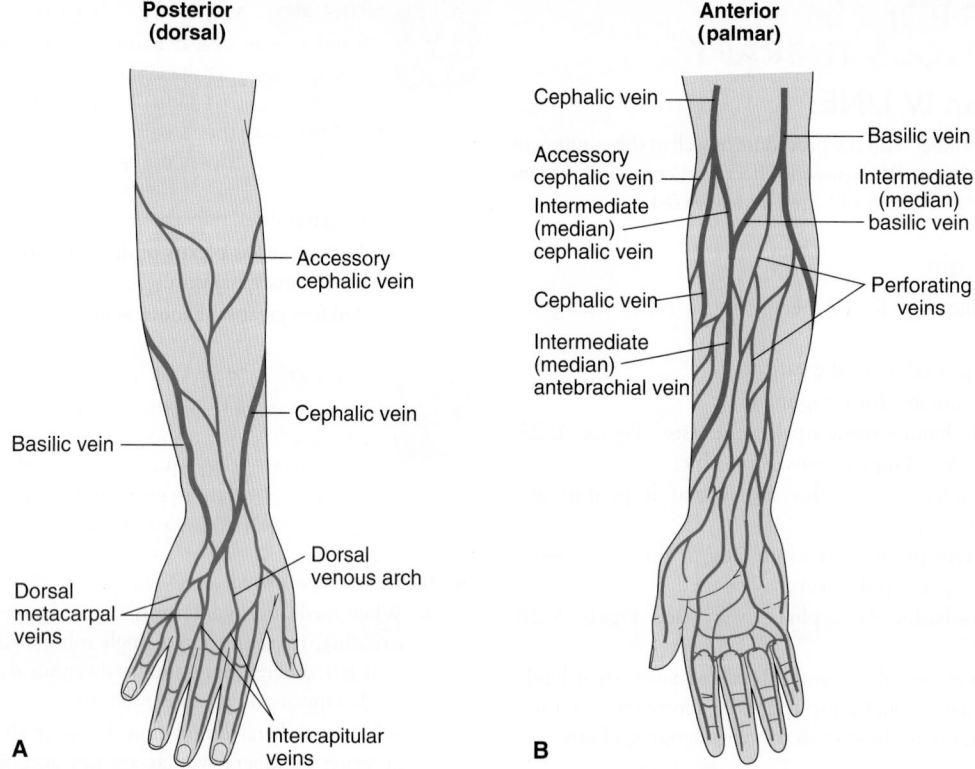

Posterior (dorsal)

- Accessory cephalic vein
- Basilic vein
- Cephalic vein
- Dorsal venous arch
- Dorsal metacarpal veins
- Intercapitular veins

A

Anterior (palmar)

- Cephalic vein
- Accessory cephalic vein
- Intermediate (median) cephalic vein
- Cephalic vein
- Intermediate (median) antebrachial vein
- Basilic vein
- Intermediate (median) basilic vein
- Perforating veins

B

Figure 6-2. **(A)** Superficial veins, dorsal aspect of the hand. **(B)** Superficial veins, forearm.

a. If a large-bore needle (greater than 18G) is being inserted in an unusually sensitive patient, 0.1 mL 1% lidocaine (without epinephrine) may be ordered and infiltrated intradermally around the site to provide local anesthesia. Topical cream may also be applied 1 hour before vein cannulation.

b. Local anesthesia is best avoided because it may cause collapse of desired veins, allergic reactions, and increased cost of the procedure.

5. For a short-term infusion of 1 hour or less, a steel needle may be used.

6. For longer-term therapy, choose a flexible catheter.

 NURSING ALERT Needlesticks are a constant risk in IV therapy. Catheter companies manufacture many protective devices such as retractable stylets in IV catheters. Facilities are strongly encouraged to stock and use these safety devices to protect employees (see Figure 6-3).

Cleaning the Infusion Site

📖 **Evidence Base** Infusion Nurses Society (INS). (2011). Infusion nursing standards of practice. *Journal of Infusion Nursing, 34*(1S), Standard 35.5.

1. If skin is dirty, clean the infusion site thoroughly with surgical soap and rinse.

2. Clean the IV site with an effective topical antiseptic according to facility protocol; the Infusion Nurses Society (INS) approves the following agents, singly or in combination:

a. Chlorhexidine solution used in a scrubbing manner following manufacturer's instructions.

b. Alcohol swabs, used one at a time, in a circular movement from the site outward for a minimum of 30 seconds; allow to dry before IV insertion. (Commonly used first in a two-step process with povidone-iodine, but three swabs may be used singly if the patient is allergic to iodine).

c. Povidone-iodine, used for 1 minute and allowed to dry completely before IV insertion. (Although rarely used because it is very irritating to skin, 1% to 2% iodine could be used first, followed by alcohol to prevent skin irritation.)

 DRUG ALERT Iodine solutions may cause allergic reactions in some patients. The patient should be assessed for iodine allergies before IV insertion. Iodine products should dry to facilitate their antimicrobial properties.

d. 2% tincture of chlorhexidine, used as a single agent antiseptic and allowed to dry, is also an appropriate agent, but is not recommended for infants under 2 months of age.

 DRUG ALERT Chlorhexidine or a combination of alcohol and povidone-iodine should be used for patients who are immunocompromised and at high risk for infection.

Before activation

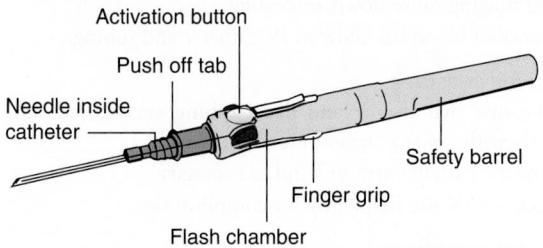

After activation

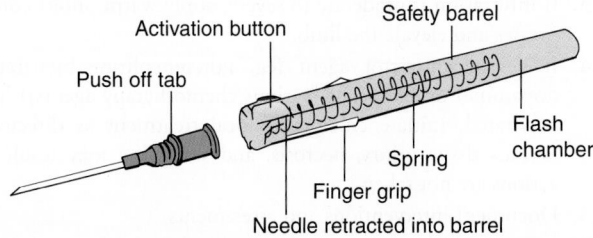

Figure 6-3. The activation button is pressed after the catheter is in the vein so that the needle will retract into the safety barrel while the needle is still in the catheter. (Courtesy of Becton Dickinson.)

Initiating the Venipuncture

Follow steps in Procedure Guidelines 6-1, pages 86 to 88.

Infusion Tubing

1. Drip chambers
   a. A "microdrip" system delivers 60 drops/mL and is used when small volumes are being delivered (eg, less than 50 mL/hour); this reduces the risk of clotting the IV line due to slow infusion rates.
   b. The "macrodrip" system delivers 10, 15, or 20 drops/mL and is used to deliver solution in large quantities or at fast rates.
2. Vents
   a. Vented tubing should be used with standard glass bottles; this permits air to enter the vacuum in the bottle and displace solution as it flows out.
   b. Nonvented tubing should be used for IV bags and glass bottles that have a built-in air vent.
3. Filters
   a. Filters help minimize the risk of contamination from certain microorganisms and particulate matter.
   b. Filters are found "in line" on conventional IV, blood, and hyperalimentation tubing and should be changed when the tubing is changed. Check your facility's equipment and protocols to see if an additional filter is warranted. (*Note:* An additional filter is needed for mannitol infusions.)
   c. "Add-on" filters should be located as close to the insertion site as possible and be changed with administration set changes. There is always a risk that bacteria may become trapped in the filter and release endotoxins, a small pyrogen capable of passing through the filter.

4. Special tubing
   a. Most mechanical infusion pumps and controllers require specialized tubing to fit their particular pumping chamber. Need for such a device should be determined before initiating infusion therapy.
   b. If added tubing length is required (especially for children and restless patients), extension tubing is available; this should be added at the time of IV setup.
   c. Secondary tubing is used for administration of intermittent "piggyback" medications that are connected to the port closest to the drip chamber.
   d. Special coated tubing, designed to prevent leaching of polyvinyl chloride, is used for delivering medications, such as nitroglycerin, paclitaxel, and cyclosporine.
5. Tubing change
   a. Check your facility protocol for time of tubing change. Standard is no more frequently than 96 hours and immediately if contamination is suspected for continuous-flow administration tubing. *Intermittent* administration tubing should be changed every 24 hours.
   b. Label new tubing with the date, the time it was hung, and your initials.
6. Dressing changes and flushing of IV—vary depending on type of IV (see Table 6-4, page 94).

Adjusting Rate of Flow

The health care provider prescribes the flow rate. The nurse is responsible for regulating and maintaining the proper rate.

Patient Determining Factors

1. Surface area of the patient—depending on the size of the patient, more fluid may be required and tolerated.
2. Condition—a patient in hypovolemic shock requires greater amounts of fluids, whereas the patient with heart or renal failure should receive fluids judiciously.
3. Age—fluids should be administered slowly in the very young and elderly.
4. Tolerance to solutions—fluids containing medications causing potential allergic reactions or intense vascular irritation (eg, potassium chloride) should be well diluted or given slowly.
5. Prescribed fluid composition—efficacy of some drugs is based on speed of infusion (eg, antibiotics); rate for other solutions is titrated to the patient's response to them (eg, dopamine, nitroprusside, heparin).

Factors Affecting Rate of Flow

1. Gauge of IV catheter.
2. Pressure gradient—the difference between two levels in a fluid system.
3. Friction—the interaction between fluid molecules and surfaces of inner wall of tubing.
4. Diameter and length of tubing.
5. Height of column of fluid.
6. Characteristics of fluid.
   a. Viscosity.
   b. Temperature—refrigerated fluids may cause diminished flow and vessel spasm; bring fluid to room temperature before infusion.

7. Vein trauma, clots, plugging of vents, venous spasm, and vasoconstriction.
8. Flow-control clamp derangement.
   a. Some clamps may slip and loosen, resulting in a rapid, or "runaway," infusion. Many tubings now have safety clamps to prevent this rapid infusion.
   b. Plastic tubing may distort, causing "creep" or "cold flow"—the inside diameter of tubing will continue to change long after clamp is tightened or relaxed.
   c. Marked stretching of tubing may cause distortions of tubing and render clamp ineffective (may occur when patient turns over and pulls on a short tubing).
9. If there is any question about the rate of fluid administration, check with the health care provider.

 GERONTOLOGIC ALERT Be aware that veins are more likely to roll within the loose tissue beneath the skin, collapse, and become irritated in older adults. Also, fluid overload may be more pronounced, making IV therapy more difficult and potentially dangerous.

Calculation of Flow Rate
1. Most infusion rates are given at a certain volume per hour.
2. Delivery of the prescribed volume is determined by calculating necessary drops per minute to deliver the volume.
3. Drops per milliliter will vary with commercial parenteral sets (eg, 10, 15, 20, or 60 drops/mL). Check the directions.
4. Calculate the infusion rate using the following formula:

$$\text{Drop/minute} = \frac{\text{total volume infused} \times \text{drops/mL}}{\text{total time for infusion in minutes}}$$

Example: Infuse 150 mL of D_5W in 1 hour (set indicates 10 drops/mL)

$$\frac{150 \times 10}{60 \text{ minutes}} = 25 \text{ drops/minute}$$

5. The nurse hanging a new IV solution should write the date, time, and her or his initials on the container label.

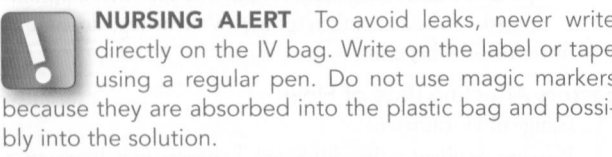 **NURSING ALERT** To avoid leaks, never write directly on the IV bag. Write on the label or tape using a regular pen. Do not use magic markers because they are absorbed into the plastic bag and possibly into the solution.

Complications of IV Therapy

Infiltration

Cause
1. Dislodgment of the IV cannula from the vein results in infusion of fluid into the surrounding tissues.

Clinical Manifestations
1. Swelling, blanching, and coolness of surrounding skin and tissues.

2. Discomfort, depending on nature of solution.
3. Fluid flowing more slowly or ceasing.
4. Absence of blood backflow in IV catheter and tubing.

Preventive Measures
1. Make sure that the IV and distal tubing are secured sufficiently with tape to prevent movement.
2. Splint the patient's arm or hand as necessary.
3. Check the IV site frequently for complications.

Nursing Interventions
1. Stop infusion immediately and remove the IV needle or catheter.
2. Restart the IV in the other arm.
3. If infiltration is moderate to severe, apply warm, moist compresses and elevate the limb.
4. If a vasoconstrictor agent (eg, norepinephrine bitartrate, dopamine) or a vesicant [various chemotherapy agents]) has infiltrated, initiate emergency local treatment as directed. Serious tissue injury, necrosis, and sloughing may result if actions are not taken.
5. Document interventions and assessments.

Thrombophlebitis

Causes
1. Injury to vein during venipuncture, large-bore needle or catheter use, or prolonged needle or catheter use.
2. Irritation to vein due to rapid infusions or irritating solutions (eg, hypertonic glucose solutions, cytotoxic agents, strong acids or alkalis, potassium, and others); smaller veins are more susceptible.
3. Clot formation at the end of the needle or catheter due to slow infusion rates.
4. More commonly seen with synthetic catheters than steel needles.

Clinical Manifestations
1. Tenderness at first, then pain along the vein.
2. Swelling, warmth, and redness at infusion site; the vein may appear as a red streak above the insertion site.

Preventive Measures
1. Anchor the needle or catheter securely at the insertion site.
2. Change the insertion site every 72 hours in adult patients (it may not be feasible to remove short-term catheters in neonates and pediatric patients every 72 hours; however, they should be removed immediately if contamination or complications are suspected). Peripheral (short-term) catheters placed during an emergency where aseptic techniques could have been compromised should be removed no later than 48 hours.
3. Use large veins for irritating fluid because of higher blood flow, which rapidly dilutes the irritant.
4. Sufficiently dilute irritating agents before infusion.

Nursing Interventions
1. Apply cold compresses immediately to relieve pain and inflammation.
2. Follow with moist, warm compresses to stimulate circulation and promote absorption.

3. Document interventions and assessments.

4. Participate in facility quality improvement activities regarding phlebitis occurrence rates. One formula that can be used is:

$$\frac{\text{Number of phlebitis incidents}}{\text{Total number of IV peripheral catheters}} \times 100$$

$$= \% \text{ peripheral phlebitis}$$

 Evidence Base Infusion Nurses Society (INS). (2011). Infusion nursing standards of practice. *Journal of Infusion Nursing, 34*(1S), Standards 7 and 47.

Bacteremia

Causes

1. Underlying phlebitis increases risk 18-fold.
2. Contaminated equipment or infused solutions (see Figure 6-4).

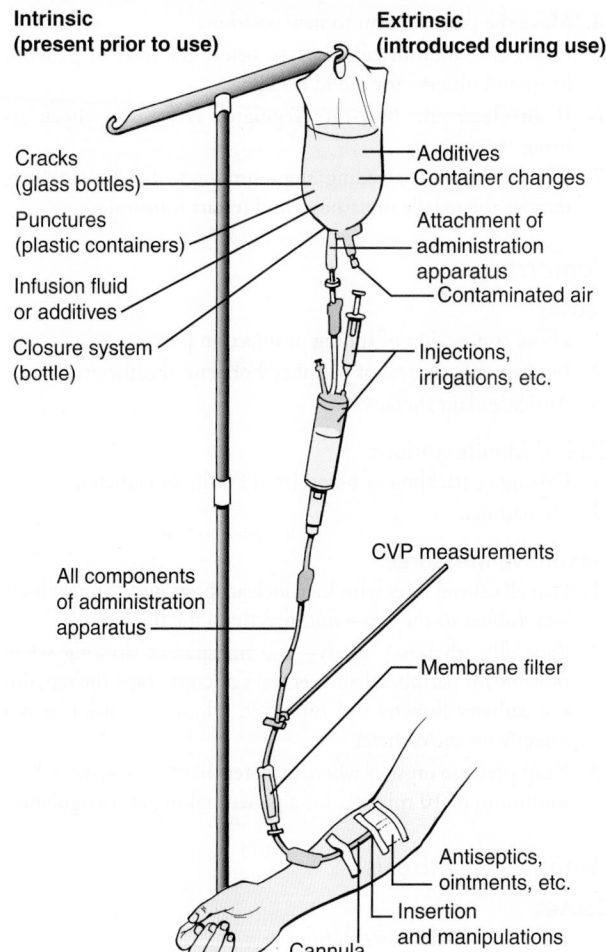

Intrinsic
(present prior to use)

Cracks
(glass bottles)

Punctures
(plastic containers)

Infusion fluid
or additives

Closure system
(bottle)

All components
of administration
apparatus

Extrinsic
(introduced during use)

Additives
Container changes

Attachment of
administration
apparatus
Contaminated air

Injections,
irrigations, etc.

CVP measurements

Membrane filter

Antiseptics,
ointments, etc.

Insertion
and manipulations
of cannula

Cannula

Figure 6-4. Potential mechanisms for contamination of IV infusion systems.

3. Prolonged placement of an IV device (catheter or needle, tubing, solution container).
4. Nonsterile IV insertion or dressing change.
5. Cross-contamination by the patient with other infected areas of the body.
6. A critically ill or immunosuppressed patient is at greatest risk of bacteremia.

Clinical Manifestations

1. Elevated temperature, chills.
2. Nausea, vomiting.
3. Elevated white blood cell (WBC) count.
4. Malaise, increased pulse.
5. Backache, headache.
6. May progress to septic shock with profound hypotension.
7. Possible signs of local infection at IV insertion site (eg, redness, pain, foul drainage).

Preventive Measures

1. Follow the same measures as outlined for thrombophlebitis.
2. Use strict sterile technique when inserting the IV or changing IV dressing.
3. Solutions should never hang longer than 24 hours.
4. Change the insertion site every 96 hours in an adult patient and within 48 hours if catheter was placed in an emergent situation.
5. Change continuous IV administration sets no more frequently than every 96 hours and intermittent IV administration sets every 24 hours.
6. Change the IV dressing on a routine basis and immediately if it becomes compromised.
   a. Gauze dressing that prevents visualization of the site should be changed every 48 hours.
   b. Transparent semipermeable dressing on a peripheral short-term site should be changed at site change or if the dressing loses its integrity.

 Evidence Base Infusion Nurses Society (INS). (2011). Infusion nursing standards of practice. *Journal of Infusion Nursing, 34*(1S), Standard 46.4.

   c. Transparent semipermeable dressing on central line sites should be changed at least every 7 days.
7. Maintain integrity of the infusion system.

Nursing Interventions

1. Discontinue infusion and IV cannula.
2. IV device should be removed and the tip cut off with sterile scissors; placed in a dry, sterile container; and immediately sent to the laboratory for analysis.
3. Check vital signs; reassure the patient.
4. Obtain WBC count, as directed, and assess for other sites of infection (urine, sputum, wound).
5. Start appropriate antibiotic therapy immediately after receiving orders.
6. Document interventions and assessments.

Circulatory Overload

Cause

1. Delivery of excessive amounts of IV fluid (greater risk exists for older patients, infants, or patients with cardiac or renal insufficiency).

Clinical Manifestations

1. Increased BP and pulse.
2. Increased CVP, venous distention (engorged jugular veins).
3. Headache, anxiety.
4. Shortness of breath, tachypnea, coughing.
5. Pulmonary crackles.
6. Chest pain (if history of coronary artery disease).

Preventive Measures

1. Know whether patient has existing heart or kidney condition. Be particularly vigilant in the high-risk patient.
2. Closely monitor the infusion flow rate. Keep accurate intake and output records.
3. Splint the arm or hand if the IV flow rate fluctuates too widely with movement.

Nursing Interventions

1. Slow infusion to a "keep-open" rate and notify the health care provider.
2. Monitor closely for worsening condition.
3. Raise the patient's head to facilitate breathing.
4. Document interventions and assessments.

Air Embolism

Causes

1. A greater risk exists in central venous lines, when air enters catheter during tubing changes (air sucked in during inspiration due to negative intrathoracic pressure).
2. Air in tubing delivered by IV push or infused by infusion pump.

Clinical Manifestations

1. Drop in BP, elevated heart rate.
2. Cyanosis, tachypnea.
3. Rise in CVP.
4. Changes in mental status, loss of consciousness.

Preventive Measures

1. Clear all air from tubing before infusion to patient.
2. Change solution containers before they run dry.
3. Ensure that all connections are secure. Always use luer-lock connections on central lines.
4. Use precipitate and air-eliminating filters unless contraindicated.
5. Change IV tubing during expiration.

Nursing Interventions

1. Immediately turn the patient on left side and lower the head of the bed; in this position, air will rise to right atrium.
2. Notify the health care provider immediately.
3. Administer oxygen as needed.
4. Reassure the patient.
5. Document interventions and assessments.

Mechanical Failure (Sluggish IV Flow)

Causes

1. Needle lying against the side of the vein, cutting off fluid flow.
2. Clot at the end of the catheter or needle.
3. Infiltration of IV cannula.
4. Kinking of the tubing or catheter.

Clinical Manifestations

1. Sluggish IV flow.
2. Alarm of flow regulator sounding.
3. May be signs of local irritation—swelling, coolness of skin.

Preventive Measures

1. Check the IV often for patency and kinking.
2. Secure the IV well with tape and an armboard, if necessary.

Nursing Interventions

1. Remove tape and check for kinking of tubing or catheter.
2. Pull back the cannula because it may bew lying against wall of vein, vein valve, or vein bifurcation.
3. Elevate or lower needle to prevent occlusion of bevel.
4. Move the patient's arm to new position.
5. Lower the solution container to below the level of patient's heart and observe for blood backflow.
6. If an electronic flow-rate regulator is in use, check its integrity.
7. If none of the preceding steps produces the desired flow, remove the needle or catheter and restart infusion.

Hemorrhage

Causes

1. Loose connection of tubing or injection port.
2. Inadvertent removal of peripheral or central catheter.
3. Anticoagulant therapy.

Clinical Manifestations

1. Oozing or trickling of blood from IV site or catheter.
2. Hematoma.

Preventive Measures

1. Cap all central lines with luer-lock adapters and connect luer-lock tubing to the cap—not directly to the line.
2. Tape all catheters securely—use transparent dressing when possible for peripheral and central catheters. Tape the remaining catheter lumens and tubing in a loop so tension is not directly on the catheter.
3. Keep pressure on sites where catheters have been removed—a minimum of 10 minutes for a patient taking anticoagulants.

Venous Thrombosis

Causes

1. Infusion of irritating solutions.
2. Infection along catheter may preclude this syndrome.
3. Fibrin sheath formation with eventual clot formation around the catheter. (This clot will eventually occlude the vein.)

Clinical Manifestations

1. Slowing of IV infusion or inability to draw blood from the central line.
2. Swelling and pain in the area of catheter or in the extremity proximal to the IV line.

Preventive Measures

1. Ensure proper dilution of irritating substances.
2. Ensure superior vena cava catheter tip placement for irritating solutions.

Nursing Interventions

1. Stop fluids immediately and notify health care provider.
2. Reassure the patient and institute appropriate therapy:
   a. Anticoagulants.
   b. Heat.
   c. Elevation of affected extremity.
   d. Antibiotics.

SELECTED REFERENCES

Agius, C. R. (2012). Intelligent infusion technologies: Integration of a smart system to enhance patient care. *Journal of Infusion Nursing, 35*(6), 364–368.

Alexander, M., Corrigan, A., Gorski, L., et al. (2010). *Infusion nursing: An evidence-based approach* (3rd ed.). St. Louis, MO: Saunders/Elsevier.

Alfaro-Leferre, R. (2010). *Applying nursing process: A tool for critical thinking.* New York: Wolters Kluwer/Lippincott Williams & Wilkins.

American Nurses Association. (2010). *Nursing scope and standards of practice* (2nd ed.). Silver Spring, MD: Author.

Charron, K. (2012). Decreasing central line infections and needlestick injury rates: Combining best practice and introducing a Luer-activated intravenous therapy system and antimicrobial intravenous connector. *Journal of Infusion Nursing, 35*(6): 370–375.

Crowley, M., Brim, C., Proehl, M., et al. (2012). Emergency nursing resource: Difficult intravenous access. *Journal of Emergency Nursing, 38*(4), 335–343.

Dargin, J. M., Rebholz, C. M., Lowenstein, R. A., et al. (2010). Ultrasonography-guided peripheral intravenous catheter survival in ED patients with difficult access. *American Journal of Emergency Medicine, 28*(1), 1–7.

Doellman, D., Pettit, J., Catudal, J. P., et al. (2010). *Best practice guidelines in the care and maintenance of pediatric central venous catheters.* Herriman, UT: Association for Vascular Access.

Edwards, C., Johnson, C. (2012). Evaluation of a Luer-activated intravenous administration system. *Journal of the Association for Vascular Access, 17*(4), 200–207.

Hadaway, L., & Richardson, D. (2010). Needleless connectors: A primer on terminology. *Journal of Infusion Nursing, 33*(1), 1–11.

Hadaway, L. (2012). Short peripheral intravenous catheters and infections. *35*(4), 230–240.

Infusion Nursing Society (INS). (2011). Infusion nursing standards of practice. *Journal of Infusion Nursing, 34*(1S).

Jarvis, W. R. (2010, July 28). Choosing the best design for intravenous needleless connectors to prevent bloodstream infections. *Infection Control Today.* For more information: *http://www.infectioncontroltoday.com/articles/2010/07/choosing-the-best-design-for-intravenous-needleless-connectors-to-prevent-bloodstream-infections.aspx.*

Phillips, L. D. (2010). *Manual of IV therapeutics: Evidence-based practice for infusion therapy* (5th ed.). Philadelphia: Davis.

Smith, J. S., Irwin, G., Viney, M., et al. (2012). Optimal disinfection times for needleless intravenous connectors. *Journal of the Association for Vascular Access, 17*(3), 137–143.

7
Perioperative Nursing

OVERVIEW AND ASSESSMENT

Introduction

Perioperative nursing is a term used to describe the nursing care provided during the total surgical experience of the patient: preoperative, intraoperative, and postoperative.

Preoperative phase—from the time the decision is made for surgical intervention to the transfer of the patient to the operating room.

Intraoperative phase—from the time the patient is received in the operating room until admitted to the postanesthesia care unit (PACU).

Postoperative phase—from the time of admission to the PACU to the follow-up evaluation.

An *anesthesia care provider* is a professional who can administer and monitor anesthesia during a surgical procedure; he or she may be a licensed physician board certified in anesthesia (anesthesiologist) or a certified registered nurse anesthetist.

Perioperative Safety

The safety and welfare of patients during surgical intervention is a primary concern. Patients entering the perioperative settings are at risk for infection, impaired skin integrity, altered body temperature, fluid volume deficit, and injury related to positioning and chemical, electrical, and physical hazards.

 Evidence Base The Joint Commission. (2012). Hospital: 2013 National Patient Safety Goals. Available: *www.jointcommission.org/standards_information/npsgs.aspx.*
    The Joint Commission. (2012). Surgical Care Improvement Project. Available at: *www.jointcommission.org/surgical_care_improvement_project/.*

Surgical Care Improvement Project

1. The Surgical Care Improvement Project (SCIP), a national quality partnership interested in improving surgical care by significantly reducing surgical complications, is a coalition of health care organizations that has developed evidence-based interventions that have proven effective.
   a. The goal is to reduce surgical complications by 25%.
   b. Implementing nursing interventions at the earliest stage possible of a developing complication is also of utmost importance.
2. SCIP measures that have been shown to be effective include:
   a. Prophylactic antibiotic received within 1 hour prior to surgical incision.
   b. Prophylactic antibiotic discontinued within 24 hours after surgery end time.
   c. Cardiac surgery patients with controlled 6:00 A.M. postoperative serum glucose.

d. Surgery patients with appropriate hair removal.

e. Urinary catheter removed on postoperative day 1 or post-operative day 2 with day of surgery being day zero.

f. Patients continue beta-blockers on day of surgery.

g. Appropriate venous thromboembolism prophylaxis and treatment.

National Patient Safety Goals

National Patient Safety Goals (2013) include:

1. Prevent infection—use hand cleaning guidelines from the Center for Disease Control or the World Health Organization.
   a. Use proven guidelines to prevent infections that are difficult to treat.
   b. Use proven guidelines to prevent infection of the blood from central lines.
   c. Use proven guidelines to prevent infection after surgery.
   d. Use proven guidelines to prevent infections of the urinary tract caused by catheters.
2. Prevent mistakes in surgery—make sure the correct surgery is done on the correct patient at the correct place on the patient's body.

a. Mark the correct place on the patient's body where the surgery is to be done.

b. Pause before surgery to make sure a mistake is not being made.

Types of Surgery

1. Elective—The scheduled time for surgery is at the convenience of the patient; failure to have surgery is not catastrophic (eg, a superficial cyst).
2. Required—The condition requires surgery within a few weeks (eg, eye cataract).
3. Urgent—Necessitates surgery as soon as possible but may be delayed for a short amount of time (eg, internal fixation of fracture).
4. Emergency—The situation requires immediate surgical attention without delay (eg, intestinal obstruction). This must be done to save life or limb or functional capacity.

Common abdominal incisions are pictured in Figure 7-1.

Ambulatory Surgery

Ambulatory surgery (same-day surgery, outpatient surgery) is a common occurrence for certain types of procedures. The office

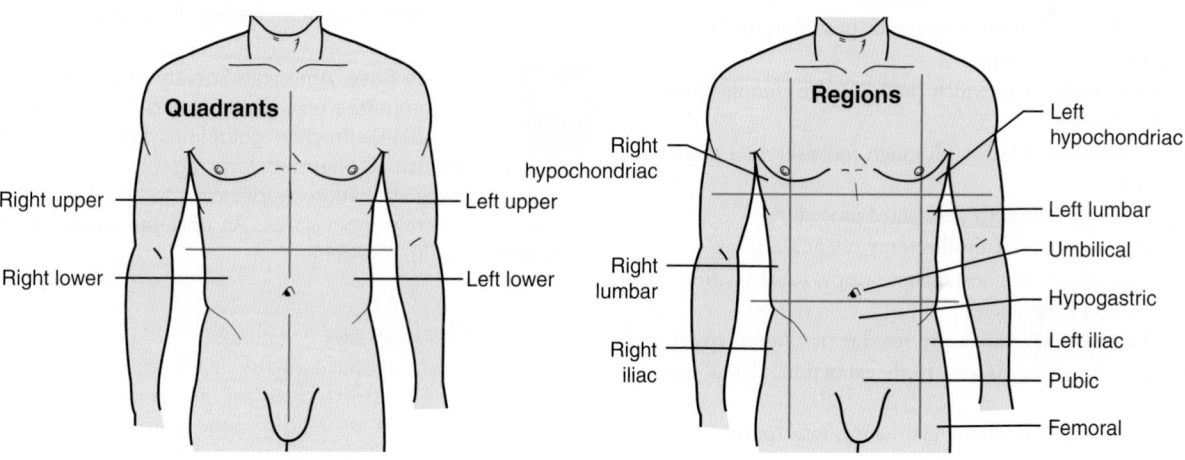

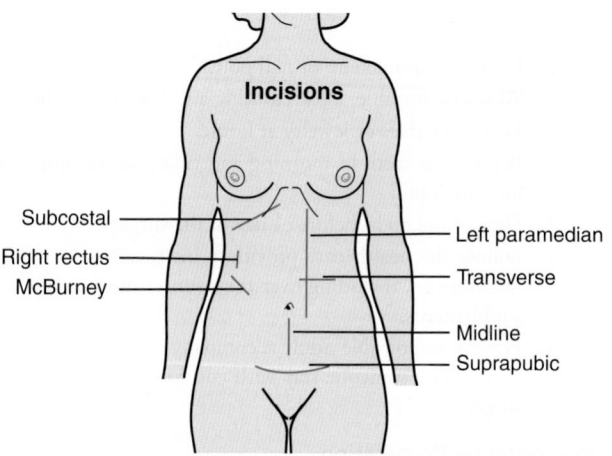

Incision site	Type of surgery
Subcostal	Gallbladder and biliary tract surgery
Paramedian	Right side - biliary tract, gallbladder
	Left side - splenectomy, gastrectomy, hiatal hernia repair
Transverse	Gastrectomy
Rectus	Right side - appendectomy, small bowel resection
	Left side - sigmoid colon resection
McBurney	Appendectomy
Midline (lower)	Female reproductive tract
Suprapubic (low-transverse, Pfannenstiel)	Gynecologic surgery

Figure 7-1. Regions and incisions of the abdomen.

nurse is in a key position to assess patient status; plan the perioperative experience; and monitor, instruct, and evaluate the patient.

Advantages

1. Reduced cost to the facility and insuring and governmental agencies.
2. Reduced psychological stress to the patient.
3. Less incidence of hospital-acquired infection.
4. Less time lost from work by the patient; minimal disruption of the patient's activities and family life.

Disadvantages

1. Less time to assess the patient and perform preoperative teaching.
2. Less time to establish rapport between the patient and health care personnel.
3. Less opportunity to assess for late postoperative complications. (This responsibility is primarily with the patient, although telephone and home care follow-up is possible.)

Patient Selection

Criteria for selection include:

1. Surgery of short duration (varies by procedure and facility).
2. Noninfected conditions.
3. Type of operation in which postoperative complications are predictably low.
4. Age usually not a factor, although too risky in a premature neonate.
5. Examples of commonly performed procedures:
   a. Ear–nose–throat (tonsillectomy, adenoidectomy)
   b. Gynecology (diagnostic laparoscopy, tubal ligation, dilation and curettage).
   c. Orthopedics (arthroscopy, fracture or tendon repair).
   d. Oral surgery (wisdom teeth extraction, dental restorations).
   e. Urology (circumcision, cystoscopy, vasectomy).
   f. Ophthalmology (cataract).
   g. Plastic surgery (mammary implants, reduction mammoplasty, liposuction, blepharoplasty, face lift).
   h. General surgery (laparoscopic hernia repair, laparoscopic cholecystectomy, biopsy, cyst removal).

Ambulatory Surgery Settings

Ambulatory surgery is performed in a variety of settings. A high percentage of outpatient surgery occurs in traditional hospital operating rooms in hospital-integrated facilities. Other ambulatory surgery settings may be hospital-affiliated or independently owned and operated. Some types of outpatient surgeries can be performed safely in the health care provider's office.

Nursing Management

Initial Assessment

1. Develop a nursing history for the outpatient; this may be initiated in the health care provider's office. The history should include the patient's physical and psychological status. You will also inquire about allergies, tobacco, alcohol, and drug use; disabilities or limitations; current medications (including over-the-counter and herbs); current health conditions (focus should be on cardiovascular and respiratory problems, diabetes, and renal impairments); and any past surgeries and/or problems with anesthesia.

2. Ensure availability of a signed and witnessed informed consent that includes correct surgical procedure and site.
3. Explain any additional laboratory studies needed and state why.
4. Begin the health education regimen. Instructions to the patient:
   a. Notify the health care provider and surgical unit immediately if you get a cold, have a fever, or have any illness before the date of surgery.
   b. Arrive at the specified time.
   c. Restrict food and fluid before surgery according to facility protocol to prevent aspiration of gastric contents. Based on scientific evidence, the American Society of Anesthesiologists has issued guidelines for elective procedures recommending the following:
      i. Clear liquids—minimum fasting of 2 hours.
      ii. Breast milk—minimum fasting of 4 hours.
      iii. Infant formula—minimum fasting of 6 hours.
      iv. Nonhuman milk—minimum fasting of 6 hours.
      v. Light meal—minimum fasting of 6 hours.

 Evidence Base American Society of Anesthesiologists Committee on Standards and Practice Parameters. (2011). Practice guidelines for preoperative fasting and the use of pharmacologic agents to reduce the risk of pulmonary aspiration: Application to healthy patients undergoing elective procedures. An updated report. *Anesthesiology, 114*(3), 495–511.

 NURSING ALERT Minimum fasting times must be followed to reduce the risk of aspiration, but patients are often instructed to fast after midnight because schedule changes the morning of surgery are possible due to cancellations, which can cause surgery time to be moved forward. Be aware that prolonged fasting before surgery may result in undue thirst, hunger, irritability, headache, and possibly dehydration, hypovolemia, and hypoglycemia.

   d. Do not wear makeup or nail polish.
   e. Wear comfortable, loose clothing and low-heeled shoes.
   f. Leave valuables or jewelry at home.
   g. Brush your teeth in morning and rinse, but do not swallow any liquid.
   h. Shower the night before or day of the surgery.
   i. Follow the health care provider's instructions for taking medications, including over-the-counter medications and supplements.
   j. Have a responsible adult accompany you and drive you home; have someone stay with you for 24 hours after the surgery.

Preoperative Preparation

1. Conduct a nursing assessment, focusing on cardiovascular and respiratory status. Determine if patient is diabetic and,

if so, follow glucose control measures. Obtain baseline vital signs, including an oxygen saturation level and current pain score.

2. Review the patient's chart for witnessed and informed consent, laterality (right or left, if applicable), lab work, and history and physical.

3. Verify correct patient, correct site, and correct procedure. Consider "time-out" and SCIP measures, including marking of incision.

4. Make sure the patient has followed food and fluid restrictions, has removed all jewelry and dentures, and is appropriately dressed for surgery.

5. Perform medication reconciliation. Certain home meds may be taken, especially beta-blockers. Check with health care provider and have patient take with a sip of water.

6. Inform anesthesia provider if patient is taking any herbal supplements.

7. Administer preprocedural medication, if applicable.

Postoperative Care

1. Check vital signs, including oxygen saturation, temperature, and pain score.

2. Administer oxygen, if necessary.

3. Change the patient's position and progress activity—head of bed elevated, dangling, walking. Watch for dizziness or nausea.

4. Ascertain, using the following criteria, that the patient has recovered adequately to be discharged:

    a. Vital signs stable and returned to preoperative level.
    b. Stands without excessive dizziness; able to walk short distances.
    c. Pain score within tolerable level (usually less than 3 required).
    d. Able to drink fluids.
    e. Oriented to time, place, and person.
    f. No evidence of respiratory distress.

g. Has the services of a responsible adult who can escort the patient home and remain with patient.

h. Understands postoperative instructions and takes an instruction sheet home (see Patient Education Guidelines 7-1).

Informed Consent (Operative Permit)

Informed consent (operative permit) is the process of informing the patient about the surgical procedure; that is, risks and possible complications of surgery and anesthesia. Consent is obtained by the surgeon. This is a legal requirement. Hospitals usually have a standard operative permit form approved by the hospital's legal department.

Purposes

1. To ensure that the patient understands the nature of the treatment, including potential complications and alternative treatment or procedures.

2. To indicate that the patient's decision was made without pressure.

3. To protect the patient against unauthorized procedures, and to ensure that the procedure is performed on the correct body part.

4. To protect the surgeon and facility against legal action by a patient who claims that an unauthorized procedure was performed.

Adolescent Patient and Informed Consent

1. An emancipated minor is usually recognized as one who is not subject to parental control. Regulations vary by jurisdiction but generally include:

    a. Married minor.
    b. Those in military service.
    c. Minor who has a child.

2. Most states have statutes regarding treatment of minors.

3. Standards for informed consent are the same as for adults.

PATIENT EDUCATION GUIDELINES 7-1

Outpatient Postanesthesia and Postsurgery Instructions and Information

- Although you will be awake and alert in the recovery room, small amounts of anesthetic will remain in your body for at least 24 hours and you may feel tired and sleepy for the remainder of the day. Once you are home, take it easy and rest as much as possible. It is advisable to have someone with you at home for the remainder of the day.

- Eat lightly for the first 12–24 hours, then resume a well-balanced, normal diet. Drink plenty of fluids. Alcoholic beverages are to be avoided for 24 hours after your anesthesia or IV sedation.

- Nausea or vomiting may occur in the first 24 hours. Lie down on your side and breathe deeply. Prolonged nausea, vomiting, or pain should be reported to your surgeon.

- Ask your surgeon or anesthesiologist when you can resume your daily medications after surgery.

- Your surgeon will discuss your postsurgery instructions with you and prescribe medication for you as indicated. You will also receive additional instructions specific to your surgical procedure before leaving the facility.

- Your family will be waiting for you in the facility's waiting room area near the outpatient surgery department. Your surgeon will speak to them in this area before your discharge.

- Do not operate a motor vehicle or any mechanical or electrical equipment for 24 hours after your anesthesia.

- Do not make any important decisions or sign legal documents for 24 hours after your anesthesia.

Procedures Requiring Informed Consent and Time-Out

1. Any surgical procedures whether major or minor.
2. Entrance into a body cavity, such as colonoscopy, paracentesis, bronchoscopy, cystoscopy, or lumbar puncture.
3. Radiologic procedures, particularly if a contrast material is required (such as myelogram, magnetic resonance imaging with contrast, angiography).
4. All procedures requiring any type of anesthesia, which includes cardioversion.

Obtaining Informed Consent

1. Before signing an informed consent document, the patient should:
   a. Be told in clear and simple terms by the surgeon what is to be done, the risks and benefits, as well as any alternatives to the surgery or procedure. The anesthesia care provider will explain the anesthesia plan and possible risks and complications.
   b. Have a general idea of what to expect in the early and late postoperative periods.
   c. Have a general idea of the time involved from surgery to recovery.
   d. Have an opportunity to ask any questions.
   e. Sign a separate form for each procedure or operation.
2. Written permission is required by law and a witness may be required according to facility policy.
3. Signature is obtained with the patient's complete understanding of what is to occur; it is obtained before the patient receives sedation and is secured without pressure or duress.
4. For a minor (or a patient who is unconscious or irresponsible), permission is required from a responsible family member—parent, legal guardian, or court-appointed guardian.
5. For a married emancipated minor, permission from the spouse is acceptable.
6. If the patient is unable to write, an "X" is acceptable.
7. In an emergency, permission by way of telephone is acceptable.

Surgical Risk Factors and Preventive Strategies

Obesity

Danger

1. Increases the difficulty involved in the technical aspects of performing surgery; risk for wound dehiscence is greater.
2. Increases the likelihood of infection because of compromised tissue perfusion.
3. Increases the potential for postoperative pneumonia and other pulmonary complications because obese patients chronically hypoventilate.
4. Increases demands on the heart, leading to cardiovascular compromise.
5. Increases the risk for airway complications.
6. Alters the response to many drugs and anesthetics.
7. Decreases the likelihood of early ambulation.

Therapeutic Approach

1. Encourage weight reduction if time permits.
2. Anticipate postoperative obesity-related complications.
3. Be extremely vigilant for respiratory complications.
4. Carefully splint abdominal incisions when moving or coughing.
5. Be aware that some drugs should be dosed according to ideal body weight versus actual weight (owing to fat content) to prevent toxicity, including digoxin, lidocaine, aminoglycoside antibiotics, and theophylline.
6. Be aware that obese patients require higher doses of antibiotics to achieve effective tissue levels.
7. Avoid intramuscular (I.M.) injections in morbidly obese individuals (IV or subcutaneous routes preferred).
8. Never attempt to move an impaired patient without assistance or without using proper body mechanics.
9. Obtain a dietary consultation early in the patient's postoperative course.

Poor Nutrition

Danger

1. Greatly impairs wound healing (especially protein and calorie deficits and a negative nitrogen balance).
2. Increases the risk of infection.

Therapeutic Approach

1. Any recent (within 4 to 6 weeks) weight loss of 10% of the patient's normal body weight or decreased serum albumin should alert the health care staff to poor nutritional status and the need to investigate as to the cause of the weight loss.
2. Attempt to improve nutritional status before and after surgery. Unless contraindicated, provide a diet high in proteins, calories, and vitamins (especially vitamins C and A); this may require enteral and parenteral feeding.
3. Review a serum prealbumin level to determine recent nutritional status.
4. Recommend repair of dental caries and proper mouth hygiene to prevent infection.

Fluid and Electrolyte Imbalance

Danger

Can have adverse effects in terms of general anesthesia and the anticipated volume losses associated with surgery, causing shock and cardiac dysrhythmias.

 NURSING ALERT Patients undergoing major abdominal operations (such as colectomies and aortic repairs) often experience a massive fluid shift into tissues around the operative site in the form of edema (as much as 1 L or more may be lost from circulation). Watch for the fluid shift to reverse (from tissue to circulation) around the third postoperative day. Patients with heart disease may develop failure due to the excess fluid "load."

Therapeutic Approach

1. Assess the patient's fluid and electrolyte status.
2. Rehydrate the patient parenterally and orally as prescribed.
3. Monitor for evidence of electrolyte imbalance, especially Na^+, K^+, Mg^{++}, Ca^{++}.
4. Be aware of expected drainage amounts and composition; report excess and abnormalities.
5. Monitor the patient's intake and output; be sure to include all body fluid losses.

Aging

Danger

1. Potential for injury is greater in older people.
2. Be aware that the cumulative effect of medications is greater in the older patient.
3. Medications in the usual dosages, such as morphine, may cause confusion, disorientation, and respiratory depression.

Therapeutic Approach

1. Consider using lesser doses for desired effect.
2. Anticipate problems from chronic disorders such as anemia, obesity, diabetes, hypoproteinemia.
3. Adjust nutritional intake to conform to higher protein and vitamin needs.
4. When possible, cater to set patterns in older patients, such as sleeping and eating.

Presence of Cardiovascular Disease

Danger

1. May compound the stress of anesthesia and the operative procedure.
2. May result in impaired oxygenation, cardiac rhythm, cardiac output, and circulation.
3. May also produce cardiac decompensation, sudden arrhythmia, thromboembolism, acute myocardial infarction (MI), or cardiac arrest.
4. Holding cardiac medications, particularly beta-blockers, may have negative impact on cardiac status.

Therapeutic Approach

1. Frequently assess heart rate and blood pressure (BP) and hemodynamic status and cardiac Rhythm, if indicated.
2. Avoid fluid overload (oral, parenteral, blood products) because of possible MI, angina, heart failure, and pulmonary edema.
3. In compliance with SCIP measures, make sure the patient has not held beta-blocker prior to surgery. Administer with a sip of water.

Evidence Base American Society of PeriAnesthesia Nurses. (2011). *2010–2012 standards of perianesthesia nursing practice.* Cherry Hill, NJ: Author.

4. Prevent prolonged immobilization, which results in venous stasis. Monitor for potential deep vein thrombosis (DVT) or pulmonary embolus.
5. Encourage position changes but avoid sudden exertion.

6. Use anti-embolism stockings and/or sequential compression device intraoperatively and postoperatively.
7. Note evidence of hypoxia and initiate therapy.

Presence of Diabetes Mellitus

Danger

1. Hypoglycemia may result from food and fluid restrictions and anesthesia.
2. Hyperglycemia and ketoacidosis may be potentiated by increased catecholamines and glucocorticoids due to surgical stress.
3. Chronic hyperglycemia results in poor wound healing and susceptibility to infection.
4. Research has shown that surgical patients have better outcomes when glucose levels are well controlled throughout the surgical process.

Therapeutic Approach

1. Recognize the signs and symptoms of ketoacidosis and hypoglycemia, which can threaten an otherwise uneventful surgical experience. Dehydration also threatens renal function.
2. Monitor blood glucose and be prepared to administer insulin, as directed, or treat hypoglycemia.
3. Confirm what medications the patient has taken and what has been held. Facility protocol and provider preference varies, but the goal is to prevent hypoglycemia. If the patient is NPO, oral agents are usually withheld and insulin may be ordered at 75% of the usual dose.
4. Reassure the diabetic patient that when the disease is controlled, the surgical risk is no greater than it is for the nondiabetic patient.

DRUG ALERT Rare reports of lactic acidosis have raised concerns about the use of metformin in the perioperative period. Metformin is usually held 48 hours before surgery and restarted when full food and fluid intake has restarted and normal renal function has been confirmed.

Presence of Alcoholism

Danger

The additional problem of malnutrition may be present in the presurgical patient with alcoholism. The patient may also have an increased tolerance to anesthetics.

Therapeutic Approach

1. Note that the risk of surgery is greater for the patient who has chronic alcoholism.
2. Anticipate the acute withdrawal syndrome within 72 hours of the last alcoholic drink.

Presence of Pulmonary and Upper Respiratory Disease

Danger

1. Chronic pulmonary illness may contribute to hypoventilation, leading to pneumonia and atelectasis.
2. Surgery may be contraindicated in the patient who has an upper respiratory infection because of the possible advance of infection to pneumonia and sepsis.
3. Sleep apnea in the perioperative patient provides a great risk to anesthesia and must be noted and assessed prior to surgery.

Therapeutic Approach

1. Patients with chronic pulmonary problems, such as emphysema or bronchiectasis, should be evaluated and treated prior to surgery to optimize pulmonary function with bronchodilators, corticosteroids, and conscientious mouth care, along with a reduction in weight and smoking and methods to control secretions.
2. Patients with obstructive sleep apnea should be evaluated by an anesthesia provider prior to surgery. General anesthesia should be avoided if possible. Patients should bring continuous positive airway pressure (CPAP) machines to the hospital for use post-anesthesia.
3. Opioids should be used cautiously to prevent hypoventilation. Patient-controlled analgesia is preferred.
4. Oxygen should be administered to prevent hypoxemia (low liter flow in chronic obstructive pulmonary disease).

Concurrent or Prior Pharmacotherapy

Danger

Hazards exist when certain medications are given concomitantly with others (eg, interaction of some drugs with anesthetics can lead to hypotension and circulatory collapse). This also includes the use of many herbal substances. Although herbs are natural products, they can interact with other medications used in surgery.

Therapeutic Approach

1. An awareness of drug therapy is essential.
2. Notify the health care provider and anesthesia provider if the patient is taking any of the following drugs:
   a. Certain antibiotics.
   b. Antidepressants, particularly monoamine oxidase inhibitors, and St. John's wort, an herbal product.
   c. Phenothiazines.
   d. Diuretics, particularly thiazides.
   e. Corticosteroids.
   f. Anticoagulants, such as warfarin or heparin, or medications or herbals that may affect coagulation, such as aspirin, feverfew, ginkgo biloba, nonsteroidal anti-inflammatory drugs, ticlopidine, and clopidogrel.

PREOPERATIVE CARE

Patient Education

Patient education is a vital component of the surgical experience. Preoperative patient education may be offered through conversation, discussion, the use of audiovisual aids, demonstrations, and return demonstrations. It is designed to help the patient understand the surgical experience to minimize anxiety and promote full recovery from surgery and anesthesia. The educational program may be initiated before hospitalization by the physician, nurse practitioner or office nurse, or other designated personnel. This is particularly important for patients who are admitted the day of surgery or who are to undergo outpatient surgical procedures. The perioperative nurse can assess the patient's knowledge base and use this information in developing a plan for an uneventful perioperative course.

Teaching Strategies

Obtain a Database

1. Determine what the patient already knows or wants to know. This can be accomplished by reading the patient's chart, interviewing the patient, and communicating with the health care provider, family, and other members of the health care team.
2. Ascertain the patient's psychosocial adjustment to impending surgery.
3. Determine cultural or religious health beliefs and practices that may have an impact on the patient's surgical experience, such as refusal of blood transfusions, burial of amputated limbs within 24 hours, or special healing rituals.

Plan and Implement Teaching Program

1. Begin at the patient's level of understanding and proceed from there.
2. Plan a presentation, or series of presentations, for an individual patient or a group of patients.
3. Include family members and significant others in the teaching process.
4. Encourage active participation of patients in their care and recovery.
5. Demonstrate essential techniques; provide the opportunity for patient practice and return demonstration.
6. Provide time for and encourage the patient to ask questions and express concerns; make every effort to answer all questions truthfully and in basic agreement with the overall therapeutic plan.
7. Provide general information and assess the patient's level of interest in or reaction to it.
   a. Explain the details of preoperative preparation and provide a tour of the area and view the equipment when possible.
   b. Offer general information on the surgery. Explain that the health care provider is the primary resource person.
   c. Notify the patient when surgery is scheduled (if known) and approximately how long it will take; explain that afterward the patient will go to the postanesthesia care unit (PACU). Emphasize that delays may be attributed to many factors other than a problem developing with this patient (eg, previous case in the operating room may have taken longer than expected or an emergency case has been given priority).
   d. Let the patient know that his or her family will be kept informed and that they will be told where to wait and when they can see the patient; note visiting hours.
   e. Explain how a procedure or test may feel during or afterward.
   f. Describe the PACU and what personnel and equipment the patient may expect to see and hear (specially trained personnel, monitoring equipment, tubing for various functions, and a moderate amount of activity by nurses and health care providers).
   g. Stress the importance of active participation in postoperative recovery.
8. Use other resource people: health care providers, therapists, chaplain, interpreters.

9. Document what has been taught or discussed as well as the patient's reaction and level of understanding.
10. Discuss with the patient the anticipated postoperative course (eg, length of stay, immediate postoperative activity, follow-up visit with the surgeon).

Use Audiovisual Aids If Available

1. Videotapes or computer programs are effective in giving basic information to a single patient or group of patients. Many facilities provide a television channel dedicated to patient instruction.
2. Booklets, brochures, and models, if available, are helpful.
3. Demonstrate any equipment that will be specific for the particular patient. Examples:
   a. Drains and drainage bags
   b. Monitoring equipment
   c. Side rails
   d. Incentive spirometer
   e. Sequential compression device

General Instructions

Preoperatively, the patient will be instructed in the following postoperative activities. This will allow a chance for practice and familiarity.

Incentive Spirometry

Preoperatively, the patient uses a spirometer to measure deep breaths (inspired air) while exerting maximum effort. The preoperative measurement becomes the goal to be achieved as soon as possible after the operation.

1. Postoperatively, the patient is encouraged to use the incentive spirometer about 10 to 12 times per hour.
2. Deep inhalations expand alveoli, which prevents atelectasis and other pulmonary complications.
3. There is less pain with inspiratory concentration than with expiratory concentration such as with coughing.

Coughing

Coughing promotes the removal of chest secretions. Instruct the patient to:

1. Interlace fingers and place hands over the proposed incision site; this will act as a splint during coughing and not harm the incision.
2. Lean forward slightly while sitting in bed.
3. Breathe, using the diaphragm.
4. Inhale fully with the mouth slightly open.
5. Let out three or four sharp "hacks."
6. With the mouth open, take in a deep breath and quickly give one or two strong coughs.
7. Secretions should be readily cleared from the chest to prevent respiratory complications (pneumonia, obstruction).

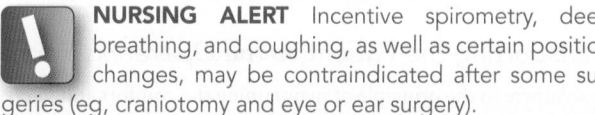 **NURSING ALERT** Incentive spirometry, deep breathing, and coughing, as well as certain position changes, may be contraindicated after some surgeries (eg, craniotomy and eye or ear surgery).

Turning

Changing positions from back to side-lying (and vice versa) stimulates circulation, encourages deeper breathing, and relieves pressure areas.

1. Help the patient to move onto his or her side if assistance is needed.
2. Place the uppermost leg in a more flexed position than that of the lower leg, and place a pillow comfortably between the legs.
3. Make sure that the patient is turned from one side to the back and onto the other side every 2 hours.

Foot and Leg Exercises

Moving the legs improves circulation and muscle tone.

1. Have the patient lie supine; instruct patient to bend a knee and raise the foot—hold it a few seconds, and lower it to the bed.
2. Repeat above about five times with one leg and then with the other. Repeat the set five times every 3 to 5 hours.
3. Then have the patient lie on one side and exercise the legs by pretending to pedal a bicycle.
4. Suggest the following foot exercise: Trace a complete circle with the great toe.

Evaluation of Teaching Program

1. Observe the patient for correct demonstration of expected postoperative behaviors, such as foot and leg exercises and special breathing techniques.
2. Ask pertinent questions to determine the patient's level of understanding.
3. Reinforce information when necessary.

Preparation of the Operative Area
Skin Antisepsis

 Evidence Base Alexander, J. W., Solomkin, J. S., & Edwards, M. J. (2011). Updated recommendations for control of surgical site infections. *Annals of Surgery, 253*, 1082–1093.

1. Human skin normally harbors transient and resident bacterial flora, some of which are pathogenic. Skin cannot be sterilized without destroying skin cells.
2. The attributes of an appropriate surgical skin antiseptic require the ability to significantly reduce microorganisms, provide broad spectrum activity, be fast acting, and have a persistent effect.
   a. Preoperative bathing with chlorhexidine reduces pathogenic organisms on the skin. Using multiple showers or showers immediately before coming to the operating room substantially reduces skin organisms.
   b. Cleansing with a bactericidal-impregnated sponge just before operation will provide additional reduction in skin bacteria.
   c. Friction enhances the action of detergent antiseptics; however, friction should not be applied over a superficial malignancy (causes seeding of malignant cells) or areas of carotid plaque (causes plaque dislodgment and emboli).

3. The Centers for Disease Control and Prevention recommends that hair not be removed near the operative site unless it will interfere with surgery. Skin is easily injured during shaving and often results in a higher rate of postoperative wound infection.
4. If required, hair removal should be done by clipping, not shaving, and should be performed within 2 hours of surgery. Scissors may be used to remove hair greater than 3 mm in length.
5. For head surgery, obtain specific instructions from the surgeon concerning the extent of shaving.

Gastrointestinal Tract

1. Preparation of the bowel is imperative for patients undergoing intestinal surgery because escaping bacteria can invade adjacent tissues and cause sepsis.
   a. Cathartics and enemas remove gross collections of stool (eg, GoLYTELY).
   b. Oral antimicrobial agents (eg, neomycin, erythromycin) suppress the colon's potent microflora.
   c. Enemas "until clear" are generally not necessary. If ordered, they are given the night before surgery. Notify the health care provider if the enemas never return clear.
2. Solid food is withheld from the patient for 6 hours before surgery. Patients having morning surgery are kept NPO overnight. Clear fluids (water) may be given up to 4 hours before surgery depending on facility protocols.

Genitourinary Tract

A medicated douche may be prescribed preoperatively if the patient is to have a gynecologic or urologic operation.

Preoperative Medication

Evidence Base Alexander, J. W., Solomkin, J. S., & Edwards, M. J. (2011). Updated recommendations for control of surgical site infections. *Annals of Surgery, 253*, 1082–1093.

With the increase of ambulatory surgery and same-day admissions, preanesthetic sedatives, skin preps, and douches are seldom ordered. Administration of systemic prophylactic perioperative antibiotics is among one of the most important steps in preventing surgical site infection, however. Recent evidence shows that the use of prophylactic antibiotics decreases the incidence of wound infections by about one half. There is a risk, however, of an increase in Clostridium difficile diarrheal infections due to antibiotic use. Redosing of antibiotics should be done every 3 hours during surgery and should be discontinued within 24 hours after surgery end time (48 hours for cardiac surgeries).

DRUG ALERT *Antibiotics should be administered just before surgery—preferably 1 hour before an incision is made—to be effective when bacterial contamination is expected.*

Administering "On Call" Medications

1. Have the medication ready and administer it as soon as the call is received from the operating room.
2. Proceed with the remaining preparation activities.
3. Indicate on the chart or preoperative checklist the time when the medication was administered and by whom.

Admitting the Patient to Surgery
Final Checklist

The preoperative checklist is the last procedure before taking the patient to the operating room. Most facilities have a standard form for this checklist. The World Health Organization Surgical Safety Checklist is available for hospital use. It does not, however, remove the nurse's responsibility for the hospital's specific checklist that may be in use (see Figure 7-2).

Identification and Verification

This includes verbal identification by the perioperative nurse while checking the identification band on the patient's wrist and written documentation (such as the chart) of the patient's identity, the procedure to be performed (laterality, if indicated), the specific surgical site marked by the surgeon with indelible ink, the surgeon, and the type of anesthesia. These are all patient safety goals as outlined by the Joint Commission.

Review of Patient Record

Check for inclusion of the fact sheet; allergies; history and physical; completed preoperative checklist; laboratory values, including most recent results, pregnancy test, if applicable; electrocardiogram (ECG) and chest x-rays, if necessary; preoperative medications; and other preoperative orders by either the surgeon or anesthesia care provider.

Consent Form

All nurses involved with patient care in the preoperative setting should be aware of the individual state laws regarding informed consent and the specific facility policy. Obtaining informed consent is the responsibility of the surgeon performing the specific procedure. Consent forms should state the procedure, various risks, and alternatives to surgery, if any. It is a nursing responsibility to make sure the consent form has been obtained with the patient or guardian's signature and that it is in the chart.

Patient Preparedness

1. NPO status.
2. Proper attire (clean gown and hair covering) and clean linen.
3. Skin preparation, if ordered.
4. IV line started with correct gauge needle.
5. Dentures or plates removed.
6. Jewelry, piercings, contact lenses, and glasses removed and secured in a locked area or given to a family member.
7. Allow the patient to void.

Transporting the Patient to the Operating Room

1. Adhere to the principle of maintaining the comfort and safety of the patient.

Surgical Safety Checklist

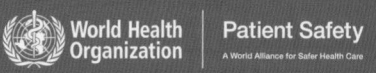

World Health Organization | Patient Safety
A World Alliance for Safer Health Care

Before induction of anaesthesia	Before skin incision	Before patient leaves operating room
(with at least nurse and anaesthetist)	(with nurse, anaesthetist and surgeon)	(with nurse, anaesthetist and surgeon)

Before induction of anaesthesia

Has the patient confirmed his/her identity, site, procedure, and consent?
☐ Yes

Is the site marked?
☐ Yes
☐ Not applicable

Is the anaesthesia machine and medication check complete?
☐ Yes

Is the pulse oximeter on the patient and functioning?
☐ Yes

Does the patient have a:

Known allergy?
☐ No
☐ Yes

Difficult airway or aspiration risk?
☐ No
☐ Yes, and equipment/assistance available

Risk of >500ml blood loss (7ml/kg in children)?
☐ No
☐ Yes, and two IVs/central access and fluids planned

Before skin incision

☐ **Confirm all team members have introduced themselves by name and role.**

☐ **Confirm the patient's name, procedure, and where the incision will be made.**

Has antibiotic prophylaxis been given within the last 60 minutes?
☐ Yes
☐ Not applicable

Anticipated Critical Events

To Surgeon:
☐ What are the critical or non-routine steps?
☐ How long will the case take?
☐ What is the anticipated blood loss?

To Anaesthetist:
☐ Are there any patient-specific concerns?

To Nursing Team:
☐ Has sterility (including indicator results) been confirmed?
☐ Are there equipment issues or any concerns?

Is essential imaging displayed?
☐ Yes
☐ Not applicable

Before patient leaves operating room

Nurse Verbally Confirms:
☐ The name of the procedure
☐ Completion of instrument, sponge and needle counts
☐ Specimen labelling (read specimen labels aloud, including patient name)
☐ Whether there are any equipment problems to be addressed

To Surgeon, Anaesthetist and Nurse:
☐ What are the key concerns for recovery and management of this patient?

This checklist is not intended to be comprehensive. Additions and modifications to fit local practice are encouraged.   Revised 1 / 2009   © WHO, 2009

Figure 7-2. World Health Organization perioperative checklist.

2. Accompany operating room attendants to the patient's bedside for introduction and proper identification.
3. Assist in transferring the patient from bed to stretcher (unless the bed goes to the operating room floor).
4. Complete the chart and preoperative checklist; include laboratory reports and x-rays as required by facility policy or the health care provider's directive.
5. Make sure that the patient arrives in the operating room at the proper time.

The Patient's Family

1. Direct the patient's family to the proper waiting room where magazines, television, and a coffee station may be available.
2. Tell the family that the surgeon will probably contact them there after surgery to inform them about the operation.
3. Inform the family that a long interval of waiting does not mean the patient is in the operating room the whole time; anesthesia preparation and induction take time, and after surgery, the patient is taken to the PACU.
4. Tell the family what to expect postoperatively when they see the patient—tubes; monitoring equipment; and blood transfusion, suctioning, and oxygen equipment.

INTRAOPERATIVE CARE
Anesthesia and Related Complications

The goals of anesthesia are to provide analgesia, sedation, and muscle relaxation appropriate for the type of operative procedure as well as to control the autonomic nervous system.

Common Anesthetic Techniques
Moderate Sedation

Evidence Base Association of periOperative Registered Nurses. (2011). *Recommended practice for managing the patient receiving moderate sedation/analgesia.* Denver, CO: Author.

1. A specific level of sedation that allows patients to tolerate unpleasant procedures by reducing the level of anxiety and discomfort; previously known as conscious sedation.
2. The patient achieves a depressed level of consciousness (LOC) and altered perception of pain while retaining the ability to respond appropriately to verbal and tactile stimuli.
3. Cardiopulmonary function and protective airway reflexes are maintained by the patient.

4. Knowledge of expected outcomes is essential. These outcomes include, but are not limited to:
   a. Maintenance of consciousness.
   b. Maintenance of protective reflexes.
   c. Alteration of pain perception.
   d. Enhanced cooperation.
5. Adequate preoperative preparation of the patient will facilitate achieving the desired effects.
6. Nurses caring for patients receiving moderate sedation should be specially trained in the agents used for moderate sedation, such as midazolam and fentanyl, and should be skilled in advanced life support. Many facilities have strict regulations and training requirements for staff handling such patients.
7. Nurses working in this setting should also be aware of the regulations from the Board of Nursing in the state they are practicing concerning the care of patients receiving anesthesia and should be compliant with state advisory opinions, declaratory rules, and other regulations that direct the practice of the registered nurse.
8. Patients who are not candidates for conscious sedation and require more complex sedation should be managed by anesthesia care providers.

Monitored Anesthesia Care

1. Light to deep sedation that is monitored by an anesthesia care provider.
2. The patient is asleep but arousable.
3. The patient is not intubated.
4. The patient may receive local anesthesia and oxygen, is monitored, and receives sedation and analgesia. Midazolam, fentanyl, alfentanil, and propofol are frequently used in monitored anesthesia care procedures.

General Anesthesia

1. A reversible state consisting of complete loss of consciousness. Protective reflexes are lost.
2. With the loss of protective reflexes, the patient's airway needs to be maintained. This can be done by endotracheal intubation or insertion of a laryngeal mask airway (LMA).
   a. For certain, short and uncomplicated surgeries (eg, myringotomies), the insertion of a breathing tube may not be necessary, and the airway is maintained manually with a jaw-thrust/chin-lift.
   b. Endotracheal (ET) intubation is facilitated by the use of a laryngoscope. The ET tube is inserted into the trachea and passed through the vocal cords. A cuff is then inflated, thus ensuring a secure airway where no secretions from the oral cavity can enter the lungs.
   c. LMA does not require a laryngoscope for insertion and is inserted only to the entrance of the trachea. Although LMA does not provide a totally protected airway, it is noninvasive and more gentle on the tissue.
3. General anesthesia consists of three phases; induction, maintenance, and emergence.
   a. Induction can be accomplished either by parenteral or inhalation route. Common agents for IV induction are propofol and phenobarbital. In addition to the induction agent, a potent analgesic is also often added (eg, fentanyl). The analgesic potentiates the induction agent as well as provides analgesia. Patients can also reach an unconscious state by inhaling a potent, short-acting volatile gas. Sevoflurane is one such example. Once the patient is asleep, and if the surgical procedure so requires, a muscle relaxant is given and the ET tube is inserted. Common muscle relaxants include vecuronium, rocuronium, and succinylcholine.
   b. Maintenance is accomplished through a continuous delivery of an inhalation agent, such as sevoflurane, isoflurane, or desflurane, or an IV infusion of an agent, such as propofol, to maintain an unconscious state. Intermittent doses of an analgesic are given as needed as well as intermittent doses of a muscle relaxant for longer surgeries.
   c. Emergence occurs at the end of the surgery when the continuous delivery of either the gas or the IV infusion is stopped and the patient slowly returns to a conscious state. If muscle relaxants are still in effect, they can be reversed with neostigmine to allow for adequate muscle strength and return of spontaneous ventilations. A nerve stimulator can be used to assess if adequate muscle control has returned before extubation of the trachea. During emergence, the patient is very sensitive to any stimuli and it is important to keep noise levels to a minimum and refrain from manipulating the patient during this stage.

Regional Anesthesia

Examples of regional anesthesia include spinal, epidural, and peripheral blocks (eg, interscalene blocks, ankle-blocks).

1. Anesthesia is achieved by injecting a local anesthetic, such as lidocaine or bupivacaine, in close proximity to appropriate nerves.
2. Nursing responsibilities include being familiar with the drug used and maximum dose that can be given, knowing signs and symptoms of toxicity, and maintaining a comfortable environment for the conscious patient.
3. *Spinal anesthesia* is the injection of a local anesthetic into the lumbar intrathecal space. The anesthetic blocks conduction in spinal nerve roots and dorsal ganglia, thereby causing paralysis and analgesia below the level of injection.
4. *Epidural anesthesia* involves injecting local anesthetic into the epidural space. Results are similar to spinal analgesia but with a slower onset.
   a. Often a catheter is inserted for continuous infusion of the anesthetic to the epidural space.
   b. The catheter may be left in place to provide postoperative analgesia as well.
5. *Peripheral nerve block* is achieved by injecting a local anesthetic into a bundle of nerves (eg, axillary plexus) or into a single nerve to achieve anesthesia to a specific part of the body (eg, hand or single finger).

Intraoperative Complications

1. Hypoventilation and hypoxemia—due to inadequate ventilatory support.
2. Oral trauma (broken teeth, oropharyngeal, or laryngeal trauma)—due to difficult ET intubation.

3. Hypotension—due to preoperative hypovolemia or untoward reactions to anesthetic agents.

4. Cardiac dysrhythmia—due to preexisting cardiovascular compromise, electrolyte imbalance, or untoward reactions to anesthetic agents.

5. Hypothermia—due to exposure to a cool ambient operating room environment and loss of normal thermoregulation capability from anesthetic agents.

6. Peripheral nerve damage—due to improper positioning of the patient (eg, full weight on an arm) or use of restraints.

7. Malignant hyperthermia.

   a. This is a rare reaction to anesthetic inhalants (notably sevoflurane, enflurane, isoflurane, and desflurane) and the muscle relaxant succinylcholine.

   b. Caused by abnormal and excessive intracellular accumulations of calcium with resulting hypermetabolism, increased muscle contraction, and elevated body temperature.

> **! NURSING ALERT** Recognize malignant hyperthermia immediately so that inhalant anesthesia can be discontinued and treatment measures started, to prevent seizures and other adverse effects.

   c. Treatment consists of discontinuing the inhalant anesthetic, administering IV dantrolene, and applying cooling techniques (eg, cooling blanket, iced saline lavages).

POSTOPERATIVE CARE

Postanesthesia Care Unit

To ensure continuity of care from the intraoperative phase to the immediate postoperative phase, the circulating nurse or anesthesia care provider gives a thorough report to the PACU nurse (see Standards of Care Guidelines 7-1). This report should include the following:

STANDARDS OF CARE GUIDELINES 7-1
PACU Care

Postanesthesia care unit (PACU) care is geared toward recognizing the signs of distress and anticipating and preventing postoperative difficulties. Carefully monitor the patient coming out of general anesthesia until:

- Vital signs are stable and are within normal range.
- The patient has no signs of respiratory distress and can maintain his or her own airway.
- Reflexes have returned to normal.
- Pain is under control and at a tolerable level for the patient.
- The patient is responsive and oriented to time and place.

This information should serve as a general guideline only. Each patient situation presents a unique set of clinical factors and requires nursing judgment to guide care, which may include additional or alternative measures and approaches.

---

1. Type of surgery performed and any intraoperative complications.

2. Type of anesthesia (eg, general, local, sedation).

3. Drains and type of dressings.

4. Presence of ET tube or type of oxygen to be administered (eg, nasal cannula, T-piece).

5. Types of lines and locations (eg, peripheral IV, central line, arterial line).

6. Catheters or tubes, such as a urinary catheter or T-tube.

7. Administration of blood, colloids, and fluids and electrolytes.

8. Drug allergies and pertinent medical history.

9. Preexisting medical conditions.

10. Intraoperative course, including any complications or instability in the patient's vital signs.

Initial Nursing Assessment

Before receiving the patient, note the proper functioning of monitoring and suctioning devices, oxygen therapy equipment, and all other equipment. The following initial assessment is made by the nurse in the PACU:

1. Verify the patient's identity, the operative procedure, and the surgeon who performed the procedure.

2. Obtain vital signs, including pulse oximetry and temperature.

3. Evaluate airway status, noting any stridor or snoring respirations. Capnography may be used to assess adequate oxygenation as well.

4. Evaluate respiratory status, including rate and effort, and auscultate breath sounds

5. Assess circulatory status, noting skin color, peripheral pulses, and ECG monitor.

6. Observe LOC and orientation to time and place.

7. Evaluate condition of surgical dressings and drains and check IV lines and infusing fluids and/or IV medications. Initial surgical dressing is usually maintained for 48 hours.

8. Determine patient's pain level using a 1 to 10 scale.

9. Review the health care provider's orders.

> **NURSING ALERT** It is important for the nurse to be able to communicate in the patient's language to provide an accurate assessment. An interpreter must be obtained when necessary.

Initial Nursing Diagnoses

- Ineffective Airway Clearance related to effects of anesthesia.
- Impaired Gas Exchange related to ventilation–perfusion imbalance.
- Risk for unstable glucose level related to uncontrolled diabetes and stress of surgery.
- Ineffective Tissue Perfusion (Cardiopulmonary) related to hypotension postoperatively.
- Risk for Imbalanced Body Temperature related to medications, sedation, and cool environment.
- Risk for Deficient Fluid Volume related to blood loss, food and fluid deprivation, vomiting, and indwelling tubes.
- Acute Pain related to surgical incision and tissue trauma.

- Impaired Skin Integrity related to invasive procedure, immobilization, and altered metabolic and circulatory state.
- Risk for Injury related to sensory dysfunction and physical environment.
- Disturbed Sensory Perception related to effects of medications and anesthesia.

Initial Nursing Interventions

Maintaining a Patent Airway

1. Closely monitor the patient arriving with an oral or nasal airway in place until fully awake.
2. Monitor for return of cough and gag reflex. When the patient is awake and able to protect his or her own airway, the oral or nasal airway can be discontinued.
3. Early initiation of CPAP in the PACU is beneficial for patients exhibiting hypoxemia, apnea, and frequent severe airway obstruction due to obstructive sleep apnea.

Maintaining Adequate Respiratory Function

1. Encourage the patient to take deep breaths to aerate the lungs fully and prevent atelectasis; use an incentive spirometer to aid in this function.
2. Assess lung fields frequently through auscultation.
3. Periodically evaluate the patient's LOC—response to name or command. *Note:* Alterations in cerebral function may suggest impaired oxygen delivery.
4. Administer humidified oxygen to reduce irritation of airways and facilitate secretion removal.

Maintaining Glycemic Control

1. Check serum glucose on arrival to PACU and monitor as indicated.
2. For patients who are diabetic, administer insulin and follow protocols to keep serum glucose levels between 120 and 160 mg/dL. Studies show that normalizing blood glucose for the first 2 to 3 days postoperatively reduces the incidence of deep wound infections comparable to that in nondiabetic patients.

 Evidence Base Alexander, J. W., Solomkin, J. S, & Edwards, M. J. (2011). Updated recommendations for control of surgical site infections. *Annals of Surgery*, 253(6), 1082–1093.

Promoting Tissue Perfusion

1. Monitor vital signs (BP, pulse, respiratory rate, and oxygen saturation) according to protocol, normally every 15 minutes while in the PACU. Monitor ECG tracing for arrhythmias.
   a. Report variations in BP, heart rate, respiratory rate, and cardiac arrhythmias.
   b. Evaluate pulse pressure to determine status of perfusion. (A narrowing pulse pressure indicates impending shock.)
2. Monitor intake and output closely.
3. Recognize the variety of factors that may alter circulating blood volume, such as blood loss during surgery and fluid shifts after surgery.

4. Recognize early symptoms of shock or hemorrhage.
   a. Cool extremities, decreased urine output (less than 30 mL/ hour), slow capillary refill (greater than 3 seconds), decreased BP, narrowing pulse pressure, and increased heart rate are usually indicative of decreased cardiac output.
5. Intervene to improve tissue perfusion.
   a. Initiate oxygen therapy or increase fraction of inspired oxygen of existing oxygen delivery system.
   b. Increase parenteral fluid infusion, as prescribed.
   c. Place the patient in the shock position with his or her feet elevated (unless contraindicated).
   d. See Chapter 35 for more detailed consideration of shock.

Stabilizing Thermoregulatory Status

1. Monitor temperature every 15 minutes and be alert for development of both hypothermia and hyperthermia.
2. Report a temperature more than 101.5° F (38.6° C) or less than 95° F (35° C).
3. Monitor for postanesthesia shivering that, although common in hypothermic patients, may also occur in normothermic patients, especially those who received inhalants during anesthesia. It represents a heat-gain mechanism, which drastically increases oxygen demand.
4. Provide warm blankets for patients feeling cold.
5. Provide active warming with forced warm air for hypothermic patients.

Maintaining Adequate Fluid Volume

1. Administer IV, as ordered.
2. Monitor intake and output.
3. Monitor electrolytes and recognize evidence of imbalance, such as nausea, vomiting, and weakness.
4. Evaluate mental status and skin color and turgor.
5. Recognize signs of fluid imbalance.
   a. Hypovolemia—decreased BP, decreased urine output, decreased central venous pressure (CVP), increased pulse.
   b. Hypervolemia—increased BP; changes in lung sounds, such as crackles in the bases; changes in heart sounds (eg, S₃ gallop); increased CVP.
6. Evaluate IV sites to detect early infiltration. Restart lines immediately to maintain fluid volume.

Promoting Comfort

1. Assess pain by observing behavioral and physiologic manifestations (change in vital signs may be a result of pain); have the patient rate pain on a scale of 1 to 10.
2. Administer analgesics and document efficacy.
3. Position the patient to maximize comfort.

Minimizing Complications of Skin Impairment

1. Perform handwashing before and after contact with the patient.
2. Inspect dressings routinely and reinforce them, if necessary.
3. Record the amount and type of wound drainage (see "Wound management," page 124).
4. Turn the patient frequently and maintain good body alignment.

Maintaining Safety

1. Keep the side rails up until the patient is fully awake.
2. Protect the extremity into which IV fluids are running so that the needle will not become accidentally dislodged.
3. Avoid nerve damage and muscle strain by properly supporting and padding pressure areas.
4. Be aware that patients who have received regional anesthesia may not be able to complain of an injury, such as the pricking of an open safety pin or a clamp that is exerting pressure.
5. Check the dressing for constriction.
6. Determine the return of motor control following regional anesthesia—indicated by how the patient responds to a request to move a body part.

Minimizing Sensory Deficits

1. Know that the ability to hear returns more quickly than other senses as the patient emerges from anesthesia.
2. Avoid saying anything in the patient's presence that may be disturbing; the patient may appear to be sleeping but still consciously hears what is being said.
3. Explain procedures and activities at the patient's level of understanding.
4. Minimize the patient's exposure to emergency treatment of nearby patients by drawing the curtains and lowering your voice and noise levels.
5. Treat the patient as a person who needs as much attention as the equipment and monitoring devices.
6. Respect the patient's feeling of sensory deprivation and overstimulation; make adjustments to minimize this fluctuation of stimuli.
7. Demonstrate concern for and an understanding of the patient and anticipate his or her needs and feelings.
8. Tell the patient repeatedly that the surgery is over and that he or she is in the PACU.

Evaluation: Expected Outcomes

- Absence of respiratory distress.
- Lung sounds clear to auscultation.
- Glucose < 160 mg/dL.
- Vital signs stable and within preoperative ranges.
- Body temperature more than 95° F (35° C) and less than 101.5° F (38.6° C).
- I.V. infusion patent; urine output 50–60 mL per hour.
- Adequate pain control.
- Wound/dressing intact without excessive drainage.
- Side rails up; positioned carefully.
- Quiet, reassuring environment maintained.
- Movement of extremities after regional anesthesia.

Transferring the Patient from the PACU

Each facility may have an individual checklist or scoring guide used to determine a patient's readiness for transfer. The above evaluation criteria must be met before transfer.

Transfer Responsibilities

1. Relay appropriate information to the unit nurse regarding the patient's condition. Use an approved method of communication such as SBAR (situation, background, assessment, and recommendations). Point out significant needs, vital signs (trends and most recent set), fluid therapy, incision and dressing requirements, intake needs, urine output, and color and amount of any drainage.
2. Physically assist in the transfer of the patient.
3. Orient the patient to the room, attending nurse, call light, and therapeutic devices.

Postoperative Discomforts

Most patients experience some discomforts postoperatively. These are usually related to the general anesthetic and the surgical procedure. The most common discomforts are nausea, vomiting, restlessness, sleeplessness, thirst, constipation, flatulence, and pain.

Postoperative Nausea and Vomiting (PONV)

Causes

1. Occurs in many postoperative patients.
2. Most commonly related to inhalation anesthetics (nitrous oxide) and opioid use.
3. Can result from an accumulation of fluid or food in the stomach before peristalsis returns.
4. May occur as a result of abdominal distention, which follows manipulation of abdominal organs.

Preventive Measures

 Evidence Base *American Society of PeriAnesthesia Nurses. (2010). 2010–2012 perianesthesia nursing standards and practice recommendations.* Cherry Hill, NJ: Author.

1. Insert a nasogastric (NG) tube intraoperatively for operations on the GI tract to prevent abdominal distention, which triggers vomiting.
2. Evaluate patient preoperatively for risk factors for PONV, such as being female, being a nonsmoker, and having a history of motion sickness.

Nursing Interventions

1. Encourage the patient to breathe deeply to facilitate elimination of anesthetic.
2. Support the wound during retching and vomiting; turn the patient's head to the side to prevent aspiration.
3. Discard vomitus and refresh the patient—provide mouthwash and clean linens.
4. Provide small sips of a carbonated beverage such as ginger ale, if tolerated or permitted.
5. Report excessive or prolonged vomiting so the cause may be investigated.
6. Maintain an accurate intake and output record and replace fluids as ordered.
7. Detect the presence of abdominal distention or hiccups, suggesting gastric retention.
8. Administer anti-emetic agents such as ondansetron or promethazine as directed; be aware that some of these drugs may potentiate the hypotensive effects of opioids.

DRUG ALERT Suspect idiosyncratic response to a drug if vomiting is worse when a medication is given (but diminishes thereafter).

Thirst

Causes
1. Inhibition of secretions by medication with atropine.
2. Fluid lost by way of perspiration, blood loss, and dehydration due to NPO status.

Preventive Measures
Unfortunately, postoperative thirst is a common and troublesome symptom that is usually unavoidable due to anesthesia. The immediate implementation of nursing interventions is most helpful.

Nursing Interventions
1. Administer fluids parenterally or orally, if tolerated and permitted.
2. Offer ice chips.
3. Apply a moistened gauze square over lips occasionally to humidify inspired air.
4. Allow the patient to rinse mouth with mouthwash.

Constipation and Gas Cramps

Causes
1. Trauma and manipulation of the bowel during surgery as well as opioid use.
2. More serious causes: peritonitis or abscess.

Preventive Measures
1. Encourage early ambulation to aid in promoting peristalsis.
2. Provide adequate fluid intake to promote soft stools and hydration.
3. Advocate proper diet to promote peristalsis.
4. Encourage the early use of nonopioid analgesia because many opiates increase the risk of constipation.
5. Assess bowel sounds frequently.

Nursing Interventions
1. Ask the patient about any usual remedy for constipation and try it, if appropriate.
2. Insert a gloved, lubricated finger and break up the fecal impaction manually, if necessary.
3. Administer an oil retention enema (180 to 200 mL), if prescribed, to help soften the fecal mass and facilitate evacuation.
4. Administer a return-flow enema (if prescribed) or a rectal tube to decrease painful flatulence.
5. Administer GI stimulants, laxatives, suppositories, and stool softeners, as prescribed.

Postoperative Pain

Pain is a subjective symptom, in which the patient exhibits a feeling of distress; stimulation of, or trauma to, certain nerve endings causes pain.

General Principles
1. Pain is one of the earliest symptoms that the patient expresses on return to consciousness.
2. Maximal postoperative pain occurs directly after surgery and usually diminishes significantly by 48 hours.

Clinical Manifestations
1. Autonomic.
   a. Elevation of BP.
   b. Increase in heart and pulse rate.
   c. Rapid and irregular respiration.
   d. Increase in perspiration.
2. Skeletal muscle.
   a. Increase in muscle tension or activity.
3. Psychological.
   a. Increase in irritability.
   b. Increase in apprehension.
   c. Increase in anxiety.
   d. Attention focused on pain.
   e. Complaints of pain.
4. The patient's reaction depends on:
   a. Previous experience.
   b. Anxiety or tension.
   c. State of health.
   d. Ability to be distracted.
   e. Meaning that pain has for the patient.

Preventive Measures
1. Reduce anxiety due to anticipation of pain.
2. Teach patient about pain management.
3. Review analgesics with patient and reassure that pain relief will be available quickly.
4. Establish a trusting relationship and spend time with patient.

Nursing Interventions

Use Basic Comfort Measures
1. Provide therapeutic environment—proper temperature and humidity, ventilation, visitors.
2. Massage patient's back and pressure points with soothing strokes—move patient gently and with prewarning.
3. Offer diversional activities, soft music, or favorite television program.
4. Provide for fluid needs by giving a cool drink; offer a bedpan.
5. Investigate possible causes of pain, such as bandage or adhesive that is too tight, full bladder, a cast that is too snug, or elevated temperature indicating inflammation or infection.
6. Instruct patient to splint the wound when moving.
7. Keep bedding clean, dry, and free from wrinkles and debris.

Recognize the Power of Suggestion
1. Provide reassurance that the discomfort is temporary and that the medication will aid in pain reduction.
2. Clarify patient's fears regarding the perceived significance of pain.
3. Assist patient in maintaining a positive, hopeful attitude.

Assist in Relaxation Techniques

Imagery, meditation, controlled breathing, self-hypnosis or suggestion (autogenic training), and progressive relaxation.

Apply Cutaneous Counterstimulation

1. Vibration—a vigorous form of massage that is applied to a nonoperative site. It lessens the patient's perception of pain. (Avoid applying this to the calf because it may dislodge a thrombus.)
2. Heat or cold—apply to the operative or nonoperative site as prescribed. This works best for well-localized pain. Cold has more advantages than heat and fewer unwanted adverse effects (eg, burns). Heat works well with muscle spasm.

Give Analgesics as Prescribed in a Timely Manner

1. Instruct the patient to request an analgesic before the pain becomes severe.
2. If pain occurs consistently and predictably throughout a 24-hour period, analgesics should be given around the clock—avoiding the usual "demand cycle" of dosing that sets up eventual dependency and provides less adequate pain relief.
3. Administer prescribed medication to the patient before anticipated activities and painful procedures (eg, dressing changes).
4. Monitor for possible adverse effects of analgesic therapy (eg, respiratory depression, hypotension, nausea, skin rash). Administer naloxone to relieve significant opioid-induced respiratory depression.
5. Assess and document the efficacy of analgesic therapy.

Pharmacologic Management

Oral and Parenteral Analgesia

1. Surgical patients are commonly prescribed a parenteral analgesic for 2 to 4 days or until the incisional pain abates. At that time, an oral analgesic, opioid, or nonopioid will be prescribed.
2. Although the health care provider is responsible for prescribing the appropriate medication, it is the nurse's responsibility to make sure the drug is given safely and assessed for efficacy.

 NURSING ALERT The patient who remains sedated due to analgesia is at risk for complications such as aspiration, respiratory depression, atelectasis, hypotension, falls, and poor postoperative course.

 DRUG ALERT Opioid "potentiators," such as hydroxyzine, may further sedate the patient.

Patient-Controlled Analgesia (PCA)

1. Benefits.
   a. Bypasses the delays inherent in traditional analgesic administration (the "demand cycle").
   b. Medication is administered by IV, producing more rapid pain relief and greater consistency in patient response.
   c. The patient retains control over pain relief (added placebo and relaxation effects).
   d. Decreased nursing time in frequent delivery of analgesics.

2. Contraindications.
   a. Generally, patients younger than age 10 or 11 (depends on the weight of the child and facility policy).
   b. Patients with cognitive impairment (delirium, dementia, mental illness, hemodynamic or respiratory impairment).
3. A portable PCA device delivers a preset dosage of opioid (usually morphine). An adjustable "lockout interval" controls the frequency of dose administration, preventing another dose from being delivered prematurely. An example of PCA settings might be a dose of 1 mg morphine with a lockout interval of 6 minutes (total possible dose is 10 mg per hour).
4. Patient pushes a button to activate the device.
5. Instruction about PCA should occur preoperatively; some patients fear being overdosed by the machine and require reassurance.

Epidural Analgesia

1. Requires injections of opioids into the epidural space by way of a catheter inserted by an anesthesiologist under aseptic conditions (see Figure 7-3, page 118).
2. Benefit: provides for longer periods of analgesia.
3. Disadvantages.
   a. The epidural catheter's proximity to the spinal nerves and spinal canal, along with its potential for catheter migration, make correct injection technique and close patient assessment imperative.
   b. Adverse effects include generalized pruritus (common), nausea, urinary retention, respiratory depression, hypotension, motor block, and sensory or sympathetic block. These adverse effects are related to the opioid used (usually a preservative-free morphine or fentanyl) and catheter position.
4. Strict sterile technique is necessary when inserting the epidural catheter.
5. Opioid-related adverse effects are reversed with naloxone.
6. The nurse ensures proper integrity of the catheter and dressing.

Postoperative Complications

Postoperative complications are a risk inherent in surgical procedures. They may interfere with the expected outcome of the surgery and may extend the patient's hospitalization and convalescence. The nurse plays a critical role in attempting to prevent complications and in recognizing their signs and symptoms immediately (see Standards of Care Guidelines 7-2, page 118).

Shock

Shock is a response of the body to decreased tissue perfusion, culminating, eventually, in cellular hypoxia and death. (See page 1216 for classification and emergency management of shock.)

Preventive Measures

1. Have blood available if there is any indication that it may be needed.
2. Accurately measure any blood loss and monitor all fluid intake and output.
3. Anticipate the progression of symptoms on earliest manifestation.
4. Monitor vital signs per facility protocol until they are stable.

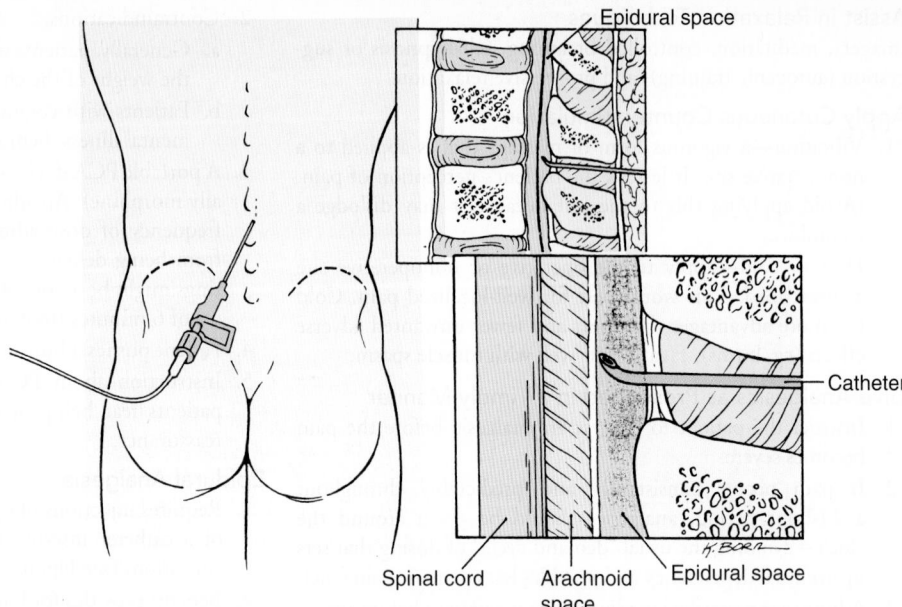

Figure 7-3. Epidural catheter placement.

5. Assess vital sign deviations; evaluate BP in relation to other physiologic parameters of shock and the patient's premorbid values. Orthostatic pulse and BP are important indicators of hypovolemic shock.
6. Prevent infection (eg, indwelling catheter care, wound care, pulmonary care) to minimize the risk of septic shock.

Hemorrhage

Hemorrhage is the escape of blood from a ruptured blood vessel. Hemorrhage from an arterial vessel may be bright red in color and come in spurts, whereas blood from a vein is dark red and comes in a steady flow. Hemorrhage may be external or internal (concealed).

Clinical Manifestations

1. Apprehension; restlessness; thirst; cold, moist, pale skin; and circumoral pallor.
2. Pulse increases, respirations become rapid and deep ("air hunger"), temperature drops.
3. With progression of hemorrhage:
   a. Decrease in cardiac output and narrowed pulse pressure.
   b. Rapidly decreasing BP, as well as hematocrit and hemoglobin (if hypovolemic shock is due to hemorrhage).

STANDARDS OF CARE GUIDELINES 7-2
Preventing and Recognizing Postoperative Complications

Care of the patient after surgery should include the following, until risk of complications has passed:

- Monitor vital signs (BP, pulse, respirations, temperature, and LOC) frequently until stable, and then periodically thereafter depending on the condition of the patient.
- Observe the wound site for drainage, odor, swelling, and redness, which could indicate infection.
- Observe the wound for intactness and stage of healing.
- Assess the patient's pain level and monitor for unusual increase in pain (which may indicate infection or other problem) as well as oversedation related to opioid administration.
- Monitor fluid status through vital signs, presence of edema, and intake and output measurements.
- Assess for presence of bowel sounds before resuming oral feedings, and monitor for abdominal distention, nausea, and vomiting, which could indicate paralytic ileus.

- Provide measures to enhance circulation of the lower extremities, such as pneumatic compression, elastic wraps, range-of-motion exercises, and early ambulation; assess for tenderness, swelling, and red streaking, which may indicate DVT.
- Assess pulmonary status including respiratory effort and rate; breath sounds; skin, mucous membrane, and nailbed color; and transcutaneous oxygen saturation.
- Make sure that the patient is voiding regularly after surgery or after catheter removal.
- Notify the surgeon if there is a significant deviation from the norm in any one of these parameters, or if a pattern of deviation is developing.

This information should serve as a general guideline only. Each patient situation presents a unique set of clinical factors and requires nursing judgment to guide care, which may include additional or alternative measures and approaches.

Nursing Interventions and Management

1. Treat the patient as described for shock (see Chapter 35).
2. Inspect the wound as a possible site of bleeding. Apply pressure dressing over an external bleeding site.
3. Increase the IV fluid infusion rate and administer blood as directed and as soon as possible.
4. Administer 100% oxygen.

 **NURSING ALERT** Numerous, rapid blood transfusions may induce coagulopathy and prolonged bleeding time. The patient should be monitored closely for signs of increased bleeding tendencies after transfusions.

Deep Vein Thrombosis

DVT occurs in pelvic veins or in the deep veins of the lower extremities in postoperative patients. The incidence of DVT varies between 10% and 40% depending on the complexity of the surgery or the severity of the underlying illness. DVT is most common after hip surgery, followed by retropubic prostatectomy and general thoracic or abdominal surgery. Venous thrombi located above the knee are considered the major source of pulmonary emboli.

Causes

1. Injury to the intimal layer of the vein wall.
2. Venous stasis.
3. Hypercoagulopathy, polycythemia.
4. High risks include obesity, prolonged immobility, cancer, smoking, estrogen use, advancing age, varicose veins, dehydration, splenectomy, and orthopedic procedures.

Clinical Manifestations

1. Most patients with DVT are asymptomatic.
2. Pain or cramp in the calf or thigh, progressing to painful swelling of the entire leg.
3. Slight fever, chills, perspiration.
4. Marked tenderness over the anteromedial surface of the thigh.
5. Intravascular clotting without marked inflammation may develop, leading to phlebothrombosis.
6. Circulation distal to the DVT may be compromised if sufficient swelling is present.

Preventive Measures and Management

1. Hydrate patient adequately postoperatively to prevent hemoconcentration.
2. Encourage leg exercises and ambulate patient as soon as permitted by surgeon.
3. Avoid restricting devices, such as tight straps, that can constrict and impair circulation.
4. Avoid rubbing or massaging calves and thighs.
5. Instruct the patient to avoid standing or sitting in one place for prolonged periods and crossing legs when seated.
6. Refrain from inserting IV catheters into legs or feet of adults.
7. Assess distal peripheral pulses, capillary refill, and sensation of lower extremities.
8. Check for positive Homans' sign—calf pain on dorsiflexion of the foot; present in nearly 30% of DVT patients.
9. Prevent the use of bed rolls or knee gatches in patients at risk because there is danger of constricting the vessels under the knee.
10. Initiate anticoagulant therapy either IV, subcutaneously, or orally as prescribed.
11. Prevent swelling and stagnation of venous blood by applying appropriately fitting elastic stockings or wrapping the legs from the toes to the groin with elastic bandage.
12. Apply external pneumatic compression intraoperatively to patients at highest risk of DVT. Pneumatic compression can reduce the risk of DVT by 30% to 50% (see Figure 7-4).

Pulmonary Complications

Causes and Clinical Manifestations

1. Atelectasis.
   a. Incomplete expansion of the lung or portion of it occurring within 48 hours of surgery.
   b. Attributed to absence of periodic deep breaths.
   c. A mucus plug closes a bronchiole, causing the alveoli distal to the plug to collapse.
   d. Symptoms are typically absent—may comprise mild to severe tachypnea, tachycardia, cough, fever, hypotension, and decreased breath sounds and chest expansion of the affected side.

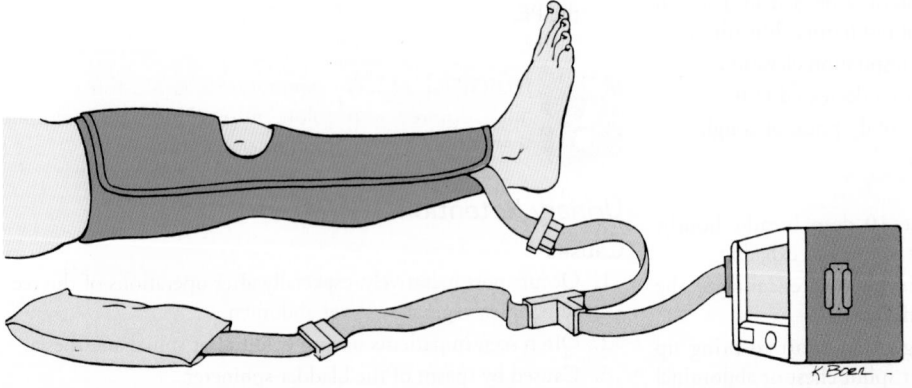

Figure 7-4. Pneumatic compression. Pressures of 35 to 20 mm Hg are sequentially applied from ankle to thigh, producing an increase in blood flow velocity and improved venous clearing.

2. Aspiration.
   a. Caused by the inhalation of food, gastric contents, water, or blood into the tracheobronchial system.
   b. Anesthetic agents and opioids depress the central nervous system, causing inhibition of gag or cough reflexes.
   c. NG tube insertion renders upper and lower esophageal sphincters partially incompetent.
   d. Gross aspiration has 50% mortality.
   e. Symptoms depend on the severity of aspiration (it may be silent); usually evidence of atelectasis occurs within 2 minutes of aspiration; other symptoms: tachypnea, dyspnea, cough, bronchospasm, wheezing, rhonchi, crackles, hypoxia, and frothy sputum.
3. Pneumonia.
   a. An inflammatory response in which cellular material replaces alveolar gas.
   b. In the postoperative patient, most commonly caused by gram-negative bacilli due to impaired oropharyngeal defense mechanisms.
   c. Predisposing factors include atelectasis, upper respiratory infection, copious secretions, aspiration, dehydration, prolonged intubation or tracheostomy, history of smoking, impaired normal host defenses (cough reflex, mucociliary system, alveolar macrophage activity).
   d. Symptoms include dyspnea, tachypnea, pleuritic chest pain, fever, chills, hemoptysis, cough (rusty or purulent sputum), and decreased breath sounds over the involved area.

Preventive Measures

1. Report evidence of upper respiratory infection to the surgeon.
2. Suction nasopharyngeal or bronchial secretions if the patient can't clear his or her own airway.
3. Use proper patient positioning to prevent regurgitation and aspiration.
4. Recognize the predisposing causes of pulmonary complications:
   a. Infections—mouth, nose, sinuses, throat.
   b. Aspiration of vomitus.
   c. History of heavy smoking, chronic pulmonary disease.
   d. Obesity.
5. Avoid oversedation.

Nursing Interventions and Management

1. Monitor the patient's progress carefully on a daily basis to detect early signs and symptoms of respiratory difficulties.
   a. Slight temperature, pulse, and respiration elevations.
   b. Apprehension and restlessness or a decreased LOC.
   c. Complaints of chest pain, signs of dyspnea, or cough.
2. Promote full aeration of the lungs.
   a. Turn the patient frequently.
   b. Encourage the patient to take 10 deep breaths hourly, holding each breath to a count of five and exhaling.
   c. Use a spirometer or other device that encourages the patient to ventilate more effectively.
   d. Assist the patient in coughing in an effort to bring up mucus secretions. Have patient splint chest or abdominal wound to minimize discomfort associated with deep breathing and coughing.
   e. Encourage and assist the patient to ambulate as early as the health care provider will allow.
3. Initiate specific measures for particular pulmonary problems.
   a. Provide cool mist or heated nebulizer for the patient exhibiting signs of bronchitis or thick secretions.
   b. Encourage the patient to take fluids to help "liquefy" secretions and facilitate expectoration (in pneumonia).
   c. Elevate the head of the bed and ensure proper administration of prescribed oxygen.
   d. Prevent abdominal distention—NG tube insertion may be necessary.
   e. Administer prescribed antibiotics for pulmonary infections.

Pulmonary Embolism

Causes

1. Pulmonary embolism (PE) is caused by the obstruction of one or more pulmonary arterioles by an embolus originating somewhere in the venous system or in the right side of the heart.
2. Postoperatively, the majority of emboli develop in the pelvic or iliofemoral veins before becoming dislodged and traveling to the lungs.

Clinical Manifestations

1. Sharp, stabbing pains in the chest.
2. Anxiousness and cyanosis.
3. Pupillary dilation, profuse perspiration.
4. Rapid and irregular pulse becoming imperceptible—leads rapidly to death.
5. Dyspnea, tachypnea, hypoxemia.
6. Pleural friction rub (occasionally).

Nursing Interventions and Management

1. Administer oxygen with the patient in an upright sitting position (if possible).
2. Reassure and calm the patient.
3. Monitor vital signs, ECG, and arterial blood gases.
4. Treat for shock or heart failure, as directed.
5. Give analgesics or sedatives, as directed, to control pain or apprehension.
6. Prepare for anticoagulation or thrombolytic therapy or surgical intervention. Management depends on the severity of the PE.

 NURSING ALERT Massive PE is life-threatening and requires immediate intervention to maintain the patient's cardiorespiratory status.

Urinary Retention

Causes

1. Occurs postoperatively, especially after operations of the rectum, anus, vagina, or lower abdomen.
2. Often seen in patients having epidural or spinal anesthesia.
3. Caused by spasm of the bladder sphincter.

4. More common in male patients due to inherent increases in urethral resistance to urine flow.

5. Can lead to urinary tract infection and possibly renal failure.

Clinical Manifestations

1. Inability to void or voiding small amounts at frequent intervals.
2. Palpable bladder.
3. Lower abdominal discomfort.

Preventive Measures and Management

1. Help patient to sit or stand (if permissible) because many patients are unable to void while lying in bed.
2. Provide patient with privacy.
3. Run tap water—frequently, the sound or sight of running water relaxes spasm of bladder sphincter.
4. Use warmth to relax sphincters (eg, a sitz bath or warm compresses).
5. Notify health care provider if the patient does not urinate regularly after surgery.

NURSING ALERT Recognize that when a patient voids small amounts (30 to 60 mL every 15 to 30 minutes), this may be a sign of an overdistended bladder with "overflow" of urine.

6. Administer bethanechol I.M., if prescribed, to reduce bladder spasm.
7. Catheterize only when all other measures are unsuccessful. SCIP recommends removing an indwelling catheter within 24 hours. Use of bladder scanner can reduce the need of catheterization by checking for residual urine noninvasively.

Evidence Base Palese, A., Buchini, S., Deroma, L., et al. (2010). The effectiveness of the ultrasound bladder scanner in reducing urinary tract infections: A meta-analysis. *Journal of Clinical Nursing, 19*(21–22), 2970–2979.

Intestinal Obstruction

Intestinal obstructions result in a partial or complete impairment to the forward flow of intestinal contents. Most obstructions occur in the small bowel, especially at its narrowest point—the ileum. (See page xxx for a full discussion of intestinal obstruction.)

Preventive Measures and Management

1. Monitor for adequate bowel sound return after surgery. Assess bowel sounds and the degree of abdominal distention (may need to measure abdominal girth); document these findings every shift.
2. Monitor and document characteristics of emesis and NG drainage.
3. Relieve abdominal distention by passing a nasoenteric suction tube as ordered.
4. Replace fluid and electrolytes.
5. Monitor fluid, electrolyte (especially potassium and sodium), and acid-base status.
6. Administer opioids judiciously because these medications may further suppress peristalsis.

7. Prepare the patient for surgical intervention if the obstruction continues unresolved.
8. Closely monitor the patient for signs of shock.
9. Provide frequent reassurance to the patient; use nontraditional methods to promote comfort (touch, relaxation, imagery).

Wound Infection

Wound infections are the second most common health care–related infection. The infection may be limited to the surgical site (60% to 80%) or may affect the patient systemically.

Causes

1. Exposed tissues during long operations, operations on contaminated structures, gross obesity, old age, chronic hypoxemia, and malnutrition are directly related to an increased infection rate.
2. The patient's own flora is most commonly implicated in wound infections (*Staphylococcus aureus*).
3. Other common culprits in wound infection include *Escherichia coli, Klebsiella, Enterobacter,* and *Proteus*.
4. Wound infections typically present 5 to 7 days postoperatively.
5. Factors affecting the extent of infection include:
   a. Type, virulence, and quantity of contaminating microorganisms.
   b. Presence of foreign bodies or devitalized tissue.
   c. Location and nature of the wound.
   d. Amount of dead space or presence of hematoma.
   e. Immune response of the patient.
   f. Presence of adequate blood supply to wound.
   g. Presurgical condition of the patient (eg, age, alcoholism, diabetes, malnutrition).

Clinical Manifestations

1. Redness, excessive swelling, tenderness, warmth.
2. Red streaks in the skin near the wound.
3. Pus or other discharge from the wound.
4. Tender, enlarged lymph nodes in the axillary region or groin closest to the wound.
5. Foul smell from the wound.
6. Generalized body chills or fever.
7. Elevated temperature and pulse.
8. Increasing pain from the incision site.

GERONTOLOGIC ALERT Older adults do not readily produce an inflammatory response to infection, so they may not present with fever, redness, and swelling. Increasing pain, fatigue, anorexia, and mental status changes are signs of infection in older patients.

NURSING ALERT Mild, transient fevers appear postoperatively due to tissue necrosis, hematoma, or cauterization. Higher sustained fevers arise with the following four most common postoperative complications: atelectasis (within the first 48 hours); wound infections (in 5 to 7 days); urinary infections (in 5 to 8 days); and thrombophlebitis (in 7 to 14 days).

Preventive Measures and Management

1. Preoperative.
   a. Encourage the patient to achieve an optimal nutritional level. Enteral or parenteral alimentation may be ordered preoperatively to reduce hypoproteinemia with weight loss.
   b. Reduce preoperative hospitalization to a minimum to avoid acquiring nosocomial infections.
2. Operative.
   a. Follow strict sterile technique throughout the operative procedure.
   b. When a wound has exudate, fibrin, desiccated fat, or non-viable skin, it is not approximated by primary closure but through secondary (delayed) closure.
3. Postoperative.
   a. Keep dressings intact, reinforcing if necessary, until prescribed otherwise.
   b. Use strict sterile technique when dressings are changed.
   c. Monitor and document the amount, type, and location of drainage. Ensure that all drains are working properly. (See Table 7-1 for expected drainage amounts from common types of drains and tubes.)
4. Postoperative care of an infected wound.
   a. The surgeon removes one or more stitches, separates the wound edges, and looks for infection using a hemostat as a probe.
   b. A culture is taken and sent to the laboratory for bacterial analysis.
   c. Wound irrigation may be done; have an aseptic syringe and saline available.
   d. A drain may be inserted or the wound may be packed with sterile gauze.

Table 7-1	Expected Drainage from Tubes and Catheters	
DEVICE	**SUBSTANCE**	**DAILY DRAINAGE**
• Foley catheter • Ileal conduit • Suprapubic catheter	Urine	500–700 mL/24 hour first 48 hour; then 1,500–2,500 mL/24 hour
• Gastrostomy tube	Gastric contents	Up to 1,500 mL/24 hour
• Chest tube	Blood, pleural fluid, air	Varies: 500–1,000 mL first 24 hour
• Ileostomy	Small bowel contents	Up to 4,000 mL in first 24 hour; then < 500 mL/24 hour
• Miller-Abbott tube	Intestinal contents	Up to 3,000 mL/24 hour
• NG tube	Gastric contents	Up to 1,500 mL/24 hour
• T-tube	Bile	500 mL/24 hour

e. Antibiotics are prescribed.
f. Wet-to-dry dressings may be applied (see page 130).
g. If deep infection is suspected, the patient may be taken back to the operating room.

Wound Dehiscence and Evisceration

Causes

1. Commonly occurs between the fifth and eighth day postoperatively when the incision has weakest tensile strength; greatest strength is found between the first and third postoperative day.
2. Chiefly associated with abdominal surgery.
3. This catastrophe is commonly related to:
   a. Inadequate sutures or excessively tight closures (the latter compromises blood supply).
   b. Hematomas; seromas.
   c. Infections.
   d. Excessive coughing, hiccups, retching, distention.
   e. Poor nutrition; immunosuppression.
   f. Uremia; diabetes mellitus.
   g. Steroid use.

Preventive Measures

1. Apply an abdominal binder for heavy or elderly patients or those with weak or pendulous abdominal walls.
2. Encourage the patient to splint the incision while coughing.
3. Monitor for and relieve abdominal distention.
4. Encourage proper nutrition with emphasis on adequate amounts of protein and vitamin C.

Clinical Manifestations

1. Dehiscence is indicated by a sudden discharge of serosanguineous fluid from the wound.
2. Patient complains that something suddenly "gave way" in the wound.
3. In an intestinal wound, the edges of the wound may part and the intestines may gradually push out. Observe for drainage of peritoneal fluid on dressing (clear or serosanguineous fluid).

Nursing Interventions and Management

1. Stay with patient and have someone notify the surgeon immediately.
2. If the intestines are exposed, cover with sterile, moist saline dressings.
3. Monitor vital signs and watch for shock.
4. Keep patient on absolute bed rest.
5. Instruct patient to bend the knees, with head of the bed elevated in semi-Fowler's position to relieve abdominal tension.
6. Assure patient that the wound will be properly cared for; attempt to keep patient calm and relaxed.
7. Prepare patient for surgery and repair of the wound.

Psychological Disturbances

Depression

1. Cause—perceived loss of health or stamina, pain, altered body image, various drugs, and anxiety about an uncertain future.

2. Clinical manifestations—withdrawal, restlessness, insomnia, nonadherence to therapeutic regimens, tearfulness, and expressions of hopelessness.
3. Nursing interventions and management.
   a. Clarify misconceptions about surgery and its future implications.
   b. Listen to, reassure, and support the patient.
   c. If appropriate, introduce the patient to representatives of ostomy, mastectomy, or amputee support groups.
   d. Involve the patient's family and support people in care; psychiatric consultation is obtained for severe depression.

Delirium

1. Cause—prolonged anesthesia, cardiopulmonary bypass, drug reactions, sepsis, alcoholism (delirium tremens), electrolyte imbalances, and other metabolic disorders.
2. Clinical manifestations—disorientation, hallucinations, perceptual distortions, paranoid delusions, reversed day–night pattern, agitation, insomnia; delirium tremens often appears within 72 hours of last alcoholic drink and may include autonomic overactivity—tachycardia, dilated pupils, diaphoresis, and fever.
3. Nursing interventions and management.
   a. Assist with the assessment and treatment of the underlying cause (restore fluid and electrolyte balance, discontinue the offending drug).
   b. Reorient the patient to environment and time.
   c. Keep surroundings calm.
   d. Explain in detail every procedure done to the patient.
   e. Sedate the patient, as ordered, to reduce agitation, prevent exhaustion, and promote sleep. Assess for oversedation.
   f. Allow extended periods of uninterrupted sleep.
   g. Reassure family members with clear explanations of the patient's aberrant behavior.
   h. Have contact with the patient as much as possible; apply restraints to the patient only as a last resort if safety is in question and if ordered by the health care provider.

WOUND CARE
Wounds and Wound Healing

A *wound* is a disruption in the continuity and regulatory processes of tissue cells; *wound healing* is the restoration of that continuity. Wound healing, however, may not restore normal cellular function.

Wound Classification

Mechanism of Injury

1. Incised wounds—made by a clean cut of a sharp instrument, such as a surgical incision with a scalpel.
2. Contused wounds—made by blunt force that typically does not break the skin but causes considerable tissue damage with bruising and swelling.
3. Lacerated wounds—made by an object that tears tissues, producing jagged, irregular edges; examples include glass, jagged wire, and blunt knife.
4. Puncture wounds—made by a pointed instrument, such as an ice pick, bullet, or nail.

Degree of Contamination

1. Clean—an aseptically made wound, as in surgery, that does not enter the alimentary, respiratory, or genitourinary tracts.
2. Clean-contaminated—an aseptically made wound that enters the respiratory, alimentary, or genitourinary tracts. These wounds have slightly higher probability of wound infection than do clean wounds.
3. Contaminated—wounds exposed to excessive amounts of bacteria. These wounds may be open (avulsive) and accidentally made, or may be the result of surgical operations in which there are major breaks in sterile techniques or gross spillage from the gastrointestinal tract.
4. Infected—a wound that retains devitalized tissue or involves preoperatively existing infection or perforated viscera. Such wounds are often left open to drain.

Physiology of Wound Healing

The phases of wound healing—inflammation, reconstruction (proliferation), and maturation (remodeling)—involve continuous and overlapping processes.

Inflammatory Phase (lasts 1 to 5 days)

1. Vascular and cellular responses are immediately initiated when tissue is cut or injured.
2. Transient vasoconstriction occurs immediately at the site of injury, lasting 5 to 10 minutes, along with the deposition of a fibrinoplatelet clot to help control bleeding.
3. Subsequent dilation of small venules occurs; antibodies, plasma proteins, plasma fluids, leukocytes, and red blood cells leave the microcirculation to permeate the general area of injury, causing edema, redness, warmth, and pain.
4. Localized vasodilation is the result of direct action by histamine, serotonin, and prostaglandins.
5. Polymorphic leukocytes (neutrophils) and monocytes enter the wound to engage in destruction and ingestion of wound debris. Monocytes predominate during this phase.
6. Basal cells at the wound edges undergo mitosis; resultant daughter cells enlarge, flatten, and creep across the wound surface to eventually approximate the wound edges.

Proliferative Phase (lasts 2 to 20 days)

1. Fibroblasts (connective tissue cells) multiply and migrate along fibrin strands that are thought to serve as a matrix.
2. Endothelial budding occurs on nearby blood vessels, forming new capillaries that penetrate and nourish the injured tissue.
3. The combination of budding capillaries and proliferating fibroblasts is called *granulation tissue*.
4. Active collagen synthesis by fibroblasts begins by the fifth to seventh day, and the wound gains tensile strength.
5. By 3 weeks, skin obtains 30% of its preinjury tensile strength, intestinal tissue about 65%, and fascia 20%.

Remodeling Phase (21 days to months or years)

1. Scar tissue is composed primarily of collagen and ground substance (mucopolysaccharide, glycoproteins, electrolytes, and water).

2. From the start of collagen synthesis, collagen fibers undergo a process of lysis and regeneration. The collagen fibers become more organized, aligning more closely to each other and increasing in tensile strength.

3. The overall bulk and form of the scar continue to change once maturation has started.

4. Typically, collagen production drops off; however, if collagen production greatly exceeds collagen lysis, keloid (greatly hypertrophied, deforming scar tissue) will form.

5. Normal maturation of the wound is clinically observed as an initial red, raised, hard immature scar that molds into a flat, soft, and pale mature scar.

6. The scar tissue will never achieve greater than 80% of its pre-injury tensile strength.

Types of Wound Healing

(See Figure 7-5.)

First Intention Healing (Primary Closure)

1. Wounds are made sterile by minor debridement and irrigation, with a minimum of tissue damage and tissue reaction; wound edges are properly approximated with sutures.

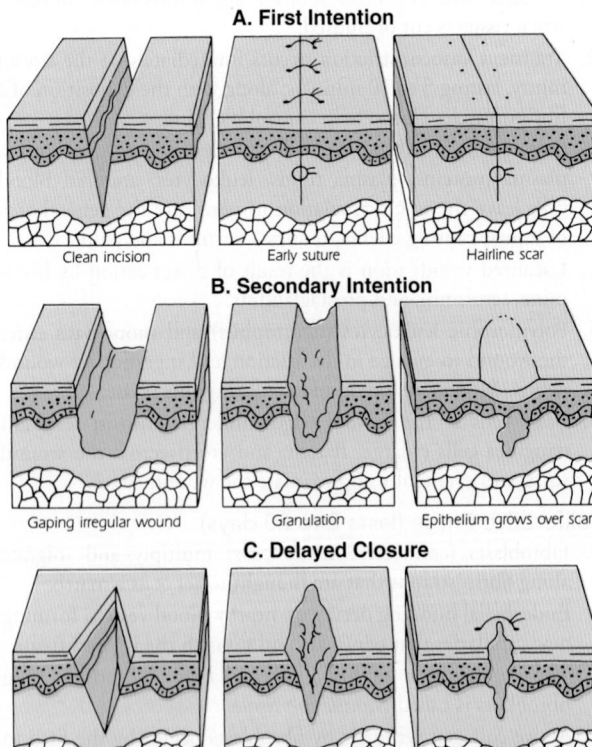

Figure 7-5. Classification of wound healing. (A) First intention: A clean incision is made with primary closure; there is minimal scarring. **(B)** Second intention: The wound is left open so that granulation can occur; a large scar results. **(C)** Delayed closure: The wound is initially left open and later closed when there is no further evidence of infection.

2. Granulation tissue is not visible and scar formation is typically minimal (keloid may still form in susceptible people).

Secondary Intention Healing (Granulation)

1. Wounds are left open to heal spontaneously or are surgically closed at a later date; they need not be infected.

2. Examples in which wounds may heal by secondary intention include burns, traumatic injuries, ulcers, and suppurative infected wounds.

3. The cavity of the wound fills with a red, soft, sensitive tissue (granulation tissue), which bleeds easily. A scar (cicatrix) eventually forms.

4. In infected wounds, drainage may be accomplished by use of special dressings and drains. Healing is thus improved.

5. In wounds that are later sutured, the two opposing granulation surfaces are brought together.

6. Secondary intention healing produces a deeper, wider scar.

Wound Management

Many factors promote wound healing, such as adequate nutrition, cleanliness, rest, and position, along with the patient's underlying psychological and physiologic state. Of added importance is the application of appropriate dressings and drains. See Procedure Guidelines 7-1 and 7-2, pages 125 to 129.

Dressings

Purpose of Dressings

1. To protect the wound from mechanical injury.

2. To splint or immobilize the wound.

3. To absorb drainage.

4. To prevent contamination from bodily discharges (feces, urine).

5. To promote hemostasis, as in pressure dressings.

6. To debride the wound by combining capillary action and the entwining of necrotic tissue within its mesh.

7. To inhibit or kill microorganisms by using dressings with antiseptic or antimicrobial properties.

8. To provide a physiologic environment conducive to healing.

9. To provide mental and physical comfort for the patient.

10. To encourage healing by applying localized subatmospheric pressure at site of wound as in negative pressure dressings.

Advantages of Not Using Dressings

When the initial dressing on a clean, dry, and intact incision is removed, it is often not replaced; this may occur within 24 hours after surgery.

1. Permits better visualization of the wound.

2. Eliminates conditions necessary for growth of organisms (warmth, moisture, and darkness).

3. Minimizes adhesive tape reaction.

4. Aids bathing.

Types of Dressings

1. Dry dressings.

   a. Used primarily for wounds closing by primary intention.

   b. Offers good wound protection, absorption of drainage, and aesthetics for the patient and provides pressure, if needed, for hemostasis.

(Text continues on page 130)

PROCEDURE GUIDELINES 7-1

Changing Surgical Dressings

GENERAL CONSIDERATIONS

1. The procedure of changing dressings, then examining and cleaning the wound, uses the principles of sterility.

2. The initial dressing change is usually done by the surgeon, especially for craniotomy, orthopedic, or thoracotomy procedures; subsequent dressing changes are the nurse's responsibility.

EQUIPMENT

Sterile
- Gloves
- Scissors, forceps (disposable packs available)
- Appropriate dressing materials
- Sterile saline solution
- Cotton-tipped swabs
- Culture tubes (if infection suspected)
- For draining a wound: add extra gauze and packing material, absorbent pads, and an irrigation set

Unsterile
- Gloves
- Plastic bag for discarded dressings
- Tape, proper size and type
- Pads to protect the patient's bed
- Gown for the nurse if the wound is purulent or infected

PROCEDURE

Nursing Action	Rationale
Preparatory phase	
1. Inform the patient of dressing change. Explain the procedure and have the patient lie in bed.	1. Enhances cooperation.
2. Avoid changing dressings near mealtime.	2. May affect appetite.
3. Ensure privacy by drawing the curtains or closing the door; expose the dressing site.	3. May reduce anxiety.
4. Respect the patient's modesty and prevent the patient from being chilled.	4–5. For protection of the patient.
5. Wash your hands thoroughly.	
6. Place dressing supplies on a clean, flat surface (overbed table).	6. Increases efficiency.
7. If linen protection is needed, place a clean towel or plastic bag under part of the body where the wound is located.	
8. Cut (or tear) off pieces of tape to be used in dressing change.	8. Having all supplies ready to use increases efficiency.
9. Place a disposable bag nearby to collect soiled dressings.	
10. Determine how many and what types of dressings are necessary. Open each dressing by peeling apart the edges of the package (maintain the sterility of the dressing). Leave each dressing within the open package.	10. Prepare enough supplies, but take care not to waste dressings.
Removing old dressing	
1. Put on gloves.	1. Unsterile gloves are sufficient if care is used not to touch wound.
2. Loosen all tape and gently pull tape ends toward the wound. It helps to hold skin taut with one hand while carefully peeling up an edge of the tape with the other hand.	2. This process is less painful and less disturbing to the healing process (avoids pulling the wound edges apart and traumatizing sensitive skin).

(continued)

PROCEDURE GUIDELINES 7-1 (continued)

Changing Surgical Dressings

PROCEDURE (continued)

Nursing Action	Rationale
3. Remove old dressings, one layer at a time, and place them in a disposable bag.	3. Hasty removal of dressing can cause trauma to the wound and dislodge existing drains.
4. Removal of adherent dressings may be facilitated by moistening dressing with sterile saline solution.	4. This process is less painful and less traumatic to the delicate healing tissues.

Obtaining a wound culture

Nursing Action	Rationale
1. Use sterile technique.	1. Prevents contamination of a clean wound or culture media, or to prevent further contamination of a "dirty" wound.
2. Open the sterile package of gloves; open the package containing the sterile syringe and needle; open the package containing a cotton-tipped culture swab. Keep all products within their sterile open packages until use.	2. Preparation for sterile procedure.
3. Put on sterile gloves.	
4. Aspirate a generous amount of drainage liquid into the syringe; inject it into an anaerobic tube. If liquid material is unobtainable, swab the desired area with a cotton-tipped culture swab, attempting to get maximum saturation.	4. It is important to collect culture specimen before wound is cleaned. The swab is the more common approach to wound cultures.
5. Make sure that specimen is properly labeled and sent to the laboratory for study.	

Cleansing the simple surgical wound

Nursing Action	Rationale
1. Use sterile technique.	
2. Open the package of sterile gloves; open the sterile cleaning supplies (cotton-tipped applicators, sterile gauze sponges, sterile solution cup, sterile saline solution).	2. Preparation for sterile procedure. Pour a sterile solution (preferably saline) into the solution cup before putting on sterile gloves.
3. Put on sterile gloves.	
4. Clean along the wound edges using a small circular motion from one end of the incision to the other; be sure to clean each side of the wound separately. Repeat the process using another moistened gauze or swab until the entire incision is clean. Do not scrub back and forth across the incision line.	4. Prevents contamination and mechanical trauma of wound.
5. Sterile saline solution is the cleansing agent of choice. Topical antiseptics (ie, povidone-iodine, chlorhexidine) may be used on intact skin surrounding the wound but should never be used within the wound.	5. Most of the antiseptic agents are caustic to tissues and impair healing. The old saying "Never put anything in a wound that you couldn't put in your eye" is a truthful one.
6. Repeat the same process with the drain site. Always clean the drain site separately from the primary incision site.	6. Reduces the risk of cross-contamination.
7. Discard used cleaning supplies in the disposable bag.	7. This will be incinerated later.
8. Pat the incision site and drain the site dry with a sterile dressing sponge.	8. Prepares the wound for final dressing.

Dressing the wound

Nursing Action	Rationale
1. Maintain sterile technique with the use of sterile gloves.	
2. After the wound is dry, apply the appropriate dressing, taking into consideration the nature of wound.	
3. Tape dressing, using only the amount of tape required for secure attachment of dressing. Applying a "skin prep" on site to be taped can facilitate fixation and reduce irritation.	3. Excessive use of tape can cause irritation and trauma to intact skin.

PROCEDURE GUIDELINES 7-1 *(continued)*

Changing Surgical Dressings

PROCEDURE *(continued)*

Nursing Action	Rationale
4. When dressing the drain site: a. Use a premade drain pad (can be prepared by making a 2-inch [5-cm] slit, with sterile scissors, in 4"× 4" gauze pad). b. Gently slip the sponge around the drain; repeat the process with the second drain sponge, placing it at a right angle to the other pad (see accompanying figure).	4. a. The slit allows gauze to fit around the drainage tube. b. Placement of the drain sponges in this manner allows for circumferential coverage of the drain site.

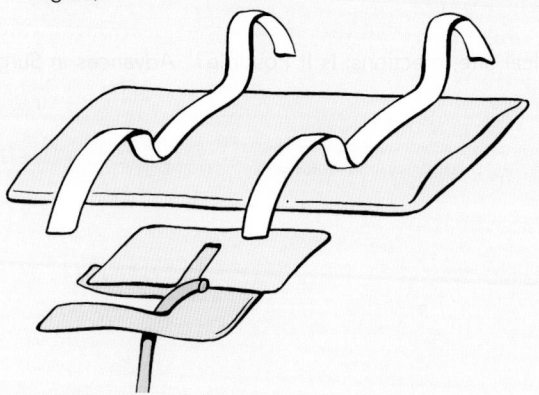

Dressing the drainage tube insertion site. Make sure that one pad is placed at a right angle to the second sponge so the slits are going in different directions. If drainage is heavy, a sterile absorbent pad or extra gauze may be placed over all.

Nursing Action	Rationale
5. When dressing an excessively draining wound: a. Consider the need for extra dressings and packing material. b. Use Montgomery straps if frequent dressing changes are required (see accompanying figure).	5. a. More dressing materials are needed to absorb excess fluid. b. Frequent dressing changes can damage surrounding, intact skin owing to the frequent application and removal of tape. Montgomery straps alleviate the problem.

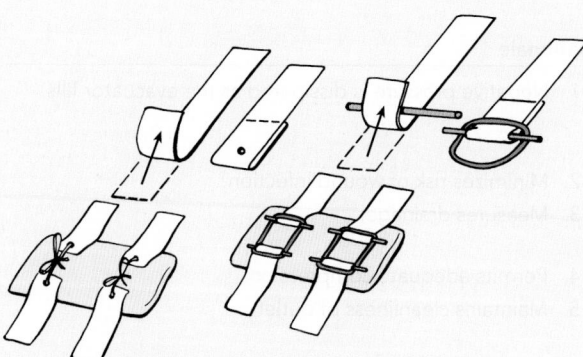

Montgomery straps; two styles are shown.

Nursing Action	Rationale
c. Excessively draining wounds may be "pouched," much like an ostomy bag. d. Protect skin surrounding wound from copious or irritating drainage (such as gastrointestinal drainage) by applying some type of skin barrier.	c. Protects surrounding skin, saves nursing time, and facilitates accurate assessment of drainage. d. Maintaining the cleanliness and integrity of surrounding tissue is essential for successful overall wound healing.

PROCEDURE GUIDELINES 7-1 *(continued)*

Changing Surgical Dressings

PROCEDURE *(continued)*

Nursing Action	Rationale
Follow-up care	
1. Assess the patient's tolerance to the procedure and help make the patient more comfortable.	
2. Discard the disposable items according to facility protocol and clean equipment that is to be reused.	2. Prevents transmission of pathogenic organisms.
3. Wash your hands.	
4. Record the nature of the procedure and the condition of the wound as well as patient reaction.	4. For continuity of care.

 Evidence Base Smith, C. Daniel. (2012). "Zero Surgical Site Infections: Is It Possible?" *Advances in Surgery* 46(1), 51–60.

PROCEDURE GUIDELINES 7-2

Using Portable Wound Suction

EQUIPMENT
- A calibrated collection container
- Nonsterile gloves

PROCEDURE

Nursing Action	Rationale
1. When the evacuator is full (200–800 mL, depending on size of evacuator), it is time to empty it. A good rule is to empty every 8 hours, or more frequently, if necessary.	1. Negative pressure is dissipated as the evacuator fills.
2. Carefully remove the plug, maintaining its sterility.	2. Minimizes risk of wound infection.
3. Empty the contents of the evacuator into the calibrated container.	3. Measures drainage.
4. Place the evacuator on a flat surface.	4. Permits adequate compression.
5. Clean the opening and the plug with an alcohol sponge.	5. Maintains cleanliness of outlet.

PROCEDURE GUIDELINES 7-2 *(continued)*

Using Portable Wound Suction

PROCEDURE *(continued)*

Nursing Action	Rationale
6. Compress the evacuator completely (see accompanying figure).	6. Removes air.

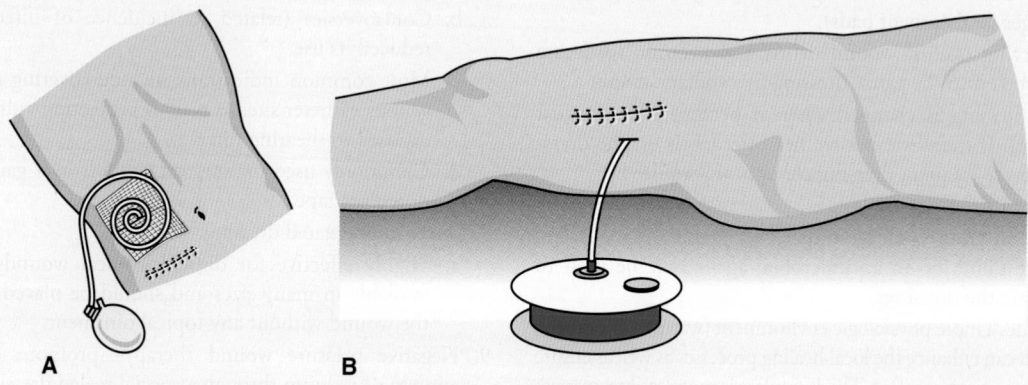

Types of surgical drains: *(**A**) Jackson-Pratt; (**B**) Hemovac. Catheters drain the incision after surgery. Drainage is drawn into the portable wound-suction unit.*

Nursing Action	Rationale
7. Replace the plug while the evacuator is compressed.	7. Reestablishes negative pressure (suction).
8. As the evacuator expands, a negative pressure of approximately 45 mm Hg is produced.	8. Any fluid and blood in tissues is sucked into the evacuator. Negative pressure is not great enough to suck the soft tissues into the holes of the drainage catheter.
9. Check system for proper operation.	9. Look for fluid entering the system; if none, look for disconnections.
10. Secure an evacuator to the patient's dressing; if the patient is ambulatory, it may be fastened to the patient's clothing.	10. Permits the patient to move without disturbing closed suction.
11. Make sure that the drainage catheters are positioned off the incisional site.	11. Minimizes the trauma and contamination of wound.
12. Wash your hands thoroughly.	12. Prevents cross-contamination with other patients and staff.
13. Record the character and amount of drainage.	13. Evaluates fluid balance.

Key Decision Point

If no drainage is observed, ensure that catheter is positioned within the wound and there are no kinks in the drain tubing. Report lack of drainage, which may signal time for removal of drain, which acts as a portal for possible wound infection.

c. Disadvantage—they adhere to the wound surface when drainage dries. (Removal can cause pain and disruption of granulation tissue.)

2. Wet-to-dry dressings.
   a. These are particularly useful for untidy or infected wounds that must be debrided and closed by secondary intention.
   b. Gauze saturated with sterile saline (preferred) or an antimicrobial solution is packed into the wound, eliminating dead space.
   c. The wet dressings are then covered by dry dressings (gauze sponges or absorbent pads).
   d. As drying occurs, wound debris and necrotic tissue are absorbed into the gauze dressing by capillary action.
   e. The dressing is changed when it becomes dry (or just before). If there is excessive necrotic debris on the dressing, more frequent dressing changes are required.

3. Wet-to-wet dressings.
   a. Used on clean open wounds or on granulating surfaces. Sterile saline or an antimicrobial agent may be used to saturate the dressings.
   b. Provides a more physiologic environment (warmth, moisture), which can enhance the local healing processes as well as ensure greater patient comfort. Thick exudate is more easily removed.
   c. Disadvantage—surrounding tissues can become macerated, there is an increased risk for infection, and bed linens become damp.

Types of Surgical Dressing Supplies

1. Hydrophobic occlusive (petroleum gauze).
   a. This is an impermeable, nonadhering dressing that protects wounds from air- and moisture-borne contamination.
   b. It is used around chest tubes and any fistula or stoma that drains digestive juices.
   c. It is relatively nonabsorptive.

2. Hydrophilic permeable (oil-based gauze, Telfa pads).
   a. Allows drainage to penetrate the dressing but remains somewhat nonadhering.
   b. For wounds with light to moderate exudate.
   c. Oil-based gauze used on abraded and open ulcerated or granulating wounds.
   d. May also be used to pack "caverns and sinuses" of large open wounds.
   e. Telfa pads are generally reserved for simple, closed, stable wounds.

3. Dressing sponges (general-use gauze sponges).
   a. Gauze sponges come in various sizes (most commonly 2″ × 2″, 4″ × 4″) and may be used for simple dry dressings, wet-to-dry dressings, or wet-to-wet dressings. Gauze allows for better absorption of drainage and necrotic wound debris.

4. All-absorbent combined dressing.
   a. Large (5″ × 9″, 8″ × 10″) cotton-filled dressing that is typically used as an "over-dressing," covering gauze or hydrophilic dressings for added wound protection, stabilization of dressings, and drainage absorption.
   b. May also be used unaccompanied over intact surgical wounds.

5. High-bulk gauze bandage ("fluffs")—primarily used for packing large wounds that are undergoing healing by secondary intention.

6. Drain sponge—a gauze sponge with a premade slit, which makes the dressing highly suitable for drain sites and tracheostomy sites.

7. Transparent film dressing.
   a. Highly elastic dressing, adjusts exceptionally well to body contours. It is permeable to oxygen and water vapor but generally impermeable to liquids and bacteria.
   b. Controversies (related to incidence of infection) have reduced its use.
   c. Most common indications include covering arterial and venous catheter sites as well as protecting vulnerable skin exposed to shearing forces.
   d. Commonly used for surgical wounds over gauze dressing to replace tape.

8. Silver impregnated dressing.
   a. Highly effective for difficult-to-heal wounds. They are available in many sizes and should be placed directly on the wound without any topical ointment.

9. Negative pressure wound therapy—promotes healing by applying a vacuum through a special sealed dressing.
   a. Evacuates wound fluid, stimulates granulation tissue and decreases bacterial colonization.
   b. Contraindicated on patients with active bleeding or taking anticoagulants.
   c. NPWT has different interface materials, safety features and recommended applications by manufacturers. Use is dependant on wound type, provider's preference for gauze or foam packing, and product available.

Drains

Purpose of Drains

1. Drains are placed in wounds only when abnormal fluid collections are present or expected.

2. Drains are placed near the incision site.
   a. Usually in compartments (eg, joints and pleural space) that are intolerant to fluid accumulation.
   b. In areas with a large blood supply (eg, the neck and kidney).
   c. In infected draining wounds.
   d. In areas that have sustained large superficial tissue dissection (eg, the breast).

3. Collection of body fluids in wounds can be harmful in the following ways:
   a. Provides culture media for bacterial growth.
   b. Causes increased pressure at surgical site, interfering with blood flow to area.
   c. Causes pressure on adjacent areas.
   d. Causes local tissue irritation and necrosis (due to fluids such as bile, pus, pancreatic juice, and urine).

Wound Drainage

1. Drains are commonly made of latex, polyvinyl chloride, or silicone and placed within either wounds or body cavities.

2. Drains placed within wounds are typically attached to portable (or, rarely, wall) suction with a collection container.

a. Examples include the Hemovac, Jackson-Pratt, and Surgivac drainage systems.

3. Drains may also be used postoperatively to form hollow connections from internal organs to the outside to drain a body fluid, such as the T-tube (bile drainage), nephrostomy, gastrostomy, jejunostomy, and cecostomy tubes.

4. Drains create a portal for entry and exit of infectious microorganisms; therefore, the risk of infection exists.

5. Drains within wounds are removed when the amount of drainage decreases over a period of days or, rarely, weeks.

6. Body fluid drains are often left in for longer periods of time.

a. Careful handling of these drains and collection bags is essential.

b. Accidental early removal may result in caustic drainage leaking within the tissues.

c. The risk is reduced within 7 to 10 days when a wall of fibrous tissue has been formed.

7. The amount of drainage varies with the procedure. Most common surgical procedures (eg, appendectomy, cholecystectomy, abdominal hysterectomy) have minimal wound drainage by the third or fourth postoperative day. Drains are not commonly used after these operations.

 NURSING ALERT The greatest amount of drainage is expected during the first 24 hours; closely monitor dressing and drains.

Nursing Process Overview

 Evidence Base Smith, C. Daniel. (2012). "Zero Surgical Site Infections: Is It Possible?" *Advances in Surgery* 46(1), 51–60.
Vancouver Island Health Authority. (2005–2008). Wound and skin care clinical guideline. Available: *www.viha.ca/ppo/learning/wound_skin_care.htm.*

Nursing Assessment

The wound should be assessed every 15 minutes while the patient is in the PACU. Thereafter, the frequency of wound assessment is determined by the nature of the wound, the degree of drainage, and the facility protocol. Assessment and documentation of the wound's status should occur at least every shift until the patient is discharged.

Determine the following, which will affect wound healing:

1. What type of surgery did the patient have?
2. Was hemostasis in the operating room effective?
3. Has the patient received blood to sustain an adequate hematocrit (and promote perfusion to wound)?
4. What is the patient's age?
5. What is the nutritional status? What was it preoperatively?

a. Is current intake of protein and vitamin C adequate?

b. Is the patient obese or cachectic?

6. What underlying medical conditions does the patient have, and what medications is he or she taking that could affect wound healing (eg, diabetes mellitus, steroids)?
7. How long has the patient been hospitalized preoperatively? (Longer preoperative facility stays can increase complications.)
8. How is the wound held together?

a. Staples, nylon sutures, adhesive strips, tension sutures, surgical skin glue.

b. If the wound is left open, how is it being treated? Is granulation tissue present?

9. Are drains in place? What kind? How many?

a. Is portable suction being used?

b. Is the amount of drainage consistent with the nature of surgery?

10. What kinds of dressings are being used?

a. Are they saturated?

b. Is the amount and type of drainage consistent with nature of the surgery?

11. How does the wound appear?

a. Is there evidence of edema, irritation, inflammation?

b. Are the wound edges well approximated?

c. Is the wound clean and dry?

12. How does the patient appear?

a. Are there signs of wound pain or discomfort?

b. Is fever or elevated white blood cell count present?

c. Does the patient express concern about the wound and potential disfigurement?

13. Does the patient understand the purpose of wound therapies, and can he or she or his or her family effectively carry out discharge instructions about wound care?

Nursing Diagnoses

- Risk for Infection related to surgical wound.
- Impaired Tissue Integrity related to surgical wound.
- Acute Pain related to wound dressing procedures.

Nursing Interventions

Preventing Infection

1. Ensure sterile technique during dressing changes.
2. Reinforce or change dressings promptly when saturated with drainage.
3. Keep drainage tubing away from the actual incision site.
4. Instruct the patient to avoid touching the incision to minimize wound contamination and injury.

Enhancing Tissue Integrity Through Healing

1. Assess the patient's nutritional intake; consult with the patient's health care provider if supplemental nutritional intake is required.
2. Minimize strain on the incision site:

a. Use appropriate tape, bandages, and binders.

b. Have the patient splint abdominal and chest incision when coughing.

c. Instruct the patient in proper way to get out of bed while minimizing incision strain (eg, for abdominal incision, have the patient turn on one side and push self up with the dependent elbow and the opposite hand).

3. Assess and accurately document the condition of the incision site each shift.

Relieving Pain

1. Give the patient prescribed medication before painful dressing changes.
2. Continue to assess for pain at incision site.
3. Consider nonpharmacologic pain relief, such as use of music therapy, relaxation exercises, and acupressure, as indicated.

Patient Education

Before discharge, instruct the patient and family on techniques and rationale for wound care.

1. Report immediately to the health care provider if the following signs of infection occur:
   a. Redness, marked swelling, tenderness, and increased warmth around wound.
   b. Pus or unusual discharge, foul odor from wound.
   c. Red streaks in skin near wound.
   d. Chills or fever (over 100° F [37.8° C]).
2. Follow the directives of the health care provider regarding activity allowances.
3. Keep the suture line clean (the patient may shower unless contraindicated by the health care provider; avoid tub bathing until wound heals); never vigorously rub near the suture line; pat dry.
4. Report to the health care provider if after 2 months the incision site continues to be red, thick, and painful to pressure (probable beginning of keloid formation).

Evaluation: Expected Outcomes

- No signs of infection.
- Wound edges well approximated without gaping.
- Pain at level 1 or 2.

POSTOPERATIVE DISCHARGE INSTRUCTIONS

It is of primary importance that the nurse makes sure that the patient has been given specific and individualized discharge instructions. These should be written by a provider and reinforced verbally by the nurse. A provider telephone contact should be included as well as information regarding follow-up care and appointments. The instructions should be signed by the patient, provider, and nurse, and a copy becomes part of the patient's chart. Forms and procedures for discharge instructions may vary per facility.

Patient Education

Rest and Activity

1. It is common to feel tired and frustrated about not being able to do all the things you want; this is normal.
2. Plan regular naps and quiet activities, gradually increasing your exercise over the following weeks.

3. When you begin to exercise more, start by taking a short walk two or three times per day. Consult your health care provider if more specific exercises are required.
4. Climbing stairs in your home may be surprisingly tiring at first. If you have difficulty with this activity, try going upstairs backward ("scooching") on your "bottom" until your strength has returned.
5. Consult your health care provider to determine the appropriate time to return to work.

Eating

1. Follow dietary instructions provided at the facility before your discharge.
2. Your appetite may be limited or you may feel bloated after meals; this problem should lessen as you become more active. (Some prescribed medications can cause this.) If symptoms persist, consult your health care provider.
3. Eat small, regular meals and make them as nourishing as possible to promote wound healing.

Sleeping

1. If sleeping is difficult because of wound discomfort, try taking your pain medication at bedtime.
2. Attempt to get sufficient sleep to aid in your recovery.

Wound Healing

1. Your wound will go through several stages of healing. After initial pain at the site, the wound may feel tingling, itchy, numb, or tight (a slight pulling sensation) as healing occurs.
2. Do not pull off any scabs because they protect the delicate new tissues underneath. They will fall off without any help when ready. Change the dressing according to the surgeon's instructions.
3. Consult your health care provider if the amount of pain in your wound increases or if you notice increased redness, swelling, or discharge from wound.

Bowels

1. Irregular bowel habits can result from changes in activity and diet or the use of some drugs.
2. Avoid straining because it can intensify discomfort in some wounds; instead, use a rocking motion while trying to pass stool.
3. Drink plenty of fluids and increase the fiber in your diet through fruits, vegetables, and grains, as tolerated.
4. It may be helpful to take a mild laxative. Consult your health care provider if you have any questions.

Bathing, Showering

1. You may get your wound wet 3 days after your operation if the initial dressing has already been changed (unless otherwise advised).
2. Showering is preferable because it allows for thorough rinsing of the wound.

3. If you are feeling too weak, place a plastic or metal chair in the shower so you can be seated during showering.

4. Be sure to dry your wound thoroughly with a clean towel and dress it as instructed before discharge.

Clothing

1. Avoid tight belts and underwear and other clothes with seams that may rub against the wound.

2. Wear loose clothing for comfort and to reduce mechanical trauma to wound.

Driving

1. Ask your health care provider when you may resume driving. Safe driving may be affected by your pain medication. In addition, any violent jarring from an accident may disrupt your wound.

Bending and Lifting

1. How much bending, stretching, and lifting you are allowed depends on the location and nature of your surgery.

2. Typically, for most major surgeries, you should avoid lifting anything heavier than 5 lb for 4 to 8 weeks.

3. It is ideal to obtain home assistance for the first 2 to 3 weeks after discharge.

SELECTED REFERENCES

Aldini, N., Fine, H., & Giordino, R. (2008). From Hippocrates to tissue engineering: Surgical strategies in wound treatment. *World Journal of Surgery, 32*(9), 2114–2121.

Alexander, J. W., Solomkin, J. S, & Edwards, M. J. (2011). Updated recommendations for control of surgical site infections. *Annals of Surgery, 253*(6), 1082–1093.

American Society of PeriAnesthesia Nurses. (2006). The American Society of PeriAnesthesia Nurses' (ASPAN) evidence-based clinical practice guideline for the prevention and/or treatment of postoperative nausea and vomiting and postdischarge nausea and vomiting in adult patients. *Journal of PeriAnesthesia Nursing, 12*(4), 230–250.

American Society of PeriAnesthesia Nurses. (2010). *2010–2012 perianesthesia nursing standards and practice recommendations*. Cherry Hill, NJ: Author.

American Society of Anesthesiologists Committee on Standards and Practice Parameters. (2011) Practice guidelines for preoperative fasting and the use of pharmacologic agents to reduce the risk of pulmonary aspiration: Application to healthy patients undergoing elective procedures. An updated report. *Anesthesiology, 114*(34), 495–511.

Association of periOperative Registered Nurses. (2011). *AORN recommended practices for monitoring the patient receiving intravenous sedation*. Denver, CO: Author.

Association of periOperative Registered Nurses. (2011). *AORN standards and recommended practices* (11th ed.). Denver, CO: Author.

Association of periOperative Registered Nurses. (2011). *Recommended practice for managing the patient receiving moderate sedation/analgesia*. Denver, CO: Author.

Association of periOperative Registered Nurses. (2012). *Perioperative standards and recommended practices* (12th ed.). Denver, CO: Author.

Berg, A., Fleisher, S., Kuss, O., et al. (2012). Timing of dressing removal in the healing of surgical wounds by primary intention. *Journal of Advanced Nursing, 68*(2):264–70.

Cohen, I. K. (2007). Lessons from the history of wound healing. *Clinical Dermatology, 25*(l), 3–8.

Dolezal, D., Cullen, L., Harp, J., et al. (2011). Implementing preoperative screening of undiagnosed obstructive sleep apnea. *Journal of PeriAnesthesia Nursing, 26*(5), 338–342

Ead, H. (2009). Meeting the challenge of obstructive sleep apnea: Developing a protocol that for the promotion of perioperative normothermia, *Journal of PeriAnesthesia Nursing, 24*(2), 103–113.

Fossum, S. A. (2011). Focus on safety: Meeting notes from the 2010 ASA Annual Meeting. *Journal of PeriAnesthesia Nursing, 26*(3), 206–210.

Godden, B. (2011). Where does capnography fit into the PACU? *Journal of PeriAnesthesia Nursing, 26*(6), 408–410.

Hooper, V. D. (2009). An introduction to the ASPAN evidence-based clinical practice guideline for the promotion of perioperative normothermia. *Journal of PeriAnesthesia Nursing, 24*(5), 269–270.

Iacono, M. V. (2009). Handoff communication: Opportunities for improvement. *Journal of Perianesthesia, 24*(5), 324–326.

The Joint Commission. (2011). National Patient Safety Goals effective July 1, 2011. Available: *www.jointcommission.org/assets/1/6/NPSG_EPs_Scoring_HAP_20110706.pdf*.

The Joint Commission. (2011). Surgical Care Improvement Project. Available: *www.jointcommission.org/surgical_care_improvement_project*.

Kibler, V. A., Hayes, R. M., Johnson, D. E., et al. (2012). Early postoperative ambulation: Back to basics. *AJN, 112*(4). 63–69.

Lakdawala, L. (2011). Creating a safer perioperative environment with an obstructive sleep apnea screening tool. *Journal of PeriAnesthesia Nursing, 26*(1), 15–24.

Lipshutz, A., & Gropper, M. (2009) Perioperative Glycemic Control. *Journal of Anesthesiology, 110*, 408–421.

Martindell, D. (2012). The safe use of negative-pressure wound therapy. *AJN, 112*(6): 59–62.

Murphy, M. J., Hooper, V. D., Sullivan, E., et al. (2006). Identification of risk factors for postoperative nausea and vomiting in the perianesthesia adult patient. *Journal of PeriAnesthesia Nursing, 21*(6), 377–384.

Palese, A., Buchini, S., Deroma, L., et al. (2010). The effectiveness of the ultrasound bladder scanner in reducing urinary tract infections: A meta-analysis. *Journal of Clinical Nursing, 19*(21–22), 2970–2979.

Pasero, C. (2009). Assessment of sedation during opioid administration for pain management. *Journal of PeriAnesthesia Nursing, 24*(3), 186–190.

Rothrock, C. J. (2011). *Alexander's care of the patient in surgery* (14th ed.). St. Louis, MO: Mosby.

Smith, C. Daniel. (2012). "Zero Surgical Site Infections: Is It Possible?" *Advances in Surgery 46*(1), 51–60.

Stewart, M. W. (2009). Obesity and the perianesthesia patient. *Journal of PeriAnesthesia Nursing, 24*(5), 332–334

Stoetling, R. K., & Miller, R. D. (2007). *Basics of anesthesia* (6th ed.). New York: Churchill Livingstone.

Tanner, J., Moncaster, K., & Woodings, D. (2011). Perioperative hair removal to reduce surgical site infection. *Cochrane Database of Systematic Reviews*, Issue 11, Article No. CD004122.

Windle, P., Ramos, E., Fairchild, A., et al. (2011). Improving postoperative outcomes for patients with obstructive sleep apnea. *Journal of PeriAnesthesia Nursing, 26*(3), 188.

World Health Organization. (2009). Surgical safety checklist. Available at *www.who.int/patientsafety/safesurgery/tools_resources/en/*.

8
Cancer Nursing

OVERVIEW AND ASSESSMENT

Cancer can be considered a chronic disease requiring ongoing management, rather than a terminal illness. It consists of more than 100 different conditions characterized by uncontrolled growth and spread of abnormal cells. Normal mechanisms of growth and proliferation are disturbed, which results in distinctive morphologic alterations of the cell and aberrations in tissue patterns (see Table 8-1).

The malignant cell is able to invade the surrounding tissue and regional lymph nodes. Primary cancer usually has a predictable natural history and pattern of spread.

Metastasis is the secondary growth of the primary cancer in another organ. The cancer cell migrates through a series of steps to another area of the body. This is the reason that cancer cannot always be cured by surgical removal alone. Most patients die as a result of metastases rather than progression of the primary cancer. Metastasis begins with local invasion followed by detachment of cancer cells that disseminate via the lymphatics and blood vessels and eventually establish a secondary tumor in another area of the body. Lymph nodes are often the first site of distant spread (see Figure 8-1).

Etiology, Detection, and Prevention

Epidemiology

 Evidence Base American Cancer Society. (2012). cancer-facts-figures-2012. Available: *www.cancer.org/Research/CancerFactsFigures/CancerFactsFigures/cancer-facts-figures-2011*.
American Cancer Society. (2008). Global facts and figures. Available: *www.cancer.org/Research/CancerFactsFigures/GlobalCancerFactsFigures/global-facts-figures-2nd-ed*.

1. According to the American Cancer Society (ACS), 1,638,910 new diagnoses of invasive cancer were diagnosed in the United States in 2012. This did not include basal and squamous cell skin cancers as well as noninvasive cancers, or DCIS (ductal carcinoma in situ).
2. According to the International Agency for Research on Cancer, there were 12.7 million new cancer cases in 2008 worldwide. This number is expected to rise as developing countries adopt Western lifestyles such as smoking and lack of exercise.
3. Although the death rate continues to decline, cancer is the second leading, under heart disease, cause of death in the United States, with 577,190 predicted for 2012.
4. Age is the most outstanding risk factor for cancer.
   a. Cancer incidence increases progressively with age.
   b. Approximately 78% of people diagnosed with cancer are over age 55.
5. Two thirds of all cancers in the United States are related to lifestyle habits (eg, smoking, alcohol consumption, diet, physical activity) and environmental carcinogens.
   a. Tobacco is the single greatest cause of cancer-related deaths and is attributed to more than 443,000 deaths annually from various cancers.
   b. Excessive alcohol intake is associated with cancers of the mouth, larynx, throat, esophagus, and liver, especially when combined with smoking. In addition, regular consumption of alcohol is associated with an increased risk of breast cancer. This may be due to alcohol-induced increases in circulating estrogens.
   c. Exposure to carcinogens, such as asbestos, benzene, and radiation, increases the risk of developing certain types of cancer.
   d. Solar ultraviolet radiation exposure is related to an increased risk of skin cancers.

Table 8-1	Differences Between Malignant and Benign Tumors	
CHARACTERISTIC	**BENIGN**	**MALIGNANT**
Growth	Slow, expansive	Invasive
Differentiation	Fully differentiated	Immature, poorly differentiated
Metastasis	Absent	Present or absent

6. There is a hereditary predisposition to specific forms of cancers that have been linked to certain events within a gene (eg, BRCA1 and BRCA2 in breast cancer; MLH1, MSH2, and MSH6 in colon cancer).

7. Infections and viruses are associated with an increased risk of certain forms of cancer.

   a. Human papilloma virus (HPV)—cervical cancer, anal cancers, upper airway cancers.

   b. Epstein-Barr virus—lymphoma, nasopharyngeal cancers, gastric cancer, Kaposi's sarcoma.

   c. Cytomegalovirus—Kaposi's sarcoma, colon cancer.

   d. Human immunodeficiency virus (HIV)—Kaposi's sarcoma, lymphoma.

   e. Human T-lymphocyte virus—T-cell lymphoma/leukemia.

   f. Hepatitis B and C—hepatocellular cancer.

   g. *Helicobacter pylori*—gastric lymphoma (possibly).

8. Five-year survival rates are increasing with improved therapy and earlier detection.

9. Ongoing genetic research is searching for the ability to correct and modify hereditary susceptibility.

10. Patterns of incidence and death rates vary with sex, age, race, and geographic location (see Table 8-2).

Nutrition, Physical Activity, and Cancer

Evidence Base Lawrence, H. K., Doyle, M. S., McCullough, M., et al. (2012). American Cancer Society guidelines on nutrition and physical activity for cancer prevention: Reducing the risk of cancer with healthy food choices and physical activity. CA: *A Cancer Journal for Clinicians*, 62:30–67.

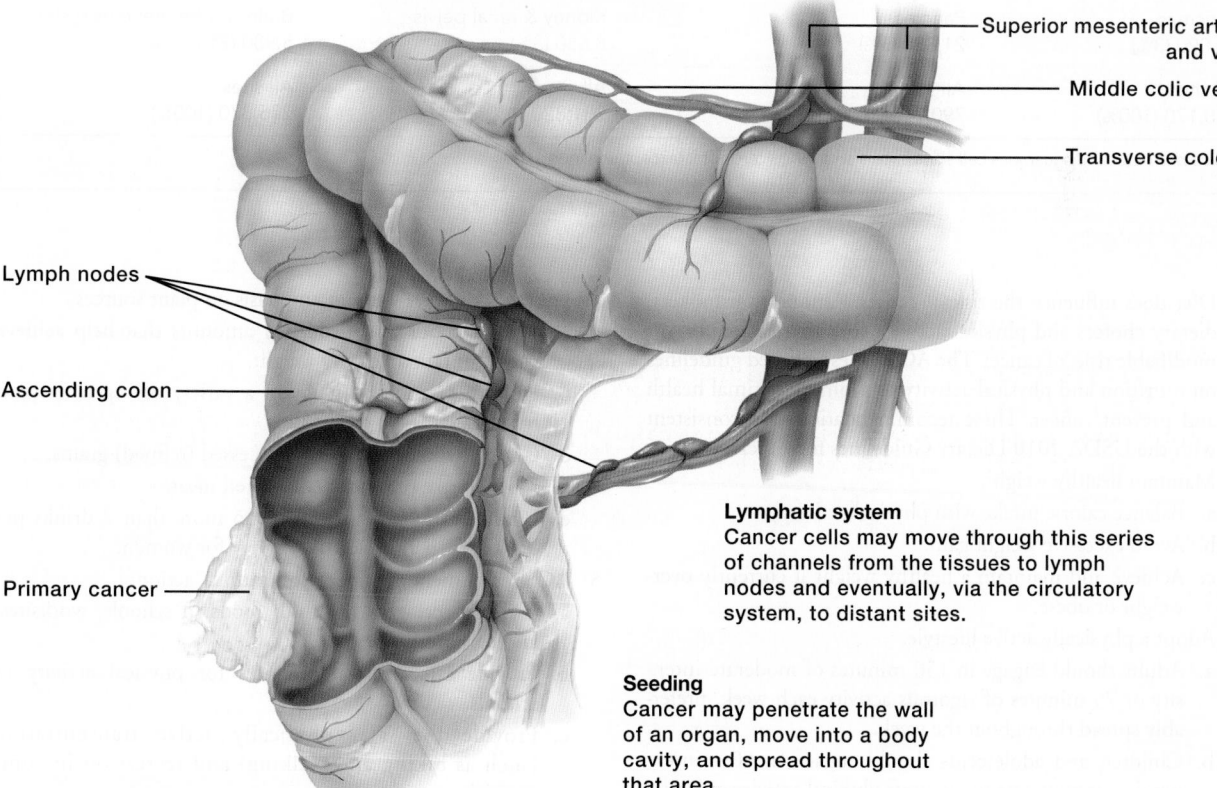

Venous system
Cancer cells may travel through the veins, often to the liver and the lungs.

Superior mesenteric artery and vein

Middle colic vein

Transverse colon

Lymph nodes

Ascending colon

Primary cancer

Lymphatic system
Cancer cells may move through this series of channels from the tissues to lymph nodes and eventually, via the circulatory system, to distant sites.

Seeding
Cancer may penetrate the wall of an organ, move into a body cavity, and spread throughout that area.

Figure 8-1. **How cancer spreads.** Cancer cells may invade nearby tissues or metastasize (spread) to other organs. Cancer cells may move to other tissues by any or all of three routes: venous, lymphatic, or seeding.

Table 8-2   Leading New Cancer Cases and Deaths – 2012 Estimates

ESTIMATED NEW CASES*		ESTIMATED DEATHS	
MALE	FEMALE	MALE	FEMALE
Prostate 241,740 (29%)	Breast 226,870 (29%)	Lung & bronchus 87,750 (29%)	Lung & bronchus 72,590 (26%)
Lung & bronchus 116,470 (14%)	Lung & bronchus 109,690 (14%)	Prostate 28,170 (9%)	Breast 39,510 (14%)
Colon & rectum 73,420 (9%)	Colon & rectum 70,040 (9%)	Colon & rectum 26,470 (9%)	Colon & rectum 25,220 (9%)
Urinary bladder 55,600 (7%)	Uterine corpus 47,130 (6%)	Pancreas 18,850 (6%)	Pancreas 18,540 (7%)
Melanoma of the skin 44,250 (5%)	Thyroid 43,210 (5%)	Liver & intrahepatic bile duct 13,980 (5%)	Ovary 15,500 (6%)
Kidney & renal pelvis 40,250 (5%)	Melanoma of the skin 32,000 (4%)	Leukemia 13,500 (4%)	Leukemia 10,040 (4%)
Non-Hodgkin lymphoma 38,160 (4%)	Non-Hodgkin lymphoma 31,970 (4%)	Esophagus 12,040 (4%)	Non-Hodgkin lymphoma 8,620 (3%)
Oral cavity & pharynx 28,540 (3%)	Kidney & renal pelvis 24,520 (3%)	Urinary bladder 10,510 (3%)	Uterine corpus 8,010 (3%)
Leukemia 26,830 (3%)	Ovary 22,280 (3%)	Non-Hodgkin lymphoma 10,320 (3%)	Liver & intrahepatic bile duct 6,570 (2%)
Pancreas 22,090 (3%)	Pancreas 21,830 (3%)	Kidney & renal pelvis 8,650 (3%)	Brain & other nervous system 5,980 (2%)
All sites 848,170 (100%)	All sites 790,740 (100%)	All sites 301,820 (100%)	All sites 275,370 (100%)

*Excludes basal and squamous cell skin cancers and in situ carcinoma except urinary bladder.

1. Diet does influence the risk of cancer. Among nonsmokers, dietary choices and physical activity are the most important modifiable risks of cancer. The ACS has established guidelines on nutrition and physical activity to promote optimal health and prevent cancer. These recommendations are consistent with the USDA 2010 Dietary Guidelines for Americans.
2. Maintain healthy weight.
   a. Balance calorie intake with physical activity.
   b. Avoid excessive weight gain.
   c. Achieve and maintain a healthy weight if currently overweight or obese.
3. Adopt a physically active lifestyle.
   a. Adults should engage in 150 minutes of moderate intensity or 75 minutes of vigorous activity each week, preferably spread throughout the week.
   b. Children and adolescents should engage in 60 minutes per day of moderate to vigorous physical activity at least 5 days per week.
4. Eat a healthy diet with an emphasis on plant sources.
   a. Choose foods and drinks in amounts that help achieve and maintain a healthy weight.
   b. Eat five or more servings of a variety of vegetables and fruits daily.
   c. Choose whole grains over processed (refined) grains.
   d. Limit intake of processed and red meats.
   e. Limit alcoholic beverages to no more than 2 drinks per day for men and 1 drink per day for women.
5. ACS recommendations for community action:
   a. Increase access to healthful foods in schools, worksites, and communities.
   b. Provide safe, enjoyable spaces for physical activity in schools.
   c. Provide for safe, physically active transportation (such as biking and walking) and recreation in communities.

Table 8-3	ACS Recommendations for the Early Detection of Cancer in Average-Risk, Asymptomatic Individuals		
CANCER SITE	**POPULATION**	**TEST OR PROCEDURE**	**FREQUENCY**
Breast	Women ages ≥20 y	BSE	It is acceptable for women to choose not to do BSE or to do BSE regularly (monthly) or irregularly. Beginning in their early 20s, women should be told about the benefits and limitations of BSE. Regardless of whether a woman ever performs BSE, the importance of prompt reporting of any new breast symptoms to a health professional should be emphasized. Women who choose to do BSE should receive instruction and have their technique reviewed on the occasion of a periodic health examination.
		CBE	For women in their 20s and 30s, it is recommended that CBE be part of a periodic health examination, preferably at least every 3 y. Asymptomatic women aged ≥40 y should continue to receive a CBE as part of a periodic health examination, preferably annually.
		Mammography	Begin annual mammography at age 40 y.[a]
Cervix	Women, ages ≥21 y	Pap test HPV DNA test	Cervical cancer screening should begin approximately 3 y after a woman begins having vaginal intercourse, but no later than aged 21 y. Screening should be done every y with conventional Pap tests or every 2 y using liquid-based Pap tests. At or after age 30 y, women who have had 3 normal test results in a row may undergo screening every 2 to 3 y with cervical cytology (either conventional or liquid-based Pap test) alone, or every 3 y with an HPV DNA test plus cervical cytology, Women aged ≥70 y who have had ≥3 normal Pap tests and no abnormal Pap tests within the last 10 y and women who have had a total hysterectomy may choose to stop cervical cancer screening.
Colorectal	Men and women, ages ≥50 y	FOBT with at least 50% test sensitivity for cancer, or FIT with at least 50% test sensitivity for cancer, or	Annual, starting at age 50 y. Testing at home with adherence to manufacturer's recommendation for collection techniques and number of samples is recommended. FOBT with the single stool sample collected on the clinician's fingertip during a DRE in the health care setting is not recommended. gFOBT tests also are not recommended. In comparison with guaiac-based tests for the detection of occult blood, immunochemical tests are more patient-friendly and are likely to be equal or better with regard to sensitivity and specificity. There is no justification for repeating FOBT in response to an initial positive finding.
		Stool DNA test, or	Interval uncertain, starting at age 50 y.
		FSIG, or	Every 5 y, starting at age 50 y. FSIG can be performed alone, or consideration can be given to combining FSIG performed every 5 y with a highly sensitive gFOBT or FIT performed annually.
		DCBE, or	Every 5 y, starting at age 50 y.
		Colonoscopy	Every 10 y, starting at age 50 y.
		CT colonography	Every 5 y, starting at age 50 y.
Endometrial	Women, at menopause		At the time of menopause, women at average risk should be informed about the risks and symptoms of endometrial cancer and strongly encouraged to report any unexpected bleeding or spotting to their physicians.
Prostate	Men, ages ≥50 y	DRE and PSA	Men who have at least a 10-y life expectancy should have an opportunity to make an informed decision with their health care provider about whether to be screened for prostate cancer, after receiving information about the potential benefits, risks, and uncertainties associated with prostate cancer screening. Prostate cancer screening should not occur without an informed decision-making process.
Cancer-related checkup	Men and women, age ≥20 y		On the occasion of a periodic health examination, the cancer-related checkup should include examination for cancers of the thyroid, testicles, ovaries, lymph nodes, oral cavity, and skin, as well as health counseling about tobacco use, sun exposure, diet and nutrition, risk factors, sexual practices, and environmental and occupational exposures.

ACS indicates American Cancer Society; BSE, breast self-examination; CBE, clinical breast examination; Pap, Papanicolaou; HPV, human papillomavirus; FOBT, fecal occult blood test; FIT, fecal immunochemical test; DRE, digital rectal examination; gFOBT, guaiac-based toilet bowl FOBT tests; FSIG, flexible sigmoidoscopy; DCBE, double-contrast barium enema; CT, computed tomography; PSA, prostate-specific antigen.
[a]Beginning at age 40 y, annual CBE should be performed prior to mammography.

Detection and Prevention

Primary prevention and secondary prevention are effective measures in decreasing mortality and morbidity of many cancers. Most cancers, however, are diagnosed after reported symptoms. The ACS recommends specific primary and secondary prevention measures to reduce an individual's risk of cancer death.

Primary Prevention

The assessment or reduction of risk factors before the disease occurs:

1. Make appropriate lifestyle changes.
2. Stop smoking.
3. Limit alcohol intake.
4. Eat a healthy diet as outlined above.
5. Be physically active: maintain a healthy weight and follow exercise guidelines outlined above.
6. Avoid sun exposure, especially during the hours of 10 A.M. and 4 P.M. and cover exposed skin with sunscreen with a skin protection factor of 15 or higher.
7. Those at high risk for certain cancers should consider genetic counseling and testing.
8. Chemoprevention—the use of natural or synthetic substances to reduce the risk of developing cancer.
   a. Aspirin—doses of at least 75 mg daily can decrease the risk of colorectal cancer.
   b. Tamoxifen and raloxifene—can reduce the risk of breast cancer in women who are at high risk by nearly 50%.
   c. Finasteride—may reduce the risk of prostate cancer.
   d. COX-2 inhibitors—may reduce the risk colorectal cancer.
   e. Vitamin D—may play a role in reducing the risk of breast cancer.
   f. Statins—may reduce the risk of prostate, lung, colorectal, and breast cancers.
9. Vaccinations—HPV is now known to cause about 70% of cervical cancers. HPV vaccines are aimed at preventing genital warts, precancerous cervical lesions, cervical cancer, and anal, penile, and oropharyngeal cancers in both men and women. The Advisory Committee on Immunization Practices in conjunction with the Centers for Disease Control and Prevention has established guidelines on the use of this vaccine.
   a. Routine HPV vaccination is recommended for males and females ages 11 to 13, may begin as early as age 9.
   b. HPV vaccination is also recommended for males and females ages 13 to 18 to "catch up" missed doses of the vaccine or complete the vaccination series.
   c. HPV vaccination is not currently recommended for persons over age 26.
   d. Screening for cervical cancer should continue in both vaccinated and unvaccinated women according to current ACS early detection guidelines.

 Evidence Base The Advisory Committee on Immunization Practices. (2012). General recommendations on immunizations. Available: *www.cdc.gov/vaccines/pubs/ACIP-list.htm.*

Secondary Prevention

 Evidence Base Smith, R. A., Cokkinides, V., Brooks, D., et al. (2012). Cancer screening in the United States, 2012: A review of current American Cancer Society guidelines and issues in cancer screening. *CA—Cancer Journal for Clinicians, 62,* 129–142.

1. The goal of screening is early detection to improve overall outcome and survival. Performing routine screening tests should be based on whether these tests are adequate to detect a potentially curable cancer in an otherwise asymptomatic person and are also cost-effective.
2. Screening should be based on an individual's age, sex, family history of cancer, ethnic group or race, previous iatrogenic factors (prior radiation therapy or drugs such as DES), and history of exposure to environmental carcinogens. See Table 8-3 for ACS recommendations for screening.
   a. The ACS has not issued guidelines for detection of early lung cancer in asymptomatic individuals, but it does recognize that patients at high risk may decide to undergo testing. Currently, the National Comprehensive Cancer Network recommends lung cancer screening in high-risk individuals using low-dose computed tomography (CT). High-risk individuals are men or women age 55 to 74 with at least a 30 pack per year history of smoking and smoking cessation for less than 15 years; or men or women at least 50 years old with a 20 or more pack per year history of smoking and one additional risk factor.

 Evidence Base Routine lung cancer screening is not recommended for low or moderate risk patients. High risk patients with no nodule on baseline low-dose CT should have annual low dose CT screening for 3 years until the age of 74.

   b. The ACS recommends that men, starting at age 50, make an informed decision with their health care providers about whether to be tested for prostate cancer. Research has not yet proven that the potential benefits of testing outweigh the harms of testing and treatment. The ACS position is that men should not be tested without learning about what we know and don't know regarding the risks and possible benefits of testing and treatment.

Diagnostic Evaluation

1. Complete medical history and physical examination.
2. Biopsy of tumor site to determine pathologic diagnosis. Biopsy results are used to determine the histology and/or grade of a tumor, which is a prerequisite for planning definitive therapy.
   a. Fine-needle aspiration (FNA)—technique in which cells are aspirated from the tumor using a needle and syringe. FNA cannot distinguish invasive from noninvasive malignancy. Negative results do not rule out malignancy. However, it is inexpensive, causes little discomfort, and can be performed in an outpatient or office setting.
   b. Needle core—needle biopsies are performed with a large-bore needle. This technique retrieves a small piece of intact tumor tissue, which yields enough tissue to adequately

diagnose most tumor types. It is highly accurate and can be performed in an office or outpatient setting.

   c. Open biopsy— may be required for some lesions to determine a definitive diagnosis. This is done in the operating room, is more expensive, and requires a longer period of recovery. The biopsy may be incisional, sampling only part of the tumor, or excisional, removing the total tumor.

3. Classification of tumor type is based on tissue and cellular staining. Differences in cytoplasmic and nuclear staining distinguish one cell type from another and identify their stage of differentiation. The grade of the tumor (rating of 1 to 4) is based on how well differentiated the tissue or cells appear. For most tumors the higher the grade, the less differentiated, which is associated with poorer prognosis.

4. Flow cytometry testing of tumor tissue determines the deoxyribonucleic acid (DNA) content and indicates potential risk of recurrence.

5. Special stains are performed to determine specific markers or proteins that may help guide treatment (ie, estrogen and progesterone receptors for breast cancer).

6. Laboratory tests—including complete blood count (CBC) with differential; platelet count; and blood chemistries, including liver function tests, blood urea nitrogen (BUN), and creatinine—are done to determine baseline values.

   a. Further testing depends on cancer diagnosis.

   b. Blood markers (carcinoembryonic antigen, PSA, CA15-3, CA125) may be appropriate to follow response to therapy.

7. Imaging procedures—chest x-ray, nuclear medicine scan, CT scanning, magnetic resonance imaging (MRI), and positron-emission tomography (PET) are used to determine evidence or extent of metastasis.

Staging

Staging is necessary at the time of diagnosis to determine the extent of disease (local versus metastatic), to determine prognosis, and to guide proper management.

1. The American Joint Committee on Cancer (AJCC) has developed a simple classification system that can be applied to all tumor types. It is a numeric assessment of tumor size (T), presence or absence of regional lymph node involvement (N), and presence or absence of distant metastasis (M) (see Box 8-1).

2. No standard evaluation exists for all cancers. Workup depends on the patient, tumor type, symptoms, and medical knowledge of the natural history of that cancer.

PROCEDURES AND TREATMENT

The method of treatment depends on the type of malignancy, the specific histologic cell type, stage, presence of metastasis, and condition of the patient. The four modalities of treatment are surgery, chemotherapy, radiation therapy, and biologic therapy or a combination of these modalities.

Surgical Management

The principles of surgical management are based on a cooperative, multidisciplinary approach to various surgical resources. This is

---

BOX 8-1	AJCC Classification System of Tumors

T—primary tumor
Tx—primary cannot be evaluated
T0—no evidence of primary tumor
Tis—carcinoma in situ
T1, T2, T3, T4—increasing size and/or local extent of primary tumor

N—presence or absence or regional lymph node involvement
Nx—regional lymph nodes are unable to be assessed
N0—no regional lymph node involvement
N1, N2, N3—increasing involvement of regional lymph nodes

M—absence or presence of distant metastasis
Mx—unable to assess
M0—absence of distant metastasis
M1—presence of distant metastasis

---

key to the management of the cancer patient. A surgical intervention usually provides the initial diagnosis; subsequent procedures may be needed for treatment.

Types of Surgical Procedures

The role of surgery can be divided into several approaches: preventive, primary surgery, cytoreductive, salvage treatment, palliative treatment, and reconstructive.

1. Preventive/prophylactic surgery—removal of lesions that, if left in the body, are at risk of developing into cancer; for example, resection of polyps in the rectum or mastectomy in women who are at high risk.

2. Primary surgery—complete surgical removal of a malignant tumor and may include regional lymph nodes and neighboring structures. This can be performed laparoscopically in some cases.

3. Cytoreductive surgery—partial removal of bulk of disease. This is performed when the spread of tumor precludes the removal of all disease. In some cases, this approach improves survival when used in combination with chemotherapy (ie, ovarian cancer).

4. Salvage treatment—use of an extensive surgical approach to treat a local recurrence.

5. Palliative treatment—attempts to relieve the complications of cancer (eg, obstruction of the GI tract, pain produced by tumor extension into surrounding nerves).

6. Reconstructive/rehabilitative surgery—repair of defects from previous radical surgical resection; can be performed early (breast reconstruction) or delayed (head and neck surgery).

Chemotherapy

Chemotherapy is the use of antineoplastic drugs to promote tumor cell destruction by interfering with cellular function and reproduction. It includes the use of various chemotherapeutic agents and hormones.

Principles of Chemotherapy Administration

1. The intent of chemotherapy is to destroy as many tumor cells as possible with minimal effect on healthy cells.
2. Cancer cells depend on the same mechanisms for cell division as normal cells. Damage to those mechanisms leads to cell death.
3. Chemotherapy is utilized in different clinical settings:
   a. Adjuvant chemotherapy is the use of systemic treatment following surgery and/or radiation therapy. Adjuvant therapy is given to patients who have no evidence of residual disease but who are at high risk for relapse. The justifications for adjuvant chemotherapy are the high recurrence rate after surgery for apparently localized tumors, the inability to identify cured patients at the time of surgery, and the failure of therapy to cure these patients after recurrence of disease.
   b. Neoadjuvant chemotherapy is the use of systemic treatment prior to primary surgery or radiation. The goal is to shrink or downstage the primary tumor to improve the effectiveness of surgery as well as control/irradicate microscopic cancer cells. For example, patients with large breast tumors can preserve the breast and undergo lumpectomy instead of mastectomy. The goal of therapy is to decrease the amount of tissue that needs to be removed as well as to attempt to maximize cure potential.
   c. High-dose/intensive therapy is the administration of high doses of chemotherapy, usually in association with growth factor support before bone marrow transplant/stem cell rescue.
   d. Palliative chemotherapy is used when a cure is not possible to control the cancer and minimize side effects from the disease.
4. Chemotherapeutic agents can be effective on any stage of the cell cycle in which cells are dividing. The cell cycle is divided into five stages:
   a. G0 (gap 0) resting phase: Cells are not dividing in this stage and, for the most part, are refractory to chemotherapy.
   b. G1 (gap one) phase: Ribonucleic acid (RNA) and protein synthesis (enzymes for DNA synthesis) are manufactured.
   c. S (synthesis) phase: During a long period, the DNA component doubles for the chromosomes in preparation for cell division.
   d. G2 (gap two) phase: This is a short period; protein and RNA synthesis occurs, and the mitotic spindle apparatus is formed.
   e. M (mitosis) phase: In an extremely short period, the cell divides into two identical daughter cells.
5. Routes of administration:
   a. Oral—capsule, tablet, or liquid.
   b. Intravenous (IV)—push (bolus) or infusion over a specified period.
   c. Intramuscular.
   d. Intrathecal/intraventricular—given by injection via an Ommaya reservoir or by lumbar puncture.
   e. Intra-arterial.
   f. Intracavitary—such as peritoneal cavity.
   g. Intravesical—into uterus or bladder.
   h. Topical.
6. Dosage is based on surface area (mg/m²) in both adults and children.
7. Most chemotherapeutic agents have dose-limiting toxicities that require nursing interventions (see Table 8-4, pages 142 to 145). Chemotherapy predictably affects normal, rapidly growing cells (eg, bone marrow, GI tract lining, hair follicles). It is imperative that these toxicities be recognized early by the nurse.

Safety Measures in Handling Chemotherapy

 Evidence Base Oncology Nursing Society. (2009). *Chemotherapy and biotherapy guidelines and recommendations for practice* (3rd ed). Pittsburgh, PA: Author.

Cytotoxic drugs are considered to be hazardous to health care workers and special handling is required to minimize the exposure and overall health risks (see Procedure Guidelines 8-1, pages 146 to 148).

Personal Protective Equipment

1. Gloves—wear gloves that are powder-free, such as nitrile, polyurethane, or neoprene, and have been tested for use with hazardous drugs. Avoid latex drugs due to potential latex sensitivity. Double gloves are recommended for all handling.
2. Gowns—wear a disposable, lint-free gown made of low-permeability fabric. The gown should have a solid front, long sleeves, tight cuffs, and back closure. The inner glove should be worn under the gown cuff and the outer glove should extend over the gown to protect the skin. Gown and gloves are meant for single use only.
3. Respirators—wear a National Institute for Occupational Health and Safety approved respirator mask when there is a risk of aerosol exposure such as when administering chemotherapy or cleaning a spill. Surgical masks do not provide adequate protection.
4. Eye and face protection—wear a face shield and/or mask that provides splash protection whenever there is a possibility of splashing.
5. Wear personal protective equipment whenever there is a risk of chemotherapy being released into the environment such as preparation or mixing of chemotherapy, spiking/priming IV tubing, administering the drug, and when handling body fluids or chemotherapy spills.

Personal Safety to Minimize Exposure

1. Prepare cytotoxic drugs in a vertical laminar flow hood.
2. Wash hands before donning PPE and change gloves after each use, tear, puncture, or medication spill or after every 60 minutes of wear. Wash hands after removing PPE.
3. Vent vials with filter needle to equalize the internal pressure or use negative-pressure techniques.
4. Wrap gauze or alcohol pads around the neck of ampules when opening to decrease droplet contamination.
5. Wrap gauze or alcohol pads around injection sites when removing syringes or needles from IV injection ports.

6. Use puncture- and leak-proof containers for noncapped, non-clipped needles.

7. Prime all IV tubing with normal saline or other compatible solution to reduce exposure.

8. Use syringes and IV tubing with luer locks (which have a locking device to hold needle firmly in place).

9. Label all syringes and IV tubing containing chemotherapeutic agents as hazardous material.

10. Place an absorbent pad directly under the injection site to absorb any accidental spillage.

11. Do not eat, drink, or chew gum while preparing or handling chemotherapy agents.

12. Keep all food and drink away from preparation area.

13. Avoid hand-to-mouth or hand-to-eye contact while handling chemotherapeutic agents or body fluids of the patient receiving chemotherapy.

14. If any contact with the skin occurs, immediately wash the area thoroughly with soap and water.

15. If contact is made with the eye, immediately flush the eye with water and seek medical attention.

16. Spill kits should be available in all areas where chemotherapy is stored, prepared, and administered.

Safe Disposal of Antineoplastic Agents, Body Fluids, and Excreta

1. Discard gloves and gown into a leak-proof container, which should be marked as contaminated or hazardous waste.

2. Use puncture- and leak-proof containers for needles and other sharp or breakable objects.

3. Linens contaminated with chemotherapy or excreta from patients who have received chemotherapy within 48 hours should be contained in specially marked hazardous waste bags.

4. Wear nonsterile nitrile gloves for disposing of body excreta and handling soiled linens within 48 hours of chemotherapy administration.

5. In the home, wear gloves when handling bed linens or clothing contaminated with chemotherapy or patient excreta within 48 hours of chemotherapy administration. Place linens in a separate, washable pillow case. Wash separately in hot water and regular detergent.

Adverse Effects of Chemotherapy

All chemotherapy drugs have adverse effects. Adverse effects are exacerbated if the patient is younger than 1 year or is elderly, has comorbid conditions, or has impaired renal or hepatic function.

Adverse effects of chemotherapy are graded on a scale of 0 to 5, with 0 being no toxicity and 5 resulting in death. Scoring of adverse effects will determine if a delay in therapy is necessary, dose modification is necessary, or cessation of therapy must occur.

Alopecia

1. Most chemotherapeutic agents cause some degree of alopecia. This is dependent on the drug dose, half-life of drug, and duration of therapy.

2. Usually begins 2 weeks after administration of chemotherapy. Regrowth takes about 3 to 5 months.

3. The use of scalp hypothermia and tourniquets is highly controversial.

Anorexia

1. Chemotherapy changes the reproduction of taste buds.

2. Absent or altered taste can lead to a decreased food intake.

3. Concurrent renal or hepatic disease can increase anorexia.

Diarrhea

1. Defined as loose or watery stool. If left untreated, can lead to severe dehydration, electrolyte imbalances, hospitalizations, and treatment delays.

2. Cause is multifactoral, but up to 90% of all patients receiving chemotherapy can experience diarrhea.

Fatigue

The cause of fatigue is generally unknown but can be related to anemia, weight loss, altered sleep patterns, and coping.

Nausea and Vomiting

1. Caused by the stimulation of the vagus nerve by serotonin released by cells in the upper GI tract.

2. Incidence depends on the particular chemotherapeutic agent and dosage.

3. Patterns of nausea and vomiting:

   a. Anticipatory—conditioned response from repeated association between therapy and vomiting; can be prevented with adequate anti-emetic control.

   b. Acute—occurs 0 to 24 hours after chemotherapy administration.

   c. Delayed—can occur 1 to 6 days after chemotherapy administration; nausea is often worse than vomiting.

Mucositis

1. Caused by the destruction of the oral mucosa, causing an inflammatory response.

2. Initially presents as a burning sensation with no changes in the mucosa and progresses to significant breakdown, erythema, and pain of the oral mucosa.

3. Consistent oral hygiene is important to avoid infection.

Neutropenia

1. Defined as an absolute neutrophil count (ANC) of 1,500/mm³ or less.

2. Primary dose-limiting toxicity of chemotherapy.

3. Risk of infection is greatest with an ANC less than 500/mm³.

4. Caused by suppression of the stem cell.

5. Usually occurs 7 to 14 days after administration of chemotherapy, but depends on the agent used.

6. Can be prolonged.

7. Patients should be taught to avoid infection through proper handwashing and hygiene and avoiding those with illness. Eliminating raw meats, seafood, eggs or unwashed vegetables is also recommended

8. Patients need to be monitored and treated promptly for fever or other signs of infection.

9. Can be prevented with the use of growth factors (eg, granulocyte colony-stimulating factor [CSF], pegfilgrastim).

Anemia

1. Caused by suppression of the stem cell or interference with cell proliferation pathways.

2. May require red blood cell transfusion or injection of erythropoietin or darbepoetin.

(Text continues on page 148)

Table 8-4   Frequently Used Chemotherapeutic Agents

CLASSIFICATION	MEDICATION NAME	ROUTE OF ADMINISTRATION	COMMON THERAPEUTIC USES
Alkylators	Cyclophosphamide	IV or P.O.	Lymphomas, leukemias, and a variety of solid tumors
	Busulfan	IV or P.O.	Chromic myleocytic leukemia, bone marrow transplantation
	Carboplatin	IV or IP	Ovarian cancer
	Chlorambucil	P.O.	Chronic lymphocytic leukemia, Hodgkin's disease
	Cisplatin	IV	Ovarian, testicular, bladder, cervical, non-small-cell lung cancer, esophageal
	Dacarbazine	IV or I.M.	Malignant melanoma, Hodgkin's lymphoma, sarcomas
	Ifosfamide	IV	Testicular, lymphoma, sarcomas, ovarian, bone
	Melphalan	IV or P.O.	Multiple myeloma, ovarian, malignant melanoma
	Oxaliplatin	IV	Colorectal cancers
	Temozolomide	P.O.	Glioblastoma, astrocytoma, melanoma
	Thiotepa	IV, I.M., SC, IT	Breast, ovarian, bladder, lymphomas, bone marrow transplantation
Antibiotics	Bleomycin	IV, SC, I.M.	Head and neck cancers, cervical, lymphomas, testicular, Hodgkin's
	Dactinomycin	IV	Ewing's sarcoma, Wilms' tumor, testicular
	Daunorubicin	IV	Leukemias
	Doxorubicin	IV	Breast, ovarian, prostate, thyroid, lung, head and neck cancers, leukemia
	Doxorubicin liposo-mal	IV	Ovarian, breast, AIDS-related sarcoma
	Epirubicin	IV	Breast cancer
	Mitomycin	IV	Pancreatic, stomach, colon, lung, bladder, esophageal
	Mitoxantrone	IV	Prostate acute myelocytic leukemia

COMMON TOXICITIES	NURSING CONSIDERATIONS
Nausea, vomiting, diarrhea, myelosuppression, alopecia, lethargy, hemorrhagic cystitis	Ensure adequate hydration (2–3 L /day) Have patients void frequently top avoid hemorrhagic cystitis
Pulmonary fibrosis, hypertension, tachycardia, myelosuppression, alopecia, skin pigmentation	Instruct patients to take on an empty stomach to decrease nausea/vomiting. Monitor blood counts
Myelosuppression particularly platelets, alopecia, hypersensitivity reaction	Have emergency medications available for possible hypersensitivity reactions
Myelosuppression, nausea, vomiting, skin reactions, seizures	Contraindications in patients with a history of seizures
Nausea, vomiting, myelosuppression, nephrotoxicity, hypersensitivity reactions, low electrolytes	Monitor renal function and electrolytes Have emergency medications available for possible hypersensitivity reactions
Nausea, vomiting, myelosuppression, alopecia, rash	Irritant—may cause tissue necrosis if extravasated.
Hemorrhagic cystitis, nausea, vomiting, myelosuppression, confusion, encephalopathy	Always given in conjunction with MESNA to decrease risk of hemorrhagic cystitis
Myelosuppression, nausea, vomiting	Vesicant—avoid extravasation
Nephrotoxicity, hypersensitivity reactions, peripheral neuropathy, nausea, vomiting, myelosuppression	Monitor for peripheral neuropathy Instruct patients to avoid consuming cold beverages for 3 to 4 days to avoid laryngopharyngeal dysesthesias
Myelosuppression, nausea, vomiting, headache, photosensitivity	Contraindicated in patients with sensitivity to dacarbazine Instruct patients to avoid sun exposure for several days
Myelosuppression, nausea, vomiting, rash, fever	
Skin reaction, pulmonary fibrosis, fever, allergic reaction, alopecia, stomatitis	Administer a test dose in patient with lymphoma as they seem to have a higher incidence of allergic reactions
Myelosuppression, nausea, vomiting, alopecia, veno-occlusive disease of the liver, skin rash and fever	Vesicant—avoid extravasation
Myelosuppression, nausea, vomiting, alopecia, cardiomyopathy, red urine, radiation recall	Vesicant—avoid extravasation Monitor cardiac function
Cardiomyopathy, alopecia, red urine, radiation recall, nausea, vomiting, red urine	Vesicant—avoid extravasation 550 mg/m^2 lifetime dose
Myelosuppression, nausea, vomiting, mucositis, diarrhea, alopecia, radiation recall	Similar to adriamycin, less cardiotoxic
Myelosuppression, nausea, vomiting, alopecia, heart failure, radiation recall, red urine	Vesicant—avoid extravasation
Delayed myelosuppression, nausea, vomiting, alopecia, mucositis, renal and pulmonary dysfunction	Vesicant—avoid extravasation
Myelosuppression, tachycardia, mucositis, nausea, vomiting, alopecia	May turn urine blue-green

Table 8-4   Frequently Used Chemotherapeutic Agents *(continued)*

CLASSIFICATION	MEDICATION NAME	ROUTE OF ADMINISTRATION	COMMON THERAPEUTIC USES
Plant alkaloids	Irinotecan	IV	Colorectal
	Topotecan	IV	Ovarian, cervical, small-cell lung cancer
	Vinblastine	IV	Hodgkin's lymphoma, Kaposi's sarcoma, testicular, bladder, prostate, renal cell
	Vincristine	IV	Lymphoma, acute leukemia, neuroblastoma, multiple myeloma, testicular
	Vinorelbine	IV	Non-small-cell lung, breast, cervical, ovarian
	Etoposide	IV or P.O.	Small-cell lung, testicular,
	Teniposide	IV	Childhood acute lymphocytic leukemia, adult neuroblastoma
Antimetabolites	Methotrexate	IV, I.M., IT, or P.O.	Lymphoma, acute lymphoblastic leukemia, breast, bladder, sarcoma
	Cytarabine	IV, SC, IT, I.M.	Hodgkin's and non-Hodgkin's lymphoma, acute myelogenous leukemia, acute lymphoblastic leukemia
	5-Fluorouracil	IV or topical	Breast, colorectal, anal, gastroesophageal, hepatocellar, pancreatic, head and neck
	Capecitabine	P.O.	Breast, colorectal, gastroesophageal, hepatocellular, pancreatic
	6-Mercaptopurin	P.O.	Acute lymphoblastic leukemia
	Thioguanine	P.O.	Acute myelogenous leukemia Acute lymphoblastic leukemia
	Fludarabine	IV or P.O.	Chronic lymphocytic leukemia, non-Hodgkin's lymphoma
	Gemcitabine	IV	Pancreatic, non-small-cell lung, breast, bladder, ovarian, sarcoma, Hodgkin's lymphoma
Taxanes	Paclitaxel	IV	Breast, ovarian, non-small-cell lung, bladder, esophagus, cervical, gastric, head and neck, sarcoma
	Docetaxel	IV	Breast, gastric, head and neck, prostate, non-small-cell lung, ovarian
	Ixabepilone	IV	Breast cancer

IV, intravenous; PO, by mouth; IP, intraperitoneal; IM, intramuscular; SQ, subcutaneous; IT, itrathecal.

COMMON TOXICITIES	NURSING CONSIDERATIONS
Diarrhea, myelosuppression	Monitor for severe diarrhea that may require delays or dose reduction
Myelosuppression, alopecia, diarrhea, headache, fatigue	
Myelosuppression, alopecia, peripheral neuropathy, bone pain	Vesicant—avoid extravasation
Constipation, nausea, vomiting, alopecia, bone pain	Vesicant—avoid extravasation, monitor for severe constipation
Alopecia, diarrhea, nausea, neuropathy	Distal neuropathies, extravasation and necrosis; should consider central access
Myelosuppression, nausea, alopecia, mucositis	Monitor renal function
Myelosuppression, nausea, vomiting, diarrhea, alopecia,	Can cause hypersensitivity reactions
Mucositis, diarrhea, myelosuppression, acute renal failure, pneumonitis	High doses require concomitant use of leucovoran and IV fluids
Nausea, vomiting, myelosuppression, cerebellar ataxia, lethargy	Side effects are dose dependent; higher doses are associated with profound myelosuppression, GI toxicity, and neurotoxicity
Nausea, vomiting, diarrhea, mucositis, myelosuppression, neurotoxicity, photosensitivity	Instruct patients to avoid sun exposure, use sunscreen Leucovorin may be used concomitantly
Diarrhea, hand-foot syndrome, stomatitis, myelosuppression,	Patient education very important. Instruction patient to stop drug and immediately report moderate hand-foot, or GI symptoms
Myelosuppression, nausea, vomiting, diarrhea, hepatotoxicity	Instruct patients to take on an empty stomach
Myelosuppression, nausea, vomiting, mucositis, diarrhea, hepatotoxicity	Instruct patients to take on an empty stomach
Myelosuppression, mild nausea, vomiting, fever, interstitial pneumonitis	Monitor pulmonary function tests
Nausea, vomiting, myelosuppression, flu-like syndrome, fever	Warn patients of flu-like symptoms that can occur the day following treatment
Myelosuppression, peripheral neuropathy, myalgias, alopecia, fatigue	Observe closely for hypersensitivity reaction; premedication required with dexamethasone, dephenydramine, and H2 blocker requires non-PVC IV tubing
Myelosuppression, edema, alopecia, nail changes, peripheral neuropathy	Treatment with dexamethasone prior to and for 2 days after can minimize edema
Myelosuppression, fatigue, neuropathy, nausea, vomiting, diarrhea, myalgias	Observe closely for hypersensitivity reaction; premedication required with dexamethasone, dephenydramine, and H2 blocker requires non-PVC IV tubing

PROCEDURE GUIDELINES 8-1

Administering IV Chemotherapy

EQUIPMENT

- Supplies to start IV infusion or a running IV line
- Alcohol swabs
- Specific antidote for extravasation (if indicated)
- Disposable plastic-backed absorbent liner
- 4" × 4" gauze pads
- Medication to be administered

PROCEDURE

Nursing Action	Rationale
Preparatory phase	

1. Prepare the patient by reviewing the treatment plan, goals, and possible adverse effects.
  a. Review strategies to manage adverse effects.
  b. Instruct patient on reportable conditions (eg, fever).
	1. Patient education will prepare the patient for adverse effects, thus increasing tolerance of the drug.

2. Double-check provider order, ideally with a second nurse, to include:
  a. Any supportive care medications, including premedications, anti-emetics, hydration, growth factors, or emergency medications.
  b. All necessary components: name of drug, route, dosing interval, date, duration of therapy, diluent type and amount, rate of infusion.
  c. Compare written orders to drug protocol. If the drug is investigational, verify informed consent.
  d. Check current laboratory values; complete blood count, differential, platelets, liver function tests, and creatinine. Notify the health care provider if values are outside acceptable limits and would preclude infusion of the drug.
  e. Review patient's medication history, including over-the-counter medications.
	2. Minimizes chemotherapy administration errors.
	
	  a. Anti-emetics are more effective if given before administration and on a regular dosing schedule thereafter.
	
	  b. Reduces or minimizes drug interactions and toxicities.
	
	  c. Ensures safe drug administration (ensure that order outside of protocol is accurate).
	  d. Drug may be withheld in severe neutropenia, thrombocytopenia, or impaired liver or kidney function.
	
	  e. Interactions may occur with prescription and over-the-counter medications and supplements.

3. Calculate the dosage according to milligrams per kilogram (mg/kg) or milligrams per meter squared (mg/m²) by body surface area (BSA).	3. Accurate dosing to maximize benefit and limit side effects.
4. Verify the patient's name and identification using two forms of identification.	4. According to Joint Commission standards.
5. Be aware of agents that cause anaphylactic reaction, such as asparaginase, paclitaxel, and docetaxel.	5. Increases awareness. Have emergency resuscitation equipment and drugs available.
Performance phase	

1. Insert IV tubing (if appropriate).
  a. Select venipuncture site free from sclerosis, thrombosis, or scar formation, if possible. If the patient has an established IV, assess the site for erythema, pain, or tenderness.
  b. Check for a blood return by aspirating at a Y-site close to the IV catheter. Do not pinch the catheter tubing.
  c. If doubt exists about patency of the IV, do not administer chemotherapy.
	1.
	  a. An optimal IV site reduces the risk of extravasation.
	
	  b. Pinching the catheter tubing may dislodge a small clot in a nonpatent IV.
	  c. Extravasation of some chemotherapeutic agents may cause severe pain and tissue injury.

2. Administration
  a. Use a disposable, absorbent, plastic-backed pad under the work area.
  b. Don personal protective equipment (PPE).
	2.
	  a. Absorbs droplets of the drug that may inadvertently spill.
	  b. Prevents injury from aerosolization/spillage of drug.

PROCEDURE GUIDELINES 8-1 (continued)

Administering IV Chemotherapy

PROCEDURE (continued)

Nursing Action	Rationale
Performance phase (continued)	
c. If possible, prime all tubing before adding antineoplastics to the bag. If priming occurs at the administration site, the IV tubing should be primed with a nondrug fluid.	c. Prevents loss of chemotherapeutic agent.
d. Monitor the patient, particularly during the first 15 minutes, for signs of hypersensitivity or anaphylaxis.	d. Change in mentation or in vital signs may indicate hypersensitivity or anaphylactic reaction.
e. Monitor the IV site through the infusion or IV push. Use a transparent (not gauze) dressing over the IV site.	e. Allows for direct visualization of IV site.
3. Monitor for pain, which may be severe, burning, and radiating along the vein, and examine the site for erythema and swelling.	3. May indicate extravasation. A vesicant causes blistering of the vein wall and tissue necrosis. An irritant causes burning along the vein with or without inflammation.

Key Decision Point

If you suspect an extravasation, stop the infusion immediately to prevent necrosis and sloughing, which may lead to permanent tissue damage. Follow the procedure for extravasation.

Management of extravasation

1. If an extravasation is suspected, stop the infusion of the chemotherapy.	1. Prevents further infusion of chemotherapy agent.
2. Disconnect the IV tubing and attempt to aspirate all residual chemotherapy in the IV catheter using a small 1–3 mL syringe.	
3. Remove the IV catheter.	
4. Assess the site and apply warm or cold packs as indicated (see below).	4. May prevent tissue necrosis.
5. Notify the health care provider.	
6. Apply local care or antidote as indicated.	

Chemotherapeutic Agent	Antidote	Local Care
Anthracyclines (doxorubicin, epirubicin, daunorubicin)	Dexrazoxane	Apply ice, but remove at least 15 minutes before dexrazoxane. Dose of dexrazoxane is based on body surface area and should be administered IV in an area other than the extravasation site, opposite arm: Day one: 1,000 mg/m^2 Day two: 1000 mg/m^2 Day three: 500 mg/m^2
Alkylating agents (nitrogen mustard, cisplatin)	Isotonic sodium thiosulfate	Prepare $\frac{1}{6}$ molar solution and inject 2 mL for each milligram of chemotherapy suspected to have extravasated. Inject solution subcutaneously in the site using a 25G needle (change the needle with each injection). Apply ice for 6–12 hours following sodium thiosulfate injection.
Vinca alkaloids (vincristine, vinblastine, vinorelbine)	Hyaluronidase	Inject 1 mL of hyaluronidase locally as five separate injections subcutaneously into the extravasated area. Apply moderate heat for 15–20 minutes at least four times daily for the first 24–48 hours to disperse drug and minimize pain.
Taxanes (paclitaxel, docetaxel)	No known antidote	Apply ice for 15–20 minutes at least four times daily for the first 24 hours.
Antibiotics	None	Apply ice for 15–20 minutes at least four times daily for the first 24 hours.

(continued)

PROCEDURE GUIDELINES 8-1 (continued)

Administering IV Chemotherapy

PROCEDURE (continued)

Nursing Action	Rationale
Follow-up phase	
1. Document drug dosage, site, and any occurrence of extravasation, including estimated amount of drug.	1. Documents extent of injury.
2. Observe regularly after administration for pain, erythema, induration, and necrosis.	2. May indicate phlebitis, which may still result from small extravasation, causing pain for several days or induration at the site that may last for weeks or months.
3. Monitor for other adverse effects of infusion.	3.
a. Patient may describe sensations of pain or pressure within the vessel, originating near the venipuncture site or extending 3–5 inches (7.5–12.5 cm) along the vein.	a. Caused by irritation to the vein.
b. Discoloration or red streak following the line of the vein (called a flare reaction) or darkening of the vein.	b. Flare reaction common with doxorubicin. Darkening of vein may occur with 5-fluorouracil (5-FU).
c. Itching, urticaria, muscle cramps, or pressure in the arm.	c. Caused by irritation of surrounding subcutaneous tissue.

 Evidence Base Oncology Nursing Society. (2009). *Chemotherapy and biotherapy guidelines and recommendations for practice.* Pittsburgh, PA: Author.

Thrombocytopenia

1. Caused by suppression of megakaryocytes.
2. Incidence depends on the agent being used.
3. Risk of bleeding is present when platelet count falls below 50,000/mm^3.
4. Risk is high when count falls below 20,000/mm^3.
5. Risk is critical when count falls below 10,000/mm^3.
6. Patient should be taught to avoid injury (eg, no razors), vaginal douches, rectal suppositories, and dental floss during the period of thrombocytopenia.
7. May require platelet transfusions if count drops below 20,000/mm^3.

Hypersensitivity Reactions

1. Nearly all of the available chemotherapeutic agents can produce hypersensitivity reactions (HSRs) in at least an occasional patient, and some cause reactions in 5% or more of patients receiving the drug. There are several agents (L-asparaginase, paclitaxel, docetaxel, teniposide, and carboplatin) for which HSRs are frequent enough to be a major form of treatment-limiting toxicity.
2. The mechanism is unknown for most of the chemotherapeutic agents.
3. Signs and symptoms include hives, pruritus, back pain, shortness of breath, hypotension, and anaphylaxis.
4. All unexpected drug reactions should be reported to the manufacturer.

Nursing Assessment

Integumentary System

1. Inspect for pain, swelling with inflammation or phlebitis, necrosis, or ulceration.
2. Inspect for skin rash and characteristics (eg, whether pruritus is general or local).
3. Assess areas of erythema and associated tenderness or pruritus. Instruct the patient to avoid irritation to skin, sun exposure, or irritating soaps.
4. Assess changes in skin pigmentation.
5. Note reports of photosensitivity, tearing of the eyes.
6. Assess condition of gums, teeth, buccal mucosa, and tongue.
   a. Determine whether any taste changes have occurred.
   b. Check for evidence of stomatitis, erythematous areas, ulceration, infection, or pain on swallowing.
   c. Determine whether the patient has any complaints of pain or burning of the oral mucosa or on swallowing.

GI System

1. Assess for frequency, timing of onset, duration, and severity of nausea and vomiting episodes before and after chemotherapy.
   a. Usually occurs from 0 to 24 hours after chemotherapy but may be delayed. Anticipatory vomiting may occur after first course of therapy. Can be initiated by various cues, including thoughts, smell, or even sight of the medical personnel.

2. Observe for alterations in hydration, electrolyte balance.
3. Assess for diarrhea or constipation.
   a. Ascertain any changes in bowel patterns.
   b. Discuss the consistency of stools.
   c. Consider the frequency and duration of diarrhea (the number of stools each day for the number of days).
   d. Evaluate dietary changes or use of medications such as opioids or 5-HT3 blockers that have had an impact on diarrhea or constipation.
4. Assess for anorexia.
   a. Discuss taste changes and changes in food preferences.
   b. Ask about daily food intake and normal eating patterns.
5. Assess for jaundice, right upper quadrant abdominal pain, changes in the stool or urine, and elevated liver function tests that indicate hepatotoxicity.
6. Monitor liver function tests and total bilirubin.

Hematopoietic System

 NURSING ALERT Fever greater than 101° F (38.3° C) in a patient with an ANC less than 500/mm3 is an emergency requiring immediate administration of antibiotics.

1. Assess for neutropenia—ANC less than 500/mm³.
   a. Assess for any signs of infection (pulmonary, integumentary, central nervous system, GI, and urinary).
   b. Auscultate lungs for adventitious breath sounds.
   c. Assess for productive cough or shortness of breath.
   d. Assess for urinary frequency, urgency, pain, or odor.
   e. Monitor for elevation of temperature above 101° F (38.3° C), chills.
2. Assess for thrombocytopenia—platelet count less than 50,000/mm³ (mild risk of bleeding); less than 20,000/mm³ (high risk of bleeding).
   a. Assess skin and oral mucous membranes for petechiae, bruises on extremities.
   b. Assess for signs of bleeding (including nose, urinary, rectal, or hemoptysis).
   c. Assess for blood in stools, urine, or emesis.
   d. Assess for signs and symptoms of intracranial bleeding if platelet count is less than 20,000/mm³; monitor for changes in level of responsiveness, vital signs, and pupillary reaction.
3. Assess for anemia.
   a. Assess skin color, turgor, and capillary refill.
   b. Ascertain whether patient has experienced dyspnea on exertion, fatigue, weakness, palpitations, or vertigo. Advise rest periods as needed.

Respiratory and Cardiovascular Systems
1. Assess lung sounds.
2. Assess for pulmonary fibrosis, evidenced by a dry, nonproductive cough with increasing dyspnea. Patients at risk include those over age 60, smokers, those receiving or having had pulmonary radiation, those receiving a cumulative dose of bleomycin, or those with any preexisting lung disease.

3. Assess for signs and symptoms of heart failure or irregular apical or radial pulses.
4. Verify baseline cardiac studies (eg, electrocardiogram, multiple-gated acquisition scan/ejection fraction) before administering cardiotoxic chemotherapy such as doxoirubicin.

Neuromuscular System
1. Determine whether the patient is having difficulty with fine motor activities, such as zipping pants, tying shoes, or buttoning a shirt.
2. Determine the presence of paresthesia (tingling, numbness) of fingers or toes.
3. Evaluate deep tendon reflexes.
4. Evaluate the patient for weakness, ataxia, or slapping gait.
5. Determine impact on activities of daily living and discuss changes.
6. Discuss symptoms of urinary retention or constipation.
7. Assess for ringing in ears or decreased hearing acuity.

Genitourinary System
1. Monitor urine output.
2. Assess for urinary frequency, urgency, or hesitancy.
3. Evaluate changes in odor, color, or clarity of urine sample.
4. Assess for hematuria, oliguria, or anuria.
5. Monitor BUN and creatinine.

Nursing Diagnoses
- Risk for Infection related to neutropenia.
- Risk for Injury related to bleeding from thrombocytopenia.
- Fatigue related to anemia.
- Imbalanced Nutrition: Less Than Body Requirements related to adverse effects of therapy.
- Impaired Oral Mucous Membranes related to stomatitis.
- Ineffective Protection and risk for hypersensitivity reaction related to chemotherapy.
- Disturbed Body Image related to alopecia and weight loss.

Nursing Interventions
Preventing Infection
1. Monitor vital signs every 4 hours; report occurrence of fever greater than 101° F (38.3° C) and chills.
2. Provide patient education.
   a. Instruct patient to report signs and symptoms of infection:
      i. Fever greater than 101° F (38.3° C) and/or chills.
      ii. Mouth lesions, swelling, or redness.
      iii. Redness, pain, or tenderness at rectum.
      iv. Change in bowel habits.
      v. Areas of redness, swelling, induration, or pain on skin surface.
      vi. Pain or burning when urinating or odor from urine.
      vii. Cough or shortness of breath.
   b. Reinforce good personal hygiene habits (routine bathing [preferably a shower], clean hair, nails, and mouth care).
   c. Avoid contact with people who have a transmittable illness.
   d. Encourage deep breathing and coughing to decrease pulmonary stasis.

3. Avoid performing invasive procedures—rectal temperatures, enemas, or insertion of indwelling urinary catheters.

4. Monitor white blood cell (WBC) count and differential.

5. Be aware that hematologic nadirs (lowest level) generally occur within 7 to 14 days after drug administration. Length of myelosuppression depends on specific drug. Institution of further therapy usually depends on an adequate WBC count and ANC.

6. Calculate ANC to determine the number of neutrophils capable of fighting an infection by:

Total WBC count × (% polys + % bands) = ANC
Example: 700 × (10% + 5%) = 105

Interpretation: 105 of the 700 WBCs are neutrophils and capable of fighting an infection (indicates severe neutropenia).

7. Administer prophylactic antibiotics, as prescribed (if WBC count is less than 500).

8. Administer growth factors, as prescribed: subcutaneous (SC) filgrastim 5 mcg/kg starting 24 hours after chemotherapy for 5 to 10 days for neutropenia prophylaxis or pegfilgrastim 6 mg SC for a single dose 24 hours after chemotherapy. Should also be administered with subsequent courses of chemotherapy to hasten neutrophil maturity.

Preventing Bleeding

1. Avoid invasive procedures when platelet count is less than 50,000/mm³, including I.M. injections, suppositories, enemas, and insertion of indwelling urinary catheters.

2. Apply pressure on injection sites for 5 minutes.

3. Monitor platelet count; administer platelets as prescribed.

4. Monitor and test all urine, stools, and emesis for blood.

5. Provide patient education.
   a. Instruct patient to avoid straight-edge razors, nail clippers, vaginal or rectal suppositories.
   b. Avoid intercourse when platelet count is less than 50,000/mm³.
   c. Encourage patient to blow his or her nose gently.
   d. Avoid dental work or other invasive procedures while thrombocytopenic.
   e. Avoid the use of nonsteroidal anti-inflammatory drugs (NSAIDs), aspirin, and aspirin-containing products.

Minimizing Fatigue

1. Monitor blood counts (hemoglobin and hematocrit).

2. Administer blood products as prescribed.

3. Administer growth factors as prescribed, such as erythropoietin or darbepoetin.

4. Provide patient education and counseling.
   a. Information about fatigue.
   b. Reassurance that treatment-related fatigue does not mean your cancer is worse.
   c. Why fatigue and shortness of breath may occur.
   d. Suggestions for ways to cope with fatigue.
      i. Encourage aerobic and strength-training exercise. Balance activity and rest.
      ii. Plan frequent rest periods between daily activities; take naps that do not interrupt nighttime sleep.
      iii. Set priorities and delegate tasks to others.

e. Stress management.
f. Explain that blood transfusions, if given, are a part of therapy and not necessarily an indication of a setback.
g. Observe skin color.
h. Monitor nutritional status.

Promoting Nutrition

 Evidence Base National Comprehensive Cancer Network. (2012). Clinical practice guidelines in oncology: Antiemesis. Available: *www.nccn.org*.

1. Prevention of nausea/vomiting is the goal. Administer anti-emetics before chemotherapy and on a routine schedule (not as needed).

2. Be aware that anti-emetic combinations are more effective than single agents.

3. For highly emetogenic chemotherapy regimens:
   a. Serotonin (5-HT3) antagonist.
      i. Ondansetron, 16 to 24 mg P.O. or 8 to 12 mg (maximum 32 mg) IV day 1, or
      ii. granisetron, 2 mg P.O. or 1 mg P.O. bid or 0.01 mg/kg (maximum 1 mg) IV day 1, or
      iii. dolasetron, 100 mg P.O., or
      iv. palonosetron, 0.25 mg IV day 1, and
   b. Corticosteroid—dexamethasone, 12 mg P.O. or IV day 1, 8 mg P.O. or IV days 2 to 4.
   c. Neurokinin 1 agonist.
      i. Aprepitant, 125 mg P.O. day 1, 80 mg P.O. daily days 2 and 3, or
      ii. Fosaprepitant, 150 mg IV day 1 only, and
      iii. ± lorazepam, 0.5 to 2 mg P.O. or IV or sublingual either every 4 or every 6 hours days 1 to 4.
   d. Include an as-needed anti-emetic, such as metoclopramide, prochlorperazine, dexamethasone, or lorazepam.

4. For moderately emetogenic regimens:
   a. Premedicate with aprepitant, 125 mg P.O. (for selected high-risk patients); dexamethasone, 12 mg P.O. or IV and a 5-HT3 antagonist, such as palonosetron, 0.25 mg IV, or ondansetron, 16 to 24 mg P.O. or 8 to 12 mg; or ± lorazepam, 0.5 to 2 mg either P.O. or IV or sublingual every 4 to 6 hours prn.
   b. On days 2 to 4: aprepitant, 80 mg P.O. on days 2 and 3 (if used on day 1); dexamethasone, 8 mg IV or P.O. daily plus a 5-HT3 agonist, such as ondansetron, P.O. b.i.d.; granisetron, 1 to 2 mg P.O. or 1 mg P.O. b.i.d.; or dolasetron, 100 mg P.O.
   c. Include an as-needed anti-emetic, such as prochlorperazine or lorazepam.

5. For low emetogenic regimens:
   a. Dexamethasone, 12 mg P.O. or IV daily, or
   b. Prochlorperazine, 10 mg P.O. or IV every 4 to 6 hours or 15 mg spansule P.O. every 8 to 12 hours, or
   c. Metoclopramide, either 20 to 40 mg P.O. every 4 to 6 hours or 1 to 2 mg/kg IV every 3 to 4 hours; ± diphenhydramine, 25 to 50 mg P.O. or IV every 4 to 6 hours; or ± lorazepam, 0.5 to 2 mg P.O. or IV every 4 to 6 hours.

6. Extrapyramidal reactions occur frequently in patients under age 30 and over age 65. Treat dystonic reactions with diphenhydramine; treat restlessness with lorazepam.
7. Consider alternative measures for relief of anticipatory nausea, such as relaxation therapy, imagery, and distraction.
8. Encourage small, frequent meals appealing to patient preferences, but including high calories and proteins. Provide a high-protein supplement as needed.
9. Discourage smoking and alcoholic beverages, which may irritate mucous membranes.
10. Encourage fluid intake to prevent constipation.
11. Monitor intake and output, including emesis.
12. Consult dietitian about patient's food preferences, intolerances, and individual dietary interventions.
13. Recognize that the patient may have alterations in taste perception, such as a keener taste of bitterness and loss of ability to detect sweet tastes.

Minimizing Stomatitis
1. Report signs of infection—erythematous areas, white patches, ulcers.
2. Encourage good oral hygiene.
   a. Soft nylon-bristled toothbrush, brush two to three times daily, rinse frequently.
   b. Floss once daily.
3. Encourage the use of oral agents to promote cleansing, debridement, and comfort. Mouthwashes with more than 25% alcohol should be avoided.
4. Assess the need for antifungal, antibacterial, or antiviral therapy (each infection has a different appearance).
5. Administer local oral therapy, such as combinations with viscous lidocaine, for symptomatic control and maintenance of calorie intake.

Preventing and Managing Hypersensitivity Reactions
1. Be alert for signs of allergic reactions such as pruritus, urticaria, and difficulty breathing as well as back pain. The situation may worsen suddenly to hypotension and anaphylaxis.
2. Stop the medication or infusion immediately, notify the health care provider, and monitor the patient closely. Treatment is supportive and dependent on type of reaction and its severity.
   a. Do not administer the agent again if there was a severe reaction resulting in significant hypotension.
   b. Premedicate the patient with antihistamine or corticosteroid, as directed, if there is a history of moderate reaction.

Strengthening Coping for Altered Body Image
1. Reassure patient that hair will grow back; however, it may grow back a different texture or different color.
2. Suggest wearing a turban, wig, or headscarf, preferably purchased before hair loss occurs. Many insurance companies will pay for a wig with a prescription.
3. Encourage patient to stay on therapeutic program.
4. Be honest with patient.

Patient Education and Health Maintenance

1. Make sure patient uses good hygiene, knows the symptoms of infection to report, and avoids crowds and people with infection while neutropenic.

2. Advise patient to avoid using a razor blade to shave, contact sports, manipulation of sharp articles, use of a hard-bristle toothbrush, and passage of hard stool to prevent bleeding while thrombocytopenic.
3. Advise women to report symptoms of vaginal infection due to opportunistic fungal or viral infection.
4. Encourage patient participation in plan for chemotherapy and to set realistic goals for work and activities.
5. Assure patient that changes in menses, libido, and sexual function are usually temporary during therapy.

Evaluation: Expected Outcomes

- Afebrile, no signs of infection.
- No bruising or bleeding noted; stool and urine heme test negative.
- Denies shortness of breath or severe fatigue.
- Tolerates small, frequent meals following anti-emetic.
- No oral lesions or pain on swallowing.
- No urticaria, shortness of breath, or change in vital signs.
- Wears turban, expresses feelings about body image.

Radiation Therapy

Radiation therapy is the treatment of benign and malignant diseases with ionizing radiation. The goal of radiation is to deliver a precisely measured dose of irradiation to a defined tumor volume with minimal damage to surrounding healthy tissue. This results in eradication of tumor, high quality of life, prolongation of survival, and allows for effective palliation or prevention of symptoms of cancer, with minimal morbidity. Over the past 20 years, advances have been made in imaging and treatment delivery, allowing for improved targeting and increased sparing of normal tissues.

General Considerations

1. Different irradiation doses are required for tumor control, depending on tumor type and the number of cells present. Varying radiation doses can be delivered to specific portions of the tumor (periphery versus central portion) or to the tumor bed in cases in which all gross tumor has been surgically removed.
2. Treatment portals must adequately cover all treatment volumes plus a margin.

Goals of Therapy
1. Curative—when there is a probability of long-term survival after adequate therapy; some adverse effects of therapy, although undesirable, may be acceptable.
2. Palliative—when there is no hope of survival for extended periods, radiation can be used to palliate symptoms, primarily pain. Lower doses of irradiation (75% to 80% of curative dose) can control the tumor and palliate symptoms without excessive toxicity.

Principles of Therapy
1. A boost is the additional dose administered through small portals to residual disease; it is given to obtain the same probability of control as for subclinical aggregates.
2. Radiosensitivity is the degree and speed of response. This measure of susceptibility of cells to injury or death by radiation depends on cancer diagnosis and its inherent biologic activity. It is directly related to reproductive capability of the cell.

3. Role of oxygen: Oxygen must be present at the time of radiation's maximal killing effect. Poor circulation with resultant hypoxia can reduce cellular radiosensitivity. Giving multiple, daily doses allows reoxygenation and enhances radiosensitivity. The dose should allow for repair of normal tissues.

4. Cellular response can be modified by changing the dose rate, manipulating the process of cell repair, recruiting cells into replication cycle, and using hyperthermia (above 104° F [40° C]).

5. Radioresistance is the lack of tumor response to radiation because of tumor characteristics (slow-growing, less responsive), tumor cell proliferation, and circulation. Radiation is most effective during the mitotic stage of the cell cycle.

6. Radioresistant tumors: Many tumors are resistant to radiation, such as squamous cell, ovarian, soft tissue sarcoma, and gliomas. Many other tumors can become resistant after a period of time. Normal radioresistant tissues include mature bone, cartilage, liver, thyroid, muscle, brain, and spinal cord.

Types of Radiation Therapy

There are generally two types of radiation and several techniques in which radiation is delivered.

1. Teletherapy is most commonly delivered through a linear accelerator machine, but there are a number of techniques used to administer teletherapy.

   a. Intraoperative radiation therapy—given during surgery for tumors that are not completely operable or are at high risk for recurrence. Examples include gynecological malignancies and colorectal cancers.

   b. Stereotactic radiation (radiosurgery)—used for brain tumors where the radiation beam is delivered precisely to the tumor itself sparing surrounding healthy brain tissue. This can be administered through gamma knife technology. The patient's head is placed into a frame that is secured to the cranium with screws. Scanning technology allows for precise and accurate delivery of radiation.

   c. Intensity-modulated radiation therapy (IMRT)—uses radiation beams of varying intensities to deliver different doses of radiation to small areas of tissue at the same time. This is used most commonly in brain, head, and neck tumors and lung tumors.

   d. Image-guided radiation therapy—uses repeated imaging scans (obtained via CT, MRI, or PET) during treatment to identify changes in a tumor's size and location due to treatment and to allow the position of the patient or the planned radiation dose to be adjusted, as needed. Repeated imaging can increase the accuracy of radiation treatment and may allow reductions in the planned volume of tissue to be treated, thereby decreasing the total radiation dose to normal tissue.

   e. Tomotherapy—type of image-guided IMRT. A tomotherapy machine is a hybrid between a CT imaging scanner and an external-beam radiation therapy machine. Tomotherapy machines can capture CT images of the patient's tumor immediately before each treatment, to allow for precise tumor targeting and sparing of normal tissue.

2. Brachytherapy uses seeds, wires, or catheters to deliver radiation directly to or adjacent to the tumor bed. This technique delivers less radiation to adjacent normal tissue, but it requires direct tumor access. It may be temporary or permanent. The permanent type remains in place with gradual decay. The implant procedure is performed under local or general anesthesia and is typically used for breast and prostate cancers.

   a. Intracavitary therapy utilizes radioactive material that is inserted into a cavity such as the vagina, as in cancer of the uterine cervix.

   b. Other forms of brachytherapy are systemic irradiation (parenteral or IV), oral ^{131}I for thyroid cancer, or intraperitoneal radiation.

Chemical and Thermal Modifiers of Radiation

1. Radiosensitization is the use of medications to enhance the sensitivity of the tumor cells.

2. Radioprotectors increase therapeutic ratio by promoting repair of normal tissues.

3. Hyperthermia is combined with radiation. Uses a variety of sources (ultrasound, microwaves) and produces a greater effect than radiation alone. It is usually applied locally or regionally immediately after radiation.

Units for Measuring Radiation Exposure or Absorption

1. Centigray (cGy) is a unit of radiation dose absorbed by the body equal to one hundredth of a gray; formerly called a rad (eg, 1 cGy equals 1 rad). Gray (Gy) is the unit of absorbed radiation dose equal to 100 rad.

2. Hyperfractionated radiation therapy is the division of the total radiation dose into smaller daily doses. Administering fractions allows treatment of tumor cells while giving healthy cells time to repair themselves.

3. Radiation dose equivalent (rem) is the product of the absorbed dose in rads and a weighting factor, W_R, which accounts for the effectiveness of the radiation to cause biological damage in human beings.

Nature and Indications for Use

Used alone or in combination with surgery or chemotherapy, depending on the stage of disease and goal of therapy.

1. Adjuvant radiation therapy—used in combination with other treatment modalities, such as chemotherapy or surgery, when a high risk of local recurrence or large primary tumor exists.

2. Curative radiation therapy—used in anatomically limited tumors (retina, optic nerve, certain brain tumors, skin, oral cavity). Course is usually longer and the dose higher.

3. Palliative—for treatment of symptoms.

   a. Provides excellent pain control for bone metastasis.

   b. Used to relieve obstruction.

   c. Relief of neurologic dysfunction for brain metastasis.

   d. Given in short, intensive courses.

Treatment Planning

1. Evaluation of tumor extent (staging), including diagnostic studies before treatment.

2. Define the goal of therapy (cure or palliation).

3. Select appropriate treatment modalities (irradiation alone or combined with surgery, chemotherapy, or both).

4. All patients undergo simulation and treatment planning.

   a. Simulation is used to accurately identify target volumes and sensitive structures. CT simulation allows for accurate three-dimensional treatment planning of target volume and anatomy of critical normal structures.

   b. Treatment aids (eg, shielding blocks, molds, masks, immobilization devices, compensators) are extremely important in treatment planning and delivery of optimal dose distribution. Repositioning and immobilization devices are critical for accurate treatment.

   c. Lead blocks are made to shape the beam and protect normal tissues.

   d. Skin markings are applied to define the target and portal. These are generally replaced later by permanent tattoos.

5. Usual schedule is Monday through Friday.

6. Actual therapy lasts minutes. Most time is spent on positioning.

7. Determine optimal dose of irradiation and volume to be treated, according to anatomic location, histologic type, stage, potential regional nodal involvement (and other tumor characteristics), and normal structures in the region.

Complications

Complications depend on the site of radiation therapy, type of radiation therapy (brachytherapy or teletherapy), total radiation dose, daily fractionated doses, and overall health of the patient. Adverse effects are predictable, depending on the normal organs and tissues involved in the field.

Acute Adverse Effects

1. Fatigue and malaise.

2. Skin: may develop a reaction as soon as 2 weeks into the course of treatment. (Skin erythema may range from mild to severe with possible dry-to-wet desquamation. Areas having folds, such as the axilla, under the breasts, groin and gluteal fold, are at an increased risk because of increased warmth and moisture.)

3. GI effects: nausea and vomiting, diarrhea, and esophagitis.

4. Oral effects: changes in taste, mucositis, dryness, and xerostomia (dryness of mouth from lack of normal secretions).

5. Pulmonary effects: dyspnea, productive cough, and radiation pneumonitis (usually occurs 1 to 3 months after radiation to the lung).

6. Renal and bladder effects: cystitis and urethritis.

7. Cardiovascular effects: damage to vasculature of organs, thrombosis (heart is relatively radioresistant).

8. Recall reactions: acute skin and mucosal reactions when concurrent or past chemotherapy (doxorubicin, dactinomycin).

9. Bone marrow suppression: more common with pelvic or large bone radiation.

Chronic Adverse Effects

After 6 months with variability in time of expression:

1. Skin effects: fibrosis, telangiectasia, permanent darkening of the skin, and atrophy.

2. GI effects: fibrosis, adhesions, obstruction, ulceration, and strictures.

3. Oral effects: permanent xerostomia, permanent taste alterations, and dental caries.

4. Pulmonary effects: fibrosis.

5. Renal and bladder effects: radiation nephritis, fibrosis.

6. Second primary cancer: patients who have received combined radiation and chemotherapy with alkylating agents have a rare risk of developing acute leukemia.

Nursing Assessment

1. Assess skin and mucous membranes for adverse effects of radiation.

2. Assess GI, respiratory, and renal function for signs of adverse effects.

3. Assess patient's understanding of treatment and emotional status.

Nursing Diagnoses

- Risk for Impaired Skin Integrity related to radiation effects.
- Ineffective Protection related to brachytherapy.

Nursing Interventions

Maintaining Optimal Skin Care

1. Inform the patient that some skin reaction can be expected, but that it varies from patient to patient. Examples include dry erythema, dry desquamation, wet desquamation, epilation, and tanning.

2. Do not apply lotions, ointments, or cosmetics to the site of radiation unless prescribed.

3. Discourage vigorous rubbing, friction, or scratching because this can destroy skin cells. Apply ointments as instructed by health professionals.

4. Avoid wearing tight-fitting clothing over the treatment field; prevent irritation by not using rough fabric such as wool and corduroy.

5. Take precautions against exposing the radiation field to sunlight and extremes in temperature.

6. Do not apply adhesive or other tape to the skin.

7. Avoid shaving the skin in the treatment field.

8. Use lukewarm water only and mild soap when bathing.

Ensuring Protection from Radiation

1. To avoid exposure to radiation while the patient is receiving therapy, consider the following:

   a. Time—exposure to radiation is directly proportional to the time spent within a specific distance to the source.

   b. Distance—amount of radiation reaching a given area decreases as resistance increases.

   c. Shield—sheet of absorbing material placed between the radiation source and the nurse decreases the amount of radiation exposure.

2. If exposed to penetrating radiation (x-ray or gamma rays), wear film badges on the front of the body.

3. Take appropriate measures associated with sealed sources of radiation implanted within a patient (sealed internal radiation).

   a. Follow directives on precaution sheet that is placed on the charts of all patients receiving radiotherapy.

   b. Do not remain within 3 feet (1 meter) of the patient any longer than required to give essential care.

4. Know that the casing material absorbs all alpha radiation and most beta radiation, but that a hazard concerning gamma radiation may exist.

5. Do not linger longer than necessary in giving patient care, even though all precautions are followed.

6. Be alert for implants that may have become loosened (those inserted in cavities that have access to the exterior); for example, check the emesis basin following mouth care for a patient with an oral implant.

7. Notify the radiation therapist of any implant that has moved out of position.

8. Use long-handled forceps or tongs and hold at arm's length when picking up any dislodged radium needle, seeds, or tubes. Never pick up a radioactive source with your hands.

9. Do not discard dressings or linens unless you are sure that no radioactive source is present.

10. After the patient is discharged from the facility, it is a good policy for the radiologist to check the room with a radiograph or survey meter to be certain that all radioactive materials have been removed.

11. Continue radiation precautions when a patient has a permanent implant, until the radiologist declares precautions unnecessary.

Evaluation: Expected Outcomes

- Skin without breakdown or signs of infection.
- Radiation precautions maintained.

Biologic Therapy

Biologic therapy is targeted cancer treatment. It has emerged as an important modality of cancer treatment and one where intensive research is actively being conducted. The goal is to produce antitumor effects through the action of natural host defense mechanisms. It is capable of altering the immune system with either stimulatory or suppressive effects.

Underlying Principles

Function

The primary function of the immune system is to detect and eliminate substances that are recognized as "nonself."

Types of Immunotherapy

Cytokines

Cytokines are soluble proteins produced by mononuclear cells of the immune system (usually the lymphocytes and monocytes) that have regulatory actions on other cells in the immune system. Cytokines produced by lymphocytes are referred to as *lymphokines*, and cytokines produced by monocytes are referred to as *monokines*.

1. Examples of cytokines include interleukins, interferons, CSFs, and tumor necrosis factor.
2. Many other biologic agents are currently under investigation.

Antibody Therapy

Monoclonal antibodies work on cancer cells in the same way natural antibodies work, by identifying and binding to the target cells. They then alert other cells in the immune system to the presence of the cancer cells.

1. Promotes targeting cells through antibody–antigen response.
2. Monoclonal antibodies may be used alone or in combination with chemotherapy.
3. Current monoclonal antibodies available:

a. Rituximab—a murine/human chimeric monoclonal antibody specific for the CD20 surface marker on B cells. It is approved for the treatment of relapsed or refractory low-grade/follicular non-Hodgkin's lymphoma.

b. Ibritumomab—combines the targeting power of monoclonal antibodies with the cell-damaging ability of localized radiation. It is developed to recognize and attach to substances on the surface of certain cells and deliver cytotoxic radiation directly to the cancerous cells.

c. Trastuzumab—a recombinant DNA–derived humanized monoclonal antibody that selectively binds with high affinity in a cell-based assay to the extracellular domain of the human epidermal growth factor receptor 2 protein (HER2). It is approved for the treatment of patients with early stage and advanced metastatic breast cancer whose tumors overexpress the HER2 protein.

d. Cetuximab—binds to extracellular EGRF resulting in inhibition of cell growth and induction of apoptosis.

e. Bevacizumab—binds to and inhibits the activity of human VEGF to its receptors blocking proliferation and formation of new blood vessels that supply tumor cells.

f. Panitumumab—inhibits the binding of ligand to the EGFR receptor resulting in inhibition of cell growth.

g. Alemtuzumab—recognizes the CD52 antigen expressed on malignant and normal B lymphocytes. It has come to be used therapeutically in B-cell malignancies.

4. Potential adverse effects of monoclonal antibodies include dyspnea and mild wheezing, fever and chills, headache, rash, nausea and vomiting, tachycardia, bleeding, and allergic reactions.

Other Targeted Therapies

1. Gefitinib—an epidermal growth factor inhibitor; has been shown to inhibit lung and bladder cancers.
2. Erlotinib—a human epidermal growth factor type 1/epidermal growth factor receptor (HER1/EGFR) inhibitor, which demonstrated an increased survival in advanced non–small-cell lung cancer patients.
3. Lapatinib—kinase inhibitor that is used for the treatment of patients with advanced or metastatic breast cancer.
4. Imatinib mesylate—inhibits tyrosine kinase thereby cell proliferation, used most commonly in chronic leukemia.

Nursing Assessment

1. Review patient's record or obtain history from the patient to determine site of cancer, previous cancer therapies, current medications, and other medical conditions.
2. Assess current cardiovascular and respiratory status.
3. Assess patient's understanding of immunotherapy and associated toxicities.

Nursing Diagnoses

- Hyperthermia as an adverse effect of immunotherapy.
- Ineffective Tissue Perfusion related to capillary permeability leak syndrome (third spacing of fluid) caused by immunotherapy.

Nursing Interventions

Controlling Hyperthermia

1. Discuss the overall goal of immunotherapy, expected adverse effects, and the method of administration.
2. Instruct the patient to report fever, chills, diarrhea, nausea and vomiting, itching, or weight gain.
3. Administer or advise self-administration of antipyretics, such as acetaminophen for fever.
4. Emphasize that adverse effects are temporary and will usually cease within 1 week after treatment ends.

Maintaining Tissue Perfusion

1. Monitor vital signs at least every 4 hours for hypotension, tachycardia, tachypnea, and fever.
   a. Instruct the patient to remain in bed if blood pressure is low.
   b. Monitor apical heart rate.
2. Assess respirations for rate and depth, and auscultate breath sounds for evidence of pulmonary edema.
3. Assess for signs of restlessness, apprehension, discomfort, or cyanosis, which may indicate respiratory distress.
4. Administer oxygen as prescribed.
5. Maintain patent IV line and administer serum albumin as prescribed.
6. Check extremities for warmth, color, and capillary refill.

Evaluation: Expected Outcomes

- Relief of fever after medication.
- Blood pressure stable, lungs clear.

SPECIAL CONSIDERATIONS IN CANCER CARE

Pain Management

Pain related to cancer may be caused by direct tumor infiltration of bones, nerves, viscera, or soft tissue or by prior therapeutic measures (surgery, radiation).

Incidence

1. Pain is the most common symptom associated with cancer.
2. The incidence of pain in cancer patients increases with progression of disease and studies report the incidence from 14% to 100% of all patients with cancer.
3. About 50% of physicians believed that they gave their cancer patients insufficient analgesic drugs for pain control, and 30% indicated they would not use maximally effective analgesic doses until they felt that the patient's life expectancy was less than 6 months.
4. Cancer pain can be controlled with medication in 80% to 95% of patients.

Causes of Pain

1. Pain induced by the disease due to direct tumor involvement of bone, nerves, viscera, or soft tissue.
2. Pain induced by treatment including surgery, chemotherapy, and immunotherapy.

Types of Pain

1. Somatic pain—caused by direct tumor involvement of sensory receptors in cutaneous and deep tissues.
   a. Usually described as dull, sharp, aching, and throbbing; usually constant and localized.
   b. Most common somatic pain is bone pain caused by metastasis.
   c. Can usually be controlled with NSAIDs or oral opioids.
2. Neuropathic pain.
   a. Results from nerve injury or compression.
   b. Includes phantom pain and postherpetic neuralgia.
   c. Described as burning, shooting, electric, and lancinating. (It can be constant or sporadic.)
   d. Usually associated with paresthesia.
   e. Treatment usually includes combinations of antidepressants, anticonvulsants, and opioids.
3. Visceral pain.
   a. Usually described as deep, dull, aching, squeezing, or pressure sensation. It can be vague or ill-defined and can be referred to cutaneous sites, making it difficult to differentiate from somatic pain.
   b. Usually caused by abnormal stretching of smooth muscle walls, ischemia of visceral muscle, and serosal irritation.
   c. Can be treated with oral opioids or surgery to remove the cause.

Other Clinical Manifestations

1. Fatigue from sleep disturbances—most patients have not slept for extended periods.
2. Loss of appetite, weight loss, anxiety, and depression.
3. Change in self-concept and quality of life.

Principles of Pain Management

1. The goal of pain management is complete relief of pain.
2. Placebos are never indicated for the treatment of pain.
3. Physical dependence and tolerance commonly occur; patients may require escalating doses of medications to control pain.
4. It is essential that physicians and nurses do not confuse addiction with tolerance. Addiction is an unrelated medical disorder with behavioral components. These facts must also be stressed with patients who are reluctant to take medications.

Pharmacologic Management

Nonopioid analgesics

1. Acetaminophen—a centrally acting analgesic; does not have anti-inflammatory or antiplatelet activities.
2. NSAIDs.
   a. Produce analgesia by decreasing levels of inflammatory mediators such as prostaglandins at the site of tissue injury.
   b. Suppress platelet function, decrease creatinine clearance, and interfere with the protective effect of prostaglandins on the gastric mucosa.
   c. Used to treat mild to moderate pain; examples include ibuprofen, 400 to 800 mg P.O. t.i.d.; nabumetone, 500 to 1000 mg P.O. b.i.d.; indomethacin, 25 to 50 mg P.O. t.i.d.

d. COX-2 inhibitors are NSAIDs that are somewhat selective for cyclooxygenase 2 (COX-2) compounds, present in most tissues but less present than COX-1 in gastric mucosa. COX-2 is induced in response to inflammation and converts arachidonic acid to prostaglandin. COX-2 inhibitors inhibit prostaglandins at the site of inflammation but cause less GI irritation and bleeding. Examples include celecoxib, 7.5 to 15 mg P.O. b.i.d.; meloxican, mg P.O. q.i.d.

3. Corticosteroids—may decrease edema associated with tumor invasion of neural tissue or bone.
   a. Typically used for headache associated with brain tumors.
   b. Examples include dexamethasone, 4 to 10 mg P.O. q.i.d. to t.i.d. (dosage varies); prednisone, 5 to 60 mg P.O. q.i.d. (dosage varies).

4. Bisphosphonates—used for lytic bone lesions to prevent fractures and may help control bone pain. Examples include zoledronic acid, 4 mg IV every 3 to 4 weeks; pamidronate, 90 mg IV every 4 weeks.

5. Anticonvulsants and antidepressants for neuropathic pain— used to enhance the effect of opioids. Examples include amitriptyline, 25 to 100 mg P.O. every h.s. (hours of sleep) (may cause drowsiness); gabapentin, 300 to 600 mg q.i.d. to t.i.d.; pregabalin, 100 to 300 mg/day.

Opioid Analgesics

1. Oral route is preferred unless patient cannot swallow or absorb medications through the GI tract. Doses should be adjusted to achieve pain relief with an acceptable level of adverse effects.

2. Most important to administer on a schedule rather than on an as-needed basis.

3. Optimal treatment approach is to treat with long-acting drugs to control baseline pain, paired with short-acting drugs, as needed, for breakthrough pain.

4. Oral opioids—primary course of treatment for moderate to severe pain; produce analgesia by binding to specific opiate receptors in the brain and spinal cord.
   a. Short-acting opioids—may be used for breakthrough pain, with relief lasting 3 to 4 hours. Examples include morphine, oxycodone, or hydromorphone.
   b. Long-acting opioids—should be equivalent to daily dose of short-acting opiates. Examples include morphine and oxycodone. Should be prescribed every 8 to 12 hours.
   c. Fentanyl—transdermal patch applied to the skin that is changed every 3 days. The peak effect is delayed for up to 3 days after applying. Should be used for patients with stable opioid requirements.

5. Parenteral administration of opioids is used for patients who cannot tolerate oral opioids or who are in an acute pain crisis.
   a. Patient-controlled analgesia (PCA)—administered by either SC or IV route using a computer-assisted drug delivery system.
   b. SC infusion of morphine should not exceed 5 mL/hour.

6. Intraspinal administration of opiates for management of acute or chronic pain:
   a. A catheter is placed into spinal epidural or subarachnoid (intrathecal) space.
   b. Catheter may be placed percutaneously and sutured in site or tunneled subcutaneously to the abdominal wall and exteriorized, or the pump system may be implanted.
   c. Catheter is positioned as near as possible to the spinal segment where the pain is projected.
   d. Preservative-free sterile morphine or other analgesic or local anesthetic drug is injected into the system at specified intervals.
   e. May be delivered by PCA pump or by continuous or intermittent infusion.
   f. Spinally administered local anesthetics produce their effects predominantly by action on axons of spinal nerve roots; produce long-lasting pain relief with relatively low doses with little or no blunting of patient's level of responsiveness.
   g. Complications of intraspinal administration include respiratory depression, urine retention, pruritus, infection, leakage, technical problems, and development of tolerance.

Nursing Assessment and Interventions

To provide effective pain management, nursing assessment, physical examination, and review of laboratory values are very important (see Standards of Care Guidelines 8-1).

1. Screen for pain at each visit. Evaluate objectively the nature of the patient's pain, including location, duration, quality, and impact on daily activities. Pain self-assessment is the most reliable guide to both cause of the pain and the effectiveness of pain treatment.

STANDARDS OF CARE GUIDELINES 8-1
Comprehensive Pain Assessment

Routinely assess pain in cancer patients using the following parameters.

- Pain Intensity (numerical scale 0–10)
  "On a scale of 0 to 10, what would be your pain rating if 0 means no pain and 10 means the worst pain you can imagine?"
  - At rest
  - With movement
- Location, referral pattern, radiation of pain
- History
  - Onset
  - Duration
  - Course
  - Aggravating or associated symptoms
- Quality
  - Persistent, intermittent
  - Aching, stabbing, throbbing, pressure—somatic pain
  - Cramping, aching, sharp—visceral pain
  - Sharp, tingling, burning, shooting—neuropathic pain
- Psychosocial
  - Family and other support
  - Cultural/spiritual beliefs about pain and pain management
- Response to pain relief and adverse effects

2. Assess patient history and physical examination findings and laboratory values to differentiate expected pain from pain due to a new problem, an oncologic complication, or worsening of the underlying process.

3. Use a pain intensity scale of 0 (no pain) to 10 (worst possible pain) or other pain scale as appropriate. Take careful history of prior and present medications, response, and adverse effects.

4. Assess relief from medications and duration of relief. (Use the same measuring scale every time.)

5. Base the initial analgesic choice on the patient's report of pain.

6. Administer drugs orally whenever possible; avoid I.M. injection.

7. Administer analgesia "around the clock" rather than as needed.

8. Convey the impression that the patient's pain is understood and that the pain can be controlled.

9. Take a careful pain history. Explore pain interventions that have been used and their effectiveness. Determine whether the intensity of the pain correlates with the prescribed analgesic.

10. Reevaluate the pain frequently. The requirement for analgesia should decrease if other treatment is given, including radiation or chemotherapy.

11. Use alternative measures to relieve pain such as guided imagery, relaxation, and biofeedback.

12. Provide ongoing support and open communication.

13. Assess bowel function and institute bowel regimen immediately.

14. Consider referral to a pain specialist for intractable pain.

15. Instruct patients that there is no benefit to suffering and that addiction is not a problem.
    a. Instruct patients that taking these medications now does not mean that they will not work later.
    b. Encourage patients to talk to their physician or nurse about their pain and effectiveness of the treatment plan.
    c. Assure patients that there are other options if the medications prescribed do not work.

Patient Education

1. Provide a complete list of each medication prescribed with instructions on how to take each one.

2. Educate patients on the adverse effects of pain medications and ways to manage them.
    a. Respiratory depression is a potentially life-threatening adverse effect of opioids; however, patients generally develop a tolerance.
    b. Constipation is expected with opioids and is treated prophylactically.
    c. Nausea is usually transitory and controllable with prophylactic anti-emetics.
    d. Sedation is common initially and is transitory.

3. Educate patients to administer medications, as necessary (ie, pump instruction and catheter and exit site care).

4. Provide home care assistance as needed.

Oncologic Emergencies

Septic Shock

Septic shock is a systemic disease associated with the presence and persistence of pathogenic microorganisms or their toxins in the blood. It is characterized by hemodynamic instability, abnormal coagulation, and altered metabolism.

Risk Factors

1. Neutropenia, ANC less than 500.
2. Patients who are neutropenic longer than 7 days most susceptible.
3. Patients with HIV and concomitant neutropenia.
4. Prolonged hospitalization.
5. Older patients.
6. Patients with comorbid conditions, such as diabetes and pulmonary diseases.

Clinical Manifestations

1. Fever greater than 100.5° F (38.3° C).
2. Warm, flushed, dry skin.
3. Hypotension.
4. Tachycardia.
5. Tachypnea.
6. Decreased level of consciousness.
7. Patients will not have the usual symptoms of infection due to the lack of neutrophils. For example, skin infections may manifest as subtle rash or erythema. Urinary tract infections may be asymptomatic and patients with lung infections may be without pulmonary infiltrates.

Diagnostic Evaluation

1. Vital signs.
2. Culture—blood, urine, stool, sputum, central and peripheral IV lines, and any open wounds to determine source and type of infection.
3. Chest x-ray—to detect underlying pneumonia.
4. CT scans as necessary.
5. Arterial blood gas analysis—decreased pH reflects acidosis.
6. BUN and creatinine—elevated due to decreased circulating blood volume.
7. CBC with differential—elevated WBC count with shift to left.

Management

1. Antibiotics are started immediately; broad-spectrum antibiotics are given until organism is identified.
2. IV fluids and plasma expanders are used to restore circulating volume.
3. CSFs are administered to increase neutrophil count.
4. Vasopressors are administered to support blood pressure.
5. Oxygen is administered, as needed, to prevent tissue hypoxia.
6. Vital signs, respiratory status, urine output, and any signs of bleeding are monitored carefully.
7. Complications, such as renal failure, respiratory failure, cardiac failure, metabolic acidosis, and disseminated intravascular coagulation, are treated aggressively.

Spinal Cord Compression

Spinal cord compression (SCC) is the result of tumor compression on the dural sac. This can result in neurologic impairment or permanent loss of function if not treated immediately.

Incidence

1. Fifty percent of diagnosed cases occur in patients with lung, multiple myeloma, breast, or colon cancer.

Clinical Manifestations

1. Cervical spine.
   a. Vertigo.
   b. Radicular pain in neck and back of head that is aggravated by neck flexion.
   c. Upper extremity weakness.
   d. Sensory loss in area of weakness (ie, paresthesia, numbness).
   e. Abnormal deep tendon reflexes.
   f. Gastric hypersecretion and paralytic ileus.
2. Thoracic spine.
   a. Local or radicular pain (or both).
   b. Lower extremity weakness.
   c. Sensory loss below the level of the lesion.
   d. Band of hyperesthesia at dermatome of tumor site.
   e. Impaired bladder or bowel control.
3. Lumbar spine.
   a. Local or radicular pain (or both).
   b. Lower extremity weakness, paralysis.
   c. Atrophy of lower extremity muscles.
   d. Sensory loss below level of the lesion.
   e. Urinary symptoms (hesitancy, retention), constipation, or bowel incontinence.
4. Weakness and unsteadiness may be noted before changes in motor function. (Progression is usually rapid with foot drop and impaired ambulation. Urgent investigation and treatment are crucial to minimize the risk of paraplegia. The degree of weakness and ability to walk at presentation are important clinical predictors of outcome.)
5. Changes in sensation—paresthesia, numbness, tingling. (Severity usually mirrors the severity of motor weakness.)

 NURSING ALERT Any abnormal neurologic symptoms in a patient with cancer should be considered an SCC until proven otherwise.

Diagnostic Evaluation

1. Neurologic examination—early diagnosis is important.
2. X-ray of the painful site—may be abnormal; can be used as an initial screen for complaints of back pain.
3. Bone scan—more sensitive to bony metastasis than x-ray to detect abnormal vertebral bodies.
4. MRI—most useful in detecting spinal cord lesions. The entire spine can be viewed. Immediately indicated if radiculopathy or myelopathy is present or x-rays are abnormal.

Management

1. Treatment is usually palliative because it is associated with metastatic disease.
2. Treatment goals are to relieve pain and preserve or restore neurologic function.
3. Corticosteroids are the initial treatment until more definitive treatment can be instituted; reduce inflammation and swelling at site, increase neurologic function, and relieve pain.
   a. A loading dose of dexamethasone is usually given followed by tapering doses over a period of weeks.
   b. Steroids must be tapered and not abruptly discontinued.
   c. Monitor patient's glucose levels during dexamethasone treatment because it can cause hyperglycemia.
4. Radiation therapy to the tumor on spinal column is the most common treatment.
   a. A common dose is 3,000 cGy, delivered in 10 fractions over 2½ weeks.
5. Surgery (laminectomy) is considered when tumors are not radiosensitive or located in an area that has been previously radiated. It is also indicated for spinal instability.

Complications

1. Respiratory impairment, including pneumonia and atelectasis.
2. Mobility impairment, footdrop, skin impairment, postural hypotension.
3. Sensory losses creating safety concerns.
4. Bladder or bowel dysfunction.

Patient Education

1. Facilitate referral to home care services for nursing assessment, nursing intervention, and rehabilitation for residual deficits.
2. Facilitate referral to appropriate outpatient services, including physical therapy, occupational therapy, and psychosocial support.
3. Provide instruction about safety issues for residual sensory deficits (eg, test bath water temperature, careful use of extreme hot or cold).

Hypercalcemia

Hypercalcemia is an elevated serum calcium level above 11 mg/dL. It results when bone resorption exceeds both bone formation and the ability of the kidneys to excrete extracellular calcium released from the bones.

Incidence

1. The most common life-threatening disorder associated with malignancy; occurs in one third of patients at some point in their illness.
2. Occurs most commonly in patients with carcinoma of the lung, breast, and renal cells; multiple myeloma; and adult lymphomas.
3. Can occur with or without skeletal metastasis, but more than 80% of patients do have bony disease.
4. Associated with a poor prognosis.

Clinical Manifestations

1. Signs and symptoms may vary, depending on the severity, and may be nonspecific and insidious.
   a. Early symptoms include anorexia, weakness, polyuria, polydipsia, and fatigue.
   b. Late symptoms include apathy, irritability, profound muscle weakness, nausea, vomiting, constipation, pruritus, vision disturbances.
2. A rapid and life-threatening increase in calcium may cause dehydration, renal failure, coma, and death.

Diagnostic Evaluation

1. Serum calcium level greater than 11 mg/dL in adults, but ionized calcium of greater than 1.29 mmol/L is the most reliable test.
2. Electrolyte levels, BUN, and creatinine are obtained to determine hydration status and renal function.
3. ECG may show shortening of the QT interval and prolongation of the PR interval.

Management

1. Management includes treating the primary malignancy with chemotherapy, surgery, or radiation.
2. Acute, symptomatic hypercalcemia should be treated as an emergency.
3. Hydration and diuresis—IV normal saline (0.9% NaCl) is the initial treatment for patients with acute hypercalcemia and clinical symptoms to dilute the calcium and promote its renal excretion. Diuresis is induced with furosemide. (Thiazide diuretics aggravate hypercalcemia and should be avoided.)
4. Pharmacotherapy includes:
   a. Bisphosphonates are primary drug therapy; administered IV, pamidronate, or zoledronic acid inhibit osteoclast resorption in the bone.
   b. Calcitonin—used in combination with glucocorticoids, inhibits bone resorption. It has a rapid onset but a short duration of action. Used most commonly in patients with multiple myeloma.
   c. Denosumab—a monoclonal antibody that is currently being used for the treatment of postmenopausal osteoporosis. It is currently under investigation for the treatment of hypercalcemia and may have application for use in hypercalcemia of malignancy in the future.

Nursing Interventions

1. Prevent and detect hypercalcemia early.
   a. Recognize patients at risk and monitor for signs and symptoms, such as nausea and vomiting, constipation, lethargy, and anorexia.
   b. Emphasize importance of mobility to minimize bone demineralization and constipation.
   c. Instruct patient on the importance of adequate hydration.
2. Administer normal saline infusions as prescribed.
3. Administer medications as prescribed.
4. Maintain accurate intake and output; observe for oliguria or anuria.
5. Take vital signs every 4 hours, especially apical pulse and blood pressure.
6. Monitor electrolyte values and renal function.
7. Assess mental status.
8. Assess cardiorespiratory status for signs of fluid overload.

Superior Vena Cava Syndrome

Superior vena cava syndrome (SVCS) is obstruction and thrombosis of the superior vena cava by a tumor or an enlarged lymph node, resulting in impaired venous drainage of the head, neck, arms, and thorax.

Incidence

1. Eighty percent to 95% of patients with SVCS are cancer patients.
2. Eighty percent of cases arise from advanced lung cancer, specifically small-cell lung cancers, and 15% from lymphoma.
3. Other malignancies associated with SVCS are thymoma and breast cancer.

Clinical Manifestations

1. Signs and symptoms may vary, depending on the degree of obstruction and how rapidly the obstruction occurs.
2. A rapid onset of SVCS is dramatic, potentially life-threatening, and requires immediate intervention.
3. Early symptoms include progressive dyspnea, cough, feeling of fullness in the head, difficulty buttoning shirt collar (Stoke's sign), dysphagia and hoarseness, and chest pain.
4. Cyanosis and edema of the head and upper extremities may be apparent. Collateral circulation with dilated chest wall veins may be visible.
5. Late symptoms include respiratory distress, headache, vision disturbances, dizziness and syncope, lethargy, irritability, and mental status changes.
6. Pleural effusion on chest x-ray may also be seen.

Diagnostic Evaluation

1. 60% of SVCS cases can be detected on plain chest x-ray, but venography may be helpful to confirm the diagnosis.
2. CT scan may be necessary to make the diagnosis for some patients, but is usually used to determine the extent of tumor and obstruction.

Management

1. Radiation therapy is the gold standard of treatment for SVCS to reduce tumor size and relieve pressure. Most patients experience a relief of symptoms within the first 4 days of therapy.
2. Chemotherapy may be used in conjunction with radiation. Specific chemotherapeutic agents depend on the tumor type.
3. Surgery is rarely used due to the associated high morbidity and mortality risks.
4. Percutaneous stent placement—an expandable stent may be placed inside the superior vena cava to keep it patent. Anticoagulants are also used in conjunction.
5. Glucocorticoids—these agents decrease the inflammatory response to tumor invasion and edema surrounding the tumor mass.
6. Thrombolytic and anticoagulant therapy may be used if a thrombus is suspected or to prevent the formation of a thrombus; must be used within the first 7 days to be effective.
7. Oxygen is given for relief of dyspnea and maintenance of tissue oxygenation.
8. Analgesics and tranquilizers are used for discomfort and anxiety.

Nursing Interventions

1. Administer oxygen, as prescribed, to relieve hypoxia.
2. Place patient in Fowler's position—facilitates gravity drainage and reduces facial edema.

3. Limit patient's activity and provide a quiet environment.
4. Reassure patient that cyanotic color and facial edema will subside with treatment.

Clinical Trials

A *clinical trial* is a scientific study designed to answer important clinical and biological questions. Trials provide a mechanism to test the effectiveness of new drug and other therapies. Clinical trials are important in the advancement of cancer treatment.

Phases of Clinical Trials

Phase I Trials

1. Phase 1 studies are offered to patients who have failed conventional therapy or for whom there is no treatment known to be superior.
2. Phase 1 trials are given to patients with various types of cancer to:
   a. Evaluate drug toxicities.
   b. Establish the maximum tolerated dose of the drug.
   c. Evaluate how the drug is metabolized or the pharmacokinetics of the drug.

Phase II Trials

1. Determine tumor activity in specific tumor types.
2. Design administration techniques.
3. Determine dose modifications.

Phase III Trials

1. Compare drugs with standard therapy.
2. Evaluate response and duration of response.

Phase IV Trials

1. Determine new ways to use the drug.
2. Determine effectiveness in the adjuvant setting.

Nursing Interventions

1. Educate patients about the clinical trial process.
2. If involved in clinical trials, follow protocol and documentation as indicated.
3. Report all adverse events during the trial period.
4. Refer patients who are interested in clinical trials to Cancer-Trials at *www.cancertrials.nci.nih.gov*.

Psychosocial Components of Care

Nursing Assessment

1. Assess lifestyle before illness. How did patient solve other problems?
2. Assess for signs of anxiety and coexistence of depression: agitation and restlessness, sleep disturbances, excessive autonomic activity, weight gain or loss, mood changes.
3. What activities of daily living can patient perform?
4. What changes in lifestyle have resulted from cancer and its treatment?
5. Determine patient's perception of the disease and treatment.
6. Evaluate available social support; who is the most significant other?

7. Ask patient if any complementary or alternative medicine (CAM) modalities are being utilized for cancer treatment. Be aware that many patients seek herbal and other remedies despite lack of scientific evidence of any benefit. Encourage patient and family to discuss CAM use with health care provider to ensure safety.
8. Try to gain a sense of emotional strengths and potential problem areas. Ask if patient and family have a plan for end-of-life care as appropriate.

Nursing Diagnoses

- Anxiety related to complex disease process, treatment options, and prognosis.
- Ineffective Coping related to life-altering disease process.
- Fear of Death and dying.

Nursing Interventions

Reducing Anxiety

1. Establish and sustain an unhurried approach to give the patient time to organize fears, thoughts, and feelings.
2. Allow patient to share feelings about having cancer.
3. Reflect and amplify insights and judgments; try to reduce anxiety through reflection and reorientation.
4. Recognize feelings of losing control.
5. Discuss methods of stress reduction (imagery, relaxation).
6. Discuss the positive aspects of treatment.
7. Encourage expression of positive emotions—emphasis on living in the here and now, greater appreciation of life.
8. Reinforce effective coping behaviors.
9. Encourage patient to join a support group. Refer to local chapter of the American Cancer Society, call 1-800-ACS-2345 or visit *www.cancer.org*.
10. Remain available as problems arise. Give patient telephone numbers of people to call when needed.
11. Initiate referrals for additional rehabilitation and psychosocial services as appropriate.

Promoting Effective Coping

1. Encourage patient and family members to enroll in cancer education program.
2. Encourage patient to learn everything about treatment plan because this promotes a sense of control.
3. Provide expert physical care and teach patient about care.
4. Assist patient in strengthening support system (family, friends, visitors, health care staff and volunteers, support groups)—strengthens self-esteem through the experience of feeling accepted and valued.
5. Help patient readjust expectations and goals to promote ongoing adjustment.
6. Support patient in coping mechanisms chosen.

Allaying Fear of Death and Dying

1. Educate patient and family about prognosis and end-of-life choices, as outlined by patient's health care provider. Be direct, stating the statistics but stressing the positive aspects of the situation.
2. Assess and respect patient's beliefs.
3. Help patient and family agree on goals.

4. Facilitate emotional support for patient.
5. Provide bereavement support to survivors.

Evaluation: Expected Outcomes

- Discusses feelings; practices stress reduction.
- Patient and family attend cancer education program.
- Asks questions about prognosis and sets goals for care.

Palliative Care

Palliative care is the active total care of patients with advanced illness. The focus is no longer on curative treatment, but on quality of life and integrating the physical, psychological, spiritual, and social aspects of care. Although palliative care is appropriate for many cancer patients, it is not limited to cancer; many neurologic, cardiac, pulmonary, and other types of disorders call for palliative care in their more severe or advanced forms.

There are facility- and community-based programs as well as inpatient facilities and home care services (including hospice). Care of patients with advanced illness, such as cancer, and dealing with death and dying is an integral part of oncology nursing. Palliative care has been added to most medical and nursing schools across the country in recent years, but the average number of hours offered in both professional programs is less than 15.

The following resources offer information pertaining to palliative and end-of-life care:
– Center to Advance Palliative Care: *www.capcmssm.org* (for health care professionals)
– End of Life/Palliative Education Resource Center: *www.eperc. mcw.edu* (for health care professionals)
– Last Acts: *www.lastacts.org* (for health care professionals and consumers)
– Hospice Foundation of America: *www.hospicefoundation.org* (for consumers)
– National Hospice and Palliative Care Organization: *www.nhpco. org* (for consumers)

Principles of Palliative Care

1. Palliative care is an interdisciplinary team approach, including experts from medicine, nursing, social work, the clergy, and nutrition. This team approach is needed to make the necessary assessments and to institute appropriate interventions.
2. The essential components of palliative care are relief of symptom distress, improved quality of life, opening of communication on a regular basis with patients to provide appropriate care on their terms, and psychosocial support for patients and families.
3. The goal is to provide comfort and maintain the highest possible quality of life for as long as possible.
4. The traditional focus of palliative care is not on death but on a compassionate, specialized care for the living. It is based on a comprehensive understanding of patient suffering and focuses on providing effective pain and symptom management to seriously ill patients while improving quality of life.

End-of-Life Care

1. Hospice and palliative care provide care during progressive illness, but hospice eligibility begins only when a patient has a life expectancy of 6 months or less. In contrast, palliative care begins when the patient has been diagnosed with a life-limiting illness. It recognizes that the goals of care may change, but the focus is always on quality of life.
2. Unfortunately, hospice is equated with care of the dying, causing it to be underutilized; thus, many patients only live a few days to a week after contacting hospice.
3. Hospice care and palliative care offer end-of-life care, which can be achieved by:
   a. Enhancing physical well-being through effective symptom management: pain, nausea, vomiting, constipation, sleeplessness.
   b. Enhancing psychological well-being through management of anxiety, depression, fear, denial, and hopelessness. Rather, happiness, enjoyment, and leisure are promoted.
   c. Enhancing social well-being by addressing financial burden, caregiver burden, roles and relationships, affection and sexual function, and concerns about appearance.
   d. Enhancing spiritual well-being through minimization of suffering and instead focusing on religious beliefs, hope, and meaning.

Management and Nursing Interventions

1. Provide pain relief, symptom control (hunger, nausea, constipation, anxiety, agitation), and prevention of complications.
2. Encourage patient and family to exceed their current situation.
   a. Encourage patient and family to pursue enjoyable activities.
   b. Assist patient and family to focus on present and past joys.
   c. Share positive and hope-inspiring stories.
3. Facilitate participation in religious or spiritual activities.
4. Encourage families to minimize social isolation.
5. Provide private time for relationships.
6. Discuss end-of-life issues early in patient's treatment plan.

> **! NURSING ALERT** It is important for health care professionals to have open and frank discussions with patients about their preferences regarding end-of-life care. This discussion should not occur during a life-threatening event when patients and families are stressed and feel rushed to make a decision.

7. Encourage patients to express their preferences about end of life in the form of a legal document.
   a. Advance directives, such as medical orders for life-sustaining treatment or healthcare proxy and durable power of attorney, allow for the refusal of further treatment or authorize a family member or friend to make decisions for the patient (see page 192).
   b. After discussion with the patient and family, the primary care provider in an inpatient setting can write orders based on the directives such as "do not resuscitate."
8. Make referrals for respite care, counseling, pastoral care, and bereavement services, as needed.
9. Assist patients and families with decisions for withholding or withdrawing life-sustaining therapies and transfer in and out of inpatient settings by explaining such therapies and clarifying how they fit with the goals of care.

10. Promote ethical practice by organizing interdisciplinary rounds on patients with end-of-life care issues, setting up a partnership in care with family members, collaborating with other nurses who have been through similar situations, and consulting with the ethics committee within your facility.

SELECTED REFERENCES

Advisory Committee on Immunization Practices. (2012). General recommendations on immunizations. Available: *www.cdc.gov/vaccines/pubs/ACIP-list.htm.*

American Cancer Society. (2011). American Cancer Society guidelines on nutrition and physical activity for cancer prevention: Reducing the risk of cancer with healthy food choices and physical activity. Available: *www.cancer.org/acs/groups/cid/documents/webcontent/002577-pdf.pdf.*

American Cancer Society (2012). Cancer facts & figures. Available: *www.cancer.org/Research/CancerFactsFigures/index.*

American Cancer Society (2008). Global facts & figures. Available: *www.cancer.org/Research/CancerFactsFigures/GlobalCancerFactsFigures/index.*

American Joint Committee on Cancer. (2010). *Cancer staging manual* (7th ed.). Philadelphia: Lippincott Raven.

Bevers, T. B. (2007). The STAR trial: Evidence for Raloxifene as a breast cancer risk reduction agent for postmenopausal women. *Journal of National Comprehensive Cancer Network,* 5(8), 719–724.

Cancer Net. Available: *www.cancernet.nci.nih.gov.*

Centers for Disease Control and Prevention (2012). Vaccine schedules. Available: *www.cdc.gov/vaccines/recs/schedules/.*

Cooper, K., Squires, H., Carroll, C., et al. (2010). Chemoprevention of colorectal cancer: Systematic review and economic evaluation. *Health Technology Assessment,* 14(32), 201–206.

Devita, V. T., Lawrence, T. S., & Rosenberg, S. A. (2011). *Cancer: Principles and practice of oncology* (9th ed.). Philadelphia: Lippinocott Williams & Wilkins.

Lawrence, H. K., Doyle, M. S., McCullough, M., et al. (2012). American Cancer Society guidelines on nutrition and physical activity for cancer prevention: Reducing the risk of cancer with healthy food choices and physical activity. CA: *A Cancer Journal for Clinicians,* 62:30–67.

Lewis, M. A., Hendrickson, A. W., & Moynihan, T. J. (2011). Oncologic emergencies: Pathophysiology, presentation, diagnosis, and treatment. *CA—Cancer Journal for Clincians,* 61, 287–314.

National Comprehensive Cancer Network. (2012). Clinical practice guidelines in oncology: Lung cancer screening. Available: *www.nccn.org.*

National Comprehensive Cancer Network. (2012). Clinical practice guidelines in oncology. Available: *www.nccn.org.*

Oncology Nursing Society. (2009). *Chemotherapy and biotherapy: Guidelines and recommendations for practice* (3rd ed.). Pittsburgh, PA: Author.

Rothwell, P. M., Wilson, M., Elwin, C. E., et al. (2010). Long-term effect of aspirin on colorectal cancer incidence and mortality: 20-year follow-up of five randomised trials. *Lancet,* 376, 1741–1750.

Ruppert, R. (2011). Radiation therapy 101. *American Nurse Today,* 6(1), 24–29.

Siegel, R., Ward, S., Brawley O., et al. (2011). Cancer statistics, 2011: The impact of eliminating socioeconomic and racial disparities on premature cancer deaths. *CA—Cancer Journal for Clinicians,* 61(17), 212–236.

Smith, R. A., Cokkinides, V., Brooks, D., et al. (2012). Cancer screening in the United States, 2012: A review of current American Cancer Society guidelines and issues in cancer screening. *CA—Cancer Journal for Clinicians,* 62, 129–142.

Vogel, V. G., Costantino, J. P., Wickerham, D. L., et al. (2006). Effects of Tamoxifen vs. Raloxifene on the risk of developing invasive breast cancer and other disease outcomes: The NSABP study of Tamoxifen and Raloxifene (STAR) P-2 Trial. *Journal of the American Medical Association,* 295(23), 2727–2784.

Yarbro, C. H., Wujciki, D., & Gobel, B. H. (2011). *Cancer nursing: Principles and practice* (7th ed.). Boston: Jones & Bartlett.

Yuen D. (2010). A clinical review of statins and cancer: Helpful or harmful? *Pharmacotherapy,* 30, 177–194.

9
Care of the Older or Disabled Adult

OVERVIEW AND ASSESSMENT

A comprehensive geriatric evaluation (CGE) is essential to fully understand the health needs of older adults. The CGE is performed by a multidisciplinary team, which typically includes a geriatric nurse, geriatric physician, and social worker. Other members of the team may include a pharmacist, physical therapist, and dietitian. The Hartford Institute for Geriatric Nursing provides many tools for assessment of older adults on their Web site (*www. consultgerirn.org/resources*).

Normal Changes of Aging

There are a number of normal age-related changes that occur in all major systems of the body. These may present at different times for different people. It is important to be able to differentiate between normal and abnormal changes in older adults and to educate patients and families about these differences.

Vision
Characteristics
1. Decreased visual acuity.
2. Decreased visual fields, thus decreased peripheral vision.
3. Decreased dark adaptation.
4. Elevated minimal threshold of light perception.
5. Presbyopia (farsightedness) due to decreased visual accommodation from loss of lens elasticity.
6. Decreased color discrimination due to the yellowing of the lens; short wavelength colors, such as blues and greens, are more difficult to see.
7. Increased sensitivity to glare.
8. Decreased depth perception.
9. Decreased tear production.

Assessment Findings
1. Arcus senilis—deposits of lipid around the eye, seen as a white circle around the iris; causes no vision impairments.
2. Cataracts—clouding of the normally clear lens of the eye. (This results in lens thickening and decreased permeability; noted on examination with an ophthalmoscope; fuzziness of vision, like looking through wax paper. Cataracts cause blurring, sensitivity to light, and/or double vision.)
3. Macular degeneration—due to damage to macula that results in loss of central vision. (Objects seem blurred, distorted, or are not seen.)
4. Glaucoma—increased intraocular pressure with tonometer testing. (Results in blurring, colored "halos" around lights, pain or redness of eyes, loss of peripheral vision.)
5. Smaller pupil size.
6. Complaints of decreased ability to read, discomfort from light, changes in depth perception, falls, collisions, difficulty handling small objects, difficulty with activities of daily living (ADLs), and tunnel vision.
7. Dry, red eyes.
8. Vitreous floaters, which are lightning flashes in the visual field.

Nursing Considerations and Teaching Points

1. Make sure objects are in the patient's visual field, and do not move objects around.
2. Use large lettering to label medications and any distributed written information.
3. Allow the person more time to focus and adjust to the environment.
4. Avoid glare—may help to wear sunglasses.
5. Use nightlights to help with dark adaptation problems.
6. Use red and yellow to stimulate vision.
7. Mark the edges of stairs and curbs to help with depth perception problems.
8. Use microspiral telescopes or magnifying glasses and high-intensity lighting.
9. Encourage yearly eye examination and/or refer for examination if vision changes worsen (flashing lights in fields or "veil over the eye").
10. Encourage use of isotonic eyedrops as needed for dry eyes.
11. Encourage use of low vision aids, such as magnifying lens, light filtering lens, telescopic lenses, or electronic devices.
12. Refer patients to the following resources for vision impairments:
    –Prevent Blindness America
    800-331-2020
    www.preventblindness.org
    –American Foundation for the Blind
    800-232-5463
    www.afb.org
    –American Council of the Blind
    800-242-8666
    www.acb.org
    –National Institutes of Health Low Vision & Blindness Educational Resources
    http://health.nih.gov/topic/LowVisionBlindness

Hearing

Characteristics

1. Approximately 30% to 50% of people older than age 65 have significant hearing loss.
2. Two major types of hearing disorders are common in the older population.
   a. Sensorineural—progressive, irreversible bilateral loss of high-tone perception often associated with aging. This results in difficulty with discriminating sounds. Sound waves reach the inner ear but are not properly transmitted to the brain.
   b. Conduction deafness—results from blockage or impairment of the mechanical movement in the outer or middle ear (also a pathologic condition). Sound waves are not conducted to the inner ear, resulting in sounds that are muffled.
3. Hearing loss in older adults is usually a combined problem. The majority of the loss is due to auditory nerve changes or deterioration of the structures of the ear. There may also be nerve damage beyond the ear. Presbycusis and central deafness can result in permanent hearing loss; conduction deafness is reversible.
4. Usual progression from high-tone or high-frequency loss to a general loss of both high and low tones.
5. Consonants (higher-pitched sounds) are not heard well.
6. Hearing loss increases with age and is greater in men.
7. Increase in the sound threshold (ie, greater sound needed to stimulate the older adult).
8. Decreased speech discrimination, especially with background noise.
9. Cerumen impaction, the most common cause of conductive hearing loss, is reversible.

Assessment Findings

1. Increased volume of patient's own speech.
2. Turning of head toward speaker.
3. Requests of a speaker to repeat.
4. Inappropriate answers, but otherwise cognitively intact.
5. The person may withdraw, demonstrate a short attention span, and become frustrated, angry, and depressed.
6. Lack of response to a loud noise.

Nursing Considerations and Teaching Points

1. Be aware that hearing loss can impact the safety and quality of life for older adults in many ways. For example, the older adult may not hear instructions, alerting signals, telephones, or oncoming traffic. Hearing loss can contribute to social isolation and lower self-esteem.
2. Suggest hearing testing with an audiologist for further evaluation and consideration of an assistive device.
3. Face the person directly so he can lip-read.
4. Use gestures and objects to help with verbal communication.
5. Touch the person to get his or her attention before talking.
6. Speak into the patient's "good ear."
7. *Do not shout.* Shouting increases the tone of the voice, and older adults are unable to hear these high tones. Try speaking in a deeper or lower tone of voice.
8. Speak slowly and clearly.
9. Suggest amplifiers on telephones and alarms.
10. Allow the person more time to answer your questions.
11. Evaluate the person's ear canals regularly and assist with cerumen removal. Cerumen removal is facilitated by:
    a. Use of ceruminolytic agents, such as carbamide peroxide, 10 drops in the affected ear twice per day for 5 days, followed by flushing the ear with warm water via a 50-mL irrigation syringe or an electronic irrigation device.
    b. Careful use of an ear spoon to mechanically remove cerumen.
12. Refer patients to the following organizations:
    –American Speech–Language–Hearing Association: *www.asha.org*
    –HearingLoss.com: *www.hearingloss.com*
    –National Institute on Deafness and Other Communication Disorders: *www.nidcd.nih.gov/health/hearing/pages/older.aspx*

Smell

Characteristics

1. Changes in smell (olfaction) are due to nasal sinus disease preventing odors from reaching smell receptors, a decrease in nerve fibers, chronic injury from infections, or bleeding.
2. Discrimination of fruity odors seems to persist the longest.
3. Generally, olfaction decreases in men more than in women.

Assessment Findings

1. Inability to notice unpleasant odors, such as fire, body odor, or excessive perfume.
2. Decreased appetite.

Nursing Considerations and Teaching Points

1. Age-related changes can impact safety and quality of life. For example, an older individual may not be able to recognize the smell of smoke or gas.
2. The inability to smell food may cause a decrease in the consumption of nutritious food.
   a. At mealtimes, name food items and give the person time to think of the smell/taste of the food.
   b. Suggest use of stronger spices and flavorings to stimulate sense of smell.

Taste

Characteristics

1. Taste buds decrease with age, especially in men. People over age 60 have lost half of their taste buds. By age 80, only one sixth of the taste buds remain.
2. Taste buds are lost from the front to the back (ie, sweet and salty tastes are lost first, whereas bitter and sour tastes remain longer).

Assessment Findings

1. Complaints that food has no taste.
2. Excessive use of sugar and salt.
3. Inability to identify foods.
4. Decrease in appetite and weight loss.
5. Decreased pleasure from food.

Nursing Considerations and Teaching Points

1. Age-related changes can impact safety. For example, the older individual may not be able to detect spoiled food.
2. Serve food attractively, and separate different types of foods.
3. Vary the texture of foods.
4. Encourage good oral hygiene.
5. Season food.

Kinesthetic Sense

Characteristics

1. With age, the receptors in the joints and muscles that tell us where we are in space lose their ability to function. Therefore, there is a change in balance.
2. Walking with shorter step length, less leg lift, a wider base, and a tendency to lean forward.
3. With age, less ability to stop a fall from occurring.

Assessment Findings

1. Alterations in posture, ability to transfer, and gait
2. Complaint of dizziness

Nursing Considerations and Teaching Points

1. Position items within reach.
2. Give person more time to move.
3. Take precautions to prevent falls.
4. Suggest physical therapy with balance training after periods of prolonged immobility.

Cardiovascular

Characteristics

1. With age, the valves of the heart become thick and rigid as a result of sclerosis and fibrosis, compounding any cardiac disease already present.
2. Blood vessels also become thick and rigid, resulting in elevated blood pressure, which is present in half of the U.S. population over age 65.
3. Maximum heart rate and aerobic capacity decrease with age.
4. Slower response to stress. Once the pulse rate is elevated, it takes longer to return to baseline.
5. Decline in maximum oxygen consumption.
6. About 50% of older adults have an abnormal resting electrocardiogram.
7. Subtle changes in artery walls result in a less flexible vasculature.
8. Decreased baroreceptor sensitivity.

Assessment Findings

1. Normal blood pressure (BP) is less than 120/80 mm Hg; prehypertension, 120 to 139/80 to 89; stage 1 hypertension, 140 to 159/90 to 99; stage 2 hypertension, 160/100 mm Hg and greater.
2. Prolonged tachycardia may occur following stress.

Nursing Considerations and Teaching Points

1. Encourage regular BP evaluation as well as lifestyle modifications and medication adherence, if indicated, for hypertension.
2. Check for postural BP changes to detect orthostatic hypotension and prevent falls. Instruct patients to rise slowly from lying to sitting to standing.
3. Encourage longer cool-down period after exercise to return to baseline cardiac function.
4. Encourage moderate physical activity: walking, biking, or swimming for 30 minutes five times per week (150 minutes per week), in addition to muscle strengthening exercises two times a week.

Pulmonary

Characteristics

1. With age, there is a weakening of the intercostal respiratory muscles, and the elastic recoil of the chest wall diminishes.
2. There is no change in total lung capacity; however, residual volume and functional residual capacity increase.
3. Partial pressure of oxygen decreases with age due to ventilation–perfusion mismatches. However, older adults are not hypoxic without coexistent disease.
4. There is a decrease in the mucus transport/ciliary system. Therefore, there is decreased clearance of mucus and foreign bodies, including bacteria.

Assessment Findings

1. Prolonged cough, inability to raise secretions.
2. Increased frequency of respiratory infections.

Nursing Considerations and Teaching Points

1. Older adults who are undergoing surgical treatment should engage in deep-breathing exercises.
2. Teach measures to prevent pulmonary infections—avoid crowds during cold and flu season, wash hands frequently, report early signs of infection.
3. Avoid smoking and exposure to secondhand smoke.
4. Encourage annual flu vaccine and pneumonia vaccine at age 65 or as needed.

Immunologic

Characteristics

1. The function of T-cell lymphocytes, such as cell-mediated immunity, declines with age due to involution and atrophy of the thymus gland.
2. Decreased T-cell helper activity; increased T-cell suppressor activity.
3. Declining B-cell function as a result of T-cell changes.

Assessment Findings

1. More frequent infections.
2. Increased incidence of many types of cancer.

Nursing Considerations and Teaching Points

1. Teach older adults that they are at increased risk of infection, cancer, and autoimmune disease; therefore, routine follow-up and screening are essential.
2. Encourage healthy lifestyle practices to maintain optimal health.

Neurologic

Characteristics

1. There is gradual loss in the number of neurons with age, but no major change in neurotransmitter levels.
2. Some brain tissue atrophy is normal and does not relate to cognitive impairment.
3. Decrease in muscle tone, motor speed, and nerve conduction velocity.
4. Decrease in gait speed of 1.6% per year after age 63; decreased step length, stride length, and arm swing.

Assessment Findings

1. Decreased position and vibration sense.
2. Diminished reflexes, possible absent ankle jerks.
3. Complaint of falls and impaired balance.
4. Wide-based gait with decreased arm swing.

Nursing Considerations and Teaching Points

1. Because of these changes in combination with sensory changes, it is essential to teach older adults fall-prevention techniques.
   a. Environmental safety techniques include nonslip surfaces, securely fastened handrails, sufficient light, glare-free lights, avoidance of low-lying objects, chairs of the proper height with armrests, skidproof strips or mats in the tub or shower, toilet and tub grab bars, elevated toilet seats.
   b. Home safety evaluations should be done on all community-dwelling older adults to reduce the risk of falls. A home safety checklist can be obtained from the National Safety Council at *www.nsc.org*.

Musculoskeletal

Characteristics

1. Declining muscle mass and endurance with age, although deconditioning may be an associated factor.
2. Decreased bone density, less so in men than in women.
3. Decreased thickness and resiliency of cartilage, with a resulting increase in the stiffness of joints.
4. Bone resorption exceeds bone formation, resulting in a decline in bone density.
5. Injuries to the cartilage accumulate with age.

Assessment Findings

1. Muscle atrophy.
2. Increased incidence of fractures.
3. Complaint of joint stiffness in absence of arthritis.
4. Decreased bone density (less than 2.5 standard deviations below normal).

Nursing Considerations and Teaching Points

1. Early intervention to encourage regular exercise (including weight-bearing exercise and resistance training) in older adults is important to prevent exacerbation of these normal changes.
2. Encourage increased intake of calcium and vitamin D and decreased alcohol and nicotine use.

Community and Home Care Considerations

1. Encourage older adults to engage in 30 minutes of moderate physical activity, including walking, biking, or swimming, at least five times per week, in addition to muscle strengthening exercises at least two times a week.
2. For older adults who will be exercising at less than 80% of the maximum heart rate (220 – age), stress testing before starting an exercise program is not needed.
3. To help with adherence to the exercise program, older adults should be encouraged to exercise at a set time, to relieve pain before exercising, and to do an activity they enjoy. Provide positive reinforcement for those who do exercise, and continually reinforce the benefits of exercise (increased bone strength, cardiovascular fitness, decreased risks of falls, overall sense of well-being).

Endocrine

Characteristics

1. Decreased secretion of trophic hormones from the pituitary gland.
2. Blunted growth hormone release during stress.
3. Elevated vasopressin (antidiuretic hormone); exaggerated response to osmotic challenge.
4. Elevated levels of follicle-stimulating hormone and luteinizing hormone because of reduced end-organ response.
5. Decreased insulin secretion after meals; this may be a function of weight or genetic factors.

Assessment Findings
Usually asymptomatic.

Nursing Considerations and Teaching Points
1. Encourage routine screening for elevated blood glucose—both fasting and postprandial.
2. Provide education about a well-balanced diet.

Reproductive
Characteristics
1. In women, menopause leads to decreases in the size of the ovaries and hormone production. This results in uterine involution, vaginal atrophy, and loss of breast mass.
2. With age, there is increased risk in females of cystocele, rectocele, and uterine prolapse.
3. In men, testosterone production and secretion decrease with age. However, serum levels may be in the low-normal range through age 80.

Assessment Findings
1. Vaginal dryness, painful intercourse.
2. Atrophic vaginitis.
3. Urinary incontinence.

Nursing Considerations and Teaching Points
1. Suggest the use of additional lubrication during sexual intercourse.
2. Advise sexually active older men that spermatogenesis may continue into advanced age.
3. Address risks and benefits of time-limited hormone replacement therapy for symptomatic relief related to menopause.

Renal and Body Composition
Characteristics
1. Increased body fat and decreased lean muscle mass, even when weight remains stable.
2. Decreased renal function, measured by the glomerular filtration rate, or creatinine clearance.
3. Despite reduced total body creatinine due to decreased muscle mass in the older adult, serum creatinine often remains within normal range. This is because of decreased elimination of creatinine by the kidneys.
4. About 10% decline in creatinine clearance per decade after age 40; however, relatively unchanged serum creatinine.

Assessment Findings
1. Usually asymptomatic.
2. Increased incidence of anemia.

Nursing Considerations and Teaching Points
1. Be aware that although serum creatinine may be within normal range, creatinine clearance may be decreased. To obtain an accurate creatinine clearance in an older adult, the following formula may be used: (140 − age)(weight [kg])/(72)(serum creatinine [mg/dL]).
2. Drugs that are cleared through the kidneys may be given in decreased dosage. Adverse effects and toxicity must be closely monitored.

3. Consider the advantages and disadvantages of drug management for anemia associated with renal disease.

Skin
Characteristics
1. Thinning of all three layers of the skin—epidermis, dermis, and subcutaneous tissue—leads to greater fragility of the skin and decreased ability of the skin to function as a barrier to external factors.
2. Fewer melanocytes and decreased tanning.
3. Less efficient thermoregulation of heat because of fewer sweat glands.
4. Drier skin because the decreased number of sebaceous glands results in reduced oil production.
5. Other changes in aging skin include reduced sensory input, decreased elasticity, and impaired cell-related immune response.

Assessment Finding
1. Dry, irritated skin.

Nursing Considerations and Teaching Points
1. Excessive use of soap, which can be drying to the skin, should be avoided.
2. Careful skin evaluation and lubrication are necessary to prevent fissures and breakdown.
3. Heat regulation needs to be controlled by proper clothing and avoidance of extreme temperatures.
4. Avoid direct application of extreme hot or cold to skin because damage may occur without feeling it.
5. Encourage use of sunscreen during all outdoor activities.

Community and Home Care Considerations
1. Xerosis (dry skin) is a common problem for older adults. Treatment should include:
   a. Drinking 2,000 mL of liquid daily.
   b. Total body immersion in warm water (90° to 105° F [32.2° to 40.6° C]) for 10 minutes.
   c. Use of nonperfumed soap without hexachlorophene.
   d. Application of emollient, particularly those with alpha-hydroxy acids, after bathing and at bedtime.

Hematopoietic
Characteristics
1. Unchanged number of stem cells of all three cell lines; however, bone marrow cellularity is decreased by 33% during adult life.
2. Declining marrow activity, especially in response to stress, such as with blood loss or infection.

Assessment Finding
Asymptomatic

Nursing Considerations and Teaching Points
1. Anemia and granulocytopenia are not normal consequences of aging and should be investigated.
2. Teach patients that there is no need to take oral iron unless there is an actual documented decrease in iron levels.
3. Encourage oral B_{12} and folate replacement to manage associated anemias.

Altered Presentation of Disease

Characteristics

1. In part due to the physiologic changes that occur with aging, the manifestations of illness in the older patient are less dramatic than in younger patients.
2. Most older adults have at least one chronic condition. These coexisting conditions can complicate the evaluation of new symptoms.
3. Some risk factors make it more likely that they will present with an altered presentation of disease: over age 85, multiple comorbid conditions, taking over five medications, and having cognitive or functional impairment.

 Evidence Base Samaras, N., Chevalley, T., Samaras, D., et al. (2010). Older patients in the emergency department: a review. *Annals of emergency medicine, 56*(3), 261–269.

Assessment Findings

1. The classic indicators of disease are usually absent or present atypically (see Table 9-1).
2. Older people are less likely to report new symptoms but, rather, attribute them to aging or existing conditions. Many older adults minimize symptoms because of fears of hospitalization or health care costs.

Nursing Considerations and Teaching Points

1. Have a high index of suspicion for underlying illness if the older adult presents with an acute change in cognition, behavior, or function.

Functional Assessment

Functional assessment is the measurement of a patient's ability to complete functional tasks and fulfill social roles, specifically addressing a patient's ability to complete tasks ranging from simple self-care to higher-level activities. It provides the nurse with objective data to help determine the older adult's needs and plan interventions.

Purpose

1. Functional assessment is essential in the care of the older adult because it:
   a. Offers a systematic approach to assessing older adults for deficits that commonly go undetected.
   b. Helps the nurse to identify problems and utilize appropriate resources.
   c. Provides a way to assess progress and decline over time.
   d. Helps the nurse evaluate the safety of the patient's ability to live alone.
2. Functional status includes the evaluation of sensory changes, ability to complete ADLs and instrumental ADLs, gait and balance problems, and elimination.

Table 9-1	Atypical Presentation of Disorders in the Older Adult
DISORDER	**ATYPICAL PRESENTATION**
Acute intestinal infection	• Abdominal pain may be absent. • May present with acute confusional state, leukocytosis, and acidosis.
Appendicitis	• Pain may be diffuse, not localized in right lower quadrant.
Biliary disease	• Confusion, declining function, and other nonspecific symptoms. • Abnormal liver function tests may be only sign.
Heart failure	• Initially, may have change in mental status and fatigue.
Hyperthyroidism	• Apathy, palpitations, weight loss, weakness.
Hypothyroidism	• Presents with weight loss.
Myocardial infarction	• Chest pain may be absent. • May present with syncope, dyspnea, vomiting, or confusion.
Perforated ulcer	• Rigidity may be absent until late.
Pneumonia	• May present with confusion. • Fever and cough may be absent.
Pulmonary embolism	• May present with change in mental status. • May not have fever, leukocytosis, or tachycardia.
Septicemia	• May be afebrile.
Systemic lupus erythematosus	• Pneumonitis, subcutaneous nodules, and discoid lesions are more common. • Malar rash, Raynaud's phenomenon, and nephritis are less common.
Urinary tract infection	• Confusion.

Instruments to Measure Functional Ability

1. Functional status may be assessed by several methods: self-report, direct observation, or family report. Direct observation is the method of choice, when possible.
2. The instrument chosen should be based on the specific goal or purpose for the evaluation. For example, if the focus is on basic self-care and mobility, the Barthel index should be used. See references, page 195 (Mahoney & Barthel).
3. The Katz Index for Activities of Daily Living and Instrumental Activities of Daily Living is another rating scale for measuring functional ability. Use this scale to determine level of independence of the older adult and repeat periodically to compare level of functioning over time. See references, page 195.
4. Performance measures, such as the Tinetti Gait and Balance measure or the Chair Rise test, can be used to evaluate higher-level functioning.

Psychosocial Assessment

Altered Mental Status

1. Assessment of mental status to detect altered cognition involves examination of memory, perception, communication, orientation, calculation, comprehension, problem solving, thought processes, language, visual–spatial abilities, abstraction, attention, aphasia, and apraxia.
2. Assessment can be facilitated by use of cognitive screening tools. A commonly utilized instrument is the Mini-Mental State Examination (MMSE), a 30-point cognitive screening instrument that assesses orientation to time and place, registration and recall, calculation, language skills, and visual–spatial abilities.
3. The total possible score is 30. A score of 24–30 suggests intact cognitive function; 20–23, mild cognitive impairment; 16–19, moderate cognitive impairment; 15 or less, severe cognitive impairment. The MMSE can help to follow the patient's cognition over time and assess for acute and/or chronic changes.
4. Although success on scales such as this has been associated with language abilities, education, and socioeconomic status, this scale continues to be used as an appropriate screening tool for abnormal cognitive function.
5. Another cognitive screening instrument is the Mini-Cog examination, which is composed of a three-item recall and the Clock Drawing Test (CDT). The Mini-Cog can be administered under 3 minutes, does not appear to be affected by the patient's education or language abilities, and has been successfully used to screen for dementia across a variety of clinical settings. The Mini-Cog can be administered as follows:
   a. Tell the patient to listen carefully and remember and repeat three unrelated words.
   b. Tell the patient to draw the face of a clock including numbers and hands to read a specific time. The CDT is considered normal if all numbers are present in the correct sequence and position and the hands display the requested time.
   c. Ask the patient to repeat the three previously stated words.
   d. Unsuccessful recall of all three items suggests dementia. Successful recall of all three items suggests intact cognition. An abnormal CDT with one to two errors on recall suggests dementia. A normal CDT with one to two errors on recall suggests no dementia.
6. Assessment of altered mental status or behavior may elicit criteria that lead to a diagnosis of dementia. It is essential to differentiate dementia from delirium (which is treatable and reversible).
   a. *Delirium* is abrupt in onset and is commonly due to an underlying medical condition, such as infection, electrolyte imbalance, medication intolerance or toxicity, and cardiac decompensation. Disorientation occurs early, and the behavior is variable hour to hour. There is a clouded, altered, or changing level of consciousness, short attention span, and disturbed sleep–wake cycle. Hallucinations are common. The condition is reversible with treatment of the underlying cause.
   b. *Dementia* has a gradual onset. Behavior is usually stable, and disorientation occurs late. Consciousness is not clouded, attention span is generally not reduced, and day–night reversal of sleep–wake cycles can occur rather than hour-to-hour variation. Delusions (fixed false beliefs) are more common than hallucinations.

Social Activities and Support

1. Social support for older adults is generally instrumental, informational, or emotional. The social environment is important with regard to recovery of acute medical problems and management of chronic illness.
2. Elicit information by asking such questions as:
   a. How often do you socialize with others?
   b. With whom do you socialize?
   c. What type of activities do you enjoy?
   d. Do you enjoy socializing?
   e. Who can you call for help?
   f. Do you know of any church or community groups you can call for help?

Emotional and Affective Status

Characteristics

1. Depression may occur for the first time in older age and has been related to the many changes that occur with aging:
   a. The independence of one's children.
   b. The reality of retirement.
   c. The loss of roles, income, spouse, friends, family, home, pets, functional ability, health, and ability to participate in leisure activities such as reading.
   d. Ageist messages from society supporting and encouraging the value of youth.
2. Depression may also be associated with underlying illnesses, such as Parkinson's disease and stroke, and by medications, such as antihypertensives (beta blockers), anti-arthritics, and anti-anxiety agents.
3. Depression is usually difficult to identify in the older adult because the presentation is different than in younger people. Obtain the following information to assess for depression:

a. Complaints of insomnia, weight loss, anorexia, and constipation (vegetative symptoms).

b. Presence of anhedonia (lack of joy in usually pleasurable activities).

c. Decrease in concentration, memory, and decision making (pseudodementia syndrome).

d. Other somatic complaints, such as decreased appetite, musculoskeletal aches and pains, chest pain, fatigue.

e. History of chronic illness or other health problems.

f. Current medications.

4. Evaluate depression using the Geriatric Depression Scale as a screening tool.

5. Suicide is sometimes associated with depression, with suicides being especially high in older white men. Assess for suicide risk.

6. Pain is underdetected and undertreated in older adults and may be contributing to depression. Assess pain by asking and observing the patient, and provide appropriate measures to make patient more comfortable.

Nursing and Patient Care Considerations

1. Treatment of depression should be given to older adults and includes drugs, psychotherapy, and, in some cases, electroconvulsive therapy.

2. Complement other therapeutic measures by providing opportunities to increase the patient's self-esteem.

   a. Encourage participation in meaningful activities.

   b. Promote the patient's positive self-image.

   c. Help the patient develop a sense of mastery.

   d. Encourage reminiscence of meaningful past events.

3. Help patient identify and use social supports.

4. For behavioral problems (agitation, combative behavior, or irritability) consider options such as aromatherapy, music therapy, pet therapy, relaxation techniques, massage, or physical activity.

Motivation in Older Adults

Characteristics

1. Motivation is an important variable in the older adult's ability to recover from any disabling event and the ability to maintain his or her highest level of wellness.

2. Understanding individual motivational factors for engaging in health promotion activities like exercise is an approach that can improve adherence. It is possible to evaluate a patient's motivation to comply with a given treatment plan and adopt interventions to help to improve the older adult's motivation.

 Evidence Base Quindry, J. C., Yount, D., O'Bryant, H., et al. (2011). Exercise engagement is differentially motivated by age-dependent factors. American Journal of Health Behavior, 35(3), 334–345.

3. Factors that influence motivation in an older adult include:

   a. Needs such as hunger.

   b. Past experiences, specifically with health care providers.

   c. Negative attitudes toward aging.

   d. Self-efficacy expectations, or the belief in one's ability to perform a specific activity.

e. Outcome expectations, or the belief that if a specific activity is performed there will be an expected outcome.

f. The cost of performing a specific activity in terms of time, money, pain, fatigue, or fear.

g. Internal factors, such as sensory changes, cognitive status, and adverse drug effects.

h. External factors, such as social norms (particularly if those norms conflict with treatment) and the influence of social supports.

4. Problems in motivation due to age-related differences include:

   a. A shift from achievement motivation to conservative motivation.

   b. Increasing difficulty in the establishment of rewards for older people, due to their many losses.

   c. A tendency to see a task as being more difficult than a younger person would.

   d. A tendency to become easily discouraged; the older adult may not initiate behavior as readily.

   e. Greater significance placed on the meaning of a task; it must be meaningful to the older person.

   f. Evidence that older adults do not do well on tasks if they are asked to do them rapidly, under a time limit, or in a stressful situation.

   g. Increased importance placed on the cost of participating in an activity; fear of failing can be expressed either as increased anxiety or decreased willingness to take risks.

   h. Increased need for older adults to get approval for their effort.

5. The Motivation Wheel (see Figure 9-1) can be used to evaluate motivation in the older adult.

   a. Motivation is influenced by beliefs about physical and emotional benefits, mastery experiences, individualized care, social support, the environment, goals, physical sensations, and new activities.

   b. Motivation can be increased by strengthening beliefs about potential benefits, providing opportunities for mastery,

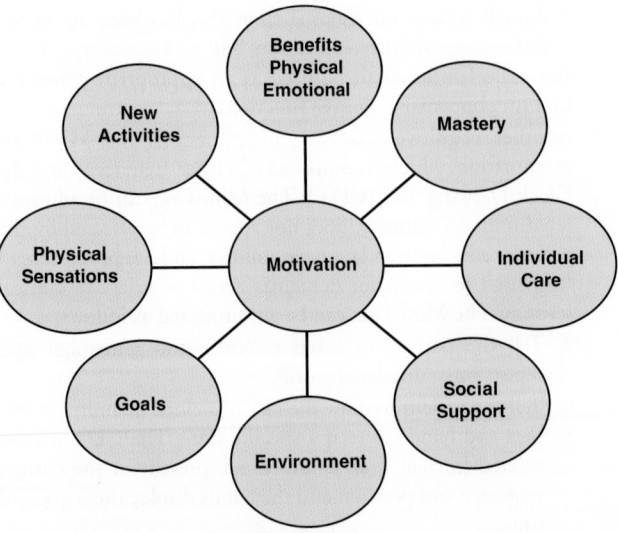

Figure 9-1. The wheel that moves.

identifying individualized care approaches and goals, using social supports, accessing supportive environments, decreasing unpleasant sensations, and trying new activities.

Nursing and Patient Care Considerations

1. Strategies to improve motivation include:
   a. Establish whose motives are being discussed—patient's, family's, or health care provider's; involve patient in setting the goals.
   b. Explore with patient any indication of fear or other unpleasant sensation associated with the activity, such as pain or fatigue, and implement interventions to decrease these unpleasant sensations.
   c. Evaluate the spokes of the wheel to consider the many factors that influence motivation and implement interventions as appropriate.
   d. Encourage patient to verbally express emotional factors associated with the activity.
   e. Examine the setting for the desired behavior to occur. Is the environment too stressful, too dark, or too noisy?
   f. Attempt to use role models. Older adult role models can change ageist attitudes and stimulate patients to perform the desired behavior.
   g. Set small goals to be met either daily or each shift. This provides frequent rewards.
   h. Do not be afraid to use yourself. Research has indicated that being nice, demonstrating caring, using humor, verbal encouragement, and support can all help motivate the older adult.
2. Educate the older adult about the benefits of the activity, whether these are physical or psychological.

HEALTH MAINTENANCE

Evidence Base United States Preventive Services Task Force. (2012). The guide to clinical preventive services: Recommendations of the U.S Preventive Services Task Force. Available: *www.uspreventiveservices taskforce.org/index.html.*

Primary Prevention

The goal of health promotion and disease prevention is to add more quality years to life. There are three levels of health promotion and disease prevention.

Primary prevention is the prevention of disease before it occurs. Primary prevention can be broken down into counseling, immunizations, and chemoprophylaxis.

Counseling

1. Encourage smoking cessation.
   a. Approximately 10% of people in the United States age 65 and older are smokers.
   b. Tobacco use has been linked to heart disease; peripheral vascular disease; cerebrovascular disease; chronic obstructive pulmonary disease; cancer such as lung, bladder, and esophageal malignancies; and numerous other health problems that decrease quality of life or cause premature death.
   c. Although much damage has been done to the lungs and blood vessels by many years of smoking, older adults can still benefit from smoking cessation by increasing quality of life.
   d. The U.S. Preventive Service Task Force recommends the "5-A" behavioral counseling framework as a useful strategy for engaging patients in smoking cessation discussions: (1) Ask about tobacco use; (2) Advise to quit through clear personalized messages; (3) Assess willingness to quit; (4) Assist to quit; and (5) Arrange follow-up and support.
2. Encourage physical activity.
   a. It has been stated that 75% of older Americans are inactive.
   b. It has been recommended that older adults participate in regular activity, especially aerobic activities that promote cardiovascular fitness, such as walking, cycling, or swimming.
   c. Refer to a physical, occupational, or rehabilitation therapist. An individualized exercise prescription should be developed and cleared with the health care provider.
3. Identify alcohol abuse in older adults.
   a. The consequences of alcoholism include liver disease, gastrointestinal (GI) bleeding, and motor vehicle accidents.
   b. Question older adults about drug or alcohol abuse. Although street drug use is rare, prescription drug abuse may be occurring or alcohol may be used for pain.
   c. Recognize the signs and symptoms of alcohol abuse in older adults (see Box 9-1).
   d. Refer for counseling.
4. Evaluate and counsel on dental health.
   a. Dental problems in older adults include missing teeth, ill-fitting dentures, periodontal disease, and tooth decay.
   b. Dental problems commonly lead to poor eating habits, apathy, and fatigue.
   c. Regular dental care should be encouraged to improve nutrition and the quality of life.

Immunizations

Evidence Base *Centers for Disease Control and Prevention. (2012). Advisory Committee for Immunization Practices (ACIP) recommendations. Atlanta, GA: CDC. Available: www.cdc.gov/vaccines/pubs/ACIP-list. htm#pcv.*

BOX 9-1	Signs of Alcohol Abuse in Older Adults

- Difficulty with gait and balance
- Acute change in cognition
- Frequent falls or accidents
- Change in drinking patterns
- Poor nutritional intake
- Poor hygiene and self-care
- Lack of physical exercise
- Social isolation

1. Pneumococcal pneumonia and influenza are significant causes of mortality and morbidity in older adults.
   a. It is recommended that a single dose of the pneumococcal vaccine be given to all people age 65 or over.
   b. A second dose is recommended for individuals aged 19 to 64 who have functional or structural asplenia or immuno-compromising conditions 5 years after the first.
   c. Influenza may cause significant complications in older adults. Annual influenza vaccination is recommended for all people over age 6 months. Several antiviral agents are effective against influenza. These agents can be effective in ameliorating symptoms if given within 48 hours of onset of illness.
2. Tetanus-diphtheria (Td) immunization is an important but frequently forgotten component of health maintenance, especially in older adults.
   a. The mortality rate of tetanus exceeds 50% in those over age 65.
   b. Combined tetanus-diphtheria boosters should be given every 10 years; no age for discontinuation has been stated.
   c. Due to an increase in pertussis cases, a single dose of acellular pertussis is also recommended as a component (Tdap) for adults aged 65 years and older who anticipate having close contact with an infant less than 12 months of age and who previously have not received Tdap. Tdap can be administered regardless of interval since the last tetanus booster.
   d. For those with no history of immunization or unknown immunization status, a primary series should be initiated, consisting of two doses of tetanus-diphtheria vaccine at least 4 weeks apart, followed by a third dose 6 to 12 months later.
3. A single dose of the herpes zoster vaccine is recommended for older adults to prevent the dermatologic reoccurrence of varicella and the possible painful sequela known as postherpetic neuralgia.
   a. Age is the most important factor in the development of herpes zoster, with a large increase beginning between age 50 and 60, and about 50% of people experience herpes zoster by age 85.

Chemoprophylaxis

1. The risk and benefits of oral anticoagulation therapy should be considered for older adults at risk of cardiovascular disease, particularly stroke. The United States Preventive Services Task Force (USPSTF) strongly recommends that clinicians discuss aspirin therapy with patients at risk for coronary heart disease.
   a. Contraindicated if patient is at risk for GI bleeding.
   b. Should be discussed with older adults with regard to prevention of deep vein thrombosis, nonvalvular atrial fibrillation, cardiomyopathy, valvular heart disease, mechanical prosthetic heart valves, and acute myocardial infarction.
2. Calcium, vitamin D, and other agents, such as selective estrogen receptor modulators or bisphosphonates, may be considered for those at risk for osteoporosis.

Secondary Prevention

Secondary prevention is the detection of disease in an early stage for best treatment outcomes, such as cancers, cardiovascular disease, osteoporosis, and tuberculosis.

Screening Recommendations

 Evidence Base United States Preventive Services Task Force. (2012). The guide to clinical preventive services: Recommendations of the U.S Preventive Services Task Force. Available: *www.uspreventiveservices-taskforce.org/index.html.*

Age alone is not a criterion as to when to stop screening. Rather, the patient and health care provider should discuss values, expectations, functional status, and quality of life. A guide to shared decision making for cancer screening is available at the USPSTF website at *www.uspreventiveservicestaskforce.org/3rduspstf/shared/sharedba.htm.*

The USPSTF has made the following recommendations for cancer screenings for older adults:

1. The precise age at which to discontinue screening mammography is uncertain. No clinical trials have been conducted on women over age 74. Furthermore, although older women face a higher probability of developing breast cancer, they also have a greater chance of dying from other causes.
2. Regarding cervical cancer, it is appropriate for older women to discontinue cervical cancer screening after age 65 only if they have had adequate recent screening with normal results and are not at high risk for cervical cancer.
3. The age to discontinue colorectal cancer screening has not been determined; however, the USPSTF recommends against routine colorectal cancer screening in adults ages 75–85, unless there are conditions that support screening for these individuals.
4. The USPSTF states that there is insufficient evidence to recommend for or against screening for prostate cancer. Older men and men with other significant medical conditions who have a life expectancy of fewer than 10 years are unlikely to benefit from the prostate-specific antigen test and digital rectal examination.

Tertiary Prevention

Tertiary prevention addresses the treatment of established disease to avoid complications and death. The major areas of focus for the older adult are preventing the complications of immobility and rehabilitation

Preventing Complications of Immobility

Positioning

1. The goal of frequent position changes is to prevent contractures, stimulate circulation and prevent pressure sores, prevent thrombophlebitis and pulmonary embolism, promote lung expansion and prevent pneumonia, and decrease edema of the extremities. Changing position from lying to sitting several times per day can help prevent changes in the cardiovascular system, which is known as *deconditioning*.
2. The recommendation is to change body position at least every 2 hours and, preferably, more frequently in patients who have no spontaneous movement.

Evidence Base Niederhauser, A., VanDeusen Lukas, C., et al. (2012). Comprehensive programs for preventing pressure ulcers: a review of the literature. *Advances in Skin and Wound Care, 25*(4), 167–188; quiz 189–190.

Proper Body Alignment

1. Dorsal or supine position
   a. The head is in line with the spine, both laterally and anteroposteriorly.
   b. The trunk is positioned so flexion of the hips is minimized to prevent hip contracture.
   c. The arms are flexed at the elbow with the hands resting against the lateral abdomen.
   d. The legs are extended in a neutral position with the toes pointed toward the ceiling.
   e. The heels are suspended in a space between the mattress and the footboard to prevent heel pressure.
   f. Trochanter rolls are placed under the greater trochanters in the hip joint areas.
2. Side-lying or lateral position
   a. The head is in line with the spine.
   b. The body is in alignment and is not twisted.
   c. The uppermost hip joint is slightly forward and supported by a pillow in a position of slight abduction.
   d. A pillow supports the arm, which is flexed at both the elbow and shoulder joints.
3. Prone position
   a. The head is turned laterally and is in alignment with the rest of the body.
   b. The arms are abducted and externally rotated at the shoulder joint; the elbows are flexed.
   c. A small, flat support is placed under the pelvis, extending from the level of the umbilicus to the upper third of the thigh.
   d. The lower extremities remain in a neutral position.
   e. The toes are suspended over the edge of the mattress.

Therapeutic Exercise

1. It has been reported that there is a daily loss of 1% to 1.5% of initial strength in an immobilized older adult.
2. The goals of therapeutic exercise are to develop and retrain deficient muscles, to restore as much normal movement as possible to prevent deformity, to stimulate the functions of various organs and body systems, to build strength and endurance, and to promote relaxation.
3. Perform passive range-of-motion (ROM) exercise.
   a. Carried out without assistance from the patient.
   b. The purpose is to retain as much joint ROM as possible and to maintain circulation.
   c. Move the joint smoothly through its full ROM (see Box 9-2, pages 174 to 177). Do not push beyond the point of pain.
4. Perform active assistive ROM.
   a. Carried out by the patient with the assistance of the nurse.
   b. The purpose is to encourage normal muscle function.

c. Support the distal part and encourage the patient to take the joint actively through its ROM.
   d. Give only the amount of assistance necessary to accomplish the action.
5. Encourage active ROM.
   a. Accomplished by the patient without assistance.
   b. The purpose is to increase muscle strength.
   c. When possible, active exercise should be done against gravity.
   d. Encourage the patient to move the joint through the full ROM without assistance.
   e. Make sure that the patient does not substitute another joint movement for the one intended.
   f. Other active forms of exercise include turning from side to side, turning from back to abdomen, and moving up and down in bed.
6. Assist with resistive exercise.
   a. Carried out by the patient working against resistance produced by either manual or mechanical means.
   b. The purpose is to increase muscle strength.
   c. Encourage the patient to move the joint through its ROM while you or someone else provides slight resistance at first and then progressively increases resistance.
   d. Weights may be used and are attached at the distal point of the involved joint.
   e. The movements should be done smoothly.
7. Teach isometric or muscle-setting exercise.
   a. Involve alternately contracting and relaxing a muscle while keeping the part in a fixed position; performed by the patient.
   b. The purpose is to maintain strength when a joint is immobilized.
   c. Teach the patient to contract or tighten the muscle as much as possible without moving the joint.
   d. The patient holds the position for several seconds, then relaxes.

Geriatric Rehabilitation and Restorative Care

Characteristics

1. The primary goal is restoring the older adult to maximum functional level.
2. Multidisciplinary service involving input from the primary care provider; nursing personnel; physical, occupational, speech, and recreational therapists; social worker; psychologist; and dietitian.
3. Rehabilitation and restorative nursing involves developing a rehabilitation philosophy of care.
   a. Patients are encouraged, and allowed sufficient time, to perform as much of their personal care as possible.
   b. Goals are set *with* the patient rather than *for* the patient.
   c. Prevention of further impairment is imperative.
   d. Focus on skin and wound care, regaining or maintaining bowel and bladder function, independent medication use, good nutritional status, psychosocial support, an appropriate activity–rest balance, and patient and family education.

(Text continues on page 177)

BOX 9-2	**Range of Motion**

SHOULDER

Flexion–Extension

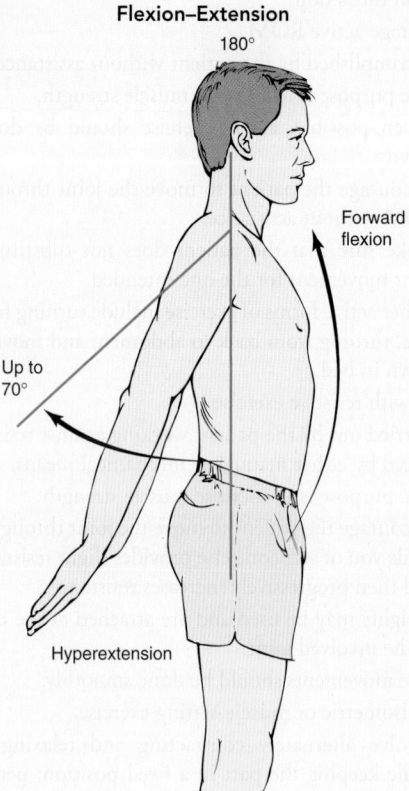

180°

Forward
flexion

Up to
70°

Hyperextension

Adduction–Abduction

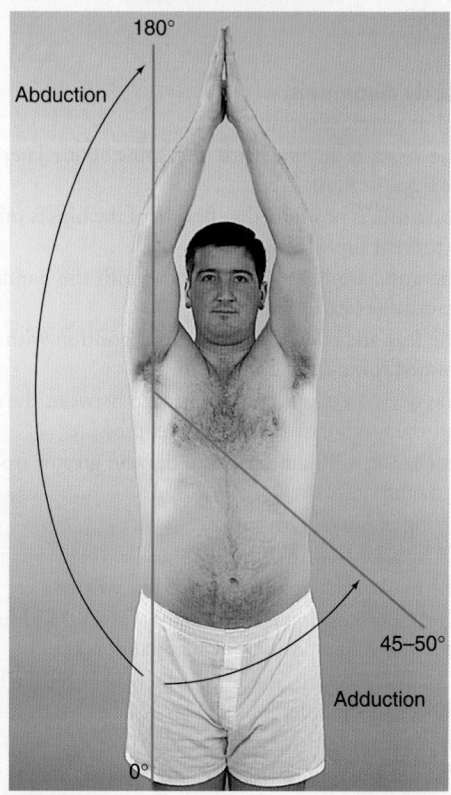

180°

Abduction

45–50°

Adduction

0°

ELBOW

Flexion–Extension

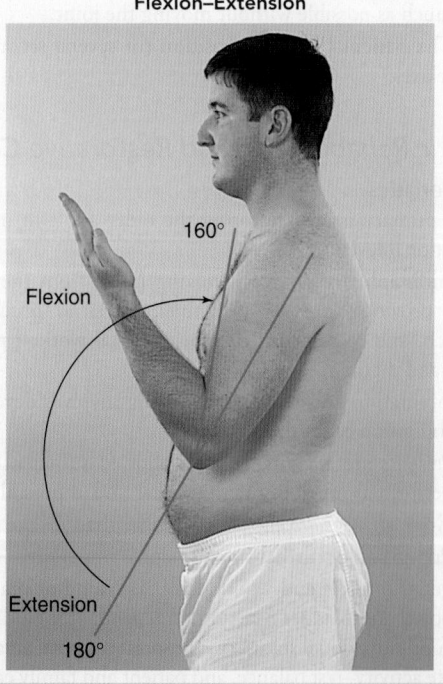

160°

Flexion

Extension

180°

Pronation–Supination

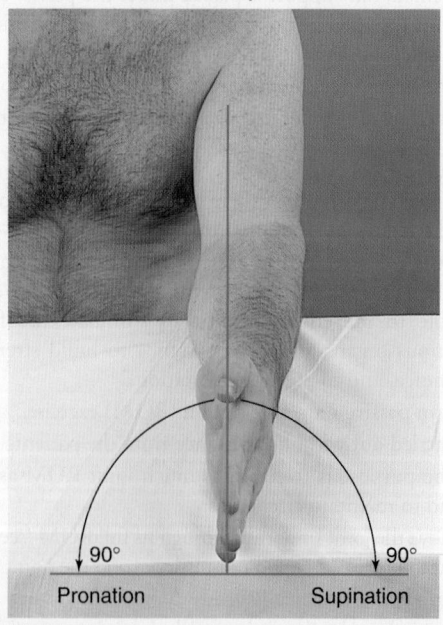

90°   90°

Pronation   Supination

BOX 9-2 Range of Motion *(continued)*

WRIST

Dorsiflexion and Palmar Flexion

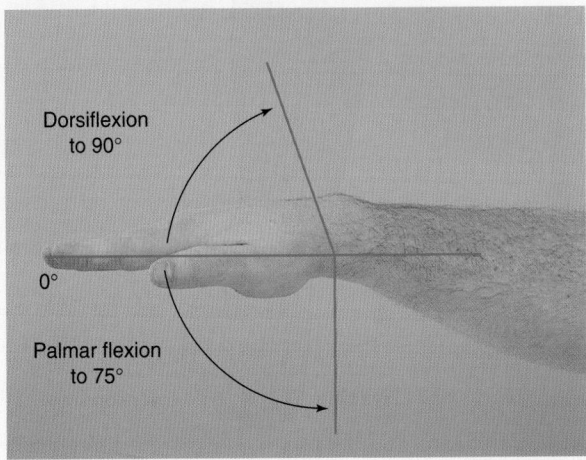

Dorsiflexion
to 90°

0°

Palmar flexion
to 75°

Ulnar–Radial Deviation

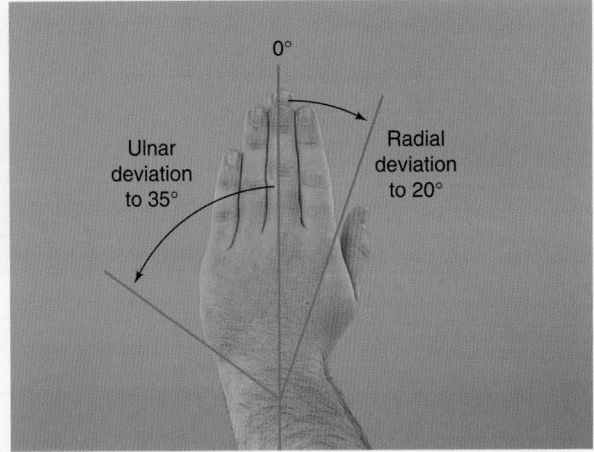

0°

Ulnar
deviation
to 35°

Radial
deviation
to 20°

THUMB

Adduction

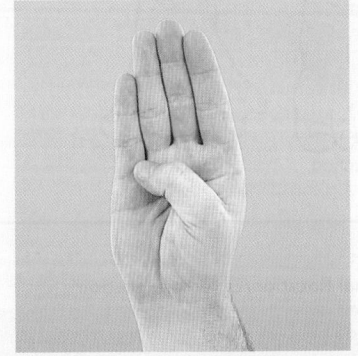

Abduction

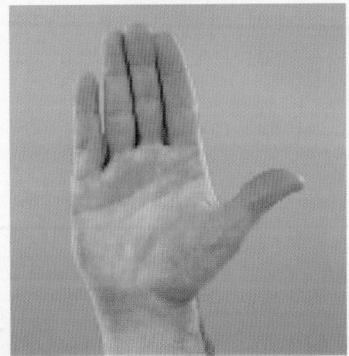

Opposition

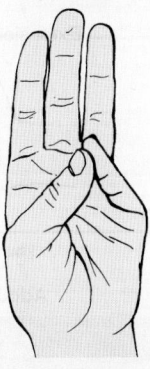

FINGERS

Adduction

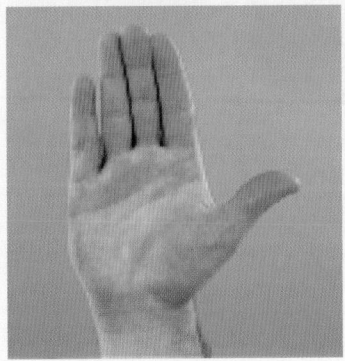

Abduction

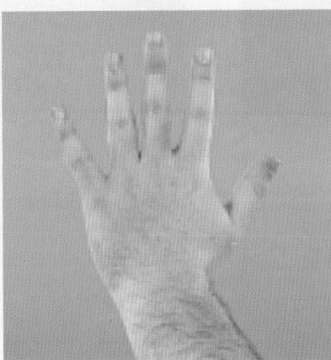

Flexion–Extension

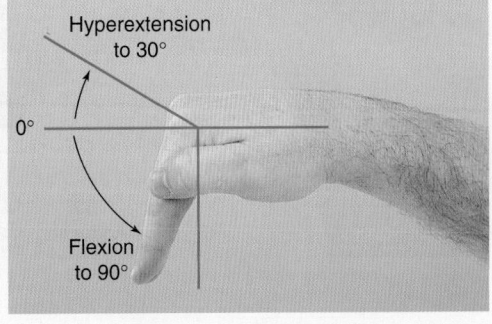

Hyperextension
to 30°

0°

Flexion
to 90°

(continued)

BOX 9-2 | **Range of Motion** (*continued*)

ANKLE

Dorsiflexion–Plantar Flexion

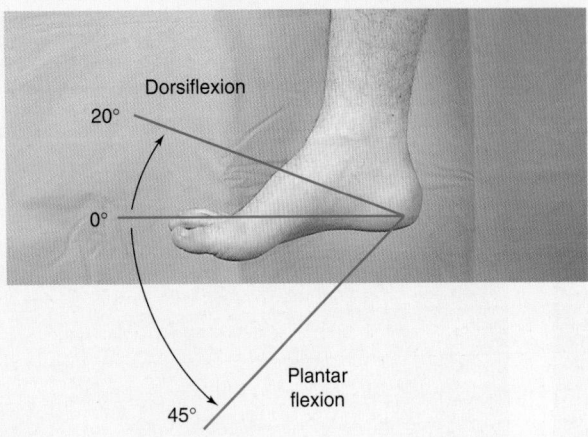

Dorsiflexion
20°
0°
45°
Plantar flexion

Flexion–Extension

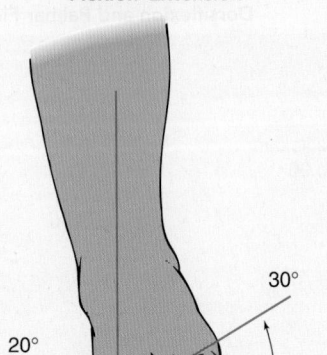

30°
20°
Eversion   Inversion

TOES

Eversion–Inversion

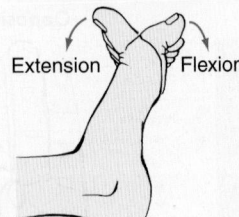

Extension   Flexion

Adduction–Abduction

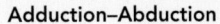
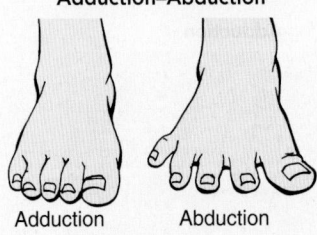

Adduction   Abduction

HIP

Adduction–Abduction

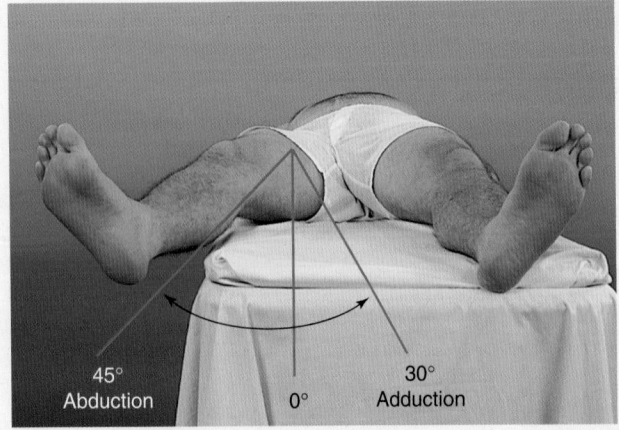

45° Abduction
0°
30° Adduction

Internal Rotation/External Rotation

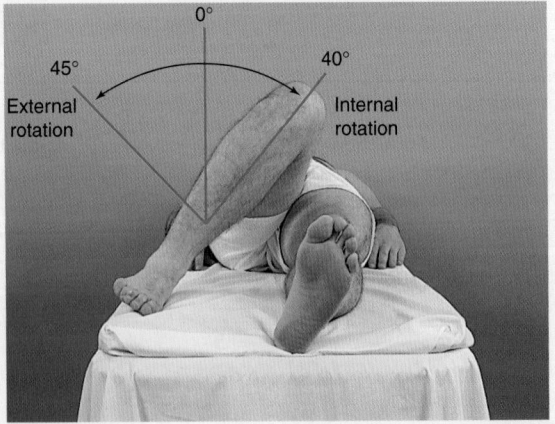

0°
45° External rotation
40° Internal rotation

BOX 9-2   Range of Motion *(continued)*

KNEE

Flexion–Hyperextension

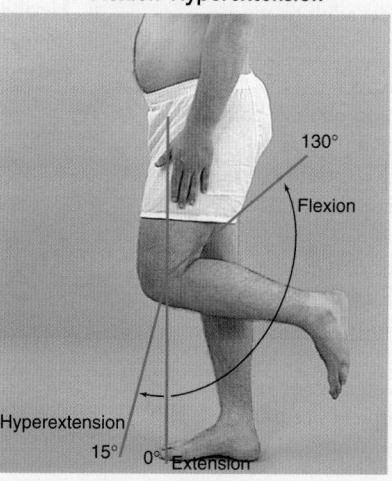

CERVICAL SPINE

Flexion/Extension/Hyperextension

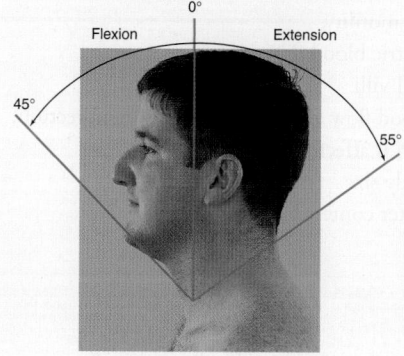

Rotation

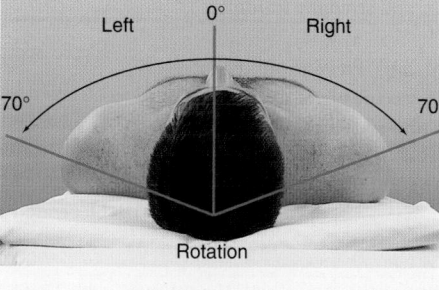

Lateral Bending

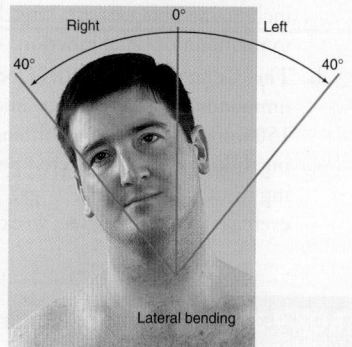

Evidence Base Resnick, B., Galik, E., Gruber-Baldini, A., et al. (2011). Testing the effect of function-focused care in assisted living. *Journal of the American Geriatrics Society, 59*(12), 2233–2240.

Nursing and Patient Care Considerations

1. Impaired cognitive function may have an impact on the quality of rehabilitation.
   a. Assess for physical problems that may exacerbate cognitive dysfunction (eg, infection, adverse drug effects, metabolic or circulatory problems, or fatigue).
   b. Provide innovative measures to encourage ambulation, active ROM, and increased function; provide frequent verbal cues and large-print reminders; focus on basic self-care abilities and activities that are consistent with the individual's past life experiences.
   c. Implement appropriate safety measures, such as bed side rails, proper lighting, appropriate staffing, and avoidance of chemical and physical restraints.
2. Disability has a tremendous impact on patient's body image and requires an adjustment by patient. Be aware of the stages of psychological reaction the patient may undergo.
   a. Period of confusion, disorganization, and denial.
   b. Period of depression or anxiety and grief.
   c. Period of adaptation and adjustment.
3. Interventions in rehabilitation nursing include:
   a. Provide an atmosphere of acceptance.
   b. Identify and encourage positive coping patterns.

c. Encourage socialization and participation in group activities.

d. Give positive reinforcement and feedback about progress.

e. Involve families as much as possible.

4. Use suggested interventions to motivate older adult to engage in functional activities and exercise.

Community and Home Care Considerations

1. Family or significant other caring for the older adult at home can have a major impact on the rehabilitation process.

a. Assist family or significant other to face the reality of the patient's disability and to set appropriate and achievable goals.

b. Involve family or significant other in decision making and in the patient's care in order for them to develop and practice the skills necessary for the patient to reach rehabilitation goals.

c. Help extend and enlarge family's or significant other's skills by teaching problem solving, treatment needs of the patient, ways to communicate to health care providers, and the use of community resources.

d. Assess the level of caregiver fatigue or burnout (see Box 9-3).

2. For the older adult living independently:

a. Encourage adherence to a regular exercise program, which includes aerobic exercise, stretching, and strength training to maintain optimal function.

b. The Centers for Disease Control and Prevention recommends that all adults should accumulate at least 150 minutes of moderate-intensity physical activity (walking, biking, swimming, etc.) per week, and strength training (heavy gardening, yoga, lifting weights, resistance exercises) at least 2 days a week.

c. Older adults can meet the physical activity recommendations with the following sample schedule:

i. Aerobic exercise: brisk walking 5 days per week for at least 30 minutes.

ii. Flexibility: stretch every day.

iii. Strength training: do strength-building activities 2 to 3 days per week that involve all major muscle groups.

d. For further information on exercise for older adults living independently, see *www.cdc.gov/physicalactivity/everyone/guidelines/olderadults.html*.

SPECIAL HEALTH PROBLEMS OF THE OLDER ADULT

Altered Response to Medication

Adults over age 65 consume 30% to 40% of all prescription drugs and an even higher proportion of over-the-counter drugs. Age-related changes predispose older adults to problems with adverse drug effects.

Pathophysiology and Etiology

1. Drug absorption is affected by such age-related changes as:

a. Decreased gastric acid.

b. Decreased GI motility.

c. Decreased gastric blood flow.

d. Changes in GI villi.

e. Decreased blood flow and body temperature in rectum.

2. Drug distribution is affected by:

a. Decreased body size.

b. Decreased water content in the body.

BOX 9-3 **Caregiver Strain Index**

Instructions given to the caregiver: I am going to read a list of things that other people have found to be difficult in caring for patients after they come home from the hospital. Would you tell me whether any of these apply to you? (Give the examples.)

Score one point for "yes" and zero for "no."

1. Sleep is disturbed (eg, because _____ is in and out of bed or wanders around at night).

2. It is inconvenient (eg, because helping takes so much time or it is a long drive over to help).

3. It is a physical strain (eg, because of lifting in and out of a chair).

4. It is confining (eg, because helping restricts free time or cannot visit).

5. There have been family adjustments (eg, because helping has disrupted routine or there has been no privacy).

6. There have been changes in personal plans (eg, had to turn down a job or could not go on vacation).

7. There have been other demands on my time (eg, from other family members).

8. There have been emotional adjustments (eg, because of severe arguments).

9. Some behavior is upsetting (eg, incontinence; _____ has trouble remembering things; _____ accuses others of taking things).

10. It is upsetting to find that _____ has changed so much from before (eg, _____ is a different person from before).

11. There have been work adjustments (eg, because of having to take time off).

12. It is a financial strain.

13. It has been completely overwhelming (eg, because of worry about _____ or concerns about how to continue to manage).

Scoring: Total score of 7 or more suggests a greater level of stress.

Robinson, B. C. (1983). Validation of a caregiver strain index. *Journal of Gerontology, 38*(3), 344–348. ©1983 The Gerontological Society of America.

c. Increased total body fat.

d. Drugs distributed in water have a higher concentration in older adults (eg, gentamicin).

e. Drugs distributed in fat have a wider distribution and less intense but prolonged effect (eg, phenobarbital).

3. Drug metabolism in the older adult:

a. Is altered by a decrease in liver size, blood flow, enzyme activity, and protein synthesis.

b. Requires more time than in younger adults. Therefore, there is increased drug activity time in drugs that are metabolized in the liver (eg, propranolol, theophylline).

4. Excretion of drugs is altered in older adults due to the following renal changes:

a. Decreased renal tubular function and blood flow.

b. This causes a decrease in renal filtration and an increase in blood levels of drugs that are excreted through the kidneys (eg, cimetidine).

 DRUG ALERT Drugs that may have severe adverse effects in elderly patients include anticholinergics (antihistamines, tricyclic antidepressants, drugs for treating urinary incontinence), nonsteroidal anti-inflammatory drugs (NSAIDs), any drug with a long half-life, and drugs with action on the central nervous system (CNS).

Nursing Assessment

1. Drug toxicities in older adults are different than they are in younger people.

2. Fewer symptoms may be identified, and they may develop slower; however, the reactions may be more pronounced and further advanced once they do present.

3. Behavioral and cognitive adverse effects are more common in older adults because the blood–brain barrier becomes less effective; the first reaction to a drug is confusion.

4. Many potential adverse drug effects are not identified because they are attributed to old age; fatigue, dementia, anorexia, or indigestion as adverse drug effects may not be reported.

5. Allergic reactions to drugs increase with age due to a greater likelihood of earlier exposure.

Nursing and Patient Care Considerations

1. Maintain awareness that the older adult is at greater risk for adverse drug reactions.

a. This risk increases from 6% when two drugs are taken to 50% when five different drugs are taken, and to 100% when eight or more drugs are taken.

2. Assess patient's ability to follow medication regimen by evaluation of:

a. Cognition.

b. Ability to read drug labels.

c. Hand and muscle coordination.

d. Swallowing difficulty.

e. Lifestyle patterns, specifically smoking and alcohol use.

f. Cultural beliefs toward medication.

g. Ability to afford medication.

h. Caregiver involvement in medication administration; assess caregiver if indicated.

3. Identify problems in the use of medications, such as:

a. Lack of knowledge about drugs.

b. Multiple medications and difficult administration techniques.

c. Caregiver misunderstanding of medication use.

4. Appropriate interventions for safe drug use include:

a. Obtain a complete drug history.

b. Reinforce verbal instructions with written instructions using large print and simple wording. If necessary, use color-coding rather than drug names.

c. Write what the drug is used for and what the adverse effects can be.

d. Make sure patient or caregiver can open the medication container.

e. Arrange medication schedules to coincide with regular activity, such as eating (if appropriate for that drug). Simplify the drug regimen as much as possible.

f. If necessary, arrange a check-off system using a chart to ensure adherence.

g. If possible, visibly evaluate all medications in the home, or ask patient to bring all medications for evaluation.

h. Encourage patient to check expirations dates and discard all old or unneeded medications.

i. Encourage patient to store medications in original containers in a dry, dark place.

j. Encourage patient to avoid over-the-counter (OTC) medication without checking with the primary care provider before use.

k. Encourage patient to report adverse drug effects.

l. Work with prescribing caregiver and patient to maintain a medication regimen that follows the principles for geriatric drug use; start dosages low and go slow, use only necessary medications, titrate the dose to patient response, simplify the regimen, and have frequent reevaluations of the medication regimen.

Community and Home Care Considerations

1. Ask the patient or family to bring in all the patient's medications for clinic or office visits or whenever the patient goes to a facility in order to obtain an accurate medication history.

2. Ask the patient what vitamins, minerals, herbal supplements, and other OTC products are being used. Many patients do not consider these medications and will not readily supply the information unless specifically asked.

3. Alert patients and family members that many "natural" products sold over the counter still may cause adverse reactions and toxicity as well as interactions with other drugs.

4. Warn patients and families that many complementary and alternative medicine (CAM) therapies do not have proven effectiveness despite advertisements. CAM should be used as an adjunct to conventional therapy, and the patient should notify all health care providers of supplements and therapies being used.

Altered Nutritional Status

 Evidence Base Morley, J. E. (2012). Undernutrition in older adults. *Family practice, 29* Suppl 1, i89–i93.

There is growing evidence that a balanced diet along with other health promotion behavior contribute to longevity. However, normal age-related changes, behavioral changes, and pathologic conditions may lead to malnutrition in the older adult

Pathophysiology and Etiology

1. Changes in the oral cavity, including loss of teeth, diminished saliva production, and difficulty with mastication, may cause decreased food intake.
2. A decrease in gastric secretion with reduced pepsin hinders protein digestion and iron, vitamin B_{12}, calcium, and folic acid absorption; there are no significant changes in the small or large bowel.
3. Sensory changes involving taste and smell cause anorexia.
4. Psychosocial factors including changes in living situation, widowhood, depression, loneliness, decreased choice of food for institutionalized older adults, need to adhere to special diets, socioeconomic status, and ability to obtain and prepare food all impact what is eaten.
5. Alcohol use interferes with the absorption of B-complex vitamins. Additionally, alcohol is high in calories and low in nutritional value.
6. Medications can alter nutrition by directly decreasing absorption and utilization of nutrients. Indirectly, medications can result in anorexia, xerostomia, dysgeusia, and early satiety.
7. Dysphagia, which commonly occurs after stroke, intubation, or head and neck surgery, or is related to Parkinson's disease and dementia, may cause decreased food intake.
8. With age, there is a decrease in energy needs because of a decrease in muscle mass (total caloric need decreases by 30%).

Nursing Assessment

1. Be alert for patients who complain of difficulty swallowing and difficulty managing saliva. Watch for coughing after swallowing, sounding "wet" after eating, and pocketing food in the cheeks.
2. Assess for absent or diminished gag reflex.
3. Assess for a 10% weight loss over 6 months (marasmus) or weight loss along with low serum albumin levels (kwashiorkor), which are signs of protein-energy malnutrition.
4. Determine if cholesterol level is below 130 mg/dL, which also may indicate malnourishment.

Nursing and Patient Care Considerations

1. Educate older adult and family or significant other about basic nutritional requirements and on overcoming barriers that interfere with optimal nutrition.
   a. The Required Dietary Allowances for healthy older adults are the same as that for younger adults, with three exceptions: decreased caloric intake, decreased protein intake (1 g/kg), and decreased iron requirements for postmenopausal women.
2. Encourage good mouth care.
3. Encourage patients to avoid alcohol if possible; refer for counseling if necessary and compensate for the nutritional consequences of alcohol abuse with liquid supplements, B vitamins.
4. Review all prescription and OTC medications with patients, and evaluate the influence of these on nutritional status.
5. If food procurement, preparation, and enjoyment are a problem, identify community resources to offer assistance in obtaining food and community meals.
6. In large facility settings, environmental factors may influence food enjoyment. Encourage socialization when eating, and try to minimize the negative effects of disruptive people and/or settings. Try to improve aesthetics.
7. To compensate for age-related changes in taste and smell, encourage use of low-sodium food additives.
8. Encourage proper body position (eg, sitting upright during mealtimes) and staying up for 30 minutes after eating to help with digestion.
9. If possible, encourage five to six small meals per day rather than three large meals.
10. If appropriate, encourage family to bring in favorite foods for patient.
11. Position food on the plate so that if there is visual neglect, or impairment, patient is best able to see the food served.
12. Identify patients with dysphagia and obtain a referral to a speech therapist.
    a. Work with the speech therapist and primary health care provider to determine what consistency of food is safe for patient to swallow. If patient is unable to swallow, thin liquids, slushes, puddings, or applesauce should be given to ensure adequate hydration.
    b. Use good compensatory techniques if indicated. These include sitting upright, tucking and turning the head, placing the food on the unaffected side of the tongue, swallowing twice to clear the pharyngeal tract, tucking the chin to the chest, and bringing the tongue up and back and holding the breath to swallow.
    c. Write out swallowing instructions for patient and family and educate family regarding the importance of maintaining these precautions.

Community and Home Care Considerations

1. Encourage the older adult at home to eat a well-balanced diet to maintain an optimal nutritional state.
2. Suggest vitamin preparations with the fewest number of minerals and vitamins needed to prevent interactions and avoid megadoses.
3. Advise taking calcium carbonate, iron, and zinc at least 2 hours apart and taking vitamins at the same time daily.
4. Advise taking iron on an empty stomach and taking fat-soluble vitamins (A, D, E, and K) with food.

5. Educate about different types of calcium preparations:
   a. Calcium carbonate is more difficult to absorb on an empty stomach; it needs an acidic environment to enhance absorption. The percent of calcium absorbed decreases as the calcium load increases; therefore calcium carbonate absorption is greatest in doses of 500 mg or less, with food.
   b. Because calcium citrate is highly soluble in acid, it is better absorbed on an empty stomach. The citrate form does not need gastric acid for absorption.
   c. Calcium lactate can be absorbed at various pHs and does not need to be taken with food for absorption.

Urinary Incontinence

 Evidence Base Talley, K. M. C., Wyman, J. F., & Shamliyan, T. A. (2011). State of the science: conservative interventions for urinary incontinence in frail community-dwelling older adults. *Nursing outlook, 59(4),* 215–220, 220.

Approximately 13 million Americans suffer from urinary incontinence, including 29% of women age 80 and over living in the community and 5% to 15% of older men living in the community. The prevalence increases significantly for older adults living in nursing homes, including 60% to 78% of women and 45% to 72% of men.

Pathophysiology and Etiology

1. There are five basic types of urinary incontinence:
   a. Stress—an involuntary loss of urine with increases in intra-abdominal pressure. Usually caused from weakness and laxity of pelvic floor musculature, or bladder outlet weakness.
   b. Urge—involves leakage of urine because of inability to delay voiding after sensation of bladder fullness is perceived. This is associated with detrusor hyperactivity, CNS disorders, or local genitourinary conditions.
   c. Overflow—due to a leakage of urine resulting from mechanical forces on an overdistended bladder. This results from mechanical obstruction or hypomobility of the detrusor muscle.
   d. Mixed—symptoms of both stress and urge incontinence secondary to both an overactive detrusor and pelvic floor/urethral incompetence.
   e. Functional—involves urinary leakage associated with inability to get to the toilet because of cognitive and/or physical functioning.

Nursing Assessment

1. Identify reversible causes of incontinence using the DRIP acronym:
   D—Delirium, especially new-onset delirium.
   R—Restricted mobility, retention.
   I—Infection (especially sudden-onset cystitis), inflammation (such as atrophic vaginitis or urethritis), impaction (fecal).
   P—Polyuria (from poorly controlled diabetes or diuretic treatment), pharmaceuticals (including psychotropics, anticholinergics, alpha agonists, beta agonists, calcium channel blockers, opioids, alpha antagonists, and alcohol).

2. Evaluate lower urinary tract function.
   a. Stress maneuvers are evaluated by asking the patient, with a full bladder, to cough three times while standing. Observe for urine leakage.
   b. Check for postvoid residual by inserting a 12- or 14-French straight catheter a few minutes after the patient voids or use a portable ultrasound bladder scanner to measure postvoid urine residual.
   c. Evaluate bladder filling by leaving the straight catheter in place and using a 50-mL syringe to fill the bladder with sterile water. Hold the syringe about 6 inches (15 cm) above the pubic symphysis. Continue to fill the bladder in 25-mL increments until the patient feels the urge to void. Observe for involuntary bladder contractions. These contractions are detected by continuous upward movement of the column of fluid in the absence of abdominal straining.

Nursing and Patient Care Considerations

1. For stress or urge incontinence, teach Kegel (pelvic muscle) exercises.
   a. Tell patient to first practice stopping the stream of urine while voiding to identify proper contraction of the pubococcygeal muscle; contraction will result in stopping flow, and relaxation allows flow.
   b. Once proper contraction is verified, advise patient to practice contraction of the muscle for 3 seconds, then relaxation of the muscle for 3 seconds in sets of 15 three times per day.
   c. The exercise can be practiced anywhere at any time because it involves contraction of an internal muscle; encourage patient to try them sitting, standing, and lying down. The abdomen should be relaxed, and no movement should be visible by doing Kegel exercises.
2. Assist with biofeedback that involves the use of bladder, rectal, or vaginal pressure recordings to train patients to contract pelvic floor muscles and relax the abdomen.
3. Institute a behavioral training program, using bladder records, biofeedback, and pelvic floor exercises for patients with stress or urge incontinence.
4. Institute other interventions such as:
   a. Bladder retraining—progressive lengthening or shortening of voiding intervals to restore the normal pattern of voiding; this is useful after period of immobility or catheterization.
   b. Scheduled toileting—using a fixed toileting schedule to prevent wetting episodes for patients with urge or functional incontinence.
   c. Habit training—involves using a variable toileting schedule based on patient's pattern of voiding; also incorporates positive reinforcement.
   d. Prompted voiding—includes regular prompts to void every 1 to 2 hours with positive reinforcement.

e. Appropriate use of incontinence aids, such as pads or diapers.

f. Judicious use of medications to help control urge incontinence. These include oxybutynin and tolterodine, among others. Contraindicated in urinary or gastric retention, myasthenia gravis, and uncontrolled glaucoma. Monitor carefully for anticholinergic effects—dry mouth, heat intolerance, urine retention, constipation, drowsiness, dry eyes, blurred vision.

Urine Retention

Evidence Base Johansson, R. M., Malmvall, B. E., Andersson-Gäre, B., et al. (2012). Guidelines for preventing urinary retention and bladder damage during hospital care. *Journal of clinical nursing.* In publication.

Urine retention is a common problem in the older adult, commonly related to a neurologic or other underlying condition.

Pathophysiology and Etiology

1. Frequently encountered in the acute care setting, postcatheterization, after stroke, in diabetics due to atonic neuropathic bladder, due to fecal impaction, and in males with prostatic enlargement.
2. The patient with urine retention may void small amounts or may be incontinent continuously due to overflow of urine.
3. Patients with urine retention will usually have incontinence during the night.
4. Urine retention may also be caused or aggravated by drugs with anticholinergic properties, such as levodopa or tricyclic antidepressants, especially amitriptyline. Other commonly prescribed drugs, such as alpha agonists, beta agonists, and calcium channel blockers, can cause urinary retention.

GERONTOLOGIC ALERT Urine retention may cause urinary tract infection, which can lead to sepsis in the older adult.

Nursing Assessment

1. Take a complete history and perform a physical examination to rule out causes of urine retention.
2. Monitor for a distended bladder and perform postvoid catheterization; there is no consensus of the upper or lower limits of a postvoid residual. However, residual of greater than 100 mL of urine is often used as a sign of urine retention.

Nursing and Patient Care Considerations

1. Remove fecal impaction to help patient regain bladder function.
2. If prostatic disease is suspected, appropriate referral is necessary.
3. Encourage male to use the standing position and female to use the sitting position to facilitate urinary flow; provide privacy.

4. Teach "double voiding." Finish voiding, then reposition oneself to void again. Also teach Credé's method: have the patient massage the area of the abdomen directly over the bladder to "milk" the bladder to express any residual urine.
5. Evaluate medication regimen and discuss with health care provider the necessity or substitution of offending medication.
6. If no underlying condition is suspected, attempt intermittent catheterizations every 8 hours, in combination with regular voiding attempts by patient. If there is no response in 2 weeks (ie, no decrease in postvoid residuals), referral to a urologist may be necessary for medical management of the urine retention.

Fecal Incontinence

Evidence Base Shah, B. J., Chokhavatia, S., & Rose, S. (2012). Fecal Incontinence in the Elderly: FAQ. *The American Journal of Gastroenterology,* *107*(11): 1635–46.

Fecal incontinence is an inability to voluntarily control the passage of gas or feces. It occurs in an estimated 15% of women and 6% to 10% of men who live in the community and in an estimated 45% of older adults who live in nursing homes.

Pathophysiology and Etiology

1. Fecal continence depends on normal rectal and anal sensation, rectal reservoir capacity, and internal and external sphincter mechanisms.
2. In institutionalized older adults, fecal impaction is a primary cause of fecal incontinence due to stool leaking around a fecal mass.
3. In noninstitutionalized older adults, fecal incontinence is commonly associated with dysfunction of one of the anorectal continence mechanisms, such as impaired contractile strength of the sphincters and lower rectal volume capacity. Stroke and spinal cord injuries cause loss of sensation in the rectal area.
4. Sometimes functional or cognitive impairment and depression may inhibit motivation and the ability to remain continent.
5. Commonly, no cause can be determined for the fecal loss, and it is believed that the incontinence may be due to a degenerative injury to the pudendal nerve.

Nursing Assessment

1. Assess overall function, cognition, and affect.
2. Perform a rectal examination to check for impaction or decreased rectal sphincter tone.
3. If the fecal incontinence is diarrheal in nature, stool evaluation for leukocytes, culture and sensitivity, ova and parasites, and *Clostridium difficile* may be indicated.

Nursing and Patient Care Considerations

1. Increase dietary fiber in an attempt to add bulk to the stool to stimulate regular defecation, if there is no infection and no impaction present.
2. Try antidiarrheals such as loperamide, as directed, for managing diarrhea.

3. Try to set up a regular bowel evacuation pattern once an impaction is detected and removed. This includes regular toileting times, set preferably after breakfast, and increased fluid and fiber intake. Use laxatives only as a last resort.

4. In bedbound patients, increased fiber in the diet is contraindicated. These patients may require a bisacodyl suppository or an enema to help with rectal evacuation two to three times per week.

5. Treat those with neurogenic fecal incontinence, such as patients with spinal cord injuries and poststroke, to induce fecal evacuation at regularly scheduled times.

6. Administer glycerin or bisacodyl suppository two to three times per week before breakfast (to use the normal gastrocolic reflex that starts after the first meal of the day) to help induce a complete rectal evacuation and decrease stool incontinence.

Community and Home Care Considerations

1. Explain to patient and family that it is not necessary to have bowel movements every day.

2. Advise avoidance of laxatives, which may induce diarrhea.

3. Encourage fibrous foods that stimulate the bowel to be eaten daily, preferably at breakfast, such as stewed prunes, citrus fruits, and bran cereals. Make sure that help is available to toilet patient when the urge to defecate is felt.

4. Recommend a home remedy to maintain regular bowel movements: 3 tbsp applesauce, 2 tbsp bran, and 1 tbsp prune juice mixed, refrigerated, and given at least 1 tbsp each morning.

Pressure Ulcers

Evidence Base Alderden, J., Whitney, J. D., Taylor, S. M., et al. (2011). Risk profile characteristics associated with outcomes of hospital-acquired pressure ulcers: A retrospective review. *Critical Care Nurse, 31*(4), 30–43.
National Pressure Ulcer Advisory Panel, European Pressure Ulcer Advisory Panel. (2009). Pressure ulcer treatment recommendations. In *Prevention and treatment of pressure ulcers: Clinical practice guideline* (pp. 51–120). Washington, DC: National Pressure Ulcer Advisory Panel.

Pressure ulcers (decubitus ulcers) are localized ulcerations of the skin or deeper structures. They most commonly result from prolonged periods of bed rest in acute- or long-term care facilities; however, they can develop within hours in the compromised individual (see Figure 9-2).

Pathophysiology and Etiology

Factors in the Development of Pressure Ulcers

1. Pressure of 70 mm Hg applied for longer than 2 hours can produce tissue destruction; healing cannot occur without relieving the pressure.

2. Friction contributes to pressure ulcer development by causing abrasion of the stratum corneum.

3. Shearing force, produced by sliding of adjacent surfaces, is particularly important in the partial sitting position. This force ruptures capillaries over the sacrum.

4. Moisture on the skin results in maceration of the epithelium.

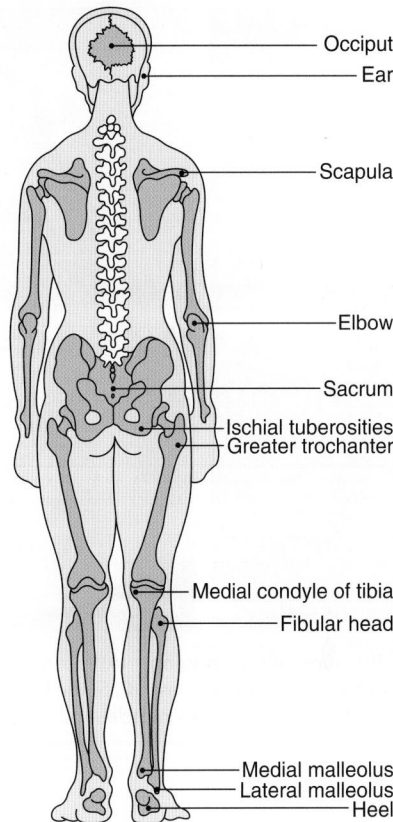

Figure 9-2. Areas susceptible to pressure ulcers.

Risk Factors for Pressure Ulcers

1. Bowel or bladder incontinence.
2. Malnourishment or significant weight loss.
3. Edema, anemia, hypoxia, or hypotension.
4. Neurologic impairment or immobility.
5. Altered mental status, including delirium or dementia.

Nursing Assessment

1. Assess for risk factors for pressure ulcer development and alter those factors, if possible.

2. Assess skin of the older adult frequently for the development of pressure ulcers. The Braden Scale for Predicting Pressure Sore Risk is one of the most commonly used instruments for predicting the development of pressure ulcers (*www.bradenscale.com*). The Braden Scale assesses pressure ulcer risk in six areas: sensory perception, skin moisture, activity, mobility, nutrition, and friction/shear.

3. Stage the ulcer so appropriate treatment can be started. The National Pressure Ulcer Advisory Panel advocates the following staging system (see Figure 9-3 on page 184):

   a. Stage I—intact skin with nonblanchable redness of a localized area, usually over a bony prominence.

   b. Stage II—partial thickness loss of dermis presenting as a shallow open ulcer with a red-pink wound bed, without

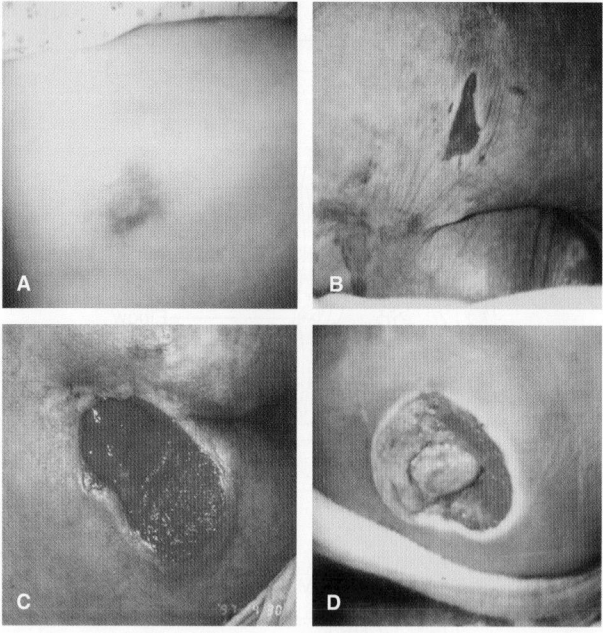

Figure 9-3. Pressure ulcer staging. (A) Stage I—erythema; **(B)** Stage II—partial thickness tissue loss; **(C)** Stage III—full-thickness skin breakdown; **(D)** Stage IV—bone, muscle, and supporting tissue exposed.

slough; may also present as an intact or open/ruptured serum-filled blister.

c. Stage III—full-thickness tissue loss, with subcutaneous fat that may be visible but bone, tendon, or muscle are not exposed; may include undermining and tunneling. Slough may be present but does not obscure the depth of tissue loss.

d. Stage IV—full-thickness tissue loss with exposed bone, tendon, or muscle; slough or eschar may be present on some parts of the wound bed; often includes undermining and tunneling.

e. Unstageable—full-thickness tissue loss in which the base of the ulcer is covered by slough and/or eschar in the wound bed.

f. Suspected deep tissue injury—a localized area of intact skin or blood-filled blister, maroon or purple in color, caused by damage of the underlying soft tissue from shear or pressure.

Nursing and Patient Care Considerations

Prevent Pressure Ulcer Development

1. Provide meticulous care and positioning for immobile patients.
   a. Inspect skin several times daily.
   b. Wash skin with mild soap, rinse, and pat dry with a soft towel.
   c. Lubricate skin with a bland lotion to keep skin soft and pliable.
   d. Avoid poorly ventilated mattress that is covered with plastic or impermeable material.

   e. Employ bowel and bladder programs to prevent incontinence.
   f. Encourage ambulation and exercise.
   g. Promote nutritious diet with optimal protein, vitamins, and iron.
2. Teach older adult and family or significant other the importance of good nutrition, hydration, activity, positioning, and avoidance of pressure, shearing, friction, and moisture.

Relieve the Pressure

1. Avoid elevation of head of bed greater than 30 degrees.
2. Reposition every 2 hours.
3. Use special devices to cushion specific areas, such as flotation rings, lamb's wool or fleece pads, convoluted foam mattresses, booties, or elbow pads.
4. Use an alternating-pressure mattress or air-fluidized bed for patients at high risk to prevent or treat pressure ulcers.
5. Provide for activity and ambulation as much as possible.
6. Advise frequent shifting of weight and occasional raising of buttocks off chair while sitting.

Clean and Debride the Wound

1. Use normal saline for cleaning and disinfecting wounds.
2. Apply wet-to-dry dressings or enzyme ointments for debridement as directed or assist with surgical debridement.

Treat Local Infection

1. Avoid obtaining wound cultures because open wounds are always colonized with bacteria, unless there is evidence of systemic infection or progressive local infection such as cellulitis.
2. Apply topical antibiotics to locally infected pressure ulcer as prescribed.

Cover the Wound

1. Cover the wound with a protective dressing as this minimizes disruption of migrating fibroblasts and epithelial cells and results in a moist, nutrient-rich environment for healing to occur.
   a. Polyurethane thin film dressings can be used for superficial low-exudate wounds. They are air and water permeable but do not absorb exudate.
   b. Hydrocolloids can provide padding to wounds but can lead to maceration; they are not oxygen permeable.
   c. Polyurethane foam/membrane dressings absorb exudate and are oxygen permeable.
   d. Hydrogel dressings are multilayered and include properties of both hydrocolloids and polyurethane (see Table 9-2 for comparison of selected occlusive dressings).

Osteoporosis

Osteoporosis is a condition in which the bone matrix is lost, thereby weakening the bones and making them more susceptible to fracture. Bone mineral density is 2.5 standard deviations below the peak bone density for young adults (T score –2.5). Decrease in bone density of 1.5 to 2.5 below young adult is termed *osteopenia* (T score –1.5 to –2.5). It is the most age-related metabolic bone disorder.

Table 9-2	Comparison of Selected Occlusive Dressing			
DRESSING TYPE	**EXAMPLES**	**APPROPRIATE USE**	**ADVANTAGES**	**DISADVANTAGES**
Absorption	Debrisan Hydrophilic Beads	• Stage II–V ulcer with drainage	• Absorbs drainage and deodorizes wound	• Need to change dressing 1–2 times daily
Hydrocolloid	DuoDerm	• Stage I–II ulcer	• Provides padding • Easy to apply • Water impermeable • No skin excoriation	• Poor absorptive capacity • Poor oxygen exchange • Messy residue • Pressure areas possible
Polyurethane	Op-Site, Tegaderm	• Nondraining wounds	• Transparent • Self-adhesive • Oxygen permeable	• No absorptive capacity • May cause excoriation • Difficult to apply
Polyurethane membrane	Mitraflex	• Skin tears • Tape burns • Blisters • Stage II ulcers • Low-moderate exudate wounds	• Good absorptive ability • Good oxygen exchange • Water impermeable • May debride	• May cause excoriation
Polyurethane foam	Epi-Lock	• Skin tears • Tape burns • Blisters • Stage II ulcers • Low to moderate exudate wounds	• Good absorptive ability • Good oxygen exchange • Water impermeable • May debride • No skin excoriation	• Nonadhesive
Hydrogel	Vigilon, Biofilm	• Stage I–III	• No skin excoriation • Transparent • Some ability to absorb drainage • Easy to apply	• Difficult to apply • Nonadherent
Debriding enzyme	Elase, Travase	• Stage III–IV	• Acts against devitalized tissue • Not appropriate for hard, dry eschar	• May damage healthy tissue

Pathophysiology and Etiology

1. The rate of bone resorption increases over the rate of bone formation, causing loss of bone mass.
2. Calcium and phosphate salts are lost, creating porous, brittle bones.
3. Occurs most commonly in postmenopausal women, but may also occur in men.
4. Other factors include:
   a. Age.
   b. Inactivity.
   c. Chronic illness.
   d. Medications, such as corticosteroids, excessive thyroid replacement, cyclosporine.
   e. Calcium and vitamin D deficiency.
   f. Family history.
   g. Smoking and alcohol use.
   h. Diet—caffeine has been linked as a risk factor.
   i. Race—whites and Asians have higher risk incidence.
   j. Body type—small frame/short stature, low body fat.

Clinical Manifestations

1. Asymptomatic until later stages.
2. Fracture after minor trauma may be first indication. Most frequent fractures associated with osteoporosis include fractures of the distal radius, vertebral bodies, proximal humerus, pelvis, and proximal femur (hip).
3. May have vague complaints related to aging process (stiffness, pain, weakness).
4. Estrogen deficiency may be noted.

Diagnostic Evaluation

1. X-rays show changes only after 30% to 60% loss of bone.
2. Dual-energy x-ray absorptiometry (DEXA) scanning shows decreased bone mineral density (T score –2.5 or worse).

3. Serum and urine calcium levels are normal.
4. Serum bone matrix Gla protein (a marker for bone turnover) is elevated.
5. Bone biopsy shows thin, porous, otherwise normal bone.

Management

Management is primarily preventive.

1. Identify patients at risk for fractures.
2. Reduce modifiable risk factors through improved diet, smoking cessation, decreased alcohol consumption, and other healthy lifestyle choices.
3. Adequate intake of calcium—1.2 g per day—may be preventive.
4. Adequate intake of vitamin D.
   a. Vitamin D plays a major role in calcium absorption and bone health. With age, there is decreased ability to take in vitamin D through the skin; therefore, replacement is recommended.
   b. Food sources are milk products, egg yolks, fish, and liver; however, dietary intake of vitamin D is limited
   c. Vitamin D can be manufactured in the skin through sunlight exposure; however, this may be limited by cloud cover, latitude, and season and skin cancer prevention methods that limit exposure.
   d. Recommended daily allowance for adults age 70 and over is 800 international units.

 Evidence Base Institute of Medicine, Food and Nutrition Board. (2010). *Dietary reference intakes for calcium and vitamin D*. Washington, DC: National Academy Press.

5. Weight-bearing exercise (eg, walking) throughout life.
6. Hormone replacement therapy is no longer recommended for osteoporosis prevention or treatment because the risks outweigh the benefits.
7. Raloxifene, an estrogen receptor agonist, is an alternative to estrogen. Not as effective as estrogen, but does show some benefit in preserving bone density. No increase in risk of breast cancer.
8. Calcitonin administered by nasal spray may help prevent spinal fracture. Adverse effect is nasal burning and a runny nose.
9. Bisphosphonates, such as risedronate, alendronate, and ibandronate, bind to and inhibit osteoclast action, remain active on bone resorptive surfaces for 3 weeks, and do not impede normal bone formation.
   a. Associated with improved bone density and decreased hip and spinal fracture rate.
   b. They must be taken with fluid but not food, and patient must remain upright for 30 minutes after taking pill to prevent esophagitis.
   c. Long-acting injectables such as zoledronic acid and teriparatide are protective for women at high risk for fractures and helpful in increasing bone mass in men who are on long-term glucocorticoid therapy.
10. Parathyroid hormone teriparatide utility is limited because it requires daily subcutaneous injections.
11. Prevention of falls in older adults helps to prevent fractures.

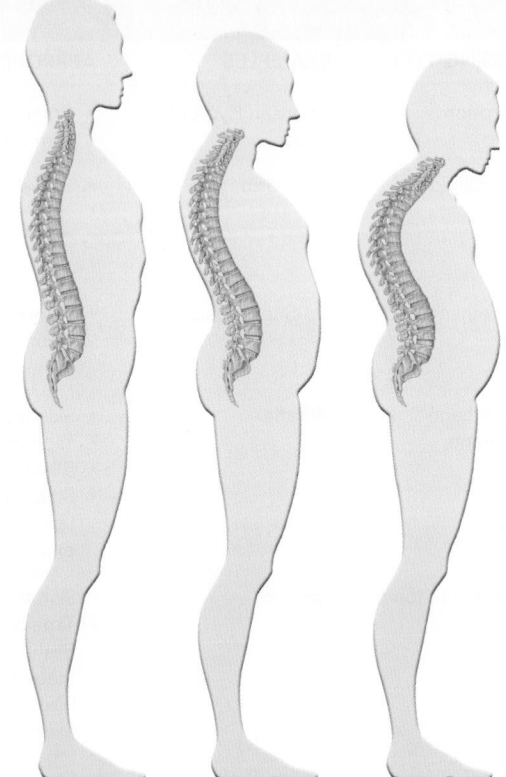

Figure 9-4. Progressive kyphosis in osteoporosis.

Complications

1. Fractures.
2. Progressive kyphosis, loss of height (see Figure 9-4).
3. Chronic back pain from compression fracture.

Nursing Assessment

1. Obtain history of risk factors for osteoporosis, fractures, and other musculoskeletal disease.
2. Assess risk for falls and fractures—sensory or motor problems, improper footwear, lack of knowledge of safety precautions, and so forth. See Table 9-3, for assessment factors and interventions.

Nursing Diagnosis

Chronic Pain related to vertebral compression fractures in late stages of osteoporosis

Nursing Interventions

Reducing Pain

1. Administer opioid analgesics, as ordered, for acute exacerbations of pain.
2. Encourage replacement with nonopioid pain relievers as soon as possible to avoid drowsiness, possible addiction.

Table 9-3	Assessment Factors and Interventions to Decrease Risk of Falls

This chart supplies specific interventions you can use to decrease the risk and incidence of falls in older or disabled patients.

KNOWN RISK FACTORS	SPECIFIC INTERVENTIONS TO DECREASE INDIVIDUAL RISK
History of falls	• Identify the patient as being at risk for falls: May use sticker on chart or door, inform families and other care providers of increased risk.
Fear of falling	• Encourage patient to verbalize feelings. • Strengthen self-efficacy related to transfers and ambulation by providing verbal encouragement about capabilities and ability to perform safely.
Bowel and bladder incontinence	• Set up regular voiding schedule (every 2 hours or as appropriate based on patient need). • Monitor bowel function and encourage sufficient fluids and fiber (eight 8-oz glasses daily and 24 g of fiber). • Utilize laxatives as appropriate.
Cognitive impairment	• Evaluate patient for reversible causes of cognitive impairment or delirium and eliminate causes as relevant. Monitor patient with cognitive impairment at least hourly with relocation of the patient such that nursing staff can observe and monitor regularly. • Encourage family member to hire staff or stay with patient continuously. • Utilize monitoring devices if available (ie, bed/chair or exit alarms) rather than restraints.
Mood	• Encourage verbalization of feelings. • Evaluate patient's ability to concentrate and learn new information. • Encourage participation in daily activities. • Utilize alternative interventions, such as massage, aromatherapy, pet and plant therapy, and music or exercise.
Dizziness	• Monitor lying, sitting, and standing blood pressures and continually evaluate for factors contributing to dizziness. • Encourage adequate fluid intake (eight 8-oz glasses daily). • Set up environment to avoid movements that result in dizziness or vertigo. • Decrease or avoid alcohol use.
Functional impairment, immobility, impaired gait	• Encourage participation in personal care activities at highest level (ie, if possible encourage ambulation to bathroom rather than use of bedpan). • Refer to physical and occupational therapy as appropriate. • Facilitate adherence to exercise program when indicated. • Maintain safe and appropriate use of assistive devices.
Medications	• Review medications with primary health care provider and determine need for each medication. • Make sure that medications are being used at lowest possible dosages to obtain desired results.
Medical problems	• Work with primary health care provider to augment management of primary medical problem, such as Parkinson's disease, heart failure, or anemia.
Environment	• Remove furniture if patient cannot be seated with feet reaching the floor. • Remove clutter. • Make sure furniture and any assistive devices used are in good condition. • Make sure lighting is adequate. • Make sure safety bars are available in bathroom.

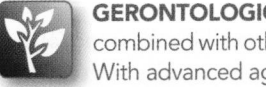 **GERONTOLOGIC ALERT** Be alert for alcohol use combined with other CNS depressants in older adults. With advanced age, there is a reduction in lean body mass, an increase in body fat, a decrease in water content, and a decrease in the gastric alcohol dehydrogenase enzyme. This results in an increase in the blood alcohol level in older individuals compared to younger individuals per unit of alcohol consumed, especially in women. Alcohol use, particularly when combined with opioids or sedative hypnotics, is commonly associated with falls in these individuals.

3. Assist with putting on back brace and ensure proper fit. Encourage use as much as possible, especially while ambulatory.
4. Encourage compliance with physical therapy appointments and practicing exercises at home to increase muscle strength surrounding bones and to relieve pain.

Patient Education and Health Maintenance

1. Encourage exercise for all age groups. Teach the value of walking daily throughout life to provide stress required for strong bone remodeling.
2. Provide dietary education in relation to adequate daily intake of calcium (1,200 mg). Calcium can be obtained through milk and dairy products, vegetables, and supplements. Anyone with a history of urinary tract calculi should consult with health care provider before increasing calcium intake.
3. Encourage use of combined calcium and vitamin D replacement. Avoid massive doses of vitamin D, however, because this may be harmful.
4. Encourage young women at risk to maximize bone mass through nutrition and exercise.
5. Suggest that perimenopausal women confer with their health care provider about the need for calcium supplements and estrogen therapy.
6. Alert patients to resources such as the National Osteoporosis Foundation (*www.nof.org*).

Community and Home Care Consideration

Evidence Base *United States Preventive Services Task Force. (2011). Update on osteoporosis screening. Available:* www.uspreventiveservicestaskforce.org/uspstf/uspsoste.htm.

1. Encourage screening according to the USPSTF guidelines for all women over age 65 and women over age 60 at increased risk through DEXA of the femoral neck, with rescreening at approximately 2-year intervals.
2. Identify women at high risk for osteoporotic fractures in the community—frail, older white or Asian women with poor dietary intake of dairy products and little exposure to sun—and provide education and safety measures to prevent falls and fracture.
3. Make sure that diet contains maximal calcium. Teach family and caregivers how to read labels, encourage dairy products, and add powdered milk to foods as possible. Use skim milk if cholesterol and fat intake is a consideration.
4. Make sure that supplements and other medications are being taken properly.
   a. Patient teaching is critical in dosing of bisphosphonates to prevent esophagitis. Patient must take this upon waking with 6 to 8 oz of water, at least 30 minutes before ingesting first food of the day, and must remain upright for 30 minutes after taking the medication. Weekly or monthly dosing increases compliance.

b. Calcitonin nasal spray dose is one spray in one nostril once per day; alternate nostrils each day.
5. Teach strategies to prevent falls. Assess home for hazards (eg, scatter rugs, slippery floors, extension cords, inadequate lighting).
6. Obtain physical and occupational therapy consultations, as needed, to encourage use of walking aids when balance is poor and to improve muscle strength.

Evaluation: Expected Outcomes

- Pain tolerable with nonopioid analgesics; no new fractures.
- Received screening and understands prevention measures.

Alzheimer's Disease

The most common form of dementia is characterized by progressive impairment in memory, cognitive function, language, judgment, perception, and learned motor skills. Ultimately, patients cannot perform self-care activities and become dependent on caregivers.

Pathophysiology and Etiology

1. Gross pathophysiologic changes in the brain include cortical atrophy most prominent in the frontal and temporal lobes, enlarged ventricles, and atrophy of the hippocampus.
2. Microscopically, changes occur in the proteins of the nerve cells of the cerebral cortex and lead to accumulation of neurofibrillary tangles composed of the tau protein and neuritic plaques composed of the amyloid protein (deposits of protein and altered cell structures on the interneuronal junctions) and granulovascular degeneration. There is loss of cholinergic nerve cells, which are important in memory, function, and cognition.
3. Biochemically, neurotransmitter systems are impaired.
4. Cause unknown, but advanced age, female gender, and family history of AD, and head trauma with a loss of consciousness are risk factors. Indeed, research has identified four specific genes involved in predisposition to Alzheimer's. Genes on chromosomes 1, 14, and 21 have been implicated in the causation of early-onset Alzheimer's disease, whereas the #4 allele of the apolipoprotein gene on chromosome 19 appears to be associated with the development of Alzheimer's disease after age 65.
5. Viruses, environmental toxins, cerebrovascular disease, and educational level may also play a role.

Clinical Manifestations

1. Disease onset is subtle and insidious. Initially, a gradual decline of cognitive function from a previously higher level may be noticed. Short-term memory impairment is commonly the first characteristic in earliest stages of the disease. Patients are forgetful and have difficulty learning and retaining new information. In addition to memory impairment, at least one of the following functional deficits is present:
   a. Language disturbance (word-finding difficulty).
   b. Visual-processing and recognition difficulty (agnosia).
   c. Inability to perform skilled motor activities, such as dressing, walking (apraxia).
   d. Poor abstract reasoning and concentration.

2. Patients may have difficulty planning meals, managing finances, using a telephone, or driving without getting lost. Other classic signs include personality changes, such as irritability and suspiciousness, personal neglect of appearance, and disorientation to time and place.

3. The following clinical manifestations are typical in the middle stage of Alzheimer's disease:
   a. Repetitive actions (perseveration).
   b. Nocturnal restlessness.
   c. Apraxia (impaired ability to perform purposeful activity).
   d. Aphasia (impaired ability to speak).
   e. Agraphia (inability to write).

4. With disease progression, signs of frontal lobe dysfunction appear, including loss of social inhibitions and loss of spontaneity. Delusions, hallucinations, aggression, and wandering behavior often occur in the middle and late stages.

5. Patients in the advanced stage of Alzheimer's disease require total care. Symptoms may include:
   a. Urinary and fecal incontinence.
   b. Emaciation.
   c. Increased irritability.
   d. Inability to walk.
   e. Decreased responsiveness to verbal and physical stimulation.
   f. Difficulty swallowing (dysphagia).

Diagnostic Evaluation

1. Detailed patient history with corroboration by an informed source to determine cognitive and behavioral changes, their duration, and symptoms that may be indicative of other medical or psychiatric illnesses.

2. Noncontrast computed tomography (CT) scan to rule out other neurologic conditions, such as a stroke or tumor. Magnetic resonance imaging and single-photon emission CT may be used.

3. Neuropsychological evaluation, including some form of mental status assessment, to identify specific areas of impaired mental functioning in contrast to areas of intact functioning.

4. Laboratory tests include complete blood count, sedimentation rate, chemistry panel, thyroid-stimulating hormone, test for syphilis, urinalysis, serum B_{12}, folate level, and test for human immunodeficiency virus to rule out infectious or metabolic disorders.

5. Commercial assays for cerebrospinal fluid tau protein and beta-amyloid are available, but their use is limited. Genetic testing is available, but its use is controversial. Three disease genes and one gene indicating susceptibility have been identified.

Management

1. Primary goals of treatment for Alzheimer's disease are to maximize functional abilities and improve quality of life by enhancing mood, cognition, and behavior. No curative treatment exists. Treatment includes pharmacologic and nonpharmacologic approaches.

2. Cholinesterase inhibitors were the first treatment for cognitive impairment of Alzheimer's disease. These drugs improve cholinergic neurotransmission to help delay decline in cognition and function over time. There is also evidence that cholinesterase inhibitors may be helpful in decreasing agitated behaviors common in dementia.
   a. Donepezil is widely used in mild to moderate cases because it can be given once daily and is well tolerated; starting at 5 mg at bedtime and increased to 10 mg after 4 to 6 weeks. Donepezil has also recently shown to be beneficial in individuals with severe dementia.
   b. Galantamine is given with food in dosage of 4 to 12 mg twice per day. Should be restarted at 4 mg bid if interrupted for several days. Dose should be reduced in cases of renal or hepatic impairment. Razadyne ER is an extended-release formula that can be given in once-daily dosing with dose ranges from 8 to 24 mg per day.
   c. Rivastigmine is given 1.5 mg twice per day with meals and increased up to 6 to 12 mg per day. Rivastigmine is also available in an oral solution and a patch form.

 DRUG ALERT Cholinesterase inhibitors were initially aimed at improving memory and cognition. These drugs, however, seem to have an important impact on the behavioral changes that occur in patients with cognitive impairment. Specifically, research studies have demonstrated that use of cholinesterase inhibitors improves the apathy, disinhibition, pacing, and hallucinations commonly noted in dementia. Be alert for drug interactions with NSAIDs, succinylcholine-type muscle relaxants, cholinergic and anticholinergic agents, drugs that slow the heart, and other drugs that are metabolized by the hepatic CYP2D6 or CYP3A4 pathways.

3. Memantine, an N-methyl D-aspartate-receptor antagonist, is approved for moderate to severe Alzheimer's disease. Dosage is 10 mg bid. The drug can be used with a cholinesterase inhibitor because it works by regulating the neurotransmitter, glutamate.

4. Studies indicate that other drugs, such as estrogen and NSAIDs, have not proven helpful in treatment and prevention of Alzheimer's disease.

5. Patients with depressive symptoms should be considered for antidepressant therapy.

6. Nonpharmacologic treatments used to optimize cognition and behavior include environmental manipulation that decreases stimulation, pet therapy, aromatherapy, massage, music therapy, and exercise.

7. If nonpharmacologic approaches have been applied consistently and have failed to adequately reduce the frequency and severity of behavioral symptoms that have the potential to cause harm to the patient or others, then the introduction of medications such as antipsychotics, benzodiazepines, anticonvulsants, antidepressants, and sedatives may be appropriate, but will still need to be carefully and routinely monitored over time.
   a. The risk and potential benefits of any medication must be discussed with the patient (when appropriate) and/or the patient's family/decision maker.
   b. The minimum amount of a medication should be used for the shortest time possible.

DRUG ALERT Be aware that no medications are specifically approved by the FDA to treat the neuropsychiatric and behavioral symptoms of individuals with dementia. Antipsychotics have been linked to higher risk of death among older adults with dementia. This led the FDA to issue a black box warning for antipsychotic use in dementia.

Complications

1. Increased incidence of functional decline.
2. Injury due to lack of insight, hallucinations, and confusion.
3. Malnutrition due to inattention to mealtimes and hunger or lack of ability to prepare meals or feed self.

Nursing Assessment

1. Perform cognitive assessment for orientation, insight, abstract thinking, concentration, memory, and verbal ability.
2. Assess for changes in behavior and ability to perform ADLs.
3. Evaluate nutrition and hydration; check weight, skin turgor, meal habits.
4. Assess motor ability, strength, muscle tone, and flexibility.

Nursing Diagnoses

- Disturbed thought processes related to physiologic disease process.
- Risk for injury due to loss of cognitive abilities.
- Insomnia secondary to disease process.
- Caregiver role strain related to physical needs and behavioral manifestations of the disease process.

Nursing Interventions

Improving Cognitive Response

1. Simplify the environment: reduce noise and social interaction to a level tolerable for the patient.
2. Maintain a predictable, structured routine, decrease the number of choices available to the patient, use pictures to identify activities, and use structured group activities.
3. Encourage active participation in care as tolerated and provide positive feedback for tasks that are accomplished.
4. Provide opportunities for physical activity alternating with rest periods.
5. Avoid confrontations and arguments. Follow the patient's direction and individualize care as much as possible.
6. Maintain consistency in interactions and introduce new people slowly.

Preventing Injury

1. Avoid restraints, but maintain observation of the patient as necessary.
2. Provide for adequate lighting to avoid misinterpretation of the environment.
3. Remove unneeded furniture and equipment from the room.
4. Provide identification tag or MedicAlert bracelet.

5. Make sure patient has nonslip shoes or slippers that are easy to put on.
6. Encourage use of assistive safety devices, such as handrails and shower chairs.
7. Ensure physical activity as tolerated and ROM exercises to maintain mobility.

Ensuring Adequate Rest

1. Attempt to limit the use of medications that act on the CNS, such as anxiolytics and antipsychotics; however, if used, monitor for clinical response and potential adverse effects, including increased confusion, excess sedation, parkinsonism, extrapyramidal symptoms, and cardiovascular events.
2. Provide periods of physical exercise to expend energy.
3. Support normal sleep habits and bedtime rituals.
   a. Keep regular bedtime.
   b. Have patient change into pajamas at bedtime.
   c. Allow desired bedtime activity, such as snack, warm non-caffeinated beverage, listening to music, or prayer.
4. Maintain quiet, relaxing environment to avoid confusion and agitation.

Supporting Caregiver

1. Encourage caregiver to discuss feelings.
2. Encourage caregiver to maintain own health and emotional well-being.
3. Stress the need for relaxation time or respite care.
4. Assist the caregiver in finding resources, such as community or church groups, social service programs, or facility-based support groups.
5. Assess caregiver's stress and refer for counseling.
6. Support decision to place patient in a long-term care facility.

Community and Home Care Considerations

1. Encourage regular medical checkups with attention to health maintenance every 3 to 6 months to provide ongoing medical surveillance of patient and stamina of caregivers. Include influenza vaccine and ensure that patient has had pneumococcal pneumonia vaccine.
2. Discuss advance directives for patients and discuss long-term placement options in anticipation of future needs to help family members adjust and plan arrangements.
3. Encourage patients to be involved in social and intellectual activities as long as possible, such as family events, exercise, and recreational activities and sharing the newspaper and other forms of media.
4. Assist caregivers to modify the home environment for safety, and advise families of safety hazards such as wandering and driving a car. Encourage use of door locks, electronic wander-alert guards, and registration with the "Safe Return" program through the Alzheimer's Association or local police department.
5. Remind family members of possible dangers around the house as patient becomes less responsible for behavior. Encourage caregivers to reduce the temperature of the hot water heater, remove dials from stove and other electrical appliances, remove matches and lighters, and safely store away tools and other potentially dangerous items.

Patient Education and Health Maintenance

1. Encourage activities that provide physical exercise and repetitive movement but that require little thought, such as dancing, painting, doing laundry, or vacuuming.

2. Teach patient and family to eliminate stimulants, such as caffeine, and maintain good nutrition.

3. Discuss with the family the need to organize finances and to make advanced directive decisions and guardianship arrangements before they are needed to allow the patient input into the process.

4. OTC products, such as ginkgo biloba, have gained popularity; however, their clinical benefits have not been demonstrated to be better than placebo in well-designed randomized clinical trials. Although high doses of vitamin E (2,000 international units) have shown to delay nursing home placement by a few months, there is no evidence of cognitive improvements, and doses higher than 400 international units have been associated with bleeding and cardiovascular events. Families should be encouraged to discuss their use with the health care provider and not abandon conventional treatment.

5. For additional information, refer families to:
   –Alzheimer's Association: *www.alz.org.*
   –Alzheimer's Disease Education and Referral Center: *www.nia.nih.gov/Alzheimers.*

Evaluation: Expected Outcomes

- Participates in ADL without agitation or resistance.
- Remains free from injury.
- Sleeps 6 to 8 hours a night with a 1-hour rest period twice per day.
- Caregiver reports using support systems and community resources.

LEGAL AND ETHICAL CONSIDERATIONS

Restraint Use

Since the Nursing Home Reform Act took effect in October 1990, long-term care facilities throughout the United States have been required to follow guidelines emphasizing individualized, less restrictive care for residents.

The goal should be to minimize restraint use. This is a challenge, yet there are many nursing strategies that can be implemented to help reduce restraint use. And, although most nurses cite the rationale for placing a restraint on a patient is for patient safety, there is little evidence that patient safety or a reduction in injuries is actually achieved.

There are many alternative approaches to care as well as how to minimize risks associated with falls, as outlined at *www.consultgerirn.org/topics/physical_restraints/want_to_know_more.*

Guidelines

1. The following are the federal requirements for the use of restraints based on the 1987 Omnibus Budget Reconciliation Act.

2. These guidelines must be met in any long-term care facility that participates in Medicare or Medicaid. However, these guidelines are useful for health care providers working with older adults in all settings.

   a. The resident has the right to be free from any physical restraints imposed or psychoactive drug administered for purposes of discipline or convenience and not required to treat the resident's medical symptoms.

   b. Physical restraints are any manual method of physical or mechanical device, material, or equipment attached or adjacent to the resident's body that the person cannot remove easily, which restricts freedom of movement or access to one's body (includes leg and arm restraints, hand mitts, soft ties or vest, wheelchair safety bars, and geriatric chairs).

   c. There must be a trial of less restrictive measures unless the physical restraint is necessary to provide life-saving treatment.

   d. The resident or legal representative must consent to the use of restraints.

   e. Residents who are restrained should be released, exercised, toileted, and checked for skin redness every 2 hours.

   f. The need for restraints should be reevaluated periodically.

   g. The specific facility will have to develop policies and procedures for the appropriate use of restraints and psychoactive drugs.

   h. Primary health care providers will have to write appropriate orders for restraints and psychoactive drugs.

3. The most frequently reported reason for nurses' use of restraints is to prevent patients from harming themselves or others. Specifically, they are used to prevent falls and prevent removal of catheters or IV lines.

4. Multiple studies have found that restraints actually increase incidence of falls, can result in patient strangulation, can increase patient confusion, can cause pressure ulcers and nosocomial infections, can decrease functional ability, and can result in social isolation.

5. In regard to the patient's personal and social integrity, restraints have resulted in emotional responses of anger, fear, resistance, humiliation, demoralization, discomfort, resignation, and denial.

Alternative Interventions Instead of Restraints

1. Evaluate those patients who are considered to be in need of a restraint. Evaluation should include physical function and cognitive status (see page 169), elimination history, history of falls, vision impairment, BP (specifically evaluating for orthostatic hypotension), and medication use.

2. Attempt to correct any problems identified in the evaluation, such as vision impairment or unsafe gait.

3. Use the evaluation to determine patients at high risk of falling (eg, those with confusion, orthostatic hypotension, multiple medication regimens, and altered gait).

4. Use interventions as alternatives to restraints as outlined in Box 9-4, page 192.

BOX 9-4	Techniques to Prevent Falls as Alternative to Restraints

FOR ALL PATIENTS

- Familiarize patient with environment (ie, identify call light or bell to ring, label the bathroom, kitchen, closet).
- Have patient demonstrate ways to obtain help if needed.
- Place bed in low position with brakes locked if possible, or mattress on the floor.
- Make sure that footwear is fitted and nonslip and is used properly.
- Determine appropriate use of side rails based on cognitive and functional status.
- Utilize nightlight.
- Keep floor surfaces clean and dry.
- Keep room uncluttered and make sure that furniture is in optimal condition.
- Make sure patient knows where personal possessions are and can safely access them.
- Ensure adequate handrails in bathroom (commode, shower, and tub), room, and hallway.
- Establish a care plan to maintain bowel and bladder function.
- Evaluate effects of medications that increase the patient's risk of falling.
- Encourage participation in functional activities and exercise at patient's highest possible level and refer to physical therapy as appropriate.
- Monitor patient regularly and encourage safe activities.

FOR PATIENTS AT HIGH RISK FOR FALLING WHEN WALKING INDEPENDENTLY

- Use beanbag chairs or specially designed chairs that make independent transfer difficult.
- Tilt the front of a chair upward by inserting a small to medium folded blanket under the anterior portion of the cushion.
- Institute physical therapy and increased exercise activities to help strengthen muscles and improve function.
- For the patient who interferes with treatment, evaluate the need for invasive treatments. When such treatments are essential, use mittens or gloves rather than restraints.
- For the patient who wanders, provide an exercise program or establish a bounded environment in which the person can ambulate freely.
- For aggressive and agitated patients, be aware that restraints may only make the behavior worse. Provide a low-stimulus environment, consistent caregivers, and appropriate medications to help control the agitation. Music therapy has also been shown to decrease aggressive behavior.

Advance Directives

The 1990 Patient Self-Determination Act, which requires that patients be asked about the existence of advanced directives at the time of enrollment into a health care facility, has increased awareness of older adults' rights to determine their own care. Based on the ethical principle of autonomy (a person's privilege of self-rule), advance directives provide a clear and detailed expression of a person's wishes for care. Providing an older adult with the opportunity to discuss their end-of-life plans is helpful. A four-step process that includes initiating a discussion, facilitating the discussion, completing the document, and updating.

Durable Power of Attorney is now called *Healthcare Proxy*. It involves the designation of another person to make health care decisions for an incapacitated person. Many states have official documents that can be downloaded from their websites with detailed information about Advanced Directives and Healthcare Proxy.

 Evidence Base Payne, K. L., Prentice-Dunn, S., & Allen, R. S. (2010). A comparison of two interventions to increase completion of advance directives. *Clinical Gerontologist, 33*(1), 49–61.

Types of Advance Directives

Living Wills

1. Living Wills were the first and most widespread type of advance directive.
2. They were proposed as a mechanism for refusing "heroic" or unwanted medical intervention for the dying person.
3. They allow a person to state in writing that certain life-sustaining treatments should be withdrawn or withheld when that person is dying and unable to directly communicate his or her wishes.
4. Living Wills only allow for the refusal of further treatment. They are not precise in terms of directives and focus only on the patient who is clearly terminally ill.

Healthcare Proxy

1. This document appoints a proxy to act on behalf of another person, provides guidance for the proxy, and endures even when the maker is incapacitated.
2. This is always a written document.
3. The document states the preferences and perhaps even the values of its maker. It outlines the types of decisions the person would want to have made on his behalf.
4. Because no Healthcare Proxy document can cover all situations, the document should name a person who has the task of ensuring that the patient's wishes are honored. The proxy has the responsibility to interpret the document and extrapolate its contents to situations not specifically covered.

Medical Orders for Life Sustaining Treatment (MOLST)

1. Many states are beginning to implement a standard health care provider order form that indicates patient choices for a variety of life-sustaining treatment, and is used across health care facilities.
2. MOLST is important for patients with serious health conditions who:
   a. Want to avoid or receive any or all life-sustaining treatment.
   b. Are residents of long-term care facilities.
   c. Might die within a year.
3. Completion of the MOLST begins with a conversation or a series of conversations between the patient, patient's health care agent or surrogate, primary care provider, and specialist care provider.

4. The health care provider should help delineate the patient's goals for care, review possible treatment options on the entire MOLST form, and facilitate informed medical decision making.

5. The completed form can then also be used as a medical order across health care settings; from emergency personnel responding to the patient at home, to the staff of an intensive care unit.

Nursing and Patient Care Considerations

1. Under the Patient Self-Determination Act, all patients who enter a Medicare- or Medicaid-certified facility, nursing home, or home health agency must:
   a. Be provided with information about the state's laws and the facility's policies regarding advance directive.
   b. Be asked if they have advance directives.
   c. Have their advance directives placed in their medical record.

2. Education of patients and families is essential in helping them to understand the difference between Living Wills, MOLST, or Healthcare Proxy and determining which document best suits their needs.

3. Patients and families need to be educated about what is involved in undergoing various life-sustaining procedures so they can make a decision regarding their future treatment.

4. Patients need to be informed that they can have more than one advance directive. That is, if a patient has a Living Will but is not terminally ill, encourage the patient to obtain a Healthcare Proxy to ensure that health care wishes will be met in any situation.

Community and Home Care Considerations

1. Information about completing advance directives can be obtained by contacting Choice in Dying at *www.choices.org*.

2. Instruct older adults that they will be allowed to record their wishes about various types of medical treatments, and let them appoint a proxy for if and when they are unable to make those decisions on their own.

Advocacy for the Disabled

There are an estimated 54 million Americans, not all of whom are older adults, with disabilities. Disability may strike any age group, ethnic or racial origin, and socioeconomic group. Nurses must not only provide skilled physical care to reduce complications and enhance the rehabilitation potential of disabled persons, they must also act as advocates to help these individuals transcend their disabilities to be as independent, functional, and self-actualized as possible. The United States Surgeon General's Call to Action to Improve the Health and Wellness of Persons with Disability requests that all health care providers do the following:

- Give each patient the information necessary to live a long and healthy life.
- Listen and respond to the patient's health concerns.
- Communicate clearly and directly.
- Take the time needed to meet the patient's health care needs.

Definition of Disability

1. A disability can be viewed as any restriction or lack of ability to perform activities in a manner that is normal for most people.

2. The Americans with Disabilities Act (1990) defines a disability as a physical or mental impairment that substantially limits one or more major life activities. A person can also be disabled if there is a record of such an impairment or is regarded as having such an impairment.

3. Handicap is an outdated term; there should be no reason for an individual with a disability to be handicapped. A handicap is a disadvantage resulting from an impairment that limits or prevents fulfillment of a role.

Disability Laws

1. There were many laws enacted in the United States in the 20th century to provide funding for health care, education, and vocational rehabilitation.
   a. Initial laws were limited and focused on groups, such as wounded soldiers, injured workers, and veterans.
   b. The Social Security Act of 1935 broadened vocational rehabilitation to cover civilians and gave rehabilitation a permanent legislative basis.
   c. Medicare and Medicaid were created in 1965 as an amendment to the Social Security Act to provide health insurance and benefits to individuals based on age, presence of disability, and low income. Medical and nursing care are covered.

2. The Rehabilitation Act of 1973 was the first federal law in the United States to protect disabled individuals from discrimination.
   a. This law focused on access to public buildings and transportation, discrimination in the workplace, and independent living situations.
   b. However, this law only applied to facilities and programs supported by the federal government and did not affect the private sector.

3. The Americans with Disabilities Act of 1990 amended previous legislation and made it illegal to discriminate against individuals with disabilities in the private sector as well as the public sector. Areas of focus are:
   a. Employers with 15 or more employees must provide qualified individuals with disabilities an equal opportunity to benefit from employment, including the hiring, training, promotion, and other privileges of employment. Employers are required to provide reasonable accommodations for the known physical or mental limitations of otherwise qualified individuals, so long as accommodations do not cause undue hardship to the employer.
   b. All state and local government institutions are required to provide equal opportunities for individuals with disabilities to take part in all programs, services, and activities, regardless of federal funding status.
   c. Public accommodations, which calls for the removal of barriers in public places that may be owned by private entities, such as restaurants, shops, hotels, and private schools. In addition, courses and examinations related

to educational programs must be provided in a manner accessible to all despite obstacles such as hearing, vision, or speech limitations.

d. Telecommunication relay services are required in all areas to allow those with hearing and speech limitations to communicate with others through a third party.

Problems for the Disabled

1. Psychosocial adaptation to a disability is an ongoing process that progresses through stages: shock, denial, depression, ambivalence, and adaptation. It may become stalled at one or more stages and not reach adaptation.

2. Caregiver and family strain due to loss of income, hopelessness, and physical and mental exhaustion from taking over roles and responsibilities from the disabled individual may impede successful rehabilitation.

3. Despite laws, disabled persons are still discriminated against when applying for jobs and educational programs. To get around the laws, employers and educational systems may list multiple physical requirements of a job or program that are meant to discourage disabled persons from applying, or that would prompt failure, even though these physical requirements may have nothing to do with the actual job.

4. In addition to physical barriers at workplaces and educational institutions, disabled persons must overcome tremendous attitude barriers. Once a disability is known, stereotyping and prejudice may overshadow a person's potential.

Nursing Interventions for Advocacy

1. Become familiar with Medicare and Medicaid regulations and coverage in the United States and assist patients with the medical forms.

a. Medicare is available to disabled individuals after 2 continuous years of disability with inability to work. Medicare is provided through the federal government and is not driven by income level.

b. Medicare does cover health care provider visits and hospitalizations, but does not cover any prescription drugs or some durable medical equipment.

c. Eligibility for Medicaid is based on income level, how many persons are in the household, and is controlled by state and local government. This may cover very-low-income disabled persons.

2. Help individuals in the United States understand the eligibility for Social Security disability income if their medical condition lasts for 1 year or longer and they are unable to perform substantial employment. The individual must have worked within the last 5 years and have adequate employment credits.

3. Become aware of social services in your geographic area, both through government and charitable programs, such as public transportation that will transport individuals who use wheelchairs to medical appointments.

4. Assist patients in obtaining prescription drugs through discounted and free programs that may be available through pharmaceutical companies to those who do not have prescription coverage. Contact pharmaceutical companies directly or

Partnership for Pharmaceutical Assistance (*www.ppaRx.com*) for eligibility requirements and applications.

5. If your facility is not fully handicapped accessible, advocate for structural changes that allow access.

6. When providing care for a disabled person, always ask if you can assist and allow the individual to direct your assistance. Most individuals with disabilities know what works for them and what causes the least amount of discomfort.

7. Be aware that an individual with an acquired disability goes through an adjustment phase that can be compared with bereavement. Allow the individual time and respect for where they are in the process. Denial can last a year or more and they must be supported, not pushed, to move on in the process.

8. Be aware of your own biases and attitudes toward disabled individuals. Refrain from stereotyping. Also be aware that not all disabilities are visible (eg, mental illness or impairment from a head injury). Treat all persons with respect and understanding.

9. Encourage sensitivity training in your facility for all employees to ensure compassionate care and polite interactions with all disabled individuals.

10. Utilize the following resources for additional information and support:
    –Americans with Disabilities Act: *www.ada.gov*
    –Centers for Disease Control and Prevention; Disability and Health: *www.cdc.gov/ncbddd/disabilityandhealth/index.html*
    –Disability Resources Monthly Guide to Disability Resources on the Internet: *www.disabilityresources.org*
    –Youreable (products, services, and information for disabled persons): *www.youreable.com*
    –National Organization on Disability: *www.nod.org*
    –National Council on Disability: *www.ncd.gov*
    –Association of Rehabilitation Nurses: *www.rehabnurse.org*
    –ExceptionalNurse.com (resources for nurses with disabilities): *www.exceptionalnurse.com*

SELECTED REFERENCES

Agency for Healthcare Research and Quality. (2011). Preventing pressure ulcers in hospitals: A toolkit for improving quality of care. Available: *www.ahrq.gov/research/ltc/pressureulcertoolkit/putool3.htm*.

Alano, G. J., Pekmezaris, R., Tai, J. Y., et al. (2010). Factors influencing older adults to complete advance directives. *Palliative and Supportive Care, 8*(3), 267–275.

Alderden, J., Whitney, J. D., Taylor, S., M., et al. (2011). Risk profile characteristics associated with outcomes of hospital-acquired pressure ulcers: A retrospective review. *Critical Care Nurse, 31*(4), 30–43.

Anderson, J., White, K. G., & Kelechi, T. J. (2010). Managing common foot problems in older adults. *Journal of Gerontological Nursing, 36*(10), 9–14.

Borson, S., Scanlan, J., Peijun, C., et al. (2003). The Mini Cog as a screen for dementia: validation in a population based sample. *Journal of the American Geriatrics Society, 51*(10), 1451–1454.

Bourdel-Marchasson, I. (2010). How to improve nutritional support in geriatric institutions. *Journal of the American Medical Directors Association, 11*, 13–20.

Brooks, P. B. (2012). Postoperative delirium in elderly patients. *AJN, 112*(9): 38–49.

Bushman, L. A., Belza, B., & Christianson, P. (2012). Older adult hearing loss and screening in primary care. *Journal for Nurse Practitioners, 8*(7): 509–514.

Centers for Disease Control and Prevention. Disability and health: Information for healthcare providers. Available: *www.cdc.gov/ncbddd/disabilityandhealth/hcp.html*.

Cocks, E., & Boaden, R. (2011). A quality framework for personalised residential supports for adults with developmental disabilities. *Journal of Intellectual Disability Research, 55*(8), 720–731.

Corbett, C. F., Setter, S. M., Daratha, K. B., et al. (2010). Nurse identified hospital to home medication discrepancies: implications for improving transitional care. *Geriatric Nursing, 31*(3), 188–196.

Davis, N. J., Hendrix, C. C., & Superville, J. G. (2011). Supportive approaches for Alzheimer's disease. *Nurse Practitioner, 36*(8), 22–29.

de Souza, D., Santos, V., Iri, H. K., et al. (2010). Predictive validity of the braden scale for pressure ulcer risk in elderly residents of long-term care facilities. *Geriatric Nursing, 31*(2), 95–104.

Dowling-Castronovo, A. (2009). Try this: Urinary incontinence assessment in older adults part 1—transient urinary incontinence. *Annals of Long Term Care, 17*(2), 15–16.

Folstein, M., Folstein, S. E., & McHugh, P. R. (1975). Mini-Mental State: A practical method for grading the cognitive state of patients for the clinician. *Journal of Psychiatric Research, 2,* 189–198.

Forsell, M., Kullberg, E., Hoogstraate, J., et al. (2011). An evidence-based oral hygiene education program for nursing staff. *Nurse Education in Practice, 11*(4), 256–259.

Galik, E. (2011). Function-focused care for long term care residents with moderate to severe dementia: a social ecological approach. *Annals of Long Term Care, 18*(6), 27–33.

Gourlay, M. I., Fines, J. P., & Preisser, J. S. (2012). Stretching the time between bone density screenings. *AJN, 112*(4): 225–233.

Hartford Institute for Geriatric Nursing. (2007). Frailty and its implications for care. Available: *http://consultgerirn.org/topics/frailty_and_its_implications_for_care_new/want_to_know_more.*

Haut, A. Kolbe, N., Strupeit, S., et al. (2010). Attitudes of relatives of nursing home residents toward physical restraints. *Journal of Nursing Scholarship, 42*(4), 448–456.

Institute of Medicine, Food and Nutrition Board. (2010). *Dietary reference intakes for calcium and vitamin D.* Washington, DC: National Academy Press.

Jamshed, N., & Schneider, E. L. (2010). Is the use of supplemental vitamin C and zinc for the prevention and treatment of pressure ulcers evidence-based? *Annals of Long Term Care, 18*(3), 28–32.

Johansson, R. M., Malmvall, B. E., Andersson-Gäre, B., et al. (2012). Guidelines for preventing urinary retention and bladder damage during hospital care. *Journal of Clinical Nursing.* In publication.

Katz, S., Ford, A. B., Moskowitz, R. W., et al. (1963). Studies of illness in the aged: The Index of ADL: A standardized measure of biologic and psychosocial function. *Journal of the American Medical Association, 185,* 914–919.

Kim, N. H. (2011). Long-term care of the aging population with intellectual and developmental disabilities. *Clinics in Geriatric Medicine, 27*(2), 291.

Luo, H., Lin, M., & Castle, N. (2011). Physical restraint use and falls in nursing homes: a comparison between residents with and without dementia. *American Journal of Alzheimer's Disease and Other Dementias, 26*(1), 44–50.

Lyketsos, C. G., Carrillo, M. C., Ryan, J. M., et al. (2011). Neuropsychiatric symptoms in Alzheimer's disease. *Alzheimer's & Dementia, 7,* 532–539.

Mahoney, F., & Barthel, D. (1965). Functional evaluation: The Barthel Index. *Maryland State Medical Journal, 14,* 62–72.

Management of osteoporosis in postmenopausal women: 2010 position statement of the North American Menopause Society. (2010). *Menopause, 17*(1), 25–54.

McCabe, D. E., Alvarez, C. D., McNulty, S. R., et al. (2011). Perceptions of physical restraints use in the elderly among registered nurses and nurse assistants in a single acute care hospital. *Geriatric Nursing, 32*(1), 39–45.

Merida, J. D., White, T. L., & Updegrove, J. D. (2010). Functional assessment of older adults with chronic obstructive pulmonary disease living at home. *Journal of the American Geriatrics Society, 58*(8), 1604–1606.

Morley, J. E. (2012). Undernutrition in older adults. *Family Practice, 29* Suppl 1, i89–i93.

National Pressure Ulcer Advisory Panel, European Pressure Ulcer Advisory Panel. (2009). Pressure ulcer treatment recommendations. In *Prevention and treatment of pressure ulcers: clinical practice guideline* (pp. 51–120). Washington, DC: National Pressure Ulcer Advisory Panel.

Newberry, A. M., & Pachet, A. K. (2008). An innovative framework for psychosocial assessment in complex mental capacity evaluations. *Psychology, Health and Medicine, 13*(4), 438–449.

Niederhauser, A., VanDeusen Lukas, C., et al. (2012). Comprehensive programs for preventing pressure ulcers: a review of the literature. *Advances in Skin and Wound Care, 25*(4), 167–188; quiz 189–190.

Nordin, C. (2011). Screening for osteoporosis: U.S. Preventive Services Task Force recommendation statement. *Annals of Internal Medicine, 155*(4), 276–276.

O'Malley, P. G. (2011). Colorectal cancer screening protocols and procedures: Comment on "overuse of screening colonoscopy in the medicare population" and "long-term outcomes following positive fecal occult blood test results in older adults." *Archives of Internal Medicine, 171*(15), 1351.

Panel on Prevention of Falls in Older Persons, American Geriatrics Society and British Geriatrics Society. (2011). Summary of the updated American Geriatrics Society/British Geriatrics Society clinical practice guideline for prevention of falls in older persons. *Journal of the American Geriatrics Society, 59*(1), 148–157.

Park, M., & Tang, J. H. (2007). Evidence-based guideline changing the practice of physical restraint use in acute care. *Journal of Gerontological Nursing, 33*(2), 9–16.

Payne, K. L., Prentice-Dunn, S., & Allen, R. S. (2010). A comparison of two interventions to increase completion of advance directives. *Clinical Gerontologist, 33*(1), 49–61.

Pfister, A. K., Welch, C. W., & Emmett, M. (2011). Screening for osteoporosis: U.S. Preventive Services Task Force recommendation statement. *Annals of Internal Medicine, 155*(4), 275–276.

Quindry, J. C., Yount, D., O'Bryant, H., et al. (2011). Exercise engagement is differentially motivated by age-dependent factors. *American Journal of Health Behavior, 35*(3), 334–345.

Resnick, B. (1994). The wheel that moves. *Rehabilitation Nursing, 19*(4), 240–241.

Resnick, B., & D'Adamo, C. (2011). Factors associated with exercise among older adults in a continuing care retirement community. *Rehabilitation Nursing, 36*(2), 47–53.

Resnick, B., Galik, E., Gruber-Baldini, A., & Zimmerman, S. (2011). Testing the effect of function-focused care in assisted living. *Journal of the American Geriatrics Society, 59*(12), 2233–2240. *doi:10.1111/j.1532-5415.2011.03699.x.*

Resnick, B., Shaughnessy, M., Galik, E., et al. (2009). Pilot testing of the PRAISEDD intervention among African American and low-income older adults. *Journal of Cardiovascular Nursing, 24*(5), 352–361.

Rich S. E., Shardell, M., Hawkes, W. G., et al. (2011). Pressure-redistributing support surface use and pressure ulcer incidence in elderly hip fracture patients. *Journal of the American Geriatrics Society, 59*(6), 1052–1059.

Richman, M. (2011). Elderly individuals with developmental disabilities and the office visit. *Clinical Geriatrics, 19*(8), 10.

Samaras, N., Chevalley, T., Samaras, D., & Gold, G. (2010). Older patients in the emergency department: a review. *Annals of emergency medicine, 56*(3), 261–269. *doi:10.1016/j.annemergmed.2010.04.015.*

Shah, B. J., Chokhavatia, S., & Rose, S. (2012). Fecal Incontinence in the Elderly: FAQ. *The American journal of gastroenterology.* doi:10.1038/ajg.2012.284

Shaughnessy, M., & Resnick, B. M. (2009). Using theory to develop an exercise intervention for patients post stroke. *Topics in Stroke Rehabilitation, 16*(2), 140–146.

Smeltzer, S., Avery, C., & Haynor, P. (2012). Interactions of people with disabilities and nursing staff during hospitalization. *AJN, 112*(4): 30–37.

Steinman, B. A., & Allen, S. M. (2012). Self-reported vision impairment and its contribution to disability among older adults. *Journal of Aging and Health, 24*(2), 307–322. *doi:10.1177/0898264311422600.*

Talley, K. M. C., Wyman, J. F., & Shamliyan, T. A. (2011). State of the science: conservative interventions for urinary incontinence in frail community-dwelling older adults. *Nursing outlook, 59*(4), 215–220, 220.e1. doi:10.1016/j.outlook.2011.05.010

U.S. Preventive Services Task Force. (2009). Aspirin for the primary prevention of cardiovascular events: An update of the evidence. Agency for Healthcare Quality and Research: Rockville, Maryland. Available: *www.uspreventiveservicestaskforce .org/uspstf09/aspirincvd/aspcvdart.htm.*

U.S. Preventive Services Task Force. (2009). Counseling and interventions to prevent tobacco use and tobacco-caused disease in adults and pregnant women: Reaffirmation recommendation statement. Agency for Healthcare Quality and Research: Rockville, Maryland. Available: *www.uspreventiveservicestaskforce.org/ uspstf09/tobacco/tobaccors2.htm.*

Van Leuven, K. A. (2012). Advanced care planning in health service users. *Journal of Clinical Nursing, 21*(21–22), 3126–3133. *doi:10.1111/j.1365-2702 .2012.04190.x.*

Voyer, P., Richard, S., Doucet, L., et al. (2010). Examination of the multifactorial model of delirium among long-term care residents with dementia. *Geriatric Nursing, 31*(2), 105–114.

White-Chu, E. F., Flock, P., Struck, B., et al. (2011). Pressure ulcers in long-term care. *Clinics in Geriatric Medicine, 27*(2), 241–258.

10
Respiratory Function and Therapy

OVERVIEW AND ASSESSMENT

Respiratory Function

The major function of the pulmonary system (lungs and pulmonary circulation) is to deliver oxygen (O_2) to cells and remove carbon dioxide (CO_2) from the cells (gas exchange). The adequacy of oxygenation and ventilation is measured by partial pressure of arterial oxygen (PaO_2) and partial pressure of arterial carbon dioxide ($PaCO_2$). The pulmonary system also functions as a blood reservoir for the left ventricle when it is needed to boost cardiac output; as a protector for the systemic circulation by filtering debris/particles; as a fluid regulator so water can be kept away from alveoli; and as a provider of metabolic functions such as surfactant production and endocrine functions.

Terminology

1. Alveolus—air sac where gas exchange takes place.
2. Apex—top portion of the upper lobes of lungs.
3. Base—bottom portion of lower lobes of lungs, located just above the diaphragm.
4. Bronchoconstriction—constriction of smooth muscle surrounding bronchioles.
5. Bronchus—large airways; lung divides into right and left bronchi.
6. Carina—location of division of the right and left main stem bronchi.
7. Cilia—hair-like projections on the tracheobronchial epithelium, which aid in the movement of secretions and removal of debris.
8. Compliance—ability of the lungs to distend and change in volume relative to an applied change in pressure (eg, emphysema—lungs very compliant; fibrosis—lungs noncompliant or stiff).
9. Dead space—ventilation that does not participate in gas exchange; also known as wasted ventilation when there is adequate ventilation but no perfusion, as in pulmonary embolus or pulmonary vascular bed occlusion. Normal dead space is 150 mL.
10. Diaphragm—primary muscle used for respiration; located just below the lung bases, it separates the chest and abdominal cavities.
11. Diffusion (of gas)—movement of gas from area of higher to lower concentration.
12. Dyspnea—subjective sensation of breathlessness associated with discomfort, often caused by a dissociation between motor command and mechanical response of the respiratory system as in:
    a. Respiratory muscle abnormalities (hyperinflation and airflow limitation from chronic obstructive pulmonary disease [COPD]).
    b. Abnormal ventilatory impedance (narrowing airways and respiratory impedance from COPD or asthma).
    c. Abnormal breathing patterns (severe exercise, pulmonary congestion or edema, recurrent pulmonary emboli).
    d. Arterial blood gas (ABG) abnormalities (hypoxemia, hypercarbia).
13. Hemoptysis—the expectoration (coughing-up) of blood or of blood-stained sputum from the larynx, trachea, bronchi, or lungs.

14. Hypoxemia—PaO_2 less than normal, which may or may not cause symptoms. (Normal PaO_2 is 80 to 100 mm Hg on room air.)
15. Hypoxia—insufficient oxygenation at the cellular level due to an imbalance in oxygen delivery and oxygen consumption. (Usually causes symptoms reflecting decreased oxygen reaching the brain and heart.)
16. Mediastinum—compartment between lungs containing lymph and vascular tissue that separates left from right lung.
17. Orthopnea—shortness of breath when in reclining position.
18. Paroxysmal nocturnal dyspnea—sudden shortness of breath associated with sleeping in recumbent position.
19. Perfusion—blood flow, carrying oxygen and CO_2 that passes by alveoli.
20. Pleura—serous membrane enclosing the lung; comprised of visceral pleura, covering all lung surfaces, and parietal pleura, covering chest wall and mediastinal structures, between which exists a potential space.
21. Pulmonary circulation—network of vessels that supply oxygenated blood to and remove CO_2-laden blood from the lungs.
22. Pulmonary hypertension—an increase in blood pressure in the pulmonary artery, pulmonary vein, or pulmonary capillaries.
23. Respiration—inhalation and exhalation; at the cellular level, a process involving uptake of oxygen and removal of CO_2 and other products of oxidation.
24. Shunt—adequate perfusion without ventilation, with deoxygenated blood conducted into the systemic circulation, as in pulmonary edema, atelectasis, pneumonia, COPD.
25. Surfactant—fluid secreted by alveolar cells that reduces surface tension of pulmonary fluids and aids in elasticity of pulmonary tissue.
26. Ventilation—is the process by which oxygen and CO_2 are transported to and from the lungs
27. Ventilation–perfusion (V/Q) imbalance or mismatch—imbalance of ventilation and perfusion; a cause for hypoxemia. V/Q mismatch can be due to:
    a. Blood perfusing an area of the lung where ventilation is reduced or absent.
    b. Ventilation of parts of lung that are not perfused.

Subjective Data

Explore symptoms retrieved from the patient's description of an event through characterization and history-taking to help anticipate needs and plan care. Encourages the patient to give a full description of the onset, the course, and the character of the problem and any factors that aggravate or relieve it.

Dyspnea

 Evidence Base Martin, D. (2011). Palliation of dyspnea in patients with heart failure. *Dimensions of Critical Care Nursing, 30*(3), 144–149.
Simonneau, G., Robbins, I. M., Beghetti, M., et al. (2009). Updated clinical classification of pulmonary hypertension. *Journal of the American College of Cardiology, 54*(1, Suppl. S).

1. Characteristics—Is the dyspnea acute or chronic? Has it occurred suddenly or gradually? Is more than one pillow required to sleep? Is the dyspnea progressive, recurrent, or paroxysmal? Walking how far leads to shortness of breath? How does it compare to the patient's baseline level of dyspnea? Ask patient to rate dyspnea on a scale of 1 to 10, with 1 being no dyspnea and 10 being the worst imaginable. What relieves and what aggravates the dyspnea?

2. Associated factors—Is there a cough associated with the dyspnea and is it productive? What activities precipitate the shortness of breath? Does it seem to be worse when upset? Is it influenced by the time of day, seasons, and/or certain environments? Does it occur at rest or with exertion? Any fever, chills, night sweats, ankle/leg swelling? Any change in body weight?

3. History—Is there a patient history or family history of chronic lung disease, cardiac or neuromuscular disease, cancer, problems with blood clotting, or immunocompromise? What is the smoking history?

4. Significance—Sudden dyspnea could indicate pulmonary embolus, pneumothorax, myocardial infarction (MI), acute heart failure, or acute respiratory failure. In a postsurgical or postpartum patient, dyspnea may indicate pulmonary embolus or edema. Orthopnea can be indicative of heart disease or COPD. If dyspnea is associated with a wheeze, consider asthma, COPD, heart failure, or upper airway obstruction. When dyspnea occurs in combination with fatigue, pulmonary hypertension may exist. Metabolic disorders, psychiatric conditions, and neuromuscular disorders may also contribute to dyspnea.

Chest Pain

1. Characteristics—Is the pain sharp, dull, stabbing, or aching? Is it intermittent or persistent? Is the pain localized or does it radiate? If it radiates, where? How intense is the pain? Are there factors that alleviate or aggravate the pain, such as position or activity?

2. Associated factors—What effect do inspiration and expiration have on the pain? What other symptoms accompany the chest pain? Is there diaphoresis, shortness of breath, nausea?

3. History—Is there a smoking history or environmental exposure? Has the pain ever been experienced before? What was the cause? Is there a preexisting pulmonary or cardiac diagnosis? Has there been recent trauma?

4. Significance—Chest pain related to pulmonary causes is usually felt on the side where pathology arises, but it can be referred. Dull persistent pain may indicate carcinoma of the lung, whereas sharp, stabbing pain usually arises from the pleura. Dyspnea with pleuritic chest pain indicates clinically significant pulmonary embolism.

Cough

Evidence Base Birring, S. (2011). Controversies in the evaluation and management of chronic cough. *American Journal of Respiratory and Critical Care Medicine, 183*(6), 708–715.

Weinberger, S., & Silverstri, R. (2011). Treatment of subacute and chronic cough in adults. *UpToDate.* Available: *www.uptodate.com/contents/treatment-of-subacute-and-chronic-cough-in-adults.*

1. Characteristics—Is the cough dry, hacking, loose, barky, wheezy, or more like clearing the throat? Is it strong or weak? How frequent is it? Is it worse at night or at any time of day? Does the intensity change on days off from work? Is there seasonal variation? Is it aggravated by food intake or exertion. Is it alleviated by any medication? How long has it been going on?

2. Associated factors—Is the cough productive? If so, what is the consistency, amount, color, and odor of the sputum? How does sputum compare to the patient's baseline? Is it associated with shortness of breath, pain, or nausea?

3. History—Is there a smoking history? Is the smoking current or in the past? Has there been any environmental or occupational exposure to dust, fumes, or gases that could lead to cough? Are there past pulmonary diagnoses, asthma, rhinitis, allergy, or exposure to allergens, such as pollen, house dust mites, animal dander, birds, mold or fungi, cockroach waste, irritants (smoke, odors, perfumes, cleaning products, exhaust, pollution, cold air)? Has there been prolonged exposure to dampness, chemical sanitizers, cobalt or other hard metals, beryllium, asbestos, dusts from coal, wood, or grains? Does the patient have a history of acid reflux or use an angiotensin-converting enzyme inhibitor with a common adverse effect of cough? Has there been a concurrent voice change? Has the patient recently traveled outside the country? Can the patient identify any specific triggers?

4. Significance—A dry, irritative cough may indicate viral respiratory tract infection. A cough at night should alert to potential left-sided heart failure, asthma, or postnasal drip worsening at night. A morning cough with sputum might be bronchitis. A cough that is less severe on days off from work may be related to occupational or environmental exposures. A patient with severe or changing cough should be evaluated for bronchogenic carcinoma. Consider bacterial pneumonia if sputum is rusty, and lung tumor if it is pink-tinged. A profuse pink frothy sputum could be indicative of pulmonary edema. A cough associated with food intake could indicate problems with aspiration. A dry cough may be associated with pulmonary fibrosis. History of recent travel may be associated with infection from a source not commonly identified in the United States.

Hemoptysis

1. Characteristics—Is the blood from the lungs? It could be from the GI system (hematemesis) or upper airway (epistaxis). Is it bright red and frothy? How much? Is onset associated with certain circumstances or activities? Was the onset sudden, and is it intermittent or continuous?

2. Associated factors—Was there an initial sensation of tickling in the throat? Was there a salty taste or burning or bubbling sensation in the chest? Has there been shortness of breath, chest pain, difficulty with exertion?

3. History—Was there any recent chest trauma or respiratory treatment (chest percussion)? Does the patient have an upper respiratory infection, sinusitis, or recent epistaxis? Has the patient used cocaine or other illicit drugs?

4. Significance—Hemoptysis can be linked to pulmonary infection, lung carcinoma, abnormalities of the heart or blood

vessels, pulmonary artery or vein abnormalities, or pulmonary emboli and infarction. Small amounts of blood-tinged sputum may be from the upper respiratory tract, and regurgitation of blood comes from a GI bleed.

Objective Data

The process in which data relating to the patient's problem are obtained through direct physical examination, including observation, palpation, percussion, auscultation; laboratory analysis; radiologic and other studies.

 Evidence Base Wilkins, R., Dexter, J. R., & Heuer, A. (2010). *Clinical assessment in respiratory care* (6th ed.). St. Louis, MO: Mosby.

Key Observations

1. What is the respiratory rate, depth, and pattern? Are accessory muscles being used? Is the patient breathing through the mouth or pursing lips during exhalation? Is sputum being raised, and what is its appearance and odor?
2. Is there an increase in the anterior to posterior chest diameter, suggesting air trapping?
3. Is there obvious orthopnea or splinting?
4. Is there clubbing of the fingers, associated with bronchiectasis, lung abscess, empyema, cystic fibrosis, pulmonary neoplasms, and various other disorders?
5. Is there central cyanosis indicating possible hypoxemia or cardiac disease? Are mucous membranes and nail beds pink?
6. Are there signs of tracheal deviation, as seen with pneumothorax?
7. Are the jugular veins distended? Is there peripheral edema or other signs of cardiac dysfunction?
8. Does palpation of the chest cause pain? Is chest expansion symmetrical? Any change in tactile fremitus?
9. Is percussion of lung fields resonant bilaterally? Is diaphragmatic excursion equal bilaterally?
10. Are breath sounds present and equal bilaterally? Are the lung fields clear or are there rhonchi, wheezing, crackles, stridor, or pleural friction rub? Does auscultation reveal egophony, bronchophony, or whispered pectoriloquy?

Laboratory Studies

Arterial Blood Gas Analysis

Description

1. A measurement of O_2, CO_2, and the pH of the blood that provides a means of assessing the adequacy of ventilation ($PaCO_2$), metabolic status (pH), and oxygenation (PaO_2).
2. Allows assessment of body's acid-base (pH) status, indicating if acidosis or alkalosis is present, whether acidosis or alkalosis is respiratory or metabolic in origin, and whether it is compensated or uncompensated.
3. Used for diagnostic evaluation and evaluation of response to clinical interventions (oxygen therapy, mechanical ventilation, etc.).

Nursing and Patient Care Considerations

1. Blood can be obtained from any artery but is usually drawn from the radial, brachial, or femoral site. It can be drawn directly by arterial puncture or accessed by way of indwelling arterial catheter (see Procedure Guidelines 10-1, pages 200 to 202). Determine facility policy for qualifications for ABG sampling and site of arterial puncture.
2. If the radial artery is used, an Allen test must be performed before the puncture to determine if collateral circulation is present.
3. Arterial puncture should not be performed through a lesion, through or distal to a surgical shunt, or in area where peripheral vascular disease or infection is present.
4. Coagulopathy or medium- to high-dose anticoagulation therapy may be a relative contraindication for arterial puncture.
5. Results may be affected by recent changes in oxygen therapy, suctioning, or positioning.
6. Interpret ABG values by looking at trends for the patient as well as the following normal values:
   a. PaO_2—partial pressure of arterial oxygen (80 to 100 mm Hg)
   b. $PaCO_2$—partial pressure of arterial carbon dioxide (35 to 45 mm Hg)
   c. SaO_2—arterial oxygen saturation (>95%)
   d. pH—hydrogen ion concentration, or degree of acid-base balance (7.35 to 7.45); bicarbonate (HCO_3^-) ion primarily a metabolic buffer (22 to 26 mEq/L).

Sputum Examination

Description

1. Sputum may be obtained for evaluation of gross appearance, microscopic examination, Gram stain, culture and sensitivity, acid-fast bacillus, and cytology.
   a. The direct smear shows presence of white blood cells and intracellular (pathogenic) bacteria and extracellular (mostly nonpathogenic) bacteria.
   b. Gram stain shows whether bacteria is gram-positive or gram-negative and can be used to guide therapy until culture and sensitivity results are available.
   c. The sputum culture is used to identify presence of specific pathogens; sensitivity determines drug efficacy and serves as a guide for drug treatment (ie, choice of antibiotic).
   d. Acid-fast smears detect presence of pathogens such as *Mycobacterium tuberculosis*.
   e. Cytology identifies abnormal and possibly malignant cells.

Nursing and Patient Care Considerations

1. Patients receiving antibiotics, steroids, and immunosuppressive agents for a prolonged time may have periodic sputum examinations because these agents may give rise to opportunistic pulmonary infections.
2. It is important that the sputum be collected correctly and that the specimen be sent to a laboratory immediately. Allowing it to stand in a warm room will result in overgrowth of organisms, making identification of pathogen difficult; this also alters cell morphology. A series of three early morning specimens is needed for acid-fast bacillus examination. Cytology samples should be collected in container with fixative solution.

(*Text continues on page 202*)

PROCEDURE GUIDELINES 10-1

Assisting with Arterial Puncture for Blood Gas Analysis

EQUIPMENT

- Commercially available blood gas kit *or*
- 2- or 3-mL syringe
- 23G or 25G needle

- 0.5 mL sodium heparin (1:1,000)
- Stopper or cap
- Sterile germicide
- Cup or plastic bag with crushed ice

- Gloves
- Goggles
- Rolled towel or washcloth

PROCEDURE

Nursing Action	Rationale
Preparatory phase	
1. Record the patient's inspired oxygen concentration.	1. Changes in inspired oxygen concentration alter the change in PaO_2. Degree of hypoxemia cannot be assessed without knowing the inspired oxygen concentration.
2. Take the patient's temperature.	2. May be considered when results are evaluated. Hyperthermia and hypothermia influence oxygen release from hemoglobin.
If not using a commercially available blood gas kit:	
3. Heparinize the 2-mL syringe.	3.
a. Withdraw heparin into the syringe to wet the plunger and fill dead space in the needle.	a. Coats the interior of the syringe with heparin to prevent blood from clotting.
b. Hold syringe in an upright position and expel excess heparin and air bubbles.	b. Air in the syringe may affect measurement of PaO_2; heparin in the syringe may affect measurement of the pH. Heparin left in the syringe can decrease the pH.
Performance phase (by health care provider, nurse or respiratory therapist with special instruction)	
1. Verify correct patient; perform hand hygiene.	1. Reduces risk of infection.
2. Put on gloves and goggles.	2. Blood and body fluid precautions.
3. Palpate the radial, brachial, or femoral artery.	3. The radial artery of the nondominant side is the preferred site of puncture, but is contraindicated if a fistula or shunt for dialysis exists. Arterial puncture is performed on areas where a good pulse is palpable.
4. If puncturing the radial artery, perform the Allen test.	4. The Allen test is a simple method for assessing collateral circulation in the hand. Ensures circulation if radial artery thrombosis occurs.
In the conscious patient:	
a. Obliterate the radial and ulnar pulses simultaneously by pressing on both blood vessels at the wrist.	a. Impedes arterial blood flow into the hand.
b. Ask the patient to clench and unclench fist until blanching of the skin occurs.	b. Forces blood from the hand.
c. Release pressure on ulnar artery (while still compressing radial artery). Watch for return of skin color within 15 seconds.	c. Documents that ulnar artery alone is capable of supplying blood to the hand because radial artery is still occluded.

Key Decision Point

If skin color does not return following the Allen test, the ulnar artery does not have sufficient blood flow to supply the entire hand. If the radial artery is compromised while obtaining arterial blood gas, circulation to the entire hand could be compromised. Make note of this and pick an alternate arterial site.

PROCEDURE GUIDELINES 10-1 *(continued)*

Assisting with Arterial Puncture for Blood Gas Analysis

PROCEDURE *(continued)*

Nursing Action	Rationale
In the unconscious patient:	
a. Obliterate the radial and ulnar pulses simultaneously at the wrist.	
b. Elevate the patient's hand above the heart and squeeze or compress hand until blanching occurs.	b. Drains blood from the hand passively in a patient who cannot cooperate by clenching the fist.
c. Lower the patient's hand while still compressing the radial artery (release pressure on ulnar artery) and watch for return of skin color.	
5. For the radial site, turn palm up and mildly hyperextend the wrist, placing a small towel roll under the patient's wrist.	5. Makes the artery more accessible. The wrist should be stabilized to allow for better control of the needle.
6. Feel along the course of the radial artery and palpate for maximum pulsation with the middle and index fingers. Prepare the skin with germicide; allow to dry completely.	6. Disinfecting the arterial site reduces the risk of infection.
7. The needle is at a 45- to 60-degree angle to the skin surface (see accompanying figure) and is advanced into the artery. Once the artery is punctured, arterial pressure will push up the hub of the syringe and a pulsating flow of blood will fill the syringe.	7. The arterial pressure will cause the syringe to be filled within a few seconds; about 2 mL will accumulate and the flow into the syringe will stop.

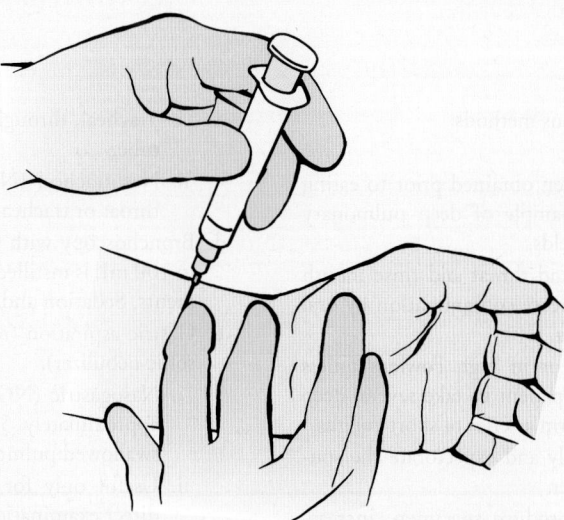

Technique of arterial puncture for blood gas analysis.

8. After blood is obtained, withdraw the needle and apply firm pressure over the puncture with a dry sponge.	8. Significant bleeding can occur because of pressure in the artery.
9. Remove air bubbles from syringe and needle. Use safety syringe system for closure.	9. Proper closure of the needle prevents room air from mixing with the blood specimen.
10. Place the capped syringe in the container of ice. Label as per facility policy.	10. Icing the syringe will prevent a clinically significant loss of oxygen.
11. Maintain firm pressure on the puncture site for 5 minutes. If the patient is on anticoagulant medication, apply direct pressure over puncture site for 10–15 minutes and then apply a firm pressure dressing.	11. Firm pressure on the puncture site prevents further bleeding and hematoma formation.

(continued)

PROCEDURE GUIDELINES 10-1 (continued)

Assisting with Arterial Puncture for Blood Gas Analysis

PROCEDURE (continued)

Nursing Action	Rationale
12. For patients requiring serial monitoring of arterial blood, an arterial catheter (connected to a flush solution of heparinized saline) is inserted into the radial or femoral artery.	12. All connections must be tight to avoid disconnection and rapid blood loss. The arterial line also allows for direct blood pressure (BP) monitoring in the critically ill patient.

Follow-up phase

1. Send the labeled, iced specimen to the laboratory immediately.	1. Blood gas analysis should be done as soon as possible because PaO_2 and pH can change rapidly.
2. Palpate the pulse (distal to the puncture site), inspect the puncture site, and assess for cold hand, numbness, tingling, or discoloration.	2. Hematoma and arterial thrombosis are complications following this procedure.
3. Change ventilator settings, inspired oxygen concentration, or type and setting of respiratory therapy equipment, if indicated by the results.	3. The PaO_2 results will determine whether to maintain, increase, or decrease the FiO_2. The PaO_2 and pH results will detect if any changes are needed in tidal volume or rate of patient's ventilator.

 Evidence Base DeWaay, D., & Gordon, J. (2011). The ABC's of ABGs: Teaching arterial blood gases to adult learners. *MedEdPORTAL.* Available: www.mededportal.org/publication/9038.

---

3. Sputum can be obtained by various methods:
   a. Deep breathing and coughing.
      i. An early morning specimen obtained prior to eating or drinking yields best sample of deep pulmonary secretions from all lung fields.
      ii. Have patient clear nose and throat and rinse mouth with plain water—to decrease contamination by oral and upper respiratory flora.
      iii. Position patient upright or in high Fowler's unless contraindicated. Instruct patient to take several deep breaths, exhale, and perform a series of short coughs.
      iv. Have patient cough deeply and expectorate the sputum into a sterile container.
      v. If patient is unable to produce specimen, increasing oral fluid intake may be useful (unless on fluid restriction).
   b. Induction through use of ultrasonic or hypertonic saline nebulization.
      i. Patient inhales mist through mouth slowly and deeply for 10 to 20 minutes.
      ii. Nebulization increases the moisture content of air going to lower tract; particles will condense on tracheobronchial tree and aid in expectoration.
   c. Suctioning—aspiration of secretions via mechanical means; must be used with caution because it may cause bleeding, cardiac dysrhythmias, and increased intracranial pressure.
      i. Tracheal, through endotracheal (ET) or tracheostomy tube.
      ii. Nasotracheal (NT), through nose and into back of throat or trachea.
   d. Bronchoscopy with bronchoalveolar lavage, in which 60 to 100 mL is instilled and aspirated from various lung segments. Sedation and/or anesthesia is required.
   e. Gastric aspiration (rarely necessary since advent of ultrasonic nebulizer).
      i. Nasogastric (NG) tube is inserted into the stomach, approximately 50 mL sterile water is instilled, and swallowed pulmonary secretions are siphoned out.
      ii. Useful only for culture of tubercle bacilli, not for direct examination.
   f. Transtracheal aspiration involves passing a needle and then a catheter through a percutaneous puncture of the cricothyroid membrane. Transtracheal aspiration bypasses the oropharynx and avoids specimen contamination by mouth flora.
4. Generally, a sputum sample of 15 mL is adequate for laboratory testing.

Pleural Fluid Analysis

Description

1. Pleural fluid is continuously produced and reabsorbed, with a thin layer normally in the pleural space. Abnormal pleural fluid accumulation (effusion) occurs in diseases

of the pleura, heart, or lymphatics. The pleural fluid is studied, with other tests, to determine the underlying cause.

2. Obtained by aspiration (thoracentesis) or by tube thoracotomy (chest tube insertion; see Procedure Guidelines 10-2).

3. The fluid is examined for cancerous cells, cellular makeup, chemical content, and microorganisms.

4. Pleural cavity usually contains less than 20 mL clear yellow (serous) fluid that lubricates the surfaces of the pleura, the thin membrane that lines the chest cavity and surrounds

(*Text continues on page 205*)

PROCEDURE GUIDELINES 10-2

Assisting the Patient Undergoing Thoracentesis

EQUIPMENT

- Thoracentesis tray (if available) *or*
- 5-, 20-, 50-mL syringes
- Needles: 22G, 26G, or 16G (3 inches long)
- Three-way stopcock and tubing
- Hemostat

- Biopsy needle
- Germicide solution
- Local anesthetic (such as lidocaine 1%)
- Sterile gauze pads (4″ × 4″ and 2″ × 2″)

- Sterile towels and drape
- Sterile specimen containers
- Sterile gloves
- Overhead table and chair

PROCEDURE

Nursing Action	Rationale

Preparatory phase

1. Determine in advance if chest x-ray or other tests have been prescribed and completed. These should be available at the bedside.

1. Localization of pleural fluid is accomplished by physical examination, chest x-ray, ultrasound localization, or fluoroscopic localization.

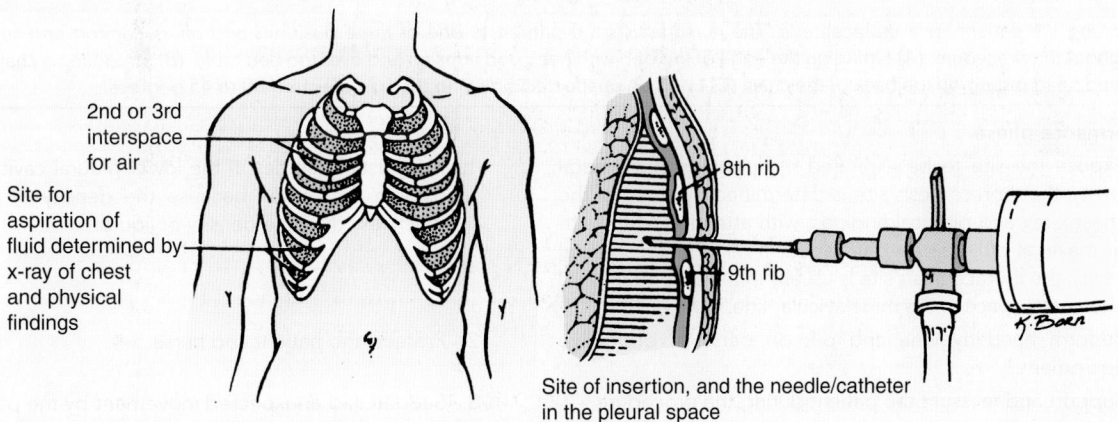

2nd or 3rd interspace for air

Site for aspiration of fluid determined by x-ray of chest and physical findings

8th rib

9th rib

Site of insertion, and the needle/catheter in the pleural space

Technique of thoracentesis

2. Check if consent form has been explained and signed.

3. Determine if the patient is allergic to the local anesthetic agent to be used. Give sedation, if prescribed.

4. Inform the patient about the procedure and indicate how the patient can be helpful. Explain:
   a. The nature of the procedure.
   b. The importance of remaining immobile and of not talking or coughing.
   c. Pressure sensations to be experienced.
   d. That no discomfort is anticipated after the procedure.

2. Invasive procedure requires informed consent.

3. Prevents allergic reaction; eases pain and anxiety.

4. An explanation helps orient the patient to the procedure, assists with coping, and provides an opportunity to ask questions and verbalize anxiety.

(continued)

PROCEDURE GUIDELINES 10-2 (continued)

Assisting the Patient Undergoing Thoracentesis

PROCEDURE (continued)

Nursing Action	Rationale
5. Assist the patient to obtain comfortable position with adequate supports. If possible, place the patient upright (see accompanying figure) and help the patient maintain this position during the procedure.	5. The upright position ensures that the diaphragm is most dependent and facilitates the removal of fluid that usually localizes at the base of the chest. A comfortable position helps the patient to relax.

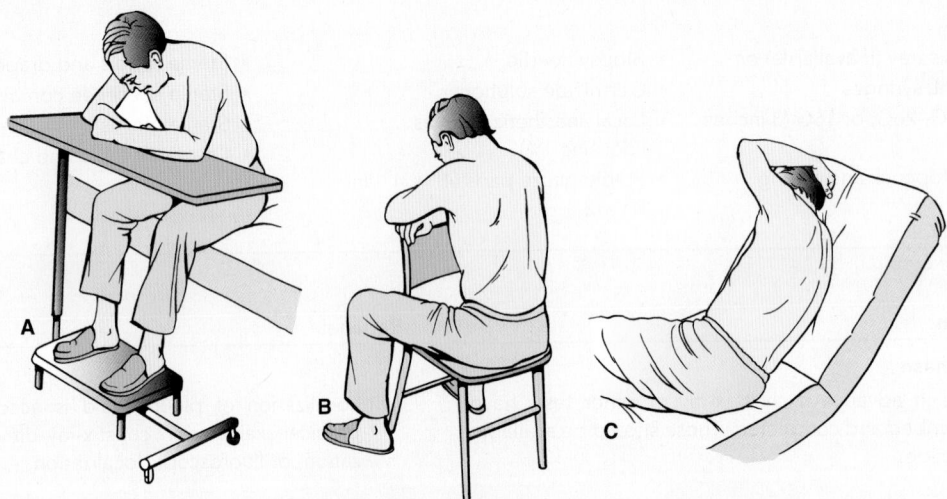

*Positioning the patient for a thoracentesis. The nurse assists the patient to one of three positions and offers comfort and support throughout the procedure. **(A)** Sitting on the edge of the bed with head and arms on and over the bed table. **(B)** Straddling a chair with arms and head resting on the back of the chair. **(C)** Lying on unaffected side with the bed elevated 30 to 45 degrees.*

Performance phase

1. Expose the site to be aspirated. If fluid is in the pleural cavity, the thoracentesis site is determined by study of the chest x-ray and physical findings, with attention to the site of maximal dullness on percussion. If air is in the pleural cavity, the thoracentesis site is usually in the second or third intercostal space in the midclavicular line.	1. Fluid usually settles in the lower pleural cavity. Air rises in the thorax because the density of air is much less than the density of liquid.
2. Perform hand hygiene and put on personal protective equipment.	2. Protects the patient and nurse.
3. Support and reassure the patient during the procedure.	3. Sudden and unexpected movement by the patient can cause trauma to the visceral pleura with resultant trauma to the lung. A local anesthetic inhibits nerve conduction and is used to prevent pain during the procedure.
a. Prepare the patient for sensations of cold from skin germicide and for pressure and sting from infiltration of local anesthetic agent.	
b. Encourage the patient to refrain from coughing, talking, or moving.	
c. Be prepared to monitor the patient's condition throughout the procedure.	
4. The procedure is done under aseptic conditions. After the skin is cleaned, the health care provider slowly injects a local anesthetic with a small-gauge needle into the intercostal space.	4. An intradermal wheal is raised slowly; rapid intradermal injection causes pain. The parietal pleura is very sensitive and should be well infiltrated with anesthetic before the thoracentesis needle is passed through it.
5. Ultrasound or direct physical examination is used to guide needle placement.	5. Prevents pneumothorax.

PROCEDURE GUIDELINES 10-2 *(continued)*

Assisting the Patient Undergoing Thoracentesis

PROCEDURE *(continued)*

Nursing Action	Rationale

6. The thoracentesis needle is advanced with the syringe attached. When the pleural space is reached, suction may be applied with the syringe.
 	
  a. A 20- or 50-mL syringe with a three-way adapter (stopcock) is attached to the needle. (One end of the adapter is attached to the needle and the other to the tubing leading to a receptacle that receives the fluid being aspirated.)
 	
  b. If a considerable quantity of fluid is to be removed, the needle is held in place on the chest wall with a small hemostat.
 	
  c. A pleural biopsy may be performed.
	6.
	
	  a. When a larger quantity of fluid is withdrawn, a three-way adapter serves to keep air from entering the pleural cavity. The amount of fluid removed depends on clinical status of the patient and absence of complications during the procedure.
	
	  b. The hemostat steadies the needle on the chest wall and prevents too deep a penetration of pleural space. Sudden pleuritic pain or shoulder pain may indicate that the visceral or diaphragmatic pleura are being irritated by the needle point.

7. After the needle is withdrawn, pressure is applied over the puncture site and a small sterile dressing is fixed in place.	7. Prevents air entry into pleural space.

Follow-up phase

1. Place the patient on bed rest. A chest x-ray is usually obtained after thoracentesis.	1. Chest x-ray verifies that there is no pneumothorax.
2. Record vital signs every 15 minutes for 1 hour.	2. Assesses for complications.
3. Administer oxygen, as directed, if the patient has cardiorespiratory disease.	3. Pulmonary gas exchange may worsen after thoracentesis in patients with cardiorespiratory disease.
4. Record the total amount of fluid withdrawn and the nature of the fluid, its color, and viscosity. If prescribed, prepare samples of fluid for laboratory evaluation (usually bacteriology, cell count and differential, determinations of protein, glucose, lactate dehydrogenase, specific gravity). A small amount of heparin may be needed for several of the specimen containers to prevent coagulation. A specimen container with preservative may be needed if a pleural biopsy is obtained.	4. The fluid may be clear, serous, bloody, or purulent. Analysis may aid in diagnosis and treatment.
5. Evaluate the patient at intervals for increasing respirations, faintness, vertigo, tightness in the chest, uncontrollable cough, blood-tinged mucus, and rapid pulse and signs of hypoxemia.	5. Pneumothorax, tension pneumothorax, hemothorax, subcutaneous emphysema, or pyogenic infection may result from a thoracentesis.
6. Encourage deep breaths.	6. Promotes lung expansion.

Evidence Base Cervini, P., Hesley, G. K., Thompson, R., et al. (2010). Incidence of infectious complications after an ultrasound-guided intervention. *American Journal of Roentgenology, 195,* 846.
    Rubins, J. (2012). Pleural effusion. *Medscape Reference.* Available: *http://emedicine.medscape.com/article/299959-overview.*

the lungs. A pleural effusion is an abnormal collection of this fluid.

5. The test is performed to determine the cause of a pleural effusion, and to relieve associated shortness of breath.

Nursing and Patient Care Considerations

1. Observe and record total amount of fluid withdrawn, nature of fluid, and its color and viscosity.

2. Prepare sample of fluid and ensure transport to the laboratory.

3. A chest x-ray may be done before or after the fluid is withdrawn.

4. Patient should not cough, breathe deeply, or move while fluid is being withdrawn.

5. Instruct patient to inform provider immediately if sharp chest pain or shortness of breath occurs.

Radiology and Imaging

Chest X-Ray

Description

1. Normal pulmonary tissue is radiolucent and appears black on film. Thus, densities produced by tumors, foreign bodies, and infiltrates can be detected as lighter or white images.
2. Commonly, two views—posterior–anterior and lateral—are obtained.
3. This test shows the position of normal structures, displacement, and presence of abnormal shadows. It may reveal pathology in the lungs in the absence of symptoms.

Nursing and Patient Care Considerations

1. Should be taken upright if patient's condition permits. Assist technician at bedside in preparing patient for portable chest x-ray.
2. Encourage patient to take deep breath, hold breath, and remain still as x-ray is taken.
3. Make sure that all jewelry, electrocardiogram (ECG) or monitor leads, and metal objects (including metal-containing transdermal patches) in x-ray field are removed so as not to interfere with film.
4. Consider the contraindication of x-rays for pregnant patients.

Computed Tomography Scan

Description

1. Cross-sectional x-rays of the lungs are taken from many different angles and processed through a computer to create three-dimensional images. This three-dimensional imaging provides more complete diagnostic information than the two-dimensional x-ray.
2. It may be used to define pulmonary nodules and pulmonary abnormalities or to demonstrate mediastinal abnormalities and hilar adenopathy.

Nursing and Patient Care Considerations

1. Describe test to patient and family, including that table will slide into doughnut-shaped scanner and patient must lie still during test. The test usually takes about 30 minutes, but may take longer.
2. Be alert to allergies to iodine or other radiographic contrast media that might be used during testing.
3. For scans performed with contrast, informed consent and IV access required. Patient should take nothing by mouth (NPO) for 4 hours prior to scan. Blood urea nitrogen and creatinine should be evaluated 24 to 48 hours before test.
4. Hydrate patient well to facilitate excretion of contrast, if used.
5. Check regarding weight limit of equipment prior to scanning bariatric patients.
6. Consider the contraindication of radiologic studies for the pregnant patient, especially computed tomography (CT) scans with contrast media.

Magnetic Resonance Imaging

Description

1. Noninvasive procedure that uses a powerful magnetic field, radio waves, and a computer to produce detailed pictures of organs, soft tissue, bone, and other internal structures.
2. Provides contrast between various soft tissues and is performed to:
   a. Assess abnormal growths, including cancer of the lungs or other tissues inadequately assessed with other imaging modalities.
   b. Determine stage of cancer, including tumor size, extent, and degree to which cancer has spread.
   c. Visualize lymph nodes and blood vessels.
   d. Assess disorders of the vertebrae, ribs, and sternum.
3. Traditional radiographic contrast media are not used but gadolinium injection or ingestion may be necessary, depending on patient's medical history and anatomy to be imaged.
4. It is helpful to synchronize the magnetic resonance imaging (MRI) picture to the ECG in thoracic studies.
5. The hazards of MRI during pregnancy are unknown, although ionizing radiation (x-ray) is not used during MRI.

Nursing and Patient Care Considerations

1. Explain procedure to patient and assess ability to remain still in a closed space; sedation may be necessary if the patient is claustrophobic. The test takes approximately 1 hour.
2. Evaluate patient for contraindications to MRI: implanted devices, such as implanted defibrillators that may malfunction; cochlear implants; or metallic surgical clips used on brain aneurysms.
3. Devices that may interfere with the exam or potentially pose a risk include artificial heart valves, implanted drug infusion ports, infusion catheters, intrauterine devices, pacemakers and neurostimulators, metallic implants such as prosthetic valves or joints, and metal pins, screws, plates, or surgical staples.
4. Make sure that all jewelry, ECG or monitor leads, hearing aids, pins/hairpins, removable dental work, and metal objects (including metal-containing transdermal patches) are removed.
5. Kidney disease and sickle cell anemia may contraindicate MRI with contrast material.
6. Check with MRI technician about the use of equipment, such as ventilator or mechanical IV pump, in MRI room.
7. Earplugs may be used to muffle loud thumping and humming noises during imaging.
8. Evaluate the patient for claustrophobia, and teach relaxation techniques to use during test or advocate for use of open MRI. Be ready to administer sedation, if necessary.
9. Check regarding size capacity of equipment prior to scanning bariatric patients.
10. It is recommended that nursing mothers not breastfeed for 36 to 48 hours after MRI with contrast.

Positron Emission Tomography Scan

Description

1. Physiologic images are obtained, based on the detection of radiation from the emission of positrons. Positrons are tiny particles emitted from a radioactive isotope–administered IV to the patient. Radioactivity localizes in the area(s) being scanned and is detected by positron emission tomography (PET). Different colors or degrees of brightness on a PET image represent different levels of tissue or organ function.

2. Radioisotope is administered 30 to 90 minutes prior to scan via IV or inhalation.
3. Distinguishes between benign and malignant lung nodules.

Nursing and Patient Care Considerations
1. Describe test to patient and family, including that table will slide into doughnut-shaped scanner and patient must lie still during test. The test usually takes 30 to 45 minutes.
2. Isotope has a short half-life and is not considered a radiologic hazard.
3. Encourage fluids to facilitate excretion of isotope.
4. Consider the contraindication of radiologic studies for the pregnant or breastfeeding patient.
5. Test results may be inaccurate for diabetic patients or for patients who have eaten within a few hours prior to the scan if blood glucose or insulin levels are not normal.

Pulmonary Angiography

Description
1. An imaging method used to study pulmonary vessels and pulmonary circulation.
2. For visualization, radiopaque medium is injected by way of a catheter in the main pulmonary artery rapidly into the vasculature of the lungs. Films are then taken in rapid succession after injection.
3. It is considered the "gold standard" for diagnosis of pulmonary embolus, but spiral CT scanning can also be effectively used.

Nursing and Patient Care Considerations
1. Determine whether patient is allergic to radiographic contrast media, describe the procedure, and obtain informed consent.
2. Patient may be kept NPO for 4 to 8 hours prior to procedure.
3. Instruct patient that injection of dye may cause flushing, cough, and a warm sensation.
4. Pulse, blood pressure (BP), and respirations are monitored during the procedure.
5. After the procedure, make sure pressure is maintained over access site and monitor pulse rate, BP, and circulation distal to the injection site.
6. Patient may be advised to keep extremity straight for up to 12 hours after the procedure.
7. Necessity of test should be carefully evaluated in patients with bleeding disorders and pregnant women.

Ventilation-Perfusion Scan

Description
1. A pair of nuclear scan tests using inhaled and injected radioisotopes to measure breathing (ventilation) and blood flow (perfusion) in all areas of the lungs. The two tests may be performed either separately or together.
2. Perfusion scan is done after injection of a radioactive isotope. It measures blood perfusion through the lungs and evaluates lung function on a regional basis.
3. Ventilation scan is done after inhalation of radioactive gas (eg, xenon with O_2), which diffuses throughout the lungs. It indicates how well air reaches all parts of the lung.
4. Usually performed to detect pulmonary embolus. Also useful in evaluating advanced pulmonary disease (COPD), detecting abnormal circulation (shunts) in the pulmonary blood vessels, evaluating lung function, and identifying fibrosis.
5. Is also referred to as *V/Q scan* because the initials are used in mathematical equations that calculate air and blood flow.

Nursing and Patient Care Considerations
1. Determine if patient is allergic to radiographic dye before V/Q scan.
2. Explain the procedure to patient and encourage cooperation with inhalation and brief episodes of breath holding.
3. Contraindicated in patients with primary pulmonary hypertension.
4. False positives may occur in patients with vasculitis, mitral stenosis, pulmonary hypertension, and when tumors obstruct a pulmonary artery with airway involvement, fatty tissues, and presence of parasites.
5. False negatives are associated with partially occluded vessels.

Other Diagnostic Tests

Bronchoscopy

Description
1. The direct inspection and observation of the upper and lower respiratory tract through fiberoptic (flexible) or rigid bronchoscope as a means of diagnosing and managing inflammatory, infectious, and malignant diseases of the airway and lungs.
2. Flexible fiberoptic bronchoscopy allows for more patient comfort and better visualization of smaller airways, including nasal passages. It is usually performed using local anesthesia with or without moderate sedation. Fluoroscopy may be needed to facilitate specimen collection. Used for therapeutic and diagnostic procedures such as:
   a. Bronchoalveolar lavage.
   b. Endobronchial or transbronchial biopsies.
   c. Cytologic wash or brush.
   d. Transbronchial needle aspiration.
   e. Endobronchial ultrasound.
   f. Autofluorescence bronchoscopy.
   g. Balloon dilation.
   h. Endobronchial laser ablation.
   i. Electrocautery.
   j. Photodynamic therapy.
   k. Brachytherapy.
   l. Some types of stent placement.
3. Rigid bronchoscopy, often performed under general anesthesia with adequate sedation and muscle relaxants, may be combined with flexible bronchoscopy for better access to distal airways. Diagnostic and therapeutic indications include:
   a. Bleeding or hemorrhage.
   b. Foreign body extraction.
   c. Deeper biopsy specimen collection than can be obtained fiber-optically.
   d. Dilation of tracheal or bronchial strictures.
   e. Relief of airway obstruction.
   f. Insertion of stents.
   g. Tracheobronchial laser therapy or other mechanical tumor ablation.

Nursing and Patient Care Considerations

1. Check that an informed consent form has been signed and that risks and benefits have been explained to patient.
2. Make sure that IV access is present and patent.
3. Absolute contraindications include uncorrectable coagulopathy, severe refractory hypoxemia, unstable hemodynamic status. Patients with increased risk are those with MI within past 6 weeks, head injuries susceptible to increased intracranial pressures (ICP), and known or suspected pregnancy (due to possible radiation exposure).
4. Review and follow facility policy and procedure for anesthesia and sedation.
5. Administer prescribed medication to reduce secretions, block the vasovagal reflex and gag reflex, and relieve anxiety. Give encouragement and nursing support.
6. Restrict fluid and food, as ordered, before procedure to reduce risk of aspiration when reflexes are blocked. Patient may be kept NPO for 4 hours prior to flexible bronchoscopy with minimal sedation; if deeper sedation is used, patient's time on NPO is extended.
7. Remove dentures, contact lenses, and other prostheses.
8. After the procedure:
   a. Monitor cardiac rhythm and rate, BP, and level of consciousness (LOC).
   b. Monitor respiratory effort and rate.
   c. Monitor oximetry.
   d. Withhold ice chips and fluids until patient demonstrates gag reflex.
   e. Monitor patient's perceptions of pain, discomfort, and dyspnea.
9. Promptly report cyanosis, hypoventilation, hypotension, tachycardia or dysrhythmia, hemoptysis, dyspnea, decreased breath sounds.
10. Provide outpatients with specific instructions regarding signs and symptoms of complications and what to do if they arise.

 NURSING ALERT After bronchoscopy, be alert for complications, such as pneumothorax, dysrhythmias, laryngospasm, and bronchospasm.

Lung Biopsy

Description

1. Procedures used for obtaining histologic material from the lung to aid in diagnosis include:
   a. Transbronchial biopsy—biopsy forceps inserted through bronchoscope and specimen of lung tissue obtained.
   b. Transthoracic needle aspiration biopsy—specimen obtained through needle aspiration under fluoroscopic guidance.
   c. Open lung biopsy—specimen obtained through small anterior thoracotomy; used in making a diagnosis when other biopsy methods have not been effective or are not possible.

Nursing and Patient Care Considerations

1. Obtain permission for consent, if required.
2. Observe for possible complications, including pneumothorax, hemorrhage (hemoptysis), and bacterial contamination of pleural space.

3. A chest x-ray should be done 1 hour after transbronchial biopsy to exclude pneumothorax.
4. See "Bronchoscopy" (page 207) or "Thoracic Surgeries" (page 263) for postprocedure care.

Pulmonary Function Tests

Description

1. Pulmonary function tests (PFTs) are used to detect and measure abnormalities in respiratory function and quantify severity of various lung diseases. Such tests include measurements of lung volumes, ventilatory function, diffusing capacity, gas exchange, lung compliance, airway resistance, and distribution of gases in the lung.
2. Ventilatory studies (spirometry) are the most common group of tests.
   a. Requires electronic spirometer, water spirometer, or wedge spirometer that plots volume against time (timed vital capacity).
   b. Patient is asked to take as deep a breath as possible and then to exhale into spirometer as completely and either slowly or as forcefully as possible, depending on the type of test.
   c. Results are compared with normals for patient's age, height, and sex (see Table 10-1).
   d. A reduction in the vital capacity, inspiratory capacity, and total lung capacity may indicate a restrictive form of lung disease (disease due to increased lung stiffness).
   e. An increase in functional reserve capacity, total lung capacity, and reduction in flow rates usually indicate an obstructive flow due to bronchial obstruction or loss of lung elastic recoil.
3. Lung volumes are determined by asking the patient to inhale a known concentration of inert gas, such as helium or 100% oxygen, and measuring concentration of inert gas or nitrogen in exhaled air (dilution method) or by plethysmography.
   a. Yields thoracic volume (total lung capacity, plus any unventilated blebs or bullae).
   b. An increased residual volume is found in air-trapping due to obstructive lung disease.
   c. A reduction in several parameters usually indicates a restrictive form of lung disease or chest wall abnormality.
4. Diffusing capacity measures lung surface effective for the transfer of gas in the lung by having patient inhale gas containing known low concentration of carbon monoxide and measuring carbon monoxide concentration in exhaled air. Difference between inhaled and exhaled concentrations is related directly to uptake of carbon monoxide across alveolar-capillary membrane. Diffusing capacity is reduced in interstitial lung disease, emphysema, pneumonectomy, pulmonary embolus, and anemia.

Nursing and Patient Care Considerations

1. Instruct patient in correct technique for completing PFTs; coach patient through test, if needed. Test results may be unreliable if patient is not cooperative or motivated to perform all maneuvers.

Table 10-1   Pulmonary Function Tests

TERM	SYMBOL	DESCRIPTION	REMARKS
Vital capacity	VC	Maximum volume of air exhaled after a maximum inspiration	• VC < 10–15 mL/kg suggests need for mechanical ventilation • VC > 10–15 mL/kg suggests ability to wean
Forced vital capacity	FVC	Vital capacity performed with a maximally forced expiratory effort	• Reduced in obstructive disease (COPD) due to air-trapping and restrictive disease • Reflects airflow in large airways
Forced expiratory volume in 1 second	FEV_1	Volume of air exhaled in the first second of the performance of the FVC	• Reduced in obstructive disease (COPD) due to air-trapping • Reflects airflow in large airways
Ratio of FEV_1/FVC	FEV_1/FVC	FEV_1 expressed as a percentage of the FVC	• Decreased in obstructive disease • Normal in restrictive disease
Forced midexpiratory flow	$FEF_{25\%-75\%}$	Average flow during the middle half of the FVC	• Reflects airflow in small airways • Smokers may have change in this test before other symptoms develop
Peak expiratory flow rate	PEFR	Most rapid flow during a forced expiration after a maximum inspiration	• Used to measure response to bronchodilators, airflow obstruction in patients with asthma
Maximal voluntary volume	MVV	Volume of air expired in a specified period (12 seconds) during repetitive maximal effort	• An important factor in exercise tolerance • Decreases in neuromuscular diseases

2. Instruct patient not to use oral or inhaled bronchodilator (eg, albuterol), caffeine, or tobacco at least 4 to 6 hours before test (longer for long-acting bronchodilators).
3. Used with caution in patients with hemoptysis of unknown origin; pneumothorax; unstable cardiovascular status; recent MI or pulmonary embolus; thoracic, abdominal, or cerebral aneurysm; or recent eye, thoracic, or abdominal surgery.
4. Using a noseclip for all spirometric maneuvers is strongly recommended.
5. Although forced expiratory volume in the first second of a forced vital capacity is the "gold standard" for diagnosing airway obstruction, there is no single cut-off value separating normal from abnormal. This determination is based more on trending of individual results.

Pulse Oximetry

Description

1. Noninvasively provides an estimate of arterial oxyhemoglobin saturation by using selected wavelengths of light to determine the saturation of oxyhemoglobin. Oximeters function by passing a light beam through a vascular bed, such as the finger or earlobe, to determine the amount of light absorbed by oxygenated (red) and deoxygenated (blue) blood.
2. Calculates the amount of arterial blood that is saturated with oxygen (SaO_2) and displays this as a percentage.
3. Provides indication only of oxygenation, not ventilation.
4. Indications include:
   a. Monitor adequacy of oxygen saturation; quantify response to therapy.
   b. Monitor unstable patient who may experience sudden changes in blood oxygen level.
   c. Evaluation of need for home oxygen therapy.
   d. Determine supplemental oxygen needs at rest, with exercise, and during sleep.
   e. Need to follow the trend and need to decrease number of ABG sample drawn.
5. The oxyhemoglobin dissociation curve allows for correlation between SaO_2 and PaO_2 (see Figure 10-1).
   a. Increased body temperature, acidosis, and increased phosphates (2,3-DPG) cause a shift in the curve to the right, thus increasing the ability of hemoglobin to release oxygen to the tissues.
   b. Decreased temperature, decreased 2,3-DPG, and alkalosis cause a shift to the left, causing hemoglobin to hold on to the oxygen, reducing the amount of oxygen being released to the tissues.
6. Increased bilirubin, increased carboxyhemoglobin, low perfusion, or SaO_2 less than 80% may alter light absorption and interfere with results.

 NURSING ALERT There is a potential error in SaO_2 readings of ±2% that can increase to greater than 2% if the patient's SpO_2 drops below 80%. Oximeters rely on differences in light absorption to determine SaO_2. At lower saturations, oxygenated hemoglobin appears bluer in color and is less easily distinguished from deoxygenated hemoglobin. ABG analysis should be used in this situation.

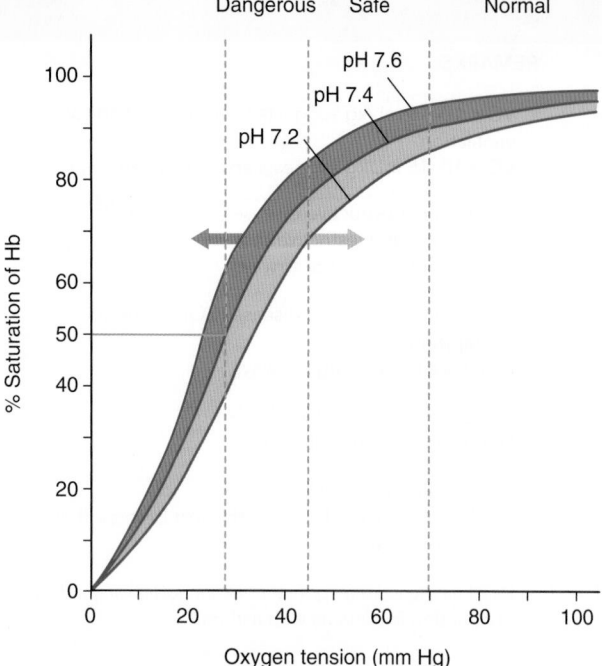

Figure 10-1. The oxyhemoglobin dissociation curve shows the relation between the partial pressure of oxygen and the oxygen saturation. At pressures greater than 60 mm Hg, the curve is essentially flat with blood oxygen content not changing with increases in the oxygen partial pressure. As oxygen partial pressures decrease in the slope of the curve, the oxygen is unloaded to peripheral tissue as the hemoglobin's affinity decreases. The curve is shifted to the right by an increase in temperature, 2,3-DPG, or $PaCO_2$, or a decrease in pH, and to the left by the opposite of these conditions.

Nursing and Patient Care Considerations

1. Assess patient's hemoglobin. SaO_2 may not correlate well with PaO_2 if hemoglobin is not within normal limits.
2. Remove patient's nail polish because it can affect the ability of the sensor to correctly determine oxygen saturation, particularly polish with blue or dark colors.
3. Correlate oximetry with ABG values and then use for single reading or trending of oxygenation (does not monitor $PaCO_2$).
4. Display heart rate should correlate with patient's heart rate.
5. To improve quality of signal, hold finger dependent and motionless (motion may alter results) and cover finger sensor to occlude ambient light.
6. Assess site of oximetry monitoring for perfusion on a regular basis because pressure ulcer may occur from prolonged application of probe. Rotate probe every 2 hours.
7. Device limitations include motion artifact, abnormal hemoglobins (carboxyhemoglobin and methemoglobin), intravenous (IV) dye, exposure of probe to ambient light, low perfusion states, skin pigmentation, nail polish or nail coverings, and nail deformities such as severe clubbing.
8. Document inspired oxygen or supplemental oxygen and type of oxygen delivery device.
9. Accuracy can be affected by decreased peripheral perfusion, ambient light, IV dyes, nail polish, deeply pigmented skin,

cold extremities, hypothermia, patients in sickle cell crisis, jaundice, severe anemia, and use of antibiotics such as sulfas.
10. In patients with COPD, oxygen saturation levels may remain unchanged, even though CO_2 levels may be rising as the patient becomes acidotic. Pulse oximetry will not detect this deterioration.
11. Contraindicated for monitoring patients who have high levels of arterial carboxyhemoglobin, such as fire victims.

Capnometry/Capnography

 Evidence Base Kodali, B. (2010). Capnography: A comprehensive educational website. Updated June 2010. Available: *www.capnography.com.*

Description

1. Used to noninvasively determine and monitor end-tidal carbon dioxide ($ETCO_2$)—the amount of CO_2 that is expired with each breath—via colorimetric indicator.
2. $ETCO_2$ is displayed as a capnogram (a waveform that may be time-based or volume-based and a numeric reading).
3. Normally 2 to 5 mm Hg less than $PaCO_2$ in adults, with the difference being greater in the presence of lung disease, or increase in dead space, and can be used as an indirect estimate of V/Q mismatching for the lung.
4. Indicated for monitoring severity of pulmonary disease and monitoring response to therapy; evaluating efficacy of mechanical ventilatory support; monitoring adequacy of pulmonary, systemic, and coronary blood flow; and assessing metabolic rate and/or alveolar ventilation.
5. A standard in anesthesia care, it is being increasingly used in the critical care setting as well as in emergency care via pocket-sized models.

Nursing and Patient Care Considerations

1. Draw ABGs initially to correlate $ETCO_2$ with $PaCO_2$ and to establish the gradient between $PaCO_2$ and $ETCO_2$.
2. Accuracy of measurement can be affected by alterations in breathing pattern or tidal volume (V_T), breathing frequency, presence of freon from metered-dose inhalers, contamination of the system by secretions or condensate, low cardiac output, use of antacids or carbonated beverages, and leaks around tracheal tube cuffs or uncuffed tubes.
3. Does not evaluate pH or oxygenation.
4. Effective for confirming ET tube placement and for monitoring CO_2 in patients who tend to retain CO_2 (eg, COPD).
5. Not a reliable method for determining inadvertent pulmonary placement of gastric tubes.
6. Clean and disinfect sensors and monitors as per manufacturer's instructions.

Exhaled Breath Condensate

 Evidence Base Shoemark, A., & Wilson, R. (2011). Exhaled breath condensate pH as a non-invasive measure of inflammation in non-cf bronchiectasis. *International Scholarly Research Network Pulmonology, 2011, 6.* Available: *http://www.hindawi.com/isrn/pulmonology/2011/169080/.*

Description

1. Emerging as a source for determining biomarkers of lung disease. Exhaled breath condensate (EBC) is a matrix of exhaled particles and droplets in which biomarkers may be identified, such as:
   a. Volatile (acetic acid, formic acid, ammonia) and nonvolatile compounds.
   b. Very-low- and low-molecular-weight compounds.
   c. Polypeptides.
   d. Proteins.
   e. Nucleic acids.
   f. Lipid mediators.
   g. Inorganic molecules.
   h. Organic molecules.
   i. Redox relevant molecules.
   j. pH relevant molecules.
   k. Cytokines and chemokines.
2. Currently, there is no gold standard—either invasively or noninvasively—for determining absolute concentrations with which EBC can be easily compared.
3. The pH of EBC depends on disease state, ranging from 3.5 to 9.0, which can affect the reactivity and stability of other biomarkers being assayed.

Nursing and Patient Care Considerations

1. Collect condensate sample. Collection methods vary, depending on specific biomarkers to be analyzed. Ten minutes of tidal breathing yields 1 to 2 mm of sample; smaller sample sizes may be adequate for analysis of only one or two biomarkers.
2. Be aware that lower airway condensate may be contaminated by particles from oral and retropharyngeal mucosa.
3. Saliva trapping systems may be used with drooling patients to reduce salivary contamination.

GENERAL PROCEDURES AND TREATMENT MODALITIES

Artificial Airway Management

Airway management may be indicated in patients with loss of consciousness, facial or oral trauma, aspiration, tumor, infection, copious respiratory secretions, respiratory distress, and the need for mechanical ventilation.

Types of Airways

1. Oropharyngeal airway—curved plastic device inserted through the mouth and positioned in the posterior pharynx to move tongue away from palate and open the airway.
   a. Usually for short-term use in the unconscious patient or may be used along with an oral ET tube.
   b. Not used if recent oral trauma, surgery, or if loose teeth are present.
   c. Does not protect against aspiration.

 NURSING ALERT Position patient on side and suction oral cavity frequently to prevent aspiration of oral secretions or vomitus when an oral airway is in place.

2. Nasopharyngeal airway (nasal trumpet)—soft rubber or plastic tube inserted through nose into posterior pharynx.
   a. Facilitates frequent nasopharyngeal suctioning.
   b. Use extreme caution with patients on anticoagulants or bleeding disorders.
   c. Select size that is slightly smaller than diameter of nostril and slightly longer than distance from tip of nose to earlobe.
   d. Check nasal mucosa for irritation or ulceration, and clean airway with hydrogen peroxide and water.

 NURSING ALERT Nasopharyngeal airways may obstruct sinus drainage and produce acute sinusitis. Be alert to fever and facial pain.

3. Laryngeal mask airway—composed of a tube with a cuffed masklike projection at the distal end; inserted through the mouth into the pharynx; seals the larynx and leaves distal opening of tube just above glottis.
   a. Easier placement than ET tube because visualization of vocal cords is not necessary.
   b. Provides ventilation and oxygenation comparable to that achieved with an ET tube.
   c. Cannot prevent aspiration because it does not separate the GI tract from the respiratory tract.
   d. May cause laryngospasm and bronchospasm.
4. Combitube—double-lumen tube with pharyngeal lumen and tracheoesophageal lumen; pharyngeal lumen has blocked distal end and perforations at pharyngeal level; tracheoesophageal lumen has open upper and lower end; large oropharyngeal balloon serves to seal mouth and nose; distal cuff seals the esophagus or trachea.
5. Endotracheal tube—flexible tube inserted through the mouth or nose and into the trachea beyond the vocal cords that acts as an artificial airway.
   a. Maintains a patent airway.
   b. Allows for deep tracheal suction and removal of secretions.
   c. Permits mechanical ventilation.
   d. Inflated balloon seals off trachea so aspiration from the GI tract cannot occur.
   e. Generally easy to insert in an emergency, but maintaining placement is more difficult so this is not for long-term use.
6. Tracheostomy tube—firm, curved artificial airway inserted directly into the trachea at the level of the second or third tracheal ring through a surgically made incision.
   a. Permits mechanical ventilation and facilitates secretion removal.
   b. Can be for long-term use.
   c. Bypasses upper airway defenses, increasing susceptibility to infection.
   d. Allows the patient to eat and swallow.

Endotracheal Tube Insertion

1. Orotracheal insertion is technically easier because it is done under direct visualization (see Procedure Guidelines 10-3, pages 212 to 214). Disadvantages are increased oral secretions, decreased patient comfort, difficulty with tube stabilization, and inability of patient to use lip movement as a communication means.

(*Text continues on page 215*)

PROCEDURE GUIDELINES 10-3

Endotracheal Intubation

EQUIPMENT

- Laryngoscope with curved or straight blade and working light source (check batteries and bulb regularly)
- Endotracheal (ET) tube with low-pressure cuff and adapter to connect tube to ventilator or resuscitation bag
- Stylet to guide the ET tube

- Oral airway (assorted sizes) or bite block to keep patient from biting into and occluding the ET tube
- Adhesive tape or tube fixation system
- Sterile anesthetic lubricant jelly (water-soluble)
- 10-mL syringe

- Suction source
- Suction catheter and tonsil suction
- Resuscitation bag and mask connected to oxygen source
- Sterile towel
- Gloves
- Face shield
- End tidal CO_2 detector

PROCEDURE

Nursing Action	Rationale
Preparatory phase	
1. Assess the patient's heart rate, level of consciousness, and respiratory status.	1. Provides a baseline to estimate the patient's tolerance of the procedure.
2. Remove the patient's dental bridgework and plates.	2. May interfere with insertion. Will not be able to remove easily from the patient once intubated.
3. Remove the headboard from the bed (optional).	3. Provides room to stand behind patient's head.
4. Prepare equipment.	4.
a. Ensure function of resuscitation bag with mask and suction.	a. The patient may require ventilatory assistance during procedure. Suction should be functional because gagging and emesis may occur during procedure.
b. Assemble the laryngoscope. Make sure the light bulb is tightly attached and functional.	
c. Select an ET tube of the appropriate size (7–9 mm for the average adult).	
d. Place the ET tube on a sterile towel.	d. Although the tube will pass through the contaminated mouth or nose, the airway below the vocal cords is sterile, and efforts must be made to prevent iatrogenic contamination of the distal end of the tube and cuff. The proximal end of the tube may be handled because it will reside in the upper airway.
e. Inflate the cuff to make sure it assumes a symmetrical shape and holds volume without leakage. Then deflate maximally.	e. Malfunction of the cuff must be determined before tube placement occurs.
f. Lubricate the distal end of the tube liberally with the sterile anesthetic water-soluble jelly.	f. Aids in insertion.
g. Have stylet available for oral intubation (user preference, although rarely used).	g. Stiffens the soft tube, allowing it to be more easily directed into the trachea. Nasal intubation does not employ use of the stylet.
5. Aspirate the stomach contents if an NG tube is in place.	5. Reduces risk of aspiration.
6. If time allows, inform the patient of the impending inability to talk and discuss alternative means of communication.	6. To alleviate fear.
7. If the patient is confused, consider requesting an order for soft wrist restraints.	7. Restraint of the confused patient may be necessary to promote patient safety and maintain sterile technique.

PROCEDURE GUIDELINES 10-3 *(continued)*

Endotracheal Intubation

PROCEDURE *(continued)*

Nursing Action	Rationale

Performance phase

1. Put on gloves and face shield.

2. During oral intubation if cervical spine is not injured, place patient's head in a "sniffing" position (raise head with folded towel to extend at the junction of the neck and thorax and flexed at the junction of the spine and skull).

3. Spray the back of the patient's throat with anesthetic spray.

4. Ventilate and oxygenate the patient with the resuscitation bag and mask before intubation.

5. Assist with intubation as needed. Anticipate the following steps:

   a. The handle of the laryngoscope is held in the left hand and the patient's mouth is held open with the right hand by placing crossed fingers on the teeth.

   b. The blade of the laryngoscope is inserted along the right side of the tongue, pushing the tongue to the left, and the right thumb and index finger are used to pull patient's lower lip away from lower teeth.

   c. The laryngoscope is lifted forward (toward opposite corner) to expose the epiglottis.

   d. The laryngoscope is lifted upward and forward at a 45-degree angle to expose the glottis and visualize vocal cords.

   e. As the epiglottis is lifted forward (toward ceiling), the vertical opening of the larynx between the vocal cords will come into view (see accompanying figure).

1. Prevents contact with patient's oral secretions.

2. Upper airway is open maximally in this position.

3. Will decrease gagging.

4. Preoxygenation decreases the likelihood of cardiac dysrhythmias or respiratory distress secondary to hypoxemia.

5.

   a. Leverage is improved by crossing the thumb and index fingers when opening the patient's mouth (scissor-twist technique).

   b. Rolling the lip away from teeth prevents injury by being caught between the teeth and the blade.

   c. The teeth should not be used as a fulcrum; this could lead to dental damage.

   d. This stretches the hypoepiglottis ligament, folding the epiglottis upward and exposing the glottis.

   e. The shoulder and arm are used to lift the epiglottis rather than the wrist.

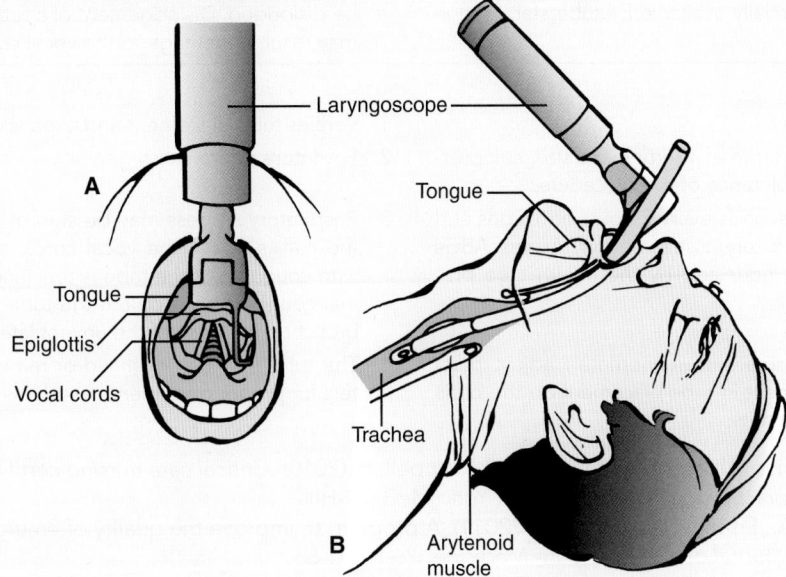

Endotracheal intubation. **(A)** *The primary glottic landmarks for tracheal intubation as visualized with proper placement of the laryngoscope.* **(B)** *Positioning the ET tube.*

(continued)

PROCEDURE GUIDELINES 10-3 *(continued)*

Endotracheal Intubation

PROCEDURE *(continued)*

Nursing Action	Rationale
f. Once the vocal cords are visualized, the tube is inserted into the right corner of the mouth and passed while keeping vocal cords in constant view.	f. Care is taken not to insert the tube into the esophagus; the esophageal mucosa is pink and the opening is horizontal rather than vertical.
g. The tube is gently pushed through the triangular space formed by the vocal cords and back wall of trachea.	g. Care is taken not to cause trauma to the vocal cords. If the vocal cords are in spasm (closed), waiting a few seconds may relieve spasm and allow passage of the tube.
h. Insertion is stopped just after the tube cuff has disappeared from view beyond the cords.	h. Advancing the tube further may lead to its entry into a mainstem bronchus (usually the right bronchus) causing collapse of the unventilated lung.
i. The laryngoscope is withdrawn while holding ET tube in place.	i. Prevents displacement.
6. Disassemble mask from resuscitation bag, attach bag to ET tube, and ventilate the patient.	6. Relieves hypoxia during the procedure.
7. Inflate the cuff with the minimal amount of air required to occlude the trachea.	7. Listen over the cuff area with a stethoscope. Occlusion occurs when no air leak is heard during ventilator inspiration or compression of the resuscitation bag.
8. Insert a bite block if necessary.	8. Keeps the patient from biting down on the tube and obstructing the airway.
9. Use a capnometer.	9. Confirms consistent exhalation of CO_2.
10. Ascertain expansion of both sides of the chest by observation and auscultation of breath sounds.	10. Observation and auscultation help in determining that tube remains in position and has not slipped into the right mainstem bronchus.
11. Auscultate over epigastrium.	11. Confirms no air movement in stomach.
12. Record distance from proximal end of tube to the point where the tube reaches the teeth.	12. Allows for detection of any later change in tube position.
13. Secure the tube to the patient's face with adhesive tape or apply a commercially available ET tube stabilization device.	13. The tube must be fixed securely to ensure that it will not be dislodged. Dislodgement of a tube with an inflated cuff may result in damage to the vocal cords.

Follow-up phase

1. Obtain a chest x-ray.	1. Verifies tube placement and expansion of both lungs.
2. Record tube type, depth of insertion and size, cuff pressure, and patient tolerance of the procedure.	2. For future reference.
3. Auscultate breath sounds every 2 hours or if signs and symptoms of respiratory distress occur. Assess ABGs after intubation if requested by the health care provider.	3. Respiratory distress may be sign of tube displacement. If the cuff is above the vocal cords, extubation may occur with coughing. If the tube is touching the carina, paroxysmal coughing will occur. If the tube slips into a mainstem bronchus, collapse of the unventilated lung may occur.
4. Measure cuff pressure with manometer; adjust pressure. Make adjustment in tube placement on the basis of the chest x-ray results.	4. The tube may be advanced or removed several centimeters for proper placement based on the chest x-ray results.

Evidence Base Ahrens, T., Prentice, D., & Kleinpell, R. (2010). *Critical care nursing certification: Preparation, review and practice exam* (6th ed.). New York: McGraw-Hill.

Hegde, A., Eisen, L., Kory, P., et al. (2011). A program to improve the quality of emergency endotracheal intubation. *Journal of Intensive Care Medicine, 26*(1), 50–56.

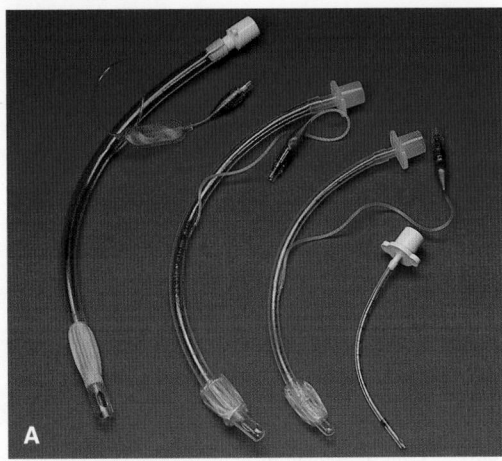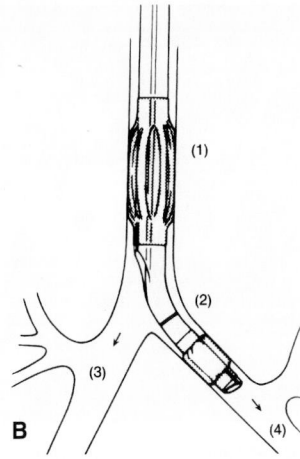

Figure 10-2. (A) Endotracheal tubes: single-lumen and double-lumen endotracheal tube. When the double-lumen tube is used (**B**), two cuffs are inflated. One cuff (1) is positioned in the trachea and the second cuff (2) in the left mainstem bronchus. After inflation, air flows through an opening below the tracheal cuff (3) to the right lung and through an opening below the bronchial cuff (4) to the left lung. This permits differential ventilation of both lungs, lavage of one lung, or selective inflation of either lung during thoracic surgery. (Marshall, B. E., Longnecker, D. E., & Fairley, H. B. (Eds.). (1988). *Anesthesia for thoracic procedures.* Boston: Blackwell Scientific).

2. NT insertion may be more comfortable to the patient and is easier to stabilize. Disadvantages are that blind insertion is required; possible development of pressure necrosis of the nasal airway, sinusitis, and otitis media.
3. Tube types vary according to length and inner diameter, type of cuff, and number of lumens.
   a. Usual sizes for adults are 6.0, 7.0, 8.0, and 9.0 mm.
   b. Most cuffs are high volume, low pressure, with self-sealing inflation valves, or the cuff may be of foam rubber.
   c. Most tubes have a single lumen; however, dual-lumen tubes may be used to ventilate each lung independently (see Figure 10-2).
4. May be contraindicated when glottis is obscured by vomitus, bleeding, foreign body, or trauma or cervical spine injury or deformity.

Tracheostomy Tube Insertion

1. Tube types vary according to presence of inner cannula and presence and type of cuff (see Figure 10-3, page 216).
   a. Tubes with high-volume, low-pressure cuffs with self-sealing inflation valves; with or without inner cannula.
   b. Fenestrated tube.
   c. Foam-filled cuffs.
   d. Speaking tracheostomy tube.
   e. Tracheal button or Passy-Muir valve.
   f. Silver tube (rarely used).
2. Vary according to length and inner diameter in millimeters. Usual sizes for an adult are 5.0, 6.0, 7.0, and 8.0.
3. Tracheostomy is usually planned, either as an adjunct to therapy for respiratory dysfunction or for longer-term airway management when ET intubation has been used for more than 14 days.
4. May be done at the bedside in an emergency when other means of creating an airway have failed (see Procedure Guidelines 10-4, pages 216 to 218).

Indications for Endotracheal or Tracheostomy Tube Insertion

1. Acute respiratory failure, central nervous system (CNS) depression, neuromuscular disease, pulmonary disease, chest wall injury.
2. Upper airway obstruction (tumor, inflammation, foreign body, laryngeal spasm).
3. Anticipated upper airway obstruction from edema or soft tissue swelling due to head and neck trauma, some postoperative head and neck procedures involving the airway, facial or airway burns, decreased LOC.
4. Need for airway protection (vomiting, bleeding, or altered mental status).
5. Aspiration prophylaxis.
6. Fracture of cervical vertebrae with spinal cord injury; requiring ventilatory assistance.

Complications of Endotracheal or Tracheostomy Tube Insertion

1. Laryngeal or tracheal injury.
   a. Sore throat, hoarse voice.
   b. Glottic edema.
   c. Trauma (damage to teeth or mucous membranes, perforation or laceration of pharynx, larynx, or trachea).
   d. Aspiration.
   e. Laryngospasm, bronchospasm.
   f. Ulceration or necrosis of tracheal mucosa.
   g. Vocal cord ulceration, granuloma, or polyps.
   h. Vocal cord paralysis.
   i. Postextubation tracheal stenosis.
   j. Tracheal dilation.
   k. Formation of tracheal–esophageal fistula.

(*Text continues on page 218*)

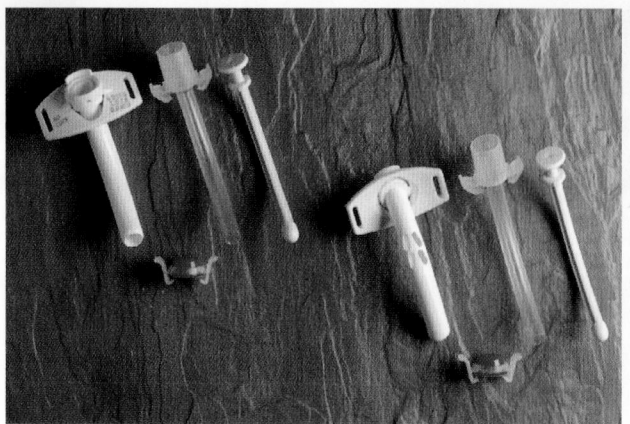

Cuffless: nonfenestrated (left) and fenestrated (right). Tracheostomy plug to allow breathing through upper airway is also shown.

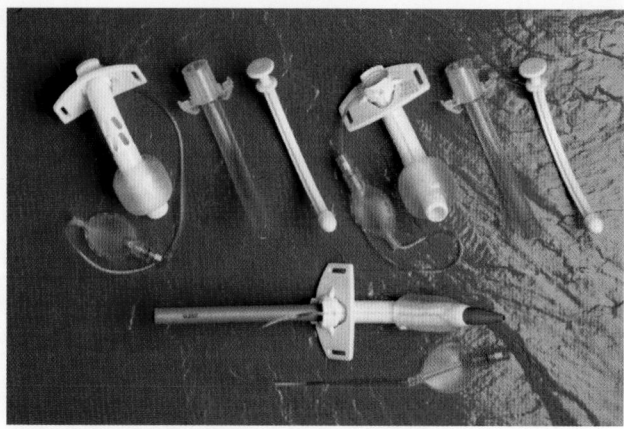

Cuffed: fenestrated (left) and nonfenestrated (right) with inner cannula and obturator for insertion. Percutaneous tracheostomy inducer (bottom).

Figure 10-3. Types of tracheostomy tubes. (Courtesy of Mallinckrodt Medical, St. Louis, MO.)

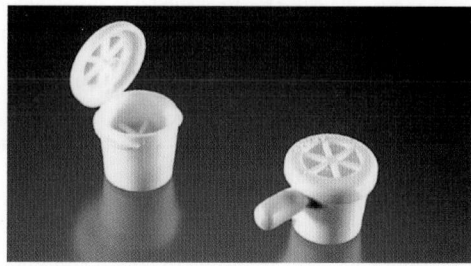

Speaking valve.

PROCEDURE GUIDELINES 10-4

Assisting with Tracheostomy Insertion

EQUIPMENT

- Tracheostomy tube (sizes 6–9 mm for most adults)
- Sterile instruments: hemostat, scalpel and blade, forceps, suture material, scissors
- Sterile gown and drapes, gloves
- Cap and face shield

- Antiseptic prep solution
- Gauze pads
- Shave prep kit
- Sedation
- Local anesthetic and syringe
- Resuscitation bag and mask with oxygen source

- Suction source and catheters
- Syringe for cuff inflation
- Respiratory support available for post-tracheostomy (mechanical ventilation, tracheal oxygen mask, CPAP, T-piece)

PROCEDURE

Nursing Action	Rationale
Preparatory phase	
1. Explain the procedure to the patient. Discuss a communication system with the patient.	1. Apprehension about inability to talk is usually a major concern of the tracheostomized patient.
2. Obtain consent for operative procedure.	2. Required.
3. Shave neck region.	3. Hair and beard may harbor microorganisms. If the beard is to be removed, inform the patient or family.
4. Assemble equipment. Using aseptic technique, inflate tracheostomy cuff and evaluate for symmetry and volume leakage. Deflate maximally.	4. Ensures that the cuff is functional before tube insertion.

PROCEDURE GUIDELINES 10-4 *(continued)*

Assisting with Tracheostomy Insertion

PROCEDURE *(continued)*

Nursing Action	Rationale
5. Position the patient (in a supine position with head extended and a support under the shoulders).	5. This position brings the trachea forward.
6. Obtain an order for and apply soft wrist restraints if the patient is confused.	6. Restraint of the confused patient may be necessary to ensure patient safety and preservation of aseptic technique.
7. Give medication, if ordered.	7. Sedation or local anesthetic may be used to decrease pain and anxiety.
8. Position the light source.	

Performance phase

1. Assist with antiseptic prep, gowning and gloving, and sterile draping.	1. Reduces the risk of infection.
2. Put on face shield.	2. Spraying of blood or airway secretions may occur during this procedure.

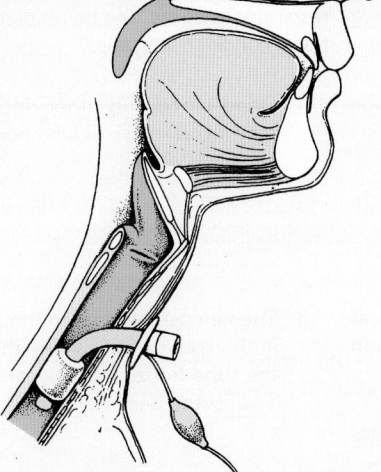

Tracheostomy tube placement.

3. During procedure, monitor the patient's vital signs, suction as necessary, give medication as prescribed, and be prepared to administer emergency care.	3. Bradycardia may result from vagal stimulation due to tracheal manipulation or hypoxemia. Hypoxemia may also cause cardiac irritability.
4. Immediately after the tube is inserted, inflate the cuff. The chest should be auscultated for the presence of bilateral breath sounds.	4. Ensures ventilation of both lungs.
5. Secure the tracheostomy tube with twill tapes or other securing device and apply dressing.	5. Prevents accidental extubation.
6. Apply appropriate respiratory assistive device (mechanical ventilation, tracheostomy, oxygen mask, CPAP, T-piece adapter).	6. Relieves hypoxia.
7. Check the tracheostomy tube cuff pressure.	7. Excessive cuff pressure may cause tracheal damage.
8. "Tie sutures" or "stay sutures" of silk may have been placed through either side of the tracheal cartilage at the incision and brought out through the wound. Each is to be taped to the skin at a 45-degree angle laterally to the sternum.	8. Should the tracheostomy tube become dislodged, the stay sutures may be grasped and used to spread the tracheal cartilage apart, facilitating placement of the new tube.

(continued)

PROCEDURE GUIDELINES 10-4 *(continued)*

Assisting with Tracheostomy Insertion

PROCEDURE *(continued)*

Nursing Action	Rationale

Follow-up phase

1. Assess vital signs and breath sounds; note tube size used, physician performing procedure, and type, dose, and route of medications given.

2. Obtain chest x-ray.

3. Assess and document condition of stoma for bleeding, swelling, or subcutaneous air. Monitor and inform the health care provider of an increase in bleeding or swelling.

1. Provides baseline.

2. Documents proper tube placement.

3. Some bleeding around the stoma site is not unusual for the first few hours, but increased bleeding, swelling, or crepitus in the subcutaneous tissue could indicate complications.

KEY DECISION POINT

When positive pressure respiratory assistive devices are used (mechanical ventilation, CPAP) before the wound is healed, air may be forced into the subcutaneous fat layer. This can be seen as enlargement of the neck and facial tissues and felt as crepitus or "crackling" when the skin is depressed. Report immediately, assess for respiratory distress, and be prepared to provide manual ventilation if condition worsens.

4. Clean the site aseptically when necessary but do not change tracheostomy ties for first 24 hours.

4. Dried blood and other debris around the surgical site may increase risk of infection.

NURSING ALERT Accidental dislodgement of the tube could result when the ties are loose, and tube reinsertion through the as-yet-unformed stoma may be difficult or impossible to accomplish.

5. An extra tube, obturator, and hemostat should be kept at the bedside. In the event of tube dislodgement, reinsertion of a new tube may be necessary.

5. The hemostat will open the airway and allow ventilation in the spontaneously breathing patient. Avoid inserting the tube horizontally because the tube may be forced against the back wall of the trachea.

6. For emergency tube insertion, place the patient in the same position as insertion, then:
   a. Spread the wound with a hemostat or stay sutures.
   b. Insert replacement tube (containing the obturator) at an angle.
   c. Point cannula downward and insert the tube maximally.
   d. Remove the obturator.

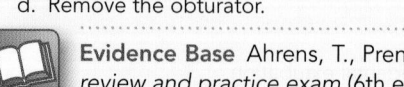

Evidence Base Ahrens, T., Prentice, D., & Kleinpell, R. (2010). *Critical care nursing certification: Preparation, review and practice exam* (6th ed.). New York: McGraw-Hill.

---

l. Formation of tracheal–arterial fistula.
m. Innominate artery erosion.

2. Pulmonary infection and sepsis.

3. Dependence on artificial airway.

Nursing Care for Patients with Artificial Airways

General Care Measures

1. Ensure adequate ventilation and oxygenation through the use of supplemental oxygen or mechanical ventilation as indicated.

2. Assess breath sounds every 2 hours. Note evidence of ineffective secretion clearance (rhonchi, crackles), which suggests need for suctioning.

3. Provide adequate humidity when the natural humidifying pathway of the oropharynx is bypassed.

4. Provide adequate suctioning of oral secretions to prevent aspiration and decrease oral microbial colonization.

5. Use clean technique when inserting an oral or nasopharyngeal airway, and take it out and clean it with hydrogen peroxide and rinse with water at least every 8 hours.

6. Perform frequent oral care with soft toothbrush or swabs and antiseptic mouthwash or hydrogen peroxide diluted with water. Frequent oral care will aid in prevention of ventilator-associated pneumonia. The patient's lips should be kept moisturized with petroleum jelly to prevent them from becoming sore and cracked.

7. Ensure that aseptic technique is maintained when inserting an ET or tracheostomy tube. The artificial airway bypasses the upper airway, and the lower airways are sterile below the level of the vocal cords.

8. Elevate the patient to a semi-Fowler's or sitting position, when possible; these positions result in improved lung compliance. The patient's position, however, should be changed at least every 2 hours to ensure ventilation of all lung segments and prevent secretion stagnation and atelectasis. Position changes are also necessary to avoid skin breakdown.

9. If an oral or nasopharyngeal airway is used, turn patient's head to the side to reduce the risk of aspiration (because there is no cuff to seal off the lower airway).

Nutritional Considerations

1. Consciousness is usually impaired in patient with an oropharyngeal airway, so oral feeding is contraindicated.

2. To enhance comfort, remove a nasopharyngeal airway in the conscious patient during mealtimes.

3. Recognize that an ET tube holds the epiglottis open. Therefore, only the inflated cuff prevents the aspiration of oropharyngeal contents into the lungs. The patient must not receive oral feeding. Administer enteral tube feedings or parenteral feedings, as ordered.

4. Administer oral feedings to a conscious patient with a tracheostomy, usually with the cuff inflated. The inflated cuff prevents aspiration of food contents into the lungs, but causes the tracheal wall to bulge into the esophageal lumen, and may make swallowing more difficult.

    Patients who are not on mechanical ventilation and are awake, alert, and able to protect the airway are candidates for eating with the cuff deflated.

5. To assess ability to protect the airway, sit the patient upright and feed the patient colored gelatin or juice. If color from gelatin can be suctioned from the tracheostomy tube, aspiration is occurring, and the cuff must be inflated during feeding and for 1 hour afterward with head of bed elevated.

6. Patients should receive thickened rather than regular liquids; this will assist in effective swallowing.

 NURSING ALERT Consider the patient's nutritional needs early in the process of intubation so nutritional status does not decline further. It is difficult to wean patients who have compromised nutritional status.

Cuff Maintenance

1. ET tube cuffs should be inflated continuously and deflated only during intubation, extubation, and tube repositioning.

2. Tracheostomy tube cuffs also should be inflated continuously in patients on mechanical ventilation or continuous positive airway pressure (CPAP).

3. Tracheostomized patients who are breathing spontaneously may have the cuff inflated continuously (in the patient with decreased LOC without ability to fully protect airway), deflated continuously, or inflated only for feeding if the patient is at risk of aspiration.

4. Monitor cuff pressure every 4 hours (see Procedure Guidelines 10-5, pages 220 to 222).

External Tube Site Care

1. Secure an ET tube so it cannot be disrupted by the weight of ventilator or oxygen tubing or by patient movement.
    a. Use strips of adhesive tape or Velcro straps wrapped around the tube and secured to tape on patient's cheeks or around the back of patient's head.
    b. Replace when soiled or insecure or when repositioning of tube is necessary.
    c. Position tubing so traction is not applied to ET tube.

2. Perform tracheostomy site care at least every 8 hours using hydrogen peroxide and water, and change tracheostomy ties at least once per day (see Procedure Guidelines 10-6, pages 223 to 224).
    a. Make sure ventilator or oxygen tubing is supported so traction is not applied to the tracheostomy tube.

3. Have available at all times at the patient's bedside a replacement ET tube in the same size as patient is using, resuscitation bag, oxygen source, and mask to ventilate the patient in the event of accidental tube removal. Anticipate your course of action in such an event.
    a. ET tube—know location and assembly of reintubation equipment including replacement ET tube. Know how to contact someone immediately for reintubation.
    b. Tracheostomy—have extra tracheostomy tube, obturator, and hemostats at bedside. Be aware of reinsertion technique, if facility policy permits, or know how to contact someone immediately for reinserting the tube.

 NURSING ALERT In the event of accidental ET or tracheostomy tube removal, use a bag/mask resuscitation device to ventilate the patient by mouth while covering tracheostomy stoma. However, if the patient has complete upper airway obstruction, a gaping stoma, or a laryngectomy, mouth-to-stoma ventilation must be performed.

Psychological Considerations

1. Assist patient to deal with psychological aspects related to artificial airway.

2. Recognize that patient is usually apprehensive, particularly about choking, inability to communicate verbally, inability to remove secretions, uncomfortable suctioning, difficulty in breathing, or mechanical failure.

3. Explain the function of the equipment carefully.

4. Inform patient and family that speaking will not be possible while the tube is in place, unless using a tracheostomy tube with a deflated cuff, a fenestrated tube, a Passy-Muir speaking valve, or a speaking tracheostomy tube.
    a. A Passy-Muir valve is a speaking valve that fits over the end of the tracheostomy tube. Air that is inhaled is exhaled through the vocal cords and out through the mouth, allowing speech.

(*Text continues on page 222*)

PROCEDURE GUIDELINES 10-5

Artificial Airway Cuff Maintenance

EQUIPMENT

- Suction catheter
- Tonsil suction
- Suction source
- 10-mL syringe
- Pressure manometer (mercury or aneroid)
- Handheld resuscitation bag with reservoir, connected to 100% O_2 at 10–15 L/minute
- Face shield

PROCEDURE

Nursing Action	Rationale
Preparatory phase	
1. Explain the procedure to the patient.	1. Decreases the patient's anxiety and promotes cooperation.
2. Put on the face shield.	2. Spraying of secretions may occur.
Performance phase	
Deflating the cuff	
1. Suction the trachea, then the oral and nasal pharynx. Replace the catheter with a second sterile suction catheter.	1. Removes secretions collected above the cuff, which could be aspirated into the lungs when the cuff is deflated. Do not reenter the trachea with the same catheter used for suctioning the mouth.
2. Deflate the cuff slowly.	2. The small test balloon at the end of the tubing remains inflated as long as the cuff at the distal end of the tube is inflated. A vacuum within the syringe is sensed when no more air can be aspirated.
3. (Concomitant with step 2.) Have the patient cough or manually inflate the lungs with the resuscitation bag. Be ready to receive secretions in a tissue or aspirate with tonsil suction.	3. Positive pressure in the airways may help force secretions upward and prevent aspiration of secretions.
4. Suction through the tracheostomy or ET tube.	4. Secretions that may have been present above the inflated cuff and around the exterior tube have now seeped downward. Coughing reflex may be stimulated, helping to mobilize secretions.

5. Provide adequate ventilation while the cuff is deflated.
   a. If the patient does not require assisted ventilation, maintain humidified oxygen, as directed.
   b. If the patient requires assisted ventilation, provide manual ventilation via a resuscitation bag. Leave cuff deflated for as long as the tube repositioning requires; then reinflate.
	5.
	
	b. Monitor the patient closely for tolerance. Loss of tidal volume or PEEP may promote hypoxemia and hypocarbia. Cuff should not be deflated for more than 30 to 45 seconds.

Inflating a cuff	

1. No leak technique.
   a. Attach air-filled syringe to cuff injection port.
   b. Slowly inject air until no air escapes from the patient's lungs around the cuff.
   c. Note amount of air injected to provide a seal.
	1. Air leakage will be heard when the intra-airway pressure is most positive (maximum peak airway pressure). For the spontaneously breathing patient, air leakage will be heard on exhalation. For the patient on positive pressure ventilation, air leakage will be heard at maximum ventilator inspiration.

PROCEDURE GUIDELINES 10-5 *(continued)*

Artificial Airway Cuff Maintenance

PROCEDURE *(continued)*

Nursing Action	Rationale
2. Minimal leak technique (for mechanical ventilation).	2. Inflates cuff at lowest possible pressure while still maintaining an adequate seal. Prevents tracheal necrosis from excessive or prolonged cuff pressure.
a. Attach air-filled syringe to cuff injection port.	
b. Slowly inject air until no leak is heard at maximum peak airway pressure.	
c. Slowly remove air from cuff until a small air leak is heard at maximum peak airway pressure.	c. Adjustment in V_T setting may be necessary to compensate for the leak.
d. Note amount of air injected.	
3. Measurement of minimal occluding volume (see accompanying figure).	3.
a. Inject sufficient air into the manometer tubing to raise the dial reading 1 cm H_2O above the zero reading.	a. This "pressurizes" the tubing and prevents loss of air from the cuff to the tubing when the reading is taken.
b. Insert male port of three-way stopcock into cuff injection port. One female port of stopcock holds the air-filled syringe, and one port holds the pressure manometer.	

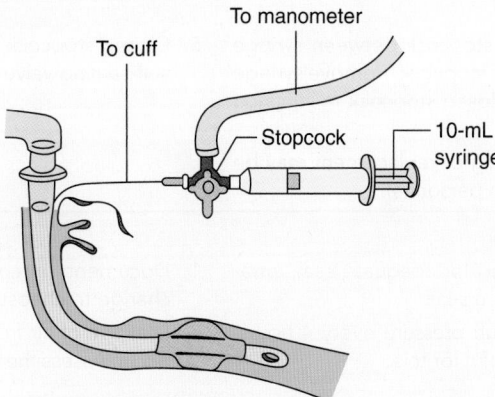

Airway cuff pressure is measured by opening stopcock to the cuff and manometer. Air is injected into the cuff by opening the stopcock to the syringe and cuff.

c. Inject air into cuff until desired intracuff pressure is reached at maximum peak airway pressure.	c. Aneroid manometer measures cuff pressure in cm H_2O: A pressure of 20–25 cm H_2O is desired. Mercury manometer pressure should be 15–20 mm Hg. Pressure greater than upper limit may cause compression of tracheal vessels, resulting in decreased blood flow to tissue. Pressure less than lower limit may allow aspiration of gastric or oral secretions.
d. Note amount of air needed to achieve the desired intracuff pressure.	
e. Remove the stopcock from the injection port.	e. Most injection ports have self-sealing valves. If not, a cap or closed stopcock may be left in the injection port (clamping of the inflation tubing is discouraged because it may result in cracking or kinking of the line permanently).

(continued)

PROCEDURE GUIDELINES 10-5 *(continued)*

Artificial Airway Cuff Maintenance

PROCEDURE *(continued)*

Nursing Action	Rationale
Monitoring cuff pressure	
1. While the cuff is inflated, monitor cuff pressure every 4 hours. Maintain cuff pressure between 20 and 25 mm Hg or 25 and 35 cm H_2O.	1. Excessive pressure will decrease blood flow to the tissue, resulting in tracheal necrosis. Insufficient cuff pressure predisposes to aspiration.
2. Document the amount of air required to maintain cuff pressure at this level.	2. Establishes a baseline for evaluation of change in pressure.
Inability to maintain a seal	
1. Assess the degree of leakage and length of time elapsed since cuff volume was replenished.	1. If an inflated cuff leaks air within 10 minutes, assessment is necessary. Possibilities may be: a. Cuff positioned above the vocal cords (direct visualization necessary for repositioning). b. Incompetence of self-sealing valve on injection port. c. Tracheal dilation (requiring larger size tube). d. Cuff may be ruptured, requiring a new tube.
2. Inflate the cuff to desired level.	
3. Disconnect syringe (and manometer, if used).	
4. Assess for leakage.	
5. If leakage recurs, place three-way stopcock between syringe and injection port, inflate cuff, close stopcock. Remove syringe (and manometer, if used) leaving closed stopcock in injection port.	5. Closed stopcock left in injection port acts as "plug" if self-sealing valve is incompetent.
6. If air leak persists, tube repositioning or replacement may be necessary. Consult with appropriate personnel.	

Follow-up phase

Nursing Action	Rationale
1. Note and record amount of air used for adequate seal, intra-cuff pressure, and inability to achieve seal.	1. Documents interventions necessary to reintubate or change tracheostomy tube to obtain a desired seal.
2. While the cuff is inflated, assess cuff pressure every 4 hours. The cuff pressure manometer is useful for this.	2. Leakage of air from the cuff or cuff injection port may occur. Assess the inflation status and adjust as needed.

 Evidence Base Ahrens, T., Prentice, D., & Kleinpell, R. (2010). *Critical care nursing certification: Preparation, review and practice exam* (6th ed.) New York: McGraw-Hill.

5. Develop with patient the best method of communication (eg, sign language, lip movement, letter boards, paper and pencil, magic slate, or coded messages).
   a. Patients with tracheostomy tubes or nasal ET tubes may effectively use orally operated electrolarynx devices.
   b. Devise a means for patient to get the nurse's attention when someone is not immediately available at the bedside, such as call bell, hand-operated bell, or rattle.
6. Anticipate some of patient's questions by discussing "Is it permanent?" "Will it hurt to breathe?" "Will someone be with me?"
7. If appropriate, advise patient that as condition improves, a tracheostomy button may be used to plug the tracheostomy

site. A tracheostomy button is a rigid, closed cannula that is placed into the tracheostomy stoma after removal of a cuffed or uncuffed tracheostomy tube. When in proper position, the button does not extend into the tracheal lumen. The outer edge of the button is at the skin surface and the inner edge is at the anterior tracheal wall (see Procedure Guidelines 10-7).

 NURSING ALERT With the use of artificial airways, remember the patient may use a call bell, he or she will not be able to communicate verbally (unless device is used to allow speech).

(Text continues on page 226)

PROCEDURE GUIDELINES 10-6

Tracheostomy Care (Routine)

EQUIPMENT

Assemble the following equipment or obtain a prepackaged tracheostomy care kit:

- Sterile towel
- Sterile gauze pads (10)
- Sterile cotton swabs

- Sterile gloves
- Hydrogen peroxide
- Sterile water
- Antiseptic solution and ointment (optional)

- Tracheostomy tie tapes or commercially available tracheostomy securing device
- Face shield

PROCEDURE

Nursing Action	Rationale
Preparatory phase	
1. Assess the condition of the stoma before tracheostomy care (redness, swelling, character of secretions, presence of purulence or bleeding).	1. The presence of skin breakdown or infection must be monitored. Culture of the site may be warranted by appearance of these signs.
2. Examine the neck for subcutaneous crepitus.	2. Indicates air leak into subcutaneous tissue.
3. Suction the trachea and pharynx thoroughly before tracheostomy care.	3. Removal of secretions before tracheostomy care keeps the area clean longer.
4. Explain the procedure to the patient.	4. Allays anxiety.
5. Wash hands thoroughly.	5. Reduces risk of infection.
Performance phase	
1. Assemble equipment:	1.
a. Place sterile towel on patient's chest under tracheostomy site.	a. Provides sterile field.
b. Open four gauze pads and pour hydrogen peroxide on them.	b. For removal of mucus and crust, which promotes bacterial growth.
c. Open two gauze pads and pour antiseptic solution on them.	c. May be applied to fresh stoma or infected stoma. Not necessary for clean, healed stoma.
d. Open two gauze pads; keep dry.	
e. Open two gauze pads and pour sterile water on them.	
f. Place tracheostomy tube tapes on field.	
g. Put on face shield and sterile gloves.	g. Face shield prevents secretions from getting into the nurse's eyes. Sterile gloves prevent contamination of the wound by nurse's hands and also protect the nurse's hands from infection.
2. Clean the external end of the tracheostomy tube with two gauze pads with hydrogen peroxide; discard pads.	2. Designate the hand you clean with as contaminated and reserve the other hand as sterile for handling sterile equipment.
3. Unlock and remove inner cannula, if present.	3. Many tracheostomies do not have an inner cannula.
4. If disposable inner cannula is used, replace with new cannula (with your clean hand), touching only external portion, and lock it securely in place.	4. To avoid contamination of inner portion.
5. If inner cannula is reusable, remove it with your contaminated hand and clean it in hydrogen peroxide solution, using brush or pipe cleaners with your sterile hand. When clean, drop it into sterile saline solution and agitate it to rinse thoroughly with your sterile hand. Tap it gently to dry it and replace it with your sterile hand.	5. Because cannula is dirty when you remove it, use your contaminated hand. It is considered sterile once you clean it, so handle it with your sterile hand.

(continued)

PROCEDURE GUIDELINES 10-6 *(continued)*

Tracheostomy Care (Routine)

PROCEDURE *(continued)*

Nursing Action	Rationale
6. Clean the stoma area with two peroxide-soaked gauze pads. Make only a single sweep with each gauze pad before discarding.	6. Hydrogen peroxide may help loosen dry, crusted secretions.
7. Loosen and remove crust with sterile cotton swabs.	
8. Repeat step 6 using the sterile water-soaked gauze pads.	8. Ensures that all hydrogen peroxide is removed.
9. Repeat step 6 using dry pads.	9. Ensures dryness of the area. Wetness promotes infection and irritation.
10. (optional) An infected wound may be cleaned with gauze saturated with an antiseptic solution, then dried. A thin layer of antibiotic ointment may be applied to the stoma with a cotton swab.	10. May help clear wound infection.

11. Change the tracheostomy tie tapes:
   a. Cut soiled tape while holding tube securely with other hand. Use care not to cut the pilot balloon tubing.
 	
   b. Remove old tapes carefully.
   c. Grasp slit end of clean tape and pull it through opening on side of the tracheostomy tube.
   d. Pull other end of tape securely through the slit end of the tape.
   e. Repeat on the other side.
   f. Tie the tapes at the side of the neck in a square knot. Alternate knot from side to side each time tapes are changed.
 	
   g. Ties should be tight enough to keep tube securely in the stoma, but loose enough to permit two fingers to fit between the tapes and the neck.
	11.
	   a. Stabilization of the tube helps prevent accidental dislodgement and keeps irritation and coughing due to tube manipulation at a minimum.
	
	   f. Prevents irritation and rotates pressure site.
	
	   g. Excessive tightness of tapes will compress jugular veins, decrease blood circulation to the skin under the tape, and result in discomfort for the patient.

12. Place a gauze pad between the stoma site and the tracheostomy tube per facility policy (see accompanying figure).	12. Gauze absorbs secretions and prevents irritation of peristomal tissue; however, it may promote infection if moisture builds up.

 NURSING ALERT If only one clinician is available, the stoma is new (less than 2 weeks), or the patient's condition is unstable, follow steps c through f before removing old tapes. Two sets of ties will be in place at the same time. After completing step f, cut and remove the old tapes. Also, a tracheostomy-securing device can be used instead of the tracheostomy ties.

Follow-up phase

1. Document procedure performance, observations of stoma (irritation, redness, edema, subcutaneous air), and character of secretions (color, purulence). Report changes in stoma appearance or secretions.	1. Provides a baseline.
2. Clean the fresh stoma every 8 hours or more frequently if indicated by accumulation of secretions. Ties should be changed every 24 hours, or more frequently if soiled or wet.	2. The area must be kept clean and dry to prevent infection or irritation of tissues.

PROCEDURE GUIDELINES 10-6 *(continued)*

Tracheostomy Care (Routine)

PROCEDURE *(continued)*

Nursing Action	Rationale

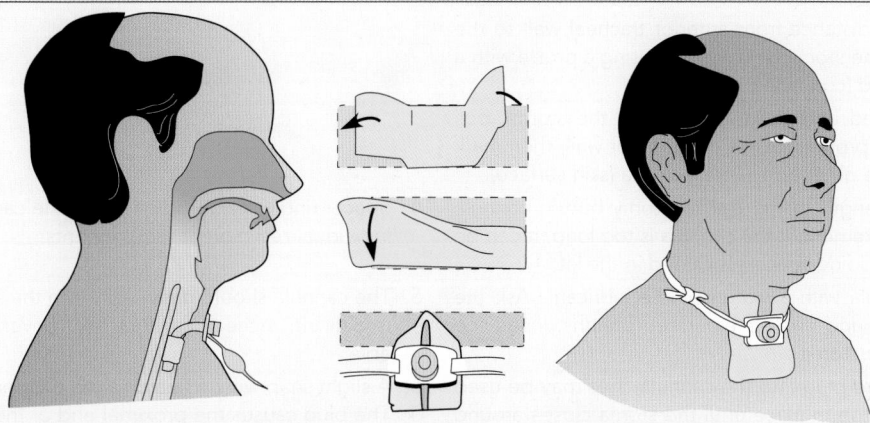

Placement of tracheostomy tube ties and elective gauze pad.

📖 **Evidence Base** Chulay, M., & Burns, S. (2010). *AACN essentials of critical care nursing.* New York: McGraw-Hill.

Johnson, W., & Meyers, A. (2012). Tracheostomy tube change. *Medscape Reference.* Available: http://emedicine.medscape.com/article/1580576-overview.

Hurst T., & Thomas A. (2010) Airway safety in adult intensive care. *Care of the Critically Ill, 25*(3–4), 65–69.

PROCEDURE GUIDELINES 10-7

Insertion of a Tracheostomy Button

EQUIPMENT

- Appropriate-size tracheostomy button kit (includes cannula, solid closure plug, spacers, universal adapter)
- Water-soluble lubricant
- Syringe for deflation of tracheostomy cuff
- Replacement of tracheostomy tube
- Flashlight
- Gloves

PROCEDURE

Nursing Action	Rationale
Preparatory phase	
1. Assess whether the patient meets the criteria for use of a tracheostomy button. Criteria include able to be adequately oxygenated with nasal cannula or face mask; able to swallow and protect the airway; able to cough up secretions; and a noninfected, nonirritated tracheal stoma.	1. If the patient does not meet these criteria, use of tracheostomy tube as airway must be continued.
2. Determine vital signs, LOC, SaO_2, or ABG.	2. Provides baseline for future assessment.
Performance phase	
1. Elevate the head of the bed 45 degrees, suction the airway, deflate the tracheostomy tube cuff, and remove the tube.	1. Protects against aspiration.

(continued)

PROCEDURE GUIDELINES 10-7 *(continued)*

Insertion of a Tracheostomy Button

PROCEDURE *(continued)*

Nursing Action	Rationale
2. Determine the distance from anterior tracheal wall to the outer edge of the stoma (skin surface) using a probe with a right-angle bend (contained in the kit).	
3. Insert the angled end of the probe into the stoma, pull gently until the probe touches the anterior wall, then mark the probe at the outer edge of the stoma (skin surface).	
4. Compare the length of the tracheostomy button cannula with this measurement. If the cannula is too long, it can be sized to fit by adding spacers included in the kit.	4. Spacer rings can be slipped over the cannula to size it for individualized patient requirements.
5. Coat the cannula with a water-soluble lubricant. Ask the patient to relax and take several deep breaths. Insert the cannula into the stoma.	5. The cannula should pass easily into the stoma. If insertion is difficult, recheck cannula size. Several sizes are available.
6. Insert the closure plug into the cannula. Ties may be used to hold the button in place until the stoma closes around the button.	6. A slight snap will be heard as the plug enters the cannula. The plug causes the proximal end of the cannula to flare, holding it in place.
7. Remove the button two times per week, clean with antibacterial soap, rinse with sterile water, and replace it.	7. Periodic removal helps to keep tissue from granulating into the distal portion of the cannula.

Follow-up phase

1. Observe immediate patient response and obtain SaO_2 or ABGs after insertion. Report changes.	1. Use of the button increases dead space, which may increase work of breathing or cause a decrease in SaO_2.
2. Determine ability of patient to cough out secretions and swallow with button in place.	2. Confirms the patient will not retain secretions or be at risk for aspiration with use of this device.

 Evidence Base Ahrens, T., Prentice, D., & Kleinpell, R. (2010). *Critical care nursing certification: Preparation, review and practice exam* (6th ed.). New York: McGraw-Hill.

Community and Home Care Considerations

1. Teach patient and/or caregiver procedure. Patient will need to use stationary mirror to visualize tracheostomy and perform procedure.
2. Suctioning patient in the home: whenever possible, patient and/or caregiver should be taught to perform procedure. Patient should use controlled cough and other secretion-clearance techniques.
3. Preoxygenation and hyperinflation before suctioning may not be routinely indicated for all patients cared for in the home. Preoxygenation and hyperinflation are based on patient need and clinical status.
4. Normal saline should not be instilled unless clinically indicated (eg, to stimulate cough).
5. Clean technique and clean examination gloves are used. At the end of suctioning, the catheter or tonsil tip should be flushed by suctioning recently boiled and cooled, or distilled, water to rinse away mucus, followed by suctioning air through the apparatus. The outer surface may be wiped with alcohol or hydrogen peroxide. The catheter and tonsil tip should be air-dried and stored in a clean, dry place. Generally, suction catheters should be discarded after 24 hours. Tonsil tips may be boiled and reused.
6. Care of tracheostomy stoma: clean with half-strength hydrogen peroxide (diluted with sterile water) and wipe with sterile water or sterile saline.

Mobilization of Secretions

The goal of airway clearance techniques is to improve clearance of airway secretions, thereby decreasing obstruction of the airways. This serves to improve ventilation and gas exchange. Patients with respiratory disorders, neuromuscular disorders, or CNS disorders, such as loss of consciousness that may impair respiratory function, typically require help with mobilization and removal of secretions. Increased amount and viscosity of secretions and/or inability to clear secretions through the normal cough mechanism may lead to pooling of secretions in lower airways. Pooling of secretions leads to infection and inadequate gas exchange. Secretions should be removed by coughing or, when necessary, by suctioning. However, routine suctioning should be avoided. Auscultation and visual inspection of the patient should be used to determine the need for suctioning. Secretions can be mobilized through the chest physical therapy measures of postural drainage, directed cough, positive expiratory pressure (PEP), high-frequency oscillation (oral devices such as Flutter or Acapella device, or chest devices such as the Vest) mucus clearance devices, autogenic drainage, intrapulmonary vibration, percussion and vibration, and other secretion-clearance measures. Research shows potentially limited benefit versus risk for percussion and vibration. Breathing exercises are done with chest physical therapy to increase the efficiency of breathing.

Nasotracheal Suctioning

1. Intended to remove accumulated secretions or other materials that cannot be moved by the patient's spontaneous cough or less-invasive procedures. Suctioning of the tracheobronchial tree in a patient without an artificial airway can be accomplished by inserting a sterile suction catheter lubricated with water-soluble jelly through the nares into the nasal passage, down through the oropharynx, past the glottis, and into the trachea (see Procedure Guidelines 10-8).

(*Text continues on page 233*)

PROCEDURE GUIDELINES 10-8

Nasotracheal Suctioning

EQUIPMENT

- Assemble the following equipment or obtain a prepackaged kit:
- Disposable suction catheter (preferably soft rubber)
- Sterile towel

- Sterile disposable gloves
- Sterile water
- Water-soluble lubricant jelly
- Suction source at −80 to −120 mm Hg

- Resuscitation bag with face mask. Connect 100% O_2 source with flow of 10 L/minute
- Oximeter

PROCEDURE

Nursing Action	Rationale
Preparatory phase	
1. Auscultate breath sounds, monitor heart rate, respiratory rate, color, ease of respirations. If the patient is on monitor, continue monitoring heart rate or arterial BP.	1. Baseline assessment is important because suctioning may cause hypoxemia, resulting in tachycardia and increased BP, and later causing cardiac ectopy, bradycardia, hypotension, and cyanosis. Vagal stimulation may result in bradycardia.

Key Decision Point

Discontinue the suctioning and apply oxygen if heart rate decreases by 20 beats/minute or increases by | 40 beats/minute, if BP increases, or if cardiac dysrhythmia is noted.

Nursing Action	Rationale
2. Make sure that the suction apparatus is functional. Place suction tubing within easy reach.	2. Ensures functionality before beginning the procedure.
3. Inform and instruct the patient about the procedure.	3. A thorough explanation will decrease patient anxiety and promote patient cooperation.
a. At a certain interval, the patient will be requested to cough to open the lung passage so the catheter will go into the lungs and not into the stomach. The patient will also be encouraged to try not to swallow because this will also cause the catheter to enter the stomach.	
b. The postoperative patient can splint the wound to make the coughing produced by NT suctioning less painful.	
4. Place the patient in a semi-Fowler's or sitting position, if possible.	4. Upright position eases breathing and helps mobilize secretions.

NURSING ALERT Avoid suctioning immediately after feeding to reduce the risk of vomiting and possible aspiration.

Nursing Action	Rationale
5. Monitor oxygen saturation via oximetry and heart rate during suctioning.	5. Detects hypoxia during the procedure.

(continued)

PROCEDURE GUIDELINES 10-8 (continued)

Nasotracheal Suctioning

PROCEDURE (continued)

Nursing Action	Rationale

Performance phase

1. Open the sterile pack containing flexible suction catheter. Maintain inside of the package as sterile, and arrange equipment after donning sterile gloves.

2. Aseptically glove both hands. Designate one hand (usually the dominant one) as "sterile" and the other hand as "contaminated."

3. Grasp the sterile catheter with the sterile hand.

3. Lubricate catheter with the water-soluble jelly and pass the catheter into the nostril and back into the pharynx.

1. Catheter entering trachea should not be contaminated.

2. The "contaminated" hand must also be gloved to protect the nurse from organisms in the sputum.

3. Lubricate adequately and proceed carefully to prevent trauma to tissue that may bleed easily.

 NURSING ALERT If obstruction is met while passing the catheter through the nose and nasopharynx, do not force the catheter. Remove it and try the other nostril.

4. Pass the catheter into the trachea. To do this, ask the patient to cough or say "ahh." If the patient is incapable of either, try to advance the catheter on inspiration. Asking the patient to stick out tongue, or hold tongue extended with a gauze pad, may also help to open the airway.

4. These maneuvers may aid in opening the glottis and allowing passage of the catheter into the trachea.

 Key Decision Point

To evaluate proper placement of the suction catheter in the trachea, listen at the catheter end for air or feel for air movement against the cheek. An increase in intensity of breath sounds or more air movement against cheek indicates nearness to the larynx. Gagging or sudden lessening of sound means the catheter is in the hypopharynx. Draw back and advance again. The presence of the catheter in the trachea is indicated by:

- Sudden paroxysms of coughing.
- Movement of air through the catheter.
- Vigorous bubbling of air when the distal end of the suction catheter is placed in a cup of sterile water.
- Inability of the patient to speak.

If three attempts to place the catheter are unsuccessful, request assistance. If a protracted amount of time is needed to position the catheter in the trachea, stop and oxygenate the patient with face mask or the resuscitation bag-mask unit at intervals.

5. Specific positioning of catheter for deep bronchial suctioning:
   a. For left bronchial suctioning, turn the patient's head to the extreme right, chin up.
   b. For right bronchial suctioning, turn the patient's head to the extreme left, chin up.
      Note: The value of turning the head as an aid to entering the right or left mainstem bronchi is not accepted by all clinicians.

6. Never apply suction until catheter is in the trachea. Once the correct position is ascertained, apply suction and gently rotate catheter while pulling it slightly upward. Do not remove catheter from the trachea.

5. Turning the patient's head to one side elevates the bronchial passage on the opposite side, making catheter insertion easier. Suctioning of a particular lung segment may be of value in patients with unilateral pneumonia, atelectasis, or collapse.

6. Because entry into the trachea is often difficult, less change in arterial oxygen may be caused by leaving the catheter in the trachea than by repeated insertion attempts.

PROCEDURE GUIDELINES 10-8 *(continued)*

Nasotracheal Suctioning

PROCEDURE *(continued)*

Nursing Action	Rationale
7. Disconnect the catheter from the suctioning source after 5–10 seconds. Apply oxygen by placing a face mask over the patient's nose, mouth, and catheter, and instruct the patient to breathe deeply.	7. Allows for reoxygenation during the procedure.
8. Reconnect the suction source. Repeat as necessary.	8. More than one suction attempt may be necessary to remove secretions; however, hypoxemia and trauma to the tissues may result from multiple suction attempts.

 NURSING ALERT No more than three to four suction passes should be made per suction episode.

Nursing Action	Rationale
9. During the last suction pass, remove the catheter completely while applying suction and rotating the catheter gently. Apply oxygen when the catheter is removed.	9. Removes secretions in the proximal airway.

 NURSING ALERT Never leave the catheter in the trachea after the suction procedure is concluded because the epiglottis is splinted open and aspiration may occur.

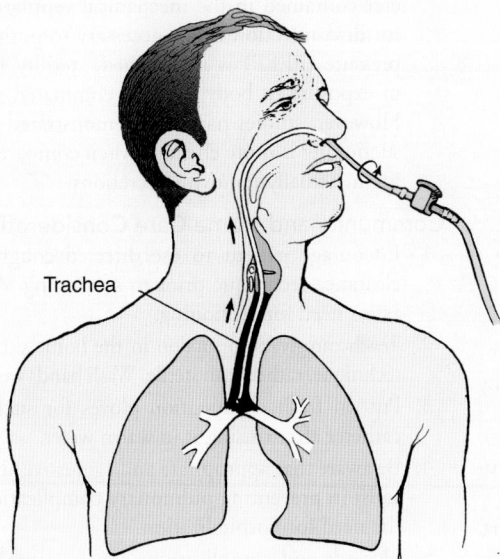

Trachea

Placement of nasotracheal catheter for suctioning the tracheobronchial tree.

Follow-up phase

1. Dispose of disposable equipment.
2. Auscultate breath sounds. Measure heart rate, BP, respiratory rate, and oxygen saturation. Record the patient's tolerance of procedure, type and amount of secretions removed, and complications.

1. Infection control.
2. Assesses for hypoxemia, trauma, or other complications.

(continued)

PROCEDURE GUIDELINES 10-8 *(continued)*

Nasotracheal Suctioning

PROCEDURE *(continued)*

Nursing Action	Rationale
3. Report any patient intolerance of procedure (changes in vital signs, bleeding, laryngospasm, upper airway noise).	3. For possible adjustment on future suctioning attempts.

 Evidence Base American Association for Respiratory Care. (2010). Clinical practice guidelines. Endotracheal suctioning of mechanically ventilated patients with artificial airways. *Respiratory Care*, 55(6), 758–764.

2. NT suction is a blind, high-risk procedure with uncertain outcome. Complications include mechanical trauma, hypoxia, dysrhythmias, bradycardia, increased BP, vomiting, increased ICP, and misdirection of catheter.
3. Contraindications include:
   a. Bleeding disorders, such as disseminated intravascular coagulation, thrombocytopenia, leukemia.
   b. Laryngeal edema, laryngeal spasm.
   c. Esophageal varices.
   d. Tracheal surgery.
   e. Gastric surgery with high anastomosis.
   f. Myocardial infarction.
   g. Occluded nasal passages or nasal bleeding.
   h. Epiglottitis.
   i. Head, facial, or neck injury.
4. May cause trauma to the nasal passages.
   a. Do not attempt to force the catheter if resistance is met.
   b. Report if significant bleeding occurs.

 **NURSING ALERT** NT suctioning should not be routinely performed. Only indicated when other methods to remove secretions from airway have failed.

5. Insert a nasal airway if repeated suctioning is necessary to protect the nasal passages from trauma.
6. Be alert for signs of laryngeal edema due to irritation and trauma.
   a. Stop if suctioning becomes difficult or if the patient develops new upper airway noise or obstruction.
   b. Duration of the suctioning should be limited to less than 15 seconds.

Suctioning Through an Endotracheal or Tracheostomy Tube

1. Ineffective coughing may cause secretion collection in the artificial airway or tracheobronchial tree, resulting in narrowing of the airway, respiratory insufficiency, and stasis of secretions.
2. Assess the need for suctioning at least every 2 hours through auscultation of the chest.
   a. Ventilation with a manual resuscitation bag will facilitate auscultation and may stimulate coughing, decreasing the need for suctioning.
3. Maintain sterile technique while suctioning (see Procedure Guidelines 10-9, pages 231 to 233).
4. Administer supplemental 100% oxygen through the mechanical ventilator or manual resuscitation bag before, after, and between suctioning passes to prevent hypoxemia.
5. Closed-system suctioning may be done with the suction catheter contained in the mechanical ventilator tubing. Ventilator disconnection is not necessary so positive end-expiratory pressure (PEEP) is maintained, sterility is maintained, risk of exposure to body fluids is eliminated, and time is saved. However, studies have not demonstrated that closed-system suctioning is more effective when compared to open suctioning in actually removing secretions.

Community and Home Care Considerations

1. Encourage patient to use directed cough or other airway-clearance technique prior to suctioning. Auscultate lungs to assess need for suctioning.
2. Teach caregivers to suction in the home situation using a clean technique, rather than sterile. Wash hands well before suctioning.
3. Put on fresh examination gloves for suctioning, and reuse catheter after rinsing it in warm water.
4. Be aware that appropriate and aggressive airway clearance will assist in preventing pulmonary complications, thus lessening the need for hospitalization.
5. Hazards and complications are the same for the home care patient as they are for a hospitalized patient.

Chest Physical Therapy

Breathing Exercises

1. Techniques used to compensate for respiratory deficits and conserve energy by increasing efficiency of breathing. Have patient breathe in through the nose and out through the mouth at a ratio of 1:2.
2. The overall purposes for doing breathing exercises are:
   a. To relax muscles, relieve anxiety, and improve control of breathing.

PROCEDURE GUIDELINES 10-9

Sterile Tracheobronchial Suction by Way of Tracheostomy or Endotracheal Tube (Spontaneous or Mechanical Ventilation)

EQUIPMENT

Assemble the following equipment or obtain a prepackaged suctioning kit:
- Sterile suction catheters—No. 14 or 16 (adult), No. 8 or 10 (child). The outer diameter of the suction catheter should be no greater than one-half the inner diameter of the artificial airway.
- Two sterile gloves

- Sterile towel
- Suction source at 80–120 mm Hg (pressure varies neonatal to adult)
- Sterile water
- Resuscitation bag with a reservoir connected to 100% oxygen source (if patient is on positive end-expiratory pressure [PEEP] or continuous positive airway pressure

[CPAP], add PEEP valve to exhalation valve on resuscitation bag in an amount equal to that on the ventilator or CPAP device)
- Normal saline solution (in syringe or single-dose packet)—optional
- Sterile cup for water
- Sterile water-soluble lubricant jelly
- Face shield

PROCEDURE

Nursing Action	Rationale
Preparatory phase	
1. Monitor heart rate and auscultate breath sounds. If the patient is monitored, continuously monitor heart rate and arterial BP. If ABG are done routinely, know baseline values.	1. Baseline assessment is important because suctioning may cause hypoxemia, initially resulting in tachycardia and increased BP, progressing to cardiac ectopy, bradycardia, hypotension, and cyanosis. Vagal stimulation may result in bradycardia.
2. Explain the procedure to the patient.	2. Thorough explanation lessens patient's anxiety and promotes cooperation.

 NURSING ALERT Instruct postoperative patients how to "splint" surgical incisions because coughing will be induced during the procedure.

Nursing Action	Rationale
3. Assemble equipment. Check function of suction and manual resuscitation bag connected to 100% O_2 source.	3. Make sure that all equipment is functional before sterile technique is instituted to prevent interruption once the procedure is begun. Use of 100% O_2 will help to prevent hypoxemia.
4. Wash hands thoroughly. Put on face shield.	4. Reduces risk of infection transmission for patient and nurse.
5. If the patient is on mechanical ventilation, test to make sure disconnection of ventilator attachment may be made with one hand.	5. If unable to disconnect and reconnect ventilator tubing with nonsterile hand, will need a second person for assistance.
Performance phase	
1. Open suction catheter package and place on flat work surface and set up a sterile field.	1. Sterile field contains suction catheter, gloves, lubricant for catheter, and sterile water/saline for rinsing catheter.
2. Put on sterile gloves. Designate one hand as contaminated for disconnecting, bagging, and working the suction control. Usually the dominant hand is kept sterile and will be used to thread the suction catheter.	2. The hand designated as sterile must remain uncontaminated so organisms are not introduced into the lungs. The contaminated hand must also be gloved to prevent sputum from contacting the nurse's hand, possibly resulting in an infection of the nurse.
3. Use the sterile hand to remove carefully the suction catheter from the package, curling the catheter around the gloved fingers.	
4. Connect suction source to the suction fitting of the catheter with the contaminated hand.	

(continued)

PROCEDURE GUIDELINES 10-9 *(continued)*

Sterile Tracheobronchial Suction by Way of Tracheostomy or Endotracheal Tube (Spontaneous or Mechanical Ventilation)

PROCEDURE *(continued)*

Nursing Action	Rationale
5. Using the contaminated hand, disconnect the patient from the ventilator, CPAP device, or other oxygen source.	5. Using one hand prevents contamination of hand used for suctioning. If closed-circuit suction catheter is being used, the patient will not need to be disconnected from the ventilator and PEEP is maintained.
6. Ventilate and oxygenate the patient with the resuscitator bag, compressing firmly and as completely as possible approximately four to five times (try to approximate the patient's tidal volume). This procedure is called "bagging" the patient. In the spontaneously breathing patient, coordinate manual ventilations with the patient's own inspiratory effort.	6. Ventilation before suctioning helps prevent hypoxemia. When possible, two nurses or a nurse and a respiratory therapist work as a team to suction. Attempting to ventilate against the patient's own respiratory efforts may result in high airway pressures, predisposing the patient to barotrauma (lung injury due to pressure).
7. Gently insert suction catheter as far as possible into the artificial airway without applying suction. Most patients will cough when the catheter touches the carina.	7. Suctioning on insertion would unnecessarily decrease oxygen in the airway.
8. Withdraw the catheter ¾ inch to 1 inch (2–3 cm) and apply suction. Quickly rotate the catheter while it is being withdrawn.	8. Failure to withdraw and rotate catheter may result in damage to tracheal mucosa. Release suction if a pulling sensation is felt.

 Key Decision Point

Limit suction time to no more than 10 seconds to avoid hypoxemia. Discontinue if heart rate decreases by 20 beats/minute (due to vagal stimulation) or increases by 40 beats/minute, or if cardiac ectopy is observed (signs of hypoxemia).

Nursing Action	Rationale
9. Bag patient between suction passes with approximately four to five manual ventilations.	9. The oxygen removed by suctioning must be replenished before suctioning is attempted again to reduce hypoxemia.
10. Rinse catheter between suction passes by inserting tip in cup of sterile water/saline and applying suction. *Note:* Evidence does not support the use of saline installation.	10. Prevents obstruction of catheter.

 Evidence Base Farnan, C., & Patrick, M. (2010). Saline instillation: Helpful or harmful? Debates over saline instillation during suctioning have raged for years. *Advances for Respiratory and Sleep Medicine.* Available: *http://respiratory-care-sleep-medicine.advanceweb.com/Editorial/Content/PrintFriendly.aspx?CC=226385.* Maureen, A. Seckel, M. (2012). Normal saline and mucous plugging. *Critical Care Nurse, 32,* 66–68.

Nursing Action	Rationale
11. Continue making suction passes, bagging the patient between passes, until the airways are clear of accumulated secretions. Limit insertions of suction catheter to as few as needed (do not exceed four passes per suction episode).	11. Repeated suctioning of a patient in a short time interval predisposes to hypoxemia, as well as being tiring and potentially traumatic to tissue.
12. Give the patient four to five "sigh" breaths with the bag.	12. Sighing is accomplished by depressing the bag slowly and completely with two hands to deliver approximately 1½ times the normal tidal volume to the patient, allowing for maximal lung expansion and prevention of atelectasis.
13. Return the patient to the ventilator or apply CPAP or other oxygen-delivery device.	
14. Suction oral secretions from the oropharynx above the artificial airway cuff.	14. Prevents possible aspiration if the cuff becomes deflated.

PROCEDURE GUIDELINES 10-9 *(continued)*

Sterile Tracheobronchial Suction by Way of Tracheostomy or Endotracheal Tube (Spontaneous or Mechanical Ventilation)

PROCEDURE *(continued)*

Nursing Action	Rationale
15. Remove suction catheter from tubing and remove gloves, folding catheter into glove in dominant hand. Dispose of equipment.	15. Controls infection.

Follow-up phase

1. Note change in vital signs or patient's intolerance to the procedure. Record amount and consistency of secretions.	1. Evaluates and documents the effectiveness of procedure and patient response.
2 Assess need for further suctioning at least every 2 hours, or more frequently if secretions are copious.	2. Copious secretions can impair oxygenation.

Evidence Base Lucchini, A., Zanella, A., Bellani, G., et al. (2011). Tracheal secretion management in the mechanically ventilated patient: Comparison of standard assessment and an acoustic secretion detector. *Respiratory Care, 56*(5), 596–603.
Fahy, J., & Dickey, B. (2010). Airway mucus function and dysfunction. *New England Journal of Medicine, 363,* 2233–2247.

---

  b. To eliminate useless, uncoordinated patterns of respiratory muscle activity.

  c. To slow the respiratory rate.

  d. To decrease the work of breathing.

  e. To improve efficiency and strength of respiratory muscles.

  f. To improve ventilation and oxygen saturation during exercise.

3. Diaphragmatic abdominal breathing is used primarily to strengthen the diaphragm, which is the main muscle of respiration. It also aids in decreasing the use of accessory muscles and allows for better control over the breathing pattern, especially during stressful situations and increased physical demands.

4. Pursed-lip breathing is used primarily to slow the respiratory rate and assist in emptying the lungs of retained CO_2. This technique is always helpful to patients, but especially when they feel extreme dyspnea due to exertion.

5. Breathing exercises are most helpful to patients when practiced and used on a regular basis.

NURSING ALERT For patients with severe COPD, evidence does not support the use of diaphragmatic breathing because this type of breathing may result in hyperinflation as a result of increased dyspnea and fatigue.

Percussion and Vibration

1. Postural drainage uses gravity and, possibly, external manipulation of the thorax to improve mobilization of bronchial secretions, to enhance matching of ventilation and perfusion, and to normalize functional residual capacity.

2. Indicated for difficulty with secretion clearance, evidence of retained secretions, and lung conditions that cause increased production of secretions such as bronchiectasis, cystic fibrosis, chronic bronchitis, and emphysema.

3. Contraindicated in undrained lung abscess, lung tumors, pneumothorax, diseases of the chest wall, lung hemorrhage, painful chest conditions, tuberculosis, severe osteoporosis, increased ICP, uncontrolled hypertension, and gross hemoptysis.

4. Percussion is movement done by "clapping" the chest wall in a rhythmic fashion with cupped hands or a mechanical device directly over the lung segments to be drained. The wrists are alternately flexed and extended so the chest is cupped or clapped in a painless manner (see Procedure Guidelines 10-10, pages 234 to 236). A mechanical percussor may be used to prevent repetitive motion injury. This technique is considered by some to have limited research-based evidence of benefit versus risk.

5. Vibration is the technique of applying manual compression with oscillations or tremors to the chest wall during the exhalation phase of respiration. This technique is considered to have limited research-based evidence of benefit versus risk.

Postural Drainage

1. Use of specific positions so the force of gravity can assist in the removal of bronchial secretions from affected lung segments to central airways by means of coughing or suctioning (see Figure 10-4).

(Text continues on page 235)

PROCEDURE GUIDELINES 10-10

Percussion (Clapping) and Vibration

EQUIPMENT

- Pillows
- Sputum cup
- Tilt table
- Paper tissues
- Emesis basin

PROCEDURE

Nursing Action	Rationale

Performance phase

1. Instruct the patient to use diaphragmatic breathing.

2. Position the patient in prescribed postural drainage positions (see page 235). The spine should be straight to promote rib cage expansion.

1. Diaphragmatic breathing helps the patient relax and helps widen airways.

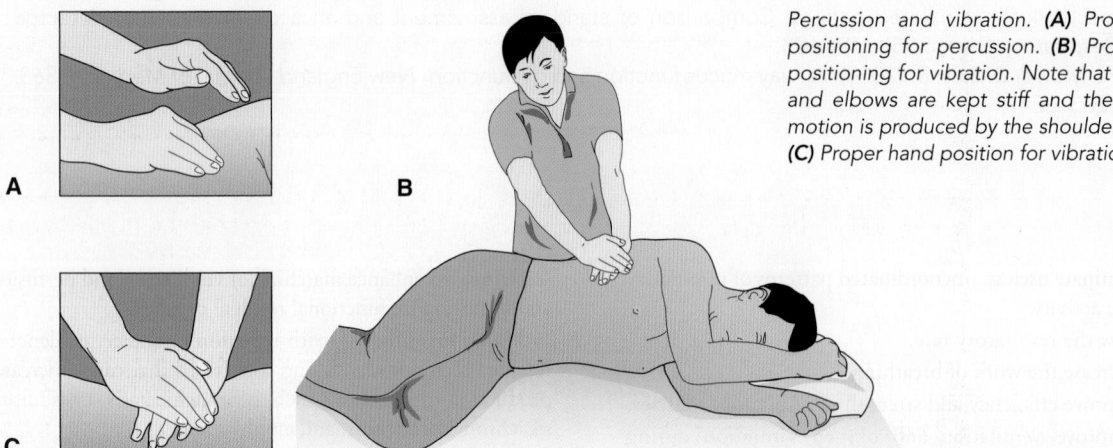

A

B

C

*Percussion and vibration. **(A)** Proper hand positioning for percussion. **(B)** Proper hand positioning for vibration. Note that the wrists and elbows are kept stiff and the vibrating motion is produced by the shoulder muscles. **(C)** Proper hand position for vibration.*

3. Percuss (or clap) with cupped hands over the chest wall for 5 minutes over each segment for cystic fibrosis (or 1–2 minutes for other conditions). Work from:
   a. The lower ribs to shoulders in the back.
   b. The lower ribs to top of chest in the front.

4. Avoid clapping over the spine, liver, kidneys, spleen, breast, scapula, clavicle, or sternum.

5. Instruct the patient to inhale slowly and deeply. Vibrate the chest wall as the patient exhales slowly through pursed lips.
   a. Place one hand on top of the other over affected area or place one hand on each side of the rib cage.
   b. Tense the muscles of the hands and arms while applying moderate pressure downward and vibrate hands and arms.
   c. Relieve pressure on the thorax as the patient inhales.
   d. Encourage the patient to cough, using abdominal muscles, after three or four vibrations.

6. Allow the patient to rest several minutes.

3. Helps dislodge mucus plugs and mobilize secretions toward the main bronchi and trachea. The air trapped between the operator's hand and chest wall will produce a characteristic hollow sound that resembles the sound of horses trotting.

4. Percussion over these areas may cause injuries to the spine or internal organs.

5. Sets up a vibration that carries through the chest wall and helps free the mucus.

b. This maneuver is performed in the direction in which the ribs move on expiration.

d. Contracting the abdominal muscles while coughing increases cough effectiveness. Coughing aids in the movement and expulsion of secretions.

PROCEDURE GUIDELINES 10-10 *(continued)*

Percussion (Clapping) and Vibration

PROCEDURE *(continued)*

Nursing Action	Rationale
7. Listen with a stethoscope for changes in breath sounds.	7. The improvement of crackles and rhonchi indicates movement of air around mucus in the bronchi.
8. Repeat the percussion and vibration cycle according to the patient's tolerance and clinical response, usually 15–30 minutes.	*Note:* Percussion and vibration are considered to have limited research-based evidence of benefit versus risk.

 Evidence Base Lester, M., & Flume P. (2010). Airway-clearance therapy guidelines and implementation. *Respiratory Care, 54*(6), 733–750.

2. The patient is positioned so the diseased areas are in a near vertical position, and gravity is used to assist drainage of the specific segments.

3. The positions assumed are determined by the location, severity, and duration of mucus obstruction.

4. The exercises are usually performed two to four times daily, before meals and at bedtime. Each position is held for 3 to 15 minutes.

5. The procedure should be discontinued if tachycardia, palpitations, dyspnea, or chest pain occurs. These symptoms may indicate hypoxemia. Discontinue if hemoptysis occurs.

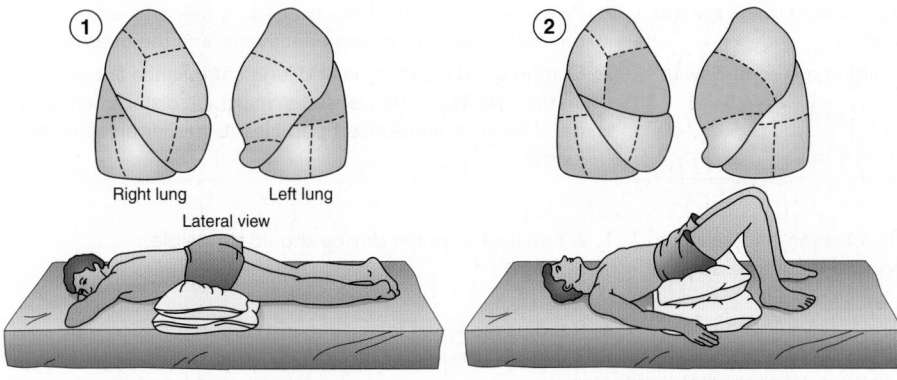

Right lung   Left lung
Lateral view

Lower lobes, superior segments

Upper lobes, anterior segment

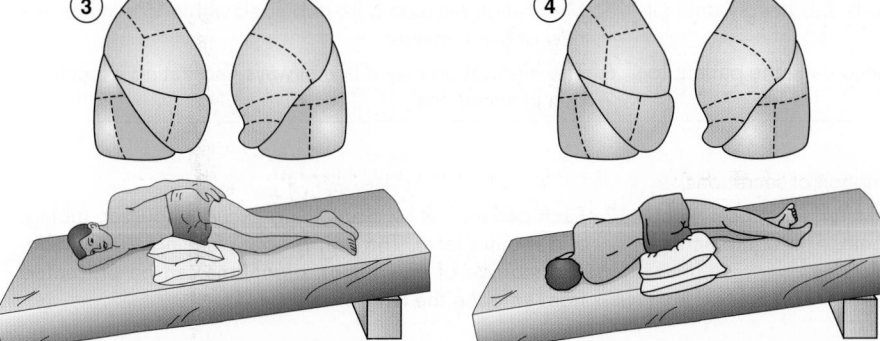

Lower lobes, anterior basal segment

Lower lobes, lateral basal segment

Figure 10-4. Postural drainage positions. Anatomic segments of the lung with four postural drainage positions. The numbers relate the position to the corresponding anatomic segment of the lung.

6. Contraindications include increased ICP, unstable head or neck injury, active hemorrhage with hemodynamic instability or gross hemoptysis, recent spinal surgery or injury, empyema, bronchopleural fistula, rib fracture, flail chest, and uncontrolled hypertension.

 NURSING ALERT Postural drainage and chest percussion may result in hypoxia and should only be used if secretions are believed to be present.

7. Bronchodilators, mucolytic agents, water, or saline may be nebulized and inhaled, or an inhaled bronchodilator may be used before postural drainage and chest percussion to reduce bronchospasm, decrease thickness of mucus and sputum, and combat edema of the bronchial walls, thereby enhancing secretion removal (see Procedure Guidelines 10-11).

8. Perform secretion-clearance procedures before eating or a minimum of 1 hour after eating.

PROCEDURE GUIDELINES 10-11

Administering Nebulizer Therapy (Sidestream Jet Nebulizer)

EQUIPMENT

- Air compressor
- Connection tubing
- Nebulizer
- Medication and saline solution

PROCEDURE

Nursing Action	Rationale
Preparatory phase	
1. Auscultate breath sounds, monitor the heart rate before and after the treatment for patients using bronchodilator drugs.	1. Bronchodilators may cause tachycardia, palpitations, dizziness, nausea, or nervousness.
2. Verify correct patient. Explain the procedure to the patient. This therapy depends on patient effort.	2. Proper explanation of the procedure helps to ensure the patient's cooperation and effectiveness of the treatment.
3. Place the patient in a comfortable sitting or a semi-Fowler's position.	3. Diaphragmatic excursion and lung compliance are greater in this position. This ensures maximal distribution and deposition of aerosolized particles to basilar areas of the lungs.
Performance phase	
1. Add the prescribed amount of medication and saline to the nebulizer. Connect the tubing to the compressor and set the flow at 6–8 L/minute.	1. A fine mist from the device should be visible.
2. Instruct the patient to exhale.	2. Readies the lungs for a deep inspiration.
3. Tell the patient to take in a deep breath from the mouthpiece, hold breath briefly, then exhale.	3. Encourages optimal dispersion of the medication. Nose clips are sometimes used if the patient has difficulty breathing only through the mouth.
4. Observe expansion of chest to ascertain that patient is taking deep breaths.	4. Ensures that medication is deposited below the level of the oropharynx.
5. Instruct the patient to breathe slowly and deeply until all the medication is nebulized.	5. Medication will usually be nebulized within 15 minutes at a flow of 6–8 L/minute.
6. On completion of the treatment, encourage the patient to cough after several deep breaths.	6. The medication may dilate airways, facilitating expectoration of secretions.
Follow-up phase	
1. Record medication used and description of secretions.	
2. Disassemble and clean nebulizer after each use. Keep this equipment in the patient's room. The equipment is changed according to facility policy.	2. Each patient has own breathing circuit (nebulizer, tubing, and mouthpiece). Through proper cleaning, sterilization, and storage of equipment, organisms can be prevented from entering the lungs.

9. Make sure patient is comfortable before the procedure starts and as comfortable as possible while he or she assumes each position.
10. Auscultate the chest to determine the areas of needed drainage.
11. Encourage the patient to deep-breathe and cough after spending the allotted time in each position (normally 3 to 15 minutes).
12. Encourage diaphragmatic breathing throughout postural drainage; this helps widen airways so secretions can be drained.

 **NURSING ALERT** Chest physical therapy (percussion, ventilation, and postural drainage) is time-consuming, requires a trained therapist or caregiver, and there is limited research-based evidence of efficacy.

Forced Expiratory Technique

1. Used to enhance effects of a spontaneous cough and compensate for physical limitations. Used for secretion clearance, atelectasis, prophylaxis against postoperative pulmonary complications, routine bronchial hygiene for cystic fibrosis, bronchiectasis, chronic bronchitis, and to obtain sputum specimen for diagnostic analysis.
2. Procedure includes a forced expiratory technique of two to three "huffs" (forced expirations), from mid- to low-lung volume, with glottis open, followed by a period of relaxed, controlled diaphragmatic breathing. Explain to the patient that to huff-cough is the same maneuver that fogs eyeglasses. The forced expiration can be augmented by brisk adduction of the upper arms to self-compress the thorax.
3. Contraindications include increased ICP or known intracranial aneurysm, as well as acute or unstable head, neck, or spinal injury.

Manually Assisted Cough

The external application of mechanical pressure to the epigastric region coordinated with forced exhalation. This procedure may improve cough efficiency in those individuals with neuromuscular weakness or structural defects of the abdominal wall.

Positive Expiratory Pressure

1. Positive back pressure is created in the airways when the patient breathes in and out 5 to 20 times through a flow resistor or fixed orifice device.
2. During prolonged exhalation against positive pressure, peripheral airways are stabilized while air is pushed through collateral pathways (pores of Kohn and canals of Lambert) into distal lung units past retained secretions.
3. Expiratory airflow moves secretions to larger airways to be removed by coughing.
4. The pressure generated can be monitored and adjusted with a manometer (usually ranges from 10 to 20 cm H_2O).
5. Active exhalation with an inspiratory-to-expiratory (I:E) ratio of 1:3 or 1:4 is suggested.
6. The cycle is repeated until secretions are expelled, usually within 20 minutes or less if patient tires.

Autogenic Drainage

1. Controlled breathing used at three lung volumes, beginning at low-lung volume to unstick mucus, moving to mid-lung volume to collect mucus, and then to high-lung volume to expel mucus.
2. This method may be difficult for some patients to learn and to perform independently.
3. Can be performed in a seated position.

Flutter Mucus Clearance Device

1. Provides PEP and high-frequency oscillations at the airway opening. Provides approximately 10 cm H_2O positive airway pressure.
2. The flutter valve is a pipe-shaped device with an inner cone and bowl loosely supporting a steel ball. The bowl containing the steel ball is covered by a perforated cap.
3. Indications include atelectasis, bronchitis, bronchiectasis, cystic fibrosis, and other conditions producing retained secretions.
4. Mucus clearance is based on:
    a. Vibration of the airways, which loosens mucus from airway walls.
    b. Intermittent increase in endobronchial pressure that keeps airways open.
    c. Acceleration of expiratory airflow to facilitate upward movement of mucus.
5. Contraindications include pneumothorax and right-sided heart failure.
6. Directions:
    a. Patient should be seated upright with chin tilted slightly upward to further open airway.
    b. Instruct patient to inhale slowly to ¾ of normal breath.
    c. Place flutter in mouth with lips firmly sealed around stem or mouthpiece.
    d. Position flutter at horizontal level or raise bulb end up to 30 degrees for greater force.
    e. Instruct patient to hold breath for 2 to 3 seconds.
    f. Exhale through flutter at moderately fast rate, keeping cheeks stiff. Urge to cough should be suppressed.
    g. Repeat for 5 to 10 more breaths.
7. Have patient perform same technique with one to two forced exhalations to generate mucus elimination and huff coughs as needed.
8. Generally used for 10 to 20 breaths with device followed by several directed coughs, repeating series four to six times or for 10 to 20 minutes up to four times daily.
9. Clean flutter device every other day by disassembling and using a liquid soap and tap water. Disinfect regularly by soaking cleaned disassembled parts in one part alcohol to three parts tap water for 1 minute; rinse, wipe, reassemble, and store.

Acapella Vibratory Positive Expiratory Pressure Device

1. Enhances movement of secretions to larger airways, prevents collapse of airways, and facilitates filling of collapsed alveoli.
2. Airway vibration provides percussive effect, disengages mucus from airway walls, causes pulsation of mucus toward larger airways, and reduces visco-elasticity of mucus.
3. Select color-coded device: green for expiratory flow ≥ 15 L/minute, blue for < 15 L/minute.

4. Place mask tightly and comfortably over patient's mouth and nose (or seal lips tight around mouthpiece if mask not used). Patient may sit, stand, or recline.

5. Instruct patient to perform diaphragmatic breathing, inhale to near total lung volume, and exhale actively but not forcefully through device fully. Set resistance to achieve I:E ratio of 1:3 to 1:4. Use inline manometer to select expiratory pressure of 10 to 20 cm H_2O.

6. Use every 1 to 6 hours, according to response.

7. Assessment: improving breath sounds, patient's report of improved dyspnea, improved chest x-ray, improved oxygenation.

8. Acapella Choice can be disassembled for cleaning in dishwasher, boiled, or autoclaved.

AeroPEP Valved Holding Chamber

1. Combines aerosol therapy from a metered-dose inhaler with a fixed orifice resister PEP therapy.

2. Place disposable mouthpiece over AeroPEP mouthpiece and attach manometer. Instruct patient to seal lips tightly around mouthpiece.

3. While performing diaphragmatic breathing, inhale fully.

4. Exhale actively and fully to achieve PEP of 10 to 20 cm H_2O. Set AeroPEP between 0 and 6 at desired pressure on manometer.

5. Repeat for up to 20 minutes four times daily, or as clinically indicated.

Intrapulmonary Percussive Ventilation or Percussionaire

1. Therapy is delivered by a percussionator, which delivers minibursts of air into the lungs at a rate of 100 to 300 per minute. Process includes delivery of a dense aerosol mist through a mouthpiece. The treatment lasts about 20 minutes.

2. Patient uses in sitting or recumbent position.

3. Instill nebulizer bowl with 20 mL of saline or aqueous water and prescribed bronchodilator.

4. Clinician or patient programs percussive cycle by holding down a button for 5 to 10 seconds for percussive inspiratory cycle and releasing to expectorate or pause during therapy.

5. Seal lips around mouthpiece with "pucker" to minimize cheek flapping.

6. Observe chest for percussive shaking.

7. Use twice daily for approximately 20 minutes with increased frequency as needed.

Mechanical Insufflation-Exsufflation

Assists in secretion clearance by applying positive pressure to the airway, then rapidly shifting to negative pressure by way of a face mask, mouthpiece, ET tube, or tracheostomy tube to increase cough effectiveness.

Electrical Stimulation of the Expiratory Muscles

Electrical stimulation of the abdominal muscles to increase cough effectiveness. An advantage is that presence of a caregiver is not required.

The Vest Airway Clearance System

1. Enhances secretion clearance through high-frequency chest wall oscillation. High-frequency compression pulses are applied to the chest wall by way of an air pulse delivery system and inflatable vest.

2. Variable-frequency large-volume air pulse delivery system attached to inflatable vest. Pressure pulses that fill the vest and vibrate the chest wall are controlled by a foot pedal. Pulse frequency ranges from 5 to 25 Hz and pressure in the vest ranges from 28 to 39 mm Hg.

3. A foot or hand control starts and stops pulsations.

4. Treatment length usually 10 to 30 minutes. Therapy should include a break at least every 10 minutes for directed cough. Use twice daily, with increased frequency as needed.

Community and Home Care Considerations

1. Nebulizer tubing and mouthpiece can be reused at home repeatedly. Recommend thorough rinsing with warm water after each use, shake off excess water, and let air-dry.

2. Twice-weekly cleaning should include washing with liquid soap and hot water, followed by 30-minute soak in one part white vinegar and two parts tap water, and then rinsing with tap water, air-drying, and storing in a clean, dry place.

Administering Oxygen Therapy

Oxygen is an odorless, tasteless, colorless, transparent gas that is slightly heavier than air. It is used to treat or prevent symptoms and manifestations of hypoxia. Oxygen can be dispensed from a cylinder, piped-in system, liquid oxygen reservoir, or oxygen concentrator. It may be administered by nasal cannula, transtracheal catheter, nasal cannula with reservoir devices, or various types of face masks, including CPAP mask. It may also be applied directly to the ET or tracheal tube by way of a mechanical ventilator, T-piece, or manual resuscitation bag. The method selected depends on the required concentration of oxygen, desired variability in delivered oxygen concentration (none, minimal, moderate), and required ventilatory assistance (mechanical ventilator, spontaneous breathing).

Methods of Oxygen Administration

1. Nasal cannula (see Procedure Guidelines 10-12)—nasal prongs that deliver low flow of oxygen.
   a. Requires nose breathing.
   b. Cannot deliver oxygen concentrations much higher than 40%.

2. Simple face mask (see Procedure Guidelines 10-13, pages 240 to 241)—mask that delivers moderate oxygen flow to nose and mouth. Delivers oxygen concentrations of 40% to 60%.

3. Venturi mask (see Procedure Guidelines 10-14, pages 242 to 243)—mask with device that mixes air and oxygen to deliver constant oxygen concentration.
   a. Total gas flow at the patient's face must meet or exceed peak inspiratory flow rate. When other mask outputs do not meet inspiratory flow rate of patient, room air (drawn through mask side holes) mixes with the gas mixture provided by the face mask, lowering the inspired oxygen concentration.
   b. Venturi mask mixes a fixed flow of oxygen with a high but variable flow of air to produce a constant oxygen concentration. Oxygen enters by way of a jet (restricted opening) at a high velocity. Room air also enters and mixes with oxygen at this site. The higher the velocity (smaller the opening), the more room air is drawn into the mask.

(Text continues on page 243)

PROCEDURE GUIDELINES 10-12

Administering Oxygen by Nasal Cannula

EQUIPMENT

- Oxygen source
- Plastic nasal cannula with connecting tubing (disposable)
- Humidifier filled with sterile water
- Flowmeter
- NO SMOKING signs

PROCEDURE

Nursing Action	Rationale
Preparatory phase	
1. Verify correct patient. Determine current vital signs, LOC, and most recent ABG.	1. Provides a baseline for future assessment. Nasal cannula oxygen administration is often used for patients prone to CO_2 retention. Oxygen may depress the hypoxic drive of these patients (evidenced by a decreased respiratory rate, altered mental status, and further $PaCO_2$ elevation).
2. Assess risk of CO_2 retention with oxygen administration.	2. If $PaCO_2$ is decreased or normal, the patient is not experiencing CO_2 retention and can use oxygen without fear of the above consequences.
3. Show the nasal cannula to the patient and explain the procedure.	3. To allay anxiety and enlist cooperation.
Performance phase	
1. Make sure the humidifier is filled to the appropriate mark.	1. Humidification may not be ordered if the flow rate is less than 4 L/minute.
2. Attach the connecting tube from the nasal cannula to the humidifier outlet.	
3. Set the flow rate at the prescribed liters per minute. Feel to determine if oxygen is flowing through the tips of the cannula.	3. Because a nasal cannula is a low-flow system (patient's tidal volume supplies part of the inspired gas), oxygen concentration will vary, depending on the patient's respiratory rate and tidal volume. Approximate oxygen concentrations delivered are:
	1 L = 24%–25% 2 L = 27%–29%
	3 L = 30%–33% 4 L = 33%–37%
	5 L = 36%–41% 6 L = 39%–45%
4. Place the tips of the cannula in the patient's nose and adjust straps around ears for snug, comfortable fit.	4. Prevents slipping out of place or creating pressure point and possible skin breakdown behind ears and across cheeks. Areas of contact may be padded to prevent pressure points.

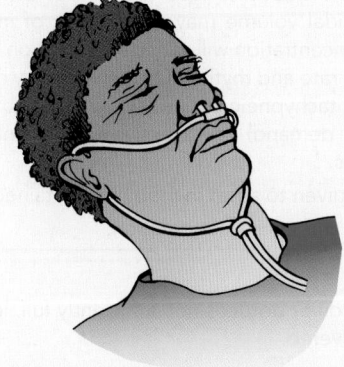

Administering oxygen by nasal cannula. Patient's inspiration consists of a mixture of supplemental oxygen supplied via the nasal cannula and room air. Oxygen concentration is variable and depends on the patient's tidal volume and ventilatory pattern.

(continued)

PROCEDURE GUIDELINES 10-12 (continued)

Administering Oxygen by Nasal Cannula

PROCEDURE (continued)

Nursing Action	Rationale
Follow-up phase	
1. Record flow rate used and immediate patient response.	1. Note the patient's tolerance of treatment. Report any intolerance noted.
2. Assess the patient's condition, ABG or SaO_2, and the functioning of equipment at regular intervals.	2. Depression of hypoxic drive is most likely to occur within the first hours of oxygen use. Monitoring of SaO_2 with oximetry can be substituted for ABG if the patient is not retaining CO_2.
3. Determine patient comfort with oxygen use.	3. Flow rates in excess of 4 L/minute may cause irritation to the nasal and pharyngeal mucosa.

 NURSING ALERT Avoid use of petroleum jelly to lubricate nares because it is flammable and may clog openings of cannula. Use saline spray or water-based gel.

 Evidence Base Dunne, P. (2010). The clinical impact of new long-term oxygen therapy technology. *Respiratory Care, 54*(10), 1413.

PROCEDURE GUIDELINES 10-13

Administering Oxygen by Simple Face Mask with or without Aerosol

EQUIPMENT

- Oxygen source
- Humidifier bottle with distilled water, if high humidity is desired for simple face mask

- Simple face mask or plastic aerosol mask
- Large-bore tubing for aerosol or small-bore tubing for simple face mask

- Flowmeter
- Nebulizer for aerosol
- Humidifier heating element

PROCEDURE

Nursing Action	Rationale
Preparatory phase	
1. Verify correct patient. Determine current vital signs, LOC, and Sao_2 or ABG, if patient is at risk for CO_2 retention.	1. Because the nebulizer face mask is a low-flow system (patient's tidal volume may supply part of inspired gas), oxygen concentration will vary depending on the patient's respiratory rate and rhythm. Oxygen delivery may be inadequate for tachypneic patients (flow does not meet peak inspiratory demand) or excessive for patients with slow respirations.
2. Assess viscosity and volume of sputum produced.	2. Aerosol is given to assist in mobilizing retained secretions.
3. Show the mask to the patient and explain the procedure.	3. Allays fear and enlists cooperation.
Performance phase	
1. Make sure the humidifier or nebulizer is filled to the appropriate mark.	1. If the humidifier bottle is not sufficiently full, less moisture will be delivered.
2. Attach the large-bore tubing from the mask to the humidifier in the heating element, if used.	

PROCEDURE GUIDELINES 10-13 *(continued)*

Administering Oxygen by Simple Face Mask with or without Aerosol

PROCEDURE *(continued)*

Nursing Action	Rationale
3. Set desired oxygen concentration and plug in the heating element, if used. If the patient is tachypneic and concentration of 50% oxygen or greater is desired, two humidifiers and flowmeters should be yoked together.	3. The inspired oxygen concentration is determined by the humidifier setting. Usual concentrations are 35%–50%. The aerosol mask is a low-flow system. Yoking two humidifiers together doubles humidifier flow but does not change the inspired oxygen concentration.
4. Adjust the flow rate until the desired mist is produced (usually 10–12 L/minute).	4. Ensures that the patient is receiving flow sufficient to meet inspiratory demand and maintains a constant, accurate concentration of oxygen.
5. Apply the mask to the patient's face and adjust the straps so the mask fits securely. Dry face around mask every 2 hours.	5. Prevents straps from slipping out of place, but not too tightly to prevent skin breakdown due to pressure and moisture.
6. Drain the tubing frequently by emptying condensate into a separate receptacle, not into the humidifier. If a heating element is used, the tubing will have to be drained more often.	6. The tubing must be kept free of condensate. Condensate allowed to accumulate in the delivery tube will block flow and alter oxygen concentration. If condensate is emptied into the humidifier, bacteria may be aerosolized into the lungs.
7. If a heating element is used, check the temperature. The humidifier bottle should be warm, not hot, to the touch.	7. Excessive temperatures can cause airway burns; patients with elevated temperature should be humidified with an unheated device.

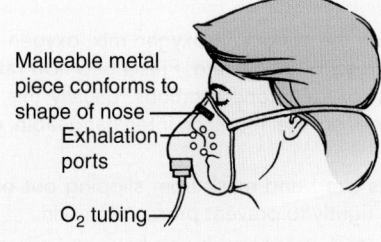

Malleable metal piece conforms to shape of nose

Exhalation ports

O₂ tubing

Simple face mask. Oxygen concentration varies with patient's tidal volume and respiratory rate.

Follow-up phase

1. Record FiO₂ and immediate patient response. Note the patient's tolerance of treatment. Notify the health care provider if intolerance occurs.	1. Documentation to guide therapy.
2. Assess the patient's condition and the functioning of equipment at regular intervals.	2. Change in mental status, diaphoresis, changes in blood pressure, and increasing heart and respiratory rates may indicate a need for change in therapy.
3. If the patient's condition changes, assess SaO₂ or ABG.	3. If the patient has a high minute ventilation or V_E, flow from the mask may not be sufficient to meet inspiratory needs without pulling in room air. Room air will dilute the oxygen provided and lower the inspired oxygen concentration, resulting in hypoxemia. A change in mask or delivery system may be indicated.
4. Record changes in volume and tenacity of sputum produced.	4. Indicates effectiveness of humidification.

Evidence Base American Association of Respiratory Care. (2002). Clinical practice guideline. Oxygen therapy for adults in the acute care facility, 2002 revision and update. *Respiratory Care, 47*(6), 717–20.
    Cranston, J. M., Crockett, A., & Currow, D. (2008). Oxygen therapy for dyspnea in adults. *Cochrane Database of Systematic Reviews*, Issue 3 (Article No. CD004769).

PROCEDURE GUIDELINES 10-14

Administering Oxygen by Venturi Mask (High Air Flow Oxygen Entrainment System)

EQUIPMENT

- Oxygen source
- Flowmeter
- Venturi mask for correct concentration (24%, 28%, 31%, 35%, 40%, 50%) or correct concentration adapter if interchangeable color-coded adapters are used

- If high humidity desired
- Compressed air source and flowmeter
- Humidifier with distilled water
- Large-bore tubing

PROCEDURE

Nursing Action	Rationale
1. Verify correct patient. Determine current vital signs, LOC, and most recent ABG.	1. Provides a baseline for future assessment. Venturi masks are used for patients prone to CO_2 retention. Oxygen may depress the hypoxic drive of these patients (evidenced by a decreased respiratory rate, altered mental status, and further $PaCO_2$ elevation).
2. Assess risk of CO_2 retention with oxygen administration.	2. Risk is greater if the patient is experiencing an exacerbation of illness.
3. Show the Venturi mask to the patient and explain the procedure.	3. Allays fear and enlists patient cooperation.

Performance phase

Nursing Action	Rationale
1. Connect the mask by lightweight tubing to the oxygen source.	
2. Turn on the oxygen flowmeter and adjust to the prescribed rate (usually indicated on the mask). Check to see that oxygen is flowing out the vent holes in the mask.	2. To ensure the correct air/oxygen mix, oxygen must be set at the prescribed flow rate. Prescribed flow rates differ for different oxygen concentrations. Usually this information is printed on the mask or interchangeable color-coded source.
3. Place Venturi mask over the patient's nose and mouth and under the chin. Adjust elastic strap.	3. Prevents strap and mask from slipping out of place, but not too tightly to prevent pressure on skin.
4. Check to make sure holes for air entry are not obstructed by the patient's bedding.	4. Proper mask function depends on mixing of sufficient amount of air and oxygen.
5. If aerosol nebulizer used:	5. When a Venturi mask is used with aerosol, an oxygen source is required. The compressed air source provides air for the air/oxygen mix. Excessive oxygen would be inspired if both tubings were connected to an oxygen source.
a. Connect the humidifier to a compressed air source.	
b. Attach large-bore tubing to the humidifier and connect the tubing to the fitting for high humidity at the base of the Venturi mask.	

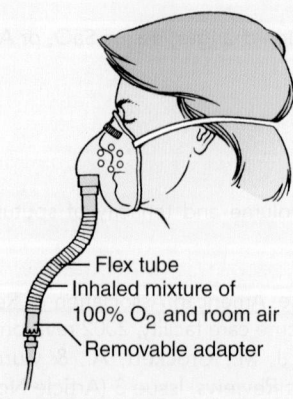

Flex tube
Inhaled mixture of
100% O_2 and room air
Removable adapter

Venturi mask. Constant high concentrations of oxygen can be delivered.

PROCEDURE GUIDELINES 10-14 *(continued)*

Administering Oxygen by Venturi Mask (High Air Flow Oxygen Entrainment System)

PROCEDURE *(continued)*

Nursing Action	Rationale

Follow-up phase

1. Record flow rate used and immediate patient response. Note the patient's tolerance of treatment. Report if intolerance occurs.

1. Depression of hypoxic drive is most likely to occur within the first hours of oxygen use.

 Key Decision Point

If CO_2 retention is present, assess ABG every 30 minutes for 1 to 2 hours or until the PaO_2 is greater than 50 mm Hg and the $PaCO_2$ is no longer increasing. Monitor for change in pH. A modest (5–10 mm Hg) increase in $PaCO_2$ may occur after initiation therapy; however, a decreasing pH indicates failure of compensatory mechanisms. Report if the pH decreases below the initial assessment value. Mechanical ventilation may be required.

2. Determine patient comfort with oxygen use.

2. Venturi masks are best tolerated for relatively short periods because of their size and appearance. They also must be removed for eating and drinking. With improvement in patient condition, a nasal cannula may often be substituted.

 Evidence Base American Association of Respiratory Care. (2002). Clinical practice guideline. Oxygen therapy for adults in the acute care facility, 2002 revision and update. *Respiratory Care, 47*(6), 717–20.
Wong, M., & Elliott, M. (2009). The use of medical orders in acute care oxygen therapy *British Journal of Nursing, 18*(8), 462–464.

---

c. Mask output ranges from approximately 24% to 50% oxygen.

d. Virtually eliminates rebreathing of CO_2. Excess gas leaves through openings in the mask, carrying with it the expired CO_2.

4. Partial rebreather mask (see Procedure Guidelines 10-15, pages 244 to 245)—has an inflatable bag that stores 100% oxygen.

   a. On inspiration, the patient inhales from the mask and bag; on expiration, the bag refills with oxygen and expired gases exit through perforations on both sides of the mask and some enters bag (see Figure 10-5).

   b. High concentrations of oxygen (50% to 75%) can be delivered.

5. Nonrebreathing mask (see Procedure Guidelines 10-15, pages 244 to 245)—has an inflatable bag to store 100% oxygen and a one-way valve between the bag and mask to prevent exhaled air from entering the bag.

   a. Has one-way valves covering one or both of the exhalation ports to prevent entry of room air on inspiration.

   b. Has a flap or spring-loaded valves to permit entry of room air should the oxygen source fail or patient needs exceed the available oxygen flow.

   c. Optimally, all the patient's inspiratory volume will be provided by the mask/reservoir, allowing delivery of nearly 100% oxygen.

6. Transtracheal catheter—accomplished by way of a small (8 French) catheter inserted between the second and third tracheal cartilage.

   a. Does not interfere with talking, drinking, or eating and can be concealed under a shirt or blouse.

   b. Oxygen delivery is more efficient because all oxygen enters the lungs.

   c. Requires surgical procedure with temporary stent until tract is healed.

7. CPAP mask (see Procedure Guidelines 10-16, pages 246 to 247)—used to provide expiratory and inspiratory positive airway pressure in a manner similar to PEEP and does not require ET intubation.

   a. Has an inflatable cushion and head strap designed to tightly seal the mask against the face.

   b. A PEEP valve is incorporated into the exhalation port to maintain positive pressure on exhalation.

   c. High inspiratory flow rates are needed to maintain positive pressure on inspiration.

8. Biphasic positive airway pressure (BiPAP) mask—a combination of inspiratory and expiratory pulmonary artery pressure (PAP) often used to avoid intubation and mechanical ventilation.

   a. Preset pressure to be delivered during inspiration and preset pressure to be maintained during expiration.

(Text continues on page 245)

PROCEDURE GUIDELINES 10-15

Administering Oxygen by Partial Rebreathing or Nonrebreathing Mask

EQUIPMENT
- Oxygen source
- Plastic face mask with reservoir bag and tubing
- Humidifier with distilled water
- Flowmeter

PROCEDURE

Nursing Action	Rationale
Preparatory phase	
1. Verify correct patient. Determine current vital signs and LOC.	1. Provides a baseline for evaluating patient response. Typically used for short-term support of patients who require a high inspired oxygen concentration.
2. Determine most recent SaO$_2$ or ABG.	2. Allows objective evaluation of patient response.
3. Show the mask to the patient and explain the procedure.	3. Allays fear and enlists patient cooperation.
Performance phase	
1. Attach tubing to flowmeter.	
2. Flush the reservoir bag with oxygen to inflate the bag and adjust flowmeter to 6–10 L/minute.	2. Bag serves as a reservoir, holding oxygen for patient inspiration.
3. Place the mask on the patient's face and adjust strap so that it fits snugly.	3. Ensures that there is an airtight seal between the mask and the patient's face for optimal performance.
4. Adjust liter flow so the rebreathing bag will not collapse during the inspiratory cycle, even during deep inspiration.	4. With a well-fitting rebreathing bag adjusted so the patient's inhalation does not deflate the bag, inspired oxygen concentration of 60%–90% can be achieved. Some patients may require flow rates higher than 10 L/minute to ensure that the bag does not collapse on inspiration.
5. Stay with the patient for a time to make the patient comfortable and observe reactions.	
6. Remove mask periodically (if the patient's condition permits) to dry the face around the mask. Apply water-based lotion to skin and massage face around the mask.	6. Reduces moisture accumulation under the mask. Massage of the face stimulates circulation and reduces pressure over the area.

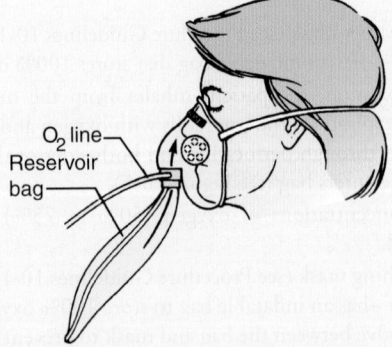

O$_2$ line
Reservoir bag

Partial rebreathing mask. 100% oxygen fills bag, but concentration delivered varies with respiration. Nonrebreathing mask is similar with the addition of a one-way valve that prevents expired air from entering bag and one-way flaps over exhalation ports.

Nursing Action	Rationale
Follow-up phase	
1. Record flow rate and immediate patient response. Note the patient's tolerance of treatment. Report if intolerance occurs. Observe the patient for change of condition.	1. Change in mental status, diaphoresis, change in BP, and increasing heart and respiratory rates may indicate need for change in therapy.
2. Assess equipment for malfunctioning and low water level in humidifier.	2. For optimal performance.

PROCEDURE GUIDELINES 10-15 *(continued)*

Administering Oxygen by Partial Rebreathing or Nonrebreathing Mask

PROCEDURE *(continued)*

Nursing Action	Rationale

 NURSING ALERT Monitor functioning of mask to ensure that side ports of mask do not get blocked. This could lead to patient inability to exhale and may lead to suffocation.

 Evidence Base Hess, D., MacIntyre, N., Mishoe, S., et al. (2012). *Respiratory care: Principles and practice* (2nd ed.). Sudbury, MA: Jones & Bartlett.

 NURSING ALERT Success of any PAP device depends on patient compliance, which can be improved by proper education, proper mask fit, and frequent follow-up care.

9. T-piece (Briggs) adapter (see Procedure Guidelines 10-17, pages 248 to 249)—used to administer oxygen to patient with ET or tracheostomy tube who is breathing spontaneously.
   a. High concentration of aerosol and oxygen delivered through wide-bore tubing.
   b. Expired gases exit through open reservoir tubing.
10. Manual resuscitation bag (see Procedure Guidelines 10-18, pages 249 to 250)—delivers high concentration of oxygen to patient with insufficient inspiratory effort.
    a. With mask, uses upper airway by delivering oxygen to mouth and nose of patient.
    b. Without mask, adapter fits on ET or tracheostomy tube.
    c. Usually used in cardiopulmonary arrest, hyperinflation during suctioning, or transport of ventilator-dependent patients.

Nursing Assessment and Interventions

1. Assess need for oxygen by observing for symptoms of hypoxia:
   a. Tachypnea.
   b. $SaO_2 < 88\%$.
   c. Tachycardia or dysrhythmias (premature ventricular contractions).
   d. A change in LOC (symptoms of decreased cerebral oxygenation are irritability, confusion, lethargy, and coma, if untreated).
   e. Cyanosis occurs as a late sign ($PaO_2 \leq 45$ mm Hg).
   f. Labored respirations indicate severe respiratory distress.
   g. Myocardial stress—increase in heart rate and stroke volume (cardiac output) is the primary mechanism for compensation for hypoxemia or hypoxia; pupils dilate with hypoxia.

(*Text continues on page 247*)

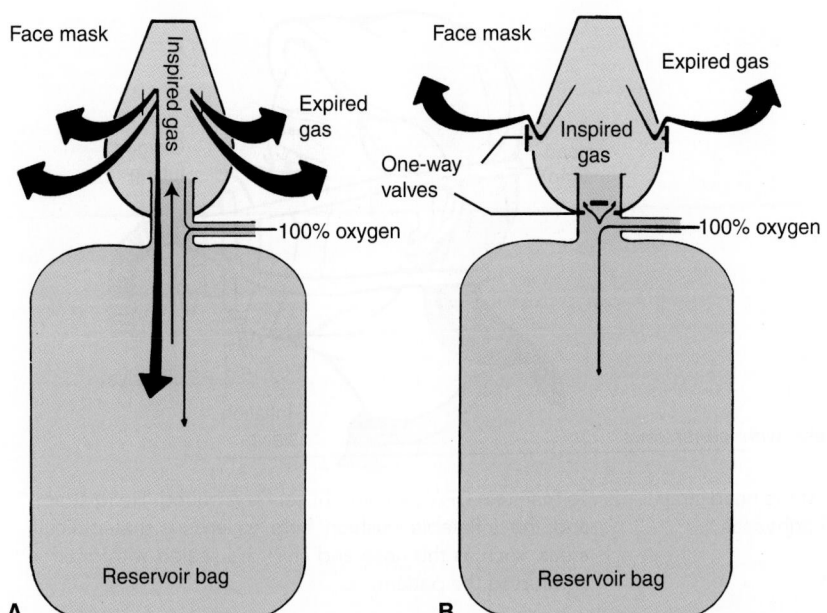

Figure 10-5. (A) Airflow diagram with partial rebreathing mask. **(B)** Airflow diagram with nonrebreathing mask. *Arrows* indicate direction of flow.

PROCEDURE GUIDELINES 10-16

Administering Oxygen by Continuous Positive Airway Pressure Mask

EQUIPMENT

- O_2 blender
- Flowmeter
- Continuous positive airway pressure (CPAP) mask
- Valve for prescribed PEEP (2.5, 5, 7.5, 10 cm H_2O)
- Nebulizer with distilled water
- Large-bore tubing
- NG tube (if ordered)
- Sealing pad to accommodate NG tube

PROCEDURE

Nursing Action	Rationale
Preparatory phase	
1. Verify correct patient. Assess the patient's LOC and gag reflex.	1. CPAP mask may lead to aspiration unless the patient is breathing spontaneously and is able to protect the airway.
2. Determine current ABGs.	2. Documents that patient meets criteria for use of this mask (normal or increased $PaCO_2$ and provides baseline to evaluate whether therapy results in CO_2 retention).

 NURSING ALERT CPAP is used when patients have not responded to attempts to increase PaO_2 with other types of masks.

Nursing Action	Rationale
3. Show the mask to the patient and explain the procedure.	3. Allays fear and enlists patient cooperation.
4. Insert NG tube if ordered. (May be used for some patients at risk for aspiration.)	4. With CPAP, the patient may swallow air, causing gastric distention or emesis. Prophylactic NG suction diminishes this risk.
Performance phase	
1. Set desired concentration of O_2 blender and adjust flow rate so it is sufficient to meet the patient's inspiratory demand.	1. O_2 blenders are devices that mix air and O_2 using a proportioning valve. Concentrations of 21%–100% may be delivered, depending on the model. Because the patient will be receiving all minute ventilation from this "closed system," it is essential that the flow rate be adequate to meet changes in the patient's breathing pattern.

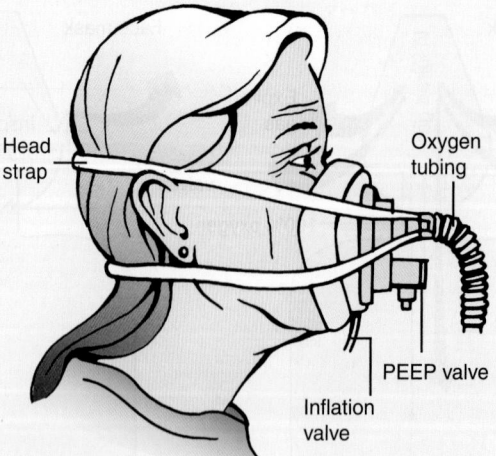

Administering oxygen by face mask with continuous positive airway pressure (CPAP).

Nursing Action	Rationale
2. Place the mask on the patient's face, adjust the head strap, and inflate the mask cushion to ensure a tight seal.	2. To maintain CPAP, an airtight seal is required. Head straps and the inflatable cushion help to ensure that difficult areas, such as the nose and chin, are sealed with greater comfort to the patient.

PROCEDURE GUIDELINES 10-16 *(continued)*

Administering Oxygen by Continuous Positive Airway Pressure Mask

PROCEDURE *(continued)*

Nursing Action	Rationale
3. Organize care to remove the mask as infrequently as possible.	3. If mask is removed (for coughing, suctioning, bathing), CPAP is not maintained and inspired O_2 concentrations drop.

Follow-up phase

1. Assess ABGs, hemodynamic status, and LOC frequently.	1. Provides objective documentation of patient response. CPAP may increase work of breathing, resulting in patient tiring and inability to maintain ventilation without intubation. CPAP may also decrease venous return, resulting in decreased cardiac output.
2. Immediately report any increase in $PaCO_2$.	2. An increase in $PaCO_2$ suggests hypoventilation, resulting from tiring of the patient or inadequate alveolar ventilation. Need for intubation and mechanical ventilation should be evaluated.
3. Assess patency of NG tube, if used, at frequent intervals.	3. May become obstructed, causing gastric distention.
4. Assess patient comfort and functioning of the equipment frequently.	4. Tight fit of the mask may predispose to skin breakdown. System may develop leaks, resulting in air escaping between the patient's face and mask.
5. Record patient response. With improvement, O_2 therapy without positive airway pressure can be substituted. With deterioration, intubation and mechanical ventilation may be required. Note the patient's tolerance of treatment. Report if intolerance occurs.	5. Face mask CPAP is usually continued only for short periods (72 hours) because of patient tiring and the necessity to remove mask for suctioning and coughing.

Note: CPAP may be used as a therapy for sleep apnea during the time the patient sleeps. A nasal CPAP mask is typically used.

Evidence Base Logan, A. G., & Bradley T. D. (2010). Sleep apnea and cardiovascular disease. *Current Hypertension Reports, 12,* 182–188.

Nouira, S., Boukef, R., Bouida, W., et al. (2011). Non-invasive pressure support ventilation and CPAP in cardiogenic pulmonary edema: a multicenter randomized study in the emergency department. *Intensive Care Medicine, 37*(2), 249–256.

Agency for Healthcare Research and Quality. (2011). Diagnosis and treatment of obstructive sleep apnea in adults (Comparative Effectiveness Review No. 32, AHRQ Publication No. 11-EHC052-EF). Rockville, MD: Author. Available: *www.effectivehealthcare.ahrq.gov/index.cfm/search-for-guides-reviews-and-reports/?pageaction=displayproduct&productid=731.*

2. Obtain ABG values and assess the patient's current oxygenation, ventilation, and acid-base status.
3. Administer oxygen in the appropriate concentration.
   a. Low concentration (24% to 28%)—may be appropriate for patients prone to retain CO_2 (COPD, drug overdose), who are dependent on hypoxemia (hypoxic drive) to maintain respiration. If hypoxemia is suddenly reversed, hypoxic drive may be lost and respiratory depression and, possibly, respiratory arrest may occur. Monitor $PaCO_2$ levels.
   b. High concentration (≥30%)—if hypoxemia is suddenly reversed, hypoxic drive may be inhibited and respiratory depression and, possibly, respiratory arrest may occur.

High concentrations are appropriate in patients not predisposed to CO_2 retention.
4. Monitor response by oximetry and/or ABG sampling.
5. Increase or decrease the inspired oxygen concentration, as appropriate.

 NURSING ALERT All Joint Commission–accredited hospitals must be smoke free; however, other health care facilities and homes where oxygen is used may allow smoking. Make sure that no smoking is permitted where oxygen is used.

(Text continues on page 251)

PROCEDURE GUIDELINES 10-17

Administering Oxygen by Way of Endotracheal and Tracheostomy Tubes with a T-Piece (Briggs) Adapter

EQUIPMENT

- Oxygen
- O_2 blender
- Flowmeter
- Nebulizer with sterile water (heating element may be used as described in aerosol masks)
- Large-bore tubing
- T-piece and reservoir tubing

PROCEDURE

Nursing Action	Rationale
Preparatory phase	
1. Verify correct patient. Assess the patient's Sao$_2$, hemodynamic status, and LOC frequently. If patient condition changes, assess ABGs.	1. Provides baseline to assess response.
2. Assess viscosity and volume of sputum produced.	2. Aerosol is given to assist in mobilizing retained secretions.
3. Show the T-tube to the patient and explain the procedure.	3. Allays fear and enlists patient cooperation.
Performance phase	
1. Make sure the humidifier is filled to the appropriate mark.	1. If humidifier is not sufficiently full, less aerosol will be delivered.
2. Attach the large-bore tubing from the T-tube to the humidifier outlet.	
3. Set desired O_2 concentration of O_2 blender or humidifier bottle and plug in heating element, if used.	3. O_2 blenders are devices that mix air and O_2 using a proportioning valve. Concentrations of 21%–100% may be delivered at flows of 2–100 L/minute, depending on the model. Used when precise control is required.
4. Adjust the flow rate until the desired mist is produced and meets the patient's inspiratory demand.	4. The aerosol mist in the reservoir tubing attached to the T-tube should not be completely withdrawn on patient inspiration. If mist is withdrawn (does not extend from reservoir tubing) on inspiration, room air may be inspired and O_2 concentration decreased.
5. Drain the tubing frequently by emptying condensate into a separate receptacle, not into the humidifier. If a heating element is used, the tubing will have to be drained more often.	5. The tubing must be kept free of condensate. Condensate allowed to accumulate in the delivery tube will block flow and alter O_2 concentration. If condensate is emptied into the humidifier, bacteria may be aerosolized into the lungs.
6. If a heating element is used, check the temperature. The humidifier bottle should be warm, not hot, to the touch.	6. Excessive temperatures can cause airway burns; patients with elevated temperatures will be better humidified with an unheated device.

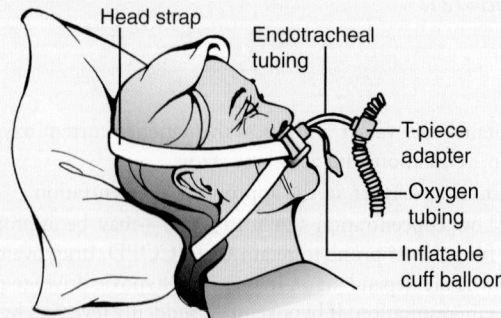

Head strap

Endotracheal tubing

T-piece adapter

Oxygen tubing

Inflatable cuff balloon

Administering oxygen via endotracheal tube with a T-piece adapter. A T-piece adapter is attached to the endotracheal tube and large-bore tubing, which serves as a source of oxygen and humidity.

PROCEDURE GUIDELINES 10-17 *(continued)*

Administering Oxygen by Way of Endotracheal and Tracheostomy Tubes with a T-Piece (Briggs) Adapter

PROCEDURE *(continued)*

Nursing Action	Rationale
Follow-up phase	
1. Record Fio$_2$ and immediate patient response. Assess functioning of equipment and patient's condition at regular intervals. Note patient's tolerance of treatment. Report if intolerance occurs.	1. Change in mental status, diaphoresis, perspiration, changes in BP, and increasing heart and respiratory rates may indicate intolerance and need to change therapy.
2. If the patient's condition changes, assess SaO$_2$ or ABGs and vital signs. Note changes suggesting increased work of breathing (diaphoresis, intercostal muscle retraction).	2. If the patient is being weaned, return to the ventilator if changes suggesting inability to tolerate spontaneous ventilation occur. (See Weaning the Patient from Mechanical Ventilation, pages 258 to 260.)
3. Record changes in volume and tenacity of sputum produced.	3. Indicates effectiveness of humidification therapy.

 Evidence Base Wiegand, D. J., & Carlson, K. K. (2010). *AACN procedure manual for critical care* (6th ed.). Philadelphia: Elsevier Saunders.

PROCEDURE GUIDELINES 10-18

Administering Oxygen by Manual Resuscitation Bag

EQUIPMENT

- O$_2$ source
- Resuscitation bag and mask
- Reservoir tubing or reservoir bag
- O$_2$ connecting tubing
- Nipple adapter to attach flowmeter to connecting tubing
- Flowmeter
- Gloves
- Face shield

PROCEDURE

Nursing Action	Rationale
Preparatory phase	
1. In cardiopulmonary arrest:	1.
a. Follow steps to establish that a cardiopulmonary arrest has occurred.	a. The steps are establish unresponsiveness; call for help; position the patient on a firm, flat surface; open the mouth and remove vomitus or debris, if visible; assess presence of respirations with the airway open; if apneic, ventilate; palpate the carotid pulse; if absent, deliver chest compressions.
b. Use caution not to injure or increase injury to the cervical spine when opening the airway.	b. If cervical spine injury is a potential, the modified jaw thrust should be used. In other situations, the head-tilt or chin-lift method can be used. These maneuvers lift the tongue off the back of the throat and, in some situations, may be all that is needed to restore breathing.
2. In suctioning or transport situation, assess patient's heart rate, level of consciousness (LOC), and respiratory status.	2. Provides a baseline to stimulate patient's tolerance of procedure.

(continued)

PROCEDURE GUIDELINES 10-18 *(continued)*

Administering Oxygen by Manual Resuscitation Bag

PROCEDURE *(continued)*

Nursing Action	Rationale

Performance phase

1. Attach connecting tubing from flowmeter and nipple adapter to resuscitation bag.

2. Turn flowmeter to "flush" position.

3. Attach reservoir tubing or reservoir bag to resuscitation bag.

4. Put on face shield and gloves.

Cardiopulmonary arrest

1. If respirations are absent after the airway is open, insert an oropharyngeal airway and ventilate twice with slow, full breaths of 1 to 1½ seconds each. Allow 2 seconds between breaths.

2. Breaths will have to be quickly interposed between cardiac compressions. If the patient needs only respiratory assistance, watch for chest expansion and listen with the stethoscope to ensure adequate ventilation.

3. A rate of approximately 10–12 breaths/minute is used.

Preoxygenation and suctioning

1. If hyperinflation is being used with suctioning, ventilate the patient before and after each suctioning pass (including after the last suction pass).

Transport

1. If hyperinflation is used in transport, suction patient before disconnection for transport; monitor heart and respiratory rates and LOC during procedure.

2. Ventilate at rate of 12–15 breaths/minute.

Follow-up phase

1. In cardiopulmonary arrest, verify return of spontaneous pulse and respirations. Initiate further support as needed.

2. In suctioning or transport, return to previous support. Note patient tolerance of procedure.

---

1. A humidifier bottle is not used because the high flow rates of oxygen required would force water into the tubing and clog it.

2. A high flow rate or "flush" position is necessary to meet the minute ventilation of the patient.

3. A high inspired O_2 concentration is required. Without a reservoir, inspired O_2 concentration will be low (28%–56%) because inspired gas will be air/O_2 mix. With a reservoir, manual resuscitation bags can achieve a FiO_2 of greater than 96% at a flow rate of 15 L/minute.

4. Body fluid precautions.

1. The airway helps prevent obstruction from prolapse of the tongue in an unconscious patient. If ventilation is difficult, confirm that airway is unobstructed.

2. Squeeze resuscitation bag with sufficient force and at the rate necessary to maintain adequate minute ventilation.

3. Continue squeezing bag at appropriate intervals until CPR is no longer required.

1. Hyperinflation before suctioning helps prevent hypoxemia. Hyperinflation after suctioning replaces O_2 removed during the procedure and helps to prevent atelectasis. The larger tidal volumes may also assist in mobilizing secretions and promote surfactant secretion.

1. Establishes a patent airway before the patient is moved. Provides information for assessing tolerance of transport.

1. Establishes the patient's need for definitive therapy (drugs, defibrillation, intensive care).

2. Note SaO_2, heart rate, rate and ease of respirations, arterial BP (if monitored), LOC. Report if intolerance occurs.

 NURSING ALERT Make sure that a good seal is maintained between face and mask so volume delivered through compression of bag is not lost.

 NURSING ALERT Airways are not appropriate in conscious patients or patients with a gag reflex because stimulation of the oropharynx could cause vomiting and aspiration. Short nasal pumps can be used in conscious patients with a gag reflex.

 Evidence Base American Heart Association. (2010). Guidelines for cardiopulmonary resuscitation and emergency cardiovascular care. *Circulation, 122*(18, Suppl. 3).

Community and Home Care Considerations

1. Indications for supplemental oxygen based on Medicare reimbursement guidelines:
   a. Documented hypoxemia: In adults: PaO_2 = 55 torr or $SaO_2 \leq 88\%$ when breathing room air, or PaO_2 56 to 59 torr or $SaO_2 \leq 89\%$ in association with cor pulmonale, heart failure, or polycythemia with hematocrit > 56%.
   b. Some patients may not qualify for oxygen therapy at rest but will qualify for oxygen during ambulation, exercise, or sleep. Oxygen therapy is indicated during these specific activities when SaO_2 is demonstrated to fall to $\leq 88\%$.
   c. Determine oxygen prescription for rest, exercise, and sleep, and instruct patient and caregiver to follow these flow rates.
2. Precautions in the home:
   a. In COPD with presence of CO_2 retention (generally due to chronic hypoxemia), oxygen administration at higher levels may lead to increased $PaCO_2$ level and decreased respiratory drive.
   b. Fire hazard is increased in presence of higher than normal oxygen concentrations. Instruct patient and caregiver of home oxygen precautions:
      i. Post NO SMOKING signs. Instruct on avoidance of cigarettes within 6 feet of oxygen.
      ii. Avoid potential electrical sparks around oxygen (shave with blade razor instead of electric razor; keep away from heat sources).
      iii. Keep oxygen at least 6 feet (1.8 m) from any source of flame.
   c. Power failure may lead to inadequate oxygen supply when an oxygen concentrator is used without backup tank.
   d. Oxygen tanks must be secured in stand to prevent falling over.
   e. Improper use of liquid oxygen (touching liquid) may result in burns.
3. Oxygen delivered by way of tracheostomy collar or T-tube should be humidified.
4. Oxygen concentrators extract oxygen from ambient air and should deliver oxygen at concentrations of 85% or greater at up to 4 L/minute.
5. Liquid oxygen is provided in large reservoir canisters with smaller portable units that can be transfilled by patient or caregiver. Liquid oxygen evaporates from canister when not in use.
6. Compressed gas may be supplied in large cylinders (G or H cylinders) or smaller cylinders (D or E cylinders) with wheels for easier movement.
7. All oxygen delivery equipment should be checked at least once daily by patient or caregiver, including function of equipment, prescribed flow rates, remaining liquid or compressed gas content, and backup supply.

Mechanical Ventilation

The mechanical ventilator device functions as a substitute for the bellows action of the thoracic cage and diaphragm. The mechanical ventilator can maintain ventilation automatically for prolonged periods. It is indicated when the patient is unable to maintain safe levels of oxygen or CO_2 by spontaneous breathing even with the assistance of other oxygen delivery devices.

Clinical Indications

Mechanical Failure of Ventilation

1. Neuromuscular disease.
2. CNS disease.
3. CNS depression (drug intoxication, respiratory depressants, cardiac arrest).
4. Inefficiency of thoracic cage in generating pressure gradients necessary for ventilation (chest injury, thoracic malformation).
5. When ventilatory support is needed postoperatively.

Disorders of Pulmonary Gas Exchange

1. Acute respiratory failure.
2. Chronic respiratory failure.
3. Left-sided heart failure.
4. Pulmonary diseases resulting in diffusion abnormality.
5. Pulmonary diseases resulting in V/Q mismatch.
6. Acute lung injury.

Underlying Principles

1. Variables that control ventilation and oxygenation include:
   a. Ventilator rate—adjusted by rate setting.
   b. V_T—volume of gas required for one breath (mL/kg).
   c. Fraction of inspired oxygen concentration (FiO_2)—set on ventilator and measured with an oxygen analyzer.
   d. Ventilator dead space—circuitry (tubing) common to inhalation and exhalation; tubing is calibrated.
   e. PEEP—set within the ventilator or with the use of external PEEP devices; measured at the proximal airway.
2. CO_2 elimination is controlled by V_T, rate, and dead space.
3. Oxygen tension is controlled by oxygen concentration and PEEP (also by rate and V_T).
4. In most cases, the duration of inspiration should not exceed exhalation.
5. The inspired gas must be warmed and humidified to prevent thickening of secretions and decrease in body temperature. Sterile or distilled water is warmed and humidified by way of a heated humidifier.

Types of Ventilators

Negative Pressure Ventilators

1. Applies negative pressure around the chest wall. This causes intra-airway pressure to become negative, thus drawing air into the lungs through the patient's nose and mouth.
2. No artificial airway is necessary; patient must be able to control and protect own airway.
3. Indicated for selected patients with respiratory neuromuscular problems or as adjunct to weaning from positive pressure ventilation.
4. Examples are the iron lung and cuirass (shell unit) ventilator.

Positive Pressure Ventilators

During mechanical inspiration, air is actively delivered to the patient's lungs under positive pressure. Exhalation is passive. Requires use of a cuffed artificial airway.

1. Pressure cycled.
   a. Delivers selected gas pressure during inspiratory phase.
   b. Volume delivered depends on lung compliance and resistance.
   c. Use of volume-based alarms is recommended because any obstruction between the machine and lungs that allows a buildup of pressure in the ventilator circuitry will cause the ventilator to cycle, but the patient will receive no volume.
   d. Exhaled tidal volume is the variable to monitor closely.
2. Volume limited.
   a. Designated volume of air is delivered with each breath regardless of resistance and compliance. Usual starting volume is 6 to 8 mL/kg.
   b. Delivers the predetermined volume regardless of changing lung compliance (although airway pressures will increase as compliance decreases). Airway pressures vary from patient to patient and from breath to breath.
   c. Pressure-limiting valves, which prevent excessive pressure buildup within the patient-ventilator system, are used. Without this valve, pressure could increase indefinitely and pulmonary barotrauma could result. Usually equipped with a system that alarms when selected pressure limit is exceeded. Pressure-limited settings terminate inspiration when reached.

Modes of Operation

Controlled Ventilation

1. Patient receives a set number and volume of breaths/minute.
2. Provides a fixed level of ventilation, but will not cycle or have gas available in circuitry to respond to patient's own inspiratory efforts. This typically increases work of breathing for patients attempting to breathe spontaneously.
3. Generally used for patients who are unable to initiate spontaneous breaths.

Assist/Control

1. Inspiratory cycle of ventilator is activated by the patient's voluntary inspiratory effort and delivers a preset full volume.
2. Ventilator also cycles at a rate predetermined by the operator. Should the patient not initiate a spontaneous breath, or breathe so weakly that the ventilator cannot function as an assistor, this mandatory baseline rate will provide a minimum respiratory rate.
3. Indicated for patients who are breathing spontaneously, but who have the potential to lose their respiratory drive or muscular control of ventilation. In this mode, the patient's work of breathing is greatly reduced.

Synchronized Intermittent Mandatory Ventilation (SIMV)

1. Allows patient to breathe at his or her own rate and volume spontaneously through the ventilator circuitry.
2. Periodically, at a preselected time, a mandatory breath is delivered. The mandatory breaths are synchronized with the patient's inspiratory effort.

3. Gas provided for spontaneous breathing flows continuously through the ventilator.
4. Ensures that a predetermined number of breaths at a selected V_T are delivered each minute.
5. Indicated for patients who are breathing spontaneously, but at a V_T and/or rate less than adequate for their needs. Allows the patient to do some of the work of breathing.

Pressure Support

1. Augments inspiration to a spontaneously breathing patient.
2. Maintains a set positive pressure during spontaneous inspiration.
3. The patient ventilates spontaneously, establishing own rate, V_T, and inspiratory time.
4. Pressure support may be used independently as a ventilatory mode or used in conjunction with CPAP or synchronized intermittent mandatory ventilation.

Positive Pressure Ventilation Techniques

Positive End-Expiratory Pressure

1. Maneuver by which pressure during mechanical ventilation is maintained above atmospheric at end of exhalation, resulting in an increased functional residual capacity. Airway pressure is therefore positive throughout the entire ventilatory cycle.
2. Purpose is to increase functional residual capacity (or the amount of air left in the lungs at the end of expiration). This aids in:
   a. Increasing the surface area of gas exchange.
   b. Preventing collapse of alveolar units and development of atelectasis.
   c. Decreasing intrapulmonary shunt.
   d. Improving lung compliance.
   e. Improving oxygenation.
   f. Recruiting alveolar units that are totally or partially collapsed.
3. Benefits:
   a. Because a greater surface area for diffusion is available and shunting is reduced, it is often possible to use a lower FiO_2 than otherwise would be required to obtain adequate arterial oxygen levels. This reduces the risk of oxygen toxicity in conditions such as acute respiratory distress syndrome (ARDS).
   b. Positive intra-airway pressure may be helpful in reducing the transudation of fluid from the pulmonary capillaries in situations where capillary pressure is increased (ie, left-sided heart failure).
   c. Increased lung compliance resulting in decreased work of breathing.
4. Hazards:
   a. Because the intrathoracic pressure is increased by PEEP, venous return is impeded. This may result in:
      i. Decreased cardiac output and decreased oxygen delivery to the tissues (especially noted in hypovolemic patients).
      ii. Decreased renal perfusion.
      iii. Increased intracranial pressure.
      iv. Hepatic congestion.

b. The decreased venous return may cause antidiuretic hormone formation to be stimulated, resulting in decreased urine output.

5. Precautions:
   a. Monitor frequently for signs and symptoms of respiratory distress—shortness of breath, dyspnea, tachycardia, chest pain.
   b. Monitor frequently for signs and symptoms of pneumothorax (increased PAP, increased size of hemothorax, uneven chest wall movement, hyperresonant percussion, distant or absent breath sounds).
   c. Monitor for signs of decreased venous return (decreased BP, decreased cardiac output, decreased urine output, peripheral edema).
   d. Abrupt discontinuance of PEEP is not recommended. The patient should not be without PEEP for longer than 15 seconds. The manual resuscitation bag used for ventilation during suction procedure or patient transport should be equipped with a PEEP device. In-line suctioning may also be used so that PEEP can be maintained.
   e. Intrapulmonary blood vessel pressure may increase with compression of the vessels by increased intra-airway pressure. Therefore, central venous pressure (CVP), PAP, and pulmonary capillary wedge pressure may be increased. The clinician must bear this in mind when determining the clinical significance of these pressures.

Continuous Positive Airway Pressure

1. Assists the spontaneously breathing patient to improve oxygenation by elevating the end-expiratory pressure in the lungs throughout the respiratory cycle.
2. May be delivered through ventilator circuitry when ventilator rate is at "0" or may be delivered through a separate CPAP circuitry that does not require the ventilator.
3. Indicated for patients who are capable of maintaining an adequate V_T, but who have pathology preventing maintenance of adequate levels of tissue oxygenation or for sleep apnea.
4. CPAP has the same benefits, hazards, and precautions noted with PEEP. Mean airway pressures may be lower because of lack of mechanical ventilation breaths. This results in less risk of barotrauma and impedance of venous return.

Newer Modes of Ventilation

Inverse Ratio Ventilation

1. I:E ratio is greater than 1, in which inspiration is longer than expiration.
2. Potentially used in patients who are in acute severe hypoxemic respiratory failure. Oxygenation is thought to be improved.
3. Very uncomfortable for patients; need to be heavily sedated.
4. Pressure-controlled inverse ratio ventilation—used in ARDS and acute lung injury.
5. Pressure-regulated volume control ventilator mode is a volume-targeted mode used in acute respiratory failure that combines the advantages of the decelerating inspiratory flow pattern of a pressure-control mode with the ease of use of a volume-control (VC) mode.

Airway Pressure Release Ventilation

1. Ventilator cycles between two different levels of CPAP.
2. The baseline airway pressure is the upper CPAP level and the pressure is intermittently released.
3. Uses a short expiratory time.
4. Used in severe ARDS/acute lung injury.

Noninvasive Positive Pressure Ventilation

1. Uses a nasal or face mask or nasal pillows. Delivers air through a volume- or pressure-controlled ventilator.
2. Used primarily in the past for patients with chronic respiratory failure associated with neuromuscular disease. Now is being used successfully during acute exacerbations. Some patients are able to avoid invasive intubation. Other indications include acute or chronic respiratory distress, acute pulmonary edema, pneumonia, COPD exacerbation, weaning, and postextubation respiratory decompensation.
3. Can be used in the home setting. Equipment is portable and relatively easy to use.
4. Eliminates the need for intubation, preserves normal swallowing, speech, and the cough mechanism.
5. May include BiPAP, which is essentially pressure support with CPAP. The system has a rate setting as well as inspiratory and expiratory pressure setting.

High-Frequency Ventilation

1. Uses very small V_T (dead space ventilation) and high frequency (rates greater than 100/minute).
2. Gas exchange occurs through various mechanisms, not the same as conventional ventilation (convection).
3. Types include:
   a. High-frequency oscillatory ventilation.
   b. High-frequency jet ventilation.
4. Theory is that there is decreased barotrauma by having small V_T and that oxygenation is improved by constant flow of gases.
5. Successful with infant respiratory distress syndrome, much less successful with adult pulmonary complications.

Nursing Assessment and Interventions

1. Monitor for complications:
   a. Airway aspiration, decreased clearance of secretions, ventilator-acquired pneumonia, tracheal damage, laryngeal edema.
   b. Impaired gas exchange.
   c. Ineffective breathing pattern.
   d. ET tube kinking, cuff failure, mainstem intubation.
   e. Sinusitis.
   f. Pulmonary infection.
   g. Barotrauma (pneumothorax, tension pneumothorax, subcutaneous emphysema, pneumomediastinum).
   h. Decreased cardiac output.
   i. Atelectasis.
   j. Alteration in GI function (stress ulcers, gastric distention, paralytic ileus).
   k. Alteration in renal function.
   l. Alteration in cognitive-perceptual status.

2. Suction the patient as indicated.

    a. When secretions can be seen or sounds resulting from secretions are heard with or without the use of a stethoscope.

    b. After chest physiotherapy.

    c. After bronchodilator treatments.

    d. Increased peak airway pressure in mechanically ventilated patients that is not due to the artificial airway or ventilator tube kinking, the patient biting the tube, the patient coughing or struggling against the ventilator, or a pneumothorax.

3. Provide routine care for patient on mechanical ventilator (see Procedure Guidelines 10-19). Provide regular oral care to prevent ventilator-associated pneumonia. Provide humidity and repositioning to mobilize secretions.

4. Assist with the weaning process, when indicated (patient gradually assumes responsibility for regulating and performing own ventilations; see Procedure Guidelines 10-20, pages 258 to 260).

    a. Patient must have acceptable ABG values, no evidence of acute pulmonary pathology, and must be hemodynamically stable.

(*Text continues on page 261*)

PROCEDURE GUIDELINES 10-19

Managing the Patient Requiring Mechanical Ventilation

EQUIPMENT

- Artificial airway (endotracheal [ET] tube or tracheostomy)
- Manual self-inflating resuscitation bag
- Pulse oximetry
- Suction equipment
- Mechanical ventilator
- Ventilation circuitry
- Humidifier

See manufacturer's directions for specific machine.

PROCEDURE

Nursing Action	Rationale
Preparatory phase	
1. Obtain baseline samples for blood gas determinations (pH, PaO_2, $PaCO_2$, HCO_3^-) and chest x-ray.	1. Baseline measurements serve as a guide in determining progress of therapy.
2. Give a brief explanation to the patient and family.	2. Allays fear and enlists cooperation. Emphasize that mechanical ventilation is a temporary measure. The patient should be prepared psychologically for weaning at the time the ventilator is first used.
3. Premedicate as needed.	3. Promotes cooperation through mild sedation.
4. Establish the airway by means of a cuffed ET or tracheostomy tube (see pages 212–216).	4. A closed system between the ventilator and patient's lower airway is necessary for positive pressure ventilation.
5. Prepare the ventilator. (Respiratory therapist does this in many facilities.)	5. Have all equipment and settings in place before applying to patient.
a. Set up desired circuitry.	
b. Connect oxygen and compressed air source.	
c. Turn on power.	
d. Set V_T (usually 6–8 mL/kg body weight [Morton]).	d. Adjusted according to pH and $PaCO_2$.
e. Set oxygen concentration.	e. Adjusted according to PaO_2.
f. Set ventilator sensitivity.	
g. Set rate at 12–14 breaths/minute (variable).	g. This setting approximates normal ventilation. These machines' settings are subject to change according to the patient's condition and response and the ventilator type being used.
h. Set inspiratory–expiratory (I:E) times (varies depending on the ventilator). Adjust flow rate (velocity of gas flow during inspiration). Usually set at 40 to 60 L/minute. Depends on rate and V_T.	h. The slower the flow, the lower the peak airway pressure will result from set volume delivery. This results in lower intrathoracic pressure and less impedance of venous return. However, a flow that is too low for the rate selected may result in inverse I:E ratios.
i. Select mode of ventilation.	
j. Check machine function—measure V_T, rate, I:E ratio, analyze oxygen, check all alarms.	j. Ensures safe function.

PROCEDURE GUIDELINES 10-19 (continued)

Managing the Patient Requiring Mechanical Ventilation

PROCEDURE (continued)

Nursing Action	Rationale
Performance phase	
1. Couple the patient's airway to the ventilator.	1. Make sure all connections are secure. Prevent ventilator tubing from "pulling" on artificial airway, possibly resulting in tube dislodgement or tracheal damage.
2. Assess patient for adequate chest movement and rate. Note peak airway pressure and PEEP.	2. Ensures proper function of equipment.
3. Set airway pressure alarms according to patient's baseline:	3.
a. High pressure alarm	a. High airway pressure is set at 10 to 15 cm H_2O above peak inspiratory pressure. An alarm sounds if airway pressure selected is exceeded. Alarm activation indicates decreased lung compliance (worsening pulmonary disease); decreased lung volume (such as pneumothorax, tension pneumothorax, hemothorax, pleural effusion); increased airway resistance (secretions, coughing, bronchospasm, breathing out of phase with the ventilator); loss of patency of airway (mucus plug, airway spasm, biting or kinking of tube).
b. Low-pressure alarm	b. Low airway pressure alarm set at 5 to 10 cm H_2O below peak inspiratory pressure. Alarm activation indicates inability to build up airway pressure because of disconnection or leak, and changing compliance and resistance.
4. Assess frequently for change in respiratory status by evaluation of ABGs, pulse oximetry, spontaneous respiratory rate, use of accessory muscles, breath sounds, and vital signs. Other means of assessing are through the use of exhaled carbon dioxide (see "Capnography," page 210, or "Oxygen saturation monitoring," page 209). If change is noted, notify health care provider.	4. Guides therapy.
5. Monitor and troubleshoot alarm conditions. Ensure appropriate ventilation at all times.	5. Priority is ventilation and oxygenation of the patient. In alarm conditions that cannot be immediately corrected, disconnect the patient from mechanical ventilation and manually ventilate with resuscitation bag.
6. Check for secure stabilization of artificial airway.	6. Reduces risk of inadvertent extubation.
7. Positioning:	7.
a. Turn patient from side to side every 2 hours, or more frequently if possible. Consider kinetic therapy as early intervention to improve outcome.	a. Repositioning may improve secretion clearance and reduce atelectasis. For patients on long-term ventilation, this may result in sleep deprivation. Follow a turning schedule best suited to a particular patient's condition.
b. Lateral turns are desirable; from right semiprone to left semiprone.	
c. Sit the patient upright at regular intervals, if possible.	c. Upright posture increases lung compliance.
d. Consider prone positioning to improve oxygenation.	d. Proning has been shown to have some beneficial effects or the improvement of oxygenation in certain populations, such as patients with ARDS.

(continued)

PROCEDURE GUIDELINES 10-19 *(continued)*

Managing the Patient Requiring Mechanical Ventilation

PROCEDURE *(continued)*

Nursing Action	Rationale

 NURSING ALERT For patients in severe compromised respiratory state or who are unstable hemodynamically, consider use of specialty bed with kinetic therapy.

8. Carry out passive range-of-motion exercises of all extremities for patients unable to do so.

8. Prevents contractures.

9. Assess for need of suctioning at least every 2 hours.

9. Patients with artificial airways on mechanical ventilation are unable to clear secretions on their own. Suctioning may help to clear secretions and stimulate the cough reflex.

10. Assess respiratory effort and breath sounds every 2 hours in all lobes bilaterally.

   a. Determine whether breath sounds are present or absent, normal or abnormal, and whether a change has occurred.

10.

   a. Auscultation of the chest is a means of assessing airway patency and ventilatory distribution. It also confirms the proper placement of the ET or tracheostomy tube.

11. Humidification:

   a. Check the water level in the humidification reservoir to ensure that the patient is never ventilated with dry gas.

   b. Empty the water that condenses in the delivery and exhalation tubing into a separate receptacle, not into the humidifier. Always wash hands before and after emptying fluid from ventilator circuitry. Humidification may also be achieved using a moisture enhancer.

11.

   a. Humidity may improve secretion mobilization.

   b. Water condensing in the inspiratory tubing may cause increased resistance to gas flow. This may result in increased peak airway pressures. Warm, moist tubing is a perfect breeding area for bacteria. If this water is allowed to enter the humidifier, bacteria may be aerosolized into the lungs. Emptying the tubing also prevents introduction of water into the patient's airways.

12. Assess airway pressures at frequent intervals.

12. May indicate changes in compliance or onset of conditions that may cause airway pressure to increase or decrease.

13. Measure delivered V_T and analyze oxygen concentration every 4 hours or more frequently, if indicated. (Respiratory therapist performs this in most facilities.)

13. Ensures that patient is receiving the appropriate ventilatory assistance.

14. Monitor cardiovascular function. Assess for abnormalities.

   a. Monitor pulse rate and arterial BP; intra-arterial pressure monitoring may be carried out.

   b. Use pulmonary artery catheter to monitor pulmonary capillary wedge pressure (PCWP), mixed venous oxygen saturation (SvO_2), and cardiac output (CO).

14. Determines patient's response to therapy and possible adverse effects.

   a. Arterial catheterization for intra-arterial pressure monitoring also provides access for ABG samples.

   b. Intermittent and continuous positive pressure ventilation may increase the PAP and decrease cardiac output.

15. Provide mouth care every 1–4 hours and assess for development of pressure areas from ET tubes.

15. For comfort and reduced risk of infection.

16. Monitor for systemic signs and symptoms of pulmonary infection (pulmonary physical examination findings, increased heart rate, increased temperature, increased count).

16. Risk of infection increases with artificial airways.

PROCEDURE GUIDELINES 10-19 (continued)

Managing the Patient Requiring Mechanical Ventilation

PROCEDURE (continued)

Nursing Action	Rationale
17. Evaluate need for sedation or muscle relaxants.	17. Sedatives may be prescribed to decrease anxiety or to relax the patient to prevent "competing" with the ventilator. At times, pharmacologically induced paralysis may be necessary to permit mechanical ventilation.

 DRUG ALERT Never administer paralyzing agents until the patient is intubated and on mechanical ventilation. Sedatives should be prescribed in conjunction with paralyzing agents because the patient may not be able to move but can still have awareness of his or her surroundings and inability to move.

Nursing Action	Rationale

18. Use "ventilator bundle" protocol, as directed, to prevent ventilator-associated complications.
 	
   a. Elevate the head of the bed to between 30 and 45 degrees.
   b. Daily "sedative interruption" and daily assessment of readiness to extubate.
   c. Peptic ulcer disease prophylaxis.
   d. Deep vein thrombosis prophylaxis (unless contraindicated).
	18. Reduces the risk of aspiration, peptic ulcer, and deep vein prophylaxis; reduces sedation that may interfere with assessment.

19. Report intake and output precisely and obtain an accurate daily weight to monitor fluid balance.	19. Positive fluid balance resulting in increase in body weight and interstitial pulmonary edema is a frequent problem in patients requiring mechanical ventilation. Prevention requires early recognition of fluid accumulation. An average adult who is dependent on parenteral nutrition can be expected to lose ½ lb (0.25 kg) per day; therefore, constant body weight indicates fluid retention.

20. Monitor nutritional status.
(Patients with ET tubes are to receive nothing by mouth [the tube splints the epiglottis open] but patients with tracheostomy tubes may take food by mouth if otherwise capable.)
   a. Weigh patient daily at same time.
   b. Assess serum prealbumin level as directed.
   c. Obtain nutritional consult with prolonged therapy.
	20. Patients on mechanical ventilation require inflation of artificial airway cuffs at all times. Enteral or parenteral nourishment is usually employed (see page 219) to prevent rapid weight loss and malnutrition.

21. Monitor for GI bleeding. a. Test all stools and gastric drainage for occult blood (if part of facility protocol).	21. Mechanically ventilated patients are at risk for development of stress ulcers, resulting in occult or frank GI bleeding.

22. Provide psychological support and assist with communication needs of patient with an artificial airway.
 	
   a. Use alternate means of communication.
   b. Orient frequently to environment and function of mechanical ventilator.
   c. Ensure that the patient has adequate rest and sleep.
	22. Mechanical ventilation may result in sleep deprivation and loss of touch with surroundings and reality, as well as inability to talk.

(continued)

PROCEDURE GUIDELINES 10-19 (continued)

Managing the Patient Requiring Mechanical Ventilation

PROCEDURE (continued)

Nursing Action	Rationale
Follow-up phase	
1. Maintain a flow sheet to record ventilation patterns, ABGs, pertinent laboratory results, fluid balance, weight, vital signs, and other clinical assessments. Notify appropriate health care provider of changes in the patient's condition.	1. Establishes means of assessing for effectiveness and progress of treatment.
2. Change ventilator circuitry per facility protocol; assess ventilator's function every 4 hours or more frequently if problem occurs.	2. Prevents contamination of lower airways.

Evidence Base Nseir, S. (2011). New tracheal tubes to prevent ventilator-associated pneumonia: Where is the evidence? *Critical Care, 15,* 459.

Chulay, M., & Burns, S. (2010). *AACN essentials of critical care nursing* (2nd ed.) New York: McGraw-Hill.

Sedgwick, M. B., Lance-Smith, M., Reeder, S., et al. (2012). Using Evidence-Based Practice to Prevent Ventilator-Associated Pneumonia. *Critical Care Nurse, 32*(4), 41–51.

PROCEDURE GUIDELINES 10-20

Weaning the Patient from Mechanical Ventilation

EQUIPMENT

- Varies according to technique used
- CPAP adapter
- Synchronized intermittent mandatory ventilation (SIMV) (set up in addition to ventilator or incorporated in ventilator and circuitry)
- Pressure support
- Briggs T piece (rarely used)

PROCEDURE

Nursing Action	Rationale
Preparatory phase	
1. For weaning to be successful, the patient must be physiologically capable of maintaining spontaneous respirations. Assessments must ensure that:	1. Provides baseline; ensures that patient is capable of having adequate neuromuscular control to provide adequate ventilation.
a. The underlying disease process is significantly reversed, as evidenced by pulmonary examination, ABGs, chest x-ray.	
b. The patient can mechanically perform ventilation. Should be able to generate a negative inspiratory pressure less than −20 cm H_2O; have a vital capacity 10–15 mL/kg; have a resting minute ventilation less than 10 L/minute, and be able to double this; have a spontaneous respiratory rate of less than 25 breaths/minute, without significant tachycardia; be normotensive; have optimal hemoglobin for condition; have adequate nutritional status.	

PROCEDURE GUIDELINES 10-20 *(continued)*

Weaning the Patient from Mechanical Ventilation

PROCEDURE *(continued)*

Nursing Action	Rationale

2. Assess for other factors that may cause respiratory insufficiency.
  a. Acid-base abnormality
  b. Nutritional depletion
  c. Electrolyte abnormality
  d. Fever
  e. Abnormal fluid balance
  f. Hyperglycemia
  g. Infection
  h. Pain
  i. Sleep deprivation
  j. Decreased LOC
	2. Weaning is difficult when these conditions are present.

3. Assess psychological readiness for weaning.	3. Patient must be physically and psychologically ready for weaning.
4. Explain procedure and that weaning is not always successful on the initial attempt.	4. Explaining procedure to patient will decrease patient anxiety and promote cooperation. The patient should not be discouraged if weaning is unsuccessful on the first attempt.
5. Prepare appropriate equipment.	
6. Position the patient in sitting or semi-Fowler's position.	6. Increases lung compliance, decreases work of breathing.
7. Pick optimal time of day, preferably early morning.	7. The patient should be rested.
8. Perform bronchial hygiene as needed (postural drainage, suctioning) before weaning attempt.	8. The patient should be in best pulmonary condition for weaning to be successful.

Performance phase

CPAP weaning (preferred)

1. Discontinue mechanical ventilation and apply CPAP adapter.	1. The patient breathes on own with 2.5–5 cm H_2O CPAP. *Note: Briggs T piece may be used instead of CPAP; however, CPAP is preferable to prevent atelectasis during the weaning process.*

2. Monitor the patient for factors indicating need for reinstitution of mechanical ventilation.
 	
  a. BP increase or decrease greater than 20 mm Hg systolic or 10 mm Hg diastolic.
  b. Heart rate increase of 20 beats/minute or greater than 110.
  c. Respiratory rate increase greater than 10 breaths/minute or rate greater than 30.
  d. V_T less than 250–300 mL (in adults).
  e. Appearance of new cardiac ectopy or increase in baseline ectopy.
  f. PaO_2 less than 60, $PaCO_2$ greater than 55, or pH less than 7.35 (may accept lower PaO_2 and pH, and higher $PaCO_2$ in patients with COPD).
	2. Indicates intolerance of weaning procedure. Stay with the patient during weaning time to decrease patient anxiety and monitor for tolerance of procedure.

3. Increase time off ventilator with each weaning attempt as the patient's condition indicates. Evaluate for toleration before moving to the next increment.	3. The patient will progress as he or she becomes mentally and physically able to perform adequate spontaneous ventilation.

(continued)

PROCEDURE GUIDELINES 10-20 *(continued)*

Weaning the Patient from Mechanical Ventilation

PROCEDURE *(continued)*

Nursing Action	Rationale

4. Institute other techniques helpful in encouraging weaning.
  a. Mental stimulation.
  b. Biofeedback.
  c. Participation in care.
  d. Provision of rewards.
  e. Contact with successfully weaned patients.
	4. Provides motivation and positive feedback.

5. When patient tolerates 40–60 minutes of continuous weaning, weaning increments can increase rapidly.	
6. When the patient can maintain spontaneous ventilation throughout day, begin night weaning.	

SIMV weaning

Nursing Action	Rationale
1. Set ventilator to SIMV mode.	
2. Set rate interval.	2. Determines the time interval between machine-delivered breaths, during which the patient will breathe on own.
3. If gas for the patient's spontaneous breath is delivered via a demand valve regulator, ensure that machine sensitivity is at maximum setting.	3. Aids in decreasing work of breathing necessary to open demand valve.
4. Evaluate for tolerance of procedure. Monitor for factors indicating need for increase or decrease of mandatory respiratory rate (see step 2 above). In rapid weaning, changes may be made approximately every 20–30 minutes.	4. If the patient does not tolerate the procedure, the $PaCO_2$ will rise and pH will fall.
5. If $PaCO_2$ and pH levels remain stable, then continue to decrease mandatory rate as patient tolerates.	5. May be done as frequently as every 20–30 minutes with ABG monitoring, pulse oximetry, documentation of successful weaning.

Pressure support

Nursing Action	Rationale
1. The amount of pressure support (cm H_2O) provided to the airway is progressively decreased over time, allowing the patient to increase role in supporting own spontaneous ventilation.	1. May be beneficial adjunct to SIMV weaning.

Follow-up phase

Nursing Action	Rationale
1. Record at each weaning interval: heart rate, BP, respiratory rate, FiO_2, ABG, pulse oximetry value, respiratory and ventilator rate (if SIMV), or length of time off ventilator (if CPAP weaning).	1. Provides record of procedure and assessment of progress.

Note: It is not within the scope of this manual to establish criteria for the use of one weaning modality as opposed to another.

 Evidence Base American Association for Respiratory Care. (2002). Clinical practice guidelines. Evidence-based guidelines for weaning and discontinuing ventilatory support (reviewed 2010). *Respiratory Care, 47*(1), 69–90.

Hess, D., & MacIntyre, N. (2011). Ventilator discontinuation: Why are we still weaning. *American Journal of Respiratory and Critical Care Medicine, 184,* 392–394.

Blackwood, B., Alderdice, F., Burns, K. E., et al. (2010). Protocolized versus non-protocolized weaning for reducing the duration of mechanical ventilation in critically ill adult patients. *Cochrane Database of Systematic Reviews,* Issue 5 (Article No. CD006904).

Conaway, M., Bleck, T., Burns, S., et al. (2012). The Relationship of 26 Clinical Factors to Weaning Outcome. *Am J Crit Care, 21,* 52–59.

b. Obtain serial ABGs and/or oximetry readings, as indicated.

c. Monitor very closely for change in pulse and BP, anxiety, and increased rate of respirations.

d. The patient is awake and cooperative and displays optimal respiratory drive.

5. Once weaning is successful, extubate and provide alternate means of oxygen (see Procedure Guidelines 10-21).

6. Extubation will be considered when the pulmonary function parameters of V_T, VC, and negative inspiratory pressure are adequate, indicating strong respiratory muscle function.

PROCEDURE GUIDELINES 10-21

Extubation

EQUIPMENT

- Tonsil suction (surgical suction instrument)
- 10-mL syringe
- Resuscitation bag and mask with oxygen flow
- Face mask connected to large-bore tubing, humidifier, and oxygen source
- Suction catheter
- Suction source
- Gloves
- Face shield

PROCEDURE

Nursing Action	Rationale
Preparatory phrase	
1. Monitor heart rate, lung expansion, and breath sounds before extubation. Record tidal volume (V_T), vital capacity (VC), negative inspiratory pressure (NIP).	1. V_T, VC, and NIF are measured to assess respiratory muscle function and adequacy of ventilation.
2. Assess the patient for other signs of adequate muscle strength.	2. Adequate muscle strength is necessary to ensure muscle strength for spontaneous breathing and coughing.
a. Instruct the patient to tightly squeeze the index and middle fingers of your hand. Resistance to removal of your fingers from the patient's grasp must be demonstrated.	
b. Ask the patient to lift head from the pillow and hold for 2–3 seconds.	

 NURSING ALERT Keep in mind that patient's underlying problems must be improved or resolved before extubation is considered. Patient should also be free from infection and malnutrition.

Nursing Action	Rationale
3. Obtain orders for extubation and postextubation oxygen therapy.	3. Do not attempt extubation until postextubation oxygen therapy is available and functioning at the bedside.
4. Explain the procedure to the patient:	4. Increases patient cooperation.
a. Artificial airway will be removed.	
b. Suctioning will occur before extubation.	
c. Deep breath should be taken on command.	
d. Instruction will be given to cough after extubation.	
5. Prepare necessary equipment. Have ready for use tonsil suction, suction catheter, 10-mL syringe, bag-mask unit, and oxygen by way of face mask.	
6. Place the patient in sitting or semi-Fowler's position (unless contraindicated).	6. Increases lung compliance and decreases work of breathing. Facilitates coughing.
Performance phase	
1. Put on face shield and gloves.	1. Spraying of airway secretions may occur.
2. Loosen tape or ET tube-securing device.	2. So that tube can be removed more easily when ready.

PROCEDURE GUIDELINES 10-21 (continued)

Extubation

PROCEDURE (continued)

Nursing Action	Rationale
3. Suction ET tube, then suction oropharyngeal airway above the ET cuff as thoroughly as possible.	3. To reduce secretions above and within the tube. Secretions not cleared from above the cuff will be aspirated when the cuff is deflated.
4. Extubate the patient: a. Ask the patient to take as deep a breath as possible (if the patient is not following commands, give a deep breath with the resuscitation bag). b. At peak inspiration, deflate the cuff completely and pull the tube out in the direction of the curve (out and downward).	4. a. At peak inspiration, the trachea and vocal cords will dilate, allowing a less traumatic tube removal.
5. Once the tube is fully removed, ask the patient to cough or exhale forcefully to remove secretions. Then suction the back of the patient's airway with the tonsil suction.	5. Frequently, old blood is seen in the secretions of newly extubated patients. Monitor for the appearance of bright red blood due to trauma occurring during extubation.
6. Apply oxygen therapy as ordered.	
7. Evaluate immediately for any signs of respiratory distress, stridor (high-pitched crowing sounds), or decreased air flow. If the patient develops any of these problems, attempt to ventilate the patient with the resuscitation bag and mask and prepare for reintubation. (Nebulized treatments may be ordered to avoid having to reintubate the patient.)	7. Evaluates for laryngospasm or edema at the cuff site, resulting in obstruction of the airway.

Follow-up phase

1. Note patient tolerance of procedure, upper and lower airway sounds postextubation, description of secretions.	1. Establishes a baseline to assess improvement/development of complications.
2. Observe the patient closely postextubation for any signs and symptoms of airway obstruction or respiratory insufficiency.	2. Tracheal or laryngeal edema may develop up to 24 hours postextubation.
3. Observe character of voice and signs of blood in sputum.	3. Hoarseness is a common postextubation complaint. Observe for worsening hoarseness or vocal cord paralysis.
4. Provide supplemental oxygen and humidification using face mask.	

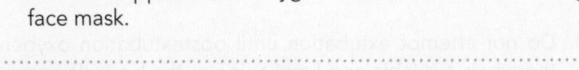 **Evidence Base** American Association for Respiratory Care. (2007). Clinical practice guidelines. Removal of endotracheal tube. *Respiratory Care, 52*(3), 81–93.
Amanullah, S. (2011). Ventilator-associated pneumonia overview of nosocomial pneumonias. Available: *http://emedicine.medscape.com/article/304836-overview.*
Amitai, A. (2011). Ventilator management. *Medscape Reference.* Available: *http://emedicine.medscape.com/article/810126-overview.*

Community and Home Care Considerations

Patients may require mechanical ventilation at home to replace or assist normal breathing. Ventilator support in the home is used to keep patient clinically stable and to maintain life.

1. Candidates for home ventilation are those patients who are unable to wean from mechanical ventilation, and/or have

disease progression requiring ventilator support. Candidates for home mechanical ventilator support:
a. Have a secure artificial airway (tracheostomy tube).
b. Have FiO_2 requirement ≤40%.
c. Are medically stable.
d. Are able to maintain adequate ventilation on standard ventilator settings.

2. Patients may choose not to receive home ventilation. Examples of inappropriate candidates for home ventilation include patients who:
   a. Have a $FiO_2 \geq 40\%$.
   b. Use PEEP > 10 cm H_2O.
   c. Require continuous invasive monitoring.
   d. Lack a mature tracheostomy.
   e. Lack able, willing, appropriate caregivers, and/or caregiver respite.
   f. Lack adequate financial resources for care in home.
   g. Lack adequate physical facilities:
      i. Inadequate heat, electricity, sanitation.
      ii. Presence of fire, health, or safety hazards.
3. For patients on mechanical ventilation in the home, a contract and relationship with a home medical equipment company and home nursing agency must be developed to provide:
   a. Care of ventilator-dependent patient.
   b. Provision and maintenance of equipment.
   c. Timely provision of disposable supplies.
   d. Ongoing monitoring of patient and equipment.
   e. Training of patient, caregivers, and clinical staff on proper management of ventilated patient and use and troubleshooting of equipment.
4. Equipment required:
   a. Appropriate ventilator with alarms (disconnect and high pressure).
   b. Power source.
   c. Humidification system.
   d. Manual resuscitation bag with tracheostomy adapter.
   e. Replacement tracheostomy tubes.
   f. Supplemental oxygen, as medically indicated.
   g. Communication method for patient.
   h. Backup charged battery to run ventilator during power failures.
5. Lay caregiver training and return demonstration must include:
   a. Proper setup, use, troubleshooting, maintenance, and cleaning and infection control of equipment and supplies.
   b. Appropriate patient assessment and management of abnormalities, including cardiopulmonary resuscitation, response to emergencies, power and equipment failure.
6. Potential complications include:
   a. Patient deterioration, need for emergency services.
   b. Equipment failure, malfunction.
   c. Psychosocial complications, including depression, anxiety, and/or loss of resources (caregiver, financial, detrimental change in family structure or coping capacity).
7. Communication is essential with local emergency medical services (fire, police, rescue) and utility (telephone, electric) companies from whom the patient would need immediate and additional assistance in event of emergency (eg, power failure, fire).

Thoracic Surgeries

 Evidence Base Mishra, E., & Davies, R. (2010). Advances in the investigation and treatment of pleural effusions. *Expert Review of Respiratory Medicine, 4*(1), 123–133.
Lewis, S., Dirksen, S. R., Heitkemper, M. M., et al. (2010). *Medical-surgical nursing* (8th ed.). St. Louis, MO: Elsevier.

Thoracic surgeries (see Table 10-2, page 264) are operative procedures performed to aid in the diagnosis and treatment of certain pulmonary conditions and when performing surgery that compromises the integrity of the thoracic cavity. Procedures include thoracotomy, video-assisted thoracoscopy, decortication, lung volume reduction surgery, lobectomy (see Figure 10-6, page 265), pneumonectomy, segmental resection, and wedge resection. These procedures may or may not require chest drainage immediately after surgery.

 NURSING ALERT Meticulous attention must be given to the preoperative and postoperative care of patients undergoing thoracic surgery. These operations are wide in scope and represent a major stress on the cardiorespiratory system.

Preoperative Management

Goal is to maximize respiratory function to improve the outcome postoperatively and reduce risk of complications.

1. Encourage the patient to stop smoking to restore bronchial ciliary action and to reduce the amount of sputum, and likelihood of postoperative atelectasis, by decreasing secretions and increasing oxygen saturation.
2. Teach an effective coughing technique.
   a. Sit upright with knees flexed and body bending slightly forward (or lie on side with hips and knees flexed if unable to sit up).
   b. Splint the incision with hands or folded towel.
   c. Take three short breaths, followed by a deep inspiration, inhaling slowly and evenly through the nose.
   d. Contract abdominal muscles and cough twice forcefully with mouth open and tongue out.
   e. Alternate technique—huffing and coughing—is less painful. Take a deep diaphragmatic breath and exhale forcefully against hand; exhale in a quick, distinct pant, or "huff."
3. Humidify the air to loosen secretions.
4. Administer bronchodilators to reduce bronchospasm.
5. Administer antimicrobials for infection.
6. Encourage deep breathing with the use of incentive spirometer (see Procedure Guidelines 10-22, pages 265 to 266) to prevent atelectasis postoperatively.
7. Teach diaphragmatic breathing.
8. Carry out chest physical therapy and postural drainage to reduce pooling of lung secretions (see page 235).
9. Evaluate cardiovascular status for risk and prevention of complication.
10. Encourage activity to improve exercise tolerance.

Table 10-2   Thoracic Surgery Types

TYPE	DESCRIPTION	INDICATIONS
Exploratory thoracotomy	*Internal view of lung* • Usually posterolateral parascapular but could be anterior incision • Chest tubes after procedure	May be used to confirm carcinoma or for chest trauma (to detect source of bleeding)
Lobectomy	*Lobe removal* • Thoracotomy incision at site of lobe removal • Chest tubes after procedure	Used when pathology is limited to one area of lung: bronchogenic carcinoma, giant emphysematous blebs or bullae, benign tumors, metastatic malignant tumors, bronchiectasis and fungal infections
Pneumonectomy	*Removal of an entire lung* • Posterolateral or anterolateral thoracotomy incision • Sometimes there is a rib resection • Normally no chest drains or tubes because fluid accumulation in empty space is desirable	Performed chiefly for carcinoma, but may be used for lung abscesses, bronchiectasis, or extensive tuberculosis *Note: Right lung is more vascular than left; may cause more physiologic problems if removed*
Segmentectomy (segmental resection)	*Only certain segment of lung removed* • Segments function as individual units	Used when pathology is localized (such as in bronchiectasis) and when the patient has preexisting cardiopulmonary compromise
Wedge resection	*Small localized section of lung tissue removed—usually pie shaped* • Incision made without regard to segments • Chest tubes after procedure	Performed for random lung biopsy and small peripheral nodules Considered when less invasive tests have failed to establish a diagnosis May be used as a therapeutic procedure
Thoracoscopy	*Direct visualization of pleura with thoracoscope via an intercostal incision* • Medical under sedation or local anesthesia; allows for visualization and biopsy • Video-assisted thoracoscopic surgery (VATS) under general anesthesia; multiple puncture sites and video screen allow for visualization and manipulation of the pleura, mediastinum, and lung parenchyma	VATS may be used for lung biopsy, lobectomy, resection of nodules, repair of fistulas
Decortication	*Removal or stripping of thick fibrous membrane from visceral pleura* • Use of chest tube drainage system postoperatively	Empyema unresponsive to conservative management
Thoracotomy not involving lungs	• Incision into the thoracic cavity for surgical procedures on other structures	Used for hiatal hernia repair, open heart surgery, esophageal surgery, tracheal resection, aortic aneurysm repair
Lung volume reduction surgery (LVRS)	• Involves reducing lung volume by multiple wedge excisions or VATS	Performed in advanced bullous emphysema, α^1-antitrypsin emphysema

11. Administer medications and limit sodium and fluid to improve heart failure, if indicated.

12. Correct anemia, dehydration, and hypoproteinemia with IV infusions, tube feedings, and blood transfusions as indicated.

13. Give prophylactic anticoagulant, as prescribed, to reduce perioperative incidence of deep vein thrombosis and pulmonary embolism.

14. Provide teaching and counseling.
    a. Orient the patient to events that will occur in the postoperative period—coughing and deep breathing, suctioning, chest tube and drainage system, oxygen therapy, ventilator therapy, pain control, leg exercises and range-of-motion (ROM) exercises for affected shoulder.

15. Make sure that patient fully understands surgery and is emotionally prepared for it; verify that informed consent has been obtained.

Postoperative Management

1. Use mechanical ventilator and/or supplemental oxygen until respiratory function and cardiovascular status stabilize. Assist with weaning and extubation.

2. Auscultate chest, monitor vital signs, monitor ECG, and assess respiratory rate and depth frequently. Arterial line, CVP, and pulmonary artery catheter are usually used.

3. Monitor ABG values and/or SaO_2 frequently.

(*Text continues on page 267*)

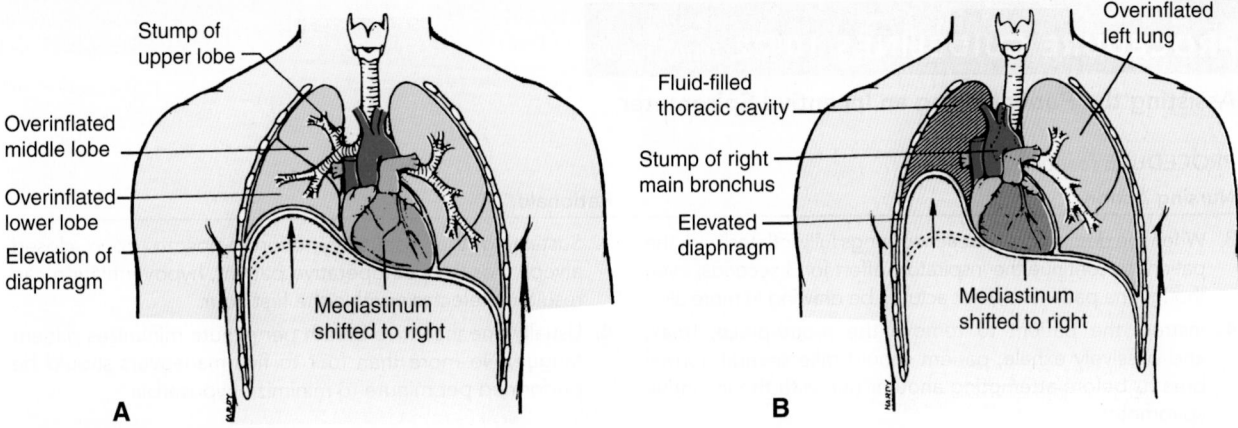

Figure 10-6. Operative procedures. (A) Lobectomy. **(B)** Pneumonectomy.

PROCEDURE GUIDELINES 10-22

Assisting the Patient Using an Incentive Spirometer

EQUIPMENT
According to the type of device used

PROCEDURE

Nursing Action	Rationale
Preparatory phase	
1. Measure the patient's normal tidal volume (V_T) and auscultate the chest, preferably preprocedure/treatment and/or preoperatively.	1. Establishes the patient's baseline.
2. Explain the procedure and its purpose to the patient. The device provides measurement and feedback related to breathing effectiveness and mimics the natural sigh and yawn, thus keeping the lungs clear.	2. Optimal results are achieved when the patient is given pretreatment or preoperative instruction.
3. Place the patient in a comfortable sitting, semi-Fowler's, or upright position.	3. Diaphragmatic excursion is greater in this position; however, if the patient is medically unable to be in this position, the exercise may be done in any position.
4. For the postoperative patient, try as much as possible to avoid discomfort. Try to coordinate treatment with administration of pain-relief medications. Instruct and assist the patient with splinting of incision.	4. Incentive spirometry is most successful when pain is controlled.
Performance phase	
1. Set the incentive spirometer V_T indicator at the desired goal the patient is to reach or exceed (500 mL is often used to start). The V_T is set according to the manufacturer's instructions.	1. The initial V_T may be prescribed, but the purpose of the device is to establish a baseline V_T and provide incentive to achieve greater volumes progressively.
2. Demonstrate the technique to the patient. a. Instruct the patient to exhale fully. b. Tell the patient to take in a slow, easy, deep breath from the mouthpiece.	2. To increase understanding and effectiveness. *Note:* Noseclips are sometimes used if the patient has difficulty breathing only through mouth. This will ensure full credit for each breath measured.

(continued)

PROCEDURE GUIDELINES 10-22 *(continued)*

Assisting the Patient Using an Incentive Spirometer

PROCEDURE *(continued)*

Nursing Action	Rationale
3. When the desired goal is reached (lungs fully inflated), ask the patient to continue the inspiratory effort for 3 seconds, even though the patient may not actually be drawing in more air.	3. Sustaining the inspiratory effort helps to open closed alveoli. For the postoperative patient, hypoventilation can result in atelectasis within the first hour.
4. Instruct the patient to remove the mouthpiece, relax, and passively exhale; patient should take several normal breaths before attempting another one with the incentive spirometer.	4. Usually one incentive breath per minute minimizes patient fatigue. No more than four to five maneuvers should be performed per minute to minimize hypocarbia.
5. Continue to monitor the patient's spirometer breaths, periodically increasing the V_T as the patient tolerates.	5. Increases lung expansion.
6. At the conclusion of the treatment, encourage the patient to cough after a deep breath.	6. The deep lung inflation may loosen secretions and enable the patient to expectorate them.
7. Instruct the patient to take 10 sustained maximal inspiratory maneuvers per hour and note the volume on the spirometer.	7. A total of 10 sustained maximal inspiratory maneuvers per hour during waking hours is a typical order. A counter on the incentive spirometer indicates the number of breaths the patient has taken.

Performance phase

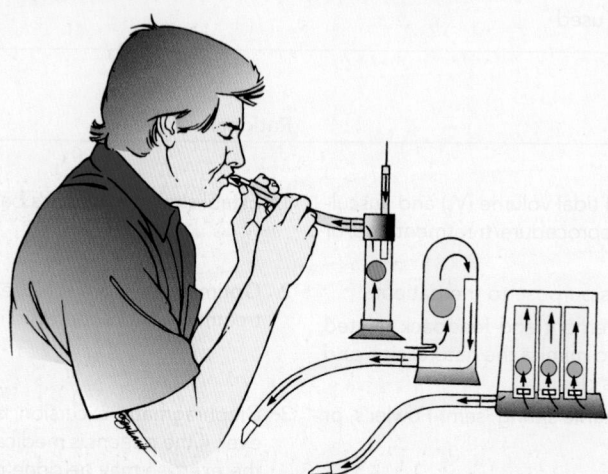

Flow incentive spirometer. Patients are instructed to inhale briskly to elevate the balls and to keep them floating as long as possible. The volume inhaled is estimated and variable.

Follow-up phase

1. Auscultate the chest. Chart any improvement or variation, the volume attained, effectiveness of cough, description of any secretions expectorated.	1. Notes the effectiveness and patient tolerance of the treatment for continuity of care.
2. Record effectiveness and frequency of use of incentive spirometer.	

 Evidence Base Restrepo, R., Wettstein, R., Wittnebel, L., et al. (2011). AARC clinical practice guideline: Incentive spirometry: 2011 *Respiratory Care, 56*(10), 1600–1604.

4. Monitor and manage chest drainage system to drain fluid, blood, clots, and air from the pleura after surgery (see page 268). Chest drainage is usually not used after pneumonectomy because it is desirable that the pleural space fills with an effusion, which eventually obliterates the space.

Complications

1. Hypoxia—assess for restlessness, tachycardia, tachypnea, and elevated BP.
2. Postoperative bleeding—monitor for restlessness, anxiety, pallor, tachycardia, and hypotension.
3. Pneumonia; atelectasis—monitor for fever, chest pain, dyspnea, changes in lung sounds on auscultation.
4. Bronchopleural fistula from disruption of a bronchial suture or staple; bronchial stump leak.
   a. Observe for sudden onset of respiratory distress or cough productive of serosanguineous fluid.
   b. Position with the operative side down.
   c. Prepare for immediate chest tube insertion and/or surgical intervention.
5. Cardiac dysrhythmias (usually occurring third to fourth postoperative day); MI or heart failure.

Nursing Diagnoses

- Ineffective Breathing Pattern related to wound closures.
- Risk for Deficient Fluid Volume related to chest drainage and blood loss.
- Acute Pain related to wound closure and presence of drainage tubes in the chest.
- Impaired Physical Mobility of affected shoulder and arm related to wound closure and the presence of drainage tubes in the chest.

Nursing Interventions

Maintaining Adequate Breathing Pattern

1. Monitor rate, rhythm, depth, and effort of respirations.
2. Auscultate chest for adequacy of air movement to detect bronchospasm, consolidation.
3. Monitor pulse oximetry and obtain ABG analysis and pulmonary function measurements as ordered.
4. Monitor LOC and inspiratory effort closely to begin weaning from ventilator as soon as possible.
5. Suction, as needed, using meticulous aseptic technique.

 NURSING ALERT Tracheobronchial secretions are present in excessive amounts in postthoracotomy patients because of trauma to the tracheobronchial tree during operation, diminished lung ventilation, and diminished cough reflex.

 NURSING ALERT Look for changes in color and consistency of suctioned sputum. Colorless, fluid sputum is not unusual; opacification or coloring of sputum may mean dehydration or infection.

6. Elevate the head of the bed 30 to 40 degrees when patient is oriented and BP is stabilized to improve movement of diaphragm and alleviate dyspnea.
7. Encourage coughing and deep-breathing exercises and use of an incentive spirometer to prevent bronchospasm, retained secretions, atelectasis, and pneumonia.
8. Provide optimal pain relief to promote deep breathing, turning, and coughing.

Stabilizing Hemodynamic Status

1. Take BP, pulse, and respiration every 15 minutes or more frequently as indicated; extend the time intervals according to the patient's clinical status.
2. Monitor heart rate and rhythm by way of auscultation and continuous ECG because dysrhythmias are frequently seen following thoracic surgery.
3. Monitor CVP for prompt recognition of hypovolemia and for effectiveness of fluid replacement.
4. Monitor cardiac output and pulmonary artery systolic, diastolic, and wedge pressures. Watch for subtle changes, especially in the patient with underlying cardiovascular disease.
5. Assess chest tube drainage for amount and character of fluid.
   a. Chest drainage should progressively decrease after first 12 hours.
   b. Prepare for blood replacement and possible reoperation to achieve hemostasis if bleeding persists.
   c. Chest tube drainage in excess of 1,000 to 1,200 mL per 24-hour period should be reported to the physician for follow-up.
6. Maintain intake and output record, including chest tube drainage.
7. Monitor infusions of blood and parenteral fluids closely because the patient is at risk for fluid overload if portion of pulmonary vascular system has been reduced.

Achieving Adequate Pain Control

1. Perform comprehensive pain assessment including onset, location, duration, characteristics, precipitating factors, and response to interventions.
2. Provide appropriate pain relief—pain limits chest excursions, thereby decreasing ventilation. Severity of pain varies with type of incision and with the patient's reaction to and ability to cope with pain. Usually a posterolateral incision is the most painful.

 NURSING ALERT Evaluate for signs of hypoxia thoroughly when anxiety, restlessness, and agitation of new onset are noted before administering as-needed sedatives.

3. Give opioids (usually by continuous IV infusion or by epidural catheter by way of patient-controlled analgesia pump) for pain relief, as prescribed, to permit patient to breathe more deeply and cough more effectively. To avoid respiratory and CNS depression, do not give too much opioid; patient should be alert enough to cough.
4. Assist with intercostal nerve block or cryoanalgesia (intercostal nerve freezing) for pain control as ordered (see page 270).

5. Position for comfort and optimal ventilation (head of bed elevated 15 to 30 degrees); this also helps residual air to rise in upper portion of pleural space where it can be removed by the chest tube.
   a. Patients with limited respiratory reserve may not be able to turn on unoperated side because this may limit ventilation of the operated side.
   b. Vary the position from horizontal to semierect to prevent retention of secretions in the dependent portion of the lungs.
6. Encourage splinting of incision with pillow, folded towel, or hands, while turning, changing position, or coughing.
7. Teach relaxation (nonpharmacologic) techniques, such as progressive muscle relaxation and imagery, to help reduce pain.

Increasing Mobility of Affected Shoulder

1. Begin ROM exercise of arm and shoulder on affected side immediately to prevent ankylosis of the shoulder ("frozen" shoulder).
2. Perform exercises at time of maximal pain relief.
3. Encourage patient to actively perform exercises three to four times per day, taking care not to disrupt chest tube or invasive lines (ie, IV).

Patient Education and Health Maintenance

1. Advise that there will be some intercostal pain for several weeks, which can be relieved by local heat and oral analgesia. Many patients experience intercostal pain up to 1 year following surgery.
2. Advise that weakness and fatigability are common during the first 3 weeks after a thoracotomy, but exercise tolerance will improve with conditioning.
3. Suggest alternating walking and other activities with frequent short rest periods. Walk at a moderate pace and gradually extend walking time and distance.
4. Encourage continuing deep-breathing exercises for several weeks after surgery to attain full expansion of residual lung tissue.
5. Instruct on maintaining good body alignment to ensure full lung expansion.
6. Advise that chest muscles may be weaker than normal for 3 to 6 months after surgery. Patient must avoid lifting more than 20 lb (9 kg) until complete healing has taken place.
7. Any activity that causes undue fatigue, increased shortness of breath, or chest pain should be stopped immediately.
8. Because all or part of one lung has been removed, warn patient to avoid respiratory irritants (smoke, fumes, high level of air pollution).
   a. Avoid irritants that may cause coughing spasms.
   b. Sit in nonsmoking areas in public places.
9. Encourage patient to receive an annual influenza vaccine and obtain a pneumococcal pneumonia vaccine.
10. Encourage patient to keep follow-up visits.
11. Instruct patient to prevent respiratory infections by frequent handwashing and avoiding others with respiratory infections.

Evaluation: Expected Outcomes

- Respirations with normal range, adequate depth; lungs clear; ABG values and SaO_2 within normal limits.
- BP, CVP, and pulse within normal limits for individual.
- Coughs and turns independently; reports relief of pain.
- Performs active ROM of affected arm and shoulder; reports improved exercise tolerance.

Chest Drainage

 Evidence Base Durai, R., Hoque, H., Davies, T. W., et al. (2010). Managing a chest tube and drainage system. *AORN Journal, 91*(2), 275–283.
Lewis, S., Dirksen, S. R., Heitkemper, M. M., et al. (2010). *Medical-surgical nursing* (8th ed.) St. Louis, MO: Elsevier.

Chest drainage is the insertion of a tube into the pleural space to evacuate air or fluid and/or help regain negative pressure. Whenever the chest is opened, there is loss of negative pressure in the pleural space, which can result in collapse of the lung. The collection of air, fluid, or other substances in the thoracic cavity can compromise cardiopulmonary function and cause collapse of the lung.

It is necessary to keep the pleural space evacuated postoperatively and to maintain negative pressure within this potential space. Therefore, during or immediately after thoracic surgery, chest tubes/catheters are positioned strategically in the pleural space, sutured to the skin, and connected to a drainage apparatus to remove the residual air and fluid from the pleural or mediastinal space. This assists in the reexpansion of remaining lung tissue.

Chest drainage can also be used to treat spontaneous pneumothorax or hemothorax/pneumothorax caused by trauma (see Table 10-3). Sites for chest tube placement are:

1. For pneumothorax (air)—second or third interspace along midclavicular or anterior axillary line.
2. For hemothorax (fluid)—sixth or seventh lateral interspace in the midaxillary line.

Principles of Chest Drainage

1. Many types of commercial chest drainage systems are in use, most of which use the water-seal principle. The chest tube/catheter and collecting tubing is attached to a chest drainage

Table 10-3	Indications for Chest Tube Use
INDICATION	**ACCUMULATING SUBSTANCE**
Pneumothorax	Air
Hemothorax	Blood
Pleural effusion	Fluid
Chylothorax	Lymphatic fluid
Empyema	Pus

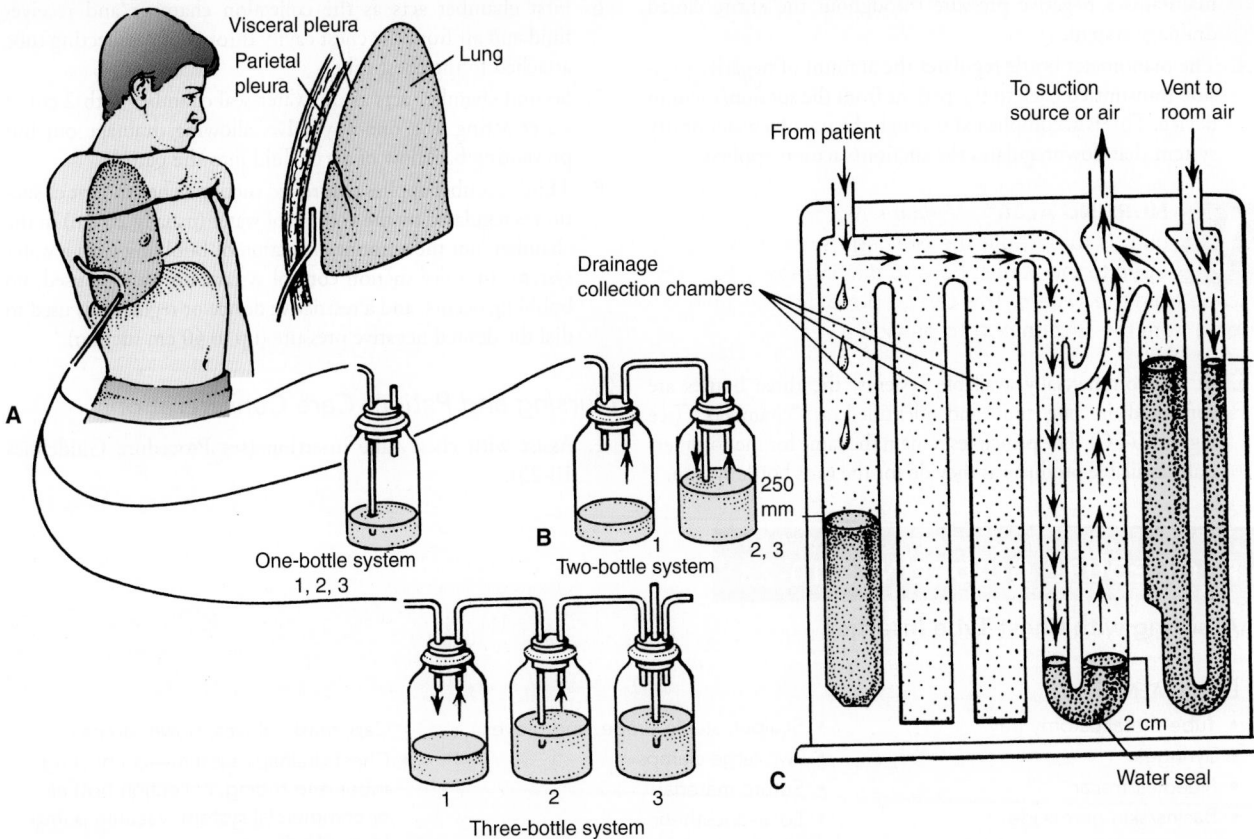

Figure 10-7. Chest drainage systems. (A) Strategic placement of a chest catheter in the pleural space. **(B)** Three types of mechanical drainage systems. **(C)** A Pleur-evac operating system: **(1)** the collection chamber, **(2)** the water-seal chamber, and **(3)** the suction control chamber. The Pleur-evac is a single unit with all three bottles identified as chambers.

system using a one-way valve principle. Water acts as a seal and permits air and fluid to drain from the chest. However, air cannot reenter the chest cavity.

2. Chest drainage can be categorized into three types of mechanical systems (see Figure 10-7). There are numerous types of chest drainage units available.

One-Bottle Water-Seal System

1. The end of the collecting tube is covered by a layer of water, which permits drainage of air and fluid from the pleural space, but does not allow air to move back into the chest. Functionally, drainage depends on gravity, on the mechanics of respiration, and, if desired, on suction by the addition of controlled vacuum.

2. The tube from the patient extends approximately 1 inch (2.5 cm) below the level of the water in the container. There is a vent for the escape of any air that may be leaking from the lung. The water level fluctuates as the patient breathes; it goes up when the patient inhales and down when the patient exhales.

3. At the end of the drainage tube, bubbling may or may not be visible. Bubbling can mean either persistent leakage of air from the lung or other tissues or a leak in the system.

Two-Bottle Water-Seal System

1. The two-bottle system consists of the same water-seal chamber, plus a fluid-collection bottle.

2. Drainage is similar to that of a single unit, except that when pleural fluid drains, the underwater-seal system is not affected by the volume of the drainage.

3. Effective drainage depends on gravity or on the amount of suction added to the system. When vacuum (suction) is added to the system from a vacuum source, such as wall suction, the connection is made at the vent stem of the underwater-seal bottle.

4. The amount of suction applied to the system is regulated by the wall gauge.

Three-Bottle Water-Seal System

1. The three-bottle system is similar in all respects to the two-bottle system, except for the addition of a third bottle to control the amount of suction applied. Recent research has shown that suction may actually prolong an air leak by pulling air through the opening that would otherwise heal on its own.

2. The amount of suction is determined by the depth to which the tip of the venting glass tube is submerged in the water and level of water in the suction chamber or setting of a dial—depending on the system in use.

3. In the three-bottle system (as in the other two systems), drainage depends on gravity or the amount of suction applied. The mechanical suction motor or wall suction creates and

maintains a negative pressure throughout the entire closed drainage system.

4. The manometer bottle regulates the amount of negative pressure transmitted back to the patient from the suction/vacuum device. This is accomplished through the use of a water or dry system that downregulates the suction/vacuum applied.

> **NURSING ALERT** When the motor or the wall vacuum is turned off, the drainage system should be open to the atmosphere so that intrapleural air can escape from the system. This can be done by detaching the tubing from the suction port to provide a vent.

5. In the commercially available systems, the three bottles are contained in one unit and identified as "chambers" (see Figure 10-7C). The principles remain the same for the commercially available products as they do for the glass bottle system.

6. First chamber acts as the collection chamber and receives fluid and air from the chest cavity through the collecting tube attached to the chest tube.

7. Second chamber acts as the water-seal chamber with 2 cm of water acting as a one-way valve, allowing drainage out but preventing backflow of air or fluid into the patient.

8. Third chamber applies controlled suction. The amount of suction is regulated by the volume of water (usually 20 cm) in the chamber, not the amount of suction or bubbling with a water system. In a dry suction control system no water is used, no bubbling occurs, and a restrictive device or regulator is used to dial the desired negative pressure (up to 40 cm suction).

Nursing and Patient Care Considerations

1. Assist with chest tube insertion (see Procedure Guidelines 10-23).

PROCEDURE GUIDELINES 10-23

Assisting with Chest Tube Insertion

EQUIPMENT

- Tube thoracostomy tray
- Syringes
- Needles/trocar
- Basins/skin germicide
- Sponges

- Scalpel, sterile drape, and gloves
- Two large clamps
- Suture material
- Local anesthetic
- Chest tube (appropriate size); connector

- Cap, mask, gloves, gown, drapes
- Chest drainage system—connecting tubes and tubing, collection bottles or commercial system, vacuum pump (if required)
- Sterile water

PROCEDURE

Nursing Action	Rationale
Preparatory phase	
1. Assess patient for pneumothorax, hemothorax, presence of respiratory distress.	
2. Obtain a chest x-ray. Other means of localization of pleural fluid include ultrasound or fluoroscopic localization.	2. Evaluates extent of lung collapse or amount of bleeding in pleural space.
3. Ensure that informed consent has been obtained.	3. Invasive procedures require written consent.
4. Verify right patient and right location/procedure.	
5. Premedicate if indicated.	5. Sedation may be required if patient is restless.
6. Assemble drainage system.	
7. Reassure the patient and explain the steps of the procedure. Tell the patient to expect a needle prick and a sensation of slight pressure during infiltration anesthesia.	7. Allays fear and enlists patient cooperation. The patient can cope by remaining immobile and doing relaxed breathing during tube insertion.
8. Position the patient as for an intercostal nerve block or according to health care provider preference.	8. The tube insertion site depends on the substance to be drained, the patient's mobility, and the presence of coexisting conditions.
Performance phase *Needle or intracath technique*	
1. Using universal precautions, the skin is prepared, anesthetized, and draped, using local anesthetic with a short 25G needle and using aseptic technique. A larger needle is used to infiltrate the subcutaneous tissue, intercostal muscles, and parietal pleura.	1. The area is anesthetized to make tube insertion and manipulation relatively painless. Use of universal precautions and aseptic technique prevent contamination of chest tube, which will be entering a sterile cavity. Patient may feel pressure while tube is inserted.

PROCEDURE GUIDELINES 10-23 (continued)

Assisting with Chest Tube Insertion

PROCEDURE (continued)

Nursing Action	Rationale
2. An exploratory needle is inserted.	2. Punctures the pleura and determines the presence of air or blood in the pleural cavity.
3. The catheter is inserted through the needle into the pleural space. The needle is removed, and the catheter is pushed several centimeters into the pleural space.	
4. The catheter is taped to the skin; may be sutured to the chest wall and covered with a dressing.	4. Prevents it from being dislodged out of the chest during patient movement or lung expansion.
5. The catheter is attached to a connector/tubing and attached to a drainage system (underwater-seal or commercial system) and all connections taped.	5. All connections are taped to prevent disconnection. The chest tube clamp is removed once the chest tube is attached to the system.

Performance phase

Trocar technique for chest tube insertion

Using universal precautions and aseptic technique, a trocar catheter is used for the insertion of a large-bore tube for removal of a moderate to large amount of air leak or for the evacuation of serous effusion.

1. A small incision is made over the prepared, anesthetized site. Blunt dissection (with a hemostat) through the muscle planes in the interspace to the parietal pleura is performed.	1. Admits the diameter of the chest tube.
2. The trocar is directed into the pleural space, the cannula is removed, and a chest tube is inserted into the pleural space and connected to a drainage system.	2. There is a trocar catheter available equipped with an indwelling pointed rod for ease of insertion.

Hemostat technique using a large-bore chest tube

Using universal precautions and aseptic technique, a large-bore chest tube is used to drain blood or thick effusions from the pleural space.

1. Using universal precautions, aseptic technique, and after skin preparation and anesthetic infiltration, an incision is made through the skin and subcutaneous tissue.	1. The skin incision is usually made one interspace below proposed site of penetration of the intercostal muscles and pleura.
2. A curved hemostat is inserted into the pleural cavity and the tissue is spread with the clamp.	2. Makes a tissue tract for the chest tube.
3. The tract is explored with an examining finger.	3. Digital examination helps confirm the presence of the tract and penetration of the pleural cavity.
4. The tube is held by the hemostat and directed through the opening up over the ribs and into the pleural cavity.	
5. The clamp is withdrawn and the chest tube is connected to a chest drainage system.	5. The chest tube has multiple openings at the proximal end for drainage of air or blood.
6. The tube is sutured in place and covered with a sterile dressing.	6. Prevents dislodgment.
7. Catheter is attached to a connector/tube and to the system. All connections are taped.	7. Clamps are removed from the chest tube once connected to the drainage system. Chest tubes open to air at the time of insertion will result in a pneumothorax.

(continued)

PROCEDURE GUIDELINES 10-23 *(continued)*

Assisting with Chest Tube Insertion

PROCEDURE *(continued)*

Nursing Action	Rationale

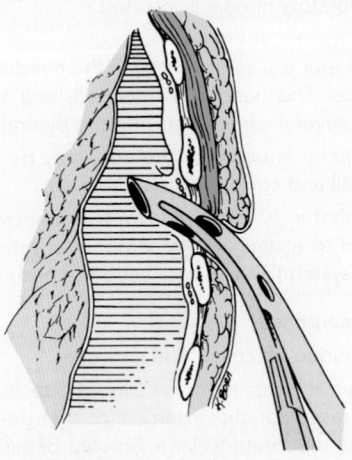

Chest tube (tube thoracostomy) inserted via hemostat technique.

Follow-up phase

1. Observe the drainage system for blood and air. Observe for fluctuation in the tube on respiration. (See page 274.)

2. Secure a follow-up chest x-ray.

3. Assess for bleeding, infection, leakage of air and fluid around the tube.

4. Maintain integrity of the chest drainage system.

1. If a hemothorax is draining through a thoracostomy tube into a bottle containing sterile normal saline, the blood is available for autotransfusion.

2. To confirm correct chest tube placement and reexpansion of the lung.

3. With too rapid removal of fluid, a vasovagal response may occur with resulting hypotension. Continued use of petroleum gauzes or ointment can irritate the skin.

4. Chest tube malposition is the most common complication.

2. Assess patient's pain at insertion site and give medication appropriately. If patient is in pain, chest excursion and lung inflation will be hampered.

3. Maintain chest tubes to provide drainage and enhance lung reinflation (see Procedure Guidelines 10-24).

4. Maintain integrity of insertion site, observing for drainage, redness, impaired healing, and subcutaneous emphysema.

NURSING ALERT Clamping of chest tubes is not recommended due to the increased danger of tension pneumothorax from rapid accumulation of air in the pleural space. Clamp only momentarily to change the drainage system. Check for leaks to assess the patient's tolerance for removal of the chest tube (perhaps up to 24 hours).

NURSING ALERT Milking and stripping of chest tubes to maintain patency is not recommended. This practice has been found to cause significant increases in intrapleural pressures and damage to the pleural tissue. New chest tubes contain a nonthrombogenic coating, thus decreasing the potential for clotting. If it is necessary to help the drainage move through the tubing, apply a gentle squeeze-and-release motion to small segments of the chest tube between your fingers.

PROCEDURE GUIDELINES 10-24

Managing the Patient with Water-Seal Chest Drainage

EQUIPMENT
- Closed chest drainage system
- Holder for drainage system (if needed) connector for emergency use
- Vacuum motor
- Sterile connector for emergency use (ie, sterile water)

PROCEDURE

Nursing Action	Rationale
Performance phase	
1. Attach the chest tube from the pleural space (the patient) to the collecting/drainage tubing and water-seal drainage system. Add sterile water to water-seal chambers, as needed. Adjust suction until bubbling is seen or set gauge as directed. Keep drainage system below level of chest.	1. Water-seal drainage provides for the escape of air and fluid into a drainage bottle. The water acts as a seal and keeps the air from being drawn back into the pleural space. Vigorous bubbling is not indicated.
2. Check the tube connections periodically. Tape, if necessary.	2. Tube connections are checked to ensure tight fit, patency of the tubes, and to prevent backflow of drainage or air.
a. The tube should be as straight as possible and coiled below level of chest without dependent loops.	
b. Do not let the patient lie on collecting/tubing drainage.	
3. Mark the original fluid level with tape on the outside of the drainage system. Mark hourly and daily increments (date and time) at the drainage level.	3. This marking will show the amount of fluid loss and how fast fluid is collecting in the drainage bottle. It serves as a basis for blood replacement, if the fluid is blood. Grossly bloody drainage will appear in the bottle in the immediate postoperative period and, if excessive, may necessitate reoperation. Drainage usually declines progressively after the first 24 hours.
4. Assess patient's clinical status at least once per shift. Observe and report immediately signs of rapid, shallow breathing, cyanosis, pressure in the chest, subcutaneous emphysema, or symptoms of hemorrhage.	4. Removal of 1,000–1,200 mL of pleural fluid at one time can result in hypotension and rebound pleural effusion. Report to physician immediately. More frequent monitoring is required at the initiation of therapy and when warranted by patient's condition. Many clinical conditions may cause these signs and symptoms, including tension pneumothorax, mediastinal shift, hemorrhage, severe incisional pain, pulmonary embolus, and cardiac tamponade. Surgical intervention may be necessary.
5. Make sure the tubing does not loop or interfere with the movements of the patient.	5. Fluid collecting in the dependent segment of the tubing will decrease the negative pressure applied to the catheter. Kinking, looping, or pressure on the drainage tubing can produce back pressure, thus possibly forcing drainage back into the pleural space or impeding drainage from the pleural space.
6. Encourage the patient to assume a position of comfort. Encourage good body alignment. When the patient is in a lateral position, place a rolled towel under the tubing to protect it from the weight of the patient's body. Encourage the patient to change position frequently.	6. The patient's position should be changed frequently to promote drainage and body kept in good alignment to prevent postural deformity and contractures. Proper positioning helps breathing and promotes better air exchange. Pain medication may be indicated to enhance comfort and deep breathing.
7. Put the arm and shoulder of the affected side through ROM exercises several times daily. Some pain medication may be necessary.	7. Exercise helps to avoid ankylosis of the shoulder and assists in lessening postoperative pain and discomfort.

(continued)

PROCEDURE GUIDELINES 10-24 (continued)

Managing the Patient with Water-Seal Chest Drainage

PROCEDURE (continued)

Nursing Action	Rationale
8. Make sure there is fluctuation ("tidaling") of the fluid level in the drainage system.	8. Fluctuation of the water level in the tube shows that there is effective communication between the pleural space and the drainage system; provides a valuable indication of the patency of the drainage system and is a gauge of intrapleural pressure.
9. Fluctuations of fluid in the tubing will stop when: a. The lung has reexpanded. b. The tubing is obstructed by blood clots or fibrin. c. A dependent loop develops.	9. Leaking and trapping of air in the pleural space can result in tension pneumothorax.
10. Watch for leaks of air in the drainage system as indicated by constant bubbling in the water-seal bottle. a. Report excessive bubbling in the water-seal change immediately.	10. Air leak prevents proper drainage and expansion of the lung.
11. Encourage the patient to breathe deeply and cough at frequent intervals. If there are signs of incisional pain, adequate pain medication is indicated.	11. Deep breathing and coughing help to raise the intrapleural pressure, which allows emptying of any accumulation in the pleural space and removes secretions from the tracheobronchial tree so the lung expands.
12. If the patient has to be transported to another area, place the drainage system below the chest level (as close to the floor as possible).	12. The drainage apparatus must be kept at a level lower than the patient's chest to prevent backflow of fluid into the pleural space.
13. If the tube becomes disconnected, cut off the contaminated tips of the chest tube and tubing, insert a sterile connector in the chest tube and tubing, and reattach to the drainage system. Otherwise, do not clamp the chest tube during transport.	13. Clamping may result in tension pneumothorax.
14. When assisting with removal of the tube: a. Administer pain medication 30 minutes before removal of chest tube. b. Instruct the patient to perform a gentle Valsalva maneuver or to breathe quietly. c. The chest tube is clamped and removed. d. Simultaneously, a small bandage is applied and made airtight with petroleum gauze covered by a 4" × 4" gauze and thoroughly covered and sealed with tape.	14. The chest tube is removed as directed when the lung is reexpanded (usually 24 hours to several days). Signs of reinflation include little or no drainage, absence of air leak, no noted respiratory distress, no fluctuations in fluid in water-seal chamber, no residual air or fluid in chest x-ray. During the tube removal, avoid a large sudden inspiratory effort, which may produce a pneumothorax.

Follow-up phase

1. Monitor the patient's pulmonary status for signs and symptoms of decompensation. Observe insertion site for signs of infection and changes in drainage.	1. Patient could have reformation of pneumothorax after removal as well as infection at injection site.

Evidence Base Bauman, M., & Handley, C. (2010). Chest-tube care: The more you know, the easier it gets. *American Nurse Today, 6*(9), 27–32.
    Durai, R., Hoque, H., Davies, T. W., et al. (2010). Managing a chest tube and drainage system. *AORN Journal, 91*(2), 275–283.

Table 10-4	Chest Drainage Units (CDU)	
TYPE	**DESCRIPTION**	**INDICATIONS FOR USE**
Standard CDU	Drainage of pleural cavity for air or any type of fluid with or without the use of suction Up to 2,000 mL capacity Replaced when full	Following surgery that impacts on the continuity of the thoracic cavity (eg, thoracic, cardiac, esophageal surgery) Pneumothorax Hemothorax Pleural effusion Pleurodesis
Smaller portable CDU	Drainage without use of suction Dry seal system that prevents air leaks No lung reexpansion occurs 500 mL maximum drainage Emptied when used in home	For ambulatory patients Home care Chronic conditions
Indwelling pleural catheter	Small-size chest tube or pigtail catheter (smaller than standard 14 French) Can be irrigated if occluded by health care provider Less traumatic	Pneumothorax Chronic drainage of fluid Not for trauma or blood Can be used for pleurodesis
Heimlich valve	One-way flutter valve Removes air as patient exhales Valve opens when pleural space pressure is greater than atmospheric pressure and closes when the reverse occurs	Evacuates air from the pleural space Used for emergency transport, home care, and long-term care units

SELECTED REFERENCES

Agency for Healthcare Research and Quality. (2011). Diagnosis and treatment of obstructive sleep apnea in adults (Comparative Effectiveness Review No. 32, AHRQ Publication No. 11-EHC052-EF). Rockville, MD: AHRQ. Available: *www.effectivehealthcare.ahrq.gov/index.cfm/search-for-guides-reviews-and-reports/?pageaction=displayproduct&productid=731*.

Agency for Healthcare Research and Quality (AHRQ). (2011). Problems and prevention: Chest tube insertion. In *Patient safety: Findings in action* (Publication No. 06-P024). Rockville, MD: Author.

Ahrens, T., Prentice, D., & Kleinpell, R. (2010). *Critical care nursing certification: Preparation, review and practice exam* (6th ed.). New York: McGraw-Hill.

Allibone, L. (2010). Assessment and management of patients with pleural effusions. *Nursing Standard, 20*(22), 55–64.

Amanullah S. (2011). Ventilator-associated pneumonia overview of nosocomial pneumonias. Available: *http://emedicine.medscape.com/article/304836-overview*.

American Association of Critical-Care Nurses. (2011). Practice alert: Prevention of aspiration. Available: *www.aacn.org/wd/practice/content/practicealerts/aspiration-practice-alert.pcms?pid=1&&menu=practice*.

American Association for Respiratory Care. (2007). Clinical practice guidelines. Bronchoscopy assisting—2007 revision and 2009 update. *Respiratory Care, 52*(1), 74–80.

American Association for Respiratory Care. (2007). Clinical practice guidelines. Removal of endotracheal tube. *Respiratory Care, 52*(1), 81–93.

American Association for Respiratory Care. (2007). Clinical practice guidelines. Removal of the endotracheal tube—2007 revision and 2009 update. *Respiratory Care, 52*(1), 81–93

American Association for Respiratory Care. (2010). Clinical practice guidelines. Endotracheal suctioning of mechanically ventilated patients with artificial airways. *Respiratory Care, 55*(6), 758–764.

American Heart Association. (2010). Guidelines for cardiopulmonary resuscitation and emergency cardiovascular care. *Circulation, 122*(18), 3.

Amitai, A. (2011). Ventilator management. *Medscape Reference*. Available: *http://emedicine.medscape.com/article/810126-overview*.

Bauman, M., & Handley, C. (2010). Chest-tube care: The more you know, the easier it gets. *American Nurse Today, 6*(9), 27–32.

Birring, S. (2011). Controversies in the evaluation and management of chronic cough. *American Journal of Respiratory and Critical Care Medicine, 183*(6), 708–715.

Blackwood, B., Alderdice, F., Burns, K. E., et al. (2010). Protocolized versus non-protocolized weaning for reducing the duration of mechanical ventilation in critically ill adult patients. *Cochrane Database of Systematic Reviews*, Issue 5 (Article No. CD006904).

Brown, M., Varia, H., Bassett, P., et al. (2007). Prospective study of sputum induction, gastric washing, and bronchoalveolar lavage for the diagnosis of pulmonary tuberculosis in patients who are unable to expectorate. *Clinical Infectious Diseases, 44*(11), 1415–1420.

Chandrasekhar, A. J. (2006). Pulmonary function test basics. Loyola University Medical Education Network. Available: *www.meddean.luc.edu/lumen/MedEd/medicine/pulmonar/fellow/pftc3.htm*.

Chulay, M., & Burns, S. (2010). *AACN Essentials of critical care nursing* (2nd ed.). New York: McGraw-Hill.

Conaway, M., Bleck, T., Burns, S., et al. (2012). The Relationship of 26 Clinical Factors to Weaning Outcome. *Am J Crit Care, 21*, 52–59.

Cranston, J. M., Crockett, A., & Currow, D. (2008). Oxygen therapy for dyspnea in adults. *Cochrane Database of Systematic Reviews*, Issue 3 (Article No. CD004769).

DeWaay, D., & Gordon, J. (2011). The ABC's of ABGs: Teaching arterial blood gases to adult learners. *MedEdPORTAL*. Available: *www.mededportal.org/publication/9038*.

Dunne, P. (2010). The clinical impact of new long-term oxygen therapy technology. *Respiratory Care, 54*(8), 1100–1111.

Durai, R., Hoque, H., Davies, T. W., et al. (2010). Managing a chest tube and drainage system. *AORN Journal, 91*(2), 275–283.

Fahy, J., & Dickey, B. (2010). Airway mucus function and dysfunction. *New England Journal of Medicine, 363*, 2233–2247.

Farnan, C., & Patrick, M. (2010). Saline instillation: Helpful or harmful? Debates over saline instillation during suctioning have raged for years. *Advance for*

Respiratory and Sleep Medicine. Available: *http://respiratory-care-sleep-medicine. advanceweb.com/Editorial/Content/PrintFriendly.aspx?CC=226385.*

Fishbach, F., & Dunning, M. (2010). *Quick reference to common laboratory and diagnostic tests* (5th ed.). Philadelphia: Lippincott Williams & Wilkins.

Gordon, C., Feller-Kopman, D., Balk, E., et al. (2010). Pneumothorax following thoracentesis: A systematic review and meta-analysis. *Archives of Internal Medicine, 170*(4), 332.

Hanania, N. A., & Marciniuk, D. D. (2011). A unified front against COPD: Clinical Practice Guidelines from the American College of Physicians, the American College of Chest Physicians, the American Thoracic Society, and the European Respiratory Society. *Chest, 140*(3), 565–566.

Hegde, A., Eisen, L., Kory, P., et al. (2011). A program to improve the quality of emergency endotracheal intubation. *Journal of Intensive Care Medicine, 26*(1), 50–56.

Hess, D. (2010). Ventilator modes: Where have we come from and where are we going? *Chest, 137,* 1256–1258.

Hess, D., & MacIntyre, N. (2011). Ventilator discontinuation: Why are we still weaning? *American Journal of Respiratory and Critical Care Medicine, 184,* 392–394.

Hess D., MacIntyre N., Mishoe S., et al. (2012). *Respiratory care: Principles and practice* (2nd ed.). Sudbury, MA: Jones & Bartlett.

Hoo, G. (2011). Noninvasive ventilation. *Medscape Reference.* Available: *http:// emedicine.medscape.com/article/304235-overview#aw2aab6b3.*

Hurst T., & Thomas A. (2010). Airway safety in adult intensive care. *Care of the Critically Ill, 25*(3–4), 65–69.

Johnson, W., & Meyers, A. (2012). Tracheostomy tube change. *Medscape Reference.* Available: *http://emedicine.medscape.com/article/1580576-overview.*

Kaufman, D. (2010). Pulmonary ventilation/perfusion scan. *Medline Plus.* Available: *www.nlm.nih.gov/medlineplus/print/ency/article/003828.htm.*

Kodali, B. (2010). Capnography.com. Available: *www.capnography.com.*

Lester, M., & Flume P. (2010). Airway-clearance therapy guidelines and implementation. *Respiratory Care, 54*(6), 733–750.

Lewis, S., Dirksen, S. R., Heitkemper, M. M., et al. (2010). *Medical-surgical nursing* (8th ed.). St. Louis, MO: Elsevier.

Logan, A. G., & Bradley T. D. (2010). Sleep apnea and cardiovascular disease. *Current Hypertension Reports, 12,* 182–188.

Lucchini A, Zanella, A., Bellani, G., et al. (2011). Tracheal secretion management in the mechanically ventilated patient: Comparison of standard assessment and an acoustic secretion detector. *Respiratory Care, 56*(5), 596–603.

Martin, D. (2011). Palliation of dyspnea in patients with heart failure. *Dimensions of Critical Care Nursing, 30*(3), 144–149.

Maureen, A., & Seckel, M. (2012). Normal Saline and Mucous Plugging. *Crit Care Nurse, 32,* 66–68.

McCoy, R. (2010). Home oxygen therapy. *Journal for Respiratory Care Practitioners, 23*(1), 14–18.

Medline Plus. (2011). Pleural fluid analysis. Available: *www.nlm.nih.gov/ medlineplus/ency/article/003624.htm.*

Medline Plus. (2011). PPD skin test. Available: *www.nlm.nih.gov/medlineplus/ency/ article/003839.htm.*

Medline Plus. (2011). Pulmonary function tests. Available: *www.nlm.nih.gov/ medlineplus/ency/article/003853.htm.*

Mishra, E., & Davies, R. (2010). Advances in the investigation and treatment of pleural effusions. *Expert Review of Respiratory Medicine, 4*(1), 123–133.

Morton, P. G., & Fontaine, D. K. (2009). *Critical care nursing: A holistic approach* (9th ed.). Philadelphia: Lippincott Williams & Wilkins.

Nouira, S., Boukef, R., Bouida, W., et al. (2011). Non-invasive pressure support ventilation and CPAP in cardiogenic pulmonary edema: A multicenter randomized study in the emergency department. *Intensive Care Medicine, 37*(2), 249–256.

Nseir, S. (2011). New tracheal tubes to prevent ventilator-associated pneumonia: Where is the evidence? *Critical Care, 15,* 459.

Oritz, G., Fritps-Vivar, F., Ferguson, N. D., et al. (2010). Outcomes of patients ventilated with synchronized intermittent mandatory ventilation with pressure support (SIMV-PS): A comparative propensity score study. *Chest, 137,* 1265–1277.

Parker, L. C. (2012). Evidence-based interventions and teamwork are crucial when caring for patients on mechanical ventilators. *American Nurse Today, 7*(3), 13–16.

RadiologyInfo.org. (2011). MRI of the chest. Available: *www.radiologyinfo.org/en/ info.cfm?pg=chestmr.*

RadiologyInfo.org. (2011). Positron emission tomography (PET imaging). Available: *www.radiologyinfo.org/en/pdf/pet.pdf.*

Restrepo, R., Wettstein, R., Wittnebel, L., et al. (2011). AARC Clinical Practice Guideline. Incentive spirometry: 2011. *Respiratory Care, 56*(10), 1600–1604.

Rubenfire, M., Bayram, M., & Hector-Word, Z. (2007). Pulmonary hypertension in the critical care setting: Classification, pathophysiology, diagnosis, and management. *Critical Care Clinics, 23*(4), 801–834.

Rubins, J. (2012). Pleural effusion. *Medscape Reference.* Available: *http://emedicine. medscape.com/article/299959-overview.*

Sedgwick, M. B., Lance-Smith, M., Reeder, S., et al. (2012). Using Evidence-Based Practice to Prevent Ventilator-Associated Pneumonia. *Crit Care Nurse, 32*(4), 41–51.

Shoemark, A., & Wilson, R. (2011). Exhaled breath condensate pH as a noninvasive measure of inflammation in non-cf bronchiectasis. *International Scholarly Research Network Pulmonology, 2011,* 6.

Simonneau, G., Robbins, I. M., Beghetti, M., et al. (2009). Updated clinical classification of pulmonary hypertension. *Journal of the American College of Cardiology, 54*(1, Suppl. S).

Smeltzer, S. C., Bare, B. G., Hinkle, J. L., et al. (2009). *Brunner & Suddarth's Textbook of Medical Surgical Nursing* (12th ed.). Philadelphia: Lippincott Williams & Wilkins.

Weinberger, S., & Silverstri, R. (2011). Treatment of subacute and chronic cough in adults. *UpToDate.* Available: *www.uptodate.com/contents/treatment-of-subacute-and-chronic-cough-in-adults.*

Wiegand, D. J., & Carlson, K. K. (2010). *AACN procedure manual for critical care* (6th ed.). Philadelphia: Elsevier Saunders.

Wilkins, R., Dexter, J. R., & Heuer, A. (2010). *Clinical assessment in respiratory care* (6th ed.). St. Louis, MO: Mosby.

Wong, M., & Elliott, M. (2009). The use of medical orders in acute care oxygen therapy. *British Journal of Nursing, 18*(8), 462–464.

World Health Organization. (2010). *M/XDR-TB Surveillance and Control: 2010 Global Update.* Geneva: Author.

11
Respiratory Disorders

ACUTE DISORDERS

Respiratory Failure

Respiratory failure is an alteration in the function of the respiratory gas exchange system in either oxygen (hypoxic respiratory failure) and/or carbon dioxide elimination (hypercapnic respiratory failure). Hypoxemic respiratory failure (type I) is characterized by arterial oxygen (PaO_2) level to fall below 60 mm Hg (hypoxemia) with a normal or low arterial carbon dioxide tension ($PaCO_2$). It is the most common form of respiratory failure, usually associated with acute diseases of the lung.

Hypercapnic respiratory failure (type II) is characterized by an arterial carbon dioxide ($PaCO_2$) level of >50 mm Hg. Hypoxemia is common while breathing room air. pH depends on the bicarbonate level, which, in turn, is dependent on the duration of hypercapnia.

Respiratory failure is classified as acute, chronic, or combined acute and chronic.

Classification

Acute Respiratory Failure

1. Characterized by hypoxemia (PaO_2 less than 50 mm Hg) and/or hypercapnia ($PaCO_2$ greater than 50 mm Hg) and acidosis (pH less than 7.35).
2. Occurs rapidly, usually in minutes to hours or days.

Chronic Respiratory Failure

1. Characterized by hypoxemia (decreased PaO_2) and/or hypercapnia (increased $PaCO_2$) with a normal pH (7.35 to 7.45).

2. Occurs over a period of days to months to years, allowing for activation of compensatory mechanisms, including bicarbonate retention with normalization of pH.

Combined Acute and Chronic Respiratory Failure

1. Characterized by an abrupt increase in the degree of hypoxemia and/or hypercapnia in patients with preexisting chronic respiratory failure.
2. May occur after an acute upper respiratory infection, pneumonia, or exacerbation or without obvious cause.
3. Extent of deterioration is best assessed by comparing the patient's present arterial blood gas (ABG) levels with previous ABG levels (patient baseline).

Pathophysiology and Etiology

Hypoxemic Respiratory Failure

Characterized by a decrease in PaO_2 and normal or decreased $PaCO_2$. Respiratory failure can be:

1. Primary problem is inability to adequately oxygenate the blood, resulting in hypoxemia, due to an abnormality in one or more parts of the respiratory system, central nervous system, respiratory muscles, or chest wall.
2. Hypoxemia occurs because damage to the alveolar–capillary membrane causes leakage of fluid into the interstitial space or into the alveoli and slows or prevents movement of oxygen from the alveoli to the pulmonary capillary blood.
   a. Typically, this damage is widespread, resulting in many areas of the lung being poorly ventilated or nonventilated.
   b. Consequences are severe ventilation–perfusion imbalance and shunt.

3. Hypocapnia may result from hypoxemia and decreased pulmonary compliance. Fluid within the lungs makes the lung less compliant or stiffer.
   a. Change in compliance reflexively stimulates the increased ventilation.
   b. Ventilation is also increased as a response to hypoxemia.
   c. Ultimately, if treatment is unsuccessful, $PaCO_2$ will increase and the patient will experience both an increase in $PaCO_2$ and a decrease in PaO_2.
4. Etiology includes:
   a. Cardiogenic pulmonary edema (left-sided heart failure; mitral stenosis).
   b. Acute respiratory distress syndrome (ARDS). Underlying causes of ARDS include shock, sepsis, pneumonia; trauma, such as fat emboli, head injury, lung trauma; aspiration, near drowning; inhaled toxins, such as oxygen in high concentrations, smoke, corrosive chemicals; hematologic conditions, such as massive transfusions, postcardiopulmonary bypass; and metabolic disorders, such as pancreatitis, uremia.

Ventilatory Failure with Normal Lungs

Characterized by a decrease in PaO_2, increase in $PaCO_2$, and a decrease in pH.

1. Primary problem is insufficient respiratory center stimulation or insufficient chest wall movement, resulting in alveolar hypoventilation.
2. Hypercapnia occurs because impaired neuromuscular function or chest wall expansion limits the amount of carbon dioxide removed from the lungs.
   a. Primary problem is not the lungs. The patient's minute ventilation (tidal volume [V_T] times the number of breaths per minute) is insufficient to allow normal alveolar gas exchange.
3. The carbon dioxide (CO_2) not excreted by the lungs combines with water (H_2O) to form carbonic acid (H_2CO_3). This predisposes to acidosis and a fall in pH.
4. Hypoxemia occurs as a consequence of inadequate ventilation and hypercapnia. When $PaCO_2$ rises, PaO_2 falls unless increased amounts of oxygen are added to the inspired air.
5. Etiology includes:
   a. Insufficient respiratory center activity (drug intoxication, such as opioid overdose, general anesthesia; vascular disorders, such as cerebral vascular insufficiency, brain tumor; trauma, such as head injury, increased intracranial pressure).
   b. Insufficient chest wall function (neuromuscular disease, such as Guillain-Barré syndrome, myasthenia gravis, amyotropic lateral sclerosis, poliomyelitis; trauma to the chest wall resulting in multiple fractures; spinal cord trauma; kyphoscoliosis).

Ventilatory Failure with Intrinsic Lung Disease

Characterized by a decrease in PaO_2, increase in $PaCO_2$, and decreased pH.

1. Primary problem is acute exacerbation or chronic progression of previously existing lung disease, resulting in CO_2 retention.
2. Hypercapnia occurs because damage to the lung parenchyma and/or airway obstruction limits the amount of CO_2 removed by the lungs.

a. Primary problem is preexisting lung disease—usually chronic bronchitis, emphysema, or severe asthma. This limits CO_2 removal from the lungs.
3. The CO_2 not excreted by the lungs combines with H_2O to form H_2CO_3. This predisposes to acidosis and a fall in pH.
4. Hypoxemia occurs as a consequence of hypoventilation and hypercapnia. In addition, damage to the lung parenchyma and/or airway obstruction limits the amount of oxygen that enters the pulmonary capillary blood.
5. Etiology includes:
   a. Chronic obstructive pulmonary disease (COPD) (chronic bronchitis, emphysema).
   b. Severe asthma.
   c. Cystic fibrosis.

Clinical Manifestations

1. Hypoxemia—restlessness, agitation, dyspnea, disorientation, confusion, delirium, loss of consciousness.
2. Hypercapnia—headache, somnolence, dizziness, confusion.
3. Tachypnea initially; then, when no longer able to compensate, bradypnea.
4. Accessory muscle use.
5. Asynchronous respirations.

 NURSING ALERT Obtain ABG levels whenever the history or signs and symptoms suggest the patient is at risk for developing respiratory failure. Initial and subsequent values should be recorded so comparisons can be made over time. The need for ABG analysis can be decreased by using an oximeter to continuously monitor oxygen saturation (SaO_2). Correlate oximeter values with ABG values and then use oximeter for trending. Be aware the oximetry does not measure $PaCO_2$ and pH, important determinants of respiratory acidosis.

Diagnostic Evaluation

1. ABG analysis—shows changes in PaO_2, $PaCO_2$, pH, and possibly HCO_3 from patient's normal; or PaO_2 less than 50 mm Hg, $PaCO_2$ greater than 50 mm Hg, pH less than 7.35.
2. Pulse oximetry—decreasing SpO_2.
3. End tidal CO_2 monitoring—elevated.
4. Complete blood count, serum electrolytes, chest x-ray, urinalysis, electrocardiogram (ECG), blood and sputum cultures—to determine underlying cause and patient's condition.

Management

1. Oxygen therapy to correct the hypoxemia.
2. Turn patient regularly and mobilize when clinically stable to improve ventilation and oxygenation.
3. Bronchodilators and possibly corticosteroids to reduce bronchospasm and inflammation.
4. Diuretics for pulmonary vascular congestion or pulmonary edema.
5. Mechanical ventilation as indicated. Noninvasive positive-pressure ventilation using a face mask may be a successful option for short-term support of ventilation.

NURSING ALERT Avoid administration of fraction of inspired oxygen (FiO_2) of 100% for COPD patients because high oxygen concentrations may cause depression of the respiratory center drive. For COPD patients, the drive to breathe may be hypoxemia.

Complications

1. Oxygen toxicity if prolonged high FiO_2 required.
2. Barotrauma from mechanical ventilation intervention.

Nursing Assessment

See Standards of Care Guidelines 11-1.

1. Note changes suggesting increased work of breathing (dyspnea, tachypnea, diaphoresis, intercostal muscle retraction, fatigue) or pulmonary edema (fine, coarse crackles or rales; frothy pink sputum).
2. Assess breath sounds.
   a. Diminished or absent sounds suggest inability to ventilate the lungs sufficiently to prevent atelectasis.
   b. Crackles may indicate ineffective airway clearance, fluid in the lungs.
   c. Wheezing indicates narrowed airways and bronchospasm.
   d. Rhonchi and crackles suggest ineffective secretion clearance.
3. Assess level of consciousness (LOC) and ability to tolerate increased work of breathing.
   a. Confusion, lethargy, rapid shallow breathing, abdominal paradox (inward movement of abdominal wall during inspiration), and intercostal retractions suggest inability to maintain adequate minute ventilation.
4. Assess for signs of hypoxemia and hypercapnia.
5. Analyze ABG and compare with previous values.
   a. If the patient cannot maintain a minute ventilation sufficient to prevent CO_2 retention, pH will fall.
   b. Mechanical ventilation or noninvasive ventilation may be needed if pH falls to 7.30 or below.
6. Determine vital capacity (VC) and respiratory rate and compare with values indicating need for mechanical ventilation:
   a. VC < 15 mL/kg.
   b. Respiratory rate > 30 breaths/minute.
   c. Negative inspiratory force < –15 to –25 cm H_2O.
   d. Refractory hypoxia.
7. Determine hemodynamic status through assessment of blood pressure (BP), heart rate, pulmonary wedge pressure, cardiac output, and SvO_2 and compare with previous values. If patient is on mechanical ventilation with positive end-expiratory pressure (PEEP), venous return may be limited, resulting in decreased cardiac output.

Nursing Diagnoses

- Impaired Gas Exchange related to inadequate respiratory center activity or chest wall movement, airway obstruction, and/or fluid in lungs.
- Ineffective Airway Clearance related to increased or tenacious secretions.

Nursing Interventions

Improving Gas Exchange

1. Administer oxygen to maintain PaO_2 of 60 mm Hg or SaO_2 greater than 90% using devices that provide increased oxygen concentrations (aerosol mask, partial rebreathing mask, non-rebreathing mask, noninvasive positive pressure ventilation or mechanical ventilation).
2. Administer antibiotics, cardiac medications, and diuretics as ordered for underlying disorder.
3. Monitor fluid balance by intake and output measurement, daily weight, and direct measurement of pulmonary capillary wedge pressure to detect presence of hypovolemia or hypervolemia.
4. Provide measures to prevent atelectasis and promote chest expansion and secretion clearance, as ordered (incentive spirometer, nebulization, head of bed elevated 30 degrees, turn frequently, out of bed when clinically stable).
5. Monitor adequacy of alveolar ventilation by frequent measurement of SpO_2, ABG levels, respiratory rate, and VC.
6. Compare monitored values with criteria indicating need for mechanical ventilation (see above in Nursing Assessment section). Report and prepare to assist with noninvasive ventilation or intubation and initiation of mechanical ventilation, if indicated.

Maintaining Airway Clearance

1. Administer medications to increase alveolar ventilation—bronchodilators to reduce bronchospasm, corticosteroids to reduce airway inflammation.

STANDARDS OF CARE GUIDELINES 11-1
Respiratory Compromise

When caring for patients at risk for respiratory compromise, consider the following assessments and interventions:

- Monitor closely and document complete assessments. Evaluate closely for any changes in clinical assessments.
- Perform thorough systematic assessment, including mental status, vital signs, respiratory status, and cardiovascular status.
- Evaluate for signs of hypoxia when anxiety, restlessness, confusion, or aggression of new onset are noted. Do not administer sedatives unless hypoxia has been ruled out by performing respiratory assessment.
- Notify appropriate health care provider of significant findings of hypoxia: SpO_2 < 92%, cyanosis, circumoral pallor, rapid and shallow respirations, abnormal breath sounds, change in behavior or level of consciousness (LOC). Request assessment and intervention by health care provider, as indicated.
- Use extreme caution in administering sedatives and opioids to patients at risk for respiratory compromise.

This information should serve as a general guideline only. Each patient situation presents a unique set of clinical factors and requires nursing judgment to guide care, which may include additional or alternative measures and approaches.

2. Teach slow, pursed-lip breathing to reduce airflow obstruction and improve oxygen levels. Chest physiotherapy may be considered for retained secretions.

3. Suction patient, if needed, to assist with removal of secretions.

4. If the patient becomes increasingly lethargic, cannot cough or expectorate secretions, cannot cooperate with therapy, or if pH falls below 7.30, despite use of the above therapy, report and prepare to assist with intubation and initiation of mechanical ventilation.

Patient Education and Health Maintenance

1. Instruct patient with preexisting pulmonary disease to seek early intervention for infections to prevent acute respiratory failure, pneumonia, and exacerbations.

2. Teach patient about medication regimen.
   a. Proper technique for inhaler use
   b. Dosage and timing of medications
   c. Monitoring for adverse effects of corticosteroids to report to health care provider: weight gain due to fluid retention, hyperglycemia, mood changes, insomnia, bruising, fragile skin; vision changes due to cataracts or glaucoma.

Community and Home Care Considerations

1. Encourage patients at risk, especially older adults and those with preexisting lung disease, to get pneumococcal pneumonia immunization.
   a. Pneumococcal vaccine protects against *Streptococcus pneumoniae* bacteria, a major cause of morbidity and mortality.
   b. If a person received their first pneumococcal vaccination before age 65, they should be revaccinated after age 65, if more than 5 years have elapsed since the previous dose.
   c. Pneumococcal polysaccharide vaccine is recommended for anyone age 2 to 64 who has heart or lung disease, sickle cell disease, diabetes, alcoholism, cirrhosis, leaks of cerebrospinal fluid or cochlear implants, lymphoma or leukemia, kidney failure, multiple myeloma, impaired immune function, or asplenia; currently a smoker; or residents of nursing homes or long-term care facilities.

 Evidence Base Centers for Disease Control and Prevention. (2010). Updated recommendations for prevention of invasive pneumococcal disease among adults using the 23-valent pneumococcal polysaccharide vaccine (PPSV23). *Morbidity and Mortality Weekly Report, 59*(34), 1102–1106. *Available: www.cdc.gov/mmwr/preview/mmwrhtml/mm5934a3.htm.*

2. Encourage annual immunization for influenza in persons 6 months and older. If vaccine is in limited supply, the Centers for Disease Control and Prevention recommends immunization of persons age 6 months to 4 years and over 49 years, and all patients with the following characteristics:
   a. Chronic pulmonary (including asthma), renal, hepatic, neurologic, hematologic, or metabolic disorders (including diabetes mellitus).
   b. Are or will be pregnant during the influenza season.

   c. Age 6 months to 18 years and receiving long-term aspirin therapy.
   d. American Indians/Alaska Natives.
   e. Morbidly obese (body mass index 40 or greater).
   f. Immunocompromised.
   g. Residents of nursing homes or chronic care facilities.
   h. Cardiovascular disease (excluding hypertension).
   i. Health care workers.
   j. Household contacts of those at risk for influenza.

3. Inactivated influenza vaccine should be given to people age 6 months to 5 years and in those age 50 and older.

4. Intranasal live attenuated vaccine is an alternative for people ages 5 to 49 without chronic conditions, human immunodeficiency virus (HIV), or asthma.

 Evidence Base Centers for Disease Control and Prevention. (2012). Prevention and control of influenza with vaccines: Recommendations of the Advisory Committee on Immunization Practices (ACIP). *Morbidity and Mortality Weekly Report, 61*(32), 613–618. Available: *www.cdc.gov/flu/professionals/acip/index.htm.*

Evaluation: Expected Outcomes

- ABG values within patient's normal limits.
- Decreased secretions; lungs clear.

Acute Respiratory Distress Syndrome

 Evidence Base Villar, J. (2011). What is acute respiratory distress syndrome? *Respiratory Care, 56*(10), 1539–1545.

Acute respiratory distress syndrome (ARDS), also called *acute lung injury*, is a clinical syndrome resulting from acute insult at the level of the alveoli causing severe hypoxemia and decreased compliance of the lungs. Hallmarks of ARDS include a risk factor for ARDS (eg, sepsis, trauma, pancreatitis), severe hypoxemia with the need for relatively high FiO$_2$, decreased lung compliance, bilateral pulmonary infiltrates, and absence of cardiogenic pulmonary edema. Mortality is 55% and is improved with early intervention.

Pathophysiology and Etiology

1. Pulmonary and/or nonpulmonary insult to the alveolar-capillary membrane causing protein-rich fluid leakage into interstitial and alveolar spaces, resulting in edema.
   a. Inflammation in the interstitium and alveolar space promote atelectasis and lung damage.
   b. This is associated with severe hypoxemia and reduced pulmonary compliance.
   c. Fibroproliferative state often accompanied by capillary thrombosis, lung fibrosis, and neovascularization follows.

2. Diffuse alveolar damage with ventilation–perfusion (V/Q) mismatch caused by shunting of blood (see Figure 11-1).

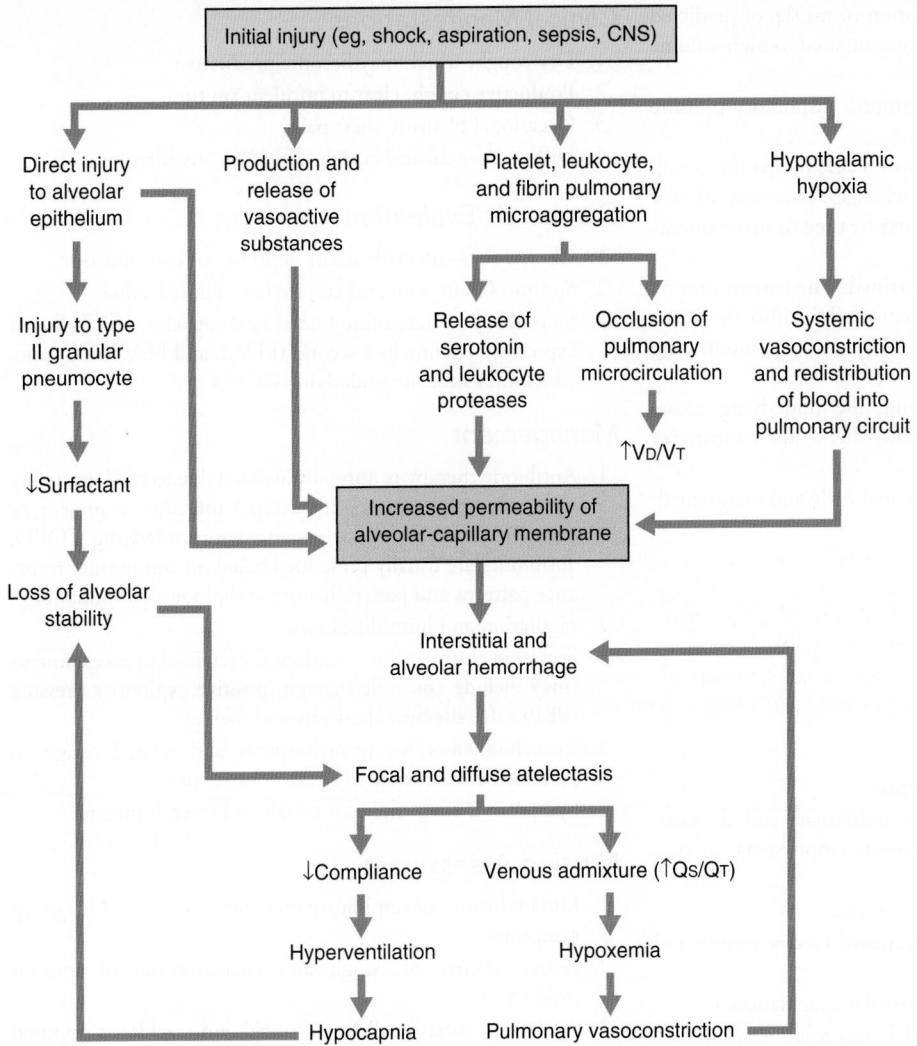

Figure 11-1. Pathogenesis of ARDS.

3. Mechanisms are unclear. Acute lung injury includes both pulmonary capillary endothelium and alveolar epithelium. Etiologies are numerous and can be pulmonary or nonpulmonary. Predisposing factors include (but are not limited to):
   a. Infections, including sepsis, pneumonia (usually bacterial or aspiration).
   b. Shock (any cause), trauma, pulmonary contusion, near drowning, direct or indirect lung injury, burns, pancreatitis.
   c. Inhaled agents—smoke, high concentration of oxygen, corrosive substances.
   d. Major surgery including coronary artery bypass graft, fat emboli, lung or bone marrow transplantation, transfusion of blood products, reperfusion pulmonary edema.

Clinical Manifestations

1. Acute onset of severe dyspnea, tachypnea, tachycardia, use of accessory muscles, cyanosis.
2. Increasing requirements of oxygen therapy. Hypoxemia refractory to supplemental oxygen therapy.

3. Scattered crackles and rhonchi heard on auscultation.
4. Decreased pulmonary compliance, evidenced by increasing pressure required to ventilate patient on mechanical ventilator.

Diagnostic Evaluation

1. Diagnosis is based on clinical, hemodynamic, and oxygen criteria. The hallmark signs for ARDS include acute-onset, severe hypoxemia, despite increasing oxygen therapy, and chest x-ray exhibiting bilateral infiltrates.
2. Pulmonary artery catheter readings show pulmonary artery wedge pressure >18 mm Hg, absence of left atrial hypertension, and no clinical signs of heart failure.

Management

1. Current ARDS treatment is primarily supportive. The underlying cause for ARDS should be determined so appropriate treatment can be initiated.
2. Mechanical ventilation is nearly always required to decrease work of breathing and improve oxygenation.

a. Low V_T by mechanical ventilation (6 mL/kg of predicted body weight) reduces mortality compared to high-volume ventilation.

b. Protective ventilation (ie, maximum inspiratory pressure of <35 cm) should be instituted.

c. PEEP should be used to improve PaO_2 (keeps the alveoli open, thereby improving gas exchange). Therefore, a lower oxygen concentration (FiO_2) may be used to maintain satisfactory oxygenation.

3. Fluid management must be maintained. The patient may be hypovolemic due to the movement of fluid into the interstitium of the lung. Pulmonary artery catheter monitoring and inotropic medication can be helpful.

4. Medications are aimed at treating the underlying cause. Corticosteroids are used infrequently due to the controversy regarding benefits of usage.

5. Adequate nutrition should be initiated early and maintained.

NURSING ALERT The treatment for ARDS is aimed at maximizing clinical stability and managing symptoms, but the underlying cause must be treated or ARDS will not resolve. Supportive measures assist the patient while the underlying cause is being treated.

Complications

1. Infections, such as pneumonia, sepsis.
2. Respiratory complications, such as pulmonary emboli, barotrauma, oxygen toxicity, subcutaneous emphysema, or pulmonary fibrosis.
3. GI complications, such as stress ulcer, ileus.
4. Cardiac complications, such as decreased cardiac output and dysrhythmias.
5. Renal failure, disseminated intravascular coagulation.
6. Multiorgan failure and sepsis, which may result in death.
7. Cognitive impairment.

Nursing Interventions

Care is similar to patient with respiratory failure (page 279) and pulmonary edema (page 291). Also see "Mechanical Ventilation" section, page 251.

Acute Bronchitis

 Evidence Base Fayyaz, J., & Mosenifar, Z. (2011). Bronchitis. *Medscape Reference.* Available: http://emedicine.medscape.com/article/297108-overview.

Acute bronchitis is an infection of the lower respiratory tract that is generally an acute sequela to an upper respiratory tract infection.

Pathophysiology and Etiology

1. Primarily viral etiology, but may also arise from bacterial agents. Exposure to irritants may also trigger bronchitis.
2. Airways become inflamed with decreased mucociliarly function. Airways may become clogged with mucus and irritated with increased mucus production.

Clinical Manifestations

1. Dry cough, which may become productive.
2. Productive cough, clear to purulent sputum.
3. Occasional pleuritic chest pain.
4. Diffuse rhonchi and crackles heard on auscultation.

Diagnostic Evaluation

1. Chest x-ray—no evidence of infiltrates or consolidation.
2. Sputum Gram stain and culture have limited value.
3. Spirometry to determine forced vital capacity (FVC), forced expiratory volume in 1 second (FEV_1), and FEV_1/FVC ratio, which may indicate underlying COPD.

Management

1. Antibiotic therapy is normally avoided due to predominantly viral cause of infection. If bacterial infection is present or strongly suspected, or for patients with underlying COPD, antibiotics are usually prescribed based on community resistance patterns and patient history and physical examination.
2. Hydration and humidification.
3. Secretion clearance interventions for retained or excess mucus (may include controlled cough, positive expiratory pressure (PEP) valve therapy, chest physical therapy).
4. Bronchodilators for bronchospasm and related cough in patients with evidence of airflow obstruction.
5. Symptom management for cough and fever, if present.

Nursing Assessment

1. Obtain history of respiratory infection, course, and length of symptoms.
2. Assess severity of cough and characteristics of sputum production.
3. Auscultate chest for diffuse rhonchi and crackles as opposed to localized crackles usually heard with pneumonia.

Nursing Diagnosis

• Ineffective Airway Clearance related to sputum production.

Nursing Interventions

Establishing Effective Airway Clearance

1. Supportive care with symptom management is usually first line in otherwise healthy patients. For those with bacterial infections or underlying COPD, administer or teach self-administration of antibiotics, as ordered.
2. Encourage mobilization of secretions through patient mobilization and, possibly, hydration, chest physical therapy, and coughing. Educate patient that beverages with caffeine or alcohol do not promote hydration.
3. If ordered, administer or teach self-administration of inhaled bronchodilators to reduce bronchospasm and enhance secretion clearance.
4. Caution patients on the use of over-the-counter cough suppressants, antihistamines, and decongestants that may cause drying and retention of secretions. Cough preparations containing the mucolytic guaifenesin may be appropriate.

Patient Education and Health Maintenance

1. Instruct patient about medication regimen, including the completion of the full course of antibiotics, if prescribed, and the effects of food on the absorption of the medications. If patient is not being treated with antibiotics, reassure patient that the majority of cases of people recover from bronchitis without antibiotic treatment, but to advise health care provider if symptoms do not improve.
2. Encourage patient to seek medical attention for shortness of breath and worsening condition.
3. Advise patient that a dry cough may persist after bronchitis due to irritation of the airways. A bedside humidifier and avoidance of dry environments may help.
4. Encourage patient to discuss complementary and alternative therapies with health care provider. When questioned, some people use garlic as an antimicrobial. Other herbs that many believe to be helpful for asthma and bronchitis are Echinacea, eucalyptus, and thyme; however, there are no definitive studies that show benefit. Since many herbal products are mixed with other ingredients and are not standardized, safety cannot be ensured.

Evaluation: Expected Outcomes

- Coughs up clear secretions effectively.

Pneumonia

 Evidence Base Infectious Disease Society of America/American Thoracic Society. (2007). Consensus guidelines on the management of community-acquired pneumonia in adults. Available: *www.guideline.gov/content.aspx?id=10560.*

Pneumonia is an inflammatory process, involving the terminal airways and alveoli of the lung, caused by infectious agents (see Table 11-1, pages 284 to 286). It may be classified according to its causative agent.

Pathophysiology and Etiology

1. The development of community-acquired pneumonia (CAP) is normally due to a defect in host defenses, exposure to a virulent microorganism, or an overwhelming exposure. An organism gains access to the lungs through aspiration of oropharyngeal contents, by inhalation of respiratory secretions from infected individuals, by way of the bloodstream, or from direct spread to the lungs as a result of surgery or trauma.
2. Risk factors for pneumonia include altered mental status, smoking, alcohol use, hypoxemia, acidosis, toxic inhalations, pulmonary edema, uremia, malnutrition, bronchial obstruction, advanced age immunosuppression, heart or lung disease (cystic fibrosis, bronchiectasis, COPD, ciliary dysfunction, lung cancer), viral respiratory infection, and history of pneumonia. Patients with bacterial pneumonia may have an underlying disease that impairs host defense; pneumonia arises from endogenous flora of the person whose resistance has been altered or from aspiration of oropharyngeal secretions.
   a. Immunocompromised patients include those receiving corticosteroids or immunosuppressants, those with cancer, those being treated with chemotherapy or radiotherapy, those undergoing organ transplantation, alcoholics, intravenous (IV) drug abusers, and those with HIV disease and acquired immunodeficiency syndrome (AIDS).
   b. These people have an increased risk of developing overwhelming infection. Infectious agents include aerobic and anaerobic gram-negative bacilli; *Staphylococcus; Nocardia;* fungi; *Candida;* viruses such as cytomegalovirus; *Pneumocystis jiroveci* (previously known as *P. carinii*); reactivation of tuberculosis (TB); and others.
3. When bacterial pneumonia occurs in a healthy person, there is usually a history of preceding viral illness.
4. Other predisposing factors include conditions interfering with normal drainage of the lung, such as tumor, general anesthesia, and postoperative immobility; depression of the central nervous system (CNS) from drugs, neurologic disorders, or other conditions, such as alcoholism; and intubation or respiratory instrumentation.
5. Pneumonia may be divided into three groups:
   a. Community acquired, due to a number of organisms.
      i. "Typical" organisms include *Streptococcus pneumoniae* (most common organism), *Haemophilus influenzae, Staphylococcus aureus,* Group A streptococci, *Moraxella catarrhalis,* anaerobes, and aerobic gram-negative bacteria.
      ii. Atypical pneumonia may be caused by *Legionella* species, *Mycobacterium pneumoniae,* and *Chlamydophila pneumoniae.*
   b. Hospital or nursing home acquired (nosocomial), due primarily to gram-negative bacilli and staphylococci.
   c. Pneumonia in the immunocompromised person.
6. People older than age 65 have a high rate of mortality, even with appropriate antimicrobial therapy.

 NURSING ALERT Recurring pneumonia commonly indicates underlying disease, such as cancer of the lung, multiple myeloma, or COPD.

Clinical Manifestations

For most common forms of bacterial pneumonia:

1. Defined by clinical signs and symptoms (fever, tachypnea, rales, cough, sputum production, pleuritic chest pain, with chest x-ray confirmation). Local epidemiology and patient travel history, history of exposures, local or national outbreaks may help in pneumonia identification.
2. Pleuritic chest pain may be aggravated by respiration/coughing.
3. Dyspnea and tachypnea may be accompanied by respiratory grunting, nasal flaring, use of accessory muscles of respiration, fatigue.
4. Tachycardia may be present.

(Text continues on page 286)

Table 11-1	Commonly Encountered Pneumonias	
TYPE	**ORGANISM RESPONSIBLE**	**MANIFESTATIONS**
Bacterial		
Streptococcal pneumonia (pneumococcal pneumonia) (60% of community-acquired pneumonia)	• *Streptococcus pneumoniae*	• May be history of previous respiratory infection • Sudden onset, with shaking and chills • Rapidly rising fever; tachypnea • Cough, with expectoration of rusty or green (purulent) sputum • Pleuritic pain aggravated by cough • Chest dull to percussion; crackles, bronchial breath sounds **GERONTOLOGIC ALERT** Confusion may be only presenting feature in older patient
Staphylococcal pneumonia	• *Staphylococcus aureus*	• Commonly, history of viral infection, especially influenza • Insidious development of cough, with expectoration of yellow, blood-streaked mucus • Onset may be sudden if patient is outpatient • Fever, pleuritic chest pain, progressive dyspnea • Pulse varies; may be slow in proportion to temperature
Pneumonia due to gram-negative enteric bacilli	• *Klebsiella* species, *Pseudomonas* organisms, *Escherichia coli*, *Serratia*, *Proteus* species	• Sudden onset with fever, chills, dyspnea • Pleuritic chest pain and production of purulent sputum
Legionella species	• *Legionella pneumophila*	• High fever, chills, cough, chest pain, tachypnea • Respiratory distress
Haemophilus influenza pneumonia *Moraxella catarrhalis* pneumonia	• *H. influenzae* • *M. catarrhalis*	• Abrupt onset of coughing, fever, chills, tachypnea
Atypical and Nonbacterial		
Mycoplasma or chlamydial pneumonia (*Legionella pneumoniae* may also be included in this category)	• *Mycoplasma pneumoniae*, *Chlamydia trachomatis*, or *L. pneumophila*	• Gradual onset; severe headache; irritating hacking cough producing scanty, mucoid sputum • Anorexia; malaise • Fever; nasal congestion; sore throat

CLINICAL FEATURES	TREATMENT*	COMPLICATIONS
• Usually involves one or more lobes • Chest x-ray shows consolidation of affected areas • Common community-acquired pneumonia as well as seen in nursing home residents, alcoholics, smokers, those with chronic obstructive pulmonary disease (COPD), IV drug use, early human immunodeficiency virus (HIV), endobronchial obstruction	• Penicillin nonresistant: MIC <2 mg/mL Penicillin G, amoxicillin • Penicillin resistant: MIC >2 mg/mL Agents chosen on the basis of susceptibility, including cefotaxime, ceftriaxone, fluoroquinolone	• Shock • Pleural effusion • Superinfections • Pericarditis • Otitis media
• Commonly seen in facility setting; during influenza epidemics; in IV drug abuse; and COPD, smokers, bronchiectasis • These infections commonly lead to necrosis and destruction of lung tissue • Treatment must be vigorous and prolonged owing to disease's tendency to destroy the lungs • Organism may develop rapid drug resistance • Prolonged convalescence usual	• Methicillin susceptible: anti-staph penicillins, cefazolin, clindamycin • Methicillin resistant: Vancomycin or TM-SMX for methicillin-resistant *S. aureus*	• Effusion/pneumothorax • Lung abscess • Empyema • Meningitis
• Infection usually occurs from aspiration of pharyngeal flora into bronchioles • Seen in persons with severe illness; among the more common causes of hospital-acquired pneumonia	• Enterobacteriaceae: Third-generation cephalosporin, carbapenem (drug of choice if extended-spectrum beta-lactamase producer) beta-lactam/beta-lactamase inhibitor, fluoroquinolone • *Pseudomonas aeruginosa:* Antipseudomonal beta-lactame *plus* ciprofloxacin or levofloxacinf or aminoglycoside Aminoglycoside *plus* ciprofloxacin or levofloxacinf	• Early necrosis of lung tissue with rapid abscess formation • High mortality
• Peak incidence in people over age 50 who are cigarette smokers and have underlying diseases that increase susceptibility to infection or who have been on a cruise ship in the past 2 weeks	• Fluoroquinolone, azithromycin Doxycycline	• Respiratory failure
• Common in smokers and former smokers • May affect healthy young adults • X-ray may show consolidation • Often seen in early HIV and may be first indication of endobronchial tumor	• Non-beta-lactam-producing organisms: amoxicillin, fluoroquinolones, doxycycline, azithromycin, clarithromycin • beta-lactam-producing organisms: 2nd- or 3rd-generation cephalosporins, amoxicillin clavulanate, fluoroquinolones, doxycycline, azithromycin, clarithromycin	• High mortality in patients with underlying disease (cancer, COPD) • Pleural effusion common
• Occurs most commonly in children and young adults, as well as in older adults in community or hospital setting • Rise in serum-complement-fixing antibodies to the organism • More common in COPD and in smokers	• For mycoplasma or *Chlamydophila pneumoniae*: macrolides, fluoroquinolones • For *Legionella*: fluoroquinolones, azithromycin, doxycycline	• Persisting cough, meningoencephalitis, polyneuritis, monoarticular arthritis, pericarditis, myocarditis • Chlamydial pneumonia has been implicated in cardiac atheromatous lesions in some patients

(continued)

Table 11-1   Commonly Encountered Pneumonias (*continued*)

TYPE	ORGANISM RESPONSIBLE	MANIFESTATIONS
Viral pneumonia	• Influenza viruses • Parainfluenza viruses • Respiratory syncytial viruses • Rhinoviruses • Adenovirus • Varicella, rubella, rubeola, herpes simplex, cytomegalovirus, Epstein-Barr virus	• Cough • Constitutional symptoms may be pronounced (severe headache, anorexia, fever, and myalgia)
Pneumocystis jiroveci pneumonia (PCP)	• *P. jiroveci*	• Insidious onset • Increasing dyspnea and nonproductive cough • Tachypnea; progresses rapidly to intercostal retraction, nasal flaring, and cyanosis • Lowering of arterial oxygen tension • Chest x-ray will reveal diffuse, bilateral interstitial pneumonia
Fungal pneumonia	• *Aspergillus fumigatus*	• Fever, productive cough, chest pain, hemoptysis • Chest x-ray reveals broad range of abnormalities from infiltration to consolidation, cavitation, and empyema

*Patients with CAP should be treated a minimum of 5 days and should be afebrile for 48–72 hours and clinically stable before discontinuing antibiotics.

Diagnostic Evaluation

1. Chest x-ray shows a discernable infiltrate and presence/extent of pulmonary disease, typically consolidation.
2. Patients with CAP should be investigated for specific pathogens that would significantly alter standard management decisions, when such pathogen is suspected on the basis of clinical and epidemiologic clues. Gram stain and culture and sensitivity tests of sputum may be indicated to determine offending organism in select cases. Endobronchial specimens should be obtained from intubated patients. Indications for sputum culture in persons with a productive cough include:
   a. Admission to intensive care unit.
   b. Antibiotic failure.
   c. Cavitary lesion on chest x-ray.
   d. Active alcohol abuse.
   e. Severe lung disease.
   f. Positive *Legionella* or pneumococcal urinary antigen test.
   g. Pleural effusion.
3. The value of sputum Gram stain and culture in nosocomial pneumonia, especially ventilator-associated pneumonia, is more universally acknowledged. Sputum Gram stain and culture are indicated for all patients with hospital-acquired pneumonia.
4. Pretreatment blood samples for culture to detect bacteremia should be obtained from patients with admission to intensive care unit, cavitary lesion on chest x-ray, leukopenia, active alcohol abuse, chronic severe liver disease, asplenia, positive pneumococcal urinary antigen test, or pleural effusion.

5. Immunologic tests may be ordered to detect microbial antigens in serum, sputum, and urine.
6. Severity-of-illness scores, such as the CURB-65 criteria (confusion, uremia, respiratory rate, low blood pressure, age 65 or greater), or pneumonia severity index can be used to identify patients with CAP who may be candidates for outpatient treatment.

 Evidence Base Ebell, M. H. (2006). Outpatient vs. inpatient treatment of community-acquired pneumonia. *Family Practice Management, 13*(4), 41–44.

Management

1. Antimicrobial therapy—depends on empiric recommendations and/or laboratory identification of causative organism and sensitivity to specific antimicrobials.
2. Oxygen therapy, if patient has inadequate gas exchange.
3. Patients with hypoxemia or respiratory distress who are refractory to oxygen should receive a cautious trial of noninvasive ventilation unless they require immediate intubation due to severe hypoxemia or acute respiratory failure.
4. Low V_T ventilation (6 mL/kg ideal body weight) for diffuse bilateral pneumonia or ARDS.
5. Early mobilization when clinically stable reduces length of facility stay.
6. Assess influenza and pneumococcal vaccination status and if not currently vaccinated, perform either at hospital discharge or during outpatient treatment.
7. Advise and assist with smoking cessation in currently smoking patients.

CLINICAL FEATURES	TREATMENT*	COMPLICATIONS
• In majority of patients, influenza begins as an acute coryza and myalgias; others have bronchitis and pleurisy, whereas still others develop GI symptoms • Risk of developing influenza related to crowding and close contact with groups	• Treat symptomatically • Prophylactic vaccination recommended for high-risk persons (over age 65; chronic cardiac or pulmonary disease, diabetes, and other metabolic disorders) • For influenza virus: oseltamivir, zanamivir	• Persons with underlying disease have increased risk of complications; primary influenzal pneumonia; secondary bacterial pneumonia • Bacterial superinfection • Pericarditis • Endocarditis
• Usually seen in host whose resistance is compromised; most common opportunistic infection in AIDS in the United States • Organism invades lungs of patients who have suppressed immune system (from AIDS, cancer, leukemia) or after immunosuppressive therapy for cancer, organ transplant, or collagen disease • Frequently associated with concurrent infection by viruses (cytomegalovirus), bacteria, and fungi	• TMP-SMX; dapsone with trimethoprim, clindamycin with primaquine • Pentamidine methanesulfonate	• Patients are critically ill • Prognosis guarded because it is usually a complication of a severe underlying disorder
• Neutropenic individual most susceptible • May develop Aspergillus as a superinfection • Often seen in late HIV disease	• Amphotericin B; Itraconazole	• High mortality rate • Invades blood vessels and destroys lung tissue by direct invasion and vascular infarction

8. Respiratory hygiene measures, including the use of hand hygiene and masks or tissues for patients with cough, should be used in outpatient settings and EDs to reduce the spread of respiratory infections.

Complications

1. Pleural effusion.
2. Sustained hypotension and shock, especially in gram-negative bacterial disease, particularly in older patients.
3. Superinfection: pericarditis, bacteremia, and meningitis.
4. Delirium—considered a medical emergency.
5. Atelectasis—due to mucus plugs.
6. Delayed resolution.

Nursing Assessment

1. Take a careful history to help establish etiologic diagnosis.
   a. History of recent respiratory illness including mode of onset, complete medical history including chronic lung or liver disease, asplenia, immunologic status including HIV infection, exposure to animals, and recent travel.
   b. Presence of purulent sputum, increased amount of sputum, fever, chills, chest pain, dyspnea, tachypnea.
   c. Any family illness.
   d. Medications (including recent antibiotics), alcohol, tobacco, or IV drug use.
2. Observe for anxious, flushed appearance, shallow respirations, splinting of affected side, confusion, disorientation.
3. Auscultate for crackles overlying affected region and for bronchial breath sounds when consolidation (filling of airspaces with exudate) is present.

Nursing Diagnoses

- Impaired Gas Exchange related to decreased ventilation secondary to inflammation and infection involving distal airspaces.
- Ineffective Airway Clearance related to excessive tracheobronchial secretions.
- Acute Pain related to inflammatory process and dyspnea.
- Risk for Injury secondary to complications.

Nursing Interventions

Improving Gas Exchange

1. Observe for cyanosis, dyspnea, hypoxia, and confusion, indicating worsening condition.
2. Follow ABG levels/SaO_2 to determine oxygen need and response to oxygen therapy.
3. Administer oxygen at concentration to maintain Pao_2 at acceptable level. Hypoxemia may be encountered because of abnormal V/Q mismatch with shunt in affected lung segments.
4. Use caution with high concentrations of oxygen in patients with COPD, particularly with evidence of CO_2 retention; use of high oxygen concentrations may worsen alveolar ventilation in some patients by depressing the patient's only remaining ventilatory drive. If high concentrations of oxygen are given, monitor alertness and PaO_2 and $PaCO_2$ levels for signs of CO_2 retention.
5. Place patient in an upright position as tolerated to obtain greater lung expansion and improve aeration. Frequent turning and increased activity (up in chair, ambulate as tolerated) should be employed.

Enhancing Airway Clearance

1. If ordered, obtain freshly expectorated sputum for Gram stain and culture, preferably early morning specimen, as directed. Instruct the patient as follows:
   a. Perform oral care and rinse mouth with water to minimize contamination by normal flora.
   b. Breathe deeply several times.
   c. Cough deeply and expectorate raised sputum into sterile container.
2. Encourage patient to cough; retained secretions interfere with gas exchange. Suction as necessary.
3. Encourage increased fluid intake, unless contraindicated, to thin mucus and promote expectoration and replace fluid losses caused by fever, diaphoresis, dehydration, and dyspnea.
4. Humidify air or oxygen therapy, which may loosen secretions and improve ventilation.
5. Employ chest wall percussion and postural drainage, when appropriate, to loosen and mobilize secretions.
6. Auscultate the chest for crackles and rhonchi.
7. Cough suppressants may be appropriate in some cases when coughing is nonproductive.
8. Mobilize patient to improve ventilation and secretion clearance and reduce risk of atelectasis and worsening pneumonia.

Relieving Pleuritic Pain

1. Place patient in a comfortable position (semi-Fowler's) for resting and breathing; encourage frequent change of position to prevent pooling of secretions in lungs and atelectasis.
2. Demonstrate how to splint the chest while coughing.
3. Avoid suppressing a productive cough.
4. Administer prescribed analgesic agent to relieve pain. Use opioids cautiously in patients with a history of COPD.

 GERONTOLOGIC ALERT Sedatives, opioids, and cough suppressants should be used cautiously in older patients because of their tendency to suppress cough and gag reflexes and respiratory drive. Also, provide or encourage frequent oral care for pneumonia prevention.

5. Use comfort measures to improve symptom control.
7. Encourage modified bed rest during febrile period.
8. Watch for abdominal distention or ileus, which may be due to swallowing of air during intervals of severe dyspnea. Insert a nasogastric (NG) or rectal tube, as directed.

Monitoring for Complications

1. Remember that fatal complications may develop during the early period of antimicrobial treatment.
2. Monitor temperature, pulse, respiration, BP, oximetry, mentation, and for evidence of dyspnea at regular intervals to assess the patient's response to therapy.
3. Auscultate lungs and heart. Heart murmurs or friction rub may indicate acute bacterial endocarditis, pericarditis, or myocarditis.
4. Employ special nursing surveillance for patients with:

   a. Alcoholism, COPD, immunosuppression—these people as well as older patients may have little or no fever.
   b. Chronic bronchitis—it may be difficult to detect subtle changes in condition because the patient may have seriously compromised pulmonary function and regular mucus production.
   c. Epilepsy—pneumonia may result from aspiration after a seizure.
   d. Delirium—may be caused by hypoxia, meningitis, delirium tremens of alcoholism.

 NURSING ALERT Delirium must be controlled to prevent exhaustion and cardiac failure. Prepare for lumbar puncture, if indicated, to rule out meningitis, which may be lethal. Mild sedation should be considered with caution.

5. Assess these patients for unusual behavior, alterations in mental status, stupor, and heart failure.
6. Assess for resistant fever or return of fever, potentially suggesting bacterial resistance to antibiotics.

Patient Education and Health Maintenance

1. Advise patient to complete entire course of antibiotics.
2. Advise patient that fatigue and weakness may be prolonged after pneumonia.
3. Once clinically stable, encourage gradual increase in activities to improve ventilation and reduce hazards of immobility.
4. Encourage breathing exercises to clear lungs and promote full expansion and function.
5. Explain that a chest x-ray is usually taken 4 to 6 weeks after recovery to evaluate lungs for clearing and detect any tumor or underlying cause.
6. Advise smoking cessation. Cigarette smoke destroys tracheobronchial cilial action, which is the first line of defense of lungs; also irritates mucosa of bronchi and inhibits function of alveolar scavenger cells (macrophages).
7. Advise the patient to keep up natural resistance with good nutrition, adequate rest, and physical activity, when tolerated. One episode of pneumonia may make the patient susceptible to recurring respiratory infections.
8. Instruct patient to avoid fatigue, sudden extremes in temperature, and excessive alcohol intake, which lower resistance to pneumonia.
9. Assess for and encourage vaccination with pneumococcal polysaccharide vaccine (see page 280).
10. Encourage annual influenza vaccination (see page 280). Influenza vaccine is associated with reduced hospitalizations for pneumonia, influenza, and death in community-dwelling older adults.
11. Advise avoidance of contact with people who have upper respiratory infections for several months after pneumonia resolves.
12. Respiratory and hand hygiene includes frequent handwashing, especially after contact with others.

Evaluation: Expected Outcomes

- Cyanosis and dyspnea reduced; ABG levels and SaO_2 improved.
- Coughs effectively; absence of crackles.
- Appears more comfortable; free of pain.
- Fever controlled, no signs of resistant infection.

Aspiration Pneumonia

Aspiration is the inhalation of oropharyngeal secretions and/or stomach contents into the lungs. It may produce an acute form of pneumonia.

Pathophysiology and Etiology

1. Patients at risk and factors associated with risk:
   a. Loss of protective airway reflexes (swallowing, cough) caused by altered state of consciousness, alcohol or drug overdose, during resuscitation procedures, seriously ill or debilitated patients, abnormalities of gag and swallowing reflexes.
   b. NG tube feedings.
   c. Obstetric patients—from general anesthesia, lithotomy position, delayed emptying of stomach from enlarged uterus, labor contractions.
   d. GI conditions—hiatal hernia, intestinal obstruction, abdominal distention.
   e. Prolonged endotracheal (ET) intubation/tracheostomy—can depress glottic and laryngeal reflexes from disuse.
2. Effects of aspiration depend on volume and character of aspirated material.
   a. Particulate matter—mechanical blockage of airways and secondary infection.
   b. Anaerobic bacterial aspiration—from oropharyngeal secretions.
   c. Gastric juice—destructive to alveoli and capillaries; results in outpouring of protein-rich fluids into the interstitial and intra-alveolar spaces. (Impairs exchange of oxygen and CO_2, producing hypoxemia, respiratory insufficiency, and respiratory failure.)

Clinical Manifestations

1. Tachycardia, fever.
2. Dyspnea, cough, tachypnea.
3. Cyanosis.
4. Crackles, rhonchi, wheezing.
5. Pink, frothy sputum (may simulate acute pulmonary edema).

Diagnostic Evaluation

1. Chest x-ray may be normal initially; with time, shows consolidation and other abnormalities.

Management

Depends on the material aspirated.
1. Clearing the obstructed airway.
   a. If foreign body is visible, it may be removed manually.
   b. Place the patient in tilted head-down position on right side (right side more commonly affected if patient has aspirated solid particles).
   c. Suction trachea/ET tube—to remove particulate matter.

2. Laryngoscopy/bronchoscopy may be performed for aspiration of solid material.
3. Fluid volume replacement for correction of hypotension.
4. Antimicrobial therapy if there is evidence of superimposed bacterial infection.
5. Correction of acidosis; respiratory acidosis and metabolic acidosis indicate a severe reaction due to aspiration of gastric contents.
6. Oxygen therapy and assisted ventilation if adequate ABG values cannot be maintained.

Complications

1. Lung abscess; empyema.
2. Necrotizing pneumonia.
3. ARDS.

Nursing Assessment

1. Assess for airway obstruction.
2. Assess for risk factors for aspiration.
3. Assess for development of fever, foul-smelling sputum, and development of congestion.

Nursing Diagnoses

- Impaired Gas Exchange related to decreased ventilation secondary to inflammation and infection involving distal airspaces.
- Ineffective Airway Clearance related to excessive tracheobronchial secretions.
- Acute Pain related to inflammatory process and dyspnea.
- Risk for Injury secondary to complications.

(See pages 287–288 for nursing interventions.)

Additional Nursing Interventions

1. Be on guard constantly and monitor patients at risk as described earlier.
2. Elevate head of bed for debilitated patients, for those receiving tube feedings, and for those with neurologic or motor diseases of the esophagus.
3. Place patients with impaired cough and/or gag reflexes in an upright position.
4. Make sure NG tube is patent.
5. Give tube feedings slowly, with patient sitting up in bed. Check for tube feeding residuals.
   a. Check position of tube in stomach before feeding.
   b. Check seal of cuff of tracheostomy or ET tube before feeding.
6. Keep the patient in a fasting state before anesthesia (at least 8 hours).
7. Feed patients with impaired swallowing slowly, and make sure that no food is retained in mouth after feeding.

 NURSING ALERT Morbidity and mortality rate of aspiration pneumonia remain high even with optimum treatment. Prevention is the key to the problem.

Pulmonary Embolism

Evidence Base Qaseem, A., Chou, R., Humphrey, L. L., et al. (2011). Venous thromboembolism prophylaxis in hospitalized patients: A clinical practice guideline from the American College of Physicians. *Annals of Internal Medicine, 155*(9), 625–632.

Pulmonary embolism refers to the obstruction of one or more pulmonary arteries by a thrombus (or thrombi) usually originating in the deep veins of the legs, the right side of the heart, or, rarely, an upper extremity, which becomes dislodged and is carried to the pulmonary vasculature.

Pulmonary infarction refers to necrosis of lung tissue that can result from interference with blood supply.

Pathophysiology and Etiology

1. Obstruction, either partial or full, of pulmonary arteries, which causes decrease or absent blood flow; therefore, there is ventilation but no perfusion (V/Q mismatch).
2. Hemodynamic consequences:
    a. Increased pulmonary vascular resistance.
    b. Increased pulmonary artery pressure (PAP).
    c. Increased right-sided heart workload to maintain pulmonary blood flow.
    d. Right-sided heart failure.
    e. Decreased cardiac output.
    f. Decreased BP.
    g. Shock.
3. Pulmonary emboli can vary in size and seriousness of consequences.
4. Predisposing factors include:
    a. Stasis, prolonged immobilization.
    b. Concurrent phlebitis.
    c. Heart failure, stroke.
    d. Injury to vessel wall.
    e. Coagulation disorders, hypercoagulable state.
    f. Malignancy.
    g. Advancing age, estrogen therapy, oral contraceptives
    h. Fracture of long boxes.
    i. Obesity.

NURSING ALERT Be aware of high-risk patients for pulmonary embolism—immobilization, trauma to pelvis (especially surgical) and lower extremities (especially hip fracture), obesity, history of thromboembolic disease, varicose veins, pregnancy, heart failure, myocardial infarction (MI), malignant disease, postoperative patients, older patients.

Clinical Manifestations

1. Rapid onset of dyspnea at rest, pleuritic chest pain, cough, syncope, delirium, apprehension, tachypnea, diaphoresis, hemoptysis.
2. Chest pain with apprehension and a sense of impending doom occurs when most of the pulmonary artery is obstructed.
3. Tachycardia, rales, fever, hypotension, cyanosis, heart gallop, loud pulmonic component of S_2 (split S_2).
4. Calf or thigh pain, edema, erythema, tenderness or palpable cord (signs suggestive of deep vein thrombosis).

NURSING ALERT Have a high index of suspicion for pulmonary embolus if there is a subtle or significant deterioration in the patient's condition and unexplained cardiovascular and pulmonary findings.

Diagnostic Evaluation

1. Thoracic imaging: V/Q scan (possibly using single-photon emission computed tomography) or helical contrast-enhanced computed tomography (CT).
2. Pulmonary angiography if noninvasive testing is inconclusive or not candidate for noninvasive testing. Contrast studies should be avoided in persons who are pregnant or have advanced renal failure.
3. D-Dimer assay for low to intermediate probability of pulmonary embolism.
4. ABG levels—decreased PaO_2 is usually found, due to perfusion abnormality of the lung.
5. Chest x-ray—normal or possible wedge-shaped infiltrate.

Management

Emergency Management

For massive pulmonary embolism, goal is to stabilize cardiorespiratory status.

NURSING ALERT Massive pulmonary embolism is a medical emergency; the patient's condition tends to deteriorate rapidly. There is a profound decrease in cardiac output, with an accompanying increase in right ventricular pressure.

1. Oxygen is administered to relieve hypoxemia, respiratory distress, and cyanosis and to dilate pulmonary vasculature.
2. An infusion is started to open an IV route for drugs and fluids.
3. Vasopressors, inotropic agents such as dopamine, and anti-dysrhythmic agents may be indicated to support circulation if the patient is unstable.
4. ECG is monitored continuously for findings suggestive of right-sided heart failure, which may have a rapid onset. Changes may include sinus tachycardia, Q waves, late T-wave inversion, S wave in lead I, right bundle-branch block, right axis deviation, atrial fibrillation, and T-wave changes.
5. Small doses of IV morphine may be given to relieve anxiety, alleviate chest discomfort (which improves ventilation), and ease adaptation to mechanical ventilator, if this is necessary.
6. Pulmonary angiography, thoracic imaging, hemodynamic measurements, ABG analysis, and other studies are carried out.

Subsequent Management–Anticoagulation and Thrombolysis

1. IV heparin—stops further thrombus formation and extends the clotting time of the blood; it is an anticoagulant and antithrombotic.
   a. IV loading dose usually followed by continuous pump or drip infusion or given intermittently every 4 to 6 hours.
   b. Dosage adjusted to maintain the partial thromboplastin time (PTT) at 1½ to 2 times the pretreatment value (if the value was normal).
   c. Protamine sulfate may be given to neutralize heparin in event of severe bleeding.
2. Oral anticoagulation with warfarin is usually used for follow-up anticoagulant therapy after heparin therapy has been established; interrupts the coagulation mechanism by interfering with the vitamin K–dependent synthesis of prothrombin and factors VII, IX, and X.
   a. Dosage is controlled by monitoring serial tests of prothrombin time (PT); desired PT is 2 to 3 times control value.
   b. Reported as international normalized ratio (INR) of 2.0 to 3.0 by most laboratories.
   c. Anticoagulation is used to prevent new clot formation but does not dissolve previously formed clots. Thrombolytics are used to dissolve clots.

 GERONTOLOGIC ALERT Consider the patient's age in dosing of anticoagulation therapy. Older patients will usually need a decreased dosing regimen.

3. Thrombolytic agents, such as streptokinase, may be used in patients with massive pulmonary embolism.
   a. Effective in lysing recently formed thrombi.
   b. Improved circulatory and hemodynamic status.
   c. Administered IV in a loading dose followed by constant infusion.
4. Newer clot-specific thrombolytics (tissue plasminogen activator, streptokinase activator complex, single-chain urokinase) are preferred.
   a. Activate plasminogen only within thrombus itself rather than systematically.
   b. Minimize occurrence of generalized fibrinolysis and subsequent bleeding.

Surgical Intervention

When anticoagulation is contraindicated or patient has recurrent embolization or develops serious complications from drug therapy.

1. Interruption of vena cava—reduces channel size to prevent lower extremity emboli from reaching lungs. Accomplished by:
   a. Ligation, plication, or clipping of the inferior vena cava.
   b. Placement of transvenously inserted intraluminal filter in inferior vena cava to prevent migration of emboli (see Figure 11-2); inserted through femoral or jugular vein by way of catheter.
2. Embolectomy (removal of pulmonary embolic obstruction).

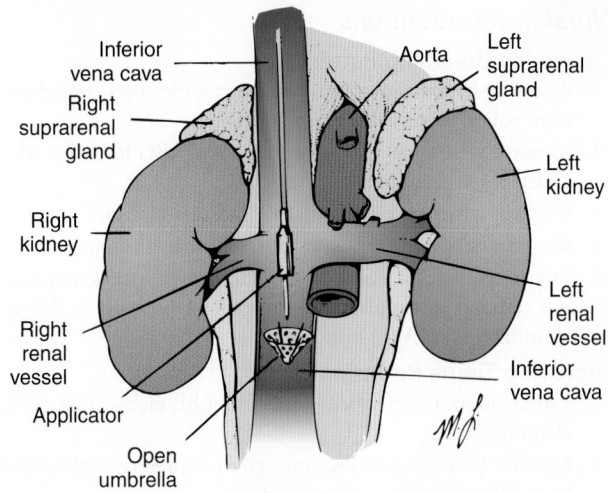

Figure 11-2. Insertion of umbrella filter in inferior vena cava to prevent pulmonary embolism. Filter (compressed within an applicator catheter) is inserted through an incision in the right internal jugular vein. The applicator is withdrawn when the filter fixes itself to the wall of the inferior vena cava after ejection from the applicator.

Complications

1. Bleeding as a result of treatment.
2. Respiratory failure.
3. Pulmonary hypertension, cor pulmonale.

Nursing Assessment

1. Take nursing history with emphasis on onset and severity of dyspnea and nature of chest pain.
2. Examine the patient's legs carefully. Assess for swelling of leg, duskiness, warmth, pain on pressure over gastrocnemius muscle, pain on dorsiflexion of the foot (positive Homans' sign), which indicate thrombophlebitis as source.
3. Monitor respiratory rate—may be accelerated out of proportion to degree of fever and tachycardia.
   a. Observe rate of inspiration to expiration.
   b. Percuss for resonance or dullness.
   c. Auscultate for friction rub, crackles, rhonchi, and wheezing.
4. Auscultate heart; listen for splitting of second heart sound.
5. Evaluate results of PT/PTT tests and INR for patients on anticoagulants and report results that are outside of therapeutic range promptly; anticipate a dosage change.

Nursing Diagnoses

- Ineffective Breathing Pattern related to acute increase in alveolar dead airspace and possible changes in lung mechanics from embolism.
- Ineffective Tissue Perfusion (Pulmonary) related to decreased blood circulation.
- Acute Pain (pleuritic) related to congestion, possible pleural effusion, possible lung infarction.
- Anxiety related to dyspnea, pain, and seriousness of condition.
- Risk for Injury related to altered hemodynamic factors and anticoagulant therapy.

Nursing Interventions

Correcting Breathing Pattern

1. Assess for hypoxia, dyspnea, headache, restlessness, apprehension, pallor, cyanosis, behavioral changes.
2. Monitor vital signs, ECG, oximetry, and ABG levels for adequacy of oxygenation.
3. Monitor patient's response to IV fluids/vasopressors.
4. Monitor oxygen therapy—used to relieve hypoxemia.
5. Prepare patient for assisted ventilation when hypoxemia does not respond to supplemental oxygen. Hypoxemia is due to abnormalities of V/Q mismatch.

Improving Tissue Perfusion

1. Closely monitor for shock—decreasing BP, tachycardia, cool, clammy skin.
2. Monitor prescribed medications given to preserve right-sided heart filling pressure and increase BP.
3. Maintain patient on bed rest during acute phase to reduce oxygen demands and risk of bleeding.
4. Monitor urinary output hourly because there may be reduced renal perfusion and decreased glomerular filtration.
5. Antiembolism compression stockings should provide a compression of 30 to 40 mm Hg.

Relieving Pain

1. Watch patient for signs of discomfort and pain.
2. Ascertain if pain worsens with deep breathing and coughing; auscultate for friction rub.
3. Give morphine, as prescribed, and monitor for pain relief and signs of respiratory depression.
4. Position with head of bed slightly elevated (unless contraindicated by shock) and with chest splinted for deep breathing and coughing.
5. Evaluate patient thoroughly for signs of hypoxia when anxiety, restlessness, and agitation of new onset are noted, before administering as-needed sedatives. Consider calling health care provider when these signs are present, especially if accompanied by cyanotic nail beds, circumoral pallor or cyanosis, and increased respiratory rate.

Reducing Anxiety

1. Correct dyspnea and relieve physical discomfort.
2. Explain diagnostic procedures and the patient's role; correct misconceptions.
3. Listen to the patient's concerns; attentive listening relieves anxiety and reduces emotional distress.
4. Speak calmly and slowly.
5. Do everything possible to enhance the patient's sense of control.

Intervening for Complications

1. Be alert for shock from low cardiac output secondary to resistance to right-sided heart outflow or to myocardial dysfunction due to ischemia.
   a. Assess for skin color changes, particularly nail beds, lips, earlobes, and mucous membranes.
   b. Monitor BP, pulse, and SpO_2.
   c. Measure urine output.
   d. Monitor IV infusion of vasopressor or other prescribed agents.

2. Bleeding—related to anticoagulant or thrombolytic therapy.
   a. Assess patient for bleeding; major bleeding may occur from GI tract, brain, lungs, nose, and genitourinary (GU) tract.
   b. Perform stool guaiac test to detect occult blood loss.
   c. Monitor platelet count to detect heparin-induced thrombocytopenia.
   d. Minimize risk of bleeding by performing essential ABG analysis on upper extremities; apply digital compression at puncture site for 30 minutes; apply pressure dressing to previously involved sites; check site for oozing.
   e. Maintain patient on strict bed rest during thrombolytic therapy; avoid unnecessary handling.
   f. Discontinue infusion in the event of uncontrolled bleeding.
   g. Notify health care provider on call immediately for change in LOC or sensation or ability to follow commands, move limbs, or respond to questions with clear articulation. Intracranial bleed may necessitate discontinuation of anticoagulation promptly to avert massive neurologic catastrophe.

Patient Education and Health Maintenance

1. Advise patient of the possible need to continue taking anticoagulant therapy for 6 weeks up to an indefinite period as well as safety considerations and drug and food interactions with anticoagulants.
2. Teach about signs of bleeding, especially of gums and nose, bruising, and blood in urine and stools.
3. For patients on anticoagulants, instruct to use soft toothbrush, avoid shaving with blade razor (use electric razor instead), and avoid aspirin-containing products. Notify health care provider of bleeding or increased bruising.
4. Warn against taking medications unless approved by health care provider because many drugs interact with anticoagulants.
5. Instruct patient to tell dentist about taking an anticoagulant.
6. Warn against inactivity for prolonged periods or sitting with legs crossed to prevent recurrence.
7. Warn against sports/activities that may cause trauma or injury to legs and predispose to a thrombus.
8. Encourage wearing a MedicAlert bracelet, identifying patient as anticoagulant user.
9. Instruct patient to lose weight, if applicable; obesity is a risk factor.
10. Discuss contraceptive methods with patient, if applicable; females with history of pulmonary embolus are advised against taking hormonal contraceptives.

Evaluation: Expected Outcomes

- Verbalizes less shortness of breath.
- Vital signs stable; adequate urinary output.
- Reports freedom from pain.
- Appears more relaxed; sleeping at long intervals.
- Progresses without complications.

Tuberculosis

Tuberculosis (TB) is an infectious disease caused by bacteria (*Mycobacterium tuberculosis*). It is usually spread from person to person through droplet aerosolization (droplet nuclei). It usually infects the lung but can occur at virtually any site in the body.

Of particular concern is the prevalence of TB among foreign-born persons residing in the United States, delays in detecting and reporting pulmonary TB, and deficiencies in identifying and screening close contacts and persons with latent TB infection (LTBI) who are at risk for progression to active TB. This population includes those who are HIV positive, who have acquired TB infection within last 2 years, in children younger than age 4, and in those with already immunocompromised conditions, such as silicosis; diabetes mellitus; chronic renal failure; leukemia; lymphoma; carcinoma of the head, neck, or lung; 10% or more below ideal body weight; prolonged corticosteroid use; use of tumor necrosis factor–alpha (TNF-α) antagonists; organ transplant; intestinal bypass or gastrectomy; and history of untreated or inadequately treated TB.

Lastly, extensively drug-resistant tuberculosis (XDR TB) is a relatively rare type of multidrug-resistant tuberculosis resistant to almost all oral drugs used to treat TB, including isoniazid, rifampin, fluoroquinolones, and at least one of three injectable drugs (ie, amikacin, kanamycin, or capreomycin). XDR TB is of special concern for persons with HIV infection and/or immunocompromised persons due to increased risk of infection and mortality.

Pathophysiology and Etiology

 Evidence Base World Health Organization. (2011). *Guidelines for the programmatic management of drug-resistant tuberculosis.* Geneva: Author. Available: *http://whqlibdoc.who.int/publications/2011/9789241501583_eng.pdf.*

Transmission

1. The term *Mycobacterium* is descriptive of the organism, which is a bacterium that resembles a fungus. The organisms multiply at varying rates and are characterized as acid-fast aerobic organisms that can be killed by heat, sunshine, and ultraviolet light.
2. TB is an airborne disease transmitted by droplet nuclei, usually from within the respiratory tract of an infected person who exhales them during coughing, talking, sneezing, or singing.
3. When a susceptible person inhales the droplet-containing air, the organism is carried into the lung to the pulmonary alveoli.
   a. About 2½ to 12 weeks after initial TB infection, TB testing (purified protein derivative [PPD] or blood test) is positive; however, most people who become infected do not develop clinical illness because the body's immune system brings the infection under control.
   b. Some bacilli remain viable in the body for years, such as with LTBI. Persons with LTBI have no symptoms and are not infectious.
4. Persons at increased risk for TB include close contacts of persons with active TB, foreign-born persons (from Africa, Asia, Eastern Europe, Latin America, and Russia), residents of high-risk congregate settings (correctional facilities, long-term care facilities, and homeless shelters), health care workers exposed to high-risk patients, infants, and children or adolescents exposed to high-risk adults.

Pathology

1. The bacilli of TB infect the lung, forming a tubercle (lesion).
2. The tubercle:
   a. May heal, leaving scar tissue.
   b. May continue as a granuloma, then heal, or be reactivated.
   c. May eventually proceed to necrosis, liquefaction, sloughing, and cavitation.
3. The initial lesion may disseminate tubercle bacilli by extension to adjacent tissues, by way of the bloodstream, the lymphatic system, or through the bronchi.
4. Extrapulmonary TB occurs more commonly in children and immunocompromised individuals and can involve lymph nodes, bones, joints, pleural space, pericardium, CNS, GI tract, GU tissue, and the peritoneum.

Clinical Manifestations

Patient may be asymptomatic or may have insidious symptoms that may be ignored.
1. Constitutional symptoms.
   a. Fatigue, anorexia, weight loss, low-grade fever, night sweats.
   b. Some patients have acute febrile illness, chills, and flu-like symptoms.
2. Pulmonary signs and symptoms.
   a. Cough (insidious onset) progressing in frequency and producing mucoid or mucopurulent sputum, hemoptysis.
   b. Chest pain; dyspnea (suggest extensive involvement).
3. Extrapulmonary TB: pain, inflammation, and dysfunction in any of the tissues infected.

Diagnostic Evaluation

1. Sputum smear—detection of acid-fast bacilli (AFB) in stained smears is the first bacteriologic clue of TB. Obtain first morning sputum on 3 consecutive days.
2. Sputum culture—a positive culture for *M. tuberculosis* confirms a diagnosis of TB.
3. Chest x-ray to determine presence and extent of disease.

 NURSING ALERT Cavitation on chest x-ray, positive sputum AFB smear, and ongoing cough increase the risk of infection transmission.

4. Tuberculin skin test (PPD or Mantoux test)—inoculation of tubercle bacillus extract (tuberculin) into the intradermal layer of the inner aspect of the forearm (see Procedure Guidelines 11-1, pages 294 to 295). It is used to detect *M. tuberculosis* infection, past or present, active or inactive (latent).
5. Interferon gamma release assays are newer (since 2005) blood assays for *Mycobacterium tuberculosis* that may serve as an alternative to PPD. The tests do not distinguish between active and latent TB and are unaffected by past exposure to BCG vaccine. Interpret negative tests with caution in immunocompromised patients, in those at high risk for TB, and children. Examples of these tests are T-SPOT and QuantiFeron TB-Gold.
6. Nonspecific screening tests, such as multiple puncture tests (tine test), should not be used.

(Text continues on page 296)

PROCEDURE GUIDELINES 11-1

Tuberculin Skin Test

EQUIPMENT

- Purified protein derivative (PPD) tuberculin antigen intermediate strength
- Tuberculin syringe
- 5/8", 27G steel needle with engineered sharps safety mechanism
- Alcohol pad
- Gloves recommended but not required as the risk of exposure to blood is minimal with intradermal injection.

PROCEDURE

Nursing Action	Rationale
Preparatory phase	
1. Administer symptom screening questionnaire.	1. Any positive response should raise the index of suspicion for TB and merits investigation regardless of the test result.
2. Determine if the patient has ever had Bacille Calmette-Guérin (BCG) vaccine, recent viral disease, immunosuppression by disease, drugs, or corticosteroids.	2. Any of these may cause false readings. Previous BCG vaccine or the other factors should not preclude PPD testing, but will be considered with the result.
3. Do not give PPD to person who has had a positive test or TB in the past.	3. Chest x-ray as indicated for screening and symptom review.
Performance phase	
1. Draw up PPD-tuberculin into tuberculin syringe.	1. Follow the manufacturer's directions. Each 0.1-mL dose should contain 5 tuberculin units (TU) of PPD-tuberculin. Use the antigen immediately to avoid absorption onto the plastic/glass syringe.
2. Put on gloves.	2. Follow standard infection control precautions.
3. Clean the skin of the inner aspect of forearm with alcohol. Allow to dry.	3. Alcohol must dry for antisepsis.
4. Stretch the skin taut.	
5. Hold the tuberculin syringe as near parallel to the skin as possible (10-degree angle) so the hub of the needle touches it as the needle is introduced, bevel up.	5. Reduces the needle angle at the skin surface and facilitates the injection of tuberculin just beneath the surface of the skin.
6. Inject the tuberculin into the superficial layer of the skin to form a wheal 6 to 10 mm in diameter. Activate engineered sharps safety mechanism.	6. If no wheal appears (because the injection was made too deep), inject again at another site at least 2 inches (5 cm) away.
7. Immediately place disposable needle and syringe into puncture-resistant sharps container.	
Follow-up phase	
To read the test	
1. Read the test within 48–72 hours.	1. Tuberculin skin tests are tests of *delayed hypersensitivity*.
2. Have a good light available. Flex the patient's forearm slightly at the elbow.	2. Relieves tension on the skin.
3. Inspect for the presence of induration; inspect from a side view against the light; inspect by direct light.	3. Induration refers to hardening or thickening of tissues.
4. Palpate: Lightly rub the finger across the injection site from the area of normal skin to the area of induration. Outline the diameter of induration.	4. Erythema (redness) without induration is generally considered to be of no significance.
5. Measure the maximum transverse diameter of induration (not erythema) in millimeters with a flexible ruler.	5. The full extent of induration is important for interpretation.

PROCEDURE GUIDELINES 11-1 *(continued)*

Tuberculin Skin Test

PROCEDURE *(continued)*

Nursing Action	Rationale
Interpretation	
1. Induration of 5 mm or more in diameter indicates positive reaction and need for treatment for latent TB infection in high-risk groups.	1. High-risk groups include: a. People with HIV. b. People who have had recent contact with active TB. c. People who have fibrotic changes on chest x-ray, consistent with healed TB. d. People with organ transplants or other causes of immunosuppression (including therapy with ≥15 mg of prednisone daily ≥1 month) or taking TNF-α antagonists.
2. Induration of 10 mm or more in diameter indicates a positive reaction and need for treatment of latent TB infection in persons at risk.	2. Persons at risk include: a. People with medical conditions, such as substance abuse, diabetes mellitus, silicosis, head and neck cancer, leukemia, end-stage renal disease, gastrectomy, intestinal bypass, prolonged corticosteroid therapy. b. Recent arrivals (<5 years) from high-prevalence countries c. Residents and employees of long-term care facilities and other congregate settings. d. Children younger than age 4; adolescents exposed to adults in high-risk categories. e. Injection drug users. f. Mycobacteriology laboratory personnel. g. All people who do not meet above criteria but who have other risk factors for TB, such as homelessness, alcoholism, malnutrition, and health care workers.
3. Induration of 15 mm in persons with no known risk factors for TB may be considered for treatment.	3. Targeted skin testing programs should be conducted among risk groups only to avoid false positives.

NURSING ALERT False-positive reaction may occur in people infected with mycobacteria other than *M. tuberculosis*, vaccination with BCG, or inaccurate testing. False-negative reactions may occur in people with HIV infection or anergy (inability to react to skin tests due to weakened immune system), recent (6 to 8 weeks of exposure) or very old TB infection (many years), very young age (<6 months), overwhelming miliary or pulmonary TB, recent measles or other viral infections, recent live-virus vaccinations (measles and smallpox), and those receiving corticosteroids or immunosuppressive drugs.

Evidence Base Centers for Disease Control and Prevention. (2011). Tuberculin skin testing. Available: *www.cdc.gov/tb/publications/factsheets/testing/skintesting.htm.*

Table 11-2   Recommended Drugs for the Initial Treatment of Tuberculosis in Adults

DRUG	DOSAGE FORMS	DAILY DOSE	TWICE WEEKLY DOSE	THRICE WEEKLY DOSE	MAJOR ADVERSE REACTIONS
Isoniazid	• Tablets: 50 mg, 100 mg, 300 mg • Syrup: 50 mg/5 mL • Vials: 1 g	5 mg/kg P.O. or I.M. (maximum 300 mg)	15 mg/kg (maximum 900 mg) (can also be given once per week)	15 mg/kg (maximum 900 mg)	Paresthesias, nausea, vomiting, elevated liver transaminases peripheral neuropathy, hepatitis, hypersensitivity, hepatotoxicity
Rifampin	• Capsules: 150 mg, 300 mg • Syrup: formulated from capsules, 10 mg/mL	10 mg/kg P.O. (maximum 600 mg)	10 mg/kg (maximum 600 mg)	10 mg/kg (maximum 600 mg)	Red-orange discoloration of secretions and urine; nausea, vomiting, anorexia, hepatitis, elevated liver transaminases, febrile reaction, purpura (rare), pruritus and rash, caution regarding drug interactions
Pyrazinamide	• Tablets: 500 mg	20–25 mg/kg P.O.	40–50 mg/kg	30–40 mg/kg (maximum 3 g)	Anorexia, rash, urticaria, nausea, vomiting, hepatotoxicity, hyperuricemia, arthralgias
Ethambutol	• Tablets: 100 mg, 400 mg	15–20 mg/kg	240–250 mg/kg	25–35 mg/kg	Optic neuritis (decreased red-green color discrimination, decreased visual acuity), joint pain, anorexia, nausea, vomiting, skin rash

Evidence Base   (2003). *Morbidity and Mortality Weekly Report, 52*(RR-11, Tables 4 and 5).

Management

See Table 11-2.

1. In patients with active TB, a combination of drugs to which the organisms are susceptible is given to destroy viable bacilli as rapidly as possible and to protect against the emergence of drug-resistant organisms.
2. Current recommended regimen of uncomplicated, previously untreated pulmonary TB is an initial phase of 2 months of bactericidal drugs, including isoniazid (INH), rifampin, pyrazinamide (PZA), and ethambutol (EMB). This regimen should be followed until the results of drug susceptibility studies are available, unless there is little possibility of drug resistance.
   a. If drug susceptibility results are known and organism is fully susceptible, EMB does not need to be included.
   b. For children whose visual acuity cannot be monitored, EMB is not normally recommended except with increased likelihood of INH resistance or if the child has upper lobe infiltration and/or cavity formation.
   c. Due to increasing frequency of global streptomycin resistance, streptomycin is not considered interchangeable with EMB unless organism is known to be susceptible to streptomycin.
   d. PZA may be withheld in patients with severe liver disease, gout, and, possibly, pregnancy.
   e. Adverse effects, including liver injury, have been noted with rifampin and pyrazinamide in a once daily or twice weekly combination; therefore, this combination is not recommended for the treatment of latent TB infection.
3. Follow with 4 months of isoniazid and rifampin. Six months of therapy is usually effective for killing the three populations of bacilli: those rapidly dividing, those slowly dividing, and those only intermittently dividing.
4. Sputum smears may be obtained every 2 weeks until they are negative; sputum cultures do not become negative for 3 to 5 months.
5. Rifabutin is used as a substitute for rifampin if the organism is susceptible to rifabutin and for patients taking medications that may interact with rifampin.
6. Second-line drugs—such as cycloserine, ethionamide, streptomycin, amikacin, kanamycin, capreomycin, para-aminosalicylic acid, and some fluoroquinolones—are used in patients with resistance, for retreatment, and in those with intolerance to other agents. Patients taking these drugs should be monitored by health care providers experienced in their use.
7. For people with suspected LTBI, treatment should begin after active TB has been ruled out (see Table 11-3). The usual treatment regimen for LTBI is isoniazid 300 mg P.O. daily for 9 months. To prevent neurotoxicity, pyridoxine 25 to 50 mg daily is also recommended.

 DRUG ALERT Adverse reactions to anti-TB drugs may be significant. Most common adverse effects are rash, GI intolerance, and liver enzyme elevation, but neurotoxicity, hepatitis, hypersensitivity reactions, and optic neuritis may occur. Liver toxicity is the most worrisome adverse reaction because toxic hepatitis may occur in patients receiving INH, RIF, or PZA. Monitor liver function tests and instruct patients to seek immediate medical attention if signs or symptoms of hepatitis occur (nausea, emesis, anorexia, jaundice, dark urine, and/or abdominal pain).

Table 11-3	Drug Therapy for Latent Tuberculosis Infection		
DRUG	**DURATION (MONTHS)**	**INTERVAL**	**MINIMUM DOSES**
Isoniazid	9	Daily	270
		Twice weekly	76
Isoniazid	6	Daily	180
		Twice weekly	52
Rifampin	4	Daily	120
Rifampin/ Pyrazinamide	Generally should not be offered for treatment of LTBI	—	—

Adapted from Centers for Disease Control and Prevention, Treatment Options for Latent Tuberculosis Infection (LTBI), updated January 2012. Available: www.cdc.gov/tb/publications/factsheets/treatment/LTBItreatmentoptions.htm.

Complications

1. Pleural effusion.
2. TB pneumonia.
3. Other organ involvement with TB.
4. Serious reactions to drug therapy.
   a. INH may produce asymptomatic elevation in liver enzymes, rare peripheral neurotoxicity, hepatitis that may, rarely, be fatal, CNS effects (dysarthria, irritability, seizures, dysphoria, diminished concentration), lupus-like syndrome, hypersensitivity reactions, and monoamine poisoning (rarely occurring with consumption of some wines and cheeses). Patients with preexisting liver disease should be monitored closely. GI adverse effects may include nausea, vomiting, and indigestion.
   b. EMB may cause retrobulbar optic neuritis with decreased visual acuity and decreased red-green discrimination in one or both eyes, although this occurs rarely with daily doses of 15 mg/kg/day. EMB may also cause peripheral neuritis and cutaneous reactions. Patients should have baseline visual acuity and color discrimination (Ishihara test) testing as well as monthly monitoring. adverse GI effects may include anorexia, nausea, and vomiting.
   c. Pyrazinamide may cause hepatotoxicity, GI symptoms, nongouty polyarthralgia, asymptomatic hyperuricemia, and acute gouty arthritis.
   d. Any anti-TB drug may cause rash. If rash occurs, withhold all medications until rash subsides. Rechallenge drugs sequentially every 3 to 4 days to find cause. Usual sequence is INH, rifampin, PZA, and EMB, using the first-line (most important) drug first.
   e. Rifampin may cause pruritus with or without rash, adverse GI effects, flu-like symptoms, hepatotoxicity, rare severe immunologic reactions, orange discoloration of body fluids, and drug interactions with hormonal contraceptives, methadone, and warfarin.

Nursing Assessment

1. Obtain history of exposure to TB.
2. Assess for symptoms of active disease—productive cough, night sweats, afternoon temperature elevation, unintentional weight loss, pleuritic chest pain.
3. Auscultate lungs for crackles.
4. During drug therapy, assess for liver dysfunction.
   a. Question the patient about loss of appetite, fatigue, joint pain, fever, tenderness in liver region, clay-colored stools, dark urine, and vision changes.
   b. Monitor for fever, right upper quadrant abdominal tenderness, nausea, vomiting, rash, and persistent paresthesia of hands and feet.
   c. Monitor results of periodic liver function studies.

Nursing Diagnoses

- Ineffective Breathing Pattern related to pulmonary infection and potential for long-term scarring with decreased lung capacity.
- Risk for superinfection related to nature of the disease and patient's symptoms.
- Imbalanced Nutrition: Less Than Body Requirements related to poor appetite, fatigue, and productive cough.
- Noncompliance related to lack of motivation particularly in LTBI, and long-term treatment associated with health risk to patient, close contacts, and public health.

Nursing Interventions

Improving Breathing Pattern

1. Administer and teach self-administration of medications as ordered.
2. Encourage rest and avoidance of exertion if acutely ill.
3. Monitor breath sounds, respiratory rate, sputum production, dyspnea, urine and stool color.
4. Provide supplemental oxygen as ordered.
5. Report adherence concerns to Department of Public Health.

Preventing Transmission of Infection

1. Be aware that TB is transmitted by respiratory droplets.
2. Provide care for hospitalized patient in a negative-pressure room to prevent respiratory droplets from escaping when door is opened.
3. Enforce rule that all staff and visitors use well-fitted standard N-95 particulate masks for contact with patient.
4. Use high-efficiency particulate masks, such as high-efficiency particulate air (HEPA) filter masks or positive air pressure respirators, for high-risk procedures, including suctioning, bronchoscopy, or pentamidine treatments.
5. Use standard precautions for additional protection: gowns and gloves for direct contact with patient, linens or articles in room, meticulous hand hygiene.
6. Educate the patient to control spread of infection through secretions.
   a. Cover mouth and nose with double-ply tissue when coughing or sneezing. Do not sneeze into bare hand.
   b. Wash hands after coughing or sneezing.
   c. Dispose of tissues promptly into closed plastic bag.
   d. Limit contact with others while infectious.

Improving Nutritional Status

1. Explain the importance of eating a nutritious diet to promote healing and improve defense against infection.
2. Provide small, frequent meals and liquid supplements during symptomatic period.
3. Monitor weight.
4. Administer vitamin supplements, as ordered, particularly pyridoxine (vitamin B_6), to prevent peripheral neuropathy in patients taking INH.

Improving Compliance

1. Educate the patient about the etiology, transmission, and effects of TB. Stress the importance of continuing to take medicine for the prescribed time because bacilli multiply slowly and thus can only be eradicated over a long period.
2. Review adverse effects of the drug therapy (see Table 11-2). Question the patient specifically about common toxicities of drugs being used and emphasize immediate reporting should these occur.
3. Participate in observation of medication taking, weekly pill counts, or other programs designed to increase compliance with treatment for TB.

 NURSING ALERT Patient compliance remains a major problem in eradicating TB. Therefore, it may be helpful and necessary to have patient take medication in observed setting. Directly observed therapy (DOT) is especially critical for patients with drug-resistant TB, HIV-infected patients, and those on intermittent treatment regimens (ie, two or three times weekly). The course of DOT is often shorter than unobserved treatment regimens.

Community and Home Care Considerations

1. Improve ventilation in the home by opening windows in room of affected person and keeping bedroom door closed as much as possible.
2. Instruct patient to cover mouth with fresh tissue when coughing or sneezing and to dispose of tissues promptly in plastic bags.
3. Discuss TB testing of people residing with patient.
4. Investigate living conditions, availability of transportation, financial status, alcohol and drug abuse, and motivation, which may affect compliance with follow-up and treatment. Initiate referrals to a social worker for interventions in these areas.
5. Report new cases of TB to public health department for screening of close contacts and monitoring.

Patient Education and Health Maintenance

1. Review possible complications: hemorrhage, pleurisy, symptoms of recurrence (persistent cough, fever, or hemoptysis).
2. Instruct patient on avoidance of job-related exposure to excessive amounts of silicone (working in foundry, rock quarry, sand blasting), which increases risk of reactivation.
3. Encourage patient to report at specified intervals for bacteriologic (smear) examination of sputum to monitor therapeutic response and compliance.

4. Instruct patient in basic hygiene practices and investigate living conditions. Crowded, poorly ventilated conditions contribute to development and spread of TB.
5. Encourage regular symptom screening. Follow-up chest x-ray is recommended if an individual with LTBI chooses not to be treated. A single posteroanterior chest x-ray annually for 2 years is sufficient. Any individual with a history of positive TB test who develops symptoms suggestive of TB (fever, night sweats, weight loss, productive cough, or hemoptysis) should be screened with chest x-ray as part of the clinical evaluation for possible recurrent TB disease.
6. Instruct patient on prophylaxis with INH for people with LTBI or for children or patients infected with HIV who are close household contacts of patients with active TB because these individuals are at high risk of becoming infected.
7. Educate asymptomatic people about PPD testing and treatment of latent TB for positive results, based on risk grouping.

Evaluation: Expected Outcomes

- Afebrile; dyspnea relieved.
- Standard precautions observed; disposes of respiratory secretions properly.
- Maintains body weight.
- Takes medications as prescribed.

Pleurisy

Pleurisy is a clinical term to describe *pleuritis* (inflammation of the pleura, both parietal and visceral).

Pathophysiology and Etiology

1. Inflammation of the pleura stimulates nerve endings, causing pain.
2. May occur in the course of many pulmonary diseases:
   a. Pneumonia (bacterial, viral).
   b. TB.
   c. Pulmonary infarction, embolism.
   d. Pulmonary abscess.
   e. Upper respiratory tract infection.
   f. Pulmonary neoplasm.

Clinical Manifestations

1. Chest pain—becomes severe, sharp, and knifelike on inspiration (pleuritic pain).
   a. May become minimal or absent when breath is held.
   b. May be localized or radiate to shoulder or abdomen.
2. Intercostal tenderness on palpation.
3. Pleural friction rub—grating or leathery sounds heard in both phases of respiration; heard low in the axilla or over the lung base posteriorly; may be heard for only a day or so.
4. Evidence of infection; fever, malaise, increased white blood cell count.

Diagnostic Evaluation

1. Chest x-ray may show pleural thickening.
2. Sputum examination may indicate infectious organism.

3. Examination of pleural fluid obtained by thoracentesis for smear and culture.
4. Pleural biopsy may be necessary to rule out other conditions.

Management

1. Treatment for the underlying primary disease (pneumonia, infarction); inflammation usually resolves when the primary disease subsides.
2. Pain relief, using pharmacologic and nonpharmacologic methods.
3. Intercostal nerve block may be necessary when pain causes hypoventilation.

Complications

1. Severe pleural effusion.
2. Atelectasis due to shallow breathing to avoid pain.

Nursing Assessment

1. Assess patient's level of pain.
2. Observe for signs and symptoms of pleural effusion (dyspnea, pain, decreased diaphragmatic excursion on affected side).
3. Auscultate lungs for pleural friction rub.

Nursing Diagnosis

- Ineffective Breathing Pattern related to stabbing chest pain.

Nursing Interventions

Easing Painful Respiration

1. Assist patient to find comfortable position that will promote aeration; lying on affected side decreases stretching of the pleura and, therefore, the pain decreases.
2. Instruct patient in splinting chest while taking a deep breath or coughing.
3. Administer or teach self-administration of pain medications, as ordered.
4. Employ nonpharmacologic interventions for pain relief, such as application of heat, muscle relaxation, and imagery.
5. Assist with intercostal nerve block if indicated.
6. Evaluate patient for signs of hypoxia (with SpO_2 or ABG) when anxiety, restlessness, and agitation of new onset are noted, before administering as-needed sedatives. Consider evaluation by a health care provider when these signs are present, especially if accompanied by cyanotic nail beds, circumoral pallor, and increased respiratory rate.

Patient Education and Health Maintenance

1. Instruct patient to seek early intervention for pulmonary diseases so pleurisy can be avoided.
2. Reassure and encourage patience because pain will subside.
3. Advise patient on reporting shortness of breath, which could indicate pleural effusion.

Evaluation: Expected Outcomes

- Respirations deep without pain.

Pleural Effusion

Pleural effusion refers to a collection of fluid in the pleural space. It is almost always secondary to other diseases.

Pathophysiology and Etiology

1. May be either transudative or exudative.
2. Transudative effusions occur primarily in noninflammatory conditions; it is an accumulation of low-protein, low-cell-count fluid.
3. Exudative effusions occur in an area of inflammation; it is an accumulation of high-protein fluid.
4. Occurs as a complication of:
   a. Disseminated cancer (particularly lung and breast), lymphoma.
   b. Pleuropulmonary infections (pneumonia).
   c. Heart failure, cirrhosis, nephrosis.
   d. Other conditions—sarcoidosis, SLE, peritoneal dialysis.

Clinical Manifestations

1. Dyspnea, pleuritic chest pain, cough.
2. Dullness or flatness to percussion (over areas of fluid) with decreased or absent breath sounds.

Diagnostic Evaluation

1. Chest x-ray or ultrasound detects presence of fluid.
2. Thoracentesis—biochemical, bacteriologic, and cytologic studies of pleural fluid indicates cause.

Management

General

1. Treatment is aimed at underlying cause (heart disease, infection, cancer).
2. Thoracentesis is done to remove fluid, collect a specimen, and relieve dyspnea.

For Malignant Effusions

1. Video-assisted thoracoscopy, chest tube drainage, radiation, and/or chemotherapy.
2. In malignant conditions, pleurodesis may be required. Thoracentesis may provide only transient benefits because effusion may reaccumulate within a few days.
3. Pleurodesis—production of adhesions between the parietal and visceral pleura accomplished by tube thoracostomy, pleural space drainage, and intrapleural instillation of a sclerosing agent (tetracycline, doxycycline, or minocycline).
   a. Drug introduced through tube into pleural space; tube clamped.
   b. Patient is assisted into various positions for 3 to 5 minutes each to allow drug to spread to all pleural surfaces.
   c. Tube is unclamped, as prescribed.
   d. Chest drainage continued for 24 hours or longer.
   e. Resulting pleural irritation, inflammation, and fibrosis cause adhesion of the visceral and parietal surfaces when they are brought together by the negative pressure caused by chest suction.

Complications

1. Large effusion could lead to respiratory failure.

Nursing Assessment

1. Obtain history of previous pulmonary condition.
2. Assess patient for dyspnea and tachypnea.
3. Auscultate and percuss lungs for abnormalities.

Nursing Diagnosis

- Ineffective Breathing Pattern related to collection of fluid in pleural space.

Nursing Interventions

Maintaining Normal Breathing Pattern

1. Institute treatments to resolve the underlying cause, as ordered.
2. Assist with thoracentesis, if indicated (see page 203).
3. Maintain chest drainage, as needed (see page 268).
4. Provide care after pleurodesis.
   a. Monitor for excessive pain from the sclerosing agent, which may cause hypoventilation.
   b. Administer prescribed analgesic.
   c. Assist patient undergoing instillation of intrapleural lidocaine if pain relief is not forthcoming.
   d. Administer oxygen as indicated by dyspnea and hypoxemia.
   e. Observe patient's breathing pattern, oxygen saturation, and other vital signs for evidence of improvement or deterioration.

Patient Education and Health Maintenance

1. Instruct patient to seek early intervention for unusual shortness of breath, especially if he or she has underlying chronic lung disease.

Evaluation: Expected Outcomes

- Reports absence of shortness of breath.

Lung Abscess

A *lung abscess* is a localized, pus-containing, necrotic lesion in the lung characterized by cavity formation.

Pathophysiology and Etiology

1. Most commonly occurs due to aspiration of vomitus or infected material from upper respiratory tract.
2. Secondary causes include:
   a. Aspiration of foreign body into lung.
   b. Pulmonary embolus.
   c. Trauma.
   d. TB, necrotizing pneumonia.
   e. Bronchial obstruction (usually a tumor) causes obstruction to bronchus, leading to infection distal to the growth.
3. The right lung is involved more frequently than the left because of dependent position of the right bronchus, the less acute angle that the right main bronchus forms within the trachea, and its larger size.
4. In the initial stages, the cavity in the lung may communicate with the bronchus.

5. Eventually, the cavity becomes surrounded or encapsulated by a wall of fibrous tissue, except at one or two points where the necrotic process extends until it reaches the lumen of some bronchus or pleural space and establishes a communication with the respiratory tract, the pleural cavity (bronchopleural fistula), or both.
6. The organisms typically seen are *Klebsiella pneumoniae* and *Staphylococcus aureus*.

Clinical Manifestations

1. Cough, fever, and malaise from segmental pneumonitis and atelectasis.
2. Headache, anemia, weight loss, dyspnea, weakness.
3. Pleuritic chest pain from extension of suppurative pneumonitis to pleural surface.
4. Production of mucopurulent sputum, usually foul-smelling; blood streaking common; may become profuse after abscess ruptures into bronchial tree.
5. Chest may be dull to percussion, decreased or absent breath sounds, intermittent pleural friction rub.

Diagnostic Evaluation

1. Chest x-ray to help diagnose and locate lesion.
2. Chest CT to locate and identify if lesion is singular or multiple areas of involvement.
3. Direct bronchoscopic visualization to exclude possibility of tumor or foreign body; bronchial washings and brush biopsy may be done for cytopathologic study.
4. Sputum culture and sensitivity tests to determine causative organisms and antimicrobial sensitivity.

Management

1. Administration of appropriate antimicrobial agent, usually by IV route, until clinical condition improves; then oral administration.
2. Percutaneous drainage by interventional radiology.
3. Bronchoscopy to drain abscess is controversial.
4. Surgical intervention only if patient fails to respond to medical management, sustains a hemorrhage, or has a suspected tumor.
5. Nutritional management is usually a high-calorie, high-protein diet.

Complications

1. Hemoptysis from erosion of a vessel.
2. Empyema, bronchopleural fistula.
3. Entrapment of lung.
4. Hemoptysis.
5. Further expansion of abscess.
6. Lung necrosis.

Nursing Assessment

1. Examine oral cavity because poor condition of teeth and gums increases number of anaerobes in oral cavity and could be source for infection. Promote frequent oral care.
2. Perform chest examination for abnormalities.

3. Monitor for foul-smelling sputum, which may indicate an anaerobic pulmonary infection.

4. Review results of laboratory and x-ray findings for location of abscess and identification of causative organism.

Nursing Diagnoses

- Ineffective Breathing Pattern related to presence of suppurative lung disease.
- Acute or Chronic Pain related to infection.
- Imbalanced Nutrition: Less Than Body Requirements related to catabolic state from chronic infection.

Nursing Interventions

Minimizing Respiratory Dysfunction

1. Monitor patient's response to antimicrobial therapy; take temperature at prescribed intervals.
2. Implement additional interventions, as indicated.
   a. Postural drainage may be recommended. Positions to be assumed depend on location of abscess.
   b. Carry out coughing and breathing exercises.
   c. Measure and record the volume of sputum to follow patient's clinical course (may be of limited use due to patient swallowing of sputum).
   d. Give adequate fluids to enhance liquefying of secretions.

Attaining Comfort

1. Use nursing measures to combat generalized discomfort: oral hygiene, positions of comfort, relaxing massage.
2. Take temperature, pulse, respirations, and BP at regular intervals to determine fever and monitor the severity and duration of the infectious process.
3. Encourage rest and limitation of physical activity during febrile periods.
4. Monitor chest tube functioning.
5. Evaluate patient thoroughly for signs of hypoxia, including SpO_2, when anxiety, restlessness, and agitation of new onset are noted before administering as-needed sedatives. Consider physician evaluation when these signs are present, especially if accompanied by cyanotic nail beds, circumoral pallor, increased respiratory rate.
6. Administer analgesics as directed. Use caution with opioids that might depress respirations.

Improving Nutritional Status

1. Provide a high-protein, high-calorie diet.
2. Offer liquid supplements for additional nutritional support when anorexia limits patient's intake.
3. Monitor weight weekly.

Patient Education and Health Maintenance

1. Teach the patient that an extended course of antimicrobial therapy (4 to 8 weeks) is usually necessary; mixed infections are common and may require multiple antibiotics.
2. Encourage patient to have periodontal care, especially in presence of gingival lesions.
3. Stress importance of follow-up x-rays to monitor abscess cavity closure.

4. Remind family that patient may aspirate if weakness, confusion, alcoholism, seizures, and swallowing difficulties are present. Train in aspiration precautions.

5. Encourage patient to assume responsibility for attaining and maintaining an optimal state of health through a planned program of nutrition, rest, and exercise.

Evaluation: Expected Outcomes

- Respirations unlabored; temperature in normal range; less purulent sputum expectorated.
- Appears more comfortable; verbalizes less pain.
- Eats better; weight stable.

Cancer of the Lung (Bronchogenic Cancer)

Bronchogenic cancer refers to an epithelial cancer, which originates in the bronchial surface epithelium or bronchial mucus glands, arising within the wall or epithelial lining of the bronchus. The lung is also a common site of metastasis by way of venous circulation or lymphatic spread. Bronchogenic cancer is classified according to cell type:

- Non-small-cell lung cancer (NSCLC) (75% to 80%) includes epidermoid (squamous cell) carcinoma, adenocarcinoma, and bronchoalveolar carcinoma.
- Small-cell lung cancer (about 13%): An aggressive cancer that can spread to other parts of the body.

Pathophysiology and Etiology

Predisposing Factors

1. Cigarette, pipe, cigar smoking, and secondhand smoke exposure—amount, frequency, and duration of smoking have positive relationship to cancer of the lung.
2. Occupational exposure to radon, asbestos, air pollution, polycyclic aromatic hydrocarbons (from incomplete combustion of carbon-based fuels, such as wood, coal, diesel, fat, tobacco, incense, or tar), arsenic, chromium, nickel, iron, radioactive substances, isopropyl oil, petroleum oil mists alone or in combination with tobacco smoke.
3. History of lung cancer.
4. Age greater than 65 years.

 NURSING ALERT Suspect lung cancer in patients who belong to a susceptible, high-risk group and who have repeated unresolved respiratory infections. The National Cancer Institute has found that low-dose spiral chest CT provides a decided benefit in screening and management of lung cancer.

Staging and Classification

1. Staging refers to anatomic extent of tumor, lymph node involvement, atelectasis, bronchus involvement, and metastatic spread, including malignant pleural effusions. Classification refers to criteria that classify pathologic type of lung cancer.
2. Staging done by the tumor, node, metastasis staging system for NSCLC is an internationally accepted system used to determine the disease stage and extent of disease, and is used

to guide management (particularly surgical) and determine prognosis.

   a. Imaging including chest CT and PET scan.

   b. Pathology including biopsy (mediastinoscopy, tissue).

3. The International Association for the Study of Lung Cancer (IASLC) has developed a classification system using standardized criteria and terminology for the pathologic diagnosis of lung cancer in small biopsies and cytology. NSCLC can be further classified into a more specific type, such as adenocarcinoma or squamous cell carcinoma, based on this system. This classification system is important since 70% of lung cancer patients present with advanced stages that are potentially unresectable.

 Evidence Base Travis, W. D., Brambilla, E., Noguchi, M., et al. (2011). The new IASLC/ATS/ERS international multidisciplinary lung adenocarcinoma classification. *Journal of Thoracic Oncology, 6,* 244–285.

Clinical Manifestations

Symptoms are related to size and location of tumor, extent of spread, and involvement of other structures.

1. Cough, especially a new type or changing cough, results from bronchial irritation.
2. Dyspnea, wheezing (suggests partial bronchial obstruction).
3. Chest pain (poorly localized and aching).
4. Excessive sputum production, repeated upper respiratory infections.
5. Hemoptysis.
6. Malaise, fever, weight loss, fatigue, anorexia.
7. Paraneoplastic syndrome—metabolic or neurologic disturbances related to the secretion of substances by the neoplasm.
8. Symptoms of metastasis—bone pain; abdominal discomfort, nausea and vomiting from liver involvement; pancytopenia from bone marrow involvement; headache from CNS metastasis.
9. Usual sites of metastasis—lymph nodes, bones, liver, central nervous system.

Diagnostic Evaluation

1. Abnormal findings seen on chest x-ray are typically followed with chest CT. If suggestive of possible cancer, a needle biopsy or bronchoscopy is typically performed to establish diagnosis, followed by a positron-emission tomography (PET) scan for staging and consideration of surgical options.
2. CT scan of chest and abdomen and whole body PET scan are indicated in most candidates for surgical resection.
3. Cytologic examination of sputum/chest fluids for malignant cells for pleural effusion.
4. Fiber-optic bronchoscopy for observation of location and extent of tumor; for biopsy or surgery.
5. PET scan—sensitive in detecting small nodules and metastatic lesions.
6. Lymph node biopsy; mediastinoscopy to establish lymphatic spread; to plan treatment.

7. Pulmonary function tests (PFTs)—to determine if patient will have adequate pulmonary reserve to withstand surgical procedure.
8. Laboratory testing, including complete blood count, metabolic panel, calcium level, liver function tests.

Management

1. Treatment depends on the cell type, stage of disease, and the physiologic status of the patient. It includes a multidisciplinary approach that may be used separately or in combination, including:

   a. Surgical resection.

   b. Radiation therapy.

   c. Chemotherapy.

   d. Biotherapy.

Complications

1. Hypercoagulable state.
2. Complications of treatment including pancytopenia, rash, hair loss.
3. Superior vena cava syndrome—oncologic complication caused by obstruction of major blood vessels draining the head, neck, and upper torso.
4. Hypercalcemia—commonly from bone metastasis.
5. Syndrome of inappropriate antidiuretic hormone (SIADH) with hyponatremia and abnormal water retention.
6. Pleural effusion.
7. Infectious complications, especially upper respiratory infections.
8. Brain metastasis, spinal cord compression, pulmonary scarring.
9. With advanced lung cancer—massive hemoptysis, central airway obstruction, malignant pleural effusion, venous thrombosis, spinal cord compression, hypercalcemia, and SIADH.

Nursing Assessment

1. Determine onset and duration of coughing, sputum production (purulent vs. bloody), and degree of dyspnea. Auscultate breath sounds. Observe symmetry of chest during respirations.
2. Take anthropometric measurements: weigh patient, review laboratory tests, and conduct appraisal of 24-hour food intake.
3. Ask about pain, including location, intensity, and factors influencing pain.
4. Monitor vital signs including oximetry.

Nursing Diagnoses

- Ineffective Breathing Pattern related to obstructive and restrictive respiratory processes associated with lung cancer.
- Imbalanced Nutrition: Less Than Body Requirements related to hypermetabolic state, taste aversion, anorexia secondary to radiotherapy/chemotherapy.
- Acute or Chronic Pain related to tumor effects, invasion of adjacent structures, toxicities associated with radiotherapy/chemotherapy.
- Anxiety and/or depression related to treatment-related side effects, uncertain outcome, and fear of recurrence.

Nursing Interventions

See also Chapter 8, page 134, for interventions related to specific cancer treatment.

Improving Breathing Patterns

1. Prepare patient physically, emotionally, and intellectually for prescribed therapeutic program.
2. For superior vena cava syndrome, elevate head of bed to promote gravity drainage and prevent fluid collection in upper body.
3. Teach breathing retraining exercises to increase diaphragmatic excursion with resultant reduction in work of breathing.
4. Give prescribed treatment for productive cough (expectorant, antimicrobial agent) and mobilize patient, as tolerated, to potentially control thickened or retained secretions and subsequent dyspnea.
5. Augment the patient's ability to cough effectively.
   a. Splint chest manually with hands.
   b. Instruct patient to inspire fully and cough two to three times in one exhalation.
   c. Provide humidifier/vaporizer to provide moisture to loosen secretions.
6. Support patient undergoing removal of pleural fluid (by thoracentesis or tube thoracostomy) and instillation of sclerosing agent to obliterate pleural space and prevent fluid recurrence.
7. Administer oxygen by way of nasal cannula as prescribed.
8. Encourage energy conservation through pacing of activities, sitting for tasks.
9. Allow patient to sleep in a reclining chair or with head of bed elevated if severely dyspneic.
10. Recognize the anxiety associated with dyspnea; teach relaxation techniques.

Improving Nutritional Status

1. Emphasize that nutrition is an important part of the treatment of lung cancer.
   a. Encourage small amounts of high-calorie, high-protein foods frequently, rather than three daily meals.
   b. Ensure adequate protein intake—milk, eggs, chicken, fowl, fish, cheese, and oral nutritional supplements if patient cannot tolerate meats or other protein sources.
2. Administer or encourage prescribed vitamin supplement to avoid deficiency states, glossitis, and cheilosis.
3. Change consistency of diet to soft or liquid if patient has esophagitis from radiation therapy.
4. Give enteral or total parenteral nutrition for malnourished patient who is unable or unwilling to eat.
5. Obtain dietitian consultation.

Controlling Pain

1. Take a history of pain complaint; assess presence/absence of support system.
2. Administer prescribed drug, usually starting with nonsteroidal anti-inflammatory drugs (NSAIDs) and progressing to adjuvant analgesic and short- and long-acting opioids.
   a. Administer regularly to control pain.
   b. Titrate to achieve pain control.
3. Consider alternative methods, such as cognitive and behavioral training, biofeedback, and relaxation, to increase patient's sense of control. Mind–body modalities (meditation, hypnosis, relaxation techniques, cognitive-behavioral therapy, biofeedback, and guided imagery) and massage therapy may be helpful for mood disorders and chronic pain. Acupuncture may improve pain control.

 Evidence Base Cassileth, B., Deng, G. E., Gomez, J. E., et al. (2007). Complementary therapies and integrative oncology in lung cancer—American College of Chest Physicians evidence-based clinical practice guidelines (2nd ed.). *Chest, 132,* 340S–354S.

4. Evaluate problems of insomnia, depression, anxiety, and so forth that may be contributing to patient's pain.
5. Initiate bowel training program because constipation is an adverse effect of some analgesic/opioid agents.
6. Facilitate referral to pain clinic/specialist if pain becomes refractory (unyielding) to usual methods of control.
7. Radiation therapy may be used to treat pain caused by bone metastasis.

Minimizing Anxiety

1. Realize that shock, disbelief, denial, anger, and depression are all normal reactions to the diagnosis of lung cancer.
2. Try to have the patient express concerns; share these concerns with health professionals. Link patient and family with cancer support groups.
3. Encourage the patient to communicate feelings to significant people in his or her life.
4. Expect some feelings of anxiety and depression to recur during illness.
5. Encourage the patient to keep active and remain in the mainstream. Continue with usual activities (work, recreation, sexual) as much as possible.
6. Antidepressants may be used to treat depression.

Patient Education and Health Maintenance

1. Teach patient to use NSAIDs or other prescribed medication, as necessary, for pain without being overly concerned about addiction.
2. Help the patient realize that not every ache and pain is caused by lung cancer; some patients do not experience pain.
3. Radiation therapy may be used for pain control if tumor has spread to bone, control of hemoptysis, bronchial obstruction, or brain metastasis.
4. Advise the patient to report new or persistent pain; it may be due to some other cause such as arthritis.
5. Suggest talking to a social worker about financial assistance or other services that may be needed.
6. For additional information, contact the American Cancer Society, 1-800-ACS-2345, *www.cancer.org*; National Comprehensive Cancer Network, *www.nccn.org*; Oncology Nurses Association, *www.ons.org*.
7. Possible referral to mental health professional.
8. Support patient and family to make decisions regarding long-term care, possibly pulmonary rehabilitation.

Evaluation: Expected Outcomes

- Performs self-care without dyspnea.
- Eats small meals four to five times per day; weight stable.
- Reports pain decreased from level 6 to level 2 or a level that patient reports as tolerable for completing activities of daily living (ADLs) when treated with medication.
- Verbalizes emotions and concerns associated with cancer diagnosis; practices relaxation techniques.

CHRONIC DISORDERS

Bronchiectasis

Bronchiectasis is a chronic inflammation and dilatation of the bronchi caused by immune defects, cystic fibrosis, aspiration and lung infections.

Pathophysiology and Etiology

1. May be a complication of respiratory infections including pneumonia, mycobacterium, and other organisms leading to damage to the bronchial wall, and buildup of thick sputum, causing obstruction.
2. Chronic coughing and excess mucus production, which is often purulent.
3. May involve a single lobe or segment or one or both lungs more diffusely.
4. As the condition progresses, there may be atelectasis and fibrosis, which lead to respiratory insufficiency.
5. Common causes include pulmonary infections (including pertussis, TB); obstruction of bronchi; aspiration of foreign bodies, vomitus, chemicals, or material from upper respiratory tract; cystic fibrosis; cilial dismotility syndrome; alpha$_1$-antitrypsin deficiency; and immunodeficiency.

Clinical Manifestations

1. Persistent cough with production of copious amounts of purulent sputum.
2. Intermittent hemoptysis; dyspnea.
3. Recurrent fever and bouts of pulmonary infection.
4. Crackles and rhonchi heard over involved lobes.
5. Finger clubbing.

Diagnostic Evaluation

1. High-resolution CT is necessary for diagnosis of bronchiectasis.
2. Chest x-ray may reveal areas of atelectasis with widespread dilation of bronchi.
3. Sputum examination may detect offending pathogens.
4. PFT to evaluate airflow obstruction and impairment.

Management

Goal is to prevent progression of disease.
1. Infection controlled by:
   a. Smoking cessation.
   b. Prompt antimicrobial treatment of exacerbations of infection.
   c. Immunization against potential pulmonary pathogens (influenza and pneumococcal vaccine).
2. Secretion clearance techniques may be helpful, such as postural drainage, devices that provide positive expiratory pressure and/or oscillations to lung walls including PEP valve, flutter valve, Acapella device, vest therapy, and, possibly, percussion and vibration or other methods.
3. Bronchodilators for bronchodilation and improved secretion clearance.
4. Mobilization and exercise such as in a pulmonary rehabilitation program.
5. Surgical resection (segmental resection) when conservative management fails.

Complications

1. Progressive excess mucus production or suppuration.
2. Hemoptysis, major pulmonary hemorrhage.
3. COPD, emphysema, chronic respiratory failure, pulmonary hypertension, cor pulmonale.

Nursing Assessment

1. Obtain history regarding amount and characteristics of sputum produced, including hemoptysis.
2. Auscultate lungs for diffuse rhonchi and crackles.

Nursing Diagnosis

- Ineffective Airway Clearance related to tenacious and copious secretions.

Nursing Interventions

Maintaining Airway Clearance

1. Encourage use of chest physical therapy techniques to empty the bronchi of accumulated secretions (see pages 230–238).
   a. Assist with postural drainage positioning for involved lung segments to drain the bronchiectatic areas by gravity, thus reducing degree of infection and symptoms. Contraindicated with increased intracranial pressure, uncontrolled hypertension, recent face or head surgery.
   b. Percussion and vibration may be used to assist in mobilizing secretions (use after bronchodilators and before meals). Contraindicated with osteoporosis, known rib or vertebral fractures.
   c. Encourage effective coughing to help clear secretions.
   d. Consider PEP valve, flutter valve, Acapella device, or Vest therapy for enhanced secretion clearance.
2. Encourage increased intake of fluids to reduce viscosity of sputum and make expectoration easier.
3. Consider vaporizer to provide humidification and keep secretions thin.

Patient Education and Health Maintenance

1. Instruct the patient to avoid noxious fumes, dust, smoke, and other pulmonary irritants.
2. Teach the patient to monitor sputum. Report if change in quantity or character occurs.
3. Instruct the patient and family about importance of pulmonary drainage.

a. Teach drainage exercises and chest physical therapy techniques.

b. Encourage postural drainage before rising in the morning because sputum accumulates during night.

c. Encourage patient to engage in physical activity throughout day to help mobilize mucus.

4. Encourage regular dental care because copious sputum production may affect dentition.

5. Emphasize the importance of influenza and pneumococcal immunizations and prompt evaluation of treatment of respiratory infections.

Evaluation: Expected Outcomes

• Decreased sputum and pulmonary infections; lungs clear after chest physical therapy.

Chronic Obstructive Pulmonary Disease

 Evidence Base Global Initiative for Chronic Obstructive Lung Disease (GOLD). (2011). Global strategy for the diagnosis, management and prevention of COPD. Available: *www.goldcopd.org.*

Chronic obstructive pulmonary disease (COPD) is a preventable and treatable disease with some significant extrapulmonary effects that may contribute to the severity in individual patients. It is characterized by airflow limitation that is not fully reversible. The airflow limitation is generally progressive and is normally associated with an inflammatory response of the lungs due to noxious particles or gases. COPD includes chronic bronchitis and emphysema. Asthma is not considered part of COPD due to its reversibility (see Chapter 28).

Chronic bronchitis is a chronic inflammation of the lower respiratory tract characterized by excessive mucus secretion, cough, and dyspnea associated with recurring infections of the lower respiratory tract.

Emphysema is a complex lung disease characterized by damage to the gas-exchanging surfaces of the lung (alveoli),

COPD is associated with changes in the proximal and peripheral airways and lung parenchyma and pulmonary vasculature. Changes include chronic inflammation and structural changes from repeated injury and repair.

Pathophysiology and Etiology

1. The person with COPD may have (see Figure 11-3) chronic cough and sputum progressing to airflow limitation and dyspnea, limiting daily activities. Dyspnea may become severe with loss of lung function as the disease progresses. Symptoms of complications such as respiratory failure, right heart failure, weight loss, and hypoxemia may develop. Patients may develop acute exacerbations associated with

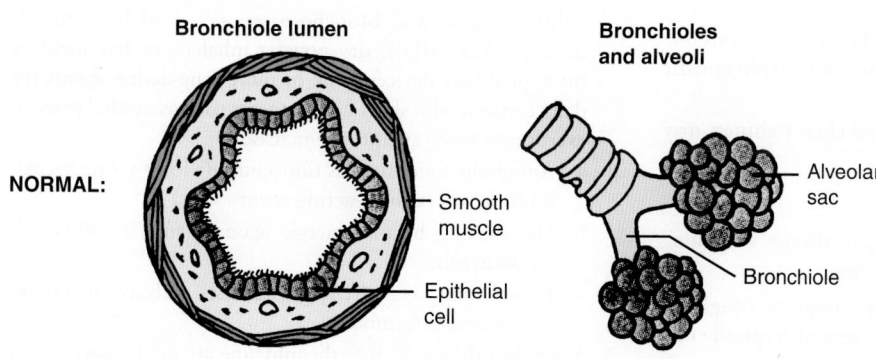

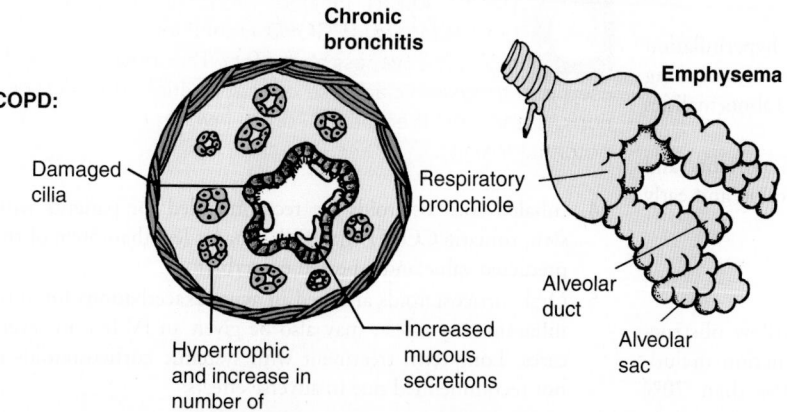

Figure 11-3. Airway changes in chronic obstructive pulmonary disease compared with normal.

worsening lung function and negative outcomes may develop.

2. Causes of COPD include:
   a. Cigarette smoking.
   b. Occupational exposure to dust from organic and inorganic substances.
   c. Indoor air pollution from heating and cooking with biomass (energy sources from organic material) in poorly ventilated areas.
   d. Infection including previous tuberculosis.
   e. Genetic predisposition, aging.

3. Alpha$_1$-antitrypsin deficiency is a genetically determined cause of emphysema and liver disease. Alpha$_1$-antitrypsin is the most common protease inhibitor in the blood and inhibits neutrophil elastase, an elastin and basement membrane-degrading protease released by neutrophils. When alveolar structures are left unprotected from exposure to elastase, progressive destruction of elastin tissues results in the development of emphysema.

Clinical Manifestations

Chronic Bronchitis and Emphysema
Usually insidious, gradual in onset, and steadily progressive.

1. Dyspnea (particularly with stairs or inclines), decreased exercise tolerance.
2. Cough, which may be productive. Purulent sputum that is a change from baseline may suggest development of an exacerbation.
3. Increased anteroposterior diameter of chest (barrel chest) due to air trapping, causing hyperinflation and diaphragmatic flattening.
4. Wheezing, decreased breath sounds, and chest tightness may be present.

Exacerbation of COPD
Episodic and often recurrent, contributing to disease worsening due to increased inflammatory airway response.

1. Acute change in the patient's baseline dyspnea, cough, or sputum, which requires a change in treatment (typically oral steroids and/or antibiotics).
2. Triggers may include viral and/or bacterial infection or environmental pollutants. One third of exacerbations have no identifiable cause.
3. Exacerbations are associated with increased hyperinflation and air trapping with decreased expiratory flow contributing to worsening dyspnea as well as worsening V/Q abnormalities leading to hypoxemia.
4. Because exacerbations have increased risk of mortality and morbidity and decreased quality of life, prevention and early detection and management are important.

Diagnostic Evaluation

1. PFTs are necessary to diagnose COPD. Airflow obstruction based on spirometry or pulmonary function including a postbronchodilator FEV$_1$/FVC of less than 70%

predicted. FEV$_1$ percent predicted is used to stage severity of COPD.
   a. Stage I (mild)—FEV$_1$/FVC < 0.7; FEV$_1$ ≥ 80% predicted.
   b. Stage II (moderate)—FEV$_1$/FVC < 0.7; FEV$_1$ 50% to 80% predicted.
   c. Stage III (severe)—FEV$_1$/FVC < 0.7; FEV$_1$ 30% to 50% predicted.
   d. Stage IV (very severe)—FEV$_1$/FVC < 0.7; FEV$_1$ < 30% predicted or FEV$_1$ > 50% predicted plus chronic respiratory failure.

2. ABG or oximetry can be used to detect hypoxemia (SaO$_2$ or SpO$_2$ < 92%). ABG can additionally detect respiratory failure (PaO$_2$ < 60 mm Hg with or without PCO$_2$ > 50 mm Hg on room air).

3. Chest x-ray—in late stages, hyperinflation, flattened diaphragm, increased retrosternal space, decreased vascular markings, possible bullae.

4. Alpha$_1$-antitrypsin assay useful in identifying genetically determined deficiency in emphysema.

Management
The goals of COPD management are to relieve symptoms, prevent disease progression, reduce mortality, improve exercise tolerance, improve health status, and prevent and treat complications and exacerbations. Goals of acute care include improving airflow obstruction. Treatment regimens are based on severity.

1. Smoking cessation is essential to reduce disease progression and improve survival.
2. Inhaled bronchodilators (see Table 11-4, pages 308 to 312) reduce dyspnea and bronchospasm; delivered by metered-dose inhalers (MDI), dry powder inhalers, or handheld or mask nebulizer devices. One or more long-acting agents for daily control, with short-acting agents used as needed prior to exertion or when symptoms increase.
   a. Anticholinergics such as tiotropium (a long-acting agent), ipratropium (a short-acting agent).
   b. Short-acting beta-adrenergic agonists such as albuterol, levalbuterols.
   c. Long-acting beta-adrenergic agonists such as salmeterol, formoterol, arformoterol.
3. Methylxanthines, such as theophylline are rarely used due to suboptimal effectiveness, side effects, and drug interactions.

 DRUG ALERT Inhaled bronchodilators are the gold standard of COPD management because of their effectiveness and safety. Theophylline is rarely used due to systemic adverse effects, multiple drug interactions, need for therapeutic drug level monitoring, and potential toxicity.

4. Inhaled corticosteroids are recommended for patients with symptomatic COPD with FEV$_1$ that is less than 50% of the predicted value and repeated exacerbations.
5. Oral corticosteroids are used in acute exacerbations for anti-inflammatory effect; may also be given an IV line in severe cases. Long-term treatment with systemic corticosteroids is not recommended due to adverse effects.

DRUG ALERT High-dose or long-term prednisone therapy is associated with significant side effects including hypertension, edema, increased intraocular pressure, hyperglycemia, depression, insomnia, gastric and esophageal ulcer, osteoporosis, and impaired wound healing. Teach patient side effects and strategies to minimize including working with medical team to taper dose as appropriate, take medication in the morning to limit insomnia, protect skin with thick fabric to reduce bruising and skin breakage. For increased appetite and weight gain, encourage eating a healthy, balanced, low-salt diet with small portions every 5 hours.

6. For retained secretions, mobilizing the patient, and for some, use of chest physical therapy, including postural drainage for secretion clearance and breathing retraining, may be used for improved ventilation and control of dyspnea.
7. Supplemental oxygen therapy for patients with hypoxemia. CO_2 must be monitored to determine increased CO_2 retention.
8. Pulmonary rehabilitation to improve function, strength, symptom control, disease self-management techniques, independence, and quality of life; and reduce health care utilization.
   a. Studies on pulmonary rehabilitation demonstrate increased strength, function, independence, ADL management, and improved symptom control, coping, well-being, and quality of life as well as decreased facility admissions and decreased length of stay.
   b. Improved survival in COPD is associated with supplemental O_2 use and smoking cessation.
9. Antimicrobial agents for episodes of respiratory infection.
10. Lung volume reduction surgery is a potential option for treatment of upper lobe emphysema in patients with poor exercise capacity.
11. Influenza (annual) and pneumococcal vaccination.
12. Lung transplantation may be considered for people with advanced COPD.
13. Self-management strategies such as prevention and management of exacerbations. Disease self-management strategies include use of action plans, frequent hand hygiene, and regular medical follow-up.
14. Treatment for alpha$_1$-antitrypsin deficiency:
    a. Regular IV infusions (normally every week) of human alpha$_1$-antitrypsin as replacement therapy to correct the antiprotease imbalance in the lungs.
    b. Smoking cessation.
    c. Lung transplantation may be considered.

Complications

1. Respiratory failure.
2. Pneumonia, overwhelming respiratory infection.
3. Right-sided heart failure, pulmonary hypertension, dysrhythmias.
4. Depression, anxiety disorder.
5. Skeletal muscle dysfunction.

Nursing Assessment

1. Determine smoking pack per year history, exposure history, positive family history of respiratory disease, onset and triggers of dyspnea.
2. Determine level of dyspnea, how it compares to patient's baseline.
3. Note amount, color, and consistency of sputum.
4. Inspect for use of accessory muscles during respiration and use of abdominal muscles during expiration; note increase of anteroposterior diameter of chest.
5. Auscultate for decreased/absent breath sounds, crackles, decreased heart sounds.
6. Determine oxygen saturation, pulse, and respiratory rate at rest and with activity.

Nursing Diagnoses

- Ineffective Breathing Pattern related to chronic airflow limitation.
- Ineffective Airway Clearance related to bronchoconstriction, increased mucus production, ineffective cough, possible bronchopulmonary infection.
- Risk for Infection related to compromised pulmonary function, retained secretions, and compromised defense mechanisms.
- Impaired Gas Exchange related to chronic pulmonary obstruction, V/Q abnormalities due to destruction of alveolar capillary membrane.
- Imbalanced Nutrition: Less Than Body Requirements related to increased work of breathing, air swallowing, drug effects with resultant wasting of respiratory and skeletal muscles.
- Activity Intolerance related to compromised pulmonary function, resulting in shortness of breath and fatigue, skeletal muscle dysfunction.
- Disturbed Sleep Pattern related to hypoxemia and hypercapnia, dyspnea, cough, and wheezing.
- Ineffective Coping related to the stress of living with chronic disease, loss of independence, depression, anxiety disorder, panic of breathlessness.

 NURSING ALERT Early in the patient's course, issues of a living will, advance directive, and resuscitation status need to be addressed. It is better to have these discussions with the patient before crisis situations.

Nursing Interventions

Improving Airway Clearance

1. Eliminate pulmonary irritants, particularly cigarette smoking.
   a. Cessation of smoking usually results in less pulmonary irritation, sputum production, and cough, slows progression of COPD, and improves survival.
   b. Keep patient's room as free from pulmonary irritants as possible.
2. Administer bronchodilators to improve dyspnea, reduce hyperinflation at rest and with activity, control bronchospasm and dyspnea, and assist with raising sputum.

(Text continues on page 312)

Table 11-4   COMMONLY USED PULMONARY DRUGS

DRUGS/ADMINISTRATION	PHARMACOLOGIC EFFECTS	INDICATIONS
Bronchodilators		
Albuterol (metered-dose inhaler [MDI], nebulized solution, oral)	• Short-acting sympathomimetic (beta$_2$-adrenergic agonist) with highly selective beta$_2$ activity	• MDI, nebulized liquid: rapid relief of bronchospasm, acute exacerbation—works within 3 to 5 minutes • *Oral:* Maintenance therapy for bronchospasm, works within 30 minutes
Pirbuterol acetate (MDI)	• Short-acting sympathomimetic with selective beta$_2$ activity	• Treatment of bronchospasm
Levalbuterol (HFA and nebulized solution)	• Short-acting sympathomimetic with selective beta$_2$ activity	• Treatment and prevention of bronchospasm
Salmeterol xinafoate (dry powder inhaler [DPI])	• Selectively stimulates beta-2 adrenergic receptors, relaxing airway smooth muscle; long-acting	• Maintenance therapy for asthma, COPD, bronchospasm, exercise-induced bronchospasm; long-acting (12 hours)
Formoterol (DPI)	• Selectively stimulates beta-2 adrenergic receptors, relaxing airway smooth muscle; long-acting	• Treatment and prevention of bronchospasm; long-acting
Indacaterol (DPI)	• Selectively stimulates beta-2 adrenergic receptors, relaxing airway smooth muscle; long-acting	• Treatment and prevention of bronchospasm; long-acting
Arformoterol (nebulized solution)	• Selectively stimulates beta-2 adrenergic receptors, relaxing airway smooth muscle.	• Maintenance therapy for COPD; long-acting
Ipratropium bromide (MDI, nebulized liquid)	• Anticholinergic	• Maintenance therapy for COPD, asthma, bronchospasm • Acts within 15 minutes
Tiotropium (DPI)	• Long-acting anticholinergic	• Maintenance therapy for COPD
Aminophylline (IV injection)	• Methylxanthine compound—relaxes smooth muscle by increasing level of cyclic adenosine monophosphate	• Acute exacerbation of asthma or bronchitis
Theophylline preparations (oral)	• Methylxanthine compound—relaxes muscle by increasing cyclic adenosine monophosphate	• Mild bronchodilator, maintenance therapy for bronchospasm, asthma, COPD maintenance
Albuterol + ipratropium combination (MDI nebulized solution)	• Sympathomimetic with selective beta$_2$ and anticholinergic activity	• Fast-acting and maintenance therapy for bronchospasm; exacerbation of COPD

ADVERSE EFFECTS	NURSING CONSIDERATIONS
• Throat irritation, URI symptoms, cough, tremor, dizziness, nervousness, tachycardia, headache, nausea, tremors • Continuous nebulization may cause hypokalemia	• Observe inhalation by patient to be certain that correct technique is used. • Caution patient not to exceed prescribed dose. Adverse effects often associated with excessive use. Does not reduce inflammation. • HFA MDIs must be primed for four puffs before initial use and after not using for long periods. Rinse MDI holder well to avoid blockage.
• Tremor, nervousness, tachycardia, headache, nausea, vomiting, diarrhea	• Observe inhalation by patient to make sure that correct technique is used.
• Tachycardia, hypertension, nervousness	• Administered by nebulization every 6–8 hours
• Headache, throat irritation, nasal congestion, rhinitis, palpitations, tachycardia, tremor, hypertension, bronchospasm • Possible increased risk of asthma-related deaths	• Observe inhalation by patient to make sure that correct technique is used. • Instruct patient that not for immediate relief of bronchospasm, dyspnea. • Maximum dose two puffs every 12 hours
• URI, dyspepsia, chest pain, back pain, fever, diarrhea, nausea, vomiting, dry mouth, dizziness, insomnia, nervousness, tremor, palpitations, bronchospasm; possible increased risk of asthma-related deaths	• Train patient for proper use of aerolizer. • Instruct patient that not for immediate relief of bronchospasm, dyspnea. • Administer twice daily or 15 minutes before exercise.
• Cough, throat irritation, headache, tremor, palpitations	• Once daily dosing.
• Pain, chest pain, back pain, diarrhea, sinusitis, leg cramps, dyspnea, rash, flu-like symptoms, bronchospasm • Possible increased risk of asthma-related deaths	• Not indicated for acute bronchospasm.
• Bronchitis, dyspnea, URI, cough, COPD exacerbation, nausea, dry mouth, flu-like symptoms. Rare: Can cause blurring of vision if sprayed into the eyes (atropine derivative) • Voice hoarseness	• Instruct patient to use spacer device with MDI or close lips around inhaler mouthpiece; close eyes during inhalation.
• Dry mouth, pharyngitis, constipation, increased heart rate, blurred vision, urinary retention, URI symptoms, chest pain, UTI, dyspepsia, rhinitis, abdominal pain, angioedema	• Not indicated for acute bronchospasm. • Eye discomfort and visual changes may indicate acute glaucoma.
• CNS: irritability, restlessness, insomnia • CV: palpitations, tachycardia, hypotension • GI: nausea, vomiting, diarrhea	• Too rapid administration can cause hypotension, extra systoles, muscle tremors. Administer at prescribed rate with an IV infusion pump.
• CNS: irritability, restlessness, insomnia, seizures in toxic ranges • CV: palpitations, tachycardia, hypotension • GI: nausea, vomiting, diarrhea	• Teach patients to take at equal intervals throughout the day. • To decrease GI irritation, take with milk or crackers. • Monitor theophylline blood level periodically as directed to ensure therapeutic range and prevent toxicity. • Be alert for drug interactions.
• See albuterol and ipratropium	• See albuterol and ipratropium. • One puff of Combivent equals one puff of albuterol and one puff of ipratropium.

(continued)

Table 11-4   COMMONLY USED PULMONARY DRUGS (*continued*)

DRUGS/ADMINISTRATION	PHARMACOLOGIC EFFECTS	INDICATIONS
Corticosteroids		
Hydrocortisone/prednisone (IV injection, oral preparation)	• Potent anti-inflammatory activity	• Acute exacerbation of asthma or bronchitis (IV preparation) • Acute exacerbation (oral preparation) of asthma or COPD.
Beclomethasone (MDI)	• Synthetic corticosteroid with potent anti-inflammatory activity; effective only by inhalation • Not effective in acute attack; must be used for 2–4 weeks to show effectiveness	• Asthma • Severe COPD with frequent exacerbations
Mometasone (DPI)	• Anti-inflammatory steroid; effective only by inhalation • Not effective in acute attack; must be used for up to 2–4 weeks to show effectiveness	• Asthma maintenance • COPD (severe COPD with frequent exacerbations)
Ciclesonide (MDI)	• Anti-inflammatory steroid; effective only by inhalation • Not effective in acute attack; must be used for up to 2–4 weeks to show effectiveness	• Asthma maintenance
Fluticasone (MDI, DPI)	• Anti-inflammatory steroid; effective only by inhalation • Not effective in acute attack; must be used for 2–4 weeks to show effectiveness	• Asthma • COPD (severe COPD with frequent exacerbations)
Budesonide (DPI)	• Anti-inflammatory steroid; effective only by inhalation • Not effective in acute attack; must be used for 2–4 weeks to show effectiveness	• Asthma • COPD (severe COPD with frequent exacerbations)
Fluticasone and salmeterol (MDI, DPI)	• Combination inhaled corticosteroid and long-acting beta-agonist bronchodilator	• Asthma maintenance • COPD maintenance • Maintenance therapy for controlled bronchospasm
Budesonide and formoterol (MDI) Mometasone and formoterol (MDI)	• Combination inhaled corticosteroid and long-acting beta agonist • Combination inhaled corticosteroid and long-acting beta agonist	• Asthma maintenance • COPD maintenance
Mast Cell Stabilizers		
Cromolyn (solution for inhalation, powder used with special inhaler)	• Inhibits activation of a variety of inflammatory cells associated with asthma, prevents bronchospasm • Not effective in acute attack; must be used for 2–4 weeks to show effectiveness	• Maintenance therapy for asthma

ADVERSE EFFECTS	NURSING CONSIDERATIONS
• CNS: depression, euphoria, mood changes, insomnia • GI: gastric irritation, peptic ulcer • Metabolic: hypernatremia, hypokalemia, hyperglycemia, water retention, and weight gain • Long-term, high dose: adrenal insufficiency, osteoporosis, muscle weakness, cataracts, glaucoma, fragile and easily bruised skin, immunosuppression	• Long-term use: Do not stop abruptly due to adrenal suppression. • Take oral form with food. • Usually given as taper from higher dose to lowest possible dose that achieves desired effect. Long-term use should be avoided if possible. • Advise patient of possible increased appetite and weight gain risk; advise to eat small, frequent meals high in protein, fruits and vegetables, and low in simple carbohydrates
• Oral candidiasis, dysphonia, cough, pharyngitis, bronchospasm, headache, sinusitis, URI, rhinitis, pain, back pain, bronchospasm • Risk for cataract, glaucoma, osteoporosis • May experience skin bruising in high doses	• Inhaled as aerosol. May precipitate bronchospasm in acute exacerbation. Not used with status asthmaticus or acute asthma episodes. • Use a spacer device with MDI; use water gargle, rinse, and spit after use to prevent oral candidiasis.
• Oral candidiasis, dysphonia • Risk for systemic adverse effects associated with oral steroids is low • May experience skin bruising in high doses • Headache, rhinitis, URI, sinusitis, bronchospasm	• Use water gargle, rinse, and spit after use to prevent oral yeast growth.
• Oral candidiasis, dysphonia • Risk for systemic adverse effects associated with oral steroids is low • May experience skin bruising in high doses • Headache, rhinitis, URI, sinusitis, bronchospasm	• Use water gargle, rinse, and spit after use to prevent oral yeast growth; avoid eyes.
• Oral candidiasis, dysphonia • Risk for systemic adverse effects associated with oral steroids is low • May experience skin bruising in high doses • URI, headache, sinusitis, bronchospasm	• Longer acting. • Use a spacer device with MDI; use water gargle, rinse, and spit after use to prevent oral candidiasis.
• Oral candidiasis • Risk for systemic adverse effects associated with oral steroids is low • May experience skin bruising in high doses • Nasopharyngitis, rhinitis, nausea, bronchospasm	• Longer acting. • Use water gargle, rinse, and spit after use to prevent oral candidiasis.
• Oral candidiasis, dysphonia, possible bruising in high doses • URI, headache, cough, sinusitis, nausea, vomiting, bronchospasm • Increased risk of asthma-related deaths	• Long-acting. • Use once or twice daily. • Use water gargle, rinse, and spit after use to prevent candidiasis.
• See budesonide and formoterol • See mometasone and formoterol	• See budesonide and formoterol
• Cough, bronchospasm	• Should not be used with status asthmaticus or acute asthma episodes. May be given in combination with bronchodilator if administration causes bronchospasm.

(continued)

Table 11-4 COMMONLY USED PULMONARY DRUGS (continued)

DRUGS/ADMINISTRATION	PHARMACOLOGIC EFFECTS	INDICATIONS
Nedocromil (MDI)	• Inhibits activation of a variety of inflammatory cells associated with asthma, prevents bronchospasm • Not effective in acute attack; must be used for 2–4 weeks to show effectiveness	• Maintenance therapy for asthma
Leukotriene Receptor Antagonists Zafirlukast	• Blocks leukotriene receptors	• Prophylaxis and chronic treatment of mild to moderate asthma for persons older than age 4
Zileuton	• Blocks leukotriene receptors	• Prophylaxis and chronic treatment of mild to moderate asthma for persons older than age 12
Montelukast	• Blocks leukotriene receptors	• Prophylaxis and chronic treatment of mild to moderate asthma for persons older than age 5 • Exercise-induced bronchospasm
Roflumilast	• Inhibits phosphodiesterase type 4 leading to increased intracellular cAMP	• Chronic bronchitis and frequent exacerbations
Omalizumab	• Inhibits IgE binding to mast cells and basophils, decreasing mediator release	• Asthma prophylaxis, aeroallergen associated

a. Train and monitor patient's inhaler technique.
b. Assess for adverse effects—tremulousness, tachycardia, cardiac dysrhythmias, CNS stimulation, hypertension.
c. Auscultate the chest after administration of aerosol bronchodilators to assess for improvement of aeration and reduction of adventitious breath sounds.
d. Observe if patient has reduction in dyspnea.
e. Monitor serum theophylline level, as ordered, to ensure therapeutic level and prevent toxicity.
3. Use controlled coughing (see page 234).
4. Mobilize the patient when stable. Use postural drainage positions to aid in clearance of secretions, if mucopurulent secretions are responsible for airway obstruction (see page 235).
5. Keep secretions thin.
a. Encourage fluid intake within level of cardiac reserve.
b. If appropriate, give continuous aerolized sterile water or nebulized normal saline to humidify bronchial tree and liquefy sputum.

Improving Breathing Pattern

1. Teach and supervise breathing retraining exercises to improve dyspnea and decrease work of breathing (see page 230).
a. Teach diaphragmatic, lower costal, and abdominal breathing, using a slow and relaxed breathing pattern to reduce respiratory rate and decrease energy cost of breathing.
b. Use pursed-lip breathing at intervals and during periods of dyspnea to reduce hyperinflation, control rate and depth of respiration, and improve respiratory muscle coordination. Pursed-lip and diaphragmatic breathing should be practiced for 10 breaths four times daily before meals and before sleep. Inspiratory to expiratory ratio should be 1: ≥2.
2. Discuss and demonstrate relaxation exercises to reduce stress, tension, and anxiety.
3. Encourage patient to assume position of comfort to decrease dyspnea. Positions might include leaning trunk forward with arms supported on a fixed object, sleeping with two or three pillows, or sitting upright.

Controlling Infection

1. Recognize early manifestations of respiratory infection—increased dyspnea, fatigue; change in color, amount, and character of sputum including purulence; anxiety, irritability; low-grade fever.
2. Obtain sputum for Gram stain and culture and sensitivity.
3. Administer prescribed antimicrobials to control bacterial infections in the bronchial tree, thus clearing the airways. Administer bronchodilators to improve ventilation.

Improving Gas Exchange

1. Monitor for hypoxemia with a typical goal of SaO_2 or SpO_2 of 92% to 93%. Watch for and report excessive somnolence, restlessness, aggressiveness, anxiety, headaches, or confusion; central cyanosis; and shortness of breath at rest, which is commonly caused by acute respiratory insufficiency and may signal respiratory failure.
2. Review ABG levels; record values on a flow sheet so comparisons can be made over time.
3. Give supplemental oxygen, as ordered, to correct hypoxemia in a controlled manner. Monitor and minimize CO_2 retention. Patients that experience CO_2 retention may need lower oxygen flow rates.

ADVERSE EFFECTS	NURSING CONSIDERATIONS
• Cough, bronchospasm • GI: nausea, vomiting	• Should not be used with status asthmaticus or acute asthma episodes. May be given in combination with bronchodilator if administration causes bronchospasm.
• Potential drug interactions, particularly warfarin, cisapride • Headache, infection, nausea, diarrhea	• Will not reverse acute bronchospasm.
• Potential drug interactions • Headache, sinusitis, nausea	• Will not reverse acute bronchospasm.
• Potential drug interactions, particularly phenobarbital, amiodarone • Headache, flu, abdominal pain	• Will not reverse acute bronchospasm.
• Diarrhea, weight loss, nausea, headache, suicidality	
• Injection site reaction, viral infection, URI, sinusitis, anaphylaxis	

! NURSING ALERT Normally, CO_2 levels in the blood provide a stimulus for respiration. However, in some patients with COPD, chronically elevated CO_2 may impair this mechanism and low oxygen levels act as stimulus for respiration. Giving a high concentration of supplemental oxygen to people who retain CO_2 may suppress the hypoxic drive, leading to worsening hypoventilation, respiratory decompensation, and the development of a worsening respiratory acidosis.

4. Be prepared to assist with noninvasive ventilation *or* intubation and mechanical ventilation if acute respiratory failure and significant CO_2 retention occur.

Improving Nutrition
1. Take nutritional history, weight, and height. Patients are at risk for cachexia and obesity due to poor nutritional intake and inactivity.
2. Encourage frequent, small meals if patient is dyspneic and/or underweight; even a small increase in abdominal contents may press on diaphragm and impede breathing. Encourage snacking on nutritious, calorie-appropriate, and high-protein snacks, such as cheese or nuts.
3. Offer liquid nutritional supplements, if needed, to improve nutrient intake and provide appropriate calorie intake.
4. Encourage foods high in potassium (including bananas, dried fruits, dates, figs, orange juice, grape juice, milk, peaches, potatoes, tomatoes) and monitor for low potassium, which may occur with CODP, corticosteroid use, and diuretic use.
5. Restrict sodium, as directed, if fluid retention is a problem.
6. Limit carbohydrates if CO_2 is retained by patient; high-carbohydrate diet may increase CO_2.
7. Avoid foods producing gas and abdominal discomfort.
8. Employ good oral hygiene before meals to sharpen taste sensations.
9. Encourage pursed-lip breathing between bites if patient is short of breath; rest after meals.
10. Give supplemental oxygen while patient is eating to relieve dyspnea as directed.
11. Monitor body weight and evaluate body mass index.

Increasing Activity Tolerance
1. Reemphasize the importance of graded exercise and physical conditioning programs (may enhance delivery of oxygen to tissues; allows a higher level of functioning and independence with greater comfort). This may be part of a pulmonary rehabilitation program or a referral to physical therapy.
   a. Discuss walking, stationary bicycling, swimming.
   b. Encourage use of portable lightweight oxygen system for ambulation for patients with hypoxemia.
2. Encourage patient to carry out regular exercise program 3 to 7 days per week to increase physical endurance, but to discuss with physician before beginning program.
3. Train patient in energy-conservation techniques and pacing of activities.

Improving Sleep Patterns
1. Maintain a balanced schedule of activity and rest.
2. Use nocturnal oxygen therapy, when appropriate.
3. Avoid use of sedatives and hypnotics that may cause respiratory depression.
4. Administer long- or short-acting inhaled anticholinergics, as directed (have been found to improve nocturnal respiratory symptoms in COPD).

Enhancing Coping

1. Recognize signs of depression and anxiety disorders, which are common and often undiagnosed and untreated in COPD. Constant shortness of breath and fatigue and loss of independence, personal identity, and quality of life may make the patient irritable, apprehensive, anxious, and depressed, with feelings of helplessness and hopelessness.

2. Assess the patient for suicide thoughts or planning and get immediate psychiatric intervention, if needed.

3. Demonstrate a positive, supportive, and interested approach to the patient.
   a. Be a good listener and show that you care.
   b. Be sensitive to patient's fears, anxiety, and depression; provide emotional support.
   c. Provide patient with control of as many aspects of care as possible.

4. Administer antidepressants and anti-anxiety agents as directed, but avoid sedation.

5. Allow the patient to express feelings. Be aware that (within a controlled degree) the mechanisms of denial and repression may be useful defense mechanisms.

6. Be aware that dyspnea, fatigue, and altered self-image may lead to discomfort with sexuality and intimacy in patients with COPD. Encourage discussion of concerns and fears and clarify misunderstandings. Encourage patient to use a bronchodilator and secretion-clearance techniques before sexual activity, plan for sexual relations at time of day when patient has highest level of energy, use supplemental oxygen, if needed, and consider alternative displays of affection to loved one.

7. Support patient and spouse/family members. Refer to local or national support groups (American Lung Association: 1-800-LUNG-USA, *www.lungusa.org*).

Community and Home Care Considerations

1. Help to relax and work at a slower pace. Obtain occupational therapy consult to help employ work simplification techniques, such as sitting for tasks, pacing activities, using dressing aids (grabber, sock aid, long-handled shoe horn), shower bench, and handheld shower head.

2. Encourage enrollment in a pulmonary rehabilitation program where available and Better Breathers club or other support group found through the American Association for Cardiovascular and Pulmonary Rehabilitation at (312) 321-5146 or *www.aacvpr.org*. Components include breathing retraining techniques, proper use of medications and inhalers, secretion-clearance techniques, prevention and management of respiratory infection, panic control, controlling dyspnea with ADLs and stair climbing, control of pulmonary irritants, monitored and supervised exercise, proper use of oxygen systems, and group support.

3. Suggest vocational counseling to help patient maintain gainful employment within physical limits for as long as possible.

4. Warn patient to avoid excessive fatigue, which is a factor in producing respiratory distress. Advise to adjust activities per individual fatigue patterns.

5. Advise in strategies and mechanisms to cope with emotional stress. Such stress triggers attacks of dyspnea. Teach coping strategies, such as relaxation techniques, meditation, and guided imagery.

7. Stress that progression of worsening lung function may be slowed through smoking cessation and prevention of exacerbations. Long-term ongoing medical follow-up is a key aspect of disease self-management.

8. For patients who use oxygen or who are hypoxic, coordinate with oxygen supplier and patient to promote safe adherence to oxygen prescription and use of appropriate oxygen system so patient can maintain activities.

9. Use community resources, such as Meals On Wheels or a home care aide, if energy level is low.

Patient Education and Health Maintenance

General Education

1. Give the patient a clear explanation of the disease, what to expect, and how to treat and live with it. Reinforce by frequent explanations, reading material, demonstrations, and question-and-answer sessions (see Patient Education Guidelines 11-1).

2. Review with the patient the objectives of treatment and nursing management.

3. Work with the patient to set goals (eg, stair climbing, return to work).

4. Encourage patient involvement in disease self-management techniques, such as identification and prompt reporting of respiratory infection or respiratory deterioration. Encourage patient to have open communication and partnership and regular follow-up with primary care provider.

Avoid Exposure to Respiratory Irritants

1. Advise patient to stop smoking and avoid exposure to secondhand smoke. Offer strategies to promote long-term cessation including use of medications, support groups, and counseling.

2. Advise patient to avoid exposure to indoor and outdoor pulmonary irritants and particulates, including dust, smog, and other respiratory irritants.

3. Advise patient to keep entire house well ventilated.

4. Warn patient to stay out of extremely hot/cold weather if exposure causes bronchospasm and dyspnea. Use a scarf over nose and mouth and drink warm beverages in cold weather.

5. Stay indoors and exercise indoors with air conditioning when air pollution level is high.

6. Shower with warm (*not hot*) water to avoid excess exposure to steam.

7. If sensitive to dry air, instruct patient to humidify indoor air in winter; maintain 30% to 50% humidity for optimal mucociliary function.

8. If the patient is sensitive to dust, pollen, and other particles, consider use of a HEPA air cleaner to remove particles from air.

Improve Airflow

1. Teach the proper technique for inhalation of medication to maximize aerosol deposition in the bronchial tree. See page 1040 for patient education on inhaler use.
   a. Use spacer device if unable to use MDI effectively.
   b. If using a dried powder inhaler, instruct in proper use according to manufacturer's instructions. Spacer devices are not necessary.

2. MDIs with HFA propellants require priming (spray four puffs of medication before first use and if not used for several

PATIENT EDUCATION GUIDELINES 11-1

Chronic Obstructive Pulmonary Disease

There are two types of chronic obstructive pulmonary disease (COPD), chronic bronchitis and emphysema, which may occur together or separately. Chronic bronchitis is diagnosed when there is a chronic cough with phlegm (sputum) for at least 3 months over a period of 2 years. With emphysema, there is a loss of elasticity of the lung tissue, leading to trapped air. Both result in inflammation of the airways, trapping air in the lung. Smoking is the leading cause.

CONTROLLING SYMPTOMS

Cough and phlegm

- Use inhalers on a regular basis as prescribed:
  - Short-acting bronchodilators, such as albuterol, albuterol with ipratropium combination, levalbuteral to open up the airways and improve shortness of breath.
  - Long-acting bronchodilators (tiotropium, salmeterol, fluticasone and salmeterol, formoterol, mometasone and formoterol, etc.) have the strongest benefit to control COPD.
  - Corticosteroids to reduce swelling inside airways (inflammation) and shortness of breath.
- Avoid irritants to the lungs, such as cigarette smoke, dust, smog, strong odors, and other irritants.
- Report worsening breathlessness and/or change in color, amount, or thickness of phlegm that could indicate an infection.
- Try to avoid respiratory infections by regular hand hygiene, limiting contact with people during cold and flu season. Get the pneumonia vaccine, as indicated, and yearly influenza vaccine and wash hands frequently.
- Drink water (8–10 glasses per day or as directed by your health care provider) to keep phlegm thin.

Shortness of breath

- Practice "pursed-lip breathing" by breathing in through the nose for a count of two and out through pursed lips (like you are whistling), with a long, slow expiration for a count of four.
- Position yourself for better breathing by leaning forward while sitting with elbows on table or resting on knees.
- Use relaxation techniques, such as listening to soft music, imagining you are in a quiet, peaceful place, or having someone give you a massage.
- If prescribed, use oxygen, as directed, especially while performing such activities as bathing, dressing, eating, and walking.

Fatigue

- Do not stop doing physical activity; instead, learn how to manage by planning activities to conserve energy.
- Start with an exercise program that is easy and progress slowly to increase your activity.
- Talk to your health care provider about joining a pulmonary rehabilitation program.
- Eat a well-balanced, nutritious diet. Consider small, frequent meals.
- Sleep with head elevated using several pillows or in a reclining chair to reduce shortness of breath and increase rest.
- If awakened by cough, sit up, sip fluid, and use inhaler to try to clear lungs of phlegm.
- Avoid overuse of short-acting bronchodilators. Discuss poor control of breathlessness with your health care provider.

Poor appetite

- Compensate by eating six or more small meals and snacks per day rather than two or three large meals.
- Eat slowly; plan at least 30 minutes per meal.
- Unless otherwise directed, try a high-protein, moderate-fat, lower-carbohydrate diet of sufficient calories to cover the increased work of breathing.
- Consider a high-calorie, high-protein drink if you do not feel like eating and are underweight.

---

days). Rinse plastic cartridge holder well daily and air dry to prevent blockage.

3. Instruct patient in proper sequence of medications, using bronchodilator first, followed by inhaled corticosteroid.

 DRUG ALERT To prevent oral candidiasis, instruct patient to use a spacer device and rinse and spit after using inhaled corticosteroid.

4. To determine how long (how many days) MDI will last, divide puffs used per day into total puffs in inhaler. If used as needed, keep track of puffs used. Write down date MDI will run out on canister and/or calendar.

Evaluation: Expected Outcomes

- Coughs up secretions easily; decreased wheezing and crackles.
- Reports less dyspnea; effectively using pursed-lip breathing.
- No fever or change in sputum.
- ABG levels and/or SpO_2 improved.
- Tolerates small, frequent meals; weight stable.
- Reports walking longer distances without tiring.
- Sleeping in 4- to 6-hour intervals; uses low-flow oxygen at night as prescribed.
- Demonstrates more effective coping; expresses feelings; seeks support group.

Cor Pulmonale

Pulmonary heart disease (cor pulmonale) is typically due to right heart strain caused by excessively high pressures in pulmonary circulation. This alteration in the structure or function of the right ventricle results from disease of lung structure or function or its vasculature, such as pulmonary hypertension (except when this alteration results from disease of the left side of the heart or from congenital heart disease). It is heart disease caused by lung disease.

Pathophysiology and Etiology

1. Cor pulmonale is often chronic (associated with right ventricular hypertrophy), but may develop acutely due to pulmonary embolism and less commonly, acute respiratory distress syndrome (ARDS) associated with right ventricular dilatation.
2. Pulmonary hypertension and subsequent cor pulmonale may develop due to pulmonary vasoconstriction due to alveolar hypoxia or blood acidemia, anatomic compromise of the pulmonary vascular bed.
3. Causes include:
   a. Pulmonary vascular disease (acute or chronic).
   b. Idiopathic pulmonary hypertension.
   c. Underlying lung disease such as COPD, cystic fibrosis, interstitial lung disease.
   d. Polycythemia vera, sickle cell disease, macroglobulinemia.
   e. Significant kyphoscoliosis.
   f. Obstructive sleep apnea.

Clinical Manifestations

1. Fatigue; tachypnea, exertional dyspnea cough.
2. Anterior chest pain, hemoptysis.
3. Distended jugular veins, peripheral edema (often associated with hypercapnia), possible cyanosis. In advanced stages, right upper abdominal discomfort, jaundice, and syncope with exertion.
4. Split-second heart sound on auscultation of chest.

Diagnostic Evaluation

1. Chest x-ray shows right-sided heart enlargement and enlargement of central pulmonary arteries.
2. ECG changes are consistent with right-sided heart hypertrophy and/or right heart strain.
3. Echocardiogram shows right-sided heart enlargement.
4. Right heart catheter examination to confirm diagnosis and evaluate for pulmonary hypertension and underlying disease.
5. ABG levels—decreased Pao_2 and pH, increased $Paco_2$.
6. PFTs to confirm underlying lung disease such as obstruction.
7. V/Q scanning or chest CT if history and physical examination suggest pulmonary thromboembolism as the cause or if other diagnostic tests do not suggest other etiologies. If interstitial lung disease is suspected, chest CT will aid in diagnosis.
8. Hematocrit for polycythemia, serum alpha$_1$-antitrypsin if deficiency is suspected, antinuclear antibody level for collagen vascular disease, such as scleroderma, coagulation studies to evaluate hypercoagulability states.

Management

Goal is the treatment of underlying lung disease and management of heart disease.

1. In cases of hypoxemia, supplemental oxygen to improve oxygen delivery to peripheral tissues, thus decreasing cardiac work and lessening sympathetic vasoconstriction. Liter flow individualized during activities, rest, and sleep.
2. Targeted therapy such as prostacyclin analogues and endothelin-receptor antagonists may be used in primary pulmonary hypertension (PPH).
   a. Epoprostenol, treprostinil, and iloprost are prostacyclin (PGI2) analogues and have potent vasodilatory properties. Epoprostenol and treprostinil are administered via the IV route and iloprost is inhaled.
   b. Bosentan is a mixed endothelin-A and endothelin-B receptor antagonist indicated for pulmonary arterial hypertension, including PPH. In clinical trials, bosentan improved exercise capacity, decreased rate of clinical deterioration, and improved hemodynamics.
   c. The PDE5 inhibitors sildenafil and tadalafil promote selective smooth muscle relaxation in lung vasculature. Their use in secondary pulmonary hypertension, such as in patients with COPD, is unclear.
3. The use of the cardiac glycoside digoxin is somewhat controversial; it can improve RV function but must be used with caution and should be avoided during acute hypoxia.
4. Oral anticoagulants in underlying thromboembolic event or primary PAH.
5. Diuretics are used if RV filling volume is markedly elevated and to manage peripheral edema.
   a. Used cautiously due to hemodynamic adverse effects with excessive volume depletion
   b. Can lead to a decline in cardiac output as well as hypokalemic metabolic alkalosis.
6. Vasodilators including calcium channel blockers, particularly oral sustained-release nifedipine and diltiazem, can lower pulmonary pressures, although these agents appear more effective in primary rather than secondary pulmonary hypertension.
7. Bronchodilators to improve lung function.
8. Mechanical ventilation, if patient in respiratory failure.
9. Sodium restriction to reduce edema.

Complications

1. Respiratory failure.
2. Dysrhythmias.

Nursing Assessment

1. Determine if patient has long-standing history of lung disease.
2. Assess degree of dyspnea, fatigue, hypoxemia.
3. Inspect for jugular vein distention and peripheral edema.

Nursing Diagnoses

- Impaired Gas Exchange related to excess fluid in lungs; increased pulmonary vascular resistance.
- Excess Fluid Volume related to right-sided heart failure.

Nursing Interventions

Improving Gas Exchange

1. Monitor ABG values and/or oxygen saturation as a guide in assessing adequacy of ventilation.
2. Use continuous low-flow oxygen as directed to reduce pulmonary artery pressure.

3. Avoid CNS depressants (opioids, hypnotics). They have depressant action on respiratory centers and mask symptoms of hypercapnia.

4. Monitor for signs of respiratory infection because infection causes CO_2 retention and hypoxemia.

Attaining Fluid Balance

1. Watch alterations in electrolyte levels, especially potassium, which can lead to disturbances of cardiac rhythm.

2. Employ ECG monitoring when necessary and monitor closely for dysrhythmias.

3. Limit physical activity until improvement is seen.

4. Restrict sodium intake based on evidence of fluid retention.

Patient Education and Health Maintenance

1. Emphasize importance of stopping cigarette smoking; cigarette smoking is a major cause of pulmonary heart disease.
   a. Ask patient about smoking habits.
   b. Inform patient of risks of smoking and benefits to be gained when smoking is stopped.
   c. Discuss use of behavior modification techniques and smoking cessation aids.

2. Teach patient to recognize and treat infections immediately.

3. Advised patient to avoid environments with poor air quality, have good ventilation, but keep windows closed and use air conditioning, if necessary.

4. Explain to patient and family that restlessness, depression, and poor sleeping as well as irritable and angry behavior may be characteristic; patient should improve with rise in oxygen and fall in CO_2 levels.

5. Explain use of supplemental oxygen, which will reduce further workload on the right side of heart.

Evaluation: Expected Outcomes

- Less dyspneic; ABG levels improved, oxygen saturation.
- Edema reduced; no dysrhythmias.

INTERSTITIAL LUNG DISEASE (PULMONARY FIBROSIS)

Interstitial lung disease is a general term that refers to a variety of chronic lung disorders, such as *idiopathic pulmonary fibrosis, sarcoidosis, asbestosis, silicosis,* and *coal worker's pneumoconiosis (CWP).* There are estimated to be 130 types of interstitial lung disease; only about one third have known causes. Causes include abnormal immune response or abnormal healing in response to a variety of causes, including connective tissue diseases, occupational exposure, environmental exposure, drugs and poisons, radiation, and infections. Pulmonary fibrosis may also be idiopathic.

Pathophysiology and Etiology

1. Unknown etiology such as idiopathic pulmonary fibrosis

2. Connective tissue diseases including scleroderma, rheumatoid arthritis, Sjogren's syndrome, systemic lupus erythematosus, polymyositis, dermatomyositis, and mixed connective tissue disease.

3. Hypersensitivity pneumonitis (acute or chronic) may be due to repeated inhalation of certain fungal, bacterial, animal protein, or reactive antigens. Susceptible persons develop immune reactions leading to pulmonary inflammation and possible scarring.

4. Sarcoidosis associated with inflamed tissue (nodules or granulomas) develop in the lungs and other tissues including skin, eyes, nose, muscles, heart, liver, spleen, bowel, kidney, testes, nerves, lymph nodes, and brain. Nodules in the lungs can lead to narrowing of the airways, inflammation, and fibrosis of lung tissue.

5. May be related to occupational exposure:
   a. Asbestosis (increased risk for lung cancer).
   b. Silicosis.
   c. CWP.

6. May be related to environmental exposure:
   a. Hypersensitivity pneumonitis.
   b. Hard metal disease (cobalt, tungsten, carbide).
   c. Gas, fumes, vapors, aerosols.
   d. Drug and poison exposure.
   e. Cancer drugs (nitrofurantoin, methotrexate, busulfan, bleomycin).
   f. Anti-inflammatory drugs (aspirin, gold, penicillamine).
   g. Cardiac drugs (amiodarone).
   h. Abused substances: heroin, methadone, propoxyphene, talc used in IV drug abuse.
   i. Exposure to radiation.
   j. Infections.

7. Chronic changes include lung tissue damage, inflammation of alveoli with scarring, and fibrosis and stiffening of the interstitium (tissue between the alveoli).

8. The damage limits oxygen transport through scarred alveolar capillary membranes into the bloodstream.

Clinical Manifestations

1. The most prevalent symptom is dyspnea, particularly with exercise.

2. Dry cough.

3. Fatigue.

4. Bibasilar crackles.

5. Connective tissue diseases may be associated with joint pain and swelling, rash, dry eyes, dry mouth, and acid reflux.

6. Symptoms may vary in severity and the course of the disease may be unpredictable. Additional information follows on idiopathic pulmonary fibrosis, interstitial lung disease due to sarcoidosis and other connective tissue diseases, and occupational lung diseases. A generalized nursing process appears on page 319.

Idiopathic Pulmonary Fibrosis

Evidence Base Raghu, G., Collard, H. R., Egan, J. J., et al. (2011). An official ATS/ERS/JRS/ALAT statement: Idiopathic pulmonary fibrosis: Evidence-based guidelines for diagnosis and management. *American Journal of Respiratory Critical Care Medicine, 183,* 788–824.

Pathophysiology and Etiology

1. *Idiopathic pulmonary fibrosis* is a chronic, progressive fibrosing interstitial pneumonia of unknown cause, occurring primarily in older adults and limited to the lungs. It is characterized by progressive worsening of dyspnea and lung function and associated with a poor prognosis.
2. Incidence is approximately 7 to 16 cases per 100,000 people, although this number is believed to be much higher than reported.
3. It is generally diagnosed between ages 50 and 70.

Clinical Manifestations

1. Most have gradual worsening of lung function over years. Progression is accompanied by worsening pulmonary function.
2. Dyspnea and hypoxia are common with physical activity and may be present at rest.
3. Chronic, dry, hacking cough.
4. Breath sounds commonly include bibasilar inspiratory crackles.
5. Finger clubbing may be present.
6. Patients may have pulmonary hypertension and gastroesophageal reflux disorder.

Diagnostic Evaluation

1. High-resolution chest CT shows usual interstitial pneumonia; progressive fibrosis is apparent as disease progresses.
2. PFTs show decreased TLC and VC, with decreased diffusion capacity.
3. ABG levels show low arterial oxygen level.
4. Exercise test shows hypoxia.
5. Chest x-ray may demonstrate patchy, nonuniform infiltrates, ground glass pattern, reticular nodular pattern, honeycomb pattern, and small lung volume.
6. Right-sided heart catheterization may be performed if pulmonary hypertension is suspected.
7. Exclusion of other causes of interstitial lung disease is important.

Management

1. There is no clearly effective medical therapy at this time; however, clinical trials are evaluating the efficacy of various therapies.
   a. Pirfenidone is an oral antifibrotic agent that has shown some benefit.
   b. N-acetylcysteine (NAC) is an amino acid that has been studied in oral and inhaled forms, alone and with prednisone and azathioprine. Combination therapy so far has not shown positive outcomes, but NAC continues to be evaluated.
   c. Warfarin therapy has not proved beneficial and may be harmful.
   d. Several promising clinical trials are developing. Patients should be informed of the National Institutes of Health registry of clinical trials at *www.clinicaltrials.gov*. The database includes information about a trial's purpose, who may participate, locations, and study contacts.

2. Supportive measures include oxygen for hypoxemia and pulmonary hypertension. Prednisone for cough (controversial), pulmonary rehabilitation to improve endurance and control shortness of breath, and management of GERD, if present.
3. Lung transplantation may offer improved symptoms, function, and survival for some patients.

 DRUG ALERT Long-term use of oral steroids may cause osteoporosis, decreased immune function, muscle wasting, glaucoma, cataracts, friable skin, mood changes, weight gain, hyperglycemia, gastric upset, and ulcers. Adverse effects are commonly related to higher doses of steroids used over an extended period. Review potential adverse effects with the patient when therapy is begun. Instruct the patient not to abruptly cease therapy. If unable to continue oral steroids, patient should notify the health care provider immediately.

Sarcoidosis and Other Connective Tissue Diseases

Pathophysiology and Etiology

1. *Sarcoidosis* is an inflammatory, multisystem disorder of unknown cause that affects the connective tissue and lungs.
   a. Granulomatous disease in which clumps of inflammatory epithelial cells occur in many organs, primarily in lungs.
   b. Lymph node enlargement seen on chest x-ray.
2. Rheumatoid arthritis is an inflammatory connective tissue disorder that causes interstitial lung disease due to pleural inflammation in about 20% of cases, mostly females between ages 50 and 60.
3. Systemic lupus erythematosus (SLE) is a multisystem autoimmune disease that causes pleural inflammation and pneumonitis.
4. Scleroderma is a connective tissue disorder that causes hardening of the skin and fibrotic changes, resulting in interstitial fibrosis.
5. Ankylosing spondylitis is a seronegative arthropathy causing back pain and possible pulmonary manifestations.

Management

Comprehensive management of the inflammatory process and multisystem effects (see Chapter 30).

Occupational Lung Diseases

Types

1. *Asbestosis* is a diffuse interstitial fibrosis of the lung caused by inhalation of asbestos dust and particles.
   a. Found in workers involved in manufacture, cutting, and demolition of asbestos-containing materials; there are more than 4,000 known sources of asbestos fiber (asbestos mining and manufacturing, construction, roofing, demolition work, brake linings, floor tiles, paints, plastics, shipyards, insulation).
   b. Asbestos fibers are inhaled and enter alveoli, which, in time, are obliterated by fibrous tissue that surrounds the asbestos particles.

c. Fibrous pleural thickening and pleural plaque formation produce restrictive lung disease, decrease in lung volume, diminished gas transfer, and hypoxemia with subsequent development of cor pulmonale.

2. *Silicosis* is a chronic pulmonary fibrosis caused by inhalation of silica dust.

   a. Exposure to silica dust is encountered in almost any form of mining because the earth's crust is composed of silica and silicates (gold, coal, tin, copper mining); also stone cutting, quarrying, manufacture of abrasives, ceramics, pottery, and foundry work.

   b. When silica particles (which have fibrogenic properties) are inhaled, nodular lesions are produced throughout the lungs. These nodules undergo fibrosis, enlarge, and fuse.

   c. Dense masses form in the upper portion of the lungs; restrictive and obstructive lung disease results.

3. *CWP* ("black lung") is a variety of respiratory diseases found in coal workers in which there is an accumulation of coal dust in the lungs, causing a tissue reaction in its presence.

   a. Dusts (coal, kaolin, mica, silica) are inhaled and deposited in the alveoli and respiratory bronchioles.

   b. There is an increase of macrophages that engulf the particles and transport them to terminal bronchioles.

   c. When normal clearance mechanisms can no longer handle the excessive dust load, the respiratory bronchioles and alveoli become clogged with coal dust, dying macrophages, and fibroblasts, which lead to the formation of the coal macule, the primary lesion of CWP.

   d. As macules enlarge, there is dilation of the weakening bronchiole, with subsequent development of focal or centrilobular emphysema.

4. Hypersensitivity pneumonitis is also considered an occupational lung disease and may be caused by a wide variety of exposures and occupations. Diagnosis can be difficult and requires good history-taking about exposure to potential occupational and environmental antigens, a detailed home and work history, as well as exposures to mold, birds, and bird products such as down.

Pathophysiology

1. Effects of inhaling organic dust (moldy hay, mushroom compost, malt, moldy maple bark, pigeon or parrot droppings, feathers, or contaminated grain), noxious particles, gases, or fumes. Development of disease depends on composition of inhaled substance, its antigenic (precipitating an immune response) or irritating properties, the dose inhaled, the length of time inhaled, and the host's response.

2. Exposure to inorganic dusts stimulates pulmonary interstitial fibroblasts, resulting in pulmonary interstitial fibrosis.

3. Acute symptoms of fever, cough, and chills may occur 4 to 12 hours after exposure and recur with repeated exposure. Chronic disease develops years later.

4. Noxious fumes may cause acute injury to alveolar wall with increasing capillary permeability and pulmonary edema.

5. Occupational lung diseases usually develop slowly (over 20 to 30 years) and are usually asymptomatic in the early stages.

 NURSING ALERT Asbestosis is strongly associated with bronchogenic cancer and mesotheliomas of the pleura and peritoneal surfaces. Smoking increases the risk of lung cancer 50 to 100 times.

Clinical Manifestations

1. Chronic cough; productive in silicosis and CWP.
2. Dyspnea on exertion; progressive and irreversible in asbestosis and CWP.
3. Susceptibility to lower respiratory tract infections.
4. Bibasilar crackles in asbestosis.
5. Expectoration of varying amounts of black fluid in CWP.

Diagnostic Evaluation

1. Chest x-ray—nodules of upper lobes in silicosis and CWP; diffuse parenchymal fibrosis, especially of lower lobes, in asbestosis.
2. High-resolution chest CT to evaluate extent of fibrosis.
3. PFTs primarily show restrictive pattern.
4. Bronchoscopy with lavage to identify specific exposure.
5. Lung tissue biopsy may be needed to rule out other disorders.

Management

1. For hypersensitivity pneumonitis, anti-inflammatory medications may be recommended if the condition is worsening, including prednisone and possibly azathioprine, mycophenolate, or cyclophosphamide.
2. For most other occupational lung diseases, there is no specific treatment; exposure is eliminated and the patient is treated symptomatically.
3. Silicosis is associated with high risk of TB; patients should receive evaluation and appropriate treatment for TB.
4. Smoking cessation measures for people who have been exposed to asbestos to decrease risk of lung cancer.
5. Keep asbestos worker under cancer surveillance; watch for changing cough, hemoptysis, weight loss, melena.
6. Bronchodilators may be of some benefit if any degree of airway obstruction is present.

Complications

1. Respiratory failure.
2. Lung cancer.

Nursing Care of the Patient with Interstitial Lung Disease

Nursing Assessment

1. Obtain occupational and environmental exposure history. Determine length and degree of exposure.
2. Obtain full medical history and family history for connective tissue disorders.
3. Obtain medication history.
4. Obtain history of smoking, respiratory infections, and other chronic lung disease.
5. Evaluate symptoms, functional capacity, and auscultate lungs for crackles.

Nursing Diagnoses

- Ineffective Breathing Pattern related to fibrotic lung tissue causing restriction.
- Impaired Gas Exchange related to fibrotic lung tissue and secretions.

Nursing Interventions

Improving Breathing Pattern

1. Administer oxygen therapy, as required.
2. If ordered, administer or teach self-administration of bronchodilators.
3. Encourage smoking cessation.

Promoting Gas Exchange

1. Encourage mobilization of secretions through hydration and breathing and coughing exercises.
2. Advise patient on pacing activities to prevent fatigue.

Patient Education and Health Maintenance

1. Provide information about the importance of smoking cessation as well as methods of smoking cessation.
2. Instruct patient in methods of health maintenance, such as adequate nutrition and exercise, so additional medical problems can be avoided.
3. Encourage participation in pulmonary rehabilitation.
4. Advise patient that compensation may be obtained for impairment related to occupational lung disease through the Worker's Compensation Act.
5. Provide information to healthy workers on prevention of occupational lung disease.
   a. Enclose toxic substances to reduce their concentration in the air.
   b. Employ engineering controls to reduce exposure.
   c. Monitor air samples.
   d. Ventilate the environment properly to reduce dust content of work atmosphere.
   e. Use protective devices, such as face masks, respirators, hoods.

Evaluation: Expected Outcomes

- Reports less dyspnea.
- Reports improved quality of life.

TRAUMATIC DISORDERS

Pneumothorax

A *pneumothorax* is air in the pleural space occurring spontaneously or from trauma (see Figure 11-4). In patients with chest trauma, it is usually the result of a laceration to the lung parenchyma, tracheobronchial tree, or esophagus. The patient's clinical status depends on the rate of air leakage and size of wound. Pneumothorax is classified as:

Spontaneous pneumothorax—sudden onset of air in the pleural space with deflation of the affected lung in the absence of trauma.

Tension pneumothorax—buildup of air under pressure in the pleural space resulting in interference with filling of both the heart and lungs.

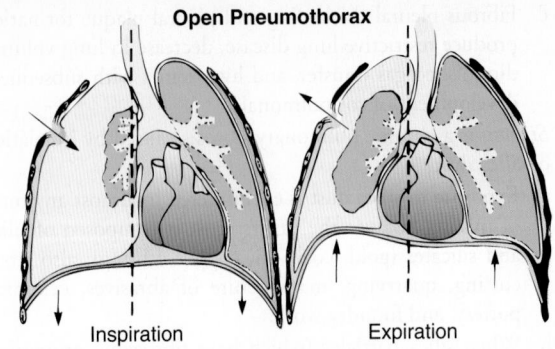

Open Pneumothorax

Inspiration   Expiration

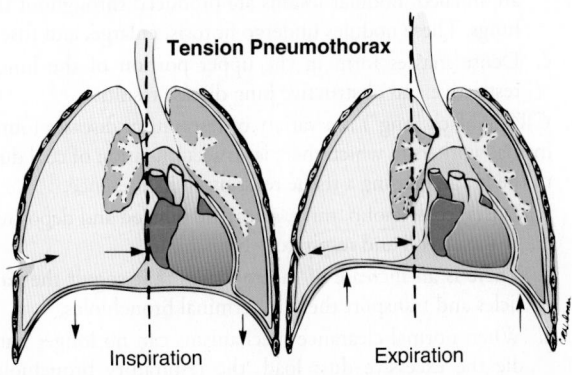

Tension Pneumothorax

Inspiration   Expiration

Figure 11-4. Open pneumothorax and tension pneumothorax. In open pneumothorax, air enters the chest during inspiration and exits during expiration. There may be slight inflation of the affected lung due to a decrease in pressure as air moves out of the chest. In tension pneumothorax, air can enter but not leave the chest. As the pressure in the chest increases, the heart and great vessels are compressed and the mediastinal structures are shifted toward the opposite side of the chest. The trachea is pushed from its normal midline position toward the opposite side of the chest, and the unaffected lung is compressed.

Open pneumothorax (sucking wound of chest)—implies an opening in the chest wall large enough to allow air to pass freely in and out of thoracic cavity with each attempted respiration.

Pathophysiology and Etiology

1. When there is a large, open hole in the chest wall, the patient will have a "steal" in ventilation of other lung.
2. A portion of the V_T will move back and forth through the hole in the chest wall, rather than the trachea as it normally does.
3. Spontaneous pneumothorax is usually due to rupture of a subpleural bleb.
   a. May occur secondary to chronic respiratory diseases or idiopathically.
   b. May occur in healthy people, particularly in thin, white males and those with family history of pneumothorax.

Clinical Manifestations

1. Moderate to very severe dyspnea and often severe chest discomfort radiating to the back.
2. Hyperresonance and diminished breath sounds on affected side.

3. Reduced mobility of affected half of thorax.
4. Tracheal deviation away from affected side in tension pneumothorax.
5. Clinical picture of open or tension pneumothorax is one of air hunger, agitation, hypotension, and cyanosis.

Diagnostic Evaluation

• Chest x-ray confirms presence of air in pleural space.

Management

Spontaneous Pneumothorax

1. Observe and allow for spontaneous resolution for less than 50% pneumothorax in otherwise healthy person.
2. Needle aspiration or chest tube if less than 50% pneumothorax.
3. Pleurodesis may be done to prevent recurrence. Chemical pleurodesis uses various solutions inserted through chest tube to irritate and thereby cause adhesion of parietal and visceral pleura. Surgical pleurodesis uses mechanical irritation to achieve adhesion, with possible removal of parietal pleura.
4. Thoracotomy to remove apical blebs in some cases.

Tension Pneumothorax

1. Immediate decompression to prevent cardiovascular collapse by chest tube insertion to let air escape.
2. Chest tube drainage with underwater-seal suction to allow for full lung expansion and healing.

Open Pneumothorax

1. Close the chest wound immediately to restore adequate ventilation and respiration.
   a. Patient is instructed to inhale and exhale gently against a closed glottis (Valsalva maneuver) as a pressure dressing (petroleum gauze secured with elastic adhesive) is applied. This maneuver helps to expand collapsed lung.
2. Chest tube is inserted and water-seal drainage set up to permit evacuation of fluid/air and produce reexpansion of the lung.
3. Surgical intervention may be necessary to repair trauma.

Complications

1. Acute respiratory failure.
2. Cardiovascular collapse with tension pneumothorax.

Nursing Assessment

1. Obtain history for chronic respiratory disease, trauma, and onset of symptoms.
2. Inspect chest for reduced mobility and tracheal deviation.
3. Auscultate chest for diminished breath sounds and percuss for hyperresonance.

Nursing Diagnoses

• Ineffective Breathing Pattern related to air in the pleural space.
• Impaired Gas Exchange related to atelectasis and collapse of lung.

Nursing Interventions

Achieving Effective Breathing Pattern

1. Provide emergency care as indicated.
   a. Apply petroleum gauze to sucking chest wound (see "Management").
   b. Assist with emergency thoracentesis or thoracostomy.
   c. Be prepared to perform cardiopulmonary resuscitation or administer medications if cardiovascular collapse occurs.
2. Maintain patent airway; suction as needed.
3. Position patient upright if condition permits to allow greater chest expansion.
4. Maintain patency of chest tubes.
5. Assist patient to splint chest while turning or coughing and administer pain medications, as needed.

Resolving Impaired Gas Exchange

1. Encourage patient in the use of incentive spirometer.
2. Monitor oximetry and ABG levels to determine oxygenation.
3. Provide oxygen as needed.

Patient Education and Health Maintenance

1. Instruct patient to continue use of the incentive spirometer at home.
2. For patients with spontaneous pneumothorax, there is an increased risk for recurrence; therefore, encourage these patients to report sudden dyspnea immediately.

Evaluation: Expected Outcomes

• Breath sounds equal bilaterally; less dyspneic.
• ABG levels improved.

Chest Injuries

Chest injuries are potentially life-threatening because of immediate disturbances of cardiorespiratory physiology and hemorrhage and later developments of infection, damaged lung, and thoracic cage. Traumatic chest injuries include *rib fracture or contusion*, *hemothorax*, *flail chest*, *pulmonary contusion*, and *cardiac tamponade or contusion*. Patients with chest trauma may have injuries to multiple organ systems. The patient should be examined for intra-abdominal injuries, which must be treated aggressively.

Pathophysiology and Clinical Manifestations

Rib Fracture

1. Most common chest injury, may be severe if several ribs are fractured or in the presence of other morbidities.
2. May interfere with ventilation and may lacerate underlying lung.
3. Causes pain at fracture site; painful, shallow respirations; localized tenderness and crepitus (crackling) over fracture site.

Hemothorax

1. Blood in pleural space as a result of penetrating or blunt chest trauma.
2. Accompanies a high percentage of chest injuries.
3. Can result in hidden blood loss, increased risk of empyema.
4. Patient may be asymptomatic, dyspneic, hypoxemic, hypotensive, apprehensive, or in shock.
5. Diminished or absent breath sounds of affected side, tracheal deviation to unaffected side.

Flail Chest

1. Loss of stability of chest wall as a result of multiple rib fractures or combined rib and sternum fractures.
   a. When this occurs, one portion of the chest has lost its bony connection to the rest of the rib cage.
   b. During respiration, the detached part of the chest will be pulled in on inspiration and moved outward on expiration (paradoxical movement).
2. Normal mechanics of breathing are impaired to a degree that seriously jeopardizes ventilation, causing dyspnea, hypoxemia, cyanosis, and risk of acute respiratory failure.
3. Generally associated with other serious chest injuries; lung contusion, lung laceration, diffuse alveolar damage. Also associated with tracheal damage, ARDS, and pneumonia.

Pulmonary Contusion

1. Injury of the lung parenchyma that results in leakage of blood and edema fluid into the alveolar and interstitial spaces of the lung. May occur with rib fracture or chest trauma.
2. May not be fully developed for 24 to 72 hours.
3. Signs and symptoms include:
   a. Tachypnea, tachycardia, hypoxemia.
   b. Crackles on auscultation.
   c. Pleuritic chest pain.
   d. Secretions may be copious.
   e. Cough—constant, loose, rattling.

Cardiac Tamponade

1. Compression of the heart as a result of accumulation of fluid within the pericardial space.
2. Caused by penetrating injuries, metastasis, cardiac rupture, cardiac surgery, pericarditis, and other disorders.
3. Signs and symptoms include:
   a. Tachycardia.
   b. Muffled heart sounds.
   c. Falling BP.
   d. Distended jugular veins, elevated central venous pressure (CVP).
   e. Pulsus paradoxus (audible BP fluctuation with respiration).
   f. Dyspnea, cyanosis, shock.

 NURSING ALERT A rapidly developing tamponade interferes with ventricular filling and causes impairment of circulation. Thus, there is a reduced cardiac output and poor venous return to the heart. Cardiac collapse can result. In the patient with hypovolemia caused by associated injuries, the CVP may not rise, thus masking the signs of cardiac tamponade.

Management and Nursing Interventions

The goal is to restore normal cardiorespiratory function as quickly as possible. This is accomplished by performing effective resuscitation if required while simultaneously assessing the patient, restoring chest wall integrity when possible, and reexpanding the lung. The order of priority is determined by the clinical status of the patient.

Rib Fracture

1. Give analgesics (usually nonopioid) to assist in effective coughing and deep breathing.
2. Encourage deep breathing with slow, full inspiration; give local support to injured area by splinting with pillow or hands.
3. Assist with intercostal nerve block to relieve pain so coughing and deep breathing may be accomplished. An intercostal nerve block is the injection of a local anesthetic into the area around the intercostal nerves to relieve pain temporarily after rib fractures, chest wall injury, or thoracotomy.
4. For multiple rib fractures, epidural anesthesia may be used.

Hemothorax

1. Assist with chest tube insertion and set up drainage system for complete and continuous removal of blood and air.
   a. Auscultate lungs and monitor for relief of dyspnea.
   b. Monitor amount of blood loss in drainage.
2. Assist with thoracentesis to aspirate blood from pleural space, if being done before a chest tube insertion.
3. Replace volume with IV fluids or blood products.
4. Trauma patients with pulmonary contusion and flail chest should receive adequate IV fluids to maintain adequate tissue perfusion. Once adequately resuscitated, unnecessary fluid administration should be meticulously avoided. A pulmonary artery catheter may be useful to avoid fluid overload.
5. The use of optimal analgesia and chest physiotherapy should be applied to minimize the likelihood of respiratory failure and ensuing ventilatory support.
6. Patients may require noninvasive positive pressure ventilation or mechanical ventilation with positive end-expiratory pressure.
7. Steroids should not be used in therapy for pulmonary contusion.
8. Diuretics may be used in the setting of hydrostatic fluid overload as evidenced by elevated pulmonary capillary wedge pressures in hemodynamically stable patients or in the setting of known concurrent heart failure.

Flail Chest

1. Analgesia for pain management. Thoracic epidural analgesia may be used for some patients to relieve pain and improve ventilation.
2. Stabilize cardiopulmonary status. If respiratory compromise or failure is present, prepare for immediate ET intubation and mechanical ventilation—treats underlying pulmonary contusion and serves to stabilize the thoracic cage for healing of fractures, improves alveolar ventilation, and restores thoracic cage stability and intrathoracic volume by decreasing work of breathing.
3. Prepare for operative stabilization of chest wall in select patients. Surgical fixation may be considered in severe unilateral flail chest or in patients requiring mechanical ventilation when thoracotomy is otherwise required.

Pulmonary Contusion

For moderate lung contusion:

1. Employ mechanical ventilation to keep lungs inflated.
2. Administer diuretics for pulmonary edema.
3. Use PAP monitoring.
4. Monitor for development of pneumonia, ARDS.

Cardiac Tamponade

For penetrating injuries:

1. Assist with pericardiocentesis (see page 364) to provide emergency relief and improve hemodynamic function until surgery can be undertaken.
2. Prepare for emergency thoracotomy to control bleeding and to repair cardiac injury.

Additional Responsibilities

1. Secure and support the airway as indicated. ET intubation or tracheostomy may be needed.
2. Assist with noninvasive CPAP or mechanical ventilation to help to clear tracheobronchial tree, help the patient breathe with less effort, and reduce paradoxical motion.
3. Secure one or more IV lines for fluid replacement and obtain blood for baseline studies, such as hemoglobin level and hematocrit.
4. Monitor serial CVP readings to prevent hypovolemia and circulatory overload.
5. Monitor ABG/SpO_2 results to determine requirements for supplemental oxygen, mechanical ventilation.
6. Obtain urinary output hourly to evaluate tissue perfusion.
7. Continue to monitor thoracic drainage to provide information about rate of blood loss, whether bleeding has stopped, and whether surgical intervention is necessary.
8. Institute ECG monitoring for early detection and treatment of cardiac dysrhythmias (dysrhythmias are a frequent cause of death in chest trauma).
9. Maintain ongoing surveillance for complications:
   a. Aspiration.
   b. Atelectasis.
   c. Pneumonia.
   d. Mediastinal/subcutaneous emphysema.
   e. ARDS.
   f. Respiratory failure.

Patient Education and Health Maintenance

1. Instruct patient in splinting techniques.
2. Make sure patient is aware of importance of seat belt use to reduce serious chest injuries caused by automobile accidents.
3. Teach patient to report signs of complications—increasing dyspnea, fever, cough.

SELECTED REFERENCES

American Association for Cardiovascular and Pulmonary Rehabilitation. (2010). *Guidelines for pulmonary rehabilitation programs* (4th ed.). Champaign, IL: Human Kinetics.

American College of Chest Physicians. (2007). Diagnosis and management of lung cancer: Evidence-based guidelines. *Chest, 132*(3) suppl: 20S–22S.

American College of Obstetricians and Gynecologists (ACOG). (2011, September). *Thromboembolism in pregnancy* (ACOG Practice Bulletin No. 123). Washington, DC: Author.

American Lung Association. (2011). Occupational lung disease. In *State of lung disease in diverse communities*. Washington, DC: Author.

Centers for Disease Control and Prevention. (2003). Treatment of latent tuberculosis infection (LTBI). *MMWR, 53*(RR-11). Available: *http://www.cdc.gov/mmwr/PDF/rr/rr5211.pdf.*

Centers for Disease Control and Prevention. (2010). Updated recommendations for prevention of invasive pneumococcal disease among adults using the 23-valent pneumococcal polysaccharide vaccine (PPSV23). *Morbidity and Mortality Weekly Report, 59*(34), 1102–1106. Available: *www.cdc.gov/mmwr/preview/mmwrhtml/mm5934a3.htm.*

Centers for Disease Control and Prevention. (2012). Prevention and control of influenza with vaccines: Recommendations of the Advisory Committee on Immunization Practices (ACIP). *Morbidity and Mortality Weekly Report, 61*(32), 613–18. Available: *www.cdc.gov/flu/professionals/acip/index.htm.*

Centers for Disease Control and Prevention. (2011). Tuberculin skin testing. Available: *www.cdc.gov/tb/publications/factsheets/testing/skintesting.htm.*

Detterbeck, F. C., Boffa, D. J., & Tanoue, L. T. (2009). The new lung cancer staging system. *Chest, 136*, 260–271.

Ebell, M. H. (2006). Outpatient vs. inpatient treatment of community-acquired pneumonia. *Family Practice Management, 13*(4), 41–44.

Fayyaz, J., & Mosenifar, Z.(2011). Bronchitis. *Medscape Reference*. Available: *http://emedicine.medscape.com/article/297108-overview.*

Global Initiative for COPD. (2011). Global strategy for the diagnosis, management, and prevention of COPD. Available: *www.goldcopd.org.*

Infectious Diseases Society of America/American Thoracic Society. (2007). Consensus guidelines on the management of community acquired pneumonia in adults. *Clinical Infectious Diseases, 44*, S27–S72.

Jereb, J. A., Goldberg, S. V., Powell, K., et al. (2011). Recommendations for use of isoniazid-rifapentine regimen with direct observation to treat latent Mycobacterium tuberculosis infection. *Morbidity and Mortality Weekly Report, 60*(48), 1650–1653.

Ley, B., Collard, H. R., King, T. E. (2011). Clinical course and prediction of survival in idiopathic pulmonary fibrosis. *Am J Respir Crit Care Med*. 183(4):431–40.

Mahler, D. A., Selecky, P., Harrod, C., et al. (2010). American College of Chest Physicians consensus statement on the management of dyspnea in patients with advanced lung or heart disease. *Chest, 137*, 674–691.

McGlothlin, D., & De Marco, T. (2010). Cor pulmonale. In R. J. Mason, V. C. Broaddus, T. R. Martin, et al. (Eds.), *Murray & Nadel's textbook of respiratory medicine* (5th ed.). Philadelphia: Elsevier.

Parshall, M. B., Schwartzstein, R. M., Adams, L., et al. (2012). An official American Thoracic Society statement: update on the mechanisms, assessment, and management of dyspnea. *Am J Respir Crit Care Med*. 185(4):435–52.

Quaseem, A., Chou, R., Humphrey, L. L., et al. (2011). Venous thromboembolism prophylaxis in hospitalized patients: A clinical practice guideline from the American College of Physicians. *Annals of Internal Medicine, 155*(9), 625–632.

Quaseem, A., Wilt, T. J., Weinberger, S. E., et al. (2011). Diagnosis and management of stable chronic obstructive pulmonary disease: A clinical practice guideline update from the American College of Physicians, American College of Chest Physicians, American Thoracic Society, and European Respiratory Society. *Annals of Internal Medicine, 155*(3), 179–191.

Raghu, G., Collard, H. R., Egan, J. J., et al. (2011). An Official ATS/ERS/JRS/ALAT Statement: Idiopathic pulmonary fibrosis: Evidence-based guidelines for diagnosis and management. *American Journal of Respiratory Critical Care Medicine, 183*, 788–824. Available: *www.thoracic.org/statements/resources/respiratory-disease-adults/ipf0311.pdf.*

Silverman, E. K., & Sandhouse, R. A. (2009). Alpha 1-antitripsyn deficiency. *New England Journal of Medicine, 360*(26), 2749–2757.

Sovari, A. A., & Ooi, H. H. (2011). Cor pulmonale: Introduction to cor pulmonale. *Medscape Reference*. Available: *http://emedicine.medscape.com/article/154062-overview#showall.*

Travis, W. D., Brambilla, E., Noguchi, M., et al. (2011). The new IASLC/ATS/ERS international multidisciplinary lung adenocarcinoma classification. *Journal of Thoracic Oncology, 6*, 244–285.

Villar, J. (2011). What is acute respiratory distress syndrome? *Respiratory Care, 56*(10), 1539–1545.

World Health Organization. (2011). *Guidelines for the programmatic management of drug-resistant tuberculosis*. Geneva: Author. Available: *http://whqlibdoc.who.int/publications/2011/9789241501582_eng.pdf.*

12

Cardiovascular Function and Therapy

OVERVIEW AND ASSESSMENT

Common Manifestations of Heart Disease

In patients with cardiac disease, chest pain is the most common manifestation and is the second most common chief complaint presenting to emergency departments. Heart disease may also be characterized by shortness of breath, palpitations, weakness, fatigue, dizziness, syncope, diaphoresis, or GI complaints.

! NURSING ALERT Older, diabetic, and female patients may not present with typical symptoms of acute coronary syndrome (ACS). Consider the diagnosis of ACS in these patients when they present with other complaints, such as back pain, nausea, fatigue, dyspnea, lightheadedness, cold sweats, jaw pain, and right arm pain (without chest pain).

Chest Pain

Characterization

1. How does the patient describe chest pain? Is it mild or severe, transient or constant? What activity or other factors make it worse, or better? Can it be characterized as tightness, discomfort, fullness, pressure-like, crushing, or searing? Does it radiate to the jaw, neck, back, or arm (particularly left)?

2. Assess chest pain systematically. See Box 12-1. Most pain management scales (visual analogues or numerical scales) are fast and easy to use, but can only be used to measure the intensity

BOX 12-1   Assessment Tips: Chest Pain

Consider all chest pain and associated symptoms to be signs of myocardial ischemia (angina pectoris or MI) until it is ruled out.

The severity of the chest pain does not correlate with the cause of the pain. Indigestion and vague symptoms in a female patient, for example, may indicate myocardial ischemia or infarction. Diabetic and older patients may present with noncardiac symptoms that, with further testing, are found to be related to ischemia.

The patient's perception of pain should also be considered, including such factors as gender, response to pain, cultural beliefs, and level of stress.

Location of perceived pain may be misleading. Referred pain occurs with many diseases—that is, pain is perceived by the patient to be in one area, but its source is actually located in another area.

The patient may present with one problem but have multiple coexisting problems. Older patients, for example, may have several health problems in addition to the reason for the present visit. Likewise, patients who delay seeking medical attention sometimes present with multisystem problems.

The patient may experience no symptoms at all.

of the pain; these scales do not measure the other essential elements for describing chest pain. In your assessment, ascertain the character and quality of the pain; location and radiation of the pain; factors that precipitate, aggravate, or relieve the pain; the duration of the pain; and any associated symptoms.

3. Use one of two popular and similar assessment mnemonics—OLDCARTS or the PQRST assessment (see Chapter 5, page 47) to evaluate chest pain.

Significance

1. Ischemia caused by an increase in demand for coronary blood flow and oxygen delivery, which exceeds available blood supply; may result from coronary artery disease (CAD) or a decreased supply without an increased demand due to coronary artery spasm or thrombus.
2. Pain that is brought on by exertion and relieved by rest suggests angina pectoris or psychogenic pain. Psychogenic pain differs from angina in that it is usually associated with other symptoms, such as headache, back pain, stomach pain, and hyperventilation. Angina is usually caused by three Es: exercise, emotion, and eating.
3. Chest pain that worsens on deep inspiration or cough is suggestive of pleural, pericardial, or chest wall type pain.
4. Chest wall tenderness and pain on inspiration is suggestive of costochondritis.
5. Chest pain that is relieved by leaning forward and aggravated by lying down suggests pericarditis.
6. Sudden onset of chest pain accompanied by dyspnea is suggestive of pulmonary emboli or pneumothorax.
7. Dissecting aortic aneurysm is likely in the hypertensive patient who complains of a sudden onset of tearing, ripping pain.
8. If the patient reports chest pain while eating, this suggests angina or esophageal spasm or biliary (cholecystitis),

pancreatic (pancreatitis), or gastric disease (gastroesophageal reflux disease or ulcers).

9. A panic attack may imitate a heart attack but is more common in younger individuals and in women more than in men.

Shortness of Breath (Dyspnea)

Characterization

1. What precipitates or relieves dyspnea?
2. How many pillows does patient sleep with at night?
3. How far can patient walk or how many flights of stairs can patient climb before becoming dyspneic?
4. Determine the type of dyspnea.
   a. Exertional—breathlessness on moderate exertion that is relieved by rest.
   b. Paroxysmal nocturnal—sudden dyspnea at night; awakens patient with feeling of suffocation; sitting up relieves breathlessness.
   c. Orthopnea—shortness of breath when lying down. Patient must keep head elevated with more than one pillow to minimize dyspnea.

Significance

1. Exertional dyspnea occurs as a result of an elevated pulmonary artery pressure (PAP) due to left ventricular dysfunction.
2. Paroxysmal (nocturnal) dyspnea, also known as cardiac asthma, is precipitated by stimuli that aggravate previously existing pulmonary congestion, resulting in shortness of breath that generally occurs at night and usually awakens the patient.
3. Orthopnea (dyspnea in the supine position) is caused by alterations in gravitational forces resulting in an elevation in pulmonary venous pressure and PAP. These, in turn, increase the pulmonary closing volume and reduce vital capacity. Orthopnea indicates advanced heart failure.

 NURSING ALERT Patients with cardiac dyspnea tend to take short, shallow breaths and patients with pulmonary dyspnea will likely breath slower and deeper.

Palpitations

Characterization

1. Does patient feel heart pounding, fluttering, beating too fast, or skipping beats?
2. Does patient experience dizziness or faintness with palpitations?
3. What brings on this sensation?
4. How long does it last?
5. What does patient do to relieve these sensations?

Significance

1. Pounding, jumping, fluttering sensations occur in the chest due to a change in the patient's heart rate or rhythm or an increase in the force of its contraction.
2. Palpitations can occur as a result of cardiac arrhythmia as well as many other cardiac and noncardiac conditions.

3. Palpitations can be a manifestation of depression and panic disorders.
4. Palpitations can be intermittent, sustained and regular, or irregular.
5. Palpitations are most significant if dizziness and difficulty breathing occur simultaneously.
6. Palpitations that have a gradual onset and terminate in a pounding heartbeat may indicate sinus tachycardia.
7. Palpitations may be caused by noncardiac causes, such as thyrotoxicosis, hypoglycemia, pheochromocytoma, and fever.
8. Certain substances, such as tobacco, coffee, tea, and alcohol, as well as certain drugs, including epinephrine, ephedrine, aminophylline, and atropine, may also precipitate arrhythmias and palpitations.

Weakness and Fatigue

Characterization
1. What activities can you perform without becoming tired?
2. What activities cause you to become tired, weak, or fatigued?
3. Is the fatigue relieved by rest?
4. Is leg weakness accompanied by pain or swelling?

Significance
1. Fatigue can be produced by low cardiac output (CO) due to right- or left-sided heart failure. The heart can't provide sufficient blood to meet the increased metabolic needs of cells.
2. As heart disease advances, fatigue is precipitated by less effort.
3. Weakness or tiring of the legs may be caused by peripheral arterial or venous disease.
4. Weakness and tiredness may be related to electrolyte imbalances, such as hypokalemia, hyperkalemia, hypercalcemia, hypernatremia, hyponatremia, hypophosphatemia, and hypermagnesemia.
5. Other disorders, such as chronic fatigue syndrome, multiple sclerosis, fibromyalgia, influenza, and Lyme disease, may also cause weakness and fatigue.

Dizziness and Syncope

Characterization
1. Is the dizziness characterized as lightheadedness, feeling faint, off balance, vertigo, or spinning?
   a. How long does the dizziness last and what relieves it?
2. How many episodes of syncope or near syncope have been experienced?
3. Did a hot room, hunger, sudden position change, defecation, or pressure on your neck precipitate the episode?

Significance
1. Patients who experience anxiety attacks and hyperventilation syndrome frequently experience faintness and dizziness.
2. Patients who suffer repeated bouts of unconsciousness may be experiencing seizures rather than syncope.
3. Syncope can be a result of hypoglycemia, anemia, or hemorrhage.
4. Vasovagal (vasodepressor or neurocardiogenic) syncope can be precipitated by a hot or crowded environment, alcohol, extreme fatigue, severe pain, hunger, prolonged standing, and emotional or stressful situations. Vasovagal syncope is caused by temporary slowing of the heart and reduction of brain perfusion.
5. Orthostatic or postural hypotension, another cause of dizziness, occurs when the patient stands up suddenly.
6. Cardiac syncope results from a sudden reduction in CO due to bradyarrhythmias and/or tachyarrhythmias.
7. Cerebrovascular disease such as carotid stenosis can cause dizziness and syncope due to reduced cerebral blood flow.

Nursing History

History of Present Illness
1. The patient's history is the single most important aspect in evaluating chest discomfort. The quality, location, duration, and modifying (ie, aggravating and relieving) factors are essential to making a correct diagnosis.
2. How long has the patient been ill? What has the course of the illness been, including current management? Obtain a characterization and review of systems (see Chapter 5).

Past Medical History

Medical and Surgical History
1. Assess childhood and adult illnesses, hospitalizations, accidents, and injuries.
   a. Does the patient have hypertension, diabetes mellitus, hyperlipidemia, chronic obstructive pulmonary disease (COPD), or other chronic illnesses (bleeding disorders or acquired immunodeficiency syndrome)? These may increase the risk of cardiac disease or aggravate disease.
   b. Review the patient's past illnesses and hospitalizations: trauma to chest (possible myocardial contusion); sore throat and dental extractions (possible endocarditis); rheumatic fever (valvular dysfunction, endocarditis); thromboembolism (MI, pulmonary embolism).

Review of Allergies
1. Ask if the patient is allergic to any drugs, foods, environmental agents, or animals, and what reaction occurred.
   a. Allergies to penicillin or other commonly used emergency drugs, such as lidocaine or morphine, may influence the choice of drug treatments, if needed.
   b. Allergies to shellfish indicate iodine allergy; many contrast dyes used in radiologic procedures contain iodine.
   c. Does the patient have allergies to aspirin or nonsteroidal anti-inflammatory drugs, such as naproxen and ibuprofen? (An upset stomach or indigestion from aspirin is not an allergy—rather, it is sensitivity; the patient may still be able to take an enteric-coated aspirin.)

Medications
1. Assess the patient's prescription drugs, if any. Many cardiac drugs must be tapered to prevent a "rebound effect," whereas other drugs affect heart rate and may cause orthostatic hypotension. Estrogen preparations may lead to thromboembolism.
2. Assess the patient's use of over-the-counter medications, which may cause an increase in heart rate and blood pressure.
3. Assess the patient's use of herbal preparations, vitamin and mineral supplements, and other alternative or complementary

therapies. Herbal preparations can interact with other drugs, anesthesia, and interfere with normal blood clotting.

Family History

1. Note the ages and health status of patient's family members (parents, grandparents, siblings, and other blood relatives).
2. A family history of CAD, MI, sudden death, hypertension, hyperlipidemia, hypercholesterolemia, or diabetes could place the patient at an increased risk for heart disease.

Personal and Social History

1. Assess the patient's health habits, such as alcohol or drug use (cocaine may cause MI), tobacco use, nutrition, obesity, pattern of recurrent weight gain after dieting, stress, sleeping patterns, and physical activity (sedentary lifestyle) (see Chapter 5 for additional information).
2. Many lifestyle choices increase the risk of acute and chronic cardiovascular disease.

Physical Examination

General Appearance

1. Is the patient awake and alert or lethargic, stuporous, or comatose?
2. Does the patient appear to be in acute distress; for example, clenching the chest (Levine's sign)? Focus the physical assessment on what is essential when examining a patient in acute distress.
3. Observe the patient's general build (eg, thin, emaciated, or obese) and skin color (eg, pink, pale, ruddy, flushed, or cyanotic).
4. Assess the patient for shortness of breath and distention of jugular veins.

Vital Signs

1. Obtain temperature and note route.
2. Determine heart rate and rhythm.
   a. Assess pulse rate and rhythm using the radial artery.
   b. Time for 1 full minute; note regularity.
   c. Compare apical and radial heart rate (pulse deficit).
   d. Rhythm should be noted as regular, regularly irregular, or irregularly irregular.
3. Monitor blood pressure.
   a. Blood pressure can be measured indirectly using a sphygmomanometer and a stethoscope, electronic devices (dynamo), or directly by way of an arterial catheter.
   b. Avoid taking blood pressure in an arm with an atrioveneous shunt or fistula or on the same side as a mastectomy site or any type of lymphedema.
   c. If possible, take pressure in both arms and note differences (5 to 10 mm Hg difference is normal). Differences of more than 10 mm Hg may indicate subclavian steal syndrome or dissecting aortic aneurysm.
   d. Determine pulse pressure (systolic pressure minus diastolic pressure), which reflects stroke volume, ejection velocity, and systemic resistance, and is a noninvasive indicator

of CO (30 to 40 mm Hg, normal; less than 30 mm Hg, decreased CO).
   e. Note presence of pulsus alternans—loud sounds alternate with soft sounds with each auscultatory beat (hallmark of left-sided heart failure).
   f. Note presence of pulsus paradoxus—abnormal fall in blood pressure more than 10 mm Hg during inspirations (cardinal sign of cardiac tamponade).
4. Assess for orthostatic hypotension.
   a. Orthostatic hypotension occurs when a patient's blood pressure drops 15 to 20 mm Hg or more (with or without an increase in heart rate of at least 20 beats/minute) when rising from a supine to sitting or standing position.
   b. Autonomic compensatory factors for upright posture are inadequate due to volume depletion; bed rest; drugs, such as beta- or alpha-adrenergic blockers; or neurologic disease; prompt hypotension occurs with assumption of the upright position.
   c. Note changes in heart rate and blood pressure in at least two of three positions: lying, sitting, standing; allow at least 3 minutes between position changes before obtaining rate and pressure.

 DRUG ALERT Note that patients taking beta-adrenergic blockers may not exhibit a compensatory increase in heart rate when changing to upright position.

 NURSING ALERT Normal vital signs change with age, sex, weight, exercise tolerance and condition, so note patient's baseline for future comparison.

Head, Neck, and Skin

1. Examination of the head includes assessment of facial characteristics and facial expressions, color of skin, and eyes, any of which can reveal underlying cardiac disease.
   a. Earlobe creases in a patient younger than age 45 may indicate a genetic tendency toward CAD.
   b. Facial color: look for a malar flush, cyanotic lips, or slightly jaundiced skin (rheumatic heart disease).
   c. De Musset's sign (head bobbing with each heartbeat) may indicate severe aortic insufficiency.
   d. Facial edema may be noted with constrictive pericarditis and associated tricuspid valve disease.
2. Examine neck for jugular venous pulse. Jugular vein distention is characteristic of heart failure and other cardiovascular disorders, such as constrictive pericarditis, tricuspid stenosis, and obstruction of the superior vena cava.
3. Examine skin for temperature, diaphoresis, cyanosis, pallor, jaundice.
   a. Warm, dry skin indicates adequate CO; cool, clammy skin indicates compensatory vasoconstriction due to low CO.
   b. Cyanosis may be central (noted on tongue, buccal mucosa, and lips) due to bronchiectasis, COPD, heart failure, lung cancer, pneumothorax, polycythemia vera, pulmonary

edema, pulmonary emboli, shock, and sleep apnea; or peripheral (noted on distal aspects of extremities, tip of nose, and earlobes) due to chronic arteriosclerotic occlusive disease, Buerger's disease, deep vein thrombosis (DVT), heart failure, acute peripheral occlusions, and Raynaud's disease and cold exposure.

   c. Jaundice may be a sign of right-sided heart failure or chronic hemolysis from prosthetic heart valve.

   d. Xanthelasmas are yellow plaque (fatty deposits) evident on skin, commonly seen along the nasal side of one or both eyelids. Xanthelasmas are associated with hyperlipidemia and CAD and may occur normally in the absence of hyperlipidemia.

   e. Pallor indicates decreased peripheral oxyhemoglobin or decreased total oxyhemoglobin. Onset may be sudden or gradual and extent may be generalized (most apparent on the face, conjunctiva, oral mucosa, and nail beds) or local (seen only in the affected limb).

Chest

See page 62.

Extremities

1. Inspect nail beds for color, splinter hemorrhages, clubbing, and capillary refill.

   a. Color—pale nail beds may be indicative of anemia, whereas cyanosis may be indicative of decreased oxygenation.

   b. Splinter hemorrhages are thin brown lines in nail bed and are associated with endocarditis. Janeway lesions (nontender, small erythematous or hemorrhagic macular or nodular lesions on the palm and soles) is indicative of infective endocarditis.

   c. Clubbing (swollen nail base and loss of normal angle) is associated with chronic pulmonary or cardiovascular disease.

   d. Capillary refill indicates an estimate of the rate of peripheral blood low.

2. Inspect and palpate for edema—if pitting edema, describe degree of edema in terms of depth of pitting that occurs with slight pressure: 1+ or mild—0 to ¼ inch (0 to 0.6 cm), 2+ or moderate—½ inch (1.3 cm), 3+ to 4+ or severe—¾ to 1 inch (2 to 2.5 cm).

3. Palpate arterial pulses (see page 68).

Laboratory Studies

Cardiovascular function and disease are evaluated by blood tests that indirectly monitor heart function and structural damage.

Enzymes and Isoenzymes

The diagnostic utilization of cardiac markers has evolved dramatically over the past 50 years. When myocardial tissue is damaged (eg, due to MI), cellular injury results in the release of intracellular enzymes and proteins (cardiac enzymes, isoenzymes, and biochemical markers) into the bloodstream, which, in turn, causes elevated peripheral blood enzyme levels (see Table 12-1).

1. Creatine kinase (CK) has a 98% sensitivity for acute myocardial infarction (AMI) 72 hours after infarction. CK is a catalyst for energy production and is found in brain, myocardium, and skeletal muscle. CK is sensitive but not specific for myocardial injury.

2. CK isoenzymes are more specific than CK. Three CK isoenzymes have been identified: CK-MM, CK-MB, and CK-BB,

Table 12-1	Cardiac Markers—Normal Values, Rise, Peak, Advantages, and Disadvantages				
ENZYME	**RISE (HRS)**	**PEAK (HRS)**	**NORMALIZATION**	**ADVANTAGES**	**DISADVANTAGES**
CK	3–12	10–36	3–4 days	• Rises fairly early	• Lacks cardiac specificity • Increases only after severe damage
CK-MB	3–8	9–30	2–3 days	• Can detect reinfarction • Low cost	• Lacks cardiac specificity • False-positive results • Increases only after severe damage
CK Isoforms	2–6	6–12	1 day	• Highly sensitive in early stages of AMI	• Elevates slowly • Lacks cardiac specificity • False-positive results
TnT	3–12	12–96	5–14 days	• Cardiac specific and sensitivity in late AMI	• Low sensitivity in early AMI • Inability to diagnose subsequent myocardial infarction (MI)
TnI	3–12	12–24	5–10 days	• Cardiac specific and sensitivity in late AMI	• Low sensitivity in early AMI • Inability to diagnose subsequent MIs
Myoglobin	1–4	6–12	1 day	• Extremely sensitive • Shows in blood before CK-MB	• Low cardiac specificity • Not beneficial in late AMIs • False-positive results

with only CK-MB related to the heart. The specificity of CK-MB is greater than 85% and in some cases as high as 100%, but false positives do occur. Two types of CK-MB assays (CK-MB mass and CK-MB activity) are presently used.

a. CK-MB mass assays are found to be more sensitive than CK-MB activity assays.

b. CK-MB mass increases about 3 hours after onset of chest pain, whereas CK-MB activity requires another hour to elevate.

c. CK-MB index is the ratio of CK-MB to the total CK and is considered abnormal when it exceeds 3% to 5%.

3. Eventually, electrophoresis further breaks down CK-MB into its isoforms or subforms ($CK-MB_1$ and $CK-MB_2$). Normally, the ratio of $CK-MB_2$ to $CK-MB_1$ is 1:1. In myocardial injury, the $CK-MB_2/MB_1$ ratio increases to greater than 1.5 within 1 to 1½ hours. CK-MB isoforms have 56% sensitivity for patients presenting within 4 hours of the onset of symptoms.

4. The troponin complex is located on the thin filament of the contractile apparatus of striated and skeletal muscle and consists of three subunits: troponin C (TnC), troponin T (TnT), and troponin I (TnI). In the presence of myocardial damage, the troponin complex on the myofibril breaks down and the subunits of troponin are slowly released into the bloodstream.

a. TnC is not sensitive or specific for myocardial injury.

b. TnT has a sensitivity of approximately 50% within 4 hours of the onset of chest pain, but increases to approximately 75% sensitivity after 6 hours of onset and approximately 100% sensitivity in 12 hours. However, its specificity for myocardial injury is lower.

c. TnI has been found to be the most sensitive and specific for myocardial injury. It has little sensitivity within 4 hours of the onset of chest pain, but increases to 96% sensitivity after 6 hours of the onset of symptoms.

> **!** **NURSING ALERT** Cardiac troponin has gained wide acceptance as the biomarker of choice in the evaluation of patients with ACS for diagnosis, risk stratification, and treatment selection.

5. Myoglobin is a small, oxygen-binding protein found in cardiac and skeletal muscles and is rapidly released into the bloodstream. Myoglobin is sensitive very early after injury, but has poor sensitivity over time and can generate many false-positive results. When myoglobin levels are assessed with CK-MB results, sensitivity increases (as high as 96%), but specificity can drop to as low as 81%.

a. Myoglobin is directly related to muscle mass and is affected by age (levels increase with age), race (blacks have higher levels), gender (women have higher levels), and physical activity.

b. Myoglobins can be elevated in the presence of reinfarction, skeletal muscle or neuromuscular disorders, trauma, severe burns, electrical shock, alcohol withdrawal delirium, metabolic disorders, systemic lupus erythematosus,

strenuous exercise, renal failure, I.M. injections, cardiac bypass surgery, seizures, and heart failure.

Other Biochemical Markers

1. Homocysteine is a toxic by-product of the metabolism of the amino acid methionine into cysteine. Homocysteine exerts a direct cytotoxic effect on the endothelium of blood vessels by blocking the production of nitrous oxide, resulting in decreased pliability of vessels and development of atherosclerotic plaque. Increased homocysteine levels ultimately result in atherosclerosis, CAD, MI, stroke, thromboembolism, and peripheral vascular disease.

a. Hyperhomocystinemia (increased homocysteine levels) are related to gender (male), advanced age, smoking, hypertension, elevated cholesterol, decreased folate, decreased levels of vitamin B_6 and B_{12}, and lack of exercise.

b. Homocysteine can also be elevated in the presence of other diseases, drug use, and caffeine intake.

2. B-type natriuretic peptide (BNP) is synthesized in the ventricular myocardium and released as a response to increased wall stress. BNP is used for diagnosis and prognosis of suspected heart failure. Plasma levels of BNP increase in the presence of left ventricular systolic and diastolic dysfunction, particularly in the presence of decompensating heart failure.

a. An increased BNP level identifies patients at the highest risk of developing sudden cardiac death and those who are in need of heart transplant. It is also associated with heart failure readmissions.

b. BNP is considered a useful marker of myocardial function and is used to guide therapy.

> **!** **NURSING ALERT** When measured at first contact or during the hospital stay the natriuretic peptides are strong predictors of both short- and long-term mortality in patients with STEMI and UA/NSTEMI.

3. C-reactive protein (CRP) is an inflammatory marker that may be an important risk factor for atherosclerosis and ischemic heart disease. CRP is produced by the liver in response to systemic cytokinesis. Elevated CRP is associated with AMI, stroke, and the progression of peripheral vascular disease. However, it can also be elevated with any inflammatory process. In addition to revealing events associated with CAD, CRP can also be used to identify patients at risk for developing CAD.

4. Lipoprotein(a) is a molecule that is similar to low-density lipoprotein cholesterol (LDL-C). It increases cholesterol deposits in the arterial wall, enhances oxidation of LDL-C, and inhibits fibrinolysis, resulting in the formation of atherosclerotic plaque and thrombosis. Treatment of elevated lipoprotein(a) is suggested only for patients with a history of premature vascular disease without other risk factors.

5. Factor I, or fibrinogen, is directly linked to increased cardiovascular risk. It is involved in the coagulation cascade (converting fibrinogen to fibrin by thrombin), stimulates smooth-muscle cell migration and proliferation, and promotes platelet aggregation, which increases blood viscosity.

Nursing and Patient Care Considerations

1. Make sure that enzymes are drawn in a serial pattern, usually on admission and every 6 to 24 hours until three samples are obtained; enzyme activity is then correlated with the extent of heart muscle damage.
2. Maintain standard precautions while obtaining blood specimens and properly dispose of all equipment.
3. Advise patient that results of blood tests will be interpreted based on time and within the context of risk factors and other diagnostic tests.

 NURSING ALERT Greater peaks in enzyme activity and the length of time an enzyme remains at its peak level are correlated with serious damage to the heart muscle and, thus, a poorer prognosis.

Radiology and Imaging

Chest X-ray

Chest x-rays can be used to assess heart size, contour, and position and may also reveal cardiac and pericardial calcification as well as physiologic alterations in pulmonary circulation. For further description and nursing considerations, see page 206.

Myocardial Imaging

Description
With the use of radionuclides and scintillation cameras, radionuclide angiograms can be used to assess left ventricular performance.

1. Thallium-201 is a radionuclide (an unstable atom that produces a small amount of energy) that behaves like potassium in the body and is distributed throughout the myocardium in proportion to blood flow.
2. Technetium-99m–labeled sestamibi is a myocardial perfusion marker used to assess cell membrane and mitochondrial integrity and to reveal myocardial perfusion.
   a. Sestamibi is not taken up by acute or chronic infarct tissue, and the amount of uptake of the radionuclide by other tissue correlates with the size of the infarction, the amount of CK released in the blood, and the postinfarction left ventricular ejection fraction (LVEF).
3. "Hot spot" or positive imaging with technetium-99m stannous pyrophosphate is used when diagnosis of MI is unclear.
4. Negative result of "cold spot" imaging with thallium-201 rules out MI. A positive result, on the other hand, is inconclusive because it cannot differentiate between old and new infarction or areas of ischemia versus infarction.
5. Radionuclide ventriculogram with technetium-99m is used to evaluate valve structure and ventricular function. In this test, a contrast medium is injected through a catheter, opacifying the ventricular cavity to enable measuring of right and LVEF. The test also distinguishes regional from global ventricular wall motion and allows subjective analysis of cardiac anatomy to detect intracardiac shunts as well as valvular or congenital abnormalities.
   a. Complications of ventriculography include arrhythmias, intramyocardial or pericardial injection of contrast medium, and, possibly, development of emboli due to injection of air or a thrombosis through the catheter.
6. Dual single-photon emission computed tomography with simultaneous imaging with 99m-Tc PYP and 201-Tl improves the accuracy of detecting 99m-Tc PYP accumulation and assessing the infarcted area. The overlap of both isotopes may reflect the presence of salvaged myocardium adjacent to necrotic tissue.

Nursing and Patient Care Considerations

1. Advise patient that a radionuclide will be injected through a central venous, Swan-Ganz, or IV catheter, or into an antecubital vein.
2. Reassure patient that the radionuclide will not cause radiation injury or affect heart function.
3. Explain to patient that hot flashes and nausea or vomiting may occur. A test dose will be administered before the dose required for contrast to assess patient's tolerance of radionuclide.
4. Results of the study will be discussed by the patient's health care provider after the study is interpreted by the radiologist.

Treadmill Stress Testing

Description
1. In treadmill stress testing, the patient walks a treadmill or rides a stationary bicycle until reaching a target heart rate, typically 70% to 80% of the maximum predicted heart rate. Treadmill stress testing has 70% sensitivity and specificity among the general population.
2. Indications for stress testing have been adapted from the American Heart Association (AHA) and the American College of Cardiology (see Box 12-2).
3. Reasons for terminating a stress test include:
   a. ST-segment elevations of 2 mm or more.
   b. 20 mm Hg drop in systolic blood pressure.
   c. Drop in heart rate or the development of heart block.
   d. Progressively increasing angina.
   e. ST-segment depression of 2 mm or greater.
   f. Three or more premature ventricular contractions (PVCs).
   g. Supraventricular arrhythmias.
   h. Severe hypertension.
   i. ST-segment depression at baseline that progresses during the test.
   j. Claudication.
   k. Fatigue, dyspnea, or feelings of light-headedness.
   l. Equipment malfunction.
   m. Sustained ventricular tachycardia.
4. Complications of stress testing include supraventricular tachyarrhythmias, bradycardias, heart failure, hypotension, ventricular ectopy (due to ventricular tachycardia), ventricular fibrillation, stroke, MI, and death.
5. Contraindications for performing a stress test include:
   a. AMI within 2 days.
   b. Unstable coronary syndrome.
   c. Wolff-Parkinson-White syndrome.
   d. Uncontrolled arrhythmias.

BOX 12-2	Indications for Stress Test

CLASS I INDICATIONS
(Clear indications for stress testing)
- Suspected or proven coronary artery disease (CAD).
- Male patients who present with atypical chest pain.
- Evaluation of functional capacity and assessment of prognosis in patients with CAD.
- Patients with exercise-related palpitations, dizziness, or syncope.
- Evaluation of recurrent exercise-induced arrhythmias.

CLASS II INDICATIONS
(Stress testing may be indicated)
- Evaluation of typical or atypical symptoms in women.
- Evaluation of variant angina.
- Evaluation of patients who are on digoxin preparations or who have a right bundle-branch block.

CLASS III INDICATIONS
(Stress testing is probably not necessary)
- Young or middle-age asymptomatic patients who have no risk factors for CAD.
- Young or middle-age asymptomatic patients who present with noncardiac chest pain.
- Evaluation of patients for CAD who have complete left bundle-branch block.
- Evaluation of patients for CAD who have preexcitation syndrome.

e. High-degree atrioventricular (AV) blocks.
f. Acute myocarditis.
g. Acute pericarditis.
h. Severe aortic stenosis.
i. Uncontrolled hypertension.
j. Acute aortic dissection.
k. Acute pulmonary embolism or pulmonary infarct.

Nursing and Patient Care Considerations
1. Explain to patient how the procedure will be done and screen for contraindications.
2. Advise patient to abstain from eating, smoking, and consuming caffeine for 2 hours before the test.
3. Inform patient that monitoring will occur throughout the test for signs of complications.
4. Advise patient to inform you of how he or she is feeling during the test.
5. Monitor patient throughout testing for color, respirations, ECG changes, and blood pressure.

Echocardiography (Ultrasound Cardiography)

Description
1. *Echocardiography* is used to visualize and assess cardiac function, structure, and hemodynamic abnormalities. It is the most commonly used noninvasive cardiac imaging tool.
2. It records high-frequency sound vibrations that are sent into the heart through the chest wall. The cardiac structures return the echoes derived from the ultrasound. The motions of the echoes are traced on an oscilloscope and recorded on film, CD, or DVD.
3. Clinical usefulness includes demonstration of valvular and other structural deformities, detection of pericardial effusion, evaluation of prosthetic valve function, and diagnosis of cardiac tumors of asymmetric thickening of interventricular septum, cardiomegaly (heart enlargement), clots, vegetations on valves, and wall motion abnormalities.
4. Types include two-dimensional (2-D), M-mode, and Doppler mode. The methods are complementary and are commonly used in conjunction.
   a. 2-D echocardiography—provides a wider view of the heart and its structures because it involves a planar ultrasound beam.
   b. M-mode—utilizes a single ultrasound beam and provides a narrow segmental view.
   c. Doppler mode—evaluates pressures and blood flow across the valves; also assesses for atrial and ventricular septal defects.

Nursing and Patient Care Considerations
1. Advise patient that traditional echocardiography is noninvasive and that no preparation is necessary.
2. Position patient on left side, if tolerated, to bring the heart closer to the chest wall. Assist patient to clean chest of transducer gel after the test.

Transesophageal Echocardiography

Description
1. In *transesophageal echocardiography (TEE)*, an ultrasound transmitter located at the end of a catheter is passed through the esophagus to the stomach, where flexion of the tip permits imaging of the heart through the stomach wall and the diaphragm, thus allowing clearer and more accurate diagnostic evaluation. It is particularly useful in evaluating valvular disease.
2. As the catheter is slowly withdrawn, views of cardiac structures are obtained at several levels in various 2-D planes.
3. TEE can be used for continuous monitoring of cardiac and noncardiac patients during surgery.
4. Atrial fibrillation is the most common indication for performing a TEE, used to evaluate for thromboembolism.

Nursing and Patient Care Considerations
1. Explain procedure to patient and provide written information, if possible.
2. This is an invasive procedure; patient will require mild sedation and must be kept on nothing-by-mouth status (NPO) for a specified time—usually 4 to 6 hours—before the procedure.
3. The entire procedure takes less than 30 minutes.
4. Results of the study will be discussed with patient by the patient's health care provider after it is interpreted by the radiologist.

Stress Echocardiography

Description
1. *Stress (treadmill) echocardiography* has been found to have better sensitivity and specificity than treadmill stress testing alone.

2. Stress echocardiography is used to evaluate changes in wall motion when the patient is at rest and under stress.

3. Stress echocardiography can be coupled with pharmacologic stress testing. Myocardial perfusion imaging with dobutamine, adenosine, and dipyridamole is an alternative for patients who cannot exercise due to degenerative joint disease, physical deconditioning, neurologic disorders, COPD, or peripheral vascular disease.

Nursing and Patient Care Considerations

1. Explain procedure to patient and provide written information, if possible.

2. Withhold caffeine-containing products for 24 hours before adenosine and dipyridamole stress testing.

3. Discuss with cardiologist which medications should be withheld before test.

4. Maintain NPO status before testing for 2 hours or according to facility policy.

5. Establish a patent IV access.

6. Results of the study will be discussed with patient by the patient's health care provider after fully interpreted.

DRUG ALERT Theophylline-containing products should be discontinued 48 to 72 hours before an adenosine or dipyridamole stress test. Patients receiving oral dipyridamole should not be given IV adenosine because of potential for precipitating severe heart block. If possible, beta-adrenergic blockers should be withheld for 48 to 72 hours before a dobutamine stress test.

Cardiac MRI

Magnetic resonance imaging (MRI) is used to evaluate diseased heart muscle. Currently three techniques are being used. Resting MRI can assess end-diastolic wall thickness and contractile function. Dobutamine MRI is used to evaluate contractile reserve. Contrast enhanced MRI allows for the visualization of the in vivo regions of microvascular obstruction. The extent of microvascular obstruction determines the magnitude of myocardial scarring. Once determined, the extent of microvascular obstruction is a strong predictor of myocardial remodeling and outcome after revascularization. It may eventually replace cardiac catheterization. Safety has been demonstrated in patients with permanent pacemakers and implantable cardioverter-defibrillators. For further description and nursing considerations, see page 206.

Phlebography (Venography)

Description

An x-ray visualization of the vascular tree after the injection of a contrast medium to detect venous occlusion.

Nursing and Patient Care Considerations

1. Inform patient that an intense burning sensation in the vessel where the solution is injected may be experienced. This will last for only a few seconds.

2. Note evidence of allergic reaction to the contrast medium; this may occur as soon as the contrast medium is injected, or it may occur after the test.

   a. Perspiring, dyspnea, nausea, vomiting.

   b. Rapid heart rate, numbness of extremities.

   c. Hives.

3. Advise patient to notify health care provider of signs of allergic reaction.

4. Observe injection site for redness, swelling, bleeding, and thrombosis.

Positron Emission Tomography

Description

1. Considered the most sensitive modality for detecting hibernating viable myocardium and predicting left ventricular recovery after coronary revascularization.

2. F-FDG, a glucose analog that is transported into cells through glucose membrane transportes is injected. It does not undergo any further metabolism (unlike glucose) and essentially is trapped within the cell.

3. Trapped F-FDG accumulates and becomes an index of cellular glucose utilization signifying ongoing cellular metabolism. Reduced FDG uptake (reduced or absent glucose metabolism) signifies myocardial scar. Also see page 206.

4. Used to determine blood flow to the heart muscle and viability of areas with decreased function due to previous MI.

5. Allows for the differentiation of nonfunctioning heart muscle from heart muscle that would benefit from a procedure.

Nursing and Patient Care Considerations

1. Inform patient not to eat for 4 hours prior to the scan.

2. Check blood glucose prior to test for diabetic patients; if greater than 200, may need to reschedule test.

3. Encourage patient to drink water following the scan to assist excretion of contrast medium.

Other Diagnostic Tests

Electrocardiogram

Basic Principles

1. Despite its limited sensitivity and specificity, the 12-lead ECG is still the standard for the evaluation of myocardial ischemia.

2. Electrical activity is generated by the cells of the heart as ions are exchanged across cell membranes.

3. Electrodes that are capable of conducting electrical activity from the heart to the ECG machine are placed at strategic positions on the extremities and chest precordium (see Figure 12-1).

4. The electrical energy sensed is then converted to a graphic display by the ECG machine. This display is referred to as the ECG.

5. Each ECG lead consists of a positive and negative pole; each lead also has an axis that represents the direction in which current flows.

6. Each lead takes a different view of the heart; therefore, the tracing will be different with each view obtained.

7. The direction in which electrical current flows determines how the waveform will appear.

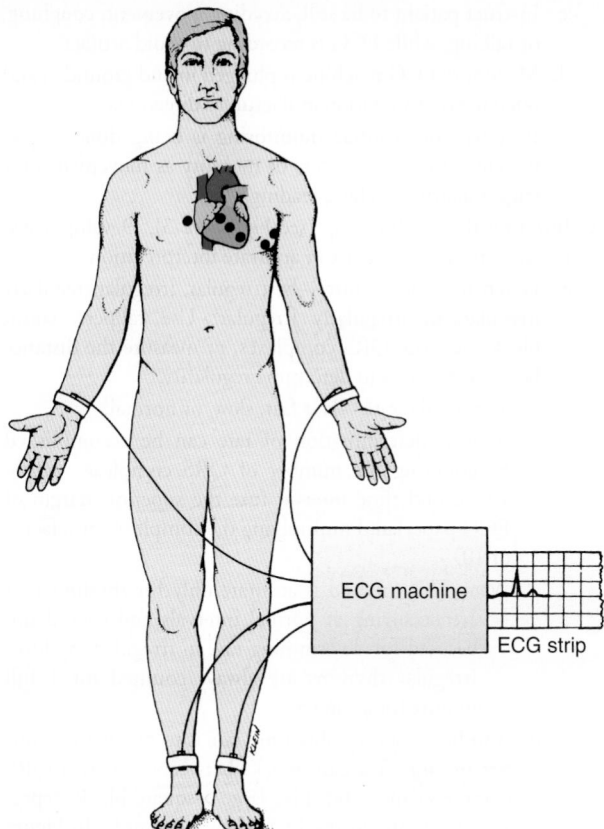

Figure 12-1. Transmission of the heart's impulse to a graphic display by ECG machine. The electrodes, which conduct electrical activity from the heart to the ECG machine, are placed at strategic positions on the extremities and chest precordium.

8. There are three sets of leads:
   a. Standard limb or bipolar leads (I, II, III) utilize three electrodes; these leads form a triangle known as Einthoven's Triangle.
   b. Augmented unipolar leads (AVR, AVL, AVF).
   c. Precordial unipolar leads (V_1, V_2, V_3, V_4, V_5, V_6).
9. A heart contraction is represented on the ECG graph paper by the designated P wave, QRS complex, and T waves.
   a. The P wave is the first positive deflection and represents atrial depolarization or atrial contraction.
   b. The PR interval represents the time it takes for the electrical impulse to travel from the sinoatrial node to the AV node and down the bundle of His to the right and left bundle branches.
   c. The Q wave is the first negative deflection after the P wave; the R wave is the first positive deflection after the P wave.
   d. The S wave is the negative deflection after the R wave.
   e. The QRS waveform is generally regarded as a unit and represents ventricular depolarization. Atrial repolarization (relaxation) occurs during the QRS complex, but cannot be seen.
   f. The T wave follows the S wave and is joined to the QRS complex by the ST segment. The ST segment represents ventricular repolarization or relaxation. The point that

represents the end of the QRS complex and the beginning of the ST segment is known as the J point.
   g. The T wave represents the return of ions to the appropriate side of the cell membrane. This signifies relaxation of the muscle fibers and is referred to as *repolarization* of the ventricles.
   h. The QT interval is the time between the Q wave and the T wave; it represents ventricular depolarization (contraction) and repolarization (relaxation).

Indications

1. The ECG is a useful tool in the diagnosis of conditions that may cause aberrations in the electrical activity of the heart. Examples of these conditions include:
   a. MI and other types of CAD such as angina.
   b. Cardiac dysrhythmias.
   c. Cardiac enlargement.
   d. Electrolyte disturbances (calcium, potassium, magnesium, and phosphorous).
   e. Inflammatory diseases of the heart.
   f. Effects on the heart by drugs, such as antiarrhythmics and tricyclic antidepressants.
2. Despite its many advantages, however, the ECG also has several shortcomings:
   a. Fifty percent of all patients with AMI have no ECG changes.
   b. A patient may have a normal ECG, present pain-free, and still have significant risk for myocardial ischemia.
   c. Several disease processes can mimic that of an AMI, including left bundle-branch blocks, ventricular paced rhythms, and left ventricular hypertrophy.

ECG Leads and Normal Waveform Interpretation
See Figure 12-2.

1. The normal amplitude of the P wave is 3 mm or less; the normal duration of the P wave is 0.04 to 0.11 second. P waves that exceed these measurements are considered to deviate from normal.

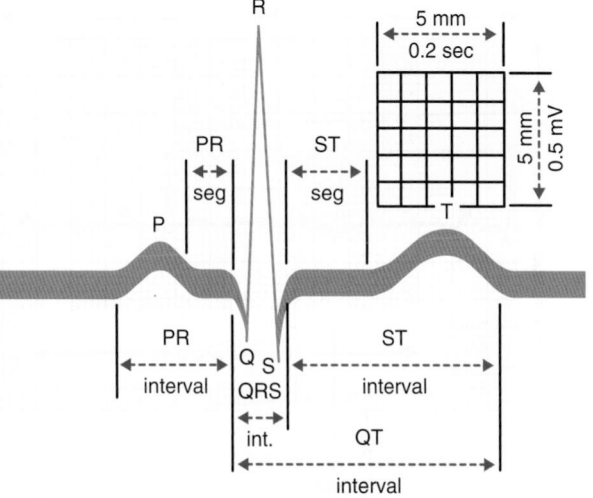

Figure 12-2. Waveform analysis.

2. The PR interval is measured from the upstroke of the P wave to the QR junction and is normally between 0.12 and 0.20 second. There is a built-in delay in time at the AV node to allow for adequate ventricular filling to maintain normal stroke volume.

3. The QRS complex contains separate waves and segments, which should be evaluated separately. Normal QRS complex should be between 0.06 and 0.10 second.

   a. The Q wave, or first downward stroke after the P wave, is usually less than 3 mm in depth. A Q wave of significant deflection is not normally present in the healthy heart. A pathologic Q wave usually indicates a completed MI.

   b. The R wave is the first positive deflection after the P wave, normally 5 to 10 mm in height. Increases and decreases in amplitude become significant in certain disease states. Ventricular hypertrophy produces very high R waves because the hypertrophied muscle requires a stronger electrical current to depolarize.

4. The ST segment begins at the end of the S wave, the first negative deflection after the R wave, and terminates at the upstroke of the T wave.

5. The T wave represents the repolarization of myocardial fibers or provides the resting state of myocardial work; the T wave should always be present.

   a. Normally, the T wave should not exceed a 5-mm amplitude in all leads except the precordial (V_1 to V_6) leads, where it may be as high as 10 mm.

6. The P, Q, R, S, and T waves all appear differently depending on which lead you are viewing.

Nursing and Patient Care Considerations

1. Perform ECG or begin continuous ECG monitoring as indicated.

   a. Provide privacy and ask patient to undress, exposing chest, wrists, and ankles. Assist with draping as appropriate. Remove large jewelry or metal from upper body to avoid interference.

   b. Place leads on chest and extremities as labeled, using self-adhesive electrodes or water-soluble gel or other conductive material.

   c. Instruct patient to lie still, avoiding movement, coughing, or talking, while ECG is recording to avoid artifact.

   d. Make sure ECG machine is plugged in and grounded and operate according to manufacturer's directions.

   e. If continuous cardiac monitoring is being done, advise patient on the parameters of mobility as movement may trigger alarms and false readings.

2. Interpret the rhythm strip (see Figure 12-3). Develop a systematic approach to assist in accurate interpretation.

   a. Determine the rhythm—Is it regular, irregular, regularly irregular, or irregularly irregular? Use calipers, count blocks between QRS complexes, or measure the distance between R waves to determine regularity.

   b. Determine the rate—Is it fast, slow, or normal?

      i. A gross determination of rate can be accomplished by counting the number of QRS complexes within a 6-second time interval (use the superior margin of ECG paper) and multiplying the complexes by a factor of 10.

         Note: This method is accurate only for rhythms that are occurring at normal intervals and should not be used for determining rate in irregular rhythms. Irregular rhythms are always counted for 1 full minute for accuracy.

      ii. Another means of obtaining rate is to divide the number of large 5-square blocks between each two QRS complexes into 300. Five large 5-square blocks represent 1 minute on the ECG paper. Example: In Figure 12-3, the number of large square blocks between complexes #5 and #6 equals 5, and 300 divided by 5 equals 60, or a rate of 60.

   c. Evaluate the P wave—Are P waves present? Is there a P for every QRS complex? If there is not a P for every QRS, do the P waves have a normal configuration?

   d. Measure and evaluate the PR interval.

   e. Evaluate the QRS complex—Measure the QRS complex and examine its configuration.

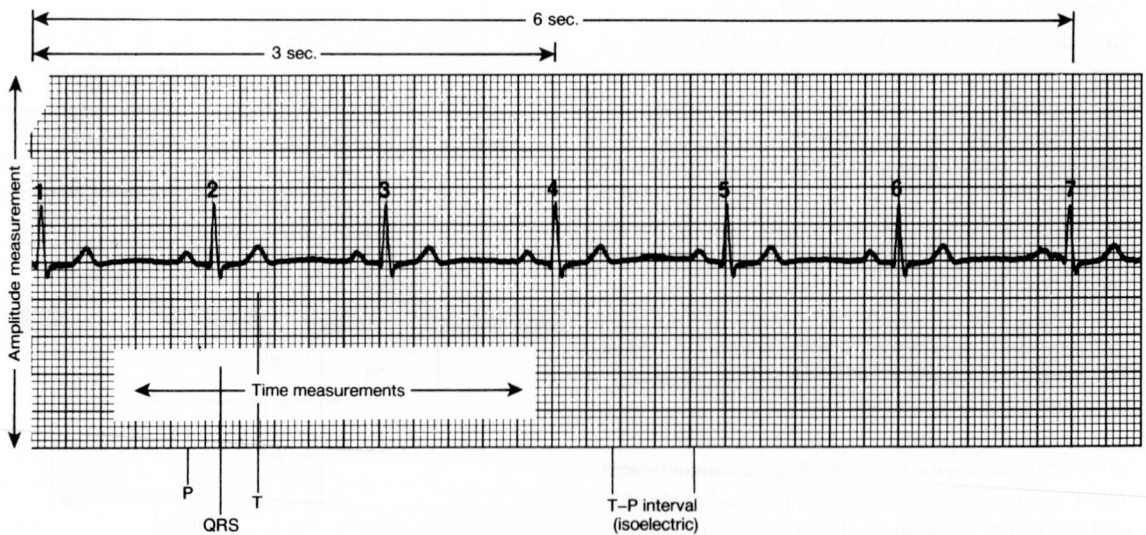

Figure 12-3. Lead II shows normal sinus rhythm on ECG paper.

f. Evaluate the ST segment—An elevated ST segment heralds a pattern of injury and usually occurs as an initial change in acute MI. ST depression occurs in ischemic states. Calcium and potassium changes also affect the ST segment.

g. Evaluate the T wave—Are T waves present? Do all T waves have a normal shape? Could a P wave be hidden in the T wave, indicating a junctional rhythm or third-degree heart block? Is it positively or negatively deflected (inverted T waves indicate ischemia) or peaked (indicative of hyperkalemia)?

h. Evaluate the QT interval—Should be less than one half the R-R interval. Prolonged QT interval may indicate digoxin toxicity, long-term quinidine or procainamide therapy, or hypomagnesemia.

See Chapter 13 for common cardiac dysrhythmias.

Angiography

Description

1. Invasive imaging procedure that enables visualization of blood vessels for their patency of blood flow versus blockage through the insertion of a catheter into an artery or vein followed by injection of contrast dye.
2. Various types include coronary, aortic, renal, peripheral, cerebral, and pulmonary angiography; lymphangiogram; ventriculography; and fluorescein angiography.
3. Provides information that may direct assessment and management of cardiovascular and cerebrovascular disease, peripheral blockage (arterial and venous), aneurysms, arterial and venous malformations, thrombosis (deep vein or pulmonary embolus), fistulae; guide mapping prior to interventional procedures; and diagnose internal bleeding.

Nursing and Patient Care Considerations
Preprocedure

1. Question patient for known allergies, particularly to iodine (shellfish). If so, notify health care provider, who may want to prepare patient with oral corticosteroids and diphenhydramine before the study.
2. Make sure there is a signed consent and that patient/family questions have been answered.
3. Make sure fasting guidelines have been followed, varying from NPO to liquid or light diet. Follow facility policy; should be in accordance with American Society of Anesthesiologists guidelines (minimum fasting 6 hours from light meal, 2 hours from clear liquids) to minimize risk of pulmonary aspiration should emesis occur.
4. Make sure laboratory testing has been ordered and results reviewed, including blood urea nitrogen (BUN) and creatinine, to evaluate kidney function for ability to clear contrast dye; hemoglobin/hematocrit; platelet count and coagulation values, to ensure clotting and anticoagulation baseline; white blood cell (WBC) count, to rule out infection that may be exacerbated by invasive procedure; electrolytes; and blood type and screen, in case blood transfusion is necessary.
5. Make sure baseline ECG is on file.
6. Ensure IV patency for medication administration.

7. Make sure patient has voided.
8. Administer premedication, if ordered.

Postprocedure

1. Record vital signs according to facility policy and stability of patient.
2. Check for bleeding or hematoma formation at insertion site.
3. Check distal extremity for normal color and intact pulses.
4. Patient may complain of discomfort in the groin or other site depending on route by which contrast medium was administered. Check for bed rest/activity progression and special fluid instructions. Encourage fluids/hydration to ensure clearance of contrast dye.
5. Provide patient with discharge instructions, including follow-up care, medications, and driving and activity restrictions.

Diagnostic Electrophysiology Studies

Description

Electrophysiology studies (EPS) are a complex invasive procedure in which flexible catheters (with 2 to 10 electrodes) are placed percutaneously in the right or left femoral vein, the subclavian vein, the internal jugular vein, or the median cephalic veins. EPS assesses pacing thresholds and measures conduction intervals in the high right atrium, the right ventricular apex, the right ventricular outflow tract, the coronary sinuses, the bundle of His, and, occasionally, the left ventricle. The test is followed by programmed stimulation protocols to evaluate the heart's conduction system.

Indications for EPS

1. Definite indications for EPS include:
   a. Sustained ventricular tachycardia.
   b. Cardiac arrest in the absence of AMI, antiarrhythmic drug toxicity, or electrolyte imbalance.
   c. Syncope of uncertain origin (for which noncardiac causes have been ruled out).
   d. Wide QRS tachycardia of uncertain etiology.
   e. To evaluate the effectiveness of a device for the detection and electrical termination of tachycardias (pacemakers or implanted defibrillators).
   f. Symptomatic Wolff-Parkinson-White syndrome.
   g. Frequent symptomatic regular supraventricular tachycardia unresponsive to medications.
2. Possible indications for EPS include:
   a. Asymptomatic Wolff-Parkinson-White syndrome.
   b. Post–myocardial infarction.
   c. Nonsustained ventricular tachycardia.
   d. Cardiomyopathy.
   e. Frequent ventricular ectopy.
   f. Supraventricular tachycardia.
3. Contraindications for EPS include:
   a. Asymptomatic sinus bradycardia.
   b. Asymptomatic bundle-branch blocks.
   c. Palpitation.
   d. Atrial fibrillation or flutter.
   e. Third-degree AV blocks.
   f. Second-degree Mobitz type II AV blocks.

Nursing and Patient Care Considerations

1. Anticoagulants (warfarin) should be discontinued at least 3 days before EPS.
2. Discuss with health care provider which cardiac medications should be discontinued and when they should be discontinued.
3. Instruct patient to fast for at least 6 hours before the study.
4. Place electrodes for a 12-lead ECG, which will be recorded during the procedure.
5. Discuss with patient any feelings about the procedure and his or her physical condition. Patients frequently experience anxiety, fear of loss of control, denial, depression, and uncertainty.
6. Explain the procedure, its purpose, and the preparation involved.
7. Inform patient that pain medication and conscious sedation will be used during the procedure.
8. Postprocedure care includes:
   a. Keeping extremity used for IV straight, restraining if necessary.
   b. Monitoring patient's groin for bleeding or hematoma formation.
   c. Monitoring vital signs as ordered.
   d. Providing emotional support to patient and family.

Cardiac Catheterization

Description

1. *Cardiac catheterization* is a diagnostic procedure in which a catheter is introduced into the heart and blood vessels to provide physiologic data to guide treatment; measure cardiovascular hemodynamics; acquire radiographic images of coronary arteries, cardiac chambers, and aorta; collect blood from various chambers for analysis; and evaluate pulmonary blood flow and shunts.
2. The access site of choice is the femoral vein; however, when there is peripheral vascular disease or morbid obesity, radial or brachial access is used, depending on distal pulses. The catheter is directed up the aorta and into the coronary vasculature to visualize coronary anatomy (right or left) and measure hemodynamics. In rare instances of aortic disease, a transseptal approach may be used.
3. Right-sided heart catheterization—right side of the heart is accessed to evaluate pulmonary shunts, cardiac anomalies, and valvular disease. A radiopaque catheter is passed from the femoral vein and through the inferior vena cava or from the basilic vein and through the superior vena cava into the right atrium, right ventricle, and pulmonary vasculature under direct visualization with a fluoroscope.
   a. Right atrium and right ventricle pressures are measured; blood samples are taken for hematocrit and oxygen saturation.
   b. After entering the right atrium, the catheter is then passed through the tricuspid valve and similar tests are performed on blood within the right ventricle.
   c. Finally, the catheter is passed through the pulmonic valve and as far as possible beyond that point; capillary samples are obtained, capillary wedge pressure is recorded, and CO can be determined.
   d. Complications include cardiac dysrhythmias, venous spasm, thrombophlebitis, infection at insertion site, cardiac perforation, and cardiac tamponade.
4. Left-sided heart catheterization—primarily done to diagnose coronary artery disease; usually done by retrograde approach by advancing the catheter up the aorta into the coronary anatomy.
   a. Retrograde approach—catheter may be introduced percutaneously by puncture of the femoral artery or by direct brachial approach and advanced under fluoroscopic control into the ascending aorta and into the left ventricle.
   b. Transseptal approach—catheter is passed from the right femoral vein (percutaneously or by saphenous vein cutdown) upward into right atrium. A long needle is passed up through the catheter and is used to puncture the septum separating the right and left atria; needle is withdrawn and the catheter is advanced under fluoroscopic control into left ventricle.
   c. The catheter tip is placed at the coronary sinus and contrast medium is injected directly into one or both of the coronary arteries to evaluate patency.
   d. Gives hemodynamic data—permits flow and pressure measurements of left side of heart.
   e. Usually performed to evaluate the patency of coronary arteries and function of the left ventricular muscle and mitral and aortic valves; may also be done to evaluate patients before surgery.
   f. Ventriculography—study of the left ventricle; catheter is passed into the left ventricle and dye is injected with a rapid, uniform rate via an injector machine to measure ejection fraction or function of the left ventricle.
   g. Complications of left-sided heart catheterization and implications for nursing assessment include dysrhythmias (ventricular fibrillation), syncope, vasospasm, pericardial tamponade, MI, pulmonary edema, allergic reaction to contrast medium, perforation of great vessels of heart, systemic embolization (stroke, MI), loss of pulse distal to arteriotomy, and possible ischemia of lower arm and hand.
5. Angiography is usually combined with heart catheterization for coronary artery visualization.
6. Contraindications for cardiac catheterization include uncontrolled ventricular irritability, electrolyte imbalance, medication toxicity (digitalis), uncontrolled heart failure, renal failure, recent stroke (within past 3 months), active GI bleeding, active infection, uncontrolled hypertension, patient's refusal, and pregnancy. Some of these conditions can be reversed or improved prior to catheterization.

Nursing and Patient Care Considerations
Preprocedure

1. Question patient for known allergies, particularly iodine (shellfish), and make health care provider aware so that premedication with corticosteroid and antihistamine may be considered.

2. Make sure that there is a signed consent form and that patient and family questions have been answered.

3. Make sure that fasting guidelines have been followed, varying from NPO to liquid or light diet. Follow facility policy; should be in accordance with American Society of Anesthesiologists guidelines (minimum fasting 6 hours from light meal, 2 hours from clear liquids).

4. Make sure laboratory testing has been ordered and results reviewed, including BUN/creatinine, to evaluate kidney function for ability to clear contrast dye; hemoglobin/hematocrit; platelet count and coagulation values, to ensure clotting and anticoagulation baseline; WBC count, to rule out infection that may be exacerbated by invasive procedure; electrolytes; and blood type and screen, in case blood transfusion is necessary.

5. Make sure baseline ECG is on file.

6. Ensure IV patency for administration of medications.

7. Mark distal pulses.

8. Explain to patient that he or she will be lying on an examination table for a prolonged period and may experience certain sensations:

   a. Occasional thudding sensations in the chest—from extrasystoles, particularly when the catheter is manipulated in ventricular chambers.

   b. Strong desire to cough, which may occur during contrast medium injection into right side of heart during angiography.

   c. Transient feeling of hot flashes or nausea as the contrast medium is injected.

9. Evaluate patient's emotional status before catheterization, dispel myths, and provide factual information.

10. Have patient void before the procedure.

11. Allow for premedication (if any) to take effect prior to procedure.

Postprocedure

1. Record vital signs according to facility protocol and patient's condition.

2. Check for bleeding or hematoma formation at insertion site.

3. Check distal extremity for normal color and intact pulses, and evaluate complaints of pain, numbness, or tingling sensation to determine signs of arterial insufficiency.

4. Assess for complaints of chest pain and respond immediately.

5. Follow activity restriction/progression directions, which are based on coagulation status and whether a vascular closure method was employed.

6. Evaluate complaints of back, thigh, or groin pain (may indicate retroperitoneal bleeding).

7. Obtain postprocedure ECG and labs according to facility protocol.

8. Be alert for signs and symptoms of vagal reaction (nausea, diaphoresis, hypotension, bradycardia); treat as directed with atropine and fluids.

9 Assess neurological status if receiving IIB/IIIA platelet inhibitors or thrombolytics according to facility protocol.

10. Provide discharge instructions, including follow-up care, medications, driving and activity restrictions, and the need to report any pain or above-listed problems.

GENERAL PROCEDURES AND TREATMENT MODALITIES

Hemodynamic Monitoring

Hemodynamic Monitoring is the assessment of the patient's circulatory status; it includes measurements of heart rate (HR), intra-arterial pressure, CO, central venous pressure (CVP), PAP, pulmonary artery wedge pressure, and blood volume. It describes the intravascular pressure and flow of blood that occurs when the heart muscle contracts and pumps blood throughout the body.

The primary purpose is the early detection, identification, and treatment of life-threatening conditions, such as heart failure, cardiac tamponade, and all types of shock (septic, cardiogenic, neurogenic, anaphylactic). See Procedure Guidelines 12-1, pages 338 to 341; Procedure Guidelines 12-2, pages 342 to 345; and Procedure Guidelines 12-3, pages 346 to 347.

Cardiac Output

Cardiac output (CO) is the amount (volume) of blood ejected by the left ventricle into the aorta in 1 minute. Normal CO is 4 to 8 L/minute.

Underlying Considerations

1. CO is determined by stroke volume (SV) and HR. Thus, CO = SV × HR. CO must be maintained to adequately oxygenate the body.

   a. HR = number of cardiac contractions per minute. The integrity of the conduction system and nervous system innervation of the heart influence functioning of this determinant.

   b. SV = amount of blood ejected from ventricle per beat (normal SV is 50 to 100 mL/beat). The amount of blood returning to the heart (preload), venous tone, resistance imposed on the ventricle before ejection (afterload), and the integrity of the cardiac muscle (contractility) influence the functioning of this determinant.

2. The body alters CO through increases or decreases in one or both of these parameters. CO is maintained if the HR falls by an increase in SV. Likewise, a decrease in SV produces a compensatory rise in HR to keep the CO normal.

3. CO will decrease if either of the determinants cannot inversely compensate for the other.

4. CO measurements are adjusted to patient size by calculating the cardiac index (CI). CI equals CO divided by body surface area (BSA); BSA is determined through standard charts based on individual height and weight. Normal CI is 2.5 to 4 L/minute/m^2.

Assessment of Cardiac Output

Signs of low CO include:

1. Changes in mental status.

2. An increase in HR.

3. Shortness of breath.

4. Cyanosis or duskiness of buccal mucosa, nail beds, and earlobes.

(Text continues on page 341)

PROCEDURE GUIDELINES 12-1

Manual Central Venous Pressure (CVP) Monitoring

EQUIPMENT

- Venous pressure tray
- Cutdown tray or percutaneous catheter insertion tray with introducer
- Infusion solution/infusion set with CVP manometer (electronic CVP monitoring does not use

- a manometer) or attached to semi-rigid pressure tubing
- IV pole
- Arm board (for antecubital insertion)
- Sterile dressing and tape
- Gowns, masks, caps, and sterile gloves

- Heparin flush system and pressure bag (if transducer to be used)
- ECG monitor
- Carpenter's level (for establishing zero point)
- Transducer and transducer cable

 NURSING ALERT A CVP line is a potential source of septicemia.

PROCEDURE

Nursing Action	Rationale
Preparatory phase (by nurse)	
1. Assemble equipment according to the manufacturer's directions. Evaluate the patient's prothrombin time, partial thromboplastin time, and complete blood count.	1. Assesses for coagulopathies or anemia.
2. Explain the procedure to the patient and ensure that informed consent is obtained.	2. Allays anxiety and enlists cooperation. Procedure is similar to an IV, and the patient may move in bed as desired after passage of catheter.
a. Explain to patient how to perform the Valsalva maneuver.	a. The Valsalva maneuver performed during catheter insertion and removal decreases risk of air emboli.
3. Position patient in supine position.	3. Anatomic access and clinical status of the patient are considered in site selection.
a. Arm vein—extend arm and secure on arm board.	a. Provides for maximum visibility of veins.
b. Jugular veins—place patient in Trendelenburg's position. Place a small rolled towel under shoulders (subclavian approach).	b. Trendelenburg's position reduces the risk of air emboli.
4. Flush IV infusion set and manometer (measuring device) or prepare heparin flush for use with transducer. Secure all connections.	4. Prevents air emboli and bleeding.
a. Attach manometer to IV pole. The zero point of the manometer should be on a level with the patient's right atrium. Mark midaxillary line with indelible ink.	a. The level of the right atrium is at the fourth intercostal space midaxillary line. Marking right atrium ensures consistency of the zero level for subsequent readings.
b. Calibrate/zero transducer and level port with patient's right atrium.	
5. Institute electrocardiogram monitoring.	5. Dysrhythmias may be noted during insertion as catheter is advanced.
Insertion phase (by health care provider)	
1. Health care provider puts on gown, cap, and mask. (Ensure that that there is a "time-out" before starting the procedure.)	1. CVP insertion is a sterile procedure. "Time-out" is Joint Commission requirement to ensure correct site, correct patient, and correct procedure.
2. The CVP site is surgically cleaned. The health care provider introduces the CVP catheter percutaneously or by direct venous cutdown.	2. Patient may be asked to perform the Valsalva maneuver to protect against risk of air embolus.

PROCEDURE GUIDELINES 12-1 *(continued)*

Manual Central Venous Pressure (CVP) Monitoring

PROCEDURE *(continued)*

Nursing Action	Rationale
3. Assist the patient in remaining motionless during insertion.	3. Prevents trauma or rupture of vessel.
4. Monitor for dysrhythmias, tachypnea, and tachycardia as catheter is threaded to great vein or right atrium.	4. These are signs of pneumothorax or arterial puncture.
5. Connect primed IV tubing/heparin flush system to catheter and allow IV solution to flow at a minimum rate to keep vein open (25 mL maximum).	5. Fluid is administered to prevent clotting of the catheter. Catheter placement must be verified before hypertonic or blood products can be administered.
6. Obtain a chest x-ray.	6. Verifies correct catheter position and absence of pneumothorax.
7. Assist with suturing the catheter in place after placement confirmation.	7. Prevents inadvertent catheter advancement or dislodgement.
8. Place a sterile occlusive dressing over site.	8. Prevents infection.

To measure CVP (by nurse)

1. Place the patient in a comfortable position.	1. This baseline position is used for subsequent readings.
2. Position the zero point of the manometer at the level of the right atrium (see accompanying figure).	2. Eliminates the effect of hydrostatic pressure on the transducer.

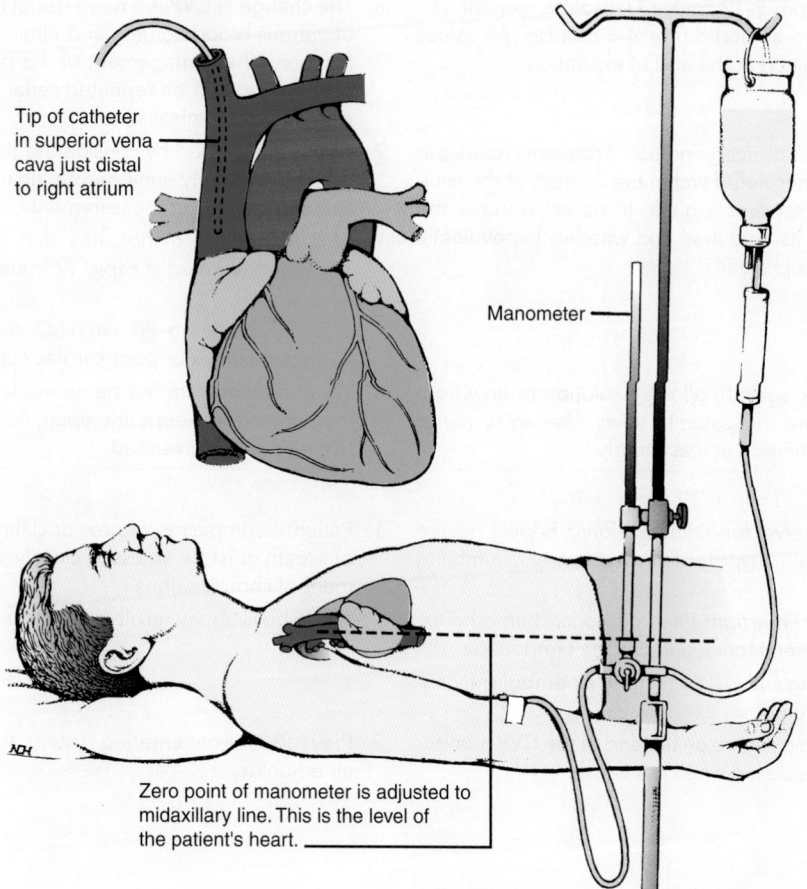

Tip of catheter in superior vena cava just distal to right atrium

Manometer

Zero point of manometer is adjusted to midaxillary line. This is the level of the patient's heart.

(continued)

PROCEDURE GUIDELINES 12-1 *(continued)*

Manual Central Venous Pressure (CVP) Monitoring

PROCEDURE *(continued)*

Nursing Action	Rationale
To measure CVP (by nurse)	
3. Turn the stopcock so the IV solution flows into the manometer, filling to about the 0- to 25-cm level. Then turn stopcock so solution in manometer flows into patient.	3. Eliminates the effects of atmospheric pressure.
4. Observe the fall in the height of the column of fluid in manometer. Record the level at which the solution stabilizes or stops moving downward. This is CVP. Record CVP and the position of the patient.	4. The column of fluid will fall until it meets an equal pressure. The CVP reading is reflected by the height of a column of fluid in the manometer when there is open communication between the catheter and the manometer. The fluid in the manometer will fluctuate slightly with the patient's respirations. This confirms that the CVP line is not obstructed by clotted blood.
5. CVP catheter may be connected to a transducer and an electrical monitor with either digital or calibrated CVP wave readout. Make sure the transducer has been zeroed to atmospheric pressure. To zero the transducer, place the stopcock so it is open between the transducer and air and press zero button on the monitor.	5. Makes sure the transducer reads zero when no pressure is against it. This procedure is like zeroing a scale before weighing something to ensure accuracy.
6. CVP may range from 5–12 cm H_2O (absolute numeric values have not been agreed on) or 2–6 mm Hg. All values should be determined at the end of expiration.	6. The change in CVP is a more useful indication of adequacy of venous blood volume and alterations of cardiovascular function. The management of the patient is not based on one reading, but on repeated serial readings in correlation with patient's clinical status.
7. Assess the patient's clinical condition. Frequent changes in measurements (interpreted within the context of the clinical situation) will serve as a guide to detect whether the heart can handle its fluid load and whether hypovolemia or hypervolemia is present.	7. CVP is interpreted by considering the patient's entire clinical picture: hourly urine output, heart rate, blood pressure, and cardiac output measurements. a. CVP near zero indicates that the patient is hypovolemic (verified if rapid IV infusion causes patient to improve). b. CVP above 15–20 cm H_2O may be due to either hypervolemia or poor cardiac contractility.
8. Turn the stopcock again to allow IV solution to flow from solution bottle into the patient's veins. Use an IV pump and monitor the infusion at least hourly.	8. When readings are not being made, IV flow bypasses the manometer but keeps line open; flow should be controlled to prevent fluid overload.
Follow-up phase	
1. Prevent and observe for complications. Report severe shortness of breath, hypotension, hypoxemia, rumbling cardiac murmur. a. *From catheter insertion:* Pneumothorax, hemothorax, air embolism, hematoma, and cardiac tamponade b. *From indwelling catheter:* Infection, air embolism, central venous thrombosis	1. Patient's complaints of new or different pain or shortness of breath must be assessed closely; may indicate development of complications. Air embolism may result in cardiac arrest.
2. Make sure the cap is secure on the end of the CVP monitor and all clamps are closed when not in use.	2. Prevents air from entering system, thereby reducing risk of air embolus.

PROCEDURE GUIDELINES 12-1 (continued)

Manual Central Venous Pressure (CVP) Monitoring

PROCEDURE (continued)

Nursing Action	Rationale
Follow-up phase	
3. If air embolism is suspected, immediately place patient in left lateral Trendelenburg's position and administer oxygen.	3. Air bubbles will be prevented from moving into the lungs and will be absorbed in 10–15 minutes in the right ventricular outflow tract.
4. Carry out ongoing nursing surveillance of the insertion site and maintain aseptic technique.	4.
a. Inspect entry site twice daily for signs of local inflammation and phlebitis. Remove the catheter immediately if there are signs of infection.	a. Local infection could spread rapidly through systemic circulation.
b. Make sure sutures are intact.	b. If catheter dislodges into right atrium, dysrhythmias may result.
c. Change dressings, as prescribed.	
d. Label to show date and time of change.	
e. Send the catheter tip for bacteriologic culture when it is removed.	e. Detects bacterial colonization.
5. When discontinued, remove central line.	5.
a. Position patient flat with head down.	a. Prevents air from entering blood vessel.
b. Remove dressing and sutures.	
c. Have patient take a deep breath and hold it while catheter is gently pulled out.	c. Prevents air emboli by creating positive chest pressure.
d. Apply pressure at catheter site and apply dressing.	d. Prevents bleeding.
e. Monitor site and vital signs for signs of bleeding or hematoma formation.	

5. Falling blood pressure.
6. Low urine output.
7. Cool, moist skin.
8. Decreased or no appetite.

Methods

1. CO is measured by various techniques. In the clinical setting, it is usually measured by the thermodilution technique in conjunction with a flow-directed balloon-tipped pulmonary artery catheter (commonly known as Swan-Ganz catheter after the inventors).
2. The Swan-Ganz catheter is positioned in its final position in a branch of the pulmonary artery; it has a thermistor (external sensing device) situated 1½ inches (4 cm) from the tip of the catheter, which measures the temperature of the blood that flows by it.
3. To ensure accuracy of hemodynamic values, the transducer must be at the appropriate level and zeroed according to facility policy.
   a. Leveling is performed to eliminate the effects of hydrostatic pressure in the transducer. It must be done with every change in bed height and elevation of the bed and prior to zeroing and calibration.

b. Zeroing is performed to eliminate the effects of atmospheric pressure in the transducer. It should be performed before connecting the pressure system to the patient, with any leveling, and whenever there is a significant change in hemodynamic variables.
c. All values should be rated at the end of expiration.

Central Venous Pressure Monitoring

1. Refers to the measurement of right atrial pressure or the pressure of the great veins within the thorax (normal range: 5 to 10 cm H_2O or 2 to 8 mm Hg).
   a. Right-sided cardiac function is assessed through the evaluation of CVP.
   b. Left-sided heart function is less accurately reflected by the evaluation of CVP, but may be useful in assessing chronic right- and left-sided heart failure and differentiating right and left ventricular infarctions.
2. Requires the threading of a catheter into a large central vein (subclavian, internal or external jugular, median basilic, or femoral). The catheter tip is then positioned in the right atrium, upper portion of the superior vena cava, or the inferior vena cava (femoral approach only).

(Text continues on page 347)

PROCEDURE GUIDELINES 12-2

Measuring Pulmonary Artery Pressure (PAP) by Flow-Directed Balloon-Tipped Catheter (Swan-Ganz Catheter)

EQUIPMENT

- Swan-Ganz catheter set
- ECG, monitor, and display unit with paper recorder
- For mixed venous oxygen saturations (SvO_2) monitoring, fiber-optic pulmonary artery catheter, optical module, and microprocessor unit
- Defibrillator

- Pressure transducer (disposable/reusable) and transducer cable
- Cutdown tray or percutaneous catheter insertion tray with introducer
- Sterile saline solution
- Pressurized bag
- Heparin infusion in plastic bag

- Continuous flush device—for general flushing and rapid flushing after blood draw
- Semi-rigid pressure tubing—attaches the catheter to transducer setup
- Local anesthetic
- Skin antiseptic
- Transparent/gauze dressing
- Tape

PROCEDURE

Nursing Action	Rationale
Preparatory phase (by nurse)	
1. Explain procedure to patient and family/significant other. Make sure that informed consent has been obtained. Explain that patient may feel the catheter moving through veins and that this is normal.	1. Allays fear and ensures understanding.
2. Check vital signs and apply electrocardiogram (ECG) electrodes. Have emergency equipment available.	2. Detects dysrhythmias or other complications.
3. Place patient in a comfortable position; this is the baseline position.	3. Note the angle of elevation if patient cannot lie flat because subsequent pressure readings are taken from this baseline position to ensure consistency. Patient may need to be in Trendelenburg's position briefly if the jugular or subclavian vein is used.

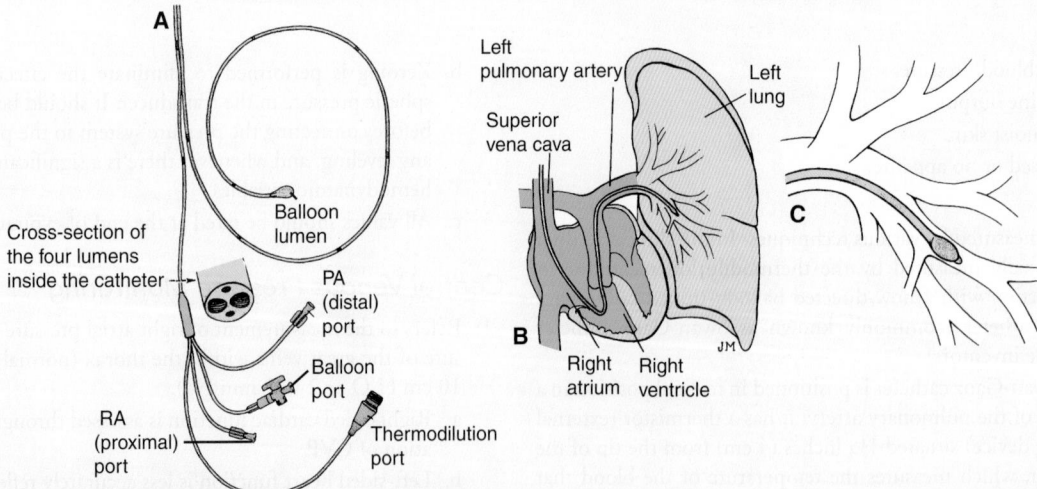

(A) Swan-Ganz catheter. (B) Location of the Swan-Ganz catheter within the heart. The catheter enters the right atrium via the superior vena cava. The balloon is then inflated, allowing the catheter to follow the blood flow through the tricuspid valve, through the right ventricle, through the pulmonic valve, and into the main pulmonary artery. Waveform and pressure readings are noted during insertion to identify location of the catheter within the heart. The balloon is deflated after the catheter is in the pulmonary artery and properly secured. (C) Pulmonary capillary wedge pressure (PCWP). The catheter floats into a distal branch of the pulmonary artery when the balloon is inflated and becomes "wedged." The wedged catheter occludes blood flow from behind, and the tip of the lumen records pressures in front of the catheter. The balloon is then deflated, allowing the catheter to float back into the main pulmonary artery.

Measuring Pulmonary Artery Pressure (PAP) by Flow-Directed Balloon-Tipped Catheter (Swan-Ganz Catheter)

PROCEDURE *(continued)*

Nursing Action	Rationale
4. Set up equipment according to manufacturer's directions:	4.
a. The pulmonary artery catheter requires a transducer and recording, amplifying, and flush systems.	a. Monitoring systems may vary greatly. The complexity of equipment requires an understanding of the equipment in use. A constant microdrip of heparin flush solution is maintained to ensure catheter patency.
b. Flush system according to manufacturer's directions.	b. Flushing of the catheter system ensures patency and eliminates air bubbles.
5. Adjust transducer to level of patient's right atrium (phlebostatic axis fourth intercostal space, midaxillary line).	5. Differences between the level of the right atrium and the transducer will result in incorrect pressure readings; the phlebostatic axis is at the level of the right atrium.
6. Calibrate pressure equipment (especially important when reusable transducers are employed).	6. A known quantity of pressure is applied to the transducer (usually by mercury manometer) to ensure accurate monitoring of pressure readings.
7. Clip excess hair. Prepare skin over insertion site.	7. The catheter is inserted percutaneously under sterile conditions.

Performance phase (by health care provider)

1. Health care provider puts on sterile gown and gloves and places sterile drapes over patient.	1. Sterile field is established to reduce risk of infection.
2. State a "time-out." (Can be done before donning gown and glove.)	2. A National Safety Patient Goal by the Joint Commission to eliminate wrong site or procedure to wrong patient.
3. The balloon is inflated with air under sterile water or saline to test for leakage (bubbles). The catheter may be flushed with saline at this time.	3. Ensures that the balloon is intact and removes air from catheter.
4. The Swan-Ganz catheter is inserted through the internal jugular, subclavian, or any easily accessible vein by either percutaneous puncture or venotomy.	4. The internal jugular vein establishes a short route into the central venous system.
5. The catheter is advanced to the superior vena cava. Oscillations of the pressure waveforms will indicate when the tip of the catheter is within the thoracic cavity. The patient may be asked to cough.	5. Catheter placement may be determined by characteristic waveforms and changes. Coughing will produce deflections in the pressure tracing when the catheter tip is in the thorax.
6. The catheter is then advanced gently into the right atrium, and the balloon is inflated with air.	6. The amount of air to be used is indicated on the catheter.
7. The inflated balloon at the tip of the catheter will be guided by the flowing stream of blood through the right atrium and tricuspid valve into the right ventricle. From this position, it finds its way into the main pulmonary artery. The catheter tip pressures are recorded continuously by specific pressure waveforms as the catheter advances through the various chambers of the heart.	7. Ventricular irritability may occur as the catheter passes into the right ventricle. Watch ECG monitor for signs of dysrhythmias and report.
8. The flowing blood will continue to direct the catheter more distally into the pulmonary tree. When the catheter reaches a pulmonary vessel that is approximately the same size or slightly smaller in diameter than the inflated balloon, it cannot be advanced further. This is the wedge position, called the pulmonary artery occlusion pressure (PAOP).	8. With the catheter in the wedge position, the balloon blocks the flow of blood from the right side of the heart toward the lungs. The sensor at the tip of the balloon detects pressures distally, which results in the sensing of retrograde left atrial pressures. PAOP is thus equal to left atrial pressures.

(continued)

PROCEDURE GUIDELINES 12-2 (continued)

Measuring Pulmonary Artery Pressure (PAP) by Flow-Directed Balloon-Tipped Catheter (Swan-Ganz Catheter)

PROCEDURE (continued)

Nursing Action	Rationale
	a. Normal PAOP is 8–12 mm Hg. Optimal left ventricular function appears to be at a wedge between 14 and 18 mm Hg.
	b. Wedge pressure is a valuable parameter of cardiac function. Filling pressures less than 10 mm Hg may indicate hypovolemia and in an acutely injured heart are commonly associated with reduction in cardiac output, hypotension, and tachycardia. Filling pressures greater than 20 mm Hg are associated with left-sided heart failure, pulmonary congestion, and hypervolemia.
9. The balloon is deflated, causing the catheter to retract spontaneously into a larger pulmonary artery. This gives continuous pulmonary artery systolic, diastolic, and mean pressure.	9. Normal systolic pulmonary pressure ranges are 20–30 mm Hg, and the diastolic pulmonary pressure ranges are 8–12 mm Hg. The normal mean PAP (average pressure in pulmonary artery throughout the entire cardiac cycle) is 15–20 mm Hg.
10. The catheter is then attached to a continuous heparin flush and transducer.	10. A low-flow continuous irrigation ensures that the catheter remains patent. The transducer converts the pressure wave into an electronic wave that is displayed on the oscilloscope.
11. The catheter is sutured in place and covered with a sterile dressing.	11. Maintains position and prevents infection.
12. A chest x-ray is obtained after Swan-Ganz insertion if fluoroscopy was not used to guide insertion.	12. Confirms catheter position and provides a baseline for future reference.

To obtain wedge pressure reading (by nurse)

1. Note amount of air to be injected into balloon, usually no more than 1.5 mL. Do not introduce more air into balloon than specified. Use the pre-calibrated 1.5 mL syringe it comes with since this has a locking guard. Maximum inflation volume only enough to see a change in waveform about 4–15 seconds.	1. Avoids rupturing balloon.
2. Inflate the balloon slowly until the contour of PAP changes to that of PAOP. As soon as a wedge pattern is observed, no more air is introduced.	2. The transducer converts the pressure wave into an electronic wave that is displayed on a screen.
a. Note the digital pressure recordings on the monitor (an average of pressure waves is displayed, but these waves are not taken at end expiration).	a. PAOP should be determined at end expiration because respiratory variation of the waveform occurs due to changes in intrathoracic pressure.
b. Obtain a strip of the pressure tracing.	b. A calibrated oscilloscope or graph paper is needed to read pressures at end expiration.
c. Determine PAOP from strip at end expiration.	
3. Deflate the balloon as soon as the pressure reading is obtained. Do not draw back with force on the syringe because too forceful a deflation may damage the balloon. Always allow for passive deflation of the balloon.	3. Segmental lung infarction may occur if the catheter balloon is left inflated for long periods. PAOP is only measured intermittently. Never wedge for more than 15 seconds, nor inflate the balloon with more than 1.5 mL of air. Do not allow catheter to remain in wedge position when patient is unattended or when not directly taking the measurement.
4. Record PAOP reading and amount of air needed to obtain wedge reading. Document recorded waveform by placing a strip of the waveform in patient's chart showing wedge tracing reverting to pulmonary artery waveform.	4. Overinflation of the balloon may cause a "superwedge" waveform and data obtained will be inaccurate. Overinflation of balloon may cause balloon to lose elastic properties and rupture. The strip provides documentation that catheter was not left in wedge position.

PROCEDURE GUIDELINES 12-2 *(continued)*

Measuring Pulmonary Artery Pressure (PAP) by Flow-Directed Balloon-Tipped Catheter (Swan-Ganz Catheter)

PROCEDURE *(continued)*

Nursing Action	Rationale

To obtain SvO$_2$ reading

1. Before insertion, perform a preinsertion calibration of the catheter.

2. After insertion, perform a calibration for light intensity and an in vivo calibration every 8 hours.

1. This calibrates the catheter to light intensity in the environment.

2. The in vivo calibration ensures that there is minimal difference, or "drift," between the actual SvO$_2$ value and the value displayed on the monitor. The light calibration adjusts for changes in light in the environment.

 NURSING ALERT Also perform in vivo calibration if the optical module is disconnected at the catheter junction, if calibration data are lost, or if the SvO$_2$ is within 4% of the SvO$_2$ value calculated from mixed venous values obtained from the pulmonary artery catheter.

3. Monitor SvO$_2$ at frequent intervals. Values of 60%–80% are normal.

3. Causes of an SvO$_2$ < 60% include decrease in CO, decrease in oxygenation, decrease in hemoglobin, or increase in O$_2$ consumption.

Causes of an SvO$_2$ > 80% include increase in oxygenation or decrease in O$_2$ consumption.

4. If the SvO$_2$ changes within 10% of the prior value, confirm that the change reflects a change in patient condition.

4. The value displayed may not be accurate if fibrin or a clot is obstructing the catheter tip (low-intensity signal), if the catheter is touching the vessel wall or in a wedged position (high-intensity signal), or if the catheter is no longer calibrated accurately.

5. If the catheter is not functioning properly, initiate steps to resolve the problem.

5. These steps may include aspiration to determine if a clot is obstructing the catheter or notifying the health care provider of the need to reposition the catheter.

6. If no catheter malfunction is identified, report changes to the physician and initiate therapy based on standard of care.

6. Prompt intervention can restore normal tissue oxygen delivery before untoward effects occur.

Follow-up phase

1. Inspect the insertion site daily. Look for signs of infection, swelling, and bleeding.

1. A foreign body (catheter) in the vascular system increases the risk of sepsis.

2. Record date and time of dressing change and IV tubing change. Note centimeter mark on catheter as it leaves the cordis.

2. The centimeter mark is a reference point in case there is catheter movement.

3. Assess contour of waveform frequently and compare with previously documented waveforms.

3 Catheter may move forward and become lodged in wedge position or drift back into right ventricle. Turn patient to left side and ask him or her to cough (may dislodge catheter from wedge position). If not dislodged, notify health care provider.

4. Assess for complications: pulmonary embolism, dysrhythmias, heart block, damage to tricuspid valve, intracardiac knotting of catheter, thrombophlebitis, infection, balloon rupture, rupture of pulmonary artery.

4. Blood coming back into syringe indicates balloon rupture. Notify health care provider immediately. Other signs of complications are dysrhythmias and change in clinical condition of the patient.

5. When indicated, assist with catheter removal without excessive force of traction; apply pressure dressing over the site. Check site periodically for bleeding.

5. Prevents trauma to tissue and excessive bleeding.

 Evidence Base Paunovic, B. (2011). Pulmonary artery catheterization. *Medscape Reference.* Available: *http://emedicine.medscape.com/article/1824547-overview.*

PROCEDURE GUIDELINES 12-3

Measurement of Cardiac Output by Thermodilution Method

EQUIPMENT

- Flow-directed thermodilution catheter in place
- Cardiac output (CO) set, which includes IV tubing
- 10-mL syringe and three-way stopcock
- Normal saline or D_5W solution bag
- Cardiac monitor with CO computation capability or stand-alone CO computer
- Temperature sensor cable

PROCEDURE

Nursing Action	Rationale

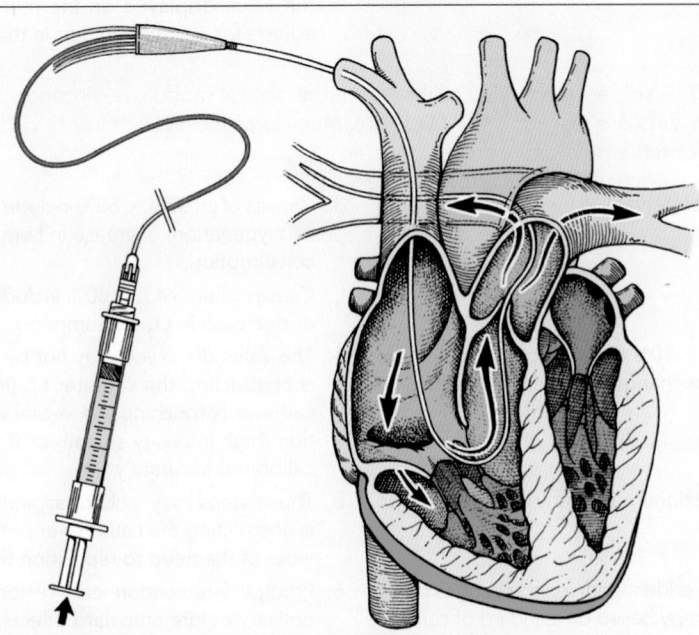

Typical equipment for a closed thermodilution cardiac output setup.

Nursing Action	Rationale
1. Explain procedure to patient.	1. Allays anxiety.
2. Connect IV solution bag and CO set maintaining aseptic technique.	2. Solution will be injected directly into the heart and must be sterile.
3. If you do not have a prepackaged CO set, attach IV solution bag to IV tubing, connect a three-way stopcock to the end of the tubing; connect a 10-mL syringe to the middle part of the three-way stopcock.	
4. Attach the three-way stopcock to the proximal injectate port of the thermodilution catheter. This port should be reserved solely for determination of CO.	4. The proximal injectate port should have its distal end in the right atrium. If medications are infusing in this port, they will be flushed through in bolus form when CO measurements are taken.
5. Another three-way stopcock may be used to allow for IV solution to run at a keep-open rate.	5. Once the CO set is connected, the system should remain closed.
6. Connect temperature sensor cable to the thermistor port of the thermodilution catheter.	6. When solution is injected through catheter, it mixes with the blood in the right side of the heart and flows to the pulmonary artery where blood temperature is detected by the thermistor.

PROCEDURE GUIDELINES 12-3 (continued)

Measurement of Cardiac Output by Thermodilution Method

PROCEDURE (continued)

Nursing Action	Rationale
7. Set cardiac monitor to CO computation format. If using a stand-alone CO computer, enter the temperature of the injectable solution and the code number for the size of thermodilution catheter in use (code will be located on the thermodilution catheter packaging).	7. The injectate solution should be 15–20 degrees cooler than the patient's body temperature. Room temperature injectate is usually adequate. Cardiac output is calculated based on change in temperature.
8. Fill 10-mL syringe with injectate solution by turning stopcock off to patient and open to syringe and solution.	
9. Turn off IV keep-open solution, if present.	9. Need closed system from syringe to catheter.
10. Turn stopcock off to injectate solution and open to patient and syringe.	
11. Press "inject" button on the CO computer or monitor and inject 10 mL rapidly (within 4 seconds) and smoothly into the proximal port.	11. Delay will interfere with results.
12. Wait for computation to be complete. Repeat the procedure two or three times to obtain an average.	12. Some monitors display a waveform for the injectate dispersal to evaluate the adequacy of dispersal and temperature sensing.
13. Turn stopcock off to the syringe and injectate and allow keep-open IV fluid to infuse through the proximal port.	13. Maintains patency of port.

3. Purposes of CVP monitoring are to serve as a guide for fluid replacement and to monitor pressures in the right atrium and central veins.
4. The CVP catheter can also be used:
   a. To obtain venous access when peripheral vein sites are inadequate.
   b. To obtain central venous blood samples.
   c. To administer blood products, total parenteral nutrition, and some drug therapies contraindicated for peripheral infusion.
   d. To insert a temporary pacemaker.

Pulmonary Artery Pressure Monitoring

Purposes
1. To monitor pressures in the right atrium (CVP), right ventricle, pulmonary artery, and distal branches of the pulmonary artery (known as *pulmonary artery occlusion pressure*, or *pulmonary artery wedge pressure*). The latter reflects the level of the pressure in the left atrium (or filling pressure in the left ventricle); thus, pressures on the left side of the heart are inferred from pressure measurement obtained on the right side of the circulation.
2. To measure CO through thermodilution.
3. To obtain blood for central venous oxygen saturation.

4. To continuously monitor mixed venous oxygen saturation (SvO_2); available on special catheters.
5. To provide for temporary atrial/ventricular pacing and intra-atrial ECG (available only on special catheters).
6. To evaluate the hemodynamic response to fluid therapy, medications, and other treatments.

Underlying Considerations
1. Left atrial pressure is closely related to left ventricular end diastolic pressure (LVEDP—filling pressure of the left ventricle) and is therefore an indicator of left ventricular function. Because there are no valves in the pulmonary arterial system when the Swan Ganz catheter is wedged, it reflects an uninterrupted flow of blood to the left atrium.
2. The pulmonary artery diastolic pressure (PADP) reflects the LVEDP in patients with normal lungs and mitral valve. The PADP can be continuously monitored as an approximation of LVEDP (limits excessive balloon inflation to obtain a PAOP and subsequent risk of balloon rupture or damage to the pulmonary artery).
3. SaO_2 is affected by four factors: CO, hemoglobin, arterial oxygen saturation (SaO_2), and tissue oxygen consumption.
4. Changes in SaO_2 alert the clinician to changes in these factors. More rapid detection of change facilitates interventions to correct problems before significant deterioration in patient's condition occurs.

5. If the amount of oxygen supplied to the tissues is inadequate to meet demands, more oxygen will be extracted from venous blood and SaO_2 will decrease. If oxygen supply exceeds demand, SaO_2 will increase.

6. Pulmonary artery (PA) catheters are associated with significant risk and disadvantages, including increased cost and mortality. Placement of a PA catheter is invasive and does not directly impact patient outcomes.

Methods

1. The Swan-Ganz catheter is a flow-directed (1.5 mL), balloon-tipped, 4- to 5-lumen catheter that is percutaneously inserted at the bedside and allows for continuous PAP monitoring as well as periodic measurement of PAOP and other parameters.

2. The catheter is 110 cm long, marked at increments of 10 cm, and is available in varying diameters.

3. Most catheters in use incorporate thermodilution for determination of CO.

4. If monitoring of $S\bar{v}O_2$ is desired, a PA catheter incorporating fiber optics is used.

5. If temporary cardiac pacing capability is desired, a catheter with a lumen for a pacing wire may be used.

6. Catheter may be inserted under fluoroscopy or at the bedside using the hemodynamic waveform as a guide to correct position.

Newer Technology for Hemodynamic Monitoring

Complications associated with insertion of invasive pulmonary artery catheters have led to the development of newer noninvasive or minimally invasive methods of hemodynamic monitoring.

1. Indirect Fick method—modification of the original Fick principle first developed in 1870.

2. Thoracic electrical bioimpedence (TEB)—noninvasive measurement of the electrical resistance of the thorax to a high-frequency, very-low-magnitude current. As thoracic fluid in the chest increases, TEB decreases; changes in CO correspond to changes in aortic blood flow.

3. Pulse contour devices—measure CO by assessing the contours of arterial pressure waveforms in relationship to the patient's stroke volume.

4. Continuous SvO_2 monitoring—measures mixed venous oxygen by means of a modified PA catheter to assess oxygen-carrying hemoglobin (oxyhemoglobin) and non-oxygen-carrying hemoglobin (deoxyhemoglobin).

5. Continuous CO monitoring—utilizes a modified PA catheter.

6. Right ventricular ejection fraction measurement—assesses the amount of blood forced from the ventricle during systole; it is an indication of the strength or contractility of the heart as determined by a special type of arterial catheter.

7. Esophageal Doppler CO monitoring—utilizes sound waves to measure aortic blood flow and thereby determine SV.

8. Exhaled CO_2 monitoring—completely noninvasive technique based on the Fick equation that measures CO.

9. Lithium dilution CO is another thermodilution method that assesses CO through injection of lithium chloride into a central or peripheral venous catheter and measurement of the concentration of lithium chloride over time using lithium-sensitive electrodes.

10. Cardiac MRI measures cardiac output by looking at blood flow generated by the picture from the magnetic current. It calculates the stroke volume, which is multiplied by heart rate.

11. Bioimpedance CO determination measures changes in the body's resistance to small electrical current. Blood volume in the chest changes during every ejection, which can be detected using eight electrical patches positioned on the neck and thorax. Based on these changes in impedance, a computer can calculate the cardiac output.

Cardiac Pacing

 Evidence Base Lynn-McHale Wiegand, D. J. (Ed.). (2011). *AACN procedure manual for critical care* (6th ed.). St. Louis, MO: Saunders.

A *cardiac pacemaker* is an electronic device that delivers direct electrical stimulation to stimulate the myocardium to depolarize, initiating a mechanical contraction. The pacemaker initiates and maintains the heart rate when the heart's natural pacemaker is unable to do so. Pacemakers can be used to correct bradycardias, tachycardias, sick sinus syndrome, and second- and third-degree heart blocks, and for prophylaxis. Pacing may be accomplished through a permanent implantable system, a temporary system with an external pulse generator and percutaneously threaded leads, or a transcutaneous external system with electrode pads placed over the chest (see Procedure Guidelines 12-4).

Clinical Indications

1. Symptomatic bradydysrhythmias.
2. Symptomatic sinus bradycardia that results from required drug therapy.
3. Symptomatic heart block.
    a. Mobitz II second-degree heart block.
    b. Complete heart block.
    c. Bifascicular and trifascicular bundle-branch blocks.
4. Hypersensitive carotid sinus syndrome and neurocardiogenic syncope.
5. Prophylaxis.
    a. After acute MI: dysrhythmia and conduction defects.
    b. Before or after cardiac surgery.
    c. During cardiac resynchronization therapy in patients with severe systolic heart failure.
    d. During diagnostic testing.
        i. Cardiac catheterization.
        ii. EPS.
        iii. PTCA.
        iv. Stress testing.
        v. Before permanent pacing.
6. Tachydysrhythmias; to override rapid rhythm disturbances.
    a. Supraventricular tachycardia.
    b. Ventricular tachycardia.

PROCEDURE GUIDELINES 12-4

Transcutaneous Cardiac Pacing

EQUIPMENT
- Disposable multifunction defibrillator/ pacing/ECG electrode pads
- External pacing module
- Resuscitative equipment

PROCEDURE

Nursing Action	Rationale
Preparatory phase	
1. Explain procedure to patient.	1. Allays anxiety.
2. Explain sensation of discomfort with external pacing.	2. Discomfort is felt with each firing but can be relieved with analgesics.
Performance phase	
1. Place multifunction electrode pads as follows:	1. Electrodes must be placed so the current passes through as much of the myocardium as possible with the least distance between the pads.
a. Anterior/posterior: The negative multifunction electrode pad is placed on the anterior chest at the V_3–V_6 position; the positive multifunction electrode pad is placed directly behind the anterior pad on the patient's back.	a. Manufacturer includes diagram on the electrode package and the electrodes themselves.
b. Anterior/lateral: The positive multifunction electrode pad is placed on the upper right chest under the clavicle; the negative multifunction electrode pad is placed at the V_3–V_6 position.	
2. Attach three-lead electrode monitoring, as required.	2. Some devices will not pace if three-lead monitoring is not attached.
3. Make sure that pacing module is off or on standby and that milliamperes (mA) output is set at the minimal level before connecting electrodes to external module.	3. Prevents accidental shock on connection.
4. Connect multifunction pacing electrode pads to external module.	
5. Determine rate setting according to instructions and patient condition. If patient's heart rate is consistently too low to maintain adequate cardiac output, set rate at 70–80. If the patient's rate falls only intermittently and the pacemaker will be used in the demand mode, set rate at 60.	5. Can be set at a fixed rate or on demand to pace only if heart rate falls below the set rate.
6. Gradually increase mA output until a pacing spike and a corresponding QRS complex is seen (perhaps as high as 70 mA or more).	6. If using the demand mode, set the rate higher than the patient's rate to establish the correct output and capture, then return the rate to 60.
7. Palpate pulse on right side to ensure adequate response to electrical event.	7. Choose either right radial or brachial pulse since muscular contractions that may be transferred down the left arm can cause misinterpretation.
8. Check pad placement frequently.	8. Patient perspiration may cause pads to loosen or slip.
Follow-up phase	
1. Check vital signs at least every 15 minutes while continuous pacing is employed. Check blood pressure in right arm.	1. Determines if cardiac output is adequate. Muscle contraction from pacing may interfere with blood pressure reading on left.
2. Monitor ECG continuously for pacer functioning.	2. Detects malfunction (may occur due to electrode loosening).
3. Assure patient that treatment is temporary and prepare patient for transvenous or permanent pacemaker insertion as indicated.	3. Should only be used continuously for 2 hours because sensation may be uncomfortable.
4. Change the multifunction electrode pads every 24 hours.	4. Decreased efficacy of gel pad after 24 hours or per manufacturer guidelines.

Evidence Base Lynn-McHale Wiegard, D. J. (Ed.). (2011). *AACN procedure manual for critical care* (6th ed.). Philadelphia: Elsevier.

Types of Pacing

Permanent Pacemakers

1. Used to treat chronic heart conditions; surgically placed utilizing a local anesthetic, the leads are placed transvenously in the appropriate chamber of the heart and then anchored to the endocardium.
2. The pulse generator is placed in a surgically made pocket in subcutaneous tissue under the clavicle or in the abdomen. Choices for types of generators include single or dual chamber devices, biventricular devices, unipolar or bipolar pacing/sensing configuration, and various types of sensors for rate response.
3. Once placed, it can be programmed externally as needed.

Temporary Pacemakers

1. Temporary pacemakers are usually placed during an emergency, such as when a patient demonstrates signs of decreased CO.
2. Indicated for patients with high-grade AV blocks, bradycardia, or low CO. They serve as a bridge until the patient becomes stable enough for placement of a permanent pacemaker.
3. Can be placed transvenously, epicardially, transcutaneously, and transthoracically.
   a. Transvenous pacemakers are inserted transvenously (into a vein, usually the subclavian, internal jugular, antecubital, or femoral) into the right ventricle (or right atrium and right ventricle for dual-chamber pacing) and then attached to an external pulse generator. This procedure may be done at the bedside or under fluoroscopy.
   b. Epicardial pacemaker wires are attached to the endocardium, brought out through a surgical incision in the thorax. These wires are then connected to an external pulse generator. This is commonly seen after cardiac surgery.
   c. With transcutaneous pacing, noninvasive multifunction electrode pads are placed either anterior-posteriorly (anterior chest wall under left nipple, slightly midaxillary, and on the patient's back directly behind anterior pad) or anterior-laterally (anterior chest wall under left nipple, slightly midaxillary, and on patient's upper right chest wall below the clavicle) (see Figure 12-4). The multifunction electrode pads are connected to an external energy source (defibrillator with pacing ability). The electrical impulses flow through the multifunction electrode pads and subcutaneous skin to the heart, thereby pacing the heart.
   d. The transthoracic pacemaker is a type of temporary pacemaker that is placed only in an emergency via a long needle, using a subxiphoid approach. The pacer wire is then placed directly into the right ventricle.

Biventricular Pacemakers

1. Biventricular pacemakers are also referred to as cardiac resynchronization therapy.
2. Biventricular pacing is used to treat moderate to severe heart failure as a result of left ventricular dyssynchrony.
3. Intraventricular conduction defects result in an uncoordinated contraction of the left and right ventricle, which causes a wide QRS complex and is associated with worsening heart failure and increased mortality.

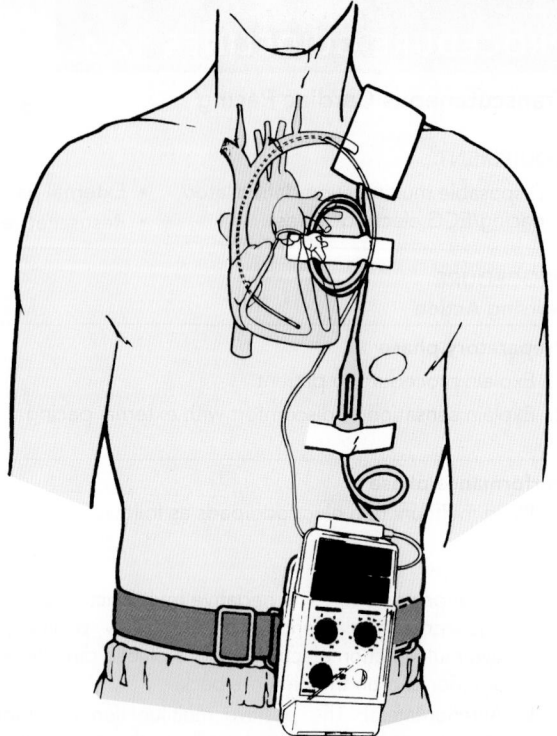

Figure 12-4. Temporary transvenous pacer wire with external pulse generator. (Courtesy of Medtronic, Inc.)

4. Biventricular pacemakers utilize three leads (one in the right atrium, one in the right ventricle, and one in the left ventricle via the coronary sinus) to coordinate ventricular contraction and improve CO.
5. Biventricular pacemakers can incorporate implantable cardioverter defibrillators or be used alone.

Pacemaker Design

Pulse Generator

Contains the circuitry and batteries to generate the electrical signal.

1. The pulse generator in a permanent pacemaker is encapsulated in a metal box that is embedded under the skin. The box protects the generator from electromagnetic interferences and trauma.
2. A temporary pacing generator is contained in a small box with dials for programming (see Figure 12-4). It is an external system.
   a. Transcutaneous pacing systems utilize an external energy source such as a defibrillator with pacing ability. Dials for programming the unit are on the device.
   b. Electromechanical interference is more likely to occur with temporary systems.
   c. Temporary pacing systems use batteries, which need replacement based on use of device. The transcutaneous system has rechargeable battery circuitry but should be plugged into an electrical outlet most of the time.
3. Permanent pacing systems use reliable power sources such as lithium batteries. Lithium batteries have a projected life span of 8 to 12 years.

Pacemaker Lead

Transmits the electrical signal from the pulse generator to the heart. One or two leads may be placed in the heart.

1. "Single-chamber" pacemaker.
   a. "Single-chamber" pacemakers have one lead in either the atrial or ventricular chamber.
   b. The sensing and pacing capabilities of the pacemaker are confined to the chamber where the lead is placed.
2. "Dual-chamber" pacemaker.
   a. A "dual-chamber" pacemaker has two leads.
   b. One lead is in the atrium and the other lead is located in the ventricle.
   c. Pacing and sensing can occur in both heart chambers, closely "mimicking" normal heart function (physiologic pacing).
3. Biventricular pacemaker.
   a. One lead is in the right atrium, one is in the right ventricle and one is in the left ventricle via the coronary sinus.
   b. In single right ventricle (traditional) pacing there is slight delay of the left ventricle contracting as the electrical impulse begins in the right ventricle and moves to the left ventricle, giving the characteristic left bundle branch block appearance. By pacing both right and left ventricle at the same time, the pacemaker can resynchronize a heart whose opposing walls do not contract in synchrony.
4. Pacemaker leads may be threaded through a vein into the right atrium and/or right ventricle (endocardial/transvenous approach) or introduced by direct penetration of the chest wall and attached to the left ventricle or right atrium (see Figure 12-5).
5. Fixation devices located at the end of the pacemaker lead allow for secure attachment of the lead to the heart, reducing the possibility of lead dislodgement.
6. Temporary leads protrude from the incision and are connected to the external pulse generator. Permanent leads are connected to the pulse generator implanted underneath the skin.

Pacemaker Function

Cardiac pacing refers to the ability of the pacemaker to stimulate either the atrium, the ventricle, or both heart chambers in sequence and initiate electrical depolarization and cardiac contraction. Cardiac pacing is evidenced on the ECG by the presence of a "spike" or "pacing artifact."

Pacing Functions

1. Atrial pacing—direct stimulation of the right atrium producing a "spike" on the ECG preceding a P wave.
2. Ventricular pacing—direct stimulation of the right or left ventricle producing a "spike" on the ECG preceding a QRS complex.
3. AV pacing—direct stimulation of the right atrium and either ventricle in sequence; mimics normal cardiac conduction, allowing the atria to contract before the ventricles. ("Atrial kick" received by the ventricles allows for an increase in CO.)

Sensing Functions

Cardiac pacemakers have the ability to "see" intrinsic cardiac activity when it occurs (sensing).

1. Demand—ability to "sense" intrinsic cardiac activity and deliver a pacing stimulus only if the heart rate falls below a preset rate limit.
2. Fixed—no ability to "sense" intrinsic cardiac activity; the pacemaker can't "synchronize" with the heart's natural activity and consistently delivers a pacing stimulus at a preset rate.
3. Triggered—ability to deliver pacing stimuli in response to "sensing" a cardiac event.
   a. "Sees" atrial activity (P waves) and delivers a pacing spike to the ventricle after an appropriate delay (usually 0.16 second, similar to PR interval).
   b. Maintains AV synchrony and increases heart rate based on increases in the body demands that occur with exercise or during stress.
   c. "Physiologic" sensors are being developed as alternatives to "trigger" a ventricular response because many patients have atrial dysfunction.
   d. "Sensor-driven" rate-responsive pacemakers do not sense atrial activity; a triggered ventricular beat occurs when the pacemaker senses either increases in muscle activity, temperature, oxygen utilization, or changes in blood pH.

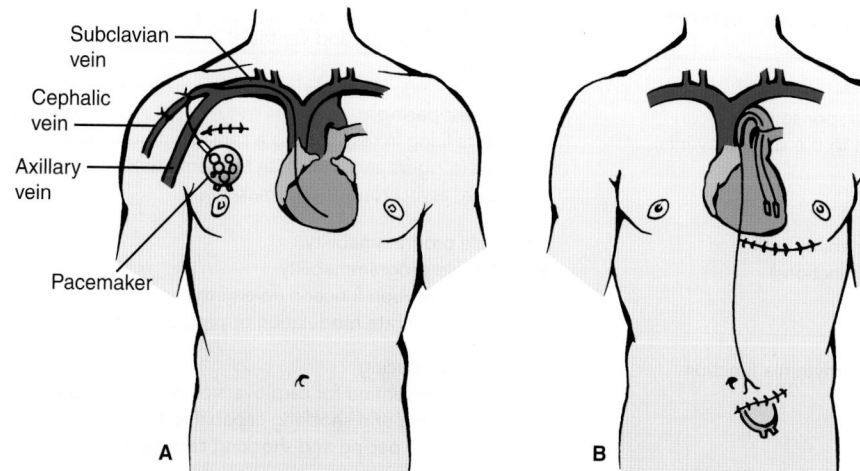

Subclavian vein

Cephalic vein

Axillary vein

Pacemaker

A

B

FIGURE 12-5. (A) The catheter is unipolar and is threaded to the apical area of the right ventricle via a major vein. **(B)** The catheter is bipolar and is passed through an opening in the chest wall and is sutured to the external surface of the left ventricle.

Capture Functions

1. The pacemaker's ability to generate a response from the heart (contraction) after electrical stimulation is referred to as capture. Capture is determined by the strength of the electrical stimulus, measured in milliamperes (mA), the amount of time the stimulus is applied to the heart (pulse width), and by contact of the distal tip of the pacing lead to healthy myocardial tissue.
   a. "Electrical" capture is indicated by a P wave or QRS following and corresponding to a pacemaker spike.
   b. "Mechanical" capture of the ventricles is determined by a palpable pulse corresponding to the electrical event.

Pacemaker Codes

The Intersociety Commission for Heart Disease (ICHD) has established a five-letter code to describe the normal functioning of today's sophisticated pacemakers. Each letter indicates the particular characteristic of the pacer (see Table 12-2).

Nursing Assessment and Preprocedure Care for Permanent Pacemaker Implantation

1. Assess patient's knowledge level of procedure.
2. Instruct patient that he or she may have nothing by mouth before the procedure.
3. Facilitate IV line insertion.
4. Explain to patient that pacemaker insertion will be performed in an operating or special procedures room with fluoroscopically and continuous ECG monitoring.
5. Describe local anesthetic that will be used to minimize discomfort; sedation.
6. Explain to patient that the usual placement for a permanent pacemaker is in the left upper chest.
7. The incision will be closed with Steri-strips (suture or staples may also be used).

Nursing Diagnoses

- Decreased Cardiac Output related to potential pacemaker malfunction and dysrhythmias.
- Risk for Injury related to pneumothorax, hemothorax, bleeding, microshock, and accidental malfunction.
- Risk for Infection related to surgical implantation of pacemaker generator and/or leads.
- Anxiety related to pacemaker insertion, fear of death, lack of knowledge, and role change.
- Impaired Physical Mobility related to imposed restrictions of arm movement.
- Acute Pain related to surgical incision and transcutaneous external pacing stimuli.
- Disturbed Body Image related to pacemaker implantation.

Nursing Interventions

Maintaining Adequate Cardiac Output

1. Record the following information after insertion of the pacemaker:
   a. Pacemaker manufacturer, model, and lead type.
   b. Operating mode (based on ICHD code).
   c. Programmed settings: lower rate limit; upper rate limit; AV delay; pacing thresholds.
   d. Patient's underlying rhythm.
   e. Patient's response to procedure.

Table 12-2	Five-Letter Code for Pacemakers	
LETTER OR POSITION	**CHARACTERISTIC**	**CODE KEY**
I	Chamber paced (Where is the pacing taking place?)	V = Ventricle A = Atrium D = Dual (Both atrium and ventricle) O = None
II	Chamber sensed (Which chamber is being sensed?)	V = Ventricle A = Atrium D = Dual (Both atrium and ventricle) O = None
III	Mode of response (Response to the sensed events)	T = Triggers pacing I = Inhibits firing in response to a sensed intrinsic event D = Dual (triggers and inhibits at the same time) O = None; asynchronous pacemaker
IV	Programmability (Program functions)	P = Single programmability M = Multiple programmability C = Communication function (telemetry) O = Absence of rate modulation or programmability
V	Antitachyarrhythmia function	P = Overdrive pacing S = Shock intervention for cardioversion or defibrillation D = Dual (Pacing and shocking capabilities) O = Absence of pacing and shocking capabilities

2. Attach ECG electrodes for continuous monitoring of heart rate and rhythm.
   a. Set alarm limits 5 beats below lower rate limit and 5 to 10 beats above upper rate limits (ensures immediate detection of pacemaker malfunction or failure).
   b. Keep alarms on at all times.
3. Analyze rhythm strips per facility protocol and as necessary.
   a. Identify presence or absence of pacing artifact.
   b. Differentiate paced P waves and paced QRS complexes from spontaneous beats.
   c. Measure AV delay (if pacemaker has dual chamber functions).
   d. Determine the paced rate.
   e. Analyze the paced rhythm for presence and consistency of capture (every pacing spike is followed by atrial and/or ventricular depolarization).
   f. Analyze the rhythm for presence and consistency of proper sensing. (After a spontaneous beat, the pacemaker should not fire unless the interval between the spontaneous beat and the paced beat equals the lower pacing rate and/or the paced beat follows the programmed AV delay.)
4. Monitor vital signs as per facility protocol, and as necessary.
5. Monitor urine output and level of consciousness—ensures adequate cardiac output achieved with paced rhythm.
6. Observe for dysrhythmias (ventricular ectopic activity can occur because of irritation of ventricular wall by lead wire).
   a. Monitor for competitive rhythms, such as runs of atrial fibrillation or flutter, accelerated junctional or idioventricular or ventricular tachycardia.
   b. Report dysrhythmias.
   c. Administer antidysrhythmic therapy, as directed.
7. Obtain 12-lead ECG, as ordered.

> **NURSING ALERT** Transport patient to other parts of facility with portable ECG monitoring and nurse. Patients with temporary pacemakers should never be placed in unmonitored areas.

Avoiding Injury

1. Note that a postpacemaker insertion chest x-ray has been taken to ensure correct lead wire position and that no fluid is in lungs.
2. Monitor for signs and symptoms of hemothorax—inadvertent punctures of the subclavian vein or artery, which can cause fatal hemorrhage; observe for diaphoresis, hypotension, shortness of breath, chest deviation, and restlessness; immediate surgical intervention may be necessary.
3. Monitor for signs and symptoms of pneumothorax—inadvertent puncture of the lung; observe for acute onset of dyspnea, cyanosis, chest pain, absent breath sounds over involved lung, acute anxiety, hypotension. Prepare for chest tube insertion.
4. Evaluate continually for evidence of bleeding.
   a. Check incision site frequently for bleeding.

   b. Apply manual pressure carefully without pushing against pacemaker generator box.
   c. Palpate for pulses distal to insertion site. (Swelling of tissues from bleeding may impede arterial flow.)
5. Monitor for evidence of lead migration and perforation of heart.
   a. Observe for muscle twitching and/or cough (may indicate chest wall or diaphragmatic pacing).
   b. Evaluate patient's complaints of chest pain (may indicate perforation of pericardial sac).
   c. Auscultate for pericardial friction rub.
   d. Observe for signs and symptoms of cardiac tamponade: distant heart sounds, distended jugular veins, pulsus paradoxus, and hypotension.
6. Provide an electrically safe environment for patient. Stray electrical current can enter the heart through temporary pacemaker lead system and induce dysrhythmias.
   a. Protect exposed parts of electrode lead terminal in temporary pacing systems per manufacturer recommendations.
   b. Wear rubber gloves when touching temporary pacing leads. (Static electricity from your hands can enter the patient's body through the lead system.)
   c. Make sure all equipment is grounded with three-prong plugs inserted into a proper outlet when using an external pacing system.
   d. Epicardial pacing wires should have the terminal needles protected by a plastic tube; place tube in rubber glove to protect it from fluids or electrical current.
7. Be aware of hazards in the facility that can interfere with pacemaker function or cause pacemaker failure and permanent pacemaker damage.
   a. Avoid use of electric razors.
   b. Avoid direct placement of defibrillator paddles over pacemaker generator; anterior placement of paddles should be 4 to 5 inches (10 to 12.5 cm) away from pacemaker; always evaluate pacemaker function after defibrillation.
   c. Electrocautery devices and transcutaneous electrical stimulator (TENS) units pose a risk.
   d. Recent studies have shown that patients may safely have an MRI with a permanent pacemaker. Check with cardiologist.

> **Evidence Base** Nazarian, S., Hansford, R., Roquin, A., et al. (2011). A prospective evaluation of a protocol for magnetic resonance imaging of patients with implanted cardiac devices. *Annals of Internal Medicine*, 155, 415–424.

   e. Caution must be used if patient will receive radiation therapy; the pacemaker should be repositioned if the unit lies directly in the radiation field.
8. Prevent accidental pacemaker malfunctions.
   a. Use clear plastic covering over external temporary generators at all times (eliminates potential manipulation of programmed settings).

b. Secure temporary pacemaker generator to patient's chest or waist; never hang it on an IV pole.

c. Transfer of patient from bed to stretcher should only be attempted with an adequate number of personnel so that patient can remain passive; caution personnel to avoid underarm lifts.

d. Evaluate transcutaneous pacing electrode pads every 2 hours for secure contact to chest wall; change electrode pads every 24 hours or if pads do not have complete contact with skin.

   Note: Transcutaneous pacing should not be utilized continuously for more than 2 hours. Transvenous pacing should then be initiated.

9. Monitor for electrolyte imbalances, hypoxia, and myocardial ischemia. (The amount of energy the pacemaker needs to stimulate depolarization may need adjustment if any of these are present.)

Preventing Infection

Permanent Pacemaker

1. Take temperature every 4 hours; report elevations. (Suspect permanent pacemaker as infection source if temperature elevation occurs.)

2. Observe incision site for signs and symptoms of local infection: redness, purulent drainage, warmth, soreness.

3. Be alert to manifestations of bacteremia. (Patients with endocardial leads are at risk for endocarditis; see page 401.)

4. Clean incision site, as directed, using sterile technique.

5. Instruct patient to keep incision site dry, which means no showers for 24 hours.

6. Evaluate patient's complaints of increasing tenderness and discomfort at incision site.

7. Administer antibiotic therapy, as prescribed, after permanent pacemaker insertion.

Temporary Pacemaker

1. Monitor temperature every 4 hours; report elevations.

2. Assess central IV site (where temporary pacing wire is inserted) for signs and symptoms of infection, such as redness and drainage.

Relieving Anxiety

1. Offer careful explanations regarding anticipated procedures and treatments, and answer the patient's questions with concise explanations.

2. Use sedation, as necessary, when inserting temporary pacemaker.

3. When using transcutaneous pacing, always sedate the patient because the level of mA used is high, and the patient may feel the uncomfortable stimulus (twitching).

4. Encourage patient and family to use coping mechanisms to overcome anxieties—talking, crying, and walking.

5. Encourage patient to accept responsibility for care.

   a. Review care plan with patient and family.

   b. Encourage patient to make decisions regarding a daily schedule of self-care activities.

   c. Engage patient in goal-setting. Establish with patient priorities of care and time frames to accomplish goals up until discharge.

6. Monitor for unwarranted fears expressed by patient and family (commonly, pacemaker failure) and provide explanations to alleviate fear. Explain to patient life expectancy of batteries and the measures taken to check for failure (see "Patient Education," page 355).

Minimizing the Effects of Immobility

1. Encourage patient to take deep breaths frequently each hour (promotes pulmonary function); however, caution against vigorous coughing because this could cause lead dislodgement.

2. Instruct patient in dorsiflexion exercises of ankles and tightening of calf muscles. This promotes venous return and prevents venous stasis. Exercises should be done hourly.

3. Restrict movement of affected extremity.

   a. Place arm nearest to permanent pacemaker implant in sling as directed. Sling use can range from 6 to 24 hours, according to prescribed order.

   b. Instruct patient to gradually resume range of motion (ROM) of extremity as directed (usually 24 hours for permanent implants); avoid over-the-head motions for approximately 5 days and limit the weight of carried items to less than 3 pounds.

   c. Evaluate patient's arm movements to ensure normal ROM progression; assist patient with passive ROM of extremity as necessary (prevents development of shoulder stiffness caused by prolonged joint immobility); consult physical therapy as directed if stiffness and pain occur.

4. Assist patient with activities of daily living (ADLs) as appropriate.

Relieving Pain

1. Prepare patient for the discomfort he or she may experience after pacemaker implant.

   a. Explain to patient that incisional pain will occur after procedure; pain will subside after the first week, but he or she may have some soreness for up to 4 weeks.

2. Administer analgesics as directed; attempt to coincide peak analgesic effect with performance of ROM exercises and ADLs.

3. Offer back rubs to promote relaxation.

4. Provide patient with diversional activities.

5. Evaluate effectiveness of pain-relieving modalities.

6. Explain to the patient about the potential for discomfort during transcutaneous pacing; however, assure patient that the lowest energy possible will be used and analgesics/anxiolytics will be given.

Maintaining a Positive Body Image

1. Encourage patient and family to express concerns regarding self-image and pacemaker implant.

2. Reassure patient and significant other that sexual activity and modes of dressing will not be altered by pacemaker implantation.

3. Offer pacemaker support group information to the patient.

4. Encourage spouse or significant other to discuss concerns of self-image with patient.

Patient Education and Health Maintenance

Anatomy and Physiology of the Heart

Use diagrams to identify heart structure, conduction system, area where pacemaker is inserted, and why the pacemaker is needed.

Pacemaker Function

1. Give patient the manufacturer's instructions (for particular pacemaker) and help familiarize patient with pacemaker.
2. If available, give patient a pacemaker to hold and identify unique features of patient's pacemaker; or, show patient picture of pacemaker.
3. Explain to patient the purpose and function of the component parts of the pacemaker: generator and lead system.

Activity

1. Reassure patient that normal activities will be able to be resumed.
2. Explain to patient that it takes about 2 months to develop full ROM of arm (fibrosis occurs around the lead and stabilizes it in heart).
3. Specific instructions include the following:
   a. Instruct patient not to lift items over 3 lb (1.4 kg) or perform difficult arm maneuvers.
   b. Tell patient to avoid activities that involve rough contact around pacemaker site.
   d. Caution patient not to fire a rifle with it resting over pacemaker implant.
   e. Sexual activity may be resumed when desired.
   f. Instruct patient not to rub or massage around pacemaker site.
4. Instruct patient to gauge activities according to sensations of moderate pain in arm or site of implant and stretching sensation in and around implant site.

Pacemaker Failure

1. Teach patient to check own pulse rate daily for 1 full minute and to keep a chart for physician visit. This pulse check should be done at rest. (Patients may check pulse daily to ensure all is well and promote a sense of control.)
2. Teach the patient to:
   a. Immediately report slowing of pulse lower than set rate, or greater than 100.
   b. Report signs and symptoms of dizziness, fainting, palpitation, prolonged hiccups, and chest pain to health care provider immediately. These signs are indicative of pacemaker failure.
   c. Take pulse while these feelings are being experienced.
3. Encourage patient to wear identification bracelet and carry pacemaker identification card that lists pacemaker type, rate, health care provider's name, and facility where the pacemaker was inserted; encourage significant other to also keep a card with patient's pacemaker information.

Electromagnetic Interference

1. Advise patient that improvements in pacemaker design have reduced problems of electromechanical interference (EMI).
2. Caution patient that EMI could interfere with pacemaker function.
   a. Inappropriate inhibition or triggering of pacemaker stimuli causing light-headedness, syncope, or death.

b. Atrial oversensing may cause inappropriate pacemaker acceleration and can cause palpitations, hypotension, or angina in patients.
   c. Rapid pacing can also result in ventricular fibrillation.
   d. Reversion to a synchronous pacing mode. A common response to transient reversion is asynchrony pacing, which can cause irregular heartbeats and/or a decrease in CO, and that may stimulate ventricular tachyarrhythmias.
   e. Reprogramming of the pacemaker or permanent damage to the pacemaker's circuitry or the electrode-tissue interface are less frequent in occurrence.
   f. Teach patient to move 4 to 6 feet away from source and to check pulse if dizziness or palpitations occur. Pulse should return to normal after moving away from interference.
3. Explain that high-energy radiation, linear power amplifiers, antennas, industrial arc welders, electrocautery equipment, TENS, unshielded motors (cars, boats), MRI equipment found in facilities, and junkyards may affect pacemaker function.
4. Tell patient that metal detectors or handheld wands may affect pacemaker function and that pacemakers will set off the alarm at metal detector gates. Therefore, patient should show pacemaker identification card and request a hand search.
5. Antitheft devices may interfere with pacemaker function if the patient remains stationary for an extended period of time near the device. Walking by the device should not interfere with pacemaker function.
6. Tell patient that household and kitchen appliances will not affect pacemaker function. Microwave ovens are no longer a threat to pacemaker operation (however, old warning signs may still be near microwave ovens). Cell phones are safe as long as they are 6 inches away from pacemaker site. Encourage patient to use the ear on the opposite side of the pacemaker site.

Care of Pacemaker Site

1. Advise patient to wear loose-fitting clothing around the area of pacemaker implantation until it has healed.
2. Watch for signs and symptoms of infection around generator and leads—fever, heat, pain, and skin breakdown at implant site.
3. Advise patient to keep incision clean and dry. Encourage tub baths rather than showers for the first 10 days after pacemaker implantation.
   a. Instruct patient not to scrub incision site or clean site with bath water.
   b. Teach patient to clean incision site with antiseptic, as directed.
4. Explain to patient that healing will take approximately 3 months.
   a. Instruct patient to maintain a well-balanced diet to promote healing.

 GERONTOLOGIC ALERT Older patients may experience delayed wound healing because of poor nutritional status. Evaluate nutritional intake carefully and offer a balanced diet to ensure proper healing.

5. Inform patient that there is no increased risk of endocarditis with dental cleaning or procedures, so antibiotic prophylaxis is not necessary.

Follow-Up

1. Make sure that the patient has a copy of ECG tracing (according to facility policy) for future comparisons. Encourage patient to have regular pacemaker checkups for monitoring function and integrity of pacemaker.
2. Inform patient that transtelephonic evaluation of implanted cardiac pacemakers for battery and electrode failure is available.
3. Review medications with patient before discharge.
4. Inform patient that the pulse generator will have to be surgically removed to replace battery and that it is a relatively simple procedure performed under local anesthesia.

Evaluation: Expected Outcomes

- Vital signs stable; pacing spikes rated on ECG tracing.
- Breath sounds noted throughout; respirations unlabored.
- Incision without drainage.
- Asks questions and participates in care.
- Affected arm and pacer site show decreased edema.
- Reports pain relief.
- Verbalizes acceptance of pacemaker.

Defibrillation and Cardioversion

 Evidence Base Link, M. S., Atkins, D. L., Passman, R. S., et al. (2010). Electrical therapies: Automated external defibrillators, defibrillation, cardioversion, and pacing. *Circulation, 122,* s706–719.

Concepts

1. *Defibrillation* is the use of electrical energy, delivered over a brief period, to temporarily depolarize the heart. When it repolarizes it has a better chance of resuming normal activity. See Procedure Guidelines 12-5.
2. *Synchronized cardioversion* is the use of electrical energy that is synchronized to the QRS complex so as not to hit the T wave during the cardiac cycle, which may cause ventricular fibrillation. See Procedure Guidelines 12-6, pages 358 to 359.
3. A *defibrillator* is an instrument that delivers an electric shock to the heart to convert the dysrhythmia to normal sinus rhythm. (Defibrillators are not used to convert other abnormal and rapid cardiac rhythms.) There are several types of defibrillators:
   a. Direct current defibrillators contain a transformer, an alternating-current–direct-current converter, a capacitor to store direct current, a charge switch, and a discharge switch to the electrodes to complete the circuit.
   b. Portable defibrillators have a battery as a power source and must be plugged in at all times when not in use.
   c. Automatic external defibrillator (AED) may be used inside the facility or in the community to deliver electric shock

to the heart before trained personnel arrive with a manual defibrillator. AEDs are accurate to be used by less trained individuals because the device has a detection system that analyzes the person's rhythm, detects the presence of ventricular fibrillation or tachycardia, and instructs the operator to discharge a shock. See Procedure Guidelines 12-7, pages 360 and 361.

Indications

Defibrillation

1. Ventricular fibrillation.
2. Ventricular tachycardia without a pulse.

Synchronized Cardioversion

1. Atrial fibrillation.
2. Atrial flutter.
3. Supraventricular tachycardia.
4. Ventricular tachycardia with a pulse.

Implantable Cardioverter-Defibrillator

The *implantable cardioverter-defibrillator (ICD)* is a device that delivers electric shocks directly to the heart muscle (defibrillation) in order to terminate lethal dysrhythmias: ventricular fibrillation and ventricular tachycardia (see Figure 12-6, page 361). The ICD is surgically placed by one of four approaches: lateral thoracotomy, median sternotomy (in conjunction with cardiac surgery), subxiphoid, or subintercostal. All ICDs have a pacing function, if needed.

Concepts

1. Sudden cardiac death as a result of ventricular tachycardia or fibrillation remains the leading cause of death in the United States.
2. ICDs terminate ventricular fibrillation and tachycardia automatically, thereby preventing sudden death.
3. Currently, ICDs can deliver high-energy or low-energy shocks, can be programmed for demand and rate-response pacing, can be programmed for antitachycardic pacing, provide noninvasive electrical stimulation to conduct EPS, can be programmed for tiered therapy, and have the ability to record and store ECGs of tachycardic episodes.

Indications

1. Cardiac arrest due to ventricular fibrillation or tachycardia not due to transient or reversible causes.
2. Spontaneous sustained ventricular tachycardia with structural heart disease.
3. Syncope of undetermined origin with clinically relevant, hemodynamically significant ventricular tachycardia or ventricular fibrillation induced by EPS when drug therapy is not effective or tolerated.
4. Nonsustained ventricular tachycardia in patients with CAD, prior MI, left ventricular dysfunction, and inducible ventricular fibrillation or sustained ventricular tachycardia at EPS that is not suppressed by Class I antiarrhythmic drugs.

(Text continues on page 359)

PROCEDURE GUIDELINES 12-5

Direct Current Defibrillation for Ventricular Fibrillation*

EQUIPMENT

- Direct current defibrillator with paddles or multifunctional defibrillator pads
- Highly conductive multipurpose electrolyte gel

PROCEDURE

Nursing Action	Rationale
Preparatory phase	
Monitored patient	
1. If ventricular fibrillation is witnessed, precordial thump may be considered.	1. Minimizes cerebral ischemia and potentially restarts cardiac rhythm.
2. Immediately implement CPR until defibrillator is available.	2. CPR is essential before and after defibrillation to ensure blood supply to the cerebral and coronary arteries.
Unmonitored patient	
1. Expose anterior chest and move jewelry and transdermal patches away from area.	1. Jewelry/transdermal patches may interfere with electrical current and cause serious burns.
2. Immediately implement CPR until defibrillator is available. If response time is greater or equal to 5 minutes, perform 2 minutes of CPR prior to defibrillation.	2. Provides oxygenated blood supply to the cerebral and coronary arteries.
3. Apply multifunctional defibrillator pads or paddles with conductive gel to patient's bare chest.	3. Multipurpose electrolyte gel provides better conduction than paddles alone. Do not allow gel to be spread across the chest because this may cause severe burns to the patient's chest and may divert the current from traveling to the heart.
4. Apply paddles or multifunctional pads.	4. The paddles/pads are placed so that the electrical current flows through as much of the myocardium as possible.
a. Anterolateral position: Apply one paddle/pad to just the right of the sternum below the clavicle and the other paddle/pad to just the left of the cardiac apex (see accompanying figure, page 358).	
b. Anteroposterior position (pads only): Apply anterior pad over left apex and posterior pad under the infrascapular region.	b. In this method, the current directly traverses the heart.

 NURSING ALERT Paddles/pads should be placed at least 5 inches (12.7 cm) away from a pacemaker to prevent damage to pacemaker circuitry.

Nursing Action	Rationale
5. Remove oxygen from immediate area.	5. Prevents danger of fire or explosion.
6. Turn on defibrillator to the prescribed setting. The American Heart Association recommends that initial defibrillation should be 200 joules for biphasic or 360 joules for monophasic.	6. Biphasic is preferred over monophasic. Means that the machine delivers current that flows in one direction for a specified duration then reverses the current to flow in the other direction. Significantly lower energy levels are required with biphasic defibrillators.
7. For paddles:	7.
a. Grasp the paddles only by the insulated handles.	a. Prevents getting shocked.
b. Charge the paddles. Once paddles are charged, give the command "ALL CLEAR." Look around quickly to make sure everyone is clear from the patient and bed.	b. Prevents shock to a person who touches the bed.
c. Push the discharge buttons located on both of the handles of the paddles while simultaneously exerting 25 lb of pressure to each of the paddles.	c. If good skin contact is not maintained, the electrical current may take the path of least resistance and arc from one paddle to the other.

(continued)

PROCEDURE GUIDELINES 12-5 *(continued)*

Direct Current Defibrillation for Ventricular Fibrillation*

PROCEDURE *(continued)*

Nursing Action	Rationale

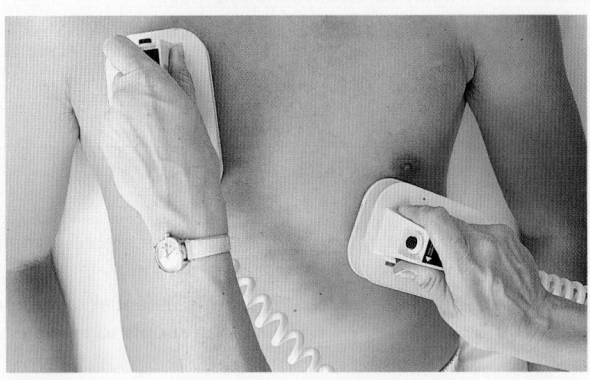

Paddle placement in ventricular defibrillation.

Nursing Action	Rationale

8. For multifunctional pads:
 	
  a. Press the charge button on the defibrillator machine. Once the charge is reached, give the command "ALL CLEAR." Look around quickly to make sure everyone is clear from the patient and bed.
 	
  b. Push the shock button on the defibrillator machine.
	8. Multifunctional pads provide hands-free defibrillation.

9. Resume CPR immediately after defibrillation.	9. Oxygenates the patient and restore circulation.

Follow-up phase

Nursing Action	Rationale
1. After the patient is defibrillated and rhythm is restored, antiarrhythmics are usually given to prevent recurrent episodes.	1. Any resultant arrhythmia may require appropriate drug intervention.
2. Continue with intensive monitoring and care.	2. The patient may remain in an unstable condition.

*Or pulseless ventricular tachycardia.

PROCEDURE GUIDELINES 12-6

Synchronized Cardioversion

EQUIPMENT

- Direct current defibrillator with paddles or multifunctional pads
- Highly conductive multipurpose electrolyte gel

PROCEDURE

Nursing Action	Rationale
1. If the procedure is elective, it is advisable to have the patient ingest nothing by mouth 12 hours before the cardioversion. Make sure to have working suction equipment available.	1. During sedation or the procedure, the patient may vomit and aspirate if the stomach is full.

2. Prepare the patient for the procedure.
 	
  a. Reassure the patient and make sure that informed consent has been obtained.
	2.
	
	  a. Allays anxiety and ensures understanding of the procedure.

PROCEDURE GUIDELINES 12-6 *(continued)*

Synchronized Cardioversion

PROCEDURE *(continued)*

Nursing Action	Rationale
b. Make sure the patient has not been taking digoxin and that serum potassium level is normal.	b. Low potassium level may precipitate postshock dysrhythmias.
3. Make sure IV line is secure.	3. An IV line is necessary for administration of emergency medications and sedation.
4. Obtain a 12-lead electrocardiogram (ECG) before and after cardioversion with the ECG machine.	4. An ECG is taken to ensure that the patient has not had a recent myocardial infarction or converted back to sinus rhythm prior to the cardioversion.
5. Make sure oxygen is readily available.	5. May be needed if arrhythmias occur after cardioversion.
6. Placement of paddles or multifunctional pads:	6. Ensures that electrical currents flows through the heart.
a. Anterolateral position: Apply one paddle/pad just to the right of the sternum below the clavicle and the other paddle/pad just to the left of the cardiac apex.	
b. Anterior position (pads only): Apply anterior pad over left apex and posterior pad under the infrascapular region.	
7. Turn the machine to the synchronize mode. Look for marking above the R wave on the machine. Set to the appropriate joules.	7. If the electrical discharge hits the T wave, ventricular fibrillation may occur.
a. Charge the machine. Then give the command "ALL CLEAR." Look around quickly to make sure everyone is clear from the patient and bed.	a. Avoids touching patient and receiving shock.
b. Push the shock button. The discharge may be delayed because it is resynchronizing with the R wave before discharging the electrical energy.	
8. If repeat cardioversion is needed, check if the machine is still in the synchronized mode.	8. Some machines reset to defibrillation mode.

 NURSING ALERT If ventricular fibrillation develops, turn synchronizer mode off, adjust joules to the appropriate setting for defibrillation and proceed with defibrillation.

9. A short-acting sedative and, possibly, an analgesic may be given.	9. Helps produce amnesia concerning the cardioversion.
10. Monitor the ECG after conversion occurs. Blood pressure should be recorded every 15 minutes for 1 hour or according to facility policy.	10. The patient may revert to previous dysrhythmias after conversion.

5. Spontaneous sustained ventricular tachycardia in patients without structural disease not amenable to other treatment.

6. Nonischemic dilated cardiomyopathy with LVEF less than or equal to 35% and who are in the NYHA functional Class II or III.

 NURSING ALERT Synchronized cardioversion is generally contraindicated when a patient has been taking a significant amount of digoxin because more lethal dysrhythmias may occur after electric discharge.

Design

The ICD is slightly larger than a pacemaker and consists of two parts:

1. Pulse generator—contains the circuitry and battery to detect dysrhythmias and generate the electric shock. The generator is usually placed in the left pectoral region and is commonly referred to as the active can or hot-can.
   a. Battery life depends on amount of shocks and pacing and is usually 5 to 6 years.

PROCEDURE GUIDELINES 12-7

Automated External Defibrillator

EQUIPMENT

- Automatic external defibrillator (AED)
- Defibrillator pads

PROCEDURE

Nursing Action	Rationale
1. Assess unresponsiveness and pulselessness.	1. Establishes need for the procedure.
2. Position patient in the supine position.	2. For access to the chest.
3. Start cardiopulmonary resuscitation (CPR) while automated external defibrillator (AED) is being applied.	3. Early restoration of oxygenation and perfusion is imperative in enhancing the resuscitative effort.

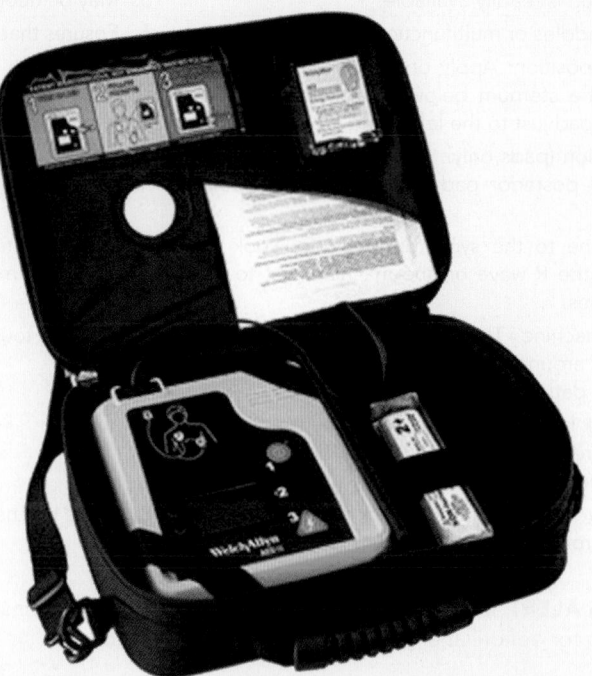

Example of an AED.

4. Place pads in the anterolateral position. Apply one paddle/pad just to the right of the sternum below the clavicle and the other paddle/pad just to the left of the cardiac apex.	4. Anterior placement is preferred because attempting anterior–posterior pad placement may delay treatment.
5. Turn on AED.	
6. Follow audio and/or visual instructions from the AED.	6. The AED will analyze the rhythm in 5 to 15 seconds and determine the need for defibrillation based on that analysis. It will then let the operator know how to proceed.
7. Suspend CPR or any movement of the patient during the analysis.	7. External movement will impair the AED's accuracy in analyzing the rhythm.

8. If, after analyzing the rhythm, a shock is advised, the AED will instruct the operator to prepare for a shock. It will charge the unit, give the warning to "STAND CLEAR," and then deliver the shock or prompt the operator to push the shock button.

9. After the first shock, resume CPR for 2 minutes before reanalyzing the rhythm per American Heart Association guidelines.

10. If no shock is indicated, continue CPR for 2 minutes, then allow the AED to analyze the rhythm. Proceed as above if a shock is now indicated. If a shock is still not indicated, continue CPR and reanalyze the rhythm every 2 minutes.

11. If the patient regains a pulse, continue to support ventilations. Keep AED pads attached and the unit on in case the patient again loses consciousness.

8. Prevents person from receiving shock if touching the patient.

9. Provides oxygenation to the patient.

10. A shock will only be delivered if ventricular fibrillation or tachycardia is present.

11. Close monitoring is necessary in case dysrhythmia recurs.

---

b. The direct current electric shock delivered is 25 to 35 joules. Depending on the device, it can be programmed up to 41 joules.

2. Lead system—consists of two components.
   a. Pace-sense component: monitors the heart rhythm and can deliver pacing output.
   b. Shocking coils: deliver the electrical shocks needed for defibrillation.

3. Most ICDs (but not all) can be noninvasively deactivated by a doughnut-shaped magnet.

Function

Electric shocks are delivered in a programmed sequence:

1. The device detects a lethal dysrhythmia, charges and reconfirms that the lethal dysrhythmia is still present, and then "defibrillates" the heart. The lethal dysrhythmia must meet two programmed criteria (rate and amount of time spent from the isoelectric line) to trigger the device to emit an initial electric shock. The number of joules necessary to convert each patient is determined during insertion and testing of the device; it is usually 15 to 25 joules.

2. Nontermination of the lethal dysrhythmia by the initial shock triggers the device to continue the sequence (detect, charge, and defibrillate) until a total of four or five shocks have been delivered (number of shocks depends on device model implanted).
   a. Subsequent shocks are slightly higher, at 30 to 32 joules.
   b. The total sequence lasts approximately 2 minutes.

3. Nontermination of the lethal dysrhythmia after the shock sequence signals the device to revert to the "detection" mode of operation and not to reinitiate the shocking sequence. The device will reinitiate the shocking sequence only if a rhythm other than the lethal dysrhythmia is detected and maintained

for at least 35 seconds. If this criterion is met and another lethal dysrhythmia is detected, the device will cycle through the shocking sequence again.

4. Termination of a lethal dysrhythmia at any time during the shocking sequence signals the device to interrupt the sequence, return to a detection mode, and reinitiate the shocking sequence if another lethal dysrhythmia is detected.

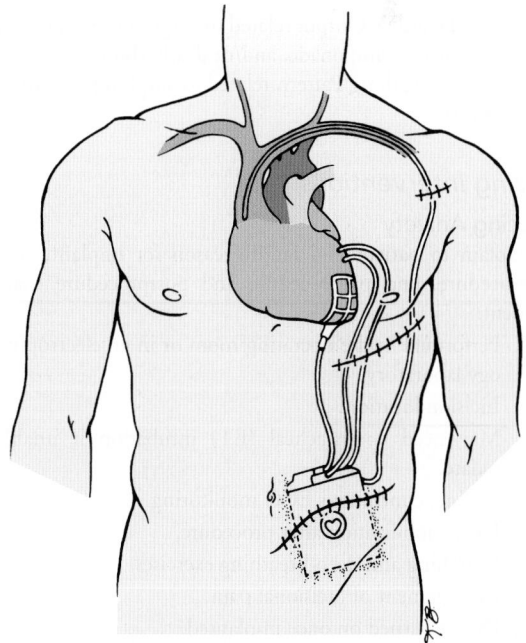

Figure 12-6. Implantable cardioverter-defibrillator.

Complications

1. Many complications that occurred previously with ICDs have been decreased by the use of the transvenous technique for implantation that is similar to that of permanent pacemaker insertion.

2. Complications associated with implantation of the ICD include:
   a. Acceleration of arrhythmias.
   b. Air emboli.
   c. Bleeding.
   d. Perforation of the myocardium.
   e. Pneumothorax.
   f. Puncture of the subclavian vein.
   g. Thromboemboli.
   h. Venous occlusion.

3. Complications that can occur after placement of an ICD:
   a. Chronic nerve damage.
   b. Diaphragmatic stimulation.
   c. Erosion of pulse generator.
   d. Formation of pocket hematoma.
   e. Fluid accumulation/seroma.
   f. Infection of pocket/system.
   g. Keloid formation.
   h. Lead dislodgement.
   i. Lead fracture and insulation breaks.
   j. Venous thrombosis.

Nursing Diagnoses

- Anxiety related to invasive procedure and fear of death.
- Risk for Infection related to invasive procedure and implanted device.
- Decreased Cardiac Output related to surgical procedure, hypotension, cardiac tamponade, and/or dysrhythmias.
- Ineffective Breathing Pattern related to surgical procedure and discomfort.

Nursing Interventions

Reducing Anxiety

1. Explain to patient and family reason for implant, surgical procedure, and preprocedure and postprocedure management:
   a. Performed in the operating room or in an electrophysiology laboratory.
   b. Incision location.
   c. May need endotracheal (ET) intubation if unable to sedate.
   d. IV line; continuous ECG monitoring.
   e. Early mobilization after procedure.
   f. Coughing and deep-breathing exercises.
   g. Management of incisional pain.
   h. Device turned on once implanted.

2. Provide emotional support to patient and family.
   a. Assess patient's and family's knowledge level, support systems, and usual coping mechanisms.
   b. Psychiatric counseling may be beneficial because patient is facing life-threatening issues.
   c. Encourage patient and family to verbalize fears and/or expectations of hospitalization, lifestyle adjustments, self-concept, body image, and device malfunction (misfiring or failure to fire).
   d. Reinforce to patient that daily activities will not increase the risk of the device misfiring.
   e. Explain the sensation that might be felt if the device fires and the patient is conscious. (Many patients will become unconscious before the device fires and therefore feel no sensations.) Sensations experienced in conscious patients vary, but are commonly described as a severe chest blow.

3. Allow patient to participate in care as much as possible.
   a. Encourage patient to dress in street clothes during hospitalization. (Loose-fitting clothes are recommended to prevent chafing and irritation at implant site.)
   b. Allow patient to look at incision site.
   c. Give patient instructional booklets about the device.

Preventing Infection

1. Check temperature every 4 hours; report elevations. (Early postoperative fever may be due to atelectasis; defibrillator system as infection source commonly occurs within 5 to 10 days of implantation.)
2. Evaluate incision site every 4 hours for signs of infection.
3. Culture drainage from incision.
4. Evaluate incision for tissue erosion.
5. Monitor WBC count and differential.
6. Clean incision and change dressing as directed, using aseptic technique.
7. Administer antibiotics, as ordered, before and after the procedure.

GERONTOLOGIC ALERT Older patients may not demonstrate abnormal temperature elevations with infections and experience prolonged wound healing.

Maintaining Adequate Cardiac Output

1. Monitor vital signs frequently until stable.
2. Evaluate incision site for evidence of bleeding or hematoma.
3. Evaluate urine output.
4. Be alert to risk for dysrhythmias postoperatively. (Manipulation of heart and swelling may induce dysrhythmias 24 to 48 hours after implant.)
5. Monitor for changes in blood pressure as a sudden drop may indicate cardiac tamponade.

NURSING ALERT Cardiopulmonary resuscitation (CPR) should be started immediately on any patient with an implantable defibrillator who becomes unconscious and has no pulse. A slight "buzz" sensation will be felt if the implanted device delivers a shock, but it is not harmful. Gloves may be worn to minimize the sensation.

6. Evaluate carefully all complaints of chest pain (noncardiac pain may be due to lead fracture or dislodgement; pain may be noted along wire pathways).
7. Auscultate heart sounds every 4 hours for presence of friction rub or muffled heart sounds.

Promoting Effective Breathing Pattern

1. Ask patient to take several deep breaths every hour to expand lung fields.
2. Encourage coughing and deep-breathing exercises frequently; medicate with analgesics before exercises and provide a pillow for splinting.
3. Monitor use of incentive spirometer.
4. Elevate head of bed to promote adequate ventilation.
5. Auscultate lung fields every 4 hours.
6. Assist with position changes every 2 hours while on bed rest.
7. Encourage early ambulation.
8. Administer analgesics, as ordered.

Patient Education and Health Maintenance

Introduction to Implantable Defibrillator

1. Review anatomy of the heart with emphasis on the conduction system, using a diagram of the heart.
2. Give accurate explanations, using correct medical terminology (allows patient to interact with the health care team more effectively), regarding reason for device implantation, components of system, and function of device.
   a. Use manufacturer's instructional booklet and video presentation about the device.
   b. Encourage family members to participate in education process.

Living with the Implantable Defibrillator

1. Instruct patient and family on actions to be taken if the device fires.
   a. Explain signs and symptoms that may be experienced if a lethal dysrhythmia occurs: palpitations, dizziness, shortness of breath, chest pain.
   b. If signs and symptoms occur, lie down and try to call 911 for help if alone.
   c. Family members should check for a pulse if patient becomes unconscious. CPR should be started immediately if no pulse is present and 911 has been called.
   d. Reinforce that shocks emitted from device are not harmful, and CPR should never be delayed to wait for device to complete the shocking sequence.
   e. If patient remains conscious or is unconscious with a pulse, family members should monitor patient during episode, continually assessing for a pulse during shocking sequence. After the episode, follow health care provider's instructions as directed.
   f. Notify health care provider immediately.
2. Explore with patient and family fears about failure of device, sensation associated with a shock, and injury to others if a shock occurs.
   a. Sensations experienced vary but are most commonly described as a severe blow to the chest.

b. No injury will occur to others if in contact with patient during a shock; a slight shock may be felt by your partner if the device fires during sexual intercourse.
   c. Battery life depends on frequency of use. The device is evaluated in 4 to 6 weeks after implantation and then every 3 months. Newer devices may allow for checks from home.
3. Review sources of EMI that should be avoided (see page 355).
4. Advise patient that there is no increased risk of endocarditis, so antibiotic prophylaxis before dental work is not necessary.
5. Review with health care provider resumption of activities, such as lifting, driving, sports, and sexual activity.

Other Instructions

1. Review care of incision site (see page 355).
2. Loose-fitting clothing should be worn until healing takes place.
3. Provide MedicAlert card; encourage carrying card at all times and obtaining a corresponding MedicAlert bracelet.
4. Explain how to keep diary of episodes and record dates of 4- to 6-month follow-up appointments.
5. Provide information to family members regarding CPR training courses.
6. Encourage use of support groups.
7. Always carry a list of current medications and name and number of physician and emergency contacts.

Evaluation: Expected Outcomes

- Verbalizes understanding of device and surgical procedure.
- Afebrile; incision without drainage.
- Vital signs stable; no dysrhythmias.
- Respirations unlabored, lungs clear.

Pericardiocentesis

Pericardiocentesis is an invasive procedure, which involves the puncture of the pericardial sac to aspirate fluid. The pericardium typically contains 10 to 50 mL of sterile fluid. Excessive fluid within the pericardial sac can cause compression of the heart chambers, resulting in an acute decrease in CO (cardiac tamponade). Fluid accumulation (pericardial effusion) can occur rapidly (acute) or slowly (subacute). The amount of excess fluid the pericardium is able to accommodate is individually based on the ability of the pericardium to stretch. Once the stretch has been maximized, intrapericardial pressure rises, possibly causing circulatory compromise.

Acute—a rapid increase of fluid into pericardial space (as little as 200 mL) causes a marked rise in intrapericardial pressure. Emergency intervention is required to prevent severe circulatory compromise.

Subacute—slow accumulation of fluid into pericardial sac over weeks or months, causing pericardium to stretch and accommodate up to 2 L of fluid without severe increases in intrapericardial pressure.

Both of these situations require intervention to remove the pericardial fluid. See Procedure Guidelines 12-8, pages 364 to 365. Pericardiocentesis is frequently performed in the cardiac catheterization laboratory under fluoroscopy or assisted by echocardiographic imaging. In the case of severely decompensated cardiac tamponade, pericardiocentesis can be safely performed at the bedside with echocardiography.

(Text continues on page 365)

PROCEDURE GUIDELINES 12-8

Assisting the Patient Undergoing Pericardiocentesis

EQUIPMENT

- Pericardiocentesis tray
- Intracath set
- Skin antiseptic
- 1%–2% lidocaine
- Sterile gloves, gown, drape, and mask

- Electrocardiograph (ECG) for monitoring purposes
- Sterile ground wire to be connected between pericardial needle and V

- lead of ECG (use alligator clip–type connectors)
- Equipment for cardiopulmonary resuscitation

PROCEDURE

Nursing Action	Rationale
Preparatory phase	
1. Administer sedation as prescribed.	1. Reduces anxiety of the patient. Depending on sedatives used, may provide amnesic effect.
2. Establish venous access.	2. Preserves a route for IV therapy in an emergency.
3. Place the patient in a comfortable position with the head of the bed or treatment table raised to a 45-degree angle.	3. Makes it easier to insert needle into pericardial sac.
4. Apply the limb leads of the ECG to the patient.	4. The patient is monitored during the procedure by ECG for arrhythmias, increased heart rate, and decreased heart rate.
5. Have defibrillator available for immediate use.	5. In the event that the patient needs to be shocked from an arrhythmia.
6. Have pacemaker available for immediate use.	6. In the event the patient becomes bradycardic.
7. Open the tray using aseptic technique.	7. Pericardiocentesis is a sterile procedure.

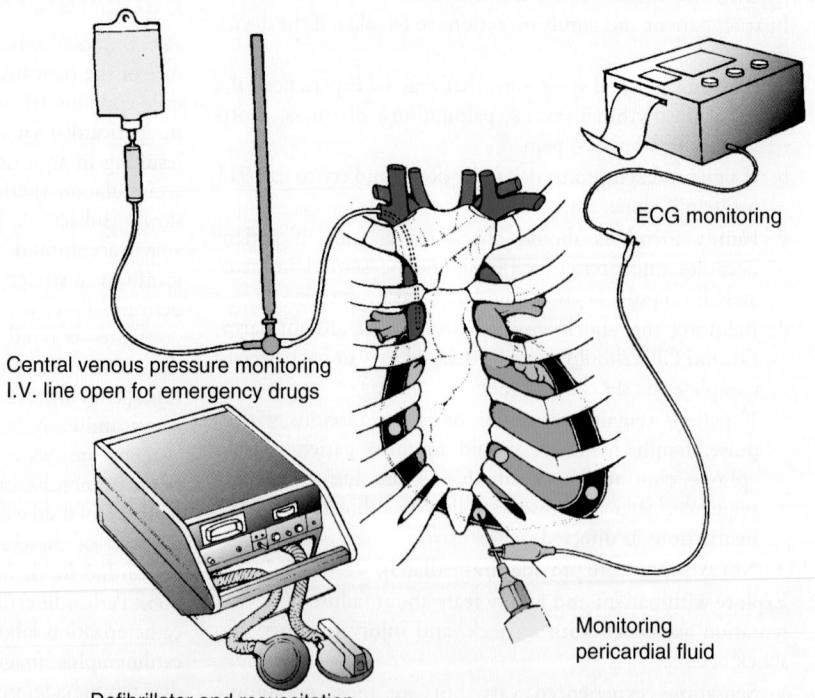

ECG monitoring

Central venous pressure monitoring
I.V. line open for emergency drugs

Monitoring
pericardial fluid

Defibrillator and resuscitation
equipment ready

Nursing support of the patient under-
going pericardiocentesis. (Yellow circles
indicate sites for pericardial aspiration.)

PROCEDURE GUIDELINES 12-8 *(continued)*

Assisting the Patient Undergoing Pericardiocentesis

PROCEDURE *(continued)*

Nursing Action	Rationale
Performance phase (by physician)	
1. The site is prepared with skin antiseptic; the area is draped with sterile towels and injected with anesthetic.	1. Cleanses and disinfects the area for pericardial needle insertion.
2. The pericardial aspiration needle is attached to a 50-mL syringe by a three-way stopcock. Lead V (precordial leadwire) of the ECG is attached to the hub of the aspirating needle by a sterile wire and alligator clips or clamp.	2. Left ventricular lead can be monitored directly. There is danger of laceration of myocardium/coronary artery and of cardiac dysrhythmias.
3. The needle is advanced slowly until fluid is obtained.	3. Fluid is generally aspirated at a depth of 1–1½ inches (2.5–4 cm).
4. When the pericardial sac has been entered, a hemostat is clamped to the needle at the chest wall just where it penetrates the skin. Pericardial fluid is aspirated slowly.	4. Prevents movement of the needle and further penetration while fluid is being removed. Aspirated fluid may be cloudy, clear, or bloody.
5. Monitor the patient's ECG, blood pressure, and venous pressure constantly.	5.
	a. The ST segment rises if the point of the needle contacts the ventricle; there may be ventricular ectopic beats.
	b. The PR segment is elevated when the needle touches the atrium.
	c. Large, erratic QRS complexes indicate penetration of the myocardium.
6. If a large amount of fluid is present, a polyethylene catheter may be inserted through a needle (an Intracath) and left in the pericardial sac. The catheter may be connected to a drainage bag or capped.	6. An indwelling catheter left in the pericardial space permits further slow drainage of fluid and prevents recurrence of cardiac tamponade.
7. Watch for presence of bloody fluid. If blood accumulates rapidly, an immediate thoracotomy and cardiorrhaphy (suturing of heart muscle) may be indicated.	7. Bloody pericardial fluid may be due to trauma. Bloody pericardial effusion fluid does not readily clot, whereas blood obtained from inadvertent puncture of one of the heart chambers does clot.
Follow-up phase	
1. Monitor patient closely.	1. After pericardiocentesis, careful monitoring of blood pressure, venous pressure, and heart sounds will be necessary to indicate possible recurrence of tamponade; repeated aspiration is necessary.
a. Watch for rising venous pressure and falling arterial pressure.	
b. Auscultate the area over the heart for pericardial friction rub, decreased intensity of heart sounds.	
2. Prepare for surgical drainage of pericardium if:	2. In the presence of these signs, the patient is probably experiencing cardiac tamponade.
a. Pericardial fluid repeatedly accumulates.	
b. Aspiration is unsuccessful.	
c. Complications develop (dysrhythmias, puncture of heart chamber, puncture of surrounding organ, laceration of coronary artery or myocardium, damage to left internal mammary artery).	c. Requires immediate intervention.

Purposes

1. To remove fluid from the pericardial sac caused by:

   a. Infection.

   b. Malignant neoplasm or lymphoma.

   c. Trauma (blunt or penetrating wounds or from cardiac surgery or procedure).

   d. Drugs and toxins.

   e. Radiation.

   f. MI.

g. Collagen vascular disease.

h. Aortic dissection extending to the pericardium.

i. Metabolic disorders, especially uremia, dialysis, and hypothyroidism.

j. Cardiac diagnostic or interventional procedures.

k. An idiopathic condition.

2. To obtain fluid for diagnosis.

3. To instill certain therapeutic drugs.

Sites for Pericardiocentesis

1. Subxiphoid—needle inserted in the angle between left costal margin and xiphoid.

2. Near cardiac apex, ¾ inch (2 cm) inside left border of cardiac dullness.

3. To the left of the fifth or sixth interspace at the sternal margin.

4. Right side of fourth intercostal space just inside border of dullness.

Percutaneous Coronary Intervention

 Evidence Base Levine, G. N., Bates, E. R., Blankenship, J. C., et al. (2011). 2011 ACCF/AHA/SCAI Guideline for percutaneous coronary intervention. *Circulation, 124,* e574–e651.

Percutaneous coronary intervention (PCI) is a broad term used to describe all invasive coronary interventions. Initially, PCI was limited to balloon angioplasty; however, it now includes intracoronary stenting and a wide spectrum of percutaneous procedures utilized to treat coronary disease. PCI has also replaced coronary artery bypass grafting (CABG) as the preferred treatment for CAD. Commonly performed PCIs include percutaneous transluminal coronary angioplasty (PTCA) with intracoronary stenting, laser-assisted PTCA, and direct coronary atherectomy (DCA).

Types of Procedures

Percutaneous Transluminal Coronary Angioplasty

Percutaneous transluminal coronary angioplasty (PTCA) accesses the femoral, brachial, or radial artery, with the right femoral artery being the most common access site. The site is anesthetized and an arterial sheath is placed into the vessel. Under fluoroscopy, a catheter is advanced through the arterial sheath and directed to the coronary lesion. To visualize the coronary anatomy, specific radiographic projections are used with the fluoroscopy tube through the use of an injection of contrast dye. Once a coronary lesion or narrowing is identified, a balloon-tipped catheter is advanced through wire to the lesion. The balloon is then inflated to displace coronary plaque against the vessel wall (see Figure 12-7). Balloon inflation and deflation may be repeated until optimal flow is achieved in the affected vessel.

Intracoronary Stenting

Intracoronary stents are small meshed metal tubes that are mounted onto a balloon angioplasty catheter. Once initial angioplasty is performed, the angioplasty catheter is removed and replaced with a stent catheter. When the balloon is inflated, the stent is deployed and pressed into the intima of the artery where the occlusion existed. The balloon is deflated and the catheter is removed; however, the stent remains. The intracoronary stent acts as a scaffold helping to hold the artery open, thereby improving blood flow and relieving symptoms once caused by the blockage. Stents may be uncoated, called bare metal stents, or coated, called drug-eluting stents (DESs). DESs are intended to limit the overgrowth of normal tissue following implantation.

Laser-Assisted Balloon Angioplasty

A laser light is directed by a percutaneously inserted flexible fiber-optic catheter and can "vaporize" atheromatous lesions in the coronary vessels. Balloon angioplasty of the vessel may then be performed. This technique may minimize damage to the intimal lining, open diseased vessels more effectively, prevent early and long-term restenosis, and expand the use of angioplasty to calcified, unusual lesions and total occlusions. The most important complication of laser-assisted balloon angioplasty involves minor to major coronary dissection of the treated lesion.

Direct Coronary Atherectomy

Direct coronary atherectomy (DCA) permits more controlled vascular injury and decreases the degree of arterial mural stretch that can occur with PTCA and balloon angioplasty. To remove plaque, DCA works by changing plaque into microscopic debris, thereby opening the diseased vessel more effectively, especially in patients who have coronary lesions not amenable to standard angioplasty. Complications associated with DCA include vascular spasm at the site of plaque removal or distal to the treated site; possible myocardial necrosis, evidenced by elevations of CK-MB; vessel perforation (infrequent but devastating); and groin complications and groin bleeding (more common with atherectomy procedures due to the size of the catheters involved).

Indications

Indications for PCI include the following (only after a comprehensive risk–benefit analysis has been reviewed): recurrent ischemia despite anti-ischemia therapy, elevated troponin levels, new ST-segment depression, symptoms of heart failure or new or worsening mitral insufficiency, depressed left ventricular systolic function, hemodynamic instability, sustained ventricular tachycardia, PCI within 6 months, prior CABG, and high-risk findings from noninvasive testing, including unprotected left main artery disease.

Contraindications

1. PCI is not indicated for patients who have no evidence of high-risk findings associated with single-vessel or multivessel CAD.

2. Procedure-related morbidity or mortality may be linked to the following relative contraindications, many of which may be avoided or reversed prior to PCI:

   a. Allergy (severe) to radiographic contrast dye.

   b. Anticoagulated state.

   c. Decompensated heart failure (eg, acute pulmonary edema).

   d. Digoxin toxicity.

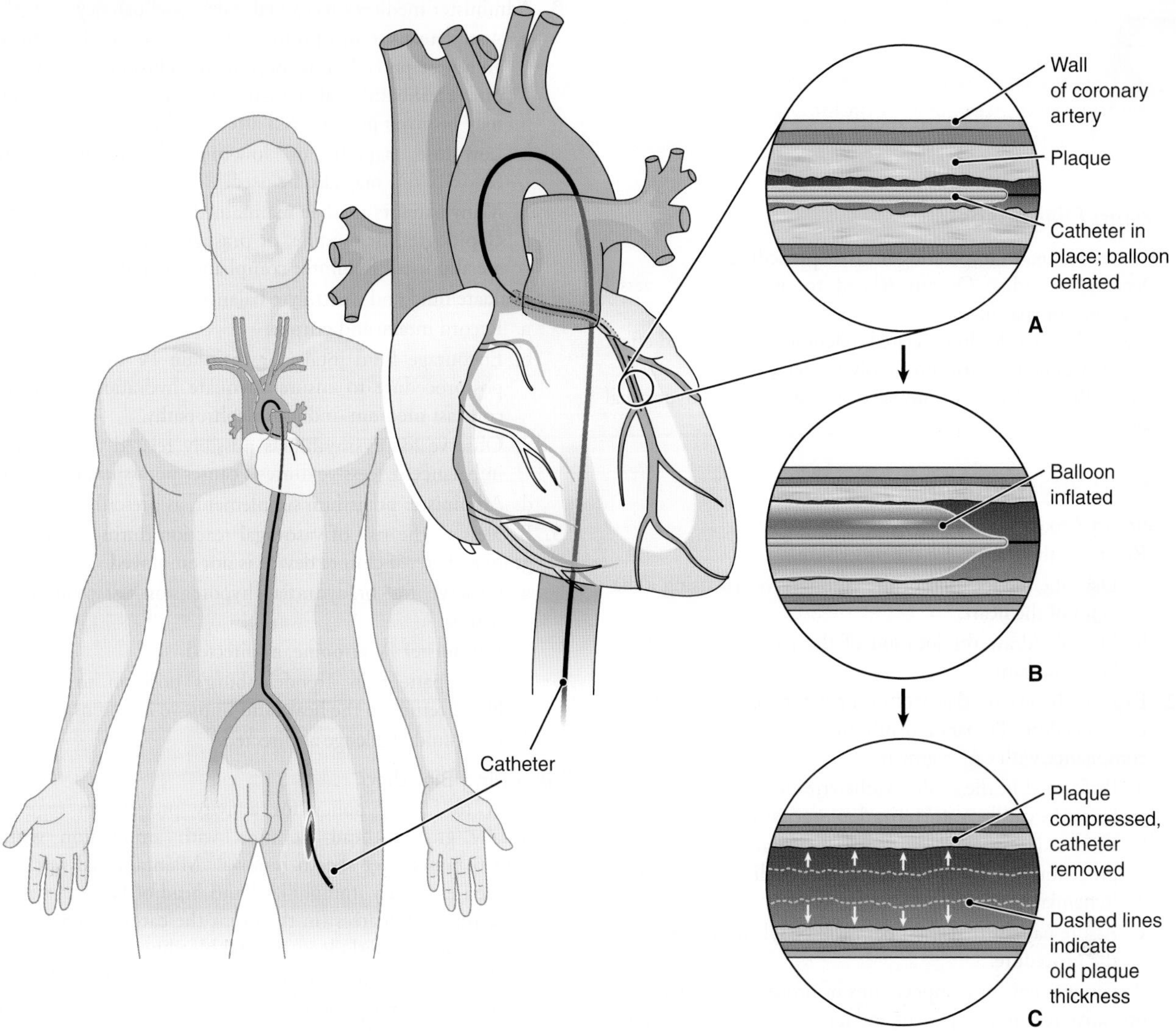

Wall
of coronary
artery

Plaque

Catheter in
place; balloon
deflated

A

Balloon
inflated

B

Plaque
compressed,
catheter
removed

Dashed lines
indicate
old plaque
thickness

C

Catheter

Figure 12-7. Percutaneous transluminal coronary angioplasty. (A) The balloon-tipped catheter is passed into the affected coronary artery. **(B)** The balloon is then rapidly inflated and deflated with controlled pressure. **(C)** The balloon disrupts the intima and causes changes in the atheroma, resulting in an increase in the diameter of the lumen of the vessel and improvement of blood flow.

e. Febrile state.
f. Severe renal insufficiency.
g. Uncorrected hypertension.
h. Uncorrected hypokalemia.
i. Ventricular irritability, uncontrolled.

Complications

1. Major complications or adverse outcomes include death, postprocedure MI, or need for emergent cardiac bypass surgery.
2. Other complications include:
   a. Anaphylaxis.
   b. Arrhythmias.
   c. Arterial dissection/coronary artery dissection.
   d. Bleeding.
   e. Cardiac perforation.
   f. Coronary occlusion, total.
   g. Hematoma at access site.
   h. Renal failure.
   i. Restenosis—occurs in 30% to 50% of PTCA and 10% to 30% of intracoronary stenting procedures.
   j. Stroke.
   k. Tamponade.

 NURSING ALERT Although the occurrence of complications from PCI has declined, immediate CABG surgery must be available with a cardiac surgical team on standby.

DRUG ALERT Missed doses of anticoagulants following intracoronary stenting procedures are clearly linked to restenosis. The patient's ability to adhere to strict anticoagulation protocol will impact on the success of the procedure.

Nursing Diagnoses

- Anxiety related to impending invasive procedure.
- Decreased Cardiac Output related to dysrhythmias, vessel restenosis, or spasm.
- Risk for Injury (bleeding) related to femoral catheter and effect of anticoagulant and/or thrombolytic therapy.
- Acute Pain related to invasive procedure or myocardial ischemia.

Nursing Interventions

Reducing Anxiety

1. Reinforce the reasons for the procedure.
   a. Describe the location of the coronary vessels using a diagram of the heart.
   b. Describe/draw the location of the patient's lesion using heart diagram.
2. Explain the events that will occur before, during, and after the procedure. Preparation minimizes anxiety and increases compliance with care regimen.
   a. Performed in the cardiac catheterization laboratory; similar to the cardiac catheterization procedure (see page 336).
   b. Mild sedation given; patient remains awake throughout procedure to report any chest pain (indicates myocardial ischemia).
   c. Assure patient that chest pain will be taken care of during the procedure.
3. Prepare patient for complications of procedure. Provide preoperative teaching to patient and family regarding procedure, potential complications, and risks associated with heart surgery (see page 374).
4. Explain the necessity of the IV, ECG monitoring, frequent vital sign and groin checks, and remaining NPO before the procedure.

Maintaining Adequate Cardiac Output

1. Check vital signs according to facility policy, typically every 15 minutes for 1 hour, then every 30 minutes for 2 hours, and subsequently every 1 to 2 hours.
2. Continually evaluate for signs and symptoms of restenosis.
   a. Emphasize importance of reporting any chest discomfort or jaw, back, or arm pain and/or nausea, abdominal distress.
   b. Perform ECG for all complaints suspicious of possible myocardial ischemia.
   c. Administer oxygen and vasodilator therapy for pain, as directed.
   d. Obtain CK and isoenzymes as directed.
   e. Keep patient NPO if prolonged chest pain occurs (patient may return to catheterization laboratory).

3. Administer medications to maintain vessel patency.
   a. Antiplatelet or antithrombin agents may be given during and after procedure to prevent reocclusion (eg, bivalirudin, eptifibatide, abciximab). Clopidogrel or prasugrel may be given prior to PCI after STEMI.
   b. Low-dose heparin or low-molecular-weight heparin (enoxaparin) may also be used.
   c. Many patients are then maintained on medications such as clopidogrel, ticlopidine, or prasugrel. Aspirin and statins are also used. Reinforce compliance with drug therapy.
4. Evaluate fluid and electrolyte balance.
   a. Record intake and output.
   b. Encourage fluid intake or maintain IV fluids pre- and postprocedure to ensure adequate hydration to prevent contrast medium–induced nephropathy.
   c. Observe for dysrhythmias possibly related to potassium imbalance. Excessive diuresis causes potassium depletion.
   d. Administer potassium supplement, as prescribed.
5. Be alert to the risk of vasovagal reaction during removal of groin catheter if closure device is not employed.
   a. Observe for bradycardia, hypotension, diaphoresis, or nausea.
   b. Administer IV atropine, as directed.
   c. Place patient in Trendelenburg's position to promote blood return to the heart and improve hypotension.
   d. Give fluid challenge as directed.

Preventing Bleeding

1. Refer to facility policy for activity progression regimen, usually gradual head elevation with ambulation within 4 to 6 hours after sheath removal. Maintain bed rest with affected extremity immobilized and head of bed elevated no more than 30 degrees (in the event the catheter remains) to prevent catheter dislodgement and bleeding.
2. Mark peripheral pulses before procedure with indelible ink.
3. Check peripheral pulse of affected extremity and insertion site with each vital sign check.
4. Observe color, temperature, and sensation of affected extremity with each vital sign check.
5. Report if extremities become cool and pale, and pulses become significantly diminished or absent.
6. Look for presence of hematoma and mark hematoma to note change in size. Report if hematoma continues to enlarge.
7. Note petechiae, hematuria, and complaints of flank pain (vessel patency is maintained by not reversing intraprocedure heparinization; chance of bleeding is increased).
8. Apply direct pressure over insertion site if bleeding is observed and report immediately.
9. Check bed linen under patient frequently for blood.
10. Ask patient to report sensation of warmth at groin area.

Relieving Pain

1. Administer analgesics and anxiolytic medication, as directed.
2. Ensure a restful environment.
   a. Provide back rubs for muscle relaxation.
   b. Minimize noise and interruptions.
   c. Offer sleep medication, as indicated.

3. Progress patient's diet as tolerated (clear liquids/full liquid diet until catheters removed); assist patient with meals.

Patient Education and Health Maintenance

Instruct patient as follows:
1. Modification of cardiac risk factors as means of controlling progression of CAD.
2. Name of medications, action, dosage, and adverse effects.
   a. Common medications to prevent clot formation.
   b. Medications to increase blood flow to heart.
   c. Medications to slow heart rate and reduce chest pain.
   d. Medications to increase blood flow and prevent coronary artery spasm.
3. Dates and importance of any follow-up tests.
4. Symptoms for which patient should seek medical attention, such as adverse effects of medication and chest pain—especially chest pain unrelieved by nitroglycerin.
5. Restenosis (with or without stent) can occur; the patient typically presents with the previous same symptoms; however, the symptoms may vary if a different lesion is involved.

Evaluation: Expected Outcomes

- Verbalizes understanding of procedure.
- Vital signs stable; urine output adequate.
- No bleeding or hematoma at insertion site.
- Verbalizes relief of pain.

Intra-Aortic Balloon Pump Counterpulsation

Counterpulsation is a method of assisting the failing heart and circulation by mechanical support when the myocardium is unable to generate adequate CO. The mechanism of counterpulsation therapy is opposite to the normal pumping action of the heart; counterpulsation devices pump while the heart muscle relaxes (diastole) and relax when the heart muscle contracts (systole).

Indications

1. Postcardiotomy support; low cardiac output after cardiopulmonary bypass.
2. Severe unstable angina that is refractory to pharmacologic therapy.
3. Cardiogenic shock/left-sided heart failure after MI, myocarditis, cardiomyopathy, myocardial contusion, and refractory heart failure.
4. Postinfarction ventricular septal defects or mitral insufficiency resulting in shock.
5. Emergency support following PTCA or high-risk percutaneous coronary interventions.
6. Hemodynamic deterioration in patients awaiting heart transplant.
7. Refractory ventricular arrhythmias.
8. Patients with severe left main coronary arterial stenosis whom surgery is pending.
9. Adjunctive therapy after fibrinolysis in patients at high-risk restenosis.

Function

Intra-Aortic Balloon Pump

1. A balloon catheter is introduced into the femoral artery percutaneously or surgically, threaded to the proximal descending thoracic aorta, and positioned 1 to 2 cm distal to the origin of the left subclavian artery (see Figure 12-8).
2. The balloon catheter is attached to an external console, allowing for inflation and deflation of the balloon with gas such as He (helium). Helium has low viscosity that allows quick travel through the long connecting tubes, and it has low potential for gas embolization should the balloon rupture.
3. The external console integrates the inflation and deflation sequence with the mechanical events of the cardiac cycle (systole–diastole) by "triggering" gas delivery in synchronization with the patient's ECG, the patient's arterial waveform, atrial/ventricular paced rhythm, or intrinsic pump rate.
   a. The most common method of "trigerring" or signalling the intra-aortic balloon pump (IABP) is from the R wave of the patient's ECG signal.
   b. The balloon is automatically set to inflate in the middle of the T wave or at the dicrotic notch of the arterial waveform. This occurs immediately after aortic valve closure.
4. Eases the workload of a damaged heart by increasing coronary blood flow (diastolic augmentation) and decreasing the resistance in the arterial tree against which the heart must pump (afterload reduction).
5. This results in an increase in CO and a reduction in myocardial oxygen requirements.
6. The balloon is inflated at the onset of diastole; this results in an increase in diastolic aortic pressure (diastolic augmentation), which increases blood flow through the coronary arteries.

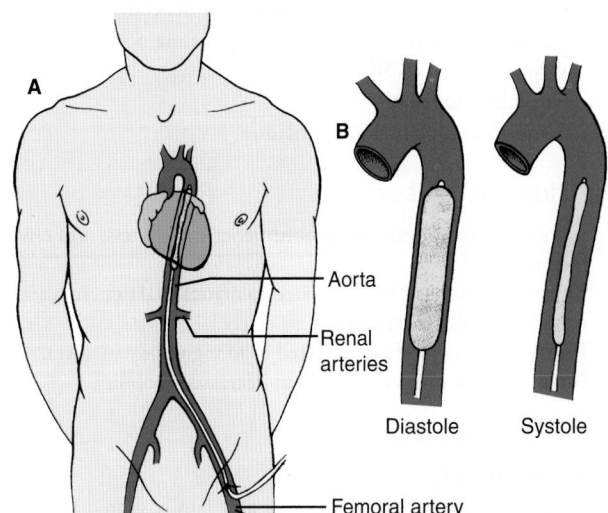

Figure 12-8. Counterpulsation. (A) Introduction of the intra-aortic balloon catheter via the femoral artery. **(B)** The intra-aortic balloon pump augments diastole, resulting in increased perfusion of the coronary arteries and myocardium and a decrease in the left ventricular workload.

7. The balloon is deflated just before the onset of systole (just before aortic valve opening), facilitating the emptying of blood from the left ventricle and decreasing pressure within the aorta. This action results in less work for the left ventricle.

Contraindications

1. Aortic insufficiency—IABP will increase aortic insufficiency.
2. Aortic aneurysm or aortic dissection—IABP catheter may perforate a weakened vessel wall leading to thrombus formation, and inflation and deflation of the catheter may cause a thrombus to break off to become an emboli.
3. Peripheral vascular disease—femoral or iliac artery insertion may be impossible in a patient with severe vascular disease.
4. Terminal illness—outcome will not be affected, unless the patient meets the criteria for heart transplantation.
5. Prosthetic graft in thoracic aorta—may disrupt graft.
6. Coagulopathy—increases the risk of bleeding.
7. Uncontrolled sepsis.

Complications

1. Vascular injuries that may occur from IABP are:
   a. Plaque dislodging.
   b. Dissection of aorta.
   c. Laceration of the aorta.
   d. Ischemia of the limb distal to the insertion site.
   e. Arterial perforation.
2. Peripheral nerve damage can occur from IABP if a cutdown was used to insert the catheter.
3. Impairment of cerebral circulation due to balloon migration occluding the subclavian artery or by embolus and impairment of renal circulation due to balloon malposition or embolus. (Impaired circulation occurs more frequently in patients with peripheral vascular occlusive disease, in women with small vessels, and in patients with insulin-dependent diabetes.)
4. Infection at the insertion site and septicemia occurs in 0.2% of patients with IABP.
5. Thrombocytopenia.
6. Hemorrhage due to anticoagulation.

Nursing Diagnoses

- Anxiety related to invasive procedure, critical illness, and environment.
- Decreased Cardiac Output related to myocardial ischemia and/or mechanical intervention.
- Impaired Tissue Perfusion related to foreign body in aorta.
- Impaired Skin Integrity related to decreased mobility.

Nursing Interventions

Relieving Anxiety

1. Explain IABP therapy to patient and family geared to their level of understanding.
   a. Review purpose of therapy and how the IABP functions.
   b. Reinforce mobility restrictions: supine position with head of bed elevated 15 to 30 degrees, no movement or flexing of leg with IABP catheter.
   c. Explain need for frequent monitoring of vital signs, rhythm, insertion site of affected extremity, and pulses.
   d. Discuss the sounds associated with functioning external console: balloon inflation and deflation and alarms.
2. Encourage family members to participate in patient's care.
   a. Allow family to visit patient frequently.
   b. Solicit family members' assistance in reinforcing mobility restrictions to patient and notifying nursing staff of patient comfort needs.
   c. Encourage family members to ask questions.
3. Allow patient to verbalize fears regarding therapy and illness.
4. Make sure that informed consent is obtained.
5. Administer anxiolytic medications as prescribed and indicated.
6. Keep the family informed of changes in the patient's condition.
7. Encourage realistic hope based on the patient's condition and discuss the patient's progress with the family.
8. Determine the family's previous coping mechanism to stressful situations.

Maintaining Adequate Cardiac Output

1. Assist during insertion of IABP catheter.
   a. Offer patient reassurance and comfort measures (patient is only mildly sedated).
   b. Ensure strict aseptic environment during insertion.
   c. Establish ECG monitoring, choosing the lead with the largest R wave (external console senses R wave of ECG to trigger gas delivery) and without artifact (integration of the patient's cardiac cycle with the inflation and deflation balloon sequence depends on a continuous clear ECG tracing).
   d. Record date, time, and the patient's tolerance to procedure.
   e. Obtain chest x-ray to ensure placement of IABP catheter.
2. Start IABP counterpulsation immediately after insertion, as directed; review manufacturer's manual for IABP equipment in use. Updated manufacturer software allows the IABP to start up with one press of a button and automatically adjust balloon inflation and/or timing. Deflation can be manually adjusted. New software automatically chooses the best trigger and mode that best suits the patient's condition.
   a. Adjust the duration of balloon deflation by the arterial waveform since inflation is timed automatically; inflation is "timed" to begin at the dicrotic notch of the arterial waveform, and deflation occurs before the next systole. Current IABPs can choose the best trigger for the patient (mostly ECG trigger and if in "auto" mode) independently from a user.
   b. Compare the patient's arterial pressure waveform with and without balloon augmentation to evaluate effectiveness of therapy. Note difference in patient's end-diastolic pressure and balloon-assisted end-diastolic pressure (the balloon-assisted end-diastolic pressure should be lower, indicating a reduction in afterload).
   c. Monitor hemodynamic parameters with Swan-Ganz catheter (see page 342). Record mean arterial pressure (MAP),

CVP, PAP, PCWP, and CO to evaluate overall effectiveness of therapy. Perform hemodynamic calculations to evaluate systemic vascular resistance and left ventricular stroke work. Use IABP MAP when titrating vasoactive medications.

   d. Assess capillary refill, pedal, and left radial pulses every 15 minutes for the first hour, then hourly. The balloon catheter or a thrombus can obstruct flow to the distal extremities. If the catheter migrates too high, it can obstruct flow of the left subclavian artery.

3. Monitor vital signs every 15 to 30 minutes for 4 to 6 hours, then hourly, if stable.
4. Monitor neurologic status at least every 2 to 4 hours.
5. Monitor urine output from indwelling catheter every hour.
6. Maintain accurate intake and output and weigh patient daily (preferably at the same time every day).
7. Report chest pain immediately.
8. Treat dysrhythmias as directed.
9. Check for blood oozing around IABP catheter every hour for 8 hours, then every 4 hours (anticoagulation therapy is used to prevent thrombus formation); apply direct pressure and report bleeding.

Maintaining Adequate Tissue Perfusion

1. Evaluate for ischemia of extremity with IABP catheter.
   a. Mark pulses with indelible ink to facilitate checks.
   b. Monitor peripheral pulses (dorsalis pedis, posterior tibial, popliteal, and left radial) for rhythm, character, and pulse quality every 15 minutes for 1 hour, then every 30 minutes for 1 hour, and then hourly.
   c. Use Doppler device for pulses difficult to palpate and to auscultate for bruits and hums.
   d. Observe skin temperature, color, sensation, and movement of affected extremity. (Dusky, cool, mottled, painful, numb/tingling extremity indicates ischemia.)
2. Observe for possible indications of thromboemboli.
   a. Note decreases in urine output after initiation of therapy— may indicate renal artery emboli.
   b. Perform neurologic checks every hour to evaluate for cerebral emboli.
   c. Auscultate bowel sounds to detect evidence of ischemia.
3. Recognize early signs and symptoms of compartment syndrome. Increased pressure in tissue reduces blood flow.
   a. Note complaints of pain, pressure, and numbness of affected extremity induced by passive stretching.
   b. Palpate affected extremity for swelling and tension.
   c. Monitor CK values. Highly elevated CK may indicate compartment syndrome.
4. Ideally, keep head of bed elevated 30 degrees versus supine to avoid aspiration, but prevent upward migration of catheter.

Maintaining Skin Integrity

1. Assess skin frequently for signs of redness or breakdown.
2. Place patient on specialty mattress or bed designed to prevent pressure ulcers (preferably before balloon insertion).
3. Pad bony prominences.

4. Implement passive ROM exercises with exception of extremity with IABP catheter.
5. Turn patient from side to side as a unit every 2 hours. Patients are usually debilitated and prone to pressure ulcers.

Evaluation: Expected Outcomes

- States activity restrictions and rationale.
- Blood pressure and CO readings improved.
- Peripheral pulses strong; extremities warm and nail beds pink.
- No skin redness or breakdown.

Heart Surgery

Open-heart surgery is most commonly performed for CAD, valvular dysfunction, and congenital heart defects. The procedure requires temporary cardiopulmonary bypass (blood is diverted from the heart and the lungs and mechanically oxygenated and circulated) to provide a bloodless field that leads to increased visibility of cardiac structures during the operation.

Newer and less invasive procedures include *minimally invasive direct coronary artery bypass (MIDCAB)* and *robotic-assisted coronary bypass and valve surgeries.* An estimated 405,000 coronary bypass graft surgeries occur yearly in the United States. Heart transplant will not be discussed. For information on percutaneous ventricular assist devices, see Box 12-3.

Types of Procedures

Coronary Artery Bypass Graft

1. CABG surgery involves anastomosis of a bypass conduit or a graft (vein or artery) with distal portion bypassing the blocked coronary vessel restoring adequate blood supply to the heart muscle. The proximal end, in some cases, is anastomosed to the aorta (when the internal mammary artery is chosen as conduit, the proximal end remains attached in its normal circulation pattern). The choice of conduit is often multifactorial. Arterial conduit has been shown to have a longer patency rate. For this reason, the internal mammary artery is often chosen if time allows for its dissection from the chest wall and the length is adequate to bypass the blocked vessel. The saphenous vein remains the most commonly used because it is easily accessed and does not require extra prepping to prevent spasm (such as the case with a radial graft).
   a. Multiple grafts can be placed to bypass multiple lesions.
   b. Traditional procedure is done through sternotomy, whereas newer procedures attempt to be less invasive.
   c. The heart is stopped (in some cases) and the patient placed on a cardiopulmonary bypass machine. In other situations, CABG is performed while the heart is beating using a stabilizer to decrease movement (off-pump CABG).
2. Primarily done to alleviate anginal symptoms and improve survival and quality of life.
3. Indications for CABG include:
   a. Left main coronary artery stenosis of 70% or greater.
   b. Proximal vessel disease greater than 50% to 70% stenosis of three main coronary arteries.
   c. Multivessel disease and decreased left ventricular function.

BOX 12-3	Percutaneous Ventricular Assist Device Therapy

The use of the percutaneous left ventricular assist device (LVAD) constitutes important advances in management of patients with severe cardiogenic shock and may serve as a bridge to recovery or heart transplantation for some patients. The immediate therapeutic benefit of the percutaneous LVAD in patients with cardiogenic shock is the restoration of normal hemodynamics and vital organ perfusion. Although the intra-aortic balloon pump (IABP) decreases preload and afterload, the percutaneous LVAD augments cardiac output and may even completely replace left ventricular function. In severe cases of cardiogenic shock, the IABP and percutaneous LVAD may be used at the same time. For the high-risk percutaneous coronary intervention patient, short-term hemodynamic stability can be provided, and the device can be implanted rapidly and percutaneously in a prophylactic or emergency setting.

There are three principal indications for percutaneous LVAD support:

- Reversible, severe left-sided heart failure (providing temporary circulatory support until recovery has ensued or revascularization has been performed).
- Large ischemic area at risk (temporary circulatory support during high-risk percutaneous or surgical revascularization procedures).
- Bridging therapy (temporary circulatory support as bridge to a permanent surgical assist device or heart transplantation).

The percutaneous LVAD works by creating a left ventricular bypass in one of two ways. One approach is to enter the left atrium transseptally by placing a catheter that pulls oxygenated blood into a centrifugal pump and then flows it back into the femoral artery, thus creating a left atrial-to-femoral bypass. The second technique is retrograde placement of a "caged" blood flow inlet in the left ventricle, which pulls oxygenated blood via catheter to a microaxial pump into the ascending aorta, thereby creating a left ventricular-to-aortic bypass. There are advantages to both systems, and selection should be patient specific.

Historically, surgically implanted right ventricular assist devices (RVAD) have been used mostly for support of cardiac surgical patients. In several reported cases, percutaneous RVADs have successfully supported patients with right ventricular infarct complicated by shock. However, further investigation of this newer therapy is warranted to determine patient outcomes and potential benefits for patients requiring RV support.

 Evidence Base Idelchik, G. M., Simpson, L., Civitello, A. B., et al. (2008). Use of the percutaneous left ventricular assist device in patients with severe refractory cardiogenic shock as a bridge to long-term left ventricular assist device implantation. *Journal of Heart and Lung Transplant, 27*, 106–111.

Windecker, S. (2007). Percutaneous left ventricular assist devices for treatment of patients with cardiogenic shock. *Current Opinion in Critical Care, 13*, 521–527.

---

  d. UA.
  e. Chronic stable angina that is lifestyle-limiting and unresponsive to medical therapies or PTCA and stenting cannot be achieved.
4. Relative contraindications for CABG include:
  a. Small coronary arteries distal to the stenosis.
  b. Severe aortic stenosis.
  c. Severe left ventricular failure with coexisting pulmonary, renal, carotid, and peripheral vascular disease.

Valvular Surgery

1. Prosthetic or biologic valves are placed in the heart as definitive therapy for incompetent heart valves. Mechanical valves are of man-made material and require a lifetime of anticoagulation therapy.
2. Valve repair or replacement can be done in conjunction with CABG surgery.
3. Usually done as an open-heart procedure through sternotomy incision or mini-thoracotomy.
4. Postoperative care of a patient with either a mitral valve or an aortic valve is similar to that of a patient who has undergone post-CABG surgery.

Congenital Heart Surgery

1. Defects of the heart can be surgically repaired and reconstructed.
2. Temporary cardiopulmonary bypass is not always required.

MIDCAB

1. Done through a left anterior small thoracotomy, a short parasternal incision, or a small incision using a port access and video-assisted technology.
2. Cardiopulmonary bypass is not needed because the heart remains beating.
3. The procedure is limited to proximal disease of the left anterior descending or right coronary artery.
4. With this procedure, there is less blood transfusion, less pain and discomfort, less infection, and less time under anesthesia; therefore, patients are moved out of the intensive care unit (ICU) more quickly.

Off-Pump CABG (Beating-Heart Bypass Surgery)

1. CABG surgery is done using a median sternotomy without the use of cardiopulmonary bypass; preferred method in high-risk patients (eg, patients with poor ventricular function or with severe aortic atherosclerosis).
2. Postaccess procedures are performed through a small anterior thoracotomy incision and a few 1-cm lateral port incisions that allow direct access to the heart and good visualization through a thoracoscope.
  a. Multiple vessel bypass can be performed as well as mitral valve surgery and repair of atrial septal defect.
  b. The heart is stopped and cardiopulmonary bypass is used in case of emergency during surgery.

c. Reduces postoperative length of stay to 1 to 3 days.

d. Contraindicated in patients with occlusion in posterior and lateral arteries, severe atherosclerosis, and aortic aneurysms.

3. Transmyocardial laser revascularization (TMLR) provides relief to patients having refractory angina that is not amendable to conventional revascularization. Indications for TMLR include severe coronary heart disease, viable myocardium with reversible ischemia, LVEF of more than 20%, and target vessels that are too small for catheter revascularization.

Preoperative Management

1. Review of patient's condition to determine status of vascular, pulmonary, renal, hepatic, hematologic, and metabolic systems.

   a. Cardiac history; circulatory studies.

   b. Pulmonary health—patients with COPD may require prolonged postoperative respiratory support. Chest computed tomography scans, baseline arterial blood gas or pulmonary function tests should be ordered and used as reliable predictors of long-term pulmonary outcomes. (Vital capacity > 2.5 L and forced expiratory volume in 1 second > 1.5 L are ideal for favorable outcomes.)

   c. Depression—can produce a serious postoperative depressive state and can affect postoperative morbidity and mortality.

   d. Present alcohol intake; smoking history.

2. Preoperative laboratory studies.

   a. Complete blood count; serum electrolytes; lipid profile; and hemoglobin A1C, if diabetic.

   b. Antibody screen, urine and other cultures.

   c. Preoperative coagulation survey (platelet count, prothrombin time, partial thromboplastin time)—extracorporeal circulation will affect certain coagulation factors.

   d. Renal and hepatic function tests.

3. Evaluation of medication regimen. These patients are usually taking multiple drugs.

   a. Digoxin—may be receiving large doses to improve myocardial contractility; may be stopped several days before surgery to avoid digitoxic dysrhythmias from cardiopulmonary bypass.

   b. Diuretics—assess for potassium depletion and volume depletion; give potassium supplement to replenish body stores.

   c. Beta-adrenergic blockers such as metoprolol and propranolol—usually continued.

   d. Psychotropic drugs such as benzodiazepines (diazepam, alprazolam)—postoperative withdrawal may cause extreme agitation.

   e. Alcohol—sudden withdrawal may produce delirium.

   f. Anticoagulant/antiplatelet aggregate drugs, such as warfarin and clopidogrel—discontinued several days before operation to allow coagulation mechanism to return to normal.

   g. Corticosteroids—if taken within the year before surgery, may lead to adrenal crisis. It is essential that these patients be dosed adequately to prevent hypotension or death.

   h. Prophylactic antibiotics—may be given preoperatively.

   i. Drug sensitivities or allergies are noted.

   j. If patients are taking herbal supplements, they should be discontinued as far in advance as possible in order to prevent interactions with certain types of anesthesia.

4. Improvement of underlying pulmonary disease and respiratory function to reduce risk of complications.

   a. Encourage patient to stop smoking.

   b. Treat infection and pulmonary vascular congestion.

 GERONTOLOGIC ALERT Older and debilitated patients are at greater risk for postoperative respiratory complications.

5. Preparation for events in the postoperative period.

   a. Take the patient and family on tour of ICU. This lessens anxiety about being in ICU.

      i. Introduce the patient to staff personnel who will be caring for him or her.

      ii. Give family a schedule of visiting hours and times for phone contact.

   b. Teach chest physical therapy procedures to optimize pulmonary function.

      i. Have the patient practice with incentive spirometer.

      ii. Show and practice diaphragmatic breathing techniques.

      iii. Have the patient practice effective coughing and leg exercises.

   c. Prepare patient for presence of monitors, chest tubes, IV lines, blood transfusion, ET tube, nasogastric (NG) tube, pacing wires, arterial line, and indwelling catheter.

      i. Explain to the patient that chest tubes will be inserted below incision into chest cavity for drainage and maintenance of negative pressure.

      ii. Explain to the patient that ET tube will prevent speaking, but communication will be possible through writing until tube is removed (usually within 6 hours when the patient is awake and able to maintain own airway).

      iii. Explain to the patient that diet will consist of liquids until 24 hours after surgery.

      iv. Explain that monitoring equipment and IV lines will restrict movement and nursing staff will position the patient comfortably every 2 hours and as necessary.

   d. Discuss with the patient the need to monitor vital signs frequently and the likelihood of frequent disturbances of the patient's rest.

   e. Discuss pain management with the patient; assure the patient that analgesics will be administered as necessary to control pain.

   f. Tell the patient that both hands may be loosely restrained for a few hours after surgery to eliminate possibility of pulling out tubes and IV lines inadvertently.

   g. Discuss with the patient the importance of physical and occupational therapy to lessen hospital stay. Patient will be assisted from the bed to chair by the morning of postoperative day 1.

6. Evaluation of emotional state to reduce anxieties.
   a. Patients undergoing heart surgery are more anxious and fearful than other surgical patients. (Moderate anxiety assists patient to cope with stresses of surgery. Low anxiety level may indicate that the patient is in denial. High anxiety may impair the patient's ability to learn and listen.)
   b. Offer support and help patient and family mobilize positive coping mechanisms.
   c. Answer questions and alleviates fears and misconceptions.
7. Surgical preparation.
   a. Shave anterior and lateral surfaces of trunk and neck; shave entire body down to ankles (for coronary bypass).
   b. Shower or bathe per facility policy. Assist patient with antiseptic scrubs used on their chest prior to surgery.
   c. Give sedative and/or antibiotics before going to the operating room, as ordered.
   d. Ensure removable dental work, jewelry, and nail polish removed.

Complications

Complications following cardiac surgery can be divided into early complications (cardiovascular, pulmonary, renal, GI, and neuropsychological) and late postoperative complications.

Early Complications

1. Cardiovascular dysfunction or low output syndrome can occur as a result of decreased preload (from bleeding or volume loss), increased afterload, arrhythmias, cardiac tamponade, or myocardial depression with or without myocardial necrosis.
2. Postoperative bleeding can occur secondary to coagulopathy, uncontrolled hypertension, or inadequate hemostasis.
3. Cardiac tamponade results from bleeding into the pericardial sac or accumulation of fluids in the sac, which compresses the heart and prevents adequate filling of the ventricles. Cardiac tamponade should be suspected when there is low CO, hypotension, tachycardia, increased CVP, or sharp drop in chest tube output postoperatively.

 GERONTOLOGIC ALERT Older patients postoperatively are more sensitive to hypovolemia, excessive bleeding, and cardiac tamponade, which affect preload and result in a decrease in CO.

4. Myocardial depression (impaired myocardial contractility), which can be reversible, occurs secondary as a result of myocardial necrosis in 15% of all CABG surgeries.
5. Perioperative MI continues to be a serious problem that can occur in 5% of patients with stable angina and up to 10% of patients with unstable angina postoperatively as a result of the surgical procedure.
6. Cardiac dysrhythmias commonly occur after heart surgery. Ischemia, hypoxia, electrolyte imbalances, alterations in autonomic nervous system, hypertension, increased catecholamine levels, among others, may attribute to dysrhythmia development.
   a. Atrial arrhythmias may occur after CABG or after valvular surgery; can occur anytime during the first 2 to 3 weeks postoperatively, but peak incidence is 3 to 5 days.

 GERONTOLOGIC ALERT Atrial fibrillation occurs in 35% of elderly patients postoperatively and may need to be treated with antiarrhythmics, anticoagulation agents, or cardioversion.

   b. PVCs occur in 8.9% to 24% of patients, most frequently after aortic valve replacement and CABG.
7. Hypotension may be caused by inadequate cardiac contractility and reduction in blood volume or by mechanical ventilation (when the patient "fights" the ventilator or positive end-expiratory pressure is used), all of which can produce a reduction in CO.
8. Pulmonary complications occur as a result of intubation and coronary pulmonary bypass.
   a. Continuous pulse oximetry, arterial blood gas (ABG) studies, and chest x-ray are done frequently in order to monitor pulmonary function of a patient after heart surgery.
   b. Noncardiac pulmonary edema can occur immediately after surgery and can occur the first several days after surgery as a result of increased pulmonary capillary permeability.
   c. Pneumothorax can occur anytime postoperatively, especially when chest tubes are removed.
   d. Phrenic nerve damage can occur, resulting in diaphragmatic paralysis.
   e. Pulmonary emboli, although uncommon, can result from atrial fibrillation, heart failure, obesity, hypercoagulability, and immobilization.
   f. Older patients are at increased risk of developing pneumonia, atelectasis, and pulmonary effusions.
   g. Be vigilant and report copious amounts of secretion or any changes in patient's secretion.
9. Renal insufficiency or failure can occur as a result of deficient perfusion (can be due to heart-lung machine), hemolysis, low CO before and after open heart surgery, hypotension, and by use of vasopressor agents to increase blood pressure.
10. GI postoperative complications can include abdominal distention, ileus, gastroduodenal bleeding, cholecystitis, hepatic dysfunction, "shock liver syndrome," pancreatitis, mesenteric ischemia, diarrhea, or constipation.
11. Neuropsychological complications postoperatively include neuropsychological dysfunction, postcardiotomy delirium, and peripheral neurologic deficits.

 GERONTOLOGIC ALERT Neurologic complications increase disproportionate to cardiac risk in elderly patients.

Late Complications

1. Late complications of cardiac surgery usually occur after the fourth day of surgery and include postpericardiotomy syndrome, cardiac tamponade, and incisional wound infections.
2. Postpericardiotomy syndrome is a group of symptoms occurring in 10% to 40% of patients several after cardiac surgery.

a. The cause of postpericardiotomy syndrome is not certain, but it may result from anticardiac antibodies, viral etiology (such as cytomegalovirus), or other causes.

b. Postpericardiotomy syndrome occurs as the result of tissue trauma, which triggers an autoimmune response and inflammation of the pericardial cavity, resulting in pericardial and severe pleural pain.

c. Manifestations—fever, malaise, arthralgias, dyspnea, pericardial effusion, pleural effusion and friction rub, pleural/pericardial pain.

d. Treatment regimen may include corticosteroids, aspirin, or colchicine. Pericardiocentesis or thoracentesis may be needed for persistent effusion.

3. Cardiac tamponade can occur in 1% to 2% of patients and is commonly associated with administration of anticoagulants or antiplatelet therapy, usually occurring after 72 hours following surgery.

4. Wound infections, including sternal wound infections and mediastinitis, occur in 0.4% to 5% of all patients having cardiac surgery. Mortality rate associated with sternal wound infection and mediastinitis can vary between 8% and 45%.

a. Wound infections usually appear 4 to 14 days postoperatively with symptoms of fever, leukocytosis, inflammation, and purulent drainage.

b. *Staphylococcus epidermidis* and *staphylococcus aureus* organisms are the most common causative organism but the infection can be caused by a number of pathogens ranging from gram positives, gram negatives, or even fungi.

5. MIs (postoperative) occur at a rate of 1.34% due to bypass time of more than 100 minutes and presence of unstable angina.

6. Constrictive pericarditis has an incidence of 0.2% to 2.0%. Risk factors reveal normal left ventricular function, warfarin administration, and inadequate drainage of early postoperative pericardial effusion as the significant causes.

7. Respiratory complications—chest wall pain, prolonged ventilation—more than 14 days of ventilatory support (morbidity rate of 9.9%).

8. Renal dysfunction—up to 40% developed transient oliguria, with 2% progressing to renal failure requiring dialysis. Postoperative renal dysfunction results from postoperative hypovolemia, anemia, hypotension, low-output syndrome, sepsis, and pericardial tamponade.

Other Complications

1. Postperfusion syndrome—diffuse syndrome characterized by systemic inflammatory response syndrome.

2. Febrile complications—probably from body's reaction to tissue trauma or accumulation of blood and serum in pleural and pericardial spaces.

3. In older patients, decreased kidney function can increase the risk of developing drug toxicities, adverse reactions, and oliguria and renal failure.

4. Failure to wean from the ventilator due to underlying pulmonary disease or postoperative pulmonary complications.

Postoperative Management

1. Adequate oxygenation is ensured; respiratory insufficiency is common after open-heart surgery.

a. Patients require intubation during cardiac surgery and the majority of them continued to require mechanical ventilation after being transported to the cardiac surgery ICU.

b. Chest x-ray taken immediately after surgery and daily thereafter to evaluate state of lung expansion and to detect atelectasis or pneumothorax and to demonstrate heart size and contour and confirm placement of central line, ET tube, and chest drains.

2. Hemodynamic monitoring during the immediate postoperative period for cardiovascular and respiratory status and fluid and electrolyte balance to prevent or recognize complications.

3. Drainage of mediastinal and pleural chest tubes is monitored.

4. Fluid and electrolyte balance is monitored closely with daily weight.

5. Hypokalemia may be caused by inadequate intake, diuretics, vomiting, excessive NG drainage, and stress from surgery.

a. Hyperkalemia may be caused by increased intake, red cell breakdown (from the pump, bleeding, or transfusion), acidosis, renal insufficiency, tissue necrosis, and adrenal cortical insufficiency.

b. Hyponatremia may be due to reduction of total body sodium or to an increased water intake, causing a dilution of body sodium.

c. Hypocalcemia may be due to alkalosis (which reduces the amount of calcium in the extracellular fluid) and multiple blood transfusions.

d. Hypercalcemia may cause dysrhythmias imitating those caused by digoxin toxicity.

6. Postoperative medications include:

a. Aspirin daily as MI prophylaxis.

b. Analgesics.

c. Antihypertensives or antiarrhythmics, if needed.

d. Beta-blockers.

e. ACE inhibitors for patients with ejection fraction less than 30%.

f. Antibiotics, if indicated.

7. Monitoring for complications.

8. Cardiac pacing, if indicated, by way of temporary pacing wires from the incision.

Nursing Diagnoses

- Anxiety related to fear of unknown, fear of death, and fear of pain.
- Impaired Gas Exchange related to alveolar capillary membrane changes, immobility, altered blood flow.
- Decreased Cardiac Output related to mechanical factors: decreased preload and impaired contractility.
- Risk for Deficient Fluid Volume related to physiologic effects of heart-lung machine.
- Acute Pain related to sternotomy and leg incisions.
- Sleep Deprivation related to intensive care environment.
- Risk for Injury related to postoperative complications.

Nursing Interventions

Minimizing Anxiety

1. Orient to surroundings as soon as patient awakens from surgical procedure. Tell patient that the surgery is over and orient to location, time of day, and your name.
2. Allow family members to visit patient as soon as condition stabilizes. Encourage family members to talk to and touch patient. (Family members may be overwhelmed by intensive care environment.)
3. As patient becomes more alert, explain purpose of all equipment in environment. Continually orient patient to time and place. Make sure patient has glasses and hearing aids, if needed.
4. Administer anxiolytics, as directed.
5. Remove lines and tubing once medically appropriate.

Promoting Adequate Gas Exchange

1. Frequently check function of mechanical ventilator, patient's respiratory effort, and ABG levels.
2. Check ET tube placement.
3. Auscultate chest for breath sounds. Crackles indicate pulmonary congestion; decreased or absent breath sounds indicate pneumothorax; rales may indicate pulmonary edema.
4. Sedate patient adequately to help tolerate ET tube and cope with ventilatory sensations.
5. Use chest physiotherapy for patients with lung congestion to prevent retention of secretions and atelectasis.
6. Promote coughing, deep breathing, and turning to keep airway patent, prevent atelectasis, and facilitate lung expansion. Have patient sit at 30 degrees unless medically contraindicated.
7. Suction tracheobronchial secretions carefully. Prolonged suctioning leads to hypoxia and possible cardiac arrest.
8. Administer diuretics, as prescribed.
9. Institute ventilatory weaning protocol when patient is awake and can initiate own breaths and assist with extubation (see page 258), when indicated.

Maintaining Adequate Cardiac Output

1. Monitor cardiovascular status to determine effectiveness of CO. Continuous monitoring of blood pressure by way of intra-arterial line, heart rate, CVP, left atrial or PAP, and PCWP from monitor modules are observed, correlated with the patient's condition, and recorded.
2. Monitor and record urine output every hour.
3. Observe buccal mucosa, nail beds, lips, earlobes, and extremities for duskiness, cyanosis—late signs of low CO.
4. Feel the skin; cool, moist skin or weak pulses reveals lowered CO. Note temperature and color of extremities.
5. Monitor neurologic status.
   a. Observe for symptoms of hypoxia—restlessness, headache, confusion, dyspnea, hypotension, and cyanosis. Obtain ABG values and core temperature.
   b. Note the patient's neurologic status hourly in terms of level of responsiveness, response to verbal commands and painful stimuli, pupillary size and reaction to light, and movement of extremities, hand-grasp ability.
   c. Monitor for and treat postoperative seizures.

Maintaining Adequate Fluid Volume

1. Administer IV fluids as ordered, but limit if signs of fluid overloading occur.
2. Keep intake and output flow sheets as a method of determining positive or negative fluid balance and the patient's fluid requirements.
   a. IV fluids (including flush solutions through arterial and venous lines) are considered intake.
   b. Measure postoperative chest drainage—should not exceed 200 mL/hour for first 4 to 6 hours.
3. Be alert to changes in serum electrolyte levels.
   a. Hypokalemia may cause dysrhythmias, digoxin toxicity, metabolic alkalosis, weakened myocardium, cardiac arrest.
      i. Watch for specific ECG changes.
      ii. Replace electrolytes, as needed.
   b. Hyperkalemia may cause mental confusion, restlessness, nausea, weakness, and paresthesia of extremities. Treatment may include administering an ion-exchange resin, sodium polystyrene sulfonate, which binds the potassium or hemodialysis. Temporary treatment includes sodium bicarbonate, insulin (with dextrose), albuterol, and calcium.
   c. Hyponatremia may cause weakness, fatigue, confusion, seizures, and coma.
   d. Hypocalcemia may cause numbness and tingling in the fingertips, toes, ears, and nose; carpopedal spasm, muscle cramps, and tetany. Give replacement therapy, as needed.
   e. Hypercalcemia may cause digoxin toxicity.
      i. Treatment may include fluids, diuretics, calcitonin, or hemodialysis.
      ii. This condition may lead to asystole and death.
4. Monitor hematocrit and hemoglobin (frequency depends on hemodynamics and evidence of bleeding) and report any significant change in findings.
   a. Ensure that patient has current blood type and screen. Transfuse blood products, as ordered.
   b. Check coagulation tests, including prothrombin time, International Normalized Ratio, and partial thromboplastin time, if patient is coagulopathic, bleeding, or anticoagulated for mechanical device.

Relieving Pain

1. Examine surgical incision sites.
2. Record nature, type, location, duration of pain, and contributing factors.
3. Differentiate between incisional pain and anginal pain. Obtain ECG and have provider confirm if there are any changes.
4. Report restlessness and apprehension not corrected by analgesics—may be from hypoxia or a low-output state.
5. Administer medications as prescribed, or monitor constant infusion to reduce amount of pain and to aid the patient in performing deep-breathing and coughing exercises more effectively.
6. Assist patient to position of comfort.
7. Encourage early mobilization.

Promoting Sleep and Recovery

1. Watch for symptoms of postcardiotomy delirium (may appear after brief lucid period).
   a. Signs and symptoms include delirium (impairment of orientation, memory, intellectual function, judgment), transient perceptual distortions, visual and auditory hallucinations, disorientation, and paranoid delusions.
   b. Symptoms may be related to sleep deprivation, increased sensory output, disorientation to night and day, prolonged inability to speak because of ET intubation, age, and preoperative cardiac status.
2. Keep the patient oriented to time and place; notify the patient of procedures and expectations of cooperation.
3. Encourage family to visit at regular times—helps patient regain sense of reality.
4. Plan care to allow rest periods, day–night pattern, and uninterrupted sleep.
5. Encourage mobility as soon as possible.
   a. Keep environment as free as possible of excessive auditory and sensory input.
   b. Prevent bodily injury.
   c. Have physical therapy work with patient and provide analgesics prior to therapy.
6. Reassure patient and family that psychiatric disorders after cardiac surgery are usually transient.
7. Remove patient from the ICU as soon as possible. Allow patient to talk about psychotic episode—helps deal with and assimilate experience.

Avoiding Complications

1. Monitor ECG continuously for arrhythmias.
   a. Evaluate possible cause of dysrhythmias—inadequate oxygenation, electrolyte imbalance, MI, mechanical irritation (eg, pacing wires, invasive lines, chest tubes), and any vasopressor or inotropic medications.
   b. Treat dysrhythmias immediately because they may lead to decreased CO. Atrial or AV pacing is used to treat sinus bradycardia or junctional rhythm with heart rates less than 70 beats/minute.
2. Assess for signs of cardiac tamponade—arterial hypotension; rising CVP; rising left atrial pressure; muffled heart sounds; weak, thready pulse; jugular vein distention; falling urine output.
   a. Check for diminished amount of drainage in the chest-collection bottle; may indicate that fluid is accumulating elsewhere.
   b. Prepare for pericardiocentesis.
   c. Assist with echocardiogram to evaluate tamponade.
3. Check cardiac enzyme levels daily. Elevations may indicate MI. (Symptoms may be masked by the usual postoperative discomfort.)
   a. Watch for decreased CO in the presence of normal circulating volume and filling pressure.
   b. Obtain serial ECGs and isoenzymes to determine extent of myocardial injury.
   c. Assess pain to differentiate myocardial pain from incisional pain.

4. Monitor for hypertension or hypotension.
   a. Mild systolic hypertension occurs in 48% to 55% of all CABG patients within the first 6 hours postoperatively.
   b. Hypotension may be caused by bleeding, hypovolemia, decreased systemic vascular resistance (eg, systemic inflammatory response syndrome), cardiogenic shock, tamponade, medications, or arrhythmias.
   c. Blood pressure goal following cardiac surgery is dependent on the patient's conditions (eg, carotid disease, renal disease, bleeding).
5. Initiate measures to prevent embolization such as anti-embolic stockings, not putting pressure on popliteal space (leg crossing, raising knee gatch), and starting passive and active exercises.
   a. Assess for signs of DVT and pulmonary embolism.
   b. Maintain integrity of all invasive lines.
6. Monitor for bleeding.
   a. Watch for steady and continuous drainage of blood.
   b. Assess for arterial hypotension, low CVP, increasing pulse rate, and low left atrial pressure and PCWP.
   c. Prepare to administer blood products, IV solutions, or protamine sulfate, antifibrinolytics, DDAVP, or vitamin K.
   d. Prepare for potential return to surgery if bleeding persists (over 300 mL/hour) for 2 hours.
   e. Monitor hemoglobin levels; if the patient's hemoglobin drops below 8 g/dL, transfusions of red blood cells or platelets may be necessary.
   f. During the first 4 to 12 hours, blood recovered from mediastinal tubes can be autotransfused to the patient.
7. Be alert for fever and signs of infection. Check blood glucose levels as ordered.
   a. Administer prophylactic antibiotics, if ordered, for the first 48 hours.
   b. Control higher degrees of fever through use of hypothermia mattress.
   c. Evaluate for atelectasis, pleural effusion, or pneumonia if fever persists. (The most common cause of early postoperative fever [within 24 hours] is atelectasis.)
   d. Evaluate for urinary tract infection and wound infection.
   e. Draw blood cultures to rule out infectious cause if fever persists.
8. Measure urine volume; less than 0.5 to 1 mL/kg/hr can indicate decreased renal function.
   a. Monitor BUN and serum creatinine levels as well as urine and serum electrolyte levels.
   b. Give rapid-acting diuretics and/or inotropic drugs (dopamine, dobutamine) to increase CO and renal blood flow.
   c. Prepare the patient for peritoneal dialysis or hemodialysis if indicated. (Renal insufficiency may produce serious cardiac dysrhythmias.)

Community and Home Care Considerations

Preparing the patient with cardiovascular disease or after cardiac surgery for the return home and/or optimizing the patient's health status in the home are important nursing functions. The key areas on which to focus include assessment, education, and evaluating responses.

1. Perform a thorough assessment of the patient's clinical condition, functional status, and home safety and support systems. Based on assessment, determine the patient's need for supportive services.
2. Coordinate services such as home health aides.
3. Refer patients to area meal delivery service as appropriate. These services provide special diets in most cases (eg, low sodium or low cholesterol).
4. Coordinate outpatient cardiac rehabilitation services as appropriate.
5. Establish outpatient or home-based physical and occupational therapy as appropriate for graduated exercise and energy-conservation techniques.
6. If therapist recommends inpatient rehabilitation, coordinate with facility social worker/discharge planner to find a rehabilitation facility suited for patient as well as his or her family.
7. Educate patient, family, and caregivers about potential complications and medication regimen.

Patient Education and Health Maintenance

Note: Specific guidelines will vary slightly among facilities and health care providers. Check facility policy and orders.
1. Instruct about activities.
   a. Increase activities gradually within limits. (Avoid strenuous activities until after exercise stress testing.)
   b. Take short rest periods.
   c. Avoid lifting more than 20 lb (9.1 kg).
   d. Participate in activities that do not cause pain or discomfort.
   e. Increase walking time and distance each day.
   f. Stairs (one to two times daily) the first week; increase as tolerated.
   g. Avoid large crowds at first.
   h. Avoid driving until after first postoperative checkup.
   i. Resumption of sexual relations parallels ability to participate in other activities.
      i. Usually may resume sexual activity 2 weeks after surgery.
      ii. Avoid sexual activity if tired or after heavy meal.
      iii. Consult health care provider if chest discomfort, difficult breathing, or palpitations occur and last longer than 15 minutes after intercourse.
   j. Return to work after first postoperative checkup, as advised by health care provider.
2. Expect some chest discomfort.
3. Advise about diet.
   a. Some patients are placed on minimum salt restriction (eg, no salt added at table); cholesterol may be limited. Have a dietitian talk to the patient and family regarding diet.
   b. Weigh daily and report weight gain of more than 5 lb (2.3 kg) per week.
   c. If the patient is taking warfarin, advise patient not to change normal dietary habits, but to maintain similar intake pattern each day to prevent changes in INR.
4. Tight blood glucose control is recommended (keeping blood sugars less than 110 mg/dL) to prevent sternal wound infection.

5. Teach patient and family about wound care and how to avoid infections.
6. Teach about medications.
   a. Label all medications; give purposes and adverse effects.
   b. Patients with prosthetic valves may continue warfarin regimen indefinitely. Explain bleeding precautions and need for periodic laboratory studies.
7. Advise patients with prosthetic valves:
   a. Pregnancy is usually discouraged due to anticoagulation therapy.
   b. Need for antibiotic coverage before dental and surgical procedures.
   c. Patients taking anticoagulants should watch for bleeding and should avoid use of aspirin (and many other drugs)—interferes with action of warfarin.
8. Advise the patient to carry an identification card stating cardiac condition and medications being taken.
9. Encourage compliance with rehabilitation and exercise program after exercise stress testing.
10. Inform the patient whom to contact (and how) in case of an emergency.
11. See also section on patient education after MI, page 394, and patient education about infective endocarditis, page 404.
12. Explore community support groups such as AHA (*www.americanheart.org*).
13. Be diligent in providing older patients with education and discharge instructions that they will be able to follow due to sensory impairments, immobility, and transportation barriers.

 GERONTOLOGIC ALERT Older patients are extremely vulnerable to complications due to decreased functional ability and the normal process of aging.

Evaluation: Expected Outcomes

- Verbalizes understanding of surgical procedure, reduction of fear.
- Extubated 24 hours postoperative; spontaneous unlabored respirations 14 to 18 per minute.
- Blood pressure and heart rate stable; adequate urine output.
- Serum electrolytes within normal range.
- Verbalizes reduced pain.
- Sleeps for 2- to 3-hour intervals during night; oriented to time and place; no hallucinations.
- No bleeding noted; afebrile; ECG shows normal sinus rhythm.

SELECTED REFERENCES

Allen, K. B. (2011). Patient characteristics and operative risk with stand-alone transmyocardial revascularization. *Journal of the American College of Cardiology, 57*(14, Suppl. S), E1140.

American Society of Anesthesiologists (ASA) Committee on Standards of Practice Parameters. (2011). Practice guidelines for preoperative fasting and the use of pharmacologic agents to reduce the risk of pulmonary aspiration: application to healthy patients undergoing elective procedures. *Anesthesiology, 114*, 495–511.

Anderson, J. L., Adams, C. D., Antman, E. M., et al. (2007). ACC/AHA 2007 guidelines for the management of patients with unstable angina/non-ST-elevation myocardial infarction. *Journal of the American College of Cardiology, 50*(7), e1–e157.

Aronson, S. (2011). Does perioperative systolic blood pressure variability predict mortality after cardiac surgery?: An exploratory analysis of the ECLIPSE trials. *Anesthesia and Analgesia, 113*(1), 19.

Chen, M. (2011). Chest pain. *Medline Plus.* Available: *www.nlm.nih.gov/medlineplus/ency/article/003079.htm.*

Desai, M., Seifalian, A. M., & Hamilton, G. (2011). Role of prosthetic conduits in coronary artery bypass grafting. *European Journal of Cardio-Thoracic Surgery, 40*(2), 394–398.

Engore, M., & Barbee, D. (2005). Comparison of cardiac output determined by bioimpedance, thermodilution, and the Fick method. *American Journal of Critical Care, 14,* 40–45.

Epstein, A. E., Dimarco, J. P., Ellenbogen, K. A., et al. (2008). ACC/AHA/HRS 2008 guidelines for device-based therapy of cardiac rhythm abnormalities: Executive Summary: A report of the American College of Cardiology/American Heart Association Task Force on Practice Guidelines (writing committee to revise the ACC/AHA/NASPE 2002 guidelines update for implantation of cardiac pacemakers and antiarrhythmia devices) developed in collaboration with the American Association for Thoracic Surgery and Society of Thoracic Surgeons. *Journal of the American College of Cardiology, 51*(21), 2085–2105.

Epstein, A. J., Polsky, D., Yang, F., et al. (2011). Coronary revascularization trends in the United States, 2001–2008. *Journal of the American Medical Association, 305*(17), 1769.

Floros, P., Sawhney, R., Vrtik, M., et al. (2011). Risk factors and management approach for deep sternal wound infection after cardiac surgery at a tertiary medical centre. *Heart, Lung and Circulation, 20*(11), 712–717.

Hall, M. J., DeFrances, C. J., Williams, S. N., et al. (2010). National hospital discharge survey: 2007 summary. *National Health Status Report, 29,* 1–20.

Imazio, M. (2011). Meta-analysis of randomized trials focusing on prevention of the postpericardiotomy syndrome. *American Journal of Cardiology, 108*(4), 575.

Johns Hopkins Medical Institutions. (2011). MRI tests can be safe for people with implanted cardiac devices, study suggests. *Science Daily.* Available: *www.sciencedaily.com/releases/2011/10/111003180423.htm.*

Kushner, F. G. (2009). 2009 focused updates: ACC/AHA guidelines for the management of patients with ST-elevation myocardial infarction (updating the 2004 guideline and 2007 focused update) and ACC/AHA/SCAI guidelines on percutaneous coronary intervention (updating the 2005 guideline and 2007 focused update). A report of the American College of Cardiology Foundation/American Heart Association Task Force on Practice Guidelines. *Circulation, 120,* 2271–2306.

Levine, G. N., Bates, E. R., & Blankenship, J. C. (2011). 2011 ACCF/AHA/SCAI guideline for percutaneous coronary intervention. *Circulation, 124,* e574–e651.

Link, M. S., Atkins, D. L., Passman, R. S., et al. (2010). Part 6: Electrical therapies automated external defibrillators, defibrillation, cardioversion, and pacing: 2010 American Heart Association guidelines for cardiopulmonary resuscitation and emergency cardiovascular care science. *Circulation, 122,* s706–s719.

Litmathe, J., Boeken, U., Bohlen, G., et al. (2011). Systemic inflammatory response syndrome after extracorporeal circulation: A predictive algorithm for the patient at risk. *Hellenic Journal of Cardiology, 52,* 493–500.

Lynn-McHale Wiegand, D. J. (Ed.). (2011). *AACN procedure manual for critical care* (6th ed.). St. Louis, MO: Saunders.

Mylonas, I., & Beanlands, R. S. B. (2011). Radionuclide imaging of viable myocardium: Is it underutilized? *Current Cardiovascular Imaging Reports, 4*(3), 251–261.

Nazarian, S., Hansford, R., Roquin, A., et al. (2011). A prospective evaluation of a protocol for magnetic resonance imaging of patients with implanted cardiac devices. *Annals of Internal Medicine, 155,* 415–424.

Onishi, T., Kobayashi, I., Onishi, Y., et al. (2010). Evaluating microvascular obstruction after acute myocardial infarction using cardiac magnetic resonance imaging and 201-thallium and 99m-technetium pyrophosphate scintigraphy. *Circulation Journal, 74,* 2633–2640.

Pannu, N. (2011). The acute kidney injury to chronic kidney disease continuum: Comment on the magnitude of acute serum creatinine increase after cardiac surgery and the risk of chronic kidney disease, progression of kidney disease, and death. *Archives of Internal Medicine, 171*(3), 233.

Pasion, E., Good, E., Tizon, J., et al. (2010). Evaluation of the monitor cursor-line method for measuring pulmonary artery and CVP. *American Journal of Critical Care, 19*(6), 511–521.

Perera, D., Stables, R., Clayton, T., et al. (2013). Long-term mortality data from the balloon pump-assisted coronary intervention study (BCIS-1): A randomized, controlled trial of elective balloon counterpulsation during high-risk percutaneous coronary intervention/clinical perspective. *Circulation, 127,* 207–212.

Perera, P., Stables, R., Thomas, M., et al. (2010). Counterpulsation during high-risk percutaneous coronary intervention. A randomized controlled trial. *Journal of the American Medical Association, 304,* 867–874.

Pompilio, G. (2011). Determinants of pericardial drainage for cardiac tamponade following cardiac surgery. *European Journal of Cardio-Thoracic Surgery, 39*(5), e107.

Reynolds, M. R., & Zimetbaum, P. (2011). Magnetic resonance imaging and cardiac devices: How safe is safe enough? *Annuals of Internal Medicine, 155*(7), 470–472.

Roger, V. L., Go, A. S., Lloyd-Jones, D. M., et al. (2011). Heart disease and stroke statistics—2011 Update. *Circulation, 123*(4), e18–e209.

Schinkel, A. F. L., Bax, J. J., Poldermans, D., et al. (2007). Hibernating myocardium: Diagnosis and patient outcomes. *Current Problems in Cardiology, 32,* 375–410.

Scirica, B. M. (2013). Therapeutic hypothermia after cardiac arrest. *Circulation, 127,* 244–250.

Szabo, G., Racz, I., & Koszegi, Z. (2010). Elective intra-aortic balloon pump placement in high risk PCI. *Journal of the American Medical Association, 304*(20), 2241.

Tricoci, P., Allen, J. M., Kramer, J. M., et al. (2009). Scientific evidence underlying the ACC/AHA clinical practice guidelines. *Journal of the American Medical Association, 301*(8), 831–841.

Vavalle, J. P., & Ohman, E. M. (2013). Left ventricular support systems for high-risk percutaneous coronary interventions: How can we improve outcomes for rare procedures? *Circulation, 127,* 162–164.

13
Cardiac Disorders

CARDIAC DISORDERS
Coronary Artery Disease

 Evidence Base Fraker, T. D., & Fihn, S. D. (2007). 2007 chronic angina focused update of the ACC/ AHA 2002 guidelines for the management of patients with chronic stable angina. *Circulation, 116*, 2762–2772.

Coronary artery disease (CAD) is the leading cause of death in the United States. CAD is characterized by the accumulation of plaque within the layers of the coronary arteries. The plaques progressively enlarge, thicken, and calcify, causing a critical narrowing (>70% occlusion) of the coronary artery lumen, resulting in a decrease in coronary blood flow and an inadequate supply of oxygen to the heart muscle.

Acute coronary syndrome (ACS) is an umbrella term that is used to describe many of the complications associated with CAD. These include unstable angina, non-ST-elevation myocardial infarction (NSTEMI), and ST-elevation myocardial infarction (STEMI).

Pathophysiology and Etiology

1. The most widely accepted cause of CAD is atherosclerosis (see Figure 13-1), which is the gradual accumulation of plaque within an artery forming an atheroma. Plaque consists of lipid-filled macrophages (foam cells), fibrin, cellular waste products, and plasma proteins, covered by a fibrous outer layer (smooth muscle cells and dense connective tissue).
    a. When the endothelium is injured by being exposed to low-density lipoproteins, by-products of cigarette smoke, hypertension, hyperglycemia, infection, and increased homocysteine, hyperfibrinogenemia, and lipoprotein(a),

an inflammatory response occurs, making the endothelium sticky and thereby attracting adhesion molecules.
    b. Over time, the plaque thickens, extends, and calcifies, causing narrowing of the lumen.
    c. Eventual hemorrhage and ulceration of the plaque may cause significant coronary obstruction.
2. Angina pectoris, caused by inadequate blood flow to the myocardium, is the most common manifestation of CAD.
    a. Angina is usually precipitated by physical exertion or emotional stress, which puts an increased demand on the heart to circulate more blood and oxygen.
    b. The ability of the coronary artery to deliver blood to the myocardium is impaired because of obstruction by a significant coronary lesion (>70% narrowing of the vessel).
    c. Angina can also occur in other cardiac problems, such as arterial spasm, aortic stenosis, cardiomyopathy, or uncontrolled hypertension.
    d. Noncardiac causes include anemia, fever, thyrotoxicosis, and anxiety/panic attacks.
3. ACS is caused by a decrease in the oxygen available to the myocardium due to:
    a. Unstable or ruptured atherosclerotic plaque.
    b. Coronary vasospasm.
    c. Atherosclerotic obstruction without clot or vasospasm.
    d. Inflammation or infection.
    e. Unstable angina due to a noncardiac cause.
    f. Thrombus formation with subsequent coronary artery occlusion (the most common cause) (see "Myocardial Infarction," page 386).
4. Risk factors for the development of CAD include:
    a. Nonmodifiable: age (risk increases with age), male sex (women typically suffer from heart disease 10 years later

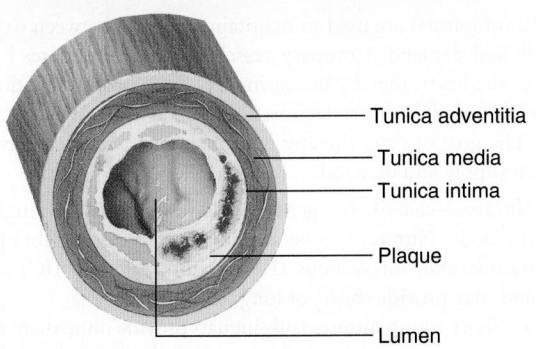

Tunica adventitia

Tunica media

Tunica intima

Plaque

Lumen

Figure 13-1. The pathogenesis of atherosclerosis.

STANDARDS OF CARE GUIDELINES 13-1
Chest Pain

- Thoroughly evaluate any complaint of chest pain.

- Be alert to those at highest risk for myocardial infarction (MI)—smokers, those with hypertension, diabetes, or hyperlipidemia—but do not discount that MI may occur in those without risk factors.

- Be alert to common alternative presentation of coronary artery disease and MI in women, diabetics, and older patients (nausea, indigestion, fatigue).

- Notify health care provider and obtain electrocardiogram for complaint of chest pain.

- For chest pain not relieved by rest or nitroglycerin, assist and advise patient to obtain emergency care immediately. Call 911 for emergency response team if pain is consistent with MI.

This information should serve as a general guideline only. Each patient situation presents a unique set of clinical factors and requires nursing judgment to guide care, which may include additional or alternative measures and approaches.

---

than men due to the postmenopausal decrease in cardiac-protective estrogen), race (nonwhite populations have increased risk), and family history.

b. Modifiable: elevated lipid levels, hypertension, obesity, tobacco use, metabolic syndrome (obesity, hypertension, and diabetes mellitus), sedentary lifestyle, and stress.

c. Recent studies have shown that there are new risk factors associated with the development of CAD. These include increased levels of homocysteine, fibrin, lipoprotein(a), and infection or inflammation (measured by C-reactive protein [CRP]).

d. The American Heart Association (AHA) also lists left ventricular hypertrophy (LVH) as a risk factor.

5. The Framingham Scoring Method is used to determine the 10-year risk of development of coronary heart disease (CHD) in men and women based on age, total cholesterol, high-density lipoprotein (HDL) level, systolic blood pressure (BP), presence of hypertension, and cigarette smoking. More information can be found at *www.nhlbi.nih.gov/guidelines/cholesterol/index.htm.*

Clinical Manifestations

See Standards of Care Guidelines 13-1.

Chronic Stable Angina Pectoris

Chest pain or discomfort that is provoked by exertion or emotional stress and relieved by rest and nitroglycerin.

1. Character—substernal chest pain, pressure, heaviness, or discomfort. Other sensations include a squeezing, aching, burning, choking, strangling, and/or cramping pain.
   a. Pain may be mild or severe and typically presents with a gradual buildup of discomfort and subsequent gradual fading.
   b. May produce numbness or weakness in arms, wrists, or hands.
   c. Associated symptoms include diaphoresis, nausea, indigestion, dyspnea, tachycardia, and increase in blood pressure.
   d. Women may experience atypical symptoms of chest pain, such as jaw pain, shortness of breath, or indigestion. Patients with diabetes or history of heart transplant may not experience chest pain.

2. Location—behind middle or upper third of sternum; the patient will generally make a fist over the site of the pain (positive Levine's sign, indicating diffuse deep visceral pain) rather than point to it with his or her finger.

3. Radiation—usually radiates to neck, jaw, shoulders, arms, hands, and posterior intrascapular area. Pain occurs more commonly on the left side than the right.

4. Duration—usually lasts 2 to 15 minutes after stopping activity; nitroglycerin relieves pain within 1 minute.

5. Other precipitating factors—exposure to weather extremes, eating a heavy meal, and sexual intercourse all increase the workload of the heart, thus increasing oxygen demand.

Unstable (Preinfarction) Angina Pectoris

Chest pain occurring at rest; no increase in oxygen demand is placed on the heart, but an acute lack of blood flow to the heart occurs because of coronary artery spasm or the presence of an enlarged plaque or hemorrhage/ulceration of a complicated lesion. Critical narrowing of the vessel lumen occurs abruptly in either instance.

1. A change in frequency, duration, and intensity of stable angina symptoms is indicative of progression to unstable angina.

2. Unstable angina pain lasts longer than 10 minutes, is unrelieved by rest or sublingual nitroglycerin, and mimics signs and symptoms of impending MI.

 NURSING ALERT Unstable angina can cause sudden death or result in MI. Early recognition and treatment are imperative to prevent complications.

Silent Ischemia

The absence of chest pain with documented evidence of an imbalance between myocardial oxygen supply and demand (ST depression of 1 mm or more) as determined by electrocardiography (ECG), exercise stress test, or ambulatory (Holter) ECG monitoring.

1. Silent ischemia most commonly occurs during the first few hours after awakening (circadian event) due to an increase in sympathetic nervous system activity, causing an increase in heart rate, blood pressure, coronary vessel tone, and blood viscosity.

Diagnostic Evaluation

1. Characteristic chest pain and clinical history.
2. Nitroglycerin test—relief of pain with nitroglycerin.
3. Blood tests.
   a. Cardiac markers, creatine kinase (CK) and its isoenzyme CK-MB, and troponin-I to determine the presence and severity if acute cardiac insult is suspected.
   b. HbA_{1C} and fasting lipid panel to rule out modifiable risk factors for CAD.
   c. Coagulation studies, CRP, homocysteine, and lipoprotein(a) (increased levels are associated with a two-fold risk in developing CAD).
   d. Hemoglobin to rule out anemia, which may reduce myocardial oxygen supply.
4. 12-lead ECG—may show LVH, ST-T wave changes, arrhythmias, and Q waves.
5. ECG stress testing—progressive increases of speed and elevation while walking on a treadmill increase the workload of the heart. ST-T wave changes occur if myocardial ischemia is induced.
6. Radionuclide imaging—a radioisotope, thallium 201, injected during exercise is imaged by camera. Low uptake of the isotope by heart muscle indicates regions of ischemia induced by exercise. Images taken during rest show a reversal of ischemia in those regions affected.
7. Radionuclide ventriculography (gated blood pool scanning)—red blood cells tagged with a radioisotope are imaged by camera during exercise and at rest. Wall motion abnormalities of the heart can be detected and ejection fraction estimated.
8. Cardiac catheterization—coronary angiography performed during the procedure determines the presence, location, and extent of coronary lesions.
9. Positron-emission tomography (PET)—cardiac perfusion imaging with high resolution to detect very small perfusion differences caused by stenotic arteries. Not available in all settings.
10. Electron-beam computed tomography (CT)—detects coronary calcium, which is found in most, but not all, atherosclerotic plaque. It is not routinely used due to its low specificity for identifying significant CAD.

Management

Drug Therapy

Antianginal medications (nitrates, beta-adrenergic blockers, calcium channel blockers, and angiotensin-converting enzyme [ACE] inhibitors) are used to maintain a balance between oxygen supply and demand. Coronary vessel relaxation promotes blood flow to the heart, thereby increasing oxygen supply. Reduction of the workload of the heart decreases oxygen demand and consumption. The goal of drug therapy is to maintain a balance between oxygen supply and demand.

1. Nitrates—caused by generalized vasodilation throughout the body. Nitrates can be administered via oral, sublingual, transdermal, intravenous (IV), or intracoronary (IC) route and may provide short- or long-acting effects.
   a. Short-acting nitrates (sublingual) provide immediate relief of acute anginal attacks or prophylaxis if taken before activity.
   b. Long-acting nitrates prevent anginal episodes and/or reduce severity and frequency of attacks.
2. Beta-adrenergic blockers—inhibit sympathetic stimulation of receptors that are located in the conduction system of the heart and in heart muscle.
   a. Some beta-adrenergic blockers inhibit sympathetic stimulation of receptors in the lungs as well as the heart ("nonselective" beta-adrenergic blockers); vasoconstriction of the large airways in the lung occurs; generally contraindicated for patients with chronic obstructive lung disease or asthma.
   b. "Cardioselective" beta-adrenergic blockers (in recommended dose ranges) affect only the heart and can be used safely in patients with lung disease.
3. Calcium channel blockers—inhibit movement of calcium within the heart muscle and coronary vessels; promote vasodilation and prevent/control coronary artery spasm.
4. ACE inhibitors—have therapeutic effects by remodeling the vascular endothelium and have been shown to reduce the risk of worsening angina.
5. Antilipid agents—reduce total cholesterol and triglyceride levels and have been shown to assist in the stabilization of plaque.
6. Antiplatelet agents—decrease platelet aggregation to inhibit thrombus formation.
7. Folic acid and B complex vitamins—treat increased homocysteine levels.

Percutaneous Coronary Interventions

1. Percutaneous transluminal angioplasty.
   a. A balloon-tipped catheter is placed in a coronary vessel narrowed by plaque.
   b. The balloon is inflated and deflated to stretch the vessel wall and flatten the plaque (see "Percutaneous Transluminal Coronary Angioplasty," page 366).
   c. Blood flows freely through the unclogged vessel to the heart.
2. IC atherectomy.
   a. A blade-tipped catheter is guided into a coronary vessel to the site of the plaque.
   b. Depending on the type of blade, the plaque is either cut, shaved, or pulverized and then removed.
   c. Requires a larger catheter introduction sheath so its use is limited to larger vessels.

3. IC stent.

a. A diamond mesh tubular device is placed in the coronary vessel.

b. Prevents restenosis by providing a "skeletal" support.

c. Drug-eluting stents contain an anti-inflammatory drug, which decreases the inflammatory response within the artery.

Other Interventional Strategies

1. Coronary artery bypass graft (CABG) surgery.

a. A graft is surgically attached to the aorta, and the other end of the graft is attached to a distal portion of a coronary vessel.

b. Bypasses obstructive lesions in the vessel and returns adequate blood flow to the heart muscle supplied by the artery (see "Heart Surgery," page 371).

2. Transmyocardial revascularization—by means of a laser beam, small channels are formed in the myocardium to encourage new blood flow.

Secondary Prevention

Evidence Base Smith, S. C., Benjamin, E. J., Bonow, R. O., et al. (2011). AHA/ACCF secondary prevention and risk reduction therapy for patients with coronary and other atherosclerotic vascular disease: 2011 update: A guideline from the American Heart Association and American College of Cardiology Foundation. *Journal of the American College of Cardiology, 58*(23), 2432–2446.

1. Cessation of smoking.

2. Control of high blood pressure (below 130/85 mm Hg in those with renal insufficiency or heart failure; below 130/80 mm Hg in those with diabetes; below 140/90 mm Hg in all others).

3. Diet low in saturated fat (<7% of calories), cholesterol (<200 mg/day), trans-fatty acids, sodium (<2 g/day), alcohol (2 or fewer drinks/day in men, 1 or fewer in women).

4. Low-dose aspirin daily for those at high risk.

5. Physical exercise (at least 30 to 60 minutes of moderate-intensity exercise most days).

6. Weight control (ideal body mass index 18.5 to 24.9 kg/m^2); waist circumference less than 40 inches for men, less than 35 inches for women.

7. Control of diabetes mellitus (fasting glucose < 110 mg/dL and HbA$_{1C}$ < 7%).

8. Control of blood lipids with low-density lipoprotein (LDL) goal less than 100 mg/dL (less than 70 mg/dL in high-risk patients).

Complications

1. Sudden death due to lethal dysrhythmias.

2. Heart failure.

3. MI.

Nursing Assessment

1. Ask patient to describe anginal attacks.

a. When do attacks tend to occur? After a meal? After engaging in certain activities? After physical activities in general? After visits of family/others?

b. Where is the pain located? Does it radiate?

c. Was the onset of pain sudden? Gradual?

d. How long did it last—Seconds? Minutes? Hours?

e. Was the pain steady and unwavering in quality?

f. Is the discomfort accompanied by other symptoms? Sweating? Light-headedness? Nausea? Palpitations? Shortness of breath?

g. Is there anything that makes it worse (such as moving, deep breathing, food)?

h. How is the pain relieved? How long does it take for pain relief?

2. Obtain a baseline 12-lead ECG.

3. Assess patient's and family's knowledge of disease.

4. Identify patient's and family's level of anxiety and use of appropriate coping mechanisms.

5. Gather information about the patient's cardiac risk factors. Use the patient's age, total cholesterol level, LDL and HDL levels, systolic BP, and smoking status to determine the patient's 10-year risk for development of CHD according to the Framingham Risk Scoring Method.

6. Evaluate patient's medical history for such conditions as diabetes, heart failure, previous MI, or obstructive lung disease that may influence choice of drug therapy.

7. Identify factors that may contribute to noncompliance with prescribed drug therapy.

8. Review renal and hepatic studies and complete blood count (CBC).

9. Discuss with patient current activity levels. (Effectiveness of anti-anginal drug therapy is evaluated by patient's ability to attain higher activity levels.)

10. Discuss patient's beliefs about modification of risk factors and willingness to change.

Nursing Diagnoses

- Acute Pain related to an imbalance in oxygen supply and demand.
- Decreased Cardiac Output related to reduced preload, afterload, contractility, and heart rate secondary to hemodynamic effects of drug therapy.
- Anxiety related to chest pain, uncertain prognosis, and threatening environment.

Nursing Interventions

Relieving Pain

1. Determine intensity of patient's angina.

a. Ask patient to compare the pain with other pain experienced in the past and, on a scale of 0 (no pain) to 10 (worst pain), rate current pain.

b. Observe for associated signs and symptoms, including diaphoresis, shortness of breath, protective body posture, dusky facial color, and/or changes in level of consciousness (LOC).

2. Position patient for comfort; Fowler's position promotes ventilation.

3. Administer oxygen, if appropriate.

4. Obtain BP, apical heart rate, and respiratory rate.

5. Obtain a 12-lead ECG.

6. Administer anti-anginal drug(s), as prescribed.

7. Report findings to health care providers.

8. Monitor for relief of pain and note duration of anginal episode.

9. Take vital signs every 5 to 10 minutes until angina pain subsides.

10. Monitor for progression of stable angina to unstable angina: increase in frequency and intensity of pain, pain occurring at rest or at low levels of exertion, pain lasting longer than 5 minutes.

11. Determine level of activity that precipitated anginal episode.

12. Identify specific activities patient may engage in that are below the level at which anginal pain occurs.

13. Reinforce the importance of notifying nursing staff when angina pain is experienced.

Maintaining Cardiac Output

1. Carefully monitor the patient's response to drug therapy.

   a. Take BP and heart rate in a sitting and a lying position on initiation of long-term therapy (provides baseline data to evaluate for orthostatic hypotension that may occur with drug therapy).

   b. Recheck vital signs as indicated by onset of action of drug and at time of drug's peak effect.

   c. Note changes in BP of more than 10 mm Hg and changes in heart rate of more than 10 beats/minute.

   d. Note patient complaints of headache (especially with use of nitrates) and dizziness (more common with ACE inhibitors).

      i. Administer or teach self-administration of analgesics, as directed, for headache.

      ii. Encourage supine position to relieve dizziness (usually associated with a decrease in BP; preload is enhanced by lying supine, thereby providing a temporary increase in BP).

   e. Institute continuous ECG monitoring or obtain 12-lead ECG as directed. Interpret rhythm strip every 4 hours and as needed for patients on continuous monitoring (beta-adrenergic blockers and calcium channel blockers can cause significant bradycardia and varying degrees of heart block).

   f. Evaluate for development of heart failure (beta-adrenergic blockers and some calcium channel blockers have negative inotropic properties).

      i. Obtain daily weight and intake and output.

      ii. Auscultate lung fields for crackles and assess for shortness of breath and decrease in oxygen saturation.

      iii. Monitor for the presence of edema.

      iv. Monitor central venous pressure (CVP), if applicable.

      v. Assess jugular vein distention.

      vi. Assess liver engorgement and check liver function studies.

   g. Monitor laboratory tests as indicated (cardiac markers).

2. Monitor for poor perfusion.

   a. Decreasing blood pressure.

   b. Weak pulses.

   c. Dizziness.

   d. Shortness of breath.

   e. Cool extremities.

   f. Pale.

   g. Diaphoretic.

3. Be sure to remove previous nitrate patch or paste before applying new paste or patch (prevents hypotension) and to reapply on different body site. To decrease nitrate tolerance, transdermal nitroglycerin may be worn only in the daytime hours and taken off at night when physical exertion is decreased.

4. Be alert to adverse reaction related to abrupt discontinuation of beta-adrenergic blocker and calcium channel blocker therapy. These drugs must be tapered to prevent a "rebound phenomenon": tachycardia, increase in chest pain, hypertension.

5. Discuss use of chromotherapeutic therapy with health care provider (tailoring of anti-anginal drug therapy to the timing of circadian events).

6. Report adverse drug effects to health care provider.

Decreasing Anxiety

1. Rule out physiologic etiologies for increasing or new-onset anxiety before administering as-needed sedatives. Physiologic causes must be identified and treated in a timely fashion to prevent irreversible adverse or even fatal outcomes; sedatives may mask symptoms delaying timely identification and diagnosis and treatment.

2. Assess patient for signs of hypoperfusion, auscultate heart and lung sounds, obtain a rhythm strip, and administer oxygen, as prescribed. Notify the health care provider immediately.

3. Document all assessment findings, health care provider notification and response, and interventions and response.

4. Explain to patient and family reasons for hospitalization, diagnostic tests, and therapies administered.

5. Encourage patient to verbalize fears and concerns about illness through frequent conversations—conveys to patient a willingness to listen.

6. Answer patient's questions with concise explanations.

7. Administer medications to relieve patient's anxiety as directed. Sedatives and tranquilizers may be used to prevent attacks precipitated by aggravation, excitement, or tension.

8. Explain to patient the importance of anxiety reduction to assist in control of angina. (Anxiety and fear put increased stress on the heart, requiring the heart to use more oxygen.) Teach relaxation techniques.

9. Discuss measures to be taken when an anginal episode occurs. (Preparing patient decreases anxiety and allows patient to describe angina accurately.)

   a. Review the questions that will be asked during anginal episodes.

   b. Review the interventions that will be employed to relieve anginal attacks.

Patient Education and Health Maintenance

Instruct Patient and Family about CAD

1. Assess readiness to learn (pain free, shows interest, and comfortable), learning style, cognition, and education level.
2. Review the chambers of the heart and the coronary artery system, using a diagram of the heart.
3. Show patient a diagram of a clogged artery; explain how the blockage occurs; point out on the diagram the location of patient's lesions.
4. Explain what angina is (a warning sign from the heart that there is not enough blood and oxygen because of the blocked artery or spasm).
5. Review specific risk factors that affect CAD development and progression; highlight those risk factors that can be modified and controlled to reduce risk.
6. Discuss the signs and symptoms of angina, precipitating factors, and treatment for attacks. Stress to patient the importance of treating angina symptoms at once.
7. Distinguish for patient the different signs and symptoms associated with stable angina versus preinfarction angina.
8. Give patient and family handouts to review and encourage questions for a later teaching session.

Identify Suitable Activity Level to Prevent Angina

Advise the patient about the following:

1. Participate in a normal daily program of activities that do not produce chest discomfort, shortness of breath, and undue fatigue. Spread daily activities out over the course of the day; avoid doing everything at one time. Begin regular exercise regimen, as directed by health care provider.
2. Avoid activities known to cause anginal pain—sudden exertion, walking against the wind, extremes of temperature, high altitude, and emotionally stressful situations, which my accelerate heart rate, raise BP, and increase cardiac workload.
3. Refrain from engaging in physical activity for 2 hours after meals. Rest after each meal, if possible.
4. Do not perform activities requiring heavy effort (eg, carrying heavy objects).
5. Try to avoid cold weather, if possible; dress warmly and walk more slowly. Wear scarf over nose and mouth when in cold air.
6. Lose weight, if necessary, to reduce cardiac load.
7. Instruct patient that sexual activity is not prohibited and should be discussed with health care provider.

Instruct about Appropriate Use of Medications and Adverse Effects

1. Carry nitroglycerin at all times.
   a. Nitroglycerin is volatile and is inactivated by heat, moisture, air, light, and time.
   b. Keep nitroglycerin in original dark glass container, tightly closed to prevent absorption of drug by other pills or pillbox.
   c. Nitroglycerin should cause a slight burning or stinging sensation under the tongue when it is potent.

2. Place nitroglycerin under the tongue at first sign of chest discomfort.
   a. Stop all effort or activity, sit, and take nitroglycerin tablet—relief should be obtained in a few minutes.
   b. Repeat dosage in 5 minutes for total of three tablets if relief is not obtained.
   c. Keep a record of the number of tablets taken to evaluate change in anginal pattern.
   d. Take nitroglycerin prophylactically to avoid pain known to occur with certain activities.

 **NURSING ALERT** Instruct patient to call 911 if chest pain persists or has worsened after the first sublingual nitroglycerin tablet was administered (5 minutes). Further instruct patient to continue to take other sublingual nitroglycerin tablets every 5 minutes until emergency medical services have arrived (instruct patient not drive self to the hospital).

3. Demonstrate for patient how to administer nitroglycerin paste correctly.
   a. Place paste on calibrated strip.
   b. Remove previous paste on skin by wiping gently with tissue. Be careful to avoid touching paste to fingertips as this will lead to increased dosing from absorption.
   c. Rotate site of administration to avoid skin irritation.
   d. Apply paste to skin; use plastic wrap to protect clothing if not provided on strip.
   e. Have patient return demonstration.
4. Instruct patient on administration of transdermal nitroglycerin patches.
   a. Remove previous patch; fold in half so that medication does not touch fingertips and will not be accessible in trash. Wipe area with tissue to remove any residual medication.
   b. Apply patch to a clean, dry, nonhairy area of body.
   c. Rotate administration sites.
   d. Instruct patient not to remove patch for swimming or bathing.
   e. If patch loosens and part of it becomes nonadherent, it should be folded in half and discarded. A new patch should be applied.
5. Teach patient about potential adverse effects of other medications. Instruct patient not to stop taking any of these without discussing with health care provider.
   a. Constipation—verapamil.
   b. Ankle edema—nifedipine.
   c. Heart failure (shortness of breath, weight gain, edema)—beta-adrenergic blockers or calcium channel blockers.
   d. Dizziness—vasodilators, antihypertensives.
   e. Impotence-decreased libido and sexual functioning—beta-adrenergic blockers
6. Ensure that patient has enough medication until next follow-up appointment or trip to the pharmacy. Warn against abrupt withdrawal of beta-adrenergic blockers or calcium channel blockers to prevent rebound effect.

Counsel on Risk Factors and Lifestyle Changes

1. Inform patient of methods of stress reduction, such as bio-feedback and relaxation techniques.
2. Review low-fat and low-cholesterol diet. Explain AHA guidelines (see *www.heart.org*), which recommend eating fish at least twice per week, especially fish high in omega-3 oils.
   a. Omega-3 oils have been shown to improve arterial health and decrease BP, triglycerides, and the growth of atherosclerotic plaque.
   b. Omega-3 oils can be found in fatty fish, such as mackerel, salmon, sardines, herring, and albacore tuna.
   c. Suggest available cookbooks (AHA) that may assist in planning and preparing foods.
   d. Have patient meet with dietitian to design a menu plan.
3. Inform patient of available cardiac rehabilitation programs that offer structured classes on exercise, smoking cessation, and weight control.
4. Instruct patient to avoid excessive caffeine intake (coffee, cola drinks), which can increase the heart rate and produce angina.
5. Tell patient not to use "diet pills," nasal decongestants, or any over-the-counter (OTC) medications that can increase heart rate or stimulate high BP.
6. Encourage patient to avoid alcohol or drink only in moderation (alcohol can increase hypotensive adverse effects of drugs).
7. Encourage follow-up visits for control of diabetes, hypertension, and hyperlipidemia.
8. Have patient discuss supplement therapy (ie, vitamins B_6, B_{12}, C, E, folic acid, and L-arginine) with health care provider.
9. For additional information, refer patient to the AHA (*www.americanheart.org*).
10. Refer patient to health care provider to discuss the use of phosphodiesterase inhibitors (PDe5) for erectile dysfunction.

 DRUG ALERT Patient should not take PDe5, such as sildenafil, concurrently with nitrates or alpha-adrenergic blockers because severe hypotension and cardiac event may occur.

Evaluation: Expected Outcomes

- Verbalizes relief of pain.
- BP and heart rate stable.
- Verbalizes lessening anxiety, ability to cope.

Myocardial Infarction

 Evidence Base Anderson, J. L., Adams, C. D., Antman, E. M., et al. (2011). 2011 ACCF/AHA focused update incorporated into ACC/AHA 2007 guidelines for the management of patients with unstable angina/non-ST elevation myocardial infarction: A report of the American College of Cardiology Foundation/American Heart Association Task Force on Practice Guidelines. *Journal of American College of Cardiology, 57*(19), 1920–1259.
    Kushner, F. G. (2009). 2009 focused updates: ACC/AHA guidelines for the management of patients with ST elevation myocardial infarction (updating the 2004 guideline and 2007 focused update) and ACC/AHA/SCAI guidelines on percutaneous coronary intervention (updating the 2005 guideline and 2007 focused update): A report of the American College of Cardiology Foundation/American Heart Association Task Force on Practice Guidelines. *Circulation, 120,* 2271–2306.

Myocardial infarction (MI) is one of the manifestations of acute coronary syndrome (ACS) and refers to a dynamic process by which one or more regions of the heart experience a prolonged decrease or cessation in oxygen supply because of insufficient coronary blood flow; subsequently, necrosis or "death" to the affected myocardial tissue occurs. The onset of the MI process may be sudden or gradual, and the progression of the event to cell death takes approximately 3 to 6 hours. MI is one manifestation of ACS.

Pathophysiology and Etiology

1. Acute coronary thrombosis (partial or total)—associated with 90% of MIs.
   a. Severe atherosclerosis (>70% narrowing of the artery) precipitates thrombus.
   b. Thrombus formation begins with plaque rupture and platelets' adhesion to the damaged area.
   c. Activation of the exposed platelets causes expression of glycoprotein IIb/IIIa receptors that bind fibrinogen.
   d. Further platelet aggregation and adhesion occurs, enlarging the thrombus and occluding the artery.
2. Other etiologic factors include coronary artery spasm, coronary artery embolism, infectious diseases causing arterial inflammation, hypoxia, anemia, and severe exertion or stress on the heart in the presence of significant CAD (ie, surgical procedures, shoveling snow).
3. Different degrees of damage occur to the heart muscle (see Figure 13-2):
   a. Zone of necrosis—death to the heart muscle caused by extensive and complete oxygen deprivation; irreversible damage.

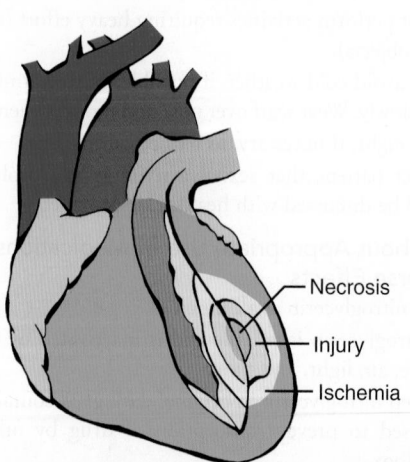

Figure 13-2. Different degrees of damage occur to the heart muscle after a myocardial infarction. This diagram shows the zones of necrosis, injury, and ischemia.

b. Zone of injury—region of the heart muscle surrounding the area of necrosis; inflamed and injured, but still viable if adequate oxygenation can be restored.

c. Zone of ischemia—region of the heart muscle surrounding the area of injury, which is ischemic and viable; not endangered unless extension of the infarction occurs.

4. Classification of MI:

a. STEMI—whereby ST-segment elevations are seen on ECG. The area of necrosis may or may not occur through the entire wall of heart muscle.

b. NSTEMI—no ST-segment elevations can be seen on ECG. ST depressions may be noted as well as positive cardiac markers, T-wave inversions, and clinical equivalents (chest pain). Area of necrosis may or may not occur through the entire myocardium.

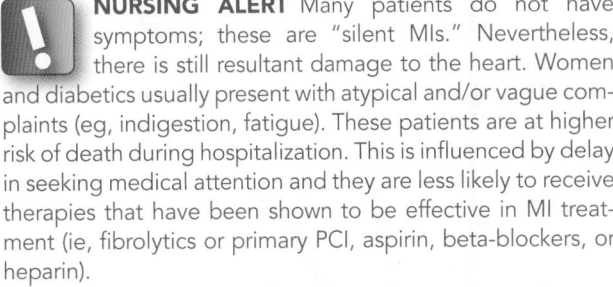

NURSING ALERT Studies have shown that with the exception of highest-risk patients, immediate catheterization or percutaneous coronary intervention (PCI) does not offer any benefit over initial medical management with subsequent catheterization/PCI in patients with NSTEMI (Anderson et al., 2011). However, NSTEMI is potentially an incomplete MI, thus careful monitoring for signs and symptoms of continuing damage to heart muscle, including arrhythmias, drop in BP, and dyspnea, is required.

5. The region(s) of the heart muscle that becomes affected depends on which coronary artery(ies) is/are obstructed (see Figure 13-3).

a. Left ventricle is a common and dangerous location for an MI because it is the main pumping chamber of the heart.

The left anterior descending artery supplies oxygen to this part of the heart.

b. Right ventricular infarctions commonly occur with damage to the inferior and/or posterior wall of the left ventricle. Occlusion in the right coronary or circumflex arteries can lead to this type of infarct.

6. The severity and location of the MI determines prognosis.

Clinical Manifestations

1. Chest pain.

a. Severe, diffuse, steady substernal pain; may be described as crushing, squeezing, or dull.

b. Not relieved by rest or sublingual vasodilator therapy such as nitroglycerine, but requires opioids (ie, morphine).

c. May radiate to the arms (usually the left), shoulders, neck, back, and/or jaw.

d. Continues for more than 15 minutes.

e. May produce anxiety and fear, resulting in increased heart rate, blood pressure, and respiratory rate.

f. Some patients, women or diabetics, may exhibit no complaints of pain (silent MI).

2. Diaphoresis; cool, clammy skin; facial pallor.

3. Hypertension or hypotension.

4. Bradycardia or tachycardia.

5. Premature ventricular and/or atrial beats.

6. Palpitations, severe anxiety, dyspnea.

7. Disorientation, confusion, restlessness.

8. Fainting, marked weakness.

9. Nausea, vomiting, hiccups.

10. Atypical symptoms: epigastric or abdominal distress, dull aching or tingling sensations, shortness of breath, extreme fatigue.

NURSING ALERT Many patients do not have symptoms; these are "silent MIs." Nevertheless, there is still resultant damage to the heart. Women and diabetics usually present with atypical and/or vague complaints (eg, indigestion, fatigue). These patients are at higher risk of death during hospitalization. This is influenced by delay in seeking medical attention and they are less likely to receive therapies that have been shown to be effective in MI treatment (ie, fibrolytics or primary PCI, aspirin, beta-blockers, or heparin).

GERONTOLOGIC ALERT Older patients are more likely to experience silent MIs or have atypical signs and symptoms, such as hypotension, low body temperature, shortness of breath, vague complaints of discomfort, mild perspiration, stroke-like symptoms, dizziness, or change in sensorium.

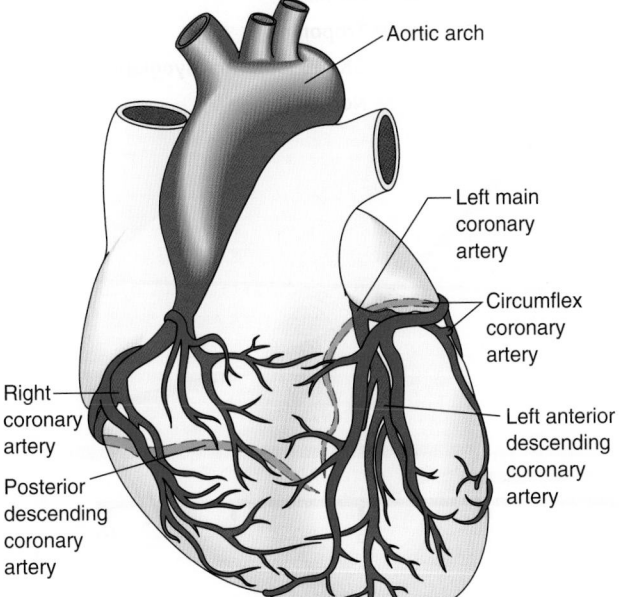

Figure 13-3. Diagram of the coronary arteries arising from the aorta and encircling the heart. Some of the coronary veins are also shown.

Labels: Aortic arch; Left main coronary artery; Circumflex coronary artery; Left anterior descending coronary artery; Right coronary artery; Posterior descending coronary artery

Diagnostic Evaluation

ECG Changes

1. Generally occurs within 2 to 12 hours, but may take 72 to 96 hours.

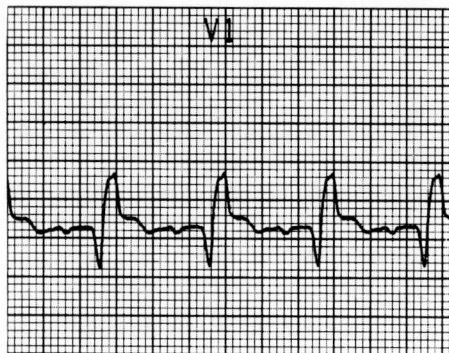

Figure 13-4. Abnormal Q wave.

2. Necrotic, injured, and ischemic tissues alter ventricular depolarization and repolarization.
   a. ST-segment depression and T-wave inversion indicate a pattern of ischemia.
   b. ST elevation indicates an injury pattern.
   c. Q waves (see Figure 13-4) indicate tissue necrosis and are permanent. A pathologic Q wave is one that is greater than 3 mm in depth or greater than one third the height of the R wave.
3. Location of the infarction (anterior, anteroseptal, inferior, posterior, lateral) is determined by the leads in which the ST changes (elevation vs. depression) are seen. Of note, the changes must be in two contiguous or related leads to be diagnostic.

> **NURSING ALERT** A normal ECG does not rule out the possibility of infarction because ECG changes can be subtle and obscured by underlying conditions (bundle-branch blocks, electrolyte disturbances).

Cardiac Markers
1. Cardiac enzymes (biochemical markers) are not diagnostic of an acute MI with a single elevation; serial markers are drawn (see page 328).
   a. Marker elevation is then correlated to the extent of heart muscle damage.
   b. Characteristic elevation over several hours confirms an MI (see Figure 13-5).

> **NURSING ALERT** It is important to note that although these markers may be abnormal in the patient presenting with unstable angina or NSTEMI, the ACCF/AHA 2011 guideline does not recommend the routine use of these markers for clinical application.

Other Findings
1. Elevated CRP and lipoprotein(s) due to inflammation in the coronary arteries.
2. Abnormal coagulation studies (prothrombin time [PT], partial thromboplastin time [PTT]).
3. Elevated white blood cell (WBC) count and sedimentation rate due to the inflammatory process involved in heart muscle cell damage.

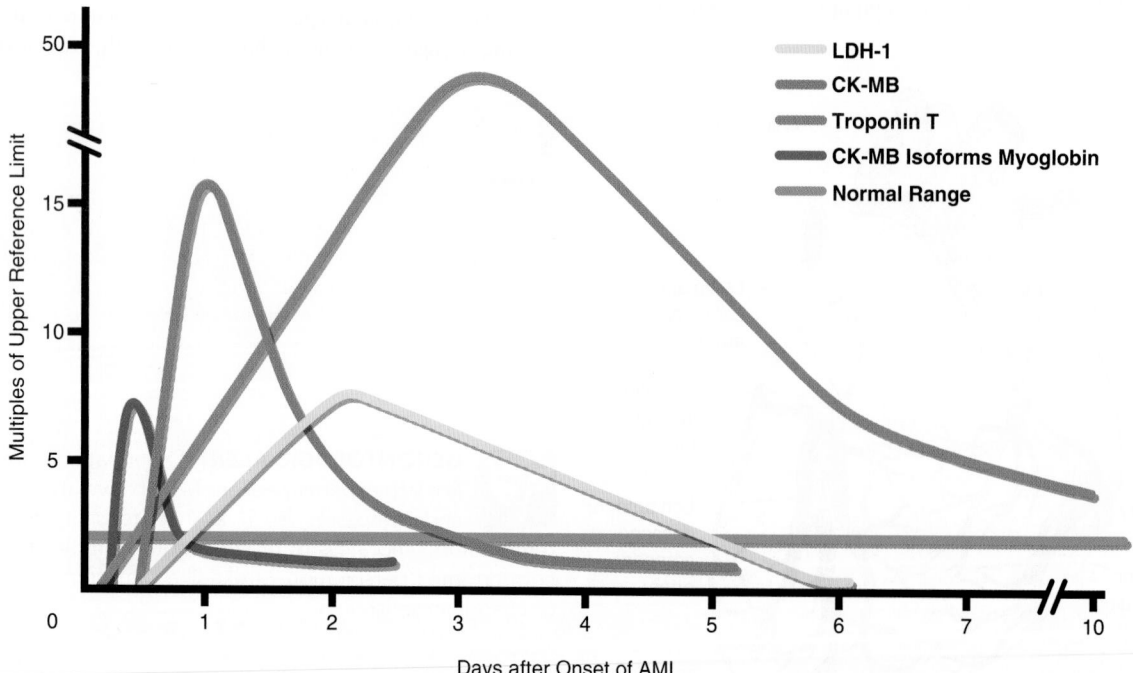

Figure 13-5. Release of cardiac markers after acute myocardial infarction (AMI). Following AMI, myoglobin and CK-MB levels rise, but the increases last only a few days. Levels of troponin T can be sustained for 4 to 10 days following AMI, allowing for more accurate diagnosis. All results are normalized to the upper reference limit. (Wu, A.H.B. [1995]. Cardiac troponins T and I in coronary artery diseases. *Endocrinology and Metabolism In-Service Training and Continuing Education, 13*, 81. © American Association for Clinical Chemistry, Inc.)

4. Radionuclide imaging allows recognition of areas of decreased perfusion.

5. PET determines the presence of reversible heart muscle injury and irreversible or necrotic tissue; extent to which the injured heart muscle has responded to treatment can also be determined.

6. Cardiac muscle dysfunction noted on echocardiography or cardiac magnetic resonance imaging (MRI).

Management

The ACCF/AHA (2011) issued "Guidelines for the Management of Patients with Unstable Angina and Non-ST-Elevation MI." These guidelines call for clinicians to begin treatment for acute chest pain immediately, based on risk level and ECG changes, rather than waiting for cardiac marker results, which was the traditional approach to diagnosis and treatment of MI.

The goals for UA/NSTEMI therapy are immediate relief of ischemia and prevention of severe outcomes such as death or myocardial infarction or reinfarction. To achieve this requires administration of anti-ischemic therapy (ie, rest, supplemental oxygen, nitroglycerin, beta blockers, ACE inhibitors); antithrombotic therapy (ie, aspirin, clopidogrel, ticlopidine); and ongoing risk stratification and use of invasive procedure (ie, cardiac catheterization) to provide early restoration of coronary blood flow.

 NURSING ALERT Prompt identification of MI and ACS as well as timely initiation of therapy is vital.

Pharmacologic Therapy

The pharmacologic therapy for MI is standard (see Table 13.1, page 390). Use the MONA acronym to outline immediate pharmacologic interventions.

1. M (morphine)—IV rather than intramuscular (I.M.) administration to prevent spurious elevation in serial biomarkers. Used to treat chest pain. Endogenous catecholamine release during pain imposes an increase in the workload on the heart, thus causing an increase in oxygen demand. Morphine's analgesic effects decrease the pain, relieve anxiety, and improve cardiac output by reducing preload and afterload.

 GERONTOLOGIC ALERT Older patients are extremely susceptible to respiratory depression in response to opioids. Titrate dose carefully and monitor respiratory status.

2. O (oxygen)—given via nasal cannula or face mask. Increases oxygenation to ischemic heart muscle.

3. N (nitrates)—given sublingually via spray or through IV administration. Vasodilator therapy reduces preload by decreasing blood return to the heart and decreasing oxygen demand.

4. A (aspirin)—immediate dosing by mouth (chewed) is recommended to halt platelet aggregation.

Other Medications

1. Fibrinolytic agents such as tissue plasma activator, streptokinase, and reteplase reestablish blood flow in coronary vessels by dissolving thrombus.
   a. No effect on the underlying stenosis that precipitated the thrombus to form.
   b. IV administration.

 **DRUG ALERT** Fibrinolytic agents are not indicated in the management of unstable angina or NSTEMI or posterior-wall MI. Studies have shown no clinical benefits in the absence of ST elevation MI or bundle branch block.

2. Anti-arrhythmics, such as amiodarone, and correction of electrolyte imbalances decrease the ventricular irritability that occurs after MI.
   a. Bolus of amiodarone is given via IV line over 10 minutes, then an infusion is given in varying doses over 24 hours (1 mg/minute for 6 hours then 0.5 mg/minute for 18 hours).

Percutaneous Coronary Interventions

1. Mechanical opening of the coronary vessel can be performed during an evolving infarction.

2. Percutaneous coronary interventions (PCIs), including percutaneous transluminal coronary angioplasty, coronary stenting, and atherectomy, can be used instead of, or as an adjunct to, fibrinolytic therapy (see "Percutaneous Transluminal Coronary Angioplasty," page 366). Fibrinolytic therapy is considered in STEMI patients if PCI is not able to be performed within 90 minutes.

3. Should be performed within 90 minutes of patient's arrival (door to balloon time).

Surgical Revascularization

1. Cardiac surgery (ie, CABG) following STEMI is associated with high mortality in the first 3 to 7 days, thus the benefit of revascularization must be weighed against the risk of cardiac surgery.

2. Benefits of this therapy include definitive treatment of the stenosis and less scar formation on the heart.

Complications

1. Dysrhythmias.
2. Sudden cardiac death due to ventricular arrhythmias.
3. Infarct expansion (thinning and dilation of the necrotic zone).
4. Infarct extension (additional heart muscle necrosis occurring after 24 hours of acute infarction).
5. Heart failure (with 20% to 35% left ventricle damage).
6. Cardiogenic shock.
7. Reinfarction.
8. Ischemic cardiomyopathy.
9. Cardiac rupture.
10. Papillary muscle rupture.
11. Ventricular mural thrombus.

Table 13-1	ACS Medications at a Glance
DRUG AND ACTION	**CLINICAL CONSIDERATIONS**
Aspirin Antiplatelet drug that blocks prostaglandin synthesis and thromboxane A_2 formation	• Administer as soon as acute coronary syndrome (ACS) is suspected. • Give patient 160–325 mg; if not already taking aspirin, patient should chew this dose. • If patient is allergic to aspirin, give clopidogrel or ticlopidine instead.
Clopidogrel, ticlopidine Antiplatelet drugs that inhibit platelet aggregation	• Alternatives for patients who cannot use aspirin. • Recent research indicates that using clopidogrel and aspirin concurrently reduces risk of myocardial infarction (MI), stroke, and death.
Unfractionated heparin, low-molecular-weight heparin (dalteparin, enoxaparin) Potentiate antithrombin III activity, inactivate thrombin, prevent conversion of fibrinogen to fibrin	*Unfractionated heparin* • Weight-adjusted dosage is given to achieve therapeutic partial thromboplastin time (PTT) and activated clotting time. • Reversible with protamine sulfate. *Low-molecular-weight heparin* • PTT is not monitored. • Give by subcutaneous injection. • Effects are not reversible.
Glycoprotein (GP) IIb/IIIa inhibitors (abciximab, tirofiban, eptifibatide) Block GP sites on platelets, preventing platelet aggregation	• Indicated for intermediate- or high-risk ACS or with percutaneous coronary intervention. • Each drug has specific indications and dosage ranges. Consult package insert for specifics.
Fibrinolytics (alteplase, tenecteplase, streptokinase, reteplase) Break up the fibrin meshwork in clots	• Indicated in ST-segment elevation ACS only. • Certain agents require weight-adjusted dose. See package inserts for details.
Beta-adrenergic blockers (metoprolol, atenolol) Reduce cardiac output and heart rate, reduce ventricular remodeling, and decrease endothelial dysfunction	• Start all ACS patients on a beta-adrenergic blocker as tolerated. • As ordered, titrate dosage to meet therapeutic goals: heart rate, 60 beats/minute; blood pressure (BP), greater than 90 mm Hg systolic.
Angiotensin-converting enzyme inhibitors (captopril, enalapril) Decrease endothelial dysfunction and prevent conversion of angiotensin I to angiotensin II	• Indicated for patients with heart failure, those with a heart rate above 100 beats/minute, and those with an anterior MI, hypertension, or diabetes. • Start with a drug with a short half-life, such as captopril, within 24 hours to treat acute MI; on discharge, switch to a longer-acting drug, such as lisinopril or enalapril.
Nitroglycerin Dilates peripheral vessels, relaxes vascular smooth muscle, and decreases preload	• Can be given sublingually, orally, or via IV line spray in an acute care setting. • Do not allow BP to drop below 90 mm Hg systolic. • Switch the patient to a topical patch or an oral form for long-term use.
Morphine Acts as an analgesic and sedative	• Indicated in acute care setting only; not for prolonged use. • Give until patient is free from chest pain or to relieve pulmonary congestion. • Monitor BP, level of consciousness, and respiratory rate.

Granger, B., & Miller, C. (2001). Acute coronary syndromes. *Nursing, 31*(11), 42.

12. Ischemic stroke.
13. Thromboemboli (deep vein thrombosis and pulmonary embolism).
14. Ventricular aneurysm.
15. Cardiac tamponade.
16. Pericarditis (2 to 3 days after MI).
17. Dissection of coronary arteries during angioplasty.
18. Psychiatric problems—depression, personality changes.

Nursing Assessment

1. Gather information regarding the patient's chest pain:
   a. Nature and intensity—describe the pain in patient's own words and compare it with pain previously experienced.
   b. Onset and duration—exact time pain occurred as well as the time pain relieved or diminished (if applicable).
   c. Location and radiation—point to the area where the pain is located and to other areas where the pain seems to travel.

d. Precipitating and aggravating factors—describe the activity performed just before the onset of pain and if any maneuvers and/or medications alleviated the pain.

2. Question patient about other symptoms experienced associated with the pain. Observe patient for diaphoresis, facial pallor, dyspnea, guarding behaviors, rigid body posture, extreme weakness, and confusion.

3. Evaluate cognitive, behavioral, and emotional status.

4. Question patient about prior health status with emphasis on current medications, allergies (opiate analgesics, iodine, shellfish), recent trauma or surgery, nonsteroidal anti-inflammatory drug (NSAID) ingestion, peptic ulcers, fainting spells, drug and alcohol use.

5. Analyze information for contraindications for fibrinolytic therapy and PCI.

6. Gather information about presence or absence of cardiac risk factors.

7. Identify patient's social support system and potential caregivers.

8. Identify significant others' reaction to the crisis situation.

Nursing Diagnoses

See also Nursing Care Plan 13-1, pages 392 to 393.
- Anxiety related to chest pain, fear of death, threatening environment.
- Activity Intolerance related to insufficient oxygenation to perform activities of daily living, deconditioning effects of bed rest.
- Risk for Injury (bleeding) related to dissolution of protective clots.
- Risk for Decreased Cardiac Tissue Perfusion related to coronary restenosis, extension of infarction.
- Ineffective Coping related to threats to self-esteem, disruption of sleep–rest pattern, lack of significant support system, loss of control, and change in lifestyle.

Nursing Interventions

Alleviating Anxiety

1. Rule out physiologic etiologies for increasing or new-onset anxiety before administering as-needed sedatives. Physiologic causes must be identified and treated in a timely fashion to prevent irreversible adverse or even fatal outcomes; sedatives may mask symptoms, delaying timely identification, diagnosis, and treatment.
   a. Autonomic signs of anxiety are increases in heart rate, BP, respiratory rate, and tremulousness, but they may also be signs of physiologic complications.
   b. Anxiety with dyspnea, tachypnea, and tachycardia may indicate pulmonary embolism; frothy pink sputum and orthopnea indicate pulmonary edema.
   c. Appearance of heart murmurs or friction rub indicates valvular dysfunction, possible intraventricular septal rupture, and pericarditis.

2. Whenever anxiety increases, assess patient for signs of hypoperfusion, auscultate heart and lung sounds, obtain a rhythm strip, and administer oxygen, as prescribed. Notify the health care provider immediately.

3. Assess and document emotional status frequently. Document all assessment findings, health care provider notification and response, and interventions and response.

4. Explain to patient and family reasons for hospitalization, diagnostic tests, and therapies administered.

5. Explain equipment, procedures, and need for frequent assessment to patient and significant others.

6. Discuss with patient and family the anticipated nursing and medical regimen.
   a. Explain visiting hours and need to limit number of visitors at one time.
   b. Offer family preferred times to phone unit to check on patient's status.

7. Administer anti-anxiety agents, as prescribed.
   a. Explain to patient the reason for sedation: undue anxiety can make the heart more irritable and require more oxygen.
   b. Assure patient that the goal of sedation is to promote comfort and, therefore, should be requested if anxious, excitable, or "jittery" feelings occur.
   c. Observe for adverse effects of sedation, such as lethargy, confusion, and/or increased agitation.

8. Maintain consistency of care with one or two nurses regularly assisting patient, especially if severe anxiety is present.

9. Offer massage, imagery, and progressive muscle relaxation to promote relaxation, reduce muscle tension, and reduce workload on the heart.

Increasing Activity Tolerance

1. Promote activity tolerance with early gradual increase in mobilization—prevents deconditioning, which occurs with bed rest.
   a. Minimize environmental noise.
   b. Provide a comfortable environmental temperature.
   c. Avoid unnecessary interruptions and procedures.
   d. Structure routine care measures to include rest periods after activity.
   e. Discuss with patient and family the purpose of limited activity and visitors—to help the heart heal by lowering heart rate and BP, maintaining cardiac workload at lowest level, and decreasing oxygen consumption.
   f. Promote restful diversional activities for patient (reading, listening to music, drawing, crossword puzzles, crafts).
   g. Encourage frequent position changes while in bed.

2. Assist patient with prescribed activities.
   a. Assist patient to rise slowly from a supine position to minimize orthostatic hypotension related to medications.
   b. Encourage passive and active range-of-motion (ROM) exercise as directed while on bed rest.
   c. Measure the length and width of the unit so patients can gradually increase their activity levels with specific guidelines (walk one width [150 ft] of the unit).
   d. Elevate patient's feet when out of bed in chair to promote venous return.

NURSING CARE PLAN 13-1

Caring for a Patient with Acute Myocardial Infarction

Mr. M. is a 60-year-old male admitted to your unit with a diagnosis of an acute inferior wall myocardial infarction (MI). From your assessment and knowledge of acute MI, you develop your care plan.

Subjective data: Mr. M. is complaining of severe, crushing chest pain unrelieved by rest, which has lasted for 2 hours. The pain is substernal and does not radiate. He tells you that he smokes two packs of cigarettes per day, is a manager at an electronics firm, and that his father died at age 59 from a heart attack.

Objective data: Vital signs: pulse, 110 and irregular; blood pressure (BP), 90/68 mm Hg; respirations, 28 breaths/minute. His cardiac monitor shows sinus tachycardia with frequent premature ventricular contractions (PVCs), and his 12-lead electrocardiogram (ECG) shows ST elevation in leads II, III, and AVF. He has no significant Q waves at this time. His heart sounds are normal except for the irregularity, and his lungs are clear. He is pale, diaphoretic, and clutching his chest.

NURSING DIAGNOSIS
Acute Pain related to an imbalance in oxygen supply and demand.

GOAL/EXPECTED OUTCOME
Pain will be reduced.

Nursing Interventions	Rationale	Actual Outcomes (Evaluation)
1. Position Mr. M. in bed in semi-Fowler's position. Handle carefully while providing initial care.	1. Allows for rest and adequate chest excursion, to increase available oxygen, and to decrease cardiac work.	1. Resting in semi-Fowler's position.
2. Administer oxygen by nasal cannula at 2 L/minute. Maintain O_2 saturation at 95% or above. Encourage slower, deep breaths as necessary.	2. Increases oxygen supply. May decrease pain and PVCs.	2. Color improved and verbalizes decreased pain.
3. Administer nitroglycerin and morphine based on vital signs and pain relief. Hold nitrate if SBP < 90, HR < 50 or > 100, suspected RV infarction, or ingestion of phosphodiesterase inhibitor such as sildenafil within 48 hours.	3. Both medications help to alleviate pain by decreasing venous return to the heart, thereby decreasing cardiac work. Morphine also helps to decrease the patient's sensation of pain. Nitrates may exacerbate hypotension.	3. Verbalizes decreased pain, from level 7 to level 3 (on scale of 0–10).
4. Monitor BP before administration and 10 minutes after each dose. Place patient in supine position to minimize hypotension.	4. Both medications may decrease BP because both decrease venous return. Continuous intra-arterial BP monitoring may be used if condition warrants.	4. BP remains stable with a mean arterial pressure of 60 mm Hg or above.
5. Attach electrodes for continuous bedside cardiac monitor. Monitor heart rate and rhythm frequently.	5. Increased rate may indicate heart block; dysrhythmias are common initially, increased frequency suggests ischemia.	5. Heart rate <90 beats/minute; normal sinus rhythm.
6. Offer support and reassurance to patient that pain relief is a priority. Encourage patient to report increasing pain. Perform pain assessment regularly.	6. Pain perception can be reduced by reducing anxiety. Increasing pain may indicate increasing ischemia.	6. Pain reduced from 10/10 to 5/10 after 30 minutes.

NURSING CARE PLAN 13-1 (continued)

Caring for a Patient with Acute Myocardial Infarction

NURSING DIAGNOSIS
Decreased Cardiac Output related to decreased cardiac contractility and dysrhythmias

GOAL (EXPECTED OUTCOME)
Cardiac output will improve.

Nursing Interventions	Rationale	Actual Outcomes (Evaluation)
1. Administer IV fluids as ordered.	1. IV fluid may be necessary to compensate for the decreased venous return caused by nitrates and morphine.	1. Improved BP.
2. Monitor closely for dyspnea, crackles, and S_3, which may indicate developing left-sided heart failure.	2. Left-sided heart failure may develop as a result of the decreased myocardial contractility and/or the administration of excess IV fluids.	2. Lungs clear; adequate respiratory rate; heart sounds normal.
3. Monitor urine output hourly.	3. A decrease in urine output may indicate a decrease in renal blood flow.	3. Urine output greater than 30 mL/hour.
4. Monitor mental status for drowsiness, confusion, restlessness, or disorientation.	4. A change in mental status may indicate a decrease in cardiac output.	4. Remains alert and oriented.
5. Evaluate skin and nailbed color and temperature and quality of major arterial pulses.	5. Pallor and cool, clammy skin are associated with vasoconstriction secondary to reduced CO. Weak pulse or presence of pulsus alternans indicate decreased CO.	5. Skin warm and dry with good capillary refill. Radial, femoral, and pedal pulses palpable.
6. Employ hemodynamic monitoring: central venous pressure (CVP) and pulmonary artery pressure (PAP) by way of a pulmonary artery catheter; calculate CO and CI and systemic vascular resistance.	6. These parameters will help to guide fluid volume administration, vasoactive drug administration, and assess cardiac performance.	6. CVP, PAP, pulmonary capillary wedge pressure, CO, CI, and systemic vascular resistance remain within normal limits.
7. Interpret rhythm strip at least every 4 hours, more frequently as condition warrants. Administer anti-arrhythmics, if indicated. Anticipate reperfusion dysrhythmias after fibrinolytic therapy. Report electrolyte values that may increase risk of dysrhythmias. Keep emergency equipment at bedside.	7. Dysrhythmias such as PVCs result in a decreased stroke volume and less coronary artery filling time. Frequent monitoring, especially during the first few hours of an acute MI and during fibrinolytic therapy administration, is necessary to prevent and treat lethal dysrhythmias.	7. PVCs decreasing in frequency.
8. Administer vasopressors as directed; titrate to goal BP and/or MAP.	8. Administration of vasopressors with acute MI is controversial in that they may cause an increase in systemic vascular resistance, which increases cardiac work.	8. BP improved without worsening chest pain or ECG changes.

e. Implement a step-by-step program for progressive activity, as directed. Typically can progress to the next step if they are free from chest pain and ECG changes during the activity.

Preventing Bleeding

1. Take vital signs every 15 minutes during infusion of fibrinolytic agent and then hourly.

2. Observe for hematomas or skin breakdown, especially in potential pressure areas such as the sacrum, back, elbows, ankles.

3. Be alert to verbal complaints of back pain indicative of possible retroperitoneal bleeding.

4. Observe all puncture sites every 15 minutes during infusion of fibrinolytic therapy and then hourly for bleeding.

5. Apply manual pressure to venous or arterial sites if bleeding occurs. Use pressure dressings for coverage of all access sites.

6. Observe for blood in stool, emesis, urine, and sputum.

7. Minimize venipunctures and arterial punctures; use heparin lock for blood sampling and medication administration.

8. Avoid I.M. injections.

9. Caution patient about vigorous tooth brushing, hair combing, or shaving.

10. Avoid trauma to patient by minimizing frequent handling of patient.

11. Monitor laboratory values: PT, International Normalized Ratio, PTT, hematocrit (HCT), and hemoglobin.

12. Check for current blood type and crossmatch.

13. Administer antacids or GI prophylaxis, as directed, to prevent stress ulcers.

14. Implement emergency interventions, as directed, in the event of bleeding: fluid, volume expanders, blood products.

15. Monitor for changes in mental status and headache.

16. Avoid vigorous oral suctioning.

17. Avoid use of automatic BP device above puncture sites or hematoma. Use care in taking BP; use arm not being used for fibrinolytic therapy.

Maintaining Cardiac Tissue Perfusion

1. Observe for persistent and/or recurrence of signs and symptoms of ischemia, including chest pain, diaphoresis, hypotension—may indicate extension of MI and/or reocclusion of coronary vessel.

2. Report immediately.

3. Administer oxygen, as directed.

4. Record a 12-lead ECG.

5. Prepare patient for possible emergency procedures: cardiac catheterization, bypass surgery, PCI, fibrinolytic therapy, intra-aortic balloon pump.

Strengthening Coping Abilities

1. Listen carefully to patient and family to ascertain their cognitive appraisals of stressors and threats.

2. Assist patient to establish a positive attitude toward illness and progress adaptively through the grieving process.

3. Manipulate environment to promote restful sleep by maintaining patient's usual sleep patterns.

4. Be alert to signs and symptoms of sleep deprivation—irritability, disorientation, hallucinations, diminished pain tolerance, aggressiveness.

5. Minimize possible adverse emotional response to transfer from the intensive care unit to the intermediate care unit:
   a. Introduce the admitting nurse from the intermediate care unit to the patient before transfer.
   b. Plan for the intermediate care nurse to answer questions the patient may have and to inform patient what to expect relative to physical layout of unit, nursing routines, and visiting hours.

Patient Education and Health Maintenance

Goals are to restore patient to optimal physiologic, psychological, social, and work level; to aid in restoring confidence and self-esteem; to develop patient's self-monitoring skills; to assist in managing cardiac problems; and to modify risk factors.

1. Inform the patient and family about what has happened to patient's heart.
   a. Explain basic cardiac anatomy and physiology.
   b. Identify the difference between angina and MI.
   c. Describe how the heart heals and that healing will not be complete for 6 to 8 weeks after infarction.
   d. Discuss what the patient can do to assist in the recovery process and reduce the chance of future heart attacks.

2. Instruct patient on how to judge the body's response to activity.
   a. Introduce the concept that different activities require varying expenditures of oxygen.
   b. Emphasize the importance of rest and relaxation alternating with activity.
   c. Instruct patient how to take pulse before and after activity as well as guidelines for the acceptable increases in heart rate that should occur.
   d. Review signs and symptoms indicative of a poor response to increased activity levels: chest pain, extreme fatigue, shortness of breath.

3. Design an individualized activity progression program for patient as directed.
   a. Determine activity levels appropriate for patient, as prescribed, and by predischarge low-level exercise stress test.
   b. Encourage patient to list activities he or she enjoys and would like to resume.
   c. Establish the energy expenditure of each activity (ie, which are most demanding on the heart) and rank activities from lowest to highest.
   d. Instruct patient to move from one activity to another after the heart has been able to manage the previous workload as determined by signs and symptoms and pulse rate.

4. Give patient specific activity guidelines and explain that activity guidelines will be reevaluated after heart heals.
   a. Walk daily, gradually increasing distance and time, as prescribed.
   b. Avoid activities that tense muscles, such as weightlifting, lifting heavy objects, isometric exercises, pushing and/or pulling heavy loads, all of which can cause vagal stimulation.
   c. Avoid working with arms overhead.
   d. Gradually return to work.
   e. Avoid extremes in temperature.
   f. Do not rush; avoid tension.
   g. Advise getting at least 7 hours of sleep each night and taking 20- to 30-minute rest periods twice per day.
   h. Advise limiting visitors to three to four daily for 15 to 30 minutes and shorten phone conversations.

5. Tell patient that sexual relations may be resumed on advice of health care provider, usually after exercise tolerance is assessed.
   a. If patient can walk briskly or climb two flights of stairs, can usually resume sexual activity; resumption of sexual activity parallels resumption of usual activities.

b. Sexual activity should be avoided after eating a heavy meal, after drinking alcohol, or when tired.

c. Discuss impotence as an adverse effect of drug therapy and phosphodiesterase contraindications.

6. Advise eating three to four small meals per day rather than large, heavy meals. Rest for 1 hour after meals.

7. Advise limiting caffeine and alcohol intake.

8. Driving a car must be cleared with health care provider at a follow-up visit.

9. Teach patient about medication regimen and adverse effects.

10. Instruct the patient to call 911 when chest pressure or pain not relieved in 5 minutes by nitroglycerin or rest.

11. Instruct the patient to notify health care provider when the following symptoms appear:

a. Shortness of breath.

b. Unusual fatigue.

c. Swelling of feet and ankles.

d. Fainting, dizziness.

e. Very slow or rapid heartbeat.

12. Assist patient to reduce risk of another MI by risk factor modification.

a. Explain to patient the major risk factors that can increase chances for having another MI.

b. Instruct patient in strategies to modify risk factors.

13. For additional information and support, refer patient to AHA (*www.americanheart.org*) and the ACC (*www.acc.org*).

Evaluation: Expected Outcomes

- No signs of anxiety or agitation.
- Activity slowly progressing and tolerated well.
- No signs of bleeding.
- No recurrent chest pain.
- Sleeps well; emotionally stable.

Hyperlipidemia

Evidence Base Grundy, S. M., Cleeman, J. I., Merz, C. N., et al. (2004). Implications of recent clinical trials for the National Cholesterol Education Program Adult Treatment Panel III guidelines. *Circulation*, *110*(2), 227–239.

Hyperlipidemia is a group of metabolic abnormalities resulting in combinations of elevated serum cholesterol. Total cholesterol (TC) and triglycerides (TG) are two of the major lipids in the body. They are transported through the bloodstream by lipoproteins. Lipoproteins are made up of a phospholipid and specific proteins called *apoproteins* or *apo lipoproteins*. There are five main classes of lipoproteins:

- Chylomicrons
- Very low-density lipoproteins (VLDLs)
- Intermediate-density lipoproteins (IDLs)
- Low-density lipoproteins (LDLs)
- High-density lipoproteins (HDLs)

Pathophysiology and Etiology

Primary Hyperlipidemias

1. Genetic metabolic abnormalities resulting in the overproduction or underproduction of specific lipoproteins or enzymes. They tend to be familial.

2. Primary hyperlipidemias include hypercholesterolemia, defective apolipoproteinemia, hypertriglyceridemia, combined hyperlipidemia, dysbetalipoproteinemia, polygenic hypercholesterolemia, lipoprotein lipase deficiency, apoprotein C-II deficiency, lethicin cholesterol acetyltransferase deficiency.

Secondary Hyperlipidemias

1. Very common and are multifactorial.

2. Etiologic factors include chronic diseases, such as diabetes, hypothyroidism, nephrotic syndrome, and liver disease.

3. Other etiologic factors are obesity, dietary intake, pregnancy, alcoholism.

4. Medications include beta-adrenergic blockers, alpha-adrenergic blockers, diuretics, glucocorticoid and anabolic steroids, and estrogen preparations.

Consequences

1. Atherosclerotic plaque formation in blood vessels.

2. Causes narrowing, possible ischemia, and may lead to thromboembolus formation.

3. Result in cardiovascular, cerebrovascular, and peripheral vascular disease.

Clinical Manifestations

1. Usually asymptomatic until significant target organ damage is done.

2. May be metabolic signs, such as corneal arcus, xanthoma, xanthelasma, pancreatitis.

3. Chest pain, MI.

4. Carotid bruit, transient ischemic attacks, stroke.

5. Intermittent claudication, arterial occlusion of lower extremities, loss of pulses.

Diagnostic Evaluation and Management

The National Cholesterol Education Program–Adult Treatment Panel III Guidelines recommend a nine-step process for the diagnosis and treatment of hypercholesterolemia.

1. Fasting (9 to 12 hours) lipoprotein profile every 5 years for people ages 20 and older, more frequent if abnormal (see Table 13-2, page 396).

2. Assess the presence of clinical atherosclerotic disease that confers high risk for CHD events or CHD risk equivalents.

a. Clinical CHD: history of MI, unstable angina, stable angina, coronary artery procedures, or evidence of clinically significant MI.

b. CHD risk equivalents: carotid artery disease, peripheral arterial disease, abdominal aortic aneurysm, diabetes. (Some experts include chronic renal insufficiency, defined by plasma creatine concentration that exceeds 1.5 mg/dL or an estimated glomerular filtration rate that is less than 60 mL/minute per 1.73 m^2.)

Table 13-2   Classification of Serum Lipids

TOTAL CHOLESTEROL (TC) mg/dL (mmol/L)

	CATEGORY
<200 (<5.2)	Normal
200 to 239 (5.2 to 6.1)	Borderline high
≥240 (≥6.2)	High

LDL-Cholesterol mg/dL (mmol/L)

<100 (<2.6)	Normal
100 to 129 (2.6 to 3.3)	Above, near optimal
130 to 159 (3.4 to 4.0)	Borderline high
160 to 189 (4.1 to 4.8)	High
≥190 (≥4.9)	Very high

HDL-Cholesterol mg/dL (mmol/L)

<40 (<1.0)	Low
≥60 (≥1.6)	High

Triglycerides (TG) mg/dL (mmol/L)

<150 (<1.7)	Normal
150 to 199 (1.7 to 2.2)	Borderline high
200 to 499 (2.3 to 5.6)	High
≥500 (≥5.6)	Very high

Management of Dyslipidemia Working Group. (2006). *VA/DoD clinical practice guideline for the management of dyslipidemia*. Washington, DC: Department of Veterans Affairs, Department of Defense, p. 140.

   d. Family history of premature CHD (first-degree relative, male under age 55, female under age 65).
   e. Age (men 45 or older, women 55 or older).
   Note: HDL ≥ 60 mg/dL counts as a negative risk factor (its presence removes one risk factor from the total count).
4. If two or more risk factors (other than LDL) are present without CHD or CHD risk equivalent, assess 10-year CHD risk using Framingham Scoring Method (see *www.nhlbi.nih.gov/guidelines/cholesterol/index.htm*). There are three levels of 10-year risk:
   a. >20%—CHD risk equivalent.
   b. 10% to 20%.
   c. <10%.
5. Determine risk category and subsequent therapy (see Table 13-3).
   a. Establish LDL goal of therapy.
   b. Determine need for therapeutic lifestyle changes (TLC)
   c. Determine level for drug consideration.
6. Initiate TLC if LDL is above goal.
   a. TLC diet.
      i. Saturated fat: <7% of total calories; trans fatty acid: <1% of total calories; cholesterol intake: <200 mg/day.
      ii. Consider increasing viscous (soluble) fiber by 10 to 25 g/day; plant stanols/sterols by 2 g/day; omega-3 oils three times per week.
   b. Smoking cessation.
   c. Weight reduction.
   d. Increased physical activity—30 minutes of moderate activity 5 days per week or 20 minutes of vigorous activity three times per week.
7. Consider adding drug therapy if LDL exceeds levels shown in Table 13-3.
   a. Consider drug simultaneously with TLC for CHD and CHD equivalents.
   b. Consider adding drug to TLC after 3 months for other risk categories.

   c. Two or more risk factors with 10-year risk for CHD greater than 20%.
3. Determine presence of major risk factors other than LDL.
   a. Cigarette smoking.
   b. Hypertension (BP ≥ 140/90 mm Hg or on antihypertensive medications).
   c. Low HDL (<40 mg/dL).

Table 13-3   LDL-C Goals and Cutpoints for Therapeutic Lifestyle Changes (TLC) and Drug Therapy in Different Risk Categories

RISK CATEGORY	LDL-C GOAL	INITIATE TLC	CONSIDER DRUG THERAPY
High risk: CHD or CHD risk equivalents (10-year risk, >20%)	<100 mg/dL (optional goal: <70 mg/dL)	≥100 mg/dL	≥100 mg/dL (<100 mg/dL: consider drug options)
Moderately high risk: 2+ risk factors (10-year risk, 10% to 20%)	<130 mg/dL	≥130 mg/dL	≥130 mg/dL (100 to 129 mg/dL: consider drug options)
Moderate risk: 2 or more risk factors (10-year risk, <10%)	<130 mg/dL	≥130 mg/dL	≥160 mg/dL
Lower risk: 0 to 1 risk factor	<160 mg/dL	≥160 mg/dL	≥190 mg/dL (160 to 189 mg/dL: LDL-lowering drug optional)

Grundy, S. M., Cleeman, J. I., Merz, C. N., et al. (2004). Implications of recent clinical trials for the National Cholesterol Education Program Adult Treatment Panel III guidelines. *Circulation, 110*(2):227–239.

8. Identify metabolic syndrome and treat, if present, after 3 months of TLC (see page 969).
9. Treat elevated TGs.
   a. Aim for LDL goal, intensify weight management, and increase physical activity.
   b. If TGs are 200 mg/dL or greater after LDL goal is reached, set secondary goal for non-HDL-C (total cholesterol minus HDL) to <130 mg/dL.
   c. If TGs are 200 to 499 mg/dL after LDL goal is reached, consider adding drug if needed to reach non-HDL goal (increase primary drug or add nicotinic acid or fibrate).
   d. If TGs are 500 mg/dL or greater, first lower TGs to prevent pancreatitis.
      i. Very-low-fat diet (15% or fewer calories from fat).
      ii. Weight management and physical activity.
      iii. Fibrate or nicotinic acid.
      iv. When TGs are less than 500 mg/dL, return to LDL-lowering therapy.
   e. Treat low HDL (<40 mg/dL) by first aiming for LDL goal, then intensifying weight management by increasing physical activity. If triglycerides of 200 to 499 mg/dL achieve non-HDL goal and, if triglycerides are <200 mg/dL (isolated low HDL) in CHD or CHD equivalent, consider adding nicotinic acid or fibrate.

Drug Classifications

See Table 13-4.
1. HMG-CoA reductase inhibitors (statins) are the most effective way to lower elevated LDL and TC. They also raise levels of HDL, lower levels of CRP, and may lower TGs. They can be used alone or in combination with other lipid-lowering drugs.
   a. Require liver function monitoring.
   b. Should not be taken with grapefruit juice; can increase risk of myopathy.
   c. Should not be taken by women who are pregnant, lactating, or plan to get pregnant.
2. Cholesterol absorption inhibitors—the newest class of lipid-lowering drugs; inhibit intestinal absorption of phytosterols and cholesterol and reduce LDL. Do not require liver function testing if given as monotherapy.
3. Bile acid sequestrants bind to cholesterol in gut, decreasing absorption Contraindicated in those with history of bile obstruction and phenylketonuria (aspartame-containing agent only).
4. Nicotinic acid (vitamin B_3)—works by inhibiting VLDL secretion, thus decreasing production of LDL. Main adverse effect is severe flushing; however, taking 81 to 325 mg of aspirin beforehand may help. Newer sustained-release forms have fewer adverse effects. Niacin should be avoided in patients with severe peptic disease.
5. Fibrinic acid derivatives—inhibit synthesis of VLDL, decrease TG, increase HDL. Liver, biliary, or kidney disease—contraindicated.

Other Treatment Considerations

1. TLC should be considered immediately for all patients with hyperlipidemia and are an important adjunct therapy for patients who receive medications.

2. Children and adolescents should be considered for screening and treatment of hyperlipidemia if they have positive family history and a family history of obesity. Other indications for screening (in these populations) include being overweight and exhibiting features of metabolic syndrome (hypertension, type 2 diabetes, central adiposity).
3. Drug therapy is recommended for boys at or older than age 10 and after the onset of menses in girls following a 6- to 12-month dietary trial. HMG-CoA reductase inhibitors are the drug class of choice.
4. Some dietary products may serve as adjunct therapy, such as omega-3 fatty acids, soy protein, plant stanols, and fiber.

Complications

1. Disability from MI, stroke, and lower-extremity ischemia.

Nursing Interventions and Patient Education

1. Teach diet basics and obtain nutritional consult.
2. Teach patient to engage in exercise.
3. Engage patient in smoking-cessation program.
4. Tell patients that for every 1% increase in HDL, there is a 2% to 3% decrease in risk for CHD.
5. Explain goal of recommended cholesterol levels. Encourage patients to keep a log of lipid results.
6. Encourage follow-up laboratory work—repeat lipoprotein analysis and liver function test monitoring every 3 months for those on HMG-CoA reductase inhibitors.
7. Teach patient taking bile acid sequestrants not to take other medications for 1 hour before or 2 hours after because it prevents absorption of many medications.
8. For more information on hyperlipidemia and TLC, refer patient to AHA (*www.heart.org*) or the National Heart, Lung, and Blood Institute diseases and conditions index (*www.nhlbi.nih.gov/health/dci*).

Cardiogenic Shock

Cardiogenic shock is the failure of the heart to pump blood adequately to meet the oxygenation needs of the body. It occurs when the heart muscle loses its contractile power. It most commonly occurs in association with, and as a direct result of, acute myocardial infarction (AMI). It is the most common cause of death in the post-AMI patient (about 5% to 10% of AMI patients develop cardiogenic shock).

Pathophysiology and Etiology

1. Impaired contractility causes a marked reduction in CO and ejection fraction.
2. Decreased CO results in a lack of blood and oxygen to the heart as well as other vital organs (brain and kidneys).
3. Lack of blood and oxygen to the heart muscle results in continued damage to the muscle, a further decline in contractile power, and a continued inability of the heart to provide blood and oxygen to vital organs.
4. MI causing extensive damage (40% or greater) to the left ventricular myocardium is the most common cause.

| Table 13-4 | Drugs Affecting Lipoprotein Metabolism | | | |

DRUG CLASS	AGENTS AND DAILY DOSES	LIPID/LIPOPROTEIN EFFECTS		ADVERSE EFFECTS	CONTRAINDICATIONS
HMG-CoA reductase inhibitors (statins)	• Lovastatin (20–80 mg) • Pravastatin (20–40 mg) • Simvastatin (20–80 mg) • Fluvastatin (20–80 mg) • Atorvastatin (10–80 mg) • Rosuvastatin (5–40 mg) • Pitavastatin (1–4 mg)	LDL HDL TG	↓ 18%–55% ↑ 5%–15% ↓ 7%–30%	• Myopathy • Increased liver enzymes	*Absolute:* • Active or chronic liver disease *Relative:* • Concomitant use of certain drugs*
Bile acid sequestrants	• Cholestyramine (4–16 g) • Colestipol (5–20 g) • Colesevelam (2.6–3.8 g)	LDL HDL TG	↓ 15%–30% ↑ 3%–5% No change or increase	• GI distress • Constipation • •	*Absolute:* • Bowel obstruction • Biliary obstruction
Nicotinic acid	• Immediate-release (crystalline) nicotinic acid (1.5–3 g); extended-release nicotinic acid (Niaspan*) (1–2 g); sustained release nicotinic acid (1-2 g)	LDL HDL TG	↓ 5%–25% ↑ 15%–35% ↓ 20%–50%	• Flushing (may be reduced by taking with aspirin) • Hyperglycemia • Hyperuricemia, gout • Upper GI distress • Hepatotoxicity	*Absolute:* • Hepatic dysfunction • Active peptic ulcer disease *Relative:* • Diabetes • Hyperphosphatemia • Gout • Unstable angina, MI
Fibric acids	• Gemfibrozil (600 mg BID) • Fenofibrate (200 mg) • Clofibrate (1,000 mg BID)	LDL *(may be increased in patients with high TG)* HDL TG	↓ 5%–20% ↑ 10%–20% ↓ 20%–50%	• Dyspepsia • Gallstones • Myopathy • Pancreatitis	*Absolute:* • Severe renal disease • Severe hepatic disease
Cholesterol absorption inhibitors	• Ezetimibe (10 mg)	LDL Apoprotein B	↓ (additional 25% over a statin when used in combination; also a TG reduction) ↓	• Back pain • Arthralgia • Diarrhea • Abdominal pain • Sinusitis	• Contraindicated in active liver disease if combined with a statin

Cyclosporine, macrolide antibiotics, various antifungal agents, and cytochrome P-450 inhibitors (fibrates and niacin) should be used with appropriate caution.

Adapted from *ATP III guidelines at a glance quick desk reference.* National Cholesterol Education Program [Electronic]. Available: www.nhlbi.nih.gov/guidelines/cholesterol/atglance.pdf.

5. End-stage cardiomyopathy, severe valvular dysfunction, drug toxicities, infection, tamponade, and ventricular aneurysm can also precipitate cardiogenic shock.

Clinical Manifestations

1. Confusion, restlessness, mental lethargy (due to poor perfusion of brain).

2. Low systolic blood pressure (90 mm Hg or 30 mm Hg less than previous levels).

3. Oliguria—urine output less than 30 mL/hour for at least 2 hours (due to decreased perfusion of kidneys).

4. Cold, clammy skin (blood is shunted from the peripheral circulation to perfuse vital organs); profoundly diaphoretic with mottled extremities.

5. Weak, thready peripheral pulses, fatigue, hypotension (due to inadequate CO).
6. Dyspnea, tachypnea, cyanosis (increased left ventricular pressures result in elevation of left atrial and pulmonary pressures, causing pulmonary congestion).
7. Dysrhythmias (due to lack of oxygen to heart muscle) and sinus tachycardia (as a compensatory mechanism for a decreased CO).
8. Chest pain (due to lack of oxygen and blood to heart muscle).
9. Decreased bowel sounds (due to paralytic ileus from decreased perfusion to GI tract).
10. Metabolic acidosis due to increased lactate production and reduced clearance (caused by anaerobic metabolism and liver dysfunction).

Diagnostic Evaluation

1. Altered hemodynamic parameters (pulmonary artery wedge pressure 15 mm Hg or greater, cardiac index [CI] less than 2.0, elevated systemic vascular resistance [SVR], decreased mixed venous oxygen saturation)
2. Chest x-ray—pulmonary vascular congestion
3. Abnormal laboratory values—elevated blood urea nitrogen (BUN) and creatinine, elevated liver enzymes, increased PTT and PT, elevated serum lactate, elevated brain natriuretic peptide (BNP). BNP may be useful as an indicator of heart failure and as an independent prognostic indicator of survival. Abnormally elevated cardiac enzymes.
4. Other tests.
   a. ECG—reveals an acute injury pattern consistent with an AMI.
   b. Echocardiogram—reveals any ventricular wall motion or surgically correctable cause, such as valvular dysfunction and tamponade.

Management

Recent studies have suggested that treatment for cardiogenic shock resulting from an AMI should focus on revascularization and thrombolytics. Reduction in mortality related to early revascularization in patients with STEMI is supported by research. Augmenting CO with devices (intra-aortic balloon pump [IABP] is method of choice) is crucial until revascularization is established. Other mechanical devices includes ventricular assist devices and extracorporeal membrane oxygenation.

The standard treatment of beta-adrenergic blockers, ACE inhibitors, analgesics, and nitrates after acute MI does little to treat cardiogenic shock and may exacerbate systolic hypotension.

Pharmacologic Therapy

Pharmacologic therapy may need to be discontinued or its use decreased when a patient has gone into cardiogenic shock. Standard therapy for a failing heart includes:

1. Positive inotropic drugs (epinephrine, dopamine, dobutamine, amrinone, milrinone) stimulate cardiac contractility. Dobutamine, amrinone, and milrinone may lower BP.

 DRUG ALERT Use vasoactive drugs with extreme caution in the presence of cardiogenic shock. They require constant vigilance and astute observation to maintain an adequate perfusion pressure while achieving afterload reduction.

2. Vasodilator therapy.
   a. Decreases the workload of the heart by reducing venous return and lessening the resistance against which the heart pumps (preload and afterload reduction).
   b. CO improves, left ventricular pressures and pulmonary congestion decrease, and myocardial oxygen consumption is reduced.
3. Vasopressor therapy may be needed to maintain adequate perfusion pressure (MAP 70 mm Hg or greater).
4. Diuretic therapy.
   a. Decreases total body fluid volume.
   b. Relieves systemic and pulmonary congestion.
   c. Nesiritide—may be considered for treatment of heart failure. Use with caution because it can cause hypotension.

Counterpulsation Therapy

See page 369.
1. Improves blood flow to the heart muscle and reduces myocardial oxygen needs.
2. Results in improved CO (1.5 L/minute increase) and preservation of viable heart tissue.

Left Ventricular Assist Device

1. Device used to unload the left ventricle as bridge to recovery, transplant, or destination.
2. May only be performed in areas where immediate access to emergency cardiac surgery is available.

Emergency Cardiac Surgery

1. Bypass graft (see page 371).
2. Heart transplantation.

Complications

1. Neurologic impairment/stroke.
2. Acute respiratory distress syndrome.
3. Renal failure.
4. Cardiopulmonary arrest.
5. Dysrhythmia.
6. Ventricular aneurysm.
7. Multiorgan dysfunction syndrome.
8. Bowel ischemia.
9. Limb ischemia.
10. Death.

Nursing Assessment

Clinical assessment begins with attention to the airway/breathing/circulation and vital signs.

1. Identify patients at risk for development of cardiogenic shock.
2. Assess for early signs and symptoms indicative of shock:
   a. Restlessness, confusion, or change in mental status.
   b. Increasing heart rate.

c. Decreasing pulse pressure (indicates impaired CO).

d. Presence of pulsus alternans (indicates left-sided heart failure).

e. Decreasing urine output, weakness, fatigue.

3. Observe for presence of central and peripheral cyanosis.

4. Observe for development of edema.

5. Identify signs and symptoms indicative of extension of MI—recurrence of chest pain, diaphoresis.

6. Identify patient's and significant other's reaction to crisis situation.

 NURSING ALERT Cardiogenic shock carries an extremely high mortality (above 50% to 80% in hospital). Astute assessments and immediate actions are essential to prevent death.

Nursing Diagnoses

- Decreased Cardiac Output related to impaired contractility due to extensive heart muscle damage.
- Impaired Gas Exchange related to pulmonary congestion due to elevated left ventricular pressures.
- Ineffective Tissue Perfusion (renal, cerebral, cardiopulmonary, GI, and peripheral) related to decreased blood flow.
- Anxiety related to intensive care environment and threat of death.

Nursing Interventions

Improving Cardiac Output

1. Establish continuous ECG monitoring to detect dysrhythmias, which increase myocardial oxygen consumption.

2. Monitor hemodynamic parameters continually with pulmonary artery catheter (see page 346) to evaluate effectiveness of implemented therapy.

   a. Obtain pulmonary artery pressure (PAP), pulmonary artery wedge pressure, and CO readings, as indicated.

   b. Calculate the CI (CO relative to body size) and SVR (estimation of afterload).

   c. Cautiously titrate vasoactive drug therapy according to hemodynamic parameters.

3. Be alert to adverse responses to drug therapy.

   a. Dopamine may cause an increase in heart rate, which may result in ischemia.

   b. Vasodilators, such as nitroglycerin and nitroprusside, may worsen hypotension.

   c. Dobutamine may result in dysrhythmias.

   d. Diuretics may cause hyponatremia, hypokalemia, and hypovolemia.

4. Administer vasoactive drug therapy through central venous access (peripheral tissue necrosis can occur if peripheral IV access infiltrates and peripheral drug distribution may be lessened from vasoconstriction).

5. Monitor blood pressure and MAP with intra-arterial line continuously during active titration of vasoactive drug therapy.

6. Maintain MAP greater than 70 mm Hg (blood flow through coronary vessels is inadequate with MAP less than 70 mm Hg).

7. Measure and record urine output every hour from indwelling catheter and fluid intake.

8. Obtain daily weight.

9. Evaluate serum electrolytes for hyponatremia, hypomagnesemia, and hypokalemia.

10. Be alert to incidence of chest pain (indicates myocardial ischemia and may further extend heart damage).

    a. Report immediately.

    b. Obtain a 12-lead ECG, check cardiac enzymes—CK, CK-MB, myoglobin, and troponin.

    c. Anticipate use of counterpulsation therapy.

11. Anticipate pump failure; evaluate need for surgical intervention (ie, ventricular assist device, extracorporeal membrane oxygenation).

Improving Oxygenation

1. Monitor rate and rhythm of respirations every hour.

2. Auscultate lung fields for abnormal sounds (coarse crackles indicate severe pulmonary congestion) every hour; notify health care provider.

3. Evaluate arterial blood gas (ABG) levels and correlate with oxygen saturation.

4. Administer oxygen therapy to increase oxygen tension and improve hypoxia.

5. Elevate head of bed 20 to 30 degrees, as tolerated (may worsen hypotension), to facilitate lung expansion.

6. Reposition patient frequently to promote ventilation and maintain skin integrity.

7. Observe for frothy pink sputum and cough (may indicate pulmonary edema); report immediately.

Maintaining Tissue Perfusion

1. Perform a neurologic check every hour using the Glasgow Coma Scale.

2. Report changes immediately.

3. Obtain BUN and creatinine blood levels and monitor urine output to evaluate renal function.

4. Auscultate for bowel sounds every 2 hours.

5. Evaluate character, rate, rhythm, and quality of arterial pulses every 2 hours.

6. Monitor temperature every 2 to 4 hours.

7. Use sheepskin foot and elbow protectors to prevent skin breakdown.

8. Obtain serum lactate to evaluate tissue perfusion and acidosis.

Relieving Anxiety

1. As with the above, always evaluate signs of increasing anxiety and/or new-onset anxiety for a physiologic cause before treating with anxiolytics.

2. Explain equipment and rationale for therapy to patient and family. Increasing knowledge assists in alleviating fear and anxiety.

3. Encourage patient to verbalize fears about diagnosis and prognosis.

4. Explain sensations patient will experience before procedures and routine care measures.

5. Offer reassurance and encouragement.
6. Utilize social worker or pastoral care for support.
7. Provide for periods of uninterrupted rest and sleep.
8. Assist patient to maintain as much control as possible over environment and care.
    a. Develop a schedule for routine care measures and rest periods with patient.
    b. Make sure that a calendar and clock are in view of patient.

Patient Education and Health Maintenance

1. Assess patient's readiness to learn.
2. Teach patients taking digoxin the importance of taking their medication as prescribed, taking pulse before daily dose, and reporting for periodic blood levels.
3. Teach signs of impending heart failure—increasing edema, shortness of breath, decreasing urine output, decreasing BP, increasing pulse—and tell patient to notify health care provider immediately.
4. See specific measures for MI (see page 394), cardiomyopathy (see page 412), and valvular disease (see page 423).
5. Teach patient importance of keeping follow-up appointments with his or her primary care physician and cardiologist.
6. Have dietitian teach patient and family about a low-sodium, low-fat diet, and reiterate the importance of adhering to this diet.
7. Explain to the patient the need to work with a physical and occupational therapist—especially if the patient has low ejection fraction—for energy conservation.

Evaluation: Expected Outcomes

- CO greater than 4 L/minute; CI greater than 2.2; PCWP less than 18 mm Hg.
- Respirations unlabored and regular; normal breath sounds throughout lung fields.
- Normal sensorium; urine output adequate; skin warm and dry.
- Verbalizes lessened anxiety and fear.

Infective Endocarditis

Infective endocarditis (IE; bacterial endocarditis) is an infection of the inner lining of the heart caused by direct invasion of bacteria or other organisms that could potentially result in myocardial abscess or heart failure and other complications.

Pathophysiology and Etiology

1. When the inner lining of the heart (endocardium) becomes inflamed, a fibrin clot (vegetation) forms.
2. The fibrin clot may become colonized by pathogens during transient episodes of bacteremia resulting from invasive procedures (venous and arterial cannulation, dental work causing gingival bleeding, GI tract surgery, liver biopsy, sigmoidoscopy), indwelling catheters, urinary tract infections, and wound and skin infections.
3. Platelets and fibrin surround the invading microorganisms, forming a protective covering and causing the infected vegetation to enlarge.
    a. The enlarged vegetation (the basic lesion of endocarditis) can deform, thicken, stiffen, and scar the free margins of valve leaflets as well as the fibrous ring (annulus) supporting the valve.
    b. The vegetations may also travel to various organs and tissues (spleen, kidney, coronary artery, brain, and lungs) and obstruct blood flow.
    c. The "protective covering" surrounding the vegetation makes it difficult for WBCs and antimicrobial agents to infiltrate and destroy the infected lesion.
4. Bacterial causes include:
    a. *Streptococcus viridans*—bacteremia occurs after dental work or upper respiratory infection.
    b. *Staphylococcus aureus*—most common cause of IE, bacteremia occurs after cardiac surgery or parenteral drug abuse.
    c. *Staphylococcus epidermidis*—bacteremia occurs due to prosthetic heart valves and IV access procedures.
    d. Enterococci (penicillin-resistant group *D. streptococci*)—bacteremia usually occurs in older patients (over age 60) with genitourinary tract infection.
    e. Gram-negative bacteria such as *Pseudomonas aeruginosa*, *Haemophilus*, *Actinobacter*, and *Cardiobacterium* are uncommon but cause serious complications.
5. Fungi (*Candida albicans*, *Aspergillus*) and rickettsiae are additional causes.
6. IE may develop on a heart valve already injured by rheumatic fever, congenital defects, on abnormally vascularized valves, normal heart valves, and mechanical and biological heart valves.
7. IE may be acute or subacute, depending on the microorganisms involved. Acute IE manifests rapidly with danger of intractable heart failure and occurs more commonly on normal heart valves.
8. Subacute IE manifests as a prolonged chronic course with a lesser risk of complications and occurs more commonly on damaged or defective valves.
9. IE may follow cardiac surgery, especially when prosthetic heart valves are used. Foreign bodies, such as pacemakers, patches, grafts, and dialysis shunts, predispose to infection.
10. High incidence among drug abusers, in whom the disease mainly affects normal valves, usually the tricuspid.
11. Hospitalized patients with indwelling catheters, those on prolonged IV therapy or prolonged antibiotic therapy, and those on immunosuppressive drugs or steroids may develop fungal endocarditis.

 NURSING ALERT The incidence of nosocomial bacteremias are commonly associated with intravascular lines and wound care may result in infective endocarditis.

12. Relapse due to metastatic infection is possible, usually within the first 2 months after completion of antibiotic regimen.

Clinical Manifestations

Severity of manifestations depends on invading microorganism.

General Manifestations

1. Fever, chills, sweats (fever may be absent in older patients or those with uremia).
2. Anorexia, weight loss, weakness.
3. Cough, back and joint pain (especially in patients over age 60).
4. Splenomegaly.

Skin and Nail Manifestations

1. Petechiae—conjunctiva, mucous membranes.
2. Splinter hemorrhages in nailbeds.
3. Osler's nodes—painful red nodes on pads of fingers and toes; usually late sign of infection and found with a subacute infection.
4. Janeway's lesions—light pink macules on palms or soles, nontender, may change to light tan within several days or fade in 1 to 2 weeks; usually an early sign of endocardial infection.
5. Clubbing of fingers and toes—primarily occurs in patients who have an extended course of untreated infective endocarditis.

Heart Manifestations

1. New pathologic or changing murmur—no murmur with other signs and symptoms may indicate right-sided heart infection.
2. Tachycardia—related to decreased CO.
3. Symptoms consistent with heart failure.

Central Nervous System Manifestations

1. Localized headaches.
2. Transient cerebral ischemia or other neurological symptoms.
3. Altered mental status, aphasia.
4. Hemiplegia.
5. Cortical sensory loss.
6. Roth's spots on fundi (retinal hemorrhages).

Pulmonary Manifestations

1. Usually occur with right-sided heart involvement.
2. Pneumonitis, pleuritis, pulmonary edema, infiltrates.

Embolic Phenomena

1. Lung—hemoptysis, chest pain, shortness of breath.
2. Kidney—hematuria, abnormal urine color.
3. Spleen—pain in left upper quadrant of abdomen radiating to left shoulder.
4. Heart—MI, aortic insufficiency, heart failure.
5. Brain—sudden blindness, paralysis, brain abscess, meningitis, CVA.
6. Blood vessels—mycotic aneurysms.
7. Abdomen—melena, acute pain.

Diagnostic Evaluation

Varied clinical manifestations and similarities to other diseases make early diagnosis of IE difficult. Accurate diagnosis is essential to guide therapy. Major and minor criteria have been used as well as the Duke criteria to help in establishing diagnosis.

Major Criteria

1. Blood cultures—at least two positive serial blood cultures (90% of IE patients have positive blood cultures).
2. Endocardial involvement (diagnosed with echocardiography)—identification of vegetations and assessment of location and size of lesions.
3. New valvular insufficiency/regurgitation.
4. Development of partial dehiscence of prosthetic valve.

Minor Criteria

1. Predisposing cardiac condition or IV drug use.
2. Fever higher than 100.4° F (38° C).
3. Vascular factors—pulmonary complication, emboli, Janeway's lesions.
4. Immunologic factors—Osler's nodes, Roth's spots, rheumatoid factor.
5. Microbiology—positive cultures, but not meeting major criteria.
6. Echocardiogram—consistent with disease, but not meeting major criteria.

Management

1. IV antimicrobial therapy, based on sensitivity of causative agent (6 weeks of therapy is recommended for most patients except uncomplicated right-sided IE in whom 2 weeks of therapy is recommended).
   a. Bactericidal serum levels of selected antibiotics are monitored by serial titers; if serum lacks adequate bactericidal activity, more antibiotic or a different antibiotic is needed.
   b. Note that missed doses of antibiotics due to the patient's unavailability while off the unit for diagnostic tests are given after return to the unit.
   c. Missed antibiotic doses may have irreversible deleterious consequences.
   d. Notify health care provider if doses will be missed to ensure that appropriate alternative measures are taken.
2. Audiogram obtained before antibiotic regimen initiated.
3. Urine cultures obtained after 48 hours to assess efficacy of drug therapy.
4. Repeat blood cultures obtained after 48 hours to assess efficacy of drug therapy.
5. Close follow-up by cardiologist.
6. Supplemental nutrition.
7. Surgical intervention for:
   a. Acute destructive valvular lesion—excision of infected valves or removal of prosthetic valve.
   b. Hemodynamic impairment, severe heart failure.
   c. Recurrent emboli.
   d. Resistant infection.
   e. Drainage of abscess or empyema.
   f. Repair of peripheral or cerebral mycotic aneurysm.

Note: Surgery should be delayed for at least a month in patients who suffered a hemorrhagic CVA, but surgery should not be delayed in patients following silent embolic event or transient ischemic attack, associated heart failure, abscess, or high embolic risk patients.

Complications

1. Severe heart failure due to valvular insufficiency.
2. Uncontrolled/refractory infection.
3. Embolic episodes (ischemia or necrosis of extremities and organs).
4. Conduction disturbances.
5. Organ dysfunction resulting from immunological process (kidneys, eyes, skin).
6. Tissue destruction by microorganism, valvular damage, mycotic aneurysms, hemorrhage and abscess formation.

Nursing Assessment

1. Identify factors that may predispose to endocarditis, such as rheumatic heart disease, congenital heart defects, idiopathic hypertrophic subaortic stenosis, IV drug abuse, prosthetic heart valves, aortic or mitral stenosis, previous history of endocarditis.
2. Determine onset of signs and symptoms of endocarditis (early treatment of infection improves prognosis).
3. Identify potential incidents that may have precipitated a transient bacteremia capable of causing endocarditis.
4. Obtain blood cultures, CBC, renal and hepatic studies, and a baseline 12-lead ECG.
5. Assess patient for allergies, with special emphasis on adverse reactions to antibiotic therapy.
6. Note if patient is currently on antibiotic therapy (may affect blood culture results).
7. Identify patient's and family's level of anxiety and use of appropriate coping mechanisms.

Nursing Diagnoses

- Decreased Cardiac Output related to structural factors (incompetent valves).
- Ineffective Tissue Perfusion (renal, cerebral, cardiopulmonary, GI, and peripheral) related to interruption of blood flow.
- Hyperthermia related to illness, potential dehydration, and aggressive antibiotic therapy.
- Imbalanced Nutrition: Less Than Body Requirements related to anorexia.
- Anxiety related to acute illness and hospitalization.

Nursing Interventions

Maintaining Adequate Cardiac Output

1. Auscultate heart to detect new murmur or change in existing murmur; presence of gallop.
2. Monitor BP and pulse.
   a. Note presence of pulsus alternans (indicative of left-sided heart failure).
   b. Evaluate pulse pressure (30 to 40 mm Hg indicates adequate CO).
3. Evaluate jugular vein distention.
4. Record intake and output.
5. Record daily weight.
6. Auscultate lung fields for evidence of crackles (rales).

7. Monitor liver function studies (elevated with liver engorgement related to right heart failure).
8. Assess skin color and temperature.

Maintaining Tissue Perfusion

1. Observe patient for altered mentation, hemoptysis, hematuria, aphasia, loss of muscle strength, and complaints of pain.
2. Monitor vital signs.
3. Monitor urine output.
4. Observe for splinter hemorrhages of nail beds, Osler's nodes, and Janeway's lesions.
5. Notify health care provider of observed changes in the patient's status.
6. Assess skin color and temperature.
7. Reposition patient frequently to prevent skin breakdown and pulmonary complications associated with bed rest.

Maintaining Normothermia

1. Observe basic principles of asepsis, good handwashing techniques, and continuity of patient care by primary nurse.
2. Employ meticulous IV care for long-term antibiotic therapy.
   a. Note the date of needle or cannula insertion on nursing care plan.
   b. If a peripheral site is used, rotate the site every 72 hours or if site becomes tender, reddened, infiltrated, or has purulent drainage.
   c. Change gauze or transparent dressing every 24 hours to prevent infection.
   d. If a continuous venous access device is used, follow facility policy for site care and dressing changes and flushing procedures.
3. Administer parenteral antibiotic therapy, as directed.
   a. Develop chart for rotation of sites for I.M. administration of antibiotic therapy.
   b. Observe for adverse reactions to antibiotic therapy (severe respiratory distress, rash, itching, fever).
   c. Observe for adverse effects of long-term antibiotic therapy—ototoxicity, renal failure.

 DRUG ALERT Rapid infusion of vancomycin (less than 1 hour) may cause red neck syndrome (intense red rash over the upper half of the body) due to histamine release. Slow the rate of infusion and the rash will clear.

4. Monitor temperature every 4 hours.
   a. Document results on graph.
   b. Note increases in heart rate and/or respirations with elevated temperatures.
   c. Provide blankets and temperature-controlled comfortable environment if patient has shaking chills; change bed linens, as necessary.
   d. Administer analgesic medications, as directed.
5. Observe patient for a general "sense of well-being" within 5 to 7 days after initiation of therapy.
6. Monitor laboratory values—HCT, BUN, creatinine, WBC, antibiotic levels, blood cultures.

7. Promote adequate hydration because diaphoresis and increased metabolic rate may cause dehydration.
   a. Encourage oral fluid intake.
   b. Administer IV fluids as directed.
   c. Observe skin turgor and mucous membranes.

Improving Nutritional Status

1. Assess patient's daily caloric intake.
2. Discuss food preferences with patient.
3. Consult with a dietitian about nutritional needs of patient and food preferences.
4. Encourage small meals and snacks throughout the day.
5. Record daily caloric intake and weight.
6. Educate family about the patient's caloric needs.
7. Encourage family to assist the patient with meals and bring in patient's favorite foods.

Reducing Anxiety

1. Rule out physiologic etiologies for increasing or new-onset anxiety before administering as-needed sedatives. Physiologic causes must be identified and treated in a timely fashion to prevent irreversible adverse or even fatal outcomes; sedatives may mask symptoms, delaying timely identification, diagnosis, and treatment.
2. Assess patient for signs of hypoperfusion, auscultate heart and lung sounds, obtain a rhythm strip, and administer oxygen, as prescribed. Notify the health care provider immediately.
3. Document assessment findings, health care provider notification and response, and interventions and response.

4. Explain to patient and family reasons for hospitalization, diagnostic tests, and therapies administered.
5. Encourage patient to verbalize fears about illness and hospitalization.
6. Explain procedures to patient before initiation.
7. Offer patient literature, if available, about the disease.
8. Encourage diversional activities for patient, such as television, reading, and interaction with other patients.
9. Encourage family to interact with patient as frequently as possible.

Patient Education and Health Maintenance

For Patients at Risk for Infective Endocarditis

1. Discuss anatomy of heart and changes that occur during endocarditis, using diagrams of the heart.
2. Give patient written literature on early signs and symptoms of disease; review these with patient.
3. Discuss with patient the mode of entry of infection.
4. Indicate that antibiotic prophylaxis is recommended prior to dental procedures that manipulate the gingival and some respiratory procedures (see Table 13-5), for patients with the following conditions:
   a. Congenital heart disease (particularly unrepaired cyanotic defects) repaired with prosthetic material (for 6 months following repair) or repaired with residual defect.
   b. Prosthetic cardiac valve.
   c. Previous IE.
   d. Heart transplantation recipient with cardiac valvular disease.

Table 13-5 Preventing Endocarditis: Regimens for a Dental Procedure

| SITUATION | AGENT | REGIMEN: SINGLE DOSE 30 TO 60 MINUTES BEFORE PROCEDURE | |
		ADULTS	CHILDREN
Oral	Amoxicillin	2 g	50 mg/kg
Unable to take oral medication	Ampicillin OR	2 g I.M. or IV	50 mg/kg I.M. or IV
	Cefazolin or ceftriaxone	1 g I.M. or IV	50 mg/kg I.M. or IV
Allergic to penicillins or ampicillin—oral	Cephalexin*† OR	2 g	50 mg/kg
	Clindamycin OR	600 mg	20 mg/kg
	Azithromycin or clarithromycin	500 mg	15 mg/kg I.M. or IV
Allergic to penicillins or ampicillin and unable to take oral medication	Cefazolin or ceftriaxone† OR	1 g I.M. or IV	20 mg/kg I.M. or IV
	Clindamycin	600 mg I.M. or IV	

*Or other first- or second-generation oral cephalosporin in equivalent adult or pediatric dosage.
†Cephalosporins should not be used in individuals with a history of anaphylaxis, angioedema, or urticaria with penicillins or ampicillin.
I.M., intramuscular; IV, intravenous.
From Nishimura, R. A., Carabello, B. A., Faxon, D. P., et al. (2008). ACC/AHA 2008 guideline update on valvular heart disease: Focused update on infective endocarditis. *Circulation, Journal of the American Heart Association, 118*, 887–896.

Evidence Base Nishimura, R. A., Carabello, B. A., Faxon, D. P., et al. (2008). ACC/AHA 2008 guideline update on valvular heart disease: Focused update on infective endocarditis. *Circulation, 118,* 887–896.

5. Identify individual steps necessary to prevent infection.
   a. Practice good oral hygiene, regular tooth brushing, and flossing.
   b. Notify health care personnel of any history of congenital heart disease or valvular disease.
   c. Discuss importance of carrying emergency identification with information of medical history at all times.
   d. Take temperature if infection is suspected, and notify health care provider of elevation.
   e. Educate patients at risk to look for and treat signs and symptoms of illness indicating bacteremia—injuries, sore throats, furuncles, and so forth.
6. Encourage at-risk individuals to receive pneumococcal and influenza vaccines.
   a. Teach that vaccines reduce the risk of severe infections that could precipitate heart failure.

For Individuals Who Have Had Endocarditis Regarding Possible Relapse

1. Discuss importance of keeping follow-up appointments after discharge (infection can recur in 1 to 2 months).
2. Review the tests that will be performed after discharge—blood cultures, physical examination.
3. Teach patient to inspect soles for Janeway's lesions (indicative of possible relapse).
4. Contact social worker to assist patient with financial planning and home discharge arrangements, if applicable.

Evaluation: Expected Outcomes

- BP stable; no change in murmur; no gallop noted.
- No change in LOC, strength, or neurologic function.
- Normal temperature; negative blood cultures; normal WBC count, BUN, and creatinine; no hearing impairments.
- Tolerates increased daily caloric intake well.
- Verbalizes decrease in anxiety.

Rheumatic Endocarditis (Rheumatic Heart Disease)

Rheumatic endocarditis is an acute, recurrent inflammatory disease that causes damage to the heart as a sequela to group A beta-hemolytic streptococcal infection, particularly the valves, resulting in valve leakage (insufficiency) and/or obstruction (narrowing or stenosis). There are associated compensatory changes in the size of the heart's chambers and the thickness of chamber walls.

See discussion of rheumatic fever in children in Chapter 45, page 1540.

Pathophysiology and Etiology

1. Rheumatic fever is a sequela to group A beta-hemolytic streptococcal infection that occurs in about 3% of untreated infections. It is a preventable disease through detection and adequate treatment of streptococcal pharyngitis.
2. Connective tissue of the heart, blood vessels, joints, and subcutaneous tissues can be affected.
3. Lesions in connective tissue are known as Aschoff bodies, which are localized areas of tissue necrosis surrounded by immune cells.
4. Heart valves, mainly the mitral valve, are affected, resulting in valve leakage and narrowing.
5. Compensatory changes in the chamber sizes and thickness of chamber walls occur.
6. Heart involvement (pancarditis) also includes pericarditis, myocarditis, epicarditis, and endocarditis.

Clinical Manifestations

1. Symptoms of streptococcal pharyngitis may precede rheumatic symptoms.
   a. Sudden onset of sore throat; throat reddened with exudates.
   b. Swollen, tender lymph nodes at angle of jaw.
   c. Headache and fever 101° to 104° F (38.3° to 40° C).
   d. Abdominal pain (children).
   e. Some cases of streptococcal throat infection relatively asymptomatic.
2. Warm and swollen joints (polyarthritis), beginning in the lower extremities (knees and ankles) and may include the large joints in the upper extremities (elbows, wrists).
3. Sydenham chorea (irregular, jerky, involuntary, unpredictable muscular movements).
4. Erythema marginatum (transient mesh-like macular rash on trunk and extremities, never on the face, in about 5% to 13% of patients).
5. Subcutaneous nodules (hard, painless nodules over extensor surfaces of extremities; rare).
6. Fever.
7. Prolonged PR interval as shown on ECG.
8. Heart murmurs; pleural and pericardial rubs.
9. History of previous rheumatic fever or rheumatic heart disease.

Diagnostic Evaluation

1. Throat culture—streptococcal organisms.
2. Sedimentation rate, WBC count and differential, and CRP—increased during acute phase of infection.
3. Elevated antistreptolysin-O (ASO) titer.
4. ECG—prolonged PR interval or heart block.
5. Echocardiography and Doppler study.
6. Cardiac catheterization to evaluate valvular damage and left ventricular function in those with severe cardiac dysfunction.

Management

1. Antimicrobial therapy—penicillin is the drug of choice.
   a. Note that missed doses of antibiotics due to the patient's unavailability while off the unit for diagnostic tests are given after return to the unit.

b. Missed antibiotic doses may have irreversible deleterious consequences.

c. Notify health care provider if doses will be missed to make sure that appropriate alternative measures are taken.

2. Rest—to maintain optimal cardiac function.

3. Salicylates or NSAIDs—to control fever and pain.

4. Prevention of recurrent episodes through long-term penicillin therapy for 5 years after initial attack in most adults; with valvular damage, periodic prophylaxis throughout life.

5. Beta blockers, ACE inhibitors, digoxin, diuretics, supplemental oxygen, rest, sodium and fluid restrictions—to manage heart failure.

6. Though chorea is self-limiting, phenobarbital and diazepam may relieve the symptom.

Complications

1. Valvular heart disease.
2. Cardiomyopathy.
3. Heart failure.
4. Atrial arrhythmias.
5. Pulmonary and systemic embolism.

Nursing Assessment

1. Ask patient about symptoms of fever or throat or joint pain.
2. Ask patient about chest pain, dyspnea, fatigue.
3. Observe for skin lesions or rash on trunk and extremities.
4. Palpate for firm, nontender movable nodules near tendons or joints.
5. Auscultate heart sounds for murmurs and/or rubs.

Nursing Diagnoses

- Hyperthermia related to disease process.
- Decreased Cardiac Output related to decreased cardiac contractility.
- Activity Intolerance related to joint pain and easy fatigability.

Nursing Interventions

Reducing Fever

1. Administer penicillin therapy, as prescribed, to eradicate hemolytic streptococcus; an alternative drug may be prescribed if patient is allergic to penicillin or sensitivity testing and desensitization may be done.

2. Give salicylates or NSAIDs, as prescribed, to suppress rheumatic activity by controlling toxic manifestations, to reduce fever, and to relieve joint pain.

3. Assess for effectiveness of drug therapy.
   a. Take and record temperature every 3 hours.
   b. Evaluate patient's comfort level every 3 hours.

Maintaining Adequate Cardiac Output

1. Assess for signs and symptoms of acute rheumatic carditis.
   a. Be alert to patient's complaints of chest pain, palpitations, and/or precordial "tightness."
   b. Monitor for tachycardia (usually persistent when patient sleeps) or bradycardia.

c. Be alert to development of second-degree heart block or Wenckebach's disease (acute rheumatic carditis causes PR-interval prolongation).

2. Auscultate heart sounds every 4 hours.
   a. Document presence of murmur or pericardial friction rub.
   b. Document extra heart sounds (S_3 gallop, S_4 gallop).

3. Monitor for development of chronic rheumatic endocarditis, which may include valvular disease and heart failure.

Maintaining Activity

1. Maintain bed rest for duration of fever or if signs of active carditis are present.
2. Provide ROM exercise program.
3. Provide diversional activities that prevent exertion.
4. Discuss need for tutorial services with parents to help child keep up with schoolwork.

Patient Education and Health Maintenance

1. Counsel patient to maintain good nutrition.
2. Counsel patient on hygienic practices.
   a. Discuss proper handwashing, disposal of tissues, laundering of handkerchiefs (decrease risk of exposure to microbes).
   b. Discuss importance of using patient's own toothbrush, soap, and washcloths when living in group situations.
3. Counsel patient on importance of receiving adequate rest.
4. Instruct patient to seek treatment immediately should sore throat or fever occur.
5. Support patients in long-term antibiotic therapy to prevent relapse (5 years for most adults).
6. Instruct patient with valvular disease to use prophylactic penicillin therapy before certain procedures and surgery (see page 404).
7. Discuss patient's ability to pay for medical treatment. If appropriate, contact social services for patient. (Financial difficulties may inhibit patient from seeking early treatment of symptoms.)

Evaluation: Expected Outcomes

- Afebrile.
- Denies chest pain; normal sinus rhythm.
- Maintains bed rest while febrile.

Myocarditis

Myocarditis is an inflammatory process involving the myocardium.

Pathophysiology and Etiology

1. Focal or diffuse inflammation of the myocardium; may be acute or chronic.
2. May follow infectious process—viral or "idiopathic" (particularly Coxsackie group B and may develop after influenza A or B, herpes simplex, parvovirus, cytomegalovirus, adenovirus, Epstein-Barr, rubella, and human immunodeficiency virus [HIV]); bacterial; parasitic; protozoal; rickettsial; spirochetal; and fungal (*Candida, Aspergillus,* and *Histoplasma*).

3. May be associated with chemotherapy (especially doxorubicin), immunosuppressive therapy, or vaccinia virus inoculation for protection against smallpox infection.

4. Systemic disorders such as sarcoidosis, celiac disease, autoimmune conditions such as systemic lupus and other collagen diseases, may cause myocarditis.

5. May be associated with exposures to certain chemicals (arsenic and hydrocarbons); allergic or toxic reactions to penicillin or sulfonamides; insect/snake bites; cocaine use.

6. Radiation exposure—most cases are the result of therapy for Hodgkin's lymphoma or breast or lung cancer. Less common are exposure to a nuclear reactor or after detonation of a nuclear device.

Clinical Manifestations

1. Symptoms depend on type of infection, degree of myocardial damage, capacity of myocardium to recover, and host resistance. Can be acute or chronic and can occur at any age. Symptoms may be minor and go unnoticed.
   a. Fatigue and dyspnea.
   b. Palpitations.
   c. Occasional precordial discomfort/vague chest pain.
2. Cardiac enlargement.
3. Abnormal heart sounds: murmur, S_3 or S_4, or friction rubs.
4. Signs of heart failure (eg, pulsus alternans, dyspnea, crackles, lower-extremity edema, low urine output).
5. Fever with tachycardia or other sign of viral infection, such as headache, joint pain, and sore throat.
6. Joint pain or swelling; leg swelling

Diagnostic Evaluation

1. Transient ECG changes—ST segment flattened, T-wave inversion, conduction defects, extrasystoles, supraventricular and ventricular ectopic beats.
2. Elevated WBC count and sedimentation rate.
3. Measurement of serum cardiac biomarkers such as CPK and troponin—may be elevated.
4. Chest x-ray—may show heart enlargement and lung congestion.
5. Elevated antibody titers (ASO titer as in rheumatic fever).
6. Stool and throat cultures isolating bacteria or a virus.
7. Endomyocardial biopsy for definitive diagnosis.
8. Echocardiogram—defines size, structure, and function of heart.
9. MRI—may be helpful to determine structural alterations.
10. Nuclear imaging using gallium or indium (antimyosin antibodies)—helps detect myocardial inflammation.

Management

Treatment objectives are targeted toward management of complications. Supportive care is the first line of treatment.
1. Diuretic and digoxin therapy for heart failure and atrial fibrillation.
2. Antidysrhythmic therapy (usually amiodarone).
3. Strict bed rest to promote healing of damaged myocardium.
4. Antimicrobial therapy if causative bacteria are isolated.
5. Anticoagulation therapy.

6. ACE inhibitor or beta-adrenergic blocker (should be used with caution; may cause hypotension)—to strengthen the heart's pumping ability and to reduce its workload, thus improve left ventricular systolic dysfunction.
7. In severe cases, aggressive therapy may be necessary: inotropes, such as dobutamine and dopamine; IABP (counterpulsation therapy); temporary artificial heart (assist device); consideration of urgent heart transplantation.
8. IV immunoglobulin has antiviral effects; immunosuppressive regimen of steroids and cyclosporine or azathioprine improves systolic function.

Complications

1. Heart failure, pericarditis.
2. Cardiomyopathy.
3. Arrhythmias.
4. Sudden cardiac death.

Nursing Assessment

1. Assess for fatigue, palpitations, fever, dyspnea, and chest pain.
2. Auscultate heart sounds.
3. Assess limbs for swelling, discoloration of skin, and temperature of skin.
4. Evaluate history for precipitating factors.

Nursing Diagnoses

- Hyperthermia related to inflammatory/infectious process.
- Decreased Cardiac Output related to decreased cardiac contractility and dysrhythmias.
- Activity Intolerance related to impaired cardiac performance and febrile illness.

Nursing Interventions

Reducing Fever
1. Administer antipyretics as directed.
2. Check temperature every 4 hours.
3. Administer antibiotics as directed.

Maintaining Cardiac Output
1. Evaluate for clinical evidence that disease is subsiding—monitor pulse, auscultate for abnormal heart sounds (murmur or change in existing murmur), check temperature, auscultate lung fields, monitor respirations.
2. Record daily intake and output.
3. Record daily weight.
4. Check for peripheral edema.
5. Elevate head of bed, if necessary, to enhance respiration. Encourage use of incentive spirometry.
6. Treat the symptoms of heart failure as prescribed (see page 414).

 DRUG ALERT Patients with myocarditis may be sensitive to digoxin. Assess for toxic signs and symptoms, such as anorexia, nausea, fatigue, weakness, yellow-green halos around visual images, prolonged PR interval.

7. Evaluate patient's pulse and apical rate for signs of tachycardia and gallop rhythm—indications that heart failure is recurring.
8. Evaluate for evidence of dysrhythmias—patients with myocarditis are prone to develop dysrhythmias.
   a. Institute continuous cardiac monitoring if evidence of a dysrhythmia develops.
   b. Have equipment for resuscitation, defibrillation, and cardiac pacing available in case of life-threatening dysrhythmia.

Reducing Fatigue

1. Ensure bed rest to reduce heart rate, stroke volume, BP, and heart contractility; also helps to decrease residual damage and complications of myocarditis and promotes healing.
   a. Prolonged bed rest may be required until there is reduction in heart size and improvement of function.
2. Provide diversional activities for patient.
3. Allow patient to use bedside commode rather than bedpan (reduces cardiovascular workload).
4. Discuss with patient activities that can be continued after discharge.
   a. Discuss the need to modify activities in the immediate future.
   b. Explore with patient lifestyle modifications and discuss adequacy of self-concept.

Patient Education and Health Maintenance

Instruct patient as follows:
1. There is usually some residual heart enlargement; physical activity may be slowly increased; begin with chair rest for increasing periods; follow with walking in the room and then outdoors.
2. Report any symptom involving rapid heartbeat.
3. Avoid competitive sports, cigarettes, illicit drugs, and alcohol. Myocardial toxic medications such as doxorubicin cannot be used.
4. Pregnancy is not advisable for women with cardiomyopathies associated with myocarditis.
5. Prevent infectious diseases with appropriate immunizations (pneumococcal and influenza vaccines).
6. Encourage family to support patient and learn about the illness.
7. Refer patient to cardiac phase II rehabilitation—a safe, monitored environment to increase patient's exercise work capacity.

Evaluation: Expected Outcomes

- Afebrile.
- BP and heart rate stable; no dysrhythmias noted.
- Maintains bed rest.

Pericarditis

Pericarditis is an inflammation of the pericardium, the membranous sac enveloping the heart. It is usually a manifestation of a more generalized disease. In healthy individuals, the pericardial cavity contains about 15 to 50 mL of an ultrafiltrate of plasma. Diseases of the pericardium present clinically in four ways:

Acute and recurrent pericarditis.
Cardiac tamponade is an acute type of pericardial effusion in which the heart is compressed, either by blood or by a penetrating injury, so that its normal function is impeded.
Pericardial effusion is an outpouring of fluid into the pericardial cavity seen in pericarditis.
Constrictive pericarditis is a condition in which a chronic inflammatory thickening of the pericardium compresses the heart so it is unable to fill normally during diastole.

Pathophysiology and Etiology

1. Acute idiopathic pericarditis is the most common and typical form; etiology unknown.
2. Infection.
   a. Viral (influenza, coxsackievirus, HIV).
   b. Bacterial—*Staphylococcus*, meningococcus, *Streptococcus*, pneumococcus, gonococcus, *Mycobacterium tuberculosis*.
   c. Fungal.
   d. Parasitic.
3. Connective tissue disorders (lupus erythematosus, periarteritis nodosa); and gastrointestinal diseases (ulcerative colitis, Crohn's and Whipple disease).
4. MI; early, 24 to 72 hours; or late, 1 week to 2 years after MI (Dressler's syndrome).
5. Malignant disease; thoracic irradiation (primary or metastatic pericardial tumors).
6. Chest trauma, heart surgery, including pacemaker implantation.
7. Drug-induced—procainamide, phenytoin, hydralazine, and isoniazid.
8. Asbestosis (may induce pericardial as well as lung lesions).
9. Metabolic disorders such as uremia; hypothyroidism may cause pericardial effusion, not necessarily pericarditis.

Clinical Manifestations

1. Pain in anterior chest, aggravated by thoracic motion—may vary from mild to sharp and severe; located in precordial area (may be felt beneath clavicle, neck, scapular region); may be relieved by leaning forward.
2. Pericardial friction rub—scratchy, grating, or creaking sound occurring in the presence of pericardial inflammation.
3. Edema, ascites, and dyspnea—from pericardial effusion and cardiac tamponade.
4. Fever, sweating, chills—due to inflammation of pericardium.
5. Dysrhythmias.

Diagnostic Evaluation

1. Echocardiogram—most sensitive method for detecting pericardial effusion.
2. Chest x-ray—may show enlarged cardiac silhouette with clear lung fields.
3. ECG—to evaluate for MI (acute stage of pericarditis, ST elevation is found in several or all leads).

4. WBC count and differential indicating infection.
5. Antinuclear antibody serologic tests elevated in lupus erythematosus.
6. Purified protein derivative test positive in tuberculosis.
7. ASO titers—elevated if rheumatic fever is present.
8. BUN—to evaluate for uremia.
9. Elevated erythrocyte sedimentation rate and serum C-reactive protein levels.
10. Elevated cardiac biomarkers –troponin and MB fraction of creatinine kinase.
11. Pericardiocentesis—for examination of pericardial fluid for etiologic diagnosis and relief from cardiac tamponade.
12. Cardiac MRI or CT.

Management

The objectives of treatment are targeted toward determining the etiology of the problem; administering pharmacologic therapy for specified etiology, when known; and being alert to the possible complication of cardiac tamponade.

1. Bacterial pericarditis—penicillin or other antimicrobials.
2. Rheumatic fever—penicillin G and other antimicrobials (see page 405).
3. Tuberculosis—antituberculosis chemotherapy (see page 296).
4. Fungal pericarditis—amphotericin B and fluconazole.
5. Systemic lupus erythematosus—corticosteroids.
6. Renal pericarditis—dialysis, biochemical control of end-stage renal disease.
7. Neoplastic pericarditis—intrapericardial instillation of chemotherapy; radiotherapy.
8. Post-MI syndrome—bed rest, aspirin, prednisone.
9. Postpericardiotomy syndrome (after open heart surgery)—treat symptomatically.
10. Emergency pericardiocentesis if cardiac tamponade develops.
11. Partial pericardiectomy (pericardial "window") or total pericardiectomy for recurrent constrictive pericarditis.
12. NSAIDs are recommended for symptom relief of acute pericarditis; colchicine and steroid regimen are used as adjunct to NSAID therapy.

Complications

1. Cardiac tamponade.
2. Heart failure.
3. Hemopericardium (especially patients receiving anticoagulants after MI).

Nursing Assessment

1. Assess chest pain.
   a. Ask the patient if pain is aggravated by breathing, turning in bed, twisting body, coughing, yawning, or swallowing.
   b. Assess for relief with sitting up and/or leaning forward.
   c. Be alert to the patient's medical diagnoses when assessing pain. Post-MI patients may experience a dull, crushing pain radiating to neck, arm, and shoulders, mimicking an extension of infarction. Report change in character of chest pain or worsening pain.

2. Auscultate heart sounds.
   a. Listen for pericardia friction rub by asking patient to hold breath briefly.
   b. Listen to the heart with patient in different positions.
   c. Assess for pulsus paradoxus.
3. Evaluate history for precipitating factors.

Nursing Diagnoses

- Acute Pain related to pericardial inflammation.
- Decreased Cardiac Output related to impaired ventricular expansion.

Nursing Interventions

Reducing Discomfort

1. Give prescribed drug regimen for pain and symptomatic relief.
2. Relieve anxiety of patient and family by explaining the difference between pain of pericarditis and pain of recurrent MI. (Patients may fear extension of myocardial tissue damage.)
3. Explain to patient and family that pericarditis does not indicate further heart damage.
4. Encourage patient to remain on bed rest when chest pain, fever, and friction rub occur.
5. Assist patient to position of comfort.

Maintaining Cardiac Output

 NURSING ALERT Normal pericardial sac contains less than 30 mL of fluid; pericardial fluid may accumulate slowly without noticeable symptoms. However, a rapidly developing effusion can produce serious hemodynamic alterations.

1. Assess heart rate, rhythm, BP, respirations at least hourly in the acute phase; continuously if hemodynamically unstable.
2. Assess for signs of cardiac tamponade—increased heart rate, decreased BP, presence of paradoxical pulse, distended jugular veins, restlessness, muffled heart sounds.
3. Prepare for emergency pericardiocentesis or surgery. Keep pericardiocentesis tray at bedside (see page 405).
4. Assess for signs of heart failure (see page 413).
5. Monitor closely for the development of dysrhythmias.

Patient Education and Health Maintenance

1. Teach patient the etiology of pericarditis.
2. Instruct patient about signs and symptoms of pericarditis and the need for long-term medication therapy to help relieve symptoms.
3. Review all medications with the patient—purpose, adverse effects, dosage, and special precautions.

Evaluation: Expected Outcomes

- Verbalizes relief of pain.
- Pulse and heart rate stable, no dysrhythmias, no friction rub.

Cardiomyopathy

Cardiomyopathy refers to disease of the heart muscle or electrical dysfunction. Causes of cardiomyopathy are classified as primary or secondary. Primary cardiomyopathies have genetic, mixed, or acquired etiologies, whereas secondary cardiomyopathies have infiltrative, toxic, or inflammatory causes. The four main types are dilated, hypertrophic, restrictive (less common), and arrhythmogenic right ventricular cardiomyopathy.

Evidence Base Gersh, B. J., Maron, B. J., Bonow, R. O., et al. (2011). ACCF/AHA guideline: 2011 ACCF/AHA guideline for the diagnosis and treatment of hypertrophic cardiomyopathy: A report of the American College of Cardiology Foundation/American Heart Association Task Force on Practice Guidelines. *Circulation, 124,* 783–831.

Hunt, S. A., Abraham, W. T., Chin, M. H., et al. (2009). 2009 focused update incorporated into the ACC/AHA guidelines for the diagnosis and management of chronic heart failure in the adult: A report of the American College of Cardiology/American Heart Association Task Force on Practice Guidelines. *Circulation, 119,* 391–479.

Pathophysiology and Etiology

Dilated Cardiomyopathy

Dilated cardiomyopathy is the most common form of cardiomyopathy. It can be divided into ischemic and nonischemic cardiomyopathy.

1. Ischemic cardiomyopathy.
   a. It is caused by inadequate oxygen supply due to obstruction in coronary arteries.
   b. The lack of oxygen interrupts both mechanical and electrical function of the cells, decreases contractility, and causes dysrhythmia.
   c. The scar formed from MI leads to systolic dysfunction.
2. Nonischemic cardiomyopathy.
   a. Cause is idiopathic (unknown).
   b. 10% to 50% of cases are identified by genetic mutation.
3. Both the right and left ventricle dilate (enlarge) significantly, causing a decrease in the ability of the heart to pump blood efficiently to the body.
4. Blood remaining in the ventricles after contraction causes increases in ventricular, atrial, and pulmonary pressures.
5. Increased pressures continue to diminish the ability of the heart to pump blood to the body, and heart failure symptoms occur after all compensatory mechanisms are exhausted.
6. Alcohol abuse; chemotherapy; chemical agents; myocarditis; pregnancy (third trimester, postpartum); valve disease; endocrine disorders such as thyroid disease; and infections, such as HIV, can cause dilated cardiomyopathy.

Hypertrophic Cardiomyopathy

1. Hypertrophic cardiomyopathy is primarily due to the abnormal thickening of the ventricular septum of the heart.
2. The thickening of the heart muscle commonly occurs asymmetrically (septum is proportionally thicker than the other ventricular walls), but may also occur symmetrically (septum and the ventricular free wall both become equally thickened).
3. The ultrastructure of the heart is also disrupted by patches of myocardial fibrosis, disorganization of myocardial fibers, and abnormalities of the coronary microvasculature.
4. The thickened heart muscle and ultrastructure disruption change the shape, size, and distensibility of the ventricular cavity and alter the normal thickness and functioning of the mitral valve; as a result, the heart's ability to relax and contract normally is impaired.
   a. Muscle stiffness impairs the filling of the ventricle with blood during relaxation.
   b. Forceful contractions eject blood from the heart too rapidly, causing abnormal pressure gradients; mechanical narrowing of the passage by which the blood leaves the heart also may occur, acutely obstructing blood flow to the body.
5. Hypertrophic cardiomyopathy is a genetically transmitted disorder.

Restrictive Cardiomyopathy

1. The heart muscle becomes infiltrated by various substances, resulting in severe fibrosis.
2. The heart muscle becomes stiff and nondistensible, impairing the ability of the ventricle to fill with blood adequately.
3. Amyloidosis and hemochromatosis (excess iron deposition) may cause restrictive cardiomyopathy.

Arrhythmogenic Right Ventricular Cardiomyopathy

1. Autosomal genetic disorder; affects 1 in 2,000 to 5,000; more common among men.
   a. Characterized by placement of the right ventricular myocytes by fibro-fatty tissue, right ventricular dysfunction, and ventricular dysrhythmias.

Clinical Manifestations

1. Exertional dyspnea.
2. Chest pain.
3. Signs of heart failure (see page 413).
4. Pulmonary edema (see page 418).
5. Dysrhythmias (frequent atrial/ventricular ectopic beats; sinus, atrial, and ventricular tachycardia).
6. Pericardial effusions (with restrictive cardiomyopathy).
7. Cardiac murmur.
8. Syncope.
9. Sudden cardiac death may be the first sign with arrhythmogenic right ventricular cardiomyopathy.

Diagnostic Evaluation

1. Chest x-ray (cardiomegaly).
2. ECG—may show dysrhythmia.
3. Echocardiogram to detect abnormalities of heart wall movements.
4. 24-hour Holter monitoring to detect dysrhythmias.
5. Radionuclide imaging to assess ventricular function.
6. Cardiac catheterization to help determine cause (ischemic or nonischemic).
7. Pulmonary artery catheter for hemodynamic monitoring.

Management

The goal of therapy is to maximize ventricular function and prevent complications.

Dilated Cardiomyopathy

1. Effective management of heart failure by conventional therapy (see page 414).
2. Oral anticoagulants may be instituted to prevent thrombus and pulmonary embolus.
3. Heart transplantation, may be considered in those eligible.
4. Mechanical circulatory support device (ie, LVAD or BiVAD) may also be considered.

 DRUG ALERT Patients with dilated cardiomyopathy and other forms of heart failure (HF) are susceptible to digoxin toxicity, especially with the concomitant use of amiodarone or verapamil and in patients with renal impairment. Monitor patient carefully for evidence of nausea, vomiting, yellow vision, and dysrhythmias.

Hypertrophic Cardiomyopathy

1. Beta-adrenergic blockers—reduce the force of the heart muscle's contraction, diminish obstructive pressure gradients, and decrease oxygen requirements. Three beta-blockers have been shown to be effective in reducing mortality in patients with chronic HF; these include metoprolol sustained release, bisoprolol, and carvedilol.
2. Calcium channel blockers—decrease heart rate and contractility and vasodilate, thereby providing symptom relief. Calcium channel blockers can worsen HF and are associated with increased risk of cardiovascular events. Only vasoselective drugs have shown not to be associated with negative impact on survival.

 **DRUG ALERT** Verapamil and diltiazem should be avoided in heart failure treatment because they depress myocardial function with increasing heart failure.

3. Antidysrhythmic therapy—Digoxin is most commonly used to slow ventricular response in patients with HF, although beta-blockers have been shown to be more effective than digoxin during exercise. Combination of beta-blockers and digoxin are more effective than either drug alone. If contraindicated, amiodarone may be an alternative.
4. Myotomy and myectomy—surgical resection of a portion of the septum to reduce muscle thickness and provide symptom relief.
5. Device implantation—pacemakers and automatic internal defibrillators may be implanted to treat severe bradycardias and lethal tachycardias.

 DRUG ALERT Chest pain experienced by patients with hypertrophic cardiomyopathy is managed by rest and elevation of the feet (improves venous return to the heart). Vasodilator therapy (nitroglycerin) may worsen chest pain by decreasing venous return to the heart and further increasing obstruction of blood flow from the heart; agents that increase contractility of the heart muscle (dopamine, dobutamine) should also be avoided or used with extreme caution.

Restrictive Cardiomyopathy

1. Therapy is palliative unless specific underlying process is established.
2. Heart failure can be controlled with fluid restriction and diuretic therapy.
3. Digoxin is beneficial for controlling atrial fibrillation.
4. Oral anticoagulants are instituted to prevent emboli.

Arrhythmogenic Right Ventricular Cardiomyopathy

Antidysrhythmic agents such as carvedilol, sotalol, amiodarone.
1. Implantable cardioverter-defibrillator.
2. Myocardial ablation or transplantation.

Complications

1. Mural thrombus (due to blood stasis in ventricles with dilated cardiomyopathy).
2. Severe heart failure.
3. Sudden cardiac death.
4. Pulmonary embolism.

Nursing Assessment

1. Evaluate patient's chief complaint, which may include fever, syncope, general aches, fatigue, palpitations, dyspnea.
2. Evaluate etiologic factors, such as alcohol abuse, pregnancy, recent infection, or history of endocrine disorders.
3. Assess for positive family history.
4. Auscultate lung sounds for crackles (pulmonary edema) or decreased sounds (pleural effusion).
5. Assess heart size through palpation of chest for point of maximal impulse (PMI) and auscultate for abnormal sounds.
6. Evaluate cardiac rhythm and ECG for evidence of atrial or ventricular enlargement and infarction.

Nursing Diagnoses

- Decreased Cardiac Output related to decreased ventricular function and/or dysrhythmias.
- Anxiety related to fear of death and hospitalization.
- Fatigue related to disease process.

Nursing Interventions

Improving Cardiac Output

1. Monitor heart rate, rhythm, temperature, and respiratory rate at least every 4 hours.
2. Evaluate CVP, pulmonary artery wedge pressure, and PCWP by pulmonary artery catheter to assess progress and effect of drug therapy.
3. Calculate CO, CI, and SVR.
4. Observe for changes in CO, such as decreased BP, change in mental status, decreased urine output.
5. Administer pharmacologic support, as directed, and observe for changes in hemodynamic and clinical status.

6. Administer medications to control or eradicate dysrhythmias, as directed.
7. Administer anticoagulants as directed, especially for patients in atrial fibrillation.
   a. Monitor coagulation studies.
   b. Observe for evidence of bleeding.

Relieving Anxiety

1. Always evaluate increasing and/or new-onset anxiety for a physiologic cause and report to the health care provider before administration of anxiolytics.
2. Explain all procedures and treatments.
3. Inform patient and visitors of visiting hours and policy and whom to contact for information.
4. Orient patient to unit, purpose of equipment, and care plan.
5. Encourage questions and voicing of fears and concerns.

Reducing Fatigue

1. Make sure that patient and visitors understand the importance of rest.
2. Assist patient in identifying stressors and reducing their effect (important for patients with hypertrophic cardiomyopathy because stress worsens the outflow obstruction).
3. Provide uninterrupted periods and assist with ambulation, as ordered.
4. Teach the use of diversional activities and relaxation techniques to relieve tension.

Patient Education and Health Maintenance

1. Medication education such as digoxin.
   a. Take daily only after taking pulse; notify health care provider if pulse is below 60 beats/minute (or other specified rate).
   b. Report signs of digoxin toxicity—anorexia, nausea, vomiting, yellow vision.
   c. Follow up for periodic blood levels.
2. Advise low-sodium diet (less than 2 g daily). Teach how to read labels.
3. Advise reporting signs of heart failure—weight gain, edema, shortness of breath, increased fatigue.
4. Make sure that family members know cardiopulmonary resuscitation (CPR) because sudden cardiac arrest is possible.

Evaluation: Expected Outcomes

- Blood pressure and hemodynamic parameters stable; urine output adequate; baseline mental status.
- Asks questions and cooperates with care.
- Rests at intervals.

Heart Failure

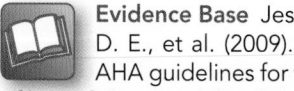

Evidence Base Jessup, M., Abraham, W. T., Casey, D. E., et al. (2009). 2009 Focused update: ACCF/AHA guidelines for the diagnosis and management of heart failure in adults: A report of the American College of Cardiology Foundation/American Heart Association Task Force on Practice Guidelines: Developed in collaboration with the International Society for Heart and Lung Transplantation. *Circulation, 119*(14), 1977–2016.

Heart failure is a clinical syndrome that results from the progressive process of remodeling, in which mechanical and biochemical forces alter the size, shape, and function of the ventricle's ability to fill with or pump enough oxygenated blood to meet the metabolic demands of the body.

Pathophysiology and Etiology

1. Cardiac compensatory mechanisms (increased heart rate, vasoconstriction, heart enlargement) initially occur to assist the struggling heart.
   a. These mechanisms are able to "compensate" for the heart's inability to pump effectively and maintain sufficient blood flow to organs and tissue at rest.
   b. Physiologic stressors that increase the workload of the heart (exercise, infection) may cause these mechanisms to fail and precipitate the "clinical syndrome" associated with a failing heart (elevated ventricular/atrial pressures, sodium and water retention, decreased CO, circulatory and pulmonary congestion).
   c. The compensatory mechanisms may hasten the onset of failure because they increase afterload and cardiac work.
2. Caused by disorders of heart muscle resulting in decreased contractile properties of the heart, such as coronary artery disease, hypertension, dilated cardiomyopathy, and valvular heart disease.
3. Risk factors include:
   a. Hypertension.
   b. Hyperlipidemia.
   c. Diabetes.
   d. CAD.
   e. Family history.
   f. Smoking.
   g. Alcohol consumption.
   h. Use of cardiotoxic drugs.
   i. Ventricular dysrhythmias.
   j. Atrial dysrhythmias.

Systolic versus Diastolic Failure

There are two types of dysfunction that may exist with heart failure (see Figure 13-6).

1. Systolic failure—poor contractility of the myocardium results in decreased CO and an elevated SVR.
2. Diastolic failure—stiff myocardium, which impairs the ability of the left ventricle to fill up with blood. This causes an increase in pressure in the left atrium and pulmonary vasculature, causing the pulmonary signs of heart failure.

Acute versus Chronic Heart Failure

1. Acute failure—sudden onset of symptoms such as acute pulmonary edema and decreased CO; requires intervention and medical attention.
2. Chronic failure—long-term process with accompanying compensatory mechanism; can progress to acute phase in the setting of dysrhythmias, ischemia, or sudden illness.

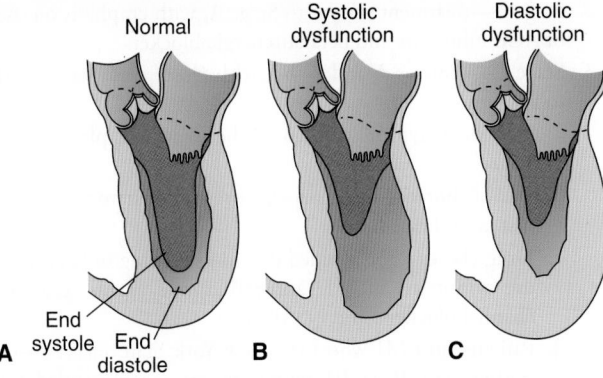

Normal   Systolic dysfunction   Diastolic dysfunction

End systole   End diastole

A   **B**   **C**

Figure 13-6. Heart failure due to systolic and diastolic dysfunction. The ejection fraction represents the difference between end-diastolic function and end-systolic volume. **(A)** Normal systolic and diastolic function with normal ejection fraction; **(B)** systolic dysfunction with decreased ejection fraction due to impaired systolic function; **(C)** diastolic dysfunction with decreased ejection fraction due to decreased diastolic filling.

Neurohormonal Compensatory Mechanisms in Heart Failure

1. Sympathetic Nervous System
   a. Increased catecholamines to compensate for low CO.
   b. Shunting of blood from nonvital to vital organs.
   c. Increased oxygen demand, decreased coronary artery perfusion, and decreased diastolic filling.
2. Renin-Angiotensin-Aldosterone System
   a. Increased fluid retention in response to decreased CO.
   b. Increased vasoconstriction (action of angiotensin II).
   c. Increased SVR.
   d. Increased workload of the heart.
   e. Further decreased CO.
3. Ventricular Hypertrophy
   a. Compensatory mechanism to overcome the increased afterload.
4. Ventricular Remodeling
   a. Change of round bowl shape of the heart as a result of compensation.

Clinical Manifestations

Initially, there may be isolated left-sided heart failure, but eventually the right ventricle fails because of the additional workload. Combined left- and right-sided heart failure is common. Heart failure may be classified according to physical activity (New York Heart Association Functional Classification) or disease progression (ACC/AHA Guidelines); see page 414.

Left-Sided Heart Failure (Forward Failure)

Altering the filling and pumping function of left ventricle, congestion occurs mainly in the lungs from blood backing up into pulmonary veins and capillaries.

1. Shortness of breath, dyspnea on exertion, tachypnea, paroxysmal nocturnal dyspnea (due to reabsorption of dependent edema that has developed during the day), orthopnea, cyanosis, pulmonary edema, and hemoptysis.
2. Cough—may be dry, unproductive; usually occurs at night.
3. Fatigability—from low CO, nocturia, insomnia, dyspnea, catabolic effect of chronic failure.
4. Insomnia, restlessness.
5. Tachycardia—ventricular gallop (S_3 and S_4).

Right-Sided Heart Failure (Backward Failure)

Altering the pumping function of right ventricle, there are signs and symptoms of elevated pressures and congestion in systemic veins and capillaries.

1. Edema of ankles; unexplained weight gain (pitting edema is obvious only after retention of at least 10 lb [4.5 kg] of fluid).
2. Liver congestion—may produce upper abdominal pain.
3. Distended jugular veins, increased CVP, pulmonary hypertension (increased PCWP).
4. Abnormal fluid in body cavities (pleural space, abdominal cavity), splenomegaly
5. Anorexia and nausea—from hepatic and visceral engorgement.
6. Nocturia—diuresis occurs at night with supine position and improved CO.
7. Weakness.

Cardiovascular Findings in Both Types

1. Cardiomegaly (enlargement of the heart)—detected by physical examination and chest x-ray.
2. Ventricular gallop—evident on auscultation.
3. Rapid heart rate.
4. Development of pulsus alternans (alternation in strength of beat).

Diagnostic Evaluation

1. Echocardiography-two-dimensional with Doppler flow studies—may show ventricular hypertrophy, dilation of chambers, and abnormal wall motion.
2. ECG (resting and exercise)—may show ventricular hypertrophy and ischemia.
3. Chest x-ray may show cardiomegaly, pleural effusion, and vascular congestion.
4. Cardiac catheterization—(left heart catheterization to rule out CAD).
   a. Right-sided heart catheterization—to measure pulmonary pressure and left ventricular function.
5. ABG studies may show hypoxemia due to pulmonary vascular congestion.
6. Bloodwork: CBC, electrolytes, Ca, Mg, renal function, glycohemoglobin, lipid profile, thyroid function, and liver function studies to fully assess patient condition that may impact heart failure.
7. Human B-type natriuretic peptide (BNP, triage BNP, N-terminal prohormone brain NP, or proBNP).
   a. As volume and pressure in the cardiac chambers rise, cardiac cells produce and release more BNP. This test aids in the differentiation of heart failure from other pulmonary

diseases (ie, chronic obstructive pulmonary disease) and establish acute exacerbation of HF.

  b. A level greater than 100/mL is diagnostic for heart failure. In addition, the higher the BNP, the more severe the heart failure.

  c. BNP is used in emergency departments to quickly diagnose and start treatment.

8. Radionuclide ventriculogram.

9. Thallium scan to rule out underlying causes.

Management

Overview Based on ACC/AHA Stage

See Table 13-6.

1. Stage A—focuses on eliminating risk factors by initiating therapeutic lifestyle changes, such as smoking cessation, increasing physical activity, and decreasing alcohol consumption. This stage also focuses on controlling chronic diseases, such as hypertension, high cholesterol, and diabetes. Beta-adrenergic blockers, ACE inhibitors, and diuretics are useful in treating this stage.

2. Stage B—treatment similar to Stage A, with emphasis on use of ACE inhibitors and beta-adrenergic blockers.

3. Stage C—same as A and B, but with closer surveillance and follow-up.

  a. Digoxin is typically added to the treatment plan in this stage.

  b. Use of diuretic, hydralazine, nitrate, aldosterone antagonist, as indicated.

  c. Drug classes to be avoided due to worsening of heart failure symptoms include anti-arrhythmic agents, calcium channel blockers, and NSAIDs.

  d. Patients post-MI who have New York State Heart Association class II or III symptoms are recommended for implantable cardioverter-defibrillator placement.

4. Stage D—may need mechanical circulatory support, continuous inotropic therapy, cardiac transplantation, or palliative care.

  a. Treatment aimed at decreasing excess body fluid.

  b. May not tolerate other classes of drugs used in previous stages.

Table 13-6   Heart Failure Guidelines and Recommendations

NEW YORK HEART ASSOCIATION CLASSIFICATION	AMERICAN COLLEGE OF CARDIOLOGY/AMERICAN HEART ASSOCIATION GUIDELINES	RECOMMENDATIONS
—	**Stage A.** People at high risk of developing heart failure but without structural heart disease or symptoms of heart failure.	• Treat hypertension, lipid disorders, diabetes • Encourage patient to stop smoking and to exercise regularly • Discourage use of alcohol, illicit drugs • Angiotensin-converting enzyme (ACE) inhibitor, if indicated
Class I. Patients with cardiac disease without limitations of physical activity. Ordinary physical activity does not cause undue fatigue, palpitations, dyspnea, or anginal pain.	**Stage B.** People who have structural heart disease but no symptoms of heart failure.	• All stage A therapies • ACE inhibitor unless contraindicated • Beta-adrenergic blocker unless contraindicated
Class II. Patients with cardiac disease who have slight limitations of physical activity. They are comfortable at rest. Ordinary physical activity results in fatigue, palpitations, dyspnea, or anginal pain. **Class III.** Patients with cardiac disease who have marked limitation of physical activity. They are comfortable at rest. Less than ordinary physical activity causes fatigue, palpitations, dyspnea, or anginal pain.	**Stage C.** People who have structural heart disease with current or prior symptoms of heart failure.	• All stage A and B therapies • Sodium-restricted diet • Diuretics • Digoxin • Avoid or withdraw anti-arrhythmic agents, most calcium channel blockers, and nonsteroidal anti-inflammatories • Consider aldosterone antagonists, angiotensin receptor blockers, hydralazine, and nitrates
Class IV. Patients with cardiac disease who cannot carry out any physical activity without discomfort. Symptoms of cardiac insufficiency or of anginal syndrome may be present even at rest. Any physical activity increases discomfort.	**Stage D.** People with refractory heart failure who require specialized interventions.	• All therapies for stages A, B, and C • Mechanical assist device, such as biventricular pacemaker or left ventricular assist device • Continuous inotropic therapy • Hospice care

Caboral, M., and Mitchell, J. (2003). New guidelines for heart failure: Focus on prevention. *Nurse Practitioner, 28*(1), 13–16, 22–23.

Drug Classes

1. Diuretics (preload reduction).
   a. Eliminate excess body water and decrease ventricular pressures.
   b. A low-sodium diet and fluid restriction complement this therapy.
   c. Some diuretics may have slight venodilator properties.
2. Positive inotropic agents—increase the heart's ability to pump more effectively by improving the contractile force of the muscle.
   a. Digoxin may be initiated at any time to reduce symptoms of HF, prevent hospitalizations, control rhythm, and improve exercise tolerance.
   b. Dopamine improves renal blood flow and urine output.
   c. Dobutamine.
   d. Milrinone and amrinone are potent vasodilators and increase contractility.
3. Vasodilator therapy—decreases the workload of the heart by dilating peripheral vessels. By relaxing capacitance vessels (veins and venules), vasodilators reduce ventricular filling pressures (preload) and volumes. By relaxing resistance vessels (arterioles), vasodilators can reduce impedance to left ventricular ejection and improve stroke volume.
   a. Nitrates (preload reducers), such as nitroglycerin, isosorbide, nitroglycerin ointment—predominantly dilate systemic veins.
   b. Hydralazine—predominantly affects arterioles; reduces arteriolar tone.
   c. Prazosin—balanced effects on both arterial and venous circulation.
   d. Sodium nitroprusside—afterload reducer, predominantly affects arterioles.
   e. Morphine—analgesic of choice because it enhances peripheral dilation, decreases venous return, and decreases anxiety, thus decreasing workload of the heart.
4. ACE inhibitors (decrease left ventricle dilation and remodeling)—inhibit the formation of angiotensin II. In doing so, produce vasodilation. Also prevent ventricular remodeling with chronic use.
   a. Studies have shown ACE inhibitors can alleviate HF symptoms and clinical status as well as overall sense of well-being among HF patients.
   b. The following ACE inhibitors have been shown to reduce morbidity and mortality: captopril, enalapril, lisinopril, perindopril, ramipril, and trandolapril.
5. Beta-adrenergic blockers—negative inotropes that decrease myocardial workload and protect against fatal dysrhythmias by blocking norepinephrine effects of the sympathetic nervous system.
   a. Metoprolol or metoprolol sustained-release are commonly used.
   b. Carvedilol is a nonselective beta- and alpha-adrenergic blocker. Patients may actually experience increase in general malaise for a 2- to 3-week period while they adjust to the medication.
6. Angiotensin II-receptor blockers—similar effects as ACE inhibitors, although mechanism of action is different. Used in patients who cannot tolerate ACE inhibitors due to cough or angioedema.
7. Aldosterone antagonists—decrease sodium retention, sympathetic nervous system activation, and cardiac remodeling.
   a. Spironolactone is most commonly used.
   b. May cause hyperkalemia, especially in those with impaired renal function, in those taking high doses of ACE inhibitors, or in those who use potassium supplements.

 DRUG ALERT Assess patient's risk for hyperkalemia when administering aldosterone antagonists, such as their use of ACE inhibitors, prescription or OTC potassium supplements, and NSAIDs; monitor serum creatinine and potassium levels closely.

8. Nesiritide (decreases pulmonary artery pressure)—used in patients with decompensated heart failure. It produces smooth muscle cell relaxation and diuresis and a reduction in afterload and dyspnea.
9. Amiodarone—to treat arrhythmias.

Diet Therapy

1. Restricted sodium.
2. Restricted fluids.

Mechanical Circulatory Support

May be used in Stage D heart failure and acute exacerbation of heart failure.

1. IABP; see page 369, helps decrease afterload.
2. Cardiac resynchronization therapy or biventricular pacing—helps to restore synchronous ventricular contractions, improves ventricular left ventricle filling, and improves CO.
3. Total artificial heart or left, right, or biventricular assist device.
4. Partial left ventriculectomy (reduction ventriculoplasty or Batista procedure)—a triangular section of the weakened heart muscle is removed to reduce ventricular wall tension. This procedure is not commonly used.
5. Endoventricular circular patch plasty or the Dor procedure—removal of diseased portion of septum or left ventricle with a synthetic or autologous tissue patch, thus providing a more normal shape and size of the heart, which improves hemodynamics.
6. Acorn cardiac support device—a polyester mesh, custom-fitted jacket is surgically placed on the epicardial surface, providing diastolic support. Over time, it decreases or halts remodeling.
7. Intubation—for pulmonary edema or respiratory distress.
8. ICD—for patients with previous cardiac arrest, sustained ventricular arrhythmias, and in those post-MI with ejection fraction less than 30%.
9. Heart transplant.

Complications

1. Intractable or refractory heart failure—becomes progressively refractory to therapy (does not yield to treatment).
2. Cardiac arrhythmias.
3. Myocardial failure and cardiac arrest.

4. Digoxin toxicity—from decreased renal function and potassium depletion.
5. Pulmonary infarction, pneumonia, and emboli.

Nursing Assessment

1. Obtain history of symptoms, onset and duration of the symptoms, limits of activity, response to rest, and history of response to drug therapy. Determine neurologic status during the history.
2. Assess heart sounds, rhythm, PMI, and blood pressure. Assess peripheral vascular system, particularly for edema (see Figure 13-7). Assess respiratory effort, auscultate chest for breath sounds and presence of wheezes and crackles, and percuss for possible pleural effusion.
3. Inspect for jugular vein distention and obtain hemodynamic measurements, as indicated, and note change from baseline.
4. Assess abdomen for ascites and determine weight and change from baseline weight.
5. Note results of serum electrolyte levels and other laboratory tests.
6. Identify sleep problems and signs of depression that is often present in patients with heart failure.

Nursing Diagnoses

- Decreased Cardiac Output related to impaired contractility and increased preload and afterload.
- Impaired Gas Exchange related to alveolar edema due to elevated ventricular pressures.

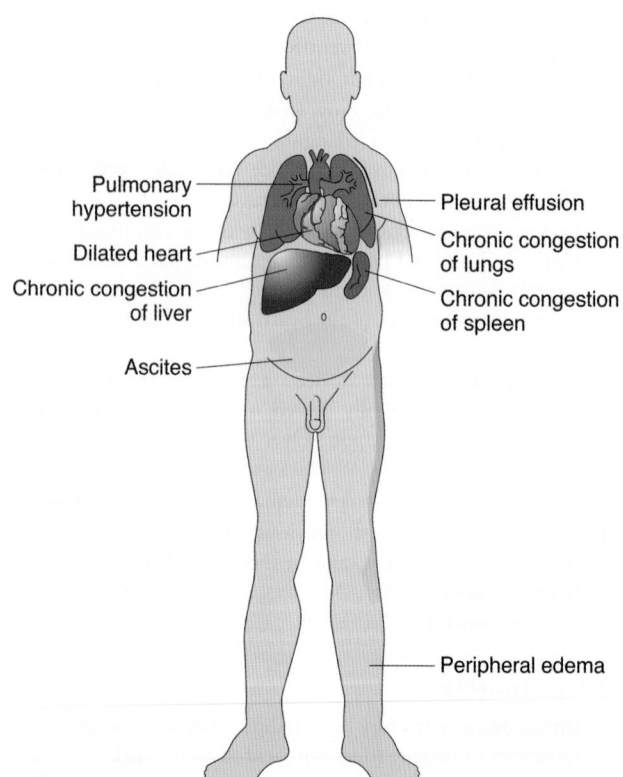

Figure 13-7. Consequences of heart failure.

- Excess Fluid Volume related to sodium and water retention.
- Activity Intolerance related to oxygen supply and demand imbalance.
- Deficient Knowledge related to lack of previous exposure to information.

Nursing Interventions

Maintaining Adequate Cardiac Output

1. Place patient at physical and emotional rest to reduce work of heart.
   a. Provide rest in semi-recumbent position or in armchair in air-conditioned environment—reduces work of heart, increases heart reserve, reduces BP, decreases work of respiratory muscles and oxygen utilization, improves efficiency of heart contraction; recumbency promotes diuresis by improving renal perfusion.
   b. Provide bedside commode—to reduce work of getting to bathroom and for defecation.
   c. Provide for psychological rest—emotional stress produces vasoconstriction, elevates arterial pressure, and speeds the heart.
      i. Promote physical comfort.
      ii. Avoid situations that tend to promote anxiety and agitation.
      iii. Offer careful explanations and answers to the patient's questions.
2. Evaluate frequently for progression of left-sided heart failure. Take frequent blood pressure readings.
   a. Watch for decreasing mean arterial pressure.
   b. Note narrowing of pulse pressure.
   c. Note alternating strong and weak pulsations (pulsus alternans).
3. Auscultate heart sounds frequently and monitor cardiac rhythm.
   a. Note presence of S_3 or S_4 gallop (S_3 gallop is a significant indicator of heart failure).
   b. Monitor for premature ventricular beats.
   c. Assess chest pain.
   d. Measure CVP.
4. Observe for signs and symptoms of reduced peripheral tissue perfusion: cool temperature of skin, facial pallor, poor capillary refill of nailbeds.
5. Administer pharmacotherapy as directed.
   a. Monitor for adverse effects and effect of drug therapy.
6. Monitor clinical response of patient with respect to relief of symptoms (lessening dyspnea and orthopnea, decrease in crackles, relief of peripheral edema).

 NURSING ALERT Watch for sudden unexpected hypotension, which can cause myocardial ischemia and decrease perfusion to vital organs.

Improving Oxygenation

1. Raise head of bed 8 to 10 inches (20 to 25 cm)—reduces venous return to heart and lungs; alleviates pulmonary congestion.

a. Support lower arms with pillows—eliminates pull of patient's weight on shoulder muscles.

b. Sit orthopneic patient on side of bed with feet supported by a chair, head and arms resting on an over-the-bed table, and lumbosacral area supported with pillows.

2. Auscultate lung fields at least every 4 hours for crackles and wheezes in dependent lung fields (fluid accumulates in areas affected by gravity).

a. Mark with indelible ink the level on the patient's back where adventitious breath sounds are heard.

b. Use markings for comparative assessment over time and among different care providers.

3. Observe for increased rate of respirations (could be indicative of falling arterial pH).

4. Observe for Cheyne-Stokes respirations (may occur in older patients because of a decrease in cerebral perfusion stimulating a neurogenic response).

5. Reposition the patient every 2 hours (or encourage the patient to change position frequently)—to help prevent atelectasis and pneumonia.

6. Encourage deep-breathing exercises every 1 to 2 hours—to avoid atelectasis.

7. Offer small, frequent feedings—to avoid excessive gastric filling and abdominal distention with subsequent elevation of diaphragm that causes decrease in lung capacity.

8. Administer oxygen, as directed.

Restoring Fluid Balance

1. Administer prescribed diuretic, as ordered.

2. Give diuretic early in the morning—nighttime diuresis disturbs sleep.

3. Keep input and output record—patient may lose large volume of fluid after a single dose of diuretic. Watch fluid intake.

4. Weigh patient daily—to determine if edema is being controlled; weight loss should not exceed 1 to 2 lb (0.5 to 1 kg)/ day.

5. Assess for signs of hypovolemia caused by diuretic therapy— thirst; decreased urine output; orthostatic hypotension; weak, thready pulse; increased serum osmolality; and increased urine specific gravity.

6. Be alert for signs of hypokalemia, which may cause weakening of cardiac contractions and may precipitate digoxin toxicity in the form of dysrhythmias, anorexia, nausea, vomiting, abdominal distention, paralytic ileus, paresthesias, muscle weakness and cramps, confusion. Check electrolytes frequently.

7. Give potassium supplements, as prescribed.

8. Be aware of disorders that may be worsened by diuretic therapy, including hyperuricemia, gout, volume depletion, hyponatremia, magnesium depletion, hyperglycemia, and diabetes mellitus. There is no evidence to support that patients who are allergic to sulfa drugs are also allergic to thiazide diuretics.

9. Watch for signs of bladder distention in older male patients with prostatic hyperplasia.

10. Administer IV fluids carefully through an intermittent access device to prevent fluid overload.

11. Monitor for pitting edema of lower extremities and sacral area. Use convoluted foam mattress and sheepskin to prevent pressure ulcers (poor blood flow and edema increase susceptibility).

12. Observe for the complications of bed rest—pressure ulcers (especially in edematous patients), phlebothrombosis, pulmonary embolism.

13. Be alert to complaints of right upper quadrant abdominal pain, poor appetite, nausea, and abdominal distention (may indicate hepatic and visceral engorgement).

14. Monitor patient's diet. Diet may be limited in sodium—to prevent, control, or eliminate edema; may also be limited in calories.

15. Caution patients to avoid adding salt to food and foods with high sodium content.

Improving Activity Tolerance

1. Increase patient's activities gradually. Alter or modify patient's activities to keep within the limits of his or her cardiac reserve.

a. Assist patient with self-care activities early in the day (fatigue sets in as day progresses).

b. Be alert to complaints of chest pain or skeletal pain during or after activities.

2. Observe the pulse, symptoms, and behavioral response to increased activity.

a. Monitor patient's heart rate during self-care activities.

b. Allow heart rate to decrease to preactivity level before initiating a new activity.

i. Note time lapse between cessation of activity and decrease in heart rate (decreased stroke volume causes immediate rise in heart rate).

ii. Document time lapse and revise patient care plan as appropriate (progressive increase in time lapse may be indicative of increased left-sided heart failure).

3. Relieve nighttime anxiety and provide for rest and sleep— patients with heart failure have a tendency to be restless at night because of cerebral hypoxia with superimposed nitrogen retention. Give appropriate sedation to relieve insomnia and restlessness.

Improving Knowledge

1. Explain the disease process, note that the term "failure" may be terrifying.

a. Explain the pumping action of the heart: to move blood through the body to provide nutrients and aid in the removal of waste.

b. Explain the difference between heart failure and heart attack.

2. Teach about the signs and symptoms of recurrence.

a. Watch for weight gain and report a gain or loss of more than 2 to 3 lb (1 to 1.4 kg) in a few days.

b. Weigh patient at same time daily to detect any tendency toward fluid retention: swelling of ankles, feet, abdomen; persistent cough; tiredness; loss of appetite; frequent urination at night.

3. Review medication regimen.

a. Medications recommended for patients with ejection fraction less than 40% include preload reductors, such as diuretics, and afterload reductors, such as ACE inhibitors.

b. Medications to control heart rate include digoxin or beta-adrenergic blockers.

c. Anticoagulation, if indicated.

Patient Education and Health Maintenance

1. Advise patient of symptoms that need to be reported to health care provider.
   a. Sudden weight gain.
   b. Increased shortness of breath, inability to lie down, wheezing, increased cough.
   c. Increased swelling of feet, legs, abdomen.
2. Help patient label all medications.
   a. Give written instructions.
   b. Make sure the patient has a pill organizer or check-off system to show that medications have been taken.
   c. Inform the patient of adverse drug effects.
   d. If the patient is taking oral potassium solution, it may be diluted with juice and taken after a meal.
   e. Tell the patient to weigh self daily at same time and log weight if on diuretic therapy.
   f. Ask whether patient is taking Coenzyme Q10 or other supplements; should discuss with health care provider.
3. Review activity program. Instruct the patient as follows:
   a. Increase walking and other activities gradually, provided they do not cause fatigue and dyspnea.
   b. In general, continue at whatever activity level can be maintained without the appearance of symptoms.
   c. Avoid excesses in eating and drinking.
   d. Undertake a weight reduction program until optimal weight is reached.
   e. Avoid extremes in heat and cold, which increase the work of the heart; air conditioning may be essential in a hot, humid environment.
   f. Keep *regular* appointment with health care provider or clinic.
4. Restrict sodium as directed.
   a. Teach restricted sodium diet (<1500 mg per day) and the DASH diet; see page 468.
   b. Give patient a written diet plan with lists of permitted and restricted foods.
   c. Advise patient to look at all labels to ascertain sodium content. Take into account serving size.
   d. Teach the patient to rinse the mouth well after using tooth cleansers and mouthwashes—some of these contain large amounts of sodium. Water softeners should be checked for salt content.
   e. Teach the patient that sodium is often hidden in foods such as bread, and in medications such as antacids, cough remedies, pain relievers, estrogens, and other drugs.
   f. Encourage use of flavorings, spices, herbs, and lemon juice.
   g. Avoid salt substitutes with renal disease.
5. Make sure patient sets up follow-up appointments.
6. Advise patient on smoking cessation, provide information, if indicated.

Evaluation: Expected Outcomes

- Normal BP and heart rate.
- Respiratory rate, 16 to 20 breaths/minute; ABG levels within normal limits; no signs of crackles or wheezes in lung fields.
- Weight decrease of 2.2 lb (1 kg) every 2 days, no pitting edema of lower extremities and sacral area.
- Heart rate within normal limits, rests between activities.
- States recurrent symptoms to watch for and knows medications and doses.

Acute Pulmonary Edema

Acute pulmonary edema refers to excess fluid in the lung, either in the interstitial spaces or in the alveoli.

Pathophysiology and Etiology

1. The presence of fluid in the alveoli impedes gas exchange, especially oxygen movement into pulmonary capillaries (see Figure 13-8).
2. May be caused by:
   a. Heart disease—acute left-sided heart failure, MI, aortic stenosis, severe mitral valve disease, hypertension, heart failure.
   b. Circulatory overload—transfusions and infusions.
   c. Drug hypersensitivity, allergy, poisoning.
   d. Lung injuries—smoke inhalation, shock lung, pulmonary embolism, or infarct.
   e. Central nervous system injuries—stroke, head trauma.
   f. Infection and fever—infectious pneumonia (viral, bacterial, parasitic).
   g. Postcardioversion, postanesthesia, postcardiopulmonary bypass.
   h. Adverse drug reaction—many drugs including heroin, cocaine, aspirin, and chemotherapy agents.
   i. Renal disease.
   j. High altitude.
   k. Near drowning.

Clinical Manifestations

1. Coughing and restlessness during sleep (premonitory symptoms).
2. Extreme dyspnea and orthopnea—patient usually uses accessory muscles of respiration with retraction of intercostal spaces and supraclavicular areas.
3. Cough with varying amounts of white- or pink-tinged frothy sputum.
4. Extreme anxiety and panic.
5. Noisy breathing—inspiratory and expiratory wheezing and bubbling sounds.
6. Cyanosis with profuse cold, clammy perspiration.
7. Distended jugular veins.
8. Tachycardia.
9. Precordial pain (if pulmonary edema secondary to MI).
10. Decreased urine output.

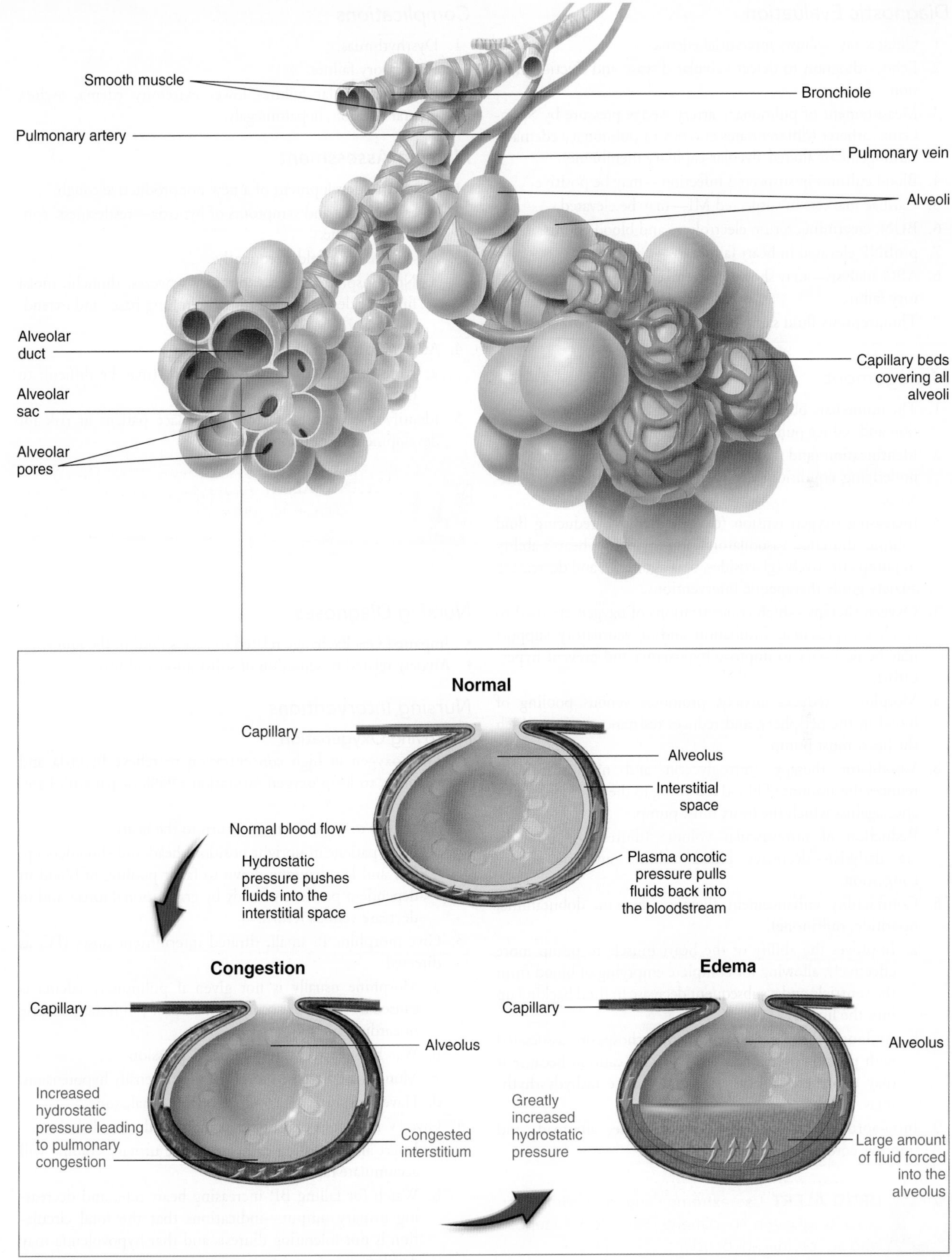

Figure 13-8. Normal alveoli and how pulmonary edema develops.

Diagnostic Evaluation

1. Chest x-ray—shows interstitial edema.
2. Echocardiogram to detect valvular disease and ejection fraction.
3. Measurement of pulmonary artery wedge pressure by Swan-Ganz catheter (differentiates etiology of pulmonary edema—cardiogenic or altered alveolar-capillary membrane).
4. Blood cultures in suspected infection—may be positive.
5. Cardiac markers in suspected MI—may be elevated.
6. BUN, creatinine, serum electrolytes and blood counts.
7. proBNP elevated in heart failure.
6. ABG analysis—may show hypoxemia and impending respiratory failure.
7. Thoracentesis-fluid sample for diagnosis and treatment.

Management

1. The immediate objective of treatment is to improve oxygenation and reduce pulmonary congestion.
2. Identification and correction of precipitating factors and underlying conditions are then necessary to prevent recurrence.
3. Increasing oxygen tension (oxygen therapy), reducing fluid volume (diuretics, vasodilators), improving the heart's ability to pump effectively (glycosides, beta agonists), and decreasing anxiety guide therapeutic interventions.
4. Oxygen therapy—high concentrations of oxygen are used to combat hypoxemia. Intubation and/or ventilatory support may be necessary to improve hypoxemia and prevent hypercarbia.
5. Morphine—reduces anxiety, promotes venous pooling of blood in the periphery, and reduces resistance against which the heart must pump.
6. Vasodilator therapy (nitroglycerin and nitroprusside)—reduces the amount of blood returning to the heart and resistance against which the heart must pump.
7. Reduction of intravascular volume (diuresis or immediate dialysis)—decreases blood volume and pulmonary congestion.
8. Contractility enhancement therapy (digoxin, dobutamine, nesiritide, milrinone).
   a. Improves the ability of the heart muscle to pump more effectively, allowing for complete emptying of blood from the ventricle and a subsequent decrease in fluid backing up into the lungs.
   b. Aminophylline may prevent bronchospasm associated with pulmonary congestion. Use with caution because it may also increase heart rate and induce tachydysrhythmias.
9. Intra-aortic balloon pump—to decrease afterload and improve coronary blood flow.

 DRUG ALERT Use extreme caution in administering nitroglycerin to patients with aortic stenosis who are preload-dependent.

Complications

1. Dysrhythmias.
2. Respiratory failure.
3. Right ventricular failure- lower extremity edema, ascites, pleural effusion, hepatomegaly.

Nursing Assessment

1. Be alert to development of a new nonproductive cough.
2. Assess for signs and symptoms of hypoxia—restlessness, confusion, headache.
3. Auscultate lung fields frequently.
   a. Note inspiratory and expiratory wheezes, rhonchi, moist fine crackles appearing initially in lung bases and extending upward.
4. Auscultate for extra heart sounds.
   a. Note presence of third heart sound (may be difficult to hear because of respiratory sounds).
5. Identify precipitating factors that place patient at risk for development of pulmonary edema.

 NURSING ALERT Acute pulmonary edema is a true medical emergency; it is a life-threatening condition. Act promptly to assess patient and notify health care provider of findings.

Nursing Diagnoses

- Impaired Gas Exchange related to excess fluid in the lungs.
- Anxiety related to sensation of suffocation and fear.

Nursing Interventions

Improving Oxygenation

1. Give oxygen in high concentration to relieve hypoxia and dyspnea, to keep oxygen saturation >94% or patient's baseline.
2. Take steps to reduce venous return to the heart.
   a. Place patient in upright position; head and shoulders up, feet and legs hanging down to favor pooling of blood in dependent portions of body by gravitational forces and to decrease venous return.
3. Give morphine in small, titrated intermittent doses (IV) as directed.
   a. Morphine usually is not given if pulmonary edema is caused by stroke or occurs with chronic pulmonary disease or cardiogenic shock.
   b. Watch for excessive respiratory depression.
   c. Monitor BP because morphine may intensify hypotension.
   d. Have morphine antagonist available—naloxone.
4. Give IV injections of diuretic or monitor during dialysis.
   a. Insert an indwelling catheter—large urinary volume will accumulate rapidly.
   b. Watch for falling BP, increasing heart rate, and decreasing urinary output—indications that the total circulation is not tolerating diuresis and that hypovolemia may develop.

c. Check electrolyte levels because potassium loss may be significant.

d. Watch for signs of urinary obstruction in men with prostatic hyperplasia.

5. Administer vasodilator if patient fails to respond to therapy.

a. Monitor by measuring BP, PAP, and CO.

6. Assist with insertion of IABP, if needed, and monitor patient according to facility's protocol.

7. Administer aminophylline, if ordered.

a. Monitor blood levels of drug.

b. Evaluate for adverse effects of drug—ventricular dysrhythmias, hypotension, headache.

8. Administer cardiac glycosides as ordered.

9. Assist with cardioversion, if indicated (pulmonary edema may precipitate tachycardias).

10. Give appropriate drugs for severe, sustained hypertension.

11. Continually evaluate the patient's response to therapy. Reevaluate lung fields and cardiac assessment and monitor urine output and laboratory values.

Decreasing Anxiety

1. Stay with patient and display a confident attitude—the presence of another person is therapeutic because the acute anxiety of the patient may tend to intensify the severity of patient's condition. (Arterial vasoconstriction diminishes as anxiety is relieved.)

2. Explain to patient in a calm manner all therapies administered and the reason for their use. Explain to patient the importance of wearing oxygen mask. Assure patient that mask will not increase sensation of suffocation.

3. Inform patient and family of progress toward resolution of pulmonary edema.

4. Allow time for patient and family to voice concerns and fears.

Patient Education and Health Maintenance

During convalescence, instruct patient as follows to prevent recurrence of pulmonary edema:

1. Remind patient of early symptoms before onset of acute pulmonary edema; these should be reported promptly.

2. If coughing develops (a wet cough), sit with legs dangling over side of bed.

3. See "Patient Education, Heart Failure," page 418.

Evaluation: Expected Outcomes

- Unlabored respirations at 12 to 20 breaths/minute, lungs clear on auscultation, pulse oximetry >94%.
- Appears calm, rests comfortably.

Acquired Valvular Disease of the Heart

 Evidence Base Nishimura, R. A., Carabello, B. A., Faxon, D. P., et al. (2008). 2008 focused update incorporated into the ACC/AHA 2006 guidelines for the management of patients with valvular heart disease. *Circulation, 118*, e523–e661.

The function of normal heart valves is to maintain the forward flow of blood from the atria to the ventricles and from the ventricles to the great vessels.

Valvular damage may interfere with valvular function by stenosis (obstruction) or by impaired closure that allows backward leakage of blood (valvular insufficiency, regurgitation, or incompetence).

Pathophysiology and Etiology

Mitral Stenosis

1. Mitral stenosis is the progressive thickening and contracture of valve cusps with narrowing of the orifice and progressive obstruction to blood flow. Rheumatic fever is the most common cause of mitral stenosis in adults. Calcium deposit around the valves is rare with mitral stenosis. In children, cause may be congenital.

2. Acute rheumatic valvulitis has "glued" the mitral valve flaps (commissures) together, thus shortening the chordae tendineae, so that the flap edges are pulled down, greatly narrowing the mitral orifice.

3. The left atrium has difficulty emptying itself through the narrow orifice into the left ventricle; therefore, it dilates and hypertrophies. Pulmonary circulation becomes congested.

4. As a result of the abnormally high PAP that must be maintained, the right ventricle is subjected to a pressure overload and may eventually fail.

Mitral Insufficiency

1. Mitral insufficiency (regurgitation or incompetence) is incomplete closure of the mitral valve during systole, allowing blood to flow back into the left atrium.

2. Left atrial pressures increase, reflected by increases in PAP and PCWP.

3. LVH may develop due to inefficient emptying.

4. May be due to myxomatous (connective tissue) degeneration, which causes stretching of leaflets and chordae tendineae, chronic rheumatic heart disease, ischemic heart disease, CAD, and infective endocarditis may also result due to medications and penetrating and nonpenetrating trauma.

Aortic Stenosis

1. Aortic stenosis is a narrowing of the orifice between the left ventricle and the aorta.

2. The obstruction to the aortic outflow places a pressure load on the left ventricle that results in hypertrophy and failure.

3. Left atrial pressure increases.

4. Pulmonary vascular pressure increases, which may eventually lead to right-sided heart failure.

5. May be caused by congenital anomalies (bicuspid aortic valve), calcification, or acute rheumatic fever.

Aortic Insufficiency

1. Due to abnormalities of aortic valve or aortic root.

2. Valve flaps fail to completely seal the aortic orifice during diastole and thus permit backflow of blood from the aorta into the left ventricle.

3. The left ventricle increases the force of contraction to maintain an adequate CO, usually resulting in hypertrophy.

4. The low aortic diastolic pressures result in decreased coronary artery perfusion.
5. May be caused by rheumatic or infective endocarditis, congenital malformation, aortic root dilation, Marfan's syndrome, Ehlers-Danlos syndrome, Reiter syndrome, hypertension, systemic lupus erythematosus, or by diseases that cause dilation or tearing of the ascending aorta (syphilitic disease, rheumatoid spondylitis, dissecting aneurysm).

Tricuspid Stenosis

1. Tricuspid stenosis is restriction or narrowing of the tricuspid valve orifice due to commissural fusion and fibrosis.
2. Usually follows rheumatic fever and is commonly associated with diseases of the mitral valve. Could be congenital in origin.

Tricuspid Insufficiency

1. Tricuspid insufficiency (regurgitation) allows the regurgitation of blood from the right ventricle into the right atrium during ventricular systole.
2. Common causes include dilation of right ventricle, rheumatic fever, and congenital anomalies.

Clinical Manifestations

1. Fatigue, weakness.
2. Dyspnea, cough, orthopnea, nocturnal dyspnea.
3. Characteristic murmur (see "Nursing Assessment").
4. Dysrhythmias, palpitations.
5. Hemoptysis (from pulmonary hypertension) and hoarseness (from compression of left recurrent laryngeal nerve by dilated left atrium) in mitral stenosis.
6. Low BP, dizziness, syncope, angina, and symptoms of heart failure in aortic stenosis.
7. Arterial pulsations visible and palpable over precordium and visible in neck; widened pulse pressure; and water-hammer (Corrigan's) pulse (pulse strikes palpating finger with a quick, sharp stroke and then suddenly collapses) in aortic insufficiency.
8. Symptoms of right-sided heart failure—edema, ascites, hepatomegaly—in tricuspid stenosis and insufficiency.

Diagnostic Evaluation

1. ECG may show dysrhythmias.
2. Echocardiography may show abnormalities of valve structure and function and chamber size and thickness.
3. Chest x-ray may show cardiomegaly and pulmonary vascular congestion.
4. Cardiac catheterization and angiocardiography confirm diagnosis and determine severity.
5. Cardiac MRI provides more information and confirms diagnosis.

Management

Medical Therapy

1. Antibiotic prophylaxis for endocarditis before invasive procedures—indicated in most cases; see page 404.
2. Treatment of heart failure—diuretics, sodium restriction, vasodilators, cardiac glycosides, as indicated.

Surgical Intervention

See page 371 for care of the patient undergoing heart surgery.

1. For mitral stenosis:
   a. Closed mitral valvotomy—introduction of a dilator through the mitral valve to split its commissures.
   b. Open mitral valvotomy—direct incision of the commissures.
   c. Mitral valve replacement.
   d. Balloon valvuloplasty—a balloon-tipped catheter is percutaneously inserted, threaded to the affected valve, and positioned across the narrowed orifice. The balloon is inflated and deflated, causing a "cracking" of the calcified commissures and enlargement of the valve orifice.
2. For mitral insufficiency—mitral valve replacement or annuloplasty (retailoring of the valve ring).
3. For aortic stenosis or insufficiency:
   a. Replacement of aortic valve with prosthetic or tissue valves.
   b. Balloon valvuloplasty (aortic stenosis).
4. For tricuspid stenosis or insufficiency—valvuloplasty or replacement may be done at time of surgical intervention for associated rheumatic mitral or aortic disease.
5. Transcatheter aortic valve implantation (TAVI)—a less invasive procedure where a bioprosthetic valve is used.

Complications

1. Left-sided heart failure.
2. Possible, right-sided heart failure.
3. Dysrhythmias.
4. Pulmonary edema.

Nursing Assessment

Mitral Stenosis

1. Auscultate for accentuated first heart sound, usually accompanied by an "opening snap" (due to sudden tensing of valve leaflets) at apex with diaphragm of stethoscope.
2. Place the patient in left lateral recumbent position. With bell of stethoscope at apex, auscultate for a low-pitched diastolic murmur (rumbling murmur). Note duration of murmur (long duration is indicative of significant stenosis).

Mitral Insufficiency

1. Auscultate for diminished first heart sound.
2. Auscultate for systolic murmur (prominent finding), commencing immediately after first heart sound at apex, and note radiation of sound to axilla and left intrascapular area.
3. Mild insufficiency may produce a pansystolic murmur (little connection between severity of mitral insufficiency and intensity of murmur auscultated).

Aortic Stenosis

1. Auscultate for prominent fourth heart sound and possible paradoxical splitting of second heart sound (suggestive of associated left ventricular dysfunction). First heart sound is normal.
2. Auscultate for a midsystolic murmur at the base of the heart (right upper sterna border) and at the apex of heart. Note

harsh and rasping quality at base of heart and a higher pitch at apex of heart.

3. There may be a palpable thrill.

Aortic Insufficiency
1. Auscultate for soft first heart sound.
2. Place the patient in sitting position, leaning forward.
3. Place diaphragm of stethoscope along left sternal border at the third and fourth intercostal space and then along the right sternal border. Auscultate for a high-pitched decrescendo diastolic murmur. To increase audibility of murmur, ask the patient to hold breath at end of deep expiration. Reauscultate for murmur.

Tricuspid Stenosis
1. Auscultate for a rumbling or blowing mid-diastolic murmur at the left sternal border (increases with inspiration).

Tricuspid Insufficiency
1. Auscultate for a third heart sound (may be accentuated by inspiration).
2. Auscultate for a pansystolic murmur in the parasternal region at the fourth intercostal space. Murmur is usually high-pitched.

Nursing Diagnoses
- Decreased Cardiac Output related to altered preload, afterload, or contractility.
- Activity Intolerance related to reduced oxygen supply.
- Ineffective Coping related to acute or chronic illness.

Nursing Interventions

Maintaining Adequate Cardiac Output
1. Assess frequently for change in existing murmur or new murmur.
2. Assess for signs of left- or right-sided heart failure; see page 413.
3. Assess for pulmonary edema.
4. Monitor and treat dysrhythmias, as ordered.
5. Prepare the patient for surgical intervention (see page 371).

Improving Tolerance
1. Maintain bed rest while symptoms of heart failure are present.
2. Allow patient to rest between interventions.
3. Begin activities gradually (eg, chair sitting for brief periods).
4. Assist with or perform hygiene needs for patient to reserve strength for ambulation.

Strengthening Coping Abilities
1. Instruct the patient about specific valvular dysfunction, possible etiology, and therapies implemented to relieve symptoms.
   a. Include family members in discussions with the patient.
   b. Stress the importance of adapting lifestyle to cope with illness.
2. Discuss with patient surgical intervention as the treatment modality, if applicable.
3. Assess the patient's use of appropriate coping mechanisms.

4. Refer the patient to appropriate counseling services, if indicated (vocational, social work, cardiac rehabilitation, substance abuse).

Patient Education and Health Maintenance
1. Review activity restriction and schedule with patient and family.
2. Instruct patient to report signs of impending or worsening heart failure—dyspnea, cough, increased fatigue, ankle swelling.
3. Review sodium and fluid restrictions.
4. Review medications—purpose, action, schedule, and adverse effects.
5. See "Patient Education, Heart Failure," page 418; "Infective Endocarditis," page 404; and "Rheumatic Endocarditis," page 406.

Evaluation: Expected Outcomes
- Blood pressure and heart rate within normal limits.
- Tolerates chair sitting for 15 minutes every 2 hours.
- Discusses ways to cope with lifestyle and activity changes.

Cardiac Dysrhythmias

Cardiac dysrhythmias are disturbances in regular heart rate and/or rhythm due to change in electrical conduction or automaticity. Dysrhythmias may arise from the sinoatrial (SA) node (sinus bradycardia or tachycardia) or anywhere within the atria or ventricles (known as ectopy or ectopic beats). Some may be benign and asymptomatic, whereas other dysrhythmias are life-threatening.

Dysrhythmias may be detected by change in pulse, abnormality on auscultation of heart rate, or ECG abnormality. Continuous cardiac monitoring is indicated for potentially life-threatening dysrhythmias.

Sinus Tachycardia

See Figure 13-9.

Etiology
1. Sympathetic nerve fibers, which act to speed up excitation of the SA node, are stimulated by underlying causes, such as anxiety, exercise, fever, shock, drugs, altered metabolic states (such as hyperthyroidism), or electrolyte disturbances.
2. The wave of impulse is transmitted through the normal conduction pathways; the rate of sinus stimulation is simply greater than normal (rate exceeds 100 beats/minute).

Analysis
Rate: 100 to 150 beats/minute.

Rhythm: R-R intervals are regular.

P wave: present for each QRS complex, normal configuration, and each P wave is identical or may be buried in previous T wave.

PR interval: falls between 0.12 and 0.20, or 0.16 second. P wave may be hidden in preceding T wave in rapid rates.

QRS complex: normal in appearance, one follows each P wave.

QRS interval: <0.11 seconds.

T wave: follows each QRS complex and is positively conducted.

QT interval: <0.48 seconds.

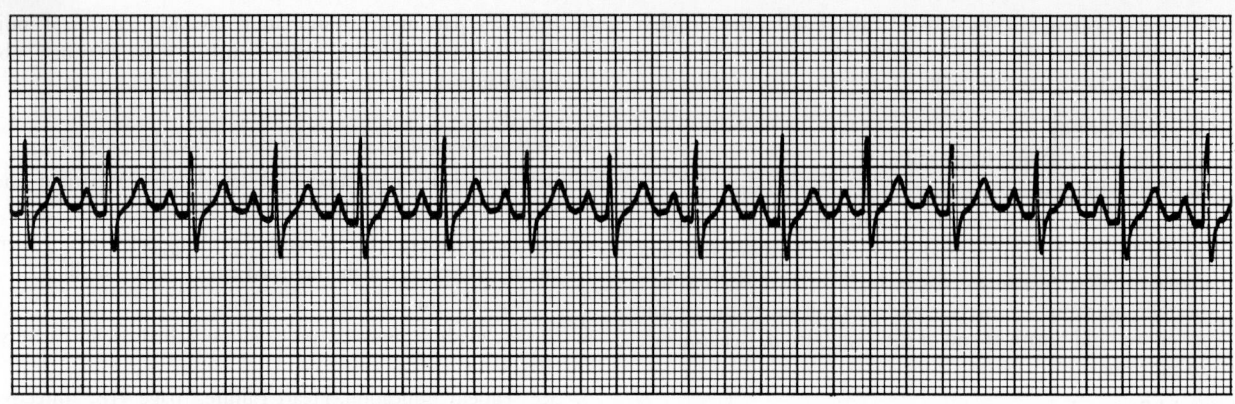

Figure 13-9. Sinus tachycardia.

Management

1. Treatment is directed toward elimination of the cause rather than the dysrhythmia.
2. Urgency is dependent on the effect of rapid heart rate on coronary artery filling time to prevent cardiac ischemia.
3. Administration of oxygen and normal saline solution should be considered as initial treatment.

Sinus Bradycardia

See Figure 13-10.

Etiology

1. The parasympathetic fibers (vagal tone) are stimulated and cause the sinus node to slow.
2. Underlying causes:
   a. Drugs.
   b. Altered metabolic states such as hypothyroidism.
   c. The process of aging, which causes increasing fibrotic tissue and scarring of the SA node.
   d. Certain cardiac diseases such as acute MI (especially inferior wall MI).

3. The wave of impulse is transmitted through the normal conduction pathways; the rate of sinus stimulation is simply less than normal (less than 60 beats/minute).

Analysis

Rate: <60 beats/minute.
Rhythm: R-R interval is regular.
P wave: present for each QRS complex, normal configuration, and each P wave is identical.
PR interval: falls between 0.12 and 0.18 second.
QRS complex: normal in appearance, one follows each P wave.
QRS interval: 0.04 to 0.11 second.
T wave: follows each QRS and is positively conducted.

Management

1. The urgency of treatment depends on the effect of the slow rate on maintenance of CO.
2. Atropine 0.5 mg IV push blocks vagal stimulation to the SA node and therefore accelerates heart rate. Dopamine or epinephrine are alternatives if atropine is ineffective.
3. If bradycardia persists, a pacemaker may be required.
4. Sinus bradycardia is common in athletic individuals and does not require treatment.

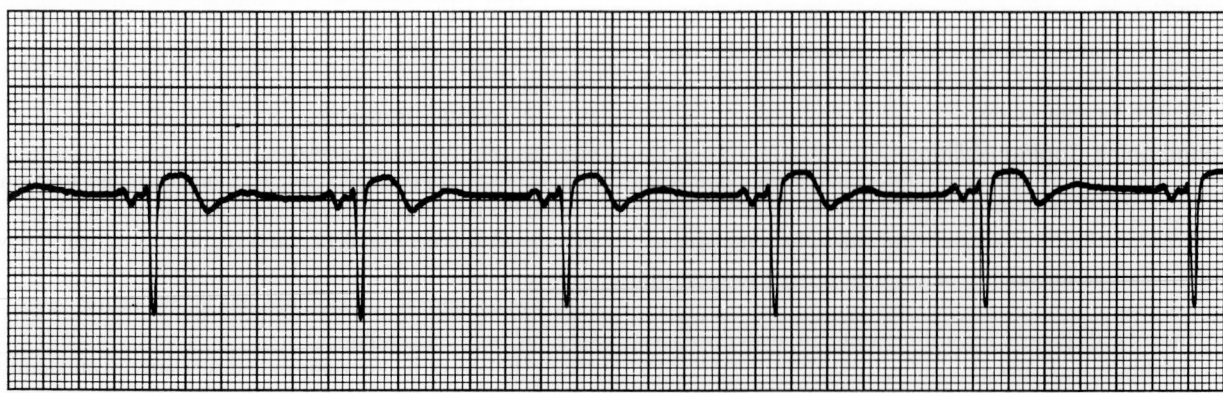

Figure 13-10. Sinus bradycardia.

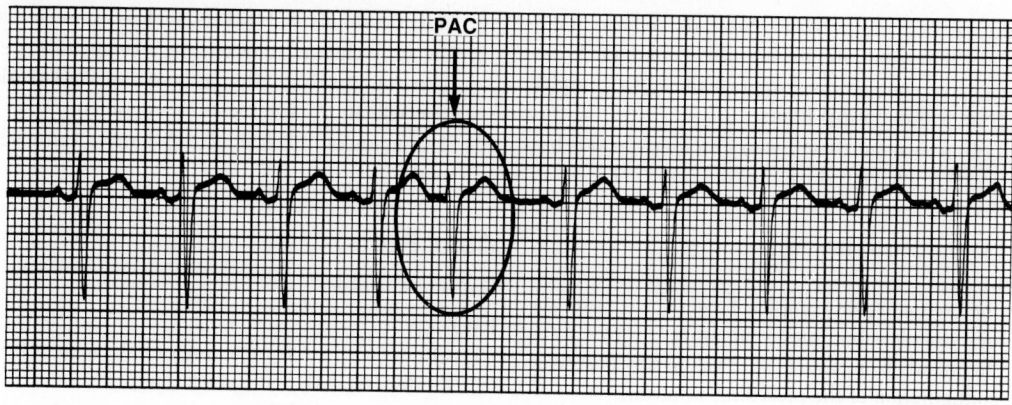

Figure 13-11. Normal sinus rhythm with premature atrial contraction.

Premature Atrial Contraction

See Figure 13-11.

Etiology

1. May occur in the healthy heart where they are idiopathic and benign.
2. In the diseased heart, premature atrial contractions (PACs) may represent ischemia and a resultant irritability in the atria. They may increase in frequency and be the precursor of more serious dysrhythmias.
3. May be caused by electrolyte abnormalities, hypoxia, MI, heart failure, and acid-base disturbances.
4. The wave of impulse of the PAC originates within the atria and outside the sinus node. Because the impulse originates within the atria, the P wave will be present, but it will be different in appearance as compared with those beats originating within the sinus node. The impulse traverses the remainder of the conduction system in a normal pattern; thus, the QRS complex is identical in configuration to the normal sinus beats.

Analysis

Rate: may be slow or fast.

Rhythm: will be irregular, caused by the early occurrence of the PAC.

P wave: will be present for each normal QRS complex; the P wave of the premature contraction will be distorted in shape.

PR interval: may be normal but can also be shortened, depending on where in the atria the impulse originated. (The closer the site of atrial impulse formation to the atrioventricular [AV] node, the shorter the PR interval will be.)

QRS complex: within normal limits because all conduction below the atria is normal.

T wave: normally conducted.

Management

1. Generally requires no treatment if laboratory values are normal.
2. PACs should be monitored for increasing frequency.

Paroxysmal Atrial Tachycardia

See Figure 13-12.

Etiology

1. Causes include:
   a. Syndromes of accelerated pathways (eg, Wolff-Parkinson-White syndrome).
   b. Syndrome of mitral valve prolapse.
   c. Ischemic CAD.
   d. Excessive use of alcohol, cigarettes, caffeine.
   e. Drugs—digoxin is a frequent cause.

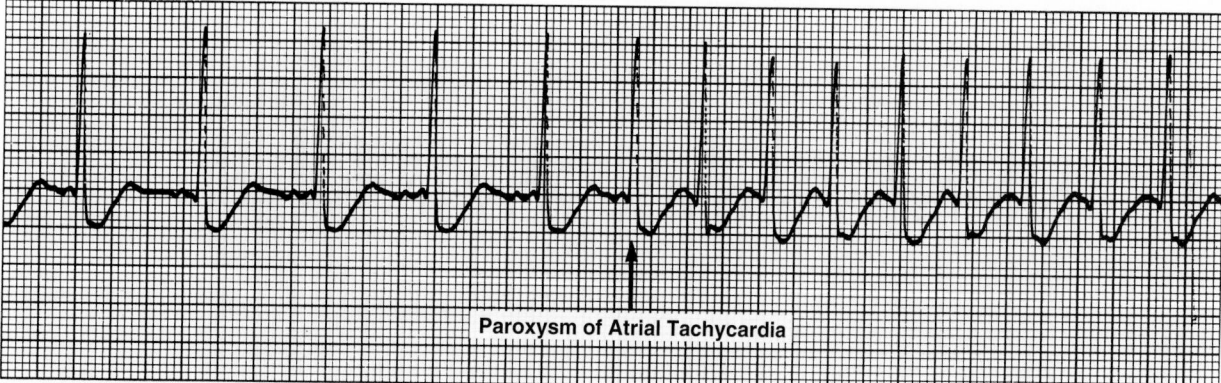

Figure 13-12. Paroxysmal atrial tachycardia.

2. An ectopic atrial focus captures the rhythm of the heart and is stimulated at a very rapid rate; the impulse is conducted normally through the conduction system so the QRS complex usually appears within normal limits.

3. The rate is often so rapid that P waves are not obvious but may be "buried" in the preceding T wave.

Analysis

Rate: between 150 and 250 beats/minute.

Rhythm: regular.

P wave: present before each QRS complex; however, the faster the rate, the more difficult it becomes to visualize P waves. (The P waves can frequently be measured with calipers by observing the varying configuration of the preceding T waves.)

PR interval: usually not measurable.

QRS complex: will appear normal in configuration and within 0.06 to 0.10 second.

T wave: will be distorted in appearance as a result of P waves being buried in them.

Management

1. Treatment is directed first to slowing the rate and, second, to reverting the dysrhythmia to a normal sinus rhythm.

2. Reducing the rate may be accomplished by having the patient perform a Valsalva maneuver. This stimulates the vagus nerve to slow the heart.

    a. A Valsalva maneuver may be done by having the patient gag or "bear down" as though attempting to have a bowel movement.

    b. The health care provider may choose to perform carotid massage.

3. Adenosine is the drug of choice for paroxysmal atrial tachycardia associated with hypotension, chest pain, or shortness of breath.

    a. The initial dose is 6 mg rapid IV push followed by a fast normal saline flush. If there is no response in 1 to 2 minutes, a second and third bolus of 12 mg may be given, each followed by fast normal saline flushes.

    b. Has a very short half-life and is therefore eliminated quickly.

4. IV beta-adrenergic blockers, such as esmolol, may be used.

5. Calcium channel blockers (eg, verapamil) are effective in reverting this dysrhythmia. Beware of hypotension, however, especially in the volume-depleted patient.

6. If drug therapy is ineffective, elective cardioversion can be used.

Atrial Flutter

See Figure 13-13.

Etiology

1. Occurs with atrial stretching or enlargement (as in AV valvular disease), MI, and heart failure.

2. An ectopic atrial focus captures the rhythm in atrial flutter and fires at an extremely rapid rate (200 to 400 beats/minute) with regularity.

3. Conduction of the impulse through the conduction system is normal; thus, the QRS complex is unaffected.

4. An important feature of this dysrhythmia is that the AV node sets up a therapeutic block, which disallows some impulse transmission.

    a. This can produce a varying block or a fixed block (ie, sometimes the AV node will transmit every second flutter wave, producing a 2:1 block, or the rhythm can be 3:1 or 4:1).

    b. If the AV node conducted 1:1, then the outcome would be a ventricular rate of about 300 beats/minute. The patient would rapidly deteriorate.

Analysis

Rate: atrial rate between 250 and 400 beats/minute; ventricular rate will depend on degree of block.

Rhythm: regular or irregular, depending on kind of block (eg, 2:1, 3:1, or a combination).

P wave: not present; instead, it is replaced by a saw-toothed pattern that is produced by the rapid. firing of the atrial focus. These waves are also referred to as "F" waves.

PR interval: not measurable.

QRS complex: normal configuration and normal conduction time.

T wave: present but may be obscured by flutter waves.

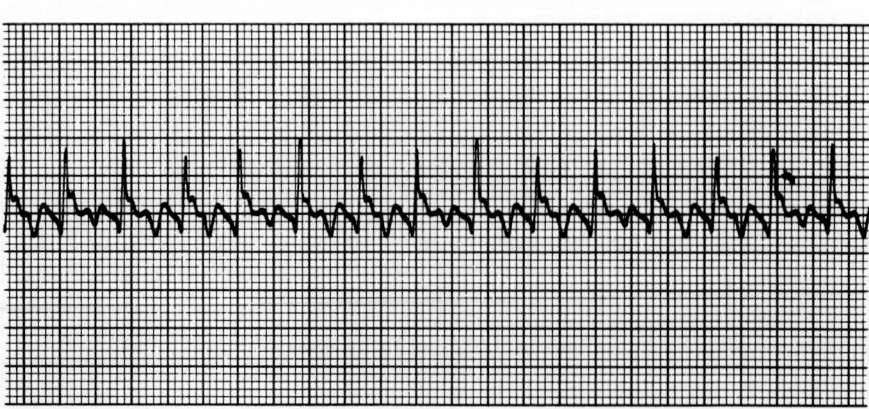

Figure 13-13. Atrial flutter.

Management

1. The urgency of treatment depends on the ventricular response rate and resultant symptoms. Too rapid or slow a rate will decrease CO.
2. A calcium channel blocker, such as diltiazem, may be used to slow AV nodal conduction. Use with caution in the patient with heart failure, hypotension, or concomitant beta-adrenergic blocker therapy.
3. Digoxin may be used.
4. An IV beta-adrenergic blocker, such as esmolol, may also be used.
5. If drug therapy is unsuccessful, atrial flutter will typically respond to cardioversion. Small doses of biphasic electrical current (50 to 100 joules) are usually successful.
6. Electrophysiologic studies and subsequent ablation therapy are highly effective because the ectopic focus is usually readily identified.

Atrial Fibrillation

See Figure 13-14.

 Evidence Base Fuster, V., Ryden, L. E., Cannom, D. S., et al. (2011). 2011 ACCF/AHA/HRS focused updates incorporated into the ACC/AHA/ESC 2006 guidelines for the management of patients with atrial fibrillation: A report of the American College of Cardiology Foundation/American Heart Association Task Force on Practice Guideline. *Circulation*, 123, e269–e367.

Etiology

1. Fibrotic changes associated with the aging process, acute MI, valvular diseases, and digoxin preparations may cause atrial fibrillation.
2. Fluid shifts in body (ie, after hemodialysis or surgery).
3. Multiple atrial foci fire impulses at rapid and disorganized rates.
4. The atria are not depolarized effectively; thus, there are no well-formed P waves.
5. Instead, the baseline between QRS complexes is filled with a "wiggly" line that is described as fine or coarse.

6. If the atrial rate is rapid enough, the line will appear almost flat. The atria are said to be firing at rates of between 300 and 500 times per minute.
7. The conduction of a QRS complex is so random that the rhythm is extremely irregular.
8. Atrial fibrillation may be described as controlled if the ventricular response is 100 beats/minute or less; the dysrhythmia is uncontrolled if the rate is above 100 beats/minute.

Analysis

Rate: atrial fibrillation is usually immeasurable because fibrillatory waves replace P waves; ventricular rate may vary from bradycardia to tachycardia.

Rhythm: classically described as an "irregular irregularity."

P wave: replaced by fibrillatory waves, sometimes called "little f" waves.

PR interval: not measurable.

QRS complex: a normally conducted complex.

T wave: normally conducted.

Management

1. Controlled atrial fibrillation of long-standing duration requires no treatment as long as the patient is experiencing no untoward effects. Most cardiologists agree that reversion of long-standing atrial fibrillation is hazardous because of the potential for a thrombus to be dislodged from the atria at the time of reversion.
2. Uncontrolled atrial fibrillation (ventricular responses of 100 beats/minute or greater) is treated with beta-adrenergic blocker or calcium channel blockers to control rate at rest and activity. If the atrial fibrillation is of recent onset, the cardiologist may choose to revert the rhythm to a sinus rhythm.
3. Digoxin is a second-line drug for rate control because it only controls rate at rest.
4. Cardioversion (electrical or pharmacologic) for recent-onset atrial fibrillation may be required starting with low amounts of biphasic electrical current (100 to 200 joules).
5. Chronic anticoagulation therapy may be warranted to prevent microemboli.

Premature Ventricular Contraction

See Figure 13-15.

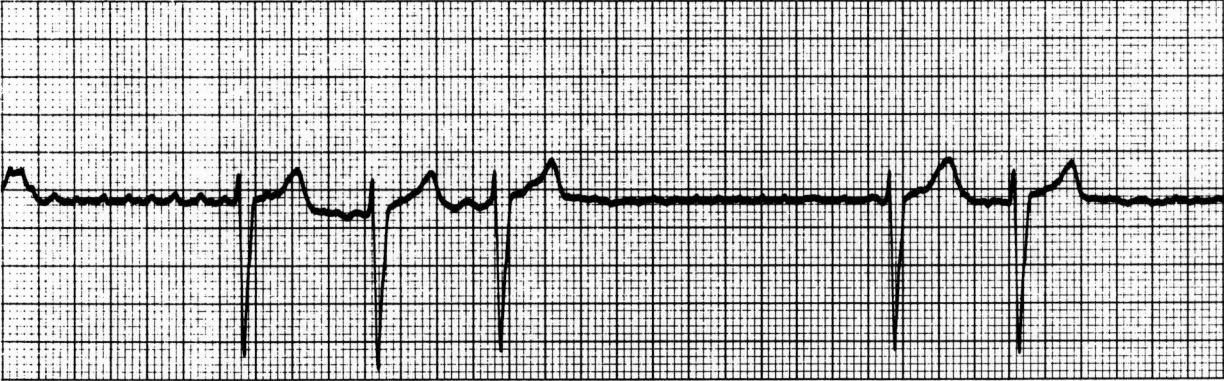

Figure 13-14. Atrial fibrillation with slow ventricular response (controlled).

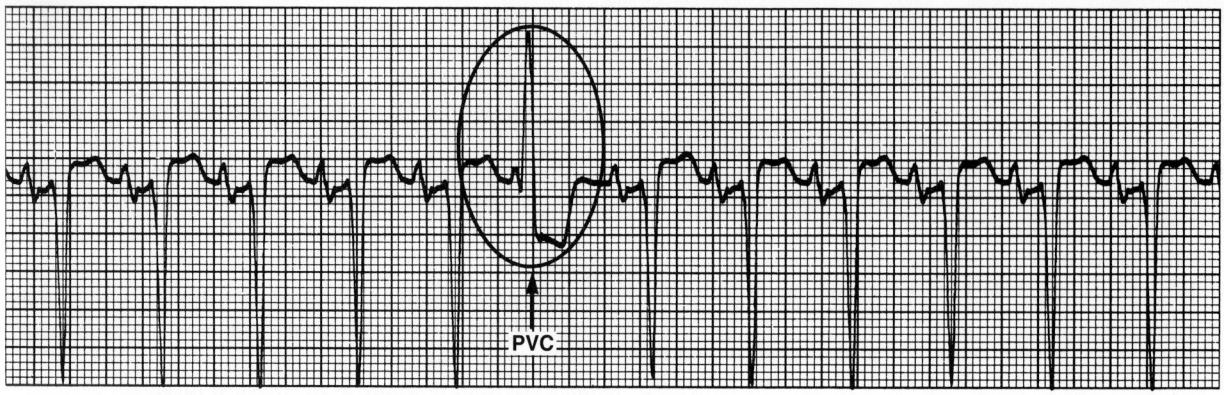

Figure 13-15. Normal sinus rhythm with premature ventricular contraction.

Etiology

1. May be caused by acute MI, other forms of heart disease, pulmonary diseases, electrolyte disturbances, metabolic instability, and drug abuse.
2. The wave of impulse originates from an ectopic focus (foci) within the ventricles at a rate faster than the next normally occurring beat.
3. Because the normal conduction pathway is bypassed, the configuration of the premature ventricular contraction (PVC) is wider than normal and is distorted in appearance. PVCs may occur in regular sequence with normal rhythm—every other beat (bigeminy), every third beat (trigeminy), and so forth (see Figure 13-16).

Analysis

Rate: may be slow or fast.

Rhythm: will be irregular because of the premature firing of the ventricular ectopic focus.

P wave: will be absent because the impulse originates in the ventricle, bypassing the atria and AV node.

PR interval: not measurable.

QRS complex: will be widened greater than 0.12 second, bizarre in appearance when compared with normal QRS complex. (The QRS of a PVC is commonly referred to as having a "sore thumb" appearance.)

T wave: the T wave of the PVC is usually deflected opposite to the QRS.

Management

1. PVCs are usually the precursors of more serious ventricular dysrhythmias. The following conditions involving PVCs require prompt and vigorous treatment, especially if the patient is symptomatic or unstable:
   a. PVCs occurring at a rate exceeding six per minute.
   b. Occur as two or more consecutively.
   c. PVCs fall on the peak or down slope of the T wave (period of vulnerability).
   d. Are of varying configurations, indicating a multiplicity of foci.
2. Historically, the standard treatment for PVCs has been lidocaine. Today, however, amiodarone IV is the preferred method due to lidocaine's risk for toxicity.
   a. Can be given by bolus of 150 mg IV over 10 minutes.
   b. IV infusion consists of a loading dose of 1 mg/minute for 6 hours, followed by a maintenance rate of 0.5 mg/minute for 18 hours.
   c. After IV load, patient may require oral dosing.
3. Lidocaine toxicities include confusion and slurred speech. It should be used with caution in older adults and in those with liver disease.

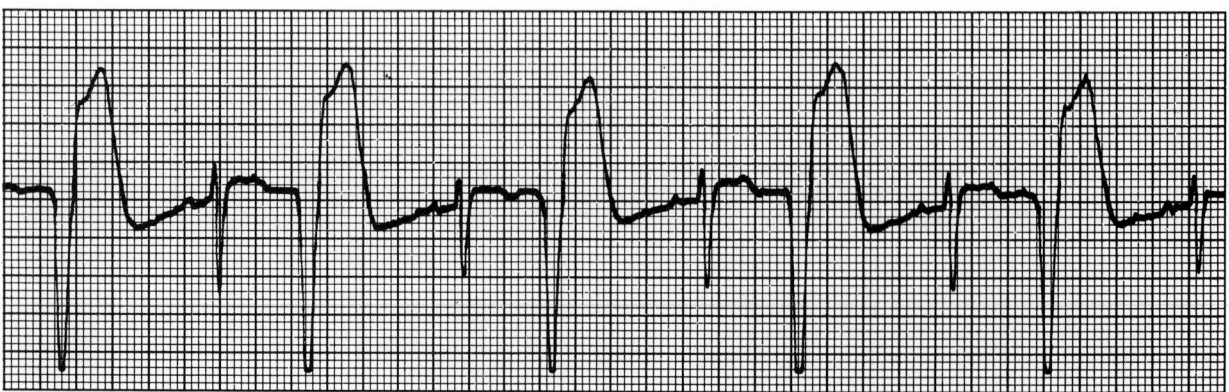

Figure 13-16. Ventricular bigeminy.

DRUG ALERT Be alert to the development of confusion, slurring of speech, and diminished mentation because lidocaine toxicity affects the central nervous system. Should these symptoms appear, slowing the lidocaine may cause them to abate.

4. Amiodarone toxicities include pulmonary fibrotic changes, hypothyroidism, and liver dysfunction.

5. If ventricular premature beats occur in conjunction with a bradydysrhythmia, atropine may be chosen to accelerate the heart rate and eliminate ectopic beats.

6. Atropine should be used with caution with acute MI. The injured myocardium may not be able to tolerate the accelerated rate.

7. Electrolyte infusions may also be needed to treat PVCs. Magnesium sulfate may be used, especially in patients with acute MI. It may be given as 1 g IV over 1 hour or according to facility policy. Potassium infusions can be given at 10 mmol/hour and should be diluted accordingly to route of IV administration.

Ventricular Tachycardia

See Figure 13-17.

Etiology

1. Occurs with:
   a. Acute MI, cardiomyopathy.
   b. Syndromes of accelerated rhythm that deteriorate (eg, Wolff-Parkinson-White syndrome).
   c. Metabolic acidosis, especially lactic acidosis.
   d. Electrolyte disturbance.
   e. Toxicity to certain drugs, such as digoxin or isoproterenol.

2. A life-threatening dysrhythmia that originates from an irritable focus within the ventricle at a rapid rate. Because the ventricles are capable of an inherent rate of 40 beats/minute or less, a ventricular rhythm at a rate of 100 beats/minute may be considered tachycardia.

Analysis

Rate: usually between 100 and 220 beats/minute.
Rhythm: usually regular but may be irregular.

P wave: not present.
PR interval: not measurable.
QRS complex: broad, bizarre in configuration, widened greater than 0.12 second.
T wave: usually deflected opposite to the QRS complex.

Management

1. Ventricular tachycardia (VT) less than 30 seconds is called nonsustained VT. VT more than 30 seconds is sustained VT and requires immediate treatment.

2. If the patient has a pulse and is hemodynamically stable, medications are the initial treatments. Amiodarone IV bolus can be given to halt the dysrhythmia. Other potential medications that may be used (if amiodarone fails) include lidocaine and procainamide. If patient becomes hemodynamically unstable, prepare for synchronized cardioversion with 200 joules of biphasic electrical current.

3. If the patient is pulseless, defibrillation is recommended with 200 joules of biphasic electrical current.

 NURSING ALERT VT is life-threatening and its presentation calls for immediate intervention by the nurse.

4. The purpose of cardioversion/defibrillation is to abolish all abnormal electrical activity and allow the intrinsic cardiac rhythm the opportunity to restart.

5. In some cases, VT may be refractory to drug therapy. Nonpharmacologic treatments, such as endocardial resection, aneurysmectomy, antitachycardia pacemakers, cryoablation, automatic internal defibrillators, and catheter ablation, are alternative treatment modalities.

6. An atypical form of VT, referred to as polymorphous VT or *torsades de pointes* (twisting of the points), can result as a consequence of drug therapy (eg, quinidine therapy) or electrolyte imbalance such as hypomagnesemia. It is important to diagnose polymorphous VT as the treatment differs from monomorphic VT.
   a. *Torsades de pointes* is characterized by a QT interval prolonged to greater than 0.60 second, varying R-R intervals, and polymorphous QRS complexes.

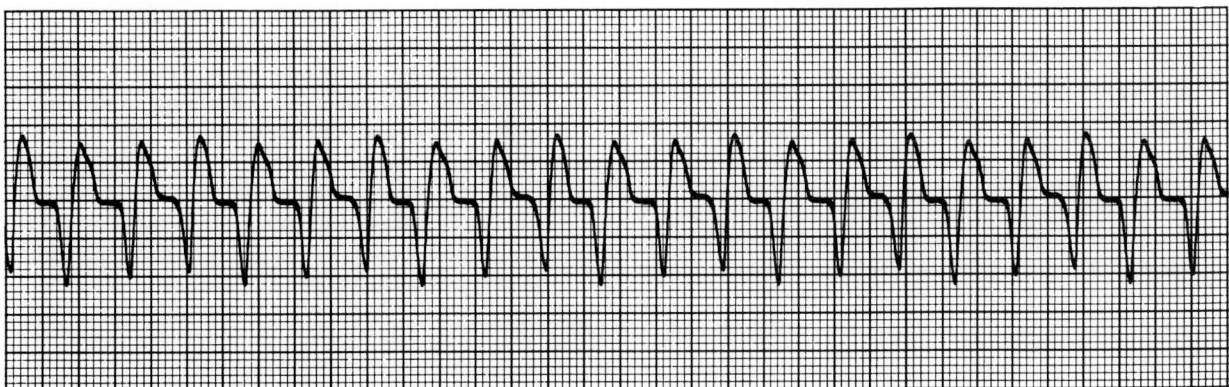

Figure 13-17. Ventricular tachycardia.

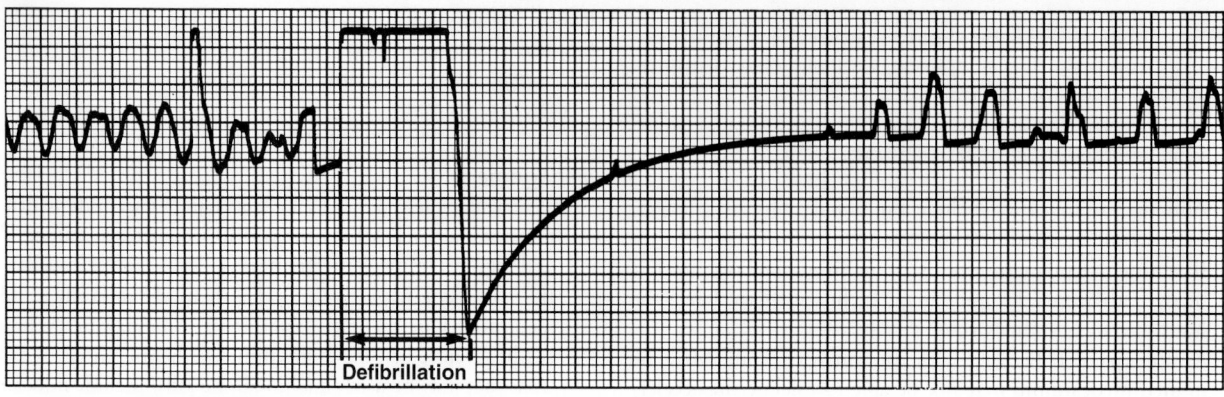

Figure 13-18. Ventricular fibrillation with defibrillation.

b. The treatment of choice is administration of magnesium sulfate 1 g IV over 5 to 60 minutes.

c. If the patient loses consciousness and pulse, defibrillate with 120 to 200 joules of biphasic electrical current.

d. Ventricular pacing to override the ventricular rate and, thus, capture the rhythm is also an acceptable treatment.

e. Procainamide should be avoided because its effect is to prolong the QT interval.

Ventricular Fibrillation

See Figure 13-18.

Etiology

1. Occurs in acute MI, acidosis, electrolyte disturbances, and other deteriorating ventricular rhythms.

2. The ventricles are firing chaotically at rates that exceed 300 beats/minute, resulting in ineffective impulse conduction. CO ceases, and the patient loses pulse, BP, and consciousness.

3. Must be reversed immediately or the patient will die.

Analysis

Rate: not measurable because of absence of well-formed QRS complexes.

Rhythm: chaotic.

P wave: not present.

QRS complex: bizarre, chaotic, no definite contour.

T wave: not apparent.

Management

1. The only treatment for ventricular fibrillation is immediate defibrillation. Defibrillate at 120 to 200 joules with a biphasic defibrillator. Current advanced cardiac life support guidelines no longer recommend three stacked shocks before initiating CPR and medication administration. Epinephrine or vasopressin are first-line drugs after defibrillation because these drugs may make the fibrillation more vulnerable to defibrillation.

2. Unsuccessful defibrillation may be a result of lactic acidosis (treatable with sodium bicarbonate).

3. Check adequacy of the high-quality CPR being performed: 100 compressions/minute at a 2 to 2½-inch depth.

Atrioventricular Block

Etiology

1. May be caused by ischemia or inferior wall MI, digoxin toxicity, hypothyroidism, or Stokes-Adams syndrome.

2. Impaired tissue at the level of the AV node prevents the timely passage of the wave of impulse through the conduction system.

3. In first-degree AV block, the impulse is transmitted normally, but it is delayed at the level of the AV node. The PR interval exceeds 0.20 second.

4. In second-degree AV block, two or more atrial impulses occur before the ventricles are stimulated.

a. Second-degree type 1 (Mobitz 1 Wenckebach)—block occurs above the AV node. There is an increase in delay of electrical impulse (increasing PR interval) with every beat until one P wave fails to conduct and is not followed by a QRS complex (beat is dropped). Mobitz type 1 is usually a temporary and benign dysrhythmia and seldom requires intervention (pacing) unless ventricular rate is slow and the patient is unstable.

b. Second-degree type 2 (Mobitz 2)—block occurs below the AV node in the bundle of His or bundle-branch system. The atria and ventricles are discharging impulses but the activity bears no relationship to each other. There is a sudden failure to conduct an atrial impulse to the ventricles without a delay of the PR interval.

5. In third-degree AV block, or complete heart block, the electrical impulse is completely blocked from the SA node to the AV node. An independent pacemaker in the ventricles takes over at a much slower rate than the atria and are firing independently of each other.

Analysis

1. First-degree AV block (see Figure 13-19).

Rate: usually normal but may be slow.

Rhythm: regular.

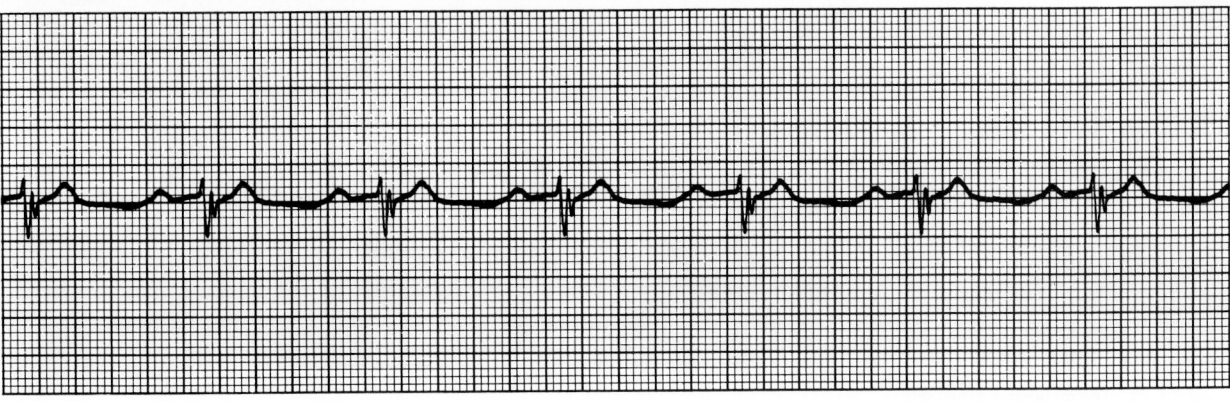

Figure 13-19. First-degree AV block.

P wave: present for each QRS complex, identical in configuration.

PR interval: prolonged to greater than 0.20 second.

QRS complex: normal in appearance and between 0.06 and 0.10 second.

T wave: normally conducted.

2. Second-degree AV block (see Figure 13-20).

   Rate: usually normal.

   Rhythm: may be regular or irregular.

   P wave: present but some may not be followed by a QRS complex. A ratio of two, three, or four P waves to one QRS complex may exist.

   PR interval: varies in Mobitz I (Wenckebach), usually lengthens until one is not conducted; constant in Mobitz II, but not all P waves conducted.

   T wave: normally conducted.

3. Third-degree AV block (complete heart block) (see Figure 13-21).

   Rate: atrial rate is measured independently of the ventricular rate; the ventricular rate is usually very slow.

   Rhythm: each independent rhythm will be regular, but they will bear no relationship to each other.

P wave: present but no consistent relationship with the QRS.

PR interval: not really measurable.

QRS complex: depends on the escape mechanism (ie, AV node will have normal QRS, ventricular will be wide and the rate will be slower).

T wave: normally conducted.

Management

Like that of other dysrhythmias, the treatment of heart blocks depends on the effect the rate is having on CO.

1. First-degree AV block usually requires no treatment.

2. Second-degree AV block, type 1 and type 2, may require treatment if the ventricular rate falls too low to maintain effective CO. Mobitz type 2 is more serious than Mobitz type 1.

3. Third-degree AV block usually requires intervention. However, some patients may be able to tolerate third-degree block for a length of time.

4. Transcutaneous pacing should be employed in the emergent situation while transvenous pacing is being set up.

5. Atropine may be given while awaiting the pacemaker, but it must be remembered that the effect of atropine is to block vagal tone, and the vagus acts on the sinus node. Because the AV node is the culprit in heart block, atropine may not be helpful.

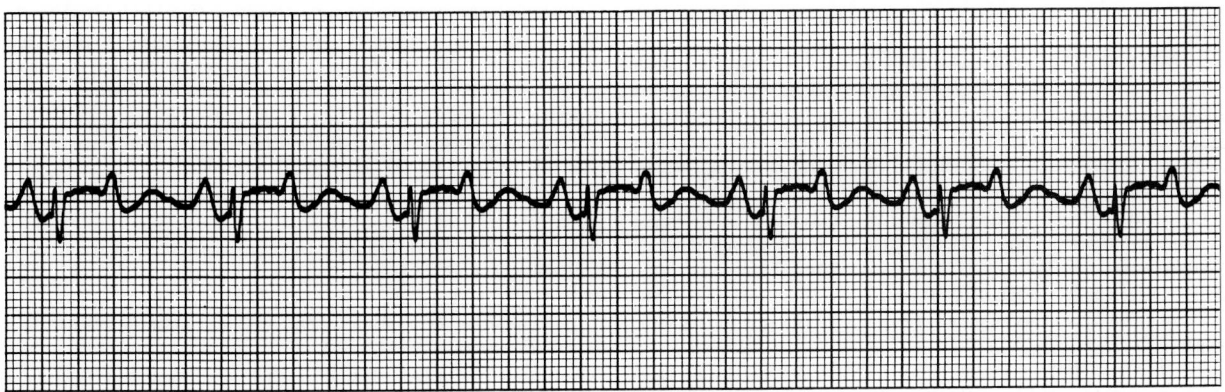

Figure 13-20. Second-degree AV block (Mobitz I).

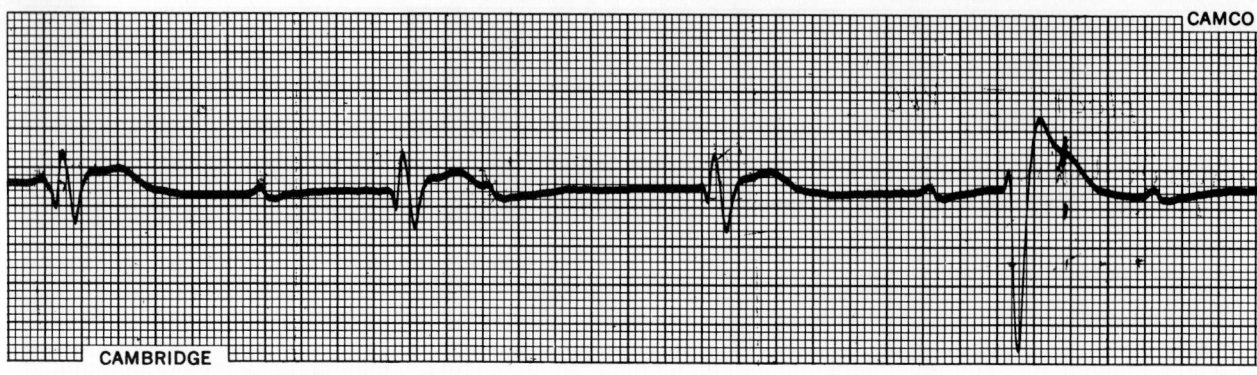

Figure 13-21. Third-degree AV block.

SELECTED REFERENCES

Allen, K. B. (2011). Patient characteristics and operative risk with stand-alone transmyocardial revascularization. *Journal of the American College of Cardiology,* 57(14, Suppl. S), E1140.

Anderson, J. L., Adams, C. D., Antman, E. M., et al. (2011). 2011 ACCF/AHA focused update incorporated into ACC/AHA 2007 guidelines for the management of patients with unstable angina/non-ST elevation myocardial infarction: A report of the American College of Cardiology Foundation/American Heart Association Task Force on Practice Guidelines. *Journal of American College of Cardiology,* 57(19), 1920–1959.

Berndt, N. C., Bolman, C., de Vries, H., et al. (2013). Smoking cessation treatment practices: recommendations for improved adoption on cardiology wards. *Journal of Cardiovascular Nursing,* 28(1), 35–47.

Brown, J. L., Bogaev, R. C., & O'Connell, J. (2011). Short-term mechanical management of cardiogenic shock. *Current Treatment Options in Cardiovascular Medicine,* 13(4), 343–353.

Byrne, J. G., Rezai, K., Sanchez, J. A., et al. (2011). Surgical management of endocarditis: The Society of Thoracic Surgeons clinical practice guideline. *Annals of Thoracic Surgery,* 91(6), 2012.

Desai, M., Seifalian, A. M., & Hamilton, G. (2011). Role of prosthetic conduits in coronary artery bypass grafting. *European Journal of Cardio-Thoracic Surgery,* 40(2), 394–398.

Epstein, A. E., Dimarco, J. P., Ellenbogen, K. A., et al. (2008). ACC/AHA/HRS 2008 guidelines for device-based therapy of cardiac rhythm abnormalities: Executive summary: A report of the American College of Cardiology/American Heart Association Task Force on Practice Guidelines (writing committee to revise the ACC/AHA/NASPE 2002 guidelines update for implantation of cardiac pacemakers and antiarrhythmia devices) developed in collaboration with the American Association for Thoracic Surgery and Society of Thoracic Surgeons. *Journal of the American College of Cardiology,* 51(21), 2085–2105

Epstein, A. J., Polsky, D., Yang, F., et al. (2011). Coronary revascularization trends in the United States, 2001–2008. *Journal of the American Medical Association,* 305(17), 1769.

Floros, P., Sawhney, R., Vrtik, M., et al. (2011). Risk factors and management approach for deep sternal wound infection after cardiac surgery at a tertiary medical centre. *Heart, Lung and Circulation,* 20(11), 712–717.

Fox, C. S. (2013). Weighty Matters: Balancing Weight Gain with Cardiovascular Risk among Patients with Type 1 Diabetes Mellitus on Intensive Insulin Therapy. *Circulation,* 127, 157–159.

Fraker, T. D., & Fihn, S. D. (2007). 2007 chronic angina focused update of the ACC/AHA 2002 guidelines for the management of patients with chronic stable angina. *Circulation,* 116, 2762–772.

Gersh, B. J., Maron, B. J., Bonow, R. O., et al. (2011). ACCF/AHA guideline: 2011 ACCF/AHA guideline for the diagnosis and treatment of hypertrophic cardiomyopathy: A report of the American College of Cardiology Foundation/

American Heart Association Task Force on Practice Guidelines. *Circulation,* 124, e783–e831.

Hall, M. J., DeFrances, C. J., Williams, S. N., et al. (2010). National hospital discharge survey: 2007 summary. *National Health Status Report,* 29, 1–20.

Head, S. J., Mokhles, M. M., Osnabrugge, R. L. J., et al. (2011). Surgery in current therapy for infective endocarditis. *Vascular Health and Risk Management,* 7, 255.

Hochman, J. S., Buller, C. E., Sleeper, L. A., et al. (2000). Cardiogenic shock complicating acute myocardial infarction—etiologies, management and outcome: A report from the SHOCK trial registry. *Journal of the American College of Cardiology,* 36(3), 1063–1070.

Hunt, S. A., Abraham, W. T., Chin, M. H., et al. (2009). 2009 focused update incorporated into the ACC/AHA guidelines for the diagnosis and management of chronic heart failure in the adult. *Circulation,* 119, e391–e479.

Imazio, M. (2011). Meta-analysis of randomized trials focusing on prevention of the postpericardiotomy syndrome. *American Journal of Cardiology,* 108(4), 575.

Jessup, M., Abraham, W. T., Casey, D. E., et al. (2009). 2009 Focused update: ACCF/AHA guidelines for the diagnosis and management of heart failure in adults. *Circulation,* 119, 1977–2016.

Kushner, F. G. (2009). 2009 focused updates: ACC/AHA guidelines for the management of patients with ST-elevation myocardial infarction (updating the 2004 guideline and 2007 focused update) and ACC/AHA/SCAI guidelines on percutaneous coronary intervention (updating the 2005 guideline and 2007 focused update). *Circulation,* 120, 2271–2306.

Leon, M., Smith, C., Mack, M., et al. (2010). Transcatheter aortic-valve implantation for aortic stenosis in patients who cannot undergo surgery. *New England Journal of Medicine,* 363(17), 1597–1607.

Levine, G. N., Bates, E. R., Blackenship, J. C., et al. (2011). 2011 ACCF/AHA/SCAI guideline for percutaneous coronary intervention. *Circulation,* 124, e574–e651.

Levy, B. (2011). Comparison of norepinephrine-dobutamine to epinephrine for hemodynamics, lactate metabolism, and organ function variables in cardiogenic shock: A prospective, randomized pilot study. *Critical Care Medicine,* 39(3), 450.

Litmathe, J., Boeken, U., Bohlen, G., et al. (2011). Systemic inflammatory response syndrome after extracorporeal circulation: A predictive algorithm for the patient at risk. *Hellenic Journal of Cardiology,* 52, 493–500.

McAtee, M. E. (2011). Cardiogenic shock. *Critical Care Nursing Clinics of North America,* 23(4), 607–615.

Moranville, M. P. (2011). Evaluation and management of shock states. *Journal of Pharmacy Practice,* 24(1), 44.

Nishimura, R. A., Carabello, B. A., Faxon, D. P., et al. (2008). ACC/AHA 2008 guideline update on valvular heart disease: Focused update on infective endocarditis. *Circulation,* 118, e887–e896.

Nishimura, R. A., Carabello, B. A., Faxon, D. P., et al. (2008). 2008 focused update incorporated into the ACC/AHA 2006 guidelines for the management of patients with valvular heart disease. *Circulation,* 118, e523–e661.

Pannu, N. (2011). The acute kidney injury to chronic kidney disease continuum: Comment on the magnitude of acute serum creatinine increase after cardiac surgery and the risk of chronic kidney disease, progression of kidney disease, and death. *Archives of Internal Medicine, 171*(3), 233.

Pompilio, G. (2011). Determinants of pericardial drainage for cardiac tamponade following cardiac surgery. *European Journal of Cardio-Thoracic Surgery, 39*(5), e107.

Ramanathan, K. (2011). Rapid complete reversal of systemic hypoperfusion after intra-aortic balloon pump counterpulsation and survival in cardiogenic shock complicating an acute myocardial infarction. *American Heart Journal, 162*(2), 268.

Reiher, A., & Sippel, R. S. (2011). Perioperative management of patients on steroids requiring surgery. In *ACS surgery: Principles and practice.* Hamilton, ON, Canada: Decker Publishing.

Roger, V. L., Go, A. S., Lloyd-Jones, D. M., et al. (2011). Heart disease and stroke statistics—2011 update 1. *Circulation, 123*(4), e18–e209.

Smith, S. C., Benjamin, E. J., Bonow, R. O., et al. (2011). AHA/ACCF secondary prevention and risk reduction therapy for patients with coronary and other atherosclerotic vascular disease: 2011 update: A guideline from the American Heart Association and American College of Cardiology Foundation. *Journal of the American College of Cardiology, 58*(23), 2432–2446.

Sonneville, R., Mourvillier, B., Bouadma, L., et al. (2011). Management of neurological complications of infective endocarditis in ICU patients. *Annals of Intensive Care, 1*(1), 10.

Staniute, M., Brozaitiene, J., Bunevicius, R. (2013). Effects of social support and stressful life events on health-related quality of life in coronary artery disease. *Journal of Cardiovascular Nursing, 28*(1), 83–89.

Starling, R.C., Naka, Y., Boyle, A.J., et al. (2011). Results of the post-US Food and Drug Administration-approval study with a continuous flow left ventricular assist device as a bridge to heart transplantation: A prospective study using the INTERMACS. *Journal of the American College of Cardiology, 57*(19), 1890.

Thomas, S. A., Chapa, D. W., Friedmann, E., et al. (2008). Depression in patients with heart failure: Prevalence, pathophysiological mechanisms and treatments. *Critical Care Nurse, 28*, 40–55.

Thornhill, M. H., Dayer, M. J., Forde, J. M., et al. (2011). Impact of the NICE guideline recommending cessation of antibiotic prophylaxis for prevention of infective endocarditis: Before and after study. *British Medical Journal, 342*, d2392.

Thuny, F., Beurtheret, S., Mancini, J., et al. (2011). The timing of surgery influences mortality and morbidity in adults with severe complicated infective endocarditis: A propensity analysis. *European Heart Journal, 32*(16), 2027–2033.

Wakefield, B. J., Boren, S. A., Groves, P. S., et al. (2013). Heart failure care management programs: A review of study interventions and meta-analysis of outcomes. *Journal of Cardiovascular Nursing, 28*(1), 8–19.

Wexler, R., Elton, T., Pleister, A., et al. (2009). Cardiomyopathy: An overview. *American Family Physician, 79*(9), 778–784.

Wilson, W. (2007). Prevention of infective endocarditis. *Circulation, 116*(15), 1736–1754.

14
Vascular Disorders

GENERAL PROCEDURES AND TREATMENT MODALITIES

Anticoagulant Therapy

Evidence Base Institute for Clinical Systems Improvement (ICSI). (2011). *Antithrombotic therapy supplement.* Bloomington, MN: Author.

Anticoagulant therapy is the administration of medications to achieve the following:

- Disrupt the blood's natural clotting mechanism when there is a risk of pathologic clotting.
- Prevent formation of a thrombus in immobile and/or postoperative patients.
- Intercept the extension of a thrombus once it has formed.
- Agents are used in the acute treatment of thromboembolic disorders, for long-term prevention of recurrent thromboembolism, or for short-term prevention following surgery for some orthopedic conditions.

Types of anticoagulants include coumarin derivatives, such as warfarin given orally; unfractionated heparin (UFH) given subcutaneously (SC) or intravenously (IV); coumadin or low-molecular-weight heparin (LMWH) given SC, particularly dalteparin and enoxaparin; factor Xa inhibitors, particularly fondaparinux given SC and rivaroxaban given orally; direct thrombin inhibitors, such as dabigatran given orally, and argatroban, bivalirudin,

or hirudin given through IV administration (see Procedure Guidelines 14-1).

 **NURSING ALERT** Anticoagulants may be contraindicated or used with extreme caution in conditions that may lead to bleeding, in patients who may have poor follow-up, and in patients with hepatic and renal insufficiency.

Anticoagulant Indications

1. LMWH (dalteparin, enoxaparin) may be given prophylactically pre- and postoperatively in specific patient populations with high-risk procedures, such as active malignancy with an abdominal surgery; following some orthopedic surgical procedures such as total hip replacement, knee replacement, or arthroscopic procedures; and for long surgical procedures or periods of immobility in high-risk patients. They are also used for the acute treatment of deep vein thrombosis (DVT) (often while warfarin is being started). Dalteparin is indicated for prevention of unstable angina or non-Q-wave infarction. The benefits over heparin include:
   a. Steady bioavailability.
   b. Longer half-life.
   c. Less platelet inhibition (than UFH).
   d. More mobility for the patient (it may be given at home).
   e. Does not cause paradoxical thrombotic events.
2. Factor Xa inhibitor fondaparinux is given prophylactically before and after some orthopedic procedures or abdominal surgery in high-risk patients and for the acute treatment of

PROCEDURE GUIDELINES 14-1

Anticoagulant Injection of Anticoagulant

PURPOSE
When prolonged therapy is indicated, unfractionated heparin, low-molecular-weight heparin (LMWH), or a factor Xa inhibitor may be given SC into fatty tissues. These anticoagulants are often given postoperatively to prevent deep vein thrombosis.

EQUIPMENT
- 1- or 2-mL disposable syringe, such as disposable tuberculin syringe, pre-filled LMWH, or fondaparinux syringe
- Fine sharp needle, #27, 5/8-inch long
- Skin antiseptic

Nursing Action	Rationale
Preparatory Phase	
1. Gather equipment and perform hand hygiene.	1. Complies with universal precautions.
2. Choose an injection site.	2.
a. Most convenient sites are along lower abdominal fat pad.	a. Avoids inadvertent intramuscular injection, injection near an incision, and hematoma formation.
b. A common site is the fatty area anterior to either iliac crest.	
c. Avoid injection sites within 2 inches (5 cm) of the umbilicus.	c. Because of possibility of entering a larger blood vessel.
3. Areas where subcutaneous layer is thin should also be avoided.	3. Ensures absorption and avoids tissue damage.

 GERONTOLOGIC ALERT The aging individual begins to lose subcutaneous fat padding. Examine patient for best site for subcutaneous administration of heparin.

PROCEDURE

Nursing Action	Rationale
Performance phase	
1. Sponge the area gently with alcohol. *Do not rub.*	1. Rubbing or pinching skin might initiate damage to the tissue; anticoagulant would aggravate any bleeding.
2. Attempt to stretch skin out, using palm of nondominant hand. Some prefer to (gently) pick up a well-defined fold of skin.	2. Try to empty blood vessels in local area to lessen likelihood of their being pierced by needle—with subsequent hematoma formation.
3. Holding the shaft of the syringe in dart fashion, insert needle directly through the skin at a right angle just into the subcutaneous fatty layer.	3. Right angle achieves adequate depth into subcutaneous tissue.
4. Move dominant hand into position to direct plunger.	4. Aspiration in a forcible manner can damage small blood vessels and frequently lead to bleeding and hematoma formation, especially in the presence of high local concentration of heparin.
a. Do not move needle tip when it is inserted.	
b. Do not pull back plunger for testing.	
5. Firmly push plunger down as far as it will go.	5. Ensures administration of total dose of medication.
6. When injection has been made, withdraw needle gently at the same angle at which it entered, releasing skin on withdrawal of needle.	6. Minimizes tissue damage.
7. Press an alcohol sponge to the site for a few seconds.	7. Minimizes oozing or bleeding.
Follow-up care	
1. Do not rub the area. Instruct patient not to rub area.	1. Rubbing would increase the likelihood of bleeding.

(continued)

PROCEDURE GUIDELINES 14-1 *(continued)*

Anticoagulant Injection of Anticoagulant

PROCEDURE *(continued)*

Nursing Action	Rationale
2. Site of injection.	2. Avoids tissue damage from repeated injection, which may alter absorption.
a. Change site of injection each time medication is administered.	
b. A chart can be marked with time, date, and measured dosage.	b. Ensures adequate rotation of sites.
3. Teach patient and family the procedure if being discharged with self-injections.	3. For continuity of therapy.

DVT (with warfarin). Rivaroxaban is indicated for treatment of acute DVT and pulmonary embolus, for prevention of DVT after hip and knee surgery, and for reducing risk of stroke in patients with nonvalvular atrial fibrillation.

3. Warfarin is used following DVT and pulmonary emboli and for long-term prophylaxis, such as prevention of thromboembolic complications of atrial fibrillation, cardiac valve replacement, or recurrent myocardial infarctions (MIs) and lower-extremity arterial bypass surgeries.

4. Direct thrombin inhibitors are the newest class of anticoagulant.
   a. Dabigatran is indicated for prevention of thromboembolic complications/stroke in patients with nonvalvular atrial fibrillation.
   b. Argatroban, bivalirudin, and hirudin are administered via IV line, so they are used on a shorter-term basis. They are indicated for patients who have a history of heparin-induced thrombocytopenia.

 DRUG ALERT Oral anticoagulants should be discontinued preoperatively to reduce the risk of hemorrhage in the intraoperative phase.

5. Perioperative considerations include discontinuing oral anticoagulants.
   a. IV UFH may be prescribed preoperatively because its half-life is short; thus, the anticoagulant effects are reversed within 30 minutes to 1 hour after discontinuation.
   b. LMWH may be given preoperatively several hours before surgery and 4 to 8 hours after surgery.
   c. It is recommended that the initial dose of fondaparinux be given 6 to 8 hours following surgery.
   d. Rivaroxaban may be given as soon as postoperative hemostasis occurs.

Nursing and Patient Care Considerations

Administering Unfractionated Heparin
1. Obtain baseline coagulation and hematologic studies before initiating anticoagulation therapy to ensure that the patient does not have an underlying bleeding or clotting disorder.

2. Weigh patient before initiating therapy because UFH, as well as some forms of LMWH, are calculated based on weight.
3. For subcutaneous administration, see page xxx.
4. For IV administration, begin continuous infusion.
   a. Use continuous infusion pump.
   b. Assess frequently to make sure the pump is functioning properly, that there are no kinks or leaks in IV tubing, and that the IV site is without signs or symptoms of infiltration.
5. Double-check concentration and dose of heparin, especially when giving high dosages.
6. Be aware that heparin may be continued for 4 to 5 days after oral anticoagulant is initiated due to the delayed onset of therapeutic effectiveness with oral anticoagulants.

 NURSING ALERT Active life-threatening bleeding is a contraindication to antithrombotic therapy. The decision for treatment in each patient should be weighed against the individual risk of bleeding.

Administering Other Anticoagulants
1. Administered low-molecular-weight heparin SC; dosage varies with drug and its intended purpose.
   a. Usually begun 1 to 24 hours before surgery or once or twice daily after surgery, limited to 7 to 14 days.
   b. If warfarin is started, continue LMWH until warfarin becomes therapeutic.
2. Administer fondaparinux once daily; dosage depends on whether it is prophylactic or treatment for thrombosis.
   a. Must be continued for at least 5 days or until warfarin level is therapeutic. May be given for longer following orthopedic procedures.
   b. Provided in preloaded syringes. (*Note:* Do not expel the air bubble from the syringe. Must not be given intramuscularly.
3. Give rivaroxaban orally at the same time every day, such as with the evening meal.
   a. Obtain a baseline creatinine level, as dosage may be decreased in patients with renal insufficiency.
   b. Usually given for 35 days post hip replacement; 12 days post knee replacement.

c. Give twice daily first 21 days then once daily in treatment of acute PE or DVT.

4. Give warfarin orally at the same time every day, usually in the afternoon or at dinnertime.

a. Therapeutic range is monitored by International Normalized Ratio (INR), usually drawn at least 16 hours after last dose.

b. Monitor frequently until stable, with any medication changes, and then monthly when stable.

5. Give dabigatran orally twice daily. Instruct patient to swallow capsules whole; do not open, crush, or chew.

 DRUG ALERT Be aware that dabigatran has a 60-day shelf life.

Monitoring Clotting Profiles

1. Partial thromboplastin time (PTT) is the coagulation test used to monitor the anticoagulation effects of UFH.

a. The patient's PTT should be 2 to 2½ times the control.

b. Obtain PTT levels daily or as ordered. Heparin dose will be adjusted to achieve the desired level of anticoagulation.

2. Prothrombin time (PT) and INR are the coagulation tests used to monitor the anticoagulation effects of warfarin.

a. The patient's INR should be 2 to 3½ times the control. *Note:* The desired levels of INR are determined by protocol for condition and risk factors being followed or by the health care provider.

b. Obtain PT/INR levels daily or as ordered. Warfarin dose will be adjusted to achieve the desired level of anticoagulation.

3. Other laboratory studies to monitor as ordered or if bleeding is suspected:

a. Platelet count—heparin-induced thrombocytopenia (HIT) may occur, particularly with UFH; 50% decrease in platelet count causing local bleeding or systemic reaction with IV.

b. Hemoglobin and hematocrit—baseline and periodically.

c. Fibrinogen—if abnormal bleeding while on UFH.

4. Be aware of drug–drug (including over-the-counter [OTC], food, and herbal supplements) and food–drug interactions that may alter the effects of warfarin. This occurs because of alterations in the clearance of the drug or the rate of intestinal absorption. See Box 14-1 for a partial list of drugs and foods that alter the metabolism of warfarin. Consult a pharmacist or medication reference book for a complete list.

5. No monitoring of PTT or other coagulation tests is required for LMWH, factor Xa inhibitors, or direct thrombin inhibitors; however, PTT may be monitored for LMWH therapy in patients with renal disease and patients weighing less than 110.2 lb (50 kg) or more than 176.4 lb (80 kg).

 DRUG ALERT Drug and food interactions can alter the effect of anticoagulants. A change in intake should prompt more frequent monitoring and, possibly, a change in dose.

Preventing Bleeding

1. Follow precautions to prevent bleeding.

a. Handle patient carefully while turning and positioning.

b. Maintain pressure on IV and venipuncture sites for at least 5 minutes. Apply ice if patient is prone to bleeding.

BOX 14-1	Selected Substances That Interact with Warfarin

SUBSTANCES THAT *DECREASE* INTERNATIONAL NORMALIZED RATIO (INR)*

- Barbiturates
- Antacids
- Oral contraceptives and estrogens
- Corticosteroids
- Quinidine
- Tamoxifen
- Rifampin
- Vitamin K–rich foods
- Grapefruit juice

SUBSTANCES THAT *INCREASE* INR*

- Aspirin
- Heparin
- Nonsteroidal anti-inflammatories
- Cimetidine
- Penicillins (high dose), macrolides, cephalosporins
- Fluconazole
- Ticlopidine
- Thyroxine
- Clopidogrel
- Sulfa compounds
- Alcohol
- Ginkgo biloba, ginseng, garlic

*Consult a pharmacist or medication reference for a complete list.

---

c. Assist with ambulation and keep walkways/hallways free from clutter to prevent falls.

2. Observe carefully for any possible signs of bleeding and report immediately so that anticoagulant dosage may be reviewed and altered, if necessary:

a. Hematuria—frank blood in urine or microhematuria as detected on test strip.

b. Melena—assess for dark/tarry stools, use test cards for occult blood.

c. Hemoptysis—assess for frank blood in emesis, use test cards for occult blood.

d. Bleeding gums—note any pink saliva or frank bleeding with dental hygiene.

e. Epistaxis—frequent/persistent nosebleeds.

f. Bruising/hematomas—inspect skin carefully.

 DRUG ALERT When epidural anesthesia or spinal puncture is employed, anticoagulants increase the risk of epidural or spinal hematoma, which may result in paralysis. Monitor these patients closely for sensory and motor dysfunction.

3. Have on hand the antidotes to reverse anticoagulants being used (see Table 14-1, page 38).

a. Heparin—protamine sulfate.

Table 14-1   Guide to Anticoagulants

DRUG	CONTRAINDICATIONS	MONITORING	ANTIDOTE	OTHER CONSIDERATIONS
Unfractionated heparin (UFH)	• Allergy • Acute major bleeding • Thrombolytic therapy given within past 24 hours in stroke victim • HIT most frequently develops 1–2 weeks after starting therapy	• Get baseline complete blood count, platelet count, prothrombin time/ INR, and creatinine before starting therapy; liver function tests and albumin with suspected liver disease. • Daily partial thromboplastin time or heparin assay. • Monitor platelet count every other day (for HIT).	• Protamine sulfate IV over 10 minutes. • Risk for anaphylaxis is 1%.	• Generally safe in pregnancy unless patient has mechanical heart valve. • Safe in the breastfeeding patient. • Monitor for HIT: reaction at injection site, systemic reaction after bolus injection, 50% decrease in platelets.
Low-molecular-weight heparins (LMWH)	• Allergy • Acute major bleeding • Thrombolytic therapy given within past 24 hours in stroke victim • HIT • Renal failure	• Same baseline as UFH. • Monitor platelet count every 2–3 days if also receiving UFH.	• No agent for complete reversal. • Protamine sulfate provides for 60%–75% reversal.	• Generally safe in pregnancy unless patient has mechanical heart valve. • Generally safe in the breastfeeding patient. • Monitor for HIT.
Factor Xa inhibitors	• Allergy • Acute major bleeding • Thrombolytic therapy given within past 24 hours in stroke victim • Renal failure	• Same baseline as UFH. • No routine monitoring of PTT or INR. • Fondaparinux: Monitor heparin assay regularly in those with renal insufficiency, body weight <50 kg, or those who are obese.	• No antidote. • Fondaparinux: Possible partial reversal with recombinant factor VIIa. • Rivaroxaban: activated charcoal to reduce absorption in overdose	• Safety unknown in the pregnant or breastfeeding patient. • Use cautiously in bacterial endocarditis, uncontrolled hypertension, and other conditions. • Increased risk of bleeding in renal or hepatic impairment. • Risk of spinal or epidural hematoma with spinal procedures
Warfarin sodium	• Allergy • Hemorrhage • Pregnancy	• Same baseline as UFH. • Monitor INR daily to every few days until stable, then monthly (best time is at least 16 hours after last dose). • If starting medication that can affect warfarin, check INR in 3–4 days.	• Vitamin K orally or IV over 30 minutes. • May lead to warfarin resistance and thromboembolism. • Transfusion of fresh frozen plasma may be given.	• Only small amount secreted in breast milk. • Hold for 4 days prior to surgery. • Increased risk of thromboembolism if INR < 1.7; increased risk of bleeding if INR > 4.0. • Purple toe syndrome may occur 3–10 weeks after starting therapy. • Numerous drug and food interactions
Direct thrombin inhibitors	• Allergy • Active bleeding	• Assess baseline renal function, and annually if creatinine clearance <50 mL/minute or age >75 years	• No known antidote • About 60% of drug may be cleared with dialysis over 3–4 hours • Transfusion of fresh frozen plasma or packed red cells may be given	• Safety not known in pregnancy or breastfeeding • Risk of bleeding increases with age • Consult medication reference for drug interactions

b. Warfarin—phytonadione (vitamin K₁, AquaMEPHYTON); dose is dependent on the INR level and/or the degree of patient bleeding.

 DRUG ALERT Vitamin K can lead to warfarin resistence and subsequently increased risk of thromboembolism.

 **NURSING ALERT** There is a risk of bleeding in any patient receiving anticoagulants. Risk of bleeding is patient related and treatment related. Recent updates for labeling on warfarin, include genetic variations that may produce resistance to drug therapeutic levels. Advanced age and hypertension add an increased risk for intracerebral hemorrhage.

Patient Education and Health Maintenance

1. Instruct patient about taking anticoagulants.
   a. Follow instructions carefully and take medications exactly as prescribed; if a dose is missed, do NOT double up dose; rather, notify health care provider.
   b. Notify all health care providers, including dentist, that you are taking anticoagulants.
   c. Avoid foods that may alter the effects of anticoagulants or, if used, should be used in the same quantity every day: green, leafy vegetables, fish, liver, green tea, tomatoes.
   d. Take medications at the same time each day and do not stop taking them unless directed by health care provider, even if symptoms of thrombus/embolus are not present.
   e. Wear a medical identification bracelet or carry a card indicating that you are taking anticoagulants; include name, address, and telephone number of health care provider.
2. Advise the patient to notify the health care provider of the following:
   a. All medications both prescribed and OTC (including vitamins and herbal supplements) that patient is currently taking.
   b. Accidents, infections, excessive diarrhea, and other significant illnesses that may affect blood clotting.
   c. Scheduled invasive procedures by other health care providers, including routine dental examinations and other dental procedures or cardiac catheterizations. If surgical care by another health care provider or dentist is needed, inform other provider that anticoagulants are being taken.
3. Advise the patient to avoid:
   a. Taking any other medications without first checking with health care provider, particularly:
      i. Vitamins, especially if they contain vitamin K.
      ii. Herbal supplements.
      iii. Aspirin or nonsteroidal anti-inflammatory drugs (NSAIDs).
      iv. Mineral oil.
      v. Cold medicines, antibiotics.
      vi. Oral contraceptives and hormones.
      vii. Antireflux medicines such as cimetidine or ranitidine.
      viii. Oral antifungals.

   b. Excessive use of alcohol; may affect clotting ability; check on acceptable limits for social drinking.
   c. Participation in activities in which there is high risk of injury.
   d. Foods that may cause diarrhea or upset stomach, rapid changes in diet.
   e. Shaving with a sharp razor.
4. Instruct the patient to be alert for these warning signs:
   a. Excessive bleeding that does not stop quickly (such as following shaving, a small cut, tooth brushing with gum injury, nosebleed).
   b. Excessive menstrual bleeding.
   c. Skin discoloration or bruises that appear suddenly—particularly on the fingers and toes or deep purple spots anywhere on the body ("blue toe syndrome").
   d. Black or bloody stools; for questionable stool discoloration, test for occult blood.
   e. Blood in urine.
   f. Faintness, dizziness, or unusual weakness.
5. Stress the importance of close follow-up and compliance with periodic laboratory work for blood clotting profiles, need to notify health care provider if unable to keep scheduled appointments, contact provider with questions about dosage.

Thrombolytic Therapy

Thrombolytic therapy is the administration of thrombolytic agents to dissolve any formed thrombus and to inhibit the body's hemostatic function. Thrombolytic agents are available for parenteral use only. Commonly used thrombolytics include streptokinase, tissue plasminogen activator and urokinase.

Thrombolytic therapy is contraindicated in conditions that may lead to bleeding and should be given only in a controlled setting, such as a cardiac catheterization laboratory or an intensive care unit (ICU). Thrombolytic therapy for deep vein or peripheral arterial thrombosis, however, may be given on step-down units or medical-surgical floors.

Clinical Indications

1. Acute MI from coronary thrombosis.
2. Pulmonary embolus.
3. Acute occlusion of peripheral arteries/prosthetic grafts.
4. DVT.

Nursing and Patient Care Considerations

1. Monitor clotting profiles every 2 to 4 hours; these are essential before the initiation of treatment to disclose any bleeding tendencies and to serve as a baseline for assessment of drug efficacy. UFH will generally be given parenterally at the same time.
2. Observe for signs of bleeding and report immediately.
   a. Have typed and crossmatched blood on hold in case bleeding is severe.
   b. Have aminocaproic acid on hand to treat bleeding.

3. Monitor for allergic reaction. A small number of patients (less than 5%) may experience an allergic reaction.
   a. Observe patient for onset of a new rash, fever, and chills.
   b. Report any suspected allergic reaction immediately.
   c. Administer corticosteroids, if ordered, to treat reaction.
4. Monitor electrocardiogram (ECG) for dysrhythmias after reperfusion if thrombolytic therapy is being used for coronary thrombus.
5. Frequently assess color, warmth, and sensation of extremity if therapy is being used for peripheral arterial occlusion.
6. Move patient as little as possible.
7. Minimize phlebotomy.
8. Observe for changes in level of consciousness or other signs of intracranial bleeding.

Care of the Patient Undergoing Vascular Surgery

Vascular surgery may involve operations of the arteries, veins, or lymphatic system. Surgery may be performed on an urgent basis, as in *embolectomy* for acute arterial embolism, or electively for *vein ligation and stripping* for varicose veins after conservative management fails. Other vascular procedures include *thrombectomy* and *vena caval filter insertion* for venous problems and *arterial bypass grafting* (aortoiliac, aortofemoral, femoropopliteal, and femoral-distal), *endarterectomy, endovascular grafting*, and *percutaneous transluminal angioplasty (PTA)* for arterial problems with or without placement of an intraluminal stent.

Preoperative Management

1. Additional health conditions, such as heart disease, hypertension, diabetes mellitus, and chronic lung disease, are fully evaluated, and management is adjusted to decrease operative risks.
2. Chronic skin and tissue changes are assessed preoperatively, and impairment is minimized through protection of the affected parts, treatment with antibiotics, and proper positioning to enhance circulation (elevated for venous and lymphatic problems, level or slightly dependent for arterial problems).
3. Nutritional status is assessed and improved preoperatively to aid in wound healing postoperatively.
4. Risk factors for vascular disease, such as smoking, obesity, and sedentary lifestyle, are reviewed, and patient teaching is initiated to prevent recurrence or progression of vascular disorder.
5. The patient is prepared emotionally and physically for surgery, with teaching focusing on positioning in bed; expected exercises and activity to be followed postoperatively; frequent checking of circulation and wound; and prevention of complications, such as bleeding, infection, and neurovascular compromise.

Postoperative Management

1. Bed rest may be maintained for 24 hours in some cases to reduce swelling and the risk of bleeding.
2. If surgery involved revascularization, peripheral pulses are assessed distal from operative site to ensure adequate tissue perfusion. (Use portable Doppler, if necessary.)
3. If surgery involved use of bypass graft, the graft site is protected and assessed for patency as well.
4. Extremity is positioned with the popliteal space supported to prevent trauma and promote circulation.
5. Anticoagulation may be continued, but it increases chance of bleeding following surgery.
6. Hydration, nutrition, and oxygenation are promoted to ensure wound healing.
7. Surgical incisions are assessed for redness, drainage, and approximation and may be covered with dry dressings.
8. Endovascular and PTA procedures are less invasive, but incision site of catheter is carefully monitored for bleeding and peripheral circulation is assessed.
9. Breathing exercises using an incentive spirometer are performed every 2 hours while patient is awake to prevent postoperative pulmonary complications if the patient is immobilized.

Nursing Diagnoses

- Ineffective Peripheral Tissue Perfusion related to underlying vascular disorder, postoperative swelling.
- Risk for Infection related to surgical incision and impaired circulation.
- Acute Pain related to surgical incision and swelling.
- Impaired Physical Mobility related to pain and imposed restrictions.

Nursing Interventions

Promoting Tissue Perfusion

1. Maintain dressing or compression bandages, as directed.
2. Monitor for bleeding through dressing—reinforce and notify surgeon, as indicated.
3. Monitor for hematoma formation beneath skin—increased pain and swelling. Apply pressure and notify surgeon.
4. Measure vital signs frequently for tachycardia and hypotension, which may indicate hemorrhage.
5. Perform frequent neurovascular checks to involved extremity. Check warmth, color, capillary refill, sensation, movement, and pulses; compare with other side.
6. Position as directed—usually legs elevated and fully supported.

Preventing Infection

1. Maintain IV infusion or heparin lock for antibiotic administration, as ordered, and assess daily for signs of infiltration and infection.
2. Check incision site for drainage, warmth, and erythema, which indicate infection.
3. Change incision dressing, as ordered and as needed, for drainage or soiling.
4. Monitor temperature for elevation.
5. Monitor hematologic profiles for elevation in white blood cell (WBC) count.

Relieving Pain

1. Assess pain level and administer analgesic as ordered.
2. If patient-controlled anesthesia is being used, instruct patient on use and make sure the pump is functioning properly.
3. Position for comfort, using pillows for support.

4. Watch for adverse effects of opioids, such as hypotension, respiratory depression, nausea and vomiting, and constipation.
5. Administer pain medication before activity.
6. Instruct patient in alternative coping methods such as visualization.

Minimizing Immobility

1. Encourage isometric and range-of-motion (ROM) exercises while on bed rest.
   a. Exercise affected extremity by pushing foot into footboard, making a fist, or simply contracting muscles without movement if approved by surgeon.
   b. Perform full ROM of other extremities.
2. Encourage ambulation as soon as allowed.
   a. Avoid dangling legs because of possible compression against the back of bed or chair.
   b. Avoid long periods of sitting or standing.
   c. Encourage short periods of walking every 2 hours.

Patient Education and Health Maintenance

1. Instruct patient and significant other in care of incision and wound at home. Make sure that patient has proper resources available.
2. Instruct patient about wearing elastic stockings or applying ace wrap, if ordered. Have patient perform return demonstration.
3. Instruct patient and significant other in signs of infection, graft failure, or worsening circulatory problem that should be reported.
4. Refer patient to vascular rehabilitation (if available), physical therapy, and occupational therapy as indicated.
5. Refer for additional support for risk factor modification, such as supervised weight loss programs, nutritional counseling, smoking cessation.
6. Instruct patient to avoid restrictive clothing (including socks, hose, shoes), especially over areas of revascularization.
7. Instruct patient to inspect feet (using a mirror, if necessary), including plantar aspect and between toes, daily and to inspect shoes for foreign objects, such as small stones, before putting them on.
8. Instruct patient to wear thick socks and well-fitting shoes with wide toe box to avoid development of breakdown/ulceration on pressure points. Instruct patient not to wear sandals.
9. Instruct patient never to walk barefoot.
10. Review any medications, especially anticoagulants (see page 439).
11. Make sure that the patient knows when and where to follow up.

Evaluation: Expected Outcomes

- Affected extremity with good color, capillary refill, and pulses; warm and sensitive to touch; moving adequately.
- Incision site is well approximated and without signs and symptoms of infection.
- Reports adequate pain control on current regimen.
- Ambulates for 10 minutes every 2 hours without difficulty or shows signs of progressing independence with the assistance of physical or occupational therapy.

	ARTERIAL	VENOUS
Table 14-2	**Comparison of Arterial and Venous Obstruction**	
FACTOR	ARTERIAL OBSTRUCTION	VENOUS OBSTRUCTION
Onset	May be sudden	Gradual
Color	Pale Later—mottled, cyanotic	Slightly cyanotic Rubescent
Skin temperature	Cold	Warm
Leg size	May be reduced	Enlarged
Leg hair and nails	Decreased hair; thick, brittle nails	No change
Edema	None to mild	Typically calf to foot
Sensation	Sensory changes	Normal sensation
Arterial pulses	Pulse deficit	Normal
Effect of elevating leg	Condition worsens	Slight improvement

CONDITIONS OF VEINS

See Table 14-2.

Venous Thrombus

 Evidence Base Institute for Clinical Systems Improvement (ICSI). (2012). *Venous thromboembolism: Diagnosis and treatment guidelines.* Bloomington, MN: Author.

There are several types of venous thrombosis:

Phlebitis is an inflammation in the wall of a vein. The term is used clinically to indicate a superficial and localized condition that can be treated with application of heat.

Superficial thrombophlebitis is a condition in which a clot forms in a vein secondary to phlebitis or because of partial obstruction of the vein. It is more commonly seen in the greater or lesser saphenous veins of the lower extremities, but may also be seen in the upper extremities, most commonly at IV sites.

Phlebothrombosis is the formation of a thrombus or thrombi in a vein; in general, the clotting is related to (1) stasis, (2) abnormality of the walls of the vein, and (3) abnormality of the clotting mechanism. Superficial or deep veins may be affected; however, deep veins of the lower extremities are most commonly involved.

DVT is thrombosis of deep rather than superficial veins. Two serious complications are pulmonary embolism and postphlebitic syndrome.

Note: While phlebothrombosis and DVT do not necessarily represent identical pathologies, for clinical purposes, they are used interchangeably when discussing the same process.

Pathophysiology and Etiology

General Points

1. Three antecedent factors are believed to play a significant role in the development of venous thromboses: (1) stasis of blood, (2) injury to the vessel wall, and (3) altered blood coagulation (Virchow's triad). Thrombosis does not occur with stasis alone.
2. Usually two of the three factors occur before thrombosis develops.

Thrombosis-Related Situations

1. Venous stasis—following operations, childbirth, or bed rest for any prolonged illness.
2. Prolonged sitting or as a complication of varicose veins.
3. Injury (bruise) to a vein; may result from direct trauma or internal trauma such as from IV catheters, infusion of medications, and/or infiltration of medications.
4. Extension of an infection of tissues surrounding the vessel.
5. Continuous pressure of a tumor, aneurysm, or excessive weight gain in pregnancy.
6. Unusual activity in a person who has been sedentary (particularly heavy lifting or prolonged holding of heavy objects—increases risk of upper-extremity thromboses.
7. Hypercoagulability associated with malignant disease, blood dyscrasias.

High-Risk Factors

1. Malignancy.
2. Previous venous insufficiency.
3. Conditions causing prolonged bed rest—MI, heart failure, sepsis, traction, end-stage cancer, human immunodeficiency virus/acquired immunodeficiency syndrome.
4. Leg trauma—fractures, cast, joint replacements.
5. General surgery—over age 40.
6. Obesity, smoking.
7. Inherited coagulopathy (eg, antithrombin III deficiency, protein C&S deficiency, Factor V Leiden thrombophilia, and others).

Clinical Manifestations

Clinical features vary with site and length of affected vein.

1. DVT may occur asymptomatically or may produce severe pain, fevers, chills, malaise, and swelling and cyanosis of affected arm or leg. The chief symptom is unilateral limb edema in which the onset is sudden.
2. Superficial thrombophlebitis produces visible and palpable signs, such as heat, pain, swelling, erythema, tenderness, and induration, along the length of the affected vein.
3. Extensive vein involvement may cause lymphadenitis or arterial compromise if the swelling is extensive enough.

Diagnostic Evaluation

1. Venous duplex/color duplex ultrasound—this commonly done, noninvasive test allows for visualization of the thrombus, including any free-floating or unstable thrombi that may cause emboli. It is to detect thrombi of the upper and lower extremities.
2. Impedance plethysmography—a noninvasive measurement of changes in calf volume corresponding to changes in blood volume brought about by temporary venous occlusion with a high-pneumatic cuff. Electrodes measure electrical impedance as cuff is deflated. Slow decrease in impedance indicates diminished blood flow associated with thrombus.
3. RF testing—radioactive fibrinogen (fibrinogen I^{125}) is administered via IV line. Images are taken through nuclear scanning at 12 to 24 hours; the RF will be concentrated at the area of clot formation.
4. Venography—IV injection of a radiocontrast agent. The vascular tree is visualized and obstruction is identified.
5. Coagulation profiles—PTT, PT/INR, circulating fibrin, monomer complexes, fibrinopeptide A, serum fibrin, D-dimer, proteins C and S, antithrombin III levels, factor V Leiden, prothrombin gene mutation. Detect intravascular coagulation or coagulopathies.

Management

Goals of management are to prevent propagation of the thrombus, prevent recurrent thrombus formation, prevent pulmonary emboli, and limit venous valvular damage.

Anticoagulation

For documented cases of DVT to prevent embolization.

1. UFH may be given IV administration initially, followed by 3 to 6 months of oral anticoagulant therapy. Rivaroxiban may also be used for acute treatment.
2. LMWH is safely given in isolated DVT and/or pulmonary embolism; when the patient is taught the proper technique, may be safely used at home. It is followed by 3 to 6 months of oral anticoagulation.
3. UFH and LMWH may also be given SC as prophylaxis for the prevention of DVT, especially in postoperative and immobile patients.
4. Fondaparinux may be used for treatment and is given SC. It is beneficial for patients with sensitivity to heparins or heparin-induced thrombocytopenia.

Thrombolytic Therapy

1. May be used in life- or limb-threatening situations.
2. Most effective in dissolving existing clots within the first 24 hours of thrombolic event.
3. Ultrasound-assisted delivery of thrombolytic works faster and with less risk of bleeding than regular infusion.

Nonpharmacologic Therapies

For superficial thrombophlebitis and as an adjunct to anticoagulation with DVT.

1. Ambulation is encouraged unless there is mobile thrombus in a proximal deep vein.
2. Elevation of effected extremity: at least 10 to 20 degrees above the level of the heart to enhance venous return and decrease swelling (see Figure 14-1).
   a. The popliteal space should be supported but not constricted.
   b. If the upper extremity is affected, a sling or stockinette attached to an IV pole may be used.

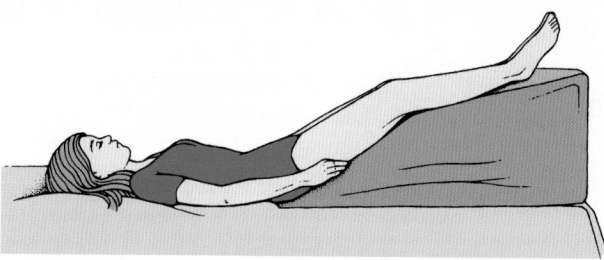

Figure 14-1. Elevation of entire legs above the level of the heart using a foam wedge.

3. Compression: promotes venous return and reduces swelling.
   a. Electrically or pneumatically controlled stockings, boots, or sleeve.
   b. Gradient compression stockings or garments after the acute phase to prevent postphlebitic syndrome or to prevent DVT during periods of immobility for high-risk patients. Level of compression ordered according to condition and severity.
      i. 8 to 15 mm Hg (light)—tired, achy legs; mild fatigue; prevention.
      ii. 15 to 20 mm Hg (therapeutic)—spider veins, minor swelling, aching, pregnancy.
      iii. 20 to 30 mm Hg (medical grade)—fatigue, low-grade varicosities, postsclerotherapy.
      iv. 30 to 40 mm Hg (medical grade)—heaviness, fatigue, postsurgery/sclerotherapy, thrombosis, complications of varicose veins, postphlebitic syndrome, treatment of edema, venous ulcers, varices with pregnancy, stasis dermatitis, lymphedema.
      v. 40 to 50 mm Hg (medical grade)—severe edema for above causes, severe chronic venous insufficiency.
4. Dry heat.
   a. Warm water bottles, heating pad.
   b. Ultrasound (acoustic vibration with frequencies beyond human ear perception).
5. Moist heat.
   a. Hydrotherapy.
   b. Whirlpool bath.
   c. Warm compresses.

Surgery

1. Placement of a filter into the inferior vena cava to prevent fatal pulmonary embolism in a patient who cannot tolerate prolonged anticoagulant therapy or who has recurrent emboli in the presence of adequate anticoagulation.
2. Thrombectomy may be necessary for severely compromised venous drainage of the extremity.
3. See page 440 for surgical care.

Complications

1. Pulmonary embolism.
2. Postphlebitic syndrome.

Nursing Assessment

1. Obtain history of risk factors for thrombophlebitis.
2. Note symmetry or asymmetry of legs. Measure and record leg circumferences daily (see Procedure Guidelines 14-2, page 444). Acute, unilateral edema may be first sign of a DVT.
3. Observe for evidence of venous distention or edema, puffiness, stretched skin, hardness to touch.
4. Examine for signs of obstruction due to occluding thrombus—swelling, particularly in loose connective tissue or popliteal space, ankle, or suprapubic area.
5. Monitor for signs of pulmonary embolus, including shortness of breath, chest pain, and tachycardia.
6. Hand-test extremities for temperature variations—use dorsum (back) of same hand; first compare ankles, then move to the calf and up to the knee.
7. Assess for calf pain, which may be aggravated when foot is dorsiflexed with the knee flexed. Unfortunately, this sign is nonspecific and has a low sensitivity for detecting thrombophlebitis.
8. Assess all IV catheter insertion sites for signs and symptoms of infection and infiltration. Rotate peripheral IV sites every 72 hours or as needed.

Nursing Diagnoses

- Acute Pain related to decreased venous blood flow.
- Risk for Bleeding related to anticoagulant therapy.
- Impaired Physical Mobility related to pain and imposed treatment.

Nursing Interventions

1. Elevate legs as directed to promote venous drainage and reduce swelling.
2. Apply warm compresses or heating pad as directed to promote circulation and reduce pain.
   a. Make sure that water temperature is not too hot.
   b. Cover plastic water bottle or heating pad with towel before applying to skin.
3. Administer acetaminophen, codeine, or other analgesic, as prescribed and as needed. Avoid the use of aspirin (or aspirin-containing drugs) and NSAIDs during anticoagulant therapy to prevent further risk of bleeding.

 NURSING ALERT Avoid massaging or rubbing calf because of the danger of breaking up the clot, which can then circulate as an embolus.

Preventing Bleeding

See page 437 for nursing interventions for patients on anticoagulant therapy.

Preventing Other Hazards of Immobility

See Procedure Guidelines 14-3, page 445.

PROCEDURE GUIDELINES 14-2

Obtaining Leg Measurements to Detect Early Swelling

PURPOSE

To obtain leg measurements for detection and monitoring of thrombophlebitis.

EQUIPMENT

- Flexible tape measure in inches/centimeters
- Black felt-tip pen

PROCEDURE

Nursing Action	Rationale
Preparatory phase	
1. Instruct patient to lie in dorsal recumbent position.	
Performance	
1. On initial assessment of the patient, measure the circumference of the ankle, calf, and thigh.	1. Provides baseline data.
2. Obtain measurements at the narrowest part of the ankle, and widest part of calf and thigh.	2. Provides a consistent anatomic place of measurement, some facilities have a predetermined starting point, such as 6–8 inches (15 or 20 cm) from the kneecap.
3. Mark the leg with a black felt-tip pen where measurements taken. Thereafter, when measuring, place the measuring tape on the marked line.	3. Promotes consistency of measurements.
4. Repeat measurements taken on admission the next morning before any patient activity.	4. Otherwise, later measurements may give a false reading because of gravitational edema.
5. Thereafter, obtain measurements at the same time of day weekly unless there is evidence of swelling, in which case it is done daily.	5. Weekly—to detect swelling. Daily—to monitor swelling and its response to treatment.
6. Record measurements:	6. Evaluates trends.

LEG MEASUREMENTS

Date: _____

Time: _____

Right	**Left**
Ankle _____ inches/cm	Ankle _____ inches/cm
Calf _____ inches/cm	Calf _____ inches/cm
Thigh _____ inches/cm	Thigh _____ inches/cm

7. Compare measurements: a. Check one leg with the other. b. Check each leg with baseline data.	*Significant Findings* Males: 1.5 cm difference between legs or compared with baseline Females: 1 cm difference between legs or compared with baseline

1. Prevent venous stasis by proper positioning in bed.
   a. Support full length of legs when they are to be elevated.
   b. Prevent pressure ulcers that may occur over bony prominences, such as sacrum, hips, knees, and heels. Be aware of bony prominence of one leg pressing on soft tissue of other leg (in side-lying position, place a soft pillow between legs).
   c. Avoid hyperflexion at knee as in jackknife position (head up, knees up, pelvis and legs down); this promotes stasis in pelvis and extremities.

PROCEDURE GUIDELINES 14-3

Applying Compression Stockings

PURPOSE

To prevent postphlebitic syndrome following deep vein thrombosis (DVT) or to prevent acute DVT or pulmonary embolism postoperatively or during periods of immobility.

EQUIPMENT

Stockings that have been properly fitted to patient (see manufacturer's information on measuring and fitting)

PROCEDURE

Nursing Action	Rationale
Preparatory Phase	
1. Make sure that stockings are clean and dry and without excessive wear.	1. Damp stockings are difficult to apply and excessive wear reduces elasticity and effectiveness.
2. Make sure patient's skin is dry. Do not apply moisturizing lotion before application; can apply a thin layer of cornstarch to reduce friction.	2. Moisture will cause difficulty with application.
3. Remove any jewelry that may get caught on stockings.	3. Could damage stockings.
Performance Phase	
1. Insert hand into stocking as far as heel pocket.	
2. Grasp center of heel pocket and pull back, turning stocking inside out as far as heel.	2. Creates shorter length to maneuver.
3. Using two hands, position stocking over foot and heel, centering heel.	3. Centering over the foot will be more difficult once application is complete.
4. Pull stocking up around ankle, then calf, then into final position (1–2 inches below knee for knee-high stockings).	4. Working it upward slowly will prevent excessive pulling, which puts stress on the elastic.
5. Run hands over stocking to smooth it into position. Do not allow top band to roll down.	5. Creases could place excessive pressure on the skin. The top band could bunch up over popliteal area, impeding venous return.
Follow-up Care	
1. Ensure that stockings are cleaned according to manufacturer's instructions. The stockings may be hand washed with mild soap and hung to dry or placed in washer and dryer on low settings.	1. Excessive heat and bleach will decrease life of elastic. Manufacturer may recommend replacement after 3–6 months of use.
2. Teach patient how to don and care for stockings at home. Refer the patient to the manufacturer's website or phone number for additional information.*	2. Manufacturers, such as Jobst and TED, offer products to help with donning and additional care information.

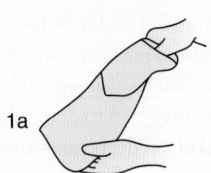 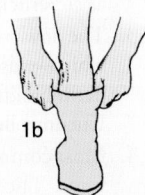 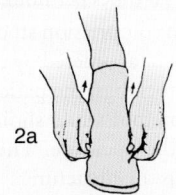 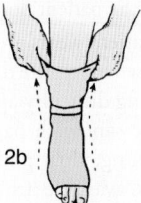

Hand positions for stocking application.

 Evidence Base National Collaborating Center for Acute Care. (2010). Venous thromboembolism: Reducing the risk. *NICE Clinical Guideline 92.* Available: *www.nice.org.uk/nicemedia/live/12695/47195/47195.pdf.*

*Manufacturer's websites such as www.jobst-usa.com; www.rescuelegs.com.

2. Initiate active exercises unless contraindicated, in which case, use passive exercises.
   a. If the patient is on bed rest:
      i. Simulate walking if lying on back—5 minutes every 2 hours.
      ii. Simulate bicycle pedaling if lying on side—5 minutes every 2 hours.
   b. If contraindicated, resort to passive exercises—5 minutes every 2 hours.
3. Encourage adequate fluid intake, frequent changes of position, and effective coughing and deep-breathing exercises.
4. Be alert for signs of pulmonary embolism—chest pain, dyspnea, anxiety, and apprehension—and report immediately.
5. After the acute phase (5 to 7 days), apply compression stockings as directed. Check color, warmth, and capillary refill through opening at toe if using open-toe stocking and remove at least once per day to look for skin changes, pressure points, and calf tenderness. Educate patient about continued use of compression stockings at home as directed.
6. Encourage walking when allowed.
   a. If permissible, have the patient sit up and move to side of bed in sitting position. Provide a foot support (stool or chair)—dangling of feet is not desirable because pressure may be exerted against popliteal vessels and may obstruct blood flow.
   b. If the patient is permitted out of bed, encourage walking 10 minutes each hour.
   c. Discourage crossing of legs and long periods of sitting because compression of vessels can restrict blood flow.

Community and Home Care Considerations

Practice preventive measures for bedridden patients who are prone to develop thrombosis:

1. Have the patient lie in bed in the slightly reversed Trendelenburg position because it is better for the veins to be full of blood than empty.
2. Place a padded footboard across the foot of the bed.
   a. Instruct the patient to press the balls of the feet against the footboard, as if rising up on toes.
   b. Have the patient relax the foot.
   c. Request that the patient do this 5 to 10 times per hour.
3. Make sure the patient wears prescription compression stockings at all times when legs are dependent or as ordered by the provider. If having difficulty applying stockings, the patient can use a plastic sandwich bag over forefoot while sliding on foot of stocking, then pull it out the open toe. There are also devices available from various manufacturers to assist with applying stockings (*www.compressionstockings.com*, *www.jobst.com*).

Patient Education and Health Maintenance

1. Teach patient signs of recurrent thrombophlebitis and pulmonary embolism to report immediately.

2. Provide thorough instructions about anticoagulant therapy (see page 439).
3. Teach patient to promote circulation and prevent stasis by applying compression stockings at home.

 NURSING ALERT Prescription compression stockings have no role in the management of the acute phase of DVT, but are of value after ambulation has begun. Their use will minimize or delay the development of postphlebitic syndrome.

4. Advise against straining or any maneuver that increases venous pressure in the leg. Eliminate the necessity to strain at bowel movement by increasing fiber and fluids in the diet.
5. Warn patient of hazards of smoking and obesity: nicotine constricts veins, decreasing venous blood flow. Extra pounds increase pressure on leg veins. Make appropriate referrals to nutritionist, smoking-cessation classes, etc., as needed.
6. Advise patient to avoid prolonged periods of sitting or standing. If necessary, perform exercises to encourage venous return.

Evaluation: Expected Outcomes
- Patient verbalizes reduced pain.
- No bleeding is observed.
- Normal respiratory status is maintained.

Chronic Venous Insufficiency

Chronic venous insufficiency may be a residual effect of phlebitis, or thrombosis, also called *postphlebitic syndrome*. It may also occur as a result of heredity. It results from chronic occlusion of the veins, destruction of the valves, congenitally weak or absent valves or weakness in the calf muscle pump of the lower extremity.

Pathophysiology and Etiology

1. In the case of venous thrombosis, smaller vessels dilate because the main channel for returning blood from the leg to the heart is blocked by a thrombus.
2. Valves of diseased connecting veins (perforators) that serve to keep blood flowing from the superficial system into the deep system can no longer prevent backflow. The result is chronic venous stasis, resulting in swelling and edema, as well as superficial varicose veins.
3. The lower leg becomes discolored because of venous stasis, which leads to edema and pigmentation changes due to hemosiderin buildup in the skin resulting in a brownish discoloration. Uncontrolled edema may lead to dermatitis and ulceration.
4. Most commonly involved deep veins are the iliac and femoral veins. The saphenous vein is the most common superficial vein affected.

Clinical Manifestations

1. Chronic edema; worse while legs are dependent.
2. Intractable induration, discoloration, pain, ulceration; area surrounding medial malleolus is the most common site.

Diagnostic Evaluation and Management

1. Doppler, plethysmography—noninvasive screening that shows obstruction and valve incompetency.
2. Best treatment is prevention of phlebitis and constant use of compression if phlebitis has occurred.
3. After this syndrome has developed, only palliative and symptomatic treatment is possible because the damage is irreparable.

Complications

1. Stasis ulcers.
2. Cellulitis.
3. Recurrent thrombosis.

Nursing Interventions and Patient Education

Instruct the patient as follows:

1. Wear prescription compression stockings to prevent edema.
2. Avoid sitting or standing for long periods or sitting with legs crossed.
3. Elevate legs on a chair for 5 minutes every 2 hours.
4. Elevate legs above level of head by lying down two or three times daily.
5. Raise foot of bed 6 to 8 inches (15 to 20 cm) at night to allow venous drainage by gravity.
6. Apply bland, oily lotions to prevent scaling and dryness of skin.
7. Avoid constricting bandages.
8. Prevent injury, bruising, scratching, or other trauma to skin of leg and foot.
9. Be alert for signs of ulceration, drainage, warmth, erythema, and pain, indicating infection.
10. Ambulate several times a day, as tolerated, to improve blood flow by contraction of the calf muscle pump of the lower leg.

Stasis Ulcers

Stasis ulcer is an excavation of the skin surface produced by sloughing of inflammatory necrotic tissue, usually caused by venous insufficiency in the lower extremity.

Pathophysiology and Etiology

1. Stasis ulcer results from inadequate oxygen and other nutrients to the tissues because of edema and decreased circulation.
2. Secondary bacterial infection occurs because of decreased microcirculation that limits the body's response to infection.
3. Postphlebitic syndrome and stasis with uncontrolled edema are responsible for most leg ulcers.

Clinical Manifestations

Severity of symptoms depends on the extent and duration of venous insufficiency.

1. Open sore that is inflamed (see Figure 14-2) (beefy red base) and has irregular edges. The ulcers are most often found in the ankle area.
2. Drainage may be present or the area may be covered by a dark crust.
3. Patient may complain of swelling, heaviness, aching, and fatigue.

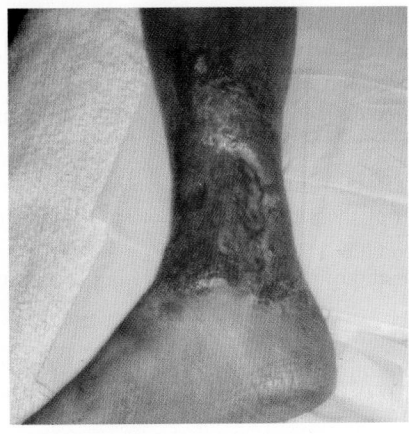

Figure 14-2. Venous ulcer.

4. Edema and pigmentation around ulcer.
5. Crusting of skin around ulcer.

 GERONTOLOGIC ALERT Most venous ulcers occur in people older than age 65.

Diagnostic Evaluation

1. Noninvasive tests, such as plethysmography and venous Doppler, may show impeded blood flow and incompetent valves.
2. Wound cultures will identify microorganisms, if infected.

Management

Removing Devitalized Tissue

1. Necrotic material is flushed out with cleaning agents to dissolve slough. These agents are chemically or naturally derived enzymes that are proteolytic or fibrinolytic.
2. Surgical excision of slough—if necrotic tissue is loose, this procedure can be done without anesthesia; if the tissue is adherent, anesthesia will be required. Some debridements may be done at the bedside or in the clinic with topical anesthetic.

Stimulating Formation of Granulation Tissue

1. Dressing of choice:
   a. Nonadherent so that removal is painless and does not damage newly forming tissue.
   b. Highly absorbent.
   c. Safe, nontoxic.
   d. Sterile, accessible, and inexpensive.
2. Application of compression over dressings, generally through the use of bandages or elastic stockings. In some circumstances, inflatable pneumatic leggings may be appropriate.
3. Unna's boot or other layered compression bandage, an effective treatment of choice, is an example of a combined dressing and compression bandage.
4. Use of human growth factor ointment to the ulcer may be appropriate to stimulate tissue growth.
5. Bed rest with leg elevation.
6. Diuretic therapy for edema reduction may improve capillary circulation.

7. Application of skin grafts.
   a. Skin grafts are used for ulcers that will not heal.
   b. They are not recommended for first-line treatment.
   c. Skin-equivalent grafts may be used particularly if skin grafts fail.

Preventing Recurrence

1. Ligation of the saphenofemoral or saphenopopliteal vessels with stripping.
2. Ligation of the lower leg communicating veins (usually endoscopic).
3. Deep vein bypass or reconstruction.
4. Injection compression sclerotherapy.
5. See page 440 for surgical care.

Complications

1. Infection.
2. Sepsis.

Nursing Assessment

1. Observe appearance and temperature of the skin.
2. Note location and appearance of ulcer.
3. Determine presence and quality of all peripheral pulses. Use Doppler, if needed.
4. Observe for drainage and signs of infection.

Nursing Diagnoses

- Impaired Tissue Integrity related to stasis ulcer.
- Acute Pain related to stasis ulcer.

Nursing Interventions

Restoring Tissue Integrity

1. Elevate affected extremity to decrease edema.
2. Place lamb's wool between toes to prevent pressure on a toe.
3. Provide overbed cradle to protect leg from pressure of bed linens.
4. Consider air-fluidized bed to provide pressure relief.
5. Administer prescribed antibiotics.
6. Apply wet-to-moist dressings, chemical beads or ointments, and topical antibiotics, as ordered. Wounds should not be allowed to completely dry out. Slight moisture aids the healing process.
7. Apply Unna's boot or other compression system to lower extremity, as ordered.
8. Ensure adequate nutritional intake to enhance wound healing.

Reducing Pain

1. Administer prescribed analgesics, such as NSAIDs, to reduce pain and inflammation.
2. Medicate 30 to 45 minutes before a dressing change.
3. Encourage short periods of ambulation after pain medication is given.

Community and Home Care Considerations

1. Make sure that all supplies are obtained for home care. Utilize social services and other resources to help with financial arrangements, as needed.
2. Assess the patient's ability to perform dressing changes at home. Include significant others in teaching to assist patient.
3. Make home visits several times per week to assess healing of ulcer, assess for infection, and assist family in carrying out dressing changes and other measures.

Patient Education and Health Maintenance

1. Stress the importance of following explicitly the recommendations of the health care provider.
2. Explain the hazards of trying other remedies without professional advice.
3. Indicate that the treatment may be long but that patience is an important aspect.
4. Encourage maintenance of healthy tissue when the ulcer has healed by continuing with the safeguards practiced before because breakdown of healed tissue frequently occurs.
5. Encourage participation in physical therapy and a regular exercise program.
6. Encourage weight control and proper dietary intake to ensure adequate amounts of protein, vitamins (A, C, E), zinc, and a reduced sodium intake.
7. Teach patient the correct method of dressing changes.
8. Instruct patient on injury prevention, including keeping hallways and walkways clear of obstacles and using a nightlight to avoid injury if awakened at night.
9. Encourage use of compression stockings when ordered.

Evaluation: Expected Outcomes

- Skin is of normal color and temperature, nontender and nonswollen, and demonstrates new epithelium.
- Verbalizes only minimal discomfort with dressing changes.

Varicose Veins

Primary varicose veins are unilateral or bilateral dilation and elongation of saphenous veins; deeper veins are normal. As the condition progresses, because of hydrostatic pressure and vein weakness, the vein walls become distended, with asymmetric dilation, and some of the valves become incompetent. The process is irreversible. *Secondary varicose veins* result from obstruction of deep veins.

Telangiectasias (spider veins) are dilated superficial capillaries, arterioles, and venules. They may be cosmetically unattractive but do not pose a threat to circulation.

Pathophysiology and Etiology

1. Dilation of the vein prevents the valve cusps from meeting; this results in increased backup pressure, which is passed into the next lower segment of the vein. The combination of vein dilation and valve incompetence produces the varicosity (see Figure 14-3).
2. Varicosities may occur elsewhere in the body (esophageal and hemorrhoidal veins) when flow or pressure is abnormally high.
3. Predisposing factors:
   a. Hereditary weakness of vein wall or valves.
   b. Long-standing distention of veins brought about by pregnancy, obesity, or prolonged standing.
   c. Advanced age—loss of tissue elasticity.

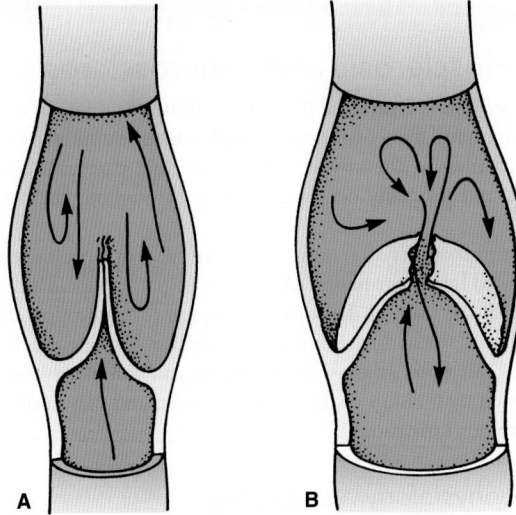

Figure 14-3. Valve incompetence develops as dilation of a vessel prevents effective approximation of valve cusps. (A) Closed venous valve. **(B)** Incompetent venous valve.

Clinical Manifestations

1. Disfigurement due to large, discolored, tortuous leg veins.
2. Easy leg fatigue, cramps in leg, heavy feeling, increased pain during menstruation, nocturnal muscle cramps.

Diagnostic Evaluation

1. Photoplethysmography—a noninvasive technique to observe venous flow hemodynamics by noting changes in the blood content of the skin; used to detect incompetence in valves located inside the vein.
2. Doppler ultrasound and duplex imaging—can detect accurately and rapidly the presence or absence of venous reflux in deep or superficial vessels.
3. Venous outflow and reflux plethysmography—able to detect deep venous occlusion.
4. Ascending and descending venography—an invasive technique that can also demonstrate venous occlusion and patterns of collateral flow. This test is expensive and may not be required if a careful history, physical examination, and laboratory testing are done.

Management

1. Conservative therapies, such as encouraging weight loss if appropriate and avoiding activities that cause venous stasis by obstructing venous flow.
2. Surgery may be considered for ulceration, bleeding, and cosmetic purposes in selected patients if patency of deep veins is ensured.
3. Surgical procedures—a single method or combination of methods is tailored to meet the needs of the individual:
   a. Sclerosing injection—may be combined with ligation or limited to treatment of isolated varicosities. The affected vessel may be sclerosed by injecting sodium

tetradecyl sulfate or similar sclerosing agent. Compression bandage is then applied without interruption for 2 to 6 weeks; inflamed endothelial surfaces adhere by direct contact.
   b. Multiple vein ligation—either by multiple incisions or ambulatory phlebectomy (veins are removed using tiny incisions and hooks to grasp the veins).
   c. Ligation and stripping of the greater and lesser saphenous systems.
   d. Laser or radiotherapy treatment—small catheter is inserted via the groin and the veins ablated.
   e. Laser therapy—eliminates small veins under the skin.

Complications

1. Hemorrhage due to weakening of and pressure on the vein wall.
2. Skin infection and breakdown, producing ulcers (rare in primary varices).
3. Skin discoloration over the veins injected.

Nursing Assessment

1. Inspect for dilated, tortuous vessel.
2. Perforating veins that are incompetent may be felt as bulging circles at intervals beneath the skin. New varices are palpated along the surface of the muscle or bone. Chronic varices create deep pockets and may feel "boggy" with deep palpation.
3. Assess for any ulceration, chronic venous insufficiency, or signs of infection.

Nursing Diagnoses

- Impaired Tissue Integrity related to chronic changes and postoperative inflammation.
- Acute Pain related to surgical incisions, inflammation.

Nursing Interventions

Promoting Tissue Integrity Postoperatively

1. Maintain compression bandages from toes to groin. Monitor neurovascular status of feet (color, warmth, capillary refill, sensation, pulses) to prevent compromise from swelling.
2. Elevate legs about 30 degrees, providing support for the entire leg. Make sure that knee gatch of the bed is positioned for straight incline. Encourage early ambulation.
3. Monitor for signs of bleeding, especially during the first 24 hours.
   a. Blood soaked through bandages.
   b. Increased pain, hematoma formation.
   c. Hypotension and tachycardia.
4. If incisional bleeding occurs, elevate the leg above the level of the heart, apply pressure over the site, and notify the surgeon.
5. Be alert for complaints of pain over bony prominences of the foot and ankle; if the elastic bandage is too tight, loosen it; later, reapply it.

6. Maintain IV infusion for fluids and antibiotics, as ordered.
7. After removal of compression bandages (about 7 days postoperatively), observe or teach patient to observe for signs of cellulitis or incisional infection.
8. Encourage use of prescription compression stockings for several weeks to months following surgery.

Relieving Pain

1. Administer analgesics, as prescribed.
2. Encourage early and frequent ambulation with legs elevated when not walking.
3. When ambulatory, advise patient to avoid prolonged standing, sitting, or crossing or dangling legs to prevent obstruction.

Patient Education and Health Maintenance

Postoperative Instructions

Instruct the patient to:

1. Wear pressure bandages or compression stockings as prescribed—usually for 3 to 4 weeks after surgery.
2. Elevate legs about 30 degrees and provide adequate support for entire leg.
3. Take analgesics for pain, as ordered.
4. Report such signs as sensory loss, calf pain, or fever to the health care provider.
5. Avoid dangling of legs.
6. Walk frequently.
7. Be aware that patchy numbness can be expected but should disappear in less than 1 year.
8. Follow conservative management instructions (below) to prevent recurrence.

Conservative Management

Instruct the patient to:

1. Avoid activities that cause venous stasis by obstructing venous flow:
   a. Wearing tight garters, tight girdle, compression around popliteal area.
   b. Sitting or standing for prolonged periods of time.
   c. Crossing the legs at knees for prolonged periods while sitting (reduces circulation by 15%).
2. Control excessive weight gain.
3. Wear firm elastic support, as prescribed, from toe to knee when in upright position.
   a. Put compression stockings on in bed before getting up.
   b. Thigh-high compression may be ordered presenting a compliance challenge.
4. Elevate foot of bed 6 to 8 inches (15 to 20 cm) or use a wedge for night sleeping.
5. Avoid injuring legs.

Evaluation: Expected Outcomes

- Skin is of normal color and temperature, nontender and nonswollen, and intact.
- Actively moves extremity; verbalizes reduced pain.

CONDITIONS OF THE ARTERIES
Arteriosclerosis and Atherosclerosis

Arteriosclerosis is an arterial disease manifested by a loss of elasticity and a hardening of the vessel wall. More commonly known as "hardening of the arteries," it is a normal part of the aging process and generally occurs uniformly throughout the arterial system.

Atherosclerosis is the most common type of arteriosclerosis, manifested by the formation of atheromas (patchy lipoidal degeneration of the intima). Lesions, or plaques, form throughout the arterial wall, reducing the size of the vessel and limiting the flow of blood. Over time, atherosclerotic lesions can completely occlude the lumen by buildup of the plaque material and may contribute to thrombus formation.

Pathophysiology and Etiology

1. Etiology thought to be a reaction to injury:
   a. Endothelial cell injury causes increased platelet and monocyte aggregation to site of injury.
   b. Smooth muscle cells migrate and proliferate.
   c. Matrix of collagen and elastic fibers forms.
2. There are two types of atherosclerotic lesions: fatty streaks and fibrous plaques (see Figure 14-4).
3. Risk factors include heredity, increasing age, male gender, cigarette smoking, hypertension, dyslipidemia, diabetes mellitus, renal disease, obesity, physical inactivity, and stress.

 NURSING ALERT Smoking is the number one risk factor for atherosclerosis.

Clinical Manifestations

1. May affect entire vascular system or one segment of the vascular tree.
2. Symptoms and signs are based on area affected:
   a. Brain (cerebroarteriosclerosis)—transient ischemic attacks (TIA); stroke; vision disturbances, such as amaurosis fugax (one type of TIA), which is described by patients as a shade over a portion of eye (see Chapter 15).
   b. Heart (coronary artery disease [CAD])—angina, MI, heart failure (see Chapter 13).
   c. GI tract (aortic occlusive disease, aortic aneurysm, and mesenteric ischemia)—abdominal pain, unintentional weight loss, lower back pain.
   d. Kidneys (renal artery stenosis)—renal insufficiency, poorly controlled hypertension.
   e. Extremities (peripheral arterial disease [PAD])—intermittent claudication (pain in a muscle associated with exercise caused by lack of oxygen to the muscle), pain at rest, tissue loss (with or without presence of infection or gangrene), embolic events.
3. Decreased or absent pulses; bruits.

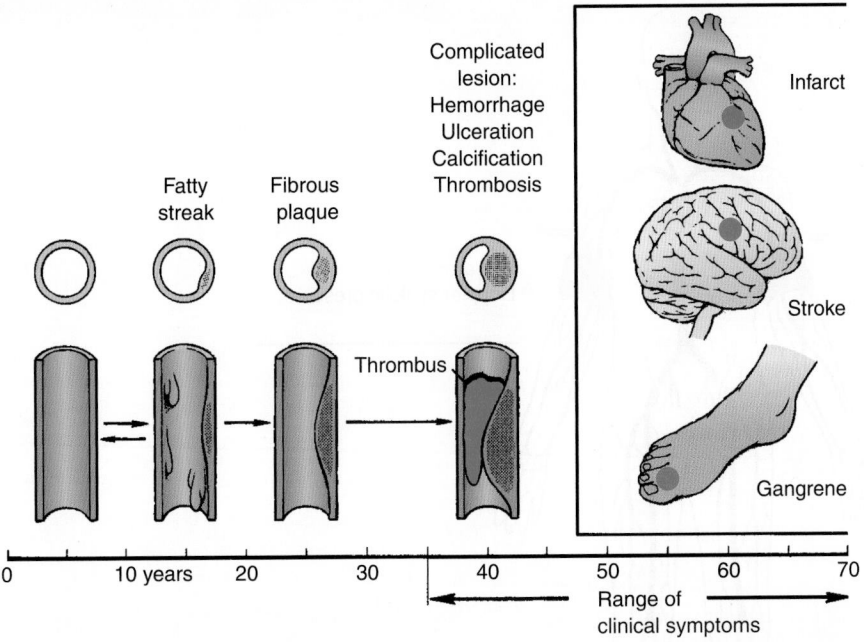

Figure 14-4. Schematic concept of the progression of atherosclerosis. Fatty streaks constitute one of the earliest lesions of atherosclerosis. Many fatty streaks regress, whereas others progress to fibrous plaques and, eventually, to atheroma, which may be complicated by hemorrhage, ulceration, calcification, or thrombosis and may produce myocardial infarction, stroke, or gangrene.

 GERONTOLOGIC ALERT Atherosclerotic cardiovascular disease afflicts 80% of the population older than age 65 and is the most common condition of the arterial system in older adults.

PAD is often undiagnosed because pain is attributed to arthritis or accepted as a normal change due to aging. It affects approximately 8 to 12 million Americans and approximately 800,000 Canadians.

Diagnostic Evaluation

Specific to body system affected:

1. Arteriography of involved area may show stenosis and increased collateral circulation.
2. Computed tomography (CT) scan.
3. Magnetic resonance imaging (MRI)/magnetic resonance angiography (MRA).
4. Noninvasive testing of the vascular system: duplex studies, sequential Doppler studies, pulse volume resistance, ankle-brachial index (ABI) (see Figure 14-5, page 452).

 Evidence Base Rooke, T. W., Hirsch, A. T., Misra, S., et al. (2011). 2011 ACCF/AHA focused update of the guideline for the management of patients with peripheral artery disease (updating the 2005 guideline). *Journal of the American College of Cardiology, 58,* 2020–2045.

5. ECG, Holter monitoring, exercise stress testing, myocardial imaging, and cardiac catheterization may be done to evaluate CAD.

Management

Medical Management

1. Modification of risk factors—stress weight loss, exercise, dietary changes, monitoring for type 2 diabetes.

2. Prescriptive management—anticoagulants, antiplatelet therapy (see Table 14-3, page 453), lipid-lowering agents, antihypertensives.
3. Specific treatment for end-organ dysfunction—see cerebrovascular insufficiency (page 497), coronary artery disease (page 380), peripheral arterial occlusive disease (page 452).
4. Vascular rehabilitation/exercise (if available).

Surgical Management

1. Endovascular procedures:
   a. PTA with or without placement of intraluminal stent—to relieve arterial stenosis when lesions are accessible, as in superficial femoral and iliac arteries, through the use of special inflatable balloon catheters and metal stents.
   b. Endovascular grafting—placement of prosthetic graft via a transluminal approach. Graft material covers a metallic stent, which may or may not be impregnated with medication to decrease failure. The stent is placed via femoral artery and is deployed. This is commonly used for abdominal aortic aneurysms, renal arteries, and iliacs.
   c. Rotational atherectomy—high-speed rotary cutter that removes lesions by abrading plaque. Benefits of this therapy are minimal damage to the normal endothelium and low incidence of complications.
   d. Laser angioplasty—amplified light waves are transmitted by fiber-optic catheters. Laser beam heats the tip of a percutaneous catheter and vaporizes the atherosclerotic plaque.
2. Surgical revascularization of the affected vessels, including:
   a. Embolectomy—removal of blood clot from the artery.
   b. Thrombectomy—removal of thrombus from the artery.
   c. Endarterectomy—removal of atherosclerotic plaque from the artery.
   d. Bypass—use of a graft, either vein graft or prosthetic material, to route blood flow around blocked area.

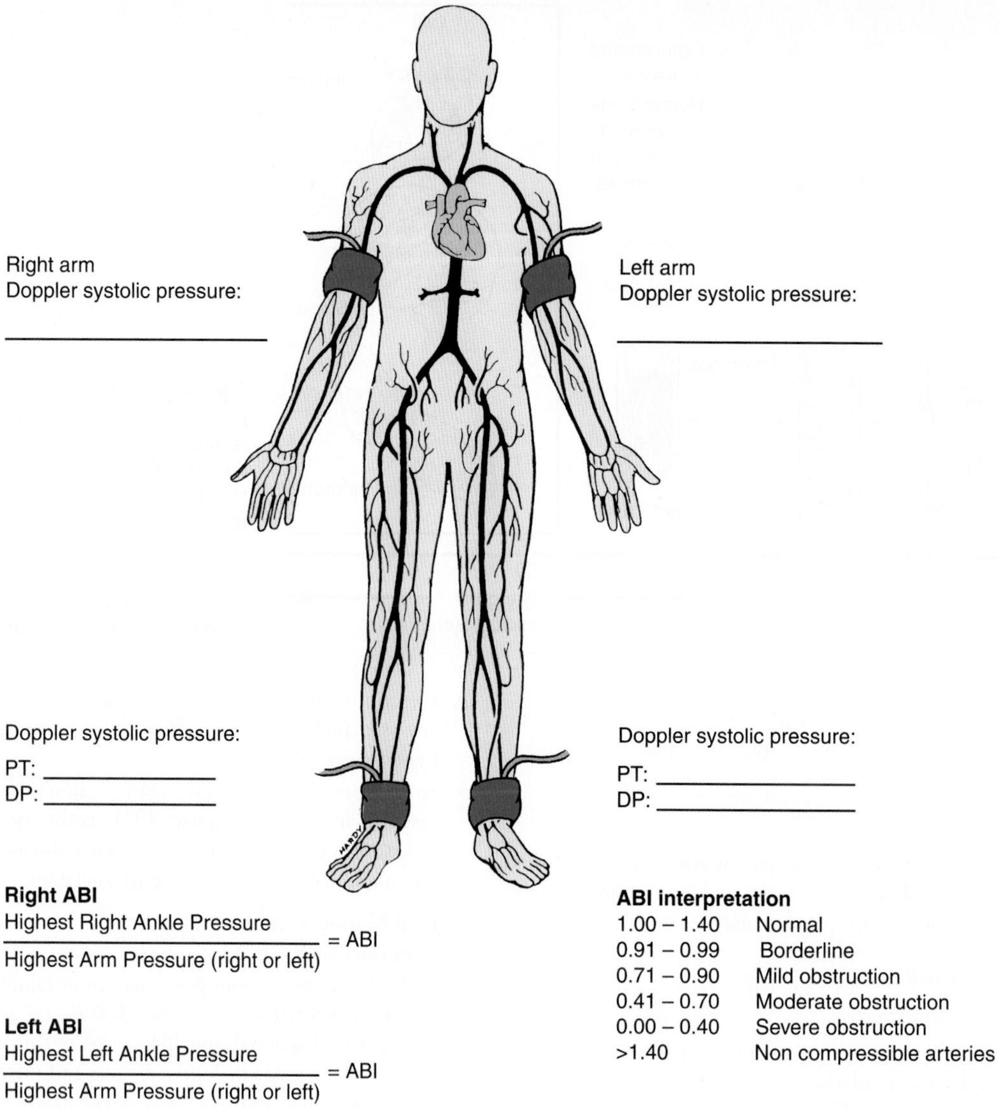

Right arm
Doppler systolic pressure:

_____

Left arm
Doppler systolic pressure:

_____

Doppler systolic pressure:

PT: _____
DP: _____

Doppler systolic pressure:

PT: _____
DP: _____

Right ABI

$$\frac{\text{Highest Right Ankle Pressure}}{\text{Highest Arm Pressure (right or left)}} = \text{ABI}$$

Left ABI

$$\frac{\text{Highest Left Ankle Pressure}}{\text{Highest Arm Pressure (right or left)}} = \text{ABI}$$

ABI interpretation

1.00 – 1.40	Normal
0.91 – 0.99	Borderline
0.71 – 0.90	Mild obstruction
0.41 – 0.70	Moderate obstruction
0.00 – 0.40	Severe obstruction
>1.40	Non compressible arteries

Figure 14-5. Determining ankle-brachial index (ABI). Pressures must be assessed using a Doppler device. PT, posterior tibial; DP, dorsalis pedis (use the higher pressure).

Complications

Long-term complications of atherosclerosis are related to the specific body system affected:

1. Brain—long- and short-term disabilities associated with stroke.
2. Heart—stable or unstable angina, MI, heart failure.
3. Aorta—ischemic bowel, aneurysms, impotence, renal failure, nephrectomy.
4. Lower extremities—intermittent claudication, nonhealing ulcers, infections or gangrene, amputation.

Nursing Interventions and Patient Education

See "Care of the Patient Undergoing Vascular Surgery," page 440. In addition, attention is directed at reducing risk factors by smoking cessation (page 32), stress reduction (page 30), weight reduction (page 31), adequate control of diabetes (Chapter 25) and/or hypertension (page 468), adjusting diet to reduce cholesterol intake (page 396) and taking lipid-lowering medications. Encourage active lifestyle to promote cardiovascular health and empower patients to manage their care.

Peripheral Arterial Occlusive Disease (Aorta and Distal Arteries)

 Evidence Base Rooke, T. W., Hirsch, A. T., Misra, S., et al. (2011). 2011 ACCF/AHA focused update of the guideline for the management of patients with peripheral artery disease (updating the 2005 guideline) *Journal of the American College of Cardiology, 58,* 2020–2045.

Table 14-3	Antiplatelet Therapy	

Antiplatelet therapy is used to prevent platelet aggregation and thrombus formation. It is used in the treatment of cerebrovascular disease, coronary artery disease, and intermittent claudication. This table lists some common antiplatelet medications, their indications, and potential contraindications/precautions.

MEDICATION	USE	CONTRAINDICATIONS/PRECAUTIONS
Aspirin	Prevention of myocardial infarction, transient ischemic attack, stroke	• Allergy to acetylsalicylic acid (ASA) • Active gastric ulcers
Ticlopidine	Prevention of stroke	• Sensitivity to drug • Neutropenia, thrombocytopenia, history of TTP, active bleeding disorders* • Liver and renal impairment • See drug–drug interactions
Ticagrelor	Decreased platelet aggregation Prevention of MI/coronary artery stent thrombosis	• Sensitivity to drug • GI and Intracranial bleeding • Liver impairment
Pentoxifylline	Treatment of intermittent claudication	• Sensitivity to drug • Recent cerebral or retinal hemorrhage • Caffeine or theophylline intolerance
Clopidogrel	Reduction of atherosclerotic events	• Sensitivity to drug • Active pathologic bleeding (eg, peptic ulcer, intracranial hemorrhage) • Severe hepatic or renal disease • See drug–drug interactions
Cilostazol	Treatment of intermittent claudication—has antiplatelet, vasodilatory, and antithrombotic effects	• Sensitivity to drug • Heart failure, liver impairment • Liver impairment • See drug–drug interactions
Dipyridamole, 200 mg; aspirin, 25 mg	Prevention of stroke	• Allergy to ASA • Active ulcer disease • Renal and hepatic impairment • Bleeding disorders • See drug–drug interactions

*Monitor complete blood count and platelet count every 2 weeks.
TTP, thrombotic thrombocytopenia.

Peripheral arterial occlusive disease (also known as peripheral artery disease or PAD) is a form of arteriosclerosis in which the peripheral arteries become blocked. Chronic occlusive arterial disease occurs much more frequently than does acute (which is the sudden and complete blocking of a vessel by a thrombus or embolus).

Pathophysiology and Etiology

Arteriosclerosis Obliterans
1. Most commonly caused by atherosclerosis with contributing factors as discussed in previous section.
2. May involve the following vessels in isolation or combination:
   a. Aortoiliac system.
   b. Femoral arteries—superficial femoral, profunda femoris.
   c. Popliteal artery.
   d. Trifurcating vessels—anterior tibial, posterior tibial, and peroneal arteries.
   e. Dorsalis pedis (DP) artery.
   f. Pedal arch.
3. Lesions tend to form at areas of bifurcation of the vessels.

4. Pattern of disease differs in nondiabetics and diabetics:
   a. Nondiabetics—disease usually involves macrocirculation (larger vessels [eg, aorta, iliac, femoral arteries]) and is more common in isolated segments.
   b. Diabetics—disease usually involves microcirculation (smaller vessels [eg, popliteal, tibial, peroneal, and small vessels in the foot/digits]) and occurs in more diffuse segments.

Thromboangiitis Obliterans (Buerger's Disease)
Inflammatory process of arterial wall, which is followed by thrombosis. Also affects adjacent veins and nerves. Associated with heavy cigarette smoking.

Clinical Manifestations
Symptoms appear gradually and are specific to the area affected.

Aortoiliac
1. Mesenteric ischemia, pain after eating that increases as disease progresses.
2. Unintentional weight loss.

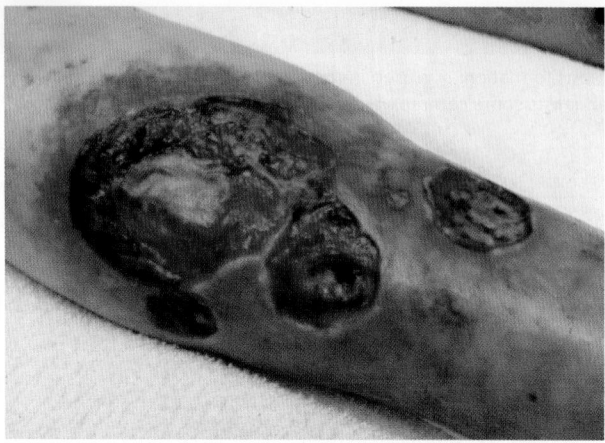

Figure 14-6. Arterial ulcer.

3. Renal insufficiency.
4. Poorly controlled hypertension.
5. Impotence.
6. Intermittent claudication (including gluteal claudication).

Femoral, Popliteal, and Distal Arteries

1. Intermittent claudication (calf, thigh, and foot).
2. Pain at rest—associated with severe arterial ischemia. Severe pain in feet aggravated by elevation of lower extremity. Pain is relieved by placing foot in dependent position.
3. Dependent rubor—dusky purple color of extremity when in dependent position; changes to pallor when elevated.
4. Numbness or tingling of feet or toes.
5. Trophic changes associated with tissue malnutrition:
   a. Hair loss.
   b. Thick toenails.
   c. Thin, shiny skin.
   d. Cool temperature of extremity.
6. Tissue loss or nonhealing ulcers, which may develop wet or dry gangrene (see Figure 14-6). Arterial ulcers are usually painful, pale, and have well-demarcated (punched-out) edges.

Diagnostic Evaluation

Noninvasive

1. Vascular physical examination.
2. ABI—comparison of systolic blood pressure (BP) in arm with that of ankle using a Doppler; may be done before and after exercise. (Normally, the systolic pressures are equal. In presence of atherosclerotic disease, the pressure below an occluded area is less than the arm pressure [see page 452].)
3. Doppler ultrasound—decreased velocity of flow through a stenotic vessel, or no flow with total occlusion.
4. Segmental plethysmography—decreased pressure distal to region of occlusion.

Invasive

1. Angiography—to confirm occlusion.
2. MRA—to confirm occlusion.
3. Spiral CT—to obtain a three-dimensional view of artery and occlusion.

Management

1. Goals:
   a. Reestablish blood flow to areas of critical ischemia.
   b. Preserve the extremity.
   c. Relieve pain associated with intermittent claudication or pain at rest.
   d. Provide sufficient blood flow for wound healing.
2. Aggressive risk factor management to prevent progression, including walking, weight reduction, smoking cessation, and control of other conditions such as hypertension, dyslipidemia, and diabetes mellitus.
3. Pharmacologic treatment with antiplatelet agents or anticoagulants to improve blood flow by increasing erythrocyte flexibility and lowering blood viscosity.
4. When conservative measures clearly are not enough, revascularization surgery (endarterectomy, arterial bypass grafting, or a combination) may be required.
5. Endovascular procedures, such as PTA with stenting, may be used alone or with revascularization surgery for dilatation of localized noncalcified segments of narrowed arteries with or without intraluminal stenting.
6. Hyperbaric oxygen therapy may be used for nonhealing wounds and gas gangrene. This is limited to centers that have a hyperbaric oxygen chamber (most commonly used for diving accidents).
   a. Increased atmospheric pressure inside the chamber combined with 100% oxygen delivery allows for greater concentration of oxygen to be delivered to all parts of the body.
   b. Typical treatment programs last 2 hours, five or six times per week for 4 weeks or more.
   c. Adverse effects include pressure or popping in ears, slight light-headedness at the end of treatment sessions, and possible temporary change in vision.
7. Amputation of affected extremity in cases of severe infection and gangrene, failed attempts at revascularization, or when revascularization is not considered a viable option.
8. See page 440 for surgical care.

Complications

1. Ulceration with slow healing.
2. Gangrene, sepsis.
3. Severe occlusion may necessitate limb or partial limb amputation.

Nursing Assessment

1. Auscultate abdomen and listen for presence of bruits.
2. Observe lower extremities for color, sensation, and temperature. Compare bilaterally for differences.
3. Palpate pulses (see Figure 14-7) and record. If pulses are nonpalpable, attempt to locate pulse with a handheld Doppler. About 10% of people have absent DP artery from birth.
4. Inspect nails for thickening and opacity; inspect skin for shiny, atrophic, hairless, and dry appearance—reflect chronic changes.

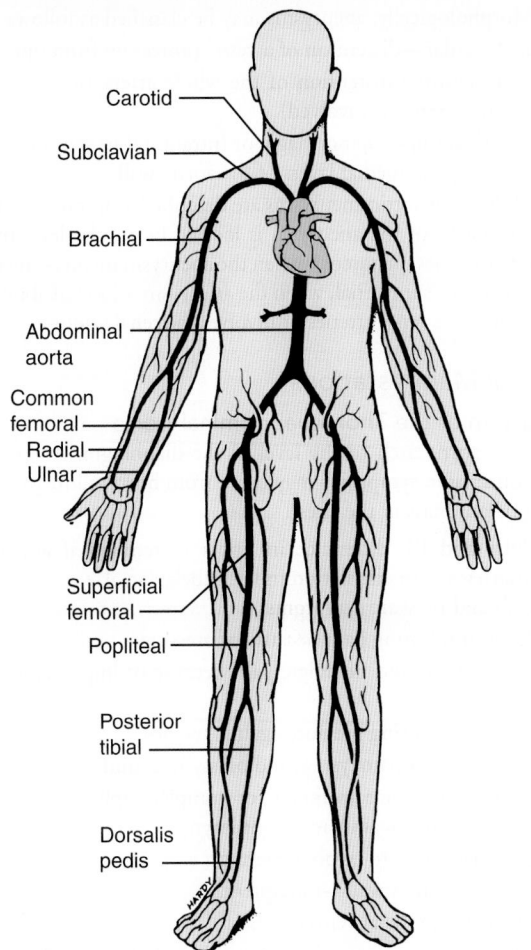

Figure 14-7. Salient points in evaluating peripheral arterial insufficiency. Reduced or absent femoral pulses indicate aortoiliac disease. Absent popliteal pulses indicate superficial femoral occlusion. Pulse deficits in one extremity, with normal pulses in the contralateral extremity, may suggest acute arterial embolus. Absent pedal pulses indicate tibioperoneal artery involvement.

Labels on figure: Carotid; Subclavian; Brachial; Abdominal aorta; Common femoral; Radial; Ulnar; Superficial femoral; Popliteal; Posterior tibial; Dorsalis pedis

5. Assess for pain:
   a. Severe abdominal pain after eating.
   b. Pain in legs with exercise.
   c. Pain in feet at rest.
6. Assess for ulcers of toes and feet.

Nursing Diagnoses

- Ineffective Peripheral Tissue Perfusion related to decreased arterial blood flow.
- Risk for Peripheral Neurovascular Dysfunction of lower extremities.
- Risk for Infection related to decreased arterial flow.

Nursing Interventions

Promoting Tissue Perfusion

1. Perform frequent neurovascular checks of affected extremity.
2. Inspect lower extremity and feet for new areas of ulceration or extension of existing ulceration.
3. Provide and encourage well-balanced diet to enhance wound healing.
4. Encourage walking or performance of ROM exercises to increase blood flow, which will increase collateral circulation.
5. Administer or teach self-administration of pain medication to achieve comfort level conducive to ambulation.

Protecting Lower Extremities

1. Encourage patient to wear protective footwear, such as rubber-soled slippers or shoes with closed, wide toe box when out of bed.
2. Instruct patient and family to keep hallways and walkways free of clutter to avoid injury.
3. Avoid tight-fitting socks and shoes.
4. Instruct patient to avoid sitting with legs crossed.
5. Avoid using adhesive tape and harsh soaps on affected skin.
6. Instruct patient to check temperature of bath water with forearm before entering tub.
7. Perform and teach foot care, including washing and carefully drying and inspecting feet daily.

Preventing Infection

1. Apply lanolin or petroleum to intact skin of lower extremities to prevent drying and cracking of skin.
2. Encourage patient to wear clean hose or socks daily: woolen socks for winter, cotton for summer.
3. Teach patient to:
   a. Trim toenails straight across after soaking the feet in warm water.
   b. Place wisps of cotton under corner of great toenail if there is a tendency toward ingrown toenails.
   c. Have a podiatrist cut corns and calluses; do not use corn pads or strong medications.
4. Teach patient signs to report:
   a. Redness, swelling, irritation, blistering, foul odor.
   b. Itching, burning; rashes.
   c. Bruises, cuts, unusual appearance of skin.
   d. New areas of ulceration.
5. Instruct patient to check with physician before using any OTC or topical lotions or creams on wound.
6. Administer antibiotics postoperatively to prevent infection around prosthetic graft material.

Patient Education and Health Maintenance

1. Instruct patient on the importance of walking to improve circulation; set up a plan for incremental increase in distance.
2. Instruct patient not to sit or stand in one position for long periods.
3. Instruct patient, when sitting, to keep knees below the level of the hips to avoid hip flexion.
4. Instruct patient to avoid tight-fitting clothing (eg, elastic-topped socks or clothing made out of Lycra/Spandex), especially over area of graft placement.
5. Instruct patient not to cross legs when sitting or lying down.
6. Instruct patient on methods to promote vasodilation by keeping extremity warm and stopping use of other vasoconstricting substances such as caffeine.
7. Instruct patient on the importance of daily foot care.

8. Encourage patient to stop smoking.
9. Encourage follow-up for control of chronic conditions and ongoing risk factor management.

Evaluation: Expected Outcomes

- No new ulcer formation.
- Verbalizes importance of wearing protective shoes and washing and inspecting feet daily.
- No signs of infection of lower extremities.

Aneurysm

An *aneurysm* is a distention of an artery brought about by a weakening/destruction of the arterial wall. They are lined with intraluminal debris, such as plaque and thrombi. Because of the high pressure in the arterial system, aneurysms can enlarge, producing complications by compressing surrounding structures; left untreated, they may rupture, causing a fatal hemorrhage. A dissection occurs when the layers of the artery become separated. Blood flows between the layers, causing further disruption of the arterial wall. Additionally, the intraluminal thrombus may totally occlude the artery, leading to acute ischemia to all arteries distal to the area of thrombosis, or they may embolize clot and/or plaque to the arteries distal to the aneurysm.

The *aorta* is the most common site for aneurysms; however, they may form in any vessel. Peripheral vessel aneurysms may involve the renal artery, subclavian artery, popliteal artery (knee), or any major artery. These produce a pulsating mass and may cause pain or pressure on surrounding structures.

Pathophysiology and Etiology

1. Aneurysms may form as the result of:
   a. Atherosclerosis.
   b. Heredity.
   c. Infection.
   d. Trauma.
   e. Immunologic conditions.
2. False aneurysms (pseudoaneurysm) are associated with trauma to the arterial wall, as in blunt trauma or trauma associated with arterial punctures for angiography and/or cardiac catheterization.
3. The ascending aorta and the aortic arch are the sites of greatest hemodynamic stress and also are the most common sites of arterial dissection.
4. Contributing factors include:
   a. Hypertension.
   b. Arteriosclerosis.
   c. Local infection, pyogenic or fungal (mycotic aneurysm).
   d. Congenital weakness of vessels.
   e. Syphilis.
   f. Trauma.

 GERONTOLOGIC ALERT Because of vascular changes that occur as a natural process of aging, all patients over age 65 are assessed for the potential for aneurysms.

5. Morphologically, aneurysms may be classified as follows:
   a. Saccular—distention of a vessel projecting from one side.
   b. Fusiform—distention of the whole artery (ie, entire circumference is involved).
   c. Dissecting—hemorrhagic or intramural hematoma, separating the medial layers of the aortic wall.
6. Abdominal aortic aneurysms are described as infrarenal, when the "neck" of the aneurysm is located below the level of the renal arteries, juxtarenal, when the aneurysm involves the renal arteries, or suprarenal, when the aneurysm is located above the level of the renal arteries or involves the renal arteries.

Clinical Manifestations

Aneurysm of the Thoracoabdominal Aorta

From the aortic arch to the level of the diaphragm. At first, no symptoms; later, symptoms may come from heart failure or a pulsating tumor mass in the chest.

1. Pulse and BP difference in upper extremities if aneurysm interferes with circulation in left subclavian artery.
2. Pain and pressure symptoms.
3. Constant, boring pain because of pressure.
4. Intermittent and neuralgic pain because of impingement on nerves.
5. Dyspnea, causing pressure against trachea.
6. Cough, often paroxysmal and brassy in sound.
7. Hoarseness, voice weakness, or complete aphonia, resulting from pressure against recurrent laryngeal nerve.
8. Dysphagia due to impingement on esophagus.
9. Edema of chest wall—infrequent.
10. Dilated superficial veins on chest.
11. Cyanosis because of vein compression of chest vessels.
12. Ipsilateral dilation of pupils due to pressure against cervical sympathetic chain.
13. Abnormal pulsation apparent on chest wall, due to erosion of aneurysm through rib cage—in syphilis.

Abdominal Aneurysm

1. Many of these patients asymptomatic.
2. Abdominal pain most common, either persistent or intermittent—often localized in middle or lower abdomen to the left of midline.
3. Lower back pain caused by pressure on the spine from enlarging aneurysm.
4. Feeling of an abdominal pulsating mass, palpated as a thrill, auscultated as a bruit.
5. Hypertension.
6. Distal variability of BP, pressure in arm greater than thigh.
7. Upon rupture, will present with hypotension and/or hypovolemic shock.

 GERONTOLOGIC ALERT Most abdominal aneurysms occur between ages 60 and 90. Rupture of the aneurysm is likely if there is coexistent hypertension or if the aneurysm is larger than 2.4 inches (5.5 to 6 cm).

Diagnostic Evaluation

1. Abdominal or chest x-ray may show calcification that outlines aneurysm.
2. CT scanning and ultrasonography are used to detect and monitor size of aneurysm.
3. MRI/MRA.
4. Spiral CT gives three-dimensional view of the aneurysm and any attendant atherosclerosis.
5. Arteriography allows visualization of aneurysm and vessel.

Management

1. May follow small aneurysms (1.6 inches [4 cm] or less) with CT scanning or ultrasound every 6 months and aggressively control BP.
2. The prognosis is poor for untreated patients as aneurysm enlarges. It is especially true if it enlarges 5 mm in 3 months or in patients with chronic obstructive pulmonary disease.
3. Surgery:
   a. Resection of the aneurysm via abdominal incision and placement of a prosthetic graft to restore vascular continuity.
   b. Endovascular grafting involves repair of aneurysm using a stent graft, which is deployed via the femoral artery. It attaches above and below the aneurysm and provides a new channel for the blood.
   c. Thoracic aneurysms are the most difficult to treat and require use of atrial–femoral circulatory bypass intraoperatively.

Complications

1. Fatal hemorrhage.
2. Myocardial ischemia.
3. Stroke.
4. Paraplegia due to interruption of anterior spinal artery.
5. Abdominal ischemia.
6. Ileus.
7. Graft occlusion.
8. Graft infections.
9. Acute renal failure.
10. Impotence.
11. Lower-extremity ischemia.
12. "Trash toes"—results from distal embolization of plaque and blood clots.

Nursing Assessment

1. In patient with thoracoabdominal aortic aneurysm, be alert for sudden onset of sharp, ripping, or tearing pain located in anterior chest, epigastric area, shoulders, or back, indicating acute dissection or rupture.
2. In patients with abdominal aortic aneurysm, assess for abdominal (particularly left lower quadrant) pain and intense lower back pain caused by rapid expansion. Be alert for syncope, tachycardia, and hypotension, which may be followed by fatal hemorrhage due to rupture.

Nursing Diagnoses

- Risk for Ineffective Gastrointestinal, Renal, Cardiac, Cerebral Tissue Perfusion (vital organs) related to aneurysm or aneurysm rupture or dissection.
- Risk for Infection related to surgery.
- Acute Pain related to pressure of aneurysm on nerves and postoperatively.

Nursing Interventions

Maintaining Perfusion of Vital Organs

Preoperatively:

1. Assess for chest pain and abdominal pain.
2. Prepare patient for diagnostic studies or surgery, as indicated.
3. Monitor for signs and symptoms of hypovolemic shock.
4. Perform mental status and neurologic assessment regularly.

Postoperatively:

1. Monitor vital signs frequently.
2. Assess for signs and symptoms of bleeding:
   a. Hypotension.
   b. Tachycardia.
   c. Tachypnea.
   d. Diaphoresis.
3. Monitor laboratory values, as ordered.
4. Monitor urine output hourly.
5. Assess abdomen for bowel sounds and distention. Observe for diarrhea, which occurs sooner than one would expect bowel function.
6. Perform neurovascular checks to distal extremities.
7. Assess feet for signs and symptoms of embolization:
   a. Cold feet.
   b. Cyanotic toes or patchy blue areas on plantar surface of feet.
   c. Pain in feet.
8. Maintain IV infusion to administer medications to control BP and provide fluids postoperatively.
9. Position patient to avoid hip flexion, keeping knees below the level of the hips when sitting in chair.
10. If thoracoabdominal aneurysm repair has been performed, monitor for signs and symptoms of spinal cord ischemia:
    a. Pain.
    b. Numbness.
    c. Paresthesia.
    d. Weakness.

Preventing Infection

1. Monitor temperature.
2. Monitor changes in WBC count.
3. Monitor incision for signs of infection.
4. Administer antibiotics, if ordered, to prevent bacterial seeding of the graft.

Relieving Pain

1. Administer pain medication, as ordered, or monitor patient-controlled analgesia.
2. Keep head of bed elevated no more than 45 degrees for the first 3 days postoperatively to prevent pressure on incision site.

3. Rarely—administer nasogastric decompression for ileus following surgery, until bowel sounds return.

4. Assess abdomen for bowel sounds and distention.

Patient Education and Health Maintenance

1. Instruct patient about medications to control BP and the importance of taking them.

2. Discuss disease process and signs and symptoms of expanding aneurysm or impending rupture, or rupture, to be reported.

3. For postsurgical patients, discuss warning signs of postoperative complications (fever, inflammation of operative site, bleeding, and swelling).

4. Encourage adequate balanced intake for wound healing.

5. Encourage patient to maintain an exercise schedule postoperatively.

6. Instruct patient that due to use of a prosthetic graft to repair the aneurysm, prophylactic antibiotics will be used for invasive procedures, including routine dental examinations and dental cleaning for 6 to 12 months after aneurysm repair.

7. Make all patients aware that a one-time screening for abdominal aortic aneurysm by ultrasound has been recommended for men ages 65 to 75 who ever smoked. If the patient has an aortic aneurysm, members of the family over age 55 should be screened with ultrasound to rule out abdominal aortic aneurysm, both male and female.

 Evidence Base U.S. Preventive Taskforce. (Revised 2010). Guide to clinical preventive services: Screening for abdominal aortic aneurysm. Available: www.ahrq.gov/clinic/pocketgd1011/gcp10s2a.htm#Abdominal.

Evaluation: Expected Outcomes

- No change in mental status, bowel sounds, vital signs, or urine output.
- Afebrile, no signs of infection.
- Reports control of pain with medication.

Acute Arterial Occlusion

Acute arterial occlusion is the sudden interruption of blood flow, which may cause complete or partial obstruction of the artery. There is no time for development of collateral circulation. Critical ischemia of the extremity develops and may result in loss of affected extremity and/or death.

Pathophysiology and Etiology

1. Embolization is the most common cause of acute arterial occlusion.

2. Emboli may consist of thrombus, atheromatous debris, or tumor.

3. Emboli most commonly originate in the heart as a result of atrial fibrillation, MI, or heart failure (about 85%), but can also occur after invasive procedures, such as cardiac catheterization, angiography, and surgery.

4. Arteriosclerosis may cause roughening or ulceration of atheromatous plaques, which can lead to emboli.

5. May also be associated with immobility, anemia, and dehydration.

6. Emboli tend to lodge at bifurcations and atherosclerotic narrowings.

7. Other causes of acute occlusion include:
   a. Trauma.
   b. Thrombus.
   c. Venous outflow obstruction, which includes compartment syndrome.

Clinical Manifestations

1. The patient may experience acute pain and loss of sensory and motor function due to emboli blocking the artery and associated vasomotor reflex.
   a. Paralysis of part.
   b. Anesthesia of part.
   c. Pallor and coldness.
   d. Edema.
   e. Rigidity of extremity.
   f. Pulselessness.

Diagnostic Evaluation

1. Neurovascular assessment of affected area.

2. Doppler ultrasonography, segmental limb pressure, and pulse volume recordings—may indicate decreased flow.

3. Radionuclide scan—may identify clot.

4. Arteriography—confirms diagnosis.

5. MRA or spiral CT—to confirm diagnosis and give a three-dimensional view of the area.

6. Digital subtraction angiography, MRA, and MRI may be done for cerebral embolization.

Management

1. Drug therapy—anticoagulants (see page 436), thrombolytics (see page 439).

2. Surgery:
   a. Embolectomy (see Figure 14-8) must be performed within 6 to 10 hours to prevent muscle necrosis and loss of extremity.
   b. Fasciotomy—incisions made over leg compartments to aid expansion of edematous tissue and relief of pressure on the arterial system.
   c. Amputation of affected limb if revascularization is inappropriate due to metabolic complications.

3. Treatment of shock.

4. Bed rest.

 NURSING ALERT Arterial embolization of a large artery, such as the iliac, and that has major systemic effects, is life-threatening and requires emergency operative intervention.

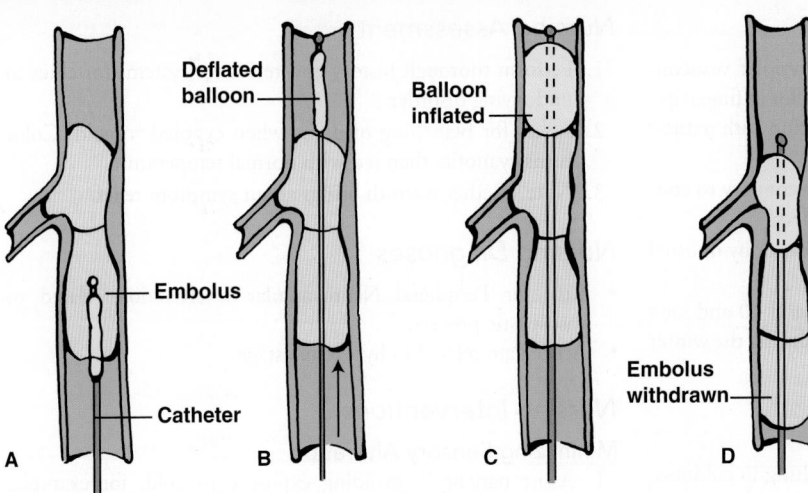

Figure 14-8. Extracting an embolus from a vessel can be done with the use of a Fogarty embolectomy catheter. The catheter, with a soft, deflated balloon near the tip, is threaded through the artery via an arteriotomy. **(A, B)** It is passed through the embolus and its thrombus; **(C)** it is then inflated. **(D)** A steady pull downward withdraws the embolus along with the catheter.

Complications

1. Irreversible ischemia and loss of extremity.
2. Metabolic complications:
   a. Acidosis.
   b. Hyperkalemia.
   c. Renal failure.
3. Shock.

Nursing Assessment

1. Assess for acute, severe pain.
2. Assess for gradual or acute loss of sensory and motor function.
3. Check for aggravation of pain by movement of and pressure on the extremity.
4. Palpate for loss of distal pulses.
5. Inspect for pale, mottled, and numb extremity.
6. Inspect for collapse of superficial veins due to decreased blood flow to the extremity.
7. Inspect for sharp line of color and temperature demarcation. This may occur distal to the site of occlusion as a result of ischemia.
8. Assess for edema.

Nursing Diagnoses

- Impaired Comfort related to impaired blood supply.
- Ineffective Peripheral Tissue Perfusion related to lack of blood flow by clot.
- Risk for Infection related to surgery.

Nursing Interventions

Protecting the Extremity

1. Protect extremity by keeping it at or below the body's horizontal plane.
2. Protect leg from hard surfaces, tight or heavy surfaces, and tight or heavy overlying bed linens.
3. Handle extremity gently and prevent pressure or friction while repositioning.
4. Administer pain medications, as ordered.

Promoting Tissue Perfusion

1. Administer UFH IV line to reduce tendency of emboli to form or expand (useful in smaller arteries).
2. Monitor thrombolytic therapy IV line to dissolve clot, as ordered.
3. Monitor patient for signs of bleeding (gums, urine, stool).
4. Monitor coagulation, hematology, and electrolyte studies.
5. Prepare the patient for surgery (see page 440).
6. Postoperatively, promote movement of extremity to stimulate circulation and prevent stasis.

Preventing Infection

1. Postoperatively, check surgical wound for bleeding, swelling, erythema, and discharge.
2. Maintain IV infusion or venous access device to administer IV antibiotics, if indicated.
3. Continue to monitor the patient for tachycardia, fever, pain, erythema, warmth, swelling, and drainage at incision site.

Patient Education and Health Maintenance

1. Teach prevention techniques, such as daily aerobic activity, observation for skin breakdown, and prevention of injury.
2. Teach patient the medical regimen and importance of taking prescribed medications, such as oral anticoagulants, to prevent reembolization (see page 436).
3. Encourage patient to report symptoms of arterial occlusion: paralysis, numbness, tingling, pallor, and coldness of extremity.

Evaluation: Expected Outcomes

- Patient reports no pain; no injury noted.
- Limb has normal color, sensation, movement, and temperature.
- No signs of infection.

Vasospastic Disorder (Raynaud's Phenomenon)

Raynaud's phenomenon or syndrome is a vasospastic disorder that is brought on by an unusual sensitivity to cold, emotional stress, or autoimmune disorders.

Pathophysiology and Etiology

1. The condition is a form of intermittent arteriolar vasoconstriction that results in coldness, pain, and pallor of fingertips, toes, or tip of the nose and a rebound circulation with redness and pain.
2. The cause is unknown, although it may be secondary to connective tissue and other immunologic disorders.
3. Episodes may be triggered by emotional factors or by unusual sensitivity to cold.
4. Most common in women between ages 16 and 40 and seen much more commonly in cold climates and during the winter months.

Clinical Manifestations

1. Intermittent arteriolar vasoconstriction resulting in coldness, pain, pallor.
2. Involvement of the fingers appears to be asymmetric; thumbs are less often involved.
3. Characteristic color changes: white–blue–red.
   a. White—blanching, dead-white appearance if spasm is severe.
   b. Blue—cyanotic, relatively stagnant blood flow.
   c. Red—a reactive hyperemia on rewarming.
4. Occasionally, there is ulceration of the fingertips (most common in autoimmune disorders).

Diagnostic Evaluation

1. Clinical symptoms must last at least 2 years to confirm the diagnosis.
2. Tests may be done to rule out secondary disease processes, such as chronic arterial occlusive or connective tissue disease.
3. Noninvasive blood flow tests for finger pressures and arterial waveforms.

Management

1. Avoidance of trigger and aggravating factors.
2. Protection of the fingers and toes with warm mittens (not gloves) and warm boots in cold weather.
3. Longer-acting calcium channel blockers are frequently used to prevent or reduce vasospasm.
4. Nitroglycerin or sympatholytics, such as reserpine, guanethidine, or prazosin, may be helpful for some. Adverse effects, such as headache, dizziness, and orthostatic hypotension, may be prohibitive.
5. Antiplatelet agents, such as aspirin or dipyridamole, may be given to prevent total occlusion.
6. Sympathectomy—removal of the sympathetic ganglia or division of their branches; may offer some improvement (extremely rare).

Complications

1. Chronic disease may cause atrophy of skin and muscles.
2. Ulceration and gangrene (rare).

Nursing Assessment

1. Perform thorough history and review of systems for clues to underlying disorder.
2. Assess for blanching of digits when exposed to cold. Color turns cyanotic, then red with normal temperature.
3. Note whether warmth brings about symptom relief.

Nursing Diagnoses

- Risk for Peripheral Neurovascular Dysfunction related to vasospastic process.
- Acute Pain related to hyperemic stage.

Nursing Interventions

Minimizing Sensory Alteration

1. Assist patient in avoiding exposure to cold; for example, use mittens to handle cold items (water pitcher, refrigerated items). Always wear mittens outside in the cold. Teach patient rewarming techniques—warm water, putting fingers in axillary or groin area.
2. Encourage patient to stop smoking.
3. Help patient to understand the need to avoid stressful situations.
4. Offer patient options for stress management.
5. Administer and teach patient about drug therapy.
6. Instruct patient about the need to take drugs every day to prevent or minimize symptoms.
7. Monitor for orthostatic hypotension precaution if taking sympatholytics.
8. Advise patient that episode may be terminated by placing hands (or feet) in warm water.

Relieving Pain

1. Explain to patient that pain may be experienced when spasm is relieved—hyperemic phase.
2. Administer or teach self-administration of analgesics.
3. Reassure patient that pain is temporary; persistent pain, ulceration, or signs of infection should be reported.

Patient Education and Health Maintenance

1. Avoid whatever provokes vasoconstriction of vessels of hands.
2. Prevent injury to hands, which can aggravate vasoconstriction and lead to ulceration.
3. Minimize exposure to cold because this precipitates a reaction. Avoid wet and windy environments.
4. Wear warm clothing—boots, mittens, and hooded jackets—when going out in cold weather and waterproof clothing when raining or snowing.
5. Avoid placing hands in cold water, the freezer, or the refrigerator unless protective mittens are worn.
6. Use extra precautions to avoid injuries to fingers and hands from needlesticks and knife cuts.

Evaluation: Expected Outcomes

- Follows medication regimen, avoiding triggers.
- Reports decreased length of painful phase with episodes.

HYPERTENSIVE DISORDERS
Hypertension

 Evidence Base Aronow, W. S., Fleg, J. L., Pepine, C. J., et al. (2011). ACCF/AHA 2011 expert consensus document on hypertension in the elderly: A report of the American College of Cardiology Foundation Task Force on Clinical Expert Consensus Documents. *Circulation, 123,* 24342506.

Joint National Committee on Prevention, Detention, Evaluation, and Treatment of High Blood Pressure. (2003). The seventh report of the Joint National Committee on Prevention, Detection, Evaluation, and Treatment of High Blood Pressure (JNC VII). Available: *www.nhlbi.nih.gov/guidelines/hypertension/jncintro.htm.*

Note: JNC VIII guideline development was delayed and not available at the time of printing.

Table 14-4	Classification of Blood Pressure for Adults	
BLOOD PRESSURE (BP) CLASSIFICATION	**SBP* (mm Hg)**	**DBP* (mm Hg)**
Normal	<120	and <80
Prehypertension	120–139	or 80–89
Stage 1 hypertension	140–159	or 90–99
Stage 2 hypertension	≥160	or ≥100

*Treatment determined by highest BP category.
Joint National Committee on Prevention, Detention, Evaluation, and Treatment of High Blood Pressure. (2003). The seventh report of the Joint National Committee on Prevention, Detection, Evaluation, and Treatment of High Blood Pressure (JNC VII). Available: www.nhlbi.nih.gov/guidelines/hypertension/jncintro.htm.
DBP, diastolic blood pressure; SBP, systolic blood pressure.

The American Heart Association defines *blood pressure* (BP) as the force of blood pushing against the arterial wall as it relates to blood viscosity (thickness) and resistance of blood vessel. Systolic blood pressure (SBP) is the highest arterial pressure when the heart contracts and empties. Diastolic blood pressure (DBP) is the lowest arterial pressure when the heart relaxes to fill with blood. *Hypertension* (high BP) is a disease of vascular regulation in which the mechanisms that control arterial pressure within the normal range are altered. The predominant mechanisms of blood pressure control are the central nervous system (CNS), the renin-angiotensin-aldosterone system, and extracellular fluid volume. Why these mechanisms fail is not known.

Pathophysiology and Etiology

Elevated diastolic pressure leads to strain on the arterial wall which over time causes thickening and calcification of the arterial media (a condition called sclerosis) and eventually narrowing of the blood vessel lumen. Elevated blood pressure is seen when there is increased cardiac output and increased peripheral resistance.

Primary or Essential Hypertension
(Approximately 95% of patients with hypertension.)

1. When the diastolic pressure is 90 mm Hg and/or the systolic pressure is 140 mm Hg or higher and other causes of hypertension are absent, the condition is said to be primary hypertension. More specifically, an individual is considered hypertensive when the average of two or more properly measured, seated BP readings taken at rest on each of two or more office visits exceeds the upper limits of normal (see Table 14-4).
2. Cause of essential hypertension is unknown; however, there are several areas of investigation:
   a. Hyperactivity of sympathetic vasoconstricting nerves.
   b. Presence of vasoactive substance released from the arterial endothelial cells, which acts on smooth muscle, sensitizing it to vasoconstriction.
   c. Increased cardiac output, followed by arteriole constriction.
   d. Excessive dietary sodium intake, sodium retention, insulin resistance, and hyperinsulinemia play roles that are not

clear. There is a growing body of evidence implicating excess sodium intake in the pathogenesis of elevated BP.
   e. Familial (genetic) tendency.
3. Systolic BP elevation in the absence of elevated diastolic BP is termed isolated systolic hypertension and is treated in the same manner.

Secondary Hypertension

1. Occurs in approximately 5% of patients with hypertension secondary to other pathology.
2. Renal pathology:
   a. Chronic kidney disease, congenital anomalies, pyelonephritis, renal artery stenosis, acute and chronic glomerulonephritis, and obstructive uropathy (hydronephrosis).
   b. Reduced blood flow to kidney causes release of renin. Renin reacts with a serum protein to form angiotensin I, which is converted to angiotenin II through the action of angiotensin-converting enzyme in the lungs, leading to vasoconstriction and increased salt and water retention.
3. Coarctation of aorta (stenosis of aorta)—blood flow to upper extremities is greater than flow to the kidneys. The kidneys release renin when they sense hypotension.
4. Endocrine disturbances:
   a. Pheochromocytoma—a tumor of the adrenal gland that causes release of epinephrine and norepinephrine and a rise in BP (extremely rare).
   b. Adrenal cortex tumors lead to an increase in aldosterone secretion (hyperaldosteronism) and an elevated BP (rare).
   c. Cushing's syndrome leads to an increase in adrenocortical steroids (causing sodium and fluid retention) and hypertension.
   d. Hyperthyroidism causes increased cardiac output.
5. Obstructive sleep apnea causes nocturnal hypertension, which leads to sustained daytime hypertension.
6. Prescription medications such as estrogens and steroids (cause fluid retention), sympathomimetics (cause vasoconstriction

and tachycardia), antidepressants (prevent the breakdown of epinephrine), appetite suppressants (cause tachycardia and vasoconstriction), and NSAIDs (cause fluid retention and can lead to renal insufficiency).

7. Nonprescription drugs and substances such as cocaine (cause vasoconstriction and tachycardia); NSAIDS; herbal agents such as St. John's wort, ginseng, ephedra (unclear etiology of hypertension); antihistamines (cause vasoconstriction and tachycardia); and nicotine (causes vasoconstriction).

8. Food substrates such as sodium chloride, ethanol, licorice, and glucose, all of which can cause increased fluid retention.

Consequences of Hypertension

1. Hypertension can cause intimal wall injury in the arteries, which can lead to arteriosclerosis in which smooth muscle cell proliferation, lipid infiltration, and calcium accumulation occur in the vascular endothelium.

2. Prolonged hypertension damages small blood vessels in the brain, eyes, heart, and kidneys.

3. The major objective in patients with high BP is to prevent target organ damage of the heart (left ventricular hypertrophy, angina, myocardial infarction, heart failure), brain (stroke, transient ischemic attack, dementia), kidneys (chronic kidney disease), eyes (retinopathy, blindness), or vasculature (aneurysm, peripheral arterial disease).

4. The Heart Disease and Stroke Statistics 2011 Update reported that compared to individuals with normal BP (120/80 mm Hg), those patients with prehypertension have a 1.5- to 2-fold risk for major cardiovascular events between the ages 60 to 80 years. Also, approximately 69% of people who have a first heart attack, 77% of those who have a first stroke, and 74% of those who have heart failure had BP of at least 140/90 mm Hg.

Prevalence and Risk Factors

Evidence Base Aronow, W. S., Fleg, J. L., Pepine, C. J., et al. (2011). ACCF/AHA 2011 expert consensus document on hypertension in the elderly: A report of the American College of Cardiology Foundation Task Force on Clinical Expert Consensus Documents. *Circulation, 123,* 2434–2506.

Rogers,V., Adams, R., Carnethon, R., et al. (2011). Heart disease and stroke statistics—2011 update. *Circulation, 123,* e18–e209.

1. Hypertension affects approximately 1 billion people worldwide and is the most common modifiable risk factor for arteriosclerosis.

2. There are an estimated 68 million Americans with hypertension (about 31% of the adult population), and this number is expected to increase due to the aging of the population. Only a fraction of these people are aware of their hypertension and are treated for it, and even fewer have gained adequate control of their BP.

3. The National Health and Nutrition Examination Surveys (NHANES), designed to monitor the health and nutritional status of the civilian U.S. population, showed that among U.S. adults with high blood pressure, the percentage of individuals with hypertension who were aware of their

condition increased from 69.6% in 1999–2000 to 80.6% in 2007–2008. The number of individuals who take antihypertensive medications and attained control of their blood pressure also increased during this period.

4. Risk factors include age between 30 and 70, African American race, overweight or obese, sleep apnea, family history, tobacco use, sedentary lifestyle, diabetes mellitus, metabolic syndrome, lower education/socioeconomic status, psychological stressors, and dietary factors (increased consumption of fats, sodium, and alcohol, with lower intake of potassium-rich foods.

 NURSING ALERT There is a higher incidence of hypertension in the African American population, along with higher mortality rate and risk for complications such as stroke, left ventricular hypertrophy, heart failure, and kidney disease.

Clinical Manifestations

1. Usually asymptomatic; known as the silent killer.

2. May cause headache, dizziness, blurred vision, chest pain, and shortness of breath when greatly elevated.

3. Elevated BP readings taken in a seated position on at least two occasions.

Diagnostic Evaluation

1. ECG—to determine effects of hypertension on the heart (left ventricular hypertrophy, ischemia) or presence of underlying heart disease.

2. Chest x-ray—may show cardiomegaly or aortic dilation by the presence of a widened mediastinum.

3. Proteinuria, elevated serum blood urea nitrogen (BUN), and creatinine levels—indicate kidney disease as a cause or effect of hypertension; first voided urine microalbumin or spot urine for albumin–creatinine ratio are earlier indicators.

4. Serum potassium—decreased in primary hyperaldosteronism; elevated in Cushing's syndrome, both are causes of secondary hypertension.

5. Urine (24-hour) for catecholamines—increased in pheochromocytoma.

6. Renal ultrasound to detect renal vascular diseases.

7. Renal artery duplex imaging to identify renal artery stenosis.

8. Outpatient ambulatory BP measurements.

9. Tests for causes of secondary hypertension are done if hypertension is resistant to treatment or specific signs and symptoms of secondary hypertension are present.

Management

Blood Pressure Target Goals

1. Blood pressure goals are based on research and published guidelines and/or consensus statements. Clinicians must be aware of their patients' target BP goals.

2. Guidelines from the 7th Report of the Joint National Commission (JNC-7):
   a. BP goals for all patients are <140/90 mm Hg.
   b. BP goals for patients with diabetes and chronic kidney disease are <130/80 mmHg.

Table 14-5 Lifestyle Modifications to Manage Hypertension*†

MODIFICATION	RECOMMENDATION	APPROXIMATE SBP REDUCTION (RANGE)
Weight reduction	Maintain normal body weight (body mass index 18.5–24.9 kg/m²).	5–20 mmHg/10 kg weight loss
Adopt DASH eating plan	Consume a diet rich in fruits, vegetables, and low-fat dairy products with a reduced content of saturated and total fat.	8–14 mmHg
Dietary sodium reduction	Reduce dietary sodium intake to no more than 100 mmol per day (2.4 g sodium or 6 g sodium chloride).	2–8 mmHg
Physical activity	Engage in regular aerobic physical activity such as brisk walking (at least 30 minutes per day, most days of the week).	4–9 mmHg
Moderation of alcohol	Limit consumption to no more than two drinks (1 oz or 30 mL ethanol; eg, 24 oz beer, 10 oz wine, or 3 oz 80-proof whiskey) per day in most men and to no more than one drink per day in women and lighter-weight persons.	2–4 mmHg

*For overall cardiovascular risk reduction, stop smoking.
†The effects of implementing these modifications are dose and time dependent, and could be greater for some individuals.
From Joint National Committee on Prevention, Detention, Evaluation, and Treatment of High Blood Pressure. (2003). The seventh report of the Joint National Committee on Prevention, Detection, Evaluation, and Treatment of High Blood Pressure (JNC VII). Available: www.nhlbi.nih.gov/guidelines/hypertension/jncintro.htm.
DASH, Dietary Approaches to Stop Hypertension.

3. Guidelines from the American Heart Association:
   a. Individuals with ischemic heart disease, CAD equivalents, and high risk for CAD have a target BP goal of <130/80 mmHg.
   b. If the patient has LV dysfunction, the target BP is < 120/80 mmHg.
4. Guidelines from the American Diabetes Association indicate that individuals with diabetes should have a target BP of < 130/80 mmHg.

Lifestyle Modifications

Lifestyle modifications reduce BP, prevent or delay the incidence of hypertension, enhance antihypertensive drug therapy, and decrease cardiovascular risk (see Table 14-5).

If, despite lifestyle changes, BP remains at or above 140/90 mm Hg (or is not at optimal level in the presence of other cardiovascular risk factors) over 3 to 6 months, drug therapy should be initiated. If BP is extremely elevated or in presence of cardiovascular risk factors, single-drug therapy may be initiated.

Drug Therapy

See Table 14-6, pages 464 to 466.

1. Considerations in selecting therapy include:
   a. Race—African Americans respond well to calcium channel blockers and thiazide diuretics, if compelling conditions are not noted. A renin–angiotensin system (RAS blocker is first line for African Americans with kidney disease, diabetes, or heart failure. Caucasians respond well to ACE inhibitors).
   b. Age—some adverse effects such as fatigue and lightheadedness may not be tolerated well by older adults. Diuretics are typically the first drug prescribed.
   c. Concomitant diseases and therapies—some agents also treat migraines, benign prostatic hyperplasia, heart failure; have beneficial effects on conditions such as renal insufficiency; or have adverse effects on such conditions as diabetes or asthma.
   d. Quality-of-life impact—tolerance of adverse effects.
   e. Cost considerations—newer agents usually more expensive.
   f. Dosing—multiple doses may be adherence issue.
2. Medications available:
   a. Diuretics—lower BP by promoting urinary excretion of water and sodium to lower blood volume.
   b. Beta-adrenergic blockers—lower BP by slowing the heart and reducing cardiac output by blocking beta adrenergic receptors that produce epinephrine.
   c. Alpha-receptor blockers—lower BP by dilating peripheral blood vessels and lowering peripheral vascular resistance. Research has indicated these medications provide little protection against heart failure but are effective in improving benign prosthetic hypertrophy.
   d. Central alpha agonists—lower BP by diminishing sympathetic outflow from the central nervous system, thereby lowering peripheral resistance.
   e. Peripheral adrenergic agents—inhibit peripheral adrenergic release of vasoconstricting catecholamines such as norepinephrine.
   f. Combined alpha and beta-adrenergic blockers—work through alpha and beta receptors.

Table 14-6   Oral Antihypertensive Drugs

CLASS	DRUG (TRADE NAME)	USUAL DOSE RANGE IN MG/DAY** (DAILY FREQUENCY)	SELECTED ADVERSE EFFECTS
Thiazide diuretics	chlorothiazide (Diuril)	500–1,000 (1–2)	Decreased potassium, sodium, magnesium; increased uric acid, calcium, glucose, cholesterol, and triglycerides. Can cause metabolic acidosis.
	chlorthalidone	12.5–25 (1)	
	hydrochlorothiazide (Microzide, HydroDI-URIL)	12.5–50 (1)	
	indapamide (Lozol)	1.25–5 (1)	
	metolazone (Zaroxolyn)	2.5–5 (1)	
Loop diuretics	bumetanide (Bumex)	0.5–2 (2–3)	Decreased potassium, sodium, and magnesium. Can cause metabolic alkalosis. At higher doses, can cause ototoxicity.
	Ethacrynic acid (Edecrin)	50 (1)	
	furosemide (Lasix)	20–80 (1–2)	
	torsemide (Demadex)	5 –10 (1)	
Potassium-sparing diuretics	amiloride (Midamor)	5–10 (1–2)	Hyperkalemia
	eplerenone (Inspra)	50–100 (1–2)	
	spironolactone (Aldactone)	50–100 (1–2)	Hyperkalemia, gynecomastia
	triamterene (Dyrenium)	50-100 (1–2)	
Beta-adrenergic blockers	atenolol (Tenormin)	25–100 (1)	Bronchospasm, bradycardia, heart failure, fatigue, hypertriglyceridemia; may mask hypoglycemia
	betaxolol (Kerlone)	5–20 (1)	
	bisoprolol (Zebeta)	5 – 20 (1)	
	metoprolol tartrate (Lopressor)	50–100 (1–2)	
	metoprolol succinate extended-release (Toprol XL)	25–100 (1)	
	nadolol (Corgard)	40–80 (1)	
	Nebivolol (Bystolic)	5 – 40 (1)	
	propranolol (Inderal)	40–120 (2)	
	propranolol long-acting (Inderal LA)	80–120 (1)	
	timolol (Blocadren)	10–40 (1–2)	
Beta-adrenergic blockers with intrinsic sympathomimetic activity	acebutolol (Sectral)	200–800 (2)	Bronchospasm, bradycardia, heart failure, fatigue, hypertriglyceridemia; may mask hypoglycemia
	penbutolol (Levatol)	10–40 (1)	
	Pindolol (Visken)	5–60 (2)	
Combined alpha- and beta-adrenergic blockers	carvedilol (Coreg)	6.25–25 (2)	Orthostatic hypotension, bronchospasm
	Carvedilol (Coreg CR)	10–80 (1)	
	labetalol (Normodyne, Trandate)	20–80 (1)	

Table 14-6   Oral Antihypertensive Drugs (*continued*)

CLASS	DRUG (TRADE NAME)	USUAL DOSE RANGE IN MG/DAY** (DAILY FREQUENCY)	SELECTED ADVERSE EFFECTS
Angiotensin-converting enzyme inhibitors	benazepril (Lotensin)	10–40 (1–2)	Cough, hyperkalemia, rash, angioedema
	captopril (Capoten)	25–50 (2–3)	
	enalapril (Vasotec)	2.5–40 (1–2)	
	fosinopril (Monopril)	10–80 (1)	
	lisinopril (Prinivil, Zestril)	10–80 (1)	
	moexipril (Univasc)	7.5–60 (1)	
	perindopril (Aceon)	4–16 (1–2)	
	quinapril (Accupril)	10–80 (1)	
	ramipril (Altace)	2.5–20 (1–2)	
	trandolapril (Mavik)	1–4 (1)	
Angiotensin receptor blockers (ARBs)	azilsartan (Edarbi)	40–80 (1)	Hyperkalemia, angioedema
	candesartan (Atacand)	8–32 (1–2)	
	eprosartan (Teveten)	400–800 (1–2)	
	irbesartan (Avapro)	150–300 (1)	
	losartan (Cozaar)	25–100 (1–2)	
	olmesartan (Benicar)	20–40 (1)	
	telmisartan (Micardis)	40–80 (1)	
	valsartan (Diovan)	80–320 (1)	
Calcium channel blockers—nondihydropyridines	diltiazem extended-release (Cardizem CD, Cardizem LA, Dilacor XR, Cartia XT, Tiazac)	180–540 (1)	Conduction defects, worsening diastolic dysfunction, gingival hyperplasia
	verapamil immediate-release (Calan, Isoptin)	80–320 (2–3)	
	verapamil long-acting (Calan SR, Isoptin SR)	100–480 (1)	
	verapamil (Covera HS, Verelan PM)	120–480 (1)	
Calcium channel blockers—dihydropyridines	amlodipine (Norvasc)	2.5–10 (1)	Ankle edema, flushing, headache
	felodipine ER (Plendil)	2.5–10 (1)	
	isradipine (DynaCirc CR)	5–20 (2)	
	nicardipine sustained-release (Cardene SR)	60–120 (2)	
	nifedipine long-acting (Adalat CC, Procardia XL)	30–60 (2)	
	nisoldipine (Sular)	17–34 (1)	
Alpha₁-blockers	doxazosin (Cardura)	1–16 (1)	Orthostatic hypotension
	prazosin (Minipress)	2–20 (2–3)	
	terazosin (Hytrin)	1–20 (1–2)	

(continued)

Table 14-6	Oral Antihypertensive Drugs (*continued*)		
CLASS	**DRUG (TRADE NAME)**	**USUAL DOSE RANGE IN MG/ DAY** (DAILY FREQUENCY)**	**SELECTED ADVERSE EFFECTS**
Central alpha$_2$-agonists and other centrally acting drugs	clonidine (Catapres)	0.1–0.6 (2)	Sedation, dry mouth, bradycardia
	clonidine patch (Catapres-TTS)	0.1–0.3 (1 weekly)	
	Guanfacine (Tenex)	1–3 (1)	
	methyldopa (Aldomet)	0.05–0.25 (1)	
	reserpine	0.5–2 (1)	
Direct vasodilators	hydralazine (Apresoline)	25–100 (2)	Headache, fluid retention, tachycardia
	minoxidil (Loniten)	2.5–80 (1–2)	
Direct renin inhibitor	aliskiren (Texturna, Rasilez)	150–300 (1)	Elevated uric acid, gout, renal stones, diarrhea, edema

These dosages may vary from those listed in the Physicians' Desk Reference. *Please review current medication reference materials for most current dosing. Many antihypertensive agents are combination medications.*
Adapted from Joint National Committee on Prevention, Detention, Evaluation, and Treatment of High Blood Pressure. (2003). The seventh report of the Joint National Committee on Prevention, Detection, Evaluation, and Treatment of High Blood Pressure (JNC VII). Available: *www.nhlbi.nih.gov/guidelines/hypertension/jncintro.htm.*

g. ACE inhibitors—lower BP by blocking the enzyme that converts angiotensin I to the potent vasoconstrictor angiotensin II and reducing sympathetic nervous system activity. These drugs also raise the level of bradykinin, a potent vasodilator, and lower aldosterone levels.

 DRUG ALERT ACE inhibitors are a drug of choice for diabetics as they delay progression to end-stage renal disease. However, they may worsen renal function in the presence of renal artery stenosis.

h. Angiotensin receptor blockers—similar in action to ACE inhibitors.
i. Calcium antagonists (calcium channel blockers, or CCB)—stop the movement of calcium into the cells; relax smooth muscle, which causes vasodilation; and inhibit reabsorption of sodium in the renal tubules. Nondihydropyridine CCB (verapamil and diltiazem) have a negative inotropic effect and may worsen heart failure.
j. Direct vasodilators—smooth muscle relaxants that primarily dilate arteries and arterioles.
k. Aldosterone inhibitors—antagonize aldosterone receptors and inhibit sodium reabsorption in the collecting duct of the nephron in the kidneys.
l. Direct renin inhibitors—inhibits renin within the renin-angiotensin system (RAS).

3. If hypertension is not controlled with the first drug within 1 to 3 months, three options can be considered:
   a. If the patient has faithfully taken the drug and not developed adverse effects, the dose of the drug may be increased.
   b. If the patient has had adverse effects, another class of drugs can be substituted.

c. A second drug from another class could be added. If adding the second agent lowers the pressure, the first agent can be slowly withdrawn or, if necessary, combination therapy can be continued.

Some patients require two medications at the time of diagnosis. This should be considered for patients who are 20 mmHg above their systolic goal or 10 mmHg above their diastolic goal.

4. The best management of hypertension is to use the fewest drugs at the lowest doses while encouraging the patient to maintain lifestyle changes. After BP has been under control for at least 1 year, a slow, progressive decline in drug therapy can be attempted. However, most patients need to resume medication within 1 year.
5. If the desired BP is still not achieved with the addition of a second drug, a third agent or a diuretic or both (if not already prescribed) could be added. 75% of individuals with hypertension require two or more antihypertensive agents to reach their BP goal.
6. Resistant hypertension is defined as an individual that requires three or more antihypertensive agents to control blood pressure.

Complications

See Figure 14-9.

1. Angina pectoris or MI due to decreased coronary perfusion.
2. Left ventricular hypertrophy and heart failure due to consistently elevated aortic pressure.
3. Renal failure due to diminished perfusion to the glomerulus.
4. TIAs, stroke, or cerebral hemorrhage due to cerebral ischemia and arteriosclerosis.

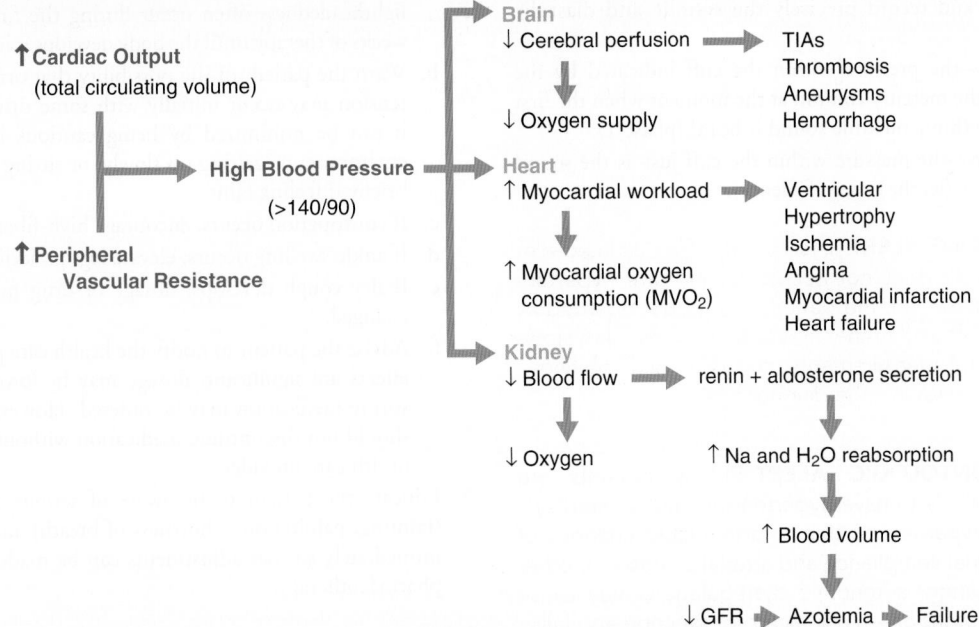

Figure 14-9. Determinants and clinical effects of high blood pressure. GFR, glomerular filtration rate; TIA, transient ischemic attack.

5. Retinopathy.
6. Accelerated hypertension (see page 469).

Nursing Assessment

Nursing History
Query the patient about the following:
1. Family history of high BP.
2. Previous episodes of high BP.
3. Dietary habits and salt intake.
4. Target organ disease or other disease processes that may place the patient in a high-risk group—diabetes, coronary artery disease, kidney disease.
5. Tobacco use.
6. Episodes of headache, weakness, muscle cramps, tingling, palpitations, sweating, vision disturbances.
7. Medication that could elevate BP (refer to "Secondary Hypertension," above):
   a. Hormonal contraceptives, corticosteroids.
   b. NSAIDs.
   c. Nasal decongestants, appetite suppressants, tricyclic antidepressants.
8. Other disease processes, such as gout, migraines, asthma, heart failure, and benign prostatic hyperplasia, which may be helped or worsened by particular antihypertensive drugs.

Physical Examination
1. Auscultate heart rate and heart sounds for the presence of an S4, indicating stiffening of the walls of the left ventricle, which may occur in hypertension.
2. If skilled in doing so, perform funduscopic examination of the eyes for the purpose of noting vascular changes. Look for edema, spasm, and hemorrhage of the eye vessels. Refer to ophthalmologist for definitive diagnosis.
3. Palpate the chest wall for a shift of the point of maximal impulse to the left, which occurs in heart enlargement. Palpate peripheral pulses for possible PAD.
4. Auscultate for bruit over the aorta, renal arteries, and peripheral arteries to determine the presence of atherosclerosis.
5. Determine mental status by asking patient about memory, ability to concentrate, and ability to perform simple mathematical calculations.

Blood Pressure Determination
1. Measure BP in both arms to determine whether there is a difference. If the systolic blood pressure (SBP) is greater than 15 mm Hg in one arm than the other, this may indicate the presence of subclavian stenosis in the arm with the lower SBP. If this BP differential is found, BP should be monitored in the arm with the highest SBP.
2. Avoid taking BP readings immediately after stressful or taxing situations. Wait 30 minutes after patient has smoked.
3. Have the patient assume position of comfort and remain silent. Make sure feet are on the floor or otherwise supported. The patient should be seated and relaxed for at least 5 minutes and the blood pressure should be taken around the same time each day it is taken to observe for trends in BP.
4. Support the bared arm; avoid constriction of arm by a rolled sleeve.
5. Use a BP cuff of the correct size.
   a. The bladder within the cuff should encircle at least 80% of the patient's arm.
   b. Many adults will require a large cuff.
   c. Two or more readings separated by 2 minutes should be averaged.
6. Be aware that falsely elevated BPs may be obtained with a cuff that is too narrow; falsely low readings may be obtained with a cuff that is too wide.

7. Auscultate and record precisely the systolic and diastolic pressures.
   a. Systolic—the pressure within the cuff indicated by the level of the mercury column at the moment when the first clear, rhythmic pulsatile sound is heard (phase 1).
   b. Diastolic—the pressure within the cuff just as the sound disappears (ie, the onset of silence).

 NURSING ALERT The finding of an isolated elevated BP does not necessarily indicate hypertension. However, the patient should be regarded as at risk for high BP until further assessment—through history-taking, repeat BP measurements, and diagnostic testing—either confirms or refutes the diagnosis.

 GERONTOLOGIC ALERT Elderly patients are more likely to have hypertension and isolated systolic hypertension due to age-related changes of decreased arterial compliance and arterial stenosis. Another age-related change, autonomic dysregulation, may cause orthostatic hypotension—a risk factor for syncope and falls.

Nursing Diagnoses

- Noncompliance with medication regimen and lifestyle changes.
- Readiness for Enhanced Self-health Management related to control of hypertension and prevention of target organ disease.

Nursing Interventions/Patient Education

Enlisting Cooperation and Compliance

1. Enlist the patient's cooperation in redirecting lifestyle in keeping with the guidelines of therapy, acknowledge the difficulty, and provide support and encouragement.
2. Develop a plan of instruction for medication self-management.
   a. Plan the patient's medication schedule so that they are given at proper and convenient times (once daily, if possible); set up a daily checklist on which the patient can record the medication taken or provide pill sorter.
   b. Be sure the patient knows the generic and brand names for all medications and throws away old medications and dosages so they will not be mixed up with current medications.
   c. Explore the cost of medications and ability for the patient to pay for prescriptions each month. Encourage the patient to discuss generic equivalents, mail-order drugs, or prescription assistance programs with the health care provider. Refer patient to Partnership for Prescription Assistance (*www.pparx.org*).
3. Stress the fact that there may be no correlation between high BP and symptoms; the patient cannot tell by the way he or she feels whether BP is normal or elevated. Because hypertension is chronic, regular follow-up is important to prevent complications and reduce more serious health care interventions in the future.
4. Assess for and try to eliminate side effects of medication regimen.
   a. Explain that antihypertensive drugs affect people differently, and side effects such as anorexia, fatigue, nausea, or

lightheadedness often occur during the first few days or weeks of therapy until the body develops tolerance to them.
   b. Warn the patient of the possibility that orthostatic hypotension may occur initially with some drug therapy, but it can be minimized by being cautious in hot, humid environments; getting up slowly; or sitting or lying down briefly if feeling faint.
   c. If constipation occurs, encourage high-fiber diet.
   d. If ankle swelling occurs, elevate legs periodically.
   e. If dry cough develops, dosage or drug may need to be changed.
   f. Advise the patient to notify the health care provider if side effects are significant, dosage may be lowered or a substitute medication may be ordered. However, the patient should not discontinue medication without notifying the health care provider.
5. Educate the patient to be aware of serious adverse effects (fainting, palpitations, shortness of breath) and report them immediately so that adjustments can be made in individual pharmacotherapy.

 GERONTOLOGIC ALERT Polypharmacy, cognitive changes, and sensory deficits in older adults may make dosage adjustment and control of BP difficult. Work with the patient, family, and home care nurse to devise a simple method for the patient to take the proper medications. Older patients are also more sensitive to therapeutic levels of drugs and may demonstrate adverse effects while on an otherwise average dosage. Monitor closely for safety and efficacy of therapy. They may be more sensitive to postural hypotension and should be cautioned to change positions with great care.

Encouraging Self-Management

1. Explain the meaning of high BP, risk factors, and their influences on the cardiovascular, cerebral, and renal systems.
2. Stress that there can never be total cure, only control, of essential hypertension; emphasize the consequences of uncontrolled hypertension.
3. Instruct the patient regarding proper method of taking BP at home and at work if health care provider so desires. Inform patient of desired range and the readings that are to be reported.
4. Determine recommended dietary plans and provide dietary education, as appropriate.
   a. Print out copy of the DASH Eating Plan and review with patient. Help patient suggest food preferences that include whole grains, fruits, vegetables, low-fat dairy, and nuts in quantities outlined in plan. Available at *www.nhlbi.nih. gov/health/health-topics/topics/dash*.
   b. Teach patient and family members how to read food labels in order to monitor sodium intake.
   c. Refer to dietitian for thorough dietary education and planning, as needed.
5. Educate patient about factors that may affect BP, such as dehydration, diarrhea, and other illnesses, so BP should be monitored closely and treatment adjusted.

6. Encourage the patient to keep follow-up appointments as directed by health care provider, have blood work drawn to monitor serum creatinine and electrolytes, and schedule eye exam by an ophthalmologist yearly.

Evaluation: Expected Outcomes

- Takes medications regularly, keeps follow-up appointments.
- Monitors BP correctly at home, able to identify sodium content on food labels.

Malignant Hypertension

Malignant hypertension, also called *accelerated hypertension*, occurs when the BP elevates extremely rapidly, threatening one or more of the target organs: brain, kidneys, or heart. Malignant hypertension is defined as blood pressure ≥180/120 mmHg or diastolic BP >130mmHg and is a medical emergency.

Pathophysiology and Etiology

1. When rapid hypertension occurs, the normal autoregulation of the artery eventually fails.
2. The rise in pressure in the arterioles and capillaries leads to damage to the vascular wall, which disrupts the endothelium and allows fibrinous material to enter the vascular wall, thereby narrowing or obliterating the vascular lumen.
3. For example, within the brain, the breakthrough vasodilation from failure of autoregulation leads to the development of cerebral edema and symptoms of hypertensive encephalopathy.
4. Etiology includes collagen vascular disorders, renal failure, renal artery stenosis, and toxemia of pregnancy.

Clinical Manifestations

1. Brain effects:
   a. Encephalopathy.
   b. Stroke.
   c. Progressive headache, stupor, seizures.
2. Kidney effects:
   a. Decreased blood flow, vasoconstriction.
   b. Elevated BUN.
   c. Increased plasma renin activity.
   d. Lowered urine-specific gravity.
   e. Proteinuria.
   f. Renal failure.
3. Cardiac effects:
   a. Left-sided heart failure.
   b. Acute MI.
   c. Right-sided heart failure.

Management

Goal is to lower BP to reduce the probability of permanent damage to target organs.

1. If diastolic BP exceeds 115 to 130 mm Hg, clinical condition is assessed very carefully.

2. Immediate hospitalization and treatment if the following are present:
   a. Seizures.
   b. Abnormal neurologic signs.
   c. Severe occipital headache.
   d. Pulmonary edema.
3. The patient is hemodynamically monitored in the ICU.
4. Antihypertensive agents are administered parenterally. Agents include:
   a. Nitroprusside—a rapidly acting arteriolar and venous dilator, given as an IV infusion. Initial dose: 0.25 to 0.5 mcg/kg per minute; maximum dose: 8 to 10 mcg/kg per minute.
   b. Nitroglycerin—a rapidly acting venous and, to a lesser degree, arteriolar dilator, given as an IV infusion. Initial dose: 5 mcg/minute; maximum dose: 200 mcg/minute.
   c. Labetalol—an alpha- and ß-adrenergic blocker, given as an IV bolus or infusion. Bolus: 20 mg initially, followed by 20 to 80 mg every 10 minutes to a total dose of 300 mg. Infusion: 0.5 to 2 mg/minute.
   d. Nicardipine—a calcium channel blocker, given as an IV infusion. Initial dose: 5 mg/hour; maximum dose: 15 mg/hour.
   e. Clevidipine—a calcium channel blocker. Initial dose: 1–2 mg/hour; 32 mg/hour maximum dose: 16 mg/hour.
   f. Fenoldopam—a peripheral dopamine-1 receptor agonist, given as an IV infusion. Initial dose: 0.01 mcg/kg per minute; the dose is titrated at 15-minute intervals, depending on the blood pressure response normal dosing: 0.01 to 1.6 mcg/kg per minute.
   g. Hydralazine—an arteriolar dilator, given as an IV bolus. Initial dose: 10 mg given every 20 to 30 minutes; maximum dose: 20 mg.
   h. Propranolol—a ß-adrenergic blocker, given as an IV infusion and then followed by oral therapy. Dose: 1 to 10 mg load, followed by 3 mg/hour.
   i. Phentolamine—an alpha-adrenergic blocker, given as an IV bolus. Dose: 5 to 10 mg every 5 to 15 minutes.
   j. Enalaprilat—an angiotensin converting enzyme inhibitor, given as an IV bolus. Dose: 1.25 to 5 mg every 6 hours.
5. Diuretics may be administered to maintain a sodium diuresis when the arterial pressure falls.
6. Vasopressor agents should be available if the BP responds too vigorously to antihypertensive agents.

Nursing Interventions

1. Record BP frequently or monitor BP via an intra-arterial line or electronically controlled cuff. Some drugs necessitate the taking of BP readings every 5 minutes or more frequently while titrating drug therapies.

 NURSING ALERT BP should be reduced gradually and wide pressure variations avoided because lowered BP may not be adequate to perfuse vital organs.

2. Monitor for adverse effects of medications—headache, tachycardia, orthostatic hypotension.
3. Measure urine output accurately.
4. Observe for hypokalemia, especially if patient is placed on diuretic therapy. Monitor for ventricular dysrhythmias.
5. Observe for CNS complications.
   a. Note signs of confusion, irritability, lethargy, and disorientation.
   b. Listen for complaints of headache, difficulty with vision.
   c. Check for evidence of nausea or vomiting.
   d. Be alert for signs of seizure activity. Provide a safe environment—padded side rails. Keep bed in lowest position.
6. Reduce activity and provide quiet environment.
7. Monitor ECG continuously.
8. Maintain constant vigilance until BP is decreased and stable and then begin a hypertension teaching program.

LYMPHATIC DISORDERS

The lymphatic system is a network of vessels and nodes that are interrelated with the circulatory system. It removes tissue fluid from intercellular spaces and protects the body from bacterial invasion. Lymph nodes are located along the course of the lymphatic vessels and filter lymph before it is returned to the bloodstream.

Lymphedema and Lymphangitis

Lymphedema is a swelling of the tissues (particularly in the dependent position) produced by an obstruction to the lymph flow in an extremity. This results in excessive accumulation of fluid in the interstitial space, which is composed of high-molecular-weight proteins.

Lymphangitis is an acute inflammation of lymphatic channels, which most commonly arises from a focus of infection in an extremity.

Pathophysiology and Etiology

Lymphedema

1. Classified as primary (congenital malformations) or secondary (acquired obstruction).
2. Swelling in the extremities occurs due to an increased quantity of lymph fluid that results from an obstruction of lymphatics.
3. Obstruction may be in both the lymph nodes and the lymphatic vessels. Eventually, subcutaneous tissue becomes fibrotic, impairing vascular flow and oxygen transfer to tissues.
4. It may be caused or aggravated by radiation therapy, trauma, cancer, morbid obesity, or surgery involving the lymph tissue (particularly radical mastectomy). It may be associated with varicose veins and chronic phlebitis.

Lymphangitis

1. Most commonly caused by infection in an extremity. The pooled protein-rich lymph fluid creates a good medium for growth of bacteria and fungi.

2. The characteristic red streak extending up an arm or leg from the infected wound outlines the course of the lymphatics as they drain.
3. Recurrent lymphangitis is typically associated with lymphedema.

Clinical Manifestations

1. Lymphedema: edema may be massive and is usually firm.
2. Lymphangitis:
   a. Displays characteristic red streaks that extend up an arm or leg from an infection that is not localized and that can lead to septicemia.
   b. Produces general symptoms—high fever, chills.
   c. Produces local symptoms—local pain, tenderness, swelling along involved lymphatics.
   d. Produces local lymph node symptoms—enlarged, red, tender (acute lymphadenitis).
   e. Produces an abscess—necrotic, pus-producing (suppurative lymphadenitis)

Diagnostic Evaluation

1. Lymphangiography—outlines lymphatic system.
2. Lymphoscintigraphy—reliable alternative to lymphangiography using radioactive colloid material; detects obstruction or inflammation.
3. CT or MRI.
4. Check feet for tinea pedis (athlete's foot), which is a common cause of bacterial entry into the skin and lymphatics.

Management

Lymphedema

1. Bed rest with leg elevation.
2. Active and passive exercises.
3. Lymphedema therapy.
   a. Massage to help move fluid and myofascial release to break up fibrotic tissue.
   b. Compression garments to help squeeze the fluid out of tissues. This may be in the form of medical-grade stockings or pneumatic compression, which provides intermittent pumping to squeeze fluid from the extremity. These may be used in upper or lower extremities.
4. Diuretics are usually not effective and can worsen edema.
5. Surgery:
   a. Excision of affected subcutaneous tissue and fascia with skin grafting.
   b. Transfer of superficial lymphatics to deep lymphatic system by buried dermal flap.
   c. Complications include flap necrosis, hematoma, abscess under flap, cellulitis.

Lymphangitis

1. Administer antibiotics.
2. Treat affected extremity by rest, elevation, and the application of hot, moist dressings.
3. Incise and drain if necrosis and abscess formation occur.
4. Treat tinea pedis, if present.

Complications

1. Abscess formation (rare with lymphangitis).
2. Firm, nonpitting lymphedema unresponsive to treatment (congenital lymphedema, called lymphedema praecox).
3. Elephantiasis secondary to parasite (filaria)—chronic fibrosis of subcutaneous tissue and chronic swelling of the extremity (rare in the United States).
4. Septicemia.

Nursing Assessment

1. Assess extremity for edema and inflammation.
   a. Palpate edema to evaluate its quality (soft and pitting or firm and nonpitting).
   b. Note any areas of abscess formation (suppurative lymphadenitis).
2. Watch for signs of fever and chills.

Nursing Diagnoses

- Risk for Impaired Skin Integrity related to edema and/or inflammation.
- Acute Pain related to incision and/or surgery.

Nursing Interventions

Maintaining Skin Integrity

1. Apply elastic bandages or prescription compression stockings (after acute attack with lymphangitis).
2. Advise the patient to rest frequently with affected part elevated—each joint higher than the preceding one.
3. Make sure the patient cleans in crevices of skin if edema has caused skin folds.
4. Administer diuretics as prescribed to control excess fluid.
5. Give antibiotics or antifungals, as prescribed.
6. Recommend isometric exercises with extremity elevated.
7. Suggest moderate sodium restriction in diet.
8. Observe postoperatively for signs of infection.

Relieving Pain Postoperatively

1. Encourage comfortable positioning and immobilization of affected area.
2. Administer or teach patient to administer analgesics, as prescribed; monitor for adverse effects.
3. Use bed cradle to relieve pressure from bed covers.

Patient Education and Health Maintenance

1. Instruct patient on proper application of compression garments.
2. Encourage compliance with therapy, which often involves frequent rewrapping of compression bandages, exercise, and massage for several months.
3. Advise patient to avoid trauma to extremity.
4. Instruct patient to use lotions that are free of perfumes, which may irritate skin.
5. Advise patient to practice good hygiene to avoid superimposed infections.
6. Instruct patient about the signs and symptoms of infection to report to health care providers.
7. Instruct patient to inspect feet and legs daily for evidence of skin breakdown, particularly between toes, and to look for tinea pedis.

Evaluation: Expected Outcomes

- Skin is normal color and temperature, nontender, nonswollen, and intact.
- Verbalizes no pain on actively moving extremity.

SELECTED REFERENCES

American Diabetes Association. (2011). Standards of medical care in diabetes 2011. *Diabetes Care, 34*(Suppl.1), 511–561.

Ansell, J., Hirsh, J., Hyleck, E., et al. (2008). The pharmacology and management of the vitamin K antagonists. The Eighth ACCP Conference on Antithrombotic and Thrombolytic Therapy. *Chest, 133*(Suppl.), 160S–198S. Available: *www.chestjournal.org/content/133/6_suppl/160S.full.pdf+html.*

Apone, J. (2012). The prevalence of peripheral arterial disease (PAD) and PAD risk factors among different ethnic groups in the US Population. *J of Vasc Nursing, 30*(2), 37–43.

Appel, L. J., Frohlich, E. D., Hall, J. E., et al. (2011). The importance of population-wide sodium reduction as a means to prevention cardiovascular disease and stroke: A call to action from the American Heart Association. *Circulation, 123,* 1138–1143.

Aronow, W. S., Fleg, J. L., Pepine, C. J., et al. (2011). ACCF/AHA 2011 expert consensus document on hypertension in the elderly: A report of the American College of Cardiology Foundation Task Force on Clinical Expert Consensus Documents. *Circulation, 123,* 2434–2506.

Banks-Gonzales, V., Ruppert, S. (2012). Thrombophilia and Hypercoagulation: Risk Assessment and Screening. *J for Nurse Practitioners, 8*(8), 649–655.

Boehringer Ingelheim. (2011). What is Pradaxa (dabigatran etexilate)? Available: *www.pradaxa.com.*

Calhoun, D., Jones, D., Textor, S., et al. (2008). Resistant hypertension: Diagnosis, evaluation, and treatment. A scientific statement from the American Heart Association Professional Education Committee of the Council for High Blood Pressure Research. *Circulation, 117,* e510–e526.

Carter, B. L., Bosworth, H. B., & Green, B. B. (2012). The hypertension team: The role of the pharmacist, nurse, and teamwork in hypertension therapy. *Journal of Clinical Hypertension, 14*(1), 51–65.

Castro-Sánchez, A. M., Matarán-Peñarrocha, G. A., Feriche-Fernández-Castanys, B., et al. (2013). A program of 3 physical therapy modalities improvise peripheral arterial disease in diabetes type 2 patients: A randomized controlled trial. *Journal of Cardiovascular Nursing, 28*(1), 74–82.

Center for Disease Control and Prevention. (CDC). (2011). May is High Blood Pressure Education Month. Atlanta, GA: Author. Available: *www.cdc.gov/Features/HighBloodPressure.*

Drozda, J., Messer, J., Spertus, J., et al. (2011). Performance measures for adults with coronary artery disease and hypertension. A report of the American College of Cardiology Foundation/American Heart Association Task Force on Performance Measures and the American Medical Association–Physician Consortium for Performance Improvement, *Circulation, 124,* 248–270.

Egberg, L., Andreassen, S., Mattiasson, A. (2012). Experiences of living with intermittent claudication. *J Vasc Nursing, 30*(1), 5–10.

Flack, J. M., Sica, D. A., Bakris, G., et al. (2010). Management of high blood pressure in blacks. An update of the International Society on Hypertension in Blacks consensus statement. *Hypertension, 56,* 780–800.

Geerts, W. H., Berqqvist, D., Pineo, G. F., et al. (2008). Prevention of venous thromboembolism: American College of Chest Physicians evidence-based clinical practice guidelines. *Chest, 133,* 381S–453S. Available: *http://chestjournal.chestpubs.org/content/133/6_suppl/381S.full.html.*

Glaxo-Smith-Kline. (2012). How ARIXTRA works. Available: *www.arixtra.com.*

Goodman, A. (2009). Ultrasound-assisted thrombolysis improves outcomes in chronic DVT. Available: *www.Medscape.com/viewarticle/712892.*

Gradman, A. H., Basile, J. N., Carter, B. L., et al. (2010). Combination therapy in hypertension. *Journal of the American Society of Hypertension, 4*(1), 42–50.

Guyatt, G., Akl, E., Crowther, M., et al. (2012). Executive Summary: Antithrombotic Therapy and Prevention of Thrombosis, 9th ed: American College of Chest Physicians Evidence-Based Clinical Practice Guidelines. *Chest, 141*(2_suppl), 7S–47S.

Hernandez, J. (2012). Prehypertension: A literature-documented public health concern. *Journal of the American Academy of Nurse Practitioners, 24*(1), 3–10.

Hirsch, A.T., Murphy, T. P., Lovell, M. B., et al. (2007). Gaps in public knowledge of peripheral arterial disease: The first national PAD public awareness survey. *Circulation, 116*, 2086–2094.

Institute for Clinical Systems Improvement (ICSI). (2011). Antithrombotic therapy supplement (Guideline). Available: *www.icsi.org/guidelines_and_more/gl_os_prot/cardiovascular/antithrombotic_therapy_supplement__guideline__14045/antithrombotic_therapy_supplement_guideline.html*.

Institute for Clinical Systems Improvement (ICSI). (2012). Health care guideline: Venous thromboembolism diagnosis and treatment. Available: *www.icsi.org/venous_thromboembolism/venous_thromboembolism_4.html*.

Janssen Pharmaceuticals. (2012). About Xarelto, evolving anticoagulation. Available: *www.xareltohcp.com*.

JBW Enterprises. (2012). Compression stocking step-by-step measuring guide. Available: *www.thelaserveincenter.com/measuring*.

Johnson, M. P. (2013). Transitions to care in patients receiving oral anticoagulants: General principles, procedures and impact of new oral anticoagulants. *Journal of Cardiovascular Nursing, 28*(1), 54–65.

Joint National Committee on Prevention, Detention, Evaluation, and Treatment of High Blood Pressure. (2003). The seventh report of the Joint National Committee on Prevention, Detection, Evaluation, and Treatment of High Blood Pressure (JNC VII). Available: *www.nhlbi.nih.gov/guidelines/hypertension/jncintro.htm*.

Kaplan, N. M., & Rose, B. D. Drug treatment of hypertensive emergencies. *UpToDate*. Available: *www.uptodate.com/contents/drug-treatment-of-hypertensive-emergencies*.

Karakurt, P., Kasikci, M. (2012). Factors affecting medication adherence in patients with hypertension. *J Vasc Nursing, 30*(4), 118–126.

Krum, H., Schlaich, M., Whitbourn, R., et al. (2009). Catheter-based renal sympathetic denervation for resistant hypertension: a multicentre safety and proof-of-principle cohort study. *Lancet, 373*, 1275–1281.

Lovell, M., Harris, K., Forbes, T., et al. (2009). Peripheral arterial disease: Lack of awareness in Canada. *Canadian Journal of Cardiology, 25*(1), 39–45.

Mancia, G., De Backer, G., Dominiczak, A., et al. (2007). 2007 guidelines for the management of arterial hypertension: The Task Force for the Management of Arterial Hypertension of the European Society of Hypertension (ESH) and of the European Society of Cardiology (ESC). *European Heart Journal, 28*(12), 1462–1536.

National Collaborating Center for Acute Care. (2010). Venous thromboembolism: Reducing the risk of venous thromboembolism (deep vein thrombosis and pulmonary embolism) in patients undergoing surgery. NICE Clinical Guideline. Available: *www.nice.org.uk/guidance/CG092*.

National Institute for Health and Clinical Excellence. (2011). Hypertension: Clinical management of primary hypertension in adults. London: National Clinical Guideline Centre at the Royal College of Physicians.

Nguyen, T., Yacoub, M., Chan, T., et al. (2012). Atrial fibrillation: Focus on anticoagulant pharmacotherapy. *The Journal for Nurse Practitioners, 8*(7), 560–565.

Nurse Practitioners' Prescribing Reference (2011). *18*(1). New York: Haymarket Media.

Registered Nurses Association of Ontario (RNAO). (2009). *Nursing management of hypertension 2009 supplement*. Toronto: Registered Nurses Association of Ontario.

Revis, D., & Geibel, J. (2011). Lymphedema. Available: *http//emedicine.medscape.com/article/191350-overview*.

Rogers, V., Adams, R., Carnethon, R., et al. (2011). Heart disease and stroke statistics–2011 update, *Circulation, 123*, e18–e209.

Rooke, T. W., Hirsch, A. T., Mirsa, S., et al. (2011). 2011 ACCF/AHA focused update of the guideline for the management of patients with peripheral artery disease (updating the 2005 guideline). *Journal of the American College of Cardiology, 58*, 2020–2045.

Rosendorff, C., Black, H. R., & Dannon, C. P. (2007). Treatment of hypertension in the prevention and management of ischemic heart disease. *Circulation, 115*, 2761–2788.

Stangier, J., & Clemens, A. (2009). Pharmacology, pharmacokinetics, and pharmacodynamics of dabigatran etexilate, an oral direct thrombin inhibitor. *Clinical and Applied Thrombosis/Hemostasis, 15*, 9S–16S.

The EINSTEIN-PE Investigators. (2012). Oral Rivaroxaban for the treatment of Symptomatic Pulmonary Embolism. *N Engl J Med, 366*(14), 1287–1297.

U.S. Preventive Services Task Force. (2010). Guide to preventive services: Screening for abdominal aortic aneurysm. Available: *www.ahrq.gov/clinic/pocketgd1011/gcp10s2a.htm#Abdominal*.

Wesley, K., & Rowe, V. (2011). Varicose vein surgery. Available: *http://emedicine.medscape.com/article/462579-overview*.

Wiley, M., Kumar, A. K., Vacek, J. L. (2012). Peripheral arterial disease. *Consultant, 52*(9), 601–610.

Yoon, S., Ostchega, Y., & Louis, T. (2010). Recent trends in the prevalence of high blood pressure and its treatment and control, 1999–2008 (NCHS Data Brief No. 48). Hyattsville, MD: National Center for Health Statistics.

15
Neurologic Disorders

OVERVIEW AND ASSESSMENT

A baseline neurologic assessment is needed to detect changes in neurologic function and includes a patient history, general physical examination, and thorough neurologic examination. An important goal of the neurologic assessment is to identify the minimum amount of stimulation required to elicit maximum response. Common manifestations of neurologic dysfunction include motor, sensory, autonomic, and cognitive deficits. By exploring these symptoms, obtaining a pertinent history, and performing a thorough neurologic examination, the reader will gain an understanding of the underlying disorder and become skilled in planning care for patients with neurologic disorders (see Standards of Care Guidelines 15-1, page 474). See Chapter 5, page 75, for neurologic examination techniques. Documentation using appropriate terminology and comparison of right to left for asymmetrical findings is important. See Box 15-1, page 475, for definitions of findings.

Radiology and Imaging

Structural and functional imaging techniques have evolved to facilitate the rapid diagnosis and treatment of neurologic disorders. Brain mapping describes the process of translating the brain into a functionally useful group of dynamic maps or patterns. The diagnosis and evaluation of neurologic disorders is increasingly guided by functional brain mapping techniques that detect changes in brain patterns associated with neuropathology. Structural or

STANDARDS OF CARE GUIDELINES 15-1
Neurologic Disorders

When caring for patients with neurologic disorders, consider the following assessments and interventions:

- Use age-appropriate assessment and examination techniques.

- Be aware of the status of the patient when assuming care so comparison can be made with subsequent assessments.

- Perform a thorough systematic assessment, including mental status, vital signs, and cardiovascular status.

- Document the patient's condition to provide a record for continuity of care.

- Provide translation services for patients who have difficulty understanding or speaking English because this may impact the interpretation of the neurologic exam.

- Evaluate for signs of worsening neurologic condition through a systematic examination. Follow the institutional guidelines and clinician's orders regarding the frequency of assessments. If the patient shows signs of neurologic deterioration, more frequent assessment and/or interventions may be necessary.

- Be cautious in the administration of sedatives, opiates, or other medications that affect neurologic functioning because these may mask signs of neurologic deterioration.

- Notify appropriate health care provider of new or worsening neurologic symptoms, such as a change in behavior or level of consciousness; a change in functioning of the cranial nerves; motor, sensory, or neurovascular deficits; or alterations in the pattern of breathing or vital signs. Implement appropriate interventions for acute changes in neurologic status.

- Institute safety precautions for patients with neurologic deficits because they may be especially prone to falls. Follow institutional guidelines for patients with seizure disorder.

- Assess the patient's level of functioning in his or her activities of daily living. For those with cranial nerve or motor deficits, assess for difficulty swallowing prior to eating. For patients with difficulty swallowing, implement appropriate institutional protocols to prevent aspiration. This may include contacting the primary clinician to obtain an evaluation from a speech therapist or changing the diet.

- Use a multidisciplinary approach to care when indicated, including medical and surgical specialists, pharmacists, dietitian/nutritional therapist, physical/occupational/ speech therapists, and rehabilitation specialists.

- Be aware that families or caretakers of patients with cognitive impairment or who are nonverbal may be able to provide assistance in the interpretation of behavioral cues.

- Assess family support and coping throughout the trajectory of the disease. Social issues (such as financial, community support systems, etc.) may require the expertise of a social worker or other clinical resource support personnel.

 Evidence Base American Association of Neuroscience Nurses. (2009). *Neurological assessment of the older adult: A guide for nurses.* Glenview, IL: Author.

---

anatomic imaging reveals information about the structure of the nervous system, including the brain and spinal cord. Functional or physiologic imaging focuses on the function of the brain and biochemical and metabolic processes in brain cells.

Computed Tomography

Description

1. Computed tomography (CT) is a structural imaging study that uses a computer-based x-ray to provide a cross-sectional image of the brain. A computer calculates differences in tissue absorption of the x-ray beams. The CT scan produces a three-dimensional view of structures in the brain and distinguishes between soft tissues and water. Intravenous (IV) contrast dye may be used to examine the integrity of the blood–brain barrier. New multidetector scanners allow for rapid imaging.

2. CT of the brain is primarily used to detect cerebral hemorrhage, whereas CT of the brain with contrast is used to detect tumors and inflammatory disorders.

3. Spinal CT may be used to evaluate lower back pain due to bony lesions or degenerative changes. CT myelography is

typically reserved for those who have had previous spinal surgery or a questionable diagnosis.

4. May be used when magnetic resonance imaging (MRI) is contraindicated (metallic or electronic implants) or not tolerated (claustrophobia).

5. *Advantages of CT:* Widespread availability, short imaging time, excellent images of bone, and 100% sensitivity for detection of cerebral hemorrhage.

6. *Disadvantages of CT:* Does not provide information about function of tissues; exposes the patient to ionizing radiation at higher doses than traditional x-rays; imposes a weight restriction of 300 pounds; if contrast is used there is the risk of contrast-induced nephropathy.

Nursing and Patient Care Considerations

1. Instruct patient to remove metal items, such as earrings, eyeglasses, and hair clips.

2. Ask whether patient has an allergy to iodine or history of previous allergy to IV dye to determine if the patient needs to be premedicated.

3. Evaluate for adequate renal function if contrast will be used.

BOX 15-1	Definitions of Neurologic Findings

Acalculia—inability to do mathematical calculations.

Agnosia—inability to recognize sensory input.

Amaurosis fugax—sudden, temporary, or fleeting blindness, not caused by disease of the eye.

Anisocoria—inequality in size of the pupils.

Apraxia—inability to perform coordinated movements.

Confabulation—fluent, nonsensical speech.

Decerebrate rigidity (extensor posturing)—dysfunction of vestibulospinal tract and the RAS of the upper brainstem; jaw clenched, neck extended, elbows extended, forearms pronated, wrists flexed, knees extended, and feet plantar flexed.

Decorticate rigidity (flexor posturing)—dysfunction of corticospinal tract above the brainstem; arms adducted, elbows and wrists flexed, legs extended and internally rotated, and feet plantar flexed.

Dyslexia—visual aphasia.

Dysarthria—difficulty speaking.

Dyspraxia—partial loss of ability to perform coordinated movements.

Fluent aphasia (Wernicke's, sensory)—comprehension is poor but speech is fluent and nonsensical.

Homonymous hemianopsia—corresponding visual field deficits in half of the visual field bilaterally.

Micrographia—change in handwriting with the script becoming smaller and more cramped.

Nonfluent aphasia (Broca's, motor)—comprehension intact but has poor expression through speech.

Nystagmus—involuntary oscillation of the eyeball, either vertical, horizontal, or rotary.

Paratonia—progressively increasing and irregular resistance to passive movements.

Table 15-1	Comparison of CT and MRI	
CONSIDERATIONS	**CT**	**MRI**
Radiation exposure	• Minimal	• None
Imaging planes	• Axial	• Axial, coronal, and sagittal
Cost	• Several hundred dollars	• Several thousand dollars, but dependent on protocol being used
Advantages	• Rapid evaluation for intracranial hemorrhage and subarachnoid hemorrhage	• Detection of stroke, multiple sclerosis, epilepsy, tumors
Disadvantages	• Poor visualization of anatomic structures; radiation exposure	• May result in claustrophobia • May need prior x-rays if metallic fragments are suspected—if identified, cannot complete study

4. Tell patient to expect a sensation of feeling flushed if contrast dye is injected through the IV catheter.

5. Inform patient that the procedure usually takes less than 5 minutes.

6. Request that patient remain as immobile as possible during the examination.

7. Tell patient to resume usual activities after the procedure.

8. Encourage increased fluid intake for the rest of the day to assist in expelling the contrast dye.

Magnetic Resonance Imaging

Description

1. Conventional MRI is a noninvasive structural imaging procedure that uses powerful magnetic field and radio frequency waves to create an image. When tissue is placed in a strong magnetic field, hydrogen atoms in the tissue line up within the field. In MRI, pulsating radio frequency waves are applied to the magnetic field to alter the tissue magnetization, creating a clear image of the tissue.

2. MRI is the imaging procedure of choice for most neurologic diseases (eg, detection of demyelinating diseases, nonacute hemorrhage, and cerebral tumors; evaluation of spinal cord injury, acute herniated disks, and cerebral infarction) and has largely replaced myelography, a more invasive procedure. See Table 15-1 for comparison to CT.

3. Specific protocols have been developed for trauma, stroke, and epilepsy.

4. MRI may be ordered with or without contrast. The contrast (gadolinium) alters the magnetic properties of tissue in order to differentiate tissue types. Contrast may be administered via IV line, by mouth, or through insertion into the rectum.

5. Closed MRI uses scanning equipment that resembles a tunnel-like chamber. Open MRI uses more sophisticated equipment that does not involve a closed chamber. During open MRI, the patient can comfortably see the surroundings from all views while the scan is in progress. This is ideal for patients who are claustrophobic or anxious, children, older adults, and the very obese.

6. Imaging orientation:
   a. Axial—slice dividing the head into upper and lower halves.
   b. Coronal—slice dividing the head into front and back halves.
   c. Sagittal—slice dividing the head into left and right halves.

7. Imaging sequences:
   a. T1—excellent tissue discrimination that provides anatomic images.
   b. T2—sensitive to the presence of increased water and visualization of edema for differentiation of normal tissue and pathologic changes.

c. MRI with gadolinium—improves specificity of normal/abnormal tissue. With blood–brain barrier disruption, there is leakage of contrast medium. The pattern of contrast uptake into brain tissue helps differentiate such conditions as central nervous system (CNS) infections, neoplasms, meningeal diseases, and noninfectious inflammatory processes.

d. Fluid attenuated inversion recovery—evaluates edema within white matter; also used to identify subarachnoid disease.

e. Diffusion-weighted imaging (DWI)—helps to evaluate the extent of a stroke and demyelinating disease and differentiates tumors from abscesses; shows increased enhancement with cytotoxic edema.

f. Apparent diffusion coefficient (ADC)—shows decreased attenuation associated with acute stroke.

g. DWI/ADC mismatch—increased enhancement on DWI in conjunction with decreased enhancement on ADC indicates acute stroke.

h. Perfusion-weighted imaging (PWI)—evaluates cerebral blood flow. It is also used to evaluate ischemia, stroke, and the penumbra of the stroke.

i. DWI/PWI mismatch—increased enhancement on DWI with flow deficit on PWI indicates acute stroke.

j. MRI single photon-emission computed tomography (SPECT)—provides assessment of neurochemicals (choline, lactate, N-acetylaspartate, glutamine/glutamate) for differentiation of brain tumors, abscess, demyelinating disease, and postradiation necrosis.

7. *Advantages of MRI:* No ionizing radiation, sensitivity to blood flow, imaging in several planes, and superior visualization of soft tissues. An important advantage is its ability to distinguish water, iron, fat, and blood. Sensitive to detection of white matter changes and valuable in detecting changes associated with Alzheimer's disease and multiple sclerosis.

8. *Disadvantages of MRI:* Contraindicated for patients with pacemakers, nontitanium aneurysm clips, or other implanted objects that could be dislodged by the magnetic field. Dental amalgam, gold, and stainless steel are generally considered safe, but may distort the image. If contrast is used, there is the risk of contrast-induced nephropathy. MRI scanner has the appearance of a tunnel-like chamber, and its constricted opening prevents its use for extremely obese people. Because of its narrow dimensions, MRI may induce claustrophobic and anxiety reactions, so anti-anxiety medication may be necessary before the procedure or an open MRI may be used.

Nursing and Patient Care Considerations

1. Encourage patient to use the bathroom before the procedure because it may take from 20 to 60 minutes, though the scan time is dependent on the protocol requested and number of scans performed.

2. Instruct patient to remove metal items, including eyeglasses, jewelry, hair clips, hearing aids, dentures, and clothing with zippers, buckles, or metal buttons.

3. Evaluate for adequate renal function if contrast will be used (see Box 15-2).

BOX 15-2	**Contrast-Induced Nephropathy**

When IV contrast medium is to be used in any radiologic study, renal function must be adequate to clear the substance. Check for risk factors for contrast-induced nephropathy:

- Renal insufficiency (creatinine level >1.5 or a glomerular filtration rate of <60 mL/minute).
- Diabetic nephropathy and other conditions that cause reduced renal perfusion.
- High total dose of contrast (<5 mL/kg or >100 mL).

If risk factors are present, hydration with normal saline starting 1 hour prior to the procedure and for 6 hours following the procedure is recommended.

Metformin should be held for 24 hours before any procedure and for 48 hours after the procedure if IV contrast is utilized.

---

4. Encourage patient to remain as still as possible during the procedure.

5. Describe the tunnel-like narrow chamber of the closed MRI scanner and inform patient it sometimes causes feelings of anxiety or claustrophobia. Evaluate the need for sedation.

6. Inform patient the scanner will make a dull, thumping noise throughout the procedure.

7. Tell patient to resume usual activities after the procedure.

Functional MRI

Description

1. Functional MRI (fMRI) is an imaging study that aids in identifying regions of the brain activated by particular stimuli and tasks. Imaging is performed during presentation of a stimulus or performance of a specific task and during rest periods. A statistical comparison is performed with images obtained during the stimulus/task periods compared with those performed during the rest periods by evaluating the conversion of oxyhemoglobin to deoxyhemoglobin and utilization of glucose, which occurs during normal brain activity. Involves IV administration of contrast material that lowers signal intensity on MRI in relation to blood flow as the material passes through the brain.

2. *Advantages of fMRI:* Does not use ionizing radiation and can be applied repeatedly in the same patient without risk. Offers potential in early detection of patients with prodromal dementia. It is also useful in preoperative evaluation of patients with lesions (tumors, seizure foci) adjacent to eloquent areas of the brain (speech center, premotor and motor cortex, and memory centers).

3. *Disadvantages of fMRI:* Same as MRI.

Nursing and Patient Care Considerations

1. Instruct patient as for MRI. Full cooperation of the patient is vital for head motion and task performance reasons. Global cognitive impairment, aphasia, neglect, substantial sensory disturbances, and severe depression are usually exclusion criteria. The performance of motor tasks during imaging should be monitored.

2. Medications that may interfere with performance of tasks during the procedure should be avoided, if possible, including benzodiazepines, sedatives, and opioids.

Positron-Emission Tomography

Description

1. Positron-emission tomography (PET) is a computer-based imaging technique that permits study of the brain's function by evaluating the metabolism, blood flow, and chemical processes within the brain. PET measures emissions of particles of injected radioisotopes—called positrons—and converts them to an image of the brain.

2. PET scanners are not frequently used or widely available due to their high cost, and PET requires sophisticated equipment to produce its radioisotopes, or positron emitter.

3. A glucose-like solution and mildly radioactive tracers are combined for injection or inhalation. After injection into the arterial bloodstream or inhalation of this radioactive compound, pairs of gamma rays are emitted into adjacent tissue during radioactive decay. The PET scanner measures the gamma rays to determine how quickly the tissues absorb the radioactive isotopes. A computer processes the data into an image that shows where the radioactive material is located, corresponding to cellular metabolism.

4. *Advantages of PET:* Provides information on patterns of glucose and oxygen metabolism. Areas of decreased metabolism indicate dysfunction. PET is useful for early detection of Alzheimer's disease and other dementias, Parkinson's disease, amyotrophic lateral sclerosis (ALS), Huntington's disease, multiple sclerosis, and psychiatric disorders, such as depression or schizophrenia. PET can also help locate/identify abnormal brain activity, such as seizure foci, and assess brain function after stroke.

5. *Disadvantages of PET:* Ionizing radiation, high initial cost.

Nursing and Patient Care Considerations

1. Inform patient that this procedure requires injection or inhalation of a radioactive substance that emits positively charged particles. Explain that the image is created when the negative particles found in the body combine with the positive particles of the imaging substance.

2. Explain that, after injection of the radioisotope, the patient will be asked to rest quietly on a stretcher for about 45 minutes to allow the substance to circulate.

3. Reassure the patient that radiation exposure is minimal.

4. Encourage patient to void before the test because the scan and associated procedures may take several hours.

5. Advise patient to increase fluid intake after the procedure to flush out the radioisotope and to resume meals.

6. Tell patient that it may take a few days to get results of the PET scan because it requires processing before it is available for interpretation.

Single-Photon Emission Computed Tomography

Description

1. SPECT is a widely available noninvasive functional imaging technique that evaluates cerebral vascular supply. A radioactive tracer is administered by inhalation or injection into the bloodstream; the tracer then decays to emit only a single photon. It uses a rotating camera to track the single photons emitted from radioactive decay and collects information from multiple views. Evaluation of the radioactive tracers creates images that show cerebral blood flow in various regions of the brain.

2. The radioactive tracer compounds used are commercially prepared and do not require the specialized equipment used in PET scanning.

3. SPECT is typically used to evaluate cerebral blood flow in patients with ischemic stroke, subarachnoid hemorrhage (SAH), migraine, dementia (including Alzheimer's disease), epilepsy, and other degenerative diseases.

4. *Advantages of SPECT:* Can perform hemodynamic, chemical, and functional imaging; widely available.

5. *Disadvantages of SPECT:* Ionizing radiation, provides only relative measurements.

Nursing and Patient Care Considerations

1. Inform patient that this is a noninvasive procedure that should cause minimal discomfort.

2. Tell patient that results of the scan are typically available for interpretation by a specialist immediately after the procedure.

Transcranial Doppler Studies

Description

1. Transcranial Doppler (TCD) ultrasonography involves noninvasive testing to measure flow changes in the form of velocities of the cerebral arteries. It helps evaluate vasospasm post-SAH, occlusion, or flow abnormalities as with stroke.

2. Bone windows (temporal, transorbital, or foramen magnum) are accessed using a fiber-optic probe after application of ultrasound gel. The fiber-optic probe is directed at a specific artery, and the velocities are then recorded.

3. Specific criteria are utilized for identification of each cerebral vessel prior to assessment of the vessel (specific bone window, depth, flow direction, and waveform).

4. *Advantages of TCD studies:* Low cost; can be performed at bedside and repeated as needed (useful in monitoring trends).

5. *Disadvantages of TCD studies:* Results are operator dependent; inability to obtain signal; limited data on sensitivity and specificity.

Nursing and Patient Care Considerations

1. Explain that the study will be done with patient in a reclining position.

2. Inform patient that the test normally takes less than 1 hour, depending on the number of arteries that are to be studied.

CT Perfusion

Description

1. CT perfusion involves rapid injection (5 to 10 mL/second) of 40 mL of iodine contrast during continuous scanning. Computer analysis of "wash-in" and "wash-out" of the contrast generates a single-slice acquisition blood flow map.

2. The test requires a large-bore catheter (14 or 16 gauge) for injection of the contrast. Contrast is cleared through the kidneys; therefore, renal function should be evaluated prior to study to reduce the risk of contrast-induced nephropathy (see Nursing Alert).

3. CT scan is programmed to analyze specific area of concern. Three 1-cm thick computer-generated images are produced that reflect relative cerebral blood flow, relative blood volume, and mean transit time.

4. *Advantages of CT perfusion:* 90% sensitivity and 100% specificity for cerebral ischemia; can be performed in conjunction with CT angiogram. Can be used in evaluating cerebral vasospasm in aneurysmal SAH, though the sensitivity and specificity is unknown.

5. *Disadvantages of CT perfusion:* Limited anatomic assessment; radiation exposure; if contrast is used there is the risk of contrast-induced nephropathy; requires large-bore catheter.

Nursing and Patient Care Considerations

1. Instruct patient about the rationale for placement of large-bore catheter.

2. Assess patient for contrast allergy and premedicate, if indicated.

3. Inform patient that radiation exposure, although present, is minimal.

Cerebral Angiography

Description

1. Following local anesthesia, a radiopaque dye is injected through a catheter in the femoral artery (or brachial artery if femoral is inaccessible) and passed through one of the major cervical blood vessels to assess cerebral circulation. Serial x-rays are taken after contrast dye illuminates the cerebral arterial and venous systems. The structure and patency of cerebral arteries are examined. Contrast is cleared through the kidneys. The test is frequently performed on an outpatient basis, unless patient is already hospitalized.

2. Three-dimensional imaging is available for more thorough evaluation of vascular abnormalities.

3. *Advantages of cerebral angiography:* Useful in detection of stenosis or occlusion, aneurysms, and vessel displacement due to pathologic processes (eg, tumor, abscess, hematoma).

4. *Disadvantages of cerebral angiography:* Involves considerable exposure to radiation. Contraindicated in patients with a stroke in evolution. Potential complications: temporary or permanent neurologic deficit, including stroke, anaphylaxis, bleeding or hematoma at the IV site, and impaired circulation in the extremity distal to the injection site, usually the femoral artery. There is risk of contrast-induced nephropathy.

Nursing and Patient Care Considerations

1. Omit the meal before the test, although clear liquids may be taken.

2. Evaluate for adequate renal function; should have recent normal serum creatinine.

3. Ask patient about allergies and specifically rule out presence of iodine allergy, which requires pretest preparation. Commonly, patients with allergy to iodine also have allergies to radiopaque contrast media that may cause severe reaction.

4. Options for pretest allergy prevention include:
   a. Elective procedure: Give prednisone 50 mg orally 13, 7, and 1 hour prior to contrast and diphenhydramine 50 mg orally 1 hour prior to contrast.

   b. Urgent procedure: Give methylprednisolone IV and diphenhydramine 50 mg orally, IM or IV 1 hour prior to contrast.

5. Mark pedal peripheral pulses.

6. Explain that a local anesthetic will be used to insert a catheter into the femoral artery (brachial artery may be used) and threaded into the required cerebral vessel.

7. Tell the patient to expect some discomfort when the catheter is inserted into the artery. Additionally, the sensation of a warm, flushed feeling and metallic taste should be expected when the dye is injected.

8. Caution the patient that he or she will need to lie still during the procedure and that he or she will be asked to hold breath intermittently during scanning.

9. After angiography:
   a. Maintain bed rest and do not flex lower extremities, as ordered, and monitor vital signs. Instruct the patient to maintain bed rest for up to 6 hours. If a closing device is utilized, the time can be reduced to 2 to 3 hours.

   b. Check the patient frequently for neurologic symptoms, such as motor or sensory alterations, reduced level of consciousness (LOC), speech disturbances, dysrhythmias, or blood pressure (BP) fluctuations.

   c. Evaluate renal function and monitor puncture site for bleeding, hematoma, and pulses, as ordered. Apply pressure if bleeding or hematoma is noted and inform physician.

   d. Evaluate renal function and monitor for adverse reaction to contrast medium (eg, restlessness, respiratory distress, tachycardia, facial flushing, nausea and vomiting).

   e. Assess skin color, temperature, and peripheral pulses of the extremity distal to the IV site—change may indicate impaired circulation due to occlusion. Inform physician, if noted.

Computed Tomographic Angiography

Description

1. CT angiography is a minimally invasive three-dimensional (3-D) imaging technique that uses multisectional spiral CT imaging in conjunction with rapid power injection of contrast (50 mL) into a large antecubital vein. Multiple, thin slices are reconstructed to provide 3-D imaging of cerebral vasculature.

2. Proper timing of contrast injection with initialization of CT scans is essential to optimize intravascular enhancement.

3. *Advantages of CT angiography:* Speed of scanning allows for unstable patients to be evaluated; increasing in availability.

4. *Disadvantages of CT angiography:* Exposure to radiation; need for large-bore (18 to 20 gauge) catheter; potential for anaphylaxis; contraindicated for patients with acute/chronic renal failure.

Nursing and Patient Care Considerations

1. Restrict food for 4 to 6 hours before procedure.

2. Assess for contrast allergy and premedicate, if indicated.

3. Evaluate renal function as contrast is cleared through kidneys. Elevated creatinine may preclude the individual from obtaining the study.

Magnetic Resonance Angiography/ Venography of the Brain

1. Magnetic resonance angiography/venography (MRA/MRV) is a 3-D phase contrast technique. The test focuses on high signal or blood flow while suppressing background nonactive tissue.
2. Two flow-opposing acquisitions are obtained and the computer subtracts the background signal to construct the cerebral vasculature.
3. *Advantages of MRA/MRV:* No exposure to radiation.
4. *Disadvantages of MRA/MRV:* Less sensitivity than CT angiography (sensitivity increases in aneurysms larger than 5 mm).

Nursing and Patient Care Considerations
1. Same as those for MRI, page 476.

Dynamic Volume Computed Tomography

Description
1. This scanning technique can include entire organs, such as the heart or brain, in a single rotation and enables dynamic processes, such as blood volume and time to peak, to be observed.
2. The scanning process takes less time and requires a smaller dose of iodinated contrast and less radiation than conventional CT, making it an ideal diagnostic test in emergency situations (heart attack or stroke) or for those who cannot tolerate large doses of iodine contrast (renal disease).

Nursing and Patient Care Considerations
1. The general considerations for conventional CT are the same.
2. Inform the patient about lying flat on the table while the tube revolves around the area to be scanned.
3. If contrast will be used, the patient will most likely have an IV catheter placed for the injection of dye. A sensation of warmth or metallic taste in the mouth may be experienced after the dye injection.

Other Diagnostic Tests

Other diagnostic tests include lumbar puncture, which provides information about the CNS through direct contact with the cerebrospinal fluid (CSF); a variety of tests that measure electrical impulses in portions of the nervous system; and neuropsychological evaluation.

Lumbar Puncture

Description
1. A needle is inserted into the lumbar subarachnoid space, usually between the third and fourth lumbar vertebrae, and CSF is withdrawn for diagnostic and therapeutic purposes.
2. Purposes include:
   a. Obtaining CSF for examination (microbiologic, serologic, cytologic, or chemical analysis).
   b. Measuring cerebrospinal pressure and assisting in detection of obstruction of CSF circulation.
   c. Determining the presence or absence of blood in the spinal fluid.
   d. Aiding in the diagnosis of viral or bacterial meningitis, subarachnoid or intracranial hemorrhage, tumors, and brain abscesses.
   e. Administering antibiotics and cancer chemotherapy intrathecally in certain cases.
   f. Determining levels of tau protein and beta-amyloid in the CSF—a new test that may be used to assist in the diagnosis of Alzheimer's disease. Elevated levels of tau protein and decreased levels of beta-amyloid are associated with Alzheimer's disease.

Nursing and Patient Care Considerations
See Procedure Guidelines 15-1, pages 480 to 481.

Electroencephalography

Description
1. EEG measures electrical activity of brain cells. Electrodes are attached to multiple sites on the scalp to provide a recording of electrical activity that is generated in the cerebral cortex. Electrical impulses are transmitted to an electroencephalograph, which magnifies and records these impulses as brain waves on a strip of paper. New devices allow for continuous EEG monitoring of selective areas of the brain, thus limited data is collected. It is useful in the intensive care unit (ICU) setting for continuous monitoring to evaluate for seizure activation.
2. Provides physiologic assessment of cerebral activity for diagnosis of epilepsy, alterations in brain activity in coma, and organic brain syndrome and sleep disorders. Particularly helpful in the investigation of patients with seizures.
3. Usually performed in a room designed to eliminate electrical interference; however, in the case of a comatose patient, it may be performed at bedside using a portable unit.
4. Restlessness and fatigue can alter brain wave patterns.
5. For a baseline recording, the patient is instructed to lie still and relax with eyes closed. After a baseline recording in a resting phase, the patient may be tested in various stress situations (eg, asked to hyperventilate for 3 minutes, look at a flashing strobe light) to elicit abnormal electrical patterns.
6. In patients with epilepsy, continuous monitoring is performed with video monitoring. This is useful for interpretation and correlation of physiologic seizure activity and clinical seizures.
   a. Grids or strips are placed intraoperatively for more accurate assessment of seizure foci.
   b. Mapping of seizure activity is performed to determine precise location of seizure foci.
   c. Once foci are located, the site is evaluated for possible surgical resection.

Nursing and Patient Care Considerations
1. For routine EEG, tranquilizers, anticonvulsants, sedatives, and stimulants should be held for 24 to 48 hours before the study.
2. Thoroughly wash and dry patient's hair to remove hair sprays, creams, or oils.
3. Explain that the electrodes will be attached to patient's skull with a special paste.

PROCEDURE GUIDELINES 15-1

Assisting the Patient Undergoing Lumbar Puncture

EQUIPMENT

- Sterile lumbar puncture set
- Skin antiseptic (avoid use of chlorhexidine)
- Sterile gloves
- Adhesive bandage
- Xylocaine 1%–2%

PROCEDURE

Nursing Action	Rationale
1. Before procedure, the patient should empty bladder and/or bowel.	1. Enhances comfort.
2. Give a step-by-step summary of the procedure. For lying position, see accompanying figure.	2. Reassures the patient and gains cooperation.

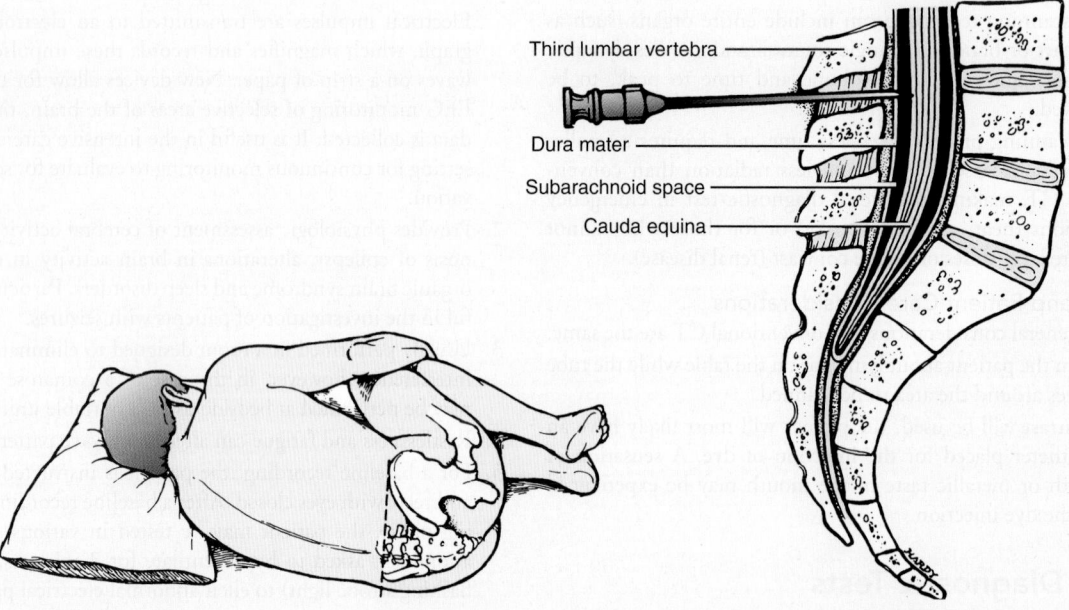

Third lumbar vertebra

Dura mater

Subarachnoid space

Cauda equina

3. If patient has signs of increased intracranial pressure, a computed tomography scan should be done to rule out mass effect.	3. Removal of cerebrospinal fluid (CSF) in the presence of mass effect may precipitate brain herniation.
4. Position the patient on side with a small pillow under head and a pillow between legs. Patient should be lying on a firm surface.	4. The spine is maintained in a horizontal position. The pillow between the legs prevents the upper leg from rolling forward.
5. Instruct the patient to arch the lumbar segment of back and draw knees up to abdomen, chin to chest, clasping knees with hands.	5. Offers maximal widening of the interspinous spaces and affords easier entry into the subarachnoid space.
6. Assist the patient in maintaining this position throughout the procedure by supporting behind the knees and upper back and neck.	6. Supporting the patient helps prevent sudden movements, which can produce a traumatic (bloody) tap and thus impede correct diagnosis.
7. Alternately, for sitting position, have the patient straddle a straight-back chair (facing the back) and rest head against arms, which are folded on the back of the chair.	7. In obese patients and those who have difficulty in assuming an arched side-lying position, this posture may allow more accurate identification of the spinous processes and interspaces.

PROCEDURE GUIDELINES 15-1 *(continued)*

Assisting the Patient Undergoing Lumbar Puncture

PROCEDURE *(continued)*

Nursing Action	Rationale
Performance phase (by the health care provider)	
1. The skin is prepared with antiseptic solution (avoiding use of chlorhexidine), and the skin and subcutaneous spaces are infiltrated with local anesthetic agent.	1. Reduces risk of contamination; decreases pain. Chlorhexidine is neurotoxic and should not come in contact with CSF.
2. A spinal needle is introduced at the L3–L4 interspace. The needle is advanced until the "give" of the ligamentum flavum is felt and the needle enters the subarachnoid space. The manometer is attached to the spinal needle.	2. L3–L4 interspace is *below* the level of the spinal cord.
3. After the needle enters the subarachnoid space, help the patient to straighten up slowly.	3. Prevents a false increase in intraspinal pressure. Muscle tension and compression of the abdomen give falsely high pressures.
4. Instruct the patient to breathe quietly (not to hold breath or strain) and not to talk.	4. Hyperventilation may lower a truly elevated pressure. Talking can elevate CSF pressure.
5. The initial pressure reading (opening pressure) is obtained by measuring the level of the fluid column after it comes to rest.	5. With respiration, there is normally some fluctuation of spinal fluid in the manometer. Normal range of spinal fluid pressure with the patient in the lateral recumbent position is 70 to 200 mm H_2O. Opening pressure exceeds normal range when hydrocephalus or increased ICP is present.
6. About 2–3 mL of spinal fluid is placed in each of three test tubes for observation, comparison, and laboratory analysis. Spinal fluid should be clear and colorless.	6. Bloody spinal fluid may indicate subarachnoid hemorrhage or a traumatic tap. If traumatic tap, blood should gradually clear with subsequent specimens.
7. Closing pressure is documented; the pressure on the manometer after the CSF specimen is collected and/or excess CSF removed.	7. Closing pressure should be within normal CSF pressure range.
Follow-up phase	
1. After the procedure, the patient is instructed to remain flat for about 2 hours.	1. Reduces pressure on tissue surfaces along the needle track to prevent CSF leakage.
2. Ensure adequate hydration with oral or parenteral fluids.	2. Facilitates replacement of CSF and prevents spinal headache.
3. Monitor for spinal headache and observe for CSF leak.	3. CSF leaks from lumbar puncture are characterized by intractable spinal headache.

 Evidence Base American Association of Neuroscience Nurses. (2011). *Care of the patient undergoing intracranial pressure monitoring/external ventricular drainage or lumbar drainage.* Glenview, IL: Author.

4. Assure patient that the electrodes will not cause shock, and encourage patient to relax during the procedure because anxiety can affect brain wave patterns.

5. Meals should be taken as usual to avoid sudden changes in blood glucose levels.

Evoked Potential Studies

Description

1. These tests measure the brain's electrical responses to visual, somatosensory, or auditory stimuli.

   a. Visual evoked potentials—produced by asking the patient to look at rapidly reversing checkerboard patterns. These assist in evaluating multiple sclerosis and traumatic injury.

   EEG electrodes are placed over the occiput and record the transmission time from the retina to the occiput.

   b. Somatosensory evoked potentials—generated by stimulating a peripheral sensory nerve and useful in diagnosing peripheral nerve disease and injury. These measure transmission time up the spinal cord to the sensory cortex.

   c. Auditory evoked potentials—produced by applying sound, such as clicks, to help locate auditory lesions and evaluate integrity of the brain stem. The transmission time up the brain stem into the cortex is measured.

2. Can be performed intraoperatively or during interventional procedures in which patient is under general anesthesia. Acute changes may indicate potential for deficits.

Nursing and Patient Care Considerations

1. Explain that the electrodes will be attached to patient's scalp to measure the electrical activity of the nervous system. Placement of the electrodes will depend on the type of evoked potentials being measured.
2. Ask patient to remove all jewelry.
3. Assure patient that the procedure is not painful and does not cause any electric shock.
4. Inform patient that the test normally takes 45 to 60 minutes.

Needle Electromyography

Description

1. In combination with nerve conduction studies, needle electromyography (EMG) is the gold standard for assessing the neurophysiologic characteristics of neuromuscular diseases. Because it is invasive and painful, its use is limited when activity from several muscles needs to be monitored simultaneously. It is the recording of a muscle's electrical impulses at rest and during contraction. A needle is attached to an electrode and inserted into a muscle. A mild electrical charge is delivered to stimulate the muscle at rest and during voluntary contraction. The response of the muscle is measured on an oscilloscope screen.
2. Useful in distinguishing lower motor neuron disorders from muscle disorders (eg, ALS from muscular dystrophy).
3. Nerve conduction time, another diagnostic test, is often measured simultaneously.

Nursing and Patient Care Considerations

1. Explain that this test measures the electrical activity of muscles.
2. Advise the patient to avoid caffeine and tobacco products for 3 hours before the test, as these substances can affect test results.
3. Inform the patient that the procedure normally takes at least 1 hour.
4. Tell the patient a needle will be inserted through the skin into select muscles and to expect some degree of discomfort when the needle is inserted.
5. Inform the patient that, after the test, a mild analgesic or warm compresses may be needed to relieve muscle soreness.
6. Inform the patient to observe the needle insertion sites for bleeding, hematoma, redness, or other signs of infection and to notify the health care provider if any of these are observed.

Nerve Conduction Studies (Electroneurography)

Description

1. A peripheral nerve is stimulated electrically through the skin and underlying tissues. A recording electrode detects the response from the stimulated nerve. The time between the stimulation of the nerve and the response is measured on an oscilloscope and speed of conduction along the nerve is calculated.
2. Used to determine lower motor neuron dysfunction, differentiating disease or injury in peripheral nerves, spinal nerve roots, or the anterior horn of the spinal cord by measuring nerve conduction velocity.

Nursing and Patient Care Considerations

1. Explain that surface-stimulating electrodes with special paste are applied and taped to the nerve site (leg, arm, or face).
2. Advise patient that an electric current is passed through the electrode and that a mild sensation or slight discomfort may be experienced while the current is applied.

Neuropsychological Testing

Description

1. A series of tests that evaluate effects of neurologic disorders on cognitive functioning and behavior.
2. A neuropsychologist selects appropriate tests to determine the extent and type of functional deficits.
3. Paper-and-pencil tests, puzzles, and word and recall games are commonly used. Testing may assess:
   a. Intelligence, attention span, memory, judgment.
   b. Motor, speech, and sensory function.
   c. Affect, coping, and adaptation.
   d. Language quality, abstraction, distractibility.
   e. Ability to sequence learned behaviors.
   f. Used in diagnosis of organic brain dysfunction and dementia.
   g. Valuable in determining vocational rehabilitation training needs.
4. Utilized in some facilities to determine competency of a patient with regard to instituting durable power of attorney or need for guardianship.

Nursing and Patient Care Considerations

1. Assure patient that these tests are not intended to evaluate mental illness.
2. Explain that testing evaluates the ability to remember, calculate numbers, and perform abstract reasoning.
3. Patient should be well rested because testing is mentally tiring and lengthy. A complete examination is a 4- to 6-hour process, depending on patient's ability to concentrate.
4. Anticipate fatigue and frustration after the examination.

Polysomnography

Description

1. Polysomnography is a noninvasive, all-night sleep study that measures character of sleep, simultaneously monitoring EEG, cardiac and respiratory function, and movements during sleep. It is used to confirm fragmented sleep patterns in narcolepsy and sleep-related epilepsy.
2. Testing is time-consuming and labor-intensive. Procedures typically include multiple physiologic measures, such as EEG, EMG, electrocardiogram [ECG]), heart rate, respiratory effort, air flow, and oxygen saturation.

Nursing and Patient Care Considerations

1. Explain that the electrodes placed on the scalp, chest, extremities, and face will be uncomfortable but do not deliver electrical current.
2. Reassure patient that a technician will be in the next room.
3. Advise patient to wear comfortable nightwear.

Multisleep Latency Test

Description

1. Multisleep latency test (MSLT) is a sleep study performed during the day. It is the most widely objective assessment of daytime sleepiness and is commonly used to confirm a diagnosis of narcolepsy.
2. Testing consists of four "napping" periods of 20 to 35 minutes, during which time the patient lies down on a bed in a darkened room and is allowed to fall asleep. The multiple short sleep periods during the MSLT increase the observation of rapid-eye-movement (REM) periods.

Nursing and Patient Care Considerations

1. Explain the time and duration of the naps.
2. Reassure patient of freedom to move about between naps.
3. Tell patient to wear comfortable clothing and to bring reading or other materials for use between naps.

GENERAL PROCEDURES AND TREATMENT MODALITIES

Nursing Management of the Patient with an Altered State of Consciousness

Unconsciousness is a condition in which there is a depression of cerebral function ranging from stupor to coma. Coma results from impairment in both the arousal and the awareness of consciousness. The arousal of consciousness is mediated by the reticular activating system (RAS) in the brain stem, while the awareness component is mediated by cortical activity within the cerebral hemispheres.

Both arousal and awareness are assessed when using the Glasgow Coma Scale (GCS) as a measure of LOC (see Table 15-2).

When using the GCS, *coma* may be defined as no eye opening on stimulation, absence of comprehensible speech, and failure to obey commands. The GCS is designed to provide a rapid assessment of LOC and does not provide a means to monitor or localize neurologic dysfunction. Facility-generated neurologic assessment tools may be used in combination with the GCS to assess, monitor, and trend neurologic function.

An altered state of consciousness may be caused by many factors, including hypoxemia, trauma, neoplasms, vascular, degenerative, and infectious disorders, as well as a variety of metabolic disorders and structural neurologic lesions. Diagnostic evaluation and management depend on the underlying cause, overall intracranial dynamics, age, comorbidities, and general state of health.

Nursing Assessment

1. Assess eye opening (level of responsiveness).
   Eye opening = arousal
   Tracking = awareness
2. Assess neurologic function using the GCS. The GCS addresses eye opening, verbal responses, and motor responses. If the patient's eyes do not open spontaneously or to your voice, then assess responses using painful stimuli by applying pressure against the nail bed, trapezius/axillary pinch, or sternum. Use the least amount of pain for the best response.

Table 15-2	Glasgow Coma Scale	
PARAMETER	**FINDING**	**SCORE**
Eye opening	Spontaneously	4
	To speech	3
	To pain	2
	Do not open	1
Best verbal response	Oriented	5
	Confused	4
	Inappropriate speech	3
	Incomprehensible sounds	2
	No verbalization	1
Best motor response	Obeys command	6
	Localizes pain	5
	Withdraws from pain	4
	Abnormal flexion	3
	Abnormal extension	2
	No motor response	1

Interpretation: Best score = 15; worst score = 3; 7 or less generally indicates coma; changes from baseline are most important.

3. Assess cognitive function.
   a. Orientation.
      i. Person, place, and time.
      ii. Where are you, why are you here.
      iii. General information—national and local current events.
   b. Speech—aphasia and other problems (see Table 15-3).
      i. Fluent aphasia (motor/Broca's)—inability to express self.
      ii. Nonfluent aphasia (sensory/Wernicke's)—inability to understand the spoken language.
      iii. Global aphasia—inability to speak or understand spoken language.
      iv. Other aphasia syndromes—amnesia, conduction.
   c. Other alterations include:
      i. Confabulation—fluent, nonsensical speech.
      ii. Preservation—continuation of thought process with inability to change train of thought without direction or repetition.
4. Assess motor function—voluntary versus reflexive:
   a. Voluntary movement.
      i. Normal complex movement—strength and symmetry in the upper extremities (UE), pronator drift proximally and grip strength distally; in the lower extremities (LE), leg lifts proximally and dorsi/plantar flexion distally.

Table 15-3 Differentiating Aphasia

APHASIA	FLUENCY	RATE	COMPREHENSION	GRAMMAR	REPETITION
Fluent (Wernicke's/receptive aphasia)	Intact, although speech is nonsensical	Normal	Absent to poor	Intact	Intact
Nonfluent (Broca's/expressive aphasia)	Poor	Slow, halting	Intact	Absent	Poor
Global	Poor	Slow	Absent	Absent	Poor
Conduction	Intact, although there is functional transposition of sounds with phonetic paraphrases	Normal	Intact	Intact	Poor
Anomic or amnesiac aphasia	Difficulty naming and finding words	Halting	Intact	Intact	Intact

ii. Localization—ability to determine location of stimuli; patient localizes area of painful stimuli.

iii. Withdrawal—abduction of the upper extremity; moving away from the stimuli.

b. Reflexive movement.

i. Abnormal flexor posturing (decorticate)—dysfunction of corticospinal tracts above the brain stem. Abnormal flexion of the UE with adduction of the UE, internal rotation of the upper extremity, wrist and extension, internal rotation and plantar flexion of the LE.

ii. Abnormal extension posturing (decerebrate)—dysfunction of vestibulospinal tract and the RAS of the upper brain stem. Abnormal extension, hyperpronation, and adduction of the UE and wrist flexion; abnormal extension and internal rotation of the LE with plantar flexion of the feet and toes.

iii. Mixed posturing—varied extensor and flexor tone in UE.

iv. Flaccid—medullary compression with complete loss of motor tone.

5. Test cranial nerve (CN) reflexes to assess for brain stem dysfunction.

a. Assess pupil size, symmetry, and reaction to light.

b. Assess extraocular movements (CNs III, IV, VI) and reflex eye movements elicited by head turning (oculocephalic response). This should not be performed on patients with suspected cervical spine injury, patients in a cervical collar, or patients known to have cervical spine injuries.

c. The oculovestibular (caloric) response (CNs III, IV, VI, VIII) is tested by medical staff when the patient is comatose and the oculocephalic response is absent, as a determination of brain death.

d. Assess CNs V and VII together to evaluate facial pain, blink, eye closure, and grimace.

e. Assess CNs IX, X, XII to evaluate gag, swallowing reflex, tongue protrusion, and patient's ability to handle own secretions.

6. Assess respiratory rate and pattern (normal, Kussmaul, Cheyne-Stokes, apneic).

7. Assess deep tendon reflexes; evaluate tone for spasticity, rigidity, and paratonia (abnormal resistance increasing throughout flexion and extension, indicating frontal lobe dysfunction).

8. Examine head for signs of trauma, and mouth, nose, and ears for evidence of edema, blood, and CSF (may indicate basilar skull fracture).

9. Monitor any change in neurologic status over time and report changes to health care provider, as indicated.

 Key Decision Point
A critical indicator of neurologic function is the LOC. A change in GCS of two or more points may be significant. If patient demonstrates deterioration, as evidenced by a change in neurologic examination, notify the health care provider without delay and reevaluate the neurologic status more often than required by orders based on nursing judgment.

Nursing Diagnoses

- Decreased Intracranial Adaptive Capacity.
- Ineffective Airway Clearance related to upper airway obstruction by tongue and soft tissues, inability to clear respiratory secretions.
- Risk for Imbalanced Fluid Volume related to inability to ingest fluids, dehydration from osmotic therapy (when used to reduce intracranial pressure [ICP]).
- Impaired Oral Mucous Membranes related to mouth breathing, absence of pharyngeal reflex, inability to ingest fluid.
- Risk for Impaired Skin Integrity related to immobility or restlessness.
- Impaired Tissue Integrity of cornea related to diminished/absent corneal reflex.
- Hyperthermia related to infectious process; damage to hypothalamic center.
- Impaired Urinary Elimination related to unconscious state.
- Bowel Incontinence related to unconscious state.

Nursing Interventions

Minimizing Secondary Brain Injury

1. Monitor for change in neurologic status, decreased LOC, onset of CN deficits.
2. Identify emerging trends in neurologic function and communicate findings to medical staff.
3. Monitor response to pharmacologic therapy, including drug levels, as indicated.
4. Monitor laboratory data, CSF cultures, and Gram stain, if applicable, and communicate findings to medical staff.
5. Assess neurologic drains/dressings for patency, security, and characteristics for drainage.
6. Institute measures to minimize risk for increased ICP, cerebral edema, seizures, or neurovascular compromise.
7. Adjust care to reduce risk of increasing ICP: body positioning in a neutral position (head aligned with shoulders) without flexing head, reduce hip flexion, distribute care throughout 24-hour period sufficiently for ICP to return to baseline.
8. Monitor temperature status; maintain normothermia. Institute cooling procedure as ordered.

Maintaining an Effective Airway

1. Position patient to prevent tongue from obstructing the airway, encourage drainage of respiratory secretions, and promote adequate exchange of oxygen and carbon dioxide.
2. Keep the airway free from secretions with suctioning. In the absence of cough and swallowing reflexes, secretions rapidly accumulate in the posterior pharynx and upper trachea and can lead to respiratory complications (eg, aspiration).
   a. Insert oral airway if tongue is paralyzed or is obstructing the airway. An obstructed airway increases ICP. This is considered a short-term measure.
   b. Prepare for insertion of cuffed endotracheal tube to protect the airway from aspiration and to allow efficient removal of tracheobronchial secretions.
   c. See page 231 for technique of tracheal suctioning.
   d. Use oxygen therapy as prescribed to deliver oxygenated blood to the CNS.
   e. Before suctioning, pretreat with sedative, opioid, or endotracheal lidocaine, if indicated.

Attaining and Maintaining Fluid and Electrolyte Balance

1. Monitor prescribed IV fluids carefully, maintaining euvolemia and minimizing large volumes of "free water," which may aggravate cerebral edema.
2. Maintain hydration and enhance nutritional status with use of enteral or parenteral fluids.
3. Measure urine output.
4. Evaluate pulses (radial, carotid, apical, and pedal) and measure BP; these parameters are a measure of circulatory adequacy/inadequacy.
5. Maintain circulation; support the BP and treat life-threatening cardiac dysrhythmias.

Maintaining Healthy Oral Mucous Membranes

1. Remove dentures. Inspect patient's mouth for dryness, inflammation, and the presence of crusting.
2. Provide mouth care by brushing teeth and cleansing the mouth with appropriate solution every 2 to 4 hours to prevent parotitis (inflammation of parotid gland).
3. Apply lip emollient to maintain hydration and prevent dryness.

Skin Integrity

1. Keep the skin clean, dry, well lubricated, and free from pressure because comatose patients are susceptible to the formation of pressure ulcers.
2. Turn the patient from side to side on a regular schedule to relieve pressure areas and help clear lungs by mobilizing secretions; turning also provides kinesthetic (sensation of movement), proprioceptive (awareness of position), and vestibular (equilibrium) stimulation.
3. Reposition carefully after turning to prevent ischemia and shearing over pressure areas.
4. Position extremities in functional position, and monitor skin underneath splints/orthosis to prevent skin breakdown and pressure neuropathies.
5. Perform range-of-motion (ROM) exercises of extremities at least four times daily; contracture deformities develop early in unconscious patients.

Maintaining Corneal Integrity

1. Protect the eyes from corneal irritation as the cornea functions as a shield. If the eyes remain open for long periods, corneal drying, irritation, and ulceration are likely to result.
   a. Make sure the patient's eye is not rubbing against bedding if blinking and corneal reflexes are absent.
   b. Inspect the condition of the eyes with a penlight.
   c. Remove contact lenses, if worn.
   d. Irrigate eyes with sterile saline or prescribed solution to remove discharge and debris.
   e. Instill prescribed ophthalmic ointment in each eye to prevent glazing and corneal ulceration.
   f. Apply eye patches, when indicated, ensuring that eyes remain closed under patch.
2. Prepare for temporary tarsorrhaphy (suturing of eyelids in closed position) if unconscious state is prolonged.

Reducing Fever

1. Look for possible sites of infections (respiratory, CNS, urinary tract, wound) when fever is present in an unconscious patient.
2. Monitor temperature frequently or continuously.
3. Control persistent elevations of temperature. Fever increases metabolic demands of the brain, decreases circulation and oxygenation, and results in cerebral deterioration.
   a. Monitor core temperature continuously and treat hyperthermia promptly. Hyperthermia increases the brain's metabolic rate and increases the risk of secondary injury. A body core temperature is 4 to 5 degrees lower than brain temperature.
   b. Maintain a cool ambient temperature. Anticipate potential for overcooling and make environmental adjustments accordingly (eg, operating room environment).
   c. Minimize excess covering on bed.

d. Administer prescribed antipyretics.

e. Use cool-water sponging and an electric fan blowing over the patient to increase surface cooling for hyperthermia resistant to antipyretics.

f. Use an external cooling device to maintain normothermia, but avoid rapid overcooling. Intravascular cooling devices may also be used.

Promoting Urinary Elimination

1. An indwelling or external urethral catheter may be used for short-term management.

2. Use intermittent bladder catheterization for distention as soon as possible to minimize risk of infection. Palpate over the patient's bladder at intervals or use a bladder scan to detect urine retention and an overdistended bladder.

3. Monitor for fever and cloudy urine.

4. Initiate a bladder-training program as soon as consciousness is regained.

Promoting Bowel Function

1. Auscultate for bowel sounds; palpate lower abdomen for distention.

2. Observe for constipation due to immobility and lack of dietary fiber. Stool softener or laxative, scheduled or as needed, may be prescribed to promote bowel elimination. The goal is bowel movement every other day.

3. Monitor for diarrhea resulting from infection, antibiotics, enteric feedings, hyperosmolar fluids, and fecal impaction.

a. Perform a rectal examination if fecal impaction is suspected.

b. Use fecal collection bags and provide meticulous skin care if patient has fecal incontinence.

Family Education and Support

1. Develop a supportive and trusting relationship with the family or significant other.

2. Provide information and frequent updates on the patient's condition and progress.

3. Involve them in routine care and teach procedures that they can perform at home.

4. Demonstrate and teach methods of sensory stimulation to be used frequently.

a. Use physical touch and reassuring voice.

b. Talk to patient in a meaningful way even when the patient does not seem to respond. Assume patient is able to hear even if unresponsive.

c. Orient the patient periodically to person, time, and place.

5. Demonstrate and teach methods frequently used to manage restlessness/agitation.

a. Eliminate distractions.

b. Reduce environmental stimuli (turn off television and radio, close door).

c. Use one-to-one communication.

d. Talk slowly and simplify information without talking down to the person.

6. Teach the family to recognize and report unusual restlessness, which could indicate cerebral hypoxia, metabolic imbalance, or pain.

7. Enlist the help of the social worker, home health agency, or other resources to assist family with such issues as financial concerns, guardianship, need for additional follow-up care (rehabilitation, long-term care facility), need for medical equipment in home, and/or respite care.

Evaluation: Expected Outcomes

- Neurologic status remains at baseline or improved.
- Maintains clear airway; coughs up secretions.
- Absence of signs of dehydration.
- Intact, pink mucous membranes.
- No skin breakdown or erythema.
- Absence of trauma to cornea.
- Core temperature within normal limits.
- Absence of urinary tract infection (UTI); maintenance of normal bladder emptying.
- Bowel movement on regular basis in response to bowel regimen.

Nursing Management of the Patient with Increased Intracranial Pressure

 Evidence Base American Association of Neuroscience Nurses. (2010). *AANN core curriculum for neuroscience nursing* (5th ed.). Glenview, IL: Author.

Intracranial pressure (ICP) is the pressure exerted by the contents inside the cranial vault—the brain tissue (gray and white matter), CSF, and the blood volume. A pressure reading at or greater than 20 mm HG is defined as increased ICP.

Pathophysiology and Etiology

1. ICP is comprised of the following components and volume ratio: brain tissue, 80%; CSF, 10%; blood volume, 10%.

2. The Monroe-Kellie doctrine states that the intracranial vault is a closed structure with a fixed intracranial volume. The intracranial contents must be kept in equilibrium and the ratio between volume and pressure must remain constant. Any increase in the volume of one component must be accompanied by a reciprocal decrease in one of the other components. When this volume–pressure relationship becomes unbalanced, ICP increases.

3. The brain attempts to compensate for rises in ICP by:

a. Displacement/shunting of CSF from the intracranial compartment to the lumbar subarachnoid space (SAS). Normally, about 500 mL of CSF are produced and absorbed in 24 hours. About 125 to 150 mL circulates throughout the ventricular system and the SAS in the following ratio: 25 mL in the ventricles, 90 mL in the lumbar SAS, and 35 mL in the cisterns and surrounding SAS.

b. Increased CSF absorption.

c. Decreased cerebral blood volume by displacement of cerebral venous blood into the venous sinuses. Compensatory measures are finite. Increased ICP will ultimately occur if the volume of the intracranial mass exceeds the volume compensated.

4. Intracranial compliance is "tightness" of the brain. Compliance is the relationship between intracranial volume and ICP. It is a nonlinear relationship; as ICP increases, compliance decreases. With functional compensatory mechanisms, an increase in volume causes a small, transient increase in ICP. As compliance decreases, small increases in volume result in moderate increases in pressure. When compensatory mechanisms are exhausted, very slight increases in volume will produce large increases in pressure. The patient's response to changes in ICP will depend on where the patient is on the volume–pressure curve.

5. Factors that influence the ability of the body to achieve this steady state include:
   a. Systemic BP.
   b. Ventilation and oxygenation.
   c. Metabolic rate and oxygen consumption (fever, shivering, physical activity).
   d. Regional cerebral vasospasm.
   e. Oxygen saturation and hematocrit.

6. Inability to maintain a steady state results in increased ICP. Traumatic brain injury, cerebral edema, intracerebral hemorrhage, ischemic stroke, abscess and infection, lesions, intracranial surgery, and radiation therapy can be potential etiologies of increased ICP.

7. Increased ICP constitutes an emergency and requires prompt treatment. ICP can be monitored by means of an intraventricular catheter, a subarachnoid screw or bolt, or an epidural pressure recording device.

8. Alterations or compromise in cerebral blood flow can be measured noninvasively by a TCD study. Increased velocities indicate vasospasm, diminished velocities indicate low blood flow, and absent velocities are consistent with no flow or brain death.

Nursing Assessment

Change in LOC
Caused by increased cerebral pressure. Assess for:

1. Change in LOC (awareness): drowsiness, lethargy.
2. Early behavioral changes: restlessness, irritability, confusion, and apathy.
3. Falling score on the GCS (see page 483).
   a. Change in orientation: disorientation to time, place, or person.
   b. Difficulty or inability to follow commands.
   c. Difficulty or inability in verbalization or in responsiveness to auditory stimuli.
   d. Change in response to painful stimuli (eg, purposeful to inappropriate or absent responses).
   e. Posturing (abnormal flexion or extension).

Changes in Vital Signs
Caused by pressure on brain stem. Assess for:

1. Rising BP or widening pulse pressure (the difference between systolic and diastolic BP). This may be followed by hypotension and labile vital signs, indicating further brain stem compromise.
2. Pulse changes with bradycardia changing to tachycardia as ICP rises.

Key Decision Point
Watch for Cushing's triad—bradycardia, hypertension (with widening pulse pressure), and irregular respirations; this is classic symptomatology related to uncompensated increased ICP and is considered a neurologic medical emergency. Alert health care provider and prepare for therapeutic intervention.

3. Respiratory irregularities: tachypnea (early sign of increased ICP); slowing of rate with lengthening periods of apnea; Cheyne-Stokes (rhythmic pattern of increasing and decreasing depth of respirations with periods of apnea) or Kussmaul (paroxysms of difficult breathing) breathing; central neurogenic hyperventilation (prolonged, deep breathing); apneustic (sustained inspiratory effort) breathing; and ataxic (incoordinated and spasmodic) breathing.

NURSING ALERT Respiratory irregularities may not be apparent if patient is mechanically ventilated.

4. Hyperthermia followed by hypothermia.

Pupillary Changes
1. Caused by increased pressure on optic and oculomotor nerves.
2. Inspect the pupils with a penlight to evaluate size, configuration, and reaction to light.
3. Compare both eyes for similarities or differences, particularly pupillary changes related to location and progression of brain stem herniation.
   a. Midbrain involvement—fixed and dilated.
   b. Pontine involvement—pinpoint pupils.
   c. Uncal herniation.
      i. Unilaterally dilating pupil ipsilateral to lesion.
      ii. Anisocoria (unequal) with sluggish light reaction in dilated pupil.
      iii. If treatment is delayed or unsuccessful, contralateral pupil becomes dilated and fixed to light.
      iv. When herniation of brain stem occurs, both pupils assume midposition and remain fixed to light.
   d. Central transtentorial herniation.
      i. Pupils are small bilaterally (1 to 3 mm).
      ii. Reaction to light is brisk but with small range of constriction.
      iii. If treatment is delayed or unsuccessful; small pupils dilate moderately (3 to 5 mm) and fix irregularly at midposition.
      iv. When herniation of brain stem occurs, both pupils dilate widely and remain fixed to light.
4. Perform funduscopic examination to inspect the retina and optic nerve for hemorrhage and papilledema.

Extraocular Movements
1. Evaluate gaze to determine if it is conjugate (paired, working together) or dysconjugate (eye deviates or movement is asymmetric).

2. Evaluate movement of eyes.
   a. Inability to abduct or adduct: deviation of one or both eyes.
   b. Alteration in vision (eg, blurred vision, diplopia, field cut).
   c. Spontaneous roving, random eye movements.
   d. Nystagmus on horizontal/vertical gaze.
3. Oculocephalic reflex (doll's eyes): brisk turning of the head left, right, up, or down with observation of eye movements in response to the stimulus. Tests brain stem pathways between CNs III, IV, VI, and VIII. This should not be performed on patients with suspected cervical spine injury, patients in a cervical collar, or patients with known cervical spine injuries unless part of the brain death exam.
4. Oculovestibular reflex (cold calorics): 30 to 60 mL of ice water instilled into the ear with the head of the bed elevated to 30 degrees. Tests brain stem pathways between CNs III, IV, VI, and VIII. Response preserved longer than the doll's eyes maneuver. Performed by health care provider as part of brain death examination.

Other Changes

Be alert for:
1. Headache increasing in intensity and aggravated by movement and straining.
2. Vomiting recurrent with little or no nausea, especially in early morning; may be projectile.
3. Papilledema from optic nerve compression.
4. Subtle changes, such as restlessness, headache, forced breathing, purposeless movements, and mental cloudiness.
5. Motor and sensory dysfunctions (proximal muscle weakness, presence of pronator drift).
6. Contralateral hemiparesis progressing to complete hemiplegia.
7. Speech impairment (nonfluent, fluent, or global aphasia) when dominant hemisphere involved.
8. Seizure activity: focal or generalized.
9. Decreased brain stem function (CN deficits, such as loss of corneal reflex, gag reflex, and ability to swallow).
10. Pathologic reflexes: Babinski, grasp, chewing, sucking.

Nursing Diagnosis

• Decreased Intracranial Adaptive Capacity.

Nursing Interventions

Decreasing ICP

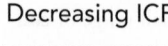 **NURSING ALERT** Increased ICP is a true life-threatening medical emergency that requires immediate recognition and prompt therapeutic intervention.

1. Establish and maintain airway, breathing, and circulation.
2. Promote normal Pco_2. Hyperventilation is not recommended for prophylactic treatment of increased ICP as cerebral circulation is reduced by 50% the first 24 hours after injury. Hyperventilation causes cerebral vasoconstriction and decreases cerebral blood flow to decrease ICP; this can potentiate secondary injury to the brain. Hyperventilation should be used only after all other treatment options have been exhausted or in an acute crisis.
3. Avoid hypoxia. Decreased PO_2 (less than 60 mm Hg) causes cerebral vasodilation, thus increasing ICP.
4. Maintain cerebral perfusion pressure (CPP) greater than 50 mm Hg. CPP is determined by subtracting the ICP from the MAP: CPP = MAP − ICP.
5. Administer mannitol (0.25 to 1 g/kg), an osmotic diuretic, if ordered. Osmotic diuretics act by establishing an osmotic gradient across the blood–brain barrier that depletes the intracellular and extracellular fluid volume within the brain and throughout the body. Mannitol will be ineffective if the blood–brain barrier is not intact.
6. Administer hypertonic saline (2% or 3%), if ordered. It creates an osmotic gradient that pulls extra fluid from the brain with an intact blood–brain barrier, lowers ICP, improves cerebral blood flow by reducing viscosity, and improves oxygen carrying capacity. Saline (23.4%) is used as a bolus to treat acute increases in ICP in conjunction with or in place of mannitol.
7. Insert an indwelling urinary catheter for management of diuresis.
8. Administer corticosteroids, such as dexamethasone, as ordered, to reduce vasogenic edema associated with brain tumors. Corticosteroids are not recommended in the treatment of cytoxic (intracellular) cerebral edema related to trauma or stroke.
9. Maintain balanced fluids and electrolytes. Watch for increased or decreased serum sodium due to the following conditions that may occur with increased ICP.
   a. Diabetes insipidus (DI) results from the absence of antidiuretic hormone (ADH); this is reflected by increased urine output with elevation of serum osmolarity and sodium.
   b. The syndrome of inappropriate antidiuretic hormone (SIADH) results from the secretion of ADH in the absence of changes in serum osmolality. This is a hypervolemic state reflected by decreased urine output with decreased serum sodium and increased free water.
   c. Cerebral salt wasting is associated with abnormal release of aldosterone resulting in increased elimination of sodium and decreased interstitial volume (hypovolemic state) (see Table 15-4).
10. Monitor effects of anesthetic agents, such as propofol, and sedatives, such as midazolam, which may be given to prevent sudden changes in ICP due to coughing, straining, or "fighting" the ventilator. Short-acting medications are preferred to allow for intermittent neurological assessment.
11. High-dose barbiturates, such as pentobarbital, may be used in patients with refractory increased ICP. (*Note:* Prophylactic use is not recommended. It is utilized when all other treatments have failed.) Dosing: 10 mg/kg over 30 minutes; then 5 mg/kg every hour for 3 hours followed by maintenance dose of 1 mg/kg/hr. (Goal serum barbiturate level of 3 to 4 mg/dL.)
    a. High-dose barbiturates induce a comatose state and suppress brain metabolism, which, in turn, reduces cerebral blood flow and ICP. Only pupillary response is assessed.
    b. Be alert to the high level of nursing support required. All responses to environmental and noxious stimuli (suctioning, turning) are abolished as well as all protective reflexes.

Table 15-4	Differentiating Etiology of Hyponatremia	
	CEREBRAL SALT WASTING	**SIADH**
Volume		
Plasma	Decreased CVP < 6	Increased
Urine output	Marked increase	Normal or decreased
Sodium		
Serum	Decreased	<135 mEq/L
Urine	Marked increase	>20 mEq/L
Osmolality		
Serum	Increased or no change	Decreased (<280 mmol/L)
Urine	Increased or no change	Increased (>100 mmol/kg)
Serum K+	Increased	Decreased or no change
Hematocrit	Increased	Decreased or no change
Treatment	Fludrocortisone	Fluid restriction Oral: Salt replacement IV: 3% saline

c. Cough or gag reflex will be absent and the patient will be unable to protect the airway, increasing susceptibility to pneumonia.

d. Monitor ICP, arterial pressure, and serum barbiturate levels, as indicated. Perform continuous EEG monitoring to document burst suppression (suppression of cortical activity) and ensure adequate dosing of barbiturates, if used.

e. Monitor temperature because barbiturate coma causes hypothermia.

f. Diminished GI motility and high risk for ileus.

12. Maintain normothermia and treat fever aggressively. Fever increases cerebral blood flow and cerebral blood volume; acute increases in ICP occur with fever spikes. Cerebral temperature is 4 to 5 degrees higher then body core temperature; therefore, small increases in body core temperature can create drastic increases in the core temperature of the brain. Infection is a common complication of ICP, and in the presence of fever, an infectious workup should be completed.

13. Avoid positions or activities that may increase ICP. Keep head in alignment with shoulders; neck flexion or rotation increases ICP by impeding venous return. Keep head of bed elevated 30 degrees to reduce jugular venous pressure and decrease ICP.

a. Minimize suctioning, keep procedure less than 15 seconds, and, if ordered, instill lidocaine via endotracheal (ET) tube before suctioning. Coughing and suctioning are associated with increased intrathoracic pressure, which is associated with ICP spikes. Inject 5 to 10 mL of lidocaine into ET tube before suctioning to dampen the cough response.

b. Minimize other stimuli, such as alarms, television, radio, and bedside conversations, which may precipitously increase ICP (stimuli that create elevation in ICP are patient-dependent).

14. Maintain normal blood sugar levels. Treat with sliding scale insulin or insulin drip as ordered.

15. Initiate treatment modalities, as ordered, for increased ICP (above 20 mm Hg or if there is a significant shift in pressure).

16. Pretreat prior to known activities that raise ICP and avoid taking pressure readings immediately after a procedure. Allow patient to rest for approximately 5 minutes.

17. Record ICP readings every hour and correlate with significant clinical events or treatments (suctioning, turning).

Evaluation: Expected Outcomes

- ICP and vital signs stable; alert and responsive.

Intracranial Monitoring

Evidence Base Raboel, P. H., Bartek, J., Andersen, M., et al. (2012). Intracranial pressure monitoring: Invasive versus noninvasive methods—A review. *Critical Care Research and Practice*, Volume 2012, Art. ID 950393. Available: *www.hndawi.com/journals/ccrp/2012/950393/abs*.

Intracranial monitoring, including ICP monitoring, is a technology that helps the nurse assess, plan, intervene, and evaluate patient responses to care. ICP monitoring is widely used.

See Figure 15-1. Also see Procedure Guidelines 15-2, pages 490 to 491.

1. External ventricular drain (EVD): catheter is inserted into lateral ventricle (right is preferred) through a drilled burr hole opening; connected to fluid-filled transducer, which converts mechanical pressure to electrical impulses and waveform; allows ventricular drainage. EVD is the most accurate method to measure ICP.

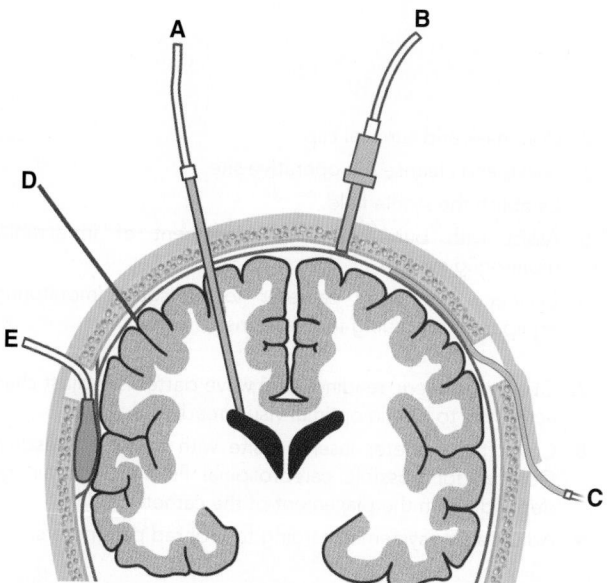

Figure 15-1. Intracranial pressure monitoring system. (A) Intraventricular; **(B)** subarachnoid; **(C)** subdural; **(D)** parenchymal; **(E)** epidural.

(Text continues on page 492)

PROCEDURE GUIDELINES 15-2

Intracranial Monitoring/Licox Monitoring System/Microdialysis System

EQUIPMENT

- Sterile gloves, mask, and surgical cap
- Monitoring system (intraventricular, subarachnoid, epidural)
- IV pole or stand on which to mount the system
- IV solutions, as ordered
- IV high-pressure tubing
- Burr hole tray for insertion or as needed
- Topical anesthetic
- Vital sign records

PROCEDURE

Nursing Action	Rationale
Preparatory phase	
1. Explain the need for extensive, continuous assessment and appropriate nursing intervention to the family and patient, if possible.	1. Explanations will decrease anxiety, allow patient and family a sense of control, and encourage compliance with procedure.
2. Gather and assemble equipment. Flush lines with ordered solution according to manufacturer's directions.	2. Availability of equipment will enhance success of procedure.
3. Calibrate equipment according to directions.	3. Accurate interpretation of intracranial pressure (ICP) values, wave patterns, cerebral temperature, and brain tissue partial pressure of oxygen will depend on appropriate baseline function.
4. Perform neurologic assessment.	4. Patient baseline must be established to determine changes and guide therapy.
5. Administer light sedation or analgesia if patient is agitated.	5. Procedure is invasive and injury may result with excessive patient movement.
Performance phase	
1. Establish head of bed at 30 degrees.	1. Head elevation is a conventional nursing intervention used to control elevated ICP and avoid complications in patients with neurotrauma.
	a. Head elevation facilitates venous drainage, decreasing intracranial volume, and prevents collapse of the ventricles if ventricular placement.
	b. However, elevating the head of the bed may decrease cerebral perfusion pressure, creating ischemia in those with low systolic BP.
2. Don mask and surgical cap.	2. Reduces risk of transmission of airborne bacteria.
3. Shave and cleanse the operative site.	3. Removes bacteria from the site, reducing the risk of infection.
4. Establish the sterile field.	4. Reduces the risk of infection.
5. Assist with burr hole and placement of intracranial monitoring system.	5. Direct monitoring of ICP allows for early detection of decompensation and management of complications.
6. Connect monitoring catheter to transducer/monitoring equipment according to directions.	6. Allows for conduction of intracranial and cerebral perfusion pressures (CPP) to the interpretive component of the system.
7. Observe numeric readings and wave patterns. Adjust characteristics to obtain optimal visual reading.	7. Changes in baseline readings indicate alterations in ICP or problems with the mechanics of the monitoring system.
8. Cover the catheter insertion site with a sterile dressing. Observe for possible cerebrospinal fluid (CSF) drainage depending on the placement of the catheter.	8. The skull and meninges have been penetrated, leaving the patient at risk for infection.
9. Adjust alarm system according to ordered parameters.	9. Alarms should be on at all times to alert the nurse of ongoing adverse changes.

PROCEDURE GUIDELINES 15-2 *(continued)*

Intracranial Monitoring/Licox Monitoring System/Microdialysis System

PROCEDURE *(continued)*

Nursing Action	Rationale

 **Key Decision Point**

Check ICP waveforms before nursing interventions such as turning or bathing the patient. The presence of an elevated P-2 wave indicates reduced cerebral compliance, meaning that the normal compensatory responses may not be effective in decreasing ICP. Thus, extra precautions and preventive actions should be taken prior to exposing the patient to additional stimuli. Nursing interventions may need to be postponed until cerebral compliance increases. Alert the health care provider if ICP greater than 20 mm Hg and prepare for therapeutic intervention.

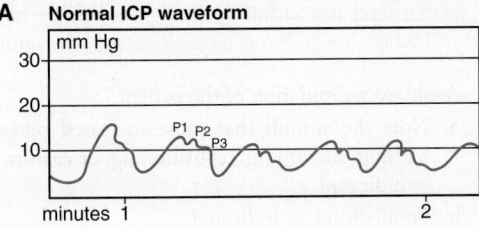

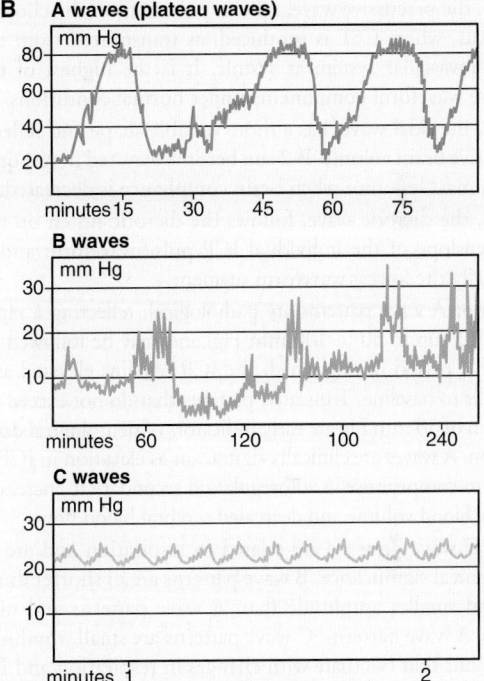

(A) Normal waveform; *(B)* A waves *(plateau waves),* B waves, and **C** waves.

Follow-up phase

1. Frequently assess the patient and the system to ascertain neurologic status, assessing ICP and CPP and patency of the system.

2. Irrigate the system using sterile technique according to policy or as needed to maintain patency.

3. Report dampened waveforms, and have 1 mL of normal saline (without preservatives) available for irrigation, if indicated.

4. Assess head dressing for CSF drainage. Change dressing according to facility policy.

5. Adjust the height of the transducer of the system to the level of the patient's ventricles (inner canthus of eye and tip of ear) with every position change for accurate readings and per orders.

1. Manipulation of the system may inadvertently close the system, leaving the patient without benefit of monitoring.

2. Irrigation helps maintain the patency of the system.

3. The tip of the catheter may have migrated against the ventricular wall or cerebral tissue depending on location, or ventricular collapse may be imminent. Irrigation is done by the health care provider in this case.

4. Because of its high glucose content, CSF is an excellent medium for bacterial growth.

5. Position of the transducer in relation to the ventricles will influence the accuracy of the readings because of fluid gradient pressures.

 Evidence Base American Association of Neuroscience Nurses. (2011). *Care of the patient undergoing intracranial pressure monitoring/external ventricular drainage or lumbar drainage.* Glenview, IL: Author.

2. Subarachnoid (bolt) hollow screw inserted into SAS beneath skull and dura through drill hole; also connected to pressure transducer system.

3. Epidural sensor inserted beneath skull but not through dura, so does not measure pressure directly; fiber-optic cable is connected directly to monitor.

4. Parenchymal device is inserted directly into brain tissue.

ICP Waveforms

ICP pulse waveforms are generated from a pressure wave transmitted through the cardiovascular system into the tissues within the intracranial cavity.

1. The normal pulse waveform consists of three identifiable components: P-1, P-2, and P-3 (see diagram A on page 491).
   a. P-1, the percussive wave, reflects pulsations of the choroid plexus, where CSF is produced, as transmitted from the cardiovascular system at systole. It is the highest of the three waveform components under normal conditions.
   b. P-2, the tidal wave, has a more variable shape and reflects relative brain volume. P-2 can become elevated in response to a mass lesion or when brain compliance is decreased.
   c. P-3, the dicrotic wave, follows the dicrotic notch on the downslope of the individual ICP pulse waveform and is usually the lowest waveform segment.

2. Plateau or A wave patterns are pathological, reflecting a rapid rise in ICP up to 50 to 100 mm Hg, and may be followed by a variable period during which the ICP remains elevated and then falls to baseline. Truncated patterns that do not exceed an elevation of 50 mm Hg are early indicators of neurological deterioration. A waves are clinically significant as elevation in ICP is related to compromise in autoregulation secondary to increased cerebral blood volume and decreased cerebral blood flow.

3. B and C wave patterns are related to respiration and are of little clinical significance. B wave patterns are of shorter duration and smaller amplitude than A wave patterns and may precede A wave patterns. C wave patterns are small, rhythmic oscillations that fluctuate with changes in respiration and BP.

Other Monitoring Systems

1. Licox Brain Oxygen Monitoring System—placed in the brain tissue through a burr hole and monitors brain tissue partial pressure of oxygen (PbrO$_2$), cerebral temperature, and indirect ICP. Continual monitoring of the cerebral temperature and oxygenation levels provides direct information on the acute changes in the intracranial tissue that can potentiate secondary brain injury.

2. Microdialysis—catheter is placed into the brain tissue through a burr hole for monitoring of cerebral oxygen, glucose, lactate, lactate-pyruvate, glutamate, and glycerol. The catheter is connected to a 2.5-mL syringe and into a micro-infusion pump. The pump is perfused with Ringer's solution. Samples are obtained periodically for analysis.

3. Jugular venous oximetry—A fiber-optic oximetric catheter is placed into the jugular bulb of the internal jugular vein for measurement of jugular venous oxygen saturation (SjvO$_2$). SjvO$_2$ is helpful in evaluating arterial saturation, cerebral metabolic rate for oxygen, and cerebral blood flow. The normal range is between 54% and 75%. A low SjvO$_2$ is suggestive of

increased brain extraction of oxygen related to systemic arterial hypoxia, decreased cerebral blood flow from hypotension or vasospasm, or an elevated ICP with a low CPP. Desaturation is thought to be associated with ischemic events and directly related to increased morbidity.

Nursing Interventions

1. Note the pattern of waveforms and any sustained elevation of pressure above 20 mm Hg.

 NURSING ALERT   The frequency of brief elevations in ICP > 20 mm Hg and CPP < 50 mm Hg correlates with worsening outcomes following traumatic brain injury. Measures to reduce increased ICP should be performed immediately and the health care provider notified when the ICP remains elevated >5 minutes.

2. Avoid overstimulation of the patient.
   a. Note the stimuli that cause increased pressure, such as bathing, suctioning, repositioning, or visitors. Adjust care, as indicated.
   b. Premedicate, as indicated.
   c. Provide rest periods between periods of care.
   d. Limit visitors as status indicates.
   e. Limit unnecessary conversation at patient's bedside.
   f. Eliminate external environmental stimuli. Close doors, turn off suction equipment when not in use, limit television or radio as status indicates.

3. Watch for developing or increasing P-2 waves and frequency of A (plateau) waves. Report these, and begin measures to lower increased ICP, as described on page 491.

Nursing Management of the Patient Undergoing Intracranial Surgery

Craniotomy is the surgical opening of the skull to gain access to intracranial structures to perform a biopsy, remove a tumor, relieve increased ICP, evacuate a blood clot, evaluate and treat the cause of intracranial hemorrhage, or remove epileptogenic tissue. Surgical approach is based on location of the lesion and may be supratentorial (above the tentorium or dural covering that divides the cerebrum from cerebellum) or infratentorial (below the tentorium, including the brain stem). Craniotomy may be performed by means of burr holes (made with a drill or hand tools) or by making a bony flap. *Craniectomy* is excision and removal of a portion of the skull. *Cranioplasty* is repair of a cranial defect by means of a plastic or metal plate. *Transsphenoidal surgery* is an approach that gains access to the pituitary gland through the nasal cavity and sphenoidal sinus (see Chapter 24).

Preoperative Management

1. Diagnostic findings, surgical procedure, and expectations are reviewed with the patient.

2. Presurgical shampoo with an antimicrobial agent may be ordered. Skull preparation is performed in the operating room.

3. Depending on primary diagnosis, corticosteroids may be ordered preoperatively to reduce vasogenic cerebral edema.

4. Depending on the type and location of lesion, anticonvulsants may be ordered to reduce risk of seizures.

5. The patient is prepared for the use of intraoperative antibiotics to reduce risk of infection.

6. Urinary catheterization is performed to assess urinary volume during operative period.

7. If cerebral edema develops, intraoperative or postoperative osmotic diuretic (mannitol) or corticosteroids may be ordered for its treatment.

8. Neurologic assessment is performed to evaluate and record the patient's neurologic baseline and vital signs for postoperative comparison.

9. Family and patient are made aware of the immediate postoperative care and where the physician will contact the family after surgery.

10. Supportive care is given, as needed, for neurologic deficits.

Postoperative Management

1. Respiratory status is assessed by monitoring rate, depth, and pattern of respirations. A patent airway is maintained.

2. Vital signs and neurologic status are monitored using a facility-based neurological assessment tool; findings are documented. Arterial line may be used for blood pressure monitoring.

3. Pharmacologic agents may be prescribed to control increased ICP.

4. Incisional and headache pain may be controlled with analgesic such as an opioid or acetaminophen, as prescribed. Monitor response to medications.

5. Position head of bed at 15 to 30 degrees, or per clinical status of the patient, to promote venous drainage. Determining appropriate position of head of bed is patient-dependent and should be adjusted based on observed changes in the patient's clinical response and ICP to positioning. A decrease in CPP is observed with raising the head of the bed to lower ICP.

6. Turn side-to-side every 2 hours; positioning restrictions will be ordered by the health care provider (craniectomy patients should not be turned on the side of the cranial defect).

7. CT scan of the brain is performed if the patient's status deteriorates.

8. Oral fluids are provided when the patient is alert and swallow reflex has returned. Intake and output are monitored. Speech therapy may be ordered for bedside swallow study or radiographic swallow study.

9. Signs of infection are monitored by checking craniotomy site, ventricular drainage, nuchal rigidity, or presence of CSF (fluid collection at surgical site).

10. Periorbital edema is controlled by such measures as elevation of head of bed and cold compresses. Removal of surgical dressing and increase in activity will assist in the resolution of periorbital edema.

Potential Complications

1. Intracranial hemorrhage/hematoma.

2. Cerebral edema.

3. Infections (eg, postoperative meningitis, pulmonary, wound).

4. Seizures.

5. CN dysfunction.

6. Decreased CPP causing cerebral ischemia.

Nursing Diagnoses

- Risk for Ineffective Cerebral Tissue Perfusion related to increased ICP.
- Risk for Aspiration related to decreased swallow reflex and postoperative positioning.
- Risk for Infection related to invasive procedure.
- Acute Pain related to surgical wound.
- Constipation related to use of opioids and immobility.

Nursing Interventions

Maintaining ICP within Normal Range

1. Closely monitor LOC, vital signs, pupillary response, and ICP, if indicated. Notify health care provider if ICP is greater than 20 mm Hg or CPP is less than 50 mm Hg.

2. Teach the patient to avoid activities that can raise ICP, such as excessive flexion or rotation of the head and Valsalva maneuver (coughing, straining with defecation).

3. Administer medications, as prescribed, to reduce ICP.

4. Eliminate noxious tactile stimuli, such as suctioning, prolonged physical assessment, turning, and ROM exercises (based on patient response).

Preventing Aspiration

1. Offer fluids only when the patient is alert and swallow reflexes have returned.

2. Have suction equipment available at bedside. Suction only if indicated. Pretreat with sedation or endotracheal lidocaine to prevent elevation of ICP.

3. Elevate head of bed to maximum of order, or per clinical status, and patient comfort.

Preventing Nosocomial Infections

1. Use sterile technique for dressing changes, catheter care, and ventricular drain management.

2. Be aware of patients at higher risk of infection—those undergoing lengthy operations, those with ventricular drains left in longer than 72 hours, and those with operations of the third ventricle.

3. Assess surgical site for redness, tenderness, and drainage.

4. Watch for leakage of CSF, which increases the danger of meningitis.

   a. Watch for sudden discharge of fluid from wound; a large leak usually requires surgical repair.

   b. Warn against coughing, sneezing, or nose blowing, which may aggravate CSF leakage.

   c. Assess for moderate elevation of temperature and neck rigidity.

   d. Note patency of ventricular catheter system.

5. Institute measures to prevent respiratory or UTI postoperatively.

Relieving Pain

1. Medicate patient as prescribed and according to assessment findings.

2. Elevate head of bed per protocol to relieve headache.
3. Provide distractive measures for pain management.
4. Darken room if patient is photophobic.

Avoiding Constipation

1. Encourage fluids when patient is able to manage liquids.
2. Ambulate as soon as possible.
3. Change to nonopioid agents for pain control as soon as possible.
4. Avoid Valsalva-like maneuvers.
5. Use stool softeners and laxatives, as ordered.

Family Education and Support

1. Keep patient and family aware of progress and plans to transfer to step-down unit, general nursing unit, subacute care, or rehabilitation facility.
2. Encourage frequent visiting and interaction of family for stimulation of patient as care allows.
3. Begin discharge planning early, and obtain referral for home care nursing, social work, or physical and occupational therapy, as needed.

Evaluation: Expected Outcomes

- Normal ICP and CPP maintained between 50 and 70 mm Hg.
- Gag reflex present; breath sounds clear.
- Afebrile without signs of infection.
- Verbalizes decreased pain.
- Passed soft stool.

CRANIAL NERVE DISORDERS

Bell's Palsy

Idiopathic *Bell's palsy* is an acute peripheral facial paralysis of the infratemporal portion of CN VII (facial nerve) that most often occurs unilaterally. The annual incidence of Bell's palsy is approximately 23 cases per 100,000 persons. It is typically a self-limiting process that improves in 3 to 6 months.

Pathophysiology and Etiology

1. Cause is unknown. Possible etiologies include sensory ganglionitis of the CNS with secondary muscle palsy, caused by inflammation, vascular ischemia, and autoimmune demyelination.
2. Most patients experience a viral prodrome (eg, upper respiratory infection, herpes simplex virus) 1 to 3 weeks before onset of symptoms.
3. Can affect anyone at any age; however, it disproportionately affects pregnant women and those who have diabetes or influenza.
4. Generally self-limiting. With or without treatment, most patients improve significantly within 2 weeks and about 80% recover completely within 3 months. In rare cases, the symptoms may never completely resolve or may recur. Risk factors thought to be associated with a poor outcome include: (1) over age 60 years, (2) complete paralysis, and (3) decreased taste or salivary flow on the side of paralysis.

Clinical Manifestations

1. Acute onset of unilateral upper and lower facial paralysis (over a 48-hour period). Paralysis of ipsilateral side of face from vertex of scalp to chin; facial muscles weak throughout forehead, cheek, and chin; can affect speech and taste, distort face, decrease tearing, and cause posterior auricular pain.
2. Involvement of all branches of facial nerve: facial weakness, diminished taste from anterior two thirds of tongue, decreased blink reflex, decreased lacrimation, inability to close eye, painful eye sensations, photophobia, drooling.
3. Hyperacusis on the affected side.

Diagnostic Evaluation

1. History to determine previous illness, onset of paralysis, and associated symptoms.
2. Exclusion of lesions that mimic Bell's palsy, such as tumor, infection (Lyme disease, meningitis), trauma, stroke, or other conditions (sarcoidosis, multiple sclerosis, Guillain-Barre syndrome) through thorough neurologic examination and CT scan.

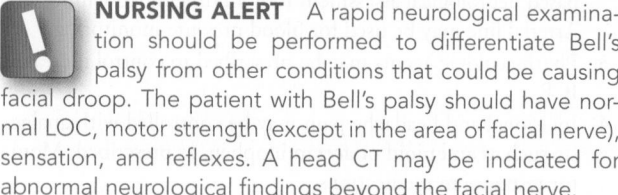 **NURSING ALERT** A rapid neurological examination should be performed to differentiate Bell's palsy from other conditions that could be causing facial droop. The patient with Bell's palsy should have normal LOC, motor strength (except in the area of facial nerve), sensation, and reflexes. A head CT may be indicated for abnormal neurological findings beyond the facial nerve.

3. Electrophysiologic testing, specifically action potentials, EMGs, and nerve conduction velocities, to evaluate nerve function.
4. Lyme disease serological testing history of tick bite or bilateral weakness. About 5% to 10% of untreated Lyme disease patients may develop Bell's palsy.

Management

1. Corticosteroid therapy may be initiated early to decrease inflammation (eg, prednisone 1 mg/kg/day for 10 to 14 days, followed by a tapering dose). Acyclovir combined with prednisone may improve facial function. When using corticosteroids for the treatment of Bell's palsy, caution should be used in patients with tuberculosis, peptic ulcer disease, diabetes mellitus, renal or hepatic dysfunction, or malignant hypertension. For patients who have a contraindication to steroid therapy, acyclovir may be given as solitary treatment.
2. Eye care to maintain lubrication and moisture if unable to close. May need to be patched during sleep.
3. Physical therapy, electrical stimulation to maintain muscle tone.
4. Biofeedback as adjunct therapy.
5. Surgery to anastomose facial nerve to other cranial nerve (CN VII to XI or CN VII to XII; although Bell's palsy is usually self-limiting); surgical closure of eyelid to protect cornea (tarsorrhaphy).

Complications

1. Corneal ulceration.
2. Impairment of vision.
3. Psychosocial adjustment to prolonged paralysis.

 NURSING ALERT Keratitis (inflammation of the cornea), ulceration, and vision loss are major threats to a patient with Bell's palsy. Protect the cornea if the eye does not close.

Nursing Assessment

1. Test motor components of facial nerve (VII) by assessing patient's smile, ability to whistle, purse lips, wrinkle forehead, and close eyes. Observe for facial asymmetry.
2. Observe patient's ability to handle secretions, food, fluids; observe for drooling.
3. Assess patient's ability to blink and speak clearly.
4. Assess effect of altered appearance on body image.

Nursing Diagnoses

- Risk for Dry Eye related to loss of protective eye closure.
- Disturbed Body Image related to facial nerve paralysis.

Nursing Interventions

Preventing Eye Dryness and Maintaining Corneal Integrity

1. Administer and teach the patient to administer artificial tears and ophthalmic ointment as prescribed.
2. Patch eye to keep shut at night, as directed.
3. Inspect eye for redness or discharge.
4. Advise the patient to report eye pain immediately.

Enhancing Body Image

1. Encourage the patient to express feelings related to body image disturbance.
2. Encourage the patient to use mirror as means to obtain feedback about actual versus perceived appearance.
3. Perform and teach the patient to perform facial massage to alleviate feelings of stiffness and enhance recovery.

Patient Education and Health Maintenance

1. Instruct the patient to wear wraparound sunglasses to decrease normal evaporation from the eye from sun and wind, to avoid eye irritants, and to increase environmental humidity.
2. Instruct the patient in use of ophthalmic drops and ointment, proper methods of lid closure, and patching of the eye.
3. Demonstrate facial exercises (eg, raise eyebrows, squeeze eyes shut, purse lips) and stress their importance to prevent muscle atrophy.
4. For further information, refer patient to Bell's Palsy Research Foundation (*www.bellspalsyresearch.com*).

Evaluation: Expected Outcomes

- Cornea without redness, pain, or discharge.
- Verbalizes adjustment to body image disturbance.

Trigeminal Neuralgia (Tic Douloureux)

 Evidence Base Obermann, M., Holle, D., & Katsarava, Z. (2011). Trigeminal neuralgia and persistent idiopathic facial pain. *Expert Review of Neurotherapeutics, 11*(11), 1619–1629.

Trigeminal neuralgia (tic douloureux) is an intensely painful neurologic condition that affects one or more branches of the fifth cranial (trigeminal) nerve. Patients experience sudden paroxysms of "lancinating" or electric shock-like facial pain (see Figure 15-2) localized to one or more branches of the nerve. The pain is often precipitated by trigger points that "fire" when the patient talks, shaves, eats, touches the face, brushes the teeth, or is exposed to cold wind. Approximately 40,000 patients in the United States suffer from this condition at any particular time. The incidence is four to five cases per 100,000. Patients who present with the disease between ages 20 and 40 are more likely to suffer from a demyelinating lesion in the pons secondary to multiple sclerosis (MS).

Pathophysiology and Etiology

1. Unknown cause, but degenerative or viral origin suspected.
2. Any of the three trigeminal nerve branches can be affected:
   a. V_1: ophthalmic branch; pain involves the eye and forehead.
   b. V_2: maxillary branch; pain involves the cheek, upper teeth, upper gums, and nose.
   c. V_3: mandibular branch; pain involves the lower jaw, side of tongue, lower teeth, lower gum, extends to ear.

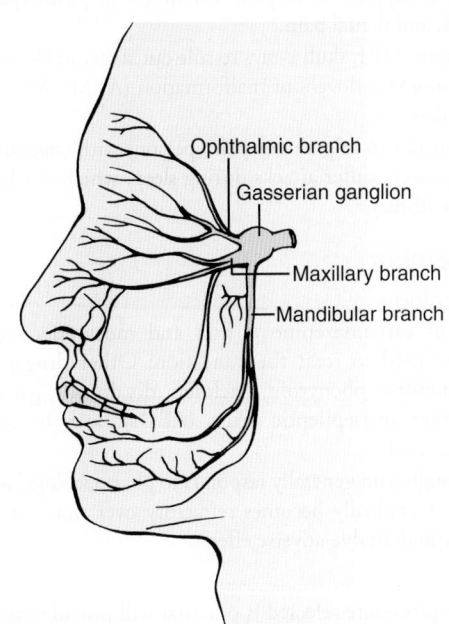

Figure 15-2. The main divisions of the trigeminal nerve are the ophthalmic, maxillary, and mandibular. Sensory root fibers arise in the gasserian ganglion.

3. Compression from artery adjacent to the nerve strips myelin from nerve when it pulsates. Loss of myelin acts like an uninsulated wire that "fires" abnormally in response to stimuli.

 GERONTOLOGIC ALERT Trigeminal neuralgia is commonly seen in older adults. Pain typically appears to be localized to one or more teeth. Patients may seek dental care for pain relief, resulting in one or more tooth extractions without alleviation of pain.

Clinical Manifestations

1. Sudden, severe episodes of intense facial pain localized to one or more of the branches of the nerve, lasting less than 30 to 60 seconds and ending abruptly.
2. Pain may occur spontaneously or be precipitated by activation of trigger points, such as touching the face, talking, chewing, yawning, and brushing the teeth, that place pressure on the terminal end of the branch affected.
3. Pain is always unilateral and does not cross the midline. Bilateral pain is sometimes seen in patients with MS and should result in a high index of suspicion for this condition. MS and hypertension are the two risk factors found in epidemiologic studies.
4. Some patients experience numbness, particularly around the mouth.

Diagnostic Evaluation

1. History of characteristic symptoms and pattern; neurologic examination is normal.
2. Quick response to pharmacologic treatment is important to rule out atypical facial pain, vasomotor or postherpetic neuralgia, and dental pain.
3. CT scan, MRI, skull x-rays to rule out structural lesions, such as tumor, arteriovenous malformation (AVM), MS, or other disorders.
4. In contrast to migrainous pain, persons with trigeminal neuralgia rarely suffer attacks during sleep, which is a key point in the history.

Management

Pharmacologic

1. Use of carbamazepine is first and most effective medication used to treat the condition. Other drugs, such as imipramine, phenytoin, baclofen, divalproex, gabapentin, or other anti-epileptic drugs (AEDs), may be added or substituted.
2. Although pain generally responds to pharmacologic intervention, it gradually becomes refractory over time, or patients suffer undesirable adverse effects.

Surgical

Operative procedure selected is one that will provide the greatest chance of long-term pain relief with the fewest complications.

1. Alcohol, phenol block, or glycerol injection for pain may last several months after injection.

2. Percutaneous radiofrequency trigeminal gangliolysis directs low-voltage stimulation of nerve by electrode inserted through foramen ovale; sensory function is destroyed with goal to preserve motor function; may cause decreased corneal sensation if V1 affected; paresthesias, jaw weakness, or undesirable, painful numbness (anesthesia dolorosa). Pain may recur as nerve regenerates, necessitating repeat procedure.
3. Rhizotomy (transection of nerve root at gasserian ganglion) causes complete loss of sensation; other complications include burning, stinging, discomfort in and around eye, herpetic lesions of face, keratitis, and corneal ulceration. Pain may recur as nerve regenerates.
4. Percutaneous balloon microcompression for selective destruction of nerve fibers that mediate light touch and trigger pain. Relieves pain in ophthalmic branch while sparing corneal sensation.
5. Microvascular decompression of trigeminal nerve (see "Nursing Management of the Patient Undergoing Intracranial Surgery," page 492). Most effective form of therapy, with 75% to 80% of patients pain-free without need for long-term medication after procedure. Treatment of choice for younger patients who are low anesthesia risk, do not want facial numbness, and are willing to accept craniotomy.
6. Gamma knife surgery is less invasive than the percutaneous procedures. It is about as effective as the percutaneous procedures; however, relief may not come for weeks to months and it is a bit more expensive.

Complications

1. Anorexia and weight loss.
2. Dehydration.
3. Anxiety, fear.
4. Depression, social isolation, and suicidal ideations in extreme cases.

Nursing Assessment

1. Take history of the pain, including duration, severity, and aggravating factors.
2. Assess nutritional status and hydration.
3. Assess for anxiety and depression, including problems with sleep, social interaction, coping ability/skills.

Nursing Diagnoses

- Chronic Pain related to physiologic changes of the disorder.
- Imbalanced Nutrition: Less Than Body Requirements related to fear of eating.
- Powerlessness related to lack of control over painful episodes.

Nursing Interventions

Relieving Pain

1. To minimize painful episodes, review with patient potential trigger factors, and develop individualized methods of coping with identified triggers.
2. Encourage the patient to take medication regularly, including "rescue" medication for breakthrough periods.
3. Help the patient maintain a method of communication without causing pain from talking.

Maintaining Adequate Nutrition

1. To maximize nutritional intake, instruct patient to take foods and fluids at room temperature and to chew on the unaffected side.
2. Have the patient consult with the dietitian for appropriate meal texture and composition.
3. Encourage small, frequent meals to avoid fatigue and pain.
4. Advise about use of nutritional supplements, if indicated.

Increasing Control

1. Support patient through treatment trials.
2. Teach relaxation exercises, such as relaxation breathing, progressive muscle relaxation, and guided imagery, to relieve tension (see page 30).
3. Encourage participation in support groups (eg, Trigeminal Neuralgia Association) and facilitate a therapeutic relationship with the health care provider.

Patient Education and Health Maintenance

1. Educate the surgical patient regarding self-care after denervation procedures.
   a. Instruct the patient to inspect the eye for redness and foreign bodies three to four times per day if corneal sensation is impaired.
   b. Instruct the patient to instill lubricating eye drops every 4 hours if corneal sensation is impaired.
   c. Instruct the patient to avoid drinking hot or very cold liquids.
   d. Instruct the patient to chew on unaffected side to avoid biting tongue, lips, and inside of mouth.
   e. Instruct the patient who wears dentures that jaw muscle will regenerate over time; avoid having dentures refitted, but maintain regular dental checkups because pain will not be felt.
   f. Instruct the patient to report any change in sensation.
2. Refer patient to the Facial Pain Association for education and support network (*www.fpa-support.org*) or the National Institute of Neurological Disorders and Stroke (*www.ninds.nih.gov*).

Evaluation: Expected Outcomes

- Verbalizes reduced pain.
- Maintains weight.
- Verbalizes decreased anxiety and depression.

CEREBROVASCULAR DISEASE
Cerebrovascular Insufficiency

Evidence Base Furie, K. L., Kasner, S. E., Adams, R. J., et al. (2011). Guidelines for the prevention of stroke in patients with stroke or transient ischemic attack: A guideline for healthcare professionals from the American Heart Association/American Stroke Association. *Stroke, 42,* 227–276.

Cerebrovascular insufficiency is an interruption or inadequate blood flow to a focal area of the brain, resulting in transient or permanent neurologic dysfunction. *Transient ischemic attack* (TIA) lasts less than 24 hours. *Ischemic stroke* is similar to myocardial infarction, in that the pathogenesis is loss of blood supply to the tissue, which can result in irreversible damage if blood flow is not restored quickly.

Pathophysiology and Etiology

1. Cerebrovascular insufficiency can be caused by atherosclerotic plaque or thrombosis, resulting in increased PCO_2, decreased PO_2, decreased blood viscosity, hyperthermia/hypothermia, increased ICP.
2. Carotid arteries, vertebral arteries, major intracranial vessels, or microcirculation may be affected.
3. Cardiac causes of emboli include atrial fibrillation, mitral valve prolapse, infectious endocarditis, and prosthetic heart valve.
4. Event may be classified as TIA—transient episode of cerebral dysfunction with associated clinical manifestations lasting usually minutes to an hour, possibly up to 24 hours.
5. Symptoms persisting longer than 24 hours are classified as stroke (also known as *brain attack*).

Risk Factors for Stroke

Medical Conditions

1. Diabetes mellitus (44% risk reduction in hypertensive diabetics with controlled BP).
2. Hypertension (30% to 40% risk reduction with treatment): goal BP is lower than 140/90; if renal insufficiency or heart failure, less than 130/85; if diabetic, less than 130/80.
3. Hyperlipidemia (20% to 30% risk reduction with those with known coronary heart disease [CHD] on statin therapy): goal LDL is less than 160 mg/dL if one or no risk factor; less than 130 if two or more risk factors and 10-year CHD risk is less than 20%; less than 100 if two or more risk factors and 10-year CHD risk is greater than 20%.
4. Coronary artery disease and cardiac disorders, such as congenital heart disease, valvular conditions, endocarditis, atrial fibrillation (68% risk reduction with oral anticoagulation; 21% with aspirin).
5. History of TIA or stroke.
6. Rare: Endothelial damage (inflammation or infection, drug-induced, fibromuscular dysplasia, carotid or vertebral artery dissections).

Behaviors

1. Cigarette smoking (smoking cessation results in a 50% risk reduction in 1 year; return to baseline in 5 years).
2. Alcohol abuse.
3. Physical inactivity.
4. Cocaine use (hemorrhagic stroke).

Nonmodifiable Factors

1. Increasing age—risk doubles for each decade over age 50.
2. Gender—men are at greater risk than women.
3. Heredity—increased risk with family history of stroke.
4. Ethnic background—blacks and Hispanics at higher risk than whites.

Other

There have been reports in the literature of increased risk due to childbirth, hormone replacement therapy or contraceptive use, and migraine headaches. Chiropractic manipulation has been associated with ischemic stroke related to dissection.

 DRUG ALERT Increased stroke risk has been noted in women who smoke and take oral contraceptives and who have a history of migraines.

Clinical Manifestations of Transient Ischemic Attacks

1. History of intermittent neurologic deficit, sudden in onset, with maximal deficit within 5 minutes and lasting less than 24 hours.
2. Carotid system involvement: amaurosis fugax, homonymous hemianopsia, unilateral weakness, unilateral numbness or paresthesias, aphasia, dysarthria.
3. Vertebrobasilar system involvement: vertigo, homonymous hemianopsia, diplopia, weakness that is bilateral or alternates sides, dysarthria, dysphagia, ataxia, perioral numbness.
4. Carotid bruit.
5. History of headaches lasting days before ischemia.

Diagnostic Evaluation

1. Cerebral angiography, digital subtraction angiography, CT angiography, MRA, Doppler ultrasound—all provide information about carotid arteries, vertebral arteries, and intracranial circulation.
2. Partial prothrombin time (PTT) and International Normalized Ratio (INR) if anticoagulation is considered. Blood levels are monitored to document therapeutic ranges and determine dosing. PTT is utilized for heparin therapy and INR is utilized for oral warfarin therapy.
3. MRI stroke protocol: consists of a standard MRI in conjunction with DWI and ADC or PWI scan (see page 476).
4. Transesophageal echocardiography to rule out emboli from heart.

Management

1. Platelet aggregation inhibitors, such as aspirin, or clopidogrel to reduce risk of stroke.
2. Surgical or endovascular intervention to increase blood flow to brain—carotid endarterectomy, extracranial/intracranial anastomosis, transarterial stenting, or angioplasty.
3. Reduction of other risk factors to prevent stroke, such as control of hypertension, diabetes, and hyperlipidemia, and smoking cessation.
4. Treatment of arrhythmias.
5. Treatment of isolated systolic hypertension.
6. Anticoagulation agents for patients who continue to have symptoms despite antiplatelet therapy (this remains controversial) and those with major source of cardiac emboli.

Complications

1. Complete ischemic stroke (30% of TIAs will progress to stroke within 5 years of initial TIA).
2. Hemorrhagic conversion of ischemic stroke.
3. Cerebral edema.

Nursing Assessment

1. Obtain history of possible TIA; hypertensive and diabetic control; hyperlipidemia; cardiovascular disease or dysrhthmias, such as atrial fibrillation; smoking.
2. Perform physical examination, including neurologic, cardiac, and circulatory systems; be sure to listen for carotid bruit.
3. Assess patient for history of headache and, if positive, for duration of headache.

Nursing Diagnoses

- Risk for Ineffective Cerebral Tissue Perfusion related to underlying arteriosclerosis.
- Risk for Injury related to surgical procedure.
- Readiness for Enhanced Therapeutic Regimen Management regarding therapeutic lifestyle changes.

Nursing Interventions

Improving Cerebral Perfusion

1. Teach patient signs and symptoms of TIA and need to notify health care provider immediately. Use the acronym FAST to know what to look for: F, face weakness; A, arm weakness; S, speech difficulties; T, time—immediately seek medical assistance.
2. Administer or teach self-administration of anticoagulants, antiplatelet agents, antihypertensives, and other medication; also teach about monitoring for adverse effects and therapeutic effect.
3. Prepare patient for surgical or endovascular intervention as indicated (see page 492).

Providing Care and Preventing Complications After Surgical Procedure

Also see "Nursing Management of the Patient Undergoing Intracranial Surgery," page 492, and "Cerebral angiography," page 478.

1. After surgical procedure, closely monitor vital signs and administer medication as prescribed to avoid hypotension (which can cause cerebral ischemia) or hypertension (which can precipitate cerebral hemorrhage).
2. Perform frequent neurologic checks, including pupil size, equality, and reaction; handgrip and plantar flexion strength; sensation; mental status; and speech. Notify the health care provider of any deficits immediately.
3. Observe operative area closely for swelling. Mild swelling is expected, but if hematoma formation is suspected, prepare patient for immediate surgery.
4. Medicate for pain and avoid agitation or sudden changes in position, which could affect BP.
5. Elevate head of bed when vital signs are stable.

6. Following carotid endarterectomy:
   a. Monitor for hoarseness, impaired gag reflex, or difficulty swallowing and facial weakness, which indicate CN injury.
   b. Keep head in neutral position to relieve stress on surgical site; monitor drainage.
   c. Keep tracheostomy tube at bedside and assess for stridor; hematoma formation can cause airway obstruction.
7. Following extracranial–intracranial anastomosis, avoid pressure over the anastomosis of the superior temporal artery (extracranial) and the middle cerebral artery (intracranial) to prevent rupture or ischemia of the site. If the patient wears glasses, remove the eyeglass arm on the operative side to avoid this possible pressure point.
8. Following transcranial stenting, administer medications, as directed.
   a. Heparin—bolus given intraprocedure, then possible continuous IV drip postprocedure to maintain PTT within ordered range; monitor PTT every 6 hours.

 NURSING ALERT In the event of an acute neurologic deficit, the heparin drip should be stopped until an acute intracerebral bleed has been ruled out.

   b. Clopidogrel before procedure, as ordered. Can be given as a loading dose of 150 mg the evening before procedure, 300-mg loading dose before procedure, 75 mg daily 48 hours before procedure, or 75 mg daily 1 week before procedure. Dosing is physician-dependent.
   c. Daily dosing of 75 mg clopidogrel for 30 to 90 days (specific duration varies), as directed.
   d. Aspirin 81 mg daily, as directed.
9. Monitor puncture site for bleeding, hematoma, and pulse, as ordered. Apply pressure if bleeding or hematoma is noted and inform physician.

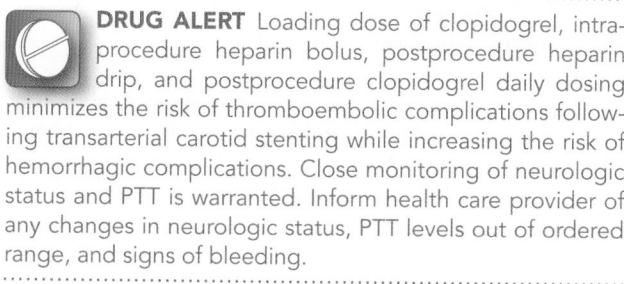 **DRUG ALERT** Loading dose of clopidogrel, intraprocedure heparin bolus, postprocedure heparin drip, and postprocedure clopidogrel daily dosing minimizes the risk of thromboembolic complications following transarterial carotid stenting while increasing the risk of hemorrhagic complications. Close monitoring of neurologic status and PTT is warranted. Inform health care provider of any changes in neurologic status, PTT levels out of ordered range, and signs of bleeding.

Encouraging Lifestyle Changes to Reduce Risk

1. Help the patient begin to formulate a plan for smoking cessation (see page 32).
2. Teach the patient and family members the basics of nutrition, how to read labels, and how to follow a low-fat diet (particularly one low in saturated fats) (see page 31).
3. Obtain a referral to a nutritionist for help with weight management and low-fat, low-sodium diet, as indicated.
4. Encourage daily activity for 30 minutes, if possible. Obtain physical therapy referral for endurance training and monitoring, as indicated.

5. Monitor INR if warfarin is prescribed and educate patient about risk of bleeding (see page 437).

Patient Education and Health Maintenance

1. Encourage the patient receiving long-term oral anticoagulants to comply with follow-up monitoring of INR and to report any signs of bleeding.
2. Encourage patients receiving antiplatelet agents to report any signs of bleeding.
3. Encourage the use of electric razors and toothbrushes to prevent bleeding.
4. Reinforce with patient and family the importance of accessing the medical system, by calling 911, when symptoms first occur.
5. Refer the patient to the American Stroke Association (*www.strokeassociation.org*) or the National Institute of Neurologic Disorders and Stroke (*www.ninds.nih.gov*) for additional information and support.

Evaluation: Expected Outcomes

- Alert without neurologic deficits.
- Respirations unlabored, vital signs stable, no swelling of neck; reports relief of pain.
- Expresses readiness to quit smoking and adhere to a low-fat diet.

Cerebrovascular Accident (Stroke, Brain Attack)

 Evidence Base American Association of Neuroscience Nurses. (2012). *Guide to the care of the hospitalized patient with ischemic stroke* (2nd ed.). Glenview, IL: Author.
Furie, K. L., Kasner, S. E., Adams, R. J., et al. (2011). Guidelines for the prevention of stroke in patients with stroke or transient ischemic attack: A guideline for healthcare professionals from the American Heart Association/American Stroke Association. *Stroke, 42*, 227–276.
Morgenstern, L. B., Hemphill, J. C. III, Anderson, C., et al. (2010). Guidelines for the management of spontaneous intracerebral hemorrhage: A guideline for healthcare professionals from the American Heart Association/American Stroke Association. *Stroke, 41*, 2108–2129.
Diringer, M. N., Bleck, T. P., Hemphill, J. C. III, et al. (2011). Critical care management of patients following aneurysmal subarachnoid hemorrhage: Recommendations from the Neurocritical Care Society's multidisciplinary consensus conference. *Neurocritical Care, 15*, 211–240.

Stroke, cerebrovascular accident (CVA), or *brain attack* is the onset and persistence of neurologic dysfunction resulting from disruption of blood supply to the brain and indicates infarction rather than ischemia. Strokes are classified as ischemic (more than 70% of strokes) or hemorrhagic (associated with greater morbidity and mortality). About 14% of strokes in the United States are of cardiac origin. About 60% of hemorrhagic strokes are the result of hypertension. Stroke is the leading cause of long-term disability and the third leading cause of death in the United States, with an annual incidence of 700,000.

Pathophysiology and Etiology

Ischemic Stroke

1. Partial or complete occlusion of a cerebral blood flow to an area of the brain due to:
   a. Thrombus (most common)—due to arteriosclerotic plaque in a cerebral artery, usually at bifurcation of larger arteries; occurs over several days.
   b. Embolus—a moving clot of cardiac origin (frequently due to atrial fibrillation) or from a carotid artery that travels quickly to the brain and lodges in a small artery; occurs suddenly with immediate maximum deficits.
2. Area of brain affected is related to the vascular territory that was occluded. Subtle decrease in blood flow may allow brain cells to maintain minimal function, but as blood flow decreases, focal areas of ischemia occur, followed by infarction to the vascular territory. See Figure 15-3 for cerebral circulation.
3. An area of injury includes edema, tissue breakdown, and small arterial vessel damage. The small arterial vessel damage poses a risk of hemorrhage. The larger the area of infarction, the greater the risk of hemorrhagic conversion.
4. Ischemic strokes are not activity-dependent; may occur at rest.

 NURSING ALERT Early detection of warning signs promotes early diagnosis and intervention aimed at lessening stroke mortality and morbidity.

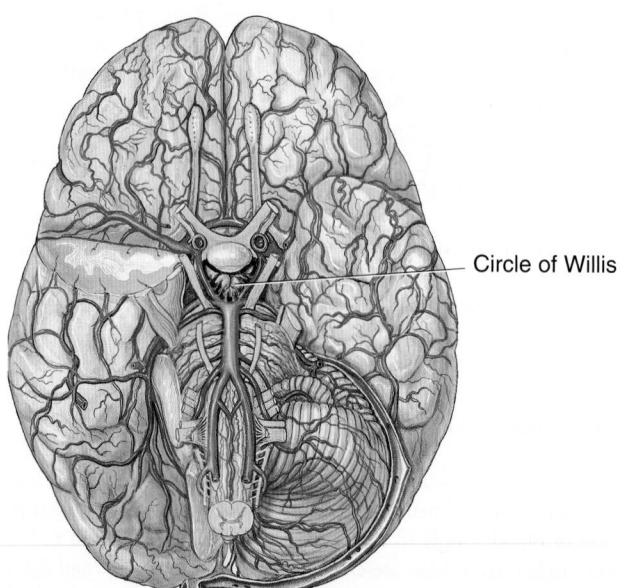

Figure 15-3. The Circle of Willis as seen at the base of a brain removed from the skull.

Hemorrhagic Stroke

1. Leakage of blood from a blood vessel and hemorrhage into brain tissue, causing edema, compression of brain tissue, and spasm of adjacent blood vessels.
2. May occur outside the dura (extradural), beneath the dura mater (subdural), in the SAS, or within the brain substance (intracerebral).
3. Causal mechanisms include:
   a. Increased pressure due to hypertension.
   b. Head trauma causing dissection or rupture of vessel.
   c. Deterioration of vessel wall from chronic hypertension, diabetes mellitus, or cocaine use.
   d. Congenital weakening of blood vessel wall with aneurysm or AVM.
4. The intracranial hemorrhage becomes a space-occupying lesion within the skull and compromises brain function.
   a. The mass effect causes pressure on brain tissue.
   b. The hemorrhage irritates local brain tissue, leading to surrounding focal edema.
   c. SAH or hemorrhage into a ventricle can block normal CSF flow, leading to hydrocephalus.
5. Hemorrhage commonly occurs suddenly while a person is active.

Clinical Manifestations

1. Clinical manifestations vary depending on the vessel affected and the cerebral territories it perfuses. Symptoms are usually multifocal. Headache may be a sign of impending cerebral hemorrhage or infarction; however, it is not always present.
2. Common clinical manifestations related to vascular territory (see Table 15-5):
   a. Numbness (paresthesia), weakness (paresis), or loss of motor ability (plegia) on one side of the body.
   b. Difficulty in swallowing (dysphagia).
   c. Aphasia (nonfluent, fluent, global).
   d. Visual difficulties of inattention or neglect (lack of acknowledgment of one side of the sensory field), loss of half of a visual field (hemianopsia), double vision, photophobia.
   e. Altered cognitive abilities and psychological affect.
   f. Self-care deficits.

Diagnostic Evaluation

1. Carotid ultrasound—to detect carotid stenosis in ischemic stroke.
2. CT scan—to determine cause and location of stroke and type of stroke, ischemic versus hemorrhagic.
3. MRA or CT angiogram—noninvasive evaluation of cerebrovascular structures in ischemic stroke.
4. Cerebral angiography—invasive evaluation of cerebrovasculature to determine the extent of cerebrovascular injury/insufficiency and to evaluate for structural abnormalities.
5. PET, MRI with DWI—to localize ischemic damage in ischemic stroke.

Table 15-5	Stroke Deficits Related to Vascular Territory	
CEREBRAL ARTERY	**BRAIN AREA INVOLVED**	**SIGNS AND SYMPTOMS***
Anterior cerebral	Infarction of the medial aspect of one frontal lobe if lesion is distal to communicating artery; bilateral frontal infarction if flow in other anterior cerebral artery is inadequate	Paralysis of contralateral foot or leg; impaired gait; paresis of contralateral arm; contralateral sensory loss over toes, foot, and leg; problems making decisions or performing acts voluntarily; lack of spontaneity, easily distracted; slowness of thought; urinary incontinence; cognitive and affective disorders
Middle cerebral	Massive infarction of most of lateral hemisphere and deeper structures of the frontal, parietal, and temporal lobes; internal capsule; basal ganglia	Contralateral hemiplegia (face and arm); contralateral sensory impairment; aphasia; homonymous hemiplegia; altered consciousness (confusion to coma); inability to turn eyes toward paralyzed side; denial of paralyzed side or limb (hemiattention); possible acalculia, alexia (visual aphasia), finger agnosia, and left–right confusion; vasomotor paresis and instability
Posterior cerebral	Occipital lobe; anterior and medial portion of temporal lobe	Homonymous hemianopia and other visual defects, such as color blindness, loss of central vision, and visual hallucinations; memory deficits; perseveration (repeated performance of same verbal or motor response)
	Thalamus involvement	Loss of all sensory modalities; spontaneous pain; intentional tremor; mild hemiparesis; aphasia
	Cerebral peduncle involvement	Oculomotor nerve palsy with contralateral hemiplegia
Basilar and vertebral	Cerebellum and brain stem	Visual disturbance such as diplopia, dystaxia, vertigo, dysphagia, dysphonia

*Dependent on hemisphere involved and adequacy of collaterals.

6. CT perfusion/MR perfusion—provides evaluation of cerebral blood flow, cerebral blood volume, and mean transient time to determine the extent of ischemic changes.

7. TCD—noninvasive method used to evaluate cerebral perfusion. Useful in the bedside evaluation and to provide a means for ongoing monitoring of cerebral blood flow to document changes and trends.

Management

Acute Treatment: Ischemic Stroke

1. Support of vital functions—maintain airway, breathing, oxygenation, circulation.
   a. Maintain pulse oximetry greater than 92%. Utilize oxygen therapy, as needed.
   b. Arrhythmias are common. Telemetry may be indicated to monitor. Atrial fibrillation is the most common arrhythmia in stroke population.

2. Astute neurologic assessment utilizing the National Institute of Health Stroke Scale (*www.ninds.nih.gov/doctors/nih/_stroke_scale_booklet.pdf*) and management of increased ICP (see page 486).

3. IV fluids (normal saline) at maintenance until able to tolerate oral diet. Colloids may be used for reperfusion and hemodilution.

4. Maintain BP within prescribed parameters. Limit BP fluctuations.
   a. Management of systemic hypertension with labetalol, nicardipine, or alternative IV antihypertensive agents to keep systolic BP (SBP) less than 200 mm Hg. Goal is to promote adequate cerebral perfusion to prevent further ischemia. Avoid lowering BP greater than 25% within the first 24 hours. Hemorrhagic conversion/transformation can occur and is associated with degree of necrotic tissue and vascular injury. Hyperglycemia and BP fluctuations or rapid increases in BP increase the risk of hemorrhagic conversion.
   b. Management of hypotension—SBP goal > 100. Vasopressor agents to maintain SBP within prescribed range. Sustained hypotensive episodes are associated with poor outcome.
   c. Pretreatment with tissue plasminogen activator (tPA)—unable to receive tPA if SBP > 185 mm Hg or diastolic BP > 110 mm Hg.
   d. Post-tPA—maintain SBP < 180 mm Hg or diastolic BP < 105 mm Hg for first 24 hours post tPA.

5. Thrombolytic therapy (see Box 15-3, page 502).
   a. Recombinant tPA administered IV is the only Food and Drug Administration (FDA)–approved medical treatment for acute ischemic stroke. Dosing: IV 0.9 mg/kg within 3 hours of onset of symptoms.
   b. Transarterial tPA within 6 hours of onset of symptoms. Benefits have been demonstrated in acute ischemic stroke related to occlusion of middle cerebral artery. Advantages include:
      i. Higher concentration delivered to clot.
      ii. Can be performed in conjunction with mechanical disruption of clot.

BOX 15-3	Inclusion and Exclusion Criteria for tPA Therapy

INCLUSION

- Onset of symptoms
  - Within 3 hours IV tPA.
  - Within 6 hours IA tPA.
- Ischemic stroke with measurable deficits using the NIH Stroke Scale (see page 501).
- No hemorrhage noted on CT scan of brain.
- Clearly defined time of symptom onset.

EXCLUSION

- Head CT demonstrates early signs of infarction or hemorrhage.
- Uncontrolled hypertensive nonresponsive to IV or oral agent (systolic > 185 or diastolic > 110 mm Hg).
- Glucose level > 400 mg/dL.
- Coagulopathy.
  - Heparin within past 48 hours.
  - Patient on warfarin.
  - Elevated PTT or prothrombin time.
  - Platelet count < 100,000.
- History of previous intracranial hemorrhage, head trauma, or stroke within past 3 months.
- GI or genitourinary tract hemorrhage in the past 3 weeks.
- History of major surgery in the past 2 weeks.

    iii. Provides precise imaging of pathology and evaluation of collateral circulation.

    iv. Defines extent of injury and recanalization.

  c. Disadvantages include:

    i. Risk of hemorrhage related to catheter manipulation.

    ii. Dislodgement of clot.

    iii. Delay in thrombolytic therapy due to access delays.

    iv. Limited facility-based accessibility.

  d. Additional treatment options (transarterial or endovascular):

    i. Abciximab—antiplatelet agent delivered intra-arterially (IA).

    ii. Verapamil—potent vasodilator injected into intracranial vessel to treat acute spasm.

    iii. Clot retrieval or manipulation of clot.

    iv. Angioplasty and stenting have been utilized in acute dissection, though data are limited.

6. Maintain normal glucose levels because hypoglycemia and hyperglycemia are associated with a poor outcome. Sliding scale insulin or insulin drip should be given to maintain normoglycemia.

7. Maintain normothermia because hyperthermia is associated with a poor neurologic outcome.

8. Deep vein thrombosis prophylaxis—sequential stockings and low-dose heparin or low-molecular-weight heparin (LMWH) should be utilized. Data does not suggest any increased risk of hemorrhage in this population.

9. Focus on early rehabilitation.

Acute Treatment: Hemorrhagic Stroke

1. Support of vital functions—maintain airway, breathing, oxygenation, circulation.

  a. Maintain pulse oximetry greater than 92%. Utilize oxygen therapy, as needed.

  b. Arrhythmias are common. Telemetry may be indicated to monitor.

  c. IV fluids (normal saline) at maintenance until able to tolerate oral diet.

2. Neurologic assessment—Facility-based neurological assessment tool should be used. Notify health care provider of clinical deterioration. Deterioration can be related to rebleed or development of cerebral edema.

3. Reversal of coagulopathies:

  a. Obtain patient's medication history. Medications to be concerned about include warfarin, aspirin, clopidogrel, ticlopidine, and dipyridamole/aspirin.

  b. Obtain INR and platelet function analyzer (PFA-100), as ordered. Elevated INR is associated with warfarin use. PFA epinephrine greater than 164 denotes platelet dysfunction related to aspirin use and PFA adenosine diphosphate greater than 116 denotes nonaspirin platelet dysfunction and has been used to determine the effectiveness of clopidogrel or ticlopidine or the presence of von Willebrand's disease.

  c. As ordered, treat with platelets, cryoprecipitate, or vitamin K to reverse coagulopathy. Prothrombin complex concentrate may be used for rapid reversal.

4. Management of BP within prescribed parameters—maintain SBP < 160 to reduce vessel wall stressors. Goal is to prevent rebleeding while promoting adequate cerebral perfusion. Labetalol, hydralazine, nicardipine, or alternative IV antihypertensive agents may be used.

5. Neurosurgical consultation for possible evacuation of intracerebral hemorrhage may be explored.

6. Prophylactic treatment of seizures with phenytoin. Seizures commonly occur within the first 24 hours of intracerebral hemorrhage.

7. Maintain normal glucose level because hypoglycemia/hyperglycemia are associated with a poor outcome. Sliding scale insulin or insulin drip should be given to maintain normoglycemia.

8. Maintain normothermia because hyperthermia is associated with a poor neurologic outcome. Current data does not support the use of therapeutic, or induced, hypothermia in patients with ischemic stroke; however, research is ongoing to determine potential applications.

9. Deep vein thrombosis prophylaxis—sequential stockings and low-dose heparin or LMWH should be utilized. Data do not suggest any increased risk of hemorrhage in this population.

10. Focus on early rehabilitation.

Subsequent Treatment

1. Anticoagulation may be instituted after hemorrhage is ruled out. However, anticoagulation remains controversial because current literature suggests acute use of heparin increases the risk of hemorrhagic conversion and use of warfarin has

demonstrated no significant benefit *unless the patient is in atrial fibrillation.* Anticoagulation is contraindicated for the first 24 hours in patients who received tPA.

2. Aspirin is the only antiplatelet agent that has been evaluated in acute ischemic stroke. Aspirin is recommended within 24 to 48 hours poststroke. (In tPA patients, aspirin should not be given until 24 hours post-tPA.) Alternative antiplatelet agents include ticlopidine, dipyridamole/aspirin 200/25, and clopidogrel.

3. Antispasmodic agents can be used for spastic paralysis.

4. Early initiation of a rehabilitation program, including physical therapy, occupational therapy, and speech therapy, and counseling, as needed.

5. Depression is common; therefore, early initiation of antidepressants can be beneficial, such as selective serotonin reuptake inhibitors.

Complications

1. Aspiration pneumonia.
2. Dysphagia in 25% to 50% of patients after stroke.
3. Spasticity, contractures.
4. Deep vein thrombosis, pulmonary embolism.
5. Brain stem herniation.
6. Poststroke depression.

Nursing Assessment

1. Maintain neurologic flow sheet (National Institutes of Health (NIH) Stroke Scale for ischemic stroke and facility-based neurological assessment tool for hemorrhagic stroke).

2. Assess for voluntary or involuntary movements, tone of muscles, presence of deep tendon reflexes (reflex return signals end of flaccid period and return of muscle tone).

3. Also assess mental status, CN function, sensation/proprioception.

4. Monitor bowel and bladder function/control.

5. Monitor effectiveness of anticoagulation therapy.

6. Frequently assess level of function and psychosocial response to condition.

7. Assess for skin breakdown, contractures, and other complications of immobility.

 DRUG ALERT Oral anticoagulants are adjusted to maintain an INR at 2 to 3 to prevent stroke associated with atrial fibrillation. Monitor for potential complications of intracranial and subdural hemorrhage. Report INRs that are elevated to reduce the risk of bleeding or decreased levels to adjust therapy to be more effective.

Nursing Diagnoses

- Risk for Injury related to neurologic deficits.
- Impaired Physical Mobility related to motor deficits.
- Impaired Environmental Interpretation Syndrome related to brain injury.
- Impaired Verbal Communication related to brain injury.
- Bathing, Dressing, Toileting Self-Care Deficit related to hemiparesis/paralysis.

- Imbalanced Nutrition: Less Than Body Requirements related to impaired self-feeding, chewing, swallowing.
- Impaired Urinary Elimination related to motor/sensory deficits.
- Disabled Family Coping related to catastrophic illness, cognitive and behavioral sequelae of stroke, and caregiving burden.

 NURSING ALERT Use of clinical pathways maximizes stroke patient outcomes. Case management models of care foster interdisciplinary utilization, timeliness of referrals, patient education, patient satisfaction, and efficient use of health care resources. The specific role of the nurse in stroke recovery integrates therapeutic aspects of coordinating, maintaining, and training.

Nursing Interventions

Preventing Falls and Other Injuries

1. Maintain bed rest during acute phase (24 to 48 hours after onset of stroke) with head of bed slightly elevated and side rails in place.

2. Administer oxygen, as ordered, during acute phase to maximize cerebral oxygenation.

3. Frequently assess respiratory status, vital signs, heart rate and rhythm, and urine output to maintain and support vital functions.

4. When patient becomes more alert after acute phase, maintain frequent vigilance and interactions aimed at orienting, assessing, and meeting the needs of the patient.

5. Try to allay confusion and agitation with calm reassurance and presence.

6. Assess patient for risk for fall status.

Preventing Complications of Immobility

Interventions to improve functional recovery require active participation of the patient and repetitive training. Functional demand and intensive training are believed to trigger CNS reorganization—responsible for late functional recovery after stroke.

1. Maintain functional position of all extremities.
   a. Apply a trochanter roll from the crest of the ilium to the midthigh to prevent external rotation of the hip.
   b. Place a pillow in the axilla of the affected side when there is limited external rotation to keep arm away from chest and prevent adduction of the affected shoulder.
   c. Place the affected upper extremity slightly flexed on pillow supports with each joint positioned higher than the preceding one to prevent edema and resultant fibrosis; alternate elbow extension.
   d. Place the hand in slight supination with fingers slightly flexion.
   e. Avoid excessive pressure on ball of foot after spasticity develops.
   f. Do not allow top bedding to pull affected foot into plantar flexion; may use tennis shoes in bed.
   g. Place the patient in a prone position for 15 to 30 minutes daily, and avoid sitting up in chair for long periods to prevent knee and hip flexion contractures.

h. Encourage neutral positioning of affected limbs to promote relaxation and to limit abnormal increases in muscular tone to enhance functional recovery (reflex-inhibiting positioning).

j. "Forced use" is an experimental treatment designed to overcome nonuse of the hemiparetic upper extremity in regaining functional use of the affected arm with selected chronic hemiparetic patients.

k. "Constraint-induced movement therapy" restricts the contralateral upper extremity in effort to force use of the affected arm.

2. Apply splints and braces, as indicated, to support flaccid extremities or on spastic extremities to decrease stretch stimulation and reduce spasticity.

   a. Volar splint to support functional position of wrist.
   b. Sling to prevent shoulder subluxation of flaccid arm.
   c. High-top sneaker for ankle and foot support.

3. Exercise the affected extremities passively through ROM four to five times daily to maintain joint mobility and enhance circulation; encourage active ROM exercise as able (see page 174).

4. Teach patient to use unaffected extremity to move affected one.

5. Assist with ambulation, as needed, with help of physical therapy, as indicated.

   a. Check for orthostatic hypotension when dangling and standing.
   b. Gradually position the patient from a reclining position to head elevated, and dangle legs at the bedside before transferring out of bed or ambulating; assess sitting balance in bed.
   c. Assess the patient for excessive exertion.
   d. Have patient wear walking shoes or tennis shoes.
   e. Assess standing balance and have patient practice standing.
   f. Help patient begin ambulating as soon as standing balance is achieved; ensure safety with a patient waist belt.
   g. Provide rest periods as patient will tire easily.

Optimizing Orientation and Awareness

1. Be aware of the patient's cognitive alterations and adjust interaction and environment accordingly.

2. Participate in cognitive retraining program—reality orientation, visual imagery, cueing procedures—as outlined by rehabilitation nurse or therapist.

3. In patients with increased awareness, use pictures of family members, clock, calendar; post schedule of daily activities where patient can see it.

4. Focus on patient's strengths and give positive feedback.

5. Be aware that depression is common and therapy should include psychotherapy and early initiation of antidepressants.

Facilitating Communication

1. Speak slowly, using visual cues and gestures; be consistent and repeat as necessary.

2. Speak directly to the patient while facing him or her.

3. Give plenty of time for response and reinforce attempts as well as correct responses.

4. Minimize distractions.

5. Use alternative methods of communication other than verbal, such as written words, gestures, or pictures.

Fostering Independence

1. Teach the patient to use nonaffected side for activities of daily living (ADL) but not to neglect affected side.

2. Adjust the environment (eg, call light, tray) to side of awareness if spatial neglect or visual field cuts are present; approach patient from uninvolved side.

3. Teach the patient to scan environment if visual deficits are present.

4. Encourage the family to provide clothing a size larger than patient wears, with front closures, Velcro, and stretch fabric; teach the patient to dress while sitting to maintain balance.

5. Make sure personal care items, urinal, and commode are nearby and that patient obtains assistance with transfers and other activities, as needed.

6. Be aware that ADL require anticipatory (automatic coordination of multiple muscle groups in anticipation of a specific movement) and reactive (adjustment of posture to stimuli) postural adjustments.

7. Be aware that patients usually have clear goals in relation to functional abilities, against which all success and forward progress will be measured; help them set realistic short- and long-term goals.

Promoting Adequate Oral Intake

1. Perform a bedside swallow screen. Follow institutional protocol. If any coughing or difficulties are noted, contact speech therapy for official consult.

2. Initiate referral for a speech therapist for individuals with compromised LOC, dyspraxic speech, or speech difficulties to evaluate swallowing function at bedside or radiographically to demonstrate safe and functional swallowing mechanisms before initiation of oral diet.

3. Help the patient relearn swallowing sequence using compensatory techniques.

   a. Place ice on tongue and encourage sucking.
   b. Progress to ice pops and soft foods.
   c. Make sure mechanical soft or pureed diet is provided, based on ability to chew.

4. Encourage small, frequent meals and allow plenty of time to chew and swallow. Dietary consults can be helpful for selection of food preferences.

5. Remind the patient to chew on unaffected side.

6. Encourage the patient to drink small sips from a straw with chin tucked to the chest, strengthening effort to swallow while chin is tucked down.

7. Inspect mouth for food collection and pocketing before entry of each new bolus of food.

8. Inspect oral mucosa for injury from biting tongue or cheek.

9. Encourage frequent oral hygiene.

10. Teach the family how to assist the patient with meals to facilitate chewing and swallowing.

    a. Reduce environmental distractions to improve patient concentration.
    b. Provide oral care before eating to improve aesthetics and afterward to remove food debris.

c. Position the patient so he or she is sitting with 90 degrees of flexion at the hips and 45 degrees of flexion at the neck. Use pillows to achieve correct position.

d. Maintain position for 30 to 45 minutes after meals to prevent regurgitation and aspiration.

Attaining Bladder Control

1. Insert indwelling bladder catheterization during acute stage for accurate fluid management; remove as soon as status stabilizes.

2. Establish regular voiding schedule—every 2 to 3 hours, correlated with fluid intake—when bladder tone returns. If the patient is unable to void, intermittent catheterization can be used to empty bladder and prevent overstretching of bladder. The bladder scan device is useful in monitoring bladder capacity and identifying individuals at risk.

3. Assist with standing or sitting to void (especially males).

4. See page 181 for bladder retraining program details.

Strengthening Family Coping

1. Consult a social worker for assistance with patient/family support, to obtain copy of durable power of attorney, address guardianship, and long-term care decisions, as needed.

2. Encourage the family to maintain outside interests.

3. Teach stress management techniques, such as relaxation exercises, use of community and faith-based support networks.

4. Encourage participation in support group for family respite program for caregivers or other available resources in area.

5. Involve as many family and friends in care as possible.

6. Provide information about stroke and expected outcome.

7. Teach the family that stroke survivors may show depression in the first 3 months of recovery.

Community and Home Care Considerations

1. Hemiplegic complications resulting from stroke commonly include "frozen" shoulder; adduction and internal rotation of arm with flexion of elbow, wrist, and fingers; external rotation of the hip with flexion of the knee and plantar flexion of the ankle.

2. Perform ROM exercises and instruct the patient and family on these as well as on proper positioning.

3. Reinforce that these muscle and ligament deformities resulting from stroke can be prevented with daily stretching and strengthening exercises.

4. Depression after stroke is a major problem because it can increase morbidity. Monitor for signs of depression, such as difficulty sleeping, frequent crying, anorexia, feelings of guilt or sadness. Notify the health care provider for possible medication therapy.

5. Continue to support family who may be caring for a hemiplegic or aphasic person at home or in long-term care for a long time. Six months after stroke, around 9% to 21% of survivors are severely disabled, fully dependent, and live in institutions.

Patient Education and Health Maintenance

1. Teach the patient and family to adapt home environment for safety and ease of use.

2. Instruct the patient of the need for rest periods throughout day.

3. Reassure the family that it is common for poststroke patients to experience emotional lability and depression; treatment can be given.

4. Encourage consistency in the environment without distraction.

5. Assist the family to obtain self-help aids for the patient.

6. Instruct the family in management of aphasia (see Box 15-4, page 506).

7. Educate those at risk for stroke about lifestyle modifications and medication therapy that can lower risk.

8. Refer the patient and family for more information and support to such agencies as the National Stroke Association (*www.stroke.org*).

Evaluation: Expected Outcomes

- No falls, vital signs stable.
- Maintains body alignment, no contractures.
- Oriented to person, place, and time.
- Communicates appropriately.
- Brushes teeth, puts on shirt and pants independently.
- Feeds self two thirds of meal.
- Voids on commode at 2-hour intervals.
- Family seeks help and assistance from others.

Rupture of Intracranial Aneurysm

 Evidence Base Bederson, J. B., Connolly, E. S., Jr., Batjer, H. H., et al. (2012). Guidelines for the management of aneurysmal subarachnoid hemorrhage: A statement for healthcare professionals from a special writing group of the Stroke Council, American Heart Association. *Stroke, 43,* 1711–1737.

Diringer, M. N., Bleck, T. P., Hemphill, J. C. III, et al. (2011). Critical care management of patients following aneurysmal subarachnoid hemorrhage: Recommendations from the Neurocritical Care Society's multidisciplinary consensus conference. *Neurocritical Care, 15,* 211–240.

An *intracranial aneurysm* is an abnormal localized dilation of the wall of a cerebral artery due to congenital absence of the muscle layer of the vessel. Constant blood flow against the weakened area results in growth of the aneurysm and thinning of the vessel wall. Aneurysms usually occur at a bifurcation of an artery or major branches of the circle of Willis. They may be of congenital, traumatic, arteriosclerotic, or infectious origin. Most are saccular and asymptomatic until rupture; other types are fusiform and berry (see Figure 15-4). When an aneurysm ruptures, sudden bleeding occurs in the SAS between the arachnoid and the pia, causing SAH, which produces symptoms related to meningeal irritation. Hemorrhage can extend into the ventricular system, causing obstruction of CSF flow (hydrocephalus) or into the brain tissue (intracerebral bleed), causing further neurologic compromise. Depending on the extent of SAH, cerebral vasospasm (transient thickening of intralumen of a vessel) can occur, producing decreased cerebral blood flow, ischemia, and potential infarction

BOX 15-4   Aphasia

Aphasia is an acquired disorder of communication resulting from brain damage due to stroke, head injury, brain tumors, or brain cysts. It may involve impairment of the ability to speak, to understand speech of others, to read, write, calculate, and understand gestures. Most aphasic individuals have difficulty with expression and comprehension to varying degrees. Fatigue has adverse effect on speech.

To enhance your communication with the patient with aphasia, keep the environment simple and relaxed, minimize distractions, and use multiple sensory channels.

Refer the family to:

American Speech-Language-Hearing Association

10801 Rockville Pike

Rockville, MD 20852

301-897-5700

www.asha.org

APHASIA SYNDROMES

- Fluent aphasia (Wernicke's or receptive aphasia): Patient retains verbal fluency but may have difficulty in understanding speech. Speech is effortless and lacks clear content, information, and direction (nonsensical).
- Nonfluent aphasia (Broca's or expressive aphasia): Varied degrees of difficulty in initiation of speech, difficulty in formation of words with poor articulation, and difficulty in finding appropriate words. Speech is slow and laborious. Auditory comprehension is preserved.
- Anomic or amnesiac aphasia: Characteristic feature is difficulty naming and finding words. However, grammar, comprehension, and repetition remain intact.
- Conduction aphasia: Major difficulty is with sequencing phonemes resulting in literal paraphrasic errors. Auditory comprehension remains intact; however, patient has difficulty repeating spoken language.
- Global aphasia: Severe disruption of communication (verbal speech, written, reading and auditory comprehension).

NURSING INTERVENTIONS

- Speak at your normal rate and volume: The patient is not hard of hearing.
- Allow plenty of time to answer.
- Do not ask questions that require complex answers.
- Rote phrases can be spontaneous.
- Provide pad and pen if the patient prefers and is able to write.
- Avoid forcing speech.
- Watch the patient for clues and gestures if his or her speech is jargon; make neutral statements.
- Allow plenty of time for response.
- Ask for minimal word response.
- Encourage the patient to speak slowly.
- Expect frustration and anger at inability to communicate.
- Keep environment simple.
- Use gestures as well as language.
- Allow the patient to manipulate objects for additional sensory input.

or delayed cerebral ischemia (DCI). Transient thickening of the vessel is believed to be in response to the circulating blood and/or its breakdown products in the CSF. Vasospasm commonly occurs 3 to 14 days after SAH and peaks on day 5.

Grading of Aneurysms

Used to determine prognosis and timing of surgical or endovascular intervention.

Hunt-Hess Scale

0, Unruptured; asymptomatic discovery.

I, Asymptomatic or minimal headache with slight nuchal rigidity.

II, Moderate to severe headache, nuchal rigidity; no neurologic deficit other than CN deficit.

III, Drowsiness, confusion, or mild focal deficit (eg, hemiparesis), or combination of these findings.

IV, Stupor, moderate to severe deficit, possibly early decerebrate rigidity and vegetative disturbances.

V, Deep coma, decerebrate rigidity, moribund appearance.

Pathophysiology and Etiology

1. Cause unknown or related to congenital abnormality, atherosclerosis, intracranial AVM, hypertensive vascular disease, infection, or head trauma. Associated with polycystic renal disease and connective tissue disorders. Increased risk of rupture with smoking, female gender, hypertension, and aneurysm greater than 6 mm.
2. May become symptomatic due to pressure of enlarging aneurysm on nearby CNs or brain tissue.
3. Rupture and hemorrhage into SAS may cause increased ICP, hydrocephalus, and ischemia.
4. Vasospasm may occur within 3 to 14 days, peak day 5 days after rupture, causing ischemia (DCI) and infarction.
5. Rebleeding may occur due to lysis of clot with greatest risk for rebleeding in the first 6 to 72 hours after initial bleed (5% to 10%). Risk is greater in Hunt-Hess grades III to IV, large aneurysms, and sentinel bleed. Immediate repair of the aneurysm reduces the risk of rebleed. Seventy percent mortality after rebleed.

Incidence

1. Of the general population, 3% to 5% have an aneurysm; 30,000 cases of SAH are reported each year in the United States.
2. Age of incidence is between ages 40 and 60 (mean of 50).
3. In the over-40 age group, prevalence is greater in women; however, prevalence is equal when under age 40.
4. The prevalence of multiple aneurysms is 10% to 15%.
5. Familial tendency is less than 2%.

Clinical Manifestations

1. Sudden onset of severe headache, often accompanied by nausea and vomiting, but no neurologic deficits; leaking of aneurysm or AVM may cause a warning bleed.
2. Sudden, severe headache (commonly described as the "worst headache of my life"), meningeal signs (nuchal rigidity, photophobia, irritability), and neurologic dysfunction (related

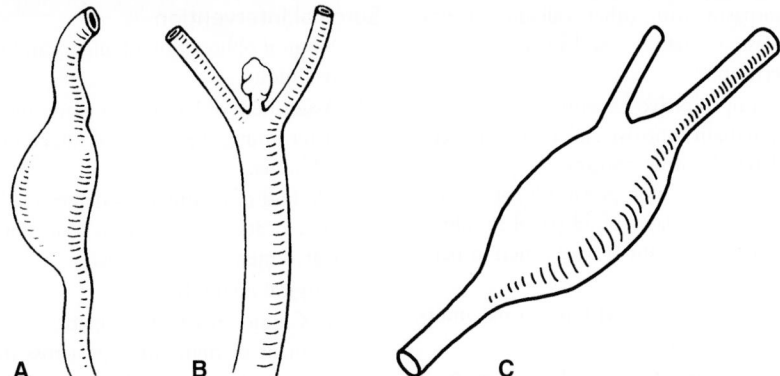

Figure 15-4. Saccular, fusiform, and berry aneurysms. (A) Saccular aneurysm; **(B)** berry aneurysm; **(C)** fusiform aneurysm.

to vascular territory) are commonly related to SAH secondary to ruptured intracranial aneurysm, which can be catastrophic.

3. Neurologic deficit related to vascular territory (see page 501); progressive CN III, IV, VI deficits due to mass effect.

4. Sentinel bleeds—10% to 20% of patients with SAH experience an acute, sudden headache that appears days or weeks before admission for SAH. Etiology of sentinel bleed is unclear. Theories include leakage of blood from the aneurysm or expansion of the aneurysm.

Diagnostic Evaluation

1. History and physical examination.
2. CT scan—to determine presence of blood in SAS, rule out other lesions, and evaluate mass effect.
   a. Fischer grade—estimates blood volume and location on CT. Assists in predicting risk for vasospasm. Grade 3 is highest risk for vasospasm.
      i. Grade 1: no subarachnoid blood.
      ii. Grade 2: diffuse or vertical layers <1 mm.
      iii. Grade 3: diffuse or vertical layers >1 mm.
      iv. Grade 4: intracerebral or intraventricular clot with diffuse or no subarachnoid hemorrhage.
3. Lumbar puncture (if no mass effect on CT)—grossly bloody CSF with more than 25,000 red blood cells (RBCs), CSF will not clear with subsequent taps as a traumatic tap would.
4. MRA or CT angiogram—noninvasive evaluation of cerebral vascular structures. Can be useful in the workup of suspected aneurysms (individuals with persistent headaches or unexplained neurologic deficits such as CN palsies). CT angiogram is the preferred study, though renal function must assessed secondary to use of contrast dye.
5. Cerebral angiogram—gold standard test; provides definitive evaluation of aneurysm etiology, presence, location, and configuration. Useful in determining the presence of vasospasm, extent of vasospasm, and collateral circulation.
6. TCD—noninvasive method to evaluate cerebral perfusion. Useful in the bedside evaluation and to provide a means for ongoing monitoring of cerebral blood flow to document changes and trends.

Management

Unruptured

1. Evaluation of diagnostic studies is key to determine need for intervention, scheduling of elective surgical clipping, or endovascular embolization, if indicated.
2. Normalize BP if hypertensive (systolic BP goal 120–140).
3. Smoking cessation.

After Rupture

1. Intracranial aneurysm precautions to minimize the risk of rebleeding and control BP—bed rest with head elevated, decreased environmental stimuli, avoidance of Valsalva maneuver and neck flexion, no caffeine, physical care as condition indicates.
2. Rapid repair of aneurysm should be performed by surgical clipping or endovascular embolization.
3. Management of systemic hypertension with labetalol, nicardipine, vasotec, hydralazine, or alternative IV antihypertensive agent can be used to maintain SBP <140 mm Hg or physician-ordered SBP goal, prior to definitive treatment. Debate continues on the precise SBP goal to be utilized. Close blood pressure monitoring should be maintained to prevent precipitous drop in BP.
4. Fluid goal is euvolemia. Prophylactic hypervolemia is not recommended. Fluid boluses should be considered prior to initiating vasopressor therapy. Close monitoring of intake and output (I&O), including running total I&O, and daily weights should be obtained to accurately assess fluid status. Routine use of central venous access for central venous pressure monitoring is not recommended.
5. Neuroprotective agents.
   a. Nimodipine, a calcium channel blocker, has demonstrated reduced incidence of delayed neurologic deficits and is felt to be neuroprotective during SAH and vasospasm. The medication is administered on admission and continues for 21 consecutive days. Dosing: 60 mg orally q4h for SBP greater than 140 mm Hg and 30 mg orally q4h for SBP 120 to 140 mm Hg, or per physician orders.
      i. Nimodipine has cerebral specificity to block the influx of calcium at the intracellular space. It is the only drug approved by the FDA for treatment of vasospasm.
      ii. For optimal effect, the nimodipine should be started within 96 hours of SAH.

b. Prevention of vasospasm with other calcium channel blockers, such as plasma expanders and hypervolemia to increase cerebral perfusion.

c. The data on the neuroprotective benefits of statins, specifically simvastatin, remain controversial, though patients on statins should have the drug continued. Statins may be considered in individuals not previously on statins. Dosing: 80 mg daily for 14 days. Lipid panel should be performed prior to institution and a liver function panel should be obtained on day 7.

d. Maintenance of magnesium level within normal limits. Hypomagnesium should be avoided.

6. Induced hypertension can be used in symptomatic vasospasm to prevent DCI. Colloids should be used initially with use of vasopressors as a secondary measure. Common vasopressor agents utilized are phenylephrine and norepinephrine. Fludrocortisone can be used as an oral agent to maintain SBP goal. No data exists on the specific SBP goal to be utilized. Neurological exam should be utilized to determine specific SBP or MAP goal.

7. Management of acute obstructive hydrocephalus related to intraventricular hemorrhage by placement of ventriculostomy or external ventricular drain (EVD) (see "Nursing Management of the Patient Undergoing Intracranial Surgery," page 492).

a. Adjustment of drain to promote drainage of CSF.

b. Intraventricular tPA-clot lysis may be used to promote CSF drainage. Current studies indicate low risk for intracranial bleeding with reduced risk for vasospasm.

c. Surgical placement of ventricular-peritoneal shunt may be necessary.

8. Witnessed seizures: Phenytoin, fosphenytoin, or levetiracetam are the preferred medications. Duration of drug therapy is variable and levels are monitored for accurate dosing. Prophylactic use of AEDs is not recommended, although it may be considered. If prophylactic AEDs are utilized, a 3- to 7-day course is recommended.

9. Cardiopulmonary complications are common, therefore it is recommended to obtain baseline cardiac enzymes, electrocardiography, echocardiography at time of admission.

10. Maintain normal glucose level because hypoglycemia and hyperglycemia is associated with a poor outcome. Sliding scale insulin or insulin drip should be utilized to maintain blood sugar at 80 to 180. Glucose level <80 and >200 should be avoided.

11. Maintain normothermia. Hyperthermia is associated with a poor neurologic outcome. Antipyretic agents are first-line treatment for the management of fever. External surface cooling devices or intravascular cooling devices should be employed when antipyretics are ineffective. Fever workup should be performed to evaluate for potential infectious etiology of fever.

12. Deep vein thrombosis prophylaxis—sequential stockings and low-dose heparin or LMWH should be utilized, although remains physician-dependent. Data does not suggest any increased risk of hemorrhage in this population. Low-dose heparin or LMWH should be held prior to and after any intracranial procedure for 24 hours.

Surgical Intervention

1. Surgical obliteration of aneurysm by clipping, ligation, or IA technique.

2. Assessment of Hunt-Hess grade and medical stability assist in determining the timing of intervention, usually within 24 to 72 hours.

3. Method of treatment is determined by evaluating aneurysm size, location, neck width, condition of the patient, and associated medical conditions.

4. Surgical methods:

a. Craniotomy is performed to access the aneurysm. Placement of titanium clips across the neck of the aneurysm or wrapping of fusiform aneurysm. Multiple-size titanium clips are available to secure aneurysm.

b. *Advantages:* removal of intracerebral hemorrhagic/subarachnoid blood; low rate of aneurysm recurrence.

c. *Disadvantage:* open procedure.

5. IA techniques:

a. Superselective angiography with placement of microcatheter into the aneurysm for evaluation.

b. Obliteration of the aneurysm.

    i. Multiple types of coils are available. Type and length of coil utilized is dependent on configuration of aneurysm. Coils fill the aneurysm and are detached using electronic heating. Multiple coils are placed until there is no blood flow noted on angiography to the aneurysm.

    ii. Coil embolization with aid of micro-stent—the micro-stent is used to form a bridge across the neck of the aneurysm and in fusiform aneurysms, allowing for placement of coils.

    iii. *Advantages:* minimally invasive treatment; shorter duration of anesthesia.

    iv. *Disadvantage:* potential for recurrence if aneurysm not completely occluded.

c. Interventional treatment of vasospasm.

    i. Balloon angioplasty—dilation of vessel by expansion of a transarterial balloon to treat vasospasm.

    ii. IA injection or verapamil or papaverine for temporary local vasodilation.

NURSING ALERT Heparin can be used intraprocedure and postprocedure, as per physician order, to minimize risk of thromboembolic events. Risks include thromboembolic complications and rupture of aneurysm with extension of SAH.

Complications

NURSING ALERT Mortality ranges from 20% to 50% (10% to 19% die before reaching the hospital, 25% die within 24 hours post-SAH, and 45% to 50% die within 30 days). Survivors are left with a 50% chance of functional disability. Rebleed and DCI secondary to vasospasm is directly related to mortality and morbidity.

1. Aneurysm rebleed—risk is 4% on day 1, then 1.5% per day on days 2 to 13, 20% within 14 days, and 50% within 6 months; highest risk within first 6 hours. Seventy percent mortality in rebleed.

2. Delayed ischemic neurological deficit occur secondary to diminished cerebral blood flow. Cerebral vasospasm and DCI are the most common cause. Greatest risk: 3 to 14 days after SAH. Current theory is that cerebral vasospasm is a reversible thickening of medial wall and smooth muscle proliferation, causing narrowing of the vessel lumen. Seventy percent to 80% of patients have radiographic vasospasm, with 30% being symptomatic or demonstrating the effects of DCI.

3. Obstructive hydrocephalus—20% to 30% of patients develop obstructive hydrocephalus. EVD placement allows for temporary CSF drainage; 18% to 26% will require placement of a ventricular-peritoneal shunt.

4. Seizures—1% to 7% at presentation. Witnessed seizures are treated with AEDs, although specific duration of treatment remains controversial. Prophylactic use of AEDs is not recommended, although it may be considered. If prophylactic AEDs are used, a 3- to 7-day course is recommended.

5. Hypernatremia related to alterations in ADH secretion or imbalance in fluid status. Close monitoring of sodium level may be indicated.

6. Hyponatremia—differentiate between SIADH and cerebral salt wasting to ensure appropriate treatment (see page 489).

7. Cardiopulmonary complications: (related to abnormal catecholamine release).
   a. Cardiovascular changes ranging from atrial fibrillation, bradycardia, and T-wave abnormalities to left ventricular dysfunction with or without myocardial failure and myocardial injury in severe cases.
   b. Neurogenic pulmonary edema.

Nursing Assessment

1. Perform and document neurologic assessment with vital signs and as patient condition warrants.

2. Monitor for changes in or decreasing LOC, CN dysfunction, pupillary abnormality, and motor deficit, which signify increased ICP, cerebral vasospasm, DCI, or expanding lesion.

3. Assess for increasing headache, which could signal rebleeding.

4. Monitor for focal neurologic deficits, which may indicate vasospasm.

Nursing Diagnoses

- Risk for Injury related to potential rebleeding, vasospasm, hydrocephalus, and seizures.
- Ineffective Tissue Perfusion (cerebral) related to disease process and vasospasm.
- Acute Pain secondary to cerebral hemorrhage, meningeal irritation, surgical procedure.
- Anxiety of patient/family related to treatment, intracranial surgery or endovascular treatment, and uncertainty of patient outcome.

Nursing Interventions

Modifying Activity to Prevent Complications

1. Prior to treatment reduce environmental stimuli, limit stress, and decrease the risk of rebleed and/or increased ICP.
   a. Maintain complete bed rest with head elevated 30 degrees to reduce cerebral edema.
   b. Maintain quiet environment with low lighting, noise control, and limit activity to prevent photophobia, agitation, and pain.
   c. Encourage the awake patient to avoid activities that increase BP or ICP: straining, sneezing, acute flexion/rotation of the neck; assist patient with position changes.
   d. Avoid Valsalva maneuver, which may increase ICP, by administering stool softeners to prevent straining; avoiding rectal temperatures, enemas, and suppositories; and teaching the awake patient to exhale through mouth during defecation.
   f. Avoid caffeinated beverages and extremes of temperatures.
   g. Provide physical care, such as bathing and feeding, as needed.

2. Implement nursing interventions to minimize ICP and cerebral swelling (eg, elevate head of bed 30 degrees, maintain proper head and neck alignment to avoid jugular vein compression, avoid prolonged suctioning procedures, keep procedure less than 15 seconds, collaborate with physicians to use lidocaine before suctioning if intubated).

3. Medicate patient, as ordered, during periods of extreme agitation.

4. Perform and document neurologic assessment with vital signs and as patient condition warrants, which includes monitoring LOC, CN function, pupillary function, and motor function.

5. Assess for signs of increased ICP, including agitation, change in LOC, bradycardia and widening pulse pressure, changes in respiratory pattern (Cheyne-Stokes pattern, apneustic, ataxic).

6. Monitor arterial blood gas (ABG) values for hypoxia and hypercapnia, which aggravate ICP.

7. Monitor ventriculostomy, if present, for patency, amount and character of drainage, and correct height level every 4 hours.

> **NURSING ALERT** There is no evidence-based data to support daily sampling of CSF. If CSF is cloudy or purulent, notify the health care provider. If ordered, obtain CSF samples from EVD using sterile technique and send for culture and Gram stains, white blood cell (WBC) count, RBC count, glucose and protein analysis.

8. Recognize need for maintenance of BP parameters based on status of treated versus untreated aneurysm (ie, treated: SBP 160 to 180; untreated: SBP 120 to 140). (BP goal post-treatment remains controversial. BP goal may vary related to physician preference or be based on clinical exam.)

9. Evaluate effectiveness of antihypertensive or vasopressor therapy.

10. Perform ongoing physical assessment, including respiratory, cardiac, GI, genitourinary (GU) function to detect potential complications.

11. Maintain safety factors based on neurologic deficits (eg, prevent sensory overload, physical injury related to vision, hearing, body awareness deficits).

Maintaining Cerebral Perfusion

1. Frequently monitor neurologic status based on condition, including LOC, pupillary reaction, motor and sensory function, CN function, speech, presence of headache.
2. Administer crystalloid to maintain euvolemia.
3. Monitor BP, hemodynamic monitoring, neurologic status, and input and output status at least every hour, or as status indicates, while in the ICU.
4. Assess for signs and symptoms of vasospasm: insidious onset of confusion, disorientation, and decreased LOC, or focal deficit associated with vascular territory associated with aneurysm bleed. Recognize that peak time for vasospasm occurrence is 5 days after bleed, with duration of 14 days.
5. Document findings and report changes; subtle change in LOC, such as drowsiness and speech slurring, or onset of pronator drift (inability to maintain unsupported position of outstretched pronated forearm), may be first sign of deterioration.
6. See "Nursing Management of the Patient with an Altered State of Consciousness," page 483.

Reducing Pain

1. Assess level of pain and pain relief; report any increase in headache.
2. Administer analgesics, as prescribed; if opioid is being given with sedative, monitor for CNS depression, decreased respirations, decreased BP. Stool softeners should be given if analgesics are utilized.
3. Administer dexamethasone, as prescribed, for headache control. May be useful for headaches as a result of inflammatory changes secondary to coils.
4. Encourage distraction and relaxation techniques to promote calming effect.
5. Explain to the patient/significant other the limited use of opioids secondary to need to assess the patient's LOC at all times.
6. Encourage elevated head of bed to minimize cerebral swelling.
7. Provide cool compresses to head.
8. Assess the patient for experiences of unrelieved or increased pain; assess for any changes in neurologic signs, nuchal rigidity, photophobia, and/or changes in vision, which could signal hemorrhage, hydrocephalus, or meningeal irritation.

Reducing Anxiety

1. Provide ongoing assessment of psychosocial issues (sexuality, anxiety, fear, depression, frustration, emotional lability).
2. Be attuned to verbal and nonverbal cues from the patient/family that signal problems with coping.
3. Inform the patient regarding all treatment modalities.
4. Encourage discussion of risks/benefits with the surgeon/interventional neuroradiologist.
5. Use reassurance and therapeutic conversation to relieve fear and anxiety.
6. Provide support to the patient/family in dealing with the stress and uncertainty of hospitalization.

7. Consult Social Services for assistance with patient/family support to obtain copy of advance directives, including durable power of attorney, address guardianship, and long-term care decisions, as needed.
8. Prepare patient and family for surgery (see "Nursing Management of the Patient Undergoing Intracranial Surgery," page 492) or endovascular treatment.

Community and Home Care Considerations

1. Assess the level of knowledge and ability of the patient/significant other to retain information.
2. Assess ongoing home care needs.
3. Assess the need for nursing home or rehabilitation center placement and obtain social service referral to help with planning.
4. Provide teaching to the family and caregivers and act as liaison between health care team and family.
5. Teach the patient and family how to deal with permanent neurologic deficits and make sure that they obtain needed supplies and services.

Patient Education and Health Maintenance

1. Instruct the patient/family on purpose and frequency of neurologic radiologic procedures.
2. Explain what an aneurysm is, signs/symptoms of rupture, and possible threats of rupture.
3. Educate the patient about activities to avoid to prevent sudden increased pressure, such as heavy lifting and straining prior to definitive treatment.
4. Encourage lifelong medical follow-up and immediate attention if severe headache develops.
5. Instruct the patient/family on need for and use of invasive monitoring and drainage systems.
6. Reinforce the need for head of bed not to be adjusted.
7. Provide educational material for procedures.
8. Set mutual goals for discharge and communicate discharge preparations with other disciplines (registered nurse, physician, physical therapist, discharge coordinator).
9. Explain medications to the patient/significant other and potential adverse effects. Explain the importance of continued nimodipine therapy and correct usage.
10. Have the patient verbalize discharge instructions regarding wound care, activity restrictions, medications, and reportable signs/symptoms.

Evaluation: Expected Outcomes

- No signs of rebleeding, increased ICP, decreased cerebral perfusion, or seizures vital signs stable; neurologic parameters stable.
- SBP goals maintained.
- Verbalizes decreased pain or control of pain to an intensity that is acceptable.
- Patient and family able to state reason for surgery/endovascular intervention, possible risks; openly discuss fears and uncertainties.

Rupture of Intracranial Arteriovenous Malformation

An *arteriovenous malformation (AVM)* is a system of dilated arteries and veins with dysplastic vessels. The normal capillary beds are absent and the arterial blood flows directly into the draining veins (fistula). AVMs are congenital lesions that can enlarge over the patient's life span; these lesions are often asymptomatic until rupture. The lifetime risk of bleed in an unruptured AVM is 2% to 4% per year throughout the patient's life span, depending on size and structural configuration of the lesion.

Pathophysiology and Etiology

1. AVMs generally contain a nidus (central core) and "red" engorged veins (oxygenated veins) and have been described as a tangled mass of discolored vessels that have the appearance of a cluster of grapes.
2. The artery to venous connection, or fistula, creates increased pressure within the venous system, resulting in vascular dilation, congestion, and hypoperfusion.
3. AVMs are generally low-pressure abnormalities at birth and can progress to a high-flow, high-pressure abnormality in adulthood.
4. Parenchymal AVMs can be located in the pia matter, subcortical tissue, paraventricular region, or a combination of these regions.
5. Approximately 50% of patients with AVMs present with hemorrhage. Other signs of AVM rupture include seizures and signs of mass effect.
6. Intracerebral bleeding in a ruptured AVM tends to be superficial; cerebral vasospasm rarely occurs. The Spetzler-Martin grading system is used as a prognostic indicator as well as a tool to define risks associated with treating AVMs. Grading scale of 1 to 5: 1 = lowest risk, 5 = greatest risk for treatment (see Table 15-6).

Table 15-6	Spetzler-Martin Grading System
	POINTS
Size of nidus	
Small	1
Medium	2
Large	3
Eloquence of brain tissue	
No	0
Yes	1
Deep vascular component	
No	0
Yes	1

Grading scale of 1 to 5: 1 = lowest risk, 5 = greatest risk for treatment.

Clinical Manifestations

1. Sudden onset of severe headache, often accompanied by nausea and vomiting, but without neurologic deficits; may be early signs of a ruptured AVM.
2. Progressively worsening headache, as well as new onset of seizure activity due to spontaneous superficial intracerebral hemorrhage, are commonly related to a ruptured AVM.
3. May present with loss of consciousness and severe deficits if massive bleed. Focal signs or deficits are dependent on the location of the bleed and compression of adjacent brain structures (visual disturbances, CN deficits, hemiparesis, etc.).

Diagnostic Evaluation

1. History and physical examination.
2. CT scan—to determine presence of blood, rule out other lesions; increased density if blood present, may also show increased ICP or mass effect.
3. MRI and MRA or CT angiogram—noninvasive evaluation of cerebral vascular structures. Useful in the diagnosis of AVM, but does not define vascular changes and flow patterns.
4. Cerebral angiogram—gold standard test and the only diagnostic tool that provides definitive evaluation of AVM presence, location, and vascular structure. Will also evaluate flow patterns, pressure gradients, and collateral circulation and identify intranidal aneurysms and feeding vessels.

Management

Unruptured

1. Aimed at diagnostic evaluation of AVM to determine appropriate intervention—surgical, endovascular, radiosurgery, or a combination.
2. Surgical resection—dependent on location, eloquence of brain tissue, and size.
3. Endovascular management with N-butyl cyanoacrylate liquid polymer, polyvinyl alcohol particles, detachable coils, balloon occlusion.
   a. Staged embolization is generally performed on larger AVMs to reduce flow patterns gradually.
   b. Initial embolization is aimed at protecting area at risk for rupture, reducing the nidus, or controlling the area at highest risk for bleeding.
   c. Can be used as primary treatment modality or as an adjunct to surgical resection and radiosurgery.
4. Radiosurgery (gamma knife/linear accelerator)—lesions less than or equal to 2.5 to 3 cm in size. Radiation creates vessel wall injury, initiating clot formation that leads to eventual blockage of vessel (this can take 1 to 3 years to occur). During this time, the AVM remains at risk for rupture.
5. AEDs for seizures as presenting symptom—fosphenytoin, phenytoin, or levetiracetam may be given initially via IV for rapid loading. Levels should be monitored for accurate dosing.
6. Normalize BP if hypertensive.
7. Smoking cessation.

After Rupture

1. Maintenance and close monitoring of SBP within prescribed limits to prevent rebleed from hypertension and ischemia from decreased cerebral perfusion with nicardipine, labetalol, vasotec, apresoline, or alternative IV antihypertensive agents.
   a. Vasopressor agents to maintain SBP within prescribed range.
2. AEDs for seizures as presenting symptom—phenytoin, fosphenytoin, and levetiracetam; duration based on provider preference and location and extent of bleed.
3. Intervention.
   a. Surgery—evacuation of hematoma with or without resection of AVM.
   b. Endovascular management—partial embolization of AVM, specifically area of suspected rupture.

Complications

1. Bleed or rebleed.
2. Hydrocephalus; obstructive initially requiring ventriculostomy, nonobstructive long-term, may require shunt.
3. Seizures.
4. Permanent deficit or deterioration and death.

Nursing Assessment

1. Perform and document neurologic assessment with vital signs and as patient condition warrants.
2. Monitor for changes in or decreasing LOC, CN function, pupillary function, and motor function, including drift (inability to maintain unsupported position).
3. Assess for increasing headache or focal neurologic deficits, which could signal rebleeding.
4. Assess vital signs and pupillary changes frequently for development of increased ICP.

Nursing Diagnoses

- Risk for Injury related to potential rebleeding, hydrocephalus, and seizures.
- Ineffective Cerebral Tissue Perfusion related to disease process.
- Acute Pain secondary to cerebral hemorrhage, meningeal irritation, surgical procedure.
- Anxiety of patient/family related to treatment, intracranial surgery or endovascular treatment, and uncertainty of patient outcome.

Nursing Interventions

Modifying Activity to Prevent Complications

1. Medicate the patient as ordered during periods of extreme agitation.
2. Institute seizure precautions by providing padded side rails, suction equipment, and oral airway at the bedside.
3. Perform and document neurologic assessment with vital signs and as patient condition warrants, which includes monitoring LOC, CN function, pupillary function, and motor function with pronator drift.

4. Assess for signs of increased ICP, including bradycardia and widening pulse pressure, changes in respiratory pattern (Cheyne-Stokes pattern, apneustic, ataxic).
5. Implement nursing interventions to minimize ICP and cerebral swelling (eg, elevate head of bed 30 degrees, maintain proper head and neck alignment to avoid jugular vein compression, avoid prolonged suctioning procedures, keep procedure less than 15 seconds, collaborate with physicians to use lidocaine presuctioning if intubated).
6. Monitor ABG values for hypoxia and hypercapnia, which aggravate ICP.
7. Monitor ventriculostomy, if present, to manage acute hydrocephalus, for patency, amount, and character of drainage, and correct height level every 4 hours.
   a. If CSF is cloudy or purulent or other signs of potential infection are present, contact the health care provider.
   b. Obtain CSF samples from the external ventricular device using sterile technique and send for culture and Gram stain, WBC count, glucose, and protein, as directed.
   c. Monitor results and report abnormal values.
   d. Administer prophylactic antibiotics, as ordered. Use of prophylactic antibiotics is controversial and provider-dependent.
8. Recognize need for maintenance of BP parameters.
9. Evaluate effectiveness of antihypertensive or vasopressor therapy.
10. Perform ongoing physical assessment including respiratory, cardiac, GI, and GU function to detect potential complications.
11. Maintain safety factors for neurologic deficits (eg, prevent sensory overload, physical injury related to vision, or hearing, body awareness deficits).

Maintaining Cerebral Perfusion

1. Frequently monitor neurologic status based on condition, including LOC, pupillary reaction, motor and sensory function, CN function, speech, presence of headache.
2. Administer vasopressive therapy, as ordered, to increase cerebral perfusion.
3. Monitor fluid and electrolytes; monitor hematocrit and hemoglobin.
4. Evaluate adequacy of therapy regimen by assessment of BP, hemodynamic monitoring, neurologic status, and input and output status at least every hour, or as status indicates, while in the ICU.
5. Assess for subjective neurologic complaints specific to decreased perfusion (eg, diplopia, headache, blurred vision).
6. Assess for signs and symptoms of rebleed: insidious onset of confusion, disorientation, and decreased LOC, or focal deficit associated with area of bleed.
7. Document findings and report changes; subtle change in LOC, such as drowsiness and speech slurring or onset of pronator drift, may be first sign of deterioration.
8. See "Nursing Management of the Patient with an Altered State of Consciousness," page 483.

Reducing Pain

1. Assess level of pain and pain relief; report any increase in headache.
2. Administer analgesics as prescribed; if opioid is being given with sedative, monitor for CNS depression, decreased respirations, decreased BP.
3. Encourage distraction and relaxation techniques to promote calming effect.
4. Explain to the patient/significant other the limited use of opioids secondary to need to assess patient's LOC at all times.
5. Encourage elevated head of bed to minimize cerebral swelling.
6. Provide cool compresses to head.
7. Assess the patient for experiences of unrelieved or increased pain; assess for any changes in neurologic signs, which could signal hemorrhage, hydrocephalus, or meningeal irritation.

Reducing Anxiety

1. Provide ongoing assessment of psychosocial issues (sexuality, anxiety, fear, depression, frustration, emotional lability).
2. Be attuned to verbal and nonverbal cues from the patient/family that signal problems with coping.
3. Inform the patient regarding all treatment modalities.
4. Encourage discussion of risks/benefits with the surgeon/interventional neuroradiologist.
5. Use reassurance and therapeutic conversation to relieve fear and anxiety.
6. Provide support to the patient/family in dealing with the stress and uncertainty of hospitalization.
7. Consult social services for assistance with the patient/family support and long-term care decisions, as needed.
8. Prepare the patient and family for surgery (see "Nursing Management of the Patient Undergoing Intracranial Surgery," page 492) or endovascular treatment.

Community and Home Care Considerations

1. Assess level of knowledge and ability of patient/significant other to retain information.
2. Assess ongoing home care needs.
3. Assess need for nursing home or rehabilitation center placement and obtain social service referral to help with planning.
4. Provide teaching to family and caregivers and act as liaison between health care team and family.
5. Teach patient and family how to deal with permanent neurologic deficits and make sure that they obtain needed supplies and services.

Patient Education and Health Maintenance

1. Instruct patient/family on purpose and frequency of neurologic/radiologic procedures.
2. Explain what an AVM is, signs/symptoms of rupture, and possible threats of rupture.
3. Educate the patient to the risk of rebleed, which is 50% within 6 months if untreated, and remains for rest of life if not definitively treated.

4. Encourage lifelong medical follow-up and immediate attention if severe headache develops.
5. Explain the need for follow-up angiograms to verify complete eradication of AVM or to define extent of eradication to facilitate treatment planning.
6. Provide educational material for procedures.
7. Set mutual goals for discharge, and communicate discharge preparations with other disciplines (registered nurse, physician, physical therapist, discharge coordinator).
8. Explain medications to the patient/significant other and potential adverse effects.
9. Have patient verbalize discharge instructions regarding wound care, activity restrictions, medications, and reportable signs/symptoms.

Evaluation: Expected Outcomes

- No signs of rebleeding, increased ICP, decreased cerebral perfusion or seizures; vital signs stable; neurologic parameters stable.
- Verbalizes decreased pain or control of pain to an intensity that is acceptable.
- Patient and family able to state reason for surgery/endovascular intervention, possible risks.
- Decrease in anxiety sufficient to allow the completion of necessary procedures and to promote recovery.

INFECTIOUS DISORDERS

Meningitis

 Evidence Base Shin, S. H., & Kim, K. S. (2012). Treatment of bacterial meningitis: An update. *Expert Opinion in Pharmacotherapy, 15*, 2189–2206.

Meningitis is an inflammation of the pia mater and arachnoid membranes that surround the brain and the spinal cord. The subarachnoid space between these two meninges contains CSF that may reflect the signs and symptoms of meningitis.

Pathophysiology and Etiology

1. Viral meningitis is the most common form. More than 10,000 cases are reported annually, but the actual incidence may be as high as 75,000. It is usually self-limiting; management is supportive. It is usually caused by a nonpolio enterovirus (90%). The incidence of viral meningitis drops with age. As a general rule, the younger the patient, the greater the risk of viral meningitis. This organism is spread by the fecal–oral route and through sewage.
2. In the United States, the incidence of acute, bacterial meningitis is approximately three cases per 100,000 per year. The mortality is 10% to 30% and many who recover are left with long-term problems (eg, hearing deficit).
3. Bacterial meningitis may cause damage to the CNS from the inflammatory process rather than the pathogen. The organisms causing these infections seem to vary depending on the

age and immune status of the patient. Bacterial meningitis is usually more serious than viral meningitis. It is typically caused by *Streptococcus pneumoniae* (pneumococcal meningitis), which is a Gram-positive diplococcus, and *Neisseria meningitidis* (meningococcal meningitis), which is a Gram-negative diplococcus.

   a. Most bacteria that cause meningitis begin by colonizing the nasopharynx, then invade the circulation and CSF, causing an inflammatory response mediated by cytokines.

   b. Bacterial meningitis can result in brain damage due to chemicals released by bacteria that kill or damage neurons, purulent exudates that may result in vasculitis and vasospasm, and increased ICP that causes cerebral edema.

4. Fungal meningitis, particularly *Cryptococcus neoformans*, affects immunosuppressed patients (eg, human immunodeficiency virus [HIV]–positive) through soil contaminated with excrement from pigeons and chickens. Cryptococcal antigen, or culture, is found in the CSF, but meningeal signs may be minimal. In HIV-positive patients, tuberculous meningitis, tuberculomas, and atypical mycobacterial infections of the brain may be noted.

5. Parasitic meningitis is usually cause by flukes, worms, or amoeba.

6. Hospital-acquired postcraniotomy meningitis, caused predominantly by Gram-negative bacilli, can result in mortalities of 30%; multiple craniotomy operations place the patient at even higher risk. It develops approximately 7 to 8 days postoperatively.

7. Neoplastic meningitis affects approximately 3% to 8% of patients who have systemic cancers. The mean survival time is approximately 5 to 8 months. In neoplastic meningitis, malignant cells infiltrate the leptomeninges as a complication of breast cancer, lung cancer, malignant melanoma, non-Hodgkin's lymphoma, and acute leukemia.

8. Meningitis is the primary intracranial complication of acute and chronic sinusitis (sphenoid sinusitis most common). *S. pneumonia* and *Staphylococcus aureus* are the most common organisms.

9. *Listeria monocytogenes*, a Gram-positive bacilli, may cause meningitis through contaminated hot dogs, cold meats, and unpasteurized dairy products.

10. The incidence of *Haemophilus influenzae* meningitis has decreased due to the haemophilus b conjugate vaccine.

Clinical Manifestations

1. Classic symptoms are fever, headache, and nuchal rigidity. Constitutional symptoms of vomiting, diarrhea, cough, and myalgias appear in more than 50% of patients. History of temperature elevation occurs in 76% to 100% of patients who seek medical attention. A common pattern is low-grade fever in the prodromal stage and higher temperature elevations at the onset of neurologic signs.

2. Altered mental status; confusion in older patients.

3. Petechial (appears like "rug" burn) or purpuric rash from coagulopathy, especially with *N. meningitidis*.

4. Photophobia.

5. Neck tenderness or a bulging anterior fontanel in infants.

6. Children may exhibit behavioral changes, arching of the back and neck, a blank stare, refusal to feed, and seizures. Viral meningitis can cause a red, maculopapular rash in children.

7. Positive Brudzinski's and Kernig's signs (see Figure 15-5).

8. Neonates may exhibit poor feeding, altered breathing patterns, or listlessness.

9. Onset may be over several hours or several days depending on the infectious agent, the patient's age, immune status, comorbidities, and other variables. Some viruses cause rapid onset of symptoms, while others may involve prodromal nonspecific flu-like symptoms, such as malaise, myalgia, and upper respiratory symptoms. In many cases, symptoms have a biphasic pattern; the nonspecific flu-like symptoms and low-grade fever precede neurologic symptoms by approximately 48 hours. With the onset of neck stiffness and headache, the fever usually returns.

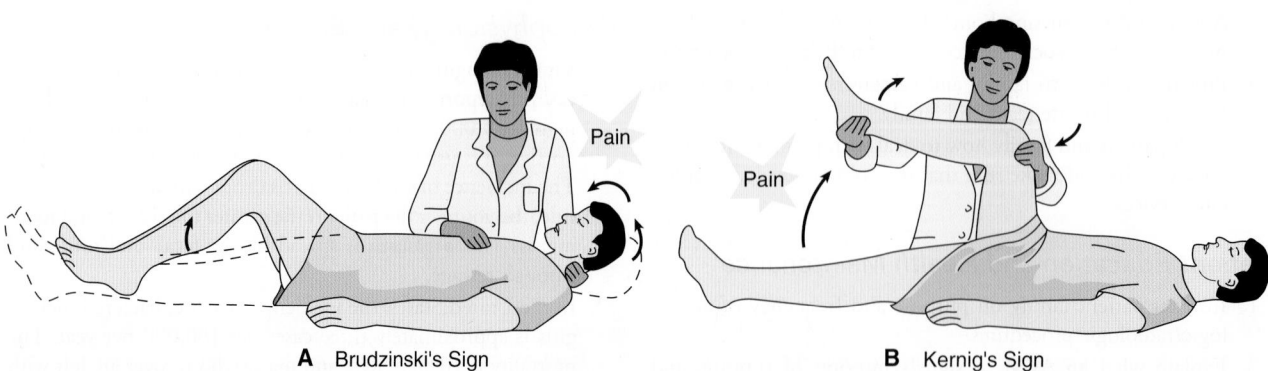

Figure 15-5. Signs of meningeal irritation include nuchal rigidity and positive Brudzinski's and Kernig's signs. (A) To elicit Brudzinski's sign, place the patient supine and flex the head upward. Resulting flexion of both hips, knees, and ankles with neck flexion indicates meningeal irritation. **(B)** To test for Kernig's sign, once again place the patient supine. Keeping the bottom leg straight, flex the other hip and knee to form a 90-degree angle. Slowly extend the upper leg. This places a stretch on the meninges, resulting in pain and spasm of the hamstring muscle. Resistance to further extension can be felt.

Key Decision Point
If patient presents with meningitis-like symptoms and appears very ill, evaluation and treatment of bacterial meningitis must be urgently initiated. Patients with bacterial meningitis are typically sicker than patients with a viral etiology, with high fever, severe headache, +/− photophobia, and mental status changes. Blood and CSF cultures should be taken as soon as possible as the goal of treatment is to administer appropriate IV antibiotics within 30 minutes of presentation.

Diagnostic Evaluation

1. Complete blood count (CBC) with differential is indicated to detect an elevated leukocyte count in bacterial and viral meningitis, with a greater percentage of polymorphonuclear leukocytes (90%) in bacterial and (less than 50%) in viral meningitis (normal 0% to 15%).
2. Blood cultures are obtained to indicate the organism.
3. CSF evaluation for pressure, leukocytes, protein, glucose—CSF normally has five or fewer lymphocytes or mononuclear cells/mm³.
   a. In acute bacterial meningitis, the CSF may indicate elevated pressure, elevated leukocytes (several thousand), elevated protein, low glucose. A culture and smear will identify the organism. WBC differential should be done by a stained smear of sediment.
   b. In viral encephalitis, the CSF may indicate normal/moderately elevated pressure, few/elevated leukocytes (fewer than 1,000), normal or slightly elevated protein, normal glucose.
4. MRI/CT with and without contrast rules out other disorders. A CT scan with contrast must be obtained to detect abscesses.
5. Latex agglutination may be positive for antigens in meningitis.
6. Low CD4+ counts indicate immunosuppression in HIV-positive patients and other patients with immunosuppressive disorders.
7. In patients with acquired immunodeficiency syndrome (AIDS), MRI is used to detect meningeal irritation, evidence of a sinus infection, or brain abscess.

Management

1. The assessment and management of meningitis should be approached through a team effort with nursing, infectious disease and otolaryngology specialists, neurology, internal medicine, and laboratory and diagnostic staff.
2. Most patients are given IV antibiotics as soon as possible until the laboratory findings determine the type of meningitis (eg, viral, bacterial). However, cultures should be taken before initiating antibiotics.

NURSING ALERT Be aware that bacterial resistance to antibiotics has been increasing, making meningitis very difficult to treat in some instances.

3. To manage inflammation, dexamethasone or another corticosteroid is given via IV line.

   a. This may result in GI bleeding and mask clinical responses to treatments (eg, resolved fever).
   b. This steroid should be used before or with the first dose of antibiotics (IV 0.6 mg/kg/day in four divided doses for the first 4 days of antibiotics) and should be confined to patients older than age 6 weeks.
   c. Plasmapheresis may be used experimentally to remove cytokines in some cases.
4. Temozolomide, a second-generation alkylating agent, is effective against many cancers that result in neoplastic meningitis. External beam radiation may be used in conjunction with chemotherapy (eg, intrathecal thiotepa or methotrexate).
5. Cochlear implantation rehabilitation due to deafness caused by meningitis should be considered. Realistic goals must be set because the patient may develop only environmental sound awareness and still have to deal with learning disabilities.
6. If meningitis is suspected after neurosurgical procedures, consider potential IV line bacteremia, CSF leak, or immunosuppression.
7. Antifungal agents, such as amphotericin B and the triazoles, fluconazole and itraconazole, are indicated for cryptococcal meningitis. Relapse is common if the patient does not have chronic suppressive therapy with fluconazole or another antifungal agent.
8. Empiric antituberculosis drugs must be initiated if infection by *Mycobacterium tuberculosis* is suspected.

Complications

1. Bacterial meningitis, particularly in children, may result in deafness, learning difficulties, spasticity, paresis, or CN disorders.
2. Increased ICP in AIDS patients with cryptococcal meningitis can result in severe visual losses.
3. Seizures occur in 20% to 30% of patients.
4. Increased ICP may result in cerebral edema, decreased perfusion, and tissue damage.
5. Severe brain edema may result in herniation or compression of the brain stem.
6. Purpura may be associated with disseminated intravascular coagulation.

Nursing Assessment

1. Obtain a history of recent infections such as upper respiratory infection and exposure to causative agents. Meticulous history taking is essential and must include evaluation of exposure to ill contacts, mosquitoes, ticks, and outdoor activities in areas of endemic Lyme disease, travel history with possible exposure to tuberculosis, as well as history of medication use, IV drug use, and sexually transmitted disease risk. Another important part of history is prior antibiotic use, which may alter the clinical picture of bacterial meningitis.
2. Assess neurologic status and vital signs.
3. Evaluate for signs of meningeal irritation.
4. Assess sensorineural hearing loss (vision and hearing), CN damage (eg, facial nerve palsy), and diminished cognitive function.

Nursing Diagnoses

- Hyperthermia related to the infectious process and cerebral edema.
- Risk for Imbalanced Fluid Volume related to fever and decreased intake.
- Ineffective Tissue Perfusion (cerebral) related to infectious process and cerebral edema.
- Acute Pain related to meningeal irritation.
- Impaired Physical Mobility related to prolonged bed rest.

Nursing Interventions

Reducing Fever

1. Administer antimicrobial agents on time to maintain optimal blood levels.
2. Monitor temperature frequently or continuously and administer antipyretics, as ordered.
3. Institute other cooling measures, such as a hypothermia blanket, as indicated.

Maintaining Fluid Balance

1. Prevent IV fluid overload, which may worsen cerebral edema.
2. Monitor intake and output closely.
3. Monitor CVP frequently.

Enhancing Cerebral Perfusion

1. Assess LOC, vital signs, and neurologic parameters frequently. Observe for signs and symptoms of increased ICP (eg, decreased LOC, dilated pupils, widening pulse pressure).
2. Maintain a quiet, calm environment to prevent agitation, which may cause an increased ICP.
3. Prepare patient for a lumbar puncture for CSF evaluation and repeat spinal tap, if indicated. Evaluate patient for ICP prior to lumbar puncture.
4. Notify the health care provider of signs of deterioration: increasing temperature, decreasing LOC, seizure activity, or altered respirations.

Reducing Pain

1. Administer analgesics, as ordered; monitor for response and adverse reactions. Avoid opioids, which may mask a decrease in LOC.
2. Darken the room if photophobia is present.
3. Assist with position of comfort for neck stiffness and turn patient slowly and carefully with head and neck in alignment.
4. Elevate the head of the bed to decrease ICP and reduce pain.

Promoting Return to Optimal Level of Functioning

1. Implement rehabilitation interventions after admission (eg, turning, positioning).
2. Progress from passive to active exercises based on the patient's neurologic status.

 DRUG ALERT Note and report any missed doses of antibiotics, osmotic diuretics, and steroids; administer necessary doses as soon as possible to avert deleterious consequences due to missed doses.

Community and Home Care Considerations

1. Prevent bacterial meningitis by eliminating colonization and infection with the offending organism.
   a. Administer vaccines against *H. influenzae* type B for children; *N. meningitidis* serogroups A, C, Y, and W135 for patients at high risk (especially college students, those without spleens, those who are immunodeficient); and *S. pneumoniae* for patients with chronic illnesses and older adults.
   b. Administer vaccines for travelers to countries with a high incidence of meningococcal disease and household contacts of someone who has had meningitis.
   c. Chemoprophylaxis for meningococcal disease, most commonly with rifampin, may be necessary for health care workers, household contacts in the community, day care centers, and other highly susceptible populations.
2. If maintenance antifungal prophylaxis is initiated for patients with low CD4+ counts, as seen in some patients with AIDS, the patient must understand the importance of long-term pharmacologic therapy.

Patient Education and Health Maintenance

1. Advise close contacts of the patient with meningitis that prophylactic treatment may be indicated; they should check with their health care providers or the local public health department.
2. Encourage the patient to follow medication regimen as directed to eradicate the infectious agent completely.
3. Encourage follow-up and prompt attention to infections in future.
4. Direct the patient and family to the Centers for Disease Control and Prevention (*www.cdc.gov/meningitis/index.html*) for support and additional information.

Evaluation: Expected Outcomes

- Afebrile.
- Adequate urine output; CVP in normal range.
- Alert LOC; normal vital signs.
- Pain controlled.
- Optimal level of functioning after resolution.

Encephalitis

 Evidence Base Long, S. S. (2011). Encephalitis diagnosis and management in the real world. *Advances in Experimental Medicine and Biology, 697*, 153–173.

Encephalitis is an inflammation of cerebral tissue, typically accompanied by meningeal inflammation. Meningoencephalitis is most commonly caused by a viral infection. Like meningitis, encephalitis can be infectious or noninfectious and acute, subacute, or chronic.

Pathophysiology and Etiology

1. In primary encephalitis, the brain or spinal cord is the predominant foci of the toxin or pathogen. Secondary encephalitis is a less serious form of encephalitis; it is caused by an infection that is spread from another part of the body.

2. Acute viral encephalitis, accounting for the vast majority of cases, is caused by a direct infection of the gray matter containing neural cells. It results in perivascular inflammation and neuronal destruction. It is more common in children and is most commonly caused by the herpes simplex virus and, to a lesser degree, by the arboviruses.

3. Brain-stem encephalitis targets the basal ganglia or CNS.

4. Postischemic inflammatory encephalitis occurs due to brain inflammation following a CVA. In patients with cerebral ischemia, inflammation can result in secondary brain injury and microvascular occlusion can be caused by activated leukocytes or a microvascular thrombus. This edema can result in increased ICP and compromised cerebral perfusion.

5. West Nile virus (WNV) is an arthropod virus (arbovirus). The mosquito is the primary vector and birds are the primary hosts. Mortality can be as high as 30%.

6. *Herpes simplex encephalitis* may result from reactivation of the virus that has been dormant in the cranial and other ganglia or to reinfection. Direct spread to the brain by the olfactory or trigeminal nerve is suspected with herpes simplex virus type 1, which is responsible for almost all cases of herpes simplex encephalitis in children and adults. Mortality is as high as 75%. Herpes simplex type 2 is more common in neonates who are born to mothers with this infection during pregnancy.

7. Herpes zoster virus (varicella) is a rare cause of encephalitis.

8. Postinfectious encephalomyelitis follows a viral or bacterial infection process, but organisms do not directly affect the neural tissue in the white matter; however, perivascular inflammation and demyelination do occur in the cerebral tissue.

   a. The incidence of postinfectious encephalomyelitis has decreased considerably with immunization against measles, mumps, and rubella and due to the eradication of smallpox. It is rare in infancy.

   b. The most common cause is respiratory or GI infection 1 to 3 weeks before the acute onset of encephalomyelitis symptoms.

   c. May be caused by specific species of mosquitoes and ticks (arthropods), which may be seasonal and geographic hosts (eg, California encephalitis, St. Louis equine encephalitis).

9. *Cytomegalovirus encephalitis* should be considered in patients who have advanced HIV infection, have evidence of the cytomegalovirus in other sites, and have progressive neurologic deterioration.

10. *Toxoplasma* encephalitis is also common in patients with AIDS.

Clinical Manifestations

1. Signs and symptoms may develop hours or weeks after exposure.

2. Classic symptoms include fever, headache, and altered mental status (eg, disorientation, neurologic deficits, seizures).

3. Increased ICP may result in alteration in consciousness, nausea, and vomiting.

4. Motor weakness, such as hemiparesis, may be detected.

5. Increased deep tendon reflexes and extensor plantar response are noted.

6. Bizarre behavior and personality changes may present at onset.

7. Hypothalamic–pituitary involvement may result in hypothermia, diabetes insipidus, SIADH (see page 488).

8. Neurologic symptoms may include superior quadrant visual field defects, aphasia, dysphagia, ataxia, and paresthesias.

9. The patient with brain-stem encephalitis may present with nystagmus, decreased extraocular movements, hearing loss, dysphagia, dysarthria, respiratory abnormalities, and motor involvement.

10. Limbic encephalitis may cause mood and personality changes that progress to severe memory loss and delirium.

11. In WNV, about two-thirds of symptomatic patients have encephalitis with signs and symptoms of fever, vomiting, headache, nuchal rigidity, decreased LOC, CN dysfunction, and an erythematous rash. Seizures are uncommon.

Diagnostic Evaluation

1. Lumbar puncture, with evaluation of CSF, is performed to detect leukocytosis, increased mononuclear cell pleocytosis, increased proteins, and normal or slightly lowered glucose.

2. Polymerase chain reaction analysis of the virus' deoxyribonucleic acid (DNA) and the detection of intrathecally produced viral antibodies are essential in diagnosing the specific virus (eg, herpes simplex virus, cytomegalovirus). Arbovirus-specific immunoglobulin (Ig)M in CSF and a four-fold change in specific IgG antibody are diagnostic for arboviral encephalitis.

3. EEG may demonstrate slow brain wave complexes in encephalitis.

4. Gadolinium-enhanced MRI differentiates postinfectious encephalomyelitis from acute viral encephalitis.

   a. Enhanced multifocal white matter lesions are seen in encephalomyelitis, which may remain for months after clinical recovery.

   b. Herpes simplex virus encephalitis typically causes medial-temporal and orbital–frontal lobe inflammation and necrosis; low-density abnormalities may be present in the temporal lobes. An MRI is preferred over a CT scan.

   c. Cytomegalovirus, seen in patients who have advanced HIV disease, may have enhanced periventricular areas.

5. Brain tissue biopsy indicates presence of infectious organisms.

6. WNV can have pleocytosis and may be seen on an MRI with enhancement of the meninges and periventricular areas. The enzyme-linked immunosorbent assay, WNV ELISA, can be done from blood or CSF; a cell culture can also be diagnostic.

Management

1. Differentiate acute viral encephalitis from noninfectious diseases, such as sarcoidosis, vasculitis, systemic lupus erythematosus, and others.

2. In patients who are immunosuppressed, such as HIV-positive patients, differentiate acute viral encephalitis from cytomegalovirus encephalitis, toxoplasmic encephalitis, and fungal infections.

   a. Patients with cytomegalovirus may be treated with ganciclovir and foscarnet, commonly used to treat cytomegalovirus retinitis in HIV-positive patients.

b. Pyrimethamine and sulfadoxine are commonly used to treat *Toxoplasma* encephalitis.

c. When encephalomyelitis develops, supportive care is indicated because there is no known treatment; corticosteroids may be used.

3. IV acyclovir over 10 to 21 days is indicated for herpes simplex virus. Mothers who have genital herpes simplex may be treated with acyclovir during the third trimester to avoid shedding the virus to their babies.

4. Anticonvulsants are used to manage seizures.

 DRUG ALERT Acyclovir, indicated for acute viral encephalitis caused by herpes simplex type 1, inhibits replication of the virus DNA. Acyclovir should be infused over 1 hour because crystalluria and renal failure may result if administration is too rapid.

Complications

1. Sequelae of the herpes simplex virus may cause temporal lobe swelling, which can result in compression of the brain stem. This virus may also cause aphasia, major motor and sensory deficits, and Korsakoff's psychosis (amnestic syndrome).

2. Relapse of encephalitis may be seen after initial improvement and completion of antiviral therapy.

3. Mortality and morbidity depend on the infectious agent, host status, and other considerations.

Nursing Assessment

1. Obtain patient history of recent infection, animal exposure, tick or mosquito bite, recent travel, exposure to ill contacts.

2. Perform a complete physical assessment.

 NURSING ALERT Although most cases of viral encephalitis only require universal precautions to prevent infection, patients that present with open lesions to the skin, as occurs in herpes simplex or herpes zoster, should have contact isolation procedures implemented.

3. Before delivery, women should be questioned regarding a history of congenital herpes simplex virus and examined for evidence of this virus; a cesarean delivery should be explored with the physician.

4. Vesicular lesions or rashes on neonates should be reported immediately because these could indicate active herpes simplex type 2 infection.

Nursing Diagnoses

- Risk for Injury related to seizures and cerebral edema.
- Ineffective Cerebral Tissue Perfusion related to disease process.
- Hyperthermia related to infectious process.
- Impaired Environmental Interpretation Syndrome related to disease process.
- Risk of Infection related to transmittal.

Nursing Interventions

Preventing Injury

1. Maintain a quiet environment and provide care gently, avoiding overactivity and agitation, which may cause increased ICP.

2. Maintain seizure precautions with side rails padded, airway, and suction equipment at bedside.

3. Administer medications, as ordered; monitor response and adverse reactions.

Promoting Cerebral Perfusion

1. Monitor neurologic status closely. Observe for subtle changes, such as behavior or personality changes, weakness, or CN involvement. Notify the health care provider.

2. In arbovirus encephalitis, restrict fluids as directed to passively dehydrate the brain.

3. Reorient the patient frequently.

4. Provide supportive care if coma develops; may last several weeks.

5. Encourage significant others to interact with the patient and participate in the patient's rehabilitation, even while the patient is in a coma.

Relieving Fever

1. Monitor temperature and vital signs frequently.

2. Administer antipyretics and other cooling measures, as indicated.

3. Monitor fluid intake and output and provide fluid replacement through IV lines as needed. Be alert to signs of other coexisting infections, such as urinary tract infection or pneumonia, and notify health care provider so cultures can be obtained and treatment started.

Managing Aberrations in Thought Processes

1. Orient to person, place, time.

2. Maintain memory book and provide cues to perform required activities.

Avoiding Infectious Disease Transmission

1. Maintain strict standard precautions.

2. Initiate and maintain isolation per your facility's policy.

Community and Home Care Considerations

1. Promote vaccination of patient, family, and significant others for measles, mumps, and rubella.

2. Pregnant women who have a history of genital herpes simplex, or their partners, should inform their physician of this history.

3. Contacts of rabies-infected patients should be offered rabies prophylaxis.

4. Direct the patient and family to the Encephalitis Society (*www.encephalitis.info*) for support and additional information.

Patient Education and Health Maintenance

1. Explain the effects of the disease process and the rationale for care.

2. Reassure significant others based on patient's prognosis.

3. Encourage follow-up for evaluation of deficits and rehabilitation progress.

4. Educate others about the signs and symptoms of encephalitis if epidemic is suspected.

5. To prevent WNV, advise the use of repellants when outdoors and removal of standing water that acts as a breeding ground for mosquitoes.

Evaluation: Expected Outcomes

- No seizures or signs of increased ICP.
- Alert with no neurologic deficits.
- Afebrile.
- Oriented, memory intact.
- No transmission of infection.

Brain and Spinal Abscesses

A *brain abscess* is a free or encapsulated collection of infectious material of brain parenchyma, between the dura and the arachnoid linings (subdural abscess) or between the dura and the skull (epidural abscess). Spinal abscesses typically occur in the epidural region.

Pathophysiology and Etiology

1. Intracranial subdural abscesses, usually due to a streptococcus organism, are caused by purulent drainage between the dura and arachnoid. It can result from pus from the meninges, middle ear or mastoid, sinuses, septicemia, or skull fracture. It occurs most frequently in children and young adults.

2. Intracranial epidural abscesses, typically involving an infection of the cranium, commonly occur due to chronic mastoiditis or sinusitis, head trauma, or craniotomy. Abscesses may be related to a subdural empyema (collection of purulent drainage originating from nasal sinuses, meninges, middle ear, or skull osteomyelitis), meningitis, or intraparenchymal abscess.

3. Spinal epidural abscesses occur in the spinal canal external to the dura. Epidural penetration may seed through the blood and occur from infected adjacent tissue (eg, infected pressure ulcer), from another infected site (eg, skin), or contamination from spinal surgery or spinal instrumentation (eg, lumbar puncture). *S. aureus* is a frequent causative agent and the midthoracic vertebrae are most commonly affected.

4. Intramedullary abscesses are more common in the pediatric population, and are associated with lumbosacral dermal sinuses. Approximately 20% to 30% are "cryptic" abscesses with no apparent source of infectious seeding.

5. In the initial inoculation period, organisms invade the brain parenchyma, resulting in local inflammation and edema. The resulting cerebritis develops into a necrotic lesion and then becomes encapsulated.

6. Fungal brain abscesses are commonly seen in HIV-positive patients and other populations that are immunosuppressed. Diffuse microabscesses may occur with infections caused by *Candida* species.

7. *M. tuberculosis* may cause abscesses of pus containing acid-fast bacilli (AFB) surrounded by a dense capsule. These abscesses are also found in patients who are HIV-positive or have other immunosuppressive diseases.

Clinical Manifestations

1. Headache is poorly localized with a dull ache.

2. Increased ICP may result in nausea, vomiting, decreased LOC.

3. Fever is found in less than 50% of cases.

4. Neurologic findings, such as hemisensory and paresis deficits, aphasia, and ataxia, may be present.

5. Seizures are frequently present.

6. Dental abscess, sinusitis, and otitis media may be present.

7. Signs and symptoms of a cerebral subdural empyema include severe headache, fever, nuchal rigidity, and signs of meningeal irritation (Kernig's and Brudzinski's sign; see page 514).

8. Patients with intracranial epidural abscess commonly present with fever, lethargy, and severe headache.

9. Spinal epidural abscesses may be evidenced by severe back pain, fever, headache, lower-extremity weakness or paralysis, nuchal rigidity, Kernig's sign, and local tenderness.

Diagnostic Evaluation

1. CT scan and MRI with contrast locate the sites of abscess and follow evolution and resolution of the suppurative process.
   a. In the inflammatory stage of cerebritis, imaging reveals high signal intensity centrally (inflammation) and peripherally (edema). When an abscess develops, the capsule becomes isointense.
   b. There may be decreased ring enhancement with patients who are immunosuppressed, which may be due to a lack of inflammatory response.
   c. Microabscesses may not be detected by the CT scan or MRI.
   d. MRI with gadolinium enhancement should be considered to detect spinal epidural abscesses.

2. Blood cultures are obtained to identify the organism; positive Gram's stain, leukocytosis, and elevated erythrocyte sedimentation rate (ESR) will be found.

3. Cultures are obtained from the suspected source of infection, using stereotaxic needle aspiration or brain surgery, to identify the organism and sensitivity to antimicrobials.

4. A metastatic brain abscess may be differentiated from a metastatic tumor by CT scan or MRI. Abscesses have hypodense centers with a smooth surrounding capsule, whereas tumors may have irregular borders and diffuse enhancement.

5. EEG detects seizure disorders.

6. Findings in cerebral subdural empyema include increased WBC count and increased pressure of the CSF.

7. In intracranial epidural abscesses, CT or MRI scans are useful; MRIs are usually more sensitive. Findings from the CSF may not be definitive. To avoid transtentorial herniation, lumbar puncture is not indicated until large cranial masses are ruled out.

8. Diagnostic findings in spinal epidural abscesses may include increased WBC count and ESR. The CSF may be cloudy.

Management

1. With cerebral subdural empyema or intracranial epidural abscesses, management consists of trephining (drilling through skull to evacuate purulent material), systemic antibiotics, and treatment of cerebral edema.

2. Closed stereotaxic needle biopsy, under CT guidance, may be used for drainage evacuation instead of craniotomy.
3. Spinal epidural abscesses may be managed with a laminectomy and surgical drainage, with antibiotics before and after the procedure. The abscess site is thoroughly irrigated with antibiotic solution and aerobic and anaerobic cultures are taken.
4. Radical surgical debridement, especially with fungal infections, may be indicated with antimicrobial therapy.
5. Initiation of empiric antimicrobial therapy is based on Gram's stain and the suspected site of origin. Because brain abscesses are frequently caused by multiple organisms, antimicrobial therapy is directed toward the most common etiologic agents: streptococci, anaerobic bacteria (eg, *Bacteroides* species).
   a. *S. aureus* may be suspected if surgical procedures have been performed.
   b. Gram-negative bacteria (eg, *Clostridium* species) should be suspected if a cranial wound has been contaminated with soil.
   c. A 6- to 8-week course of parenteral antibiotics is typical, followed by a 2- to 3-month course of oral antimicrobial therapy.
   d. Penicillin G, metronidazole, and third-generation cephalosporins are common therapeutic agents.
6. Antifungal therapy, such as amphotericin B, is initiated for candidiasis and other fungal infections.
7. Antituberculosis pharmacotherapy, such as rifampin, isoniazid, and pyrazinamide, should be used to treat abscesses containing AFB.
8. Adjunctive therapy includes corticosteroids and osmotic diuretics to reduce cerebral edema and anticonvulsants to manage seizures.

 **NURSING ALERT** If a subdural drain is used to provide continuous drainage of the abscess, the patient should be placed in a supine position to prevent rapid fluid shifts into the drainage device.

Complications

1. The brain abscess can rupture into the ventricular space, causing a sudden increase in the severity of the patient's headache. This complication is often fatal.
2. Papilledema may occur in less than 25% of cases, indicating intracranial hypertension.
3. Lumbar puncture may be contraindicated if there is a spinal epidural abscess because pus may be transferred into the subarachnoid space.
4. Permanent neurologic deficits, such as seizure disorders, visual defects, hemiparesis, and CN palsies, may be present.
5. There is greater mortality if the patient has acute onset of symptoms with severe mental status changes and has rapid progression of neurologic impairment.
6. Delayed treatment of a spinal epidural abscess may result in transection syndrome, in which flaccid paraplegia with sensory loss occurs at the level of the abscess.

7. In chronic otitis media, intracranial and intratemporal complications frequently result from progressive bony erosion, which may expose the dura, labyrinth, and facial nerves.

Nursing Assessment

1. Obtain history of previous infection, immunosuppression, headache, and related symptoms.
2. Perform neurologic assessment, including CN evaluation, motor, and cognitive status.

Nursing Diagnoses

- Acute Pain related to cerebral mass.
- Impaired Environmental Interpretation Syndrome related to disease process.
- Risk for Injury related to neurologic deficits.
- Anxiety related to surgery, prognosis, and relapse.

Nursing Interventions
Relieving Pain

1. Administer pain medications, as ordered.
2. Provide comfort measures, such as quiet environment, positioning with head slightly elevated, and assistance with hygiene needs.
3. Provide passive relaxation techniques, such as soft music and back rubs.

Promoting Thought Processes

1. Frequently monitor vital signs, LOC, orientation, and seizure activity.
2. Report changes, which can signal increased ICP, to health care provider.
3. Administer medications, as ordered, noting response and adverse reactions.
4. Prepare patient for repeated diagnostic tests to evaluate response to therapy and surgery.

Minimizing Neurologic Deficits

1. Maintain a safe environment with side rails up, call light within reach, and frequent observation.
2. Evaluate other CN function and report changes.
3. Refer to occupational therapist, speech therapist, or other rehabilitation specialist to provide adjunct to nursing rehabilitation.

Reducing Anxiety

1. Prepare patient and family for surgery when indicated. Encourage discussion with surgeon to understand risks and benefits of the procedure.
2. Explain postoperative progression and nursing care (see page 493).

Community and Home Care Considerations

1. Patient follow-up is essential for sinusitis, otitis media, respiratory infections, and other infectious processes that may result in a brain abscess.
2. Continue with rehabilitation to regain or compensate for neurologic deficits.
3. Continue with pharmacologic regimen in community setting.
4. Observe for recurrence of brain and spinal abscesses.

Patient Education and Health Maintenance

1. Maintain wellness with vaccinations, immunizations, and overall health.
2. Reinforce need for dental procedure prophylaxis to avoid dental abscesses.
3. Instruct on need for immediate assessment of head wounds.

Evaluation: Expected Outcomes

- Verbalizes reduced pain.
- Oriented to person, place, and time; follows simple commands.
- No injury related to neurologic deficits.
- Reduced anxiety regarding disease process and procedures.

DEGENERATIVE DISORDERS
Parkinson's Disease

 Evidence Base Jankovic, J., & Poewe, W. (2012). *Therapies in Parkinson's disease. Current Opinion in Neurology, 25,* 433–447.

Parkinson's disease is a chronic, progressive neurologic disease affecting the brain centers responsible for control and regulation of movement. It is characterized by tremor, bradykinesia, rigidity, and postural abnormalities. Parkinson's can complicate the diagnosis, clinical course, and recovery from other illness. Approximately 1% of the total U.S. population older than age 60 is affected by idiopathic Parkinson's disease, and it less commonly affects people of younger ages. It is the second most common neurodegenerative disease.

Pathophysiology and Etiology

1. A deficiency of dopamine, due to degenerative changes in the substantia nigra of the brain, is thought to be responsible for the symptoms of Parkinson's disease.
2. Underlying etiology may be related to a virus; genetic susceptibility; toxicity from pesticides, herbicides, methyl-phenyl-tetrahydropyridine, or welding fumes; repeated head injuries; or other unknown cause.
3. The clinical diagnosis of Parkinson's disease may be difficult because older patients may have other causes of rigidity, bradykinesia, and tremor.

Clinical Manifestations

1. Bradykinesia (slowness of movement), loss of spontaneous movement, and delay in initiating movements.
2. Resting ("pill-rolling") tremor of 4 to 5 Hz. The tremor may be worse on one side of the body, affecting the limbs and sometimes involving the head, neck, face, and jaw.
3. Rigidity in performance of all movements. Rigidity is always present but increases during movement. May lead to sensations of pain, especially in the arms and shoulders.
4. Poor balance when moving abruptly or suddenly changing body position. May lead to falls.
5. Autonomic disorders—sleeplessness, salivation, sweating, orthostatic hypotension, dizziness.

6. Depression, dementia.
7. Mask-like facies secondary to rigidity.
8. Gait difficulties characterized by a decreased or nonexistent arm swing; short, shuffling steps (festination); difficulty in negotiating turns; and sudden freezing spells (inability to take the next step).
9. Verbal fluency may be impaired.
10. Finger-tapping responses are slowed.
11. Micrographia (change in handwriting, with the script becoming smaller).
12. Problems with speech, breathing, swallowing, and sexual function.

Diagnostic Evaluation

1. Observation of clinical symptoms; may perform imaging studies to rule out other disorders.
2. Physical examination of upper-extremity elbow flexion/extension reveals rigidity on extension.
3. Sensorimotor assessment of grip reveals abnormally high grip forces and longer than normal to complete object lift, particularly with lighter loads.
4. Favorable response to a single dose of levodopa or apomorphine helps confirm the diagnosis.

Management
Pharmacologic

1. Anticholinergics, including trihexyphenidyl, benztropine, and procyclidine, to reduce transmission of cholinergic pathways, which are thought to be overactive when dopamine is deficient. These medications are most effective in controlling tremor, but are known to cause confusion and hallucinations.
2. Amantadine, originally an antiflu medication, blocks the reuptake of dopamine or increases the release of dopamine by neurons in the brain, thereby increasing the supply of dopamine in the synapses. Widely used as an early monotherapy, its effect may be augmented by drug-free days.
3. Levodopa, a dopamine precursor, combined with carbidopa, a decarboxylase inhibitor, to inhibit destruction of L-dopa in the bloodstream, making more available to the brain.

 DRUG ALERT History of melanoma and angle-closure glaucoma are contraindications to levodopa therapy; patients should have suspicious skin lesions removed before initiating therapy.

4. The combination of levodopa–carbidopa is usually used. The addition of carbidopa prevents levodopa from being metabolized in the gut, liver, and other tissues and allows more to get to the brain. Therefore, a smaller dose of levodopa is required to treat symptoms and the unpleasant adverse effects are greatly reduced.
5. Bromocriptine, pramipexole, and ropinirole are dopaminergic agonists that activate dopamine receptors in the brain. Can be taken alone or in combination with levodopa–carbidopa.

6. Use of the monoamine oxidase inhibitor selegiline or deprenyl boosts the effect of levodopa–carbidopa when levodopa becomes less effective.

7. Tolcapone and entacapone are in a new drug class (catechol-O-methyltransferase inhibitors) for adjunct treatment. They prolong the duration of symptom relief by blocking the action of an enzyme that breaks down levodopa before it reaches the brain. Must be taken with levodopa.

 GERONTOLOGIC ALERT Older patients may have reduced tolerance to anti-Parkinson's drugs and may require smaller doses. Watch for and report psychiatric reactions, such as anxiety, confusion, and hallucinations; cardiac effects, such as dizziness, orthostatic hypotension, and pulse irregularity; and blepharospasm (twitching of the eyelid), an early sign of toxicity. Other adverse effects may include dry mouth, nausea, drowsiness, and insomnia.

Surgery

1. New surgical treatments for Parkinson's disease and essential tremor are promising.

2. Medial pallidotomy (electrode destroys cells in the globus pallidus) often improves long-standing symptoms, such as dyskinesia, akinesia, rigidity, and tremor, and for patients who have developed dyskinetic movements in reaction to their medications.

3. Deep brain stimulation of the thalamus decreases tremor and uncontrollable movements unresponsive to medication. Electrodes are implanted in the thalamus or globus pallidus and connected to a pacemaker-like device, which the patient can switch on or off as symptoms dictate.

4. Brain tissue transplants are still in the experimental stages but have produced encouraging results using stem cells and genetically engineered animal cells that can be made to produce dopamine.

Complications

1. Dementia.
2. Aspiration.
3. Injury from falls.

Nursing Assessment

1. Obtain history of symptoms and their effect on functioning. Mobility, feeding, communication, and self-care difficulties will have many nursing implications (see Figure 15-6).
2. Assess CNs, cerebellar function (coordination), motor function.
3. Observe gait and performance of activities.
4. Assess speech for clarity and pace.
5. Assess for signs of depression.
6. Assess family dynamics, support systems, and access to social services.

Nursing Diagnoses

- Impaired Physical Mobility related to bradykinesia, rigidity, and tremor.
- Imbalanced Nutrition: Less Than Body Requirements related to motor difficulties with feeding, chewing, and swallowing.
- Impaired Verbal Communication related to decreased speech volume and facial muscle involvement.

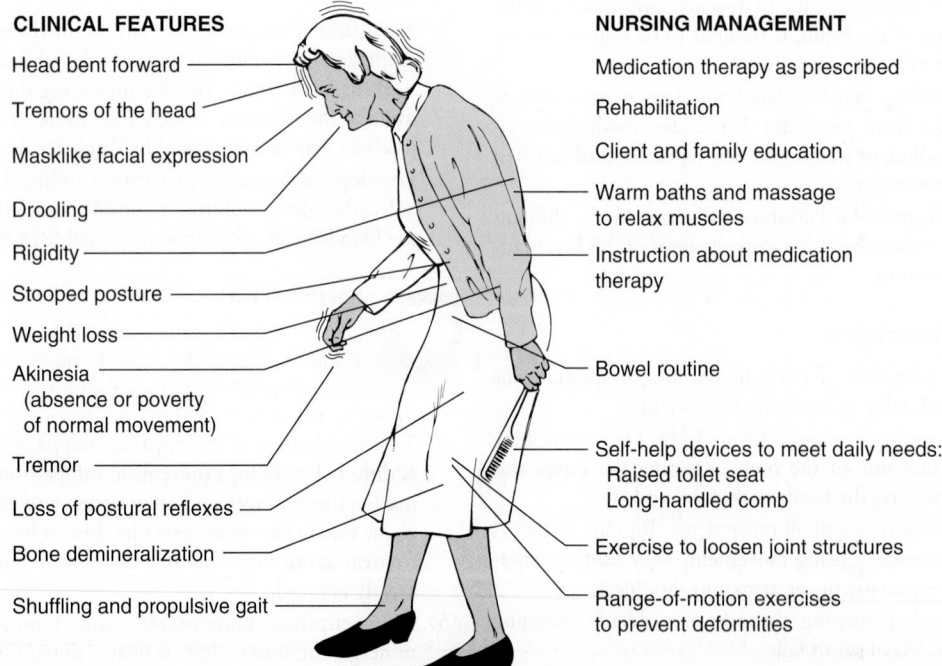

CLINICAL FEATURES

- Head bent forward
- Tremors of the head
- Masklike facial expression
- Drooling
- Rigidity
- Stooped posture
- Weight loss
- Akinesia (absence or poverty of normal movement)
- Tremor
- Loss of postural reflexes
- Bone demineralization
- Shuffling and propulsive gait

NURSING MANAGEMENT

- Medication therapy as prescribed
- Rehabilitation
- Client and family education
- Warm baths and massage to relax muscles
- Instruction about medication therapy
- Bowel routine
- Self-help devices to meet daily needs: Raised toilet seat Long-handled comb
- Exercise to loosen joint structures
- Range-of-motion exercises to prevent deformities

Figure 15-6. Appearance of female with Parkinson's disease.

- Constipation related to diminished motor function, inactivity, and medications.
- Ineffective Coping related to physical limitations and loss of independence.

Nursing Interventions

Improving Mobility

1. Encourage the patient to participate in daily exercise, such as walking, riding a stationary bike, swimming, or gardening.
2. Advise the patient to do stretching and postural exercises as outlined by a physical therapist.
3. Encourage the patient to take warm baths and receive massages to help relax muscles.
4. Instruct the patient to take frequent rest periods to overcome fatigue and frustration.
5. Teach postural exercises and walking techniques to offset shuffling gait and tendency to lean forward.
   a. Instruct the patient to use a broad-based gait.
   b. Have the patient make a conscious effort to swing arms, raise the feet while walking, use a heel-toe gait, and increase the width of stride.
   c. Tell the patient to practice walking to marching music or sound of ticking metronome to provide sensory reinforcement.

Optimizing Nutritional Status

1. Teach the patient to think through the sequence of swallowing—close lips with teeth together; lift tongue up with food on it; then move tongue back and swallow while tilting head forward.
2. Instruct the patient to chew deliberately and slowly, using both sides of mouth.
3. Tell the patient to make conscious effort to control accumulation of saliva by holding head upright and swallowing periodically.
4. Have the patient use secure, stabilized dishes and eating utensils.
5. Suggest smaller meals and additional snacks.
6. Monitor weight.

Maximizing Communication Ability

1. Encourage compliance with medication regimen.
2. Suggest referral to speech therapist.
3. Teach the patient facial exercises and breathing methods to obtain appropriate pronunciation, volume, and intonation.
   a. Take a deep breath before speaking to increase the volume of sound and number of words spoken with each breath.
   b. Exaggerate pronunciation and speak in short sentences; read aloud in front of a mirror or into a tape recorder to monitor progress.
   c. Exercise facial muscles by smiling, frowning, grimacing, and puckering.

Preventing Constipation

1. Encourage foods with moderate fiber content—whole grains, fruits, and vegetables.
2. Increase water intake.
3. Obtain a raised toilet seat to encourage normal position.

4. Encourage the patient to follow regular bowel regimen.

Strengthening Coping Ability

1. Help the patient establish realistic goals and outline ways to achieve goals.
2. Provide emotional support and encouragement.
3. Encourage use of all resources, such as therapists, primary care provider, social worker, and social support network.
4. Encourage open communication, discussion of feelings, and exchange of information about Parkinson's disease.
5. Have the patient take an active role in activity planning and evaluation of treatment plan.
6. Observe for changes in depression to determine if the patient is responding to antidepressants.

Community and Home Care Considerations

1. Recommend interdisciplinary home health care program. Requires skilled assessment of needs of patient, professional nursing and therapeutic services, patient and family education, and case management to optimize patient outcomes.
2. Encourage use of soothing music to reduce pain and depression.
3. Assess safety in environment to reduce risk of falls.
4. Utilize physical therapy services to encourage safe ambulation and reduce fear of falls.
5. Encourage use of social services, respite care and health visitors, mental health counselors, and support groups to prevent caregiver strain.
6. Use occupational therapy aids to ensure mobility and safety, such as grab rails in the tub or shower, raised toilet seat, hand rails on both sides of the stairway, rope secured to foot of bed to achieve sitting position, and straight-backed wooden chairs with armrests.

 NURSING ALERT Bowel and bladder management is an extremely important factor in the decision to keep the patient at home. Techniques to reduce incontinence episodes, such as having frequently scheduled toileting time, and handle episodes of incontinence, such as having cleaning supplies and a change of clothes/briefs in the bathroom, should be taught to decrease caregiver burden.

Patient Education and Health Maintenance

1. Instruct the patient to avoid sedatives, unless specifically prescribed, which have additive effect with other medications.
2. Instruct the patient in medication regimen, signs of toxicity, and adverse reactions, such as orthostatic hypotension, dry mouth, dystonia, muscle twitching, urine retention, impaired glucose tolerance, anemia, and elevated liver function tests.
3. Encourage follow-up and monitoring for diabetes, glaucoma, hepatotoxicity, and anemia while undergoing drug therapy. Increasing episodes of freezing should be reported.

4. Teach the patient ambulation cues to avoid "freezing" in place and possibly avoid falls by doing one of the following:
   a. Raise head, raise toes, then rock from one foot to another while bending knees slightly.
   b. Raise arms in a sudden short motion.
   c. Take a small step backward, then start forward.
   d. Step sideways, then start forward.
5. Instruct the family not to pull patient during episodes of "freezing," which increases the problem and may cause falling.
6. Refer the patient/family for more information and support to such agencies as National Parkinson's Foundation (*www.parkinson.org*) and National Institute of Neurologic Disorders and Stroke (*www.ninds.nih.gov*).

Evaluation: Expected Outcomes

- Attends physical therapy sessions, does facial exercises 10 minutes twice per day.
- Eats three small meals and two snacks, no weight loss.
- Enunciation clear, speaking in four to five words per breath.
- Passes soft stool every day.
- Asks questions about Parkinson's, obtains help from family and/or friends.

Multiple Sclerosis

 Evidence Base American Association of Neuroscience Nurses, the Association of Rehabilitation Nurses, & the International Organization of Multiple Sclerosis Nurses. (2011). *Nursing management of the patient with multiple sclerosis.* Glenview, IL: Author.

Multiple sclerosis (MS) is a chronic, frequently progressive neurologic disease of the CNS of unknown etiology and uncertain trajectory. MS is characterized by the occurrence of small patches of demyelination of the white matter of the optic nerve, brain, and spinal cord. MS is distinguished by exacerbations and remissions of symptoms over the course of the illness. MS is the most common CNS disease among young adults and the third leading cause of disability in the United States. It is estimated that 400,000 Americans have this disorder of the brain and spinal cord, causing disruption of electrical messages from the brain to the peripheral nervous system.

Pathophysiology and Etiology

1. *Demyelination* refers to the destruction of the myelin, the fatty and protein material that covers certain nerve fibers in the brain and spinal cord (see Figure 15-7).
2. Demyelination results in disordered transmission of nerve impulses.
3. Inflammatory changes lead to scarring of the affected nerve fibers.
4. Cause is unknown but may possibly be related to autoimmune dysfunction, genetic susceptibility, or an infectious process.
5. More prevalent in the northern latitudes and among whites.

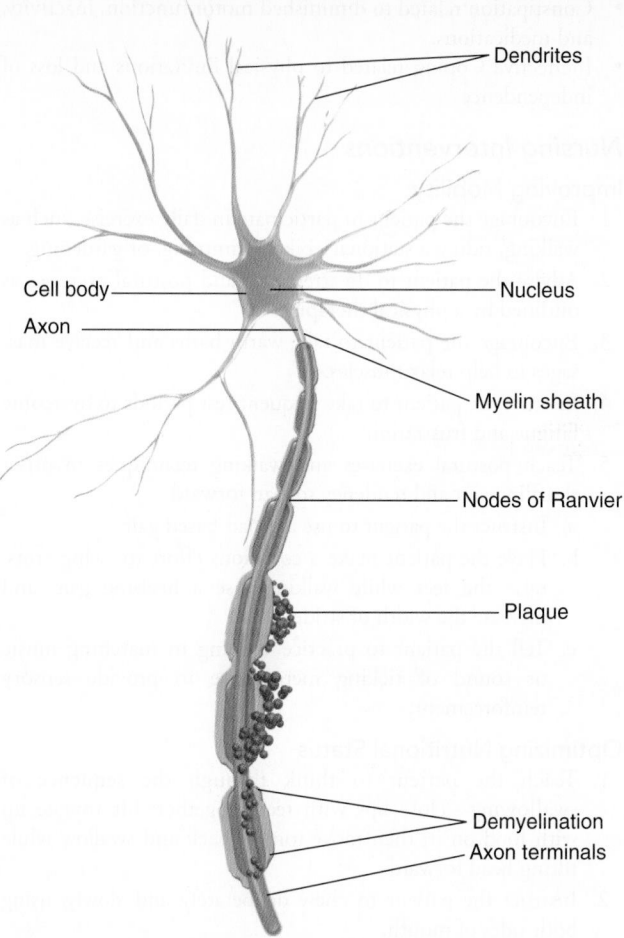

Figure 15-7. Myelin destruction of the nerve cell axon in multiple sclerosis.

Classification

The National Multiple Sclerosis Advisory Committee recognizes four clinical forms of MS:

1. Relapsing remitting (RR)—clearly defined acute attacks evolve over days to weeks. Partial recovery of function occurs over weeks to months. Average frequency of attacks is once every 2 years and neurologic stability remains between attacks without disease progression. (At the time of onset, 90% of cases of MS are diagnosed as RR.)
2. Secondary progressive (SP)—always begins as RR but clinical course changes with increasing relapse rate, with a steady deterioration in neurologic function unrelated to the original attack. (Fifty percent of those with RR will progress to SP within 10 years; 90% will progress within 25 years.)
3. Primary progressive (PP)—characterized by steady progression of disability from onset without exacerbations and remissions. More prevalent among males and older individuals. Worst prognosis for neurologic disability. (Ten percent of cases of MS are diagnosed as PP.)
4. Progressive relapsing (PR)—the same as PP except that patients experience acute exacerbations along with a steadily progressive course (rarest form).

Clinical Manifestations

Lesions can occur anywhere within the white matter of the CNS. Symptoms reflect the location of the area of demyelination.

1. Fatigue and weakness.
2. Abnormal reflexes—absent or exaggerated.
3. Vision disturbances—impaired and double vision, nystagmus.
4. Motor dysfunction—weakness, tremor, incoordination.
5. Sensory disturbances—paresthesias, impaired deep sensation, impaired vibratory and position sense.
6. Impaired speech—slurring, scanning (dysarthria).
7. Urinary dysfunction—hesitancy, frequency, urgency, retention, incontinence; upper UTI. Urinary dysfunction affects about 90% of patients with MS and may exacerbate relapse of MS.
8. Neurobehavioral syndromes—depression, cognitive impairment, emotional lability.
9. Symptoms of MS are often unpredictable, varying from person to person and from time to time in the same person.

Diagnostic Evaluation

1. Establishing a definitive diagnosis is often difficult, with much uncertainty concerning prognosis once the diagnosis is made.
2. Serial brain MRI studies have proved to be useful for diagnosing and monitoring patients with MS—show small plaques scattered throughout white matter of CNS.
3. Magnetic resonance spectroscopy is now being studied to monitor specific pathophysiology of evolving MS plaques.
4. Electrophoresis study of CSF shows abnormal IgG antibody.
5. Visual, auditory, and somatosensory evoked potentials—slowed conduction is evidence of demyelination.

Management

MS treatment is dynamic and rapidly evolving, covering two main areas: direct treatment of MS and treatment of the effects or symptoms resulting from MS. Treatment is aimed at relieving symptoms and helping the patient function. However, a therapeutic relationship between the patient and nurse creates a critical and strong bond that is essential across the long trajectory of the illness.

Current Disease-Modifying Drugs

1. Corticosteroids or adrenocorticotropic hormone are used to decrease inflammation and shorten duration of relapse or exacerbation.
2. Immunosuppressive agents may stabilize the course.
3. Interferon beta-1a and interferon beta-1b are being used for treatment of rapidly progressing symptoms in some patients.
4. Glatiramer acetate, fingolimod, and natalizumab are immunomodulators used in RR disease.
5. Mitoxantrone, a chemotherapeutic agent used for the treatment of SP (chronic), PR, or worsening RR MS not responding to other disease-modifying drugs.

Treating Exacerbations

1. A true exacerbation of MS is caused by an area of inflammation in the CNS.
2. The treatment most commonly used to control exacerbations is IV, high-dose corticosteroids. Methylprednisolone is one of the most commonly used corticosteroids in MS.
3. Plasmapheresis (plasma exchange) is only considered for the 10% who do not respond well to standard corticosteroid treatment.

Chronic Symptom Management

1. Treatment of spasticity with such agents as baclofen, dantrolene, diazepam; physical therapy; nerve blocks and surgical intervention.
2. Control of fatigue with amantadine and lifestyle changes.
3. Treatment of depression with antidepressant drugs and counseling.
4. Bladder management with anticholinergics, intermittent catheterization for drainage, prophylactic antibiotics.
5. Bowel management with stool softeners, bulk laxative, suppositories.
6. Multidisciplinary rehabilitation management with physical therapy, occupational therapy, speech therapy, cognitive therapy, vocational rehabilitation, and complementary and alternative medicine, as indicated, to restore or maintain functions essential to daily living in individuals who have lost these capacities through the disease process.
7. Control of dystonia with carbamazepine.
8. Management of pain syndromes with carbamazepine, phenytoin, perphenazine/amitriptyline, and nonpharmacologic modalities.

Complications

1. Dysphagia and respiratory dysfunction.
2. Infections: bladder, respiratory, sepsis.
3. Complications from immobility.
4. Speech, voice, and language disorders such as dysarthria.

Nursing Assessment

1. Observe motor strength, coordination, and gait.
2. Perform CN assessment.
3. Evaluate elimination function.
4. Explore coping, effect on activity and sexual function, emotional adjustment.
5. Assess patient and family coping, support systems, available resources.
6. Assess for anxiety, depression, sleep disturbances, cognitive impairment, and pain, which commonly occur in patients with MS.

Nursing Diagnoses

- Impaired Physical Mobility related to muscle weakness, spasticity, and incoordination.
- Fatigue related to disease process and stress of coping.
- Risk for Injury related to motor and sensory deficits.
- Risk for Aspiration related to dysphagia.
- Impaired Urinary Elimination related to the disease process.

- Interrupted Family Processes related to inability to fulfill expected roles.
- Sexual Dysfunction related to disease process.

Nursing Interventions

Promoting Motor Function

1. Perform muscle-stretching and -strengthening exercises daily, or teach patient or family to perform, using a stretch–hold–relax routine to minimize spasticity and prevent contractures.
2. Apply ice packs before stretching to reduce spasticity.
3. Tell patient to avoid muscle fatigue by stopping activity just short of fatigue and to take frequent rest periods.
4. Encourage walking and activity and teach patient how to use such devices as braces, canes, and walkers, when necessary.
5. Inform the patient to avoid sudden changes in position, which may cause falls due to loss of position sense, and to walk with a wide-based gait.
6. Encourage frequent change in position while immobilized to prevent contractures; sleeping prone will minimize flexor spasm of hips and knees.

Minimizing Fatigue

1. Help patient and family understand that fatigue is an integral part of MS.
2. Plan ahead and prioritize activities. Take brief rest periods throughout the day.
3. Avoid overheating, overexertion, and infection.
4. Encourage energy-conservation techniques, such as sitting to perform activity, limiting trips up and down stairs, pulling, or pushing rather than lifting.
5. Help patient develop healthy lifestyle with balanced diet, rest, exercise, and relaxation.

Preventing Injury

1. Suggest use of an eye patch or frosted lens (alternate eyes) for patients with double vision.
2. Encourage regular ophthalmologic consultation to maximize vision and be aware of potential for hearing changes and assess as needed.
3. Provide a safe environment for patient with any sensory alteration.
   a. Orient patient to the environment and keep arrangement of furniture and personal articles constant.
   b. Make sure floor is free from obstacles, loose rugs, or slippery areas.
   c. Teach the use of all senses to maintain awareness of environment.

Managing Dysphagia

1. Initiate referrals to speech/language pathologist and dietician for evaluation and treatment of swallowing problems.
2. Ensure that patient is alert and distractions are minimized at mealtimes: provide supervision, as indicated.
3. Use safe swallowing practices, including proper positioning, double swallow, and chin tuck.
4. Monitor patient for signs and symptoms of choking or aspiration; use suctioning as indicated.
5. Educate and counsel patients and care partners about feeding options as disease progresses.

Maintaining Urinary Elimination

1. Ensure adequate fluid intake to help prevent infection and stone formation.
2. Assess for urine retention and catheterize for residual urine, as indicated.
3. Teach patient to report signs of UTI immediately.
4. Set up bladder training program to reduce incontinence.
   a. Encourage fluids every 2 hours.
   b. Follow regular schedule of voiding, every 1 to 2 hours, lengthening as tolerated.
   c. Restrict fluid volume and salty foods 1 to 2 hours before bedtime.
5. See pages 182 to 183 for more information on urine retention and incontinence.

Normalizing Family Processes

1. Encourage verbalization of feelings of each family member.
2. Encourage counseling and use of church or community resources.
3. Suggest dividing up household duties and childcare responsibilities to prevent strain on one person.
4. Explore adaptation of some roles so patient can still function in family unit.
5. Expand treatment efforts to include the whole family.
6. Support mothers with MS who often face fatigue and episodic exacerbations during their childrearing years.

Promoting Sexual Function

1. Encourage open communication between partners.
2. Discuss birth control options, if appropriate.
3. Suggest sexual activity when patient is most rested.
4. Suggest consultation with sexual therapist to help obtain greater sexual satisfaction.

Community and Home Care Considerations

1. The nurse case manager functions as care provider, facilitator, advocate, educator, counselor, and innovator aimed at intervening in a wide variety of settings to improve patient function and mobility.
2. Teach the patient receiving interferon beta-1a and interferon beta-1b to expect adverse effects of flu-like symptoms, fever, asthenia, chills, myalgias, sweating, and local reaction at the injection site. Liver function test elevation and neutropenia may also occur. Adverse effects may persist for up to 6 months of treatment before subsiding.
3. Instruct the patient receiving interferon beta-1a and interferon beta-1b in self-injection technique.

 DRUG ALERT Ensure rotation of subcutaneous injection site of disease-modifying drugs to prevent skin reactions. Avoid injections into an area of skin that is sore, reddened, infected, or damaged. Injection sites include the inner thigh, outer surface of the upper arm, stomach, or buttocks. If the patient is thin, thigh and arm sites are preferred. Use a diagram or log of the date and site location for each injection.

4. Teach the patient and family to use their own judgment, knowledge, and ingenuity to control MS symptoms.

5. Teach the patient and family how to conduct periodic self-assessment of daily functioning so that home care team can continue to make modifications in treatment plan.

Patient Education and Health Maintenance

1. Encourage the patient to maintain previous activities, although at a lowered level of intensity, and reinforce appropriate and safe use of adaptive equipment and aides.

2. Teach the patient to respect fatigue and avoid physical overexertion and emotional stress; remind patient that activity tolerance may vary from day to day.

3. Advise the patient to avoid exposure to heat and cold or infectious agents.

4. Encourage a nutritious diet that is high in fiber to promote health and good bowel elimination.

5. Advise the patient that some medications may accentuate weakness, such as some antibiotics, muscle relaxants, anti-arrhythmics and antihypertensives, antipsychotics, oral contraceptives, and antihistamines; check with health care provider or pharmacist before taking any new medications.

8. Try to include children in the education of MS and the relationship of fatigue and functional status.

9. Refer the patient/family for more information and support to such agencies as the National Multiple Sclerosis Society (*www.nmss.org*).

Evaluation: Expected Outcomes

- Performs exercises correctly without spasm.
- Rests at intervals, tolerates activity well.
- Moves about in environment without injury.
- No episodes of aspiration.
- Voids every 2 hours with no incontinent episodes.
- Family sharing care, discussing feelings.
- Reports satisfaction with sexual activity.

Amyotrophic Lateral Sclerosis

 Evidence Base Clark, K., & Levine, T. (2011). Clinical recognition and management of amyotrophic lateral sclerosis: The nurse's role. *Journal of Neuroscience Nursing, 43*, 205–214.

Blackhall, L. J. (2012). Amyotrophic lateral sclerosis and palliative care: Where we are, and the road ahead. *Muscle & Nerve, 45*, 311–318.

Amyotrophic lateral sclerosis (ALS), also known as Lou Gehrig disease, is an incapacitating, fatal neuromuscular disease that affects as many as 20,000 Americans, with 5,000 new cases occurring in the United States each year. ALS results in progressive muscle weakness and progressive wasting and paralysis of the muscles. It is accompanied by other lower motor neuron signs, such as atrophy or fasciculations. Approximately 80% of cases begin between ages 40 and 70. The life expectancy of an ALS patient averages 2 to 5 years.

Pathophysiology and Etiology

1. Degeneration of upper motor neurons (nerves leading from the brain to medulla or spinal cord) and lower motor neurons (nerves leading from the spinal cord to the muscles of the body).

2. Results in progressive loss of voluntary muscle contraction and functional capacity, involving the legs, feet, arms, and hands, and those that control swallowing and breathing. Patients develop variable hyperreflexia, clonus, spasticity, extensor plantar responses, and limb or tongue fasciculations. Extraocular muscles and bladder and anal sphincter muscles typically are spared. ALS rarely affects cognitive functions.

3. Cause is unknown. Usually affects men in the fifth or sixth decade of life.

4. Nearly 10% of ALS cases are familial; the disease is transmitted in an autosomal dominant fashion. The copper/zinc SOD1 gene is mutated in 10% to 20% of these familial cases. Although the primary mechanism of SOD1-mediated neural injury is currently unknown, apoptosis, excitotoxicity, and oxidative stress are thought to play major roles in pathogenesis. Sporadic ALS shares clinical features with familial ALS. However, no SOD1 mutations or polymorphisms have been identified in these patients. Common pathways of disease pathogenesis may play a role, with different molecular abnormalities that lead to similar phenotypes.

5. Several studies have shown an inflammatory component to the affected spinal cord regions, with the presence of activated microglia, reactive astrocytes, and IgG deposition. Whether this reaction precedes or accompanies the molecular events that promote neuronal cell death is unknown.

Clinical Manifestations

1. Progressive weakness and wasting of muscles of arms, trunk, and legs.

2. Fasciculations and signs of spasticity.

3. Progressive difficulty swallowing (sialorrhea [drooling], regurgitation of liquids through nose), speaking (nasal and unintelligible), and, ultimately, breathing.

4. CN deficits (bulbar symptoms) are present in 20% of cases (prevalence increases with age), along with dysarthria, voice deterioration, and dysphagia. (Patients with bulbar presentation have poorer prognosis; these symptoms also have a profound impact on quality of life due to nutritional risk factors, aspiration, and respiratory complications.)

Diagnostic Evaluation

1. Electromyography to evaluate denervation and muscle atrophy.

2. Nerve conduction study to evaluate nerve pathways.

3. Pulmonary function tests to evaluate respiratory function.

4. Barium swallow to evaluate ability to achieve various phases of swallowing mechanisms.

5. MRI, CT to rule out other disorders.

6. Laboratory tests: creatine kinase, heavy metal screen, thyroid function tests, CSF evaluation to rule out other causes of muscle weakness.

Management

1. There is no cure for ALS; nor is there a proven therapy that will prevent or reverse the course of the disorder.
2. Riluzole has been shown to prolong the survival of ALS patients, but its effects are limited.
3. Most treatment is palliative and symptomatic.
4. Botulinum toxin B injections into the parotid and submandibular glands, amitriptyline therapy, or low-dose radiation therapy to the salivary glands may be used to treat drooling.
5. There is insufficient data to support or refute any specific intervention for the treatment of cramps, spasticity, depression, anxiety, insomnia, pain, dyspnea, or cognitive/behavioral impairments in ALS.
6. Neuropsychological screening may be conducted to assess for cognitive and behavioral impairments.
7. Feeding gastrostomy.
8. Tracheostomy and mechanical ventilation eventually become necessary and should be discussed prior to need in order to ascertain the patient's wishes regarding these measures.

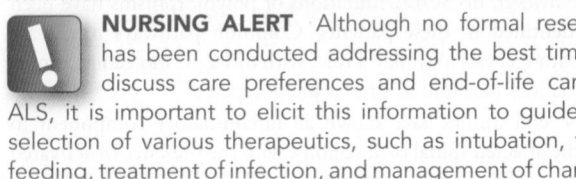

NURSING ALERT Although no formal research has been conducted addressing the best time to discuss care preferences and end-of-life care in ALS, it is important to elicit this information to guide the selection of various therapeutics, such as intubation, tube feeding, treatment of infection, and management of changes in LOC. Having the family or significant other present when these discussions occur can help to alleviate miscommunication or disagreements in the plan of care.

Complications

1. Respiratory failure.
2. Aspiration pneumonia.
3. Cardiopulmonary arrest.
4. Locked-in syndrome—fully conscious but unable to respond in any way.

Nursing Assessment

1. Evaluate respiratory function: rate, depth, tidal volume.
2. Perform CN assessment, particularly gag reflex and swallowing.
3. Assess voluntary motor function and strength.

Nursing Diagnoses

- Ineffective Breathing Pattern related to respiratory muscle weakness.
- Impaired Physical Mobility related to disease process.
- Imbalanced Nutrition: Less Than Body Requirements related to inability to swallow.
- Fatigue related to denervation of muscles.
- Social Isolation related to fatigability and decreased communication skills.
- Risk for Infection related to inability to clear airway.

Nursing Interventions

Maintaining Respiration

1. Monitor vital capacity frequently. Document pattern and report any decrease below patient's baseline.
2. Position patient upright, suction upper airway, and perform chest physical therapy to enhance respiratory function.
3. Encourage use of incentive spirometer to exercise respiratory muscles.
4. Assess for signs of hypoxia, such as tachypnea, hypopnea, restlessness, poor sleep, and excessive fatigue.
5. Obtain ABG values as ordered.
6. Establish the wishes of the patient in terms of life-support measures; obtain copy of advance directive for chart, if applicable.
7. Assist with intubation, tracheostomy, and mechanical ventilation when indicated (see Chapter 10).
8. Provide suctioning and routine care of a patient with artificial airway and mechanical ventilation.

Optimizing Mobility

1. Encourage the patient to continue usual activities as long as possible but modify exertion to avoid fatigue.
2. Encourage physical therapy exercises to strengthen unaffected muscles and perform ROM exercises to prevent contractures.
3. Encourage energy-conservation techniques.
4. Obtain assistive devices, as needed, to help patient maintain independence, such as special feeding devices, remote controls, and a motorized wheelchair.

Meeting Nutritional Requirements

1. Provide high-calorie, small, frequent feedings.
2. Provide meals that are of a texture the patient can handle; semisolid food is usually easiest to swallow.
   a. Avoid easily aspirated, pureed, and mucus-producing foods (eg, milk).
   b. Try warm or cold foods that stimulate temperature receptors in mouth and may help in swallowing.
   c. Do not wash down solids with fluids—may cause choking and aspiration.
3. Allow the patient to make his or her own food selection.
4. Provide assistive devices for self-feeding when possible.
5. Make mealtimes a pleasant experience in a bright room, with quiet company so the patient may concentrate on eating and avoid undue embarrassment.
6. Examine oral cavity for food debris before and after meals, and assess swallowing function and buildup of saliva.
7. Encourage rest periods before meals to alleviate muscle fatigue.
8. Place the patient upright for meals with neck flexed to partially protect the airway.
9. Instruct the patient to take a breath before swallowing, hold breath to swallow, exhale or cough after swallow, and swallow again.
10. Tell the patient to avoid talking while eating.
11. Prepare the patient for gastrostomy or other alternate feeding methods when appropriate.

Minimizing Fatigue

1. Encourage activity alternating with frequent naps.
2. Encourage the patient to accomplish most important activities early in day.
3. Consult with occupational therapist about energy-conservation techniques in performing ADL.

Maintaining Social Interaction

1. Use mechanical speech aids or communication board.
2. Use an environmental control board.
3. Eye movements/blinks may be the last voluntary movement; develop a code system to serve as a communication method.
4. Because standard call lights cannot be activated by the severely debilitated ALS patient, provide adaptive call light (environmental control unit) and/or some type of constant monitoring and surveillance to meet patient's needs.
5. Allow the patient to select which social activities are meaningful.
6. Refer to counselor or psychologist for coping with communication barriers and inevitability of losses.

Preventing Aspiration and Infection

1. Consult with a speech therapist for techniques and devices to assist swallowing.
2. Discourage bed rest to prevent pulmonary stasis.
3. Perform chest physiotherapy, as tolerated.
4. Monitor for fever and tachycardia and obtain sputum, urine, and other cultures, as indicated.

Community and Home Care Considerations

1. Teach caregivers how to perform suctioning, tracheostomy care, and ventilator care in the home, as indicated. Clean technique will be used rather than sterile.
2. Teach caregivers how to perform gastrostomy feedings and care of tube.
3. Assess for adequate supplies for care and ability of caregivers to carry out procedures.
4. Encourage cleanliness in home environment and avoidance of contact with anyone with respiratory infection. Give influenza and pneumonia vaccines, as indicated.

Patient Education and Health Maintenance

1. Stress the importance of maintaining physical exercise.
2. Review with the patient and family proper eating mechanics to avoid fatigue and aspiration.
3. Inform the patient of right to make decisions early in the disease process regarding an Advance Directive.
4. Encourage the family to seek support and respite care.
5. Remind the family that the patient with ALS maintains full alertness, sensory function, and intelligence. Encourage them to maintain interaction, socialization, and stimulation and to seek out technology such as mind-activated computer-driven communication devices.
6. Refer the patient/family for more information and support to such agencies as the Amyotrophic Lateral Sclerosis Association (*www.alsa.org*).

Evaluation: Expected Outcomes

- Normal respiratory rate and rhythm, shallow, unlabored at rest.
- Does active ROM exercises for 15 minutes twice per day; uses assistive utensils to feed self.
- Tolerates small, frequent feedings without aspiration.
- Naps twice per day for 1 to 2 hours.
- Communicates needs effectively to staff and family.
- No signs of respiratory or urinary infection.

NEUROMUSCULAR DISORDERS

Guillain-Barré Syndrome (Polyradiculoneuritis)

Evidence Base Shahrizaila, N., & Yuki, N. (2011). The role of immunotherapy in Guillain-Barre syndrome: Understanding the mechanism of action. *Expert Opinion in Pharmacotherapy, 12*(10), 1551–1560.

Guillain-Barré syndrome (GBS) is an acute, rapidly progressing, ascending inflammatory demyelinating polyneuropathy of the peripheral sensory and motor nerves and nerve roots. GBS is most often, but not always, characterized by muscular weakness and distal sensory loss or dysesthesias. GBS is the most frequently acquired demyelinating neuropathy. It affects 1 in 100,000 people and must be identified quickly to initiate treatment and decrease life-threatening complications. Usually, GBS occurs a few days or weeks following symptoms of a respiratory or GI viral infection. Occasionally, surgery or vaccinations will trigger the syndrome. The disorder can develop over the course of hours, days, or weeks. Maximum weakness usually occurs within the first 2 weeks after symptoms appear, and by the third week of the illness, 90% of all patients are at their weakest. About 30% of those with GBS have residual weakness after 3 years and the recurrence rate is approximately 3%.

Mortality results from respiratory failure, autonomic disturbances, sepsis, and complications of immobility and occurs at a rate of about 5% despite intensive medical care.

Pathophysiology and Etiology

1. Believed to be an autoimmune disorder that causes acute neuromuscular paralysis due to destruction of the myelin sheath surrounding peripheral nerve axons and subsequent slowing of transmission.
2. Viral infection, immunization, or other event may trigger the autoimmune response.
3. About 30% to 40% of cases are preceded by *Campylobacter* infection, an acute infectious diarrheal illness.
4. Cell-mediated immune reaction is aimed at peripheral nerves, causing demyelination and, possibly, axonal degeneration.

Clinical Manifestations

1. Paresthesias and, possibly, dysesthesias.
2. Acute onset of symmetric progressive muscle weakness, most often beginning in the legs and ascending to involve the trunk, upper extremities, and facial muscles; paralysis may develop.

3. Difficulty with swallowing, speech, and chewing due to CN involvement.
4. Decreased or absent deep tendon reflexes, position and vibratory perception.
5. Autonomic dysfunction (increased heart rate and postural hypotension).
6. Decreased vital capacity, depth of respirations, and breath sounds.
7. Occasionally spasm and fasciculations of muscles.

Diagnostic Evaluation

1. History and neurologic exam. Progressive weakness, decreased sensation, decreased deep tendon reflexes.
2. Lumbar puncture for CSF examination—reveals low blood cell count, high protein.
3. Electrophysiologic studies—nerve conduction velocity shows decreased conduction velocity of peripheral nerves.

Management

1. Plasmapheresis produces temporary reduction of circulating antibodies to reduce the severity and duration of the GBS episode.
2. High-dose Ig therapy and corticosteroids are used to reduce the severity of the episode.
3. ECG monitoring and treatment of cardiac dysrhythmias.
4. Analgesics and muscle relaxants, as needed.
5. Intubation and mechanical ventilation if respiratory paralysis develops.

Complications

1. Respiratory failure.
2. Cardiac dysrhythmias.
3. Complications of immobility and paralysis.
4. Anxiety and depression.

Nursing Assessment

1. Assess pain level due to muscle spasms and dysesthesias.
2. Assess cardiac function including orthostatic BPs.
3. Assess respiratory status closely to determine hypoventilation due to weakness.
4. Perform CN assessment, especially CN IX for gag reflex.
5. Assess motor strength.

Nursing Diagnoses

- Ineffective Breathing Pattern related to weakness/paralysis of respiratory muscles.
- Impaired Physical Mobility related to paralysis.
- Imbalanced Nutrition: Less Than Body Requirements, related to CN dysfunction.
- Impaired Verbal Communication related to intubation, CN dysfunction.
- Chronic Pain related to disease pathology.
- Anxiety related to communication difficulties and deteriorating physical condition.

Nursing Interventions

Maintaining Respiration

1. Monitor respiratory status through vital capacity measurements, rate and depth of respirations, breath sounds.
2. Monitor level of weakness as it ascends toward respiratory muscles.
3. Watch for breathlessness while talking, a sign of respiratory fatigue.
4. Maintain calm environment and position the patient with head of bed elevated to provide for maximum chest excursion.
5. As much as possible, avoid opioids and sedatives that may depress respirations.
6. Monitor the patient for signs of impending respiratory failure; heart rate above 120 or below 70 beats/minute; respiratory rate above 30 breaths/minute; prepare to intubate.
7. Long-term respiratory management may be necessary with placement of a tracheostomy.

Avoiding Complications of Immobility

1. Position the patient correctly and provide ROM exercises (see page 174).
2. Encourage physical and occupational therapy exercises to regain strength during the rehabilitative period.
3. Assess for complications, such as contractures, pressure ulcers, edema of lower extremities, and constipation.
4. Provide assistive devices, as needed, such as cane or wheelchair, for patient to take home.
5. Recommend referral to rehabilitation services or physical therapy for evaluation and treatment.

Promoting Adequate Nutrition

1. Assess chewing and swallowing ability by testing CN V, IX, and X; if function is inadequate, provide alternate nutrition through enteral or parenteral methods.
2. During rehabilitation period, encourage a well-balanced, nutritious diet in small, frequent feedings with vitamin supplement, if indicated.
3. Recommend referral to dietitian for evaluation and proper diet therapy.

Maintaining Communication

1. Develop a communication system with the patient who cannot speak.
2. Have frequent contact with the patient and provide explanation and reassurance, remembering that the patient is fully conscious.
3. Provide some type of patient call system. Because standard call lights cannot be activated by the severely weak patient, provide adaptive call light and/or some type of constant monitoring and surveillance to meet patient's needs.
4. Recommend referral to speech therapy for evaluation and treatment.
5. Refer to counselor, social worker, or psychologist to develop/enhance coping skills and regain sense of control.

Relieving Pain

1. Administer analgesics, as required; monitor for adverse reactions, such as hypotension, nausea and vomiting, and respiratory depression.

2. Provide adjunct pain management therapies, such as therapeutic touch, massage, diversion, guided imagery.
3. Provide explanations to relieve anxiety, which augments pain.
4. Turn the patient frequently to relieve painful pressure areas.

Reducing Anxiety
1. Get to know the patient and build a trusting relationship.
2. Discuss fears and concerns while verbal communication is possible.
3. Reassure the patient that recovery is probable.
4. Use relaxation techniques such as listening to soft music.
5. Provide choices in care and give the patient a sense of control.
6. Enlist the support of significant others.

Community and Home Care Considerations

1. Be aware that GBS is a significant cause of new long-term disability for at least 1,000 people per year in the United States, necessitating long-term rehabilitation and community reintegration. Outcome can range from mild paresthesias to death. The chance of recovery is significantly affected by age, antecedent gastroenteritis, disability, electrophysiologic signs of axonal degeneration, latency to nadir, and duration of active disease.
2. Given the young age at which GBS sometimes occurs, the patient and family must be treated as an integral unit, assessing family communication, knowledge, adjustment, and use of support systems.
3. Include in caregiver training strategies the need for exercise, positioning, and activity to prevent secondary complications, such as contractures, deep vein thrombosis (DVT), hypercalcemia, and pressure ulcers.

Patient Education and Health Maintenance

1. Advise the patient and family that acute phase lasts 1 to 4 weeks, then the patient stabilizes and rehabilitation can begin; however, convalescence may be lengthy, from 3 months to 2 years.
2. Instruct the patient in breathing exercises or use of incentive spirometer to reestablish normal patterns.
3. Teach the patient to wear good supportive and protective shoes while out of bed to prevent injuries due to weakness and paresthesia.
4. Instruct the patient to check feet routinely for injuries because trauma may go unnoticed due to sensory changes.
5. Reinforce maintenance of normal weight; additional weight will further stress motor abilities.

6. Encourage the use of scheduled rest periods to avoid over-fatigue.
7. Refer the patient/family for more information and support to such agencies as Guillain-Barré Syndrome Foundation International (*www.gbsfi.com*).

Evaluation: Expected Outcomes

- Normal respiratory rate and rhythm, shallow, unlabored.
- Performs assistive ROM exercises every 2 hours; no pressure ulcers or edema present.
- Gag reflex present, eating small meals without aspiration.
- Uses short phrases and head nodding to communicate effectively.
- Verbalizes decreased pain.
- Verbalizes reduced anxiety.

Myasthenia Gravis

 Evidence Base Silvestri, N. J., & Wolfe, G. I. (2012). Myasthenia gravis. *Seminars in Neurology, 32*, 215–226.

Myasthenia gravis (MG) is a chronic autoimmune disorder affecting the neuromuscular transmission of impulses in the voluntary muscles of the body. MG is characterized by fluctuating weakness increased by exertion. Weakness increases during the day and improves with rest. Presentation and progression vary due to an antibody-mediated attack against acetylcholine receptors at the neuromuscular junction. Loss of acetylcholine receptors leads to a defect in neuromuscular transmission. Cardinal features are muscle weakness and fatigue. Evidence suggests that the frequency and recognition of MG is increasing.

Pathophysiology and Etiology

1. MG is idiopathic in most patients. Penicillamine is known to induce various autoimmune disorders, including MG.
2. Depletion of acetylcholine receptors at neuromuscular junctions brought about by an autoimmune attack (see Figure 15-8). In about 90% of patients, no specific cause can be identified, but genetic makeup is a predisposing factor, suggesting environmental factors may be involved in development of this disorder.
3. The reduced number of acetylcholine receptors results in diminished amplitude of end-plate potentials. Failed transmission of nerve impulses to skeletal muscle at the myoneural

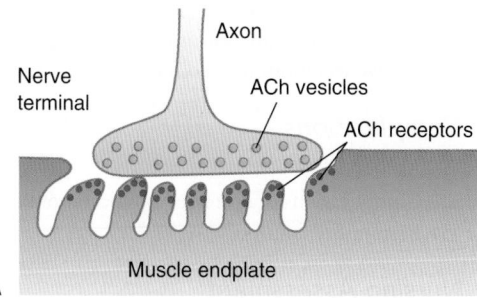
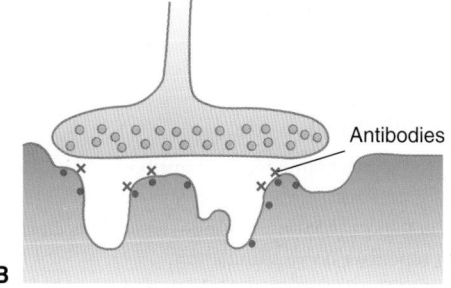

Figure 15-8. Myasthenia gravis. (A) Normal acetylcholine receptor site; **(B)** acetylcholine receptor site in myasthenia gravis.

junction results in decreased muscle power, clinically manifested as extreme fatigue and weakness. The pattern of muscle involvement varies among individuals.

4. About 80% to 90% of patients with MG have serum antibodies to acetylcholine.

5. Thyroid gland abnormalities are present in 80% of patients. Thymic tumor is the most important known cause; 10% of patients with MG have a thymoma.

6. *Cholinergic crisis* can result from overmedication with anticholinergic drugs, which release too much acetylcholine at the neuromuscular junction.

7. *Brittle crisis* occurs when the receptors at the neuromuscular junction become insensitive to anticholinesterase medication.

8. Women are three times more susceptible to developing MG than men.

9. Spontaneous remissions are rare. Long and complete remissions are even less common. Most remissions (with treatment) occur during the first 3 years of disease.

Clinical Manifestations

1. Extreme muscular weakness and easy fatigability.

2. Vision disturbances—diplopia and ptosis from ocular weakness. Extraocular muscle weakness or ptosis is present initially in 50% of patients and occurs during the course of illness in 90%. Bulbar muscle weakness is also common, along with weakness of head extension and flexion.

3. Facial muscle weakness causes a mask-like facial expression. Patients may present a snarling appearance when attempting to smile.

4. Dysarthria and dysphagia from weakness of laryngeal and pharyngeal muscles.

5. Proximal limb weakness, with specific weakness in the small muscles of the hands. Patients progress from mild to more severe disease over weeks to months. Weakness tends to spread from the ocular to facial to bulbar muscles and then to truncal and limb muscles. The disease remains ocular in only 16% of patients. About 87% of patients generalize within 13 months after onset.

6. Respiratory muscle weakness can be life-threatening. Intercurrent illness or medication can exacerbate weakness, quickly precipitating a myasthenic crisis and rapid respiratory compromise.

7. Impending myasthenic crisis may be triggered by respiratory infection, aspiration, physical/emotional stress, and changes in medications. Symptoms include:
   a. Sudden respiratory distress.
   b. Signs of dysphagia, dysarthria, ptosis, and diplopia.
   c. Tachycardia, anxiety.
   d. Rapidly increasing weakness of extremities and trunk.

Diagnostic Evaluation

1. Serum test for acetylcholine receptor antibodies—positive in up to 90% of patients.

2. Electrophysiologic (EMG) testing—reveals decremental response to repetitive nerve stimulation.

3. Edrophonium (Tensilon) test—IV injection of this short-acting anticholinesterase relieves symptoms temporarily. After injection, a marked but temporary improvement in muscle

strength identified by performance of repetitive movements or EMG testing suggests MG. It also differentiates myasthenic crisis from cholinergic crisis.

4. Thyroid function tests should be done to evaluate for coexistent thyroid disease and CT scan to assess enlargement of thymus gland. Chest CT scan is mandatory to identify thymoma in all cases of MG. This is especially true in older individuals.

Management

1. With treatment, most patients can lead fairly normal lives.

2. Oral anticholinesterase drugs, such as neostigmine and pyridostigmine, are first-line treatments for mild MG, enhancing neuromuscular transmission.

3. Immunosuppressive drugs, such as prednisone, are the mainstay of treatment when weakness is not adequately controlled by anticholinergic medication. Azathioprine may be added as a steroid-sparing agent. Immunosuppressant treatment is often permanent.

4. Plasmapheresis removes antibodies from the blood and is used for patients in myasthenic crisis or for short-term treatment of patients undergoing thymectomy. IV Ig is also an option and has less side effects.

5. Thymectomy is indicated for patients with tumor or hyperplasia of the thymus gland (thymectomy is not usually beneficial in late-onset patients).

6. Interventions for myasthenic crisis:
   a. Immediate hospitalization and may require intensive care.
   b. Edrophonium to differentiate crisis and treat myasthenic crisis; temporarily worsens cholinergic crisis; unpredictable results with brittle crisis.
   c. Airway management—mechanical ventilation, vigorous suctioning, oxygen therapy, postural drainage with percussion and vibration. Tracheostomy may be required, depending on duration of intubation. Maintain semi-Fowler's position, especially in obese patients.
   d. Plasmapheresis, IV Ig, and high-dose parenterally administered corticosteroids are used to reduce symptoms.

 DRUG ALERT Plasmapheresis must be carried out before IV Ig therapy because plasmapheresis will remove the IV Ig proteins that are effective in symptom reduction.

   e. Neostigmine IV for myasthenic crisis.
   f. Discontinuation of anticholinergic medications until respiratory function improves; atropine to reduce excessive secretions for cholinergic crisis.

Complications

1. Aspiration.
2. Complications of decreased physical mobility.
3. Respiratory failure.

Nursing Assessment

1. Expect the patient to complain of extreme muscle weakness and fatigue.

2. Assess CN function, motor fatigability with repetitive activity, and speech. Observe eye muscles (usually affected first) for ptosis, ocular palsy, diplopia.

3. Assess respiratory status—breathlessness, respiratory weakness, tidal volume, and vital capacity measurements.

4. Assess complications secondary to drug treatment—long-term immunomodulating therapies may predispose patients with MG to various complications.

   a. Long-term steroid use may lead to or aggravate many conditions, such as osteoporosis, cataracts, hyperglycemia, weight gain, avascular necrosis of hip, hypertension, and gastritis or peptic ulcer disease. To decrease the risk of ulcer, patients should take an H2 blocker or antacid.

   b. Increased risk for infection from immunomodulating therapy, especially if the patient is on more than one agent. Such infections include tuberculosis, systemic fungal infections, and *Pneumocystis carinii* pneumonia.

   c. Risk of lymphoproliferative malignancies may be increased with chronic immunosuppression.

   d. Immunosuppressive drugs may have teratogenic effects. In addition, risk of congenital deformity (arthrogryposis multiplex) is increased in offspring of women with severe MG.

 DRUG ALERT Neonates born to women with MG need to be monitored for respiratory failure for 1 to 2 weeks after birth. Discuss these aspects with women in reproductive years prior to beginning therapy with these drugs.

Nursing Diagnoses

- Fatigue related to disease process.
- Risk for Aspiration related to muscle weakness of face and tongue.
- Impaired Social Interaction related to diminished speech capabilities and increased secretions.

Nursing Interventions

Minimizing Fatigue

1. Plan exercise, meals, and other ADL during energy peaks. Time administration of medications 30 minutes before meals to facilitate chewing and swallowing.

2. Assist the patient in developing realistic activity schedule.

3. Provide an eye patch and alternate eyes for the patient with diplopia to allow safe participation in activity.

4. Allow for rest periods throughout the day.

5. Obtain assistive devices to help patient perform ADL.

 DRUG ALERT Many medications can accentuate the weakness experienced by the patient with MG, including some antibiotics (such as ciprofloxacin, aminoglycosides, chloroquine, and procaine), anti-arrhythmics (such as procainamide, beta-adrenergic blockers, and quinidine), local and general anesthetics, muscle relaxants, and analgesics such as nonsteroidal anti-inflammatory drugs (NSAIDs). Assess function after administering any new drug, and report deterioration in condition.

Preventing Aspiration

1. Assess the patient's oral motor strength before each meal.

2. Teach the patient to position his or her head in a slightly flexed position to protect airway during eating.

3. Modify diet, as needed, to minimize risk of aspiration; for instance, soft, solid foods instead of liquids. Teach the patient that eating warm foods (not hot foods) can ease swallowing difficulties.

4. Have suction available that the patient can operate.

5. Administer IV fluids and nasogastric tube feedings to the patient in crisis or with impaired swallowing; elevate head of bed after feeding.

6. Suction the patient frequently if on a mechanical ventilator; assess breath sounds and check chest x-ray reports because aspiration is a common problem.

Maintaining Social Interactions

1. Encourage the patient to use an alternate communication method, such as flash cards or a letter board, if speech is affected.

2. Instruct the patient to speak in a slow manner to avoid voice strain; refer to speech therapy, as needed.

3. Show the patient how to cup chin in hands during speech to support lower jaw and assist with speech.

4. Teach the patient to tilt head and to carry a handkerchief to manage secretions in public.

5. Encourage family participation in care.

6. Refer the patient to the Myasthenia Gravis Foundation of America (*www.myasthenia.org*) to meet other patients with the disease who lead productive lives.

Community and Home Care Considerations

1. Assess the home environment for physical and emotional stressors, such as uncomfortable temperature, draft, or loud noises.

2. Emphasize continued follow-up and compliance with treatment regimen.

3. Identify the need for additional home care services such as respiratory therapy, physical therapy, and nutritional services.

4. Assess the patient frequently for fluctuation in condition and inform caregivers that this is common.

5. Teach the patient and family how to use home suction in case of aspiration. Make sure everyone in household knows Heimlich maneuver.

Patient Education and Health Maintenance

1. Instruct the patient and family regarding the symptoms of crisis. Intercurrent infection or treatment with certain drugs may worsen symptoms of MG temporarily. Mild exacerbation of weakness is possible in hot weather.

2. Review the peak times of medications and how to schedule activity for best results. For patients on anticholinesterase therapy:

   a. Stress accurate dosage and times; take anticholinesterase drugs 30 to 45 minutes before meals.

   b. Tell the patient not to skip medication.

c. Instruct the patient to avoid taking medication with fruit, coffee, tomato juice, or other medications.

d. Inform the patient of adverse effects such as GI distress.

3. Stress the importance of activity with scheduled rest periods before fatigue develops.

4. Teach the patient ways to prevent crisis and aggravation of symptoms.

a. Avoid exposure to colds and other infections.

b. Avoid excessive heat and cold.

c. Inform the dentist of condition because use of procaine is not well tolerated.

d. Avoid emotional upset; plan ahead to minimize stress.

5. Encourage the patient to wear a MedicAlert bracelet.

6. Stress the importance of adequate nutrition; instruct to chew food thoroughly and eat slowly.

7. Advise the patient to avoid alcohol, tonic water.

8. Refer the patient/family for more information to the Myasthenia Gravis Foundation of America (*www.myasthenia.org*).

Evaluation: Expected Outcomes

- Demonstrates optimal self-care in bathing, eating, toileting, and dressing without fatigue.
- Breathes effectively, cough is effective, suctioning own secretions, lungs clear.
- Visits with friends, participates in social activities, uses alternative method of communications.

TRAUMA

Traumatic Brain Injury

Evidence Base American Association of Neuroscience Nurses and the Association of Rehabilitation Nurses. (2011). *Care of the patient with mild traumatic brain injury.* Glenview, IL: Author.

English, S. W., Turgeon, A. F., Owen, E., et al. (2012). Protocol management of severe traumatic brain injury in intensive care units. A systematic review. *Neurocritical Care,* published online August 2012.

Traumatic brain injury (TBI), also known as head injury, is the disruption of normal brain function due to trauma-related injury. TBI produces compromised neurologic function, resulting in focal or diffuse symptoms. Falls are the most common etiology of injury, followed by motor vehicle accidents. TBI is the leading cause of trauma-related deaths and accounts for 40% of trauma-related injuries. The goal of treatment is to prevent secondary brain injury by providing supportive care (see Chapter 35, page 1208, for emergency management of TBI).

Pathophysiology and Etiology

Types of Traumatic Brain Injury

1. Concussion—transient interruption in brain activity; no structural injury noted on radiographic studies.

2. Cerebral contusion—bruising of the brain with associated swelling. Coup injury is the site of initial trauma; the contra

coup injury is the site of rebound injury. Temporal and frontal lobes are common sites.

3. Intracerebral hematoma—bleeding into the brain tissue commonly associated with edema.

4. Epidural hematoma (EDH)—blood between the inner table of the skull and dura. Frequently associated with injury or laceration of the middle meningeal artery secondary to a temporal bone fracture. EDH is commonly associated with a lucid interval, followed by unresponsiveness.

5. Subdural hematoma—blood between the dura and arachnoid caused by venous bleeding; commonly associated with additional cerebral injuries: contusion or intracerebral hematoma.

6. Diffuse axonal injury (DAI) or shear injury—axonal tears within the white matter of the brain. Frequently occurs within the corpus callosum or brain stem and at the junction of the frontal/temporal poles. Associated with prolonged coma and poor prognosis.

Mechanism of Injury and Effects

1. Mechanism of injury is related to acceleration and deceleration of the brain (soft gelatin matter) within the skull (hard external surface with sharply edged internal surface). May be caused by blunt or penetrating injury.

2. The initial insult is the primary injury and the injury related to the sequela is the secondary injury. Cellular changes (release of oxygen-free radicals and neurotransmitters, calcium loss, and increase in lactate acid) and systemic instability (hypotension, anemia, hypoxia, hypercarbia, hypovolemia) potentiate secondary injury.

3. Neurologic deficits result from primary brain injury (contusion, hematoma, DAI, or shearing of white matter) or secondary injury (ischemia and mass effect from hemorrhage and cerebral edema of surrounding brain tissue).

4. Second impact syndrome (SIS) occurs in repetitive concussion when there is insufficient time for the brain to recover from the previous injury. SIS is common in sports-related injuries and is associated with cerebral injury and cerebral edema, which can be severe.

5. Studies have shown that mild TBI with a positive CT scan is more indicative of moderate injury, resulting in a more pronounced neurobehavioral presentation and extended neurologic recovery time beyond the typical 3 months.

6. Coagulopathy may result from increased release of intracranial thromboplastin, causing elevation in PTT, prothrombin time, and fibrinogen levels, which in turn results in mild clotting dysfunction to disseminating intravascular coagulation.

7. Paroxysmal sympathetic hyperactivity (PSH) or sympathetic storming may result from uncontrolled release of sympathetic hormones spontaneously or in response to some stressor. PSH results in tachycardia, tachypnea, hyperthermia, diaphoresis, agitation, and dystonia.

8. DI—reduced secretion of ADH with excessive fluid and electrolyte loss through the kidneys due to edema or compression of the pituitary/hypothalamic region; may cause severe dehydration.

9. SIADH—oversecretion of ADH with normal to increased intravascular volume (hypervolemic state) and dilutional hyponatremia (see page 488).

10. Cerebral salt wasting—increase in urinary secretion of sodium accompanied by volume depletion (hypovolemic state) (see page 488).

Classification

See page 483 for GCS.

1. Mild (GCS 13 to 15, with loss of consciousness to 15 minutes).

2. Moderate (GCS 9 to 12, with loss of consciousness for up to 6 hours).

3. Severe (GCS 3 to 8, with loss of consciousness greater than 6 hours).

Associated Injuries: Extracranial Trauma

1. Facial trauma and skull fractures—occur in 20% of major TBI. Temporal skull is thinnest; frontal and occipital bones are the thickest.

    a. Linear fracture—fracture through entire thickness of bone that runs in linear pattern.

    b. Basilar skull fracture.

        i. Anterior fossa results in contusions around the eyes (raccoon eyes) and risk of rhinorrhea.

        ii. Posterior fossa results in contusions around the ears (Battle sign) and risk of otorrhea.

    c. Depressed fracture—displacement of fracture past the inner table of the skull; risk of dural tear, CSF leak, and intracranial injury; may be closed or open.

    d. Facial fractures—orbital (LeForte I-II), mandible, zygoma, maxillary, nasal fractures.

2. Vascular injuries—vertebral or carotid artery dissection.

3. Spine fracture with or without spinal cord injury (SCI).

4. Soft tissue injuries.

Clinical Manifestations

1. Disturbances in consciousness: confusion to coma.

2. Headache, vertigo.

3. Agitation, restlessness.

4. Respiratory irregularities.

5. Cognitive deficits (confusion, aphasia, reading difficulties, writing difficulties, acalculi [inability to perform simple arithmetic], memory deficits such as retrograde and antegrade amnesia and difficulty learning new information).

6. Pupillary abnormalities.

7. Sudden onset of neurologic deficit.

8. Coma and coma syndromes; persistent vegetative state.

9. Otorrhea may indicate leakage of CSF from ear (otorrhea) due to posterior fossa skull fracture; rhinorrhea may indicate leakage of CSF from nares (rhinorrhea) due to anterior fossa skull fracture.

10. Raccoon eyes and Battle sign indicate skull base fractures.

11. Episodes of altered LOC, tachycardia, tachypnea, hyperthermia, agitation due to sympathetic storming (aggravated stress response).

12. Abnormal bleeding due to coagulopathy.

13. Cardiac arrhythmias due to increased release of catecholamines in stress response.

Diagnostic Evaluation

1. CT scan to identify and localize lesions, edema, bleeding.

2. Skull and cervical spine films to identify fracture, displacement.

3. Neuropsychological tests during rehabilitation phase to determine extent of cognitive deficits.

4. MRI to identify and diagnose DAI (rarely performed because it does not alter medical management).

5. CBC, coagulation profile, electrolyte levels, serum osmolarity, ABG values, and other laboratory tests to monitor for complications and guide treatment.

Management

1. Airway—assess and maintain patent airway.

    a. Intubate for GCS less than 8 (comatose) or clinical signs of respiratory failure.

    b. Placement of nasogastric tube with intubation to prevent aspiration.

2. Breathing—all intubated patients should have ventilatory support.

    a. Oxygen, as needed, to maintain PaO_2 greater than 100 mm Hg.

    b. Maintain $Paco_2$ 35 to 45 mm Hg.

    c. Avoid use of hyperventilation.

    d. Consider early tracheostomy if anticipate intubation greater than 2 weeks.

3. Circulation—prevent hypotension.

    a. Maintain SBP above 90 mm Hg. This may be maintained with use of fluid or vasopressors.

    b. Maintain normovolemia.

    c. Treat symptomatic anemia with packed RBC.

    d. Treat symptomatic arrhythmias.

4. Management of increased ICP (see page 486) and cerebral edema.

5. Management of PSH with medications, such as oxycodone (opiate), propranolol (beta-adrenergic blocker), clonidine (alpha-adrenergic antagonist), dantrolene (muscle relaxant), and bromocriptine (dopamine-receptor agonist). (Response to medications varies.)

6. Supportive care—rehabilitation services, skin care.

7. Nutritional support should be initiated within 3 to 5 days; 25 kcal/kg via nasogastric feeding tube. Conversion to gastrostomy tube if anticipate need for alternative feeds is >1 to 2 weeks.

8. Antibiotics, as ordered, to prevent infection with open skull fractures or penetrating wounds.

9. Surgery to evacuate intracranial hematomas, debridement of penetrating wounds, elevation of skull fractures, or repair of CSF leaks.

10. Treatment of hypernatremia (due to DI, dehydration, diaphoresis) with fluid replacement, vasopressin therapy.

11. Treatment of hyponatremia.
    a. Cerebral salt wasting: monitor daily fluid status, fluid administration, oral salt replacement, and IV saline 0.9% or 3% (250 to 500 mL over 3 to 5 hours).
    b. SIADH: monitor daily fluid status, fluid restriction, oral salt replacement, IV saline 2% or 3% bolus over 3 to 5 hours.
12. Seizure prophylaxis is not recommended to prevent posttraumatic seizures, as it has been shown to inhibit cognitive recovery; however, prophylactic AEDs are ordered in some cases; duration is 7 days.
    a. If seizure activity is witnessed and there is associated temporal lobe injury or penetrating injuries, AEDs are recommended.
    b. AEDs are given IV for rapid loading and should be converted to enteric route. Commonly used AEDs include phenytoin, fosphenytoin sodium, or levetiracetam. Levels should be monitored for accurate dosing.

Complications

1. Infections: systemic (respiratory, urinary), neurologic (meningitis, ventriculitis).
2. Increased ICP, hydrocephalus, brain herniation.
3. Posttraumatic seizures and seizure disorder.
4. Permanent neurologic deficits: cognitive, motor, sensory, speech.
5. Neurobehavioral alterations: impulsivity, uninhibited aggression, emotional lability.
6. Persistent PSH.
7. Disseminated intravascular coagulation.
8. DI, SIADH, cerebral salt wasting.
9. Death.

Nursing Assessment

1. Monitor for signs of increased ICP—altered LOC, abnormal pupil responses, vomiting, increased pulse pressure, bradycardia, hyperthermia.
2. Monitor for signs of PSH—altered LOC, diaphoresis, tachycardia, tachypnea, hypertension, hyperthermia, agitation, and dystonia. PSH is generally seen in severe TBI (GCS 3 to 8) or minimally responsive patients.
3. Monitor cardiac status for hypotension and arrhythmias (bradycardia, elevated T waves, premature ventricular contractions, premature atrial contractions, and sinus arrhythmias)—common and frequently asymptomatic. Tachycardia with hypotension is indicative of hypovolemia; patient should be evaluated for additional source of blood loss.
4. Be alert for DI—excessive urine output, dilute urine (specific gravity less than 1.005), hypernatremia.
5. Be alert for hyponatremia and assess etiology (SIADH or cerebral salt wasting); see page 488.
6. Monitor laboratory findings and report abnormal values:
    a. Abnormal PTT, PT, and fibrinogen levels indicating coagulopathy.
    b. Electrolyte imbalance—alterations in serum potassium (hypokalemia) and sodium (hypernatremia/hyponatremia) levels are common.

c. Anemia—related to additional trauma or may be dilutional.
    d. Elevated WBC count—indicating infection related to trauma or invasive procedures.
    e. Hypoxia or hypercarbia.
7. Perform CN, motor, sensory, and reflex assessment.
8. Assess for behavior that warrants potential for injury to self or others.

 **NURSING ALERT** Regard every patient who is unresponsive with a brain injury as having a potential spinal cord injury. Cervical collar and spine precautions should be maintained until spinal fracture has been ruled out. A significant number of patients are under the influence of alcohol at the time of injury, which may mask the nature and severity of the injury.

Nursing Diagnoses

- Ineffective Cerebral Tissue Perfusion related to increased ICP.
- Ineffective Breathing Pattern related to increased ICP or brain stem injury.
- Imbalanced Nutrition: Less Than Body Requirements related to compromised neurologic function and stress of injury.
- Impaired Environmental Interpretation Syndrome related to physiology of brain injury.
- Risk for Injury related to altered thought processes.
- Compromised Family Coping related to unpredictability of outcome.

Nursing Interventions

Maintaining Adequate Cerebral Perfusion

1. Maintain a patent airway.
2. Monitor ICP, as ordered (see page 490).
3. Monitor cerebral oxygenation, temperature, or neurochemicals, as ordered. Provide oxygen therapy to maintain PaO_2 above 100 and carbon dioxide within normal range.
4. Maintain SBP above 90 to enhance cerebral perfusion and administer treatment for arrhythmias if patient is symptomatic. Evaluate for source of blood loss if patient is tachycardic and hypotensive.
5. Monitor LOC, CN function, and motor and sensory function as per GCS or neurologic flow sheet; identify emerging trends in neurologic function; and communicate findings to medical staff.
6. If patient has severe TBI, monitor for signs of PSH (abnormal stress response) and identify triggers and effective treatment modalities. Institute nursing measures that have been found to be helpful, such as maintaining normothermia, pretreating before known trigger, applying cool compress to forehead, and providing relaxing music.

 NURSING ALERT PSH places the patient at high risk for secondary brain injury, cardiac abnormalities, weight loss, skin breakdown, and infection. Be alert to triggers (suctioning, turning, hyperthermia, infection, auditory stimuli) and treat promptly to control symptoms.

7. Monitor response to pharmacologic therapy, including AED levels, as directed.

8. Monitor laboratory data, CSF cultures, and Gram stains, if applicable, and institute prompt antibiotic therapy, as directed.

9. Monitor for hypernatremia and administer fluid replacement, as directed. If due to DI, vasopressin may be utilized.

10. Monitor for hyponatremia. Determine if hyponatremia is related to SIADH or cerebral salt wasting (see page 488). Administer fluids/restrict fluids and administer oral or IV salt replacement, as directed. Administer 250 to 500 mL 3% saline solution over 3 to 5 hours via central venous access to prevent damage to peripheral vein wall.

 NURSING ALERT Severe states of hypernatremia and hyponatremia can cause further neurologic compromise (seizures, nausea, confusion, irritability/agitation, coma). Close monitoring of laboratory values is indicated to evaluate trends and maintain normal range. Hypernatremia and hyponatremia should not be reversed quickly because the rapid change can create rebound cerebral edema and be detrimental to the patient. Rapid increase in serum sodium level can cause central pontine myelinolysis and results in severe damage of myelin sheath of white matter in pons.

11. Monitor coagulation panel and replace clotting factors at room temperature, as directed.

12. Assess dressings and drainage tubes after surgery for patency, security, and characteristics of drainage.

13. Institute measures to minimize increased ICP, ischemic changes, cerebral edema, seizures, or neurovascular compromise, such as careful positioning, to avoid flexing head, reducing hip flexion (can reduce venous drainage, causing congestion), and spreading out care evenly over 24-hour period.

Maintaining Respiration

1. Monitor respiratory rate, depth, and pattern of respirations; report any abnormal pattern, such as Cheyne-Stokes respirations or periods of apnea.

2. Assist with intubation and ventilatory assistance, if needed.

3. Obtain frequent ABG values to maintain Pao_2 greater than 100 mm Hg and $Paco_2$ 35 to 45 mm Hg.

4. The use of positive end-expiratory pressure (PEEP) in the care of critically ill patients after TBI remains controversial. PEEP (5 to 10 cm) is felt to be physiological and not detrimental; however, excessive PEEP can create increases in intrathoracic pressure, diminish venous drainage, reduce mean arterial pressure (MAP), and increase ICP.

5. Turn patient every 2 hours and assist with coughing and deep breathing.

6. Suction patient, as needed.

Meeting Nutritional Needs

1. Begin nutritional support as soon as possible after a head injury; provide 140% of energy requirements (100% in paralyzed patient), with 15% in the form of protein. Supplements should provide 25 kcal/kg.
   a. Continuous enteric feedings.
      i. Elevate the head of the bed during feedings.
      ii. Check residuals to prevent aspiration.
      iii. Monitor for diarrhea.
   b. Consider IV hyperalimentation—for patients unable to tolerate nasogastric feedings.
   c. Oral feeding—started when adequate swallowing mechanism is demonstrated.

2. Administer H_2-blocking agents to prevent gastric ulceration and hemorrhage from gastric acid hypersecretion.

3. Consult with dietitian to provide adequate calories and nitrogen supplement.

4. Monitor glucose levels frequently, utilizing fingerstick samples and glucometer. Insulin (IV drip/sliding scale) may be required to regulate serum glucose levels within a normal range to avoid hypoglycemia and hyperglycemia, which worsens the effects of secondary brain injury.

 NURSING ALERT Caloric needs of a patient with a head injury increase by 100% to 200%. Consult your dietitian to institute nutritional support within the first 2 to 3 days after injury to support the recovery process. Weight loss is generally in the form of muscle loss and can be as much as 25 to 30 lb (11.3 to 13.6 kg).

5. Perform bedside dysphagia screen to evaluate swallow function before initiation of oral foods. Consult speech therapist for bedside or radiographic swallow study if patient fails swallow screen or appears at risk for dysphagia. Recognize that any patient with coma is at risk for swallowing difficulties. Assessment of swallowing function decreases risk of aspiration. Speech therapy is essential for retraining and developing adaptive techniques.

Promoting Cognitive Function

1. Periodically assess the patient's LOC and compare to baseline.

2. Be aware of the patient's cognitive alteration and adjust interaction and environment accordingly.

3. Provide meaningful stimulation using all senses—visual, olfactory, gustatory, acoustic, and tactile.

4. Observe the patient for fatigue or restlessness from overstimulation.

5. Involve the family in sensory stimulation program to maximize its effectiveness.

6. Decrease environmental stimuli when the patient is in agitated state.

7. Reorient to surroundings using repetition, verbal and visual cues, and memory aids; routinely orient the patient after awakening.

8. Use pictures of family members, clock, and calendar as outlined by occupational and speech therapist.

9. Encourage the family to provide items from home to increase sense of identity and security.

10. Anticipate the need for additional help with toileting, eating, and performing ADL due to cognitive impairment.

11. Break down ADL into simple steps that patient can progressively take part in.

12. Structure the environment and care activities to minimize distraction and provide consistency.

13. Identify and maintain usual patterns of behavior—sleep, medication use, elimination, food intake, and self-care routine.

14. Refer the patient for cognitive retraining, if appropriate.

Preventing Injury

1. Instruct the family regarding the behavioral phases of recovery from brain injury, such as restlessness and combativeness.

2. Investigate for physical sources of restlessness, such as uncomfortable position, signs of UTI, or pressure ulcer development.

3. Reassure the patient and family during periods of agitation and irrational behavior.

4. Pad side rails and wrap hands in mitts if patient is agitated. Maintain constant vigilance and avoid restraints, if possible.

5. Keep environmental stimuli to a minimum to avoid confusion and agitation. Veil beds can be useful in reducing injury in the agitated patient.

6. Provide adequate light if patient is hallucinating.

7. Avoid sedatives to avoid medication-induced confusion and altered states of cognition.

Strengthening Family Coping

1. Refer the family to community support services, such as respite care, faith-based groups, city and state social services, and resources on the Internet. Suggest the Brain Injury Association of America (*www.biausa.org*) for further information.

2. Assist the family members to establish stress management techniques that can be integrated into their lifestyle, such as ventilation of feelings, use of respite care, relaxation techniques.

3. Consult with social worker or psychologist to assist the family in adjusting to patient's permanent neurologic deficits.

4. Help the family assist the patient to recognize current progress and not focus on limitations.

Community and Home Care Considerations

1. Observe for signs of postconcussion syndrome (PCS), which include headache, decreased concentration, irritability, dizziness, insomnia, restlessness, diminished memory, anxiety, easy fatigability, and alcohol intolerance.

2. Be aware that persistence of these symptoms can interfere with relationships and employability of the patient.

3. Encourage the patient and family to report these symptoms and obtain additional support and counseling, as needed. PCS may persist as long as 2 years.

4. Act as liaison to coordinate all home care services the patient will need while keeping in touch with the patient's primary care provider, neurologist, and neurosurgeon.

5. Provide the necessary education to caregivers in tube feedings, positioning, ROM exercises, and so forth.

6. Make sure that coaches and parents from community recreation programs and schools are familiar with and follow guidelines for sports-related concussion (see Table 15-7).

Table 15-7	American Academy of Neurology Guidelines for Sports-Related Concussion
SEVERITY	**RECOMMENDATIONS**
Grade 1 Transient confusion without loss of consciousness and resolution of symptoms within 15 minutes	• Removal from game and only returned to the game if remains asymptomatic after 15 minutes • If second grade 1 concussion occurs, removal from sports activity until asymptomatic for 1 week
Grade 2 Transient confusion without loss of consciousness and symptoms persisting longer than 15 minutes	• Removal from sporting event and further workup if symptoms do not resolve in 1 week • No sporting activity for 1 week • If grade 2 occurs after a grade 1 concussion, removal from sporting event and no sporting activities for 2 weeks
Grade 3 Loss of consciousness	• Removal from sporting event • Return to sporting activities if asymptomatic for 1 week (brief loss of consciousness) • Return to sporting activities if asymptomatic for 2 weeks (prolonged loss of consciousness) • Unconsciousness with neurologic findings should be transported to nearest emergency for full evaluation • Removal from sporting activity for 1 year and discouraged from future participation in contact sports if any structural findings on computed tomography scan or magnetic resonance imaging

Patient Education and Health Maintenance

1. Review the signs of increased ICP with the family.
2. Reinforce the lability of cognitive, language, and physical functioning of the person with brain injury and the lengthy recovery period.
3. Teach the family techniques to calm the agitated patient.
   a. Therapeutic use of touch, massage, and music.
   b. Elimination of distractions (television, radio, alarms, crowds).
   c. Provide one-on-one communication.
   d. Distract patients.

Evaluation: Expected Outcomes

- No signs of increased ICP.
- Respirations—24 breaths/minute, regular.
- Tube feedings tolerated well without residual.
- Oriented to person, place, and time.
- Less agitated; side rails maintained.
- Family reports using respite care.

Spinal Cord Injury

 Evidence Base SCIRE Project. (2010). Spinal Cord Injury Rehabilitation Evidence. Available: *www .scireproject.com.*

Spinal cord injury (SCI) is a traumatic injury to the spinal cord that may vary from a mild cord concussion with transient numbness to immediate and complete tetraplegia. The most common sites are the cervical areas C5, C6, and C7, and the junction of the thoracic and lumbar vertebrae, T12 and L1. Injury to the spinal cord may result in loss of function below the level of cord injury (see Figure 15-9). SCI requires comprehensive and specialized care. The Model Spinal Cord Injury System is a network of comprehensive, federally funded, regional SCI centers in the United States. The Department of Veterans Affairs operates 23 SCI centers. (Also see Chapter 35, page 1211, for emergency management of SCI.)

Pathophysiology and Etiology

1. The estimated annual incidence of SCI is about 11,000 new cases per year, and the prevalence is approximately 183 cases per 230,000 people in the United States. The average age is 32 and approximately 80% are males. The primary etiologies are motor vehicle accidents, violence (mainly gunshot), falls, and sports injuries. Most injuries result in tetraplegia, and more patients with SCI are incomplete than complete. (A complete SCI is absence of motor and sensory function at the lowest sacral segment affected; see below for a description of incomplete SCI.) About 90% of these patients are discharged to noninstitutional settings.
2. The life expectancy for an individual with SCI is lower (80% to 85%) than that of a person without SCI. The leading causes of death are pneumonia, emboli, and septicemia.

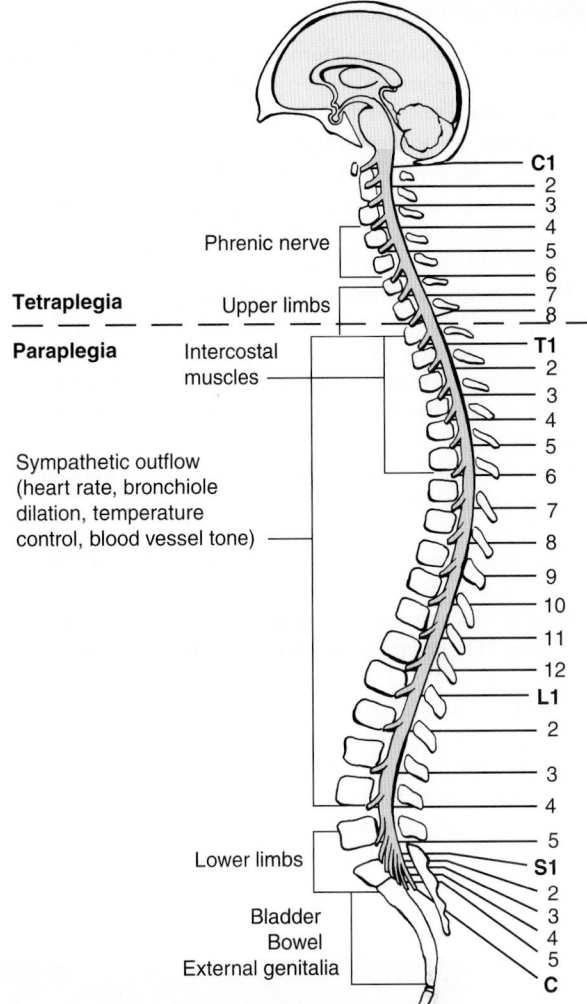

Figure 15-9. Levels of spinal cord innervation.

3. SCI may result from trauma, vascular disorders, infectious conditions, tumor, and other insults.
4. SCI can affect upper motor neurons (UMNs) or lower motor neurons (LMNs). UMNs extend from the motor strip in the cerebral cortex of the brain through the corticospinal tract in the spinal cord, where they synapse with interneurons in the ventral horn. LMNs originate in the ventral horn, exit the spinal cord at each segment, and extend to the neuromuscular junction. Each LMN innervates 10 to 2,000 muscle fibers. UMN lesions at T12 and above result in spasticity. LMN lesions at L1 and below result in flaccidity and reflex loss.

 GERONTOLOGIC ALERT Older patients are at greater risk for altered glucose metabolism, loss of bone minerals leading to fractures, musculoskeletal pain and weakness, and greater loss of function with spinal cord injury.

Clinical Manifestations

1. Patients with tetraplegia (formerly called quadriplegia) have damage to the cervical segments of nerves (C1–C8) in the spinal canal. Function may be impaired in the upper extremities, trunk, pelvic organs, and lower extremities.

2. Patients with paraplegia have damage to the thoracic, lumbar, or sacral segments of nerves in the spinal cord. The arms are unaffected, but function may be impaired in the trunk, pelvic organs, and lower extremities.

3. The International Standards for Neurological Classification of Spinal Cord Injury, promoted by the American Spinal Injury Association (ASIA), are used (available at *www.asia-spinalinjury.org/publications/index.html*). The ASIA Impairment Scale is based on completeness of injury and motor/sensory function.

   ASIA A—complete; absent sensory and motor function in the sacral segments S4–5.

   ASIA B—incomplete; intact sensory but absent motor function below the neurologic level of injury (LOI) and includes level S4–5.

   ASIA C—incomplete; intact motor function distal to neurologic LOI, and more than half of key muscles distal to LOI have muscle grade less than 3.

   ASIA D—incomplete; intact motor function distal to neurologic LOI, and more than half of key muscles distal to LOI have muscle grade greater than or equal to 3.

   ASIA E—normal; intact motor and sensory function.

4. Sacral sensation is intact if there is deep sensation and sensation at the anal mucocutaneous junction; sacral motor is intact if the patient has voluntary contraction of the external anal sphincter with digital stimulation.

5. The zone of partial preservation (ZPP) indicates areas of partial sensory/motor innervation below the LOI; the ZPP is applicable only to complete injuries.

6. The neurologic level of injury is the lowest neural level with normal sensory and motor function on both sides of the body. When describing the LOI, the neurologic level is noted unless stated specifically that the skeletal LOI, which is the level of greatest vertebral damage, is being discussed.

7. Various syndromes (incomplete injuries) may characterize the clinical presentation (see Table 15-8).

8. Sensation function (eg, sensitivity of pinprick/light touch) is tested on each of the 28 dermatomes on both sides of the body. The following grading is suggested: 0 = Absent; 1 = Impaired; 2 = Normal. The external anal sphincter should also be tested (sensory incomplete if sensate).

9. Motor function is tested on each of the 10 paired myotomes on both sides of the body. The following grading is suggested: 0 = Total paralysis; 1 = Contraction visible or palpable; 2 = Active movements and full ROM without gravity; 3 = Active movement and full ROM against gravity; 4 = Active movement and full ROM with moderate resistance; 5 = Normal motor with active movement and full ROM against full resistance. The external anal sphincter tone should also be tested (motor incomplete if contraction).

10. Most recovery occurs within 6 months of injury; patients with incomplete injuries have greater recovery than patients with complete injuries.

Table 15-8	Incomplete Spinal Cord Clinical Syndromes		
SYNDROME	**AFFECTED SITE**	**DEFICIT**	**PRESERVATION**
Central cord	Central cervical spinal cord	More motor deficit in upper extremities than lower extremities caused by medial damage of corticospinal tract	Sacral sensory; lower extremities have better motor function than upper extremities due to lateral sparing of corticospinal tract
Brown-Sequard	Hemisection of spinal cord	Ipsilateral motor function and fine touch, vibration, and proprioception (posterior tract); contralateral sensory function pain and temperature (spinothalamic tract)	Ipsilateral sensory function of pain and temperature (spinothalamic tract); contralateral motor function, fine touch, vibration, and proprioception (posterior tract)
Anterior cord	Main anterior spinal artery of anterior spinal cord affecting anterior two thirds of spinal cord	Variable motor deficit; variable sensory deficit of pain and temperature (spinothalamic tract)	Posterior one third of spinal cord (posterior spinal artery); sensory function of proprioception, light touch, vibration (posterior tract)
Conus medullaris	Conus and lumbar nerve roots in spinal cord	Variable motor deficit; bowel, bladder, and lower-extremity reflexes (flaccid)	Lesions of proximal conus may be reflexic (eg, butocavernosa, micturition)
	Lumbosacral nerve roots in spinal cord (distal from conus medullaris)	Variable motor deficit; bowel, bladder, and lower-extremity reflexes (flaccid)	Lesions proximal to level of injury may be reflexic (eg, bulbocavernosa, micturition)

11. Instability exists when ligamentous structures and vertebra cannot protect the vulnerable spinal cord and movement can further damage the injured spinal cord; stability exists when ligamentous structures and vertebra can protect the spinal cord from further neurologic injury.

12. Vertebral fractures may be simple, compressed or wedge, dislocated (vertebra overrides another vertebra), subluxed (vertebra partially dislocated over another vertebrae), comminuted (vertebrae shattered), or teardrop (vertebrae chipped). Jefferson's fractures, which may occur with head injuries, involve the C1 level.

Diagnostic Evaluation

1. X-ray of spinal column—include open mouth studies for adequate visualization of C1 and C2.

2. MRI of spine—to detect soft tissue injury, hemorrhage, edema, bony injury; syringomyelia (cystic degeneration in spinal cord) may present as cord compression, syrinx (cavity) at the fracture site, and kyphosis at fracture site.

3. Electrophysiologic monitoring to determine function of neural pathways.

4. Urodynamic studies may include urine flow to detect bladder outlet obstruction and/or impaired bladder contractility; cystometrogram to determine bladder sensation, compliance, and capacity; sphincter EMG and other studies. The gold standard in urodynamics is to measure bladder and urethral pressure under fluoroscopy monitoring.

5. If DVT or pulmonary emboli are suspected, an ultrasound of the lower extremity or ventilation/perfusion scan is performed.

6. Heterotopic ossification may be diagnosed in the inflammatory stages using ultrasound. Alkaline phosphatase and ESR are typically elevated.

7. Nutritional status should be assessed using nutritional history, anthropometric measurements, prealbumin (half-life 12 to 36 hours), and transferrin (half-life 6 to 10 days).

8. Total lymphocyte count and creatinine height index are also used to establish nutritional risk.

Management

Requires a multidisciplinary approach because of multiple-system involvement and the psychosocial aspects of catastrophic injuries.

 NURSING ALERT Patients sustaining an SCI have better outcomes when treated by a multidisciplinary SCI team. Once the patient is stabilized, the option of transferring the patient to an SCI facility should be provided to the patient and/or family.

Immediately After Trauma (Less Than 1 Hour)

1. Immobilization with rigid cervical collar, sandbags, and rigid spine board to transport from the field to acute care facility.

2. Monitor for respiratory failure, hypotension, and/or bradycardia and treat appropriately.

Acute Phase (1 to 24 Hours)

1. Maintenance of pulmonary and cardiovascular stability.
   a. Intubation and mechanical ventilation, if needed.
   b. Vasopressors to maintain adequate perfusion to sustain mean arterial BP > 90 mm Hg.
   c. Medical stabilization before spinal stabilization and decompression.

2. Spinal cord immobilization—use of skeletal tongs.
   a. Crutchfield and Vinke tongs require predrilled holes in the skull under local anesthesia; Gardner-Wells and Heifitz tongs do not.
   b. Weight is added to traction gradually to reduce the vertebral fracture; weight maintained at a level to ensure vertebral alignment. Lateral spine films are taken after the addition of weight to assess spinal alignment.

3. Rigid kinetic turning bed can be used to immobilize patients with thoracic and lumbar injuries.

4. Surgical interventions are considered when the patient has vertebral instability that may result in further neurologic damage; an injury that is incomplete at onset may become complete if instability exists. The objectives are to remove all of the bony and soft tissues that are compressing the spinal cord, thereby minimizing the possibility of deteriorating neurologic status, and stabilize the vertebra surrounding the spinal cord so that rehabilitation may begin as soon as possible. Goals of treatment of the spinal fractures are aimed at protecting the neural elements and preventing deformity and instability.
   a. Decompression, typically using the anterior approach in cervical instances, may be accomplished by removing the bony structures and soft tissues (eg, fusion, decompression laminectomy). Realignment of the soft tissues and vertebral column is required.
   b. Stabilization, typically done using the posterior approach, involves the use of wires, bone grafts, plates, screws, and other fixation devices to prevent movement at the damaged bony site.

5. Methylprednisolone sodium succinate may be administered within 8 hours of injury.
   a. Bolus 30 mg/kg administered over 15 minutes; maintenance infusion of 5.4 mg/kg/hr infused for 23 hours.
   b. Additional benefit may be achieved by administering the maintenance dose for 48 hours.

6. Management of neurogenic bladder—Foley catheter.

7. Pressure ulcer prevention—pressure reduction mattress or kinetic turning frame.

8. Prevention of DVT and its sequelae is an important aspect of the treatment of patients who have sustained SCI due to the high risk of thromboembolic complications.
   a. Adjusted-dose heparin or LMWH for anticoagulant prophylaxis within 72 hours of SCI, except in those with active bleeding, evidence of head injury, or coagulopathy.
   b. Low-dose heparin therapy, external pneumatic devices, or compression stockings provide inadequate protection when used alone, but they have proved beneficial when used in combination in patients with SCI.

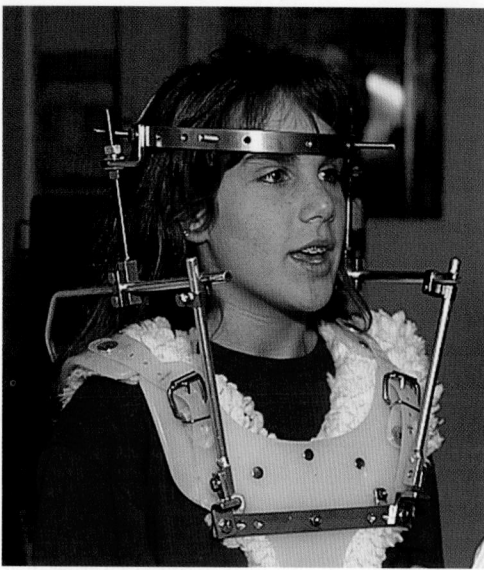

Figure 15-10. Halo brace.

Subacute Phase (within 1 Week)

1. Stiff orthosis is utilized for external stabilization of cervical fractures. Devices include the Halo brace, Minerva collar, extended Philadelphia collar, and fabricated orthosis. Device is selected based on the type of fracture and extent of instability. Average length of time in a halo brace is 12 weeks, followed by a Philadelphia collar for 4 weeks. Halo brace is used for cervical injuries (see Figure 15-10).

   a. Graphite rings are MRI compatible, lightweight, and radiolucent.

   b. Some halos are now open posteriorly, which reduces the incidence of cervical fracture displacement.

   c. The ring is attached to stainless steel pins (two anterior pins, two posterior pins) and attached to a vest by four connecting rods (also MRI compatible and radiolucent).

   d. Torque wrenches connect the rods to the ring and vest; pressures are typically 8 inches/lb for pins (2 to 5 inches/lb in children) and locking bolts are 28 inches/lb.

   e. Pins and locking bolts must be retightened approximately 24 to 48 hours after placement and periodically thereafter.

   f. Pin sites should be cleaned daily with half-strength hydrogen peroxide or soap and water.

2. H_2-receptor blockers to prevent gastric irritation and hemorrhage.

3. Early mobilization and passive exercise as soon as patient is surgically and medically stable.

4. Hyperalimentation, if unable to tolerate enteric feeds, to retard negative nitrogen balance.

5. Interventions to help prevent thromboembolism include compression hose, compression boots, range of motion, adjusted-dose heparin, or LMWH.

   a. Prior to applying mechanical compression, tests to exclude the presence of lower-extremity DVT should be performed if thromboprophylaxis has been delayed for more than 72 hours after injury.

   b. Vena cava filters are indicated in patients who have not achieved success with anticoagulant prophylaxis or who have a contraindication to anticoagulation. They are not a substitute for thromboprophylaxis due to morbidity related to DVT (eg, postphlebitic syndrome) and propagation of venal caval embolism.

Chronic Phase (Beyond 1 Week)

1. Segmental instrumentation systems are used in conjunction with a body jacket and are used for patients with thoracolumbar injuries.

2. To prevent thrombophlebitis in the chronic phase, compression boots should be continued for 2 weeks; anticoagulants should also be continued based on risk category.

   a. Minimum of 8 weeks from time of injury for those with incomplete or complete motor injury with no additional risk factors.

   b. For those with complete motor injury with additional risk factors, anticoagulants should be continued for 12 weeks.

3. Management of complications may include treatment of infections with antibiotics; treatment of respiratory compromise with phrenic nerve pacing, mechanical ventilation, and other methods; pressure ulcer treatment; management of heterotopic ossification with calcium chelators and anti-inflammatory agents; drainage of syringomyelia; management of spasticity with oral or intrathecal antispasmodics, surgical procedure, or spinal cord stimulation; and management of central neuropathic pain with anticonvulsants, minor sedatives, antidepressants, nerve block, or surgical procedure.

4. Spasticity should be managed by:

   a. Maintaining calm, stress-free environment.

   b. Allowing ample time for activities such as positioning and transferring.

   c. Performing joint ROM exercises with slow, smooth movements.

   d. Avoiding temperature extremes.

   e. Administering muscle relaxants, such as baclofen (via pump or orally), diazepam, and dantrolene, as prescribed.

   f. Botulism toxin injections can be utilized.

   g. Clonidine has been used to manage spasticity and facilitate walking in patients with incomplete injuries.

6. External sphincterotomy may be used for detrusor–sphincter dyssynergia. Other options include urethral stents and balloon dilatation.

7. Resistive inspiratory muscle training shows promise in promoting respiratory muscle strength and reducing sleep-induced breathing disturbances in patients with tetraplegia. Resistive training devices are used to perform respiratory maneuvers at scheduled times during the day.

8. Rehabilitation includes medical and psychosocial support, physical therapy, urologic evaluation, occupational therapy, and multiple other interventions to facilitate an increased level of function and community participation.

Complications

1. Spinal shock lasting a few hours to a few weeks noted by loss of all reflex, motor, sensory, and autonomic activity below the level of the lesion.
2. Respiratory arrest, pneumonia, atelectasis requiring mechanical ventilation with cervical injury.
3. Cardiac arrest may result from initial trauma, worsening of initial injury from edema, concomitant injuries, and other illnesses.
4. Thromboembolic complications—in 15% of patients.
5. Infections—respiratory, urinary, pressure ulcers, sepsis.
6. Autonomic dysreflexia—exaggerated autonomic response to stimuli below the level of the lesion in patients with lesions at or above T_6 is a medical emergency and can result in dangerous elevation of BP.
7. Autonomic dysfunction resulting in orthostatic hypotension, thermodysregulation, and vasomotor abnormalities.
8. Urologic—bladder storage pressure greater than 35 to 40 cm due to neurogenic bladder may result in renal deterioration; SCI patients who have indwelling urinary catheters are at increased risk of bladder cancer.
9. Paralytic ileus—common in subacute and acute stage.
10. Heterotopic ossification—bony overgrowth that occurs below the level of injury any time after SCI.
11. Syringomyelia—cystic formation in the spinal cord may occur any time after SCI.
12. Depression—occurs in 25% of men and 47% of women with SCI.
13. Pressure ulcers may occur in up to 35% of patients with SCI.
14. Spasticity may result in contractures.
15. Amenorrhea occurs in 60% of women with SCI, usually temporary.
16. Neuropathic pain occurs in 34% to 94% of patients with SCI.
17. Complications can arise from the halo apparatus in persons with cervical injuries.
    a. Pin/ring loosening—can result from bone reabsorption. Signs and symptoms include increased pain, altered pin position, and drainage.
    b. Infection—can result from bacterial infections. Signs and symptoms include drainage and erythema.
    c. Skull/dural penetration—can result from inner table penetration, usually due to a fall. Signs and symptoms include a headache, visual disturbances, and CSF leak from the pin site.
    d. Dysphagia and respiratory problems—can result from halo or vest positioning. Signs and symptoms include difficulty swallowing and respiratory distress.

Nursing Assessment

1. Assess cardiopulmonary status and vital signs to help determine degree of autonomic dysfunction, especially in patients with tetraplegia.
2. Determine LOC and cognitive function indicating TBI or other pathology.
3. Perform frequent motor and sensory assessment of trunk and extremities—extent of deficits may increase due to edema and hemorrhage. Later, increasing neurologic deficits and pain may indicate development of syringomyelia.
4. Note signs and symptoms of spinal shock, such as flaccid paralysis, urine retention, absent reflexes.
5. Assess bowel and bladder function.
6. Assess quality, location, and severity of pain.
7. Perform psychosocial assessment to evaluate motivation, support network, financial, or other problems.
8. Assess for indicators of powerlessness, including verbal expression of no control over situation, depression, nonparticipation, dependence on others, passivity.

Nursing Diagnoses

- Ineffective Breathing Pattern related to paralysis of respiratory muscles or diaphragm.
- Impaired Physical Mobility related to motor dysfunction.
- Risk for Impaired Skin Integrity related to immobility and sensory deficit.
- Urinary Retention related to neurogenic bladder.
- Constipation or Bowel Incontinence related to neurogenic bowel.
- Risk for Injury related to autonomic dysreflexia and orthostatic hypotension.
- Powerlessness related to loss of function, long rehabilitation, depression.
- Sexual Dysfunction related to erectile dysfunction and fertility changes.
- Chronic Pain related to neurogenic changes.

Nursing Interventions

Attaining an Adequate Breathing Pattern

1. For patients with high-level lesions, continuously monitor respirations and maintain a patent airway. Be prepared to intubate if respiratory fatigue or arrest occurs.
2. Frequently assess cough and vital capacity. Teach effective coughing, if patient is able (see Box 15-5).
3. Provide adequate fluids and humidification of inspired air to loosen secretions.
4. Suction, as needed; observe vagal response (bradycardia—should be temporary).
5. When appropriate, implement chest physiotherapy regimen to assist pulmonary drainage and prevent infection.
6. Monitor results of ABG values, chest x-ray, and sputum cultures.
7. Tape halo wrench to body jacket or halo traction in the event the jacket must be removed for basic or advanced life support or respiratory distress.

Promoting Mobility

1. Place the patient on firm bed until spinal cord stabilization. After stabilization, turn every 2 hours on a pressure reduction surface, ensuring good alignment. Specialized beds, such as a kinetic turning bed, may be used.
2. Logroll the patient with unstable SCI.
3. Perform ROM exercises to prevent contractures and maintain rehabilitation potential.

BOX 15-5 Assisted Coughing

Many patients with tetraplegia have an impairment of the diaphragmatic and intercostal muscles. The result is a weak or ineffective cough. To increase the mechanical effectiveness of the patient's cough, perform or teach the assisted cough technique.

1. Place the patient in supine, low semi-Fowler's position.
2. Place the heels of your hands on the costophrenic angle of the patient's rib cage.
3. With the patient's head turned away, ask the patient to hyperventilate and exhale once or twice. Allow your hands to move with the patient.
4. During the next breath, ask the patient to take a deep breath and cough while exhaling.
5. As the patient coughs, thrust your hands down and in (inferiorly and medially) to add power to the diaphragm during exhalation.
6. Allow one or two normal breaths and repeat the procedure.

 NURSING ALERT Incorrect hand placement may cause injury to the internal organs, ribs, and xiphoid process.

4. Monitor BP with position change in the patient with lesions above midthoracic area to prevent orthostatic hypotension.
5. Encourage physical therapy and practicing of exercises as tolerated. Functional electrical stimulation may facilitate independent standing and walking.
6. Encourage weight-bearing activity to prevent osteoporosis and risk of kidney stones.

 NURSING ALERT Never attempt to reposition the patient by grasping a halo or any other stabilization device. This may result in severe damage to the brain, head, or vertebra.

Protecting Skin Integrity

1. Pay special attention to pressure points when repositioning patient. Seating and mobility requirements must be determined.
2. Obtain pressure relief mattress and appropriate wheelchair and cushion.
3. Inspect for pressure ulcer development daily over bony prominences, including the back of head, ears, trunk, heels, and elbows. Observe under stabilization devices for pressure areas, particularly on the scapulae. Use a risk assessment tool to determine risk of developing pressure ulcer.
4. Keep skin clean, dry, and well lubricated.
5. Turn the patient a minimum of every 2 hours and instruct him to perform wheelchair weight shifts every 15 minutes. Place the patient in prone position at intervals, unless contraindicated.
6. Institute treatment for pressure ulcers immediately and relieve pressure to promote healing.

Promoting Urinary Elimination

1. Consider use of intermittent catheterization, typically beginning every 4 hours, as an alternative to an indwelling catheter.
2. If the patient has an upper motor neuron lesion (above L1) and no indwelling catheter, promote reflex voiding by tapping the bladder, gently pulling the patient's pubic hair, or stroking the patient's inner thigh.
3. If the patient has a lower motor neuron lesion (L1 or below) and no indwelling catheter, promote voiding by using a bladder Credé's method by gently compressing the suprapubic area to promote voiding.
4. Encourage fluid intake of 3,000 to 4,000 mL of fluid per day (2,000 mL per day if intermittent catheterization is used) to prevent infection and urinary calculi. Space fluids out over 24-hour period to avoid bladder overdistention. Juices should be encouraged to help decrease urinary pH (inhibiting stone production) and bacterial adherence to a catheter.
5. Monitor for urine retention by percussing the suprapubic area for dullness, catheterizing for residual urine after voiding, or using noninvasive devices such as the BladderScan.
6. Prophylactic antibiotics for prevention of recurrent UTIs are not supported due to the increase in resistant organisms.
7. The use of biofilms and other materials that inhibit adhesion of pathogens to catheters is being explored.

Promoting Bowel Elimination

1. Assess bowel sounds and note abdominal distention. Paralytic ileus is common immediately after injury.
2. Encourage intake of high-calorie, high-protein, and high-fiber (15 g) diet when food is tolerated.
3. Assess for loose stool oozing from rectum and perform rectal examination to check for fecal impaction; remove fecal matter, if necessary.
4. Institute a bowel program as early as possible.
   a. Schedule bowel care at the same time of day to develop a predictable outcome.
   b. Stimulate the gastrocolic reflex 30 minutes before bowel care with food or liquid intake.
   c. Perform bowel care with the patient in a bowel chair or in left side-lying position; the procedure should not take more than 2 hours.
   d. Use abdominal massage, deep breathing, warm fluids, and leaning forward in the chair to enhance success.
5. For patients with upper motor neuron lesions, perform reflexic bowel care.
   a. Insert a glycerin or bisacodyl suppository or mini-enema (4 mL).
   b. Alternatively, use digital stimulation with gloved, lubricated finger—perform a semicircular motion against posterior rectal wall. Repeat every 5 to 10 minutes until evacuation is complete.
6. For patients with lower motor neuron lesions, perform areflexic bowel care.
   a. Perform manual stool elimination.

7. Have the patient perform Valsalva maneuver (after urinary elimination to prevent vesicoureteral reflux of urine).

8. For chronic constipation without relief from more conservative approaches, consider a bulk-forming agent or laxative 8 hours before bowel care.

Preventing Autonomic Dysfunction and Orthostatic Hypotension

1. Be alert to signs of autonomic dysreflexia (see Box 15-6), try to avoid triggers, assess for causes, and treat, as directed.

2. Be alert for, prevent, and manage orthostatic hypotension, especially in patients with cervical SCI.

3. Use tilt table, as ordered, to gradually increase the patient's ability to tolerate sitting after acute SCI.

4. Other conservative strategies consist of use of embolic hose, abdominal binder, and high-salt diet.

5. Administer a sympathomimetic, such as ephedrine or pseudoephedrine, as ordered, before the patient is transferred to wheelchair.

 DRUG ALERT Caution should be exercised for patients with SCI who are taking tricyclic antidepressants because of autonomic dysfunction. SCI patients are more vulnerable to anticholinergic adverse effects and orthostatic hypotension. In addition, numerous potential drug reactions are associated with monoamine oxidase inhibitors and SCI.

Empowering the Patient

1. Explain all procedures to the patient. Answer questions.

2. Make sure that the patient plays an integral part in decision making about care plan. Allow the patient to make modifications to treatment plan when possible.

3. Schedule procedures and planning sessions when the patient is rested and experiencing decreased anxiety.

4. Praise the patient for incremental gains in function or participation.

5. Discuss stress management techniques, such as relaxation therapy, counseling, and problem solving.

6. Refer to vocational training program if the patient expresses an interest.

7. Use peer counseling for patient to gain support from others with SCI.

8. Be alert for signs of depression (problems with sleep, loss of interest, guilt, loss of energy, lack of concentration, change in appetite, feeling sad) or risk for suicide and refer to mental health counselor. Administer antidepressant medications, as directed.

9. Explore the use of hands-free environmental control units to control environment (eg, turn on television).

Minimizing Alteration in Sexuality and Fertility

1. Encourage the patient to discuss alternate expression of feelings with partner.

2. Advise bowel care and urinary elimination before intercourse.

BOX 15-6 | **Autonomic Dysreflexia**

Be aware of and try to prevent common causes of autonomic dysreflexia whenever possible:

- Bladder distention, UTI, bladder or kidney stones.
- Urinary abnormalities or procedures.
- Bowel distention, bowel impaction.
- Constrictive clothing, shoes, or apparatus.
- Noxious stimuli such as pain, strong smells, pressure.

Be alert for signs and symptoms of autonomic dysreflexia:

- Sudden and significant increase in systolic and diastolic BP 20–40 mm Hg above the patient's baseline. (Normal systolic BP for a person with tetraplegia is 90–110 mm Hg.) In children and adolescents, a systolic increase of >15–20 mm Hg above baseline is significant.
- Pounding headache.
- Bradycardia and/or cardiac arrhythmias.
- Profuse sweating, piloerection, and flushing above the level of injury (LOI).
- Blurred vision and spots in visual field.
- Nasal congestion.
- Apprehension and anxiety.

Take the following actions if autonomic dysreflexia occurs:

- Check BP; if elevated, call health care provider immediately.
- Immediately sit the patient up.
- Loosen clothing and other constrictive apparatus.

- Monitor BP every 2–5 minutes.
- Check the urinary system—catheterize patient (use 2% lidocaine jelly and wait 2 minutes); if catheter in place, check for kinks in tubing obstructing drainage; if catheter blockage suspected, gently irrigate with 10–15 mL normal saline (use 5–10 mL in children younger than age 2); replace catheter if not draining adequately.
- If BP remains > 150 mm Hg systolic, check for impaction (use 2% lidocaine jelly and wait 2 minutes). Remove stool.
- If BP remains > 150 mm Hg systolic, administer immediate-release nifedipine 10 mg (bite and swallow), nitroglycerin ointment 2% 1 inch (2.5 cm) above the LOI, or another antihypertensive agent.
- If autonomic dysreflexia is still unresolved, check for additional causes (eg, pressure ulcer, ingrown toenail).

After the episode of autonomic dysreflexia, document the following:

- Monitor BP for at least 2 hours for recurrent hypertension or symptomatic hypotension. Notify the health care provider as indicated.
- Provide patient teaching for prevention and treatment of complication.
- Make sure all caregivers understand autonomic dysreflexia and that the patient carries an identification card indicating LOI and emergency information.

3. Advise women that 90% regain regular menstrual cycles by 1 year. Pregnancy can occur and delivery occurs in 40% before 37 weeks' gestation. Autonomic dysreflexia may occur as a complication of delivery.
4. Refer the patient to a urologist or other health care provider to explore sexuality options.
   a. Women with SCI experience little sensation during sexual intercourse, but fertility and ability to bear children are usually not affected.
   b. Men with SCI may consider implantation of a penile prosthesis or an assistive device to obtain an erection. Sildenafil has been used to manage erectile dysfunction in men with SCI. Ejaculation is more common with lower motor neuron or incomplete injuries; men with injuries at T_{10} and above may ejaculate with vibrostimulation.

Reducing Pain

1. Assess pain using consistent pain scale. Report changes from baseline or new location or type of pain.
2. Manage neurogenic pain with pharmacologic agents, as directed.
3. Help the patient assess the effects of nonpharmacologic treatment such as acupuncture.

Community and Home Care Considerations

Promoting Optimal Function

1. Determine short- and long-term functional goals. Expected outcomes should relate to motor recovery, level of functional independence, social integration, and quality of life.
2. Monitor neurologic status, including functional outcomes, periodically throughout the patient's life span. Functional outcomes may relate to:
   a. Respiratory, bowel, bladder, and skin.
   b. Bed/wheelchair mobility, transfers, positioning.
   c. Standing and ambulation.
   d. Independent ADL, such as eating, grooming, bathing, and dressing.
   e. Communication, including speech, computer skills, handwriting, telephone.
   f. Transportation, including driving, adapted vehicle use, public transportation.
   g. Homemaking, including meal planning and preparation and chores.
3. Periodically evaluate the need for an increased level of assistance and equipment as the patient with an SCI ages.
4. Assist the patient in arranging modifications necessary to his or her home and in obtaining financial assistance for modifications to the environment.
5. Coordinate continued rehabilitation effort to ensure social support, ongoing pharmacologic treatment, and monitoring for long-term complications, such as depression; vocational training; and adaptation to home and work environments. Use Functional Independence Measure or other instrument to set and achieve goals with the patient in ADL, transferring, locomotion, and other functional aspects.
6. Teach bowel care and urinary elimination procedures to the patient and all caregivers to ensure continuity.

7. Teach care of traction and immobilization devices.
8. Enlist help of occupational therapist, physical therapist, vocational therapist, recreational therapist, and other specialists, as needed.
9. Alert caregivers that autonomic dysreflexia is a complication that may occur up to several years after SCI involving T6 and above. Teach the patient and caregivers preventive and emergency treatment measures.

Patient Education and Health Maintenance

1. Teach the patient and family about the physiology of nerve transmission and how the SCI has affected normal function, including mobility, sensation, and bowel and bladder function.
2. Reinforce that rehabilitation is lengthy and involves compliance with therapy to increase function.
3. Explain that spasticity may develop 2 weeks to 3 months after injury and may interfere with routine care and ADL.
4. Teach the patient to protect skin from pressure ulcer development by frequent repositioning while in bed, weight-shifting and liftoffs every 15 minutes while in a wheelchair, and avoiding shear forces and friction.
5. Teach inspection of skin daily for development of pressure ulcers, using a mirror, if necessary.
6. Encourage sexual counseling, if indicated, to promote satisfaction in personal relationships.
7. Teach importance of seat belts.

Evaluation: Expected Outcomes

- Respirations adequate, ABG values within normal limits.
- Repositioning hourly, no orthostatic changes.
- No evidence of pressure ulcers or DVT.
- Reflex (or areflexic) voiding without retention.
- Bowel evacuation controlled.
- No episodes of autonomic dysreflexia.
- Verbalizes feeling of control over condition.
- Patient and partner exploring sexuality and sexual options.
- Reports pain at or lower than 2 to 3 level on a scale of 1 to 10.

Vertebral Compression Fractures

 Evidence Base Ensrud, K. E., & Schousboe, J. T. (2011). Vertebral fractures. *New England Journal of Medicine, 364,* 1634–1642.

Vertebral fractures commonly occur with trauma, but can also be associated with osteoporosis or cancer.

Pathophysiology and Etiology

1. The vertebral body is made up of cancellous (soft) and outer cortical (hard) bone. The fracture creates an area of weakness within the vertebral column.
2. This weakness is further stressed and compressed with normal biomechanical stresses (weight-bearing activities from standing, sitting, and lifting). Over time, the fracture loses height, compressing the vertebral body.

3. The periosteum layer of the bone contains many pain receptors and with weight-bearing activities that apply pressure on the fractured bone, stimulates the nerve endings, thereby producing pain.

4. Risk factors include:
   a. Osteoporosis—women over age 50; men over age 70; prolonged use of steroids.
   b. Metastatic cancer—breast, lung, renal, prostrate, melanoma, multiple myeloma.

5. Other risk factors include:
   a. Smoking.
   b. Inactivity.
   c. Poor nutrition.

Clinical Manifestations

General Considerations

1. A vertebral body may fracture without causing debilitating pain.

2. Symptoms depend on location, extent of fracture, progression of fracture, and effect on surrounding structures.

3. Most symptomatic fractures result in pain, although the development of instability can result in sensory changes, loss of reflex, and muscle weakness from canal compromise.

Cervical

1. Pain and stiffness in the neck, top of shoulders, and region of the scapula.

2. Pain with rotation, flexion, and extension.

3. Paresthesias and numbness of upper extremities.

4. Weakness of upper extremities.

Thoracic/Lumbar

1. Middle to lower back pain at site of fracture.

2. Pain aggravated with activity and relieved with rest and flexion.

3. Progressive kyphosis or postural deformity of the lumbar spine. Progressive thoracic kyphosis decreases lung capacity and can compromise pulmonary function.

4. Point tenderness to palpation on clinical examination.

Diagnostic Evaluation

1. Plain x-rays (anterior–posterior and lateral views)—evaluate vertebral structure, height loss, and alignment.

2. CT scan—evaluation of extent of fracture and canal involvement.

3. MRI—differential diagnosis includes infectious process or metastatic lesion. MRI has greater sensitivity for soft-tissue abnormalities.

4. Bone scan—evaluation of microscopic changes within the bone. Identification of additional metastatic lesions, infectious process, microscopic fractures.

Management

Conservative Treatment

1. Orthosis/brace; heat or ice to affected area.

2. Physical therapy.

3. Anti-inflammatory drugs.

4. Analgesics, opioids may be necessary during acute phase.

5. Treatment and prevention of osteoporosis.

Surgical/Invasive Intervention

1. Surgical intervention—spinal instrumentation is not considered an option in patients with advanced osteoporosis secondary to the risk of nonfusion and hardware failure.

2. Vertebroplasty—injection of methylmethacrylate (bone cement) with barium (radiopaque) into vertebral body aimed at providing stabilization of vertebral body.

3. Kyphoplasty—partial restoration of vertebral height using percutaneous placement of a balloon into vertebral body, inflation of the balloon with radiopaque solution (creates a cavity), and deflation and removal of the balloon followed by insertion of methylmethacrylate with barium. May be done under moderate sedation or general anesthesia. Reduced risk of glue leakage secondary to creation of the cavity.

Complications

1. Pulmonary embolus due to leakage of cement into venous system following vertebroplasty or kyphoplasty.

2. Spinal cord or nerve root compromise due to leakage of cement following vertebroplasty or kyphoplasty.

3. Muscular spasms related to preprocedure deconditioning and postprocedure change in posture.

Nursing Assessment

1. Perform repeated assessments of motor function and sensation.

2. Assess for localized tenderness.

3. Assess pain level on scale of 1 to 10.

Nursing Diagnoses

- Acute Pain related to area of compression.
- Risk for Injury related to invasive procedure and recovery.

Nursing Interventions

Minimizing Pain

1. Administer or teach self-administration of analgesics as prescribed; inform patient about potential adverse effects (sedation, constipation, GI upset). Advise use of over-the-counter stool softeners.

2. Administer or teach self-administration of anti-inflammatories, as prescribed; advise taking with food or antacid to prevent GI upset.

3. Teach self-administration of muscle relaxants, as prescribed; inform patient about potential adverse effects of sedation.

4. Instruct in proper application and use of orthosis, if ordered.

5. Apply moist ice or heat to affected area of back, per patient-defined relief of pain.

6. Inspect skin several times a day, especially under stabilization devices, for redness and evidence of pressure sore development. Pressure ulcers can cause severe pain.

7. Educate the patient about vertebroplasty or kyphoplasty, as indicated.
   a. One to two small punctures with a large-bore needle will be made at site of vertebral body to be treated. Level will be verified using fluoroscopy before insertion of bone cement.
   b. Routine postprocedure care will include assessment of vital signs and neurologic function, pain control, and ambulation, as ordered.
8. Encourage compliance with physical therapy treatments, as ordered.

Preventing Injury Postoperatively

1. Monitor vital signs and assess movement and sensation of extremities. Report any new deficit. CT of spine may be ordered if encroachment on spinal cord or nerve root is suspected.
2. Assess respiratory status and report any breathing difficulties. Chest x-ray or CT of chest (PE protocol) may be ordered if pulmonary embolus is suspected.
3. Administer analgesics and NSAIDs to control pain from incision and muscular inflammation due to procedure.
4. Enforce bed rest for 2 to 3 hours; patient may turn side to side, as directed; gradually increase activity, as tolerated.
5. Position for comfort. May apply heat or ice to affected muscles if spasm occurs and administer muscle relaxant, as indicated.
6. Report any increasing pain, weakness, or breathing difficulties.

Patient Education and Health Maintenance

1. Advise the patient of 10- to 25-lb lifting restriction for 1 week after vertebroplasty/kyphoplasty, as ordered, and to avoid strenuous activities; level of activity may be increased gradually as status indicates.
2. Demonstrate proper body mechanics to be used for bending, reaching, lifting in all activities.
3. Alternate ice and heat for 20-minute intervals five to six times per day, as needed.
4. No soaking baths for 1 week to enhance wound healing of puncture sites.
5. Encourage the patient to do stretching and strengthening exercises for back and aerobic exercise for endurance on a daily basis.
6. Physical therapy may be indicated for reconditioning, heat therapy, and massage.
7. Instruct the patient to report any changes in neurologic function or recurrence of pain.

Evaluation: Expected Outcomes

- Verbalizes reduced pain.
- Vital signs stable, respirations unlabored, out of bed without difficulty.

Peripheral Nerve Injury

Peripheral nerve injury (PNI) is an injury to nerves in the upper extremity (eg, radial, ulnar, median) or lower extremity (eg, peroneal, sciatic, femoral, tibial). PNI may include damage to major nerves, the nerve root, the plexus (eg, brachial or lumbar), and other peripheral sites.

Pathophysiology and Etiology

1. The incidence of PNI is approximately 2% to 3% in populations with multiple injuries. Males have higher incidence than females.
2. PNI damage may occur by congenital, traumatic, chemical, pathologic, thermal, or mechanical means. Focal trauma is the most common of all PNI. Injuries can be direct (eg, gunshot) or indirect (eg, casting).
3. The most frequently injured site is the upper extremity, specifically the upper arm. Childhood PNIs occur predominantly in the lower extremities.
4. Injury to the nerve causes impairment in axonal function and, possibly, disruption of myelination. Approximately 50% of motor nerves and 75% of cutaneous nerves are myelinated. Schwann cells contain multiple axons. Myelinated axons enhance conduction between nodes, accelerating transmission compared to nonmyelinated axons. Fibers are classified according to diameter, conduction speed, myelination, and target.
5. Sensory regeneration, as opposed to motor regeneration, may take years following a PNI.
6. Nerve injuries are classified according to the Sunderland system, which establishes grades of nerve function on which to base recovery and need for surgery.
   a. First-degree PNI (neurapraxia)—there is a conduction impairment but the anatomy is intact. Complete recovery is anticipated in 3 months.
   b. Second-degree PNI (axonotmesis)—Wallerian degeneration occurs distal to the PNI site and axons disintegrate. Complete recovery is anticipated.
   c. Third-degree PNI—scarring occurs in the endoneural tube. Axons recover 1 inch (2.5 cm) per month. Incomplete recovery is anticipated.
   d. Fourth-degree PNI (eg, crush injury)—axonal regeneration is blocked by scar tissue. Surgical repair is typically required.
   e. Fifth-degree PNI (eg, penetrating trauma)—the peripheral nerve is severed. Surgical intervention is required.
7. Compression neuropathy depends on the amount and extent of compression force. Edema, connective tissue thickening, and segmental demyelization of large fibers occur.
8. Useful function can be achieved when up to 75% of axons are damaged.

Clinical Manifestations

1. Flaccid paralysis.
2. Absent deep tendon reflexes.
3. Atonic/hypotonic muscles.
4. Progressive muscle atrophy.
5. Fasciculations peak 2 to 3 weeks after injury.
6. Trophic changes: skin is warm and dry 3 weeks after injury, then becomes cold and cyanotic with loss of hair, brittle fingernails, and ulceration.
7. Causalgia (chronic pain syndrome): Neuropathic pain may be crawling, electric, tingling, or burning. (It typically follows the cutaneous sensory nerve distribution of the PNI.)

8. Specifics to area affected:

a. Radial nerve injury—weakness in extension, possible wrist drop, inability to grasp objects/make a fist, impaired sensation over posterior forearm and dorsum of the hand.

b. Brachial plexus—difficulty in abduction of shoulder, weakness with supination and flexion of the forearm (upper trunk) or extension of the forearm (middle trunk), or paralysis and atrophy of small muscles of the hand (lower trunk).

c. Median and ulnar nerve injuries—sensory (median nerve) and motor (ulnar) loss of function in the hand (pronation, opposition of thumb, paralysis of finer flexor muscles).

d. Femoral—weakness of knee and hip extension, atrophy of quadriceps, absence of knee jerk, loss of sensation of anterior aspect of the thigh.

e. Common peroneal—foot drop, sensory loss on dorsum of foot, difficulty with eversion.

f. Sciatic—foot drop, pain across gluteus and thigh, loss of knee flexion, weakness/paralysis of muscles below knee.

9. Chronic nerve compression may begin with intermittent signs and symptoms; these may only occur in specific maneuvers such as digital pressure or position. For example, damage to the brachial plexus, entrapped at the supra/infraclavicular junction, may elicit symptoms following arm elevation for 1 minute. In carpal tunnel syndrome (compression of the median nerve), wrist flexion or external pressure applied proximally to the carpal tunnel may evoke symptoms.

Diagnostic Evaluation

1. The electrodiagnostic examination consists of nerve conduction studies (sensory, motor, mixed) and needle electrode examination.

a. The electrodiagnostic examination tests only large myelinated axons; it does not assess pain, temperature, or paresthesia.

b. It can confirm PNI occurrence and determine the type of axon, pathophysiology, severity, location, and injury prognosis.

2. Muscle ultrasonography evaluates the extent of muscle involvement and assesses acute nerve injuries.

3. MRI and electrophysiologic studies such as electroneurography and EMG detect the site and degree of nerve injury.

4. Muscle imaging may detect atrophy and mesenchymal alteration of skeletal muscles.

5. Tinel's sign (tapping the axons of the regenerating nerve produces a paresthesia in the normal distribution of the nerve) reveals the rate of axonal regeneration.

Management

1. Microsurgery reapproximates the severed peripheral nerve endings. The sooner the repair is performed, the better the chance of recovery. Microsurgical repair can be done with tension-free coaptation using technology such as carbon dioxide laser welding, fibrin gluing, and ring coupling. Autogenous nerve grafts are the gold standard.

2. Primary nerve repair (neurorrhaphy) may be done within 1 week of injury (eg, open wounds—except gunshots). Secondary nerve repair is performed after 1 week (eg, crush injury with soft tissue damage). In partially transected nerves, surgery may be delayed 2 to 3 months to determine whether regeneration will take place.

a. Nerve grafting—Two neurorrhaphy sites are used. Thin, cutaneous nerve grafts with large fascicles and minimal connective tissue are optimal. Common donor sites include the sacral nerve (lateral aspect of the foot), lateral antebrachial cutaneous nerve (lateral forearm), and the median antebrachial cutaneous nerve (medial arm and elbow). Small segments of nerve grafts may be placed to create a bridge to facilitate axonal and Schwann cell growth. Nerve "conduits," connectors of nerve sites, may be composed of bone, vein, artery, silicone, or other material.

b. End-to-side neurorrhaphy—the severed nerve's distal end is attached to the side of a healthy nerve.

c. Nerve transfer—Ideally, the donor nerve fascicles are in close proximity to the target muscle motor end plate or target sensory nerve. If the patient has multiple nerve injuries, such as a complete brachial plexus injury, nerve transfer priority is given to promoting elbow flexion, shoulder abduction, and external rotation, respectively. Sensory nerve priorities are given to the ulnar thumb and radial index finger.

3. Tissue expansion is used to compensate for tissue deficit.

4. Insulin-like growth factor and acidic fibroblast growth factor have enhanced regeneration when administered systemically or topically and other factors are being investigated.

5. Corticosteroids may be used to decrease edema.

6. Occupational therapy may be consulted to splint or cast the patient. Splinting (eg, hands) or casting may be indicated to reduce tension on the PNI site and facilitate healing. Day splints are typically functional splints; night splints are positioning splints. Splint material depends on the amount of resistance to be exerted by the orthosis, the splint size, and the patient's compensatory movements.

a. Radial nerve splint—volar or dorsal cock-up splints are indicated if wrist extension is impaired.

b. Median nerve splint—a thumb opposition splint preserves the function of the hand grip.

c. Ulnar nerve splint—this functional and positioning splint prevents "claw hand" deformity and contractures of fingers four and five.

7. Flexibility is primarily due to connective tissues stretching as opposed to muscle contraction. Passive and active ROM exercises are essential to provide stretch and prevent contractions. Ultrasound diathermy may be used on deep muscles, and topical heat may be used for superficial muscles to promote stretching. Progressive resistance and strengthening, including isometric activities, are used to restore function. Functional electrical stimulation may also be used.

8. Fibrosis, caused by edema, may be minimized by elevating the affected limb. Using static graduated compression devices (eg, sleeves, gloves, hose) or sequential compression devices, distal to proximal wrapping, may also minimize edema. Likewise, massage may reduce edema.

9. Desensitization techniques (eg, scheduled exposure to irritating textures, vibration) may be used to manage hyperesthesia. Sensory reeducation may be protective (compensatory). Sensory restoration is progressive, with temperature and pain returning first, followed by transient light touch and vibration.

10. Neuropathic pain may be managed by traditional analgesics, antidepressants (eg, tricyclic), anticonvulsants (eg, gabapentin), topical and transdermal agents (eg, capsaicin), NSAIDs, alpha-adrenergic agonists (eg, clonidine), calcium channel blockers (eg, nicardipine), or transcutaneous electrical stimulation.

11. Carpal tunnel syndrome management may include activity modification, NSAIDs, serial steroid injections, vitamin B_6, diuretics, and a wrist splint for 6 months. Endoscopic surgical release of the ligament may also be an option.

12. Complex peripheral injuries, such as injury to the brachial plexus, may require multimodal treatment, including surgery, pain management, and functional rehabilitation. A multidisciplinary team approach is most effective in maximizing outcomes.

Complications

1. Infection, if injury is penetrating and site becomes contaminated.
2. Compartment syndrome due to edema or positioning.
3. Muscle atrophy/flaccid paralysis; disuse syndrome.
4. Sensory deficit.
5. Contractures.
6. Chronic pain.
7. Nerve damage resulting from surgical repair.

Nursing Assessment

1. Perform frequent neurovascular checks of the affected extremity (pressure, vibration, and two-point discrimination sensation; motor function, strength; pulses; temperature; capillary refill; degree of swelling).
2. Assess degree of pain on a scale of 0 to 10.
3. Test reflexes of affected extremity.
4. Observe for signs of infection if there is an open wound.
5. Assess for concomitant injuries such as head or skeletal trauma.

Nursing Diagnoses

- Risk for Peripheral Neurovascular Dysfunction.
- Chronic Pain related to injury.
- Risk for Infection secondary to tissue disruption, surgery.

Nursing Interventions

Protecting Neurovascular Function

1. Administer corticosteroids and diuretics, as ordered, to decrease swelling and development of compartment syndrome.
2. Keep extremity elevated to promote venous drainage.
3. Perform neurovascular check to evaluate status of injury.
   a. Incorporate Tinel's sign into assessment.
   b. Report any changes in condition.

4. Postoperatively assist rehabilitation team in reeducating nerves and muscles to achieve function.
5. Observe for paresthesias, pain, or altered skin integrity in areas of splinting and casting.

Promoting Comfort

1. Administer and teach self-administration of analgesics, as ordered.
2. Elevate extremity.
3. Avoid exposing denervated areas to temperature extremes.
4. Apply such devices as splints and slings, as ordered.
5. Maintain mobility with ROM exercises. Perform gently, following administration of analgesics.

Preventing Infection

1. Assess wound and dressing frequently for erythema, warmth, swelling, odor, and drainage.
2. Monitor temperature with vital signs for hyperthermia and tachycardia, indicating infection.
3. Encourage deep-breathing exercises and ambulation to prevent pulmonary complications.

Patient Education and Health Maintenance

1. Teach management of wound and dressing and casts or splints.
2. Review analgesia schedule and need for elevation of injured area.
3. Teach exercises for involved area.
4. Suggest assistive devices to promote independence.
5. Stress the importance of complying with long-term rehabilitation, physical therapy, and follow-up evaluations.
6. Support a community accident prevention program, including the use of seat belts, industrial regulations, and sports and recreational safety measures.

Evaluation: Expected Outcomes

- Stable neurovascular status; functional use of extremity.
- Patient reports adequate relief of pain.
- Wound/surgical site free of erythema, drainage, odor.

CENTRAL NERVOUS SYSTEM TUMORS

Brain Tumors

Intracranial neoplasms are the result of abnormal proliferation of cells within the CNS. A *tumor* is a mass of cancerous cells within the brain. It is believed that there is a 2- to 3-cm surrounding area of cancer cells with the potential to develop into a tumor. Tumors require blood to grow and recruit a vascular supply to support the metabolic needs of the tumor. Intracranial tumors are primary or metastatic tumors and malignancy depends on cell type and location. Primary tumors include tumors of the brain itself, the skull or meninges, the pituitary gland, and the blood vessels. Metastatic tumors spread from the primary site of cancer (breast, lung, prostate, kidney) through the vascular supply and lymphatic systems. Defining primary cancer cell type determines the treatment modality and influences the overall prognosis.

Primary CNS tumor etiology remains unknown. Glioma research has identified a genetic mutation of p53 on chromosome 17 occurs in 50% of all cancers. Loss of heterozygosity of chromosome arm 10q also has been reported in gliomas, although research continues into potential genetic mutation and growth factors, as well as attempting to identify a tumor marker. No known environmental risks have been identified. Primary CNS tumors rarely metastasize outside the CNS.

Pathophysiology and Etiology

1. May originate in the CNS or metastasize from tumors elsewhere in the body (see Figure 15-11).
2. May be benign or malignant; all tumors produce effects of space-occupying lesion (edema, increased ICP). Malignancy may be related not only to cell type and invasiveness but also to location and operative accessibility (ie, the tumor is located in an area of the brain that will not tolerate compression of the brain structures or is not surgically accessible). The World Health Organization grading scale is currently used to classify gliomas, although other grading scales are available. The grading system evaluates the probability of tumor recurrence and malignancy from low (Grades I to II) to high (Grades III to IV).
3. May arise from any tissue of the CNS.
4. Common tumor types:
   a. Gliomas—tumors of the neuroepithelial/glial cells (supportive tissue of the brain; account for 40% to 50% of intracranial neoplasms):
      i. Astrocytoma—overgrowth of the astrocyte cells (connective tissue) of the brain. Tumors are graded on a scale from I to IV that defines growth pattern, invasiveness, infiltration, cell differentiation, margination, and necrosis. Grade I (polycystic astrocytoma)—slow-growing tumor with well-defined cells and minimal infiltration; Grade II (astrocytoma)—some atypical cells with higher rate of recurrence and risk of advancing to Grade III or IV with recurrence; Grade III (anaplastic astrocytoma) that is highly invasive and infiltrative, with poorly marginated cells and a rapid growth pattern and risk of advancing to Grade IV with

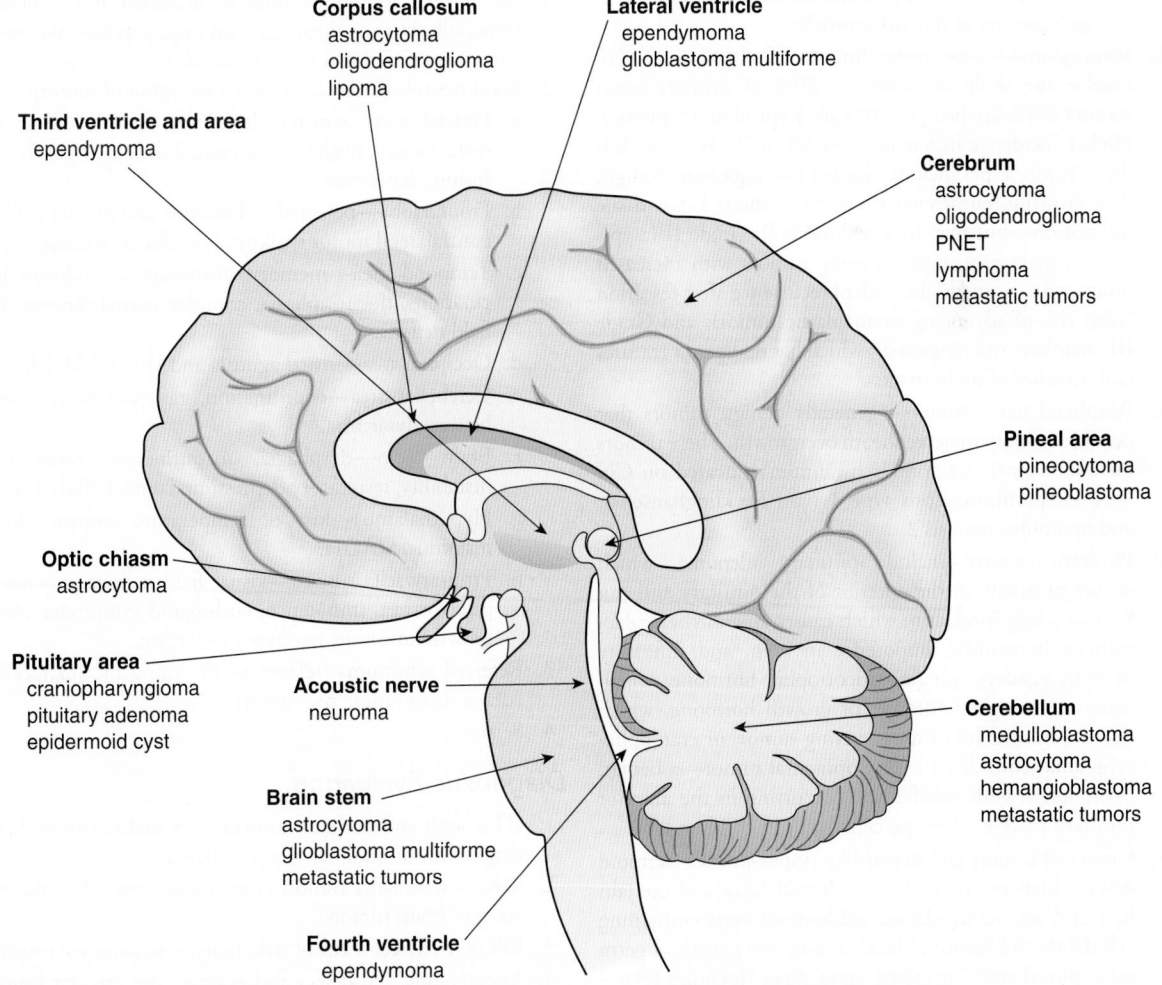

Corpus callosum
astrocytoma
oligodendroglioma
lipoma

Lateral ventricle
ependymoma
glioblastoma multiforme

Third ventricle and area
ependymoma

Cerebrum
astrocytoma
oligodendroglioma
PNET
lymphoma
metastatic tumors

Pineal area
pineocytoma
pineoblastoma

Optic chiasm
astrocytoma

Pituitary area
craniopharyngioma
pituitary adenoma
epidermoid cyst

Acoustic nerve
neuroma

Cerebellum
medulloblastoma
astrocytoma
hemangioblastoma
metastatic tumors

Brain stem
astrocytoma
glioblastoma multiforme
metastatic tumors

Fourth ventricle
ependymoma

Figure 15-11. Common brain tumor sites.

recurrence; Grade IV (glioblastoma multiforme)—a malignant tumor that is highly invasive, infiltrative, and poorly marginated with necrosis and a very rapid growth pattern (accounts for 55% of gliomas).

ii. Oligodendroglioma—overgrowth of oligodendroglial cells with calcification. Begins as a less invasive tumor but demonstrates malignancy as it progresses. The frontal and temporal lobes of the cerebrum are common locations. Rare in children.

iii. Ependymoma (5% to 6% of intracranial gliomas)—overgrowth of the ependymal cells of the brain. Slow growing; commonly occurs in the floor of the 4th ventricle; presents with signs and symptoms of increased ICP and hydrocephalus; 69% of cases occur in children.

iv. Mixed gliomas—two or more cell types within a tumor.

v. Medulloblastoma—most common pediatric malignant tumor. Commonly located in the 4th ventricle/cerebellar vermis; rapid growth pattern, highly invasive; high risk for metastasis within CSF.

vi. Hemangioblastoma—rare, benign tumor commonly located in the posterior fossa. von Hippel-Lindau disease is multiple hemangiomas within CNS.

vii. Colloid cyst—a rare cyst that contains neuroepithelial cells; occurs in the 3rd ventricle.

b. Meningioma—arise from linings of the brain. Can involve the skull; accounts for 20% of primary brain tumors (90% are benign; 10% are atypical or anaplastic). Higher incidence in females ages 40 to 70. Rare in children. Tumor types include Grade I meningiomas (benign, slow-growing, encapsulated lesions without brain tissue infiltration—but may have a dural tail); Grade II (atypical meningiomas), rapid-growing tumors with increased miotic activity and higher risk of recurrence after resection (with risk of advancing to anaplastic tumor); and Grade III (anaplastic meningioma), which has malignant features and invasion of brain tissue.

c. Peripheral nerve tumors—generally benign tumors that occur secondary to nerve sheath overgrowth. These tumors include acoustic neuroma/schwannoma (located on CN VIII); neurofibromatosis type 1 (von Recklinghausen's); and neurofibromatosis 2.

d. Pituitary tumors—include pituitary adenoma, which occurs primarily in the anterior of the pituitary and can be a secreting (prolactin, which causes amenorrhea/galactorhhea in women, impotence in men, and infertility in both genders; adrenocorticotrophic hormone, which causes Cushing's syndrome; or growth hormone, which causes acromegaly) or nonsecreting tumor; or craniopharyngioma (considered a developmental tumor—a benign cystic lesion with calcification, occurring in the anterior pituitary margin. (Fifty percent occur in children.)

e. Germ cell tumors and tumor-like cysts—include dermoid cysts, which occur in the ectodermal layer and contain hair and sebaceous glands; epidermoid cysts containing cell debris and keratin; pineal tumor, overgrowth of germ cells, pineal cells, or mixed germ types (includes teratomas) within the pineal region (more common in children

and males); and cordoma, a rare neoplasm that contains embryonic remnant occurring along the neuraxis.

f. Hematopoietic tumors—include primary malignant lymphoma (rare, diffusely infiltrating tumor of the brain, occurs in adults, high rate of recurrence), and secondary lymphoma associated with AIDS.

g. Secondary CNS tumors/metastatic lesions—commonly from lung cancer (40% to 50%), breast cancer (14% to 20%), melanoma (10%), renal (5%), and undetermined primary sites (10% to 15%). Single lesions common with lung and breast cancer, can have multiple lesions that are unresectable. Indicate systemic spread of primary cancer. Metastatic lesions account for 50% of all brain tumors.

Clinical Manifestations

Manifestations depend on the location and biologic nature of the tumor. If the tumor is in a noneloquent area of the brain or is slow-growing, specific symptoms may not develop until the late stages of the process. Instead, the tumor may produce generalized symptoms related to the increasing size of the tumor and the expanding area of cerebral edema surrounding the margins of the tumor. This is referred to as the "mass" effect of the tumor.

1. Generalized symptoms (due to increased ICP)—headache (especially in the morning), vomiting, papilledema, malaise, altered cognition and consciousness.
2. Focal neurologic deficits (related to region of tumor):
   a. Parietal area—sensory alterations, speech and memory disturbances, neglect, visuospatial deficits, right–left confusion, depression.
   b. Frontal lobe—personality, behavior, and memory changes; contralateral motor weakness; nonfluent aphasia.
   c. Temporal area—memory disturbances, auditory hallucinations, fluent aphasia, complex partial seizures, visual field deficits.
   d. Occipital area—visual agnosia and visual field deficits.
   e. Cerebellar area—coordination, gait, and balance disturbances, dysarthria.
   f. Brain stem—dysphagia, incontinence, cardiovascular instability, respiratory depression, coma, CN dysfunction.
   g. Hypothalamus—loss of temperature control, diabetes insipidus, SIADH.
   h. Pituitary/sella turcica—visual field deficits, amenorrhea, galactorrhea, impotence, cushingoid symptoms, elevated growth hormone, panhypopituitarism.
3. Referred symptoms (related to the vasogenic [extracellular] edema surrounding the tumor).
4. Seizures.

Diagnostic Evaluation

1. CT—with and without contrast to visualize tumor, hemorrhage, shift of midline, cerebral edema.
2. MRI—to visualize tumor; more useful than CT in the evaluation of brain tumors.
3. EEG—to detect locus of irritability, if seizures are present.
4. Angiography—to detect and evaluate the vascular supply of the tumor.

5. MR spectroscopy—evaluates the neurochemicals located within a core segment of the lesion; useful in differentiating tumors from infectious lesions.

6. Functional MRI—evaluates the functional eloquence of the brain tissue affected by the tumor, and the tissue at risk, for mass effect.

7. Skull radiography—to determine bone involvement, identify pineal shift, helpful in children.

8 Stealth guided surgery or stereotactic biopsy surgery—needed for definitive diagnosis, cell type.

Management

Effectiveness of treatment depends on tumor type and location, capsulation, or infiltrative status. Tumors in vital areas, such as the brain stem, or nonencapsulated and infiltrating tumors, may not be surgically accessible and treatment may produce severe neurologic deficits (blindness, paralysis, mental impairment). Treatment is usually multimodal.

 NURSING ALERT Treatment of gliomas is palliative. There is no current treatment modality that provides a definitive cure. Treatment is aimed at improving duration of survival.

1. Surgery—removal/debulking by way of craniotomy, stealth guidance, laser resection, or ultrasonic aspiration.
   a. Craniotomy: goal is gross total resection of the tumor for maximum removal of tumor cells. Biopsy may be performed on tumors in eloquent locations; whereas surgery may not be an option for some tumors secondary to location. Gross total resection is associated with longer survival compared with subtotal resection in glioblastoma multiforme; 10% are inoperable based on location of the tumor.
   b. Awake craniotomy—allows intraoperative brain mapping.
   c. Image-guided surgery—computer-generated intraoperative localization of lesion.
   d. Laser resection or ultrasonic aspiration—may augment surgical resection.
   e. Endovascular treatment—useful in embolization of the arterial feeders to the meningiomas to reduce surgical risk related to blood loss.

2. Radiation therapy—external radiation to tumor bed with 2- to 3-cm border.
   a. Conventional therapy daily for 6 weeks; shorter to brain stem.
   b. Prophylactic radiation to brain stem for other brain tumors with high risk of metastasis.
   c. Brachytherapy—can use radioisotopes implanted through interstitial catheters to permit high doses for high-grade malignant tumors.

3. Radiosurgery—stereotactic radiosurgery by way of linear accelerator scalpel, proton beam, or gamma knife delivers a single, high dose of radiation to a precisely targeted tumor area. Destroys only targeted abnormal tissue, limiting damage to surrounding brain tissue.

4. Chemotherapy (the blood–brain barrier limits the effectiveness of chemotherapy agents).
   a. Metastatic tumors—single or combination drug therapy; may require autologous bone marrow transplantation (aspirated before chemotherapy and reinfused afterward to treat bone marrow depression).
   b. Primary glioma—may be used as adjunct to surgery and radiation.
      i. Temozolomide, an oral agent, is considered first line in chemotherapy for glioblastoma multiforme.
      ii. Carmustine (BCNU) wafers are biodegradable chemotherapy wafers that are surgically placed into the tumor bed during tumor debulking. Up to 8 wafers are placed in the space where the tumor was located and they slowly break down over time.
      iii. Bevacizumab, an anti-angiogenic agent that is used in recurrent colorectal cancer, has been used in recurrent glioblastoma multiforme. Preliminary date demonstrates a 20% to 26% tumor response.
      iv. Immunotherapy (epidermal growth factor receptor variant III) remains investigational, though has shown promising results in phase II studies.

5. Shunting procedure—to manage hydrocephalus, which may be obstructive or nonobstructive depending on location, tumor type, degree of necrosis, and associated edema and inflammation.

6. Supportive therapy and medications.
   a. AEDs for treatment of seizure activity. AEDs may be utilized for seizure prophylaxis (see page 553).
   b. Dexamethasone to reduce swelling and reduce radiation edema; also given during end stage to enhance quality of life.

7. Investigational therapies currently in progress:
   a. ICT-107, an immune-based cancer treatment, is currently in phase III of evaluation.
   b. Sunitinib, currently in phase II of evaluation.
   c. Ongoing studies include gene therapy, second messenger inhibition, O-6-methylguanine-DNA methyltransferase, targeted toxins, and intratumor dosing of chemotherapy via glial balloon.

Complications

1. Increased ICP and brain herniation; death.
2. Neurologic deficits from expanding tumor or treatment.

Nursing Assessment

1. Assess vital signs and signs of increased ICP (see page 487).
2. Assess CN function, LOC, mental status, affect, and behavior.
3. Monitor for seizures.
4. Assess level of pain using visual analogue scale (0 to 10) or face scale, as indicated.
5. Assess level of anxiety.
6. Assess patient and family patterns of coping, support systems, and resources.
7. If treated with chemotherapy, assess bone marrow function by monitoring neutrophil and platelet counts.

Nursing Diagnoses

- Acute Pain related to brain mass, surgical intervention.
- Risk for Injury related to altered LOC, possible seizures, increased ICP, and sensory and motor deficits.
- Anxiety related to diagnosis, surgery, radiation, and/or chemotherapy.
- Imbalanced Nutrition: Less Than Body Requirements related to compromised neurologic function and stress of injury.
- Disabled Family Coping related to changes in roles and structure.

Nursing Interventions

Relieving Pain

1. Provide analgesics around the clock at regular intervals that will not mask neurologic changes.
2. Maintain the head of the bed at 15 to 30 degrees to reduce cerebral venous congestion.
3. Provide a darkened room or sunglasses if the patient is photophobic.
4. Maintain a quiet environment to increase patient's pain tolerance.
5. Provide scheduled rest periods to help patient recuperate from stress of pain.
6. Instruct the patient to lie with the operative side up.
7. Alter diet, as tolerated, if patient has pain on chewing.
8. Collaborate with patient on alternative ways to reduce pain such as use of music therapy.

Preventing Injury

1. Report any signs of increased ICP or worsening neurologic condition to health care provider immediately.
2. Adjust care to reduce risk of increased ICP; body positioning without flexion of head, reduce hip flexion, distribute care throughout the 24-hour period to allow ICP to return to baseline.
3. Monitor laboratory data, CSF cultures, and Gram stains and communicate results to medical staff.
4. Monitor intake and output, osmolality studies, and electrolytes; prevent overhydration, which can worsen cerebral edema.
5. Monitor response to pharmacologic therapy, including drug levels.
6. Initiate seizure precautions; pad the side rails of the bed to prevent injury if seizures occur; have suction equipment available.
7. Maintain availability of medications for management of status epilepticus (see page 562).
8. Initiate fall precautions; side rails up at all times, call light within reach at bedside, assist with toileting on a regular basis.
9. Gradually progress patient to ambulation with assistance as tolerated, enlist help from physical therapist, occupational therapist early, as indicated, to prevent falls.
10. If the patient is dysphagic or unconscious, initiate aspiration precautions: elevate head of the bed 30 degrees and position patient's head to the side to prevent aspiration.
11. If dysphagic, position the patient upright and instruct in sequenced swallowing to maintain feeding function (see page 504).

12. Maintain oxygen and suction at the bedside in case of aspiration.
13. For the patient with visual field deficits, place materials in visual field.
14. Provide appropriate care and teaching for patient receiving chemotherapy (see page 149).
15. Provide appropriate care and teaching for the patient receiving radiation (see page 153).
16. Provide routine postoperative care for the patient undergoing craniotomy (see page 492).

Minimizing Anxiety

1. Provide a safe environment in which the patient may verbalize anxieties.
2. Help the patient to express feelings related to fear and anxiety.
3. Answer questions and provide written information.
4. Include the patient/family in all treatment options and scheduling.
5. Introduce stress management techniques.
6. Provide consistency in care and continually provide emotional support.
7. Assess the patient's usual coping behaviors and provide support in these areas.
8. Consult with social worker for community resources.

 NURSING ALERT Anxiety and depression prior to and following surgery is associated with shorter postsurgical survival in patients with glioblastoma multiforme. Screening assessments can be performed with standard instruments and levels indicating a high risk of anxiety or depression should be reported to the health care provider.

Optimizing Nutrition

1. Medicate for nausea before position changes, radiation, or chemotherapy, and as needed.
2. Maintain adequate hydration within guidelines for cerebral edema.
3. Offer small, frequent meals as tolerated.
4. Consult with dietitian to evaluate food choices and provide adequate caloric needs through enteral or parenteral nourishment if unable to take oral nutrition.
5. Alter consistency of diet, as necessary, to enhance intake.

Strengthening Family Coping

1. Recognize stages of grief.
2. Foster a trusting relationship.
3. Provide clear, consistent explanations of procedures and treatments.
4. Encourage family involvement in care from the beginning.
5. Establish a means of communication for family with patient when verbal responses are not possible.
6. Consult with social worker and mental health provider if the family needs assistance in adjusting to neurologic deficits.
7. Assist the family to use stress management techniques and community resources such as respite care.

8. Encourage discussion with health care provider about prognosis and functional outcome.

9. Discuss development of advance directive and durable power of attorney (DPA). Maintain positive attitude and define that rationale as a way to allow for patient-defined extent of care in the advent of deterioration.

Patient Education and Health Maintenance

1. Explain the adverse effects of treatment.

2. Encourage close follow-up after diagnosis and treatment.

3. Explain the importance of continuing corticosteroids and how to manage adverse effects, such as weight gain and hyperglycemia.

4. Encourage the use of community resources for physical and psychological support, such as transportation to medical appointments, financial assistance, and respite care.

5. Refer the patient/family for more information and support to such agencies as the National Institute of Neurologic Disorders and Stroke (*www.ninds.nih.gov*) and the National Brain Tumor Foundation (*www.braintumor.org*).

Evaluation: Expected Outcomes

- Reports satisfactory comfort level.
- No new neurologic deficits, seizures, falls, or other injuries.
- Expresses decreased anxiety.
- Nutritional intake meeting metabolic demands.
- Patient and family verbalize understanding of treatment and available resources.

Tumors of the Spinal Cord and Canal

Tumors of the spinal cord and canal may be extradural (existing outside the dural membranes), including chordoma and osteoblastoma; intradural–extramedullary (within the SAS), including meningiomas, neurofibromas, and schwannomas; or intramedullary (within the spinal cord), including astrocytomas, ependymomas, and neurofibromatosis "dumbbell tumors." Vascular tumors can affect any part of the spinal cord or canal.

Pathophysiology and Etiology

1. Astrocytomas, characterized by asymmetrical expansion in the spinal cord, are more common in children than adults. Ependymomas, usually with a cyst, are the most common intramedullary tumor in the adult, but are rare in children. These tumors are central in the spinal cord.

2. Vascular tumors can affect the spinal cord in various ways. Hemangioblastomas often cause edema and syrinx formation. Cavernomas are located on the dorsal surface of the spinal cord.

3. Approximately 85% of all patients with cancer develop bony metastasis, with the spinal column as the primary site. Spinal cord compression due to cancer typically presents with incomplete paraplegia involving the thoracic spine.

4. Cause for abnormal cell growth is unknown.

5. Extradural tumors spread to the vertebral bodies.

6. Spinal cord and/or nerve compression can result.

Clinical Manifestations

Depends on location and type of tumor and extent of spinal cord compression.

1. Back pain that is localized or radiates; may be absent in more than 50% of patients.

2. Weakness of extremity with abnormal reflexes.

3. Sensory changes.

4. Bladder, bowel, or sexual dysfunction.

Diagnostic Evaluation

1. A plain x-ray or CT scan can detect a pathologic fracture, collapse, or destruction resulting from a mass.

2. MRI is sensitive to tumor detection.

3. CT myelography with lumbar puncture is sensitive to tumor detection but may be uncomfortable and result in complications from lumbar puncture.

Management

1. Two surgical approaches may be used to manage spinal cord tumors:

    a. Anterior decompression is typically indicated because most spinal cord tumors are anterior.

    b. The posterolateral approach may be used for excision of thoracic tumors. Endoscopy, or other surgical techniques using instrumentation, can be used to visualize the anterior part of the cord. In thoracic tumors above T_5, posterolateral decompression negates the need for an anterior thoracotomy or sternotomy.

2. Intraoperative somatosensory-evoked potentials and motor-evoked potentials can be used to "map" the optimal spinal cord site for incision and identify sensory and motor tracts within the spinal cord. This mapping reduces the neurologic deficits that are frequently associated with tumor incisions.

3. Various techniques are used to remove spinal cord tumors, including the following:

    a. Intramedullary tumors are totally resected. Corticosteroids are administered before and after surgery. MRI verifies tumor characteristics preoperatively (eg, exact level). Microsurgical laser techniques, ultrasound, and x-rays may be used intraoperatively. In surgery, every effort must be made to keep the anterior spinal artery intact.

    b. Vascular tumors may be managed in different ways. Hemangioblastomas are usually removed from the outside inward by exterior coagulation and progressive tumor shrinkage before removal. Cavernomas are usually removed by exterior coagulation and progressive tumor shrinkage before removal, but from the inside outward.

    c. Neoplastic tumors may be treated with radiation or surgically excised using an anterior approach because these tumors typically cause anterior cord compression.

4. Radiation therapy may be used over 2 to 4 weeks; dosing protocols vary. Spinal radiation before surgical decompression may adversely affect wound healing. In patients who have a good functional status, radiotherapy to a malignant spinal cord tumor can significantly improve survival time.

5. Corticosteroids, such as dexamethasone and prednisone in moderate to high doses, are indicated for use before radiation therapy to improve the ambulation rate in the paretic patient.
   a. Corticosteroids are not typically used in nonparetic ambulatory patients.
   b. They are tapered over 2 weeks before discontinuing.
6. When compared to patients with traumatic SCI, the rehabilitation of patients with spinal cord tumors is shorter; however, cancer patients have more limited functional improvement than SCI patients.

Complications

1. Spinal cord infarction secondary to compression.
2. Nerve or spinal compression from tumor expansion.
3. Tetraplegia or paraplegia due to spinal cord compression.

Nursing Assessment

1. Perform motor and sensory components of the neurologic examination.
2. Assess pain using scale of 0 to 10, as indicated.
3. Assess autonomic nervous system relative to level of lesion—pupillary responses, vital signs, bowel, and bladder function.
4. Assess for spinal or nerve compression—progressive increase in pain, paralysis or paresis, sensory loss, loss of rectal sphincter tone, and sexual dysfunction.

Nursing Diagnoses

- Anxiety related to surgery and outcome.
- Pain related to nerve compression.
- Risk for Peripheral Neurovascular Dysfunction related to nerve compression.
- Impaired Urinary Elimination related to spinal cord compression.
- Risk for Injury related to surgery.

Nursing Interventions

Relieving Anxiety
1. Provide a safe environment for patient to verbalize anxieties.
2. Provide explanations regarding all procedures. Answer questions or refer the patient to someone who can answer questions.
3. Refer to cancer and SCI support groups, as needed.
4. Provide the patient/family with written information regarding disease process and medical interventions.
5. Reduce environmental stimulation.
6. Promote periods of rest to enhance coping skills.
7. Involve the family in distraction techniques.
8. Provide options in care when possible.

Relieving Pain
1. Administer analgesics, as indicated, and evaluate for pain control.
2. Instruct the patient in the use of patient-controlled analgesia, if available.
3. Instruct the patient in relaxation techniques, such as deep breathing, distraction, and imagery.
4. Position patient off surgical site postoperatively.

Compensating for Sensory Alterations
1. Reassure the patient that the degree of sensory/motor impairment may decrease during the postoperative recovery period as the amount of surgical edema decreases.
2. Instruct the patient with sensory loss to visually scan the extremity during use to avoid injury related to lack of tactile input.
3. Instruct the patient with painful paresthesias in appropriate use of ice, exercise, and rest.
4. Assess the patient with sensory and motor alterations and refer to physical therapy for assistance with ADL, ambulation.

Achieving Urinary Continence
1. Assess the urinary elimination pattern of the patient.
2. Instruct the patient in the therapeutic intake of fluid volume and relationship to elimination.
3. Instruct the patient in an appropriate means of urinary elimination and bowel management (see page 505).

Providing Additional Postoperative Care
1. Provide routine postoperative care to prevent complications.
2. Monitor surgical site for bleeding, CSF drainage, signs of infection.
3. Keep surgical dressing clean and dry.
4. Clean surgical site, as ordered.
5. Pad the bed rails and chair if the patient experiences numbness or paresthesias to prevent injury.
6. Support the weak/paralytic extremity in a functional position.

Patient Education and Health Maintenance

1. Encourage the patient with motor impairment to use adaptive devices.
2. Demonstrate proper positioning and transfer techniques.
3. Instruct the patient with sensory losses about dangers of extreme temperatures and the need for adequate foot protection at all times.
4. If the patient has suspected or confirmed neurofibromatosis, suggest referral to genetic counselor. Also, encourage follow-up for MRI every 12 months to monitor disease progression.
5. Refer to cancer and SCI support groups, as needed.

Evaluation: Expected Outcomes

- Asks questions and discusses care options.
- Reports that pain is relieved.
- Reports decreased paresthesias; ambulatory postoperatively.
- Voids at intervals without residual urine.
- Incision healing, skin intact.

OTHER DISORDERS
Seizure Disorders

Seizures (also known as *epileptic seizures* and, if recurrent, *epilepsy*) are defined as a sudden alteration in normal brain activity that causes distinct changes in behavior and body function. Seizures are thought to result from disturbances in the cells of the brain that cause cells to give off abnormal, recurrent, uncontrolled electrical discharges.

Pathophysiology and Etiology

Altered Physiology

1. The pathophysiology of seizures is unknown. It is known, however, that the brain has certain metabolic needs for oxygen and glucose. Neurons also have certain permeability gradients and voltage gradients that are affected by changes in the chemical and humoral environment.
2. Factors that change the permeability of the cell population (ischemia, hemorrhage) and ion concentration (Na^+, K^+) can produce neurons that are hyperexcitable and demonstrate hypersynchrony, producing an abnormal discharge.
3. A seizure may manifest itself as an altered behavior, motor, or sensory function relating to any anatomic location in the brain.

Classification

The International League Against Epilepsy developed an international classification of epileptic seizures that divides seizures into two major classes: partial-onset seizures and generalized-onset seizures. Partial-onset seizures begin in one focal area of the cerebral cortex, whereas generalized-onset seizures have an onset recorded simultaneously in both cerebral hemispheres.

1. *Simple-partial seizures* can have motor, somatosensory, psychic, or autonomic symptoms *without impairment* of consciousness.
2. *Complex-partial seizures* have an *impairment* (but not a loss) of consciousness with simple-partial features, automatisms, or impairment of consciousness only.
3. *Generalized seizures* have a loss of consciousness with convulsive or nonconvulsive behaviors.
4. Simple-partial seizures can progress to complex-partial seizures and complex-partial seizures can secondarily become generalized.

Etiology

The etiology may be unknown or due to one of the following:

1. Trauma to head or brain resulting in scar tissue or cerebral atrophy.
2. Tumors.
3. Cranial surgery.
4. Metabolic disorders (hypocalcemia, hypoglycemia/hyperglycemia, hyponatremia, anoxia).
5. Drug toxicity, such as theophylline, lidocaine, penicillin.
6. CNS infection.
7. Circulatory disorders.
8. Drug withdrawal states (alcohol, barbiturates).
9. Congenital neurodegenerative disorders.
10. Nonepileptogenic behaviors, which can emulate seizures but have a psychogenic, rather than an organic, origin.

Clinical Manifestations

Manifestations are related to the area of the brain involved in the seizure activity and may range from single abnormal sensations, aberrant motor activity, altered consciousness or personality to loss of consciousness and convulsive movements.

1. Impaired consciousness.
2. Disturbed muscle tone or movement.
3. Disturbances of behavior, mood, sensation, or perception.
4. Disturbances of autonomic functions.

Diagnostic Evaluation

1. EEG with or without video monitoring—locates epileptic focus, spread, intensity, and duration; helps classify seizure type.
2. MRI, CT scan—to identify lesion that may be cause of seizure.
3. SPECT or PET scan—additional tests to identify seizure foci.
4. Neuropsychological studies—to evaluate for behavioral disturbances.
5. Serum laboratory studies or lumbar puncture—to evaluate for infectious, hormonal, or metabolic etiology.

Management

1. Pharmacotherapy—AED selected according to seizure type (see Table 15-9, pages 558 to 561).
2. Biofeedback—useful in the patient with reliable auras.
3. Surgery—resective and palliative operations (temporal lobectomy, extratemporal resection, corpus callosotomy, hemispherectomy).
4. Vagal nerve stimulation.

Complications

1. Status epilepticus (see Box 15-6).
2. Injuries due to falls, especially head injuries.

Nursing Assessment

1. Obtain seizure history, including prodromal signs and symptoms, seizure behavior, postictal state, history of status epilepticus.
2. Document the following about seizure activity:
   a. Circumstances before attack, such as visual, auditory, olfactory, or tactile stimuli; emotional or psychological disturbances; sleep; hyperventilation.
   b. Description of movement, including where movement or stiffness started; type of movement and parts involved; progression of movement; whether beginning of seizure was witnessed.
   c. Position of the eyes and head; size of pupils.
   d. Presence of automatisms, such as lip smacking or repeated swallowing.
   e. Incontinence of urine or feces.
   f. Duration of each phase of the attack.
   g. Presence of unconsciousness and its duration.
   h. Behavior after attack, including inability to speak, any weakness or paralysis (Todd's paralysis), sleep.
3. Investigate the psychosocial effect of seizures.
4. Obtain history of drug or alcohol abuse.
5. Assess compliance and medication-taking strategies.

 DRUG ALERT Nonadherence to medication regimen as well as toxicity of anti-epileptic medications can increase seizure frequency. Obtain drug levels before implementing medication changes.

(Text continues on page 562)

Table 15-9 | Anti-Epileptic Drugs

GENERIC NAME	DOSAGE FORMS	USUAL DOSES	HALF-LIFE
Carbamazepine	• Suspension 100 mg/5 mL • Tablet 200 mg • Chewtab 100 mg • Extended-release tablets 100 mg, 200 mg, 400 mg • Extended-release sprinkle capsules 200 mg, 300 mg	• 10–40 mg/kg/day divided b.i.d. for extended-release; t.i.d. to q.i.d. for immediate-release	Initial 20–50, then 5–14 hours; induces own metabolism over first 2 weeks
Clonazepam	• Tablets 0.5 mg, 1 mg, 2 mg	• 0.01–0.3 mg/kg/day divided TID or given QHS • 0.5 mg PO TID—adults maximum 20 mg/day	20–40 hours
Diazepam (rectal)	• Pediatric rectal gel 2.5 mg, 5 mg, 10 mg • Adult rectal gel 10 mg, 15 mg, 20 mg	• 2–5 y/o—0.5 mg/kg • 6–11 y/o—0.3 mg/kg • >12 y/o—0.2 mg/kg	30–60 hours
Ethosuximide	• Capsule 250 mg • Solution 250 mg/5 mL	• 15–40 mg/kg/day divided b.i.d.	30–60 hours
Felbamate	• Tablets 400 mg, 600 mg • Suspension 600 mg/5 mL	• 15–45 mg/kg/day (or 1,200–3,600 mg) divided t.i.d. to q.i.d.; usual maximum 60 mg/kg/day	14–23 hours
Gabapentin	• Capsule 100 mg, 300 mg, 400 mg • Tablets 600 mg, 800 mg • Solution 250 mg/5 mL	• Initially 10–20 mg/kg/day divided t.i.d. to q.i.d.; titrate up to 40–60 mg/kg/day; usual maximum 90 mg/kg/day	5–9 hours
Lamotrigine	• Tablets 25 mg, 100 mg, 150 mg, 200 mg • Chew tablets 2 mg, 5 mg, 25 mg	• 200–500 mg/day divided b.i.d. • 2–15 mg/kg/day; start dose slowly	12–50 hours up to 70 hours with VPA
Levetiracetam	• Tablets 250 mg, 500 mg, 750 mg	• Initially 10 mg/kg P.O. divided b.i.d. or 500 mg P.O. b.i.d.; increase every 2 weeks to 40–60 mg/kg/day	Adults 7 hours
Lorazepam	• Tablets 0.5 mg, 1 mg, 2 mg • Solution 2 mg/mL • Injection 2 mg/mL, 4 mg/mL	• 0.05–0.1 mg/kg/dose; 4 mg/dose maximum may repeat in 10–15 minutes	10–20 hours

USUAL TARGET RANGE	MECHANISM OF ACTION	INDICATIONS	DOSE-RELATED ADVERSE EFFECTS
4–12 mcg/mL	Modulates sodium channels	• Simple partial • Complex partial • Generalized tonic/clonic seizures	Double or blurred vision, lethargy (reduced by slow-dose titration)
20–70 mcg/mL	Enhances GABA	• Myoclonic • Lennox-Gastaut syndrome • Atonic • Absence	Drowsiness (50%), ataxia (30%), behavioral disturbances (25%), movement disorders, slurred speech, hypersecretion
Not applicable	Enhances GABA	• Acute repetitive seizures	Sedation
40–100 mcg/mL	Reduces current in the T-type calcium channels	• Absence	GI distress, drowsiness, hiccups, sedation
30–100 mcg/mL	Blocks glycine binding to the NMDA receptors, modulates sodium channel, enhances GABA	• Lennox-Gastaut syndrome • Complex partial seizures	Anorexia, weight loss, vomiting, insomnia, headache, somnolence; rare cases of aplastic anemia (25 cases per 100,000) and liver failure (8 cases per 100,000) have also been seen
4–20 mcg/mL	Not known	• Partial seizures with or without secondary generalized tonic/clonic seizures	Somnolence, dizziness, ataxia, nystagmus, weight gain, nausea, vomiting, blurred vision, tremor, slurred speech, peripheral edema, dyspepsia, hiccups
3–20 mcg/mL	Blocks sodium channels and blocks release of glutamate	• Simple partial seizures • Complex partial seizures • Generalized tonic/clonic seizures • Lennox-Gastaut syndrome • Absence	Fatigue, drowsiness, ataxia, dizziness, headache, nausea, vomiting, double or blurred vision, nystagmus
5–50 mcg/mL	Inhibits propagation of seizure by unknown mechanism	• Partial-onset seizures	Somnolence (14.8%), asthenia (14.7%), coordination difficulties (3.4%), dizziness, nervousness, behavioral problems, decreased blood counts
50–240 mcg/mL	Enhances GABA	• Status epilepticus	Sedation with risk of respiratory depression, amnesia, abnormal behavior, withdrawal reactions

(continued)

Table 15-9   Anti-Epileptic Drugs (*continued*)

GENERIC NAME	DOSAGE FORMS	USUAL DOSES	HALF-LIFE
Oxcarbazepine	• Tablets 150 mg, 300 mg, 600 mg	• Adult initially 300 mg P.O. b.i.d., increase weekly to a usual maintenance dose of 1,200–2,400 mg/day • Child initially 10 mg/kg/day; titrate to a dose of 30–60 mg/kg/day	Parent 1–2½ hours Metabolite 8–15 hours
Phenobarbital C-IV	• Capsule 16 mg • Elixir 15 mg/5 mL, 20 mg/5 mL • Tablet 8 mg, 15 mg, 16 mg, 30 mg, 32 mg, 60 mg, 65 mg, 100 mg • Injection 30 mg/mL, 60 mg/mL, 65 mg/mL, 130 mg/mL	• 2–6 mg/kg/day divided q.i.d. to b.i.d. (high end of range for infants/young children)	40–140 hours
Phenytoin, Fosphenytoin	• Injection 50 mg/mL (Fosphenytoin is 50 mg/mL phenytoin equivalent) • Suspension 125 mg/5 mL, 30 mg/5 mL • Chew tablets 50 mg • Capsules 30 mg, 100 mg	• 4–12 mg/kg/day divided b.i.d. to t.i.d. for children getting P.O.; q.i.d.–b.i.d. for adults getting P.O.; divided q6h for IV dosing	5–34 hours
Primidone	• Suspension 250 mg/5 mL • Tablets 50 mg, 250 mg	• 10–25 mg/kg/day divided b.i.d. to t.i.d.; maximum 2 mg/day	4–20 hours (PEMA ½ 30–36 hours)
Tiagabine	• Tablets 2 mg, 4 mg, 12 mg, 16 mg, 20 mg	• Adult 32–56 mg/day divided b.i.d.–q.i.d. (start with a 4 mg P.O. q.i.d., adjust weekly) • Child 0.1 mg/kg/day divide t.i.d., increase to 0.6 mg/kg/day (1 mg/kg/day with enzyme inducers)	2–9 hours
Topiramate	• Tablets 25 mg, 100 mg, 200 mg • Sprinkle capsules 15 mg, 25 mg	• Children initiate at 0.5–1 mg/kg/day divided b.i.d.; usual dose is 6–12 mg/kg/day divided b.i.d.–t.i.d. • Adult: 200–800 mg/day divided b.i.d.; initiate slowly with 25 mg q.h., increase weekly	12–30 hours
VPA/divalproex sodium	• Solution 250 mg/5 mL • Capsule 250 mg • Sprinkle 125 mg • Extended-release 500 mg • Tablet 125 mg, 200 mg, 500 mg	• 15–60 mg/kg/day divided b.i.d. to t.i.d.	7–20 hours
Vigabatrin	• Tablet 500 mg scored	• Adult: 2–4 mg/day divided b.i.d. • Children: 1–2 mg/day or 40–100 mg/kg/day	5–7 hours
Zonisamide	• Capsule 100 mg	• Adult 200–400 mg/day P.O. b.i.d. (max 600 mg), initially 100 mg P.O. q.i.d. and adjust every 2 weeks • Children initially 1 mg/kg/day, adjust every 2 weeks (maximum 15 mg/kg/day)	27–60 hours

GABA, gamma- aminobutyric acid; NMDA, N-methyl-D-aspartate; PEMA, phenylethylmalonamide; VPA, valproic acid.

USUAL TARGET RANGE	MECHANISM OF ACTION	INDICATIONS	DOSE-RELATED ADVERSE EFFECTS
10–35 mcg/mL for the monohydroxy derivative	Modulates sodium channels	• Partial-onset seizures	Headache, drowsiness, fatigue, nausea, dizziness, hyponatremia (hematologic toxicity not observed to date); dermatological reactions (rash)
15–40 mcg/mL	Enhances GABA	• Generalized tonic/clonic seizures • Simple partial seizures • Complex partial seizures	Sedation, mental dullness, cognitive impairment, hyperactivity, ataxia
10–20 mcg/mL total 1–2 mcg/mL free (for patients with protein binding)	Modulates sodium channels	• Generalized tonic/clonic seizures • Complex partial seizures • Simple partial seizures	Nystagmus, ataxia, lethargy, propylene glycol in IV preparation can cause myocardial depression, bradycardias, other electrocardiogram changes, hypotension, rash
5–20 mcg/mL	Enhances GABA	• Generalized tonic/clonic seizures • Simple partial seizures • Complex partial seizures	Same as phenobarbital
5–70 mcg/mL	Inhibits neuronal and glial uptake of GABA	• Partial-onset seizures	Sedation, dizziness, memory impairment, inattention, emotional lability, headache, abdominal pain, anorexia, tremor
2–25 mcg/mL	Modulates sodium channels, enhances GABA activity, and modulates NMDA receptor	• Partial-onset seizures • Lennox-Gastaut syndrome • Generalized tonic/clonic • Juvenile myoclonic epilepsy	Speech and language problems, difficulty with concentration and attention, confusion, fatigue, paresthesias, weight loss
50–150 mcg/mL	Unknown (may modulate sodium channel, enhance GABA)	• Generalized tonic/clonic seizures • Absence • Myoclonic • Partial-onset seizures • Lennox-Gastaut syndrome	GI upset, lethargy, changes in menstrual cycle, thrombocytopenia
Not known	Inhibits GABA-transaminase (preventing GABA metabolism)	• Infantile spasms due to tuberous sclerosis	Drowsiness, fatigue, ataxia, behavioral changes, weight gain, psychosis (in predisposed patients and upon abrupt withdrawal), hematologic, visual field problems
15–40 mcg/mL	Modulates sodium and T-type calcium channels	• Partial-onset seizures • Generalized seizures • Absence • Myoclonic • Lennox-Gastaut • Infantile spasms	Drowsiness, psychosis (2%)

BOX 15-7 Emergency Management of Status Epilepticus

Status epilepticus (acute, prolonged, repetitive seizure activity) is a series of generalized seizures without return to consciousness between attacks. The term has been broadened to include continuous clinical and/or electrical seizures lasting at least 5 minutes, even without impairment of consciousness. Status epilepticus is considered a serious neurologic emergency. It has high mortality and morbidity (permanent brain damage, severe neurologic deficits). Factors that precipitate status epilepticus in patients with preexisting seizure disorder include medication withdrawal, fever, metabolic or environmental stresses, alcohol or drug withdrawal, and sleep deprivation.

NURSING INTERVENTIONS

- Establish airway and maintain blood pressure (BP).
- Obtain blood studies for glucose blood urea nitrogen, electrolytes, and anticonvulsant drug levels to determine metabolic abnormalities and serve as a guide for maintenance of biochemical homeostasis.
- Administer oxygen—there is some respiratory depression associated with each seizure, which may produce venous congestion and hypoxia of brain.

- Establish IV lines and keep open for blood sampling, drug administration, and infusion of fluids.
- Administer IV anticonvulsant (lorazepam, phenytoin, diazepam) *slowly* to ensure effective brain tissue and serum concentrations.
  - Give additional anticonvulsants, as directed—effects of lorazepam are of short duration.
  - Monitor anticonvulsant drug levels regularly.
- Monitor the patient continuously; depression of respiration and BP induced by drug therapy may be delayed.
- Use mechanical ventilation, as needed.
- If initial treatment is unsuccessful, general anesthesia may be required.
- Assist with search for precipitating factors.
  - Monitor vital and neurologic signs on a continuous basis.
  - Use electroencephalographic monitoring to determine nature and abolition (after diazepam administration) of epileptic activity.
  - Determine (from family member) if there is a history of epilepsy, alcohol/drug use, trauma, recent infection.

Nursing Diagnoses

- Ineffective Cerebral Tissue Perfusion related to seizure activity.
- Risk for Injury related to seizure activity.
- Ineffective Coping related to psychosocial and economic consequences of epilepsy.

Nursing Interventions

Maintaining Cerebral Tissue Perfusion

1. Maintain a patent airway until the patient is fully awake after a seizure.
2. Provide oxygen during the seizure if color change occurs.
3. Stress the importance of taking medications regularly.
4. Monitor serum levels for therapeutic range of medications.
5. Monitor the patient for toxic adverse effects of medications.
6. Monitor platelet and liver functions for toxicity due to medications.

Preventing Injury

1. Provide a safe environment by padding side rails and removing clutter.
2. Place the bed in a low position.
3. Do not restrain the patient during a seizure.
4. Do not put anything in the patient's mouth during a seizure.
5. Place the patient on his or her side during a seizure to prevent aspiration.
6. Protect the patient's head during a seizure. If seizure occurs while ambulating or from chair, cradle head or provide cushion/support for protection against head injury.
7. Stay with the patient who is ambulating or who is in a confused state during seizure.
8. Provide a helmet to the patient who falls during seizure.
9. Manage the patient in status epilepticus.

Strengthening Coping

1. Consult with social worker for community resources for vocational rehabilitation, counselors, support groups.
2. Teach stress-reduction techniques that will fit into the patient's lifestyle.
3. Initiate appropriate consultation for management of behaviors related to personality disorders, brain damage secondary to chronic epilepsy.
4. Answer questions related to use of computerized video EEG monitoring and surgery for epilepsy management.

Community and Home Care Considerations

1. Counsel patients with uncontrolled seizures about driving or operating dangerous equipment. Be familiar with state laws regarding driving while on or tapering AEDs.
2. Assess home environment for safety hazards in case the patient falls, such as crowded furniture arrangement, sharp edges on tables, glass. Soft flooring and furniture and padded surfaces may be necessary.
3. Provide instructions on safety precautions while performing activities alone to prevent injury, drowning, or choking.
4. Support patient in discussion about seizures with employer, school, and so forth.

NURSING ALERT Sudden unexpected death in epilepsy can be reduced by decreasing the number of seizures that a patient experiences and taking medications, as prescribed. Although multiple medications may be required to reduce seizure frequency, it should be considered within the context of quality of life and risk reduction.

Patient Education and Health Maintenance

1. Encourage the patient to determine existence of trigger factors for seizures (eg, skipped meals, lack of sleep, emotional stress, menstrual cycle).
2. Remind the patient of the importance of following medication regimen.
3. Tell the patient to avoid alcohol because it interferes with metabolism of anti-epileptic medications.
4. Encourage the patient and family to discuss feelings and attitudes about epilepsy.
5. Encourage patient to carry or wear a MedicAlert card or bracelet.
6. Encourage a moderate lifestyle that includes exercise, mental activity, and nutritional diet.
7. For the surgical candidate, reinforce instructions related to surgical outcome of the specific surgical approach (temporal lobectomy, corpus callosotomy, hemispherectomy, and extratemporal resection).
8. Refer the patient/family for more information and support to such agencies as the Epilepsy Foundation of America (*www.efa.org*).

Evaluation: Expected Outcomes

- Takes medication as ordered, drug level within normal range.
- No injuries observed.
- Reports using support services and stress-management techniques.

Narcolepsy

Narcolepsy is a neurologic disorder characterized by abnormalities of REM sleep, some abnormalities of non-REM sleep, and excessive daytime sleepiness.

Pathophysiology and Etiology

1. Recent advances suggest that this common sleep disorder may be a neurodegenerative or autoimmune disorder resulting in the loss of hypothalamic neurons that contain a peptide, hypocretin (orexin). Hypocretin plays a central role in the timing of sleep and wakefulness and inhibits REM sleep. The deficiency in hypocretin contributes to the abnormalities of sleep and wakefulness in narcolepsy.
2. Genetic susceptibility—associated with class II human leukocyte antigens.
3. Although considered a hypersomnia disorder, the person does not experience excessive amounts of sleep in a 24-hour period. Typically, patients with narcolepsy have a normal amount of sleep over 24 hours. They have abnormal REM sleep that intrudes into wakefulness.
4. Onset is usually between ages 15 and 25.

Clinical Manifestations

1. Four classic symptoms (all symptoms not present in all patients):
   a. Excessive daytime sleepiness is usually the first symptom.
   b. Cataplexy (abrupt loss of muscle tone after emotional stimulation such as laughter, anger).
   c. Sleep paralysis (powerless to move limbs, speak, open eyes, or breathe deeply while fully aware of condition).
   d. Hypnagogic hallucinations (drowsiness before sleep, usually visual or auditory).
2. Symptoms enhanced by high temperature, indoor activity, and idleness.
3. Clinical manifestations may abate, but never phase out completely.
4. Patient may complain of inability to focus vision or thought process rather than have a feeling of sleepiness.
5. Nocturnal sleep disturbance—occurs 2½ to 3 hours after falling asleep.
   a. After being awake for 45 to 60 minutes, the patient will fall back to sleep for another 2½ to 3 hours and then awaken again.
   b. This is believed to be the source of the daytime somnolence.

Diagnostic Evaluation

1. An overnight polysomnogram in a sleep disorders lab is included in the evaluation to assess nighttime sleep—indicates the underlying cause for the complaint of sleepiness. The polysomnogram helps evaluate sleep quality and excludes other disorders, such as sleep apnea.
2. The polysomnogram is followed the next day by a multiple sleep latency test to assess daytime sleepiness—indicates severity of the problem. Patients are given four or five opportunities to nap every 2 hours. Patients with narcolepsy typically fall asleep more rapidly than the norm of 10 to 15 minutes.

Management

1. Long-term treatment is required. Mutual goal-setting is imperative because not everyone derives benefit from treatment. Even with medication, patients may never attain normal levels of alertness.
2. Nonpharmacologic therapy includes support groups, short naps (10 to 20 minutes, three times daily), caffeinated beverages, exercise, sleep hygiene techniques, and avoidance of heavy meals.
3. Stimulants prescribed may include pemoline, methylphenidate, dextroamphetamine, methamphetamine.
4. Antidepressants for cataplexy; protriptyline, desipramine, fluoxetine.

Complications

1. Injury related to falling asleep.
2. Psychosocial problems such as disturbed relationships, loss of employment, depression.

Nursing Assessment

1. Obtain history of sleep and activity pattern.
2. Assess emotional status and social interactions.
3. Assess response to medication and lifestyle treatment.

Nursing Diagnoses

- Disturbed Sleep Pattern related to disease process.
- Fatigue related to disrupted nighttime sleep.
- Ineffective Coping related to interference with activity.

Nursing Interventions

Promoting Normal Sleep–Wake Cycle

1. Review daily schedule to determine periods of sleep and cataplexy. Advise to wake at the same time daily.
2. Help the patient establish nondrug therapies (exercise, diet) that will fit into lifestyle.
3. Make sure that the bedroom is dark, cool, and quiet to facilitate sleep.
4. Administer or teach self-administration of prescribed medications.
   a. Advise of adverse effects of amphetamines, such as nervousness, irritability, tremors, and GI upset.
   b. Warn the patient to take only as prescribed and not to increase dosage because of tolerance and drug dependence.

Reducing Fatigue

1. Schedule 10- to 20-minute rest periods two or three times per day. Help the patient incorporate naps into lifestyle.
2. Encourage the patient to incorporate small amounts of caffeinated beverages at intervals and smaller, more frequent meals rather than large, heavy meals during the day to maintain energy.
3. Plan diversional activities and relaxation during fatigued periods.

Strengthening Coping

1. Encourage active participation in selection of treatment modalities.
2. Assist the patient in identifying trigger factors of worsening symptoms.
3. Teach problem-solving strategy to promote sense of control over activities and symptoms during the day.
4. Review patient coping mechanisms and reinforce positive ones.
5. Assist the patient to discuss information about narcolepsy with friends, family, school, and employers to help reduce anxiety and/or embarrassment about his or her condition.
6. Encourage the use of support groups and community resources, such as the American Sleep Association (*www.sleepassociation.org*).

Patient Education and Health Maintenance

1. Review the normal sleep cycle and the pathophysiology of narcolepsy.
2. Stress the importance of nonpharmacologic measures as an adjunct to treatment.
3. Inform the patient of rights of employment conditions under the Americans with Disabilities Act (see page 193).
4. Advise caution with using alcohol, working with machinery, or using dangerous equipment to prevent injury to self or others during sleepiness or cataplexy.
5. If the patient drives, advise using caution and avoiding lengthy trips.
6. Encourage the patient to wear a MedicAlert bracelet.
7. Encourage follow-up with health care provider, specialist, and mental health counselor, as needed.

Evaluation: Expected Outcomes

- Complies with medication regimen.
- Reports working without undue fatigue.
- Identifies trigger factors.

Headache Syndromes

Headaches are one of the most common complaints of people seeking health care. Pain in the head is a symptom of underlying pathology. The International Headache Society instituted a classification system that is the standard for defining various types of headaches. It divides headaches into two categories: primary headache disorders, which include migraine, tension-type headache, and cluster headache, and secondary headache disorders. Identifying the etiology of headaches requires an understanding of the characteristics of each type of headache.

Pathophysiology and Etiology

Primary Headaches

Diagnosis is generally based on the characteristic clinical history and elimination of other pathology such as stroke, intracranial bleed, AVM, or brain tumor.

1. Migraine headache—consists of initial vasospasm followed by dilation of intracranial and extracranial arteries; occurs in about 10% of the population.
   a. Caused by hyperactivity to the neurotransmitter serotonin; familial predisposition.
   b. Attack may consist of any of five phases: prodrome, aura, headache, resolution, and postdrome.
   c. Classified with or without aura (usually visual); aura is due to reduced cortical neuronal activity.
2. Tension headache—due to irritation of sensitive nerve endings in the head, jaw, and neck from prolonged muscle contraction in the face, head, and neck; mild or moderate intensity that does not prohibit activity.
   a. Precipitating factors include fatigue, stress, poor posture.
   b. Characterized by hatband distribution.
3. Cluster headache—release of increased histamine results in vasodilation.
   a. Usually unilateral, recurring.
   b. Occurs more often in men.

Secondary Headaches

Headache due to a neurologic or systemic disease.

1. Mass lesion (tumor, abscess, AVM, subdural or epidural hematoma).
2. Intracranial infection (bacterial/viral/fungal meningitis or encephalitis).
3. Inflammation (giant cell arteritis, vasculitis).
4. Cerebrovascular disease (subarachnoid hemorrhage, intracranial hemorrhage, occlusive vascular disease).
5. Increased ICP.
6. Low-pressure headache (postlumbar puncture, trauma-induced).
7. Sinus infection, viral infection such as influenza, systemic illness.

Clinical Manifestations

1. Migraine: sensory, motor, or mood alterations precede headache; gradual onset of severe unilateral, throbbing headache; may become bilateral.
   a. Migraine with aura (classic migraine), characteristic aura may include scintillating scotoma (area of decreased vision surrounded by area of less abnormal or normal vision with zigzag appearance), hemianopsia (loss of half of field of vision), and paresthesias; headache follows aura in less than 1 hour; usually lasts less than a day.
   b. Migraine without aura (common migraine), nausea, vomiting, and photophobia may accompany moderate to severe headache; worsened by activity; may last 4 to 72 hours and greatly impair activities.
   c. Either type of migraine may be triggered in women by hormonal fluctuations (menses, pregnancy), excess or lack of sleep, change in eating habits, and certain food additives.
2. Tension/muscle contraction: dull, band-like, constricting, persistent pain and pressure in the back of the head and neck, across forehead, bitemporal areas; may be tender points of head or neck.
   a. Not aggravated by activity, but may be worsened by noise and light.
   b. No nausea and vomiting, but may be associated with anorexia.
3. Cluster headache: sudden, sharp, burning, excruciating, unilateral pain; always involving facial area from neck to temple and often occurs during the evening or night; more frequent in men.
   a. Occurs in clusters of 2 to 8 weeks followed by headache-free periods.
   b. Associated with unilateral excessive tearing, redness of the eye, stuffiness of nostril on affected side, facial swelling, flushing, and sweating.
   c. Attacks last several minutes to several days. Multiple attacks may occur in 1 day.

Diagnostic Evaluation

1. Skull/sinus films to rule out lesions, sinusitis.
2. CT scan/MRI to rule out lesions, hemorrhage, chronic sinusitis.

> **! NURSING ALERT** "Red flags" for possible serious cause of headache (hemorrhage, stroke, tumor, infection) include altered level of consciousness; neurological findings such as weakness, facial droop, dysarthria, or aphasia; nausea and vomiting; new onset of or change in characteristic headaches; and patient reporting that it is "the worst headache of my life." These patients should be evaluated with a brain CT scan.

3. Erythrocyte sedimentation rate and other blood studies to help determine inflammatory process with temporal arteritis.

Management

Pharmacologic Treatment

Medications are intended to reduce the frequency, severity, and duration of the headache. Effectiveness of medication is individualized. Some persons may need a combination of medications.

1. Aspirin, acetaminophen, and NSAIDs for mild to moderate pain of tension, sinus, or mild vascular headaches.
2. Some drugs may abort vascular headaches if taken at the onset, including methysergide, a serotonin antagonist; ergotamine, a vasoconstrictor; or 5HT-agonists such as sumatriptan.
3. Sumatriptan is available in subcutaneous injection and nasal inhalation, as well as in oral form.
4. Other oral 5HT-agonists include zolmitriptan, naratriptan, and rizatriptan.

> **DRUG ALERT** Vasoconstrictors and 5HT-agonists used to abort vascular headaches are contraindicated in patients with uncontrolled hypertension, coronary artery disease, and peripheral vascular disease.

5. Inhalation of 100% oxygen may abort a cluster headache.
6. Some drugs may be used continuously as prophylactic treatment for recurrent migraines, including beta-adrenergic blockers, calcium channel blockers, and antidepressants.
7. Antihistamines and decongestants may be effective for sinus headaches.
8. Corticosteroids may be used for temporal arteritis.
9. Occasionally, opioid analgesics, muscle relaxants, and anti-anxiety agents may be needed for severe pain.

Nonpharmacologic Management

1. Relaxation techniques, guided imagery, paced breathing.
2. Biofeedback, cognitive therapy.
3. Trigger identification and control of such factors as intake of alcohol (red wine), skipped meals, oversleeping, or undersleeping.
4. To prevent migraine: avoidance of monosodium glutamate, mixed spices such as "seasoned salt," nitrates and nitrites commonly contained in bacon, hot dogs, or deli meats.
5. Rest in a quiet, dark room at onset of headache.
6. If caffeine user, spread caffeine intake evenly over the day.
7. Routine exercise program.

Complications

1. Usually none from primary headaches.

Nursing Assessment

1. Obtain a history of related symptoms, triggering factors, degree of pain, and medications used.
2. Perform a complete neurologic examination to detect any focal deficits or signs of increased ICP that indicate tumor or hemorrhage.
3. Assess coping mechanisms and emotional status.

Nursing Diagnoses

- Acute Pain related to headache.
- Ineffective Coping related to chronic and/or disabling pain.

Nursing Interventions

Controlling Pain

1. Reduce environmental stimuli: light, noise, and movement to decrease severity of pain.
2. Suggest light massage for tight muscles in neck, scalp, or back for tension headaches.
3. Apply warm, moist heat to areas of muscle tension.
4. Encourage patient to lie down and attempt to sleep.
5. Teach progressive muscle relaxation to treat and prevent tension headaches.
   a. Alternately tense and relax each group of muscles for a count of five, starting with the forehead and working downward to the feet.
   b. Try to maintain a state of relaxation of each muscle group until the whole body feels relaxed.
   c. Relaxation of just head and neck may also be helpful if time is limited.
6. Teach patient the cause of headache and proper use of medication.
7. Encourage adequate rest once headache is relieved to recover from fatigue of the pain.

Promoting Positive Coping

1. Encourage patient to become aware of triggering factors and early symptoms of headache, so it can be prevented or promptly treated. Hunger, lack of exercise, and erratic sleep schedules may trigger headaches.
2. Encourage adequate nutrition, rest and relaxation, and avoidance of stress and overexertion to better cope with headaches.
3. Implement problem solving to help patient manage problems that arise in social or work situations related to headaches.
4. Review coping mechanisms and strengthen positive ones.

Patient Education and Health Maintenance

1. Teach proper administration of medication.
   a. Self-injection of sumatriptan given subcutaneously with autoinjector.
   b. Oral inhalation technique of ergotamine through metered-dose inhaler.
   c. Nasal spray dosing of sumatriptan.
2. Teach about adverse effects of medications.
   a. GI upset, gastritis, and possible ulcer formation with NSAIDs—take with food.
   b. Numbness, coldness, paresthesias, and pain of extremities with ergot derivatives—report to health care provider.
   c. Chest pain, wheezing, flushing with sumatriptan—report to health care provider.
   d. Hypotension with beta-adrenergic blockers and calcium channel blockers—arise slowly, do not exceed prescribed dosage, do not discontinue beta-adrenergic blockers abruptly.
3. Advise avoidance of alcohol, which can worsen headaches.

4. Teach about foods that are high in tyramine, which may trigger migraines—aged cheese, red wine, some processed meats. Some food additives such as nitrates may also trigger migraines, and many people identify their own individual triggers.
5. Teach patient how to perform relaxation techniques to reduce stress and promote inner well-being.
6. Refer patient for more information to the International Headache Society (*www.i-h-s.org*).

Evaluation: Expected Outcomes

- Reports fewer, less-severe headaches.
- Describes use of positive coping mechanisms.

Herniated Intervertebral Disk (Ruptured Disk)

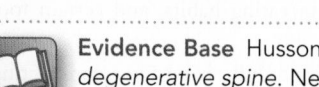

Evidence Base Husson, J. (2012). *Thoraco-lumbar degenerative spine.* New York: Springer. American Association of Neuroscience Nurses. (2012). *Thoracolumbar spine surgery: A guide to preoperative and postoperative patient care.* Glenview, IL: Author.

Herniation of the intervertebral disk is a protrusion of the nucleus of the disk into the annulus (fibrous ring around the disk) with subsequent nerve compression. The herniation may occur in any portion of the vertebral column (see Figure 15-12). The pressure on spinal nerve roots or the spinal cord causes severe, chronic, or recurrent back and leg pain.

Pathophysiology and Etiology

1. The intervertebral disk is a cartilaginous plate made up of gelatinous material in the center, known as the nucleus pulposus, and is encapsulated in the fibrous annulus.
2. About 90% of herniated disks involve the lumbar and lumbosacral spine. The most common site is the L4–L5 disk

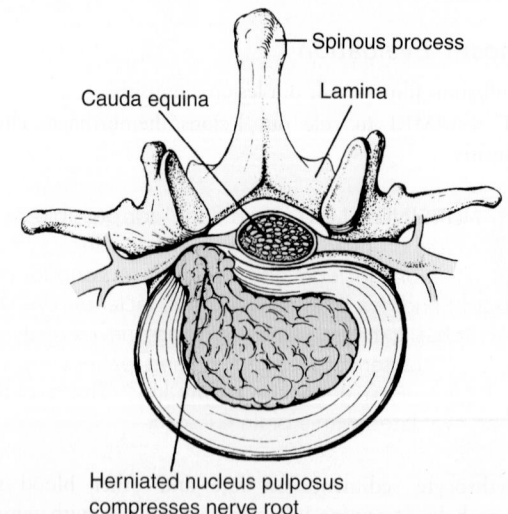

Figure 15-12. Ruptured vertebral disk.

space. The cause of a herniated lumbar disk is usually a flexion injury, but many patients do not recall experiencing a traumatic event. Cervical herniation is less common; but when it does occur, it is usually in individuals age 45 or older.

3. Risk factors for herniation include:
   a. Degeneration (aging), trauma, and congenital predisposition.
   b. Biomechanical factors, such as twisting and repetitive motions in occupational settings.
   c. Sedentary occupations.
   d. Obesity.
   e. Smoking.
4. The herniation compresses the spinal nerve root, usually restricted to one side and, with further degeneration of the disk, may eventually produce pressure on the spinal cord.
5. This sequence may take months to years, producing acute and chronic symptoms.

Clinical Manifestations

General Considerations
1. An intervertebral disk may herniate without causing symptoms.
2. Symptoms depend on location, size, rate of development, and effect on surrounding structures.
3. Most symptomatic disk herniations result in pain, sensory changes, loss of reflex, and muscle weakness that resolve without surgery.

Cervical
1. Pain and stiffness in the neck, top of shoulders, and region of the scapula.
2. Pain in upper extremities and head.
3. Paresthesias and numbness of upper extremities.
4. Weakness of upper extremities.

Lumbar
1. Lower back pain with varying degrees of sensory and motor dysfunction.
2. Pain radiating from the lower back into the buttocks and down the leg, referred to as sciatica.
3. A stiff or unnatural posture.
4. Some combination of paresthesias, weakness, and reflex impairment.
5. Positive straight-leg raise test: pain occurs in leg below the knee when leg is raised from a supine position.

 NURSING ALERT Cauda equina syndrome is an urgent condition caused by an acute compression of the cauda equina area of the spinal cord by massive disk extrusion. Symptoms include progressive sensory and motor loss of lower extremities, saddle anesthesia (loss of sensation around perineum), bowel and/or bladder incontinence, or sexual dysfunction. It must be recognized early and compression must be relieved to prevent permanent loss of these functions. If patients report such symptoms, emergent assessment and intervention is indicated.

Diagnostic Evaluation
1. CT scan or MRI—demonstrates herniation; MRI has greater sensitivity.
2. Electromyography—localizes specific spinal nerve involvement.
3. Myelogram—rarely done, but demonstrates herniation and pressure on spinal cord or nerve roots.

Management

Nonpharmacologic Measures
1. Bed rest on a firm mattress (2 days usually sufficient) usually results in improvement in 80% of patients.
2. Heat or ice massage to affected area.
3. Cervical collar or possibly cervical traction are widely used, although efficacy is not proven.
4. Physical therapy may be prescribed to maximize function and assist the patient in recovery.
5. Epidural steroid injection may be administered by interventional radiologist, particularly with the presence of radiculopathy, radiating/shooting pain down the extremity, to relieve symptoms.
6. Nonpharmacologic and pharmacologic measures may be used together for 4 to 6 weeks as conservative management if there is no progressive neurologic deficit.
   a. More than 90% of low back pain episodes resolve completely by 4 to 6 weeks and those with herniated disc may experience spontaneous remission of pain.
   b. Surgical intervention is reserved for those with neurological deficits or persistent symptoms over 6 weeks and is designed to relieve radicular (sciatic) pain.

Pharmacotherapy
1. Anti-inflammatory drugs, such as ibuprofen or prednisone.
2. Muscle relaxants, such as diazepam or cyclobenzaprine.
3. Analgesics; opioids may be necessary for several days during acute phase.

Surgical Intervention
1. May be done if there is progression of neurologic deficit or failure to improve with conservative management.
2. Surgical procedures include discectomy (decompression of nerve root), laminectomy, spinal fusion, microdiscectomy, and percutaneous discectomy.
3. Hemilaminectomy with excision of the involved disk is the surgical procedure most often indicated for lumbar disk disease.

Chemonucleolysis
1. Less common invasive treatment for lumbar disk herniation.
2. Injection of chymopapain into herniated disk that produces loss of water and proteoglycans from the disk, reducing the size of the disk and subsequent pressure on the nerve root.
3. May cause severe complications, such as transverse myelitis, allergic reactions, persistent muscle spasm.

Alternative and Complementary Measures
1. Acupuncture.
2. Manipulative therapy.
3. Massage therapy for adjunct pain relief.

4. Homeopathic remedies.
5. Various nutritional supplements.

Complications

1. Permanent neurologic dysfunction (weakness, numbness).
2. Chronic pain with associated psychosocial issues.
3. Cauda equina syndrome.

Nursing Assessment

1. Perform repeated assessments of motor function, sensation, and reflexes to determine progression of condition.
2. Assess level at which straight-leg raise test is positive; generally, radiation of pain below knee at 45 degrees of elevation is considered positive for nerve root involvement; positive at lesser elevation may indicate worsening condition.
3. Assess pain level on scale of 1 to 10.

Nursing Diagnoses

- Acute Pain related to area of compression.
- Impaired Physical Mobility related to pain and disease physiology.
- Deficient Knowledge related to impending surgery.
- Risk for Injury related to surgical procedure.

Nursing Interventions

Minimizing Pain

1. Administer or teach self-administration of anti-inflammatory drugs, as prescribed, and with food or antacid to prevent GI upset.
2. Administer or teach self-administration of prescribed muscle relaxant; observe safety because drowsiness may result.
3. Administer or teach self-administration of analgesics, as prescribed; be prepared for sedation.
4. Encourage regular activity with limits of pain.
5. Apply dry or moist heat to affected area of back, as desired.
6. Encourage relaxation techniques, such as imagery and progressive muscle relaxation.

Maintaining Mobility

1. Encourage ROM exercises while in bed.
2. Properly fit and use a cervical collar (if appropriate to level of injury).
3. Apply a back brace or cervical skin traction, if ordered.
4. Inspect skin several times a day, especially under stabilization devices, for redness and evidence of pressure ulcer development.
5. Provide good skin care to pressure-prone areas.
6. Assist the patient with activities at bedside and discourage lifting or straining of any kind.
7. Encourage compliance with physical therapy treatments and activity restrictions, as ordered.

Preparing the Patient for Surgery

1. Educate the patient about surgical procedure.
   a. Procedure is generally short.
   b. Small incision will be made on front or back of neck for cervical herniation; second incision may be on hip if a bone graft is taken from iliac crest for spinal fusion.
   c. Routine postoperative care will include frequent assessment of vital signs and neurologic function, frequent turning and deep breathing, pain control, and ambulation on the first postoperative day.
2. Document baseline neurologic assessment to compare with after surgery.
3. Explain your actions to the patient as you prepare operative area, administer preoperative medications, and perform any other preoperative order.

Preventing Complications Postoperatively

1. Monitor vital signs and surgical dressing frequently because hemorrhage is a possible complication.
2. If the patient has a wound drainage system, check tubing frequently for patency and secure vacuum seal.
3. Assess movement and sensation of extremities regularly, report new deficit.
4. Administer analgesics and steroid medications to control pain from incision and swelling around nerve roots and spinal cord due to surgery.
5. Maintain cervical collar, if ordered.
6. Logroll the patient to reposition frequently and encourage coughing and deep breathing.
7. Position the patient for comfort with a small pillow under his or her head (but avoid extreme neck flexion) and pillow under knees to take pressure off lower back.
8. Provide fluids as soon as gag reflex and bowel sounds are noted.
9. Assess for hoarseness, which suggests that cervical surgery resulted in a recurrent laryngeal nerve injury; this injury may cause an ineffective cough.
10. Watch for dysphagia due to edema of the esophagus and provide dietary modifications, as necessary.
11. Make sure that the patient voids after surgery; report urine retention.
12. Encourage ambulation as soon as possible by having the patient lie on the side close to the edge of the bed and push up with arms while swinging legs toward floor in one motion; alternate walking with bed rest, discourage sitting.
13. Report any sudden reappearance of radicular pain (may indicate nerve root compression from slipping of bone graft or collapsing of disk space) or burning back pain radiating to buttocks (may indicate arachnoiditis).

Community and Home Care Considerations

1. Demonstrate and encourage back strengthening, aerobic exercise (walking, biking, swimming), and endurance exercises.
2. Make sure that the patient avoids heavy lifting and bending/twisting from the waist and uses proper body mechanics in all activities.
3. Discourage prolonged bed rest and inactivity.
4. Refer for vocational counseling, if indicated.
5. If cervical skin traction is ordered for home use, teach the patient how to apply the chinstrap and head halter. The weight should hang freely over the back of a chair or doorknob near the head of the bed. Make sure the patient maintains proper alignment of the neck and removes traction before moving the head.

Patient Education and Health Maintenance

1. Educate the patient regarding lifestyle changes—smoking cessation, increased activity, weight loss.

2. Provide instructions regarding back anatomy and back care to reduce symptoms.

3. Teach the patient the importance of cervical collar use and other conservative measures to try to reduce inflammation and heal disk herniation.

4. Tell the patient who has had a cervical disk herniation to avoid extreme flexion, extension, or rotation of the neck and to keep the head in neutral position during sleep.

5. Encourage the patient with a lumbar disk herniation to maintain ADL within pain limits, but lifting and sitting for prolonged periods are discouraged.

6. Encourage the patient to do stretching and strengthening exercises of extremities and abdomen after acute symptoms have subsided. The back can be gently stretched by lying on the back and bringing the knees up toward the chest.

7. Teach the patient about proper body mechanics and the use of leg and abdominal muscles rather than the back. Knees should be bent on lifting and load should be carried close to midtrunk.

8. Encourage follow-up with physical therapy, as indicated, for reconditioning and work hardening.

9. Tell the patient to avoid the prone position, long car rides, and sitting in a soft chair.

10. Instruct the patient to report any changes in neurologic function or recurrence of radicular pain.

11. Encourage good nutrition, avoidance of obesity, and proper rest to reduce risk of recurrence.

Evaluation: Expected Outcomes

- Verbalizes reduced pain.
- Maintains mobility with active lifestyle.
- Expresses understanding of preoperative preparation and postoperative care.
- Incision healing without signs of infection; patient ambulating with minimal pain.

SELECTED REFERENCES

American Academy of Neurology. (2012). Evidence-based guideline update: Steroids and antivirals for Bell palsy: Report for the guideline development subcommittee of the American Academy of Neurology. Minneapolis, MN: Author.

American Association of Neuroscience Nurses, the Association of Rehabilitation Nurses, & the International Organization of Multiple Sclerosis Nurses. (2011). Nursing management of the patient with multiple sclerosis. Glenview, IL: American Association of Neuroscience Nurses.

American Association of Neuroscience Nurses. (2009). Neurological assessment of the older adult; A guide for nurses. Glenview, IL: Author.

American Association of Neuroscience Nurses. (2009). Nursing management of Adults with severe traumatic brain injury. Glenview, IL: Author.

American Association of Neuroscience Nurses. (2010). AANN Core Curriculum for neuroscience nursing (5th ed.). Glenview, IL: Author.

American Association of Neuroscience Nurses. (2011). Care of the patient undergoing intracranial pressure monitoring/external ventricular drainage or lumbar drainage. Glenview, IL: Author.

American Association of Neuroscience Nurses. (2012). Guide to the care of the hospitalized patient with ischemic stroke (2nd ed.). Glenview, IL: Author.

American Association of Neuroscience Nurses. (2012). Thoracolumbar spine surgery: A guide to preoperative and postoperative patient care. Glenview, IL: Author.

American Association of Neuroscience Nurses and the Association of Rehabilitation Nurses. (2011). Care of the patient with mild traumatic brain injury. Glenview, IL: Author.

American Heart Association. (2012). Guidelines for the management of aneurysmal subarachnoid hemorrhage. Stroke, 43, 1711–1737.

American Medical Director's Association. (2010). Clinical practice guideline: Parkinson's disease. Columbia, MD: Author.

Andrews, C. M., Jauch, E. C., Hemphill, J. C., Smith, W. S., & Weingart, S. D. (2012). Emergency neurological life support: Intracerebral hemorrhage. Neurocritical Care, 17:S37–S46.

Bederson, J. B., Connolly Jr., E. S., Batjer, H. H., et al. (2012). Guidelines for the management of aneurysmal subarachnoid hemorrhage: A statement for healthcare professionals from a special writing group of the Stroke Council, American Heart Association. Stroke, 43, 1711–1737.

Bendok, B. R., Naideck, A. M., Walker, M. T., et al. (2011). Hemorrhagic and ischemic stroke: Medical, imaging, surgical and interventional approaches. New York: Thieme.

Bertorini, T. (2010). Neuromuscular disorders: Treatment and management. New York: Saunders.

Bhardwaj, A., & Mirski, M. A. (2010). Handbook of neurocritical care (2nd ed.). New York: Springer-Verlag.

Birch, R. (2011). Surgical disorders of the peripheral nerves (2nd ed.). New York: Thieme.

Blackhall, L. J. (2012). Amyotrophic lateral sclerosis and palliative care: Where we are, and the road ahead. Muscle & Nerve, 45, 311–318.

Blissitt, P. (2012) Controversies in the management of adults with severe traumatic brain injury. Advance Critical Care, 23(2), 188–203.

Campagnolo, D. I., Nash, M. S., Heary, R. F., et al. (2011). Spinal cord medicine. Philadelphia: Lippincott, Williams & Wilkins.

Carney, P. R., Berry, R. B., & Geyer, J. D. (2011). Clinical sleep disorders. New York: Lippincott, Williams & Wilkins.

Clark, K., & Levine, T. (2011). Clinical recognition and management of amyotrophic lateral sclerosis: The nurse's role. Journal of Neuroscience Nursing, 43, 205–214.

Consortium for Spinal Cord Medicine. (2008). Early acute management in adults with spinal cord injury: a clinical practice guideline for health-care professionals. Journal of Spinal Cord Medicine, 31(4), 403–479.

D'Arcy, C. (2012). Multiple sclerosis: Symptom management. Nursing & Residential Care, 14, 405–409.

Diringer, M. N., Bleck, T. P., Hemphill, J. C. III, et al. (2011). Critical care management of patients following aneurysmal subarachnoid hemorrhage: Recommendations from the Neurocritical Care Society's multidisciplinary consensus conference. Neurocritical Care, 15, 211–240.

Easton, J. D. (2009). Definition and evaluation of transient ischemic attack. Stroke, 40, 2276–2293.

Edlow, J. A., Samuels, O., Smith, W. S., & Weingart, S. D. (2012). Emergency neurological life support: Subarachnoid hemorrhage. Neurocritical Care, 17: S47–S53.

English, S. W., Turgeon, A. F., Owen, E., et al. (2012). Protocol management of severe traumatic brain injury in intensive care units. A systematic review. Neurocritical Care, published online August 2012.

Ensrud, K. E., & Schousboe, J. T. (2011). Vertebral fractures. New England Journal of Medicine, 364, 1634–1642.

Ferrara, A. R. (2011). Brain arteriovenous malformations. Radiological Technology, 82(6), 543–556.

Furie, K. L., Kasner, S. E., Adams, R. J., et al. (2011). Guidelines for the prevention of stroke in patients with stroke or transient ischemic attack: A guideline for healthcare professionals from the American Heart Association/American Stroke Association. Stroke, 42, 227–276.

Gilhus, N. E., Owe, J. F., Hoff, J. M., et al. (2011). Myasthenia gravis: A review of available treatment approaches. Autoimmune Diseases, 2011, 847393.

Giorgio, A., Battaglini, M., Rocca, M. A., et al. (2013). Location of brain lesions predicts conversion of clinically isolated syndromes to multiple sclerosis. Neurology, 80, 234–241.

Goldszmidt, A. J., & Caplan, L. R. (2010). *Stroke essentials* (2nd ed.). Boston: Jones & Bartlett.

Gross, H., Sung, G., & Weingart, S. D. (2012). Emergency neurological life support: Acute ischemic stroke. *Neurocritical Care, 17*:S29–S36.

Haddad, S. H., & Arabi, Y. M. (2012). Critical care management of severe traumatic brain injury in adults. *Scandanavian Journal of Trauma, Resuscitation, and Emergency Medicine, 20*(12). Available: *http://www.sjtrem.com/content/20/1/12.*

Haines, D. (2013). Fundamental neuroscience for basic and clinical applications. New York: Saunders.

Hardiman, O., & Doherty, C. P. (2011). *Neurodegenerative disorders: A clinical guide.* New York: Springer.

Hauser, S., & Josephson, S. (2010). *Harrison's neurology in clinical medicine* (2nd ed.). New York: McGraw-Hill.

Hayat, M. A. (2011). *Tumors of the central nervous system* (Vol. 3). New York: Springer.

Hayat, M. A. (2012). *Tumors of the central nervous system* (Vol. 6). New York: Springer.

Jallo, J., & Loftus, C. M. (2009). *Neurotrauma and critical care of the brain.* New York: Thieme.

Jankovic, J., & Poewe, W. (2012). *Therapies in Parkinson's disease. Current Opinion in Neurology, 25,* 433–447.

John, C. A., & Day, M. W. (2012). Central neurogenic diabetes insipidus, syndrome of inappropriate secretion of antidiuretic hormone, and cerebral salt-wasting syndrome in traumatic brain injury. *Critical Care Nursing, 32*(2): e1–8.

Khoo, T. K., Yarnall, A. J., Duncan, G. W., et al. (2013). The spectrum of nonmotor symptoms in early Parkinson disease. *Neurology, 80,* 276–281.

Laakso, A., Hernesniemi, J., Yonekawa, Y., et al. (2010). *Surgical management of cerebrovascular disease.* New York: Springer.

Long, S. S. (2011). Encephalitis diagnosis and management in the real world. *Advances in Experimental Medicine and Biology, 697,* 153–173.

Martelletti, P., & Steiner, T. J. (2011). *Handbook of headache: Practical management.* New York: Springer.

Miller, R. G., Jackson, C. E., Kasarskis, E. J., et al. (2009). Practice parameter update: The care of the patient with amyotrophic lateral sclerosis: Multidisciplinary care, symptom management, and cognitive/behavioral impairment (an evidenced-based review): Report of the Quality Standards Subcommittee of the American Academy of Neurology. *Neurology, 73*(15), 1227–1233.

Morgenstern, L. B., Hemphill, J. C., Anderson, C., et al. (2010). Guidelines for the management of spontaneous intracerebral hemorrhage: A guideline for healthcare professionals from the American Heart Association/American Stroke Association. *Stroke, 41,* 2108–2129.

Obermann, M., Holle, D., & Katsarava, Z. (2011). Trigeminal neuralgia and persistent idiopathic facial pain. *Expert Review of Neurotherapeutics, 11*(11), 1619–1629.

Pfaff, D. W. (2013). Neuroscience in the 21st century: From basic to clinical. New York: Springer.

Powell, R., McLauchlan, D. J. (2012). Acute symptomatic seizures. *Practical Neurology, 12,* 154–165.

Qureshi, A. I., & Georgiadis, A. L. (2011). *Textbook of interventional neurology.* New York: Cambridge University Press.

Raboel, P. H., Bartek, J., Andersen, M., et al. (2012). Intracranial pressure monitoring: Invasive versus noninvasive methods—A review. *Critical Care Research and Practice,* Volume 2012, Art. ID 950393. Available: *www.hndawi.com/journals/ccrp/2012/950393/abs.*

Rae-Grant, A., & Cohen, J. A. (2010). *Handbook of multiple sclerosis.* New York: Springer.

Rosen, B. A. (2012). Guillain-barre syndrome. *Pediatrics in Review, 33,* 164–171.

Samuels, M. A., & Ropper, A. H. (2010). *Samuels's manual of neurologic therapeutics* (8th ed.). Philadelphia: Lippincott, Williams & Wilkins.

SCIRE Project. (2010). Spinal Cord Injury Rehabilitation Evidence. Available: *www.scireproject.com.*

Shahrizaila, N., & Yuki, N. (2011). The role of immunotherapy in Guillain-Barre syndrome: Understanding the mechanism of action. *Expert Opinion in Pharmacotherapy, 12*(10), 1551–1560.

Shin, S. H., & Kim, K. S. (2012). Treatment of bacterial meningitis: An update. *Expert Opinion in Pharmacotherapy, 15,* 2189–2206.

Silvestri, N. J., & Wolfe, G. I. (2012). Myasthenia gravis. *Seminars in Neurology, 32,* 215–226.

Stein, D. M., Roddy, V., Marx, J., Smith, W. S., & Weingart, S. D. (2012). Emergency neurological life support: Traumatic spinal injury. *Neurocritical Care, 17*:S102–S111.

Theroux, N., Phipps, M., Zimmerman, L., et al. (2013). Neurologic complications associated with HIV and AIDS: Clinical implications for nursing. *Journal of Neuroscience Nursing, 45*(1), 5–13.

Thompson, C., Kneen, R., Riordan, A., Kelly, D., Pollard, A. J. (2012). Encephalitis in children. *Archives of Disease in Childhood, 97,* 150–161.

Tonn, J., Westphal, M., & Rutka, J. T. (2010). *Oncology of CNS tumors.* New York: Springer.

Winn, H. R. (2011). *Youmans Neurological Surgery.* Philadelphia: Elsevier.

Woehrl, B., Klein, M., Grandgirard, D., et al. (2011). Bacterial meningitis: Current therapy and possible future treatment options. *Expert Review of Anti-infective Therapies, 9*(11), 1053–1065.

Wuchner, S., Bakas, T., Adams, G., Buelow, J., & Cohn, J. (2012). Nursing Interventions and assessments for aneurysmal subarachnoid hemorrhage patients: A mixed methods study involving practicing nurses. *Journal of Neuroscience Nursing, 44*(4): 177–185.

Yousem, D. M., & Grossman, R. I. (2010). *Neuroradiology: The requisites* (3rd ed.). Philadelphia: Elsevier.

16
Eye Disorders

INTRODUCTION
Definitions of Terms

1. *Accommodation:* Focusing apparatus of the eye that adjusts to objects at different distances by means of increasing the convexity of the lens (brought about by contraction of the ciliary muscles).
2. *Ametropia:* Abnormal vision.
   a. *Myopia:* Nearsightedness: rays of light coming from an object at a distance of 20 feet or more are brought to a focus in front of the retina.
   b. *Hyperopia:* Farsightedness: rays of light coming from an object at a distance of 20 feet or more are brought to a focus in back of the retina.
3. *Astigmatism:* Uneven curvature of the cornea causing the patient to be unable to focus horizontal and vertical rays of light on the retina at the same time.
4. *Emmetropia:* Normal vision: rays of light coming from an object at a distance of 20 feet (6 m) or more are brought to focus on the retina by the lens (see Figure 16-1).
5. *Presbyopia:* The elasticity of the lens decreases with increasing age; an emmetropic person with presbyopia will read the paper at arm's length and will require prescription lenses to correct the problem.
6. *Strabismus:* Deviation of the eye so that the visual axes are not physiologically coordinated.
7. *Vision:* Passage of rays of light from an object through the cornea, aqueous humor, lens, and vitreous humor to the retina and its appreciation in the cerebral cortex.
8. *Visual acuity:* Measurement of a person's ability to see at a distance or near (reading distance) and is measured against a standard of a normal person's visual ability.

Common Abbreviations

OD (oculus dexter) or RE—right eye
OS (oculus sinister) or LE—left eye
OU (oculus unitas)—both eyes
IOP—intraocular pressure
IOL—intraocular lens
EOL—extraocular lens
VA—visual acuity

Eye Care Specialists

1. **Ophthalmologist:** Physician specializing in diagnosis, surgery, and treatment of the eye; may specialize in a specific part of the eye or disorder, such as a cornea specialist or glaucoma specialist.

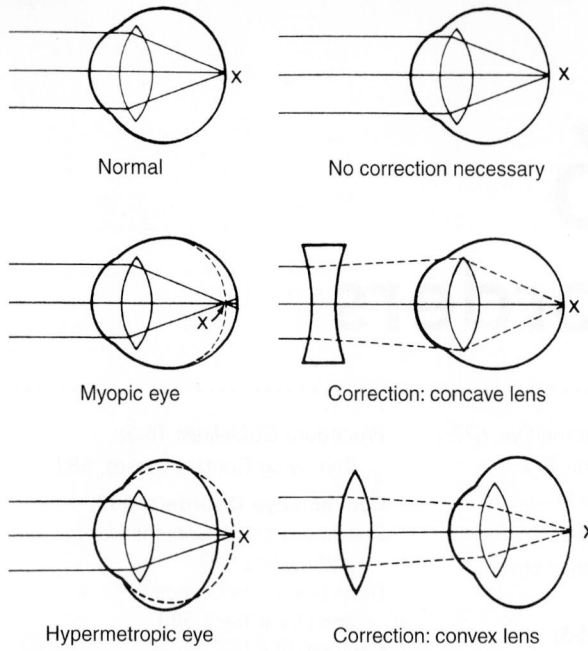

Figure 16-1. Normal vision and refractory errors.

2. **Optometrist:** Doctor of optometry who can examine, diagnose, and manage visual problems and diseases of the eye, but does not perform surgery.
3. **Optician:** Technician who fits, adjusts, and gives eyeglasses or other devices on the written prescription of an ophthalmologist or optometrist.
4. **Ocularist:** Technician who makes ophthalmic prostheses.

Subjective Data

 Evidence Base American Society of Ophthalmologic Registered Nurses. (2008). *Core curriculum for ophthalmic nursing* (3rd ed.). Dubuque, IA: Kendall/Hunt.

Subjective data for eye assessment include complaints of altered vision or other symptoms, associated lifestyle and other factors, and recent and past health history.

Presenting Symptoms

1. Explore the chief complaint from patient by asking the following questions:
   a. Is there pain, foreign body sensation (scratchy, something in the eye), photophobia, dryness, redness, itchiness, lacrimation, or drainage?
   b. Is there blurred vision, double vision, loss of vision, or change in vision in a portion of the visual field?
   c. Are there other visual symptoms such as glare, halos, floaters?
   d. Is there difficulty in functioning, such as driving or reading, due to visual problem?

2. Review related systems.
   a. Neurologic: Are there scintillations, scotomas, transient ischemic attacks, headache, sensory or motor dysfunction?
   b. Ear, nose, and throat: Any nasal congestion, rhinitis, sinus pain, dry mouth?
   c. Integumentary: Are there changes in skin and mucus membranes?
   d. Endocrine: Any complaints of polyuria, polydipsia; signs of hyperthyroidism (see page 922)?
   e. Musculoskeletal: Is there joint pain or swelling?

History

1. Review ocular history.
   a. Have there been previous eye injuries, surgeries, and ocular procedures?
   b. Is patient using glasses or contact lenses?
   c. Was there childhood poor vision or patching of the eye?
   d. Are there current visual problems such as glaucoma, cataracts, macular degeneration, or diabetic retinopathy?
2. Obtain medication history, including nonprescription, herbal, topical, and inhalant products.
3. Determine allergies to medications; note type of reaction.
4. Determine history of systemic conditions such as diabetes, cardiovascular disease, arthritis, Marfan's syndrome, albinism, sickle cell anemia.
5. Obtain family history of ocular condtions such as glaucoma, cataracts, macular degeneration, color blindness, retinitis pigmentosa, retinoblastoma, nystagmus, keratoconus, choroideremia, corneal dystrophies, and other chronic diseases.
6. Perform functional assessment.
   a. Depending on the patient's circumstance, administer the National Eye Institute Visual Function Questionnaire (VFQ-25) available at *www.rand.org/health/surveys_tools/vfq.html*, or other valid visual functioning questionnaires such as the VF-14.
   b. This helps determine the need for surgery based on the extent to which the eye disorder interferes with the patient's ability to carry out a visually dependent activity of daily living such as driving and reading.

 GERONTOLOGIC ALERT Question older patients about driving. Change in driving pattern, such as avoidance of night driving and less rush-hour driving, may indicate visual dysfunction as well as impaired reflexes and ability to concentrate in complex situations. A common complaint is not being able to read road signs in time to respond to them.

Ocular Examination

See Figure 16-2. Also see "Adult Physical Assessment," page 52.

 NURSING ALERT Every patient who seeks medical attention for an eye complaint should have visual acuity tested.

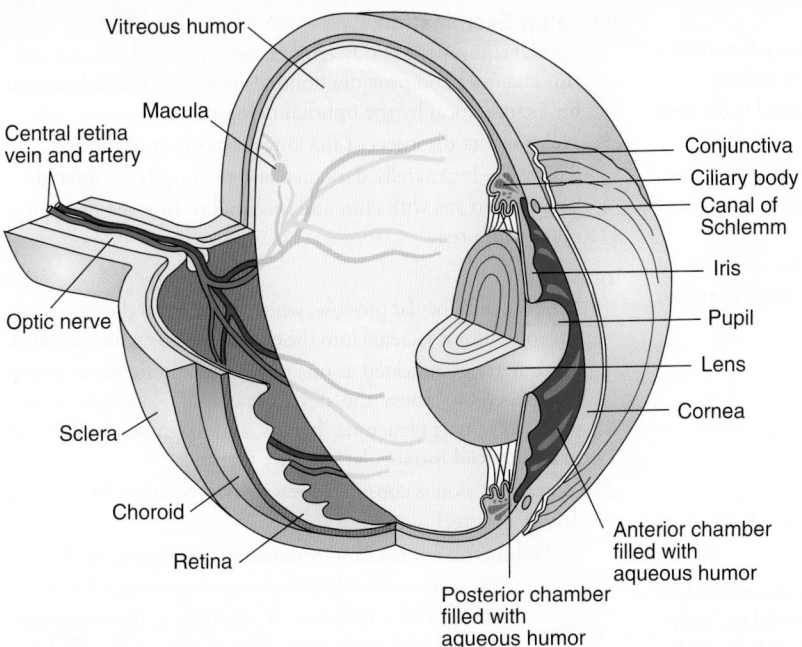

Vitreous humor

Macula

Central retina
vein and artery

Optic nerve

Sclera

Choroid

Retina

Posterior chamber
filled with
aqueous humor

Conjunctiva

Ciliary body

Canal of
Schlemm

Iris

Pupil

Lens

Cornea

Anterior chamber
filled with
aqueous humor

Figure 16-2. Three-dimensional cross section of the eye.

External Examination

Includes examination of the eye and accessory organs without the aid of special apparatus.

Visual Acuity at Distance (Snellen Chart and Other Methods)

1. Letters and objects are of different sizes that can be seen by the normal eye at a distance of 20 feet (6 m) from the chart.
2. Letters appear in rows and are arranged so the normal eye can see them at distances of 30, 40, and 50 feet (9, 12, and 15 m), and so forth.
3. Each eye is tested separately, with and without correction (glasses or contact lenses) while the nontesting eye is completely occluded.
4. Test the right eye (OD) first and then the left eye (OS)
5. A person who can identify letters of the size 20 at 20 feet (6 at 6 m) is said to have 20/20 (6/6) vision.
6. If vision is less than 20/200 (6/60), additional tests may be recorded as:
   a. Counting fingers (CF)—at feet (meters).
   b. Hand motion (HM)—ability to detect hand movement at a certain distance.
   c. Light perception and projection (LP).
   d. Light perception only.
   e. No light perception.

Visual Acuity at Near (Jaeger Chart and Other Methods)

1. Letters and objects are of different sizes that can be seen by the normal eye at a reading distance of 14 inches from the chart.
2. Letters appear in rows and are arranged so the normal eye can read them at different levels on the Jaeger chart.

3. Each eye is tested separately, with and without correction (glasses or contact lenses) while the nontesting eye is completely occluded.
4. Test the right eye (OD) first and then the left eye (OS).
5. The vision is documented in Jaeger or Snellen notation where J1+ is equivalent to 20/20, J2 equivalent to 20/30 and so forth.

Visual Fields

Determines function of optic pathways and identifies loss of visual field and functional capacity.

1. Equipment—light source and test objects. May be performed manually or as automated visual fields.
2. Peripheral field—useful in detecting decreased peripheral vision in one or both eyes.
   a. Patient is seated 18 to 24 inches (45.5 to 61 cm) in front of the examiner.
   b. The left eye is covered while the patient focuses with the right eye on a spot about 12 inches (30.5 cm) from the eye.
   c. A test object is brought in from the side at 15-degree intervals, through a complete 360 degrees.
   d. The patient signals when he or she sees the test object and again when the object disappears through the 360 degrees.

Color Vision Tests

These tests are done to determine the person's ability to perceive primary colors and shades of colors. It is particularly significant for people whose occupation requires discerning colors, such as artists, interior decorators, transportation workers, surgeons, and nurses. (Useful in diagnosing diffuse retinal dysfunction and various types of optic neuropathies.)

1. Equipment.
   a. Polychromatic plates—dots of primary colors printed on a background of similar dots in a confusion of colors.
   b. Individual colored disks—each disk is matched to its next closest color.
2. Procedure.
   a. Various polychromatic plates are presented to the patient under specified illumination.
   b. The patterns may be letters or numbers that the normal eye can perceive instantly, but that are confusing to the person with a perception defect.
3. Outcome.
   a. Color blindness—person can't perceive the figures.
   b. Red-green blindness—8% of males, 0.4% of females.
   c. Blue-yellow blindness—rare.

Refraction

Refraction is a clinical measurement of the error of focus in an eye.

1. Refraction and internal examination may be accomplished by instilling a medication with cycloplegic and mydriatic properties into the conjunctiva of the eye. Tropicamide or cyclopentolate are two such medicines that cause ciliary muscle relaxation, pupil dilation (mydriasis), and lowered accommodative power (cycloplegia).
2. In older children and adults, refraction without the use of drugs is preferred.
3. Visual screening through a multiple pinhole card can help refractive causes of decreased vision versus decreased vision secondary to organic disease.
4. The refractive state of the eye can be determined in two ways:
   a. Objectively—through retinoscopy or by automatic refraction (special instrument that measures, computes, and prints out refraction errors of each eye).
   b. Subjectively—trial of lenses to arrive at the best visual image.

Internal Examination

Ophthalmoscopic Examination

1. Direct ophthalmoscopy—uses a strong light reflected into the interior of the eye through an instrument called an ophthalmoscope.
2. Indirect ophthalmoscopy—allows the examiner to obtain a stereoscopic view of the retina. Light source is from a head-mounted light. The examiner views the retina through a convex lens held in front of the eye and a viewing device on the head mount. The image appears inverted. This method of examination allows the examiner to use binocular vision with depth perception and a wider viewing field.
3. Clinical significance:
   a. Detection of cataracts, vitreous opacities, corneal scars.
   b. Close examination for the pathologic changes in retinal blood vessels that may occur with diabetes or hypertension.
   c. Examination of the choroid for tumors or inflammation.
   d. Examination of the retina for retinal detachment, scars, or exudates and hemorrhages.

Slit-Lamp Examination

1. Special equipment that magnifies the cornea, sclera, and anterior chamber and provides oblique views into the trabeculum for examination by the ophthalmologist.
2. Helps detect disorders of the anterior portion of the eye.
3. The room is generally darkened and the pupils are dilated.
4. The patient sits with chin and forehead resting against equipment supports.

Tonometry

1. Measures intraocular pressure, which depends on the amount of aqueous humor secreted into the eye and ease by which it leaves.
2. Tonometry is indicated as one of the measurements to screen for glaucoma, assess the development of glaucoma if suspected, evaluate glaucoma therapy, and diagnose phthisis and drug-induced intraocular pressure increase.
3. Normal tension is considered less than or equal to 20 mm Hg.
4. Tonometry techniques.
   a. Goldmann applanation tonometry (see Figure 16-3).
      i. This is the most effective measuring method for determining IOP; however, it requires a biomicroscope and a trained interpreter. May be part of the slit-lamp examination or done by handheld device.
      ii. After instillation of topical anesthesia, the cornea is flattened by a known amount (3.14 mm).
      iii. The pressure necessary to produce this flattening is equal to the IOP, counterbalancing the tonometer.

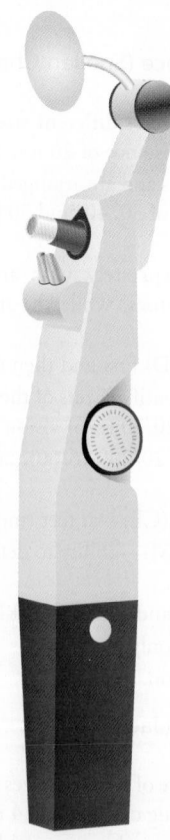

Figure 16-3. Example of an applanation tonometer.

b. Schiotz tonometry (rarely used in ophthalmology).

c. Electronic tonometer that provides a digital reading of intraocular pressure, such as the Tono-Pen.

d. Pneumotonometer or air applanation tonometry—requires no topical anesthesia and measures tension by sensing deformation of the cornea in reaction to a puff of pressurized air.

e. Perkins hand-held tonometer.

f. Finger tension—pressure determined by use of digital pressure.

Radiology and Imaging

Several imaging studies beyond the basic eye examination may be done to further evaluate eye disease.

Fluorescein Angiography

Description

1. Provides information concerning vascular obstructions, microaneurysms, abnormal capillary permeability, and defects in retinal pigment permeability.

2. Introduction of sodium fluorescein IV administration over several minutes, usually through a brachial vein.

3. Indirect ophthalmoscopy using a blue filter may be done and photographs of the ocular fundus are obtained.

Nursing and Patient Care Considerations

1. Advise the patient that a series of eye drops will be given to dilate the pupil for better visualization of the retina. The patient will be positioned in a special chair with head immobilized.

2. Dye will be injected into the arm over several minutes. Photographs will be taken during injection and up to 1 hour after injection.

3. Adverse effects include nausea due to dye injection, burning in eye from eye drop instillation, blurred vision and photophobia for 4 to 8 hours due to pupil dilation, and possible yellow skin and urine discoloration for up to 48 hours after dye injection.

 DRUG ALERT Serious reactions, such as hoarseness, respiratory obstruction, tachycardia, and anaphylactic reaction leading to death may result from sodium fluoroscein IV administration.

Eye and Orbit Sonography

Description

Sound waves are used in the diagnosis of intraocular and orbital lesions. Three types of ultrasonography are used in ophthalmoscopy:

1. A-scan—uses stationary transducers to measure the distance between changes in acoustic density. This is used to differentiate between benign and malignant tumors and to measure the length of the eye to determine the power of an IOL.

2. B-scan—moves linearly across the eye; increases in acoustic density are shown as an intensification on the line of the scan that presents a picture of the eye and the orbit.

3. IOL Master technology—evaluates the length of the eye, surface curvature, and IOL power; has increased the accuracy of biometry by five-fold. It is also less technician-dependent for accuracy.

Abnormal patterns are seen in alkali burns, detached retina, keratoprosthesis, thyroid ophthalmopathy, foreign bodies, vascular malformations, benign and malignant tumors, and a variety of other conditions.

Nursing and Patient Care Considerations

1. Advise the patient that topical anesthetic drops are applied to the eye before the procedure so the patient will not feel the transducer contacting the eye.

2. The procedure may take as little as 8 to 10 minutes or 30 minutes or longer, if a lesion is detected, to locate the lesion.

3. Warn patient not to rub eyes until the anesthetic has worn off to avoid trauma to the eye.

Electroretinography

Description

Used to evaluate hereditary and acquired disorders of the retina; an electrode is placed over the eye to evaluate the electrical response to light.

Nursing and Patient Care Considerations

1. Advise the patient that the eyes are propped open and patient will be positioned lying or sitting down.

2. Topical anesthetic drops are instilled.

3. A cotton wick electrode saturated in saline is applied to the cornea.

4. Various intensities of light are produced and the electrical potential is measured.

5. Caution the patient not to rub eyes for up to 1 hour after procedure to avoid trauma while eyes are anesthetized.

GENERAL PROCEDURES AND TREATMENT MODALITIES

Instillation of Medications

See Procedure Guidelines 16-1, pages 576 to 577.

Ophthalmic medications may be used for diagnostic and therapeutic purposes:

1. To dilate or contract the pupil.
2. To relieve pain, discomfort, itching, and inflammation.
3. To act as an antiseptic in cleansing the eye.
4. To combat infection.

See Table 16-1, pages 578 and 579, for ophthalmic pharmacologic agents.

Irrigation of the Eye

See Procedure Guidelines 16-2, page 580.

Ocular irrigation is often necessary for the following:

1. To irrigate chemicals or foreign bodies from the eyes.
2. To remove secretions from the conjunctival sac.
3. To treat infections.

PROCEDURE GUIDELINES 16-1

Instillation of Eye Medications

EQUIPMENT

- Sterile solution or medication (most medications have accompanying dropper or are in squeeze bottle or tube)
- Small gauze squares or tissues

PROCEDURE

Nursing Action	Rationale
Preparatory phase	
1. Inform the patient of the need and reason for instilling drops or ointment.	1. Allays fear and enlists cooperation.
2. Allow the patient to sit with head tilted backward or to lie in a supine position.	2. Provides a position of comfort and safety for the patient and accessibility for the nurse.
3. Verify the patient's identification.	3. Prevents error.
4. Check written prescription and bottle, vial, or tube for correct medication.	4. Avoids medication error.
5. Check prescription, designating eye requiring drops.	5. Order may be written with abbreviation. OD (oculus dexter)—right eye OS (oculus sinister)—left eye OU (oculus uterque)—both eyes
6. Wash hands before instilling medication.	6. Prevents transfer of microorganisms to patient.
Performance phase	
1. Remove cap from container and place on clean surface.	1. Prevents contamination of lid.
2. If eyedropper is used, fill eyedropper with medication by squeezing bulb.	2. Eye droppers are used less frequently than dropper bottles.
3. Using forefinger, pull on skin below lower lid	3. Exposes inner surface of lid and cul-de-sac.
4. Instruct patient to look upward.	4. Prevents medication from hitting sensitive cornea and prevents blephorospasm.
5. Drop medication amount prescribed into center of lower lid (cul-de-sac) (see Figure A).	5. Prevents medication from hitting sensitive cornea.

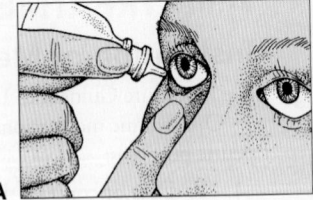 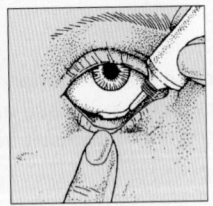

A   B

6. If ointment is to be instilled, squeeze out $\frac{1}{8}$-inch ribbon of medication (size of grain of rice) from the tube into the lower lid without touching the eye with the end of the tube (see Figure B).	6. Prevents contamination of the tube. Avoids dispensing excessive ointment; clouds vision.
7. Instruct patient to close eyes slowly but not to squeeze or rub them. Open eye.	7. Squeezing or rubbing would express medication from eye and increase lacrimal drainage from the eye; closing allows medication to be distributed evenly over eye.
8. Clear any excess medication with gauze or tissues.	8. Prevents possible skin irritation.
9. If additional eye drops are ordered, wait 30 seconds between each drop.	9. Allows time for absorption of medication.

 NURSING ALERT Parietal occlusion (place finger over lacrimal duct for 1 minute) may be necessary after instilling drops if systemic absorption is to be avoided, prolonged corneal contact is desired, or taste or smell of medication is distressing.

PROCEDURE GUIDELINES 16-1 (continued)

Instillation of Eye Medications

PROCEDURE (continued)

Nursing Action	Rationale
Follow-up phase	
1. Wash hands after instilling medication.	1. Prevents transfer of microorganisms to self or other patients.
2. Record time, type, strength, and amount of medication and the eye into which medication was instilled.	2. Provides documentation in the medication record.

 Evidence Base American Society of Ophthalmologic Registered Nurses. (2011). *Ophthalmic procedures in the office and clinic* (3rd ed.). Dubuque, IA: Kendall/Hunt.

4. To relieve itching.
5. To provide moisture on the surface of the eyes of an unconscious patient.

Application of Dressing or Patch

See Procedure Guidelines 16-3, page 581.

One or both eyes may need shielding for the following:

1. To keep an eye at rest, thereby promoting healing.
2. To prevent the patient from touching eye.
3. To absorb secretions.
4. To protect the eye.
5. To control or lessen edema.

Removing a Particle from the Eye

See Procedure Guidelines 16-4, pages 582 to 583.

1. Typically, removing a foreign body from the eye is an uncomplicated first-aid measure.
2. However, if the object appears to be embedded, medical intervention is required, that is, local anesthetic, antibiotic therapy, and clinical expertise in using other instruments.
3. The cornea should be evaluated for abrasion from the foreign body by use of fluorescein staining, even if a foreign body cannot be found.

Removing Contact Lenses

Because contact lenses need regular cleaning and changing, if a person is injured and incapacitated because of an accident, sickness, or other cause, the lenses should be removed. See Procedure Guidelines 16-5, pages 583 to 584.

1. Contact lenses should be removed in conjunction with a thorough eye exam. An optometrist or ophthalmologist may have to be notified.
2. Determine the type of lens from the patient or family.
   a. Soft corneal lenses are widely used. The diameter covers the cornea plus a portion of the sclera of the eye. Extended- and daily-wear soft lenses are available.
   b. Rigid or gas-permeable lenses are usually smaller than the cornea of the eye, although some are made to extend beyond the cornea onto the sclera of the eye. These lenses need to be removed promptly.
3. Do not remove lenses if the iris is not visible on opening the eyelids; await the arrival of an ophthalmologist. If patient is to be transported, note that contacts are in the eyes. (Write out the message and tape it to the patient or send with transporter.)

Ocular Surgery

Follow this nursing process overview for any patient having ocular surgery. Specific nursing interventions are listed in the next section for particular types of surgical procedures.

Nursing Assessment

1. Collect subjective and objective data about patient's general state of health.
2. Ascertain what symptoms the patient has been having (eye pain, visual loss, drainage, history of trauma) and how that has impacted usual activity.
3. Assess the patient's mobility and self-care ability.
4. Assess visual and other sensory impairments.
5. Gather data regarding usual support systems used by patient. Is family near? Do friends visit regularly?
6. Review the patient's daily schedule.
7. Record pertinent data in patient's record.

Nursing Diagnoses

- Deficient Knowledge of postoperative expectations and continuing care.
- Risk for Injury related to altered vision.
- Impaired Environmental Interpretation Syndrome related to visual disturbance.
- Fear of blindness related to invasive procedure to eye.
- Bathing, Dressing, Feeding Self Care Deficit related to reduced or altered vision.

(Text continues on page 584)

Table 16-1   Ophthalmic Pharmacologic Agents*

PHARMACOLOGY	ACTION	PRODUCTS
Sympathomimetics	Given topically for the treatment of glaucoma. Immediate effect is decrease in production of aqueous humor. Long-term effect is an increase in outflow facility. May be used in combination with miotics, beta-adrenergic blockers, carbonic anhydrase inhibitors, or hyperosmotic agents.	• Epinephrine, dipivetrin, phenylephrine
Miotics, direct-acting	Cholinergic agents given topically that affect the muscarinic receptors of the eye; results include miosis and contraction of the ciliary muscle. In narrow-angle glaucoma, miosis opens the angle to improve aqueous outflow. Contraction of the ciliary muscle enhances the outflow of aqueous humor by indirect action of the trabecular network—the exact mechanism is unknown. Primary use of miotics is in glaucoma but can be used to counter the effects of cycloplegics/mydriatics.	• Acetylcholine • Carbachol • Pilocarpine
Miotics, cholinesterase inhibitors	Topical agents that inhibit the enzyme cholinesterase, causing an increase in the activity of the acetylcholine already present in the body. Causes intense miosis and contraction of the ciliary muscle. Decrease in intraocular pressure that is seen is a result of increased outflow of aqueous humor. Used for treatment of open-angle glaucoma, conditions where the outflow of aqueous is obstructed; postiridectomy problems; and accommodative esotropia (inward deviation of one eye).	• Demecarium bromide • Isoflurophate • Physostigmine
Beta-adrenergic blockers	Act on the beta receptors of the adrenergic nervous system. Two types of beta sites: B_1 and B_2. B_1 site primarily the myocardium resulting in decreased heart rate and cardiac output. B_2 primarily bronchial and vascular smooth muscle resulting in bronchoconstriction, decreased blood pressure. There are two types of ophthalmic beta-adrenergic blockers: cardioselective blocker (betaxolol) acts only on B_1 sites and may on rare occasions cause cardiac effects if absorbed systemically. All other nonselective blockers act on B_1 and B_2 sites and cause significant cardiac and pulmonary effects if absorbed systemically. Used for treatment of increased intraocular pressure by decreasing the formation of aqueous humor and causing a slight increase in the outflow facility.	• Betaxolol • Levobunolol • Timolol • Carteolol
Carbonic anhydrase inhibitors	Oral agents that act to inhibit the action of carbonic anhydrase. Suppression of this enzyme results in a decreased production of aqueous humor. Used in combination regimen to treat glaucoma and postoperative rise in IOP.	• Acetazolamide • Methazolamide
Osmotic diuretics	Osmotic agents given intravenously used for reduction of IOP in acute attack of glaucoma or before ocular surgery where preoperative reduction of IOP is indicated.	• Mannitol • Glycerin
Prostaglandin analogues	Newer agents used in the lowering of IOP presumably by increasing transuveal flow or filtration of aqueous. Used in open-angle glaucoma resistant to other agents.	• Latanoprost • Travoprost • Bimaprost • Unoprostone
Mydriatics	Topical agents that result in dilation of the pupil, vasoconstriction, and an increase in the outflow of aqueous humor. Used for pupillary dilatation for surgery and examination.	• Phenylephrine
Cycloplegic mydriatics	Topical agents that block the reaction of the sphincter muscle of the iris and the muscle of the ciliary body to cholinergic stimulation, resulting in dilatation of the pupil (mydriasis) and paralysis of accommodation (cycloplegia). Used in conditions requiring pupil to be dilated and kept from accommodation.	• Atropine • Homatropine • Scopolamine • Cyclopentolate • Tropicamide
Ophthalmic anti-infectives	Topical agents used for treatment of ophthalmic infections. Commercial products are intended for treatment of superficial ocular problems, such as conjunctivitis and blepharitis. Extemporaneous (compounded) drops are used for more serious topical infections (ie, corneal ulcer, endophthalmitis [intraocular infection]).	*Antibiotics* • Bacitracin • Chloramphenicol • Ciprofloxacin • Erythromycin

Table 16-1	Ophthalmic Pharmacologic Agents* *(continued)*	
PHARMACOLOGY	**ACTION**	**PRODUCTS**
		• Gentamycin • Gatafloxacin • Levofloxacin • Moxifloxacin • Neomycin/polymyxin/bacitracin • Norfloxacin • Sulfacetamide • Tobramycin *Antifungal* • Amphotericin B • Fluconazole • Natamycin *Antiviral* • Trifluridine • Vidarabine
Local anesthetics	Block the transmission of nerve impulses. Used topically to provide local anesthetic for tests, such as tonometry, and for procedures of short duration. Injections used in ophthalmology for retrobulbar blocks.	*Topical* • Proparacaine • Tetracaine injection • Lidocaine
Ophthalmic steroid anti-inflammatories	Mostly corticosteroids. Used topically to relieve pain and photophobia as well as suppress other inflammatory processes of the conjunctiva, cornea, lid, and interior segment of the globe.	• Dexamethasone • Fluorometholone • Loteprednol • Prednisolone acetate
Nonsteroidal anti-inflammatory drugs (NSAIDs)	Act by inhibiting an enzyme involved in the synthesis of prostaglandins, which are key in the body's response to inflammation. These drugs, given topically, are analgesics and anti-inflammatories.	• Diclofenac sodium • Flurbiprofen • Ketorolac • Suprofen
Anti-allergy medications	There are a number of different types of drugs, given topically, in this category, including antihistamine, mast cell stabilizers, NSAID anesthetic, and astringents (some in combination).	*Antihistamines* • Emedastine • Levocabastine • Olopatadine • Pheniramine *Mast cell stabilizers* • Cromolyn • Lodoxamide *Astringent* • Zinc sulfate
Vasoconstrictors	Topical agents that contract local blood vessels, resulting in less redness and irritation.	• Naphazoline
Alpha-selective adrenergic agonist agents	Topical agents that mimic the effects of endogenous adrenergic compounds by selectively binding to alpha-2 receptors, resulting in aqueous formation, pupil diameter, and ocular flow. Commonly used for lowering elevated IOP.	• Apraclonidine hydrochloride • Brominidine tartate
Anti-VEGF agents	Slow growth of abnormal blood vessels under the retina by blocking the effects of VEGF to slow vision loss and possibly improve vision in wet age-related macular degeneration.	• Bevacizumab • Pegaptanib • Ranibizumab

*All pharmacologic agents should be reviewed from manufacturer's information or drug reference source before administration for contraindications, adverse reactions, and cautions.

IOP, intraocular pressure; VEGF, vascular endothelial growth factor.

PROCEDURE GUIDELINES 16-2

Irrigating the Eye (Conjunctival Irrigation)

EQUIPMENT

- An eyedropper, aseptic bulb syringe, or plastic bottle with prescribed solution depending on the extent of irrigation needed (usually more than 1,000 mL for each eye)
- For copious use (ie, chemical burns), sterile normal saline or prescribed solution and IV setup with attached tubing
- Irrigating lens for chemical injury (contraindicated for particulate matter)
- Litmus paper
- Basin, towels

PROCEDURE

Nursing Action	Rationale
Preparatory phase	
1. Verify the eye to be irrigated and the solution and amount of irrigant. Work as quickly as possible and have equipment ready ahead of time if chemical injury is suspected.	1. Prevents error.
2. The patient may sit with head tilted back or lie in a supine position.	2. Facilitates flow of solution over the eye.
3. Instruct the patient to tilt head toward the side of the affected eye.	3. Prevents fluid from draining into unaffected eye.

 DRUG ALERT Topical anesthetic drops may be instilled prior to irrigation according to policy or order. If used, do not allow patient to rub eye for 45 minutes to avoid injury.

Nursing Action	Rationale
Performance phase	
1. Test pH using plain litmus paper in cul-de-sac of affected eye.	1. Serves as a baseline. Alkaline (pH > 7) is more damaging than acidic (pH < 7).
2. Wash eyelashes and lids with prescribed solution at room temperature; a curved basin should be placed on the affected side of the face to catch the outflow.	2. Any materials on the lids and lashes should be washed off before exposing conjunctiva.
3. Evert the lower conjunctival sac. (If feasible, have the patient pull down lower lid with index finger.)	3. Exposes inner surfaces of lower lid and conjunctival sac (involves the patient and gives a sense of control).
4. Instruct the patient to look up; avoid touching eye with equipment.	4. Prevents injury to the sensitive cornea.
5. Allow irrigating fluid to flow from the inner canthus to the outer canthus along the conjunctival sac.	5. Prevents solution from flowing toward the unaffected eye.
6. Use only enough force to flush secretions from conjunctiva. (Allow patient to hold receptacle near the eye to catch fluid.)	6. Prevents eye injury (involves the patient in the treatment).
7. Occasionally, have patient close eyes.	7. Allows upper lid to meet lower lid with the possibility of dislodging additional particles.
8. Wait 1 minute after irrigation and retest pH.	8. If pH is not 7, repeat irrigation.
Follow-up phase	
1. Pat eye dry and dry the patient's face with a soft cloth.	1. Provides comfort.
2. Record kind and amount of fluid used as well as its effectiveness.	2. Provides documentation of nursing actions.

 Evidence Base American Society of Ophthalmic Registered Nurses. (2011). *Ophthalmic procedures for the office and clinic* (3rd ed.). Dubuque, IA: Kendall/Hunt.

PROCEDURE GUIDELINES 16-3

Application of an Eye Patch, Eye Shield, and Pressure Dressing to the Eye

EQUIPMENT

- Eye covering to be used (shield, oval patches)
- Tape
- Scissors
- Tincture of benzoin or skin protectant (optional)

PROCEDURE

Nursing Action	Rationale
Preparatory phase	
1. Wash hands.	1. Prevents contamination.
2. Explain procedure to patient.	2. Allays fear and ensures cooperation.
3. Verify patient and eye to be patched.	3. Prevents error.
4. Instill ointment, if directed, prior to patching.	4. May be ordered to protect cornea from abrasion or prevent infection.
5. Shave the male face and apply tincture of benzoin, as indicated.	5. Enhances ability for tape to stick and protect the skin from tape.
Performance phase	
1. For eye patch:	
a. Instruct patient to close both eyes.	a. It may be difficult to close only the affected eye.
b. Place patch over affected eye.	b. May need two or more patches, depending on the depth of the eye compared with the surrounding bones.
c. Secure the patch with two or more strips of tape applied downward and diagonally from midforehead to cheek.	c. Although transparent tape is easy to remove and adhesive tape is most secure, hypoallergenic tape should be used if patient has had reaction to tape in past.
2. For eye shield:	
a. Apply over dressings or directly over the undressed eye, fastening with two or more strips of tape.	a. Used primarily to protect the eye. Some shields may be bent to rest over bony prominences. Tape placed around edges of the shield will not obstruct vision through holes in the shield.
b. Be sure there are no rough edges against the skin.	b. Prevents abrasion. Use skin protectant, as indicated.
3. For pressure dressing:	
a. Have the patient close both eyes tightly.	a. Prevents eye from opening before dressing is secured.
b. Fold patch in half (short end to short end) and place over closed eyelid (with fold line at eyebrow). Cover with additional unfolded patches.	b. Provides pressure dressing bulk.
c. Apply strips of tape firmly from check to forehead, overlapping each strip.	c. Secures dressing and applies pressure.
Follow-up phase	
1. Trim tape and monitor for security of patch or shield.	1. For patient's safety and comfort.
2. Advise patient that because depth perception will be impaired, he or she should perform activities carefully and report any foreign body sensation.	2. Prevent accidents or corneal abrasion if eyelid opens and patch rubs against cornea.

 Evidence Base American Ophthalmic Association of Registered Nurses. (2011). *Ophthalmic procedures for the office or clinic* (3rd ed.). Dubuque, IA: Kendall/Hunt.

PROCEDURE GUIDELINES 16-4

Removing a Particle from the Eye and Fluorescein Staining

EQUIPMENT

- Local anesthesia
- Hand lens
- Sterile fluorescein strips and illumination source
- Cotton applicator
- Normal saline
- Antibiotic solution

PROCEDURE

Nursing Action	Rationale

Preparatory phase

 NURSING ALERT It is important to take a patient history to determine the nature of the foreign body. If the particle is metal or entered the eye with projectile force, trauma to the eye could result. It may be necessary for the ophthalmologist to remove the foreign body immediately without attempting this method to prevent further injury.

Nursing Action	Rationale
1. Perform hand hygiene.	1. Prevents contamination.
2. Explain procedure to patient.	2. Allays fear and ensures cooperation.
3. Instill anesthetic eye drops, as directed.	3. Facilitates comfort.

Performance phase

Removal of Particle

Nursing Action	Rationale
1. As patient looks upward, place your finger below the lower lid and pull downward to expose the conjunctival sac. Inspect for particles using a hand lens.	1. Particles are often washed downward by the upper lid.
2. With small cotton applicator dipped in saline, remove particle by gently wiping across conjunctival surface.	2. Prevents trauma. Saline promotes adherence of a particle.
3. If offending particle is not found, proceed to examine upper lid.	3.
a. Have the patient look downward.	a. Moves sensitive cornea down and away from area of activity.
b. Encourage the patient to relax; move slowly and reassure patient that procedure will not be painful.	b. Relaxation prevents squeezing the lids shut, a maneuver that contracts the obicularis muscle, making eversion of lid impossible.
c. Place cotton applicator stick horizontally on outer surface of upper lid. Apply pressure about 1 cm above lid margin (see Figure A).	c. Because the upper tarsal plate extends 0.4–0.5 inch (10–12 mm) above the lid margin, pressure must be applied at least ½ inch (1 cm) above the lid margin for easy eversion of lid.
d. Grasp upper eyelashes with forefinger and thumb and pull the upper lid outward and upward over cotton applicator (see Figure B). Remove particle, if present.	d. Because particles may be washed under the lid, visual exposure assists in detection. Eyelid will remain everted by itself during inspection and removal.
e. Ask the patient to look up and blink.	e. Returns eyelid to neutral position.

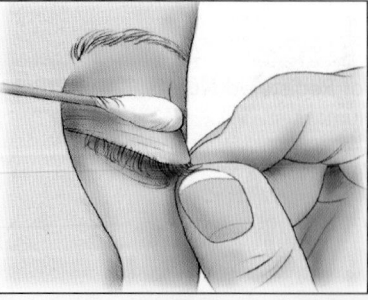

A

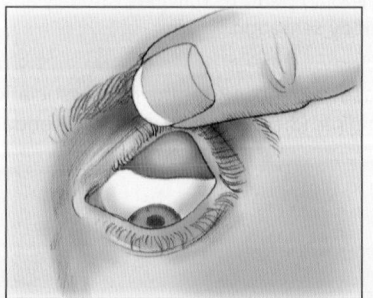

B

PROCEDURE GUIDELINES 16-4 (continued)

Removing a Particle From the Eye and Fluorescein Staining

PROCEDURE (continued)

Nursing Action	Rationale
Fluorescein Staining	
1. Use fluorescein strip to detect corneal abrasion.	1. Green stain will indicate if abrasion is present.
2. Apply a drop of saline to the strip; pull the lower eyelid down and gently touch the tip of the strip to the inner aspect of the eyelid.	2. Moistening the strip enhances release of the dye.
3. Ask the patient to blink several times to distribute the dye.	3. Dye will be dispersed over the conjunctive and cornea.
4. Cornea is viewed through a slit lamp, Woods lamp, or other blue filter light to best illuminate area of abrasion and ulceration.	4. Breaks in the epithelium will cause aqueous humor to color the fluorescein dye green under blue light.

Follow-up phase

1. Apply antibiotic ointment, as directed.	1. Prevents potential serious infection from break in cornea.
2. Apply patch, if indicated.	2. Rest eye and protect cornea for healing.

 Evidence Base American Society of Ophthalmic Registered Nurses. (2011). *Ophthalmic procedures for the office and clinic* (3rd ed.). Dubuque, IA: Kendall/Hunt.

PROCEDURE GUIDELINES 16-5

Removing Contact Lenses

EQUIPMENT

- Containers
- Labels
- Normal saline
- Towel
- Good lighting
- Eye suction cup (optional)

PROCEDURE

Nursing Action	Rationale
Preparatory phase	
1. If patient is able, have him or her sit upright with towel in lap. If patient is incapacitated, use recumbent position.	1. Towel will catch lens if it slips away.
2. Perform hand hygiene.	2. Prevents contamination of conjunctiva.
3. Explain procedure to patient.	3. Allays fear if patient is conscious.
Performance phase	
1. For hard lens with patient sitting:	
a. Open eyelids with two fingers and determine if lens is in normal position; if not, gently manipulate it over pupil.	a. Will need to be removed through area of greatest lid opening.
b. Place one finger at the outer canthus (temporal) and have the patient open both eyes widely.	
c. While applying traction toward the ear, ask the patient to look toward nose and blink.	c. Lens should become dislodged or pop out when blinks.

(continued)

PROCEDURE GUIDELINES 16-5 *(continued)*

Removing Contact Lenses

PROCEDURE *(continued)*

Nursing Action	Rationale
2. For hard lens with patient lying recumbent and use of suction cup:	2. If patient is incapacitated and not able to cooperate with steps in #1, use of suction cup may be necessary.
a. Make sure suction cup has been properly cleaned and disinfected.	a. Should be washed with soap and water and wiped with alcohol after each use and stored in clean container.
b. Moisten suction cup with normal saline.	b. Attracts lens.
c. Separate eyelids with your fingers and gently manipulate lens over pupil, if necessary.	c. Will remove more easily and without trauma if centered.
d. Apply suction cup to lens to obtain suction and gently lift to remove lens.	d. Lifting will maintain suction and prevent trauma. Tilting will break suction.
3. For soft lens:	
a. Open eyelids and determine position of lens.	a. Soft lens may be difficult to see and may be creased and displaced.
b. Retract the lower lid and place your index finger on the lower edge of the lens and attempt to slide it off the cornea onto the sclera.	b. Lens should be removed from the sclera to avoid trauma. Having the patient look up (if possible) will facilitate this.
c. If the lens is adherent to eye or misshaped, apply normal saline drops or commercial rewetting solution.	c. Will loosen lens and prevent trauma with manipulation.
d. Pinch the lens between your thumb and index finger and gently remove it from the eye.	d. Soft lenses will not pop out on their own.

Follow-up phase

1. Retrieve lens and put lens (lenses) in containers containing solution labeled right and left.	1. So patient may be able to use lenses again after proper cleaning.
2. Make sure patient is comfortable following the procedure.	2. Eyes should not be dry or lids retracted. Cool compress may be soothing.
3. Perform hand hygiene.	3. Prevents contamination to nurse or other patients.
4. Ensure safe disposition of the lenses.	4. So lenses will not be lost or thrown away.

 Evidence Base American Society of Ophthalmic Registered Nurses. (2011). *Ophthalmic procedures in the office and clinic* (3rd ed.). Dubuque, IA: Kendall/Hunt.

Nursing Interventions

Preparing for Surgery

1. Explain to the patient preoperative orders as well as postoperative expectations. (These will be specific for each type of surgery and particular health care provider.)
   a. Postoperatively, a specific position in bed may be maintained for a few hours; for example, the patient may lie on unoperated side.
   b. Postoperatively, a small pillow may be used while the patient is in supine position.
2. Instruct the patient to wash hair the evening before surgery; long hair of female patients should be arranged so it is off the face. There may be restrictions on using makeup and the patient may have self-image issues with this restriction. Explain that the reason for the restriction is that makeup flakes may enter the operative site as a foreign body, thereby increasing the risk for infection and inflammation.

3. Check agency surgical policy regarding skin preparation. Patients may be requested to shower with antibacterial soap the evening before or morning of surgery.
4. Check that operative permit is correct and signed with specified eye having surgery noted. Ask patient which eye (do not suggest an eye). Verification can prevent two thirds of wrong site incidents.
5. Remove dentures, contact lenses, or artificial eye and metal objects before patient goes to the operating room. (Wedding band can usually be taped in place.) For monitored anesthesia care or regional anesthesia, these requirements are usually waived.

6. Inform the patient if eye bandages are necessary postoperatively.

7. Administer preoperative medications, including eye drops, as prescribed.

8. Position bed side rails (up) after administering medications and place the call bell next to the patient.

9. Be available to answer questions the patient may have relating to the surgery or postoperative period.

 NURSING ALERT For patients requiring bed rest (ie, after keratoplasty, injury, retinal detachment surgery), measures should be taken to prevent pulmonary and/or circulatory complications. This may include range-of-motion exercises, anti-embolism stockings, and pneumatic compression devices.

 DRUG ALERT Be aware that anticoagulant therapy is usually stopped around the time of retinal surgery; however, anticoagulants are usually continued for patients undergoing cataract surgery.

Preventing Injury Postoperatively

1. Position the patient, as permitted, for specific surgery.

2. Position side rails (up) to offer the patient a sense of security.

3. Place the call bell next to the patient; have the patient call the nurse rather than risk increased IOP from the stress and strain of attempting to be self-sufficient.

4. Advise the patient to avoid bending over or straining that may cause increase in IOP. (May be waived for modern, small-incision cataract surgery.)

5. Instruct caregivers to tell the patient when they enter and leave the room.

6. Avoid activities such as combing hair that will disturb the patient's head or cause tension on sutures or operative site.

Compensating for Altered Vision

1. Orient the patient to any new environment—room arrangement and people.

2. Encourage self-care within the patient's limits.

3. Supervise attempts of the patient to feed him- or herself and in other self-care activities.

 GERONTOLOGIC ALERT Be aware that older people may have additional sensory/perceptual alterations, such as hearing loss and decreased position sense, which increases their risk of falls and feeling of isolation.

Reducing Fear

1. Recognize that dependence on sight is exaggerated when one faces diminishment or loss of sight.

2. Recognize that patients' concern of surgical outcome may be manifested differently, for example, fear, depression, tension, resentment, anger, or rejection.

3. Encourage the patient to express feelings.

4. Demonstrate interest, empathy, and understanding.

5. Reassure the patient that rehabilitative programs and personnel are available.

Increasing Self-Care Activities

1. Provide diversional and occupational therapy to keep the patient occupied mentally within the limits of decreased vision.

2. Provide rest periods, as necessary.

3. Provide adequate diet and fluids to promote proper elimination and decreased straining.

4. Discourage the patient from smoking, reading, and self-shaving for safety reasons.

5. Caution the patient against rubbing eyes or wiping them with soiled tissues.

6. Instruct the patient to wear dark glasses if eyes are light-sensitive.

7. Maintain safe environment—doors should be completely open or closed, floors kept clear of articles.

Patient Education and Health Maintenance

1. Advise the patient to consult ophthalmologist before undertaking diversional or recreational therapy that may be fatiguing to the eyes—no reading; television in moderation.

2. Emphasize that lights should not be too bright or glaring.

3. Before the patient leaves the hospital, inform him or her about medications, eyeglasses, and follow-up visits.

4. Instruct the patient and family on instillation of eye medications and proper cleansing of eyes.
   a. Instillation of eye drops.
   b. Application of an eye shield or patch.

5. Educate the patient about talking books, records, tapes, and machines available from most public libraries without charge.

6. Confirm the following with the patient and family before discharge:
   a. Is a return appointment date with health care provider confirmed?
   b. Are patient's medications properly identified and labeled?
   c. Do the patient and family member know how to use the prescribed medications?
   d. Does the patient understand the restrictions placed on him or her and the reasons for them?
   e. Do the patient and family know what signs and symptoms to report to health care provider between appointments (ie, pain, temperature above 101° F [38.3° C], discharge)?

Evaluation: Expected Outcomes

- Complies with preoperative routine; asks appropriate questions.
- Describes precautions that must be taken as safety measures, carries cane to prevent possible falls.
- Demonstrates improved vision in accordance with expectations of the surgery.
- Appears relaxed and positive concerning outcome of surgery.
- Manages self-care with minimal assistance.

Corneal Transplantation (Keratoplasty)

Description

The transplantation of a donor cornea, usually obtained at autopsy, to repair a corneal scar, burn, deformity, or dystrophy.

1. Types of grafts.
   a. Full-thickness (6.5 to 8 mm)—most common.
   b. Partial-thickness-lamellar.
2. Fresh cornea is the preferred tissue; it is removed from the donor within 12 hours after death and used within 24 hours.
3. Special solutions for storage of fresh cornea are available, which may extend storage up to 3 days.
4. *Cryopreservation* is the care and handling of a corneal graft by freezing to retain its transparency.

Preoperative Management and Nursing Care

1. Discuss psychological, cultural, and spiritual concerns with patient and health care personnel.
2. Advise the patient that the surgery is usually performed under local anesthesia and that he or she will be awake and must remain still during procedure.
3. Clean the face thoroughly with antibacterial solution, as ordered.
4. Administer preoperative medications, as ordered.

Postoperative Management and Nursing Care

1. Assess for:
   a. Anxiety—healing may be slow.
   b. Security of the eye patch—patch helps protect the eye from disruption of sutures or injury due to increased inflammation.
   c. Level of discomfort—pain may be symptomatic of complication. Headache may be symptom of increased IOP in both ocular and monocular surgery.
   d. Bowel and bladder habits—to prevent straining, which may raise IOP, or urine retention, which may result in urinary tract infection.
   e. Activity—avoid activities that increase IOP (sneezing, coughing, quick movement of the head).
2. Administer medications, as prescribed (ie, pain medication, steroid eye drops).
3. Prevent infection—use aseptic technique with medication administration and dressing change.
4. Instruct the patient to avoid touching dressing and eyes.

Complications

1. Hemorrhage.
2. Graft dislocation.
3. Infection.
4. Postoperative glaucoma.
5. Graft rejection—may occur 10 to 14 days postoperatively.
   a. Signs and symptoms include decreased vision, ocular irritation, corneal edema, red sclera.

Patient Education and Health Maintenance

1. Teach the patient signs of graft rejection occurring between 10 and 14 days postoperatively.
2. Instruct the patient to monitor the eye daily for graft rejection. Recommend assessment be done at the same time daily for comparison.
3. Teach the patient that vision varies and that functional vision does not return until sutures are removed.
4. Emphasize the importance of follow-up visits.

Refractive Surgery

Types of Procedures

 Evidence Base U.S. Food and Drug Administration. (2011). LASIK. Available: *www.fda.gov/MedicalDevices/ProductsandMedicalProcedures/SurgeryandLifeSupport/LASIK/default.htm.*

1. Radial keratotomy.
   a. Procedure designed to provide correction of myopia (nearsightedness).
   b. The cornea is anesthetized topically and, under a microscope, the surgeon marks the visual axis.
   c. Eight to 16 radial incisions are made into the corneal surface to flatten it. This permits images to fall on the retina instead of in front of it.
   d. Time to optimal correction is about 3 months. (Procedure is being performed much less frequently now with the development of laser surgery for refraction.)
2. Excimer photorefractive keratectomy.
   a. Limited to correcting myopia and some astigmatism.
   b. The front surface of the corneal epithelium is removed (by laser, manual scraping, or both).
   c. The laser is then used to change the corneal curvature by vaporizing the tissue (reshaping or sculpting the cornea).
   d. Optimal visual recovery about 6 months.
3. Laser-assisted in-situ keratomileusis (LASIK); also laser-automated lamellar keratoplasty (laser ALK).
   a. Procedure is designed to treat a wider range of prescriptions than the other refractive procedures.
   b. Microsurgical instrument (microkeratome) is used to create a corneal flap.
   c. A cool laser beam (using an excimer laser) reshapes the cornea and the flap is then closed.
   d. The excimer laser can remove corneal tissue with an accuracy of up to 0.25 microns.
   e. Only about 50 microns of tissue are removed to achieve the desired correction.
   f. Refractive recovery about 3 months.
4. Holmium laser thermokeratoplasty (Holmium LTK).
   a. Tissue is heated, not vaporized.
   b. Cornea is marked to pinpoint where to aim the laser.
   c. The laser heats only selected portions of the cornea to shrink collagen fibers around the cornea edges.

Patient Education and Nursing Care

1. Procedure performed in physician's office or clinic.
2. Specific procedures used to correct nearsightedness, farsightedness, astigmatism.
3. May eliminate need for glasses, especially with aging.
4. No guarantee of desired effects.

5. May not be appropriate for patients with corneal disease, retinal disease, glaucoma, severe diabetes, uncontrolled vascular disease, autoimmune diseases, pregnancy.
6. Elective procedure may be costly.
7. Frequent concerns:
   a. Pain—generally no pain with most procedures.
   b. Length of procedure—laser itself 15 to 40 seconds; entire procedure as little as 30 minutes.
   c. Activity—minor restriction, resume full activity in 1 to 3 days.
   d. Postoperative instructions—differ with physician and procedure; include antibiotic drops, anti-inflammatory drops, eye protection.

Note: Many new procedures that have not yet received Food and Drug Administration (FDA) approval, including new lasers and implanted contact lenses, are being developed.

Vitrectomy

Description
1. This procedure is performed for conditions such as unresolved hemorrhage with diabetic retinopathy, intraocular foreign body, and vitreoretinal adhesions.
2. It involves the removal of all or part of the vitreous humor, the transparent, gelatin-like substance behind the lens.
3. As the vitreous is removed, saline is infused to replace the vitreous. At the end of the procedure, gas, air, or silicone oil may be introduced into the eye to keep the retina in place.

Preoperative Management and Nursing Care
1. Provide explanations of procedure and answer any questions the patient may have.
2. Assess the patient's baseline visual acuity and level of function.
3. Give preoperative medication, as ordered.
4. Advise the patient that if gas is used he or she may be restricted to prone position for 1 to 6 weeks until the SF6 gas is absorbed.

Postoperative Management and Nursing Care
1. Place pressure patch on one or both eyes after surgical closure.
2. Assist with activities to ensure patient safety.
3. Apply cold compresses to control edema and associated discomfort.
4. Restrict activity to bed rest with bathroom privileges.
5. Medicate for pain, nausea, and vomiting, as indicated.
6. Monitor vital signs and patient's underlying medical condition such as glucose levels in diabetic patients.
7. Monitor for activities that increase IOP (ie, sneezing, coughing, straining, bending).
8. Instill eye medications, as ordered.
9. Properly position the patient—if the eye was injected with air during surgery, he or she will remain face down to keep the air/gas bubble over the retina. If not, a semi-Fowler's position is appropriate to keep the visual axis clear.
10. Evaluate drainage—a moderate amount is to be expected for about 2 postoperative days. Unusual amounts of color should be reported immediately.
11. Encourage patience because the patient will be anxious to witness immediate improvement in vision.

Enucleation

Description
1. Complete removal of the eyeball, usually performed due to trauma, infection, tumor such as melanoma, or prevention of sympathetic ophthalmia.
2. At surgery, the eye is removed by opening the conjunctiva and extraocular muscles, severing the optic nerve, and removing the eyeball.
3. A ball implant is then covered by the muscles and maintains the contour of the eye. The conjunctiva is then closed and a plastic conformer is placed to maintain the integrity of the eyelid.
4. An individualized prosthesis can be fitted 4 to 6 weeks later and a second procedure may be done to improve ocular motility.

Preoperative Management and Nursing Care
1. Review the procedure with the patient and family.
2. Describe postoperative expectations in detail.
3. Begin teaching preoperatively in care of enucleated eye socket and prosthesis.
   a. Inspecting eye and lid.
   b. Instilling medication.
   c. Irrigating site to remove mucus.
   d. Removing the prosthesis.
   e. Using aseptic technique when performing procedures.
4. Assess fear and anxiety associated with loss of body part.
5. Advise the patient and family of support systems available and make appropriate referrals.
6. Prepare the patient for surgery and give preoperative medications, as ordered.

Postoperative Management and Nursing Care
1. Instill medications, usually antibiotic and steroid ointments, to prevent infection.
2. Apply pressure/ice dressings, as ordered, to reduce swelling.
3. Irrigate conformer area to reduce mucus.
4. Clean the eyelid to reduce chance of infection.
5. Assist the patient in adjusting to body image change.
6. Assist the patient in adjusting to monocular vision—especially with loss of peripheral vision and depth perception.
7. Review that in 4 to 6 weeks after surgery, the patient will receive an ocular prosthesis (artificial eye).
8. Continue to assess fear and anxiety associated with loss of body part. Provide supportive care.

Complications
1. Hemorrhage.
2. Infection.
3. Implant extrusion.

COMMON EYE DISORDERS
Conditions of the Conjunctiva and Eyelids

The *eyelids* are the outermost defense mechanisms of the eyes, functioning as a physical barrier as well as to maintain moisture and dispersement of tears. The *palpebral conjunctiva* lines the upper and lower lids and the bulbar conjunctiva forms a protective

Table 16-2	Conditions of the Eyelids and Conjunctiva
CONDITION	**TREATMENT AND NURSING CONSIDERATIONS**
Blepharitis An inflammatory reaction of the eyelid margin caused by bacteria (usually *Staphylococcus aureus*) or seborrheic skin condition, resulting in flaking, redness, irritation, and possibly recurrent styes of the upper or lower lid, or both.	Diagnostic culture usually not necessary. Mild cases treated with eyelid margin scrub at least once daily (baby shampoo may be used). If *S. aureus* is likely, antibiotic ointment is prescribed one to four times per day to eyelid margin. Teach patient to scrub eyelid margin with cotton swab to remove flaking and then apply ointment with cotton swab, as directed.
Hordeolum (Stye)/Chalazion The term "stye" refers to an inflammation or infection of the glands and follicles of the eyelid margin. External hordeolum involves the hair follicles of the eyelashes; chalazion is a granulomatous (chronic) infection of the meibomian glands. Bacteria, usually staphylococcus, and seborrhea are the causes. Pain, redness, foreign body sensation, and a pustule may be present.	Treatment usually consists of warm soaks to help promote drainage, good handwashing and eyelid hygiene, and possible application of antibiotic ointment. In some cases, incision and drainage in the office with local anesthetic may be necessary. Teach patient how to clean eyelid margins and not to squeeze the stye.
Conjunctivitis Inflammation or infection of the bulbar (covering the sclera and cornea) or palpebral (covering inside lids) conjunctiva. May be allergic, bacterial (*S. aureus*, *Streptococcus pneumoniae*, *Haemophilus influenzae*, and others), gonococcal, viral (adenovirus, herpes simplex, coxsackievirus, and others), or irritative (topical medication, chemicals, wind, smoke, contact lenses, ultraviolet light) causes. Trachoma is caused by *Chlamydia trachomatis* and is a major cause of blindness worldwide, but is rare in North America. Symptoms of conjunctivitis vary from mild pruritus and tearing to severe drainage, burning, hyperemia, and chemosis (edema). The term "pink eye" usually refers to infectious conjunctivitis.	Fluorescein staining may be done to rule out ulceration or keratitis (involvement of cornea). Culture if purulent exudate; special culture for *Neisseria gonorrhoeae*. Warm soaks (10 minutes four times per day) used when crusting and drainage present; cold compresses helpful for allergic and irritative causes. If topical antibiotic ordered, teach patient instillation technique. Urge good handwashing to prevent spread. Allergic conjunctivitis treated with topical or oral antihistamines, vasoconstrictors, and mast cell stabilizers.

coating over the sclera. The conjunctiva responds to infections, inflammatory disorders, and environmental irritants. Blood vessels in the conjunctiva dilate readily, causing redness, and pain receptors respond to inflammatory changes. Inflammatory disorders are outlined in Table 16-2. Structural disorders that may be amenable to surgery include:

- Entropion—inward turning of the eyelid margin.
- Ectropion—outward turning of the eyelid margin.
- Ptosis—drooping of the upper eyelid.
- Lagophthalmos—inadequate closure of the eyelids.
- Ptyerygium—overgrowth of tissue on the conjunctiva.

Disorders of the Cornea and Uveal Tract

The *cornea* is the outermost tissue that functions in vision. It must remain clear and smooth to admit light to the retina. Blood vessels are contained in the *limbus* (periphery). Epithelial layers of the cornea repair rapidly, but if they are penetrated, infection can rapidly spread inward and vision may be lost.

The *uveal tract* is made up of the iris, which controls pupil size; ciliary body, which secretes aqueous humor and controls accommodation; and choroid layer, which provides vasculature to the anterior uveal tract. Disorders of the uveal tract may cause pupil changes, problems with accommodation, clouding of the anterior chamber or vitreous, and more serious problems due to adhesions (see Table 16-3).

Cataract

Clouding or opacity of the crystalline lens that impairs vision.

Pathophysiology and Etiology

1. Senile cataract—commonly occurs with aging.
2. Congenital cataract—occurs at birth.
3. Traumatic cataract—occurs after injury.
4. Aphakia—absence of crystalline lens.
5. Additional risk factors for cataract formation include diabetes; ultraviolet light exposure; high-dose radiation; and drugs such as corticosteroids, phenothiazines, and some chemotherapy agents.

Clinical Manifestations

1. Blurred or distorted vision.
2. Glare from bright lights.
3. Gradual and painless loss of vision.
4. Previously dark pupil may appear milky or white.

Table 16-3   Conditions of the Cornea and Uveal Tract

CONDITION	TREATMENT AND NURSING CONSIDERATIONS
Corneal Abrasion and Ulceration (Keratitis)	
Loss of epithelial layers of cornea due to some type of trauma—contact with fingernail, tree branch, spark or other projectile, or overwearing contact lens. May lead to corneal ulceration and secondary infection into cornea (keratitis), which may lead to blindness. Symptoms are pain, redness, foreign body sensation, photophobia, increased tearing, and difficulty opening eye.	Treatment is urgent. Fluorescein staining and examination with Woods lamp or slit lamp to identify the abrasion or ulceration. Antibiotic ointment may be instilled and eye patched for 24 hours. No benefit to patching has been found for simple abrasions, however. Cycloplegic drops may also be used in large abrasions or ulcers. Abrasion heals in 24–48 hours. Ulceration should be followed by an ophthalmologist. Make sure that patch is secure enough so patient cannot open eyelid, but not so tight that patient "sees stars." Teach patient to use topical antibiotic (or antiviral in cases of herpes simplex dendritic keratitis) after patch is removed, and follow up as directed. Review safety practices, such as wearing protective eye shields, not rubbing eyes, using contact lenses properly, and washing hands frequently.
Iritis/Uveitis	
Uveitis is an inflammation of the intraocular structures. It is classified by involved structures (1) anterior uveitis—iris (iritis) or iris and ciliary body (iridocyclitis), (2) intermediate uveitis—structures posterior to the lens (pars plantis or peripheral uveitis), and (3) posterior uveitis—choroid (choroiditis), retina (retinitis), or vitreous near the optic nerve and macula. Anterior uveitis is most common and is usually unilateral. Posterior uveitis is usually bilateral. Causes of uveitis are infections; immune-mediated disorders, such as ankylosing spondylitis, Crohn's disease, Reiter's syndrome, lupus; trauma; or it may be idiopathic. Onset is acute with deep eye pain, photophobia, conjunctival redness, small pupil that does not react briskly, ciliary flush (redness around limbus), and decreased visual acuity.	Urgent ophthalmology evaluation is needed. Inflammation is treated with a topical corticosteroid and a cycloplegic agent. Teach patient how to instill medications and adhere to dosing schedule to prevent permanent eye damage. Suggest sunglasses to decrease pain from photophobia. Encourage follow-up for IOP measurements because corticosteroids can increase IOP.

IOP, intraocular pressure.

Diagnostic Evaluation

1. Slit-lamp examination—to provide magnification and visualize opacity of lens.
2. Tonometry—to determine IOP and rule out other conditions.
3. Direct and indirect ophthalmoscopy to rule out retinal disease.
4. Perimetry—to determine the scope of the visual field (normal with cataract).

Management

General

1. Surgical removal of the lens is indicated.
   a. When a cataract interferes with activities, the patient may request cataract surgery.
   b. Because cataract often occurs in both eyes, surgery is recommended when vision in the better eye causes problems in daily activities. Surgery is done on only one eye at a time.
2. Cataract surgery is usually done under either regional block or topical anesthesia, with or without IV sedation, and on an outpatient basis.
3. Oral medications may be given to reduce IOP.

4. IOL implants are usually implanted at the time of cataract extraction, replacing thick glasses that may provide suboptimal refraction.
5. In the rare instance that intraocular lens implant is not used, the patient will be fitted with appropriate eyeglasses or a contact lens to correct refraction after the healing process.

Surgical Procedures

1. There are two types of extractions:
   a. Intracapsular extraction—the lens as well as the capsule are removed through a small incision. (This technique is rarely used in the United States.)
   b. Extracapsular extraction—the lens capsule is incised and the nucleus, cortex, and anterior capsule are extracted.
      i. The posterior capsule is left in place and is usually the base to which an IOL is implanted.
      ii. A conservative procedure of choice, simple to perform, is usually done under local anesthesia.
2. Phacoemulsification is usually used to remove the lens.
   a. A hollow needle vibrating at ultrasonic speed is used to emulsify the lens.
   b. Then the emulsified particles are irrigated and aspirated from the anterior chamber.

3. Cryosurgery is rarely used to remove the lens. A pencil-like instrument with a metal tip is supercooled (−35° C), then touched to the exposed lens, freezing to it so the lens is easily lifted out.

Intraocular Lens Implantation

1. The implantation of a synthetic lens (IOL) is designed for distance vision; the patient may wear prescription glasses for reading and near vision. Intraocular lens implant restores binocular vision.
2. Previously, most IOLs were spherical with the front surface curved. Aspheric IOLs increase contrast sensitivity.
   a. In 2003, the FDA approved the use of the multifocal IOL. The lens incorporates more than one optical power to permit focusing at different distances.
   b. In 2004, the FDA approved an aspheric IOL. The lens can reduce postoperative spherical aberrations and, therefore, improve the ability to see in varying light conditions, such as rain, snow, fog, twilight, and nighttime darkness.
   c. In 2005, the FDA approved the first toric IOL, which is designed to correct astigmatism.
   d. Sophisticated calculations are required to determine the prescription for the lens.
   e. Numerous types of IOLs are available. Designs and materials change as new developments occur.
3. Advantages of the IOL include:
   a. Provides an alternative for the person who cannot wear contact lenses.
   b. Cannot be lost or misplaced like conventional glasses.
   c. Provides superior vision correction and better depth perception than glasses.
4. Complications (specific to implantation):
   a. Pain from inflammation of various eye structures—usually controlled by nonsteroidal anti-inflammatories, but systemic antibiotics and immunosuppression may be required.
   b. Rosy vision (glare) due to keeping pupil from full constriction; excessive light enters pupil, causing a dazzling of macula (minute corneal opacity).
   c. Degeneration of the cornea.
   d. Malpositioning or dislocation of lens.
5. Implants may not be advisable for patients with severe myopia, history of chronic iritis, retinal detachment, diabetic retinopathy, glaucoma, and complications during surgery.

Contact Lens

Extended-wear contact lens is an option for those who do not receive IOL implants. They restore binocular vision and result in magnification of images in the range of 7% to 10%.

The patient will need to take the lens out for cleaning periodically or, if the patient is an older adult or debilitated, will need to follow up at intervals for cleaning at the ophthalmologist's office.

Complications

1. Blindness.

Nursing Assessment

Preoperative

1. Assess knowledge level regarding procedure.

2. Assess level of fear and anxiety.
3. Determine visual limitations.

Postoperative

1. Assess pain level.
   a. Sudden onset—may be due to ruptured vessel or suture and may lead to hemorrhage.
   b. Severe pain—accompanied by nausea and vomiting; may be caused by increased IOP and may require immediate treatment.
2. Assess visual acuity in unoperated eye.
3. Assess for signs of infection—fever, inflammation, pain, drainage.
4. Assess the patient's level of independence.

Nursing Diagnoses

- Deficient Knowledge of operative course.
- Risk for Injury related to surgical complications.

Nursing Interventions

Preparing the Patient for Surgery

1. Orient the patient and explain procedures and care plan to decrease anxiety.
2. Instruct the patient not to touch eyes to decrease contamination.
3. Obtain conjunctival cultures, if requested, using aseptic technique.
4. Administer preoperative eye drops—antibiotic, mydriatic-cycloplegic, and other medications—mannitol solution IV, sedative, anti-emetic, and opioid, as directed. Explain medication actions to patient.

Preventing Complications Postoperatively

1. Medicate for pain, as prescribed, to promote comfort.
2. Administer medication to prevent nausea and vomiting, as needed.
3. Notify the health care provider of sudden pain associated with restlessness and increased pulse, which may indicate increased IOP, or fever, which may indicate infection.
4. Caution the patient against coughing or sneezing to prevent increased IOP.
5. Advise the patient against rapid movement or bending from the waist to minimize IOP. The patient may be more comfortable with head elevated 30 degrees and lying on the unaffected side.
6. Allow the patient to ambulate as soon as possible and to resume independent activities.
7. Assist the patient in maneuvering through environment with the use of one eye while eye patch is on (1 to 2 days).
8. Encourage the patient to wear eye shield at night to protect operated eye from injury while sleeping.

Patient Education and Health Maintenance

Promoting Independence

1. Advise the patient to increase activities, as tolerated, unless given restrictions by the surgeon.
2. Caution against activities that cause patient to strain (eg, lifting heavy objects, straining at defecation, and strenuous activity) for up to 6 weeks, as directed.

3. Instruct the patient and family about proper eyedrop or ointment instillation.
4. Advise the patient to bring all medications to follow-up visits to permit dosage adjustments by ophthalmologist. Discontinued medications can then be discarded to prevent confusion.

Adjusting to Visual Change

1. Inform the patient receiving corrective lenses that fitting for temporary corrective lenses for the first 6 weeks will occur several days after surgery.
   a. Prescription for permanent lenses will be determined 6 to 12 weeks after surgery.
   b. Prescription for a permanent contact lens will be determined about 3 to 6 weeks after surgery.
2. Encourage the patient to wear dark glasses after eye dressings are removed to provide comfort from photophobia due to lack of pupil constriction from mydriatic-cycloplegic drops.

Adjusting to the Eyeglasses

1. Stress the importance of patience in the coming weeks of adjustment—it is easy to become frustrated.
2. Tell the patient that if glasses are to be worn, they will cause the perceived image to be about one third larger than normal. Glasses cannot restore binocular vision as an intraocular lens implant or contact lens will because of the discrepancy of image size between the treated eye and untreated eye.
3. If glass is used in the prescription, it is heavier and thicker than the more expensive plastic cataract eyeglass lenses.
4. Instruct the patient to look through the center of corrective glasses and to turn head when looking to the side because peripheral vision is markedly distorted.
5. It is necessary to relearn space judgment—walking, using stairs, reaching for articles on the table (such as a cup of coffee), and pouring liquids—due to loss of binocular vision and peripheral distortion.
6. Advise patients to use handrails while walking and doing steps and to reach out slowly for objects to be picked up.

Becoming Familiar with Contact Lenses

Teach the patient that:

1. With contact lenses, magnification is only about 7% to 10%; peripheral vision is not distorted so binocular vision is achieved and spatial distortion is usually not an issue.
2. Patients do need to learn how to remove daily-wear and extended-wear lenses or return to the ophthalmologist's office for replacement of extended-wear lens periodically.

Becoming Familiar with Intraocular Lens

1. Teach the patient that with an intraocular lens, magnification problems are negligible. Both the operated eye and the unoperated eye can work together after cataract surgery with lens implantation, and the preoperative glasses can usually be worn in the recuperative period.
2. Advise the patient that eyeglasses may not be required for distance but may be needed for reading and writing.
3. Caution the patient against straining of any type. Bend knees only if necessary to reach for something on the floor.
4. Recommend sponge bathing. Avoid getting soap in the eyes.

5. Advise avoidance of tilting head forward when washing hair; tilt head slightly backward. Vigorous shaking of the head is to be avoided.

Evaluation: Expected Outcomes

- Vision maximized and distortions or limitations in vision described by patient.
- Independent activities demonstrated, denies discomfort.

Acute (Angle-Closure) Glaucoma

A condition in which an obstruction occurs at the access to the trabecular meshwork and the canal of Schlemm. IOP is normal when the anterior chamber angle is open, and glaucoma occurs when a significant portion of that angle is closed. Glaucoma is associated with progressive visual field loss and eventual blindness if allowed to progress. This is most commonly an acute painful condition (about 10% of glaucoma cases), not to be confused with chronic open-angle glaucoma (about 90% of cases).

Pathophysiology and Etiology

1. Mechanical blockage of anterior chamber angle results in accumulation of aqueous humor (fluid).
2. Anterior chamber is anatomically shallow in most cases.
3. The shallow chamber with narrow anterior angles is more prone to physiologic events that result in closure.
4. Angle closure occurs because of pupillary dilation or forward displacement of the iris.
5. Angle closure can occur in subacute, acute, or chronic forms.
6. Episodes of subacute closure may precede an acute attack and cause transient blurred vision and pain but no increased IOP.
7. Acute angle closure causes a dramatic response with sudden elevation of IOP and permanent eye damage within several hours if not treated.
8. Within several days, scar tissue forms between the iris and cornea, closing the angle. The iris and ciliary body begin to atrophy, the cornea degenerates because of edema, and the optic nerve begins to atrophy.

Clinical Manifestations

1. Pain in and around eyes due to increased ocular pressure; may be transitory attacks.
2. Rainbow of color (halos) around lights.
3. Vision becomes cloudy and blurred.
4. Pupil mid-dilated and fixed.
5. Nausea and vomiting may occur.
6. Hazy-appearing cornea due to corneal edema.
7. Although onset may have initial subclinical symptoms, severity of symptoms may progress to cause acute symptoms of increased IOP—nausea and vomiting, sudden onset of blurred vision, severe pain, profuse lacrimation, and ciliary injection.

 NURSING ALERT Acute angle-closure glaucoma is a medical emergency and requires immediate treatment. Untreated, it can result in blindness in less than 1 week.

Diagnostic Evaluation

1. Tonometry—elevated IOP, usually greater than 50 mm Hg.
2. Ocular examination may reveal a pale optic disk.
3. Gonioscopy (using special instrument called gonioscope) to study the angle of the anterior chamber of the eye.

> **NURSING ALERT** Dilatation of pupils is avoided if the anterior chamber is shallow. This is determined by oblique illumination of the anterior segment of the eye. A flashlight is shined across the iris from the temporal side. If the iris is bulging (with a shallow anterior chamber), a crescent shadow appears on the nasal side of the iris.

Management

Pharmacologic

1. Emergency pharmacotherapy is initiated to decrease eye pressure before surgery.
2. Medications are based on the patient's condition but may include:
   a. Parasympathomimetic drugs used as miotic drugs—pupil contracts; iris is drawn away from cornea; aqueous humor may drain through lymph spaces (meshwork) into canal of Schlemm.
   b. Carbonic anhydrase inhibitor—restricts action of enzyme that is necessary to produce aqueous humor.
   c. Beta-adrenergic blockers—nonselective—may reduce production of aqueous humor or may facilitate outflow of aqueous humor.
   d. Hyperosmotic agents—to reduce IOP by promoting diuresis.

Surgery

1. Surgery is indicated if:
   a. IOP is not maintained within normal limits by medical regimen.
   b. There is progressive visual field loss with optic nerve damage.
2. Types of surgery include:
   a. Peripheral iridectomy—excision of a small portion of the iris whereby aqueous humor can bypass pupil; treatment of choice. Typically a laser procedure.
   b. Trabeculectomy—partial-thickness scleral resection with small part of trabecular meshwork removed and iridectomy. Necessary if peripheral anterior adhesions (synechiae) have developed due to repeated glaucoma attacks.
   c. Laser iridotomy—multiple tiny laser incisions to iris to create openings for aqueous flow; may be repeated.
3. Other eye is usually operated on eventually as a preventive measure.

Complications

Uncontrolled IOP that can lead to optic atrophy and total blindness.

Nursing Assessment

1. Evaluate the patient for severe pain, nausea and vomiting, signs of increased IOP.
2. Assess visual symptoms.

3. Establish history of onset of attack and previous attacks.
4. Assess the patient's level of anxiety and knowledge base.

Nursing Diagnoses

- Acute Pain related to increased IOP.
- Fear related to pain and potential loss of vision.

Nursing Interventions

Relieving Pain

1. Notify the health care provider immediately of the patient's condition.
2. Administer opioids and other medications, as directed. Medications that may cause nausea and vomiting are avoided. The patient may be medicated with anti-emetic if nausea occurs.
3. Explain to the patient that the goal of treatment is to reduce IOP as quickly as possible.
4. Explain procedures to the patient.
5. Reassure the patient that, with reduction in IOP, pain and other signs and symptoms should subside.
6. Explain adverse effects of medications:
   a. Mannitol (IV)—transient blurred vision, rhinitis, thirst, nausea, transient circulatory overload, and headache.
   b. Acetazolamide or methazolamide (oral)—drowsiness, anorexia, paresthesia, stomach upset, tinnitus, fluid and electrolyte imbalance, rare kidney or liver dysfunction.
   c. Pilocarpine (topical)—burning and redness of eye, headache, constricted pupil, poor vision in dim light, retinal detachment, rare lens opacity.

Relieving Fear

1. Provide reassurance and calm presence to reduce anxiety and fear.
2. Prepare the patient for surgery, if necessary.
3. Describe procedure to the patient; surgery will likely be done on outpatient basis.
   a. Patch will be worn for several hours and sunglasses may help with photophobia.
   b. Vision will be blurred for first few days after the procedure.
   c. Frequent initial follow-up will be necessary for tonometry to make sure control of IOP.

Patient Education and Health Maintenance

1. Instruct the patient in use of medications. Stress the importance of long-term medication use to control this chronic disease. Patients commonly forget that eye drops are medications and that glaucoma is a chronic illness.
2. Remind the patient to keep follow-up appointments.
3. Instruct the patient to seek immediate medical attention if signs and symptoms of increased IOP return—severe eye pain, photophobia, and excessive lacrimation.
4. Advise the patient to notify all health care providers of condition and medications and to avoid use of medications that may increase IOP, such as corticosteroids and anticholinergics (such as antihistamines), unless the benefit outweighs the risk (see Table 16-4).

Table 16-4 Drugs That Elevate Intraocular Pressure

MEDICATION	ROUTE	EFFECT
Corticosteroids	Oral, inhalant, intravenous, intravitreal, periocular topical solutions (creams and drops)	Elevates IOP
Viscoelastic agents	Intraocular	Elevates IOP
Alpha-chymotrypsin	Intraocular	Transient elevation of IOP
Topomax (anticonvulsant)	Oral	Elevates IOP
Anticholinergics	Topical	Causes angle-closure glaucoma
Sulfonamides	Oral	Causes angle-closure glaucoma
Tricyclic antidepressants	Oral	Causes acute angle-closure glaucoma
Monoamine oxidase inhibitors	Oral	Causes acute angle-closure glaucoma
Antihistamines	Oral	Causes acute angle-closure glaucoma
Antiparkinsonian	Oral	Causes acute angle-closure glaucoma
Antipsychotics	Oral	Causes acute angle-closure glaucoma
Antispasmolytic	Oral	Causes acute angle-closure glaucoma
Cycloplegic agents	Topical	Contraindicated in narrow-angle glaucoma
Mydriatric agents	Topical	Contraindicated in narrow-angle glaucoma
Sympathomimetic agents	Topical	Contraindicated in narrow-angle glaucoma

IOP, intraocular pressure.

Evaluation: Expected Outcomes

- Pain is decreased.
- Describes treatment regimen and verbalizes reduced fear.

Chronic (Open-Angle) Glaucoma

Glaucoma is characterized as a disorder of increased IOP, degeneration of the optic nerve, and visual field loss. Incidence increases with age—2% at age 40, 7% at age 70, 8% at age 80.

Pathophysiology and Etiology

1. Degenerative changes occur in the trabecular meshwork and canal of Schlemm, causing microscopic obstruction.
2. Aqueous fluid cannot be emptied from the anterior chamber, increasing IOP.
3. IOP varies with activity and some people tolerate elevated IOP without optic damage (ocular hypertension), whereas others exhibit visual field defects and optic damage with minimal or transient IOP elevation.
4. The risk of eye damage increases with age, family history of glaucoma, diabetes, and hypertension.

Clinical Manifestations

1. Mild, bilateral discomfort (tired feeling in eyes, foggy vision).
2. Slowly developing impairment of peripheral vision—central vision unimpaired.
3. Progressive loss of visual field.
4. Halos may be present around lights with increased ocular pressure.

Diagnostic Evaluation

1. Tonometry—IOP usually greater than 24 mm Hg but may be within normal limits.
2. Ocular examination—to check for clipping and atrophy of the optic disk.
3. Visual fields testing for deficits.

 NURSING ALERT Because of the relative ease of developing chronic glaucoma asymptomatically, encourage people of all ages to have an eye examination that includes measurement of eye pressure (tonometry) periodically to facilitate early detection and treatment to prevent loss of eyesight.

Management

1. Commonly treated with a combination of topical miotic agents (increase the outflow of aqueous humor by enlarging the area around trabecular meshwork) and oral carbonic

anhydrase inhibitors and beta-adrenergic blockers (decrease aqueous production).

2. Remission may occur; however, there is no cure. The patient should continue to see health care provider at 3- to 6-month intervals for control of IOP.

3. If medical treatment is not successful, surgery may be required, but is delayed as long as possible.

4. Types of surgery include:
   a. Laser trabeculoplasty.
      i. An outpatient procedure, treatment of choice if increased ocular pressure unresponsive to medical regimen only.
      ii. As many as 100 superficial surface burns are placed evenly at junction of pigmented and nonpigmented trabeculum meshwork for 360 degrees in anesthetized eye, which allows increased outflow of aqueous humor.
      iii. Maximum decrease in IOP is achieved in 2 to 3 months, but IOP may rise again in 1 to 2 years.
   b. Iridencleisis—an opening is created between anterior chamber and space beneath the conjunctiva; this bypasses the blocked meshwork and aqueous humor is absorbed into conjunctival tissues.
   c. Cyclodiathermy or cyclocryotherapy—the ciliary body's function of secreting aqueous humor is decreased by damaging the body with high-frequency electrical current or supercooled probe applied to the surface of the eye over the ciliary body.
   d. Corneoscleral trephine (rarely done)—a permanent opening at the junction of the cornea and sclera is made through the anterior chamber so aqueous humor can drain.

 DRUG ALERT Using beta-adrenergic blocker eye drops in the treatment of glaucoma can cause an adverse reaction in patients taking beta-adrenergic blockers for cardiovascular disease. Monitor vital signs because the risk for bradycardia exists.

Nursing Assessment

1. Assess frequency, duration, and severity of visual symptoms.
2. Assess the patient's knowledge of disease process and anxiety about the diagnosis.
3. Assess the patient's motivation to participate in long-term treatment.

Nursing Diagnosis

• Deficient Knowledge about glaucoma and surgical procedure.

Nursing Interventions

Providing Information About Glaucoma

1. Review the normal anatomy and physiology of the eye as well as the changes that occur in the drainage of aqueous humor with glaucoma.
2. Make sure that the patient understands that, although asymptomatic, IOP could still be elevated and damage to the eye could be occurring. Therefore, ongoing use of medication and follow-up are essential.

3. Teach the patient the action, dosage, and adverse effects of all medications. Make sure of adequate administration of eye drops by watching the patient give return demonstration.
   a. Timolol and betaxolol—adverse effects include headache, eye irritation, decreased corneal sensitivity, blurred vision, bradycardia, palpitations, bronchospasm, hypotension, and heart failure.
   b. Pilocarpine—adverse effects include eye irritation, blurring, and redness; headache; pupil constriction; poor vision in dim light; possible hypertension and tachycardia; and rare retinal detachment and lens opacity.
   c. Acetazolamide and methazolamide—adverse effects include drowsiness, anorexia, paresthesia, stomach upset, tinnitus, fluid and electrolyte imbalance, and rare kidney and liver dysfunction.

4. Discuss visual defects with the patient and ways to compensate. Vision loss is permanent and treatment is aimed at stopping the process.

5. Inform the patient that surgery is done on outpatient basis and recovery is quick. Prolonged restrictions are not required.
   a. After surgery, elevation of head 30 degrees will promote aqueous humor drainage after a trabeculectomy.
   b. Additional medications after surgery include topical steroids and cycloplegics to decrease inflammation and to dilate the pupil.

Patient Education and Health Maintenance

1. Patient must remember that glaucoma cannot be cured, but it can be controlled.
2. Remind the patient that periodic eye checkups are essential because pressure changes may occur.
3. Alert the patient to avoid, if possible, circumstances that may increase IOP:
   a. Upper respiratory infections.
   b. Emotional upsets—worry, fear, anger.
   c. Exertion, such as snow shoveling, pushing, heavy lifting.
4. Recommend the following:
   a. Continuous daily use of eye medications as prescribed.
   b. Moderate use of the eyes.
   c. Exercise in moderation to maintain general well-being.
   d. Unrestricted fluid intake: alcohol and coffee may be permitted unless they are noted to cause increased IOP in the particular patient.
   e. Maintenance of regular bowel habits to decrease straining.
   f. Wearing a medical identification tag indicating the patient has glaucoma

Evaluation: Expected Outcomes

• Verbalizes understanding of glaucoma as a chronic disease; demonstrates proper instillation of ophthalmic medications.

Retinal Detachment

Detachment of the sensory area of the retina (rods and cones) from the pigmented epithelium of the retina. A break in the continuity of the retina may first occur from small degenerative holes and tears, which may lead to detachment.

Pathophysiology and Etiology

1. Spontaneous detachment may occur due to degenerative changes in the retina or vitreous.
2. Trauma, inflammation, or tumor causes detachment by forming a mass that mechanically separates the retinal layers.
3. Diabetic retinopathy commonly leads to retinal degeneration and tears disrupting the integrity of the retina.
4. Myopia and loss of a lens from a cataract (aphakia) also predisposes to retinal tears and detachment because the posterior chamber is enlarged, leading to vitreous pull.
5. After detachment occurs, that portion of the retina cannot perceive light because the blood and oxygen supply is cut off; hence, part of visual field is lost.
6. Detachment occurs most commonly in patients over age 40.

Clinical Manifestations

1. Retinal detachment may occur slowly or rapidly, but without pain.
2. The patient complains of flashes of light or blurred, "sooty" vision due to stimulation of the retina by vitreous pull.
3. The patient notes sensation of particles moving in line of vision (more so than usual—"floaters" that a person can see floating across field of vision when looking at a light background).
4. Delineated areas of vision may be blank.
5. A sensation of a veil-like coating coming down, coming up, or coming sideways in front of the eye may be present if detachment develops rapidly.
   a. This veil-like coating, or shadow, is commonly misinterpreted as a drooping eyelid or elevated cheek.
   b. Straight-ahead vision may remain good in early stages.
6. Unless the retinal holes are sealed, the retina will progressively detach; ultimately there will be a loss of central vision as well as peripheral vision, leading to legal blindness.

Diagnostic Evaluation

Indirect ophthalmoscopy shows gray or opaque retina. The retina is normally transparent. Slit-lamp examination and three-mirror gonioscopy magnify the lesion.

Management

General

1. Sedation, bed rest, and eye patch may be used to restrict eye movements.
2. Surgical intervention may be indicated.
3. Return of visual acuity with a reattached retina depends on:
   a. Amount of retina detached before surgery.
   b. Whether the macula (area of central vision) was detached.
   c. Length of time the retina was detached.
   d. Amount of external distortion caused by the scleral buckle.
   e. Possible macular damage as a result of diathermy of cryocoagulation.
4. Surgical reattachment is successful approximately 90% to 95% of the time. If the retina remains attached 2 months postoperatively, the condition is likely to be corrected and unlikely to recur.

Surgical Procedures

1. Photocoagulation—a light beam (either laser or xenon arc) is passed through the pupil, causing a small burn and producing an exudate between the pigment epithelium and retina.
2. Electrodiathermy—an electrode needle is passed through the sclera to allow subretinal fluid to escape. An exudate forms from the pigment epithelium and adheres to the retina.
3. Cryosurgery or retinal cryopexy—a supercooled probe is touched to the sclera, causing minimal damage; as a result of scarring, the pigment epithelium adheres to the retina.
4. Scleral buckling—a technique whereby the sclera is shortened to allow a buckling to occur, which forces the pigment epithelium closer to the retina (often accompanied by vitrectomy).

Complications

1. Glaucoma.
2. Infection.

Nursing Assessment

Preoperative

1. Assess for history of trauma or other risk factors.
2. Assess level of anxiety and knowledge level regarding procedures.
3. Determine visual limitations and obtain visual description from patient to determine assistance needed.

Postoperative

1. Assess pain level.
2. Assess visual acuity if unoperated eye not patched.
3. Determine the patient's ability to ambulate and assume independent activities, as tolerated.

Nursing Diagnoses

- Anxiety related to visual deficit and surgical outcome.
- Risk for Injury related to eye surgery.

Nursing Interventions

Reducing Anxiety Before Surgery

1. Instruct the patient to remain quiet in prescribed position. (Detached area of retina remains in dependent position.) Assist with all activities and offer frequent reassurance.
2. Patch both eyes. Make sure that the patient is oriented to surroundings and can call for assistance.
3. Describe preoperative procedures before carrying them out.
4. Wash the patient's face with antibacterial solution.
5. Administer preoperative medications, as ordered.
6. Instruct the patient not to touch eyes.

Preventing Postoperative Complications

1. Caution the patient to avoid bumping head.
2. Encourage the patient not to cough or sneeze or to perform activities that will increase IOP.
3. Assist the patient with activities, as needed.
4. Encourage ambulation and independence.
5. Administer medications for pain, nausea, and vomiting, as prescribed.

6. Provide sedate, diversional activities such as radio, audio books.
7. If the patient's anticoagualtion therapy has been stopped, carefully monitor for signs and symptoms of embolism and stroke.

Patient Education and Health Maintenance

1. Encourage self-care at discharge, if done in an unhurried manner. (Avoid falls, jerks, bumps, or accidental injury.)
2. Instruct the patient about the following:
   a. Rapid eye movements should be avoided for several weeks.
   b. Driving is restricted.
   c. Within 3 weeks, light activities may be pursued.
   d. Within 6 weeks, heavier activities and athletics are possible. Define such activities for the patient.
   e. Avoid straining and bending head below the waist.
   f. Use meticulous cleanliness when instilling eye medications.
   g. Apply a clean, warm, moist washcloth to eyes and eyelids several times a day for 10 minutes to provide soothing and relaxing comfort.
   h. Symptoms that indicate a recurrence of the detachment: floating spots, flashing light, progressive shadows. Recommend that the patient contact health care provider if they occur.
3. Advise the patient to follow up. The first follow-up visit to the ophthalmologist should occur in 2 weeks, with other visits scheduled thereafter.

Evaluation: Expected Outcomes

- Verbalizes understanding of treatment.
- Follows activity restrictions.

Other Problems of the Retina and Vitreous

The retina is a multilayered structure that receives images and transmits them to the brain. It is nourished by retinal arteries and veins. Problems result from inflammation, trauma, vascular changes, congenital defects, and aging. Central lesions affect the macula, impairing central vision, near vision, and color discrimination. Peripheral lesions impair peripheral vision, causing blind spots, night blindness, and eventual tunnel vision. See Table 16-5 for treatment of individual disorders.

Nursing Assessment

1. Take history of eye problems, general health, and family history of eye disease.
2. Obtain functional history of how eye problem may be impairing work, recreation, and other activities.
3. Assess bilateral visual acuity, peripheral vision, and color discrimination.
4. Assist with pupil dilation and ophthalmoscopy, as directed.

Nursing Diagnoses

- Bathing, Dressing, Feeding Self-Care Deficit related to sudden visual loss.
- Readiness for Enhanced Self Care related to gradual visual loss.

- Risk for Injury related to visual impairment.
- Anxiety related to fear of further visual loss.

Nursing Interventions

Compensating for Sudden Loss of Vision

1. Orient the patient to the layout of the facility and explain procedures.
2. Assist with self-care activities.
3. Have personal articles placed nearby and take care not to move things without alerting the patient.

Compensating for Gradual Loss of Vision

1. Discuss strategies/modifications to carry out usual activities.
2. Engage support people in assistance with patient activity.
3. Refer patients with vision less than 20/70 to the Blind Association or other resource for assistive devices.
4. Advise patient to memorize environment while some vision is intact, then do not rearrange furniture or change environment.

Ensuring Safe Activities

1. Help the patient understand visual weaknesses, such as where blind spots are and how to compensate by turning head to scan environment, using magnifying glass, having environment brightly lit.
2. Discourage use of throw rugs, furniture placed in the middle of room or in cramped spaces.
3. Encourage arranging of frequently used items (kitchen wares, clothing, personal care items) in accessible areas.
4. Use side rails, as needed, and make sure that patient can call for help, if needed.
5. Assist the patient on stairs, make sure wearing good footwear, and obtain order for assistive devices, as needed.

Relieving Anxiety

1. Keep the patient informed during the diagnostic process.
2. Educate about resources.
3. Encourage participation in support groups.

Patient Education and Health Maintenance

1. Encourage frequent follow-up with ophthalmologist.
2. Advise the patient to use corrective lenses, as directed, keep lens prescription up-to-date, and to have a spare pair of glasses available.
3. Warn the patient against straining eyes by excessive exposure to the sun, reading, or computer work.
4. Rest eyes, as needed.
5. Report sudden deterioration in vision or other changes: sudden loss of vision, increase in floaters, flashes of light, sharp pain.

Evaluation: Expected Outcomes

- Bathes and dresses with assistance.
- Performs self-care activities independently.
- No falls or other injuries.
- Reports understanding of disease and acceptance of treatment plan.

Table 16-5   Other Conditions of the Retina and Vitreous

CONDITION	TREATMENT AND NURSING CONSIDERATIONS
Vitreous Hemorrhage Bleeding into the vitreous may occur due to trauma, sickle cell disease, hypertension, diabetic retinopathy, retinal tear or detachment, intraocular lens displacement, and clotting abnormalities. It causes decrease or loss of vision in affected eye.	The underlying cause is treated and surgery to repair the retina may include photocoagulation, cryotherapy, scleral buckle, or vitrectomy. (See "Retinal Detachment," page 594.) Assist the patient with visual deficit and activity and position restrictions before surgery. Maintain eye patches, activity restriction, and medication administration after surgery.
Central Retinal Artery Occlusion Sudden occlusion of the central retinal artery causes painless loss of vision in one eye with loss of light perception. It may have been preceded by episodes of transient blindness (amaurosis fugax) for 10–15 minutes. It is caused by an embolus, usually from the ipsilateral carotid artery.	**NURSING ALERT** Central retinal artery occlusion is a medical emergency. Vision may be salvaged if treated within 24 hours of onset. Treatment consists of massaging the globe in an attempt to break up the embolus or move it distally, inhalation of a mixture of 95% oxygen and 5% CO_2 to get the retinal vessels to dilate, and IV infusion of acetazolamide to lower intraocular pressure. Place the patient in Trendelenburg's position and monitor vital signs, as directed. Offer reassurance and assist with additional testing and treatment, as indicated.
Central Retinal Vein Occlusion Occlusion of the central retinal vein or a branch causes sudden (over several hours), painless decrease in visual acuity. Usually occurs in people with hypertension or other vascular disorders.	Urgent ophthalmologic evaluation is needed. Photocoagulation may be used to prevent local hemorrhage and promote neovascularization. Corticosteroids are used to treat retinal edema and an aspirin or anticoagulant may be used to prevent further occlusive disease. Encourage regular screening for glaucoma in follow-up as a complication from scar tissue formation after photocoagulation.
Macular Degeneration Age-related changes in the choroid deprive the fovea centralis of blood supply, causing a dry (atrophic) form (onset over several years) or wet (exudative) form (onset over several days to weeks with neovascularization and hemorrhaging). Central and near vision are affected, but some peripheral vision remains bilateral.	Support patient and family. Be realistic about prognosis—there is no cure but treatment may include laser, anti-VEGF therapy, diet, and vitamins (AREDS formulation) to slow the progression of the disease. Anti-VEGF therapy involves intraocular injection of medication every few weeks; can be painful and may raise the risk of infection. Refer patient to the local chapter of The Lions Club or other agencies for vision rehabilitation in order to assist with adaptive devices for low vision.
Retinitis Inflammation of the retina, usually caused by cytomegalovirus as a complication of human immunodeficiency virus disease. Symptoms include blurred vision, floaters and/or flashes in the eye, and loss of peripheral vision and eventually blindness. Determination of the progression of the disease is made by direct and indirect ophthalmoscopy and intravenous fluorescein angiography.	Antiviral medications can help control the symptoms and slow the progression of retinitis. Other treatment modalities include vitrectomy, silicone oil injection, and retinal detachment repair. Nursing interventions focus on patient education of drug side effects, care of central venous lines for intravenous medication, and monitoring blood count and for signs of kidney damage. Patient may be referred to community resources for low-vision assistance.
Diabetic Retinopathy A vascular disorder of the retina that leads to diminished vision as a complication of diabetes mellitus. Classified as nonproliferative or proliferative and typically occurs in four stages.	See page 958. Untreated diabetic retinopathy may cause complications such as retinal detachment, vitreous hemorrhage, clinically significant macular edema, glaucoma, and blindness.

AREDS, Age-Related Eye Disease Study; IOP, intraocular pressure; VEGF, vascular endothelial growth factor.

Eye Trauma

Trauma to the eye may be caused by blunt or sharp injury or chemical or thermal burns. The eyelids, protective layers, surrounding soft tissue, or the globe itself may be injured. Vision may be impaired by direct injury or latent scarring. See Table 16-6 for specific conditions.

Nursing Assessment

1. Obtain history of mechanism of injury as well as extent of other injuries.
2. Assess level of pain and visual symptoms.
3. Perform neurologic assessment and assess vital signs.
4. Assess visual acuity.

Table 16-6   Eye Trauma

CONDITION	CLINICAL MANIFESTATIONS	MEDICAL MANAGEMENT
Blunt Contusion Bruising of periorbital soft tissue	• Swelling and discoloration of the tissue • Bleeding into the tissue and structures of the eye • Pain • Diagnosis: Tests must determine if injury to parts of eye and systemic trauma	• Treatment to reduce swelling • Pain management dependent on structures involved *Note:* If there is any possibility of a ruptured globe, a loose patch and shield should be placed and ocular manipulation discouraged until ophthalmologist assessment completed.
Hyphema Presence of blood in the anterior chamber	• Pain • Blood in anterior chamber • Increased intraocular pressure	• Usually spontaneous recovery • If severe, bed rest or chair rest with bathroom privileges, eye shield, interior chamber paracentesis, topical steroids, and cycloplegics
Orbital Fracture Fracture and dislocation of walls of the orbit, orbital margins, or both	• May be accompanied by other signs of head injury • Rhinorrhea • Contusion • Diplopia • Diagnosis: x-ray, computed tomography	• May heal on own if no displacement or impingement on other structures • Surgery (repair the orbital floor with plate freeing entrapped orbital tissue)
Foreign Body On cornea (25% all ocular injuries), conjunctiva Intraocular particles penetrate sclera, cornea, globe	• Severe pain • Lacrimation • Foreign body sensation • Photophobia • Redness • Swelling *Note:* Wood and plant foreign body may cause severe infection within hours.	• Medical emergency • Removal of foreign body through irrigation, cotton-tipped applicator, or magnet • Treatment of intraocular foreign body depends on size, magnetic properties, tissue reaction, location • Surgical removal
Laceration/Perforation Cutting or penetration of soft tissue or globe	• Pain • Bleeding • Lacrimation • Photophobia	• Medical emergency • Surgical repair—method of repair depends on severity of injury • Antibiotics—topically and systemically
Ruptured Globe Concussive injury to globe with tears in the ocular coats, usually the sclera	• Pain • Altered intraocular pressure • Limitation of gaze in field of rupture • Hyphema • Hemorrhage (poor prognostic sign) • Diagnosis: computed tomography, ultrasound	• Medical emergency • Surgical repair • Vitrectomy • Scleral buckle • Antibiotics • Steroids • Enucleation

Table 16-6   Eye Trauma (continued)

CONDITION	CLINICAL MANIFESTATIONS	MEDICAL MANAGEMENT
Burns		
Chemical—caused by alkali or acid agent	• Pain • Burning • Lacrimation • Photophobia	• Medical emergency • Copious irrigation until pH is 7 • Severe scarring may require keratoplasty • Antibiotics
Thermal—usually burn to eyelids—may be first-, second-, or third-degree	• Pain • Burned skin • Blisters	• First aid—apply sterile dressings • Pain control • Leave fluid blebs intact • Suture eyelids together to protect eye—if perforation a possibility • Skin grafting with severe second- and third-degree burns
Ultraviolet—excessive exposure to sunlight, sunlamp, snow blindness, welding	• Pain—delayed several hours after exposure • Foreign body sensation • Lacrimation • Photophobia Note: Symptoms occur sometime after exposure.	• Pain relief • Condition self-limiting • Bilateral patching with antibiotic ointment and cycloplegics

Nursing Diagnoses

- Acute Pain from tissue trauma.
- Fear related to loss of vision.

Nursing Interventions

Relieving Pain

1. Medicate for pain, as directed; however, monitor for respiratory depression, hypotension, and decreased level of consciousness if opioid analgesic is used.
   Note: Medications that depress the central nervous system may be contraindicated if head injury is suspected.
2. Provide ice and cool compresses to relieve swelling and pain.
3. Provide additional comfort measures, such as positioning, dimmed lights, and quiet environment.
4. Irrigate and patch eye, as directed.
5. Monitor vital signs and neurologic status, as indicated.
6. Watch for and report signs of infection, such as fever, drainage, increased pain, warmth, and redness.

Reducing Fear

1. Provide psychological support and assist with self-care activities, as needed.
2. Describe procedures and treatments to the patient and family.
3. Maintain safe environment.
4. Prepare the patient for surgery, as indicated.

Patient Education and Health Maintenance

1. Teach the patient how to administer medications such as topical antibiotics.
2. Instruct on use of patch or shield.
3. Advise the patient to report increase in pain, decrease in vision, redness, fever.
4. Teach safety measures with decreased visual acuity.
5. Advise the use of corrective lenses, as prescribed.
6. Stress follow-up care.
7. Attempt to prevent future trauma with protective eyewear.

Evaluation: Expected Outcomes

- Rests comfortably, reports less pain.
- Cooperates with procedures.

Resources

For further information regarding eye disorders and resources, contact:

- American Council of the Blind (*www.acb.org*)
- American Macular Degeneration Foundation (*www.macular.org*)
- Wilmer Eye Institute at Johns Hopkins (*www.wilmer.jhu.edu*)
- National Eye Institute, Eye Health Information (*www.nei.nih.gov/health*)
- Common Eye Problems & Conditions (*www.eyecaresource.com*)
- Royal National Institute of Blind People (*www.rnib.org.uk*)
- American Academy of Ophthalmology (*www.geteyesmart.org, www.eyecareamerica.org*)

SELECTED REFERENCES

American Foundation for the Blind. (2011). Home modifications for people who are blind or have low vision. Vision Aware. Available: *www.visionaware.org/home_modifications*.

American Society of Ophthalmologic Registered Nurses. (2011). *Ophthalmic procedures in the office and clinic* (3rd ed.). Dubuque, IA: Kendall/Hunt.

American Society of Ophthalmologic Registered Nurses. (2008). *Core curriculum for ophthalmic nursing* (3rd ed.). Dubuque, IA: Kendall/Hunt.

American Society of Ophthalmologic Registered Nurses. (2011). *Care and handling of ophthalmic microsurgical instruments* (3rd ed.). Dubuque, IA: Kendall/Hunt.

Barnes, S., Chock, L., Sabell, P., et al. (2011). Cataract extraction: one area of infection risk and surveillance focus. *Insight (American Society of Ophthalmic Registered Nurses), 36*(3), 16–17, 32.

Chew, M., Pei-Chia Chiang, P., Zheng, Y., et al. (2012). The Impact of Cataract, Cataract Types, and Cataract Grades on Vision-Specific Functioning Using Rasch Analysis. *American Journal of Ophthalmology, 154*(1), 29–38.

Clark, A., Morlet, N., Ng, J. Q., et al. (2012). Retinal Detachment Risk Decreases after Phacoemulsification. *Arch Ophthalmol., 130*:882–888.

Dayani, P. N., & Grand, M. G. (2006). Maintenance of warfarin anticoagulation for patients undergoing vitriretinal surgery. *Archives in Ophthalmology, 124*, 1558–1565.

Fong, D. S., Poon, K. (2012). Recent Statin Use and Cataract Surgery. *American Journal of Ophthalmology, 153*(2), 222–228.

Heier, J. S., Brown, D. M., Chong, V., and the VIEW 1 and VIEW 2 Study Groups. (2012). Intravitreal aflibercept (VEGF Trap-Eye) in wet age-related macular degeneration. *Ophthalmology*. Published online October 18.2012. pii: S0161–6420(12)00865–2.

Hirschman, D. R., & Morby, L. J. (2006). Safety of continued anticoagulation therapy for cataract surgery patients. *Nursing Forum, 41*(1), 30–37.

Hooper, N. (2012, January). Low vision managing loss when vision fails. Presented at a Competency-based Approach to Geriatric Ophthalmology CME Course, The Methodist Hospital Research Institute, Houston, TX.

Lemp, M. A., & Nichols, K. K. (2009). Blepharitis in the United States 2009: A survey-based perspective on prevalence and treatment. *Ocular Surface, 7*(2, Suppl.), S1–S14

Mangione, C. M., Lee, P. P., Gutierrez, P. R., et al. (2001). Development of the 25-item National Eye Institute Visual Function Questionnaire (VFQ-25). *Archives of Ophthalmology, 119*, 1050–1058.

Niyadurupola, N., & Astbury, A. (2008). Endophthalmitis: controlling infection before and after cataract surgery. *Community Eye Health Journal, 21*(65), 9–10.

Ramulu, P., van Landingham, S., Massof, R., et al. (2012). Fear of Falling and Visual Field Loss from Glaucoma. *Ophthalmology, 119*(7), 1352–1358.

Shukla, A. N., Daly, M. K., & Legutko, P. (2011). Informed consent for cataract surgery: patient understanding of verbal, written, and videotaped information. *Journal of Cataract Refraction Surgery, 38*(1), 80–84.

Tseng, V. L., Yu, F., Lum, F., et al. (2012). Risk of fractures following cataract surgery in Medicare beneficiaries. *JAMA. 308*:493–501.

U.S. Food and Drug Administration. (2011). LASIK. Available:

www.fda.gov/MedicalDevices/ProductsandMedicalProcedures/SurgeryandLifeSupport/LASIK/default.htm.

17

Ear, Nose, and Throat Disorders

OVERVIEW AND ASSESSMENT

History

Obtaining a history, including the patient's signs and symptoms, current health patterns, and previous past medical history, will help in identifying ear, nose, and throat (ENT) problems and developing an individualized plan of care.

Key Signs and Symptoms

1. Epistaxis.
   a. When did the bleeding first begin? Did it occur spontaneously or occur after facial or nasal trauma, nose blowing, digital manipulation, or recent nasal or sinus surgery? In many cases, anterior bleeding commonly flows from the nasal vestibule and, in reclining position, will drip into the throat. Posterior bleeding commonly causes dripping in to the oropharynx when upright or supine. Nasal endoscopy or examination via anterior rhinoscopy is performed to confirm the site of bleeding.
   b. Unilateral or bilateral? What side of the nose is the bleeding coming from, and if bilateral, on what side did it begin? Ask patient about measures employed to control the bleeding thus far.
   c. Assess current medication history: Is the patient taking acetylsalicylic acid (ASA, aspirin), antiplatelet agents, or anticoagulants? When was the last dose taken?
   d. Is there a history of current oxygen therapy? Is there a history of chronic bleeding disorders? Obtain results of recent bloodwork: complete blood count (CBC), prothrombin time (PT), International Normalized Ratio (INR), or partial prothrombin time (PTT).
2. Headache.
   a. Exactly what parts of the head or face hurt? Is it pain or a pressure sensation? Use the PQRST Method of Pain Assessment with emphasis on location, duration, and symptom onset.
   b. Assess for associated neck, dental, or jaw pain, nausea, vomiting, visual changes, and/or sensitivity to light or sound.

Assess for associated nasal congestion, postnasal drip, or clear or purulent rhinorrhea. Assess for history of migraine disease.

3. Sore throat. Assess onset and duration of symptoms, previous medical treatment, and symptom response.
   a. Is it accompanied by swollen glands, high fever, nasal congestion, and postnasal drip? Assess for associated weight loss; head, neck, or ear pain; voice changes; neck mass; trismus; or difficulty breathing. Has the patient been able to eat or drink?
   b. Is it acute or chronic? Was there any exposure to others with throat infection?

4. Nasal congestion.
   a. Is it acute or chronic? Accompanied by fever and purulent drainage? Assess severity and duration of symptoms, associated purulent or clear rhinorrhea, fever, facial pain or sinus tenderness, itchy eyes, sneezing, or postnasal drip. If symptoms are chronic, assess if worsened with changes in barometric pressure, vary with seasons, or brought on by odors or allergen exposure.
   b. Assess for current/chronic history of use of nasal sprays containing oxymetazoline, or if the patient is experiencing anosmia/microsmia (loss of sense of smell or diminished sensitivity). Ask if the patient has had previous history of nasal polyps, previous nasal or sinus surgery, or nasal fracture.

5. Hoarseness.
   a. Assess history of recent surgical procedures involving the head or neck, recent endotracheal intubation, radiation treatment to the head/neck, history of tobacco/alcohol use, occupation as vocal performer, or history of lung disease with use of inhaled steroids, chronic or recent antibiotic therapy, symptoms of gastroesophageal reflux.
   b. Is it acute (less than 2 weeks), recurrent, or chronic (more than 2 weeks)? Assess onset and duration of symptoms, subjective impairment in communication or voice-related quality.

 NURSING ALERT Hoarseness for longer than 2 weeks in a smoker is an indication for ENT evaluation and laryngoscopy.

   c. Assess for recent URI symptoms, associated dysphagia, odynophagia, globus sensation (sensation of something in the throat), throat pain, weight loss, ear pain, neck mass or enlarged lymph nodes in neck, hemoptysis, or shortness of breath.

6. Earache (otalgia).
   a. Is it worsened by manipulation of the auricle or is it a deep, throbbing pain? Is there otorrhea? Assess onset and duration of pain using the PQRST Pain Scale. Assess for associated erythema or edema of the external ear canal or external auricle, pruritis, hearing loss, or otorrhea. Is the pain intermittent or constant?
   b. Were there preceding upper respiratory infection symptoms? Is the pain associated with hearing loss, aural fullness, vertigo, headache, or fluctuation of hearing? Has there been any recent dental procedures?

   c. Assess history for nighttime bruxism, clenching of the jaw or teeth, malocclusion, or pain worsened with movement of the jaw, dental pain, or swelling of the muscles of mastication.
   d. Assess for ear pain that occurs with swallowing and associated symptoms of head and neck cancer.

7. Hearing loss.
   a. Was it sudden or gradual in onset? Assess subjective onset of hearing loss. Did the patient experience sudden or gradual onset of the hearing loss? Is there associated tinnitus, vertigo, aural fullness, or ear pain?
   b. Unilateral or bilateral? Assess for history of noise exposure; recreational shooting, occupational, acoustic trauma, or history of chronic otitis media. Assess for history of familial/hereditary hearing loss.

8. Dizziness.
   a. Is the patient light-headed or experiencing vertigo (as if the room or self is spinning). Assess for subjective light-headedness, room spinning, or imbalance. Are symptoms acute or chronic and associated with symptoms of fluctuation of hearing, aural fullness, or tinnitus (symptoms of Ménière's disease).
   b. Is the dizziness associated with a change in head or body position? Do symptoms occur with rolling over in bed, looking up or bending over, or when going from sitting to standing? Are there feelings of presyncope, history of syncopal episode when rising from sitting to standing? Are there changes in blood pressure associated with lying, sitting, and standing?
   c. Assess for duration of symptoms and associated nausea, vomiting, headache, or focal neurological symptoms.

Current Health Patterns

1. Inquire about nutrition, dental care, normal mouth care habits, dental caries, use of partial or full dentures, stress-related grinding, clenching, or clamping of teeth.
2. Ask about history of alcohol, smoking, use of a pipe, and smokeless tobacco. Is there a personal history of human immunodeficiency virus (HIV), sexually transmitted disease, recreational drug use, or human papillomavirus (HPV)?
3. Determine personal hygiene about ears. Are cotton swabs or other objects used for cleaning or to relieve itching? Does the patient wear hearing aids or ear plugs?
4. Is there any loud noise exposure? Is there history of noise exposure via recreational shooting, or in the patient's occupation? Ask about use of noise protection when exposed to prolonged and loud noise. Is there family history of hearing loss?
5. Does the patient frequently strain voice through talking, singing, or shouting? Is the patient a singer?
6. What medications is the patient taking? Have antibiotics been used? For how long?

Past Medical History

1. Is there a history of allergic rhinitis, other allergy symptoms, immunotherapy, chronic or recurrent sinusitis, previous nasal surgery, chronic otitis media, chronic pharyngitis, history of snoring, or obstructive sleep apnea?

2. Is there any immunosuppressive illness, such as diabetes mellitus, cancer, HIV infection, autoimmune disease, recent radiation or chemotherapy?
3. Is there a history of previous thyroid, carotid artery, or other surgery involving the laryngeal nerve?
4. Any history of previous or recent head, facial, or nasal trauma?

See Chapter 5, page 57, for physical assessment of the ears, nose, throat, and neck.

Diagnostic Tests

Audiometry

Description

1. Audiometry is the most basic and accurate testing to determine and measure hearing ability. The results are plotted on a graph known as an audiogram. Testing is performed by an audiologist. The following points below describe aspects of audiometry:
   a. Pure tone threshold audiometry is the lowest level at which sound is heard across various sound frequencies. This is compared to normative data to measure hearing loss and used to monitor hearing sensitivity over time.
   b. Speech audiometry provides information about the patient's communication ability. Speech reception threshold is defined as the softest level at which the patient can repeat a word. Speech recognition or speech discrimination is the percentage of words that a patient can repeat accurately at the comfortable listening level. This helps to determine ability to understand conversational speech.
   c. Pure tune testing is performed by presenting pure tones via air and bone conduction. Air conduction testing is done by presenting pure tones at various octave levels from 250 to 8,000 Hz through a transducer, such as insert earphone or cushion headphone. The patient sits in a soundproof booth and the audiologist presents tones and the patient is asked to indicate when the sound is heard. Testing by bone conduction is done with use of a bone oscillator, which is placed on the mastoid of the test ear and pure tones are presented at 500, 1,000, 2,000, and 4,000 Hz.
   d. Immitance testing includes tympanometry and acoustic reflex testing.
      i. Acoustic reflex testing measures the response of the stapedius muscle in response to auditory signals. It provides information about the acoustic and the facial nerves, as well as information about a conductive or sensioneural hearing loss.
      ii. Tympanometry measures the changes that occur to the tympanic membrane and middle ear when changes in air pressure are introduced into the ear canal. It can provide information about eustachian tube dysfunction, middle ear fluid, tympanic membrane perforation, patency of pressure-equalizing tubes, and middle ear disease such as otosclerosis.

Nursing and Patient Care Considerations

1. The patient wears earphones and signals upon hearing a tone.
2. A soundproof room is used to increase accuracy.
3. No special patient preparation or participation is necessary for tympanometry.

Cineradiography

Description

1. This motion study is performed to study the functional dynamics of the pharynx and esophagus.
2. It provides a more physiologic examination than esophagram (barium swallow). Mucosal detail is seen better with cineradiography, whereas video capture allows more dynamic evaluation with less radiation.
3. "Modified barium swallow" evaluates laryngotracheal aspiration while a speech pathologist provides various consistencies of food and swallowing techniques. An esophagram evaluates the pharyngeal and esophageal mucosa.

Nursing and Patient Care Considerations

1. The patient is usually kept NPO the night before surgery.
2. The patient will be given radioprotective gear to prevent radiation from reaching other parts of the body.

Electronystagmography

Description

1. *Electronystagmography* is the recording of eye movements, specifically nystagmus, during various oculomotor and vestibular testing. Videonystagmography is the recording of eye movements using infrared video image analysis in three dimensions. The pattern of nystagmus, in conjunction with the patient's neurotological examination and clinical history, may provide information about the underlying etiology of the patient's symptoms.
2. Used to establish the diagnosis of Ménière's disease, vestibular neuronitis or labyrinthitis, benign paroxysmal positional vertigo (BPPV), or migraine-associated vertigo and to assist in ruling out vestibular pathology in a patient with symptoms of dizziness.
3. The test takes place in a dimly lit room, with the patient on an examination table, and lasts for 60 to 90 minutes.
4. Electrodes are placed on the forehead and lateral to each eye in electronystagmogram (ENG) testing. Video goggles are used in videonystagmography. Eye movements are recorded in response to various position changes and visual stimuli, with eyes open and eyes closed.
5. Caloric testing is the evaluation of nystagmus induced by warm or cold water irrigation into the external ear canals. Caloric testing can also be obtained by instilling cool and warm air into the ear canal. Caloric testing is used to measure the degree of vestibular dysfunction. Testing of patients with a normally functioning vestibular system will induce vertigo.
6. The audiologist may perform the vertebral artery test with older adults, patients who have history of neck trauma, or patients in which vertebral artery disease is suspected. Patients that elicit symptoms when the head is hyperextended may not be able to have portions of the positional testing completed.

Nursing and Patient Care Considerations

1. Patient preparation includes avoiding a heavy meal before the procedure and avoiding caffeine and alcohol for 48 hours before the procedure.

2. Medications that may affect the vestibular system, such as sedatives, anti-anxiety agents, narcotics, and medications ordered for dizziness, may be held for several days before the procedure.

3. The patient will receive instructions from the facility/provider who will be administering the test for specific medications that will need to be held and for how long before testing is performed. The patient should be counseled in the importance of following these preprocedure instructions, as they may affect the accuracy of the testing.

GENERAL PROCEDURES AND TREATMENT MODALITIES

Nasal Surgery

Types of Surgery and Indications

Facial Trauma and Nasal Fractures

1. Nasal bone fractures are common after blows to the nose during sports activities, interpersonal altercations, motor vehicle accidents, or falls. These can be diagnosed via physical examination or nasal/facial images, including x-rays or computed tomography (CT) scans.

2. Techniques of repair of nasal fractures include closed reduction or open reduction.
   a. Closed reduction may be performed by ENT surgeon by applying force, internally and externally, to move the septum back into proper position. This may be done under local/general anesthesia, in operating room, or in office with local anesthesia. Closed reductions are ideally performed 5 to 10 days after the injury when the bones are still mobile.
   b. Open reduction can also be done for older, healed fractures several months after the injury.

3. Repair and stabilization of other maxillofacial fractures usually require an operating room procedure for wiring or plating.

Nasal Septal Surgery

1. Septoplasty is an intranasal procedure performed under general anesthesia to remove portions of, straighten, or trim the septal bone and/or cartilage. Silastic splints are sutured on either side of the septum to stabilize the repositioned septum. The splints are removed several days postoperatively. This surgery is performed to treat chronic nasal obstruction and may be done in conjunction with sinus surgery to promote a clear nasal airway.

2. Submucosal turbinate reduction or excision of middle turbinate concha bullosa is an intranasal procedure performed under local or general anesthesia in the operating room to surgically trim, excise, or reduce tissue in the nasal cavity that contributes to nasal obstruction. May be done in conjunction with septoplasty.

Rhinoplasty

1. Involves changing the nose's external appearance. Grafted cartilage or bone harvested from other parts of the body may be used.

2. A septorhinoplasty may be done when there are external and internal nasal deformities.

Sinus Surgery

1. Functional endoscopic sinus surgery (FESS) is corrective sinus surgery performed under general anesthesia in the operating room using direct visualization via a rigid nasal endoscope or, more recently, with assistance of image-guided systems. Image-guided systems utilize CT scans to provide surgeon with intraoperative landmarks and map.

2. Diseased mucosa is removed and the natural sinus ostia are widened to facilitate the normal sinus drainage patterns.

3. In addition to nasal and sinus conditions, surgery may also be used to treat traumatic optic neuropathy, cerebrospinal leaks, nasolacrimal duct obstruction, dysthyroid orbitopathy, posterior orbital lesions, and choanal atresia.

4. Packing may be placed intraoperatively depending on surgeon's preference and amount of bleeding. Packing is usually very small, filling only the area adjacent to the sinus ostia, so is not visible except for a retrieval string extending outside the nasal ala.

5. Balloon catheter sinuplasty: The procedure uses a small balloon catheter to open blocked sinus passageways. The procedure is done to widen and restructure the blocked passageways without surgical removal of bone and tissue (see Figure 17-1).

6. Other approaches to the sinuses, such as the Caldwell-Luc procedure (opening under lip to enter maxillary sinus and strip out diseased mucosa), may be performed but newer techniques are more often utilized. A nasoantral window (creating an opening between the maxillary sinus and the anterior inferior nose), and anterior/posterior ethmoidectomies may be perfomed, as well as opening and draining the frontal or sphenoid sinuses. The patient with historically extensive postoperative nasal and sinus packing is rarely seen and is now used only in selected complicated cases with extensive bleeding.

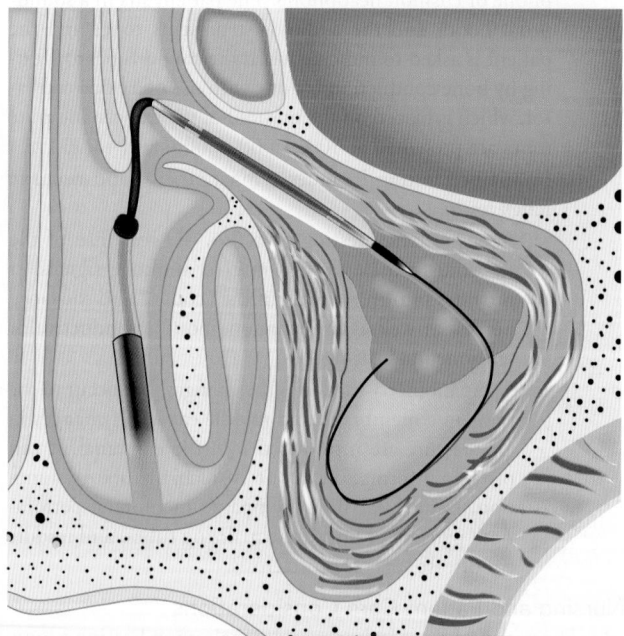

Figure 17-1. Balloon catheter sinus surgery. A catheter is introduced through the nose and into the sinus ostia, where the balloon is inflated to enlarge the sinus opening and promote drainage.

Preoperative Management

1. The head of bed should be raised to promote drainage, lessen edema, and make patient more comfortable.
2. Intermittent cold compresses and pain medications should be utilized, as ordered.
3. Antibiotics may be used preoperatively to reduce bacterial colonization of nose and sinuses.
4. The patient should be advised that a sensation of pressure may be felt in the nasal area during surgery performed under local anesthetic.
5. The patient should be counseled about the possible use of packing with some surgeries, which may be removed several days postoperatively
6. Instructions for stopping aspirin, nonsteroidal anti-inflammatory medications and antiplatelet and anticoagulant medications will be provided by the surgeon and individualized after collaboration with the patient's cardiologist or primary care provider.

 NURSING ALERT In most cases, the patient should avoid use of aspirin, nonsteroidal anti-inflammatory drugs, anticoagulants, antiplatelet agents, and herbal medications such as *Ginkgo biloba*, garlic, green tea, and any other drugs that may affect platelet function before surgery. If patient has taken these medications within a week of surgery, make sure surgeon is notified.

Complications

1. Hematoma/hemorrhage: Septal hematoma or postoperative bleeding. A septal hematoma will need to be drained by surgeon immediately if this should occur.
2. Local infection—contaminated nasal packing is an excellent culture medium for pathogens. Most patients are treated postoperatively with antibiotics, but this is surgeon-specific.
3. Aspiration.
4. Pressure necrosis (from packing) may occur, but the current trend is toward less packing.
5. Blindness from orbital hematoma or unintended orbital involvement in endoscopic sinus surgery.
6. Cerebrospinal fluid (CSF) rhinorrhea from unintended or traumatic violation of the cribriform plate. This is commonly referred to as a CSF leak.
7. Pulmonary decompensation.

Nursing Diagnoses

- Ineffective Breathing Pattern (nasal airway clearance) related to nasal packing and swelling.
- Risk for Aspiration related to bleeding, inability to blow nose.
- Deficient Knowledge related to performance of nasal hygiene.
- Impaired Oral Mucous Membrane related to mouth breathing.
- Risk for Infection related to alterations in nasal/sinus mucous membranes and drainage patterns.

Nursing Interventions

Facilitating Breathing and Comfort

1. Keep head elevated (three to four pillows) day and night to minimize swelling. This also promotes comfort.
2. Apply cold compresses or ice packs intermittently for 24 hours to lessen edema and discoloration and to promote comfort. (Use great caution and only with approval of surgeon after rhinoplasty.)
3. Advise the patient that packing will be removed within 1 week of placement.
4. Encourage the use of a humidifier to relieve crusting of nasal mucosa and prevent irritation from dryness in nose and throat.
5. Encourage relaxation techniques and deep-breathing exercises for anxiety associated with nasal passages being blocked.
6. Be alert for worsening pulmonary conditions, such as asthma, chronic obstructive pulmonary disease, and sleep apnea, when the nose is congested or packed.
7. Encourage use of analgesics but caution overuse, which may cause respiratory depression. Medicate with analgesics as prescribed. Topical decongestants may be prescribed to relieve nasal congestion in the first few days postoperatively. Pain after nasal surgery is usually mild to moderate.

Preventing Bleeding and Aspiration

1. Monitor closely for bleeding; check for increased swallowing, blood dripping down back of throat (use flashlight and tongue blade), expectoration of large amounts of clots and blood.
2. Change the 4 × 4 gauze pad under the nose as it becomes soaked with blood; bleeding should gradually decrease. Teach family and patient that blood will be bright red at first and will gradually lessen over the next several days.
3. Notify the surgeon if bleeding increases. Expect a temporary minor increase in bleeding with vomiting, sneezing, ambulation, or crying in the first 48 hours.
4. Teach the patient that mild nausea is normal postoperatively and may be from anesthesia, pain medications, swallowing of blood; however, be alert for continuous trickle of blood postnasally.
5. Instruct the patient not to blow nose but to blot secretions with tissue and "sniff and spit."
6. Regularly observe and document visible packing retrieval strings external to nose, taped to cheek, if present. Postoperative instructions should be given upon discharge with appointments for postoperative splint removal or sinus debridement, if indicated. Surgeon will discuss activity and work restrictions specific to the patient.

Ensuring Proper Nasal Hygiene

1. Encourage the patient to use a vaporizer to help relieve crusting of nasal mucosa from dryness.
2. Remind the patient that sneezing, straining, and nose blowing increase venous pressure and can result in bleeding/hematoma.

3. Advise the patient to keep the mouth open while sneezing if unable to control sneezing.

4. Teach the patient an appropriate method of nasal hygiene as approved by surgeon. After FESS, the patient will need regular appointments for sinus debridement by the surgeon. Advise the patient sinus irrigation will need to be done to control nasal crusting and to facilitate healing (see Patient Education Guidelines 17-1).

5. In general, the patient may gently clean nasal ala area with saline and/or peroxide for comfort, but large crusts should be removed by surgeon or allowed to work themselves free.

6. Instruct the patient to avoid environmental irritants, especially smoke.

Protecting Oral Mucous Membranes

1. Administer frequent mouth care because the patient is forced to breathe through the mouth.

2. Use flexible straw to sip mouthwash for rinsing purposes.

3. Encourage fluid intake and use of lip protectant.

Preventing Infection

1. Be alert for uncontrolled postoperative pain, fever, foul odor or taste in mouth, or unusual drainage.

2. Administer or encourage prophylactic antibiotics on time, if ordered.

3. Advise patient to keep follow-up appointment for splint removal, packing removal, and sinus debridement.

Patient Education and Health Maintenance

1. Tell the patient to notify the surgeon immediately for uncontrolled postoperative pain, any visual changes postoperatively, fever, unilateral clear nasal discharge with leaning the head forward, uncontrolled excessive nasal bleeding, dyspnea, or blanching or necrosis of the external nasal tissues or the palate while packing is in place.

2. After Caldwell-Luc procedure or rhinoplasty, advise the patient that numbness in operative area may be present for several weeks to months.

3. Instruct the patient to avoid strenuous activity, lifting, and trauma to nose.

4. After splint removal, avoid trauma to nose and sleep in supine position. Operating surgeon will provide more specific postoperative instructions.

5. Excessive sun exposure should also be avoided after rhinoplasty for 1 year due to a tendency for hyperpigmentation.

6. If a nasal splint is present, tell patient to avoid getting it wet; do not attempt to remove it.

7. Advise the patient that postoperative follow-up may need to continue for several weeks to months to monitor for excess scar formation or cosmetic deformity.

Evaluation: Expected Outcomes

- Mouth breathing without difficulty.
- No excessive bleeding, protects airway without aspiration.

PATIENT EDUCATION GUIDELINES 17-1

Nasal Saline Irrigation

This procedure will help clear nasal passages of crusted drainage that may be blocking the sinus opening. Perform this once or twice per day to feel less nasal congestion and to help sinuses drain.

1. Prepare saline solution right before irrigation. *Commercially prepared sinus irrigation kits are readily available that contain packets and sinus rinse bottle.*

2. Mix ½ tsp table salt and ¼ tsp baking soda with 8 oz warm distilled or sterilized water until well dissolved.

3. Lean forward from the waist over a sink.

4. Fill a bulb syringe (1 oz infant ear or nasal bulb) or rinse bottle with the saline solution by squeezing it in the solution and letting it fill by suction. If using sinus rinse kit, follow instructions.

5. Insert the tip of the filled syringe into one nostril, aimed toward the eye away from the nasal septum.

6. Squeeze the syringe gently and feel the solution run backward in the nose and out the other nostril and possibly down the back of the throat and out of the mouth.

7. When comfortable with this procedure, you may be able to rotate head forward, backward, and from side to side to irrigate the sinuses as well as the nose.

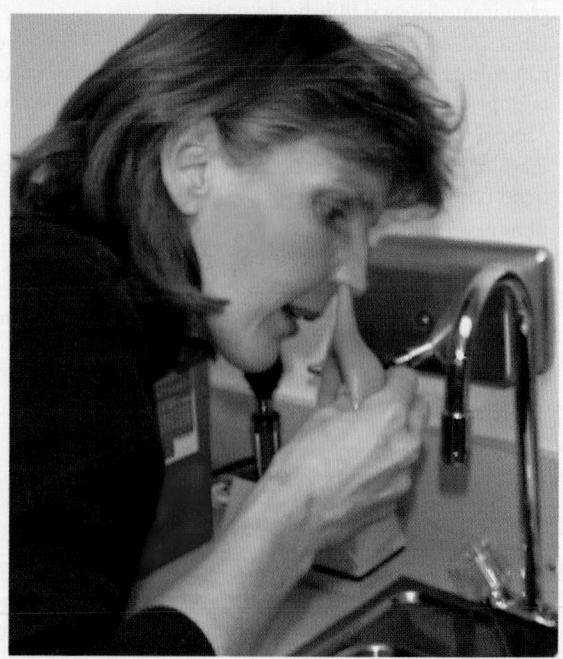

Nose irrigation with bulb syringe or sinus irrigation kit.

- Nasal and palatal tissues free from blanching or darkening.
- Oral mucous membranes dry, but pink and intact.
- Afebrile, no signs of infection.

Ear Surgery

Ear surgery may involve the tympanic membrane, the middle ear cavity, the mastoid, or the inner ear. It may be done for perforation of the eardrum to facilitate drainage and remove diseased tissue in cases of infection or cholesteotoma, to relieve vertigo, or to treat hearing loss.

Types of Surgery

1. Myringotomy—creating a surgical opening into tympanic membrane (with knife or laser) for possible drainage tube insertion.
2. Tympanoplasty—reconstruction of diseased or deformed middle ear components (see Table 17-1).
   a. Type I (myringoplasty)—purpose is to close perforation by placing a graft over it to create a closed middle ear to improve hearing and decrease risk of infection and cholesteatoma. Perforation is closed using one of the following:
      i. Fascia from temporalis muscle (this is the most commonly used material).
      ii. Vein grafts from hand or forearm.
      iii. Epithelium from auditory canal (eustachian tube).
   b. Type II to V—suitable replacement (polyethylene, Teflon or titanium prosthesis, bone, cartilage) is used to maintain continuity of conduction sound pathway. The necessity of a two-stage procedure is determined.
      i. First stage—eradication of all diseased tissues; area is cleaned out to achieve a dry, healed middle ear.
      ii. Second stage—performed 4 to 6 months after first stage; reconstruction, using grafts.

3. Mastoidectomy—removal of mastoid process of temporal bone.
   a. Simple or cortical mastoidectomy is done via a postauricular approach but the bony ear canal is left intact.
   b. Modified radical mastoidectomy or canal wall down mastoidectomy is done with a meatoplasty for the best results. A wide excision of the mastoid and diseased middle ear contents through a postauricular incision is performed with the bony canal being drilled out. A new larger ear canal is created that gives better access to the areas where cholesteatoma usually occurs (the attic and antrum).
4. Stapedectomy—removal of footplate of stapes and insertion of a graft or prosthesis
5. Stapedotomy—removal of the stapes suprastructure, allowing a hole to be created with a laser in the stapes footplate. The base of the prosthesis will be inserted into the opening and the other end will be crimped around the incus.
6. Labyrinthectomy—destruction of the labyrinth (inner ear) through the middle ear and aspiration of the endolabyrinth.
7. Endolymphatic decompression and shunt—release of pressure on the endolymphatic system in the labyrinth and creation of a shunt for fluid to the subarachnoid space or the mastoid.
8. Cochlear implant—implantation of electronic device that bypasses the damaged cochlea and stimulates auditory nerve.
9. Osseointegrated implantation for placement of a hearing implant for single-sided deafness or for conductive hearing loss (Baha system or Oticon implantable hearing system).

Preoperative Management

1. Hearing function is fully evaluated.
2. Antibiotics are given to treat infection.
3. The patient is prepared emotionally for the effects of surgery.
4. Careful assessment for signs of acute infection is performed, which may delay surgery.

Table 17-1	Types of Tympanoplasty		
	MIDDLE EAR DAMAGE		**REPAIR PROCESS**
Type	**Tympanic Membrane**	**Ossicles**	
I	Perforated	Normal	• Close perforation—myringoplasty
II	Perforated	Erosion of malleus and/or incus	• Close perforation; graft against incus or whatever remains of malleus
III	Tympanic membrane destroyed or widely perforated	Rest of ossicular chain destroyed but stapes are intact and mobile	• Grafts implanted to contact the normal stapes • Tympanostapedopexy
IV	Tympanic membrane destroyed or widely perforated	Ossicular chain destroyed. Head, neck, and crura of stapes destroyed. Stapes footplate mobile.	• Expose mobile stapes footplate—graft implanted. Air pocket between graft and round window provides protection • The cavum minor operation
V	Tympanic membrane destroyed or widely perforated	Ossicular chain destroyed. Head, neck, and crura of stapes destroyed. Stapes footplate fixed.	• Make opening in horizontal semicircular canal; graft seals off middle ear to give sound protection for round window • Tympanoplasty and fenestration of lateral semicircular canal

Postoperative Management

1. Antibiotics may be continued to prevent local and central nervous system (CNS) infection.
2. Patients are advised to have limited activity for the first 24 hours to decrease symptoms of nausea and vertigo (if the inner ear was disturbed) or to prevent disruption of prosthesis.
3. Analgesics, anti-emetics, and antihistamines are given, as needed.
4. The patient is positioned to promote drainage but maintain some immobility. Using two extra pillows to elevate the head, thereby preventing edema for 2 weeks, is a good idea.
5. Patient is often seen 7 to 10 days after surgery to remove any metal stent placed. Additional packing may be removed up to 6 weeks postoperatively if prosthesis or graft procedure was performed. Often an ear drop will be used to slowly dissolve remaining packing over a period of 6 to 8 weeks to give some weight to the grafted tympanic membrane.
6. Hearing will be reevaluated after edema has subsided and healing has occurred. The time frame for this varies by procedure but may be as long as 3 to 4 months after surgery to allow for healing.
7. With an osseointegrated implant, a fitting of the outer processor is usually delayed by 2 to 3 months to allow the bone to osseointegrate around the implant. In children, or in radiated bone, this may be done in two stages separated by 6 months to allow for a slower rate of bone growth.
8. Cochlear implant activation and placement of the outer speech processor and external transmitter occurs approximately 4 weeks after surgery to allow for healing.

Complications

1. Infection: local, CNS (meningitis, brain abscess).
2. Hearing loss.
3. Facial nerve paralysis—rare.
4. Dizziness—usually temporary.

Nursing Diagnoses

- Acute Pain related to surgical incision and swelling.
- Risk for Infection related to invasive procedure.
- Risk for Injury related to vertigo.

Nursing Interventions

Relieving Pain

1. Administer or teach self-administration of analgesic, as indicated, postoperatively.
2. Tell the patient to expect pain to subside within first few hours with simple procedures or within first day or two with major procedures.
3. Position the patient for comfort following the instructions from the surgeon.
   a. On side with surgical ear upward to maintain graft position and immobility.
   b. Lying on side with surgical ear down to promote drainage from ear canal.
   c. Position of patient preference.

4. Elevate the head of bed to reduce swelling and pressure.
5. Advise the patient to avoid sudden movement. Use pillows for support.

Preventing Infection

1. Reinforce external dressings, as needed, until after first changed by surgeon, then change when saturated to prevent bacterial growth in damp dressings.
2. Loosely pack cotton or gauze in ear canal, as indicated, without causing increased pressure.
3. Do not probe or insert anything into ear canal.
4. Administer or teach self-administration of antibiotics, as prescribed. Do not use eardrops unless specifically ordered postoperatively.
5. Wash hands before ear care and instruct the patient not to touch ear.
6. Take care not to get the dressing or ear wet.
7. Advise the patient not to blow nose, which could cause nasopharyngeal secretions to be forced up eustachian tube into middle ear.
8. Instruct the patient to report any increased pain, fever, ear inflammation, or drainage, indicating local infection.
9. Be alert for headache, fever, stiff neck, or altered level of consciousness, which may indicate CNS infection.

Ensuring Safety

1. Be aware that dizziness or vertigo may occur for the first several days postoperatively.
2. Maintain side rails up while the patient is in bed.
3. Assist the patient with ambulation for the first time after surgery and as needed thereafter.
4. Encourage the patient to move slowly because sudden movements may exacerbate vertigo.
5. Administer or teach self-administration of anti-emetics and antihistamines, as ordered and as needed; watch for sedation.
6. Instruct the patient not to blow nose, cough, lean forward, or perform Valsalva's maneuver to avoid disrupting graft or prosthesis, aggravating vertigo, or forcing bacteria up the eustachian tube. If coughing or blowing nose is necessary, do so with open mouth to relieve pressure.

Patient Education and Health Maintenance

1. Advise the patient that there may be a temporary hearing loss for a few weeks after surgery because of tissue edema, packing, and so forth. The effects of a hearing restoration operation will not be known for several weeks and additional rehabilitation may be necessary to optimize results.
2. Advise the patient to protect the ear, perform dressing changes, or place loose cotton in outer ear, as indicated. Replace cotton twice daily or sooner if saturated by drainage.
3. Encourage follow-up for packing removal, as directed.
4. Instruct the patient to avoid sudden pressure changes in the ear.
   a. Do not blow nose.
   b. Do not fly in a small plane. The date for which a patient may fly is individualized by their surgery and surgeon's preference.
   c. Do not dive.

5. Advise against smoking.
6. Tell the patient to protect ears when going outdoors for the first week. A cotton ball is all that is needed.
7. Tell the patient to avoid getting ear wet until completely healed.
8. Tell the patient to avoid crowds or exposure to colds so upper respiratory infection is prevented.
9. Instruct the patient about signs and symptoms of complications to report.
   a. Return of tinnitus.
   b. Vertigo.
   c. Fluctuations of hearing ability.
   d. Fever, headache, ear inflammation, increased pain, stiff neck.
   e. Facial drooping or numbness.
10. Advise the patient that facial nerve paralysis may be temporary and to increase fluid intake through a straw during this time.

Evaluation: Expected Outcomes

- Verbalizes relief of pain.
- No signs of infection.
- Ambulates without difficulty.

CONDITIONS OF THE MOUTH AND JAW

Candidiasis

 Evidence Base Pappas, P., Kauffman C. A., & Andes, D. (2009). Clinical management guidelines for the management of candidiasis: 2009 update by the Infectious Disease Society of America. *Clinical Infectious Diseases, 48,* 503–535.

Candidiasis is an opportunistic fungal infection commonly caused by *Candida albicans*. It may be localized in the mouth and pharynx, but may also occur in the esophagus. Candidiasis can become a source of systemic dissemination, particularly in high-risk persons.

Pathophysiology and Etiology

1. Commonly seen in individuals with immunosuppression from disease states or treatment regimens such as diabetes, cancer, or HIV and those receiving radiation therapy and/or chemotherapy.
2. May be caused by altered oral environment from xerostomia, use of inhaled steroids for asthma and COPD, or chronic antibiotic therapy, preexisting infections, poor oral hygiene or nutritional status, or wearing dentures.

Clinical Manifestations

1. Oral examination reveals diffuse, white, painless plaques. Underlying mucosa may be erythematous.
2. May be asymptomatic but may result in mild oral discomfort, burning, or alterations in taste.
3. Patients with disease spread beyond the oral cavity may present with chest pain, pain and difficulty with swallowing, or hoarseness.

Diagnostic Evaluation

1. Microscopic smear of plaques shows characteristic hyphae.
2. Oral fungal culture positive for *C. albicans.*
3. Occasionally, biopsy of lesions may be necessary to rule out leukoplakia (premalignant plaques).

Management

1. Topical antifungal medications such as nystatin suspension or clotrimazole troches are most often used.
2. Systemic treatment is indicated if topical agents fail or for esophageal cases with fluconazole, ketoconazole, or amphotericin B.
3. Topical oral rinses or preparations containing combinations of hydrocortisone, diphenhydramine, antifungals, or antibiotics may be used to enhance healing and to lessen discomfort.
4. Viscous lidocaine may be used topically to coat the oral mucosa before meals to lessen pain and enhance oral intake.
5. Oral prostheses may also be treated to avoid harboring and reintroducing infection.

Complications

1. Candidal infection throughout the GI tract.
2. Candidal sepsis in patients who are immunocompromised.

Nursing Assessment

1. Carefully examine oral cavity daily to monitor lesions as well as response to prescribed antifungal therapy.
2. Assess level of pain; administer analgesics, as prescribed; and monitor response to analgesics.
3. Assess nutritional status and effect of pain on oral intake. Monitor oral intake, nutritional and hydration status, weight loss/gain, signs of dehydration.
4. Teach patients that are prescribed inhaled steroid therapy for asthma/COPD to rinse mouth after each use to prevent oropharyngeal candidiasis.

Nursing Diagnoses

- Imbalanced Nutrition: Less Than Body Requirements related to oral discomfort.
- Deficient Knowledge related to antifungal therapy.

Nursing Interventions

Attaining Adequate Nutrition

1. Administer analgesics, as prescribed, 30 to 60 minutes before meals.
2. Provide soft foods, soothing liquids; avoid temperature extremes.
3. Provide gentle suctioning if pain becomes so severe that patient cannot handle secretions and provide intravenous (IV) fluids.

Ensuring Adequate Therapy

1. Administer antifungal agents, as prescribed. Observe the patient for proper use of topical preparation.
   a. Make sure that mouth is clean and free of food debris before administering drug.

b. For swish-and-swallow preparations, tell the patient to swish and hold in mouth for at least 5 minutes before swallowing.

c. For troches, have the patient suck until dissolved.

2. Observe for signs and symptoms of systemic drug adverse effects: nausea, vomiting, diarrhea. Renal, bone marrow, cardiovascular, hepatic, or neurologic toxicities may occur in patients receiving systemic therapy with underlying chronic disease states.

3. Explain the importance of continuing therapy for duration prescribed.

Patient Education and Health Maintenance

1. Instruct high-risk patients about daily oral examination and signs and symptoms to observe.

2. Teach the patient to avoid highly seasoned foods, extremes in temperature, alcoholic beverages, and smoking, all of which irritate the oral mucosa.

3. Encourage good oral hygiene.

4. May need to refrain from wearing dentures due to oral discomfort.

5. Encourage the patient on long-term systemic antifungal therapy to follow up for liver function test monitoring, as directed.

Evaluation: Expected Outcomes

- Adequate intake of liquids and soft foods as evidenced by stable body weight, signs of dehydration.
- Swishes oral suspension for 10 minutes before spitting or swallowing.

Herpes Simplex Infection (Type 1)

Also known as *cold sores* or *fever blisters*, herpes simplex virus (HSV; usually type 1) is commonly associated with lip and oral lesions 80% of the time. HSV-1 causes genital outbreaks in 20% of the cases.

Pathophysiology and Etiology

1. After a primary infection and the patient produces antibodies, the virus remains latent in the sensory ganglia.

2. Recurrent herpes labialis may by precipitated by sun exposure, fever, oral trauma, fatigue, emotional upset, hormonal changes, and other factors.

3. The spread of HSV-1 is through respiratory droplets or exposure to infected saliva via a break in the skin or mucous membranes.

4. HSV type 2 (and rarely HSV type 1) is associated with genital lesions and is sexually transmitted.

Clinical Manifestations

1. Prodromal period—tingling, soreness, burning in area where lesion will develop.

2. Small vesicles appear on erythematous, edematous base, frequently near the mucocutaneous junction of the lips and adjacent skin.

3. May also occur in oral mucosa, especially in immunocompromised persons.

4. Vesicles rupture, causing ulcerations.

5. Lesions heal spontaneously in 7 to 14 days.

Diagnosis and Management

1. No diagnostic tests are necessary but serologic testing may be done. The diagnoses of herpes simplex is made from viral culture from skin vesicles, serology, or monoclonal antibody testing.

2. Treatment may not be necessary if cases are mild and are usually short lived.

3. Comfort measures, such as mild oral or topical analgesics.

4. Good hygiene to prevent spread to self and others.

5. Antiviral agents are available to decrease the duration of symptoms.

6. Penciclovir 1% cream—FDA approved; applied every 2 hours while awake at earliest sign. If used within 1 hour of outbreak, will decrease duration of viral shedding.

7. Acyclovir 5% cream may be used on topical lesions. Oral or IV antivirals may also be used if clinically indicated.

Nursing Interventions and Patient Education

1. Advise adequate rest and nutrition and avoidance of identified triggers.

2. Advise that virus is transmitted through close contact, such as kissing and sharing food and cups, so avoid these from prodromal period until well healed.

3. Recommend good handwashing and hygiene.

4. Apthous ulcers or canker sores—not caused by HSV-1.

Temporomandibular Disorders

Temporomandibular disorders are conditions affecting the jaw joint that consist of one or more of the following:

1. Myofascial pain—pain in the muscles serving the jaw (temporalis, masseter, medial and lateral pterygoids), neck, and shoulder.

2. Internal derangement of the jaw joint (dislocated or displaced joint disk or injured condyle).

3. Degenerative joint disease (eg, arthritis).

Pathophysiology and Etiology

1. Causes include rheumatoid or osteoarthritis; scleroderma; ankylosing spondylitis; trauma; teeth clenching or bruxism (teeth grinding). Neoplasms and acute infections such as parotitis, dental infections, and peritonsillar abscesses cause referred ear pain and should be differentiated from temporomandibular disorders.

2. Any mental and physical stresses can induce or exacerbate symptoms.

3. Above factors result in inflammation and muscle spasm of TMJ.

Clinical Manifestations

1. Pain at the joint, temples, mandible, or masticatory muscles may worsen with jaw movement. Referred muscle spasm of the neck, trapezius, and sternocleidomastoid muscle causes discomfort.

2. Clicking or crepitus from opening and closing of the jaw or popping of the joint.

3. Limitation of movement, dislocation, or jaw locking.

4. May be associated with headaches, earaches, or tinnitus.

5. Change in the bite where the upper and lower teeth do not match in the normal comfortable way.

6. May experience deteriorating oral hygiene or halitosis from limited oral opening (trismus), making dental hygiene difficult.

7. May experience difficulty chewing due to limited jaw excursion, resulting in altered diet and weight loss.

8. Jaw clicking alone is common and requires no workup or intervention if asymptomatic.

Diagnostic Evaluation

1. Diagnosis can usually be achieved by history and physical examination without extensive testing. Provocative maneuvers performed on physical examination that reproduce pain with opening and closing of the jaw are generally suggestive of TMJ arthralgia.

2. Dental and TMJ x-rays may or may not be helpful.

3. Occlusal analysis evaluates for malocclusion of the jaw and teeth in a bite position.

4. CT scan and magnetic resonance imaging (MRI) are usually normal unless there is underlying degenerative changes, fracture, or neoplasm of jaw or cervical spine.

5. Arthrography (joint x-rays using dye).

6. Arthroscopy (endoscopic invasive joint examination).

Management

1. Initial management employs jaw rest (soft, no-chew diet for 2 weeks, plus avoiding extreme jaw movements, such as wide yawning and gum chewing).

2. Anti-inflammatory/analgesic medications such as ibuprofen.

3. Application of warm, moist heat or ice packs.

4. Muscle relaxants may be prescribed.

5. Therapeutic nightguard or splint—to realign malocclusion or joint disk and to optimize muscle relaxation.

6. Physical therapy for gentle stretching and relaxing exercises with or without ultrasound (deep-heat) therapy—to enhance analgesia and muscle relaxation and to promote local tissue metabolism.

7. Check that transcutaneous electrical nerve stimulation reduces muscle spasm of head, neck, and back and reduces pain.

8. In general, conservative reversible measures above are employed as long as possible before progressing to invasive/surgical management.

  a. Arthroscopy—investigational procedure to visualize joint, reposition disk, lyse adhesions, or debride joint.

    i. Reserved for conditions not improved by medical management.

    ii. Complications include cranial nerve (CN) VII damage with facial paralysis and paresis, perforation of the external auditory canal, piercing of the middle cranial fossa.

  b. Surgery—to remove the disk or reshape bony prominences.

9. Complications include malocclusion, CN VII damage, infection.

Nursing Interventions and Patient Education

1. Assess the character, frequency, location, and duration of pain. Evaluate what triggers and relieves the pain. Determine how effective previous treatments have been.

2. Explore the effect of the disorder on the patient's lifestyle, especially eating habits. Assist the patient to alter methods of oral hygiene and eating if severe trismus is present.

3. Instruct the patient on the indications, dosages, and adverse effects of analgesics and anti-inflammatory medications.

4. Teach the patient proper use of heat therapies. Cold applications may be preferred by some patients to reduce pain and spasm.

5. Encourage the patient to perform active mouth opening, protrusion, and lateral movement exercises of the jaw for 5 minutes, four to five times per day, as prescribed, to stretch muscles and reduce spasm.

6. Encourage the use of soft food and liquid supplements during times of acute pain exacerbated by eating. Advise reduction of foods that require excessive chewing, such as raw vegetables, tough meat, nuts. Discourage gum chewing.

7. Explore tension-reducing modalities with the patient, especially progressive muscle relaxation to reduce muscle tension and spasm.

8. Encourage follow-up with dentist, oral surgeon, ENT specialist, or other caregiver, as indicated.

9. Encourage proper use of the night guard or dental splint, including periodic appointments to assess fit.

10. May need MedicAlert bracelet and preoperative anesthesia consultation for elective surgeries if maximum jaw opening is less than 30 mm, limiting access for airway intubation.

Maxillofacial and Mandibular Fractures

Fractures of the maxillofacial bones or mandible may occur as the result of industrial, athletic, and vehicular accidents; violent acts; and falls.

Pathophysiology and Etiology

1. Maxillofacial fractures usually occur due to blow to the cheek or face.

2. Mandibular fractures frequently occur due to blow to the chin.

3. May be nondisplaced or displaced, usually closed, and includes soft tissue injury.

4. May also occur as part of planned surgical reconstruction for jaw problems.

5. Injuries sustained in altercations or motor vehicle accidents may be associated with alcohol intoxication or recreational drug use.

Clinical Manifestations

1. Malocclusion, asymmetry, abnormal mobility, crepitus (grating sound with movement), pain, or tenderness.
2. Tissue injury: swelling, ecchymosis, bleeding, pain.

Diagnostic Evaluation

1. X-rays (posteroanterior, oblique, occlusal, panorex)—to show fracture and possible displacement.
2. CT scan—to evaluate extent of complicated injuries.

Management

1. Maintenance of adequate respiratory functioning—may include oxygen support, endotracheal intubation, or tracheostomy. See Chapter 35, page 1197.
2. Control of bleeding—usually accomplished with direct pressure.
3. Reduction of the fracture—usually closed reduction.
4. Immobilization—depends on location, type, and severity of the fracture.
   a. Barton's bandage with a Kling or stockinette bandage.
   b. Interdental fixation with rubber bands or wiring.
   c. Intermaxillary fixation with rubber bands or wiring.
   d. Interosseous fixation with open reduction.
5. Maintenance of adequate nutritional intake with liquid or soft diet—to maintain immobilization of fracture site.
6. Pain control—to promote comfort.
7. Control of infection with antibiotics in the presence of positive cultures.

Complications

1. Airway obstruction, aspiration.
2. Hemorrhage, infection.
3. Disfigurement.
4. Extraocular muscle entrapment/orbital globe displacement with resultant visual disturbance.
5. Acute drug or alcohol withdrawal.

Nursing Assessment

1. Obtain description of injury and review chart and diagnostic tests for extent of injury.
2. Continually assess respiratory status.
3. Assess level of pain.
4. Assess visual acuity and extraocular movement.
5. Assess for tremors, delirium or hallucinations, anxiety, and seizure activity related to alcohol or drug withdrawal.

Nursing Diagnoses

- Risk for Aspiration related to immobilization of jaw.
- Imbalanced Nutrition: Less Than Body Requirements related to pain, injury, and immobilization.
- Acute Pain related to injury and surgical intervention.
- Disturbed Body Image related to disfigurement of injury or surgical repair.
- Risk for Injury related to complications of surgery.

Nursing Interventions

Preventing Aspiration

1. Maintain effective airway.
   a. Elevate head of bed 30 to 45 degrees or position leaning over a bedside stand to reduce edema and improve handling of secretions.
   b. Make sure suctioning equipment is readily accessible; teach patient oral and nasal suctioning; position on side or upright during suctioning.
   c. Administer anti-emetic, as prescribed, for nausea and vomiting to prevent aspiration.
   d. Make sure wire cutters or scissors are present for immediate removal of the wires or rubber bands if the airway becomes obstructed. (Vertical rubber bands or wires should be cut.)
   e. Make sure that a method for calling the nurse (call bell) is within easy access for the patient at all times in case of emergency.
2. Monitor blood pressure, pulse, respirations, and temperature to note early onset of infection or aspiration.

Maintaining Nutritional Status

1. Administer liquid diet, as prescribed; place straw against teeth or through any gaps in the teeth. Teeth may initially be sensitive to hot and cold.
2. Position in upright position before, during, and for 45 to 60 minutes after all feedings.
3. Evaluate ongoing nutritional and hydration status; weight; intake, output, and specific gravity; laboratory values—24-hour urea nitrogen, transferrin level, electrolytes, and albumin.
4. Advance to blenderized diet, as tolerated.
5. Make environment as pleasant as possible to enhance appetite—remove all sources of odor, decrease interruptions, position comfortably.

Increasing Comfort

1. Administer liquid or a suspension of analgesics, as prescribed—avoid opioids on an empty stomach, which may cause nausea and vomiting.
2. Administer diazepam as prescribed to reduce anxiety and control reflex muscle spasm.
3. Apply paraffin wax to the ends of wire fixation devices to decrease irritation to the gums and oral mucosa.
4. Apply petroleum jelly to the lips to decrease dryness and prevent cracking.

Strengthening Body Image

1. Provide firm reassurance regarding progress to reduce anxiety and allay fears.
2. Avoid unrealistic promises in relation to scars or disfigurement.
3. Allow the patient to choose the first time for looking in the mirror.
4. Provide privacy, as requested. The patient may be sensitive to appearance.

Preventing Complications

1. Provide mouth care every 2 hours while awake for the first several days, then four to six times per day.

2. Initially, provide mouth care with warm normal saline mouth swishes.

3. As diet is progressed, remove collected debris with a pressurized water stream cleaner and encourage the patient to brush teeth with a soft, child-size toothbrush.

4. Observe facial injuries for swelling, erythema, pain, or warmth to detect onset of infection.

5. Change facial dressings as needed to prevent soiling with secretions, food, or drainage, which may promote bacterial growth.

6. Provide alternative form of communication, such as magic slate or picture board, because maxillomandibular fixation limits articulating ability, making speech difficult to understand.

Patient Education and Health Maintenance

1. Encourage adequate nutrition—inform the patient and family that foods can be blenderized and thinned with juices or broths to a consistency that can be taken through a straw.

2. Explore with the patient options for maintaining proper oral care; encourage the patient to practice the options of choice.

3. Discuss the use of anti-emetic medications to prevent nausea and vomiting, stressing the complications this could cause.

4. Make sure the patient has wire cutters or scissors at all times and knows how to use them should airway obstruction occur.

5. Encourage follow-up health care visits, including counseling for alcohol or drug abuse.

Evaluation: Expected Outcomes

- No evidence of aspiration.
- Tolerates fluids through straw; maintains adequate body weight.
- Expresses relief of pain.
- Views self in mirror; notices improvement in appearance.
- No signs of infection; oral hygiene maintained.

PROBLEMS OF THE NOSE, THROAT, AND SINUSES

Rhinopathies

Evidence Base Distler, J. W. (2011). Environmental allergens: Diagnoses and management of Ig-E mediated disorders. *American Journal of Nurse Practitioners, 15*(9/10).

Rhinopathies are disorders of the nose that interrupt its normal functions of olfaction and warming, filtering, and humidifying inspired air. These include *allergic rhinitis, nonallergic rhinitis, vasomotor rhinitis,* and other conditions.

Pathophysiology and Etiology

1. Allergic rhinitis—immunoglobulin E (IgE)–mediated response causing release of vasoactive substances from mast cells (see page 1020).

2. Non-IgE-mediated allergy/sensitivity—exposure to irritants such as tobacco smoke, perfumes, soaps, hairsprays, air pollution, or certain foods may produce symptoms of nasal congestion, postnasal drip, or rhinorrhea but are not caused by inhalant allergy.

3. Nonallergic rhinitis includes infectious rhinitis, rhinitis medicamentosa, rhinitis of pregnancy, or vasomotor rhinitis.

   a. Infectious—viral (common cold), bacterial (purulent rhinitis).

   b. Drug-induced (rebound rhinitis; rhinitis medicamentosa)—caused by excessive use of topical nasal decongestants. These products include oxymetazoline and phenylephrine. Many systemic medications may induce nasal congestion and stuffiness and include specific beta blockers, antihypertensives, and antidepressants.

   c. Vasomotor rhinitis—consists of symptoms caused by autonomic instability with disruption of the normal balance of sympathetic and parasympathetic innervation. This produces nasal congestion, rhinorrhea, and postnasal drip. Symptoms may be manifested on exposure to cold weather or eating spicy, hot, or cold foods (gustatory rhinitis).

   d. Rhinitis of pregnancy—nasal congestion resulting from estrogen-mediated mucosal engorgement, especially in the last trimesters of pregnancy, may also occur with oral contraceptive use, postmenopausal estrogen therapy, and during the last portion of the menstrual cycle. Edema of the nasal mucosa and turbinate congestion occur.

   e. Nonallergic rhinitis with eosinophilia syndrome—patients have symptoms of rhinitis, negative allergy testing, but large number of eosinophils in nasal secretions. Treatment is similar to those with vasomotor rhinitis.

Manifestations of Allergic Rhinitis

1. Hypersecretion—wet, running/dripping nose or postnasal drip.

2. Eyes—edema of the conjunctivae, tearing and itching of the eyes, increase in vascularity, fine allergic shiners or dark staining under eyes.

3. Nasal cavity—congestion, pressure, or stuffiness (see Figure 17-2). Chronic nasal crusting and erythema around outer nares, turbinates are often swollen, edematous with pale or bluish hue. Allergic salute often seen in children caused by upward lifting of the tip of the nose with the hand.

4. Oral cavity—chronic mouth breathing, enlarged lymph tissue in the oropharynx, prominent vascularity or cobblestoning in posterior pharynx.

Management

1. Treatment of underlying cause.

   a. Allergy—antihistamines (see Chapter 28).

   b. Nonallergic rhinitis—treatment modalities can include avoidance if caused by chemical, food, or other irritants.

2. Topical decongestants (for short-term use); systemic decongestants—topical or systemic decongestants may be used for short-term usage only, no more than 2 to 3 days, in patients with various forms of nonallergic rhinitis.

A. Rhinitis

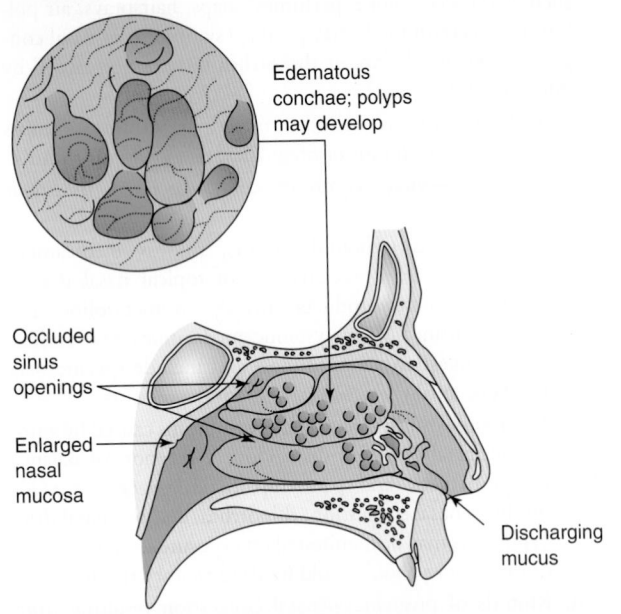

Edematous conchae; polyps may develop

Occluded sinus openings

Enlarged nasal mucosa

Discharging mucus

B. Sinusitis

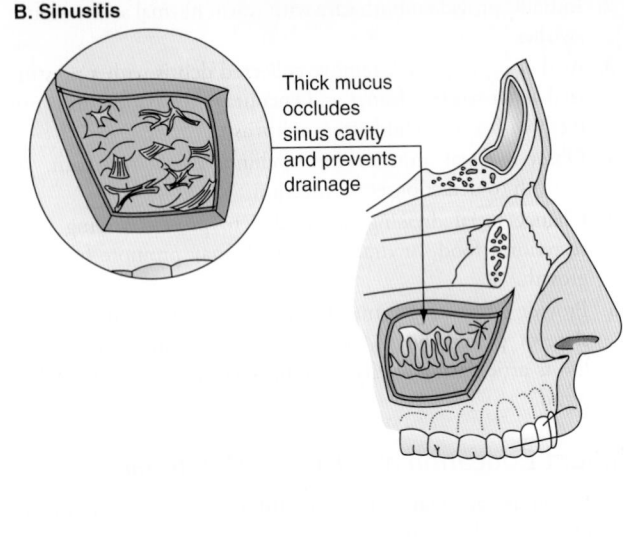

Thick mucus occludes sinus cavity and prevents drainage

Figure 17-2. Rhinitis and sinusitis. (A) The mucous membranes lining the nasal passages become inflamed, congested, and edematous, blocking sinus openings and obstructing air passage. **(B)** The sinus cavity mucous membranes are also marked by inflammation and congestion, with thickened mucous secretions filling the sinus cavities and further occluding the openings.

 DRUG ALERT Severe rebound nasal obstruction may occur with overuse of topical decongestants. Stress the importance of only using for 2 to 3 days, as directed.

3. Intranasal corticosteroids—used in the treatment of allergic and nonallergic rhinitis because of their antiinflammatory effects.
4. Vasomotor rhinitis—treated with ipratropium, which blocks vagally mediated reflexes that cause congestion.

Nursing Interventions and Patient Education

1. Avoid irritating inhalants, especially smoke, aerosols, noxious fumes.
2. Do not overuse topical nasal sprays and drops.
3. Advise about adverse effect of systemic decongestants is stimulation of sympathetic nervous system—insomnia, nervousness, palpitations.
4. Be aware that intranasal corticosteroids do not cause significant systemic absorption in usual doses, but occasionally may cause nasal fungal infections and in rare cases cause nasal septal perforation and epistaxis.
5. Educate patients about correct administration technique for nasal sprays, particularly to direct the tip of the spray bottle away from the septum, toward the outward corner of the eye or toward the ear.

Epistaxis

Epistaxis refers to nosebleed or hemorrhage from the nose. It most commonly originates in the anterior portion of the nasal cavity.

Pathophysiology and Etiology

1. Local causes:
   a. Dryness leading to crust formation—bleeding occurs with removal of crusts by nose picking, rubbing, or blowing.
   b. Trauma—direct blows.
2. Systemic causes are less common—hypertension, arteriosclerosis, renal disease, bleeding disorders. Episodic epistaxis is mostly commonly seen with patients on antiplatelet, anticoagulant, and antithrombolytic agents. Osler-Weber-Rendu syndrome or hereditary hemorrhagia telangiectasia, hemophilia, von Willebrand disease, and liver disease are examples of bleeding disorders that can predispose patients to frequent episodes of epistaxis.
3. Most nosebleeds are anterior; posterior bleeds are more difficult to control.

Diagnostic Evaluation

1. Inspection with nasal speculum to determine site of bleeding or nasal endoscopy by otolaryngologist. Important to determine which side bled first.
2. Laboratory evaluation to exclude blood dyscrasias and coagulopathy.

Management

Depends on severity and source of bleeding in nasal cavity.

1. The patient is placed in an upright posture, leaning forward to reduce venous pressure, and instructed to breathe gently through the mouth to prevent swallowing of blood. The patient is asked to sit on a 90-degree angle, while the nasal ala, or the

soft part of the anterior nose, is pinched and pressure is applied for 10 to 15 minutes, or as needed to control the bleeding.

2. With anterior bleeds, the patient is instructed to compress the soft part of nose with index finger and thumb for 5 to 10 minutes to maintain pressure on the nasal septum.

3. A cotton pledget soaked with a vasoconstricting agent may be inserted into each nostril and pressure is applied if bleeding is not controlled. After 5 to 10 minutes, the cotton is removed and the site of bleeding is identified. Oxymetazoline, in combination with a topical anesthetic agent such as lidocaine, may be sprayed directly into the nasal cavity or applied on pledgets or cotton balls. Suction may be used to evacuate the bloody contents of the nasal cavity to visualize the source of bleeding.

4. The blood vessel may be cauterized with use of silver nitrate sticks or with electrocautery.

5. If bleeding continues despite use of pressure or cautery, anterior or posterior packing may be placed into the nasal cavity or nasopharynx. Packing is usually kept in for 72 hours or more. Balloon tamponade may be required to apply pressure over a larger area.

 NURSING ALERT Monitor the patient for a vasovagal episode during insertion and with removal of nasal packing. This is best prevented with reclining the patient back when symptoms first occur.

6. Surgical ligation of vessels may be required if bleeding is unable to be controlled with above measures.

Complications

1. Rhinitis, maxillary and frontal sinusitis.
2. Orthostatic hyptension from sudden blood loss.

Nursing Interventions and Patient Education

1. Monitor vital signs and assist with control of bleeding. Assess for changes in blood pressure and pulse indicative of hypovolemia.

2. Be aware that packing is uncomfortable and painful and may be in place for 48 to 72 hours. Analgesics may be prescribed but generally acetylsalicylic acid (ASA) should be avoided.

3. Nosebleed precautions and postprocedure instructions should be given to the patient. Instructions for holding specific antiplatelet and anticoagulant medications will be coordinated in conjunction with the patients' clinical history. Patient should be advised to avoid sneezing with mouth closed, blowing nose, removing the packing, and avoiding any strenuous activity.

4. Monitor patient with posterior packing for hypoxia (from aspiration of blood, sedation, and preexisting pulmonary dysfunction). Patients who require posterior balloon packing are admitted for observation and monitoring. These patients are at risk for soft palate necrosis and airway obstruction. If coagulopathies are found on bloodwork, these are corrected while the patient is hospitalized. Monitor PT, INR and PTT, if ordered.

5. Instruct the patient as follows for self-management of minor bleeding episodes:
   a. Sit up and lean forward while compressing the soft part (lower half) of nose between index finger and thumb.

   b. If bleeding continues, moisten a small piece of cotton with vasoconstricting nose drops (phenylephrine or oxymetazoline) and place inside nose.
   c. Apply pressure to the bleeding site 5 to 10 minutes.

6. Instruct the patient to avoid blowing or picking nose after a nosebleed.

7. Advise patients prone to nosebleeds to:
   a. Apply a lubricant to nasal septum twice daily to reduce dryness. Nasal saline spray may also be advised a few days after nasal cautery is performed and on a regular basis if patient has recurrent episodes.
   b. A bedside humidifier is recommended, especially if the environmental air is dry.
   c. If the patient uses chronic oxygen therapy or CPAP, a humidifier may be recommended on the oxygen delivery or CPAP delivery system.

Sinusitis

Rhinosinusitis is defined as a symptomatic inflammation of the sinuses and nasal cavity. It may be precipitated by congestion from viral upper respiratory infection and/or nasal allergy. A patient with chronic allergic disease may be prone to recurrent episodes of sinusitis or chronic rhinosinusitis. Obstruction of the sinus ostia (resulting from mucosal swelling and/or mechanical obstruction) leads to retention of secretions and is the usual precursor to sinusitis.

Rhinosinusitis is classified by duration as acute (less than 4 weeks), subacute (4 to 12 weeks), or chronic (more than 12 weeks). Acute rhinosinusitis can be classified as bacterial or viral.

Clinical Manifestations

Acute Sinusitis

1. Defined as up to 4 weeks of purulent, nonclear nasal drainage with nasal congestion and/or facial pain/pressure/fullness (see Figure 17-3). There may be both symptoms of nasal congestion and facial pain, and symptoms are present for 10 days or more. There may be chronic exacerbations of symptoms within the 4 weeks.

2. Nasal congestion or obstruction is defined as subjective symptoms of difficulty breathing through nose and/or red and edematous nasal mucosa visualized on physical examination.

3. Anosmia (lack of smell) may be reported.

4. Other symptoms that may be present include fever, cough, ear pressure, maxillary dental pain, and fatigue.

5. Viral rhinosinusitis is differentiated from bacterial by duration—symptoms for 10 days or less without worsening symptoms. Bacterial rhinosinusitis manifests for 10 days with worsening symptoms.

Chronic Rhinosinusitis

1. Mucopurulent nasal drainage, nasal obstruction, facial pain/pressure/fullness and/or decreased sense of smell. May also have malaise and ear pain or pressure and cough. Patients may have recurrent episodes or continued symptoms for 12 weeks or more.

2. Symptoms may or may not be present, but are nondiagnostic of chronic rhinosinusitis.

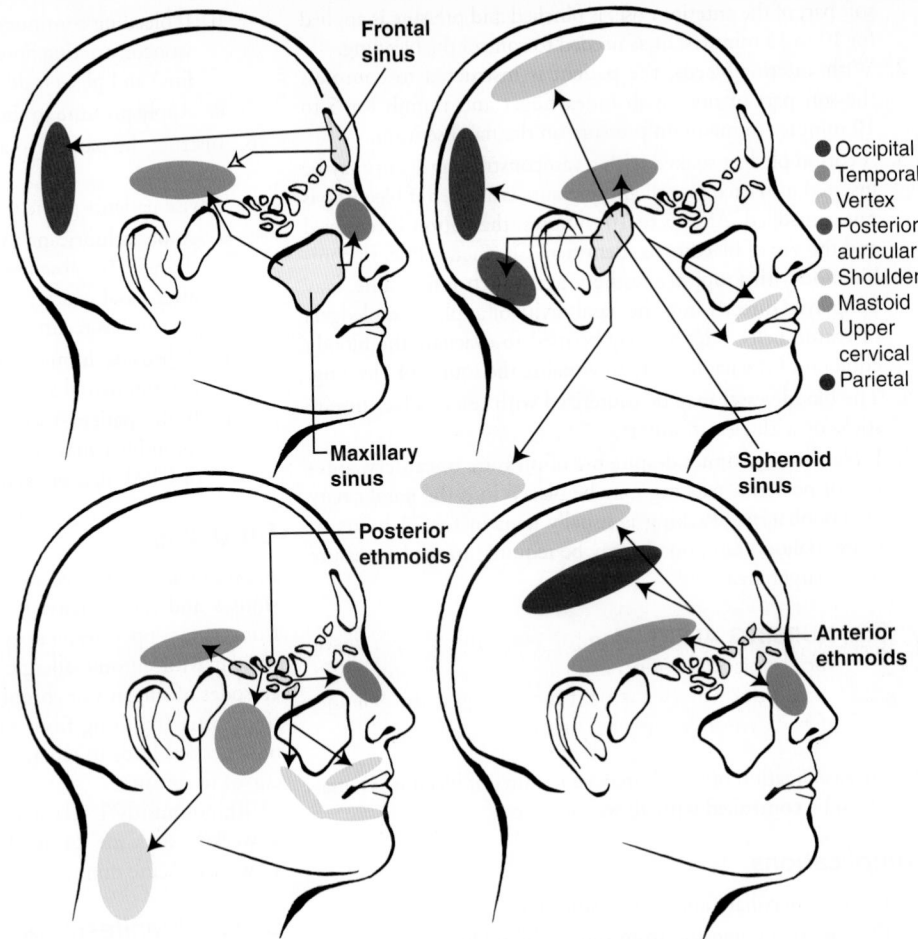

Figure 17-3. Referred pain from the paranasal sinuses.

Diagnostic Evaluation

1. Sinus plain film consisting of Caldwell, Water's, and lateral views may be obtained but not routinely recommended for acute, isolated, or noncomplicated cases. X-rays may reveal air-fluid level, mucosal thickening, or opacification of one or more sinus cavities.
2. CT scanning recommended when complication is suspected or in patients with chronic sinus disease.
3. Nasal endoscopy, performed by an ENT specialist, is used to evaluate the nasal and sinus cavity and to obtain cultures of material for the purpose of directing appropriate antibiotic therapy.
4. CT with contrast or MRI with gadolinium may be obtained if cranial extension suspected.

Management

1. Topical decongestant spray or drops or systemic decongestants may be used to treat the nasal congestion associated with rhinosinusitis. Topical therapy should be limited to no more than 3 successive days of use as increased use beyond 3 days may cause rebound nasal congestion (rhinitis medicamentosa).
2. Topical nasal corticosteroids are frequently used in chronic sinusitis and may be used in acute cases. Nasal corticosteroids have been shown to decrease severity of symptoms when used with appropriate antibiotic therapy.
3. Antibiotics—amoxicillin is the initial drug of choice in adults with acute rhinosinusitis. For penicillin-allergic patients, sulfamethoxazoletrimethoprim or macrolide antibiotics may also be used as first-line therapy. The most common organisms identified in patients with acute bacterial rhinosinusitis are *Streptococcus pneumoniae*, *Haemonopilus influenzae*, and *Moraxella catarrhalis*. Other less common organisms include *Staphloccocus ureas* and anaerobes.
4. Usually 10- to 14-day course for acute sinusitis; azithromycin may be prescribed for 3 to 5 days.
5. Prolonged therapy for chronic sinusitis (up to several months).
6. Analgesics—pain may be significant.
7. Warm compresses; cool vapor humidity for comfort and to promote drainage; nasal saline irrigation.
8. Surgical interventions (for chronic sinusitis when conservative treatment is unsuccessful).
   a. Endoscopic sinus surgery—endoscopic removal of diseased tissue from affected sinus; used to treat chronic sinusitis of maxillary, ethmoid, and frontal sinuses.

b. Nasal antrostomy (nasal-antral window)—surgical placement of an opening under inferior turbinate to provide aeration of the antrum and to permit exit for purulent materials.

c. For nursing care, see page 605.

Complications

1. Extension of infection to the orbital contents and eyelids.

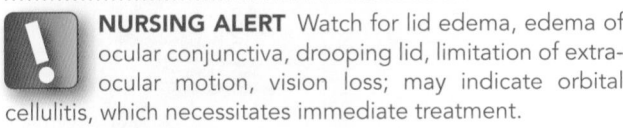 **NURSING ALERT** Watch for lid edema, edema of ocular conjunctiva, drooping lid, limitation of extraocular motion, vision loss; may indicate orbital cellulitis, which necessitates immediate treatment.

2. Bone infection (osteomyelitis) may spread by direct extension or through blood vessels. Frontal bone commonly affected.

3. CNS complications include meningitis, subdural and epidural purulent drainage, brain abscess, cavernous sinus thrombosis (acute thrombophlebitis originating from an infection in an area having venous drainage to cavernous sinus).

Nursing Interventions and Patient Education

1. Teach the patient signs and symptoms of acute, bacterial rhinosinusitis versus signs and symptoms of rhinitis. Educate the patient in regard to symptoms that prompt medical attention.

2. Advise the patients about adverse reactions of antibiotic therapy including side effects, drug interactions, and symptoms that prompt medical attention.

3. Stress the importance of complying with antibiotic therapy for complete duration and following up for recurrence.

4. Teach the patient with recurrent sinusitis how to irrigate nasal passages with saline to remove crusted mucus near the sinus openings and enhance drainage. (See Patient Education Guidelines 17-1, page 606.)

Pharyngitis

Pharyngitis is an inflammation of the pharynx, including palate, tonsils, and posterior wall of the pharynx, most commonly caused by acute infection, usually transmitted through respiratory secretions. Streptococcal pharyngitis (*strep throat*) and rhinoviruses (the common cold) are frequent causes. Pharyngitis is diagnosed in 11 million emergency rooms and outpatient office visits per year.

Pathophysiology and Etiology

1. Acute bacterial pharyngitis is usually caused by group A betahemolytic streptococci.

2. Other bacterial causes include *Haemophilusinfluenzae, Moraxella catarrhalis, Corynebacteriumdiphtheriae* (diphtheria), *Neisseria gonorrhoeae* (gonorrhea), and other groups of streptococcus. Transmission of *N. gonorrhoeae* is through oral contact with genital secretions; it is a sexually transmitted disease.

3. Viral pharyngitis is common and causes include rhinovirus, adenovirus, parainfluenza virus, coxsackievirus, coronavirus, and others.

4. More chronic causes are irritation from postnasal drip of allergic rhinitis and chronic sinusitis, chemical irritation, and systemic diseases.

Clinical Manifestations

1. For acute bacterial infections, abrupt onset of sore throat and fever, usually above 100.4° F (38.0° C), and exposure to *Streptococcus* within the preceding 2 weeks is suggestive of streptococcal pharyngitis.
   a. Throat pain is aggravated by swallowing.
   b. Pharynx appears reddened with edema of uvula; tonsils enlarged and reddened; pharynx and tonsils may be covered with exudate (see Figure 17-4).
   c. Palatal petechiae and a scarlatiniform rash are highly specfic but uncommonly seen.

2. Varying degrees of sore throat, nasal congestion, fatigue, and fever with other bacterial and viral causes.

3. Cough, conjunctivitis, and diarrhea are common with viral causes.

4. Swollen, palpable, and tender cervical lymph nodes in most cases. Anterior cervical lymph node swelling and enlargement is common.

Diagnostic Evaluation

1. Throat culture or rapid streptococcal antigen detection test to rule out streptococci. Rapid strep tests provide results within 5 minutes; false-negative rate is higher than with culture method.

2. Gonococcal antigen detection test to rule out gonococcal pharyngitis, if genital gonococcal infection or positive sexual contact is suspected.

3. Viral testing is not practical and viral causes are self-limiting.

Management

1. For streptococcal pharyngitis, penicillin V 250 mg four times a day orally for 10 days or penicillin G benzathine in a single intramuscular (I.M.) dose of 2.4 million units appears to shorten duration of symptoms and prevents rheumatic fever.

2. Erythromycin for patient who is allergic to penicillin.

3. Other penicillins, macrolides, and cephalosporins are also used.

Complications

1. Acute rheumatic fever.
2. Peritonsillar abscess/cellulitis.
3. Acute glomerulonephritis.
4. Scarlet fever.
5. Sinusitis, otitis media, mastoiditis.

 NURSING ALERT Acute rheumatic fever, a complication of streptococcal pharyngitis, can be prevented if patient is treated adequately with penicillin and, possibly, another antibiotic. Unfortunately, there is no evidence that antibiotic therapy will prevent acute glomerulonephritis.

Nursing Interventions and Patient Education

1. Advise the patient to have any sore throat with fever evaluated, especially in the absence of cold symptoms.

2. Encourage compliance with full course of antibiotic therapy, despite feeling better in several days, to prevent complications.

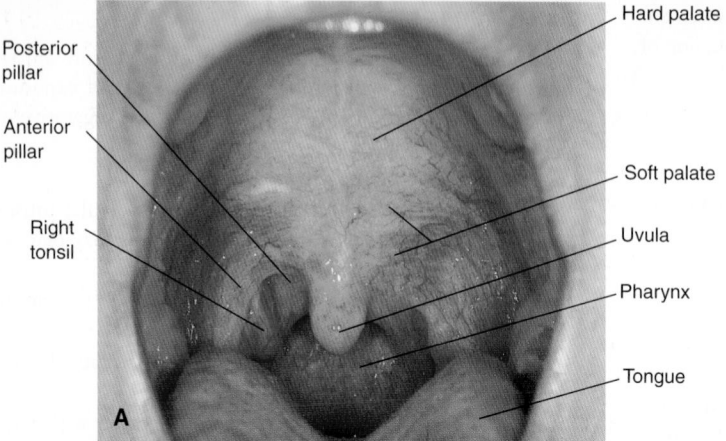

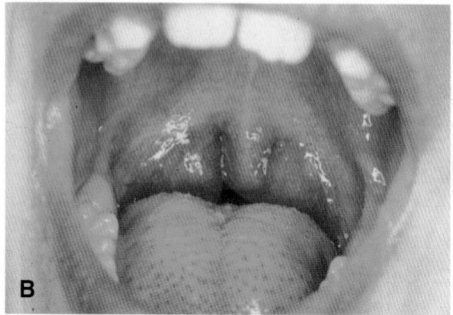

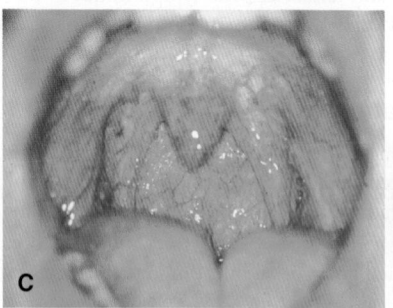

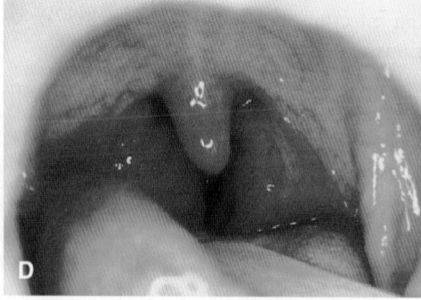

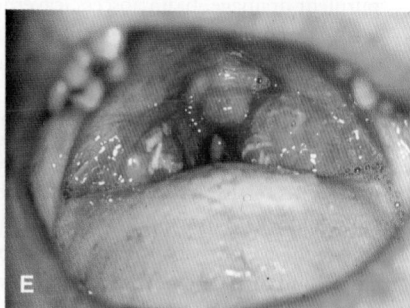

Figure 17-4. Assessment of pharyngitis. (A) Normal throat. **(B)** Normal large tonsils without redness. **(C)** Mild redness without exudate. **(D)** Intense redness without exudate. **(E)** Redness with exudate on tonsils (probably indicates group A streptococcal infection).

3. Advise lukewarm saline gargles and use of antipyretic/analgesics, as directed, to promote comfort.
4. Encourage bed rest with increased fluid intake during fever.

EAR DISORDERS

Hearing Loss

Hearing loss ranks high as a health disability. There are multiple causes, and the range of hearing loss varies from mild hearing loss to profound hearing loss with complete inability to understand the spoken word. Two major types of hearing loss are conductive and sensorineural. There are 20 million Americans with hearing loss.

Classification of Hearing Loss

1. Conductive loss—any condition interfering with sound transmission through the external auditory canal or transmission of tympanic membrane vibrations through the middle ear ossicles to the inner ear.
2. Sensorineural (perceptive) loss—hearing loss due to disease of the inner ear or nerve pathways; sensitivity to and discrimination of sounds are impaired. Hearing aids usually are helpful.
3. Combined or mixed hearing loss—combination of the above.
4. Sudden sensioneural hearing loss—30-decibel hearing loss in one or both ears in three contiguous frequencies that

occurs within 3 days or less. It can be caused by an acute viral infection or vascular event.

See Table 17-2 for tuning fork tests that assist in differentiating conductive from sensorineural hearing loss.

Presbycusis

A progressive, bilaterally perceptive hearing loss of older adults, usually involving high frequencies, that occurs with the aging process.

1. An audiogram should be obtained by a professional audiologist to evaluate the degree of hearing loss, word discrimination

Table 17-2	Tuning Fork Tests	
EAR CONDITION	**WEBER'S TEST**	**RINNE TEST**
Normal, no hearing loss	No shifting of sounds laterally	Sound perceived longer by *air* conduction
Conductive loss	Shifting of sounds to poorer ear	Sound perceived as long or longer by *bone* conduction
Sensorineural loss	Shifting of sounds to better ear	Sound perceived longer by *air* conduction

ability, and identification of any hearing loss suggestive of a retrocochlear etiology.

2. The patient should be counseled by an otolaryngologist in collaboration with an audiologist, who can make recommendations for hearing amplification.

3. Helpful aids should be considered, such as a telephone amplifier, radio and television earphone attachments, and a buzzer instead of a doorbell.

4. Understanding and help from family members are important.

Otosclerosis

Otosclerosis is defined as an abnormal growth of bone of the middle ear that prevents the ossicles, or middle ear bones, from working properly and impeding movement of the stapes. Causes chronic and progressive hearing loss, either in one ear or both.

The cause is unknown, but there is a familial tendency, and women are affected more often than men.

Clinical Manifestations

1. Young adults present with a history of slow, progressive hearing loss of soft-spoken tones, with no signs of middle ear infection. In women of childbearing age, often progresses during pregnancy.

2. Audiometry findings substantiate conductive or mixed hearing loss.

Management

1. No known medical treatment exists for this form of deafness, but amplification with a hearing aid may be helpful.

2. Surgery—stapedotomy or stapedectomy.

   a. The removal of otosclerotic lesions at the footplate of stapes or complete removal of the stapes and the creation of a tissue implant with prosthesis to maintain suitable conduction.

   b. To perform such delicate surgery, an otologic binocular microscope is used.

Cochlear Implant

A *cochlear implant* is a device that emits auditory signals for profoundly deaf people (see Figure 17-5). The single-electrode system bypasses the damaged cochlear system and stimulates the remaining auditory nerve fibers. This results in the perception of sound.

Description

1. Purpose is for the patient to detect louder environmental sounds, but will not restore normal hearing. Many recipients continue to rely on lip reading to make sense of the sound input being received. Some patients are able to rely entirely on hearing with their cochlear implant device and may even be able to use the telephone.

2. The microphone and sound processor are positioned externally; the electrode array is implanted internally and inserts into the cochlea. The receiver-stimulator is inserted into a bony well created in the mastoid behind the ear.

3. Electrical stimuli converted from the sound processor are sent inside the body to the implanted electrode. These electrical signals stimulate the auditory nerve fibers, which are interpreted by the brain.

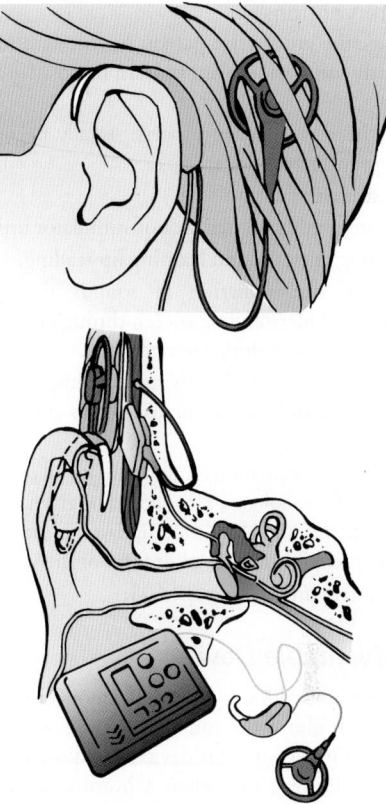

Figure 17-5. Nucleus 24 cochlear implant system. Sounds are picked up by the small, directional microphone located in the headset at the ear. A thin cord carries the sound from the microphone to the speech processor, a powerful miniaturized computer. The speech processor filters, analyzes, and digitizes the sound into coded signals that are sent from the speech processor to the transmitting coil. The transmitting coil sends the coded signals as FM radio signals to the cochlear implant under the skin. The cochlear implant delivers the appropriate electrical energy to the array of electrodes, which have been inserted into the cochlea. The electrodes along the array stimulate the remaining auditory nerve fibers in the cochlea. The resulting electrical sound information is sent through the auditory system to the brain for interpretation. The entire process takes microseconds.

4. Success rate is highly variable, which has made the cochlear implant controversial. About 30,000 cochlear implants have been inserted worldwide.

Patient Criteria

There are no standardized criteria for patient selection. Some data that are considered include:

1. Severe to profound sensorineural hearing loss in both ears.

2. Little to no benefit with hearing aids.

3. No medical contraindications.

4. Physically healthy adult or child as young as age 8 months.

5. No evidence of brain impairment that would prevent useful processing of the information delivered. Some would argue that implantation in those with mental impairment would still allow more awareness of environmental sounds, making them safer.

6. Reasonable expectations and optimism; motivation must be present.

Nursing Interventions

1. Encourage the prospective patient to visit with someone who is currently using an implant to learn its positive and negative results.
2. Explain the rehabilitation process; usually begins 2 months after surgery. Included are:
   a. Adjustment of controls.
   b. Operation and maintenance of stimulator unit.
   c. Listening critically and learning lip reading.
   d. Learning discrimination of sounds through cochlear implant. Understanding speech through cochlear implant is not possible with this device alone.
   e. Many people trained with such an implant can lip read more easily and can distinguish voices and environmental sounds.
3. Pneumococcal vaccination is important for all cochlear implant candidates and recipients. This should be given at least 2 weeks prior to surgery and should be updated as the child reaches age 2 and is eligible for the adult form of the vaccine.
4. For care after surgery, see page 608.

Other Implantable Devices

1. Osseointegrated devices transmit sound from an external device, worn above the ear, through the skin and into the skull to the inner ear. This device is indicated in those with conductive hearing loss when a hearing aid is contraindicated such as chronic ear infection, those with aural atresia or microtia without the normal ear canal needed to carry sound to the middle ear, and those with single-sided deafness.
2. Semi-implantable hearing aids are being tested for conductive and mixed hearing loss.

Maximizing Communication with the Person Who is Hearing Impaired

When hearing loss is permanent or not amenable to medical or surgical intervention, aural rehabilitation is necessary for the patient to maintain communication and prevent isolation. Aural rehabilitation is a multifaceted process that includes auditory training (listening skills), speech reading (formerly called lip reading), and the use of hearing aids. Nurses strive to maintain effective communication with patients. These suggestions promote better communication.

When the Person Is Hearing Impaired and Able to Lip-Read

1. Face the person as directly as possible when speaking.
2. Place yourself in good light so the person can see your mouth.
3. Do not chew, smoke, or have anything in your mouth when speaking.
4. Speak slowly and enunciate distinctly.
5. Provide contextual clues that will assist the person in following your speech. For example, point to a tray if you are talking about the food on it.
6. To verify that patient understands your message, write it for him or her to read (ie, if you doubt that patient is understanding you).

When the Person is Hearing Impaired and Difficult to Understand

1. Pay attention when the person speaks; facial and physical gestures may help you understand what person is saying.
2. Exchange conversation with person when it is possible to anticipate replies. This is particularly helpful in your initial contact with person and may help you become familiar with speech peculiarities.
3. Anticipate context of speech to assist in interpreting what the person is saying.
4. If unable to understand person, resort to writing or include in your conversation someone who does understand; request that person repeat that which is not understood.

Organizations That Help the Hearing Impaired

- Alexander Graham Bell Association for the Deaf (*www.agbell.org*)
- American Speech-Language-Hearing Association (*www.asha.org*)
- National Association of the Deaf (*www.nad.org*)

Community and Home Care Considerations

1. Prevention of hearing loss should be discussed in the community—in schools, the workplace, and community gatherings.
2. Preventable hearing loss includes:
   a. Noise-induced hearing loss—long periods of exposure to loud noise from machinery or engines.
   b. Acoustic trauma—single exposure to intense noise such as an explosion or amplified music.
3. Prevention involves avoidance of both types of noise, generally noise above 85 or 90 decibels.
4. Teach people to be aware of their surroundings and avoid noisy places or turn off sources of noise in the environment whenever possible.
5. Teach proper use of ear protection including earplugs and headsets both in the workplace and elsewhere.
6. Advise people that the Occupational Safety and Health Administration requires ear protection when noise exposure is above the legal limits, so workers have a right to protective equipment.

Otitis Externa

 Evidence Base Baugher, K. M, Somers Hemme, T., Harkshaw, M., et al. (2011). MRSA otorrhea: A case series and review of the literature. *Ear, Nose, and Throat Journal, 90*(2), 60–79.

Otitis externa is an inflammation/infection of the external ear, pinna, and/or ear canal.

Pathophysiology and Etiology

1. Bacterial causes: Most common causes are *Pseudomonas aeruginosa*, *Proteus mirabilis*, and *Staphylococcus aureus*.
2. May be caused by fungal source: *Aspergillus niger*, *Candida albicans*.

3. Commonly caused by chronic dermatologic conditions, such as seborrhea, psoriasis, eczema, or contact dermatitis. Allergic reaction to topical otic such as neomycin/polymixin preparations may also occur in some patients.
4. Trauma to the ear canal, usually from cleaning the canal.
5. Stagnant water in ear canal after swimming or from water irrigation for cerumen removal are common etiologies.
6. Necrotizing malignant otitis externa is a serious infection into deeper tissue adjacent to the ear canal, including cellulitis and osteomyelitis. It is usually caused by *Pseudomonas* and may be seen in diabetic patients, older patients, debilitated patients, or patients with compromised immune systems.
7. Methicillin-resistant Staphylococcus aureus otorrhea has been a common cause of chronic ear drainage. Treatment is based on culture and sensitivity of the ear drainage.

Clinical Manifestations

1. Otalgia or ear pain, increased by manipulation of auricle or tragus; hearing loss and aural fullness. Itching may also be present.
2. Periauricular lymphadenopathy.
3. Foul-smelling white to purulent drainage otorrhea. Drainage may be thick and purulent or thin and white, depending on the causative organism.
4. Red, swollen ear canal with discharge on otoscopic examination; ear canal can be swollen shut.

Management

1. Instillation of isopropyl alcohol drops (dries moisture), acetic acid solution (restores acidity), or topical antibiotics (curbs infection). A combination of these treatments may be used depending on the cause. Antifungal agents, either in ointment, powder, or drop form, may be used.
   a. Prophylactic use of alcohol drops or acetic acid solution by swimmers or those prone to otitis externa may be indicated.
   b. Antibiotic drops include combination products containing polymyxin, neomycin, and hydrocortisone; ciprofloxacin; and ofloxacin. Tobramycin preparations may be used with methicillin-resistant infections (confirmed by culture and sensitivity).
   c. A 10-day course of treatment is usually indicated.
   d. Parenteral antibiotics will be used for necrotizing otitis externa.

2. If canal is swollen and tender, an antibiotic solution containing a corticosteroid is chosen to reduce inflammation and swelling. If acute inflammation and closure of the ear canal prevent drops from saturating canal, a wick may need to be inserted by an ENT specialist so drops will gain access to walls of entire ear canal.
3. Burow's solution (aluminum acetate solution) or topical corticosteroid cream or lotion may be used in otitis externa caused by dermatitis.
4. Fungal infections may be treated with a topical antifungal such as nystatin or ketoconazole.
5. In chronic otitis externa, debris from ear canal may need to be removed through suction after pain and swelling have subsided. Avoid water irrigation, as this promotes bacterial and fungal growth from stagnant moisture.
6. Warm compresses and analgesics may be needed.

Nursing Interventions and Patient Education

1. Demonstrate proper application of eardrops. See Patient Education Guidelines 17-2.
2. Advise the patient that otitis externa can be prevented or minimized by thoroughly drying the ear canal after coming into contact with water or moist environment.
3. Teach the patient to use prophylactic eardrops after swimming to assist in preventing swimmer's ear, as directed by health care provider.
4. Advise the use of properly fitting earplugs for recurrent cases.
5. Teach proper ear hygiene: clean auricle and outer canal with washcloth only; do not insert anything smaller than finger wrapped in washcloth in ear canal. Avoid inserting cotton swabs or sharp objects into ear canal because:
   a. Cerumen may be forced against the tympanic membrane, causing impaction.
   b. The canal lining may be abraded, making it more susceptible to infection.
   c. The tympanic membrane may be injured.

Impacted Cerumen and Foreign Bodies

Cerumen impaction is defined as accumulation of cerumen, or "ear wax," that causes symptoms of ear pain, fullness, or hearing loss and/or prevents visualization of the tympanic membrane.

PATIENT EDUCATION GUIDELINES 17-2

Instilling Ear Drops

1. Hold the medication bottle between your hands for 1–2 minutes to warm drops before administering.
2. Lie on side with affected ear facing upward. Shake drops. Pull ear up and back, and then instill drops by sqeezing the bulb the ordered number of times.
3. Pump tragus by pushing on the flap of skin protecting the ear canal five to six times to ensure drops reach eardrum.
4. Remain on side for 1–2 minutes. Repeat, if necessary, on opposite ear.

Etiology and Clinical Manifestations

1. Cerumen is a mixture of glandular secretions from the ear canal mixed with squamous epithelium. Cerumen builds up over a period of time, causing a decrease in hearing acuity and a feeling that the ear is plugged.
   a. May be underlying seborrhea or other dermatologic condition that causes flaking of skin that mixes with cerumen and becomes obstructive.
   b. Cerumen may be pushed back into external canal and cover tympanic membrane by action of cotton swab.
2. Insect may fly or crawl into ear, causing initial low rumbling sound; later, feeling that ear is plugged and decreased hearing acuity. Foreign bodies may be placed into the ear canal, especially by children, and include food particles, small objects, or tips of cotton swabs.
3. The patient often seeks treatment for symptoms related to the foreign body or impacted cerumen.

Management

1. Accumulated cerumen does not have to be removed unless it causes symptoms, interferes with examination of the ear drum, or interferes with hearing. May be removed by currette or by irrigation (see Figure 17-6). See also Procedure Guidelines 17-1.
2. Foreign bodies may be removed by instrumentation or irrigation by health care provider.
   a. Insects—treat by instilling oil drops to smother insect, which then can be removed with ear spatula or irrigation.
   b. Vegetable foreign bodies (eg, peas)—irrigation is contraindicated because vegetable matter absorbs water, which would further wedge it in the canal.
   c. Only a skilled person should attempt to remove foreign body to prevent tympanic membrane perforation and trauma to canal.
   d. General anesthesia may be required to remove foreign bodies from young children, if they are unable to cooperate.

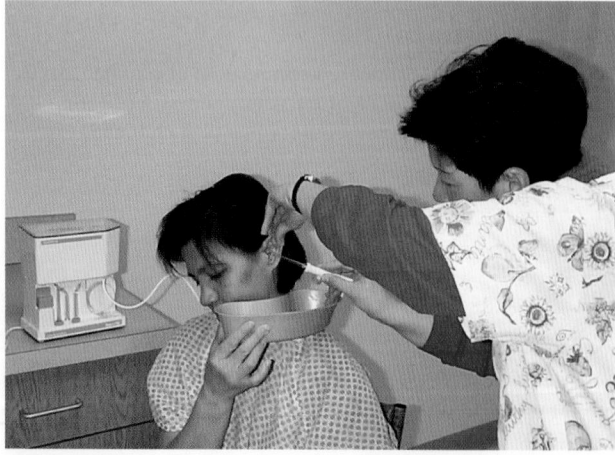

Figure 17-6. Using a dental irrigation device to irrigate the external auditory cavity.

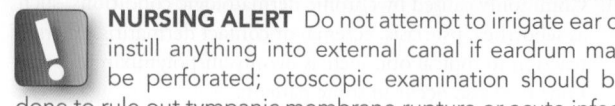

NURSING ALERT Do not attempt to irrigate ear or instill anything into external canal if eardrum may be perforated; otoscopic examination should be done to rule out tympanic membrane rupture or acute infection. If the tympanic membrane is unable to be visualized and perforation is suspected, do not irrigate and refer to ENT specialist. If acute infection is suspected, do not irrigate and refer to ENT specialist for further care. Some antibiotic eardrops are contraindicated if the tympanic membrane is not intact.

Nursing Interventions and Patient Education

1. Teach proper ear hygiene, especially not putting anything in ears.
2. Explain the normal protective function of cerumen.
3. If patient has a problem with cerumen buildup and has been advised by health care provider to use a ceruminolytic periodically, make sure that patient is getting cerumen out of ear before more medication is instilled. A bulb syringe may be used by the patient at home to help remove softened cerumen.
4. Advise patient to report persistent fever, pain, drainage, or hearing impairment.

Acute Otitis Media

Acute otitis media is an inflammation and infection of the middle ear caused by the entrance of pathogenic organisms, with rapid onset of signs and symptoms. Acute otitis media or acute suppurative otitis media is infection of the middle ear caused by contamination from bacteria from the middle ear fluid through the eustachian tube.

Pathophysiology and Etiology

1. Pathogenic organisms gain entry into the normally sterile middle ear, usually through a dysfunctional eustachian tube.
2. Organisms include *Streptococcus pneumoniae, H. influenzae, M. catarrhalis,* and *S. aureus.*
3. In serous (secretory) otitis media, no purulent infection occurs, but blockage of the eustachian tube causes negative pressure and transudation of fluid from blood vessels and development of effusion in the middle ear.

Clinical Manifestations

1. Pain is usually the first symptom.
2. Fever may rise to 104° F to 105° F (40° C to 40.6° C).
3. Purulent drainage (otorrhea) is present if tympanic membrane is perforated.
4. Irritability may be noted in the young person.
5. Headache, hearing loss, anorexia, nausea, and vomiting may be present.
6. Purulent effusion may be visible behind tympanic membrane or tympanic membrane may be reddened and bulging on otoscopic examination.

(Text continues on page 624)

PROCEDURE GUIDELINES 17-1

Irrigating the External Auditory Canal

PURPOSES

1. To facilitate removal of cerumen or foreign body and improve hearing.

 NURSING ALERT Ask if patient has a history of draining ears, has ever had perforation, has current myringotomy tube, history of mastoid surgery, or complications from a previous ear irrigation. If the reply is "yes," check with the health care provider before proceeding with the irrigation.

EQUIPMENT AND SOLUTIONS

- Kind and amount of solution desired (usually warm water)
- Ear syringe and irrigation device
- Protective towels
- Cotton balls and cotton-tipped applicators
- Solution bowl or emesis basin
- Bag for disposable items

PROCEDURE

Nursing Action	Rationale
Preparatory phase	
1. After explaining procedure to the patient, place in a position of sitting or lying with head tilted forward and toward affected ear.	1. Ear should be accessible and able to drain into basin.
2. Position protective towels.	2. Water often runs down neck onto clothing.

Performance phase

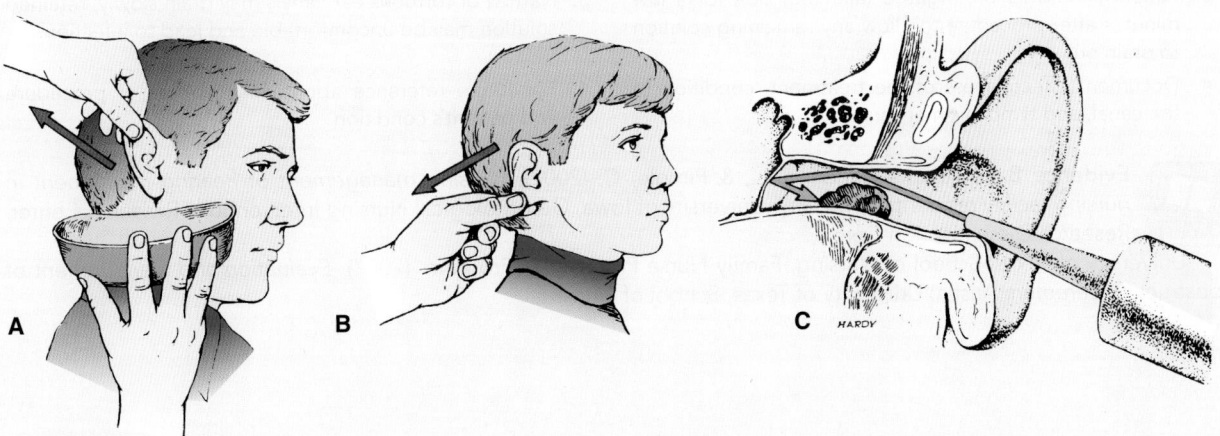

Ear irrigation. (A) *The external auditory canal in the adult can best be exposed by pulling the earlobe upward and backward.* (B) *The same exposure can be achieved in the child by gently pulling the auricle of the ear downward, outward, and backward.* (C) *An enlarged diagram showing the direction of irrigating fluid against the side of the canal.*

Note: *This is more effective in dislodging cerumen than if the flow of solution were directed straight into the canal.*

1. Use a cotton applicator to remove any discharge on outer ear.	1. Prevents carrying discharge deeper into canal.
2. Place basin close to the patient's head and under the ear.	2. Provides a receptacle to receive irrigating solution.
3. Test temperature of solution. It should be comfortable to the inner aspect of wrist area (approximately 98.6° F [37° C] or body temperature).	3. Solutions that are hot or cold are most uncomfortable and may initiate a feeling of dizziness.

(continued)

PROCEDURE GUIDELINES 17-1 *(continued)*

Irrigating the External Auditory Canal

PROCEDURE *(continued)*

Nursing Action	Rationale

 GERONTOLOGIC ALERT Take special care not to irrigate an older adult's ear with cool water because dizziness may be pronounced.

Nursing Action	Rationale
4. Ascertain whether impaction is due to a foreign hydroscopic (attracts or absorbs moisture) body before proceeding.	4. If water contacts such a substance, it may cause it to swell and produce intense pain.
5. Gently pull the outer ear upward and backward (adult) or downward and outward (child).	5. Straightens the ear canal (see Figure A).
6. Place tip of syringe or irrigating catheter just inside canal (no more than 8 mm); gently direct stream of fluid against sides of canal.	6. Decreases direct force of irrigation against eardrum and possibility of rupturing it.
7. Observe for signs of pain or dizziness.	7. Discontinue treatment if they occur.
8. If irrigating does not dislodge the wax, instill several drops of prescribed cerumenolytic and repeat as directed.	8. Softens and loosens impaction; may be effective in as little as 15 minutes.

Follow-up phase

Nursing Action	Rationale
1. Dry external ear.	
2. Remove soiled equipment and make the patient comfortable.	2. Large amount of brown cerumen may be returned in irrigation solution.
3. Patient should lie on irrigated (affected) side for a few minutes after procedure to allow any remaining solution to drain out.	3. Narrow or tortuous ear canals may drain slowly; retained solution may be uncomfortable and lead to infection.
4. Document effectiveness of the treatment, condition of the canal, and tympanic membrane.	4. For future reference about effectiveness of procedure and patient's condition.

 Evidence Base Adams-Wendling, L., & Pimple, C. (2007). *Nursing management of hearing impairment in nursing facility residents.* Iowa City: University of Iowa, Gerontological Nursing Interventions Research Center, Research Dissemination Core.
University of Texas, School of Nursing, Family Nurse Practitioner Program. (2007). *Evaluation and management of obstructing cerumen.* Austin: University of Texas, School of Nursing.

---

7. History may reveal previous upper respiratory infection, allergic rhinitis, eustachian tube dysfunction, history of reflux, adenoid hypertrophy, history of cleft palate, smoking in household, sibling otitis media in children, or child in daycare. Patients who have received radiation therapy of head and neck or experienced barotrauma or those with nasopharyngeal tumor may develop middle ear effusions.

Diagnostic Evaluation

1. Pneumatic otoscopy shows a tympanic membrane that is full, bulging, and opaque with impaired mobility (or retracted with impaired mobility).

2. Cultures of discharge through ruptured tympanic membrane may suggest causative organism.

Management

1. Antibiotic treatment—amoxicillin is first-line treatment; cephalosporins, macrolides, or trimpethoprim-sulfamethoxazole may be used in patients with penicillin allergy.
2. Amoxicillin/clavulanate and cephalosporins are used for treatment failure due to increasing rate of beta-lactamase-producing bacteria that inactivate penicillin and other antibiotics.
3. Usual treatment course is 10 days.
4. Follow-up is indicated to determine effectiveness of therapy.

5. Nasal or topical decongestants and antihistamines have a limited role in promoting eustachian tube drainage.
6. Surgery—myringotomy with placement of pressure-equalizing tubes.
   a. An incision is made into the posterior inferior aspect of the tympanic membrane for relief of persistent effusion. A pressure-equalizing tube may be inserted to prevent recurrent episodes.
   b. Performed in selected patients to prevent recurrent episodes or in patients with middle ear effusion for 3 months or more.
   c. May be done because of failure of patient to respond to antimicrobial therapy; for severe, persistent pain; and for persistent conductive hearing loss.

Complications

1. Perforation of tympanic membrane.
2. Chronic otitis media and mastoiditis.
3. Conductive hearing loss.
4. Meningitis, brain abscess.

Nursing Assessment

1. Obtain history of upper respiratory infection, previous ear infections, allergies, and progression of symptoms.
2. Assess fever and level of pain.
3. Obtain baseline hearing evaluation, if indicated.

Nursing Diagnosis

- Acute Pain related to inflammation and increased middle ear pressure.

Nursing Interventions

Relieving Pain
1. Administer or teach self-administration of anti-inflammatories and other analgesics, as prescribed.
2. Administer or teach self-administration of antibiotics, as prescribed. Oral corticosteroids may be prescribed, as well as nasal steroids.
3. Encourage the use of local warm compresses or heating pad to promote comfort and help resolve infectious process.
4. Be alert for such symptoms as headache, slow pulse, vomiting, and vertigo, which may be significant for sequelae that involve the mastoid or the brain.

Patient Education and Health Maintenance

1. Encourage follow-up after treatment to ensure resolution.
2. Advise the patient that sudden relief of pain may indicate tympanic membrane rupture. Do not instill anything in ear and call health care provider.
3. Instruct the patient to follow up for recurrence of symptoms, such as pain, fever, ear congestion.

Evaluation: Expected Outcomes

- Verbalizes relief of pain at follow-up visit.

Chronic Otitis Media and Mastoiditis

Chronic otitis media is a chronic inflammation of the middle ear with tissue damage, usually caused by repeated episodes of acute otitis media. It may be caused by an antibiotic-resistant organism or a particularly virulent strain of organism. It may be associated with tympanic membrane perforation. *Mastoiditis* is inflammation of the mastoid air cells of the temporal bone adjacent to the ear.

Pathophysiology and Etiology

1. The accumulation of pus inflammatory exudate under pressure in the middle ear cavity may result in necrosis of tissue, with damage to the tympanic membrane and possibly the ossicles.
   a. The most common organisms are *Streptococcus pneumonia, H. influenzae,* and *Moxarella caterallis.*
   b. Other organisms may be present, such as *Pseudomonas, Proteus,* and *Bacteroides* species.
2. Persistent rupture of the tympanic membrane and damage to the ossicles lead to conductive hearing loss.
3. Extension of infection may occur into the mastoid cells (mastoiditis).
4. Cholesteatoma may form (mass of squamous epithelium and desquamated debris in the middle ear), which may cause erosion of the ossicles or inner ear.

Clinical Manifestations

1. Painless or dull ache and tenderness of mastoid.
2. Otorrhea may be odorless or foul smelling.
3. Vertigo and pain may be present if CNS complications have occurred.
4. History will indicate several episodes of acute otitis media, possible rupture of tympanic membrane.
5. Fever and postauricular erythema and edema.

Diagnostic Evaluation

1. Conductive hearing loss is present through audiometric tests.
2. CT of temporal bone may show mastoid pathology, for example, cholesteatoma or opacification of mastoid cells.
3. Culture of exudate from middle ear (through ruptured tympanic membrane or at time of surgery).

Management

Note: If advanced chronic ear disease is left untreated, inner ear and life-threatening CNS complications may develop because of erosion of surrounding structures.

Medical Therapy
1. Antibiotic and steroid eardrops may control middle ear infection and inflammation, but when mastoiditis develops, parenteral antibiotic therapy is necessary.
2. Eardrops containing neomycin, garamycin, tobramycin, and quinolones, such as ciprofloxacin, are instilled into the middle ear when the tympanic membrane is ruptured. Otic drops containing antibiotics or antibiotic powder preparations may be used for infection and otorrhea. Local cleaning using

microscope and instrumentation is mainstay of treatment and done by ENT specialist.

3. IV antibiotics must cover beta-lactamase-producing organisms—ampicillin-sulbactam, cefuroxime—based on culture results.

Surgical Interventions

1. Indicated when cholesteatoma is present.
2. Indicated when there is pain, profound deafness, dizziness, sudden facial paralysis, or stiff neck (may lead to meningitis or brain abscess).
3. Types of procedures:
   a. Simple mastoidectomy—removal of diseased bone and insertion of a drain; indicated when there is persistent infection and signs of intracranial complications.
   b. Radical mastoidectomy—removal of posterior wall of ear canal, remnants of the tympanic membrane, and the malleolus and incus.
   c. Posteroanterior mastoidectomy—combines simple mastoidectomy with tympanoplasty (reconstruction of middle ear structures).

Complications

1. Acute and chronic mastoiditis.
2. Cholesteatoma.
3. CNS infection (meningitis, intracranial abscess).
4. Postoperatively—facial nerve paralysis, bleeding, vertigo.

Nursing Assessment

1. Assess for history of ear infection and treatment compliance. Identify factors that may prevent compliance with treatment in future—lack of money/prescription coverage, lack of transportation, lack of knowledge on severity of infection, and so forth.
2. Assess for ear drainage, patency of tympanic membrane.
3. Assess for hearing loss.
4. Palpate for mastoid tenderness.

For nursing process related to patients undergoing surgical treatment, see "Care Related to Ear Surgery," page 608.

Patient Education and Health Maintenance

1. Teach the patient to keep ear dry—use ENT-approved or molded ear plugs during showering, washing hair, and swimming—to prevent any water from gaining access to middle ear.
2. Encourage the patient to follow up for frequent ear cleaning.
3. Stress the importance of adhering to antibiotic schedule and to notify the home care nurse or health care provider if there is any problem with venous access or a dose is missed for any reason.
4. Advise of complications and to report headache, change in mental status or arousal, or increased ear pain.
5. Stress the importance of follow-up hearing evaluations and early intervention for any signs of ear infection in the future.

Ménière's Disease

Ménière's disease (or *endolymphatichydrops*) is a chronic inner ear disease characterized by spontaneous episodes of vertigo, fluctuating hearing loss, aural fullness, and tinnitus.

Pathophysiology and Etiology

1. Cause is unknown.
2. Fluid distention of the endolymphatic spaces of the labyrinth destroys cochlear hair cells. Pathology of the disease is endolymphatichydrops, which is thought to be caused by overaccumuulation of endolymphatic fluid and distention of the endolymphatic-containing areas in the cochlea and vestibular organs.
3. Usually unilateral, later may become bilateral. Diagnoses primarily based on clinical symptoms but audiometry and ENG are traditionally obtained.
4. Occurs most frequently between ages 30 and 60.
5. Severity of attacks may diminish over the years, but hearing loss increases.

Clinical Manifestations

1. Sudden attacks occur, in which patient feels that the room is spinning (vertigo); may last 30 minutes to several hours or days.
2. Aural fullness, tinnitus, and reduced hearing or fluctuating hearing loss occur on involved side.
3. Headache, nausea, vomiting, and disequilibrium may be present.
4. The most comfortable position for the patient is lying down.
5. After multiple attacks, tinnitus and impaired hearing may be continuous.

Diagnostic Evaluation

1. ENG or EcOG (see page 603), along with the patients' history and neurotologic exam, is used to establish diagnosis of Ménière's disease.
2. Audiogram may reveal low-frequency sensorineural hearing loss in affected ear.
3. CT scan, MRI to rule out acoustic neuroma. Only MRI of internal auditory canal with gadolinium can differentiate Ménière's disease symptoms from the symptoms of an intracranial lesion.

Management

Medical

1. The patient can be asked to keep a diary noting presence of aural symptoms (eg, tinnitus, distorted hearing) when episodes of vertigo occur.
2. Administration of a vestibular suppressant to control symptoms.
   a. Meclizine up to 25 mg four times a day.

 DRUG ALERT In general, meclizine is not recommended a long-term basis, as it prevents central nervous system compensation. Meclizine may be used for symptomatic relief on a short-term basis.

   b. Diphenhydramine 25 to 50 mg three or four times a day
   c. Lorazepam may be helpful as vestibular suppressant.

3. Intratympanic dexamethasone injection can be used for temporary control of vertigo and for some patients provides symptomatic relief of flare of vertigo.

4. Streptomycin (I.M.) or gentamicin (transtympanic injection) may be given to selectively destroy vestibular apparatus if vertigo is uncontrollable.

5. An anti-emetic, such as promethazine, may be needed to reduce nausea, vomiting, and resistant vertigo.

Surgical

1. Conservative—endolymphatic subarachnoid or mastoid shunt to relieve symptoms without destroying function.

2. Destructive surgery.
   a. Labyrinthectomy—recommended if the patient experiences progressive hearing loss and severe vertigo attacks so normal tasks cannot be performed; results in total deafness of affected ear.
   b. Vestibular nerve section—neurosurgical suboccipital approach to the cerebellopontine angle for intracranial vestibular nerve neurectomy.

Complications

1. Irreversible hearing loss.
2. Disability and social isolation due to vertigo and hearing loss.
3. Injury due to falls.

Nursing Assessment

1. Assess for frequency and severity of attacks.
2. Provide screening hearing tests.
3. Evaluate effect on the patient's activities, potential for fall or injury.

Nursing Diagnoses

- Risk for Injury related to sudden attacks of vertigo.
- Social Isolation related to fear of attack and hearing loss.

Nursing Interventions

For care related to labyrinth surgery, see page 607.

Ensuring Safety

1. Help the patient recognize an aura so that he or she has time to prepare for an attack.
2. Encourage the patient to lie down during attack, in safe place, and lie still.
3. Put side rails up on bed if in hospital.
4. Have the patient close eyes if this lessens symptoms.
5. Inform the patient that the dizziness may last for varying lengths of time. Maintain safety precautions until attack is complete.

Minimizing Feelings of Isolation

1. Provide encouragement and understanding. Show the patient that you understand the seriousness of this disorder, even though there is little that can be done to ease the discomfort.
2. Assist the patient to identify specific triggers to control attacks.
   a. Remind the patient to move slowly because jerking or making sudden movements may precipitate an attack.

b. Avoid noises and glaring, bright lights, which may initiate an attack.
   c. Control environmental factors and personal habits that may cause stress or fatigue.
   d. If there is a tendency to allergic reactions to foods, eliminate those foods from the diet.

3. Avoid oversedation of the patient through polypharmacy with sedatives, anticholinergics, and opioids that may increase risk of falling if attack occurs.

4. Teach the patient to be aware of other sensory cues from the environment, visual, olfactory, and tactile, if hearing is affected.

Patient Education and Health Maintenance

1. Teach about medication therapy, including adverse effects of vestibular suppressants—drowsiness, dry mouth.
2. Advise sodium restriction as adjunct to vestibular suppressant therapy.
3. Advise the patient to keep a log of attacks, triggers, and severity of symptoms.
4. Encourage follow-up hearing evaluations and provide information about surgical care if planned.
5. Teach the patient hearing-conservation methods—avoid loud noises, wear earplugs if necessary, avoid smoking, and avoid use of ototoxic drugs, such as aspirin, quinine, and some antibiotics.

Evaluation: Expected Outcomes

- Lays down with side rails up and eyes closed during attack; resolves without injury.
- Identifies dietary triggers and follows treatment plan.

Vestibular Labyrinthitis

Labyrinthitis is an inflammation of the inner ear caused by a viral or bacterial infection. It is characterized by hearing loss, vertigo, and usually nausea and vomiting.

See Box 17-1, page 628, for other causes of vertigo, including benign paroxysmal positional vertigo.

Pathophysiology and Etiology

1. Bacterial labyrinthitis is usually associated with acute otitis media or cholesteatoma. Infectious organisms may enter the inner ear through the oval or round window. Bacterial meningitis can cause labyrinthitis by spread of the bacterial infection via the cochlear aqueduct and internal auditory canal.

2. Viral labyrinthitis can occur as a result of viral illnesses of the respiratory tract system and may include measles, mumps, rubella, or herpetic infections of the facial or acoustic nerve. This may be seen in Ramsey-Hunt syndrome.

3. Vestibular neuronitis or neuritis is a disorder of the vestibular nerve (CN XII) characterized by severe, sudden onset of vertigo with normal hearing. Etiology most commonly from viral illness, but may be attributed to other causes. The course is usually self-limiting. The patient may have an unsteady gait but is able to walk. (This is differentiated by cerebellar disease, in which the patient has vertigo and nystagmus and is usually

BOX 17-1 Vertigo

Vertigo is a type of dizziness characterized by the illusion of movement: either a perception that the surroundings are moving while the body remains still, or that one's body is moving while the surroundings remain still. It is caused by vestibular dysfunction—either in the peripheral vestibular system (inner ear) or the central vestibular system (brain stem and cerebellum).

- Common causes of vertigo of peripheral origin include Ménière's disease, labyrinthitis, acoustic neuroma, and benign paroxysmal positional vertigo (BPPV).

- Causes of central vertigo include multiple sclerosis, basilar migraine, transient ischemic attack or stroke of the basilar artery, brain tumor, trauma, and cerebral hemorrhage.

- Other causes of dizziness are vaso-vagal syncope, hypovolemia, autonomic neuropathy of diabetes, severe anemia, aortic stenosis, hypoglycemia, hypoxia, hypocarbia, multiple sensory deficits, adverse drug effects, and emotional illness.

BPPV is the most common cause of vertigo. Its onset is sudden, it can be severe in intensity, and it is always related to change in position of the head. It can be diagnosed by thorough history and physical examination, including some provocative maneuvers such as the Dix-Hallpike maneuver. Diagnostic tests are required only to rule out central vestibular dysfunction and dizziness caused by other disorders. Patients with BPPV may be very concerned about their symptoms and are at risk for injury due to imbalance.

NURSING CONSIDERATIONS

- Ensure safety by creating an uncluttered environment, using side rails and handrails as necessary, using proper footwear, and encouraging the patient to call for help.

- Teach patient to avoid sudden position changes, including simple head movements, such as looking up or turning over in bed.

- Discourage use of alcohol and sedating drugs, which may further impair safe ambulation.

- Most episodes of BPPV last seconds to minutes and completely resolve within 3 months; however, if severe or prolonged, suggest referral to a physical therapist for vestibular rehabilitation.

imaging may include CT of temporal bone, MRI of internal auditory canal with gadolinium, and lumbar puncture, if bacterial meningitis suspected.

2. Viral and physiologic causes are treated with symptomatic support. In patients with viral labyrinthitis, management may include antiviral therapy, anti-emetics, vestibular suppressants, and later in illness, vestibular rehabilitation.

3. Vestibular suppressant and anti-emetic medication as with Ménière's disease (meclizine, diazepam, promethazine).

4. Audiometric evaluation should be obtained with all patients with vertigo to differentiate between vestibular labyrinthitis and vestibular neuronitis. MRI of brain and internal auditory canal is obtained when assymetrical hearing loss is present to rule out acoustic neuroma.

Complications

1. Permanent hearing loss.
2. Injury from fall.

Nursing Assessment

1. Assess frequency and severity of attacks and how patient handles them.
2. Assess for fever related to bacterial infection.
3. Assess for additional neurologic symptoms—visual changes, change in mental status, sensory and motor deficits—that may indicate CNS pathology.
4. Assess for effectiveness of vestibular stimulants and anti-emetics.
5. If fall occurs, assess for injury.

Nursing Diagnoses

- Risk for Injury related to gait disturbance secondary to vertigo.
- Anxiety related to sudden onset of symptoms.
- Risk for Deficient Fluid Volume related to vomiting and impaired intake.
- Bathing and Hygiene Self-Care Deficit related to vertigo.

Nursing Interventions

Preventing Injury

1. At onset of attack, have the patient lie still in darkened room with eyes closed or fixed on stationary object until the vertigo passes.
2. Make sure that the patient can obtain help at all times through use of call system, close proximity to staff, or companion.
3. Remove obstacles in the patient's environment.
4. Make sure that sensory aids are available—glasses, hearing aid, proper lighting.
5. Use side rails while the patient is in bed.
6. Administer medications, as directed; assess for and avoid oversedation.

Minimizing Anxiety

1. Explain the physiology behind vertigo and the possible triggers.
2. Support patient and family through the diagnostic process.

unable to walk.) Treatment is supportive with meclizine, benzodiazapines, anti-emetics, or vestibular rehabilitation.

Clinical Manifestations

1. Sudden onset of incapacitating vertigo, with varying degrees of nausea and vomiting, hearing loss, and tinnitus.
2. Persists; does not occur in episodic attacks like Ménière's disease.

Management

1. The rare cases of bacterial labyrinthitis are treated with antibiotics, as with the suspected predisposing infection. Bacterial labyrinthitis is treated by antibiotics, anti-emetics, vestibular suppresssants, and vestibular rehabilitiation. Diagnostic

3. Assist the patient to adjust activities to minimize the impact.
4. Teach stress-reduction techniques, such as deep breathing, talking and asking questions, and distraction.

Ensuring Adequate Fluid

1. Keep diet light while vertigo is present.
2. Administer anti-emetics, as directed.
3. Assess intake and output, as indicated.
4. Encourage fluids and small feedings while patient is feeling better.

Encouraging Safe Self-Care

1. Encourage activity while vertigo is minimal; rest during attacks.
2. Set up environment for the patient's safety and convenience—chair near sink, walker to hold on to while walking, if necessary, and so forth.
3. Assist the patient with hygiene and other care, as needed.

Patient Education and Health Maintenance

1. Teach patients with viral labyrinthitis that attacks are self-limiting, will become less severe, and should leave no permanent disability.
2. Teach safety measures during vertigo attacks.
3. Tell the patient that vertigo is best tolerated while lying flat in bed in a darkened room, with eyes closed or looking at stable object.
4. Teach patients how to take medications and to avoid other CNS depressants such as alcohol.
5. Encourage follow-up.

Evaluation: Expected Outcomes

- Rests in bed during attack with side rails up.
- Verbalizes feelings and questions about treatment.
- Takes fluids, light diet every 4 hours, after medication administration.
- Performs appropriate hygiene and dressing by him- or herself at bedside.

MALIGNANT DISORDERS

Cancer of the Oral Cavity, Oropharynx, Nasopharynx, and Paranasal Sinuses

Cancer of the oral cavity may arise from the lips, buccal mucosa, gums, hard palate, floor of the mouth, salivary glands, and anterior two thirds of the tongue. Cancer of the oropharynx may arise from the tonsillar fossa, pharyngeal wall, and palatal arch (soft palate, uvula, and anterior border of the anterior tonsillar pillar). Cancer of the nasopharynx may arise from the fossa of Rosenmueller. Cancer of the paranasal sinuses may arise from the maxillary sinuses (80%) or, less commonly, in the ethmoid, frontal, and sphenoid sinuses.

Pathophysiology and Etiology

1. Oral and oropharyngeal cancer: accounts for approximately 2% of all cancers diagnosed annually in the United States. About 40,000 people will be diagnosed with oral cancer each year and about 7,850 will die from this disease. Occurs more in males, with a ratio of 2:1. Most prevalent in ages 55 to 64; approximately 90% are squamous cell carcinoma.
   a. High-risk factors include use of tobacco and alcohol (particularly in combination), use of smokeless tobacco (snuff), pipe smoking, marijuana use, exposure to HPV, (causes 40 to 80% of all oropharyngeal cancers in the U.S.), poor oral hygiene, and genetic factors.
   b. Overall survival rate depends on the primary location of the tumor and the stage of the disease at diagnosis. On average, 60% of those with this disease will survive more than 5 years.

 Evidence Base D'Souza, G., & Dempsey, A. (2011). The role of HPV in head and neck cancer and review of the HPV vaccine. *Preventative Medicine*, 53(Suppl. 1), S5–S11.

2. Nasopharyngeal carcinoma is most prevalent in persons from China, Hong Kong, and Southeast Asia because of a diet high in perseveration (eg, salted fish). These types of cancers have a high genetic predisposition.
   a. Has a strong association with the Epstein-Barr virus.
   b. Occurs 75% of the time in males, usually between age 30 and 60. Overall survival rate is 50% to 90%, depending on the stage of disease at diagnosis.
3. Malignant paranasal sinus tumors are rare and have relatively poor survival outcomes. They are usually squamous cell in origin.
   a. Other types include soft tissue sarcomas, inverting papillomas, and esthesioneuroblastomas.
   b. Overall survival rate is 50% to 80%, depending on the stage of disease at diagnosis.

Clinical Manifestations

1. Commonly asymptomatic in early stages.
2. Oral cancer—nonhealing, nonpainful crusting and ulcerated leukoplakic and erythemic lesions.
3. Cancer of the lip—presence of a lesion that fails to heal.
4. Cancer of the tongue—swelling, ulceration, areas of tenderness or bleeding, abnormal texture, or limited movement of the tongue.
5. Floor-of-the-mouth cancer—red, slightly elevated, mucosal lesion with ill-defined borders, leukoplakia, indurated, ulceration, or wartlike growth.
6. Cancer of the tonsil—swelling, neck mass, wartlike growth, odynophagia, otalgia.
7. Cancer of the retromolar trigone area—trismus, otalgia, dysphagia, odynophagia.
8. Cancer of the pharyngeal wall—dysphagia, odynophagia, otalgia, neck mass.
9. Cancer of the nasopharynx—epistaxis, unilateral serous otitis, unilateral nasal blockage, loss of sense of smell (CN I), eye movements (CN III, IV, and V), and tongue movement impairment and dysphagia (CN IX, X and XII).
10. More advanced stages characterized by ulceration, bleeding, pain, induration, CN impairments, dysphagia, odynophagia, weight loss, and/or cervical lymphadenopathy (neck mass).

Diagnostic Evaluation

1. Careful inspection of the oral cavity with indirect mirror examination of pharynx.
2. Flexible or rigid nasopharyngoscopy to directly examine the nasopharynx and pharynx.
3. Staining of the oral lesion with toluidine blue—the lesion stains dark blue after rinsing with acetic acid (normal tissue does not absorb stain).
4. Excisional biopsy of suspected tissue.
5. Radiologic studies: chest x-ray, CT, MRI, and positron emission tomography to determine local invasiveness and metastasis.
6. Gray-scale and Doppler ultrasonography of the neck to determine presence of lymphadenopathy of the neck.

Management

Selection of treatment depends on the size and site of lesion and how extensively surrounding tissues are involved.

1. Early-stage lesions can be treated with a combination of surgery, radiation, and chemotherapy.
2. Large lesions of the oral cavity or oropharynx may be excised widely and/or treated by radical neck dissection for extensive lymphatic involvement, followed by external irradiation to decrease recurrence rate but maintain appearance.
3. Surgical resection of nasopharyngeal cancer and base of tongue cancer may be difficult due to the location and the relationship to many important structures.
   a. Radiation therapy is the treatment of choice in early-stage cancers of these areas.
   b. Locally advanced oropharyngeal cancer is treated with surgery and adjuvant radiation with or without concurrent cisplatin, or concurrent chemoradiation to preserve speech and swallowing function.
4. Paranasal sinus cancer treatment usually consists of minimally invasive or open surgery followed by radiation; chemotherapy may also be involved.

Complications

1. Second primary cancers of the larynx, hypopharynx, esophagus, and lungs.
2. Secondary to treatment:
   a. Surgery—transient salivary outflow obstruction, infection, voice changes, fistula formation, loss of swallowing, cosmetic defects.
   b. Radiation (early effects)—taste alterations, mucositis, xerostomia, dysphagia, odynophagia, anorexia, dermatitis, fatigue, pain.
   c. Radiation (late effects)—thyroid dysfunction, radiation caries, osteoradionecrosis, xerostomia, nasopharyngeal stenosis, cerebrospinal fluid leak and other neurolgic complications, tissue fibrosis, trismus, laryngeal edema, vascular complications.
   d. Chemotherapy—nausea, vomiting, dehydration, skin reaction, mucositis, hyperuremia, liver abnormalities, weight loss, anorexia, myelosuppression, peripheral neuropathy, hypomagnesemia, ototoxicity, nephrotoxicity, alopecia, and cognitive effects.

Nursing Assessment

1. Obtain complete history, noting risk factors such as smoking and alcohol use, exposure to Epstein-Barr virus, diet, high-risk sexual behavior, and exposure to environmental toxins.
2. Question the patient regarding changes in swallowing, smell or taste, salivation, discomfort when eating, sore throat, foul breath odor, weight loss, epistaxis, unilateral nasal obstruction, changes in hearing, neck mass, changes in tongue movement, and changes in vision.
3. Note the quality of voice patterns and odor of breath.
4. Inspect the oral cavity: erythema, red velvety areas; white patches; crusting, bleeding; swelling; record the size, location, and description.
5. Use nasal speculum to inspect the nares for obstruction.
6. Palpate the cervical lymph nodes for size, firmness, or tenderness.

Nursing Diagnoses

- Acute Pain related to malignant infiltration, lesions, difficulty swallowing, surgery, radiation therapy.
- Imbalanced Nutrition: Less Than Body Requirements related to pain, difficulty in chewing or swallowing, history of alcohol abuse, dysphagia, xerostomia.
- Disturbed Body Image related to changes in facial contour, cosmetic defect from surgery, CN deficits.

Nursing Interventions

Also see page 632 if radical neck dissection has been performed.

Achieving an Acceptable Level of Comfort

1. Provide systemic analgesics or analgesic gargles, as prescribed.
2. If the patient can tolerate it, provide mouth care with soft toothbrush and flossing between teeth.
3. If the patient cannot tolerate brushing and flossing:
   a. Gently lavage oral cavity with a catheter inserted between the patient's cheek and gums with warm water or salt water and/or sodium bicarbonate solution rinses.
4. Provide management of excessive salivation and mouth odors.
   a. Insert a gauze wick in corner of mouth; place basin conveniently to catch drooling; replace frequently to absorb and direct excess saliva.
   b. Suction secretions with a soft rubber catheter, if not allergic to latex, as needed; instruct the patient on suctioning methods.
5. Provide management of decreased salivation, if necessary.
   a. Encourage intake of fluids, if not contraindicated.
   b. Instruct the patient to avoid dry, bulky, and irritating foods.
   c. Offer lemon lozenges or chewing gum to stimulate salivation.
   d. Encourage use of humidifier.
   e. Suggest foods with sauces and gravies to make them moist and easier to swallow.
6. Maintain a clean and odor-free environment by removing soiled dressings, tissues, and gauzes, and providing room deodorants.

Improving Nutritional Status

1. Handle feeding problems in one or a combination of the following ways, as ordered:
   a. IV fluid to prevent dehydration.
   b. Nasogastric (NG) tube feedings or prophylactic placement of gastrostomy tube for feedings.
   c. Orally—serve meals high in protein and vitamin content, low in acidity and salt.
2. Provide mouth care before and after eating.
3. Allow the patient to have meals in privacy, if desired.
4. Offer easily chewed foods; mash or blenderize, if necessary.
5. Add herbs or sweeteners to enhance flavor.
6. If swallowing difficulties persist, see Procedure Guidelines 18-7, pages 671 to 672, or consult the speech-language pathologist.
7. Monitor weight, intake and output, and laboratory tests, such as 24-hour urine for urea nitrogen, C-reactive protein, albumin, prealbumin, transferring level, and electrolytes.
8. Have patient carry a bottle of water whenever traveling.

Strengthening Body Image

1. Assess the patient's reaction to condition.
   a. Evaluate the patient's apprehension and offer emotional support.
   b. Correct misinformation.
   c. Determine therapeutic care plan for the patient's rehabilitation.
2. Recognize that face and neck surgery can be disfiguring and the patient often is embarrassed, withdrawn, and depressed.
3. Assist the patient in caring for personal appearance.
4. Observe closely for indications of the patient's needs, which may be communicated in other ways, such as acting out or withdrawn behavior.
5. Allow verbalization of fears, anger, distaste with body changes in a nondefensive manner.
6. Communicate acceptance of appearance in an honest manner.
7. Encourage the patient's family and friends to visit so patient is aware that others care about him or her.
8. Provide diversional activities.

Community and Home Care Considerations

1. Teach mouth care procedure and dressing care to maintain cleanliness and prevent odor.
2. Emphasize adequate nutrition—proper consistency, proper seasoning, and right temperature. Show the family how to prepare food in blender or food processor, as necessary. Teach tube feeding procedure, if applicable.
3. If suctioning is required, instruct as to method, use, and care of equipment and obtain supplies for family.
4. Provide detailed instructions and demonstration to the patient and caregiver on incisional care.
5. Assess for signs of obstruction, hemorrhage, infection, and depression and teach caregivers what to do about them if they occur.

6. If the patient is undergoing radiation therapy, encourage them to perform appropriate skin care, avoid exposure to potential chemical irritants, limit direct sun exposure, and avoid application of lotions, ointments, or fragrances to the head and neck region, which might alter the depth at which the maximum radiation dose is delivered.
7. Encourage the radiated patient to use sialogogues such as hard candy to stimulate saliva flow. Pilocarpine may be prescribed to prevent xerostomia for patients who have completed radiation therapy.

Patient Education and Health Maintenance

1. Encourage follow-up with speech-language pathologist, if indicated.
2. Encourage cessation of high-risk behaviors to all—smoking, alcohol consumption, use of smokeless tobacco, pipe smoking.
3. Emphasize the need for routine follow-up examinations with specialist, dentists (for the use of fluoride trays during radiation), and speech pathologists.

Evaluation: Expected Outcome

- Reports adequate comfort levels, is pain-free, handles secretions adequately.
- Achieves adequate nutritional status, able to eat prescribed diet.
- Verbalizes acceptance of body image, demonstrates behaviors that reflect self-esteem (eg, shaves, dresses, applies makeup).

Neck Dissection for Head and Neck Malignancy

Systematic removal of lymph nodes with their surrounding fibrofatty tissue from the various compartments of the neck. The goal of neck dissection is to eradicate metastases involving the cervical lymph nodes. Metastases originate from primary lesions involving the oral cavity, pharynx, and larynx. The cervical lymph nodes are grouped into six major levels (I to VI) with additional division into two sublevels (A and B) of levels I, II, and V.

Surgical Procedures

1. Resection of lesion is the primary intervention.
2. Radical neck dissection— removal of lymph nodes in levels I through V and internal jugular vein (IJ), sternocleidomastoid muscle (SCM), and the spinal accessory nerve (CN XI).
3. Modified radical neck dissection— removal of lymph nodes in levels I through V, and preservation of one or more of IJ, SCM, CN XI.
4. Selective neck dissection—en bloc removal of one or more lymph node (LN) groups that are at greatest risk for harboring metastasis.
5. Commonly followed by postoperative radiation therapy. In some instances where resection is impossible, radical radiation therapy is the sole treatment for head and neck malignancy.
6. Surgical reconstruction may be performed with a rotational flap, skin graft, or free flap to promote healing and improve aesthetics.

Preoperative Management

1. Interventions to improve nutritional status preoperatively include nutritional supplements, hyperalimentation, alcohol withdrawal, and counseling.
2. The patient's general health status is evaluated and underlying conditions, such as cirrhosis and obstructive pulmonary or cardiovascular disease, are identified and treated, if possible.
3. The patient is evaluated for level of understanding of disease process, treatment regimen, and follow-up care.
4. Emotional preparation for major surgery, long rehabilitation, and change in body image is provided.

Postoperative Management

1. A major goal of postoperative management is protection of the airway. After the patient has fully recovered from anesthesia, the endotracheal tube is removed (unless respiratory compromise occurs).
2. The patient is closely monitored for hemorrhage. Wound drainage is facilitated with a negative pressure drain. The drain is removed when output is less than 25 mL in a 24-hour period.
3. Prophylactic antibiotics are given to prevent infection because of extensive incision, lymph node resection, and close proximity to oral secretions.

Evidence Base Steinberg, J. P., Braun, B. I., Hellinger, W. C., et al. (2009). Timing of antimicrobial prophylaxis and the risk of surgical site infections: Results from the Trial to Reduce Antimicrobial Prophylaxis Errors. *Annals of Surgery, 250*(1), 10–16.

4. Oral nutritional supplements, enteral feedings, or hyperalimentation is provided until oral intake is adequate and nutritional status is improved.
5. Pain management is also an important postoperative intervention.

Complications

1. Surgery—air leaks, bleeding, chylous fistula, facial or cerebral edema, blindness, carotid artery rupture, and damage to nerves such as the phrenic, vagus, brachial plexus, and cutaneous nerves and the mandibular branch of the facial, hypoglossal, or lingual nerves.
2. Radiation.
   a. Early—radiation mucositis, xerostomia erythema, desquamation, dysphagia, secondary infection, oral pain.
   b. Long-term—atrophy, fibrosis, salivary dryness, hoarseness, difficulty swallowing, bone pain, osteonecrosis, pathologic fractures, limitation of movement, poor wound healing.

Nursing Diagnoses

- Ineffective Breathing Pattern related to laryngeal edema, secretions, presence of a tracheostomy.
- Risk for Infection related to surgery, proximity of secretions to suture line, radiation.
- Imbalanced Nutrition: Less Than Body Requirements related to anorexia, inability to swallow, pain on swallowing.
- Disturbed Body Image related to surgical therapy, radiation changes.

Nursing Interventions
Maintaining Effective Breathing Pattern

1. Place the patient in Fowler's position.
2. Observe for signs of respiratory embarrassment, such as dyspnea, cyanosis, edema, hoarseness, or dysphagia.
3. Provide supplemental oxygen by face mask, if necessary; if tracheostomy is present, provide humidified air or oxygen by tracheostomy collar or adequate ambient humidification.
4. Auscultate for decreased breath sounds, crackles, wheezes; auscultate over the trachea in the immediate postoperative period to assess for stridor indicative of edema.
5. Encourage deep breathing and coughing.
6. Assist the patient in assuming a sitting position to bring up secretions (the nurse's hands support the patient's neck).
7. Suction secretions orally or aseptically through a tracheostomy if patient is unable to cough them up.

Preventing Infection

1. Assess vital signs for indication of infection—increased heart rate, elevation of temperature.
2. Inspect wound for hemorrhage, drainage, or tracheal constriction; reinforce dressings, as needed.
3. Inspect incision for signs of infection—redness, warmth, swelling, drainage.
4. If a drain is used, expect approximately 80 to 120 mL of serosanguineous secretions to be drawn off during the first postoperative day; this diminishes with each day. Ensure that the drain is stripped at the insertion site at least three times per day to prevent clotting. Assess for color and amount of drainage.
   a. The initial output will be serosanguineous and eventually will turn serous. If the fluid appears milky, the surgeon should be notified right away as this may be indicative of a chyle leak.
   b. A high output of several hundred milliliters or more per day may also indicate chyle leak. If the output is less than 600 mL of chyle per day, the leak is initially managed conservatively with closed-wound drainage, pressure dressings, and zero-fat nutritional support. Parenteral alimentation through a central line may also be utilized to further reduce chylous output.
5. Aseptically clean skin area around drain exit, using saline or prescribed solution.
6. Make sure that the incision site remains clean and dry; remove secretions immediately.

Improving Nutritional Status

1. Postoperatively provide IV fluids and hyperalimentation, tube feedings through NG tube or gastrostomy tube, or oral feedings as soon as swallowing is established.
2. Provide mouth care before and after meals.
3. Assess for excessive or decreased salivation, which may impair swallowing.

4. Make sure that emergency suctioning and airway equipment is available at the bedside during meals in the event of choking or aspiration. Utilize speech-language therapist to evaluate dysphagia.

5. Position the patient in an upright position, supporting shoulders and neck with pillows, if necessary.

6. Ask whether the patient would prefer privacy during meals.

7. Provide an environment that is clean and free from interruptions and odor.

8. Assist with oral intake, providing easily chewed foods. Mash or blenderize meals, if necessary.

Strengthening Body Image

1. Respect the patient's desire for privacy during treatments, dressing changes, and feedings.

2. Prepare visitors for the patient's change in appearance.

3. If the patient has difficulty speaking, assist with alternate communication methods and allow adequate time for communication.

4. Observe for lower facial paralysis; this may indicate facial nerve injury.

5. Watch for shoulder dysfunction, which may follow resection of spinal accessory nerves.
   a. Use muscle exercises provided by the physical therapist and muscle reeducation postoperatively.
   b. Work with the patient to obtain good functional range of motion.

6. Encourage the patient to verbalize concerns and feelings.
   a. Consult the health care provider to determine the nature and extent of explanation and prognosis that has been given to the patient.
   b. Encourage the patient to seek confirmation of personal philosophy and religious beliefs because this may provide answers.
   c. Accentuate the positive.
   d. Encourage the patient to participate in the plan of care.
   e. Recognize that a great effort has to be made in behavior modification to change a lifestyle that included alcohol consumption and cigarette smoking. Provide educational material and support.

Community and Home Care Considerations

If patient has a permanent tracheostomy or laryngectomy, instruct the patient and family about:

1. Need for increased humidification in home environment.
2. Protective stoma cover to help filter air.
3. Avoiding activities that may cause aspiration (eg, swimming).
4. Referral for speech-language pathologist and social worker to meet ongoing communication needs.

Patient Education and Health Maintenance

Exercises

Instruct the patient and family regarding exercises to prevent limited range of motion and discomfort (see Figure 17-7).

1. Perform exercises morning and evening. Initially, exercises are done only once; the number is increased by one each day until each exercise is done 10 times.

2. After each exercise, the patient is instructed to relax.

3. For neck:
   a. Gently rotate head to each side as far as possible.
   b. Tilt head to the right side as far as possible; repeat for left side.
   c. Drop chin to chest, and then raise chin as high as possible.

4. For shoulder:
   a. Standing beside bed, place hand from unoperated side on bed for support.
   b. Gradually swing arm on operated side up and back as far as is comfortable for the patient.
   c. Each day, work toward finishing a complete circle.

Follow-Up Visits

1. Emphasize the need for frequent follow-up visits and completion of radiation therapy, if prescribed.

2. Recommend a dental follow-up to ensure good oral hygiene and dental rehabilitation, if indicated.

Evaluation: Expected Outcomes

- Maintains adequate breathing pattern; absence of dyspnea, shortness of breath; is able to handle secretions.
- Is free from signs and symptoms of infection; vital signs stable; incision is clean, dry, without redness or drainage.
- Is adequately hydrated, maintains stable nutrition and weight, can tolerate diet without choking or aspiration.
- Discusses concerns about condition, verbalizes positive aspects of self.

Cancer of the Larynx

Cancer of the larynx is a malignant growth of the vocal cords. The supraglottic larynx refers to the area above the vocal cords including the epiglottis. The subglottic larynx refers to the area below the vocal cords to about the first tracheal ring. When treated early, the likelihood of cure is great. The National Cancer Institute at the National Institutes of Health estimate that in 2012, 12,360 new cases will be diagnosed in the United States and 3,650 persons will die from the disease.

Pathophysiology and Etiology

1. Occurs predominantly in men older than age 60.

2. Most patients have a history of smoking and heavy alcohol intake. Other risk factors include laryngopharyngeal reflux; industrial exposure to diesel exhaust, asbestos, organic solvents, sulfuric acid, mustard gas, certain mineral oils, metal dust, asphalt, wood dust, stone dust, mineral wool, cement dust; genetic susceptibility; and diet.

3. In North America, about two thirds of carcinomas of the larynx arise in the glottis, almost one third arise in the supraglottic region, and about 3% arise in the subglottic region of the larynx.

4. When limited to the vocal cords, spread is slow because of lessened blood supply.

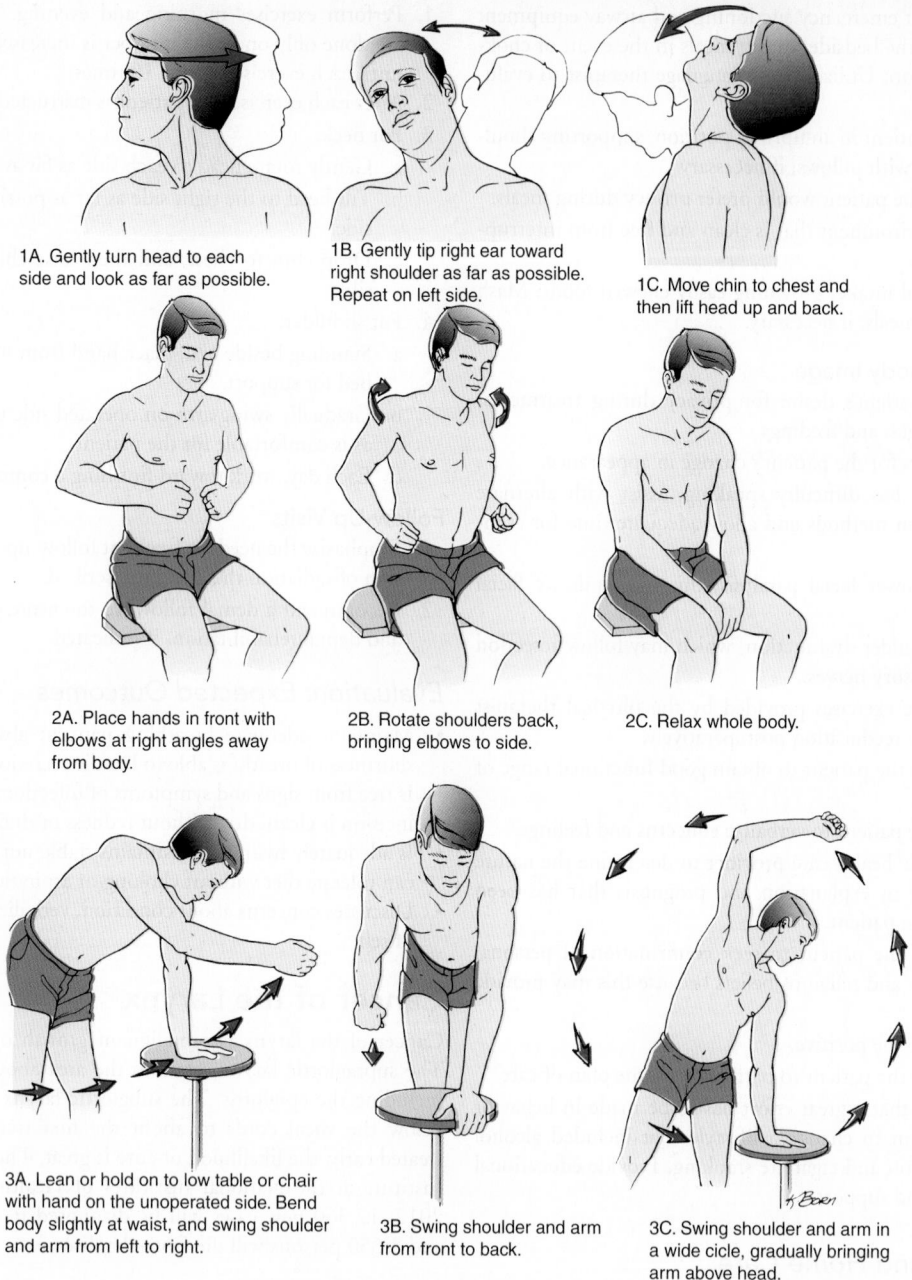

1A. Gently turn head to each side and look as far as possible.

1B. Gently tip right ear toward right shoulder as far as possible. Repeat on left side.

1C. Move chin to chest and then lift head up and back.

2A. Place hands in front with elbows at right angles away from body.

2B. Rotate shoulders back, bringing elbows to side.

2C. Relax whole body.

3A. Lean or hold on to low table or chair with hand on the unoperated side. Bend body slightly at waist, and swing shoulder and arm from left to right.

3B. Swing shoulder and arm from front to back.

3C. Swing shoulder and arm in a wide cicle, gradually bringing arm above head.

Figure 17-7. Rehabilitation exercises after head and neck surgery to regain maximum shoulder function and neck motion.

5. When cancer involves the supraglottis, cancer spreads more rapidly to the lymph nodes of the neck than does glottis cancer.

Clinical Manifestations

Depend on tumor location; sequence in appearance related to pattern and extent of tumor growth.

Supraglottic Cancer

1. Tickling sensation in throat.
2. Dryness and fullness (lump) in throat.
3. Painful swallowing (odynophagia) associated with invasion of extralaryngeal musculature.
4. Coughing on swallowing.
5. Pain radiating to ear (late symptom).

Glottic Cancer (Cancer of the Vocal Cord)

1. Most common cancer of the larynx.
2. Hoarseness or aphonia (loss of voice).
3. Aspiration
4. Dyspnea.
5. Pain (in later stages).

Subglottic Cancer (Uncommon)

1. Coughing.
2. Short periods of difficulty in breathing.
3. Hemoptysis; fetid odor, which results from ulceration and disintegration of tumor.

Diagnostic Evaluation

1. Indirect mirror examination of larynx may indicate lesion.
2. Direct laryngoscopy and biopsy to identify lesion.
3. CT scan and other special radiologic tests to detect tumor.
4. The T, N, M classification system is used for staging (see page 139). In larynx cancer, prognosis can be predicted by the tumor size and nodal involvement. If lymph nodes are involved, the prognosis is usually poorer than when no lymph nodes are involved.

Management

General Considerations

Depends on sites and stages of cancer. Early malignancy may be removed endoscopically.

1. Early glottic squamous cell carcinoma (SCC, defined as stage I or II disease) may be treated with either radiation therapy or surgery, without the need to treat the neck. Surgical treatment goal of early glottic SCC is to preserve the larynx and is referred to as conservation laryngeal surgery or partial laryngectomy.
2. Advanced glottic SCC (stage III or IV disease) is associated with poor prognosis. T3 glottic carcinomas have a low risk of nodal metastasis. Typically, T3 tumors have been treated with total laryngectomy as single-modality therapy. Radiation therapy offers a local control rate of approximately 50% for these tumors.
3. T4 glottic carcinoma is treated with total laryngectomy (usually with postoperative radiation therapy or chemotherapy, near-total laryngectomy, or primary CRT in selected low-volume disease) with limited cartilage destruction to preserve the larynx. Near-total laryngectomy may be performed in selected cases with limited subglottic extension and no interarytenoid involvement. Primary radiation therapy for T4 glottic carcinoma has poor local control rates.
4. According to the National Comprehensie Cancer Network, the patient should be examined every 1 to 3 months for the first year after treatment, every 2 to 4 months in the second year, every 4 to 6 months in the third, fourth, and fifth years, and every 6 to 12 month thereafter.

Surgery

1. Carbon dioxide laser for early-stage disease.
2. Partial laryngectomy—removal of small lesion on true cord, along with a substantial margin of healthy tissue.
3. Open supraglottic laryngectomy (OSGL)—removal of all laryngeal structures superior to the floor of the ventricle, maintaining both true vocal cords, both arytenoids, the base of the tongue, and the hyoid bone. Is performed for T1, T2, or selected T3 supraglottic tumors. An acceptable alternative to OSGL is transoral laser microsurgery for T1–T2 and selected T3 tumors.
4. Hemilaryngectomy—removal of one true vocal cord, false cord, one half of thyroid cartilage, arytenoid cartilage.
5. Total laryngectomy—removal of entire larynx (epiglottis, false or true cords, cricoid cartilage, hyoid bone; two or three tracheal rings are usually removed when there is extrinsic cancer of the larynx [extension beyond the vocal cords]). A radical neck dissection may also be performed because of metastasis to cervical lymph nodes.
6. Total laryngectomy with tracheo-esophageal puncture. During surgery, a puncture is made in the posterior wall of the trachea, which is also the anterior wall of the esophagus. A voice prosthesis or a red rubber catheter is inserted into the puncture. The red rubber catheter serves two purposes: to mature the track until a voice prosthesis is inserted and to provide enteral feedings until the patient is allowed to swallow. If a voice prosthesis is inserted at the time of surgery, the patient is fed through either a nasogastric or gastrostomy tube.

Complications

1. Pharyngocutaneous fistula may develop after any surgical procedure that involves entering the pharynx or esophagus.
   a. Monitor for saliva collecting beneath the skin flaps or leaking through suture line or drain site.
   b. Management—NG tube feeding, meticulous local wound care with frequent dressing changes, promotion of drainage.
2. Hemorrhage (carotid artery rupture) or hematoma formation.
   a. A major postoperative complication (eg, skin necrosis or salivary fistula) usually precedes carotid artery rupture.
   b. Management—immediate wound exploration in operating room.
3. Drain failure.
4. Infection.
5. Wound dehiscence—patients who have been radiated prior to surgery and/or who are malnourished are more at risk for wound dehiscence.
6. Complications of radiation—edema of the larynx, soft tissue and cartilage necrosis, skin reaction, chondritis.
7. Long-term complications:
   a. Stomal stenosis.
   b. Pharyngoesophageal stenosis and stricture.
   c. Hypothyroidism.

Nursing Assessment

1. Ask about alcohol intake, smoking and drug history, and chronic illnesses.

2. Take a nutrition history and 24-hour food intake recall. Review results of laboratory test. Weigh the patient.

3. Observe ability to swallow.

4. Review recommendations of speech-language pathologist and social worker.

5. Assess for independence, self-assuredness, and willingness to try new things; these are strengths on which to build.

6. Assess reality of the patient's expectations.

7. Assess the patient's social support system. Who will be home with the patient after discharge?

Nursing Diagnoses

- Readiness for Enhanced Knowledge about laryngectomy.
- Ineffective Breathing Pattern related to artificial airway, accumulation of secretions, inability to cough secondary to surgical procedure.
- Imbalanced Nutrition: Less Than Body Requirements related to impaired swallowing secondary to surgical alteration of pharynx and larynx; laryngeal edema and pain; radiation-induced mucositis.
- Impaired Verbal Communication related to surgery or absence of larynx; presence of artificial airway.
- Deficient Knowledge related to stoma care and living with effects of laryngectomy.

Nursing Interventions

Preparing for Total Laryngectomy

1. Collaborate with the surgeon in preparing the patient; interpret and amplify what surgeon and speech-language pathologist have explained.
   a. Inform the patient that breathing will occur through an opening (tracheostoma) in the neck.
   b. Advise the patient that speech will be altered by surgery.
2. Expect reactions of anxiety and depression because the psychosocial effects of voice loss are substantial.
3. Practice a means of communication (pad and pencil, sign language, pictures, word cards, artificial larynx) that can be used until speech therapy begins.
4. Arrange for the patient to be visited by laryngectomee (one who has had larynx removed) for support.
5. Provide portable battery-operated suction machine, suction catheter kits, and other supplies from a home care company and educate patient on suctioning procedure prior to the patient's discharge. Initiate referral for home care nursing and other community services.
6. Provide information about other community support services such as the International Association of Laryngectomees or Supporting Patients with Oral Head and Neck Cancer.
7. Reinforce information about alternative modes of communication.
   a. Artificial larynx, using either neck or intraoral placement: Electrolarynx provides communication assistance in early postoperative period or later to those unable to learn alternative method.
   b. Tracheoesophageal puncture with voice prosthesis: A one-way valved voice prosthesis is inserted through tracheoesophageal puncture to allow the patient to shunt pulmonary air into esophagus for voice production (see Figure 17-8).

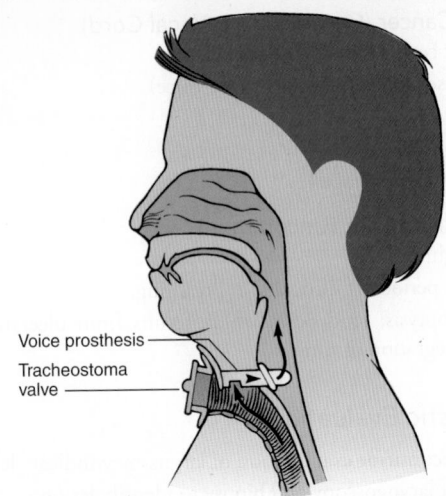

Voice prosthesis

Tracheostoma valve

Figure 17-8. Schematic representation of tracheoesophageal puncture speech. When the patient plugs the stomal opening, air is forced from the lungs through a one-way valve voice prosthesis. Air travels into the esophagus and out the mouth, creating speech.

   c. Esophageal speech is accomplished by training the patient to force air down the esophagus and release it in a controlled manner.

Improving Breathing Pattern

1. Monitor for signs of difficult breathing—suprasternal and intercostal retractions, tachypnea, dyspnea, tachycardia, and changes in sensorium.
2. Auscultate trachea/chest for evidence of stridor or wheezing and for absence of breath sounds.
3. Make sure the patient uses a specific signal to indicate need for suctioning; enter on nursing care plan.
4. Suction secretions according to the prescriber's orders to prevent accumulation of mucus and to prevent mucus plugging.
   a. Also suction nasal secretions because the patient is unable to blow nose.
   b. Remove crusts from stoma at least three times daily to prevent webbing of mucus across the stoma.
5. Use chest physical therapy, as necessary, to remove secretions.
6. Remember that postoperative patient is unable to cough.
   a. Teach the patient to bend forward until stoma is below lung level and to exhale rapidly. This aids in secretion removal from lungs.
   b. Teach the patient to wipe resultant secretions away from tracheostoma with a handkerchief.
7. Encourage breathing exercises because most patients have been heavy smokers.
8. Supply constant humidification to moisten tracheostoma and avoid viscous secretions; tracheal air will require additional warmth and moisture.
9. Keep calm and maintain sense of security.
   a. Reassure the patient that someone is always near to assist.
   b. Have call bell within reach.
10. In the event of clogging or obstruction of the stoma, follow Procedure Guidelines 17-2.

PROCEDURE GUIDELINES 17-2

Emergency First Aid for the Laryngectomee

EQUIPMENT (IF AVAILABLE)

- Suction equipment
- Sterile disposable catheter
  - # 14 to # 16 F (adult)
- Sterile gloves
- Sterile saline
- Portable mask and bag

Nursing Action	Rationale
Performance phase	
1. Place the patient on his or her back on a firm surface, head straight, chin up. Bare the neck down to the sternum.	1. Facilitates access to the laryngeal stoma and observation of thoracic movement.
2. Position a blanket or any article of clothing under the shoulders.	2. Promotes extension of the neck area, permitting access.
3. Make a rapid assessment of the situation:	3.
a. Is victim wearing a tracheostomy or laryngectomy tube?	a. In a laryngectomee, tube removal cannot cause immediate danger.
b. Has patient been operated on recently?	b. If so, tracheostomy tube cannot be removed.
c. Check for tracheal obstruction. Clean stomal opening of mucus and encrusted matter.	c. Mucus and other material may account for obstruction. Use clean cloth or handkerchief—never tissue.
4. Start mouth-to-neck breathing promptly: Position yourself at side of victim. Place your mouth and lips/mask tightly over neck opening or around the tracheal tube if the person is wearing one.	4. Seconds count. Do not remove the tube.
5. If suction equipment is available, insert a soft rubber tube 3–5 inches (7.5–12.5 cm) into opening for a few seconds.	5. A partially open airway transporting air to the victim is infinitely better than a clean airway that does not supply air at this crucial time.
6. Blow in a sufficient amount of air to see chest rise; then release and allow chest to fall.	6. Indicates ventilation.
7. For the first 5 seconds, repeat every 1–2 seconds; then slow down to a steady pace of every 4–5 seconds (12–20 times per minute).	7. Allows air to exhale passively.
8. Continue until spontaneous breathing returns.	
Follow-up phase	
1. When spontaneous breathing occurs, provide oxygen from a portable supply.	1. Relieves hypoxemia.
2. If breathing fails again, resume mouth-to-neck breathing.	
3. You can also use a manual resuscitation bag with an infant-size mask.	3. Attach infant-size mask; be sure there is a tight seal against neck opening. Because a tight seal is difficult to maintain and because pressure of the mask on the major blood vessels of the neck may interfere with blood supply to the brain, mouth-to-neck breathing is safer and better.
4. Watch the chest rise.	4. Easiest way to detect spontaneous breathing.
5. Observe the patient constantly.	

Facilitating Adequate Nutrition

1. Monitor IV fluids during first few postoperative days.
2. Administer fluids and nutrients by NG or gastrostomy tube.
   a. Tube feedings may be started after bowel sounds are heard and continued until sufficient healing of pharynx has occurred (approximately 7 to 14 days) and patient is ready to resume oral feedings.
   b. Avoid manipulating NG tube as it is resting on or near suture line.
   c. Clean nostrils and lubricate with water-soluble lubricant.
   d. Clean crust on outside of tube.
   e. Pay attention to oral hygiene, with regular toothbrushing and prescribed antiseptic mouthwashes.
3. Assure the patient that swallowing is safe and may feel a little differently than before surgery. Some structures and muscles removed during surgery may cause the patient to "work harder" to swallow.
   a. Patients may need more liquids to wash down foods.
   b. It may be easier to eat smaller, more frequent meals.
   c. A modified barium swallow may be ordered several days after surgery to be sure adequate healing has occurred and that there are no leaks or fistulas opening into the airway.
   d. After a total laryngectomy, there is a separation of the airway (trachea) from the esophagus and theoretically there is no risk for aspiration. However, if a tracheo-esophageal puncture (TEP) is present occupied by either a voice prosthesis or red rubber catheter, leakage around the TEP site could occur.
4. The speech-language pathologist will educate the patient and family about the presence, care, and maintenance of the TEP and any potential problems.

Providing Alternative Communication

1. Advise the patient to communicate by writing or with artificial larynx until voice work can begin with speech-language pathologist.
2. Discourage forced whispering, which increases pharyngeal tension.
3. Encourage the patient to join local laryngectomy support group (eg, Lost Chord Club, New Voice Club, International Association of Laryngectomees) which gives opportunity to practice new speech and serves as a bridge between therapy and return to social life.
4. Inform the patient of the various communication methods:
   a. An electromechanical device, which is placed against the neck, cheek, or in the mouth for a monotone, mechanical sound, can be used immediately after surgery. The speech-language pathologist will provide instruction on the use of the device.
   b. Esophageal speech is the act of air charging, which is achieved by thrusting the tongue back and forcing a bolus through the cricopharyngeus. The air bolus then is regurgitated through the pharyngoesophageal segment, which vibrates to produce sound.
   c. Tracheo-esophageal speech, which is the most common voice restoration option, involves placing a one-way valve voice prosthesis into the tracheo-esophageal puncture. The patient takes a breath and occludes the stoma with either a finger or stoma button. This air is forced through the voice prosthesis into the pharynx, which vibrates and produces sound.

Providing Information About Laryngectomy

1. Inform the patient that it is very important to keep the stoma clear of mucus. This is accomplished through regular tracheal suctioning and by cleaning mucus from the stoma several times per day.
2. A laryngectomy or tracheostomy tube may be worn if there is neck edema and narrowing of the stoma. The tube is not always permanent. The type of tube used is determined by the provider or speech-language pathologist.
3. Demonstrate procedure for cleaning and changing tube.
   a. See page 223 for tracheostomy tube care. A laryngectomy tube is cleaned the same way as an inner cannula.
   b. Place gauze dressing under tube to absorb secretions, as prescribed. Change when it becomes soiled to prevent skin irritation and odor.
   c. Encourage the patient to change the laryngectomy or tracheostomy fastener when soiled.
4. Tracheostoma care—teach the patient to:
   a. Wash hands before touching stoma to prevent infection.
   b. Wet washcloth with warm water; wring dry and gently wipe stoma. Do not use soap, tissues, or cotton balls because these may enter airway.
   c. Apply petroleum around exterior of stoma to prevent skin irritation.
   d. Report excessive redness, swelling, purulent secretions, or bleeding.
5. Stoma cover.
   a. Stoma cover is necessary to filter air and increase humidity of air; also necessary for hygienic purposes.
   b. Stoma cover can be crocheted, made of cotton cloth, or commercially available as foam filters.
   c. For men: ascot or turtleneck sweaters may be worn. When a regular shirt is worn, the second button from the top can be sewed over the buttonhole as though it were fastened. This leaves a wide opening through which a handkerchief can be inserted when coughing.
   d. For women: a variety of fashionable scarves, jewelry, high-neck dresses, and turtleneck sweaters can be |worn.
6. Bowel care: discuss high-fiber diet and use of stool softener because patient with tracheostoma is usually not able to hold breath to "bear down" for bowel movement.
7. If the patient snored before surgery, they will no longer snore after laryngectomy since air no longer passes through the nose and mouth. For the same reason, the patient may have difficulty sniffing and blowing his or her nose. The speech-language pathologist can provide techniques for briefly sniffing through the nose.

8. Swallowing after laryngectomy will resume no sooner than 7 days after surgery. A barium swallow may be ordered to detect a leak in the internal incision line. Swallowing may be a little slower and or more difficult. The speech-language pathologist will provide swallowing therapy.

Community and Home Care Considerations

1. Provide humidification in the home; use pans of water in the rooms, a humidifier, or cool-mist vaporizer, especially in bedroom and when dry heat is used.
2. Tell the patient to avoid cold air; cover tracheostoma with thin layer of foam or other cover to warm and humidify air.
3. Encourage the patient to drink fluids liberally (2 to 3 qt [2 to 3 L]) to help liquefy secretions.
4. Have the patient always keep stoma covered for hygienic management of secretions and to keep dust and foreign matter from entering trachea.
5. Place a protective shield over stoma before bathing, showering, or shampooing hair and while getting a haircut or shaving. Use an electric razor instead of blade because shaving cream can irritate.
6. Swimming is not recommended as there is no way to prevent water from entering the stoma.
7. Ensure working smoke detectors are available in the home as the sense of smell is decreased.

Patient Education and Health Maintenance

1. Tell the patient to expect some loss of smell and taste sensation.
2. Advise the patient to check with health care provider before taking medication because many drugs (such as antihistamines and cold products) tend to dry the mucous membranes of the stoma.
3. Warn the patient to seek immediate attention for pain, difficulty breathing or swallowing, appearance of pus or blood-streaked sputum.

Evaluation: Expected Outcomes

- Verbalizes understanding of tracheostoma and communication options.
- Breathes quietly; no evidence of noisy secretions.
- Swallows soft foods; maintains weight.
- Makes needs known; speech therapy has started.
- Manages tracheostomal care; has made provisions for home humidification and tracheostomal supplies.

SELECTED REFERENCES

Armstrong, W. B., Vokes, D. E., & Marsel, R. H. (2010). Malignant tumors of the larynx. In P. W. Flint, B. H. Haughey, V. J. Lund, et al. (Eds.), *Cummings otolaryngology head and neck surgery* (5th ed.), 1482–1511. Philadelphia: Elsevier.

Baugher, K. M, Somers Hemme, T., Harkshaw, M., et al. (2011). MRSA otorrhea: A case series and review of the literature. *Ear, Nose, and Throat Journal, 90*(2), 60-79.

Bozetti, R. (2011). Nutritional support in oncologic patients: Where are we and where are we going? *Clinical Nutrition, 30*(6), 714-717.

Branstetter, I. V., & Barton, F. (2010). Diagnostic imaging of the pharynx and esophagus. In P. W. Flint, B. H. Haughey, V. J. Lund, et al. (Eds.), *Cummings otolaryngology head and neck surgery* (5th ed.), 1393–1420. Philadelphia: Elsevier.

Distler, J. W. (2011). Environmental allergens: Diagnoses and management of Ig-E mediated disorders. *American Journal of Nurse Practitioners, 15*(9/10), 14–24.

Gulya, A. J., Minor, L. B., Poe, D. S. People's Medical Publishing House (2010). *Glasscock-Shambaugh surgery of the ear* (6th ed.). Shelton, CT: People's Medical.

Gillison, M., Alemany, L., Snijders, P., et al. (2012). Human papillomavirus and diseases of the upper airway: head and neck cancer and respiratory papillomatosis. *Vaccine, 30S*, F34–54.

Hain, T. C. (2009). Vestibular neuritis and labyrinthitis. Available: *www.dizziness-and-balance.com/disorders/unilat/vneurit.html*.

Hamid, M., & Bookler, K. H. (2007). Tympanometry. *Ear, Nose, and Throat Journal, 86*(11), 668–669.

Harreus, U. (2012). Malignant neoplasms of the oropharynx, in Flint, P.W., et al., Cummings Otolaryngology Head and Neck Surgery (5th ed.). Philadelphia: Elsevier.

Harris, L. L., & Huntoon, M. B. (2008). *Core curriculum for otolrhinolaryngology and head and neck nursing* (2nd ed.). New Smyrna Beach, FL: Society of Otorhinolaryngology and Head and Neck Nurses.

Harvey, R., Hannan, S. A., Badia, L., et al. (2007). Nasal saline irrigations for the symptoms of chronic rhinosinusitis. *Cochrane Database of Systematic Reviews*, Issue 3. Available: *http://summaries.cochrane.org/CD006394/nasal-irrigation-with-saline-salt-water-for-the-symptoms-of-chronic-rhinosinusitis*.

Jensen, G. L., Hsiao, P. Y., & Wheeler, D. (2012). Nutritional screening and assessment. In Mueller, C. M., Kovacevich, D. S., McClave, S. A., et al. (eds), *The A.S.P.E.N. Adult Nutrition Support Core Curriculum* (2nd ed.). USA: American Society for Parenteral Enteral Nutrition, 155–169.

Kellman, R. M. (2010). Maxillofacial trauma. In P. W., Flint, B. H. Haughey, V. J. Lund, et al. (Eds.), *Cummings otolaryngology head and neck surgery* (5th ed.), 318–341. Philadelphia: Elsevier.

Maragos, C. S. (2009). Improving quality of life with FESS. *OR Nurse, 3*(4), 4–29.

Marur, S., D'Souza, G., Westra, W., et al. (2010). HPV-associated head and neck cancer: a virus-related cancer epidemic. *Lancet, 11*(8), 781–789.

Mitchell, T., & Turton, P. (2011). 'Chemobrain': Concentration and memory effects in people receiving chemotherapy—A descriptive phenomenolgical study. *European Journal of Cancer Care, 20*, 539–548.

Mueller, C. (2012). Nutritional screening and assessment In N. M. Gottschlich, M. H. DeLegge, T. Mattox, et al. (Eds.), *The ASPEN Nutrition Support Core Curriculum: A case-based approach–The Adult patient.* Silver Spring, MD: American Society for Parenteral and Enteral Nutrition.

Niparko, J. K., Mellon, N. K., & Kirk, K. I. (2009). Cochlear implants: Principles and practices (2nd ed.). Philadelphia: Wolters Kluwer/ Lippincott, Williams & Wilkins.

Pichichero, M. E., Sexton, D., & Edwards, M. (2011). Treatment and prevention of streptococcal tonsillopharyngitis. Available: *www.uptodate.com/contents/treatment-and-prevention-of-streptococcal-tonsillopharyngitis*.

Popovtzer, A., & Eisbruch, A. (2010). Radiotherapy for head and neck cancer:Radiation physics, radiobiology and clinical principles. In P. W., Flint, B. H. Haughey, V. J. Lund, et al. (Eds.), *Cummings otolaryngology head and neck surgery* (5th ed.), 1030–1050. Philadelphia: Elsevier.

Robbins, K.T., Samant, S., & Ronewn, O. (2010). Neck dissection. In P. W., Flint, B. H. Haughey, V. J. Lund, et al. (Eds.), *Cummings otolaryngology head and neck surgery* (5th ed.), 1702–1725. Philadelphia: Elsevier.

Roland, P. S., Smith, T. L., Schwartz, S. R. (2008). Clinical practice guidelines: Cerumen impaction. *Otolaryngology and Head and Neck Surgery, 139*, S1–S21.

Rosenfield, R. M., Andes, D., Bhattacharyya, N., et al. (2007). AAOHNS clinical practice guideline: Adult sinusitis. *Otolarynogology and Head and Neck Surgery, 137*, S1–S31.

Rosenfield, R. M., Culpepper, L., & Doyle, K. J. (2004). Clinical practice guideline: Otitis media with effusion. *Otolaryngology and Head and Neck Surgery, 130*, S95–118.

Rosenfield, R. M, Singer, M., & Jones, S. (2007). AAOHNS Clinical practice guideline: Systematic Review of antimicrobial therapy in patients with acute rhinosinusitis. *Otolaryngology and Head and Neck Surgery, 137*, S32–45.

Rossekh, C. H., & Haughey, B. H. (2010). Total laryngectomy and laryngopharyngectomy. In P. W., Flint, B. H. Haughey, V. J. Lund, et al. (Eds.), *Cummings otolaryngology head and neck surgery* (5th ed.), 1563–1576. Philadelphia: Elsevier.

Rotter, B. E. (2010). Temporomnandibular joint disorders. In P. W., Flint, B. H. Haughey, V. J. Lund, et al. (Eds.), *Cummings otolaryngology head and neck surgery* (5th ed.). Philadelphia: Elsevier.

Ship, J. A., & Turner, M. D. (2010) Oral manifestations of systemic disease. In P. W., Flint, B. H. Haughey, V. J. Lund, et al. (Eds.), *Cummings otolaryngology head and neck surgery* (5th ed.), 1245–1258. Philadelphia: Elsevier.

Tan, L., & Loh, T. (2010). Benigns and malignant tumors of the neopharynx. In P. W., Flint, B. H. Haughey, V. J. Lund, et al. (Eds.), *Cummings otolaryngology head and neck surgery* (5th ed.), 1348–1357. Philadelphia: Elsevier.

Tardy, M. E., & Thomas, J. R. (2010). Rhinoplasty. P. W., Flint, B. H. Haughey, V. J. Lund, et al. (Eds.), *Cummings otolaryngology head and neck surgery* (5th ed.), 508–544. Philadelphia: Elsevier.

University of Texas, School of Nursing, Family Nurse Practitioner Program.(2007). Evaluation and management of obstructing cerumen. Austin: University of Texas, School of Nursing. Available: *www.guidelines.gov.*

U.S. Food and Drug Administration. Is Rinsing Your Sinuses Safe? FDA Consumer Health Information. August 2012. Available: *www.FDA.gov/consumer/consumer news.*

Weymuller, E. A., & Davis, G. E. (2010). Malignancies of the paranasal sinuses. In P. W., Flint, B. H. Haughey, V. J. Lund, et al. (Eds.), *Cummings otolaryngology head and neck surgery* (5th ed.). Philadelphia: Elsevier.

18
Gastrointestinal Disorders

OVERVIEW AND ASSESSMENT

The gastrointestinal (GI) system is comprised of the alimentary canal and its accessory organs. The alimentary canal begins at the mouth and extends through the pharynx, esophagus, stomach, small intestine, colon, and rectum, and ends at the anus. The accessory organs include the teeth, salivary glands, liver, pancreas, and spleen.

The functions of the GI system include ingestion and propulsion of food; mechanical and chemical digestion of food; synthesis of nutrients, such as vitamin K; absorption of nutrients into the bloodstream; and the storage and elimination of nondigestible waste products from the body through feces.

See Standards of Care Guidelines 18-1, page 642.

Subjective Data

A comprehensive health history should be obtained to elicit subjective data related to major manifestations of GI problems. Common manifestations include nutritional problems, abdominal pain, indigestion, nausea, vomiting, diarrhea, constipation, bloody bowel movements, change in bowel habits, weight loss, and dysphagia.

STANDARDS OF CARE GUIDELINES 18-1
Gastrointestinal Dysfunction

When caring for a patient after abdominal surgery or with any type of GI disorder:

- Make sure that adequate bowel sounds are present before allowing anything by mouth. Periodically reassess for bowel sounds, bloating, nausea, vomiting, and abdominal distension or tenderness.
- Monitor food/fluid intake and output as indicated.
- Periodically monitor weight, and watch for trend in weight loss or weight gain.
- Assess stools for frequency, consistency, color, and amount.
- Report increase in pain, fever, nausea, vomiting, bloating, change in stools, or signs of wound infection to health care provider promptly.
- Monitor complete blood count, electrolytes, albumin, and protein as directed.

This information should serve as a general guideline only. Each patient situation presents a unique set of clinical factors and requires nursing judgment to guide care, which may include additional or alternative measures and approaches.

Nutritional Problems

1. Characteristics: What is your typical 24-hour food intake? What is your usual weight? Has there been a recent weight gain or loss? If a recent weight change, how many pounds and over what time period? How is your appetite?
2. Associated factors: Explore other factors that may influence weight changes—food preferences; family/individual routines associated with eating; cultural and religious values; psychological factors, such as depression, anxiety, stress; physical factors, such as activity level, health status, dental problems, allergies; access/transportation to grocery stores; eating habits, self-imposed dietary restrictions; body image; nutritional knowledge; finances.
3. History: Any history of eating disorders? Any family history of ulcer, GI cancer, inflammatory bowel disease, obesity?

Abdominal Pain

1. Characteristics: Can you describe the pain (sharp, dull, superficial, or deep)? Is the pain intermittent or continuous? Was the onset sudden or gradual? Can you point to where the pain is located? What makes the pain better, worse?
2. Associated factors: Are there other symptoms associated with the pain—fever, chills, night sweats, nausea, vomiting, diarrhea, constipation, anorexia, weight loss, dyspepsia, black tarry stools or blood in the stool?
3. History: Any family history of GI cancer, ulcer disease, inflammatory bowel disease? Any previous history of tumors, malignancy, ulcers?

Indigestion (Dyspepsia)

1. Characteristics: Have you experienced any of the following symptoms—a feeling of fullness, heartburn, excessive belching, flatus, nausea, a bad taste, mild or severe pain? How is your appetite? If pain or tenderness, where is it located? Does the pain radiate to any other areas? What precipitating factors are associated with the pain? What makes the symptoms better, worse? Are the symptoms associated with food intake? If associated with food, the amount and type?
2. Associated factors: Is there nausea, vomiting, dysphagia, blood in bowel movements, or diarrhea? Is there a history of alcohol, nonsteroidal anti-inflammatory drug (NSAID), bisphosphonate, or aspirin use?
3. History: Any family history of cancer, inflammatory bowel disease? Any history of bowel obstruction? Any previous abdominal surgeries?

Nausea and Vomiting

1. Characteristics: Is the nausea or vomiting associated with certain stimuli, such as specific foods, odors, activity, or a certain time of day? Does it occur before or after food intake? How many times per day does vomiting occur? What specific fluids/foods can be tolerated when vomiting occurs? What is the amount, color, odor, and consistency of the vomitus (see Table 18-1)?
2. Associated factors: Is there fever, headache, dizziness, weakness, or diarrhea? Missed menstrual period? Any weight loss? Any new medications? Any psychological stress, depression, or emotional problems?
3. History: Any history of gallbladder disease? Ulcer disease? GI cancer? Unprotected intercourse?

Diarrhea

1. Characteristics: How long has the diarrhea been present? Determine the frequency, consistency, color, quantity, and odor of stools. Are there blood, mucus, pus, or food particles in the stools? Does this represent a change in bowel habits?

Table 18-1   Nature of Vomitus

COLOR/TASTE/CONSISTENCY	POSSIBLE SOURCE
Yellowish or greenish	• May contain bile • Medication—senna
Bright red (arterial)	• Hemorrhage, peptic ulcer
Dark red (venous)	• Hemorrhage, esophageal or gastric varices
"Coffee grounds"	• Digested blood from slowly bleeding gastric or duodenal ulcer
Undigested food	• Gastric tumor • Ulcer, obstruction • Gastric paresis
"Bitter" taste	• Bile
"Sour" or "acid"	• Gastric contents
Fecal components	• Intestinal obstruction

BOX 18-1　Causes of Diarrhea and Constipation

CAUSES OF DIARRHEA

- Infectious agents (*Escherichia coli, Salmonella, Shigella, Campylobacter, Giardia, Amoeba, Clostridium difficile, Yersinia, Cyclospora, Cryptosporidium, Rotavirus*)
- Drugs (antibiotics, magnesium)
- Fecal impaction
- Bowel disease (irritable bowel syndrome, ulcerative colitis, Crohn's disease)
- Malabsorption syndromes (lactose intolerance, celiac sprue, fat malabsorption)
- Short bowel syndrome
- Malignant syndromes (Zollinger-Ellison syndrome, carcinoid syndrome)

CAUSES OF CONSTIPATION

- Inadequate fluid intake
- Psychological factors
- Electrolyte imbalances
- Hormonal abnormalities, such as hypothyroidism
- Mechanical bowel obstruction, ileus
- Drugs (laxative abuse, anticholinergic agents, calcium channel blockers, opiates)
- Loss of innervation (Hirschsprung's disease)
- Neuromuscular (paralysis, spinal cord injury or sacral lesion, multiple sclerosis)
- Anorectal disorders (hemorrhoids, fecal impaction, cancer, abscess, fissures)
- Sedentary lifestyle

Any nocturnal diarrhea? What makes the diarrhea worse, better? Any associated weight loss? (see Box 18-1).

2. Associated factors: Any fever, nausea, vomiting, abdominal pain, abdominal distention, flatus, cramping, urgency with straining? Is the patient taking antibiotics? Has there been any recent travel to foreign countries? (Mexico, South America, Africa, and Asia are countries with the highest risk of traveler's diarrhea.) Is the patient experiencing emotional stress or anxiety? Are there any recently prescribed medications?

3. History: Is there a history of celiac disease, colon cancer, ulcerative colitis, Crohn's disease, malabsorption syndrome? Has the patient undergone surgery recently (eg, bariatric surgery)?

DRUG ALERT Obtain history of over-the-counter (OTC), herbal, or "natural" products the patient may be taking. Ginger is commonly used as an antiemetic and, although generally safe, it can cause heartburn. Licorice root is used for upset stomach and to soothe ulcers, but can cause sodium and fluid retention and loss of potassium. Goldenseal is used as an antidiarrheal, but can cause a number of adverse reactions, including skin and mucous membrane irritation, interference with anticoagulation, and cardiac and nervous system excitability. Also, many herbs can impair absorption of other medicines. Remind patients that herbal products are not found naturally in the body or in significant amounts in the daily diet, so should be treated like drugs.

Constipation

1. Characteristics: What is the frequency, consistency, color of the stools? Is this a change in bowel habits? If a change, has this been gradual or sudden? What is the size of the stools? Have there been dietary changes? Is there blood or mucus in the stools? Any laxative use?

2. Associated factors: Are there periods of diarrhea? Is there abdominal pain or distention? Is the patient experiencing stress? Is there a change in activity level? Does the patient have a regular time for defecation? Does the patient use antacids containing calcium or an anticholinergic? Have there been any fevers, chills, night sweats, or weight loss?

3. History: Any family history of colorectal cancer? Any history of depression or metabolic disorders, such as hypothyroidism or hypercalcemia?

Dysphagia

1. Characteristics: Is the onset acute or gradual? Is the problem with swallowing intermittent or continuous? Is this associated with solid foods, liquids, or both? Has there been any nasal regurgitation? Where does the food stick: neck (cricopharyngeal), midesophagus, or sternal xiphoid process?

2. Associated factors: Is there any regurgitation, heartburn, chest or back pain, weight loss? Any hoarseness, voice change, or sore throat? Have there been any fevers, chills, night sweats, or weight loss?

3. History: Is there a family history of esophageal cancer? Is there a history of stroke, palsy, or any other neurologic conditions? Is there a history of alcohol or tobacco intake?

Physical Examination

When performing a physical examination of the abdomen, include the following: inspection of the abdomen, auscultation of all four abdominal quadrants, percussion for tympany or dullness, light and deep palpation.

NURSING ALERT Auscultation should be performed before percussion and palpation, which may stimulate bowel sounds. Deep palpation in noted areas of tenderness or pain should be performed last.

Key Findings

1. Tenting of the skin when skin is rolled between thumb and index finger. Tenting may indicate dehydration.

2. Mouth lesions, missing teeth, swollen or bleeding gums may contribute to weight loss and nutritional deficiencies.

3. Body weight may indicate obesity or such problems as anorexia nervosa or malignancy.

4. Palpable mass may indicate an enlarged organ, inflammation, malignancy, hernia.

5. Rebound tenderness, guarding, and rigidity may indicate appendicitis, cholecystitis, peritonitis, pancreatitis, duodenal ulcer.

6. Protuberant or bulging abdomen or flanks can indicate ascites. Two physical assessment skills that may help to confirm the

presence of ascites are testing for shifting dullness and testing for a fluid wave.

7. Distention and absence of bowel sounds may indicate intestinal obstruction.

Characteristics of Stool

1. The appearance of blood in stool may be characteristic of its source.
   a. Upper GI bleeding—tarry black (melena).
   b. Lower GI bleeding—bright red blood.
   c. Lower rectal or anal bleeding—blood streaking on surface of stool or on toilet paper.
2. Other characteristics of stool may indicate a particular GI problem.
   a. Bulky, greasy, foamy, foul smelling, gray with silvery sheen—steatorrhea (fatty stool).
   b. Light gray "clay-colored" (due to absence of bile pigments, acholic)—biliary obstruction.
   c. Mucus or pus visible—chronic ulcerative colitis, shigellosis.
   d. Small, dry, rocky-hard masses—constipation, obstruction.
   e. Marble-size stool pellets—irritable bowel syndrome.

Laboratory Tests

Laboratory tests for GI disorders include a variety of stool studies and blood tests.

 Evidence Base Rex, D. K., Johnson, D. A., Anderson, J. C., et al. (2009). American College of Gastroenterology guidelines for colorectal cancer screening 2009 (corrected). *American Journal of Gastroenterology, 104,* 739–750.

Fecal Immunochemical Test (FIT) for Occult Blood Detection

Description

An immunochemical test card has antibodies that detect human hemoglobin in stool. This test is used to screen for colon cancer and is preferred over the stool guaiac tests due to higher sensitivity and ease of use (eg, no dietary restrictions).

Nursing and Patient Care Considerations

1. Advise patient not to collect specimen during menstruation or if hemorrhoidal bleeding is present. Usually, at least 2 stool specimens need to be collected, on separate occasions.
2. Collect specimen or advise patient regarding proper collection of specimen.
   a. Place collection paper on top of water in toilet.
   b. Sit on toilet and proceed with bowel movement so that stool will be on top of collection paper.
   c. Use the sample probe and brush across the stool sample so that groove of probe is filled with stool (obtain sample from several different locations within the stool).
   d. Insert probe back into sample container and tighten lid of container.
   e. Write date on sample container label.

3. Put container with stool sample into plastic bag and deliver to lab within 7 days (or if point-of-service test, follow manufacturer instructions for processing).

Stool Guaiac Tests for Occult Blood

Description

Commercially available guaiac-impregnated slides or wipes test feces for blood. May be used as another option for colon cancer screening.

Nursing and Patient Care Considerations

1. Advise patient about the test preparation procedure. Common practices are listed below. For 3 days before the test and during the stool collection period:
   a. Diet should have a high fiber content.
   b. Avoid red meat in the diet.
   c. Avoid foods with a high peroxidase content, such as turnips, cauliflower, broccoli, horseradish, and melon.
   d. Avoid iron preparations, iodides, bromides, aspirin, NSAIDs, or vitamin C supplements greater than 250 mg/day.
   e. Avoid enemas or laxatives before stool specimen collection.
2. Collect sample or advise patient on collection procedure.
   a. A wooden applicator is used to apply a stool specimen to the slide, or a special wipe is used and placed in the packet.
   b. Avoid urine or toilet tissue contamination.
3. When hydrogen peroxide (denatured alcohol-stabilizing mixture) is added to samples, any blood cells present liberate their hemoglobin, and a bluish ring appears on the electrophoretic paper. Read precisely at 30 seconds.
4. Three stool samples are taken because of the possibility of intermittent bleeding and false-negative results.
   a. A single positive test is an indication for further diagnostic evaluation for GI lesions.
   b. False-positive results occur in about 10% of tests.
   c. Test may become false-negative in 10% of specimens tested 4 or more days after streaking on paper.

Stool DNA Test

Description

This test detects DNA associated with colon cancer. Cells are shed from the tumor into the intestinal lumen as stool passes through. Procedure is similar to guaiac tests.

Other Common Stool Studies

Description

There are multiple types of stool analyses that are helpful in detecting conditions affecting the GI tract, liver, and pancreas. Basic stool examination is for amount, consistency, and color. Normal color varies from light to dark brown, but various foods and medications may affect stool color. Additional testing may include tests for ova and parasistes; stool cultures that can identify viruses and bacteria; fecal leukocytes; fecal fat, which can help in the diagnosis of malabsorption syndromes; and stool for *Helicobacter pylori,* which is performed about 4 weeks after treatment to confirm eradication.

Nursing and Patient Care Considerations

1. Use a tongue blade to place a small amount of fresh stool in a container. The container may be sterile or may have a preservative depending on which test has been ordered. Remind patient not to mix urine or toilet paper in specimen.
2. Save a sample of fecal material if unusual in appearance, contains worms or blood, blood streaked, unusual in color, or has excess mucus; show to health care provider.
3. For accurate specimen results, the vials must be sent to the laboratory as soon as possible. Certain stool studies allow for refrigeration of the sample, but this is test dependent.
4. Send specimens to be examined for parasites to the laboratory immediately so the parasites may be observed under a microscope while viable, fresh, and warm.
5. Test for occult blood or to confirm grossly visible melena or blood—Hemoccult guaiac test.
6. Consider that barium, bismuth, mineral oil, and antibiotics may alter the results.

Hydrogen Breath Test

Description

1. The hydrogen breath test is used to evaluate carbohydrate malabsorption and maldigestion, detect the presence of excess bacteria in the small intestine, and to estimate small bowel transit time.
2. A substance, such as lactulose, lactose, or another carbohydrate is ingested and, after a certain time period, exhaled gases are measured.
3. The test measures the amount of hydrogen, methane, and carbon dioxide produced in the colon, absorbed in the blood, and then exhaled in the breath. The levels of hydrogen and methane are indicators of bacterial metabolism in the small intestine.
4. This test is diagnostic for lactose intolerance, other carbohydrate malabsorption syndromes, and small intestine bacterial overgrowth (SIBO).

Nursing and Patient Care Considerations

1. Patient should have nothing-by-mouth (NPO) for 12 hours before the procedure.
2. Patient should not smoke after midnight before the test.
3. Antibiotics and laxatives/enemas should not be used for 1 week before the test. These products may alter the laboratory results.
4. Appropriate diet instructions should be given before discharge if the test is positive.

Helicobacter pylori *Testing*

Description

1. Diagnostic tests for *H. pylori* include a serum antibody test, urea breath test, and fecal antigen test. Alternatively, if an endoscopy is being performed, then biopsies of the gastric mucosa can be evaluated for *H. pylori* with rapid urea testing, histology review by a pathologist, or culture, or polymerase chain reaction testing.
2. A positive serum antibody test may not differentiate between current or past disease.
3. The urea breath test and fecal antigen test are useful in detecting active *H. pylori* prior to treatment with antibiotics. Both of these tests can be used to confirm eradication after antibiotic therapy has been completed.

Nursing and Patient Care Considerations

1. Symptomatic patients and patients with an active or past history of ulcer disease or with gastric MALT lymphoma should be tested for *H. pylori*. Endoscopy may be necessary for patients with symptoms of weight loss, anemia, or occult blood loss and for patients older than age 50.
2. It is recommended that negative *H. pylori* test results in a patient with ulcer-related complications be confirmed by a second test.
3. Describe the procedure for urea breath testing to the patient.
   a. Antibiotics, proton-pump inhibitors, and bismuth preparations must be held for 2 weeks prior to testing.
   b. Food and fluids should be held for at least 1 hour prior to testing.
   c. A baseline breath sample will be taken by having the patient breathe into a container, then patient will ingest a carbon-labeled urea substance, and a final breath sample will be taken shortly after ingestion.
   d. The whole process takes about 40 minutes.

 Evidence Base Quest Diagnostics. (2012). *Helicobacter pylori* urea breath test. Available: *www.questdiagnostics.com/hcp/topics/gastroent/hpylori_breath.html*.

4. When confirming eradication of *H. pylori*, testing should not be done earlier than 4 weeks posttreatment.
5. False-positive results from *H. pylori* breath testing may be caused by achlorhydria or urease production associated with other GI disorders.

Radiology and Imaging Studies
Upper GI Series and Small-Bowel Series

Description

1. Upper GI series and small-bowel series are fluoroscopic x-ray examinations of the esophagus, stomach, and small intestine after the patient ingests barium sulfate.
2. As the barium passes through the GI tract, fluoroscopy outlines the GI mucosa and organs.
3. Spot films record significant findings.
4. Double-contrast studies administer barium first, followed by a radiolucent substance, such as air, to produce a thin layer of barium to coat the mucosa. This allows for better visualization of any type of lesion.

Nursing and Patient Care Considerations

1. Explain procedure to patient.
2. Instruct patient to maintain low-residue diet for 2 to 3 days before test and a clear liquid dinner the night before the procedure.
3. Emphasize NPO after midnight before the test.
4. Encourage patient to avoid smoking before the test.
5. Explain that the health care provider may prescribe all opioids and anticholinergics to be withheld 24 hours before the test because they interfere with small-intestine motility. Other medications may be taken with sips of water, if ordered.
6. Explain that the patient will be instructed at various times throughout the procedure to drink the barium (480 to 600 mL).

7. Explain that a cathartic will be prescribed after the procedure to facilitate expulsion of barium.

8. Instruct patient that stool will be light in color for the next 2 to 3 days from the barium.

9. Instruct patient to notify health care provider if he has not passed the barium in 2 to 3 days because retention of the barium may cause obstruction or fecal impaction.

10. Note that a water-soluble iodinated contrast agent (eg, Gastrografin) may be used for a patient with a suspected perforation or colonic obstruction. Barium is toxic to the body if it leaks into the peritoneum with perforation. It can also worsen an obstruction, thus it is not used if an obstruction is suspected.

Barium Enema

Description

1. Fluoroscopic x-ray examination visualizing the entire large intestine is administered after the patient is given an enema of barium sulfate.

2. Can visualize structural changes, such as tumors, polyps, diverticula, fistulas, obstructions, and ulcerative colitis.

3. Air may be introduced after the barium to provide a double-contrast study.

Nursing and Patient Care Considerations

1. Explain to patient:
   a. What the x-ray procedure involves.
   b. That proper preparation provides a more accurate view of the tract and that preparations may vary.
   c. That it is important to retain the barium so all surfaces of the tract are coated with opaque solution.

2. Instruct patient on the objective of having the large intestine as clear of fecal material as possible:
   a. Patient may be given a low-fiber, low-fat diet 1 to 3 days before the examination.
   b. The day before examination, intake may be limited to clear liquids (no drinks with red dye).
   c. The day before the examination, an oral laxative, suppository, and/or cleansing enema may be prescribed.

3. Patient will be NPO after midnight the day of the procedure.

4. An enema or cathartic may be ordered after the barium enema to cleanse bowel of barium and prevent impaction.

5. Inform patient that barium may cause light-colored stools for several days after the procedure.

NURSING ALERT If barium enema and upper GI series are both ordered, the upper GI series is done last so that barium traveling down the digestive tract does not interfere with the results of the barium enema.

Ultrasonography (Ultrasound)

Description

1. A noninvasive test that focuses high-frequency sound waves over an abdominal organ to obtain an image of the structure.

2. Ultrasound can detect small abdominal masses, fluid-filled cysts, gallstones, dilated bile ducts, ascites, and vascular abnormalities.

3. Doppler ultrasonography may be ordered for vascular assessment.

Nursing and Patient Care Considerations

1. An ultrasound should be done prior to barium studies, or at least 24 hours after barium administration because it may interfere with the images.

2. Abdominal ultrasound usually requires patient to be NPO for at least 6 hours before the procedure.

3. Change position of patient, as indicated, for better visualization of certain organs.

Computed Tomography (CT)

Description

1. CT is an x-ray technique that provides excellent anatomic definition and is used to detect tumors, cysts, and abscesses.

2. The CT scan can also reveal masses, dilated bile ducts, pancreatic inflammation, and some gallstones.

3. It identifies changes in intestinal wall thickness and mesenteric abnormalities.

4. Ultrasound and CT can be used to perform guided needle aspiration of fluid or cells from lesions anywhere in the abdomen. The fluid or cells are then sent for laboratory tests (eg, cytology or culture).

Nursing and Patient Care Considerations

1. Instruct patient to fast for 4 hours before the procedure. Patient can take usual medications with a sip of water, but should hold diabetic medications.

2. A pregnancy test should be obtained on females of childbearing potential. If pregnant, do not proceed with scan and notify health care provider.

3. Ask if there are known allergies to iodine or contrast media. Intravenous (IV) administration of contrast medium may be performed to provide better visualization of body parts. If allergic, notify the technician and health care provider immediately.

4. Instruct patient to report symptoms of itching or shortness of breath if receiving contrast media, and observe patient closely.

Endoscopic Procedures

 Evidence Base Scholten, S. R. (2010). Endoscopy: A guide for the registered nurse. *Critical Care Nursing Clinics of North America, 22*(1), 19–32.

Endoscopy is the use of a flexible tube (the fiber-optic endoscope) to visualize the GI tract and to perform certain diagnostic and therapeutic procedures. Images are produced through a video screen or telescopic eyepiece. The tip of the endoscope moves in four directions, allowing for wide-angle visualization. The endoscope can be inserted through the rectum or mouth, depending on which portion of the GI tract is to be viewed. Capsule endoscopy utilizes an ingestible camera device rather than an endoscope.

Endoscopes contain multipurpose channels that allow for air insufflation, irrigation, fluid aspiration, and the passage of special instruments. These instruments include biopsy forceps, cytology brushes, needles, wire baskets, laser probes, and electrocautery snares.

Endoscopic functions other than visualization include biopsy or cytology of lesions, removal of foreign objects or polyps, control of internal bleeding, and opening of strictures.

Capsule Endoscopy

Description

1. Adjunctive diagnostic tool used to detect abnormalities of the small bowel (angiodysplasias, areas of active bleeding, polyps, ulcerations, tumors or causes of diarrhea, and nutritional malabsorption).
2. The procedure involves swallowing a capsule (camera device), which passes through the digestive system while taking pictures of the intestine.
3. Images are transmitted to sensor array abdominal leads, which are attached to a Walkman-like recording device belted to the patient's waist.
4. After approximately 8 hours, the recording device is removed and is connected to a computer to download the images for review. The capsule will be excreted naturally through the digestive tract.

 NURSING ALERT Capsule endoscopy is contraindicated for patients with small bowel obstruction, dysphagia, fistulas, severe delayed gastric emptying, gastrectomy with gastrojejunostomy, or GI stricture. There is a risk of trapping the capsule, delayed passage, or impaired peristalsis. Pacemakers or implanted defibrillators may alter the quality and quantity of study information.

Nursing and Patient Care Considerations

1. Give patient instructions on bowel prep. Inform patient that a good bowel prep allows for better pictures. Patient will be NPO for about 12 hours before swallowing the camera.
2. Oral medications are discontinued 2 hours before the study. Antispasmodics, bismuth preparations, and antidiarrheal medications should be held for 24 hours before the study. Iron preparations and Carafate should be held 5 days before the study to prevent mucosal staining.
3. Instruct patient not to smoke 24 hours before the procedure to prevent mucosal staining.
4. Instruct patient to avoid strenuous activity, heavy lifting, bending or stooping, or immersion in water while wearing the leads and recorder. This is to prevent detachment of the leads or damage of the recorder.
5. After ingesting the capsule, patient is instructed not to eat or drink for at least 2 hours, then can advance to clear liquids. After 4 hours, patient can have a light snack and medications. When the procedure is completed, patient can resume a normal diet.
6. During the capsule endoscopy procedure, instruct the patient to check the blinking light on the top of the data recorder every 15 minutes. Avoid radio equipment (ham radio or broadcasting towers), which may interfere with the capsule's signal.
7. The capsule is naturally excreted within 1 to 3 days. Patient should be instructed to call the physician for the following symptoms: abdominal bloating or pain, chest pain, vomiting, or fever. These symptoms may indicate that the capsule has obstructed the GI tract.

NURSING ALERT The patient should verify excretion of the capsule before undergoing MRI.

Esophagogastroduodenoscopy (EGD)

Description

1. Allows for visualization of the esophagus, stomach, and duodenum.
2. EGD can be used to diagnose acute or chronic upper GI bleeding, esophageal or gastric varices, polyps, malignancy, ulcers, gastritis, esophagitis, esophageal stenosis, and gastroesophageal reflux.
3. Instruments passed through the scope can be used to perform a biopsy or cytologic study, remove polyps or foreign bodies, control bleeding, or open strictures.

Nursing and Patient Care Considerations

1. Ensure that patient is NPO for 6 to 12 hours before the procedure to prevent aspiration and allow for complete visualization of the stomach.
2. Remove dentures and partial plates to facilitate passing the scope and preventing injury.
3. As an outpatient, advise that someone must accompany the patient to drive home due to the patient being sedated.
4. Inform the health care provider of any known allergies and current medications. Medications may be held until after the test is completed.
5. Obtain prior x-rays, and send with patient.
6. Describe what will occur during and after the procedure:
   a. The throat will be anesthetized with a spray or gargle.
   b. An IV sedative will be administered.
   c. Patient will be positioned on the left side with a towel or basin at the mouth to catch secretions.
   d. A plastic mouthpiece will be used to help relax the jaw and protect the endoscope. Emphasize that this will not interfere with breathing.
   e. Patient may be asked to swallow once while the endoscope is being advanced. Then patient should not swallow, talk, or move tongue. Secretions should drain from the side of the mouth, and the mouth may be suctioned.
   f. Air is inserted during the procedure to permit better visualization of the GI tract. Most of the air is removed at the end of the procedure. Patient may feel bloated, burp, or pass flatus from remaining air.
   g. Keep patient NPO according to protocol until patient is alert and gag reflex has returned.
   h. May resume regular diet after gag reflex returns and fluids are tolerated.
   i. May experience a sore throat for 24 to 36 hours after the procedure. When the gag reflex has returned, throat lozenges or warm saline gargles may be prescribed for comfort.
7. Monitor vital signs every 30 minutes for 3 to 4 hours, and keep the side rails up until patient is fully alert.
8. Monitor patient for abdominal or chest pain, cervical pain, dyspnea, fever, hematemesis, melena, dysphagia, lightheadedness, or a firm distended abdomen. These may indicate complications.
9. Instruct patient on the above listed signs and symptoms and advise to report immediately should any occur, even after discharge.
10. Possible complications include perforation of the esophagus or stomach, pulmonary aspiration, hemorrhage, respiratory depression or arrest, infection, cardiac arrhythmias or arrest.

! NURSING ALERT Perforation of the GI tract is a complication of endoscopy. Assess for abdominal or chest pain, dyspnea, fever, tachycardia, light-headedness, and distended abdomen. Report immediately.

Flexible Sigmoidoscopy and Colonoscopy

1. Sigmoidoscopy is the visualization of the anal canal, rectum, sigmoid colon, and proximal colon through a fiber-optic sigmoidoscope.
2. Colonoscopy is the visualization of the entire large intestine, sigmoid colon, rectum, and anal canal. It is used as a screening test for colon cancer because it can be used to identify and remove potentially precancerous and cancerous polyps.

3. Sigmoidoscopy or colonoscopy can be used to diagnose malignancy, polyps, inflammation, or strictures.
4. Colonoscopy is used for surveillance in patients with a history of chronic ulcerative colitis, previous colon cancer, or colon polyps.
5. Lower GI endoscopy can be used to perform biopsy, remove foreign objects, or obtain diagnostic specimens.
6. Colonoscopy requires bowel preparation for a couple of days before the procedure and use of conscious sedation during the procedure. The bowel preparation includes approximately 1 gallon of iso-osmolar electrolyte solution to consume over a 3- to 4-hour period the day before the procedure, a clear liquid diet the day before, and an oral laxative the night before (protocols vary). See Patient Education Guidelines for a

PATIENT EDUCATION GUIDELINES

Colonoscopy Instructions

You have been scheduled for a colonoscopy to examine your large bowel (colon). It will be necessary for you to prepare your bowel before the procedure by drinking a substance called CoLyte, GoLYTELY, or NuLytely. It is not absorbed by your body; rather, it rinses solid matter from your colon. You should expect to empty your bowel frequently.

During the procedure, you will receive medication to keep you comfortable. You will be ready to leave the facility in 1 to 3 hours. The medication you will receive may affect your memory. You must bring a competent adult driver with you. Your driver will be responsible for signing you out and must receive the discharge instructions.

Do not take aspirin, aspirin-containing products, or iron supplements for 7 days before your exam. If you take a blood-thinning medication, such as Coumadin, call the health care provider who prescribed it for you for further instructions.

The day before your procedure
1. Begin clear liquid diet for the entire day (see below). NO SOLID FOOD. Make sure to drink plenty of fluids so you do not get dehydrated.

2. At 3 PM, start drinking one gallon of bowel prep (CoLyte, GoLYTELY, or NuLytely). You may have it on ice or refrigerated. You may add one package of lemon-lime Crystal Light to the entire gallon. Drink one glass every 10 to 15 minutes, completing the entire gallon in 2 hours. Slow down if you begin to feel bloated or nauseated (sick to your stomach). It is normal to feel chills while drinking the prep. Warm clothing may help. If you cannot drink the prep, call your health care provider for instructions.
3. You may continue to take clear liquids until midnight.
4. Do not eat or drink anything after midnight.

The day of your procedure
1. Take your heart and blood pressure medications with a small sip of water.
2. Insulin doses should be cut in half. If you are on a sliding scale, please bring your insulin with you.
3. Do not forget to bring an adult driver with you.

CLEAR LIQUID DIET
Remember: NO SOLID FOOD

Food Group	Foods Included	Foods Excluded
Fruit Juices	All clear or strained fruit juices	• Red or orange juices • Juices with pulp or that you cannot see through
Soup	Clear broth, bouillon, and consommé	• All other soups or stews
Desserts	Clear flavored gelatin, ice pops, fruit-flavored ices, hard candy	• Red or orange desserts, pudding, gelatin with fruit or whipped cream
Beverages	Coffee, tea, carbonated beverages, beverages, such as Kool-aid and Gatorade	• Red or orange beverages, dairy products, or other beverages

Adapted from SHANDS at the University of Florida.

sample preparation. If unable to tolerate CoLyte, GoLYTELY, or NuLytely, an alternate prep may be used.

 DRUG ALERT Sodium phosphate preps should be avoided in people with congestive heart failure, renal impairment, and in others that may be more sensitive to electrolyte imbalances.

7. CT colonography, also known as virtual colonoscopy, is evolving as a noninvasive screening method.

Endoscopic Ultrasound (EUS)

Description

1. This procedure is a combination of endoscopy and ultrasonography to visualize the GI tract and can be used to evaluate the upper GI tract or the lower GI tract.
2. An ultrasonic transducer is built into the distal end of the endoscope.
3. This procedure allows for high-quality resolution and imaging of the walls of the esophagus, stomach, duodenum, small intestines, and colon. Adjacent abdominal structures can also be studied.
4. EUS is also indicated to evaluate and stage lesions of the GI tract.

Nursing and Patient Care Considerations

1. Verify patient's compliance with the pretest bowel preparation the day before the procedure, usually an oral laxative (such as magnesium citrate) and a clear liquid diet.
2. Patient must be NPO after midnight.
3. Explain to patient that a feeling of fullness will occur when water is introduced into the GI tract. This eliminates air space and provides for high resolution.
4. If an upper EUS is performed, maintain the NPO status until the gag reflex returns. A lower EUS can be performed using a rectal approach.
5. Observe patient for a change in vital signs, bleeding, pain, vomiting, and abdominal distention or rigidity.
6. Make sure that patients who have had endoscopic procedures requiring sedation have a caregiver to drive them home after the procedure.

GENERAL PROCEDURES AND TREATMENT MODALITIES

Relieving Constipation and Fecal Impaction

One method of evacuating the lower bowel is an enema, the installation of a solution into the rectum and sigmoid colon. See Procedure Guidelines 18-1. If fecal impaction is discovered

PROCEDURE GUIDELINES 18-1

Administering an Enema

EQUIPMENT

- Prepackaged enema or enema container
- Disposable gloves
- Water-soluble jelly
- Waterproof pad
- Bath blanket
- Bedpan or commode
- Washcloth and towel
- Basin
- Toilet tissue

PROCEDURE

Nursing Action	Rationale
Preparatory phase	
1. Assess the patient's bowel habits (last bowel movement, laxative usage, bowel patterns) and physical condition (hemorrhoids, mobility, external sphincter control).	1. Helps distinguish chronic constipation from new or acute condition. Enema should not be given if there is a suspicion of appendicitis or bowel obstruction.
2. Provide for privacy and explain procedure to patient.	2. Provides comfort and cooperation.
Performance phase	
1. Wash hands.	1. Promotes hygiene.
2. Place patient on left side with right knee flexed (Sims' position). Place waterproof pad underneath patient and cover with bath blanket.	2. Allows for enema solution to flow by gravity along the natural curve of the sigmoid colon and rectum.
3. Place bedpan or bedside commode in position for patients who cannot ambulate to the toilet or who may have difficulty with sphincter control.	3. Allows for easy accessibility.

(continued)

PROCEDURE GUIDELINES 18-1 *(continued)*

Administering an Enema

PROCEDURE *(continued)*

Nursing Action	Rationale
4. Remove plastic cover over tubing, and lubricate tip of enema tubing 3–4 inches (7.5–10 cm) unless prepackaged (tip is already lubricated). Even prepackaged enema may need more lubricant.	4. Prevents trauma and eases application.
5. Apply disposable gloves.	5. Standard precautions.
6. Separate buttocks and locate rectum.	
7. Instruct patient that you will be inserting tubing and to take slow, deep breaths.	7. Allows for patient relaxation and readiness.
8. Insert tubing 3–4 inches for adult patients.	8. Prevents tissue trauma of rectum.
9. Slowly instill the solution using a clamp and the height of the container to adjust flow rate if using an enema bag and tubing. For high enemas, raise enema container 12–18 inches (30.5–45.5 cm) above anus; for low enemas, 12 inches. If using a prepackaged enema, slowly squeeze the container until all solution is instilled.	9. Rapid infusion can cause colon distention and cramping. Container elevated past 12–18 inches and controller on tubing not regulated contribute to rapid infusion.
10. Lower container or clamp tubing if patient complains of cramping.	10. Slows instillation and allows fluid time to disperse.
11. Withdraw rectal tubing after all enema solution has been instilled and instruct patient to hold solution as long as possible and that a feeling of distention may be felt.	11. Promotes better results.
12. Discard supplies in the appropriate trash receptacle.	12. Maintains hygiene; minimizes patient embarrassment.
13. Assist patient on the bedpan or to the bedside commode or toilet when urge to defecate occurs.	13. Prompt action will prevent soiling.
14. Observe enema return for amount, fecal content. Instruct patient not to flush toilet until the nurse has seen the results.	14. If enema has not had sufficient time to absorb, result may be mostly clear with little fecal material. One or two repeat enemas may be ordered, if much fecal matter is expected, and discontinued when return turns clear.

Follow-up phase

1. Document the type of enema given, volume, and results on the appropriate chart forms.	1. For continuity of care.
2. Assess and document presence or absence of abdominal distention after enema was given.	2. Relief of abdominal distention indicates success of gas relief.
3. Assist the patient with washing perineum and rectal area, if indicated; may also need a clean gown or linen change.	3. Fecal soiling may result, especially in bedridden patients.

 NURSING ALERT Enemas should not be given routinely to treat constipation because they disrupt normal defecation reflexes, and the patient becomes dependent.

on exam, manual disimpaction may be performed to remove stool and promote bowel elimination (see Figure 18-1). However, it is best to try to prevent constipation by using fiber, laxatives, or stool softeners so that enemas and manual disimpaction are not needed.

Purposes of Enema Administration

1. Bowel preparation for diagnostic tests or surgery to empty the bowel of fecal content.

2. Delivery of medication into the colon (such as enemas containing steroids to treat ulcerative proctitis or a sodium polystyrene sulfonate enema to decrease the serum potassium level).

3. To soften the stool (oil-retention enemas).

4. To relieve gas (tidal, milk and molasses, or Fleet's enemas).

5. To promote defecation and evacuate feces from the colon for patients with constipation or an impaction (not a first-line therapy).

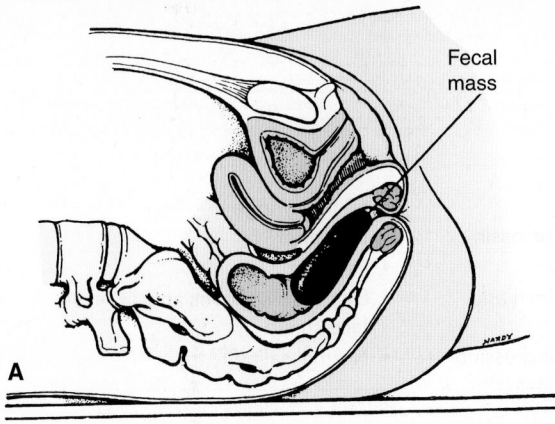

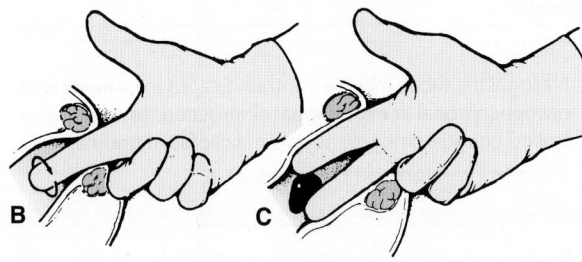

Figure 18-1. Fecal Impaction. (**A**) Note shaded area inside rectal sphincter, which indicates fecal impaction. (**B**) By gently stimulating the rectal wall with a gloved index finger and using a circular motion, it is possible to loosen fecal material. (**C**) It may be necessary to gently insert two fingers in an attempt to crush the fecal mass. A scissorlike motion is used.

Nursing and Patient Care Considerations

1. Consider manual removal of fecal impaction in the following patients at risk:
   a. Older adults with chronic constipation or insufficient hydration, or who are inactive.
   b. Orthopedic patients who have been in traction or in body casts.
   c. When barium has not been adequately removed after radiologic examination.
   d. Patients with neurologic or psychotic disorders.
2. Fecal impaction can occur with a descending/sigmoid colostomy. The fingers may be used to break up feces through the stoma, followed by cleansing irrigation.
3. Contraindications of manual removal of fecal impaction include:
   a. Pregnancy.
   b. After genitourinary, rectal, perineal, abdominal, or gynecologic surgery.
   c. Myocardial infarction, coronary insufficiency, pulmonary embolus, heart failure, heart block.
   d. GI or vaginal bleeding.
   e. Blood dyscrasias, bleeding disorders.
   f. Hemorrhoids, fissures, and rectal polyps.

 NURSING ALERT Be aware that manual removal of fecal impaction may cause syncope due to stimulation of the vagus nerve.

Nasogastric and Nasointestinal Intubation

 Evidence Base Niv, E., Fireman, Z., & Vaisman, N. (2009). Post-pyloric feeding. *World Journal of Gastroenterology, 15*(11), 1281–1288.

Nasogastric (NG) intubation refers to the insertion of a tube through the nasopharynx into the stomach (see Procedure Guidelines 18-2 and Procedure Guidelines 18-3, pages 652 to 655). NG intubation has multiple purposes including stomach decompression, stomach lavage (irrigation due to active bleeding or poisoning), medication administration, and short-term feeding.

Nasointestinal (NI) intubation is performed by inserting a small-bore, weighted tube that is carried by way of peristalsis into the duodenum or jejunum. Insertion of this type of tube can be done manually, endoscopically, or fluoroscopically. Using fluoroscopy is considered the "gold standard" or preferred method of insertion. NI intubation is primarily used for administering feedings and maintaining nutritional intake (see Procedure Guidelines 18-4, page 656).

Nursing and Patient Care Considerations

1. If patient is unconscious, advance the tube between respirations to make sure it does not enter the trachea.
   a. You will need to stroke the unconscious patient's neck to facilitate passage of the tube down the esophagus.
   b. Watch for cyanosis while passing the tube in an unconscious patient. Cyanosis indicates the tube has entered the trachea.
2. If patient has a nasal condition that prevents insertion through the nose, the tube is passed through the mouth.
   a. Remove dentures, slide the distal end of the tube over the tongue, and proceed the same way as a nasal intubation.
   b. Make sure to coil the end of the tube and direct it downward at the pharynx.
3. Pain or vomiting after the tube is inserted indicates tube obstruction or incorrect placement.
4. If the NG tube is not draining, the nurse should reposition tube by advancing or withdrawing it slightly (with a physician's order). After repositioning, always check for placement.
5. Recognize the complications when the tube is in for prolonged periods: nasal erosion, sinusitis, esophagitis, esophagotracheal fistula, gastric ulceration, and pulmonary and oral infections.
6. Extended-use NG tubes are made of a flexible, soft plastic material with manufacturer's recommendations that may include leaving the tube in place for up to 30 days before changing the tube.
7. Assess the color, consistency, and odor of gastric contents. Coffee ground–like contents may indicate GI bleeding. Report findings immediately.
8. The tube should be irrigated before and after medication administration through the tube.
   a. Medications should be given in liquid form, if possible.
   b. Clamp the tube for 30 to 45 minutes to ensure medication absorption before reconnecting to suction, if ordered.
9. Check GI function by auscultating for bowel sounds on a regular basis after the tube has been clamped for 30 minutes.

(*Text continues on page 654*)

PROCEDURE GUIDELINES 18-2

Nasogastric Intubation

EQUIPMENT

- Nasogastric (NG) tube—usually single-lumen Levin or double-lumen Salem sump tube
- Anesthetic jelly or spray or water-soluble lubricant
- Suction equipment, if ordered
- Clamp for tubing
- Towel, tissues, and emesis basin
- Glass of water and straw
- Hypoallergenic tape: ½ inch and 1 inch
- Bio-occlusive transparent dressing
- 60 mL syringe
- pH paper
- Penlight
- Disposable gloves and face shield
- Normal saline

PROCEDURE

Nursing Action	Rationale
Preparatory phase	
1. Ask if patient has ever had nasal surgery, trauma, a deviated septum, or bleeding disorder.	1. Nasogastric tubes may be contraindicated in patients with nasopharyngeal or esophageal obstruction, severe uncontrolled coagulopathy, or severe maxillofacial trauma.
2. Explain procedure to the patient, and tell how mouth breathing, panting, and swallowing will help in passing the tube.	2. Improves comfort and compliance.
3. Place the patient in a sitting or high-Fowler's position; place a towel across chest.	3. Facilitates passage of tube into esophagus.
4. Determine with the patient what sign he might use, such as raising the index finger, to indicate "wait a few moments" because of gagging or discomfort.	4. Provides a method of communication, which is reassuring to the patient.
5. Remove dentures; place emesis basin and tissues within the patient's reach.	5. Dentures may become loose and interfere with tube insertion.
6. Inspect the tube for defects; look for partially closed holes or rough edges.	6. Irrigation and suction may be affected by defective tube.
7. Determine the length of the tube needed to reach the stomach (see accompanying figure).	7. Prevents coiling of tube in stomach or tube ending in esophagus.
8. Have the patient blow nose to clear nostrils.	8. Facilitates passage through the nose.
9. Inspect the nostrils with a penlight, observing for any obstruction. Occlude each nostril, and have the patient breathe.	9. Helps determine which nostril is more patent.
10. Wash your hands. Put on disposable gloves (face shield should also be considered).	10. Protects nurse from patient's secretions.
11. Hold the end of the NG tube at the tip of the patient's nose, extend the tube to the earlobe and then down to the xiphoid process. Mark this distance on the tubing with tape.	11. The measurement will help ensure that the end of the tube reaches the stomach.

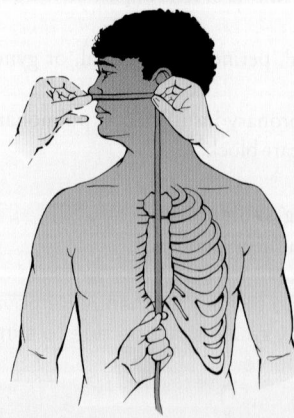

Measuring nasogastric tube length.

PROCEDURE GUIDELINES 18-2 *(continued)*

Nasogastric Intubation

PROCEDURE *(continued)*

Nursing Action	Rationale

Performance phase

1. Lubricate the first 2 to 3 inches of the tube with water-soluble lubricant. Avoid occluding the tube's holes with lubricant.

2. With patient's head in a neutral position, insert tube into nostril and gently pass tube into the posterior nasopharynx, directing downward and backward toward the ear.

3. When tube reaches the pharynx, the patient may gag; allow patient to rest for a few moments.

4. Have the patient tilt head slightly forward. Offer several sips of water through a straw, or permit patient to suck on ice chips, unless contraindicated. Advance tube as patient swallows.

5. Gently rotate the tube 180 degrees to redirect the curve.
6. Continue to advance tube gently each time the patient swallows.

1. Lubrication reduces friction between the mucous membranes and tube and prevents injury to the nasal passages. Using a water-soluble lubricant prevents oil aspiration pneumonia if the tube accidentally slips into trachea.

2. The passage of the tube is facilitated by following the natural contours of the body. The slower the advancement of the tube at this point, the less likelihood of putting pressure on the turbinates, which could cause pain and bleeding.

3. Gag reflex is triggered by the presence of the tube.

4. Flexed head position partially occludes the airway, and the tube is less likely to enter trachea. Swallowing closes the epiglottis over the trachea and facilitates passage of tube into the esophagus. Actually, when the tube passes the cricopharyngeal sphincter into the esophagus, it can be slowly and steadily advanced even if the patient does not swallow.

5. Prevents the tube from entering the patient's mouth.
6. Facilitates forward movement and prevents trauma and discomfort.

 Key Decision Point

Be especially cautious with tube insertion in patients with craniofacial trauma, reduced cough and gag reflexes, confusion, presence of endotracheal tube, decreased consciousness, and uncooperative behavior. If obstruction appears to prevent tube from passing, do not use

force. Rotating tube gently may help. If unsuccessful, remove tube and try another nostril.

If there are any signs of distress while passing the tube, such as gasping, coughing, or cyanosis, immediately remove tube. The tube may have entered the trachea.

7. Continue to advance the tube when the patient swallows, until the tape mark reaches the patient's nostril.

8. To check whether the tube is in the stomach:
   a. Ask the patient to talk.
   b. Obtain aspirate with 60-mL syringe and check for gastric fluid characteristics. If stomach contents cannot be aspirated, reposition the patient. Attempt to aspirate again.
   c. X-rays may be obtained to confirm tube placement.

7. Reference point where the tube was measured.

8.
   a. If the patient cannot talk, the tube may be coiled in throat or passed through vocal cords.
   b. Gastric fluid characteristics: $pH \leq 5$ and gastric fluid characteristics of grassy green, clear and colorless, or brown.
   c. Consider x-ray confirmation of tube placement in patients with risk factors for malpositioning of tubes.

! NURSING ALERT Never place the end of the tube in water while checking placement. If the tube is in the trachea, the patient could aspirate.

9. After tube is passed and the correct placement is confirmed, attach the tube to suction or clamp the tube.

9. Clamping can be done using a clamp, plastic plug, or folding the tube over and slipping the bend into the tube end.

(continued)

PROCEDURE GUIDELINES 18-2 *(continued)*

Nasogastric Intubation

PROCEDURE *(continued)*

Nursing Action	Rationale
10. Anchor tube with: a. Hypoallergenic tape; split lengthwise and only halfway, attach unsplit end of tape to nose, and cross split ends around tubing. Apply another piece of tape to bridge of nose. b. Bio-occlusive transparent dressing where it exits the nose.	10. Prevents the patient's vision from being disturbed; prevents tubing from rubbing against nasal mucosa. This will ensure tape being secure. Do not tape to forehead, which could cause necrosis of the nostril.
11. Anchor the tubing to the patient's gown. Use a rubber band to make a slipknot to anchor the tubing to the patient's gown. Secure the rubber band to the patient's gown using a safety pin.	11. Permits mobility of patient. This prevents tugging on the tube when the patient moves.
12. Clamp the tube until the purpose for inserting the tube takes place.	
13. Attach the larger lumen of the Salem sump tube to suction equipment if ordered. Low continuous suction or high intermittent suction may be used with the Salem sump tube. If the Levin tube is used, low intermittent suction is recommended.	13. Prevents gastric mucosal damage, if a vacuum forms and the tube adheres to the gastric wall.

Follow-up phase

1. Assure the patient that most discomfort will lessen with time.	
2. Irrigate the tube at regular intervals (every 4 hours unless otherwise indicated) with small volumes of prescribed fluid. Remember to always check placement first. a. If the tube is a Salem sump, it will require periodic placing of 10 to 20 cc of air through the vent port (blue port or smaller lumen). Do not instill water into the vent and, if the vent is draining fluid, instill air to clear it. b. Check the Salem sump tube patency by placing the vent port next to your ear.	2. Ensures tube patency. b. A soft hissing sound is heard if the tube is patent. If the port hangs downward and the tube backs up, stomach contents will spill over the patient.
3. Cleanse nares and provide mouth care every shift.	3. Promotes patient comfort and decreases risk of infection.
4. Apply petroleum jelly to nostrils, as needed, and assess for skin irritation or breakdown.	4. Keeps tissue soft and prevent crusting and skin breakdown.
5. Keep head of bed elevated at least 30 degrees.	5. Minimizes gastroesophageal reflux.
6. Record the time, type, and size of tube inserted. Document placement checks after each assessment, along with amount, color, consistency of drainage.	6. Ensures proper tube and placement at all times, and assists in evaluation of tube effectiveness.

 Evidence Base Simons, S. R., & Abdallah, L. M. (2012). Bedside assessment of enteral tube placement: Aligning practice with evidence. *American Journal of Nursing, 112*(2), 40–46.

Caring for the Patient Undergoing Gastrointestinal Surgery

Types of Procedures

Gastric Surgeries
See page 679.
1. Total gastrectomy—complete excision of the stomach with esophageal–jejunal anastomosis.

2. Subtotal or partial gastrectomy—a portion of the stomach excised:
   a. Billroth I procedure—gastric remnant anastomosed to the duodenum.
   b. Billroth II procedure—gastric remnant anastomosed to the jejunum.
3. Gastrostomy (Janeway or Spivak)—rectangular stomach flap created into abdominal stoma, used for intermittent tube feedings.

PROCEDURE GUIDELINES 18-3

Nasogastric Tube Removal

EQUIPMENT

- Towel
- Disposable gloves
- Lip pomade
- Mouth hygiene materials

PROCEDURE

Nursing Action	Rationale
Preparatory phase	
1. Make sure that gastric or small bowel drainage is not excessive in volume.	1–3. Tube may not be discontinued unless drainage is minimal, bowel sounds are present, and patient is passing flatus.
2. Make sure, by auscultation, that audible peristalsis is present.	
3. Determine whether the patient is passing flatus, which indicates peristalsis.	
4. Verify the health care provider's order for removal.	4. Complies with the Joint Comission National Patient Safety Goals.
Performance phase	
1. Place a towel across the patient's chest and inform about the withdrawal.	1. No doubt, the patient will be happy to have progressed to this stage.
2. Apply disposable gloves.	2. Provides protection from contaminated body fluids.
3. Turn off suction; disconnect and clamp tube.	3. Prevents fluids from leaking from tube.
4. Remove the tape from the patient's nose.	
5. Instruct the patient to take a deep breath and hold it.	5. This maneuver closes the epiglottis.
6. Slowly, but evenly, withdraw tubing and cover it with a towel as it emerges. (As the tube reaches the nasopharynx, you can pull quickly.)	6. Covering the tubing helps dispel patient's nausea.
7. Provide the patient with materials for oral care and lubricant for nasal dryness.	7. Mouthwash and a nasal lubricant will be appreciated by the patient.
8. Dispose of equipment in appropriate receptacle.	
9. Document time of tube removal and the patient's reaction.	
10. Document tube removal and color, consistency, and amount of drainage in suction canister.	9–10. For continuity of care.
11. Continue to monitor the patient for signs of GI difficulties.	11. Recurrence of nausea or vomiting may require reinsertion of nasogastric tubing. Changes in vital signs may suggest infection.

Hernia Surgeries

1. Herniorrhaphy—surgical repair of a hernia with suturing of the abdominal wall.
2. Hernioplasty—reconstructive hernia repair with mesh sewn over the defect for reinforcement.

Bowel Surgeries

1. Appendectomy—excision of the vermiform appendix.
2. Bowel resection—segmental excision of small and/or large bowels with varied approaches:
   a. Anastomosis of proximal and distal ends of bowel.
   b. Anastomosis of proximal and distal ends of bowel with temporary diverting loop ostomy.
   c. Both ends of bowel exteriorized to the abdominal wall with proximal ostomy and distal mucous fistula.
   d. Hartmann's procedure—proximal large bowel as ostomy; distal end of large bowel oversewn inside abdomen as Hartmann's pouch.
3. Low-anterior resection—subtotal resection of the rectum with colorectal or coloanal anastomosis.
4. Abdominoperineal resection—a combined abdominal and perineal approach for removal of the rectum and anus with permanent colostomy.
5. Subtotal colectomy—partial removal of the large bowel or colon.

PROCEDURE GUIDELINES 18-4

Nasointestinal Intubation (Small-Bore Feeding Tubes)

EQUIPMENT

- Type of tube ordered by health care provider
- 30-mL or 60-mL luer-lock or tip syringe
- Water-soluble lubricant
- Tape, rubber band, clamp, safety pin
- Glass of water
- Stethoscope

 NURSING ALERT Intestinal feeding tubes are soft, flexible, small-diameter (8 or 12 French) tubes with a longer length than gastric feeding tubes (measuring up to 47 inches [120 cm] as compared with approximately 30 inches [76 cm] for a gastric feeding tube). Some tubes are weighted at the distal end of the tube. All tubes should be routinely pretested for patency and function before passage.

PROCEDURE

Nursing Action	Rationale
Preparatory and performance phases (by health care provider—nurse assisted)	
1. Tube preparation:	1.
a. Do not ice plastic tubes.	a. Become too stiff to work with.
b. Inject 10 mL of water into the tube.	b. Removes air that may cause gas.
c. Insert guide wire or stylet into tube, making sure it is positioned snugly against tube.	c. Aids in insertion.
d. Dip weighted tip into glass of water.	d. Activates lubricant.
2. Similar to passing a short nasogastric tube and taping to patient (see Procedure Guidelines 18-2, pages 652 to 654).	
3. After the tube enters the stomach, it passes by peristalsis and gravity into the small intestine. Change patient's position from Fowler's to a position in which the patient is lying on his or her right side.	3. Assists in advancing the tubing to and through the pylorus; tilting to the right is helpful.
4. Obtain an x-ray of the abdomen after tube insertion. Stylet should remain in place until position is confirmed.	4. Confirms placement.
5. When tube placement has been confirmed, mark the tube at the nare exit site.	5. Helpful in reassessment of tube position. Check that the mark on the tube remains at the exit site.
Nursing/patient care considerations	
1. Be aware of risk of aspiration in an unconscious patient.	1. Inserted tube prevents total closure of airway.
2. Instruct patient on complications associated with tube feedings, such as nausea, vomiting, diarrhea.	2. Feedings that are too large or too fast cause these symptoms.
3. A continuous drip infusion delivered with an infusion pump may lessen the risk of aspiration, abdominal distention, and/or diarrhea.	3. Controls the volume and rate of infusion.
4. If abdominal distention, vomiting, or diarrhea occurs, notify the health care provider; the rate of infusion may need to be adjusted.	4. May indicate paralytic ileus.

6. Total colectomy—complete removal of the large bowel or colon with varied approaches:
   a. Ileorectal anastomosis—colon removal with ileum anastomosed to rectum.
   b. Proctocolectomy—colon removal including the rectum and anus with permanent ileostomy.
   c. Ileal reservoir—anal anastomosis. (Colon removal, subtotal proctectomy, possible distal rectal mucosectomy, creation of pelvic reservoir from two, three, or four loops of ileum with anastomosis at anal canal. Usually a temporary loop ileostomy is performed as fecal diversion to protect the reservoir and the ileal–anal anastomosis. After takedown of

temporary loop ileostomy [2 to 3 months postoperatively], the reservoir stores feces and patient eliminates under voluntary control through the anus [see page 694].)

    d. Kock or Barnett continent internal reservoir (BCIR) procedures—proctocolectomy, creation of a continent small bowel reservoir with nipple valve abdominal stoma used for stool removal through routine intubation. (Continence is provided through the nipple valve.)

7. Roux-en-Y jejunostomy—jejunum severed with distal end exteriorized as permanent stoma for intermittent tube feedings; proximal end reanastomosed to GI tract distal to stoma to reestablish pathway.

Laparoscopic Surgery

1. GI surgical procedures are increasingly being assisted by the use of a laparoscope, either partially or totally. The laparoscope is usually inserted through a 1-cm umbilical incision with additional trocars used for visualization and assistance. Dissection is performed with endocautery, scissors, or laser.

2. Advantages may include reduction in postoperative pain, shorter hospital and recuperative periods, decreased risk of infection, and improved cosmetic outcome. The direct cost of a laparoscopic procedure may be greater than an open procedure; however, the overall cost of the procedure and recuperative period may be lower due to a more rapid recovery.

3. Contraindications may include obesity, internal adhesions, and bowel obstruction with distention.

4. Cholecystectomies and appendectomies are routinely done through laparoscopy; hernia repairs can be done using the laparoscope. Other GI surgeries, including ostomies and bowel resections (may include select cancer patients), are increasingly being done through this surgical approach.

Preoperative Management

1. All diagnostic tests and procedures are explained to promote cooperation and relaxation.

2. The patient is prepared for the type of surgical procedure as well as postoperative care (IV, patient-controlled analgesia pump, NG tube, surgical drains, incision care, possibility of ostomy).

3. Measures to prevent postoperative complications are taught, including coughing, turning, and deep breathing; using the incentive spirometer; and splinting the incision.

4. IV fluids or total parenteral nutrition (TPN) before surgery may be ordered to improve fluid and electrolyte balance and nutritional status.

5. Intake and output is monitored.

6. Preoperative laboratory studies are obtained.

7. Bowel cleansing will be initiated 1 to 2 days before surgery for better visualization. Preparation may include diet modifications, such as liquid or low residue, oral laxatives, suppositories, enemas, or polyethylene glycoelectrolyte solution (CoLyte, GoLYTELY).

8. Antibiotics are ordered to decrease the bacterial growth in the colon.

9. An ostomy specialty nurse is consulted if patient is scheduled for an ostomy to initiate early understanding and management of postoperative care.

10. Patient may not have anything by mouth after midnight the night before surgery. Medications may be withheld, if ordered. This will keep the GI tract clear.

Postoperative Management and Nursing Care

1. Physical assessment is completed at least once per shift, or more frequently, as indicated.

    a. Monitor vital signs for signs of infection and shock—fever, hypotension, tachycardia.

    b. Monitor intake and output for signs of imbalance, dehydration, and shock. Include all drains in evaluating intake and output.

    c. Assess abdomen for increased pain, distention, rigidity, and rebound tenderness because these may indicate postoperative complications. Report abnormal findings.

    d. Expect diminished or absent bowel sounds in the immediate postoperative phase.

    e. Evaluate dressing and incision. Check for purulent or bloody drainage, odor, and unusual tenderness or redness at incision site, which may indicate bleeding or infection.

    f. Evaluate for passing of flatus or feces.

    g. Monitor for nausea and vomiting. Note the presence of fecal smell or material in vomitus because it may indicate an obstruction.

    h. Check NG aspirate, vomitus, and stools for signs of bleeding. Record and report findings if present.

2. Laboratory values are monitored and patient is evaluated for signs and symptoms of electrolyte imbalance.

3. Wound drains, IV lines, and all other catheters are monitored and evaluated for signs of infection or infiltration.

4. To maintain patency of NG tube, the tube may be irrigated with 30 mL of normal saline solution every 2 hours and as needed. If there are large amounts of NG output, IV replacement may be necessary.

 NURSING ALERT Due to the type of abdominal surgery and location of the suture line, the health care provider may order not to irrigate or manipulate the NG tube.

5. Subcutaneous heparin may also be ordered to prevent embolus. Antiembolism stockings may be used.

6. Turning, coughing, deep breathing, and incentive spirometry are performed every 2 hours. Dangling at bedside is encouraged the night of surgery and an attempt at ambulation the first postoperative day is made, unless ordered otherwise.

7. Patient-controlled analgesia for pain control or other analgesics, as ordered, are administered to promote comfort.

8. Wound dressing is changed every day or as needed, maintaining aseptic technique.

9. Diet is advanced, as ordered, after presence of bowel sounds indicates GI tract has regained motility. After 1 to 2 days of NPO postoperatively, the usual diet progression is ice chips, sips of water, clear liquids, full liquids, soft or regular diet.

10. Dietary education includes fiber, avoiding gas-producing foods, and maintaining adequate fluid intake.

11. Reinforcement of teaching and assistance with ostomy care, if indicated.
12. Administration of medications, as ordered, which may include a stool softener or laxative when bowel function has returned.

Complications

1. Paralytic ileus or obstruction.
2. Peritonitis or sepsis.
3. Anastomotic leakage, which may result in peritonitis.

Nursing Diagnoses

- Acute Pain related to surgical incision.
- Imbalanced Nutrition: Less Than Body Requirements related to dietary modifications after surgery.
- Impaired Skin Integrity related to surgical incision.
- Constipation related to surgery.
- Risk for Infection related to surgical incision.
- Deficient Fluid Volume related to surgical procedure.

Nursing Interventions

Promoting Comfort

1. Assess pain location, intensity, and characteristics, and make sure they are appropriate for postoperative stage.
2. Administer prescribed pain medications, and provide instructions if using a patient-controlled analgesia pump, to keep patient comfortable.
3. Assess the effectiveness of the pain medications. If ordered, promethazine can potentiate the effectiveness of pain medication.
4. Encourage the patient to change positions frequently and to splint incision when turning, coughing, or deep breathing to minimize discomfort.

Improving Nutritional Status

1. Monitor intake and output each shift, or more frequently if indicated, to maintain fluid balance.
2. Advance diet as tolerated.
3. Weigh the patient daily to ensure adequate calorie intake.
4. Provide snacks or high-protein, high-calorie supplements and assist in menu selection, if needed.
5. Instruct the patient to avoid gas-producing foods, and encourage ambulation.

Improving Skin Integrity

1. Assess wound for signs of erythema, swelling, and purulent drainage, which may indicate infection.
2. Change surgical dressing every 24 hours, and as needed, to protect skin from drainage and decrease risk of infection.
3. Apply dressings around drains and tubes to protect skin from leakage, if indicated.
4. Turn the patient frequently or encourage position changes to prevent skin breakdown over bony prominences.

Promoting Bowel Elimination

1. Assess for presence of bowel sounds to evaluate return of bowel function.
2. Ask the patient if passing flatus rectally or through an ostomy—also indicative of return of bowel function.
3. Evaluate for abdominal distention, nausea, or vomiting, which may indicate obstruction.
4. Monitor stool for frequency, amount, and consistency.
5. Administer stool softener or laxative, as ordered, to promote comfort with elimination.
6. Encourage diet with adequate fiber and fluid content for natural laxative effect.
7. Encourage and assist with ambulation to promote peristalsis.

Preventing Infection

1. Monitor temperature every shift or as ordered, and review previous readings to recognize early increases.
2. Change surgical dressings every 24 hours, or more frequently, as indicated. Maintain aseptic technique to avoid contamination.
3. Monitor wound for signs and symptoms of infection, such as redness, swelling, purulent drainage, odor, and pain.
4. Obtain a wound culture, as ordered.
5. Monitor the patient with a Foley catheter for signs and symptoms of urinary tract infection (UTI), such as concentrated, cloudy urine; hematuria; fever. If Foley discontinued, monitor for the above plus complaints of burning and frequency.
6. Assist the patient in washing perineum daily and as needed if incontinence is present, for increased comfort and hygiene.
7. Assess breath sounds and monitor for crackles.
8. Instruct the patient to turn, cough, deep-breathe, and use incentive spirometer every 2 hours to minimize complications.
9. Encourage early ambulation to initiate bowel function and reduce risk of embolus.
10. Administer antibiotics, as ordered, to maintain constant blood level.

Maintaining Fluid Volume

1. Monitor intake and output every 8 hours, or more frequently, if ordered, to assess recent status. Include amount of wound drainage from dressing changes and drains that may be in place.
2. Assess the patient for signs of dehydration—flushed, dry skin; tenting of skin; oliguria; tachycardia, hypotension, and rapid respirations; increase in hematocrit, blood urea nitrogen (BUN), electrolytes; fever; weight loss.
3. Monitor laboratory results and report abnormal findings.
4. Assess the patient for signs of electrolyte imbalance—nausea or vomiting, cardiac dysrhythmia, tremor, seizures, anorexia, malaise, weakness, irregular pulse; changes in behavior, mental status.
5. Weigh the patient daily to ensure adequate caloric intake.
6. Administer parenteral fluids, enteral feedings, and blood products, as ordered, to maintain volume during period of decreased oral intake.

Community and Home Care Considerations

1. Reinforce discharge instructions and the importance of postoperative regimen to include health provider follow-up appointments and laboratory and other scheduled tests or therapies.
2. A person who has undergone a total gastrectomy needs lifelong parenteral administration of vitamin B_{12} to prevent pernicious anemia. This may also apply to people with the terminal ileum removed, and sometimes for those with ileostomies.

3. Change dressing and reinforce ostomy care as directed by health care provider. Report any signs of infection—unusual drainage, redness, warmth, increased pain, swelling.

4. Instruct to gradually increase activities of daily living. No heavy lifting (more than 10 lb), pushing, pulling, or driving for 6 to 8 weeks postoperatively.

5. Referral to additional community resources if applicable (support groups, meal programs, social services).

Patient Education and Health Maintenance

1. Review signs and symptoms of wound infection so early intervention may be instituted.

2. Explain signs and symptoms of other postoperative complications to report—elevated temperature, nausea or vomiting, abdominal distention, changes in bowel function and stool consistency or color.

3. Instruct the patient to report promptly blood in the stool or the coughing up of blood.

4. Teach the patient regarding wound and/or ostomy care, if applicable, to promote healing and self-confidence.

5. Encourage the patient to turn, cough, deep-breathe; to use incentive spirometer; and ambulate. Discuss the importance of these functions during the recovery period.

6. Review dietary changes, such as increased fiber content and fluid intake, and their importance in improving bowel function.

7. Review actions and adverse effects of prescribed medications to encourage compliance and understanding of management.

8. Assess the need for home health follow-up and initiate appropriate referrals if indicated.

Evaluation: Expected Outcomes

- Verbalizes increased comfort (using a 0-to-10 pain scale, with 0 being no pain and 10 being the highest score to measure pain).
- Consumes 50% to 75% of each meal; no weight loss.
- Incisional flaps approximated and healing ridge present.
- Passing flatus and stool.
- No signs and symptoms of infection.
- Vital signs stable, fluid and electrolytes in balance.

Caring for the Patient Undergoing Ostomy Surgery

See Standards of Care Guidelines 18-2.

Types of Fecal Ostomies

Colostomy
See Figure 18-2.

1. A surgically created opening between the colon and the abdominal wall to allow fecal elimination. It may be a temporary or permanent diversion.

2. A colostomy may be placed in any segment of the large intestine (colon), which will influence the nature of fecal discharge. The more right-sided the colostomy, the looser the stool. Transverse and descending/sigmoid colostomies are the most common types.

STANDARDS OF CARE GUIDELINES 18-2
Care of the Patient with an Ostomy

- Prepare patient and patient's family preoperatively by explaining the surgical procedure, stoma characteristics, and ostomy management with a pouching system.
- Have ostomy specialty nurse mark an optimal stoma site.
- Postoperatively, monitor the stoma color and amount and color of stomal output every shift; document and report any abnormalities.
- Periodically change a properly fitting pouching system over the ostomy to avoid leakage and protect the peristomal skin. Use this time as an opportunity for teaching.
- Assess peristomal skin with each pouching system change, document findings, and treat any abnormalities (skin breakdown due to leakage, allergy, or infection) as indicated.
- Teach patient and/or caregiver self-care skills of routine pouch emptying, cleansing skin and stoma, and changing of the pouching system until independence is achieved.
- Instruct patient and family in lifestyle adjustments regarding gas and odor control; procurement of ostomy supplies; and bathing, clothing, and travel tips.
- Encourage patient to verbalize feelings regarding the ostomy, body image changes, and sexual issues.
- Inform patient of community resources, such as United Ostomy Association, local and mail-order ostomy supply dealers, ostomy specialty nurses, American Cancer Society, and Crohn's & Colitis Foundation.

This information should serve as a general guideline only. Each patient situation presents a unique set of clinical factors and requires nursing judgment to guide care, which may include additional or alternative measures and approaches.

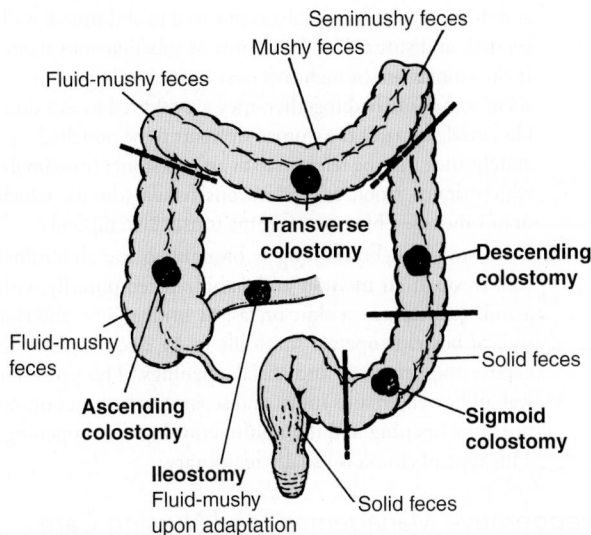

Figure 18-2. A diagrammatic representation of the placement of fecal ostomies and nature of discharge at these sites.

3. A colostomy may be performed as part of an abdominoperineal resection for rectal cancer; a fecal diversion for unresectable cancer; a temporary measure to protect an anastomosis; or surgical treatment for inflammatory bowel diseases, trauma, perforated diverticulitis, ischemic bowel, cancer, and congenital conditions.

Ileostomy

1. A surgically created opening between the ileum of the small intestine and the abdominal wall to allow elimination of small bowel effluent.
2. An ileostomy is usually formed at the terminal ileum of the small bowel and is usually placed in the right lower quadrant of the abdomen. Stool from an ileostomy drains frequently (average four to five times per day) and contains proteolytic enzymes, which can be harmful to skin.
3. Diagnoses that may require a temporary or permanent ileostomy include ulcerative colitis, Crohn's disease, familial polyposis, cancer, congenital defects, and trauma.

Characteristics of Stomas

1. A stoma is the part of the intestine (small or large) that is brought above the abdominal wall to become the outlet for discharge of intestinal waste. Stoma is often used interchangeably with "ostomy."
2. Normal stomal characteristics: pink-red, moist, bleeds slightly when rubbed, no feeling to touch, stool functions involuntary, and postoperative swelling gradually decreases over several months.
3. Stoma classifications:
   a. End stoma: After bowel is divided, the proximal bowel is exteriorized to abdominal wall, everted (which exposes mucosal lining), and sutured to dermis or subcutaneous tissue. There is only one opening that drains stool. The distal bowel is either surgically removed or sutured closed within abdominal cavity.
   b. Double-barrel stoma: After bowel is divided, the proximal and distal ends of bowel are exteriorized to abdominal wall, everted, and sutured to the dermis or subcutaneous tissue. If the stomas are brought up next to each other requiring them to be pouched together, they are referred to as a double-barrel stoma; if the stomas are apart to be pouched separately, they may be referred to as an end stoma (proximal), which drains stool, and a mucous fistula (distal), which drains mucus. This type of stoma is usually temporary.
   c. Loop stoma: A bowel loop is brought to the abdominal wall through an incision and stabilized temporarily with a rod, catheter, or a skin or fascial bridge. The anterior wall of bowel is opened surgically or by electrocautery to expose the proximal and distal openings. The posterior wall of bowel remains intact and separates the functioning proximal opening and the nonfunctioning distal opening. This type of stoma is usually temporary.

Preoperative Management and Nursing Care

1. Prepare the patient for general abdominal surgery (see page 657). Have the patient see an ostomy specialty nurse.

   a. An ostomy specialty nurse has the title of certified ostomy care nurse or certified wound, ostomy, and continence nurse (CWOCN, previously known as a certified enterostomal therapy nurse). These nurses play a vital role in the rehabilitation of patients with ostomies and related problems.
   b. The Wound Ostomy and Continence Nurses Society has an official publication called the *Journal of Wound, Ostomy, and Continence Nursing* (*www.wocn.org*).
2. Administer replacement fluid, as ordered, before surgery due to possible increased output during the postoperative phase.
3. Provide low-residue diet before NPO status.
4. Explain that the abdomen may be marked by the ostomy specialty nurse or surgeon to ensure proper positioning of the stoma. *Note:* The abdominal location of the stoma is usually determined by anatomical location of the bowel segment (eg, a sigmoid colostomy is ideally located in left lower abdominal quadrant).
5. Other considerations when selecting a stoma include:
   a. Positioning within rectus muscle.
   b. Avoidance of bony prominences, such as iliac crest and costal margin.
   c. Clearance from umbilicus, scars, and deep creases, observed in lying, sitting, and standing positions.
   d. Positioning on a flat pouching surface.
   e. Avoidance of beltline when possible.
   f. Positioning within patient's visibility to optimize independent ostomy care.
6. Support the patient and family with the many psychosocial considerations of ostomy surgery.

Postoperative Management and Nursing Care

1. Administer general abdominal surgery care (see page 657).
2. Assess stoma every shift for color and record findings:
   a. Normal color: pink-red.
   b. Dusky: dark red; purplish hue (ischemic sign).
   c. Necrotic: brown or black; may be dry (notify health care provider to determine extent of necrosis).
3. Apply pouching system as close to stoma as possible without it being rubbed. It is acceptable to have a $\frac{1}{16}$- to $\frac{1}{8}$-inch clearance to prevent constriction, which can contribute to edema (see Box 18-2).
4. Check for abdominal distention, which reduces blood flow to stoma through mesenteric tension.
5. Evaluate and empty drains and ostomy pouch frequently to promote patency and maintain seal.
6. Monitor intake and output with extreme accuracy because output may remain high during early postoperative period.
7. Suction and irrigate NG tube frequently, as ordered, to relieve pressure and decrease gastric contents.
8. Offer continued support to patient and family.

Complications

1. Mucocutaneous separation (between skin and stoma).
2. Stomal ischemia.

BOX 18-2	Fecal Ostomy Pouching Systems

- Pouching systems are varied according to manufacturer and patient needs. Systems are classified as one-piece or two-piece and disposable or reusable. A disposable, one-piece pouch is commonly used with backing as adhesive tape, skin barrier, or both. A disposable two-piece system consists of a skin barrier wafer with or without a tape border and a pouch. Disposable systems are popular and are discarded after one use. Reusable systems are declining in use and are made of heavier material, allowing use for weeks to months. They require the use of double-backed adhesive disks, cement, or belt to provide a seal.
- Pouching systems are available in precut sizes and cut-to-fit options as well as with a flat backing versus degrees of convexity. Convex pouching systems are used with flush or retracted stomas to increase stomal protrusion and reduce undermining of feces.
- Fecal pouches are available in closed-end and drainable styles. Drainable pouches require the use of a tail closure and may be used more than once. Closed-end pouches may contain a built-in filter to release gas and require no tail closure. A closed-end pouch is discarded after one use. Pouch selection depends on the patient's preference or ability to manipulate the volume and frequency of fecal output.
- Many accessory products are available to assist in the management of a fecal ostomy. They include skin sealants, skin barrier powders, pastes, washers, adhesive removers, tapes, belts, pouch covers, and deodorants.
- The goal is to change a pouching system on a routine basis to prevent leakage. Usually, this is every 3 to 7 days and will vary per individual needs. Routine changes allow for examination of the peristomal skin for breakdown. Schedule the change when the bowel is least active, usually early morning before breakfast, 2 to 4 hours after a meal, or before bedtime. At times, the pouching system may need to be changed immediately if leakage is imminent, itching or burning of peristomal skin is present, odor is detected with a closed system, or the wafer is dissolving.

3. Stomal stricture or stenosis (usually a long-term complication).
4. Stomal prolapse.
5. Peristomal hernia.
6. Peristomal skin breakdown from exposure to fecal output, allergic reaction to products, or infection, such as candidiasis.

Nursing Diagnoses

- Deficient Knowledge related to surgical procedures and ostomy management.
- Disturbed Body Image related to change in structure, function, and appearance.
- Anxiety related to loss of bowel control and autonomy.
- Impaired Skin Integrity related to irritation of peristomal skin by drainage and equipment.
- Imbalanced Nutrition: Less Than Body Requirements related to increased output and inadequate intake.
- Sexual Dysfunction related to altered body structure.

Nursing Interventions
Educating the Patient

1. Review the surgical procedure with the patient and discuss the information that the surgeon and other providers have given. Clarify any misunderstandings.
2. Avoid overwhelming the patient with information.
3. Include family in discussions, when appropriate.
4. Use available educational materials, including pictures and drawings, if the patient is receptive.
5. Involve the ostomy specialty nurse (CWOCN) in ostomy teaching and reinforce information, including lifestyle modifications.
6. Use a team approach; the need for information may come from many disciplines.
7. Assess the patient's response to teaching. If the patient is not interested, provide alternative times for teaching and review.
8. Consider the psychosocial issues of the patient and their effect on learning.

Promoting a Positive Self-Image

1. Encourage the patient to verbalize feelings about the surgical outcome.
2. Provide support during initial viewing of the stoma and encourage the patient to touch the area.
3. Encourage spouse or significant other to view the stoma.
4. Arrange a visit by a United Ostomy Association ostomy visitor if the patient desires. This is preferably done preoperatively.
5. Offer counseling, as necessary, and encourage the patient to use normal support systems, such as family, church, community groups.

Reducing Anxiety

1. Provide information regarding expected outcomes, such as the type and consistency of bowel function.
2. Introduce gradual steps toward achieving independent ostomy management. The patient may progress through the following steps:
   a. Observe stoma, pouch change, and emptying procedure.
   b. Learn tail closure application and removal.
   c. Empty and rinse pouch.
   d. Assist with pouching system change until independent. See Procedure Guidelines 18-5, pages 662 to 663.
   Note: Some patients may have decreased vision or dexterity and may require additional assistance and encouragement.
3. Teach colostomy irrigation procedure, if appropriate. See Procedure Guidelines 18-6, pages 664 to 665.
   a. Review that irrigating involves inserting an enema into a descending or sigmoid colostomy.
   b. Reinforce its purposes of cleansing the colon and stimulating the colon to move at a desired time regularly to regain control of fecal elimination.
   c. It is a patient preference whether colostomy irrigations are attempted for control. Irrigation may occur every day or every other day depending on bowel pattern. It usually takes 1 to 2 months to establish control. Patients with a preoperative history of regular, formed bowel movements are more likely to realize success.

PROCEDURE GUIDELINES 18-5

Changing a Two-Piece Drainable Fecal Pouching System

EQUIPMENT
- Duplicate wafer and pouch
- Washcloth and towel
- Tail closure
- Mild, nonoily soap (optional)
- Accessory products prescribed for patient

PROCEDURE

Nursing Action	Rationale
Preparatory phase	
1. Have patient assume a relaxed position and provide privacy. The best position may be sitting, reclining, or standing.	1. Patient must see stoma site to learn care.
Performance phase	
1. To remove pouching system:	1.
a. Wear nonsterile gloves.	a. Maintains universal precautions.
b. Push down gently on skin while lifting up on the wafer (ostomy adhesive remover may be used).	b. Minimizes skin trauma.
c. Discard soiled pouch and wafer in odorproof plastic bag. Save tail closure for reuse.	c. Removes room odor and maintains universal precautions.
2. To cleanse skin:	2.
a. Use toilet tissue to remove feces from stoma and skin if needed.	a. Stoma may function during the change.
b. Cleanse stoma and peristomal skin with soft cloth and water, soap optional. The patient may shower with or without pouching system in place. Clip or shave peristomal hair if appropriate.	b. Minimizes skin breakdown and promotes hygiene.
c. Rinse and dry skin thoroughly after cleansing. It is normal for the stoma to bleed slightly during cleaning and drying.	c. Removes residue, which may interfere with adhesion of wafer.
3. To apply wafer:	3.
a. Use measuring guide or pattern to determine stoma size.	a. This step is omitted when stomal shrinkage is complete, about 2 months postoperatively.
b. Trace correct size onto back of wafer and cut to stoma size. It is acceptable to cut $\frac{1}{16}$ to $\frac{1}{18}$ inch larger than stoma.	b. Avoids wafer rubbing stoma; omit this step if the wafer is precut.
c. Apply a line of skin barrier paste around stoma or on lip of wafer opening. Allow to set according to manufacturer's instructions. (Other barrier may be used in place of paste, such as strips or washer. Some may find the paste too difficult to see or have developed an allergy to the alcohol within the paste.)	c. Extra skin protection is imperative for ileostomy and right-sided colostomy. A left-sided colostomy may not need a secondary barrier because formed stool is less harmful to skin. Paste acts as "caulking" to prevent undermining of feces.
d. Remove paper backing from the wafer, center opening over stoma, and press wafer down onto peristomal skin.	d. Ensures adherence.
4. Snap pouch onto the flange of the wafer according to manufacturer's directions (see accompanying figure).	4. If attached properly, there will be no leakage or odor.
5. Apply tail closure to pouch tail.	5. Proper closure controls odor.

PROCEDURE GUIDELINES 18-5 (continued)

Changing a Two-Piece Drainable Fecal Pouching System

PROCEDURE (continued)

| Nursing Action | Rationale |

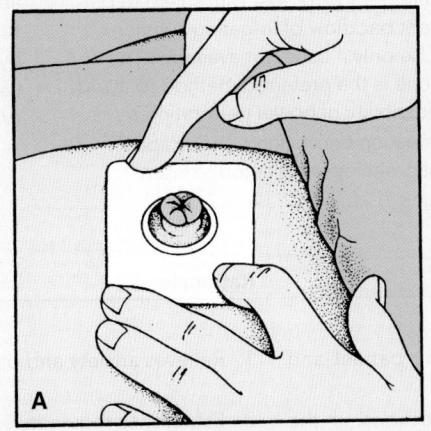 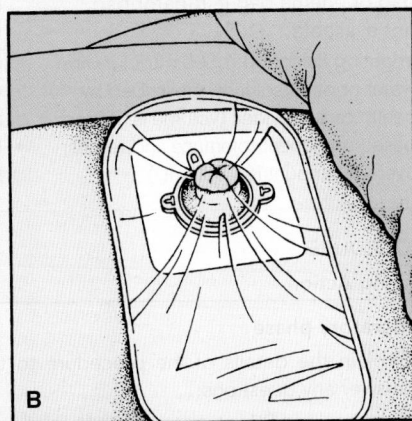

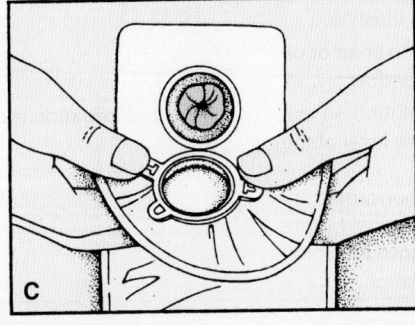 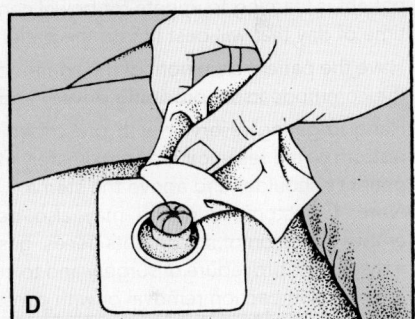

(A) A wafer with flange (1½", 1¾", 2¼", 2¾", 4") is applied after cleaning and drying of peristomal skin. **(B)** A transparent or opaque drainable pouch is positioned over stoma at desired angle. **(C)** Pouch may be removed without removal of wafer. **(D)** Stoma may be assessed without removing wafer. (Adapted with permission from Convatec, a Bristol-Myers, Squibb Company.)

Follow-up phase

1. Dispose of plastic bag with waste materials.
2. Clean drainable pouch with soap and water, if appropriate. Drainable pouches may be reused several times.
3. A commercial deodorant can be placed in the pouch to reduce odor.
4. Gas can be released from the pouch by releasing the tail closure or by snapping off an area on the pouch flange. Never make a pinhole in the pouch to release gas.

1. Complies with universal precautions.
2. Controls odor; reduces cost.

4. Destroys the odorproof seal.

---

d. Disadvantages to colostomy irrigation: it is time-consuming, requires consistency, and bowel dependence may occur.

e. Only a patient with a descending or sigmoid colostomy is an irrigation candidate for fecal control. A colostomy more proximal than descending has too much liquid and too high a volume of fecal output to be managed through irrigation.

f. If a patient discontinues colostomy irrigations after months or years of performance, due to illness, hospitalization, or preference, a bulk laxative or other stimulant may be routinely necessary to maintain regular bowel function.

4. Acknowledge that it is normal to have negative feelings toward ostomy surgery; empathize with the patient.

5. Describe behaviors to attain a sense of control such as resuming activities of daily living (ADLs).

Maintaining Skin Integrity

1. Select pouching system based on type of ostomy and condition of stoma and skin (see page 661).
2. Empty pouch when one third to one half full to avoid overfilling, which interferes with pouch seal.

PROCEDURE GUIDELINES 18-6

Irrigating a Colostomy

EQUIPMENT

- Reservoir for irrigating fluids; irrigator bag or enema bag if irrigator bag not available
- Irrigating fluid: 500–1,500 mL lukewarm water or other solution prescribed by health care provider. (Volume is titrated based on patient tolerance and results; average amount is 1,000 mL.)

- Irrigating tip: Cone tip or soft rubber catheter #22 or #24 with shield to prevent backflow of irrigating solution. (Use only if cone not available. The cone is the preferred method to avoid possibility of bowel perforation.)
- Irrigation sleeve (long, large-capacity bag with opening at top to insert

cone or catheter into stoma); available in different styles: snap-on, self-adhering to skin, or held in place by belt
- Large tail closure
- Water-soluble lubricant

PROCEDURE

Nursing Action	Rationale
Preparatory phase	
1. Explain the details of the procedure to the patient and answer any questions.	1. Relieves anxiety and promotes compliance.
2. Select a consistent time, free from distractions. If the patient is learning to irrigate for bowel control, choose the time of day that will best fit into the patient's lifestyle.	2. Establishes regularity.
3. Have the patient sit in front of the commode on chair or on the commode itself, providing privacy and comfort.	
4. Hang irrigating reservoir with prescribed solution so the bottom of the reservoir is approximately at the level of the patient's shoulder and above the stoma. *Note:* Colostomy irrigation may also be performed to empty the colon of its contents (feces, gas, mucus) before a diagnostic procedure or surgery and to cleanse the colon after fecal impaction removal or with constipation.	4. Height of irrigation bag regulates pressure of irrigant.
Performance phase	
1. Remove pouch or covering from stoma and apply irrigation sleeve, directing the open tail into the commode.	1. Allows water and feces to flow directly into commode.
2. Open tubing clamp on the irrigating reservoir to release a small amount of solution into the commode.	2. Removes air from the setup; avoids air from being introduced into the colon, which can cause crampy pain.
3. Lubricate the tip of the cone/catheter, and gently insert into the stoma. Insert catheter no more than 3 inches (7.5 cm). Hold cone/shield gently, but firmly, against stoma to prevent backflow of water.	3. Prevents intestinal perforation and irritation of mucous membranes.
4. If catheter does not advance easily, allow water to flow slowly while advancing catheter. NEVER FORCE CATHETER. Dilating the stoma with lubricated, gloved pinky finger may be necessary to direct cone/catheter properly.	4. Slow rate relaxes bowel to facilitate passage of catheter.
5. Allow water to enter colon slowly over a 5- to 10-minute period. If cramping occurs, slow flow rate or clamp tubing to allow cramping to subside. If cramping does not subside, remove cone/catheter to release contents.	5. Cramping may occur from too rapid flow, cold water, excess solution, or colon ready to function.
6. Hold cone/shield in place 10 seconds after water is instilled, then gently remove cone/catheter from stoma.	6. Discourages premature evacuation of fluid.
7. As feces and water flow down sleeve, periodically rinse sleeve with water. Allow 10–15 minutes for most of the returns, then dry sleeve tail and apply tail closure.	7. Prevents caking of feces on the sleeve.

PROCEDURE GUIDELINES 18-6 (continued)

Irrigating a Colostomy

PROCEDURE (continued)

Nursing Action	Rationale
8. Leave sleeve in place for approximately 20 more minutes while patient gets up and moves around.	8. Ambulation stimulates peristalsis and completion of irrigation return.
9. When returns are complete, clean stomal area with mild soap and water; pat dry; reapply pouch or covering over stoma.	9. Cleanliness and dryness promote comfort.

Follow-up phase

1. Clean equipment with soap and water; dry and store in well-ventilated area.	1. This will control odor and mildew, prolonging the life of equipment.
2. If applicable, the patient should use a pouch until the colostomy is sufficiently controlled.	2. It may take several months to establish control. The patient can then use minipouch, stoma cap, or gauze covering as desired.

---

a. Remove tail closure from pouch tail.

b. Cuff bottom of pouch tail.

c. Drain stool from pouch.

d. Clean pouch tail with toilet tissue or wipe (may rinse pouch if desired).

e. Uncuff pouch and reapply tail closure.

3. Treat peristomal skin breakdown as needed.

a. Dust skin breakdown with skin barrier powder (eg, Stomahesive powder).

b. Seal powder with water or skin sealant (eg, Skin Prep). May be applied one to three times per day, depending on the severity of the skin breakdown.

c. Allow skin to dry before applying pouching system.

> **NURSING ALERT** When peristomal skin is exposed to excess moisture, candidiasis can occur. It presents as an erythematous rash, which may include papules, pustules, or white patches. Patients may complain of pruritus. The treatment procedure is the same as treating skin breakdown, using a prescribed antifungal powder (nystatin) in place of the skin barrier powder. The antifungal powder should be used at each pouching system change and continued 2 weeks after the condition has cleared. Positive identification of *Candida albicans* can be done through a culture or microscopic visualization. Treatment is usually initiated without culture or scraping if the signs and symptoms are classic.

Maximizing Nutritional Intake

1. Review dietary habits with the patient to determine patterns, preferences, and bowel irritants.

2. Advise the patient to avoid foods that stimulate elimination, such as nuts, seeds, and certain fruits.

3. Recommend consistency in dietary habits as well as moderation.

4. Coordinate consult with nutritionist, as needed.

5. Weigh daily; monitor vital signs and electrolytes to determine patient's nutritional status.

Achieving Sexual Well-Being

1. Encourage the patient and significant other to express feelings about the ostomy.

2. Discuss ways to conceal pouch during intimacy, if desired: pouch covers, special ostomy underwear. May briefly use small-capacity pouch (minipouch or cap).

3. Recommend different positions for sexual activity to decrease stoma friction and skin irritation.

4. Review, when appropriate, that an ostomy in a woman does not prevent a successful pregnancy.

5. Recommend counseling as needed.

Patient Education and Health Maintenance

Skin Care

1. Instruct the patient to inspect peristomal skin with each pouching system change.

2. Review techniques for treating peristomal skin problems.

3. Recommend alternative products if patient develops allergic reaction to an ostomy product.

4. Teach the patient to notify health care provider when skin care problems do not resolve by usual methods.

Odor Control

1. Encourage pouch hygiene through rinsing, keeping pouch tail free of stool, airing of reusable pouches, discarding odor-impregnated pouches.

2. Recommend the use of pouch deodorants, room deodorizers, and oral deodorizers, such as bismuth subgallate or parsley.

3. Avoid use of pinholes in pouch.

Gas Control

1. Suggest avoidance of straws, excessive talking while eating, chewing gum, and smoking to reduce swallowed air.

2. Instruct about gas-forming foods, such as beans and cabbage, and eliminate when appropriate. It takes about 6 hours for gas to travel from mouth to colostomy.

3. Recommend using arm over stoma to muffle gas sounds when appropriate.

ADLs

Educate the patient about the following:

1. Resumption of normal bathing habits (tub or shower) with or without pouching system.

2. Picture framing the edges of the pouching system with water-proof tape, if needed, for bathing or swimming.

3. Clothing modifications usually minimal. Girdles without stays and pantyhose are acceptable.

4. Carrying an ostomy supply kit during work or travel in case of an emergency.

5. Participating in sports as desired. Caution must be exercised with contact sports. During vigorous activities, a belt or binder may provide extra security.

6. For additional information and support, refer to the United Ostomy Association, a self-help group for ostomates and other interested people, at *www.uoa.org*. The official membership publication is the *Ostomy Quarterly*. Encourage ostomy patients to participate in a local chapter. Chapters usually publish a local newsletter, conduct monthly meetings, and provide trained ostomy visitors on request by health care providers.

7. Ostomy manufacturers offer literature covering a wide variety of ostomy-related topics.

8. Encourage the patient to maintain contact with health care providers.

Evaluation: Expected Outcomes

- Verbalizes knowledge regarding ostomy surgery.
- Can view ostomy.
- Demonstrates skills for care of the ostomy.
- No skin breakdown around ostomy.
- Plans menus with nutritionist; weight stable.
- Discusses intimacy concerns with partner.

ESOPHAGEAL DISORDERS

Esophageal varices are covered in Chapter 19, page 721.

Gastroesophageal Reflux Disease and Esophagitis

Gastric contents flow back into the esophagus in gastroesophageal reflux disease (GERD) due to incompetent lower esophageal sphincter (LES). Esophagitis, or inflammation of the esophageal mucosa, may result.

Pathophysiology and Etiology

1. Gastroesophageal reflux associated with an incompetent LES—gastric contents reflux (flow backward) through the LES into the esophagus.

2. Can be the result of impaired gastric emptying from gastroparesis or partial gastric outlet obstruction.

3. The acidity of gastric content and amount of time in contact with esophageal mucosa are related to the degree of mucosal damage.

4. Inflammation and ulceration of the esophagus may result, causing esophagitis.

5. May be caused by motility disorders (scleroderma, esophageal spasm).

Clinical Manifestations

GERD

1. The most common symptom is heartburn (pyrosis), typically occurring 30 to 60 minutes after meals and in reclining positions. May have complaints of spontaneous reflux (regurgitation) of sour or bitter gastric contents into the mouth.

2. Other typical symptoms include globus (sensation of something in throat), mild epigastric pain, dyspepsia, and nausea and/or vomiting.

3. Dysphagia is a less common symptom.

4. Atypical symptoms include chest pain, hoarseness, recurrent sore throat, frequent throat clearing, chronic cough, dental enamel loss, bronchospasm (asthma/wheezing), and odynophagia (sharp substernal pain on swallowing).

5. Symptoms that may suggest other disease etiologies need further evaluation: atypical chest pain (rule out possible cardiac causes), dysphagia, odynophagia, GI bleeding, shortness of breath, or weight loss (rule out cancer or esophageal stricture).

Esophagitis

1. Esophagitis is an acute or chronic inflammation of the esophagus. Severity of symptoms may be unrelated to the degree of esophageal tissue damage.

2. Symptoms vary according to etiology of esophagitis. Symptoms include dysphagia, odynophagia, severe burning, chest pain.

3. Causes of esophagitis other than GERD:
   a. Infectious—*Candida*, herpes, human immunodeficiency virus, cytomegalovirus.
   b. Chemical (alkali or acid) or radiation therapy.
   c. Medication-induced—may include doxycycline, ascorbic acid, quinidine, potassium chloride, bisphosphonates, tetracycline.

Diagnostic Evaluation

1. Uncomplicated GERD may be diagnosed on patient history of typical symptoms.

2. Endoscopy can visualize inflammation, lesions, or erosions. Biopsy can confirm diagnosis.

3. Esophageal manometry measures LES pressure and determines if esophageal peristalsis is adequate. This study should be used before patients undergo surgical treatment for reflux. This test is also done before a pH probe for determination of correct catheter placement.

4. Acid perfusion (Bernstein test)—onset of symptoms after ingestion of dilute hydrochloric acid and saline is considered positive. This test differentiates between cardiac and noncardiac chest pain.

5. Ambulatory 24-hour pH monitoring is frequently performed for diagnosing GERD or reflux esophagitis. It determines

the amount of gastroesophageal acid reflux and has a 70% to 90% specificity rate. The Bravo pH capsule system is a catheter-free system in which a capsule containing a radiotelemetry pH sensor is inserted into the esophagus. This sensor transmits signals to an external pager-size receiver, allowing the patient to be catheter-free during the 24 hours of pH testing.

NURSING ALERT The Bravo pH capsule system is contraindicated for patients with pacemakers, implantable defibrillators, or neurostimulators. It is also contraindicated for patients with a history of severe esophagitis, varices, obstructions, bleeding diatheses, or strictures.

NURSING ALERT The patient should not undergo MRI within 30 days of Bravo capsule pH monitoring.

6. Barium esophagography—use of barium with radiographic studies to diagnose mechanical and motility disorders. This test is rarely useful in diagnosing GERD.

Management

Treatment goals include symptom elimination, healing esophageal damage (if present), and preventing complications and relapse.

Lifestyle Modifications

1. Head of bed raised 6 to 8 inches (15 to 20 cm).
2. Do not lie down for 3 to 4 hours after eating—time frame for greatest reflux.
3. Bland diet—avoid garlic, onion, peppermint, fatty foods, chocolate, coffee (including decaffeinated), citrus juices, colas, and tomato products.
4. Avoid overeating—causes LES relaxation.
5. No tight-fitting clothes.
6. Weight control.
7. Smoking cessation.
8. Reduce alcohol.

Pharmacologic Treatment

1. Antacids—reduce gastric acidity. Use on an as-needed basis. Provide symptomatic relief but do not heal esophageal lesions.
2. Histamine-2 (H_2)-receptor antagonists, such as ranitidine, cimetidine, famotidine, nizatidine—decrease gastric acid secretions. Provide symptomatic relief. May require lifelong therapy.

DRUG ALERT Patients with renal insufficiency and older patients may need decreased dosing of H_2-receptor antagonists.

3. If symptoms do not respond to H_2-receptor antagonist, change to a once-per-day proton pump inhibitor (PPI), such as omeprazole, esomeprazole, pantoprazole, rabeprazole, or lansoprazole, to block gastric acid secretion.

DRUG ALERT PPIs should be taken 30 to 60 minutes before a meal for optimal control of gastric acidity.

4. PPIs have been shown to be more effective than H_2-receptor antagonists in achieving faster healing rates for erosive esophagitis.
5. Drug maintenance therapy may be needed depending on the severity of disease and recurrence of symptoms after initial drug therapy is stopped.
6. Use the lowest effective drug dose of H_2-receptor blocker or PPI.

Antireflux Surgery

1. May be indicated for patients who do not respond to medical management. Common procedure is Nissen fundoplication.
   a. Upper portion of the stomach is wrapped around the distal esophagus and sutured, creating a tight LES.
   b. This procedure can be performed laparoscopically.
   c. Combined with vagotomy-pyloroplasty if associated with gastroduodenal ulcer.
   d. Antireflux surgery may not eliminate the need for future pharmacologic treatment.

Endoscopic Treatments for GERD

1. The Stretta procedure is a radiofrequency energy delivery system used to provide a thermal burn to the gastroesophageal junction.
2. The EndoCinch procedure uses an endoscopic sewing device to create pleats with a series of sutures passed through adjoining folds at the proximal fundus.
3. These procedures are designed to decrease reflux symptoms by tightening the LES.
4. Enteryx, an endoscopically implanted device, prevents reflux of gastric acid into the throat. The device is permanently placed and may eliminate the need for pharmacologic treatment of GERD symptoms.

Complications

1. Esophageal stricture formation.
2. Ulceration of the esophagus, with or without fistula formation.
3. Aspiration, may be complicated by pneumonia.
4. Development of Barrett's esophagus—presence of columnar epithelium above the gastroesophageal junction associated with adenocarcinoma of the esophagus.

Nursing Interventions and Patient Education

1. Teach the patient about prescribed medications, adverse effects, and when to notify the health care provider. PPIs may interact with carbamazepine, cyclosporine, diazepam, diclofenac, digoxin, iron, ketoconazole, lidocaine, methotrexate, metoprolol, nifedipine, phenytoin, propranolol, quinidine, theophylline, and warfarin.
2. Inform the patient about medications that may exacerbate symptoms.
3. Advise the patient to sit or stand when taking any solid medication (pills, capsules); emphasize the need to follow the drug with at least 100 mL of liquid.
4. Familiarize the patient and family with foods and activities to avoid, such as fatty foods, garlic, onions, alcohol, coffee, chocolate, and peppermint.

5. Caution the patient against straining, bending over, tight-fitting clothes, and smoking.
6. Encourage the patient to sleep with the head of the bed elevated (not pillow elevation).
7. Encourage a weight-reduction program, if the patient is overweight, to decrease intra-abdominal pressure.

 DRUG ALERT Anticholinergics may further impair functioning of the LES, allowing reflux; antihistamines, antidepressants, antihypertensives, antispasmodics, and some neuroleptics and antiparkinsonian drugs decrease saliva production, which may decrease acid clearance from the esophagus.

Hiatal Hernia

A hiatal hernia is a protrusion of a portion of the stomach through the hiatus of the diaphragm and into the thoracic cavity.

Pathophysiology and Etiology

1. There are two types of hiatal hernias (see Figure 18-3):
   a. Sliding hernia: Stomach and gastroesophageal junction slip up into the chest (most common).
   b. Paraesophageal hernia (rolling hernia): Part of the greater curvature of the stomach rolls through the diaphragmatic defect.
2. Caused by muscle weakening due to aging or other conditions, such as esophageal carcinoma or trauma, or following certain surgical procedures.

Clinical Manifestations

1. May be asymptomatic.
2. Heartburn (with or without regurgitation of gastric contents into the mouth).
3. Dysphagia, chest pain.

Diagnostic Evaluation

1. Barium study of the esophagus outlines hernia.
2. Endoscopic examination visualizes defect.

Management

1. Elevation of head of bed (6 to 8 inches [15 to 20 cm]) to reduce nighttime reflux.
2. Antacid therapy to neutralize gastric acid.
3. H_2-receptor antagonist (cimetidine, ranitidine) if patient has esophagitis.
4. Surgical repair of hernia if symptoms are severe.

Complications

1. Aspiration of reflux contents.
2. Ulceration, hemorrhage.
3. Gastritis.
4. Stricture.
5. Incarceration of the portion of the stomach in the chest.

Nursing Interventions and Patient Education

1. Instruct the patient on the prevention of reflux of gastric contents into the esophagus by:
   a. Eating smaller meals.
   b. Avoiding stimulation of gastric secretions by omitting caffeine and alcohol.
   c. Refraining from smoking.
   d. Avoiding fatty foods: promote reflux and delay gastric emptying.
   e. Refraining from lying down for at least 1 hour after meals.
   f. Losing weight, if obese.
   g. Avoiding bending from the waist and/or wearing tight-fitting clothes.
2. Advise the patient to report to health care facility immediately for the onset of acute chest pain, which may indicate incarceration of a large paraesophageal hernia.

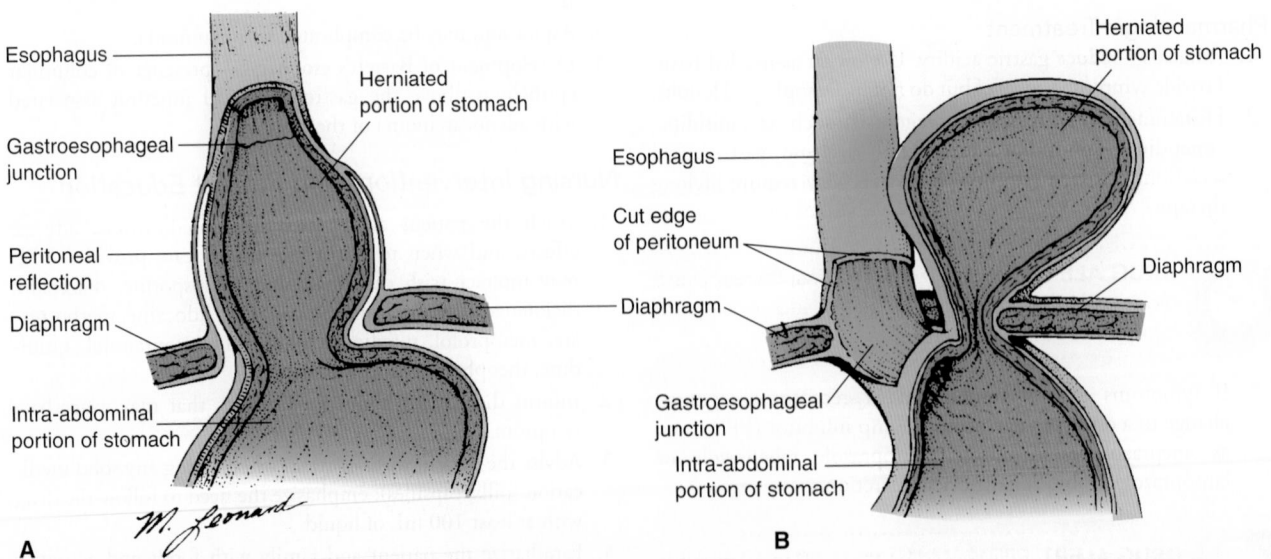

Figure 18-3. Hiatal hernia. (A) Sliding hernia. **(B)** Paraesophageal hernia.

Esophageal Trauma and Perforations

Esophageal trauma or perforations are injuries to the esophagus caused by external or internal insult.

Pathophysiology and Etiology

1. External: Stab or bullet wounds, crush injuries, blunt trauma.
2. Internal:
   a. Swallowed foreign objects (coins, pins, bones, dental appliances, caustic poisons).
   b. Spontaneous or postemetic rupture—usually in the presence of underlying esophageal disease (reflux, hiatal hernia).
   c. Mallory-Weiss syndrome—nonpenetrating mucosal tear at the gastroesophageal junction. Caused by an increase in transabdominal pressure from lifting, vomiting, or retching. Alcoholism is a predisposing condition.

Clinical Manifestations

1. Pain at the site of injury or impaction, aggravated by swallowing—chest pain, may be severe.
2. Dysphagia or odynophagia.
3. Persistent foreign object sensation.
4. Subcutaneous emphysema and crepitus of face, neck, or upper thorax—noted in cervical, thoracic, and esophageal perforations.
5. Temperature elevation occurring within 24 hours of trauma.
6. Blood-stained saliva or excessive salivation.
7. Hematemesis; previous history of vomiting or retching—Mallory-Weiss syndrome.
8. Respiratory difficulty if there is pressure on the tracheobronchial tree from injury or edema.

Diagnostic Evaluation

1. History of recent esophageal trauma.
2. Chest x-ray to look for foreign body.
3. Esophagogram to outline trauma.
4. Endoscopy to directly visualize trauma.

Management

1. Maintenance of adequate respiratory functioning; may require oxygen support or endotracheal intubation—to ensure an open airway in the presence of edema of the neck.
2. Replacement of fluids. May need blood transfusion. Bleeding may stop spontaneously; if not, endoscopic hemostatic therapy or surgery is indicated.
3. Restoration of the continuity of the esophagus by removing the cause.
4. For external wound injury, emergency first-aid wound care and surgical repair may be indicated.
5. For swallowed foreign bodies:
   a. Barium swallow determines location of foreign body; usually removed through endoscopy.
   b. Some patients with a history of food impaction may be treated with a spasmolytic such as IV glucagon.

6. For chemical ingestion:
   a. If lye or other caustic or organic solvent was swallowed, do NOT try to induce vomiting.
   b. Treat with IV fluids and analgesics.
   c. A gastrostomy may be performed, either as a temporary or a permanent means of feeding the patient.
   d. Resulting strictures may be relieved by dilating the narrow esophagus.
   e. Reconstructive surgery may be necessary to create a new passageway for food between pharynx and stomach.

Complications

1. Airway occlusion.
2. Shock.
3. Perforation with mediastinitis or pleural effusion.
4. Stricture formation.
5. Abscess or fistula formation.

Nursing Assessment

1. Assess the following to determine status of patient:
   a. Vital signs.
   b. Respiratory status.
   c. Bleeding.
   d. Ability to swallow—choking, gagging.
2. Monitor the patient for hypovolemic shock.

Nursing Diagnoses

- Deficient Fluid Volume related to blood loss from injury.
- Imbalanced Nutrition: Less Than Body Requirements related to esophageal injury.
- Ineffective Breathing Pattern related to pain and trauma.
- Acute Pain related to injury.

Nursing Interventions

Maintaining Fluid Volume

1. Administer IV fluids and blood transfusion for volume replacement, if indicated.
2. Monitor intake and output. Urine output should be greater than 30 mL/hour.
3. Monitor laboratory results (electrolytes, hemoglobin, and hematocrit) and report abnormal findings.

Maintaining Nutritional Status

1. Monitor daily weights and skin turgor.
2. Administer parenteral hyperalimentation as prescribed—to prevent gastric reflux into the esophagus, which may occur with enteral feedings.
3. Encourage progression of diet through NG, esophagostomy, or oral feedings when esophagoscopy or esophagogram reveals healing of the esophagus.
4. Continue to monitor intake and output.

Maintaining Respiratory Function

1. Auscultate the lungs and trachea for stridor, crackles, or wheezes. Assess respiratory rate, depth, use of accessory muscles, and skin color.

2. Position the patient in semi-Fowler's position to facilitate breathing and reduce neck edema.
3. Monitor vital signs frequently for signs and symptoms of shock and infection.
4. Administer oxygen as prescribed.
5. Have emergency airway equipment at bedside.

Reducing Pain

1. Administer analgesics as prescribed—IV analgesia may be required to control pain and allow the esophagus to rest.
2. Provide reassurance and support.
3. Assess and record pain relief.
4. Evaluate for symptoms that may indicate spillage of digestive contents into the mediastinum, pleura, or abdominal cavity—sudden onset of acute pain.

Patient Education and Health Maintenance

1. Instruct the patient on the indications and adverse effects of analgesics.
2. Inform the patient on the signs and symptoms to report on possible complications: increase in severity or nature of pain; difficulty breathing or swallowing.
3. See Procedure Guidelines 18-7. This assists the patient who has difficulty swallowing after injury or surgical correction of the oropharynx or upper esophagus (also helpful with neurologic deficit or stroke).
4. Teach the patient about tests or surgical procedures that may be performed.

Evaluation: Expected Outcomes

- Urine output greater than 30 mL/hour; electrolytes stable.
- No further weight loss, tolerating parenteral feedings well.
- Lungs clear, respirations unlabored.
- States pain decreased to level of 2 or 3 on 0-to-10 scale.

Motility Disorders of the Esophagus

Primary motility disorders include achalasia, diffuse esophageal spasm, and those of nonspecific origin. Secondary motility disorders may be caused by neuromuscular, GI, endocrine, or connective tissue disorders.

Pathophysiology and Etiology

Primary Motility Disorders

1. Achalasia refers to excessive resting tone of the LES, incomplete relaxation of the LES with swallowing, and failure of normal peristalsis in the lower two thirds of the esophagus. The pathology is related to defective innervation of the myenteric plexus innervating the involuntary muscles of the esophagus.
2. Diffuse esophageal spasm is a motor disorder in which high-amplitude, nonpropulsive, nonperistaltic tertiary contractions (a form of aperistalsis) are present. LES functioning is frequently normal.

Secondary Motility Disorders

1. Neuromuscular dysfunction includes myasthenia gravis, Parkinson's disease, muscular dystrophy, amyotrophic lateral sclerosis, and cerebral palsy.
2. Connective tissue disorders include scleroderma.
3. GI causes include GERD.
4. Other secondary causes include the autonomic neuropathy of diabetes mellitus.

Clinical Manifestations

Achalasia

1. Gradual onset of dysphagia with solids and liquids.
2. Substernal discomfort or a feeling of fullness.
3. Regurgitation of undigested food during a meal or within several hours after a meal.
4. Weight loss.

Diffuse Esophageal Spasm

1. Intermittent dysphagia for solids or liquids—does not progress to continuous dysphagia.
2. Aggravation of symptoms (large volume of food and hot or cold liquids).
3. Anterior chest pain.

Secondary Motility Disorders

Symptoms of esophagitis from gastroesophageal reflux.

Diagnostic Evaluation

Achalasia

1. Chest x-ray, which may show an enlarged, fluid-filled esophagus.
2. Barium esophagography showing dilation, decreased or absence of peristalsis, decreased emptying, and a "bird beak" narrowing of the distal esophagus.
3. Esophageal manometry to confirm the diagnoses suspected.
4. EUS or a chest CT for suspected tumor.

Diffuse Esophageal Spasm

1. Barium esophagography showing simultaneous contractions of the esophagus having a "corkscrew" or "rosary bead" appearance.
2. Esophageal manometry showing intermittent contractions with episodes of normal peristalsis.

Secondary Motility Disorders

Diagnostic workup may include barium esophagography or manometry.

Management

Achalasia

1. Drug therapy using calcium channel blockers such as nifedipine to reduce LES pressure. This type of treatment is usually best for patients presenting with mild symptoms and a non-dilated esophagus or patients who are medically unstable to undergo invasive therapies.
2. Esophageal dilation using a balloon-tipped catheter is the preferred treatment for most patients.
3. Surgical therapy (Heller's myotomy of the LES) may be used on patients who do not respond to balloon dilation. This surgery requires a laparotomy or thoracotomy or may be done through a thoracoscope.

PROCEDURE GUIDELINES 18-7

Teaching the Patient with Dysphagia How to Swallow

EQUIPMENT

- Suction
- Face mask
- Glass with straw
- Oxygen
- Selected foods

PROCEDURE

Nursing Action	Rationale
Preparation	
1. Explain to the patient that you plan to work with him or her in developing an effective swallow.	1. The patient's cooperation, concentration, and directed participation are essential to the success of this learning experience.
2. Make sure that emergency equipment—including suction, oxygen, and face mask—is at the bedside.	2. For use in the event that the patient chokes, vomits, or aspirates.
3. Place the patient in an upright sitting position in a chair or support with pillows in high-Fowler's position if unable to get out of bed—for about 20 minutes before and 45–60 minutes after meals.	3. Allows time to adjust and relax in this position before meals; allows gravity to assist the swallowing procedure during meals; helps prevent reflux or regurgitation after meals.
4. Provide mouth care before meals. Suction the patient if secretions are present. If the patient's mouth is dry, provide a lemon wedge or pickle to suck on.	4. Increases patient's ability to taste and enjoy the sensation of eating.
5. Prepare an environment that is pleasant, peaceful, and without interruptions. Remove distractions, such as TV and radio.	5. Patient must be able to concentrate on the process of swallowing in a relaxed manner.
Food and fluid selection	
1. Foods that hold some shape should be chosen; moist enough to prevent crumbling but dry enough to hold a bolus shape—casseroles, custards, scrambled eggs.	1. Foods that crumble may be aspirated when they fall apart; foods that are too moist may be drooled through the lips.
2. Mugs and glasses with spouts or a straw should be used for liquids.	2. These utensils help prevent liquids from leaking out of corners of patient's mouth.
3. Avoid sticky foods—peanut butter, chocolate, milk, ice cream.	3. These foods stimulate thick mucus and will make swallowing more difficult.
4. Dry foods can be moistened with margarine, gravy, or broths. If liquids are a problem, juices can be thickened with sherbets.	4. Foods need to be of a consistency that will hold a bolus form until swallowed.
5. Avoid tepid or room-temperature foods.	5. Hot and cold foods are thought to maximally stimulate receptors that activate swallowing mechanism.
Instructions during meals	
1. Have patient position head in the midline and forward, chin pointed toward chest.	1. Improves ability to consciously swallow without food falling down the posterior pharynx. Support patient's forehead with your hand if the patient lacks neck control.
2. Instruct the patient to smell the food before each bite; hold each bite for a few seconds; hold lips together firmly; concentrate on swallowing; then swallow.	2. Concentrating on each step before swallowing will increase the effectiveness of the swallow.
3. If the patient has an increase in saliva during the meal, instruct the patient to collect the saliva with the tongue and consciously swallow it between bites throughout the meal.	3. Helps prevent aspiration of saliva between mouthfuls.
4. If the patient complains of a dry mouth during meals, instruct him to move his tongue in a circular fashion against the insides of the cheeks.	4. Helps stimulate salivation.
5. Caution the patient against talking during the meal or with the mouth full of food.	5. Talking or laughing during eating is a common cause of airway obstruction.

(continued)

PROCEDURE GUIDELINES 18-7 *(continued)*

Teaching the Patient with Dysphagia How to Swallow

PROCEDURE *(continued)*

Nursing Action	Rationale
Feeding the patient with an affected side of the mouth (facial paralysis, hemiplegia)	
1. Turn the patient to the unaffected side.	1. Helps prevent food from falling down the weaker/paralyzed part of the oral cavity, a possible cause of aspiration.
2. Place food on the unaffected side of mouth rather than in the middle of the mouth.	2. Permits food to be managed more effectively.
3. Encourage the patient to form a bolus by moving the food around the mouth with the tongue.	3. Assists in placing food in a proper position for swallowing, rather than permitting food to collect near the cheek.
Follow-up care	
1. Provide mouth care after meals.	1. Food particles may collect in the mouth or cheeks.
2. Record the amount of intake, the patient's taste and food preferences, progress, and any special tactics that were effective in helping the swallowing process.	2. Progress notes will assist in moving toward self-care.
3. Encourage family members to participate in the patient's feeding program.	3. Helps provide continuity on discharge.

Diffuse Esophageal Spasm

1. Drug therapy using nitrates and calcium channel blockers is the primary treatment.
2. Dilation may provide some symptom relief.
3. Surgical myotomy is used rarely for patients with a debilitating disorder who are able to withstand a surgical procedure.

Other Motility Disorders

1. Treatment of the gastroesophageal reflux.
2. Dilation may be required for peptic stricture.

Complications

1. Malnutrition.
2. Pneumonia, lung abscess, bronchiectasis from nocturnal regurgitation causing aspiration.
3. Esophagitis, esophageal diverticula.
4. Perforation from dilation procedure.
5. Peptic stricture or Barrett's esophagus from severe erosive esophagitis.

Nursing Assessment

1. Assess for difficulty with swallowing, vomiting, weight loss, chest pain associated with eating.
2. Inquire as to what facilitates passage of food, such as position changes, use of liquids.

Nursing Diagnoses

- Imbalanced Nutrition: Less Than Body Requirements related to dysphagia.
- Acute Pain related to heartburn or surgical procedure.

Nursing Interventions

Improving Nutritional Status

1. Direct the patient to eat sitting in an upright position; eat slowly and chew food thoroughly.
2. Avoid food and beverages that precipitate symptoms.
3. Suggest that the patient sleep with head elevated to avoid reflux or aspiration.
4. Provide a bland diet and tell the patient to avoid alcohol as well as spicy, very hot, and very cold foods, to minimize symptoms.
5. Eliminate sources of tension as a precipitating factor producing stress during mealtimes.
6. Administer pharmacologic agents as prescribed.

Promoting Comfort

1. Assess the patient for discomfort, chest pain, regurgitation, and cough. If a surgical procedure was performed, assess for incisional pain.
2. Provide appropriate postoperative care. Incisional approach determines nature of postoperative care (eg, an incision through chest implies nursing care similar to that given to a patient with a thoracotomy [see page 263]).
3. Administer analgesics as ordered.
4. Assess for effectiveness of pain medication.

Patient Education and Health Maintenance

1. Encourage lifestyle activity changes similar to those for patients with reflux (see page 667).
2. See Procedure Guidelines 18-7 to help the patient with dysphasia with swallowing.
3. Provide information on all diagnostic procedures or surgery performed.

Evaluation: Expected Outcomes

- Demonstrates proper positioning for eating; describes dietary habits that minimize symptoms; compliant with medications regimen.
- States pain decreased to 2 or 3 on 0-to-10 scale.

Esophageal Diverticulum

An esophageal diverticulum is an outpouching of the esophageal wall, usually in the cervical posterior side, secondary to an obstructive or inflammatory process.

Pathophysiology and Etiology

1. *Zenker's diverticulum*—protrusion of pharyngeal mucosa at the pharyngoesophageal junction between the interior pharyngeal constrictor and cricopharyngeal muscle.
2. Mid or distal esophageal diverticula may develop above strictures or may be secondary to motility disorders.

Clinical Manifestations

Zenker's Diverticulum

1. Difficulty in swallowing, fullness in neck, throat discomfort, a feeling that food stops before it reaches the stomach, and regurgitation of undigested food.
2. Belching, gurgling, or nocturnal coughing brought about by diverticulum becoming filled with food or liquid, which is regurgitated and may irritate the trachea.
3. Halitosis and foul taste in mouth caused by food decomposing in a pouch (diverticulum).
4. Weight loss due to nutritional depletion.

 GERONTOLOGIC ALERT Hoarseness, asthma, and pneumonitis may be the only signs of esophageal diverticula in older adults.

Mid or Distal Esophageal Diverticula
Generally no symptoms.

Diagnostic Evaluation

1. Barium esophagogram outlines diverticulum.
2. Endoscopy is not indicated and may be dangerous due to the possibility of rupture.

Management

Zenker's Diverticulum

1. Small diverticula may not be treated, but the underlying cause is treated with dilatation or myotomy.
2. A transverse cervical diverticulectomy or diverticuloplexy with suspension and cricopharyngeal myotomy may be done.
   a. Caution is taken to avoid injury to common carotid artery and internal jugular vein.
   b. Sac is dissected free and then excised flush with esophageal wall.

Mid or Distal Esophageal Diverticula
Underlying primary condition must be treated.

Complications

1. Aspiration pneumonia.
2. Malnutrition.
3. Lung abscess.

Nursing Assessment

1. Obtain history of dysphagia, coughing, throat discomfort, choking, regurgitation of food.
2. Evaluate for halitosis.
3. Determine what measures assist the patient with food intake; what foods and fluids the patient can tolerate.
4. Evaluate weight loss and dietary habits.

Nursing Diagnoses

- Imbalanced Nutrition: Less Than Body Requirements related to dysphagia.
- Acute Pain related to symptoms and surgical procedure.

Nursing Interventions

Improving Nutritional Status

1. Provide frequent, small meals, which are better tolerated.
2. Elevate head of bed for 2 hours after eating.
3. Monitor intake and output.
4. Weigh daily.

Maintaining Comfort and Preventing Complications

1. Preoperatively, or if the condition is nonoperative, implement nursing interventions similar to those for esophagitis.
2. Postoperatively, wound care is similar to that of other surgical incisions of the same anatomical position (eg, thoracotomy [see page 263] or neck surgery).
3. Administer appropriate pain medications and assess effectiveness.
4. Patient may need oral suctioning to control drooling.
5. Maintain NG tube if in place.
   a. Irrigate tube as ordered.
   b. Do not manipulate NG tube due to location of tube and suture line.

Patient Education and Health Maintenance

1. Instruct patient regarding treatment of esophagitis caused by gastroesophageal reflux (see page 667).
2. Instruct patient on importance of good oral hygiene.

Evaluation: Expected Outcomes

- Tolerates oral feedings; maintains weight.
- States pain decreased to 2 or 3 on 0-to-10 scale.

Cancer of the Esophagus

Malignant lesions of the esophagus occur in four types worldwide: squamous cell, adenocarcinoma, carcinosarcoma, and sarcoma.

Pathophysiology and Etiology

Incidence

1. Incidence of adenocarcinoma of the distal and middle third of the esophagus appears to be increasing in the Western world.

2. Squamous cell carcinoma, most often originating in the upper half of the esophagus, appears to have an incidence equal to adenocarcinoma.

3. Highest rate in the United States occurs in men, who are usually older than age 60; more common in nonwhite males.

Associated Factors

Cause is unknown but has been associated with:

1. Barrett's esophagus.
2. Achalasia.
3. Chronic use of alcohol and tobacco (squamous cell carcinoma).
4. Genetic predisposition—nonwhite male population.
5. Ingestion of caustic substances (such as lye), which cause esophageal strictures.
6. Other head and neck cancers.

Clinical Manifestations

1. Dysphagia is the usual presenting symptom, although it is a late sign, by which time there often is regional or systemic involvement.
2. Mild, atypical chest pain associated with eating precedes dysphagia but is rarely significant enough for the patient to seek health care.
3. Pain on swallowing (odynophagia).
4. Progressive weight loss.
5. Hoarseness (if laryngeal involvement).
6. Lymphadenopathy (supraclavicular or cervical) or hepatomegaly with metastatic involvement.
7. Later symptoms—hiccups, respiratory difficulty, foul breath, regurgitation of food and saliva.

Diagnostic Evaluation

1. Chest x-ray may show adenopathy, mediastinal widening, metastasis, or a tracheoesophageal fistula.
2. Endoscopy with cytology and biopsy.
3. Surveillance endoscopy of Barrett's esophagus is beneficial for early detection of malignant changes.
4. Barium esophagram may show polypoid, infiltrative, or ulcerative lesion requiring biopsy.
5. CT scanning may be helpful in delineating the extent of the tumor as well as in identifying presence of adjacent tissue invasion and metastases.

Management

1. The goal of treatment may be cure or palliation, depending on the staging of the tumor and the patient's overall condition in relation to nutritional, cardiovascular, pulmonary, and functional status.
2. The wide variability in treatment reflects the overall poor results from any one approach.
3. Surgery.
   a. Lesions of the middle and lower esophagus are excised with use of the thoracotomy approach with esophagogastrectomy or colon interposition (section of colon is used to replace the excised portion of the esophagus).
   b. Lesions of the cervical esophagus are excised with a bilateral neck dissection and esophagogastrectomy; laryngectomy and thyroidectomy may be necessary.

   c. A two-step approach may be selected when resection with a cervical esophagostomy and feeding gastrostomy are performed initially; subsequent reconstructive surgery is performed.
4. Radiation, chemotherapy, or their combination; combination therapy appears to have better results.
5. Palliative treatment of dysphagia through dilation done by endoscopy or laser therapy.
6. The goal of palliative treatment is to reduce the complications of the tumor to improve quality of life. Any one or a combination of the aforementioned therapies can be used for palliative treatment.

Complications

1. Preoperatively: Malnutrition, aspiration pneumonitis, hemorrhage, sepsis, tracheoesophageal fistula.
2. Postoperatively: Pneumonia, dumping syndrome, nutritional deficiencies, reflux esophagitis, anastomosis leakage.

Nursing Assessment

1. Obtain history of symptoms, such as dysphagia, pain, cough, hoarseness.
2. Evaluate for weight loss and dietary changes.
3. Assess support system and personal coping mechanisms.

Nursing Diagnoses

- Imbalanced Nutrition: Less Than Body Requirements related to disease process and treatment.
- Risk for Infection related to chronic disease, invasive procedures, and treatment.
- Ineffective Coping related to dealing with cancer.

Nursing Interventions

Improving Nutritional and Fluid Status

1. Provide the preoperative patient with a high-protein, high-calorie diet as tolerated. Nutritional supplements may be indicated. TPN may be ordered if unable to take food or fluids orally.
2. Postoperatively, administer IV fluids as prescribed. Initially, the patient may require large volumes if extensive excision of lymph nodes was performed. TPN may be ordered.
3. Assess for bowel sounds; administer fluids per NG tube and liquid feedings through jejunostomy, as prescribed.
4. Encourage patient in advancing diet from liquids to soft foods.
5. Remind patient to remain in upright position for approximately 2 hours after eating to avoid reflux.
6. Provide mouth care for patient comfort and hygiene.

Monitoring for Complications

1. Monitor blood pressure (BP), pulse, respiration, and temperature to note early onset of hemorrhage, infection, dysrhythmias, aspiration, or anastomosis leakage.
2. Observe drainage from incision and/or chest tube for bleeding or purulence.
3. Monitor arterial blood gas (ABG) levels, manage pain, suction, provide chest physiotherapy, and provide oxygen as indicated.

Strengthening Individual Coping

1. Encourage patient to utilize support system during treatment and recovery process.
2. Provide information about laryngectomy, gastrostomy, and other procedures related to surgery, as indicated.
3. Provide training in relaxation techniques and diversional therapy for anxiety and pain control after surgery.
4. Refer to the American Cancer Society (*www.acs.org*) for additional information and sources of support.

Patient Education and Health Maintenance

1. Encourage the patient to avoid overeating, take small bites, chew food well; avoid chunks of meat and stringy raw vegetables and fruit.
2. Depending on type of surgery, small, frequent meals may be better tolerated.
3. Encourage rest postoperatively and advancing activities as tolerated.
4. Instruct the patient regarding signs and symptoms of complications to report: nausea, vomiting, elevated temperature, cough, difficulty swallowing.

Evaluation: Expected Outcomes

- Good skin turgor; eating small, frequent meals; gaining weight.
- Vital signs stable, incision without drainage.
- Performing self-care with help of support people.

GASTRODUODENAL DISORDERS

Gastrointestinal Bleeding

GI bleeding is not just a gastroduodenal disorder but may occur anywhere along the alimentary tract. Bleeding is a symptom of an upper or lower GI disorder. It may be obvious in emesis or stool, or it may be occult (hidden).

Pathophysiology and Etiology

1. Trauma anywhere along the GI tract.
2. Erosions or ulcers.
3. Rupture of an enlarged vein such as a varicosity (esophageal or gastric varices).
4. Inflammation, such as esophagitis (caused by acid or bile), gastritis, inflammatory bowel disease (chronic ulcerative colitis, Crohn's disease), and bacterial infection.
5. Alcohol and drugs (aspirin-containing compounds, NSAIDs, anticoagulants, corticosteroids).
6. Diverticular disease.
7. Cancers.
8. Vascular lesions or disorders, such as bowel ischemia, aortoenteric fistula, arteriovenous malformations.
9. Mallory-Weiss tear.
10. Anal disorders, such as hemorrhoids or fissures.

Clinical Manifestations

Characteristics of Blood

1. Bright red: vomited from high in esophagus (hematemesis); passed from rectum or distal colon (coating stool).
2. Dark red: higher up in colon and small intestine; mixed with stool.
3. Shades of black ("coffee ground"): vomited from esophagus, stomach, and duodenum.
4. Tarry stool (melena): occurs in patient who accumulates excessive blood in the stomach.

Signs and Symptoms of Bleeding

1. Massive bleeding.
   a. Acute, bright red hematemesis or large amount of melena with clots in the stool.
   b. Rapid pulse, drop in BP, hypovolemia, and shock.
2. Subacute bleeding.
   a. Intermittent melena or coffee-ground emesis.
   b. Hypotension.
   c. Weakness, dizziness.
3. Chronic bleeding.
   a. Intermittent appearance of blood.
   b. Increased weakness, paleness, or shortness of breath.
   c. Occult blood.
   d. Iron-deficiency anemia.

Diagnostic Evaluation

1. It is not difficult to diagnose bleeding, but it may be difficult to locate the source of bleeding.
2. History: change in bowel pattern, presence of pain or tenderness, recent intake of food and what kind (eg, red beets), alcohol consumption, drugs (eg, aspirin or steroids).
3. Complete blood count (CBC) (hemoglobin, hematocrit, platelets) and coagulation studies (partial thromboplastin time, prothrombin time with international normalized ratio) may show abnormalities.
4. Endoscopy: identifies source of bleeding, determines risk of rebleeding, and provides endoscopic therapy, if needed.
5. Imaging may detect etiology of bleeding.
6. Test of stool for occult blood.

Management

Based on Etiology

1. If aspirin or NSAIDs are the cause, discontinue medication and treat bleeding.
2. If ulcer is the cause, assess medications, dietary and lifestyle modifications, and for *Helicobacter pylori*.
3. Therapeutic endoscopic procedure (cautery, injection).
4. Surgery may be indicated for cancers, inflammatory diseases, and vascular disorders.

Emergency Intervention

1. Patient remains on NPO status.
2. IV lines and oxygen therapy initiated.
3. If life-threatening bleeding occurs, treat shock, administer blood replacement, intra-arterial vasopressin or embolization.
4. Surgical therapy, if indicated.

Nasogastric Intubation

1. An NG tube should be in place for most patients with acute or upper GI bleeding.
2. If the aspirate continues to be bloody after 2 to 3 L of tap water lavage, the patient may have an active bleed requiring more emergent intervention or endoscopic therapy.

Other Measures

1. Electrocoagulation using a heater probe.
2. Injection of sclerosant or epinephrine.

 NURSING ALERT Because of the action of topical thrombin, it is used only on the surface of bleeding tissue and is never injected into the blood vessels, where intravascular clotting could occur.

3. Endoscopy used in conjunction with management measures as well as in diagnostic evaluation.
4. Pharmacotherapy depends on cause; can include histamine blockers—as either continuous IV (preferred) or bolus infusion to block the acid-secreting action of histamine—or IV pantoprozole (Protonix). Intra-arterial vasopressin can be used to slow or stop active bleeding from diverticulum or vascular ectasia.
5. Surgery is indicated when more conservative measures fail.

Complications

1. Hemorrhage.
2. Shock.
3. Death.

Nursing Assessment

1. Obtain history regarding:
   a. Change in bowel patterns or hemorrhoids.
   b. Change in color of stools (dark black, red, or streaked with blood).
   c. Alcohol consumption.
   d. Medications, such as aspirin, NSAIDs, antibiotics, anticoagulants, corticosteroids.
   e. Hematemesis.
   f. Other medical conditions.
2. Evaluate for presence of abdominal pain or tenderness.
3. Monitor vital signs and laboratory tests for changes that indicate bleeding (hemoglobin, hematocrit, platelet count, coagulation studies).
4. Test for occult blood, if indicated.

Nursing Diagnoses

• Deficient Fluid Volume related to blood loss.
• Imbalanced Nutrition: Less Than Body Requirements related to nausea, vomiting, diarrhea.

Nursing Interventions

Attaining Normal Fluid Volume

1. Maintain NG tube and NPO status to rest GI tract and evaluate bleeding.
2. Monitor intake and output, as ordered, to evaluate fluid status.
3. Monitor vital signs, as ordered.
4. Observe for changes indicating shock, such as tachycardia, hypotension, increased respirations, decreased urine output, change in mental status.
5. Administer IV fluids and blood products, as ordered, to maintain volume.

Attaining Balanced Nutritional Status

1. Weigh daily to monitor caloric status.
2. Administer IV fluids, TPN, if ordered, to promote hydration and nutrition while on oral restrictions.
3. Begin liquids when patient is no longer NPO. Advance diet as tolerated. Diet should be high-calorie, high-protein. Small, frequent feedings may be indicated.
4. Offer snacks; high-protein supplements.

Patient Education and Health Maintenance

1. Discuss the cause and treatment of GI bleeding with patient.
2. Instruct patient regarding signs and symptoms of GI bleeding: melena, emesis that is bright red or "coffee ground" color, rectal bleeding, weakness, fatigue, shortness of breath.
3. Instruct patient on how to test stool or emesis for occult blood, if applicable.

Evaluation: Expected Outcomes

• Intake and output equal, vital signs stable.
• Tolerates small feedings, weight stable.

PEPTIC ULCER DISEASE

Peptic ulcer disease refers to ulcerations in the mucosa of the lower esophagus, stomach, or duodenum (see Figure 18-4).

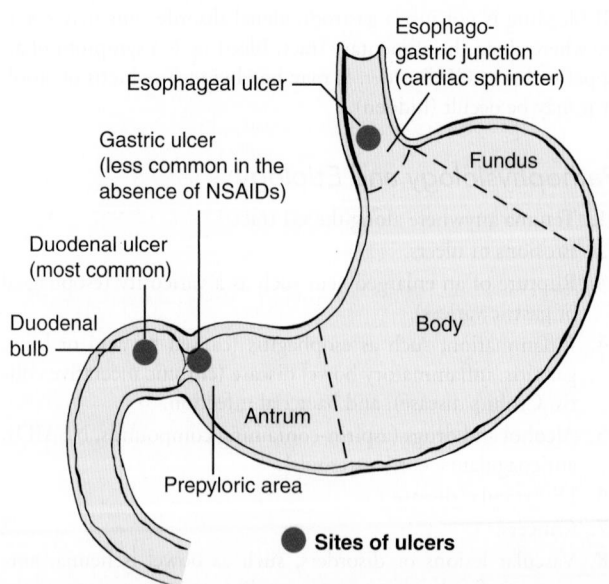

Figure 18-4. Esophageal, gastric, and duodenal ulcer sites.

Pathophysiology and Etiology

1. Etiology of peptic ulcer disease is multifactorial.
   a. *H. pylori* infection—present in most patients with peptic ulcer disease.
   b. NSAID-induced injury—presents as a chemical gastropathy.
   c. Acid secretory abnormalities (especially in duodenal ulcers).
   d. Zollinger-Ellison syndrome (hypersecretory syndrome) should be considered in refractory ulcers.
2. Risk factors may include drugs (NSAIDs, prolonged high-dose corticosteroids), family history, Zollinger-Ellison syndrome, cigarettes, stress, O blood type, and lower socioeconomic status.
3. Studies are inconclusive in determining an association between ulcer formation and diet or the intake of alcohol and caffeine.

Clinical Manifestations

1. Gnawing or burning epigastric pain occurring 1½ to 3 hours after a meal.
2. Nocturnal epigastric, abdominal pain or burning; may awaken patient at night, usually around midnight to 3 AM.
3. Epigastric tenderness on examination.
4. Early satiety, anorexia, weight loss, heartburn, belching (may indicate reflux disease).
5. Dizziness, syncope, hematemesis, or melena (may indicate hemorrhage).
6. Anemia.

 NURSING ALERT Sudden, intense midepigastric pain radiating to the right shoulder may indicate ulcer perforation.

Diagnostic Evaluation

1. Upper GI endoscopy with possible tissue biopsy and cytology.
   a. PyloriTek, a biopsy urea test, is up to >97% specific and >96% sensitive for detection of *H. pylori*.
   b. Point of service test with results within 1 hour.

 Evidence Base Serim Research Corporation. (2012). PyloriTek for *H.pylori*. Available: *www.serim. com/products_overview.aspx?fid=2*.

2. Upper GI radiographic examination (barium study).
3. Serial stool specimens to detect occult blood.
4. Gastric secretory studies (gastric acid secretion test and serum gastric level test)—elevated in Zollinger-Ellison syndrome.
5. Serology to test for *H. pylori* antibodies or stool test to assess for *H. pylori* antigen.
6. C-urea breath test to detect *H. pylori*.

 DRUG ALERT Stop antisecretory proton pump inhibitor at least 2 weeks before the C-urea breath test. It can cause false-negative test result.

Management

General Measures

1. Eliminate use of NSAIDs or other causative drugs.
2. Eliminate cigarette smoking (impairs healing).
3. Well-balanced diet with meals at regular intervals. Avoid dietary irritants.

Drug Therapy

Multiple drug regimens are used to treat *H. pylori* (see Table 18-2, page 678), usually involving triple therapy with two antibiotics and a proton-pump inhibitor for 10 to 14 days to eradicate the bacteria.

 DRUG ALERT Antibiotic resistance is a problem that has led to longer therapy and research into alternative drug regimens.

Surgery

1. Surgical interventions may be indicated for hemorrhage, obstruction, perforation, and acid reduction (see Figure 18-5, page 679). Surgery may also be indicated with ulcer disease of long duration or severity or difficulty with medical regimen compliance.
2. Gastroduodenostomy (Billroth I).
   a. Partial gastrectomy with removal of antrum and pylorus of stomach.
   b. The gastric stump is anastomosed with the duodenum.
3. Gastrojejunostomy (Billroth II).
   a. Partial gastrectomy with removal of antrum and pylorus of stomach.
   b. The gastric stump is anastomosed with the jejunum.
4. Antrectomy.
   a. Gastric resection includes a small cuff of duodenum, the pylorus, and the antrum (lower half of stomach).
   b. The duodenal stump is closed and the jejunum is anastomosed to the stomach.
5. Total gastrectomy.
   a. Also called an esophagojejunostomy.
   b. Removal of the stomach with attachment of the esophagus to the jejunum or duodenum.
6. Pyloroplasty.
   a. A longitudinal incision is made in the pylorus, and it is closed transversely to permit the muscle to relax and to establish an enlarged outlet.
   b. Often, a vagotomy is performed at the same time.
7. Vagotomy.
   a. The surgical division of the vagus nerve to eliminate the impulses that stimulate HCL secretion.
   b. There are three types: *selective vagotomy*, which severs only the branches that interrupt acid secretion; *truncal vagotomy*, which severs the anterior and posterior trunks to decrease acid secretion and gastric motility; and *parietal vagotomy*, which severs only the part of vagus that innervates the parietal acid-secreting cells.
   c. Traditionally performed by laparotomy, the vagotomy procedure can also be done using a laparoscope.

Table 18-2 Medication Considerations for *H. pylori* Therapy

COMMON DRUG REGIMEN	DOSING	NURSING CONSIDERATIONS
Omeprazole 20 mg **A**moxicillin 1000 mg **C**larithromycin 500 mg	b.i.d. × 10 days b.i.d. × 10 days b.i.d. × 10 days	• Antibiotics: Metronidazole and clarithromycin may cause unpleasant metallic taste, nausea and vomiting; it may help to eat small, frequent meals, suck on sugar-free candy, take with food.
Bismuth subsalicylate 525 mg Metronidazole 250 mg Tetracycline 500 mg Ranitidine 150 mg	q.i.d. × 14 days q.i.d. × 14 days q.i.d. × 14 days b.i.d. × 4 weeks following initial three- drug regimen	Avoid alcohol within 72 hours of taking metronidazole; can cause severe reaction. Clarithromycin may interact with lovastatin, salmeterol, phenytoin, and other medications; do drink grapefruit juice during therapy. Tetracycline may increase sensitivity to sun; food and dairy products decrease absorption. Report inability to take antibiotic or vomiting doses. Report watery or bloody diarrhea, which may indicate pseudomembranous colitis.
Lansoprazole 30 mg Amoxicillin 1000 mg Clarithromycin 500 mg	b.i.d. × 10 or 14 days b.i.d. × 10 or 14 days b.i.d. × 10 or 14 days	• Proton pump inhibitors: Once daily dose may be substituted. May cause dizziness, headache, stomach upset. Best taken before meals. Do not take with certain drugs such as anti-epileptics and warfarin.

DRUG ALERT Avoid treatment if patient may be pregnant.

• Bismuth subsalicylate: Interacts with many drugs such as anti-epileptics, salicylates, corticosteroids.
    May turn stool black.
    May interfere with radiologic testing of the GI tract.
    Report ringing in the ears, may indicate salicylate toxicity.

Complications

1. GI hemorrhage.
2. Ulcer perforation.
3. Gastric outlet obstruction.

Nursing Assessment

1. Determine location, character, radiation of pain, factors aggravating or relieving pain, how long it lasts, when it occurs.
2. Ask about eating patterns, regularity, types of food, eating circumstances.
3. Ask about medications (especially aspirin, steroids, or anti-inflammatory drugs).
4. Inquire about a history of illnesses, including previous GI bleeds.
5. Obtain psychosocial history.
6. Perform physical assessment with documentation of positive abdominal findings.
7. Take vital signs, including lying, standing, and sitting BPs and pulses, to determine if orthostasis is present due to bleeding.

Nursing Diagnoses

• Deficient Fluid Volume related to hemorrhage.
• Acute Pain related to epigastric distress secondary to hypersecretion of acid, mucosal erosion, or perforation.
• Diarrhea related to GI bleeding.
• Imbalanced Nutrition: Less Than Body Requirements related to the disease process.
• Deficient Knowledge related to physical, dietary, and pharmacologic treatment of disease.

Nursing Interventions

Avoiding Fluid Volume Deficit

1. Monitor intake and output continuously to determine fluid volume status.

2. Monitor stools for blood and emesis.
3. Monitor hemoglobin and hematocrit and electrolytes.
4. Administer prescribed IV fluids and blood replacement, as prescribed.
5. Insert NG tube as prescribed, and monitor the tube drainage for signs of visible and occult blood.
6. Administer medications through the NG tube to neutralize acidity, as prescribed.
7. Prepare the patient for saline lavage, as ordered.
8. Observe the patient for an increase in pulse and a decrease in BP (signs of shock).
9. Prepare the patient for diagnostic procedure or surgery to determine or stop the source of bleeding.

Achieving Pain Relief

1. Administer prescribed medication.
2. Provide small, frequent meals to prevent gastric distention if not NPO.
3. Advise the patient about the irritating effects of certain drugs and foods.

Decreasing Diarrhea

1. Monitor the patient's elimination patterns to determine effects of medications.
2. Monitor vital signs and watch for signs of hypovolemia.
3. Administer antidiarrheal medication as prescribed.
4. Watch for signs and symptoms of impaired skin integrity (erythema, pain, pruritus) around anus to promote comfort and decrease risk of infection.

Achieving Adequate Nutrition

1. Eliminate foods that cause pain or distress; otherwise, the diet is usually not restricted.
2. Provide small, frequent meals that neutralize gastric secretions and may be better tolerated.

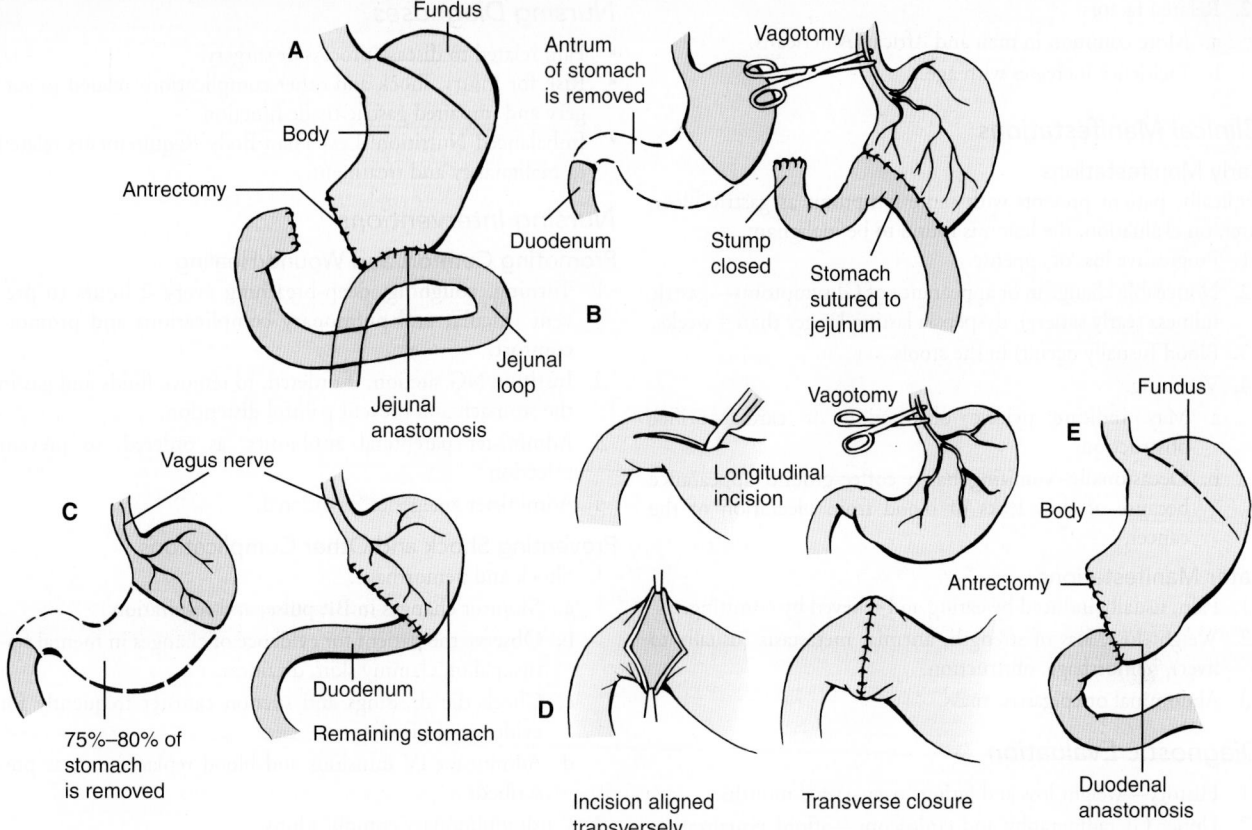

Figure 18-5. Surgical procedures for peptic ulcer. (A) Gastrojejunostomy (Billroth II). The jejunum is anastomosed to the gastric stump after a partial gastrectomy (removal of antrum and pylorus). **(B)** Antrectomy and vagotomy. The resected portion includes a small cuff of duodenum, the pylorus, and the antrum (about one half of the stomach). The stump of the duodenum is closed by suture, and the side of the jejunum is anastomosed to the cut end of the stomach. **(C)** Subtotal gastrectomy. The resected portion includes a small cuff of the duodenum, the pylorus, and from two thirds to three quarters of the stomach. The duodenum or side of the jejunum is anastomosed to the remaining portion of the stomach. **(D)** Vagotomy and pyloroplasty. A longitudinal incision is made in the pylorus, and it is closed transversely to permit the muscle to relax and to establish an enlarged outlet. This compensates for the impaired gastric emptying produced by vagotomy. **(E)** Gastroduodenostomy (Billroth I). The duodenum is anastomosed to the gastric stump after removal of the antrum and pylorus (partial gastrectomy).

3. Provide high-calorie, high-protein diet with nutritional supplements, as ordered.
4. Administer parenteral nutrition, as ordered, if bleeding is prolonged and patient is malnourished.

Educating the Patient About the Treatment Regimen

1. Explain all tests and procedures to increase knowledge and cooperation and minimize anxiety.
2. Review the health care provider's recommendations for diet, activity, medication, and treatment. Allow time for questions and clarify any misunderstandings.
3. Give the patient a chart listing medications, dosages, times of administration, and desired effects to promote compliance.

Patient Education and Health Maintenance

1. Teach the patient the signs and symptoms of bleeding and when to notify the health care provider.
2. Promote healthy lifestyle changes to include adequate nutrition, cessation of smoking, decreased alcohol consumption, stress reduction strategies.

3. Explain the purpose, dosage, and adverse effects of each medication prescribed.

Evaluation: Expected Outcomes

- Vital signs stable; fluid volume maintained.
- Pain free.
- No more than two to three loose stools per day.
- Eats small, frequent meals each day; reports no loss of weight.
- Describes peptic ulcer disease, its treatment, and complications; complies with treatment regimen.

Gastric Cancer

Malignant tumor of the stomach.

Pathophysiology and Etiology

1. Risk factors include:
   a. Chronic atrophic gastritis with intestinal metaplasia.
   b. Pernicious anemia or having had gastric resections (more than 15 years).
   c. Adenomatous polyps.

2. Related factors:
   a. More common in men and African Americans.
   b. Incidence increases with age.

Clinical Manifestations

Early Manifestations

Typically, patient presents with same symptoms as gastric ulcer; later, on evaluation, the lesion is found to be malignant.

1. Progressive loss of appetite.
2. Noticeable change in or appearance of GI symptoms—gastric fullness (early satiety), dyspepsia lasting longer than 4 weeks.
3. Blood (usually occult) in the stools.
4. Vomiting.
   a. May indicate pyloric obstruction or cardiac–orifice obstruction.
   b. Occasionally, vomiting has a coffee-ground appearance because of slow leaks of blood from ulceration of the cancer.

Later Manifestations

1. Pain, usually induced by eating and relieved by vomiting.
2. Weight loss, loss of strength, anemia, metastasis (usually to liver), hemorrhage, obstruction.
3. Abdominal or epigastric mass.

Diagnostic Evaluation

1. History—weight loss and fatigue over several months.
2. Upper GI radiography and endoscopy—afford visualization and provide means for obtaining tissue samples for histologic and cytologic review.
3. Imaging, such as bone or liver scan—may determine extent of disease.

Management

1. The only successful treatment of gastric cancer is surgical removal. Gastric resection is surgical removal of part of the stomach.
2. If tumor has spread beyond the area that can be excised surgically, cure is not possible.
   a. Palliative surgery, such as subtotal gastrectomy with or without gastroenterostomy, may be performed to maintain continuity of the GI tract.
   b. Surgery may be combined with chemotherapy to provide palliation and prolong life.

Complications

1. If surgery is performed, possible risk of hemorrhage or infection.
2. Dumping syndrome following gastrectomy.
3. Metastasis and death.

Nursing Assessment

1. Assess for anorexia, weight loss, GI symptoms (gastric fullness, dyspepsia, vomiting).
2. Evaluate for pain, noting characteristics/location.
3. Check stool for occult blood.
4. Monitor CBC to assess for anemia.

Nursing Diagnoses

- Pain related to disease process or surgery.
- Risk for Injury, shock and other complications related to surgery and impaired gastric tissue function.
- Imbalanced Nutrition: Less Than Body Requirements related to malignancy and treatment.

Nursing Interventions

Promoting Comfort and Wound Healing

1. Turning, coughing, deep-breathing every 2 hours to prevent vascular and pulmonary complications and promote comfort.
2. Institute NG suction, if ordered, to remove fluids and gas in the stomach and prevent painful distention.
3. Administer parenteral antibiotics, as ordered, to prevent infection.
4. Administer analgesics, as ordered.

Preventing Shock and Other Complications

1. Shock and hemorrhage.
   a. Monitor changes in BP, pulse, and respiration.
   b. Observe the patient for evidence of changes in mental status, pallor, clammy skin, dizziness.
   c. Check the dressings and suction canister frequently for evidence of bleeding.
   d. Administer IV infusions and blood replacement, as prescribed.
2. Cardiopulmonary complications.
   a. Encourage the patient to cough and take deep breaths to promote ventilatory exchange and enhance circulation.
   b. Assist the patient to turn and move, thereby mobilizing secretions.
   c. Promote ambulation, as prescribed, to increase respiratory exchange.
3. Thrombosis and embolism.
   a. Initiate a plan of self-care activities to promote circulation.
   b. Encourage early ambulation to stimulate circulation.
   c. Prevent venous stasis by use of elastic stockings, if indicated.
   d. Check for tight dressings or binder that might restrict circulation.
4. Dumping syndrome—a complex reaction that may occur because of excessively rapid emptying of gastric contents. Manifestations include nausea, weakness, perspiration, palpitation, some syncope, and possibly diarrhea. Instruct the patient as follows:
   a. Eat small, frequent meals rather than three large meals.
   b. Suggest a diet high in protein and fat and low in carbohydrates, and avoid meals high in sugars, milk, chocolate, salt.
   c. Reduce fluids with meals, but take them between meals.
   d. Take anticholinergic medication before meals (if prescribed) to lessen GI activity.
   e. Relax when eating; eat slowly and regularly.
   f. Take a rest after meals.
5. Phytobezoar formation (formation of gastric concretion composed of vegetable matter) can be seen with partial

gastrectomy and vagotomy. After a gastric resection, the remaining gastric tissue is not able to disintegrate and digest fibrous foods. This undigested fiber congeals to form masses that become coated by mucus secretions of the stomach.

a. Avoid fibrous foods, such as citrus fruits (skins and seeds), because they tend to form phytobezoars.

b. Stress the importance of adequate chewing.

Attaining Adequate Nutritional Status

1. Administer parenteral nutrition, if ordered.
2. Follow prescribed diet progressions.
   a. Give fluids by mouth when audible bowel signs are present.
   b. Increase fluids according to the patient's tolerance.
   c. Offer a diet with vitamin supplements when the patient's condition permits.
   d. Avoid high-carbohydrate foods, such as milk, which may trigger dumping syndrome.
   e. Offer diet, as prescribed—usually high in protein and calories to promote wound healing.

Patient Education and Health Maintenance

1. Emphasize the importance of coping with stressful situations. Provide information about support groups.
2. Review nutritional requirements with the patient.
3. Stress the importance of I.M. vitamin B_{12} supplements after gastrectomy to prevent surgically induced pernicious anemia.
4. Encourage follow-up visits with the health care provider.

5. Recommend annual blood studies and medical checkups for any evidence of pernicious anemia or other problems.
6. Instruct on measures to prevent dumping syndrome.

Evaluation: Expected Outcomes

- States pain decreased to 2 or 3 on 0-to-10 scale.
- Vital signs stable; no evidence of complications.
- Tolerating small, frequent meals.

INTESTINAL CONDITIONS
Abdominal Hernias

An abdominal hernia occurs when the contents of the abdomen, usually the small intestine, push through a weak point in the muscular wall of the abdomen. The weakness of the abdominal wall can be congenital in nature, due to acquired weakness (eg, aging or trauma), or due to increased intra-abdominal pressure (eg, due to heavy lifting, obesity, pregnancy, straining, coughing, ascites, or proximity to tumor).

Pathophysiology and Etiology

Classification by Site

1. Inguinal—a hernia into the inguinal canal that is more common in males (see Figure 18-6). This type of hernia is further differentiated based on the causative factor.
   a. Indirect inguinal—congenital hernia that occurs when the entrance of the inguinal canal does not close after birth, causing a weakness in the abdominal wall. Through this

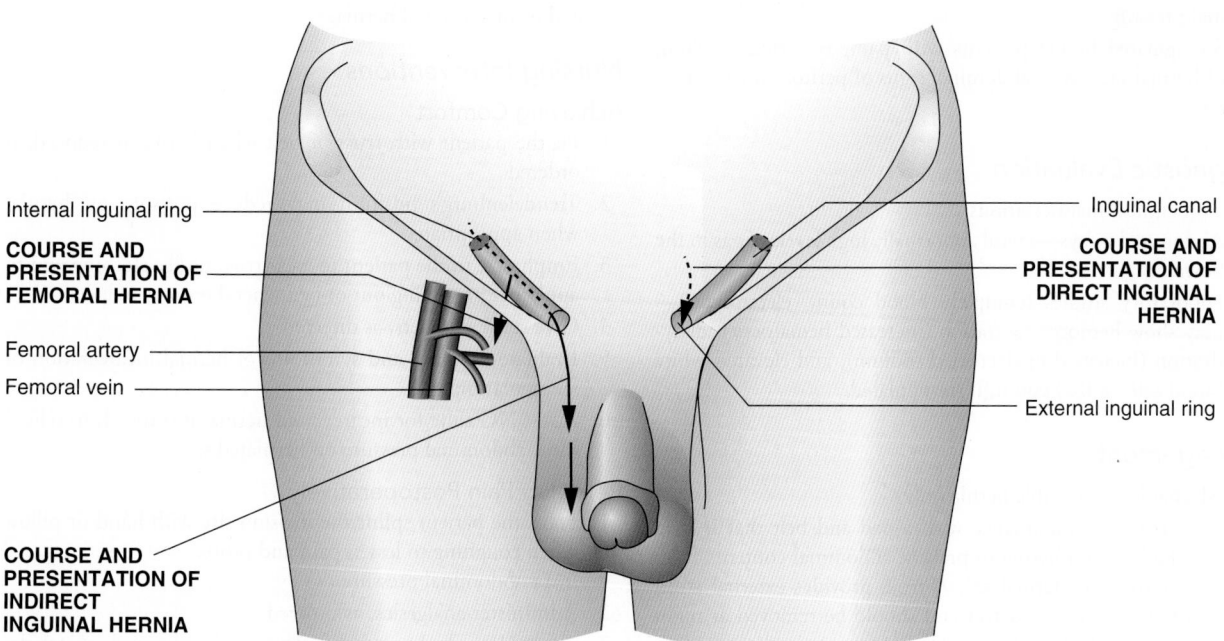

Figure 18-6. Direct and indirect inguinal hernia.

weakened area, the hernia extends down the inguinal canal and often into the scrotum or labia.

b. Direct inguinal—caused by degeneration of the abdominal muscles allowing small intestine to pass through the posterior inguinal wall into the groin.

2. Femoral—hernia follows the tract below the inguinal ligament through the femoral canal.

3. Umbilical—intestinal protrusion at the umbilicus due to failure of umbilical orifice to close. Occurs most often in obese women, children, and in patients with increased intra-abdominal pressure from cirrhosis and ascites.

4. Ventral or incisional—intestinal protrusion due to weakness at the abdominal wall; may occur after impaired incisional healing due to infection or drainage.

5. Peristomal—hernia through the fascial defect around a stoma and into the subcutaneous tissue.

Classification by Severity

1. Reducible—the protruding mass can be placed back into abdominal cavity.

2. Irreducible—the protruding mass cannot be moved back into the abdomen.

3. Incarcerated—an irreducible hernia in which the intestinal flow is completely obstructed.

4. Strangulated—an irreducible hernia in which the blood and intestinal flow are completely obstructed; develops when the loop of intestine in the sac becomes twisted or swollen and a constriction is produced at the neck of the sac.

Clinical Manifestations

1. Bulging over herniated area appears when the patient stands or strains and disappears when supine.

2. Hernia tends to increase in size and recurs with intra-abdominal pressure.

3. Strangulated hernia presents with pain, vomiting, swelling of hernial sac, lower abdominal signs of peritoneal irritation, fever.

Diagnostic Evaluation

Based on clinical manifestations:

1. Abdominal x-rays—reveal abnormally high levels of gas in the bowel.

2. Laboratory studies (complete blood count, electrolytes)—may show hemoconcentration (increased hematocrit), dehydration (increased or decreased sodium), and elevated white blood cell (WBC) count, if strangulated.

Management

1. Mechanical (reducible hernia only).
   a. A truss is an appliance with a pad and belt that is held snugly over a hernia to prevent abdominal contents from entering the hernial sac. A truss provides external compression over the defect and should be removed at night and reapplied in the morning before patient arises. This nonsurgical approach may be used only when a patient is not a surgical candidate.

b. Peristomal hernia is often managed with a hernia support belt with Velcro, which is placed around an ostomy pouching system (similar to a truss).

c. Conservative measures—no heavy lifting, straining at stool, or other measures that would increase intra-abdominal pressure.

2. Surgical—recommended to correct hernia before strangulation occurs, which then becomes an emergency situation.
   a. Herniorrhaphy—removal of hernial sac; contents replaced into the abdomen; layers of muscle and fascia sutured. Laparoscopic herniorrhaphy is a possibility and often performed as outpatient procedure.
   b. Hernioplasty involves reinforcement of suturing (often with mesh) for extensive hernia repair.
   c. Strangulated hernia requires resection of ischemic bowel in addition to repair of hernia.

Complications

1. Bowel obstruction.
2. Recurrence of hernia.

Nursing Assessment

1. Ask the patient if hernia is enlarging and uncomfortable, reducible or irreducible; determine relationship to exertion and activities.

2. Assess bowel sounds and determine bowel pattern.

3. Determine if the patient is exhibiting signs and symptoms of strangulation, such as distention, fever, nausea, and vomiting.

Nursing Diagnoses

• Chronic Pain related to bulging hernia (mechanical).
• Acute Pain related to surgical procedure.
• Risk for Infection related to emergency procedure for strangulated or incarcerated hernia.

Nursing Interventions

Achieving Comfort

1. Fit the patient with truss or belt when hernia is reduced, if ordered.

2. Trendelenburg's position may reduce pressure on hernia, when appropriate.

3. Emphasize to the patient to wear truss under clothing and to apply before getting out of bed when hernia is reduced.

4. Give stool softeners, as directed.

5. Evaluate for signs and symptoms of hernial incarceration or strangulation.

6. Insert NG tube for incarcerated hernia, if ordered, to relieve intra-abdominal pressure on herniated sac.

Relieving Pain Postoperatively

1. Have the patient splint the incision site with hand or pillow when coughing to lessen pain and protect site from increased intra-abdominal pressure.

2. Administer analgesics, as ordered.

3. Teach about bed rest, intermittent ice packs, and scrotal elevation as measures used to reduce scrotal edema or swelling after repair of an inguinal hernia.

4. Encourage ambulation as soon as permitted.

5. Advise the patient that difficulty in urinating is common after surgery; promote elimination to avoid discomfort, and catheterize if necessary.

Preventing Infection

1. Check dressing for drainage and incision for redness and swelling.

2. Monitor for other signs and symptoms of infection: fever, chills, malaise, diaphoresis.

3. Administer antibiotics, if appropriate.

Patient Education and Health Maintenance

1. Advise that pain and scrotal swelling may be present for 24 to 48 hours after repair of an inguinal hernia.
   a. Apply ice intermittently.
   b. Elevate scrotum and use scrotal support.
   c. Take medication prescribed to relieve discomfort.

2. Teach to monitor self for signs of infection: pain, drainage from incision, temperature elevation. Also, report continued difficulty in voiding.

3. Inform that heavy lifting should be avoided for 4 to 6 weeks. Athletics and extremes of exertion are to be avoided for 8 to 12 weeks postoperatively, per provider instructions.

Evaluation: Expected Outcomes

- Hernia effectively reduced with truss or belt; patient comfortable.
- Verbalizes pain decreased to 2 or 3 on 0-to-10 scale.
- No swelling present; afebrile, no drainage from incision.

Intestinal Obstruction

Intestinal obstruction is an interruption in the normal flow of intestinal contents along the intestinal tract. The block may occur in the small or large intestine, may be complete or incomplete, may be mechanical or paralytic, and may or may not compromise the vascular supply. Obstruction most frequently occurs in the young and the old.

Pathophysiology and Etiology

Types and Causes

1. Mechanical obstruction—a physical block to passage of intestinal contents without disturbing blood supply of bowel. High small-bowel (jejunal) or low small-bowel (ileal) obstruction occurs four times more frequently than colonic obstruction (see Figure 18-7). Causes include:
   a. Extrinsic—adhesions from surgery, hernia, wound dehiscence, masses, volvulus (twisted loop of intestine). Up to 70% of small-bowel obstructions are caused by adhesions.
   b. Intrinsic—hematoma, tumor, intussusception (telescoping of intestinal wall into itself), stricture or stenosis, congenital (atresia, imperforate anus), trauma, inflammatory diseases (Crohn's, diverticulitis, ulcerative colitis).
   c. Intraluminal—foreign body, fecal or barium impaction, polyp, gallstones, meconium in infants.

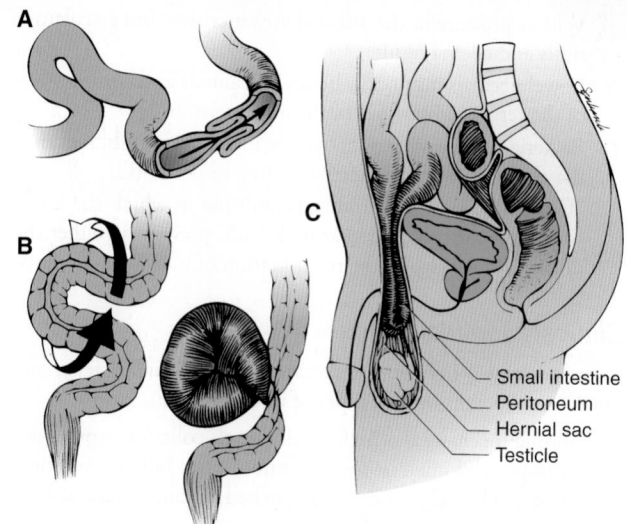

Figure 18-7. Three causes of intestinal obstruction. (A) Intussusception. Note shortening of the colon by the movement of one segment of bowel into another. **(B)** Volvulus of the sigmoid colon. The twist is counterclockwise in most cases of sigmoid volvulus. **(C)** Hernia (inguinal). Note that the sac of the hernia is a continuation of the peritoneum of the abdomen and that the hernial contents are intestine, omentum, or other abdominal contents that pass through the hernial opening into the hernial sac.

Labels: Small intestine, Peritoneum, Hernial sac, Testicle

   d. In postoperative patients, approximately 90% of mechanical obstructions are due to adhesions. In nonsurgical patients, hernia (most often inguinal) is the most common cause of mechanical obstruction.

2. Paralytic (adynamic, neurogenic) ileus.
   a. Peristalsis is ineffective (diminished motor activity perhaps because of toxic or traumatic disturbance of the autonomic nervous system).
   b. There is no physical obstruction and no interrupted blood supply.
   c. Disappears spontaneously after 2 to 3 days.
   d. Causes include:
      i. Spinal cord injuries; vertebral fractures.
      ii. Postoperatively after any abdominal surgery.
      iii. Peritonitis, pneumonia.
      iv. Wound dehiscence (breakdown).
      v. GI tract surgery.

3. Strangulation—obstruction compromises blood supply, leading to gangrene of the intestinal wall. Caused by prolonged mechanical obstruction.

Altered Physiology

1. Increased peristalsis, distention by fluid and gas, and increased bacterial growth proximal to obstruction. The intestine empties distally.

2. Increased secretions into the intestine are associated with diminution in the bowel's absorptive capacity.

3. The accumulation of gases, secretions, and oral intake above the obstruction causes increasing intraluminal pressure.

4. Venous pressure in the affected area increases and circulatory stasis and edema result.
5. Bowel necrosis may occur because of anoxia and compression of the terminal branches of the mesenteric artery.
6. Bacteria and toxins pass across the intestinal membranes into the abdominal cavity, thereby leading to peritonitis.
7. "Closed-loop" obstruction is a condition in which the intestinal segment is occluded at both ends, preventing either the downward passage or the regurgitation of intestinal contents.

Clinical Manifestations

Fever, peritoneal irritation, increased WBC count, toxicity, and shock may develop with all types of intestinal obstruction.

1. Simple mechanical—high small-bowel: colic (cramps), mid- to upper abdomen, some distention, early bilious vomiting, increased bowel sounds (high-pitched tinkling heard at brief intervals), minimal diffuse tenderness.
2. Simple mechanical—low small-bowel: significant colic (cramps), midabdominal, considerable distention, vomiting slight or absent, later feculent, increased bowel sounds and "hush" sounds, minimal diffuse tenderness.
3. Simple mechanical—colon: cramps (mid- to lower abdomen), later-appearing distention, then vomiting may develop (feculent), increase in bowel sounds, minimal diffuse tenderness.
4. Partial chronic mechanical—may occur with granulomatous bowel in Crohn's disease. Symptoms are cramping, abdominal pain, mild distention, and diarrhea.
5. Strangulation symptoms are initially those of mechanical obstruction, but progress rapidly—pain is severe, continuous, and localized. There is moderate distention, persistent vomiting, usually decreased bowel sounds and marked localized tenderness. Stools or vomitus become bloody or contain occult blood.

Diagnostic Evaluation

1. Fecal material aspiration from NG tube.
2. Abdominal and chest x-rays.
   a. May show presence and location of small or large intestinal distention, gas or fluid.
   b. "Bird beak" lesion in colonic volvulus.
   c. Foreign body visualization.
3. Contrast studies.
   a. Barium enema may diagnose colon obstruction or intussusception.
   b. Ileus may be identified by oral barium or Gastrografin.
4. Laboratory tests.
   a. May show decreased sodium, potassium, and chloride levels due to vomiting.
   b. Elevated WBC counts due to inflammation; marked increase with necrosis, strangulation, or peritonitis.
   c. Serum amylase may be elevated from irritation of the pancreas by the bowel loop.
5. Flexible sigmoidoscopy or colonoscopy may identify the source of the obstruction such as tumor or stricture.

Management

Nonsurgical Management

1. Correction of fluid and electrolyte imbalances with normal saline or Ringer's solution with potassium as required.
2. NG suction to decompress bowel and decrease risk of perforation.
3. Treatment of shock and peritonitis.
4. TPN may be necessary to correct protein deficiency from chronic obstruction, paralytic ileus, or infection.
5. Analgesics and sedatives, avoiding opiates due to GI motility inhibition.
6. Antibiotics to prevent or treat infection.
7. Ambulation for patients with paralytic ileus to encourage return of peristalsis.

Surgery

Consists of relieving obstruction. Options include:

1. Closed bowel procedures: lysis of adhesions, reduction of volvulus, intussusception, or incarcerated hernia.
2. Enterotomy for removal of foreign bodies or bezoars.
3. Resection of bowel for obstructing lesions, or strangulated bowel with end-to-end anastomosis.
4. Intestinal bypass around obstruction.
5. Temporary ostomy may be indicated (see "Caring for the Patient Undergoing Ostomy Surgery," page 659).

Complications

1. Dehydration due to loss of water, sodium, and chloride.
2. Peritonitis.
3. Shock due to loss of electrolytes and dehydration.
4. Death due to shock.

Nursing Assessment

1. Assess the nature and location of the patient's pain, the presence or absence of distention, flatus, defecation, emesis, obstipation.
2. Listen for high-pitched bowel sounds, peristaltic rushes, or absence of bowel sounds.
3. Assess vital signs.

 GERONTOLOGIC ALERT Watch for air-fluid lock syndrome in older patients, who typically remain in the recumbent position for extended periods. Fluid collects in dependent bowel loops and peristalsis is too weak to push fluid "uphill." Conduct frequent checks of the patient's level of responsiveness; decreasing responsiveness may offer a clue to an increasing electrolyte imbalance or impending shock.

Nursing Diagnoses

- Acute Pain related to obstruction, distention, and strangulation.
- Risk for Deficient Fluid Volume related to impaired fluid intake, vomiting, and diarrhea from intestinal obstruction.
- Diarrhea related to obstruction.
- Ineffective Breathing Pattern related to abdominal distention, interfering with normal lung expansion.

- Risk for Injury related to complications and severity of illness.
- Fear related to life-threatening symptoms of intestinal obstruction.

Nursing Interventions

Achieving Pain Relief

1. Administer prescribed analgesics.
2. Provide supportive care during NG intubation to assist with discomfort.
3. To relieve air-fluid lock syndrome, turn the patient from supine to prone position every 10 minutes until enough flatus is passed to decompress the abdomen. A rectal tube may be indicated.

Maintaining Electrolyte and Fluid Balance

1. Measure and record all intake and output.
2. Administer IV fluids and parenteral nutrition as prescribed.
3. Monitor electrolytes, urinalysis, hemoglobin, and blood cell counts, and report any abnormalities.
4. Monitor urine output to assess renal function and to detect urine retention due to bladder compressions by the distended intestine.
5. Monitor vital signs; a drop in BP may indicate decreased circulatory volume due to blood loss from strangulated hernia.

Maintaining Normal Bowel Elimination

1. Collect stool samples to test for occult blood, if ordered.
2. Maintain adequate fluid balance.
3. Record amount and consistency of stools.
4. Maintain NG tube as prescribed to decompress bowel.

Maintaining Proper Lung Ventilation

1. Keep the patient in Fowler's position to promote ventilation and relieve abdominal distention.
2. Monitor ABG levels for oxygenation levels, if ordered.

Preventing Injury Due to Complications

1. Prevent infarction by carefully assessing the patient's status; pain that increases in intensity or becomes localized or continuous may herald strangulation.
2. Detect early signs of peritonitis, such as rigidity and tenderness, in an effort to minimize this complication.
3. Avoid enemas, which may distort an x-ray or make a partial obstruction worse.
4. Observe for signs of shock—pallor, tachycardia, hypotension.
5. Watch for signs of:
   a. Metabolic alkalosis (slow, shallow respirations; changes in sensorium; tetany).
   b. Metabolic acidosis (disorientation; deep, rapid breathing; weakness; and shortness of breath on exertion).

Relieving Fears

1. Recognize the patient's concerns and initiate measures to provide emotional support.
2. Encourage presence of support person.

Patient Education and Health Maintenance

1. Explain the rationale for NG suction, NPO status, and IV fluids initially. Advise the patient to progress diet slowly as tolerated once home.
2. Advise plenty of rest and slow progression of activity as directed by surgeon or other health care provider.
3. Teach wound care, if indicated.
4. Encourage the patient to follow up as directed and to call surgeon or health care provider if increasing abdominal pain, vomiting, or fever occur prior to follow-up.

Evaluation: Expected Outcomes

- Maintains position of comfort, states pain decreased to 3 or 4 on 0-to-10 scale.
- Urine output greater than 30 mL/hour; vital signs stable.
- Passed flatus and small, formed brown stool; negative occult blood.
- Respirations 24 breaths per minute and unlabored with head of bed elevated 45 degrees.
- Alert, lucid, vital signs stable, abdomen firm, not rigid.
- Appears relaxed and reports feeling better.

Appendicitis

Appendicitis is inflammation of the vermiform appendix caused by an obstruction of the intestinal lumen from infection, stricture, fecal mass, foreign body, or tumor.

Pathophysiology and Etiology

1. Obstruction is followed by edema, infection, and ischemia.
2. As intraluminal tension develops, necrosis and perforation usually occur.
3. Appendicitis can affect any age group; most common in adolescents/young adults, especially males.

Clinical Manifestations

1. Generalized or localized abdominal pain in the epigastric or periumbilical areas and upper right abdomen. Within 2 to 12 hours, the pain localizes in the right lower quadrant and intensity increases.
2. Anorexia, moderate malaise, mild fever, nausea, and vomiting.
3. Usually constipation occurs, occasionally diarrhea.
4. Rebound tenderness, involuntary guarding, generalized abdominal rigidity.

Diagnostic Evaluation

1. Physical examination consistent with clinical manifestations.
2. WBC count reveals moderate leukocytosis (10,000 to 16,000/mm^3) with shift to the left (increased immature neutrophils).
3. Urinalysis to rule out urinary disorders.
4. Abdominal x-ray may visualize shadow consistent with fecalith in appendix; perforation will reveal free air.
5. Abdominal ultrasound or CT scan can visualize appendix and rule out other conditions, such as diverticulitis and Crohn's disease. Focused appendiceal CT can quickly evaluate for appendicitis.

 GERONTOLOGIC ALERT In older adults, be aware of vague symptoms: milder pain, less pronounced fever, and leukocytosis with shift to the left on differential.

Management

1. Surgery (appendectomy) is indicated.
   a. Simple appendectomy or laparoscopic appendectomy in absence of rupture or peritonitis.
   b. An incisional drain may be placed if an abscess or rupture occurs.
2. Preoperatively maintain bed rest, NPO status, IV hydration, possible antibiotic prophylaxis, and analgesia.

Complications

1. Perforation (in 95% of cases).
2. Abscess.
3. Peritonitis.

Nursing Assessment

1. Obtain history for location and extent of pain.
2. Auscultate for presence of bowel sounds; peristalsis may be absent or diminished.
3. On palpation of the abdomen, assess for tenderness anywhere in the right lower quadrant, but usually localized over McBurney's point (point just below midpoint of line between umbilicus and iliac crest on the right side). Assess for rebound tenderness in the right lower quadrant as well as referred rebound when palpating the left lower quadrant.
4. Assess for positive psoas sign by having the patient attempt to raise the right thigh against the pressure of your hand placed over the right knee. Inflammation of the psoas muscle in acute appendicitis will increase abdominal pain with this maneuver.
5. Assess for positive obturator sign by flexing the patient's right hip and knee and rotating the leg internally. Hypogastric pain with this maneuver indicates inflammation of the obturator muscle.

Nursing Diagnoses

- Acute Pain related to inflamed appendix.
- Risk for Infection related to perforation.

Nursing Interventions

Preoperative nursing care is listed; for postoperative care, see "Caring for the Patient Undergoing Gastrointestinal Surgery," page 657.

Relieving Pain

1. Monitor pain level, including location, intensity, pattern.
2. Assist patient to comfortable positions, such as semi-Fowler's and knees up.
3. Restrict activity that may aggravate pain, such as coughing and ambulation.
4. Apply ice bag to abdomen for comfort.
5. Give antiemetics and analgesics, as ordered, and evaluate response.
6. Avoid indiscriminate palpation of the abdomen to avoid increasing the patient's discomfort.

 DRUG ALERT Do not give analgesics/antipyretics to mask fever, and do not administer cathartics because they may cause rupture.

Preventing Infection

1. Monitor frequently for signs and symptoms of worsening condition indicating perforation, abscess, or peritonitis: increasing severity of pain, tenderness, rigidity, distention, ileus, fever, malaise, tachycardia.
2. Administer antibiotics, as ordered.
3. Promptly prepare the patient for surgery.

Patient Education and Health Maintenance

1. Instruct the patient to avoid heavy lifting for 4 to 6 weeks after surgery.
2. Instruct the patient to report symptoms of anorexia, nausea, vomiting, fever, abdominal pain, incisional redness or drainage postoperatively.

Evaluation: Expected Outcomes

- Verbalizes decreased pain to 2 or 3 on 0-to-10 scale with positioning and analgesics.
- Afebrile; no rigidity or distention.

Diverticular Disease

 Evidence Base Hall, J., Hammerich, K., & Roberts, P. (2010). New paradigms in the management of diverticular disease. *Current Problems in Surgery*, 47(9), 680–735.

Diverticular disease is a wide-spectrum disease encompassing all problems that can be caused by diverticula. A *diverticulum* is a pouch or saccular dilatation of the colon wall. *Diverticulosis* is a condition exhibiting multiple diverticula without inflammation. *Diverticulitis* is inflammation and infection of one or more diverticula. Diverticular disease is usually categorized into complicated or uncomplicated disease.

Pathophysiology and Etiology

Diverticulosis

1. Marks the formation of diverticula, which are herniations of the mucosal and submucosal layers of the colon developing at weak points where nutrient blood vessels penetrate the colon wall (see Figure 18-8).
2. Causes for diverticular disease are unclear, but data suggest excessive intraluminal pressure plays a key role. A contributing factor may be a low-residue diet, which reduces fecal residue, narrows the bowel lumen, and leads to higher pressure intra-abdominally during defecation.
3. The risk of developing diverticulosis is about 40% by age 60 and more than 60% of those 80 years and older.

Diverticulitis

1. Results when one or more diverticula become inflamed and usually perforate the thin diverticular wall, which consists of mucosal and serosal layers. The exact cause is unknown, but postulated to be caused by stasis or obstruction of the diverticula leading to bacterial overgrowth, inflammation, and ischemia.

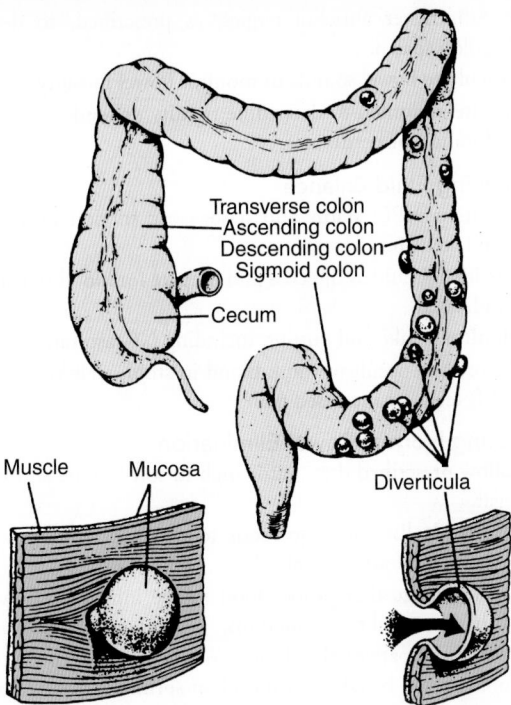

Figure 18-8. Diverticula are most common in the sigmoid colon; they diminish in number and size as the colon approaches the cecum. Diverticula are rarely found in the rectum.

2. Complicated diverticulitis refers to diverticular disease that has led to abscess, perforation, fistula, stricture, or obstruction.
3. Uninflamed or minimally inflamed diverticula may erode adjacent arterial branches causing acute massive rectal bleeding.
4. It is estimated that 10% to 25% of people with diverticulosis will develop diverticulitis.

Clinical Manifestations

Diverticulosis
1. May be asymptomatic.
2. Crampy abdominal pain.
3. Bowel irregularity—constipation or diarrhea.
4. Periodic abdominal distention.
5. Sudden massive hemorrhage may be first symptom.

Diverticulitis
1. Left lower quadrant pain.
2. Low-grade fever, chills, leukocytosis.
3. Sometimes an abdominal mass is palpable.
4. Urinary frequency and dysuria are associated with bladder involvement in the inflammatory process.
5. Ruptured diverticula produce abscesses or peritonitis with abdominal rigidity; signs of shock and sepsis (hypotension, chills, high fever). Near a blood vessel, a rupture may cause massive hemorrhage.
   a. Sepsis may spread through portal vein to liver, causing liver abscesses.
   b. Sometimes, fistulae form with the bladder, the adjacent small bowel, the vagina, and the perianal area or skin.

c. Chronic diverticulitis may cause adhesions that narrow the bowel's opening and can cause partial or complete bowel obstruction.

Diagnostic Evaluation

1. Laboratory studies: WBC may show leukocytosis with shift to the left; hemoglobin/hematocrit may be low with chronic or acute bleeding.
2. CT scan is the preferred imaging study since it is the most accurate in correctly identifying diverticulitis and in staging its severity. CT guidance can also be used if an abscess needs to be drained.
3. Sigmoidoscopy/colonoscopy—to rule out carcinoma and confirm diagnosis. These studies should not be done during an acute attack. A waiting period of 6 weeks after resolution of symptoms is preferred.
4. Barium enema (after infection subsides)—may visualize diverticular sacs, narrowing of colonic lumen, partial or complete obstruction, or fistulae.

> **NURSING ALERT** In patients with acute diverticulitis, a barium enema may rupture the bowel.

Management

Diverticulosis
1. High-fiber diet with possible avoidance of large seeds or nuts, which may obstruct diverticular sac.
2. Bran therapy, psyllium preparation, or stool softeners, such as docusate sodium (Colace), to avoid constipation.
3. Encourage adequate fluid intake.
4. Intestinal diverticulosis with pain usually responds to a liquid or low-residue diet and stool softeners to relieve symptoms, minimize irritation, and reduce progression to diverticulitis.

Uncomplicated Diverticulitis
1. Medical management.
   a. If symptoms are mild, treatment can occur as an outpatient. Usually a broad-spectrum antibiotic is given for 7 to 14 days.
   b. If fever or systemic symptoms, patient should be treated in hospital with intravenous broad-spectrum antibiotic.
2. Surgical management.
   a. Elective resection may be considered, but this is dependent on severity of disease, risk of subsequent attacks, age, comorbidities, and complications of the disease.

Complicated Diverticulitis
Treatment is dependent upon the associated complication that has occurred.
1. Abscess—may be managed with bowel rest and antibiotics while under close observation, however, percutaneous drainage may be needed if patient becomes septic. Sigmoid resection may also be recommended.
2. Perforation—surgical resection of the diseased area with colostomy (Hartmann procedure) is the most widely accepted treatment. Surgical resection with primary anastomosis may be done if patient is a good candidate. Recent studies show

that laparoscopic lavage may be an alternative to resection, but further studies are needed.

3. Fistulae—usually require surgical resection depending on type of fistula and its associated symptoms.
4. Stricture/obstruction—if the obstruction is complete, surgery is required. If a partial obstruction has occurred, bowel rest, intravenous hydration, and antibiotics may successfully treat symptoms, however, surgery may be required later.
5. Hemorrhage—NPO, IV therapy, blood transfusion as necessary, NG tube placement. Colonoscopy to identify source of bleeding.
   a. If colonoscopy is not successful in identifying source of bleeding, a technetium 99–labeled red blood cell scan will be done.
   b. Mesenteric angiography is an alternative study that may be used and has potential to be therapeutic, since the bleeding source can be thrombosed if identified.
   c. Surgical resection is not typical, since this type of hemorrhage is usually self-limited.

Complications

1. Hemorrhage from colonic diverticula, usually in the right colon.
2. Bowel obstruction.
3. Fistula formation (colovesical fistula is the most common).
4. Septicemia.

Nursing Assessment

1. Have the patient describe amount of fiber and fluid intake per day and past and present bowel patterns. Any constipation, diarrhea, or alternating of both?
2. Ask if experiencing abdominal cramping or pain, bloody stools, or stool/gas passage from vagina or in urine.
3. Watch for signs and symptoms of peritonitis: increasing abdominal pain, guarding, rebound tenderness, abdominal distention, nausea/vomiting.
4. Monitor vital signs: temperature may be elevated; tachycardia and hypotension may indicate peritonitis/massive bleeding.

Nursing Diagnoses

- Acute Pain related to intestinal discomfort, diarrhea, and/or constipation.
- Risk for Deficient Fluid Volume related to diarrhea, fluid and electrolyte loss, nausea, and vomiting.
- Constipation or Diarrhea related to the disease process.
- Deficient Knowledge of the relationship between diet and diverticular disease.

Nursing Interventions

Achieving Pain Relief

1. Observe for signs and location of pain, type, and severity, and intervene when appropriate.
   a. Administer nonopiate analgesics as prescribed (opiates may mask signs of perforation).
   b. Administer anticholinergics, as prescribed, to decrease colon spasm.
2. Auscultate bowel sounds to monitor bowel motility.
3. Palpate abdomen to determine rigidity or tenderness due to perforation or peritonitis.

Maintaining Fluid Balance

1. Maintain NPO status and nasogastric suction until bowel sounds return.
2. Provide IV fluid as directed and prepare for blood transfusion if indicated.
3. Monitor intake and output, including NG aspirate.
4. Report any occult or frank blood in stool, tachycardia, drop in BP, fever, or increased pain.

Promoting Normal Bowel Elimination

1. Follow prescribed diet that is high in soft residue and low in sugar.
   a. Provide lists of these foods to enhance familiarity with proper dietary control.
   b. Emphasize that proper food intake influences how well the intestinal tract functions.
2. Inform the patient that bran products will add bulk to the stool and can be taken with milk or sprinkled over cereal.
3. Monitor food intake and weight periodically to determine caloric status.
4. Advise the patient to establish regular bowel habits to promote regular and complete evacuation.
5. Observe and record color, consistency, and frequency of stools.
6. Encourage fluids if constipated to promote bowel stimulation.

Increasing Understanding of Disease

1. Explain the disease process to the patient and its relationship to diet.
2. Have the patient continue periodic medical supervision and follow-up; report problems and untoward symptoms.
3. Refer to nutritionist, as needed.

Patient Education and Health Maintenance

1. Instruct on high-residue diet choices.
2. Emphasize the importance of establishing regular bowel habits.
3. Advise the patient to report left lower quadrant pain, generalized abdominal tenderness, and fever.

Evaluation: Expected Outcomes

- Expresses relief of pain and has a decrease in symptoms.
- No change in vital signs, stool negative for occult blood.
- Reports near-normal bowel function; no diarrhea or constipation.
- Delineates the general nature of diverticulosis and can list dietary regimen that helps or aggravates the condition.

Peritonitis

Peritonitis occurs when bacteria or other microorganisms cause a generalized or localized inflammation of the peritoneum, the membrane lining the abdominal cavity and abdominal organs (see Figure 18-9).

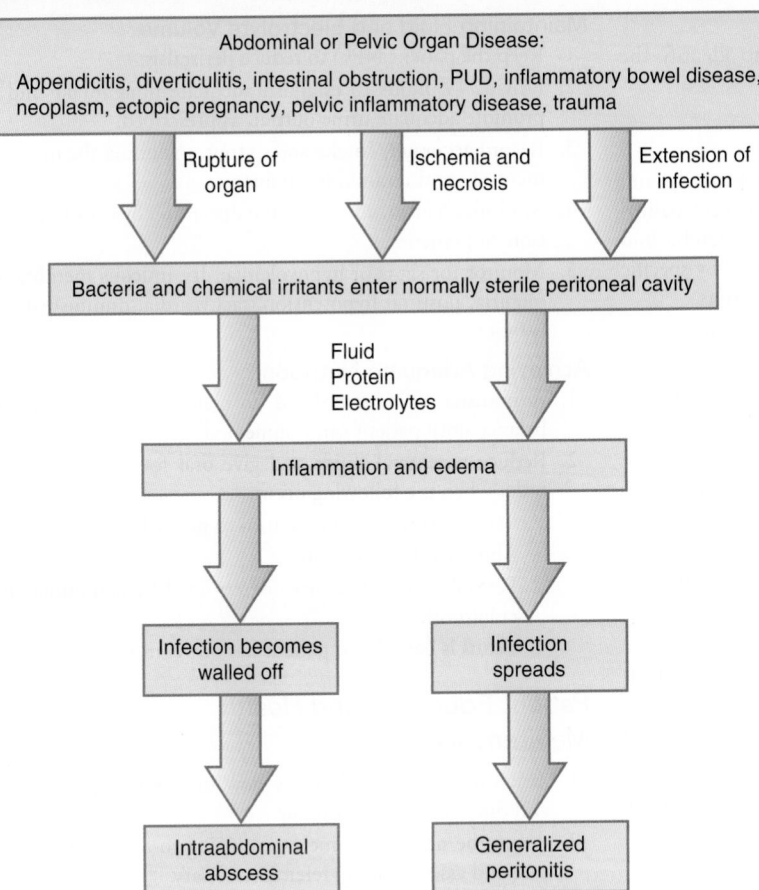

Figure 18-9. Pathophysiology of peritonitis.

Pathophysiology and Etiology

Primary Peritonitis

Also known as spontane+ous bacterial peritonitis (SBP). This occurs when bacteria cross through the intestinal wall into the peritoneum, causing infection. SBP can occur in patients with cirrhosis, nephrotic syndrome, and ovarian diseases (eg, cancer).

Secondary Peritonitis

This type of peritonitis is due to perforation, rupture of an organ, trauma, or peritoneal dialysis.

Clinical Manifestations

1. Initially, local type of abdominal pain tends to become constant, diffuse, and more intense.
2. Abdomen becomes extremely tender and muscles become rigid; rebound tenderness and ileus may be present; the patient lies very still, usually with legs drawn up.
3. Percussion: Resonance and tympany due to paralytic ileus; loss of liver dullness may indicate free air in abdomen.
4. Auscultation: Decreased bowel sounds.
5. Nausea and vomiting often occur; peristalsis diminishes; anorexia is present.
6. Elevation of temperature and pulse as well as leukocytosis.
7. Fever; thirst; oliguria; dry, swollen tongue; signs of dehydration.
8. Weakness, pallor, diaphoresis, and cold skin are a result of the loss of fluid, electrolytes, and protein into the abdomen.
9. Hypotension, tachycardia, and hypokalemia may occur.
10. With generalized peritonitis, large volumes of fluid may be lost into abdominal cavity (ascites). Shallow respirations may result from abdominal distention and upward displacement of the diaphragm.

Diagnostic Evaluation

1. WBC count to determine if leukocytosis is present (leukopenia if severe).
2. ABG levels may show hypoxemia or metabolic acidosis with respiratory compensation.
3. Urinalysis may indicate urinary tract problems as primary source.
4. Peritoneal aspiration (paracentesis) to demonstrate blood, pus, bile, bacteria (Gram's stain), amylase.
5. Abdominal x-rays may show free air in peritoneal cavity, gas and fluid collection in small and large intestines, generalized bowel dilation, intestinal wall edema.
6. CT scan of abdomen or sonography may reveal intraabdominal mass, abscess, ascites.
7. Radionuclide scans (gallium, hepatobiliary iminodiacetic acid, and liver/spleen scan) may identify an intra-abdominal abscess.

8. Chest x-ray may show elevated diaphragm.
9. Exploratory laparotomy may be performed to identify the underlying cause.

Management

1. Treatment of inflammatory conditions preoperatively and postoperatively with antibiotic therapy may prevent peritonitis. Broad-spectrum antibiotic therapy to cover aerobic and anaerobic organisms is initial treatment, followed by specific antibiotic therapy after culture and sensitivity results.
2. Bed rest, NPO status, respiratory support, if needed.
3. IV fluids and electrolytes, possibly TPN.
4. Analgesics for pain; antiemetics for nausea and vomiting.
5. NG intubation to decompress the bowel.
6. Possibly rectal tube to facilitate passage of gas.
7. Operative procedures to close perforations, remove infection source (ie, inflamed organ, necrotic tissue), drain abscesses, and lavage peritoneal cavity.
8. Abdominal paracentesis may be done to remove accumulating fluid.
9. Blood transfusions, if appropriate.
10. Oral feedings after return of bowel sounds and passage of gas and/or feces.

Complications

1. Intra-abdominal abscess formation (ie, pelvic subphrenic space).
2. Septicemia.
3. Hypovolemic problems.
4. Renal or liver failure.
5. Respiratory insufficiency.

Nursing Assessment

1. Assess for abdominal distention and tenderness, guarding, rebound, hypoactive or absent bowel sounds to determine bowel function.
2. Observe for signs of shock—tachycardia and hypotension.
3. Monitor vital signs, ABG levels, CBC, electrolytes, and central venous pressure to monitor hemodynamic status and assess for complications.

Nursing Diagnoses

- Acute Pain related to peritoneal inflammation.
- Deficient Fluid Volume related to vomiting and interstitial fluid shift.
- Imbalanced Nutrition: Less Than Body Requirements related to GI symptomatology.

Nursing Interventions

Achieving Pain Relief

1. Place the patient in semi-Fowler's position before surgery to enable less painful breathing.
2. After surgery, place the patient in Fowler's position to promote drainage by gravity.
3. Provide analgesics as prescribed.

Maintaining Fluid and Electrolyte Volume

1. Keep the patient NPO to reduce peristalsis.
2. Provide IV fluids to establish adequate fluid intake and to promote adequate urine output, as prescribed.
3. Record accurately intake and output, including the measurement of vomitus and NG drainage.
4. Minimize nausea, vomiting, and distention by use of NG suction, antiemetics.
5. Monitor for signs of hypovolemia: dry mucous membranes, oliguria, postural hypotension, tachycardia, diminished skin turgor.

Achieving Adequate Nutrition

1. Administer TPN, as ordered, to maintain positive nitrogen balance until patient can resume oral diet.
2. Reduce parenteral fluids and give oral food and fluids per order when the following occur:
   a. Temperature and pulse return to normal.
   b. Abdomen becomes soft.
   c. Peristaltic sounds return (determined by abdominal auscultation).
   d. Flatus is passed and patient has bowel movements.

Patient Education and Health Maintenance

1. Teach the patient and family how to care for open wounds and drain sites, if appropriate.
2. Assess the need for home care nursing to assist with wound care and assess healing; refer as necessary.

Evaluation: Expected Outcomes

- Minimal analgesics needed; abdomen soft, nontender, and no distention.
- Balanced intake and output, no evidence of dehydration or electrolyte imbalances.
- Bowel sounds present; tolerating soft diet.

Irritable Bowel Syndrome

Irritable bowel syndrome (IBS) is a functional bowel disorder characterized by abdominal pain and altered bowel function. It is the most common functional GI disorder and is estimated to affect 20% of Americans.

Pathophysiology and Etiology

The exact etiology of IBS is unknown. Pathophysiologic processes include abnormal GI motility, heightened visceral hypersensitivity, and abnormal central nervous system processing. IBS is not a life-threatening disorder, and surgery is not necessary. It does not transform into inflammatory bowel disease and does not increase the risk for colorectal cancer. Occurs in 70% of females, with greatest prevalence in youth and middle age.

Clinical Manifestations

1. Functional abnormalities vary and may come and go, leading to a chronic problem.

2. Symptoms may include:
   a. Lower abdominal pain.
   b. Diarrhea, constipation, or alternating of both.
   c. Bloating, distention.
   d. Mucous drainage.
   e. Fecal urgency, feeling of incomplete evacuation.
3. Patients usually have a characteristic pain pattern ranging from pain in the postprandial period, occurring before or at the time of bowel movement, or arising during times of stress or anxiety.
4. Symptoms that occur after eating may be associated with certain foods.

Diagnostic Evaluation

Overview
Diagnosis can be made based on symptom criteria alone.

1. Careful medical history.
2. Rectal examination—normal or tenderness at left lower quadrant abdomen, which may reflect a spasm in the sigmoid colon.
3. If patient fulfills the Rome III diagnostic criteria for IBS (see below), and there are no warning signs of other disease processes, the diagnosis is confirmed.
4. Traditional warning signs, which could signal other organic diseases include fever, chills, night sweats, bleeding, obvious anemia, weight loss, and onset occurring in patients older than age 50.

Rome III Diagnostic Criteria
1. Recurrent abdominal pain or discomfort at least 3 days per month in the past 3 months associated with two or more of the following:
   a. Improvement with defecation.
   b. Onset associated with a change in frequency of stool.
   c. Onset associated with a change in form (appearance) of stool.
2. Symptoms described above for the past 3 months with symptom onset at least 6 months prior to diagnosis.
3. Discomfort means an uncomfortable sensation not described as pain. In pathophysiology research and clinical trials, a pain/discomfort frequency of at least 2 days a week during screening evaluation for subject eligibility.

Evidence Base Drossman, D. A. (2006). The functional gastrointestinal disorders and the Rome III Process. *Gastroenterology, 130,* 1377–1390.

Tests to Rule Out Other Disease Processes
1. CBC to test for anemia.
2. Sedimentation rate, C-reactive protein to detect inflammation.
3. Stool testing for ova and parasites; fecal occult blood testing.
4. Serology testing for celiac disease.
5. Barium enema—should be done when warning signs are present.
6. Flexible sigmoidoscopy/colonoscopy—should be done when warning signs are present.

Management
Treatment is focused on relieving symptoms. Treating the patient's most predominant symptoms determines the most successful therapy.

1. Pain—predominant symptom:
   a. Anticholinergic drugs: dicyclomine or hyoscyamine taken before meals; should be used only for limited periods such as during a flare-up.
   b. Combination agents: phenobarbital, hycosamine, atropine, and scopolamine or chlordiazepoxide and clidinium bromide are second-line agents.
   c. Nonopioid agents: acetaminophen, tramadol, gabapentin, carbamazepine, and anti-inflammatory agents.
   d. Tricyclic antidepressants: desipramine, doxepin, and amitriptyline.

DRUG ALERT Opioids should not be used to treat abdominal pain in patients with IBS due to possibility of drug interaction or dependency leading to addiction.

2. Constipation—predominant symptom:
   a. Fiber: psyllium, ispaghula husk, polycarbophil.
   b. Osmotic laxatives: lactulose, sorbitol, lubiprostone.
3. Diarrhea—predominant symptom:
   a. Loperamide—reduces stool consistency and improves stool consistency.
   b. Cholestyramine—binds bile salts.
4. Eliminate irritating dietary substances, such as caffeine, fatty foods, fructose, or lactose, which may cause such symptoms as spasms, cramps, bloating, and/or diarrhea.
5. A regular exercise routine can improve gastric emptying and relieve constipation and stress.

Complications
1. This disorder is associated with:
   a. Psychological distress.
   b. Sexual dysfunction.
   c. Interference with work and sleep.
   d. Decreased quality of life.
2. Unnecessary surgery due to misdiagnosis (such as cholecystectomy, appendectomy, or partial colectomy).

Nursing Assessment
1. Assess the patient for contributing factors that may affect symptoms: diet, emotions, professional and personal relationships, fears and concerns, and precipitating events, such as financial stress or problems at work or at home.
2. Record specific symptoms that the patient is experiencing in order to determine best treatment options.
3. Explore pain characteristics: frequency, duration, location, timing, and intensity.

Nursing Diagnoses
- Chronic Pain related to functional disorder.

- Constipation or Diarrhea related to change in bowel motility.
- Ineffective Coping related to anxiety, stress, and depression.

Nursing Interventions

Minimizing Pain or Discomfort

1. Assess and evaluate abdominal pain using a pain scale.
2. Review pain medications for proper usage and possibility of adverse effects—drowsiness and dry mouth with anticholinergics, combination agents, and tricyclic antidepressants; bloating, abdominal pain, gas, diarrhea, or constipation with other medications.

Decreasing Diarrhea or Constipation

1. Monitor amount, consistency, and frequency of stool.
2. Encourage exercise and adequate fluid/fiber intake to promote bowel motility for constipation.
3. Encourage adequate fluid intake to prevent fluid volume deficit and electrolyte imbalance for diarrhea.

Providing Supportive Care

1. Validate the patient's complaints and express interest in diagnosis.
2. Follow-up and reassess the patient's complaints and status of treatment goals.
3. Refer the patient for pain management, psychological counseling, or behavior management therapy if indicated.

Patient Education and Health Maintenance

1. Educate the patient on the diagnosis and the natural course of IBS.
2. Instruct the patient about all prescribed medications, including purpose, dosage, and adverse effects.
3. Encourage the patient to participate in stress-reducing activities, such as exercise, relaxation techniques, and music therapy.
4. Encourage participation in counseling sessions to deal with anxiety and depression.
5. Suggest ways for the patient to learn coping skills and stress management.

Evaluation: Expected Outcomes

- Expresses pain is controlled for ADLs.
- Relates that bowel symptoms are manageable with treatment plan.
- Verbalizes strategies to deal with the psychological components of disorder.

Ulcerative Colitis

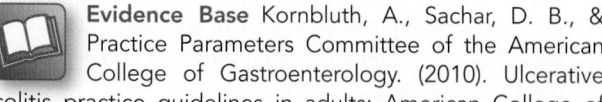

Evidence Base Kornbluth, A., Sachar, D. B., & Practice Parameters Committee of the American College of Gastroenterology. (2010). Ulcerative colitis practice guidelines in adults: American College of Gastroenterology, practice parameters committee. *American Journal of Gastroenterology,* 105(3), 501–523.

Ulcerative colitis is a chronic, idiopathic, diffuse inflammatory disease of the mucosa and, less frequently, the submucosa of the colon and rectum. If only the rectum is involved, it may be called ulcerative proctitis.

Pathophysiology and Etiology

1. The exact cause of ulcerative colitis is unknown. Possible theories include:
   a. Genetic predisposition.
   b. Environmental factors (viral or bacterial pathogens, dietary).
   c. Immunologic imbalance or disturbances.
   d. Defect in intestinal barrier causing hypersensitive mucosa and increased permeability.
   e. Defect in repair of mucosal injury, which may develop into a chronic condition.
2. Multiple crypt abscesses develop in intestinal mucosa that may become necrotic and lead to ulceration and perforation (see Figure 18-10).
3. May manifest as a systemic disease with inflammatory changes of connective tissue. Most common in young adulthood and middle age, peak incidence at ages 20 to 40.
4. Incidence greatest in whites of Jewish descent.

Clinical Manifestations

1. Bloody diarrhea is a key symptom.
2. Tenesmus (painful straining), sense of urgency, and frequency.
3. Increased bowel sounds; abdomen may appear flat, but, as condition continues, abdomen may appear distended.
4. There often is weight loss, fever, dehydration, hypokalemia, anorexia, nausea and vomiting, iron-deficiency anemia, and cachexia (general lack of nutrition and wasting with chronic disease).
5. Crampy abdominal pain.
6. The disease usually begins in the rectum and sigmoid and spreads proximally, at times, involving the entire colon. Anal area may be irritated and reddened; left lower abdomen may be tender on palpation.
7. There is a tendency for the patient to experience remissions and exacerbations.
8. Increased risk of developing colorectal cancer.
9. May exhibit extracolonic manifestations of eye (iritis, uveitis), joint (polyarthritis), and skin complaints (erythema nodosum, pyoderma gangrenosum).

Diagnostic Evaluation

Diagnosis is based on a combination of laboratory, radiologic, endoscopic, and histologic findings.

Laboratory Tests

1. Stool examination to rule out enteral pathogens; fecal analysis positive for blood during active disease.
2. CBC—hemoglobin and hematocrit may be low due to bleeding; WBC may be increased.
3. Elevated erythrocyte sedimentation rate (ESR).
4. Decreased serum levels of potassium, magnesium, and albumin may be present.

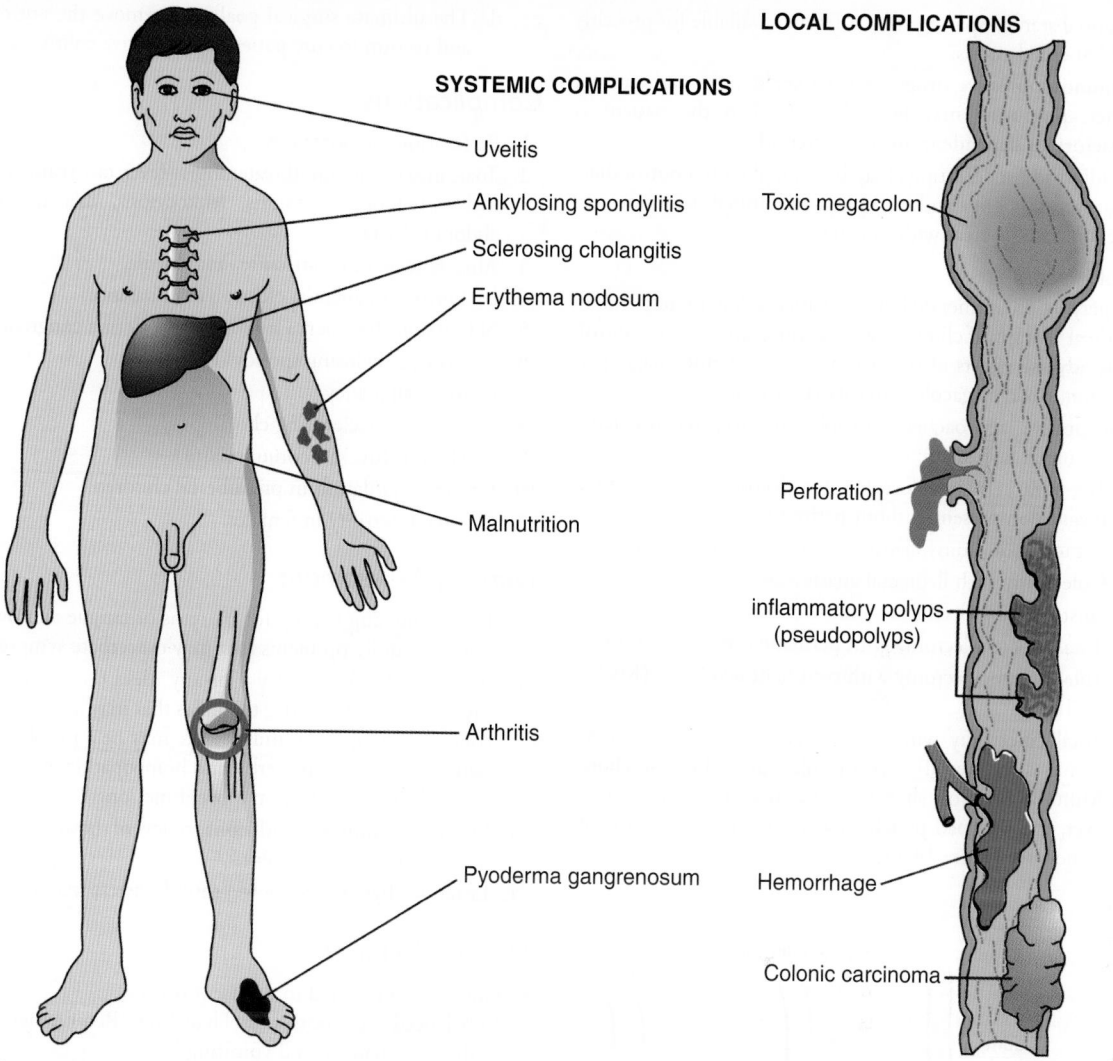

Figure 18-10. GI and systemic complications of ulcerative colitis.

Other Diagnostic Tests

1. Barium enema to assess extent of disease and detect pseudopolyps, carcinoma, and strictures. May show absence of haustral markings; narrow, lead-pipe appearance; superficial ulcerations.
2. Flexible proctosigmoidoscopy/colonoscopy findings reveal mucosal erythema and edema, ulcers, inflammation that begins distally in the rectum and spreads proximally for variable distances. Pseudopolyps and friable tissue may be present.
3. Histological findings from biopsies of the colon include changes in crypt height, loss of crypts, and neutrophils infiltrates in the crypts.
4. CT scan can identify complications such as toxic megacolon.
5. Rectal biopsy—differentiates from other inflammatory diseases or cancer.

Management

General Measures

1. Bed rest, IV fluid replacement, clear liquid diet.

2. For patients with severe dehydration and excessive diarrhea, TPN may be recommended to rest the intestinal tract and restore nitrogen balance.
3. Treatment of anemia—iron supplements for chronic bleeding, blood replacement for massive bleeding.

Drug Therapy

1. Sulfasalazine—mainstay drug for acute and maintenance therapy. Given orally and is systemically absorbed. Dose-related adverse effects include vomiting, anorexia, headache, skin discoloration, dyspepsia, and lowered sperm count.
2. Oral salicylates, such as mesalamine, olsalazine—appear to be as effective as sulfasalazine but are not systemically absorbed and are used when patients are allergic to sulfa.
3. Mesalamine enema available for proctosigmoiditis; suppository for proctitis.
4. Corticosteroids—primary agent used in the management of inflammatory disease. Should be treated concomitantly with 5-aminosalicylic acid preparations to benefit from their

potential steroid-sparing effects. Enema available for proctitis and left-sided colitis.

5. Immunosuppressive drugs—purine analogues, azathioprine, 6-mercaptopurine may be indicated when the patient is refractory or dependent on corticosteroids.

6. Antidiarrheal medications may be prescribed to control diarrhea, rectal urgency and cramping, abdominal pain; not routinely ordered—treat with caution.

Surgical Measures

1. Surgery is recommended when patients fail to respond to medical therapy, if clinical status is worsening, for uncontrollable adverse effects of medications, severe hemorrhage, perforation, toxic megacolon, dysplasia, or cancer.

2. Noncurative approaches (possible curative, reconstructive procedure at later date):
   a. Temporary loop colostomy for decompression if toxic megacolon present without perforation.
   b. Subtotal colectomy, ileostomy, and Hartmann's pouch.
   c. Colectomy with ileorectal anastomosis.

3. Reconstructive procedures—curative:
   a. Total proctocolectomy with permanent end-ileostomy.
   b. Total proctocolectomy with continent ileostomy (Kock or BCIR).
   c. Total colectomy with ileal reservoir—anal (or ileal reservoir–distal rectal) anastomosis—procedure of choice. Multiple reservoir shapes can be surgically created; however, the J-shaped pouch (reservoir) is the easiest to construct (see Figure 18-11).

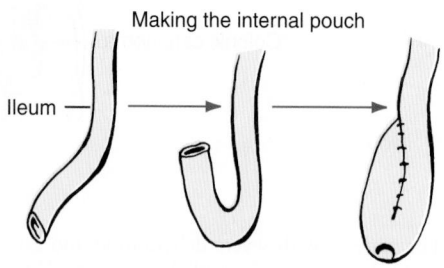

Making the internal pouch

Ileum

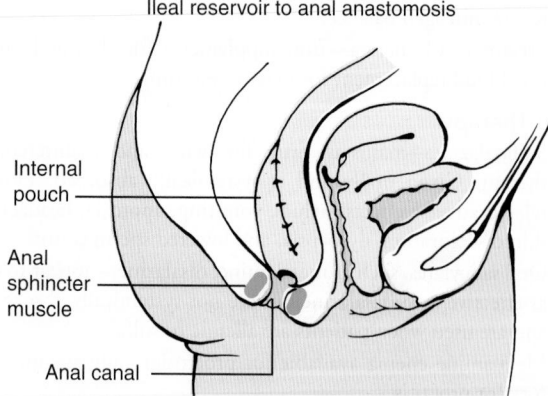

Ileal reservoir to anal anastomosis

Internal pouch

Anal sphincter muscle

Anal canal

Figure 18-11. Ileal reservoir–anal anastomosis. This reservoir is constructed of two loops of small intestine forming a J configuration (J pouch).

d. The ultimate surgical goal is to remove the entire colon and rectum to cure patient of ulcerative colitis.

Complications

1. Perforation, hemorrhage.
2. Toxic megacolon (life-threatening)—fever, tachycardia, abdominal distention, peritonitis, leukocytosis, dilated colon on abdominal x-ray.
3. Abscess formation, stricture, anal fistula.
4. Malnutrition, anemia, electrolyte imbalance.
5. Skin lesions (erythema nodosum, pyoderma gangrenosum).
6. Arthritis, ankylosing spondylitis.
7. Colon malignancy.
8. Liver disease (sclerosing cholangitis).
9. Eye lesions (uveitis, conjunctivitis).
10. Growth retardation in prepubertal children.
11. Possible infertility in females.

Nursing Assessment

1. Review nursing history for patterns of fatigue and overwork, tension, family problems that may exacerbate symptoms.
2. Assess food habits and use of any dietary or herbal supplements used as alternative therapies that may have a bearing on triggering symptoms (milk intake may be a problem). Many patients use vitamins, herbs, and homeopathic remedies without realizing the effect on bowel function.
3. Determine number and consistency of bowel movements, any rectal bleeding present.
4. Listen for hyperactive bowel sounds; assess weight.

Nursing Diagnoses

- Chronic Pain related to disease process.
- Imbalanced Nutrition: Less Than Body Requirements related to diarrhea, nausea, and vomiting.
- Deficient Fluid Volume related to diarrhea and loss of fluid and electrolytes.
- Risk for Infection related to disease process, surgical procedures.
- Ineffective Coping related to fatigue, feeling of helplessness, and lack of support system.

Nursing Interventions

Promoting Comfort

1. Follow prescribed treatment of reducing or eliminating food and fluid and instituting parenteral feeding or low-residue diets to rest the intestinal tract.
2. Give sedatives and tranquilizers, as prescribed, not only to provide general rest but also to slow peristalsis.
3. Be aware of skin breakdown around anus.
   a. Cleanse the skin gently after each bowel movement.
   b. Apply a protective emollient, such as petroleum jelly, skin sealant, or moisture-barrier ointment.
4. Relieve painful rectal spasms (produced by frequent diarrheal stools) with anodyne suppositories, as prescribed.
5. Report any evidence of sudden abdominal distention—may indicate toxic megacolon.

6. Reduce physical activity to a minimum, or provide frequent rest periods.

7. Provide commode or bathroom next to bed because urgency of movements may be a problem.

Achieving Nutritional Requirements

1. Maintain an acutely ill patient on parenteral replacement of vitamins, fluids, and electrolytes (potassium), as prescribed.

2. When resuming oral fluids and foods, select those that are nonirritating to the mucosa (mechanically, thermally, and chemically). If this fails, an elemental diet may be prescribed to provide low residue to rest the lower intestinal tract.

3. Avoid dairy products if the patient is lactose intolerant.

4. Provide a well-balanced, low-residue, high-protein diet to correct malnutrition.

5. Determine which foods the patient can tolerate and modify diet plan accordingly.

6. Bolster with supplemental vitamin therapy, including vitamins C, B complex, and K, as prescribed.

7. Possibly avoid cold fluids, which may increase intestinal motility.

8. Administer prescribed medications for symptomatic relief of diarrhea.

Maintaining Fluid Balance

1. Maintain accurate intake and output records.

2. Weigh daily; rapid increase or decrease may relate to fluid imbalance.

3. Monitor serum electrolytes and report abnormalities.

4. Observe for decreased skin turgor, dry skin, oliguria, decreased temperature, weakness, increased hemoglobin, hematocrit, BUN, and specific gravity, all of which are signs of fluid loss leading to dehydration.

Minimizing Infection and Complications

1. Give antibacterial drugs as prescribed.

2. Administer corticosteroids as prescribed.

3. Provide conscientious skin care after severe diarrhea.

4. For severe proctitis, instill rectal steroids, as prescribed, to produce a remission of symptoms.

5. Administer prescribed therapy to correct existing anemia.

6. Observe for signs of colonic perforation and hemorrhage—abdominal rigidity, distention, hypotension, tachycardia.

Providing Supportive Care

1. Recognize psychological needs of the patient.
   a. Fear, anxiety, and discouragement.
   b. Hypersensitivity may be evident.

2. Acknowledge the patient's complaints.

3. Encourage the patient to talk; listen and offer psychological support.

4. Answer questions about the permanent or temporary ostomy, if appropriate.

5. Initiate patient education about living with chronic disease.

6. Include the patient as part of the health care team to provide continuity of care, communication, and periodic evaluation.

7. Offer educational and emotional support to family members.

8. Refer for psychological counseling, as needed.

Community and Home Care Considerations

Pouchitis

1. Patients undergoing one of the continent restorative procedures (Kock, BCIR, or ileal reservoir–anal anastomosis) must be alert for a common late-postoperative complication called pouchitis.

2. The symptoms include increased stool output, cramps, and malaise.

3. It is thought to be related to stasis within the pouch/reservoir and usually responds to metronidazole.

4. Assess for these symptoms and notify health care provider.

Food Blockage

1. Patients with a temporary or permanent ileostomy must be alert for signs and symptoms of a food blockage.
   a. This is a mechanical blockage of undigested foodstuffs at the level of the fascia.
   b. It is most likely to occur in the first 6 weeks postoperatively when the bowel is edematous; however, patients with an ileostomy must be aware that it can occur at any time if precautions are not taken.

2. Symptoms may include spurty, watery stool with strong odor, decreased or no stool output, abdominal discomfort, cramping or bloating, and stomal swelling. Nausea and vomiting are late symptoms and require immediate attention.

3. Treatment includes:
   a. Avoiding solid foods and drinking clear liquids when symptoms occur. Patients with ileostomies must never take laxatives.
   b. Applying a pouching system with a larger opening to allow for stomal swelling.
   c. Gently massaging the abdomen around the stoma and/or pulling the knees to chest and rocking the body back and forth.
   d. A warm shower or bath may help with relaxation.
   e. If the blockage lasts for more than 2 to 3 hours or if nausea/vomiting occurs, seek medical attention immediately. Usually, an ileostomy lavage is done by the health care provider or ostomy specialty nurse to relieve the blockage.

4. It is best to instruct the patient how to prevent a food blockage by limiting certain foods the first few months after surgery—Chinese vegetables, skins and seeds, fatty meats, bean hulls, popcorn, and other foods that do not digest well.

5. Instruct the patient to avoid problem foods, chew food well, drink plenty of fluids while eating, eat possible problem foods in small amounts, and reintroduce problem foods slowly into the diet.

6. Some patients may need to avoid problem foods permanently.

Patient Education and Health Maintenance

1. Teach the patient about chronic aspects of ulcerative colitis and each component of care prescribed.

2. Encourage self-care in monitoring symptoms, seeking annual checkup, and maintaining health (eg, immunizations).

3. Alert the patient to possible postoperative problems with skin care, aesthetic difficulties, and surgical revisions.

4. Inform patients that early indications of relapse, such as bleeding or increased diarrhea, should be reported immediately so treatment may be initiated.

5. If the patient has an ileostomy, provide information about the local chapter of the United Ostomy Association (*www.uoa .org*).

6. Encourage the patient to share experiences with others undergoing similar procedures.

7. For further information and support, refer to the Crohn's and Colitis Foundation of America at *www.ccfa.org*.

Evaluation: Expected Outcomes

- Reports lessening of pain; functions well with minimal analgesics.
- Demonstrates improved food and fluid intake; avoids roughage intake.
- Controls diarrhea; maintains fluid and electrolyte balance.
- Afebrile, no skin breakdown, vital signs stable, no abdominal rigidity.
- Shows improved psychological outlook; participates in counseling, if desired; uses support systems.

Crohn's Disease

Crohn's disease is a chronic, idiopathic inflammatory disease that can affect any part of the GI tract. It is predominantly a transmural disease of the bowel wall. Other names for this disease include *regional enteritis, granulomatous colitis, transmural colitis, ileitis,* and *ileocolitis.*

Pathophysiology and Etiology

1. Exact etiology is unknown for this disease. It is thought to be multifactorial with the following theories:
   a. Genetic predisposition.
   b. Environmental agents, such as infections (viral or bacterial overload) or dietary factors, may trigger the disease.
   c. Immunologic imbalance or disturbances.
   d. Defect in the intestinal barrier that increases the permeability of the bowel.
   e. Defect in the repair of mucosal injury, leading to chronic condition.
   f. Cigarette smoking is a risk factor in developing disease and increases exacerbations. In contrast, cigarette smoking seems to have a protective effect with ulcerative colitis.

2. Intestinal tissue is thickened and edematous; ulcers enlarge, deepen, and form transverse and longitudinal linear ulcers that intersect, resembling a cobblestone appearance. The deep penetration of these ulcers may form fissures, abscesses, and fistulae. The healing and fibrosis of these lesions may lead to stricture (see Figure 18-12).

3. The rectum is typically spared from disease, and "skip lesions" are discontinuous areas of diseased bowel.

4. Transmural inflammation is a characteristic finding of this disease as well as granulomas.

5. Involvement of the upper GI tract (mouth, esophagus, stomach, and duodenum) is rare and, if present, there is usually disease elsewhere.

6. May occur at any age; however, peak incidence is in the third decade, with a smaller peak in the fifth decade.

7. Most common in whites and those of Jewish descent.

8. The clinical presentation can be divided into three patterns:
   a. Inflammatory.
   b. Fibrostenotic (stricturing).
   c. Perforating (fistulizing).

9. Recurrences tend to fall into the same pattern for each individual patient and may provide an approach to treatment.

Clinical Manifestations

These are characterized by exacerbations and remissions—may be abrupt or insidious.

1. Crampy intermittent pain.
2. Chronic diarrhea—usual consistency is soft or semiliquid. Bloody stools or steatorrhea (due to malabsorption) may occur.
3. Fever may indicate infectious complication such as abscess.
4. Fecal urgency and tenesmus.
5. Other symptoms include anorexia, weight loss, malaise, nausea, arthralgias, and hematochezia.
6. Rectal examination may reveal a perirectal abscess, fistula, fissure, or skin tags (which represent healed perianal lesions).
7. The *inflammatory pattern* may display malabsorption, weight loss, and less abdominal pain; *fibrostenotic pattern* may display a partial small bowel obstruction, diffuse abdominal pain, nausea, vomiting, and bloating; *perforating pattern* may display a sudden profuse diarrhea due to enteroenteric fistula, fever, and localized tenderness due to abscess, or other fistulizing symptoms, such as pneumaturia and recurrent UTIs.

Diagnostic Evaluation

1. The diagnosis is based on a combination of laboratory, radiologic, endoscopic, and histologic findings.
2. CBC may show mild leukocytosis, thrombocytosis, anemia.
3. Elevated ESR, hypoalbuminemia.
4. Stool analysis may reveal leukocytes but no enteric pathogens; guaiac-positive stool.
5. Upper GI and small-bowel follow-through barium studies may show the classic "string sign" at the terminal ileum, which suggests a constriction of an intestinal segment.
6. A barium enema may permit visualization of lesions in the large intestine and terminal ileum.
7. CT of the abdomen and pelvis are helpful with diagnosis but are more often used to evaluate complications, such as abscess or fistulae.
8. Colonoscopy is the procedure of choice. Typical findings include presence of skip lesions, cobblestoning, ulcerations, and rectal sparing.
9. Biopsy may reveal granulomas, infiltration of lymphocytes, and monocytes.

Management

Medical Management

1. The goals of medical management include managing symptoms, reducing complications, inducing remissions, improving nutrition, and avoiding surgical interventions when possible. Management is also based on location and severity of disease and extraintestinal complications.

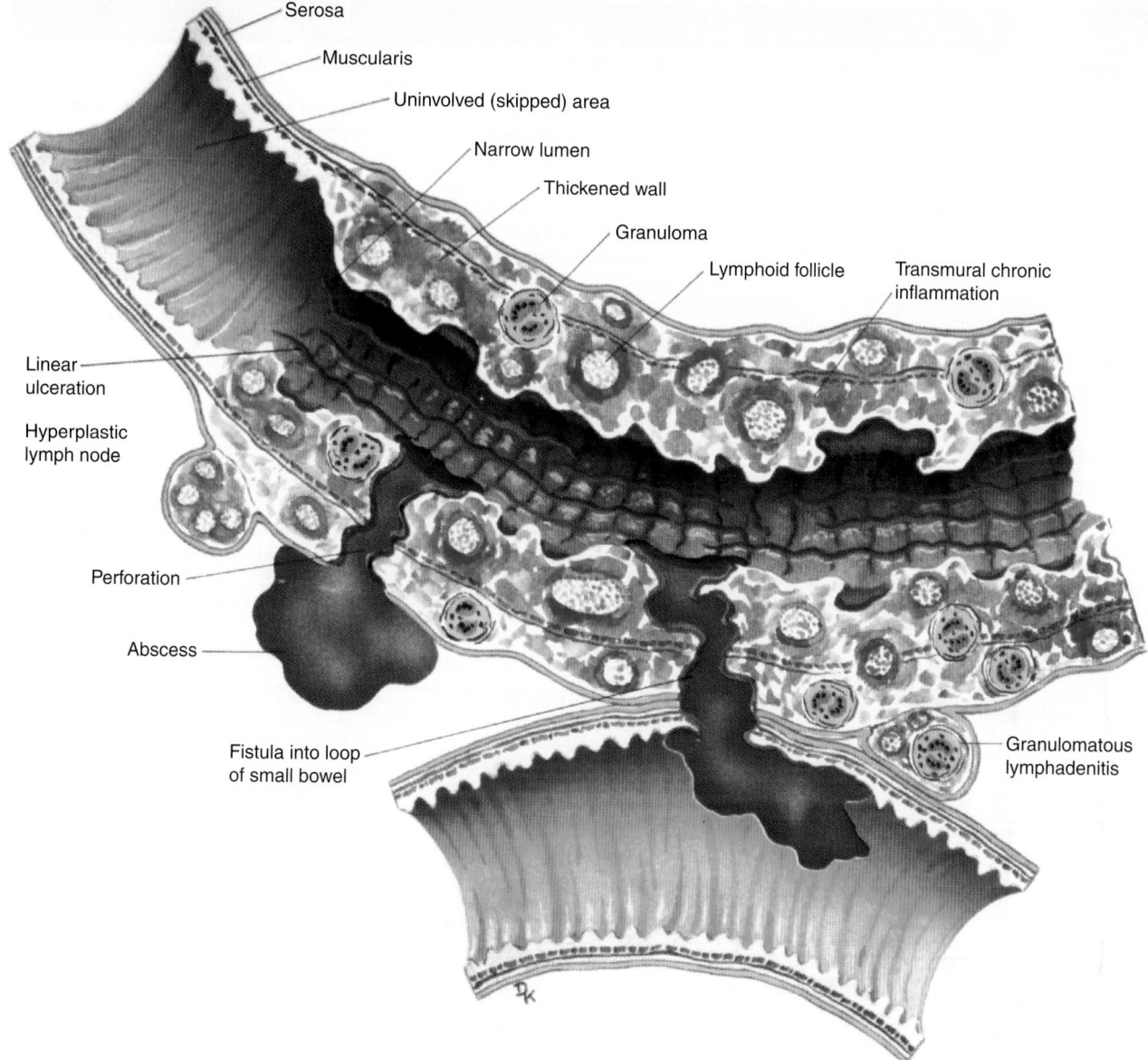

Figure 18-12. Transmural intestinal changes in Crohn's disease.

2. Weight loss, water and electrolyte imbalances, and iron, vitamin, mineral, and protein deficiencies occur in 80% of patients.

3. During acute episodes, bowel rest is usually required.

4. Nutritional replacements may include an elemental diet (Vivonex) administered orally or through an NG tube.

5. TPN may be ordered.

6. For milder cases, a low-residue diet may be indicated and avoidance of untolerated foods. Nutritional supplements may be ordered to provide additional nutrients and calories.

Drug Therapy

1. There is no known cure for this disease; it is primarily treated with medications. The disease severity and the area of the GI tract influence drug therapy (see Table 18-3, pages 698 to 699).

2. 5-Aminosalicylic acid (5-ASA)—first-line drug to induce and maintain remission. Has anti-inflammatory effect locally without systemic absorption. Asacol releases mesalamine in the terminal ileum and colon. Pentasa releases mesalamine throughout the GI tract.

3. Topical 5-ASA (Rowasa suppositories or enemas)—used for distal colitis.

4. Sulfasalazine—one third absorbed systemically; remaining two thirds splits into 5-ASA (acts locally) and sulfapyridine (absorbed). It is a first-line agent but may have unfavorable adverse effects.

5. Antibiotics (metronidazole, ciprofloxacin)—may be used in conjunction with 5-ASA or sulfasalazine to induce remission.

Table 18-3   Drugs Used to Treat Inflammatory Bowel Disease

CATEGORY	ROUTE	DRUG	ADVERSE EFFECTS	CONSIDERATIONS
5-ASA drugs	Oral	Sulfasalazine	Headache, diarrhea, abdominal pain, abdominal cramping, malaise, hair loss, rash, orange discoloration of urine, bone marrow suppression, photosensitivity, and decreased sperm motility in men.	• Monitor CBC for signs of bone marrow suppression. • Recommend daily sunscreen use. • Decreased sperm motility is reversible upon drug discontinuation. • Urine discoloration is harmless.
	Oral	Olsalazine	Headache, diarrhea, abdominal pain, abdominal cramping, malaise, rash, joint pain, and nephrotoxicity. Rare cases of hepatitis have been reported to the FDA.	• Use with caution in patients with renal insufficiency.
	Oral	Mesalamine and balsalazide	Headache, diarrhea, abdominal pain, abdominal cramping, malaise, rash, arthralgias, and nephrotoxicity.	• Use mesalamine with caution in patients with renal insufficiency. Researchers have yet to determine the safety of balsalazide in patients with renal impairment. • Asacol tablets may be excreted whole in stool. Ask patients to report frequent passage of whole tablets.
	Rectal	Mesalamine	Abdominal pain, cramping, rectal bleeding, fever, and nephrotoxicity.	• Effective for distal disease (inflammation in the rectum and sigmoid colon). • Most adverse effects are mild and transient. • Available in both enema and suppository form for topical treatment of distal disease. The enema form allows coverage from the rectum to the sigmoid colon; suppositories suppress rectal inflammation.
Corticosteroids	Oral	Prednisone, methylprednisolone, and budesonide	Cushingoid appearance, hypertension, acne, water retention, weight gain, hair loss, increased appetite, hypokalemia, gastric irritation, ulcer formation, adrenal suppression, decreased resistance to infection. Complications associated with prolonged use include osteoporosis, cataract development, growth retardation, peptic ulceration, hyperglycemia, hypertension, aseptic joint necrosis, and glaucoma.	• May be administered in IV form when the gastrointestinal tract isn't able to absorb drugs properly. • Budesonide is approved for treating mild to moderately active Crohn's disease of the terminal ileum. Because of budesonide's first-pass metabolism, systemic adverse effects are less common than those that occur with conventional steroids. • Corticosteroids aren't indicated for maintenance therapy in treating IBD secondary to associated long-term adverse effects.
	IV	Hydrocortisone and methylprednisolone		
	Rectal	Hydrocortisone/pramoxine and hydrocortisone		
Immune-modulating agents	Oral	6-mercaptopurine and azathioprine	Bone marrow suppression, increased vulnerability to infection, rash, fever, malaise, arthralgias, hepatic dysfunction, nausea, vomiting, diarrhea, pancreatitis, hair loss, and neoplasm development.	• Monitor for bone marrow suppression. • Pregnancy category D. • Testing available that evaluates the patient's ability to metabolize the drug, determines therapeutic levels, and monitors for hepatotoxicity.

Table 18-3   Drugs Used to Treat Inflammatory Bowel Disease (*continued*)

CATEGORY	ROUTE	DRUG	ADVERSE EFFECTS	CONSIDERATIONS
Biologic agents	IV	Infliximab	Infusion-related reactions: pruritus, rash, chest pain, hypotension, hypertension, dyspnea, headache, nausea, vomiting, fatigue, and fever.	• Infusion reactions usually resolve with decreasing the rate of infusion.
	S.Q	Adalimumab	Other potential adverse effects (rare): autoantibody development (lupuslike syndrome) and increased susceptibility to infection.	• Perform tuberculosis (TB) skin test prior to first dose because of the drug's ability to allow latent TB to become active; a positive skin test (>5 mm induration) indicates the need for treatment for latent TB, before initiation of infliximab therapy. • Do not administer to patients with an active infection.

Adapted with permission from Rayhorn, N., & Rayhorn, D. (2002). Inflammatory bowel disease: Symptoms in the bowel and beyond. *The Nurse Practitioner, 27*(11), 24–25.

6. Corticosteroids—to reduce inflammation; given orally, by IV line, or by suppository, retention enema, or foam, depending on the severity of disease. Steroids should be tapered off whenever possible.

7. Immunomodulators (6-mercaptopurine, azathioprine, methotrexate, cyclosporine, and tacrolimus)—used in patients who are steroid-dependent or steroid-refractory. Assists with fistula improvement or healing.

8. Antidiarrheals (loperamide, diphenoxylate and atropine, opium tincture, and codeine)—decrease stool frequency in mild to moderate disease; use with caution.

9. Fish oil—may be used in maintaining remission. The adverse effects (diarrhea, flatulence, halitosis, heartburn) may limit patient use, however.

10. Miscellaneous drugs—antispasmodics (dicyclomine), bulking agents (psyllium), or tricyclic antidepressants (amitriptyline) for treatment of abdominal pain.

11. Infliximab, adalimumab—monoclonal antibodies that block the activity of the inflammatory agent, tumor necrosis factor. They are indicated for moderate to severe disease not responding to traditional therapies and for patients with draining fistulae.

Surgery

Indicated only for the complications of Crohn's disease. Approximately 70% of Crohn's disease patients will eventually require one or more operations to relieve obstruction, close fistulae, drain abscesses, repair perforations, manage hemorrhage, or widen strictures. Depending on the patient, surgical options include:

1. Segmental bowel resection with anastomosis.
2. Subtotal colectomy with ileorectal anastomosis.
3. Total colectomy with ileostomy for severe disease in colon and rectum (see page 659 for care of the ostomy patient).
4. Kock pouch and ileal reservoir–anal anastomosis are contraindicated in Crohn's patients. These procedures require the use of the small intestine in which Crohn's disease may develop.

Complications

1. Abscess (occurs in 20%) and fistulae (occur in 40%).
2. Strictures—may result from inflammation, edema, abscess, and adhesions, but usually from fibrostenosis.
3. Hemorrhage, bowel perforation, intestinal obstruction.
4. Nutritional deficiencies: poor caloric intake due to food avoidance, malabsorption of bile salts and fat, vitamin B_{12} deficiency with ileal disease, short-gut syndrome after extensive surgical resections.
5. Dehydration and electrolyte disturbances.
6. Peritonitis and sepsis.

Nursing Assessment

1. Assess frequency and consistency of stools to evaluate volume losses and effectiveness of therapy.
2. Have the patient describe the location, severity, and onset of abdominal cramping or pain.
3. Ask the patient about weight loss and anorexia; weigh daily to monitor changes.
4. Have the patient describe foods eaten to elicit dietary exacerbations.
5. Determine if the patient smokes, including duration and amount.
6. Ask about family history of GI diseases.

Nursing Diagnoses

• Imbalanced Nutrition: Less Than Body Requirements related to pain, nausea.
• Deficient Fluid Volume related to diarrhea.
• Chronic Pain related to the inflammatory disease of the small intestine.
• Ineffective Coping related to feelings of rejection and embarrassment.

Nursing Interventions

Achieving Adequate Nutritional Balance

1. Encourage a diet that is low in residue, fiber, and fat and high in calories, protein, and carbohydrates, with vitamin and mineral supplements.
2. Monitor weight daily.
3. Provide small, frequent feedings to prevent distention.
4. Have the patient participate in meal planning to encourage compliance and increase knowledge.
5. Prepare the patient for elemental diet or TPN if the patient is debilitated.

Maintaining Fluid and Electrolyte Balance

1. Monitor intake and output.
2. Provide fluids, as prescribed, to maintain hydration (1,000 mL/24 hours is minimum intake to meet body fluid needs).
3. Monitor stool frequency and consistency.
4. Monitor electrolytes (especially potassium) and acid-base balance because diarrhea can lead to metabolic acidosis.
5. Watch for cardiac dysrhythmias and muscle weakness due to loss of electrolytes.

Controlling Pain

1. Administer medications for control of inflammatory process, as prescribed.
2. Observe and record changes in pain—frequency, location, characteristics, precipitating events, and duration.
3. Monitor for distention, increased temperature, hypotension, and rectal bleeding—all signs of obstruction due to the inflammation.
4. Clean rectal area and apply ointments, as necessary, to decrease discomfort from skin breakdown.
5. Prepare the patient for surgery if response to medical and drug therapy is unsatisfactory.
6. Surgery is determined specifically for each patient.
7. Recurrence of the disease is possible after surgery.

Providing Psychosocial Support

1. Offer understanding, concern, and encouragement—this person is often embarrassed about frequent and malodorous stools and often is fearful of eating.
2. Facilitate supportive psychological counseling, if appropriate.
3. Encourage the patient's usual support people to be involved in management of the disease and seek additional support groups as needed.
4. Encourage health-promoting behavior.

Patient Education and Health Maintenance

1. Provide comprehensive education about anatomy and physiology of the GI system, the chronic disease process, drug therapy, potential complications, and potential surgery.
2. Instruct patient about all prescribed medications, including the purpose, dosage, and adverse effects as well as to discuss use of any OTC drugs with health care provider.
3. Encourage regular follow-up and to report signs of complications: increasing abdominal distention, cramping pain, diarrhea, malaise, anorexia, fever, and passing stool through urethra or vagina.
4. Explain the importance of adequate hydration and nutrition (based on individual tolerance) and monitoring weight.
5. Encourage the patient to participate in stress-reducing activities, such as exercise, relaxation techniques, music therapy.
6. For further information and support, refer to Crohn's & Colitis Foundation at *www.ccfa.org*.

Evaluation: Expected Outcomes

- Improved nutritional intake; weight stable.
- Adequate fluid intake; no evidence of dehydration; electrolyte levels within normal limits.
- Demonstrates relief of pain and manageable symptoms.
- Verbalizes improved attitude toward ways to live with the disease.

Colorectal Cancer

Colorectal cancer refers to malignancies of the colon and rectum. This type is the third leading cause of death in the United States. Colorectal tumors are nearly all adenocarcinomas. Lymphoma, carcinoid, melanoma, and sarcomas account for only 5% of colorectal lesions.

Pathophysiology and Etiology

1. Risk factors include:
   a. Age: Risk increases sharply after age 45 in African Americans, 50 in others.
   b. Previous history of resected colorectal cancer or adenomatous polyps.
   c. Family history of colorectal cancer or adenomatous polyps, especially if one first-degree relative diagnosed before age 60 or two first-degree relatives diagnosed at any age.
   d. Familial adenomatous polyposis (FAP; also a variant called Gardner's syndrome) is an inherited condition characterized by multiple adenomatous polyps of the colon, in which cancer will inevitably develop in all affected individuals.
   e. Hereditary nonpolyposis colorectal cancer (HNPCC)—hereditary condition with a markedly increased risk of developing colorectal cancer as well as other cancers, such as endometrial, ovarian, renal, pancreatic, gastric, and small intestinal. There are few or no adenomatous polyps, and the bowel may undergo rapid change from normal tissue to polyp to cancer.
   f. Chronic ulcerative colitis—increasing risk after 10-year history.
   g. Incidence is higher in industrialized countries and lower in underdeveloped countries. Reason unclear but may be related to diet. The Western diet, which is high in refined grains, processed and red meats, high-fat dairy products, desserts, and fried foods, has been shown to increase risk of colorectal cancer.
   h. Immunodeficiency disease.

Evidence Base Institute for Clinical Systems Improvement (ICSI). (2010). *Colorectal cancer screening.* Bloomington, MN: Author.

Lieberman, D. A., Rex, D., Winawer, S. J., et al. (2012). Guidelines for colonoscopy surveillance after screening and polypectomy: A consensus update by the US Multi-Society Task Force on Colorectal Cancer. *Gastroenterology, 143,* 844–857.

2. Colorectal lesions occur most frequently in the rectum and sigmoid areas; however, it appears there is a trend toward increasing frequency of right-sided lesions.

3. Most adenocarcinomas are ulcerative in appearance. A left-sided lesion tends to be annular and scarlike; a right-sided lesion tends to be a cauliflower-like mass that protrudes into the bowel lumen.

4. A lesion starts in the mucosal layers of the colonic wall and eventually penetrates the wall and invades surrounding structures and organs (bladder, prostate, ureters, vagina). Cancer spreads by direct invasion, lymphatic spread, and through the bloodstream. The liver and lungs are the most common metastatic sites.

Clinical Manifestations

Colorectal cancer is often asymptomatic. If present, symptomatology varies according to the location of the lesion and the extent of involvement.

1. Right-sided lesions—change in bowel habits, usually diarrhea; vague abdominal discomfort; black, tarry stools; anemia; weakness; weight loss; palpable mass in right lower quadrant.

2. Left-sided lesions—change in bowel habits, often increasing constipation with bouts of diarrhea due to partial obstruction; bright, streaked red blood in stool; cramping pain; weight loss; anemia; palpable mass.

3. Rectal lesions—change in bowel habits with possible urgent need to defecate, alternating constipation and diarrhea, and narrowed caliber of stool; bright red blood in stool; feeling of incomplete evacuation; rectal fullness progressing to dull constant ache.

Diagnostic Evaluation

1. Fecal occult blood test (FOBT)—can detect bleeding when the patient is otherwise asymptomatic.

2. Barium enema—useful in detecting smaller tumors.

3. Colonoscopy with biopsy—diagnostic procedure of choice after strong suspicious clinical history or abnormal barium enema. CT colonography, also known as virtual colonoscopy, may be used for screening.

4. Pelvic MRI and endorectal ultrasonography—provide information about cancer penetration and pararectal lymph nodes.

5. Carcinoembryonic antigen (CEA)—70% of patients have elevated CEA levels. The CEA level monitors possible recurrence or metastasis.

6. CT scan of abdomen, liver, lungs, and brain—may reveal metastatic disease.

Management

Blood Replacement

Administration of whole blood or packed red blood cells if severe anemia exists.

Surgical Resection

Treatment of choice for those with resectable lesions. Regional lymph node dissection determines staging and guides decisions regarding adjuvant therapy. Surgical options include:

1. Laparotomy with wide segmental bowel resection of tumor, including regional lymph nodes and blood vessels (right hemicolectomy, transverse colectomy, left hemicolectomy, or sigmoid resection).

2. Transanal excision—select people with tumors less than 1¼ inches (3 cm) and well differentiated less than 3 inches (7.5 cm) from the anal verge, and localized to the rectal wall may avoid laparotomy.

3. Low anterior resection for upper rectal lesions—may include temporary loop colostomy to protect anastomosis with second procedure for takedown of colostomy.

4. Colonic J pouch—may be offered as a new surgical technique for rectal cancer (see page 694).

5. Select patients may be offered laparoscopic cancer surgery, although this remains controversial.

6. Abdominoperineal resection with permanent end colostomy for lower rectal lesions when adequate margins cannot be obtained, or there is involvement of anal sphincters. Due to improved stapling devices used deep in the pelvis, abdominoperineal resection accounts for fewer than 5% of colorectal resections.

7. Temporary loop colostomy to decompress bowel and divert fecal stream, followed by later bowel resection, anastomosis, and takedown of colostomy.

8. More extensive surgery involving the removal of other organs if cancer has spread, such as liver wedge, bladder, uterus, and/or small intestine, may be performed.

9. Unresectable colorectal cancer—diverting colostomy or ileostomy as palliation for obstructing tumor, laser fulguration, or the placement of an expandable wire stent.

10. Total proctocolectomy or ileal reservoir–anal anastomosis procedure for patients with FAP and chronic ulcerative colitis before colorectal cancer develops.

Radiation Therapy

1. May be used preoperatively to improve resectability of the tumor.

2. May be used postoperatively as adjuvant therapy to treat residual disease.

Chemotherapy

1. May be used as adjuvant therapy to improve survival time.

2. May be used for residual disease, recurrence of disease, unresectable tumors, and metastatic disease.

3. Drug combinations may include 5-fluorouracil plus levamisole or 5-fluorouracil plus leucovorin. A newer drug, irinotecan, is being used in protocols for advanced colorectal cancer.

Complications

1. Obstruction.

2. Hemorrhage.

3. Anemia.

4. Metastasis.

Nursing Assessment

1. Interview patient regarding dietary habits and family and medical history to identify risk factors.

2. Question the patient regarding symptomatology of colorectal cancer, changes in bowel habits, rectal bleeding, tarry stools, abdominal discomfort, weight loss, weakness, and anemia.

3. Palpate abdomen for tenderness (usually not tender), presence of mass.

4. Test stool for occult blood.

Nursing Diagnoses

- Imbalanced Nutrition: Less Than Body Requirements related to malignancy effects and weight loss.

- Constipation and/or Diarrhea related to change in bowel lumen.

- Chronic pain related to malignancy, inflammation, and possible intestinal obstruction.

- Fatigue related to anemia, radiation, chemotherapy, and metastatic disease.

- Fear related to diagnosis, prognosis, potential for complications.

Nursing Interventions

Achieving Adequate Nutrition

1. Meet the patient's nutritional needs by serving a high-calorie, low-residue diet for several days before surgery, if condition permits.

2. Observe and record fluid losses, such as may be sustained by vomiting and diarrhea.

3. Maintain hydration through IV therapy and record urine output. Metabolic tissue needs are increased, and more fluids are needed to eliminate waste products.

4. Serve smaller meals spaced throughout the day to maintain adequate calorie and protein intake if not NPO.

5. Encourage the patient to participate in meal planning to promote compliance.

6. Adjust diet before and after treatments, such as chemotherapy or radiation. Serve clear liquids, bland diet, or NPO, as prescribed.

7. Instruct the patient to take prescribed anti-emetic, as needed, especially if receiving chemotherapy.

Relieving Constipation or Diarrhea

1. Monitor amount, consistency, frequency, and color of stool.

2. For constipation, use laxatives or enemas, as needed, and encourage exercise and adequate fluid/fiber intake to promote bowel motility.

3. For diarrhea, encourage adequate fluid intake to prevent fluid volume deficit and electrolyte imbalance.

4. For diarrhea related to radiation or chemotherapy, administer antidiarrheal medications and discuss foods that may slow transit time of bowel, such as bananas, rice, peanut butter, and pasta.

 NURSING ALERT Antidiarrheal medications and foods to control diarrhea are contraindicated for the patient with an obstructing lesion. Use these measures only postoperatively after lesion resection for control of diarrhea related to cancer therapy.

Relieving Pain

1. Assess type and severity of pain and administer analgesics, as needed.

2. Evaluate effectiveness of analgesic regimen.

3. Investigate different approaches, such as relaxation techniques, repositioning, imaging, laughter, music, reading, and touch, for control or relief of pain.

Maintaining Energy Level

1. Institute an individualized activity plan after assessing the patient's activity level and tolerance, noting shortness of breath or tachycardia.

2. Allow for frequent rest periods to regain energy.

3. Administer blood products or recombinant human erythropoietin, as ordered, if fatigue is related to severe anemia.

Minimizing Fear

1. Encourage the patient and family to express feelings and fears together and separately.

2. Acknowledge that it is normal to have negative feelings toward cancer, surgery, colostomy, and treatment options.

3. Provide information and answer questions regarding disease process, treatment modalities, and complications. Offer diverse educational materials, such as brochures and videotapes.

4. Refer for counseling, if desired.

5. Genetic testing can confirm a hereditary diagnosis such as FAP or HNPCC.

Patient Education and Health Maintenance

1. Provide detailed information or resources about treatment modalities of radiation and chemotherapy.

2. Teach and demonstrate to the patient and/or family the skills necessary for colostomy management, which may include colostomy irrigation. The ostomy specialty nurse can provide formal education in this area.

3. Initiate a home care nursing referral to assist with wound care, to manage treatment adverse effects, and to continue teaching colostomy care.

4. Become an advocate for colon cancer prevention by educating the public about screening. Beginning at age 45 for African Americans and age 50 for others, men and women should follow one of the following American Cancer Society guidelines for early detection of colon cancer.

   a. Flexible sigmoidoscopy every 5 years.

   b. Colonoscopy every 10 years.

   c. Double-contrast barium enema every 5 years.

   d. Computed tomographic colonography (CTC) every 5 years.

   e. Alternately, stool-based testing can be done annually, but if positive, a colonoscopy must follow. Tests include guaiac-based fecal occult blood test (gFOBT) with high sensitivity for cancer, fecal immunochemical test (FIT) with high sensitivity for cancer, and stool DNA (sDNA) with high sensitivity for cancer (interval uncertain pending further research).

 Evidence Base Smith, R. A., Cokkinides, V., Brooks, D., et al. (2012). Cancer screening in the United States 2012: A review of current American Cancer Society Guidelines and issues in cancer screening. *CA-A Cancer Journal for Clinicians*, 61, 8–30.

5. For additional information and support, refer to the American Cancer Society at *www.cancer.org*.

Evaluation: Expected Outcomes

- Exhibits weight gain and improves nutritional status by adequate dietary intake.
- Has regular soft bowel movements.
- Minimal pain, controlled with analgesics or other techniques.
- Able to perform ADLs with adequate amounts of energy; no shortness of breath on exertion.
- Sleeping well; able to discuss feelings and fears related to surgery, prognosis, and treatment options.

ANORECTAL CONDITIONS

Hemorrhoids

Hemorrhoids are vascular masses in the lower rectum or anus. External hemorrhoids appear outside the external sphincter, whereas internal hemorrhoids appear above the internal sphincter (see Figure 18-13). When blood within the hemorrhoids becomes clotted due to obstruction, the hemorrhoids are referred to as thrombosed.

Pathophysiology and Etiology

1. The exact pathogenesis remains controversial. Theories include:
   a. Abnormal dilation of veins of internal hemorrhoidal venous plexus.
   b. Abnormal distension of the arteriovenous anastomoses.
   c. Downward displacement or prolapse of anal cushions.
   d. Destruction of the anchoring connective tissue system.
2. Predisposing factors include:
   a. Pregnancy, prolonged sitting/standing.
   b. Straining at stool, chronic constipation/diarrhea.
   c. Anal infection, rectal surgery, or episiotomy.
   d. Hereditary factor.
   e. Exercise.
   f. Coughing, sneezing, vomiting.
   g. Loss of muscle tone due to age.
   h. Anal intercourse.
3. Increased intra-abdominal pressure causes engorgement in the vascular tissue lining the anal canal.
4. Loosening of vessels from surrounding connective tissue occurs with protrusion or prolapse into anal canal.

Clinical Manifestations

1. Bleeding during or after defecation, bright red blood on stool due to injury of mucosa covering hemorrhoid (most common).
2. Visible (if external) and palpable mass.
3. Constipation, anal itching.
4. Sensation of incomplete fecal evacuation.
5. Infection or ulceration, mucus discharge.
6. Pain noted more in external hemorrhoids.
7. Sudden rectal pain due to thrombosis in external hemorrhoids.

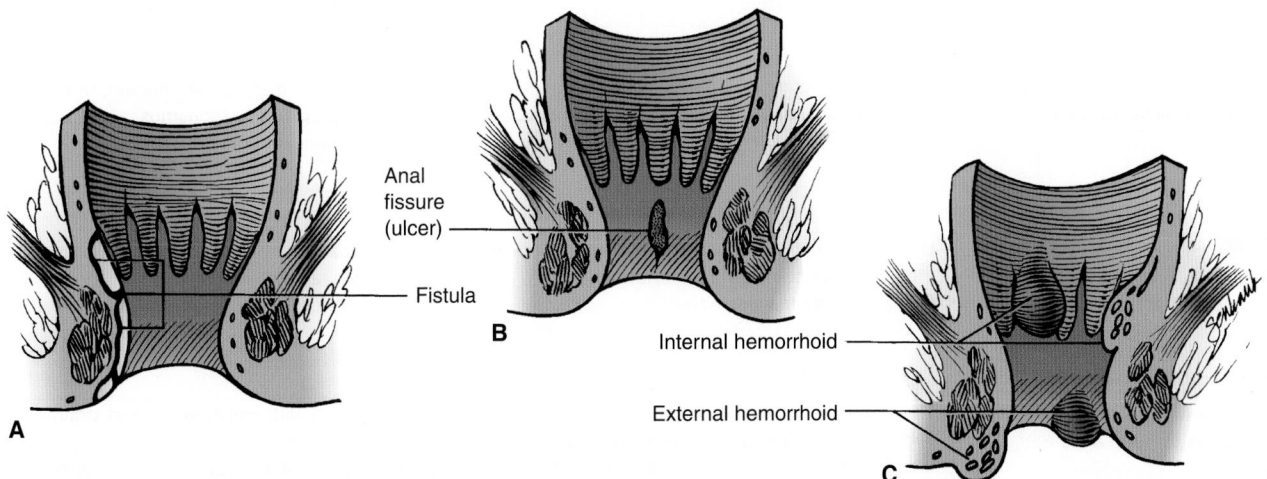

Figure 18-13. Various types of anal lesions. (**A**) Fistula. (**B**) Fissure. (**C**) External and internal hemorrhoids.

Diagnostic Evaluation

1. History and visualization by external examination through anoscopy or proctosigmoidoscopy.
2. Barium enema or colonoscopy to rule out more serious colonic lesions causing rectal bleeding.

Management

Asymptomatic hemorrhoids require no treatment.

Medical

1. Bowel habits should be regulated with nonirritating stool softeners and high-fiber diet to keep stools soft.
2. Frequent, warm sitz baths to ease pain and combat swelling.
3. Analgesics as needed.
4. Topical creams, lotions, and suppositories to provide comfort (Tucks pads, Anusol cream/suppositories, Balneol lotion, ProctoFoam, Preparation H).
5. Control of itching by improved anal hygiene measures and control of moisture.
6. Avoid prolonged use of topical anesthetics on hemorrhoids or fissures because they often produce hypersensitive (allergic) perianal skin rashes with severe itching.
7. Manual reduction of external hemorrhoids if prolapsed.

Table 18-4 Anorectal Disorders

CONDITION	ETIOLOGY	CLINICAL MANIFESTATIONS
Fissure Linear laceration of anal epithelium; typically located in the posterior midline	• Constipated stools may tear anal lining • Perineum strain during childbirth • Tuberculosis, syphilis, Crohn's disease are less common causes	• Tearing acute pain during and after bowel movement; discomfort may continue several hours after bowel movement • Spotting of bright red blood with stool; spasm of anal canal; burning
Abscess Localized area of pus from inflammation of anorectal tissue	• Infection develops from abrasion from foreign object, such as enema tip or fishbone • Acute phase of anal fistula, suspect Crohn's disease • Tuberculosis or actinomycosis	• Painful, reddened bulge or swelling near anus; pain increases with sitting; moderate to severe pain • Purulent drainage
Fistula Abnormal tubelike passage from skin near anus into anal canal	• Often preceded by anal abscess • May be associated with inflammatory bowel disease, cancer, or foreign body • Hidradenitis suppurativa	• Purulent drainage from opening • Itching and pain
Anal condylomas; Venereal warts	• Infectious cauliflower-like papillomas; probably sexually transmitted papillomavirus • Differentiate from syphilitic warts, hemorrhoids, and anal/skin cancers	• Thrive in moist, macerated surfaces, as with purulent drainage • Often recur • Rarely invade urethra, bladder, or rectum
Proctitis Acute or chronic inflammation of rectal mucosa	• Common infecting organisms: *Neisseria gonorrhoeae*, *Chlamydia*, herpes simplex virus, *Treponema pallidum* (syphilis) • Radiation	• Anorectal pain; purulent, mucoid, or bloody discharge; pruritus; tenesmus • Diarrhea and/or constipation
Stricture Narrowing of the anorectal lumen, preventing dilation of sphincter	• Usually results from scarring after anorectal surgery (hemorrhoidectomy) or inflammation • Congenital anomalies	• Constipation, ribbon stools, may not completely evacuate stools • Pain with bowel movement; itching
Rectal Prolapse Mucosal membrane protrudes through anus	• The support structures are weakened (sphincters and muscles), leading to rectal intussusception • Conditions may include neurologic disorders, chronic diseases, aging	• Associated with constipation and straining; rectal fullness • Bloody diarrhea; rectal ulcer secondary to intussusception

8. Injection of sclerosing solutions (phenol 5%) to produce scar tissue and decrease prolapse.
9. Cryodestruction (cryosurgery)—freezing of hemorrhoids.
   a. Profuse drainage and swelling occurs.
   b. Foul-smelling discharge may last for 7 to 10 days after cryosurgery.
10. Other procedures include infrared coagulation (infrared radiation) and bipolar diathermy (heat).

Surgical

1. Surgery may be indicated when the following conditions exist:
   a. Prolonged bleeding.
   b. Disabling pain.
   c. Intolerable itching.
   d. Prolapse.
2. Rubber ring ligation is treatment of choice.
   a. During anoscopy, the apex of the hemorrhoid is grasped and drawn through a drum.
   b. A trigger device expels two rubber bands, which encircle the base of the hemorrhoid.
   c. After a period of time, the hemorrhoid sloughs away.
3. Dilatation of the anal canal and lower rectum under general anesthesia is another treatment.
   a. This procedure is not advocated for patients whose main complaints are prolapse or incontinence.

MANAGEMENT	NURSING CONSIDERATIONS
• Promotion of regular, soft bowel movements through stool softeners, suppositories, high-fiber diet, bulking agents • Topical creams • Fissurectomy; sphincterotomy	• Assist with warm sitz baths and local application of anesthetic ointment to reduce pain • Instruct to eat high-fiber foods and drink fluids to prevent constipation
• Incision and drainage of purulent exudate • Placement of drainage catheter for 7–10 days; possible packing dressing • Warm sitz baths; pulsed lavage	• Wound assessment • Pain medications as needed • Alert for passage of bowel movements, postoperatively
• Fistulotomy • Fistulectomy • Bowel rest to allow fistula to heal; possible fecal diversion temporarily	• Wound assessment • Pain medications as needed • Alert for passage of bowel movements, postoperatively
• Application of podophyllum resin (may be painful) • Electrofulguration • Alpha-interferon injections/synergistic with podophyllum resin • Fluorouracil	• Encourage good anal hygiene and frequent use of talc dusting powder • Schedule follow-up visits to assess area periodically for recurrence
• Treatment specific to isolated organism—antibiotics, antivirals • Bulking agents, antispasmodics	• Review medications • Assist with examination and treatment
• Treatment of inflammatory cause • Dilation by digital, instrumentation, or balloon methods • If stenosis severe, may need plastic surgery to anal canal	• Prevention of stenosis after anal surgery facilitated by anal hygiene, warm sitz baths, and dilation • Postoperative care includes stool softeners, warm sitz baths, and wound care
• Treatment depends on underlying cause • Sclerosing agent injection may fix rectum in place • Surgery may include sphincter repair or resection of prolapsed tissue	• Diet/fluid instructions to avoid constipation • Teach perineum-strengthening exercises

b. It also is not recommended for aging patients with weak sphincters.

4. Incision and removal of clot from acutely thrombosed hemorrhoid.

5. Hemorrhoidectomy—excision of internal/external hemorrhoids.

Complications

1. Hemorrhage, anemia.
2. Incontinence.
3. Prolapse and strangulation.

Nursing Interventions and Patient Education

1. After thrombosis or surgery, assist with frequent positioning, using pillow support for comfort.
2. Provide analgesics, warm sitz baths, or warm compresses to reduce pain and inflammation.
3. Apply anal pads, creams, or suppositories, as ordered, to relieve discomfort.
4. Observe anal area postoperatively for drainage and bleeding; report if excessive.
5. Administer stool softener/laxative to assist with bowel movements soon after surgery to reduce risk of stricture.
6. Encourage regular exercise, high-fiber diet, and adequate fluid intake (8 to 10 glasses per day) to avoid straining and constipation.
7. Discourage regular use of laxatives—firm, soft stools dilate the anal canal, decreasing stricture formation.
8. Determine the patient's normal bowel habits, and identify predisposing factors in order to educate patient about changes necessary to prevent recurrence of symptoms.

Other Conditions of the Anorectum

See Table 18-4, pages 704 to 705.

SELECTED REFERENCES

Chey, W. D., & Wong, B. C. (2007). American College of Gastroenterology guideline on the management of *Helicobacter pylori* infection. *American Journal of Gastroenterology, 102*, 1808–1825.

Ellett, M. L. (2006). Important facts about intestinal feeding tube placement. *Gastroenterology Nursing, 29*(2), 112–124.

Fletcher, J. (2011). Nutrition: Safe practice in adult enteral tube feeding. *British Journal of Nursing, 20*(19), 1234–1239.

Hall, J., Hammerich, K., & Roberts, P. (2010). New paradigms in the management of diverticular disease. *Current Problems in Surgery, 47*(9), 680–735.

Institute for Clinical Systems Improvement (ICSI). (2010). *Colorectal cancer screening.* Bloomington, MN: Author.

Jones, T., Springfield, T., Brudwick, M., et al. (2011). Fecal ostomies: management for the home health clinician. *Home Healthcare Nurse, 29*(5), 306–317.

Kornbluth, A., & Sachar, D.B. (2010). Ulcerative colitis practice guidelines in adults: American College of Gastroenterology, practice parameters committee. *American Journal of Gastroenterology, 105,* 501–523.

Korownyk, C., & Kolber, M. R. (2012). Is quadruple therapy the new triple therapy for *H. pylori? Canadian Family Physician, 58*(1), 58.

Kozell, K., Abrams, H., Barton, P., et al. (2009). Ostomy care and management. *National Guideline Clearinghouse.* Available: www.guideline.gov.

Lieberman, D. (2010). Progress and challenges in colorectal cancer screening and surveillance. *Gastroenterology, 138,* 2115–2126.

Lieberman, D. A., Rex, D., Winawer, S. J., et al. (2012). Guidelines for colonoscopy surveillance after screening and polypectomy: A consensus update by the US Multi-Society Task Force on Colorectal Cancer. *Gastroenterology, 143,* 844–857.

Lindberg, D.A. (2009). Hydrogen breath testing in adults: What is it and why is it performed? *Gastroenterology Nursing, 32*(1), 19–24.

Locke, G. R., Pemberton, J. H., & Phillips, S. F. (2000). AGA technical review on constipation. *Gastroenterology, 119*(6), 1766–1778.

Longo, A. (2011). Best evidence: nasogastric tube placement verification. *Journal of Pediatric Nursing, 26,* 373–376.

Lopez, N., Kobayashi, L., & Coimbra, R. (2011). A comprehensive review of abdominal infections. *World Journal of Emergency Surgery, 6*(7). Available: www.wjes.org/content/6/1/7.

McKay, S. L., Fravel, M., & Scanlon, C. (2009). Management of constipation. *National Guideline Clearinghouse.* Available: www.guideline.gov.

Meier, J., & Sturm, A. (2011). Current treatment of ulcerative colitis. *World Journal of Gastroenterology, 17*(27), 3204–3212.

Mowat, C., Cole, A., Windsor, A., et al. (2011). Guidelines for the management of inflammatory bowel disease in adults. *Gut, 60,* 571–607.

Niv, E., Fireman, Z., & Vaisman, N. (2009). Post-pyloric feeding. *World Journal of Gastroenterology, 15*(11), 1281–1288.

Pavlidis, T. E., Pavlidis, E. T., & Sakantamis, A. K. (2010). Current management of diverticular disease of the colon. *Techniques in Coloproctology, 14*(1), 79–81.

Proehl, J. A., Heaton, K., Naccarato, M. K., et al. (2011). Emergency nursing resource: Gastric tube placement verification. *Journal of Emergency Nursing, 37,* 357–362.

Rex, D. K., Johnson, D. A., Anderson, J. C., et al. (2009). American College of Gastroenterology guidelines for colorectal cancer screening 2008. *American Journal of Gastroenterology, 104,* 739–750.

Scholten, S. R. (2010). Endoscopy: A guide for the registered nurse. *Critical Care Nursing Clinics of North America, 22*(1), 19–32.

Serim Research Corporation. (2012). PyloriTek for *H.pylori.* Available: www.serim.com/products_overview.aspx?fid=2.

Smith, A., Young, G. P., Cole, S. R., et al. (2006). Comparison of a brush-sampling fecal immunochemical test for hemoglobin with a sensitive guaiac-based fecal occult blood test in detection of colorectal neoplasia. *Cancer, 107*(9), 2152–2159.

Smith, R. A., Cokkinides, V., Brooks, D., et al. (2012). Cancer screening in the United States 2012: A review of current American Cancer Society Guidelines and issues in cancer screening. *CA-A Cancer Journal for Clinicians, 61,* 8–30.

Tack, J. (2011). Current and future therapies for chronic constipation. *Best Practice and Research Clinical Gastroenterology, 25,* 151–158.

Viale, P. H. (2010). Incorporating new data on colorectal cancer in nursing. *Clinical Journal of Oncology Nursing. 14*(1), 92–100.

19
Hepatic, Biliary, and Pancreatic Disorders

OVERVIEW AND ASSESSMENT
Assessment of Accessory Organ Dysfunction

The liver and its bile ducts, the gallblader, and the pancreas are called accessory glands in the GI system. Their function is to aid digestion through the delivery of bile and enzymes to the small intestine. The liver plays additional roles in detoxification of chemicals and synthesis and storage of important nutrients. The pancreas also functions as an endocrine gland, as discussed in Chapter 24.

Effects of Aging on Liver and Gallbladder

Liver function tests generally remain within normal range, but a number of other physiologic changes occur within the hepatic and biliary systems with aging.

1. Decline in liver volume and size.
2. Decrease in blood flow.
3. Reduced drug metabolism.
4. Decline in capability of drug clearance.
5. Slower repair of damaged liver cells after injury.
6. Decreased production and flow of bile with decline in gall-bladder contraction after meals.

7. Atypical clinical presentation of gallbladder and bile duct disorders.
8. Increased cholesterol secretion in bile leading to increased occurrence of gallstones.
9. Slower clearance of hepatitis B surface antigen, if infected.
10. Rapid progression of hepatitis C infection with lower response rate to therapy.

 GERONTOLOGIC ALERT *Use caution with administering potentially hepatotoxic drugs, such as acetaminophen, to older adults.*

Common Manifestations

1. Jaundice—any yellow color of sclerae and skin, pruritus, dark tea-colored urine, light gray or clay-colored (acholic) stool?
2. Any dyspepsia, anorexia, nausea, vomiting, right upper quadrant or epigastric pain, or pain radiating to the back or shoulder blade? What is the relationship of pain to eating or to position?
3. Has there been fatigue, malaise, loss of vigor and strength, easy bruising, or weight loss?
4. Any fever, chills, headache, myalgias, arthralgias, photophobia?
5. Any steatorrhea—stools that are loose, greasy, foamy, orange in color, foul smelling, and that float?

History

1. Have there been recent blood transfusions? Are there known blood disorders? GI bleeding?
2. Has there been contact with a person who has an infection such as hepatitis? Any unprotected sexual activity or ingestion of potentially contaminated food?
3. Has there been drug or chemical toxicity, such as carbon tetrachloride, chloroform, phosphorus, arsenicals, ethanol, halothane, isoniazid, or acetaminophen? Have amanita mushrooms been ingested recently? Are certain medications being taken, such as phenothiazine derivatives, sulfonamides, antidiabetic drugs, propylthiouracil, monoamine oxidase inhibitors, methyldopa, azathioprine, corticosteroids, thiazide diuretics, estrogens, valproic acid? Any antiviral medications taken for acquired immunodeficiency syndrome such as didanosine or antineoplastic agents, as many of these drugs can cause hepatic, biliary, and pancreatic gastrointestinal symptoms?
4. Is there a history of nonsterile needle puncture, as in intravenous (IV) drug use or tattoos?
5. Does medical history include gallstones, hepatitis, pancreatitis, Wilson's disease, Budd-Chiari syndrome, biliary cirrhosis, liver surgery, or transplantation?
6. Any family history of gallstones, pancreatitis, gallbladder, or pancreatic cancer or related cancers such as breast or ovarian cancer?
7. How much alcohol, if any, is or has been ingested during the patient's life and what specific type of alcohol (beer, wine, whiskey)?

Physical Examination Findings

1. Skin—yellow sclerae or skin? Rashes or scratches on body from severe scratching because of pruritus? Any signs of bruising or petechiae on body, palmar erythema, or overt bleeding?
2. Abdomen—any tenderness or liver enlargement in the right upper quadrant? Any ascites? Any palpable masses in the abdomen? Any fluid wave?
3. Peripheral vascular—any edema, anasarca, or telangiectasia?
4. Neurologic—what is the level of consciousness (LOC)? Any asterixis (flapping tremor elicited when the arms are extended and wrists dorsiflexed)?

Laboratory Tests

 Evidence Base Sturgeon, C. M., Duffy, M. J., Hofman, B. R., et al. (2010). National Academy of Clinical Biochemistry Laboratory Medicine practice guidelines for the use of tumor markers in liver, bladder, cervical, and gastric cancers. *Clinical Chemistry, 50,* e1–48.

See Table 19-1.

CA 19-9
Description
A tumor antigen found in serum; used as a marker to assess the efficacy of treatment in pancreatic cancer.

Nursing and Patient Care Considerations
1. Tell patient a blood test will be taken and the results will be ready in 1 to 3 days.
2. Not a screening test for pancreatic cancer, this is an adjunct with other tests to provide support for a diagnosis of pancreatic cancer and to better measure the recurrence of pancreatic cancer after treatment.
3. Acute pancreatitis also causes elevated levels of the antigen.

Alpha-fetoprotein
Description
An oncofetal antigen found in serum that appears when a tumor returns to a more primitive state. Alpha-fetoprotein (AFP) is elevated in 70% to 95% of hepatocellular carcinomas (primary liver cancer).

Nursing and Patient Care Considerations
1. Tell patient a blood test will be taken and the results will be ready in 1 to 3 days.
2. Not a screening test for primary liver cancer, this is an adjunct with other tests to provide support for a diagnosis of primary liver cancer and to better measure the recurrence of primary liver cancer after treatment.
3. AFP may also be elevated in certain tumors of the gonads (testes and ovaries), retroperitoneum, and mediastinum.

Radiology and Imaging Studies

Ultrasonography
Description
1. A noninvasive test that focuses high-frequency sound waves over an area in the abdomen to generate an image of the structure.
2. Ultrasound of the abdomen can detect gallstones, dilated bile ducts, fluid-filled cysts, ascites, and small abdominal masses.
3. This test has replaced oral cholecystography as the preferred diagnostic procedure as it is rapid and accurate and can be used in patients with liver dysfunction and jaundice.
4. It is reported to be able to detect gallstones with 95% accuracy.
5. Ultrasound with Doppler can assess the patency of the portal vein, hepatic artery, hepatic vein, and direction of blood flow. It can be used to diagnose patients with Budd-Chiari syndrome or vessel thrombosis after major liver surgery or liver transplant.

Nursing and Patient Care Considerations
1. No patient preparation is required.
2. Explain to patient that a gel is applied to the skin over the selected area and a wandlike transducer is swept across the area of interest.
3. Radiographic pictures will be obtained.

Hepatobiliary Scan
Description
1. A noninvasive nuclear medicine study (also referred to as a hepatobiliary iminodiacetic acid [HIDA] scan based on isotope used) using radioactive materials to evaluate gallbladder function

Table 19-1 Liver Diagnostic Studies

TEST AND PURPOSE	NORMAL	NURSING CONSIDERATIONS
Bile Formation and Secretion		
Serum Bilirubin		
Measures bilirubin in the blood; this determines the ability of the liver to take up, conjugate, and excrete bilirubin. Bilirubin is a product of the breakdown of hemoglobin.		
Direct (conjugated)—soluble in water	0–0.3 mg/dL	• Abnormal in biliary and liver disease, causing jaundice clinically.
Indirect (unconjugated)—insoluble in water	0–1 mg/dL	• Abnormal in hemolysis and in functional disorders of uptake or conjugation.
Total serum bilirubin	0.1–1.2 mg/dL	• Used as screening test for liver or biliary dysfunction.
Urine Bilirubin		
Not normally found in urine, but if direct serum bilirubin is elevated, some spills into urine.	None (0)	• Tea-colored urine; when specimen is shaken, yellow-green tinted foam can be observed. • If phenazopyridine is being taken, there may be a false-positive bilirubin result. (Mark laboratory slip if this medication is being taken.)
Urobilinogen		
Formed in small intestine by action of bacteria on bilirubin. Related to amount of bilirubin excreted into bile.	Urine urobilinogen <1 mg in 2-hour specimen or 0.5–4 mg/dL in 24–hour specimen Fecal urobilinogen 50–300 mg/24 hours	• Urine specimen is collected over 24 hours or 2-hour period after lunch. • Place specimen in dark brown container and send it to laboratory immediately or refrigerate to prevent decomposition. • If the patient is receiving antimicrobials, mark laboratory slip to this effect because production of urobilinogen can be falsely reduced.
Protein Studies		
Albumin and Globulin Measurement		
Is of greater significance than total protein measurement.		• As one increases, the other decreases.
Albumin—produced by liver cells	3.5–5.5 g/dL	• Albumin ↓ (decrease) in cirrhosis, chronic hepatitis
Globulin—produced in lymph nodes, spleen, bone marrow, and Kupffer's cells of liver	2.5–5.9 g/dL	• Globulin ↑ (increase) in cirrhosis, chronic obstructive jaundice, viral hepatitis
Coagulation		
Prothrombin Time (PT)		
Prothrombin and other clotting factors are manufactured in the liver; its rate is influenced by the supply of vitamin K. International Normalized Ratio (INR)	100% of control 9.6–12.5 seconds 0.8–1.2	• PT may be prolonged in liver disease, in which case it will not return to normal with vitamin K. It may also be prolonged in malabsorption of fat and fat-soluble vitamins, in which case it will return to normal with vitamin K.
Fat Metabolism		
Cholesterol		
It is possible to measure lipid metabolism by determining serum cholesterol levels.	140–200 mg/dL	• Serum cholesterol level is decreased in parenchymal liver disease. • Serum lipid level is increased in biliary obstruction.

(continued)

Table 19-1 Liver Diagnostic Studies *(continued)*

TEST AND PURPOSE	NORMAL	NURSING CONSIDERATIONS
Liver Detoxification		
Serum Alkaline Phosphatase		
Because bile disposes this enzyme, any impairment of liver cell excretory function will cause an elevation. In cholestasis or obstruction, increased synthesis of enzyme causes very high levels in blood.	30–120 IU/L	• Elevated to more than three times normal in extrahepatic obstructive jaundice, intrahepatic cholestasis, liver metastasis, or granulomas. Also elevated in osteoblastic diseases, Paget's disease, and hyperparathyroidism.
Enzyme Production		
These enzymes are found in high concentration in the liver as well as some other tissues. Liver injury results in enzyme release into blood.		
Aspartate aminotransferase (AST)	0–37 IU/L	• An elevation in these enzymes indicates liver cell damage.
Alanine aminotransferase (ALT)	0–40 IU/L	• Some drugs such as opioids may also cause a rise in AST and ALT.
Lactate dehydrogenase (LDH)	105–333 IU/L	• LDH is found in liver, heart, kidney, muscle, and blood cells.
Gamma glutamyl transpeptidase (GGT)	0–51 IU/L	• GGT is also found in kidney, pancreas, and bile ducts, but is most sensitive to alcohol-induced liver damage.
Ammonia (serum)	0–32 mmol/L	• Ammonia levels rise when the liver is unable to convert ammonia to urea.

and aid in the diagnoses of hepatobiliary disorders, such as common bile duct obstruction, acute and chronic cholecystitis, bile leaks, bile reflux, and hepatocellular dysfunction after liver transplantation.

2. A radioactive agent is administered in an IV line. It is taken up by the hepatocytes and excreted rapidly through the biliary tract.
3. The biliary tract is scanned and images of the gallbladder and biliary tract are obtained.

Nursing and Patient Care Considerations
1. Patient should have nothing by mouth (NPO) for at least 4 hours before the procedure.
2. If possible, no opiates should be administered for at least 6 hours before the procedure.
3. Inform patient that the scan takes approximately 2 hours and additional images may need to be taken up to 24 hours later.

Endoscopic Retrograde Cholangiopancreatography

Description
1. Endoscopic retrograde cholangiopancreatography (ERCP) involves visualization of the common bile, pancreatic, and hepatic ducts with a flexible fiber-optic endoscope inserted into the esophagus, passed through the stomach, and into the duodenum.

2. The common bile duct and the pancreatic duct are cannulated and contrast medium is injected into the ducts, permitting visualization and radiographic evaluation.
3. Done to detect extrahepatic biliary obstruction, such as calculi, tumors of the bile duct, strictures or injuries to the bile duct; intrahepatic biliary obstruction caused by stones or tumor; and pancreatic disease, such as chronic pancreatitis, pseudocyst, pancreatic duct anomalies, or tumor.
4. May be combined with a therapeutic biliary or pancreatic procedure, such as endoscopic sphincterotomy, placement of biliary or pancreatic stents, tissue biopsy, removal of fluid for cytology, or retrieval of retained gallstones from the common bile duct.

Nursing and Patient Care Considerations
Preprocedure

1. Assess for allergies to iodine, seafood, or contrast media to determine the need for premedication with antihistamines or steroids (per facility protocol) to prevent a reaction.
2. Patient must be NPO for at least 6 hours before the procedure. Withhold medications according to facility protocol.
3. Any patient receiving heparin should have the infusion stopped for 4 to 6 hours before the procedure. If patient is receiving warfarin, aspirin, clopidogrel, or other platelet-inhibiting or blood-thinning medication, a recent International Normalized Ratio (INR)/partial prothrombin time must be available.

4. Make sure that dentures are removed; instruct patient to gargle and swallow topical anesthetic to decrease gag reflex, as ordered.
5. Verify that patient has a signed consent form before sedation is given.
6. Establish baseline vital signs.
7. Establish IV access.
8. Administer antibiotic prophylaxis, as ordered.
9. If outpatient procedure, patient must have a responsible adult to drive him or her home as patient is not allowed to drive or operate machinery for 24 hours due to the effects of mild sedation.

Postprocedure

1. Monitor and document vital signs.
2. Observe for and report abdominal distention and signs of perforation, GI bleeding, or possible pancreatitis, including chills, fever, pain, vomiting, hypotension, tachycardia. Notify health care provider immediately.
3. Maintain NPO status until gag reflex returns. Check for gag reflex by applying gentle pressure with a tongue depressor placed on the back of the tongue.

Endoscopic Ultrasound

Description

1. In endoscopic ultrasound (EUS), a high-frequency ultrasound probe is placed at the tip of an endoscope to assess the pancreas through the GI lumen. This helps to provide images of the pancreas and adjacent organs.
2. It is useful in staging pancreatic tumors; establishing the size of the tumor, its extension into adjacent structures, local and regional nodal involvement, and any blood vessels that may be involved.
3. Tissue may also be obtained by fine-needle aspiration through EUS guidance to confirm the diagnosis of a pancreatic malignancy.

Nursing and Patient Care Considerations

1. Instruct patient that tissue may be obtained for analysis.
2. Verify that patient has a signed consent form for the procedure and tissue aspiration before sedation is given.
3. Preprocedure and postprocedure care are the same as for ERCP.

Magnetic Resonance Cholangiopancreatography

Description

1. A noninvasive, nonradiation radiologic technique that produces images of the pancreatic ducts and biliary tree similar in appearance to those obtained from an ERCP with the advantage of providing images of the surrounding parenchyma.
2. Magnetic resonance cholangiopancreatography (MRCP) can detect the level and presence of biliary obstruction, but cannot offer therapeutic intervention.
3. MRCP does not require the administration of contrast material and provides ideal imaging for patients with allergies to iodine-based contrast materials. Noniodine contrast agent may be given to enhance the picture of the biliary anatomy or secretin may be given as it stimulates exocrine secretion of the pancreas and improves visualization of the pancreatic duct by increasing its caliber.

Nursing and Patient Care Considerations

Preprocedure

1. Confirm that patient does not have a pacemaker or internal defibrillator because the magnetic field could cause malfunction.
2. Confirm that patient does not have any metal hardware in or on the body, such as intracranial aneurysm clips, intraocular metal fragments, surgically placed inner ear devices, metal joint replacements, or steel sutures, because this will cause artifact and a distorted picture from the magnetic pull by the metal.
3. Remove all metal attachments from patient, such as watch, rings, IV poles, and infusion devices.
4. Patient must be NPO for at least 4 hours before the procedure.
5. Inform patient that the test takes about 10 to 30 minutes.

Postprocedure

Patient may resume usual activities.

Positron Emission Tomographic Scan

Description

1. Positron emission tomography (PET) is an imaging technique that uses positively charged radioactive particles to detect subtle changes in the body's metabolism and chemical activities.
2. Fluorodeoxyglucose 18F (18F-FDG) is injected via IV line as a radiotracer and has a short half-life of 110 minutes and is cleared rapidly from the body.
3. The radiotracer used most often for PET scan has a glucose component; because malignant tumors use glucose and grow at a faster rate than normal tissue, PET scans are able to locate areas of high tracer uptake, which represents tumor growth.
4. A PET scan provides a black-and-white or color-coded image of the function of a particular area of the body, rather than its structure. Functional change precedes structural change in tissues and organs; therefore, PET scans can detect abnormalities earlier than a computed tomography (CT) scan or magnetic resonance imaging (MRI).
5. Current PET scan application in hepatic, biliary, and pancreatic disease includes the detection of cancer—particularly when other conventional imaging findings are negative—and response to cancer treatment. The use of PET scanning in exploring the physiology of other diseases is under investigation.

Nursing and Patient Care Considerations

Preprocedure

1. Patient must be NPO, except for plain water, for at least 4 hours before the procedure. Patient may drink several glasses of water before the scan to ensure hydration.
2. Patients with diabetes or patients with glucose-intolerance may require adjustments in diet and oral hypoglycemic or insulin dosage on the day of the test as blood glucose levels

must be no higher than 150 mg/dL. Adjustments should be made on an individual basis.

3. Advise patient to remove jewelry or other items containing metal.

4. Inform patient that scanning time varies from 15 minutes to 2 hours, depending on the areas to be scanned, but the total time in the imaging center is longer (2 to 3 hours).

5. Caution patient that it is essential to arrive on time for this test because the FDG tracer is radioactive only for a short time. Some centers order the tracer on a per case basis, scheduling delivery of the radiotracer to coincide with patient's time of arrival.

6. Inform patient that an IV line will be used to inject the radiotracer. To allow the radiotracer to disperse throughout the body, the scan will be performed 30 to 60 minutes after the injection.

7. Make sure that a bowel preparation has been carried out, if ordered. A urinary catheter may be inserted for a pelvic PET scan.

8. Inform patient that the radiotracer is rapidly cleared from the body and that the test has no adverse effects.

Postprocedure

1. Patient may resume usual activities.

2. Patient may be encouraged to increase fluid intake to assist in flushing out the radiotracer.

Percutaneous Transhepatic Cholangiography

Description

1. Percutaneous transhepatic cholangiography (PTC) is a fluoroscopic examination of the intrahepatic and extrahepatic biliary ducts after injection of contrast medium into the biliary tree through percutaneous needle injection.

2. Helps to distinguish obstructive jaundice caused by liver disease from jaundice caused by biliary obstruction, such as from a tumor, injury to the common bile duct, stones within the bile ducts, or sclerosing cholangitis.

3. A biliary catheter may be placed during the procedure to drain the biliary tree, called percutaneous transhepatic biliary drainage (PTBD). This relieves jaundice, decreases pruritus, improves nutritional status, allows easy access into the biliary tree for further procedures, and can be used as an anatomic landmark and stent of a surgical anastomosis to allow for healing.

Nursing and Patient Care Considerations

Preprocedure

1. Assess for allergies to iodine, seafood, or contrast media to determine need to be premedicated with antihistamines or steroids (per facility protocol) to prevent reaction.

2. Patient must be NPO for at least 4 hours before the procedure.

3. Verify that patient has a signed consent form before sedatives are given.

4. Establish baseline hemoglobin, hematocrit, and platelet count.

5. Make sure prothrombin time (PT) or INR is within normal limits.

6. Establish baseline vital signs.

7. Establish an IV line.

8. Administer antibiotic prophylaxis, as ordered.

Postprocedure

1. Monitor and document vital signs and assess puncture site for bleeding, hematoma, or bile leakage.

2. Check for and report signs of peritonitis from bile leaking into the abdomen: fever, chills, diffuse abdominal pain, tenderness, distention, or cholangitis (infection in the biliary tree) from bacteria in the bile being released into the GI tract and then into the bloodstream.

3. Continue antibiotic prophylaxis per facility protocol.

4. If patient has a PTBD, monitor catheter exit site for bleeding or bile drainage and monitor drainage in bile bag for color, amount, and consistency. The drainage initially may have some blood mixed with bile but should clear within a few hours. The liver makes 700 to 1,000 mL of bile in 24 hours and there should be adequate drainage when bile is draining into a bile bag (called external drainage).

   a. Report frank blood and blood clots that appear in the bile bag.

   b. Large amounts of bile drainage may require fluid replacement.

   c. Maintain patency and security of biliary catheter; perform routine care and dressing at catheter exit site.

   d. Perform routine flushing of biliary catheter per order.

 NURSING ALERT Do not aspirate from a PTBD catheter because this draws bacteria from the bowel back through the liver and may cause cholangitis. Gently push solution into the PTBD catheter to prevent increased pressure within the biliary tree.

   e. Cap off end of biliary catheter to allow internal drainage of bile, if indicated. Teach patient the care and flushing of biliary catheter and signs of complications, if indicated.

5. Signs of complications include fever, chills, persistent jaundice, inability to flush the catheter, bleeding from the catheter, leakage around the exit site of the catheter, and dislodgment of the catheter.

6. Notify health care provider immediately if patient complains of abdominal bloating and exquisite abdominal tenderness as patient may be bleeding into the abdomen.

Other Diagnostic Tests

 Evidence Base Rockey, D. C., Caldwell, S. H., Goodman, Z. D., et al. (2009). Liver biopsy. *Hepatology*, 49, 1017–1044.

Liver Biopsy

Description

Sampling of liver tissue through needle aspiration to establish a diagnosis of liver disease through histologic review.

Nursing and Patient Care Considerations

Preprocedure

1. Establish baseline hemoglobin level, hematocrit, and platelet count.
2. Make sure INR is within normal limits.
3. Verify informed consent.
4. Establish baseline vital signs.
5. Inform the patient that cooperation in holding their breath for about 10 seconds during the procedure is important to obtain biopsy without damaging the diaphragm.
6. An IV may be inserted for sedation, as needed.

Postprocedure

1. Position patient on right side with pillow supporting lower rib cage for several hours.
2. Check vital signs and observe biopsy site frequently for bleeding or drainage.
3. Report increasing pulse, decreasing blood pressure (BP), increasing pain, and apprehension, which may indicate hemorrhage.

Fine-Needle Aspiration

Description

1. The removal of fluid from a cyst or the removal of cells from a mass to establish a diagnosis through histologic review.
2. A fine needle is inserted into the suspicious area and a small sample is withdrawn.
3. The needle is guided by fluoroscopy, CT scan, or ultrasound and can usually reach most internal organs with minimal risk to the patient.

Nursing and Patient Care Considerations

Preprocedure

1. Establish baseline hemoglobin, hematocrit, and platelet count.
2. Verify informed consent.
3. Establish baseline vital signs.
4. Tell patient that a mild sedative may be given and a pain block may be performed in the area where the needle will be placed.
5. Encourage patient to cooperate with body position to obtain the necessary cells.
6. An IV may be inserted for sedation, as needed. If performed as an outpatient procedure, patient must have a responsible adult to drive him or her home as patient is not allowed to drive or operate machinery for 24 hours after procedure due to the effects of mild sedation.

Postprocedure

1. Monitor vital signs per facility protocol.
2. Assess patient for any signs of complications, including pain, hypotension, tachycardia, and abdominal distention or hematoma at the biopsy site.
3. Inform patient that bruising or some discomfort may be experienced at the biopsy site.
4. Instruct patient on resuming anticoagulants based on health care provider directions.

HEPATIC DISORDERS

Functions of the liver include:

- Storage of vitamins A, B, D; iron; and copper.
- Synthesis of plasma proteins, including albumin and globulins.
- Synthesis of the clotting factors vitamin K and prothrombin.
- Storage of glycogen and synthesis of glucose from other nutrients (gluconeogenesis).
- Breakdown of fatty acids for energy.
- Production of bile.
- Detoxification and excretion of waste products.

Hepatitis

 Evidence Base Lok, A. S., & McMahon, B. J. (2009). American Association for the Study of Liver Diseases practice guideline update: Chronic hepatitis B: Update 2009. *Heptology, 50,* 661–662.

Ghany, M. G., Nelson, D. R., Strader, D. B., et al. (2011). An update on treatment of genotype 1 chronic hepatitis C virus infection: 2011 practice guideline by the American Association for the Study of Liver Diseases. *Hepatology, 54,* 1433–1444.

Pascarella, S., & Negro, F. (2011). Hepatitis D virus: an update. *Liver International, 31,* 7–21.

Hepatitis is a viral infection of the liver associated with a broad spectrum of clinical manifestations from non-symptom-producing infection through icteric hepatitis to hepatic necrosis. Five types of viral hepatitis have been identified.

Pathophysiology and Etiology

Type A Hepatitis

1. Hepatitis A (HAV) is caused by a ribonucleic acid (RNA) virus of the enterovirus family.
2. Mode of transmission is primarily fecal–oral, usually through the ingestion of food or liquids contaminated with the virus.
   a. Prevalent in underdeveloped countries or in instances of overcrowding and poor sanitation.
   b. Infected food handler can spread the disease and people can contract it by consuming water or shellfish from contaminated waters.
   c. Commonly spread by person-to-person contact and, rarely, by blood transfusion.
3. Incubation period is 3 to 5 weeks, with the average being 4 weeks.
4. Occurrence is worldwide, usually among children and young adults.
5. Mortality is 0% to 1%, with recovery as the rule.

Type B Hepatitis

1. Hepatitis B (HBV) is a double-shelled particle containing deoxyribonucleic acid. This particle is composed of the following:
   a. HBcAg—hepatitis B core antigen (antigenic material in an inner core).
   b. HBsAg—hepatitis B surface antigen (antigenic material in an outer coat).
   c. HBeAg—an independent protein circulating in the blood.

2. Each antigen elicits a specific antibody:
   a. Anti-HBc—persists during the acute phase of illness; may indicate continuing HBV in the liver.
   b. Anti-HBs—detected during late convalescence; usually indicates recovery and development of immunity.
   c. Anti-HBe—usually signifies reduced infectivity.
3. Significance:
   a. HBcAg—found only in liver cells, not serum.
   b. HBsAg—usually detected transiently in blood of 80% to 90% of infected people; may be noted in blood for months or years, indicating that the patient has acute or chronic hepatitis B or is a carrier.
   c. HBeAg—if absent, the patient is an asymptomatic carrier. If present, it indicates highly infectious period of acute, active hepatitis. If it persists, it indicates progression to chronic state.
4. Mode of transmission is primarily through blood (percutaneous and permucosal route).
   a. Oral route through saliva or through breastfeeding.
   b. Sexual activity through blood, semen, saliva, or vaginal secretions. Hepatitis B is recognized as a sexually transmitted disease.
   c. Homosexual men are at high risk.
5. Incubation period is 2 to 5 months.
6. Occurrence is for all ages, but mostly affects young adults worldwide.
7. Mortality can be as high as 10%, with another 10% of patients progressing to carrier status or developing chronic hepatitis. It is the main cause of cirrhosis and hepatocellular carcinoma worldwide.

Type C Hepatitis

1. Hepatitis C (HCV) was formerly called non-A, non-B hepatitis; an RNA virus.
2. Mode of transmission in most cases is through blood or blood products; prior to 1992, commercial blood was not routinely tested; now, the rate of transmission through blood transfusions is less than 1%.
   a. Found among IV drug users and renal dialysis patients.
   b. Can be transmitted through sexual intercourse and from mother to fetus (vertical transmission).
   c. Can theoretically be transmitted through contaminated piercing and tattooing tools and ink, but transmission by this route has not been proven.
3. Incubation period varies from 1 week to several months.
4. Occurs in all age groups.
   a. Most common form of posttransfusion hepatitis.
   b. May occur sporadically or in epidemic proportions.

Type D Hepatitis (Delta Hepatitis)

1. Hepatitis D virus (HDV) is a defective RNA agent that appears to replicate only with the hepatitis B virus. It requires HBsAg to replicate.
   a. Occurs along with HBV or may superinfect a chronic HBV carrier.
   b. Cannot outlast a hepatitis B infection.
   c. May be acute or chronic.

2. Mode of transmission and incubation are the same as for HBV.
3. Occurrence in the United States is primarily in IV drug abusers or multiple-transfused patients. The highest incidence exists in the Mediterranean, Middle East, and in South America.
4. Mortality—causes about 50% of fulminant hepatitis, which has a high mortality.

Type E Hepatitis

1. A recently identified, nonenveloped, single-strand RNA virus.
2. Mode of transmission is fecal–oral, but because this virus is inconsistently shed in feces, detection is difficult.
3. Incubation is the same as for HAV.
4. Occurrence is primarily in India, Africa, Asia, and Central America, but may be found in recent travelers to these areas and is more common in young adults and more severe in pregnant women.

Autoimmune Hepatitis

1. In addition to viral hepatitis, autoimmune hepatitis (AIH) has also been identified. It is a chronic form of hepatitis that is progressive and fluctuates with degree of liver damage.
2. Although the cause of AIH is unknown, it is thought to be self-antigen mediated.
3. Treatment usually consists of anti-inflammatory or immunosuppressive agents, which may need to be taken throughout the patient's life.
4. AIH may lead to chronic or fulminant liver failure and transplantation.

Clinical Manifestations

Type A Hepatitis

1. May have no symptoms.
2. Prodromal symptoms: fatigue, anorexia, malaise, headache, low-grade fever, nausea, and vomiting.
3. Highly contagious during this period, usually 2 weeks before the onset of jaundice.
4. Icteric phase: jaundice, tea-colored urine, clay-colored stool, and right upper quadrant tenderness.
5. Symptoms may be mild in children; adults are more likely to have severe symptoms and a prolonged course of disease.

Type B Hepatitis

1. Symptom onset usually more insidious and prolonged compared with HAV.
2. May be asymptomatic.
3. One week to 2 months of prodromal symptoms: fatigue, anorexia, transient fever, abdominal discomfort, nausea and vomiting, headache.
4. Extrahepatic manifestations may include myalgias, photophobia, arthritis, angioedema, urticaria, maculopapular eruptions, skin rashes, vasculitis.
5. Jaundice in icteric phase.
6. In rare cases, it may progress to fulminant hepatic failure, also called fulminant hepatitis.
7. May become chronic active or chronic persistent (asymptomatic) hepatitis.

Type C Hepatitis

1. Similar to those associated with HBV but usually less severe.
2. Symptoms usually occur 6 to 7 weeks after transfusion but may be attributed to another viral infection and not diagnosed as hepatitis.
3. Approximately 60% to 85% of people infected with HCV go on to develop a chronic infection. (Complications of chronic HCV include cirrhosis, decompensated liver disease, and hepatocellular carcinoma.)
4. In patients with HCV, the estimated risk of developing hepatocellular carcinoma after 20 years is 1% to 5%.
5. It is recommended that high-risk individuals be tested for HCV because many may remain asymptomatic for approximately 20 years.

Type D Hepatitis

1. Similar to HBV but more severe.
2. With superinfection of chronic HBV carriers, causes sudden worsening of condition and rapid progression of cirrhosis.

Diagnostic Evaluation

1. Elevated serum transferase levels (aspartate transaminase [AST], alanine transaminase [ALT]) for all forms of hepatitis.
2. Radioimmunoassays that reveal immunoglobulin (Ig)M antibodies to hepatitis virus in the acute phase of HAV.
3. Radioimmunoassays to include HBsAg, anti-HBc, and anti-HBsAg detected in various stages of HBV (see Figure 19-1).
4. Hepatitis C antibody—may not be detected for 3 to 6 months after onset of HCV illness; antibody test used for screening purposes.
5. Polymerase chain reaction test to confirm viral activity in HIV illness.

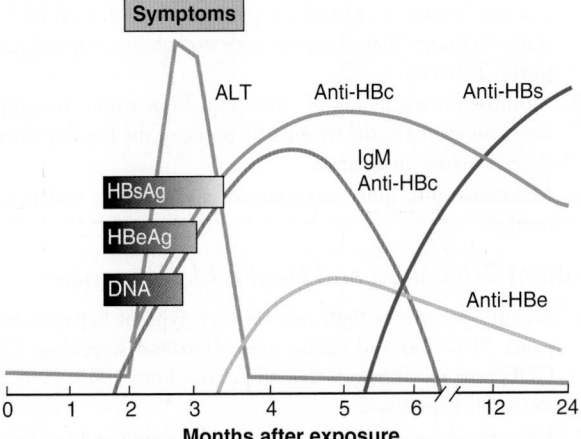

Figure 19-1. Time course for clinical, laboratory, and virologic features of acute hepatitis B infection. ALT, alanine aminotransferase; anti-HBc, antibody to hepatitis B core antigen; anti-HBe, antibody to hepatitis Be antigen; anti-HBs, antibody to hepatitis B surface antigen; HBeAg, hepatitis Be antigen; HBsAg, hepatitis B surface antigen.

6. Antidelta antibodies of HBsAg for HDV or the detection of IgM in acute disease and IgG in chronic disease.
7. Hepatitis E antigen (with HCV ruled out).
8. Liver biopsy to detect chronic active disease, progression, and response to therapy.

Management

All Types of Hepatitis

1. Rest according to patient's level of fatigue.
2. Therapeutic measures to control dyspeptic symptoms and malaise.
3. Hospitalization for protracted nausea and vomiting or life-threatening complications; enteral feedings may be necessary.
4. Small, frequent feedings of a high-calorie, low-fat diet; proteins are restricted when the liver cannot metabolize protein by-products, as demonstrated by symptoms.
5. Vitamin K injected subcutaneously if PT is prolonged.
6. IV fluid and electrolyte replacement, as indicated.
7. Administration of antiemetic for nausea.
8. After jaundice has cleared, gradual increase in physical activity. This may require many months.

Patients with HBV

1. First-line therapy is pegylated interferon, entecavir, or tenofovir. Treatment with nucleoside analogues is no longer considered first-line therapy due to drug resistance and viral breakthrough.
2. All patients should be vaccinated for hepatitis A.

Patients with HCV

1. Treatment of the virus with long-acting injectable interferons, such as peginterferon alfa-2a, in combination with the oral antiviral ribavirin may induce a sustained response of undetectable viral levels in about 41% to 50% of people with genotype 1 and 70% to 80% of people with genotypes 2 and 3.
2. Direct-acting antiviral agents recently received FDA approval for use in patients with chronic hepatitis C. These drugs include boceprevir and telaprevir and are used in addition to pegylated interferon and ribavirin to improve viral response and clearance.

Evidence Base Lok, A. S., Gardiner, D. F., Lawitz, E., et al. (2012). Preliminary study of two antiviral agents for hepatitis C genotype 1. *New England Journal of Medicine, 19,* 216–224.

3. Close monitoring, including complete blood count, liver function tests, and HCV viral load during the long treatment period is imperative.
4. Patients should be vaccinated against hepatitis A and B if they do not have immunity.

Complications

1. Dehydration, hypokalemia.
2. Chronic "carrier" hepatitis or chronic active hepatitis.

3. Cholestatic hepatitis.
4. Fulminant hepatitis (liver transplantation may be necessary).
5. HBV and HCV carriers have a higher risk of developing hepatocellular carcinoma.

Nursing Assessment

1. Assess for systemic and liver-related symptoms.
2. Obtain history, such as IV drug use, sexual activity, travel, and ingestion of possible contaminated food or water to assess for any mode of transmission of the virus.
3. Assess size and texture of liver to detect enlargement or characteristics of cirrhosis.
4. Obtain vital signs, including temperature.

Nursing Diagnoses

All Types of Hepatitis
• Imbalanced Nutrition: Less Than Body Requirements related to effects of liver dysfunction
• Deficient Fluid Volume related to nausea and vomiting.
• Activity Intolerance related to anorexia and liver dysfunction.
• Deficient Knowledge related to transmission.

Patients with HBV
• Risk for Bleeding related to coagulopathy because of impaired liver function.
• Acute confusion related to encephalopathy because of impaired liver function.

Nursing Interventions

Maintaining Adequate Nutrition
1. Encourage frequent small feedings of high-calorie, low-fat diet. Avoid large quantities of protein during acute phase of illness.
2. Encourage eating meals in a sitting position to decrease pressure on the liver.
3. Encourage taking pleasing meals in an environment with minimal noxious stimuli (odors, noise, interruptions).
4. Administer or teach self-administration of anti-emetics, as prescribed.

DRUG ALERT Avoid the use of phenothiazines as an anti-emetic in patients with liver dysfunction, such as prochlorperazine, which have a cholestatic effect and may cause or worsen jaundice.

Maintaining Adequate Fluid Intake
1. Provide frequent oral fluids, as tolerated.
2. Administer IV fluids for patients with inability to maintain oral fluids.
3. Monitor intake and output.

Maintaining Adequate Rest and Activity
1. Promote periods of rest during symptom-producing phase, according to level of fatigue.
2. Promote comfort by administering or teaching self-administration of analgesics as prescribed.

3. Provide emotional support and diversional activities when recovery and convalescence are prolonged.
4. Encourage gradual resumption of activities and mild exercise during convalescent period.

Ensuring Prevention of Disease Transmission
1. Educate patient about disease and about disease transmission.
2. Emphasize the self-limiting nature of most forms of hepatitis and the need for follow-up of liver function tests.
3. Stress importance of proper public and home sanitation and of proper preparation and dispensation of foods.
4. Encourage specific protection for close contacts.
   a. Immune globulin as soon as possible to household contacts of HAV patients.
   b. Hepatitis B immune globulin as soon as possible to blood or body fluid contacts of HBV patients, followed by HBV vaccine series.
5. Explain precautions to patient and family about transmission and prevention of transmission to others.
   a. Good handwashing and hygiene after using bathroom.
   b. Avoidance of sexual activity (especially for HBV) until free of HBsAg.
   c. Avoidance of sharing needles, eating utensils, and toothbrushes to prevent blood or body fluid contact (especially for HBV and HCV).
6. Report all cases of hepatitis to public health officials.

Preventing and Controlling Bleeding
1. Monitor and teach patient to monitor and report signs of bleeding.
2. Monitor PT and administer vitamin K, as ordered.
3. Avoid trauma that may cause bruising, limit invasive procedures, if possible, and maintain adequate pressure on needlestick sites.

Monitoring Thought Processes
1. Monitor for signs of encephalopathy—lethargy and somnolence with mild confusion and personality changes, such as excessive sexual or aggressive activity and loss of usual inhibitions. Lethargy may alternate with excitability, euphoria, or unruly behavior.
2. Monitor for worsening of condition, from stupor to coma; assess for asterixis, the irregular flapping of the forcibly dorsiflexed outstretched hands.
3. Maintain calm, quiet environment and reorient patient, as needed.

Patient Education and Health Maintenance

1. Identify persons at high risk for each type of hepatitis (see pages 713–714) and advise prevention and screening. The CDC now recommends that all persons born 1945–1965 be tested for hepatitis C.
2. Educate adolescents about the risk of piercing and tattooing in transmission of HCV.

Evidence Base Smith, B. D., Morgan, R. L., Beckett, G. A., et al. (2012). Recommendations for the identification of chronic hepatitis C virus infection in persons born during 1945–1965. *MMWR, 61*(RR05), 1–18.

3. Encourage vaccination for HBV with series of three shots (initial shot at birth, 1, and 6 months) for high-risk patients, such as health care workers or institutionalized persons, as well as vaccination of all children from birth or at adolescence.

4. Instruct all patients who have received a blood transfusion to refrain from donating blood for 6 months (the incubation period of HBV). After hepatitis infection, blood should never be given if patient is an HBV carrier or was infected with HCV.

5. Stress the need to follow precautions with blood and secretions until the patient is deemed free of HBsAg.

6. Explain to HBV carriers that their blood and secretions will remain infectious.

7. For additional information, refer to the local public health department or the Centers for Disease Control and Prevention (*www.cdc.gov*).

Evaluation: Expected Outcomes

- Tolerates small carbohydrate feedings.
- No vomiting, tolerates fluids.
- Maintains self-care and light ambulation.
- Family members seek active immunization.

- No signs of bleeding.
- Lethargic but oriented, no tremor.

Hepatic Cirrhosis

 Evidence Base O'Shea, R. S., Dasarathy, S., & McCullough, A. J. (2010). Alcoholic liver disease: Practice guideline of the American Association for the Study of Liver Diseases, American College of Gastroenterology practice guideline. *Hepatology, 1,* 307–328.

Cirrhosis of the liver is characterized by scarring. It is a chronic disease in which there has been diffuse destruction and fibrotic regeneration of hepatic cells (see Figure 19-2). As necrotic tissue is replaced by fibrotic tissue, normal liver structure and vasculature is altered, impairing blood and lymph flow, resulting in hepatic insufficiency and portal hypertension.

Pathophysiology and Etiology

1. Laënnec's cirrhosis (macronodular), also known as alcoholic cirrhosis.
   a. Fibrosis—mainly around central veins and portal areas.
   b. Usually due to chronic alcohol toxicity and malnutrition.

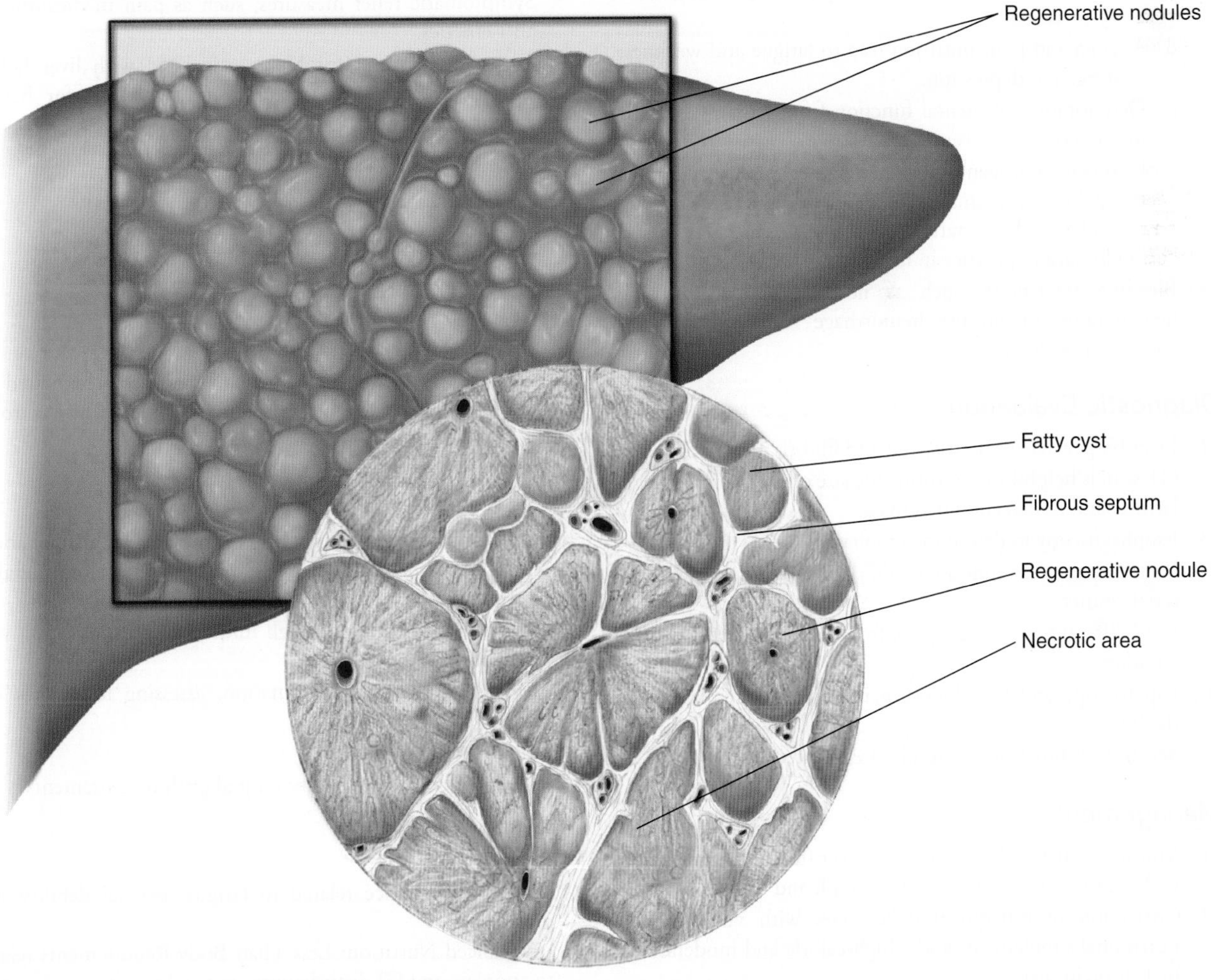

Regenerative nodules

Fatty cyst

Fibrous septum

Regenerative nodule

Necrotic area

Figure 19-2. Fibrotic changes to liver tissue in cirrhosis.

2. Postnecrotic cirrhosis (micronodular).
   a. Broad bands of scar tissue.
   b. Because of previous acute viral hepatitis or drug-induced massive hepatic necrosis.
3. Biliary cirrhosis.
   a. Scarring around bile ducts and lobes of the liver.
   b. Results from chronic biliary injury and obstruction of the intrahepatic or extrahepatic biliary system.
   c. Partial or total obstruction of the bile ducts can lead to infectious cholangitis and cirrhosis, which is much rarer than Laënnec's and postnecrotic cirrhosis.

Clinical Manifestations

1. Onset is insidious; may take years to develop.
2. Early complaints include fatigue, anorexia, ankle edema in the evening, epistaxis and bleeding gums, and weight loss.
3. Later complaints because of chronic failure of the liver and obstruction of portal circulation.
   a. Chronic dyspepsia, constipation, or diarrhea.
   b. Esophageal varices, dilated cutaneous veins around the umbilicus (caput medusa), internal hemorrhoids, ascites, splenomegaly, and pancytopenia.
   c. Plasma albumin is reduced, leading to edema and contributing to ascites.
   d. Anemia and poor nutrition lead to fatigue and weakness, wasting, and depression.
   e. Deterioration of mental function from lethargy to delirium to coma and eventual death.
   f. Estrogen–androgen imbalance causes spider angiomata and palmar erythema; menstrual irregularities in females; testicular and prostatic atrophy, gynecomastia, loss of libido, and impotence in males.
4. Bleeding tendencies, such as nosebleeds, easy bruising, hematemesis, or profuse hemorrhage from stomach and esophageal varices.

Diagnostic Evaluation

1. Liver biopsy detects destruction and fibrosis of hepatic tissue.
2. CT scan is helpful to determine the size of the liver, its irregularities, and in detection of a mass.
3. Esophagoscopy to determine esophageal varices.
4. Paracentesis to examine ascitic fluid for cell, protein, and bacterial counts.
5. PTC differentiates extrahepatic from intrahepatic obstructive jaundice.
6. Laparoscopy and liver biopsy permit direct visualization of the liver.
7. Serum liver function test results are elevated.

Management

1. Minimize further deterioration of liver function through the withdrawal of toxic substances, alcohol, and drugs.
2. Correction of nutritional deficiencies with vitamins and nutritional supplements and a high-calorie and moderate- to high-protein diet.

3. Treatment of ascites and fluid and electrolyte imbalances.
   a. Restrict sodium and water intake, depending on amount of fluid retention.
   b. Bed rest to aid in diuresis.
   c. Diuretic therapy, frequently with spironolactone, a potassium-sparing diuretic that inhibits the action of aldosterone on the kidneys. Furosemide, a loop diuretic, may also be used in conjunction with spironolactone to help balance potassium depletion.
   d. Abdominal paracentesis to remove fluid and relieve symptoms (see Procedure Guidelines 19-1); ascitic fluid may be ultrafiltrated and reinfused through a central venous access device.
   e. Administration of albumin to maintain osmotic pressure.
4. Transjugular intrahepatic portosystemic shunt (TIPS), an interventional radiologic procedure, may be performed in patients whose ascites is resistant to other forms of treatment. TIPS is a percutaneously created connection within the liver between the portal and systemic circulations. A shunt is placed to reduce the portal pressure in patients with complications related to portal hypertension.
   a. Complications include bacterial infections, shunt obstruction, encephalopathy, and increase in coagulopathies.
5. Symptomatic relief measures, such as pain medication and anti-emetics.
6. Treatment of other problems associated with liver failure. Administer lactulose, rifaximin, or neomycin for hepatic encephalopathy.
7. Liver transplantation may be necessary.

Complications

1. Hyponatremia and water retention.
2. Bleeding esophageal varices.
3. Coagulopathies.
4. Spontaneous bacterial peritonitis.
5. Hepatic encephalopathy, which may be precipitated by the use of sedatives, high-protein diet, sepsis, or electrolyte imbalance.

Nursing Assessment

1. Obtain history of precipitating factors, such as alcohol abuse, hepatitis, or biliary disease. Establish present pattern of alcohol intake.
2. Assess mental status through interview and interaction with patient.
3. Perform abdominal examination, assessing for ascites (see Figure 19-3, page 719).
4. Observe for bleeding.
5. Assess daily weight and abdominal girth measurements.

Nursing Diagnoses

- Activity Intolerance related to fatigue, general debility, and discomfort.
- Imbalanced Nutrition: Less Than Body Requirements related to anorexia and GI disturbances.

PROCEDURE GUIDELINES 19-1

Assisting with Abdominal Paracentesis

EQUIPMENT

- Sterile paracentesis tray and gloves
- Local anesthetic
- Drape or cotton blankets
- Collection bottle (vacuum bottle)
- Skin preparation tray with antiseptic
- Specimen bottles and laboratory forms

PROCEDURE

Nursing Action	Rationale
Preparatory phase	
1. Explain procedure to the patient. Make sure that consent form has been signed.	1. Ensures patient's understanding and consent for the procedure and reduces patient's fear and anxiety.
2. Record the patient's vital signs.	2. Provides baseline values for later comparison.
3. Have the patient void before treatment is begun.	3. Lessens the danger of accidentally piercing the bladder with the needle or trocar.
4. Position patient in Fowler's position with back, arms, and feet supported.	4. Patient is more comfortable and a steady position can be maintained.
5. Drape patient with sheet exposing abdomen.	5. Minimizes exposure of patient and keeps patient warm.
Performance phase	
1. Assist in preparing skin with antiseptic solution.	1. This is considered a minor surgical procedure that requires aseptic precautions.
2. Open sterile tray and package of sterile gloves; provide anesthetic solution.	
3. Have collection bottle and tubing available.	
4. Assess pulse and respiratory status frequently during procedure; watch for pallor, cyanosis, or syncope (faintness).	4. Indicates shock. Keep emergency drugs available.
5. Provider administers local anesthesia and introduces needle or trocar.	
6. Needle or trocar is connected to tubing and vacuum bottle or syringe; fluid is slowly drained from peritoneal cavity.	6. Drainage is usually limited to 1–2 L to relieve acute symptoms and minimize risk of hypovolemia and shock.
7. Apply dressing when needle is withdrawn.	7. Elasticized adhesive patch is effective, serving as waterproof adhering dressing.
8. Usually, a dressing is sufficient; however, if the trocar wound appears large, the provider may close the incision with sutures.	8. Prevents blood loss and aids healing.
Follow-up phase	
1. Assist patient to a comfortable position after treatment.	1. There may be minor pain at incision site.
2. Record amount and characteristics of fluid removed, number of specimens sent to laboratory, and patient's condition during treatment.	2. Documentation is important for continuity of care.
3. Check blood pressure and vital signs every ½ hour for 2 hours, every hour for 4 hours, and every 4 hours for 24 hours.	3. Close observation will detect poor circulatory adjustment and possible development of shock.
4. Watch for leakage or scrotal edema after paracentesis.	4. Indicates complication. If seen, report at once.

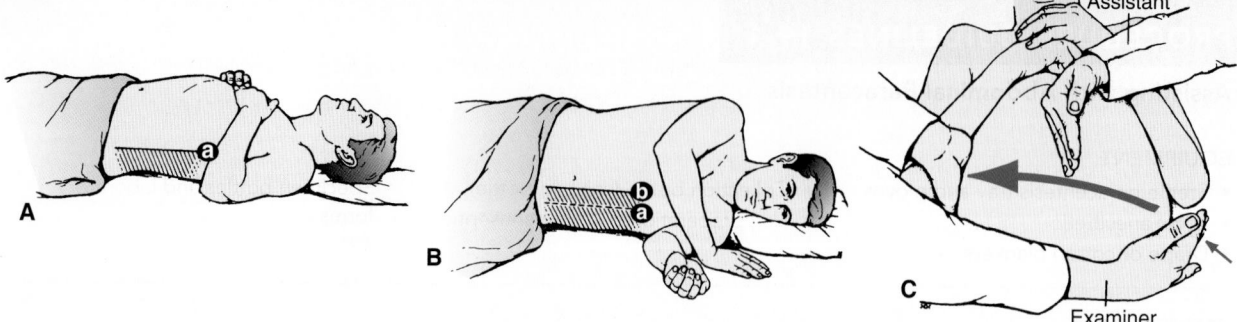

Figure 19-3. Assessing for ascites. (A) To percuss for shifting dullness, each flank is percussed with patient in a supine position. If fluid is present, dullness is noted at each flank. The most medial limits of the dullness should be marked as indicated in **a**. Patient should then be shifted to the side. **(B)** Note what happens to the area of dullness if fluid is present; the area of dullness begins at **b**. **(C)** To detect the presence of a fluid wave, the examiner places one hand alongside each flank. A second person then places a hand, ulnar side down, along patient's midline and applies light pressure. The examiner then strikes one flank sharply with one hand, while the other hand remains in place to detect any signs of a fluid impulse. The assistant's hand should dampen any wave impulses traveling through the abdominal wall, unless fluid is present.

- Impaired Skin Integrity related to edema, jaundice, and compromised immunologic status.
- Risk for Injury related to altered clotting mechanisms.
- Acute Confusion related to deterioration of liver function and increased serum ammonia level.

Nursing Interventions

Promoting Activity Tolerance

1. Encourage alternating periods of rest and ambulation.
2. Maintain some periods of bed rest with legs elevated to mobilize edema and ascites.
3. Encourage and assist with gradually increasing periods of exercise.

Improving Nutritional Status

1. Encourage patient to eat high-calorie, moderate-protein meals and to have supplementary feedings.
2. Suggest small, frequent feedings and attractive meals in an aesthetically pleasing setting at mealtimes.
3. Encourage oral hygiene before meals.
4. Administer or teach self-administration of medication for nausea, vomiting, diarrhea, or constipation.

Protecting Skin Integrity

1. Note and record degree of jaundice of skin and sclerae and scratches on the body.
2. Encourage frequent skin care, bathing without soap, and massage with emollient lotions.
3. Advise patient to keep fingernails short.

Preventing Injury Through Bleeding

1. Observe stools and emesis for color, consistency, and amount; test each one for occult blood.
2. Be alert for symptoms of anxiety, epigastric fullness, weakness, and restlessness, which may indicate GI bleeding.
3. Observe for external bleeding: ecchymosis, leaking needle-stick sites, epistaxis, petechiae, and bleeding gums.

4. Keep patient quiet and limit activity if signs of bleeding are exhibited.
5. Administer vitamin K, as prescribed.
6. Stay in constant attendance during episodes of bleeding.
7. Institute and teach measures to prevent trauma:
   a. Maintain safe environment.
   b. Gentle blowing of nose.
   c. Use of soft toothbrush.
8. Encourage intake of foods with high vitamin C content.
9. Use small-gauge needles for injections and maintain pressure over site until bleeding stops.
10. Management of bleeding from esophageal varices can include endoscopic variceal ligation (banding) or injection sclerotherapy.

Promoting Improved Thought Processes

1. Restrict high-protein loads while serum ammonia is high to prevent hepatic encephalopathy. Monitor ammonia levels.
2. Protect from sepsis through good handwashing and prompt recognition and management of infection.
3. Monitor fluid intake and output and serum electrolyte levels to prevent dehydration and hypokalemia (may occur with the use of diuretics), which may precipitate hepatic coma.
4. Keep environment warm and limit visitors.
5. Pad the side rails of the bed and provide careful nursing surveillance to ensure patient's safety.
6. Assess LOC and frequently reorient, as needed.

 DRUG ALERT Opioids, sedatives, and barbiturates are used cautiously in the restless patient with cirrhosis to prevent precipitation of hepatic coma.

7. Administer lactulose or neomycin through a retention enema or nasogastric (NG) tube, as ordered, for elevated ammonia levels and decreasing LOC.

Patient Education and Health Maintenance

1. Stress the necessity of giving up alcohol completely.
2. Urge acceptance of assistance from a substance abuse program.
3. Provide written dietary instructions.
4. Encourage daily weighing for self-monitoring of fluid retention or depletion.
5. Discuss adverse effects of diuretic therapy.
6. Emphasize the importance of rest, a sensible lifestyle, and an adequate, well-balanced diet.
7. Advise patient to avoid substances (over-the-counter medications, herbs, illicit drugs, toxins) that may affect liver function.
8. Involve the person closest to the patient because recovery usually is not easy and relapses are common.
9. Stress the importance of continued follow-up for laboratory tests and evaluation by a health care provider.

Evaluation: Expected Outcomes

- Ambulates for 10 minutes each hour.
- Tolerates small, frequent feedings.
- Skin without breakdown or scratches.
- No bleeding or bruising; results of stool tests are negative for occult blood.
- Drowsy but easily aroused and oriented.

Bleeding Esophageal Varices

Esophageal varices are dilated tortuous veins usually found in the submucosa of the lower esophagus; however, they may develop higher in the esophagus or extend into the stomach.

Pathophysiology and Etiology

1. Nearly always because of portal hypertension, which may result from obstruction of the portal venous circulation and cirrhosis of the liver.
   a. Because of increased obstruction of the portal vein, venous blood from the intestinal tract and spleen seeks an outlet through collateral circulation, which creates new pathways of return to the right atrium and causes an increased strain on the vessels in the submucosal layer of the lower esophagus and upper part of the stomach.
   b. These collateral vessels are tortuous and fragile and bleed easily.
2. Other causes of varices are abnormalities of the circulation in the splenic vein or superior vena cava and hepatic venothrombosis.
3. Mortality is high because of further deterioration of liver function to hepatic coma and complications, such as aspiration pneumonia, sepsis, and renal failure.

Clinical Manifestations

1. Hematemesis—vomiting of bright red blood.
2. Melena—passage of black, tarry stools, which indicates that blood has been in the GI tract for at least 14 hours.
3. Bright red rectal bleeding from hypermotility of the bowel or rectal varices.
4. Blood loss may be sudden and massive, causing shock.

Diagnostic Evaluation

1. Upper GI endoscopy for patients with a suspected upper GI source of bleeding.
2. Hemoglobin may be decreasing and liver function tests can be elevated.

Management

Treatment

1. Restoration of circulating blood volume with blood and IV fluids.
2. Use of IV vasoconstrictors, such as octreotide or vasopressin to control bleeding. These drugs may be used to reduce portal pressure by decreasing splanchnic blood flow and to increase clotting and hemostasis. Vasopressin has a significant negative (vasoconstrictive) effect on other organs, such as the heart and intestine.
3. Gastric lavage to remove blood from the GI tract and to enhance visualization for endoscopic examination.
4. Esophageal balloon tamponade, whereby balloons are inflated in the distal esophagus and the proximal stomach to collapse the varices and induce hemostasis (see Procedure Guidelines 19-2, pages 722 to 724).
   a. Complications include esophageal necrosis, perforation, aspiration, asphyxiation, and stricture.
   b. This procedure should be reserved for patients who are known, without a doubt, to be bleeding from esophageal varices and in whom all forms of conservative therapy have failed.
5. Endoscopic sclerotherapy.
   a. A sclerosing agent is injected directly into the varix with a flexible fiber-optic endoscope to promote thrombosis and sclerosis of bleeding sites.
   b. To control bleeding and reduce the frequency of subsequent variceal hemorrhages, but repeated treatments may be required.
   c. Complications include esophageal ulceration, stricture, and perforation.
6. Endoscopic esophageal ligation (variceal banding) may be urgent or nonurgent and is usually the first-line treatment to control acute bleeding. The procedure may need to be repeated until all varices are obliterated.
7. TIPS procedure, or surgical type of shunt (portocaval or portorenal), can be used to create a portal systemic shunt to treat portal hypertension and bleeding.
8. Beta-adrenergic blocker therapy to reduce the resting pulse.
9. Consider high-dose proton pump inhibitor (PPI) therapy for long-term management of erosive gastropathy.
10. If TIPS or surgical shunt do not control portal hypertension, the patient may be evaluated for liver transplantation.

Complications

1. Exsanguination or recurrent hemorrhage.
2. Portal systemic encephalopathy.

(Text continues on page 724)

PROCEDURE GUIDELINES 19-2

Using Balloon Tamponade to Control Esophageal Bleeding (Sengstaken-Blakemore Tube Method, Minnesota Tube Method)

EQUIPMENT

- Esophageal balloon (Sengstaken-Blakemore or Minnesota)
- Basin with cracked ice
- Clamps for tubing
- Water-soluble lubricant

- Syringe (50 mL with catheter tip)
- Towel and emesis basin
- Glass of water and straw
- Adhesive tape

- Device to apply traction (eg, football helmet)
- Large scissors (for emergency deflation)
- Manometer (to measure balloon pressure)

PROCEDURE

Nursing Action	Rationale
Preparatory phase	
1. Explain procedure, provide support, and reassure patient that bleeding will be controlled.	1. Should allay fear and anxiety.
2. Advise patient to breathe through the mouth and swallow periodically. (See accompanying figure.)	2. Assists with passing of the tube.
3. Elevate head of bed slightly, unless patient is in shock.	3. Elevating head may worsen shock.

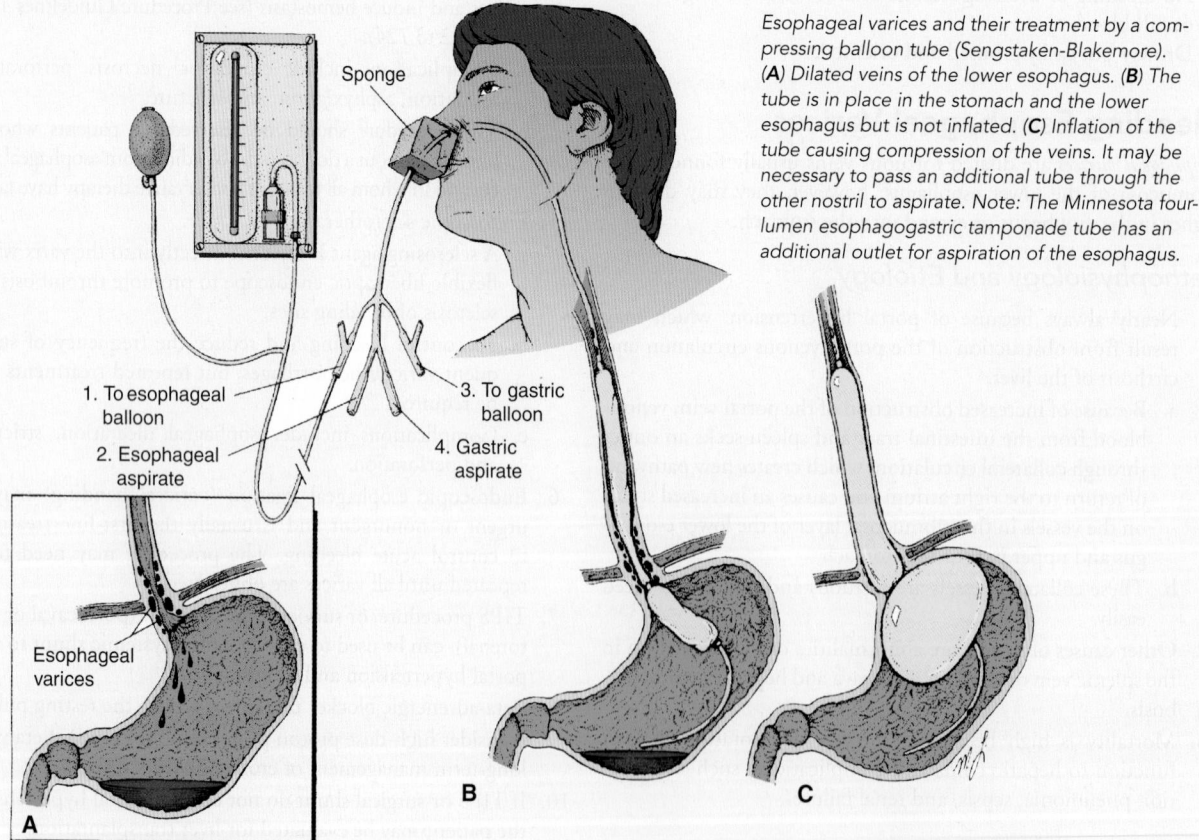

Sponge

1. To esophageal balloon
2. Esophageal aspirate
3. To gastric balloon
4. Gastric aspirate

Esophageal varices

A   B   C

Esophageal varices and their treatment by a compressing balloon tube (Sengstaken-Blakemore). (A) Dilated veins of the lower esophagus. (B) The tube is in place in the stomach and the lower esophagus but is not inflated. (C) Inflation of the tube causing compression of the veins. It may be necessary to pass an additional tube through the other nostril to aspirate. Note: The Minnesota four-lumen esophagogastric tamponade tube has an additional outlet for aspiration of the esophagus.

PROCEDURE GUIDELINES 19-2 *(continued)*

Using Balloon Tamponade to Control Esophageal Bleeding (Sengstaken-Blakemore Tube Method, Minnesota Tube Method)

PROCEDURE *(continued)*

Nursing Action	Rationale
Performance phase	
1. Check balloons by trial inflation under water to detect leaks.	1. This is best done under water because it is easier to see escaping air bubbles.
2. Chill the tube, then lubricate it before the provider passes it via mouth or nose (preferable).	2. Chilling makes the tube more firm and lubrication lessens friction.
3. Provide the patient with a few sips of water.	3. Helps pass the tube more easily.
4. After the tube has entered the stomach, verify its placement by irrigating the gastric tube with air while auscultating over the stomach.	4. It is imperative that the tube is in the stomach so that the gastric tube is not inflated in the esophagus.
5. After obtaining x-ray film of the lower chest and upper abdomen to verify placement in the stomach, inflate gastric balloon (200–250 mL) with air; gently pull tube back to seat balloon against gastroesophageal junction.	5. Exerts force against the cardia.
6. Clamp gastric balloon; mark tube location at nares.	6. Prevents air leakage and tube migration. The mark on the tube allows easy visualization of movement of the tube.
7. Apply gentle traction to the balloon tube and secure it with a foam rubber cube at the nares or tape it to the faceguard of a football helmet.	7. Prevents the tube from migrating with peristalsis and assists in exerting proper pressure.
8. Attach Y-connector to esophageal balloon opening. Attach syringe to one arm of the Y-connector and manometer to the other. Inflate esophageal balloon to 25–35 mm Hg. Clamp esophageal balloon.	8. Maintains enough pressure to tamponade bleeding while preventing esophageal necrosis.
9. Apply suction to gastric aspiration opening. Irrigate at least hourly.	9. Suctioning and irrigating the tube can remove old blood from the stomach and prevent hepatic encephalopathy; allows monitoring of bleeding status.
10. *[If using Sengstaken-Blakemore tube]* Insert a nasogastric (NG) tube, positioning it above the esophageal balloon and attach to suction.	10. Suctions saliva accumulated above the esophageal balloon, which may be aspirated, and checks for bleeding above the esophageal balloon.
11. *[If using a Minnesota tube]* Attach fourth port, esophageal suction port, to suction.	11. Removes esophageal secretions.
a. Label each port.	a. Prevents accidental deflation or irrigation.
b. Tape scissors to head of bed.	b. Airway occlusion may occur if the esophageal balloon is pulled into the hypopharynx. If this occurs, the esophageal balloon tube must be cut and removed immediately.

ADDITIONAL NURSING RESPONSIBILITIES

1. Maintain *constant* vigilance while balloons are inflated in the patient.
2. Keep balloon pressures at required level to control bleeding. (Clamps help to maintain pressure.)
3. Observe and record vital signs; monitor color and amount of NG lavage fluid (subtracting lavage input) for evidence of bleeding.
4. Be alert for chest pain—may indicate injury or rupture of esophagus.
5. Irrigate suction tube, as prescribed; observe and record nature and color of aspirated material.
6. Keep head of bed elevated to avoid gastric regurgitation and to diminish nausea and a sensation of gagging.
7. Maintain nutritional and electrolyte levels parenterally.
8. Maintain NG suction or suction to esophageal suction port to aspirate any collected saliva.
9. Note nature of breathing; if counterweight pulls the tube into oropharynx, the patient may be asphyxiated.

(continued)

PROCEDURE GUIDELINES 19-2 *(continued)*

Using Balloon Tamponade to Control Esophageal Bleeding (Sengstaken-Blakemore Tube Method, Minnesota Tube Method)

PROCEDURE *(continued)*

Nursing Action	Rationale

Key Decision Point

Patient must be monitored closely in an intensive care unit because of the risk of serious complications. Precaution must be taken to ensure the patient does not pull or inadvertently displace the tube. Keep scissors taped to the head of the bed.

In the event of *acute respiratory distress*, use the scissors to cut across tubing (to deflate both balloons) and remove tubing.

Note: This procedure should be reserved for patients who are known, without a doubt, to be bleeding from esophageal varices and in whom all forms of conservative therapy have failed.

Evidence Base Cat, T. B., & Liu-DeRyke, X. (2010). Medical management of variceal hemorrhage. *Critical Care Nursing Clinics of North America, 22,* 381–393.

Christensen, T., & Christen, M. (2007). The implementation of a guideline of care for patients with a Sengstaken-Blakemore tube in situ in a general intensive care unit using transitional change theory. *Intensive and Critical Care Nursing, 23*(4), 234–242.

Nursing Assessment

1. Monitor vital signs and respiratory function.
2. Assess LOC and impending signs of liver failure.

Nursing Diagnoses

- Ineffective Tissue Perfusion related to GI bleeding.
- Risk for Aspiration related to GI bleeding and intubation.
- Anxiety related to fear of unknown procedures and consequences of GI bleeding.

Nursing Interventions

Maintaining Adequate Tissue Perfusion

1. Assess BP, heart rate, skin condition, and urine output for signs of hypovolemia and shock.
2. Monitor patient frequently having vasopressin infusion for complications: hypertension, bradycardia, abdominal cramps, chest pain, or water intoxication.
3. Observe patient for straining, gagging, or vomiting; these increase pressure in the portal system and increase risk of further bleeding.
4. Check all GI secretions and feces for occult and frank blood.
5. Monitor infusion of blood products.
6. Administer vitamin K, as prescribed.

Preventing Aspiration

1. Assess respirations and monitor oxygen saturation of blood.
2. Note and report occurrence of signs of obstructed airway or ruptured esophagus from the esophageal balloon: changes in skin color, respirations, breath sounds, LOC, or vital signs; chest pain.
3. Check location and inflation of esophageal balloon; maintain traction on tubes, if applicable.
4. Have scissors readily available. Cut tubing and remove esophageal balloon immediately if patient develops acute respiratory distress.
5. Keep head of bed elevated to avoid gastric regurgitation and aspiration of gastric contents.
6. When using the Sengstaken-Blakemore esophageal balloon tube, ensure removal of secretions above the esophageal balloon: position NG tube in the esophagus for suctioning purposes; provide intermittent oropharyngeal suctioning.
7. Inspect nares for skin irritation; clean and lubricate frequently to prevent bleeding.

Reducing Anxiety and Fear

1. Provide care in a concerned, nonjudgmental manner.
2. Explain all procedures to patient.
3. Remain with patient or maintain close observation and place call bell within patient's reach.
4. Work swiftly and confidently, not hurriedly and anxiously.
5. Provide alternate means of communication if tubes or other equipment interfere with patient's ability to talk.
6. Use touch and other tactile stimuli to provide reassurance to the patient.
7. Use protective restraints to prevent dislodging of tubes in a confused, combative patient.

Patient Education and Health Maintenance

1. Discuss signs and symptoms of recurrent bleeding and the need to seek emergency medical treatment if these occur.

2. Instruct patient to avoid behaviors that increase portal system pressure: straining, gagging, Valsalva's maneuver.

3. Explain to patient that high-protein diets and alcohol consumption can cause further complications.

4. Encourage patient to abstain from alcohol consumption; discuss support organizations such as Alcoholics Anonymous.

Evaluation: Expected Outcomes

- BP stable; urine output adequate.
- Airway maintained without aspiration.
- Cooperates and indicates understanding of treatment.

Liver Cancer

 Evidence Base National Comprehensive Cancer Network. (2011). NCCN clinical practice guidelines in oncology: Hepatobiliary cancer, version 2.2012. Available: *www.nccn.org/professionals/physician_gls/pdf/hepatobiliary.pdf*.

Cancer of the liver, or *hepatocellular carcinoma*, is a primary cancer of the liver and is relatively uncommon in the United States. It is, however, one of the most common malignancies in the world, particularly in Africa and Asia. *Cholangiocarcinoma* is a primary malignant tumor of the bile ducts, which can be intrahepatic or extrahepatic. This type of cancer is uncommon in the United States but is more commonly seen in Asia. These two types of cancer are typically combined for reporting purposes and make the incidence data harder to interpret.

Liver metastasis may occur from a primary site, which is found in about one half of all late cancer cases. Neoadjuvant therapy is being given to shrink metastatic liver tumor to make them more amenable to resection.

Pathophysiology and Etiology

 Evidence Base Cho, L. Y., Yang, J. J., Ko, K. P., et al. (2011). Coinfection of hepatitis B and C viruses and risk of hepatocellular carcinoma: Systematic review and meta-analysis. *International Journal of Cancer, 128*, 176–184.

1. Incidence of primary cancer of the liver is increasing in the United States in the younger population and in females.

2. Cirrhosis, HBV, and HCV have been implicated in its etiology.

3. Rarer associated causes are hemochromatosis; alpha$_1$-antitrypsin deficiency; aflatoxins; chemical toxins, such as vinyl chloride and Thorotrast; carcinogens in herbal medicines; nitrosamines; and ingestion of hormones, as in oral contraceptives.

4. Arises in normal tissue as a discrete tumor or in end-stage cirrhosis in a multinodular pattern.

5. Liver metastasis reaches the liver by way of the portal system or the lymphatic channels or by direct extension from an abdominal tumor.

Clinical Manifestations

1. Depends on the state of the liver in which it arises; without cirrhosis and with good liver function, carcinoma of the liver may grow to huge proportions before becoming symptomatic, but in a cirrhotic patient, the lack of hepatic reserve usually leads to a more rapid course.

2. Most common presenting symptom is right upper quadrant abdominal pain, usually dull or aching, and may radiate to the right shoulder.

3. A right upper quadrant mass, weight loss, abdominal distention with ascites, fatigue, anorexia, malaise, and unexplained fever.

4. Jaundice is present only in a minority of patients at diagnosis in primary cancer of the liver. In cholangiocarcinoma, the presenting symptom is usually painless obstructive jaundice.

5. With portal vein obstruction, ascites and esophageal varices occurs.

Diagnostic Evaluation

1. Increased levels of serum bilirubin, alkaline phosphatase, and liver enzymes.

2. AFP is the principal tumor marker for hepatocellular carcinoma and is elevated in 70% to 95% of patients with the disease.

3. Ultrasonography and CT along with MRI are the most useful noninvasive tests to detect liver cancer and assess if the tumor can be surgically removed.

4. PET scan to look for recurrent or metastatic disease.

5. As the newer CT scans and MRI can demonstrate necessary vascular involvement of any tumor, invasive studies, such as arteriography, are no longer needed to determine resectability.

6. Percutaneous needle biopsy or biopsy assisted by ultrasonography or CT scan may be done.

7. Laparoscopy with liver biopsy may be performed.

Management

 Evidence Base Bruix, J., & Sherman, M. (2011). Management of hepatocellular carcinoma: An update. American Association for the Study of Liver Diseases. *Hepatology, 53*, 1020–1022.

Nonsurgical Treatment

Varying degrees of success with chemotherapy and radiation. These therapies may prolong survival and improve patient's quality of life by reducing pain, but the overall effect is palliative.

1. Neoadjuvant therapies for liver cancer, including transarterial chemoembolization, combination chemotherapy, chemotherapy along with radiotherapy, hepatic artery infusion of chemotherapeutic agents, and radioimmunotherapy, are being investigated for use before surgical resection. These therapies are used to reduce the size of the tumor and make surgical excision possible.

2. Liver cancer is radiosensitive, but treatment is restricted by the limited radiation tolerance of the normal liver.

3. Radiation therapy can help reduce pain and discomfort of large unresectable tumors.
4. Chemotherapy is used as an adjuvant therapy after surgical resection of liver cancer.
   a. Systemic chemotherapy is the only treatment applicable when the cancer has spread outside the liver.
   b. Regional infusion chemotherapy by implantable pump has been used to deliver a high concentration of chemotherapy directly to the liver through the hepatic artery. This method is employed for a large amount of tumor burden or tumors spread throughout the liver.
5. Hyperthermia has been used to treat hepatic metastasis.
6. Hepatic artery occlusion and embolization with the use of chemotherapeutic agents is another method used for unresectable liver tumors.

 Evidence Base Oliveri, R. S., Wetterslev, J., & Gluud, C. (2011). Transarterial (chemo)embolism for unresectable hepatocellular carcinoma. *Cochrane Database of Systematic Reviews*, Issue 16 (Article No. CD004787).

7. Immunotherapy is under investigation by itself and in combination with chemotherapy and radiotherapy.
8. Percutaneous alcohol injection is an ablative procedure that is safe and effective for treating small liver tumors.
9. PTBD is used to drain obstructed biliary ducts in patients with inoperable tumors or in patients considered poor surgical risks.
10. Percutaneous or endoscopic placement of internal stents may also palliate a patient with obstructed bile ducts with a terminal diagnosis.

 Evidence Base Cho, Y. K., Rhim, H., & Noh, S. (2011). Radiofrequency ablation versus surgical resection as primary treatment of hepatocellular carcinoma meeting the Milan criteria: A systematic review. *Journal of Gastroenterology and Hepatology*, *26*(9), 1354–1360.

Surgical Treatment

 Evidence Base Jarnagin, W., Chapman, W. C., Curley, S., et al. (2010). Surgical treatment of hepatocellular carcinoma: Expert consensus statement. American Hepato-Pancreato-Biliary Association; Society of Surgical Oncology; Society for Surgery of the Alimentary Tract. *HPB*, *12*, 301–310.

Surgery is the best treatment but is limited to those patients whose tumor size is less than 5 cm and confined to the liver with no vascular invasion. The 5-year survival rate is only 40% to 50%; recurrence and metastasis are frequent.

1. Surgery is an option only after the extent of the tumor and hepatic reserve have been considered.
2. Surgical resection may be along anatomic divisions of the liver or nonanatomic resections.

3. Percutaneous portal vein embolization may be performed prior to surgery of large liver tumors. Cutting off blood supply to the diseased portion of the liver allows enlargement of the nondiseased portion of the liver. An adequate amount of liver is needed to sustain a patient and prevent postoperative complications.
4. Radiofrequency ablation uses heat produced by a radiofrequency electrode to kill tumors. This can be performed by the percutaneous or laparoscopic approach and is used for relatively small tumors.
5. Liver transplantation is an accepted treatment for liver cancer, especially if hepatic reserve is low (as with concurrent cirrhosis due to HCV or HBV). Tumor size must be less than 5 cm and have no vascular involvement for the best patient outcomes. The United Network of Organ Sharing allows additional points to their Model for End Stage Liver Disease (MELD) score for patients diagnosed with HCCA within these parameters. There is only a 10% risk of recurrence of hepatocellular carcinoma (HCCA) after transplant if the tumor size restrictions are taken into consideration and there is no vascular involvement. Many times, patients are treated with chemo-embolization while waiting for a liver transplant.
6. Care of the patient after liver surgery is similar to general abdominal surgery (see page 657).

Complications

1. Malnutrition, biliary obstruction with jaundice.
2. Sepsis, liver abscesses.
3. Fulminant liver failure, metastasis.

Nursing Assessment

1. Obtain history of hepatitis, alcoholic liver disease and cirrhosis, exposure to toxins, or other potential causes.
2. Assess for signs and symptoms of malnutrition, including recent weight loss, loss of strength, anorexia, and anemia.
3. Assess for abdominal pain, any right shoulder pain, and enlargement of the liver.
4. Assess for fever, jaundice, ascites, or bleeding.
5. Note any change in mental status as precipitating hepatic encephalopathy.

Nursing Diagnoses

- Acute and Chronic Pain related to growth of tumor.
- Imbalanced Nutrition: Less Than Body Requirements related to anorexia.
- Excess Fluid Volume related to ascites and edema.

Nursing Interventions

Controlling Pain

1. Administer pharmacologic agents, as ordered, to control pain, considering metabolism through a liver with decreased function.
   a. Use caution; do not administer doses more frequently than prescribed.
   b. Monitor for signs of drug toxicity.

2. Provide nonpharmacologic methods of pain relief, such as massage and guided imagery.

3. Position patient for comfort, usually in semi-Fowler's position.

4. Assess patient's response to pain-control measures.

Improving Nutritional Status

1. Encourage patient to eat small meals and take oral supplementary feedings such as Ensure.

2. Assess and report changes in factors affecting nutritional needs: increased body temperature, pain, signs of infection, stress level. Encourage additional calories, as tolerated.

3. Monitor daily weight.

Relieving Excess Fluid Volume

1. Monitor vital signs and record accurate fluid intake and output.

2. Restrict sodium and fluid intake, as prescribed.

3. Administer diuretics and replacement potassium and phosphate, as prescribed.

4. Administer albumin and protein supplements, as prescribed, to draw fluid from interstitial to intravascular space.

5. Measure and record abdominal girth daily.

6. Weigh daily, watching for increases that indicate increased fluid retention such as abdominal and lower-extremity edema.

7. Monitor laboratory values pertinent to liver function.

Patient Education and Health Maintenance

1. Instruct patient and family on preparation for surgery, reinforce and clarify surgical procedure proposed, and review postoperative instructions.

2. Instruct patient and family on nonsurgical treatment, if appropriate.

3. Explore pain management options.

4. Inform patient of signs and symptoms of complications.

5. Instruct patient in continued surveillance for recurrence.

6. Instruct patient and family in care of tubes or drains.

Evaluation: Expected Outcomes

- Verbalizes reduced pain.
- Tolerates small feedings; no weight loss.
- Abdominal girth decreased; urine output greater than intake.

Fulminant Liver Failure

Fulminant liver failure is acute necrosis of the liver cells without preexisting liver disease, resulting in the inability of the liver to perform its many functions.

Pathophysiology and Etiology

1. Viral hepatitis is the most common cause.

2. Poisons, chemicals, and such drugs as acetaminophen, tetracycline, isoniazid, halogenated anesthetics, monoamine oxidase inhibitors, valproate, amiodarone, methyldopa, and amanita mushrooms may cause liver toxicity.

3. Ischemia and hypoxia because of hepatic vascular occlusion, hypovolemic shock, acute circulatory failure, septic shock, or heat stroke may be causes.

4. Miscellaneous causes include hepatic vein obstruction, Budd-Chiari syndrome, acute fatty liver of pregnancy, autoimmune hepatitis, partial hepatectomy, complication of liver transplantation.

5. Progression of hepatocellular injury and necrosis is rapid, with development of hepatic encephalopathy within 8 weeks of onset of disease.

6. Mortality is high, 60% to 85%, despite intensive treatment.

Clinical Manifestations

1. Malaise, anorexia, nausea, vomiting, fatigue.

2. Jaundice, especially mucous membranes.

3. Urine is tea-colored and frothy when shaken.

4. Pruritus caused by bile salts deposited on skin.

5. Steatorrhea and diarrhea because of decreased fat absorption.

6. Peripheral edema as the fluid moves from the intravascular to the interstitial spaces, secondary to hypoproteinemia.

7. Ascites from hypoproteinemia or portal hypertension.

8. Easy bruising, petechiae, overt bleeding because of clotting deficiency.

9. Altered LOC, ranging from irritability and confusion to stupor, somnolence, and coma.

10. Change in deep tendon reflexes—initially hyperactive, become flaccid, asterixis (tremor).

11. Fetor hepaticus—breath odor of acetone.

12. Portal systemic encephalopathy, also known as hepatic coma or hepatic encephalopathy, can occur in conjunction with cerebral edema.

13. Cerebral edema is commonly the cause of death because of brain stem herniation or because of respiratory arrest.

Diagnostic Evaluation

1. Prolonged PT/INR, decreased platelet count.

2. Elevated ammonia, amino acid, and mercaptan levels.

3. Hypoglycemia or hyperglycemia.

4. Dilutional hyponatremia or hypernatremia, hypokalemia, hypocalcemia, and hypomagnesemia.

Management

1. Oral or rectal administration of lactulose to minimize formation of ammonia and other nitrogenous by-products in the bowel.

2. Rectal administration of neomycin to suppress urea-splitting enteric bacteria in the bowel and decrease ammonia formation.

3. Low-molecular-weight dextran or albumin followed by a potassium-sparing diuretic (spironolactone) to enhance fluid shift from interstitial back to intravascular spaces.

4. Pancreatic enzymes, if diarrhea and steatorrhea are present, to permit better tolerance of fats in the diet.

5. Mannitol IV for management of cerebral edema, when indicated.

6. Cholestyramine to promote fecal excretion of bile salts to decrease itching.
7. Antacids, PPIs, and histamine-2 (H_2) antagonists to reduce the risk of bleeding from stress ulcers.
8. Restriction of dietary protein and sodium while maintaining adequate caloric intake with diet or hypertonic dextrose solutions.
9. Supplemental vitamins (A, B complex, C, and K) and folate.
10. Infusion of fresh frozen plasma to maintain PT/INR; cryoprecipitate, as needed.
11. Additional medical interventions, depending on the patient's condition, may include hemodialysis, hemofiltration, hemoperfusion, or plasmapheresis.
12. Liver transplantation has become the treatment of choice.

Complications

1. Acute respiratory failure.
2. Infections and sepsis.
3. Cardiac dysfunction, hypotension.
4. Hepatorenal failure.
5. Hemorrhage.

Nursing Assessment

1. Obtain history of exposure to drugs, chemicals, or toxins; exposure to infectious hepatitis; and course of illness.
2. Assess respiratory status, breath, LOC, and vital signs.
3. Assess for ascites, edema, jaundice, bleeding, asterixis, presence or absence of reflexes.
4. Assess results of arterial blood gas (ABG) tests, electrolytes, INR, hemoglobin level, and hematocrit.

Nursing Diagnoses

- Deficient Fluid Volume related to hypoproteinemia, peripheral edema, ascites.
- Ineffective Breathing Pattern related to anemia and decreased lung expansion from ascites.
- Imbalanced Nutrition: Less Than Body Requirements related to GI adverse effects and decreased absorption, storage, and metabolism of nutrients.
- Risk for Impaired Skin Integrity related to malnutrition, deposition of bile salts, peripheral edema, decreased activity.
- Risk for Infection related to altered immune response.
- Risk for Injury related to encephalopathy.

Nursing Interventions

Maintaining Adequate Fluid Volume
1. Monitor vital signs frequently.
2. Weigh patient daily and keep an accurate intake and output record; record frequency and characteristics of stool.
3. Measure and record abdominal girth daily.
4. Assess and record peripheral edema.
5. Restrict sodium and fluids; replace electrolytes, as directed.
6. Administer low-molecular-weight dextran or albumin and diuretics, as prescribed.
7. Assess for signs and symptoms of hemorrhage or bleeding.

Improving Respiratory Status
1. Monitor respiratory rate, depth, use of accessory muscles, nasal flaring, and breath sounds.
2. Evaluate ABG values, hemoglobin level, and hematocrit.
3. Elevate head of the bed to lower diaphragm and decrease respiratory effort.
4. Turn patient frequently to prevent stasis of secretions.
5. Administer oxygen therapy, as directed.

Improving Nutritional Status
1. Enlist a nutrition specialist to help evaluate nutritional status and needs.
2. Encourage patient to eat in a sitting position to decrease abdominal tenderness and feeling of fullness.
3. Provide small, frequent meals or dietary supplements of complex carbohydrates to avoid protein loading to conserve patient's energy.
4. Provide mouth care if patient has bleeding gums or fetor hepaticus.
5. Restrict intake of sodium and protein (usually between 1.0 and 1.5 g/kg) based on ammonia levels and symptoms of encephalopathy.
6. Provide enteral and parenteral feedings, as needed.

Maintaining Skin Integrity
1. Inspect skin for alteration in integrity.
2. Provide good skin care.
3. Bathe without soap and apply soothing lotions.
4. Keep patient's fingernails short to prevent scratching from pruritus.
5. Administer medications, as prescribed, for pruritus.
6. Assess for signs of bleeding from broken areas on the skin.
7. Turn patient frequently to prevent pressure ulcers.
8. Avoid trauma and friction to the skin.

Preventing Infection
1. Be alert for signs of infection, such as fever, cloudy urine, abnormal breath sounds.
2. Use good handwashing and aseptic technique when caring for a break in the skin or mucous membranes.
3. Restrict visits with anyone who may have an infection.
4. Encourage the patient not to scratch skin.

Preventing Injury
1. Maintain close observation, bed side rails up, and nurse call system within reach.
2. Assist with ambulation, as needed, and avoid obstructions to prevent falls.
3. Have well-lit room and frequently reorient patient.
4. Observe for subtle changes in behavior (such as unkempt appearance), worsening of sample of handwriting, and change in sleeping pattern to detect increasing encephalopathy.

Patient Education and Health Maintenance

1. Teach patient and family to notify health care provider of increased abdominal discomfort, bleeding, increased edema or ascites, hallucinations, or lapses in consciousness.

2. Instruct patient to avoid activities that increase the risk of bleeding: scratching, falling, forceful nose blowing, aggressive toothbrushing, use of straight-edged razor.
3. Advise limiting activities when fatigued and encourage use of frequent rest periods.
4. Maintain close follow-up for laboratory testing and evaluation by health care provider.

Evaluation: Expected Outcomes

- BP stable, urine output adequate.
- Respirations unlabored.
- Tolerates three to four small feedings per day.
- Skin intact without abrasions.
- No fever or signs of infection.
- No falls.

BILIARY DISORDERS

The gallbladder and bile ducts comprise the biliary system. The gallbladder stores and concentrates bile produced by the liver. The hormone cholecystokinin, secreted by the small intestine, stimulates contraction of the gallbladder and relaxation of the sphincter of Oddi for delivery of bile into the small intestine.

Bile assists in the emulsification (breakdown) of fat; absorption of fatty acids, cholesterol, and other lipids from the small intestine; and excretion of conjugated bilirubin from the liver.

Common terms related to the gallbladder and bile ducts are:

Cholecyst—gallbladder.
Cholecystitis—inflammation of the gallbladder.
Cholelithiasis—presence or formation of gallstones in the gallbladder.
Cholecystectomy—removal of the gallbladder.
Cholecystostomy—drainage of the gallbladder through a tube.
Choledocho—common bile duct.
Choledochotomy—incision into the common bile duct.
Choledocholithiasis—presence of stones in the common bile duct.
Choledocholithotomy—incision of the common bile duct for the extraction of an impacted gallstone.
Choledochoduodenostomy—surgical formation of a communication between the common bile duct and the duodenum.
Choledochojejunostomy—surgical formation of a communication between the common bile duct and the jejunum.

Cholelithiasis, Cholecystitis, Choledocholithiasis

These conditions refer to stones or inflammation of the biliary system (see Figure 19-4). Cholecystitis may be acute or chronic.

Pathophysiology and Etiology

Cholelithiasis

1. Stones occur when cholesterol supersaturates the bile in the gallbladder and precipitates out of the bile. The

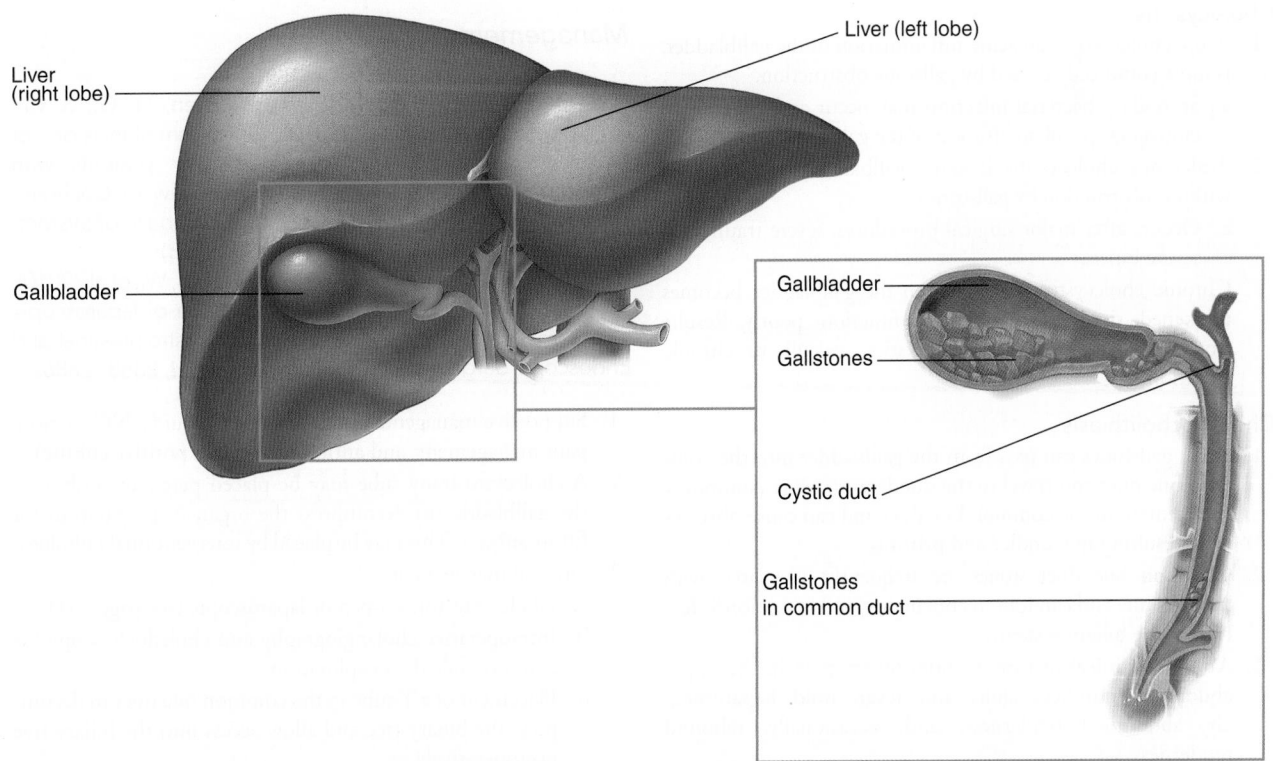

Figure 19-4. Cholelithiasis and choledocholithiasis.

cholesterol-saturated bile predisposes to the formation of gallstones and acts as an irritant, producing inflammatory changes in the gallbladder.

a. Cholesterol stones are the most common type of gallstones found in the United States.

b. Four times more women than men develop cholesterol stones.

c. Women are usually older than age 40, multiparous, and obese.

d. Stone formation increases in users of contraceptives, estrogens, and cholesterol-lowering drugs, which are known to increase biliary cholesterol saturation.

e. Bile acid malabsorption, genetic predisposition, and rapid weight loss are also risk factors for cholesterol gallstones.

2. Pigment stones occur when free bilirubin combines with calcium.

a. Found in patients with cirrhosis, hemolysis, and infections in the biliary tree.

b. These stones cannot be dissolved.

3. An estimated 25 million people in the United States have gallstones, with 1 million new cases discovered each year.

a. Incidence of stone formation increases with age because of increased hepatic secretion of cholesterol and decreased bile acid synthesis.

b. Increased risk in patients with malabsorption of bile salts with GI disease, bile fistula, gallstone ileus, carcinoma of the gallbladder, or in those who have had ileal resection or ileal bypass.

Cholecystitis

1. Acute cholecystitis, an acute inflammation of the gallbladder, is most commonly caused by gallstone obstruction.

a. Secondary bacterial infection may occur and progress to empyema (purulent effusion of the gallbladder).

2. Acalculous cholecystitis is acute gallbladder inflammation without obstruction by gallstones.

a. Occurs after major surgical procedures, severe trauma, or severe burns.

3. Chronic cholecystitis occurs when the gallbladder becomes thickened, rigid, and fibrotic and functions poorly. Results from repeated attacks of cholecystitis, calculi, or chronic irritation.

Choledocholithiasis

1. Small gallstones can pass from the gallbladder into the common bile duct and travel to the duodenum. More commonly they remain in the common bile duct and can cause obstruction, resulting in jaundice and pruritus.

2. Common bile duct stones are frequently associated with infected bile and can lead to cholangitis (inflammation/infection in the biliary system).

3. A typical clinical picture includes biliary pain in the upper abdomen, jaundice, chills and fever, mild hepatomegaly, abdominal tenderness, and, occasionally, rebound tenderness.

Clinical Manifestations

1. Gallstones that remain in the gallbladder are usually asymptomatic.

2. Biliary colic can be caused by gallstones.

a. Steady, severe, aching pain or sensation of pressure in the epigastrium or right upper quadrant, which may radiate to the right scapular area or right shoulder.

b. Begins suddenly and persists for 1 to 3 hours until the stone falls back into the gallbladder or passes through the cystic duct.

3. Acute cholecystitis causes biliary colic pain that persists more than 4 hours and increases with movement, including respirations.

a. Also causes nausea and vomiting, low-grade fever, and jaundice (with stones or inflammation in the common bile duct).

b. Right upper quadrant guarding and Murphy's sign (inability to take a deep inspiration when examiner's fingers are pressed below the hepatic margin) are present.

4. Chronic cholecystitis causes heartburn, flatulence, and indigestion. Repeated attacks of symptoms may occur resembling acute cholecystitis.

Diagnostic Evaluation

1. Oral cholecystography, ultrasonography, and HIDA scan may show stones or inflammation.

2. ERCP or PTC to visualize location of stones and extent of obstruction.

3. Elevated conjugated bilirubin and alkaline phosphatase because of obstruction.

Management

 Evidence Base Keus, F., Gooszen, H. G., & van Laarhoven, C. J. (2010). Open, small-incision, or laparoscopic cholecystectomy for patients with symptomatic cholecystolithiasis. An overview of Cochrane Hepato-Biliary Group review. *Cochrane Database of Systematic Reviews*, Issue 20 (Article No. CD008318).

Overby, D. W., Apelgren, K. N., Richardson, W., et al. (2010). SAGES guidelines for the clinical application of laparoscopic biliary tract surgery. Society of American Gastrointestinal and Endoscopic Surgeons. *Surgical Endoscopy, 24*, 2368–2386.

1. Supportive management may include IV fluids, NG suction, pain management, and antibiotics (with a positive culture).

2. A cholecystostomy tube may be placed percutaneously into the gallbladder to decompress the organ in preparation for future surgery. This may be placed by interventional radiology.

3. Surgical management.

a. Cholecystectomy, open or laparoscopic (see page 731).

b. Intraoperative cholangiography and choledochoscopy for common bile duct exploration.

c. Placement of a T-tube in the common bile duct to decompress the biliary tree and allow access into the biliary tree postoperatively.

4. Oral therapy with chenodeoxycholic acid, ursodeoxycholic acid, or a combination of both to decrease the size of existing cholesterol stones or to dissolve small ones.
   a. Indicated for patients at high risk for surgery because of comorbid conditions.
   b. Major adverse effects include diarrhea, abnormal liver function tests, increases in serum cholesterol.
5. Direct contact therapy by which a local cholelitholytic agent is infused by a catheter directly into the gallbladder or through a percutaneous transhepatic biliary catheter.
   a. Indicated for a symptomatic, high-risk patient whose gallbladder can be visualized by a radiographic study.
   b. Adverse effects include pain from the catheter, nausea, and transient elevations of liver function tests and white blood cell (WBC) count.
6. After cholecystectomy, intracorporeal lithotripsy may be used to fragment retained stones in the common bile duct by pulsed laser or hydraulic lithotripsy applied through an endoscope directly to the stones. The stone fragments are removed by irrigation or aspiration. Retained stones may also be removed by basket retrieval through the endoscopic or percutaneous transhepatic biliary approach.

Complications

1. Cholangitis.
2. Necrosis, empyema, or perforation of the gallbladder.
3. Biliary fistula through the duodenum.
4. Gallstone ileus.
5. Adenocarcinoma of the gallbladder.

Nursing Assessment

1. Obtain history and demographic data that may indicate risk factors for biliary disease.
2. Assess patient's pain for location, description, intensity, relieving and exacerbating factors.
3. Assess for signs of dehydration: dry mucous membranes, poor skin turgor, low urine output with elevated specific gravity.
4. Assess sclera and skin for jaundice.
5. Monitor temperature and WBC count for indications of infection.

Nursing Diagnoses

- Acute Pain related to biliary colic or stone obstruction.
- Deficient Fluid Volume related to nausea and vomiting and decreased intake.

Nursing Interventions

Relieving Pain

1. Assess pain location, severity, and characteristics.
2. Administer medications or monitor patient-controlled analgesia (PCA) to control pain.
3. Assist in attaining position of comfort.

Restoring Normal Fluid Volume

1. Administer IV fluids and electrolytes, as prescribed.
2. Administer anti-emetics, as prescribed, to decrease nausea and vomiting.
3. Maintain NG decompression, if needed.
4. Begin food and fluids, as tolerated, after acute symptoms subside or postoperatively.
5. Observe and record amount of biliary tube drainage, if applicable.

Patient Education and Health Maintenance

1. Instruct patient in care of tubes or catheters that may be in place at discharge.
   a. Observe for bleeding or drainage around insertion site.
   b. Replace dressing per facility protocol.
   c. Report change or decrease in drainage.
2. Review discharge instructions for activity, diet, medications, and follow-up.
3. Emphasize symptoms of complications to be reported, such as increased or persistent pain, fever, abdominal distention, nausea, anorexia, jaundice, unusual drainage.
4. Encourage follow-up, as indicated.

Evaluation: Expected Outcomes

- Verbalizes reduced pain level.
- Tolerates oral fluids and solid food; adequate urine output.

Care of the Patient Undergoing Cholecystectomy

 Evidence Base Keus, F. Gooszen, H.G., & van Laarhoven, C.J. (2010). Open, small-incision, or laparoscopic cholecystectomy for patients with symptomatic cholecystolithiasis. An overview of Cochrane Hepato-Biliary Group reviews. *Cochrane Database of Systematic Reviews,* Issue 1 (Article No. CD008318).

Society of American Gastrointestinal and Endoscopic Surgeons (SAGES). (2010). SAGES guidelines for the clinical application of laparoscopic biliary tract surgery. Available: *www.sages.org/publication/id/06/.*

Cholecystectomy is surgical removal of the gallbladder for acute and chronic cholecystitis. It is one of the most frequent surgical procedures, with more than 1 million performed each year in the United States.

Procedure

1. Open laparotomy—gallbladder removed after making an abdominal incision.
2. Laparoscopy—gallbladder removed from a small opening just above the umbilicus through the use of a laparoscope (also called an endoscope) for viewing (see Figure 19-5).

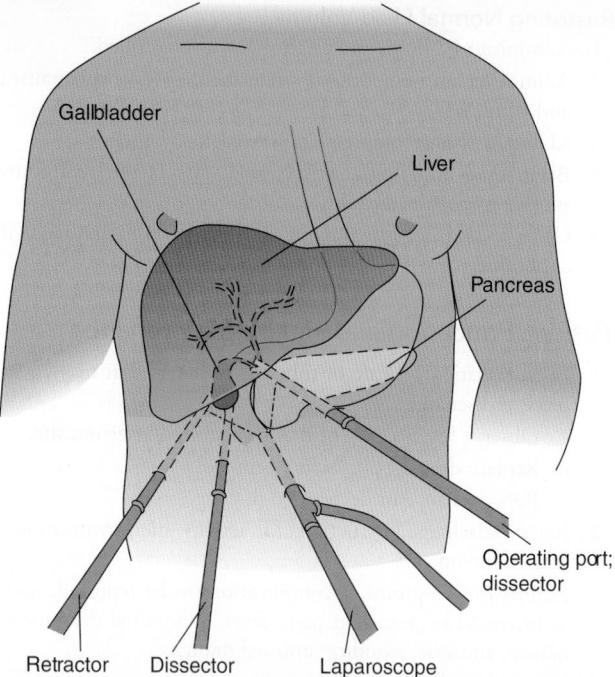

Retractor   Dissector   Laparoscope

Figure 19-5. Laparoscopic cholecystectomy. The surgeon makes four small incisions (less than ½ inch each) in the abdomen and inserts a laparoscope with a miniature camera into the opening. The camera apparatus displays the gallbladder and adjacent tissues on a screen allowing the surgeon to visualize the organ for removal.

    a. Three other small punctures are made in the abdomen to place other special instruments used to assist in the manipulation and removal of the gallbladder.

    b. The organs in the abdomen can be viewed through the laparoscope and via a television monitor through a camera attached to the laparoscope.

3. If patient is scheduled for a laparoscopic cholecystectomy, consent is also obtained for a traditional open cholecystectomy in case the gallbladder is not accessible through the laparoscopic technique.

4. After cholecystectomy, bile ducts will eventually dilate to accommodate the volume of bile once held by the gallbladder to aid in the digestion of fats.

Preoperative Management

1. IV fluids are given before surgery to improve hydration status if patient has been vomiting.

2. Antibiotics are ordered for acute cholecystitis.

3. Educate patient about the procedure and what to expect postoperatively.

4. Patient must remain NPO from midnight the night before surgery and must void before surgery.

Postoperative Management

1. Postoperatively, the patient is evaluated for:
    a. Vital signs, LOC.
    b. Level of pain.

    c. Appearance of wound or puncture sites: wound drain or T-tube patency (if common bile duct exploration also performed), security and drainage (if present).

    d. Intake and output.

2. Early ambulation is encouraged to prevent thromboembolus, to facilitate voiding, and to stimulate peristalsis.

3. Complications to be alert for include incisional infection, hemorrhage, and bile duct injury (persistent pain, fever, abdominal distention, nausea, anorexia, or jaundice).

Potential Complications

1. Deep vein thrombosis or pulmonary embolism.

2. Pneumonia or atelectasis.

3. Infection, hemorrhage, or bile duct injury.

Nursing Diagnoses

• Acute Pain related to surgical procedure.
• Risk for Infection related to surgical procedure.
• Impaired Skin Integrity related to surgical procedure.
• Imbalanced Nutrition: Less Than Body Requirements related to surgical procedure, wound pain, or tube drainage.

Nursing Interventions

Relieving Pain

1. Assess pain location, level, and characteristics.

2. Administer prescribed pain medications or monitor PCA.

3. Encourage splinting of incision when moving.

4. Encourage ambulation as soon as prescribed to decrease flatus and abdominal distention and to promote bowel motility.

5. Instruct patient that usual activities can normally be resumed within 5 to 7 days after laparoscopic cholecystectomy or within 4 to 6 weeks of open cholecystectomy.
    a. Sexual activity may be resumed when pain has abated.
    b. Obtain specific instructions for wound care; activity, such as heavy lifting; strenuous activity; showers and tub baths; and driving per surgeon's protocol.

Preventing Infection

1. Assess wound dressings for any increased or purulent drainage.

2. Assess wound drain or T-tube site for drainage, and note amount, color, and odor.

3. Assess bile drainage from T-tube into bile bag:
    a. Report decrease in drainage.
    b. Maintain T-tube patency and security.

4. Report right upper quadrant pain, abdominal distention, fever, chills, or jaundice, as these may indicate a bile duct injury.

5. Administer antibiotics, as prescribed.

6. Encourage use of incentive spirometer, coughing and deep breathing, and ambulation to decrease risk of pulmonary infection.

Maintaining Skin Integrity

1. Assess wounds for healing.

2. Perform wound care as prescribed.

3. Assess for adequate hydration.

4. Assess and report any signs of redness, swelling, pain, or drainage from the wounds.

Providing Adequate Nutrition

1. Assess for nausea and vomiting and administer anti-emetics, as prescribed.

2. Encourage fluid intake and advance to regular diet, as tolerated.

3. Administer replacement fluids for bile drainage from T-tube, if indicated.

4. Clamp T-tube, when indicated, and assess tolerance of food and color of stools.

Patient Education and Health Maintenance

1. Teach patient and family that rapid postoperative recovery should be expected.

2. Advise patient and family to notify the surgeon immediately of any subtle change in patient's postoperative course or persistent symptoms. A bile duct injury should be suspected after a laparoscopic cholecystectomy in patients who do not show the expected recovery during the early postoperative period.

3. Advise patient to advance diet, as tolerated. Fats can be taken *as tolerated* because the bile ducts dilate to accommodate storage of bile, as needed.

Evaluation: Expected Outcomes

- Verbalizes decreased pain.
- No fever or signs of infection.
- Wound healing without drainage.
- Tolerates fluids and small solid feedings.

PANCREATIC DISORDERS

The pancreas secretes pancreatic enzymes, including amylase and lipase, through the pancreatic duct when stimulated by cholecystokinin and secretin to aid in digestion of carbohydrates and fat in the small intestine. The pancreas also secretes hormones, such as insulin and glucagon, which help to regulate and maintain normal serum glucose.

Acute Pancreatitis

Acute pancreatitis is an inflammation of the pancreas, ranging from mild edema to extensive hemorrhage, resulting from various insults to the pancreas. It is defined by a discrete episode of abdominal pain and serum enzyme elevations. The structure and function of the pancreas usually return to normal after an acute attack. Chronic pancreatitis occurs when there is persistent cellular damage to the pancreas (see Table 19-2 for comparison).

Pathophysiology and Etiology

1. Excessive alcohol consumption is the most common cause in the United States.

2. Also commonly caused by biliary tract disease, such as cholelithiasis, acute and chronic cholecystitis.

3. Less common causes are bacterial or viral infection, blunt abdominal trauma, peptic ulcer disease, ischemic vascular disease, hyperlipidemia, and hypercalcemia; the use of corticosteroids, thiazide diuretics, and oral contraceptives; surgery on or near the pancreas or after instrumentation of the pancreatic duct by ERCP; tumors of the pancreas or ampulla; and a low incidence of hereditary pancreatitis.

4. Mortality is high (10%) because of shock, anoxia, hypotension, or multiple organ dysfunction.

5. Attacks may resolve with complete recovery, may recur without permanent damage, or may progress to chronic pancreatitis.

6. Autodigestion of all or part of the pancreas is involved, but the exact mechanism is not completely understood.

Clinical Manifestations

(Depends on severity of pancreatic damage.)

1. Abdominal pain, usually constant, midepigastric or periumbilical, radiating to the back or flank. Patient assumes a fetal position or leans forward while sitting (known as "proning") to relieve pressure of the inflamed pancreas on celiac plexus nerves. Pain can be mild to incapacitating.

2. Nausea and vomiting.

3. Fever.

4. Involuntary abdominal guarding, epigastric tenderness to deep palpation, and reduced or absent bowel sounds.

5. Dry mucous membranes; hypotension; cold, clammy skin; cyanosis; and tachycardia, which may reflect mild to moderate dehydration from vomiting or capillary leak syndrome (third space loss).

6. Shock may be the presenting manifestation in severe episodes, with respiratory distress and acute renal failure.

7. Purplish discoloration of the flanks (Turner's sign) or of the periumbilical area (Cullen's sign) occurs in extensive hemorrhagic necrosis of the pancreas.

Diagnostic Evaluation

1. Serum amylase, lipase, glucose, bilirubin, alkaline phosphatase, lactate dehydrogenase, AST, ALT, potassium, and cholesterol may be elevated.

2. Serum albumin, calcium, sodium, magnesium, and, possibly, potassium may be low due to dehydration, vomiting, and the binding of calcium in areas of fat necrosis.

3. Abdominal x-ray to detect an ileus or isolated loop of small bowel overlying pancreas. Pancreatic calcifications or gallstones may suggest an alcohol or biliary etiology.

4. CT scan is the most definitive study for determining pancreatic changes.

5. Chest x-ray for detection of pulmonary complications. Pleural effusions are common, especially on the left, but may be bilateral.

Management

Depending on severity of episode, management focuses on alleviation of symptoms and support of patient to prevent complications.

Table 19-2   Acute Versus Chronic Pancreatitis: Comparing Findings

	ACUTE PANCREATITIS	CHRONIC PANCREATITIS
Definition	• Inflammation that leads to swelling of the pancreas • Autodigestion—enzymes normally secreted by the pancreas become activated inside the pancreas and start to digest the pancreatic tissue	• Associated with widespread scarring and destruction of pancreatic tissue • Affects more men than women
Etiology	• Gallstones passing through the common bile duct • Alcohol abuse • Viral infection, hereditary conditions, traumatic injury, certain medications (especially estrogens, corticosteroids, thiazide diuretics, and azathioprine), pancreatic or common bile duct surgical procedures, or ERCP • Underlying pancreatic tumor • Hypercalcemia • Hyperlipidemia • Idiopathic	• Alcohol abuse (70% of patients) • Hereditary pancreatitis • Ductal destruction (from trauma, stones, tumors) • Tropical pancreatitis • Systemic diseases (cystic fibrosis, systemic lupus erythematosus, hyperparathyroidism) • Congenital conditions such as pancreas divisum • Hypercalcemia • Hyperlipidemia • Idiopathic
Symptoms	• Sudden attack of constant, severe upper abdominal pain that may radiate to the back • Pain that is sudden and steady • Pain that may be aggravated by walking or lying down and relieved by sitting or leaning forward (proning) • Other possible symptoms: nausea, vomiting, diarrhea, bloating, fever, diaphoresis, and jaundice	• Constant, dull mid- to upper-abdominal pain; may also have back pain • Pain that worsens with eating food or drinking alcohol; lessens with sitting or leaning forward (proning) • As disease progresses, attacks of pain that last longer and occur more frequently • May have nausea, vomiting • Weight loss
Course	• Mild disease in 85% of patients with rapid recovery within a few days of onset of illness	• Destruction of pancreatic tissue that slowly progresses from chronic inflammatory damage
Diagnosis	• Medical history • Serum amylase and lipase • Serum triglycerides • Ultrasound, CT scan, MRI	• Medical history • Liver function tests • Fecal elastase test • Abdominal x-ray that may reveal calcium deposits in the pancreas • Imaging studies, such as ultrasound, CT scan, ERCP, EUS, MRI/MRCP • CEA and CA 19-9 to assess for pancreatic cancer
Treatment	• Depends on severity as acute pancreatitis may be mild, moderate, or severe • IV fluids • Pain medication • NPO • Surgery for such complications as necrosis, infection, bleeding	• Pain management • Nutritional support and diet modification with smaller, frequent, low-fat meals • Pancreatic enzymes • Diabetes control • Pancreatic duct drainage procedures or excision of damage of all or part of the pancreas • Alcohol abstinence

Complications	• Severe acute pancreatitis may lead to:
	  • Multiple organ system failure, such as lung, liver, kidney, and heart
	  • Infected pancreatic necrosis
	  • Pancreatic abscess
	  • Pseudocysts
	  • Pancreatic fistula
	  • Pancreatic ascites
	  • Damage to surrounding organs, such as small bowel, colon, and duodenum (due to inflammation)
		• Malnutrition from poor absorption of nutrients, especially fats
		• Frequent bowel movements that are loose, greasy, foul-smelling (steatorrhea)
		• Insulin-dependent diabetes
		• Increased risk of pancreatic cancer
		• Pseudocyst
		• Bleeding from the stomach
		• Increased risk of blood clots
		• Possible bouts of acute pancreatitis

Prognosis	• Can usually fully recover without recurrence if cause is removed	• Can maintain quality of life with supportive care and adherence to medical regimen

1. Restoration of circulating blood volume with IV crystalloid or colloid solutions or blood products.
2. Maintenance of adequate oxygenation reduced by pain, anxiety, acidosis, abdominal pressure, or pleural effusions.
3. Pain control to alleviate pain and anxiety, which increases pancreatic secretions.
4. Rest of the GI tract.
   a. Withhold oral feedings to decrease pancreatic secretions.
   b. NG intubation and suction to relieve gastric stasis, distention, and ileus, if needed.
5. Maintenance of alkaline gastric pH with PPI or H_2-receptor antagonists and antacids to suppress acid drive of pancreatic secretions and to prevent stress ulcer complications of acute illness.
6. Nutrition provided or treatment of malnutrition with parenteral feedings, as needed.

 Evidence Base Grant, J. P. (2011). Nutritional support in acute and chronic pancreatitis. *Surgical Clinics of North America, 91*, 805–820.

7. Pharmacotherapy.
   a. Electrolyte replacements, as needed.
   b. Sodium bicarbonate to reverse metabolic acidosis.
   c. Insulin to treat hyperglycemia.
   d. Antibiotic therapy for documented infection or sepsis.
8. Surgical intervention if complications occur.
   a. Incision and drainage of infection and pseudocysts.
   b. Debridement or pancreatectomy to remove necrotic pancreatic tissue.
   c. Cholecystectomy for gallstone pancreatitis.

Complications

1. Pancreatic ascites, abscess, or pseudocyst.
2. Pulmonary infiltrates, pleural effusion, acute respiratory distress syndrome.
3. Hemorrhage with hypovolemic shock.
4. Acute renal failure.
5. Sepsis and multiple-organ dysfunction syndrome.

Nursing Assessment

1. Obtain history of gallbladder disease, alcohol use, or precipitating factors.
2. Assess GI distress, including nausea and vomiting, diarrhea, and passage of stools containing fat.
3. Assess characteristics of abdominal pain.
4. Assess nutritional and fluid status.
5. Assess respiratory rate and pattern and breath sounds.

 **GERONTOLOGIC ALERT** The incidence of severe, systemic complications of pancreatitis increases with age. Assess for any changes in mental status in an older person with pancreatitis as an indicator of an underlying complication. Acute pancreatitis in an older person without other precipitating factors may indicate an underlying pancreatic tumor obstructing the pancreatic duct.

Nursing Diagnoses

- Acute Pain related to disease process.
- Deficient Fluid Volume related to vomiting, self-restricted intake, fever, and fluid shifts.
- Ineffective Breathing Pattern related to severe pain and pulmonary complications.

Nursing Interventions

Controlling Pain

1. Administer opioid analgesics, as ordered, to control pain.
2. Assist patient to a comfortable position.
3. Maintain NPO status to decrease pancreatic enzyme secretion.
4. Maintain patency of NG suction to remove gastric secretions and to relieve abdominal distention, if indicated.
5. Provide frequent oral hygiene and care.
6. Administer antacids, PPI or H_2-receptor antagonists, as prescribed.
7. Report increase in severity of pain, which may indicate hemorrhage of the pancreas, rupture of a pseudocyst, or inadequate dosage of the analgesic.

Restoring Adequate Fluid Balance

1. Monitor and record vital signs, skin color, and temperature.
2. Monitor intake and output and weigh daily.
3. Evaluate laboratory data for hemoglobin, hematocrit, albumin, calcium, potassium, sodium, and magnesium levels and administer replacements, as prescribed.
4. Observe and measure abdominal girth if pancreatic ascites is suspected.
5. Report trends in falling BP or urine output or rising pulse because this may indicate hypovolemia and shock or renal failure.

Improving Respiratory Function

1. Assess respiratory rate and rhythm, effort, oxygen saturation, and breath sounds frequently.
2. Position in upright or semi-Fowler's position to enhance diaphragmatic excursion.
3. Administer oxygen supplementation, as prescribed, to maintain adequate oxygen levels.
4. Report signs of respiratory distress immediately.
5. Instruct patient in coughing and deep breathing to improve respiratory function.

Patient Education and Health Maintenance

1. Instruct patient to gradually resume a low-fat diet.
2. Instruct patient to increase activity gradually, providing for daily rest periods.
3. Reinforce information about disease process and precipitating factors. Stress that subsequent bouts of acute pancreatitis may destroy the pancreas, cause additional complications, and lead to chronic pancreatitis.
4. If pancreatitis is a result of alcohol abuse, patient needs to be reminded of the importance of eliminating all alcohol; advise about Alcoholics Anonymous or other substance abuse counseling.

Evaluation: Expected Outcomes

- Verbalizes reduced pain level.
- BP stable; urine output adequate.
- Respirations unlabored; breath sounds clear.

Chronic Pancreatitis

 Evidence Base Braganza, J. M., Lee, S. H., McCloy, R. F., et al. (2011). Chronic pancreatitis. *Lancet, 377,* 1184–1197.

Chronic pancreatitis is defined as the persistence of pancreatic cellular damage after acute inflammation and decreased pancreatic endocrine and exocrine function.

Pathophysiology and Etiology

1. Alcohol abuse is the most common cause; less common causes are hyperparathyroidism, hereditary pancreatitis, malnutrition, and trauma to the pancreas.
2. With chronic inflammation, destruction of the secreting cells of the pancreas causes maldigestion and malabsorption of protein and fat and possibly diabetes mellitus if islet cells of the pancreas have been affected.
3. As cells are replaced by fibrous tissue, obstruction of the pancreatic and common bile ducts and duodenum may result.

Clinical Manifestations

1. Pain is usually located in the epigastrium or left upper quadrant, frequently radiating to the back; similar to that observed in acute pancreatitis, but more constant and occurring at unpredictable intervals. As the disease progresses, recurring attacks of pain will be more severe, more frequent, and of longer duration.
2. Weight loss, nausea, vomiting, anorexia.
3. Malabsorption and steatorrhea occur late in the course of the disease.
4. Diabetes mellitus.

Diagnostic Evaluation

1. Serum amylase and lipase may be normal to low because of decreased pancreatic exocrine function.
2. Fecal fat analysis determines need for pancreatic enzyme replacement.
3. Bilirubin and alkaline phosphatase may be elevated if biliary obstruction occurs.
4. Secretin and cholecystokinin stimulatory test results are abnormal.
5. Plain abdominal x-ray to determine diffuse calcification of the pancreas.
6. CT scan identifies pancreatic structural changes, such as calcifications, masses, ductal irregularities, enlargement, and pseudocysts.
7. ERCP defines ductal anatomy and localizes complications, such as pancreatic pseudocysts and ductal disruptions.

Management

1. Pain management.
2. Correction of nutritional deficiencies.
3. Pancreatic enzyme replacement.
4. Treatment of diabetes mellitus.
5. Endoscopic placement of pancreatic stent allowing free flow of pancreatic juices through distorted and irregular/narrowed pancreatic duct.
6. Surgical interventions to reduce pain, restore drainage of pancreatic secretions, correct structural abnormalities, and manage complications. Care is similar to the patient undergoing abdominal surgery (see page 657).
   a. Pancreaticojejunostomy—side-to-side anastomosis of pancreatic duct to jejunum to drain pancreatic secretions into jejunum.
   b. Revision of sphincter of ampulla of Vater by a sphincteroplasty, in which the sphincter is sewn open to allow free flow of pancreatic juices.
   c. Drainage of pancreatic pseudocyst into nearby structures or by external drain.
   d. Resection of part of pancreas (Whipple procedure, distal pancreatectomy) or removal of entire pancreas (total pancreatectomy).
   e. Autotransplantation of islet cells.

Complications

1. Pancreatic pseudocyst.
2. Pancreatic ascites and pleural effusions.
3. GI hemorrhage.
4. Biliary tract obstruction.
5. Pancreatic fistula.

Nursing Assessment

1. Assess level of abdominal pain.
2. Assess nutritional status.
3. Assess for steatorrhea and malabsorption.
4. Assess for signs and symptoms of diabetes mellitus.
5. Assess current level of alcohol intake and motivation and resources available to abstain from drinking such as Alcoholics Anonymous.

Nursing Diagnoses

- Acute and Chronic Pain related to chronic and unrelenting insult to pancreas.
- Imbalanced Nutrition: Less Than Body Requirements related to fear of eating, malabsorption, and glucose intolerance.
- Anxiety related to surgical intervention or not knowing when pain may recur.

Nursing Interventions

Controlling Pain

1. Assess and record the character, location, frequency, and duration of pain.
2. Determine precipitating and alleviating factors of the patient's pain.

3. Explore the effect of pain on patient's lifestyle and eating habits.

4. Administer or teach self-administration of analgesics (opioids), as ordered, to control pain.

5. Use nonpharmacologic methods to promote relaxation, such as distraction, imagery, and progressive muscle relaxation.

6. Assess response to pain-control measures and refer to chronic pain management clinic, if indicated.

Improving Nutritional Status

1. Assess nutritional status, history of weight loss, and dietary habits, including alcohol intake.

2. Administer pancreatic enzyme replacement with meals, as prescribed.

3. Administer antacids, PPI or H$_2$-receptor antagonists to prevent neutralization of enzyme supplements, as indicated.

4. Monitor intake and output and daily weight.

5. Assess for GI discomfort with meals and character of stools.

6. Monitor blood glucose levels and teach balanced, low-concentrated carbohydrate diet and insulin therapy, as indicated.

 DRUG ALERT Warn the patient that dangerous hypoglycemic reaction may result from use of insulin while drinking alcohol and skipping meals.

7. Identify foods that aggravate symptoms and teach low-fat diet.

Relieving Anxiety About Surgical Intervention

1. Describe planned surgical intervention and the expected results.
   a. Decreased pain.
   b. Ability to eat better and improve general condition.

2. Prepare patient for adverse effects and complications of surgery.
   a. Total pancreatectomy will cause permanent diabetes mellitus, dependence on insulin, severe malabsorption, and the need for lifelong pancreatic enzyme replacement. Consultation and close monitoring by endocrinologist and diabetic educator.
   b. Malnutrition and debility increase patient's risk for poor healing and complications of surgery.

3. Assist patient to prepare for surgery by encouraging abstinence of alcohol and intake of nutritional and vitamin supplements.

4. Encourage patient to enlist help of support network and strengthen appropriate coping mechanisms.

5. After surgery, provide meticulous care to prevent infection, promote wound healing, and prevent routine complications of surgery (see page 124).

Patient Education and Health Maintenance

1. Instruct patient regarding correct use of analgesics.

2. Instruct in proper administration of pancreatic enzyme replacement.
   a. Take just before or during meals.
   b. May be enteric coated. Do not crush or chew tablets; powder may be obtained if swallowing tablets is difficult.

   c. Take with antacid, PPI, or H$_2$-receptor antagonist, as directed, to prevent pancreatic enzyme from being destroyed by gastric acid secretions.

3. Advise patient to monitor number and characteristics of stools; report increased stools or food intolerance.

4. Diabetic teaching with follow-up to monitor progression of condition, if applicable.

5. Stress that no treatment will be effective if alcohol consumption is continued.

Evaluation: Expected Outcomes

- Verbalizes reduced pain level.
- Weight stabilized or weight gain noted.
- Verbalizes understanding of effects of surgical procedure.

Pancreatic Cancer

 Evidence Base National Comprehensive Cancer Network (NCCN). (2011). NCCN clinical practice guidelines in oncology: Pancreatic adenocarcinoma, version 2.2012. Available: www.nccn.org/professionals/physician_gls/pdf/pancreatic.pdf.

Cancer of the pancreas may arise in the head (70%) or body and tail (30%) of the pancreas. Adenocarcinoma of the cells that line the ducts of the pancreas is the most common (80%) type. Pancreatic cancer is the fourth-leading cause of cancer deaths in the United States because 90% of tumors are not resectable at the time of diagnosis.

Pathophysiology and Etiology

1. Incidence is increasing.

2. Usually occurs between ages 60 and 80, but can be found in younger patients.

3. Smoking, prolonged exposure to industrial chemicals, high-fat diet, diabetes mellitus, and chronic pancreatitis are considered risk factors. Small percentage of pancreatic cancer is inherited.

4. Excessive weight and physical inactivity are now considered risk factors for pancreatic cancer.

5. Obstruction of bile flow may occur with tumors in the head of the pancreas because of compression of the distal common bile duct.

6. Obstruction of pancreatic duct produces pain and exocrine dysfunction.

Clinical Manifestations

1. Symptoms are commonly vague and nonspecific, preventing early detection.

2. Weight loss, abdominal pain, anorexia, nausea, vomiting, and weakness may occur.

3. Pain usually occurs in the upper abdomen and is gnawing or boring and may radiate around the flank to the back.
   a. Pain is usually worse at night, and patients tend to lie with legs drawn up in the fetal position or may lean forward when seated (proning).
   b. Pain may become more localized, severe, and unremitting as the disease progresses.

4. Early satiety and a feeling of bloating after eating may occur.
5. Biliary obstruction produces jaundice, dark tea-colored urine, clay-colored stools, and pruritus.
6. Depression and lethargy may be present.

Diagnostic Evaluation

Evidence Base Hariharan, D., Constantinides, V. A., Froeling, F. E., et al. (2010). The role of laparoscopy and laparoscopic ultrasound in the preoperative staging of pancreatico-biliary cancers—a meta-analysis. *European Journal of Surgical Oncology, 36,* 941–948.

1. Ultrasonography and CT scan—detect tumors larger than 1 cm.
2. ERCP defines anatomy and allows placement of biliary stent for unobstructive flow of bile by tumor in the head of the pancreas prior to surgery or as palliation in patients not deemed surgical candidates.
3. MRCP—defines anatomy without contrast dye.
4. PET scan to differentiate cancer from cyst as well as to assess for recurrence or metastatic disease.
5. Liver function tests elevated; coagulation studies may be prolonged.
6. Carcinoembryonic antigen (CEA) and CA 19-9—may be elevated.
7. Percutaneous fine-needle aspiration or biopsy through ultrasonography or CT scan guidance to determine malignancy.
8. EUS for preoperative staging and facilitates fine needle aspiration for cytology to confirm diagnosis.

Management

The goal of treatment may be cure or palliation, depending on the staging of the tumor. Most cases are usually too far advanced for cure. Longer palliation is now being achieved.

Surgery

1. Whipple procedure (pancreaticoduodenectomy) is the removal of the head of the pancreas, distal portion of the common bile duct including the gallbladder, duodenum, and the distal stomach with anastomosis of the remaining pancreas, stomach, and common bile duct to the jejunum (see Figure 19-6). If the gallbladder is present, it is also removed.
   a. Stomach and pylorus may be preserved—pylorus-preserving Whipple procedure.
   b. Performed for carcinoma of the head of the pancreas, periampullary area, chronic pancreatitis of the head of the pancreas, and trauma.
2. Total pancreatectomy, including a splenectomy, may be performed for diffuse tumor throughout the pancreas.
3. Distal pancreatectomy is the removal of the distal pancreas and spleen for tumors localized in the body and tail.
4. Palliative bypass for nonresectable tumors: choledochojejunostomy or cholecystojejunostomy for obstructive jaundice or gastrojejunostomy for gastric outlet obstruction.

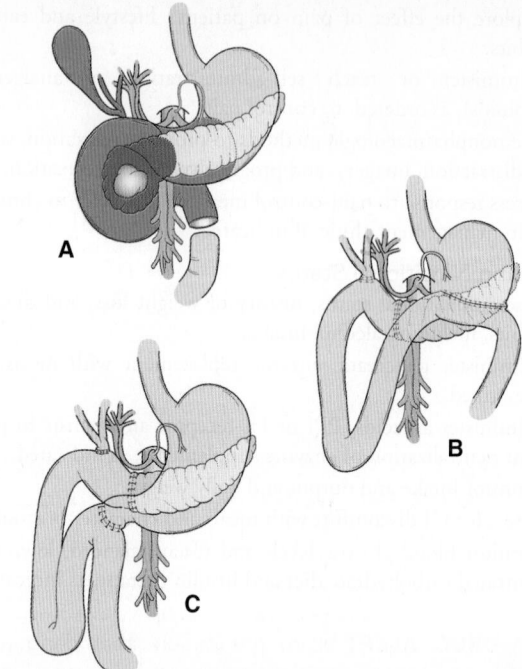

Figure 19-6. Pancreaticoduodenectomy. (A) The standard pancreaticoduodenectomy (Whipple procedure) involves a wide area of resection around the tumor, including the gallbladder, distal stomach including the pyloric region, duodenum, and head of the pancreas, as indicated. **(B)** Indicates anastomoses of the common bile duct, fundus of the stomach, and body and tail of the pancreas to the jejunum. **(C)** Pylorus-sparing variant involves preservation of the stomach, including the pyloric valve anastomosed to the jejunum.

5. Care is similar to that of patient undergoing abdominal surgery (see page 657).

Other Measures

1. Chemotherapy alone or may be used in combination with radiation therapy as neoadjuvant therapy may be given before surgery to shrink tumors that involve major blood vessels.
2. Chemotherapy combined with radiation therapy may be given for resectable tumors after surgery for microscopic or undetectable disease left behind.
3. Chemotherapy and radiation therapy may be given for tumors deemed unresectable at the time of surgery and after palliative bowel bypass surgery.
4. Chemotherapy may be given alone for treatment of unresectable or metastatic disease.
5. Radiation therapy may be used alone.
   a. External beam irradiation for local control, to reduce pain, and to palliate obstruction.
   b. Intraoperative radiation therapy given after the panceas resection has also been used in some centers.
6. Endoscopic or percutaneous stent placement for relief of biliary obstruction. (Metal stents may be placed for patients near the end of life.)
7. Endoscopic stent for relief of duodenal obstruction (usually for patients near end of life).

8. Chemical splanchnicectomy, injection of alcohol into the celiac plexus, numbs the nerves in the area of the pancreas for pain relief.
   a. May be performed intraoperatively by the surgeon or percutaneously under CT guidance as an outpatient procedure by an anesthesia pain service.
   b. Provides temporary pain relief and can be repeated.

 Evidence Base Arcidiacono, P. G., Calori, G., Carrara, S., et al. (2011). Celiac plexus block for pancreatic cancer pain in adults. *Cochrane Database of Systematic Reviews*, Issue 16 (Article No. CD007519).

9. Novel therapies, including immunotherapy and gene and vaccine therapies, are being investigated.
10. Clinical investigations combining various treatments are aimed at improving the prognosis of pancreatic cancer.

Complications

1. Biliary, gastric, and duodenal obstruction.
2. Metastasis and liver failure secondary to metastasis.
3. Portal hypertension and pain because of encasement of major blood vessels and celiac nerve plexus in the area of the pancreas.

Nursing Assessment

1. Obtain history for risk factors, pain, and symptoms of pancreatic dysfunction.
2. Assess nutritional status, including diet history, anorexia, weight loss, nausea and vomiting, steatorrhea, skin turgor.
3. Evaluate laboratory results for alterations in glucose, pancreatic enzymes, liver function, and coagulation studies.
4. Assess psychosocial status to determine depression, usual coping strategies, support systems, and experience with past serious illness.
5. Assess use of alternative therapies or over-the-counter medications.

 DRUG ALERT The efficacy of herbal medications to treat or cure pancreatic cancer has not been proven. Little is known about the interaction of herbal medications with conventional medications or treatments. Herbal medications may interact with chemotherapy drugs and compromise treatment. If a patient is using alternative treatments or herbal medications, this must be known to all health care providers. Complementary and alternative therapies, other than those that are ingested, may be of benefit to a patient with pancreatic cancer if used adjunctly; however, much research is needed.

Nursing Diagnoses

- Acute Pain related to pancreatic tumor or surgical incision.
- Imbalanced Nutrition: Less Than Body Requirements related to disease process and surgical intervention.
- Deficient Fluid Volume related to hypoproteinemia, surgical alterations.
- Impaired Tissue Integrity related to malnutrition, surgical incisions, and altered pancreatic or bile drainage.

Nursing Interventions

Controlling Pain

1. Administer opioids, as ordered, or monitor PCA.
2. Teach relaxation techniques, such as relaxation breathing, progressive muscle relaxation, and imagery, as adjuncts for pain relief.
3. Assist with frequent turning and comfortable positioning.
4. Administer adjuvant medications, such as antidepressants, as prescribed.
5. Assess patient's response to pain and symptom-control measures.
6. Consider palliative care or hospice services for symptom management if patient no longer benefits from therapy.

Improving Nutritional Status

1. Administer parenteral nutrition, as prescribed, preoperatively and postoperatively, if indicated.
2. Monitor serum glucose level for hyperglycemia or hypoglycemia.
3. Progress diet slowly when oral intake is tolerated; observe for nausea, vomiting, and gastric distention.
4. Administer high-protein, high-carbohydrate diet with vitamin supplements and pancreatic enzymes, as prescribed.
5. Encourage use of spices to stimulate taste buds, provide cool foods to decrease odor, use plastic utensils if patient complains of metallic taste from treatments, and offer small, frequent meals.
6. Provide appetite stimulant, such as megestrol, as needed.
7. Monitor serum albumin.
8. Weigh daily.
9. Assess for fat and protein malabsorption; stools that float, have greasy appearance, are orange in color, and are foul smelling.

Attaining Adequate Fluid Volume

1. Monitor vital signs and record accurate intake and output.
2. Monitor wound drain output.
3. Evaluate laboratory values for hypoalbuminemia, hyponatremia, hypochloremia, and metabolic alkalosis; replace electrolytes, as prescribed.
4. Administer fluid replacement, as indicated.
5. Report change in vital signs or increased pain; may indicate hemorrhage, leak from anastomosis, or tumor progression.

Maintaining Tissue Integrity

1. Observe skin for jaundice, breakdown, irritation, or excoriation.
2. Administer antipruritics, provide frequent skin care without soap and with thorough rinsing, apply emollient lotions, trim fingernails short to prevent scratching.
3. Inspect skin around drains for irritation and protect skin from leakage of fluids from drains or tubes.
4. Inspect surgical dressings and incision for bleeding, drainage, or signs of infection.
5. Prevent tension on anastomoses by monitoring for abdominal distention and maintaining patency of surgically placed tubes and drains.
6. Maintain aseptic technique in handling wound dressings and drainage of all secretions.

Community and Home Care Considerations

1. Educate patient and family about course of disease and support them through the process.
2. Provide assistive devices and direct care to help with energy conservation. Patients who die of pancreatic cancer may have progressive weight loss from anorexia leading to severe cachexia, fatigue, and muscle wasting, which is refractory to any intervention.
3. Assess for bowel obstruction, which may also deplete energy and lower nutritional status. Notify health care provider of reduced bowel activity, increased pain.
4. Emphasize to patient and family that pain can always be managed and patients need not die in pain. The plan for pain management should be aggressive and should provide the patient an optimal quality of life.
5. Encourage family to take advantage of palliative care or hospice services.

Patient Education and Health Maintenance

1. Instruct patient and family on self-care measures for pancreatic insufficiency.
   a. Glucose monitoring, insulin administration, signs and symptoms of hypoglycemia and hyperglycemia.
   b. Pancreatic enzyme replacement, high-protein, high-carbohydrate diet.
2. Teach wound and drain care, as needed.
3. Explore options for pain management.
4. Coordinate referral for home care for any wound or drain care, new diabetic management, new medications, change in diet, or referral for palliative care or hospice services.

Evaluation: Expected Outcomes

- Verbalizes reduced pain.
- Weight stable.
- Vital signs stable; urine output adequate.
- Incision intact without drainage or bleeding

For more information on hepatic, biliary, and pancreatic disorders, the following websites are recommended.

INTERNET RESOURCES

Gallbladder and Liver Diseases
- *www.acg.gi.org* (American College of Gastroenterology)
- *www.digestive.niddk.nih*.gov (National Digestive Diseases Information Clearinghouse)
- *www.gastro.org* (American Gastroenterological Assocation)
- *www.nlm.nih.gov* (National Library of Medicine)

Liver Diseases
- *www.liverfoundation.org* (American Liver Foundation)
- *www.cdc.gov/ncidod/diseases/hepatitis/c* (Centers for Disease Control and Prevention: viral hepatitis)

Pancreatic Disease
- *www.american-pancreatic-association.org* (American Pancreatic Assocation)
- *www.pancreasfoundation.org* (National Pancreas Foundation)

Pancreatic Cancer
- *www.cancer.org* (American Cancer Society)
- *www.cancer.gov* (National Cancer Institute)
- *www.cancercare.org* (Cancer Care Inc.)
- *www.nccn.org* (National Comprehensive Cancer Network)
- *www.nlm.nih.gov/medlineplus/pancreaticcancer.html* (MedlinePlus: pancreatic cancer)
- *www.pancan.org* (Pancreatic Cancer Action Network)
- *www.pathology.jhu.edu/pancreas* (Johns Hopkins Medicine: The Sol Goldman Pancreatic Cancer Research Center)

SELECTED REFERENCES

Arcidiacono, P. G., Calori, G., Carrara, S., et al. (2011). Celiac plexus block for pancreatic cancer pain in adults. *Cochrane Database of Systematic Reviews,* Issue 16 (Article No. CD007519).

ASGE Standards of Practice Committee, Maple. J. T., Ikenberry, S. O., et al. (2011). The role of endoscopy in the management of choledocholithiasis. *Gastrointestinal Endoscopy, 74*, 731–744.

Aspinall, E. J., Hawkins, G., Fraser, A., et al. (2011). Hepatitis B prevention, diagnosis, treatment and care: a review. *Occupational Medicine, 61*, 531–540.

Bernal, W., Auzinger, G., Dhawan, A., et al. (2010). Acute liver failure. *Lancet, 376*, 190–201.

Bonder, A., & Afdhal, N. (2012). Evaluation of liver lesions. *Clinics in Liver Disease, 16*, 271–283.

Braganza, J. M., Lee, S. H., McCloy, R. F., et al. (2011). Chronic pancreatitis. *Lancet, 377*, 1184–1197.

Brisinda, G., Vanella, S., Crocco, A., et al. (2011). Severe acute pancreatitis: Advances and insights in assessment of severity and management. *European Journal of Gastroenterology and Hepatology, 23*, 541–551.

Brody, J. R., Witkiewicz, A. K., & Yeo, C. J. (2011). The past, present, and future of biomarkers: A need for molecular beacons for the clinical management of pancreatic cancer. *Advances in Surgery, 45*, 301–321.

Bruix, J., & Sherman, M. (2011). Management of hepatocellular carcinoma: An update. American Association for the Study of Liver Diseases. *Hepatology, 53*, 1020–1022.

Buck, A. K., Herrmann, K., Eckel, F., et al. (2011). Pancreatic and hepatobiliary cancers. *Methods in Molecular Biology, 727*, 243–264.

Carr, B. I. (2012). Some new approaches to the management of hepatocellular carcinoma. *Seminars in Oncology, 39*, 369–373.

Cat, T. B., & Liu-DeRyke, X. (2010). Medical management of variceal hemorrhage. *Critical Care Nursing Clinics of North America, 22*, 381–393.

Chen, C. P., & Haas-Kogan, D. (2010). Neoplasms of the hepatobiliary system: clinical presentation, molecular pathways and diagnostics. *Expert Reviews in Molecular Diagnostics, 10*, 883–895.

Choi, G., & Runyon, B. A. (2012). Alcoholic hepatitis: a clinician's guide. *Clinics in Liver Disease, 1*, 371–385.

Cho, L. Y., Yang, J. J., Ko, K. P., et al. (2011). Coinfection of hepatitis B and C viruses and risk of hepatocellular carcinoma: Systematic review and meta-analysis. *International Journal of Cancer, 128*, 176–184.

Cho, Y. K., Rhim, H., & Noh, S. (2011). Radiofrequency ablation versus surgical resection as primary treatment of hepatocellular carcinoma meeting the Milan criteria: A systematic review. *Journal of Gastroenterology and Hepatology, 26*(9), 1354–1360.

DuBray, B. J. Jr., Chapman, W. C., & Anderson, C. D. (2011). Hepatocellular carcinoma: A review of the surgical approaches to management. *Missouri Medicine, 108*, 195–198.

Faingold, R., Albuquerque, P. A., & Carpineta, L. (2011). Hepatobiliary tumors. *Radiology Clinics of North America, 49*, 679–687.

Farci, P., & Niro, G. A. (2012). Clinical features of hepatitis D. *Seminars in Liver Disease, 32*, 228–236.

Gao, B., & Bataller, R. (2011). Alcoholic liver disease: pathogenesis and new therapeutic targets. *Gastroenterology. 141*, 1572–1585.

García-Pagán, J. C., Reverter, E., Abraldes, J. G., et al. (2012). Acute variceal bleeding. *Seminars in Respiratory and Critical Care Medicine, 33*, 46–54.

Ghany, M. G., Nelson, D. R., Strader, D. B., et al. (2011). An update on treatment of genotype 1 chronic hepatitis C virus infection: 2011 practice guideline by the American Association for the Study of Liver Disease. *Heptology, 54*, 1433–1444.

Gossard, A. A., & Lindor, K. D. (2012). Autoimmune hepatitis: a review. *Journal of Gastroenterology, 47*, 498–503.

Grant, J. P. (2011). Nutritional support in acute and chronic pancreatitis. *Surgical Clinics of North America, 91*, 805–820.

Hackert, T., Büchler, M. W., & Werner, J. (2009). Surgical options in the management of pancreatic cancer. *Minerva Chirurgica, 64*, 465–476.

Hall, T. C., Dennison, A. R., Bilku, D. K., et al. (2012). Single-incision laparoscopic cholecystectomy: a systematic review. *Archives of Surgery, 147*, 657–666.

Han, Y. F., Zhao, J., Ma, L. Y., et al. (2011). Factors predicting occurrence and prognosis of hepatitis B-virus-related hepatocellular carcinoma. *World Journal of Gastroenterology, 17*, 4258–4270.

Hariharan, D., Constantinides, V. A., Froeling, F. E., et al. (2010). The role of laparoscopy and laparoscopic ultrasound in the preoperative staging of pancreatico-biliary cancers—a meta-analysis. *European Journal of Surgical Oncology, 36*, 941–948.

Hughes, S. A., Wedemeyer, H., & Harrison, P. M. (2011). Hepatitis delta virus. *Lancet, 378*, 73–85.

Ilyas, J. A., & Vierling, J. M. (2011). An overview of emerging therapies for the treatment of chronic hepatitis C. *Clinics in Liver Disease, 15*, 515–536.

Jarnagin, W., Chapman, W. C., Curley, S., et al. (2010). Surgical treatment of hepatocellular carcinoma: Expert consensus statement. American Hepato-Pancreato-Biliary Association: Society of Surgical Oncology; Society for Surgery of the Alimentary tract. *HPB, 12*, 301–310.

Jiang D. (2011). Care of chronic liver disease. *Primary Care, 38*, 483–498; viii–ix.

Jothimani, D., Cramp, M. E., Mitchell, J. D., et al. (2011) Treatment of autoimmune hepatitis: A review of current and evolving therapies. *Journal of Gastroenterology and Hepatology, 26*, 619–627.

Keus, F., Gooszen, H. G., & van Laarhoven, C. J. (2010). Open, small-incision, or laparoscopic cholecystectomy for patients with symptomatic cholecystolithiasis. An overview of Cochrane Hepato-Biliary Group review. *Cochrane Database of Systematic Reviews,* Issue 20 (Article No. CD008318).

Koretz, R. L., Avenell, A., Lipman, T. O. (2012). Nutritional support for liver disease. *Cochrane Database Systematic Review, 16; 5*:CD008344.

Kwon, H., & Lok, A. S. (2011). Hepatitis B therapy. *National Reviews. Gastroenterology and Hepatology, 8*, 275–284.

Lee, L. S., & Conwell, D. L. (2012). Update on advanced endoscopic techniques for the pancreas: endoscopic retrograde cholangiopancreatography, drainage and biopsy, and endoscopic ultrasound. *Radiologic Clinics of North America, 50*, 547–561.

Lok, A. S., Gardiner, D. F., Lawitz, E., et al. (2012). Preliminary study of two antiviral agents for hepatitis C genotype 1. *New England Journal of Medicine, 19*, 216–224.

Lok, A. S., & McMahon, B. J. (2009). Chronic hepatitis B: Update 2009. *Heptology, 50*, 661–662.

Maccioni, F., Martinelli, M., Al Ansari, N., et al. (2010). Magnetic resonance cholangiography: Past, present and future: A review. *European Review for Medical and Pharmacological Sciences, 14*, 721–725.

Malik, T. A., & Saeed, S. (2010). Autoimmune hepatitis: A review. *Journal of Pakistan Medical Association, 60*, 381–387.

Marsh, Rd, W., Alonzo, M., Bajaj, S., et al. (2012). Comprehensive review of the diagnosis and treatment of biliary tract cancer 2012. Part I: diagnosis-clinical staging and pathology. *Journal of Surgical Oncology, 106*, 332–338.

Marsh Rd, W., Alonzo, M., Bajaj, S., et al. (2012). Comprehensive review of the diagnosis and treatment of biliary tract cancer 2012. Part II: Multidisciplinary management. *Journal of Surgical Oncology, 106*, 339–345.

Mathurin, P., Moreno, C., Samuel, D., et al. (2011). Early liver transplantation for severe alcoholic hepatitis. *New England Journal of Medicine, 365*, 1790–1800.

National Comprehensive Cancer Network (NCCN). (2011). NCCN clinical practice guidelines in oncology: Hepatobiliary cancer, version 2.2012. Available: *www.nccn.org/professionals/physician_gls/pdf/hepatobiliary.pdf.*

National Comprehensive Cancer Network (NCCN). (2011). NCCN clinical practice guidelines in oncology: Pancreatic adenocarcinoma, version 2.2012. Available: *www.nccn.org/professionals/physician_gls/pdf/pancreatic.pdf.*

Neuzillet, C., Sauvanet, A., & Hammel, P. (2011). Prognostic factors for resectable pancreatic adenocarcinoma. *Journal of Visceral Surgery, 148*, e232–243.

Oliveri, R. S., Wetterslev, J., & Gluud, C. (2011). Transarterial (chemo)embolism for unresectable hepatocellular carcinoma. *Cochrane Database Systematic Reviews,* Issue 16 (Article No. CD004787).

O'Shea, R. S., Dasarathy, S., & McCullough, A. J. (2010). Alcoholic liver disease. Practice Guidelines Committee of the American Association for the Study of Liver Diseases: Practice Parameters Committee of the American College of Gastroenterology. *Hepatology, 1*, 307–328.

Overby, D. W., Apelgren, K. N., Richardson, W., et al. (2010). SAGES guidelines for the clinical application of laparoscopic biliary tract surgery. Society of American Gastrointestinal and Endoscopic Surgeons. *Surgical Endoscopy, 24*, 2368–2386.

Pascarella, S., & Negro, F. (2011). Hepatitis D virus: An update. *Liver International, 31*, 7–21.

Peddu, P., Quaglia, A., Kane, P. A., et al. (2009). Role of imaging in the management of pancreatic mass. *Critical Reviews in Oncology Hematology, 70*, 12–23.

Rahimi, R. S., & Rockey, D. C. (2011). Complications and outcomes in chronic liver disease. *Current Opinions in Gastroenterology, 27*, 204–209.

Rockey, D. C., Caldwell, S. H., Goodman, Z. D., et al. (2009). Liver biopsy. *Hepatology, 49*, 1017–1044.

Rosen, H. R. (2011). Clinical practice. Chronic hepatitis C infection. *New England Journal of Medicine, 364*, 2429–2438.

Săftoiu A. (2011). State-of-the-art imaging techniques in endoscopic ultrasound. *World Journal of Gastroenterology, 17*, 691–696.

Sharma, C., Eltawil, K. M., Renfrew, P. D., et al. (2011). Advances in diagnosis, treatment and palliation of pancreatic carcinoma: 1990–2010. *World Journal of Gastroenterology, 17*, 867–897.

Smith, B. D., Morgan, R. L., Beckett, G. A., et al. (2012). Recommendations for the identification of chronic hepatitis C virus infection in persons born during 1945–1965. *MMWR, 61*(RR05), 1–18.

Society of American Gastrointestinal and Endoscopic Surgeons (SAGES). (2010). SAGES guidelines for the clinical application of laparoscopic biliary tract surgery. Available: *www.sages.org/publication/id/06/.*

Stampfl, U., Hackert, T., Radeleff, B., et al. (2011). Percutaneous management of postoperative bile leaks after upper gastrointestinal surgery. *Cardiovascular Interventional Radiology, 34*, 808–815.

Sturgeon, C. M., Duffy, M. J., Hofman, B. R., et al. (2010). National Academy of Clinical Biochemistry Laboratory Medicine practice guidelines for the use of tumor markers in liver, bladder, cervical, and gastric cancers. *Clinical Chemistry, 50*, e1–48.

Takeda, K., Yokoe, M., Yakada, T., et al. (2010). Assessment of severity of acute pancreatitis according to new prognostic factors and CT grading. *Journal of Hepatobiliary Pancreatic Sciences, 17*, 37–44.

Takada, T, Hirata, K., Mayumi, T., et al. (2010). Cutting-edge information for the management of acute pancreatitis. *Journal of Hepatobiliary Pancreatic Sciences, 17*, 3–12.

Tannpfel, A., Dienes, H. P., Lohse, A. W., et al. (2012). The indications for liver biopsy. *Deutsches Arzteblatt International, 109*, 477–483.

Thalheimer, U., Triantos, C., Goulis, J., et al. (2011). Management of varices in cirrhosis. *Expert Opinion on Pharmacotherapy, 12*, 721–735.

Trikudanathan, G., Navaneethan, U., Vege., S. (2012). Modern treatment of patients with chronic pancreatitis. *Gastroenterology Clinics of North America, 41*, 63–76.

Tulchinsky, M., Colletti, P. M., Allen. T. W. (2012). Hepatobiliary scintigraphy in acute cholecystitis. *Seminars in Nuclear Medicine, 42*, 84–100.

Vachon, M. L., & Dieterich, D. T. (2011). The HIV/HCV-coinfected patient and new treatment options. *Clinics in Liver Disease, 15*, 585–596.

Ward, J. W., & Lok, A. S. (2012). Report on a single-topic conference on "Chronic viral hepatitis: Strategies to improve effectiveness of screening and treatment." *Hepatology, 55*, 307–315.

Wilkins, T., Malcolm, J. K., Raina, D., et al. (2010). Hepatitis C: Diagnosis and treatment. *American Family Physician, 81*, 1351–1357.

20
Nutritional Problems

OVERVIEW AND ASSESSMENT

Nutrition Overview

Knowledge of nutrients and the basic principles of nutrition are important in the role of patient teaching for disease prevention and health promotion. The principles also help to provide an understanding and background to diseases affected by a person's nutritional status. The basic food groups and their placement on a plate help to serve as a guide to basic, healthy nutrition.

Key Principles

1. Nutrients, including carbohydrates, fats, proteins, vitamins, and minerals, have specific functions within the body. They work together to provide energy, regulate metabolic processes, and synthesize tissues.
2. Nutrition influences all body systems favorably and unfavorably. Examples of unfavorable effects include the link between cholesterol and heart disease or salt intake and high blood pressure (BP). Favorable effects are many, such as the association of fiber intake with improved GI function and the role of folic acid in preventing neural tube defects.
3. Nutritional needs vary in response to metabolic changes, age, sex, growth periods, stress (trauma, disease, pregnancy, lactation), and physical condition.
4. Nutritional supplements may be needed depending on disease states, dietary intake, and other factors.
5. The types of foods eaten and eating patterns are developed during a lifetime and are determined by psychosocial, cultural, religious, and economic influences.
6. The nurse works with the registered dietitian to promote optimum nutrition for each patient.

MyPlate and the Dietary Guidelines for Americans

1. Dietary guidelines were first developed in 1958 and were based on four basic food groups: grains, vegetables and fruits, meat, and milk. In 2010 the Department of Health and Human Services and U.S. Department of Agriculture (USDA) Dietary Guidelines for Americans were restructured and divided the four basic food groups into five food groups, which now consist of grains, fruits, vegetables, protein, and dairy. Although the guidelines have been reformatted, it still holds true that a well-balanced diet consists of foods from each of these groups and is composed of foods low in fat, cholesterol, and sodium and high in fiber (*www.dietaryguidelines.gov*). See Chapter 3, page 26, for more specific information about the guidelines.
2. In response to growing scientific knowledge regarding the linkage of diet and disease, the USDA developed the MyPlate Plan (see Figure 20-1). It reflects making food choices for a healthy lifestyle and includes basic information on how to build a healthy plate by cutting back on foods high in solid fats, added sugars, and salt; eating the right amount of calories; and being physically active.

Nutritional Assessment

Nutrition assessment is an ongoing process designed to identify a person's nutritional status and the significance on the person's well-being. Although there are many methods and tools for assessing nutritional status, there is no universal method or "gold standard." Indeed, multiple factors must be evaluated and considered to determine risk for or degree of malnutrition. One such factor is determining nutritional intake.

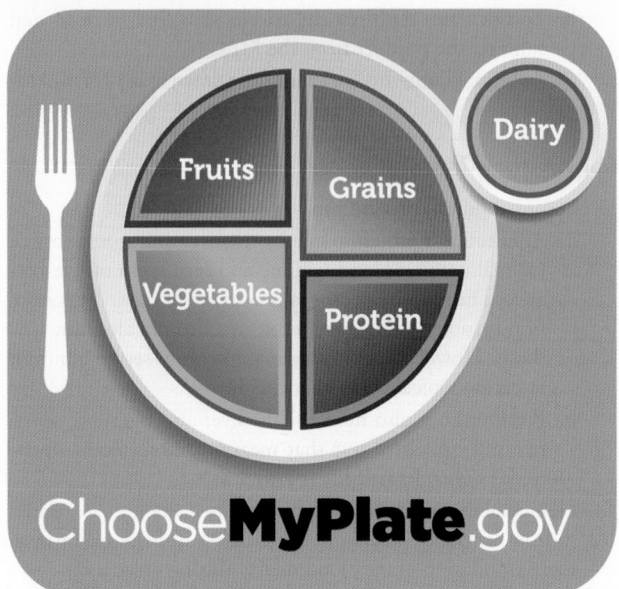

Figure 20-1. MyPlate illustrates healthy eating. (U.S. Department of Agriculture.)

There are many methods to assess the type and amount of food consumed, including a 24-hour recall of foods eaten, a food diary kept by the patient for several days, and a food frequency questionnaire that reflects food-intake patterns. In addition to these specific tools, the following information is useful to determine nutritional patterns and status.

Key History Points

1. General background information—name, age, sex, family composition, socioeconomic status, occupation.
2. General health status and any chronic conditions, including diabetes and associated dietary restrictions.
3. Cultural and religious factors influencing dietary patterns.
4. Family history of diseases, including diabetes and obesity.
5. Current medications, over-the-counter products, and herbal supplements.
6. Food habits.
   a. Typical daily intake, including meal frequency, meal timing, meal location.
   b. Snacking patterns.
   c. Food intolerance or dislikes.
   d. Nutritional supplements, including vitamins, minerals, fortified beverages, and foods.
   e. Alcohol consumption.
   f. Use of specific diets or dietary restrictions.
7. Food purchase and preparation.
   a. Who purchases and prepares food and where food is purchased.
   b. Facilities for food storage and preparation.
   c. Factors influencing the types of food purchased.
8. Nutritionally related problems.
   a. General well-being, energy level.
   b. Weight change during the past 6 months.
   c. Difficulty chewing or swallowing, use of dentures.

   d. Change in sense of taste or smell.
   e. Eructation, flatulence, nausea, vomiting, diarrhea, constipation, or abdominal pain or swelling in relation to food intake.
   f. Bowel habits.

Physical Examination and Anthropometrics

1. Perform a systematic physical examination, observing for a wide variety of physical findings associated with nutritional status.
   a. Listlessness, apathy.
   b. Poor muscle tone.
   c. Dull, brittle hair; hair may be thin or sparse, easily plucked.
   d. Rough, dry, and scaly skin or dermatitis.
   e. Cheilosis (fissures at angles of mouth).
   f. Stomatitis (inflammation of mouth).
   g. Inflammation and easy bleeding of gums.
   h. Glossitis (inflammation of tongue).
   i. Dental caries and poor dentition.
   j. Spoon-shaped, brittle, ridged nails.
   k. Skeletal deformities such as bowlegs.
2. Perform anthropometry, as indicated. (Anthropometry comes from the word *anthropology* and is the science that studies the size, weight, and proportions of the human body to determine body fat mass, lean mass, and nutritional status.) Types of anthropometric measurements include height and weight, skin-fold thickness, and circumferentialtests.
3. Height and weight are determined on patient admission and are later used as a baseline for comparisons in nutritional status.
   a. Weight should be measured using a consistent and reliable scale and at a consistent time.
   b. Unintended weight loss of more than 10% of body weight during 6 months is considered clinically significant and may be associated with physiologic abnormalities and increased morbidity and mortality.
4. Body mass index (BMI) is weight in kilograms divided by height in meters squared (see Table 20-1 on page 744).
   a. BMI of less than 18.5 is classified as underweight.
   b. BMI of 18.5 to 24.9 is classified as normal weight.
   c. BMI of 25 to 29.9 is classified as overweight.
   d. BMI of 30 to 39.9 is classified as obese.
   e. BMI greater than 40 is classified as extremely obese.
5. Metabolism is generally faster in younger people and for this reason, babies and children have higher energy requirement needs than adults. Requirement needs are based on many factors including age, gender, activity level, and disease state. Exact measurements of caloric requirements for infants can be obtained by using charts; these estimate the body surface area by height and weight and the standard basal metabolic rate for a given weight (see Appendix B).
6. Skin-fold thickness provides an estimate of body fat based on the amount of fat in subcutaneous tissue (see Figure 20-2 on page 744).
   a. Triceps skin-fold thickness:
      i. At the midpoint of the nondominant upper arm (halfway between the tip of the shoulder and tip of the elbow), grasp skin and subcutaneous fat, pulling it away from the underlying muscle, and place the caliper jaws over the skin-fold flap.

Table 20-1   Body Mass Index (BMI)*

WEIGHT	5'	5'3"	5'6"	5'9"	6'	6'3"
140	27	25	23	21	19	18
150	29	27	24	22	20	19
160	31	28	26	24	22	20
170	33	30	28	25	23	21
180	35	32	29	27	25	23
190	37	34	31	28	26	24
200	39	36	32	30	27	25
210	41	37	34	31	29	26
220	43	39	36	33	30	28
230	45	41	37	34	31	29
240	47	43	39	36	33	30
250	49	44	40	37	34	31

*Body mass index = weight (kg)/height (m^2).

ii. Take the reading within 2 to 3 seconds and without using excessive pressure.

iii. Repeat the reading twice and take an average of the three readings to increase accuracy.

b. Subscapular skin-fold thickness: Grasp the skin and subcutaneous tissue just below the inferior border of the left scapula and measure with calipers, as noted.

7. Circumferential tests provide information on the amount of skeletal muscle and adipose tissue. Mid-upper arm circumference (MAC)—an indirect estimate of the body's muscle mass:

   a. Place a tape measure around the midpoint of the nondominant upper arm and secure it snugly.

b. To calculate, multiply the triceps skin fold by 3.14 and subtract the product from the MAC.

c. Adult standards are 16.5 mm for women and 12.5 mm for men.

Laboratory Tests

1. Serum albumin, prealbumin.

   a. Albumin is a protein made by the liver and is responsible for maintaining blood volume and serum electrolyte balance. The half-life of albumin is about 21 days. A decrease in nutritional status may result in a drop in albumin synthesis. However, in chronic malnutrition, serum albumin levels are typically normal or high.

   b. Prealbumin is also made by the liver and is a more sensitive but expensive test that measures more recent nutritional status. Its half-life is 2 to 3 days.

2. Hemoglobin—made by the liver; decreased amounts are related to iron-deficiency anemia or other defect in hemoglobin synthesis or dilution of the blood such as during pregnancy.

3. Serum transferrin—another transport protein made by the liver; responsible for binding iron to plasma and transporting it to the bone marrow. Reduced levels are found in catabolic states and some chronic diseases.

4. Twenty-four-hour urine creatinine—an increase in this measure indicates increased tissue breakdown.

5. Twenty-four-hour urine urea nitrogen or total urinary nitrogen—this test can be used to determine nitrogen balance.

NURSING ALERT Serum albumin, prealbumin, and transferrin levels measure visceral proteins that inversely correlate with metabolic stress, such as inadequate nutrition, but do not directly measure nutritional status.

General Procedures and Treatment Modalities

The inability to take nutrients through the oral route either totally or in part may require alternative means to enhance and maintain

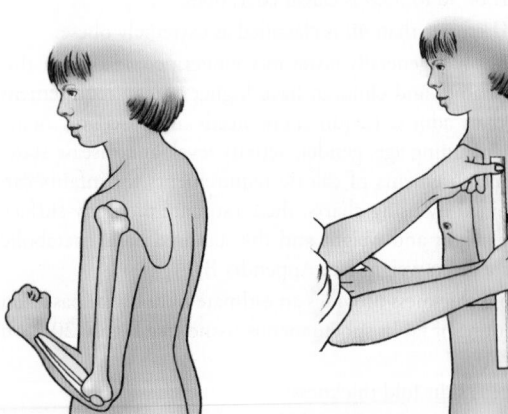
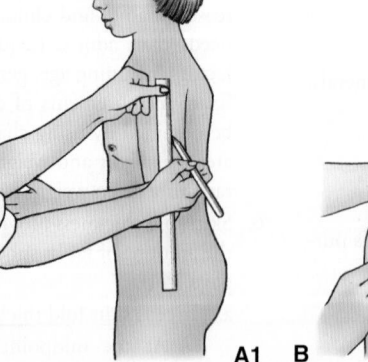
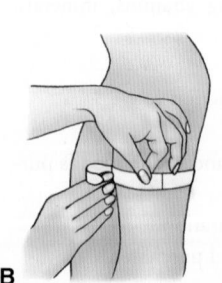
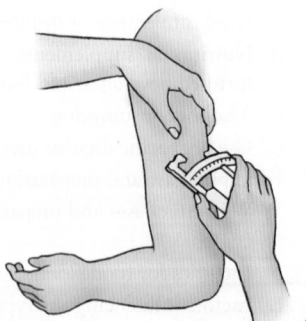

A   A1   B   C

Figure 20-2. Anthropometric measurements. (A) Marking the midpoint of the upper arm; **(B)** obtaining the mid–upper arm circumference; **(C)** measuring triceps skin-fold thickness.

nutritional status. Alternative methods of nutritional support include enteral feeding and parental nutrition. The decision as to which method is used will depend on many factors including the patient's acuity and nutritional status.

Enteral Feeding

See Procedure Guidelines 20-1.

Administration of nutrients directly into the stomach, duodenum, or jejunum through a tube is more physiologically beneficial and cost-effective than parenteral feeding. Enteral feeding carries less risk of infection than parenteral feeding and maintains a functional GI tract by preventing mucosal atrophy and biliary and hepatic dysfunction. Enteral therapy is appropriate for patients with at least a minimally functional GI tract who cannot take adequate nutrition by mouth.

Enteral therapy has become utilized more frequently as more commercially available enteral formulas have been developed and long-term enteral feeding tubes have become safer and more easily inserted.

Clinical Indications

1. Increased metabolic needs and inability to take adequate oral diet—trauma, burns, cancer, sepsis.
2. Coma or mechanical ventilation.

PROCEDURE GUIDELINES 20-1

Administration of Enteral (Tube) Feedings: Intermittent or Continuous

EQUIPMENT

- Tube feeding formula
- Graduated containers
- 60-mL catheter-tipped syringe
- Water

- Stethoscope
- Gavage feeding bag (optional)
- Gloves

For continuous tube feeding:
- Tube feeding bag and tubing and feeding pump

PROCEDURE

Nursing Action	Rationale
Preparatory phase	
1. Remove formula from refrigerator and allow to warm to room temperature. Check expiration date.	1. Room temperature formula is less likely to cause intolerance; use prepared dietary formulas within 24 hours.
2. Explain procedure to patient.	2. Promotes patient trust and allays patient anxiety.
3. Wash hands. Don gloves.	3. Prevents bacterial contamination of formula.
4. Protect patient from spillage.	4. Protects exposed areas of skin and/or clothing from damage with formula.
5. Shake formula container.	5. Shaking eliminates separation of formula.
6. Elevate head of bed 30 to 45 degrees.	6. Prevents aspiration.
7. Using the catheter-tipped syringe, inject 30 cc of air while listening with a stethoscope positioned at the epigastric area (for nasogastric [NG] tubes). For nasointestinal tubes, 20 mL of air may be injected, but auscultation site may be displaced laterally and inferiorly.	7. Auscultation of a "whooshing" or bubbling sound assists in confirmation of proper tube placement. Should patient burp immediately after injection of air, suspect esophageal placement of tube.
8. If NG tube is used, aspirate stomach contents to check gastric residual. Also observe the position of the tube in the nose or mouth to ensure proper placement.	8. If residual gastric contents exceed 200 mL for intermittent tube feedings, hold feeding and notify health care provider. Residual should not be obtained with intestinal placement.
9. If residual is within normal limits and stomach or intestinal placement has been confirmed, return gastric contents to stomach through syringe using gravity to assist flow. If residual is >200 mL, replace 200 mL and discard the rest. Flush tube with 30 mL of water. If there is a question about the tube placement, notify the health care provider and obtain an order for an x-ray.	9. Returning gastric contents to stomach prevents acidbase and electrolyte imbalance.
Performance phase	
1. For intermittent or bolus tube feeding, attach barrel of catheter-tipped syringe to pinched-off feeding tube.	1. Pinching off the feeding tube prevents air from entering the stomach and causing distention.
2. Fill catheter-tipped syringe with formula and allow fluid to flow in by gravity.	2. The rate of flow is regulated by raising or lowering the syringe.

(continued)

PROCEDURE GUIDELINES 20-1 (continued)

Administration of Enteral (Tube) Feedings: Intermittent or Continuous

PROCEDURE (continued)

Nursing Action	Rationale
3. Pour additional formula into barrel of syringe when it is three-quarters empty.	3. Prevents air from entering stomach.
4. After administering the prescribed amount of formula, flush tubing with at least 30 cc of water.	4. Prevents clogging of feeding tube.
5. If using a gavage bag for intermittent feeding, fill bag with prescribed amount of feeding, purge feeding bag tubing of air, attach distal end to feeding tube, and regulate to run over at least 10–20 minutes.	5. Prevents distention from air in stomach or too rapid administration.
6. For continuous tube feeding, fill bag with 4 hours of tube feeding (or prepare ready-to-hang container), flush tubing, attach to volume control infuser according to manufacturer's instructions, attach distal end to feeding tube, and start. Flush with 30–60 ml of water every 4 hours after first checking residual.	6. Prevents bacterial contamination. Maintains tube patency.
7. After intermittent feeding is completed, cover end of feeding tube with plug or clamp.	7. Prevents leakage.

Follow-up phase

1. Rinse equipment with warm water, and dry. Replace every 24 hours or per facility policy.	1. Limits bacterial contamination.
2. Maintain head of bed elevation for 30–60 minutes after feeding is completed. If continuous feeding, maintain head elevation continuously.	2. Prevents aspiration.
3. Document type and amount of feeding, amount of water given, and patient tolerance of procedure.	3. Ensures continuity of care. Sensation of fullness, nausea, or vomiting may indicate intolerance.
4. Monitor breath sounds, bowel sounds, gastric distention, diarrhea or constipation, intake and output, daily weight, and serum chemistry results.	4. Evaluates for aspiration, effect on GI system, and therapeutic effect of feedings.

GASTROSTOMY OR JEJUNOSTOMY CARE

Nursing Action	Rationale

Performance phase

1. Special care of ostomy tube insertion site should include:	1.
a. Cleaning around tube with prescribed cleansing solution every shift and as needed.	a. Prevent peristomal infection.
b. Applying sterile 4″ × 4″ gauze pad and taping in place.	b. Collects any drainage.
c. Applying skin barrier should peristomal skin become excoriated.	c. Prevent breakdown of peristomal tissue.
d. Taping of tube to skin or skin barrier with hypoallergenic tape.	d. Anchor and secure tube.

 Evidence Base Bankhead, R., Boullata, J., Brantley, S., et al. (2009). A.S.P.E.N. enteral nutrition practice recommendations. *Journal of Parenteral and Enteral Nutrition, 33*(2), 122–167.

3. Head/neck surgery.
4. Malabsorption.
5. Obstruction of esophagus or oropharynx.
6. Severe anorexia nervosa.
7. Dysphagia.

Sites of Tube Insertion

Short-Term Nutritional Support (<30 days)

1. Nasogastric (NG) feeding—tubes are passed through the nose or mouth (orogastric) into the stomach and secured in place.
   a. Tube placement must be verified by x-ray before use. Aspiration of contents for pH or auscultation of air injected through tube has been shown to be of limited value. New techniques that are available include colorimetric carbon dioxide detectors and electronic capnographics, both of which measure end-tidal carbon dioxide to determine if the tube has gone into the trachea.
   b. If there is a question about tube placement in the respiratory tract, the tube should be removed.
2. Nasoenteric feeding (ie, nasoduodenal or nasojejunal)—tube is passed through the nose into duodenum or jejunum and secured in place. X-ray is usually needed to verify correct tube placement.

Long-Term Nutritional Support (>30 days)

1. Gastrostomy—insertion of a tube surgically, radiologically, or by a percutaneous endoscopic procedure into the stomach.
2. Gastrostomy button—small device inserted through gastrostomy stoma to allow for long-term feeding with minimal effect on body image.
3. Jejunostomy—insertion of a tube directly into the jejunum either surgically or by a percutaneous endoscopic procedure. Jejunostomy feedings are generally by continuous infusion using a feeding pump.

Types of Tubes

1. Large-bore NG polyurethane tube—size 12 to 18F, used very short term (eg, Salem Sump).
2. Small-bore NG tube—made of polyurethane, silicone, or polyvinyl chloride with a tungsten-weighted tip or nonweighted tip, size 8 to 12F and 30 to 36 inches (76 to 91.5 cm) long.
3. Nasointestinal tube—made of silicone, polyurethane, or polyvinyl chloride with tungsten-weighted tip or a nonweighted tip, size 8 to 12F and 40 to 60 inches (101.5 to 152.5 cm) long.
4. Gastrostomy tube—catheter made of silicone, polyurethane, polyvinyl chloride, or latex; a balloon on the distal end to stabilize tube may be used and ranges from 5 to 30 mL capacity, size 14 to 28F. Adults usually have 20F tubes and children usually start with 14F.
5. Gastrostomy button—silicone; ranging from 18 to 28F and 1 inch (2.5 cm) long; useful for person wanting minimal alteration in body image.
6. Jejunostomy tube—size ranging from 5 to 14F with or without a balloon (a balloon may obstruct lumen of jejunum). A plain red rubber catheter is occasionally used as a short-term jejunostomy tube and some gastrostomy tubes may be used for jejunostomy.

Delivery Systems for Feeding Solution

1. Intermittent or continuous infusion of feeding solution by gravity is accomplished by hanging container of feeding solution from an intravenous (IV) pole and adjusting delivery rate by flow regulator.
2. Continuous feeding by controller feeding pump allows uniform flow, particularly of viscous solutions.
3. Bolus feeding involves enteral formula poured into barrel of a large (60 mL) syringe attached to a feeding tube and allowed to infuse by gravity.

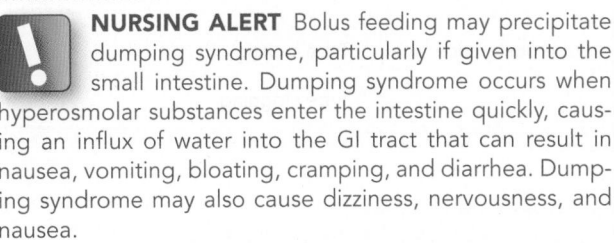

NURSING ALERT Bolus feeding may precipitate dumping syndrome, particularly if given into the small intestine. Dumping syndrome occurs when hyperosmolar substances enter the intestine quickly, causing an influx of water into the GI tract that can result in nausea, vomiting, bloating, cramping, and diarrhea. Dumping syndrome may also cause dizziness, nervousness, and nausea.

Community and Home Care Considerations

Teach patient and family:

1. Technique for administration of tube feeding outlined in Procedure Guidelines 20-1.
2. Signs and symptoms of potential complications.
3. Need to assess tube placement and residual before each feeding (for gastric feedings only).
4. Principles of medical asepsis, including careful handwashing, refrigeration of formula, cleaning of equipment with soap and water and thorough drying between feedings.
5. When the gastrostomy or jejunostomy tube insertion site is well healed, surrounding skin can be cleaned with soap and water.
6. Gauze dressing can be applied, as needed.
7. Leakage around tube or signs of peristomal skin irritation should be reported.

Complications

See Table 20-2.

Parenteral Nutrition

See Procedure Guidelines 20-2, pages 750 to 751.

Parenteral nutrition is the introduction of nutrients, including amino acids, lipids, dextrose, vitamins, minerals, and water, through a venous access device (VAD) directly into the intravascular fluid to provide nutrients required for metabolic functioning of the body.

Clinical Indications

1. Patient cannot tolerate enteral nutrition due to:
   a. Paralytic ileus.
   b. Intestinal obstruction.
   c. Acute pancreatitis and enteral feedings not possible.

Table 20-2 Complications of Enteral Feeding and Treatment

COMPLICATIONS	CAUSES	INTERVENTIONS
Tube displacement	Tube migration into esophagus	• Observe for eructation of air when injecting air to test for tube placement in stomach. • Aspirate gastric contents; if none is obtained, suspect esophageal placement.
	Tube placement into respiratory tract	• Observe for gagging, dyspnea, inability to speak, coughing when tube insertion attempted. • Obtain chest x-ray.* • Withdraw tube and attempt reinsertion with patient's head flexed forward.*
Tube obstruction	Tube kinking	• Obtain chest x-ray to confirm and withdraw and reinsert new tube.*
	Tube clogging	• Flush tube every 4 hours with 30 mL of water and after administration of intermittent feeding and medication administration. • Administer medications in liquid form if possible. Crush medications finely (if crushable). • Attempt to declog by administering water first. If unsuccessful, then administer pancreatic enzyme/bicarbonate mixture.
Aspiration	Patient lying flat	• Elevate HOB 30–45 degrees during continuous feedings or for 30–60 minutes after bolus feeds.
	Absent or depressed gag reflex	• Elevate HOB 30–45 degrees during continuous feedings or for 30–60 minutes after bolus feeds.
	Reflux	• Elevate HOB 30–45 degrees during continuous feedings or for 30–60 minutes after bolus feeds. • Administer proton pump inhibitor per MD's orders.
	Improper tube placement	• Confirm proper placement with x-ray imaging. • Tape tube in place.
Vomiting	Tube migration into esophagus	• See interventions for tube displacement above.
	Decreased absorption	• Auscultate for decreased bowel sounds, observe for abdominal distention. • Consider decreasing amount of tube feeding.* • Consider administration on a continuous basis.* • Consider placement of a small-bore, weighted-tip nasointestinal tube.*
	Rapid rate of infusion	• Administer no faster than 200–300 mL during 10–20 minutes. • Consider administration on a continuous basis.*
	Excessive infusion of air	• If giving a bolus feeding, pinch tubing off when refilling syringe with formula. • If giving continuous feeding, make certain bag does not empty before closing off tubing.
	Patient position	• Maintain patient at 30- to 45-degree angle of head elevation during and 30–60 minutes after feeding. If administering continuous feeding, maintain head elevation at all times.
	Nausea	• Anti-emetics.
	Obstruction	• Assess for distention and decreased bowel sounds; obtain x-ray.
	Constipation	• Assess for impaction and review frequency of bowel movements.

Table 20-2 Complications of Enteral Feeding and Treatment *(continued)*

COMPLICATIONS	CAUSES	INTERVENTIONS
Diarrhea	Drug therapy	• Evaluate drug regimen for possible causes of drug-induced diarrhea from antibiotics, elixirs with high osmolarity, elixirs with sorbitol, magnesium-containing antacids.
	High osmolarity of formula	• Begin administration of formula at slow rate.* • Consider continuous feeding rather than intermittent.*
	Lactose intolerance	• Administer lactose-free formula. (Few commercial formulas contain lactose.)
	Bacterial contamination of formula	• Change administration set daily or per facility protocol. • Maintain strict medical asepsis, including careful handwashing before administration of formula. • Allow formula to hang no longer than 8 hours (unless it is a "ready-to-hang" container that can hang for 24–48 hours).
	Rapid infusion rate	• Administer slowly; consider continuous rather than intermittent infusion.*
	Fecal impaction	• Manually clear the impaction.
	Clostridium difficile	• Administer antibiotics.
Constipation	Lack of fiber	• Ensure that patient is not impacted and administer formula with fiber.*
	Decreased fluid intake	• Increase intake of water.*
	Drug therapy	• Evaluate drug regimen for possible cause, including aluminum-containing antacids or lack of stool softener.
Hyperglycemia	Diabetes Impaired metabolism	• Monitor serum glucose, assess for dehydration caused by hyperosmotic diuresis; observe for symptoms of hyperglycemia, including polyuria, polydipsia. • Administer insulin.* • Observe for hypercapnia (increased respirations, elevated Pco_2).
Hypernatremia	Dehydration	• Assess for signs and symptoms of dehydration (I&O, daily weight, skin turgor, blood urea nitrogen, CVP, tachycardia, hypotension). • Rehydrate with extra water via the feeding tube or, if patient is severely hypernatremic, use IV route. • Rehydrate with D_5W or hypotonic saline solutions.*
Hyponatremia	Overhydration Excessive sodium loss (diaphoresis, nasogastric suction)	• Observe for signs and symptoms of hypervolemia (shortness of breath, rales, I&O, daily weight, peripheral edema, elevated CVP). • Observe for signs and symptoms of hyponatremia (lethargy, headaches, mental status change, nausea, vomiting, abdominal cramping). • Replace sodium, administer diuretics, or, depending on the cause of hypernatremia, restrict fluids.*
Hyperkalemia	Metabolic acidosis/renal insufficiency	• Observe for signs and symptoms of hyperkalemia (dysrhythmias, nausea, diarrhea, muscle weakness). • Treat underlying cause. • Administer exchange resin, glucose, and insulin.* • Choose lower potassium formula.
Hypokalemia	Diarrhea Refeeding syndrome	• See interventions for diarrhea. • If severe, replace potassium.*

Obtain orders from health care provider.
H_2, histamine; HOB, head of bed; I&O, intake & output; CVP, central venous pressure.

PROCEDURE GUIDELINES 20-2

Administration of Parenteral Nutrition

EQUIPMENT

- Volume control infuser
- Bag of parenteral nutrition (PN)
- Bag of IV lipids (if not using 3-in-1 nutrient admixture [NA])
- Administration tubing with Luer-lock connections

- 1.2 um filter for solutions containing albumin or lipids, 0.22 um filter for solutions without lipids
- Hypoallergenic tape, 1 inch
- Clean gloves

Sterile dressing kit to include:
- Alcohol swab sticks (3)
- Povidone-iodine sticks (3)
- Sterile gloves
- Transparent dressing

PROCEDURE

Nursing Action	Rationale
To change bag and bottle:	
Preparatory phase	
1. Remove NA from refrigerator at least 1 hour before hanging. Check date and patient's name.	1. Decreases incidence of hypothermia, pain, and venospasm.
2. Inspect fluid for cracking or creaming. Verify that PN/ NA matches current orders.	2. Indicates fluid separation, do not use. If infusing PN, solution should be clear without clouding.
3. Wash hands.	3. Prevents bacterial contamination.
Performance phase	
1. Using strict sterile technique, attach I.V. tubing (with filter) to NA bag and purge of air.	1. Prevents air embolus. *Note:* Tubing should be changed on a regular basis (every 2–3 days). Filter will be different for PN because lipids are not included.
2. Close all clamps on new tubing. Insert tubing into volume control infuser.	2. Prevents free flow of PN fluid.
3. If venous access device (VAD) has a clamp at proximal end, clamp tubing.	3. Prevents air embolus if VAD is inserted in a central vein.
4. If no clamp is available on central VAD, instruct patient to perform Valsalva's maneuver (bear down and hold breath) while new tubing is connected.	4. Valsalva maneuver creates positive pressure, preventing air from being sucked into tubing.
5. Sterilely connect tubing to hub of VAD, making sure the connection is securely fastened using Luer-lock connections.	5. Prevents disconnection of tubing.
6. Open all clamps and regulate flow through volume control infuser.	6. Ensures appropriate administration rate.
Follow-up phase	
1. Monitor administration hourly, assess integrity of fluid and administration system and patient tolerance and complications.	1. See Table 20-3, page 753, for complications of PN.
2. Document tubing change and rate of fluid administration, presence of complications, and any treatment given.	2. For continuity of care.
Patient education	
1. Teach patient signs and symptoms of complications, including sepsis, phlebitis, extravasation, and to report changes to nursing personnel.	1. Patient can assist nursing personnel in monitoring therapy and in detecting complications.
2. If patient is to be discharged to home with NA, begin instruction regarding proper storage, handling, and administration of NA. Include family members as appropriate.	2. Long-term therapy may be indicated in burns, emaciation due to cancer treatment, and other conditions. Home care nurses will reinforce your teaching.

PROCEDURE GUIDELINES 20-2 *(continued)*

Administration of Parenteral Nutrition

PROCEDURE *(continued)*

Nursing Action	Rationale
To change central venous catheter dressing:	
Preparatory phase	
1. Obtain equipment.	1. Have all equipment readily available.
2. Explain procedure to patient.	2. Allays anxiety and enlist cooperation.
3. Place patient in a comfortable supine position and turn head away from site.	3. Turning patient's head away from site will decrease possible microbial contamination of site.
4. Wash hands.	4. All precautions are taken to prevent contamination.
5. Put on mask (optional).	5. Helps prevent possible microbial contamination of site.
Performance phase	
1. Put on clean gloves and carefully remove old dressing.	1. Protects nurse from contamination.
2. Inspect insertion site for complications.	2. Observe for edema, erythema, tenderness, and leakage of fluid.
3. Clean insertion site with each alcohol swab beginning at insertion site and moving outward in a circular pattern.	3. Moves potential contaminants away from insertion site.
4. Repeat using each povidone-iodine swab.	4. Removes bacteria from insertion site.
5. Allow to dry.	5. Allows adhesive dressing to adhere securely.
6. Remove adhesive backing of transparent dressing. Center dressing over site.	6. Application of transparent dressing provides a bacterial barrier while allowing full visualization of insertion site.
7. Loop and tape tubing to skin using hypoallergenic tape. Do not tape over dressing.	7. Prevents dislodgment of tubing.
Follow-up phase	
1. Document dressing change and observation of insertion site.	1. For continuity of care.
2. Observe insertion site frequently for signs of complications.	2. Observe for edema, erythema, tenderness, and leakage of fluid.
Patient education	
1. Teach patient signs and symptoms of infection, phlebitis, and fluid extravasation and to report changes to nursing personnel.	1. Patient may be first to notice complications.
2. If patient is to be discharged to home with NA, begin instruction regarding sterile dressing change. Include family members as appropriate.	2. Because risk of sepsis is so great, sterile technique is still required for home dressing changes.

 Evidence Base Mirtallo, J. (2009). *Assessment tools and guidelines: Parenteral nutrition therapy.* New York: McMahon.

---

d. Severe malabsorption.

e. Persistent vomiting and jejunal route not possible.

f. Enterocutaneous fistula and enteric feeding not possible.

h. Inflammatory bowel disease.

i. Short bowel syndrome.

2. Hypermetabolic states for which enteral therapy is either not possible or inadequate, such as burns, trauma, or sepsis.

3. In these situations, additional components are added to the enteral therapy or individualized solutions are developed to meet the nutritional needs of the patient.

Methods of Parenteral Nutrition

Total Nutrient Admixture

1. Given through a central vein, commonly into the superior vena cava, total nutrient admixture (TNA) is a parenteral

formula that combines carbohydrates in the form of a concentrated (20% to 70%) dextrose solution; proteins in the form of amino acids (3% to 15%); lipids in the form of an emulsion (10% to 30%), including triglycerides, egg phospholipids, glycerol, and water; and vitamins and minerals.

2. Central TNA is indicated for patients requiring parenteral feeding for 7 or more days.

Peripheral Parenteral Nutrition

1. Given through a peripheral vein, this parenteral formula combines a less concentrated dextrose solution with amino acids, vitamins, minerals, and lipids.

2. Unlike TNA given centrally, peripheral parenteral nutrition provides fewer calories and, occasionally, a larger percentage of calories is supplied by lipids rather than by carbohydrates.

3. Indicated for patients requiring parenteral nutrition for fewer than 7 days who do not already have enteral access.

Total Parenteral Nutrition

1. Total parenteral nutrition (TPN) combines dextrose, amino acids, vitamins, and minerals and is given through a central IV line.

2. If lipids are needed, they are given intermittently or mixed with the TPN solution through a central IV line.

Fat Emulsion (Lipids)

1. Ten percent, 20%, or 30% emulsion composed of triglycerides, egg phospholipids, glycerol, and water. It also contains vitamin K.

2. May be given centrally or peripherally.

Complications

See Table 20-3 on page 753.

Delivery Systems for Parenteral Nutrition

1. Central VADs:
   a. Insertion of long-term VADs, such as Hickman, Broviac, or Groshong catheters.
   b. Peripherally inserted central catheters (peripherally inserted central catheter lines) may be used.
   c. If multilumen, these VADs can allow concomitant administration of TNA and other solutions, including medications or blood, each running through a separate lumen.

2. Peripheral IV access:
   a. Insertion of an angiocatheter into a vein in the arm or leg.
   b. Midline catheters of longer length and with the ability to remain in place for more than 3 days.

3. Delivery of parenteral nutrition should be controlled by a volume control infuser.

4. Filters should be used whenever possible.
   a. A 0.22-micron filter may be used for TPN (without added fat emulsion).
   b. A 1.2-micron filter may be used for TNA or fat emulsion.

NUTRITIONAL DISORDERS

Nutritional disorders can have a negative impact on the health and well-being of a person. In addition, some nutritional disorders may in turn lead to the development of other diseases or health issues. If not identified and treated in a timely fashion, these disorders can have a devastating effect.

Obesity

Obesity is a local, national, and global epidemic that impacts all ages, religions, socioeconomic classes, and both genders. *Obesity* is an overabundance of body fat and is typically measured by a person's BMI (weight in kilograms divided by height in meters squared). A BMI greater than 30 is considered obese. About 32.9% of Americans are obese (up from 15% in 1976–1980) with 72% of men and 64% of women either overweight or obese.

 Evidence Base Flegal, K. M., Carroll, M. D., Ogden, C. L., et al. (2010). Prevalence and trends in obesity among U.S. adults, 1999–2008. *Journal of the American Medical Association*, 303(3), 235–241.

Pathophysiology and Etiology

Increasing evidence reveals that obesity is a multifactorial disease and may be the result of several different factors. Such factors may include:

1. Heredity and genetic factors.
   a. Identical twins raised separately are more likely to have similar amounts of body fat than are fraternal twins raised separately.
   b. Genetic defects in certain disorders such as Bardet-Biedl syndrome and Prader-Willi syndrome can directly cause obesity.

2. Environmental factors.
   a. Some evidence shows that children reared by obese parents have an increased tendency toward obesity.
   b. Increased availability of high-fat, high-calorie foods.
   c. Reduction in physical activity.
   d. Modern-day conveniences (ie, riding lawnmowers, escalators, elevators, etc.).

3. Psychological factors.
   a. Depression.
   b. Anxiety.
   c. Anger.
   d. Posttraumatic stress.
   e. Boredom.

4. Physiologic factors.
   a. Endocrine abnormalities (rare causes of obesity)—Cushing's syndrome, polycystic ovary syndrome, hypothyroidism, hypogonadism, or hypothalamic lesions.
   b. Age—advancing age may be associated with obesity, usually due to changes in activity level and metabolic rate, or in women because of hormonal changes; early childhood and the start of puberty may also be associated with obesity.

5. Pharmacologic factors.
   a. Corticosteroids.
   b. Antidepressants.
   c. Hormones and other medications.

Table 20-3 Complications of Total Parenteral Nutrition and Treatment

COMPLICATIONS	CAUSES	INTERVENTIONS
Sepsis	• High glucose content of fluid • Venous access device contamination	• Monitor temperature, white blood cell count, insertion site for signs and symptoms of infection. • Maintain strict surgical asepsis when changing dressing and tubing. • Consider removal of venous access device with replacement in alternate site.* • If blood cultures positive, consider institution of antibiotic therapy.*
Electrolyte imbalance	• Iatrogenic • Effect of underlying diseases (ie, fistula, diarrhea, vomiting) • Blood sample contaminated by parenteral nutrition	• Monitor electrolyte levels at least daily initially. • Monitor signs and symptoms of electrolyte imbalance. • Treat underlying cause.* • Change concentration of electrolytes in total parenteral nutrition (TPN) as necessary to address blood levels.*
Hyperglycemia	• Insufficient insulin secretion • High glucose content of fluid • Blood sample contaminated by parenteral nutrition	• Monitor blood glucose frequently. • Administer exogenous insulin per addition to TPN, subcutaneously or through a separate IV drip.* • Decrease glucose content of fluid if warranted.*
Hypoglycemia	• Abrupt discontinuation of parenteral nutrition administered through a central vessel	• Reduce rate of parenteral nutrition by 50% × 2 hours, then discontinue. • If TPN/peripheral parenteral nutrition must be stopped abruptly, hang a separate dextrose solution if insulin has been administered.
Hypervolemia	• Iatrogenic • Underlying disease (ie, heart failure, renal failure)	• Monitor intake and output, daily weights, central venous pressure (CVP), breath sounds, peripheral edema. • Consider administering more concentrated solution.*
Hyperosmolar diuresis	• High osmolarity of parenteral nutrition	• Monitor intake and output, daily weights, CVP. • Consider decreasing concentration or increasing amount of fluid administered.*
Hepatic dysfunction	• IV nutrition	• Monitor liver function tests, triglyceride levels, presence of jaundice. • Consider alteration in macronutrients.*
Hypercapnia	• Excessive calorie delivery	• Consider reducing total calories.*
Lipid intolerance	• Low birth weight or premature neonate • History of liver disease • History of elevated triglycerides	• Monitor for bleeding (check stools for occult blood, coagulation studies, platelet levels). • Monitor oxygen levels for impaired oxygenation. • Monitor for fat overload syndrome: monitor triglyceride levels and liver function tests, hepatosplenomegaly, decreased coagulation, cyanosis, dyspnea. • Monitor allergic reaction: nausea, vomiting, headache, chest pain, back pain, fever. • Administer lipid-containing solutions slowly initially, while observing for symptoms.
Lipid particulate aggregation	• Unstable mixture of dextrose solution with lipid emulsion	• Observe for cracking or creaming of fluid and discontinue use of fluid with these characteristics.

*Obtain orders from health care provider.

Clinical Manifestations

1. BMI greater than 30, depending on body composition.
2. Increased weight is correlated with increased incidence of comorbid conditions.
   a. Cardiovascular disease.
   b. Type 2 diabetes mellitus.
   c. Hypertension.
   d. Obstructive sleep apnea.
   e. Osteoarthritis.
   f. Gastroesophageal reflux disease.
   g. Gallbladder disease.
   h. Cancer of the breast, endometrium, prostate, and colon.
   i. Stroke.
   j. Dyslipidemia.
   k. Stress urinary incontinence.
   l. Infertility.
   m. Depression (may be a cause of obesity as well as caused by obesity).

3. Metabolic syndrome (insulin resistance syndrome)—a group of characteristics that when co-occur increase the risk of coronary artery disease, stroke, and type 2 diabetes.
   a. Obesity.
   b. Hypertension.
   c. Insulin resistance.
   d. High triglycerides.

Diagnostic Evaluation

1. Nutritional assessment—a systematic method for obtaining, verifying, and interpreting data needed to identify nutrition-related problems and their causes and significance.
2. Anthropometric and physical assessment—to evaluate increased body fat and effects of obesity on body.
3. Selected hormonal studies (thyroid, adrenal)—to assess for potential underlying cause.

Management

Conservative Measures

1. Diet therapy—has been controversial, but a well-balanced diet containing all the major food groups is still advised and recommended as a first-step therapy.
   a. A 1,000-calorie deficit per day is required to lose 2.2 lb (1 kg) of body weight per week.
   b. Diet therapy should be individualized to the patient; however, the overall goal is to create a calorie deficit through reduced calorie intake or increased calorie expenditure.
   c. A balance of food groups is essential to maintain vitamin and nutrient balance. Nutrient supplementation may be necessary (calcium, vitamin D, iron, B₆, zinc, and folate).
   d. Food preparation should include seasoning with herbs, onion, garlic, and pepper, and foods should be baked, broiled, steamed, or sautéed using minimal oil.
   e. Food attractively arranged on smaller plates, using whole rather than processed foods and eaten slowly, will assist the overall process.
   f. Eliminating entire food groups from the diet, such as carbohydrates (in many popular protein- and fat-based diets), will eventually result in craving of those foods eliminated, disruption of normal metabolic processes, and quick weight gain when the food is added to the diet.
2. Exercise—Regular physical activity is an important component in weight loss and weight maintenance along with reduced caloric intake. In addition, physical activity may add other health benefits if done on a regular basis such as improved cardiovascular status and emotional well-being.
3. Behavior modification is a cornerstone of any successful diet.
   a. Identify and eliminate situations or cues leading to over-eating or high-calorie foods with use of a food diary.
   b. Provide positive reinforcement of proper dietary habits.
   c. Should a lapse in diet habits occur, focus on a prompt and positive return to appropriate dietary habits.
   d. Stress-reduction techniques, such as visual imagery or progressive muscle relaxation; peer support may be helpful.

Pharmacotherapy

1. Anorexia medications include amphetamines, sympatho-mimetics, and norepinephrine-releasing agents or reuptake inhibitors; reduce appetite and stimulate weight loss initially.
   a. However, tolerance may develop and weight may be regained when the drugs are discontinued.
   b. Numerous long-term studies have failed to show long-term success with these agents.
2. Phentermine products are available in prescription form and primarily act on chemicals in the brain to decrease appetite. Phentermine products also have a stimulant component and should not be used in uncontrolled hypertension, advanced heart disease, history of drug abuse, or with monoamine oxidase (MAO) inhibitors.
3. Phentermine-topiramate extended release is a newly FDA approved drug available in prescription form. This drug combines the effects of phentermine with the weight loss effects of topiramate (a medication used to treat seizures).
4. Lorcaserin works on the chemicals in the brain to help decrease appetite. Although this medication is FDA approved, it is not yet available.
5. Orlistat, a pancreatic lipase inhibitor, blocks the breakdown of fat in the GI system; about 30% of dietary fat is eliminated.
   a. Adverse effects include oily or fatty stool, flatulence, and GI distress.
   b. Long-term safety of the drug has not been determined, but addition of a fat-soluble vitamin supplement (vitamins A, D, E, and K and beta carotene) taken 1 hour before or 2 hours after orlistat will prevent a theoretical vitamin deficiency.
   c. Should not be used in cases of cholestasis or malabsorption.
   d. Orlistat is available over the counter in a lower dosage than originally prescribed.
   e. These medications are only adjunct to diet and exercise therapy.
6. Several other medications used to treat depression, seizures, and/or diabetes have been prescribed off-label to help promote weight loss. These medications have not been approved by the FDA for the treatment of obesity:
   a. Bupropion—an antidepressant medication.
   b. Topiramate—an anticonvulsant medication.
   c. Zonisamide—an anticonvulsant medication.
   d. Metformin—an oral medication used to treat diabetes.
7. Sibutramine is no longer available in the United States due to studies that identified an increased risk of developing cardiovascular events such as heart attack or stroke.

Bariatric Surgery

Numerous surgical procedures have been used to help treat obesity and metabolic disorders. Although gastric bypass has been considered the gold standard for years, many new surgical treatment options have emerged, lending to a greater availability of treatment options (see Figure 20-3). These surgical therapies are generally reserved for extremely obese patients who cannot lose weight and maintain weight loss through the above therapies. Bariatric surgery has proven to be a safe and effective means for weight loss when performed by an experienced surgeon within a multidisciplinary center. In addition to the anatomical and mechanical changes created by the various procedures, there is increasing evidence of metabolic or hormonal changes that lead to weight loss. Metabolic/hormonal changes seen with these surgeries include a decrease in

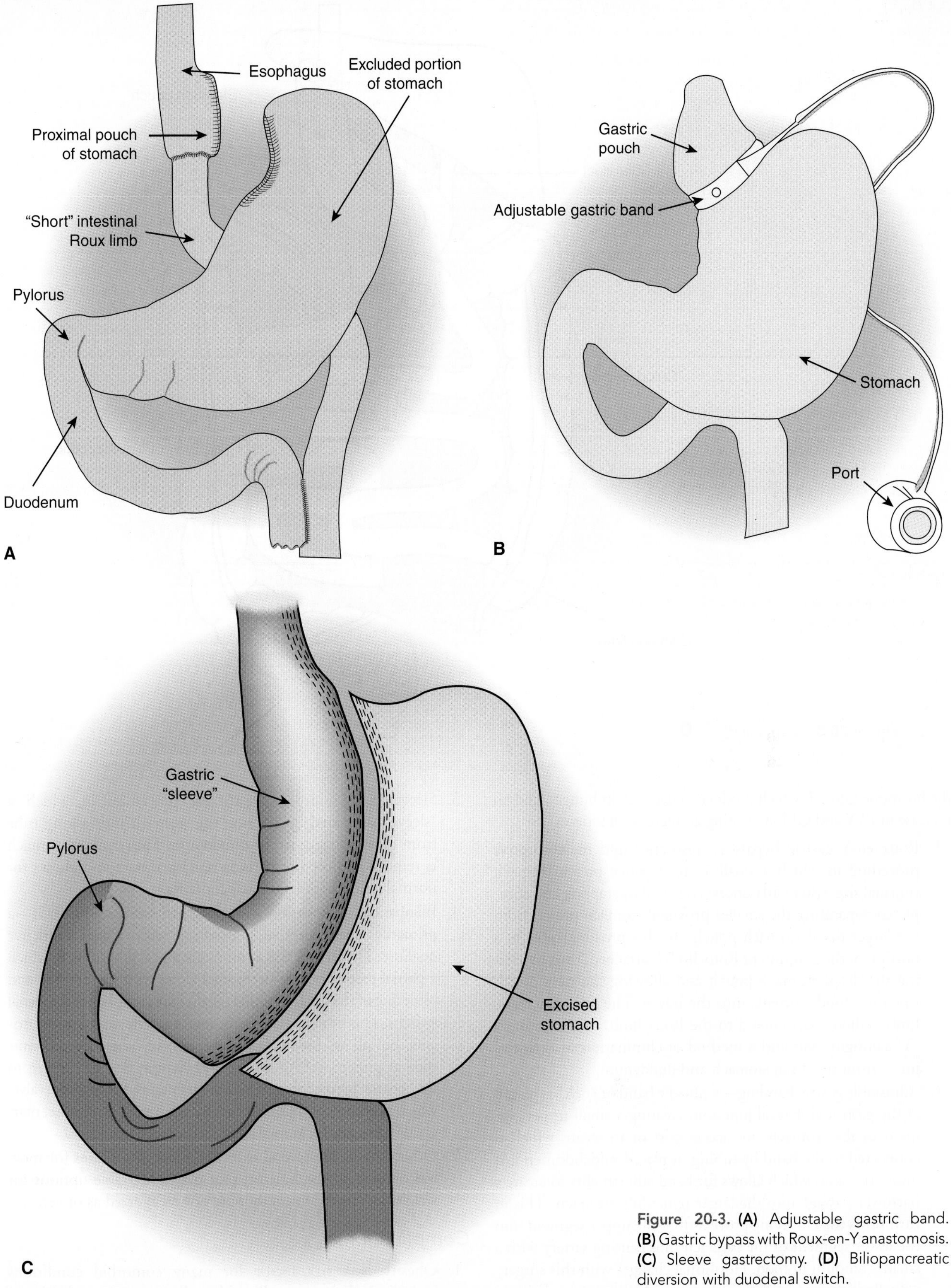

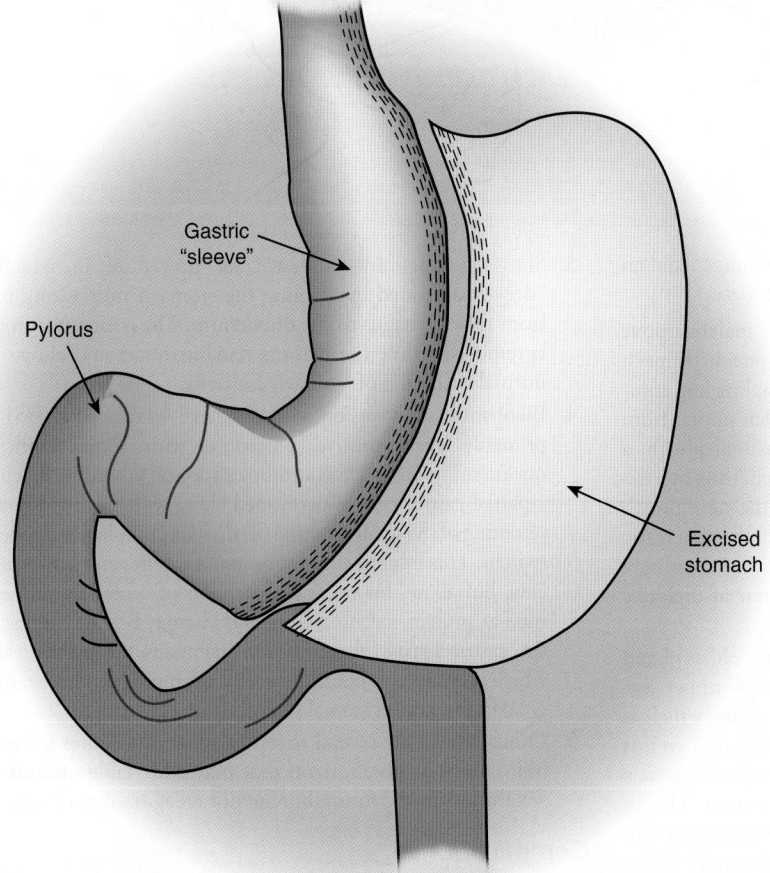

A

Esophagus

Excluded portion of stomach

Proximal pouch of stomach

"Short" intestinal Roux limb

Pylorus

Duodenum

B

Gastric pouch

Adjustable gastric band

Stomach

Port

C

Gastric "sleeve"

Pylorus

Excised stomach

Figure 20-3. (A) Adjustable gastric band. **(B)** Gastric bypass with Roux-en-Y anastomosis. **(C)** Sleeve gastrectomy. **(D)** Biliopancreatic diversion with duodenal switch.

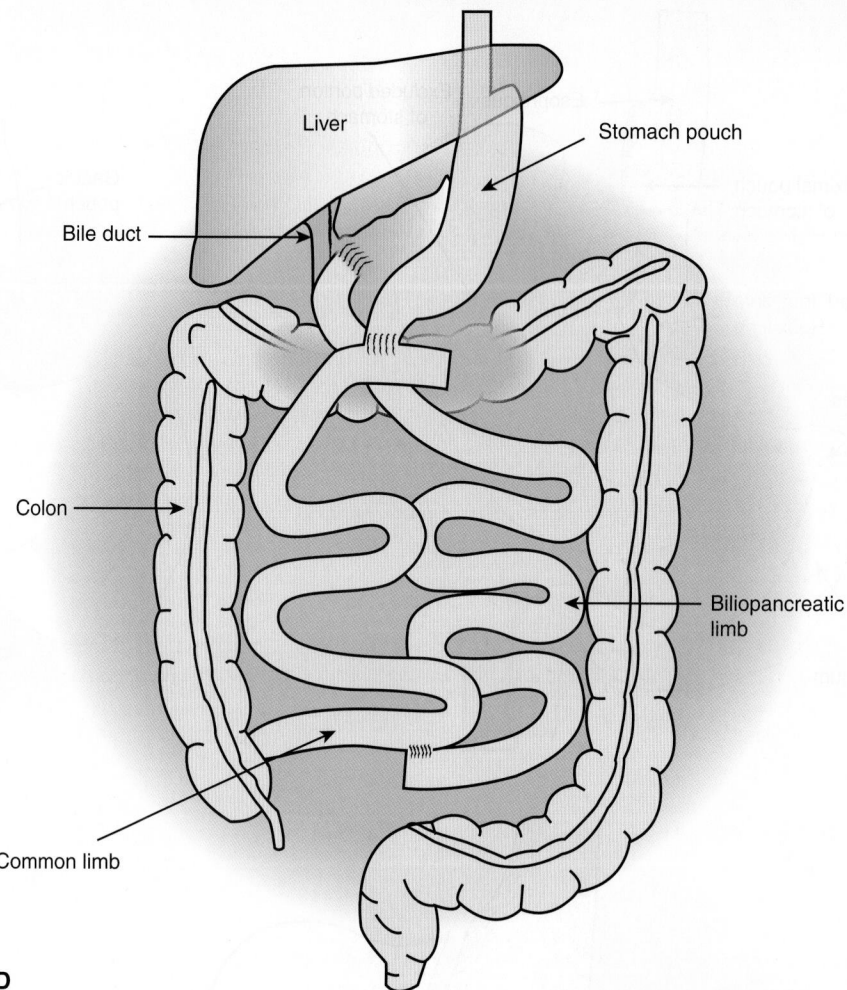

Figure 20-3. *(Continued)* **D**

the hormone Ghrelin which produces a decrease in hunger, and an increase in PYY and GLP-1 creating an increase in satiety.

1. Roux en-Y gastric bypass—a restrictive and malabsorptive procedure in which a small 1- to 2-ounce pouch/stomach (normal size = 30 to 50 ounces) is created by stapling and completely separating the smaller proximal stomach pouch from the larger distal stomach pouch. To this proximal pouch, a portion of the jejunum or Roux limb is attached, thus bypassing the distal stomach pouch and allowing the new pouch to empty food contents into the bowel. The biliopancreatic limb is then anastomosed to the Roux limb, thus creating a "Y" configuration and a method of elimination of digestive juices from the distal stomach and duodenum.

2. Adjustable gastric banding—a silicone band or "belt" is placed at the gastroesophageal junction, creating a small upper segment of the stomach. An access port or reservoir, which is connected to the band by tubing, is placed midabdomen just under the skin, which allows for band adjustments to create a narrower passage into the larger remaining stomach. This in turn slows the emptying process from the upper segment into the lower segment of the stomach thus causing satiety with a smaller amount of food. Hormonal changes with this surgery actually increase Ghrelin production which increases hunger.

3. Sleeve gastrectomy—a restrictive procedure in which a "sleeve" is created by stapling the stomach into a long tube from the esophagus to the duodenum. The remnant stomach is removed, while the pylorus remains intact and allows for normal emptying of stomach contents.

4. Biliopancreatic diversion with duodenal switch (BPD/DS)—a primarily malabsorptive procedure with some restrictive qualities. The BPD/DS is a complex surgical procedure in which a partial gastrectomy is performed along with the division and rerouting of the small intestine (ie, duodenum—hence duodenal switch). This inhibits the absorption of calories and some nutrients, but allows for normal absorption of other key nutrients such as protein, calcium, iron, and vitamin B$_{12}$. In contrast to the gastric bypass, the BPD/DS maintains the pyloric valve, which prevents complications such as dumping syndrome, marginal ulcers, and/or stomal stenosis from occurring.

5. Other—there are several investigational procedures for morbid obesity on the horizon that may add viable options for weight loss in the future but are not recognized as of yet.

Complications

1. Obesity is a risk factor for many comorbid conditions including diabetes, gallbladder disease, osteoarthritis of

weight-bearing joints, hypertension, CAD, obstructive sleep apnea, metabolic syndrome, and so on.

2. Obesity has become a global health issue affecting both rich and poor countries. Current global estimates find that nearly 500 million adults are obese, with a projected increase to 1 billion obese adults by 2030.

3. Vitamin and mineral deficiencies because of surgical intervention, severely restricted diet, or noncompliance with recommended regimen.
   a. A moderate, well-balanced weight reduction diet will generally not cause deficiencies, although a multiple vitamin/mineral supplement may be used.
   b. A low-calorie diet (fewer than 800 to 1,000 calories per day) will require careful monitoring and vitamin/mineral supplements.
   c. Complications of bariatric surgery may include marginal ulcers, anastomotic leaks, fistulas, infection, pulmonary emboli, chronic nausea and vomiting, vitamin D and B_{12} deficiency, thiamine, copper, and iron deficiency. A daily vitamin and mineral supplement is necessary.

Nursing Assessment

1. Obtain a complete nutritional assessment (may be in collaboration with a registered dietitian).
2. Assess behavioral and emotional components of eating, coping mechanisms, and past successes and failures with dieting.

Nursing Diagnoses

- Imbalanced Nutrition: More Than Body Requirements related to high-calorie, high-fat diet, and limited exercise.
- Deficient Fluid Volume related to weight loss surgery.
- Readiness for Enhanced Self-Concept related to appearance and weight.

Nursing Interventions

Modifying Nutritional Intake

1. Assist patient in assessing current dietary habits and identifying poor dietary habits.
2. Assist patient in developing appropriate diet plan based on likes and dislikes, activity level, and lifestyle.
3. Suggest behavior-modification strategies, such as exercise (ie, walking) during lunch break, preventing access to quick snacks, eating only at mealtimes at the table.
4. Provide emotional support to patient during weight-reduction efforts through positive reinforcement and creative problem solving.
5. Provide patient with alternative coping mechanisms, including stress-reduction techniques such as progressive relaxation and guided imagery.
6. Assess patient's ability to tolerate exercise through measurement of vital signs before, during, and after exercise and ask about symptoms of shortness of breath and chest pain.
7. Discourage fad dieting.

Preventing Complications Postoperatively

1. Provide initial postoperative care as for gastrointestinal surgery (see page 657).
2. Administer IV fluids, as directed. Record intake and output.

3. Start oral fluids per surgeon's protocol (this will vary from facility to facility and surgeon to surgeon). General progression for most patients will be to start with small sips and gradually advance to larger sips of clear liquids.
4. Advance diet as per surgeon's protocol. Confirmation of the bariatric diet stages with the facility's bariatric program and/or surgeon is crucial, as this will vary from facility to facility and surgeon to surgeon.
5. Observe for and report increased abdominal pain, distention, or alteration in abdominal drain output (if utilized), which may indicate leakage or bleeding at anastomosis or staple sites or obstruction.
6. Monitor vital signs and wound for signs of wound infection and dehiscence.
7. Watch for and report signs of dehydration (thirst, oliguria, dry mucous membranes) and hypokalemia (muscle weakness, anorexia, nausea, decreased bowel sounds, and dysrhythmias).
8. Warn patient that overeating may cause vomiting, painful esophageal distention, and/or dumping syndrome. Dumping syndrome may also occur with food products that are high in fat or high in sugar.
9. Stress the importance of good dietary habits and behavior modification to lose weight because bariatric surgery is only an adjunct to treatment.
10. Encourage close, long-term follow-up for monitoring of weight loss and nutritional status. Additional long-term complications may include marginal ulcers, hernias, strictures, and/or malnutrition.

Strengthening Self-Concept

1. Direct patient education and conversation in a nonjudgmental manner.
2. Get to know patient and point out the positive aspects of patient's health and well-being.
3. Encourage patient to make change in weight for the positive health aspects, not just for cosmetic reasons.
4. Be a good role model—show a healthy attitude toward sensible eating, exercise, and other healthy practices.
5. Be sensitive to discrimination, behaviors, and attitudes toward obese people.

Patient Education and Health Maintenance

1. Discuss fat, carbohydrate, and protein, their inclusion in common foods, and their calories per gram.
2. Describe the five basic food groups and their placement in the MyPlate plan.
3. Explain the purpose of a balanced diet and the need for vitamins and minerals from food sources; supplement needed following bariatric surgery.
4. Review the health hazards of obesity.
5. Advise patient of plateau period that may occur without weight loss for some time, but advise patient not to get discouraged.
6. Tell patient to keep a food diary to show to nutritionist and to weigh self no more than once per week.
7. If patient is interested in liquid diets or herbal supplements to lose weight, encourage discussion with health care provider. Some preparations may contain ephedra, a powerful stimulant that may cause increased BP, significant adverse effects, and many drug interactions.

8. Refer to such organizations as Obesity Action Coalition (*www.obesityaction.org*) and the National Institutes of Diabetes and Digestive and Kidney Disease: Weight-control Information Network (*http://win.niddk.nih.gov/publications/gastric.htm*) for further information on weight loss options.

Evaluation: Expected Outcomes

- Loses 10–15% excess body weight during the first month.
- No abdominal distention, nausea or vomiting, or wound infection.
- Verbalizes feeling good about self, secondary to change in diet and exercise habits.

Anorexia Nervosa

Anorexia nervosa is an eating disorder characterized by self-induced weight loss greater than 15% of normal weight for age and height and is associated with many factors including psychological and endocrine abnormalities. Anorexia usually begins during the teen years or young adulthood and is more common in females. The disorder is characterized by periods of starvation and may be mixed with episodes of binging and purging.

Pathophysiology and Etiology

1. A semistarvation state with glucose and protein sparing, fat utilization, endocrine changes, and fluid and electrolyte disturbances is induced, causing:
   a. Loss of fat stores.
   b. Decreased protein synthesis.
   c. Hypothalamic or pituitary dysfunction—decrease in follicle-stimulating hormone (FSH), luteinizing hormone (LH), and estrogen.
   d. Decrease in thyroid hormone.
   e. Decrease in catecholamines.
2. The biopsychosocial etiologic components are not well known but seem to play a significant role in this disease and vary from one person to the next.
   a. Biological or genetic predisposition remains unclear.
   b. Psychological components.
      i. Distorted body image.
      ii. Intense fear of gaining weight or becoming fat.
      iii. Self-esteem dependent on body image.
      iv. Ability to achieve weight loss viewed as a sign of self-control.
      v. Denial of problem.
   c. Social influences.
      i. Most patients are between ages 14 and 24 and 90% are female.
      ii. Seen most commonly in the middle- and upper-class social strata.
      iii. Patients may relate high family expectations.
      iv. Frequent peer and social pressure to strive toward an esthetic of thinness.

Clinical Manifestations

1. Symptoms vary widely and are commonly dependent on the severity of illness.
2. Physical signs and symptoms include loss of adipose tissue and weight loss of greater than 15% of ideal body weight, bradycardia, hypotension, cold intolerance, hypothermia, dry skin, thinning scalp hair, lanugo, amenorrhea for 3 consecutive months, decreased libido, constipation, and abdominal pain.
3. Psychological manifestations include perfectionistic or obsessive–compulsive behavior with high performance expectations, anxiety, increased exercise activity, inhibited or destructive social interactions, sleep disturbance, depression, and diminished sexual interest.

Diagnostic Evaluation

1. Serum chemistry may show electrolyte imbalances that may be life-threatening (decreased chloride, potassium, phosphate, magnesium, zinc levels); increased blood urea nitrogen (BUN), creatinine, liver function tests, bicarbonate, amylase; and decreased albumin levels.
2. Hormone studies may show decreased LH, FSH, estrogen, testosterone (in men), and thyroid hormone and decreased response to LH-releasing hormone.
3. Complete blood count may show decreased white blood cells and hematocrit, indicating starvation's effect on immunity and anemia.
4. Electrocardiogram to detect dysrhythmias or signs of electrolyte imbalance.
5. Urinalysis may show ketonuria.

Management

A multidisciplinary clinical approach including nurses, nutritionists, psychologists, and physicians who specialize in treating patients with eating disorders is most effective.

1. Dietary modification to achieve gradual weight gain and normal eating habits.
2. Enteral or parenteral feeding may be necessary if prescribed diet cannot be maintained by patient and physical status warrants. Enteral feeding is preferred and is used more frequently.
3. Individual counseling focuses on patient's need to control weight, alteration in body image, and associated diagnoses, including depression and suicidal ideation.
4. Antidepressants and other pharmacologic agents for associated psychiatric problems may be tried.
5. Inpatient treatment (preferably on specialized eating disorder unit) is recommended if weight is less than 75% ideal; marked orthostatic hypotension; bradycardia less than 40; sustained tachycardia greater than 100; inability to maintain core body temperature of 98.6° F (37° C); suicidal or no response to outpatient therapy.

Complications

1. Severe electrolyte disturbances, especially hypokalemia; dehydration; and anemia.
2. Cardiac dysrhythmias, hypotension, cardiac arrest.
3. Seizures due to fluid loss from frequent diarrhea and vomiting.
4. Increased risk of infection related to a decrease in white blood cells.
5. Severe malnutrition.

6. Amenorrhea and other endocrine dysfunctions.
7. Comorbid psychiatric conditions, such as depression, anxiety disorders, and high risk for suicide.

Nursing Assessment

1. Obtain detailed dietary history and complete review of systems, including psychological, gynecologic, endocrine, GI systems, activities of daily living, and exercise history.
2. Perform physical examination, including vital signs, height and weight, heart rate and rhythm, bowel sounds, and observation for hematemesis and dental caries (which may indicate self-induced vomiting).

Nursing Diagnoses

- Imbalanced Nutrition: Less Than Body Requirements related to self-restricted intake.
- Disturbed Body Image related to weight.
- Risk for Suicide related to psychological distress.

Nursing Interventions

Promoting Weight Gain

1. Monitor daily intake and output and weight (before breakfast).
2. Assess bowel function. Promote fluids and activity to prevent constipation if the patient cannot tolerate food high in fiber.
3. Encourage small, frequent meals or snacks of high-calorie foods and beverages. Liquid nutritional supplements may be best tolerated.
4. Provide positive reinforcement for improved intake and weight gain.

Fostering a Healthy Body Image

1. Establish a trusting relationship and provide for patient's safety and security needs.
2. Be alert for lying and manipulation that patient may display to preserve control.
3. Involve patient in the treatment plan, offering choices to increase patient's sense of control.
4. Encourage patient to verbalize feelings about body image, self-concept, fears, and frustrations.
5. Emphasize the importance of counseling, stress management, assertiveness training, and other therapies.

Preventing Suicide

1. Assess level of risk by obtaining history of past suicide attempts, recent suicidal thoughts, and current ideation, plan, and possible method.
2. Maintain level of observance called for by situation.
3. Make sure that access to sharp objects is prohibited.
4. Make sure that a crisis intervention team is on call, if needed.

Patient Education and Health Maintenance

1. Teach principles of nutrition and healthful diet and eating habits. Discuss food matter-of-factly to avoid reinforcing patient's preoccupation with food.
2. Teach the effect of starvation on both physiologic and psychological functioning.
3. Involve patient's family and significant others in the treatment plan, as appropriate.
4. Describe the dangers of using laxatives and diuretics in weight control, such as electrolyte imbalances, dehydration, and bowel atony.
5. Refer to such agencies as American Anorexia-Bulimia Association (*www.aba.org*).

Evaluation: Expected Outcomes

- Gains 1 lb (0.5 kg) during first week.
- Verbalizes satisfaction with body image and weight.
- Denies suicidal thoughts.

Bulimia Nervosa

Bulimia nervosa is an eating disorder characterized by recurrent episodes of binge eating and a feeling of loss of control over eating behavior during these episodes, The binging episodes lead to self-disgust and are typically followed by inappropriate methods to prevent weight gain, including self-induced vomiting, excessive use of laxatives, diuretics, fasting, or excessive exercise. Eating binges may occur as often as several times per day and be present for many months. Although the exact cause of bulimia is not known, it appears that many different factors such as genetics, trauma, family, society, and cultural factors may all play a role. Psychological factors, such as self-image, are significantly influenced by body weight and shape.

Pathophysiology and Etiology

1. Onset of illness typically occurs in late adolescence or early 20s and is approximately 10 times more common in young women than in young men.
2. Bulimia may be associated with a personal or family history of obesity, substance abuse, depression, anxiety, or mood disorders.
3. Self-induced vomiting may result in electrolyte imbalance (hypokalemia, hyponatremia, hypochloremia, elevated bicarbonate), esophageal tears, gastric rupture, and/or poor dental hygiene.
4. Starvation and its physiologic effects may be as evident as they are in anorexia nervosa.

Clinical Manifestations

1. The course of the disease may be chronic or intermittent during many years.
2. Weight is usually maintained within normal range or may be significantly elevated or decreased.
3. Binge eating may be followed by inappropriate compensatory mechanisms, including self-induced vomiting, self-induced diarrhea through the use of laxatives or cathartics, the use of diuretics, excessive fasting, and excessive exercise.
4. Physical signs may include calluses or skin changes on hands and fingers, loss of dental enamel, swollen lymph nodes, and bad breath or mouthwash smell on breath because of self-induced vomiting.
5. Endocrine changes, such as amenorrhea, may be present.

Diagnostic Evaluation

1. Serum chemistry for electrolytes, BUN, and creatinine and bicarbonate—may be abnormal, indicating fluid and electrolyte imbalances.
2. Additional tests may include thyroid function tests, LH, FSH, estrogen, and electrocardiogram to determine effects of bulimia on body.

Management

1. Nutritional plan to accomplish weight goal (gain or loss).
   a. Balanced diet with incremental inclusion of foods previously perceived by patient as "fattening."
   b. Exercise.
2. Psychological counseling and support.
   a. Assist patient to develop insight into behavior and a more realistic body image.
   b. Assist patient to develop effective coping strategies and problem-solving mechanisms.

Complications

1. Fluid and electrolyte disturbances, particularly hypokalemia, metabolic alkalosis, and associated cardiac dysrhythmias.
2. Obesity or anorexia nervosa.
3. Dental erosion.
4. Esophageal tear or gastric rupture.

Nursing Assessment

1. Perform complete nutritional assessment.
2. Evaluate fluid and electrolyte status and manifestations of associated problems.
3. Assess for signs and symptoms of depression, anxiety, personality disorder, and associated eating behaviors and history of family dysfunction.

Nursing Diagnoses

• Imbalanced Nutrition: More or Less Than Body Requirements related to binge/purge behavior.
• Ineffective Coping related to lack of control over eating habits.

Nursing Interventions

Attaining Appropriate Weight

1. Assist patient to select well-balanced diet and maintain appropriate eating habits.
2. Provide positive reinforcement for appropriate eating behaviors.
3. Teach patient the risks associated with abnormal eating behavior and the benefits of maintaining healthful nutritional and exercise habits.
4. Assess daily weight, intake and output, urine for ketones, and serum electrolytes to determine physical response to nutritional interventions.

Improving Coping

1. Encourage patient to set realistic goals for weight and appearance.
2. Assist patient to identify and implement alternative coping strategies in times of stress, including expression and exploration of feelings, problem solving, appropriate use of exercise, and relaxation techniques.
3. Include family in counseling and teaching sessions, as appropriate.
4. Set limits so patient will feel in control of self.

Patient Education and Health Maintenance

1. Stress the importance of maintaining follow-up visits and counseling.
2. Refer to such agencies as American Anorexia-Bulimia Association (*www.aaba.org*), Eating Disorder Information Center (*www.nedic.ca*), Eating Disorders Awareness and Prevention (*www.edap.org*), National Association of Anorexia Nervosa and Associated Disorders (*www.anad.org*), and National Eating Disorder Association (*www.nationaleatingdisorders.org*).

Evaluation: Expected Outcomes

• Well-balanced dietary intake without evidence of vomiting.
• Verbalizes correct problem-solving approach.

Malabsorption Syndrome

Malabsorption syndrome is a group of symptoms and physical signs that occur because of poor nutrient absorption in the small intestine, particularly fat absorption, with a resultant decrease in absorption of fat-soluble vitamins A, D, E, and K. Poor absorption of other nutrients, including carbohydrates, minerals, and other vitamins and proteins, may also occur. *Celiac sprue* and *lactose intolerance* are common types of malabsorption syndromes.

Pathophysiology and Etiology

Malabsorption has multiple etiologies, including gallbladder, liver, or pancreatic disease, lymphatic obstruction, vascular impairment, and bowel resection. Two common causes:

1. Celiac sprue—malabsorption of nutrients resulting from atrophy of villi and microvilli of the small intestine because of an intolerance to gluten found in common grains, such as wheat, rye, oats, and barley (see Chapter 48).
2. Lactose intolerance—typically of genetic origin, this digestive enzyme deficiency prevents the digestion of lactose found in milk, causing osmosis of water into the lumen of the intestine.

Clinical Manifestations

1. Steatorrhea.
2. Abdominal distention and pain.
3. Flatulence.
4. Anorexia, weight loss, edema.
5. Vitamin deficiency—fat soluble (A, D, E, K).
6. Protein deficiency and negative nitrogen balance.
7. Anemia, weakness, and fatigue due to poor absorption of iron, folic acid, and vitamin B_{12}.

Diagnostic Evaluation

1. Fecal fat analysis—72-hour stool collection; fecal fat may be increased.
2. M2A Imaging System—a device that provides images via a receiver and recorder tracing the transit of a capsule that is

swallowed by the patient. Used to evaluate and diagnose malabsorption syndromes as well as other gastrointestinal diseases.

3. Lower GI series (barium enema)—may be used to evaluate the colon.
4. Serum measurement of vitamin levels, total protein, and albumin may be decreased.
5. Prothrombin time may be prolonged because of vitamin K deficiency.

Management

1. Treatment of the underlying cause, if possible, by eliminating causative agents, such as grains or milk.
2. Promotion of adequate nutritional intake through a carefully designed diet that substitutes alternatives to the offending agent and that ensures replacement of deficient nutrients through oral, enteral, or parenteral therapy.
3. Medications such as pancreatic enzymes.

Complications

1. Dehydration.
2. Electrolyte imbalance with possible cardiac dysrhythmias.
3. Protein deficiency with muscle atrophy and edema.
4. Vitamin deficiency with tetany, bleeding, anemia, and osteoporosis.
5. Skin breakdown.

Nursing Assessment

1. Assess fluid and electrolyte status through careful monitoring of intake and output, daily weight, serum electrolytes, vital signs, and other signs and symptoms of dehydration and electrolyte imbalance.
2. Assess GI function through observation of frequency and characteristics of stool, bowel sounds, and distention, pain, and other associated symptoms.
3. Assess nutritional status.

Nursing Diagnoses

- Imbalanced Nutrition: Less Than Body Requirements related to malabsorption of nutrients.
- Deficient Fluid Volume related to loss of fluid through stool.
- Acute Pain related to abdominal distention and cramps.
- Risk for Impaired Skin Integrity related to irritation of anal area by stool.

Nursing Interventions

Improving Nutritional Status

1. Ensure that diet is free from causative agents, such as dairy or wheat products.
2. Provide diet high in missing nutrients, including proteins, carbohydrates, fats, vitamins, and minerals.
3. Teach patient to use substitute products for causative agents, such as gluten-free flour, corn, soybean, and lactose-free milk substitutes.
4. Monitor weight and characteristics of stool closely.

Restoring Fluid Balance

1. Monitor intake and output and urine-specific gravity.
   a. Include watery stool in output.
   b. Be aware that edema is caused by low serum proteins, not fluid overload.

2. Monitor vital signs frequently, based on condition.
3. Be alert for dehydration—orthostatic hypotension, tachycardia, decreased skin turgor, dry mucous membranes, thirst, oliguria.
4. Observe for signs and symptoms of potential electrolyte disturbances—nausea, vomiting, dysrhythmias, tremors, seizures, anorexia, weakness—and report abnormal results of serum electrolytes.
5. Administer IV fluids or parenteral or enteral nutrition, as ordered.

Relieving Pain

1. Assess timing, frequency, and character of pain and its relationship to food.
2. Encourage Fowler's position and frequent change in position for comfort.
3. Administer analgesics, antidiarrheals, and antiflatulents, as ordered.

Maintaining Tissue Integrity

1. Provide meticulous perineal care after each stool with application of hydrophobic ointments, if necessary, to prevent skin breakdown.
2. Give careful attention to general skin condition, assessing for redness, breakdown, and poor turgor, and maintain general skin integrity through cleanliness, lubrication, padding of bony prominences, frequent turning, and adequate hydration and nutrition.

Patient Education and Health Maintenance

1. Provide nutritional counseling for patient and family, particularly if symptoms are secondary to food intolerance; stress which foods to avoid and the importance of carefully reading all food labels, recommend appropriate food substitutions, and necessary nutritional supplements.
2. Advise regarding signs and symptoms that indicate worsening of disease—increased frequency of stool, diarrhea or steatorrhea, increased pain.
3. Suggest such support groups as the Celiac Sprue Association (*www.csaceliacs.org*) and the Crohn's and Colitis Foundation of America (*www.ccfa.org*).

Evaluation: Expected Outcomes

- Maintains weight and energy level.
- Vital signs stable; urinary output adequate.
- Verbalizes decreased pain after meals.
- No skin breakdown noted.

Vitamin and Mineral Deficiencies

Vitamins are organic compounds found in food needed for growth, reproduction, good health, and resistance to infection. Minerals are inorganic compounds found in nature and serve a variety of physiologic functions. Specific requirements depend on age, activity, metabolic rate (increased fever), and special processes, such as pregnancy, lactation, and disease processes.

See Table 20-4 on pages 762 to 767 for vitamin and mineral needs for healthy adults age 19 or older. Needs are different for children and pregnant or lactating women.

Dietary reference intakes tables have been developed by the Food and Nutrition Board at the Institute of Medicine of the National Academies and include the following:

(Text continues on page 768)

Table 20-4   Vitamin and Mineral Requirements and Imbalances

VITAMIN, RDA, AND EAR	FUNCTION	CLINICAL MANIFESTATIONS OF IMBALANCE
Vitamin A (Retinol) RDA: 700–900 mcg EAR: 500–625 mcg Fat soluble	• Tissue maintenance via antioxidant ability • Helps regulate the immune system • Skeletal and soft tissue growth and development • Visual adaptation to light and dark • Supports reproductive function	*Deficiency:* Night blindness, xerophthalmia, keratinization, generalized mucosa dryness/damage, vomiting, diarrhea, weight loss, urinary and vaginal infections, tooth decay, follicular hyperkeratosis, fatigue. *Toxicity:* Hair loss, joint pain, dry skin, mouth soreness, anorexia, vomiting, liver damage.
Vitamin B$_1$ (Thiamine) RDA: 1.1–1.2 mg EAR: 0.9–1.0 mg Water soluble	• Carbohydrate metabolism • Necessary for neurologic, gastric, cardiac, and musculoskeletal function	*Deficiency:* Appetite loss, constipation, dyspnea, fatigue, irritability, nervousness, memory loss, paresthesias, muscle pain, beriberi, blurred or double vision, difficulty swallowing, nausea, vomiting. *Toxicity:* Large doses may be given generally without difficulty, although anaphylaxis has been reported.
B$_2$ (Riboflavin) RDA: 1.1–1.3 mg EAR: 0.9–1.1 mg Water soluble	• Carbohydrate metabolism • Promotes growth, red blood cell formation, and healthy eyes and skin	*Deficiency:* Sore throat, cheilosis, dermatitis, burning and itching of eyes, tearing and vascularization of corneas; late-stage symptoms include neuropathy and growth retardation. *Toxicity:* None known.
B$_6$ (Pyridoxine) RDA: 1.3–1.7 mg EAR: 1.1–1.4 mg Water soluble	• Required for protein metabolism • Maintains neurologic function and RBC production	*Deficiency:* Anemia, weakness, glossitis, cheilosis, irritability, seizures. *Toxicity:* Neuromuscular damage, peripheral neuropathy.
B$_{12}$ (Cobalamin) RDA: 2.4 mcg EAR: 2.0 mcg Water soluble	• Maintains neurologic function and RBC development via hemoglobin synthesis	*Deficiency:* Megaloblastic anemia, memory impairment, confusion, depression, fatigue, nervousness, decreased reflex response, balance impairment, speech difficulties, demyelination of the large fibers of the spinal cord, anorexia, vomiting, weight loss, yellowing of skin, abdominal pain, dyspnea, diarrhea, glossitis, burning of lips or mouth, palpitations, tachycardia, sore tongue, weakness. *Toxicity:* None.
Biotin RDA: 30 mcg EAR: Not established Water soluble	• Metabolism of proteins, fats, and carbohydrates	*Deficiency:* Dry skin, fatigue, grayish skin discoloration, muscle pain, depression, insomnia, anorexia. *Toxicity:* None.
Folate (Folic Acid) RDA: 400 mcg EAR: 320 mcg Water soluble	• RBC formation • DNA and RNA synthesis and support of cell growth and reproduction • Prevention of birth defects	*Deficiency:* Glossitis, diarrhea, megaloblastic anemia, digestive problems, fatigue, palpitations, restless leg syndrome. *Toxicity:* Inactivation of anticonvulsants, masking of vitamin B$_{12}$ deficiency.
Niacin RDA: 14–16 mg EAR: 11–12 mg Water soluble	• Metabolism of carbohydrates, fats, and proteins • Works with thiamine and riboflavin for the production of cellular energy • Promotes skin, neurologic, and GI function	*Deficiency:* Apathy, fatigue, appetite loss, headaches, indigestion, muscle weakness, nausea, insomnia, dermatitis, diarrhea, confusion, disorientation, memory impairment, glossitis, stomatitis, pellagra. *Toxicity:* Liver damage, flushing.
Pantothenic Acid RDA: 5 mg EAR: Not established Water soluble	• Vital for overall metabolism • Aids in formation of carbohydrates, proteins, and fats • Aids in cortisone production, ATP production, stress tolerance, vitamin utilization, hemoglobin synthesis	*Deficiency:* Diarrhea, hair loss, respiratory infections, nervousness, muscle cramps, premature aging, intestinal disorders, eczema, kidney disorders. *Toxicity:* None.

DIAGNOSTIC EVALUATION	MANAGEMENT
Deficiency: • History and physical findings are helpful in diagnosis of most vitamin imbalances. • Serum level less than 35 mg/dL suggests vitamin deficiency.	*Deficiency:* • Replacement therapy of 30,000 international units to treat night blindness. • Good dietary sources of vitamin A are green and yellow fruits and vegetables and liver. • In patients with malabsorption of fat-soluble vitamins and patients with low dietary intake of vitamin A, IV supplements are required.
Deficiency: • Erythrocyte transketolase activity less than 15%–20%.	*Deficiency:* • Treat underlying cause. • High-protein diet with supplemental B complex vitamins. • Food sources rich in thiamine are brewer's yeast, meat, wheat germ, enriched grains and beans. • Parenteral therapy with 50–100 mg/day followed by 5–10 mg/day P.O.
Deficiency: • Erythrocyte glutathione activity greater than 1.2–1.3. • Decreased urinary riboflavin levels.	*Deficiency:* • Good dietary sources of B_2 are dairy products, vegetables, enriched grains, eggs, nuts, liver. • Oral supplements of 5–15 mg/day.
Deficiency: • Pyridoxal phosphate levels less than 50 ng/mL.	*Deficiency:* • Oral supplementation: 10–20 mg. • Good dietary sources of B_6 are bananas, brewer's yeast, fish, meat, whole grains, liver. • Individuals taking oral contraceptives or isoniazid may need to supplement their diets with pyridoxine. • Pregnancy also increases need.
Deficiency: • Serum levels of less than 100 pg/mL. • Decreased hematocrit with elevation of MCV. • Schilling test also measures absorption of radioactive B_{12}.	*Deficiency:* • B_{12} 200 mcg/day I.M. for 1 week, then every month for life if deficiency is due to pernicious anemia. • Oral vitamin B_{12} may be necessary for strict vegetarians. • Good dietary sources of B_{12} are eggs, fish, organ meats, lean meat, dairy products.
—	*Deficiency:* • Good sources of biotin are egg yolks, vegetables, yeast, milk, grains.
Deficiency: • Serum level less than 3 ng/mL.	*Deficiency:* • Nutritional supplementation: 1 mg/day P.O. • Avoid alcohol. • Good sources of folate are citrus fruits, eggs, milk, green leafy vegetables, dairy products, organ meats, seafood, whole grains, yeast.
Deficiency: • Serum levels less than 30 mcg/100 mL. • Diminished or absent metabolites in urine.	*Deficiency:* • Good sources of niacin are eggs, lean meats, organ meats, poultry, seafood, fish, dairy products, nuts, whole and enriched grains, brewer's yeast. • Nutritional supplementation: 10–150 mg. • Supplemental niacin may also be necessary when taking oral contraceptives.
—	*Deficiency:* • This vitamin is widely available in foods, especially organ meats, legumes, vegetables, fruits.

(continued)

Table 20-4   Vitamin and Mineral Requirements and Imbalances *(continued)*

VITAMIN, RDA, AND EAR	FUNCTION	CLINICAL MANIFESTATIONS OF IMBALANCE
Vitamin C RDA: 75–90 mg EAR: 60–75 mg Water soluble	• Antioxidant action decreases cellular dysfunction • Promotes wound healing • Aids in connective tissue, bone, tooth, and cartilage formation • Promotes capillary integrity • Promotes nonheme iron absorption	*Deficiency:* Bleeding gums, tooth decay, nosebleeds, low infection resistance, bruising, anemia, delayed wound healing, anorexia, joint pain, lethargy, perifollicular hemorrhage. *Toxicity:* GI distress.
Vitamin D RDA: 15 mcg EAR: 10 mcg Fat soluble	• Regulates calcium and phosphate absorption and metabolism and bone formation • Aids in renal phosphate clearance, myocardial function, nervous system maintenance, and normal blood clotting	*Deficiency:* Rickets, osteomalacia, weakness, spasm/twitching of eyes, burning in mouth, sweating. *Toxicity:* Hypercalcemia, bone pain, nausea, vomiting, itching, thirst, agitation, weakness. Calcifications in soft tissue can be fatal.
Vitamin E (Tocopherol) RDA: 15 mg EAR: 12 mg Fat soluble	• Antioxidant action decreases cellular dysfunction • Aids in RBC formation	*Deficiency:* Neuromuscular disturbances, including decreased reflexes, vibratory and position sense, ataxia, night blindness, fatigue, leg weakness or cramps, dry skin. *Toxicity:* Interference with vitamin K.
Vitamin K RDA: 90–120 mcg EAR: Not established Fat soluble	• Promotes coagulation through the formation of prothrombin and other clotting factors	*Deficiency:* Abnormal bleeding times, hemorrhage, epistaxis, hematemesis, and bleeding at any orifice or puncture site are possible. *Toxicity:* No tolerable upper limit has been established.
Minerals		
Calcium AI: 1,000–1,200 mg EAR: 800–1,000 mg	• Aids in bone and tooth formation, muscle contraction, blood coagulation, nerve impulse transmission, cardiac function, cell membrane permeability, enzyme activation	*Deficiency:* Tooth decay, muscle cramps, tetany, nervousness and delusion, cardiac palpitations, heart failure, and paresthesia. *Toxicity:* Constipation, loss of appetite, nausea, vomiting, dry mouth, renal calculi.
Chloride AI: 2,000–2,300 mg	• Helps keep the body's acid-base balance • Helps with metabolism	*Deficiency:* Extremely rare but can cause loss of appetite, weakness and lethargy. *Toxicity:* May result in fluid retention.
Chromium AI: 20–35 mcg EAR: Not established	• Maintains serum glucose levels Maintains fat metabolism	*Deficiency:* Glucose intolerance, vertigo, abdominal pain, shock, convulsions, anuria, dermatitis. *Toxicity:* Unknown.
Copper RDA: 900 mcg EAR: 700 mcg	• Hemoglobin synthesis • Maintenance of hemostasis • Energy production	*Deficiency:* Hypochromic anemia, bone disease, weakness, skin lesions, altered respiratory status. *Toxicity:* Nausea, vomiting, diarrhea, abdominal pain, malaise.
Iodine RDA: 150 mcg EAR: 95 mcg	• Thyroid hormone synthesis	*Deficiency:* Hypothyroidism or goiter, nervousness, irritability, obesity, cold hands and feet, chills, brittle hair, fatigue, bradycardia, decreased cardiac output, thick tongue, hoarseness, poor memory, hearing loss, anorexia. *Toxicity:* Goiter.

DIAGNOSTIC EVALUATION	MANAGEMENT
Deficiency: • Serum levels less than 0.2 mg/100 dL.	*Deficiency:* • Nutritional supplementation: 100–1,000 mg/day of vitamin C. • Good sources of vitamin C are citrus fruits, green leafy vegetables, broccoli, tomatoes, peppers, potatoes, strawberries. • Avoid smoking.
Deficiency: • Low levels of vitamin D (Serum 25 [OH] D). • Radiographic bone deformities. • Abnormal bone densitometry.	*Deficiency:* • Nutritional supplementation: Ergocalciferol, 25 mcg/day P.O. • Good sources of vitamin D are egg yolks, yeast, enriched milk, fish liver oils. • Exposure to sunlight.
Deficiency: • Serum levels less than 0.5 mg/dL.	*Deficiency:* • Nutritional supplementation: 100–400 international units/day P.O. • Parenteral therapy may be necessary to treat neurologic symptoms. • Good sources of vitamin E are vegetable oils, milk, eggs, meat, fish, green leafy vegetables.
Deficiency: • Prothrombin time extended longer than PTT.	*Deficiency:* • Administration of vitamin K 15 mg subcutaneously. • Good sources of vitamin K are green leafy vegetables, liver, wheat germ, cheeses, egg yolks, soybean oil.
Deficiency: • Dual-energy x-ray absorptiometry (DEXA) for bone mineral density *Toxicity:* • Serum level greater than 10.5 mg/dL.	*Deficiency:* • Oral supplements of 1–2 g/day of elemental calcium. • In severe hypocalcemia, 10 mL of 10% calcium gluconate IV administered no faster than 2 mL/minute. • Good sources of calcium are milk products, green leafy vegetables, legumes, tofu processed with calcium. *Toxicity:* • Force fluids, diuretics, and limit dietary intake. Administration of phosphate salts and glucocorticoids may also be necessary.
Deficiency: • Serum levels less than 98. *Toxicity:* • Serum levels greater than 108.	• No specific treatment.
Deficiency: • Serum levels less than 0.3 mg/mL.	*Deficiency:* • Nutritional supplementation: 50–200 mg/day. • Good sources of chromium are brewer's yeast, whole grains, cereals.
Deficiency: • In addition to diminished serum levels, 24-hour urine samples showing levels of urinary excretion of copper below 15–60 mcg/24 hours.	*Deficiency:* • Nutritional supplementation: 0.1 mg/kg/day P.O. • IV supplementation: 1–2 mg/day. • Good sources of copper are nuts, seeds, organ meats, seafood.
Deficiency: • Low T_3 and T_4 levels. • Thyroid scan.	*Deficiency:* • Nutritional supplementation: 50–100 mg daily P.O. • Good sources of iodine are iodized salt, seafood.

(continued)

Table 20-4	Vitamin and Mineral Requirements and Imbalances (*continued*)

VITAMIN, RDA, AND EAR	FUNCTION	CLINICAL MANIFESTATIONS OF IMBALANCE
Minerals (*continued*)		
Iron RDA: 8–18 mg EAR: 5–8.1 mg	• Hemoglobin synthesis • Cellular oxidation • Transportation of oxygen	*Deficiency:* Iron-deficiency anemia, fatigue, tachycardia, palpitations, dyspnea, susceptibility to infection, brittle nails. *Toxicity:* Iron poisoning; nausea, vomiting, gastrointestinal irritation, constipation, diarrhea.
Magnesium RDA: 310–420 mg EAR: 265–350 mg	• Parathyroid hormone regulation • Acid-base balance • Enzyme activation • Smooth muscle regulation • Metabolism of carbohydrates and protein • Cell growth and reproduction	*Deficiency:* Tetany, tremors, confusion, depression, tachycardia, dysrhythmias, seizures. *Toxicity:* Nausea, vomiting, drowsiness, muscle weakness, decreased deep tendon reflexes, hypotension, respiratory depression.
Phosphorus RDA: 700 mg EAR: 580 mg	• Nerve and muscle activity • Vitamin utilization • Kidney function • Metabolism of carbohydrates, proteins, and fats • Cell growth and repair • Myocardial contraction • Energy production • Bone and tooth formation • Acid-base balance • Red blood cell function	*Deficiency:* Anorexia, weakness, tremor, paresthesias, anemia, mental status change, hypoxia, osteomalacia. *Toxicity:* Tetany, soft tissue calcification, seizures, renal damage.
Potassium AI: 4,700 mg	• Muscle contraction • Cardiac function • Protein synthesis • Nerve impulse transmission • Carbohydrate metabolism • Acid-base balance • Major intracellular cation	*Deficiency:* Muscle weakness, fatigue, malaise, flaccidity, mental confusion, irritability, depression, dysrhythmias, hypotension, nausea, vomiting, anorexia, decreased GI motility, muscle cramps, paresthesias, hyperglycemia, polyuria, metabolic alkalosis. *Toxicity:* Muscle weakness, paralysis, paresthesias, nausea, vomiting, diarrhea, metabolic acidosis, prolonged cardiac conduction, ventricular dysrhythmias.
Sodium AI: 1,300–1,500 mg	• Maintains fluid balance • Cell membrane permeability and absorption of glucose • Bioelectric potential of tissues • Cardiac function • Acid-base balance • Regulation of neuromuscular function	*Deficiency:* Muscle weakness, irritability, headache, seizures, nausea, vomiting, malaise, abdominal cramping, hypotension, tachycardia. *Toxicity:* Flushed skin, oliguria, agitation, thirst, dry mucous membranes, seizures.
Zinc RDA: 8–11 mg EAR: 6.8–9.4 mg	• Cellular metabolism • Maintenance of taste and smell • Burn and wound healing • Gonadal function • Maintenance of serum vitamin A concentration • Acid-base balance • Protein digestion • Promotion of growth	*Deficiency:* Fatigue, hair loss, poor wound healing, impaired growth, bone deformities, loss of taste, anorexia, iron-deficiency anemia, hypogonadism, hyperpigmentation. *Toxicity:* Diminished deep tendon reflexes, malaise, decreased level of consciousness, diarrhea, leukopenia.

AI, Adequate intake; EAR, estimated average requirement; DRI, dietary reference intake; IV, intravenous; P.O., by mouth; RBC, red blood cell; MCV, mean corpuscular volume; I.M., intramuscular; ATP, adenosine triphosphate; PTT, partial thromboplastin time; t.i.d., three times per day; ADH, antidiuretic hormone; RDA, recommended daily allowance.

DIAGNOSTIC EVALUATION	MANAGEMENT
Deficiency: • Decreased hemoglobin, hematocrit, iron, and ferritin levels and increased total iron-binding capacity.	*Deficiency:* • Nutritional supplementation: ferrous sulfate 325 mg P.O. t.i.d.; Imferon 250 mg/day I.M. for each gram of hemoglobin below normal. • IV supplementation: 1.5–2 g over 4 to 6 hours. • Good sources of iron are egg yolks, fish, organ meats, wheat germ, beef, peas, chicken, turkey, legumes, spinach.
Deficiency: • Serum levels less than 1.3 mEq/L. *Toxicity:* • Serum levels greater than 2.1 mEq/L.	*Deficiency:* • Nutritional supplementation: 1–2 g IV during 15 minutes. • Good sources of magnesium are nuts, meat, whole grains, green vegetables, seafood, dairy products. *Toxicity:* • Supportive measures.
Deficiency: • Serum levels less than 2.5 mg/dL. *Toxicity:* • Serum levels greater than 4.5 mg/dL.	*Deficiency:* • Nutritional supplementation: P.O. or IV phosphate. • Good sources of phosphate are dairy products, eggs, fish, grains, meat, poultry, cheeses, beans, cocoa, chocolate, liver, milk, peas, nuts. *Toxicity:* • Administration of phosphate-binding agents. • Hemodialysis or peritoneal dialysis.
Deficiency: • Serum levels less than 3.5 mEq/L. *Toxicity:* • Serum levels greater than 5 mEq/L.	*Deficiency:* • Nutritional supplementation: P.O. or IV, IV replacement generally at a rate of 10 mEq/hour with careful cardiac monitoring and frequent measurements of serum potassium levels. • Good sources of potassium are bananas, oranges, beef, prunes, beans, seafood, raisins. *Toxicity:* • Infuse calcium gluconate 10% (10 mL). • Sodium bicarbonate infusion. • Insulin and glucose infusion. • Oral or rectal exchange resins. • Hemodialysis or peritoneal dialysis.
Deficiency: • Serum levels less than 135 mEq/L. *Toxicity:* • Serum levels greater than 145 mEq/L.	*Deficiency:* • Restrict free water intake. • Infuse 0.9% saline solution if patient is hypovolemic. • Infuse 3% saline and administer diuretic if sodium levels significantly low. • Demeclocycline may be used to block ADH in the renal tubules to promote water excretion. *Toxicity:* • Administer salt-free solutions such as D_5W followed by 0.45% saline solution. • Low-sodium diet. • Administer vasopressin if diminished ADH is the cause.
Deficiency: • Serum levels less than 75 mcg/dL.	*Deficiency:* • Nutritional supplementation: zinc sulfate 200 mg P.O. t.i.d. • Good sources of zinc are liver, seafood, beans, lentils, oatmeal, wheat bran, egg yolks, peas, chicken, and milk. *Toxicity:* • Supportive measures.

Recommended dietary allowance—the average daily dietary intake level sufficient to meet the nutrient requirements of nearly all (97% to 98%) healthy individuals in a group.

Adequate intake—amount believed to cover the needs of all healthy individuals in the groups, but lack of data or uncertainty in the data prevent being able to specify with confidence the percentage of individuals covered by this intake.

Estimated average requirement—average daily nutrient intake level estimated to meet the requirements of half of the healthy individuals in a group.

SELECTED REFERENCES

Bankhead, R., Boullata, J., Brantley, S., et al. (2009). A.S.P.E.N. Enteral Nutrition Practice Recommendations. *Journal of Parenteral and Enteral Nutrition, 33*(2), 122–167.

Barker, L. A., Gout, B. S., Growe, T. C., et al. (2011). Hospital malnutrition: Prevalence, identification and impact on patients and the healthcare system. *International Journal of Environmental Research and Public Health, 8*(2), 514–527.

Bourgault, A., Ipe, L., Weaver, J., et al. (2007). Development of evidence-based guidelines and critical care nurses' knowledge of enteral feeding. *Critical Care Nurse, 27*(4), 17–29.

Division of Nutrition, Physical Activity, and Obesity [Internet]. Atlanta (GA): Centers for Disease Control and Prevention (US): [updated 2012 May, cited 2012]. Overweight and obesity. Available from: *http://www.cdc.gov/obesity/adult/index.html.*

Flegal, K., Carroll, M. D., Ogden, C. L., et al. (2010). Prevalence and trends in obesity among US adults, 1999–2008. *Journal of the American Medical Association, 303*(3), 235.

Flegal, K. (2010). Prevalence and trends in obesity among US adults, 1999–2008. *JAMA, 303*(3):235.

Fletcher, J. (2010). Nutrition: safe practice in adult enteral tube feeding. *Br J Nurs, 20*(19):1234–1239.

Gagnon, L. E., & Sheff, E. J. (2012). Outcomes and complications after bariatric surgery. *AJN 112*(9), 26–36.

Holmes, S. (2012). Enteral nutrition: an overview. *Nurs Standard, 26*(39): 41–46.

Jia, H., & Lubetkin, E. (2010). Obesity-related quality-adjusted life years lost in the U.S. from 1993 to 2008. *American Journal of Preventive Medicine, 39*(3), 220–227.

Litchford, M. D. (2011). Laboratory assessment of nutritional status: bridging theory & practice. Greensboro: Case Software.

Litchford, M. D. (2012). Nutrition focused physical assessment: making clinical connections. Greensboro: Case Software.

Mirtallo, J. (2009). *Assessment tools and guidelines: Parenteral nutrition therapy.* New York: McMahon.

Mueller, C., Compher, C., Ellen, D. M., et al. (2011). A.S.P.E.N. clinical guidelines. Nutrition screening, assessment and intervention in adults. *Journal of Parenteral and Enteral Nutrition, 35*(1), 16–24.

National Heart, Lung, Blood Institute Obesity Education Initiative Expert Panel. (2011). *Clinical guidelines on the identification and evaluation, and treatment of overweight and obesity in adults.* Bethesda, MD: Author.

National Agricultural Library [Internet]. Beltsville (MD): United States Department of Agriculture (US): [modified 2012 September, cited 2012]. DRI tables. Available from: http://fnic.nal.usda.gov/dietary-guidance/dietary-reference-intakes/dri-tables.

Rickers, L., McSherry C. (2012). Bariatric surgery: nutritional considerations for patients. *Nurs Standard, 26*(49): 41–48.

Shikora, S. A., Claros, L., & Furtado, M. (2008). Bariatric surgery. In M. Marian, S. A. Shikora, & M. K. Russell (Eds.), *Clinical nutrition for surgical patients.* Sudbury, MA: Jones & Bartlett.

Simmons, S. R., Abdallah, L. M. (2012). Bedside assessment of enteral tube placement: Aligning practice with evidence. *American Journal of Nursing, 112*(2), 40–46.

The Obesity Prevention Source [Internet]. Boston (MA): Harvard School of Public Health; [c. 2012, The President and Fellows of Harvard College, cited 2012]. Adult Obesity. Available from: *http://www.hsph.harvard.edu/obesity-prevention-source/obesity-trends/obesity-rates-worldwide/index.html.*

U.S. Departments of Agriculture and Health and Human Services. (2010). Dietary guidelines for Americans, 2010. Washington, DC: U.S. Government Printing Office.

21
Renal and Urinary Disorders

OVERVIEW AND ASSESSMENT
Subjective Data

Subjective data include characterization of symptoms, history of present illness, past medical and surgical history, demographic data, and lifestyle factors. Signs and symptoms involving the urinary tract may be due to disorders of the kidneys, ureters, or bladder; surrounding structures; or disorders of other body systems. See Standards of Care Guidelines 21-1.

Changes in Micturition (Voiding)

Changes in Amount or Color of Urine
1. Hematuria—blood in the urine, may be gross (visible by color change) or microscopic.
   a. Considered a serious sign and requires evaluation.
   b. Color of bloody urine depends on several factors including the amount of blood present and the anatomical source of the bleeding.

STANDARDS OF CARE GUIDELINES 21-1
Renal Impairment

- Be aware that systemic factors, urologic status, and renal function affect urine output. Notify health care provider of decreased urine output.
- Patients at risk for renal impairment include those with cardiovascular disease, diabetes, and hypertension; postoperative patients; hypotensive patients; and those with prostate and other diseases of the urinary tract.
- Thorough assessment of the urinary tract includes:
  - Hourly intake and output measurement.
  - Assessment of color, clarity, and specific gravity of the urine.
  - Palpation of the abdomen for suprapubic tenderness.
  - Percussion of the flanks for costovertebral angle tenderness.
  - Prostate examination.
  - Subjective assessment for symptoms, such as urgency, frequency, nocturia, hesitancy, dribbling, decreased force of stream, hematuria, and incontinence.
- Be alert to drugs or agents that may impair urinary and renal function, such as nonsteroidal anti-inflammatory drugs, anticholinergics, sympathomimetics, aminoglycoside antibiotics, antifungals, calcineurin inhibitors, angiotensin-converting enzyme inhibitors, angiotensin receptor blockers, chemotherapeutic agents, and contrast media.
- Report abnormal urinalysis, urine culture, and renal function test results to health care provider promptly.

This information should serve as a general guideline only. Each patient situation presents a unique set of clinical factors and requires nursing judgment to guide care, which may include additional or alternative measures and approaches.

---

c. Microscopic hematuria is the presence of red blood cells (RBCs) in urine, which can be seen only under a microscope; urine appears normal.
d. Hematuria may be due to a systemic cause, such as blood dyscrasias, anticoagulant therapy, or extreme exercise.
e. Painless hematuria may indicate neoplasm in the urinary tract.
f. Hematuria is common in patients with urinary tract stone disease, malignancy, acute infection, glomerulonephritis, trauma to the kidneys or urinary tract, thrombosis and embolism involving renal artery or vein, and polycystic kidney disease.
2. Polyuria—large volume of urine voided in given time.
   a. Volume is out of proportion to usual voiding pattern and fluid intake.
   b. Demonstrated in diabetes mellitus, diabetes insipidus, chronic renal disease, use of diuretics.

3. Oliguria—small volume of urine.
   a. Output between 100 and 500 mL/24 hours.
   b. May result from acute renal failure, shock, dehydration, fluid and electrolyte imbalance, or obstruction.
4. Anuria—absence of urine output.
   a. Output less than 50 mL/24 hours.
   b. Indicates serious renal dysfunction requiring immediate medical or surgical intervention.

Symptoms Related to Irritation of the Lower Urinary Tract

1. Dysuria—painful or uncomfortable urination.
   a. Burning sensation seen in wide variety of inflammatory and infectious urinary tract conditions.
2. Frequency—voiding occurs more frequently than usual when compared with patient's usual pattern or with a generally accepted norm of once every 3 to 6 hours.
   a. Determine if habits governing fluid intake have been altered—it is essential to know normal voiding pattern to evaluate frequency.
   b. Increasing frequency can result from a variety of conditions, such as infection and diseases of urinary tract, metabolic disease, hypertension, medications (diuretics).
3. Urgency—strong desire to urinate that is difficult to postpone.
   a. Due to inflammatory conditions of the bladder, prostate, or urethra; acute or chronic bacterial infections; neurogenic voiding dysfunctions; chronic prostatitis or bladder outlet obstruction in men; overactive bladder; and urogenital atrophy in postmenopausal women.
4. Nocturia—urination at night that interrupts sleep.
   a. Causes include urologic conditions affecting bladder function, poor bladder emptying, bladder outlet obstruction, or overactive bladder.
   b. Metabolic causes include decreased renal concentrating ability or heart failure, hyperglycemia, and remobilization of dependent edema.
5. Strangury—slow and painful urination; only small amounts of urine voided. Wrenching sensation at end of urination produced by spasmodic muscular contraction of the urethra and bladder.
   a. Blood staining may be noted.
   b. Seen in numerous urological conditions, including severe cystitis, interstitial cystitis, urinary calculus, and bladder cancer.

Symptoms Related to Obstruction of the Lower Urinary Tract

1. Weak stream—decreased force of stream when compared to usual stream of urine when voiding.
2. Hesitancy—undue delay and difficulty in initiating voiding.
   a. May indicate compression of urethra, outlet obstruction, neurogenic bladder.
3. Terminal dribbling—prolonged dribbling or urine from the meatus after urination is complete. May be caused by bladder outlet obstruction.

4. Incomplete emptying—feeling that the bladder is still full even after urination. Indicates either urinary retention, overactive bladder, or a condition that prevents the bladder from emptying well; may lead to infection.
5. Urinary retention—inability to void.

Involuntary Voiding
1. Urinary incontinence—involuntary loss of urine; may be due to pathologic, anatomical, or physiologic factors affecting the urinary tract (see page 181).
2. Nocturnal enuresis—involuntary voiding during sleep. May be physiologic during early childhood; thereafter, may be functional or symptomatic of obstructive or neurogenic disease (usually of lower urinary tract) or dysfunctional voiding.

Urinary Tract Pain
1. Kidney pain—may be felt as a dull ache in costovertebral angle or may be a sharp, colicky pain felt in the flank area that radiates to the groin or testicle. Due to distention of the renal capsule; severity related to how quickly it develops.
2. Ureteral pain—felt in the back and/or abdomen and can radiate to groin, urethra, penis, scrotum, or testicle.
3. Bladder pain (lower abdominal pain or pain over suprapubic area)—may be due to bladder infection, overdistended bladder, or bladder spasms.
4. Urethral pain—from irritation of bladder neck, from foreign body in canal, or from urethritis due to infection or trauma; pain increases when voiding.
5. Pain in scrotal area—due to inflammatory swelling of epididymis or testicle, torsion of the testicle, testicular mass, or scrotal infection. May also be referred pain from neurological, renal, or gastrointestinal source.
6. Testicular pain—due to injury, mumps, orchitis, torsion of spermatic cord, testes, or testes appendix.
7. Perineal or rectal discomfort—due to acute or chronic prostatitis, prostatic abscess, or trauma.
8. Pain in glans penis—usually from prostatitis; penile shaft pain results from urethral problems; may also be referred pain from ureteral calculus.

Related Symptoms
1. GI symptoms related to urologic conditions include nausea, vomiting, diarrhea, abdominal discomfort, paralytic ileus.
2. Occur with urologic conditions because the GI and urinary tracts have common autonomic and sensory innervation and because of renointestinal reflexes.
3. Fever and chills may also occur with infectious processes.

History
Seek the following historical data related to urinary and renal function:
1. What are patient's present and past occupations? Look for occupational hazards related to the urinary tract—contact with chemicals, plastics, tar, rubber; also truck or school bus drivers, dry cleaners, farmers.
2. What is patient's smoking history?
3. What is the past medical and surgical history, especially in relation to urinary problem?
4. Is there any family history of renal disease?
5. What childhood diseases did patient have?
6. Is there a history of urinary tract infections (UTIs)? Did any occur before age 12?
7. Did enuresis continue beyond the age when most children gain control?
8. Any history of genital lesions or sexually transmitted diseases (STDs)?
9. For the female patient: Number of children? Vaginal or cesarean delivery? Any forceps deliveries? When? Any signs of vaginal discharge? Vaginal/vulvar itch or irritation? Family history of pelvic organ prolapse ("dropped" bladder or uterus) or urinary incontinence?
10. Does patient have diabetes mellitus? Hypertension? Allergies? Neurologic disease or dysfunction? Vascular disease?
11. Has patient ever been hospitalized for a UTI? What diagnostic tests were performed? Cystoscopy? Urodynamics? Kidney x-ray procedures? Was patient catheterized for a time? Were antibiotics administered via intravenous (IV) or oral route?
12. Has patient ever had surgery for bladder or prostate problems or traumatic injuries involving the pelvis?
13. Is patient taking any prescription or over-the-counter (OTC) drugs or herbal preparations that may affect renal or urinary function? Have any drugs been prescribed for renal or urinary problems?
14. Is patient at risk for UTI?

Objective Data
Objective data should focus on physical examination of the abdomen and the genitalia. Complete body system assessment may be indicated in some conditions such as renal failure. See Chapter 5, pages 70 and 72, for examination of the abdomen and male genitalia and page 73 for female pelvic examination.

Laboratory Tests
Common laboratory studies pertaining to renal and urologic disorders include blood and urinary excretion tests for renal function, prostate-specific antigen, and urinalysis.

Tests of Renal Function
Description
1. Renal function tests are used to determine effectiveness of the kidneys' excretory functioning, to evaluate the severity of kidney disease, and to follow patient's progress.
2. There is no single test of renal function; rather, optimal results are obtained by combining a number of clinical tests.

Nursing and Patient Care Considerations
Renal function may be within normal limits until about 50% of renal function has been lost (see Table 21-1).

Table 21-1 Tests of Renal Function

There is no single test of renal function because this function is subject to variation. The rate of change of renal function is more important than the result of a single test.

TEST	PURPOSE/RATIONALE	TEST PROTOCOL
Renal concentration test • Specific gravity • Osmolality of urine	• Both tests evaluate the ability of the kidney to dilute or concentrate urine. • Values are elevated in prerenal states, including dehydration. Concentration ability is lost (resulting in low values) in CKD and some types of AKI despite changes in volume status.	• Fluids may be withheld 12 to 24 hours to evaluate the concentrating ability of the tubules under controlled conditions. Specific gravity measurements of urine are taken at specific times to determine urine concentration.
Creatinine clearance	• Provides a reasonable approximation of rate of glomerular filtration. • Measures volume of blood in mL cleared of creatinine in 1 minute. • Most sensitive indication of early renal disease. • Useful to follow progress of the patient's renal status.	• Collect all urine over 24-hour period. • Draw one sample of blood within the period.
Serum creatinine	• A test of renal function reflecting the balance between production and filtration by renal glomerulus. • Most sensitive test of renal function.	• Obtain sample of blood serum.
Serum urea nitrogen (blood urea nitrogen [BUN])	• Serves as index of renal excretory capacity. • Serum urea nitrogen depends on the body's urea production and on urine flow. (Urea is the nitrogenous end-product of protein metabolism.) • Affected by protein intake, hydration status, and catabolism.	• Obtain sample of blood serum.
Protein	• Random specimen may be affected by dietary protein intake. Proteinuria > 300 mg/24 hours may indicate renal disease.	• Collect all urine over 24-hour period.
Microalbumin/creatinine ratio	• Sensitive test for the subsequent development of proteinuria; >25 mg/g for females and >17 mg/g for males predicts early nephropathy.	• Collect random urine specimen.
Urine casts	• Mucoproteins and other substances present in renal inflammation; help to identify type of renal disease (eg, red cell casts present in glomerulonephritis, fatty casts in nephrotic syndrome, white cell casts in pyelonephritis).	• Collect random urine specimen.

Prostate-Specific Antigen

Description

1. Prostate-specific antigen (PSA) is an amino acid glycoprotein that is measured in the serum by a simple blood test.
2. An elevated PSA indicates the presence of prostate disease, but is not exclusive to prostate cancer.
3. Level rises continuously with the growth of prostate cancer.
4. Normal serum PSA level is less than 4 ng/mL.
5. Patients who have undergone treatment for prostate cancer are monitored yearly with PSA levels for recurrence. These levels should be 0.00 ng/mL; any rise may indicate recurrence or metastasis of prostate cancer.

Nursing and Patient Care Considerations

1. No patient preparation is necessary.
2. Current or recent UTI, prostatitis, digital rectal exam, or urethral instrumentation can cause an artificial elevation of PSA.
3. Clinical laboratories may differ slightly in methods used for determining PSA; patients having serial PSA should be sent to the same laboratory.

Urinalysis

Description

Involves examination of the urine for overall characteristics, including appearance, pH, specific gravity, and osmolality as well as microscopic evaluation for the presence of normal and abnormal cells.

1. Appearance—normal urine is clear. Cloudy urine may or may not be pathologic.
   a. Nonpathologic causes: normal urine may develop cloudiness on refrigeration, from standing at room temperature, or from precipitation of phosphates in alkaline urine (phosphaturia).
   b. Pathologic causes: due to pus (pyuria), blood, epithelial cells, bacteria, fat, colloidal particles, phosphate, or lymph fluid (chyluria).
2. Odor—normal urine has a faint aromatic odor.
   a. Characteristic odors produced by ingestion of asparagus.
   b. Cloudy urine with ammonia odor: urea-splitting bacteria such as *Proteus*, causing UTIs.
   c. Offensive odor: may be due to bacterial action in presence of pus.
3. Color—varies with urine concentration and if affected by metabolites, medications, and certain foods.
   a. Normal urine is clear yellow or amber because of the pigment urochrome.
   b. Dilute urine is pale yellow or clear.
   c. Concentrated urine is tea-colored, may be a sign of insufficient fluid intake.
   d. Blue, blue-green: medication, namely amitriptyline, propofol, indomethacin, and methenamine; pseudomonas infection.
   e. Red or red-brown: due to blood pigments, porphyria, bleeding lesions in urogenital tract, some drugs such as phenazopyridine and foods (beets).
   f. Yellow-brown, green-brown, or tea colored: may reveal obstructive lesion of bile duct system, obstructive jaundice, or hepatitis.
   g. Dark brown or black: due to malignant melanoma, leukemia, methemoglobin; or medications, namely methyldopa, levodopa.
4. pH of urine—reflects the ability of kidney to maintain normal hydrogen ion concentration in plasma and extracellular fluid; indicates *acidity* or *alkalinity* of urine.
   a. pH should be measured in fresh urine because the breakdown of urine to ammonia causes urine to become alkaline.
   b. Normal pH is 4.5 to 8.0.
   c. Urine acidity (pH < 4.5) or alkalinity (pH > 8.0) has relatively little clinical significance unless the patient is being treated for renal calculous disease or being evaluated for renal tubular acidosis.
5. Specific gravity (SG)—reflects the kidney's ability to concentrate or dilute urine; may reflect degree of hydration or dehydration.
   a. Normal specific gravity ranges from 1.005 to 1.030.
   b. Specific gravity is low and matches the specific gravity of plasma at 1.010 (isosthenuria) in late stages of chronic kidney disease.
   c. Volume depletion will cause the SG to be elevated and volume overload will result in a low SG.
6. Osmolality—indication of the amount of osmotically active particles in urine (number of particles per unit volume of water). It is similar to specific gravity, but is considered a more precise test and only 1 to 2 mL of urine are required. Osmolality can range from 20 to 1,350 mOsm/kg.

Nursing and Patient Care Considerations

1. Freshly voided urine provides the best results for routine urinalysis; some tests may require first morning specimen.
2. Obtain sample of about 30 mL.
3. Urine culture and sensitivity tests are typically performed using the same specimen obtained for urinalysis; therefore, use clean-catch (see Procedure Guidelines 21-1) or catheterization techniques.
4. Patients with urinary diversions, especially ileal conduit diversions, require catheterized urine specimen. The urinalysis will demonstrate bacteria as the specimen is collected from intestinal diversion.

Radiology and Imaging Studies

These tests include simple x-rays, x-rays with the use of contrast media, ultrasound, nuclear scans, and imaging via computed tomography (CT) and magnetic resonance imaging (MRI). Patient age and pregnancy status help dictate imaging choice.

 Evidence Base Mandeville, J. A., Gnessin, E., & Lingeman, J. E. (2011). Imaging evaluation in the patient with renal stone disease. *Seminars in Nephrology, 31,* 254–258.

X-ray of Kidneys, Ureters, and Bladder

Description

1. Consists of plain film of the abdomen.
2. Delineates size, shape, and position of kidneys.
3. Reveals deviations, such as calcifications (stones), tumors, or kidney displacement.
4. Not reliable as sole imaging modality to diagnose stones as it will not show radiolucent stones.

Nursing and Patient Care Considerations

1. No preparation is needed.
2. Usually done before other testing.
3. Patient will be asked to wear a gown and remove all metal from the x-ray field.

Intravenous Pyelogram (Intravenous Urogram)

Description

1. IV introduction of a radiopaque contrast medium that concentrates in the urine and thus facilitates visualization of the kidneys, ureter, and bladder. Rarely used test as CT urogram is now the radiographic modality of choice.
2. The contrast medium is cleared from the bloodstream by renal excretion.

Nursing and Patient Care Considerations

1. Contraindicated in patients with renal failure, uncontrolled diabetes, multiple myeloma, or creatine levels >1.6.
2. In patients taking metformin, the drug must be stopped the day of the test and held for 2 days.
3. Patients with known iodine/contrast material allergy must have corticosteroid/antihistamine medication; in some cases, an anesthesiologist must be available.

PROCEDURE GUIDELINES 21-1

Technique for Obtaining Clean-Catch Midstream Voided Specimen

A *clean-catch midstream specimen* is the most clinically effective method of securing a voided specimen for urinalysis. Because it is not a simple procedure, it requires thorough patient education as well as active assistance of the *female* patient.

EQUIPMENT

- Antiseptic solution or liquid soap solution
- Sterile water
- 4" × 4" gauze pads

- Disposable gloves for nurse assisting female patient
- Sterile specimen container

PROCEDURE

Nursing Action	Rationale
Male patient	
1. Instruct patient to expose glans and cleanse area around meatus. Wash area with mild antiseptic solution or liquid soap. Rinse thoroughly. If uncircumcised, retract foreskin.	1. The urethral orifice is colonized by bacteria. Urine readily becomes contaminated during voiding. Rinse antiseptic solution or soap solution thoroughly because these agents can inhibit bacterial growth in a urine culture.
2. Allow the initial urinary flow to escape.	2. The first portion of urine washes out the urethra and contains debris.
3. Collect the midstream urine specimen in a sterile container.	3. The midstream sample reflects the status of the bladder.
4. Avoid collecting the last few drops of urine.	4. Prostatic secretions may be introduced into urine at the end of the urinary stream in men.

Female patient

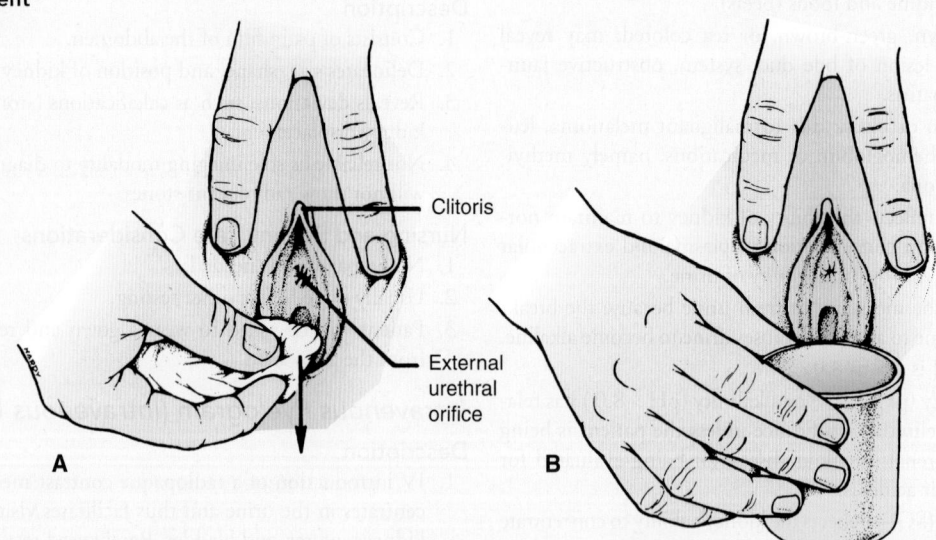

Clitoris

External urethral orifice

A   B

Obtaining a clean-catch midstream urine specimen in the female patient. (A) Instruct the patient to hold the labia apart and wash from high up front toward the back with gauze soaked in soap. (B) The collection cup is held so that it does not touch the body, and the sample is obtained only while the patient is voiding with the labia held apart. Note: If the nurse is assisting the patient, gloves are worn.

Nursing Action	Rationale
1. Ask patient to separate her labia to expose the urethral orifice. If no one is available to assist patient, she may sit backward on the toilet seat facing the water tank or sit on (straddle) the wide part of the bedpan.	1. Keeping the labia separated prevents labial or vaginal contamination of the urine specimen. By straddling the toilet seat or bedpan, patient's labia are spread apart for cleansing.
2. Clean the area around the urinary meatus with pads soaked with antiseptic/soap solution. Rinse thoroughly.	2. The urethral orifice is colonized by bacteria. Urine readily becomes contaminated during voiding.
	a. Avoids contamination from the anus.

PROCEDURE GUIDELINES 21-1 *(continued)*

Technique for Obtaining Clean-Catch Midstream Voided Specimen

PROCEDURE *(continued)*

Nursing Action	Rationale
3. While patient keeps the labia separated (see accompanying figure), instruct her to void forcibly.	3. Helps wash away urethral contaminants.
4. Allow initial urinary flow to drain into bedpan (toilet) and then catch the midstream specimen in a sterile container, making sure that the container does not come in contact with the genitalia.	4. The first portion of urine washes out the urethra. Have patient remove the container from the stream while she is still voiding.

Follow-up phase

1. Send specimen to laboratory immediately.	1. A culture should be performed as soon as possible to avoid multiplication of urinary bacteria and lysis of cells.

4. Bowel preparation may be needed in patients with constipation issues:
   a. Cathartics/laxatives may be given the evening before the examination.
   b. Nothing by mouth (NPO) after midnight the day of the examination (if scheduled for afternoon, clear liquids only in the morning).
5. May not be done after barium studies or oral contrast studies because barium will obscure view of intravenous pyelography (IVP).

Retrograde Pyelography

Description
1. Injection of radiopaque contrast material through ureteral catheters, which have been passed into ureters by means of cystoscopic manipulation. The radiopaque solution is introduced by syringe injection. May require sedation.
2. May be done when IVP is contraindicated or if IVP provides inadequate visualization of the collecting system.

Nursing and Patient Care Considerations
1. Contraindicated in patients with UTI.
2. May require sedation.
3. Allergic reactions are rare.

Cystourethrogram

Description
1. Visualization of urethra and bladder by x-ray after retrograde instillation of contrast material through a catheter. An examination of only the bladder is a *cystogram*, of only the urethra is a *urethrogram*.
2. Used to identify injuries, vesicoureteral reflux, tumors, or structural abnormalities of the urethra or bladder or to evaluate emptying problems or incontinence (voiding cystourethrogram).

Nursing and Patient Care Considerations
1. Carries risk of infection due to instrumentation.
2. Allergy to contrast material is not a contraindication.

3. Additional x-rays may be taken after catheter is removed and patient voids (voiding cystourethrogram).
4. Provide reassurance to allay patient's embarrassment.

Renal Angiography

Description
1. IV catheter is threaded through the femoral and iliac arteries into the aorta or renal artery.
2. Contrast material is injected to visualize the renal arterial supply.
3. Evaluates blood flow dynamics, demonstrates abnormal vasculature, and differentiates renal cysts from renal tumors.
4. May be done prior to renal transplant or to embolize a kidney before nephrectomy for renal tumor.

Nursing and Patient Care Considerations
1. Clear liquids only after midnight before the examination; adequate hydration is essential.
2. Continue oral medications (special orders needed for diabetic patients).
3. IV access required.
4. May not be done on the same day as other studies requiring barium or contrast material.
5. Maintain bed rest for 8 hours after the examination, with the leg kept straight on the side used for groin access.
6. Observe frequently for hematoma or bleeding at access site. Keep sandbag at bedside for use if bleeding occurs.

Renal Scan

Description
1. Radiopharmaceuticals (also called radiotracers or isotopes) are injected intravenously.
   a. Tc-DTPA, Tc^{99m}-DMSA is used for anatomical or MAG3 visualization and evaluation of glomerular filtration.
   b. Other radiopharmaceuticals may also be used depending on the purpose of the scan.

2. Assesses renal function and not used to assess for renal anatomy, mass, or stones.

3. Studies are obtained with a scintillation camera placed posterior to the kidney with patient in a supine, prone, or sitting position.

Nursing and Patient Care Considerations

1. Patient should be well hydrated. Give several glasses of water or IV fluids, as ordered, before scan.

2. Furosemide or captopril may be administered in conjunction with the scan to determine their effects.

Ultrasound

Description

1. Uses high-frequency sound waves passed into the body and reflected back in varying frequencies based on the composition of soft tissues. Organs in the urinary system create characteristic ultrasonic images that are electronically processed and displayed as an image.

2. Abnormalities, such as masses, malformations, stones, or obstructions, can be identified; useful in differentiating between solid and fluid-filled masses.

3. A noninvasive technique without the use of radiation.

Nursing and Patient Care Considerations

1. Ultrasound examination of the prostate is performed using a rectal probe. A Fleet enema may be ordered just within hours of the examination.

2. Ultrasound examination of the bladder requires that the bladder be full.

3. Patient should not have had any studies using barium for 2 days before ultrasound of the kidney or bladder.

Computed Tomography and Magnetic Resonance Imaging

See descriptions on page 206.

Other Tests

Other tests that may be done to evaluate disorders of the renal and urologic systems include cystoscopy, urodynamic testing, and needle biopsy of the kidney.

Cystoscopy

Description

1. *Cystoscopy* is a method of direct visualization of the urethra and bladder by means of a cystoscope that is inserted through the urethra into the bladder. It has a self-contained optical lens system that provides a magnified, illuminated view of the bladder.

2. Uses include:
   a. To inspect bladder wall directly for tumor, stone, or ulcer and to inspect urethra for abnormalities or to assess degree of prostatic obstruction.
   b. To allow insertion of ureteral catheters for radiographic studies or before abdominal or GU surgery.
   c. To see configuration and position of ureteral orifices.
   d. To remove calculi from urethra, bladder, and ureter.
   e. To diagnose and treat lesions of bladder, urethra, and prostate.
   f. To perform endoscopic prostate surgeries including transurethral resection of the prostate (TURP) (see page 793).

Nursing and Patient Care Considerations

1. Simple cystoscopy is usually performed in an office setting. More complicated cystoscopies, involving resections or ureteral catheter insertions, are done in the operating room suite, where IV sedation or spinal or general anesthesia may be used.

2. Patient's genitalia are cleaned with an antiseptic solution just before the examination. A local topical anesthetic (lidocaine gel) is instilled into the urethra before insertion of cystoscope.

3. Because fluid flows continuously through the cystoscope, patient may feel an urge to urinate during the examination.

4. Contraindicated in patients with known UTI.

5. Nursing interventions after cystoscopic examination:
   a. Monitor for complications: urinary retention, urinary tract hemorrhage, infection within prostate or bladder.
   b. Expect patient to have some burning on voiding, blood-tinged urine, and urinary frequency from trauma to mucous membrane of the urethra.
   c. Administer or teach self-administration of antibiotics prophylactically, as ordered, to prevent UTI.
   d. Advise warm sitz baths or analgesics, such as ibuprofen or acetaminophen, to relieve discomfort after cystoscopy. Increase hydration.
   e. Provide routine catheter care if urine retention persists and an indwelling catheter is ordered.

Urodynamics

Description

Urodynamics is a term that refers to any of the following tests that provide physiologic and functional information about the lower urinary tract. They measure the ability of the bladder to store and empty urine. Most urodynamic equipment uses computer technology with results visible in real time on a monitor.

1. Uroflowmetry (flow rate)—a record of the volume of urine passing through the urethra per unit of time (mL/s). It is shown on graph paper and gives information about the rate and flow pattern of urination. It is used to evaluate obstructive voiding. Minimum volume of urine needed for accurate test is 150 mL.

2. Cystometrography—recording of the pressures exerted during filling and emptying of the urinary bladder to assess its function. Data about the ability of the bladder to store urine at low pressure and the ability of the bladder to contract appropriately to empty urine are obtained.
   a. A small catheter is placed through the urethra (or suprapubic area) into bladder. The residual volume is measured if patient recently voided and the catheter is left in place.
   b. The catheters are connected to urodynamic equipment designed to measure pressure at the distal end of the catheter.

c. Water, saline, or contrast material is infused at a slow rate into the bladder.

d. When the bladder feels full, patient is asked to "void." A normal detrusor contraction of the bladder appears as a sharp rise in bladder pressure on the graph. If the patient is unable to void, the test may be considered normal because it is difficult to void normally with catheters in place.

3. Sphincter electromyelography (EMG)—measures the activity of the pelvic floor muscles during bladder filling and emptying. EMG activity may be measured using surface (patch) electrodes placed around the anus or with percutaneous wire or needle electrodes.

4. Pressure-flow studies—involve all of the above components, along with the simultaneous measurement of intra-abdominal pressure by way of a small tube with a fluid-filled balloon that is placed in the rectum. This permits better interpretation of actual bladder pressures without the influence of intra-abdominal pressure.

5. Video urodynamics—use all of the above components. The fluid used to fill the bladder is contrast material and the entire study is performed under fluoroscopy, providing radiographic pictures in combination with the recording of bladder and intra-abdominal pressures. Video urodynamics are reserved for patients with complicated voiding dysfunction.

Nursing and Patient Care Considerations

1. Contraindicated in patients with UTI.

2. Frequently performed by nurses; essential to provide information and support throughout the test to ensure clinically significant results.

3. Patients may have burning on urination afterward (due to instrumentation); encourage fluids.

4. Short-term antibiotics are commonly given to prevent infection.

Needle Biopsy of Kidney

Description

Performed by percutaneous needle biopsy through renal tissue with ultrasound guidance or by open biopsy through a small flank incision; useful in securing specimens for electron and immunofluorescent microscopy to determine diagnosis, treatment, and prognosis of renal disease.

Nursing and Patient Care Considerations

1. Prebiopsy nursing management.

    a. Ensure that coagulation studies, platelet count, and hematocrit results are reported to provide baseline values and to identify patients at risk for postbiopsy bleeding.

    b. Ensure that patient is NPO for several hours before the procedure, as ordered.

    c. Establish an IV line, as ordered.

    d. Describe the procedure to patient, including holding breath (to prevent movement of the thorax) during insertion of the biopsy needle.

2. Postbiopsy nursing management.

    a. Place patient in a supine position immediately after biopsy and on bed rest for 8 to 24 hours to minimize bleeding.

    b. Take vital signs every 5 to 15 minutes for the first hour and then with decreasing frequency if stable to assess for hemorrhage, which is a major complication.

    c. Watch for rise or fall in blood pressure (BP), anorexia, vomiting, or development of dull, aching discomfort in abdomen.

    d. Assess for flank pain (usually represents bleeding into the muscle) or colicky pain (clot in the ureter).

    e. Assess for backache, shoulder pain, or dysuria.

    f. Persistent bleeding may be suspected when an enlarging hematoma is palpable through the abdomen.

    g. If perirenal bleeding develops, avoid palpating or manipulating the abdomen after the first examination has determined that a hematoma exists.

    h. Collect serial urine specimens to evaluate for hematuria.

    i. Assess for any patient complaints, especially frequency and urgency on urination.

    j. Keep fluid intake at 3,000 mL daily, if tolerated, unless patient has renal insufficiency.

    k. Check results of hematocrit and hemoglobin (done the following morning) to assess for anemia, unless vital signs change before then.

    l. Prepare for transfusion and surgical intervention for control of hemorrhage, which may necessitate surgical drainage or nephrectomy.

3. Instruct patient on the following after biopsy:

    a. Avoid strenuous activity, strenuous sports, and heavy lifting for at least 2 weeks.

    b. Notify health care provider if any of the following occur: flank pain, hematuria, light-headedness and fainting, rapid pulse, or any other signs and symptoms of bleeding.

    c. Report for follow-up 1 to 2 months after biopsy; will be checked for hypertension and the biopsy area is auscultated for a bruit.

GENERAL PROCEDURES AND TREATMENT MODALITIES

Catheterization

Catheterization may be done to relieve acute or chronic urinary retention, to drain urine preoperatively and postoperatively, to determine the amount of residual urine after voiding, or to determine accurate measurement of urinary drainage in critically ill patients. See Procedure Guidelines 21-2, pages 778 to 780. Also see Procedure Guidelines 21-3, pages 780 to 783.

Suprapubic catheterization establishes drainage from the bladder by introducing a catheter percutaneously or by an incision through the anterior abdominal wall into the bladder. It may be done for acute urinary retention when urethral catheterization is not possible; for urethral trauma, stricture, or fistula to divert flow of urine from the urethra; or for obtaining an uncontaminated urine specimen for culture. See Procedure Guidelines 21-4, pages 784 to 785.

(Text continues on page 785)

PROCEDURE GUIDELINES 21-2

Catheterization of the Urinary Bladder

EQUIPMENT

- Sterile gloves
- Disposable sterile catheter set with single-use packet of lubricant
- Antiseptic solution for periurethral cleaning (sterile)
- Sterile container for culture
- Gloves, drape, pads
- Bath blanket or sheet for draping
- Standing lamp (preferred) or flashlight

Selection of catheter size
Use the smallest catheter capable of providing adequate drainage.

PROCEDURE

Nursing Action	Rationale
Female patient	
Preparatory phase	
1. Wash hands. Explain procedure to patient.	1. Patient will feel reassured if the procedure is explained and if she is handled gently and considerately.
2. Open catheter tray using aseptic technique. Place waste receptacle in accessible place.	2. Catheterization requires the same aseptic precautions as a surgical procedure. The principal danger of catheterization is urinary tract infection, which is associated with increased morbidity and longer, more costly hospitalization.
3. Place patient in a supine position with knees bent, hips flexed, and feet resting on bed in a "frog's-legs" position. Drape the patient.	3. Position should allow visualization of the vulva.
4. Direct light for visualization of genital area.	
5. Position moisture-proof pad under patient's buttocks.	5. Absorb urine, if necessary.
6. Put on sterile gloves.	6. Prevents bacterial contamination.

Performance phase

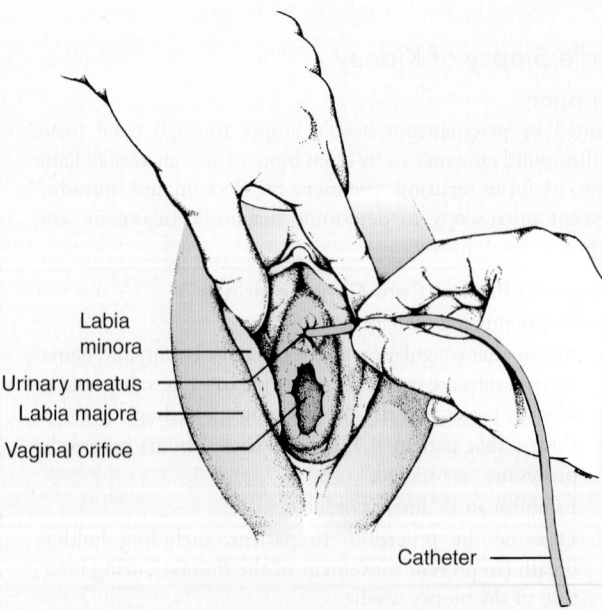

Labia minora
Urinary meatus
Labia majora
Vaginal orifice
Catheter

Catheterization of urinary bladder in the female patient.

PROCEDURE GUIDELINES 21-2 (continued)

Catheterization of the Urinary Bladder

PROCEDURE (continued)

Nursing Action	Rationale
1. Separate labia minora so urethral meatus is visualized; one hand is to maintain separation of the labia until catheterization is finished.	1. Helps prevent labial contamination of the catheter (see accompanying figure).
2. Clean around the urethral meatus with a povidone–iodine solution, unless patient is allergic to iodine—in which case, clean with soap and water.	2. Bacteria that normally colonize the distal urethra may be introduced into the bladder during or immediately after catheter insertion. Inadequate preparation of the urethral meatus is a major cause of infection.
a. Manipulate cleaning pads or cotton balls with forceps, cleaning with downward strokes from anterior to posterior.	a. Prevents introducing bacteria from the perineum into the urethra.
b. Dispose of cotton pad after each use.	
c. If patient is sensitive to iodine, benzalkonium chloride or other cleaning agent such as chlorhexidine may be used.	
3. Introduce well-lubricated catheter 2–3 inches (5–7.5 cm) into urethral meatus using strict aseptic technique.	3. A well-lubricated catheter reduces friction and trauma to the meatus. The female urethra is a relatively short canal, measuring 1¼ to 1½ inches (3–4 cm) in length.
a. Avoid contaminating surface of catheter.	
b. Make sure that catheter is not too large or too tight at urethral meatus.	b. Too large a catheter may cause painful distention of the meatus and cause damage to the uroepithelium.
4. Allow some bladder urine to flow through catheter before collecting a specimen.	4. Obtains representative bladder sample.

Male patient

Preparatory phase

Nursing Action	Rationale
1. Lubricate the catheter well with lubricant or prescribed topical anesthetic.	1. Prevents urethral trauma (decreasing the opportunity for bacterial invasion).
2. Wash off glans penis around urinary meatus with an iodophor solution using forceps to hold cleaning pads. Clean urethral meatus from tip to foreskin with downward stroke on one side. Discard pad. Repeat as required. Keep the foreskin retracted.	2. Reduces risk of bacterial transmission when catheter enters urethra. Use of forceps maintains sterility of dominant hand.
3. Grasp shaft of penis (with nondominant hand) and elevate it. Apply gentle traction to penis while catheter is passed.	3. Straightens the penile urethra and facilitates catheterization. Maintaining a grasp of the penis prevents contamination and retraction of penis.
4. Using sterile gloves, insert catheter into the urethra; advance catheter 6–10 inches (15–25 cm) until urine flows	4. The male urethra length varies within wide limits; the average length is about 8 inches (20 cm).

> **Key Decision Point**
>
> If resistance is felt at the external sphincter while trying to advance the catheter, increase the traction on the penis slightly and apply steady, gentle pressure on the catheter. Ask patient to strain gently (as if passing urine) to help relax sphincter. Some resistance may be due to spasm of external sphincter, which should subside. If you are unable to pass the catheter at all, there may be a urethral stricture or other form of urethral pathology. Withdraw catheter and notify health care provider. Consultation with a urologist for possible dilation is indicated.

Nursing Action	Rationale
5. When urine begins to flow, advance the catheter another 1 inch (2.5 cm).	5. Advancing the catheter ensures its position in the bladder.
6. Replace (or reposition) the foreskin.	6. Paraphimosis (retraction and constriction of the foreskin behind the glans penis), secondary to catheterization, may occur if the foreskin is not replaced.

(continued)

PROCEDURE GUIDELINES 21-2 *(continued)*

Catheterization of the Urinary Bladder

PROCEDURE *(continued)*

Nursing Action	Rationale
Follow-up phase	
1. Remove catheter gently when urine ceases to flow.	1. Minimizing trauma to the urethra and time the catheter is in contact with the urethral mucosa will minimize chance of infection.
2. Dry area; make patient comfortable.	2. Some urine may have leaked while withdrawing catheter or lubricating gel may need to be cleared.
3. Send specimen to laboratory, as indicated.	3. Proper processing of specimen will assure accuracy of test.
4. Record time, procedure, amount, and appearance of urine.	4. For continuity of care.

COMMUNITY AND HOME CARE CONSIDERATIONS

- Caregiver or patient can catheterize using clean technique, however, Medicare guidelines now allow for reimbursement of sterile catheters for each catheterization to prevent UTI.
- Assemble catheter (usually flexible, red rubber catheter; clear plastic, firmer catheter may be used by men), lubricant, and liquid soap.
- Clean area around urethral meatus with liquid soap, if desired.
- Wash hands; wear unsterile gloves if desired.
- Catheterize; remove catheter when drainage ceases.
- Wash catheter with soap and water; rinse and dry well with paper towel.
- Store in new sealable plastic bag.
- Nurse catheterizing patient in home usually maintains sterile technique.
- Replace catheters as often as possible, at least once per month.

 Evidence Base Gould, C. V., Umscheid, C. A., Agarwal, R. K., et al. (2009). Guideline for prevention of catheter associated urinary tract infections. Atlanta, GA: Centers for Disease Control and Prevention. Available: *www.cdc.gov/hicpac/pdf/CAUTI/CAUTIguideline2009final.pdf.*
Wein, A. J., Kavoussi, L. R., Novick, A. C., et al. (Eds.). (2012). *Campbell-Walsh urology* (10th ed., Vols. 1–3). Philadelphia: W.B. Saunders.

PROCEDURE GUIDELINES 21-3

Management of the Patient with an Indwelling (Self-Retaining) Catheter and Closed Drainage System

EQUIPMENT

- Catheter tray with closed system of urinary drainage
- Gauze pads
- Antibacterial solution for cleaning
- Single-use packet of lubricant

PROCEDURE

Nursing Action	Rationale
General considerations	
1. Catheterize the patient (pages 778–780) using a catheter that is preconnected to a closed drainage system.	1. A closed drainage system is one that is closed to outside air.
a. Advance catheter almost to its bifurcation (for male patient).	a. Prevents the balloon from becoming trapped in the urethra.
b. Inflate the balloon according to manufacturer's directions. Make sure catheter is draining properly before inflating balloon, then withdraw catheter slightly.	b. Inadvertent inflation of the balloon within the urethra is painful and causes urethral trauma.

PROCEDURE GUIDELINES 21-3 *(continued)*

Management of the Patient with an Indwelling (Self-Retaining) Catheter and Closed Drainage System

PROCEDURE *(continued)*

Nursing Action	Rationale
2. Secure the indwelling catheter to patient's thigh using tape, strap, adhesive anchor, or other securement device.	2. Properly securing the catheter prevents catheter movement and traction on the urethra.
a. Allow some slack of the tubing to accommodate the patient's movements.	
b. Keep the tubing over the patient's leg.	b. This tubing position helps prevent kinking or forming loops of stagnant urine.

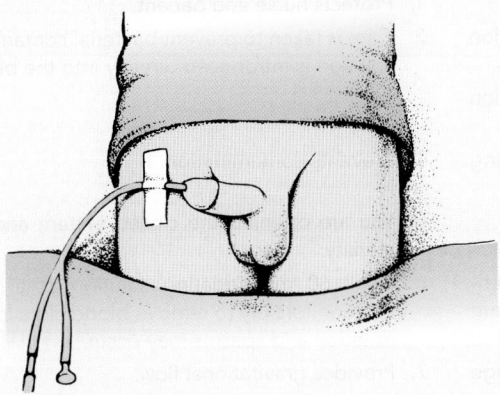

In the male patient, the indwelling catheter is taped to the thigh to straighten the angulation of the peno-scrotal junction, thus reducing pressure on the urethra exerted by the catheter.

Care of the indwelling catheter

1. Clean around the area where catheter enters urethral meatus (meatal–catheter junction) with soap and water during the daily bath to remove debris.	1. Suppurative drainage and encrustation occur at the exit of any tube. Infectious organisms can migrate to the bladder along the outside of any indwelling catheter; however, excessive manipulation of the catheter may promote migration of bacteria.
2. Avoid using powders and sprays on the perineal area.	2. Powder can encrust and cause soreness and infection.
3. Avoid pulling on the catheter during cleaning.	3. Pulling on the catheter may be painful. Backward and forward displacement of the catheter introduces contaminants into the urinary tract.

To obtain urine for culture

1. Clamp the drainage tubing below the aspiration (sampling) port for a few minutes to allow urine to collect.	1. Avoid separating catheter and connecting tube. Disconnection of the catheter and tubing is a major cause of urinary tract infection (UTI).
2. Clean the aspiration port with povidone–iodine or 70% alcohol.	2. Prevents introduction of contaminants into closed system.
3. Insert a needleless syringe into the aspiration port of the catheter tubing and aspirate a small volume of urine for culture.	
4. Remove from syringe and release urine carefully into sterile specimen container.	4. Prevents contamination of specimen, which will alter the results.
5. Unclamp the drainage tube.	5. Prevents retention of urine and potential infection.
6. Send specimen to laboratory immediately.	6. The specimen should be marked as a "catheterized specimen" because the presence of any number of colonies of an organism indicates a UTI.

(continued)

PROCEDURE GUIDELINES 21-3 *(continued)*

Management of the Patient with an Indwelling (Self-Retaining) Catheter and Closed Drainage System

PROCEDURE *(continued)*

Nursing Action	Rationale
To irrigate the catheter	
Note: This is not done unless ordered to relieve obstruction or if persistent gross hematuria is anticipated (bleeding after bladder or prostate surgery). If frequent irrigations are necessary to keep the catheter open, the catheter may need to be changed to a larger size.	
1. Wash hands. Put on gloves.	1. Protects nurse and patient.
2. Using aseptic technique, pour sterile irrigating solution into sterile container.	2. Care is taken to prevent bacterial contamination because solution is introduced directly into the bladder.
3. Clean around catheter and drainage tubing connection with alcohol swabs.	
4. Disconnect catheter from drainage tubing. Cover tubing with a sterile cap.	4. Prevents contamination.
5. Place a sterile drainage basin under the catheter.	5. You are opening the closed system and must maintain sterility.
6. Connect a large-volume syringe to the catheter and irrigate catheter using prescribed amount of sterile irrigant.	6. Instill 60 mL irrigating solution at a time. Instill the solution forcibly to remove blood clots from the bladder; irritation and spasms may occur.
7. Remove syringe and place end of catheter over drainage basin, allowing returning fluid to drain into basin.	7. Provides gravitational flow.
8. Repeat irrigation procedure until fluid is clear or according to order. For clot irrigation, pull back gently on syringe.	8. After prostatic surgery, the goal of irrigation is to clear bloody fluid that may clot.
9. Disinfect the distal end of the catheter and end of drainage tubing; reconnect the catheter and tubing. Dispose of irrigation solution and syringe. Remove gloves. Wash hands.	9. Prevents contamination of catheter and transfer of any bacteria to another patient.
10. Document type and amount of irrigating solution, color and character of returning fluid, presence of sediment/blood clots, and patient's reaction.	10. For continuity of care.
Changing the catheter	
Change catheter according to the needs of patient.	Facility policy may vary.
Maintaining a closed drainage system	
1. Wash hands immediately before and after handling any part of the system. Wear clean, disposable gloves when handling the drainage system.	1. Hands are the major route of transmission of Gram-negative bacteria.
2. Maintain unobstructed urine flow.	2. Urine flow must be downhill.
a. Keep the drainage bag in a dependent position, below the level of the bladder.	a. Raising the bag will cause reflux of contaminated urine from the bag into patient's bladder.
b. Urine should not be allowed to collect in the tubing because a free flow of urine must be maintained to prevent infection.	b. Improper drainage occurs when the tubing is kinked or twisted, allowing pools of drainage to collect in the loops of tubing.
c. Keep the bag off the floor.	c. Prevents bacterial contamination.

PROCEDURE GUIDELINES 21-3 *(continued)*

Management of the Patient with an Indwelling (Self-Retaining) Catheter and Closed Drainage System

PROCEDURE *(continued)*

Nursing Action	Rationale

3. Empty the bag at regular intervals, making sure that the drainage valve/spout is not contaminated.
 	
  a. Wash hands; put on gloves.
  b. Disinfect spigot. Empty the bag in a separate collecting receptacle for each patient. Disinfect spigot again.
  c. Avoid letting the drainage bag touch the floor.
  d. Change the drainage bag if contamination occurs, if the urine flow becomes obstructed, or if the connecting junctions start to leak.
	3. Care is taken to maintain a closed system to prevent catheter-acquired infection and to prevent transmission of infection to other patients.
	
	  b. Each patient should have own collecting receptacle that is labeled and kept in the bathroom, not on the floor—to prevent cross-contamination.

Preventing cross-contamination 1. Wash hands before and after handling the catheter and drainage system and between patients. 2. Identify patients at risk.	1. Many UTIs are due to extrinsically acquired organisms transmitted by cross-contamination. 2. Female, older, debilitated, and critically ill patients, those in the postpartum state, and patients with obstructed or neurologically impaired bladders are at risk for infection.

COMMUNITY AND HOME CARE CONSIDERATIONS

For care of catheter at home, instruct patient to:

- Wash hands before and after handling the catheter.
- Wash around urinary opening daily, taking care to avoid pulling on the catheter during cleaning and removing encrustation around the catheter.
- Drink 8 to 12 glasses of fluids daily; increase fluid intake if urine becomes dark and concentrated.
- Wipe all connecting junctions with alcohol before changing from leg-bag drainage to overnight drainage bag.
- Keep the drainage bag at a lower level than the bladder; do not place the bag on your chair.
- Avoid letting the bag lay on its side because urine may flow back into the drainage tube.

- Usually, the catheter is changed every 4–6 weeks or when obstruction or malfunction occurs.
- The interval between catheter cleaning and changes may be decreased if there is heavy encrustation.
- Call health care provider if fever or cloudy, bloody, or odoriferous urine develops. In the male patient, the indwelling catheter is taped to the thigh to straighten the angulation of the penoscrotal junction, thus reducing pressure on the urethra exerted by the catheter.

 Evidence Base Wein, A. J., Kavoussi, L. R., Novick, A. C., et al. (Eds.). (2012). *Campbell- Walsh urology* (10th ed., Vols. 1–3). Philadelphia: W.B. Saunders.

PROCEDURE GUIDELINES 21-4

Assisting the Patient Undergoing Suprapubic Bladder Drainage

EQUIPMENT

- Sterile suprapubic drainage system package (disposable)
- Skin germicide for suprapubic skin preparation; sterile gloves
- Local anesthetic agent, if needed

PROCEDURE

Nursing Action	Rationale
Preparatory phase	
1. Place patient in a supine position with one pillow under head.	1. Allows access to suprapubic area but reduces muscle tension.
2. Expose the abdomen.	
Performance phase (by health care provider)	
1. The bladder is distended with 300–500 mL sterile saline in a urethral catheter, which is removed, or patient is given fluids (P.O. or via IV line) before the procedure.	1. Distention of the bladder makes the bladder easier to locate by the suprapubic route.
2. The suprapubic area is surgically prepared. After the skin is dried, the needle entry point is located.	2. The needle entry point is in the midline, ¾ to 1¼ inches (2–3 cm) above the symphysis pubis and directly over the palpable bladder.
3. The skin and subcutaneous tissues are infiltrated with local anesthesia.	3. An adequate level of local anesthesia is achieved to facilitate catheter introduction.
4. A small incision may be made.	
5. The catheter is introduced via a guide wire, needle, or cannula through the incision and advanced in a slightly caudal direction.	5. Entrance into the bladder is usually felt and can be verified by free flow of urine.
6. The catheter is advanced until the flange is against the skin where it is secured with tape, a body seal system, or sutures.	6. Another method is to advance a long needle into the bladder until urine flow verifies the needle is in the bladder.
7. The catheter is connected to a sterile drainage system.	7. Aseptic technique must be maintained to prevent infection.
8. Secure drainage tubing to lateral abdomen with tape.	8. Prevents undue tension on the catheter.
9. If the catheter is not draining properly, withdraw the catheter 1 inch (2.5 cm) at a time until urine begins to flow. Do not dislodge catheter from bladder.	9. Catheter tip may be pinned against the wall of the bladder.
10. Drainage may be maintained continuously for several days.	10. Due to risk of infection, this is not a long-term option for urinary drainage.
11. If a "trial of voiding" is requested, the catheter is clamped for 4 hours.	11. Usually, patients will void earlier after surgery with suprapubic drainage than with indwelling catheters.
a. Have patient attempt to void while the catheter is clamped.	
b. After patient voids, unclamp the catheter and measure residual urine.	b. Determines the effectiveness of voiding.
c. Usually, if the amount of residual urine is less than 100 mL on two separate occasions (AM and PM), the catheter may be removed.	c. If larger residual, the patient is not ready for catheter removal.
d. If the patient reports pain or discomfort, or if the residual urine is over the prescribed amount, the catheter is usually left open.	d. Facilitates urinary drainage and prevent infection due to urinary stasis.

PROCEDURE GUIDELINES 21-4 *(continued)*

Assisting the Patient Undergoing Suprapubic Bladder Drainage

PROCEDURE *(continued)*

Nursing Action	Rationale
12. When the catheter is removed, a sterile dressing is placed over the site. Usually the tract will close within 48 hours.	12. Suprapubic drainage is considered more comfortable than an indwelling urethral catheter. It allows greater patient mobility and there is less risk of bladder infection.
13. Monitor for complications.	13. Complications of this procedure: inadvertent peritoneal and bowel damage, leakage around catheter, kinking of catheter, hematuria, abdominal wall abscess.

Evidence Base Wein, A. J., Kavoussi, L. R., Novick, A. C., et al. (Eds.). (2012). *Campbell-Walsh urology* (10th ed., Vols. 1–3). Philadelphia: W.B. Saunders.

Dialysis

Dialysis refers to the diffusion of solute molecules through a semipermeable membrane, passing from the side of higher concentration to that of lower concentration. The purpose of dialysis is to maintain fluid, electrolyte, and acid-base balance and to remove endogenous and exogenous toxins. It is a substitute for some kidney excretory functions but does replace the kidneys' endocrine functions. Methods of dialysis include:

1. Peritoneal dialysis.
   a. Intermittent peritoneal dialysis (IPD).
   b. Continuous ambulatory peritoneal dialysis (CAPD).
   c. Continuous cycling peritoneal dialysis (CCPD)—uses automated peritoneal dialysis machine overnight with prolonged dwell time during day.
2. Hemodialysis (see page 786).
3. Continuous renal replacement therapy (CRRT)—this includes slow continuous ultrafiltration, continuous venovenous hemofiltration, continuous venovenous hemodialysis, and continuous venovenous hemodiafiltration. These use extracorporeal blood circulation through a small-volume, low-resistance filter to provide continuous removal of solutes and fluid in the intensive care setting. Historically, CRRT required arterial and venous access ("atriovenous") and was driven by the patient's mean arterial pressure (MAP). This approach is rarely practiced today as pump-assisted equipment that only requires venous access is the standard of care.
   a. CRRT is indicated for hemodynamically unstable patients who cannot tolerate the rapid fluid shifts that occur with intermittent dialysis and in oliguric patients who require large amounts of hourly IV fluids or parenteral nutrition. CRRT is often better tolerated by critically ill patients because it is a slower and less aggressive process for removal of fluid and solutes than hemodialysis.
   b. CRRT is accomplished by insertion of a large-gauge double-lumen catheter into the internal jugular, subclavian, or femoral vein. A roller-type pump is used to propel blood through the system and anticoagulation may be used to prevent clotting. This is the current standard of care because of consistent blood flow rates.
   c. Care for the patient on CRRT is provided in an intensive care setting, with special attention given to assessing and calculating fluid and electrolyte balance, aggressively managing hypotension, preventing hemorrhage, monitoring for heat loss through the extracorporeal circulation, assessing for infection, and preventing clotting.

Continuous Ambulatory Peritoneal Dialysis

Continuous ambulatory peritoneal dialysis (CAPD) is a form of intracorporeal dialysis that uses the peritoneum as the semipermeable membrane (see Figure 21-1, page 786).

Procedure

1. A permanent indwelling catheter is implanted into the peritoneum; the internal cuff of the catheter becomes embedded by fibrous ingrowth, which stabilizes it and minimizes leakage.
2. A tube for connecting the catheter to an administration set is attached via a locking mechanism to the distal end of the peritoneal catheter, called the transfer set. It remains with the patient (attached to the catheter tubing) and must be changed at regular intervals per manufacturer recommendations and with contamination. Specific transfer sets may only fit administration tubings from the same manufacturer, but there are devices available to make the transfer set compatible with other PD systems.
3. There are many types of administration sets, the most common being the double bag system. The double bag system has a preattached bag of dialysate solution and drainage, which has been shown to reduce peritonitis rates.

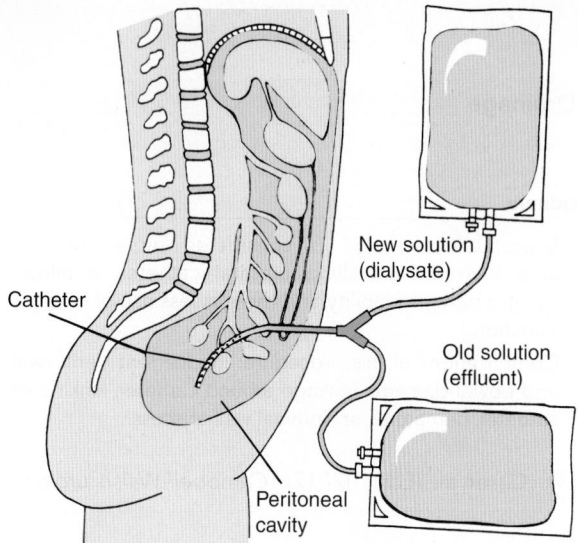

Figure 21-1. Continuous ambulatory peritoneal dialysis. The peritoneal catheter is implanted through the abdominal wall. Fluid infuses into the peritoneal cavity and drains after a prescribed time.

4. In CAPD, a patient is prescribed a set number of exchanges (fill, drain, and dwell) throughout the day.
5. During the fill, the dialysate bag is raised to shoulder level and infused by gravity into the peritoneal cavity (approximately 10 minutes for a 2-L volume).
6. During the dwell time, diffusion and osmosis occurs. The typical dwell time is 4 to 6 hours.
7. At the end of the dwell time, the dialysate fluid is drained from the peritoneal cavity by gravity. Drainage of 2 L plus ultrafiltration takes about 10 to 20 minutes if the catheter is functioning optimally.
8. After the dialysate is drained, a fresh bag of dialysate solution is infused using aseptic technique and the procedure is repeated.
9. Patient performs four to five exchanges daily, 7 days per week, with an overnight dwell time allowing uninterrupted sleep; most patients become unaware of fluid in the peritoneal cavity.

Advantages Over Hemodialysis
1. Physical and psychological freedom and independence.
2. More liberal diet and fluid intake.
3. Relatively simple and easy to use.
4. Satisfactory biochemical control of uremia.

Complications
1. Infectious peritonitis, exit-site and tunnel infections.
2. Noninfectious catheter malfunction, obstruction, dialysate leak.
3. Peritoneal–pleural communication, hernia formation.
4. GI bloating, distention, nausea.
5. Hypervolemia, hypovolemia.
6. Bleeding at catheter site.

7. Bloody effluent secondary to internal bleeding. In female patients, this may occur during menstruation.
8. Obstruction may occur if omentum becomes wrapped around the catheter or the catheter becomes caught in a loop of bowel.

Patient Education
1. The use of CAPD as a long-term treatment depends on prevention of recurring peritonitis.
   a. Use strict aseptic technique when performing bag exchanges.
   b. Perform bag exchanges in clean, closed-off area without pets and other activities.
   c. Wash hands before touching bag.
   d. Inspect bag and tubing for defects and leaks.
2. Do not omit bag changes—this will cause inadequate control of renal failure.
3. Some weight gain may accompany CAPD—the dialysate fluid contains a significant amount of dextrose, which adds calories to daily intake.
4. Report signs and symptoms of peritonitis—cloudy peritoneal fluid, abdominal pain or tenderness, malaise, fever.

Intermittent Peritoneal Dialysis

Intermittent peritoneal dialysis (IPD) is an option for treating acute kidney injury when access to the bloodstream is not possible or hemodialysis/CRRT is not available. It also may be used in cases of poisoning, congestive heart failure, or hypothermia. It is similar to CAPD in that it involves access to the peritoneal cavity, either with a newly inserted rigid stylet catheter or, in chronic peritoneal patients, the existing chronic catheter can be used. In IPD, an exchange ranges between 30 minutes and 2 hours. Exchanges are repeated continuously for a prescribed period of time, which varies between 12 and 36 hours. Due to the rapid exchanges, patients are on bedrest. As with all peritoneal dialysis procedures, aseptic technique is essential during catheter insertion, exchanges, and dressing changes to prevent peritonitis.

Hemodialysis

Hemodialysis is a process of cleansing the blood of accumulated waste products. It is used for patients with end-stage renal failure or for acutely ill patients who require short-term dialysis.

Procedure
1. Patient's access is prepared and cannulated.
2. Heparin is administered (unless contraindicated).
3. Heparinized blood flows through a semipermeable dialyzer in one direction and dialysis solution surrounds the membranes and flows in the opposite direction.
4. Dialysis solution consists of highly purified water to which sodium, potassium, calcium, magnesium, chloride, and dextrose have been added. Bicarbonate is added to achieve the proper pH balance.
5. Through the process of diffusion, solute in the form of electrolytes, metabolic waste products, and acid-base components can be removed or added to the blood.
6. Excess water is removed from the blood (ultrafiltration).
7. The blood is then returned to the body through patient's access.

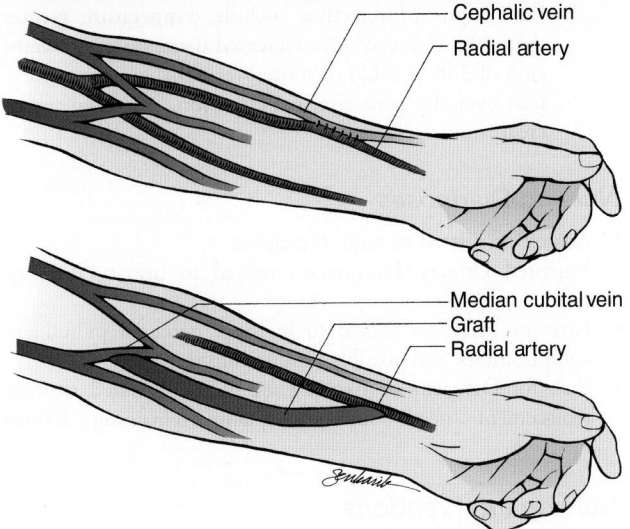

Figure 21-2. An internal arteriovenous fistula (*top*) is created by a side-to-side anastomosis of the artery and vein. A graft (*bottom*) can also be established between the artery and vein.

Requirements for Hemodialysis
1. Access to patient's circulation.
2. Dialysis machine and dialyzer with semipermeable membrane.
3. Appropriate dialysate bath.
4. Time—approximately 4 hours, three times weekly.
5. Place—dialysis center or home (if feasible).

Methods of Circulatory Access
1. Arteriovenous fistula (AVF)—creation of a vascular communication by suturing a vein directly to an artery (see Figure 21-2).
   a. Usually, radial artery and cephalic vein are anastomosed in nondominant arm; vessels in the upper arm may also be used.
   b. After the procedure, the superficial venous system of the arm dilates.
   c. By means of two large-bore needles inserted into the dilated venous system, blood may be obtained and passed through the dialyzer. The arterial end is used for arterial flow and the distal end for reinfusion of dialyzed blood.
   d. Healing of AVF requires at least 6 to 8 weeks; a central vein catheter is used in the interim.
2. Arteriovenous graft—arteriovenous connection consisting of a tube graft made from autologous saphenous vein or from polytetrafluoroethylene. Ready to use in 3 to 4 weeks.
3. Central vein catheters—direct cannulation of veins (subclavian, internal jugular, or femoral); may be used as temporary or permanent dialysis access.

Complications of Vascular Access
1. Infection.
2. Catheter clotting.
3. Central vein thrombosis or stricture.
4. Stenosis or thrombosis.
5. Ischemia of the hand (steal syndrome).
6. Aneurysm or pseudoaneurysm.

Monitoring During Hemodialysis
1. Involves constant monitoring of hemodynamic status, electrolyte, and acid-base balance as well as maintenance of sterility and a closed system.
2. Performed by a specially trained nurse and dialysis technician who are familiar with the protocol and equipment being used.

Lifestyle Management for Chronic Hemodialysis
1. Dietary management involves restriction or adjustment of protein, sodium, potassium, phosphorous, or fluid intake.
2. Ongoing health care monitoring includes careful adjustment of medications that are normally excreted by the kidney or are dialyzable.
3. Surveillance for complications.
   a. Arteriosclerotic cardiovascular disease, heart failure, disturbance of lipid metabolism (hypertriglyceridemia), coronary heart disease, stroke.
   b. Intercurrent infection, including monitoring for hepatitis B.
   c. Anemia and fatigue.
   d. Gastric ulcers and other problems.
   e. Bone problems (renal osteodystrophy)—from disturbed mineral metabolism.
   f. Hypertension.
   g. Psychosocial problems: depression, anxiety, suicide, alteration in body image, and sexual dysfunction.
4. Support agencies are American Association of Kidney Patients (*www.aakp.org*), National Kidney Foundation (*www.kidney. org*), National Kidney and Urologic Diseases Information Clearing House (*www.niddk.nih.gov*).

Kidney Surgery

Evidence Base Wein, A. J., Kavoussi, L. R., Novick, A. C., et al. (Eds.). (2012). *Campbell-Walsh urology* (10th ed., Vols. 1–3). Philadelphia: W.B. Saunders. Nankivell, B., & Kuypers, D. (2011). Diagnosis and prevention of chronic kidney allograft loss. *Lancet, 15*, 1428–1437.

Kidney surgery may include partial or total nephrectomy (removal of the kidney), kidney transplantation for end-stage renal disease (ESRD), procedures to remove stones or tumors, and procedures to insert drainage tubes (nephrostomy). Incisional approaches vary but may involve the flank, thoracic, and abdominal regions. Nephrectomy is most commonly performed for malignant tumors of the kidney but may also be indicated for trauma and kidneys that no longer function due to obstructive disorders and other renal disease. Nephrectomy is also the procedure of choice to remove a healthy kidney for donation to a transplant recipient. The absence of one kidney does not result in impaired renal function when the remaining kidney is normal and healthy.

Many surgical procedures were previously performed as "open" procedures, but are now being done with laparoscopic "keyhole" surgeries. An endoscope is introduced and the abdomen is inflated with carbon dioxide. Instruments are passed through other sites or a sleeve may be used, which allows a hand to be introduced at the operative site. Advantages are decreased postoperative pain, decreased blood loss, and, in some cases, decreased length of hospital stay.

Preoperative Management

1. Patient is prepared for surgery, and consent is witnessed. Preoperative antibiotics and bowel cleansing regimen may be prescribed.
2. Risk factors for thromboembolism are identified (smoking, oral contraceptive use, varicosities of lower extremities), and anti-embolism stockings may be applied. Leg exercises are taught, and the patient is prepared for pneumatic/sequential compression stockings that will be used postoperatively.
3. Pulmonary status is assessed (presence of dyspnea, productive cough, other related cardiac symptoms) and deep-breathing exercises, effective coughing, and use of incentive spirometer are taught.
4. If embolization of the renal artery is being done preoperatively for patients with renal cell carcinoma, the following symptoms of postinfarction syndrome are observed for (may last up to 3 days):
   a. Flank pain.
   b. Fever.
   c. Leukocytosis.
   d. Hypertension.

Postoperative Management

1. Vital signs are monitored and incisional area is assessed for evidence of bleeding or hemorrhage.

 **NURSING ALERT** Use frequent and close observation of BP, pulse, and respiration to recognize hemorrhage (and shock)—chief danger after renal surgery. Watch for pain, sanguineous drainage from drain sites, or expanding pulsatile flank mass. Prepare for rapid blood and fluid replacement and reoperation.

2. Possible pulmonary complications of atelectasis, pneumonia, and pneumothorax are observed. Pulmonary clearance through deep breathing, percussion, and vibration is maintained. Chest tube drainage may be used in patients who have an open procedure (the proximity of the thoracic cavity to the operative area may result in the need for chest tube drainage postoperatively).
3. Patency of urinary drainage tubes is maintained (nephrostomy, suprapubic, or urethral catheter). Ureteral stents may be used.
4. Respiratory status and lower extremities are assessed for thromboembolic complications.
5. Bowel sounds, abdominal distention, and pain are monitored, which may indicate paralytic ileus and need for nasogastric decompression.
6. For kidney transplantation patients, immunosuppressant drugs are ordered.
   a. A combination of medications is used, including a corticosteroid; calcineurin inhibitor, such as tacrolimus or cyclosporine; and mycophenolate mofetil.

   b. Early signs of rejection include temperature greater than 100.4° F (38° C), decreased urine output, weight gain of 3 lb (1.5 kg) or more overnight, pain or tenderness over the graft site, hypertension, increased serum creatinine.

Nursing Diagnoses

- Acute Pain related to surgical incision.
- Impaired Urinary Elimination related to urinary drainage tubes or catheters.
- Risk for Infection related to incision, potential pulmonary complications, and possibly immunosuppression.
- Risk for Deficient or Excess Fluid Volume related to fluid replacement needs and transplanted/remaining kidney function.

Nursing Interventions

Relieving Pain

1. Assess pain location, level, and characteristics. Transient renal colic-like pain may be caused by passage of blood clots down the ureter; however, report any persistent increasing or unrelievable pain, which may indicate obstruction of urinary drainage or hemorrhage.
2. Administer pain medications; evaluate effectiveness of patient-controlled analgesia (PCA).
3. Encourage patient to ambulate; splint incision to move or cough.

Promoting Urinary Elimination

1. Maintain patency of urinary drainage tubes and catheters while in place. Prevent kinking or pulling.
2. Use handwashing and asepsis when providing care and handling urinary drainage system (especially important for patient taking immunosuppressants).
3. Make sure indwelling catheter is dependent and draining.
   a. Report decrease in output or excessive clots.
   b. Be alert for signs of urinary infection, such as cloudy urine, fever, or bladder or flank ache.
4. Intervene to encourage removal of catheter when patient becomes ambulatory.
5. Maintain adequate fluid intake, IV or oral, when allowed.

Preventing Infection

1. Monitor for fever, elevated leukocyte count, abnormal breath sounds.
2. Administer antibiotics, as prescribed.
3. Assist patient with use of incentive spirometer, coughing and deep breathing, and ambulation to decrease risk of pulmonary infection. Provide meticulous care to chest tube sites.
4. Change dressings promptly if drainage is present—drainage is an excellent culture medium for bacteria.
5. Obtain specimens for bacteriologic testing of urine, wounds, sputum, and discontinued catheters, drains, and IV lines as indicated. Before removing catheters or urinary drains, disinfect skin around entry site, then remove. Using aseptic technique, cut off tip of catheter or drain and place in sterile container for laboratory culture.

6. Monitor vascular access to hemodialysis to ensure patency and watch for evidence of infection.

7. For kidney transplantation patients, provide antimicrobial therapy.
   a. Oral antifungals to prevent mucosal candidiasis, which commonly occurs due to immunosuppression.
   b. Antiviral medications are routinely used to prevent cytomegalovirus infection.

8. Provide regular skin care and assist with hygiene.

Maintaining Fluid Balance

1. Closely monitor intake and output, especially after kidney transplantation.
   a. Expect normal urine output to be 30 to 100 mL/hour.
   b. Report oliguria with less than 30 mL/hour or polyuria of 100 to 500 mL/hour.

2. Monitor serum electrolyte results and electrocardiogram (ECG) for changes associated with electrolyte imbalance.
   a. Report arrhythmias or other cardiac symptoms immediately.

3. Monitor BP and heart rate, central venous pressure (CVP), and pulmonary artery pressure (if indicated) to anticipate adjustment of fluid replacement.

4. Avoid using dialysis access extremity for IV lines, intra-arterial monitoring, or restraints.

5. Although rare, hemodialysis may be required in the postoperative period if the transplanted kidney does not function immediately.

Patient Education and Health Maintenance

After Nephrectomy

1. Provide information about continued recovery from surgery, including engaging in regular exercise, refraining from heavy lifting or strenuous activities, and resuming normal dietary intake.

2. Promote wearing a MedicAlert bracelet and inform all health care providers of solitary kidney status.

3. Encourage close follow-up and need to seek medical attention for any signs of urinary infection, urinary obstruction, or urinary tract disease if there is only one kidney present to prevent damage to that kidney.

After Kidney Transplantation

1. Explain and reinforce symptoms of rejection—fever, chills, sweating, lassitude, hypertension, weight gain, peripheral edema, decrease in urine output.
   a. Hyperacute rejection—occurs within minutes or hours of transplantation and is rarely treatable.
   b. Accelerated rejection—occurs 24 hours to 5 days after transplantation and is treated by plasmapheresis and IV immunoglobulin G.
   c. Acute T-cell-mediated rejection (90% of all rejection episodes)—occurs days to weeks after transplantation and is treated by IV steroids or additional immunosuppression.
   d. Chronic rejection—occurs months to years after transplantation and results in slowly declining function of the allograft.

2. Observe for symptoms of urine leak, such as sudden loss of kidney function, pain over transplant site, and copious drainage of yellow fluid from the wound.

3. Explain continued protection of vascular access graft, which may still be enlarged, tender to palpation, and associated with edema of overlying tissues.

4. Encourage compliance with laboratory tests (blood urea nitrogen [BUN], creatinine, serum chemistry, hematology, bacteriology, cyclosporine, or tacrolimus levels) to monitor patient's immune status and detect early signs of rejection.

5. Instruct patient and family about prescribed immunosuppressants and complications of therapy—infection or incomplete control of rejection.
   a. Review immunosuppressive medications in detail, including color identification of pills, dose schedules, adverse effects, and the necessity for taking the medication.
   b. Review other medications, such as histamine-2 (H_2) blockers or proton pump inhibitors (PPIs), to prevent stress ulcers and prophylaxis for *Candida* and community-acquired infections.

6. Review in detail postoperative self-care regimen (may be inpatient or outpatient), including adequate fluid intake, daily weight, measurement of urine, stool test for occult blood, prevention of infection, exercise.

7. Instruct to report immediately:
   a. Decrease in urinary output.
   b. Weight gain, edema.
   c. Malaise, fever.
   d. Graft swelling and tenderness (visible and palpable below the skin).
   e. Changes in BP readings.
   f. Respiratory distress.
   g. Anxiety, depression, change in appetite or sleep.

8. Discuss with health care provider the feasibility of participating in contact sports because of the risk of trauma to the transplanted kidney.

9. Stress that follow-up care after transplantation is a lifelong necessity.

10. For additional support and information, refer to American Association of Kidney Patients (*www.aakp.org*) and the United Network for Organ Sharing (*www.unos.org*).

Evaluation: Expected Outcomes

- Verbalizes relief of pain.
- Urinary drainage clear without clots.
- Absence of fever or signs of infection.
- Vital signs stable; urine output 50 mL/hour.

Urinary Diversion

Evidence Base Wein, A. J., Kavoussi, L. R., Novick, A. C., et al. (Eds.). (2012). *Campbell-Walsh urology* (10th ed., Vols. 1–3). Philadelphia: W.B. Saunders.

Urinary diversion refers to diverting the urinary stream from the bladder so that it exits by way of a new avenue. A number of operative procedures may be performed to achieve this (see Figure 21-3). Methods of urinary diversion include:

1. Ileal conduit (or "Bricker's loop")—most common; transplants the ureters into an isolated section of the terminal ileum, bringing one end through the abdominal wall to create a stoma. Urine flows from the kidney into the ureters, then through the ileal conduit, and exits through urinary stoma. The ureters may also be transplanted into a segment of the transverse colon (colon conduit).

2. Nephrostomy—insertion of a catheter into the renal pelvis by way of an incision into the flank or by percutaneous catheter placement into the kidney. They are rarely placed for long periods of time; they are a short-term method of diverting urine away from an obstruction or lesion below the level of the renal pelvis.

3. Continent urinary diversion procedures—create a urinary reservoir from an intestinal segment that is either brought to the skin using a valve mechanism that permits catheterization, or is anastomosed directly to the proximal urethra.

   a. Continent urinary reservoir (Kock pouch, Indiana pouch, Mainz pouch, and others)—transplants the ureters into a pouch created from small bowel or large and small bowel. Mechanisms to discourage ureteral reflux are used to implant the ureters into the pouch, including an intussuscepted nipple valve or tunneling the ureters through the taeniae of the bowel. The existing ileocecal valve, or a surgically created intussuscepted nipple valve, provides the continence mechanism. Patient does not have to wear an external appliance, but the procedure does require intermittent self-catheterization of the pouch.

   b. Orthotopic bladder replacement (Hemi-Kock pouch, Neobladder, and others)—pouch created from small or large and small bowel is anastomosed to urethral stump; voiding is through the urethra. Patient usually has nocturnal incontinence; not all patients are candidates for this procedure.

Types of Cutaneous Diversions

A	B	C	D
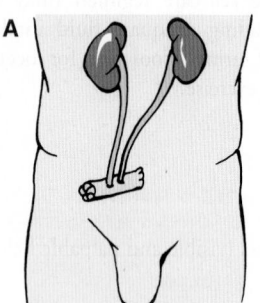	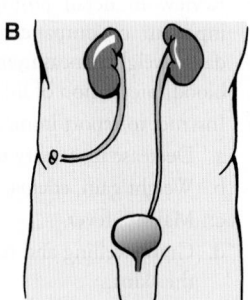	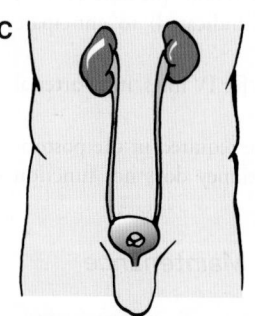	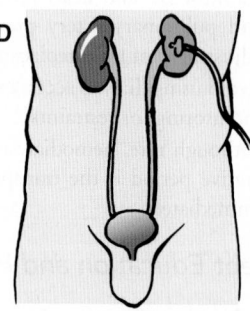

A Conventional ileal conduit. The surgeon transplants the ureters to an isolated section of the terminal ileum (ileal conduit), bringing one end to the abdominal wall. The ureter may also be transplanted into the transverse sigmoid colon (colon conduit) or proximal jejunum (jejunal conduit).

B Cutaneous ureterostomy. The surgeon brings the detached ureter through the abdominal wall and attaches it to an opening in the skin.

C Vesicostomy. The surgeon sutures the bladder to the abdominal wall and creates an opening (stoma) through the abdominal and bladder walls for urinary drainage.

D Nephrostomy. The surgeon inserts a catheter into the renal pelvis via an incision into the flank or by percutaneous catheter placement, into the kidney.

Types of Continent Urinary Diversions

A	B	C	D
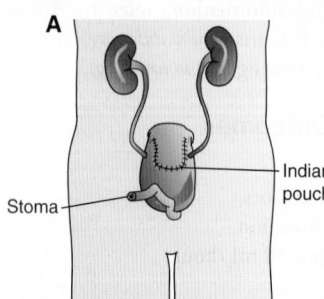	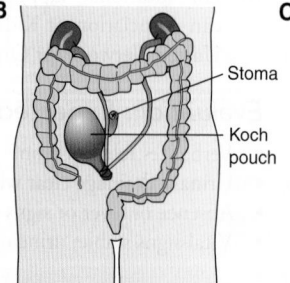	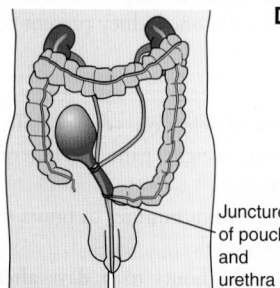	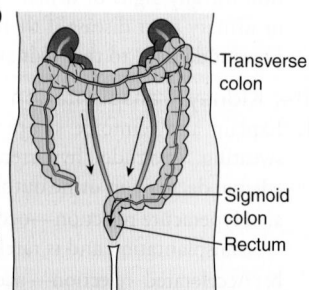

A Indiana pouch. The surgeon introduces the ureters into a segment of ileum and cecum. Urine is drained periodically by inserting a catheter into the stoma.

B Continent ileal urinary diversions (Koch pouch). The surgeon transplants the ureters to an isolated segment of small bowel, ascending colon, or ileocolonic segment and develops an effective continence mechanism or valve. Urine is drained by inserting a catheter into the stoma.

C In male patients, the Koch pouch can be modified by attaching one end of the pouch to the urethra, allowing more normal voiding. The female urethra is too short for this modification.

D Ureterosigmoidostomy. The surgeon introduces the ureters into the sigmoid, thereby allowing urine to flow through the colon and out of the rectum.

Figure 21-3. Methods of urinary diversion.

Preoperative Management

1. Functional assessment should be performed including degree of manual dexterity and visual acuity along with cognitive function—essential for stoma care or self-catheterization postoperatively.
2. Patient's psychosocial resources are evaluated, including available support persons, education, occupation, and economic resources (including insurance coverage of ostomy supplies, if needed), coping strengths, attitudes toward urinary diversion.
3. Bowel preparation is performed to prevent fecal contamination during surgery and the potential complication of infection.
   a. Clear liquids only and prescribed laxatives for mechanical cleansing of the bowel.
   b. Antibiotics, as prescribed (nonabsorbable; active against enteric organisms), to reduce bacterial count in the bowel lumen.
4. Adequate hydration is ensured, including IV infusions, to ensure urine flow during surgery and to prevent hypovolemia.
5. The procedure is explained by the surgeon and the WOCN (wound, ostomy, continence nurse) before surgery.
   a. For ileal or colon conduit, the stoma site is planned preoperatively with patient standing, sitting, and lying—to place the stoma away from bony prominences, skin creases, and scars, and where the patient can see it.
   b. Stoma site may also be marked even though continent urinary diversion procedure is planned, in case findings during surgery prevent continent procedure and standard ileal or colon conduit is necessary.

Postoperative Management

1. Patient is assessed for immediate postoperative complications; wound or UTI, urinary or fecal anastomotic leakage, small bowel obstruction, paralytic ileus, deep vein thrombosis, pulmonary embolism, and necrosis of stoma.
2. Intake and output are monitored including amount of urinary output, patency of drainage catheters, and degree of hematuria.
3. Pelvic gravity or suction drains are evaluated—sudden increase in drainage suggests an anastomotic leak; send specimen of drainage for creatinine, if ordered. (Presence of measurable creatinine in the drainage indicates urine in drainage, confirming a urine leak.)
4. Ureteral stents are used to protect ureterointestinal anastomoses; stents will emerge from stoma or through separate wound (stents are not visible in orthotopic bladder replacement patients). They are removed in 3 weeks.

Nursing Diagnoses

- Impaired Urinary Elimination related to urinary diversion.
- Acute Pain related to surgery.
- Disturbed Body Image related to urinary diversion.
- Sexual Dysfunction related to reconstructive surgery and impotence (in men).

Nursing Interventions

Achieving Urinary Elimination

For ileal or colon conduit patients:

1. Maintain a transparent urostomy pouch over the stoma postoperatively to allow for easy assessment.
2. Inspect the stoma for color and size; whether it is flush, nippled, or retracted; and the condition of the skin around the stoma. Document baseline information for subsequent comparison.
   a. Stoma should be red, wet with mucus, soft, and slightly rubbery to the touch (stoma lacks nerve ending, so feeling in stoma is absent).
   b. Cyanotic stoma indicates poor circulation.
   c. Necrotic stoma is blue-black or tan-brown.
3. Report bleeding, necrosis, sloughing, suture separation.
4. Check patency of ureteral stents.
5. Keep the pouch on at all times, and observe normal urine (but not fecal) drainage at all times.
   a. Connect pouches to drainage bag when patient is in bed and record urine volume hourly.
   b. Initial urostomy pouch remains in place for several days postoperatively; it is changed every 3 to 4 days when patient teaching begins.

For continent urinary diversion patients:

1. Maintain patency of drainage catheters placed into internal urinary pouch during surgery; irrigate with 30 mL saline every 2 to 4 hours to prevent obstruction from mucous accumulation.
2. Assess stoma—should be very small and flush.
3. Record urine output and character of urine.
4. Monitor output of pelvic drain (on gentle suction or gravity drainage) every 8 hours.
5. Advise patient that approximately 3 weeks after surgery the drainage catheter is removed from the pouch after a radiographic study ("pouch-o-gram") confirms healing of all anastomoses.

Controlling Pain

1. Administer analgesic medications or teach use of and monitor PCA (IV or epidural).
2. Assess response to pain control.
3. Provide positioning for comfort, alternating with ambulation, as able.

Resolving Body Image Issues

1. Assess patient's reaction to looking at new urinary stoma, if applicable; provide reassurance and support.
2. Accept patient's depression, which may be manifested in irritability or lack of motivation to learn.
   a. Give extra support until patient can cope.
   b. Reinforce the concept that the stoma will be manageable.
   c. Acknowledge feelings of fear and anxiety as normal.
3. Encourage patient to participate gradually in care of stoma or catheters.
4. Encourage verbalization of feelings and concerns related to urinary diversion.

5. If possible, arrange for patient to speak with another patient who has undergone the same surgery; this provides realistic expectations and support for a positive outcome.

6. Help patient and family to gain independence through learning to manage the ostomy. Provide for demonstrations, supervised practice, written instructions, and return demonstrations until patient is independent in self-care.

Coping with Sexual Dysfunction

1. Be aware that many men experience impotence as a result of surgery; provide information or referrals about options including medications, pharmacologic erection programs, and penile prostheses.

2. Allow patient to express feelings related to loss of sexual function and encourage discussion with partner.

3. Tell women that they may usually resume sexual activity after healing is complete.

Patient Education and Health Maintenance

For Ileal or Colon Conduit Patients

1. Obtain and familiarize patient with the appropriate equipment. Most urostomy pouching systems are disposable. The choice of pouch is determined by location of stoma, patient activity, body build, and economic status.
   a. Two-piece pouches consist of a skin barrier (or wafer) that fits around the stoma and adheres to the skin and a pouch that snaps onto the skin barrier.
   b. One-piece pouches may be precut for the correct stoma size and include the adhesive; the pouch is applied directly to the peristomal skin.

2. Assist patient to determine stoma size (for ordering correct appliance). The stoma will shrink considerably as edema subsides and the size is recalibrated several times during the first 3 to 6 weeks postoperatively.
   a. Measuring guides are included with most urostomy pouches.
   b. The inside diameter of the skin barrier should not be more than 1/16 inch larger than the diameter of the stoma.

3. Teach how to change the pouch.
   a. Change pouch early in morning before taking fluids or before evening meal—urine output is lower at these times.
   b. Prepare the new pouching system according to manufacturer's directions.
   c. Wash the peristomal skin with non-cream-based soap and water. Rinse and pat dry. *The skin must be dry or appliance will not adhere.*
   d. A gauze or tissue wick may be applied over the stoma to absorb urine while the appliance is being changed. Keep the skin free from direct contact with urine. Suggest the use of tampons to soak up urine from stoma while changing pouch at home, if desired; however, do not insert into stoma.
   e. Center the skin barrier directly over the stoma and apply it carefully. Apply gentle pressure around appliance for secure adherence.
   f. Apply a belt to keep pouch in place, if desired; it is especially useful in patients with soft abdomens.

4. Advise that additional adhesives, such as pastes or cements, are not usually necessary with a well-fitting pouch.

5. Tell patient that frequency of pouch changes depends on the type of pouch used—generally pouches should be changed every 3 to 4 days.

6. Advise emptying the pouch when it is one third to one half full to prevent weight of urine from loosening adhesive seal—open drain valve (spigot) for periodic emptying.

7. Teach how to attach outlet on pouch to a bedside urinary drainage container with plastic tubing (at least 5 feet to allow turning) and how to secure tubing to leg to prevent twisting or kinking.
   a. Position the drainage bottle lower than the level of the bed to enhance flow by gravity.
   b. Clean nighttime drainage equipment with vinegar and water. Rinse well.

8. Advise patient to drink liberal amounts of fluids to flush the conduit free of mucus and reduce possibility of urinary infection.

9. Teach that the stoma may bleed if it is bumped or rubbed; report bleeding that continues for several hours.

10. Advise carrying spare pouches in handbag or pocket and bringing an extra pouch to every visit with health care provider.

11. Advise wearing cotton (rather than nylon) underwear or the use of specially made underwear for ostomy patients that prevents contact between plastic pouch and skin. Heavy girdles are not allowed because they may cause chafing of the stoma and prevent free flow of urine.

12. Advise reporting problems with peristomal skin or with leakage from the pouch or the development of fever, chills, pain, change in color of urine (cloudy, bloody), diminishing urine output.

13. For additional information and support, refer to United Ostomy Associations of America (*www.ostomy.org*).

For Continent Ileal Urinary Reservoir Patients

1. Teach irrigation of catheter; this must be done every 4 to 6 hours at home.

2. Teach how to change stoma dressing.

3. Instruct in use of leg bag or bedside urinary drainage bag while catheter remains in place.

4. Teach how to catheterize continent urinary diversion when healing is verified:
   a. Red rubber or plastic, straight or coudé catheters are used.
   b. Apply a small amount of water-soluble lubricant to the tip of the catheter.
   c. Use clean technique; wash hands before each catheterization.
   d. Maintain schedule of catheterizations during initial "training" period to allow the pouch to adapt gradually to holding larger amounts of urine (every 2 hours during day and every 3 hours at night; increase by 1 hour each week for 5 weeks).
   e. After training period, catheterize four to five times per day; pouch should not hold more than 400 to 500 mL.
   f. Irrigate pouch with saline through catheter once per day to clear it of accumulated mucus.

5. Teach patient to report problems such as leakage of urine from stoma between catheterizations.

6. Tell patient to shower or bathe normally, wear normal clothing; only a small dressing or an adhesive bandage needs to be worn over the stoma.

7. Advise patient to drink 8 to 10 glasses of water daily.

For Orthotopic Bladder Replacement

1. Teach patient to irrigate Foley catheter that will stay in place for 3 weeks after surgery; irrigate with 30 mL saline every 4 to 6 hours.

2. Instruct in use of leg bag or bedside drainage bag while catheter remains in place.

3. Instruct on how to change dressing.

4. After healing of pouch is confirmed and catheter is removed, teach patient to "void."
   a. Voiding is accomplished by abdominal straining; mucus is expected in voided urine.
   b. Voiding schedule must be maintained for first 5 to 6 weeks (every 2 hours during day and every 3 hours at night; increase by 1 hour each week).
   c. Incontinence is anticipated after catheter is removed; usually more pronounced when patient is asleep and muscles are relaxed.

5. Teach patient to perform pelvic floor exercises, which must be done faithfully for the rest of his or her life; as pelvic floor sphincter muscles strengthen, incontinence subsides. Most patients continue to have small amounts of nocturnal incontinence.
   a. Contract pelvic floor muscles (as if stopping stream of urine or flatus) for 5 seconds, then relax for 5 to 10 seconds.
   b. Repeat approximately 15 to 20 times for one set, and do three sets per day.
   c. May require referral to physical therapist to assist in the process.

6. Provide information about absorbent products that may be used temporarily; also teach about preventive skin care.

7. Instruct in clean self-catheterization, which may be needed if urethra becomes obstructed with mucus; pouch should be irrigated with saline if catheterization is necessary.

8. Reassure patient that time, patience, and continued adherence to voiding and exercise schedule will result in continence.

Evaluation: Expected Outcomes

- Urine draining by way of urinary diversion.
- Verbalizes good pain control.
- Discusses feelings about change in body image; seeks support through family.
- Verbalizes reasonable expectations about sexual function.

Prostatic Surgery

Prostatic surgery may be done for begin prostatic hyperplasia (BPH) or prostate cancer. Surgical approach depends on size of the gland, severity of obstruction, age, underlying health, and prostatic disease.

Surgical Procedures

 Evidence Base Wein, A. J., Kavoussi, L. R., Novick, A. C., et al. (Eds.). (2012). *Campbell-Walsh urology* (10th ed., Vols. 1–3). Philadelphia: W.B. Saunders.

1. TURP (formerly the most common procedure) is done without an incision by means of endoscopic instrument.

2. Photovaporization of the prostate (PVP) is starting to replace TURP; it is done through a cystoscope, using a laser to vaporize diseased prostatic tissue.

3. Transurethral microwave thermotherapy of the prostate (TUMT) and transurethral needle ablation of the prostate (TUNA) are both office-based procedures that use heat to destroy diseased prostatic tissue.

4. Indigo interstitial laser therapy of the prostate is another procedure that is done on an outpatient basis.

5. Open prostatectomy.
   a. Suprapubic—incision into suprapubic area and through bladder wall; commonly done for BPH.
   b. Perineal—incision between scrotum and rectal area; may be done for poor surgical risk patients, but causes highest incidence of urinary incontinence and impotence.
   c. Radical retropubic—incision at level of symphysis pubis; may preserve nerves responsible for sexual function; done for prostate cancer.

6. Robotic radical prostatectomy uses a laparoscopic approach for removal of cancerous prostate.

Preoperative Management

1. Information about the procedure and the expected postoperative care, including catheter drainage, irrigation, and monitoring of hematuria, is discussed.

2. Complications of surgery are discussed.
   a. For radical and laparoscopic prostatectomy, incontinence or dribbling of urine may occur for up to 1 year after surgery; pelvic floor (Kegel) exercises help regain urinary control.
   b. For TURP and PVP, retrograde ejaculation—seminal fluid released into bladder and eliminated in the urine rather than through the urethra during intercourse, occurs in 75% or patients; impotence is usually not a complication but occurs in 5% to 10% of TURP and PVP patients and can be as high as 75% in those undergoing radical prostatectomy.

3. Bowel preparation is given or patient is instructed in home administration and fasting after midnight.

4. Optimal cardiac, respiratory, and circulatory status should be achieved to decrease risk of complications.

5. Prophylactic antibiotics are ordered.

Postoperative Management

1. Urinary drainage is maintained and observed for signs of hemorrhage.

2. Wound care is provided to prevent infection.

3. Pain is controlled and early ambulation is promoted.

4. Surveillance is maintained for complications.
   a. Wound infection and dehiscence.
   b. Urinary obstruction or infection.
   c. Hemorrhage.
   d. Thrombophlebitis, deep vein thrombosis, and pulmonary embolism.
   e. Urinary incontinence, sexual dysfunction.

Nursing Diagnoses

- Impaired Urinary Elimination related to surgical procedure and urinary catheter.
- Risk for Infection related to surgical incision, immobility, and urinary catheter.
- Acute Pain related to surgical procedure.
- Anxiety related to urinary incontinence, difficulty voiding, and erectile dysfunction.

Nursing Interventions

Facilitating Urinary Drainage

1. Maintain patency of urethral catheter placed after surgery.
   a. For TURP and open prostatectomy for BPH, monitor flow of three-way closed irrigation and drainage system (see Figure 21-4) if used. Continuous irrigation helps prevent clot formation, which can obstruct catheter, cause painful bladder spasms, and lead to infection.
   b. If Foley is obstructed and with a health care provider order, manually irrigate with 50 to 60 mL irrigating fluid using aseptic technique.

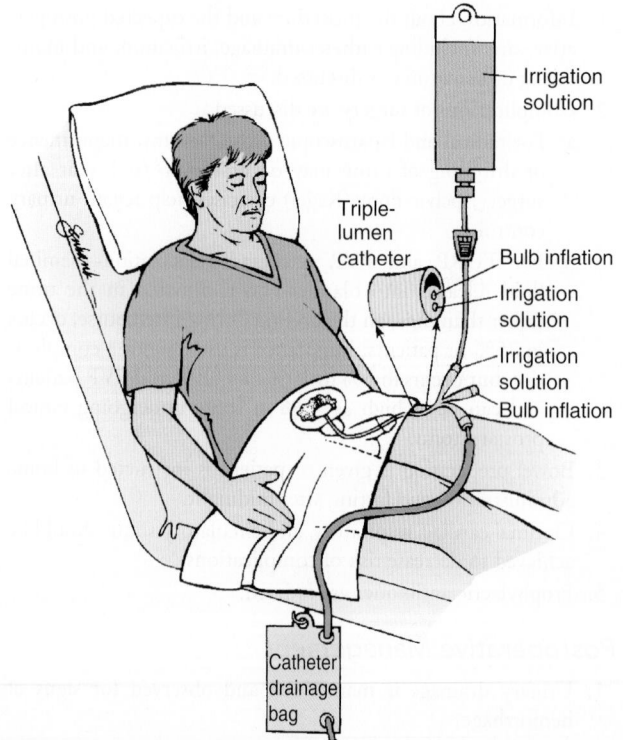

Figure 21-4. A three-way system for bladder irrigation.

c. Avoid overdistention of bladder, which could lead to hemorrhage.
d. Administer anticholinergic medications to reduce bladder spasms, as ordered.

 DRUG ALERT Anticholinergic medications are contraindicated in patients with narrow angle-closure glaucoma.

2. Assess degree of hematuria and any clot formation; drainage should become light pink within 24 hours.
   a. Report bright red bleeding with increased viscosity (arterial)—may require surgical intervention.
   b. Report increase in dark red bleeding (venous)—may require traction of the catheter so the inflated balloon applies pressure to prostatic fossa.
   c. Prepare for blood transfusion if bleeding persists.
3. Administer IV fluids, as ordered, and encourage oral fluids when tolerated to ensure hydration and urine output.

Preventing Infection

1. After open prostatectomy, provide frequent monitoring of vital signs, intake and output, and observation of incisional dressing, if present.
2. Encourage ambulation to prevent venous thrombosis, pulmonary embolism, and pneumonia.
3. Observe urine for cloudiness or odor and obtain urine for evaluation of infection, as ordered.
4. Administer antibiotics, as prescribed.
5. Report testicular pain, swelling, and tenderness, which could indicate epididymitis from spreading infection.
6. Assist with perineal care if perineal incision is present to prevent contamination by feces.

Relieving Pain

1. Administer pain medication or monitor PCA, as directed.
2. Position patient for comfort and tell him or her to avoid straining, which will increase pelvic venous congestion and may cause hemorrhage.
3. Administer stool softeners to prevent discomfort from constipation.
4. Make sure catheter is secured to patient's thigh and tubing is not creating traction on catheter, which will cause pain and potential hemorrhage.

 NURSING ALERT Avoid rectal temperatures, enemas, or rectal tubes postoperatively to prevent hemorrhage or disruption of healing.

Reducing Anxiety

1. Provide realistic expectations about postoperative discomfort and overall progress.
   a. Tell patient to avoid sexual intercourse, straining at stool, heavy lifting, and long periods of sitting for 6 to 8 weeks after surgery.
   b. Advise follow-up visits after treatment because urethral stricture or bladder neck contracture may occur.

2. Reassure patient that urinary incontinence and frequency, urgency, and dysuria are expected after removal of catheter and should gradually subside.

3. Reassure patient that there may be measures to help.

4. Reinforce the risks for impotence as told by the surgeon. Remind patient that erectile function may not return for 12 months.

5. Encourage patient to express fears and anxieties related to potential loss of sexual function and to discuss concerns with partner.

6. Advise that options are available to restore sexual function if impotence persists.

Patient Education and Health Maintenance

1. Advise patient that PVP is commonly done on an outpatient basis; patient may go home the evening of surgery.

2. Reinforce instructions provided on catheter care, maintaining patency, and catheter irrigation.
   a. For open, radical, and laparoscopic prostatectomy patients, the catheter will be removed in 2 to 3 weeks. A cystogram may be performed to confirm healing of anastomosis prior to removing catheter.
   b. Advise that stress incontinence may occur after catheter is removed and is more pronounced when abdominal pressure is increased, such as with coughing, laughing, straining.
   c. For patients who experience urgency before surgery, caution that they may have urge incontinence for several weeks postoperatively.
   d. Discuss the use of absorbent products to contain urine leakage around catheter and after catheter is removed.

3. Teach measures to regain urinary control. Teach patient to perform pelvic floor exercises correctly. Have patient squeeze the pelvic floor muscles (as if stopping stream of urine or flatus) for 5 seconds and then relax for 5 to 10 seconds. This should be done 15 to 20 times, three times per day. Caution against using abdominal muscles (straining or Valsalva maneuver), which increases incontinence.

4. Reinforce availability of options such as medications for urinary urgency and oral medicine such as sildenafil, vacuum erectile device, penile injections, and penile prosthesis to restore sexual function.

5. Encourage prostate cancer patients to have a PSA blood test 3 months after surgery and yearly thereafter.

Evaluation: Expected Outcomes

- Clear yellow drainage by way of catheter.
- Incision without drainage; afebrile.
- Verbalizes good pain relief.
- Verbalizes realistic expectations for urinary and sexual functioning.

RENAL AND UROLOGIC DISORDERS

Acute Kidney Injury

Acute kidney injury (AKI) is a clinical syndrome in which there is a sudden decline in renal function. This results in disturbances in fluid and electrolyte balance, acid-base homeostasis, blood pressure regulation, erythropoiesis, and mineral metabolism. It is frequently associated with an increase in BUN and creatinine, oliguria (less than 500 mL urine/24 hours), hyperkalemia, and sodium and fluid retention.

Pathophysiology and Etiology

Causes

See Figure 21-5, page 796.

1. Prerenal causes—result from conditions that decrease renal blood flow (hypovolemia, shock, hemorrhage, burns, impaired cardiac output, diuretic therapy, and renal artery disorders).

2. Intrarenal causes—result from injury to renal tissue and are usually associated with intrarenal ischemia, toxins, immunologic processes, systemic disorders, trauma, and vascular disorders.

3. Postrenal causes—arise from obstruction or disruption to urine flow anywhere along the urinary tract.

Clinical Course

1. Onset: begins when the kidney is injured and lasts from hours to days.

2. Oliguric–anuric phase: urine volume less than 400 to 500 mL/24 hours.
   a. Accompanied by rise in serum concentration of elements usually excreted by kidney (urea, creatinine, organic acids, and the intracellular cations—potassium and magnesium).
   b. There can be a decrease in renal function with increasing nitrogen retention even when patient is excreting more than 2 to 3 L of urine daily—called nonoliguric or high-output renal failure.

3. Diuretic phase: begins when the 24-hour urine volume exceeds 500 mL and ends when the BUN and serum creatinine levels stop rising.

4. Recovery phase.
   a. Usually lasts several months to 1 year.
   b. Probably some scar tissue remains, but the functional loss is not always clinically significant.

Clinical Manifestations

1. Prerenal—signs and symptoms consistent with hypovolemia may be present such as decreased tissue turgor, dryness of mucous membranes, weight loss hypotension, oliguria or anuria, reduced jugular venous distention, and tachycardia. However, if the prerenal cause is related to vasodilation, third-spacing of fluid, or cardiovascular disease, signs/symptoms of increased extracellular fluid may be present.

2. Intrarenal—presentation based on cause; edema usually present.

3. Postrenal—findings may include a distended bladder, an abdominal mass, and an enlarged prostate. Renal colic may be present with nephrolithiasis.

Diagnostic Evaluation

1. Urinalysis—reveals proteinuria, hematuria, casts.

2. Rising serum creatinine and BUN levels.

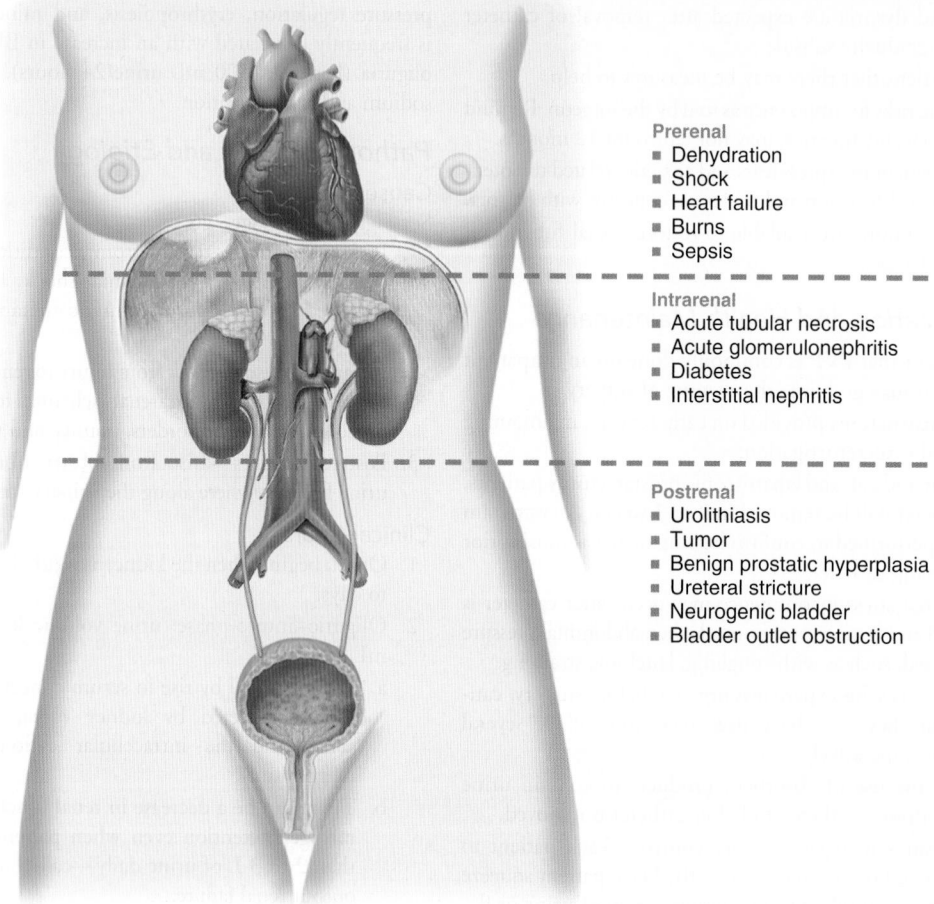

Prerenal
- Dehydration
- Shock
- Heart failure
- Burns
- Sepsis

Intrarenal
- Acute tubular necrosis
- Acute glomerulonephritis
- Diabetes
- Interstitial nephritis

Postrenal
- Urolithiasis
- Tumor
- Benign prostatic hyperplasia
- Ureteral stricture
- Neurogenic bladder
- Bladder outlet obstruction

Figure 21-5. Causes of acute renal failure.

3. Urine chemistry examinations to distinguish various forms of acute renal failure; decreased sodium.
4. Renal ultrasonography—for estimate of renal size and to exclude a treatable obstructive uropathy.

Management

Preventive Measures

1. Identify patients with preexisting renal disease.
2. Initiate adequate hydration before, during, and after any procedure requiring NPO status.
3. Avoid exposure to nephrotoxins. Be aware that the majority of drugs or their metabolites are excreted by the kidneys.

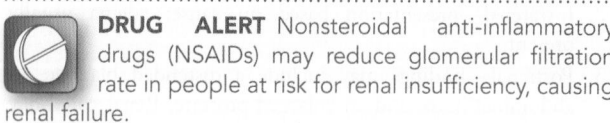 **DRUG ALERT** Nonsteroidal anti-inflammatory drugs (NSAIDs) may reduce glomerular filtration rate in people at risk for renal insufficiency, causing renal failure.

4. Monitor chronic analgesic use—some drugs may cause interstitial nephritis and papillary necrosis.
5. Prevent and treat shock with blood and fluid replacement. Prevent prolonged periods of hypotension.

6. Monitor urinary output and CVP in critically ill patients to detect onset of renal failure at the earliest moment.
7. Schedule diagnostic studies requiring dehydration so there are "rest days," especially in older patients who may not have adequate renal reserve.
8. Pay special attention to draining wounds, burns, and so forth, which can lead to dehydration and sepsis and progressive renal damage.
9. Avoid infection; give meticulous care to patients with indwelling catheters and IV lines.
10. Take every precaution to make sure that the right person receives the right blood to avoid severe transfusion reactions, which can precipitate renal complications.

Corrective and Supportive Measures

1. Correct reversible cause of acute renal failure (eg, improve renal perfusion, maximize cardiac output, surgical relief of obstruction).
2. Be alert for and correct underlying fluid excesses or deficits.
3. Correct and control biochemical imbalances—treatment of hyperkalemia.
4. Restore and maintain BP.

5. Maintain nutrition.
6. Initiate hemodialysis, peritoneal dialysis, or continuous renal replacement therapy for patients with renal failure.

Complications

1. Infection.
2. Arrhythmias due to hyperkalemia.
3. Electrolyte and mineral (sodium, potassium, calcium, phosphorus, magnesium) abnormalities.
4. GI bleeding due to stress ulcers.
5. Multiple organ systems failure.

Nursing Assessment

1. Determine if there is a history of cardiac disease, malignancy, sepsis, or intercurrent illness.
2. Determine if patient has been exposed to potentially nephrotoxic drugs (antibiotics, NSAIDs, contrast agents, solvents).
3. Conduct an ongoing physical examination for tissue turgor, pallor, alteration in mucous membranes, BP, heart rate changes, pulmonary edema, and peripheral edema.
4. Monitor intake and output.

Nursing Diagnoses

- Risk for Imbalanced Fluid Volume.
- Risk for Electrolyte Imbalance related to kidney injury.
- Risk for Infection related to alterations in the immune system and host defenses.
- Imbalanced Nutrition: Less Than Body Requirements related to catabolic state, anorexia, and malnutrition associated with acute kidney injury.
- Risk for Bleeding related to gastrointestinal stress ulcers.
- Acute Confusion related to the effects of uremic toxins on the central nervous system (CNS).

Nursing Interventions

Achieving Fluid and Electrolyte Balance

See Table 21-2.
1. Monitor for signs and symptoms of hypovolemia or hypervolemia because the regulating capacity of kidneys is inadequate.
2. Monitor urinary output and urine-specific gravity, as ordered; measure and record intake and output including urine, gastric suction, stool, and wound drainage,
3. Monitor serum and urine electrolyte concentrations.
4. Weigh patient daily to provide an index of fluid balance.
5. Adjust fluid intake to avoid volume overload and volume depletion.
   a. Fluid restriction is usually initiated in oliguric patients.
   b. During oliguric–anuric phase, give only enough fluids to replace losses (usually 400 to 500 mL/24 hours plus measured fluid losses).
   c. Fluid allowance should be distributed throughout the day.
   d. Restrict salt and water intake if there is evidence of extracellular excess.
6. Measure BP regularly with patient in supine, sitting, and standing positions.
7. Auscultate lung fields for rales.
8. Inspect neck veins for engorgement and extremities, abdomen, sacrum, and eyelids for edema.

Maintaining Electrolyte and Acid-Base Balance

1. Evaluate for signs and symptoms of hyperkalemia and monitor serum potassium levels.
   a. Notify health care provider of value above 5.5 mg/L.
   b. Watch for ECG changes—tall, tented T waves; depressed ST segment; wide QRS complex.

Table 21-2	Signs and Symptoms of Fluid and Electrolyte Imbalances	
	DEFICIT	EXCESS
Volume	Acute weight loss (>5%), drop in body temperature, dry skin and mucous membranes, postural hypotension, longitudinal wrinkles or furrows of tongue, oliguria or anuria	Acute weight gain (>5%), edema, hypertension, distended neck veins, dyspnea, rales
Sodium	Abdominal cramps, apprehension, convulsions, fingerprinting on sternum, oliguria or anuria	Dry, sticky mucous membranes, flushed skin, oliguria or anuria, thirst, rough and dry tongue
Potassium	Anorexia, abdominal distention, intestinal ileus, muscle weakness, tenderness, and cramps	Diarrhea, intestinal colic, irritability, nausea, paresthesias; flaccid paralysis, cardiac arrhythmias and arrest
Calcium	Abdominal cramps, positive Chvostek's and Trousseau's signs, tingling of extremities, tetany	Anorexia, nausea, vomiting, abdominal pain and distention, mental confusion
Bicarbonate	Deep, rapid breathing (Kussmaul), shortness of breath on exertion, stupor, weakness (metabolic acidosis)	Depressed respirations, muscle hypertonicity, tetany (metabolic alkalosis)
Magnesium	Positive Chvostek's sign, seizures, disorientation, hyperactive deep tendon reflexes, tremor	Hypotension, flushing, lethargy, dysarthria, hypoactive deep tendon reflexes, respiratory depression

c. Administer sodium bicarbonate or glucose and insulin to shift potassium into the cells, as ordered.

d. Administer cation exchange resin (sodium polystyrene sulfonate) orally or rectally to provide more prolonged correction of elevated potassium, as ordered.

e. Instruct patient about the importance of following prescribed diet, avoiding foods high in potassium.

f. Prepare for dialysis when rapid lowering of potassium is needed.

g. Administer blood transfusions *during* dialysis to prevent hyperkalemia from stored blood.

2. Watch for cardiac arrhythmias and heart failure from hyperkalemia, electrolyte imbalance, or fluid overload. Have resuscitation equipment on hand in case of cardiac arrest.

3. Monitor arterial blood gas (ABG) levels, as necessary.

4. Prepare for ventilator therapy if severe acidosis is present or respiratory problems develop.

5. Administer oral alkalizing medications or IV sodium bicarbonate as directed.

6. Be prepared to implement dialysis for uncontrolled acidosis.

Preventing and Monitoring for Infection

1. Monitor for all signs of infection. Be aware that renal failure patients do not always demonstrate fever and leukocytosis.

2. Remove bladder catheter as soon as possible; monitor for UTI.

3. Use intensive pulmonary hygiene—high incidence of lung edema and infection.

4. Carry out meticulous wound care.

5. If antibiotics are administered, care must be taken to adjust the dosage for renal impairment.

Maintaining Adequate Nutrition

1. Work collaboratively with dietitian to regulate protein intake according to impaired renal function because metabolites that accumulate in blood derive almost entirely from protein catabolism.

2. Protein should be of high biologic value—rich in essential amino acids (dairy products, eggs, meat)—so that the patient does not rely on tissue catabolism for essential amino acids.

3. Offer high-carbohydrate feedings because carbohydrates have greater protein-sparing power and provide additional calories.

4. Weigh patient daily.

5. Monitor BUN, creatinine, electrolytes, serum albumin, prealbumin, total protein, and transferrin.

6. Be aware that food and fluids containing large amounts of sodium, potassium, and phosphorus may need to be restricted.

Monitoring For and Preventing GI Bleeding

1. Examine all stools and emesis for gross and occult blood.

2. Administer H_2-receptor antagonist or PPIs, as directed as prophylaxis for gastric stress ulcers. If an H_2-receptor antagonist is used, care must be taken to adjust the dose for the degree of renal impairment.

3. Prepare for endoscopy when GI bleeding occurs.

Maintaining Neurologic Function

1. Speak to the patient in simple orienting statements, using repetition when necessary.

2. Maintain predictable routine and keep change to a minimum.

3. Watch for and report mental status changes—somnolence, lassitude, lethargy, and fatigue progressing to irritability, disorientation, twitching, seizures.

4. Correct cognitive distortions.

5. Use seizure precautions—padded side rails, airway and suction equipment at bedside.

6. Encourage and assist patient to turn and move because drowsiness and lethargy may prevent activity.

7. Use music tapes to promote relaxation.

8. Prepare for dialysis, which may help prevent neurologic complications.

Patient Education and Health Maintenance

1. Explain that the patient may experience residual defects in kidney function for long period after acute illness.

2. Encourage reporting for routine urinalysis and follow-up examinations.

3. Advise avoidance of any medications unless specifically prescribed.

4. Recommend resuming activity gradually because muscle weakness will be present from excessive catabolism.

Evaluation: Expected Outcomes

- BP stable, no edema or shortness of breath.
- Serum electrolytes and arterial blood gas values within normal range.
- No signs of infection.
- Food intake adequate, maintaining weight.
- Stools heme negative.
- Appears more alert, sleeps less during the day.

Chronic Renal Failure (End-Stage Renal Disease)

Chronic renal failure (CRF; ESRD; chronic kidney disease, CKD) is a progressive deterioration of renal function, which ends fatally in uremia (an excess of urea and other nitrogenous wastes in the blood) and its complications unless dialysis or a kidney transplantation is performed. According to the National Kidney Foundation, approximately 26 million Americans have some type of chronic kidney disease. Most cases are asymptomatic until later stages.

Pathophysiology and Etiology

Causes

1. Hypertension, prolonged and severe.
2. Diabetes mellitus.
3. Glomerulopathies (from lupus or other disorders).
4. Interstitial nephritis.
5. Hereditary renal disease, polycystic disease.
6. Obstructive uropathy.
7. Developmental or congenital disorder.

Consequences of Decreasing Renal Function

1. Rate of progression varies based on underlying cause and severity of that condition.
2. Stages: decreased renal reserve → renal insufficiency → renal failure → ESRD.
3. Retention of sodium and water causes edema, heart failure, hypertension, ascites.
4. Decreased glomerular filtration rate (GFR) causes stimulation of renin–angiotensin axis and increased aldosterone secretion, which raises BP.
5. Metabolic acidosis results from the kidney's inability to excrete hydrogen ions, produce ammonia, and conserve bicarbonate.
6. Decreased GFR causes increase in serum phosphate with reciprocal decrease in serum calcium and subsequent bone resorption of calcium.
7. Erythropoietin production by the kidney decreases, causing profound anemia.
8. Uremia affects the CNS, causing altered mental function, personality changes, seizures, and coma.

Clinical Manifestations

1. GI—anorexia, nausea, vomiting, hiccups, ulceration of GI tract, and hemorrhage.
2. Cardiovascular—hyperkalemic ECG changes, hypertension, pericarditis, pericardial effusion, pericardial tamponade.
3. Respiratory—pulmonary edema, pleural effusions, pleural rub.
4. Neuromuscular—fatigue, sleep disorders, headache, lethargy, muscular irritability, peripheral neuropathy, seizures, coma.
5. Metabolic and endocrine—glucose intolerance, hyperlipidemia, sex hormone disturbances causing decreased libido, impotence, amenorrhea.
6. Fluid, electrolyte, acid-base disturbances—usually salt and water retention but may be sodium loss with dehydration, acidosis, hyperkalemia, hypermagnesemia, hypocalcemia (see page 797).
7. Dermatologic—pallor, hyperpigmentation, pruritus, ecchymoses, uremic frost.
8. Skeletal abnormalities—renal osteodystrophy resulting in osteomalacia.
9. Hematologic—anemia, defect in quality of platelets, increased bleeding tendencies.
10. Psychosocial functions—personality and behavior changes, alteration in cognitive processes.

Diagnostic Evaluation

1. Complete blood count (CBC)—anemia (a characteristic sign).
2. Elevated serum creatinine, BUN, phosphorus.
3. Decreased serum calcium, bicarbonate, and proteins, especially albumin.
4. ABG levels—low blood pH, low carbon dioxide, low bicarbonate.
5. 24-hour urine for creatinine, protein, creatinine clearance

Management

Goal is to conserve renal function as long as possible.

1. Detection and treatment of reversible causes of renal failure (eg, bring diabetes under control; treat hypertension).
2. Dietary regulation—low-protein diet supplemented with essential amino acids or their keto analogues to minimize uremic toxicity and to prevent wasting and malnutrition.
3. Treatment of associated conditions to improve renal dynamics.
   a. Anemia—erythropoiesis-stimulating agents, such as epoetin alfa and darbepoetin.
   b. Acidosis—replacement of bicarbonate stores by infusion or oral administration of sodium bicarbonate.
   c. Hyperkalemia—restriction of dietary potassium; administration of cation exchange resin.
   d. Phosphate retention—decrease in dietary phosphorus (chicken, milk, legumes, carbonated beverages); administration of phosphate-binding agents because they bind phosphorus in the intestinal tract.
4. Maintenance dialysis or kidney transplantation when symptoms can no longer be controlled with conservative management.

Complications

Death.

Nursing Assessment

1. Obtain history of chronic disorders and underlying health status.
2. Assess degree of renal impairment and involvement of other body systems by obtaining a review of systems and reviewing laboratory results.
3. Perform thorough physical examination, including vital signs, cardiovascular, pulmonary, GI, neurologic, dermatologic, and musculoskeletal systems.
4. Assess psychosocial response to disease process including availability of resources and support network.

Nursing Diagnoses

- Excess Fluid Volume related to disease process.
- Imbalanced Nutrition: Less Than Body Requirements related to anorexia, nausea, vomiting, and restricted diet.
- Impaired Skin Integrity related to uremic frost and changes in oil and sweat glands.
- Constipation related to fluid restriction and ingestion of phosphate-binding agents.
- Risk for Injury while ambulating related to potential fractures and muscle cramps due to calcium deficiency.
- Ineffective Therapeutic Regimen Management related to restrictions imposed by CRF and its treatment.

Nursing Interventions

Maintaining Fluid and Electrolyte Balance
See interventions related to acute kidney injury, page 789.

Maintaining Adequate Nutritional Status
See interventions related to acute kidney injury, page 789.

Maintaining Skin Integrity

1. Keep skin clean while relieving itching and dryness.
   a. Soap for sensitive skin.
   b. Sodium bicarbonate added to bath water.
   c. Oatmeal baths.
   d. Bath oil added to bath water.
2. Apply ointments or creams for comfort and to relieve itching.
3. Keep nails short and trimmed to prevent excoriation.
4. Keep hair clean and moisturized.
5. Administer antihistamines for relief of itching, if indicated, but discourage patient from taking any OTC drugs without discussing with health care provider.

Preventing Constipation

1. Be aware that phosphate binders cause constipation that cannot be managed with usual interventions.
2. Encourage high-fiber diet, bearing in mind the potassium content of some fruits and vegetables.
   a. Commercial fiber supplements may be prescribed.
   b. Use stool softeners, as prescribed.
   c. Avoid laxatives and cathartics that cause electrolyte toxicities (compounds containing magnesium or phosphorus).
   d. Increase activity, as tolerated.

Ensuring a Safe Level of Activity

1. Monitor serum calcium and phosphate levels; watch for signs of hypocalcemia or hypercalcemia (see page 797).
2. Inspect patient's gait, range of motion, and muscle strength.
3. Administer analgesics, as ordered, and provide massage for severe muscle cramps.
4. Monitor x-rays and bone scan results for fractures, bone demineralization, and joint deposits.
5. Increase activity as tolerated—avoid immobilization because it increases bone demineralization.
6. Administer medications, as ordered.
   a. Phosphate-binding medications, such as sevelamer or calcium carbonate, with meals and snacks to lower serum phosphorus.
   b. Calcium supplements between meals may be used in instances of hypocalcemia.
   c. Vitamin D to increase absorption and utilization of calcium.

Increasing Understanding of and Compliance with Treatment Regimen

1. Prepare patient for dialysis or kidney transplantation.
2. Offer hope tempered by reality.
3. Assess patient's understanding of treatment regimen as well as concerns and fears.
4. Explore alternatives that may reduce or eliminate adverse effects of treatment.
   a. Adjust schedule so rest can be achieved after dialysis.
   b. Offer smaller, more frequent meals to reduce nausea and facilitate taking medication.
5. Encourage strengthening of social support system and coping mechanisms to lessen the impact of the stress of chronic kidney disease.
6. Provide social work referral.
7. Contract with patient for behavioral changes if noncompliant with therapy or control of underlying condition.
8. Discuss option of supportive psychotherapy for depression.
9. Promote decision making by patient.
10. Refer patients and family members to renal support agencies.

Patient Education and Health Maintenance

1. To promote adherence to the therapeutic program, teach the following:
   a. Weigh self every morning to avoid fluid overload.
   b. Drink limited amounts of fluids only when thirsty.
   c. Measure allotted fluids and save some for ice cubes; sucking on ice is thirst-quenching.
   d. Eat food before drinking fluids to alleviate dry mouth.
   e. Use hard candy or chewing gum to moisten mouth.
2. For further information and support, refer to the National Kidney Foundation (*www.kidney.org*).
3. Encourage all people in the following at-risk patient groups to obtain screening for chronic kidney disease: older adults, Native Americans, African Americans, Latinos, people with diabetes, people with hypertension, those with autoimmune disease, and those with family history of kidney disease. More information on the National Kidney Foundation's Clinical Practice Guidelines for Chronic Kidney Disease can be obtained from *www.kidney.org/professionals/kdoqi/index.cfm*.

Evaluation: Expected Outcomes

- BP stable, no excessive weight gain.
- Tolerates small feedings of low-protein, high-carbohydrate diet.
- No skin excoriation; reports some relief of itching.
- Passes small, firm stool daily.
- Ambulates without falls.
- Asks questions and reads education materials about dialysis.

Acute Glomerulonephritis

Acute *glomerulonephritis (GN)* refers to a group of kidney diseases in which there is an inflammatory reaction in the glomeruli.

Pathophysiology and Etiology

1. Occurs after an infection elsewhere in the body or may develop secondary to systemic disorders.
2. An antigen–antibody reaction produces immune complexes that lodge in the glomeruli, producing thickening of glomerular basement membrane; the renal vasculature, interstitium, and tubular epithelium may also be affected.
3. Immune complexes activate a variety of secondary mediators, such as complement pathways, neutrophils, macrophages, prostaglandins, and leukotrienes. These affect vascular tone and permeability, resulting in tissue injury.
4. Eventual scarring and loss of filtering surface may lead to renal failure.

Clinical Manifestations

1. Mild disease is frequently discovered accidentally through a routine urinalysis.
2. History of infection (in post-infectious GN): pharyngitis or impetigo from group A streptococcus, such viral infections as Epstein-Barr and hepatitis B.
3. Tea-colored urine, oliguria.
4. Puffiness of face, edema of extremities.
5. Fatigue and anorexia, possible headache.
6. Hypertension (mild, moderate, or severe), headache.

Diagnostic Evaluation

1. Urinalysis for hematuria (microscopic or gross), proteinuria, cellular elements, and various casts.
2. Twenty-four-hour urine for protein (increased) and creatinine clearance (may be reduced) outline the degree of renal function.
3. Elevated BUN and serum creatinine levels, low albumin level, increased antistreptolysin titer (increased in postinfectious GN from reaction to streptococcal organism) and, in some cases, decreased serum complement.
4. Needle biopsy of the kidney reveals obstruction of glomerular capillaries from proliferation of endothelial cells.

Management

1. Management is symptomatic and includes antihypertensives, diuretics, drugs for management of hyperkalemia (due to renal insufficiency), H_2 blockers (to prevent stress ulcers), and phosphate-binding agents (to reduce phosphate and elevate calcium).
2. Antibiotic therapy is initiated to eliminate infection (if still present).
3. Fluid intake is restricted.
4. Dietary protein is restricted moderately if there is oliguria and BUN is elevated. It is restricted more drastically if acute renal failure develops.
5. Carbohydrates are increased liberally to provide energy and reduce catabolism of protein.
6. Potassium and sodium intake is restricted in presence of hyperkalemia, edema, or signs of heart failure.

Complications

1. Hypertension and heart failure. Endocarditis can occur in postinfectious GN.
2. Fluid and electrolyte imbalances in the acute phase, hyperkalemia, hyperphosphatemia, hypervolemia.
3. Malnutrition.
4. Hypertensive encephalopathy, seizures.
5. ESRD.

Nursing Assessment

1. Obtain medical history; focus on recent infections or symptoms of chronic immunologic disorders (systemic lupus erythematosus, scleroderma).
2. Assess urine specimen for blood, protein, color, and amount.

3. Perform physical examination, specifically looking for signs of edema, hypertension, and hypervolemia (engorged neck veins, elevated jugular venous pressure, adventitious lung sounds, cardiac arrhythmia).
4. Evaluate cardiac status and serum laboratory values for electrolyte imbalance.

Nursing Diagnoses

- Ineffective Renal Perfusion related to damage to glomerular function.
- Excess Fluid Volume related to compromised renal function.

Nursing Interventions

Promoting Renal Function

1. Monitor vital signs, intake and output, and maintain dietary restrictions during acute phase.
2. Administer medications, as ordered, and evaluate patient's response to antihypertensives, diuretics, H_2 blockers, phosphate-binding agents, and antibiotics, if indicated.

Improving Fluid Balance

1. Carefully monitor fluid balance; replace fluids according to patient's fluid losses (urine, respiration, feces) and daily body weight, as prescribed.
2. Monitor pulmonary artery pressure and CVP, if indicated, during acute hospitalizations.
3. Monitor for signs and symptoms of heart failure: distended neck veins, tachycardia, gallop rhythm, enlarged and tender liver, crackles at bases of lungs.
4. Observe for hypertensive encephalopathy and any evidence of seizure activity.

 NURSING ALERT Hypertensive encephalopathy is a medical emergency and treatment is aimed at reducing BP without impairing renal function.

Patient Education and Health Maintenance

1. Explain that patient must have follow-up evaluations of BP, urinary protein, and BUN concentrations to determine if there is exacerbation of disease activity.
2. Encourage patient to treat any infection promptly.
3. Tell patient to report any signs of decreasing renal function and to obtain treatment immediately.

Evaluation: Expected Outcomes

- Urine output adequate; vital signs stable.
- No edema, shortness of breath, or adventitious heart or lung sounds.

Nephrotic Syndrome

Nephrotic syndrome is a clinical disorder characterized by marked increase of protein in the urine (proteinuria), decrease in albumin in the blood (hypoalbuminemia), edema, and excess lipids in the blood (hyperlipidemia). These occur as a consequence of excessive leakage of plasma proteins into the urine because of increased permeability of the glomerular capillary membrane.

Pathophysiology and Etiology

1. Seen in any condition that seriously damages the glomerular capillary membrane.
    a. Chronic glomerulonephritis.
    b. Diabetes mellitus with intercapillary glomerulosclerosis.
    c. Amyloidosis of kidney.
    d. Systemic lupus erythematosus.
    e. Renal vein thrombosis.
    f. Secondary to malignancy (older adults).
2. Hypoalbuminemia results in decreased oncotic pressure, causing generalized edema as fluid moves out of the vascular space (see Figure 21-6).
3. Decreased circulating volume then activates the renin–angiotensin system, causing retention of sodium and further edema.
4. Mechanism for increased lipids is unknown.

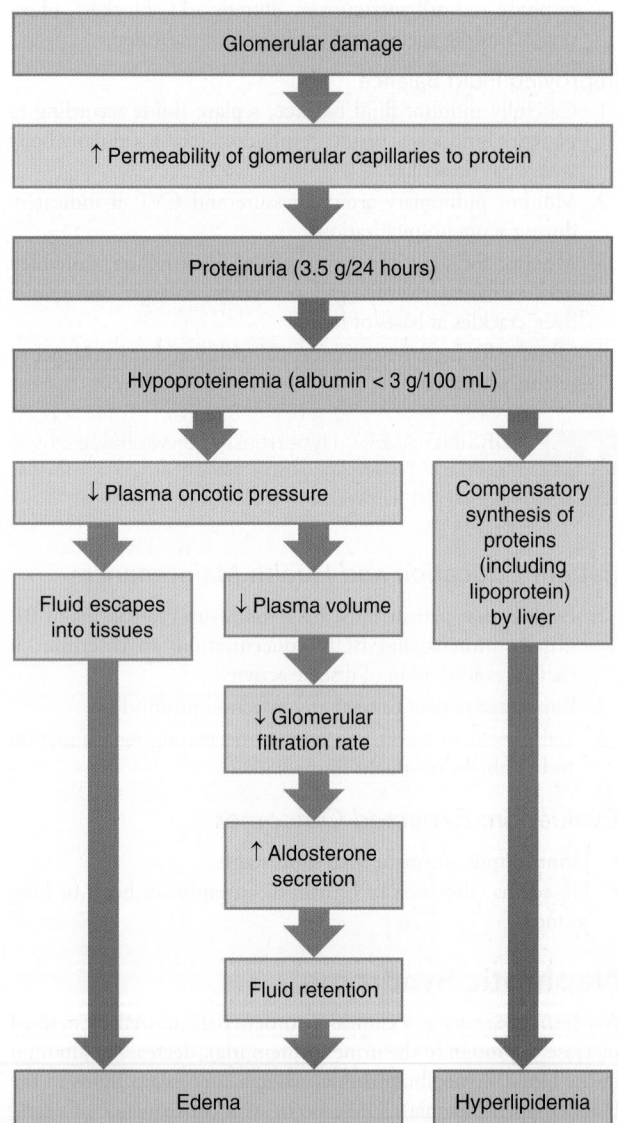

Figure 21-6. Pathophysiology of the nephrotic syndrome.

Clinical Manifestations

1. Insidious onset of pitting dependent edema, periorbital edema, and ascites; weight gain.
2. Fatigue, headache, malaise, irritability.
3. Marked proteinuria—leading to depletion of body proteins.
4. Hyperlipidemia—may lead to accelerated atherosclerosis.

Diagnostic Evaluation

1. Urinalysis—marked proteinuria, microscopic hematuria, urinary casts, appears "foamy."
2. Twenty-four-hour urine for protein (increased) and creatinine clearance (may be decreased).
3. Protein electrophoresis and immunoelectrophoresis of the urine to categorize the proteinuria.
4. Needle biopsy of kidney—for histologic examination of renal tissue to confirm diagnosis.
5. Serum chemistry—decreased total protein and albumin, normal or increased creatinine, increased triglycerides, and altered lipid profile.

Management

1. Treatment of causative glomerular disease.
2. Diuretics (used cautiously) and angiotensin-converting enzyme inhibitors to control proteinuria.
3. Corticosteroids or immunosuppressive agents to decrease proteinuria.
4. General management of edema.
    a. Sodium and fluid restriction.
    b. Infusion of salt-poor albumin.
    c. Dietary protein supplements.
5. Diet low in saturated fats.

Complications

1. Hypovolemia.
2. Thromboembolic complications—renal vein thrombosis, venous and arterial thrombosis in extremities, pulmonary embolism, coronary artery thrombosis, cerebral artery thrombosis secondary to loss of hemostasis control proteins such as anti-thrombin III, protein S, and protein C.
3. Altered drug metabolism due to decrease in plasma proteins.
4. Progression to end-stage renal failure.

Nursing Assessment

1. Obtain history of onset of symptoms including changes in characteristics of urine and onset of edema.
2. Perform physical examination looking for evidence of edema and hypovolemia.
3. Assess vital signs, daily weights, intake and output, and laboratory values.

Nursing Diagnoses

- Risk for Deficient Fluid Volume related to disease process.
- Risk for Infection related to treatment with immunosuppressive agents.

Nursing Interventions

Increasing Circulating Volume and Decreasing Edema

1. Monitor daily weight, intake and output, and urine-specific gravity.
2. Monitor CVP (if indicated), vital signs, orthostatic BP, and heart rate to detect hypovolemia.
3. Monitor serum BUN and creatinine to assess renal function.
4. Administer diuretics or immunosuppressive agents, as prescribed, and evaluate patient's response.
5. Infuse IV albumin, as ordered.
6. Encourage bed rest for a few days to help mobilize edema; however, some ambulation is necessary to reduce risk of thromboembolic complications.
7. Enforce mild to moderate sodium and fluid restriction if edema is severe.

Preventing Infection

1. Monitor for signs and symptoms of infection.
2. Monitor temperature routinely; check laboratory values for neutropenia.
3. Use aseptic technique for all invasive procedures and strict handwashing by patient and all contacts; prevent contact by patient with persons who may transmit infection.

Patient Education and Health Maintenance

1. Teach patient signs and symptoms of nephrotic syndrome; also review causes, purpose of prescribed treatments, and importance of long-term therapy to prevent ESRD.
2. Instruct patient in adverse effects of prescribed medications and methods of preventing infection if taking immunosuppressive agents.
3. Carefully review with patient and family dietary and fluid restrictions; consult dietitian for assistance in meal planning.
4. Discuss the importance of maintaining exercise, decreasing cholesterol and fat intake, and changing other risk factors, such as smoking, obesity, and stress, to reduce risk of severe thromboembolic complications.
5. In patients with severe disease, prepare for dialysis and possible transplantation.

Evaluation: Expected Outcomes

- Vital signs remain stable; edema decreased.
- No signs of infection.

URINARY DISORDERS

Lower Urinary Tract Infections

Evidence Base Gupta, K., Hooton, T. M., Naber, K. G., et al. (2011). International clinical practice guidelines for the treatment of acute uncomplicated cystitis and pyelonephritis in women: A 2010 update by the Infectious Diseases Society of America and the European Society for Microbiology and Infectious Diseases. *Clinical Infectious Diseases, 52*(5), 103–120.

A *urinary tract infection (UTI)* is caused by the presence of pathogenic microorganisms in the urinary tract with or without signs and symptoms. Lower UTIs may predominate at the bladder (cystitis) or urethra (urethritis).

Bacteriuria refers to the presence of bacteria in the urine (10^3 bacteria/mL of urine or greater generally indicates infection).

In *asymptomatic bacteriuria*, organisms are found in urine, but patient has no symptoms.

Recurrent UTIs may indicate the following:

Unresolved—bacteria fails to respond to antimicrobial therapy.

Recurrent—reinfection after eradication of pathogens.

Pathophysiology and Etiology

1. Ascending infection after entry by way of the urinary meatus.
   a. Women are more susceptible to developing acute cystitis because of shorter length of urethra; anatomical proximity to vagina, periurethral glands, and rectum (fecal contamination); and the mechanical effect of coitus.
   b. Women with recurrent UTIs typically have gram-negative organisms at the vaginal introitus; there may be some defect of the mucosa of the urethra, vagina, or external genitalia of these patients that allows enteric organisms to invade the bladder.
   c. Poor voiding habits may result in incomplete bladder emptying, increasing the risk of recurrent infection.
   d. Acute infection in women most commonly arises from organisms of the patient's own intestinal flora (*Escherichia coli*).
2. Although *E. coli* causes 86% of UTIs, other pathogens, such as *Klebsiella* species, *Proteus* species, and *Staphylococcus saprophyticus*, may also cause these infections.
3. In men, obstructive abnormalities (strictures, prostatic hyperplasia) are the most frequent cause.
4. UTI is a considerable source of nosocomial infection and sepsis in older adults.
5. Upper urinary tract disease may occasionally cause recurrent bladder infection.

Clinical Manifestations

1. Dysuria, frequency, urgency, nocturia.
2. Suprapubic pain and discomfort.
3. Microscopic or gross hematuria.

GERONTOLOGIC ALERT The only sign of UTI in the older patient may be mental status changes.

Diagnostic Evaluation

1. Urine dipstick may react positively for blood, white blood cells (WBCs), and nitrates, indicating infection.
2. Urine microscopy shows RBCs and many WBCs per field without epithelial cells.

> **NURSING ALERT** Urinalysis showing many epithelial cells is likely contaminated by vaginal secretions in women and is therefore inaccurate in indicating infection. Urine culture may be reported as contaminated as well. Obtaining a clean-catch, midstream specimen is essential for accurate results, and catheterization may be necessary in some patients.

3. Urine culture is used to detect presence of bacteria and for antimicrobial sensitivity testing; however, it is not necessary in all cases.
4. Patients with indwelling catheters may have asymptomatic bacterial colonization of the urine without UTI. In these patients, UTI is diagnosed and treated only when symptoms are present.

Management

1. Antibiotic therapy according to sensitivity results.
   a. A wide variety of antimicrobial drugs are available.
   b. Urinary infections usually respond to drugs that are excreted in urine in high concentrations; a potentially effective drug should rapidly sterilize the urine and thus relieve the patient's symptoms.
2. For uncomplicated infection:
   a. First-line therapy for women with uncomplicated cystitis includes a 5-day course of nitrofurantoin or a 3-day course of co-trimoxazole. A 3-day course of a fluoroquinolone such as ciprofloxacin is also effective, but consideration should be given to side effects and reserving this class of drug for other, more serious infections.
   b. Seven to 10 days of therapy are recommended for women over age 65.
   c. Men are treated with 7 to 10 days of antibiotic therapy.
   d. Follow-up culture to prove treatment effectiveness may be indicated.
   e. Adverse effects include nausea, diarrhea, drug-related rash, and vaginal candidiasis.
3. Pregnant women are usually treated for 7 to 10 days.
4. Women with recurrent infections may be treated longer, undergo diagnostic testing to rule out a structural abnormality, or be maintained on a daily dose of antibiotic as prophylaxis.
5. For complicated infection, see treatment of pyelonephritis (see page 807).
6. For severe discomfort with voiding, phenazopyridine may be ordered three times per day for 2 days.

Complications

1. Pyelonephritis.
2. Hematogenous spread resulting in sepsis.

Nursing Assessment

1. Determine if patient has a history of UTIs in childhood, during pregnancy, or has had recurrent infections.
2. Question about voiding habits, personal hygiene practices, and methods of contraception (use of diaphragm or spermicides is associated with development of cystitis).
3. Ask if patient has any associated symptoms of vaginal discharge, itching, or irritation—dysuria may be prominent symptom of vaginitis or infection from sexually transmitted pathogens, rather than UTI.
4. Examine for suprapubic tenderness, as well as abdominal tenderness, guarding, rebound, or masses that may indicate more serious process.

Nursing Diagnoses

- Acute Pain related to inflammation of the bladder mucosa.
- Deficient Knowledge related to prevention of recurrent UTI.

Nursing Interventions

Relieving Pain

1. Administer or teach self-administration of antibiotic—eradication of infection is usually accompanied by rapid resolution of symptoms.
2. Encourage patient to take prescribed analgesics and antispasmodics, if ordered.
3. Encourage rest during the acute phase if symptoms are severe.
4. Encourage plenty of fluids to promote urinary output and to flush out bacteria from urinary tract.

Increasing Understanding and Practice of Preventive Measures

1. For women with recurrent UTIs, give the following instructions:
   a. Reduce vaginal introital concentration of pathogens by hygienic measures.
   b. Wash genitalia in shower or while standing in bathtub—bacteria in bath water may gain entrance into urethra.
   c. Cleanse around the perineum and urethral meatus after each bowel movement, with front-to-back cleansing to minimize fecal contamination of periurethral area.
2. Drink liberal amounts of water to lower bacterial concentrations in the urine.
3. Avoid bladder irritants—coffee, tea, alcohol, cola drinks, and aspartame.
4. Decrease the entry of microorganisms into the bladder during intercourse.
   a. Void immediately after sexual intercourse.
   b. A single dose of an oral antimicrobial agent may be prescribed after sexual intercourse.
5. Avoid external irritants such as bubble baths, talcum powders, perfumed vaginal cleansers or deodorants.
6. Patients with persistent bacteria may require long-term antimicrobial therapy to prevent colonization of periurethral area and recurrence of UTI.
   a. Take antibiotic at bedtime after emptying bladder to ensure adequate concentration of drug overnight because low rates of urine flow and infrequent bladder emptying predispose to multiplication of bacteria.
   b. Use self-monitoring tests (dipsticks) at home to monitor for UTI.

Patient Education and Health Maintenance

1. Advise women with simple, uncomplicated cystitis that they do not require follow-up as long as symptoms are completely resolved with antibiotic therapy. Men usually need follow-up cultures and possibly additional testing if more than one episode of infection.
2. Instruct patient to void frequently (every 2 to 3 hours) and to empty bladder completely because this enhances bacterial clearance, reduces urine stasis, and prevents reinfection. Infrequent voiding distends the bladder wall, leading to hypoxia of bladder mucosa, which is then more susceptible to bacterial invasion.
3. Instruct patients who have had UTIs during pregnancy to have follow-up studies.
4. Female patients with uncomplicated but recurrent cystitis may self-administer a 2- or 3-day course of antibiotics when symptoms begin, if prescribed.
5. Cranberry juice or capsules may help to prevent cystitis by altering the bladder mucosa so that the bacteria cannot attach. Acidophilus and cranberry capsules are available in health food and vitamin stores.

Evaluation: Expected Outcomes

- Verbalizes relief of symptoms.
- Verbalizes self-care measures to prevent recurrence.

Interstitial Cystitis/Bladder Pain Syndrome

Evidence Base Whitmore, K, & Theoharides, T. (2011). When to suspect interstitial cystitis. *Journal of Family Practice, 60,* 340–348.
Rovner, E. S., & Kim, E. D. (2011). Interstitial cystitis. *Medscape Reference.* Available: http://emedicine.medscape.com/article/441831-overview#a0112.

Interstitial cystitis (also called *painful bladder syndrome*) is a syndrome of chronic, cystitis-like symptoms in the absence of bacterial infection. It is a diagnosis of exclusion.

Pathophysiology and Etiology

1. The etiology of interstitial cystitis in unknown. However, theories include an inflammatory or autoimmune process that alters the normal configuration of cells in the bladder epithelium, although infectious, neurological, psychological, and vascular origins are also considered possible.
   a. One plausible theory is a neurogenic origin, in which an initial peripheral inflammatory response later activates the sacral nerves to continue to respond without evidence of continued inflammation.
   b. Mast cell involvement in the inflammatory response also seems a plausible etiology, with many patients having a concomitant history of allergies.
2. The bladder is normally lined with a gel-like substance composed of glycosaminoglycans (heparin, hyaluronic acid, and chondroitin) that acts as an impermeable barrier to irritating solutes such as potassium.

3. Disruption to the bladder epithelium leads to irritant seepage, which produces the symptoms.
4. The bladder wall is chronically inflamed with no evidence of bacterial infection.
5. Occurs far more frequently in women than in men.

Clinical Manifestations

1. History of slow, progressive increase in urinary frequency and urgency. Urgency may be extreme; frequency (as many as 16 times per day) and nocturia increase with duration of symptoms.
2. Symptoms of suprapubic pain and pressure occurring for at least 3 to 6 months.
   a. Bladder pain may be continuous; may increase prior to voiding when the bladder is full; or may present as diffuse perineal, vaginal, suprapubic, or lower back pain.
   b. Pain is usually relieved by voiding.
3. Symptoms are exacerbated by sexual intercourse and at the time of menstruation.
4. Symptoms may be present for 5 to 7 years before diagnosis is made.

Diagnostic Evaluation

1. Tender bladder base during pelvic examination, assessed by palpation of the anterior vaginal wall.
2. Urinalysis and urine culture to rule out infection
3. Cystoscopy under anesthesia with bladder biopsies and bladder distention; presence of bleeding or ulcerations on bladder distention is characteristic of some cases of interstitial cystitis.
4. Urodynamic tests commonly reveal a small bladder capacity with early sensation of urgency and, in some cases, poor detrusor function with incomplete bladder emptying.
5. In potassium sensitivity testing, symptoms are produced when potassium is placed in bladder; however, the use of this test is controversial as inflammation also produces a positive test.
6. Diagnosis is usually made by ruling out other potential causes of symptoms, including radiation or chemical cystitis, gynecologic or urologic malignancies, STD, and urolithiasis.

Management

1. Treatment is individualized and focused on symptom control.
2. Dietary modification to identify foods that act as triggers can be accomplished through an elimination diet. Possible triggers are citrus fruits, tomatoes, caffeinated beverages, carbonated beverages, chocolate, and spicy foods.
3. Bladder retraining (increasing intervals between voiding) is commonly necessary to increase bladder capacity that has been diminished by frequent voiding; pelvic floor strengthening with Kegel exercises can help with urgency and frequency.
4. Oral administration of pentosan polysulfate relieves symptoms in some patients, with maximal effect seen after 3 to 6 months; many continue this therapy for years. If no improvement after 3 to 6 months the drug is discontinued.

> **DRUG ALERT** Pentosan polysulfate has anticoagulant properties; therefore, it should not be used by patients taking other anticoagulant drugs or in conditions associated with increased risk for bleeding. Reversible alopecia may occur as well but resolves once the drug is discontinued.

5. Antihistamines may be beneficial for patients who have allergies. Hydroxyzine has been beneficial in patients.
6. Tricyclic antidepressants such as amitriptyline may be helpful for their analgesic, anticholinergic, and antihistaminic effects. Gabapentin is also used for chronic pain.
7. Bladder distention during cystoscopy under general anesthesia relieves symptoms in 30% to 50% of patients, especially those with small bladder capacity. Relapse commonly occurs 3 months' posttreatment, however, and the effectiveness of this treatment diminishes with repeated use.
8. Intravesical therapy with various substances, including silver nitrate and dimethyl sulfoxide, may be used.
9. Transcutaneous electrical nerve stimulation has demonstrated some relief for the pain syndrome associated with interstitial cystitis.
10. Stress management techniques such as yoga and meditation.

Complications

1. Psychosocial problems related to pain, urgency, and frequency.
2. Secondary bacteriuria.

Nursing Assessment

1. Assess voiding patterns including frequency, nocturia, urgency (a voiding diary is helpful). Determine if symptoms increase in relation to certain foods, menstrual cycle, or sexual intercourse.
2. Assess level of pain using a scale of 1 to 10; determine if pain increases during or after voiding and if bladder spasms occur. Some practitioners may use a symptom questionnaire such as the O'Leary-Sant Interstitial Cystitis Symptom and Problem Index or the Pelvic Pain and Urgency/Frequency questionnaire.
3. Perform abdominal examination and assist with pelvic examination, if indicated, to rule out gynecologic causes and to identify location of pain on palpation.
4. Assess impact on relationships and quality of life.

Nursing Diagnoses

- Chronic Pain related to disease process.
- Impaired Urinary Elimination related to frequency, urgency, dysuria, and nocturia.
- Ineffective Coping related to interruption of lifestyle and chronic, unrelenting symptoms.

Nursing Interventions

Controlling Pain

1. Administer pharmacologic agents, as ordered, to relieve pain and other symptoms. Counsel patient on adverse effects, such as drowsiness, with antihistamines and tricyclic antidepressants.
2. Instruct patient in comfort and preventive measures, such as application of heating pad, avoidance of bladder irritants (caffeine, alcohol, chocolate, and acidic or spicy foods), and avoidance of known allergens.
3. If prescribed, teach patient self-catheterization and the self-administration of intravesical medications.

Improving Urinary Elimination

1. Encourage patient to use a voiding diary as well as a dietary record to make associations between intake of certain foods or fluids and increase in symptoms.
2. Set up bladder retraining program to increase bladder capacity and reduce symptoms.
   a. Have patient start with every 10- to 15-minute voiding intervals during the day.
   b. Instruct patient to gradually (every week or two) increase intervals by 15 minutes.
   c. The ultimate goal (over a period of about 3 months) should be voiding intervals of 3½ hours during the day.
   d. Teach Kegel exercises to help strengthen supporting muscles. Warm baths and perineal massage may help with relaxation before exercises.
   e. Make a referral for biofeedback training, if needed, to enhance Kegel exercises.
3. Advise patient to restrict fluids only when necessary due to impending limited access to toilet facilities; normal fluid intake should be encouraged otherwise.
4. Assess patient's response to pharmacologic therapy.

Strengthening Coping

1. Inquire about patient's ability to work and carry on roles as spouse, parent, etc., based on frequency and discomfort.
2. Explore with patient positive coping strategies for self and family in dealing with chronic illness.
3. Encourage counseling, as needed.

Patient Education and Health Maintenance

1. Teach patient mechanism of action and adverse effects of pharmacologic therapies.
2. Teach self-catheterization using clean technique, if needed, to self-administer medications or accomplish complete bladder emptying.
3. Provide information about food and fluids known to be bladder irritants.
4. Refer for additional information and support to agencies such as Interstitial Cystitis Association (*www.ichelp.org*).

Evaluation: Expected Outcomes

- Verbalizes some relief of pain.
- Verbalizes less urgency, frequency, and nocturia.
- Identifies coping strategies.

Acute Bacterial Pyelonephritis

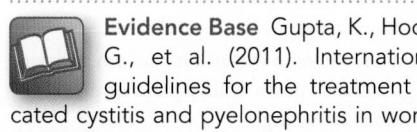 **Evidence Base** Gupta, K., Hooton, T. M., Naber, K. G., et al. (2011). International clinical practice guidelines for the treatment of acute uncomplicated cystitis and pyelonephritis in women: A 2010 update by the Infectious Diseases Society of America and the European Society for Microbiology and Infectious Diseases. *Clinical Infectious Diseases, 52*(5), 103–120.

Bacterial pyelonephritis is an acute infection and inflammatory disease of the kidney and renal pelvis involving one or both kidneys.

Pathophysiology and Etiology

1. Enteric bacteria, such as *E. coli*, is most common pathogen; other Gram-negative pathogens include *Proteus* species, *Klebsiella*, and *Pseudomonas*. Gram-positive bacteria are less common, but include *Enterococcus* and *Staphylococcus aureus*.
2. Bacterial infection usually ascends from the lower urinary tract; however, hematogenous migration is possible (particularly with *S. aureus*).
3. Pyelonephritis can result from urinary obstruction such as vesicoureteral reflux (incompetence of ureterovesical valve, which allows urine to regurgitate into ureters, usually at time of voiding), other renal disease, trauma, or pregnancy.
4. Low-grade inflammation with interstitial infiltrations of inflammatory cells may lead to tubular destruction and abscess formation.
5. Chronic pyelonephritis may result in scarred, atrophic, and nonfunctioning kidneys.

Clinical Manifestations

1. Fever, chills.
2. Flank pain (with or without radiation to groin).
3. Nausea, vomiting, anorexia, abdominal pain, diarrhea.
4. Costovertebral angle tenderness (unilateral or bilateral).
5. Urgency, frequency, and dysuria may be present.

 GERONTOLOGIC ALERT Older patients may exhibit GI or pulmonary symptoms and not show the usual febrile response to pyelonephritis.

Diagnostic Evaluation

1. Urinalysis (dipstick or microscopic) to identify leukocytes, bacteria, nitrites, and RBCs and WBCs in urine; white cell casts may also be seen.
2. Urine culture to identify causative bacteria.

3. CBC shows elevated WBC count consisting of neutrophils and bands.
4. CT scan of abdomen—with contrast—is the imaging study of choice. Other studies include intravenous urography (IVU) or renal ultrasound to evaluate for urinary tract obstruction; other radiologic or urinary tests may be conducted, as necessary.
5. Blood cultures may be drawn, if indicated.

Management

1. For severe infections (dehydrated, cannot tolerate oral intake) or complicating factors (suspected obstruction, pregnancy, advanced age, immunocompromised), inpatient antibiotic therapy is recommended.
   a. Usually immediate treatment is started with an IV fluoroquinolone, aminoglycoside, or extended-spectrum cephalosporin to cover the prevalent Gram-negative pathogens; may be subsequently adjusted according to culture results.
   b. An oral antibiotic may be started 24 hours after fever has resolved and oral therapy continued for 2 weeks.
2. Oral antibiotic therapy is acceptable for outpatient treatment.
   a. A fluoroquinolone or co-trimazole is used—10 to 14 days is the usual length of treatment.
3. Repeat urine cultures should be performed after the completion of therapy.
4. Supportive therapy is given for fever and pain control and hydration.

Complications

1. Bacteremia with sepsis.
2. Papillary necrosis leading to renal failure.
3. Renal abscess requiring treatment by percutaneous drainage or prolonged antibiotic therapy.
4. Perinephric abscess.
5. Paralytic ileus.

Nursing Assessment

1. Monitor symptoms and assess ability to tolerate oral fluids and food.
2. Obtain urologic history that could suggest recurrent infections or urinary tract obstruction.
3. Obtain vital signs; monitor for impending sepsis.
4. Assess bowel sounds for possible paralytic ileus.

Nursing Diagnoses

- Hyperthermia due to infection.
- Acute Pain related to renal swelling and edema.

Nursing Interventions

Reducing Body Temperature

1. Administer or teach self-administration of antibiotics, as prescribed, and monitor for effectiveness and adverse effects.

2. Assess vital signs frequently and monitor intake and output; administer anti-emetic medications to control nausea and vomiting.

3. Administer antipyretic medications, as prescribed and according to temperature.

4. Report fever that persists beyond 72 hours after initiating antibiotic therapy; further testing for complicating factors will be ordered.

5. Use measures to decrease body temperature, if indicated: cooling blanket, application of ice to armpits and groins, and so forth.

6. Correct dehydration by replacing fluids, orally if possible, or via IV administration.

7. Monitor CBC, blood cultures, and urine studies for resolving infection.

Relieving Pain

1. Administer or teach self-administration of analgesics and monitor their effectiveness.

2. Use comfort measures, such as positioning, for local relief of flank pain.

3. Assess patient's response to pain-control measures.

Patient Education and Health Maintenance

1. Explain to patient possible causes of pyelonephritis and its signs and symptoms; also review signs and symptoms of lower UTI.

2. Review antibiotic therapy and importance of completing prescribed course of treatment and having follow-up urine cultures.

3. Explain preventive measures, including good fluid intake, personal hygiene measures, and healthy voiding habits.

Evaluation: Expected Outcomes

• Afebrile within 48 hours.
• Verbalizes reduced pain.

Nephrolithiasis and Urolithiasis

Nephrolithiasis refers to renal stone disease; *urolithiasis* refers to the presence of stones in the urinary system. Stones, or calculi, are formed in the urinary tract from the kidney to bladder by the crystallization of substances excreted in the urine.

Pathophysiology and Etiology

1. Most stones (75%) are composed mainly of calcium oxalate crystals; the rest are composed of calcium phosphate salts, uric acid, struvite (magnesium, ammonium, and phosphate), or the amino acid cystine.

2. Causes and predisposing factors:
   a. Hypercalcemia and hypercalciuria caused by hyperparathyroidism, renal tubular acidosis, multiple myeloma, and excessive intake of vitamin D, milk, and alkali.
   b. Chronic dehydration, poor fluid intake, and immobility.
   c. Diet high in purines and abnormal purine metabolism (hyperuricemia and gout).
   d. Genetic predisposition for urolithiasis or genetic disorders (cystinuria).
   e. Chronic infection with urea-splitting bacteria (*Proteus vulgaris* and *mirabilis*).
   f. Chronic obstruction with stasis of urine, foreign bodies within the urinary tract.
   g. Excessive oxalate absorption in inflammatory bowel disease and bowel resection or ileostomy.
   h. Living in mountainous, desert, or tropical areas.

3. Stones may be found anywhere in the urinary system and vary in size from mere granular deposits (called sand or gravel) to bladder stones the size of an orange.

4. One of three patients with stones are men; in both sexes, the peak age of onset is 40 to 60 years.

5. Most stones migrate downward (causing severe colicky pain when the stone obstructs the ureter) and are discovered in the lower ureter. Spontaneous stone passage can be anticipated in 80% to 90% of patients with calculus less than 5 mm in size.

6. Some stones may lodge in the renal pelvis, ureters, or bladder neck, causing obstruction, edema, secondary infection, and, in some cases, nephron damage.

7. Those with stones for the first time have a 50% risk of recurrence within the next 7 to 10 years.

Clinical Manifestations

1. Pain pattern depends on site of obstruction (see Figure 21-7).
   a. Renal stones produce an increase in hydrostatic pressure and distention of the renal pelvis and proximal ureter causing renal colic. Pain relief is immediate after stone passage.
   b. Ureteral stones produce symptoms due to obstruction as they pass down the ureter (ureteral colic).
   c. Bladder stones may be asymptomatic or produce symptoms similar to cystitis.

2. Obstruction—stones blocking the flow of urine will produce symptoms of colic, chills, and fever.

3. GI symptoms include nausea, vomiting, diarrhea, abdominal discomfort—due to renointestinal reflexes and shared nerve supply (celiac ganglion) between the ureters and intestine.

Diagnostic Evaluation

1. Kidney, ureters, and bladder radiography may show stone.

2. IVU—to determine site and evaluate degree of obstruction.

3. Regular ultrasound may be as sensitive with good technique; however, it won't show radiolucent stones.

4. Spiral CT scan stone study—special non-contrast CT technique to assess for stone in ureter; it is the study of choice and will show all stones.
   a. Requires no preparation and is noninvasive.
   b. Takes only 10 minutes.

5. Analysis of available stone material—crystals can be identified by polarization microscopy, x-ray diffraction, and infrared spectroscopy.

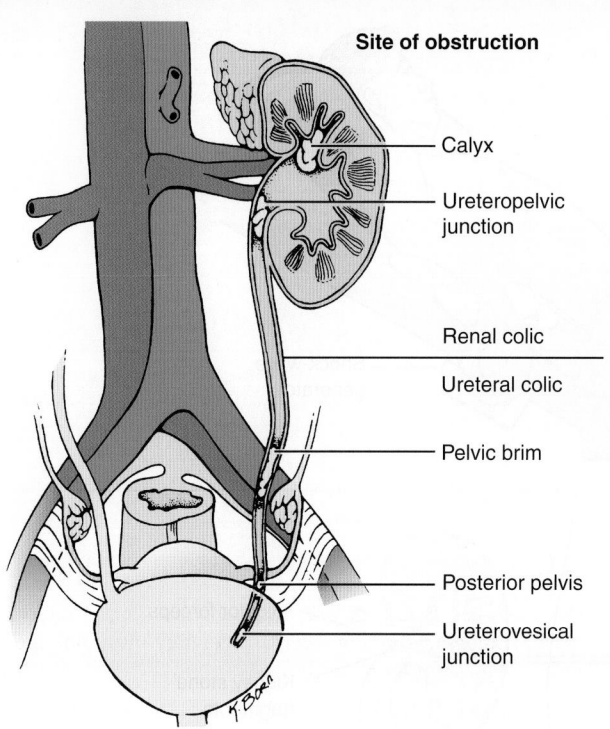

Site of obstruction

- Calyx
- Ureteropelvic junction
- Renal colic
- Ureteral colic
- Pelvic brim
- Posterior pelvis
- Ureterovesical junction

Clinical manifestations

Flank or costovertebral angle pain, hematuria, abdominal distention

Pain at flank or costovertebral angle, migrating to groin and testicle/labia minora

Pain in lateral flank and suprapubic area

Urgency, frequency, genital pain

Figure 21-7. Areas where calculi may obstruct the urinary system. The ensuing clinical manifestations depend on the site of obstruction. Stones that have broken loose may obstruct the flow of urine, cause severe pain, and injure the kidney.

6. Urinalysis—hematuria and pyuria; pH less than 5.5 may indicate uric acid stone; more than 7.5 may indicate struvite stone; urine culture and drug sensitivity studies to detect infection.

7. Serum kidney function tests, electrolytes, calcium, phosphorus, uric acid, and magnesium levels; serum parathyroid hormone may also be evaluated.

Management

General Principles

1. If it is a small stone (<5 mm) and able to treat as outpatient, 80% to 90% of patients will pass stone spontaneously with hydration, pain control, and reassurance.

2. Patient may be hospitalized for intractable pain, persistent vomiting, high-grade fever, obstruction with infection, bilateral ureteral calculi, and solitary kidney with obstruction.

Extracorporeal Shock Wave Lithotripsy

1. Noninvasive technique and treatment of choice for radiopaque stones less than 2 cm in diameter and greater than 4 mm and located in the kidney or ureter above the iliac crest. For stones below the iliac crest, ureteroscopy may be performed.

2. Extracorporeal shock wave lithotripsy (ESWL) can be used for both renal and ureteral stones <2 cm. ESWL is a noninvasive procedure that utilizes shock waves to break up stones into small pieces, allowing the patient to pass stone fragments. Under conscious sedation and with the assistance of fluoroscopy, the offending stone is identified and fragmented with shock waves. Contraindications to ESWL include pregnancy and uncorrected bleeding disorders.

3. High-energy shock waves are directed at the kidney stone, disintegrating it into minute particles that pass in the urine. (A shock wave is a large, condensed wave of energy produced by high-speed motion.)

4. Patient is placed on specially designed table and immersed in a water bath or placed on an adjustable stretcher positioned over a cushion of water.
   a. In water bath model, shock waves travel through water surrounding the patient.
   b. In cushion model, a layer of gel lies between the stretcher and water; shock waves move through the cushion and gel.

5. Position of the kidney stone is located by fluoroscopy and the shock waves are targeted directly at the stone. The shock waves do not affect soft tissue.

6. Eliminates need for surgery in majority of patients and can be repeated for recurrent stones with no apparent risk to kidney structure or function. Long-term adverse effects may include increased risk of hypertension or diabetes.

7. Complications include pain from both the procedure and passing stone fragments, urinary infection, and perirenal hematoma (bleeding around kidney).

Percutaneous Nephrolithotomy

For stones in renal collecting system or upper portion of ureter and larger than 2 cm in diameter (see Figure 21-8, page 810).

1. Under fluoroscopic guidance, a needle is advanced into collecting system; guide wire is advanced into renal pelvis or ureter.

2. Tract is dilated with mechanical dilators or high-pressure balloon dilator until nephroscope can be inserted up against stone.

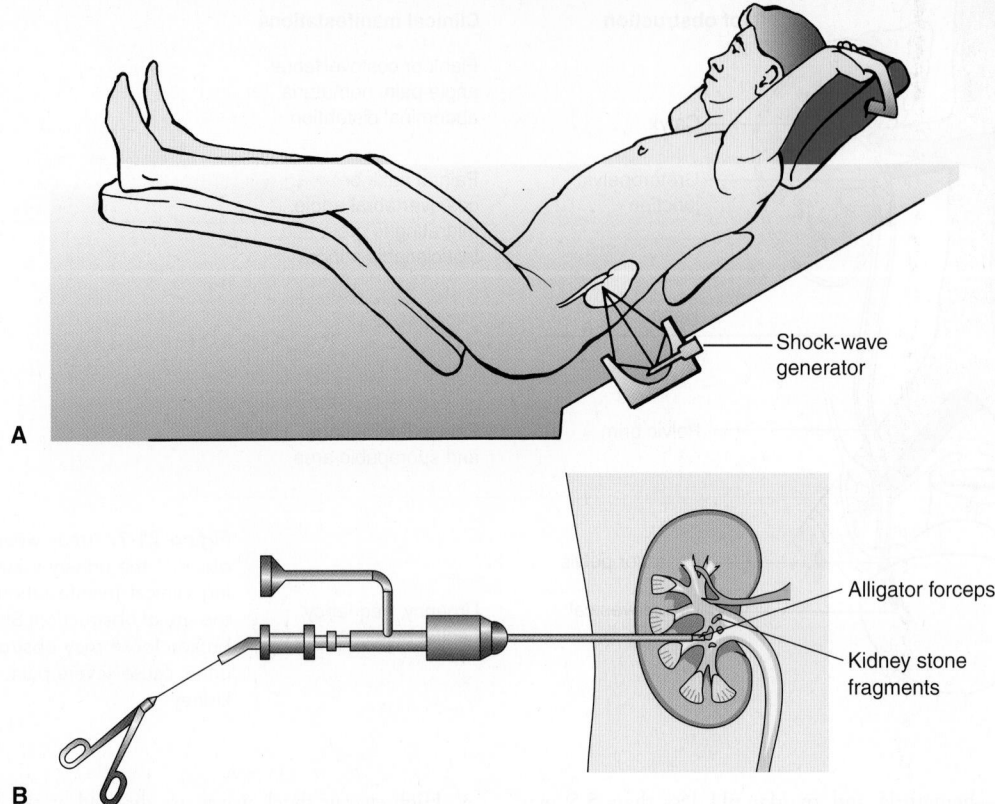

Figure 21-8. (**A**) Extracorporeal shock wave lithotripsy for renal calculi dissolution. (**B**) A percutaneous nephrostomy tract permits access to the collecting system of the kidney for removal of renal calculi under direct vision via a nephroscope.

3. Stones can be broken apart with hydraulic shock waves or a laser beam administered by way of nephroscope; fragments are removed using forceps, graspers, or basket.
4. May be combined with extracorporeal shock wave lithotripsy.
5. Complications include hemorrhage, infection, and extravasation of urine.

Ureteroscopy

1. Used for distal ureteral calculi; may be used for midureteral calculi.
2. Flexible or rigid ureteroscopes are used in conjunction with baskets or graspers.
3. Electrohydraulic, ultrasonic, or laser equipment may also be used to fragment stone.
4. A stent may be inserted and left in place after surgery to maintain patency of ureter.

Open Surgical Procedures

Indicated for only 1% to 2% of all stones; rarely performed, most likely to be done percutaneously or laparoscopically, if indicated.

1. Pyelolithotomy—removal of stones from kidney pelvis.
2. Nephrolithotomy—incision into kidney for removal of stone.
3. Nephrectomy—removal of kidney; indicated when kidney is extensively and irreparably damaged and is no longer a functioning organ; partial nephrectomy sometimes done.
4. Ureterolithotomy—removal of stone in ureter.
5. Cystolithotomy—removal of stone from bladder.

Complications

1. Obstruction—from remaining stone fragments.
2. Infection—from dissemination of infected stone particles or bacteria resulting from obstruction.
3. Impaired renal function—from prolonged obstruction before treatment and removal.
4. Perirenal hematoma—from bleeding around the kidney caused by trauma of shock waves or laser treatments.

Nursing Assessment

1. Obtain history, focusing on history of calculi, family history of calculi, episodes of dehydration, prolonged immobility, UTI, dietary, bleeding history, and medication history.
2. Assess pain location and radiation; assess level of pain using a scale of 1 to 10. Observe for presence of associated symptoms: nausea, vomiting, diarrhea, abdominal distention.
3. Monitor for signs and symptoms of UTI, such as chills, fever, dysuria, frequency. Examine urine for hematuria.
4. Observe for signs and symptoms of obstruction, such as frequent urination of small amounts, oliguria, anuria.

Nursing Diagnoses

- Acute Pain related to inflammation, obstruction, and abrasion of urinary tract by migration of stones.
- Impaired Urinary Elimination related to blockage of urine flow by stones.
- Risk for Infection related to obstruction of urine flow and instrumentation during treatment.

Nursing Interventions

Controlling Pain

1. Give prescribed NSAID or opioid analgesic (usually via IV line or intramuscular [I.M.]) until cause of pain can be removed.
   a. Monitor patient closely for increasing pain; may indicate inadequate analgesia.
   b. Large doses of opioids are typically required to relieve pain; so, monitor for respiratory depression and drop in BP.
2. Encourage patient to assume position that brings some relief.
3. Reassess pain frequently using pain scale.
4. Administer anti-emetics (I.M. or rectal suppository), as indicated, for nausea.

Maintaining Urine Flow

1. Administer fluids orally or via IV line (if vomiting) to reduce concentration of urinary crystalloids and ensure adequate urine output.

 NURSING ALERT Avoid overhydration, which may result in increased distention at stone location, causing an increase in pain and associated symptoms.

2. Monitor total urine output and patterns of voiding. Report oliguria or anuria.
3. Strain all urine through strainer or gauze to harvest the stone; uric acid stones may crumble. Crush clots and inspect sides of urinal/bedpan for clinging stones or fragments.
4. For outpatient treatment, patient may use a coffee filter to strain urine.
5. Help patient to walk, if possible, because ambulation may help move the stone through the urinary tract.

Controlling Infection

1. Administer parenteral or oral antibiotics, as prescribed during treatment, and monitor for adverse effects.
2. Assess urine for color, cloudiness, and odor.
3. Obtain vital signs and monitor for fever and symptoms of impending sepsis (tachycardia, hypotension).

Patient Education and Health Maintenance

Recovery from Surgical Interventions for Stone Disease

1. Encourage fluids to accelerate passing of stone particles.
2. Teach about analgesics that still may be necessary for colicky pain, which may accompany passage of stone debris.
3. Warn that some blood may appear in urine for several weeks.
4. Encourage frequent walking to assist in passage of stone fragments.

5. Teach patient to strain urine through a coffee filter or stone strainer and to save stone for analysis.
6. Teach patient to take alpha-adrenergic blockers to help dilate ureter, thus improve stone passage.

Prevention of Recurrent Stone Formation

1. For patients with calcium oxalate stones:
   a. Instruct on diet—avoid excesses of calcium and phosphorus; maintain a low-sodium diet (sodium restriction decreases amount of calcium absorbed in intestine). (*Note:* Patient should not decrease calcium intake; rather, should maintain regular intake.)
   b. Teach purpose of drug therapy—thiazide diuretics to reduce urine calcium excretion, allopurinol therapy to reduce uric acid concentration.
2. For patients with uric acid stones:
   a. Teach methods to alkalinize urine to enhance urate solubility.
   b. Instruct on testing urine pH.
   c. Teach purpose of taking allopurinol—to lower uric acid concentration.
   d. Provide information about reduction of dietary purine intake (low protein—red meat, fish, fowl).
3. For patients with infected (struvite) stones:
   a. Teach signs and symptoms of urinary infection (in patients with neurologic or spinal cord disease, teach use of dipsticks to evaluate urine for nitrites and leukocytes); encourage patient to report infection immediately; must be treated vigorously.
   b. Try to avoid prolonged periods of recumbency—slows renal drainage and alters calcium metabolism.
4. For patients with cystine stones (occur in *cystinuria*, a hereditary disorder of amino acid transport):
   a. Teach patient to alkalinize urine by taking sodium bicarbonate tablets to increase cystine solubility; instruct patient how to test urine pH with a pH indicator.
   b. Teach patient about drug therapy with D-penicillamine—to lower cystine concentration or dissolution by direct irrigation with thiol derivatives.
   c. Explain importance of maintaining drug therapy consistently.
5. For all patients with stone disease:
   a. Explain need for consistently increased fluid intake (24-hour urinary output greater than 2 L)—lowers the concentration of substances involved in stone formation.
      i. Drink enough fluids to achieve a urinary volume of 2,000 to 3,000 mL or more every 24 hours.
      ii. Drink larger amounts during periods of strenuous exercise and in hot, humid weather due to perspiration.
   b. Encourage a diet low in sugar and animal proteins—refined carbohydrates appear to lead to hypercalciuria and urolithiasis; animal proteins increase urine excretion of calcium, uric acid, and oxalate.
   c. Increase consumption of fiber—inhibits calcium and oxalate absorption.

d. Save any stone passed for analysis. (Only patients with more than one episode of urolithiasis are advised to have a metabolic evaluation.)

e. Can discontinue urine straining once stone is passed.

Evaluation: Expected Outcomes

- Verbalizes reduced pain level.
- Urine output adequate with low specific gravity.
- Afebrile; urine clear.

Renal Cell Carcinoma

Renal cell carcinoma accounts for 85% of primary malignant renal tumors, occurring twice as more frequently in men than in women. Most renal cell tumors are found in the renal parenchyma and develop with few (if any) symptoms.

Pathophysiology and Etiology

1. Unknown etiology; tobacco exposure, through use of cigarettes or chew, causes a twofold increase in risk. Obesity and hypertension are additional risk factors for developing renal cell cancer. Exposure to asbestos, solvents, and cadmium also increases risk.
2. Occurs most frequently in persons between ages 50 and 70.
3. Early-stage renal cancer usually diagnosed incidentally during CT scan or sonogram for an unrelated health problem.
4. Incidence is 10% to 20% higher in African American men.

Clinical Manifestations

1. Many renal tumors produce no symptoms.
2. Weight loss, fever, and night sweats—from systemic effects of renal cancer.
3. Classic triad (late symptoms, occurs in only 7% to 10% of patients):
   a. Hematuria—intermittent or continuous, microscopic or gross.
   b. Flank pain—from distention of renal capsule, invasion of surrounding structures.
   c. Palpable mass in flank or abdomen.
4. Hematuria, dyspnea, cough, and bone pain with advanced disease.

Diagnostic Evaluation

1. Ultrasonography—helpful in differentiating renal cyst from renal tumor.
2. Three-phase CT scan with and without IV contrast—primary technique for detecting, diagnosing, categorizing, and staging a renal mass.
3. IVP—used as a screening procedure and rarely performed, IVP alone may fail to detect some renal tumors.
4. MRI—determines if thrombosis is in renal vein and evaluates for vascular extension.

Management

Goal is to eradicate the tumor and prevent metastasis.

Radical Nephrectomy

Removal of kidney and associated tumor, adrenal gland, surrounding perirenal fat, Gerota's fascia, and possibly regional lymph nodes—provides maximum opportunity for disease control.

1. Performed through a vertical midline, subcostal, thoracoabdominal, or flank incision.
2. See page 788 for care of patient after renal surgery.
3. Increasingly done laparoscopically.
4. Partial nephrectomy is done for localized tumors as nephron sparing.

Renal Artery Embolization

Preoperative occlusion of renal artery followed by nephrectomy—limited to patient with large vascular tumor in which the renal artery may be difficult to reach early in procedure.

1. Catheter is advanced into renal artery.
2. Embolizing material (Gelfoam, steel coils) is injected into artery and carried with arterial blood flow to occlude the tumor vessels.
3. Monitor for postinfarction syndrome (lasts 2 to 3 days)—severe abdominal pain, nausea, vomiting, diarrhea, fever.
4. Complications—arterial obstruction, bleeding, diminution of renal function.

Chemotherapy and Immunotherapy

Renal cell carcinomas are generally refractory to chemotherapeutic agents, radiation, and hormonal manipulation.

1. Interleukin-2—lymphokine that stimulates growth of T lymphocytes—may offer some benefit to patients with metastatic renal cancer, although toxicity is severe.
2. Sunitinib and sorafenib inhibit vascular endothelial growth factor and platelet-derived growth factors.
   a. Main adverse effects include rash, diarrhea, and hand-foot skin rash.
   b. Possible 3- to 5-month increase in survival.

Cryoablation

1. Freezing of tumor with liquid nitrogen or argon gas through percutaneous needles placed into tumors, using ultrasound guidance.
2. Appropriate for tumors 3.5 cm or less in size.

Thermal Ablation

1. Use of heat through percutaneous needles to cause tissue necrosis, thus killing tumor cells.
2. Appropriate for tumors 3.5 cm or less in size.

Complications

Metastasis to the lung, bone, liver, brain, and other areas.

Nursing Assessment

1. Assess for clinical manifestations of systemic disease—fatigue, anorexia, weight loss, pallor, fever, bone pain—as well as evidence of metastasis.
2. Assess cardiopulmonary and nutritional status before surgery.
3. Monitor for adverse effects and complications of diagnostic tests and treatment.
4. Assess pain control and coping ability.

Nursing Diagnoses

- Anxiety related to diagnosis of cancer and possibility of metastatic disease.
- Acute Pain and Hyperthermia related to postinfarction syndrome.

Also see page 788 for nursing diagnoses and interventions related to renal surgery.

Nursing Interventions

Reducing Anxiety

1. Explain each diagnostic test, its purpose, and possible adverse reactions. Ensure that informed consent has been obtained, as indicated.
2. Assess patient's understanding about diagnosis and treatment options. Answer questions, and encourage more thorough discussion with health care provider, as needed.
3. Encourage patient to discuss fears and feelings; involve family and significant others in teaching.

Controlling Symptoms of Postinfarction Syndrome

1. Administer analgesics, as prescribed, to control flank and abdominal pain.
2. Encourage rest and assist with positioning for 2 to 3 days until syndrome subsides.
3. Obtain temperature every 4 hours and administer antipyretics, as indicated.
4. Restrict oral intake and provide IV fluids while patient is nauseated.
5. Administer anti-emetics, as ordered.

Patient Education and Health Maintenance

1. Ensure that patient understands where and when to go for follow-up (surgeon, primary care provider, oncologist, and radiologist for metastatic workup and treatment).
2. Explain the importance of follow-up for hypertension and renal function, even if patient feels well.
3. Advise patient with one kidney to wear a MedicAlert bracelet and notify all health care providers because potentially nephrotoxic medications and procedures must be avoided.

Evaluation: Expected Outcomes

- Asks questions and verbalizes fears.
- Afebrile; states reduced pain.

Injuries to the Kidney

Trauma to abdomen, flank, or back may produce renal injury. Suspicion is high in a patient with multiple injuries.

Pathophysiology and Etiology

1. *Blunt trauma* (falls, sporting accidents, motor vehicle accidents) can suddenly move the kidney out of position and in contact with a rib or lumbar vertebral transverse process, resulting in injury. This is the most common injury to the kidney, accounting for 80% to 85% of all renal injuries.
2. *Penetrating trauma* (gunshot and stab wounds) can injure the kidney if it lies in the path of the wound.

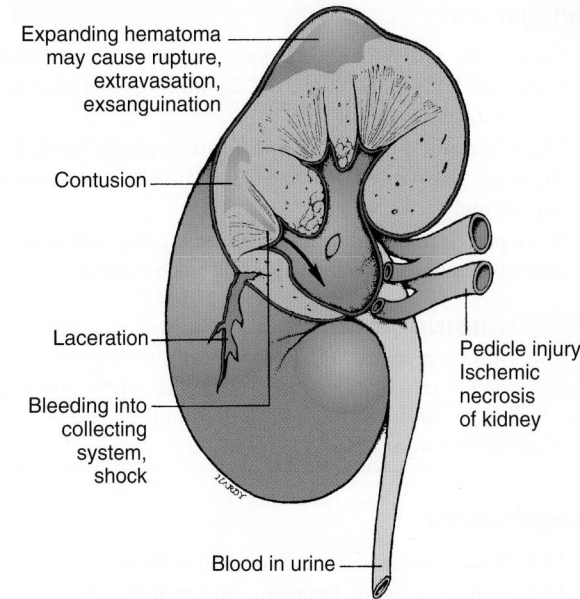

Figure 21-9. Types and physiologic effects of renal injuries: contusion, laceration, rupture, and pedicle injury.

3. Renal trauma is classified according to severity of injury (see Figure 21-9):
   a. Grade I (most common): renal contusion or bruising with normal radiographic imaging.
   b. Grade II: perirenal hematoma or laceration that extends into renal cortex.
   c. Grade III: laceration extends into renal cortex and renal medulla.
   d. Grade IV: laceration extends into collecting system, urine extravasation; requires surgical management.
   e. Grade V: shattered kidney or avulsion of renal artery or renal vein/artery injury; requires surgical management.
4. 80% of patients with renal trauma will have injuries to other organ systems also necessitating treatment.

Clinical Manifestations

1. Hematuria is common but not indicative of severity of injury.
2. Flank pain; perirenal hematoma.
3. Nausea, vomiting, abdominal rigidity—from ileus (seen when there is retroperitoneal bleeding).
4. Shock—from severe or multiple injuries.

Diagnostic Evaluation

1. History of injury—determine if injury was caused by blunt or penetrating trauma.
2. IVU with nephrotomograms—to define extent of injury to involved kidney and the function of contralateral kidney.
3. CT scan with IV contrast—differentiates between major and minor injuries.
4. Arteriography—to evaluate the renal artery, if necessary.

Management

1. Contusions and minor lacerations are managed conservatively with bed rest, IV fluids, and monitoring of serial urines for clearing of hematuria.
2. Major lacerations (Grades IV and V) are surgically repaired.
3. Ruptures are surgically repaired, usually by partial nephrectomy.
4. Renal pedicle injury is a hemorrhagic emergency and requires immediate surgical repair and possible nephrectomy.

 NURSING ALERT If there is a history consistent with renal injury and patient presents in shock, suspect a renal pedicle injury. This is a hemorrhagic emergency, requiring immediate treatment of shock and preparation for surgery.

Complications

1. Hemorrhage, shock with cardiovascular collapse.
2. Hematoma or urinoma formation, abscess formation.
3. Hypertension.
4. Pyelonephritis.
5. Nephrolithiasis.
6. Hydronephrosis.
7. Arteriovenous fistula.

Nursing Assessment

1. Obtain history of traumatic event and any history of renal disease.
2. Inspect for any abrasions, lacerations, or entrance and exit wounds to upper abdomen or lower thorax.
3. Monitor BP and pulse to assess for bleeding and impending shock; perirenal hemorrhage may cause rapid exsanguination.
4. Assess for presence and degree of hematuria.

 NURSING ALERT Watch for any *sudden* change in patient's condition—drop in BP, increasing flank or abdominal pain and tenderness, or palpable mass in flank. May indicate hemorrhage, which requires surgical intervention.

Nursing Diagnoses

- Risk for Ineffective Renal Perfusion related to injury.
- Impaired Urinary Elimination related to injury.
- Acute Pain related to injury.

Nursing Interventions

Restoring and Maintaining Renal Perfusion

1. Assess vital signs frequently, including BP, heart rate, and CVP to monitor for hemorrhage and impending shock.
2. Assess abdomen and back for local tenderness and palpable mass, swelling, and ecchymosis, indicating hemorrhage or urine extravasation.
3. Outline original mass with marking pen for future comparison of size.
4. Establish IV access for support of BP with fluids or vasopressors, replacement of blood, and perfusion of kidneys.
5. Monitor serial hematocrit determinations to be sure that bleeding has stopped.

Preserving Urinary Elimination

1. Save, inspect, and compare each urine specimen—to follow the course and degree of hematuria.
   a. Label each specimen with date and time.
   b. If specimen is not grossly bloody, dipstick for blood or send to laboratory for microscopic examination.
2. Monitor intake and output carefully.
3. Give antibiotics, as directed, to discourage infection from perirenal hematoma or urinoma or severely contaminated wounds.
4. Monitor for paralytic ileus (lack of bowel sounds) caused by retroperitoneal bleeding.
   a. Keep patient NPO until bowel sounds return.
   b. Administer IV fluids to maintain urine output.

Controlling Pain

1. Administer analgesic medication, as prescribed; exercise caution with drugs that may aggravate hypotension or mask complications of hemorrhage.
2. Encourage bed rest and positioning of comfort until hematuria clears to facilitate healing of minor injuries.
3. Expect a low-grade fever with retroperitoneal hematomas as absorption of the clot occurs; administer antipyretics, as ordered, for comfort.

Patient Education and Health Maintenance

1. Instruct patient not to engage in strenuous activity for at least 1 month after blunt trauma to minimize incidence of delayed or secondary bleeding.
2. Teach patient signs and symptoms of late complications—infection and nephrolithiasis.
3. Advise patient to have BP measured frequently and consistently to monitor for hypertension.
4. Review safety precautions to prevent future injuries.

Evaluation: Expected Outcomes

- Vital signs stable.
- Serial urines clearing.
- Reports decreased pain.

Injuries to the Bladder and Urethra

Injuries to the bladder and urethra commonly occur along with pelvic fracture or may be due to surgical interventions.

Pathophysiology and Etiology

1. Bladder injuries are classified as follows:
   a. Contusion of bladder.
   b. Intraperitoneal rupture.
   c. Extraperitoneal rupture.
   d. Combination intraperitoneal and extraperitoneal bladder rupture.

2. Urethral injuries (occurring almost exclusively in men) are classified as follows:
   a. Partial or complete rupture.
   b. Anterior or posterior urethral rupture.
3. Injuries to the bladder and urethra are commonly associated with pelvic fractures and multiple trauma.
4. Certain surgical procedures (endoscopic urologic procedures, gynecologic surgery, surgery of the lower colon and rectum) also carry a risk of trauma to the bladder and urethra.
5. Intraperitoneal bladder rupture occurs when the bladder is full of urine and the lower abdomen sustains blunt trauma. The bladder ruptures at its weakest point, the dome. Urine and blood extravasate into the peritoneal cavity.
6. Extraperitoneal bladder rupture occurs when the lower bladder is perforated by a bony fragment during pelvic fracture or with a sharp instrument during surgery. Urine and blood extravasate into the pelvic cavity.
7. Urethral rupture occurs during pelvic fracture (posterior) or when the urethra or penis is manipulated accidentally during surgery or injury (anterior).

Clinical Manifestations

1. Inability to void.
2. Gross hematuria; presence of blood at urinary meatus may indicate ruptured urethra.
3. Shock and hemorrhage—pallor, rapid and increasing pulse rate.
4. Suprapubic pain and tenderness.
5. Rigid abdomen—indicates intraperitoneal rupture.
6. Absence of prostate on rectal examination in posterior urethral rupture.
7. Swelling or discoloration of penis, scrotum, and anterior perineum in anterior urethral rupture.

Diagnostic Evaluation

1. Retrograde urethrogram—to detect rupture of urethra.

 **NURSING ALERT** If ruptured urethra is suspected and/or blood at meatus observed, do NOT catheterize because doing so may complete a partial urethral rupture. A urethrogram must be obtained first to determine patency of urethra.

2. Cystogram—to detect and localize perforation/rupture of bladder.
3. Plain film of abdomen—may show associated pelvic fracture.
4. Abdominal CT with contrast—best study to evaluate extent of kidney injury.
5. Excretory urogram—to survey the kidneys and ureters for injury.

Management

Bladder Injury
1. Treatment instituted for shock and hemorrhage.
2. Surgical intervention carried out for intraperitoneal bladder rupture. Extravasated blood and urine will first be drained and urine diverted with suprapubic cystostomy or indwelling catheter.
3. Small extraperitoneal bladder ruptures will heal spontaneously with indwelling suprapubic or urethral catheter drainage.
4. Large extraperitoneal bladder ruptures are repaired surgically.

Urethral Injury Management—Controversial
1. Immediate repair—urethra is manipulated into its correct anatomical position with reanastomosis after evacuation of hematoma.
2. Delayed repair—suprapubic cystostomy drainage for 6 to 12 weeks allows the urethra to realign itself while hematoma and edema resolve; then surgical reanastomosis.
3. Two-stage urethroplasty—reconstruction of the urethra occurs in two separate surgeries with urinary elimination diverted until final procedure.

Complications

1. Shock, hemorrhage, peritonitis.
2. UTI.
3. Urethral stricture disease.
4. Impotence.
5. Incontinence.

Nursing Assessment

1. Obtain vital signs; assess for evidence of shock.
2. Obtain detailed history of injury, if possible.
3. Inspect urinary meatus for evidence of bleeding. If present do not insert Foley until retrograde urethrogram verifies patent urethra.
4. Perform physical examination for symptoms of bladder rupture; dullness to palpation; rebound tenderness or rigidity.

Nursing Diagnoses

- Risk for Deficient Fluid Volume related to trauma and resulting hemorrhage.
- Impaired Urinary Elimination related to disruption of intact lower urinary tract.
- Acute Pain related to traumatic injury.
- Fear related to traumatic injury and uncertain prognosis.

Nursing Interventions

Stabilizing Circulatory Volume
1. Monitor vital signs and CVP frequently, as indicated by condition.
2. Establish IV access and replace blood and fluids, as ordered.

Facilitating Urinary Elimination
1. Inspect urethral meatus for blood and, if present, do not catheterize but prepare for diagnostic evaluation and suprapubic cystostomy.
2. Obtain urine specimen, if possible, and assess for degree of hematuria and presence of infection.
3. Prepare patient for surgical repair by assisting with preoperative workup and describing postoperative experiences.

4. Postoperatively, maintain patency and flow of indwelling urinary catheters.
5. Inspect suprapubic incision and Penrose drains from perivesical areas for bleeding, extravasation of urine, or signs of infection.

Controlling Pain

1. Administer analgesics, as ordered (when patient's vital signs are stable).
2. Assess patient's response to pain-control medications.
3. Position for comfort (usually semi-Fowler's position), if not contraindicated by other injuries, and prevent pulling of catheter tubing.

Relieving Fear

1. Provide information to the conscious patient throughout the stabilization and evaluation phase; prepare for surgery, if impending.
2. Keep patient's family or significant others informed of condition and progress.
3. Provide information on long-term outcome of treatment.

Patient Education and Health Maintenance

1. Teach patient to care for indwelling catheters that will remain in place during healing or after surgery.
   a. Empty catheter frequently.
   b. Clean catheter and insertion area with soap and water.
   c. Inspect urine for blood, cloudiness, or concentration.
   d. Drink plenty of fluids to keep urine flowing.
2. Teach patient to report signs and symptoms of UTI.
3. Instruct patient (after surgical repair of bladder rupture) that bladder capacity may be temporarily decreased, causing frequency and nocturia; this resolves over time.
4. Explain possibility of recurrent urethral stricture disease to patients with urethral injury; instruct in daily self-catheterization to dilate urethra, if prescribed.
5. Support patient (after severe urethral injury) if there is a chance of impotence or incontinence.

Evaluation: Expected Outcomes

- Vital signs stable.
- Adequate urine output by way of catheter.
- Verbalizes relief of pain.
- Verbalizes reduction in fear.

Cancer of the Bladder

Cancer of the bladder is the second most common urologic malignancy. Approximately 90% of all bladder cancers are transitional cell carcinomas, which arise from the epithelial lining of the urinary tract; transitional cell tumors can also occur in the ureters, renal pelvis, and urethra. The remaining 10% of bladder cancers are adenocarcinoma, squamous cell carcinoma, or sarcoma.

Pathophysiology and Etiology

1. Many bladder tumors are diagnosed when the lesions are superficial, papillary tumors are easily resected.
2. One fourth of patients with bladder cancer present with non-papillary, muscle-invasive disease.
3. Bladder tumors tend to be either low-grade superficial tumors or high-grade invasive cancers.
4. Metastasis occurs in the bladder wall and pelvis; para-aortic or supraclavicular nodes; in liver, lungs, and bone.
5. Although the specific etiology is unknown, it appears that multiple agents are linked to the development of cancer of the bladder, including:
   a. Cigarette smoking—the risk of developing bladder cancer is up to four times higher in smokers.
   b. Prolonged exposure to aromatic amines or their metabolites—generally dyes manufactured by the chemical industry and used by other industries.
   c. Exposure to cyclophosphamide, radiation therapy to the pelvis, chronic irritation of the bladder (as in long-term indwelling catheterization), and excessive use of the analgesic drug phenacetin, which has been taken off the market.
6. Bladder cancer is the fourth most common cancer in men; it occurs four times more frequently in men than in women; peak incidence occurs in the sixth to eighth decades.

Clinical Manifestations

1. Painless hematuria, either gross or microscopic—most characteristic sign.
2. Dysuria, frequency, urgency—bladder irritability.
3. Pelvic or flank pain—obstruction or distant metastases.
4. Leg edema—from invasion of pelvic lymph nodes.

Diagnostic Evaluation

1. Cystoscopy for visualization of number, location, and appearance of tumors; for biopsy
2. Urine and bladder washing for cytologic study
3. Urine for flow cytometry—uses a computer-controlled fluorescence microscope to scan and image the nucleus of each cell on a slide; based on the fact that cancer cells contain abnormally large amounts of deoxyribonucleic acid.
4. IVU—may reveal filling defect indicative of bladder tumor; also determines status of upper tracts.
5. CT urography (three-phase CT scan)—replacing IVU or IVP as the test of choice to evaluate kidneys, ureter, and bladder.
6. To evaluate for metastatic disease:
   a. CT scan or MRI—to evaluate extent of disease and tumor responsiveness.
   b. Chest x-ray—to evaluate for pulmonary metastases.
   c. Pelvic lymphadenectomy (during cystectomy)—most accurate for staging.

Management

Surgery

1. Transurethral resection and fulguration—endoscopic resection for superficial tumors.
   a. May be followed by intravesical chemotherapy to prevent tumor recurrence.
   b. Complications include hemorrhage, infection, bladder perforation, and temporary irritative voiding.

c. Laser irradiation of bladder tumors is also used to destroy tumors; however, it does not allow for tumor specimen collection for pathologic analysis.

2. Partial cystectomy when lesions are located only in the dome of the bladder, away from the ureteral orifices.

3. Radical cystectomy (removal of bladder) for invasive or poorly differentiated tumors.
   a. Requires diversion of the urinary stream (see page 789).
   b. In men, includes removal of bladder, prostate and seminal vesicles, proximal vas deferens, and part of proximal urethra.
   c. Men may be impotent.
   d. In women, consists of anterior exenteration with removal of bladder, urethra, uterus, fallopian tubes, ovaries, and segment of anterior wall of the vagina.
   e. May be combined with chemotherapy and radiation.

Intravesical (within the Bladder) Chemotherapy and Immunotherapy

1. Instillation of immunotherapeutic agent bacillus Calmette-Guérin (BCG) stimulates immune response to prevent recurrence of transitional cell bladder tumors. BCG is attenuated mycobacterium initially developed as a vaccine for tuberculosis and has demonstrated antitumor activity in selected cancers.

2. Instillation of antineoplastic agent, such as thiotepa, mitomycin-C, doxorubicin; allows a high concentration of drug to come in contact with the tumor and urothelium with minimal systemic toxicity.

3. Patient is instructed as follows:
   a. Minimize fluid intake and avoid taking diuretic medications for several hours before the instillation period to maximize concentration of drug treatment period.
   b. Change position, as directed during instillation, in an effort to have drug contact as much of urothelial surface as possible.
   c. Wash hands and perineal area after voiding the medication to prevent contact dermatitis.
   d. Do not void for 2 hours after instillation; then increase fluid intake and void frequently.
   e. When using BCG, place 2 cups of bleach into toilet with each void for 6 hours after starting voiding to neutralize the chemotherapeutic agent and prevent possible contamination to others.
   f. Course of treatment involves weekly instillations for 6 weeks followed by monthly instillations.

4. Complications from intravesical chemotherapy and immunotherapy include UTI, irritative voiding symptoms, allergic reaction, bone marrow suppression, or systemic BCG reaction. A systemic BCG reaction occurs when fever higher than 100° F (37.8° C) persists for more than 24 hours; it is treated with antituberculosis agents.

Systemic Chemotherapy

Metastatic bladder cancer is a chemotherapeutically responsive disease; gemcitabine and cisplatin have lower toxicity, improved tolerability, and similar overall survival to the MVDC combination (methotrexate, vinblastine, doxorubicin, and cisplatin), which had been in wide use.

Radiation Therapy

External beam radiation therapy is commonly used in combination with chemotherapy.

Complications

Regional metastasis through the pelvis as well as metastasis to the lung, liver, and bone.

Nursing Assessment

1. Assess for hematuria, irritative voiding symptoms, risk factors (especially smoking history), weight loss, fatigue, and signs of metastasis.

2. Assess coping ability and knowledge of the disease and explore feelings about impotence.

Nursing Diagnoses

- Impaired Urinary Elimination related to hematuria and transurethral surgery.
- Acute Pain related to irritative voiding symptoms and catheter-related discomfort.
- Anxiety related to diagnosis of cancer.

Nursing Interventions

Maintaining Urinary Elimination After Transurethral Surgery

1. Maintain patency of indwelling urinary drainage catheter; manual irrigation is not recommended due to dangers of bladder perforation; continuous bladder irrigation may be used, if necessary.

2. Ensure adequate hydration either orally or via IV line.

3. Monitor intake and output, including irrigation solution.

4. Monitor urine output for clearing of hematuria.

Controlling Pain

1. Administer analgesic medication for pelvic discomfort.

2. Administer anticholinergic medications or belladonna and opium suppositories to relieve bladder spasms.

3. Ensure patency of catheter drainage; do not irrigate unless specifically ordered.

4. Remove indwelling catheter as soon as possible after procedure.

Relieving Anxiety

1. Allow patient to verbalize fears and concerns about altered sexuality.

2. Provide realistic information about diagnostic studies, surgery, and treatments.

Patient Education and Health Maintenance

1. Advise patient that irritative voiding symptoms and intermittent hematuria are possible for several weeks after transurethral resection of bladder tumors.

2. Teach patient with superficial bladder cancer importance of vigilant adherence to follow-up schedule: After initial 6-week induction course of BCG they need cystoscopy and three weekly instillations of BCG at 3 and 6 months then

every 6 months thereafter for 3 years. Yearly cystoscopy is required as 70% of superficial tumors will recur.

3. Review purpose and adverse effects of intravesical chemotherapy treatments (usually not given until after recurrence).

Evaluation: Expected Outcomes

- Urine output adequate and clear.
- Verbalizes relief of pain and bladder spasms.
- Verbalizes lessened anxiety.

CONDITIONS OF THE MALE REPRODUCTIVE TRACT

Urethritis

 Evidence Base Centers for Disease Control and Prevention. (2010). *Sexually transmitted diseases.* Available: *www.cdc.gov/STD/treatment.*

Urethritis is inflammation of the urethra. It is usually an ascending infection in men. In women, it is usually associated with cystitis (see page 804) or vaginitis (see page 858).

Pathophysiology and Etiology

1. Nongonococcal urethritis—urethritis not caused by gonococcus; may be sexually transmitted:
   a. Chlamydia trachomatis—most clinically significant of the pathogens, three cases of chlamydia diagnosed for every one case of gonorrhea. Usually asymptomatic.
   b. *Ureaplasma urealyticum* and *Mycoplasma genitalium*—responsible for up to one third of cases.
   c. *Trichomonas vaginalis* and herpes simplex virus are other sexually transmitted organisms causing urethritis in men and women.
   d. Incubation period of 1 to 5 weeks depending on the organism; in some cases, infection may be subclinical for a period of time, particularly in men.
2. Gonococcal urethritis—caused by *Neisseria gonorrhoeae*, sexually transmitted; usually most virulent and destructive.
   a. Incubation period usually 3 to 10 days.
   b. Urethritis in homosexual men is more commonly gonococcal than nongonococcal.
3. Gonococcal and nongonococcal urethritis can both be present.
4. Nonsexually transmitted.
   a. Bacterial urethritis—may be associated with UTI.
   b. From trauma—secondary to passage of urethral sounds, repeated cystoscopy, indwelling catheter.

Clinical Manifestations

1. Can be asymptomatic.
2. Itching and burning around area of urethra.
3. Urethral discharge: may be scant or profuse; thin, clear, or mucoid; or thick and purulent (gonococcal).
4. Dysuria and frequency.
5. Penile discomfort.

Diagnostic Evaluation

1. Gram stain—*N. gonorrhoeae* is detected as Gram-positive diplococci on microscopic examination of urethral discharge or urine.
2. Culture of urethral discharge on selective medium.
3. Deoxyribonucleic acid (DNA) amplification tests on urethral voided specimen or other DNA/antibody tests of urethral discharge (currently, primary test)—to detect *C. trachomatis* and *N. gonorrhoeae*.
4. Wet mount microscopic examination of fresh urethral discharge—trichomonads may be visible and motile.
5. First voided urine for screening—either positive leukocyte esterase test by dipstick or greater than 10 WBC per high-power field by microscopy indicates urethritis.
6. In rare cases, urethroscopy may be necessary to isolate a lesion such as warts caused by human papillomavirus (HPV).

Management

1. Gonococcal urethritis: one dose oral antibiotic of cefixime 400 mg; or one-dose I.M. treatment with ceftriaxone 125 mg.

 DRUG ALERT Fluoroquinolones are now avoided in the treatment of gonococcal infections due to drug resistance.

2. Chlamydial urethritis: single dose of oral antibiotic azithromycin 1 g or doxycycline 100 mg orally twice per day for 7 days.
3. Unless proven otherwise by negative testing, treatment for chlamydia is given along with treatment for gonorrhea.
4. Recurrent urethritis despite appropriate treatment for nongonococcal urethritis or confirmed presence of *Trichomonas vaginalis* one dose oral metronidazole 2 gm.

Complications

Depends on cause, but may include:

1. Prostatitis, epididymitis, urethral stricture, sterility due to vas epididymal duct obstruction.
2. Rectal infection, pharyngitis, conjunctivitis, skin lesions, arthritis with gonococcal infection.
3. Long-term complications of these infections in women include pelvic inflammatory disease and infertility.

Nursing Assessment

1. Obtain history of unprotected sexual contact and assess patient's understanding of risk.
2. Assess for signs and symptoms involving urinary and reproductive tracts.
3. Perform genital and abdominal examination to assess for extent of infection.

Nursing Diagnoses

- Risk for Infection related to ascending or systemic spread of pathogens.
- Risk for Infection related to high-risk sexual activity.

Nursing Interventions

Resolving Infection and Preventing Complications

1. Collect urethral swab of discharge, urine, and blood, as ordered, for laboratory examination.
2. Use standard precautions when handling specimens.
3. Administer antibiotics, as prescribed.
   a. Usually ordered based on presumptive diagnosis before test results are obtained.
   b. Monitor for and advise patient of adverse effects or allergic reactions.

Preventing Spread of Infection

1. Encourage compliance with antimicrobial regimen for the prescribed time period.
2. Advise abstinence from sexual activity until treatment is complete and cure is established (usually 7 to 10 days).
3. Instruct the patient to avoid sexual activity with previous sexual partner until that person has been tested and treated for infection as well.
4. The use of condoms may prevent transmission, but depends on technique.

Patient Education and Health Maintenance

1. Advise safer sex practices, such as abstinence, mutual monogamy, and use of male or female condom to prevent transmission of sexually transmitted organisms as well as unintended pregnancy.
2. Emphasize the need for follow-up care if symptoms persist or return.
3. Advise patient that reporting of gonorrhea to the public health department is required by law in all of the United States and Canada.
4. Tell patient that he or she will be called on to name all sexual partners within the past 60 days and that the process will be confidential.
5. Provide written information about all STDs and ensure that patient understands the dangers of high-risk sexual behavior.

Evaluation: Expected Outcomes

- Signs of infection resolved.
- Reports sexual contacts have been treated.

Benign Prostatic Hyperplasia

 Evidence Base Armando, J., Plata, M., Kazzazi, A., et al. (2012). American Urological Association and European Association of Urology guidelines in the management of benign prostatic hypertrophy: Revisited. *Current Opinion in Urology, 22,* 34–39.

Benign prostatic hyperplasia (BPH) is enlargement of the prostate that constricts the urethra, causing urinary symptoms. One in four men who reach age 80 will require treatment for BPH.

Pathophysiology and Etiology

1. The process of aging and the presence of circulating androgens are required for the development of BPH.
2. The prostatic tissue forms nodules as enlargement occurs.
3. The normally thin and fibrous outer capsule of the prostate becomes spongy and thick as enlargement progresses.
4. The prostatic urethra becomes compressed and narrowed, requiring the bladder musculature to work harder to empty urine.
5. Effects of prolonged obstruction cause trabeculation (formation of cords) of the bladder wall, decreasing its elasticity.

Clinical Manifestations

1. In early or gradual prostatic enlargement, there may be no symptoms because the bladder musculature can initially compensate for increased urethral resistance.
2. Obstructive symptoms—hesitancy, diminution in size and force of urinary stream, terminal dribbling, sensation of incomplete emptying of the bladder, urinary retention.
3. Irritative voiding symptoms—urgency, frequency, nocturia.

Diagnostic Evaluation

1. American Urologic Association Symptom Index score greater than 7 (uses rating of questions about the obstructive and irritative symptoms): 0 to 7, mild; 8 to 19, moderate; 20 to 35, severe.
2. Rectal examination—smooth, firm, symmetric or asymmetric enlargement of the prostate.
3. Urinalysis—to rule out hematuria and infection.
4. Serum creatinine and BUN—to evaluate renal function.
5. Serum PSA—may be elevated in patients with BPH.
6. Optional diagnostic studies for further evaluation:
   a. Urodynamics—measures peak urine flow rate, voiding time and volume, and status of the bladder's ability to effectively contract
   b. Measurement of postvoid residual urine; by ultrasound or catheterization
   c. Cystourethroscopy—to inspect urethra and bladder and evaluate prostatic size
   d. Uroflow—graphically demonstrates voiding pattern and can help characterize the severity of obstruction.

Management

1. Patients with mild symptoms (in the absence of significant bladder or renal impairment) are followed annually; BPH does not necessarily worsen in all men.
2. Pharmacologic management.
   a. Alpha-adrenergic blockers, such as doxazosin, tamsulosin, terazosin, and alfuzosin—relax smooth muscle of bladder neck and prostate to facilitate voiding.

 DRUG ALERT Although prescribed for their effect on prostatic smooth muscle, alpha-adrenergic blockers (except for tamsulosin and alfuzosin) also have an antihypertensive effect. Dosage is usually titrated up from an initial small dose. It is commonly recommended that the first dose, or all once-per-day doses, be taken at bedtime.

DRUG ALERT Patients who are taking tamsulosin and need cataract surgery should contact ophthalmologist because taking tamsulosin prior to cataract surgery may increase risk of floppy iris syndrome.

b. 5-alpha-reductase inhibitors such as finasteride and dutasteride—exert anti-androgen effect on prostatic cells and can reverse or prevent hyperplasia. These drugs decrease the size of the prostate and improve urinary symptoms. Effect of drug may take up to 6 months. Women should not handle drug because it can be absorbed through skin and is pregnancy category X. In addition, patients taking dutasteride cannot donate blood.

 DRUG ALERT Finasteride present in semen may have deleterious effects on the fetus of pregnant women.

3. Surgery (also see page 793)—options include TURP (formerly most common procedure), transurethral incision of the prostate, or open prostatectomy for very large prostates, usually by suprapubic approach.
4. PVP is starting to replace TURP; it is done through a cystoscope, using a laser to vaporize diseased prostatic tissue.
5. TUMT and TUNA are both office-based procedures that use heat to destroy diseased prostatic tissue.
6. Indigo interstitial laser therapy of the prostate is another procedure that is done on an outpatient basis.

Complications

1. Acute urinary retention, involuntary bladder contractions, bladder diverticula, and cystolithiasis.
2. Vesicoureteral reflux, hydroureter, hydronephrosis.
3. Gross hematuria, UTI.

Nursing Assessment

1. Obtain history of voiding symptoms, including onset, frequency of day and nighttime urination, presence of urgency, dysuria, sensation of incomplete bladder emptying, and decreased force of stream. Determine impact on quality of life.
2. Perform rectal (palpate size, shape, and consistency) and abdominal examination to detect distended bladder, degree of prostatic enlargement.
3. Perform simple urodynamic measures—uroflowmetry and measurement of postvoid residual, if indicated.

Nursing Diagnosis

• Impaired Urinary Elimination related to obstruction of urethra.

Also see page 794 for care of the patient undergoing prostatic surgery.

Nursing Interventions

Facilitating Urinary Elimination

1. Provide privacy and time for patient to void.

2. Assist with catheter introduction with guide wire or by way of suprapubic cystotomy, as indicated.
   a. Monitor intake and output.
   b. Maintain patency of catheter.
3. Administer medications, as ordered, and monitor for and teach patient about adverse effects.
   a. Alpha-adrenergic blockers—hypotension, orthostatic hypotension, syncope (especially after first dose), potential impotence, potential retrograde ejaculation, blurred vision, rebound hypertension if discontinued abruptly.
   b. Finasteride and dutasteride—hepatic dysfunction, potential impotence, interference with PSA testing, presence in semen with potential adverse effect on fetus of pregnant woman.

 DRUG ALERT Treatment with finasteride and dutasteride decreases the PSA by half so this should be taken into account when obtaining PSA to monitor for prostate cancer.

4. Assess for and teach patient to report hematuria, signs of infection.

Patient Education and Health Maintenance

1. Explain to patient symptoms and complications of BPH—urinary retention, hydronephrosis, cystitis, increase in irritative voiding symptoms. Encourage reporting these problems and maintaining close follow-up.
2. Advise patients with BPH to avoid certain drugs that may impair voiding (see Table 21-3), particularly OTC cold medicines containing sympathomimetics such as phenylpropanolamine.
3. Advise patient that irritative voiding symptoms do not immediately resolve after relief of obstruction; symptoms diminish over time.
4. Tell patient postoperatively to avoid sexual intercourse, straining at stool, heavy lifting, and long periods of sitting for 6 to 8 weeks after surgery, until prostatic fossa is healed.
5. Advise follow-up visits after treatment because urethral stricture may occur and regrowth of prostate is possible after TURP.
6. Be aware of herbal or "natural" products marketed for "prostate health."
   a. Advise patients that saw palmetto has shown some efficacy in reducing symptoms of BPH in a number of clinical trials.
   b. The active ingredient in commercial preparations is lipidosterol extract of *Serenoa repens*; dosage is 160 mg twice per day.
   c. It should be taken with breakfast and an evening meal to minimize GI adverse effects.
   d. Although it appears safe and there are no known drug interactions, tell patients they must discuss use of saw palmetto with their health care providers.

Evaluation: Expected Outcomes

• Voiding adequate without residual urine.

Table 21-3   Bladder Function and Drug Actions

FUNCTION	DRUG GROUPS	EXAMPLES
Detrusor Muscle		
Increased tone and contraction	Cholinergic drugs (stimulate parasympathetic receptors that cause detrusor muscle contraction)	• Bethanechol • Neostigmine
Decreased tone, possible retention	Anticholinergic drugs (block parasympathetic receptors that cause detrusor muscle contraction)	• Methantheline • Propantheline • Oxybutynin • Darifenacin • Solifenacin • Trospium
Relaxes bladder tone	Calcium channel blocking drugs (may interfere with influx of calcium to support detrusor muscle tone)	• Nifedipine • Verapamil • Diltiazem • Tolterodine tartrate
Internal Sphincter		
Increased tone, possible retention	Alpha$_1$-adrenergic agonists (activate alpha receptors that cause contraction of muscles of the internal sphincter)	• Phenylephrine • Ephedrine • Phenylpropanolamine
Decreased tone	Alpha$_1$-adrenergic blockers	• Alfuzosin • Prazosin • Doxazosin • Terazosin • Tamsulosin
External Sphincter		
Decreased tone, possible retention	Skeletal muscle relaxants	• Baclofen • Dantrolene • Diazepam

Prostatitis

 Evidence Base Touma, N., & Nickel, C. (2011). Prostatitis and chronic pelvic pain syndrome in men. *Medical Clinics of North America, 95,* 75–86.

Prostatitis is an inflammation of the prostate gland. It is classified as bacterial prostatitis (acute or chronic) or chronic pelvic pain syndrome (without presence of bacterial invasion).

Pathophysiology and Etiology

Acute and Chronic Bacterial Invasion of Prostate

1. From reflux of infected urine into ejaculatory and prostatic ducts.
2. From hematogenous (bloodstream) origin, lymphogenous spread, or direct extension from the rectum.
3. Secondary to urethritis—from ascent of bacteria from urethra.
4. May be stimulated by urethral instrumentation or rectal examination of the prostate when bacteria are present.
5. May be caused by Gram-negative enteric bacteria, such as *Pseudomonas aeruginosa*, *E. coli*, and *Klebsiella pneumonia*, and Gram-positive cocci, such as *Streptococcus* and *Staphylococcus*; may also be caused by *Chlamydia trachomatis*.

Chronic Pelvic Pain Syndrome
Pain or discomfort without other signs of infection and no known etiologic cause; difficult to diagnose and manage.

Clinical Manifestations

1. Sudden chills and fever (moderate to high fever) and body aches with acute prostatitis.
2. Symptoms are more subtle with chronic prostatitis and chronic pelvic pain syndrome.
3. Bladder irritability—frequency, dysuria, nocturia, urgency, hematuria to varying degrees.

4. Pain in perineum, rectum, lower back, lower abdomen, and tip of penis.
5. Pain after ejaculation, symptoms of urethral obstruction.

Diagnostic Evaluation

1. Urinalysis.
2. Urine culture and sensitivity tests.
   a. Prostate massage is inadvisable because it can precipitate frank sepsis or bacteremia.
   b. In acute bacterial prostatitis, there are numerous WBCs and a positive culture; in chronic bacterial prostatitis, there is a lower bacterial colony count; in chronic pelvic pain syndrome, there may be WBCs but a negative culture.
3. Rectal examination commonly reveals exquisitely tender, painful, swollen (boggy) prostate that is warm to the touch (with acute bacterial prostatitis).
4. Serum WBC count is elevated in acute bacterial prostatitis.
5. Bladder scan for postvoid residual evaluates bladder emptying.
6. Transrectal ultrasound detects prostate abscess.

Management

Acute Bacterial Prostatitis

1. Antimicrobial therapy generally for 2 to 4 weeks based on drug sensitivity; commonly a fluoroquinolone or sulfatrimethoprim.
2. IV therapy with ampicillin or an aminoglycoside in the hospitalized patient. Patients are hospitalized if there is suspected abscess, urosepsis, or immunocompromise.
3. Urinary retention is managed with suprapubic cystostomy; urethral catheterization usually is avoided.
4. Antipyretics, analgesics, hydration, stool softeners, and sitz baths for symptom relief.

Chronic Bacterial Prostatitis

1. Usually 4 to 6 weeks of oral antibiotic therapy with ability to diffuse into prostate.
   a. Quinolones such as ciprofloxacin, levofloxacin, ofloxacin, or norfloxacin.
   b. Sulfonamide such as sulfamethoxazole trimethoprim.
2. Oral antispasmodic agents may provide relief from urinary frequency and urgency.
3. Alpha-adrenergic blockers may help with urination.

Chronic Pelvic Pain Syndrome

1. Usually requires multiple modalities.
2. Alpha-adrenergic blockers and skeletal muscle relaxants may provide some relief of symptoms.
3. Aggressive diagnostic intervention should take place to rule out other conditions, such as cancer of the prostate or interstitial cystitis.
4. Anti-inflammatory medications such as NSAIDS are helpful.
5. Tricyclic antidepressants may be helpful for pain control.
6. Pentosan may be helpful to relieve discomfort.
7. Quinoline antibiotics may be taken for 4 to 6 weeks.
8. Pelvic floor massage and biofeedback may help relieve perineal muscle spasms.

Complications

1. Bacteriuria, urethritis, epididymitis, prostatic abscess, bacteremia, septicemia.
2. Acute urinary retention.
3. Constipation.

Nursing Assessment

1. Obtain history of previous lower UTIs or STDs, recent voiding patterns.
2. Perform examination of genitalia for urethral discharge; rectal examination (except in acute bacterial prostatitis due to tenderness and possibility of disseminating infection) to assess tenderness of prostate.
3. Collect specimens: urine for culture and expressed prostatic secretions. To help distinguish urethral, bladder, and prostate infections, have the patient collect the first 10 mL of urine and label this voided bladder-1. This will be a urethral specimen. Next have the patient collect a midstream urine specimen and label this voided bladder-2. This is a bladder specimen. Have the patient urinate after a prostatic massage and label this voided bladder-3. This is a prostatic specimen.

Nursing Diagnoses

- Hyperthermia related to infectious process.
- Acute Pain related to prostatic inflammation.
- Chronic Pain related to chronic prostatitis, chronic pelvic pain syndrome.

Nursing Interventions

Reducing Fever

1. Start antibiotic therapy as soon as specimens are obtained for culture.
2. Administer antipyretic medications; use cooling measures, if necessary.
3. Keep patient well hydrated, via IV administration or orally, due to fluid loss through fever; however, avoid overhydration, which increases urine volume and reduces antibiotic concentration in urine.

Relieving Pain

1. Administer analgesic or anti-inflammatory medication, as ordered.
2. Maintain bed rest in acute prostatitis to relieve perineal and suprapubic pain.
3. Maintain high-fiber diet and give stool softeners, as needed, to prevent constipation, which increases pain.

Controlling Chronic Pain

1. Administer or teach self-administration of analgesics, anti-inflammatory agents, alpha-adrenergic blockers, or skeletal muscle relaxants as ordered.
2. Advise warm sitz baths to relieve pain and promote muscular relaxation of pelvic floor and reduce potential for urinary retention.
3. Assess patient's response to supportive measures and coping with chronic pain.

Patient Education and Health Maintenance

1. Instruct patient to take antibiotic, as prescribed; emphasize importance of completing long course of therapy to prevent recurrence and resistance of organisms.
2. Teach patient symptoms of recurrence and of disseminated spread of infection.
3. Instruct patient in comfort measures: sitz baths (10 to 20 minutes) several times daily, continued use of stool softeners, and not sitting for long periods.
4. Advise patient to avoid sexual arousal and intercourse during period of acute inflammation; sexual intercourse may be beneficial in the treatment of chronic prostatitis to stimulate the secretion of prostatic fluid and relieve prostate congestion; chronic prostatic infection is not sexually transmittable.
5. Encourage prescribed follow-up because recurrence is possible.

Evaluation: Expected Outcomes

- Afebrile.
- Verbalizes relief of pain after analgesic.
- Verbalizes reduction of chronic pain.

Cancer of the Prostate

Cancer of the prostate is the leading cause of cancer and second leading cause of cancer death among American men and is the most common carcinoma in men older than 65.

Pathophysiology and Etiology

1. The incidence of prostate cancer is 30% higher in African American men.
2. The majority of prostate cancers arise from the peripheral zone of the gland.
3. Prostate cancer can spread by local extension, by lymphatics, or by way of the bloodstream.
4. The etiology of prostate cancer is unknown; however, there is an increased risk for persons with a family history of the disease.
5. The influences of dietary fat intake, serum testosterone levels, and industrial exposure to carcinogens are under investigation.

Clinical Manifestations

1. Most early-stage prostate cancers are asymptomatic.
2. Symptoms due to obstruction of urinary flow:
   a. Hesitancy and straining on voiding, frequency, nocturia.
   b. Diminution in size and force of urinary stream.
3. Symptoms due to metastasis:
   a. Pain in lumbosacral area radiating to hips and down legs (from bone metastases).
   b. Perineal and rectal discomfort.
   c. Anemia, weight loss, weakness, nausea, oliguria (from uremia).
   d. Hematuria (from urethral or bladder invasion, or both).
   e. Lower-extremity edema—occurs when pelvic node metastases compromise venous return.

Diagnostic Evaluation

1. Digital rectal examination—prostate can be felt through the wall of the rectum; hard nodule may be felt (see Figure 21-10).
2. Transrectal ultrasound-guided needle biopsy (through anterior rectal wall or through perineum) for histologic study of biopsied tissue, includes Gleason tumor grade if carcinoma is present.
3. Transrectal ultrasonography—sonar probe placed in rectum.
4. PSA—a protease produced by both benign and malignant prostate tissue. An elevated PSA may be due to benign prostatic hyperplasia, prostatitis, or prostate cancer.
   a. Prostate cancer is suspected if PSA is above 4; however, prostate cancer may also occur at levels under 4.0.
   b. A free PSA level can be used to help stratify the risk of an elevated PSA. The lower the free PSA level, the higher the risk for prostate cancer.
   c. PSA velocity: PSA increases of 0.75 ng in 1 year could indicate prostate cancer.
   d. Age-specific PSA can help stratify risk for prostate cancer as well.
5. Guidelines vary among The American Cancer Society, National Comprehensive Cancer Network (NCCN), United States Preventive Services Task Force (USPSTF), and the American Urological Association (AUA) regarding prostate cancer screening. The USPSTF states that there is insufficient evidence to recommend screening. ACS is not in favor of routine screening until an informed discussion with those patients wanting to be screened takes place. NCCN recommends baseline DRE/PSA at 40 years of age and annual screening at age 50. AUA recommends baseline DRE/PSA at 40 years of age. All recommend informed discussion with patients.

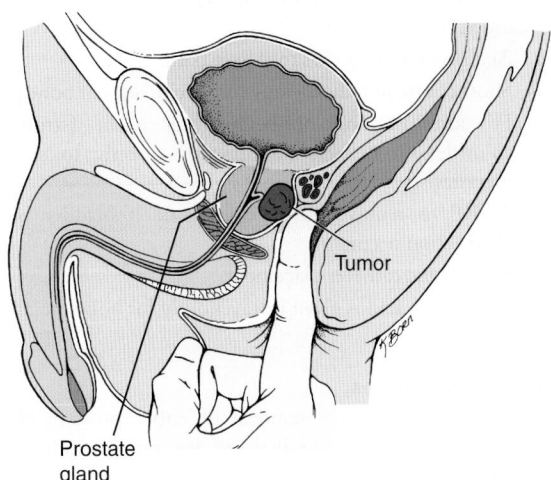

Figure 21-10. The prostate gland can be felt through the wall of the rectum. The size of the gland, overall consistency, and the presence of any firm areas and nodules are noted.

Evidence Base Gomella, L., Liu, X., Trabulsi, E., Kelly, W., Myers, R., Showalter, T., Dicker, A., & Wender, R. (2011). Screening for prostate cancer: the current evidence and guidelines controversy. *The Canadian Journal of Urology, 18*(5), 5875–5883.

National Cancer Institute. (2012). Prostate Cancer Screening. PDQ. Available: *http://www.cancer.gov/cancertopics/pdq/screening/prostate/HealthProfessional/page1/AllPages.*

6. Staging evaluation—skeletal x-rays, CT scan, MRI, bone scan, analysis of pelvic lymph nodes provide accurate staging information.
7. Newer imaging study called the ProstaScint scan uses an IV infusion of monoclonal antibody to prostate-specific membrane antigen.
   a. Immediate and delayed images at 48 and 72 hours may identify soft tissue and bone metastasis for staging.
   b. Radiation is excreted through urine and feces and body fluids but is very low and not a risk to others.
   c. Patient is monitored for signs of allergic reactions following test.
8. Research is being conducted on numerous genetic and chromosomal abnormalities. Overexpression of the *AMACR* gene was found in 90% of prostate cancer patients. Testing for this gene could result in identifying prostate cancer at an earlier stage.

Management

Conservative Measures
1. Watchful waiting/active surveillance may be indicated in men with Gleason 6 or lower-stage prostate cancer or life expectancy of 10 years or less because prostate cancer may be slow growing and it is expected that many men will die from other causes. It is commonly recommended that these patients be followed closely with periodic PSA determinations and examination for evidence of metastases.
2. Symptom control for advanced prostatic cancer in which treatment is not effective:
   a. Analgesics and opioids to relieve pain.
   b. Short course of radiotherapy for specific sites of bone pain.
   c. IV administration of beta-emitter agent (strontium chloride 89) delivers radiotherapy directly to sites of metastasis.
   d. TURP to remove obstructing tissue if bladder outlet obstruction occurs.
   e. Suprapubic catheter placement.
   f. Zoledronic acid is given intravenously for bone metastasis pain.

Surgical Interventions
1. Radical prostatectomy—removal of entire prostate gland, prostatic capsule, and seminal vesicles; may include pelvic lymphadenectomy.
   a. Procedure is used to treat stage T_1 and T_2 prostate cancers.
   b. Complications may include urinary incontinence and impotence, possible rectal injury.

c. Newer nerve-sparing techniques may preserve sexual potency and continence.
2. Cryosurgery of the prostate freezes prostate tissue, killing tumor cells without removing the gland.

Radiation
1. External beam radiation or intensity modulated radiotherapy focused on the prostate—to deliver maximum radiation dose to tumor and minimal dose to surrounding tissues.
2. Brachytherapy—interstitial implantation of radioactive substances into prostate, which delivers doses of radiation directly to tumor while sparing uninvolved tissue.
3. Used to treat stages T_1, T_2, and T_3, especially if patient is not a good surgical candidate. Both forms of radiation are used in some patients; external beam followed by brachytherapy.
4. Complications include radiation cystitis (urinary frequency, urgency, nocturia), urethral injury (stricture), radiation enteritis (diarrhea, anorexia, nausea), radiation proctitis (diarrhea, rectal bleeding), impotence, skin reaction, and fatigue.

Hormone Manipulation (Palliative)
1. Prostate cancer is a hormone-sensitive cancer. The aim of hormonal treatment is to deprive tumor cells of androgens or their by-products and thereby alleviate symptoms and retard progress of disease.
2. Bilateral orchiectomy (removal of testes) results in reduction of the major circulating androgen, testosterone. A small amount of androgen is still produced by adrenal glands.
3. Pharmacologic methods of achieving androgen deprivation—also used to reduce tumor volume before surgery or radiation therapy.
   a. Luteinizing hormone-releasing hormone (LHRH) agonists (such as leuprolide and goserelin acetate) reduce testosterone levels as effectively as orchiectomy.
   b. Anti-androgen drugs (flutamide, bicalutamide, nilutamide) block androgen action directly at the target tissues (testes and adrenals) and block androgen synthesis within the prostate gland and adrenal glands.
   c. Combination therapy with LHRH agonist and an anti-androgen blocks the action of all circulating androgen.
4. Complications of hormonal manipulation include hot flashes, nausea and vomiting, gynecomastia, sexual dysfunction, and osteoporosis.

Complications
1. Bone metastasis—vertebral collapse and spinal cord compression, pathologic fractures.
2. Complications of treatment.

Nursing Assessment
1. Obtain history of current symptoms; assess for family history of prostate cancer.
2. Palpate lymph nodes, especially in supraclavicular and inguinal regions (may be first sign of metastatic spread); assess for flank pain and distended bladder.
3. Assess comorbidities, nutritional status, and coping before treatment.

Nursing Diagnoses

- Anxiety related to fear of disease progression and treatment options.
- Sexual Dysfunction related to effects of therapy.
- Chronic Pain related to bone metastasis.
  Also see page 794 for care of the patient after prostatectomy.

Nursing Interventions

Reducing Anxiety

1. Help patient assess the impact of the disease and treatment options on quality of life.
2. Give repeated explanations of diagnostic tests and treatment options; help patient gain some feeling of control over disease and decisions.
3. Help patient and family set achievable goals.
4. Convey a sense of caring and reassurance in your physical care.

Achieving Optimal Sexual Function

1. Although patient may be ill while experiencing the effects of therapy, he may wonder about sexual function. Give him the opportunity to communicate his concerns and sexual needs.
2. Let patient know that decreased libido is expected after hormonal manipulation therapy and impotence may result from some surgical procedures and radiation.
3. Expect patient's behavior to reflect depression, anxiety, anger, and regression. Encourage expression of feelings and communication with partner.
4. Suggest such options as sexual counseling, learning other methods of sexual expression, and consideration of implant, pharmacologic agents, and other options for treatment of erectile dysfunction.
5. Have patient ask urologist about penile rehabilitation after radical open or laparoscopic prostatectomy. The early incorporation of PDE5 inhibitors, vacuum erectile device, or intracavernosal injections may increase the return of post-prostatectomy erections.

> **DRUG ALERT** Yohimbine is an herbal preparation sold OTC as an aphrodisiac and treatment for male erectile dysfunction. Caution patients that it is considered an unsafe herb by the U.S. Department of Agriculture due to its many drug and food interactions and adverse effects, including hypertension, tachycardia, and tremor.

Controlling Pain

1. Administer and teach self-administration of opioid analgesics, as ordered; oral sustained-release opioids, sustained-release transdermal patches, and subcutaneous or epidural patient-controlled infusion pumps are among the many options.
2. Encourage patient to take prescribed aspirin, acetaminophen, or NSAIDs for reduction of mild pain or to supplement opioid pain-control regimen.
3. Make sure that patient is not undermedicated; help patient and family understand that addiction is not a concern in hormonally refractory or metastatic prostate cancer.

4. Teach relaxation techniques, such as imagery, music therapy, progressive muscle relaxation.
5. Use safety measures to prevent pathologic fractures from falls.
6. Encourage follow-up and palliative treatment such as radiation therapy to bony lesions for pain improvement.

Community and Home Care Considerations

 Evidence Base Smith, R. A., Cokkinides, V., Brawley, O. W. (2012). Cancer screening in the United States 2012: A review of current American Cancer Society guidelines and current issues in cancer screening, 62(2), 129–142.

Encourage awareness of prostate cancer in the community.

1. Risks include being African American, over age 50, and having a first-degree relative with prostate cancer. High-fat diet has also been linked to prostate cancer.
2. Asymptomatic men with at least a 10-year life expectancy should have the opportunity to make an informed decision about screening.
3. If screening is desired after a detailed discussion between patient and health care provider, digital rectal examination and PSA blood testing begin at age 50 for men at average risk; at age 45 for African American men and those with a first-degree relative with history of prostate cancer; or at age 40 if a man has multiple relatives diagnosed with prostate cancer before age 65.
4. There is insufficient and conflicting evidence whether prostate cancer screening saves lives.
5. PSA less than 2.5 ng/mL indicates low risk for prostate cancer; therefore, recommendation is to repeat in 2 years.

Patient Education and Health Maintenance

1. Teach patient importance of follow-up for check of PSA levels (every 3 months to 1 year depending on pathology and recommendation of urologist) and evaluation for disease progression through periodic bone scan or CT scan.
2. Teach I.M. or subcutaneous administration of hormonal agents, as indicated.
3. If bone metastasis has occurred, encourage safety measures around the home to prevent pathologic fractures such as removal of throw rugs, use of handrail on stairs, use of nightlights.
4. Advise reporting symptoms of worsening urethral obstruction, such as increased frequency, urgency, hesitancy, and urinary retention.
5. Advise patient to monitor for signs of metastasis, such as fatigue, weight loss, weakness, pain, and bowel and bladder dysfunction.
6. For additional information and support, refer to agencies such as Us TOO International (*www.ustoo.com*); Man to Man, a program of the American Cancer Society (*www.cancer.org*); and American Urological Association Foundation (*www.urologyhealth.org*).

Evaluation: Expected Outcomes

- Discusses treatment options, asks questions.
- Verbalizes understanding of sexual dysfunction and interest in seeking sexual counseling.
- Reports pain relief after opioid administration.

Testicular Cancer

Testicular cancer is a disease that occurs in younger men between age 15 and 35. It is relatively uncommon, affecting 9 of 100,000 men annually. It is the most treatable form of urologic cancer.

Pathophysiology and Etiology

1. The majority of testicular cancers are of germ cell origin; the most common germinal tumors in adults are seminoma, embryonal carcinoma, teratoma, and choriocarcinoma (the latter three are also called *nonseminomas*).
2. The etiology of testicular tumors is unknown, but there is a relationship between cryptorchidism (failure of the testes to descend into the scrotum) and tumor occurrence.
3. Testicular tumors metastasize in a stepwise fashion to the retroperitoneal lymph nodes with subsequent involvement of the mediastinal lymph nodes, lungs, and liver.
4. Testicular germ cell tumors are considered potentially curable; seminomas are extremely responsive to radiation therapy; nonseminomas are sensitive to platinum-based chemotherapy.

Clinical Manifestations

1. Painless swelling or enlargement of the testis; accompanied by sensation of heaviness in scrotum.
2. Pain in the testis (if patient has epididymitis or bleeding into tumor).
3. Symptoms of metastatic disease: cough or dyspnea, lymphadenopathy, back pain, GI symptoms, lower-extremity edema, or bone pain.

Diagnostic Evaluation

1. Elevated serum markers of human chorionic gonadotropin, lactic acid dehydrogenate, and alpha-fetoprotein; assay of tumor markers also used for diagnosis, detection of early recurrence, staging, and monitoring response to therapy.
2. Scrotal ultrasonography—to identify location of lesion and differentiate between solid and cystic lesion.
3. Chest x-ray—to seek pulmonary or mediastinal metastasis.
4. CT scanning of chest, abdomen, and pelvis—to evaluate retroperitoneal lymph nodes and to follow progress of therapy.

Management

Choice of treatment depends on tumor histology and stage of disease.

Surgery

1. Inguinal orchiectomy—removal of testis and its tunica and spermatic cord.

2. Retroperitoneal lymph node dissection (RPLND) may be performed after orchiectomy in nonseminomas for staging and therapeutic purposes.
3. Complications of surgery:
   a. RPLND causes infertility due to ejaculatory dysfunction.
   b. Modified nerve-sparing unilateral lymphadenectomy can be done on selected patients, thus preserving ejaculation.
   c. Unilateral orchiectomy eliminates half of germinal cells, thus reducing sperm count.
   d. Libido and ability to attain an erection are preserved.

Radiation Therapy

1. Radiation therapy to lymphatic drainage pathways (after orchiectomy in seminomas); cure rate is close to 99%.
2. Other testicle is shielded, usually preserving fertility.

Chemotherapy

1. Cisplatin combination therapy is used in treatment of non-seminomatous primary tumor and regional lymphatic metastases and in managing distant metastatic disease.
2. Discomforts of chemotherapy include significant nausea and vomiting, alopecia, myalgia, GI cramping, and mucositis.

Complications

1. Infertility; loss of testicle.
2. Retrograde ejaculation after retroperitoneal lymphadenectomy.
3. Death from metastatic disease.

Nursing Assessment

1. Examine testicular mass; ascertain when it was discovered and if it has changed or enlarged since initial discovery.
2. Examine supraclavicular and inguinal lymph nodes for enlargement.
3. Assess for symptoms of metastatic disease.

Nursing Diagnoses

- Anxiety related to diagnosis of cancer and impending treatments.
- Disturbed Body Image related to loss of testicle and fertility.
- Risk for Injury related to complications of treatment.

Nursing Interventions

Reducing Anxiety

1. Provide realistic information about impending surgery or treatment; dispel myths associated with testicular disease, emphasize positive cure rates.

Preserving Body Image

1. Reassure patient that orchiectomy will not diminish virility and RPLND will alter fertility and ejaculation but not libido, erection, and sensation.
2. Advise patient that testicular prosthesis can preserve look and feel of scrotum.
3. Refer the patient for counseling, as needed, for problems and concerns with relationships, peers, or work life.
4. Discuss possible donation of sperm due to infertility issues.

Preventing Complications of Treatment

1. Provide routine postoperative care, including early ambulation, respiratory care, and administration of pain medication.
2. After RPLND, monitor for paralytic ileus, which is common after extensive resection.
   a. Auscultate bowel sounds frequently and observe for abdominal distention.
   b. Withhold oral fluids until bowel sounds have returned.
   c. Report complaints of nausea and vomiting.
   d. Begin nasogastric decompression, if indicated.
3. For nursing care involving radiation and chemotherapy, see pages 151 and 139.

Patient Education and Health Maintenance

1. Teach all young men to perform monthly testicular self-examination; after orchiectomy, patient should examine remaining testicle monthly (see Patient Education Guidelines 21-1).
2. Review schedule for radiation treatments or chemotherapy; teach patient and family possible adverse effects; discuss expectations for treatment period.
3. Provide information about retrograde ejaculation after RPLND and alternatives for fertility.

Evaluation: Expected Outcomes

- Verbalizes understanding of treatment and complications.
- No abdominal distention noted.

- Discusses concerns about sexual function with staff and partner.

Epididymitis

Epididymitis is an infection of the epididymis that usually spreads from the urethra or bladder to the epididymis by way of the ejaculatory duct and vas deferens.

Pathophysiology and Etiology

1. Occurs as a complication of UTI, urethral stricture disease, bacterial prostatitis, gonococcal or nongonococcal bacterial urethritis.
2. In men under age 35, sexually transmitted organisms are the main etiologic agents, usually *C. trachomatis* and *N. gonorrhoeae*.
3. In homosexual men, *E. coli* is a common cause.
4. In older men, the main causes are bladder outlet obstruction and urinary bacteria (*E. coli*, *P. aeruginosa*).

Clinical Manifestations

1. Unilateral scrotal pain and tenderness.
2. Edema, redness, and tenderness of scrotum.
3. Dysuria, frequency.
4. Fever, nausea, vomiting.
5. Pyuria, bacteriuria, leukocytosis.

PATIENT EDUCATION GUIDELINES 21-1

Testicular Self-Examination

1. Examine for testicular tumor once per month, at a convenient time such as the first of the month or your birth date every month, preferably while showering or bathing.
2. Use both hands to feel the testes through the scrotal tissue.
3. Locate the epididymis; this is the irregular cordlike structure on the top and at the back of the testicle that stores and transports sperm. The spermatic cord (and vas) extends upward from the epididymis.
4. Feel each testis between the thumb and first two fingers of each hand. The testes lie freely in the scrotum, are oval shaped, and measure 4–5 cm in length, 3 cm in width, and about 2 cm in thickness.
5. Note size, shape, abnormal tenderness. An abnormality may be felt as a firm area on the front or side of the testicle.
6. Stand in front of mirror and look for changes in size/shape of scrotum. It is normal to find one testis larger than the other.
7. Report any evidence of a small, pea-size lump or other abnormality.

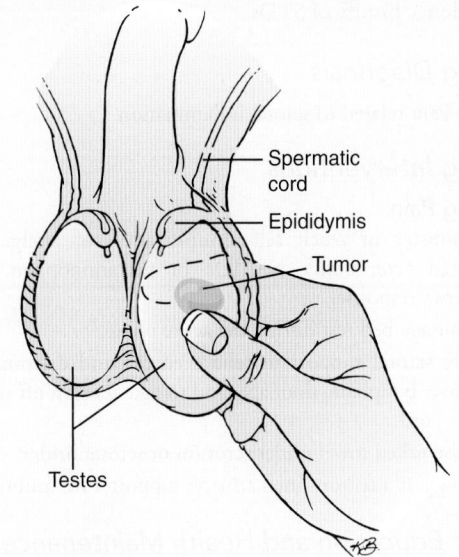

Using the fingertips and thumb, the epididymis, testes, and spermatic cord are located bilaterally.

Diagnostic Evaluation

1. Urine culture and sensitivity.
2. Examination (Gram stain, culture, gonorrhea and *Chlamydia* testing) of urethral discharge and expressed prostatic secretions to establish causative organism.
3. Ultrasound with Doppler to rule out testicular torsion.

Management

1. Antimicrobial therapy after collection of specimens.
   a. Treatment of choice for presumed sexually transmitted infections is combination ceftriaxone 250 mg I.M. in a single dose with doxycycline 100 mg orally twice per day for 10 days.
   b. For presumed *E. coli* and other infections, a quinolone, such as ciprofloxacin 500 mg orally twice a day for 10 days or co-trimoxazole for 10 days, is recommended.
2. Analgesics for pain relief.
3. Bed rest with the scrotum elevated on a towel to allow for lymphatic drainage.
4. In some cases, the spermatic cord is injected with a local anesthetic to relieve pain.

Complications

1. Spread of infection to testicle—epididymo-orchitis.
2. Infertility; risk is greater when infection is bilateral.

Nursing Assessment

1. Obtain history of STDs (or symptoms); UTI or prostatitis; recent urologic instrumentation or surgery.
2. Assess for elevated temperature; pain level; swollen, tender scrotum.
3. Assess for sexual behavior risk—multiple partners, nonuse of condoms, history of STDs.

Nursing Diagnosis

- Acute Pain related to scrotal inflammation.

Nursing Interventions

Relieving Pain

1. Administer or teach self-administration of analgesics, as ordered—commonly NSAIDs or acetaminophen. Assess patient's response.
2. Encourage bed rest during the acute phase.
3. Apply scrotal support to relieve edema and discomfort, to improve lymphatic drainage, and to take tension off the spermatic cord.
   a. Use rolled towel under scrotum or scrotal bridge.
   b. Suggest a cotton-lined athletic supporter for ambulation.

Patient Education and Health Maintenance

Instruct the patient as follows:
1. Avoid straining (lifting, straining at stool, and sexual activity) until infection is under control.

2. Sexual partners within the past 60 days of patients with chlamydial or gonorrheal urethritis or epididymitis should be examined and treated.
3. Follow up with health care provider, as directed—it may take 2 to 4 weeks or longer for epididymitis to resolve completely.
4. Report signs of infection in the reproductive tract immediately to obtain treatment and prevent spread.
5. Obtain follow-up care to ensure complete resolution of infection; uncontrolled infection may impair fertility.
6. Use safer sex practices, such as abstinence, mutual monogamy, and condoms, to prevent further infection associated with sexual activity.

Evaluation: Expected Outcomes

- Verbalizes relief of pain.

Genital Lesions Caused by Sexually Transmitted Diseases

 Evidence Base Centers for Disease Control and Prevention. (2010). Sexually transmitted diseases. Available: *www.cdc.gov/std/treatment.*

Genital lesions are ulcerations or other skin or mucous membrane lesions that indicate infection with an STD and may actively shed the infecting organism.

Pathophysiology and Etiology

Causes include:
1. Syphilis—*Treponema pallidum.*
2. Chancroid—*Haemophilus ducreyi.*
3. Lymphogranuloma venereum—specific subtypes of *C. trachomatis.*
4. Genital herpes—herpes simplex virus.
5. Condylomata acuminata (genital warts)—specific subtypes of HPV.

Clinical Manifestations

See Table 21-4, for clinical manifestations, diagnosis, and treatment of genital lesions.

Patient Education and Health Maintenance

1. Explain transmission of STDs and preventive measures, such as male or female condoms, abstinence, and mutual monogamy.
2. Encourage compliance with treatment regimen and follow-up to ensure cure before resuming sexual activity.
3. Explain that some shedding of herpes virus may occur even while asymptomatic, so patient must discuss this with partner; consider use of condoms at all times; reduce risk of transmission by abstaining at the first sign of an outbreak (tingling sensation) until 1 to 2 weeks after resolution of symptoms.
4. For additional information and support, refer to STD National Hotline at (800) 227-8922.

Table 21-4	Characteristics and Management of Genital Lesions Caused by STDs	
DISORDER AND INCUBATION	CLINICAL MANIFESTATIONS	DIAGNOSIS AND TREATMENT
Herpes Genitalis 2–20 days	Clustered vesicles on erythematous, edematous base that rupture, leaving shallow, painful ulcer that eventually crusts; mild regional lymphadenopathy; recurrent and may be brought on by stress, infection, pregnancy, sunburn.	• Diagnostic tests include Tzanck smear, viral culture, antigen test of tissue or exudate from lesion, or serum antibody tests. • No cure, but symptomatic period is diminished by acyclovir or other antiherpetic started with each recurrence; or recurrences greatly reduced or prevented by continuous treatment. • Analgesics and sitz baths promote comfort.
Syphilis 10–90 days for primary; up to 6 months following lesion (chancre) for secondary	*Caused by bacteria T. pallidum Primary:* Nontender, shallow, indurated, clean ulcer; mild regional lymphadenopathy. *Secondary:* Maculopapular rash including palms and soles, mucous patches, and condylomatous lesions; fever, generalized lymphadenopathy.	• VDRL test or RPR blood test with confirmation by specific treponemal antibody tests. • Preferred treatment is benzathine penicillin G 2.4 million units I.M. in a single dose; erythromycin or aftrioxone may be used in penicillin allergy.
Chancroid 3–14 days	Bacterial disease caused by *H. ducreyi.* Vesiculopustule that erodes, leaving a tender, painful, shallow or deep, well-circumscribed ulcer with ragged, undermined borders and a friable base covered by purulent exudate; unilateral or bilateral large, tender inguinal lymph nodes (buboes) in 50% of patients.	• Identification of *H. ducreyi* on special culture media. • Treated with azithromycin, ciprofloxacin, erythromycin, or ceftriaxone I.M. Single-dose regimens are available. • Apply warm soaks to buboes.
Lymphogranuloma Venereum 3–30 days	Small, transient, nontender papule or superficial ulcer precedes firm, adherent unilateral inguinal and femoral lymph nodes (buboes) with characteristic groove in between (groove sign); may suppurate.	• Microimmunofluorescence testing of bubo aspirate, if possible. Clinical diagnosis after ruling out other causes for genital lesions and lymphadenopathy. • Treatment of choice is doxycycline, but erythromycin may be effective. • Incision and excision of buboes should be avoided: aspiration may be helpful.
Condyloma Acuminatum Genital warts caused by HPV; 3 weeks to 3 months, possibly years before grossly visible	Single or multiple, soft, fleshy, flat or vegetating growths may occur on penis, anal area, urethra; no lymphadenopathy.	• Diagnosed by inspection or biopsy. • Topical therapy with podofilox 0.5% for external warts, podophyllin 10%–25% solution or trichloroacetic acid 80%–90% imiquimod. May require multiple applications. • Cryotherapy, electrodissection, electrocautery, carbon dioxide laser, and surgical excision may also be done. • Recurrence is common.

IM, intramuscular; HPV, human papilloma virus; RPR, rapid plasma reagin; VDRL, Venereal Disease Research Laboratory.

Carcinoma of the Penis

 Evidence Base Letendre, J., Saad, F., & Lattouf J. (2011). Penile cancer: What's new? *Current Opinion in Supportive and Palliative Care, 5,* 185–191.

Carcinoma of the penis occurs primarily on the glans of the penis. Risk factors include uncircumcised, phimosis, HPV, lichen sclerosus, balanitis xerotica obliterans, increasing age, smoking, poor personal hygiene, and the accumulation of smegma under the skin of an uncircumcised penis. It primarily occurs in men older than age 50 and represents 0.5% of malignancies in men in the United States.

Pathophysiology and Etiology

1. Several types of penile lesions are potentially premalignant.
   a. Condylomata acuminate.
   b. Giant condylomata acuminata (Buschke-Löwenstein tumor).
   c. Kaposi's sarcoma.
   d. Leukoplakia.
2. Erythroplasia of the glans (erythroplasia of Queyrat) is a carcinoma in situ of the penis and may involve the glans, prepuce, or penile shaft, or may spread to the remainder of the genitalia and perineal region. It appears as a red, velvety lesion with ulcerations.
3. Bowen disease is a squamous cell carcinoma in situ resembling a red plague. Commonly involving the shaft of penis.
4. Malignant lesions that ulcerate metastasize quickly to the regional femoral and iliac lymph nodes.
5. Distant metastasis occurs in the inguinal lymph nodes; in rare cases to lungs, liver, bone, or brain.

Clinical Manifestations

1. Can present as a painless, wartlike growth or ulcer on the glans or prepuce or with painful, bleeding, or exudative lesion.
2. Phimosis (constriction of foreskin with inability to retract over glans) may obscure a lesion, preventing detection until advanced stages.
3. Lymphadenopathy; secondary infection of lesions or metastatic disease.
4. Malodorous and persistent discharge from the penis is a late symptom.

Diagnostic Evaluation

1. Biopsy of penile lesion and lymph nodes.
2. Ultrasonography and MRI of inguinal lymph nodes.
3. Chest x-ray, CT or MRI scan, bone scan to assess for distant nodal metastases.
4. Positron emission tomography (PET) scans assist in primary staging or to assess for lymph node metastases.
5. Sentinel node biopsy to determine whether nonenlarged inguinal lymph nodes contain cancer.

Management

1. Localized lesions are surgically removed by partial penectomy, laser or cryotherapy, or Mohs' micrographic surgery; total penectomy with perineal urethrostomy is necessary for more involved tumors.
2. Because inguinal lymphadenopathy may be due to inflammation and not malignancy, patients are prescribed a 4- to 6-week course of antibiotics after partial or total penectomy and are reassessed. If lymphadenopathy remains, then a bilateral lymphadenectomy is performed for cancer control.
3. Radiation therapy to small superficial tumors and lymph nodes may control the disease.

Complications

1. Disfigurement due to ulceration or treatment.
2. Complications of lymphadenectomy—necrosis and infection of skin flap, chronic edema of lower extremities.

Nursing Assessment

1. Obtain history of current lesion, history of STDs, and hygiene.
2. Perform genital examination for characteristics of lesion, phimosis, inguinal lymph node enlargement.
3. Assess support system and personal coping mechanisms.

Nursing Diagnoses

- Fear related to diagnosis of cancer.
- Disturbed Body Image related to partial or total penectomy.

Nursing Interventions

Resolving Fears

1. Provide patient with opportunity to acquire information about causes and prognosis of disease.
2. Interpret diagnostic and staging results to patient.
3. Encourage realistic expectations regarding outcome of treatment.

Enhancing Coping with Body Image Changes

1. Maintain a nonjudgmental approach; allow patient to ventilate feelings about loss of part or all of penis.
2. Provide routine postoperative care confidently, watching for bleeding, monitoring urination, and anticipating pain.
3. Provide opportunity for patient to discuss alternative methods of sexual expression with knowledgeable professional.
   a. About 40% of patients are able to participate in sexual activity and stand erect to void after partial penectomy.
4. Monitor patient for symptoms of depression requiring intervention.

Patient Education and Health Maintenance

1. Instruct the uncircumcised patient about proper hygiene—importance of daily removal of all retained smegma.
2. Explain expected postoperative function of the penis in patient undergoing partial penectomy.
3. Describe how voiding will occur to patient undergoing perineal urethroplasty.
4. Provide information about follow-up and monitoring for recurrences or radiation and chemotherapy, as appropriate.

Evaluation: Expected Outcomes

- Verbalizes understanding and acceptance of diagnosis and treatment plan.
- Discusses feelings and interest in seeking counseling.

SELECTED REFERENCES

American Cancer Society. (2011). *Cancer facts and figures 2011*. Atlanta, GA: Author.

Black, A., Copland, M., Sondrup, B., et al. (2011). Medication considerations for patients with chronic kidney disease who are not yet on dialysis. *Nephrology Nursing Journal, 38*(6), 491–497.

Borden, P., Dixon, J., Kaneko, T., et al. (2011). Multidisciplinary CKD care enhances outcomes at dialysis initiation. *Nephrology Nursing Journal, 38*(2), 165–171.

Brill, J. (2010). Sexually transmitted infections in men. *Primary Care Clinics Office Practice, 37,* 509–525.

Centers for Disease Control and Prevention. (2010). Guidelines for treatment of sexually transmitted diseases. Available: *www.cdc.gov/std/treatment.*

Counts, C. S. (Ed.). (2008). *Core curriculum for nephrology nursing* (5th ed.). New Jersey: Anthony Janetti.

Coyne, D. (2010). It's time to compare anemia management strategies in hemodialysis. *Clinical Journal of the American Society of Nephrology, 5*(4), 740–742.

Cupples, S., & Ohler, L. (2008). *Core curriculum for transplant nurses.* St. Louis, MO: Mosby.

Dirkes, S. (2011). Acute kidney injury: Not just acute renal failure anymore? *Critical Care Nurse, 31*(1), 37–49.

Dirkes, S., & Hodge, K. (2007). Continuous renal replacement therapy in the adult intensive care unit: History and current trends. *Critical Care Nurse, 27*(2), 62–80.

Eskridge, M. (2010). Hypertension and chronic kidney disease: The role of lifestyle modification and medication management. *Nephrology Nursing Journal, 37*(1), 55–60, 99.

Grey, M., & Moore, K. (2009). *Urologic disorders: Adult and pediatric care.* St. Louis, MO: Mosby.

Golestaneh, L., Richter, B., & Amato-Hayes, M. (2012). Logistics of renal replacement therapy: Relevant issues for critical care nurses. *American Journal of Critical Care, 21*(2), 126–130.

Gupta, K., Hooton, T. M., Naber, K. G., et al. (2011). International clinical practice guidelines for the treatment of acute uncomplicated cystitis and pyelonephritis in women: A 2010 update by the Infectious Diseases Society of America and the European Society for Microbiology and Infectious Diseases. *Clinical Infectious Diseases, 52*(5), 103–120.

Hoffman, R. (2011). Screening for prostate cancer. *New England Journal of Medicine, 365,* 2013–2019.

Juliao, A., Plata, M., Kazzazi, A., et al. (2012). American urological association and European association of urology guidelines in the management of benign prostatic hypertrophy: revisited. *Current Opinion in Urology, 22,* 34–39.

Letendre, J., Saad, F., & Lattouf, J. (2011). Penile cancer: what's new? *Current Opinion in Supportive and Palliative Care, 5,* 185–191.

Li, P.-K., Szeto, C. C., Piraino, B., et al. (2010). Peritoneal dialysis-related infection recommendations: 2010 update. *Peritoneal Dialysis International, 30,* 393–423.

Liles, A. (2011). Medication considerations for patients with chronic kidney disease who are not yet on dialysis. *Nephrology Nursing Journal, 38*(3), 263–270.

Mandeville, J., Gnessin, E., & Lingeman, J. (2011). Imaging evaluation in the patient with renal stone disease. *Seminars in Nephrology, 31,* 254–258.

National Kidney Foundation. (2012). KDOQI Clinical Practice Guidelines for Diabetes and CKD: 2012 Update. *Am J Kidney Dis., 60*(5), 850–886.

Roth-Kauffman, M. (2011). Prostate cancer. *Clinician Reviews, 21,* 28–33.

Rovner, E. S., & Kim, E. D. (2011). Interstitial cystitis. *Medscape Reference.* Available: *http://emedicine.medscape.com/article/441831-overview#a0112.*

Scheel, P., & Choi, M. (2008). *Oxford American handbook of nephrology and hypertension.* New York: Oxford University Press.

Tanagho, E., & McAninch, J. (Eds.). (2008). *Smith's general urology* (17th ed.). New York: McGraw-Hill/Lange.

Touma, N., & Nickle, J. (2011). Prostatitis and chronic pelvic pain syndrome in men. *Medical Clinics of North America, 95,* 75–86.

Turek, P. J., Hedayati, T., & Stehman, C. R. (2011). Prostatitis. *Medscape Reference.* Available: *http://emedicine.medscape.com/article/785418-overview.*

Weidenhold, D., Langer, G., & Landenberger, M. (2011). Ambivalent lived experiences and instruction need of patients in the early period after kidney transplantation: A phenomenological study. *Nephrology Nursing Journal, 38*(5), 417–423.

Wein, A. J., Kavoussi, L. R., Novick, A. C., et al. (Eds.). (2012). *Campbell-Walsh urology* (10th ed., Vols. 1–3). Philadelphia: W.B. Saunders.

Whitmore, K., & Theoharides, T. (2011). When to suspect interstitial cystitis. *Journal of Family Practice, 60,* 340–348.

Wolf, A. M., Wender, R. C., Ruth, B. E., et al. (2010). American Cancer Society guideline for the early detection of prostate cancer update 2010. *CA—A Cancer Journal for Clinicians, 60*(2), 71–98.

22
Gynecologic Disorders

OVERVIEW AND ASSESSMENT

The Menstrual Cycle

The *menstrual cycle* is the cyclical pattern of ovarian hormone secretion (estrogen and progesterone) under the control of pituitary hormones (luteinizing hormone [LH] and follicle-stimulating hormone [FSH]) that results in thickening of the uterine endometrium, ovulation, and menstruation. Cycle length varies among women.

Phases of the Menstrual Cycle

The menstrual cycle is generally divided into two phases: follicular (or proliferative) and luteal (or secretory). See Figure 22-1. Further subdivisions of the cycle are:

1. Menstrual or bleeding phase (or early follicular phase): starts day 1 of the cycle and lasts approximately 5 days; endometrial sloughing and discharge occur due to low levels of estrogen and progesterone.
2. Postmenstrual phase (or early follicular phase); approximately days 5 to 8—thin endometrium. Ovarian follicles grow.
3. Proliferative phase (or mid- to late follicular phase): approximately days 8 to 15; estrogen starts to increase the thickness of the endometrium. A selected ovarian follicle continues to grow. A surge in LH occurs. Transition from proliferative phase to secretory phase occurs with ovulation, the expulsion of a mature follicle (or ovum) from the ovary.
4. Secretory phase (or luteal phase, which lasts 14 days after LH surge in most women): approximately days 16 to 23; endometrium thickens because of increased progesterone; after ovulation, a corpus luteum forms and then regresses unless pregnancy occurs.
5. Premenstrual phase (or late luteal phase): days 24 to 28; levels of estrogen and progesterone begin to fall.

Characteristics of Menstruation

See Table 22-1.

Subjective Data

Explore patient's gynecologic history, current symptoms and general history to elicit important data. Provide a private

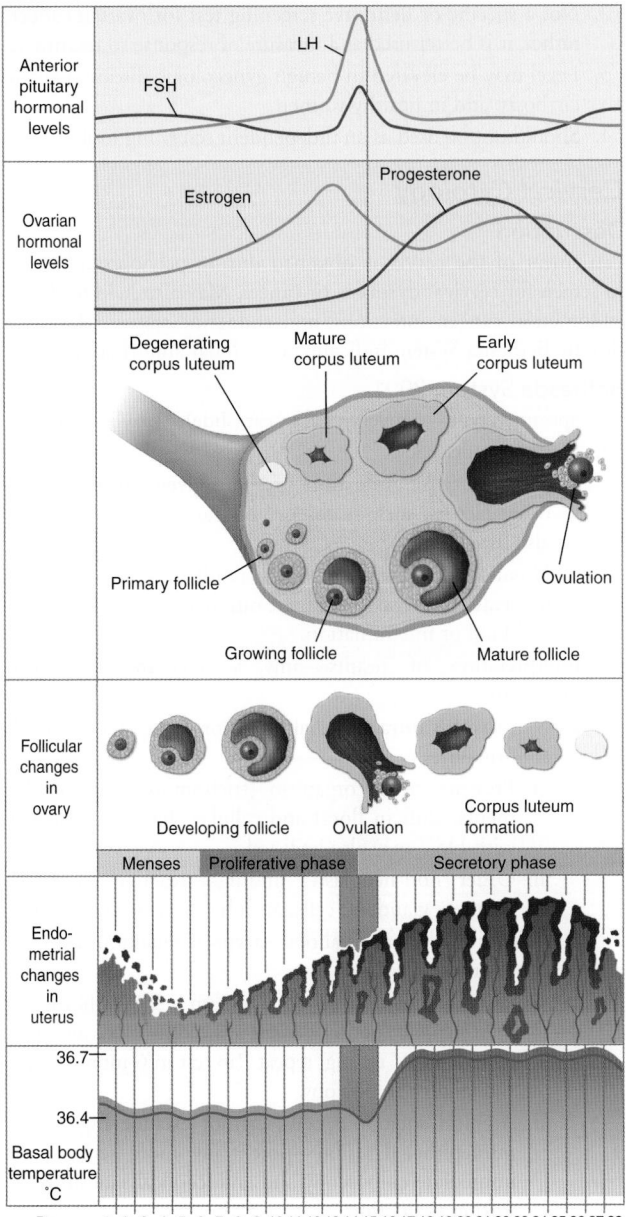

Figure 22-1. The menstrual cycle.

Table 22-1	Characteristics of Menstruation	
CHARACTERISTIC	**RANGE**	**AVERAGE**
Menarche (age at onset)	9–17 years	12.5 years
Cycle length	21–35 days	28 days
Flow—duration	2–8 days	3–5 days
Flow—amount	10–80 mL	35 mL
Menopause (age at onset)	45–55 years	51 years

and comfortable setting for history-taking before the patient undresses. Reassure the patient about confidentiality and rationale for history-taking (see Chapter 5, page 46).

Gynecological Review of Systems

1. Menstrual history: date of start of last menstrual period (LMP) or age at last menses. Documented in this manner: age at menarche × cycle length × number of days of bleeding (eg, 13 × 28 × 4). Symptoms of dysmenorrhea? Symptoms of premenstrual syndrome? Intermenstrual spotting/bleeding, postcoital bleeding, or postmenopausal bleeding.

2. Obstetric history: gravida (number of pregnancies), para (number of term births, preterm births, miscarriages/abortions, living children) (eg, G2P1102). Difficulty conceiving or assisted reproduction? For each pregnancy, list date; gestational age at delivery; mode of delivery; maternal complications (gestational diabetes, hypertension); and fetal, delivery, or neonatal complications.

3. Cervical cytology/Papanicolaou (Pap) test history: date and result of most recent test? Diagnosis and follow-up of abnormal Pap tests? History of HPV vaccination (as age-appropriate)?

4. Sexual history: sexual concerns? Partner preference (men, women, or both)? Activity type? Satisfaction? Frequency? Number of partners in past year and during lifetime?

5. Methods of contraception and sexually transmitted disease (STD) prevention: desire for pregnancy testing or STD screening? Desire for other methods? Desire for preconceptual counseling?

6. Screening for intimate partner violence and previous emotional, physical, or sexual abuse.

Irregular Bleeding

1. Characteristics: date of LMP? Frequency, duration, and amount of flow for most recent several cycles? Previous menstrual pattern and change? What is the color and consistency of blood? What are the sizes of the clots? Significant change in quantity or quality of menstrual flow? Bleeding or spotting between periods, postcoital bleeding, or postmenopausal bleeding? Pain with bleeding? Age at menarche? Age at menopause?

2. Associated factors: pregnancy and childbirth history? Is patient sexually active? What method of contraception is used? Is patient taking hormone replacement or hormonal contraceptives? Any other medications? Is patient obese or underweight? Does patient have acne and hirsutism? History of amenorrhea? Coagulation disorders?

3. Significance: may indicate infection of the vagina or cervix; malignancy of the vulva, vagina, cervix, or uterus; benign tumor of the uterus; ovarian cyst; pregnancy; endometriosis; polycystic ovary syndrome; thyroid disorder; or perimenopausal phase.

Vaginal Discharge

1. Characteristics: color, amount, and duration of the discharge? Any odor, itching, burning, urinary symptoms, or pain? Fever? Dyspareunia (painful intercourse—vulvar, vaginal, or internal pain with intercourse)? Onset related to menses or to intercourse?

2. Associated factors: LMP? What is the sexual history, such as number of partners or new partner within the past 6 months, type of sexual activity, symptoms in partner? Is barrier method of contraception used? Is patient menopausal or postmenopausal? Environmental factor changes? Vaginal dryness? Does patient take estrogen replacement? Recent use of antibiotics? Recent douching? Recent over-the-counter product use or herbal/natural remedies? History of sexually transmitted diseases?

3. Significance: may indicate normal or pathologic discharge, bacterial vaginosis, candidal vaginitis, cervicitis, gonorrhea, chlamydia, trichomoniasis, pelvic inflammatory disease (PID), or genital malignancy.

Pelvic Pain

1. Characteristics: frequency, duration, severity, and location of pain? Does the pain radiate? Was the onset sudden or gradual? What aggravates and what relieves it? Relationship to menstrual cycle, eating, physical exercise, bowel, or bladder function? Any dyspareunia? Does it feel like heaviness in the pelvis? Intensity and effect on daily activities?

2. Associated factors: LMP? Fever, nausea, vomiting, dizziness, abnormal bleeding? Urinary symptoms? Back pain? Recent significant weight loss or gain? Use of estrogen preparations? Difficulty conceiving? Did patient perform a home pregnancy test? Use of an intrauterine device (IUD)? Any change in bowel habits or diarrhea? History of sexual abuse? Use of pain medications and home remedies?

3. Significance: may indicate condition arising from relaxed pelvic muscles, PID, endometriosis, interstitial cystitis, urinary tract infection, irritable bowel syndrome, history of sexual abuse (posttraumatic stress disorder), ectopic pregnancy, miscarriage, uterine fibroids, cervical or uterine cancer.

Physical Examination

Physical examination for a patient with a gynecologic disorder should focus on the abdomen and genitalia. Palpate the abdomen for masses or tenderness. Request verbal permission before starting the pelvic examination. Consider using a chaperone during the examination. If the patient has presented as a victim of sexual assault, then do not ask the patient to undress nor examine the patient but ensure immediate transfer to a local emergency department with sexual assault nurse examiners or other professionals with expertise in forensic evidence collection and supportive services after assault. See Chapter 35, page 1233.

The nurse in a gynecologic or obstetric setting may perform a vaginal examination to obtain specimens for diagnostic studies and assess the patient's condition (see Procedure Guidelines 22-1).

Laboratory Tests

CA 125

Description
Tumor antigen used as a marker for ovarian cancer.

Nursing and Patient Care Considerations
1. Tell patient a blood test will be performed and the results will be ready in 1 to 3 days.

2. Not a specific or definitive screening test for ovarian cancer; rather, it is better used as a measure of response to treatment.

3. Level may be elevated in benign gynecologic disease, hepatic cirrhosis, and in healthy women.

4. Should not be used as an independent screening tool.

Cervical Cytology

Description
Pap smear of the cervix is obtained during pelvic examination to screen for cervical dysplasia or cancer. May also help to detect endometrial cancer, infections, and endocrine status. Classification by Bethesda System indicates any cellular abnormalities.

Bethesda System 2001
1. Specimen type—conventional smear (slide) versus liquid based.
2. Specimen adequacy.
   a. Satisfactory for evaluation—result is given but presence of other factors, such as absence of transformation zone, is also listed.
   b. Unsatisfactory for evaluation—result may not be given; lists reason, such as inadequate number of cells or obscured by blood or inflammation.
3. Interpretation of results—only a screening tool, not diagnostic.
   a. Negative for intraepithelial lesion or malignancy: no cell abnormalities.
      i. Presence of an organism (trichomonas, fungal elements, shift in flora) and cellular changes consistent with HSV may also be listed.
      ii. Other non-neoplastic findings (reactive reparative changes, glandular cells, atrophy) may be described.
   b. Epithelial cell abnormalities—atypical squamous cells are common.
      i. Atypical squamous cells of undetermined significance—management options based on population and can include HPV testing, repeat Pap test in 6-month intervals, and/or colposcopy.
      ii. Atypical squamous cells, cannot exclude high-grade intraepithelial lesion—potentially more serious; do immediate colposcopy and endocervical sampling for further evaluation.
      iii. Low-grade squamous intraepithelial lesion—management options based on population and can include repeat Pap test in 6-month intervals, HPV testing, and/or colposcopy.
      iv. High-grade squamous intraepithelial lesion—management options based on population and can include colposcopy with biopsy and endocervical curettage.
      v. Squamous cell carcinoma—colposcopy and biopsy.
   c. Glandular cell abnormalities—atypical, not otherwise specified (NOS) or atypical, favor neoplastic (require further evaluation); colposcopy, and HPV testing. Endometrial biopsy is performed if over 35 years of age and on younger women with risk factors for endometrial neoplasia such as unexplained uterine bleeding or chronic anovulation.
   d. Endocervical adenocarcinoma in situ; colposcopy, cervical biopsy, conization and possible referral to oncologist.

(*Text continues on page 838*)

PROCEDURE GUIDELINES 22-1

Vaginal Examination by the Nurse

EQUIPMENT

- Perineal drape or other drape
- Vaginal speculum of appropriate size (the smaller, the more comfortable; medium or large should be reserved for multiparous and/or obese women)
- Warm water
- Water-soluble lubricant

- Gloves
- Long swab sticks
- Adequate lighting

As needed:
- Papanicolaou (Pap) smear equipment (spatula, cervical brush, cytology slide and fixative; or cervical broom and liquid-based preparation)

- Microscope slide equipment (microscope, glass slides and covers, dropper bottles of normal saline and potassium hydroxide [KOH])
- pH paper with range from 3.5 to 5.5
- Specimen collection swabs and containers for gonorrhea, chlamydia, or other organisms.

PROCEDURE

Nursing Action	Rationale
Preparatory phase	
1. Have patient void before examination. Collect urine specimen. Patient to remove clothing from waist to knees.	1. A full bladder may cause discomfort during examination. Urine testing may be required for pregnancy detection, dipstick urinalysis, or DNA probe for gonorrhea or chlamydia.
2. Help to position patient on examining table.	2. Exposes vulva and tilts pelvis for easier positioning of speculum.
a. Have buttocks extend beyond the edge of table.	
b. Position feet in stirrups to assume dorsal lithotomy position.	
c. Make patient as comfortable as possible with a small pillow under her head or slightly raising the head of the table.	c. Positioning to enable eye contact with the examiner will decrease patient anxiety. Raising the head of the table will help to relax abdominal muscles.
d. Drape patient to permit minimal exposure; press the drape down between legs to permit eye contact between examiner and patient.	d. Patient will feel less exposed with waist and anterior thighs covered.
3. Encourage patient to relax; tell her what you are doing and what she may feel.	3. Explanation elicits cooperation.
4. Adjust light for maximum focus.	4. A light source is necessary to visualize vagina.
5. Offer patient a mirror to watch the examination to teach vulvar self-examination and to teach about contraceptives, as appropriate.	5. Education increases a sense of control over one's body and contraceptive options.
6. Lubricate speculum with warm water.	6. If warm water can be reached during the examination, this step may occur immediately before inserting the speculum.
Performance phase	
1. Be gentle and take your time; wash hands; put on clean gloves.	1. Standard precautions. A calm approach promotes relaxation of patient, making the procedure easier for both. *Caution:* The examination should be performed efficiently and carefully: taking too long may prolong patient discomfort. Address patient discomfort by stopping the exam or changing technique.
2. Observe external genitalia for apparent abnormalities such as lesions, discharge, or bulging from the vagina. Gently separate labia and continue visual inspection.	2. Note evidence of irritation, infection, or abnormalities, such as swelling, bleeding, erythema, discharge (other than clear and odorless).
3. Gently place the tip of one or two fingers into introitus. Say to patient, "Tighten your muscles and squeeze my fingers—try hard—then relax."	3. Encourages relaxation. If the patient demonstrates extreme anxiety or has suffered from previous sexual abuse or trauma, the exam may need to be delayed in order to seek assistance from another professional.

(continued)

PROCEDURE GUIDELINES 22-1 (continued)

Vaginal Examination by the Nurse

PROCEDURE (continued)

Nursing Action	Rationale
4. Identify cervix manually and depress the perineum downward with the fingers of one hand.	4. Downward pressure is away from the more sensitive anterior structures.
5. Lubricate speculum with warm water with your other hand.	5. Any lubricant other than water may interfere with cytology results.
6. Gently insert warm speculum horizontally with downward pressure, passing it over your fingers and aiming it toward the cervix.	6. If it is preferred not to initially insert gloved fingers, the speculum is introduced vertically using a downward pressure; after entering the vestibule, the speculum is slowly rotated to the horizontal position.

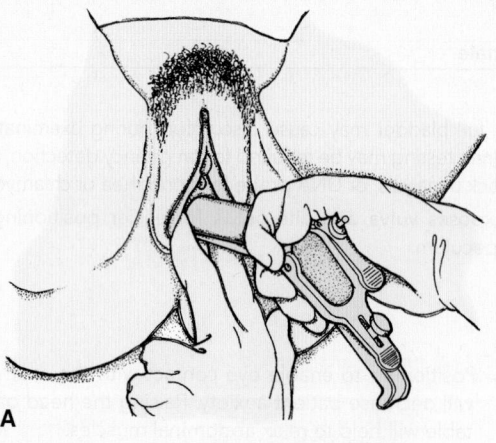

A

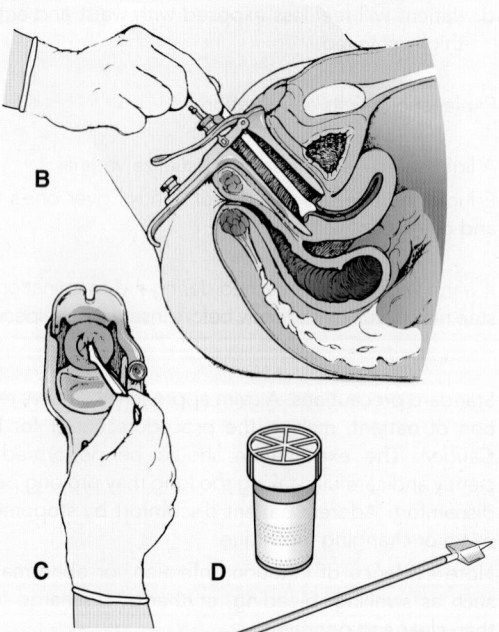

B

C   D

(A) Insertion of vaginal speculum during pelvic examination. (B) Cervical cytology specimen collection: either conventional or liquid-based preparations are acceptable for cervical cancer screening. A scraping of endocervical and exocervical cells is obtained using a spatula and cervical brush or using a cervical broom. (C) The spatula, which obtains exocervical cells (inserted with the longer end in the cervical os), and cervical brush, which obtains endocervical cells, are rotated in the os, smeared on a microscope slide, and finished with a fixative. (D) The cervical broom obtains samples from both the endocervix and the exocervix by rotation in the os. The handle is detached and the broom is sent in liquid medium for processing; or the brush is rinsed in the preservative with 15 strokes and the liquid then sent for processing.

PROCEDURE GUIDELINES 22-1 *(continued)*

Vaginal Examination by the Nurse

PROCEDURE *(continued)*

Nursing Action	Rationale
7. Slowly open the speculum while inserting. With slow manipulation, the speculum can be turned to permit visualization of the vaginal walls. Lock into place.	7. Careful opening and manipulation prevents discomfort and achieves good visualization. Walls normally are pink and moist. A pale white or clear secretion may be noted.
8. Inspect the cervix, which should be pink. Normally, the os is a closed, round indentation, unless the woman has had children, in which case a slit is noted. A cervical transformation zone may be visible, especially in adolescents, and may appear as a darker, coarse-textured pink entering the os.	8. If woman is taking a hormonal contraceptive, the cervix may be deep pink to purplish. A thread coming out of the cervix would suggest presence of an intrauterine device. Abnormal cervical signs include erosion, lacerations, speckling, and polyps.
9. If Pap test is to be done, follow procedure in accompanying figure.	
10. When removing speculum, hold it open until cervix is cleared, then withdraw speculum downward, applying pressure to posterior vaginal wall and allowing speculum to close as it is withdrawn.	10. By the time speculum is completely withdrawn, it will be closed.
11. For palpation (bimanual examination), see accompanying figure.	

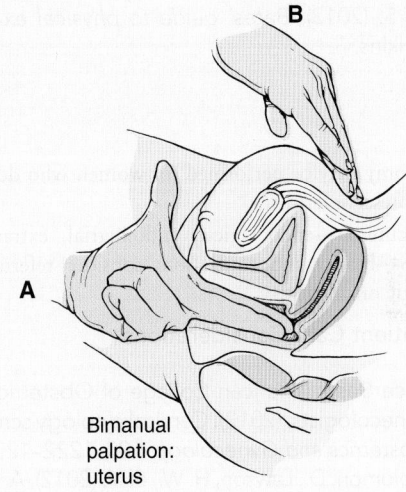

Bimanual palpation: uterus

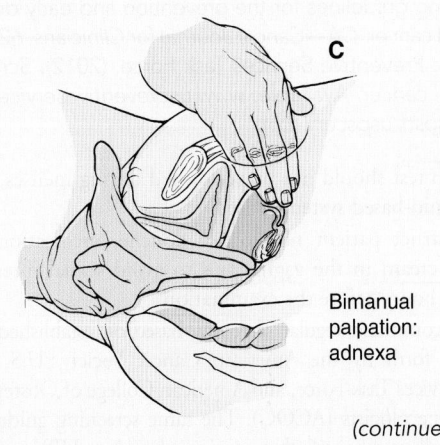

Bimanual palpation: adnexa

Bimanual examination of the pelvic organs. **(A)** *Insert two fingers of dominant hand into vagina.* **(B)** *Place second hand over midline lower abdomen. Gently capture the uterus between your two hands to feel the contour and size and to elicit tenderness.* **(C)** *Move hands to either side of midline to palpate the adnexa, feeling for swelling, masses, or tenderness of the ovaries and fallopian tubes. Source: From Fuller J and Schaller-Ayers J.* Health Assessment: A Nursing Approach, *2nd ed. Philadelphia: J.B. Lippincott Company, 1994.*

(continued)

PROCEDURE GUIDELINES 22-1 *(continued)*

Vaginal Examination by the Nurse

PROCEDURE *(continued)*

Nursing Action	Rationale

Follow-up phase

1. Gently wipe the perineal area with soft tissue or gauze, using firm strokes from the pubic area back to beyond the rectum. Cover patient with drape.
2. Instruct and assist patient to remove feet from stirrups.
3. Elevate the lower third of the examining table to receive legs. Keep patient covered with a sheet.
4. Assist patient in sliding toward head end of table then in slowly rising to sitting; provide a wide-based stool for her to step on as she gets off table.
5. Assist patient in dressing, if necessary. Answer any questions she may have.

1. Removes secretions and liquid lubricant. Provide the patient with a tissue or wipe for the patient to wipe, as desired.
2. Be aware that it may be difficult or uncomfortable.
3. Permits patient to assume dorsal recumbent position.
4. Cervical manipulation and sudden shifting from recumbent to sitting position may cause vasovagal response resulting in dizziness.

Evidence Base Saslow, D., Solomon, D., Lawson, H. W., et al. (2012). American Cancer Society, American Society for Colposcopy and Cervical Pathology, and American Society for Clinical Pathology screening guidelines for the prevention and early detection of cervical cancer. *CA—Cancer Journal for Clinicians, 62,* 147–172.
Bickley, L. S. (2012). *Bates' guide to physical examination and history taking* (11th ed.). Philadelphia: Lippincott Williams & Wilkins.

Hysterectomy may be performed for women who do not desire to preserve fertility.

e. Adenocarcinoma—endocervical, endometrial, extrauterine, NOS—biopsy and conization; consider referral to gynecologic oncologist.

Nursing and Patient Care Considerations

Evidence Base American College of Obstetricians and Gynecologists. (2012). Cervical cytology screening. *Obstetrics and Gynecology, 120,* 1222–1230.
Saslow, D., Solomon, D., Lawson, H. W., et al. (2012). American Cancer Society, American Society for Colposcopy and Cervical Pathology, and American Society for Clinical Pathology screening guidelines for the prevention and early detection of cervical cancer. *CA—Cancer Journal for Clinicians, 62,* 147–172.
U.S. Preventive Services Task Force. (2012). *Screening for cervical cancer.* Available: *www.uspreventiveservicestaskforce.org/uspstf/uspscerv.htm.*

1. Pap test should not be performed during menses, unless the liquid-based system is used.
2. Instruct patient not to use douche, medication, tampon, or cream in the vagina and to avoid sexual intercourse for 48 hours before the examination.
3. Recommend regular screening based on established guidelines set forth by the American Cancer Society, U.S. Preventive Services Task Force, and American College of Obstetricians and Gynecologists (ACOG). The same screening guidelines apply to all women whether vaccinated against HPV or not. More

frequent testing is recommended if the woman has human immunodeficiency virus (HIV), is immunosuppressed, was exposed to diethylstilbestrol in utero, or has been treated for cervical intraepithelial neoplasia (CIN) 2, CIN 3, or cervical cancer.

a. Recommend starting Pap testing at age 21.
b. Recommend testing every 3 years from ages 21–65 for women without risk factors such as DES exposure.
c. For those aged 30–65 wanting to extend the screening interval, screen with a combination of HPV testing and cytology every 5 years.
d. Discontinue screening after age 65 if adequate negative prior screening and no history of CIN 2 or greater within the last 20 years.
e. Discontinue after total hysterectomy if no dysplasia or cancer.

4. Make sure that patient obtains results. If patient has an abnormal smear, explain that this is not always conclusive but requires further testing based on age, such as repeat Pap test, HPV testing, colposcopy, biopsy, or conization. Encourage patient to return for further testing.
5. Yearly examination for breast cancer screening, detection of other genital cancers, infections, reproductive problems, and contraception management may be indicated.

Tests for Gonorrhea and Chlamydia

Evidence Base *Centers for Disease Control and Prevention. (2010). Sexually transmitted diseases treatment guidelines, 2010.* Available: www.cdc.gov/std/treatment/2010/STD-Treatment-2010-RR5912.pdf.

Description

1. Commonly known as deoxyribonucleic acid (DNA) probe or antigen detection tests, a single specimen can detect both STD-causing organisms. Will detect even subclinical infection; can be used as screening test.
2. Can also be done by culture method, but takes longer and requires separate specimens and special processing for each.
3. Screening for chlamydia and gonorrhea can also be done on urine specimen using amplified DNA technology. This method is more expensive, but saves time in specimen collection (especially for women) in screening centers.

Nursing and Patient Care Considerations

1. Explain the procedure to patient before taking the specimen.
2. Specimens should be taken from the cervix without douching for 24 hours or from the male urethra before urinating.
3. Obtain specimen with cotton-tipped swab inserted and rotated in the cervical os for 10 seconds or urethral meatus in a male patient. Small-tipped swabs are available for the urethra. Send swab to laboratory in provided container with preservative.
4. For urine testing, ask the patient to provide the first 10 to 20 mL of voided urine in a specimen container (this represents a urethral specimen that is more likely to contain the organism, if present, without being diluted by a larger amount of urine from the bladder).
5. May also use ThinPrep as a testing vehicle.

Radiology and Imaging Studies

Hysterosalpingography

Description

1. This fluoroscopic x-ray study of the uterus and fallopian tubes is used to determine tubal patency, detect pathology in the uterine cavity, and identify peritoneal adhesions, and for treatment of unexplained fertility.
2. A bivalve speculum is introduced while patient is in the lithotomy position and contrast medium is injected into the uterine cavity; the medium will enter the peritoneum in 10 to 15 minutes if tubes are patent.

Nursing and Patient Care Considerations

1. Determine date of last menstrual period; the test is done a few days after menses ends, before ovulation. Obtain pregnancy test if patient is within childbearing years, as indicated.
2. Verify that the patient does not have a history of allergy to contrast media or iodine.
3. Administer prescribed antibiotic and analgesic.
4. After procedure, apply perineal pad for drainage of excess contrast medium or blood and instruct patient to notify health care provider if bloody drainage continues after 3 days or if signs of infection are present.
5. Inform patient that pain medication may be necessary for shoulder discomfort because of dye irritation of the phrenic nerve.

Pelvic Ultrasonography

 Evidence Base American College of Radiology. (2009). ACR–ACOG–AIUM–SRU practice guideline for the performance of pelvic ultrasound. Available: www.acr.org/SecondaryMainMenuCategories/quality_safety/guidelines/us/us_pelvic.aspx.

Description

A noninvasive test that uses high-frequency sound waves to form images of the interior pelvic cavity; used to detect uterine, tubal, ovarian, and pelvic cavity pathology, to measure organ size, and to evaluate pregnancy.

Nursing and Patient Care Considerations

1. Inform patient that a full bladder may be necessary to make the uterus easier to visualize.
2. Instruct patient to drink 16 to 32 ounces of water (may differ among facilities) before the procedure and not to void. If transvaginal ultrasound will be performed, inform patient that a vaginal probe will be inserted to obtain more accurate measurements from internal organs. Have patient empty her bladder prior to insertion of probe. (Probe is not used if patient is virginal.)
3. After the procedure, help patient wipe off ultrasound gel from abdomen and allow her to empty her bladder.
4. Abnormalities are represented as different densities that differentiate solid from cystic masses and can help make a diagnosis; however, explain to patient that further testing may be necessary.

Other Diagnostic Procedures

See Standard of Care Guidelines 22-1, page 840.

Colposcopy

Description

Examination of the cervix with a bright light and magnification of 10 to 40 times; done to determine distribution of abnormal squamous epithelium and to pinpoint areas from which biopsy tissue can be taken; may be done with cervicography (photographing the cervix).

Nursing and Patient Care Considerations

1. Procedure is preferably done when cervix is least vascular (usually 1 week after the end of the menstrual flow). Obtain pregnancy test if patient is within childbearing years, as indicated.
2. Explain that a vaginal speculum will be inserted and that a biopsy may be taken, causing only slight discomfort.
3. Help patient into lithotomy position, drape her appropriately, and provide emotional support throughout the procedure. Provide distraction techniques, such as music and posters (hung on the ceiling), as appropriate.
4. After the cervix and vagina are swabbed with acetic acid solution and inspected through the colposcope, biopsies may be taken. Biopsy tissue is preserved in 10% formalin, labeled, and sent to the laboratory. Saline may be used to rinse the area, and bleeding may be stopped with silver nitrate or ferric subsulfate (Monsel's solution).
5. After procedure, assist patient to rise slowly and give the following discharge instructions:
   a. Avoid heavy lifting for 24 hours.
   b. There may be some bleeding and cramping; however, more than that of a normal period must be reported to health care provider.
   c. Obtain health care provider's instructions regarding douching and sexual intercourse.

STANDARDS OF CARE GUIDELINES 22-1
Caring for a Patient
Undergoing Gynecologic Surgery

When caring for a patient undergoing gynecologic surgery, the following care is essential to prevent complications and to promote healthy adaptation:

- Discuss procedure with patient before surgery—does she know why surgery is being done? Does she know which organs will be removed or altered? Does she understand the implications for childbearing, sexuality, menopause? Answer questions and contact surgeon, if necessary.

- After the procedure, assess vital signs as frequently as indicated for signs of shock, infection, fluid overload, and atelectasis.

- Assess incision for drainage and signs of infection (redness, oozing, warmth, increased pain).

- Assess vaginal area for excessive bleeding or foul-smelling drainage.

- Monitor intake and output.

- If patient has an indwelling catheter, ensure that it is draining clear urine greater than 30 to 50 mL/hour.

- After catheter has been removed, ensure that patient voids in adequate amounts and monitor for urinary retention or signs of infection.

- Ensure adequate IV and then oral fluids, but monitor for edema and shortness of breath, signs of fluid overload.

- Monitor level of pain and relief with analgesics but watch for oversedation, hypotension, and decreased bowel sounds as adverse effects of opioids.

- Provide comfort measures, such as positioning, splinting incision during position changing, or coughing, applying ice pack to perineum.

- Auscultate bowel sounds for return, signaling progression of diet. Report nausea, vomiting, and loss of or decrease in bowel sounds immediately; intervention for bowel obstruction may be needed.

- Institute thromboembolism prevention, as ordered, and monitor for calf tenderness.

- Encourage ambulation as early as possible but encourage gradual resumption of activities, according to surgeon instructions.

- Notify surgeon of fever, shortness of breath, increased pain, excessive bleeding or drainage, foul odor, change in vital signs, urinary retention, decreased urine output, nausea and vomiting, or tender, swollen calf.

This information should serve as a general guideline only. Each patient situation presents a unique set of clinical factors and requires nursing judgment to guide care, which may include additional or alternative measures and approaches.

Conization

Description

Excision of a cone-shaped piece of tissue from the cervix, including the area where the squamous and columnar epithelial tissue meet (transformation zone) for diagnostic and therapeutic purposes. The transformation zone is the area of most cervical cancers. The procedure can be done via scalpel, laser, or electrosurgery techniques.

Nursing and Patient Care Considerations

1. Explain to patient that this test can be a minor surgical procedure that requires local or general anesthesia. Obtain pregnancy test if patient is within childbearing years, as indicated.

2. After excision, bleeding is controlled by cauterization or suturing and packing.

3. Patient should be observed for several hours after the procedure for excessive bleeding.

4. Instruct patient to avoid tampons, douching, and intercourse as well as not to immerse herself in water (no swimming, hot tub, tub bath) for 2 weeks, or as directed by health care provider, to allow healing.

Hysteroscopy

Description

Endoscopic visualization of the uterine cavity used to evaluate endometrial cancer, check tubal patency, determine the cause of uterine bleeding, remove polyps or fibroids, and observe the placement and appearance of IUDs.

Nursing and Patient Care Considerations

1. Obtain pregnancy test prior to the procedure if patient is within childbearing years, as indicated.

2. Administer prescribed sedative before the procedure and explain that a local anesthetic will also be injected into the cervix in the operating room.

3. Patient will be assisted into the lithotomy position and the perineum and vagina will be cleaned immediately before sterile draping.

4. Explain that instruments called sounds are inserted into the cervical canal for dilation before insertion of the hysteroscope. With the scope in place, normal saline or CO_2 gas is slowly infused into the endometrial cavity to distend it and allow for viewing.

5. Observe patient for several hours and give discharge instructions.
   a. Over-the-counter analgesics may be needed for minor discomfort if analgesic has not been prescribed.
   b. Notify the health care provider of severe cramping or bleeding, fever, or unusual discharge.

Endometrial Biopsy

Description

1. Procedure is done with or without local anesthesia to obtain cells from the uterine lining to assist in the diagnosis of endometrial cancer, menstrual disorders, and infertility.

2. During speculum examination, a uterine sound is placed, followed by a curette or Pipelle suction device to withdraw specimen.

Nursing and Patient Care Considerations

1. Obtain pregnancy test if patient is within childbearing years, as indicated.
2. Administer prostaglandin inhibitor to decrease postoperative uterine cramping.
3. Assist patient into the dorsal lithotomy position and explain procedure.
4. Label specimen, place in formalin, and send to laboratory.
5. Inform patient that she may experience light bleeding and occasional cramping for a few days.
6. Instruct patient to report fever, chills, and increased bleeding; no tampons, douching, or intercourse for 2 to 3 days.

GENERAL PROCEDURES AND TREATMENT MODALITIES

Fertility Control

Nurses who work with women in the gynecologic setting or in any setting may be involved in contraceptive counseling.

Basic Principles

1. *Contraception* is the prevention of fertility on a temporary basis.
2. *Sterilization* is the permanent prevention of fertility. Female and male sterilization procedures can be performed. Some procedures can be reversed but with possible complications and variable success rates.
3. Contraception effectiveness depends on motivation, which is a result of education, culture, religious beliefs, and personal situation. It is best to include both partners in any contraception decision.
4. Nurses should be familiar with contraceptive methods and educate patients without moral judgment.
5. Failure rate (pregnancy) is determined by experience of 100 women for 1 year and is expressed as pregnancies per 100 woman-years.

Contraceptive Methods

See Table 22-2.

(Text continues on page 844)

Table 22-2	Contraceptive Methods			
METHODS	**DEFINITION**	**PROCEDURE**	**ADVANTAGES**	**DISADVANTAGES**
Natural Methods				
Periodic abstinence	• Abstain from intercourse during fertile period of each cycle.	Determine fertile period by: • Calendar method—ovulation occurs 14 days before next menstrual period. • Cervical mucus method—increase in mucus at time of ovulation; clear and stringy. • Basal body temperature—drops immediately before ovulation and rises 24–72 hours after ovulation. • Symptothermal method—combines mucus and temperature.	• No health hazards. • Inexpensive. • May be religiously acceptable. • Increased knowledge of cycles.	• 20% failure rate. • Requires consistent record-keeping. • Decrease in spontaneity.
Coitus interruptus (withdrawal method)	• Withdrawal of penis from vagina when ejaculation is imminent.	• Must withdraw before ejaculation so that ejaculation occurs away from female genitalia.	• No cost. • No health hazards. • Always available.	• Failure rate of 19%; preejaculatory fluid may contain sperm. • Interruption of sexual act.
Lactation	• Breastfeeding has a contraceptive effect due to prolactin's inhibition of luteinizing hormone, which maintains menstrual cycle.	• Breast-feed on demand, around the clock, without formula supplementation.	• No health hazards. • No cost.	• Unreliable. • Need to use other method such as spermicide or barrier, which has no effect on breast milk.

(continued)

Table 22-2 Contraceptive Methods (*continued*)

METHODS	DEFINITION	PROCEDURE	ADVANTAGES	DISADVANTAGES
Barrier Methods				

> **! NURSING ALERT** Warn patients who use condoms, diaphragms, and the cervical cap that latex sensitivity may be a problem—watch for itching, swelling, generalized reactions.

METHODS	DEFINITION	PROCEDURE	ADVANTAGES	DISADVANTAGES
Condom—male and female	• Latex or polyurethane or processed collagenous tissue sheaths, placed over erect penis to prevent semen from entering vagina. • Female condom is placed in the vagina.	• Place condom over erect penis. • Leave dead space at tip of condom (from which air has been expelled) to allow room for ejaculate. • Use spermicide on exterior for added protection. • Grasp ring around condom at withdrawal to avoid leaving condom in vagina.	• Failure rate is low with proper use (2%–3%). • Prevention of STD. • Inexpensive. • No health hazard. • May help premature ejaculation by decreasing sensitivity. • Increases male involvement in contraception.	• Decreased sensitivity. • Interruption of sexual act. • Sensitivity to latex may be a problem. • Failure rate with typical use is 12%. • Female condoms are more expensive, made of polyurethane.
Diaphragm	• Rubber cap shaped like a dome with a flexible rim.	• Check for holes. • Place spermicide inside dome. • Place diaphragm against and covering cervical opening, behind lower edge of pubic bone. • Leave in place for 6–8 hours after intercourse.	• Failure rate with perfect use is 6%; 16% with typical use. • May reduce the risk of developing cervical cancer.	• Occasional toxic shock or allergic reactions. • May experience pelvic discomfort. • Possible increase in urinary tract infections (UTIs). • Must be properly cleaned with soap and water, dried and stored to preserve integrity of rubber.
Cervical cap	• Rubber cap, shaped like a cup with a tall dome and flexible rim.	• Place spermicide inside cap and place cap over cervical opening prior to intercourse.	• Failure rate similar to diaphragm. • Can be left in place for up to 48 hours.	• Risk of toxic shock, cervicitis, and PID. • Requires frequent follow-up. • Must be properly cleaned with soap and water, dried, and stored.
Spermicides				
Nonoxynol-9 or octoxynol-9	• Available in a variety of forms: foam, jelly, cream, suppository, tablet.	• Place next to cervix before intercourse; better if used with a barrier method.	• Available in a variety of forms. • Sold over-the-counter.	• Less effective if not used with barrier method; generally, 28% failure rate. • Some patients are allergic. • Increases risk of UTI. • Frequent use may cause genital lesions, increasing risk of HIV transmission.
Intrauterine Devices				
	• Small device made of plastic with exposed copper or progesterone-release system; acts to inhibit uterine wall implantation.	• Health care provider inserts device; slowly and usually at time of menses. • Check intrauterine device string regularly—at least once per month—or after each intercourse when it is first inserted.	• Failure rate low, 2% or less. • Convenient; permits spontaneous intercourse. • Replace every 5–10 years, depending on manufacturer recommendations.	• Risk of PID for first month and resultant tubal damage and infertility. • May cause spotting, bleeding, or pain. • Risk of spontaneous abortion. • Risk of uterine rupture (rare).

Table 22-2   Contraceptive Methods (*continued*)

METHODS	DEFINITION	PROCEDURE	ADVANTAGES	DISADVANTAGES
Hormones				
Combination oral contraceptives	• Tablets containing estrogen to inhibit ovulation and progestin to make cervical mucus impenetrable to sperm; lowest effective doses are used.	• Take daily in a cyclical or continuous manner.	• Less than 1% failure rate in the first year with correct use. • Decreased pelvic pain due to endometriosis, decreased risk of ovarian and endometrial cancer, decreased bleeding due to uterine fibroids. • Aids in menstrual disorders • Improves acne	• Serious adverse reactions include thromboembolism, stroke, myocardial infarction, and cerebral embolism, especially for those who smoke cigarettes or are overweight. • Questionable risk of breast, cervical cancer. • May experience nausea, vomiting, headache, bloating, and weight gain. • Must remember to take at same time daily.
Progestin-only oral contraceptive (mini-pill)	• Smaller doses of progestins than in combined oral contraceptives.	• Take daily.	• As low as <1% failure rate during the first year with correct use. • Avoids estrogen-related adverse effects and possibly cardiovascular risks. • The thickened cervical mucus may reduce the risk of ascending infection with development of PID. • Safe in breastfeeding.	• May cause irregular menses, spotting, amenorrhea. • Must be taken at the same time daily (no more than 3 hours late) or protection is lost.
Combination transdermal contraceptive patch	• Estrogen and progesterone are absorbed systemically; as efficacious as oral hormones.	• Apply weekly to buttocks, inner aspect of upper arms, or abdomen for 3 weeks, then off for 1 week for menses.	• Same as oral hormones but administered weekly. • Avoids first-pass metabolism through liver.	• Same as oral hormones. • May become loose or cause minor skin reaction. • Increased risk of DVT compared to oral method.
Hormonal vaginal contraceptive	• Vaginal ring containing estrogen and progesterone, as effective as oral contraceptive.	• Insert ring into vagina on day 5 of cycle, remove after 3 weeks for 1 week for menses.	• Same as oral contraceptives except is administered monthly. • Avoids first-pass metabolism through the liver.	• Same as oral contraceptives. • Requires vaginal insertion and retrieval. • May cause vaginitis, leukorrhea.
Postcoital contraception (morning-after pill)	• May be combined estrogen and progestin, high-dose estrogen, or progestin.	• More effective if started within 24–72 hours after intercourse, may be used up to 5 days after intercourse.	• Very effective.	• May be religiously opposed. • Can cause nausea. • May cause birth defects.
Progesterone implant	• Progesterone release system made up of silastic rod.	• Implanted in subcutaneous fat of upper arm.	• Long-term (up to 3 years). • Convenient. • Only 0.4% failure rate.	• May cause irregular bleeding, spotting, amenorrhea, acne, headaches. • May be difficult to remove. • High initial expense.

(continued)

Table 22-2   Contraceptive Methods (continued)

METHODS	DEFINITION	PROCEDURE	ADVANTAGES	DISADVANTAGES
Hormones (continued)				
Progesterone injection	• I.M. injection of long-acting progesterone.	• Initial injection within first 5 days of menses, then every 3 months.	• Convenient. • Less than 1% failure rate with correct use.	• Requires every 3-month follow-up. • May cause irregular bleeding, spotting, amenorrhea, weight gain. • Long-term effects still unknown. • High discontinuation rate in adolescents due to adverse effects and missed appointments.
Progesterone Antagonist				
RU-486; mifepristone	• Drug that prevents implantation and leads to menses (medical abortion).	• Given orally within 10 days of a missed period; may be combined with prostaglandin suppository.	• Causes abortion in 95% of users up to 5 weeks after conception.	• Is an abortifacient; not a contraceptive in most cases. • May cause nausea, bleeding, incomplete abortion.

STD, sexually transmitted disease.

Sterilization Procedures

Tubal sterilization is frequently performed for birth control. Hysterectomy and oophorectomy, performed for other reasons, also result in sterility. Male sterilization by vasectomy is another option.

General Considerations

1. Approaches.
   a. Abdominal is most frequently used: may be postpartum laparotomy, minilaparotomy, or laparoscopy. Laparoscopy with electrocoagulation is frequently performed. It is a safe and effective procedure.
   b. Vaginal incision in posterior vagina (colpotomy) with the uterine tube pulled through it; rarely done due to higher rate of complications—infection.
   c. Uterine approach utilizing hysteroscopy to visualize the tubal ostia and insert coils or plugs.
2. Techniques vary by surgeon preference.
   a. Electrocoagulation: burn section of tube with or without excision; low reversal rate.
   b. Pomeroy: the tube is tied in midsection and section removed; may be reversed.
   c. Fimbriectomy: the fimbriated end removed and end tied; irreversible.
   d. Cornual resection: removal of the section of tube nearest uterus and suture cornual opening closed.
   e. Silastic bands: plastic or metal clips to occlude tube; may be reversed, although rare.
   f. Coils or plugs inserted in the tubal ostia through hysteroscopy.

Complications

   a. Failure to successfully block the tubes—pregnancy or tubal pregnancy.
   b. Hemorrhage, infection, uterine perforation, damage to bowel, bladder, or aorta.

Nursing and Patient Care Considerations

1. Assess motivation for sterilization and level of knowledge about the procedure. Informed consent is needed. The couple should be thoroughly counseled about the permanence of the procedure.
   a. Teach patient there is no effect on hormones and menstruation will continue.
   b. Teach patient there should not be any adverse effect on sexual response.
2. Birth control methods are discontinued immediately before the procedure.
3. Prepare patient to expect some abdominal soreness for several days; instruct her to report any bleeding, increasing pain, or fever.
4. Sexual intercourse and strenuous activity should be avoided for 2 weeks.

Dilation and Curettage

Dilation and curettage is a common gynecologic surgery for diagnostic and therapeutic purposes consists of widening the cervical canal with a dilator and scraping the uterine cavity with a curette. Performed to control uterine bleeding, secure endometrial and endocervical tissue for cytologic examination, and treat missed, incomplete, or induced abortion.

Nursing and Patient Care Considerations

1. Prepare patient for the procedure—answer questions; request that she void; administer an enema, if ordered; and administer nonsteroidal anti-inflammatory drug (NSAID) or a sedative, as directed.
2. Immediately postoperatively, monitor vital signs at frequent intervals; potential for hemorrhage exists.
3. Monitor perineal pads and the bed for amount of bleeding; report excessive amounts.
4. Offer prescribed analgesics for lower back and pelvic pain; cramping may occur for 2 to 3 days because of dilation of the cervix.
5. Instruct patient to maintain decreased activity for remainder of day to decrease cramping and bleeding.
6. Instruct patient to use perineal pads at home and to report fever (more than 100.4°F), heavy bleeding (saturating a pad within 1 hour more than once), cramps lasting longer than 48 hours, increasing pain, prolonged or a foul-smelling vaginal discharge.
7. Instruct patient to avoid strenuous activity until bleeding stops.
8. Inform patient that the procedure does not affect sexual functioning, but that she should refrain from sexual intercourse, douching, and tampons for at least 2 weeks, according to preference of health care provider.

Laparoscopy

Laparoscopy is the endoscopic visualization of the pelvic and abdominal cavities through a small incision below the umbilicus. It is used to diagnose pelvic pain and infertility; differentiate between ovarian, tubal, and uterine masses; evaluate genital anomalies; treat endometriosis, ectopic pregnancy, and adhesions; perform tubal sterilizations and as a major surgical tool used to treat a multitude of gynecologic indications including laparoscopically assisted hysterectomy.

Nursing and Patient Care Considerations

1. Obtain pregnancy test if patient is within childbearing years, as indicated.
2. Prepare patient by ensuring that she has taken nothing by mouth (NPO), answering questions about the procedure, and administering a sedative and enema, if ordered.
3. Inform patient that she may experience shoulder or abdominal discomfort after the procedure from the infusion of carbon dioxide given to separate the intestines from pelvic organs. Elevation of feet higher than shoulders after the procedure helps relieve this.
4. Patient will receive local, general, or regional anesthesia and will be placed in Trendelenburg's position to displace the intestines for better visualization.
5. After procedure, monitor bleeding and vital signs and administer analgesics, as indicated.
6. Inform patient that passing gas and bowel movements may be difficult initially because of the manipulation of the intestines; ambulation and fluids will be helpful.

7. Advise patient not to have intercourse or to perform strenuous activity for 2 to 3 days and to report bleeding, cramping, or fever. For more complex procedures, return to normal activities, as directed by the health care provider.

Hysterectomy

Hysterectomy is the surgical removal of the uterus. It is the second most common operation in the United States among reproductive-age women.

Types of Hysterectomy

1. Abdominal.
   a. Subtotal/supracervical hysterectomy—corpus of uterus is removed, but cervical stump remains.
   b. Total hysterectomy—entire uterus is removed, including cervix; tubes and ovaries remain.
   c. Total hysterectomy with bilateral salpingo-oophorectomy—entire uterus, tubes, and ovaries are removed.
2. Vaginal—removal of uterus and cervix through vagina.
3. Laparoscopically assisted vaginal hysterectomy—allows for the removal of pelvic adhesions that would otherwise prevent vaginal hysterectomy.
4. Laparoscopic supracervical hysterectomy—laparoscopic removal of the uterus that spares the cervix.
5. Laparoscopic total hysterectomy—laparoscopic removal of the entire uterus and cervix.

Indications

1. Uterine fibroids, endometriosis and adenomyosis, dysfunctional uterine bleeding—most common.
2. Uterine prolapse, chronic pelvic pain.
3. Cancer of the vagina, cervix, uterus, ovaries, or fallopian tubes.
4. Obstetric complications—rare.

Preoperative Management

1. Procedure and reason for hysterectomy, what the procedure involves, and what to expect postoperatively are explained.
2. Patient must remain NPO from midnight the night before surgery and must void before surgery.
3. An enema may be administered before surgery to evacuate the bowel and prevent contamination and trauma during surgery.
4. Vaginal irrigation is performed before surgery and skin preparation is done, if ordered.
5. Implement the Universal Protocol for Preventing Wrong Site, Wrong Procedure, Wrong Person Surgery (see Chapter 7).
6. Preoperative medication is given to help the patient relax.

Postoperative Management

1. Postoperatively, the following assessments are made:
   a. Wound appearance and drainage.
   b. Vital signs, level of consciousness.
   c. Level of pain and comfort to include nausea and vomiting.

d. Vaginal drainage (serous, bloody).

e. Intake and output.

f. Urge to void, bladder distention, residual urine (if appropriate).

g. Clarity, color, and sediment of urine.

h. Homans' sign or impaired circulation.

i. Return of bowel sounds, passage of flatus, first bowel movement.

2. Exercise and ambulation are encouraged to prevent thromboembolus, facilitate voiding, and stimulate peristalsis.

Complications

1. Incisional/pelvic infection.
2. Hemorrhage.
3. Urinary tract injury.
4. Bowel obstruction.
5. Thrombophlebitis/venous thrombus emboli.

Nursing Diagnoses

- Acute Pain related to surgical procedure.
- Impaired Urinary Elimination related to decreased sensation and stimulation.
- Risk for Infection related to surgical procedure.
- Disturbed Body Image related to alteration in female organs and hormones.
- Sexual Dysfunction related to alteration in reproductive organs and function.

Nursing Interventions

Relieving Pain

1. Assess pain location, level, and characteristics.
2. Administer prescribed pain medications. Ensure that patient knows how to use patient-controlled analgesia pump and is using it properly.
3. Encourage patient to splint incision when moving.
4. Encourage patient to ambulate as soon as possible to decrease flatus and abdominal distention.
5. Institute sitz baths or ice packs, as prescribed, to alleviate perineal discomfort.
6. Monitor level of sedation related to opioid administration—may interfere with ambulation and elimination.

Promoting Urinary Elimination

1. Monitor intake and output, bladder distention, signs and symptoms of bladder infection.
2. Maintain patency of indwelling catheter if one is in place.
3. Catheterize patient intermittently if uncomfortable or if she has not voided in 8 hours.
4. Catheterize to check for residual urine after patient voids; should be less than 100 mL. Continue to check if more than 100 mL, or bladder infection may develop.
5. Encourage patient to empty bladder around the clock, not only when feeling the urge, because of loss of sensation of bladder fullness.
6. Encourage fluid intake to decrease risk of urinary infection.

Preventing Infection

1. Assess vaginal drainage amount, color, and odor, incision site, and temperature.
2. Administer antibiotics, as prescribed.
3. Assist use of incentive spirometer, coughing and deep breathing, and ambulation to decrease risk of pulmonary infection. Monitor respirations and breath sounds for compromise.

Strengthening Body Image

1. Allow patient to discuss her feelings about herself as a woman.
2. Reassure patient she is still feminine.
3. Encourage patient to discuss her feelings with her spouse or significant other.
4. Reassure patient that she will not go through premature menopause if her ovaries were not removed.

Regaining Sexual Function

1. Discuss changes regarding sexual functioning, such as shortened vagina and possible dyspareunia because of dryness.
2. Offer suggestions to improve sexual functioning.
   a. Use of water-soluble lubricants.
   b. Change position—female-dominant position offers more control of depth of penetration.

Patient Education and Health Maintenance

1. Advise patient that a total hysterectomy with bilateral salpingo-oophorectomy produces a surgical menopause. Patient may experience hot flashes, vaginal dryness, and mood swings unless short-term hormonal replacement therapy is instituted.
2. Advise patient against sitting too long at one time, as in driving long distances, because of the possibility of blood pooling in the lower extremities, which increases the risk of thromboembolism.
3. Suggest that patient delay driving a car until the third postoperative week because even pressing the brake pedal puts stress on the lower abdomen. Avoid hazardous activities when taking opioid analgesics.
4. Tell patient to expect a tired feeling for the first few days at home and not to plan too many activities for the first week. She can perform most of her usual daily activities within 4 to 6 weeks or per provider instruction. Teach patient that the recovery period differs for each individual and is dependent on medical history and any complications that may have occurred. Inform her that it may be 2 to 3 months or even a year "to feel like herself again."
5. Tell patient not to feel discouraged if, at times during convalescence, she experiences depression, feels like crying, and seems unusually nervous. This is common but will not last. Tell patient to call her provider if the feelings persist.
6. Remind patient to ask her surgeon about strenuous or lifting activities, which are usually restricted for 4 to 6 weeks.
7. Reinforce instructions given by the surgeon on intercourse, douching, and use of tampons, which are usually discouraged for 6 to 8 weeks. Sexual intercourse should be resumed cautiously to prevent injury and discomfort. Showers are permitted, but tub baths are deferred until healing is sufficient.

8. Instruct patient to report fever higher than 100°F (37.8°C), heavy vaginal bleeding, drainage, increased pain or cramping, foul odor of discharge, and bleeding or increased drainage from incision site.

9. Emphasize the importance of follow-up visits and routine physical and gynecologic examinations.

Evaluation: Expected Outcomes

- Verbalizes decreased pain.
- Voids every 4 to 6 hours of sufficient quantity.
- No fever or signs of infection.
- Verbalizes positive statements about self and positive outlook on recovery.
- Verbalizes understanding of possible changes in sexual functioning and what to do about it.

MENSTRUAL CONDITIONS

Dysmenorrhea

 Evidence Base University of Texas at Austin, School of Nursing, Family Nurse Practitioner Program. (2010). *An evidence based practice guideline for the treatment of primary dysmenorrhea.* Austin: University of Texas at Austin, School of Nursing.

Dysmenorrhea is painful menstruation; most common of gynecologic dysfunctions.

Pathophysiology and Etiology

Primary Dysmenorrhea

1. No pelvic lesion; usually intrinsic to uterus.
2. Current research supports increased prostaglandin production by the endometrium as the chief cause.
3. May also be because of hormonal, obstructive, and psychological factors.

Secondary Dysmenorrhea

1. Caused by lesion, such as endometriosis, pelvic infection, congenital abnormality, uterine fibroids, or ovarian cyst or may be caused by passage of a clot through undilated cervix.

Clinical Manifestations

1. Pain may be caused by increased uterine contractility and uterine hypoxia.
2. Characteristics of pain—recurrent, crampy, colicky or dull, usually in lower midabdominal region; spasmodic or constant.
3. Nausea, vomiting, diarrhea, headache, chills, tiredness, nervousness, and lower backache may be experienced.
4. Usually self-limiting without complications.

Diagnostic Evaluation

Tests to rule out underlying cause:

1. Chlamydia and gonorrhea tests—may show infection.
2. Pelvic ultrasound—may detect tumor, endometriosis, cysts.

3. Serum or urine pregnancy test—to rule out ectopic pregnancy.
4. Possibly, hysteroscopy and laparoscopy—primarily to detect endometriosis.

Management

The following measures are for primary dysmenorrhea; treatment of secondary dysmenorrhea is aimed at underlying pathology.

1. Nonsteroidal anti-inflammatory agents, such as ibuprofen or naproxen sodium for their antiprostaglandin action. Most effective with loading dose 1 to 2 days before onset of menses and taken on a regular schedule for 2 to 3 days.
2. Local heat, such as heating pad, to increase blood flow and decrease spasms, for 20-minute intervals More effective in combination with other therapies.
3. Hormonal contraceptives to decrease contractility and menstrual flow. Evidence supports decreased dysmenorrhea symptoms with monthly oral contraceptives, extended-cycle oral contraceptives, intravaginal hormonal devices, and intrauterine hormonal systems.
4. Possibly—exercise to increase endorphin release, which decreases pain perception, and to suppress prostaglandin release. More evidence is needed to support this intervention.

Nursing Assessment

1. Obtain menstrual and gynecologic history that could suggest underlying pathology.
2. Assess level of pain using scale of 1 to 10; assess patient's emotional response to pain, coping mechanisms, and ability to carry out activities.
3. Obtain vital signs, including temperature, to rule out infection.
4. Perform abdominal and pelvic examination (if indicated) to obtain specimens.

Nursing Diagnoses

- Acute Pain related to uterine contractions.
- Risk for Activity Intolerance related to pain severity and associated symptoms.
- Readiness for Enhanced Coping related to chronic, recurrent condition.

Nursing Interventions

Controlling Pain

1. Administer pharmacologic agents, as ordered, to control pain and menstrual flow.
2. Apply heating pad to lower back or abdomen, as indicated, for 20-minute intervals.
3. Assess patient's response to pain-control measures.
4. Encourage verbalization of feelings and reassure patient through the evaluation process.
5. Encourage activity and exercise, as tolerated.

Decreasing Risk for Activity Intolerance

Instruct patient that tolerance will increase with increased activity. The more active that she is, the better that she will feel.

Enhancing Coping Skills

Instruct patient in stress-reduction techniques, breathing techniques, and lifestyle changes that may improve symptoms such as exercise, healthy eating habits, adequate sleep, and smoking cessation.

Patient Education and Health Maintenance

1. Explain to patient possible causes of dysmenorrhea.
2. Teach patient nonpharmacologic methods to reduce pain.
   a. Apply heating pad to lower midabdomen or back or take warm tub baths for 20-minute intervals.
   b. Exercise regularly (30 minutes, five or more times per week).
   c. Healthy eating habits; see *www.myplate.gov*.
   d. Smoking cessation.
3. Teach patient to use prescribed medications effectively by taking medication at beginning of discomfort and repeating as necessary, especially on first day of menses.
4. Teach patient adverse effects of medications.
5. Encourage patient to reduce stress through adequate sleep, good nutrition, exercise, smoking cessation, and coping with stressors.
6. Discuss patient's feelings toward menstruation (hygienic issues, inconvenience, female identity).

Evaluation: Expected Outcomes

- Verbalizes reduced pain level.
- Demonstrates participation in functional activities of daily living without intolerance.
- Describes methods to reduce pain and to increase coping skills.

Premenstrual Syndrome

Evidence Base Biggs, W., & DeMuth, R. (2011). Premenstrual syndrome and premenstrual dysphoric disorder. *American Family Physician, 84*(8), 918–924.

Premenstrual syndrome (PMS) is a group of behavioral, psychological, and physical symptoms that include headache, irritability, depressed mood, breast tenderness, and abdominal bloating that are clearly related to onset of menstruation.

Pathophysiology and Etiology

1. Etiologic theories include hormonal imbalances, such as ovarian steroid interaction; dysfunction of neurotransmitters (such as serotonin), prostaglandins, or endorphins; psychological factors, such as attitudes and beliefs related to menstruation; and environmental factors, such as nutrition and pollution.
2. Most common in women in their 30s.
3. May occur in 20% to 32% of menstruating women. Up to 80% of women experience one or more of the symptoms during the luteal phase of their menstrual cycle.

Clinical Manifestations

1. Symptoms may begin 7 to 14 days before onset of menstrual flow; may diminish 1 to 2 days after menses begins.
2. Physical—edema of extremities, abdominal fullness, breast swelling and tenderness, headache, vertigo, palpitations, acne, backache, constipation, thirst, weight gain.

3. Psychological and behavioral—labile mood, irritability, fatigue, lethargy, depressed mood, anxiety, crying spells, changes in appetite, decreased concentration.
4. Diagnosis based on clinical manifestations; usually neither diagnostic laboratory nor radiological evaluation is necessary.
5. Usually self-limiting without complications.

Management

1. First-line pharmacological therapy for severe PMS or PMDD includes selective serotonin reuptake inhibitors (SSRIs) such as citalopram, escitalopram, fluoxetine, and sertraline; and serotonin-norepinephrine reuptake inhibitors such as venlafaxine.

DRUG ALERT Paroxetine should be avoided in women of childbearing age because of increased risk of congenital abnormalities.

2. Drospirenone (a spironolactone derivative diuretic) combined with low-dose estrogen in oral contraceptives helps symptoms. Theoretically, longer cycles of oral contraceptives with shorter inactive phases would ameliorate symptoms by suppressing natural hormones.
3. Calcium supplementation of 1,200 mg elemental calcium per day has good evidence that supports decreased mood swings, irritability, depression, and anxiety.
4. Vitamin B_6 supplements of 50 to 100 mg daily (should not exceed 100 mg/day).
5. Cognitive-behavioral therapy has some limited evidence supporting relief of symptoms.
6. Healthy lifestyle changes, such as restriction of sodium, caffeine, tobacco, alcohol, and refined sweets, and inclusion of aerobic exercise, while are often recommended, have insufficient evidence to support their efficacy in treatment of PMS symptoms.
7. High-dose daily vitamin D intake is supported by some evidence.
8. Prostaglandin inhibitors such as ibuprofen will decrease dysmenorrhea-related symptoms.
9. Spironolactone, a diuretic with androgenic effect, may decrease fluid retention and weight gain.
10. With great caution because of abuse potential, anxiolytic agents may be prescribed for use during the luteal phase for patients with anxiety symptoms.
11. Chasteberry, an herbal supplement, 20 mg daily was shown to be effective in one randomized controlled trial.

Nursing Assessment

1. Ask patient to describe symptoms, their onset, and means of relief.
2. Assess patient's diet, activity, and rest habits.
3. Assess patient's emotional response to symptoms and methods of coping.

Nursing Diagnoses

- Deficient knowledge related to self-care measures.
- Anxiety related to symptoms and difficulty coping with condition.

Nursing Interventions

Increasing Knowledge and Coping Skills

Use patient education as a tool to help patient increase control over symptoms.

Reducing Anxiety

1. Administer medications, as ordered; warn patient that diuretics will cause increased urination and anxiolytics may cause drowsiness or cognitive impairment.
2. Provide emotional support for patient and significant others.
3. Teach stress management and relaxation measures such as imagery and progressive muscle relaxation (see Chapter 3).
4. Suggest counseling, as indicated.

Patient Education and Health Maintenance

1. Encourage patient to keep a diary for several consecutive months, which includes dates, cycle days, stressors, symptoms, and their severity, to determine if therapy is effective.
2. Instruct patient in the use and adverse effects of prescribed medications.
3. Teach patient possible causes of syndrome and nonprescription methods to alleviate distress, such as calcium and vitamin B$_6$ intake.
4. Refer for further resources and support to such groups as the National Association for Premenstrual Syndrome (UK) (*http://pms.org.uk*) or womenshealth.gov, a project of the U.S. Department of Health and Human Services Office on Women's Health (*www.womenshealth.gov*).

Evaluation: Expected Outcomes

- Verbalizes increased knowledge and sense of control over condition.
- Reduced signs and symptoms of anxiety.

Amenorrhea

Amenorrhea is the absence of menstrual flow.

Pathophysiology and Etiology

Primary Amenorrhea

1. Menarche does not occur by age 16 with pubertal development or by age 14 with absence of secondary sex characteristics.
2. May be caused by chromosomal disorders, such as Turner's syndrome, agenesis of the uterus, or constitutional delay of growth and puberty.
3. Transverse vaginal septum or imperforate hymen.

Secondary Amenorrhea

1. Menstruation stops for 3 months in women with previously established regular menstrual cycles or 9 months in a woman with previously established oligomenorrhea (infrequent or longer menstrual cycles).
2. May be caused by pregnancy, lactation, menopause, or corpus luteal ovarian cysts.
3. Excessive exercise, inadequate nutrition with decreased body fat stores, and excessive weight loss may cause amenorrhea in young athletes (included in the female athlete triad: an eating disorder, amenorrhea, and osteoporosis).
4. Amenorrhea and anovulation secondary to polycystic ovary syndrome (PCOS) commonly occurs in obese women but may be seen in women with normal body mass index (BMI).
5. Ovarian, adrenal, or pituitary tumors and thyroid disorders are hormonal causes.
6. Some medications, such as antipsychotics (phenothiazines), antidepressants, antihypertensives, histamine H2 blockers, opiates, chemotherapy, and hormonal contraceptives, may also induce amenorrhea.
7. It may be a result of severe depression, severe psychological trauma, physical trauma, or radiation.

Diagnostic Evaluation

1. Pregnancy test.
2. Prolactin level (elevated) with pituitary tumor.
3. Thyroid-stimulating hormone (TSH)
4. Progesterone challenge test in secondary amenorrhea if both prolactin and TSH are normal.
   a. Positive result—bleeding occurs; chronic anovulation is most likely.
   b. Negative result—no bleeding occurs; may indicate ovarian failure; other tests are needed.
5. Hormonal levels—LH and FSH—to determine type of hypogonadism in primary amenorrhea or to detect ovarian failure in secondary amenorrhea.
6. Genetic karyotyping to detect chromosome abnormalities in primary amenorrhea.
7. Ultrasound to identify presence of uterus and/or outflow obstruction.

Management

Treatment is based on causative factor.

1. Discontinue causative medications if benefit of discontinuance outweighs risk.
2. Nutritional, exercise, or psychological counseling, as indicated.
   a. Recommend decreased exercise in athletes to increase body fat stores and restore normal BMI.
   b. Recommend weight reduction if obese.
3. Low-dose hormonal contraceptives to regulate cycle after underlying cause has been determined.
4. In polycystic ovarian syndrome, insulin-sensitizing agents decrease androgen levels, improve ovulation rate, and improve glucose tolerance. Clomiphene citrate is first-line for ovulation induction. Laser treatment plus eflornithine is indicated for hirsutism in PCOS.
5. Treatment of tumor or other underlying cause. Surgery, as indicated.

Complications

1. Amenorrhea increases risk for osteoporosis and endometrial hyperplasia, which may lead to atypia and cancer of the endometrium.
2. PCOS conveys risk of metabolic syndrome, type 2 diabetes, and cardiovascular disease. Improvement in ovulation rate increases the risk of pregnancy.

Nursing Assessment

1. Assess for signs of chromosomal disorders, such as abnormal genitalia, masculinization, short stature, and characteristic facies.
2. Assess for signs of pituitary tumor, such as headache, vision disturbances, dizziness, and galactorrhea.
3. Assess weight and body build, BMI, change in weight, and nutritional and exercise habits that may indicate anorexia or loss of body fat because of exercise.
4. Assess for signs of PCOS: elevated blood pressure, elevated BMI, waist circumference, stigmata of insulin resistance, hirsutism.
5. Assess emotional status, areas of stress, and coping ability.

Nursing Diagnoses

- Imbalanced Nutrition: Less Than Body Requirements related to inadequate nutritional intake and/or rigorous exercise.
- Imbalanced Nutrition, More Than Body Requirements related to obesity or PCOS.
- Disturbed Body Image related to lack of menses, perception of inappropriate weight.

Nursing Interventions

Meeting Nutritional Requirements

1. Explore knowledge of the food groups, behavior regarding meals, and exercise routine; point out misconceptions, dangerous behavior, and ideas for improvement.
2. Monitor weight and BMI and return of menstrual cycles.

Improving Body Image

1. Explore patient's body image and coping strategies. Provide emotional support for patient and family.
2. Describe diagnostic tests and who will give results to patient.
3. Point out ineffective coping mechanisms and teach more positive coping mechanisms such as assertiveness. Instruct in relaxation techniques.

Patient Education and Health Maintenance

1. Teach patient the physiology of the normal menstrual cycle and possible causes in diagnostic workup for amenorrhea.
2. Teach proper use and adverse effects of prescribed medications.
3. Teach patient to chart menstrual periods on a calendar and maintain regular gynecologic and medical follow-up visits.
4. Teach patients with PCOS that they should be screened for type 2 diabetes and cardiovascular risk factors such as fasting lipid levels and body mass index.

Evaluation: Expected Outcomes

- Verbalizes adequate dietary intake and appropriate exercise regimen.
- Achieves normal body mass index with restoration of menses.
- Verbalizes understanding of diagnostic tests and improved body image.

Abnormal Uterine Bleeding

 Evidence Base Sweet, M., Schmidt-Dalton, T., & Weiss, P. (2012). Evaluation and management of abnormal uterine bleeding in premenopausal women. *American Family Physician, 85*(1), 35–43.

Abnormal uterine bleeding (AUB) is irregular or excessively heavy menstrual bleeding. *Dysfunctional uterine bleeding (DUB)* is a subcategory of AUB. Specifically, it is anovulatory abnormal uterine bleeding that has no organic cause, such as tumor, infection, or pregnancy.

Pathophysiology and Etiology

Causes of AUB are subdivided into anovulatory and ovulatory patterns.

Anovulatory AUB

1. Common causes of anovulatory AUB include polycystic ovarian syndrome (PCOS), uncontrolled diabetes mellitus, thyroid disorders (hypo- and hyperthyroidism), hyperprolactinemia, or medications (such as antipsychotics and anti-epileptics).
2. In adolescents, AUB is frequently caused by immature hypothalamic–pituitary–ovarian axis.
3. Ovarian failure in perimenopausal women frequently causes DUB. Recurrent irregular menstrual cycles are considered abnormal if they occur 8 years before menopause.
4. Anovulation may be related to hypothalamic or pituitary dysfunction, impaired follicular formation or rupture, or corpus luteum dysfunction.
5. Temporary estrogen withdrawal at ovulation may cause mid-cycle ovulatory bleeding.

Ovulatory AUB

1. Excessive bleeding or duration may be related to hypothyroidism, late-stage liver disease, or bleeding disorders (such von Willebrand disease).
2. Structural abnormalities, such as submucosal fibroids or endometrial fibroids, may cause AUB.
3. Approximately one half of women with ovulatory AUB have no identifiable cause.

Clinical Manifestations

Anovulatory AUB Patterns/Dysfunctional Bleeding

1. Amenorrhea—no bleeding for three cycles or more (see page 849).
2. Oligomenorrhea—significantly diminished menstrual flow; infrequent intervals (greater than 35 days) or irregular intervals.
3. Metrorrhagia—bleeding from uterus between regular menstrual periods; significant because it is usually a symptom of disease.
4. Menometrorrhagia—excessive bleeding at the usual time of menstruation and at other irregular intervals.

Ovulatory Patterns

1. Menorrhagia—excessive bleeding during regular menstruation cycles; can be increased in duration or amount.
2. Polymenorrhea—frequent menstruation occurring at intervals of less than 21 days.
3. Menometrorrhagia—excessive bleeding at the usual time of menstruation and at other irregular intervals.

Diagnostic Evaluation

Tests to rule out pathologic causes of abnormal bleeding include:

1. Pregnancy test.
2. Complete blood count (CBC) to detect anemia and platelet count.
3. TSH to rule out thyroid disorder; prolactin to rule out pituitary adenoma.
4. Thorough history and examination to look for anovulatory medical conditions (such as obesity and hirsutism—signs of PCOS) and to rule out enlarged uterus, trauma or foreign body.
5. Other tests that may be done during physical exam include a Pap smear to rule out cervical dysplasia or malignancy; chlamydia and gonorrhea tests to rule out PID.
6. Endometrial biopsy to determine hormonal effect on uterus and rule out malignancy.
7. Transvaginal ultrasound to rule out ovarian or uterine pathology or structural abnormality. Saline infusion sonohysterography is more sensitive and specific than transvaginal ultrasound.
8. Coagulation screen to rule out blood dyscrasias in adolescents with menorrhagia. Iron studies are not first-line, but are recommended if hematocrit and hemoglobin are low.
9. If cause is still undetermined, then hysteroscopy is recommended to detect uterine fibroids, polyps, and other lesions.

Management

Treatment is based on underlying cause.

1. Hormonal contraceptives (birth control pills or hormone-releasing IUD) to control chronic bleeding or induce regular withdrawal bleeding. Endometrial biopsy should be repeated after 3 to 6 months of treatment to monitor endometrial hyperplasia. Combination estrogen–progesterone oral contraceptives, while commonly prescribed first-line, lack adequate evidence for treatment of AUB.
2. In women who cannot take estrogen due to an increased thrombotic risk, progesterone-only administration can be effective. Cyclical oral progesterone for 21 days significantly reduces menorrhagia. For patients with menorrhagia, levonorgestrel-releasing intrauterine system is superior to oral contraceptives. Long-acting progestin injections may reduce bleeding but cause irregular spotting.
3. In emergencies, parenteral conjugated estrogen may be used to stop acute bleeding. Due to increased risk of thromboembolism, concomitant use of low-molecular-weight heparin may be considered.
4. Treat underlying anemia with iron, possible transfusions.
5. NSAIDs are useful to decrease menstrual flow volume in menorrhagia.
6. Tranexamic acid, an antifibrinolytic agent, has demonstrated efficacy in decreasing menorrhagia. In an underlying bleeding disorder (such as von Willebrand disease), intranasal desmopressin may be indicated.
7. Androgen therapy with a gonadotropin-releasing hormone, such as leuprolide acetate), to reduce menstrual blood loss in perimenopausal women or to reduce the size of uterine fibroids before surgery.
8. Surgical procedures, such as hysteroscopic polypectomy or resection of uterine submucosal fibroids.
9. Hysteroscopic endometrial resection (removal of diseased or abnormal tissue) or endometrial ablation (application of heat to endometrium to induce scarring) when above methods are not helpful.
   a. By 5 years postablation, one third of patients require another surgery.
   b. Uterus is preserved but it results in infertility.
10. Hysterectomy in refractory cases.

Complications

1. Recurrent anovulation in anovulatory AUB increases the risk of endometrial cancer due to the impact of unopposed estrogen on the endometrium. Women with regular ovulation and AUB have no greater risk of endometrial cancer because the endometrium regularly sloughs.
2. Severe anemia may result from menorrhagia or menometrorrhagia.

Nursing Assessment

1. Ask patient for menstrual and gynecologic history, sexual activity, and possibility of pregnancy.
2. Assess frequency, duration, and amount of menstrual flow.
3. Assess for other symptoms of underlying pathology, such as systemic hormonal conditions, pelvic pain, fever, and abdominal masses or tenderness.
4. Assess for signs and symptoms of anemia—fatigue, shortness of breath, pallor, tachycardia.

Nursing Diagnoses

- Fatigue related to excessive blood loss.
- Fear of bleeding through clothing related to excessive or unpredictable bleeding.

Nursing Interventions

Increasing Energy Level

1. Administer medications, as ordered. Teach patient indications and side effects.
2. Encourage good dietary intake with increased sources of iron-fortified cereals and breads, meat (especially red meat), and green, leafy vegetables.
3. Administer oral iron preparations with meals to prevent nausea and with vitamin C–rich foods or drinks to enhance absorption. Treat constipation, as necessary.
4. Monitor hemoglobin and infuse packed red blood cells, as ordered.
5. Encourage activity, as tolerated.

Relieving Fear

1. Review pattern of menstrual flow with patient and help her plan for excessive bleeding.
2. Suggest wearing double tampons (if able) and double sanitary pads.
3. Tell patient to expect heavy gush of blood on arising from lying or reclining position.
4. Prepare patient to carry an adequate supply of sanitary products and a change of clothing until bleeding is under control.

Patient Education and Health Maintenance

1. Teach patient the causes of AUB and about the diagnostic process to rule out pathologic causes of abnormal bleeding.
2. Teach patient to prevent anemia by eating a diet high in iron and by consuming vitamin C or citrus fruit to enhance absorption of iron.
3. Teach about hormonal therapy, related adverse effects, and what adverse effects to expect and what to expect of bleeding. Bleeding should stop within first week of hormonal contraceptives but should start again in fourth week as regular menstrual period would with cyclical contraceptives.
4. Advise patient to keep a calendar or log of menses.

Evaluation: Expected Outcomes

- Verbalizes adequate energy to perform activities.
- Verbalizes more confidence in ability to conceal bleeding.

Menopause

Evidence Base Goodman, N. F., Cobin, R. H., Ginzburg, S. B., et al. (2011). American Association of Clinical Endocrinologist medical guidelines for clinical practice for the diagnosis and treatment of menopause. *Endocrine Practice, 17*(Suppl. 6), 1–25.

Menopause is described as the physiologic cessation of menses. Climacteric or perimenopause is the period during which there is decline in ovarian function and the woman experiences symptoms of estrogen deficiency and, possibly, irregular cycles. Menopause has occurred if menses has not occurred for 12 months.

Pathophysiology and Etiology

1. Menopause is caused by the cessation of ovarian function and decreased estrogen production by the ovary; average age range is 45 to 55, with the average age of 51.
2. Anovulation may occur during perimenopause, disrupting menstrual cycles.
3. Artificial or surgical menopause may occur secondary to surgery or radiation involving the ovaries. Some chemotherapeutic agents also cause a chemical menopause.
4. Hysterectomy without ovary removal may result in earlier menopause due to disruption of the blood supply to the ovaries.

Clinical Manifestations

1. Genitalia—atrophy of vulva, vagina, urethra results in dryness, bleeding, itching, burning, dysuria, thinning of pubic hair, loss of labia minora, decreased secretions during intercourse.
2. Sexual function—vaginal dryness, discomfort, dyspareunia, decreased intensity and duration of sexual response, but can still have active and satisfactory function.
3. Vasomotor—60% to 75% of women experience "hot flashes," which may be preceded by an anxious feeling and accompanied by sweating. These may occur at night, causing "night sweats."
   a. Psychological—insomnia, irritability, anxiety, memory loss, fear, and depression may be experienced.
   b. Some women experience palpitations.
   c. Symptoms, severity, and personal/cultural meanings vary with each individual.

Diagnostic Evaluation

Levels of LH and FSH will increase, and estradiol will decrease; however, levels may fluctuate often during perimenopause, so diagnosis is based on symptoms. FSH greater than 30 to 40 IU/L indicates menopause; greater than 100 IU/L indicates complete ovarian failure. Laboratory studies of FSH are not necessary to diagnose the perimenopausal phase or menopause itself.

Management

Menopausal Hormone Therapy/Estrogen Replacement Therapy

1. Indicated at the smallest possible dose for the shortest time period (less than 5 years) to reduce vasomotor symptoms (with the added benefit to prevent osteoporosis). Common systemic routes of administration include oral and transdermal.
2. Progesterone co-therapy preparations (oral, transdermal; or in combination products with estrogen) are required in a cyclical dosage pattern if the uterus is intact in order to prevent endometrial hyperplasia and possible cancer. Continuous progesterone therapy is no longer recommended because of association with adverse breast outcomes.
3. Vaginal preparations are most effective for atrophic vaginitis. Concomitant progesterone is not indicated with vaginal estrogen due to minimal systemic absorption of estrogen.
4. Available as synthetic, animal based, and natural (plant source) products.
5. Menopausal hormone therapy is contraindicated with the following conditions:
   a. Increased risk of thromboembolic disease, previous or current idiopathic deep vein thrombosis or pulmonary embolism.
   b. Past, current, or suspected breast cancer.
   c. Estrogen-sensitive cancers (uterine, ovarian), untreated endometrial hyperplasia, undiagnosed genital bleeding.
   d. Active or recent angina or myocardial infarction.
   e. Untreated hypertension.
   f. Active liver disease.
   g. Hypersensitivity to active substances in menopausal hormone therapy.
   h. Porphyria cutanea tarda (absolute contraindication).
6. Data is lacking to support progesterone or progestin alone for treatment of hot flashes.

Other Measures

1. Vaginal lubricants to decrease vaginal dryness and dyspareunia.
2. Calcium and vitamin D supplements to prevent bone loss.

3. Nonhormonal treatment of menopausal symptoms that may be considered include SSRIs for depressive symptoms, clonidine (central alpha blocker) for vasomotor symptoms, and gabapentin for hot flashes. These therapies are supported by evidence.

4. Dietary supplements (considered natural products by consumers)—limited data is available on efficacy and safety. Patient should discuss potential benefits and risks with a health care provider.

   a. Soy products (isoflavones)—inconsistent relief of hot flashes. May cause headache, oily skin. Contraindicated as a phytoestrogen in women with strong personal or family history of hormone-dependent cancers (breast, uterine, ovarian), thromboembolic events, or cardiovascular events.

   b. Black cohosh—has demonstrated some relief of hot flashes, but has contraindications (as above) as a phytoestrogen. Nausea, hypotension, spontaneous abortion are adverse effects. No safety studies were conducted beyond 6 months, thus recommended use should not exceed 6 months.

   c. Vitamin E—400 IU daily has demonstrated minimal relief of hot flashes.

 DRUG ALERT Clinical trial data on the following commonly used herbal supplements has not demonstrated improved symptom relief over placebo: evening primrose, ginseng, dong quai, red clover.

Complications

1. Osteoporosis has been clearly linked to estrogen depletion in menopause.
2. Coronary artery disease (CAD) rarely develops in women before menopause and may be associated with the effects of estrogen depletion on blood vessels.
3. Vaginal atrophy related to a dry, estrogen-depleted epithelium increases the risk for dyspareunia, recurrent vulvovaginitis, and urinary tract infections. More research is required related to the etiology and treatment of postmenopausal stress and urge urinary incontinence.
4. Psychosocial issues of menopause: risk of depression increases.

Nursing Assessment

1. Obtain history of patient's current symptoms and menstrual cycle.
2. Obtain history for other risk factors for CAD, osteoporosis, stroke, depression, breast cancer, and uterine cancer.
3. Assess genitalia for atrophy, dryness, and elasticity.
4. Assess patient's emotional response to menopause.

Nursing Diagnoses

- (Risk for) Sexual Dysfunction related to menopausal symptoms and psychological impact of menopause.
- Readiness for Enhanced Self Health Management.

Nursing Interventions
Maintaining Sexuality Patterns

1. Explore with patient her feelings about menopause, clear up misconceptions about sexual functioning, and encourage her to discuss her feelings with her partner.
2. Tell patient that sexual functioning may decrease during menopause but may even increase because of loss of fear of pregnancy and increased time if children are grown.
3. Instruct patient how to use water-based lubricant for intercourse to decrease dryness or discuss vaginal estrogen replacement therapy.

Increasing Self Health Management

1. Provide patient with information related to estrogen replacement therapy, including dosage schedule, route, adverse effects, and what to expect of menstrual bleeding.

   a. Women who still have a uterus can expect a period at the end of every month if they take hormones cyclically. Progesterone cyclical co-therapy is indicated to prevent endometrial hyperplasia.

   b. Systemic preparations (oral, transdermal) are indicated for systemic symptoms, such as hot flashes and mood swings.

   c. Vaginal preparations are indicated for vaginal atrophy and may help to reduce recurrent UTIs.

2. Help patient to understand the risks versus benefits of menopausal hormone therapy, formulate questions, and initiate discussion with her health care provider about treatment options for vasomotor symptoms. Refer patient to clinical trial results from the Women's Health Initiative (www.nhlbi.nih.gov/whi).

Patient Education and Health Maintenance

1. Teach patient about foods that are high in calcium and vitamin D—dairy products, dark-green vegetables, salmon, and fortified foods. Encourage her to maintain weight-bearing activities several times weekly to prevent osteoporosis.
2. Counsel patient on reducing risk factors for CAD, including smoking cessation.
3. Encourage patient to keep regular medical and gynecologic follow-up visits, including all age-appropriate screenings, such as mammography, pelvic exam, DEXAscan for osteoporosis, lipid panel, and colonoscopy.
4. Advise patient that vulvovaginal infection and trauma are possible because of the dryness of the tissue and to seek prompt evaluation if pain and discharge occur or increases.
5. Encourage patients to talk to their health care providers about concerns such as breast cancer with hormonal therapy. Also refer patient for information on postmenopausal hormone therapy to *www.nhlbi.nih.gov/health/women*.
6. Encourage patients to report all use of supplements to their health care providers so they can use these preparations appropriately and safely.

GERONTOLOGIC ALERT In the postmenopausal woman, if vaginal bleeding not associated with hormone replacement occurs, encourage patient to see her health care provider immediately because cancer may be suspected.

Evaluation: Expected Outcomes

- Verbalizes confidence in sexual function and identity.
- Verbalizes satisfactory coping with menopausal symptoms and appropriate self health management behaviors..

INFECTIONS AND INFLAMMATION OF THE VULVA, VAGINA, AND CERVIX

Vulvitis

Vulvitis is inflammation of the vulva.

Pathophysiology and Etiology

Causative Factors

1. Infections—*Trichomonas*, molluscum contagiosum, bacteria, fungi, herpes simplex virus (HSV), human papilloma virus (HPV; genital warts). Also see pages 861–864.
2. Irritants.
   a. Urine, feces, vaginal discharge.
   b. Close-fitting, synthetic fabrics.
   c. Chemicals, such as laundry detergents, vaginal sprays, deodorants, perfumes, some soaps, chlorine, dryer sheets, and bubble bath.
3. Carcinoma.
4. Chronic dermatologic conditions, such as psoriasis or eczema.

Predisposing Factors

1. Illnesses, such as diabetes mellitus and dermatologic disorders.
2. Atrophy due to menopause.

Clinical Manifestations

1. Pruritus—more acute at night, aggravated by warmth, often associated with candidal infections.
2. Reddened, edematous tissue, possible ulceration.
3. Pain, burning, dyspareunia.
4. Exudate—possibly profuse and purulent—involving vaginitis.
5. Lesions of molluscum contagiosum are multiple, from 1 mm to 1 cm in size, and filled with white caseous material.
6. Lesions of HSV are vesicles with an erythematous base, clustered in a somewhat linear pattern.
7. Lesions of HPV are flesh-colored, irregular, raised, soft warty-like growths.

Diagnostic Evaluation

1. Vulvar smears and cultures—may show infectious organism.
2. Biopsy of vulvar tissue—may be necessary to rule out malignancy and chronic dermatologic conditions.

Management

1. Oral or topical anti-infectives (antibiotics, antifungals, antivirals) to treat infectious agents.
2. Extremely low-dose topical steroids to treat inflammation in some cases.
3. Vaginal estrogen to treat vaginal atrophy associated with menopause.
4. Treatment of underlying disorder.
5. Molluscum contagiosum may be treated by scalpel excision, silver nitrate, electrical cautery, or curette or may be left untreated, allowing spontaneous resolution.

Complications

1. Scarring and chronic discomfort.
2. Transmission of STD to partner.

Nursing Assessment

1. Question patient about medical history, symptoms, sexual activity.
2. Determine use of chemical-containing products on undergarments or directly on vulva.
3. Examine the genitalia and lymph nodes.

Nursing Diagnosis

- Acute Pain related to vulvar inflammation.

Nursing Interventions

Relieving Pain

1. Administer prescribed medications and instruct patient on their use, method of application, and adverse effects.
2. Instruct use of sitz baths, sitting in or over warm water for 15 to 20 minutes, three to four times daily. May also use cool compresses to soothe and clean vulva.
3. Instruct patient about nature of condition (eg, chronic recurrent or curable) and expectations for symptoms after treatment.

Patient Education and Health Maintenance

1. Teach patient hygienic principles.
   a. Wipe from front to back after voiding.
   b. Use cotton with warm water and bland soap for cleansing, rinse, and pat dry. May also use fragrance-free hypoallergenic wet wipes.
2. Teach patient to avoid chemical irritants, such as sprays, perfumed and deodorant soaps, new laundry detergents, static-control dryer sheets, and bubble bath.
3. Teach patient to avoid mechanical irritants, such as tight clothing, synthetic fabrics and undergarments; replace these with loose-fitting cotton undergarments. Avoid chronic moisture; change bathing suit after swimming.
4. Teach patient how to use sitz bath and cool compresses at home and to avoid scratching.
5. Teach patient that some infections, such as *Trichomonas*, molluscum contagiosum, and HSV, are sexually transmitted; so partner needs to seek treatment before intercourse is resumed.

BOX 22-1   Sexually Transmitted Disease Prevention Counseling

Sexually transmitted diseases can be prevented through interactive, client-centered counseling approaches that address personal risk. Key techniques to facilitate rapport include use of open-ended questions and understandable language. Most effective strategies are performed in nonjudgmental and empathetic ways, incorporating the patient's culture, language, gender, sexual orientation, age, and developmental level. Motivational interviewing techniques and assessing for readiness to change are also helpful. The first step in counseling is taking a sexual history, including:

- Type and number of partners.
- Methods for prevention of pregnancy.
- Methods for prevention of STDs.
- Past history of STDs.
- Exposure to intravenous drug use or sex workers.

An individualized prevention plan may incorporate one or more of the following specific methods of prevention:

- Abstinence from oral, vaginal, and anal sex. Encourage abstinence until beginning a mutually monogamous lifetime relationship.
- Monogamy: to be in a long-term, mutually monogamous relationship with an uninfected person. Before starting a mutually monogamous sexual relationship, individuals may consider screening for STDs.
- Reduce the number of lifetime sexual partners.
- Pre-exposure vaccination:

- HPV vaccine (ages 9–26)
- Hepatitis B vaccine (plus Hepatitis A vaccine for men who have sex with men and IV drug users)
- Proper use of male condoms (latex or polyurethane; not "natural" or "lambskin" condoms, which do not protect against viral transmission) with correct use:
  - A new condom with each new sex act.
  - Carefully handle the condom so as not to puncture it.
  - Put condom on after penis is erect.
  - Ensure adequate lubrication.
  - Use only water-based lubricants; oil-based lubricants (petroleum jelly, massage oil, cooking oils) will weaken condom.
  - Hold condom firmly at base during withdrawal to avoid slipping off.
  - Condoms with spermicidal lubricants are not recommended to prevent STDs.
- Proper use of female condoms (lubricated polyurethane or nitrile sheath with a ring on each end that is inserted into the vagina): Use as a protective barrier before intimate contact.
- Adolescents and women who use nonbarrier methods of contraception (hormones, IUDs, surgery) should be counseled about barrier methods to prevent STDs because they may incorrectly perceive that they are not at risk for STDs.
- Spermicides do not prevent STD/HIV transmission; they may increase it by disrupting normal epithelium.

 Evidence Base Centers for Disease Control and Prevention. (2010). Sexually transmitted diseases (STDs). Treatment. Available: *www.cdc.gov/std/treatment*.

Assist patient with health communication techniques to inform partner.

6. Educate about STD prevention and encourage screening (see Box 22-1).

Evaluation: Expected Outcomes

- Verbalizes increased comfort level and control of symptoms.

Bartholin Cyst or Abscess

 Evidence Base Wechter, M., Wu, J., Marzano, D., et al. (2009). Management of Barthlin duct cysts and abscesses: A systematic review. *Obstetrical and Gynecological Survey, 64*(6), 395–404.

Bartholin cyst or *abscess*, also called *bartholinitis*, is an infection of the greater vestibular gland, causing cyst or abscess formation.

Pathophysiology and Etiology

1. These glands lie on both sides of the vagina at the base of the labia minora; they lubricate the vagina.
2. If they become obstructed secondary to infection, abscess or cyst formation may occur (see Figure 22-2).

3. Abscess or cyst may spontaneously rupture or enlarge and become painful.
4. Most are sterile or abscess/cellulitis caused by mixed vaginal flora.
5. May also be caused by sexual transmission of infection (gonorrhea or chlamydia).

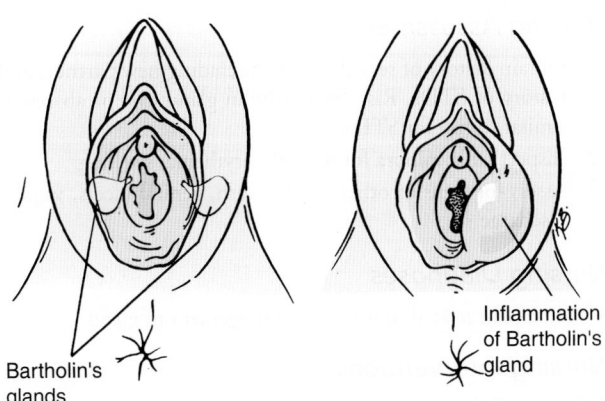

Bartholin's glands

Inflammation of Bartholin's gland

Figure 22-2. Site and infection of vestibular gland.

Clinical Manifestations

1. Asymptomatic cyst.
2. Pain, erythema, tenderness, swelling.
3. Edema, cellulitis, possible abscess formation.

Diagnostic Evaluation

1. Culture, if draining or upon excision, to identify infectious organisms.
2. If older than age 40, or recurrent, carcinoma must be ruled out by biopsy.

Management

1. May be treated conservatively with warm soaks or sitz baths if small or asymptomatic; antibiotics used if cellulitis is present.
2. May need incision and drainage; provides immediate relief, but may recur. Procedures are generally done under local anesthesia and take about 20 minutes in an outpatient office.
   a. Contents are opened and drained; culture sent. Then, sutures are closed.
      i. As an alternative, a Word catheter, Foley catheter, or Jacobi ring is inserted to keep cavity open (called fistulization).
      ii. Healing occurs around catheter and it is removed 2 to 4 weeks later to provide a new opening to the gland.
3. Marsupialization, for recurrent abscesses.
   a. Cyst is incised and sutured open to incision edges.
   b. Healing occurs from within the area of the abscess.
4. Other acceptable methods of treatment include silver nitrate gland ablation, cyst or abscess ablation or excision with a carbon dioxide laser, and needle aspiration with or without alcohol sclerotherapy.
5. Complete excision under general anesthesia if carcinoma is suspected.
6. All treatment methods heal within 2 weeks or less. Recurrence may occur in up to 20% of patients with all treatment methods. No method has been demonstrated to be superior in healing rate or recurrence rate.

Complications

Scarring from recurrent infection and rupture.

Nursing Assessment

1. Obtain history of sexual activity, including new partners and history of STDs. Risk for Bartholin gland cyst or abscess is similar to risk for STDs.
2. Inspect labia minora for warmth, erythema, swelling.
3. Assess for signs of other STDs—rash, genital ulcers, vaginal discharge.

Nursing Diagnoses

• Acute pain related to infection, enlargement of gland.

Nursing Interventions

Relieving Pain

1. Administer pain medications and antibiotics, as ordered; explain adverse effects to patient.

2. Instruct patient to apply warm soaks or to use sitz bath three to four times per day for 15 to 20 minutes to promote comfort and drainage.
3. Encourage patient to limit activity as much as possible because pain is exacerbated by activity.
4. Prepare patient for incision and drainage, if indicated. Gather supplies for procedure; assist during procedure, as necessary.
5. For marsupialization: apply ice packs intermittently for 24 hours to reduce edema and provide comfort; thereafter, warm sitz baths, a perineal heat pack, or a lamp provide comfort.

Patient Education and Health Maintenance

1. If STD is the suspected cause of infection, advise patient to instruct her partner to be tested and treated prophylactically.
2. Advise patient to abstain from intercourse until cyst or abscess has resolved, partner has been examined and treated, and patient has completed all her antibiotics (approximately 2 weeks).
3. Review principles of perineal hygiene with patient.
4. Discuss STDs and methods of prevention—abstinence, monogamy, proper use of female or male condoms. See page 855.
5. Encourage patient to follow up for recurrent abscess to rule out malignant lesions. Surgical treatment is commonly necessary for recurrences.

Evaluation: Expected Outcomes

• Verbalizes relief of pain.

Vaginal Fistula

A *vaginal fistula* is an abnormal, tortuous opening between the vagina and another hollow organ (see Figure 22-3).

Pathophysiology and Etiology

Causes

1. Obstetric injury, especially in long labors and in countries with inadequate obstetric care (rarely occurs in developed nations).
2. Pelvic surgery (rare)—hysterectomy or vaginal reconstructive procedures.

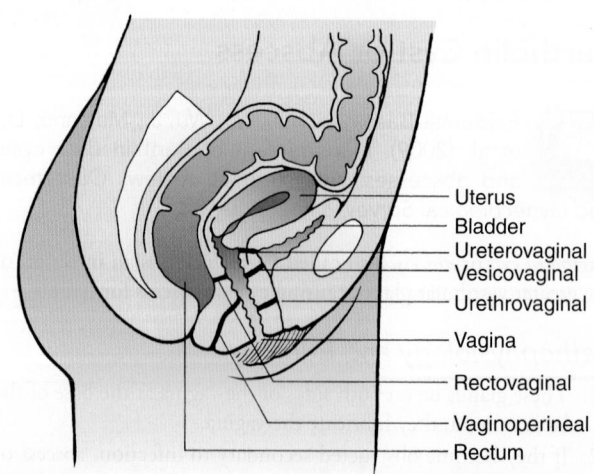

Figure 22-3. Sites of vaginal fistulas.

3. Carcinoma (rare)—extensive disease or complication of treatment such as radiation therapy.

Types

1. *Vesicovaginal* fistula is an opening between the bladder and vagina.
2. *Rectovaginal* fistula is an opening between the rectum and vagina.
3. *Ureterovaginal* fistula is an opening between the ureter and vagina.
4. *Urethrovaginal* fistula is an opening between the urethra and vagina.
5. *Vaginoperineal* fistula is an opening between the vagina and perineum.

Clinical Manifestations

1. Vesicovaginal—most common type of fistula.
   a. Constant trickling of urine into vagina.
   b. Loss of urge to void because bladder is continuously emptying.
   c. May cause excoriation and inflammation of vulva.
2. Rectovaginal.
   a. Fecal incontinence and flatus through the vagina; malodorous.
   b. May present as vulvar cancer.
3. Ureterovaginal fistula—rare.
   a. Urine in vagina but patient still voids regularly.
   b. May cause severe UTIs.
4. Urethrovaginal fistula.
   a. Dysuria.
   b. Urine in vagina on voiding.
5. Vaginoperineal fistula—pain and inflammation of perineum.

Diagnostic Evaluation

1. Methylene blue test—after instillation of this dye in bladder via catheter, place tampon in vagina. Remove after the woman has ambulated.
   a. Methylene blue appears in vagina in vesicovaginal fistula.
   b. Methylene blue does not appear in vagina in ureterovaginal fistula.
2. Indigo carmine test—after a methylene blue test shows negative results, indigo carmine is injected intravenously (IV). If dye appears in vagina, this indicates ureterovaginal fistula.
3. Cystoscopy with retrograde pyelography.
4. Intravenous pyelography (IVP)—helps to detect ureteral fistulas.

Management

1. Fistulas recognized at time of delivery should be corrected immediately.
2. Historically, surgeries were delayed for 8 to 12 weeks to allow recovery from infection or inflammation. However, early excision and repair within 1 to 2 weeks of urine leakage has become common.
3. Surgical closure of opening via vaginal route is most common in developing nations. In developed nations, laparoscopic, vaginal, or abdominal, or robot-assisted routes may be used.
4. Fecal or urinary diversion procedure may be required for large fistulas.
5. Rarely, a fistula may heal without surgical intervention.
6. Medical approach.
   a. Prosthesis to prevent incontinence and allow tissue to heal; done for patients who are not surgical candidates.
   b. Prosthesis is inserted into vagina; it is connected to drainage tubing leading to a leg bag.

Complications

1. Hydronephrosis, pyelonephritis, and possible renal failure with ureterovaginal fistula.
2. Risk for vaginal infection and pelvic organ infection from rectovaginal fistula.

Nursing Assessment

1. Obtain obstetric, gynecologic, and surgical history.
2. Monitor intake and output and voiding pattern.
3. Assess drainage on perineal pads.
4. Watch for signs of infection (fever, chills, flank pain).

Nursing Diagnoses

- Risk for Infection related to contamination of urinary tract by vaginal flora or contamination of the vagina by rectal organisms.
- Impaired Urinary Elimination related to fistula.

Nursing Interventions

Preventing Infection

1. Encourage frequent sitz baths.
2. Perform vaginal irrigation, as ordered, and teach patient the procedure.
3. Before repair surgery, administer prescribed antibiotics to reduce pathogenic flora in the intestinal tract. A single injectable dose of gentamycin before surgery is as effective as extended use of amoxicillin, chloramphenicol, or cotrimoxazole.
4. After rectovaginal repair:
   a. Maintain patient on clear liquids, as prescribed, to limit bowel activity for several days.
   b. Encourage rest.
   c. Administer warm perineal irrigations to decrease healing time and increase comfort.

Maintaining Urinary Drainage

1. Suggest the use of perineal pads or incontinence products preoperatively.
2. After vesicovaginal repair:
   a. Maintain proper drainage from indwelling catheter (intermittent flushing with sterile normal saline) to prevent pressure on newly sutured tissue (usually for about 7 days postoperatively).
   b. Administer vaginal or bladder irrigations gently because of tenderness at operative site.

c. Maintain strict intake and output records. IV fluids or copious oral fluid intake may be recommended to maintain good bladder flow.

d. Prophylactic antibiotics to prevent infection may be recommended.

3. If medical management is indicated, teach patient the use of prosthetic device.

4. Encourage patient to express feelings about her altered route of elimination and share them with a significant other.

Patient Education and Health Maintenance

1. Teach patient to report signs of infection early.

2. Teach patient to clean perineum gently and to follow surgeon's instructions on when to resume sexual intercourse and strenuous activity.

3. Advise patient to keep regular follow-up appointments.

Evaluation: Expected Outcomes

- No signs of infection—afebrile, no complaints of flank pain or difficulty voiding.
- Clear urine flows from catheter postoperatively; voids without difficulty after catheter removal.

Vaginitis

 Evidence Base Centers for Disease Control and Prevention. (2010). Sexually transmitted diseases treatment guidelines. Available: *www.cdc.gov/std/treatment*.

Vaginitis is inflammation of the vagina caused by infectious pathogens.

Pathophysiology and Etiology

1. May be caused by sexually transmitted organisms or overgrowth of vaginal flora.

2. Normal vaginal secretions because of estrogen secretion and acidity inhibit the growth of pathogens.

3. Such conditions as diabetes, pregnancy, stress, coitus, and menopause alter normal vaginal environment.

4. Types of vaginitis (see Table 22-3).
   a. Simple (contact).
   b. Bacterial vaginosis (most often caused by *Gardnerella*).
   c. *Trichomonas*.
   d. *Candida albicans*.
   f. Atrophic.

Table 22-3	Types of Vaginitis	
DESCRIPTION	**MANIFESTATIONS**	**MANAGEMENT**
Simple Vaginitis (Contact Vaginitis)		
• An inflammation of the vagina, with discharge; due to mechanical, chemical, allergic, or other noninfectious irritation, poor hygiene, imbalance in vaginal flora. • Urethritis commonly accompanies vaginitis because of the proximity of the urethra to the vagina. • Predisposing factors: contact allergens, excessive perspiration, synthetic underclothing, poor hygiene, foreign bodies (tampons, condoms, spermicides, condoms with spermicides, diaphragms that have been left in too long).	• Increased (yet minimal) vaginal discharge with itching, redness, burning, and edema. • Voiding and defecation aggravate the above symptoms.	• Stimulate the growth of lactobacilli (Döderlein's bacilli) through consumption of yogurt with live active cultures. • Current evidence does not support douching. • Foster cleanliness by meticulous care after voiding and defecation. • Discontinue use of causative agent.
Bacterial Vaginosis		
• An inflammation of the vagina commonly referred to as nonspecific vaginitis because it is *not* caused by *Trichomonas*, *Candida*, or gonorrhea. It is not considered an STD. • Increased levels of *Gardnerella vaginalis* are usually responsible for symptoms.	• Vaginal discharge with odor. • Itching and burning may suggest concomitant organisms present. • It is benign in that when the discharge is wiped away, underlying tissue is healthy and pink. • Vaginal pH is >4.5. • May be asymptomatic. • Presence of "clue" cells on microscopic examination of saline slide. • Positive KOH "whiff" test (fishy odor).	• Treatment only recommended for symptomatic women. • Metronidazole taken orally for 7 days or topical clindamycin or metronidazole. • Alcohol intake should be avoided during Flagyl treatment and for 24 hours after completion to avoid nausea and vertigo. Studies have demonstrated that metronidazole is not teratogenic. • Treating partners is not recommended. • Clindamycin cream weakens latex condoms. • Data does not support douching.

Table 22-3 Types of Vaginitis

DESCRIPTION	MANIFESTATIONS	MANAGEMENT
Trichomonas Vaginalis		
• STD. A condition produced by a protozoan (pear-shaped and motile) that thrives in an alkaline environment. Recurrence may occur due to low levels of antimicrobial resistance.	• Copious malodorous discharge; may be frothy and yellow-green in color. • May have pruritus, dyspareunia, and spotting. • Red, speckled (strawberry) punctate hemorrhages on the cervix. • May also have vulvar edema, dysuria, and hyperemia secondary to irritation of discharge. • Motile organisms visible on saline microscopy. • Point of care rapid test and cultures are available.	• Destroy infective protozoa by taking oral metronidazole 2 g or tinidazole 2 g. • *Note:* Treatment during pregnancy is acceptable. • Prevent reinfection by treating partner concurrently, even though male may be asymptomatic. • Avoid alcohol during treatment. • Rescreen after three months due to possibility of low-level antimicrobial resistance.
Candida Albicans		

• A fungal infection caused by *Candida albicans.* Associated factors include:
  • Steroid therapy
  • Obesity
  • Pregnancy
  • Antibiotic therapy
  • Diabetes mellitus
  • Oral contraceptives
  • Frequent douching
  • Chronic debilitative diseases
• Characteristics
  • *C. albicans* is a normal inhabitant of the intestinal tract and therefore a frequent contaminant of the vagina.
  • Because this fungus thrives in an environment rich in carbohydrates, it is seen commonly in patients with poorly controlled diabetes.
  • This infection is observed in patients who have been on antibiotic or steroid therapy for a while (reduces natural protective organisms in vagina).
	• Vaginal discharge is thick and irritating; white or yellow patchy, cheese like particles adhere to vaginal walls.
	• Itching is the most common complaint.
	• May also experience burning, soreness, vulvar edema, excoriations, fissures, dyspareunia, frequency, and dysuria.
	• Microscopic examination will reveal hyphae, buds, pseudohyphae.
	• Vaginal pH is normal (<4.5).
		• Eradicate the fungus by applying antifungal vaginal cream (clotrimazole, miconazole, or ketoconazole), suppository, or tablet for 1–14 nights, as ordered; or take oral fluconazole in single dose.
		• Oral fluconazole is contraindicated in pregnancy; topical creams may be used.
		• Side effects of topical vaginal creams include burning and irritation. Systemic fluconazole is associated with GI intolerance, headaches, and rare and transitory elevations in liver function tests.
		• Azole antifungals have clinically important interactions with many medications.
		• Incorporate live-culture yogurt into diet to enhance lactobacillus colonization and improve microorganism balance in vagina.
		• Treat the symptomatic or uncircumcised partner with balanitis by applying antifungal cream under the foreskin nightly for 7 nights.
		• For severe or recurrent cases, use systemic antifungal, such as weekly fluconazole for suppression therapy.

Atrophic Vaginitis		
• A common postmenopausal occurrence due to atrophy of the vaginal mucosa secondary to decreased estrogen levels; more susceptible to infection.	• Vaginal itching, dryness, burning, dyspareunia, and vulvar irritation. • May also have vaginal bleeding. • Vaginal mucosa appears dry and slightly paler. 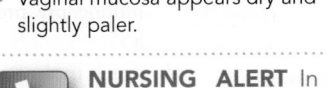 **NURSING ALERT** In the postmenopausal woman, if vaginal bleeding occurs, encourage patient to see her health care provider immediately because bleeding is a warning sign of cancer.	• Vaginal estrogen treatment is most effective. • The condition reverses itself under treatment, which must be maintained. • If infection is also present, this is treated. • If uterus is intact and systemic estrogen therapy is used to treat additional menopausal symptoms, progesterone must be added to prevent endometrial hyperplasia due to unopposed estrogen.

STD, sexually transmitted disease.

Clinical Manifestations

Signs and symptoms vary with etiology or causative organism.

1. Vaginal itching, irritation, burning.
2. Odor, increased or unusual vaginal discharge.
3. Dyspareunia, pelvic pain, dysuria.
4. Asymptomatic.

Diagnostic Evaluation

1. History and physical examination.
2. Wet smear for microscopic examination.
   a. Saline slide: discharge mixed with saline; useful in detecting *Gardnerella* and *Trichomonas* organisms.
   b. Potassium hydroxide (KOH): useful in detecting *C. albicans*. Whiff test: if fishy odor is noted when KOH is applied, suspect *Gardnerella* organisms causing bacterial vaginosis.
3. Vaginal pH (not diagnostic, but may indicate infection)—use Nitrazine paper.
   a. Normal pH: 4.0 to 4.5.
   b. Bacterial vaginosis: >4.5.
   c. *Trichomonas*: >4.5.
4. Chlamydia and gonorrhea cultures or DNA probe—to rule out chlamydia or gonorrhea cervicitis.
5. Pap smear—not considered a diagnostic tool for vaginitis: it has low sensitivity and specificity to detect bacterial vaginosis and *Trichomonas*.

Management

1. Anti-infectives (oral or vaginal preparations).
2. Estrogen replacement (systemic or vaginal preparation) for atrophic vaginitis.
3. Evaluation and treatment of sexual partners for STDs, such as *Trichomonas*.
4. Vaginal recolonization with lactobacilli through ingestion of yogurt with active cultures.

Nursing Assessment

1. Obtain a health history including questions specific to the condition.
   a. Nature of discharge: cheese-like, frothy, pus-like, thick or thin, scant? Onset? Color? Odor? Other symptoms: dysuria, itching, dyspareunia?
   b. Menstrual history.
   c. Disease history: diabetes mellitus and its control? Previous vaginal infections? STDs?
   d. Obstetric history.
   e. Sexual history: age of onset of sexual activity? Numbers of current and lifetime partners? Frequency of sexual activity? Its nature? Urogenital symptoms or infections in partner? Current barrier use?
   f. Medications, allergies. Current contraceptive use?
   g. Vaginal hygiene: use of douches, deodorants, sprays, ointments; types of tampons, bubble bath, shower/bath soap, nature of clothing (tight-fitting)?

2. Perform a physical examination, including a vaginal examination, and obtain vaginal and/or cervical discharge specimens, as indicated.

Nursing Diagnoses

- Acute or Chronic Pain related to vaginal irritation.
- Impaired Tissue Integrity related to vaginal infection.
- Risk prone health behavior related to sexual activity and transmission of infection.

Nursing Interventions

Relieving Pain

1. Instruct patient to discontinue use of irritating agents, such as bubble baths and vaginal douches.
2. Suggest patient take cool baths or sitz baths and pat dry or dry with hair dryer on low setting.
3. Encourage patient to wear loose cotton undergarments.
4. Encourage patient to take analgesics.
5. Provide emotional support.

Restoring Tissue Integrity

1. Teach patient to clean perineum and pat dry before applying medication.
2. Demonstrate application of prescribed medication.
3. Emphasize importance of taking prescribed medication for full length of therapy and as directed; teach patient adverse effects.
4. Stress importance of follow-up visits.

Reducing Risk

1. Emphasize importance of sexual abstinence and vaginal rest (nothing in vagina) until therapy is complete and sexual partner has been treated, if indicated.
2. Tell patient use of condoms may be protective but may produce irritation.
3. Instruct patient in the use of water-soluble lubricant if vagina is dry and atrophic.
4. Instruct patient that some oil-based vaginal medications may decrease the efficacy of condoms to protect against STDs and pregnancy.

Patient Education and Health Maintenance

1. Teach causes of vaginitis and its symptoms so patient can seek treatment promptly.
2. Discuss STDs and methods of prevention—abstinence, monogamy, proper use of female or male condoms. See page 855.
3. Teach measures to prevent vaginitis.
   a. Wipe from front to back after toilet use.
   b. Keep area clean and dry.
   c. Wear loose cotton clothing to absorb moisture and provide good circulation.
   d. Change sanitary pads, tampons frequently so they do not become saturated.
   e. Avoid bubble baths, vaginal deodorants, sprays, and douches.

f. If patient insists on using douches (not recommended), use a mild vinegar solution (2 teaspoons white vinegar to 1 quart water) at the end of a menstrual cycle. Teach proper technique: to infuse gently to lightly bathe tissues; to avoid using a forceful stream that could push bacteria higher inside pelvis.

4. For recurrent *Candida* infections, encourage good control if patient has diabetes or encourage patient to be tested for diabetes. Teach all patients to eliminate concentrated carbohydrates from diet to prevent recurrence.

Evaluation: Expected Outcomes

- Verbalizes relief of pain.
- Vaginal mucosa pink, with normal amount and color of secretions.
- Reports practice of prevention methods.

Human Papillomavirus Infection

Evidence Base Centers for Disease Control and Prevention. (2010). Sexually transmitted diseases treatment guidelines. Available: *www.cdc.gov/std/treatment*.

Human papillomavirus (HPV) infection may be asymptomatic but frequently causes *Condyloma acuminatum* or genital warts.

Pathophysiology and Etiology

1. Sexually transmitted; highly contagious.
2. More than 40 types of HPV can infect the genital tract, many are asymptomatic, and multiple types may coexist.
3. Ninety percent of visible genital warts are caused by HPV types 6 and 11.
4. Other types (16, 18, 31, 33, 35) have been strongly associated with cervical neoplasia.
5. Incubation period of up to 8 months.

Clinical Manifestations

1. Single or multiple soft, fleshy painless growths of the vulva, vagina, cervix, urethra, or anal area that may be irritating or uncomfortable (see Figure 22-4).
2. May be subclinical infection and still contagious.
3. Occasional vaginal bleeding, discharge, odor, and dyspareunia.

Diagnostic Evaluation

1. Pap smear—shows characteristic cellular changes (koilocytosis).
2. Acetic acid swabbing on vaginal examination will whiten lesions and make them more identifiable in genital mucosa. However, this test is not specific to HPV and is not recommended for screening.
3. Viral DNA tests to detect subclinical cases; however, the significance of positive and negative results has not been determined. HPV testing can be done from a liquid Pap smear cervical cancer screening for women older than

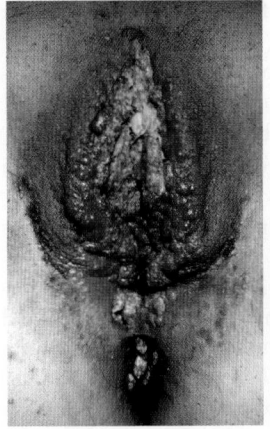
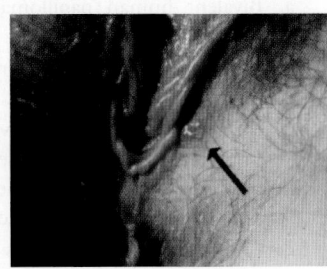

A   **B**

Figure 22-4. Genital lesions. (A) Condyloma acuminatum. **(B)** Genital herpes.

30 years, if the Pap smear is abnormal (known as reflex testing), to confirm the presence of HPV causing cellular changes on cervix. HPV testing is not recommended for genital wart diagnosis.
4. Colposcopy is also used to diagnose subclinical HPV infection.
5. Anoscopy or urethroscopy may be necessary to identify anal and urethral lesions.
6. Genital warts are usually diagnosed on physical exam through visual inspection.

Management

Therapies are likely to reduce HPV infectivity but do not eradicate HPV. Treatment method is guided by provider and patient preferences.

1. External lesions may be treated by patient with multiple applications of a topical preparation.
   a. Podofilox—applied with cotton swab or finger to visible warts twice per day for 3 days, then no treatment for 4 days; may be repeated for up to four cycles of therapy.
   b. Imiquimod—applied by finger three times per week for up to 16 weeks; may be washed off 6 to 10 hours after application.
   c. Sinecatechins ointment—applied by finger three times daily for up to 16 weeks; not washed off after use.
   d. Safety of these products during pregnancy is unknown and therefore is not recommended.
2. Noncervical lesions may be treated by health care provider with topical preparations, such as podophyllin resin, trichloroacetic acid, or bichloroacetic acid.
   a. Requires multiple visits for repeat treatments.
   b. May require washing off several hours later.
3. Cryotherapy with liquid nitrogen or cryoprobe, electrocautery, laser treatment, or local excision of large warts or cervical lesions.

4. Highly recurrent, particularly in first 3 months—may require retreatment.

5. Subclinical genital HPV infection typically clears spontaneously and treatment is not recommended.

6. Two vaccines for HPV are available in the United States.

   a. Bivalent human papillomavirus vaccine types 16, 18; recombinant.

   b. Quadrivalent vaccine human papillomavirus vaccine types 6, 11, 16, 18; recombinant.

   c. Both HPV vaccines are given as a series of three injections over 6 months. The Centers for Disease Control and Prevention (CDC) recommends both vaccines for females ages 11 or 12 to 26 (licensed for ages 9 to 26).

   d. The quadrivalent vaccine is recommended for males ages 11 or 12 to 26 (licensed for ages 9 to 26).

   e. They are effective when all doses are administered before onset of sexual activity.

Complications

1. Implicated in cervical intraepithelial neoplasia.
2. May cause neonatal laryngeal papillomatosis if infant born through infected birth canal.
3. Obstruction of anal canal, vagina by enlarging lesions.
4. Scarring and pigment changes if treatment not employed properly.

Nursing Assessment

1. Obtain history of STDs, Pap test results, sexual partners.
2. Inspect external genitalia for lesions, perform vaginal examination.

Nursing Diagnosis

• Disturbed Body Image related to genital warts.

Nursing Interventions

Improving Body Image

1. Explain to patient that the goal of therapy is to remove visible lesions; however, HPV will not be cured or eliminated. Genital warts are not life-threatening.

2. Encourage patient to comply with treatment schedule and inspect areas for resolution of lesions or redevelopment of new lesions.

3. Advise patient of high recurrence rate; 3-month follow-up visit is advisable; if lesions redevelop, patient should follow up for retreatment.

4. Advise patient about proper use of male or female condoms to reduce the risk of transmission, although not fully because HPV can infect areas not covered by the condom. Condom use, abstinence, and monogamy will protect against other STDs.

5. Encourage female patients to follow up regularly for Pap tests because HPV has been associated with cervical neoplasia.

6. Advise patient of risk to neonate during delivery; patient should receive close prenatal care if pregnant.

Patient Education and Health Maintenance

1. Advise patient to discuss HPV with her partner. He should receive treatment for visible lesions. Screening for other STDs in both patient and partner is recommended.

2. Make sure patient realizes that even though lesions may be gone, she may still transmit HPV to new sexual partners. Abstinence, monogamy, and condoms are advisable to prevent transmission of all STDs. See page 855.

Evaluation: Expected Outcomes

• Presents with no visible lesions at follow-up visit.

Herpes Genitalis

 Evidence Base Centers for Disease Control and Prevention. (2010). Sexually transmitted diseases treatment guidelines. Available: *www.cdc.gov/std/treatment.*

Herpes genitalis is a viral infection that causes lesions of the cervix, vagina, and external genitalia.

Pathophysiology and Etiology

1. Caused by HSV, usually type 2, but may be type 1.
2. Sexually transmitted.
3. An estimated 50 million people are infected in the United States.
4. Recurrent infection; virus lies dormant in dorsal root ganglia of spinal nerves between outbreaks.

Clinical Manifestations

1. Lesions occur 2 to 30 days after initial exposure, sometimes with fever, malaise, lymphadenopathy, and headache for primary infection (see Figure 22-4, page 861).

2. Lesions are preceded by sensation of tingling; proceed from vesicles on erythematous, edematous base to painful ulcers that crust and heal without scars.

3. Internal lesions may cause watery discharge, dyspareunia.

4. Recurrent lesions may be stimulated by fever, stress, illness, local trauma, menses, sunburn.

5. Infection can be asymptomatic.

Diagnostic Evaluation

1. PCR assay for HSV DNA and viral culture are preferred tests. Failure to detect HSV by PCR or culture does not rule out HSV infection because viral shedding is intermittent.

2. Pap smear and Tzanck smear are neither sensitive nor specific for HSV and therefore not recommended.

3. Type-specific glycoprotein G (gG) serological tests—to detect HSV-1 or HSV-2 antibodies in the following cases: recurrent or atypical genital symptoms with negative viral culture; clinical diagnosis of genital herpes without laboratory confirmation; partner with genital herpes; persons presenting for STD evaluation; persons with HIV.

4. Screening in the general population for HSV-1 and HSV-2 is not recommended.

Management

1. Systemic antivirals, such as acyclovir, famciclovir, and valacyclovir, suppress virus and decrease length, severity, and shedding of infection.
   a. Oral therapy may be episodic—started as soon as the first episode is diagnosed and, whenever the first signs of a recurrence are recognized (within 24 hours of onset of prodromal symptoms or lesion onset).
   b. Oral therapy may be given continuously to suppress recurrences and viral shedding, which reduces transmission, especially within the first 12 months of disease onset.
   c. IV administration (acyclovir) may be necessary for severe infections (disseminated infections, pneumonitis, hepatitis, meningoencephalitis) or for immunocompromised patients.
   d. Topical treatment (acyclovir) is the least effective and not recommended.

2. Pain medication—ranges from acetaminophen and NSAID drugs to oral opioids.

3. Local comfort measures, such as lidocaine gel, sitz baths, compresses, and use of a hair dryer to area on cool setting.

4. Immunization has been under investigation See *www .clinicaltrials.gov.*

Complications

1. Disseminated infection, meningitis, pneumonitis, hepatitis.
2. Neonatal infection if neonate born through infected canal.

Nursing Assessment

1. Question patient about frequency and type of sexual activity and discomfort noted.
2. Question patient about pruritus, burning, tenderness, urinary symptoms, unusual discharge.
3. Assess patient's view of herpes, transmission, stigmas, misconceptions, fears.
4. Inspect genitalia for lesions, erythema, edema. Use speculum to examine vagina and cervix, as indicated.

Nursing Diagnoses

- Acute Pain related to HSV outbreak.
- Impaired Skin Integrity related to herpetic lesions.
- Anxiety related to stigma attached to herpes.
- Sexual Dysfunction related to potential transmission of herpes.

Nursing Interventions

Relieving Pain

1. Demonstrate and encourage the use of warm sitz baths to increase blood supply to the areas and facilitate healing.
2. Instruct patient to keep the area clean and dry. Pat dry with a clean towel or use blow dryer on cool setting. Wear loose cotton undergarments and loose clothing.
3. Encourage bed rest if case is severe.
4. Administer pain medications, as prescribed.
5. Encourage patient to void in a warm sitz bath if urination is painful.
6. Insert indwelling catheter if urination is extremely painful or if retention occurs.
7. Encourage fluid intake.

Restoring Skin Integrity

1. Administer antiviral agent and teach patient proper use and adverse effects.
2. Keep lesions clean and dry.
3. Teach patient not to rub or to scratch lesions.

Relieving Anxiety

1. Explore with patient her feelings about herpes and its effects on relationships.
2. Reiterate that when patient is feeling better physically, her feelings about herself will improve.
3. Encourage patient to discuss antiviral suppressive therapy to reduce the risk of transmission and to reduce frequency and duration of recurrent outbreaks.
4. Discuss effects of stress on future outbreaks. Assist patient to identify stressors in her life and how to cope with them. Review stress-reduction methods, such as relaxation, breathing, and imagery.
5. Encourage patient to discuss her feelings with family and significant others.
6. Refer patient to support groups, such as the American Social Health Association (*www.ashastd.org* or 919-361-8488).

Restoring Satisfying Sexual Function

1. Teach patient to avoid intercourse from first sign of active outbreak (often a tingling sensation) to resolution of lesions (at least 2 weeks after primary infection, approximately 1 week after recurrent outbreaks).
2. Teach patient that shedding of virus through genital secretions is possible even during asymptomatic period, so partner must be notified.
3. Inform patient that she and partner should use condoms for intercourse, but condoms may not be fully protective. Encourage patient to discuss suppressive antiviral therapy with her health care provider.
4. Explore possibility of noncoital aspects of sexual relationship.
5. Teach patient that virus may be spread through the genital–oral route.

Patient Education and Health Maintenance

1. Inform patient that initial outbreak is usually more painful than recurrent outbreaks and that outbreaks vary from monthly to only a few times per year.
2. Teach patient to recognize precipitating factors and change lifestyle to prevent potential triggers, if possible.
3. Remind patient of the effects on a neonate and the importance of notifying her health care provider if she becomes pregnant.
4. Instruct patient in methods to decrease risk of sexual transmission: abstinence, monogamy, male or female condom use, antiviral suppressive therapy. See patient page 855. The patient must inform partner of the risk of transmission to a potential sexual partner before any intimate contact. Viral shedding is highest during the prodromal and active lesion stages.
5. Tell patient that oral lesions can occur with HSV-2 because of transmission by oral intercourse, but that most oral cold sores are caused by HSV-1 infection.
6. Refer patient to support groups, such as the American Social Health Association (*www.ashastd.org* or 800-227-8922).

Evaluation: Expected Outcomes

- Verbalizes decreased pain.
- Skin intact, without signs of secondary infection, scarring.
- Verbalizes reduced anxiety and more confidence.
- Reports satisfying sexual activity.

Chlamydial Infection

 Evidence Base Centers for Disease Control and Prevention. (2010). Sexually transmitted diseases treatment guidelines. Available: *www.cdc.gov/std/treatment*.

Chlamydia infection is the most common STD that occurs in women and men, particularly in adolescents and young adults. Women are asymptomatic or present with cervicitis; men are commonly asymptomatic but may present with urethritis.

Pathophysiology and Etiology

1. Chlamydia infection in women is the result of sexual intercourse, with infection entering the vagina, infecting the cervix and, possibly, spreading up through the endometrium and fallopian tubes.
2. Adolescents and young women ages 15 to 24 are at highest risk for infection, possibly because of susceptibility of cervical tissue to the organism and higher-risk sexual behaviors in this age group.
3. *C. trachomatis* is the most common sexually transmitted pathogen in men and women in the United States, with an incidence of more than 347.8 cases per 100,000 people.

Clinical Manifestations

1. May be asymptomatic or have vaginal discharge—may be clear mucoid to creamy discharge.
2. May have dysuria and mild pelvic discomfort.
3. Cervix may be covered by thick mucopurulent discharge and be tender, erythematous, edematous, and friable.

Diagnostic Evaluation

1. Cervical swab specimen or urine sample (DNA amplification method, also known as nucleic acid amplification test [NAAT])—most sensitive and specific test.
2. Chlamydia culture from cervical exudate and cervical mucosa.
3. The CDC recommends annual screening for all sexually active women younger than age 25 and for older women at high risk (multiple sex partners or new partner).

Management

1. Antibiotic regimens include:
   a. Azithromycin 1 g orally in a single dose.
   b. Doxycycline 100 mg orally twice per day for 7 days.
   c. Alternatives include erythromycin, levofloxacin, or ofloxacin.
2. Current and/or most recent sexual partners (during 60 days or more preceding onset) should be tested and treated despite test results.

 NURSING ALERT Because chlamydia infection and gonorrhea frequently coexist, especially in adolescents and young adults, treatment of both STDs is recommended.

Complications

1. PID.
2. Ectopic pregnancy or infertility secondary to untreated or recurrent PID.
3. Transmission to neonate born through infected birth canal.

Nursing Assessment

1. Obtain history of sexual activity and symptoms or infections in partner.
2. Perform abdominal and pelvic examination for tenderness caused by possible spread to pelvic organs.

Nursing Diagnosis

- Risk for Infection related to sexual activity.

Nursing Interventions

Preventing Infection Transmission

1. Advise abstinence from sexual intercourse until 7 days after treatment has been completed.
2. Ensure that partner is treated at the same time; recent partners should receive treatment despite lack of symptoms and negative chlamydia test result. Abstinence should continue until 7 days after partners have completed treatment.
3. Report case to local public health department (chlamydia is a reportable infectious disease in most of the United States).
4. Ensure that patient begins treatment and will have access to prescription and transportation for follow-up. Single-dose azithromycin as directly observed therapy is often a good choice for patients with limited access to healthcare resources.
5. Retesting for chlamydia is recommended 3 months after treatment to detect reinfection, particularly in adolescents and young women.

Patient Education and Health Maintenance

1. Teach about all STDs, mode of transmission, symptoms, and complications. Clarify misconceptions.
2. Explain the treatment regimen to patient and advise her of adverse effects and the importance of informing her partner about the need for treatment.
3. Discuss STDs and methods of prevention—abstinence, monogamy, proper use of female or male condoms. See page 855.
4. Stress the importance of follow-up examination and retesting. Recurrence rates are highest in younger patients.
5. Encourage screening periodically for at-risk women.
6. For further information on STDs, refer patients to such agencies as the American Social Health Association (*www.ashastd. org* or 800-227-8922).

Evaluation: Expected Outcomes

- Returns for follow-up; states complied with abstinence during treatment of self and partner; verbalizes use of measures to prevent STD transmission.

Gonorrhea

 Evidence Base Centers for Disease Control and Prevention. (2010). Sexually transmitted diseases treatment guidelines. Available: *www.cdc.gov/std/ treatment.*

Gonorrhea is a common STD that affects men and women, causing cervicitis in women and urethritis in men. In women it can easily ascend to the uterus and fallopian tubes, if untreated.

Pathophysiology and Etiology

1. Gonorrhea is caused by the Gram-positive diplococci *Neisseria gonorrhoeae*.
2. Infection occurs through sexual transmission, causing cervicitis in women and possible conjunctivitis, pharyngitis, and proctitis.
3. Untreated infection may lead to PID, generalized dissemination, or gonococcal arthritis.
4. Approximately 700,000 new gonococcal infections arise in the United States each year; teens and young adults are most commonly affected.

Clinical Manifestations

1. Frequently asymptomatic in women.
2. May cause mucopurulent vaginal discharge or a painful burning sensation when urinating.
3. Vaginal speculum examination may reveal cervical discharge and inflammation.
4. Cervical motion tenderness and tender pelvic organs on bimanual examination if infection has begun to ascend.

Diagnostic Evaluation

1. DNA testing (or nucleic acid hybridization tests or NAATs) of cervical swab, vaginal swab, urine, or male urethral swab (most sensitive and specific; can be done simultaneously for chlamydia).
2. Endocervical culture should be performed in order to provide antimicrobial susceptibility results.
3. Pharyngeal or conjunctival secretions can be tested if pharyngitis or conjunctivitis is suspected. Follow laboratory specifications for these tests.
4. Joint aspiration and blood cultures may be necessary if disseminated infection is suspected.

Management

1. Uncomplicated gonococcal infection of the cervix, urethra (in men), or rectum (in men or women) can be treated with a single-dose antibiotic, such as the following (plus treatment for coinfection with chlamydia):
   a. Cefixime 400 mg orally.
   b. Ceftriaxone 250 mg I.M.
   c. Alternative regimens involving other cephalosporins are also approved.
2. Pharyngeal infections should be treated for coinfection with chlamydia with the following:
   a. Ceftriaxone 250 mg I.M. single dose *plus*
   b. Azithromycin 1 g orally single dose or doxycycline 100 mg orally twice daily × 7 days.
3. Gonococcal conjunctivitis should be treated with ceftriaxone 1 gm I.M. single dose plus concomitant chlamydial treatment.
3. Disseminated infections require IV or I.M. therapy, such as:
   a. Ceftriaxone 1 g I.M. or IV every 24 hours.
   b. Cefotaxime 1 g IV every 8 hours.
   c. Ceftizoxime 1 g IV every 8 hours.
4. For IV or I.M. therapy, patient is switched to oral therapy 24 to 48 hours after improvement, then takes cefixime 400 mg orally twice daily to complete 7 days of antimicrobial therapy.
5. In all cases of suspected gonorrhea, concomitant treatment of chlamydia is recommended with appropriate second antibiotic agent.

 DRUG ALERT Fluoroquinolone therapy is no longer recommended for treatment of gonorrhea in the United States due to resistance.

Complications

1. PID, ectopic pregnancy, and infertility.
2. Disseminated infection.
3. Ophthalmia neonatorum and sepsis (rare) caused by infant born through infected birth canal.

Nursing Assessment

1. Question patient on history of STDs, STD protection, sexual activity, usual women's health self-care practices.
2. Obtain history of symptoms in patient and partner—incubation period is usually 3 to 7 days in men, but symptoms are typically overlooked in women.

3. Assess for ability to change lifestyle practices that may have led to STD.

Nursing Diagnosis

• Risk for Infection related to sexual activity.

Nursing Interventions

Stopping Transmission of STD

1. Administer antibiotics, as prescribed, explaining adverse effects to patient.
2. Make sure that patient can obtain prescription medication at discharge.
3. Monitor for relief of pain, discharge, and other symptoms.
4. Explain importance of sexual abstinence until symptoms are resolved completely and until 7 days after therapy is complete in patient and partner.
5. Report to public health department and tell patient that information will be obtained to ensure testing of sexual contacts.

Patient Education and Health Maintenance

1. Teach patient about all possible STDs, their prevalence, and their mode of transmission. Clarify misconceptions.
2. Advise patient of complications of gonorrhea and chlamydia.
3. Discuss STDs and methods of prevention—abstinence, monogamy, proper use of female or male condoms. See page 855.
4. Stress the importance of follow-up examination and testing to ensure eradication of infection. Encourage follow-up for routine women's health care and periodic STD screening.
5. For additional information, refer to the American Social Health Association (*www.ashastd.org*) or Centers for Disease Control and Prevention (*www.cdc.gov/std/default.htm*).

Evaluation: Expected Outcomes

• Reports resolution of symptoms and use of condoms, abstinence, or other prevention measures at follow-up visit.

PROBLEMS RESULTING FROM RELAXED PELVIC MUSCLES

Pelvic Organ Prolapse Cystocele and Urethrocele

Cystocele is a downward displacement (protrusion) of the bladder into the vagina (see Figure 22-5). *Urethrocele* is downward displacement of the urethra into the vagina.

Pathophysiology and Etiology

1. Associated with obstetric trauma to fascia, muscle, and ligaments during childbirth (results in poor support).
2. Typically becomes apparent years later, when genital atrophy associated with aging occurs.
3. May also be caused by congenital defect or may appear after hysterectomy.

Clinical Manifestations

1. May be asymptomatic in early stages.
2. Pelvic pressure or heaviness, backache, nervousness, fatigue.
3. Urinary symptoms—urgency, frequency, incontinence, incomplete emptying.
4. Aggravated by coughing, sneezing, standing for long periods, and obesity, which increase intra-abdominal pressure.
5. Relieved by resting or by lying down.

Diagnostic Evaluation

1. Pelvic examination identifies condition.
2. Urinalysis and culture are done to rule out infection.

Management

1. Vaginal pessary—silicone (can be latex or polycarbonate) device inserted into vagina as temporary treatment to support pelvic organs.
   a. Prolonged use may lead to necrosis and ulceration.
   b. Should be removed and cleaned at least once weekly.
2. Estrogen therapy after menopause to decrease genital atrophy.
3. Pelvic floor muscle exercises to improve symptoms.

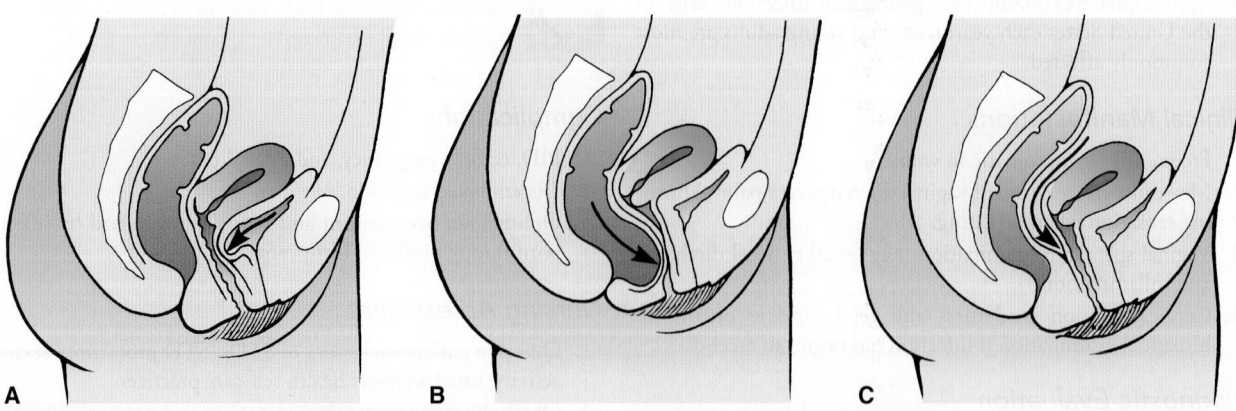

Figure 22-5. Pelvic support disorders. (A) Cystocele. **(B)** Rectocele. **(C)** Enterocele.

4. Surgery—if cystocele is large and interferes with bladder functioning.
   a. May do anterior vaginal colporrhaphy (repair of anterior vaginal wall).
   b. Complications of surgery include urinary retention, bleeding (requires vaginal packing).

Complications

Urinary incontinence and infection.

Nursing Assessment

1. Obtain history of obstetric trauma, abdominal surgery, menopause, use of estrogen.
2. Ask about urinary symptoms, pain.
3. Observe perineum while patient bears down or is in upright position for bulge from vagina.

Nursing Diagnoses

- Acute Pain related to pelvic pressure.
- Stress Urinary Incontinence related to relaxed pelvic muscles, displaced organs.
- Urinary Retention related to displaced organs.

Nursing Interventions

Relieving Pain
1. Encourage periods of rest with legs elevated to relieve strain on pelvis.
2. Advise use of mild analgesics, as necessary.
3. Provide postoperative care.
   a. Encourage voiding every 4 to 8 hours to reduce pressure so that no more than 150 mL will accumulate in bladder—intermittent catheterization or use of an indwelling catheter may be required.
   b. Administer perineal care to patient after each voiding and defecation.
   c. Use available sprays for anesthetic and antiseptic effects.
   d. Apply an ice pack locally to relieve congestion and discomfort.
   e. Administer analgesics, as prescribed, for relief of pain.

Controlling Incontinence
1. Teach patient Kegel pelvic floor exercises to regain muscle tone.
   a. Practice while voiding by stopping the flow of urine for 3 to 5 seconds, then releasing for 5 seconds.
   b. Patient can tighten pelvic floor muscle at any time, repeat 10 times, three times per day, increase as able.
2. Encourage patient to void frequently, respond to the urge to void promptly.
3. Warn patient to avoid straining to prevent incontinence.

Preventing Urinary Retention
1. Encourage fluids to decrease bacterial flora in the bladder.
2. Catheterize patient if retention is suspected.
3. Obtain urine specimen for culture and sensitivity if infection is suspected.

Patient Education and Health Maintenance

1. Teach women to avoid straining, remain active, avoid obesity, and perform Kegel exercises to minimize pelvic relaxation in their older years.
2. Encourage prompt attention to symptoms of UTI—dysuria urgency, frequency, foul-smelling urine.

Evaluation: Expected Outcomes

- Verbalizes reduced pain.
- Reports decreased frequency of incontinence.
- Voids regularly without symptoms of infection.

Rectocele and Enterocele

Rectocele is displacement (protrusion) of the rectum into the vagina. *Enterocele* is displacement of intestine into the vagina (see Figure 22-5).

Pathophysiology and Etiology

1. Posterior vaginal wall becomes weakened, allowing displacement.
2. Weakening caused by obstetric trauma, childbirth, pelvic surgery, aging.

Clinical Manifestations

1. Pelvic pressure or heaviness, backache, perineal burning.
2. Constipation—may have difficulty in fecal evacuation; patient may use fingers in vagina to push feces up so defecation may occur.
3. Incontinence of feces and flatus—if tear between rectum and vagina.
4. Visible protrusion into vagina.
5. Symptoms are aggravated by standing for long periods.

Diagnostic Evaluation

1. Vaginal examination reveals condition.
2. May use Sims speculum to uplift cervix and fully evaluate condition.

Management

1. Pessary—plastic device inserted into vagina to aid pelvic support.
2. Estrogen replacement vaginally to prevent atrophy.
3. Pelvic floor muscle exercises to improve symptoms.
4. Surgery, if rectocele is large enough to interfere with bowel functioning: posterior colpoplasty (perineorrhaphy)—repair of posterior vaginal wall.

Complications

Total fecal incontinence.

Nursing Assessment

1. Obtain history of childbirth, pelvic surgery, symptoms of bowel function.

2. Observe for bulge into vagina while patient bears down or is in upright position.
3. Monitor bowel movements.

Nursing Diagnoses

- Acute Pain related to pelvic pressure.
- Constipation related to displaced rectum or bowel.

Nursing Interventions

Relieving Pain

1. Encourage periods of rest with legs elevated to relieve pelvic strain.
2. Encourage use of mild analgesics, as needed; avoid opioids, which may worsen constipation.
3. Postoperative care:
   a. Suggest low-Fowler's position to reduce edema and discomfort.
   b. Administer perineal care to patient after each voiding and defecation.
   c. Beware heat may enhance the healing process but may cause burns.
   d. Use ice packs locally to relieve congestion and discomfort.
   e. Administer analgesics and stool softeners, as ordered.

Relieving Constipation

1. Teach patient to increase fluid and fiber in diet.
2. Encourage use of stool softeners or bulk laxatives to make passage of stool easier.

Patient Education and Health Maintenance

1. Advise patient to follow surgeon's instructions for resuming activity and to avoid heavy lifting, straining, and intercourse until cleared.
2. Educate patient for the future to avoid straining and obesity, which may cause return of rectocele or enterocele.

Evaluation: Expected Outcomes

- Verbalizes reduced pain.
- Passes soft stool daily.

Uterine Prolapse

Uterine prolapse is an abnormal position of the uterus in which the uterus protrudes downward.

Pathophysiology and Etiology

1. Uterus herniates through pelvic floor and protrudes into vagina (prolapse) and possibly beyond the introitus (procidentia).
2. Usually caused by obstetric trauma and overstretching of musculofascial supports.
3. Degrees (see Figure 22-6).
   a. First degree—cervix prolapses into vaginal canal.
   b. Second degree—cervix is at the introitus.
   c. Third degree—cervix extends over the perineum.
   d. Marked procidentia—the entire uterus protrudes outside vaginal cavity.

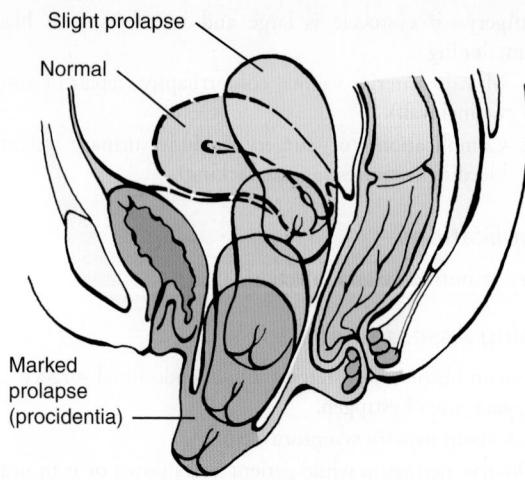

Figure 22-6. Degrees of uterine prolapse.

Clinical Manifestations

1. Low backache or dyspareunia.
2. Pressure and heaviness in pelvic region.
3. Bloody discharge because of cervix rubbing against clothing or inner thighs.
4. Urinary frequency, urgency, or repeated bladder infections.
5. Symptoms are aggravated by obesity, standing, straining, coughing, or lifting a heavy object because of increased intra-abdominal pressure.

Diagnostic Evaluation

Pelvic examination identifies condition.

Management

1. Hysterectomy or surgical correction.
2. Vaginal pessary—plastic device inserted into vagina as temporary or palliative measure if surgery cannot be done.
3. Pelvic floor muscle exercises to improve symptoms.
4. Estrogen cream—to decrease genital atrophy.

Complications

1. Necrosis of cervix, uterus.
2. Infection.

Nursing Assessment

1. Obtain history of childbirth and surgery.
2. Ask about symptoms and aggravating factors.
3. Examine patient in lying or standing position; if cervix not readily visible, spread labia gently, do not attempt to insert speculum.

Nursing Diagnoses

- Acute Pain related to downward pressure and exposed tissue.
- Impaired Tissue Integrity related to exposed cervix and uterus.
- Sexual Dysfunction related to loss of vaginal cavity.

Nursing Interventions

Relieving Pain
1. Administer sitz baths and explain procedure to patient.
2. Provide heating pad for lower back or lower abdomen.
3. Administer pain medications, as ordered.
4. Check for proper placement of pessary.
5. Increase fluid intake and encourage patient to void frequently to prevent bladder infection.

Maintaining Cervical and Uterine Mucosal Integrity
1. For second- and third-degree prolapse, apply saline compresses frequently.
2. Provide postoperative care.
   a. Administer perineal care to patient after each voiding and defecation.
   b. If urinary retention occurs, catheterize or use indwelling catheter until bladder tone is regained.
   c. Apply an ice pack locally to relieve congestion.
   d. Promote ambulation but prevent straining to reduce pelvic pressure.

Restoring Sexual Function
1. Discuss with patient noncoital sexual activity before treatment is instituted.
2. Explain to patient that sexual intercourse is possible with pessary; however, vaginal canal may be shortened.
3. Reinforce surgeon's instructions postoperatively about waiting to have vaginal penetration.
4. Encourage patient to explore with partner ways to engage in sexual activity without strain and with greatest comfort.

Patient Education and Health Maintenance
1. Encourage patient with pessary to follow up, as directed, for removal and cleaning of pessary and evaluation of any vaginal irritation or trauma.
2. Encourage all patients to report vaginal discharge, pain, or bleeding before or after treatment.

Evaluation: Expected Outcomes
- Verbalizes reduced pain.
- Cervix and uterus without ulceration.
- Verbalizes satisfying sexual activity.

GYNECOLOGIC TUMORS

Cancer of the Vulva

Cancer of the vulva is most commonly carcinoma of the labia majora, labia minora, or clitoris; it may also originate as a urethral tumor. It is the fourth most common gynecologic cancer.

Pathophysiology and Etiology
1. Most common in postmenopausal women, with an average age of 65. Although there has recently been increased incidence in women ages 40 to 50 (which may be related to HPV screening), many new cases have been diagnosed because of increase in older population.
2. Represents 5% of gynecologic cancers.
3. The cause is unknown, but HPV has been shown to be responsible for 60% of vulvar cancers.
4. Spreads primarily through local, direct extension and lymphatic system; distant metastasis can occur late in the disease process.

Clinical Manifestations
1. Lump or mass present for several months—first is leukoplakic (white plaque or mild ulceration); becomes reddened, pigmented, ulcerated.
2. Vulvar pruritus is a common complaint,
3. Discharge or bleeding; may be foul-smelling because of secondary infection.
4. Dysuria because of invasion of urethra with bacteria.
5. Edema of tissues.
6. Lymphadenopathy.
7. Pain or dyspareunia.

Diagnostic Evaluation

Biopsy of lesion and lymph nodes. If small, lesion may be excised at time of biopsy. Most lesions are squamous cell carcinoma.

Management

 Evidence Base National Cancer Institute. (2011). Vulvar cancer treatment (PDQ). Bethesda, MD: Author. Available: http://cancer.gov/cancertopics/pdq/treatment/vulvar/HealthProfessional.

Choice of surgical methods depends on the site and extent of the primary lesion and the risk of lymph node involvement. The most conservative operation that is consistent with cure of disease is chosen.

1. Precancerous lesions—vulvar intraepithelial neoplasia.
   a. Simple vulvectomy is seldom indicated.
   b. Skinning vulvectomy with possible grafting.
   c. Local excision or laser therapy or a combination.
   d. Fluorouracil Cream 5% (response rate 50% to 60%).
2. Carcinoma in situ—noninvasive.
   a. Simple vulvectomy is seldom indicated.
   b. Skinning vulvectomy with possible grafting.
   c. Local excision or laser therapy or a combination.
   d. Fluorouracil Cream 5% (response rate 50% to 60%).
3. Invasive carcinoma—radical or modified radical vulvectomy with bilateral groin lymph node resection.
   a. Pelvic nodes may also be removed if involvement is suspected.
   b. If cancer is confined to the vulva, there is a 70% to 93% 5-year survival rate after surgery (for patients with negative nodes).
4. Advanced carcinoma—pelvic exenteration or surgery and radiation as a palliative measure.
   a. Radiation therapy has an increased role in the preoperative and postoperative management.
   b. Preoperative radiation therapy can decrease the volume of disease and decrease need for radical surgery.

c. Postoperative radiation therapy is used for patients with positive lymph nodes and close surgical margins.

d. Long-term outcomes of treatment compared to morbidity associated with treatment are being studied.

5. Chemotherapy alone or in combination with radiation may shrink lesion so surgery can be less extensive.

6. Cisplatin and/or 5 FU used as radiation sensitizers have been shown to increase efficacy of radiation treatment.

Complications

1. Lymphatic spread.

2. Complications after vulvectomy are common—wound infection, wound breakdown, lymphedema, leg cellulitis, and introital stenosis.

Nursing Assessment

1. Obtain history of lesion, including when the patient first noticed it and any change in appearance.

2. Obtain gynecologic history, especially about past infections.

3. Assess overall health for tolerance of treatment.

4. Assess support systems and personal coping skills.

Nursing Diagnoses

• Fear related to cancer and radical surgery.
• Impaired Tissue Integrity related to surgery.
• Sexual Dysfunction related to vulvectomy.

Nursing Interventions

Relieving Fear Preoperatively

1. Have patient describe what her understanding is about the problem; answer questions and clear up misconceptions.

2. Emphasize the positive outcomes of the prescribed treatment plan; reinforce what the surgeon has already described to her.

3. Prepare patient for surgery and describe to her the postoperative appearance of the wound, use of drains, urinary catheter (see Figure 22-7).

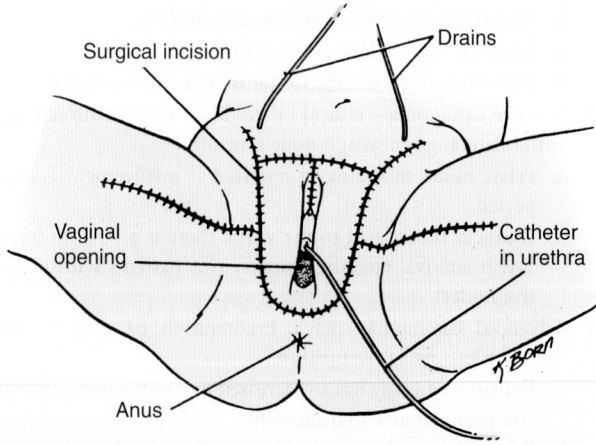

Figure 22-7. Postoperative appearance after radical vulvectomy.

a. Provide skin preparation as directed and cleanse the vulva via a chlorhexidine shower the night before surgery; 2% chlorhexidine gluconate antiseptic solution may also be ordered.

b. Administer bowel preparation, as ordered, to evacuate intestinal tract before surgery; there will be no bowel movement for 2 to 3 days postoperatively.

Promoting Tissue Healing Postoperatively

1. Maintain drainage and compression of tissues to remove fluid that could cause edema and prevent wound healing. Empty drains, as needed (at least every 8 hours).

2. Keep wound clean and dry.

a. Perform sterile dressing changes, as prescribed.

b. Apply heat lamp, if prescribed, to decrease moisture and increase circulation and healing.

c. Perform perineal care or sitz baths after each bowel movement or voiding (after catheter is removed).

d. Maintain patency of urinary catheter, as ordered, to prevent wound contamination with urine.

e. Encourage low-Fowler's position to promote comfort and reduce tension on sutures.

f. Prevent straining with defecation by providing a low-residue diet initially and stool softeners later, as ordered.

g. Provide deep vein thrombosis prophylaxis (anticoagulant or sequential compression device), as prescribed, and encourage leg exercises to prevent thrombus/embolus formation. Encourage careful ambulation when allowed while preventing perineal tension.

Restoring Sexual Function

1. Encourage patient to ventilate feelings about sexual mutilation, altered functioning.

2. Tell patient that if vagina is still intact, vaginal intercourse is still possible.

3. Inform patient of changes that may occur because of surgery—loss of sexual arousal if clitoris is removed, shortening of vagina, decreased lubrication.

4. Help patient explore alternate methods of sexual intimacy and encourage her to discuss feelings with her partner.

Patient Education and Health Maintenance

1. Encourage follow-up visits for additional therapy, if required.

2. Encourage regular health checkups and screening for cancer and other age-related illnesses.

3. Encourage early evaluation of any suspicious lesions, bleeding, or discharge.

Evaluation: Expected Outcomes

• Verbalizes reduced fear.
• Perineum healed without complications.
• Verbalizes understanding of anatomic changes and sexual function.

Cancer of the Cervix

Cancer of the cervix is the third most common gynecologic malignancy. There are about 12,000 new cases and 4,000 deaths each year in the United States.

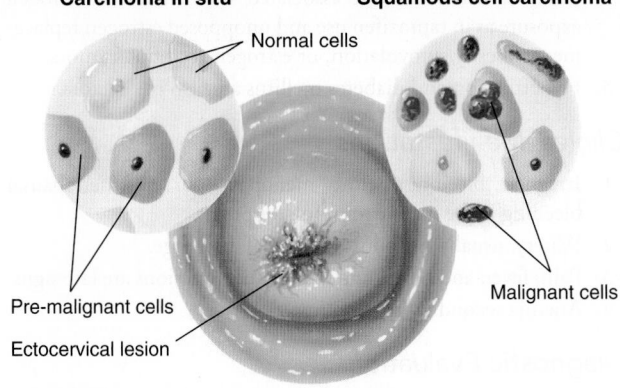

Carcinoma in situ   **Squamous cell carcinoma**

Normal cells

Pre-malignant cells

Ectocervical lesion

Malignant cells

FIGURE 22-8. Cervical cancer.

Pathophysiology and Etiology

1. Early sexual activity, multiple sexual partners, a high-risk sexual partner, history of HIV and other STDs—especially HPV—and a history of vulvar or vaginal squamous intraepithelial neoplasia or cancer, immunosuppression are major risk factors. There also appears to be an increased risk of cervical cancer associated with the use of oral contraceptives.
2. Incidence is higher in lower socioeconomic status and in Hispanics, African Americans, American Indians, and Alaska Natives—presumably related to decreased access to health care and screening.
3. Decreased mortality in United States, but most frequent malignancy among women in developing countries.
4. Types (see Figure 22-8):
   a. Dysplasia (precancer)—atypical cells with some degree of surface maturation.
   b. Carcinoma in situ—cytology similar to invasive carcinoma, but confined to epithelium.
   c. Invasive carcinoma—stroma is involved; 69% are of the squamous cell type. Spreads by local invasion and lymphatics to vagina and beyond.

Clinical Manifestations

1. Early disease is usually asymptomatic, although patient may notice watery, vaginal discharge.
2. Initial symptoms include postcoital bleeding, irregular vaginal bleeding or spotting between periods or after menopause, and malodorous discharge.
3. As disease progresses, bleeding becomes more constant and is accompanied by pain that radiates to buttocks and legs as well as urinary and rectal symptoms that may be due to invasion of these organs.
4. Weight loss, anemia, edema of lower extremities, and fever signal advanced disease.

Diagnostic Evaluation

1. Pap smear—routine screening measure; abnormal results warrant further diagnostic tests, such as colposcopy and biopsy or conization.

2. Staging is done clinically rather than surgically as with other cancers. Based on physical findings on abdominal and pelvic examination.
3. Supplemental imaging can include chest x-ray, IVP, urography, colposcopy, cystoscopy, proctosigmoidoscopy, computed tomography (CT) scan with IV contrast, and barium studies of the lower colon and rectum.

Management

 Evidence Base National Cancer Institute. (2012). Cervical cancer Treatment (PDQ). Bethesda, MD: Author. Available: *www.cancer.gov/cancertopics/pdq/treatment/cervical/HealthProfessional*.

Dysplasia to Carcinoma in Situ
1. Techniques to destroy abnormal cells in the cervical transformation zone.
2. Cryosurgery, laser therapy, electrocautery (loop electrosurgical excision procedure), or conization may be performed on outpatient basis.
3. Vaginal discharge, bleeding, pain, and cramping result from these procedures in various degrees, but postoperative convalescence is minimal.

Microinvasive Stage
1. Surgical conization—large excision of cervical tissue, may be done under local or general anesthesia.
2. Invasive cervical cancer—extent is staged and treated with hysterectomy, radiotherapy, or chemotherapy.

Other Management
1. Radiotherapy.
   a. Intracavitary (localized for earlier stage) or external (more generalized dosage to pelvis for stages IIB through IVB).
   b. Cisplatin, a radiation sensitizer, is used to improve survival.
2. Chemotherapy—cisplatin may be used in combination with radiation for locally advanced disease or for metastatic disease in which recurrence is common. Other agents that may be used include ifosfamide, carboplatin, and topotecan.
3. Surgery.
   a. Total hysterectomy, conization, modified radical hysterectomy and intracavitary radiation therapy may be performed for stage IA with or without oophorectomy and/or lymph node dissection.
   b. Radical hysterectomy and bilateral lymph node resections for stage IB and IIA. Radiation and chemotherapy may also be considered for these stages after hysterectomy.
   c. Pelvic exenteration for advanced cases if the patient is a candidate. Usually done for patients with isolated central recurrence.
      i. Removal of the vagina, uterus, uterine tubes, ovaries, bladder, rectum, and supporting structures and the creation of an ileal conduit and fecal stoma.
      ii. Performed for pelvic recurrence after radiation or chemotherapy.

Complications

1. Spread to bladder and rectum; metastasis to lungs, mediastinum, bones, and liver.
2. Complications of intracavitary radiotherapy include cystitis, proctitis, vaginal stenosis, uterine perforation.
3. Complications of external radiation include bone marrow depression, bowel obstruction, fistula.

Nursing Assessment

1. Obtain history of Pap tests, sexual activity, past STDs.
2. Obtain history of symptoms.
3. Assess understanding of disease and responses, such as guilt, fear, denial, anxiety.

Nursing Diagnoses

- Anxiety related to cancer and treatment.
- Disturbed Body Image related to surgical treatment.

Nursing Interventions

Relieving Anxiety

1. Assist patient to seek information on stage of cancer, treatment options.
2. Prepare patient for hysterectomy or other surgery (see page 845 for nursing interventions for hysterectomy).
3. Prepare patient for radiation therapy to the uterus (see page 873 for nursing interventions for radiation therapy).

Enhancing Body Image

1. Provide emotional support during treatment.
2. Encourage patient to take pride in appearance by dressing, putting on makeup as able.
3. Encourage activity and socialization when patient is able.

Patient Education and Health Maintenance

1. Explain the importance of lifelong follow-up, regardless of treatments, to determine the response to treatment and detect spread of cancer.
2. Refer to cancer support group in community.
3. Encourage all women to discuss cervical cancer screening guidelines with their health care providers (see page 834).

Evaluation: Expected Outcomes

- Reports decreased anxiety, increased decision-making ability.
- Reports continued interest in appearance and femininity.

Endometrial Cancer

Cancer of the uterus is usually adenocarcinoma of the endometrium of the fundus or body of the uterus. Most common gynecologic cancer in the United States.

Pathophysiology and Etiology

1. Most patients are postmenopausal with an average age of early 60s at time of diagnosis.
2. Cause is unknown but associated with increased estrogen exposure as in tamoxifen use and unopposed estrogen replacement, obesity, anovulation, or estrogen-secreting tumors.
3. Hypertension and diabetes mellitus are also risk factors.

Clinical Manifestations

1. Irregular bleeding before menopause or postmenopausal bleeding is the most common complaint.
2. Watery, usually malodorous vaginal discharge.
3. Pain, fever, and bowel and bladder dysfunctions are late signs.
4. Anemia secondary to bleeding.

Diagnostic Evaluation

1. Pelvic and rectovaginal examination—enlarged uterus may be palpated.
2. Endometrial biopsy is preferred as the initial diagnostic test; however, if less than 50% of the endometrium is affected, malignancy can be missed.
3. Transvaginal ultrasound to measure endometrial thickness.
4. Dilation and curettage—if endometrial sampling cannot be performed in office, hysteroscopy may also be helpful.
5. Atypical glandular cells may be found on cervical cytology.
6. Metastatic workup—includes CA 125 (which may be elevated, especially in papillary serous carcinomas), x-ray studies, and cystoscopy.

Management

Evidence Base National Cancer Institute. (2012). Endometrial cancer treatment (PDQ). Bethesda, Maryland: Author. Available: www.cancer.gov/cancertopics/pdq/treatment/endometrial/HealthProfessional.

1. Staging for endometrial cancer is based on surgical aspects versus clinical staging.
   a. Emphasis is placed on histologic grade, depth of myometrial invasion, and cervical involvement.
   b. These parameters assist in prediction of lymph node involvement and help determine need for lymph node dissection.
2. Early stage I requires total abdominal hysterectomy with bilateral salpingo-oophorectomy (TAH/BSO).
3. Advanced stage I and stage II require TAH/BSO and selective lymph node dissection.
4. Radiation therapy (intracavitary or external) may be added after surgery or chosen instead of surgery for more advanced stages or for patients who are high-risk surgical candidates.
   a. Acute complications include hemorrhagic cystitis, vaginitis, enteritis, proctitis.
   b. Chronic complications include vaginal dryness, vaginal stenosis, cystitis, bladder dysfunction, proctitis, small bowel obstruction, fistulas, strictures, leg edema.
5. Hormonal therapy—progestational agents may alter receptor sites in endometrium for estrogen and thus decrease growth (for metastatic disease); may provide stabilization of disease.
6. Chemotherapy—for metastatic and recurrent disease; using cisplatin, doxorubicin, and possibly paclitaxel.

Complications

Spread throughout the pelvis; metastasis to lungs, liver, bone, and brain.

Nursing Assessment

1. Obtain history of menses, pregnancy, estrogen replacement.
2. Ask about irregular or postmenopausal bleeding and other symptoms.
3. Assess patient's response to possible diagnosis of cancer—fear, guilt, denial.

Nursing Diagnoses

- Fear related to cancer, treatment options.
- Acute Pain related to disease process and surgical treatment.

Nursing Interventions

Relieving Fear

1. Support patient through the diagnostic process and reinforce information given by health care provider about treatment options.
2. Prepare patient for radiation therapy, if indicated (see below).
3. Prepare patient for hysterectomy, if indicated (see page 845).
4. Provide complete and concise explanations for all care you provide; emphasize the positive aspects of patient's recovery.

Relieving Pain

1. Administer pain medications, as prescribed, and monitor patient's response.
2. Encourage use of relaxation techniques, such as deep breathing, imagery, and distraction, to help promote comfort.

Patient Education and Health Maintenance

1. Explain importance of reporting postmenopausal bleeding.
2. Encourage keeping follow-up visits.
3. Explain that surgery or radiation treatment does not prevent satisfying sexual activity.
4. Refer to local cancer support group or American Cancer Society (*www.acs.org*).

Evaluation: Expected Outcomes

- Verbalizes understanding of diagnosis and treatment chosen.
- Verbalizes decreased pain.

Care of the Patient Receiving Intracavitary Radiation Therapy

Procedural Considerations

1. An applicator (tandems and ovoids are most common) is positioned in the endocervical canal and vagina in the operating room with the patient under anesthesia. (High-dose remote brachytherapy is also used. This is an outpatient procedure and the treatment takes just minutes. The radioactive source is removed between treatments.)
2. After recovery from anesthesia, x-rays are taken to check correct placement.

3. Radiologist inserts radioactive material (radium or cesium) into applicator, which remains in place 24 to 72 hours. Therapy is individualized according to the stage of disease and patient's response to and tolerance of radiation.
4. External radiation over pelvis may be supplemented to eliminate cancer spread via lymphatic system.

Nursing Interventions

Patient Preparation

1. Patients require a thorough medical evaluation before treatment to evaluate risks and precautions related to preexisting medical problems or special needs.
2. An indwelling catheter is placed in the operating room.
3. Encourage patient to bring diversional activities because she will remain on bed rest during radiation treatment.
4. Instruct patient on radiation safety measures:
   a. Neither patient nor her secretions are radioactive, but the applicator is.
   b. Do not touch source of radiation.
   c. Notify someone immediately if source is dislodged.
   d. When applicators are removed, no radioactivity remains.
   e. Radioactivity is monitored by specially trained personnel.
   f. No pregnant women or children younger than age 18 are allowed to visit.
   g. Lead shields may be used to decrease radiation that emanates from the patient.
5. Reinforce that help is readily available.

During Radiation Treatment

1. Maintain patient on strict bed rest on her back with head of bed elevated 15 to 30 degrees. Patient may be log-rolled three or four times per day. Use convoluted foam mattress.
2. Have patient bathe upper body. Perineal care and linen changes are done by the nursing staff.
3. Maintain patient on a low-residue diet to prevent bowel movements, which could dislodge the apparatus. Encourage patient to eat several small portions rather than few large servings. Medication to induce constipation is given.
4. Inspect indwelling catheter frequently to ensure proper drainage. A distended bladder may cause severe radiation burns.
5. Encourage fluids to prevent bladder infection.
6. Observe for signs and symptoms of radiation sickness—nausea, vomiting, fever, diarrhea, abdominal cramping.
7. Check applicator position every 8 hours and monitor amount of bleeding and drainage (a small amount is normal).
8. Check patient frequently to minimize anxiety, but minimize time spent at bedside to reduce radiation exposure.
9. Mild sedatives or pain medication may be given for patient comfort.

 NURSING ALERT Long-handled forceps and a lead-lined container are left in the room after loading in the event the radioactive sources are dislodged. Maintain cardinal rules of time, distance, shielding when caring for the patient.

During Radiation Removal

1. Before removal of the applicator, patient is medicated with appropriate analgesic.
2. The radioactive sources are removed by radiation personnel and safely stored for transport.
3. The indwelling catheter is removed and then the applicator is removed.
4. The patient is given an enema or suppository to reverse the induced constipation.
5. Patient should be evaluated for safe ambulation because of prolonged bed rest before discharge.

 **NURSING ALERT** Rules and regulations regarding radiation safety are strictly enforced to protect patients and health care workers.

Myomas of the Uterus

Myomas (fibroids, leiomyomas, fibromyomas) are benign tumors of the uterine myometrium (smooth muscle).

Pathophysiology and Etiology

1. The most common pelvic tumor in women. Approximately 80% of women have fibroids but many are not symptomatic.
2. May spontaneously regress after menopause.
3. Unknown cause; increased incidence in black women.

Clinical Manifestations

1. Small myomas do not cause symptoms.
2. First indication may be palpable mass.
3. Irregular bleeding—usually menorrhagia.
4. Pain may come from pressure on adjacent organs—possible heavy feeling in pelvis or degeneration associated with vascular occlusion.
5. Secondary symptoms include fatigue because of anemia, urinary disturbances, and constipation.

Diagnostic Evaluation

1. Transvaginal ultrasound or hysteroscopy—to identify size and location of myomas.
2. Magnetic resonance imaging (MRI) may be helpful in clarifying anatomy and myoma location; however, it is expensive and best reserved for surgical planning of difficult procedures.

Management

1. Myomectomy may be done for small or accessible tumor, may be done through hysteroscope, laparoscope, or laparotomy. If fertility preservation is desired, abdominal myomectomy is preferred for symptomatic women.
2. Hysterectomy for large or numerous tumors.
3. Medical therapies for management of symptoms include gonadotropin-releasing hormone antagonist therapy to create hypoestrogenic environment and to try to shrink tumors. Hormonal birth control, NSAIDs, or antifibrinolytic agents are used for heavy menstrual bleeding.

4. Frequently resolve on their own postmenopausally.
5. Uterine artery embolization—transvenous procedure in which the blood supply to the myoma is obstructed and the myoma degenerates.

Complications

1. Infertility with hysterectomy.
2. Habitual abortion.

Nursing Assessment

1. Ask about pain, menstrual irregularity, possible urinary symptoms, and constipation.
2. Assess patient's understanding of condition as benign.

Nursing Diagnosis

- Acute and Chronic Pain related to tumor growth.

Nursing Interventions

Relieving Pain

1. Teach patient proper use and adverse effects of analgesics and use of heating pad, as desired.
2. Encourage patient to avoid long periods of standing; rest with pelvis in dependent position periodically to achieve comfort.
3. Encourage patient to void frequently to avoid increased pressure from distended bladder.
4. Advise a high-fiber diet to prevent constipation.
5. Prepare patient for surgery, if indicated.

Patient Education and Health Maintenance

1. Tell patient to report increased symptoms and worsening bleeding because myomas may be enlarging and treatment may be indicated.
2. Reassure patient that myomas do not become malignant, but she should keep regular follow-up visits for cancer screening.

Evaluation: Expected Outcomes

- Verbalizes control of pain.

Ovarian Cysts

Ovarian cysts are growths arising from ovarian components, usually benign.

Pathophysiology and Etiology

1. Commonly arise from functional changes in the ovary—from graafian follicle or from persistent corpus luteum.
2. Dermoid cysts may develop from abnormal embryonic epithelium.
3. Frequently found during childbearing years.

Clinical Manifestations

1. May be asymptomatic or cause minor pelvic pain.
2. Possible menstrual irregularity.
3. Tender, palpable mass.

4. Rupture causes acute unilateral lower abdominal pain and tenderness; may mimic mittelschmerz, PID, appendicitis, or ectopic pregnancy.

5. Discomfort during bowel movement or pressure on the bowel.

Diagnostic Evaluation

1. Pelvic sonogram to determine size and characteristics.
2. Pregnancy test to rule out ectopic pregnancy.
3. Biopsy (at time of surgery) is done for suspicious cysts.
4. Other tests that may be ordered: CBC with diff., CA-125.

Management

1. Cysts without malignant characteristics and cysts that measure <10 cm in diameter can be observed with repeat ultrasound in 2 to 3 months.
2. Surgery for large, complex, or leaking cyst by laparoscopy or laparotomy.

Complications

Rupture may cause peritoneal inflammation.

Nursing Assessment

1. Obtain history of sexual activity, use of contraception, past episodes of PID to rule out ectopic pregnancy.
2. Obtain history of recent menses—irregular bleeding and spotting commonly signal follicular cyst; delayed menses and prolonged bleeding signal corpus luteal cyst.
3. Perform vital signs and abdominal examination for tenderness, guarding, and rebound, which may indicate rupture.

Nursing Diagnoses

- Acute Pain related to abnormal growth.
- Risk for Deficient Fluid Volume related to rupture of cyst or postoperative change in intra-abdominal pressure.

Nursing Interventions

Relieving Pain

1. Encourage the use of analgesics, as prescribed, and of heating pad, if desired.
2. Teach patient the proper use of hormonal contraceptives, if prescribed, with adverse effects; encourage monthly follow-up visits to determine if cyst is resolving.
3. Tell patient that heavy lifting, strenuous exercise, and sexual intercourse may increase pain.

Maintaining Fluid Volume

1. Monitor for nausea, vomiting, rigid abdomen, and change in vital signs related to rupture of cyst. Administer IV fluids, as directed, and maintain NPO status until abdominal rigidity resolves.
2. Reassure patient that symptoms will resolve.
3. Prepare patient with large or nonresponsive cyst for surgery, as indicated.
4. Postoperatively monitor vital signs frequently and maintain IV infusion while NPO.

5. Assess frequently for abdominal distention because of fluid and gas pooling in abdominal cavity.

6. Place the patient in semi-Fowler's position for greatest comfort and encourage early ambulation to reduce distention (help patient arise slowly to prevent orthostatic hypotension).

7. Administer anti-emetics and insert a nasogastric tube, as ordered, to prevent vomiting.

8. As distention resolves, assess bowel sounds and advance oral intake slowly.

Patient Education and Health Maintenance

1. Reassure patient that in most cases ovarian function remains and she remains fertile.
2. Reassure patient about low malignancy rate of cysts.
3. Encourage patient to report recurrent symptoms or worsening of pain if cyst is being treated medically.

Evaluation: Expected Outcomes

- Verbalizes reduced pain.
- Vital signs stable, no orthostasis.

Ovarian Cancer

Ovarian cancer is a gynecologic malignancy with high mortality because of advanced disease by time of diagnosis. It is the leading cause of morbidity of gynecologic cancers.

Pathophysiology and Etiology

1. Median age is 60 years. One of 70 women will develop ovarian cancer.
2. Cause is unknown but about 10% of cases are associated with family history of breast, endometrial, colon, or ovarian cancer.
3. Smoking and personal history of breast, colon, or endometrial cancer are also risk factors.
4. There is also higher incidence in nulliparous women.

Clinical Manifestations

1. No early manifestations.
2. First manifestations—(vague) bloating, increased abdominal size, urinary urgency or frequency, difficulty eating or feeling full, and abdominal or pelvic pain, which may occur with other symptoms, almost daily and are more severe than expected.
3. Late manifestations—abdominal pain, ascites, pleural effusion, intestinal obstruction.

Diagnostic Evaluation

1. Pelvic examination to detect enlargement, nodularity, immobility of the ovaries.
2. Pelvic sonography (transabdominal and transvaginal) is the most useful diagnostic test and CT scan is done to determine metastatic spread.
3. Color Doppler imaging may be used to detect vascular changes within the ovaries.
4. Paracentesis or thoracentesis if ascites or pleural effusion is present.

5. Laparotomy to stage the disease and determine effectiveness of treatment.

6. Increase of CA 125 signifies progression, but not as useful as diagnostic or screening tool because level can be elevated due to inflammation and other causes.

Management

1. TAH/BSO and omentectomy is usual treatment because of delayed diagnosis. Optimal debulking to less than 1 cm is goal.

2. Chemotherapy is more effective if tumor is optimally debulked (less than 1 cm residual disease); usually follows surgery because of frequency of advanced disease; may be given IV or intraperitoneal.

3. Radiation therapy is not usually valuable.

4. Second-look laparotomy may be done after adjunct therapies to take multiple biopsies and determine effectiveness of therapy. Practice is controversial because it does not affect survival.

5. Immunotherapy is being investigated in clinical trials as stand-alone treatment or in conjunction with other modalities.

Complications

Direct intra-abdominal or lymphatic spread, peritoneal seeding

Nursing Assessment

1. Obtain history of irregular menses, pain, postmenopausal bleeding.

2. Ask about vague GI-related complaints.

3. Ask about history of other malignancy and family history of breast or ovarian cancer.

4. Assess patient's general health status in terms of tolerating surgical and adjuvant therapy.

 NURSING ALERT A combination of a long history of ovarian dysfunction and persistent undiagnosed GI complaints raises the suspicion for ovarian cancer. A palpable ovary in a postmenopausal woman is abnormal and should be evaluated as soon as possible.

Nursing Diagnoses

- Ineffective Coping related to advanced stage of cancer.
- Imbalanced Nutrition: Less Than Body Requirements related to nausea and vomiting from chemotherapy.
- Disturbed Body Image related to hair loss from chemotherapy.
- Acute Pain related to surgery.

Nursing Interventions

Strengthening Coping

1. Provide emotional support through diagnostic process; allow patient to express feelings and encourage positive coping mechanisms.

2. Administer anxiolytic and analgesic medications, as prescribed, and teach patient and caregivers the potential adverse effects.

3. Refer patient to cancer support group locally or American Cancer Society (*www.acs.org*) or National Cancer Institute (*www.cancer.org*).

Maintaining Adequate Nutrition

1. Administer or teach patient or caregiver to administer anti-emetics, as needed, for nausea and vomiting.

2. Encourage small, frequent, bland meals or liquid nutritional supplements as able.

3. Assess the need for IV fluids if patient is vomiting.

4. Monitor for passage of gas and bowel movements after surgery. Bowel dysfunction related to surgery may cause nausea and anorexia.

Maintaining Body Image

1. Prepare patient for body image changes with chemotherapy (ie, hair loss).

2. Encourage patient to prepare ahead of time with turbans, wigs, hats.

3. Encourage patient to enhance appearance with makeup, clothing, jewelry as she is used to doing.

4. Stress the positive effects of patient's treatment plan.

Relieving Pain

1. Prepare patient for surgery, as indicated; explain the extent of incision, IV, catheter, packing, and drain tubes expected (see page 845 for a discussion of hysterectomy).

2. Postoperatively, administer analgesics, as needed, and explain to patient that she may be drowsy.

3. Reposition frequently and encourage early ambulation to promote comfort and prevent adverse effects.

Patient Education and Health Maintenance

1. Explain to patient the onset of menopausal symptoms with ovary removal.

2. Tell patient that disease progression will be monitored closely by laboratory tests and second-look laparoscopy may be necessary.

3. Female relatives of patient should notify their physicians; biannual pelvic examinations may be necessary.

Evaluation: Expected Outcomes

- Openly discusses prognosis, asks appropriate questions, makes plans for short-term future.
- Maintains weight.
- Verbalizes satisfaction in appearance with wig.
- Verbalizes good control over pain.

OTHER GYNECOLOGIC CONDITIONS

Pelvic Inflammatory Disease

 Evidence Base Centers for Disease Control and Prevention. (2010). Sexually transmitted diseases treatment guidelines. Available: *www.cdc.gov/std/treatment*.

Pelvic inflammatory disease (PID) includes several inflammatory disorders of the upper female genital tract, often with infection that may involve the fallopian tubes, ovaries, uterus, or peritoneum.

Pathophysiology and Etiology

1. Incidence has been increasing; high recurrence rate because of reinfections.
2. Commonly polymicrobial; causative agents include *N. gonorrhoeae*, *C. trachomatis*, anaerobes (*Gardnerella vaginalis*), Gram-negative bacteria, and *streptococci*. Cervical infection ascends through the endometrium, into the fallopian tubes, and possibly into the peritoneal cavity.
3. Predisposing factors include multiple sexual partners, early onset of sexual activity, use of IUDs (the wick promotes ascension of bacteria), and procedures such as therapeutic abortion, cesarean sections, and hysterosalpingograms.

Clinical Manifestations

1. Pelvic pain—most common presenting symptom; usually dull and bilateral.

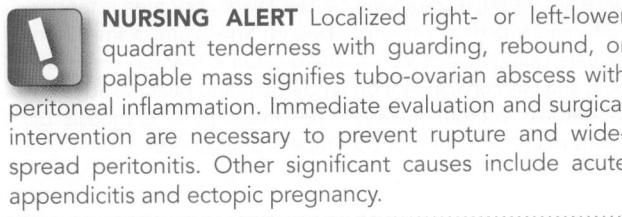 **NURSING ALERT** Localized right- or left-lower quadrant tenderness with guarding, rebound, or palpable mass signifies tubo-ovarian abscess with peritoneal inflammation. Immediate evaluation and surgical intervention are necessary to prevent rupture and widespread peritonitis. Other significant causes include acute appendicitis and ectopic pregnancy.

2. Fever >101° F—especially with gonococcal infections.
3. Cervical discharge—mucopurulent.
4. Irregular bleeding.
5. GI symptoms—nausea, vomiting, acute abdomen usually signify abscess.
6. Urinary symptoms—dysuria, frequency.
7. Presentation with chlamydia may be mild.

Diagnostic Evaluation

1. Diagnostic criteria for empiric treatment of PID in women at risk for STDs is warranted if no cause for pelvic pain can be identified or if any of the following three minimum criteria are present:
    a. Cervical motion tenderness.
    b. Uterine tenderness.
    c. Adnexal tenderness.
       In addition to the presence of the minimum criteria, sign/symptoms of lower genital tract infection (such as cervical exudate, a friable cervix, and white blood cells on microscopic examination of cervical secretions) improve the specificity of the diagnosis.
2. Endocervical DNA testing or culture to identify organisms (*Gonorrhea* or *chlamydia*).
3. CBC may show elevated leukocytes.
4. Elevated C-reactive protein or elevated erythrocyte sedimentation rate show inflammation.
5. Some cases may warrant endometrial biopsy, hysterosalpingostomy, transvaginal ultrasound, MRI, or laparoscopic visualization of the fallopian tubes.

Management

1. Patients with mild to moderate symptoms can be treated on an outpatient basis with oral antimicrobial regimens and timely follow-up at 48 to 72 hours after initiation of antibiotic and at completion of 2-week antibiotic course.
2. Inpatient treatment is required for surgical emergencies; abscess; pregnancy; severe infection with nausea, vomiting, and high fever; cannot take oral fluids; immunodeficient patient; or more aggressive antibiotics required to preserve fertility.
3. Parenteral antimicrobial regimens recommended by the CDC during hospitalization include the following:
    a. Cefotetan 2 g IV every 12 hours or cefoxitin 2 g IV every 6 hours *plus* doxycycline 100 mg IV or orally every 12 hours. *Note:* IV doxycycline infusion is painful; oral doxycycline should be administered whenever possible because IV and oral bioavailability of doxycycline is similar.
    b. Clindamycin 900 mg IV every 8 hours *plus* gentamicin 2 mg/kg of body weight IV or I.M. as loading dose, followed by 1.5 mg/kg every 8 hours as maintenance dosage. (A single daily dose [3 to 5 mg/kg] of gentamicin may be substituted.)
4. Outpatient, oral antimicrobial regimens recommended by the CDC include:
    a. Ceftriaxone 250 mg I.M. single dose *plus* doxycycline 100 mg orally twice per day for 14 days, with or without metronidazole 500 mg orally twice per day for 14 days.
    b. Cefoxitin 2 g I.M. single dose *and* probenecid 1 g orally administered concurrently as a single dose *plus* doxycycline 100 mg orally twice daily for 14 days, with or without metronidazole 500 mg orally twice daily for 14 days.
    c. Other I.M. third-generation cephalosporin (ceftizoxime or cefotaxime) *plus* doxycycline 100 mg orally twice a day for 14 days, with or without metronidazole 500 mg twice a day for 14 days.
5. Parenteral therapy can be switched to oral therapy 24 to 48 hours after improvement is shown (reduced fever, decreased pain, resolution of nausea and vomiting). Ongoing oral therapy after parenteral therapy may be one of the following regimens:
    a. Doxycycline 100 mg orally twice per day to complete a total of 14 days.
    b. Clindamycin 450 mg orally four times per day to complete a total of 14 days.
    c. With or without addition of metronidazole 500 mg orally twice per day to complete 14 days.

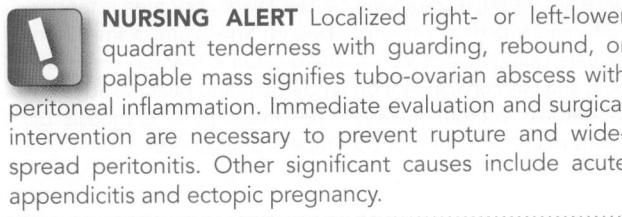 **NURSING ALERT** If patient with PID is to be treated at home, stress the importance of follow-up, usually in 48 hours, to determine if oral antibiotic treatment is effective. Advise patient to report worsening of symptoms immediately.

6. Surgical treatment or interventional drain placement may be necessary to drain abscess or later to treat adhesions or tubal damage.

Complications

1. Abscess rupture and sepsis.
2. Infertility because of adhesions to fallopian tubes and ovaries.
3. Ectopic pregnancy caused by inability of fertilized egg to pass stricture.
4. Dyspareunia because of adhesions.

Nursing Assessment

1. Obtain history of menstruation, contraception, sexual activity (including number of partners and new partner), STD history, symptoms in sexual partner.
2. Assess level of pain, fever; evaluate vital signs for hypotension and increased pulse, indicating hypovolemia.
3. Perform abdominal and pelvic examinations, if indicated; be alert for abdominal tenderness, rebound, guarding, or a mass.
4. Assess patient's feelings about having an STD.

Nursing Diagnoses

- Acute Pain related to pelvic inflammation and infection.
- Deficient Fluid Volume related to fever and decreased oral intake.
- Risk for Infection related to STDs.

Nursing Interventions

See Nursing Care Plan 22-1.

NURSING CARE PLAN 22-1

Care of the Patient with Pelvic Inflammatory Disease

Janice Smith is a 17-year-old female admitted with acute pelvic inflammatory disease (PID).

Subjective data: Janice tells you she has severe lower abdominal pain, vaginal discharge, fever, and nausea and vomiting that have made her unable to eat or drink for 2 days. She feels weak and dizzy. She has a new sexual partner, is not using condoms, and is taking hormonal contraceptives. Her last menstrual period was 1 week ago.

Objective data: Temperature 102.2° F (39° C), pulse 98, blood pressure 94/60, respirations 24. Her lower abdomen is tender with mild guarding without rebound. Speculum examination reveals purulent cervical discharge. On bimanual examination, she has cervical motion tenderness and bilateral adnexal tenderness without masses. The presumptive diagnosis of PID is made and antibiotic therapy is prescribed.

NURSING DIAGNOSIS
Acute Pain related to pelvic inflammation and infection.

GOAL/EXPECTED OUTCOME
Pain will be reduced.

Nursing Interventions	Rationale	Evaluation: Actual Outcome
Administer analgesics as prescribed. Alert patient to adverse effect of drowsiness.	Analgesics provide pain relief. Knowledge of adverse effects enhances patient compliance.	Pain reduced from level 10 to level 3.
Assist patient to position of pelvic dependence, with head and feet elevated slightly.	Promotes drainage of infection without strain on pelvic structures.	Resting in pelvic-dependent position.
Encourage patient to apply heating pad to lower abdomen or low back.	Promotes circulation and relief of inflammation, promotes comfort.	Uses heating pad for 20-minute intervals.

NURSING DIAGNOSIS
Deficient Fluid Volume related to fever and decreased oral intake.

GOAL/EXPECTED OUTCOME
Fluid balance will be restored.

Nursing Interventions	Rationale	Evaluation: Actual Outcome
Maintain IV fluids as ordered.	IV fluids replace circulating fluid volume.	Denies dizziness. BP 106/64, pulse 88.
Administer anti-emetics, as prescribed.	Anti-emetics prevent vomiting.	No vomiting.

NURSING CARE PLAN 22-1 (continued)

Care of the Patient with Pelvic Inflammatory Disease

Nursing Interventions	Rationale	Evaluation: Actual Outcome
Monitor intake and output.	Provides feedback on fluid replacement.	Intake equals output.
Restart oral intake with ice chips and sips of water when vomiting has ceased for 2 hours.	Will not distend stomach and produce vomiting.	Ice chips and sips of water tolerated without vomiting.

NURSING DIAGNOSIS
Risk for Infection, Reinfection, and Transmission to partners related to sexual activity.

GOAL/EXPECTED OUTCOME
Infection will not be transmitted or recur.

Nursing Interventions	Rationale	Evaluation: Actual Outcome
Administer and teach self-administration of antibiotics to patient. Advise patient to inform partner to seek evaluation and empiric treatment immediately.	Simultaneous treatment for prescribed length of therapy without missed doses ensures microbiologic cure.	No skipped doses of antibiotics.
Advise abstinence until completion of patient's and partner's antimicrobial regimens.	Abstinence is the only sure method of preventing transmission of organisms.	Reports understanding of abstinence, need for follow-up.
Tell patient to advise all partners within past 60 days to seek treatment.	All partners must receive treatment to break the chain of transmission.	All partners have been advised by patient.
Teach patient methods of preventing STDs—abstinence, monogamy, proper use of male and female condoms. Encourage patient to consider monogamy or abstinence until in a mutually monogamous relationship.	Safe sexual behavior reduces risk of STDs.	Verbalizes monogamy. Describes proper use of condoms.

Patient Education and Health Maintenance

1. Encourage compliance with antibiotic therapy for full length of prescription.
2. Stress the need for sexual abstinence and pelvic rest (nothing in vagina, including no douching or tampons) until completion of patient's and partner's antimicrobial regimens, resolution of patient's and partner's symptoms, and follow-up visit.
3. Advise testing and empiric treatment of gonorrhea and chlamydia for all sexual partners (within past 60 days or more). Tell patient that diagnosis of chlamydia or gonorrhea necessitates reporting to public health department and partners will be traced.
4. Repeat patient and partner testing for gonorrhea and chlamydia is recommended 3 to 6 months after treatment completion.
5. Discuss STDs and methods of prevention—abstinence, monogamy, proper use of female or male condoms. See page 855.

Evaluation: Expected Outcomes

- Verbalizes relief of pain.
- Vital signs stable; intake equals output.
- Reports abstinence during treatment period for self and partner and continued plan to prevent STDs.

Endometriosis

 Evidence Base American College of Obstetrics and Gynecology. (2010). Medical management of endometriosis. *ACOG Practice Bulletin*, No. 114.

Endometriosis is the abnormal proliferation of uterine endometrial tissue outside the uterus.

Pathophysiology and Etiology

1. May also be found outside the pelvic cavity; an intact uterus is not needed to have endometriosis (see Figure 22-9, page 880).

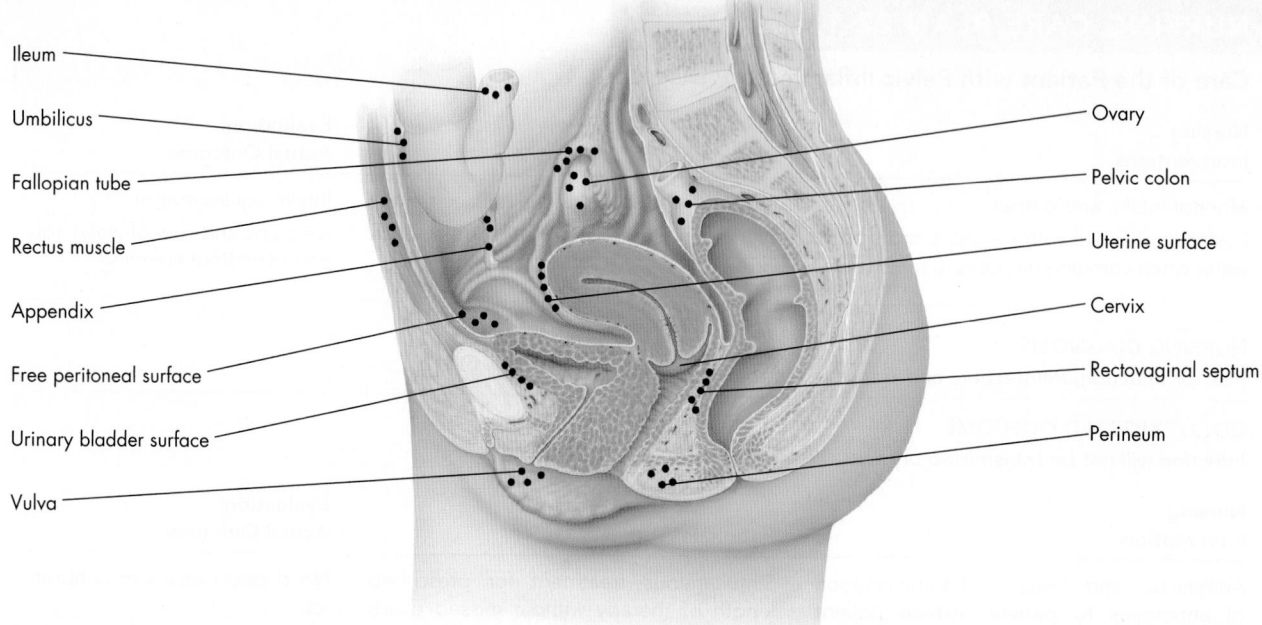

Ileum

Umbilicus

Fallopian tube

Rectus muscle

Appendix

Free peritoneal surface

Urinary bladder surface

Vulva

Ovary

Pelvic colon

Uterine surface

Cervix

Rectovaginal septum

Perineum

Figure 22-9. Common sites of endometriosis. Ectopic endometrial tissue can implant almost anywhere in the pelvic peritoneum. It can even invade distant sites such as the lungs.

2. Peaks in women ages 25 to 45; may occur at any age. Increased risk in siblings, women with shorter menstrual cycles, and longer duration of flow. More common in white women than black women, in women who do not exercise, and in obese women.
3. Responds to ovarian hormonal stimulation—estrogen increases it; progestins decrease it.
   a. Bleeds during uterine menstruation, resulting in accumulated blood and inflammation and subsequent adhesions and pain.
   b. Regresses during amenorrhea (ie, pregnancy and menopause) and hormonal contraceptive and androgen use.
4. Theories of origin:
   a. May be embryonic tissue remnants that differentiate as a result of hormonal stimulation and spread via lymphatic or venous channels.
   b. May be transferred via surgical instruments.
   c. May be caused by retrograde menstruation through fallopian tubes into peritoneal cavity (but this theory does not account for some types of endometriosis)
   d. Genetic predisposition may increase the likelihood in women with a first-degree relative with endometriosis.
   e. Lymphatic or vascular distribution of endometrial tissue.

Clinical Manifestations

1. Depends on sites of implantation; may be asymptomatic.
2. Pelvic pain—especially during or before menstruation.
3. Dyspareunia.

4. Painful defecation—if implants are on sigmoid colon or rectum.
5. Abnormal uterine bleeding.
6. Persistent infertility (in 30% to 40% of women with endometriosis).
7. Hematuria, dysuria, flank pain—if bladder involved.

Diagnostic Evaluation

1. Pelvic and rectal examinations—tender, fixed nodules or ovarian mass or uterine retrodisplacement; nodules may not be palpable.
2. Transvaginal ultrasound—diagnostic tool of choice to first assess for endometriosis. MRI and CT are reserved for inconclusive ultrasound results.
3. Laparoscopy—for definitive diagnosis to view implants, obtain tissue for histologic analysis, and determine extent of disease.

Management

Medical

Goal of medical suppressive therapy is to decrease pain. However, if therapy is stopped, pain recurs. Medical therapies are ineffective for infertility associated with endometriosis.

1. Hormonal contraceptives—such as combination oral contraceptives (OCs); use small amount of estrogen, maximum amount of progestin and androgen effect to decrease implant size. OC use for more than 24 months effectively decreases

endometrioma recurrence and decreases the frequency and intensity of dysmenorrhea.

2. Progestins—such as depot medroxyprogesterone acetate; create a hypoestrogenic environment. Efficacy is equivalent to OCs.

3. Nonsteroidal anti-inflammatory drugs—such as ibuprofen, naproxen sodium—decrease dysmenorrhea with antiprostaglandin action

4. If after 3 months of OCs and NSAIDs treatment has not provided adequate pain relief, then gonadotropin-releasing hormone (GnRH) agonist (leuprolide) injections may be administered during a 6-month period—create hypoestrogenic environment. Menopausal-like side effects, such as hot flashes and vaginal dryness, may not be tolerable to some women. If GnRH therapy will continue later, then norethindrone acetate add-back therapy will be added to prevent bone mineral loss and alleviate some symptoms. Calcium, vitamin D, and bisphosphonates may be added also.

5. Aromatase inhibitors, such as letrozole—inhibits the action of aromatase, which converts androgens to estrogen, thereby reducing estrogen levels in all tissues including the endometriosis (currently under study for endometriosis, but have been used in postmenopausal women).

6. Danazol—synthetic androgen suppresses endometrial growth. Rarely used secondary to intolerable adverse effects (increased facial hair, acne, weight gain, vasomotor symptoms) and other drugs are available with better side effect profiles. Contraindicated in pregnancy.

Surgical

1. Laparoscopic surgery—preferred procedure to remove implants and lyse adhesions by excision; not curative; high recurrence rate.

2. Carbon dioxide laser laparoscopy—for minimal to moderate disease; vaporizes tissue; may be done at same time as diagnosis; good pregnancy rate.

3. Laparotomy—rarely performed; involves a larger abdominal incision than laparoscopy; for severe endometriosis or persistent symptoms.

4. Presacral neurectomy—rarely performed; to decrease central pelvic pain; preserves fertility; limited efficacy in relieving pain; severe constipation results.

5. Hysterectomy—if fertility is not desired and symptoms are severe; greater pain relief is achieved when ovaries are also removed.

Complications

1. Infertility.
2. Rupture of cyst—mimics ruptured appendix.
3. Chronic pelvic pain.
4. Dyspareunia.
5. Bowel or ureter obstruction.

Nursing Assessment

1. Obtain history of symptoms to determine spread and severity of disease.
2. Assess pain—level, location, frequency, duration, characteristics, impact on functioning.
3. Perform abdominal examination to assess for areas of tenderness, nodules.
4. Assess for impact of endometriosis and/or infertility on patient and her relationship with significant other.

Nursing Diagnoses

- Acute and Chronic Pain related to hormonal stimulation, adhesions.
- Readiness for Enhanced Self-Care related to difficult management of disease, infertility.

Nursing Interventions

Reducing Pain

1. Teach use of analgesics and other prescribed medication, with adverse effects.
2. Encourage use of heating pad to painful areas, as needed.
3. Teach patient relaxation techniques to control pain, such as deep breathing, imagery, and progressive muscle relaxation.
4. Encourage patient to try position changes for sexual intercourse if experiencing dyspareunia.

Fostering Enhanced Self-Care

1. Include patient in treatment planning; answer questions about drug and surgical treatment so she can make informed choices.
2. Encourage adequate rest and nutrition.
3. Provide emotional support and encourage patient to discuss treatment of infertility with her physician.
4. Prepare patient for surgery, as indicated.

Patient Education and Health Maintenance

1. Instruct patient in the adverse effects of prescribed medication.
2. Refer patient to support groups such as Endometriosis Association (*www.endometriosisassn.org*) and reliable resources for information such as Endometriosis.org (*http://endometriosis.org*).

Evaluation: Expected Outcomes

- Verbalizes reduced pain.
- Verbalizes increased self-care measures.

Toxic Shock Syndrome

Toxic shock syndrome (TSS) is a rare condition caused by a bacterial toxin from *Staphylococcus aureus* or sometimes by group A *Streptococcus pyogenes* in the bloodstream; it can be life-threatening.

Pathophysiology and Etiology

1. Cause is uncertain, but 70% of cases historically were associated with menstruation and super-absorbent tampon use. Menstrual cases have declined since the withdrawal of superabsorbent tampons from the market around 1986. Now, half of TSS cases are not menstrually related.

2. TSS does occur in nonmenstruating or postmenopausal females, males, and children with conditions such as cellulitis, surgical wound infections, subcutaneous abscesses, vaginal

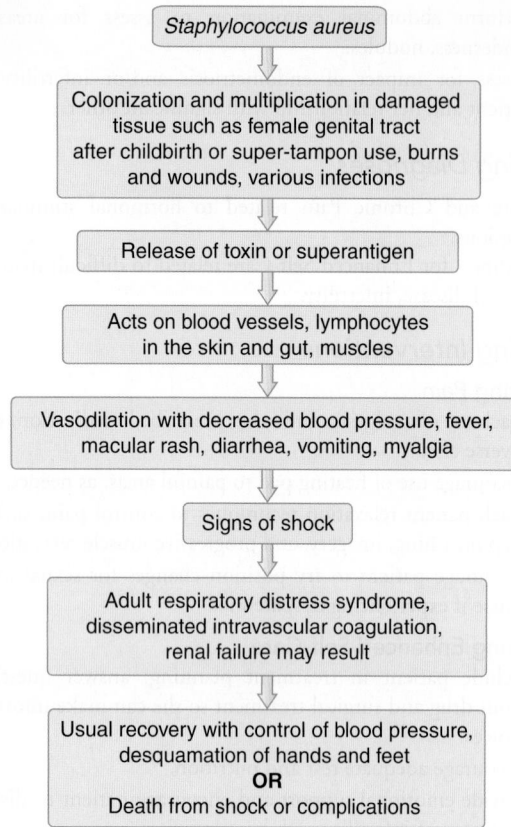

Figure 22-10. Pathophysiology of toxic shock syndrome.

infections, after childbirth, and with the use of contraceptive sponge or diaphragm.

3. See Figure 22-10 for pathophysiology.

Clinical Manifestations

1. Patients may initially present with fever, hypotension, and diffuse rash.
2. May have sudden onset of fever greater than 102° F (38.9° C), often with flu-like symptoms (myalgias, headache, sore throat).
3. Hypotension and rapid progression to shock within 72 hours of onset.
4. Rash (similar to sunburn) that is diffuse, red, and macular; followed by desquamation, particularly of the palms and soles, 1 to 2 weeks after illness onset.
5. Mucous membrane hyperemia.
6. Vomiting and profuse watery diarrhea.
7. Rapid progression to multisystem involvement.

Diagnostic Evaluation

1. Blood, urine, throat, and vaginal or cervical cultures; possibly cerebrospinal fluid culture to detect or rule out infectious organism.
2. Tests to rule out other febrile illnesses—Rocky Mountain spotted fever, Lyme disease, meningitis, Epstein-Barr, or Coxsackie virus.

3. CBC, electrolytes, blood urea nitrogen, creatinine, coagulation studies, and other tests to monitor condition.

Management

Management will be achieved in an intensive care unit due to the nature of the rapidly progressing shock, circulatory compromise, impending potential acute renal failure, and multisystem organ failure.

1. Fluid and electrolyte replacement to increase blood pressure and prevent renal failure.
2. Inotropes and vasopressor medications (ie, dopamine), as needed.
3. Intravenous antibiotics (ie, penicillins, cephalosporins, vancomycin); methicillin-resistant *Staphylococcus aureus* has been reported in some cases of TSS.
4. Mechanical ventilation in acute respiratory distress and lactic acidosis.
5. The use of steroids and immunoglobulins is controversial and under investigation.
6. Surgery may be employed to remove causative infectious site or to debride skin and soft tissue.

Complications

Cardiovascular collapse and renal failure because of shock.

Nursing Assessment

1. Determine menstrual history, use of tampons, or whether there has been recent skin infection, childbirth, or surgery.
2. Determine vital signs quickly; hemodynamic monitoring may be needed.

Nursing Diagnoses

- Hyperthermia related to infectious process.
- Deficient Fluid Volume related to toxin effects.
- Impaired Skin Integrity related to latent desquamation.

Nursing Interventions

Reducing Fever

1. Administer antipyretics and antibiotics, as ordered.
2. Use cooling measures, such as sponge baths and hypothermia blanket, if indicated.
3. Monitor core body temperature frequently.

Restoring Fluid Volume

1. Perform hemodynamic monitoring, as indicated (ie, arterial line, central venous pressure, or pulmonary artery pressure).
2. Maintain strict intake and output measurement.
3. Insert indwelling catheter to monitor urine output.
4. Administer IV fluids and vasopressors, as ordered, to control hypotension.
5. Monitor respiratory status for pulmonary edema and respiratory distress syndrome because of fluid overload from increased fluid replacement or from lactic acidosis from acute renal failure. Mechanical ventilation may be required.
6. Administer diuretics, as ordered, if edema results.

Restoring Skin Integrity

1. Tell patient to expect desquamation of skin, as in peeling sunburn.
2. Protect skin and avoid use of harsh soaps and alcohol that cause drying.
3. Tell patient to apply mild moisturizer and avoid direct sunlight until healed.
4. Advise patient that reversible hair loss may occur 1 to 2 months after TSS.

Patient Education and Health Maintenance

1. Tell patient to expect fatigue for weeks to months after TSS.
2. Tell patient not to use tampons in future to reduce risk of recurrence.
3. Encourage follow-up examination and cultures.
4. Teach prevention of TSS.
   a. Avoid use of tampons if menstrual flow is light. Use pads whenever possible.
   b. Alternate use of pads with tampons; avoid super-absorbent tampons.
   c. Change tampons frequently and do not wear one longer than 8 hours—4 hours maximum in heavy discharge time.
   d. Be careful of vaginal abrasions that can be caused by some applicators.
   e. Be alert to symptoms of TSS.

Evaluation: Expected Outcomes

- Afebrile.
- Normotensive, good urine output.
- Skin heals without scar.

SELECTED REFERENCES

American College of Obstetricians and Gynecologists. (2009). Cervical cytology screening. *Obstetrics and Gynecology, 120*, 1222–1230.

American College of Obstetricians and Gynecologists. (2009). Polycystic ovarian syndrome. *ACOG Practice Bulletin,* No. 108. Washington, DC: Author.

American College of Obstetricians and Gynecologists. (2010). Medical management of endometriosis. *ACOG Practice Bulletin,* No. 114. Washington, DC: Author.

American College of Radiology. (2009). ACR–ACOG–AIUM–SRU practice guideline for the performance of pelvic ultrasound. Available: *www.acr.org/SecondaryMainMenuCategories/quality_safety/guidelines/us/us_pelvic.aspx.*

Biggs, W., & DeMuth, R. (2011). Premenstrual syndrome and premenstrual dysphoric disorder. *American Family Physician, 84*(8), 918–924.

Centers for Disease Control and Prevention. (2010). Sexually transmitted diseases treatment guidelines. Available: *www.cdc.gov/std/treatment/2010/STD-Treatment-2010-RR5912.pdf*

Cesario, S. (2010). Advances in the early detection of ovarian cancer. *Nursing for Women's Health, 14*(3), 222–234.

Chen, L. M., & Berek, J. S. (2011). Endometrial cancer: Epidemiology, risk factors, clinical features, diagnosis, and screening. Available: *www.uptodate.com.*

Chura, J. C., & Axtell, A. E. (2011). Ovarian cancer. *Epocrates.* Available: *https://online.epocrates.com/noFrame/showPage.do?method=diseases&MonographId=260&ActiveSectionId=23.*

DeRidder, D. (2011). An update on surgery for vesicovaginal and urethrovaginal fistulae. *Current Opinion in Urology, 21*, 297–300.

Ducher, G., Turner, A., Kukulian, S., et al. (2011). Obstacles in the optimization of bone health outcomes in the female athletic triad. *Sports Medicine, 41*(7), 587–607.

Feldman, S. (2011). Making sense of the new cervical-cancer screening guidelines. *New England Journal of Medicine, 365*(23), 2145–2147.

Goodman, N. E., Cobin, R. H., Ginzburg, S. B., et al. (2011). American Association of Clinical Endocrinologist medical guidelines for clinical practice for the diagnosis and treatment of menopause. *Endocrine Practice, 17*(Suppl. 6), 1–25.

Hopkins, M. P., & Schnettle, W. T. (2011). Ovarian cyst. *Epocrates.* Available: *https://online.epocrates.com/noFrame/showPage.do?method=diseases&MonographId=660&ActiveSectionId=42.*

Hurd, W. W. (2011). Gynecologic laparoscopy. *Medscape Reference.* Available: *http://emedicine.medscape.com/article/265201-overview#showall.*

Master-Hunter, T., & Heiman, D. (2006). Amenorrhea: Evaluation and treatment. *American Family Physician, 73*, 1374–1382, 1387.

National Cancer Institute. (2011). Vulvar cancer treatment (PDQ). Bethesda, MD: Author. Available: *http://cancer.gov/cancertopics/pdq/treatment/vulvar/HealthProfessional.*

National Cancer Institute. (2012). PDQ cervical cancer treatment. Bethesda, MD: Author. Available: *www.cancer.gov/cancertopics/pdq/treatment/cervical/HealthProfessional*

National Cancer Institute. (2012). Endometrial cancer treatment (PDQ). Bethesda, MD: Author. Available: *www.cancer.gov/cancertopics/pdq/treatment/endometrial/HealthProfessional*

National Institute for Health and Clinical Excellence, National Collaborating Centre for Women's and Children's Health. (2007). Heavy menstrual bleeding. NICE Clinical Guideline 44. Available: *http://publications.nice.org.uk/heavy-menstrual-bleeding-cg44.*

North American Menopause Society. (2010). Estrogen and progesterone use in postmenopausal women: 2010 position statement of the North American Menopause Society. *Menopause: The Journal of the North American Menopause Society, 17*(2), 242–255.

North American Menopause Society. (2012). The 2012 hormone therapy position statement of the North American Menopause Society. *Menopause, 19*(3), 257–271.

Nyirjesy, I. Conization of cervix treatment and management. Medscape Reference. Available: *http://emedicine.medscape.com/article/270156-treatment#a1133.*

Pinkerton, J. (2011). Pharmacotherapy for abnormal uterine bleeding. *Menopause: The Journal of the North American Menopause Society, 18*(4), 453–461.

Roush, K. (2012). Managing menopausal symptoms. *AJN, 28*(6), 28–35.

Saslow, D., Solomon, D., Lawson, H. W., et al. (2012). American Cancer Society, American Society for Colposcopy and Cervical Pathology, and American Society for Clinical Pathology screening guidelines for the prevention and early detection of cervical cancer. *CA—Cancer Journal for Clinicians, 62*, 147–172.

Society of Obstetricians and Gynaecologists of Canada. (2009). Menopause and osteoporosis update 2009. *Journal of Obstetrics and Gynaecology Canada, 31*(1, Suppl. 1).

Sweet, M., Schmidt-Dalton, T., & Weiss, P. (2012). Evaluation and management of abnormal uterine bleeding in premenopausal women. *American Family Physician, 85*(1), 35–43.

Tilanus, A., de Geus, H., Rijnders, B., et al. (2010). Severe group A streptococcal toxic shock syndrome presenting as primary peritonitis: a case report and brief review of the literature. *International Journal of Infectious Diseases, 14S*, e208–e212.

University of Texas at Austin, School of Nursing, Family Nurse Practitioner Program. (2010). *An evidence based practice guideline for the treatment of primary dysmenorrheal.* Austin: University of Texas at Austin, School of Nursing.

U.S. Preventive Services Task Force. (2012). Screening for cervical cancer, topic page. Available: *www.uspreventiveservicestaskforce.org/uspstf/uspscerv.htm.*

Wechter, M., Wu, J., Marzano, D., et al. (2009). Management of Bartholin duct cysts and abscesses: A systematic review. *Obstetrical and Gynecological Survey, 64*(6), 395–404.

Welt, C. (2012). Physiology of the normal menstrual cycle. *UpToDate.* Available: *www.uptodate.com.*

23
Breast Conditions

OVERVIEW AND ASSESSMENT

Subjective Data

Obtain a nursing history about specific breast complaints and general health information from the patient to plan care and appropriate patient teaching.

Breast Manifestations

1. Palpable lumps—date noted; affected by menstruation; changes noted since detection.
2. Nipple discharge—date of onset, color, unilateral or bilateral, spontaneous or provoked.
3. Pain or tenderness—localized or diffuse, cyclic or constant, unilateral or bilateral.
4. Date of last mammogram and result.
5. Patient's practice of breast self-examination (BSE).

History

General Information
1. Age.
2. Past medical-surgical history; injuries; bleeding tendencies.
3. Medications, including current or prior use of hormonal contraceptives and hormones, over-the-counter (OTC) products, vitamins, and herbal supplements.

Gynecologic and Obstetric History
1. Menarche.
2. Date of last menses.
3. Pregnancies, miscarriages, abortions, deliveries.
4. Lactation history.
5. Prior breast history, including previous history of irradiation involving breast region.
6. Family history of breast cancer.

Physical Examination

Perform a breast examination, as outlined in Procedure Guidelines 23-1. Remind all women of the importance of routine checkups with breast examination. Although BSE is a first step in prevention of breast cancer, it has not been shown to be effective in reducing mortality. However, it does allow women to become more comfortable and familiar with their own bodies.

Guidelines for Early Detection

 Evidence Base Smith, R., Cokkinides, V., Brooks, D., et al. (2012). Cancer screening in the United States, 2012: A review of current American Cancer Society guidelines and issues in cancer screening. *CA—A Cancer Journal for Clinicians, 62*, 129–142.

Women at Average Risk
1. Begin annual mammography at age 40. Annual clinical breast examination should be performed prior to mammography.
2. For women in their 20s and 30s, it is recommended that clinical breast examination be part of a periodic health examination, preferably at least every 3 years. Asymptomatic

PROCEDURE GUIDELINES 23-1

Examination of the Breast by the Nurse

PURPOSE
1. To detect abnormalities in the breasts
2. To teach a woman how to perform breast self-examination

EQUIPMENT
- Good lighting and a private, warm setting

PROCEDURE

Nursing Action	Rationale

 GERONTOLOGIC ALERT Normal breast changes in older patients include drooping, flaccid breasts caused by decreased subcutaneous tissue from decreased estrogen levels. Nipple size and erection are also reduced.

Sitting position

Nursing Action	Rationale
1. Wash your hands under warm water and dry them. Apply powder if they feel "sticky."	1. The breast is sensitive to cold. Powder reduces friction.
2. Have patient undress to her waist and sit comfortably facing the examiner. Observe breast for abnormalities.	2. Provides an opportunity to observe breasts for lack of symmetry and for gross signs such as redness, irritated nipple, dimpling, orange-peel skin.
3. Have patient raise arms overhead.	3. Changes in lower half of breast are more visible.
4. Palpate cervical and supraclavicular area.	4. Note whether lymph nodes are enlarged, fixed, movable, or difficult to locate.
5. Palpate axillary nodes; hold patient's forearm in your left palm while you check nodes with your right fingertips. Repeat on other side.	5. Same as 4 above.
6. Have patient place hands on hips and press.	6. Flexes pectoral muscles, accentuates skin dimpling or masses.

Lying position

Nursing Action	Rationale
1. Instruct the patient to lie down with her right arm under her head. Place a small pillow under the right shoulder.	1. Spreads breast tissue evenly over chest wall.
2. With the finger pads of two or three fingers, gently palpate breast tissue beginning at the upper outer quadrant.	2. The sensitive fingers, proceeding in a kneading fashion, can detect thickened, lumpy, or "buckshot" tissue between the patient's skin and chest wall. Because most breast lesions are in the upper outer quadrant, this segment is double-checked.
a. Proceed in an orderly pattern around the breast and repeat the first quarter examined.	
b. Repeat procedure for other breast.	
3. Recognize that there is a prolongation of the axillary extension of normal breast tissue that may extend high into axilla.	3. This is normal if symmetrical and may be abnormal if asymmetrical.
4. Check areolar area for crustiness, nipple discharge, signs of infection. If nipple discharge is observed, note if from single or multiple ducts. Hemoccult test may be used to check for hidden blood.	4. A nipple discharge may be benign or may be related to cancer.

(continued)

PROCEDURE GUIDELINES 23-1 *(continued)*

Examination of the Breast by the Nurse

PROCEDURE *(continued)*

Nursing Action	Rationale
5. Record findings and report abnormalities to the health care provider.	5. Diagram may be useful for future reference.
6. Instruct the patient in performing self-examination. Encourage her to ask questions; provide her with appropriate literature.	6. Ninety percent of women discover their own abnormalities.

Evidence Base American Cancer Society. (2012). Can breast cancer be found early? Available: *www.cancer.org/cancer/breastcancer/detailedguide/breast-cancer-detection*.

women age 40 and older should continue to receive a clinical breast examination as part of a periodic health examination, preferably annually.

3. Beginning in their 20s, women should be told about the benefits and limitations of BSE. The importance of prompt reporting of any new breast symptoms to a health care professional should be emphasized. Women who choose to do BSE should receive instruction and have their technique reviewed on the occasion of a periodic health examination.

Older Women

1. Screening decisions in older women should be individualized by considering the potential benefits and risks of mammography in the context of current health status and estimated life expectancy. As long as a woman is in reasonably good health and would be a candidate for treatment, she should continue to be screened with mammography.

GERONTOLOGIC ALERT Many older women may not be aware of newer treatments for breast cancer and may fear radical mastectomy, therefore avoiding breast cancer screening. Provide information about incidence, screening, and treatment and encourage discussion with a health care provider.

Women at Increased Risk

Evidence Base Bevers, T., Banu, A., Cowan, K. H., et al. (2010). Breast cancer risk reduction. *Journal of the National Comprehensive Cancer Network, 10,* 1112–1146.

1. Women at increased risk for breast cancer might benefit from additional screening strategies beyond those offered to women of average risk, such as earlier initiation of screening, shorter screening intervals, or the addition of screening modalities other than mammography and physical examination, such as ultrasound or magnetic resonance imaging (MRI).

2. Screening MRI is recommended for women with an approximately 20% to 25% or greater lifetime risk of developing breast cancer, including women with a strong family history of breast or ovarian cancer and women who were treated for Hodgkin's disease. Other women at high risk include those over the age of 35 with a 5-year risk of invasive breast cancer >1.7% risk per the Gail model, women with a history of LCIS and atypical hyperplasia, and those with a prior history of breast cancer. Annual MRI should be considered in these women. The Gail model is available on the National Cancer Institute website at *www.cancer.gov* or at *www.breastcancer-prevention.com*.

Laboratory Tests

Nipple Discharge Cytology

Description
Secretions are smeared on a slide, fixed, and submitted for cytologic examination. There is a high rate of false-negative test results with this method.

Nursing and Patient Care Considerations
1. Wash nipple area with water and pat dry before obtaining specimen if crusting of drainage is present.
2. Gently milk breast or ask woman to express fluid to obtain a large drop on nipple.
3. Carefully touch slide to drop and draw slide across nipple to obtain smear. Spray with fixative or drop into container with fixative.
4. Inform patient of results promptly to reduce anxiety and explain that other tests may be needed.

Ductal Lavage

Description
A procedure that targets asymptomatic women at increased risk for breast cancer. Breast duct epithelial cells are collected from the nipple for cytological analysis.

Nursing and Patient Care Considerations

Advise patient to discuss questions with health care provider. This test is not widely used and there is insufficient data at this time to recommend its use for screening.

Additional Laboratory Tests

Tumor-Specific Tests

Tests to evaluate the characteristics of a tumor and/or its potential to regrow.

1. Estrogen and progesterone receptors identify patients most likely to benefit from hormonal forms of therapy. Approximately 75% are estrogen receptor positive. A negative result is associated with a less favorable prognosis.
2. HER2—human epidermal growth factor receptor that has been demonstrated in 15% to 30% of breast cancers. Found by many investigators to be associated with poorer survival, regardless of clinical stage. May affect treatment decisions.
3. Histologic grade is reported using an Elston-Ellis modification of the Scarf-Bloom Richardson Scale. It is a combination of nuclear grade, mitotic rate, and tubule formation with scores given for each. A low score equates to a low grade (grade I), and a higher score to a higher grade (grade III). In general, high-grade tumors are more likely to recur when compared to low-grade tumors.
4. Multiparameter gene assays (eg, Oncotype DX and MammaPrint) quantify the likelihood of distant breast cancer recurrence and measure how chemotherapy may assist with planning treatment. The OncotypeDX assay is included in the National Comprehensive Cancer Network guideline treatment decision pathway. A similar assay for ductal carcinoma in situ (DCIS) is under investigation. Breast cancer diagnostic and treatment guidelines are available at *www.nccn.org*.
5. Cancer subtyping—as determined by gene expression profiling—is currently under investigation.
6. Pathologists may use other special stains to aid in diagnosis.

Tests to Detect Metastasis

1. Increased values on liver function tests may indicate possible liver metastasis.
2. Increased calcium and alkaline phosphatase levels may indicate possible bony metastasis.
3. Additional metastatic workup may include chest x-ray, bone scan, computed tomography (CT) scan, and positron emission tomography (PET) scan.
4. Biological markers (ie, CA15.3 and CA27.29) may be used for monitoring patients with metastatic disease in conjunction with diagnostic imaging, history, and physical examination. Present data are insufficient to recommend their use alone for screening, diagnosis, or staging. However, they may be used to indicate treatment failure.

Radiology and Imaging

Mammography

Description

1. Low-dose x-ray of breast used to screen for breast abnormalities or may be used when a lump is found on physical examination. Can detect patients with clustered microcalcifications.

2. Compression of the breast is used to reduce the amount of radiation absorbed by the breast tissue and separate overlapping tissue.
3. Two views are taken routinely: craniocaudal and mediolateral; other views are done as necessary.
4. Best performed at a facility that is accredited by the American College of Radiology. The machines and staff at these facilities have met specific criteria. Computer-aided detection has been developed to aid radiologists in detecting abnormalities. Assessment categories have been developed to describe the results and provide follow-up recommendations.
   a. Category 1 is a negative result (normal mammogram) with nothing on which to comment.
   b. Category 2 is a normal mammogram but there is a benign finding on which to comment.
   c. Category 3 is probably benign, but short interval follow-up may be recommended to determine stability of the finding.
   d. Category 4 describes a suspicious abnormality and biopsy should be considered.
   e. Category 5 is highly suggestive of malignancy requiring appropriate action.
   f. Category 6 describes a known, biopsy-proven malignancy requiring appropriate action.

 Evidence Base American College of Radiology. (2003). *Bi-rads-mammography: Assessment categories* (4th ed.). Reston, VA: Author.

5. Mammography is not routinely done if a woman is pregnant.
6. The breasts of young women tend to be extremely dense and are poorly suited to mammography.
7. False-negative results occur even in the best facilities; figure may reach 10%.
8. Both screen film and digital mammography use x-rays to obtain images. With digital mammography, a film image is replaced with an electronic image similar to digital photography. For younger women under age 50, women with radiographically dense breasts, and premenopausal and perimenopausal women, digital mammography is more accurate than film mammography. For all other women, there is no significant advantage to using digital mammography.

Nursing and Patient Care Considerations

1. Recommend regular screening based on established guidelines (see page 884). Tell patients that routine screening mammography has been shown to reduce mortality from breast cancer. Procedure takes approximately 15 minutes.
2. Remind patients not to apply deodorant, cream, or powder to breast, nipple, or underarm areas on examination day.
3. Advise that some discomfort may be felt from compressing the breast.
4. Patients should have an opportunity to become informed about the benefits, limitations, and potential harms associated with regular screening. Overdiagnosis of clinically insignificant disease is possible. Benefits are thought to outweigh the exposure to low dose of radiation.
5. Alert patient that extra views do not imply that the patient has breast cancer.

NURSING ALERT Because health teaching is an important nursing role, nurses should educate women about the importance of routine screening.

Ultrasonography

Description

1. Uses high-frequency sound waves to get an image of the breast.
2. Helps determine if a lump is a cyst or a solid mass.
3. May be used if patient is pregnant or is younger than age 35.

Nursing and Patient Care Considerations

1. Advise that this test is painless and noninvasive.
2. No preparation is necessary.

Additional Imaging Studies

Galactography/Ductogram

1. A contrast mammogram is obtained by injection of water-soluble contrast medium into a duct for patient with persistent bloody nipple discharge. It is a time-consuming procedure that is not routinely used.
2. It may outline an intraductal papilloma.
3. Its ability to differentiate benign from malignant lesions is limited.
4. Other tests such as tomosynthesis (3D mammography) and thermography may be useful in some women; however, these are not often used.

Magnetic Resonance Imaging

1. Produces images from the combination of a magnetic field, radio waves, and computer processing.
2. May be used in newly diagnosed breast cancer patients for presurgical planning. May help in determining extent of disease, multifocality, and unsuspected disease in the contralateral breast.
3. Useful in high-risk women, those with dense breasts, and in those with silicone implants.
4. Because MRI is less accessible and more expensive than mammography, it is not useful for generalized screening. There may be increased false-positive results. MRI-guided biopsy is not widely available.
5. See page 206 for description of MRI.

Other Tests

In addition to laboratory tests and imaging studies, biopsy methods are commonly used to evaluate breast conditions. A biopsy is the only certain way to learn whether a breast lump or suspicious area seen on a mammogram is cancerous.

Fine-Needle Aspiration

Description

1. Uses a thin needle and syringe to collect tissue or to drain lump after using a local anesthetic. If it is a cyst, removing the fluid will collapse it; no other treatment may be needed. Ultrasound may be used to locate a nonpalpable cyst.
2. Normal cyst fluid appears straw-colored or greenish. Fluid should be sent for cytology if it appears suspicious (clear or bloody); otherwise, it is discarded.
3. This office procedure uses local anesthetic with results usually within 24 hours.
4. It has limited sensitivity, possibly because of insufficient acquisition of cytologic material.

Nursing and Patient Care Considerations

1. Inform patient of small risk of hematoma and infection.
2. Adhesive bandage applied after procedure; usually no discomfort.
3. Solid lesions may warrant an excisional biopsy.

Needle Biopsy

Description

1. Office procedure uses local anesthetic and removes a small piece of breast tissue using a needle with a special cutting edge.
2. For palpable lesions with a high suspicion of malignancy. May provide a tissue diagnosis quickly—usually approximately 24 hours—without doing an excisional biopsy to plan definitive surgery.
3. Ultrasound guidance may be used for nonpalpable lesions.

Nursing and Patient Care Considerations

1. Inform patient of small risk of hematoma and infection.
2. Tell patient that several passes may be necessary to obtain specimen, with minor discomfort.
3. Pressure dressing applied after procedure.
4. Recommend use of acetaminophen or ibuprofen for postprocedure discomfort—usually minimal, if any.

Stereotactic Core Needle Biopsy

Description

1. An x-ray-guided method for localizing and sampling nonpalpable lesions detected on mammography with 90% to 95% sensitivity in detecting breast cancer.
2. Performed as an outpatient procedure with the patient lying prone on a special table using an automated biopsy gun with a vacuum system to draw tissue into a sampling chamber and rotate cutter to excise tissue.
3. After local anesthetic is administered, a needle is placed in the lesion with confirmation of its position on stereotactic x-ray views. Multiple samples are taken from different portions of the lesion. Allows harvesting of larger quantities of tissue with a single needle insertion. A tiny clip may be left in place at the end of the procedure to mark the area.
4. The procedure is quicker and less expensive than mammographically guided needle localization followed by surgical excisional biopsy and is an alternative to surgical excisional biopsy to make a diagnosis.

Nursing and Patient Care Considerations

1. Inform patient that it is a 1-hour outpatient procedure that requires no special preparation.
2. The patient should dress comfortably and will need to remain still during the procedure.

3. Complications may include minor bleeding, hematoma, and infection.

4. Explain that nonspecific, suspicious, or atypical findings may result in proceeding to excisional biopsy.

5. Remind patient that area in question will not be removed, only sampled.

> *Note:* Many nonpalpable abnormalities that require breast biopsy are being identified because of increased use of screening mammography.

Excisional Biopsy

Description

1. Surgical removal of a palpable or nonpalpable lesion. A frozen section may be done for immediate tissue diagnosis.

2. Excisional biopsy or lumpectomy entails entire removal of a mass; incisional biopsy entails partial removal of a mass.

3. This outpatient procedure may be performed under local or general anesthesia.

4. Curvilinear incision is usually made directly over the mass, which is excised en bloc including a 1-cm grossly free margin of tissue.

Nursing and Patient Care Considerations

1. Pressure dressing is placed, which can be removed in 24 to 48 hours.

2. Inform patient to watch for bleeding, hematoma, and signs of infection.

3. Recommend analgesics for discomfort and a support bra for comfort.

4. May take several days to get results, a stressful time for patients.

Needle Localization with Biopsy

Description

1. Performed when there is a nonpalpable mammographic finding.

2. Mammogram is used as a guide for placing a needle at the site of the breast change after injecting some local anesthetic.

3. A wire may be left in place for the surgeon and dye may be injected to mark the site.

4. Excisional biopsy is then done (see above) removing the area around the tip of the wire.

Nursing and Patient Care Considerations

Inform patient that this may be a tedious procedure because she must remain immobile while the breast is compressed in the mammogram machine and different views are obtained.

Sentinel Lymph Node Biopsy

Description

1. A diagnostic surgical procedure utilizing selective lymph node sampling.

2. Pathologic study of the first (sentinel) axillary lymph node to receive drainage from a tumor; predicts the status of the remainder of the lymph nodes in the axilla.

3. Localization accomplished by injection of a blue dye and/or radioactive particles around a tumor to identify lymph nodes with afferent drainage.

4. The excised sentinel lymph nodes are subjected to routine pathologic examination and, possibly, immunohistochemical staining to detect micrometastasis.

5. The status of the sentinel lymph node is used to determine whether to proceed with full axillary dissection and/or determine treatment modalities.

6. If the sentinel lymph node tests negative, no further axillary surgery is indicated.

7. If test result is positive, further axillary dissection may be needed. There is currently debate regarding optimal treatment for node-positive disease in women undergoing breast-conserving surgery and having fewer than three involved lymph nodes. The omission of completion axillary lymph node dissection in selected patents has increased with no difference in overall survival. There are no clear-cut guidelines at this time.

Nursing and Patient Care Considerations

1. This is a reliable procedure, which is usually performed at the same time as definitive surgery—in conjunction with a breast-preserving procedure or mastectomy.

2. There is less morbidity and cost than with axillary dissection.

GENERAL PROCEDURES AND TREATMENT MODALITIES

Breast Self-Examination

Breast self-examination (BSE) is an inexpensive, risk-free method to detect cancer. When lumps are discovered at an early stage, patients have a better chance for long-term survival (see Patient Education Guidelines 23-1, page 890).

Patient Education

General Points to Emphasize

1. Examine breasts once per month, just after the menstrual period because breasts are less engorged and a tumor is easier to detect, and at regular monthly intervals after the cessation of menses.

2. Compare findings with the opposite breast.

3. Remind patient that 90% of breast lumps are not cancerous.

4. Do not neglect men when teaching BSE—1% of breast cancers occur in men.

 NURSING ALERT Nurses play an important role in promoting BSE. Women report increased frequency of BSE when taught by a nurse.

5. It is acceptable for women to choose not to do BSE or to do BSE irregularly.

Suggestions for Patients Who Find BSE Difficult

1. Tenderness—gentle self-examination may be more effective and less painful than examination by someone else.

2. Cystic breasts—recommend professional examination annually, and instruct patient to compare changes in breasts from one month to the next.

3. Large, pendulous breasts—encourage woman to support her breast with her hand to palpate thoroughly; lying down may help to flatten breasts.

PATIENT EDUCATION GUIDELINES 23-1

Breast Self-Examination

1. Look for changes.

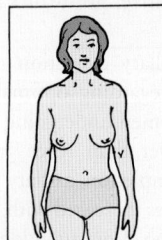 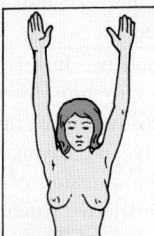 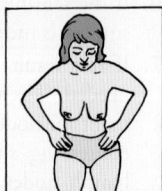

Hands at side.
Compare for symmetry.
Look for changes in:
• shape
• color
Check for:
• puckering
• dimpling
• skin changes
• nipple changes

Hands over head.
Check front and
side view for:
• symmetry
• puckering
• dimpling

Hands on hips,
press down,
bend forward.
Check for:
• symmetry
• nipple direction
• general
  appearance

2. Feel for changes.
3. Check your left breast with your right hand in the same way.

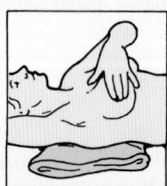 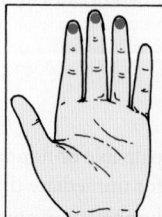 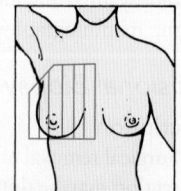

Lie down with a towel
under right shoulder;
raise right arm above
the head.

Use the pads of the
three middle fingers
of the left hand.
Hold hand in
bowed position.
Move fingers in
dime-size circles.

Examine area from:
• underarm to lower
  bra line
• across to breast
  bone
• up to collar bone
• back to armpit

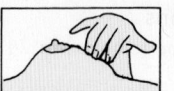 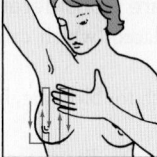

Use three levels
of pressure:
• light
• medium
• firm

Examine entire area
using vertical strip
pattern.

4. If you detect any changes, lumps, or knots, notify your
   health care provider immediately.

Evidence Base American Cancer Society. (2012). How to perform a breast self-exam. Available: *www.cancer.org/cancer/breastcancer/detailedguide/breast-cancer-detection.*

Community Health Education

Implement patient teaching of BSE on a community level by:

1. Teaching BSE to women in the community—schools, churches, women's groups.
2. Reinforcing that early detection is associated with decreased mortality.
3. Helping patients and families establish and maintain support networks.
4. Tailoring patient education messages to patients of different cultures.
5. Knowing the resources available and making people aware of them.
   a. National Cancer Institute—answers questions and provides booklets about cancer. Call 800-4-CANCER or go to *www.cancer.gov.*
   b. American Cancer Society—offers many services to patients and their families. Call 800-ACS-2345 for local chapter or go to *www.cancer.org.*

Surgery for Breast Cancer

Surgery for breast cancer may involve *mastectomy* or a *breast-preserving procedure.* The objective of breast-preserving procedures is a cosmetically acceptable breast after complete excision of the tumor. Research studies that compare breast conservation with mastectomy have demonstrated equivalent patient survival. Contraindications to breast conservation include multifocal disease; diffuse, extensive DCIS; inability to tolerate radiation therapy; and persistent positive margins. The evolving field of oncoplastic surgery uses techniques to allow the removal of large volumes of breast tissue while avoiding deformity. Although mastectomy rates have remained stable, risk-reducing contralateral prophylactic mastectomy has risen. See Table 23-1 for the surgical approach options that are available. The following discussion covers mastectomy and axillary node dissection.

Preoperative Management

See Chapter 7 for routine preoperative care. In addition:

Table 23-1	Types of Surgery for Breast Cancer	
PROCEDURE	**DESCRIPTION**	**INDICATIONS**
Tumor ablation	Insertion of probe that destroys cancer cells by heating or freezing	Done in research setting for some localized breast cancers.
Lumpectomy (excisional biopsy)	Removal of tumor and surrounding tissue	For diagnosis of an abnormal mammographic finding or palpable breast lump if needle biopsy not performed. Further surgery may be needed.
Quadrantectomy (partial mastectomy)	Removal of a breast quadrant that includes the tumor area and possibly overlying skin	Normal- to large-sized breasts. Usually done at the same time as axillary surgery.
Sentinel lymph node biopsy	Removal of only a few gatekeeper lymph nodes	Performed to predict status of lymph nodes—if negative for tumor, axillary dissection is not performed. May be done in conjunction with quadrantectomy or mastectomy.
Axillary dissection	Surgical removal of the axillary lymph nodes	Performed when lymph node is positive for tumor, mainly for prognosis, staging, and local/regional disease control.
Simple mastectomy*	Surgical removal of the entire breast	Large or multifocal tumors; women with very small breasts in whom local excision of tumor will be cosmetically unacceptable; ineligibility for radiation therapy; patient preference; prophylaxis.
Modified radical mastectomy*	Surgical removal of the entire breast and the axillary lymph nodes (simple mastectomy plus axillary dissection)	Positive lymph nodes; advanced disease.
Radical mastectomy*	Removal of entire breast, pectoral muscles, axillary nodes	Rarely done today—may be performed for advanced disease.

* Mastectomy may be followed by immediate or delayed reconstruction.

1. The nature of the procedure is explained, along with expected postoperative care that includes drain care, location of the incision, and mobility of the arm.
2. Information is clarified about diagnosis and possibility of further therapy.
3. Measures are taken to recognize the extreme anxiety and fear that the patient, family, and significant others experience.
   a. Discuss patient's concerns and usual coping mechanisms.
   b. Explore support systems with patient.
   c. Discuss concerns regarding body-image changes.
4. Evaluate the patient's overall medical condition to guide preoperative care, help determine how well the patient will tolerate surgery, and help prepare for complications that may occur postoperatively.

 GERONTOLOGIC ALERT Assessment of preoperative mental status of the older patient will help determine if a cognitive change occurs postoperatively.

Potential Complications

1. Infection.
2. Hematoma, seroma.
3. Lymphedema.
4. Paresthesia, pain of axilla and arm.
5. Impaired mobility of arm.

Postoperative Management and Nursing Care

See Chapter 7 for routine postoperative care. In addition:

1. Dressing is removed and the wound is assessed for erythema, hematoma (fluid under incision), edema, tenderness, odor, and drainage. Report suspected hematoma promptly.
   a. Initial dressing may consist of gauze held in place by elastic, tape, or clear occlusive dressing wrap.
   b. Usually removed within 24 hours.
   c. Incision may remain open to air or elastic wrap may be replaced if patient prefers.
2. Suction drain from wound is maintained.
   a. May have 100 to 200 mL serous to serosanguineous drainage in the first 24 hours.
   b. Report if grossly bloody or excessive in amount.
3. Arm on affected side is observed for edema, erythema, and pain.
4. Patient teaching about drain care, exercises, surgical outcome, and BSE occurs.
5. Female relatives, especially sisters, daughters, and mother, who may need closer breast cancer surveillance are discussed.

 NURSING ALERT Mastectomy patients may have an elastic wrap bandage that should fit snugly but not so tightly that it hinders respiration. It should fit comfortably and support unaffected breast.

Nursing Diagnoses

- Impaired Physical Mobility related to impaired movement of arm on operative side.
- Deficient Knowledge related to care of incision, arm, and performance of BSE.
- Ineffective Tissue Perfusion of affected arm related to lymphedema.
- Disturbed Body Image related to loss of breast (for mastectomy patient).
- Anxiety related to diagnosis of cancer.
- Sexual Dysfunction related to loss of breast and diagnosis of breast cancer.
- Compromised Family Coping related to diagnosis of cancer.

Nursing Interventions

In addition to routine postoperative interventions, provide the following care.

Mobilizing Affected Arm

1. Assess patient's ability to perform self-care and factors impeding performance.
2. Encourage wrist and elbow flexion and extension initially. Encourage use of arm for washing face, combing hair, applying lipstick, and brushing teeth. Encourage patient to gradually increase use of arm.
3. Encourage patient to avoid abduction initially to help prevent seroma formation.
4. Support arm in sling, if prescribed, to prevent abduction of the arm.
5. Instruct and provide patient with exercises to do when permitted (see Table 23-2).

Increasing Knowledge

1. Explain how wound will gradually change and that the newly healed wound may have less sensation because of severed nerves.
2. Instruct patient on signs of infection, hematoma, or seroma formation to be reported.
3. Teach patient to bathe incision gently and to blot carefully to dry, and later, with approval, massage the healed incision gently with cocoa butter to encourage circulation and increase skin elasticity.
4. Teach care of drains, if appropriate; empty contents, measure, and record.
5. Teach importance of BSE, mammograms, and regular follow-up visits.
6. Encourage discussion with health care provider about pregnancy after breast cancer, if indicated.

 GERONTOLOGIC ALERT Signs and symptoms of infection may not be obvious in older patients. Assess patients for mental status changes or urinary incontinence.

Promoting Lymphatic Drainage

1. Instruct patient in potential problem of lymphedema—at particular risk are patients who undergo axillary node dissection in combination with radiation therapy to axilla.

Table 23-2	Exercises for the Rehabilitation of the Patient Following Mastectomy
EXERCISE	**EQUIVALENT DAILY ACTIVITIES**
1. Stand erect. • Lean forward at waist. • Allow arms to hang. • Swing arms from side to side together; then in opposite direction. • Next, swing arms from front to back together; then in opposite direction.	• Broom sweeping • Vacuum cleaning • Mopping floor • Pulling out and pushing in drawers • Weaving • Playing golf
2. Stand erect facing wall with palms flat against wall, arms extended. • Relax arms and shoulders and allow upper part of body to lean forward against hands. • Push away to original position; repeat.	• Pushing self out of bath tub • Kneading bread • Breaststroke—swimming • Sawing or cutting types of crafts
3. Stand erect facing wall with palms flat against wall. • Climb the wall with the fingers; descend, repeat.	• Raising windows • Washing windows • Hanging clothes on line • Reaching to an upper shelf
4. Stand erect and clasp hands at small of back; raise hands; lower; repeat. • Clasp hands back of neck; reach downward; upward; repeat.	• Fastening brassiere • Buttoning blouse or dress • Pulling up a dress zipper • Fastening beads • Washing the back
5. Toss a rope over a shower curtain rod. • Hold the ends of the rope (knotted) in each hand and alternately pull on each end. • Using a seesaw motion and with arms outstretched, slide the rope up and down over the rod.	• Drying the back with a bath towel • Raising and lowering a window blind • Closing and opening window drapes
6. Flex and extend each finger in turn.	• Sewing, knitting, crocheting • Typing, painting, playing piano or other musical instrument

Explain that lymphedema may occur years postoperatively. May present as arm heaviness, decreased flexibility, aching, or swelling.

2. Do not take blood pressure, draw blood, inject medications, or start intravenous lines in affected arm. Post sign over bed.
3. Elevate affected arm on pillows, above level of heart, and hand above elbow to promote gravity drainage of fluid.

PATIENT EDUCATION GUIDELINES 23-2

Prevention of Lymphedema

To reduce the risk of lymphedema of your arm after the removal of lymph nodes, follow these general guidelines to prevent infection and obstruction of blood and lymph fluid.

- Take care of your skin to prevent dryness, cracking, and irritation that may lead to infection.
- Keep your arm clean and cover any open areas.
- Take care of your fingernails to avoid ripped cuticles and nails.
- Avoid using a razor for underarm hair removal.
- Protect hands and fingers from injury while gardening, sewing, cooking, and other chores.
- Avoid constricting clothing around arms.
- Avoid having blood drawn or needles inserted into affected arm.
- Avoid having blood pressure taken on affected arm.
- Prevent insect bites and stings through use of repellent and protective clothing.

For more information, refer to American Cancer Society (*www.cancer.org*).

 Evidence Base Lymphedema: What every woman with breast cancer should know from the American Cancer Society (2012). Available: *http://www.cancer.org/cancer/breastcancer/detailedguide/breast-cancer-detection*.

---

4. Teach patient to massage affected arm, if prescribed, which will increase circulation and decrease edema. Treatment for severe lymphedema may also include the application of elastic bandages and/or intermittent pneumatic compression. Compressive sleeves and exercises may be recommended to prevent lymphedema.
5. Teach patient care of the affected arm to prevent lymphedema and infection (see Patient Education Guidelines 23-2.

Enhancing Body Image

1. Assess mastectomy patient's knowledge of prosthesis and reconstruction options and provide information, as needed.
2. Discuss patient's views on her altered body image.
3. Suggest clothing adjustments to camouflage loss of breast.
4. Assist patient to obtain a temporary prosthesis (may be provided by Reach to Recovery [see below]). First prosthesis should be light and soft to allow incision to heal. She may wear heavier type usually 4 to 8 weeks after surgeon's approval has been secured. Provide information regarding where to obtain permanent prosthesis and bras.
5. Encourage patient to discuss feelings with partner.
6. Encourage patient to allow herself to experience the grief process over the loss of her breast and to learn to cope with these feelings.

Reducing Anxiety

1. Familiarize patient with Reach to Recovery (*www.cancer.org*, then click on Support Programs), an American Cancer Society program that consists of volunteers who have had mastectomies or breast-preserving procedures and who make postoperative hospital visits to provide support and information. Clear first with patient's care provider.
2. Discuss patient's usual coping mechanisms.
3. Encourage and assist family to support patient.

4. Assist patient to maintain control by planning care with her and incorporating her usual routines.
5. Refer patient for postmastectomy support group, as needed and desired.
6. Offer list of community resources.
7. Remind patient that stress related to breast cancer and mastectomy may persist for a year or more and to seek help.
8. Include family in supportive interventions and measures to increase coping skills.

Maintaining Sexual Activity

1. Discuss effect of diagnosis and surgery on view of self as a woman.
2. Explore alternative means of sexual activity, such as changing position during intercourse, to decrease pressure on incision.
3. Encourage patient to discuss concerns with partner.
4. Assist patient and partner to look at incision when ready.

Facilitating Family Coping

1. Allow family members to acknowledge their feelings.
2. Approach family with warmth, respect, and support.
3. Acknowledge family strengths.
4. Involve family in care of patient.
5. Discuss stresses.
6. Direct family to community agencies, as indicated.

Community and Home Care Considerations

Because of short stays (1 to 2 days) after mastectomy, many patients can achieve the following benefits from home care:

1. Assess incision and drain tubes for proper healing and no signs of infection.
2. Teach patient drain tube and dressing care.
3. Support patient with adjustment back into home and community.

4. Monitor for lymphedema and reinforce teaching about arm care and exercises.

5. Help identify those patients who may require longer hospitalizations and, possibly, a short stay in a subacute unit for rehabilitation before going home because of age and comorbid conditions.

6. Goals of home care for these patients are to provide assessment of cardiovascular status and to ensure return of energy and proper healing.

Patient Education and Health Maintenance

1. Advise patient to call surgeon for signs of infection, increased pain, or edema of arm.

2. Make sure that patient knows schedule for follow-up with surgeon.

3. Provide resources for patient for ongoing information and support: The American Cancer Society (800-ACS-2345 or *www.cancer.org*) has numerous pages of information about surgery, nutrition and cancer, lymphedema, psychosocial issues, and other concerns.

4. Stress the importance of continued yearly mammogram, clinical breast exam, and monthly BSE.

Evaluation: Expected Outcomes

- Moves affected arm within prescribed limits.
- States care of incision, drains, follow-up guidelines.
- No infection or swelling in affected arm.
- Expresses positive body image.
- Exhibits minimal anxiety.
- Reports satisfactory sexual activity and sexuality.
- Maintains a functional support system.

Breast Reconstruction After Mastectomy

Breast reconstruction (mammoplasty) may be performed immediately or as long after surgery as desired. Benefits include improved psychological coping because of improved body image and self-esteem. Cost is usually covered by insurance. Reconstruction selection is based on an assessment of cancer treatment, patient body type, smoking history, comorbidities, and patient concerns. An advantage of immediate reconstruction is a smaller scar through the use of a skin-sparing mastectomy. Current data are inadequate to support the use of nipple-sparing mastectomy outside the confines of a clinical trial. Reconstruction does not interfere with the detection of tumors.

NURSING ALERT Because breast reconstruction does not affect disease recurrence or survival, the expectations and desires of the patient are paramount in the decision-making process. Collaboration among members of the breast cancer team is essential.

Implants

Indicated for patients with inadequate breast tissue and skin of good quality.

Description

1. Uses prosthetic implants placed in pocket under skin or pectoralis muscle. A variety of implants are available that contain saline, silicone gel, or a combination of both.

2. If opposite breast is ptotic (protruding downward), mastopexy may be necessary for symmetry.

3. A dermal matrix may be used at surgery to help provide a foundation for the tissue expander and/or implant.

4. Complications include capsular contracture resulting in firmness; may be painful, cause infection.

5. Tissue expanders may be necessary before implants are inserted.
   a. Inflatable envelope is placed under muscle or skin and is filled with saline when incision is healed (about 4 weeks).
   b. Saline is instilled every 1 to 3 weeks until the expander is beyond desired size.
   c. Later, expander is removed and a permanent implant is placed.
   d. Some types of expanders may be left in permanently.

6. Advantages of implant reconstruction over other methods: only one incision; less fibrosis.

7. Disadvantages are may take months and may not be as cosmetically pleasing as other methods.

Nursing and Patient Care Considerations

1. Teach signs and symptoms of infection, hematoma, migration, and deflation.

2. Teach patient to massage breast to decrease capsule formation around implant.

3. Teach patient she may feel discomfort with expanders, if used.

Flap Grafts

Description

1. Transfer of skin, muscle, and subcutaneous tissue from another part of the body to the mastectomy site.

2. Types:
   a. Latissimus dorsi—skin, fat, and muscles of back between shoulder blades—are tunneled under skin to front of chest. Usually, an implant is also needed.
   b. Transverse rectus abdominis myocutaneous flap—muscle, fat, skin, and blood supply are tunneled to breast area.
   c. Perforator flap reconstruction; ie, deep inferior epigastric perforator (DIEP) or superior gluteal artery perforator (SGAP), uses tissue as above without using muscle. Due to its complexity, offered by few breast centers.

3. Disadvantages include cost, slow process (done in stages), increased morbidity.

4. Complications include flap loss, hematoma, infection, seroma, and abdominal hernia.

 NURSING ALERT Smoking increases the risk of complications for all types of reconstruction. Patients who smoke should be made aware of increased rates of wound infections and healing complications.

Nursing and Patient Care Considerations

1. Assess flap and donor site for color, temperature, and wound drainage.
2. Control pain.
3. Provide support with bra or abdominal binder to maintain position of prosthesis.
4. Teach patient to perform BSE monthly and that she may have some asymmetry.

Nipple-Areolar Reconstruction

1. Usually done at a separate time from breast reconstruction.
2. Uses skin and fat from reconstructed breast for nipple and upper thigh for areola; tanning or tattoo done to obtain appropriate color.

Other Surgeries of the Breast

Reduction mammoplasty may be done for cosmetic purposes or to relieve uncomfortable symptoms. Augmentation mammoplasty is considered a cosmetic procedure.

Reduction Mammoplasty

Description

1. Removal of excess breast tissue, which also involves a reduction in skin and possible transposition of nipple–areolar complex.
2. Used for alleviation of symptoms that may include back and neck pain, muscle spasm, and grooving at the shoulders secondary to bra straps.
3. Complications include hematoma, infection, necrosis of skin flap, and nipple inversion.

Nursing and Patient Care Considerations

1. Explore reasons patient may desire surgery.
2. Discuss postoperative expectations with patient.
3. Nursing interventions are similar to those in patient undergoing reconstruction.

Augmentation Mammoplasty

Description

1. Enlarging of the breasts with the use of implants.
2. Implants may be made of silicone or saline. In most cases, this is a self-pay procedure if for cosmetic purpose.
3. Complications include hematoma, wound infection, diminished sensation of the nipple, and capsular contracture, resulting in firmness of the breast.
4. Breast implants are not associated with an increased incidence of breast cancer.

Nursing and Patient Care Considerations

1. Discuss patient's expectations preoperatively.
2. Nursing interventions are similar to those in the patient undergoing reconstruction with implants.

DISORDERS OF THE BREAST

See Standard of Care Guidelines 23-1.

> ## STANDARDS OF CARE GUIDELINES 23-1
> ### Problems of the Breast
>
> When caring for any patient undergoing evaluation, diagnostic testing, treatment, or counseling for a breast-related problem, ensure optimal outcome by adhering to the following guidelines:
>
> - Explain the mammogram procedure or other diagnostic test and make sure patient knows when and how she will obtain results.
> - Perform breast examination according to American Cancer Society guidelines and teach procedure to patient.
> - Inform health care provider and patient of any suspicious findings on breast examination—asymmetry of breasts, dimpling, skin changes, nipple discharge, fixed or hard mass.
> - Inform health care provider and patient of abnormal mammogram or other test result and make sure that follow-up is arranged.
>
> **AFTER SURGERY FOR BREAST CANCER**
>
> - Assess for evidence of bleeding from the incision or flaps, including increase in pain, and notify surgeon promptly for increased pain or bleeding.
> - Assess drainage from suction drain for amount, color, and odor. Report if grossly bloody, purulent, or excessive in amount (may have 100–200 mL in the first 24 hours).
> - Assess newly reconstructed breast flaps for viability by color, warmth, and wound drainage. Notify surgeon promptly for increased warmth, change in color, purulent or excessive drainage.
> - Maintain proper protective positioning (avoid abduction to prevent edema) of arm and follow precautions for lymphedema.
> - Assess patient's emotional response and provide support throughout the diagnostic and treatment process.
>
> ---
>
> This information should serve as a general guideline only. Each patient situation presents a unique set of clinical factors and requires nursing judgment to guide care, which may include additional or alternative measures and approaches.

Fissure of the Nipple

A *fissure* is a type of ulcer that develops in the nipple of a nursing mother.

Etiology and Clinical Manifestations

1. May be caused by lack of preparation of nipples in the prenatal period.
2. Condition aggravated by sucking infant.
3. Nipple appears sore and irritated.
4. Nipple bleeds.
5. Infection may result.

Management and Nursing Interventions

1. Wash nipples with sterile saline solution.
2. Use artificial nipple for nursing.
3. If above does not initiate healing process, stop nursing and use breast pump.
4. Teach proper breastfeeding techniques to prevent fissures.
   a. Wash, dry, and lubricate nipples in prenatal period in preparation for nursing.
   b. Make sure infant's mouth covers areola.
   c. Keep nipple clean by washing and drying after each nursing period.
   d. Use lanolin cream to prevent cracking; must remove before breastfeeding.

Nipple Discharge

Nipple discharge may be serous, serosanguineous, bloody, purulent, or multicolored. It is commonly associated with benign conditions; rarely, malignancy is responsible. It may be spontaneous or nonspontaneous (occurs only when breast compressed) and it is important to differentiate between the two.

Etiology and Clinical Manifestations

1. Galactorrhea—bilateral, nonspontaneous, multiple ducts, milky gray or green discharge usually seen in patients in childbearing years.
   a. Commonly seen after pregnancy and can last for 1 to 2 years.
   b. May also be secondary to excessive breast manipulation, increased production of prolactin, medication, an endocrine anovulatory syndrome, or pituitary adenoma.
2. Mastitis—usually unilateral, purulent (see below).
3. Discharge containing blood—usually caused by intraductal papilloma (wart) or other benign lesion, but, in rare cases, may be malignant.

Diagnostic Evaluation

1. Evaluate a spontaneous nipple discharge with clinical examination, test for occult blood, mammography, and/or ultrasonography. MRI is not usually helpful.
   a. Use of a Hemoccult card gently pressed against the nipple when expressing discharge will help determine if the discharge is bloody, which warrants further workup.
   b. May get prolactin level; if elevated, may indicate pituitary adenoma.
2. Nonspontaneous milky gray or green discharge generally is not of pathologic significance and may not require workup.

Management and Nursing Interventions

1. Nursing interventions are aimed at alleviating anxiety and providing support to patient undergoing diagnostic testing. Reassure woman that nipple discharge rarely indicates cancer.
2. Bromocriptine may be given to suppress galactorrhea.
3. Treat for mastitis if purulent (see below).

4. Surgery may be indicated to treat cause of bloody and some other discharges caused by breast lesions.
   a. Most commonly because of wartlike intraductal papilloma in one of larger collecting ducts at edge of areola. May be secondary to fibrocystic changes or duct ectasia.
   b. Excisional biopsy and histologic examination may be done to rule out cancer.
   c. Ductoscopy, an image-guided excision using direct visualization of the ductal system and an intraductal biopsy, is being investigated at some larger centers.
5. Pituitary surgery for excision of adenoma (see page 918).

Acute Mastitis

Acute mastitis is inflammation of the breast secondary to infection. Breast infections may be lactational or nonlactational.

Pathophysiology and Etiology

1. Lactational infections usually occur at beginning of lactation in first-time, breastfeeding mothers. May also occur later in chronic lactation mastitis and central duct abscesses.
2. Milk stasis may lead to obstruction, followed by noninfectious inflammation, then infectious mastitis.
3. Source of infection may be from hands of patient, personnel caring for patient, baby's nose or throat, or bloodborne.
4. Nonlactational infections usually present with central subareolar inflammation.
5. Most common pathogens: *Staphylococcus aureus*, *Escherichia coli*, and *Streptococcus*.

Clinical Manifestations

1. Redness, warmth, edema; breast may feel doughy, tough. Fever may be present.
2. Patient may complain of dull pain in affected area and may have nipple discharge.
3. Complication is mammary abscess (see below).

Management and Nursing Interventions

1. Diagnosis is usually made by characteristic manifestations.
2. Antibiotics are given—10- to 14-day course of penicillinase-resistant antibiotic.
   a. Dicloxacillin—250 to 500 mg every 6 hours.
   b. Clindamycin—150 to 300 mg every 6 hours.
   c. Co-trimazole every 12 hours. (If this is used must dump breast milk in babies less than 8 weeks).
3. May have patient stop breastfeeding (controversial).
4. Apply heat to resolve tissue reaction; may cause increased milk production and worsen symptoms.
5. May apply cold to decrease tissue metabolism and milk production.
6. Have the patient wear firm breast support.
7. Encourage the breastfeeding patient to practice meticulous personal hygiene to prevent mastitis.
8. Consider lactation consult.

Mammary Abscess

Mammary abscess is a localized collection of pus in a cavity of breast tissue. About 3% of patients with mastitis may develop a breast abscess.

Etiology and Clinical Manifestations

1. May follow acute mastitis if untreated. Some patients may develop a chronic subareolar abscess thought to be caused by a plugging of major mammary ducts in the nipple with infection of obstructed secretions. This usually occurs in smokers.
2. Patient may have fever, chills, and malaise.
3. Affected area is sensitive and erythematous; may have palpable mass.
4. Pus may be expressed from nipple.

Management and Nursing Interventions

1. May perform needle aspiration if superficial mass.
2. Incision and drainage may be done, if deep.
3. A biopsy of the cavity wall may be done at time of incision and drainage to rule out breast carcinoma associated with abscess.
4. Administer antibiotics and analgesics, if ordered.
5. Apply hot, wet dressings to increase drainage and hasten resolution. Pack wound, as directed.
6. A diagnostic mammogram and sonogram may be ordered after resolution of the abscess to rule out cancer.

Fibrocystic Change/Breast Pain

Fibrocystic change is a general term that includes various changes in the breast, namely, fibrosis and cystic dilation of the ducts. May be present in up to 50% of women.

Pathophysiology and Etiology

1. Pathogenesis is not known but is related to the cyclic stimulation of the breast by estrogen and represents a change from the normal stimulation and regression pattern of this process.
2. Occurs usually in women between ages 35 and 50 and is a source of considerable discomfort in a sizable percentage of women.
3. Hormone replacement therapy (HRT) may be associated with fibrocystic changes in a woman who has never experienced this previously.

Clinical Manifestations

1. Increased generalized breast lumpiness or excessive nodularity with tenderness, pain, and breast swelling. Symptoms may decrease after menses.
2. Lumps or cysts—soft or firm; single or multiple; smooth, round, and movable. Cysts may enlarge and become tender and painful. There may be many cysts of different sizes; some may be palpable.
3. Possible nipple discharge—may be milky, yellow, or greenish.

Diagnostic Evaluation

1. Physical examination detects changes.
2. Mammography or ultrasound.
3. Aspiration—if a palpable, symptomatic mass exists or the cyst is complex.
4. Cytology of cyst fluid is not cost-effective and rarely of clinical value in fibrocystic breast changes.

Management

There is no satisfactory treatment and management is usually geared toward relief of symptoms.

Surgical Management

1. Needle aspiration and conservative medical follow-up if:
   a. The aspirate appears like normal cyst fluid and is not blood-stained.
   b. Cyst completely resolves after aspiration.
   c. No indication of an underlying neoplasm.
2. Surgical excision—indicated if a cyst keeps recurring after several aspirations or if a single solid discrete lump is present.

Medical Management

1. Sporadic discomfort may be relieved by OTC analgesics, including topical nonsteroidal anti-inflammatory drugs (ie, diclofenac).
2. Bromocriptine, a dopamine agonist.
   a. May help with mastalgia by decreasing serum prolactin levels.
   b. Adverse effects include nausea, vomiting, headache, dizziness, and fatigue; used rarely because of intolerable adverse effects.
3. Contraceptives or supplemental progestins during the secretory phase of the menstrual cycle may help with pain control.
   a. Mastalgia that begins after initiating hormonal contraceptive pills may resolve after a few cycles.
   b. Switching to a lower estrogen/higher progesterone ratio may help.
4. Danazol, a synthetic androgen used for severe fibrocystic changes to decrease hormonal stimulation of the breast by suppressing gonadotropins.
   a. Adverse effects include a deepening of the voice, which may be permanent, menstrual irregularity, weight gain, depression, bloating, and acne.
   b. Tamoxifen is currently being investigated.

Other Measures

1. Diet modifications.
   a. Eliminating caffeine (coffee, tea, cola drinks, and chocolate) from the diet may help reduce symptoms in some women.
   b. Decreasing fat intake may improve swelling, tenderness, and nodularity.
2. Stopping tobacco use has been suggested to relieve symptoms.
3. Prophylactic lumpectomy—rarely indicated for intractable pain not relieved with medical therapy in women with multiple previous biopsies or biopsy evidence of a precancerous lesion.

Nursing Interventions and Patient Teaching

1. Emphasize importance of monthly BSE—cysts may mask underlying cancer.
2. Reinforce patient's confidence in BSE by rechecking her findings.
3. Offer suggestions for alternative methods if BSE is difficult to do (ie, tender breasts).
4. Encourage patient to see health care provider regularly for examinations.
5. Recommend that patient wear a well-fitted support bra.
6. Offer emotional support for her anxiety and fear of cancer.
7. Reassure that discomfort is common to many women and that it is rarely the only presenting sign of cancer.

Benign Tumors of the Breast

Benign tumors of the breast are characterized clinically as benign lesions that are distinct and persistent over time. Approximately 90% of breast lumps are benign.

Pathophysiology and Etiology

1. Fibrocystic changes—solid lumps may be fatty or fibrous tissue or fluid-filled cysts (see above).
2. Galactocele—a milk-filled cyst.
3. Fibroadenoma—a benign breast tumor composed of epithelial and stromal components.
   a. Common in young women.
   b. A slight increase in the risk of breast cancer among women with fibroadenomas.
4. Other benign tumors include adenosis, intraductal papillomas, lipomas, and neurofibromatosis that may produce a palpable mass.

Clinical Manifestations

1. Gross cysts—may be tender or nontender. Consistency depends on pressure of fluid within cyst and breast tissue around them; may be soft and fluctuant or may feel like a solid tumor if dense.
2. Galactocele—firm, nontender mass.
3. Fibroadenoma—may be a firm, smooth, movable lump that is usually painless. Size does not usually fluctuate with menstrual cycle changes but tends to enlarge over time.

Diagnostic Evaluation

1. Physical examination, mammography, and ultrasound identify and characterize lesion.
2. Cyst aspiration—diagnostic aspiration is usually curative in a galactocele or breast cyst.
3. If a lump does not respond to cyst aspiration, excisional biopsy remains the "gold standard" to rule out cancer.

Management and Nursing Interventions

1. Nonsuspicious or indeterminate masses in young women may be observed through one or two menstrual cycles for resolution of the mass.

2. In general, any distinct and persistent solid lump should have biopsy and possibly excision.
3. Nursing care is directed toward support as woman goes through diagnostic process.

Disorders of the Male Breast

Disorders of the male breast include gynecomastia (benign) and malignant breast cancer.

Clinical Features

Gynecomastia

1. Overdevelopment of breast tissue, usually bilateral.
2. Common in infants, adolescents, and men older than age 50.
3. Usually results from hormonal alterations—idiopathic systemic disorders, such as endocrine disorders, disease of the liver, pituitary adenoma, and chronic renal failure; such drugs as cimetidine, thiazides, spironolactone, omeprazole, phenytoin, reserpine, nifedipine, and theophylline; such neoplasms as testicular tumors and in association with lung and prostate cancer (may be related to therapy).
4. Pubertal gynecomastia has an onset in boys ages 10 to 12 and generally regresses within 18 months. Need to rule out illicit drugs in teens. Marijuana, alcohol, amphetamines, heroin, LSD, and methadone can cause gynecomastia.

 DRUG ALERT Question teenage boys presenting with gynecomastia about illicit drug use.

5. Asymptomatic and pubertal gynecomastia does not require further tests, but should be reevaluated in 6 months. There is no evidence that links gynecomastia with male breast cancer.
6. Investigation is warranted if the drugs used by the patient do not explain the gynecomastia and the breast is tender or the diameter of the breast tissue is more than 4 cm.
7. Reduction subcutaneous nipple-sparing mammoplasty is considered for patients with long-standing gynecomastia for cosmetic and accompanying psychosocial reasons.

Breast Cancer

1. Resembles cancer of the breast in women.
2. Less than 1% of all breast cancers—incidence greatest in men in their 60s.
3. Carries poor prognosis because men may delay seeking treatment until disease is advanced.
4. Risk factors: family history (20% of men with breast cancer have a first-degree relative with the disease), occupation, and some genetic syndromes, such as Cowden and Klinefelter's. Men chronically exposed to hot environments, such as steel mills, have been shown to be at increased risk as well those employed in the soap and perfume industry and those exposed to petroleum and exhaust fumes.
5. There are no specific screening recommendations for men.
6. Nursing care and treatment is essentially the same as for female breast cancer, including tamoxifen, chemotherapy, and/or radiation therapy.

Cancer of the Breast

Breast cancer is the most common cancer in women in the United States and is second only to lung cancer as a cause of cancer death.

Pathophysiology and Etiology

1. Most breast cancer (85% to 90%) begins in the lining of the milk ducts, sometimes in the lobule. Eventually it grows through the wall of the duct and into the fatty tissue. (See Table 23-3 for types of breast cancer.)
2. Family history accounts for approximately 7% of all breast cancers.
   a. Current genetic models attribute 5% to 10% of all breast cancer to dominantly inherited breast cancer susceptibility genes.
   b. Two breast/ovarian susceptibility genes have been identified and named BRCA-1 and BRCA-2. Testing may be performed for those patients diagnosed before age 50 with breast and/or ovarian cancer who also have two first-degree relatives with a similar diagnosis or a combination of three or more relatives (including males) with breast cancer

regardless of age at diagnosis. Women of Ashkenazi Jewish descent have an increased likelihood of BRCA mutations. Knowledge of a mutation can help patients make informed decisions to manage their risk for future breast cancers. It is important to have genetic counseling before the test because of its implications. Screening is not warranted for general population.

 Evidence Base U.S. Preventive Services Task Force. (2005). Genetic risk assessment and BRCA mutation testing for breast and ovarian cancer susceptibility: Recommendation statement; 2005. Available: *www.ahrq.gov/downloads/pub/prevent/pdfser/brcagensyn .pdf.*

3. Present knowledge does not indicate that carcinogens play an important role in the development of breast cancer.
4. Several models exist that attempt to predict the short-term or lifetime risk of breast cancer for women with identifiable factors associated with the disease. These include the Breast Cancer Pro Statistical Model, and the Gail model (*www.bcra.nci.nih.gov*).

Table 23-3	Types of Breast Cancer		
CELL TYPE	**DESCRIPTION**	**INCIDENCE***	**COMMENTS**
In situ			
DCIS	Abnormal cells in duct	28% Frequently found in combination with invasive cancer	A noninvasive breast cancer; the majority found by mammogram
LCIS	Solid proliferation of small cells within breast lobules	3%–5% More frequent in premenopausal women	Nonpalpable mammographic finding; a marker that indicates increased risk of developing cancer in either breast
Invasive			
Ductal	Classified on basis of microscopic appearance as ductal or lobular	85–90%	Characterized by stony hardness on palpation
Lobular	As above	5%–10%	Relatively uncommon; tends to be more infiltrative
Others			
Tubular Medullary Mucinous Papillary Sarcoma	Types frequently associated with above; cell type must dominate to be assigned	<10% of all breast cancers	Axillary metastasis uncommon in tubular; medullary associated with fast growth rate and favorable prognosis
Inflammatory	Applies to distinctive inflamed appearance of skin; no consistent histologic type	1%–4%	Presents with erythema, warmth, tenderness, and edema; may be treated with chemotherapy or radiation therapy first
Paget's Disease of Nipple	Usually associated with underlying intraductal or invasive carcinoma	2%	Presents as scaly, erythematous, periareolar eruption

DCIS, ductal carcinoma in situ; LCIS, lobular carcinoma in situ.
*Percent greater than 100—infiltrating carcinoma frequently includes small areas containing other special types or a combination of in situ and infiltrating carcinoma is seen.

Epidemiology of Breast Cancer

 Evidence Base Siegel, R., Naishadham, D., Jemal, A., et al. (2012). Cancer statistics, 2012. *CA—A Cancer Journal for Clinicians, 62,* 10–29.

Incidence

1. The American Cancer Society estimates that 229,060 (2,190 male) new cases of breast cancer will be diagnosed in 2012 in the United States, with approximately 39,920 deaths. Breast cancer incidence rates appear to be decreasing primarily in white women and in younger women.
2. There are expected to be 63,300 cases of DCIS in 2012.

Survival Rates

1. Five-year overall survival rates:
   Localized: 97%.
   Regional: 78.7%.
   Distant: 23.3%.
2. In the general population, the relative survival rate is lower among black women than white women.
3. Lymph node status is the most important prognostic indicator of disease-free survival.
4. Age, comorbidity, staging (tumor size, lymph node status, and distant metastasis), nuclear grade, histologic differentiation, possibly HER2 status, and treatment are important prognostic factors for survival (see Table 23-4). Adjuvant! Online at *www.adjuvantonline.com* is available for estimating 10-year overall survival.
5. Mortality is declining 1% to 2% in the United States. This may be related to:
   a. Change in lifestyle such as diet.
   b. Early diagnosis—increased use of screening mammography.
   c. Improved treatment.

Table 23-4	Staging of Breast Cancer
STAGE	**DESCRIPTION**
0	Carcinoma in situ
I	Tumor 2 cm or less in greatest dimension, no axillary lymph node metastasis other than micrometastasis; no evidence of distant metastasis.
II	Tumor less than 2 cm in greatest dimension but with one to three positive lymph nodes, a tumor 2–5 cm with or without axillary lymph node metastasis, or a tumor >5 cm without spread to lymph nodes; no evidence of distant metastasis.
III	Any size tumor with four or more positive axillary lymph nodes or with direct extension to the chest wall or skin; inflammatory breast cancer; no evidence of distant metastasis.
IV	Any of the above plus distant metastasis (ie, liver, lungs, bone, brain).

Based on information from the National Cancer Institute and the American Joint Committee on Cancer (2010).

 NURSING ALERT Black women are more likely than white women to be diagnosed with large tumors and distant-stage disease. Learn about the demographics of your patient population.

Risk Factors

A woman's lifetime risk of developing breast cancer is 12.5% based on a life span of 80 years.

1. Major—female gender, increased age, a diagnosis of lobular carcinoma in situ, a prior history of breast or ovarian cancer, and family history (especially mother, sisters). Approximate twofold risk in women with affected sister or mother; this increases if more relatives were affected or if affected close relatives developed breast cancer before menopause.
2. Probable—nulliparity, older age at first live childbirth, late menopause, early menarche, benign proliferative breast disease, diagnosis of atypical ductal hyperplasia on biopsy, long-term use of estrogen replacement therapy that increases with duration of use and previous exposure to chest wall irradiation.
3. Controversial—hormonal contraceptive use (estrogen and progestin may stimulate tumor growth with long-term use), alcohol use, obesity, and increased dietary fat intake.
4. Results of breast cancer prevention trials have shown a reduction in incidence of breast cancer in high-risk women treated with tamoxifen, exemestane, or raloxifene.

 GERONTOLOGIC ALERT Age is the greatest single risk factor for the development of cancer. Cancer warning signals may be unheeded in older women, so thorough history-taking and physical examination is essential.

Clinical Manifestations

See Figure 23-1.

1. A firm lump or thickening in breast, usually painless; 50% located in upper outer quadrant of breast. Enlargement of axillary or supraclavicular lymph nodes may indicate metastasis.
2. Nipple discharge—spontaneous, may be bloody, clear, or serous.
3. Breast asymmetry—a change in the size or shape of the breast or abnormal contours. As woman changes positions, compare one breast to other.
4. Nipple retraction or scaliness, especially in Paget's disease.
5. Late signs—pain, ulceration, edema, orange-peel skin (peau d'orange) from interference of lymphatic drainage.
6. Inflammatory breast cancer may present with erythema.
7. Many small invasive breast cancers as well as noninvasive breast cancer (DCIS) do not present with a palpable mass, but are found on mammography.

 NURSING ALERT Pain is not usually an early warning sign of breast cancer.

Diagnostic Evaluation

See page 887.

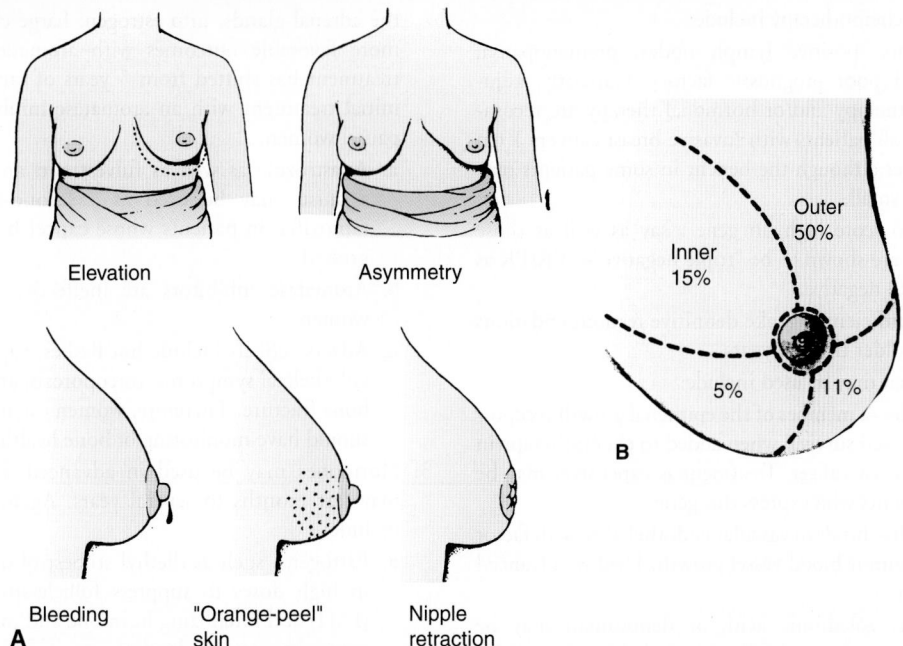

Figure 23-1. (A) Signs of cancer of the breast. **(B)** Distribution of carcinomas in different areas of breast.

Management

Based on type and stage of breast cancer, receptors, and menopausal status. For women with localized breast cancer, information from clinical trials indicates that treatment with a breast-preserving procedure has similar survival rates, as does simple modified radical mastectomy. Surgery for DCIS may involve only a lumpectomy, but mastectomy may be necessary for extensive disease.

Surgery

See page 890 for a discussion of surgery for breast cancer.

Radiation Therapy

1. In conjunction with breast-preserving procedure as adjuvant (additional) therapy to decrease incidence of local recurrence for invasive breast cancer and DCIS. May be used preoperatively to shrink a large tumor to operable size.
2. May be used after a mastectomy in patients with large tumors that involve the chest wall and/or many positive axillary lymph nodes, may delay reconstruction.
3. Contraindications to a breast-preserving procedure include two primary tumors in separate quadrants of the breast, history of previous radiation therapy to the breast or chest wall, pregnancy, and positive margins.
4. Treatment may be individualized in pregnancy—ie, appropriate surgery followed by chemotherapy in the second or third trimester and delayed irradiation in order to preserve the breast.
5. May also be used to alleviate bone pain in metastatic breast cancer.
6. Radiation directed to breast, chest wall, and remaining lymph nodes.
   a. Usually five treatments per week for 6 or 7 weeks.
   b. A booster or second phase of treatment may be given.
   c. May include implants of radioactive material after external treatment completed.
7. Adverse effects include mild fatigue, sore throat, dry cough, nausea, anorexia; later, skin will look and feel sunburned. Eventually, the breast may become firmer. Complications include increased arm edema, decreased arm mobility, pneumonitis, and brachial nerve damage. See page 891 for care of patient undergoing radiation therapy.
8. The FDA has approved a device called MammoSite that delivers partial breast irradiation through a balloon temporarily surgically implanted in the breast. Treatment is twice per day for 5 days. Early data suggest acceptable locoregional disease control with this approach; however, long-term follow-up studies are needed. Partial breast irradiation should be performed only as part of a prospective trial.
9. A one-time dose of radiation intraoperatively is also under investigation.

Chemotherapy

1. Major use is in adjuvant systemic treatment postoperatively; usually begins 4 weeks after surgery (stressful for patient who just finished major surgery).
2. Treatments are given every 2 to 4 weeks for 6 to 9 months. Because the drugs differ in their mechanisms of action, combinations of agents are used to treat cancer.
3. Main drugs used for breast cancer include cyclophosphamide, methotrexate, 5-fluorouracil (5-FU), doxorubicin, and paclitaxel. For advanced cancer, docetaxel, vinorelbine, capecitabine, mitoxantrone, and fluorouracil by continuous infusion and oral forms of fluorouracil are used.

4. Indications for chemotherapy include:

a. Large tumors, positive lymph nodes, premenopausal women, and poor prognostic factors. Currently, adjuvant chemotherapy and/or hormonal therapy are recommended for all patients with invasive breast cancers 1 cm wide or larger although the benefit in some patients may be relatively small.

b. Patients who score high on gene assay as well as those tumors that are shown to be "triple negative"—ER/PR as well as HER2 negative.

c. Data are insufficient to make definitive recommendations for patients older than 70 years.

5. Other agents that may be used include:

a. Trastuzumab—a member of the epithelial growth receptor family; increased survival when added to chemotherapy in metastatic breast cancer. Treatment is expensive; may be given to patients who express this gene.

b. Bevacizumab—binds to vascular endothelial growth factor and blocks tumor blood vessel growth. Used in advanced breast cancer.

c. Pamidronate, zoledronic acid, or denosumab may be added if bone metastasis present to help reduce pain. Patients should undergo dental exam prior to initiation of this therapy.

d. Poly ADP ribose polymerase inhibitors, such as olaparib, are enzymes that help repair DNA, may be helpful in triple negative cancers.

6. Adverse effects include bone marrow suppression, cardiotoxicity, nausea and vomiting, alopecia, weight gain or loss, fatigue, stomatitis, anxiety, depression, and premature menopause (see page 146 for nursing care of patient undergoing chemotherapy). Childbearing after treatment of invasive breast cancer does not increase rates of breast cancer recurrence or death.

7. Chemotherapy may also be used as primary treatment in inflammatory breast cancer and occasionally in large tumors; otherwise, preoperative chemotherapy remains investigational.

8. Hope for the future is the development of specific targeted biologic therapies and more individualized treatment.

Endocrine Therapy

1. Selective estrogen receptor modulators, such as tamoxifen and raloxifene, bind estrogen receptors, thereby blocking effects of estrogen.

a. Adjuvant systemic therapy after surgery.

b. Benefits estrogen receptor–positive patients, regardless of menopausal status.

c. Given for at least 5 years; oral administration once or twice per day.

d. Adverse effects include hot flashes, irregular periods, vaginal irritation, nausea and vomiting, headaches, increased risk of endometrial cancer and thromboembolic events.

e. Women on tamoxifen should have an annual gynecologic assessment if uterus present.

2. Aromatase inhibitors, such as anastrozole, exemestane, and letrozole, block conversion of androgen, which is secreted by the adrenal glands, into estrogen. Large clinical trials report more favorable outcomes with aromatase inhibitors, and treatment has shifted from 5 years of tamoxifen therapy to initial treatment with an aromatase inhibitor in postmenopausal women.

a. Anastrozole as well as fulvestrant, an estrogen receptor agonist, may be used as a second-line therapy after tamoxifen in patients whose cancer has returned or progressed.

b. Aromatase inhibitors are ineffective in premenopausal women.

c. Adverse effects include hot flashes, vaginal dryness, musculoskeletal symptoms, osteoporosis, and increased rate of bone fracture. Therefore, women on aromatase inhibitors should have monitoring of bone health.

3. Hormones may be used in advanced disease. Remissions may last months to several years. Agents commonly used include:

a. Estrogens, such as diethyl stilbestrol or ethinyl estradiol, in high doses to suppress follicle-stimulating hormone (FSH) and luteinizing hormone and may decrease endogenous estrogen production.

b. Progestins may decrease estrogen receptors.

c. Androgens may suppress FSH and estrogen production.

d. Aminoglutethimide suppresses estrogen production by blocking adrenal steroids; "medical adrenalectomy," especially useful for women with bone and soft tissue metastasis.

4. Corticosteroids suppress estrogen and progesterone secretion from the adrenals.

 DRUG ALERT Traditionally, breast cancer survivors have not been considered candidates for estrogen. However, debates and studies continue to be conducted regarding the safety of estrogen in this population.

Bone Marrow Transplant

1. Autologous method after high-dose chemotherapy.

2. Clinical trials have shown it to be ineffective for breast cancer.

Oophorectomy

Removal of ovaries.

1. Treatment for recurrent or metastatic disease in estrogen receptor–positive premenopausal women.

2. Deprives tumor of primary estrogen source—remissions of 3 months to several years.

3. Medical ablation with tamoxifen has been compared to surgical oophorectomy in estrogen receptor–positive postmenopausal women and response rates are similar.

4. Surgical ablation is now considered second choice because of its increased risks.

5. The benefits of tamoxifen in combination with oophorectomy are the subject of ongoing research.

Adrenalectomy

Removal of adrenal glands to eliminate androgen production (which converts to estrogen).

1. Rarely done because of need for long-term steroid replacement therapy.
2. Remissions may last 6 months to several years.
3. Medical ablation with drugs being studied.

Complications

1. Metastasis—most common sites: lymph nodes, lung, bone, liver, and brain.
2. Signs and symptoms of metastasis may include bone pain, neurologic changes, weight loss, anemia, cough, shortness of breath, pleuritic pain, and vague chest discomfort.

Nursing Assessment

1. Assess general health status and underlying chronic illnesses that may have an impact on patient's response to treatment.

 NURSING ALERT Evidence suggests that active lifestyle and achieving and maintaining an ideal body weight (20 to 25 BMI) may lead to optimal breast cancer outcomes.

2. Identify what the patient and family need to know regarding breast cancer and its treatment and take measures to decrease their impact. Base education on patient and family needs.
3. Determine level of anxiety, fears, and concerns.
4. Identify coping ability and availability of support systems.

Nursing Diagnoses

Also see page 892 for breast surgery care and Chapter 8, Cancer nursing.

- Anxiety related to diagnosis of cancer.
- Deficient Knowledge related to disease process and treatment options.
- Ineffective Coping by patient or family related to diagnosis, prognosis, financial stress, or inadequate support.

Nursing Interventions

 Evidence Base Carlson, R. W., Allred, C., Anderson, B. O., et al. (2011). Invasive breast cancer: Clinical practice guidelines in oncology. *Journal of the National Comprehensive Cancer Network, 9,* 136–221.

Reducing Anxiety

1. Realize that diagnosis of breast cancer is a devastating emotional shock to patient. Support patient through the diagnostic process. Many women must make challenging decisions in a brief period of time. Some communities have developed nursing navigators as a way of assisting and supporting individuals through the process. Check if there is a nurse navigator in your community.
2. Interpret the results of each test in language patient can understand.
3. Stress the advances made in earlier diagnosis and treatment options.

Providing Information About Treatment

1. Involve patient in treatment planning.
2. Describe surgical procedures.
3. Prepare patient for the effects of chemotherapy; encourage patient to plan ahead for the common adverse effects of chemotherapy.
4. Educate patient about the effects of radiation therapy.
5. Teach patient about hormonal therapy. Patient may develop hot flashes with the start of hormonal therapy or with the discontinuation of HRT at the time of diagnosis of breast cancer (see Chapter 22 for information on menopausal symptoms). Measures that may help with symptoms of hot flashes include:
   a. Clonidine, belladonna/ergotamine/phenobarbital, antidepressants.
   b. Various supplements and herbs have been used but have not been rigorously tested. Soy has been suggested, but there is no compelling evidence that phytoestrogens help menopausal symptoms. Indeed, concerns have been raised regarding stimulating breast cancer cell growth and, therefore, should not be used.
   c. Progesterone may be helpful, but the possible effect on breast cancer needs further study.

Strengthening Coping

1. Repeat information and speak in calm, clear manner.
2. Display empathy and acceptance of patient's emotions.
3. Explore coping mechanisms.
4. Evaluate where patient is in stages of acceptance.
5. Help patient identify and use support persons.
6. Obtain visit from support group member.
7. Refer for counseling, financial aid, and so forth.
8. Resources include American Cancer Society (800-ACS-2345 or *www.cancer.org*), National Cancer Institute (*www.cancer.gov*), National Alliance of Breast Cancer Organizations (*www.nabco.org*), and the Susan G. Komen Breast Cancer Foundation (*www.komen.com*).

Patient Education and Health Maintenance

1. Encourage patient to continue close follow-up and to report any new symptoms. Most women will be seen every 3 months for the first 2 years, every 6 months for the next 3 years, and once per year after 5 years.
2. Stress importance of continued yearly mammogram.
3. Inform patient that yearly laboratory work, bone scan, and chest x-ray may be performed when clinically indicated.
4. Suggest to patient that psychological intervention may be necessary for anxiety, depression, or sexual problems.

Evaluation: Expected Outcomes

- Verbalizes less anxiety.
- Verbalizes understanding of all treatment options and their adverse effects.
- Identifies appropriate coping mechanisms and support systems.

SELECTED REFERENCES

American Cancer Society. (2012). Can breast cancer be found early? Available: *http://www.cancer.org/cancer/breastcancer/detailedguide/breast-cancer-detection.*

American Cancer Society. (2012). How to perform a breast self-exam. Available: *http://www.cancer.org/cancer/breastcancer/detailedguide/breast-cancer-detection.*

American Cancer Society. (2012). Lymphedema: What every woman with breast cancer should know. Available: *http://www.cancer.org/treatment/treatmentsandsideeffects/physicalsideeffects/lymphedema/whateverywomanwithbreastcancershouldknow/lymphedema-what-every-woman-with-breast-cancer-should-know-toc.*

American College of Radiology. (2003). Bi-rads-mammography: Assessment Categories, 4th ed. Reston, VA: Author.

American Joint Committee on Cancer. (2010). *AJCC cancer staging manual* (7th ed.). New York: Springer.

Bevers, T. B., Banu, A., Cowan, K. H., et al. (2010). Breast cancer risk reduction. *Journal of the National Comprehensive Cancer Network, 8,* 1112–1146.

Carlson, R. W., Allred, C., Anderson, B. O., et al. (2011). Invasive breast cancer: Clinical practice guidelines in oncology. *Journal of the National Comprehensive Cancer Network, 9,* 136–221.

Giuliano, A. E., Hunt, K. K., Ballman, K. V., et al. (2011). Axillary dissection versus no axillary dissection in women with invasive breast cancer and sentinel node metastasis: A randomized clinical trial. *Journal of the American Medical Association, 305,* 569–575.

Hamilton, R. (2012). Being young, female, and BRCA positive. *AJN, 112*(10), 26–31.

Korber, S. F., Padula, C., Gray, D., et al. (2011). A breast navigator program: barriers, enhancers, and nursing interventions. *Oncology Nursing Forum, 38*(1), 44–50.

National Comprehensive Cancer Network (NCCN) 2012. Clinical practice guidelines in oncology breast cancer. Available: *www.nccn.org.*

National Comprehensive Cancer Network. (2012). Clinical practice guidelines in oncology: Breast cancer screening and diagnosis. Version 1. 2012. Available: *www.nccn.org.*

Nye, L., Huyck, T. K., Gradishar, W. J. (2012). Diagnostic and treatment considerations when newly diagnosed breast cancer coincides with pregnancy: a case report and review of the literature. *Journal of the National Comprehensive Cancer Network, 10,* 1145–1148.

Patterson, S. K., & Noroozian, M. (2012). Update on emerging technologies in breast imaging. *Journal of the National Comprehensive Cancer Network, 10,* 1355–1360.

Quirion, E. (2010). Recognizing and treating upper extremity lymphedema in postmastectomy/lumpectomy patients: A guide for primary care providers. *Journal of the American Academy of Nurse Practitioners, 22,* 450–459.

Robinson-White, S., Conroy, B., Slavish, K., et al. (2010). Patient navigators in breast cancer: A systematic review. *Cancer Nursing, 33,* 127–140.

Siegel, R., Naishadham, D., Jemal, A., et al. (2012). Cancer statistics, 2012. *CA—A Cancer Journal for Clinicians, 62,* 10–29.

Smith, R. A., Cokkinides, V., Brooks, D., et al. (2011). Cancer screening in the United States, 2011. A review of current American Cancer Society guidelines and issues in cancer screening. *CA—A Cancer Journal for Clinicians, 61,* 8–30.

U.S. Preventive Services Task Force. (2005). Genetic risk assessment and BRCA mutation testing for breast and ovarian cancer susceptibility: Recommendation statement. *Annals of Internal Medicine, 143*(5), 355–361.

Weaver, D. L., Ashikaga, T., Krag, D. N., et al. (2011). Effect of occult metastases on survival in node-negative breast cancer. *New England Journal of Medicine, 364,* 412–421.

24
Endocrine Disorders

OVERVIEW AND ASSESSMENT
The Function of Hormones

The endocrine system and the nervous system maintain homeostasis. The endocrine glands produce hormones, chemical substances that are secreted into the bloodstream and that exert a stimulatory or inhibitory effect on target tissues or on glands. Hormones achieve their effect by binding with specific receptors located on the membrane on the target cell (eg, catecholamines) or by penetrating the cell membrane and forming a complex that influences cellular metabolism (eg, steroids). The target cell response may be reflected through the production and secretion of a second hormone or through a change in cell metabolism that alters the concentration of electrolytes or other substances in the bloodstream.

General Effects of Hormone Action

1. Regulate the overall metabolic rate and the storage, conversion, and release of energy.
2. Regulate fluid and electrolyte balance.
3. Initiate coping responses to stressors.
4. Regulate growth and development.
5. Regulate reproduction processes.

Regulation of Hormones

1. Hormone secretion is typically controlled through a negative feedback system.
   a. Fall in blood concentration of hormone leads to activation of the regulator endocrine gland and to release of its stimulator hormones.
   b. Elevations in blood concentration of target cell hormones or of changes in blood composition resulting from target cell activity can cause inhibition of hormone secretion.
2. Endocrine disorders are manifested as states of hormone deficiency or hormone excess. The underlying pathophysiology may be expressed as:
   a. *Primary*—the secreting gland releases inappropriate hormone because of disease of the gland itself.

b. *Secondary*—the secreting gland releases abnormal amounts of hormone because of disease in a regulator gland (eg, pituitary).

c. *Tertiary*—the secreting gland releases inappropriate hormone because of hypothalamic dysfunction, resulting in abnormal stimulation by the pituitary.

3. Abnormal hormone concentrations may also be caused by hormone-producing tumors (adenomas) located at a remote site.

History

Patients with diseases of the endocrine system commonly report nonspecific complaints. Commonly, symptoms may reflect changes in general well-being, such as fatigue, weakness, weight change, appetite, sleep patterns, or psychiatric status. A thorough review of systems is necessary to detect changes in various body systems caused by an endocrine disorder (see Table 24-1).

Physical Examination

Objective findings may be obvious and related to the patient's complaints or may be "silent signs" of which the patient is completely unaware. Thorough physical examination of all body systems, particularly the integumentary, cardiovascular, and neurologic systems, may reveal key findings for endocrine dysfunction (see Chapter 5).

Tests of Thyroid Function

Total Thyroxine

Description

1. This is a direct measurement of the concentration of total thyroxine (T_4) in the blood, using a radioimmunoassay technique.
2. It is an accurate index of thyroid function when T_4-binding globulin (TBG) is normal.
3. Low plasma-binding protein states (malnutrition, liver disease) may give low values.
4. High plasma-binding protein values (pregnancy, estrogen therapy) may give high values.
5. It is used to diagnose hypofunction and hyperfunction of the thyroid and to guide and evaluate thyroid hormone replacement therapy.

Nursing and Patient Care Considerations

1. The test to monitor thyroid hormone therapy should be performed 6 to 8 weeks after dosage adjustment because of the time required for thyroid-stimulating hormone (TSH) to reflect the body's response to the new dose.
2. Interpretation of test results:
   a. Hypothyroidism—below normal.
   b. Hyperthyroidism—above normal.
3. Iodides can affect the results of thyroid tests; therefore, it is important to determine if patient has had any recent tests that used iodine as a contrast medium.

Free Thyroxine

Description

1. Direct measurement of free T_4 concentration in the blood using a two-step radioimmunoassay method.

2. Accurate measure of thyroid function independent of the variable influence of thyroid-binding globulin levels.
3. Used to aid in the diagnosis of hyperthyroidism and hypothyroidism.
4. Used to monitor and guide thyroid hormone replacement therapy, particularly with pituitary disease.

Nursing and Patient Care Considerations

1. Interpretation of test results:
   a. Hyperthyroidism—above normal.
   b. Hypothyroidism—below normal.
2. Results best interpreted in conjunction with TSH levels for diagnostic purposes.
3. When used to monitor thyroid hormone replacement therapy, levels meaningful only after 6 to 8 weeks of therapy to evaluate adequacy of dosage because of long half-life of T_4.

Thyroid-Binding Globulin

Description

1. This measures the concentration of the carrier protein for T_4 in the blood.
2. Because most T_4 is protein bound, changes in TBG will influence values of T_4.
3. Helpful in distinguishing between true thyroid disease and T_4 test abnormalities caused by TBG excess or deficit.

Nursing and Patient Care Considerations

Determine if patient is taking estrogen or is pregnant, both of which can elevate TBG; results may be depressed by malnutrition or by liver disease.

Triiodothyronine

Description

1. Directly measures concentration of triiodothyronine (T_3) in the blood using a radioimmunoassay technique.
2. T_3 is less influenced by alterations in thyroid-binding proteins.
3. T_3 has a shorter half-life than T_4 and occurs in minute quantities in the active form.
4. Useful to rule out T_3 thyrotoxicosis, hyperthyroidism when T_4 is normal, and to evaluate effects of thyroid replacement therapy.

Nursing and Patient Care Considerations

1. T_3 can be transiently depressed in the acutely ill patient.
2. Interpretation of test results:
   a. Hypothyroidism—below normal.
   b. Hyperthyroidism—above normal.

T_3 Resin Uptake

Description

1. This is an indirect measure of thyroid function, based on the available protein-binding sites in a serum sample that can bind to radioactive T_3.
2. The radioactive T_3 is added to the serum sample in the test tube and will bind with available protein-binding sites. The unbound T_3 binds to resin for T_3 uptake, reflecting the amount of T_3 left over because of lack of binding sites.
3. Estrogen and pregnancy produce an increase in binding sites, thus causing a lowered T_3 resin uptake.

Table 24-1   Clinical Manifestations of Endocrine Dysfunction

SIGN OR SYMPTOM	POSSIBLE CAUSES	SIGN OR SYMPTOM	POSSIBLE CAUSES
Cardiovascular		Weight loss	• Hyperthyroidism • Hyperparathyroidism • Pheochromocytoma
Tachycardia or tachyarrhythmia	• Hyperthyroidism • Pheochromocytoma • Adrenal insufficiency	Hyperdefecation	• Hyperthyroidism
Bradycardia	• Hypothyroidism	Abdominal pain	• Addisonian crisis • Hyperparathyroidism
Orthostatic hypotension	• Adrenal insufficiency	**Musculoskeletal**	
Hypertension	• Pheochromocytoma • Hyperaldosteronism • Cushing's syndrome • Hyperparathyroidism • Hypothyroidism	Weakness	• Hyperthyroidism • Hypothyroidism • Cushing's syndrome • Adrenal insufficiency • Hyperparathyroidism • Hypoparathyroidism • Hyperaldosteronism
Heart failure	• Hyperthyroidism • Hypothyroidism • Cushing's syndrome	Pathologic fractures	• Hyperparathyroidism
Neurologic		Joint pain	• Hypothyroidism • Acromegaly
Fatigue	• Adrenal insufficiency • Hypothyroidism • Hyperparathyroidism	Bone pain	• Hyperparathyroidism
		Bone thickening	• Acromegaly
Nervousness, tremor	• Pheochromocytoma • Hyperthyroidism	**Urologic**	
Confusion, lethargy, or coma	• Diabetic ketoacidosis • Hypothyroidism • Syndrome of inappropriate antidiuretic hormone	Polyuria	• Diabetes insipidus • Diabetes mellitus
		Kidney stones	• Hyperparathyroidism • Acromegaly • Cushing's syndrome
Paresthesia	• Hypothyroidism • Hypoparathyroidism • Diabetes mellitus	**Integumentary**	
Headache	• Acromegaly • Pituitary tumor • Pheochromocytoma	Hirsutism	• Adrenal hyperfunction • Acromegaly
Psychosis	• Hyperaldosteronism • Hypothyroidism • Hyperthyroidism • Cushing's syndrome • Adrenal insufficiency • Hyperparathyroidism	Hair loss	• Hypoparathyroidism • Hypothyroidism • Cushing's syndrome
		Sparse body hair	• Pituitary insufficiency • Adrenal insufficiency • Hypogonadism
Chvostek's sign, Trousseau's sign	• Hypoparathyroidism	Hyperpigmentation	• Addison's disease • Hyperthyroidism • Ectopic corticotropin production
Increased reflexes	• Hyperthyroidism		
Decreased reflexes	• Hypothyroidism	Profuse diaphoresis	• Hyperthyroidism • Pheochromocytoma
Peptic ulcer	• Cushing's syndrome	Thin skin	• Cushing's syndrome
Diarrhea	• Adrenal insufficiency	Coarse hair	• Hypothyroidism
Constipation	• Hypothyroidism • Hyperparathyroidism • Pheochromocytoma	Fine hair	• Hyperthyroidism
		Edema	• Cushing's syndrome

(continued)

Table 24-1	Clinical Manifestations of Endocrine Dysfunction (*continued*)		
SIGN OR SYMPTOM	**POSSIBLE CAUSES**	**SIGN OR SYMPTOM**	**POSSIBLE CAUSES**
Reproductive		**Ophthalmic/Visual**	
Amenorrhea	• Hyperthyroidism • Hypogonadism • Cushing's syndrome • Acromegaly • Pituitary tumor	Exophthalmos	• Graves' disease
		Diplopia	• Graves' disease • Pituitary tumor
		Visual field deficit	• Pituitary tumor
Gynecomastia	• Hypogonadism • Pituitary tumor	Periorbital swelling	• Hypothyroidism • Graves' disease
		Body Habitus	
Loss of libido, impotence	• Hypogonadism • Hypothyroidism • Adrenal insufficiency • Diabetes mellitus	Round face, "buffalo hump"	• Cushing's syndrome
		Abnormally tall stature	• Prepubertal growth • Acromegaly

Nursing and Patient Care Considerations

1. Results may be altered if patient has been taking estrogens, androgens, salicylates, or phenytoin.
2. Interpretation of test results:
   a. Hypothyroidism—below normal.
   b. Hyperthyroidism—above normal.

Free Thyroid Index

Description

The free thyroid index is a laboratory estimate of free T_4 concentration with calculated adjustment for variations in patient's TBG concentration.

Nursing and Patient Care Considerations

Interpretation of test results:

1. Below normal—hypothyroidism.
2. Above normal—hyperthyroidism.

Thyrotropin, Thyroid-Stimulating Hormone

Description

1. Direct measure of TSH, the hormone secreted by the pituitary gland that regulates the production and secretion of T_4 by the thyroid gland.
2. Blood sample is analyzed by radioimmunoassay.
3. Preferred test differentiates between thyroid disorders caused by disease of the thyroid gland itself and disorders caused by disease of the pituitary or hypothalamus. Also useful to detect early stages of hypothyroidism (subclinical hypothyroidism) and to monitor hormone replacement therapy (HRT). Patient must be on a stable dose of thyroxine for 6 to 8 weeks for TSH levels to accurately reflect adequacy of treatment.
4. Morning samples are preferred.

Nursing and Patient Care Considerations

1. Interpretation:
   a. In primary hypothyroidism, TSH levels are elevated.
   b. In secondary hypothyroidism (failure of the pituitary gland), TSH levels are low.
   c. In hyperthyroidism, TSH levels are low.

Thyrotropin-Releasing Hormone Stimulation Test

Description

1. The thyrotropin-releasing hormone (TRH) stimulation test evaluates the patency of the pituitary–hypothalamic axis. Once used primarily to distinguish between primary and central hypothyroidism, this test is rarely used for that purpose with the advent of more sensitive TSH assays. Now, its primary use is to distinguish between secondary and tertiary hypothyroidism and evaluate acromegaly.
2. A baseline sample is drawn, then TRH is administered via intravenous (IV) injection and blood samples are drawn to determine TSH levels at 30, 90, and 120 minutes.

Nursing and Patient Care Considerations

1. Interpretation:
   a. Increased TSH should be seen within 30 minutes.
   b. No rise in secondary hypothyroidism.
   c. Blunted rise in hyperthyroidism.
   d. Delayed rise (90-minute sample) associated with tertiary hypothyroidism.
   e. Elevated growth hormone levels associated with acromegaly.
2. A subnormal response can occur in patients taking L-dopa or cortisol.

Thyroid Autoantibodies

Description

Used to detect selected autoantibodies associated with some thyroid diseases and the levels of those autoantibodies.

1. Thyroid-stimulating immunoglobulin (TSI)—autoantibodies that stimulate the TSH receptor on the thyroid gland,

causing hyperfunction of the thyroid. Helpful in the diagnosis of Graves' disease.

2. Thyroid peroxidase antibodies—associated with Hashimoto's thyroiditis and Graves' disease.

3. Thyroglobulin antibodies—elevated with Hashimoto's thyroiditis and Graves' disease.

Tests of Parathyroid Function

Parathyroid Hormone

Description

1. Test is a direct measurement of parathyroid hormone (PTH) concentration in the blood, using radioimmunoassay technique.

2. Results are usually compared with results of total serum calcium to determine likely cause of parathyroid dysfunction.

3. Range of normal values may vary by laboratory and method.

Nursing and Patient Care Considerations

Elevated PTH in hyperparathyroidism; decreased PTH in hypoparathyroidism.

Serum Calcium, Total

Description

1. This is a direct measurement of protein-bound and "free" ionized calcium.

2. Ionized calcium fraction is the best indicator of changes in calcium metabolism.

3. Results can be affected by changes in serum albumin, the primary protein carrier.

4. Used to detect alterations in calcium metabolism caused by parathyroid disease or malignancy.

Nursing and Patient Care Considerations

1. Sample may be obtained from fasting patient and should be collected in tube with heparin as anticoagulant.

2. Test may be repeated to confirm parathyroid disease.

3. Elevations in serum calcium can be caused by dehydration, vitamin D intoxication, thiazide diuretics, immobilization, hyperthyroidism, or lithium therapy.

4. Low values may be seen in renal failure, chronic disease states, malabsorption syndrome, and vitamin D deficiency.

5. Interpretation of test results:
   a. Hyperparathyroidism, malignancy—elevated.
   b. Hypoparathyroidism—below normal.

Serum Calcium, Ionized

Description

1. Approximately 45% to 50% of total serum calcium is in biologically active ionized form.

2. This is preferred method of testing changes in calcium metabolism caused by parathyroid disease, malignancy, or neck surgery.

Nursing and Patient Care Considerations

1. Sample should be collected in tube with heparin as anticoagulant.

2. Test should be repeated on three different occasions to confirm parathyroid disease.

a. Hyperparathyroidism, malignancy—elevated.
b. Hypoparathyroidism—below normal.

 NURSING ALERT Tourniquet use during blood sample collection for calcium studies should be kept to a minimum. Prolonged constriction will cause migration of plasma proteins into the bloodstream locally; this results in spuriously high serum calcium values and pseudohypercalcemia.

Serum Phosphate

Description

1. Test measures the level of inorganic phosphorus in the blood.

2. Alteration in parathyroid function tends to have opposite effects on calcium and phosphorus metabolism.

3. Used to confirm metabolic abnormalities that affect calcium metabolism.

Nursing and Patient Care Considerations

Elevated in hypoparathyroidism; low values in hyperparathyroidism.

Tests of Adrenal Function

Plasma Cortisol

Description

1. This is a direct measure of the primary secretory product of the adrenal cortex by radioimmunoassay technique.

2. Serum concentration varies with circadian cycle so normal values vary with time of day and stress level of patient (8:00 A.M. levels typically double that of 8:00 P.M. levels).

3. Useful as an initial step to assess adrenal dysfunction, but further workup is usually necessary.

4. A sample collected at midnight (while the patient is asleep) that yields a result of less than 2 mcg/dL may be considered diagnostic of Cushing's syndrome.

Nursing and Patient Care Considerations

1. A fasting sample is preferred.

2. Blood samples should coincide with circadian rhythm with draw time indicated on laboratory slip.

3. Interpretation of test results:
   a. Decreased values seen in Addison's disease, anterior pituitary hyposecretion, and secondary hypothyroidism.
   b. Increased values seen in hyperthyroidism, stress (eg, trauma, surgery), carcinoma, Cushing's syndrome, hypersecretion of corticotropin by tumors (oat cell cancer), adrenal adenoma, and obesity.

Salivary Cortisol

Description

1. Because cortisol binding globulin (CBG) is normally absent from saliva, it does not interfere with cortisol levels. Therefore, salivary cortisol can be more reliably measured without variation due to fluctuating CBG levels.

Nursing and Patient Care Considerations

1. A mouth swab is collected from patient at midnight.

2. A result of more than 2.0 ng/mL is diagnostic for Cushing's syndrome.

Twenty-Four-Hour Urinary Free Cortisol Test

Description

1. Test measures cortisol production during a 24-hour period.
2. Useful to establish diagnosis of hypercortisolism.
3. Less influenced by diurnal variations in cortisol.

Nursing and Patient Care Considerations

1. Instruct patient in appropriate collection technique.
2. Collection jug should be kept on ice and sent to laboratory promptly when collection completed.
3. Interfering factors:
   a. Elevated values—pregnancy, hormonal contraceptives, spironolactone, stress.
   b. Recent radioisotope scans can interfere with test results.

Dexamethasone Suppression Tests

Description

1. The dexamethasone suppression test (DST) is a valuable method to evaluate adrenal hyperfunction.
2. Adrenal production and secretion of cortisol is stimulated by adrenocorticotropic hormone (ACTH; corticotropin) from the pituitary gland.
3. Dexamethasone is a synthetic steroid effective in suppressing corticotropin secretion.
4. In a healthy patient, the administration of dexamethasone will inhibit corticotropin secretion and will cause cortisol levels to fall below normal.
5. Certain drugs (rifampin, phenytoin) increase metabolic clearance of dexamethasone and may contribute to false-positive test results.

Nursing and Patient Care Considerations

Explain the procedure to patient.

1. Overnight low-dose (1 mg) DST (used primarily to identify those *without* Cushing's syndrome).
   a. Administer dexamethasone 1 mg orally at 11:00 P.M.
   b. Draw cortisol level at 8:00 A.M. before patient rises.
   c. Expect suppressed cortisol levels (<5 mcg/dL). Test is highly sensitive when a 2-mg cut-off is used for diagnosis.
2. Forty-eight-hour low-dose (2 mg) DST.
   a. Patient is instructed to take 0.5 mg of dexamethasone every 6 hours for a 2-day period.
   b. Plasma cortisol sample is collected 9 hours after first dose is administered and again at 48 hours.
   c. It is essential that patient have clearly written instructions for compliance with dosing and blood sampling schedule for test to be valid.
3. High-dose overnight DST (helpful to distinguish Cushing's disease from other forms of Cushing's syndrome).
   a. Give patient dexamethasone 8 mg orally at 11:00 P.M.
   b. Draw cortisol level at 8:00 A.M. before patient rises.
   c. Suppressed cortisol levels (less than 50% of baseline value) indicative of patient with corticotropin-secreting pituitary adenoma (Cushing's disease).
   d. Unsuppressed cortisol levels are associated with ectopic corticotropin secretion (malignancy) or adrenal tumors.
4. Encourage patient to take dexamethasone with milk because it may cause gastric irritation.

Adrenocorticotropic Stimulation Test

Description

1. ACTH stimulates the production and secretion of cortisol by the adrenal cortex.
2. Demonstrates the ability of the adrenal cortex to respond appropriately to ACTH.
3. This is an important test to evaluate adrenal insufficiency, but may not distinguish primary insufficiency from secondary insufficiency.

Nursing and Patient Care Considerations

1. Obtain baseline cortisol level.
2. Administer 0.25 mg ACTH (cosyntropin IV or intramuscularly [I.M.]).
3. Collect cortisol levels at times ordered (usually at 30 and 60 minutes).
4. Interpretation of test results:
   a. Range of normal responses may vary; however, typically a rise in cortisol of double baseline value is considered normal.
   b. Diminished response—adrenal insufficiency with low cortisol values.

 DRUG ALERT Infusion of cosyntropin can cause flushing or slight reduction in blood pressure (BP). Warn patients about these effects, monitor BP, and ensure safety.

Corticotropin-Releasing Hormone Stimulation Test

Description

1. Test measures responsiveness of pituitary gland to corticotropin-releasing hormone (CRH)—a hypothalamic hormone that regulates pituitary secretion of ACTH.
2. Useful to differentiate the cause of excess cortisol secretion when ectopic source of ACTH is suspected.
3. In general, CRH will stimulate ACTH secretion in the pituitary, but not in nonpituitary corticotropin-secreting tissues.

Nursing and Patient Care Considerations

1. Describe procedure to patient.
   a. Patient is given CRH (1 mcg/kg or 100 mcg) via IV line.
   b. Catheters are advanced through the femoral veins to areas near the adrenal glands, so sampling can take place near ACTH secretion.
   c. Blood samples for ACTH test are collected at 2, 5, 10, and 15 minutes.
2. Normal response is a rise in ACTH to at least double the baseline value.
3. Interpretation of test results:
   a. Brisk rise in ACTH double baseline value—Cushing's disease.
   b. No response in ACTH—corticotropin-independent Cushing's syndrome (adrenal tumor) or ectopic source of corticotropin secretion (ectopic tumor).
   c. Test can produce false-negative response.

Urine Vanillylmandelic Acid and Metanephrine

Description

1. Direct measure of metabolites of catecholamines secreted by the adrenal medulla.
2. Metanephrine is a more reliable measure of catecholamine secretion.
3. Preferred method to diagnose pheochromocytoma.

Nursing and Patient Care Considerations

1. Obtain proper urine collection jug with hydrochloride preservative and explain 24-hour urine collection to patient.
2. A wide range of medications and foods may alter test performed by some laboratories. Verify with the laboratory and health care provider the need to hold some medications, such as sympathomimetics and methyldopa, and such foods as coffee, tea, vanilla extract, and bananas before and during urine collection.
3. Interpretation—pheochromocytoma: vanillylmandelic acid greater than 10 mcg/mg of creatinine or greater than 10 mg/24 hours; metanephrine greater than 0.7 mcg/mg of creatinine or greater than 0.7 mg/24 hours.

Plasma Catecholamines

Description

Direct measure of circulating catecholamines using radioimmunoassay technique; more sensitive test than urine test, but more prone to false-positive results.

Nursing and Patient Care Considerations

1. Collect sample from IV catheter 20 to 30 minutes after venipuncture, if possible, to reduce the rise in catecholamine levels from pain and anxiety.
2. Collect the sample in a heparinized tube.
3. Interpretation—levels higher than 2,000 ng/L diagnostic for pheochromocytoma.

Clonidine Suppression Test

Description

1. Based on the principle that catecholamine production by pheochromocytomas is autonomous, as opposed to other causes of excess catecholamines, which are regulated by the sympathetic nervous system.
2. Clonidine, as a central alpha-adrenergic agonist, suppresses production of catecholamines.
3. Useful to differentiate pheochromocytoma from essential hypertension when test results are inconclusive.

Nursing and Patient Care Considerations

1. Collect baseline catecholamine sample from IV catheter 20 to 30 minutes after venipuncture, if possible, to reduce the rise in catecholamine levels from pain and anxiety.
2. Give clonidine 0.3 mg orally.
3. After 3 hours, collect second catecholamine sample.
4. Interpretation—in patients without pheochromocytoma, a significant drop in catecholamines should be seen at 3 hours (less than 500 pg/mL or reduction of total catecholamines by 50%), whereas in patients with pheochromocytoma, no drop in catecholamines will be evident.

 DRUG ALERT Warn patients not to rise quickly and monitor for orthostatic hypotension after clonidine administration.

Aldosterone (Urine or Blood)

Description

1. Direct measure, using radioimmunoassay technique, of aldosterone, a hormone secreted by the adrenal cortex that regulates renal control of sodium and potassium.
2. May be measured in the blood or in 24-hour urine collection specimen.
3. Urine test is more reliable because it is less influenced by short-term fluctuations in the bloodstream.
4. Useful to diagnose primary aldosteronism.

Nursing and Patient Care Considerations

1. Test results can be elevated by stress, strenuous exercise, upright posture, and medications such as diazoxide, hydralazine, and nitroprusside.
2. Test results may be decreased by excessive licorice ingestion and the medication, fludrocortisone and propranolol.

Tests of Pituitary Function

Serum Growth Hormone

Description

1. Direct radioimmunoassay measurement of human growth hormone (GH), secreted by the anterior pituitary gland; useful to diagnose acromegaly, gigantism, pituitary tumors, pituitary-related growth failure in children, or GH deficiency in adults.
2. Because GH secretion is episodic, single fasting samples may not be reliable to detect GH excess or deficiency.
3. These conditions are best evaluated by using a stimulation test (for deficiency states) or a suppression test (for hormone excess conditions).

Nursing and Patient Care Considerations

1. Blood sample is taken after an overnight fast (caloric intake will lower GH blood levels).
2. Patient should be restful and calm before blood sample collection.
3. Normal range: males—less than 5 ng/mL; females—less than 8 ng/mL.
4. May be elevated by the following medications: alcohol, L-dopa, hormonal contraceptives, alpha-antagonists, and beta-adrenergic blockers.

Serum Prolactin

Description

Direct radioimmunoassay measurement of prolactin, secreted by the anterior pituitary gland; helps diagnose pituitary tumors.

Nursing and Patient Care Considerations

1. Blood sample is taken after an overnight fast.
2. Normal values: men—1 to 20 ng/mL; women—1 to 25 ng/mL.
3. Values above 300 ng/mL highly suggestive of pituitary tumor.
4. Elevated values may be caused by exercise or by breast stimulation, such as from friction.

5. Medications that will elevate test results include pheno-thiazines, reserpine, estrogens, tricyclic antidepressants, methyldopa, antihypertensive medications, and selective serotonin reuptake inhibitors.

Adrenocorticotropic Hormone

Description

1. Direct measurement of ACTH concentration in the blood-stream by radioimmunoassay technique.
2. One measure of pituitary gland function useful to provide important information regarding adrenal gland dysfunction.
3. Useful to identify cause of adrenal abnormalities when com-pared with serum cortisol levels.

Nursing and Patient Care Considerations

1. Because ACTH is rapidly degraded, blood samples should be centrifuged and frozen promptly to avoid falsely low results.
2. High stress levels in patient can invalidate results.
3. Interpretation of test results:
   a. Elevated levels with elevated cortisol—Cushing's disease or ectopic production of ACTH.
   b. Elevated levels with low cortisol—Addison's disease.
   c. Low levels with elevated cortisol—adrenal tumor.
   d. Low levels with low cortisol—hypopituitarism.

Insulin Tolerance Test

Description

1. Dynamic test measures pituitary response to induced hypo-glycemia, particularly GH secretion and ACTH-stimulated cortisol production by the adrenal gland.
2. Useful to diagnose functional hypopituitarism that is caused by pituitary disease or that appears after pituitary surgery.
3. Considered the "gold standard" for diagnosis of GH deficiency.

Nursing and Patient Care Considerations

1. After overnight fast, insulin 0.1 unit/kg body weight is given via IV line.
2. Blood samples are collected, usually at baseline, 30, 60, and 90 minutes after insulin dose.
3. The test is considered valid if blood glucose falls to half of baseline or less than 40 mg/dL.
4. Peak response is seen at 60 to 100 minutes.
5. For adrenal response, a rise in cortisol by a factor of at least 1.5 is necessary to show normal response.
6. GH deficiency is present if growth hormone levels fail to rise above 3 mcg/L.
7. This test is contraindicated in people with epilepsy or heart disease. In people with suspected adrenal insufficiency, ACTH stimulation test should be done first.
8. For people in whom the insulin tolerance test is contraindicated, other agents may be used, such as clonidine, arginine, glucagon, L-dopa, or GH-releasing hormone, to stimulate GH secretion.

NURSING ALERT Test should be performed with health care provider present. Dextrose 50% solution should be available at bedside to treat hypoglycemia, if needed.

Glucose Suppression Test

Description

Postprandial elevations of glucose inhibit the secretion of GH by the pituitary gland. Failure to suppress GH levels after ingestion of glucose suggests a GH-secreting tumor.

Nursing and Patient Care Considerations

1. Patient should fast for this test.
2. Seventy-five to 100 g of concentrated glucose is administered by mouth.
3. Blood samples are collected at baseline, 30, and 60 minutes.
4. Interpretation of test results:
   a. GH levels less than 2 mcg/L are considered normal.
   b. GH levels that are not suppressed are suggestive of acro-megaly.
5. Failure of GH suppression may also be caused by starvation or protein calorie restriction.
6. Patients may complain of nausea after ingesting Glucola.

Water Deprivation Test

Description

1. Functional test of the adequacy of posterior pituitary secre-tion of antidiuretic hormone (ADH) and its ability to con-centrate urine and to maintain serum osmolality in the face of water deprivation.
2. Useful to determine the diagnosis and etiology of diabetes insipidus (DI).

Nursing and Patient Care Considerations

1. The test is begun by obtaining patient's weight, serum, and urine osmolality at time 0.
2. Patient weight, urine output volume, and osmolality are determined hourly.
3. Deprivation is continued until urine osmolality "plateaus," as evidenced by a change of less than 10% in urine osmolality between consecutive measurements and a 2% reduction in patient's body weight. At this time, samples are collected for serum sodium, osmolality, and vasopressin.
4. The test may be stopped if patient loses more than 3% of his or her body weight or if cardiac instability occurs.
5. If urine osmolality remains below that of serum (usually 300 mOsm/kg), the diagnosis of DI is confirmed and the sec-ond stage of the test, which distinguishes central and nephro-genic DI, is begun.
6. Artificial ADH (desmopressin acetate [DDAVP]) 2 mcg is given SubQ or I.M. to determine changes in urine osmolality at 30, 60, and 120 minutes in response to the injected hormone.
7. If the highest urine osmolality value obtained after injection is more than 50% higher than the preinjection value, DI is caused by pituitary failure. If the osmolality value is less than 50% of preinjection value, then DI is caused by renal disease.

NURSING ALERT Patients with suspected DI who undergo the water deprivation test must be moni-tored closely because dehydration may occur rap-idly in people with severe disease.

Radiology and Imaging

Radioactive ¹³¹I Uptake

Description
Measures thyroid uptake patterns of iodine as a whole or within specified areas of the gland.

Nursing and Patient Care Considerations
1. A solution of sodium iodide 131 (^{131}I) is administered orally to fasting patient.
2. After a prescribed interval, usually 24 hours, measurements of radioactive counts per minute are taken with a scintillator.
3. Normal thyroid will remove 15% to 50% of the iodine from the bloodstream.
4. Hyperthyroidism may result in the removal of as much as 90% of the iodine from the bloodstream (eg, Graves' disease); it may also cause a low uptake with some forms of thyroiditis.
5. Hypothyroidism—reflected in low uptake.

Thyroid Scan

Description
1. Rapid imaging of thyroid tissue, particularly suspicious nodules, as contrast imaging agent is rapidly taken up by functioning tissue.
2. Useful to diagnose thyroid carcinoma.
3. Contrast media is usually administered via IV line.
   a. Technetium (^{99m}Tc) pertechnetate or ^{123}I is used for best images.
4. Images can be obtained from gamma counter within 20 to 60 minutes.

Nursing and Patient Care Considerations
1. May interfere with serum radioimmunoassay tests; contact laboratory to determine when blood test can be done.
2. Benign adenomas may be visualized as "hot" nodules, indicating increased uptake of iodine, or as "cold" nodules, indicating decreased uptake.
3. Malignant nodules usually take the form of "cold" nodules.

GENERAL PROCEDURES AND TREATMENT MODALITIES

See Standards of Care Guidelines 24-1.

Steroid Therapy

Steroid therapy is a treatment used in some endocrine disorders and in various other conditions. Steroids are hormones that affect metabolism and many body processes.

Classification of Steroids

(By major metabolic effects on body.)

Mineralocorticoids
1. Concerned with sodium and water retention and potassium excretion.
2. Example—aldosterone and 11-desoxycorticosterone.

STANDARDS OF CARE GUIDELINES 24-1
Endocrine Disorders

When caring for a patient with an endocrine disorder, remember that important metabolic functions may be disrupted, such as fluid and electrolyte balance, glucose and protein metabolism, energy production, calcium ionization, blood pressure (BP) control, thermoregulation, cardiac contractility, intestinal peristalsis, and ability of the body to react to stress.

- Monitor closely for electrolyte imbalance—sodium, potassium, chloride, bicarbonate—by checking laboratory test results, changes in the electrocardiogram pattern, and signs of particular excess or deficit (see Chapter 21, page 797).
- Check fingerstick or serum glucose periodically for patients on corticosteroids or for patients with adrenal disease; watch for signs of hyperglycemia (polydipsia, polyphagia, polyuria, blurred vision) or hypoglycemia (nervousness, tremor, difficulty concentrating, lethargy).
- Monitor for hypocalcemia after thyroidectomy, parathyroidectomy, or with hypoparathyroidism by checking serum calcium and phosphorus levels; watch for muscular twitching, anxiety, apprehension, spasms, and tetany. Check Chvostek's sign and Trousseau's sign.
- Monitor vital signs for heart rate, BP, and presence of arrhythmias.
- Monitor temperature and respiratory rate changes in thyroid and adrenal disease.
- Monitor intake and output, weight changes, and edema.
- Maintain a calm, quiet environment and provide meticulous care to prevent infection or dehydration in patients with adrenal hypofunction or patients on corticosteroid replacement.
- After surgery, check for bleeding, signs of infection, changes in vital signs. Monitor respiratory status carefully after thyroidectomy.
- Report worsening condition or development of suspicious signs and symptoms promptly to prevent serious complications, such as myxedema coma, thyroid storm, hypocalcemic tetany, adrenal crisis.
- Provide support and explain care slowly and repeatedly because patient may have mental slowness, confusion, or lethargy due to his or her condition. Ask patient to restate important information to verify understanding.

This information should serve as a general guideline only. Each patient situation presents a unique set of clinical factors and requires nursing judgment to guide care, which may include additional or alternative measures and approaches.

Glucocorticoids (Corticosteroids, Steroids)
1. Concerned with metabolic effects, including carbohydrate metabolism.
2. Example—cortisol.

Sex Hormones
1. Important when secreted in large amounts or when the growth of hormone-sensitive cancers is stimulated.

2. Examples:
  a. Androgens—testosterone.
  b. Estrogens—estradiol.
  c. Progestins—progesterone.

Effects of Glucocorticoids

1. Antagonize action of insulin; promote gluconeogenesis, which provides glucose.
2. Increase breakdown of protein (inhibit protein synthesis).
3. Increase breakdown of fatty acids.
4. Suppress inflammation, inhibit scar formation, block allergic responses.
5. Decrease number of circulating eosinophils and leukocytes; decrease size of lymphatic tissue.
6. Exert a permissive action (allow the full effects) on catecholamines.
7. Exert a permissive action on functioning of central nervous system (CNS).
8. Inhibit release of adrenocorticotropin.
9. In summary, glucocorticoids are necessary to resist noxious stimuli and environmental change.

Uses of Steroids

1. Physiologically—to correct deficiencies or malfunction of a particular endocrine organ or system (eg, Addison's disease).
2. Diagnostically—to determine proper functioning of the endocrine system.
3. Pharmacologically—to treat the following:
  a. Asthma and obstructive lung disease.
  b. Acute rheumatic fever.
  c. Blood conditions, such as idiopathic thrombocytopenic purpura, leukemia, hemolytic anemia.
  d. Allergic conditions—allergic rhinitis, anaphylaxis (after epinephrine).
  e. Dermatologic problems—drug rashes, contact dermatitis, atopic dermatitis.
  f. Ocular diseases—conjunctivitis, uveitis.
  g. Connective tissue disorders—systemic lupus erythematosus, rheumatoid arthritis.
  h. GI problems—ulcerative colitis.
  i. Organ transplant recipients—as an immunosuppressive agent.
  j. Neurologic conditions—cerebral edema, multiple sclerosis.

Preparing the Patient to Receive Steroid Therapy

1. Determine contraindications/precautions for such therapy.
  a. Peptic ulcer.
  b. Diabetes mellitus.
  c. Viral infections.
2. Administer a tuberculin test, if indicated, before therapy because steroids may suppress response to the test.
3. Assess the patient's own level of steroid secretion, if possible.
4. Explain the nature of the therapy, what is required of the patient, how long therapy will last, adverse effects to watch for, and answer any questions.

Choice of Steroid and Method of Administration

1. May be given by various methods—orally, parenterally, sublingually, rectally, by inhalation, or by direct application to skin or mucous membrane.
2. Combinations of steroids with other drugs should be avoided.
3. To help avoid steroid adverse effects, alternate-day therapy may be used; dose is taken in the morning.
4. May be given in initial high doses, then reduced; if the patient has been taking steroids for several weeks, doses must be tapered gradually to prevent addisonian crisis.

Nursing Interventions
Preventing Infection

1. Steroids may affect the circulating blood, resulting in decreased eosinophils and lymphocytes, increased red cells, and increased incidence of thrombophlebitis and infection.
2. Encourage the patient to avoid crowds and the possibility of exposure to infection.
3. Encourage exercise to prevent venous stasis.
4. Be aware that signs of infection/inflammation may be masked—fever, redness, swelling.
5. Practice and encourage good handwashing technique and asepsis.

Preventing Nutritional and Metabolism Complications

1. Determine whether the patient needs assistance in dietary control. Steroids may cause weight gain and an increase in appetite.
2. Encourage a high-protein diet. Because steroids affect protein metabolism, there may be negative nitrogen balance.
3. Encourage the patient to take steroids with milk or with food. Because steroids increase secretion of gastric acid and have an inhibiting effect on secretion of mucus in the stomach, they may cause peptic ulcer.
4. Be on guard for early evidence of gastric hemorrhage, such as melena, blood in vomitus.
5. Check fasting blood glucose levels.
  a. Steroids precipitate gluconeogenesis and insulin antagonism, which results in hyperglycemia, glucosuria, decreased carbohydrate tolerance.
  b. Temporary insulin injections may be necessary.

Observing for Bone Complications

1. Be on the alert for the possibility of pathologic fractures. Stress safety measures to prevent injury.
  a. Steroids affect the musculoskeletal system, causing potassium depletion and muscular weakness.
  b. Steroids cause increased output of calcium and phosphorus, which may lead to osteoporosis.
2. Administer a diet high in calcium and protein.
3. Recommend activities of daily living (ADLs) and weight-bearing program; recommend normal range of motion and safe repositioning for those that are bedridden.

Avoiding Electrolyte Disturbance

1. Restrict sodium intake and increase potassium intake.
  a. Mineralocorticoids differ from other steroids, resulting in sodium retention and potassium depletion; edema, weight gain.

b. Lemon juice is high in potassium and low in sodium.

c. Avoid saline as a diluent in preparing injectable medications.

2. Check BP frequently and weigh the patient daily.

3. Observe for edema.

Monitoring Behavioral Reactions

1. Watch for convulsive seizures (especially in children). Steroids may alter behavior patterns, increase excitability, and may affect the CNS.

2. Avoid overstimulating situations.

3. Recognize and report any mood that deviates from the usual behavior patterns.

4. Report unusual behavior, haunting dreams, withdrawal, or suicidal tendencies.

Preventing Stress Reactions

1. Recommend that the patient carry an identification card that indicates steroid therapy and name of health care provider.

2. Be aware that steroids affect the hypothalamic–pituitary–adrenal system, which affects the patient's ability to respond to stress.

3. Advise the patient to avoid extremes of temperature, infections, and upsetting situations.

Preventing Injury and Promoting Healing

1. Instruct the patient to avoid injury; stress safety precautions. Because steroids interfere with fibroblasts and granulation tissue, altered response to injury results in impaired growth and delayed healing.

2. Observe daily the healing process of wounds, particularly surgical wounds, to recognize the potential for wound dehiscence.

Patient Education and Health Maintenance

1. Teach patient that steroids are valuable and useful medications, but that if taken for longer than 2 weeks, they may produce certain adverse effects.

   a. Acceptable adverse effects may include weight gain (due to increased appetite and water retention), acne, headaches, fatigue, and increased urinary frequency.

   b. Unacceptable adverse effects that are to be reported to the health care provider include dizziness when rising from chair or bed (orthostatic hypotension indicative of adrenal insufficiency), nausea, vomiting, thirst, abdominal pain, or pain of any type.

   c. Additional reportable adverse effects include convulsive seizures, feelings of depression or nervousness, or development of an infection.

2. Advise patient that a fall or an automobile accident may precipitate adrenal failure. This requires an immediate injection of hydrocortisone phosphate.

3. Tell patients on long-term therapy that they should wear a MedicAlert bracelet and carry a kit with hydrocortisone, as prescribed.

4. Instruct patient to inform any physician, dentist, or nurse about steroid therapy.

5. Tell patient that regular follow-up visits to health care provider are required.

Care of the Patient Undergoing Fine-Needle Aspiration Biopsy

 Evidence Base American Thyroid Association Guidelines Task Force on Thyroid Nodules and Differentiated Thyroid Cancer. (2009). Revised American Thyroid Association management guidelines for patients with thyroid nodules and differentiated thyroid cancer. *Thyroid, 19*(11), 1167–1214.

Gharib, H., Papini, E., & Paschke, R. (2010). American Association of Clinical Endocrinologists, Associazione Medici Endocrinologi, and European Thyroid Association medical guidelines for clinical practice for the diagnosis and management of thyroid nodules. *Endocrine Practice, 16*(Suppl. 1), 1–43.

Fine-needle aspiration (FNA) biopsy is a procedure by which tissue from within a thyroid nodule is removed to detect malignancy. This procedure can easily be performed on an outpatient basis and requires no special patient preparation. Complications are uncommon, but may include hematoma, tracheal perforation, and infection.

Preparation and Procedure

1. No special patient preparation activities are necessary for this procedure.

2. The procedure is explained to patient and consent is obtained.

3. Patient is positioned comfortably on an examination table in the supine position with the neck fully exposed.

4. A rolled towel or sheet is placed beneath the patient's shoulder to hyperextend the neck, allowing ease of access to the biopsy site.

5. The biopsy site area is cleaned with alcohol and/or an antibacterial cleaning agent.

6. One percent lidocaine may be injected intracutaneously for local anesthetic to promote patient comfort.

7. A 25G needle is inserted into the thyroid nodule and manipulated by the physician until a small amount of bloody material is seen on the hub of the needle.

8. The needle is removed and attached to a syringe. The contents of the needle are expressed onto a clean glass slide. A second slide is placed on top of the first slide and then pulled apart quickly to create a thin smear.

9. The slides are placed in a fixative and transported to a cytologist for interpretation.

Postprocedure Management

1. The biopsy site may be dressed with an adhesive bandage or other small dressing.

2. Follow-up visit for patient should be arranged to discuss results.

Nursing Considerations

1. Prevent infection by making sure that biopsy area is prepped appropriately before procedure.

2. Employ comfort measures during procedure, as necessary.

3. Assure patient that most thyroid nodules are determined to be benign and that most thyroid malignancies have a high cure rate.

4. Advise patient that some soreness at the biopsy site should be expected for a brief time.

5. Make sure that patient follows up for results and definitive treatment.

Care of the Patient Undergoing Thyroidectomy

Thyroidectomy involves the partial or complete removal of the thyroid gland to treat thyroid tumors, hyperthyroidism, or hyperparathyroidism.

Types of Procedures

1. Thyroidectomy can be total (removal of the entire thyroid gland); subtotal (95% of gland removed)—to prevent damage to the parathyroid glands; and partial (one lobe or isthmus removed)—to treat nodular disease.

2. The parathyroid glands are usually spared to prevent hypocalcemia.

3. Indications for thyroidectomy include Graves' disease refractory to ^{131}I therapy, large goiters, adenoma (thyroid cancer), and some nodules.

Preoperative Management

1. The patient must be euthyroid at time of surgery, so thioamides are administered to control hyperthyroidism.

2. Iodide is given to increase firmness of thyroid gland and to reduce its vascularity after blood loss.

3. An attempt is made to counteract the effects of hypermetabolism by maintaining a restful and therapeutic environment and by providing a nutritious diet.

4. The patient is prepared for surgery physically and emotionally in the following ways:

   a. Make a special effort to ensure that patient has a good night's rest preceding surgery.

   b. Explain to patient that speaking is to be minimized immediately postoperatively and that oxygen may be administered to facilitate breathing.

   c. Explain that postoperatively, fluids may be given via IV line to maintain fluid, electrolyte, and nutritional needs; IV glucose may also be given in the hours before the administration of anesthetic agents.

Postoperative Management

1. The patient is monitored for bleeding and respiratory distress that indicates laryngeal edema, secondary to swelling in the area of surgery.

2. Signs of hypocalcemia are watched for—irritability, twitching, spasms of hands and feet.

   a. Calcium levels are monitored. If in 48 hours level falls below 7 mg/100 mL (3 mEq), IV calcium (gluconate, lactate) replacement is given.

   b. IV calcium is used cautiously in patients who have renal disease or who are taking digoxin.

3. Thyroid function is monitored after surgery.

Complications

1. Hemorrhage, edema of the glottis, damage to laryngeal nerve.

2. Hypothyroidism following subtotal thyroidectomy occurs in 5% of patients in first postoperative year; increases at rate of 2% to 3% per year.

3. Hypoparathyroidism occurs in about 4% of patients and is usually mild and transient; requires calcium supplements via IV administration and orally when more severe.

Nursing Diagnoses

- Risk for Injury related to invasive procedure of the neck.
- Risk for Injury related to possible removal of parathyroid glands.

Nursing Interventions

Observing for Hemorrhage and Airway Edema

1. Administer humidified oxygen, as prescribed, to reduce irritation of airway and to prevent edema.

2. Move patient carefully; provide adequate support to the head so that no tension is placed on the sutures.

3. Place patient in semi-Fowler's position, with the head elevated and supported by pillows; avoid flexion of neck.

4. Monitor vital signs frequently, watching for tachycardia and hypotension that indicates hemorrhage (most likely between 12 and 24 hours postoperatively).

5. Observe for bleeding at sides and back of the neck, and anteriorly, when patient is in dorsal position.

6. Watch for repeated clearing of the throat or for complaint of smothering or difficulty swallowing, which may be early signs of hemorrhage.

7. Watch for irregular breathing, swelling of the neck, and choking—other signs pointing to the possibility of hemorrhage and tracheal compression.

8. Reinforce dressing, if indicated.

9. Be alert for voice changes, which may indicate damage to laryngeal nerve.

10. Keep a tracheostomy set in patient's room for 48 hours for emergency use.

Preventing Tetany

1. Watch for the development of tetany caused by removal or disturbance of parathyroid glands through a progression of signs:

   a. Tingling of toes and fingers and around the mouth; apprehension.

   b. Positive Chvostek's sign—tapping on the cheek over the facial nerve causes a twitch of the lip or facial muscles (see Figure 24-1A).

   c. Positive Trousseau's sign—carpopedal spasm induced by occluding circulation in the arm with a BP cuff (see Figure 24-1B).

2. Be prepared to treat hypocalcemic tetany.

   a. Position patient for optimal ventilation; remove pillow to prevent head from bending forward and compressing trachea.

   b. Keep side rails padded and elevated and position the patient to prevent injury if a seizure occurs; do not use

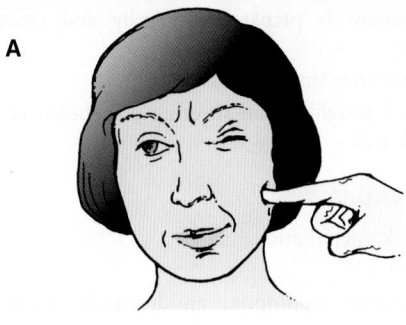

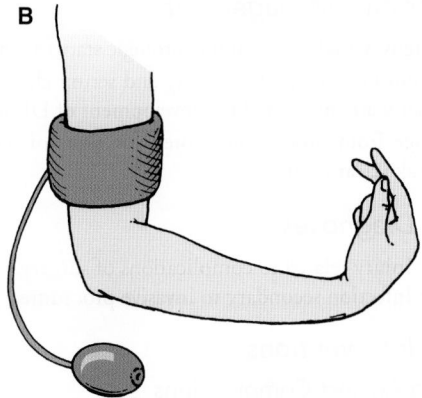

Figure 24-1. **(A)** Chvostek's sign. **(B)** Trousseau's sign.

restraints because they only aggravate the patient and may result in muscle strain or fractures.

   c. Have equipment available to treat respiratory difficulties that includes airway suction equipment, tracheostomy, and cardiac arrest equipment.

3. Administer IV calcium, as directed.

Patient Education and Health Maintenance

1. Teach patient about complications to look for if discharge occurs within a day or two of surgery.
2. Advise patient to rest at home and to prevent any strain on suture line, as directed by surgeon.
3. Advise nutritious diet; report difficulty swallowing.
4. Encourage follow-up for monitoring and thyroid hormone replacement after surgery.

Evaluation: Expected Outcomes

- No signs of hemorrhage or edema.
- No signs of hypocalcemia.

Care of the Patient Undergoing Adrenalectomy

Adrenalectomy may be unilateral or bilateral to treat adrenal tumors, Cushing's syndrome, or hyperaldosteronism. It is accomplished through abdominal or flank incision. Careful manipulation of the gland is necessary—if surgery is indicated for pheochromocytoma—to prevent excessive release of epinephrine causing hypertensive crisis.

Preoperative Management

1. BP and fluid volume are optimized.
2. Surgery and nursing care are explained to patient. Patient is shown where adrenal glands lie on top of kidneys and where incision may be on abdomen or loin area.
3. BP will be checked frequently before and after surgery and glucocorticoids will be given to cover period of stress (surgery) because at least one adrenal gland will be removed.
4. Patient is prepared as for major abdominal surgery (see page 654).

Complications

Hemorrhage, adrenal crisis.

Postoperative Management

1. Usual postoperative care for abdominal surgery includes frequent check of vital signs; assessment for hemorrhage; turning, coughing, and deep breathing; early ambulation; slow progression of diet when bowel sounds return; and control of pain with scheduled opioid administration or patient-controlled analgesia (see page 658).
2. IV hydrocortisone is given, as directed, to prevent adrenal crisis.
3. Nonstressful environment is maintained, rest is promoted, and meticulous care is given to protect patient from infection and from other complications that could cause adrenal crisis.
4. Serum sodium, potassium, and glucose are monitored for abnormality.
    a. Sodium and potassium may normalize or potassium may become elevated (because of transient adrenal insufficiency after surgery).
    b. Electrolyte imbalances may persist for 4 to 18 months after surgery.
    c. Hypertension may persist for 3 to 6 months after surgery.
5. Hydrocortisone treatment causes glucose to rise and worsens control in patients with diabetes; may require additional treatment.

Nursing Diagnoses

- Risk for Injury related to nature of surgery.
- Readiness for Enhanced Knowledge about corticosteroid replacement.

Nursing Interventions

Ensuring Healing

1. Assess dressing for leakage initially and after it has been changed, assess wound for signs of infection.
2. Perform dressing changes, wound care, and teach family how to do wound care at home.

Providing Patient Education

1. Teach patient with bilateral adrenalectomy that glucocorticoid and mineralocorticoid replacement is necessary for rest of life.
2. Administer additional doses I.M. in times of stress.

3. Administer oral glucocorticoids after unilateral adrenalectomy and teach patient that this treatment will be needed for 6 months to 2 years after surgery until remaining adrenal gland can compensate.

4. Encourage wearing or carrying this information at all times so that proper treatment can be instituted if patient becomes unconscious.

5. Encourage follow-up to monitor for signs of adrenal insufficiency.

Care of the Patient Undergoing Transsphenoidal Hypophysectomy

Procedure

1. Transsphenoidal approach to pituitary removal is carried out through the nasal cavity, sphenoid sinus, and into the sella turcica (see Figure 24-2).
2. Advantages over intracranial approach to hypophysectomy include:
   a. No need to shave head.
   b. No visible scar.
   c. Low blood loss, less need for transfusions.
   d. Lower infection rate.
   e. Well tolerated by frail and older patients.
   f. Good visualization of tumor field.
3. Disadvantages include:
   a. Restricted field of surgery.
   b. Potential cerebrospinal fluid (CSF) leak.

Preoperative Management

1. Sinus infection is assessed and treated, if necessary.
2. Hydrocortisone may be given preoperatively because the source of ACTH is being removed.

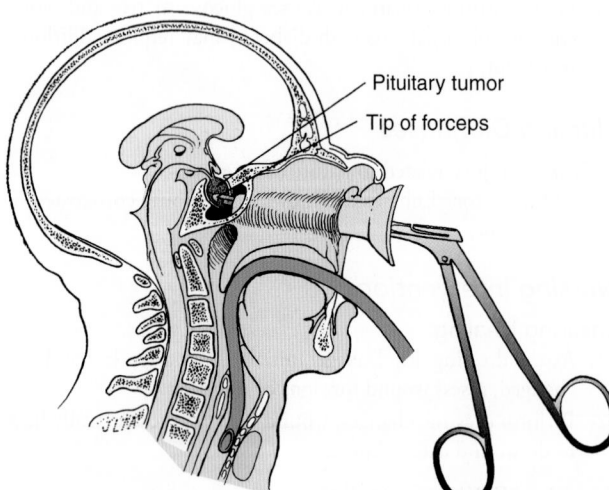

Figure 24-2. Transsphenoidal approach to the pituitary. A special nasal speculum is used to view the sinus cavity. After the dura is opened, the tumor is removed using microcurettes or other specially designed instruments.

Labels in figure: Pituitary tumor / Tip of forceps

3. The patient is prepared physically and emotionally for surgery.
   a. Deep-breathing exercises.
   b. Avoid coughing and sneezing postoperatively to prevent CSF leak.

Complications

1. CSF leak, meningitis.
2. Transient DI.
3. Syndrome of inappropriate antidiuretic hormone (SIADH).

Postoperative Management

1. Vital signs, visual acuity, and neurologic status are monitored.
2. Urine output and specific gravity and serum electrolytes and osmolality are monitored for development of DI or SIADH.
3. Drainage from nose is monitored for signs of infection or CSF leak (clear fluid).

Nursing Diagnoses

- Risk for Injury related to complications of surgery.
- Risk for Infection secondary to invasive procedure.

Nursing Interventions

Protecting Against Complications

1. Monitor vital signs, visual acuity, and neurologic status frequently for signs of increasing intracranial pressure.
2. Monitor fluid intake and output and report any increase in output and decrease in specific gravity, which may indicate DI.
3. Report persistent clear fluid from nose and increasing headache; could signal CSF leak.
4. Teach patient signs of complications and to report them immediately and to follow up as scheduled.
5. Assess level of pain and administer analgesic or supervise patient-controlled analgesia.

Preventing Infection

1. Observe for signs of infection. Check incision within inner aspect of upper lip for drainage or bleeding.
2. Note frequency of nasal dressing changes and character of drainage. Prepare patient for packing removal one to several days postoperatively.
3. Encourage the use of a humidifier to prevent drying from mouth breathing.

Evaluation: Expected Outcomes

- Vital signs stable, urine-specific gravity 1.010, no clear drainage from nose.
- No purulent drainage noted.

DISORDERS OF THE THYROID GLAND

The thyroid gland affects the metabolic rate of all tissues, including the speed of chemical reactions, the volume of oxygen consumed, and the amount of heat produced. The stimulating effect is through the production and distribution of two hormones:

1. Levothyroxine (T_4)—contains four iodine atoms; maintains body's metabolism in a steady state; T_4 serves as a precursor of T_3.
2. Triiodothyronine (T_3)—contains three iodine atoms; approximately five times as potent as T_4; has a more rapid metabolic action and utilization than T_4 does.
3. Most conversion of T_4 to T_3 occurs at the cellular level in the periphery. Some T_3 is produced in the thyroid gland.

Hypothyroidism

Hypothyroidism is a condition that arises from inadequate amounts of thyroid hormone in the bloodstream.

Pathophysiology and Etiology

1. Primary hypothyroidism is the most common form of this condition and is generally caused by (in order of frequency):
   a. Autoimmune disease (Hashimoto's thyroiditis).
   b. Use of radioactive iodine.
   c. Destruction, suppression, or removal of all or some of the thyroid tissue by thyroidectomy.
   d. Dietary iodide deficiency.
   e. Subacute thyroiditis.
   f. Lithium therapy.
   g. Overtreatment with antithyroid drugs.
2. Secondary hypothyroidism is caused by inadequate secretion of TSH caused by disease of the pituitary gland (ie, tumor, necrosis, head trauma).
3. Inadequate secretion of thyroid hormone leads to a general slowing of all physical and mental processes.
4. General depression of most cellular enzyme systems and oxidative processes occurs.
5. The metabolic activity of all cells of the body decreases, reducing oxygen consumption, decreasing oxidation of nutrients for energy, and producing less body heat.
6. The signs and symptoms of the disorder range from vague, nonspecific complaints that make diagnosis difficult to severe symptoms that may be life-threatening if unrecognized and untreated.

Clinical Manifestations

1. Fatigue and lethargy.
2. Weight gain.
3. Complaints of cold hands and feet.
4. Temperature and pulse become subnormal; patient cannot tolerate cold and desires increased room temperature.
5. Reduced attention span; impaired short-term memory.
6. Severe constipation; decreased peristalsis.
7. Generalized appearance of thick, puffy skin; subcutaneous swelling in hands, feet, and eyelids.
8. Thinning hair; loss of the lateral one third of eyebrow.
9. Menorrhagia or amenorrhea; may have difficulty conceiving or may experience spontaneous abortion; decreased libido.
10. Neurologic signs include polyneuropathy, cerebellar ataxia, muscle aches or weakness, clumsiness, prolonged deep tendon reflexes (especially ankle jerk).
11. Hyperlipoproteinemia and hypercholesterolemia.
12. Enlarged heart on chest x-ray.
13. Increased susceptibility to all hypnotic and sedative drugs and anesthetic agents.
14. Syndrome of subclinical hypothyroidism: state in which the patient is asymptomatic and the free T_4 level is within the normal range; however, the TSH level is elevated, suggesting impending thyroid gland failure. Therefore, many clinicians may elect to treat this condition as if the patient were symptomatic.

Diagnostic Evaluation

1. Low T_3 and T_4 levels.
2. Elevated TSH levels in primary hypothyroidism.
3. Elevation of serum cholesterol.
4. Electrocardiogram (ECG)—sinus bradycardia, low voltage of QRS complexes, and flat or inverted T waves.
5. Elevation of thyroid peroxidase antibodies and antithyroglobulin antibodies.

Management

Approach

1. Depends on severity of symptoms; may necessitate replacement therapy in mild cases or lifesaving support and treatment in severe hypothyroidism and myxedema coma.
2. As thyroid hormone levels gradually return to normal, the patient is monitored closely to prevent complications resulting from sudden increases in metabolic rate and oxygen requirements.

Restoration of Normal Metabolic State (Euthyroid)

1. Thyroid hormone: T_4-levothyroxine; T_3-liothyronine; T_3 and T_4 mixed. T_4 replacement therapy is typically the treatment of choice.
   a. Because T_3 acts more quickly than T_4, it is given via nasogastric tube if patient is unconscious (myxedema coma).
   b. Sodium levothyroxine is administered parenterally (until consciousness is restored) to restore T_4 level.
   c. Later, patient is continued on oral thyroid hormone therapy.
   d. With rapid administration of thyroid hormone, plasma T_4 levels may initiate adrenal insufficiency; hence, steroid therapy may be started.
   e. Mild symptoms in alert patient or asymptomatic cases (with abnormal laboratory results only) require only initiation of low-dose thyroid hormone given orally.
2. Monitoring to anticipate treatment effects.
   a. Diuresis, decreased puffiness.
   b. Improved reflexes and muscle tone.
   c. Accelerated pulse rate.
   d. A slightly higher level of total serum T_4.
   e. All signs of hypothyroidism should disappear in 3 to 12 weeks.
   f. Decreasing TSH level.

GERONTOLOGIC ALERT When starting thyroid hormone replacement, care must be taken with older patients and with those who have coronary artery disease to avoid coronary ischemia because of increased oxygen demands of the heart. It is preferable to start with much lower doses and increase gradually, taking 1 to 2 months to reach full replacement doses.

Complications

1. Myxedema coma—hypotension, unresponsiveness, bradycardia, hypoventilation, hyponatremia, (possibly) convulsions, hypothermia, cerebral hypoxia.
2. High mortality in myxedema coma.

Nursing Assessment

1. Obtain history of symptoms, medication program, and past history of thyroid disease, surgery, or treatment.
2. Perform multisystem assessment, including cardiac, respiratory, neurologic, and GI systems.

Nursing Diagnosis

In addition, see Nursing Care Plan 24-1.
- Decreased Cardiac Output related to decreased metabolic rate and decreased cardiac conduction.

Nursing Interventions

Increasing Cardiac Output

1. Monitor vital signs frequently to detect changes in cardiovascular status and ability to respond to stress.
2. Monitor ECG tracings to detect arrhythmias and deterioration of cardiovascular status.
3. Prevent chilling to avoid increasing metabolic rate, which, in turn, places strain on the heart. Provide bed socks, bed jacket, warm environment.
4. Avoid rapid rewarming techniques (warmed IV fluids, hypothermia blanket) because the resulting increased oxygen requirements and peripheral vasodilation may worsen cardiac failure.
5. Administer fluids cautiously, even though hyponatremia is present.
6. Administer all prescribed drugs with caution before and after thyroid replacement begins.
   a. Monitor the effects of sedatives, opioids, and anesthetics closely because patient is more sensitive to these agents.
   b. After thyroid replacement is initiated, the thyroid hormones may increase the effects of digoxin (monitor pulse) and anticoagulants (watch for signs of bleeding).
7. Report occurrence of angina and be alert for signs and symptoms of myocardial infarction and cardiac failure.
8. Monitor arterial blood gas levels to assess cardiopulmonary function.

Patient Education and Health Maintenance

Instruct the patient about the following:
1. The need to receive lifelong thyroid hormone replacement therapy.
2. How and when to take medications.
3. Signs and symptoms of insufficient and excessive medication; reinforce teaching by providing written instructions.
4. The necessity of having blood evaluations periodically to determine thyroid levels.
5. Energy-conservation techniques and the need to increase activity gradually.
6. Fluid intake and use of fiber to prevent constipation.

NURSING CARE PLAN 24-1

Care of the Patient with Hypothyroidism

You see Mrs. White in the clinic. She is a 45-year-old woman with a history of hypothyroidism, who has been treated with L-thyroxine 0.15 mg daily.

From your assessment and knowledge of hypothyroidism, develop your care plan.

Subjective data: Mrs. White tells you that she has been feeling tired lately and finds it hard to manage even the simplest chores around the house. She complains of constipation that gives her a feeling of fullness and affects her appetite. When asked about her medication, she states, "Oh, I ran out of those a few months ago, and I never refilled the prescrip-

tion. I was feeling fine, so I didn't see any need to keep taking medicine."

Objective data: Vital signs are temperature 98.2° F (36.8° C), pulse 58, blood pressure 100/60, respirations 12. On examination, you notice her skin is cool and dry to the touch. She is wearing a sweater even though it is a warm day outside. Bowel sounds are hypoactive. Knee jerk reflexes are sluggish.

Laboratory results: T_4-3.4 mcg/dL (normal range 5–12 mcg/dL), thyroid-stimulating hormone 25 μU/mL (normal range < 7 μU/mL)

NURSING DIAGNOSIS

Constipation related to decreased bowel motility caused by hypofunction of the thyroid gland.

GOAL/EXPECTED OUTCOME

The patient will resume normal bowel function.

NURSING CARE PLAN 24-1 (continued)

Care of the Patient with Hypothyroidism

Nursing Intervention	Rationale	Evaluation: Actual Outcome
Encourage increased intake of fluids.	Promotes passage of soft stools.	Drinks 8–10 glasses of fluid per day.
Recommend foods high in fiber.	Increases bulk of stools and promotes more frequent bowel movements.	Identifies and consumes foods high in fiber.
Recommend patient monitor bowel function by recording frequency and consistency of stools.	Documents patient response to nursing interventions.	Reports bowel pattern has returned to normal.
Encourage increased mobility within patient's exercise tolerance.	Promotes evacuation of the bowel.	Gradually increases exercise.

NURSING DIAGNOSIS

Activity Intolerance related to reduced metabolic rate.

GOAL/EXPECTED OUTCOME

Exercise tolerance and participation in activities will increase.

Nursing Intervention	Rationale	Evaluation: Actual Outcome
Teach patient to space activities to promote rest and exercise as tolerated.	Promotes activity without overly stressing the patient.	Reports increased participation in activities of daily living.
Teach patient to keep a record of physical activity, noting duration, intensity, and level of fatigue.	Promotes patient participation in care and promotes independence.	Provides reports of exercise tolerance and performance in daily activities.
Gradually increase level of activity as tolerated.	Demonstrates changes in patient activity tolerance.	Reports successful increases in activity tolerance.

NURSING DIAGNOSIS

Deficient Knowledge related to self-care needs for thyroid hormone replacement therapy.

GOAL/EXPECTED OUTCOME

Patient will demonstrate knowledge appropriate for self-care in thyroid replacement therapy.

Nursing Intervention	Rationale	Evaluation: Actual Outcome
Teach patient about the nature of chronic hypothyroidism and the purpose of thyroid hormone replacement therapy.	Provides rationale for adherence to prescribed hormone replacement.	Describes reason for thyroid hormone replacement therapy and describes regimen correctly.
Describe effects of thyroid hormone medication to patient.	Allows patient to appreciate benefits of therapy from the standpoint of her current physical complaints.	States physiologic effects of thyroid hormone replacement therapy.
Describe signs and symptoms of underdosage and overdosage of medication. • Underdosage—fatigue, slow pulse, constipation • Overdosage—increased pulse or palpitations, sweating, difficulty sleeping, feeling jittery	Allows patient to be an active participant in monitoring her therapy.	Identifies signs and symptoms indicative of overdosage and underdosage that should be reported to her health care provider promptly.

BOX 24-1	Endocrine Internet Resource Web Sites for Patients and Nurses

GENERAL
- The Endocrine Society: *www.endo-society.org*
- Endocrine Nurses Society: *www.endo-nurses.org*
- National Endocrine and Metabolic Diseases Information Service: *www.endocrine.niddk.nih.gov/index.htm*

The Hormone Foundation: *www.hormone.org*

THYROID
- American Thyroid Association: *www.thyroid.org*

ADDISON'S DISEASE
- National Adrenal Diseases Foundation: *www.nadf.us*

CUSHING'S SYNDROME
- National Endocrine and Metabolic Diseases Information Service: *www.endocrine.niddk.nih.gov/pubs/cushings/cushings.htm*

PITUITARY DISORDERS
- Pituitary Network Association: *www.pituitary.org*

7. Control of dietary intake to limit calories and reduce weight.
8. Assist patient in identifying sources of information and support available in the community (see Box 24-1).

Evaluation: Expected Outcomes

- BP and pulse rate stable.

Hyperthyroidism

 Evidence Base American Thyroid Association and American Association of Clinical Endocrinologists Taskforce on Hyperthyroidism and Other Causes of Thyrotoxicosis. (2011). Hyperthyroidism and other causes of thyrotoxicosis: Management guidelines of the American Thyroid Association and American Association of Clinical Endocrinologists. *Thyroid, 121*(6), 593–646.

Hyperthyroidism is a hypermetabolic condition is characterized by excessive amounts of thyroid hormone in the bloodstream.

Pathophysiology and Etiology

1. More common in women than in men; occurs in about 2% of the female population.
2. Graves' disease (most prevalent)—diffuse hyperfunction of the thyroid gland with autoimmune etiology and associated with ophthalmopathy; most common in younger women; may subside spontaneously.
   a. TSI, an immunoglobulin found in the blood of patients with Graves' disease, is capable of reacting with the receptor for TSH on the thyroid plasma membrane and of stimulating thyroid hormone production and secretion.
   b. May appear after an emotional shock, an infection, or emotional stress.
3. Toxic nodular goiter (single or multiple)—more common in older women with preexisting goiter; will continue to be overactive unless eradicated or kept under suppressive therapy.

4. Hyperthyroidism is characterized by hypertrophy and hyperplasia of the thyroid gland, which is accompanied by increased vascularity and blood flow and enlargement of the gland.
5. Most of the clinical manifestations result from increased metabolic rate, excessive heat production, increased neuromuscular and cardiovascular activity, and hyperactivity of the sympathetic nervous system.
6. Hyperthyroidism ranges from a mild increase in metabolic rate to the severe hyperactivity known as thyrotoxicosis, thyroid storm, or thyroid crisis.
7. Hyperthyroidism can also be the result of ingestion of excessive amounts of thyroid hormone medication (factitious hyperthyroidism).

Clinical Manifestations

1. Nervousness, emotional lability, irritability, apprehension.
2. Difficulty sitting quietly.
3. Rapid pulse at rest and on exertion (ranges between 90 and 160); palpitations.
4. Heat intolerance; profuse perspiration; flushed skin (eg, hands may be warm, soft, moist).
5. Fine tremor of hands; change in bowel habits—constipation or diarrhea.
6. Increased appetite and progressive weight loss; frequent stools.
7. Muscle fatigability and weakness; amenorrhea.
8. Atrial fibrillation possible (cardiac decompensation common in older patients).
9. Bulging eyes (exophthalmos)—seen only in Graves' disease.
10. Thyroid gland may be palpable and a bruit may be auscultated over gland.
11. Course may be mild, characterized by remissions and exacerbations.
12. May progress to emaciation, extreme nervousness, delirium, disorientation, thyroid storm or crisis, and death.
13. Thyroid storm or crisis, an extreme form of hyperthyroidism, is characterized by hyperpyrexia, diarrhea, dehydration, tachycardia, arrhythmias, extreme irritation, delirium, coma, shock, and death if not adequately treated.
14. Thyroid storm may be precipitated by stress (surgery, infection) or inadequate preparation for surgery in a patient with known hyperthyroidism.

Diagnostic Evaluation

1. Elevated T_3 and T_4.
2. Elevated serum T_3 resin uptake and free thyroid index.
3. Low TSH levels.
4. Presence of TSI antibodies (if Graves' disease is the cause).
5. ^{131}I uptake scan may be elevated or below normal depending on the underlying cause of the hyperthyroidism.

Management

Approach to Management

1. Treatment depends on causes, age of patient, severity of disease, and complications.
2. Remission of hyperthyroidism (Graves' disease) occurs spontaneously within 1 to 2 years; however, relapse can be

expected in half the patients. Antithyroid drugs, radiation, or surgery may be used for treatment.

3. Nodular toxic goiter—surgery or use of radioiodine is preferred.
4. Thyroid carcinoma—surgery or radiation is used.
5. Goal of therapy is to bring the metabolic rate to normal as soon as possible and to maintain it at this level.

Pharmacotherapy

1. Drugs that inhibit hormone formation:
   a. Thioamides—propylthiouracil and methimazole.
   b. Act by depressing the synthesis of thyroid hormone by inhibiting thyroid peroxidase.
   c. Propylthiouracil given in divided daily doses, methimazole may be given in a single daily dose.
   d. Duration of treatment is determined by clinical criteria.
      i. Thyroid gland becomes smaller.
      ii. Treatment continued until patient becomes clinically euthyroid; this varies from 3 months to 2 years; if euthyroidism cannot be maintained without therapy, then radiation or surgery is recommended.
      iii. Therapy is withdrawn gradually to prevent exacerbation.
2. Drugs to control peripheral manifestations of hyperthyroidism:
   a. Propranolol, a beta-adrenergic blocking agent.
      i. Inhibits peripheral conversion of T_4 to T_3.
      ii. Abolishes tachycardia, tremor, excess sweating, nervousness.
      iii. Controls hyperthyroid symptoms until antithyroid drugs or radioiodine can take effect.
   b. Glucocorticoids—decrease the peripheral conversion of T_4 to T_3, a more potent thyroid hormone.

Radioactive Iodine

1. Action—limits secretion of thyroid hormone by destroying thyroid tissue.
2. Dosage is controlled so that hypothyroidism does not occur.
3. Chief advantage over thioamides is that a lasting remission can be achieved.
4. Chief disadvantage is that permanent hypothyroidism can be produced.

Surgery

1. Used for those with large goiters, or for those for whom the use of radioiodine or thioamides is contraindicated.
2. Subtotal thyroidectomy involves removal of most of the thyroid gland (see page 916).

 DRUG ALERT Observe the patient for evidence of iodine toxicity: swelling of buccal mucosa, excessive salivation, coryza, skin eruptions. If these occur, iodides are discontinued.

Emergency Management of Thyroid Storm

1. Inhibition of new hormone synthesis with thioamides (PTU).
2. Inhibition of thyroid hormone release using iodine (Lugol's solution).
3. Inhibition of peripheral effects of thyroid hormones with propranolol, corticosteroids, and propylthiouracil (PTU).
4. Treatment aimed at systemic effects of thyroid hormones and prevention of decompensation.
   a. Hyperthermia—cooling blanket, acetaminophen.
   b. Dehydration—administration of IV fluids and electrolytes.
5. Treatment of precipitating event.

Complications

1. Thioamide toxicity—agranulocytosis may occur suddenly.
2. Hypothyroidism if overtreated with antithyroid medication or if radiation treatment is used.
3. Radiation thyroiditis (a transient exacerbation of hyperthyroidism) may occur as a result of leakage of thyroid hormone into the circulation from damaged follicles.
4. Infiltrative ophthalmopathy.
   a. Occurs in 50% of patients with Graves' disease.
   b. Features include exophthalmos, weakness of extraocular muscles, lid edema, lid lag.

Nursing Assessment

1. Obtain history of symptoms, family history of thyroid disease, medications, any recent physical stress, particularly infection.
2. Perform multisystem assessment that includes cardiac, respiratory, neurologic, and GI systems.
3. Closely monitor patient's temperature for thyroid storm.

Nursing Diagnoses

- Imbalanced Nutrition: Less Than Body Requirements related to hypermetabolic state and fluid loss through diaphoresis.
- Risk for Impaired Skin Integrity related to diaphoresis, hyperpyrexia, restlessness, and rapid weight loss.
- Disturbed Thought Processes related to insomnia, decreased attention span, and irritability.
- Anxiety related to condition and concern about upcoming surgery/radioiodine treatment.

Nursing Interventions

Providing Adequate Nutrition

1. Determine patient's food and fluid preferences.
2. Provide high-calorie foods and fluids consistent with the patient's requirements.
3. Provide a quiet, calm environment at meals.
4. Restrict stimulants (tea, coffee, alcohol); explain rationale of requirements and restrictions to patient.
5. Encourage and permit patient to eat alone if embarrassed or if otherwise disturbed by voracious appetite.
6. Monitor IV infusion when prescribed to maintain fluid and electrolyte balance.
7. Monitor fluid and nutritional status by weighing patient daily and by keeping accurate intake and output records.
8. Monitor vital signs to detect changes in fluid volume status.
9. Assess skin turgor, mucous membranes, and neck veins for signs of increased or decreased fluid volume.

Maintaining Skin Integrity

1. Assess skin frequently to detect diaphoresis.
2. Bathe frequently with cool water; change linens when damp.
3. Avoid soap to prevent drying and apply lubricant skin lotions to pressure points.
4. Protect and relieve pressure from bony prominences while immobilized or while hypothermia blanket is used.

Promoting Normal Thought Processes

1. Explain procedures to patient in an unhurried, calm manner.
2. Limit visitors; avoid stimulating conversations or television programs.
3. Reduce stressors in the environment; reduce noise and lights.
4. Promote sleep and relaxation through use of prescribed medications, massage, and relaxation exercises.
5. Minimize disruption of patient's sleep or rest by clustering nursing activities.
6. Use safety measures to reduce risk of trauma or falls (padded side rails, bed in low position).

Relieving Anxiety

1. Encourage patient to verbalize concerns and fears about illness and treatment.
2. Support patient who is undergoing various diagnostic tests.
   a. Explain the purpose and requirements of each prescribed test.
   b. Explain results of tests if unclear to patient or if questions arise.
3. Clear up misconceptions about treatment options.

Patient Education and Health Maintenance

1. Instruct patient as follows:
   a. When to take medications.
   b. Signs and symptoms of insufficient and excessive medication.
   c. Necessity of having blood evaluations periodically to determine thyroid levels.
   d. Signs of agranulocytosis (fever, sore throat, upper respiratory infection) or rash, fever, urticaria, or enlarged salivary glands caused by thioamide toxicity.
   e. Signs and symptoms of thyroid storm (ie, tachycardia, hyperpyrexia, extreme irritation) and predisposing factors to thyroid storm (ie, infection, surgery, stress, abrupt withdrawal of antithyroid medications and adrenergic blockers).
2. Reinforce teaching by providing written instructions as well.
3. Assist patient in identifying sources of information and support available in the community (see Box 24-1, page 922).

Evaluation: Expected Outcomes

- Food and fluid intake adequate, gaining weight.
- Skin cool, dry, and intact.
- Maintains concentration, follows conversation, and responds appropriately.
- Verbalizes concerns and questions about illness, treatment, and surgery.

Subacute Thyroiditis

Subacute thyroiditis is a self-limiting, painful inflammation of the thyroid gland, usually associated with viral infections.

Pathophysiology and Etiology

1. Affects younger women predominantly.
2. Acute inflammation results in sudden release of preformed T_3 and T_4, commonly causing symptoms of hyperthyroidism initially.
3. A clinical variant of this disorder, "silent thyroiditis," has been described as similar to subacute thyroiditis; however, the symptoms may be milder and the thyroid gland is not painful.
4. Subacute thyroiditis has been associated with onset within 6 months of the postpartum period in women.

Clinical Manifestations

1. Pain, swelling, thyroid tenderness lasts several weeks or months and then disappears.
2. Fever, sore throat.
3. Pain referred to the ear, making swallowing difficult and uncomfortable.
4. Fever, malaise, chills.
5. May develop clinical manifestations of hyperthyroidism (irritability, nervousness, insomnia, and weight loss) or hypothyroidism, depending on the point of time in the natural course of the disease when patient presents.

Diagnostic Evaluation

1. TSH level is low.
2. ^{131}I uptake is low.
3. Serum T_3 and T_4 levels are elevated.
4. Erythrocyte sedimentation rate is increased.

Management

1. Analgesics and mild sedatives.
2. The patient may be placed on beta-adrenergic blockers to reduce the symptoms of thyrotoxicosis.
3. Steroids may be administered for pain, fever, and malaise.
4. Aspirin or nonsteroidal anti-inflammatory drugs may be used in mild cases to treat the symptoms of inflammation.

 DRUG ALERT Aspirin should be avoided if the patient exhibits signs of hyperthyroidism because it displaces thyroid hormone from its binding site and may increase the amount of free circulating hormone, resulting in exacerbation of the symptoms of hyperthyroidism.

Complications

In about 10% of patients, permanent hypothyroidism occurs and long-term T_4 therapy is needed.

Nursing Assessment

1. Assess for signs and symptoms of hyperthyroidism (see page 922).

2. Assess for level of discomfort.

3. Evaluate patient's coping skills regarding pain.

Nursing Diagnosis

- Pain related to inflammation of thyroid gland.

Nursing Interventions

Reducing Pain

1. Explain all tests and procedures to patient/family.
2. Administer or teach self-administration of pain relief medication, as prescribed.
3. Provide a restful environment.
4. Assess for degree of pain relief.
5. Notify health care provider if pain relief medications are inadequate for acceptable pain control.

Patient Education and Health Maintenance

1. Explain all medications patient is to continue at home.
2. Reassure patient that subacute thyroiditis usually resolves spontaneously during weeks to months.
3. Teach patient signs and symptoms of hypothyroidism (ie, fatigue and lethargy, weight gain, cold intolerance) that may be experienced. These should be reported as inflammation of the gland subsides.
4. Assist patient in identifying sources of information and support available in the community (see Box 24-1, page 922).

Evaluation: Expected Outcomes

- Verbalizes acceptable pain relief.

Hashimoto's Thyroiditis (Lymphocytic Thyroiditis)

Hashimoto's thyroiditis is a chronic progressive disease of the thyroid gland caused by infiltration of lymphocytes; it results in progressive destruction of the parenchyma and hypothyroidism if untreated.

Pathophysiology and Etiology

1. Cause is unknown; believed to be an autoimmune disease, genetically transmitted and perhaps related to Graves' disease.
2. Ninety-five percent of cases occur in women in their 40s or 50s.
3. Possibly the most common cause of adult hypothyroidism.
4. Appears to be increasing in incidence.

Clinical Manifestations

1. Marked by a slowly developing, firm enlargement of the thyroid gland.
2. Usually no gross nodules.
3. Basal metabolic rate is usually low.
4. Periods of hyperthyroidism caused by large amounts of T_3 and T_4 being released into bloodstream.

Diagnostic Evaluation

1. T_3 and T_4 may be normal but usually become subnormal as the disease progresses.
2. TSH level is usually elevated.
3. Antithyroglobulin antibodies and antimicrosomal antibodies are virtually always present.
4. Normal or high concentration of thyroglobulin-binding protein.

Management

1. Thyroid medications to maintain a normal level of circulating thyroid hormone; this is done to suppress production of TSH, to prevent enlargement of the thyroid, and to maintain a euthyroid state.
2. Surgical resection of goiter if tracheal compression, cough, or hoarseness occur.
3. Careful follow-up to detect and treat hypothyroidism.

Complications

1. Progressive hypothyroidism.
2. Without treatment, Hashimoto's thyroiditis may progress from goiter and hypothyroidism to myxedema.

Nursing Assessment

1. Assess for signs and symptoms of hyperthyroidism and hypothyroidism.
2. Assess size of thyroid gland and symptoms of compression—neck tightness, cough, hoarseness.

Nursing Diagnosis

- Anxiety related to enlargement of neck/thyroid gland.

Nursing Interventions

Reducing Anxiety

1. Explain physiology of the disorder and the reason for enlarging gland. Show anatomic pictures of thyroid gland, if possible.
2. Administer or teach self-administration of thyroid hormone to suppress stimulation on gland and possibly reduce size.
3. Reassure regarding slow progression of gland enlargement (during months) and the option of surgical resection, if necessary.
4. Suggest wearing loose-necked clothing, avoiding jewelry or scarves around neck, and avoiding excessive neck flexion or hyperextension, which may aggravate feeling of compression.

Patient Education and Health Maintenance

1. Teach signs of tracheal compression that should be reported to health care provider as soon as possible—difficulty breathing, cough, hoarseness.
2. Explain outcome of hypothyroidism and necessity of taking thyroid hormones every day for life.
3. Explain the need for regular medical follow-up visits to monitor thyroid hormone and TSH levels.
4. Assist patient in identifying sources of information and support available in the community (see Box 24-1, page 922).

GERONTOLOGIC ALERT Careful and regular follow-up of older patients with Hashimoto's thyroiditis is especially important because the progression to hypothyroidism is usually subtle in older people and is unlikely to be recognized promptly.

Evaluation: Expected Outcomes

• Verbalizes reduced anxiety, appears more relaxed, sleeps better.

Cancer of the Thyroid

Cancer of the thyroid is a malignant neoplasm of the gland.

Pathophysiology and Etiology

1. Incidence increases with age. The average age at time of diagnosis is 45.
2. There appears to be an association between external radiation to the head and neck in infancy and childhood and subsequent development of thyroid carcinoma. (Between 1949 and 1960, radiation therapy was commonly given to shrink enlarged tonsil and adenoid tissue, to treat acne, or to reduce an enlarged thymus.)
3. Papillary and well-differentiated adenocarcinoma (most common).
   a. Growth is slow and spread is confined to lymph nodes that surround thyroid area.
   b. Cure rate is excellent after removal of involved areas.
4. Follicular (rapidly growing, widely metastasizing type).
   a. Occurs predominantly in middle-aged and older persons.
   b. Brief encouraging response may occur with irradiation.
   c. Progression of disease is rapid; high mortality.
5. Parafollicular–medullary thyroid carcinoma.
   a. Rare, inheritable type of thyroid malignancy, which can be detected early by a radioimmunoassay for calcitonin.
6. Undifferentiated anaplastic carcinoma.
   a. The most aggressive and lethal solid tumor found in humans.
   b. Least common of all thyroid cancers.
   c. Usually fatal within months of diagnosis.

Clinical Manifestations

1. On palpation of the thyroid, there may be a firm, irregular, fixed, painless mass or nodule.
2. The occurrence of signs and symptoms of hyperthyroidism is rare.

Diagnostic Evaluation

1. A thyroid scan with ^{99m}Tc will detect a "cold" nodule with little uptake.
2. FNA biopsy.
3. Surgical exploration.

Management

1. Surgical removal is extensive, as required.
   a. Postoperative radiation therapy is commonly done to reduce chances of recurrence.
   b. Follow-up includes periodic ^{131}I uptake scan to detect evidence of recurrence.
2. Thyroid replacement.
   a. Thyroid hormone is administered to suppress secretion of TSH.
   b. Such treatment is continued indefinitely and requires annual checkups.
3. For unresectable cancer, patient is referred for treatment with ^{131}I, chemotherapy, or radiation therapy.

Complications

Untreated thyroid carcinoma can be fatal.

Nursing Assessment

Explore patient's feelings and concerns regarding the diagnosis, treatment, and prognosis.

Nursing Diagnosis

• Anxiety related to concern about cancer, upcoming surgery.

Nursing Interventions

Also see "Care of the Patient Undergoing Thyroidectomy," page 916.

Allaying Anxiety

1. Provide all explanations in a simple, concise manner and repeat important information, as necessary, because anxiety may interfere with patient's processing of information.
2. Stress the positive aspects of treatment and high cure rate, as outlined by health care provider.
3. Encourage support by significant other, clergy, social worker, nursing staff, as available.

Patient Education and Health Maintenance

1. Instruct the patient on thyroid hormone replacement and follow-up blood tests.
2. Stress the need for periodic evaluation for recurrence of malignancy.
3. Supply additional information or suggest community resources dealing with cancer prevention and treatment.
4. Assist patient in identifying sources of information and support available in the community (see Box 24-1, page 922).

Evaluation: Expected Outcomes

• Discusses concerns with family, hospital, clergy.

DISORDERS OF THE PARATHYROID GLANDS

The *parathyroid glands* are small, bean-size structures embedded in the posterior section of the thyroid gland. Functions include the production, storage, and release of PTH in response to the serum level of ionized calcium. PTH increases serum calcium by decreasing elimination of calcium ions in the urine by the kidney, increasing absorption of calcium ions from the gut, and increasing bone contribution of calcium ions to the plasma.

Hyperparathyroidism

Hyperparathyroidism is hypersecretion of PTH.

Pathophysiology and Etiology

1. Disorder is most common among women older than age 50.
2. Primary hyperparathyroidism.
   a. Single parathyroid adenoma is the most common cause (approximately 80% of cases).
   b. Parathyroid hyperplasia accounts for approximately 20% of cases.
   c. Parathyroid carcinoma accounts for less than 1% of cases.
3. Secondary hyperparathyroidism.
   a. Primarily the result of renal failure.
4. Excess secretion of PTH results in increased serum calcium levels (see Figure 24-3).

Clinical Manifestations

1. Decalcification of bones.
   a. Skeletal pain, backache, pain on weight-bearing, pathologic fractures, deformities, formation of bony cysts.
   b. Formation of bone tumors—overgrowth of osteoclasts.
   c. Formation of calcium-containing renal calculi.
2. Depression of neuromuscular function.
   a. The patient may trip, drop objects, show general fatigue, lose memory for recent events, experience emotional instability, have changes in level of consciousness, with stupor and coma.
   b. Cardiac arrhythmias, hypertension, cardiac standstill.

Diagnostic Evaluation

1. Persistently elevated serum calcium (11 mg/100 mL); test is performed on at least two occasions to determine consistency of results.
2. Exclusion of other causes of hypercalcemia—malignancy (usually bone or breast), vitamin D excess, multiple myeloma,

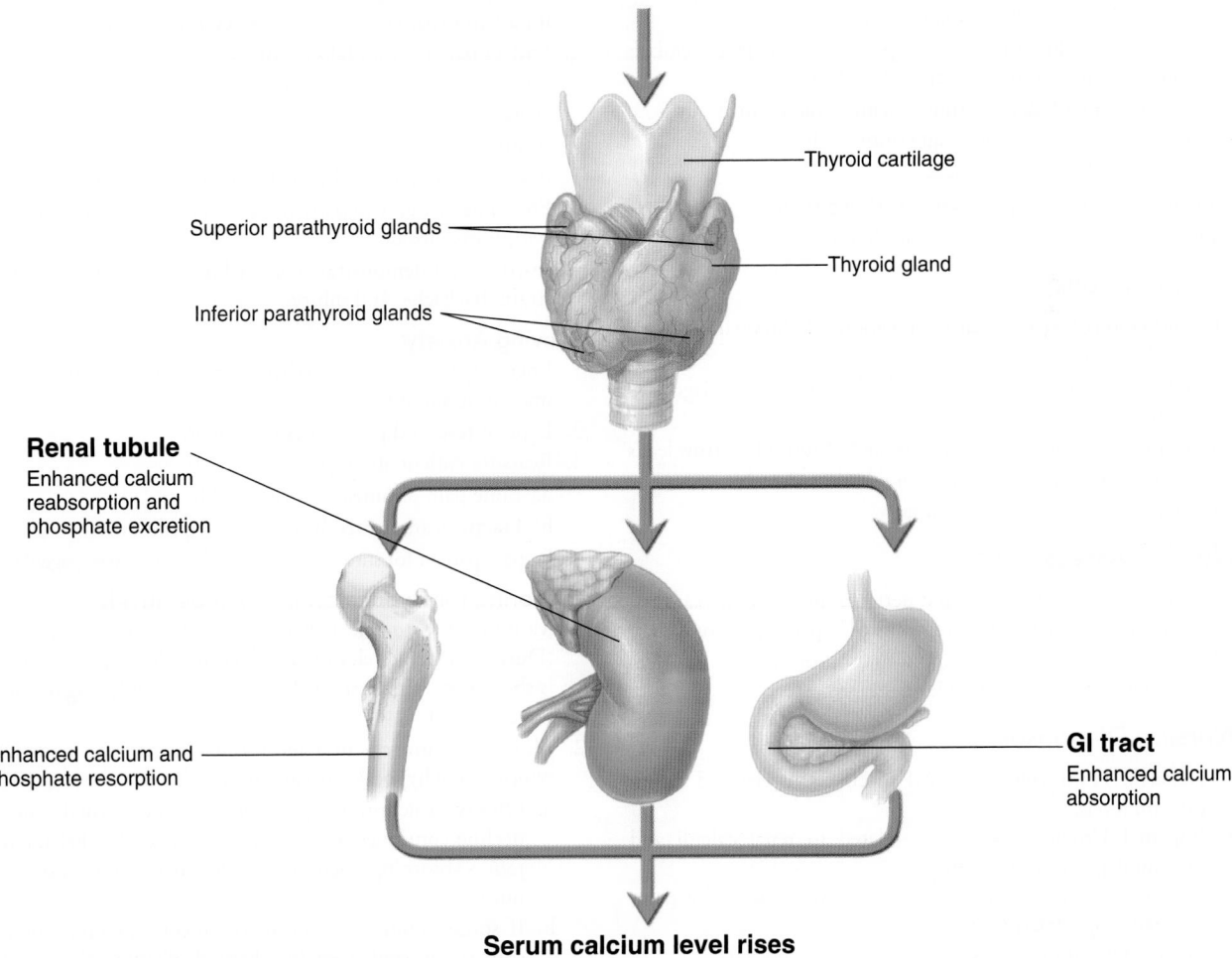

Tumor or hyperplastic tissue secretes excess PTH

Thyroid cartilage

Superior parathyroid glands

Thyroid gland

Inferior parathyroid glands

Renal tubule
Enhanced calcium reabsorption and phosphate excretion

Enhanced calcium and phosphate resorption

GI tract
Enhanced calcium absorption

Serum calcium level rises

Figure 24-3. Pathogenesis of hyperparathyroidism.

sarcoidosis, milk-alkali syndrome, such drugs as thiazides, Cushing's disease, hyperthyroidism.
3. PTH levels are increased.
4. Serum calcium and alkaline phosphatase levels are elevated and serum phosphorus levels are decreased.
5. Skeletal changes are revealed by x-ray.
6. Cine computed tomography (CT) will disclose parathyroid tumors more readily than x-ray.
7. Sestamibi scan is used to evaluate location of the tumor prior to surgery.

Management
Treatment of Hypercalcemia
1. Hydration with IV saline, loop diuretics such as furosemide and ethacrynic acid—to increase urinary excretion of calcium in patients not in renal failure.
2. Oral phosphate may be used as an antihypercalcemic agent.
3. In patients developing osteoporosis, Pamidronate, calcitonin, or etidronate disodium are effective in treating hypercalcemia by inhibiting bone resorption.
4. Dietary calcium is restricted and all drugs that might cause hypercalcemia (thiazides, vitamin D) may be discontinued.
5. Dialysis may be necessary in patients with resistant hypercalcemia or those with renal failure.
6. Digoxin is reduced because the patient with hypercalcemia is more sensitive to toxic effects of this drug.
7. Monitoring of daily serum calcium, blood urea nitrogen (BUN), potassium, and magnesium levels.
8. Removal of underlying cause.

Treatment of Primary Hyperparathyroidism
Surgery for removal of abnormal parathyroid tissue.

Complications
1. Formation of renal calculi, calcification of kidney parenchyma, renal shutdown.
2. Ulceration of upper GI tract leading to hemorrhage and perforation.
3. Demineralization of bones, cysts, and fibrosis of marrow leads to fractures, especially of vertebral bodies and ribs.
4. Hypoparathyroidism after surgery.

Nursing Assessment
1. Obtain review of systems and perform multisystem examination to detect signs and symptoms of hyperparathyroidism.
2. Closely monitor patient's input and output and serum electrolytes, especially calcium level.

Nursing Diagnoses
- Deficient Fluid Volume related to effects of elevated serum calcium levels.
- Impaired Urinary Elimination related to renal calculi and calcium deposits in the kidneys.
- Impaired Physical Mobility related to weakness, bone pain, and pathologic fractures.
- Anxiety related to surgery.
- Risk for Injury related to hypocalcemia.

Nursing Interventions
Achieving Fluid and Electrolyte Balance
1. Monitor fluid intake and output.
2. Provide adequate hydration—administer water, glucose, and electrolytes orally or via IV line, as prescribed.
3. Prevent or promptly treat dehydration by reporting vomiting or other sources of fluid loss promptly.
4. Help patient understand why and how to avoid dietary sources of calcium—dairy products, broccoli, calcium-containing antacids.

Promoting Urinary Elimination
1. Strain all urine to observe for calculi.
2. Increase fluid intake to 3,000 mL/day to maintain hydration and prevent precipitation of calcium and formation of calculi.
3. Instruct patient about dietary recommendations for restriction of calcium.
4. Observe for signs of urinary tract infection (UTI), hematuria, and renal colic.
5. Assess renal function through serum creatinine and BUN levels.

Increasing Physical Mobility
1. Assist patient in hygiene and activities if bone pain is severe or if patient experiences musculoskeletal weakness.
2. Protect patient from falls or injury.
3. Turn patient cautiously and handle extremities gently to avoid fractures.
4. Administer analgesia, as prescribed.
5. Assess level of pain and patient's response to analgesia.
6. Encourage patient to participate in mild exercise gradually as symptoms subside.
7. Instruct and demonstrate correct body mechanics to reduce strain, backache, and injury.

Relieving Anxiety
1. Encourage patient to verbalize fears and feelings about upcoming surgery.
2. Explain tests and procedures to patient.
3. Reassure patient about skeletal recovery.
   a. Bone pain diminishes fairly quickly.
   b. Fractures are treated by orthopedic procedures.
4. Prepare patient for surgery as for thyroidectomy (see page 916).

Monitoring for Hypocalcemia Postoperatively
1. Monitor ECG to detect changes secondary to hypercalcemia. (During moderate elevations of serum calcium, QT interval is shortened; with extreme hypercalcemia, widening of the T wave is seen.)
2. Monitor serum calcium level and evaluate for signs and symptoms of hypocalcemia and onset of tetany (see page 916).
   a. Observe calcium levels—if well below normal, and if decline continues into the second week, the skeletal system is absorbing calcium and calcium administration may not be necessary.
   b. If some significant bone involvement was noted before surgery, as evidenced by elevated alkaline phosphatase level, elemental calcium may be ordered.

Patient Education and Health Maintenance

1. Instruct patient about calcium-reducing medications.
   a. Calcitonin is given subcutaneously—teach proper technique.
   b. Etidronate disodium—calcium-rich foods should be avoided within 2 hours of dose; therapeutic response may take 1 to 3 months.
   c. Pamidronate—monitor hypercalcemia-related parameters when treatment begins. Adequate intake of calcium and vitamin D is necessary to prevent hypocalcemia. Bisphosphonates should be used with caution in patients with active upper GI problems.
2. Teach signs and symptoms of tetany that patient may experience postoperatively and should report to health care provider (numbness and tingling in extremities or around mouth).
3. Assist patient in identifying sources of information and support available in the community (see Box 24-1, page 922).

Evaluation: Expected Outcomes

- Output equals intake, normal skin turgor, moist mucous membranes.
- No signs and symptoms of renal calculi or UTI; serum creatinine and BUN levels normal.
- Reports less bone and joint pain; uses correct body mechanics.
- Verbalizes concerns and fears about surgery; appears less anxious.
- ECG without QT, T-wave changes; no numbness or tingling reported.

Hypoparathyroidism

Hypoparathyroidism results from a deficiency of PTH and is characterized by hypocalcemia and neuromuscular hyperexcitability.

Pathophysiology and Etiology

1. The most common cause is accidental removal or destruction of parathyroid tissue or its blood supply during thyroidectomy or radical neck dissection for malignancy.
2. Decrease in gland function (idiopathic hypoparathyroidism); may be autoimmune or familial in origin.
3. Malignancy or metastasis from a cancer to the parathyroid glands.
4. Resistance to PTH action.
5. With inadequate PTH secretion, there is decreased resorption of calcium from the renal tubules, decreased absorption of calcium in the GI tract, and decreased resorption of calcium from bone.
6. Blood calcium falls to a low level, causing symptoms of muscular hyperirritability, uncontrolled spasms, and hypocalcemic tetany.
7. In response to decreased serum calcium levels and lack of PTH, the serum phosphate level rises and phosphate excretion by the kidneys decreases.

Clinical Manifestations

1. Tetany—general muscular hypertonia; attempts at voluntary movement result in tremors and spasmodic or uncoordinated movements; fingers assume classic tetanic position.
   a. Chvostek's sign—a spasm of facial muscles that occurs when muscles or branches of facial nerve are tapped.
   b. Trousseau's sign—carpopedal spasm within 3 minutes after a BP cuff is inflated 20 mm Hg above patient's systolic pressure.
   c. Laryngeal spasm.
2. Severe anxiety and apprehension.
3. Renal colic is usually present if patient has history of calculi; preexisting calculi loosen and migrate into the ureter.

Diagnostic Evaluation

1. Phosphorus level in blood is elevated.
2. Decrease in serum calcium level to a low level (7.5 mg/100 mL or less).
3. PTH levels are low in most cases; may be normal or elevated in pseudohypoparathyroidism.
4. In chronic hypoparathyroidism, bone density may be increased as seen on radiography.

Management

IV Calcium Administration

1. A syringe and an ampule of a calcium solution (calcium chloride, calcium glucepate, calcium gluconate) are to be kept at the bedside at all times.
2. Most rapidly effective calcium solution is ionized calcium chloride (10%).
3. For rapid use to relieve severe tetany, infusion carried out every 10 minutes.
   a. All IV calcium preparations are administered slowly. It is highly irritating, stings, and causes thrombosis; patient experiences unpleasant burning flush of skin and tongue.

 DRUG ALERT Too-rapid calcium administration may cause cardiac arrest.

   b. Typical doses are as follows:
      i. Calcium chloride—500 mg to 1 g (5 to 10 mL) as indicated by serum calcium; administer at rate of less than 1 mL/minute of 10% solution.
      ii. Calcium gluconate—500 mg to 2 g (10 to 20 mL) at a rate of less than 0.5 mL/minute of a 10% solution.
      iii. Calcium glucepate—1 to 2 g (5 to 10 mL) at a rate of less than 1 mL/minute.
4. A slow drip of IV saline containing calcium gluconate is given until control of tetany is ensured; then I.M. or oral administration of calcium is prescribed.
5. Later, vitamin D is added to calcium intake—increases absorption of calcium and also induces a high level of calcium in the bloodstream. Thiazide diuretics may also be added because of their calcium-retaining effect on the kidney; doses of calcium and vitamin D may be lowered.
6. Administration of IV calcium seems to cause rapid relief of anxiety.

Other Measures

1. Treat renal calculi.
2. Monitor patient for hypercalciuria.

3. Monitor blood calcium level periodically; variations in vitamin D may affect calcium levels.

Complications

1. Acute complications related to hypocalcemia include seizures, tetany, and mental disorders, all of which can be reversed with calcium therapy.
2. If onset of hypocalcemia is acute, the major concerns are laryngeal spasm, acute airway obstruction, and cardiovascular failure.
3. Long-term complications include subcapsular cataracts, calcification of the basal ganglia, and papilledema (caused by precipitation of calcium out of serum and deposition in tissue); shortening of the fingers and toes; and bowing of the long bones (caused by inadequate PTH and additional genetic abnormalities). Of these complications, only papilledema is reversible.

Nursing Assessment

1. Perform multisystem assessment, focusing on neuromuscular system.
2. Closely monitor patient's input and output and serum electrolytes, especially calcium level.
3. Assess anxiety.

Nursing Diagnosis

• Imbalanced Nutrition: Less Than Body Requirements related to decreased calcium.

Nursing Interventions

Maintaining Normal Serum Calcium Levels

1. Assess neuromuscular status frequently in patients with hypoparathyroidism and in those at risk for hypocalcemia (patients in the immediate postoperative period after thyroidectomy, parathyroidectomy, radical neck dissection).
2. Check for Trousseau's and Chvostek's signs and notify health care provider if test results are positive.
3. Assess respiratory status frequently in acute hypocalcemia and postoperatively.
4. Monitor serum calcium and phosphorus levels.
5. Promote high-calcium diet, if prescribed—dairy products; green, leafy vegetables.
6. Instruct the patient about signs and symptoms of hypo- and hypercalcemia that should be reported.
7. Use caution in administering other drugs to the patient with hypocalcemia.
   a. The hypocalcemic patient is sensitive to digoxin; as hypocalcemia is reversed, the patient may rapidly develop digoxin toxicity.
   b. Cimetidine interferes with normal parathyroid function, especially with renal failure, which increases the risk of hypocalcemia.

Patient Education and Health Maintenance

1. Explain to patient and family the function of PTH and the roles of vitamin D and calcium in maintaining good health.

2. Discuss the importance of each medication prescribed for the control of hypocalcemia including vitamin D, calcium, and thiazide diuretic.
   a. Take medications, as prescribed.
   b. Do not substitute with over-the-counter preparations without the advice and supervision of the health care provider.
3. Provide patient with a written list about hypercalcemia and hypocalcemia and advise the patient to contact the health care provider immediately should signs of either condition develop.
4. Advise patient to wear a MedicAlert bracelet.
5. Explain the need for periodic medical follow-up for life.

Evaluation: Expected Outcome

• Verbalizes understanding of diet and medications; calcium level within normal limits.

DISORDERS OF THE ADRENAL GLANDS

The *adrenal medulla*, or inner portion of the gland, is not necessary to maintain life, but enables a person to cope with stress. It secretes two hormones:

• *Epinephrine* (adrenalin) acts on alpha and beta receptors to increase contractility and excitability of heart muscle, leading to increased cardiac output; facilitates blood flow to muscles, brain, and viscera; enhances blood sugar by stimulating conversion of glycogen to glucose in liver; and inhibits smooth-muscle contraction.
• *Norepinephrine* (noradrenaline) acts primarily on alpha receptors to increase peripheral vascular resistance, leading to increases in diastolic and systolic BP.

The adrenal cortex, or outer portion of the gland, is essential to life. It secretes adrenocortical hormones—synthesized from cholesterol.

• *Glucocorticoids* (cortisone and hydrocortisone) enhance protein catabolism and inhibit protein synthesis; antagonize action of insulin and increase blood sugar; increase synthesis of glucose by liver; influence defense mechanism of body and its reaction to stress; and influence emotional reaction.
• *Mineralocorticoids* (aldosterone and desoxycorticosterone) regulate reabsorption of sodium; regulate excretion of potassium by renal tubules.
• *Adrenosterones* (adrenal androgens) exert minimal effect on sex characteristics and function.

Primary Aldosteronism

Primary aldosteronism refers to excessive secretion of aldosterone by the adrenal cortex.

Pathophysiology and Etiology

1. Excessive secretion of aldosterone results in the conservation of sodium and excretion of potassium primarily in the renal tubules, but also in the sweat glands, salivary glands, and in the GI tract.
2. Usually caused by a cortical adenoma; also caused by bilateral adrenal hyperplasia.

3. Secondary aldosteronism occurs in conjunction with heart failure, renal dysfunction, or cirrhosis of the liver.
4. Women constitute 70% of patients with aldosterone-secreting adenomas and the incidence of primary aldosteronism is four times higher among blacks than among the general population.

Clinical Manifestations

1. Hypertension (1% to 2% of cases of hypertension are a result of primary aldosteronism, which usually can be treated successfully by surgical removal of the adenoma).
2. A profound decline in blood levels of potassium (hypokalemia) and hydrogen ions (alkalosis) results in muscle weakness and inability of kidneys to acidify or concentrate urine, leading to excess volume of urine (polyuria).
3. A decline in hydrogen ions (alkalosis) results in tetany, paresthesia.
4. An elevation in blood sodium (hypernatremia) results in excessive thirst (polydipsia) and arterial hypertension.

Diagnostic Evaluation

1. Suspected in all hypertensive patients with spontaneous hypokalemia; also if hypokalemia develops concurrently with start of diuretics and remains after diuretics are discontinued.
2. The screening test of choice is the aldosterone/renin ratio, which is suggestive of primary aldosteronism if the ratio is greater than 20:1.
3. Salt loading may be used as a confirmatory test—ingestion of at least 200 mEq/day (approximately 12 g salt) for 4 days does not influence the serum potassium level without aldosteronism, but will cause a decrease of serum potassium to less than 3.5 mEq/L in a patient with aldosteronism.
4. CT scanning to determine and localize cortical adenoma.

Management

1. Removal of adrenal tumor if the tumor is localized to one side—unilateral adrenalectomy.
2. If the cause is bilateral adrenal hyperplasia—spironolactone is used to treat both hypertension and potassium-depleted stages; therapy is needed 4 to 6 weeks before the full effect on BP is seen.
   a. Adverse effects include reduced testosterone in men (decreased libido, impotence, gynecomastia) and GI discomfort.
   b. Amiloride may be used instead in sexually active men or in cases of GI intolerance.
   c. Sodium restriction is necessary—no saline infusions, low-sodium diet.
   d. Potassium supplementation is usually necessary, based on severity of deficit.
3. Addition of antihypertensive agent—thiazide diuretic such as triamterene.
4. Management of underlying causes of secondary aldosteronism.

Complications

Long-term effects of untreated hypertension—stroke, renal failure, heart failure.

Nursing Assessment

1. Obtain history of symptoms, such as muscle weakness, paresthesia, thirst, and polyuria.
2. Perform multisystem physical examination.
3. Evaluate BP.

Nursing Diagnosis

- Excess Fluid Volume related to sodium retention.

Nursing Interventions

Also see "Care of the Patient Undergoing Adrenalectomy," page 917.
Maintaining Normal Fluid and Sodium Balance
1. Monitor fluid intake and output, daily weight, ECG changes for hypokalemia.
2. Teach low-sodium diet, administration of potassium supplements, as ordered; evaluate serum sodium and potassium results.
3. Monitor BP; administer or teach self-administration of antihypertensives, as ordered.
4. Assess for dependent edema; encourage activity, frequent repositioning, and elevation of feet periodically.

Patient Education and Health Maintenance

1. Instruct patient about the nature of illness, the necessary treatment, and the need for continued medical care after discharge.
2. Instruct patient on the importance of following prescribed medical treatments.
   a. For medical management, patient must remain on spironolactone for life.
   b. Patient should report significant adverse effects that interfere with sexual performance and quality of life.
   c. Glucocorticoid administration may be temporary after subtotal or unilateral adrenalectomy, chronic for bilateral adrenalectomy; dose may need to be increased during times of illness or stress.
3. Teach patient and family members how to take BP readings, if indicated.

Evaluation: Expected Outcomes

- Intake equals urine output, daily weight stable.

Cushing's Syndrome

Cushing's syndrome is a condition in which the plasma cortisol levels are elevated, causing signs and symptoms of hypercortisolism.

Pathophysiology and Etiology

1. Is 10 times more common in women than in men.
2. The normal feedback mechanisms that control adrenocortical function are ineffective, resulting in secretion of adrenal

cortical hormones despite adequate amounts of these hormones in the circulation.

3. The manifestations of Cushing's syndrome are the result of excess hormones (glucocorticoids).

4. Excess of one hormone or all the hormones can occur; the predominant hormone secreted in excess (usually glucocorticoids) determines the predominant symptoms.

5. Pituitary Cushing's syndrome (Cushing's disease)—hyperplasia of both adrenal glands caused by overstimulation of the adrenal cortex by ACTH, usually from a pituitary adenoma or hyperplasia.
   a. Most common cause of Cushing's syndrome.
   b. Affects mostly women between ages 20 and 40.

6. Adrenal Cushing's syndrome.
   a. Associated with tumors of the adrenal cortex—adenoma or carcinoma.

7. Ectopic.
   a. Results from autonomous ACTH secretion by extrapituitary neoplasms.
   b. Tumors elsewhere in body (such as lung) producing excess ACTH.

8. Iatrogenic Cushing's syndrome caused by exogenous glucocorticoid administration.

Clinical Manifestations

Manifestations Caused by Excess Glucocorticoids
1. Weight gain or obesity (see Figure 24-4).
2. Heavy trunk; thin extremities.
3. "Buffalo hump" (fat pad) in neck and supraclavicular area.
4. Rounded face (moon face); plethoric, oily.
5. Fragile and thin skin, striae and ecchymosis, acne.
6. Muscles wasted because of excessive catabolism.
7. Osteoporosis—characteristic kyphosis, backache.
8. Mental disturbances—mood changes, psychosis.
9. Increased susceptibility to infections.

Manifestations Caused by Excess Mineralocorticoids
1. Hypertension.
2. Hypernatremia, hypokalemia.
3. Weight gain.
4. Expanded blood volume.
5. Edema.

Manifestations Caused by Excess Androgens
1. Women experience virilism (masculinization).
   a. Hirsutism—excessive growth of hair on the face and midline of trunk.
   b. Breasts—atrophy.
   c. Clitoris—enlargement.
   d. Voice—masculine.
   e. Loss of libido.
2. If exposed in utero—possible hermaphrodite.
3. Males—loss of libido.

Diagnostic Evaluation
1. Excessive plasma cortisol levels.
2. An increase in blood glucose levels and glucose intolerance.
3. Decreased serum potassium level.

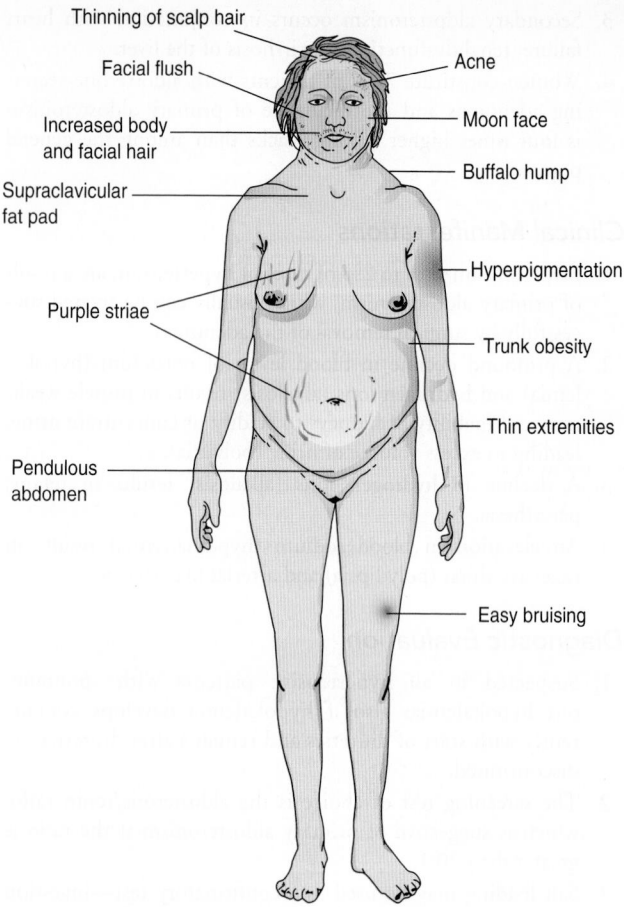

Figure 24-4. Clinical manifestations of Cushing's syndrome.

Thinning of scalp hair
Facial flush
Increased body and facial hair
Supraclavicular fat pad
Purple striae
Pendulous abdomen
Acne
Moon face
Buffalo hump
Hyperpigmentation
Trunk obesity
Thin extremities
Easy bruising

4. Reduced eosinophils.
5. Elevated urinary 17-hydroxycorticoid and 17-ketogenic steroid levels.
6. Elevation of plasma ACTH in patients with pituitary tumors.
7. Low plasma ACTH levels with adrenal tumor.
8. Loss of diurnal variation of cortisol secretion.
9. X-rays of the skull may detect erosion of the sella turcica by a pituitary tumor.
10. Overnight DST or 48-hour low-dose DST, possibly with cortisol urinary excretion measurement.
11. Elevated levels of cortisol measured in saliva are significant.
12. CT scan and ultrasonography detect location of tumor.

Management

Surgery and Radiation
Tumor (adrenal or pituitary) is removed or treated with irradiation.
1. An important development in the management of pituitary Cushing's syndrome in adults is transsphenoidal adenomectomy or hypophysectomy (pituitary removal) (see page 918).
2. Transfrontal craniotomy may be necessary when pituitary tumor has enlarged beyond sella turcica (see page 492).
3. Hyperplasia of adrenals—bilateral adrenalectomy.

Replacement Therapy Postoperatively

1. Adrenalectomy patients require lifelong replacement therapy with the following:
   a. A glucocorticoid—cortisone.
   b. A mineralocorticoid—fludrocortisone.
2. After pituitary irradiation or hypophysectomy, patient may require adrenal replacement, plus thyroid, posterior pituitary, and gonadal replacement therapy.
3. After transsphenoidal adenomectomy, patient requires hydrocortisone replacement therapy for periods of 12 to 18 months and additional hormones if excessive loss of pituitary function has occurred.
4. Protein anabolic steroids may be given to facilitate protein replacement; potassium replacement is usually required.

Medical Treatment

1. If patients cannot undergo surgery, cortisol synthesis-inhibiting medications may be used.
   a. Mitotane, an agent toxic to the adrenal cortex (dichloro-diphenyltrichloroethane derivative)—known as medical adrenalectomy. Nausea, vomiting, diarrhea, somnolence, and depression may occur with use of this drug.
   b. Metyrapone to control steroid hypersecretion in patients who do not respond to mitotane therapy.
   c. Aminoglutethimide blocks cholesterol conversion to pregnenolone, effectively blocking cortisol production. Adverse effects include GI disturbances, somnolence, and skin rashes.

Complications

Possibility of recurrence in patients with adrenal carcinoma.

Nursing Assessment

1. Observe patient for signs and symptoms of Cushing's disease.
2. Perform multisystem physical examination.
3. Monitor intake and output, daily weights, and serum electrolytes.

Nursing Diagnoses

- Impaired Skin Integrity related to altered healing, thin and fragile skin, and edema.
- Dressing, Grooming, Toileting Self-Care Deficit related to muscle wasting, osteoporosis, weakness, and fatigue.
- Disturbed Body Image related to altered physical appearance and emotional instability.
- Anxiety related to surgery.
- Risk for Injury related to surgical procedure.

Nursing Interventions

Maintaining Skin Integrity

1. Assess skin frequently to detect reddened areas, breakdown or tearing of skin, excoriation, infection, or edema.
2. Handle skin and extremities gently to prevent trauma; protect from falls by use of side rails.
3. Avoid use of adhesive tape to reduce risk of trauma to skin on its removal.
4. Encourage patient to turn in bed frequently or to ambulate to reduce pressure on bony prominences and areas of edema.
5. Use meticulous skin care to reduce injury and breakdown.
6. Provide foods low in sodium to minimize edema formation.
7. Assess intake and output and daily weight to evaluate fluid retention.

Encouraging Active Participation in Self-Care

1. Assist patient with ambulation and hygiene when weak and fatigued.
2. Assist patient in planning schedule to permit exercise and rest.
3. Encourage patient to rest when fatigued.
4. Encourage gradual resumption of activities as patient gains strength.
5. Identify for patient the signs and symptoms indicating excessive exertion.
6. Instruct patient in correct body mechanics to avoid pain or injury during activities.
7. Use assistive devices during ambulation to prevent falls and fractures.
8. Encourage foods high in potassium (bananas, orange juice, tomatoes) and administer potassium supplement, as prescribed, to counteract weakness related to hypokalemia.

Strengthening Body Image

1. Encourage patient to verbalize concerns about illness, changes in appearance, and altered role functions.
2. Identify situations that are disturbing to patient and explore with patient ways to avoid or modify those situations.
3. Be alert for evidence of depression; in some instances, this has progressed to suicide; alert health care provider of mood changes, sleep disturbance, change in activity level, change in appetite, or loss of interest in visitors or other experiences.
4. Refer for counseling, if indicated.
5. Explain to patient who has benign adenoma or hyperplasia that, with proper treatment, evidence of masculinization can be reversed.

Reducing Anxiety

1. Answer questions about surgery and encourage thorough discussion with health care provider if patient is not well informed.
2. Describe nursing care to expect in postoperative period.
3. Prepare the patient for abdominal surgery (see page 654) or hypophysectomy (see page 918) as indicated.

Providing Postoperative Care

1. Provide routine postoperative care for patient with abdominal surgery (see page 657) or hypophysectomy (see page 918).
2. Monitor closely for infection because glucocorticoid administration interferes with immune function; maintain sterile technique, clean environment, and good handwashing.
3. Monitor thyroid function tests and provide HRT, as ordered, after hypophysectomy.
4. Monitor fluid intake and output and urine-specific gravity to detect DI caused by ADH deficiency after hypophysectomy.

Patient Education and Health Maintenance

1. Instruct patient on lifetime HRT and the need to follow up at regular intervals to determine if dosage is appropriate or to detect adverse effects.
2. Instruct patient in proper skin care and in the prompt reporting of trauma or infection for medical treatment.
3. Teach patient to monitor urine or blood glucose or to report for blood glucose tests, as directed, to detect hyperglycemia.
4. Help patient prevent hyperglycemia and obesity by teaching about a low-calorie, low-concentrated carbohydrate, and low-fat diet and to increase activity, as tolerated.
5. Encourage diet high in calcium (dairy products, broccoli) and weight-bearing activity to prevent osteoporosis caused by glucocorticoid replacement.
6. Assist patient in identifying sources of information and support available in the community (see Box 24-1, page 922).

Evaluation: Expected Outcomes

- Skin intact without evidence of breakdown, excoriation, infection, or trauma.
- Participates safely in ADLs.
- Verbalizes concerns about appearance, interacts well with visitors.
- Verbalizes understanding of surgery.
- Vital signs stable, pain controlled, no signs of infection.

Adrenocortical Insufficiency

Adrenocortical insufficiency occurs with inadequate secretion of the hormones of the adrenal cortex, primarily the glucocorticoids and mineralocorticoids.

Pathophysiology and Etiology

1. Primary adrenocortical insufficiency (Addison's disease)—destruction and subsequent hypofunction of the adrenal cortex, usually caused by autoimmune process.
2. Secondary adrenocortical insufficiency—ACTH deficiency from pituitary disease or suppression of hypothalamic–pituitary axis by corticosteroid treatment for nonendocrine disorders causes atrophy of adrenal cortex.
3. Inadequate aldosterone produces disturbances of sodium, potassium, and water metabolism.
4. Cortisol deficiency produces abnormal fat, protein, and carbohydrate metabolism; no cortisol during a period of stress can precipitate addisonian crisis, an exaggerated state of adrenal cortical insufficiency, and can lead to death.

Clinical Manifestations

1. Hyponatremia and hyperkalemia.
2. Water loss, dehydration, and hypovolemia.
3. Muscular weakness, fatigue, weight loss.
4. GI problems—anorexia, nausea, vomiting, diarrhea, constipation, abdominal pain.
5. Hypotension, hypoglycemia, low basal metabolic rate, increased insulin sensitivity.
6. Mental changes—depression, irritability, anxiety, apprehension caused by hypoglycemia and hypovolemia.
7. Normal responses to stress lacking.
8. Hyperpigmentation.

Diagnostic Evaluation

1. Blood chemistry—decreased glucose and sodium; increased potassium, calcium, and BUN levels.
2. Increased lymphocytes on complete blood count.
3. Low fasting plasma cortisol levels; low aldosterone levels.
4. Twenty-four-hour urine studies—decreased 17-ketosteroid, 17- hydroxycorticoid, and 17-ketogenic steroid levels.
5. ACTH stimulation test—no rise or minimal rise in plasma cortisol and urinary 17-ketosteroid levels.

Management

1. Restoration of normal fluid and electrolyte balance: high-sodium, low-potassium diet and fluids.
2. Treatment of glucocorticoid deficiency with such agents as hydrocortisone or prednisone. Patients with chronic obstructive pulmonary disease and heart failure may require preparations with low mineralocorticoid activity, such as methylprednisolone, to prevent fluid retention.
3. Mineralocorticoid deficiency is treated with fludrocortisone.

 NURSING ALERT Overtreatment may be manifested by hypertension, edema from sodium and water retention, and weakness caused by potassium loss.

4. Cardiovascular support, if indicated.
5. Immediate treatment if addisonian (adrenal) crisis or circulatory collapse is imminent:
   a. IV sodium chloride solution to replace sodium ions.
   b. Hydrocortisone.
   c. Injection of circulatory stimulants, such as atropine sulfate, calcium chloride, epinephrine.
6. Diagnosis and treatment of underlying cause of adrenocortical insufficiency or addisonian crisis (eg, antibiotic therapy to treat infection if this is a factor in crisis).

Complications

1. Adrenal crisis—hypotension, nausea, vomiting, weakness, lethargy, and possibly coma.
2. May be precipitated by physiologic stress, such as surgery, infection, trauma, dehydration.

Nursing Assessment

1. Obtain recent or past history of corticosteroid therapy, including length of treatment, dosage, and compliance.
2. Review history for sources of stress, such as surgical procedures, infection, or development of other illness.
3. Perform thorough physical examination for manifestations of adrenocortical insufficiency or contributing factors.

Nursing Diagnoses

- Deficient Fluid Volume related to renal losses of sodium and water.
- Risk for Injury related to ineffective stress response.
- Activity Intolerance related to decreased cortisol production and fatigue.

Nursing Interventions

Achieving Normal Fluid and Electrolyte Balance

1. Assess fluid intake and output and serial daily weights.
2. Monitor vital signs frequently; a drop in BP may suggest an impending crisis.
3. Monitor results of serum sodium and potassium.
4. Assess skin turgor and mucous membranes for dehydration.
5. Encourage diet high in sodium and fluid content; administer or teach self-administration of potassium supplements, if prescribed.
6. Administer or teach self-administration of prescribed glucocorticoids and mineralocorticoids; document response.
7. Administer IV infusions of sodium, water, and glucose, as indicated.

Protecting Well-Being

1. Minimize stressful situations.
2. Protect patient from infection.
   a. Control patient's contacts so that infectious organisms are not transmitted.
   b. Protect patient from drafts, dampness, exposure to cold.
   c. Prevent overexertion.
   d. Use meticulous handwashing and sterile techniques.
3. Assess comfort and emotional status of patient.
   a. Control the temperature of the room to avoid sharp deviations in patient's temperature.
   b. Maintain a quiet, peaceful environment; avoid loud talking and noisy radios.
4. Observe and report early signs of addisonian crisis (sudden drop in BP, nausea and vomiting, fever).

Increasing Activity Tolerance

1. Assist the patient with ADLs.
2. Provide for periods of rest and activity to avoid overexertion.
3. Provide for high-calorie, high-protein diet.

Patient Education and Health Maintenance

1. Instruct patient about the necessity for long-term therapy for adrenocortical insufficiency and medical follow-up visits.
   a. Inform patient that therapy must be continued throughout his or her life.
   b. Emphasize the importance of taking more hormones when under stress.
   c. Suggest that patient carry an identification card that indicates the type of medication being taken and health care provider's telephone number.
2. Instruct patient about manifestations of excessive use of medications and reportable symptoms.
3. Identify actions to take to avoid factors that may precipitate addisonian crisis (infection, extremes of temperature, trauma).
4. Assist patient in identifying sources of information and support available in the community (see Box 24-1, page 922).

Evaluation: Expected Outcomes

- Normal skin turgor, moist mucous membranes, stable vital signs.
- No signs of infection or stress.
- Completes daily activities with minimal assistance.

Pheochromocytoma

Pheochromocytoma is a catecholamine-secreting neoplasm associated with hyperfunction of the adrenal medulla. It may appear wherever chromaffin cells are located; however, most are found in the adrenal medulla.

Pathophysiology and Etiology

1. Pheochromocytoma can occur at any age, but is most common between the ages of 30 and 60; it is uncommon in people older than age 65.
2. Most pheochromocytoma tumors are benign; 10% are malignant with metastasis.
3. Tumors located in the adrenal medulla produce both increased epinephrine and norepinephrine; those located outside the adrenal gland tend to produce epinephrine only.
4. May occur as component of multiple endocrine neoplasia IIA, an autosomal-dominant syndrome characterized by pheochromocytoma, thyroid cancer, and hyperparathyroidism.

Clinical Manifestations

1. Variation in signs and symptoms depends on the predominance of norepinephrine or epinephrine secretion and on whether secretion is continuous or intermittent.
2. Excess secretion of norepinephrine and epinephrine produces hypertension, hypermetabolism, and hyperglycemia.
3. Hypertension may be paroxysmal (intermittent) or persistent (chronic).
   a. Chronic form mimics essential hypertension; however, antihypertensives are not effective.
   b. Headaches and vision disturbances are common.
4. The hypermetabolic and hyperglycemic effects produce excessive perspiration, tremor, pallor or face flushing, nervousness, elevated blood glucose levels, polyuria, nausea, vomiting, diarrhea, abdominal pain, and paresthesia.
5. Emotional changes, including psychotic behavior, may occur.
6. Symptoms may be triggered by allergic reactions, physical exertion, emotional upset, or may occur without identifiable stimulus.

Diagnostic Evaluation

1. Metanephrine (metabolites of epinephrine and norepinephrine) are elevated in 24-hour urine specimen.
2. Epinephrine and norepinephrine in urine and blood are elevated while patient is symptomatic.
3. CT scan and magnetic resonance imaging (MRI) of the adrenal glands or of the entire abdomen are done to identify tumor.

Management

Medical Control of BP and Preparation for Surgery

1. Alpha-adrenergic blocking agents, such as phentolamine or phenoxybenzamine, inhibit the effects of catecholamines on BP.
   a. Effective control of BP and blood volume may take 1 or 2 weeks.
   b. Surgery is delayed until BP is controlled and blood volume has been expanded.
2. Catecholamine synthesis inhibitors, such as metyrosine, may be used preoperatively or for long-term management of inoperable tumors.
   a. Adverse effects include sedation and crystalluria.

Surgery

Unilateral or bilateral adrenalectomy or other tumor removal.

Complications

Metastasis of tumor.

Nursing Assessment

1. Obtain history of signs and symptoms patient has been experiencing.
2. Assess for predisposing factors that may be triggering signs and symptoms (ie, physical exertion, emotional upset, allergies).
3. Perform thorough physical examination to determine effects of hypertension.

Nursing Diagnoses

- Anxiety related to the systemic effects of epinephrine and norepinephrine.
- Ineffective Tissue Perfusion related to hypotension during the postoperative period.

Nursing Interventions

Reducing Anxiety

1. Remain with patient during acute episodes of hypertension.
2. Ensure bed rest and elevate the head of bed 45 degrees during severe hypertension.
3. Carry out tasks and procedures in calm, unhurried manner when with patient.
4. Instruct patient about use of relaxation exercises.
5. Reduce environmental stressors by providing calm, quiet environment. Restrict visitors.
6. Eliminate stimulants (coffee, tea, cola) from the diet.
7. Reduce events that precipitate episodes of severe hypertension—palpation of the tumor, physical exertion, emotional upset.
8. Administer sedatives, as prescribed, to promote relaxation and rest.
9. Monitor for orthostatic hypotension after administration of phentolamine.
10. Encourage oral fluids and maintain IV infusion preoperatively to ensure adequate volume expansion going into surgery.

Maintaining Tissue Perfusion Postoperatively

1. Monitor vital signs, ECG, arterial BP, neurologic status, and urine output closely postoperatively.
2. Assess for and report complications of hypertension, hypotension, and hyperglycemia.
3. Maintain adequate hydration with IV infusion to prevent hypotension. (Because reduction of catecholamines immediately postoperatively causes vasodilation and enlargement of vascular space, hypotension may occur.)
4. Monitor intake and output and laboratory results for BUN, creatinine, and glucose levels.

Patient Education and Health Maintenance

1. Instruct patient how and when to take medications. Warn patients who take metyrosine of sedation and need to avoid taking other CNS depressants and participating in activities that require alertness; need to increase fluid intake to at least 2,000 mL/day to prevent renal calculi.
2. Inform patient regarding the need for continued follow-up for:
   a. Recurrence of pheochromocytoma.
   b. Assessment of any residual renal or cardiovascular injury related to preoperative hypertension.
   c. Documentation that catecholamine levels are normal 1 to 3 months postoperatively (by 24-hour urine test).
3. Help patient identify sources of information and support available in the community (see Box 24-1, page 922).

Evaluation: Expected Outcomes

- Reports less anxiety during hypertensive episodes.
- BP stable, adequate urine output.

DISORDERS OF THE PITUITARY GLAND

The pituitary gland (hypophysis) exerts prime control over the body's hormonal functions. It is located in the sella turcica at the base of the brain. Its function is regulated by the hypothalamus. The pituitary consists of two parts that are structurally and functionally separate: the anterior pituitary and the posterior pituitary. Hypothalamic control of the anterior pituitary is mediated by releasing factors secreted by the hypothalamus; the posterior pituitary is regulated through direct neural stimulation. See Table 24-2 for hormones of the pituitary gland.

Diabetes Insipidus

Diabetes insipidus (DI) is a disorder of water metabolism caused by deficiency of ADH, also called vasopressin, secreted by the posterior pituitary or by inability of the kidneys to respond to ADH (nephrogenic DI).

Pathophysiology and Etiology

1. Primary: idiopathic.
2. Secondary: head trauma, neurosurgery, tumors (intracranial or metastatic), vascular disease (aneurysms, infarct), infection (meningitis, encephalitis).

Table 24-2	Hormones of the Pituitary Gland
HORMONE	**TARGET TISSUE**
Anterior Pituitary	
Growth hormone	Multiple sites
Thyroid-stimulating hormone	Thyroid gland
Adrenocorticotropic hormone	Adrenal glands
Prolactin	Breasts
Luteinizing hormone	Ovaries, testes
Follicle-stimulating hormone	Ovaries, testes
Melanocyte-stimulating hormone	Melanocytes (skin)
Posterior Pituitary	
Oxytocin	Uterus, breasts
Antidiuretic hormone	Kidneys

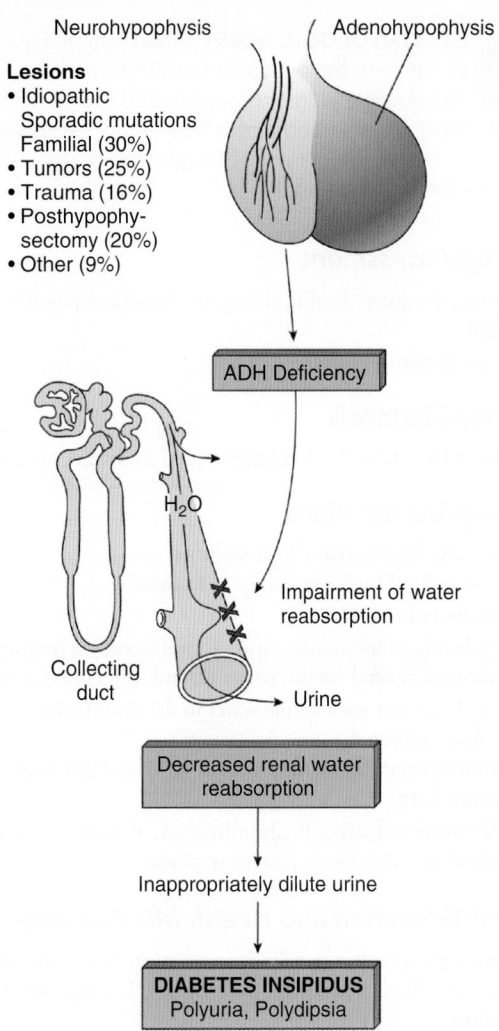

Figure 24-5. The mechanisms of diabetes insipidus.

3. Nephrogenic DI: long-standing renal disease, hypokalemia, some medications.
4. Deficiency of ADH results in decreased renal water reabsorption; it may be partial or complete (see Figure 24-5).
5. DI may be transient or permanent.

Clinical Manifestations

1. Marked polyuria—daily output of 5 to 20 L of dilute urine; appearance of urine like that of water, with a specific gravity of 1.000 to 1.005, corresponding to a urine osmolality of 50 to 200 mOsm/kg.
2. Polydipsia (intense thirst)—drinks 4 to 40 L of fluid daily; has craving for cold water.
3. High serum osmolality (above 295 mOsm) and high serum sodium level (greater than 145 mEq/L).

Diagnostic Evaluation

1. Serum osmolality—high; urine osmolality—low.
2. Water deprivation test determines central and nephrogenic DI.
3. Measurements of serum and urine ADH—decreased to absent.

Management

1. Administration of ADH or its derivative.
   a. DDAVP—vasopressin derivative administered intravenously, into the nose through a soft, flexible nasal tube, by nasal spray, or orally in tablet form. Potency varies by form of preparation (eg, IV form almost 10 times more potent than nasal spray).
      i. Duration of action 8 to 12 hours.
      ii. For patients who have some residual hypothalamic ADH (determined by low levels of circulating ADH).
      iii. Dosage may be reduced in older adults and in individuals with renal impairment.
   b. Chlorpropamide—potentiates action of vasopressin on renal-concentrating mechanism.
   c. Tricyclic antidepressants and selective serotonin reuptake inhibitor antidepressants may potentiate the action of DDAVP.
   d. Carbamazepine—potentiates action of endogenous vasopressin.
2. For patients with nephrogenic DI—chlorpropamide or thiazide diuretics may be of value. Reversible by discontinuing causative medication if cause is drug related.

Complications

1. If untreated, may result in death.
2. Overtreatment of DDAVP may cause hyponatremia and water intoxication.

GERONTOLOGIC ALERT Older patients are more sensitive to the effects of DDAVP, so make sure that overdosage does not occur and watch for early signs of hyponatremia and water intoxication—drowsiness, confusion, headache, anuria, weight gain—to prevent seizures, coma, and death.

Nursing Assessment

1. Obtain complete health history to determine possible cause of DI.
2. Assess hydration status.

Nursing Diagnosis

- Risk for Deficient Fluid Volume related to disease process.

Nursing Interventions

Maintaining Adequate Fluid Volume

1. Measure fluid intake and output accurately.
2. Obtain daily weights.
3. Monitor hemodynamic status, as indicated, via frequent BP, heart rate, central venous pressure, and other measurements.
4. Provide patient with ample water to drink and administer IV fluids as indicated.
5. Monitor results of serum and urine osmolality and serum sodium tests.
6. Administer or teach self-administration of medication, as prescribed, and document patient response.

Patient Education and Health Maintenance

1. Inform patient that metabolic status must be monitored on a long-term basis because the severity of DI changes from time to time.
2. Advise patient to avoid limiting fluids to decrease urine output; thirst is a protective function.
3. Advise patient to wear a MedicAlert bracelet stating that the wearer has DI.
4. Teach patient to be alert for signs of dehydration—decreased weight, decreased urine output, increased thirst, dry skin and mucous membranes; and overhydration—increased weight and edema; report these to the health care provider.
5. Tell patient to consider eliminating coffee and tea from diet—may have an exaggerated diuretic effect.
6. Give written instruction on vasopressin administration. Have patient demonstrate intranasal and injection technique.

Evaluation: Expected Outcomes

- Fluid intake equals output, weight stable.

Pituitary Tumors

Pituitary tumors represent various cell types. Symptoms reflect tumor effects on target tissues or on local structures surrounding the pituitary gland.

Pathophysiology and Etiology

1. The cause of pituitary tumors is unknown.
2. Typically, pituitary tumors are characterized by size and by what hormones, if any, are secreted.
   a. Size.
      i. Microadenoma—less than 10 mm wide.
      ii. Macroadenoma—greater than 10 mm wide.
   b. Functional status.
      i. Hormone secreting—exaggerated hormone activity; may secrete multiple hormones.
      ii. Nonsecreting—usually diminished hormone activity.
3. Malignancy in pituitary tumors is rare.

Clinical Manifestations

1. Mass effects—effects of tumor on surrounding structures.
   a. Headache.
   b. Nausea and vomiting (in some cases).
   c. Impairment of cranial nerves II, III, IV, and VI on testing because of bilateral hemianopsia, which results from pressure on the optic chiasm.
   d. Vision disturbances, such as visual field defects and diplopia.
2. Endocrine effects—effects of hormone imbalances caused by tumor (see Table 24-3).

Table 24-3	Clinical Manifestations Associated with Hormone Effects of Pituitary Tumors	
HORMONE	**HYPERPITUITARISM (INCREASED SECRETION)**	**HYPOPITUITARISM (DIMINISHED SECRETION)**
Growth hormone	• Gigantism (child) • Acromegaly (adult)	• Shortness of stature (child) • Silent (adult)
Prolactin	• Infertility and galactorrhea (female)	• Postpartum lactation failure
Adrenocorticotropic hormone	• Cushing's disease	• Adrenocortical insufficiency
Thyroid-stimulating hormone	• Hyperthyroidism	• Hypothyroidism
Luteinizing hormone and follicle-stimulating hormone	• Gonadal dysfunction	• Hypogonadism

Diagnostic Evaluation

1. Skull films (usually normal).
2. MRI using sella protocol shows mass.
3. Serum hormone levels to identify suspected abnormalities based on clinical evaluation.
4. Provocative testing to detect hormone secretion abnormalities of the pituitary, such as glucose tolerance test and DST.

Management

Hypophysectomy Removal of Pituitary

1. Considered first line of treatment for pituitary adenomas.
2. Transsphenoidal hypophysectomy—direct approach through the sinus and nasal cavity to sella turcica (see page xxx).
3. Frontal craniotomy—uncommon approach except where tumor occupies broad area (see page 492).

Other Methods of Pituitary Ablation

1. Cryogenic destruction or stereotaxic radiofrequency coagulation (may be used in conjunction with surgery or drug therapy).
2. Radiation therapy.
3. Drug therapy.
   a. Bromocriptine for prolactinomas and, in some instances, GH-secreting tumors is given daily.
   b. Cabergoline, a dopamine agonist, is administered twice per week for the treatment of acromegaly.
   c. Somatostatin analogues (octreotide, lanreotide) used in the treatment of acromegaly.
   d. GH antagonist (pegvisomant) used in the treatment of acromegaly.
   e. HRT for hypopituitarism.

Complications

1. Hypothyroidism and adrenocortical insufficiency after ablation, requiring hormone replacement.
2. Menstruation ceases and infertility occurs almost always after total or nearly total ablation.
3. Transient or permanent DI after surgery.
4. Without treatment—death or severe disability caused by stroke, blindness, or imbalances of ACTH, TSH, or ADH.

Nursing Assessment

1. Obtain history of signs and symptoms.
2. Perform thorough neurologic examination and general physical examination to identify signs of hormone deficiency or excess.
3. Assess patient's understanding of the management plan, coping with the diagnosis, and support from others.

Nursing Diagnoses

- Anxiety related to ablation treatment.
- Readiness for Enhanced Management of Therapeutic Regimen.

Nursing Interventions

Also see "Care of the Patient Undergoing Transsphenoidal Hypophysectomy," page 918.

Reducing Anxiety

1. Provide emotional support through the diagnostic process and answer questions about treatment options.
2. Prepare patient for surgery or other treatment by describing nursing care thoroughly.
3. Stress likelihood of positive outcome with ablation therapy.

Promoting Management of the Therapeutic Regimen

1. Teach patient the nature of hormonal deficiencies after treatment and the purpose of replacement therapy.
2. Instruct patient about the early signs and symptoms of cortisol or thyroid hormone deficiency or excess and the need to report them.
3. Describe and demonstrate the correct method of administering prescribed medications.
4. Encourage patient in assuming active role in self-care through information seeking and problem solving.

Patient Education and Health Maintenance

1. Advise patient on temporary limitations in activities.
2. Teach patient the need for frequent initial follow-up visits and lifelong medical management when on hormonal therapy.
3. If applicable, advise patient on the need for postsurgery radiation therapy and periodic follow-up MRI and visual field testing.
4. Teach patient to notify health care provider if signs of thyroid or cortisol imbalance become evident.
5. Advise patient to wear MedicAlert bracelet.
6. Help patient identify sources of information and support available in the community (see Box 24-1, page 922).

Evaluation: Expected Outcomes

- States rationale for treatment, asks appropriate questions.
- Demonstrates correct medication administration.

SELECTED REFERENCES

American Thyroid Association and American Association of Clinical Endocrinologists Taskforce on Hyperthyroidism and Other Causes of Thyrotoxicosis. (2011). Hyperthyroidism and other causes of thyrotoxicosis: Management guidelines of the American Thyroid Association and American Association of Clinical Endocrinologists. *Thyroid, 121*(6), 593–646.

American Thyroid Association Guidelines Task Force on Thyroid Nodules and Differentiated Thyroid Cancer. (2009). Revised American Thyroid Association Management guidelines for patients with thyroid nodules and differentiated thyroid cancer. *Thyroid, 19*(11), 1167–1214.

Alexander, E. L., Rothrock, J. C., & McEwen, D. R. (Eds.). (2011). *Alexander's care of the patient in surgery* (14th ed.). St. Louis, MO: Mosby/Elsevier.

Axelrod, L. (2010). Glucocorticoid therapy. In L. J. DeGroot, J. L. Jameson, et al. (Eds.), *Endocrinology* (6th ed.). Philadelphia: W.B. Saunders; pp. 1493–1511.

Blum, M. (2010). Thyroid imaging. In L. J. DeGroot, J. L. Jameson, et al. (Eds.), *Endocrinology* (6th ed.). Philadelphia: W.B. Saunders.

Burton, J. (2012). Primary hypothyroidism. *Medical Surgical Nursing, 21*(3), 169–170.

Cappabianca, P., Cavallo, L., & DeDevitiis, O. (2010). Pituitary surgery. In L. J. DeGroot, J. L. Jameson, et al. (Eds.), *Endocrinology* (6th ed.). Philadelphia: W.B. Saunders; pp. 358–376.

Chen, H., Sippel, R. S., O'Dorisio, M.S., et al. (2010). The North American Neuroendocrine Tumor Society consensus guideline for the diagnosis and management of neuroendocrine tumors: Pheochromocytoma, paraganglioma, and medullary thyroid cancer. *Pancreas, 39*(6), 775–783.

Chung, T., Grossman, A., & Clark, A.J., (2010). Adrenal insufficiency. In L. J. DeGroot, J. L. Jameson, et al. (Eds.), *Endocrinology* (6th ed.). Philadelphia: W.B. Saunders; pp. 1853–1863.

Crawford, A., Harris, H. (2012). Adrenal cortex disorders: hormones out of kilter. *Nursing, 42*(10), 32–38.

Daniels, R., & Nicoll, L. (Eds.). (2012). *Contemporary medical-surgical nursing* (2nd ed.). Clifton Park, NY: Delmar/Cengage Learning.

Gharib, H., Papini, E., & Paschke, R. (2010). American Association of Clinical Endocrinologists, Associazione Medici Endocrinologi, and European Thyroid Association medical guide lines for clinical practice for the diagnosis and management of thyroid nodules. *Endocrine Practice, 16*(Suppl. 1), 1–43.

Guimares, V. (2010). Subacute and Reidel's thyroiditis. In L. J. DeGroot, J. L. Jameson, et al. (Eds.), *Endocrinology* (6th ed) Philadelphia: W.B. Saunders; pp. 1595–1606.

Ignatavicius, D. D., & Workman, M. L. (Eds.). (2010). *Medical surgical nursing: Patient centered collaborative care* (6th ed). St. Louis, MO: Saunders.

Kapustin, J. F. (2010). Hypothyroidism: An evidence-based approach to a complex disorder. *Nurse Practitioner, 35*(8), 44–53.

Kapustin, J. F., Schofield, D. L. (2012). Hyperparathyroidism: an incidental finding. *Nurse Practitioner, 37*(11), 9–11.

Katznelson, L., Atkinson, J. L., Cook, D. M., et al. (2011). American Association of Clinical Endocrinologists medical guidelines for clinical practice for the diagnosis and treatment of acromegaly—2011 update. *Endocrine Practice, 17*(Suppl. 4), 1–44.

Kee, J. L., Hayes, E. R., & McCuistan, L. E. (Eds.). (2012). *Pharmacology: A nursing process approach* (7th ed.). St. Louis, MO: Elsevier Saunders.

Khan, M. I., Waguespack, S. G., & Hu, M. I. (2011). Medical management of postsurgical hypoparathyroidism. *Endocrine Practice, 17*(Suppl. 1), 18–25.

Laws, E. R., & Lanzino, G. (2010). *Transsphenoidal surgery*. Philadelphia: Saunders.

Lazarus, J. L. (2010). Chronic (Hashimoto's) thyroiditis. In L. J. DeGroot, J. L. Jameson, et al. (Eds.), *Endocrinology* (6th ed.). Philadelphia: W.B. Saunders; pp. 1583–1594.

LeMone, P., Burke, K., & Bauldoff, G. (Eds.). (2011). *Medical-surgical nursing: Critical thinking in patient care* (5th ed.). Upper Saddle River, NJ: Pearson.

Lewis, S. L., Dirksen, S. R., Heitkemper, M. M., et al. (Eds.). (2011). *Medical surgical nursing: Assessment and management of clinical problems* (8th ed.). St. Louis, MO: Elsevier/Mosby.

Mertens, L., & Bogaert, J. (2010). *Handbook of hyperthyroidism: Etiology, diagnosis, and treatment*. New York: Nova Science.

Monahan, F. D., Neighbors, M., & Green, C. J. (Eds.). (2011). *Swearingen's manual of medical-surgical nursing* (7th ed.). Maryland Heights, MO: Mosby.

Morris, D. G., Crossman, A., & Nieman, L. K. (2010). Cushings syndrome. In L. J. DeGroot, J. L. Jameson, et al. (Eds.), *Endocrinology* (6th ed.). Philadelphia: W.B. Saunders; pp. 282–311.

Osborn, K. S., Wraa, C. E., & Watson, A. B. (Eds.). (2010). *Medical surgical nursing: Preparation for practice*. Boston: Pearson.

Nakamoto, J., Salameh, W. A., & Carlton, E. (2010). Endocrine testing. In L. J. DeGroot, J. L. Jameson, et al. (Eds.), *Endocrinology* (6th ed.). Philadelphia: W.B. Saunders; pp. 2801–2834.

Rosig, J. H., & Norton, J. A. (2010). Surgical management of hyperparathyroidism. In L. J. DeGroot, J. L. Jameson, et al. (Eds.), *Endocrinology* (6th ed.). Philadelphia: W.B. Saunders; pp. 1212–1222.

Silverberg, S. J., & Bilezikian, J. P. (2010). Primary hyperparathyroidism. In L. J. DeGroot, J. L. Jameson, et al. (Eds.), *Endocrinology* (6th ed.). Philadelphia: W.B. Saunders; pp. 1176–1197.

Stowasser, M., Taylor, P. J., Pimenta, E., et al. (2010). Laboratory investigation of primary aldosteronism. *Clinical Biochemist Reviews, 31*(2), 39–56.

Weiss, R. E., & Reftoff, S. (2010). Thyroid function testing. In L. J. DeGroot, J. L. Jameson, et al. (Eds.) *Endocrinology* (6th ed.). Philadelphia: W.B. Saunders; pp. 1444–1492.

Wiersinga, W. M. (2010). Hypothyroidism and myxedema coma. In L. J. DeGroot, J. L. Jameson, et al. (Eds.), *Endocrinology* (6th ed.). Philadelphia: W.B. Saunders; pp. 1607–1622.

Woodhouse, K. N. (2012). Thyrotoxicosis: evaluation and treatment of a multinodualr goiter. *Nurse Practitioner, 37*(7), 6–10.

25
Diabetes Mellitus and Related Disorders

OVERVIEW AND ASSESSMENT

Evidence Base Centers for Disease Control and Prevention (CDC). (2011). National diabetes fact sheet: National estimates and general information on diabetes and prediabetes in the United States, 2011. Available: *www.cdc.gov/diabetes/pubs/pdf/ndfs_2011.pdf.*

In 2010, diabetes mellitus was estimated to affect almost 26 million Americans. This is more than 8% of the U.S. population. Unfortunately, this number is expected to double, if not triple, by 2050.

It is thought that the factors contributing to the explosion of diabetes are an aging population, increased prevalence of type 2 diabetes mellitus in youth, growing numbers of ethnic minorities, and the increasing trend of obesity (>65% of American adults are overweight or obese).

The cost of caring for people with diabetes is staggering. In 2007, the United States spent $174 billion on diabetes care alone. This is two to three times more than the health care costs of those without diabetes. By 2030, it is estimated that the United States will spend more than $333 billion on diabetes mellitus.

Diabetes mellitus is the leading cause of blindness, kidney failure, and lower limb amputations. People with diabetes are two to four times more likely to be diagnosed with heart disease, three times more likely to have dental disease, and twice as more likely to suffer from depression.

This is a very serious disease with even more serious consequences. All nurses must stay current on the latest care recommendations. Screening for this disease is essential because early treatment leads to a reduction of morbidity and mortality.

Insulin Secretion and Function

1. Insulin is a hormone secreted by the beta cells of the islet of Langerhans in the pancreas.
2. Small amounts of insulin are released into the bloodstream in response to changes in blood glucose levels throughout the day (basal secretion).
3. Increased secretion or a bolus of insulin, released during meals, helps maintain euglycemia.
4. Through an internal feedback mechanism that involves the pancreas and the liver, circulating blood glucose levels are maintained at a normal range of 60 to 100 mg/dL.
5. Insulin is essential for the utilization of glucose for cellular metabolism as well as for the proper metabolism of protein and fat.
   a. Carbohydrate metabolism—insulin affects the conversion of glucose into glycogen for storage in the liver and skeletal muscles, and allows for the immediate release and utilization of glucose by the cells.
   b. Protein metabolism—amino acid conversion occurs in the presence of insulin to replace muscle tissue or to provide needed glucose (gluconeogenesis).

c. Fat metabolism—storage of fat in adipose tissue and conversion of fatty acids from excess glucose occurs only in the presence of insulin.

6. Glucose can be used in the endothelial and nerve cells without the aid of insulin.

7. Without insulin, plasma glucose concentration rises and glycosuria results.

   a. Absolute deficits in insulin result from decreased production of endogenous insulin by the beta cell of the pancreas.

   b. Relative deficits in insulin are caused by inadequate utilization of insulin by the cell.

Classification of Diabetes

 Evidence Base American Association of Clinical Endocrinologists (AACE). (2011). Medical guidelines for clinical practice for developing a diabetes mellitus comprehensive care plan. *Endocrine Practice, 17*(Suppl. 2), 1–53.

American Diabetes Association (ADA). (2013). Standards of medical care in diabetes (position statement). *Diabetes Care, 36*(Suppl. 1), S11–S66.

Type 1 Diabetes Mellitus

Type 1 diabetes mellitus (T1DM) was formerly known as insulin-dependent diabetes mellitus and juvenile diabetes mellitus.

1. Little or no endogenous insulin, requiring injections of insulin to control diabetes, prevent ketoacidosis and sustain life.

2. Only 5% to 10% of all people with diabetes have T1DM.

3. Etiology is not well understood: includes autoimmune, viral, and certain histocompatibility antigens as well as genetic components.

4. Clinical manifestation is abrupt with classic symptoms of polydipsia, polyphagia, polyuria, and weight loss.

5. Most commonly seen in patients under age 30 but can be seen in older adults.

Type 2 Diabetes Mellitus

Type 2 diabetes mellitus (T2DM) was formerly known as non-insulin-dependent diabetes mellitus or adult-onset diabetes mellitus.

1. Caused by a combination of insulin resistance and relative insulin deficiency—some individuals have predominantly insulin resistance, whereas others have predominantly deficient insulin secretion, with little insulin resistance.

2. Approximately 90% to 95% of people with diabetes have T2DM.

3. Etiology: strong hereditary component, commonly associated with obesity.

4. Usual presentation is slow and typically insidious with symptoms of fatigue, weight loss, poor wound healing, and recurrent infection.

5. Found primarily in adults over age 30; however, it is now more frequently seen in younger adults and adolescents who are overweight.

6. People with this type of diabetes may be treated with insulin, but are still referred to as having T2DM.

Gestational Diabetes Mellitus

Gestational diabetes mellitus (GDM) is defined as the onset of carbohydrate intolerance that initially presents during pregnancy and resolves upon delivery.

1. Affects approximately 2% to 10% of pregnancies; however, the new diagnostic criteria may yield that as many as 18% of pregnancies are affected by GDM.

2. Women with GDM have a 35% to 60% chance of developing T2DM diabetes in the next 10 to 20 years. They should be screened for diabetes 6 to 12 weeks postpartum and continue to have lifelong screening at least every 3 years.

3. GDM is associated with significant risk of maternal and fetal complications.

4. Due to the worldwide increases of both obesity and diabetes rates, the American Diabetes Association (ADA) made the recommendation that all pregnant women should be screened for the presence of T2DM at the initial prenatal visit using the standard diagnostic criteria (2011). Women who are negative for T2DM at that time should then be screened for GDM at 24 to 28 weeks of gestation.

5. Screening for GDM is done using a 75-g 2-hour oral glucose tolerance test (2-h OGTT).

6. The American College of Obstetricians and Gynecologists (ACOG) issued a Committee statement asserting that they have not yet adopted the new diagnostic criteria for gestational diabetes (as listed on page 944) and will continue to use the diagnostic criteria established by either Carpenter and Coustan or the National Diabetes Data Group. Both of these screening methods utilize a 100-g 3-h OGTT, require two abnormal results and the threshold for these results is higher than the newer criteria.

Diabetes Due to Other Causes

1. Genetic defects of insulin secretion and/or insulin action.

2. Pancreatic diseases (such as cystic fibrosis, pancreatitis, and pheochromocytoma).

3. Drug-induced (such as corticosteroids and medications used to treat HIV/AIDS).

Prediabetes

1. *Prediabetes* is an abnormality in glucose values intermediate between normal and overt diabetes.

2. Associated with obesity, dyslipidemia, and hypertension; prediabetes is a potent risk factor for developing T2DM and cardiovascular disease.

3. Every effort should be made to assist the patient with aggressive lifestyle modifications (diet, exercise, and weight loss) to prevent the progression from prediabetes to overt T2DM.

4. There are two forms of prediabetes, based on when glucose is elevated. Patients that simultaneously have both forms of prediabetes have a very high risk of developing T2DM.

   a. Impaired fasting glucose (IFG)—defined as having fasting blood glucose levels of 100 to 125 mg/dL.

   b. Impaired glucose tolerance (IGT)—defined as blood glucose measurement of 140 to 199 mg/dL using a 2-hour OGTT.

Laboratory Tests

 Evidence Base American Association of Clinical Endocrinologists (AACE). (2011). Medical guidelines for clinical practice for developing a diabetes mellitus comprehensive care plan. *Endocrine Practice, 17*(Suppl. 2), 1–53.

American Diabetes Association (ADA). (2013). Standards of medical care in diabetes (position statement). *Diabetes Care, 36*(Suppl. 1), S11–S66.

Global International Diabetes Federation (IDF)/International Society of Pediatric and Adolescent Diabetes (ISPAD). (2011). Guideline for diabetes in childhood and adolescence. Available: *www.ispad.org/NewsFiles/IDF-ISPAD_Diabetes_in_Childhood_and%20Adolescence_Guidelines_2011.pdf.*

Laboratory tests include those tests used to make the diagnosis as well as measures to monitor short- and long-term glucose control. See Box 25-1 for details of when and how often to screen adults, adolescents, and children for T2DM.

BOX 25-1	Risk Factors and Screening for Type 2 Diabetes

ADULTS

Begin screening at any age if overweight (BMI ≥ 25 kg/m²) *plus* any *one* of the following risk factors; otherwise begin screening all adults at age 45.

Screening should occur at least every 3 years.

- Family history of diabetes (first-degree relative).
- Sedentary lifestyle/habitual inactivity.
- Race/ethnicity (ie, black, Hispanic American, Native American, Alaskan American, and Pacific Islander).
- Diagnosis of prediabetes (IFG or IGT or A1C ≥ 5.7%).
- Prior history of GDM or baby weighing >9 lbs at birth.
- HTN ≥ 140/90 mm Hg.
- HDL cholesterol < 35 mg/dL and/or triglyceride level >250 mg/dL.
- History of insulin resistance (ie, polycystic ovary disease, acanthosis nigricans).
- History of cardiovascular disease.

CHILDREN

Begin screening at age 10 or onset of puberty (whichever first) and continuing at least every 3 years if:

Overweight (BMI > 85th percentile for age, gender OR weight for height > 85th percentile, OR weight > 120% of ideal height) *plus* any *two* of the following risk factors:

- Family history of type 2 diabetes in first- or second-degree relative.
- Race/ethnicity (ie, Native American, black, Latino, Asian American, Pacific Islander).
- Signs of insulin resistance or conditions associated with insulin resistance (ie, acanthosis nigricans, hypertension, dyslipidemia, or PCOS).
- Maternal history of T2DM or GDM during child's gestation.

Blood Glucose

Description

1. Fasting blood sugar (FBS), drawn after at least an 8-hour fast, to evaluate circulating amounts of glucose.
2. Postprandial test, drawn usually 2 hours after a well-balanced meal, to evaluate glucose metabolism.
3. Random glucose, drawn at any time, without regard to the time of last caloric intake.

Nursing and Patient Care Considerations

1. For fasting glucose, make sure that patient has maintained 8-hour fast overnight; sips of water are allowed.
2. Advise patient to refrain from smoking before the glucose sampling because this affects the test results.
3. For postprandial glucose, advise patient that no additional food or caloric beverages should be consumed during the 2-hour interval.
4. For random blood glucose, note the time and content of the last meal.

Diagnostic Criteria and Treatment Goals for Blood Glucose Values

1. American Diabetes Association (ADA) and American Association of Clinical Endocrinologists (AACE) diagnostic blood glucose values for diabetes mellitus in children, adolescents, and nonpregnant adults are:
   a. FBS greater than or equal to 126 mg/dL, confirmed with a repeat test on another day.
   b. Random blood sugar (regardless of time of last caloric intake) 200 mg/dL or higher *and* presence of classic symptoms of diabetes (polyuria, polydipsia, polyphagia, and weight loss). This test does not need to be repeated nor does the diagnosis need to be confirmed with another test.
   c. Fasting blood glucose result of 100 to 125 mg/dL is prediabetes (IFG) and demands close follow-up and repeat monitoring at least every 3 years.
2. Blood glucose treatment goals for many nonpregnant adults with diabetes mellitus:
   a. Premeal: 70 to 130 mg/dl (ADA) or <110 mg/dL (AACE).
   b. 1 to 2 hours postmeal: less than 180 mg/dL (ADA) or <140 mg/dL (AACE).
3. The International Diabetes Federation (IDF)/International Society of Pediatric and Adolescent Diabetes (ISPAD) blood glucose treatment goals for children and adolescents:
   a. Premeal: 90 to 145 mg/dL.
   b. Postmeal: 90 to 180 mg/dL.
   c. Bedtime: 120 to 180 mg/dL.
4. ADA and AACE blood glucose treatment goals for women with gestational diabetes:
   a. Premeal: 95 mg/dL or lower.
   b. 1 hour postmeal: 140 mg/dL or lower.
   c. 2 hours postmeal: 120 mg/dL or lower.
5. ADA and AACE blood glucose treatment goals for pregnant women with preexisting diabetes:
   a. Premeal, bedtime: 60 to 99 mg/dL.
   b. 1 hour postmeal: 100 to 129 mg/dL.

NURSING ALERT Capillary blood glucose values obtained by fingerstick samples tend to be higher than values in venous samples. Diagnostic tests are always to be conducted in a laboratory using venous samples.

Oral Glucose Tolerance Test

Description

The *oral glucose tolerance test (OGTT)* evaluates insulin response to glucose loading. FBS is obtained before the ingestion of a glucose load and blood samples are drawn at timed intervals.

Nursing and Patient Care Considerations

1. Advise patient that for accuracy in results, certain instructions must be followed:
   a. Usual diet and exercise pattern must be followed for 3 days before OGTT.
   b. During OGTT, patient must refrain from smoking and remain seated.
   c. Hormonal contraceptives, salicylates, diuretics, phenytoin, and nicotinic acid can impair results and may be withheld before testing based on the advice of the health care provider.

Diagnostic Criteria Using the 75-g 2-h OGTT

1. ADA and AACE diagnostic OGTT values when screening for diabetes mellitus in children, adolescents, and nonpregnant adults:
   a. 200 mg/dL or higher at the 2-hour interval.
   b. 140 to 199 mg/dL at the 2-hour interval is prediabetes (IGT) and demands close follow-up and repeat monitoring at least every 3 years.
2. ADA and AACE diagnostic blood glucose values for gestational diabetes performed 24 to 28 weeks gestation: (only need to meet the limits of *one* of the following values):
   a. Fasting of 92 mg/dL or higher, or
   b. 180 mg/dL or higher at the 1-hour interval, or
   c. 153 mg/dL or higher at the 2-hour interval.

Glycated Hemoglobin (Glycohemoglobin, HbA$_{1c}$, A1c)

Description

Measures glycemic control over a 60- to 120-day period by measuring the irreversible reaction of glucose to hemoglobin through freely permeable erythrocytes during their 120-day life cycle. Currently used to screen for diabetes as well as to monitor control.

Nursing and Patient Care Considerations

1. No prior preparation, such as fasting or withholding insulin/medications, is necessary.
2. Test results can be affected by red blood cell disorders (eg, thalassemia, sickle cell anemia), room temperature, ionic charges, and ambient blood glucose values.
3. Many methods exist for performing the test, making it necessary to consult the laboratory for normal values.
4. Should be performed at least twice yearly in patients whose diabetes is stable and well controlled. Quarterly (every 3 months)

testing is recommended for patients who have had treatment changes/adjustments or whose diabetes is not well controlled.

Diagnostic Criteria and Treatment Goals for A1c Values

1. ADA and AACE diagnostic A1c values when screening for diabetes mellitus in children, adolescents, and nonpregnant adults:
   a. 6.5% or higher (should be confirmed with repeat A1c or fasting glucose or OGTT).
   b. 5.7% to 6.4% (ADA) or 5.5% to 6.4% (AACE) is considered prediabetes and demands close follow-up and repeat monitoring at least every 3 years.
2. The joint position statement (2009) of the ADA, the American College of Cardiology Foundation, and the American Heart Association asserts that in general, the A1c goal for nonpregnant adults is less than 7%, but that this must be individualized based on life expectancy, duration of diabetes, history of hypoglycemia, presence of microvascular complications, and presence of cardiovascular disease.
3. The IDF/ISPAD treatment A1c goal for children is between 7.5% and less than 9% based on age and ability to detect hypoglycemia.
4. The ADA and AACE treatment A1c goal of pregnant women with preexisting type 1 or type 2 diabetes is less than 6% (if without excessive hypoglycemia).
5. Because GDM is diagnosed late in pregnancy, the A1c is not a reliable marker of control (3-month average) and the fructosamine value (2- to 3-week average) may be more meaningful.

Fructosamine Assay

Description

Glycated protein with a much shorter half-life than glycated hemoglobin, reflecting control over a shorter period, approximately 14 to 21 days. May be advantageous in patients with hemoglobin variants that interfere with the accuracy of glycated hemoglobin tests.

Nursing and Patient Care Considerations

1. Note if patient has hypoalbuminemia or elevated globulins because test may not be reliable.
2. Should not be used as a diagnostic test for diabetes mellitus.
3. No special preparation or fasting is necessary.

C-Peptide Assay (Connecting Peptide Assay)

Description

Cleaved from the proinsulin molecule during its conversion to insulin, C-peptide acts as a marker for endogenous insulin production.

Nursing and Patient Care Considerations

1. Test can be performed after an overnight fast or after stimulation with Sustacal, intravenous (IV) glucose, or 1 mg of Glucagon SubQ.
2. Absence of C-peptide indicates no beta cell function, reflecting possible T1DM or insulinopenia in T2DM.

Autoantibody Testing

Description

An *autoantibody* is an antibody (a type of protein) manufactured by the immune system that is directed against one or more of the individual's own proteins. Islet cell autoantibodies are strongly associated with the development of T1DM. The appearance of autoantibodies to one or several of the autoantigens—GAD65, IA-2, or insulin—signals an autoimmune pathogenesis of β-cell destruction. The positivity of any or all of these autoantibodies in the presence of hyperglycemia is used to confirm the diagnosis of T1DM. Because T1DM affects such a small number of the population, generalized screening would be costly and therefore is not recommended.

Nursing and Patient Care Considerations

1. No special preparation or fasting is necessary.
2. Screen patients with T1DM for other autoimmune disorders such as hypothyroidism and celiac disease.

GENERAL PROCEDURES AND TREATMENT MODALITIES

Blood Glucose Monitoring

 Evidence Base American Association of Clinical Endocrinologists (AACE). (2011). Medical guidelines for clinical practice for developing a diabetes mellitus comprehensive care plan. *Endocrine Practice, 17*(Suppl. 2), 1–53.

American Diabetes Association. (2013). Standards of medical care in diabetes (position statement). *Diabetes Care, 36*(Suppl. 1), S11–S66.

Klonoff, D. C., Blonde, L., Cembrowski, G., et al. (2011). Consensus report: The current role of self-monitoring of blood glucose in non-insulin-treated type 2 diabetes. *Journal of Diabetes Science and Technology, 5*(6), 1529–1548.

Polonsky, W., Fisher, L., Schikman, C. H., et al. (2011). Structured self-monitoring of blood glucose significantly reduces A1C levels in poorly controlled, noninsulin-treated type 2 diabetes. Results from the Structured Testing Program study. *Diabetes Care, 34*(2), 262–267.

Accurate determination of capillary blood glucose assists patients in the control and daily management of diabetes mellitus. Blood glucose monitoring helps evaluate effectiveness of medication; reflects glucose excursion after meals; assesses glucose response to exercise regimen; and assists in the evaluation of episodes of hypoglycemia and hyperglycemia to determine appropriate treatment.

Procedure

1. Guidelines for glucose monitoring are included in Procedure Guidelines 25-1, pages 946 to 947.
2. The most appropriate schedule for glucose monitoring is determined by the patient and health care provider.
   a. Medication regimens and meal timing are considered to set the most effective monitoring schedule.
   b. Scheduling of glucose tests should reflect cost-effectiveness for the patient. Glucose meter test strips may cost up to $1 each.
   c. Glucose monitoring is intensified during times of stress or illness or when changes in therapy are prescribed.

3. Patients with T2DM who are not being treated with insulin should be testing blood glucose using a structured format where information obtained is used to guide treatment.
4. Patients with T1DM as well as those with T2DM who are using a multiple-dose insulin regimen should test blood sugar at least three times a day. Those times should include before/after meals, at bedtime, and occasionally at 2:00 to 3:00 A.M.
5. Alternate-site testing has been recommended by some clinicians for patients who complain of painful fingers and for individuals such as musicians, who use their fingertips for occupational activities. However, testing in such sites as the forearm, palm, thigh, and calf have not proved as accurate as fingertip testing in most studies.
   a. If alternate site is used, the area should be rubbed until it is warm before testing.
   b. Do not use an alternate site when:
      i. Glucose levels are rapidly changing (postprandial, hypoglycemia, reaction to exercise/activity).
      ii. Accuracy is critical (hypoglycemia is suspected, before exercise, or before driving).
   c. Check with the glucometer manufacturer to see if it is approved for alternate-site testing.
6. Continuous glucose monitoring (CGM) is a supplemental tool for use in selected patients, such as type 1 diabetics with frequent hypoglycemia or hypoglycemia unawareness. Fingerstick glucose is required at least twice daily to calibrate the device. CGM data require confirmation with fingerstick glucose before any action is taken (ie, treatment of hypoglycemia or hyperglycemia).

Insulin Therapy

 Evidence Base American Association of Clinical Endocrinologists (AACE). (2011). Medical guidelines for clinical practice for developing a diabetes mellitus comprehensive care plan. *Endocrine Practice, 17*(Suppl. 2), 1–53.

American Diabetes Association. (2012). Standards of medical care in diabetes (position statement). *Diabetes Care, 35*(Suppl. 1), S11–S63.

Frid, A., Hirsch, L., Gaspar, R., et al. (2010). New injection recommendations for patients with diabetes. *Diabetes and Metabolism, 36*(Suppl. 2), S3–S18. Available: ISPAD_Diabetes_in_Childhood_and%20Adolescence_Guidelines_2011.pdf.

Hanson, B., & Matytsina, I. (2011). Insulin administration: Selecting the appropriate needle and individualizing the injection technique. *Expert Opinion on Drug Delivery, 8*(10), 1395–1406.

Insulin therapy involves the subcutaneous injection of rapid-, short-, intermediate-, or long-acting insulin at various times to achieve the desired effect (see Table 25-1). Short-acting regular insulin as well as some of the rapid-acting analogs can also be administered intravenously. Currently, there are approximately 10 types of insulin available in the United States; most of these are human insulin manufactured synthetically (analogs). Beef and pork insulins are no longer available in the United States.

PROCEDURE GUIDELINES 25-1

Blood Glucose Monitoring Technique

 NURSING ALERT *Because of variation among glucose monitors, please refer to the operating instructions of the glucose monitoring device used in your facility.*

EQUIPMENT

- Blood glucose meter
- Lancet/lancing device
- Test strip
- Alcohol wipe
- Disposable gloves
- 2" × 2" gauze or clean tissue
- Cotton ball*

PROCEDURE

Nursing Action	Rationale
1. Prepare the finger to be lanced by having the patient wash hands in warm water and soap. Dry thoroughly. For convenience, an alcohol wipe may be used to cleanse the finger. Alcohol must dry thoroughly before finger is lanced.	1. Washing in warm water will increase the blood flow to the finger and remove superficial contaminants that could cause erroneous readings. Alcohol is not needed when patient is testing at home. Alcohol not completely dry will yield inaccurate results.
2. Don disposable gloves.	2. Complies with Centers for Disease Control and Prevention standards for blood-borne pathogens.
3. Turn on the glucose meter. Prepare the meter by validating the proper calibration with the strips to be used. (This usually involves matching a code number on the strip bottle to the code registered on the meter.)	3. Errors in glucose readings can result from miscalibrated or improperly coded meters. (Some meters do not require calibration.)
4. The meter will indicate its readiness for testing blood glucose by message or symbol. Some meters require that the glucose test strip be inserted at this time.	
5. Prick the patient's finger lateral to the fingertip using lancet/lancing device, obtaining a drop of blood large enough to satisfy the requirements of the testing strips being used. Almost all glucose meters available today require very small amounts, ranging from 0.3 microliters to 4 microliters.	5. Avoids the most sensitive area of the fingertip. Most inaccurate readings of blood glucose result from insufficient blood samples.
6. Apply the blood carefully to the strip test area (varies by glucose meter model).	6. Some glucose meters require that the test area be covered completely for accurate results. Others use only a small drop of blood inserted at the side of the test strip.

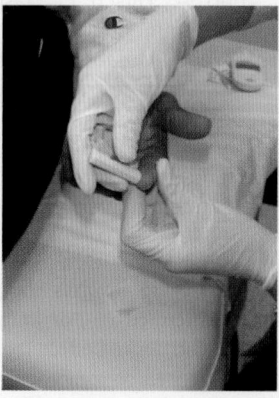

Obtaining blood from a finger using a lancet device

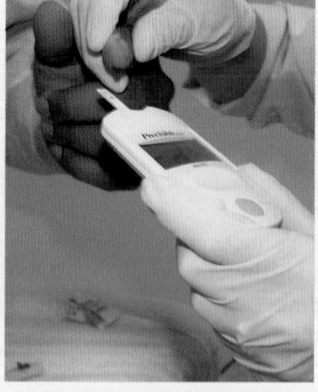

Applying drop of blood to test strip

PROCEDURE GUIDELINES 25-1 (continued)

Blood Glucose Monitoring Technique

PROCEDURE (continued)

Nursing Action	Rationale

7. Completing the test:
  a. The blood remains on the strip as the meter processes the result.
	7.
	  a. Processing time varies between meters, but will be programmed to display result at the appropriate time.

8. The lanced finger is covered with gauze or a tissue until bleeding subsides. If necessary, an adhesive bandage is then applied.	

Note: Standard precautions should be used throughout the procedure. All blood-contaminated items should be disposed of properly.

Table 25-1	Insulin Products Available in the United States and Their Onset, Peak, Duration, Route, Pregnancy Category

TYPE	ONSET	PEAK	DURATION	ROUTE	PREGNANCY CATEGORY
Rapid-Acting Analogs					
Insulin aspart (Novolog)	<15 minutes	1–3 hours	3–5 hours	SQ, pump, IV	B
Insulin glulisine (Apidra)	<15 minutes	1 hour	2–4 hours	SQ, pump, IV	C
Insulin lispro (Humalog)	<15 minutes	1 hour	3 ½ –4½ hours	SQ, pump	B
Short-Acting Human Insulin					
Insulin injection Humulin R	30 minutes	2–4 hours	6–8 hours	SQ, IV	B
Novolin R	30 minutes	2½–5 hours	8 hours	SQ, IV	B
Intermediate-Acting Basal					
Insulin isophane susp. (NPH)	1–2 hours	6–12 hours	18–24 hours	SQ	B
Humulin N	1.5 hours	4–12 hours	24 hours	SQ	B
Novolin N					
Long-Acting Basal Analogs					
Insulin detemir (Levemir)	1 hour	None	12–24 hours	SQ	B
Insulin glargine (Lantus)	1 hour	None	≥24 hours	SQ	C
Premixed Insulin					
Analog Preparations					
Novolog Mix 70/30	<15 minutes	2–4 hours	24 hours	SQ	B
Humalog Mix 75/25	<15 minutes	0½–1.5 hours	24 hours	SQ	B
Humalog Mix 50/50	<15 minutes	1 hour	16 hours	SQ	B
NPH and Regular Suspensions					
Humulin 70/30	30 minutes	2–12 hours	24 hours	SQ	B
Novolin 70/30	30 minutes	2–12 hours	24 hours	SQ	B

Notes: No FDA-approved insulins derived from beef are available in the United States. They were discontinued in 1998 because of concerns about bovine spongiform encephalopathy (BSE; "mad cow disease.")
Iletin II Regular (Pork), Iletin II NPH (Pork), Humulin Lente, and Humulin Ultralente were all discontinued by the manufacturer (Lilly) in 2005 because of reduced demand and high cost.
Exubera (inhaled insulin) was discontinued by Pfizer in late 2007 because of poor sales.

DRUG ALERT The following insulin types can be used during pregnancy (Category B): human Regular, human NPH, aspart, lispro, and detemir. Glargine and glulisine remain Category C and should not be used during pregnancy if other alternatives are available.

Self-Injection of Insulin

1. Teaching of self-injection of insulin should begin as soon as the need for insulin has been established.
2. Teach the patient and another family member or significant other.
3. Use written and verbal instructions and demonstration techniques.
4. Teach injection first because this is the patient's primary concern; then teach loading the syringe.
5. See Procedure Guidelines 25-2 for instructions on technique.
6. For patients who have difficulty with the injection procedure, insulin pens are available that use a prefilled cartridge that delivers the set dose of insulin. A few devices also deliver the insulin by jet stream without a needle.

Community and Home Care Considerations

1. Assist the patient in deciding whether to reuse insulin syringe at home. The patient may decide to do so due to cost; however, reuse has become controversial because the newer, finer needles may become dull or bent after one or two injections, causing tearing of tissue, which can lead to lipodystrophy.
   a. Needles should not be reused if painful injection or irritated site results.
   b. Needle should be recapped by patient and stored in a clean place if it is going to be reused.
2. Assist the patient in obtaining the appropriate syringe size and needle length for injections.
   a. Determine if there are visual or dexterity issues that make a syringe with gradations farther apart more desirable.
   b. There is no medical reason to use needles >8 mm in length, even in obese patients. Needle lengths of 4, 5, and 6 mm are reliable to deliver medication into the subcutaneous space. To prevent inadvertent intramuscular injection in patients who are thin, the needle can be inserted at a 45-degree angle (rather than at a 90-degree angle) and/or the skin should be folded prior to needle insertion.

PROCEDURE GUIDELINES 25-2

Teaching Self-Injection of Insulin and Other Injectable Diabetes Medications

EQUIPMENT

- Prescribed bottle of insulin or insulin pen or other injectable diabetes medication
- Disposable insulin syringe and needle or pen injection device and pen needle
- Cotton ball and alcohol or alcohol wipe (only in the institutionalized setting, not required for most patients at home)

PROCEDURE

Nursing Action	Rationale
To inject insulin using a syringe	
1. Give the patient the syringe or insulin pen device containing the prescribed dose of insulin.	1. Patient must see stoma site to learn care.
2. Have patient select a clean area of skin.	2. Preparation with alcohol is not necessary, but if used must completely dry before injection to reduce pain.
3. Instruct the patient to hold the syringe as he or she would a pencil or a dart.	3. Helps to accurately target the injection site.
4. Show the patient how to select an area of skin from the anterior thighs and form a skin fold by picking up subcutaneous tissue between the thumb and forefinger if the patient is thin. The skin fold should not be squeezed so tight that it would cause pain or blanching of the area.	4. Using a skin fold and injecting at a 45-degree angel is recommended for thin people; injecting at a 90-degree angle into taut skin is recommended for heavier people. Avoid pinching the skin tightly to avoid pain, bleeding, and trauma.
5. Select areas of upper arms, abdomen, and upper buttocks for injection after patient becomes proficient with needle insertion (see figure).	5. The skin is loose and there is more subcutaneous fat in these areas. Systematic rotation of sites will keep the skin supple and favor uniform absorption of insulin. Use of the same body part for each time of day dosage will make absorption more consistent.

PROCEDURE GUIDELINES 25-2 *(continued)*

Teaching Self-Injection of Insulin and Other Injectable Diabetes Medications

PROCEDURE *(continued)*

Nursing Action	Rationale

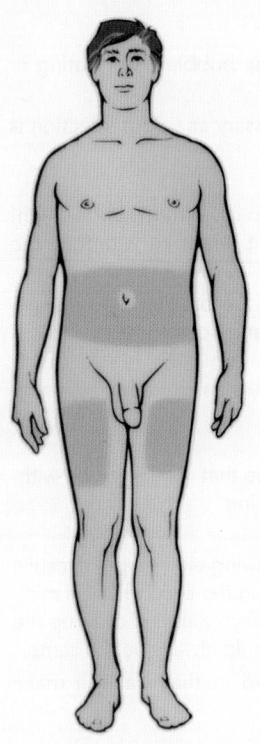
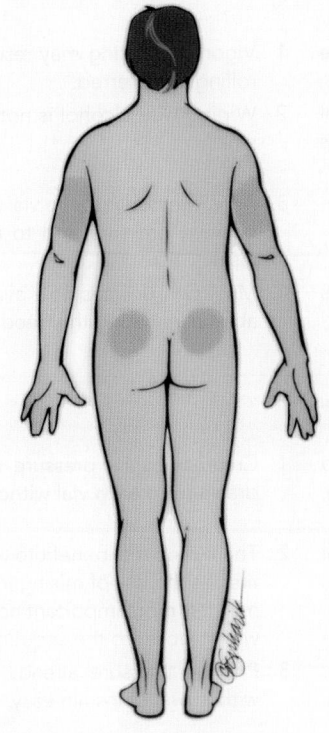

Rotate sites within each body part and use the same body part for the same injection time each day. Absorption is quicker from the abdomen and arms than the thighs and buttocks. Exercising a body part will hasten insulin absorption, so exercise should be consistent.

6. Assist the patient to insert the needle with a quick thrust to the hub at a 45- to 90-degree angle to the skin surface.

6. The needle is inserted into deep subcutaneous tissue.

7. Inject the insulin slowly and then withdraw the needle from the skin.

7. The insulin is injected into the subcutaneous tissue and the risk of bruising is reduced.

8. Instruct the patient to release the skin fold and dispose of the needle safely.

To inject insulin/other DM medication using a pen device

All non-insulin-injectable diabetes medications are only available in prefilled pen devices.

1. Pen devices must be primed according to manufacturer's instructions before use. Once primed, the desired dose should be dialed.

1. Ensures no obstruction and clears any air in the needle.

2. Inserting the pen needle into the skin is the same procedure used for inserting a needle of a syringe and is described above.

2. 90 degree angle for most individuals.

3. Once the needle is inserted into the skin up to the hub, the patient will administer the medication by pushing the thumb button at the end of the pen device.

4. After completely pushing the thumb button, the patient will continue to hold the needle in place for a slow count of 10 before withdrawing the needle.

4. Unlike when using a syringe, the full dose takes longer to be fully dispensed from a pen device.

5. Remove the needle from the pen and dispose of it safely.

5. Leaving the needle attached to the pen will allow for air and possibly other contaminants to enter the cartridge or for the medication to leak out.

(continued)

PROCEDURE GUIDELINES 25-2 *(continued)*

Teaching Self-Injection of Insulin and Other Injectable Diabetes Medications

PROCEDURE *(continued)*

Nursing Action	Rationale
To load the syringe	
1. If insulin is in a suspension (NPH), gently rotate or roll the insulin bottle to mix well.	1. Vigorous shaking may result in air bubbles, so rotating or rolling is preferred.
2. Do not instruct the patient to wipe off the top of the vial with alcohol; instead, make sure that the vial is stored in its original carton and is kept clean.	2. Wiping with alcohol is not necessary as risk of infection is small.
3. Inject approximately the same volume of air into the insulin vial as the volume of insulin to be withdrawn.	3. Air is injected into the vial to keep its contents under slight positive pressure and to make it easier to withdraw the insulin.
4. If insulin pen device is being used, follow manufacturer's instructions for dialing the dosage and changing cartridges (if not using a prefilled pen device).	4. Most pen devices now available are prefilled and disposable, eliminating the need to change cartridges.
To fill a syringe with NPH and short-acting or rapid-acting insulin mixture	
1. Inject air equal to the number of units to be injected into each vial. Use the same sequence each time, for example, always NPH insulin first.	1. Creates positive pressure in vial so that insulin will be withdrawn from each vial without mixing.
2. After injecting air into the second vial, keep needle in vial and withdraw prescribed amount of that type of insulin, then withdraw needle.	2. There is no real benefit to withdrawing either type of insulin first, as the risk of mixing insulins in the second vial is minimal. It is more important not to switch vials and draw up the wrong dose, so the sequence should always be the same.
3. Withdraw prescribed amount of insulin from the second vial.	3. Positive pressure already created in that vial will make withdrawal of insulin easy.

DRUG ALERT Lantus and Levemir insulins must never be mixed with any other insulin in the same syringe.

Evidence Base Frid, A., Hirsch, L., Gaspar, R., et al. (2010). New injection recommendations for patients with diabetes. *Diabetes and Metabolism, 36*(Suppl. 2), S3–S18.

Hanson, B., & Matytsina, I. (2011). Insulin administration: Selecting the appropriate needle and individualizing the injection technique. *Expert Opinion on Drug Delivery, 8*(10), 1395–1406.

3. Advise the patient that it is not necessary to use alcohol to wipe off the top of the vial or prepare the skin before injection. It has not proved to result in lower rate of infection and adds cost and time to the procedure. The patient should maintain good hygiene.

4. Instruct the patient to store insulin currently in use in a clean, secure place away from direct sunlight and heat. In-use insulin does not require refrigeration. Check manufacturer recommendations for when to discard insulin vials and pens; recommendations may vary from 10 to 28 days after opening. All unopened vials/pens must be stored in the refrigerator until initial use.

5. Check manufacturer's recommendations before teaching the patient how to mix insulin; for example, the patient should know that insulin glargine and insulin detemir must never be mixed with any other insulin. Other manufacturers' websites containing recommendations are Aventis (*www.aventis.com*), Eli Lilly (*www.lilly.com*), and Novo Nordisk (*www.novonordisk.com*).

6. Avoid prefilling syringes if at all possible because manufacturers have no data on the stability of insulin stored in syringes for long periods. If prefilling is the only option, store in refrigerator or suggest an insulin pen injection device.

7. Help the patient develop a plan for the disposal of needles. There are no federal regulations for discarding needles used at home; however, needles and lancets can pose a risk for injury. The rules and regulations regarding sharps disposal are different in towns and counties around the country, so advise the patient to check with local sanitation or health departments.

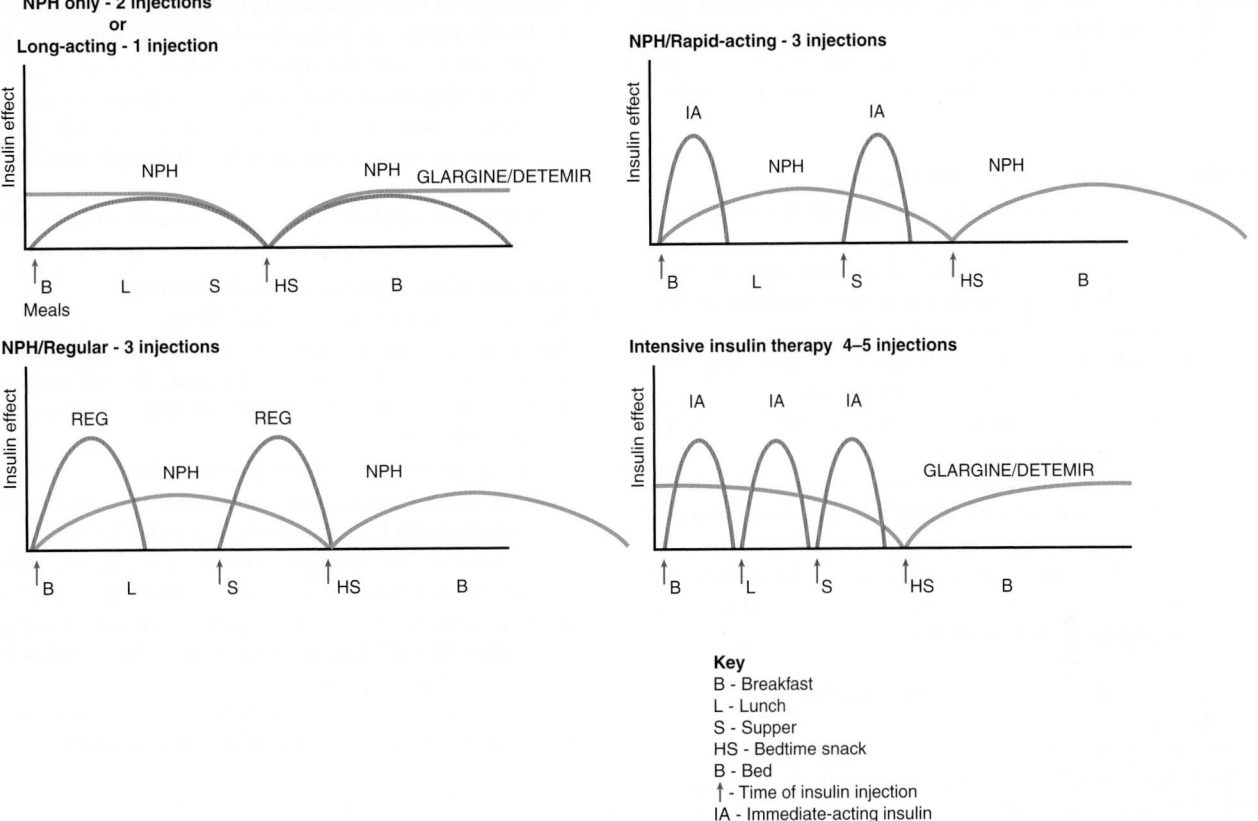

Figure 25-1. Insulin regimens.

a. Sharps can be placed in a hard plastic or metal container with a tightly secured lid after use.

b. More information on disposal can be obtained from the Environmental Protection Agency (*www.epa.gov/osw/nonhaz/industrial/medical/med-home.pdf*) or by contacting the Coalition for Safe Community Needle Disposal (800-643-1643 or *www.safeneedledisposal.org*).

Insulin Regimens

See Figure 25-1.

NPH or Long-Acting Analog Only

1. NPH is not used as frequently as basal insulin because of the availability of the newer analog basal insulins that are more reliable and associated with less hypoglycemia.

2. Used as monotherapy only in T2DM as a supplement for better glucose control when patients are still capable of producing some exogenous insulin.

3. Traditionally, administered at bedtime to assist with controlling early-morning hyperglycemia.

4. Can be given as a morning dosage to assist with normalization of glucose during the afternoon and evening.

5. NPH can also be given twice daily (morning and bedtime) to eliminate afternoon hypoglycemia yet provide nighttime coverage. Typically, ⅔ to ¾ of the daily dosage is given before breakfast and ⅓ to ¼ is given at bedtime.

NPH/Regular or NPH/Rapid-acting Insulin

1. Short-acting regular insulin or rapid-acting lispro, glulisine, or aspart insulin is added to NPH to promote postprandial glucose control.

2. Short- or rapid-acting insulin added to morning NPH controls glucose elevations after breakfast.

3. Increased blood glucose levels after supper can be controlled by the addition of short- or rapid-acting insulin before supper.

4. NPH and regular, lispro, glulisine, or aspart insulin given before breakfast and before supper is termed a "split-mix" regimen, providing 24-hour insulin coverage. However, there is an increased risk of nocturnal hypoglycemia (2:00 to 3:00 A.M.) when NPH is given before supper.

Intensive Insulin Therapy

1. Designed to mimic the body's normal insulin responses to glucose.

2. Uses multiple (four to five) daily injections of insulin.

3. Analog long-acting detemir or glargine insulin is used for basal insulin control. These are shown in Figure 25-1, to be administered once daily at bedtime; however, any time of the day can be used for the once-daily administration.

4. Regular insulin acts as a premeal bolus given 30 minutes before each meal. However, analog rapid-acting insulin (lispro, glulisine, or aspart) are used more frequently instead

of regular. The rapid-acting insulin is taken within 1 to 15 minutes before eating.

5. Twenty-four-hour insulin coverage designed in this way can be flexible to accommodate mealtimes and physical activity.

Sliding Scale versus Algorithm Therapy

1. Sliding scale therapy uses short- or rapid-acting insulin to retrospectively correct hyperglycemia.

2. Algorithm therapy prospectively determines short- or rapid-acting insulin dosages, taking into account meal content, premeal blood glucose level, and physical activity.

3. Individualization of insulin dosages is the most important aspect of sliding scale and algorithm therapy.
   a. The patient is encouraged to test blood glucoses to analyze insulin dose response.
   b. A pattern of increased blood glucose associated with certain foods (eg, pasta, pizza) can help determine the appropriate regimen of insulin dosage.
   c. Physical activity, which enhances insulin activity and decreases serum glucose, may indicate the need to reduce the dosage of premeal insulin.

Continuous Subcutaneous Insulin Infusion (Insulin Pump Therapy)

Pump therapy is more commonly considered for treatment of T1DM, but it is becoming more common in the treatment of T2DM when multiple daily injections/intensive insulin management is required.

1. Continuous subcutaneous insulin infusion (CSII) or insulin pump therapy provides continuous infusion of regular, lispro, glulisine, or aspart insulin via subcutaneous catheter inserted in the abdomen.

2. The catheter should be replaced every 72 hours or sooner if the site becomes painful or inflamed.
   a. Usually, the insulin pump is removed for bathing and tubing and catheter are changed at that time.
   b. To reduce tubing and catheter blockage, diluted insulin may be used. However, this is less of a problem with the newer insulin analogs (lispro, glulisine, and aspart).

3. Intensive insulin management by pump therapy requires patient motivation.
   a. Blood glucose monitoring must be done at least four to six times per day.
   b. Frequent contact with health care team is necessary to adjust insulin dosage.
   c. Careful recordings of diet, insulin, and activity are required to evaluate adjustments.
   d. Increased cost of insulin pump and infusion set compared to usual syringe method.
   e. Heightened risk of hypoglycemia with tighter glucose control.
   f. Danger of hyperglycemia exists should insulin pump fail to deliver correct insulin dosage.
   g. Increased visibility of diabetes by use of an external device, although newer pumps are smaller and more discreet.

4. Advantages of CSII in improving blood glucose control:
   a. Insulin pump can deliver basal insulin at individualized programmed rates throughout a 24-hour period.
   b. Bolus injections of short-acting insulin given 30 minutes before eating or rapid-acting insulin no more than 15 minutes before a meal allow for flexibility in meal content and timing.
   c. Correction supplements of short- or rapid-acting insulin are easily given to rapidly correct elevated glucose levels.

Combination Oral Agent and Insulin Therapy

1. Appropriate only for patients with T2DM.

2. Intermediate-acting insulin (NPH) or long-acting glargine or detemir is given in the evening and an oral sulfonylurea agent in the morning—called BIDS (bedtime insulin, daytime sulfonylurea) therapy.
   a. No oral antidiabetic agent is given at bedtime.
   b. Controlling hepatic glucose production overnight with evening insulin helps to start the day with a lower FBS.
   c. Daytime antidiabetic agent (usually sulfonylurea), along with diet and exercise, controls daytime blood glucose levels.
   d. Some patients may require regular or immediate-acting insulin injected before supper to assist with elevated postprandial evening glucoses.

3. Combination therapy may also include the use of other diabetes medications that are FDA approved for use with insulin.

DIABETES MELLITUS AND RELATED DISORDERS

Diabetes Mellitus

Diabetes mellitus is a metabolic disorder characterized by hyperglycemia and results from defective insulin production, secretion, or utilization.

Pathophysiology and Etiology

1. There is an absolute or relative lack of insulin produced by beta cells, resulting in hyperglycemia.

2. Defects at the cell level, impaired secretory response of insulin to rises in glucose, and increased nocturnal hepatic glucose production (gluconeogenesis) are seen in type 2 diabetes.

3. Etiology of type 1 diabetes is not well understood; viral, autoimmune, and environmental theories are under review.

4. Etiology of type 2 diabetes involves heredity, genetics, and obesity.

5. Risk factors for type 2 diabetes in adults and children include family history and ethnicity and a variety of other factors (see page 943).

Clinical Manifestations

1. Onset is usually abrupt with T1DM and insidious with T2DM.

2. Classic symptoms of hyperglycemia include polyuria, polydipsia, polyphagia, weight loss, fatigue, and blurred vision.

3. Chronic hyperglycemia often presents as disorders of altered tissue response, evidenced by poor wound healing and recurrent infections of the skin and genitourinary tract.

Diagnostic Evaluation

See page 947.

Management

 Evidence Base American Association of Diabetes Educators (AADE). (2012). Diabetes and physical activity (AADE position statement). *The Diabetes Educator, 38*(1), 129–132.

Colagiuri, S. (2012). Optimal management of type 2 diabetes: the evidence. *Diabetes, Obesity and Metabolism, 14*(Suppl. 1), 3–8.

Franz, M. J. (2012). Nutrition therapy for diabetes: effectiveness, carbohydrates and alcohol. *Expert Review of Endocrinology & Metabolism, 7*(6), 647–657.

Diet

1. The goal of meal planning is to meet nutritional requirements essential for healthy growth/development, achieve/maintain healthy weight, and control blood glucose and lipid levels (see Table 25-2).
2. Weight reduction is a primary treatment for T2DM.
3. Medical nutrition therapy should be conducted by a registered dietitian, preferably one who is also a certified diabetes educator.

Exercise

Regularly scheduled, moderate exercise performed 30 to 60 minutes at least every other day promotes the utilization of carbohydrates, assists with weight control, enhances the action of insulin, and improves cardiovascular fitness.

Medication

1. Oral and injectable antidiabetic agents for patients with T2DM who do not achieve glucose control with diet and exercise only (see Table 25-3, pages 954 to 955).
2. Insulin therapy is essential for patients with T1DM who require replacement (see page 943). Insulin therapy may also be used for T2DM when unresponsive to diet, exercise, and oral anti-diabetic therapy as well as when β-cell failure progresses.

Table 25-2	Meal-Planning Guidelines
PRINCIPLE	**ACTION**
Each meal should consist of a balance of carbohydrates, proteins, and fats.	• Carbohydrates should be varied to include fruits, starches, and vegetables. • Protein selections that are lean will help reduce fat and cholesterol intake. • Fats should be used sparingly with <10% of total calories derived from saturated fats. High in calories, fats contribute to weight gain in type 2 diabetes mellitus (DM).
Consistency in timing of meals and amounts of food eaten on a day-to-day basis help regulate blood glucose levels.	• Avoid skipping or delaying meals. • Measure portion sizes using a scale or measuring cups. • Know the equivalent amounts of commonly used foods within a food group (eg, 1 slice of bread = ½ cup cooked pasta).
Increase the intake of soluble and insoluble fiber.	• Substitute foods high in fiber for processed foods when possible (eg, whole-grain bread in place of white bread). • Eat fresh fruits and vegetables in place of juices.
Avoid salt whenever possible.	• Do not season foods with salt or salt-containing spices. • Limit use of foods with "hidden" sodium content (eg, crackers, pickled foods, cheese, processed meats). • Use salt-containing condiments sparingly (ketchup, soy sauce, gravies, bouillon).
Prepare foods to retain vitamins and minerals and reduce fats.	• Do not fry foods. • Bake, broil, or boil foods and discard fat. • Eat raw fruits and vegetables or steam vegetables to retain fiber. • Avoid adding calories with butter or cream sauces, fatback, and bacon. • Trim all visible fat from meat; skim off fat from stews or other prepared dishes.
Distribute snacks in the meal plan depending on insulin/medication regimens, physical activity, and lifestyle.	• Smaller, more frequent meals may enhance glucose control in type 2 DM. • Unplanned activity may call for an additional snack to avoid hypoglycemia.
Use alcohol only in moderation.	• Always consume alcohol with food to avoid hypoglycemia. • Do not omit food from meal plan in exchange for alcohol. • Limit intake to 1–2 drinks per week (4 oz dry wine, 12 oz beer, or 1.5 oz distilled liquor = 1 alcohol serving).
Use alternative non-nutritive, noncaloric sweeteners in moderation.	• Limit "diet" soda intake to 2 L/day. • Avoid frequent use of foods and beverages with concentrated sucrose.

Table 25-3	Antidiabetic Medications

AGENT	HOW GIVEN
Insulin-Secreting Agents	
Second-Generation Sulfonylureas	
• Glyburide	1.25–20 mg P.O. in single or divided doses with meals
• Glyburide, micronized	0.75–12 mg P.O. in single or divided dose
• Glipizide	2.5–40 mg P.O. in single or divided doses with meals
• Glipizide, long-acting	2.5–20 mg P.O. in single dose, usually before breakfast
• Glimepiride	1–8 mg P.O. in single dose with first main meal
Meglitinide Analogue	
• Repaglinide	0.5–16 mg P.O. in 2–4 divided doses, 1–30 minutes before meals Do not take if meal is skipped.
Amino Acid Derivative	
• Nateglinide	120–360 mg P.O. in 3 divided doses, 1–30 minutes before meals Do not take if meal is skipped.
Insulin-Sensitizing Agents	
Biguanides	
• Metformin	500–2,550 mg P.O. in 2–3 divided doses
• Metformin, long-acting	500–2,000 mg P.O. in single or two divided doses
Thiazolidinediones	
• Pioglitazone	15–45 mg P.O. once daily
• Rosiglitazone*	4–8 mg P.O. in single or two divided doses
Glucose Absorption-Delaying Agents	
Alpha-glucosidase inhibitors	
• Acarbose	50–300 mg P.O. in 3 divided doses before meals
• Miglitol	50–300 mg P.O. in 3 divided doses before meals
Glucagon-Suppressing Agents	
DPP-4 Inhibitors	
• Sitagliptin	25–100 mg P.O. once daily
• Linagliptin	5 mg P.O. once daily
• Saxagliptin	2.5–5 mg P.O. once daily
Incretin Mimetics	
• Exenatide	5–10 mcg subcutaneously, twice daily 1–60 minutes before meals
• Liraglutide	1.2–1.8 mg subcutaneously, once daily
• Exenatide extended-release	2 mg subcutaneously every 7 days
Amylin analogue	
• Pramlintide	Type 1: 15–60 mcg subcutaneously with each main meal Type 2: 60–120 mcg subcutaneously with each main meal
Other Agents	
Bile Acid Sequestrant	
• Colesevelam	625 mg tablets: 3 tabs P.O. twice daily or 6 tabs P.O. once daily
Dopamine Agonist	
• Bromocriptine	0.8–4.8 mg P.O. once daily in the morning
Combination Agents	
• Metaglip (glipizide + metformin)	Up to 20 mg/2,000 mg P.O. in single or divided doses
• Glucovance (glyburide + metformin)	Up to 20 mg/2,000 mg P.O. in single or divided doses

Table 25-3 Antidiabetic Medications (*continued*)

AGENT	HOW GIVEN
Combination Agents (*continued*)	
• ACTOplus met (pioglitazone + metformin)	Up to 45 mg/2,550 mg P.O. in divided doses
• ACTOplus met XR (pioglitazone + metformin XR)	Up to 45 mg/ 2,000 mg P.O. once daily
• Avandamet (rosiglitazone* + metformin)	Up to 8 mg/2,000 mg P.O. in divided doses
• Duetact (pioglitazone + glimepiride)	Up to 30 mg/4 mg P.O. once daily
• Avandaryl (rosiglitazone* + glimepiride)	Up to 8 mg/4 mg P.O. in single or divided doses
• Janumet (sitagliptin + metformin)	Up to 100 mg/2,000 mg P.O. in divided doses
• Kombiglyze XR (saxagliptin + metformin XR)	Up to 5 mg/2,000 mg P.O. in divided doses
• PrandiMet (repaglinide + metformin)	Up to 10 mg/2,500 mg P.O. in divided doses

DPP-4, dipeptidyl peptidase-4; P.O., by mouth.
*Due to FDA restrictions, rosiglitazone is only available through a distribution program form the manufacturer.

DRUG ALERT Hypoglycemia may result from insulin therapy as well as rebound hyperglycemia (Somogyi effect). Insulin therapy commonly results in increased appetite and weight gain.

3. Sulfonylurea compounds promote the increased secretion of insulin by the pancreas and partially normalize both receptor and postreceptor defects.
   a. Many drug interactions exist, so patient should alert all health care providers of use.
   b. Potential adverse reactions include hypoglycemia, photosensitivity, GI upset, allergic reaction, reaction to alcohol, cholestatic jaundice, and blood dyscrasias.

4. Metformin, a biguanide compound, appears to diminish insulin resistance. It decreases hepatic glucose production and intestinal reabsorption of glucose and increases insulin reception and glucose transport in cells.
   a. Many drug interactions exist, so patient should alert all health care providers of its use.
   b. Metformin must be used cautiously in renal insufficiency, conditions that may cause dehydration, and hepatic impairment.
   c. Potential adverse reactions include GI disturbances, metallic taste, and lactic acidosis (rare). Riomet is the only formulation available as an oral solution.

DRUG ALERT Lactic acidosis is a rare but potentially fatal complication of metformin. The drug should be discontinued for conditions that predispose to lactic acidosis, including dehydration, alteration in renal function, vomiting and diarrheal illnesses, fasting for surgery and other procedures, imaging studies requiring IV iodinated contrast media, septicemia, heavy alcohol use, and hemodynamic instability.

5. Alpha-glucosidase inhibitors (acarbose and miglitol delay the digestion and absorption of complex carbohydrates (including sucrose or table sugar) into simple sugars, such as glucose and fructose, thereby lowering postprandial and fasting glucose levels.
   a. Contraindicated in inflammatory bowel disease and other conditions of the intestinal tract. They are used cautiously in renal insufficiency and with several other drugs.
   b. Flatulence, abdominal pain, and diarrhea are common.
   c. If these medications are taken in conjunction with insulin-secretagogues (ie, sulfonylureas) and hypoglycemia occurs, patient must use a monosaccharide (glucose tablets) to treat hypoglycemia because sucrose will not be broken down to an absorbable sugar.

6. Thiazolidinedione (TZD) derivatives (rosiglitazone and pioglitazone) primarily decrease resistance to insulin in skeletal muscle and adipose tissue without increasing insulin secretion. Secondarily, they reduce hepatic glucose production.
   a. They should be used cautiously in liver disease and heart failure. Liver function tests should be monitored periodically.
   b. Ovulation may occur in anovulatory premenopausal women.
   c. Adverse reactions include edema, weight gain, anemia, elevation in serum transaminases, and increased incidence of bone fracture.
   d. Rosiglitazone is associated with increased risk of myocardial infarction; therefore, it is available only through a restricted distribution program from the manufacturer.
   e. Thiazolidinediones themselves do not cause hypoglycemia; when administered with insulin or oral medications that increase the secretion of insulin, however, they increase the risk of hypoglycemia. Be aware that insulin requirements will drop with therapy, so glucose monitoring and insulin adjustments should be done regularly.

DRUG ALERT Both pioglitazone and rosiglitazone can cause or worsen heart failure and are contraindicated for use in patients with New York Heart Association Class III or Class IV heart failure.

7. Meglitinide analogues (repaglinide) and amino acid derivatives (nateglinide) stimulate pancreatic release of insulin in response to a meal. They have a more rapid onset and shorter duration than sulfonylureas.
   a. Should not be taken when a meal is skipped or missed.
   b. Should be used cautiously in patients with renal and hepatic dysfunction and may cause hypoglycemia.

8. Dipeptidyl peptidase-4 inhibitors (sitagliptin, linagliptin, saxagliptin) inhibit the breakdown of glucagon-like peptide-1 (GLP-1). GLP-1 stimulates insulin release from the pancreas and decreases glucagon secretion, which inhibits glycogenolysis and gluconeogenesis. These agents are most effective at controlling postprandial blood glucose and, when used alone or in combination with metformin or TZD, do not cause hypoglycemia.

   a. Dose is based on renal function.
   b. Generally well tolerated and weight-neutral. Adverse reactions include upper respiratory infections, nasopharyngitis, and headaches.

DRUG ALERT Acute pancreatitis has been reported with sitagliptin and should not be used if patient has a prior history of pancreatitis.

9. Bile acid sequestrant (colesevelam) is traditionally a cholesterol-lowering agent that has now been indicated for the treatment of T2DM. The exact mechanism of action is unclear but may have effect on sensitizing the liver to insulin, reducing hepatic glucose production. May also work by reducing intestinal absorption of glucose.

   a. Side effects include nausea, bloating, and constipation.

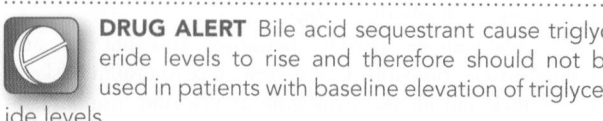

DRUG ALERT Bile acid sequestrant cause triglyceride levels to rise and therefore should not be used in patients with baseline elevation of triglyceride levels.

10. Dopamine agonist (bromocriptine) is another agent in which the mechanism of action is unclear and its role in diabetes management ill defined. It is believed it acts to reduce glucose levels by reducing the effects of insulin resistance on the central nervous system.

   a. Side effects include hypotension and syncope, especially with dose titrations. Proceed slowly and cautiously, especially in older patients.

11. GLP-1 incretin mimetics (exenatide, liraglutide) work to lower blood glucose by enhancing first-phase insulin secretion by the pancreas, slowing gastric emptying, suppressing glucagon secretion, and reducing appetite, which can facilitate weight loss.

   a. Exenatide is injected twice daily within 1 to 60 minutes before breakfast and dinner.
   b. Liraglutide is injected once daily without regard to meals.
   c. These are used as add-on therapy to metformin, metformin + TZD, metformin + sulfonylurea, TZD, or TZD + sulfonylurea; not to be used as a substitute for insulin.

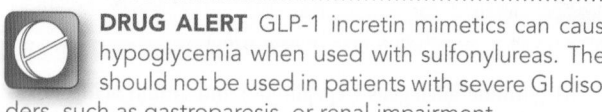

DRUG ALERT GLP-1 incretin mimetics can cause hypoglycemia when used with sulfonylureas. They should not be used in patients with severe GI disorders, such as gastroparesis, or renal impairment.

   d. Most common adverse effects are nausea and vomiting. Other adverse reactions include GI upset, headache, and pancreatitis.
   e. Both are available in a disposable pen device.

DRUG ALERT GLP-1 incretin mimetics have been associated with pancreatitis. Additionally, exenatide has been associated with renal insufficiency and liraglutide has been associated with medullary thyroid cancer in rodents.

12. Amylin analog (pramlintide). Amylin is co-secreted by the B cells of the pancreas to assist with postprandial glucose control. Its actions are similar to GLP-1 incretin mimetics (reduced gastric emptying, suppression of glucagon, increased satiety, and weight loss). It is indicated for patients with either type 1 or type 2 diabetes who require a mealtime insulin bolus.

   a. It is not a substitute for insulin, but must be administered immediately prior to meals that must consist of at least 250 kcal or at least 30 g of carbohydrates.
   b. If used with insulin, mealtime dose of insulin must be reduced by 50%. Pramlintide cannot be mixed with insulin and must be injected at least 1 inch (2.5 cm) away from insulin injection site.
   c. It is contraindicated in patients with confirmed gastroparesis and should be used with caution in patients who require the use of drugs to stimulate gastric motility.
   d. The most common adverse effects are GI related (nausea/vomiting). It is available in a disposable pen device.

DRUG ALERT Pramlinitide may cause severe insulin-induced hypoglycemia and is contraindicated in patients with hypoglycemia unawareness.

General Health

Evidence Base American Association of Clinical Endocrinologists. (2011). Medical guidelines for clinical practice for developing a diabetes mellitus comprehensive care plan. *Endocrine Practice, 17*(Suppl. 2), 1–53.
American Diabetes Association. (2013). Standards of medical care in diabetes (position statement). *Diabetes Care, 36*(Suppl. 1), S11–S66.

In addition to the glycemic and A1C goals discussed previously, rigid prevention and management guidelines have been established for blood pressure (BP), lipid values, and kidney function to prevent complications. Several authoritative groups recommend the following goals of treatment for nonpregnant adults, adolescents, and children with diabetes mellitus.

Adults:

1. BP < 130/80 mm Hg.
2. Lipid control.
   a. Low-density lipoprotein < 100 mg/dL.
   b. High-density lipoprotein > 40 mg/dL; > 50 mg/dL women.
   c. Triglycerides < 150 mg/dL.
3. Microalbumin (spot urine) < 30 mg/g creatinine.

Children and adolescents:

1. BP < 130/80 or below the 90th percentile for sex, age, and height.
2. Lipid control.

a. Low-density lipoprotein < 100 mg/dL.

b. High-density lipoprotein > 35 mg/dL (regardless of sex).

c. Triglycerides < 150 mg/dL.

Complications

Acute

1. Hypoglycemia occurs as a result of an imbalance in food, activity, and insulin/oral antidiabetic agent.

2. Diabetic ketoacidosis (DKA) occurs primarily in type 1 diabetes during times of severe insulin deficiency or illness, producing severe hyperglycemia, ketonuria, dehydration, and acidosis (see page 966).

3. Hyperosmolar hyperglycemic state (HHS) primarily affects patients with type 2 diabetes, causing severe dehydration, hyperglycemia, hyperosmolarity, and stupor (see page 968).

Chronic

See Table 25-4.

1. In type 1 diabetes, chronic complications usually appear about 10 years after the initial diagnosis.

2. The prevalence of microvascular complications (retinopathy, nephropathy, and neuropathy) is higher in type 1 diabetes.

3. Because of its insidious onset, chronic complications can appear at any point in type 2 diabetes. Approximately 50% will have at least one complication at time of diagnosis.

4. Macrovascular complications—in particular cardiovascular disease, occurring in type 1 and type 2 diabetes—are the leading cause of morbidity and mortality among persons with diabetes.

Nursing Assessment

1. Obtain a history of current problems, family history, and general health history.

   a. Has the patient experienced polyuria, polydipsia, polyphagia, and any other symptoms?

   b. Number of years since initial diagnosis of diabetes.

   c. Family members diagnosed with diabetes, their subsequent treatment, and complications.

2. Perform a review of systems and physical examination to assess for signs and symptoms of diabetes, general health of patient, and presence of complications.

   a. General: recent weight loss or gain, increased fatigue, tiredness, anxiety.

   b. Skin: skin lesions, infections, dehydration, evidence of poor wound healing.

   c. Eyes: changes in vision—floaters, halos, blurred vision, dry or burning eyes, cataracts, glaucoma.

   d. Mouth: gingivitis, periodontal disease.

   e. Cardiovascular: orthostatic hypotension, cold extremities, weak pedal pulses, leg claudication.

   f. GI: diarrhea, constipation, early satiety, bloating, increased flatulence, hunger or thirst.

   g. GU: increased urination, nocturia, impotence, vaginal discharge.

   h. Neurologic: numbness and tingling of the extremities, decreased pain and temperature perception, changes in gait and balance.

Nursing Diagnoses

- Imbalanced Nutrition: More than Body Requirements related to intake in excess of activity expenditures.
- Fear related to medication injection.
- Risk for Unstable Blood Glucose Level related to effects of insulin, inability to eat.
- Activity Intolerance related to poor glucose control.
- Deficient Knowledge related to use of oral hypoglycemic agents and injectable agents.
- Risk for Impaired Skin Integrity related to decreased sensation and circulation to lower extremities.
- Ineffective Coping related to chronic disease and complex self-care regimen.

Nursing Interventions

See Standards of Care Guidelines 25-1, page 962.

Improving Nutrition

1. Assess current timing and content of meals.

2. Advise patient on the importance of an individualized meal plan in meeting weight-loss goals. Reducing intake of carbohydrates may benefit some patients; however, fad diets or diet plans that stress one food group and eliminate another are generally not recommended.

3. Discuss the goals of dietary therapy for the patient. Setting a goal of a 10% (of patient's actual body weight) weight loss over several months is usually achievable and effective in reducing blood sugar and other metabolic parameters.

4. Assist patient to identify problems that may have an impact on dietary adherence and possible solutions to these problems. Emphasize that lifestyle changes should be maintainable for life.

5. Explain the importance of exercise in maintaining/reducing body weight.

   a. Caloric expenditure for energy in exercise.

   b. Carryover of enhanced metabolic rate and efficient food utilization.

6. Assist patient to establish goals for weekly weight loss and incentives to assist in achieving them.

7. Strategize with patient to address the potential social pitfalls of weight reduction.

Teaching About Insulin

1. Assist patient to reduce fear of injection by encouraging verbalization of fears regarding insulin injection, conveying a sense of empathy, and identifying supportive coping techniques.

2. Demonstrate and explain thoroughly the procedure for insulin self-injection (see page 948).

3. Help patient to master technique by taking a step-by-step approach.

   a. Allow patient time to handle insulin and syringe to become familiar with the equipment.

   b. Teach self-injection first to alleviate fear of pain from injection.

   c. Instruct patient in filling syringe when he or she expresses confidence in self-injection procedure.

(Text continues on page 962)

Table 25-4   Chronic Complications of Diabetes Mellitus

CONDITION	ASSESSMENT
Macrovascular Complications	
Cerebrovascular Disease	
• *Incidence*: Two to four times more likely in diabetes. • Hypertension, increased lipids, smoking, uncontrolled blood glucose, increase risk of stroke and transient ischemic attack.	• Increased BP • Change in mental status • Hemiparesis • Aphasia • Clinical presentation mimics that of nondiabetic patient.
Coronary Artery Disease	
• *Incidence*: Increased vessel disease with more vessels affected in diabetes. Higher incidence of "silent" myocardial infarctions (MIs). • Hyperglycemia contributes to atherosclerosis and vessel deterioration.	• Severe CAD is commonly asymptomatic, seen only in ECG changes. ECG changes may indicate silent MI. • Symptoms can also present as pain in the jaw, neck, or epigastric area.
Peripheral Vascular Disease	
• *Incidence*: 50% of nontraumatic amputations are related to diabetes. • Intermittent claudication, absent pedal pulses, and ischemic gangrene are increased in diabetes.	• Physical examination of the lower extremities may reveal changes in skin integrity associated with diminished circulation. • Decreased lower leg hair, absent or decreased anterior tibial or dorsal pedis pulses, poor capillary refill of toenails may occur. The extremity may appear pale/cool. Further examination for neurologic changes is indicated.
Microvascular Complications	
Retinopathy	
• *Incidence*: Type 1—10 years postdiagnosis 60% have some degree of retinopathy. Type 2—approximately 20% present with retinopathy at diagnosis, which increases to 60% to 85% after 15 years. DM is the leading cause of blindness in the United States. • Appearance of hard exudates, blot hemorrhages, and microaneurysms on the retina in background retinopathy. Progresses to neurovascularization in proliferative diabetic retinopathy.	• Usually asymptomatic in the early stages. Symptoms occurring with acute visual problems—"floaters," flashing lights, blurred vision may indicate hemorrhage or retinal detachment. Funduscopic examination should be done by an ophthalmologist for full retinal visualization.
Nephropathy	
• *Incidence*: Type 1—with >20 years history of diabetes, approximately 40% will have renal disease. Type 2—5 to 10 years after diagnosis 5% to 10% of patients develop nephropathy, with higher incidence in Native Americans, Hispanics, and blacks. DM is the leading cause of kidney failure in the United States. • Thickening of the glomerular basement membrane, mesangial expansion, and renal vessel sclerosis are caused by diabetes. • Subsequently, diffuse and nodular intercapillary glomerulosclerosis diminishes renal function.	• Evidence of increased glomerular filtration rate. • Microalbuminuria is the first clinical sign of renal disease. • Elevation in blood urea nitrogen and creatinine levels indicates advanced renal disease. • Gross proteinuria is further indication of renal deterioration.
Peripheral Neuropathy	
• In general, neuropathy affects 60% to 70% of persons with diabetes, with nearly 100% showing signs and symptoms of slowing nerve conduction velocity. • It can affect almost every organ system with varying specific symptoms.	• Decreased light touch, vibratory, temperature sensation. Loss of foot proprioception, followed by ataxia, gait disturbances. • Diminished ankle jerk response. • Formation of "hammer toes," Charcot joint disease, which predispose patient to new pressure-point areas.

INTERVENTION	PREVENTION/TEACHING
• Check blood glucose level to differentiate signs and symptoms of stroke versus hypoglycemia. If stroke is suspected, do not give fast-acting carbohydrate as increased levels contribute to recurrence and high mortality of strokes in patients with diabetes. Monitor for bleeding if aspirin or other platelet-active medicine is used.	• Maintain target goals of blood glucose, avoiding severe hypoglycemia and hyperglycemia, which predispose the patient to stroke. In hypoglycemia, increased levels of adrenalin and catecholamines can produce cardiac arrhythmias. • Hyperglycemia can lead to dehydration, which affects platelet aggregation.
• Usual medical treatment for angina prevails—sublingual nitroglycerin, oral nitrates. Beta-adrenergic blockers and calcium channel blockers can also be used.	• Emphasis must be placed on reducing cardiac risk factors (eg, cigarette smoking, hypertension, hyperlipidemia). Avoid wide fluctuations in blood glucose. Patients with autonomic neuropathy, which can cause orthostatic hypotension, should be carefully monitored when cardiac drug therapies are introduced. Beta-adrenergic blockers can blunt or eliminate the clinical signs and symptoms of hypoglycemia.
• Any lesion, decrease in peripheral pulses, or change in skin color, temperature, or sensation should be evaluated within 24–48 hours. To ensure proper healing and prevent infection, treatment should begin as soon as possible and be carefully monitored. Mild antiseptics/antibiotic preparations are used to avoid further damage to the surrounding skin. Avoid the use of surgical tape to skin. Rest affected leg to promote circulation and wound healing.	• Foot care guidelines and smoking cessation must be stressed. Safe exercise guidelines and weight reduction, as appropriate, will further reduce risk of foot injury.
• Laser therapy (photocoagulation) can be helpful in macular edema (focal laser) and proliferative retinopathy (panretinal laser). Reduction of active neovascularization by laser therapy reduces the risk of vitreous hemorrhage. Vitrectomy may be needed to treat retinal detachment or remove vitreous hemorrhage. • During the acute phase, before laser therapy, patients must avoid activities that increase the chances of vitreous hemorrhage (eg, weight-lifting, high-impact aerobics).	• Stress importance of annual eye examination with an ophthalmologist (preferably retina specialist). Optimal glucose control can prevent or slow the progression of retinopathy. Maintaining normal BP also reduces the risk of retinopathy.
• Hypertension control, blood glucose control, and reduction of protein and sodium are essential. Angiotensin-converting enzyme inhibitors are the drugs of choice to control BP. Calcium channel blockers may also be used. In end-stage renal disease, dialysis or transplantation may be necessary.	• Frequent hypertension screening, noting any deviation from patient's normal reading. Early initiation of BP control to prevent kidney damage. Excellent glucose control with insulin/oral agent adjustment to compensate for reduced kidney function, which predisposes the patient to hypoglycemia. Avoidance of nephrotoxic drugs, dyes, or renal procedures that may cause infection. Immediate treatment for any urinary tract infections.
• All foot wounds or injuries are immediately evaluated. Culture and sensitivity tests ordered for any drainage present. Affected foot is elevated—avoid weight-bearing. Wet to dry dressings applied as ordered. Avoid use of caustic chemicals, dressing tapes. • Use of systemic antibiotics, as needed.	• In general, blood glucose control is recommended, avoiding wide fluctuations. In patients who are poorly controlled, care must be taken to correct glucoses slowly to avoid increasing symptoms of neuropathy. • Foot care guidelines. • Smoking cessation.

(continued)

Table 25-4	Chronic Complications of Diabetes Mellitus (*continued*)
CONDITION	**ASSESSMENT**

Peripheral Neuropathy (*continued*)

• Distal symmetrical polyneuropathy involving the lower extremities is most commonly seen. • In conjunction with peripheral vascular disease, neuropathy to the feet increases susceptibility to trauma and infection. The more severe forms of peripheral neuropathy are a major contributing cause of lower-extremity amputations. • Three clinical syndromes of distal symmetrical polyneuropathy are seen: acute painful, small-fiber, and large-fiber neuropathy.	• Hypersensitivity or other dysesthetic symptoms are experienced, followed by hypnoanesthesia or anesthesia, which is not reversible.

Autonomic Neuropathy

Gastroparesis

• *Incidence*: Occurs in 25% of people with diabetes. • *Characteristics*: Delayed gastric emptying, prolonged pylorospasms, and loss of the powerful contractions of the distal stomach to grind and mix foods.	• Typical symptoms may include nausea/vomiting, early satiety, abdominal bloating, epigastric pain, change in appetite. Wide fluctuations in blood glucoses and postmeal hypoglycemia caused by poor glucose absorption. Visualization of the gut by upper GI barium series may show retained food after an 8-to 12-hour fast.

Diarrhea

• *Incidence*: Approximately 5% of diabetic patients. • *Characteristics*: Frequent, watery movements. • Mild steatorrhea. • Can be intermittent, persistent, or alternate with constipation.	• Diarrhea occurs without warning, frequently at night or after meals. Fecal incontinence may be caused by loss of internal sphincter control and anorectal sensation. Other causes, such as celiac sprue, pancreatic insufficiency, and lactose intolerance, must be investigated. Bacterial overgrowth in the bowel is also suspected.

Impotence/Sexual Dysfunction

• Incidence is not well documented due to inhibitions about reporting this problem to health care providers. • Sexual dysfunction can involve changes in erectile ability, ejaculation, or libido.	• *Men*: History of poor erectile function despite stimulation. Absence of early morning erection in response to increased hormonal levels. • *Women*: May experience decreased vaginal lubrication and dyspareunia. • Screening for use of ethanol or other medications associated with impotence (eg, antidepressants, antihypertensives).

Orthostatic Hypotension

• One of three syndromes associated with cardiovascular autonomic neuropathy, orthostatic hypotension occurs when the "postural reflex," which increases heart rate and peripheral vascular resistance, is dysfunctional.	• Patients may report episodes of syncope, weakness, or visual impairment, particularly with positional changes. Evaluate BP and pulse in lying and standing position at each visit. BP changes that indicate neuropathic involvement: fall in systolic pressure of >30 mm Hg or fall in diastolic pressure of >10 mm Hg with change from lying to standing position.

Hypoglycemia Unawareness

• *Incidence*: 17% of type 1 diabetic patients. • Condition in which the usual warning signs of hypoglycemia are no longer experienced. The symptoms may be different (and therefore not recognized), less pronounced, or even absent.	• Patients may exhibit irrational thought; unprovoked anger or irritability; insisting that they "feel fine" in the midst of very unusual behavior; inappropriate laughing/silliness/giddiness.

INTERVENTION	PREVENTION/TEACHING
• Medication for painful neuropathy may include use of the tricyclic antidepressant drugs (eg, amitriptyline, a serotonin and epi-nephrine reuptake inhibitor (duloxetine), or topical application of capsaicin ointment.	• Frequent evaluation by podiatrist for modified foot wear (eg, orthotics, extra-depth shoes). • Safe exercise guidelines. • Weight reduction, as necessary.
• Excellent glucose control to avoid hyperglycemia, which interferes with gut contractility. Avoidance of severe postmeal hypoglycemia by small, frequent meals, low fat and low fiber. This diet is also helpful in bloating/early satiety. Medication to improve gut motility is metoclopramide.	• Maintenance of excellent glucose control. Regular exercise improves/maintains GI motility. Avoid use of laxatives. Small, frequent meals may help.
• Dietary changes may include increased fiber, elimination of milk products. Sphincter-strengthening exercises may help. Medica-tions: For diarrhea, hydrophilic fiber supplement, cholestyramine, or synthetic opiates are used. • Tetracycline, ampicillin are used for bacterial overgrowth.	• Routine bowel elimination habits. • Maintenance of adequate hydration. • Excellent blood glucose control reduces dehydration. • Inclusion of dietary fiber in the daily diet. • Daily exercise program that includes walking or swimming has been effective in encouraging bowel regularity.
• *Men*: Referral to urologist for full examination is indicated. Treat-ment options may include injection of alprostadil (a prostaglandin), inflatable penile prosthesis, or oral sildenafil. • *Women*: Increase lubrication with use of water-based lubricant or estrogen creams, which may also help thicken the vaginal mucosa, affecting dyspareunia.	• Reduce consumption of alcohol, which may hasten or contribute to neuropathy. • Maintain target ranges of blood glucose control to reduce likelihood of vaginal infections. • Discuss alternative ways of maintaining intimacy.
• Improvement in blood glucose control to prevent fluid loss from glycosuria. Moderate amounts of sodium may be used in the diet to encourage fluid retention during hot weather or strenuous exercise. Mechanical devices such as support stockings (full hose to waist) may decrease venous pooling. Drugs to enhance volume expansion may be used (eg, fludrocortisone).	• Encourage increased fluid intake to maintain hydration. • Caution should be used in changing position from lying to standing. Sitting on side of bed with feet dan-gling is recommended until BP stabilizes. • Avoid standing in one position, which may increase venous pooling.
• Can be reversed by avoiding frequent low blood sugars. Raising target blood sugar (ie, 140 mg/dL) by easing up on aggressive/intensive insulin treatment for a few weeks will allow the counter-regulatory hormone response to return to normal.	• Increase frequency of blood glucose monitoring and stay alert to physical warning signs for 48 hours follow-ing low blood sugar. Keeping a glucose log will help patients predict when lows are more likely to occur. An occasional 2:00 A.M. blood glucose test can help with identifying unrecognized nocturnal hypoglycemia.

(continued)

| Table 25-4 | Chronic Complications of Diabetes Mellitus (*continued*) |

CONDITION	ASSESSMENT
Autonomic Neuropathy	
• *Causes:* Long-standing diabetes; reduced glucagon excretion; frequent low blood sugars; alcohol consumption within the previous 12 hours; previous low blood sugar within the last 24 to 48 hours; certain medications (ie, beta-adrenergic blockers) • Women more susceptible because of reduced counterregulatory response and reduced symptoms. • More likely to occur in patients with other types of autonomic neuropathy.	• Grand mal seizures can occur if hypoglycemia is not recognized and treated.

BP, blood pressure; CAD, coronary artery disease; ECG, electrocardiography.

STANDARDS OF CARE GUIDELINES 25-1
Caring for Patients with Diabetes Mellitus

When caring for patients with diabetes mellitus:

- Assess level of knowledge of disease and ability to care for self.
- Assess adherence to diet therapy, monitoring procedures, medication treatment, and exercise regimen.
- Assess for signs of hyperglycemia: polyuria, polydipsia, polyphagia, weight loss, fatigue, blurred vision.
- Assess for signs of hypoglycemia: sweating, tremor, nervousness, tachycardia, light-headedness, confusion.
- Perform thorough skin and extremity assessment for peripheral neuropathy or peripheral vascular disease and any injury to the feet or lower extremities.
- Assess for trends in blood glucose and other laboratory results.
- Make sure that appropriate insulin dosage is given at the right time and in relation to meals and exercise.
- Make sure patient has adequate knowledge of diet, exercise, and medication treatment.
- Immediately report to health care provider any signs of skin or soft tissue infection (redness, swelling, warmth, tenderness, drainage).
- Get help immediately for signs of hypoglycemia that do not respond to usual glucose replacement.
- Get help immediately for patient presenting with signs of either ketoacidosis (nausea and vomiting, Kussmaul's respirations, fruity breath odor, hypotension, and altered level of consciousness) or hyperosmolar hyperglycemic nonketotic syndrome (nausea and vomiting, hypothermia, muscle weakness, seizures, stupor, coma).

This information should serve as a general guideline only. Each patient situation presents a unique set of clinical factors and requires nursing judgment to guide care, which may include additional or alternative measures and approaches.

 GERONTOLOGIC ALERT Assess older patients for sensory deficits, such as impaired vision, hearing, fine touch, and tremors that may have an impact on learning and ability to self-administer insulin. Suggest use of an insulin pen or magnifying glass to assist with drawing up insulin. Pen must be inverted 10 times to ensure mixing.

4. Review dosage and time of injections in relation to meals, activity, and bedtime based on patient's individualized insulin regimen.

Preventing Injury Secondary to Hypoglycemia

1. Closely monitor blood glucose levels to detect hypoglycemia.
2. Instruct patient in the importance of accuracy in insulin preparation and meal timing to avoid hypoglycemia.
3. Assess patient for the signs and symptoms of hypoglycemia.
   a. Adrenergic (early symptoms)—sweating, tremor, pallor, tachycardia, palpitations, nervousness from the release of adrenalin when blood glucose falls rapidly.
   b. Neurologic (later symptoms)—light-headedness, headache, confusion, irritability, slurred speech, lack of coordination, staggering gait from depression of central nervous system as glucose level progressively falls.
4. Treat hypoglycemia promptly using the 15-gm/15-minute rule according to the ADA with 15 g of rapidly absorbed carbohydrates.
   a. One-half cup (4 oz) juice, 1 cup skim milk, three glucose tablets, four sugar cubes, five to six pieces of hard candy may be taken orally.
   b. Wait 15 minutes.
   c. Repeat blood glucose; if less than 70 mg/dL, repeat the treatment.
   d. If more than 70 mg/dL and more than 3 hours since last dose of rapid-acting insulin, no further treatment required.
   e. If more than 70 but less than 3 hours since last dose of rapid-acting insulin, follow with a snack of 75 to 100 calories.

INTERVENTION	PREVENTION/TEACHING
• Injected glucagon is the best treatment when the patient resists treatment, becomes unconscious, or has seizures due to hypoglycemia.	• Carry glucose tablets/gel at all times to quickly and appropriately raise blood sugar levels. • All patients using intensive insulin management should have glucagon emergency kits and their family members must know how and when to administer. • Patients will need to closely match insulin doses to diet and exercise. They may need to reduce their insulin doses during and for several hours following increased physical activity. • Avoid alcohol or limit to no more than 1 to 2 drinks per day and never drink on an empty stomach. • Patients should wear a MedicAlert ID at all times to facilitate appropriate treatment by emergency personnel.

f. If using a "split-mix" or REG/NPH insulins and more than 30 minutes before next planned meal/snack, have snack now.

i. Nutrition bar specially designed for diabetics—supplies glucose from sucrose, starch, and protein sources with some fat to delay gastric emptying and prolong effect; may prevent relapse. Used after hypoglycemia treated with fast-acting carbohydrate.

g. Glucagon 1 mg (SubQ or I.M.) is given if the patient cannot ingest a sugar treatment. Family member or staff must administer injection.

h. IV bolus of 50 mL of 50% dextrose solution can be given if the patient fails to respond to glucagon within 15 minutes.

5. Encourage patient to carry a portable treatment for hypoglycemia at all times.

 DRUG ALERT If the patient is taking an alpha-glucosidase inhibitor, must use a monosaccharide (glucose tablets) to treat hypoglycemia because sucrose will not be broken down to an absorbable sugar.

6. Assess patient for cognitive or physical impairments that may interfere with ability to accurately administer insulin.

7. Between-meal snacks as well as extra food taken before exercise should be encouraged to prevent hypoglycemia.

8. Encourage patients to wear an identification bracelet or card that may assist in prompt treatment in a hypoglycemic emergency.
   a. Identification bracelet can be obtained from MedicAlert Foundation International (*www.medicalert.org*).
   b. Identification card may be requested from the ADA (*www.diabetes.org*).

9. If hypoglycemia occurs frequently, please discuss with health care provider. Dose adjustments of insulin and/or oral medications may be necessary.

10. Address safety issues if patient has hypoglycemic attacks—driving, operating machinery, and exertional activity. Cognitive recovery takes 45 to 75 minutes following blood glucose levels of less than 50 mg/dL.

Improving Activity Tolerance

1. Advise patient to assess blood glucose level before and after strenuous exercise.
2. Instruct patient to plan exercises on a regular basis each day.
3. Encourage patient to eat a carbohydrate snack before exercising to avoid hypoglycemia.
4. Advise patient that prolonged strenuous exercise may require increased food at bedtime to avoid nocturnal hypoglycemia.
5. Instruct patient to avoid exercise whenever blood glucose levels exceed 250 mg/day and urine ketones are present. Patient should contact health care provider if levels remain elevated.
6. Counsel patient to inject insulin into the abdominal site on days when arms or legs are exercised.

Providing Information About Oral Antidiabetic Agents

1. Identify barriers to learning, such as visual or hearing impairments, low literacy, distractive environment.
2. Encourage active participation of the patient and family in the educational process.
3. Teach the action, use, and adverse effects of oral antidiabetic agents (see page 954).
4. Identify financial barriers to accessing medications and follow-up care. Offer resources such as Partnership for Prescription Assistance (*www.PPARx.org*).

Maintaining Skin Integrity

1. Assess feet and legs for skin temperature, sensation, soft tissue injuries, corns, calluses, dryness, hammertoe or bunion deformation, hair distribution, pulses, deep tendon reflexes.
   a. Use a monofilament to test sensation of the feet and detect early signs of peripheral neuropathy (see Figure 25-2).
   b. Test vibratory sense over interphalangeal joints of the feet using a low-frequency (128 Hz) tuning fork. Vibratory sense is typically lost before tactile sensation. The test is considered abnormal if the vibratory sensation is felt for less than 10 seconds.

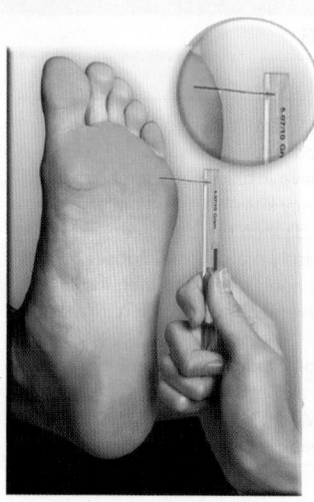 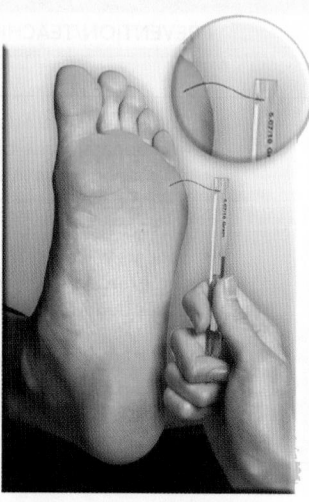 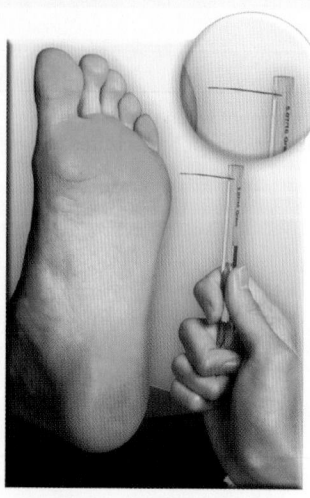 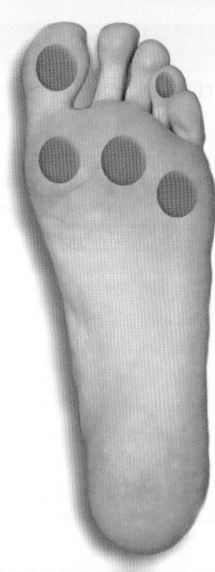

1 Holding the monofilament perpendicular to the skin, touch an area to be tested.

2 Apply pressure so that the monofilament buckles.

3 Release the monofilament from skin within 1.5 seconds.

Repeat on the other testing areas (above) in random order, returning to an area if it did not receive a "yes" response.

Figure 25-2. The Semmes-Weinstein 5.07 (10-gm) monofilament test.

2. Maintain skin integrity by protecting feet from breakdown.
   a. Use heel protectors, special mattresses, foot cradles for patients on bed rest.
   b. Avoid applying drying agents to skin (eg, alcohol).
   c. Apply skin moisturizers (preferably creams) to maintain suppleness and prevent cracking and fissures.
3. Instruct patient in foot care guidelines (see Procedure Guidelines 25-3).
4. Advise the patient who smokes to stop smoking, or reduce if possible, to reduce vasoconstriction and enhance peripheral blood flow. Help patient to establish behavior modification techniques to eliminate smoking in the hospital and to continue them at home for smoking-cessation program.

Improving Coping Strategies
1. Discuss with the patient the perceived effect of diabetes on lifestyle, finances, family life, occupation.
2. Explore previous coping strategies and skills that have had positive effects.
3. Encourage patient and family participation in diabetes self-care regimen to foster confidence.
4. Identify available support groups to assist in lifestyle adaptation. Refer to a certified diabetes educator.
5. Assist family in providing emotional support.

Community and Home Care Considerations
1. A home care or visiting nurse referral can be initiated to follow up on patient education initiated in the hospital or clinic and ensure that the patient has the resources to care for self at home.
2. Patient should be checking fingerstick glucose at home, and glucometer should be checked by home care or clinic nurse periodically to make sure it is properly calibrated and correlates with meter used at clinic or hospital.
3. As long as the home is clean and the patient uses reasonable hygiene, procedures for glucose self-monitoring and insulin injection do not need to be sterile. No alcohol preparation of the skin or insulin vial is needed.
4. Assist patients with choosing the diabetes self-care products and devices that best meet their needs/circumstances. An annual update is available at *www.forecast.diabetes.org/consumerguide.*
5. Insulin syringes may be reused, so long as the needle is kept clean and no pain or signs of skin irritation develop after multiple uses.
6. Although urine glucose testing is no longer recommended to monitor diabetic condition, the patient may benefit from urine ketone testing, especially when ill. Teach the patient how to test urine with ketone test strip and to notify health care provider if ketosis persists.
7. Make sure that all patients have a handy source of glucose for hypoglycemic episodes. A small tube of glossy decorating gel for cakes, easily carried in a pocket or purse, contains about 15 g glucose and can be squirted in the mouth for fast absorption during a hypoglycemic attack.
8. Draw blood for analysis on a fasting basis (no food or fluids other than water for 8 hours) or ensure that patients attend laboratory appointments for drug monitoring.
   a. For patients taking thiazolidinediones, serum transaminases (aspartate aminotransferase and alanine aminotransferase) should be monitored every 2 months for a year and then periodically. If levels rise, more frequent monitoring and, possibly, drug discontinuation will be necessary.

PROCEDURE GUIDELINES 25-3

Foot Care Guidelines

Perform foot care and teach the patient the following guidelines.

EQUIPMENT

- Mirror (optional)
- Moisturizing lotion
- Scissors and nail file
- Magnifying glass (optional)
- Lamb's wool

PROCEDURE

Teaching Action	Rationale/Comment
1. Inspect the feet carefully and daily for calluses, corns, blisters, abrasions, redness, and nail abnormalities.	1. a. Use a small mirror to check bottom of each foot. b. Use a magnifying glass under good light if eyesight is poor, or have someone else check feet.
2. Bathe the feet daily in warm (never hot) water.	2. a. Do not soak the feet for prolonged periods (soaking is drying). b. Dry feet carefully, especially between the toes.
3. Massage the feet with an absorbable agent.	3. a. Use lanolin or a cream moisturizer, but avoid between the toes to prevent maceration.
4. Prevent moisture between the toes to prevent maceration of the skin.	4. a. Insert lamb's wool between overlapping toes. b. Use foot powder, especially if feet perspire.
5. Wear well-fitting, noncompressive shoes and socks—long enough, wide enough, soft, supple, and low-heeled.	5. a. Buy shoes with a wide toe box for room to wiggle toes without friction. b. Buy shoes in the afternoon—feet are larger in the afternoon than in the morning. c. Have each foot measured before buying shoes—feet enlarge with age. d. Have the measurement taken while standing because foot is larger in the standing position. e. Do not "break in" shoes all at one time. f. Avoid rubber- or plastic-soled shoes or vinyl shoes, which cause the feet to perspire and aggravate fungal infections. g. Avoid walking in soft-soled bedroom slippers or other nonsupportive footwear.
6. Go to a podiatrist on a regular basis if corns, calluses, and ingrown toenails are present.	6. a. Trim toenails straight across to prevent ingrown toenails. b. File any rough corners with an emery board.
7. Avoid heat, chemicals, and injuries to the feet.	7. a. Do not go barefoot or expose feet to hot-water bottles, heating pads, caustic solutions. b. Check bath temperature with thermometer or elbow before bathing if neuropathy is present. c. Switch off electric blanket before going to bed; wear socks at night to keep feet warm, if necessary. d. Avoid sitting too close to a fire.
8. Inspect inside of shoes for foreign objects or areas of roughness.	8. a. Inspect seams and lining of shoes for possible areas of pressure or abrasion. b. Avoid the use of constricting sandals, high heels, or boots, which are more likely to cause injury.
9. Take action if an injury occurs to the foot.	9. a. Wash the area with mild soap and water. b. Cover with a dry sterile dressing without adhesive. c. Wear white cotton socks; dye in colored socks and wool may serve as irritants when skin is already irritated. d. Call health care provider.

PATIENT EDUCATION GUIDELINES 25-1

Diabetes Sick-Day Guidelines

- Never omit insulin dosage. Check with health care provider about oral medication. For instance, metformin should be withheld if vomiting or in danger of becoming dehydrated.
  - Take at least the usual dosage of insulin.
  - Keep regular insulin on hand for supplemental doses, as prescribed by health care provider.
- Monitor blood glucose and urine ketones every 2–4 hours.
  - Whenever blood glucose is >240 mg/dL, test urine ketones.
  - Record all test results.
- Drink plenty of fluids.
  - Six to 8 oz of fluid every hour is recommended, every third hour the fluid should include sodium (ie, broth).

- If unable to eat, drink fluids that contain carbohydrates (eg, fruit juices, regular soda); patient must consume 150–200 g of carbohydrates/day.
- Contact health care provider or report to nearest ER if illness becomes severe or unmanageable.
  - Fever, nausea, vomiting (>1 episode), and diarrhea (>5 episodes or for longer than 6 hours) increase risk of dehydration.
  - Signs and symptoms of infection—redness, swelling, drainage—need immediate attention.
  - Large amount of urine ketones or other signs and symptoms of diabetic ketoacidosis: call health care provider immediately.

---

b. Renal function tests (blood urea nitrogen [BUN] and serum creatinine) and urine for microalbumin or microalbumin/creatinine ratio will be monitored periodically.

c. Fasting plasma glucose and glycated hemoglobin are followed regularly.

d. Fasting lipid panel (12 to 14 hours fasting) is done periodically.

Patient Education and Health Maintenance

1. Ongoing education of patient to include advanced skills and rationales for treatment, prevention, and management of complications.

2. Educational focus—lifestyle management issues, to include sick-day management (see Patient Education Guidelines 25-1), exercise adjustments, travel preparations, foot care guidelines, intensive insulin management, and dietary considerations for dining out.

3. For additional information and support, refer to drug manufacturers' websites for special programs for diabetics and to agencies, such as ADA (*www.diabetes.org*) and American Dietetic Association (*www.eatright.org*).

Evaluation: Expected Outcomes

- Maintains ideal body weight with body mass index less than 25.
- Demonstrates self-injection of insulin with minimal fear.
- Hypoglycemia identified and treated appropriately.
- Exercises daily.
- Verbalizes appropriate use and action of oral hypoglycemic agents.
- No skin breakdown.
- Verbalizes initial strategies for coping with diabetes.

Diabetic Ketoacidosis

 Evidence Base Kitabchi, A. E., Guillermo, E. U., Miles, J. M., & Fisher, N. F. (2009). Hyperglycemic crises in adult patients with diabetes. *Diabetes Care*, *32*(7): 1335–1343.

Wolfsdorf, J., Glaser, N., & Sperling, M. A. (2006). Diabetic Ketoacidosis in infants, children and adolescents. A consensus statement from the American Diabetes Association. *Diabetes Care*, *29*(5), 1150–1159.

Diabetic ketoacidosis (DKA) is an acute complication of diabetes mellitus (usually type 1 diabetes) characterized by hyperglycemia, ketonuria, acidosis, and dehydration. Underlying infection is the most common cause of this acute complication.

Pathophysiology and Etiology

1. Insulin deficiency prevents glucose from being used for energy, forcing the body to metabolize fat for fuel.

2. Free fatty acids, released from the metabolism of fat, are converted to ketone bodies in the liver.

3. Ketone bodies are organic acids that cause metabolic acidosis.

4. Increase in the secretion of glucagon, catecholamines, growth hormone, and cortisol, in response to the hyperglycemia caused by insulin deficiency, accelerates the development of DKA.

5. Osmotic diuresis caused by hyperglycemia creates a shift in electrolytes, with losses in potassium, sodium, phosphate, and water.

6. Caused by inadequate amounts of endogenous or exogenous insulin.

   a. Commonly occurs due to failure to increase the dose of insulin during periods of stress (eg, infection, surgery, pregnancy).

   b. May occur in previously undiagnosed or untreated diabetics.

Clinical Manifestations

Early

1. Polydipsia, polyuria.
2. Fatigue, malaise, drowsiness.
3. Anorexia, nausea, vomiting.
4. Abdominal pain, muscle cramps.

Later

1. Kussmaul's respirations (deep respirations).
2. Fruity, sweet breath.

3. Hypotension, weak pulse.

4. Stupor and coma.

Diagnostic Evaluation

1. Serum glucose level is elevated over 250 mg/dL.

2. Serum and urine ketone bodies are present.

3. Serum bicarbonate and pH are decreased due to metabolic acidosis, and partial pressure of carbon dioxide is decreased as a respiratory compensation mechanism.

4. Serum sodium and potassium levels may be low, normal, or high due to fluid shifts and dehydration, despite total body depletion.

5. BUN, creatinine, hemoglobin, and hematocrit are elevated due to dehydration.

 NURSING ALERT Severity of DKA is not determined by serum glucose levels; the degree of acidosis determines severity of DKA.

6. Urine glucose is present in high concentration and specific gravity is increased, reflecting osmotic diuresis and dehydration.

Management

1. IV fluids to replace losses from osmotic diuresis, vomiting.

2. IV insulin drip—regular insulin infused only to increase glucose utilization and decrease lipolysis.

3. Electrolyte replacement—sodium chloride and phosphate as required, potassium chloride and bicarbonate based on laboratory results.

Complications

1. Premature discontinuation of IV insulin or the failure to initiate subcutaneous insulin injections prior to discontinuing IV insulin will result in rebound of DKA.

2. Too-rapid infusion of IV fluids in cases of severe dehydration can cause cerebral edema and death.

Nursing Assessment

1. Assess skin for dehydration—poor turgor, flushing, dry mucous membranes.

2. Observe for cardiac changes reflecting dehydration, metabolic acidosis, and electrolyte imbalance—hypotension; tachycardia; weak pulse; electrocardiographic changes, including elevated P wave, flattened T wave, or inverted, prolonged QT interval.

3. Assess respiratory status—Kussmaul's respirations, acetone breath characteristic of metabolic acidosis.

4. Perform GI assessment—nausea, vomiting, extreme thirst, abdominal bloating and cramping, diarrhea.

5. Determine GU symptoms—nocturia, polyuria.

6. Observe for neurologic signs—crying, restlessness, twitching, tremors, drowsiness, lethargy, headache, decreased reflexes.

7. Interview family or significant other regarding precipitating events to episode of DKA.

   a. Patient self-care management before hospitalization.

   b. Unusual events that may have precipitated episode (eg, chest pain, trauma, illness).

Nursing Diagnoses

- Deficient Fluid Volume related to hyperglycemia.
- Ineffective Therapeutic Regimen Management related to failure to increase insulin during illness.

Nursing Interventions

Restoring Fluid and Electrolyte Balance

1. Assess BP and heart rate frequently, depending on patient's condition; assess skin turgor and temperature.

2. Monitor intake and output every hour.

3. Replace fluids, as ordered, through peripheral IV line.

4. Monitor urine-specific gravity to assess fluid changes.

5. Monitor blood glucose frequently.

6. Assess for symptoms of hypokalemia—fatigue, anorexia, nausea, vomiting, muscle weakness, decreased bowel sounds, paresthesia, arrhythmias, flat T waves, ST-segment depression.

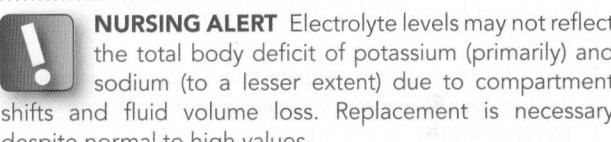 **NURSING ALERT** Electrolyte levels may not reflect the total body deficit of potassium (primarily) and sodium (to a lesser extent) due to compartment shifts and fluid volume loss. Replacement is necessary despite normal to high values.

7. Administer replacement electrolytes and insulin, as ordered. Flush the entire IV infusion set with solution containing insulin and discard the first 50 mL because plastic bags and tubing may absorb some insulin and the initial solution may contain decreased concentration of insulin.

 DRUG ALERT Interruption in insulin administration may result in reaccumulation of ketone bodies and worsening acidosis. Glucose will normalize before acidosis resolves, so IV insulin is continued until bicarbonate levels normalize and subcutaneous insulin takes effect and the patient starts eating.

8. Monitor serum glucose, bicarbonate, and pH levels periodically.

9. Provide reassurance about improvement of condition and that correction of fluid imbalance will help reduce discomfort.

Preventing Further Episodes of DKA

1. Review with patients precipitating events and causes of DKA.

2. Assist patient in identifying warning signs and symptoms of DKA.

3. Instruct patient on sick-day guidelines (see page 966).

Patient Education and Health Maintenance

1. Make sure that patient and caretakers can demonstrate drawing up and administering insulin in the proper dose, blood glucose monitoring, and urine ketone testing.

2. Make sure that patient and caretakers know whom to notify in the event of hyperglycemia, stressful situation, or symptoms of DKA.

Evaluation: Expected Outcomes

- BP and heart rate stable; glucose and bicarbonate levels improving.
- Verbalizes sick-day guidelines correctly.

Hyperosmolar Hyperglycemic State

 Evidence Base Kitabchi, A. E., Guillermo, E. U., Miles, J. M., & Fisher, N. F. (2009). Hyperglycemic crises in adult patients with diabetes. *Diabetes Care, 32*(7): 1335–1343.

The International Society of Pediatric and Adolescent Diabetes (ISPAD). (2009). ISPAD clinical practice consensus guidelines 2009 compendium. *Pediatric Diabetes, 10*(Suppl. 12).

Hyperosmolar hyperglycemic state (HHS) is an acute complication of diabetes mellitus (particularly type 2 diabetes) characterized by hyperglycemia, dehydration, and hyperosmolarity, with little or no ketosis. Underlying infection is the most common cause of this acute complication.

Pathophysiology and Etiology

1. Prolonged hyperglycemia with glucosuria produces osmotic diuresis.
2. Loss of water, sodium, and potassium results in severe dehydration, causing hypovolemia and hemoconcentration.
3. Hyperosmolarity is a result of excessive blood sugar and increasing sodium concentration in dehydration.
4. Insulin continues to be produced at a level that prevents ketosis.
5. Increased blood viscosity decreases blood flow to the organs, creating tissue hypoxia.
6. Intracellular fluid and electrolyte shifts produce neurologic signs and symptoms.
7. Caused by inadequate amounts of endogenous/exogenous insulin to control hyperglycemia.
   a. Precipitating event may occur, such as cardiac failure, burn, or chronic illness that increases need for insulin.
   b. Use of therapeutic agents that increase blood glucose levels (eg, glucocorticoids, immunosuppressive agents).
   c. Use of therapeutic procedures that cause stress or increase blood glucose levels (eg, hyperosmolar hyperalimentation, peritoneal dialysis).

Clinical Manifestations

Early
1. Polyuria, dehydration.
2. Fatigue, malaise.
3. Nausea, vomiting.

Later
1. Hypothermia.
2. Muscle weakness.
3. Seizures, stupor, coma.

Diagnostic Evaluation

1. Serum glucose and osmolality are greatly elevated, with glucose values usually >600 mg/dL.
2. Serum and urine ketone bodies are minimal to absent.
3. Serum sodium and potassium levels may be elevated, depending on degree of dehydration, despite total body losses.
4. BUN and creatinine may be elevated due to dehydration.
5. Urine-specific gravity is elevated due to dehydration.

Management

1. Correct fluid and electrolyte imbalances with IV fluids.
2. Provide insulin via IV drip to lower plasma glucose.
3. Evaluate complications, such as stupor, seizures, or shock, and treat appropriately.
4. Identify and treat underlying illnesses or events that precipitated HHNKS.

Complications

1. Too rapid infusion of IV fluids can cause cerebral edema and death.
2. HHS is a medical emergency that, if not treated properly, can cause death (10% to 50% mortality).
3. Patients who become comatose will need nasogastric (NG) tubes to prevent aspiration.

Nursing Assessment

1. Assess level of consciousness (LOC).
2. Assess for dehydration—poor turgor, flushing, dry mucous membranes.
3. Assess cardiovascular status for shock—rapid, thready pulse; cool extremities; hypotension; electrocardiogram changes.
4. Interview family or significant other regarding precipitating events to episode of HHS.
   a. Evaluate patient's self-care regimen before hospitalization.
   b. Determine events, treatments, or drugs that may have caused the event.

Nursing Diagnoses

- Deficient Fluid Volume related to severe dehydration.
- Risk for Aspiration related to reduced LOC and vomiting.

Nursing Interventions

Restoring Fluid Balance
1. Assess patient for increasing signs and symptoms of dehydration, hyperglycemia, or electrolyte imbalance.
2. Institute fluid replacement therapy, as ordered (usually normal or half-strength saline initially), maintaining patent IV line.
3. Assess patient for signs and symptoms of fluid overload and cerebral edema as IV therapy progresses.
4. Administer regular insulin IV, as ordered, and add dextrose to IV infusion as blood glucose falls below 300 mg/dL, to prevent hypoglycemia.
5. Monitor hydration status by monitoring hourly intake and output and urine-specific gravity.

Preventing Aspiration
1. Assess patient's LOC and ability to handle oral secretions.
   a. Cough and gag reflex.
   b. Ability to swallow.
2. Properly position patient to reduce possibility of aspiration.
   a. Elevate head of bed unless contraindicated.
   b. If nausea is present, use side-lying position.
3. Suction as frequently as needed to maintain patent airway.
4. Withhold oral intake until patient is no longer in danger of aspiration.
5. Insert NG tube as indicated for gastric decompression.

6. Monitor respiratory rate and breath sounds for signs of aspiration pneumonia.

7. Provide mouth care to maintain adequate mucosal hydration.

Patient Education and Health Maintenance

1. Advise patient and family that it may take 3 to 5 days for symptoms to resolve.

2. Instruct patient and family in signs and symptoms of hyperglycemia and use of sick-day guidelines (see page 966).

3. Explain possible causes of HHS.

4. Review changes in medication, activity, meal plan, or glucose monitoring for home care. It may not be necessary to continue insulin therapy following HHS; many patients can be treated with diet and oral agents.

Evaluation: Expected Outcomes

- BP stable, dehydration resolved.
- No evidence of aspiration.

Metabolic Syndrome

Metabolic syndrome (also known as syndrome X, insulin resistance syndrome, and dysmetabolic syndrome) has been used to characterize a state of insulin resistance. It is believed to be a major contributing factor to the development of a variety of significant health problems to include T2DM and cardiovascular disease.

The National Cholesterol Education Program's Adult Treatment Panel III criteria for metabolic syndrome—three or more of the following:

- Abdominal obesity: waist circumference > 102 cm (>40") in men; >88 cm (>35") in women.
- Hypertriglyceridemia: ≥150 mg/dL.
- Low HDL cholesterol: <40 mg/dL in men and <50 mg/dL in women.
- Elevated BP: ≥130/85 mm Hg.
- Elevated fasting glucose: ≥110 mg/dL.

 Evidence Base National Cholesterol Education Program (NCEP) Expert Panel on Detection, Evaluation, and Treatment of High Blood Cholesterol in Adults (Adult Treatment Panel III). (2002, Updated 2004). Third Report of the National Cholesterol Education Program (NCEP) Expert Panel on Detection, Evaluation, and Treatment of High Blood Cholesterol in Adults (Adult Treatment Panel III). final report. *Circulation, 106*, 3143–421.

Pathophysiology and Etiology

1. The central feature of this metabolic disorder is the diminished responsiveness of peripheral tissues to circulating insulin.

2. The typical physiological response of the body to this condition is the increased production and secretion of insulin, leading to a state of compensatory hyperinsulinemia in order to maintain glucose homeostasis.

3. Although this response is beneficial from the standpoint of glucose metabolism, it is now believed that the state of hyperinsulinemia necessary to prevent glucose intolerance gives rise to other abnormalities that can also have significant health consequences.

4. In addition to increased risk of type 2 diabetes associated with insulin resistance, hyperinsulinemia has also been associated with the development of hypertension, hyperlipidemia, atherosclerotic cardiovascular disease, cerebrovascular disease, polycystic ovary syndrome (PCOS), and acanthosis nigricans.

5. Because these clinical features are associated with insulin resistance, the term "syndrome" has been applied to signify that these conditions are linked to a common problem.

6. Although the pathogenesis of insulin resistance is not fully understood, genetic factors and environmental factors, such as obesity and physical inactivity, are believed to play an important role in the development and natural course of this condition.

Risk Factors

1. Diagnosis of type 2 diabetes, cardiovascular disease, PCOS, hypertension, hyperlipidemia, or acanthosis nigricans.

2. History of glucose intolerance or gestational diabetes.

3. Family history of type 2 diabetes, cardiovascular disease, or hypertension.

4. Sedentary lifestyle.

5. Obesity.

Management

1. Treatment of metabolic syndrome involves measures that are directed at treating any diagnosed disease resulting from insulin resistance (diabetes, hypertension, hypercholesterolemia) as well as the underlying insulin resistance. This is accomplished by interventions that improve insulin sensitivity.

2. Nonpharmacologic interventions effective in reducing insulin resistance include lifestyle changes that can have a direct impact on insulin sensitivity and include regular physical activity and nutritional management designed to reduce body weight.

3. No pharmacologic agents have been FDA-approved for use in the treatment of metabolic syndrome. However, metformin is being used more frequently, especially if the risk for develop T2DM is very high. Other agents currently available with known insulin-sensitizing effects (ie, thiazolidinedione compounds) have shown effectiveness in treating individuals with PCOS and type 2 diabetes. The potential role of these agents in the management of metabolic syndrome is under investigation.

SELECTED REFERENCES

ACCORD (Action to Control Cardiovascular Risk in Diabetes) Study Group. (2008). Effects of intensive glucose lowering in type 2 diabetes. *New England Journal of Medicine, 358*(24), 2545–2559.

ADVANCE (Action in Diabetes and Vascular Disease: Preterax and Diamicron Modified Release Controlled Evaluation) Collaborative Group. (2008). Intensive blood glucose control and vascular outcomes in patients with type 2 diabetes. *New England Journal of Medicine, 358*(24), 2560–2572.

American Association of Clinical Endocrinologists. (2011). Medical guidelines for clinical practice for developing a diabetes mellitus comprehensive care plan. *Endocrine Practice, 17*(Suppl. 2), 1–53.

American Association of Diabetes Educators (AADE). (2012). Diabetes and physical activity (AADE position statement). *The Diabetes Educator, 38*(1), 129–132.

American College of Obstetricians and Gynecologists (ACOG). (2011). Screening and diagnosis of gestational diabetes mellitus: Committee Opinion No. 504. *Obstetrics & Gynecology, 118*(3), 751–753.

American Diabetes Association. (2012). Standards of medical care in diabetes (position statement). *Diabetes Care, 35*(Suppl. 1), S1–S110.

Beneck, J. (2011). Management of diabetic ketoacidosis in adults. *The Clinical Advisor, 14*(11), 33–40.

Blount, A., & Largay, J. (2011). Insulin pump therapy for the patient with diabetes. *Clinician Reviews, 21*(11), 26–31.

Centers for Disease Control and Prevention. (2010). National chronic kidney disease fact sheet: General information and national estimates on chronic kidney disease in the United States, 2010. Available: *www.cdc.gov/diabetes/pubs/factsheets/kidney.htm*.

Centers for Disease Control and Prevention. (2011). National diabetes fact sheet: National estimates and general information on diabetes and prediabetes in the United States, 2011. Available: *www.cdc.gov/diabetes/pubs/pdf/ndfs_2011.pdf*.

Chau, P. H., Woo, J., Lee, C. H., et al. (2011). Older people with diabetes have higher risk of depression, cognitive and functional impairments: Implications for diabetes services. *Journal of Nutrition, Health and Aging, 15*(9), 751–755.

Chobanian, A. V., Bakris, G. L., Black, H. R., et al. (2003). The seventh report of the Joint National Committee on Prevention, Detection, Evaluation, and Treatment of High Blood Pressure: The JNC 7 report. *Journal of the American Medical Association, 289*, 2560–2572.

Colagiuri, S. (2012). Optimal management of type 2 diabetes: the evidence. *Diabetes, Obesity and Metabolism, 14*(Suppl. 1), 3–8.

D'Adamo, E., & Caprio, S. (2011). Type 2 diabetes in youth: Epidemiology and pathophysiology. *Diabetes Care, 34*(Suppl. 2), S161–S165.

Diabetes Prevention Program Research Group. (2002). Reduction in the incidence of type 2 diabetes with lifestyle intervention of metformin. *New England Journal of Medicine, 346*(6), 393–403.

Dickman, K., Pintz, C., Gold, K., et al. (2012). Behavior changes in patients with diabetes and hypertension after experiencing shared medical appointments. *Journal of the American Academy of Nurse Practitioners, 24*, 43–51.

Duckworth, W., Abraira, C., Moritz, T., et al. (2009). Glucose control and vascular complications in veterans with type 2 diabetes. *New England Journal of Medicine, 360*(2), 129–139.

Fowler, M. (2011). Microvascular and macrovascular complications of diabetes. *Clinical Diabetes, 29*(3), 116–122.

Franciosi, M., Lucisano, G., Pellegrini, F., et al. (2011). ROSES: Role of self-monitoring of blood glucose and intensive education in patients with type 2 diabetes not receiving insulin. A pilot randomized clinical trial. *Diabetic Medicine, 28*(7), 789–796.

Franz, M. J. (2012). Nutrition therapy for diabetes: effectiveness, carbohydrates and alcohol. *Expert Review of Endocrinology & Metabolism, 7*(6), 647–657.

Frid, A., Hirsch, L., Gaspar, R., et al. (2010). New injection recommendations for patients with diabetes. *Diabetes and Metabolism, 36*(Suppl. 2), S3–S18.

Giugliano, D., Maiorino, M. I., Bellastella, G., et al. (2011). Treatment regimens with insulin and haemoglobin A1C target of < 7% in type 2 diabetes: A systematic review. *Diabetes Research and Clinical Practice, 92*(1), 1–10.

Global International Diabetes Federation (IDF)/International Society of Pediatric and Adolescent Diabetes (ISPAD). (2011). Guideline for diabetes in childhood and adolescence. Available: *www.ispad.org/NewsFiles/IDF-ISPAD_Diabetes_in_Childhood_and%20Adolescence_Guidelines_2011.pdf*

Hanson, B., & Matytsina, I. (2011). Insulin administration: Selecting the appropriate needle and individualizing the injection technique. *Expert Opinion on Drug Delivery, 8*(10), 1395–1406.

Hemmingsen, B, Lund, S. S., Gluud, C., et al. (2011). Targeting intensive glycaemic control versus targeting conventional glycaemic control for type 2 diabetes mellitus. *Cochrane Database of Systematic Reviews*, Issue 6 (Article No. CD008143)

Hughes, L. (2012). Think "SAFE": Four crucial elements for diabetes education. *Nursing, 42*(1), 58–61.

Kitabchi, A. E., Guillermo, E. U., Miles, J. M., & Fisher, N. F. (2009). Hyperglycemic crises in adult patients with diabetes. *Diabetes Care, 32*(7): 1335–1343.

Kitabchi, A., & Rose, B. (2012). Clinical features and diagnosis of diabetic ketoacidosis and hyperosmolar hyperglycemic state in adults. In D. Basow (Ed.), *UpToDate*. Available: *www.uptodateonline.com*.

Klonoff, D. C., Blonde, L., Cembrowski, G., et al. (2011). Consensus report: The current role of self-monitoring of blood glucose in non-insulin-treated type 2 diabetes. *Journal of Diabetes Science and Technology, 5*(6), 1529–1548.

Kruegel, G., Keers, J. C., Kerstens, M. N., et al. (2011). Randomization trial on the influence of the length of two insulin pen needles on glycemic control and patient preference in obese patients with diabetes. *Diabetes Technology and Therapeutics, 13*(7), 737–741.

Laffel, L., & Svoren, B. (2012). Management of type 2 diabetes mellitus in children and adolescents. In D. Basow (Ed.), *UpToDate*. Available: *www.uptodateonline.com*.

Laffel, L., & Svoren, B. (2012). Comorbidities and complications of type 2 diabetes mellitus in children and adolescents. In J. Wolfsdorf (Ed.), *UpToDate*. Available: *www.uptodateonline.com*.

Laffel, L., & Svoren, B. (2012). Epidemiology, presentation, and diagnosis of type 2 diabetes mellitus in children and adolescents. In D. Basow (Ed.), *UpToDate*. Available: *www.uptodateonline.com*.

Marette, A., & Sweeney, G. (2011). Cardiovascular complications of diabetes: Recent insights in pathophysiology and therapeutics. *Expert Review of Endocrinology and Metabolism, 6*(5), 689–696.

Mayer-Davis, E. J., Bell, R. A., Dabelea, D., et al. (2009). The many faces of diabetes in American youth: Type 1 and type 2 diabetes in five race and ethnic populations. *Diabetes Care, 32*(Suppl. 2), S99–S101.

McCoy, E., & Wright, B. (2010). A review of insulin pen devices. *Postgraduate Medicine, 122*(3), 81–88.

McCrindle, B. W, Urbina, E. M., Dennison, B. A., et al. (2007). Drug therapy of high-risk lipid abnormalities in children and adolescents: A scientific statement from the American Heart Association Atherosclerosis, Hypertension, and Obesity in Youth Committee, Council of Cardiovascular Disease in the Young, with the Council on Cardiovascular Nursing. *Circulation, 115*, 1948–1967.

National Cholesterol Education Program (NCEP) Expert Panel on Detection, Evaluation, and Treatment of High Blood Cholesterol in Adults (Adult Treatment Panel III). (2002, Update 2004). Third Report of the National Cholesterol Education Program (NCEP) Expert Panel on Detection, Evaluation, and Treatment of High Blood Cholesterol in Adults (Adult Treatment Panel III). Final report. *Circulation, 106*, 3143–3421. Available: *www.nhlbi.nih.gov/guidelines/cholesterol/atp3_rpt.htm*.

National Kidney Foundation. KDOQI™. (2007). Clinical practice guidelines and clinical practice recommendations for diabetes and chronic kidney disease. *American Journal of Kidney Disease, 49*(Suppl. 2), S1–S180. Available: *www.kidney.org/professionals/kdoqi*.

Pickup, J. (Ed.). (2009). *Insulin pump therapy and continuous glucose monitoring*. New York: Oxford University Press.

Polonsky, W., Fisher, L., Schikman, C. H., et al. (2011). Structured self-monitoring of blood glucose significantly reduces A1C levels in poorly controlled, noninsulin-treated type 2 diabetes. Results from the Structured Testing Program study. *Diabetes Care, 34*(2), 262–267.

Pornet, C., Bourdel-Marchasson, I., Lecomte, P., et al. (2011). Trends in the quality of care for elderly people with type 2 diabetes: The need for improvements in safety and quality (the 2001 and 2007 ENTRED Surveys). *Diabetes and Metabolism, 37*(2), 152–161.

Rewers, M., Pihoker, C., Donaghue, K., et al. (2009). Assessment and monitoring of glycemic control in children and adolescents with diabetes. *Pediatric Diabetes, 10*(Suppl. 12), 71–81.

Reynolds, K., & Helgeson, V. (2011). Children with diabetes compared to peers: Depressed? Distressed? A meta-analytic review. *Annals of Behavioral Medicine, 42*(1), 29–41.

Segal, A. R., Brunner, J. E., Burch, F. T., et al. (2010). Use of concentrated insulin human regular (U-500) for patients with diabetes. *American Journal of Health-System Pharmacy, 67*(18), 1526–1535.

Shane-McWhorter, L. (2012). Dietary supplements and probiotics for diabetes. *AJN, 112*(7), 47–53.

Skyler, J., Bergenstal, R., Bonow, R. O., et al. (2009). Intensive glycemic control and the prevention of cardiovascular events: Implications of the ACCORD, ADVANCE, and VA Diabetes trials: A position statement of the American Diabetes Association and a scientific statement of the American College of Cardiology Foundation and the American Heart Association. *Diabetes Care, 32*(1), 187–192.

UK Prospective Diabetes Study Group. (1998). Intensive blood-glucose control with sulfonylureas or insulin compared with conventional treatment and risk of complications in patients with type 2 diabetes (UKPDS 33). *Lancet, 352*, 837–853.

Wolfsdorf, J., Glaser, N., & Sperling, M. A. (2006). Diabetic Ketoacidosis in infants, children and adolescents. A consensus statement from the American Diabetes Association. *Diabetes Care, 29*(5), 1150–1159.

Writing Group for the SEARCH for Diabetes in Youth Study Group, Dabelea, D., Bell, R. A., et al. (2007). Incidence of diabetes in youth in the United States. *Journal of the American Medical Association, 297*(24), 2716–2724.

Zinszer, K., Mulhern, J. L., & Kareem, A. A. (2011). The implementation of the chronic care model with respect to dealing with the biopsychosocial aspects of the chronic diseaseof diabetes. *Skin and Wound Care, 24*(10), 475–484.

Zisser, H., Gong, P., Kelley, C. M., et al. (2011). Exercise and diabetes. *International Journal of Clinical Practice, 65*(Issue Suppl.), 71–75.

26
Hematologic Disorders

OVERVIEW AND ASSESSMENT

Blood, the body fluid circulating through the heart, arteries, capillaries, and veins, consists of plasma and cellular components. The average male adult has about 5.5 L of blood, the average female 4.5 L. Plasma, the fluid portion, accounts for 55% of the blood volume and is composed of 92% water, 7% protein, and 1% inorganic salts; nonprotein organic substances such as urea; dissolved gases; hormones; and enzymes. Plasma proteins include albumin, fibrinogen, and globulins. Cellular components include erythrocytes (red blood cells [RBCs]), leukocytes and lymphocytes (white blood cells [WBCs]), and platelets. These cells are derived from pluripotent stem cells in the bone marrow, a process known as hematopoiesis (see Figure 26-1). Under normal conditions, only mature cells are found in circulating blood. The cellular components of blood account for 45% of the blood volume.

Characteristics of Cellular Components

Blood has multiple functions that are carried out by plasma or the cellular components (see Table 26-1, page 973).

Erythrocytes (RBCs)

1. Enucleated, biconcave disc.
2. Approximately 5 million erythrocytes per cubic millimeter of blood.
3. Cell contents consist primarily of hemoglobin, essential for oxygen transport. Whole blood contains 14 to 15 g of hemoglobin per 100 mL of blood.
4. Circulate about 115 to 130 days before elimination by reticuloendothelial system, primarily in spleen and liver.

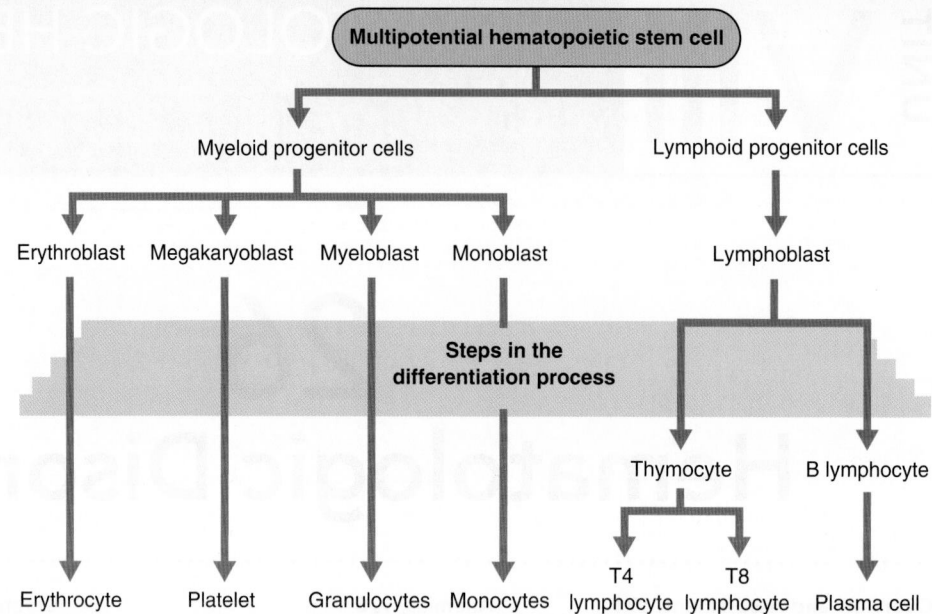

Figure 26-1. Steps in differentiation of blood cells.

Leukocytes (WBCs)

See Table 26-2.

1. Approximately 5,000 to 10,000 leukocytes (WBCs) per cubic millimeter of blood.
2. Classified as granulocytes or mononuclear leukocytes.
   a. Granulocytes account for about 70% of all WBCs; have abundant granules in cytoplasm; include neutrophils, basophils, and eosinophils.
   b. Mononuclear leukocytes have single-lobed nucleus and granule-free cytoplasm; include monocytes and lymphocytes.

Platelets (Thrombocytes)

1. Approximately 150,000 to 450,000 platelets per cubic millimeter of blood.
2. Small particles without nuclei arise as a result of budding from giant cells (megakaryocytes) in bone marrow.
3. Primary function is to control bleeding through hemostasis.

Subjective and Objective Data

The patient who presents with a hematologic disorder may have a disruption of the hematologic, immune, or coagulation system, producing a diverse array of symptoms and physical examination findings. Patients commonly present with vague complaints of fatigue, frequent infections, swollen glands, and bleeding tendencies. Characterize these complaints and obtain a review of systems, concentrating on the neurologic, respiratory, cardiovascular, GI, genitourinary (GU), and integumentary systems to look for more clues of hematologic dysfunction. Perform a systematic physical examination, paying careful attention to the cardiovascular, respiratory, and integumentary systems.

Review of Systems

1. Skin and mucous membranes: Any bruises, infections, drainage, or bleeding from wound sites?
2. Neurologic: Any dizziness, tingling or numbness (paresthesia), headache, forgetfulness or confusion, difficulty walking (disturbance in gait), tiredness (fatigue), weakness?
3. Respiratory: Experiencing shortness of breath, especially on exertion?
4. Cardiovascular: Chest pain or feelings of funny heartbeats (palpitations)?
5. GI: Any bleeding from gums, abdominal pain, black stools, or blood-streaked vomit (emesis)? Any mouth sores, rectal pain, or diarrhea?
6. GU: Excessive menstrual flow? Any blood in urine or discomfort on urination?

Key History Questions

1. What are your present medications? Do you take over-the-counter (OTC) medications, vitamins, herbals, or nutritional supplements? What else have you taken in the past several months?
2. What medical problems have you had in the past? Any surgeries? Ask specifically about partial or total gastrectomy, splenic injury or splenectomy, tendency to bleed (eg, with dental procedures), infectious diseases, human immunodeficiency virus (HIV) infection, cancer.
3. What is your occupation? Ask about exposure to substances such as benzene, pesticides, and ionizing radiation.
4. Do you have a family history of hematologic or malignant disorder?
5. Determine the social history and lifestyle. Do you use illicit drugs or alcohol? What is your pattern of sexual activity?

Table 26-1 Functions of Blood

METHOD	INVOLVED	CELLS AND SUBSTANCES FUNCTION
Oxygen and carbon dioxide transport	Binding to hemoglobin; dissolved in plasma	• Erythrocyte • Hemoglobin • Plasma
Nutrient and metabolite transport	Bound to plasma proteins; dissolved in plasma	• Plasma proteins • Plasma
Hormone transport	In plasma	• Plasma
Transport of waste products to kidneys and liver	In plasma	• Plasma
Transport of cells and substances involved in immune reactions	In plasma to site of infection or foreign body	• Granulocytes • Monocytes • Lymphocytes • Immunoglobulins • Other substances
Clotting at breaks in blood vessels	Hemostasis	• Platelets • Clotting factors
Maintenance of fluid balance	Blood volume regulation	• Water • Electrolytes
Body temperature regulation	Peripheral vasoconstriction or dilation	—
Maintenance of acid-base balance	Acid-base regulation	• Electrolytes

Table 26-2 Characteristics of White Blood Cells

CELL	MAJOR FUNCTION	PHYSICAL CHARACTERISTICS
Neutrophil	Ingest and destroy microorganisms (phagocytosis)	Small cell, multilobed nucleus, most plentiful leukocyte
Eosinophil	Host resistance to helminthic infections; also allergic response	Bi-lobed nucleus; red-staining granules
Basophil	Allergic response	Bi-lobed nucleus; granules containing heparin and histamine
Monocyte	Phagocytosis	Large cell, kidney-shaped nucleus
B lymphocyte	Produce antibodies (immunoglobulins); humoral immunity	Small, agranular
T lymphocyte	Regulation of immune response; cellular immunity	Small, agranular; include cytotoxic, helper (T4) and suppressor (T8) T cells; identified by surface markers

Key Examination Findings

1. Dyspnea; shiny smooth tongue; ataxia; pallor of conjunctivae, nail beds, lips, and oral mucosa—suggest anemia.
2. Decreased blood pressure (BP), tachycardia, possibly altered level of consciousness (LOC)—suggest anemia or altered blood clotting.
3. Hematuria, tarry stools, petechiae, bleeding sites—suggest altered clotting.
4. Fever; tachycardia; abnormal breath sounds; delirium; oral lesions; erythema, swelling, tenderness, and drainage of the skin—suggest infection.

Laboratory Studies

Laboratory studies routinely done for patients with hematologic disorders include complete blood count (CBC), blood smear, and iron profile. Blood samples for these tests are most accurate when obtained by venipuncture (see Procedure Guidelines 26-1, pages 974 to 975).

Complete Blood Count

Description

1. Generally includes absolute numbers or percentages of erythrocytes, leukocytes, platelets, hemoglobin, and hematocrit in blood sample.
   a. Erythrocyte (RBC) indices—can be done to provide information on the size, hemoglobin concentration, and hemoglobin weight of an average RBC; aids in diagnosis and classification of anemias.
   b. Leukocyte (WBC) differential—can be done to determine the percentage of each type of granulocyte (neutrophils, eosinophils, and basophils) and nongranulocytes (lymphocytes and monocytes).
2. Absolute value of each is determined by multiplying the percentage by the total number of WBCs.
3. Used to evaluate infection or potential for infection and identify various types of leukemia.

Nursing and Patient Care Considerations

Blood sample can be drawn at any time without fasting or patient preparation.

Blood Smear

Description

Blood sample prepared for microscopic viewing using appropriate stains, allowing visual analysis of numbers and characteristics of cells; can identify abnormal cells of certain anemias, leukemias, and other disorders that affect the bloodstream.

PROCEDURE GUIDELINES 26-1

Obtaining Blood by Venipuncture

EQUIPMENT

- Chlorhexidine-alcohol (if blood cultures will be obtained) or 70% alcohol
- Dry sterile gauze pads
- Vacutainer or syringe

- 20G needles or equivalent "needleless" supplies
- Blood tubes
- Disposable gloves

PROCEDURE

Nursing Action	Rationale
Performance phase	
1. Reassure the patient. Explain that relatively little blood will be taken.	1. Allays anxiety and enlists cooperation.
2. Wash hands and put on gloves.	2. Universal precautions.
3. Instruct the patient to extend arm; the arm should be held straight at the elbow.	3. Exposes antecubital area.
4. Apply the tourniquet directly above the elbow (or targeted vein) with just sufficient pressure to prevent venous return.	4. Increases venous pressure and makes the vein more prominent and easier to enter.
5. Inspect the area to visualize the vein, including the antecubital area, wrist, dorsum (back) of hand, and top of foot (if necessary). Palpate the vein.	5. Select a vein that is visible, palpable, and well fixed to surrounding tissue so that it does not roll away. (Some veins may be deep and can only be palpated.)
6. Clean the skin with chlorhexidine-alcohol or alcohol. Allow to dry.	6. Sterile procedures.
7. Fix chosen vein with the thumb and draw the skin taut immediately below the site before inserting needle to stabilize the vein.	7. The vein may roll beneath the skin when the needle approaches its outer surface (especially in older and extremely thin patients).
8. Hold the syringe or Vacutainer between the thumb and last three fingers with the bevel of the needle up and directly in line with the course of the vein. Insert the needle quickly and smoothly under the skin and into the vein.	8. A pop may be felt as the needle enters the vein.

 Key Decision Point

If a pop is not heard, gently reposition the needle. If a pop is still not heard, a hematoma becomes visible, or blood does not flow into tube when inserted into vacutainer, release the tourniquet and remove the needle. Try an alternate site.

Nursing Action	Rationale
9. Insert tube into Vacutainer and allow to fill. For syringe, gently pull back on the plunger until desired amount of blood is obtained.	9. Use minimal suction on syringe to prevent hemolysis of blood and collapse of the vein.
10. Release the tourniquet as soon as specimen is obtained, then remove tube from Vacutainer.	
11. Withdraw the needle slowly.	11. Slow withdrawal of the needle is less painful.
12. Apply a dry sterile gauze pad to puncture site and request patient to apply gentle but firm pressure to site for 2–4 minutes.	12. Firm pressure over the puncture site prevents leakage of blood into surrounding tissues with subsequent hematoma development.
13. Make a blood smear from the needle, if ordered.	13. Physical characteristics of blood cells can be observed under the microscope.
14. If blood was obtained in a syringe, use needleless supplies per facility procedure and gently eject the blood sample into tubes.	14. Slow transfer of blood into the test tube without forming bubbles prevents hemolysis, which may alter results.

PROCEDURE GUIDELINES 26-1 *(continued)*

Obtaining Blood by Venipuncture

PROCEDURE *(continued)*

Nursing Action	Rationale
15. Invert the tube gently several times to mix blood with anticoagulant, if present.	15. For some tests, the blood is allowed to coagulate in the test tube.
16. Label samples correctly and send to laboratory immediately.	16. Samples should be sent to the laboratory with a minimum of delay for optimum reliability.
17. Dispose needle and syringe in appropriate containers to avoid possible spread of blood-borne viral diseases. Clean spills with 10% bleach solution. Remove gloves and wash hands.	17. Bleach will kill any pathogens, such as HIV.

Nursing and Patient Care Considerations

Can be done from blood sample drawn for CBC; no additional sample or patient preparation is necessary.

Iron Profile

Description

Test completed on blood sample that generally includes levels of serum ferritin, iron, total iron-binding capacity, folate, vitamin B_{12}; used to determine type and severity of anemia.

Nursing and Patient Care Considerations

Recent administration of chloramphenicol, hormonal contraceptives, iron supplements, and corticotropin may affect results of serum iron and iron-binding capacity. No patient preparation needed.

Other Diagnostic Procedures

Bone Marrow Aspiration

Description

1. Aspiration of bone marrow from the iliac crest or (rarely) sternum to obtain specimen to examine microscopically and to perform a biopsy (see Procedure Guidelines 26-2, page 976).
2. Purposes include diagnosis of hematologic disorders; monitoring of course of illness and response to treatment; diagnosis of other disorders, such as primary and metastatic tumors, infectious diseases, and certain granulomas; and isolation of bacteria and other pathogens by culture.

Nursing and Patient Care Considerations

1. Give medication for pain and anxiety before or after the procedure, as ordered. A bone marrow aspiration with biopsy is more painful and may require use of mild to moderate sedation with appropriate monitoring.
2. Watch for bleeding and hematoma formation after procedure.

Lymph Node Biopsy

Description

1. Surgical excision or needle aspiration usually of a superficial lymph node in the cervical, supraclavicular, axillary, or inguinal region.
2. Performed to determine the cause of lymph node enlargement, to distinguish between benign and malignant lymph node tumors, and to stage metastatic carcinoma.

Nursing and Patient Care Considerations

1. Local anesthetic is usually given.
2. Specimen is placed in normal saline or 10% formaldehyde solution for transportation to the laboratory for cytologic and histologic evaluation.

GENERAL PROCEDURES AND TREATMENT MODALITIES

Splenectomy

The *spleen* is a fist-size organ located in the upper left quadrant of the abdomen. It includes a central "white pulp" where storage and some proliferation of lymphocytes and other leukocytes occurs and a peripheral "red pulp" involved in fetal erythropoiesis, and later in erythrocyte destruction and the conversion of hemoglobin to bilirubin. It may be surgically removed because of trauma or to treat certain hemolytic or malignant disorders with accompanying splenomegaly. A laparoscopic technique, usually with a lateral approach, is preferred to remove a normal to slightly enlarged spleen in benign conditions, such as idiopathic thrombocytopenic purpura, hemolytic anemia, or sickle cell disease. Compared to open surgery, laparoscopic splenectomies have a shortened hospital stay, decreased postoperative pain, and decreased risk of wound complications such as adhesions and infections.

Preoperative Management

1. For general aspects of preoperative nursing management, see Chapter 7.
2. Stabilization of preexisting condition:
   a. For trauma: volume replacement with intravenous (IV) fluids, evacuation of stomach contents via nasogastric tube to prevent aspiration, urinary catheterization to monitor urine output, assessment for pneumothorax or hemothorax and possible chest tube placement.

PROCEDURE GUIDELINES 26-2

Bone Marrow Aspiration and Biopsy

EQUIPMENT

- Bone marrow aspiration tray
- Marrow aspiration needles with stylets
- Towels
- 25G and 22G needles
- Two 25-mL syringes
- Three 5-mL syringes

- Local anesthetic (1% procaine or lidocaine)
- Sterile gauze squares
- Sterile gloves, drape
- Skin antiseptic
- Masks and protective eyewear for physician and nurse (check your facility's policy)

- Laboratory equipment
- Coverslips
- Microscopic slides
- Test tubes (plain and heparinized)
- Scalpel blade and handle

PROCEDURE

Nursing Action	Rationale
1. Explain the procedure to the patient. Tell patient when the skin will be marked, antiseptic applied, and the needle puncture performed.	1. Allays anxiety and enlists cooperation. Tactile sensations (pressure, cold) can be misinterpreted as pain unless the patient is forewarned.
2. Give analgesic or tranquilizer, as requested, 30 minutes before procedure. May not be necessary for aspiration.	2. May minimize pain, discomfort, and anxiety during procedure.
3. Place the patient in prone or supine position for desired site: a. Posterior superior iliac crest—prone b. Anterior iliac crest (if patient is very obese)—supine	3. Exposes desired site.

Iliac Crest Aspiration/Biopsy

Performance phase (nurse assists)

1. If patient cannot tolerate prone position, assist patient to side-lying position with top knee flexed.	1.
a. The posterior iliac crest is located and marked.	a. The iliac crest provides a large marrow cavity at the posterior superior iliac spine away from nearby abdominal organs.
b. The skin area is prepared and draped. The marked area is infiltrated with local anesthetic through the skin and subcutaneous tissue to the periosteum of the bone.	b. Tell the patient to expect a needle prick followed by a burning sensation. The periosteum is the region of greatest sensitivity.
c. A small incision may be made.	c. The biopsy needle is large and a small incision facilitates insertion.
d. The bone marrow needle, with stylet in place, is introduced through the incision.	d. The needle is pointed toward the anterior superior iliac spine and brought into contact with the posterior iliac spine.
e. The needle is advanced and rotated by using firm and steady pressure. When the needle is felt to enter the outer cortex of the bone marrow cavity, the stylet is removed and the syringe attached. Negative pressure is applied and a small volume of blood and marrow is aspirated.	e. There is usually decreased resistance when the bone marrow cavity is entered. The actual aspiration may cause brief pain and the patient should be forewarned.
f. A biopsy is taken by using a special needle equipped with a sharp cutting edge and a hollow core.	f. Bone marrow appears rusty-red and normally has a thick, fluidlike consistency.
g. After removal of needle, apply pressure to site and dressing.	g. Prevents bleeding from puncture site. Dressing keeps site clean and dry until healed.

b. For hemolytic or malignant disorder with accompanying thrombocytopenia: coagulation studies, administration of coagulation factors (eg, vitamin K, fresh-frozen plasma, cryoprecipitate), platelet and red cell transfusions.

3. Preoperative pulmonary evaluation and teaching.

4. For patient undergoing elective splenectomy, vaccination against pneumococcus, *Haemophilus influenzae* type B, and meningococcus are given at least 2 weeks before surgery.

Postoperative Management

1. For general aspects of postoperative nursing management, see Chapter 7.

2. Prevention of respiratory complications: hypoventilation and limited diaphragmatic movement, atelectasis of left lower lobe, pneumonia, left pleural effusion.

3. Monitoring for hemorrhage.

4. Pharmacologic DVT prophylaxis, begun in operating room or if patient is at increased bleeding risk, as soon as bleeding risk subsides.

5. Administration of opioids for pain and observance for adverse effects.

6. Monitoring for fever.
   a. Postsplenectomy fever—mild, transient fever is expected.
   b. Persistent fever may indicate subphrenic abscess or hematoma.

7. Monitoring daily platelet count: thrombocytosis (elevation of platelet count) may appear a few days after splenectomy and may persist during first 2 weeks.

Potential Complications

1. Pancreatitis and fistula formation: tail of pancreas is anatomically close to splenic hilum.

2. Hemorrhage.

3. Atelectasis and pneumonia.

4. Overwhelming postsplenectomy infection (OPSI)—increased risk of developing a life-threatening bacterial infection with encapsulated organisms, such as *Streptococcus pneumoniae*, *Neisseria meningitidis*, or *H. influenzae* type b. The incidence of OPSI is 0.23% to 0.42% per year with a lifetime risk of 5%. An OPSI is a medical emergency and requires immediate IV antibiotics in an intensive care setting. IV immunoglobulins are also used.

NURSING ALERT The risk of OPSI is highest soon after splenectomy and in patients whose splenectomy occurred during childhood or for a malignant disease. Early symptoms include fever and malaise; the infection may progress within hours to sepsis and death, with mortality as high as 50% to 70%. Patient education before and after splenectomy should include the risks of OPSI, recognition of early symptoms and prompt medical attention, MedicAlert bracelet, immunization against *S. pneumoniae*, *H. influenzae* type b, and *N. meningitidis*, and, in some cases, prophylactic and standby antibiotics.

Nursing Diagnoses

- Ineffective Breathing Pattern related to pain and guarding of surgical incision.
- Risk for Deficient Fluid Volume related to hemorrhage caused by surgery of highly vascular organ.
- Risk for Injury (thromboembolism) related to thrombocytosis.
- Risk for Infection related to surgical incision and removal of the spleen.
- Acute Pain related to surgical incision.

Nursing Interventions

Maintaining Effective Breathing

1. Assess breath sounds and report absent, diminished, or adventitious sounds.

2. Assist with aggressive chest physiotherapy and incentive spirometry.

3. Encourage early and progressive mobilization.

Monitoring for Hemorrhage

1. Monitor vital signs frequently and as condition warrants.

2. Measure abdominal girth and report abdominal distention.

3. Assess for pain and report increasing pain.

4. Prepare patient for surgical re-exploration if bleeding is suspected.

Avoiding Thromboembolic Complications

1. Monitor platelet count daily, report abnormal result promptly.

2. Administer DVT prophylaxis, as ordered.

3. Assess for possible thromboembolism.
   a. Assess skin color, temperature, and pulses.
   b. Advise patient to report chest pain, shortness of breath, pain, or weakness.

4. Report signs of thromboembolism immediately.

Preventing Infection

1. Assess surgical incision daily or if increased pain, fever, or foul smell.

2. Maintain meticulous handwashing and change dressings using sterile technique.

3. Teach patient to report signs of infection (fever, malaise) immediately.

4. Educate patient and family regarding OPSI, including plan for postsplenectomy immunizations, recognition of symptoms, use of prophylactic and standby antibiotics.

Relieving Pain

1. Administer opioids or teach self-administration, as prescribed and as necessary, to maintain level of comfort.

2. Warn patient of adverse effects, such as nausea and drowsiness; watch for hypotension and decreased respirations.

3. Teach the use of nonpharmacologic methods, such as music, relaxation breathing, progressive muscle relaxation, distraction, and imagery to help manage pain.

4. Document dosage of medications and response to medication.

5. Make sure patient has analgesics for use postdischarge.

Patient Education and Health Maintenance

1. Teach care of incision.
2. Encourage to gradually increase activity according to guidelines given by surgeon.
3. Advise proper rest, nutrition, and stress avoidance while recovering from surgery.
4. Encourage follow-up as directed by surgeon and primary care provider to maintain immunizations.
5. Encourage patient to seek prompt medical attention for any infections and to contact health care provider immediately for high fever.

Evaluation: Expected Outcomes

- Respirations unlabored, breath sounds clear.
- Vital signs stable, abdominal girth unchanged.
- Pulses strong, extremities warm and without pallor or cyanosis.
- Afebrile, no purulent drainage from incision.
- Verbalizes decreased pain.

ANEMIAS

Anemia is the lack of sufficient circulating hemoglobin to deliver oxygen to tissues. Anemia has multiple causes and is commonly associated with other diseases and disorders (eg, renal disease, cancer, Crohn's disease, alcoholism). Anemia may be caused by inadequate production of RBCs, abnormal hemolysis and sequestration of RBCs, or blood loss. Iron-deficiency anemia, pernicious anemia, folic acid–deficiency anemia, and aplastic anemia are the anemias most commonly seen in adults. Hereditary hemolytic disorders include spherocytosis, hemoglobinopathies (eg, sickle cell), and enzymatic deficiencies such as glucose 6-phosphate dehydrogenase (G6PD). Treatments for anemia include nutritional counseling, supplements, RBC transfusions, and, for some patients, administration of exogenous erythropoietin (epoetin alfa or darbepoetin alfa), a growth factor stimulating production and maturation of erythrocytes. New erythropoiesis-stimulating agents are under development. Erythropoietin is used to stimulate RBC production in anemias associated with chronic renal failure, chemotherapy treatment, and HIV.

 DRUG ALERT Erythropoietic-stimulating agents, such as epoetin alfa and darbepoetin alfa, have been associated with increased risk of death and serious cardiovascular events. Use the lowest possible dose and monitor for such potential problems as hypertension—particularly in patients with chronic kidney disease—and deep venous thrombosis.

Iron-Deficiency Anemia (Microcytic, Hypochromic)

Iron-deficiency anemia is a condition in which the total body iron content is decreased below a normal level, affecting hemoglobin synthesis. RBCs appear pale and are small.

Pathophysiology and Etiology

1. The most common cause is chronic blood loss (GI bleeding including occult colorectal cancers, excessive menstrual bleeding, hookworm infestation), but anemia may also be caused by insufficient intake of iron (weight loss, inadequate diet), iron malabsorption (end-stage renal disease, small-bowel disease, gastroenterostomy), or increased requirements (pregnancy, periods of rapid growth).
2. Decreased hemoglobin may result in insufficient oxygen delivery to body tissues.
3. The incidence of iron-deficiency anemia, the most common type of anemia, varies widely by age, sex, and race. In the United States, it is more than twice as common in women as compared to men, affecting 10% of non-Hispanic white women and 20% of black and Hispanic women. It is a major health problem in developing countries.
4. Symptoms generally develop when hemoglobin has fallen to less than 11 g/100 mL.

Clinical Manifestations

1. Headache, dizziness, fatigue, tinnitus.
2. Palpitations, dyspnea on exertion, pallor of skin and mucous membranes.
3. In developing world: smooth, sore tongue; cheilosis (lesions at corners of mouth), koilonychia (spoon-shaped fingernails), and pica (craving to eat unusual substances).

Diagnostic Evaluation

1. CBC and iron profile—decreased hemoglobin, hematocrit, serum iron, and ferritin; elevated red cell distribution width and normal or elevated total iron-binding capacity (transferrin).
2. Determination of source of chronic blood loss may include sigmoidoscopy, colonoscopy, upper and lower GI studies, stools and urine for occult blood examination.

Management

1. Diagnosis and correction of chronic blood loss.
2. Oral or parenteral iron therapy.
   a. Oral ferrous sulfate preferred and least expensive; treatment continues until hemoglobin level is normalized and iron stores replaced (up to 6 months).
   b. Parenteral therapy may be used when patient cannot tolerate or is noncompliant with oral therapy. May use sodium ferric gluconate, iron sucrose, or iron dextran.

Complications

1. Severe compromise of the oxygen-carrying capacity of the blood may predispose to ischemic organ damage, such as myocardial infarction or stroke.
2. Anaphylaxis to parenteral iron therapy, especially with iron dextran.

Nursing Assessment

1. Obtain history of symptoms, dietary intake, past history of anemia, possible sources of blood loss.
2. Examine for tachycardia, pallor, dyspnea, and signs of GI or other bleeding.

Nursing Diagnoses

- Imbalanced Nutrition: Less Than Body Requirements related to inadequate intake of iron.
- Activity Intolerance related to decreased oxygen-carrying capacity of the blood.
- Ineffective Tissue Perfusion related to decreased oxygen-carrying capacity of the blood.

Nursing Interventions

Promoting Iron Intake

1. Assess diet for inclusion of foods rich in iron. Arrange nutritionist referral, as appropriate.
2. Administer iron replacement, as ordered. Monitor iron levels of patients on chronic therapy.

 DRUG ALERT Anaphylactic reactions may occur after parenteral iron administration. A test dose is required for iron dextran and recommended for iron sucrose or sodium ferric gluconate. Monitor patient closely for hypotension, angioedema, and stridor after injection. Do not administer with oral iron.

Increasing Activity Tolerance

1. Assess level of fatigue and normal sleep pattern; determine activities that cause fatigue.
2. Assist in developing a schedule of activity, rest periods, and sleep.
3. Encourage conditioning exercises to increase strength and endurance.

Maximizing Tissue Perfusion

1. Assess patient for palpitations, chest pain, dizziness, and shortness of breath; minimize activities that cause these symptoms.
2. Elevate head of bed and provide supplemental oxygen, as ordered.
3. Monitor vital signs and fluid balance.

Patient Education and Health Maintenance

1. Educate patient on proper nutrition and good sources of iron: select well-balanced diet that includes animal proteins, iron-fortified cereals and bread, beans, dried fruits, legumes, tofu (see Table 26-3). The daily requirement of iron for adult females age 19 to 50 is 18 mg, for men 8 mg; however, more is needed to build iron stores in those who have been anemic and for those who are at risk for anemia.
2. Teach patient about iron supplementation.
   a. Take iron on empty stomach, with full glass of water or fruit juice.
   b. Liquid forms may stain teeth; mix well with water or fruit juice and use a straw.
   c. Anticipate some epigastric discomfort, change in color of stools to green or black, and, in some cases, nausea, constipation, or diarrhea. Prevent and treat constipation with increased fiber, fluids, and exercise. Report GI intolerance to health care provider.
   d. Keep iron medications away from children as overdose may be fatal.

Table 26-3	Dietary Sources of Iron	
FOOD	**SERVING SIZE**	**MG PER SERVING**
Cereal (fortified)	1 oz	1.8–21
Chicken liver	3.5 oz	12.8
Oatmeal (fortified)	1 cup	10
Soybeans	1 cup	8.8
Beef liver	3 oz	7.5
Lentils	1 cup	6.6
Beans (kidney, lima, navy, pinto)	1 cup	3.6–5.2
Oysters	6 pieces	4.5
Pumpkin seeds, roasted	1 oz	4.2
Beef (various cuts)	3–3.5 oz	2–3.9
Molasses	1 tbsp	3.5
Tofu	1/2 cup	3.4
Spinach, cooked	1/2 cup	3.2
Clams	3/4 cup	3.0
Sardines	3 oz	2.5
Turkey	3.5 oz	1.6–2.3
Macaroni (enriched, cooked)	1 cup	1.9
Bread (enriched)	2 slices	1.8
Rice (cooked)	1 cup	1.8
Apricots (dried)	10 pieces	1.7
Raisins	1/2 cup	1.5
Prune juice	1/2 cup	1.5
Pork	3–3.5 oz	1.2–1.5
Peas	1/2 cup	1.3
Chicken	3–3.5 oz	1.1–1.3

3. Encourage follow-up laboratory studies and visits to health care provider.

Evaluation: Expected Outcomes

- Incorporates several foods high in iron into diet; takes prescribed iron supplementation, as ordered.
- Tolerates increased activity; obtains sufficient rest.
- Vital signs stable without complaints of chest pain, palpitations, or shortness of breath.

Megaloblastic Anemia: Pernicious (Macrocytic, Normochromic)

A *megaloblast* is a large, nucleated erythrocyte with delayed and abnormal nuclear maturation. *Pernicious anemia* is a type of megaloblastic anemia associated with vitamin B_{12} deficiency.

Pathophysiology and Etiology

1. Vitamin B_{12} is necessary for normal deoxyribonucleic acid synthesis in maturing RBCs.
2. Pernicious anemia demonstrates familial incidence related to autoimmune gastric mucosal atrophy.
3. Normal gastric mucosa secretes a substance called intrinsic factor, necessary for absorption of vitamin B_{12} in ileum. If a defect exists in gastric mucosa, or after gastrectomy or small-bowel disease, intrinsic factor may not be secreted and orally ingested B_{12} may not be absorbed.
4. Some drugs interfere with B_{12} absorption, notably ascorbic acid, cholestyramine, colchicine, neomycin, cimetidine, and hormonal contraceptives.
5. Lower-serum vitamin B_{12} concentrations are associated with aging, but the evidence linking subnormal vitamin B_{12} to anemia in older people remains limited and inconclusive.

Clinical Manifestations

1. Of anemia—pallor, fatigue, dyspnea on exertion, palpitations. May be angina pectoris and heart failure in older adults or those predisposed to heart disease.
2. Of underlying GI dysfunction—sore mouth, glossitis, anorexia, nausea, vomiting, loss of weight, indigestion, epigastric discomfort, recurring diarrhea or constipation.
3. Of neuropathy (occurs in high percentage of untreated patients)—paresthesia that involves hands and feet, gait disturbance, bladder and bowel dysfunction, psychiatric symptoms caused by cerebral dysfunction.

Diagnostic Evaluation

1. CBC and blood smear—decreased hemoglobin and hematocrit; marked variation in size and shape of RBCs with a variable number of unusually large cells.
2. Folic acid (normal) and B_{12} levels (decreased).
3. Gastric analysis—volume and acidity of gastric juice diminished.
4. Schilling test for absorption of vitamin B_{12} uses small amount of radioactive B_{12} orally and 24-hour urine collection to measure uptake—decreased.

Management

Parenteral replacement with hydroxocobalamin or cyanocobalamin (B_{12}) is necessary by intramuscular (I.M.) injection from health care provider, generally every month.

Complications

Neurologic: paresthesia, gait disturbances, bowel and bladder dysfunction, and cerebral dysfunction may be persistent.

Nursing Assessment

1. Assess for pallor, tachycardia, dyspnea on exertion, exercise intolerance to determine patient's response to anemia.
2. Assess for paresthesia, gait disturbances, changes in bladder or bowel function, altered thought processes indicating neurologic involvement.
3. Obtain history of gastric surgery or GI disease.

Nursing Diagnoses

- Chronic Confusion related to neurologic dysfunction in absence of vitamin B_{12}.
- Impaired Comfort related to neurologic dysfunction in absence of vitamin B_{12}.

Nursing Interventions

Improving Thought Processes

1. Administer parenteral vitamin B_{12}, as prescribed.
2. Provide patient with quiet, supportive environment; reorient to time, place, and person, if needed; give instructions and information in short, simple sentences and reinforce frequently.

Minimizing the Effects of Paresthesia

1. Assess extent and severity of paresthesia, imbalance, or other sensory alterations.
2. Refer patient for physical therapy and occupational therapy, as appropriate.
3. Provide safe, uncluttered environment; make sure personal belongings are within reach; provide assistance with activities, as needed.

Patient Education and Health Maintenance

1. Advise patient that monthly vitamin B_{12} administration should be continued for life.
2. Instruct patient to see health care provider approximately every 6 months for hematologic studies and GI evaluation; may develop hematologic or neurologic relapse if therapy inadequate.

 NURSING ALERT Patients with pernicious anemia have higher incidence of gastric cancer and thyroid dysfunction; therefore, periodic stool examinations for occult blood, gastric cytology, and thyroid function tests should be done.

Evaluation: Expected Outcomes

- Oriented, cooperative, and follows instructions.
- Carries out activities without injury.

Megaloblastic Anemia: Folic Acid Deficiency

Chronic *megaloblastic anemia* is caused by folic acid (folate) deficiency.

Pathophysiology and Etiology

1. Dietary deficiency, malnutrition, marginal diets, excessive cooking of foods; commonly associated with alcoholism.
2. Impaired absorption in jejunum (eg, with small-bowel disease).
3. Increased requirements (eg, with chronic hemolytic anemia, exfoliative dermatitis, pregnancy).
4. Impaired utilization from folic acid antagonists (methotrexate) and other drugs (phenytoin, broad-spectrum antibiotics, sulfamethoxazole, alcohol, hormonal contraceptives).

Clinical Manifestations

1. Of anemia: fatigue, weakness, pallor, dizziness, headache, tachycardia.
2. Of folic acid deficiency: sore tongue, cracked lips.

Diagnostic Evaluation

1. Vitamin B_{12} and folic acid level—folic acid will be decreased.
2. CBC will show decreased RBC, hemoglobin, and hematocrit with increased mean corpuscular volume and mean corpuscular hemoglobin concentration.

Management

Oral folic acid replacement on daily basis.

Complications

Folic acid deficiency has been implicated in the etiology of congenitally acquired neural tube defects.

Nursing Assessment

1. Obtain nutritional history.
2. Monitor level of dyspnea, tachycardia, and development of chest pain or shortness of breath for worsening of condition.

Nursing Diagnosis

- Imbalanced Nutrition: Less Than Body Requirements related to inadequate intake of folic acid.

Nursing Interventions

Improving Folic Acid Intake

1. Assess diet for inclusion of foods rich in folic acid: beef liver, peanut butter, red beans, oatmeal, broccoli, asparagus.
2. Arrange nutritionist referral, as appropriate.
3. Administer folic acid supplement.
4. Assist alcoholic patient to obtain counseling and additional medical care, as needed.

Community and Home Care Considerations

1. Encourage pregnant patient to maintain prenatal care and to take folic acid supplement.
2. Provide alcoholic patient with information about treatment programs and Alcoholics Anonymous meetings in the community.

Patient Education and Health Maintenance

1. Teach patient to select balanced diet that includes green vegetables (asparagus, broccoli, spinach), yeast, liver and other organ meats, some fresh fruits; avoid overcooking vegetables.
2. Encourage patient to follow up periodically to monitor CBC.

Evaluation: Expected Outcomes

- Eats appropriate and nutritious diet; takes folic acid supplements, as prescribed.

Aplastic Anemia

Aplastic anemia is a rare disorder characterized by bone marrow hypoplasia or aplasia resulting in pancytopenia (insufficient numbers of RBCs, WBCs, and platelets).

Pathophysiology and Etiology

Destruction of hematopoietic stem cells is thought to be through an immune-mediated mechanism.

1. Most often (70% to 80% of patients) characterized as idiopathic because no cause is found.
2. May be caused by exposure to chemical toxins (eg, benzene); ionizing radiation; viral infections, particularly hepatitis; certain drugs (eg, chloramphenicol).
3. May be congenital (eg, Fanconi's anemia, Diamond-Blackfan anemia, and Shwachman-Diamond syndrome).
4. Clinical course is variable and dependent on degree of bone marrow failure; severe aplastic anemia is almost always fatal if untreated.

Clinical Manifestations

1. From anemia: pallor, weakness, fatigue, exertional dyspnea, palpitations.
2. From infections associated with neutropenia: fever, headache, malaise; adventitious breath sounds; abdominal pain, diarrhea; erythema, pain, exudate at wounds or sites of invasive procedures.
3. From thrombocytopenia: bleeding from gums, nose, GI or GU tracts; purpura, petechiae, ecchymoses.

Diagnostic Evaluation

1. CBC and peripheral blood smear show decreased RBC, WBC, platelets (pancytopenia).
2. Bone marrow aspiration and biopsy: bone marrow is hypocellular or empty with greatly reduced or absent hematopoiesis.

Management

1. Removal of causative agent or toxin.
2. Allogeneic bone marrow transplantation (BMT)—treatment of choice for patient with severe aplastic anemia (see page 1013). This treatment option provides long-term survival for 75% to 90% of patients, depending on the age of the patient, history of prior blood transfusions, and source of marrow.

3. Immunosuppressive treatment with cyclosporine and antithymocyte globulin or cyclophosphamide. This treatment option provides long-term survival for 60% to 70% of patients.

4. Androgens (oxymetholone or testosterone enanthate) may stimulate bone marrow regeneration; significant toxicity encountered. They may be used when other treatments have failed.

5. Supportive treatment includes platelet and RBC transfusions, antibiotics, and antifungals. Blood components should be irradiated for patients eligible for BMT and this approach is also recommended for patients receiving immunosuppressive therapy.

Complications

1. Untreated severe aplastic anemia is almost always fatal, generally because of overwhelming infection. Even with treatment, morbidity and mortality caused by infections and bleeding are high.

2. Late complications, even after successful treatment, include clonal hematologic diseases such as paroxysmal nocturnal hemoglobinuria, myelodysplasia, and acute myelogenous leukemia.

Nursing Assessment

1. Obtain thorough history that includes medications, past medical history, occupation, hobbies.

2. Monitor for signs of bleeding and infection.

Nursing Diagnoses

• Risk for Infection related to granulocytopenia secondary to bone marrow aplasia.

• Risk for Bleeding related to disease process.

Nursing Interventions

Minimizing Risk of Infection

1. Care for patient in protective environment while hospitalized (eg, private room with strict handwashing and avoidance of any contaminants).

2. Encourage good personal hygiene, including daily shower or bath with mild soap, mouth care, and perirectal care after using the toilet.

3. Monitor vital signs, including temperature, frequently; notify health care provider of oral temperature of 101° F (38.3° C) or higher.

4. Minimize invasive procedures or possible trauma to skin or mucous membranes.

5. Obtain cultures of suspected infected sites or body fluids.

Minimizing Risk of Bleeding

1. Use only soft toothbrush or toothette for mouth care and electric razor for shaving; keep nails short by filing.

2. Avoid I.M. injections and other invasive procedures.

3. Prevent constipation with stool softeners, as prescribed.

4. Restrict activity based on platelet count and active bleeding.

5. Monitor pad count for menstruating patient; avoid use of vaginal tampons.

6. Control bleeding by applying pressure to site, using ice packs and prescribed topical hemostatic agents.

7. Administer blood product replacement, as ordered; monitor for allergic reaction, anaphylaxis, and volume overload.

Patient Education and Health Maintenance

1. Teach patient how to minimize risk of infection (see Patient Education Guidelines 26-1):
   a. Wash hands after contact with possible source of infection.
   b. Immediately clean any abrasion or wound of mucous membranes or skin.
   c. Monitor temperature and report fever or other sign of infection immediately.
   d. Avoid crowds and people with illnesses.
   e. Avoid raw or undercooked foods.
   f. Use condoms and other safe-sex practices.

2. Teach patient how to minimize risk of bleeding (see Patient Education Guidelines 26-2, page 984):
   a. Avoid falls or other injury.
   b. Use electric razor rather than plain razor.
   c. Use nail clippers or file rather than scissors.
   d. Avoid blowing nose.
   e. Use soft toothbrush or toothette for mouth care.
   f. Use water-soluble lubricants, as needed, during sexual activity.

3. Advise patient to avoid exposure to potential bone marrow toxins: solvents, sprays, paints, pesticides.

4. Teach patient to take only prescribed medications; avoid aspirin and nonsteroidal anti-inflammatory drugs (NSAIDs), which may interfere with platelet function. As some vitamins and herbs may also affect platelet function, instruct patient to check with physician before using any supplements.

5. Resources for patient and family include the Aplastic Anemia & MDS International Foundation (*www.aamds.org*).

Evaluation: Expected Outcomes

• Remains afebrile with no signs or symptoms of infection.
• Episodes of bleeding rapidly controlled.

MYELOPROLIFERATIVE DISORDERS

Myeloproliferative disorders are disorders of the bone marrow that result from abnormal proliferation of cells from the myeloid line of the hematopoietic system. They include polycythemia vera, acute lymphocytic and acute myelogenous leukemia, and chronic myelogenous leukemia.

Polycythemia Vera

Polycythemia vera is a chronic myeloproliferative disorder that involves all bone marrow elements, resulting in an increase in RBC mass and hemoglobin.

PATIENT EDUCATION GUIDELINES 26-1

Preventing, Recognizing, and Treating Infection

What kinds of infections am I at risk for?
Because some of your white blood cells (called neutrophils) are not present in their normal numbers, you are at risk for infections. Neutrophils attack bacteria and other organisms that cause infections. You are at risk for infections from bacteria (eg, wound infections, urinary tract infections, pneumonia) and some viral infections (eg, cold sores) and fungal infections (eg, thrush, fungal pneumonia).

How do I know when I have an infection?
With low numbers of neutrophils, some of the normal signs of infection, such as pus, may not be present. If you have a fever greater than 100° F (37.8° C), you should contact your health care provider immediately. Other signs of infection include chills and sweating, redness near a wound or a catheter, white patches in your mouth, or shortness of breath.

How can I protect myself from infection?
The most important thing you can do is to wash your hands thoroughly after using the bathroom or after any other "dirty" activity (such as taking out the trash). You should keep your mouth clean by brushing your teeth with a soft toothbrush after every meal or snack and by rinsing with a mild mouth rinse. You should shower daily using a mild soap.

Can I have visitors? Can I go out?
It is important to ask friends and family not to visit if they are not feeling well. You can certainly go out (unless your physician or nurse gives you different instructions), but you should avoid crowded, poorly ventilated places. You may be taught how to wear a special mask when you are outside.

Do I need to get rid of my pet?
If you have pets and gardens, you can still enjoy them. If possible, find someone else who will clean your cat's litter box or scoop your dog's waste. Wear gloves when gardening and be careful not to get cuts and abrasions.

Should I stop having sexual intercourse?
With your low neutrophil count, you are also at higher risk for sexually transmitted diseases. However, this does not mean you have to stop having sexual intercourse. It is important to use a condom and make sure your sexual practice is safe. Depending on your general health, your physician or nurse may recommend that you avoid sexual intercourse.

If I get an infection, how will it be treated?
A new infection typically requires hospital admission to diagnose it and to begin treatment. You may be given many tests to find out exactly what infection you have. Blood will be drawn and examined for infection, x-rays and computed tomography scans may be done, and you may need a lumbar puncture to look for an infection in your spinal fluid. Before the results of all the tests are available, your physician will begin treatment with IV antibiotics. If your infection does not get better (eg, if you still have a fever in a couple of days), your antibiotics may be changed or other medications may be added. When your infection begins to improve, it is usually possible to go home and continue taking IV or oral antibiotics at home.

Pathophysiology and Etiology

1. Hyperplasia of all bone marrow elements results in:
   a. Overproduction of all three blood cell lines, most prominently RBCs.
   b. Increased red cell mass.
   c. Increased blood volume and viscosity.
   d. Decreased marrow iron reserve.
   e. Splenomegaly.
2. Increased mass of blood cells increases viscosity and leads to engorgement of blood vessels and possible thrombosis.
3. Underlying cause is unknown.
4. Usually occurs in middle and later years.

Clinical Manifestations

Result from increased blood volume and viscosity.

1. Reddish purple skin and mucosa, pruritus (especially after bathing).
2. Splenomegaly, hepatomegaly.
3. Epigastric discomfort, abdominal discomfort.
4. Painful fingers and toes from arterial and venous insufficiency, paresthesia.
5. Headache, fullness in head, dizziness, visual abnormalities, altered mentation from disturbed cerebral circulation.
6. Weakness, fatigue, night sweats, bleeding tendency.
7. Hyperuricemia from increased formation and destruction of erythrocytes and leukocytes and increased metabolism of nucleic acids.
8. Itching related to histamine release from basophils.

Diagnostic Evaluation

1. CBC—elevated RBC and hemoglobin and hematocrit (> 60%); elevated platelets.
2. Bone marrow aspirate and biopsy—hyperplasia.
3. Elevated uric acid.

Management

1. Of hyperviscosity: phlebotomy (withdrawal of blood) at intervals determined by CBC results to reduce RBC mass; generally, 250 to 500 mL removed at a time to maintain hematocrit less than 45%. The British Committee for Standards in Hematology recommendations also include aspirin at 75 mg/day unless contraindicated.

PATIENT EDUCATION GUIDELINES 26-2

Preventing, Recognizing, and Treating Bleeding

Why am I at risk for bleeding?

You could be at risk for bleeding because you do not have enough platelets (cells that help make clots), because your platelets are not working properly, or because you do not have enough clotting factors in your blood (substances that help make clots). Some people need treatment with drugs, such as heparin and coumadin, to prevent dangerous clots in the legs and lungs. These drugs increase the risk of bleeding.

How will I know if I have bleeding?

You might have visible bleeding, such as a nosebleed or bleeding from your gums. You might have very heavy bleeding with your menses (period), which might go on longer than usual. You might notice blood in your stools or black stools (black stools can also occur if you take iron). You might see blood streaks or black flecks in your emesis (vomit). The color of your urine might be pink or red, or you might see red streaks in it. You might have small bruises appear on your skin or redness in the white part of your eyes. If you have bleeding internally you might have symptoms, such as pain, swelling, shortness of breath (bleeding in the lungs), or confusion or stroke symptoms (bleeding in the brain).

What should I do to stop something from bleeding?

If your nose is bleeding, you can apply pressure by squeezing the bridge of the nose. If you have a wound that is bleeding, apply pressure to the site with a clean or sterile pad. Ice packs can also help; apply ice for 20 minutes at a time, then remove and reapply every hour or two, if needed. If you have bleeding in the mouth, biting on a tea bag may also help. If bleeding does not stop quickly or seems to be a lot, you should contact your health care provider or go to an emergency department.

You should also seek help right away if you are coughing up blood or vomiting blood, if you feel weak or confused, or if you are worried that it is serious.

What can I do to prevent bleeding?

There are lots of things you can do to decrease the risk of bleeding. Avoid activities where you have a high risk of injury (eg, contact sports). Use a soft toothbrush (you can floss gently if it does not cause bleeding). Avoid blowing your nose. Use an electric razor instead of a regular razor. Keep your fingernails and toenails short and smooth using a nail clipper and file rather than scissors. Make sure you do not get constipated—straining may cause bleeding. Do not take aspirin, ibuprofen, or naproxen. Acetaminophen is a safe alternative to these types of medications. Other medications and several vitamins and herbs can increase your risk of bleeding. Do not take over-the-counter medications or herbal and nutritional supplements and vitamins until you have checked with your health care provider. Take medicine to suppress your menses (period) as ordered. Use water-soluble lubricants during sexual activity to decrease the risk of abrasions.

What else should I do?

Talk with your health care provider and nurse about your activities. If you are at high risk for bleeding, you may need to restrict or change your exercise and activities. You may need to change sexual practices. Keep your appointments with your health care providers and take medications, as prescribed. If you visit another physician, dentist, or need surgery, be sure to tell health care providers about your risk of bleeding. Wear a MedicAlert bracelet if you will be at risk for bleeding for some time.

Evidence Base Tefferi, A. (2012). Polycythemia vera and essential thrombocythemia: 2012 update on diagnosis, risk stratification, and management. *American Journal of Hematology, 87,* 285–293.

2. Of marrow hyperplasia: chronic myelosuppressive therapy, generally using hydroxycarbamide (formerly known as hydroxyurea) or IV radioactive phosphorus; biologic response modifier (ie, alpha-interferon). Aggressive chemotherapy is not recommended because of increased risk of secondary leukemia.

3. Of hyperuricemia: allopurinol.

4. Of pruritus: antihistamines (cimetidine or cyproheptadine); low-dose aspirin; certain antidepressants (doxepin, paroxetine); phototherapy; cholestyramine; alpha-interferon.

Complications

1. Thromboembolic events caused by hyperviscosity, including deep vein thrombophlebitis, myocardial and cerebral infarction, transient ischemic attacks, pulmonary embolism, retinal vein thrombosis, and thrombotic occlusion of the splenic, hepatic, portal, and mesenteric veins.

2. Spontaneous hemorrhage caused by venous and capillary distention and abnormal platelet function.

3. Gout caused by hyperuricemia.

4. Heart failure caused by increased blood volume and hypertension.

5. Myelofibrosis or acute myeloid leukemia may be terminal complications.

Nursing Assessment

1. Obtain history of symptoms, including changes in skin, epigastric discomfort, bleeding tendencies, circulatory problems, or painful, swollen joints.

2. Monitor for signs of bleeding or thromboembolism.

3. Monitor for hypertension and signs and symptoms of heart failure, including shortness of breath, distended neck veins.

Nursing Diagnosis

- Ineffective Tissue Perfusion (multiple organs) related to hyperviscosity of blood.

Nursing Interventions

Preventing Thromboembolic Complications

1. Encourage or assist with ambulation. Employ thromboembolism precautions during periods of immobility.
2. Assess for early signs of thromboembolic complications—swelling of limb, increased warmth, pain, shortness of breath, chest pain. Report immediately.
3. Monitor CBC and assist with phlebotomy, as ordered.

Patient Education and Health Maintenance

1. Educate patient about risk of thrombosis; encourage patient to maintain normal activity patterns and avoid long periods of bed rest.
2. Advise patient to avoid taking hot showers or baths because rapid skin cooling worsens pruritus; use skin emollients; take antihistamines, as prescribed; may find starch baths helpful.
3. Instruct patient to take only prescribed medications.
4. Encourage patient to report at prescribed intervals for follow-up blood (hematocrit) studies and phlebotomies.
5. Instruct patient in technique of subcutaneous injection for alpha-interferon.

Evaluation: Expected Outcomes

- Hematocrit less than 45%; no signs or symptoms of thromboembolism, heart failure, or bleeding.

Acute Lymphocytic and Acute Myelogenous Leukemia

See Nursing Care Plan 26-1.

NURSING CARE PLAN 26-1

Care of the Patient with Acute Leukemia

You are assigned Charles Wintry, a 48-year-old with acute myelogenous leukemia (AML) who has been admitted with neutropenia and thrombocytopenia following chemotherapy. From your assessment and your knowledge of AML, you develop your care plan.

Subjective data: Charles tells you he has felt very tired during the past week and has stopped working at his part-time store manager job. Since yesterday evening, he has had a low-grade fever and pain in his chest with inspiration. He has

also noticed new bruises on his lower legs and abdomen. This morning he had a nosebleed.

Objective data: Vital signs are temperature 101° F (38.3° C), pulse 104, blood pressure 145/90, respirations 32. On examination, you notice extensive petechiae; dried blood around the nares and gingival bleeding; warm, dry skin; and crackles heard in the bases of both lungs. Complete blood count reveals 30,000 platelets, 1,200 white blood cells with 450 neutrophils, and hematocrit of 32%.

NURSING DIAGNOSIS
Risk for Infection related to granulocytopenia secondary to leukemia or its treatment with chemotherapy or radiation.

GOAL/EXPECTED OUTCOME
Risk of infection will be minimized.

Nursing Intervention	Rationale	Evaluation: Actual Outcome
Place patient in private room with handwashing precautions strictly enforced.	Meticulous handwashing is the single most important method of preventing transmission of endogenous and exogenous nosocomial infections.	Staff and visitors comply with handwashing precautions.
Avoid exposure to all sources of stagnant water (eg, flower vases, denture cups, water pitchers, humidifiers) and plants.	Stagnant water and soil are good media for anaerobic bacterial growth.	No visible sources of bacterial growth found in room.
Encourage or assist with personal hygiene—mouth care, perirectal care, daily shower or bath with mild soap. Inspect skin and mucous membranes daily for possible signs of infection.	Skin care and good oral hygiene may help prevent skin, oral, respiratory, and GI infections. Signs of infection may be minimal in neutropenic patient.	Skin remains clean and lubricated. Oropharynx has no lesions, plaques, or erythema.
Monitor vital signs every 4 hours. Obtain baseline pulse oximeter reading (SaO_2).	Infections may progress rapidly in immunocompromised patient.	Vital signs stable with no changes to report to health care provider.

(continued)

(Text continues on page 988)

NURSING CARE PLAN 26-1 (continued)

Care of the Patient with Acute Leukemia

Nursing Intervention	Rationale	Evaluation: Actual Outcome
Assess respiratory function every 4 hours while symptoms present, otherwise every 8 hours. Encourage ambulation, deep breathing, and coughing.	Neutropenic patient may have significant bacterial or fungal pneumonia with minimal changes on chest x-ray or physical examination.	Ambulates and uses incentive spirometer every 4 hours.
Assess for changes in mental status at least every 8 hours, including restlessness, irritability, confusion, headache, or changes in level of consciousness.	Mental status changes are commonly first subtle signs of sepsis.	Mental status remains stable; appears alert and oriented.
Avoid invasive procedures if possible (eg, urinary catheterization). Use strict sterile technique if procedure unavoidable.	Risk of infection from invasive procedure is high.	No invasive procedures initiated. Injections given via IV line.
Prevent rectal trauma by avoiding rectal temperatures, enemas, or suppositories. Use sitz bath and barrier cream for patient with diarrhea and hemorrhoids. Use stool softeners, as needed, to prevent constipation.	Perianal area is high-risk site for infection, including rectal abscesses.	Perianal area remains clean and intact.
Obtain cultures of suspected infected sites or body fluids.	Pus may not be present with neutropenia. Cultures may reveal bacterial, fungal, or viral pathogens.	Sputum sent for culture.
Report: (1) fever = 101° F (38.3° C) once or 100.4° F (38° C) two times; (2) significant change in vital signs, particularly hypotension, tachycardia, or tachypnea; (3) chills or rigors; (4) mental status changes.	Fever may be only response to infection in neutropenic patient. Patient is at risk for sepsis due to lack of normal immunologic response.	Fever of 101.2° F (38.4° C) reported.
Teach patient measures to prevent infection: avoid crowds; avoid raw or undercooked food; use condoms.	Potential for infection remains after discharge.	States preventive measures.

NURSING DIAGNOSIS
Risk for Injury related to bleeding secondary to thrombocytopenia, disseminated intravascular coagulation, or leukostasis associated with leukemia.

GOAL/EXPECTED OUTCOME
Risk of bleeding will be minimized.

Nursing Intervention	Rationale	Evaluation: Actual Outcome
Assess for signs of bleeding at least every 8 hours.	Overt and covert spontaneous bleeding is possible at platelet counts <50,000/mm³.	No further bleeding noted.
Provide soft toothbrush or toothettes and mild mouthwash for mouth care.	Minimize damage to mucous membranes.	Uses soft toothbrush after meals for gentle cleansing.
Use only an electric razor for shaving. Keep fingernails and toenails short and smooth. Lubricate skin with mild lotion.	Minimize skin excoriation.	Family member or spouse brings electric razor from home.
Avoid I.M. injections, invasive procedures, rectal procedures. Use stool softeners to prevent constipation.	Minimize risk of bleeding.	Invasive procedures minimized. Injections given via IV line.
Restrict activity based on assessment of platelet count and presence of active bleeding.	Injury to muscles or spontaneous bleeding may be minimized by restricting activity at lower platelet counts.	Ambulates within room with assistance until bleeding controlled and platelet count stabilized.

NURSING CARE PLAN 26-1 (continued)

Care of the Patient with Acute Leukemia

Nursing Intervention	Rationale	Evaluation: Actual Outcome
Menstrual suppression may be necessary for females. Monitor pad count/amount. Avoid use of vaginal tampons.	Menorrhagia may be severe in thrombocytopenic patient.	Menstrual bleeding not exceeding 4–5 pads per day.
Control bleeding by applying pressure to site, ice packs, and prescribed topical hemostatic agents, such as microfibrillar collagen hemostat or thrombin.	Topical interventions generally adequate to control most bleeding episodes.	No further bleeding episodes.
Administer blood product replacement, as ordered. Monitor for signs and symptoms of allergic reactions, anaphylaxis, and volume overload.	Platelet transfusions may be necessary when platelet count <20,000/mm³ or with active bleeding. Other blood products (red blood cells, fresh frozen plasma, cryoprecipitate) may also be required.	Platelet products given every 2–3 days until thrombocytopenia resolved.
Teach patient to avoid activities likely to cause injury (eg, contact sports) and other methods to prevent bleeding.	Risk of bleeding remains after discharge.	States preventive measures.

NURSING DIAGNOSIS
Acute pain related to tumor growth, infection, or adverse effects of chemotherapy.

GOAL/EXPECTED OUTCOME
Pain will be controlled.

Nursing Intervention	Rationale	Evaluation: Actual Outcome
Assess at least every 4 hours for presence, location, intensity, and characteristics of pain.	Pain is potentially distressing symptom. Pain may be symptom of infection.	Rates pain between 1 and 3 on scale of 0–10 after first day.
Administer analgesics, as ordered, to control pain. Administer on regular schedule rather than as needed. Avoid aspirin and nonsteroidal anti-inflammatory drugs (NSAIDs) in thrombocytopenic patients. If oral analgesics in optimal doses are not effective or not tolerated, consider IV route.	Analgesics on regular schedule at appropriate doses should be used to control pain. Aspirin and NSAIDs interfere with platelet function. I.M. and SubQ injections should be avoided in thrombocytopenia.	Oral analgesia (codeine 30 mg every 4 hours) well tolerated.
Teach and use nonpharmacologic measures, such as the use of music, relaxation breathing, progressive muscle relaxation, distraction, and imagery to help manage pain.	Nonpharmacologic measures may be useful adjunctive treatments for patients with pain.	Heat packs to right chest area provide additional relief.

NURSING DIAGNOSIS
Powerlessness related to diagnosis and perceived lack of support/resources.

GOAL/EXPECTED OUTCOME
Patient and family will be empowered to seek appropriate help.

Nursing Intervention	Rationale	Evaluation: Actual Outcome
Encourage verbalization of feelings regarding diagnosis, treatment plan, and anticipated course of illness.	Nurse–patient relationship allows appropriate discussion of concerns.	Verbalizes feelings through discussion, crying.
Refer, as needed, to social worker, psychiatric liaison nurse, psychologist.	Further assistance and support may be needed.	Referred to social worker for assistance with financial concerns.
Share information regarding national and local resources.	National and local organizations may be significant sources of support for patients and families.	Attends American Cancer Society support group after discharge.

Leukemias are malignant disorders of the blood and bone marrow that result in an accumulation of dysfunctional, immature cells that are caused by loss of regulation of cell division. They are classified as acute or chronic based on the development rate of symptoms, and further classified by the predominant cell type. Acute leukemias affect immature cells and are characterized by rapid progression of symptoms. When lymphocytes are the predominant malignant cell, the disorder is *acute lymphocytic leukemia (ALL)*; when monocytes or granulocytes are predominant, it is *acute myelogenous leukemia (AML)*, sometimes called *acute non-lymphocytic leukemia*. *Biphenotypic leukemia* is an acute leukemia with both lymphocytic and myelogenous cell characteristics.

Pathophysiology and Etiology

1. The development of leukemia has been associated with:
   a. Exposure to ionizing radiation.
   b. Exposure to certain chemicals and toxins (eg, benzene, alkylating agents).
   c. Human T-cell leukemia—lymphoma virus (HTLV-1 and HTLV-2) in certain areas of the world, including the Caribbean and southern Japan.
   d. Familial susceptibility.
   e. Genetic disorders (eg, Down syndrome, Fanconi's anemia).
2. Approximately one half of new leukemias are acute. Approximately 85% of acute leukemias in adults are AML. ALL is most common in children, with peak incidence between ages 2 and 9.
3. Childhood ALL is usually cured with chemotherapy alone (>75%), whereas only 30% to 40% of adults with ALL are cured.
4. AML is a disease of older people, with a median age at diagnosis of 67. Even in the young-old (patients who are younger than age 60), AML is difficult to treat, with a median survival of 5 to 6 months, despite intensive therapy.

Clinical Manifestations

1. Common symptoms include pallor, fatigue, weakness, fever, weight loss, abnormal bleeding and bruising, lymphadenopathy (in ALL), and recurrent infections (in ALL).
2. Other presenting symptoms may include bone and joint pain, headache, splenomegaly, hepatomegaly, neurologic dysfunction.

Diagnostic Evaluation

1. CBC and blood smear—peripheral WBC count varies widely from 1,000 to 100,000/mm³ and may include significant numbers of abnormal immature (blast) cells; anemia may be profound; platelet count may be abnormal and coagulopathies may exist.
2. Bone marrow aspiration and biopsy—cells also studied for chromosomal abnormalities (cytogenetics) and immunologic markers to classify type of leukemia further.
3. Lymph node biopsy—to detect spread.
4. Lumbar puncture and examination of cerebrospinal fluid for leukemic cells (especially in ALL).

Management

1. National Comprehensive Cancer Network (NCCN; *www.nccn.org*) guidelines provide recommendations for workup, management, and supportive care of patients with various subtypes of AML.
   a. Evidence-based treatment guidelines for management of ALL are published by the National Cancer Institute (*www.cancer.gov/cancertopics/pdq/treatment/adultALL/HealthProfessional*).
2. Management of AML and ALL is designed to eradicate leukemic cells and allow restoration of normal hematopoiesis.
   a. High-dose chemotherapy given as an induction course to obtain remission (disappearance of abnormal cells in bone marrow and blood) and then in cycles as consolidation or maintenance therapy to prevent recurrence of disease (see Table 26-4).
   b. Leukapheresis (or exchange transfusion in infants) may be used when abnormally high numbers of white cells are present to reduce the risk of leukostasis and tumor burden before chemotherapy.
   c. Radiation, particularly of central nervous system (CNS) in ALL.
   d. Autologous or allogeneic bone marrow or stem cell transplantation.
3. Supportive care and symptom management.

Complications

1. Leukostasis: in setting of high numbers (greater than 50,000/mm³) of circulating leukemic cells (blasts), blood vessel walls are infiltrated and weakened, with high risk of rupture and bleeding, including intracranial hemorrhage.
2. Disseminated intravascular coagulation (DIC).
3. Tumor lysis syndrome: rapid destruction of large numbers of malignant cells leads to alterations in electrolytes (hyperuricemia, hyperkalemia, hyperphosphatemia, and hypocalcemia), renal failure, and other complications.
4. Infection, bleeding, organ damage.

 DRUG ALERT Allopurinol is commonly used as part of a regimen to prevent tumor lysis syndrome. In rare cases, it causes severe, even lethal, skin reactions (toxic epidermolysis syndrome). Allopurinol should be discontinued for any patient who develops a new skin rash.

Nursing Assessment

1. Take nursing history, focusing on weight loss, fever, frequency of infections, progressively increasing fatigability, shortness of breath, palpitations, visual changes (retinal bleeding).
2. Ask about difficulty in swallowing, coughing, rectal pain.
3. Examine patient for enlarged lymph nodes, hepatosplenomegaly, evidence of bleeding, abnormal breath sounds, skin lesions.
4. Look for evidence of infection: mouth, tongue, and throat for reddened areas or white patches. Examine skin for breakdown, which is a potential source of infection.

Table 26-4 Common Chemotherapeutic Drugs Used in Acute Leukemias

DRUG	MAJOR ADVERSE EFFECTS	CLASSIFICATION	PRIMARY USE
All-trans retinoic acid	Dry skin and mucous membranes, headaches, eyesight changes, bone pain, flulike symptoms, bone marrow suppression, retinoic acid syndrome (includes weight gain, peripheral edema, dyspnea, and fever)	Retinoid	Therapy for AML subtype M3 (APL)
Cyclophosphamide	Bone marrow suppression, alopecia, nausea and vomiting, diarrhea, hemorrhagic cystitis, cardiomyopathy	Alkylating agent	Induction and consolidation therapy for ALL
Cytarabine	Bone marrow suppression, nausea and vomiting, pulmonary toxicity, mucositis, lethargy, cerebellar toxicity, dermatitis, keratoconjunctivitis	Antimetabolite	Induction and consolidation therapy for AML
Daunorubicin	Bone marrow suppression, nausea and vomiting, alopecia, cardiotoxicity, vesicant	Antibiotic	Induction and consolidation therapy for AML
Doxorubicin	Leukopenia, nausea and vomiting, alopecia, cardiotoxicity, photosensitivity, vesicant	Antibiotic	Induction and consolidation therapy for AML
Imatinib mesylate	Edema, nausea and vomiting, musculoskeletal pain, rash	Tyrosine kinase inhibitor	Induction and consolidation therapy for Philadelphia chromosome positive adult ALL
L-asparaginase	Liver dysfunction, nausea and vomiting, hypersensitivity reaction, depression, lethargy	Miscellaneous: enzyme	Induction therapy for ALL
6-Mercaptopurine	Mild bone marrow suppression, GI disturbances, hepatotoxicity	Antimetabolite	Maintenance therapy for ALL
Methotrexate	Bone marrow suppression, stomatitis, nausea, diarrhea, hepatotoxicity, neurotoxicity with intrathecal doses	Antimetabolite	Intrathecal central nervous system treatment and prophylaxis for ALL; maintenance therapy for ALL
Prednisone	Appetite stimulation, mood alteration, Cushing's syndrome, hypertension, diabetes, peptic ulcer	Corticosteroid	Induction therapy for ALL
Vincristine	Neurotoxicity, alopecia, vesicant	Plant alkaloid	Induction therapy for ALL

ALL, acute lymphocytic leukemia; AML, acute myelogenous leukemia; APL, acute promyelocytic leukemia.

Nursing Diagnoses

- Risk for Infection related to granulocytopenia of disease and treatment.
- Risk for bleeding secondary to bone marrow failure and thrombocytopenia.

Nursing Interventions

Preventing Infection

1. Especially monitor for pneumonia, pharyngitis, esophagitis, perianal cellulitis, urinary tract infection, and cellulitis, which are common in leukemia and which carry significant morbidity and mortality.
2. Monitor for fever, flushed appearance, chills, tachycardia; appearance of white patches in mouth; redness, swelling, heat, or pain of eyes, ears, throat, skin, joints, abdomen, and rectal and perineal areas; cough, changes in sputum; skin rash.
3. Check results of granulocyte counts. Concentrations less than 500/mm^3 put the patient at serious risk for infection. Administer granulocyte-stimulating and erythropoiesis-stimulating agents, as ordered (eg, epoetin alfa or darbepoetin alfa).
4. Avoid invasive procedures and trauma to skin or mucous membrane to prevent entry of microorganisms.
5. Use the following rectal precautions to prevent infection:
   a. Avoid diarrhea and constipation, which can irritate the rectal mucosa.
   b. Avoid use of rectal thermometers.
   c. Keep perianal area clean.

6. Care for patient in private room with strict handwashing practice. Patients with prolonged neutropenia may benefit from high-efficiency particulate air filtration.
7. Encourage and assist patient with personal hygiene, bathing, and oral care.
8. Obtain cultures and administer antimicrobials promptly, as directed. Prophylactic antimicrobials, antifungals, and antivirals serve to protect the patient from life-threatening infections.

Preventing and Managing Bleeding

1. Watch for signs of minor bleeding, such as petechiae, ecchymosis, conjunctival hemorrhage, epistaxis, bleeding gums, bleeding at puncture sites, vaginal spotting, heavy menses.
2. Be alert for signs of serious bleeding, such as headache with change in responsiveness, blurred vision, hemoptysis, hematemesis, melena, hypotension, tachycardia, dizziness.
3. Monitor urine, stools, emesis for gross and occult blood.
4. Monitor platelet counts daily.
5. Administer blood components, as directed.
6. Keep patient on bed rest during bleeding episodes.

Patient Education and Health Maintenance

1. Teach infection precautions (see Patient Education Guidelines 26-1, page 983).
2. Teach signs and symptoms of infection and advise whom to notify.

3. Encourage adequate nutrition to prevent emaciation from chemotherapy.
4. Teach avoidance of constipation with increased fluid and fiber and good perianal care.
5. Teach bleeding precautions (see Patient Education Guidelines 26-2, page 984).
6. Encourage regular dental visits to detect and treat dental infections and disease.
7. Provide patient and family with information about resources in the community, such as the Leukemia Society of America and the American Cancer Society (see Box 26-1).

Evaluation: Expected Outcomes

- Afebrile, without signs of infection.
- No signs of bleeding.

Chronic Myelogenous Leukemia

Chronic myelogenous leukemia (CML) (ie, involving more mature cells than acute leukemia) is characterized by proliferation of myeloid cell lines, including granulocytes, monocytes, platelets, and, occasionally, RBCs.

Pathophysiology and Etiology

1. Specific etiology unknown, associated with exposure to ionizing radiation and family history of leukemia. Results from malignant transformation of pluripotent hematopoietic stem cell.

BOX 26-1	Resources for Patients with Hematologic Malignancies

American Cancer Society
250 Williams Street NW
Atlanta, GA 30303
(404) 320-3333 or (800) 227-2345
www.cancer.org
Patient education materials, Can Surmount and I Can Cope educational and support programs, durable medical equipment loans

Corporate Angel Network, Inc.
Westchester County Airport, 1 Loop Road
White Plains, NY 10604
(914) 328-1313 or (866) 328-1313
www.corpangelnetwork.org
Use of corporate aircraft to provide free travel to cancer patients going to checkups, treatments, or consultations

Leukemia and Lymphoma Society
1311 Mamaroneck Avenue
Suite 310
White Plains, NY 10605
(914) 949-5213 or (800) 955-4572
www.lls.org
Patient education materials, support groups, financial assistance (patient aid) program for patients with leukemia, Hodgkin's and non-Hodgkin's lymphoma, and multiple myeloma

National Coalition for Cancer Survivorship
1010 Wayne Ave., Suite 707
Silver Spring, MD 20910

(301) 650-9127
www.canceradvocacy.org
Network related to survivorship issues, sponsors National Cancer Survivors' Day, publishes Cancer Survivors Almanac of Resources

National Marrow Donor Program
3001 Broadway Street NE, Suite 100
Minneapolis, MN 55413
(800) 507-5427
www.marrow.org
Information for patients and volunteer donors regarding unrelated bone marrow transplant

National Cancer Institute
National Institutes of Health
Bethesda, MD 20892
(800) 4-CANCER
www.cancer.gov
National telephone hotline for information, patient education materials, research reports

Blood & Marrow Transplant Information Network
2900 Skokie Valley Road, Suite B
Highland Park, IL 60035
(888) 597-7674
www.bmtinfonet.org
Resources, support, and educational materials for patients and families

2. First cancer associated with chromosomal abnormality (the Philadelphia [Ph] chromosome), present in more than 90% of patients.

3. Accounts for 25% of adult leukemias and less than 5% of childhood leukemias. Generally presents between ages 25 and 60 with peak incidence in the mid-40s.

4. May progress to an accelerated phase or blast crisis, resembling an acute leukemia.

Clinical Manifestations

1. Insidious onset, may be discovered during routine physical examination.

2. About 70% of patients have symptoms at diagnosis such as fatigue, pallor, activity intolerance, fever, weight loss, night sweats, abdominal fullness (splenomegaly).

Diagnostic Evaluation

1. CBC and blood smear: large numbers of granulocytes (usually more than 100,000/mm^3), platelets may be decreased.

2. Bone marrow aspiration and biopsy: hypercellular, usually demonstrates Philadelphia (Ph^1) chromosome.

Management

Treatment guidelines for the management of CML are provided by NCCN (*www.nccn.org*).

Chronic Phase

1. Tyrosine kinase inhibitors are oral agents used as primary treatment for most patients with CML. They include imatinib mesylate, dasatinib, and nilotinib. These agents work by inhibiting proliferation of abnormal cells and inducing cell death (apoptosis) in abnormal cells. Adverse effects vary based on the agent used but include edema, diarrhea, headache, muscle cramps, muscle and bone pain, rash, and, rarely, hepatotoxicity, pleural or pericardial effusion, and myelosuppression.

2. For patients who do not respond to tyrosine kinase inhibitors, allogeneic (related or unrelated) BMT may be an option.

Accelerated Phase or Blast Crisis

1. High-dose tyrosine kinase inhibitors or chemotherapy (ALL or AML regimens) may be used to attempt to regain chronic phase.

2. Supportive care and palliative care may be appropriate because this phase is usually terminal.

Complications

1. Leukostasis.
2. Infection, bleeding, organ damage.
3. If untreated, CML is a terminal disease with unpredictable survival, on average 3 years.

Nursing Assessment

1. Obtain health history, focusing on fatigue, weight loss, night sweats, activity intolerance.
2. Assess for signs of bleeding and infection.
3. Evaluate for splenomegaly, hepatomegaly.
4. Assess for weight gain and edema in patients taking tyrosine kinase inhibitors.

Nursing Diagnosis

• Fear related to disease progression and death.

Nursing Interventions

For patient with CML in blast crisis, see Nursing Care Plan 26-1, pages 985 to 987.

Allaying Fear

1. Encourage appropriate verbalization of feelings and concerns.
2. Provide comprehensive patient teaching about disease, using methods and content appropriate to patient's needs.
3. Assist patient in identifying resources and support (eg, family and friends, spiritual support, community or national organizations, support groups).
4. Facilitate use of effective coping mechanisms.

Patient Education and Health Maintenance

1. Teach patient to take medications, as prescribed, and monitor for adverse effects.
2. Teach patient method of subcutaneous injection for self-administration of alpha interferon and teach strategies for managing such adverse effects as fatigue and fever.
3. Provide patient and family with information about resources in the community, such as the Leukemia and Lymphoma Society and the American Cancer Society (see Box 26-1).

Evaluation: Expected Outcomes

• Demonstrates effective coping skills.

LYMPHOPROLIFERATIVE DISORDERS

Lymphoproliferative disorders result from proliferation of cells from the lymphoid line of the hematopoietic system. They include chronic lymphocytic leukemia, Hodgkin's lymphoma, non-Hodgkin's lymphomas, and multiple myeloma.

Chronic Lymphocytic Leukemia

Chronic lymphocytic leukemia (CLL) (ie, involving more mature cells than acute leukemia) is characterized by proliferation of morphologically normal but functionally inert B-lymphocytes. In CLL the abnormal lymphocytes are found in the bone marrow and blood, whereas in *small lymphocytic lymphoma (SLL)* the same abnormal lymphocytes are found predominantly in lymph nodes. The differential diagnosis includes *hairy cell leukemia* and *Waldenström's macroglobulinemia*.

Pathophysiology and Etiology

1. Specific etiology unknown. Tends to cluster in families, much more common in Western hemisphere. Male hormones may play role.
2. Most common adult leukemia in United States and Europe. Disease of later years (90% over age 50); 1.5 times more common in men than in women.

3. Lymphocytes are immunoincompetent and respond poorly to antigenic stimulation.
4. In late stages, organ damage may occur from direct lymphocytic infiltration of tissue.
5. Variable course, may be indolent for years, with gradual transformation to more malignant or aggressive disease with 1- to 2-year course.

Clinical Manifestations

1. Insidious onset; may be discovered during routine physical examination.
2. Early symptoms may include painless lymph node swelling, commonly in cervical area, history of frequent skin or respiratory infections, mild splenomegaly and hepatomegaly, fatigue.
3. Symptoms of more advanced disease include fever, night sweats, weight loss, pallor, activity intolerance, easy bruising, skin lesions, bone tenderness, abdominal discomfort.

Diagnostic Evaluation

1. CBC and blood smear: large numbers of lymphocytes (10,000 to 150,000/mm^3); may also be anemia, thrombocytopenia, hypogammaglobulinemia.
2. Bone marrow aspirate and biopsy: lymphocytic infiltration of bone marrow.
3. Lymph node biopsy to detect spread.

Management

Symptom Control and Treatments

1. Patient with newly diagnosed and indolent CLL is generally observed and followed closely until symptoms develop. Treatment is individualized; NCCN guidelines suggest clinical trial or various chemotherapy and monoclonal antibody combinations (*www.nccn.org*).
2. Lymphocyte proliferation can be suppressed with chlorambucil, cyclophosphamide, and prednisone.
3. The purine analogue fludarabine has significant activity in CLL alone or in combination with rituximab and/or cyclophosphamide.
4. Monoclonal antibodies, such as alemtuzumab and rituximab, may be used.
5. Hairy cell leukemia, a distinctive type of B-cell leukemia with hairlike projections of cytoplasm from lymphocytes, may be successfully treated with cladribine, pentostatin, or alpha interferon.
6. Splenic irradiation or splenectomy for painful splenomegaly or platelet sequestration, hemolytic anemia.
7. Irradiation of painful enlarged lymph nodes.
8. Allogeneic bone marrow transplant is also used to treat CLL.

Supportive Care

1. Transfusion therapy to replace platelets and RBCs.
2. Antibiotics, antivirals, and antifungals, as needed, to control infections.
3. IV immunoglobulins or gamma globulin to treat hypogammaglobulinemia.

Complications

1. Thrombophlebitis from venous or lymphatic obstruction caused by enlarged lymph nodes.
2. Infection, bleeding.
3. Median survival depends on severity of disease; varies from 2 to 7 years.

Nursing Assessment

1. Obtain health history, focusing on history of infections, fatigue, bruising and bleeding, swollen lymph nodes.
2. Assess for signs of anemia, bleeding, or infection.
3. Evaluate for splenomegaly, hepatomegaly, lymphadenopathy.

Nursing Diagnoses

- Acute Pain related to tumor growth, infection, or adverse effects of chemotherapy.
- Activity Intolerance related to anemia and adverse effects of chemotherapy.

Nursing Interventions

Reducing Pain

1. Assess patient frequently for pain and administer or teach patient to administer analgesics on regular schedule, as prescribed; monitor for adverse effects.
2. Teach patient the use of nonpharmacologic methods, such as music, relaxation breathing, progressive muscle relaxation, distraction, and imagery to help manage pain.

Improving Activity Tolerance

1. Encourage frequent rest periods alternating with ambulation and light activity, as tolerated.
2. Assist patient with hygiene and physical care, as necessary.
3. Encourage balanced diet or nutritional supplements, as tolerated.
4. Teach patient to use energy-conservation techniques while performing activities of daily living, such as sitting while bathing, minimizing trips up and down stairs, using shoulder bag or push cart to carry articles.

Patient Education and Health Maintenance

1. Teach patient to minimize risk of infection (see Patient Education Guidelines 26-1, page 983).
2. Teach patient use of medications, as ordered, and possible adverse effects and their management; also teach patient to avoid aspirin and NSAIDs, which may interfere with platelet function.
3. Provide patient and family with information about resources in the community, such as the Leukemia and Lymphoma Society and the American Cancer Society (see Box 26-1, page 990).

Evaluation: Expected Outcomes

- States pain relief.
- Performs activities without complaints of fatigue.

Hodgkin's Lymphoma

Lymphomas are malignant disorders of the reticuloendothelial system that result in an accumulation of dysfunctional, immature lymphoid-derived cells. They are classified according to the predominant cell type and by the degree of malignant cell maturity (eg, well differentiated, poorly differentiated, or undifferentiated). Hodgkin's lymphoma originates in the lymphoid system and involves predominantly lymph nodes. It accounts for about 12% of all lymphomas.

Pathophysiology and Etiology

1. Etiology is unknown.
2. Characterized by appearance of "Reed-Sternberg" multinucleated giant cell in tumor.
3. Generally spreads via lymphatic channels, involving lymph nodes, spleen, and ultimately extralymphatic sites. May also spread via bloodstream to such sites as GI tract, bone marrow, skin, upper air passages, and other organs.
4. Incidence demonstrates two peaks, between ages 20 and 30 and after age 55. Risk is increased in males, for patients with HIV, in individuals with previous Epstein-Barr viral infection, and in individuals with first-degree relative with Hodgkin's lymphoma.

Clinical Manifestations

1. Common symptoms include painless enlargement of lymph nodes (generally unilateral cervical or supraclavicular), splenomegaly, fever, chills, night sweats, weight loss, pruritus.
2. Various symptoms may occur with pulmonary involvement, superior vena cava obstruction, hepatic or bone involvement.

Diagnostic Evaluation

Tests are used to determine extent of disease involvement before treatment and followed at regular intervals to assess response to treatment.

1. CBC—determines abnormal cells.
2. Lymph node biopsy—determines type of lymphoma.
3. Bilateral bone marrow aspirate and biopsy—determine whether bone marrow is involved.
4. Radiographic tests (eg, x-rays, positron emission tomography [PET] scan, computed tomography [CT] scan, magnetic resonance imaging [MRI])—detect deep nodal involvement.
5. Gallium-67 scan—detects areas of active disease and may be used to determine aggressiveness of disease.
6. Liver function tests—determine hepatic involvement; liver biopsy may be indicated if results abnormal.
7. Lymphangiogram—detects size and location of deep nodes involved, including abdominal nodes, which may not be readily seen via CT scan.
8. Surgical staging (laparotomy with splenectomy, liver biopsy, multiple lymph node biopsies)—in selected patients.

Management

Choice of treatment depends on extent of disease, histopathologic findings, and prognostic indicators. Hodgkin's lymphoma is more readily cured than other lymphomas, with a 5-year survival rate of 80%. The NCCN guidelines for Hodgkin's lymphoma (*www.nccn.org*) provide recommendations for diagnosis and treatment with chemotherapy, chemotherapy and radiation, and/or hematopoietic

stem cell transplant for select patients. Hodgkin's lymphoma arising in presence of HIV requires specialized treatment.

1. Radiation therapy.
   a. Treatment of choice for localized disease.
   b. Areas of body where lymph node chains are located can generally tolerate high radiation doses.
   c. Vital organs are protected with lead shielding during radiation treatments.
2. Chemotherapy.
   a. Initial treatment commonly consists of ABVD regimen of doxorubicin (Adriamycin), bleomycin, vinblastine (Velban), and dacarbazine; or MOPP regimen of nitrogen mustard (Mustargen), vincristine (Oncovin), procarbazine, and prednisone.
   b. Three or four drugs may be given in intermittent or cyclical courses with periods off treatment to allow recovery from toxicities.
3. Autologous or allogeneic bone marrow or stem cell transplantation.

Complications

1. Adverse effects of radiation or chemotherapy (see pages 151 and 139).
2. Dependent on location and extent of malignancy, but may include splenomegaly, hepatomegaly, thromboembolic complications, spinal cord compression.

Nursing Assessment

1. Obtain health history, focusing on fatigue, fever, chills, night sweats, swollen lymph nodes.
2. Evaluate splenomegaly, hepatomegaly, lymphadenopathy.

Nursing Diagnoses

- Impaired Tissue Integrity related to high-dose radiation therapy.
- Impaired Oral Mucous Membrane related to high-dose radiation therapy.

Nursing Interventions

Maintaining Tissue Integrity

1. Avoid rubbing, powders, deodorants, lotions, or ointments (unless prescribed) or application of heat and cold to treated area.
2. Encourage patient to keep treated area clean and dry, bathing area gently with tepid water and mild soap.
3. Encourage wearing loose-fitting clothes.
4. Advise patient to protect skin from exposure to sun, chlorine, temperature extremes.

Preserving Oral and GI Tract Mucous Membranes

1. Encourage frequent small meals, using bland and soft diet at mild temperatures.
2. Teach patient to avoid irritants, such as alcohol, tobacco, spices, extreme food temperatures.
3. Administer or teach self-administration of pain medication or anti-emetic before eating or drinking, if needed.

4. Encourage mouth care at least twice per day and after meals using gentle flossing, soft toothbrush or toothette, and mild mouth rinse.

5. Assess for ulcers, plaques, or discharge that may be indicative of superimposed infection.

6. For diarrhea, switch to low-residue diet and administer anti-diarrheals, as ordered.

Patient Education and Health Maintenance

1. Teach patient about risk of infection (see Patient Education Guidelines 26-1, page 983).

2. Teach patient how to take medications, as ordered, and instruct about possible adverse effects and management.

3. Explain to patient that radiation therapy may cause sterility; men should be given opportunity for sperm banking before treatment; women may develop ovarian failure and require hormone replacement therapy.

4. Reassure patient that fatigue will decrease after treatment is completed; encourage frequent naps and rest periods.

5. Provide patient and family with information about resources in the community, such as the Leukemia and Lymphoma Society and the American Cancer Society (see Box 26-1, page 990).

Evaluation: Expected Outcomes

- Skin intact without erythema or swelling.
- Oral mucosa intact, patient eating.

Non-Hodgkin's Lymphomas

Non-Hodgkin's lymphomas are a group of malignancies of lymphoid tissue arising from T or B lymphocytes or their precursors; it includes both indolent and aggressive forms. In the United States B-cell lymphomas represent about 80% of all cases. Types of Non-Hodgkin's lymphomas include chronic lymphocytic leukemia or small lymphocytic lymphoma (CLL/SLL; see page 991), follicular lymphoma, diffuse large B-cell lymphoma, and primary cutaneous B-cell lymphoma.

Pathophysiology and Etiology

1. Association with defective or altered immune system; higher incidence in patients receiving immunosuppression for organ transplant, in HIV-positive people, and in people with some viruses (eg, HTLV-1 and Epstein-Barr). Other risk factors include family history, male gender, white ethnicity, autoimmune diseases such as rheumatoid arthritis, history of *Helicobacter* gastritis (for gastric B-cell lymphoma), history of Hodgkin's lymphoma, history of radiation therapy, diet high in meats and fat, exposure to certain pesticides.

2. Arise from malignant transformation of lymphocyte at some stage during development; level of differentiation and type of lymphocyte influences course of illness and prognosis.

3. Incidence rises steadily from age 40.

Clinical Manifestations

1. Common symptoms include painless enlargement of lymph nodes (generally unilateral); fever; chills; night sweats; weight loss; unexplained pain in chest, abdomen, or bones. Unlike Hodgkin's lymphoma, is more likely to be advanced disease at presentation.

2. Various symptoms may occur with pulmonary involvement, superior vena cava obstruction, hepatic or bone involvement.

Diagnostic Evaluation

1. Incisional or excisional lymph node biopsy to detect type.

2. CBC, bone marrow aspirate, and biopsy to detect bone marrow involvement.

3. CT scan of the chest, abdomen, and pelvis with oral and intravenous contrast or PET with CT scan to detect deep nodal involvement.

4. Liver function tests, liver scan to detect liver involvement. Hepatitis B testing is recommended due to risk of reactivation.

5. Lumbar puncture to detect CNS involvement (for some lymphoma types).

6. Surgical staging (laparotomy with splenectomy, liver biopsy, multiple lymph node biopsies).

Management

1. The NCCN guidelines for non-Hodgkin's lymphomas (*www.nccn.org*) describe a variety of regimens, using radiation therapy, chemotherapy, monoclonal antibodies, radioimmune therapy, and hematopoietic stem cell transplant. Precise diagnosis and staging is needed to ensure appropriate treatment.

2. Radiation therapy is generally palliative, not curative.

3. Chemotherapy: various regimens available, including CHOP regimen of cyclophosphamide, doxorubicin (Adriamycin), vincristine (Oncovin), and prednisone; or BACOP regimen of bleomycin, doxorubicin (Adriamycin), cyclophosphamide, vincristine (Oncovin), and prednisone.

4. Monoclonal antibody therapy: rituximab may be given alone or with chemotherapy to patients with CD20 positive lymphomas. Hepatitis B–positive patients receiving rituximab are at high risk for reactivation and need antiviral prophylaxis and close monitoring.

5. Radioimmune therapies, such as Yttrium-90-labeled ibritumomab tiuxetan and ^{131}I tositumomab, have been effective for patients with certain lymphomas who do not respond to rituximab.

6. Autologous or allogeneic bone marrow or stem cell transplantation.

Complications

1. Of radiation therapy and chemotherapy (see pages 151 and 139).

2. Of disease: depends on location and extent of malignancy, but may include splenomegaly, hepatomegaly, thromboembolic complications, spinal cord compression.

Nursing Assessment

1. Obtain health history, focusing on fatigue, fever, chills, night sweats, swollen lymph nodes, and history of illness or therapy causing immunosuppression.

2. Evaluate splenomegaly, hepatomegaly, lymphadenopathy.

Nursing Diagnosis

- Risk for Infection related to altered immune response because of lymphoma and leukopenia caused by chemotherapy or radiation therapy.

Nursing Interventions

Minimizing Risk of Infection

1. Care for patient in protected environment with strict handwashing observed.
2. Avoid invasive procedures, such as urinary catheterization, if possible.
3. Assess temperature and vital signs, breath sounds, LOC, and skin and mucous membranes frequently for signs of infection.
4. Notify health care provider of fever greater than 101° F (38.3° C) or change in condition.
5. Obtain cultures of suspected infected sites or body fluids.

Patient Education and Health Maintenance

1. Teach patient infection precautions (see Patient Education Guidelines 26-1, page 983).
2. Encourage frequent follow-up visits for monitoring of CBC and condition.
3. Provide patient and family with information about resources in the community, such as the Leukemia and Lymphoma Society and the American Cancer Society (see Box 26-1, page 990).

Evaluation: Expected Outcomes

- Remains afebrile with no signs or symptoms of infection.

Multiple Myeloma

Multiple myeloma is a malignant disorder of plasma cells accounting for approximately 13% of all hematologic malignancies.

Pathophysiology and Etiology

1. Etiology unknown; genetic and environmental factors, such as chronic exposure to low levels of ionizing radiation and agricultural exposures to herbicides, may play a part.
2. Characterized by proliferation of neoplastic plasma cells derived from one B lymphocyte (clone) and producing a homogeneous immunoglobulin (M protein or Bence-Jones protein) without any apparent antigenic stimulation.
3. Plasma cells produce osteoclast-activating factor leading to extensive bone loss, severe pain, and pathologic fractures.
4. Abnormal immunoglobulin affects renal function, platelet function, resistance to infection, and may cause hyperviscosity of blood.
5. Generally affects older people (median age at diagnosis is 68) and is twice as common among African Americans as among Caucasians.

Clinical Manifestations

1. Constant, usually severe bone pain caused by bone lesions and pathologic fractures; sites commonly affected include thoracic and lumbar vertebrae, ribs, skull, pelvis, and proximal long bones.
2. Fatigue and weakness related to anemia caused by crowding of marrow by plasma cells.
3. Proteinuria and renal insufficiency.
4. Electrolyte disturbances, including hypercalcemia (bone destruction), hyperuricemia (cell death, renal insufficiency).

Diagnostic Evaluation

1. Bone marrow aspiration and biopsy—demonstrate increased number and abnormal form of plasma cells.
2. CBC and blood smear—changes reflect anemia.
3. Urine and serum analysis for presence and quantity of abnormal immunoglobulin.
4. Skeletal x-rays—osteolytic bone lesions.

Management

1. Patients with "smoldering" multiple myeloma do not require treatment.
2. The NCCN guidelines for symptomatic multiple myeloma (*www.nccn.org*) and other clinical guidelines currently recommend two treatment approaches: either melphalan plus thalidomide or melphalan plus bortezomib as initial treatment. Melphalan is a chemotherapy agent. Thalidomide is an anti-angiogenesis agent and bortezomib is a proteasome inhibitor. Another option is low-dose dexamethasone plus lenalidomide, a structural analogue of thalidomide.
2. Autologous bone marrow or peripheral blood stem cell transplant in selected cases (usually younger than age 65 with no renal failure, few bone lesions, and good organ function).
3. Supportive care options:
   a. Plasmapheresis to treat hyperviscosity or bleeding.
   b. Radiation therapy for bone lesions.
   c. Biphosphonates (eg, pamidronate), potent inhibitors of bone resorption, to treat hypercalcemia and alleviate bone pain.
   d. Allopurinol and fluids to treat hyperuricemia.
   e. Hemodialysis to manage renal failure.
   f. Surgical stabilization and fixation of fractures.

 DRUG ALERT Pamidronate and other biphosphonates may cause transient temperature elevations, hypophosphatemia, hypomagnesemia, hypocalcemia, and local reactions at the site of IV administration, such as thrombophlebitis, pain, and erythema. Biphosphonates are administered as IV infusions, generally during 4 or more hours; rapid IV administration may cause renal failure. Long-term biphosphonate use has been associated with jaw osteonecrosis—patients should be monitored closely and advised to maintain good oral health and avoid invasive dental procedures.

Complications

1. Pathologic fractures, spinal cord compression.
2. Recurrent infections, particularly bacterial.
3. Electrolyte abnormalities (hypercalcemia, hypophosphatemia).
4. Renal failure, pyelonephritis.
5. Bleeding.

6. Thromboembolic complications caused by hyperviscosity.
7. Patients with multiple myeloma treated by chemotherapy have a median survival of 2 to 3 years; the impact of newer treatment options on survival is still unknown.

Nursing Assessment

1. Obtain health history, focusing on pain, fatigue.
2. Evaluate for evidence of bone deformities and bone tenderness or pain.
3. Assess patient's support system and personal coping skills.

Nursing Diagnoses

- Acute Pain related to destruction of bone and possible pathologic fractures.
- Impaired Physical Mobility related to pain and possible fracture.
- Fear related to poor prognosis.
- Risk for Injury related to complications of disease process.

Nursing Interventions

Controlling Pain

1. Assess for presence, location, intensity, and characteristics of pain.
2. Administer pharmacologic agents, as ordered, to control pain. Use adequate doses of regularly scheduled, around-the-clock analgesics.
3. Teach the use of nonpharmacologic methods, such as music, relaxation breathing, progressive muscle relaxation, distraction, and imagery, to help manage pain.
4. Assess effectiveness of analgesics and adjust dosage or drug used, as necessary, to control pain.

Promoting Mobility

1. Encourage patient to wear back brace for lumbar lesion.
2. Recommend physical and occupational therapy consultation.
3. Discourage bed rest to prevent hypercalcemia but ensure safety of environment to prevent fractures.
4. Assist patient with measures to prevent injury and decrease risk of fractures. Advise avoidance of lifting and straining; use walker and other assistive devices, as appropriate.

Relieving Fear

1. Develop trusting, supportive relationship with patient and his or her significant others.
2. Encourage patient to discuss medical condition and prognosis with health care provider when patient is ready.
3. Assure patient that you are available for support, to provide comfort measures, and to answer questions.
4. Encourage use of patient's own support network, religious and community services, and national agencies (see Box 26-1, page 990).

Monitoring for Complications

1. Report sudden, severe pain, especially of back, which could indicate pathologic fracture.
2. Watch for nausea, drowsiness, confusion, polyuria, which could indicate hypercalcemia caused by bony destruction or immobilization. Monitor serum calcium levels.

3. Check results of blood urea nitrogen (BUN) and creatinine and urine protein tests to detect renal insufficiency, caused by nephrotoxicity of abnormal proteins in multiple myeloma.
4. Increase fluid intake, monitor intake and output, and weigh patient daily.

Community and Home Care Considerations

1. Make sure patient has appropriate housing and equipment to support decreased mobility and risk of pathologic fractures (eg, stair handrails, cane or walker, commode chair).
2. Inspect home environment for throw rugs, cluttered furnishings, dark hallways, or difficult stairs that may cause a fall and possible fracture.

Patient Education and Health Maintenance

1. Teach patient about risk of infection caused by impaired antibody production and chemotherapy (see Patient Education Guidelines 26-1, page 983).
2. Teach patient to take medications, as prescribed, and monitor for possible adverse effects; avoid aspirin and NSAIDs unless prescribed by health care provider because these drugs may interfere with platelet function.
3. Teach patient to minimize risk of fractures. Use proper body mechanics and assistive devices, as appropriate; avoid bed rest, remain ambulatory.
4. Advise patient to report new onset of pain, new location, or sudden increase in pain intensity immediately. Report new onset or worsening of neurologic symptoms (eg, changes in sensation) immediately.
5. Encourage the patient to maintain high fluid intake (2 to 3 L/day) to avoid dehydration and prevent renal insufficiency; also not to fast before diagnostic tests.
6. Provide patient and family with information about resources in the community, such as the Leukemia and Lymphoma Society and the American Cancer Society (see Box 26-1, page 990).

Evaluation: Expected Outcomes

- States decreased pain.
- Ambulates without injury.
- Asks questions about disease; contacts support group.
- No development of complications.

BLEEDING DISORDERS

Bleeding disorders may be congenital or acquired and may be caused by dysfunction in any phase of hemostasis (clot formation and dissolution). Bleeding disorders seen in adults include thrombocytopenia, idiopathic thrombocytopenic purpura (ITP), DIC, and von Willebrand disease.

Thrombocytopenia

Thrombocytopenia is characterized by a decreased platelet count (less than $150,000/mm^3$), the most common cause of bleeding disorders.

Pathophysiology and Etiology

Classification by Etiology

1. Decreased platelet production—infiltrative diseases of bone marrow, leukemia, aplastic anemia, myelofibrosis, myelosuppressive therapy, radiation therapy; may include inherited disorders, such as Fanconi's anemia and Wiskott-Aldrich syndrome.
2. Increased platelet destruction—infection (eg, HIV or hepatitis C), drug-induced (eg, heparin or quinidine), ITP, DIC.
3. Abnormal distribution or sequestration in spleen.
4. Dilutional thrombocytopenia—after hemorrhage, RBC transfusions.

Clinical Manifestations

1. Usually asymptomatic.
2. When platelet count drops below 20,000/mm³:
   a. Petechiae occur spontaneously.
   b. Ecchymoses occur at sites of minor trauma (venipuncture, pressure).
   c. Bleeding may occur from mucosal surfaces, nose, GI and GU tracts, respiratory system, and within CNS.
   d. Menorrhagia is common.
3. Excessive bleeding may occur after procedures (dental extractions, minor surgery, biopsies).
4. Thrombotic complications (arterial and venous) and areas of skin necrosis are associated with heparin-induced thrombocytopenia.

Diagnostic Evaluation

1. CBC with platelet count—decreased hemoglobin, hematocrit, platelets.
2. Bleeding time, prothrombin time (PT), partial thromboplastin time (PTT)—prolonged.
3. Platelet aggregation test for heparin-dependent platelet antibodies—positive.

Management

1. Treat underlying cause.
2. Platelet transfusions.
3. Steroids or IV immunoglobulins may be helpful in selected patients.
4. Heparin-induced thrombocytopenia: discontinue heparin, use alternate anticoagulant therapy due to high risk of venous and arterial thromboses in these patients (direct thrombin inhibitors, such as lepirudin or argatroban hirudin), avoid platelet transfusions. Although incidence varies dependent upon patient population and heparin preparation, any exposure to heparin can precipitate this serious autoimmune syndrome.

Complications

Severe blood loss or bleeding into vital organs may be life-threatening.

Nursing Assessment

1. Obtain health history, focusing on prior illnesses and episodes of bleeding, past surgical experiences, exposure to toxins or ionizing radiation, family history of bleeding.
2. Obtain list of current and recent medications (including OTC preparations, herbal and dietary supplements).
3. Perform complete physical examination for signs of bleeding.

Nursing Diagnosis

- Risk for Injury related to bleeding due to thrombocytopenia.

Nursing Interventions

Minimizing Bleeding

1. Institute bleeding precautions.
   a. Avoid use of plain razor, hard toothbrush or floss, I.M. injections, tourniquets, rectal procedures, suppositories.
   b. Administer stool softeners, as necessary, to prevent constipation.
   c. Restrict activity and exercise when platelet count is less than 20,000/mm³ or when active bleeding occurs.
2. Monitor pad count and amount of saturation during menses; administer or teach self-administration of hormones to suppress menstruation, as prescribed.
3. Administer blood products, as ordered. Monitor for signs and symptoms of allergic reactions, anaphylaxis, and volume overload.
4. Evaluate urine, stools, and emesis for gross and occult blood.

Patient Education and Health Maintenance

1. Teach patient bleeding precautions (see Patient Education Guidelines 26-2, page 984).
2. Demonstrate the use of direct, steady pressure at bleeding site if bleeding develops.
3. Encourage routine follow-up for platelet counts.

Evaluation: Expected Outcomes

- Episodes of bleeding rapidly controlled; platelet count maintained at goal (usually 20,000/mm³).

Immune (Idiopathic) ThrombocytopeniA

Immune thrombocytopenia (ITP), historically known as idiopathic thrombocytopenic purpura, is an acute or chronic bleeding disorder that results from immune destruction of platelets by antiplatelet antibodies.

Pathophysiology and Etiology

1. Proteins on the platelet cell membrane stimulate production of autoantibodies that bind to circulating platelets, leading to destruction of platelets in spleen, liver.
2. Acute disorder more common in childhood, typically following viral illness; has good prognosis, with 80% to 90% recovering uneventfully within 6 months.
3. Chronic disorder (more than 6-month course) most common between ages 20 and 50, three times more common in women, may last for years or even indefinitely. May be associated with pregnancy or with development of systemic lupus erythematosus, thyroid disease, infections (eg, *Helicobater pylori*, cytomegalovirus, varicella zoster, hepatitis C and HIV) or malignancy (eg, CLL).

Clinical Manifestations

May have no signs and symptoms with mild disease (platelet counts 30,000 to 100,000/mm^3) Platelet counts less than 30,000/mm^3: bruising, petechiae, bleeding from nares and gums, menorrhagia.

Diagnostic Evaluation

1. CBC demonstrates platelet count less than 100,000/mm^3; may also be lymphocytosis and eosinophilia.
2. Testing for Hepatitis C, HIV, *Helicobacter pylori*, and Epstein-Barr virus, which have been found to be associated with ITP.
3. Bone marrow aspirate (not necessary for most patients with typical features of ITP) shows increased numbers of young megakaryocytes, sometimes increased numbers of eosinophils.
4. Assay for platelet autoantibodies sometimes helpful.
5. Bleeding times are typically normal.

Management

1. Supportive care: judicious use of platelet transfusions, control of bleeding.
2. High-dose corticosteroids, IV immunoglobulins, parenteral anti-D (for Rhesus-positive patients with spleens). Thrombopoietin receptor agonists may be used to treat patients at risk for bleeding with chronic or relapsed ITP.
3. Splenectomy (see page 975) removes potential site for sequestration and destruction of platelets and is used to treat chronic refractory ITP in adults.

Complications

Severe blood loss or bleeding into vital organs may be life-threatening.

Nursing Assessment

1. Obtain history of bleeding episodes, including bruising and petechiae, bleeding of gums, and heavy menses.
2. Perform physical examination for signs of bleeding.

Nursing Diagnosis

• Risk for bleeding due to thrombocytopenia.

Nursing Interventions

Minimizing Bleeding

1. Institute bleeding precautions.
2. Monitor pad count and amount of saturation during menses; administer or teach self-administration of hormones to suppress menstruation, as prescribed.
3. Administer blood products, as ordered. Monitor for signs and symptoms of allergic reactions, anaphylaxis, and volume overload.
4. Evaluate all urine and stools for gross and occult blood.

Patient Education and Health Maintenance

1. Teach patient bleeding precautions (see Patient Education Guidelines 26-2, page 984).

2. Demonstrate the use of direct, steady pressure at bleeding site if bleeding does develop.
3. Encourage routine follow-up for platelet counts.

Evaluation: Expected Outcomes

• Episodes of bleeding rapidly controlled.

Disseminated Intravascular Coagulation

Disseminated intravascular coagulation (DIC) is an acquired thrombotic and hemorrhagic syndrome characterized by abnormal activation of the clotting cascade and accelerated fibrinolysis. This results in widespread clotting in small vessels with consumption of clotting factors and platelets, so that bleeding and thrombosis occur simultaneously.

Pathophysiology and Etiology

1. A syndrome arising secondary to an underlying disorder or event.
   a. Overwhelming infections, particularly bacterial sepsis.
   b. Obstetric complications: abruptio placentae, eclampsia, amniotic fluid embolism, retention of dead fetus.
   c. Massive tissue injury: burns, trauma, fractures, major surgery, fat embolism, organ destruction (eg, severe pancreatitis, hepatic failure).
   d. Malignancy: particularly lung, colon, stomach, pancreas.
   e. Vascular and circulatory collapse, shock.
   f. Severe toxic or immunologic reactions: hemolytic transfusion reaction, snake bites, recreational drugs.

Clinical Manifestations

1. Signs of abnormal clotting:
   a. Coolness and mottling of extremities.
   b. Acrocyanosis (cold, mottled extremities with clear demarcation from normal tissue).
   c. Dyspnea, adventitious breath sounds.
   d. Altered mental status.
   e. Acute renal failure.
   f. Pain (eg, related to bowel infarction).
2. Signs of abnormal bleeding:
   a. Oozing, bleeding from sites of procedures, IV catheter insertion sites, suture lines, mucous membranes, orifices.
   b. Internal bleeding leading to changes in vital organ function, altered vital signs.

Diagnostic Evaluation

1. Platelet count—diminished.
2. PT, PTT, and thrombin time—prolonged.
3. Fibrinogen—decreased level.
4. Fibrin split (degradation) products—increased level.
5. D-dimer fibrin degradation product—increased level.
6. Antithrombin III—decreased level.
7. Protein C—decreased level.

Management

1. Treat underlying disorder.
2. Replacement therapy for serious hemorrhagic manifestations:
   a. Fresh-frozen plasma replaces clotting factors.
   b. Platelet transfusions.
   c. Cryoprecipitate replaces clotting factors and fibrinogen.
3. Supportive measures including fluid replacement, oxygenation, maintenance of BP and renal perfusion.
4. Heparin or other anticoagulant therapy (controversial) inhibits clotting component of DIC.

Complications

1. Thromboembolic: pulmonary embolism; cerebral, myocardial, splenic, or bowel infarction; acute renal failure; tissue necrosis or gangrene.
2. Hemorrhagic: cerebral hemorrhage is most common cause of death in DIC.

Nursing Assessment

1. Be aware that seriously ill patients are at risk; monitor condition closely.
2. Assess for signs of bleeding and thrombosis, including chest pain, shortness of breath, hematuria, abdominal pain, headache, numbness and coolness of an extremity.

Nursing Diagnoses

- Risk for bleeding due to thrombocytopenia.
- Ineffective Tissue Perfusion (all tissues) related to ischemia due to microthrombi formation.

Nursing Interventions

Minimizing Bleeding

1. Institute bleeding precautions.
2. Monitor pad count and amount of saturation during menses; administer or teach self-administration of hormones to suppress menstruation, as prescribed.
3. Administer blood products, as ordered. Monitor for signs and symptoms of allergic reactions, anaphylaxis, and volume overload.
4. Avoid dislodging clots. Apply pressure to sites of bleeding for at least 20 minutes, use topical hemostatic agents. Use tape cautiously.
5. Maintain bed rest during bleeding episode.
6. If internal bleeding is suspected, assess bowel sounds and abdominal girth.
7. Evaluate fluid status and bleeding by frequent measurement of vital signs, central venous pressure, intake and output.

Promoting Tissue Perfusion

1. Keep patient warm.
2. Avoid vasoconstrictive agents (systemic or topical).
3. Change patient's position frequently and perform range-of-motion exercises.
4. Monitor electrocardiogram and laboratory tests for dysfunction of vital organs caused by ischemia—arrhythmias,

abnormal arterial blood gas levels, increased BUN and creatinine levels.
5. Monitor for signs of vascular occlusion and report immediately.
   a. Brain—decreased LOC, sensory and motor deficits, seizures, coma.
   b. Eyes—visual deficits.
   c. Bone—bone pain.
   d. Pulmonary vasculature—chest pain, shortness of breath, tachycardia.
   e. Extremities—cold, mottling, numbness.
   f. Coronary arteries—chest pain, arrhythmias.
   g. Bowel—pain, tenderness, decreased bowel sounds.

Patient Education and Health Maintenance

Explain the syndrome and its management to patient and family members as part of reassurance and support during this critical illness.

Evaluation: Expected Outcomes

- Episodes of bleeding rapidly controlled.
- Alert, vital signs stable, urine output adequate, no complaints of chest pain or shortness of breath.

von Willebrand Disease

Von Willebrand disease is an inherited (autosomal dominant) or acquired bleeding disorder characterized by decreased level of von Willebrand factor and prolonged bleeding time.

Pathophysiology and Etiology

1. von Willebrand factor synthesized in vascular endothelium, megakaryocytes, and platelets; enhances platelet adhesion as first step in clot formation, also acts as carrier of factor VIII in blood.
2. von Willebrand is most common inherited bleeding disorder, with estimated incidence as high as 1 in 90 people; includes multiple subtypes with varying severity; affects males and females.
3. Acquired form is rare, generally appears late in life, typically in association with lymphoma, leukemia, multiple myeloma, or autoimmune disorder.

Clinical Manifestations

1. Mucosal and cutaneous bleeding (eg, bruising, gingival bleeding, epistaxis, menorrhagia).
2. Prolonged bleeding from cuts or after dental and surgical procedures.

Diagnostic Evaluation

1. Bleeding time—prolonged.
2. Ristocetin cofactor—abnormal.
3. von Willebrand factor—decreased.
4. von Willebrand factor multimers—demonstrate defective von Willebrand factor in some types.
5. Factor VIII—generally decreased.

Management

1. Replacement of von Willebrand factor and factor VIII using clotting factor concentrates.
2. Antifibrinolytic medications (aminocaproic acid, tranexamic acid) to stabilize clot formation before dental procedures and before minor surgery.
3. Desmopressin acetate, a synthetic analogue of vasopressin, may be used to manage mild to moderate bleeding.
4. Estrogen and progesterone stimulate production of von Willebrand factor and factor VIII and may be particularly helpful in control of menorrhagia.

Complications

Severe blood loss or bleeding into vital organs may be life-threatening.

Nursing Assessment

1. Obtain history of bleeding episodes such as menstrual flow. Ask quantitative questions (eg, how many nosebleeds do you have each year?) as patient may not realize his or her experience is abnormal.
2. Perform physical examination for signs of bleeding.

Nursing Diagnosis

- Risk for Bleeding due to decreased level of von Willebrand factor and factor VIII.

Nursing Interventions

Minimizing Bleeding

1. Institute bleeding precautions:
   a. Avoid use of plain razor, hard toothbrush, or floss.
   b. Avoid I.M. injections, tourniquets, rectal procedures, or suppositories.
   c. Administer stool softeners, as necessary, to prevent constipation.
   d. Restrict activity and exercise when platelet count less than 20,000/mm³ or when active bleeding occurs.
2. Monitor pad count and amount of saturation during menses; administer or teach self-administration of hormones to suppress menstruation, as prescribed.
3. Administer blood products, as ordered. Monitor for signs and symptoms of allergic reactions, anaphylaxis, and volume overload.
4. Use topical hemostatic agents, such as absorbable gelatin, oxidized cellulose, topical adrenaline, or phenylephrine, if pressure and use of ice does not stop bleeding.

Patient Education and Health Maintenance

1. Teach patient bleeding precautions (see Patient Education Guidelines 26-2, page 984).
2. Demonstrate the use of direct, steady pressure at bleeding site if bleeding develops.

Evaluation: Expected Outcomes

- Episodes of bleeding rapidly controlled.

SELECTED REFERENCES

Aguilar, R. B., Keister, K. J., & Russell, A. C. (2010). Prevention of sepsis after splenectomy. *Dimensions of Critical Care Nursing, 29*(2), 65–68.

Bauer, K., Rancea, M., Schmidtke, B., et al. (2011). Thirteenth annual report of the Cochrane Haematological Malignancies Group: Focus on multiple myeloma. *Journal of the National Cancer Institute, 103*(17), E1–E19.

Belavik, J. M. (2010). New treatment for von Willebrand disease. *The Nurse Practitioner, 35*(9), 13–14.

Blaisdel, F. W. (2012). Causes, prevention, and treatment of intravascular coagulation and disseminated intravascular coagulation. *Journal of Trauma and Acute Care Surgery, 72*(6), 1719–1722.

Cornell, R. F. & Palmer, J. (2012). Adult acute leukemia. *Disease-A-Month, 58,* 219–238.

Den Elzen, W. P., Willems, J. M., Westendorp, R. G., et al. (2010). Subnormal vitamin B12 concentrations and anaemia in older people: A systematic review. *BMC Geriatrics, 10*(42), 1–11.

Feldman, L. S. (2011). Laparoscopic splenectomy: Standardized approach. *World Journal of Surgery, 35,* 1487–1495.

Hunt, C. W. (2010). Immune thrombocytopenia purpura. *Medical-Surgical Nursing, 19*(4), 237–239.

Kauffman, J. (2011). Recombinant infusion therapies indicated for bleeding disorders. *Journal of Infusion Nursing, 34*(1), 29–35.

Kojima, S., Nakao, S., Young, N., et al. (2011). The Third Consensus Conference on the treatment of aplastic anemia. *International Journal of Hematology, 93,* 832–837.

Marsh, J. C. W., Ball, S. E., Cavenagh, J., et al. (2009). Guidelines for the diagnosis and management of aplastic anaemia. *British Journal of Haematology, 147,* 43–70.

Meenaghan, T., Dowling, M., & Kelly, M. (2012). Acute leukaemia: Making sense of a complex blood cancer. *British Journal of Nursing, 21*(2), 76–83.

Neunert, C., Lim, W., Crowther, M., et al. (2011). The American Society of Hematology 2011 evidence-based practice guideline for immune thrombocytopenia. *Blood, 117,* 4190–4207.

Tefferi, A. (2012). Polycythemia vera and essential thrombocythemia: 2012 update on diagnosis, risk stratification, and management. *American Journal of Hematology, 87,* 285–293.

Watmough, S., & Flynn, M. (2011). A review of pain management interventions in bone marrow biopsy. *Journal of Clinical Nursing, 20,* 615–623.

Weiss, J. A. (2012). Just heavy menses or something more? Raising awareness of von Willenbrand disease. *American Journal of Nursing, 112*(6), 38–44.

Zelenetz, A. D., Abramson, J. S., Advani, R. H., et al. (2011). Non-Hodgkin's lymphomas. *Journal of the National Comprehensive Cancer Network, 9,* 484–560.

27

Transfusion Therapy and Blood and Marrow Stem Cell Transplantation

TRANSFUSION THERAPY

Principles of Transfusion Therapy

Due to the potentially life-threatening consequences of blood type ABO incompatibility and disease transmission through blood products, transfusion therapy is limited to occasions when it is absolutely necessary and stringent screening techniques are required before transfusion begins. Alternatives to transfusion therapy should also be considered, as appropriate, such as erythropoietin-stimulating agents, iron supplementation, blood loss prevention during surgery, and volume replacement with other solutions. Blood product procurement, storage, preparation, and testing are regulated by the Food and Drug Administration (FDA), the American Association of Blood Banks, and the Joint Commission.

Blood Compatibility

Antigens
1. The surface membrane of the red blood cell (RBC) is characterized by glycoproteins known as antigens.
2. More than 400 different antigens have been identified on the RBC membrane.
3. There are fewer than a dozen clinically significant antigens, and of these, only two antigenic systems (ABO and Rh) require routine prospective matching before the transfusion.

4. The ABO blood group system is clinically the most significant because A and B antigens elicit the strongest immune response.
5. The presence or absence of A and B antigens on the RBC membrane determines the person's ABO group (see Table 27-1). The ability to make A or B antigens is inherited.
6. Antibody formation without specific exposure to the antigen is unique to the ABO system. Antibody directed against the missing antigens is produced in neonates by 3 months of age.

Antibodies
1. Antibodies (or immunoglobulins) are proteins produced by B lymphocytes; they consist of two light and two heavy chains that form a Y shape.
2. Antibodies generally have a high degree of specificity and interact only with the antigen that stimulated their production.
3. The five classes of immunoglobulins are determined by differences in their heavy chains: immunoglobulin (Ig) G, IgA, IgM, IgD, IgE.
4. The interaction of antibodies and antigens triggers the humoral immune response.
5. Antibodies against the A and B antigens are large IgM molecules. When they interact with and coat the A and B antigens on the RBC surface, the antibody/RBC complexes clump together (agglutinate).

Table 27-1	Blood Group Antigens and Antibodies of ABO System		
BLOOD GROUP	**ANTIGEN ON RBC**	**ANTIBODY IN PLASMA**	**APPROXIMATE FREQUENCY OF OCCURRENCE IN POPULATION**
A	A	anti-B	45%
B	B	anti-A	8%
AB	A and B	None	3%
O	None	anti-A and anti-B	44%

6. Antibody/RBC complexes also activate the complement cascade, resulting in the release of numerous active substances and RBC lysis. The large antibody/RBC complexes also become trapped in capillaries, where they may cause thrombotic complications to vital organs, and in the reticuloendothelial system, where they are removed from circulation by the spleen.

7. The extent of the humoral response elicited by anti-A and anti-B interaction with A and B antigens depends on the quantity of antibody and antigen.

Other Red Blood Cell Antigens

1. Non-ABO RBC antigen–antibody reactions usually do not produce powerful immediate hemolytic reactions, but several have clinical significance.

2. After A and B, D is the most immunogenic antigen. It is part of the Rhesus system, which includes C, D, and E antigens.

   a. D (Rh)-negative people do not develop anti-D without specific exposure, but have a high incidence of antibody development (alloimmunization) after exposure to D.

   b. Two common methods of sensitization to these RBC antigens are by transfusion or fetomaternal hemorrhage during pregnancy and delivery.

   c. Anti-D can complicate future transfusions and pregnancies. For the D (Rh)-negative person, exposure to D should be avoided by the use of Rh-negative blood products. In the case of Rh-negative mother and Rh-positive fetus, prophylaxis for exposure to D uses Rh immunoglobulin (RhoGAM), which will prevent anti-D formation.

   d. Exposure to RBC antigens from other antigenic systems (such as Lewis, Kidd, or Duffy) may also cause alloimmunization, which becomes clinically significant in people who receive multiple blood products for extended periods of time.

Blood Transfusion Options

Autologous Transfusion

1. Before elective procedures, the patient may donate blood to be set aside for later transfusion. Patients may donate up to 3 days prior to surgery provided hemoglobin is greater than 11 g/dL.

2. Autologous RBCs can also be salvaged during some surgical procedures or after trauma-induced hemorrhage by use of automated cell-saver devices or by manual suction equipment.

3. Autologous blood products must be clearly labeled and identified.

4. Autologous transfusion eliminates the risks of alloimmunization, immune-mediated transfusion reactions, and transmission of disease, making it the safest transfusion choice.

 NURSING ALERT Patients who do not meet standard criteria for blood donation may still be eligible to donate autologous blood before elective surgeries. The nurse should encourage suitable candidates to consider this underused option.

Homologous Transfusion

1. With this most common option, volunteer donors' blood products are assigned to patients randomly.

2. Before donation, volunteer donors receive information about the process, potential adverse effects, tests that will be performed on donated blood, postdonation instructions, and education regarding risk of human immunodeficiency virus (HIV) infection and signs and symptoms.

3. Donors are screened against eligibility criteria designed to protect donor and recipient (see Table 27-2).

Table 27-2	General Blood Donor Eligibility Criteria
Age	≥17 years *or* 16 years with parental consent if state law allows
Weight	Minimum 110 lb (49.9 kg) (additional rules apply for donors ≤ 18 years)
Vital signs	Afebrile, normotensive, pulse 50–100, blood pressure < 180/100 mm Hg
Hemoglobin	≥12.5 g/dL
History	Travel, exposures, and past illnesses or events may defer or disallow blood donation. *Examples*: travel to malarial areas, living in areas exposed to bovine spongiform encephalopathy, blood transfusion or tattoo within 12 months, recent surgery or pregnancy, corneal transplant, history of hepatitis or unexplained jaundice, history of blood cancer or recent cancer, history of behaviors at high risk for human immunodeficiency virus.
Immunizations	Recent attenuated and live vaccines generally result in deferral.
Illnesses	A variety of current illnesses may defer or disallow blood donation. *Examples*: clotting disorders, sickle cell disease, systemic lupus erythematosus, multiple sclerosis, Lyme disease, tuberculosis, chronic fatigue syndrome.
Medications	Blood thinners, such as heparin and warfarin, disallow donation. Some other medications may result in deferral.

Evidence Base American Red Cross. (2012). Donate blood: Eligibility requirements. Available: *www.redcrossblood.org/donating-blood/eligibility-requirements*.

Directed Transfusion

1. In directed transfusion, blood products are donated by a person for transfusion to a specified recipient.
2. This option may be used in certain circumstances (eg, a parent who provides sole transfusion support for a child), but in general, no evidence exists that directed donation reduces transfusion risks.

Blood Product Screening

Serologic Testing

1. Routine laboratory testing is performed to assess the compatibility of a particular blood product with the recipient before release of the blood product from the blood bank (see Table 27-3).
   a. ABO group and Rh type: determines the presence of A, B, and D antigens on the surface of the patient's RBCs.
   b. Direct Coombs' test: determines the antibody attached to the patient's RBCs.
   c. Crossmatch (compatibility test): detects agglutination of donor RBCs caused by antibodies in the patient's serum.
   d. Indirect Coombs' test: identifies lower molecular-weight antibodies (IgG) directed against blood group antigens.

Screening for Infectious Diseases

1. Routine laboratory testing is performed to identify antigens or antibodies in donor blood that may indicate prior exposure to specific blood-borne diseases.
2. Such testing supplements other principles of donation designed to decrease the risk of disease transmission via blood products, including the use of volunteer donors, the exclusion of high-risk populations, and the screening of donors via health and social history.
3. Through the use of donor screening and blood testing, the risk of infections transmitted with donated blood is less than 1% and continues to decline.
4. Specific conditions screened for include:
   a. Hepatitis: Per FDA recommendations, each unit of blood is tested for the presence of hepatitis B core antibody, surface antigen, and more recently hepatitis B viral DNA through nucleic acid testing (NAT). Hepatitis C antibody and viral DNA tests (NAT) are also completed.
   b. HIV-1 and HIV-2: tests for prior exposure to the virus.
      i. All blood products in the United States have been screened since the test first became available in 1985. Current tests include testing for antibodies with enzyme-linked immunosorbent assay or enzyme immunoassay or antigen with the P24 test. NAT is becoming more widely used and provides a mechanism to look for the presence of HIV-1 and HIV-2 before antibody formation.
      ii. Because antibody to the virus is not produced until at least 6 weeks after exposure, diligent donor screening

---

Table 27-3 — ABO and Rh Compatibility Chart

This chart identifies ABO and Rh compatibility when transfusing whole blood, red blood cells, and plasma. Components suspended in plasma, such as platelets and cryoprecipitate, usually follow plasma compatibility rules if the total volume exceeds 120 mL for an adult patient.

WHOLE BLOOD

Recipient	A	B	O	AB	Rh positive	Rh negative
A	✔					
B		✔				
O			✔			
AB				✔		
Rh positive					✔	✔
Rh negative						✔

RED BLOOD CELLS

Recipient	A	B	O	AB	Rh positive	Rh negative
A	✔		✔			
B		✔	✔			
O			✔	✔		
AB	✔	✔	✔			
Rh positive					✔	✔
Rh negative						✔

PLASMA

Recipient	A	B	O	AB	Rh positive	Rh negative
A	✔			✔		
B		✔		✔		
O	✔	✔	✔	✔		
AB				✔		
Rh positive					✔	✔
Rh negative					✔	✔

and exclusion of high-risk groups (eg, homosexual men, intravenous [IV] drug abusers, prostitutes, and sexual partners of high-risk people) remain important parts of preventing transmission of HIV via blood products.

   iii. A low risk of HIV transmission (estimated to be less than 1/2,000,000 units of blood) remains.

c. Cytomegalovirus (CMV): tests for the antibody against CMV.

   i. Approximately 50% to 75% of blood donors have been exposed to CMV and 10% to 20% carry CMV virus in their white blood cells (WBCs).

   ii. Patients with impaired immune function (eg, bone marrow and organ transplant recipients, premature babies) are at risk for CMV infection from transfused blood. It is recommended that these patients receive CMV sero-negative blood or leukoreduced products.

d. Syphilis: tests for the presence of antibody against the spirochete.

e. Bacteria: contamination of blood products with bacteria may occur during and after collection of blood. This risk is managed by adherence to sterile technique during phlebotomy and blood-processing procedures, correct storage techniques, visual inspection of blood products, and limitations on shelf life.

f. Other infections that may be transmitted via blood transfusions include West Nile virus, human T-cell lymphoma virus (HTLV) 1 and 2, human herpes virus-8 (implicated as the causative agent of Kaposi's sarcoma), malaria, babesiosis, Chagas' disease, and yersinia. Variant Creutzfeldt-Jacob disease has also been transmitted via blood transfusions, which has led to restrictions on donation by individuals who have lived in areas with bovine spongiform encephalopathy or "mad cow" disease.

Administration of Whole Blood and Blood Components

Whole blood and blood components are administered to increase the amount of oxygen being delivered to the tissues and organs, to prevent or stop bleeding because of platelet defects or because of deficiencies or coagulation abnormalities, and to combat infection caused by decreased or defective WBCs or antibodies (see Procedure Guidelines 27-1, and Standards of Care Guidelines 27-1, page 1007).

General Considerations

1. A unit of whole blood is usually separated into its various components shortly after collection.
2. Less than 3% of the blood collected nationwide is transfused as whole blood.
   a. The use of blood components conserves the limited supply of blood, provides optimal therapeutic benefit, and reduces the risk of circulatory overload.
   b. Due to the risks, blood components should be administered only with informed consent and meticulous identification procedures.

Whole Blood

Description

1. Consists of RBCs, plasma, plasma proteins, and approximately 60 mL anticoagulant/preservative solution in a total volume of approximately 500 mL.
2. Indications include acute, massive blood loss of greater than 1,000 mL, requiring the oxygen-carrying properties of RBCs and the volume expansion provided by plasma. In general, even acute loss of as much as one third of a patient's total blood volume (1,000 to 1,200 mL) can be safely and rapidly replaced with crystalline or colloidal solutions.

Nursing and Patient Care Considerations

1. For rapid infusions of large volumes of whole blood, additional steps may be taken to deliver product rapidly and safely.
   a. A small-pore (20 to 40 mm) filter may be used to remove microaggregates (platelets, WBCs) that have been identified in the lungs of massively transfused patients.
   b. An approved blood warmer may be indicated to prevent hypothermia and cardiac arrhythmias associated with the rapid infusion of refrigerated solutions.
   c. Electromechanical infusion devices to deliver blood at high flow rates can hemolyze RBCs and should be used with caution.
2. Observe closely for the most common acute complication associated with whole blood transfusion—circulatory overload (rise in venous pressure, distended neck veins, dyspnea, cough, crackles at bases of lungs).

Packed RBCs

Description

1. Consist primarily of RBCs, a small amount of plasma, and approximately 100 mL anticoagulant/preservative solution in a total volume of approximately 250 to 300 mL/unit.
2. Packed RBCs may be contaminated with WBCs that may increase the risk of minor transfusion reactions and alloimmunization. For patients who receive multiple blood products during a specific period (eg, patients with leukemia or aplastic anemia), packed RBCs may be further manipulated to remove WBCs (leukoreduced) by washing or freezing the product in the blood bank or by the use of small-pore (20 to 40 mm) leukoreduction filters during administration.
3. Indications include restoration or maintenance of adequate organ oxygenation with minimal expansion of blood volume.
4. Dosage: average adult dose administered is 2 units; pediatric doses are generally calculated as 5 to 15 mL/kg.

Nursing and Patient Care Considerations

1. Infuse at the prescribed rate. Generally, a unit can be given to an adult in 90 to 120 minutes. Pediatric patients are usually transfused at a rate of 2 to 5 mL/kg per hour.
2. To reduce the risk of bacterial contamination and sepsis, RBCs must be transfused within 4 hours of leaving the blood bank.
3. Observe closely (particularly during first 15 to 30 minutes) for the most common acute complications associated with

PROCEDURE GUIDELINES 27-1

Administering Blood and Blood Components

EQUIPMENT

- Tourniquet
- Iodine-containing skin antiseptic
- Needle or venous catheter
- Y-type blood infusion set
- 170-μm filter
- Normal saline
- Blood product as described

PROCEDURE

Nursing Action	Rationale

Preparatory phase

1. Verify patient has given informed consent for the procedure.

2. Inform the patient of the procedure, blood product to be given, approximate length of time, and desired outcome.

1. Transfusions have known risks and complications. The patient has the right to know these risks and alternatives to transfusions. The patient has the right to consent or refuse.

2. Allays fear and anxiety.

 DRUG ALERT Crystalloid solutions other than 0.9% saline and all medications are incompatible with blood products. They may cause agglutination or hemolysis.

3. Obtain and record baseline vital signs.

4. Prepare infusion site. Select a large vein that allows patient some degree of mobility. Start the prescribed IV infusion.

5. Obtain blood product from blood bank. Inspect for abnormal color, cloudiness, clots, and excess air. Read instructions on the product label regarding storage and infusion. Check expiration date. If the transfusion cannot begin immediately, return product to blood bank.

6. Verify patient identification.

   a. Ask the patient to state full name and date of birth or other identifier and compare with information on the wristband. If the patient is unable to provide two identifiers, verify identity with an individual familiar with the patient.

   b. Compare the name, date of birth, and ID number on the wristband with the bag tag, transfusion form, and medical order.

   c. Confirm ABO and Rh compatibility by comparing the bag label, bag tag, medical record, and transfusion form.

   d. Check bag labels for expiration date and satisfactory serologic testing.

3. If the patient's clinical status permits, delay transfusion if baseline temperature is greater than 101.7° F (38.7° C).

4. Antecubital veins are not recommended for lengthy infusions. Prolonged restriction of arm movement is uncomfortable and inconvenient for the patient. In the event of an acute reaction, the IV catheter should be maintained with normal saline.

5. Platelets are normally cloudy. Blood out of proper storage (above 50° F [10° C]) for more than 30 minutes cannot be reissued. Never store blood in unauthorized refrigerators, such as those on the nursing unit, because proper storage conditions cannot be verified.

6. The majority of acute fatal transfusion reactions are caused by clerical errors. Patient and product verification is the single most important function of the nurse. It is strongly recommended that two qualified individuals perform this task.

 Key Decision Point
Do not proceed with the transfusion if there is a discrepancy in labeling, patient identification, or expiration date. Contact the blood bank immediately.

(continued)

PROCEDURE GUIDELINES 27-1 (continued)

Administering Blood and Blood Components

PROCEDURE (continued)

Nursing Action	Rationale

Performance phase

1. Start infusion slowly (ie, 2 mL/minute). Remain at bedside 15–30 minutes. If there are no signs of adverse effect, increase flow to the prescribed rate.

1. Institutional policy may vary regarding flow rates and patient monitoring. Signs of a severe transfusion reaction (ie, acute hemolytic, anaphylactic) are usually manifested during infusion of the initial 50–100 mL.

2. Observe the patient closely and check vital signs at least hourly until 1 hour after transfusion.

2. Acute reactions may occur at any time during the transfusion.

Key Decision Point

Observe for fever, chills, flushing, urticaria, difficulty breathing, anxiety, change in vital signs. Stop transfusion and report signs of adverse effect to health care provider immediately if acute reaction is suspected.

3. Record the following information on the patient's chart:
   a. Time and names of individuals starting and ending the transfusion.
   b. Names of individuals verifying patient ID.
   c. Unique product identification number.
   d. Product and volume infused.
   e. Immediate response—for example, "no apparent reaction."

3. Facts relating to the transfusion should be charted exactly.

   c. It must be possible to trace each transfusion product to the original blood donor.

---

packed RBCs, allergic and febrile transfusion reactions. Signs and symptoms of the more serious, but rare, hemolytic transfusion reactions are usually manifested during infusion of the first 50 mL.

Platelet Concentrates

Description

1. Consist of platelets suspended in plasma. Products vary according to the number of units (each unit is a minimum of 5.5×10^{10} platelets) and the volume of plasma (50 to 400 mL).

2. Platelets may be obtained by centrifuging multiple units of whole blood and expressing off the platelet-rich plasma (multiple-donor platelets) or from a single volunteer platelet donor using automated cell-separation techniques (apheresis). The use of single donor products decreases the number of donor exposures, thus decreasing the risk of alloimmunization and transfusion-transmitted disease.

3. Patients may become alloimmunized to human leukocyte antigens (HLAs) through exposure to multiple platelet products. When this occurs, apheresis products from HLA-matched platelet donors may be necessary. However, HLA-matched transfusions are commonly difficult to obtain

because of the vast number of possible HLA combinations among the human population.

4. Indications include prevention or resolution of hemorrhage in patients with thrombocytopenia or platelet dysfunction.

5. Platelet transfusions are generally contraindicated in heparin-induced thrombocytopenia, where they may precipitate arterial thrombosis, and in immune (idiopathic) thrombocytopenia, where they may worsen this autoimmune destruction of platelets.

6. Dosage: average dose is generally 1 unit of platelets for each 10 kg of body weight; however, patients who are actively bleeding or undergoing surgical procedures may require more.

Nursing and Patient Care Considerations

1. Infuse at the rate prescribed. Generally, the infusion can be completed within 20 to 60 minutes, depending on total volume.

2. Observe closely for the most common acute complications associated with platelet transfusions, allergic and febrile transfusion reactions.

3. Platelets are stored at 68° F to 75° F (20° C to 24° C), a warmer environment than other blood products and more conducive to bacterial growth. This increases the risk of bacterial contamination of a platelet product, which occurs in 4 to 10 per 10,000 units, limiting their shelf life.

STANDARDS OF CARE GUIDELINES 27-1
Blood Transfusion

When administering whole blood or blood components, ensure the following:

- Follow up on results of complete blood count (CBC) and report to health care provider so appropriate blood product can be ordered based on patient's condition.
- Verify informed consent.
- Contact the blood bank with health care provider's order and ensure timely delivery of blood product.
- Establish a patent IV line with compatible IV fluid.
- Use appropriate administration setup, filter, warmer, etc.
- Obtain baseline vital signs.
- Ensure proper blood product is given to the right patient by verifying at least two identifiers (eg, full name and date of birth) with patient, blood product, and original order.
- Transfuse at prescribed rate during prescribed time, as tolerated by patient.
- Observe for acute reactions—allergic, febrile, septic, hemolytic, air embolism, and circulatory overload—by assessing vital signs, breath sounds, edema, flushing, urticaria, vomiting, headache, back pain.
- Stop transfusion and notify patient's health care provider or available house officer if signs of reaction or other abnormalities occur.
- Be aware of delayed reactions and educate patient on risk and what to look for: hemolytic, iron overload, graft-versus-host disease, hepatitis, and other infectious diseases.

This information should serve as a general guideline only. Each patient situation presents a unique set of clinical factors and requires nursing judgment to guide care, which may include additional or alternative measures and approaches.

Plasma (Fresh or Fresh-Frozen)

Description
1. Consists of water (91%), plasma proteins including essential clotting factors (7%), and carbohydrates (2%). Each unit is the volume removed from a unit of whole blood (200 to 250 mL).
2. May be stored in a liquid state or frozen within 6 hours of collection.
3. Indications include treatment of blood loss or blood clotting disorders related to liver disease and failure, disseminated intravascular coagulation (DIC), over-anticoagulation with warfarin, all congenital or acquired clotting factor deficiencies, and dilutional coagulopathy resulting from massive blood replacement. Storage in liquid state results in the loss of labile clotting factors V and VIII, so that only plasma that has been fresh-frozen can be used to treat factor V and VIII deficiencies.
4. Dosage: depends on the clinical situation and assessment of prothrombin time, partial thromboplastin time, or specific factor assays.

Nursing and Patient Care Considerations
1. Infuse at the rate prescribed. Generally, the infusion can be completed within 15 to 30 minutes, depending on total volume.
2. Observe closely for the most common acute complication associated with plasma infusion, volume overload.

Cryoprecipitate

Description
1. Consists of certain clotting factors suspended in 10 to 20 mL plasma. Each unit contains approximately 80 to 120 units of factor VIII (antihemophilic and von Willebrand factors), 250 mg fibrinogen, and 20% to 30% of the factor XIII present in a unit of whole blood.
2. Indications include correction of deficiencies of factor VIII (ie, hemophilia A and von Willebrand disease), factor XIII, and fibrinogen (ie, DIC).
3. Dosage: adult dosage is generally 10 units, which may be repeated every 8 to 12 hours until the deficiency is corrected or until hemostasis is achieved.

Nursing and Patient Care Considerations
Infuse at the rate prescribed. Generally, the infusion can be completed within 3 to 15 minutes.

Fractionated Plasma Products

Description
1. Various highly concentrated plasma protein products are commercially prepared by pooling thousands of single plasma units and by extracting the desired protein. Most techniques involve heat or chemical treatments, which eliminate the risk of transmitting blood-borne viruses, such as hepatitis B and HIV.
2. Colloid solutions provide volume expansion in situations where crystalloid solutions are not adequate, such as therapeutic plasma exchange, shock, and massive hemorrhage. They may also be used in the treatment of acute liver failure, burns, and hemolytic disease of the neonate.
   a. Albumin is available as a 5% solution, which is oncotically equivalent to plasma, and as a concentrated 25% solution.
   b. Plasma protein fraction (PPF) is available as a 5% solution. Rapid infusion of PPF has been associated with hypotension.
   c. Albumin and PPF are pasteurized and carry no risk of viral disease. They do not contain preservatives and should be used immediately after opening.
3. Immune serum globulins (ISGs) are concentrated aqueous solutions of gamma globulin that contain high titers of antibody.
   a. Must be administered by deep intramuscular (I.M.) injection.
   b. Nonspecific ISG is prepared from random donor plasma and is used to increase gamma globulin levels and to enhance general immune response in mild inherited or acquired immune disorders such as hypogammaglobulinemia.
   c. Specific ISG is prepared from donors who have high antibody titers to known antigens and is used to treat specific disorders or conditions. Hepatitis B immunoglobulin,

varicella zoster immunoglobulin, and Rh immunoglobulin are examples of specific ISGs.

   d. ISGs carry no risk of hepatitis B, HIV, or other blood-borne infections.

   e. Problems associated with use include pain at the injection site, limitations on volume administered, loss of IgG into extravascular tissue, or by degradation at the injection site.

4. IV immunoglobulins (IVIGs) are aqueous solutions of immunoglobulins at a higher concentration and are given in larger volumes than ISGs.

   a. Like ISGs, they may be nonspecific or specific.

   b. Indications include chronic replacement therapy in patients with congenital or acquired immunodeficiency syndromes, acute autoimmune disorders such as immune (idiopathic) thrombocytopenia, and the treatment of chronic lymphocytic leukemia. Also, there are numerous investigational uses, such as Guillain-Barré syndrome, myasthenia gravis, rheumatoid arthritis, multiple sclerosis, lupus, and viral infections such as CMV, adenovirus, and influenza. IVIGs may also be used to treat platelet alloimmunization.

   c. IVIGs do not appear to transmit HIV, but have been reported to transmit hepatitis C.

   d. Administration of IVIG should be closely monitored because of the possibility of anaphylactic reactions. Dosage and rate of infusion depend on the manufacturer's formulation.

5. Factor VIII concentrate is a lyophilized concentrate used to treat moderate to severe hemophilia A and severe von Willebrand's disease.

6. Factor IX concentrate is a lyophilized concentrate used to treat factor IX deficiency (Christmas disease).

Nursing and Patient Care Considerations

1. These products are often distributed by a pharmacy rather than by a blood bank.

2. Check order and product insert to ensure proper dosage and administration route.

Granulocyte Concentrates

Description

1. Consist of a minimum of 1×10^{10} granulocytes, variable amounts of lymphocytes (usually less than 10% of the total number of WBCs), 6 to 10 units of platelets, 30 to 50 mL RBCs, and 200 to 400 mL plasma.

2. Obtained via apheresis, generally of multiple donors.

3. Indications include treatment of life-threatening bacterial or fungal infection unresponsive to other therapy in a patient with severe neutropenia.

4. Dosage: generally 1 unit daily for approximately 5 to 10 days, discontinuing if no therapeutic response.

Nursing and Patient Care Considerations

1. Product must be ABO compatible and, if possible, Rh compatible because of the high erythrocyte content. Granulocytes are irradiated prior to transfusion to prevent the risk of graft-versus-host disease.

2. Transfuse granulocytes as soon as they are available. WBCs have a short survival time and therapeutic benefit is directly related to dose and viability.

3. Premedicate per order to prevent adverse effects, generally with antihistamine and acetaminophen. Steroids may also be required.

4. Begin the transfusion slowly and increase to the rate prescribed and as tolerated. The recommended length of infusion is 1 to 2 hours.

5. Observe the patient closely throughout the transfusion for signs and symptoms of febrile, allergic, and anaphylactic reactions, which may be severe. Have emergency medications and equipment readily available.

6. Agitate the bag approximately every 15 minutes to prevent granulocytes from clumping at the bottom of the bag.

7. Do not administer amphotericin products immediately before or after granulocyte transfusion because pulmonary insufficiency has been reported with concurrent administration of amphotericin and granulocytes. Many institutions recommend a 4-hour gap to avoid this risk.

Modified Blood Products

Purpose

1. To reduce the risk of specific transfusion-related complications, blood products may receive further processing or treatment.

   a. Leukocytes are removed from blood products through filtration, washing, and freezing to reduce the risk of febrile, nonhemolytic transfusion reactions and alloimmunization to HLA.

   b. Function and proliferation of donor lymphocytes are inhibited by irradiation, to decrease the risk of posttransfusion graft-versus-host disease (GVHD) in immunocompromised patients including oncology patients, lung or heart transplant patients, and pediatric patients under age 6.

Methods

1. Filtration.

   a. Standard filters (170 µm) effectively remove gross fibrin clots.

   b. Microaggregate filters (approximately 40 µm) remove microscopic aggregates of fibrin, platelets, and leukocytes that accumulate in RBC products during storage. Their use is recommended during rapid, massive transfusion of whole blood or packed RBCs to prevent pulmonary complications. They reduce the risk of CMV transmission and may also decrease the incidence of febrile transfusion reactions by removing many of the leukocytes present.

   c. Special leukocyte-depletion filters have been developed for use with platelet products that remove 80% to 95% of leukocytes and that retain 80% of the platelets. These filters also reduce the risk of CMV transmission.

   d. A product may be filtered before release from the blood bank, but more commonly is released with the appropriate filter that must be attached to the standard infusion set at the bedside per manufacturer's or blood bank's instructions.

2. Washing.

a. Washing RBCs or platelets with a normal saline solution removes 80% to 95% of the WBCs and virtually all of the plasma to reduce the incidence of febrile, nonhemolytic transfusion reactions.

b. Washing requires an additional hour of processing time, and the shelf life of the product is reduced to 24 hours after this additional manipulation.

3. Freezing.

a. RBCs can be frozen within 7 days of blood collection and then remain viable for 7 to 10 years.

b. Removal of the hypertonic freezing preservative (glycerol) before transfusion eliminates all of the plasma and 99% of WBCs.

c. Thawing and deglycerolization of RBCs requires an additional 90 minutes of preparation time and reduces shelf life to 24 hours after this additional manipulation.

d. Freezing is also an effective method of storing rare blood types and autologous RBCs.

4. Irradiation.

a. Exposure of blood products to a measured amount of gamma irradiation inhibits lymphocyte function and proliferation without damaging RBCs, platelets, or granulocytes. This eliminates the ability of transfused lymphocytes to engraft in the immunocompromised transfusion recipient and the accompanying risk of posttransfusion GVHD.

b. Patients at risk for posttransfusion GVHD include bone marrow and peripheral stem cell transplant recipients, lung or heart transplant patients, premature neonates, and patients with congenital immunodeficiency disorders, Hodgkin's and non-Hodgkin's lymphomas, and HIV.

Transfusion Reactions

Every transfusion of blood components can result in an adverse effect. Reactions can be placed into two general categories: acute and delayed.

Acute Reactions

1. Acute reactions may occur during the infusion or within minutes to hours after the blood product has been infused.

2. Acute reactions include allergic, febrile, septic, and hemolytic reactions, air embolism, and circulatory overload. Patients who also receive multiple blood products within a short time frame may also be at risk for hyperkalemia, hypocalcemia, and hypothermia.

3. Because reactions may exhibit similar clinical manifestations, every symptom should be considered potentially serious and the transfusion should be discontinued until the cause is determined.

4. When a reaction is suspected, the health care provider should be notified immediately and blood bags with tubing from all products recently transfused should be returned to the blood bank for evaluation.

5. The following samples should also be obtained if an acute reaction is suspected.

a. A clotted blood specimen to examine serum for hemoglobin and confirm RBC group and type.

b. An anticoagulated blood sample for a direct Coombs' test to determine the presence of antibody on the RBCs.

c. The first voided urine specimen to test for hemoglobinuria (this does not need to be a clean-catch specimen).

6. Precautions must be taken to avoid the hemolysis of RBCs during venipuncture and sample collection because this could lead to invalid test results. Whenever possible, blood samples should be drawn from a fresh venipuncture and not from existing needles or catheters.

7. If the only symptoms are those resulting from a mild allergic reaction (eg, urticaria), extensive evaluation may not be necessary. In the event of a severe reaction (eg, hypotension, tachypnea), more tests may be required to determine the cause of the reaction.

8. Causes, clinical manifestations, management, and prevention of acute reactions are summarized in Table 27-4, pages 1010 and 1011.

Delayed Reactions

1. Delayed reactions occur days to years after the transfusion.

2. Delayed reactions include delayed hemolytic reactions, iron overload (hemosiderosis), GVHD, infectious diseases (eg, hepatitis B, hepatitis C, CMV, Epstein-Barr virus, malaria, HIV, HTLV).

3. Symptoms of a delayed reaction can vary from mild to severe. Diagnosis may be complicated by the long incubation period between transfusion and reaction and the complexity of diagnostic tests.

4. Causes, clinical manifestations, management, and prevention of delayed reactions are summarized in Table 27-5, pages 1011 and 1012.

BLOOD AND MARROW STEM CELL TRANSPLANTATION

Blood and marrow stem cell transplantation are potentially lifesaving treatments with application in many malignant and nonmalignant disorders. Decades of research have advanced this technology from an experimental treatment of last resort to the preferred method of intervention for selected diseases. Although the basic procedures are now well established, this field continues to grow rapidly through ongoing research in areas such as nonmyeloablative ("mini") allogeneic transplants, the application of biologic response modifiers to modulate the immune response, and the use of donor lymphocyte infusions to prevent or treat posttransplant relapse.

Principles of Blood and Marrow Stem Cell Transplantation

Types of Stem Cell Transplant

The type of transplant selected is contingent on a variety of factors, such as the underlying disorder, the availability of a

(Text continues on page 1013)

Table 27-4   Acute Reactions to Blood Transfusion

ACUTE REACTION	CAUSE	CLINICAL MANIFESTATIONS	MANAGEMENT	PREVENTION
Allergic	Sensitivity to plasma protein or donor antibody, which reacts with recipient antigen.	• Flushing • Itching, rash • Urticaria, hives • Asthmatic wheezing • Laryngeal edema • Anaphylaxis	• Stop transfusion immediately. Keep vein open (KVO) with normal saline. Notify health care provider and blood bank. • Give antihistamine, as directed (diphenhydramine). • Observe for anaphylaxis—prepare epinephrine if respiratory distress is severe. • If hives are the only clinical manifestation, the transfusion can sometimes continue at a slower rate. • Send blood samples and blood bags to blood bank. Collect urine specimens for testing.	• Before transfusion, ask patient about past reactions. If patient has history of anaphylaxis, alert health care provider, have emergency drugs available, and remain at bedside for the first 30 minutes.
Febrile, nonhemolytic	Hypersensitivity to donor white blood cells, platelets, or plasma proteins.	• Sudden chills and fever • Headache • Flushing • Anxiety	• Stop transfusion immediately and KVO with normal saline. Notify health care provider and blood bank. • Send blood samples and blood bags to blood bank. Collect urine specimens for testing. • Check temperature 30 minutes after chill and as indicated thereafter. • Give antipyretics, as prescribed—treat symptomatically.	• Give antipyretic (acetaminophen or aspirin) before transfusion as directed. • Leukocyte-poor blood products may be recommended for future transfusions.
Septic reactions	Transfusion of blood or components contaminated with bacteria.	• Rapid onset of chills • High fever • Vomiting, diarrhea • Marked hypotension	• Stop transfusion immediately and KVO with normal saline. Notify health care provider and blood bank. • Obtain cultures of patient's blood and return blood bags with administration set to blood bank for culture. • Treat septicemia, as directed—antibiotics, IV fluids, vasopressors, steroids.	• Do not permit blood to stand at room temperature longer than necessary. Warm temperatures promote bacterial growth. • Inspect blood for gas bubbles, clotting, or abnormal color before transfusion. • Complete infusions within 4 hours. Change administration set after 4 hours of use.

Table 27-4   Acute Reactions to Blood Transfusion (continued)

ACUTE REACTION	CAUSE	CLINICAL MANIFESTATIONS	MANAGEMENT	PREVENTION
Circulatory overload	Fluid administered at a rate or volume greater than the circulatory system can accommodate. Increased blood in pulmonary vessels and decreased lung compliance.	• Rise in venous pressure • Distended neck veins • Dyspnea • Cough • Crackles at base of lungs	• Stop transfusion and KVO with normal saline. Notify health care provider. • Place patient upright with feet in dependent position. • Administer prescribed diuretics, oxygen, morphine, and aminophylline.	• Concentrated blood products should be given whenever positive. • Transfuse at a rate within the circulatory reserve of the patient. • Monitor central venous pressure of patient with heart disease.
Hemolytic reaction	Infusion of incompatible blood products: • Antibodies in recipient's plasma attach to transfused red blood cells (RBCs), hemolyzing the cells either in circulation or in the reticuloendothelial system. • Antibodies in donor plasma attach to recipient RBCs, causing hemolysis (may result from infusion of incompatible plasma—less severe than incompatible RBCs).	• Chills; fever • Lower back pain • Feeling of head fullness; flushing • Oppressive feeling • Tachycardia, tachypnea • Hypotension, vascular collapse • Hemoglobinuria, hemoglobinemia • Bleeding • Acute renal failure	• Stop transfusion immediately—KVO with 0.9% saline. • Notify health care provider and blood bank. • Treat shock, if present. • Draw testing samples, collect urine specimen. • Maintain blood pressure with IV colloid solutions. Give diuretics, as prescribed, to maintain urine flow, glomerular filtration, and renal blood flow. • Insert indwelling catheter to monitor hourly urine output. Patient may require dialysis if renal failure occurs.	• Meticulously verify patient identification—from sample collection to product infusion. • Begin infusion slowly and observe closely for 30 minutes—consequences are in proportion to the amount of incompatible blood transfused.

Table 27-5   Delayed Reactions to Transfusion Therapy

DELAYED REACTION	CAUSE	CLINICAL MANIFESTATIONS	MANAGEMENT	PREVENTION
Delayed hemolytic reaction	The destruction of transfused red blood cells by antibody not detectable during crossmatch, but formed rapidly after transfusion. Rapid production may occur because of antigen exposure during previous transfusions or pregnancy.	• Fever • Mild jaundice • Decreased hematocrit	• Generally, no acute treatment is required, but hemolysis may be severe enough to cause shock and renal failure. If this occurs, manage as outlined under acute hemolytic reactions.	• The crossmatch blood sample should be drawn within 3 days of blood transfusion. Antibody formation may occur within 90 days of transfusion or pregnancy.
Iron overload (hemosiderosis)	Deposition of iron in the heart, endocrine organs, liver, spleen, skin, and other major organs as a result of multiple, long-term transfusions (aplastic anemia, thalassemia).	• Diabetes • Decreased thyroid function • Arrhythmias • Heart failure and other symptoms related to major organ failure	• Treat symptomatically. • Deferoxamine, which chelates and removes accumulated iron through the kidneys; administered via IV line, I.M., or SubQ.	—

(continued)

Table 27-5   Delayed Reactions to Transfusion Therapy (*continued*)

DELAYED REACTION	CAUSE	CLINICAL MANIFESTATIONS	MANAGEMENT	PREVENTION
Graft-versus-host disease	Engraftment of lympho-cytes in the bone marrow of immunosuppressed patients, setting up an immune response of the graft against the host.	• Erythematous skin rash • Liver function test abnormalities • Profuse, watery diarrhea	• Immunosuppression with corticosteroids, cyclosporine A. • Symptomatic manage-ment of pruritus, pain. • Fluid and electrolyte replacement for diarrhea.	• Transfuse with irradiated blood products.
Hepatitis B	Hepatitis B virus transmit-ted from blood donor to recipient via infected blood products.	• Elevated liver enzymes (ALT/AST) • Anorexia, malaise • Nausea and vomiting • Fever • Dark urine • Jaundice	• Usually resolves spontaneously within 4–6 weeks. Can result in permanent liver damage. Treat symp-tomatically.	• Screen blood donors, tem-porarily rejecting those who may have had contact with the virus. Those with a his-tory of hepatitis after age 11 are permanently deferred; pretest all blood products (EIA).
Hepatitis C (formerly non-A, non-B hepatitis)	Hepatitis C virus transmit-ted from blood donor to recipient via infected blood products.	• Similar to serum B hepatitis, but symp-toms are usually less severe. Chronic liver disease and cir-rhosis may develop.	• Symptoms usually mild. Interferon and ribavirin may be used to treat chronic liver disease.	• Pretest all blood donors (ALT, anti-HBc antibody, anti-hepatitis C antibody).
Epstein-Barr virus, cytomeg-alovirus, malaria	Transmitted through infected blood products.	• Fever • Fatigue • Hepatomegaly • Splenomegaly	• Rest and supportive management.	• Question prospective blood donors regarding colds, flu, foreign travel.
Acquired immu-nodeficiency syndrome (AIDS)	Human immunodeficiency virus (HIV) transmitted from blood donor to recipient via infected blood prod-ucts.	• Night sweats • Unexplained weight loss • Lymphadenopathy • Pneumocystis pneumonia • Kaposi's sarcoma • Diarrhea	• Combination antiret-roviral therapy.	• Test each donor for HIV antibody. • Reject prospective high-risk donors: males who have had sex with another male since 1977; users of self-injected IV drugs; male or female partners of prostitutes; hemophiliacs or their sexual partners; sexual partners of those with AIDS or high risk for AIDS; immigrants from Haiti or sub-Saharan Africa.
Human T-lymphotropic virus type 1 (HTLV-1) associ-ated myelopathy and tropical spastic parapare-sis (HAM/TSP) Adult T-cell leukemia	HTLV-1 transmitted from blood donor to recipient via blood products.	• Signs of neuromus-cular disease • Signs of T-cell leukemia	• HTLV-1-infected indi-viduals have a low risk of developing disease (3%–5%). Incubation period 10–20 years. • Should disease occur, treat symptomatically.	• Screen all prospective blood donors for anti-HTLV-1 antibody.
Syphilis	Spirochetemia caused by *Treponema pallidum*. Incu-bation 4–18 weeks.	• Presence of chancre • Regional lymphad-enopathy • Generalized rash	• Penicillin therapy	• Test blood before transfu-sion (rapid plasma reagin). Organism will not remain viable in blood stored 24–48 hours at 39.2° F (4° C).

histocompatible (HLA-matched) donor, and the clinical condition of the patient. Stem cells may come from the patient (autologous), an identical twin (syngeneic), or another donor (allogeneic). Stem cells are found in bone marrow, in peripheral blood (especially if the donor is treated to increase the numbers of circulating stem cells), and in umbilical cord blood.

Autologous Bone Marrow Transplantation

1. Bone marrow is removed from the patient during an operative harvesting procedure, frozen, and reinfused after the patient has undergone high-dose chemotherapy and possibly radiotherapy.
2. Advantages: readily available, usually lower morbidity and mortality than allogeneic bone marrow transplantation (BMT).
3. Disadvantages: operative procedure, marrow must be disease-free, sufficient quantity of cellular marrow must be aspirable, in most cases has higher rate of relapse than allogeneic BMT.

Syngeneic Bone Marrow Transplantation

1. Bone marrow is removed from an identical twin during an operative harvesting procedure and infused into the recipient, who has undergone high-dose chemotherapy and possibly radiotherapy.
2. Advantages: recipient's marrow does not need to be harvestable (as in hypocellular or tumor-contaminated bone marrow), generally lower morbidity and mortality than allogeneic BMT.
3. Disadvantages: higher disease relapse rate than in allogeneic BMT.

Allogeneic Bone Marrow Transplantation

1. Bone marrow is removed from a donor who is most commonly a sibling or other close relative (related) but may be a volunteer donor (unrelated).
   a. Identical or mismatched HLA phenotypes may be used, though identical phenotypes are often preferred. HLA mismatches require additional immunosuppression and GVHD prophylaxis and can be associated with higher morbidity and mortality.
   b. Bone marrow is removed from the donor during an operative harvesting procedure and infused into the recipient, who has undergone high-dose chemotherapy and possibly radiotherapy.
   c. Allogeneic bone marrow may be treated in various ways before infusion, including removing RBCs if ABO incompatible and removing T lymphocytes to reduce the risk of GVHD.
2. Advantages: recipient's marrow does not need to be harvestable (as in hypocellular or tumor-contaminated bone marrow), lowest rate of relapse.
3. Disadvantages: risk for GVHD, generally higher morbidity and mortality than other types of BMT. Unrelated and HLA-mismatched transplants have higher risk of GVHD and infectious complications and some risk of graft rejection or failure.

Autologous, Syngeneic, or Allogeneic Peripheral Blood Stem Cell Transplantation

1. Although hematopoietic stem cells are primarily found in the bone marrow, they can also be found in the peripheral circulation in smaller numbers.

2. Peripheral blood stem cells are collected using one or more apheresis procedures after the patient or donor has been treated to increase the number of circulating stem cells. This is done by methods such as timed administration of chemotherapy (patient only) and stem cell growth factors. After the collection, the cells are frozen and stored for reinfusion into the patient after high-dose chemotherapy and possibly radiotherapy.
3. Advantages: patient's marrow does not need to be harvestable (as in hypocellular or tumor-contaminated bone marrow); there is no operative risk to the patient or donor.
4. Disadvantages: for allogeneic donors, the long-term risks of boosting healthy bone marrow production with growth factors, and in some cases chemotherapy, are not yet known. Research has shown that allogeneic peripheral blood stem cell transplant may be associated with a higher incidence of chronic GVHD than allogeneic bone marrow transplant.

Umbilical Cord Blood Stem Cell Transplantation

1. Umbilical cord blood is rich in stem cells and may be stored at birth for later autologous use, related allogeneic use, or unrelated allogeneic use. Cord blood transplantation requires less stringent HLA-matching because mismatched cord blood stem cells are less likely to cause GVHD than mature stem cells from other sources.
2. Advantages: may provide lifesaving allogeneic stem cells from new sibling to older child at no risk to the donor. Cord blood banks provide options for unrelated donor transplantation when there is an urgent need.
3. Disadvantages: may have higher risk of graft failure than other types of transplants; number of stem cells may be insufficient for older patients.

Nonmyeloablative or "Mini" Transplants

1. Conventional conditioning for blood and marrow stem cell transplants requires high doses of chemotherapy and radiotherapy (myeloablative) to destroy existing bone marrow cells. This results in significant morbidity and mortality, particularly in certain patient populations (eg, older patients, those with poor organ function).
2. Research has demonstrated that under certain conditions, individuals can exist with bone marrow stem cells from two sources (self and allogeneic donor), a state known as *mixed chimerism*. These changes in the immune system appear to enhance the antitumor immune response, creating a desired graft-versus-tumor effect.
3. The goals of nonmyeloablative conditioning regimens are to prevent graft rejection and promote mixed chimerism. The nonmyeloablative preparative regimen uses combinations of agents such as cyclophosphamide, fludarabine, antithymocyte globulin, and low-dose total body irradiation. Alemtuzumab is often considered as well. After the completion of the reduced-intensity regimen, the allogeneic bone marrow or peripheral blood stem cells are then infused.
4. Donor lymphocytes may also be given at specific intervals following transplant to enhance the immune antitumor effect further.
5. Advantages: patients otherwise ineligible for allogeneic transplant due to age, comorbid conditions, or organ function

are more likely to tolerate the less-toxic preparative regimen. Patients do not usually experience significant neutropenia, thrombocytopenia, anemia, and other complications that typically accompany myeloablative therapy. Patients generally have shorter episodes of neutropenia and a reduced need for RBC and platelet transfusions, allowing an opportunity for outpatient transplants to be performed.

6. Disadvantages: Increased risk of graft failure.

The Human Leukocyte Antigen System and Transplantation

1. The human leukocyte antigen (HLA) system is part of the major histocompatability complex.

2. The immune-mediated recognition of the differences in each individual's HLA system is the first step in the rejection of a transplanted organ or graft or in GVHD.

3. The HLA antigens are complex proteins expressed on the surface of all nucleated cells (A, B, C antigens – Class I) or cells of the immune system (D antigens – Class II).
   a. More than 100 different antigens have been identified.
   b. Antigens are classified according to their location on chromosome 6, which encodes them.
   c. A person's genetically inherited mixture of antigens expressed on cell surfaces is their individual phenotype or tissue type.

4. Determination of an individual's HLA type is completed by complex DNA phenotyping or gene sequencing.
   a. The gold standard for HLA typing in bone marrow transplantation is to complete the above testing at high resolution (allelic level), identifying both the Class I (A, B, C) and Class II (D) groups.
   b. A phenotypically identical donor is considered to be one who matches at all 10 antigens at their associated allelic level—A, B, C, DR, and DQ.

4. Siblings have a 1-in-4 chance of having identical sets of HLA antigens. With a decreasing national birthrate, however, only 35% of people in the United States can anticipate having an HLA-identical sibling.

5. Due to the complexity of the HLA system, unrelated people have less than a 1-in-5,000 chance of being HLA identical.

6. The National Bone Marrow Donor Program (BeTheMatch Registry), established in 1987, maintains a computerized list of potential HLA-matched peripheral blood stem cell and bone marrow donors, providing assistance to patients who seek an unrelated donor. Information on becoming a volunteer bone marrow donor or on initiating a computerized search for a donor can be obtained by calling the National Marrow Donor Program (see Box 26-1, page 990, for additional resources for patients undergoing blood and marrow stem cell transplantation).

Indications

1. If an HLA-matched related donor is available, allogeneic bone marrow or stem cell transplantation is generally considered the treatment of choice in certain disorders, including:
   a. Severe aplastic anemia.

> **BOX 27-1 Indications for Blood and Marrow Stem Cell Transplantation**
>
> **Allogeneic**
> **Nonmalignant**
> - Aplastic anemia
> - Myelofibrosis
> - Wiskott-Aldrich syndrome
> - Thalassemia
> - Severe combined immunodeficiency diseases
> - Mucopolysaccharidoses
> - Sickle cell disease
>
> **Malignant**
> - Acute myeloid leukemia
> - Acute lymphocytic leukemia
> - Hodgkin's lymphoma
> - Non-Hodgkin's lymphoma
> - Myelofibrosis
> - Multiple myeloma
> - Selected solid tumors
>
> **Autologous**
> - Hodgkin's lymphoma
> - Non-Hodgkin's lymphoma
> - Multiple myeloma
> - Selected solid tumors

---

   b. Inherited immunodeficiency disorders, such as severe combined immunodeficiency disease and Wiskott-Aldrich syndrome.
   c. Allogeneic bone marrow and peripheral blood stem cell transplantation have also been used with varying success in the treatment of other genetic disorders (eg. thalassemia, sickle cell disease).

2. Allogeneic, syngeneic, and autologous bone marrow and peripheral blood stem cell transplantation are also widely applied in the treatment of malignancies, where success rates depend largely on factors such as the age of the patient, disease status at time of transplant, the extent of prior treatment, and existing comorbidities.

3. Autologous peripheral blood stem cell transplantation is used in the treatment of certain lymphomas, multiple myeloma, and solid tumors such as Ewing's sarcoma and neuroblastoma. Allogeneic bone marrow and peripheral blood stem cell transplantation are generally used in the treatment of leukemias as well as certain lymphomas.

4. Diseases and disorders treated with this technology are summarized in Box 27-1.

Harvesting of Bone Marrow and Peripheral Blood Stem Cells

Evaluation of Recipient

1. Eligibility criteria include age (generally younger than age 65 for allogeneic myeloablative transplants and autologous and syngeneic transplants and younger than age 75 for allogeneic nonmyeloablative transplants) and availability of suitable donor and stem cell source.

2. Before undergoing transplantation, an extensive workup is completed to ensure that the patient's disease is treatable with the selected type of transplant and that the patient has no limitations that will increase the risk of mortality.

3. Specific criteria may vary among transplant centers and treatment protocols, but generally include:
   a. Disease-specific evaluation of severity and extent of current disease manifestations.
   b. Adequate cardiac function: generally left ventricular ejection fraction greater than 45%.
   c. Adequate pulmonary function: generally, forced expiratory capacity and forced vital capacity greater than 50%.
   d. Adequate renal function: generally, creatinine less than 2 mg/dL.
   e. Adequate hepatic function: generally, bilirubin less than 2 mg/dL.
   f. No active infections (including HIV).
   g. No coexisting severe or uncontrolled medical conditions.

Evaluation of Blood and Marrow Donors

1. Because bone marrow donation for allogeneic or syngeneic BMT is an elective procedure with no benefit to the donor, great care is taken to ensure that the potential donor is fit for surgery and understands the potential risks. Autologous bone marrow donors must generally meet the same criteria. Evaluation includes:
   a. Thorough medical history and physical examination.
   b. Chest x-ray.
   c. Electrocardiogram.
   d. Laboratory evaluation (CBC; chemistry profile; testing for CMV, hepatitis B and C, HIV, HTLV, and syphilis; ABO and Rh determination; coagulation studies).

2. Informed consent including potential donor complications must be obtained.

3. Relatively common complications include:
   a. Bruising.
   b. Pain at aspiration sites.
   c. Mild bleeding.

4. Rare complications include:
   a. Adverse effects of anesthesia (general, spinal, or epidural).
   b. Infection of aspiration sites.
   c. Persistent pain.
   d. Transient neuropathies.

5. Because of the significant loss of blood volume and RBCs during the harvest procedure, donors are advised to give one or two units of autologous blood 1 to 3 weeks before surgery, which may be reinfused during marrow collection, if needed.

6. Evaluation of donors for peripheral blood stem cell transplantation is similar, but less stringent as there is generally no anesthesia required. The apheresis procedure is similar to donating platelets.

Stem Cell Collection Procedure

Bone Marrow Harvest (Autologous, Syngeneic, or Allogeneic)

1. Performed under epidural, spinal, or general anesthesia under sterile conditions in operating room.

2. An aspiration needle is used to puncture the skin and puncture the iliac crest multiple times without exiting the skin, removing marrow in 2- to 5-mL aliquots (samples).

3. Marrow is drawn up into heparinized syringes and filtered to remove fibrin clots and other debris.

4. Marrow may be infused immediately, treated and infused, or frozen in a preservative solution containing dimethyl sulfoxide (DMSO) until needed.

5. Bone marrow donation is a relatively safe operative procedure with few serious complications.

Postharvest Care of the Bone Marrow Donor

1. Procedure is generally done as same-day care, with discharge after recovery from anesthesia.

2. Observe for potential complications (bleeding, hypotension caused by fluid loss).

3. Instruct patient to resume normal activities gradually during the week after donation.

4. Instruct patient to keep aspiration sites clean and dry and observe for signs of infection (redness, swelling, warmth or discharge at sites, fever, malaise).

5. Provide adequate analgesia and instruct patient about pain management.

Harvesting of Peripheral Blood Stem Cells

1. Involves donor preparation by "priming" hematopoietic system with timed chemotherapy (autologous stem cell collection only) and sequential growth factor administration to increase number of circulating stem cells.

2. Large-bore central catheter suitable for apheresis procedures is inserted.

3. One to ten apheresis procedures may be needed to collect sufficient numbers of suitable cells.

4. Cells are frozen in a preservative solution that contains DMSO until needed.

5. Acute complications of apheresis include citrate toxicity, which may be managed by increasing dietary calcium intake 2 to 3 days before procedure and by using calcium-based antacids during procedure. Blood calcium levels are carefully monitored throughout the procedure and IV calcium given, as needed.

Preparation and Performance of the Transplant

Preparation of Recipient

1. A long-term central catheter is inserted for multiple IV treatments, including blood products, total parenteral nutrition, and blood-drawing.

2. High-dose chemotherapy or radiotherapy is administered to:
   a. Destroy residual tumor cells.
   b. Suppress immune response against new stem cells.
   c. Create space within recipient's marrow for the new stem cells.

3. Symptoms immediately associated with high-dose chemotherapy or radiotherapy regimens used in blood and marrow stem cell transplantation may include:
   a. Severe nausea and vomiting (with most regimens).
   b. Cardiomyopathy, hemorrhagic cystitis (with cyclophosphamide).

c. Seizures (with busulfan).

d. Fever, generalized erythema, parotitis (with total body irradiation).

Infusion of Bone Marrow or Peripheral Blood Stem Cells

See Table 27-6.

 NURSING ALERT Unlike all other blood products administered to transplant recipients, stem cells should never be irradiated. In addition, infusion pumps and filters should be avoided because they may remove or damage stem cells.

Posttransplant Care

General Considerations

1. Significant complications that require specialized medical and nursing care may occur during the first few weeks and months after blood and marrow stem cell transplantation.
   a. Risk is highest in mismatched unrelated allogeneic BMT.
   b. Followed by matched unrelated and mismatched related allogeneic BMT.
   c. Followed by matched related allogeneic BMT.
   d. Followed by syngeneic BMT.
   e. Followed by autologous BMT.
   f. Followed by autologous peripheral blood stem cell transplantation (lowest risk).

2. Nursing care is aimed at early identification and treatment of problems and includes:
   a. Comprehensive physical and psychosocial assessment.
   b. Immediate notification of health care provider of any abnormal assessment parameters found.
   c. Early recognition and intervention for life-threatening complications, such as sepsis, respiratory failure, GI bleeding, renal and hepatic failure, and veno-occlusive disease (VOD).
   d. Prevention of infection.
   e. Prevention of bleeding.
   f. Expert symptom management of problems that may occur after blood and marrow stem cell transplantation, such as nausea, vomiting, diarrhea, pain, fatigue, anxiety, and delirium.

Hematopoietic Complications

1. Blood and marrow stem cell transplant patients, particularly allogeneic recipients, are at risk for life-threatening bacterial, viral, and fungal infections because of their profound neutropenia and prolonged immunosuppression.
   a. Transplant recipients are usually cared for in a protective environment, most commonly single HEPA-filtered rooms.
   b. In an ambulatory or home setting, the patient and family must pay strict attention to methods of preventing infection, including wearing high-filtration masks, handwashing, safe food handling, and avoidance of crowded areas and exposure to illnesses.

Table 27-6 Infusion Guidelines for Bone Marrow or Peripheral Blood Stem Cells

TYPE OF STEM CELLS	PROCESSING PRIOR TO INFUSION	VOLUME	POTENTIAL ADVERSE EFFECTS	NURSING CONSIDERATIONS
ABO-compatible untreated allogeneic bone marrow	Filtered to remove large particles	500–2,000 mL	Volume overload, allergic reactions, pulmonary compromise (fat emboli, cell aggregates)	Emergency medications available, close monitoring
ABO-incompatible bone marrow	Removal of red blood cells and plasma	200–600 mL	Allergic reactions, intravascular hemolysis (rare)	Prehydrate to ensure adequate renal perfusion and alkaline urine, emergency medications available, close monitoring
Autologous bone marrow	Filtered and frozen with DMSO as preservative, thawed in warm water bath immediately prior to infusion	100–500 mL	Related to DMSO: histamine-release reaction (flushing, chest tightness, abdominal cramping, nausea), cardiac arrhythmias, anaphylaxis	Emergency medications available, close monitoring, cardiac monitoring recommended
Peripheral blood stem cells	Frozen with DMSO as preservative, thawed in warm water bath immediately prior to infusion.	100–1,000 mL	Related to DMSO: histamine-release reaction (flushing, chest tightness, abdominal cramping, nausea), cardiac arrhythmias, anaphylaxis	Administer as tolerated (may be high volume and DMSO content), premedicate with antihistamine and anti-emetic, emergency medications available, close monitoring, cardiac monitoring recommended

DMSO, dimethyl sulfoxide.

c. Blood and marrow stem cell recipients are at high risk for nosocomial bloodstream infections related to long-term central venous catheters, neutropenia, and immunosuppression. Strict adherence to an evidence-based procedure for insertion and management of central venous catheters is essential in this population.

d. Colony-stimulating factors such as G-CSF and GM-CSF have been shown to reduce the duration of neutropenia, though the optimal timing for administration has not been determined.

e. Additional preventive interventions vary widely and include elaborate disinfection procedures; modified or sterile diets; prophylactic antibiotics, antivirals, and antifungals; surveillance cultures.

2. The megakaryocyte is generally the last cell produced by new stem cells and platelet counts may take months to return to normal.

a. Blood and marrow stem cell transplant patients require frequent assessment for signs and symptoms of overt or covert bleeding, protection from injury, and support with platelet products.

3. Anemia is a common complication caused by loss of RBCs through aging, destruction, bleeding, and routine phlebotomy. Blood and marrow stem cell transplant patients require frequent RBC transfusions. Erythropoietin alfa and darbepoetin alfa may also be used to stimulate RBC production. Delayed erythropoiesis and immune hemolytic anemia are complications of ABO-incompatible allogeneic stem cell transplants.

GI Complications

1. Mucositis may develop because of high-dose chemotherapy and radiation therapy that destroy rapidly dividing cells, including cells lining the mouth, esophagus, and GI tract. Management includes meticulous oral hygiene, local and systemic analgesia, and antimicrobial therapy.

2. Nausea and vomiting may arise from multiple causes, including high-dose chemotherapy, infection, GI bleeding, acute GVHD, and medications. Management includes pharmacologic and nonpharmacologic interventions, adequate replacement of fluids and electrolytes, and support of nutritional requirements.

3. Diarrhea may have multiple causes, including high-dose chemotherapy, infection, GI bleeding, GVHD, and medications. Management includes cautious use of antidiarrheals, adequate replacement of fluids and electrolytes, support of nutritional requirements, and protection of perirectal skin from excoriation.

Renal and Genitourinary Complications

1. Renal failure may arise from multiple factors, including drug toxicity, infection, and ischemia. Management includes maintenance of fluid and electrolyte balance, monitoring of drug levels, and hemodialysis or continuous venovenous hemodialysis.

2. Hemorrhagic cystitis may occur as a result of high-dose cyclophosphamide or with certain viral infections, such as adenovirus and BK virus (a polyoma virus, named for the first patient). Management includes hydration, blood product support, continuous bladder irrigation, and rare invasive procedures, such as instillation of alum or formalin, or surgery.

Hepatic Complications

Sinusoidal obstruction syndrome or VOD may occur as a result of damage to the liver from high-dose chemotherapy and radiation therapy; incidence is approximately 30%.

1. Signs and symptoms include hepatomegaly (generally painful), hyperbilirubinemia, and weight gain.

2. May progress to hepatic encephalopathy, coagulopathies, coma, and death in up to 50% of patients with VOD.

3. Management is generally aimed at preventing further damage and at treating symptoms. The antithrombotic and thrombolytic agent defibrotide may be administered for severe VOD; however, the risk of bleeding is high with the administration of this agent; other agents being studied include heparin, recombinant tissue plasminogen activator, and ursodeoxycholic acid.

Pulmonary Complications

1. Life-threatening pulmonary infections in stem cell recipients include bacterial pneumonias, fungal infections including aspergillosis, viral infections such as CMV (especially in allogeneic recipients), respiratory syncytial virus, parainfluenza, and, less commonly, *Pneumocystis carinii* pneumonia (PCP), legionnaires' disease, toxoplasmosis, and tuberculosis.

a. Preventive measures include hand hygiene, encouragement of exercise, deep breathing, and coughing; routine CMV polymerase chain reaction monitoring if recipient or donor is CMV IgG positive at time of transplant, administration of CMV-screened and/or leukoreduced blood products, high-dose acyclovir or ganciclovir, and IVIG for allogeneic BMT patients at high risk for CMV; prophylactic cotrimoxazole for patients at risk for PCP. Staff, patient, and family education regarding risk factors and transmission of these infectious agents may help prevent primary and nosocomial infections.

b. Supportive care if symptomatic includes pulmonary hygiene, oxygen therapy, and mechanical ventilation.

2. Noninfectious pulmonary disease includes idiopathic pneumonitis, diffuse alveolar hemorrhage, pulmonary fibrosis, and bronchiolitis obliterans.

Graft-Versus-Host Disease

1. Acute GVHD occurs in 40% to 60% of allogeneic recipients even with HLA-matching, generally within first 3 months after transplant as a manifestation of the immune system's response to activated donor T lymphocytes against the recipient's cells and organs.

a. Primarily affects the skin, liver, and GI tract; may also affect conjunctivae and lungs.

b. Severity ranges from mild and self-limited erythematous rash to widespread blistering of skin, profuse watery diarrhea, and liver failure.

c. Prophylaxis generally includes immunosuppression with such medications as cyclosporine, tacrolimus, and methotrexate; may also include T-cell depletion of bone marrow.

d. Recently, research has demonstrated that administration of high-dose cyclophosphamide a few days after the stem cell transplant decreases the rate of acute GVHD.

e. Treatment generally includes increased doses of routine immunosuppressive drugs and additional drugs, such as corticosteroids, antithymocyte globulin, and monoclonal antibodies.

2. Chronic GVHD occurs in approximately 20% of long-term survivors; usually appears within first year after allogeneic blood and marrow stem cell transplant.

   a. It has many similarities to autoimmune disorders such as scleroderma.

   b. It affects the skin, mouth, salivary glands, eyes, musculoskeletal system, liver, esophagus, GI tract, and vagina.

   c. Treatment generally consists of corticosteroids and other immunosuppressive drugs, such as mycophenolate and thalidomide.

   d. Immune system frequently suppressed beyond the effects of medications; patient is at risk for infections, particularly from encapsulated bacteria, and should receive prophylaxis with suitable antibiotic such as penicillin.

Long-Term Sequelae and Survivorship Issues

1. Long-term, disease-free survival varies from 5% to 20% for patients with resistant, aggressive leukemias or lymphomas to 75% to 80% for aplastic anemia.

2. Long-term complications of blood and marrow stem cell transplantation include:

   a. Relapse of original disease.

   b. Secondary malignancy, including skin, oral mucosa, brain, thyroid, bone, and acute leukemia.

   c. Sterility.

   d. Endocrine dysfunction, including reduced levels of human growth hormone, estrogens, and testosterone.

   e. Cataracts (risk increased with radiation therapy, corticosteroids).

   f. Chronic GVHD (allogeneic).

   g. Aseptic necrosis and osteoporosis (risk increased with corticosteroids).

   h. Encephalopathy (risk increased with cranial irradiation and intrathecal chemotherapy).

3. Survivorship issues after this intensive and potentially life-threatening treatment include:

   a. Feelings of isolation, guilt, and loss.

   b. Altered family dynamics.

   c. Delayed puberty, decreased libido, early menopause, and other physical problems that have an impact on sexual relationships.

   d. Readjustment to school or work setting.

   e. Financial burden of blood and marrow stem cell transplantation.

   f. Chronic health problems and fatigue.

   g. Difficulty obtaining adequate health insurance.

4. Despite the complex issues blood and marrow stem cell transplant survivors face, several quality-of-life studies have demonstrated that the majority rate their quality of life highly and would choose to undergo transplant again.

SELECTED REFERENCES

Armand, P., Gibson, C. J., Cutler, C., et al. (2012). A disease risk index for patients undergoing Allogeneic stem cell transplantation. *Blood, 120,* 905–913.

Brodsky, R. A., Luznik, L., Bolanos-Meade, J., et al. (2008). Reduced intensity HLA-haploidentical BMT with post transplantation cyclophosphamide in nonmalignant hematologic diseases. *Bone Marrow Transplantation, 42,* 523–527.

Copelan, E. A., Malik, S., & Avalos, B. R. (2011). Peripheral blood hematopoietic stem cell mobilization for autologous transplantation. *US Oncology and Hematology, 7*(1), 75–77.

Davis, R., Murphy, M. F., Sud, A., et al. (2012). Patient involvement in blood transfusions safety: patients' and healthcare professionals' perspective. *Transfusion Medicine, 22*(4), 251–256.

Dunn, P. J. J. (2011). Human leucocyte antigen typing: Techniques and technology, a critical appraisal. *International Journal of Immunogenetics, 38,* 463–473.

Ezzone, S., & Schmit-Pokomy, K. (2007). *Blood and marrow stem cell transplantation: Principles, practice, and nursing insights* (3rd ed.). Pittsburgh, PA: Jones & Bartlett.

Hart, D. P., & Peggs, K. S. (2007). Current status of allogeneic stem cell transplantation for treatment of hematologic malignancies. *Clinical Pharmacology and Therapeutics, 82*(3), 325–329.

Hijji, B., Parahoo, K., Hussein, M. M., & Barr, O. (2012). Knowledge of blood transfusion among nurses. *Journal of Clinical Nursing,* July 25m 2012 (epub ahead of print) doi: 10.1111/j.1365–2702.2012.04078.x.

Jenkins, C., Ramirez-Arcos, S., Goldman, M., et al. (2011). Bacterial contamination in platelets: Incremental improvements drive down but do not eliminate risk. *Transfusion, 51,* 2555–2565.

Krimmel, T., & Williams, L. A. (2008). Hepatic sinusoidal obstruction syndrome following hematopoietic stem cell transplantation. *Oncology Nursing Forum, 35*(1), 37–39.

Mattson, M. R. (2007). Graft-versus-host disease: Review and nursing implications. *Clinical Journal of Oncology Nursing, 11*(3), 325–328.

Miraflor, E., Yeung, L., Strumwasser, A., Liu, T. H., Gregory. V. (2012). Emergency uncrossmatched transfusion effect on blood type allow antibodies. *Journal of Trauma and Acute Care Surgery, 72*(1), 48–53.

Petersdorf, E. W., Hansen, J. A., Martin, P. J., et al. (2011). Major histocompatibility complex class I alleles and antigens in hematopoietic cell transplantation. *New England Journal of Medicine, 345*(25), 1794–1800.

Price, T. H. (2006). Granulocyte transfusion therapy. *Journal of Clinical Apheresis, 21,* 65–71.

Ringden, O., Labopin, M., Beelen, D. W., et al. (2012). Bone marrow or peripheral blood stem cell transplantation from unrelated donors in adult patients with acute myeloid leukaemia, an Acute Leukaemia Working Party analysis in 2262 patients. *Journal of International Medicine, 272*(5), 472–483.

Scherf, R., & White-Reid, K. (2008). Giving intravenous immunoglobulin. *RN Journal, 71*(2), 29–34.

Stroncek, D. F., & Rebulla, P. (2007). Platelet transfusions. *Lancet, 370,* 427–438.

Tolich, D. J. (2008). Alternatives to blood transfusion. *Journal of Intravenous Nursing, 31*(1), 46–51.

Vasiliki, K. (2011). Enhancing transfusion safety: Nurse's role. *International Journal of Caring Sciences, 4*(3), 114–119.

28
Asthma and Allergy

OVERVIEW AND ASSESSMENT
The Allergic Reaction

An allergic reaction results from antigen–antibody reaction on sensitized mast cells or basophils, causing the release of chemical mediators. The reaction may be characterized by inflammation, increased secretions, and bronchoconstriction.

Definitions

1. Antigen—protein that stimulates an immune reaction, causing the production of antibodies.
2. Antibody—globulin (protein) secreted by B cells as a defense mechanism against foreign materials.
3. Atopy—term that refers to the ability to produce immunoglobulin E antibodies to common allergens.
4. Immunity:
   a. Humoral—process by which B lymphocytes produce circulating antibodies to act against antigens.
   b. Cell-mediated—portion of the immune system in which the participation of T lymphocytes and macrophages is predominant.
5. Mast cell—tissue cell similar to peripheral blood basophil, which contains granules with chemical mediators.
6. Basophil—leukocyte with large granules that contain histamine.
7. Hypersensitivity—reaction to an antigen after reexposure (there are four types); type I (immediate) and type IV (delayed) are considered allergic reactions.

Immunoglobulins

Antibodies that are formed by lymphocytes and plasma cells in response to an immunogenic stimulus comprise a group of serum proteins called *immunoglobulins*.

1. The abbreviation for immunoglobulin is Ig.
2. Antibodies combine with antigens in lock-and-key style.
3. There are five major classes of immunoglobulins.
   a. IgM—constitutes 10% of immunoglobulin pool; found mostly in intravascular fluid and primarily engaged in initial defense; levels elevated with recent infection.
   b. IgG—major immunoglobulin that accounts for 70% to 75% of secondary immune responses and combats tissue infection.
   c. IgA—15% to 20% of immunoglobulins; predominantly found in seromucous secretions (such as saliva, tears) in which it provides a primary defense mechanism.
   d. IgD—less than 1% of immunoglobulin pool; found on circulating B lymphocytes, and signals B cells to become activated.
   e. IgE—only a trace found in serum; attaches to surface membrane of basophils and mast cells; responsible for immediate types of allergic reactions.

Immunologic Reactions

Immediate Hypersensitivity (Type I)

1. Characterized by:
   a. IgE-mediated allergic reaction (see Figure 28-1).
   b. Occurs immediately after contact with the antigen.
   c. Causes release and neo-synthesis of preformed chemical mediators.
2. Examples—anaphylaxis, allergic rhinitis, urticaria.

Products of Immediate Hypersensitivity (Chemical Mediators)

1. Histamine—bioactive amine stored in granules of mast cells and basophils.
2. Leukotrienes—newly synthesized potent bronchoconstrictors; cause increased venous permeability.
3. Prostaglandins—potent vasodilators and potent bronchoconstrictors.
4. Platelet-activating factor—has many properties; causes the aggregation of platelets.
5. Cytokines—control and regulate immunologic functions (eg, interleukins, tumor necrosis factor).
6. Proteases—enzymes, such as tryptase and chymase, increase vascular permeability.
7. Eosinophil chemotactic factor of anaphylaxis—causes an influx of eosinophils into the area of allergic inflammation.

Effects of Chemical Mediators and Their Manifestations

1. Generalized vasodilation, hypotension, flushing.
2. Increased permeability.
   a. Capillaries of the skin—edema.
   b. Mucous membranes—edema.
3. Smooth muscle contraction.
   a. Bronchioles—bronchospasm.
   b. Intestines—abdominal cramps, diarrhea.
4. Increased secretions.
   a. Nasal mucous glands—rhinorrhea.
   b. Bronchioles—increased mucus in airways.
   c. GI—increased gastric secretions.
   d. Lacrimal—tearing.
   e. Salivary—salivation.
5. Pruritus (itching).
   a. Skin.
   b. Mucous membrane.

Delayed Hypersensitivity (Type IV)

1. Characterized by a cell-mediated reaction between antigens and antigen-responsive T lymphocytes.
2. Maximal intensity occurs between 24 and 48 hours.
3. Usually consists of erythema and induration.
4. Examples—tuberculin skin test; contact dermatitis such as poison ivy.

Allergy Assessment

Subjective and Objective Data

1. Evaluate for symptoms related to hay fever, asthma, skin reactions, insect allergy, and food allergy.
2. Determine exacerbating factors such as contact with pets, outdoor exposure, a certain season, contact with mold, exposure to dust.
3. Obtain complete medical history for past illnesses, medication allergies, family history, medications that have been tried, exercise, smoking, and work environment.
4. Perform physical examination based on patient presentation and specific allergy condition, usually skin, head, chest, eye, ear, nose, and throat examination.

REACTION TO ALLERGEN EXPOSURE

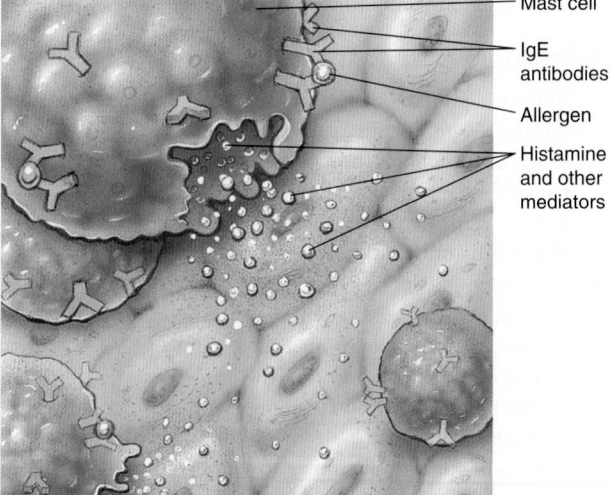

Figure 28-1. Type I immediate hypersensitivity. During the initial exposure, T cells recognize foreign allergens and release chemicals to instruct B cells to produce immunoglobulin (Ig) E. These antibodies attach themselves to mast cells. Upon reexposure, the allergen comes in contact with the IgE antibodies attached to mast cells, causing degranulation and release of chemical mediators.

Skin Testing

The purpose of skin testing is to identify antigens responsible for immediate hypersensitivity. The types of skin tests used in clinical allergy are epicutaneous (prick, puncture, or scratch) and intradermal methods. The skin test remains unequaled as a sensitive, specific, and effective test for the diagnosis of allergies. See Procedure Guidelines 28-1, page 1022, and Procedure Guidelines 28-2, pages 1023 and 1024.

Epicutaneous (Prick) Method

1. Advantages:
   a. Efficient—results within 15 minutes.
   b. Little discomfort to the patient.
   c. Only rare instances of anaphylaxis because of minimal systemic absorption.
2. Disadvantages:
   a. Old or thick, leathery skin decreases reactivity.
   b. Drops have a tendency to run together, which would affect the accuracy of the test.

Intradermal Method

1. Advantages:
   a. Useful to confirm equivocal epicutaneous results with some antigens.
2. Disadvantages:
   a. Less specific than prick testing.
   b. Increased possibility for anaphylactic reactions.
   c. Requires more time and skill to perform.
   d. Increased discomfort to the patient.

In Vitro Testing

Description

1. In vitro—using blood samples—tests for IgE antibodies to specific allergens. Instead of looking for a reaction in vivo (with the patient's body—as in skin testing), in vitro testing measures the IgE response to specific antigens added to blood samples. Advantages over skin testing include the following:
   a. Can be done without special knowledge of skin testing or availability of allergen extract.
   b. Patient does not need to stop antihistamine before testing.
   c. Can be done even with severe eczema.
   d. There is no risk of systemic reaction.
2. An immunofluorescent process is preferred for specific IgE testing because of high degree of sensitivity and specificity.
3. Some labs may offer a radioallergosorbent test (RAST); measures the allergen-specific IgE antibodies in serum samples after panel of allergens have been added to samples.

Nursing and Patient Care Considerations

1. Tell the patient that it is allergy testing without the risk of causing severe allergic reaction.
2. Obtain adequate venous blood for each allergen panel to be tested.
3. A positive result depends on the standards for that particular laboratory. The test does not indicate clinical significance of symptoms and must be interpreted with patient's history.

4. Arrange for a follow-up visit for the patient with the health care provider to discuss test results.

GENERAL PROCEDURES AND TREATMENT MODALITIES
Immunotherapy

 Evidence Base Cox, L. S., Nelson, H. A., Lockey, R., et al. (2010). Allergen immunotherapy: A practice parameter third update. *Journal of Allergy and Clinical Immunology, 127*(1, Suppl.), S1–S55.

Immunotherapy is the modulation of the immune system to develop tolerance to a known allergen that causes IgE, type I (immediate) hypersensitivity. Given in appropriate doses, it can significantly decrease patient symptoms in most patients. It is indicated for significant symptoms of allergic rhinitis, conjunctivitis, asthma, and stinging insect allergy that cannot be controlled by avoidance of the allergen. Considerable compliance and time commitment are essential for successful therapy. See Procedure Guidelines 28-3, pages 1025 to 1026.

Features of Immunotherapy

1. Specific allergens are identified by skin or blood testing.
2. Serial injections are begun that contain extracts from identified allergens (allergy vaccine).
3. Initially, a small amount of dilute allergy vaccine is given, usually at weekly intervals.
4. Amount and concentration are slowly increased to maximum tolerable dose.
5. The maintenance dose is injected every 2 to 4 weeks for a period of several years to achieve maximal benefit.
6. Several allergens are now standardized (dust mite, cat, grass and ragweed pollens, Hymenoptera venoms [yellow jacket, yellow and white-faced hornet, honey bee, wasp]).

Precautions and Considerations

1. Anaphylaxis rarely occurs after injection but risk remains.
   a. Should be given only in health care facility with epinephrine, trained personnel, and emergency equipment available. See Standards of Care Guidelines 28-1, page 1026.
   b. Patient should remain in office for 30 minutes after injection, after which the risk of anaphylaxis is greatly reduced.
   c. If large, local reaction (erythema, induration) occurs after an injection, the next dose should not be increased without checking with prescribing health care provider because a systemic reaction may occur.
2. If several weeks are missed, dosage may need to be decreased to prevent a reaction.
3. Medication, such as antihistamines and decongestants, should be continued until significant symptom relief occurs (may take 12 to 24 months).
4. Environmental controls should be maintained to enhance effectiveness of therapy.

(Text continues on page 1024)

PROCEDURE GUIDELINES 28-1

Epicutaneous Skin Testing

EQUIPMENT

- Antigens for testing
- Controls
  Positive—histamine 1 mg/mL
  Negative—glycerol saline
- Disposable pricking devices (sterile needles or lancets)
- Alcohol swabs
- Paper tissues
- Skin-marking pencil
- Millimeter ruler
- Tourniquet
- Epinephrine 1:1,000 aqueous solution for injection for emergency use

PROCEDURE

Nursing Action	Rationale
Preparatory phase	
1. Explain the procedure to the patient. Ask if patient has taken antihistamines in the past 72 hours.	1. Oral antihistamines taken within 72 hours of skin testing are likely to prevent a reaction from occurring. Desloratadine can affect skin testing up to 7 days.
2. Prepare the site (volar surface of forearm or back) by cleansing with alcohol.	2. The forearm is usually preferable because in the event of a significant local or systemic reaction, a tourniquet may be placed proximal to the skin test to slow the diffusion of the antigen into the circulation.
3. Mark the test sites with a skin-marking pencil approximately 3–4 cm apart.	3. Sites need to be spaced appropriately so that reactions will remain distinct from one another, thus allowing an accurate reading.
Implementation phase	
1. Apply positive (histamine) and negative (saline) controls next to the appropriate markings. Apply pricking device to skin per manufacturer's instructions. Discard pricking device after each puncture.	1. Because of interpatient variability in cutaneous reactivity, it is necessary to include positive and negative controls whenever skin testing is performed. A response to the positive control confirms an immunologic ability to react. A response to the negative control indicates reactivity to the diluting solution or mechanical trauma. Care must be taken to prevent cross-contamination between antigens.
2. Apply small drops of antigens next to the skin markings and prick the drops as described above.	2. Large drops may run and cross-contaminate, affecting interpretation.
3. Instruct the patient not to scratch the test area during the 15-minute waiting interval before the reactions are graded.	3. It is normal for sensitive individuals to have a pruritic sensation at the testing site because of the histamine released by the mast cells.
4. Observe the patient closely for signs of impending anaphylaxis (such as itching, flushing, abnormal sensation in throat).	4. General systemic or anaphylactic reactions are rare, but do occur. If suspected, apply tourniquet above test site and administer epinephrine 1:1,000 subcutaneously in a dose of 0.01 mL/kg (maximum 0.3 mL).
Follow-up phase	
1. Fifteen minutes after pricking the antigens, measure the diameter of induration (wheal) and erythema (flare) in two perpendicular axes through the center of the reaction; record in millimeters.	1. Amount of induration indicates the extent of reaction, but erythema is noted as well.
2. Document the procedure, test results, patient tolerance, and any other pertinent observations.	2. Continuity of care.

PROCEDURE GUIDELINES 28-2

Intradermal Skin Testing

EQUIPMENT

- Antigens for testing
- Controls
  Positive—histamine 0.1 mg/mL
  Negative—human serum albumin/saline
- 1-mL syringes with 26G or 27G intradermal needle
- Alcohol swabs
- Paper tissues
- Skin-marking pencil
- Millimeter ruler
- Tourniquet
- Gloves
- Epinephrine for emergency use

PROCEDURE

Nursing Action	Rationale
Preparatory phase	
1. Explain the procedure to the patient. Ask if patient has taken antihistamines in the past 72 hours.	1. Oral antihistamines taken 72 hours before skin testing are likely to prevent a reaction from occurring. Desloratadine should be held for 7 days.
2. Prepare the site (volar surface of forearm or upper arm) by cleansing with alcohol. Allow to dry.	2. Allowing alcohol to dry ensures antisepsis.
3. Mark the test sites with a skin-marking pencil approximately 3–4 cm apart.	3. Sites need to be spaced appropriately so that reactions will remain distinct from one another, thus allowing an accurate reading.
Implementation phase	
1. Using sterile technique, draw up 0.05 mL of each testing material. All bubbles must be carefully expelled to avoid "splash reactions," which reduce precision. While wearing gloves, place syringe at a 10- to 15-degree angle to the skin with the bevel up. Stretch the skin taut and insert 0.02 mL of the positive and negative controls. The bevel should penetrate the skin entirely and end between the layers of skin. A bleb approximately 2 mm in diameter should be produced.	1. Gloves should be worn when there is any possibility of exposure to blood or body fluids. Only a small amount needs to be deposited into skin—enough to raise a bleb.
2. Inject approximately 0.02 mL of test antigens intradermally next to the skin markings. A different syringe and needle must be used for each antigen.	2. Avoids antigen and microbial contamination.

(A) Intradermal injection producing a wheal.

(B) Measuring area of induration.

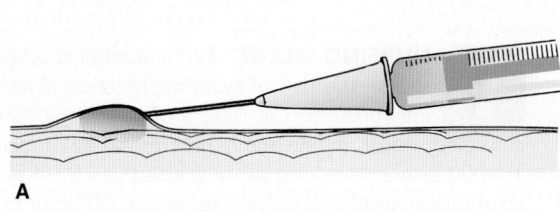

A

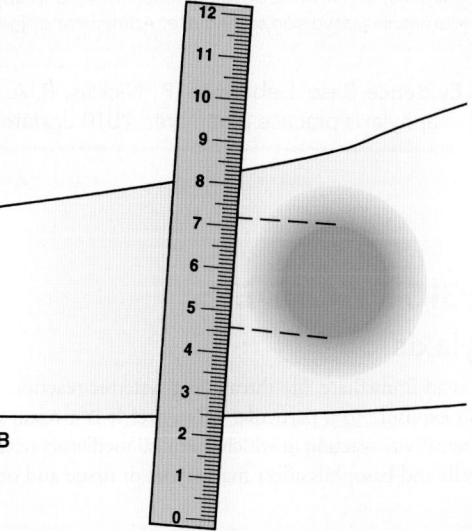

B

(continued)

PROCEDURE GUIDELINES 28-2 (continued)

Intradermal Skin Testing

PROCEDURE (continued)

Nursing Action	Rationale
3. Instruct the patient not to scratch the test area during the 15-minute waiting interval before the reaction is graded.	3. It is normal for sensitive individuals to have a pruritic sensation at the testing site because of the histamine released by the mast cells.
4. Observe the patient closely for signs of impending anaphylaxis (itching, flushing, lump in throat).	4. There is an increased possibility of anaphylactic reactions with intradermal skin testing. If suspected, apply tourniquet above test site and administer epinephrine 1:1,000 I.M. in a dose of 0.3 mL (0.01 mL/kg in children <30 kg)
5. Fifteen minutes after applying antigens, measure the diameter of induration (wheal) and erythema (flare) in two perpendicular axes through the center of the reaction and record in millimeters.	

Follow-up phase

1. Document the procedure, test results, patient tolerance, and any other pertinent observations.	1. For continuity of care.
2. Monitor for the following complications during and following testing:	2. Any significant reaction may be anxiety-provoking for the patient, but anaphylaxis occurs suddenly and may be life-threatening.

Local Reactions—unusually large reactions (>25 mm in duration)

   a. Apply prescribed steroid cream to affected area.

   b. If no relief, administer prescribed oral antihistamine.

Vasovagal Reactions—fainting episode

   a. Monitor vital signs.

   b. Reassure the patient.

   c. Finish skin testing, if possible.

Systemic Anaphylaxis

Key Decision Point

If signs of anaphylaxis develop, stop testing and apply tourniquet above skin testing site. Administer epinephrine I.M. (using vastus lateralis muscle) and administer oxygen. Alert provider or emergency responders.

Evidence Base Lieberman, P., Nicklas, R. A., Oppenheimer, J., et al. (2010). Diagnosis and management of anaphylaxis practice parameter: 2010 update. *Journal of Allergy and Clinical Immunology, 126,* 477–480.

ALLERGIC DISORDERS

Anaphylaxis

Anaphylaxis is an immediate, life-threatening systemic reaction that can occur on exposure to a particular substance. It is a result of a type I hypersensitivity reaction in which chemical mediators released from mast cells and basophils affect many types of tissue and organ systems.

NURSING ALERT With immunotherapy (allergy shots), the risk of systemic reaction is always present, occurring in 0.02% of injections. Skin testing can also result in systemic reactions. Have epinephrine 1:1,000 available during these procedures (with syringe and tourniquet) and have patient remain in office or clinic for at least 30 minutes after administration.

PROCEDURE GUIDELINES 28-3

Giving an Allergy Injection

EQUIPMENT

- individualized allergy vaccine
- 1-mL syringe
- 25G to 27G ½- to ⅝ -inch needle
- Gauze or cotton ball
- Alcohol sponges

 NURSING ALERT   Because of the risk of anaphylaxis, have epinephrine 1:1,000 readily available for injection, as well as oxygen, parenteral diphenhydramine, and IV supplies.

PROCEDURE

Nursing Action	Rationale
Preparatory phase	
1. Check record and ask patient about reaction to last injection. Note how many weeks since last shot.	1. Local erythema and induration may have occurred during observation period or later.
2. Check order for prescribed dosage and any special instructions based on reaction history.	2. Significant reaction (greater than 2–3 cm and lasting 24 hours) may require injection at same or lower dose. Missed weeks may require dosage adjustment.
3. Draw up dose, checking strength of allergy vaccine and amount (usually 0.05–0.5 mL)	3. Vaccine will be replaced periodically with a stronger preparation.
4. Verify correct dose for the patient.	4. Incorrect vaccine or dose may cause anaphylaxis.
Performance phase	
1. Select the appropriate site for subcutaneous injection, usually the midlateral upper arms. If two injections are necessary, give in opposite arms.	1. Because injections are usually only given once per week, no need to use abdomen or thighs. Using different arms for two injections allows for determining which vaccine may have caused reaction if one occurs.
2. Wear gloves if pressure is applied to patient's arm.	2. Prevents contact with patient's blood.
3. Cleanse site with alcohol and allow to dry.	3. Disinfects skin.
4. Grasp upper arm with nondominant hand so that tissue is elevated slightly.	4. Secures arm and subcutaneous tissue beneath outer skin.
5. Insert needle at a 45- to 90-degree angle, depending on thickness of subcutaneous tissue at the site.	5. Thickness of subcutaneous tissue varies among individuals.
6. Aspirate for blood return and if none occurs, inject serum.	6. If blood enters syringe, dispose of it and begin again rather than injecting into a blood vessel.
7. Withdraw syringe, cover site with alcohol sponge, and dispose of needle and syringe. Check site for bleeding or bruising.	7. Follow facility policy; do not resheath needle.
Follow-up phase	
1. Have patient wait 30 minutes before leaving the facility. Check for local reaction periodically and tell patient to report any sudden swelling, itching, or respiratory difficulty.	1. Significant local or systemic reaction may occur; most likely with increased dose or new vaccine vial.

 Key Decision Point

If angioedema, respiratory distress, or hypotension develop, institute emergency actions, including administration of oxygen, application of tourniquet above the injection site, and injection of epinephrine 1:1000 0.3–0.5 mL in the opposite arm.

(continued)

PROCEDURE GUIDELINES 28-3 *(continued)*

Giving an Allergy Injection

PROCEDURE *(continued)*

Nursing Action	Rationale

Follow-up phase

2. Record amount and concentration of vaccine, site given, and appearance of site after 30 minutes.

2. Flow sheet serves as official documentation of medication given and may be reviewed by allergist when evaluating therapy.

3. Dismiss patient with instructions on who to call if reaction occurs and when to return for next injection.

3. May call allergist or primary care provider, or go to emergency department if systemic reaction occurs.

 Evidence Base Joint Task Force on Practice Parameters for Allergy and Immunology. (2010). Allergen immunotherapy: A practice parameter third update. *Journal of Allergy and Clinical Immunology.*

Pathophysiology and Etiology

1. May be caused by:
   a. Immunotherapy.
   b. Stinging insects.
   c. Skin testing.
   d. Medications.
   e. Contrast media infusion.
   f. Foods.
   g. Exercise.
   h. Latex.
2. Release of chemical mediators results in massive vasodilation, increased capillary permeability, bronchoconstriction, and decreased peristalsis.

Clinical Manifestations

1. Respiratory—laryngeal edema, bronchospasm, cough, wheezing, dyspnea, lump in throat.
2. Cardiovascular—hypotension, tachycardia, palpitations, syncope.
3. Cutaneous—urticaria (hives), angioedema, pruritus, erythema (flushing).
4. GI—nausea, vomiting, diarrhea, abdominal pain, bloating.

 DRUG ALERT Before administering any drug, ask if the patient has ever had a reaction to it. Do not rely on the chart alone.

Management

Prompt identification of signs and symptoms and immediate intervention are essential; a reaction that occurs quickly tends to be more severe.

Immediate Treatment

1. Place patient supine and check vital signs.
2. Immediately administer epinephrine 1:1,000—adolescents and adults, 0.3 to 0.5 mL; children, 0.01 mL/kg via intramuscular (I.M.) route into vastus lateralis muscle. This may be repeated every 5 to 10 minutes if necessary—causes vasoconstriction, decreases capillary permeability, relaxes airway smooth muscle, and inhibits mast cell mediator release.

STANDARDS OF CARE GUIDELINES 28-1
Immunotherapy

To perform immunotherapy or allergy testing, have epinephrine 1:1,000 available with a 1-mL syringe and a 1-inch (2.5 cm) needle.

- Make sure that the patient remains under observation for at least 30 minutes after injection and assess for local reaction and respiratory distress before the patient leaves.
- If a significant reaction occurred after the last injection or if the patient is late for his or her dosage, follow written protocol for those cases or call the patient's health care provider for instructions.
- Be prepared to inject 0.3–0.5 mL (or 0.01 mL/kg for children <30 kg) of epinephrine I.M. as directed by health care provider present or facility protocol if signs of anaphylaxis develop. Call for immediate help and transfer to an acute care facility.

This information should serve as a general guideline only. Each patient situation presents a unique set of clinical factors and requires nursing judgment to guide care, which may include additional or alternative measures and approaches. I.M., intramuscular.

3. Monitor vital signs continuously. Administer oxygen, if needed.
4. A tourniquet is applied above site of antigen injection (allergy injection, insect sting, etc.) or skin test site to slow the absorption of antigen into the system.

Subsequent Treatment

1. An adequate airway is established and albuterol is administered by inhalation, as needed.
2. Hypotension and shock are treated with fluids and vasopressors.
3. Additional bronchodilators are given to relax bronchial smooth muscle.
4. Histamine-1 (H_1) antihistamines, such as diphenhydramine, and, possibly, H_2 antihistamines, such as ranitidine, are given to block the effects of histamine.
5. Corticosteroids are given to decrease vascular permeability and diminish the migration of inflammatory cells; may be helpful in preventing late-phase responses.

Complications

1. Cardiovascular collapse.
2. Respiratory failure.

Nursing Assessment

1. Promptly assess airway, breathing, and circulation (ABCs) with severe presentation and intervene with cardiopulmonary resuscitation, as appropriate.
2. When ABCs are stable, assess vital signs, degree of respiratory distress, and angioedema.
3. Obtain a history of onset of symptoms and of exposure to allergen.

Nursing Diagnoses

- Ineffective Breathing Pattern related to bronchospasm and laryngeal edema.
- Decreased Cardiac Output related to vasodilation.
- Anxiety related to respiratory distress and life-threatening situation.

Nursing Interventions

Restoring Effective Breathing

1. Establish and maintain an adequate airway.
   a. If epinephrine has not stabilized bronchospasm, assist with endotracheal intubation, emergency tracheostomy, or cricothyroidotomy, as indicated.
   b. Continually monitor respiratory rate, depth, and breath sounds for decreased work of breathing and effective ventilation.
2. Administer nebulized albuterol or other bronchodilators, as ordered. Monitor heart rate (increased with bronchodilators).
3. Provide oxygen via nasal cannula at 2 to 5 L/minute or by alternative means, as ordered.
4. Administer intravenous (IV) corticosteroids, as ordered.

Increasing Cardiac Output

1. Monitor blood pressure (BP) by continuous automatic cuff, if available.
2. Administer rapid infusion of IV fluids to fill vasodilated circulatory system and raise BP.
3. Monitor central venous pressure (CVP) to ensure adequate fluid volume and to prevent fluid overload.
4. Insert indwelling catheter and monitor urine output hourly to ensure kidney perfusion.
5. Initiate and titrate vasopressor, as ordered, based on BP response.

Reducing Anxiety

1. Provide care in a prompt, calm, and confident manner.
2. Remain responsive to the patient, who may remain alert but not completely coherent because of hypotension, hypoxemia, and effects of medication.
3. Keep family or significant others informed of patient's condition and the treatment being given.
4. When patient is stable and alert, give a simple, honest explanation of anaphylaxis and the treatment that was given.

Community and Home Care Considerations

1. Make sure that patient who has experienced anaphylaxis or severe local reactions obtains a prescription for self-injectable epinephrine to have available at all times.
   a. Instruct the patient and family members in the injection technique upon exposure to known antigen or at the first signs of a systemic reaction.
   b. Provide patient with information on epinephrine, including dose, drug action, possible adverse effects, the importance of prompt administration at the first sign of a systemic reaction, storage conditions, and replacement of outdated syringe.
   c. Ensure day care providers and school personnel are aware of patient's potential for anaphylaxis and have access to and are able to administer epinephrine.
2. Even if treatment is given successfully at home, the patient should follow up with the health care provider immediately.
3. Make sure that the patient with history of anaphylaxis has access to emergency medical system and does not spend time alone if risk of reaction is present.

Patient Education and Health Maintenance

1. Teach the patient at risk for anaphylaxis about the potential seriousness of these reactions.
2. Educate patient to recognize the early signs and symptoms of anaphylaxis and have epinephrine available.
3. People allergic to venom stings should avoid wearing brightly colored or black clothes, perfumes, and hair spray. Shoes should be worn at all times.
4. For exercise-induced anaphylaxis, patient should exercise in moderation, preferably with another person, and in a controlled setting, where assistance is readily available.
5. Instruct patient to wear a MedicAlert-type bracelet at all times.

6. For potential drug allergies, teach the patient to:
   a. Read labels and be familiar with the generic name of the drug thought to cause a reaction.
   b. Discard all unused drugs. Make sure any drug kept in the medicine cabinet is clearly labeled.
   c. Become familiar with drugs that may cross-react with a drug to which patient is allergic.
   d. Always know the name of every drug taken.
   e. Clear all herbals and nutraceuticals with health care provider.
7. Advise patient with a known sensitivity to a food product to be extremely careful about everything he or she eats—allergen compounds may be hidden in a preparation (such as caseinate, lactalbumin).
8. Advise that if food is associated with exercise-induced anaphylaxis, wait at least 2 hours after eating to exercise.

Evaluation: Expected Outcomes

- Respirations unlabored with clear lung fields, minimal wheezing.
- BP and CVP within normal range; urine output adequate.
- Responsive and cooperative.

Allergic Rhinitis

Allergic rhinitis is an inflammation of the nasal mucosa caused by an allergen that affects 10% to 30% of the population and up to 40% of children.

Pathophysiology and Etiology

1. Type I hypersensitivity causes local vasodilation and increased capillary permeability.
2. Caused by airborne allergens.
3. IgE-mediated inflammatory process is now believed to be the same disease process for asthma and allergic rhinitis.
4. Allergic rhinitis was formerly classified as seasonal or perennial; current classifications are intermittent or persistent.
   a. Intermittent—symptoms present less than 4 days per week and less than 4 weeks per year.
   b. Persistent—symptoms present more than 4 days per week and more than 4 weeks per year.
5. Severity is classified as mild (no interference with daily activities or troublesome symptoms) or moderate-severe (presence of at least one: impaired sleep, daily activity, work, or school; troublesome symptoms).

Clinical Manifestations

1. Nasal—mucous membrane congestion, edema, itching, rhinorrhea with clear secretions, sneezing.
2. Eyes—edema, itching, burning, tearing, redness, dark circles under eyes (allergic shiners).
3. Ears—itching, fullness.
4. Other—postnasal drainage, palatal itching, throat itching, nonproductive cough.

Diagnostic Evaluation

1. Skin testing—confirms a hypersensitivity to certain allergens.
2. Nasal smear—increased number of eosinophils suggests allergic disease.
3. ImmunoCAP or other in vitro IgE-specific antigen testing—positive test result for offending allergens.
4. Rhinoscopy—allows better visualization of the nasopharynx; helps rule out physical obstruction (septal deviation, nasal polyps).
5. Evaluation for asthma.

Management

Avoidance

1. Patient should minimize contact with offending allergens, regardless of other treatment.
2. Patient may be instructed to reduce dust mite exposure by encasing bed pillows and mattress in allergen-proof covering; however, studies have not shown that this alone improves symptoms. Use of allergen-proof bedding should be carried out in conjunction with broad environmental controls (see Patient Education Guidelines 28-1).

Medications: Antihistamines

H_1 antihistamines—block the effects of histamine on smooth muscle and blood vessels by blocking histamine receptor sites, thereby preventing the symptoms of allergic rhinitis.

1. Loratadine, fexofenadine, and cetirizine are long-acting antihistamines sold OTC and are considered nonsedating (cetirizine is considered less sedating).
2. Long-acting, nonsedating antihistamines available by prescription include desloratadine and levocetirizine.
3. Topical antihistamine nasal spray available by prescription (azelastine or olopatadine).
4. Older, sedating antihistamines (diphenhydramine, chlorpheniramine) are inexpensive, available OTC, short-acting, and effective if tolerated by the patient. They also have an anticholinergic effect—inhibit mucous secretions, act as drying agents.

Medications: Controllers

1. Intranasal corticosteroids:
   a. Reduce inflammation of nasal mucosa.
   b. Prevent mediator release.
   c. Can be used safely every day.
   d. May be given systemically for a short course during a disabling attack.
2. Mast cell stabilizers—such as intranasal cromolyn sodium or ophthalmic cromolyn and lodoxamide hinder the release of chemical mediators. These medications are used before and during allergen season.
3. Leukotriene receptor antagonists, including montelukast and zafirlukast, are systemic agents used for asthma; montelukast also has an indication in allergic rhinitis and reduces the inflammation, edema, and mucous secretion of allergic rhinitis.

PATIENT EDUCATION GUIDELINES 28-1

Environmental Control for Allergic Rhinitis

The following environmental modifications may help reduce symptoms of allergic rhinitis (hay fever):

- Encase pillows and mattress in allergen-proof covers.
- Wash all bed linens (mattress pad, sheets, blanket, comforter, and bedspread) in hot water weekly.
- Keep clothing in a closet with door shut or in dresser drawers that are kept closed.
- Use easily cleaned shades, blinds, and curtains.
- Avoid stuffed animals and other items that collect dust.
- Vacuum and damp-dust weekly; wear a mask while doing it.
- If you have severe symptoms of dust allergy, leave the house during cleaning. Allergic reaction is possible for about 30 minutes after vacuuming because dust mite feces and other allergens become airborne. Fine-filtering face masks may provide some protection.

- Eliminate upholstered furniture, carpets, and draperies.
- Use air conditioning and keep windows closed during high pollen and mold seasons to reduce antigen load indoors.
- Change furnace and air conditioner filters frequently.
- Using a high-efficiency air filtering system may help.
- Avoid smoking and smoke-filled areas.
- Avoid rapid changes in temperature.
- If you are allergic to animal dander, you should not have household pets. If pets are present in your household, keep them out of the bedroom and run a high-efficiency particulate air filter (place on table).
- Avoid mold growth by dehumidification (<45% ambient humidity) and use of a fungicide in bathrooms, damp basements, food storage areas, and garbage containers.
- Avoid outdoor activities when pollen or other pollutants are in the air.

Medications: Symptom Relief

1. Oral corticosteroids may be given systematically for a short course during a disabling attack.
2. Decongestants—shrink nasal mucous membrane by vasoconstriction; oral and topical, many available OTC and in combination with antihistamines, pain relievers, and anticholinergics.
3. Topical eye preparations—sold OTC and by prescription reduce inflammation and relieve itching and burning.

Immunotherapy

1. Regimen consists of administering subcutaneous injections of increasing amounts of an allergen to which the patient is sensitive to decrease sensitivity and reduce the severity of symptoms (see page 1025).
2. Immunotherapy produces the following immunologic changes:
   a. Production of IgG-blocking antibody that combines with antigen before it reacts with IgE antibodies.
   b. Decreases IgE antibodies against specific antigens.
   c. Modulation from T helper (Th) 2 to Th1 T lymphocytes (Th2 associated with allergy).
3. Possible adverse effects of immunotherapy.
   a. Systemic reactions—anaphylaxis is rare, but potentially fatal.
   b. Local reactions—consist of erythema and induration at the site of injection.

! NURSING ALERT Immunotherapy should be administered with caution to patients taking beta-adrenergic blockers and should not be given to patients whose asthma is not controlled.

Complications

1. Allergic asthma.
2. Chronic otitis media, hearing loss.
3. Chronic nasal obstruction, nasal polyps, sinusitis.
4. Orthodontic malocclusion in children.

Nursing Assessment

1. Obtain history of severity and seasonality of symptoms.
2. Inspect for characteristic tearing, conjunctival erythema, pale nasal mucous membranes with clear discharge, allergic shiners, and mouth breathing.
3. Auscultate lungs for wheezing or prolonged expiration characteristic of asthma.

Nursing Diagnosis

- Ineffective Breathing Pattern related to nasal obstruction.

Nursing Interventions

Facilitating Normal Breathing Pattern

1. Reassure patient that suffocation will not occur because of nasal obstruction; mouth breathing will occur.
2. Use intranasal saline to soothe irritating mucous membranes and increase oral fluid intake to prevent drying of mucous membranes and increased insensible loss through mouth breathing.
3. Administer and teach self-administration of antihistamines, decongestants, intranasal corticosteroids and antihistamine, and other medications, as directed.
   a. Instruct patients on proper use of nasal sprays—clear mucus from nose first, exhale, flex neck to point nose downward, direct spray away from the nasal septum

(toward the eye), activate inhaler, and gently sniff while releasing medication. Report any nasal irritation or nose bleeds to provider.

b. Warn patient to avoid driving or other situations that require alertness if sedating antihistamines, such as diphenhydramine or chlorpheniramine, are being used.

c. Do not use OTC nasal decongestants for more than 4 to 5 days because their effect is short term and a rebound effect, which causes nasal mucosal edema, commonly occurs.

 DRUG ALERT Long-term use of nasal corticosteroids may cause nasal septum rupture. Teach patients to direct spray or aerosol away from septum.

Patient Education and Health Maintenance

1. Provide information on purpose, administration method, time frame of expected results, and possible risks involved (local reactions, anaphylaxis) with immunotherapy.
2. Inform the patient that close observation for 30 minutes is essential after each injection.
3. Alert patient to the possibility of a delayed reaction during immunotherapy that should be reported to the nurse or health care provider.
4. Teach lifestyle and environmental changes to reduce exposure to allergens.
5. For additional information and support, refer to American Academy of Allergy, Asthma, and Immunology (*www.aaaai. org*), American College of Allergy, Asthma & Immunology (*www.acaai.org*), and National Institute of Allergy and Infectious Diseases Office of Communications (*www.niaid.gov*).

Evaluation: Expected Outcomes

Decreased eye and nasal symptoms, mouth breathing; no complaints of dry mouth.

Urticaria and Angioedema

Urticaria, or hives, may affect 25% of the population at any given time. *Angioedema* is a similar lesion, but involves deep dermis and subcutaneous tissues. Urticaria and angioedema can occur individually or in combination.

Pathophysiology and Etiology

1. Acute urticaria:
   a. Hives that last less than 6 weeks.
   b. A detectable cause is often determined.
2. Chronic urticaria:
   a. Hives that last 6 weeks or longer.
   b. Up to 50% of cases may be autoimmune chronic urticaria with autoantibodies against high-affinity IgE receptor or IgE.
   c. At least 50% are idiopathic.
3. Cause may be undetermined or may include:
   a. Ingested substances—food, food additives, drugs.
   b. Infections—viral, bacterial, parasitic.

c. Physical factors—heat, sun, cold, pressure, emotional stress.
d. Insect stings.

Clinical Manifestations

1. Raised, red, edematous wheals.
2. Intense pruritus.
3. May affect any body region.
4. Diffuse swelling with angioedema, especially of the lips, eyelids, cheeks, hands, and feet.
5. Symptoms may develop within seconds or over 1 to 2 hours and may last up to 24 to 36 hours.

Diagnostic Evaluation

1. Laboratory—serum tryptase is elevated in the acute phase, complement study results can be abnormal, total serum IgE elevated.
2. Challenge testing to determine physical cause.
   a. Dermographism present (most common).
   b. Exercise challenge.
   c. Ice cube challenge.
   d. Heat challenge.
   e. Pressure challenge.

Management

Acute Urticaria

1. Identification and elimination of causative factors.
2. Medications.
   a. H_1 antihistamines, such as diphenhydramine and cetirizine.
   b. Corticosteroids—limited to severe cases; unresponsive to antihistamines.
   c. Epinephrine 1:1,000 (0.3 to 0.5 mL I.M.) for severe angioedema or urticaria.

Chronic Urticaria

1. Avoid causative factors.
2. Medications.
   a. H_1 antihistamines.
   b. H_2 antihistamines, such as ranitidine, may be of some value.
   c. Tricyclic antidepressants, such as doxepin, given for antihistaminic effect.
   d. Topical agents to relieve itching (moisturizer or oatmeal baths).
3. Severe, unremitting urticarial treatment may include low-dose cyclosporine, tacrolimus, or omalizumab therapy.

Complications

1. Neurovascular impairment because of swelling.
2. Rarely, edema of the larynx or bronchi.

Nursing Assessment

1. Assess for time frame during which lesions appear and disappear.
2. Assess for triggering factors.
3. Assess for family history of angioedema; may indicate hereditary angioedema rather than allergic reaction.

Nursing Diagnosis

- Impaired comfort related to pruritus.

Nursing Interventions

Relieving Pruritus

1. Administer or teach self-administration of antihistamines, corticosteroids, and additional medications, as prescribed.
2. Encourage the proper use of topical and OTC agents, as directed.
3. Advise patient to avoid exposure to heat, exercise, sunburn, and alcohol and to promptly control fever and anxiety—factors that may aggravate reactions caused by vasodilation.
4. Warn patient to avoid identified triggers.
5. Teach relaxation techniques and methods of distraction to enhance coping.
6. Assess effectiveness of therapy.

Patient Education and Health Maintenance

1. Warn the patient to monitor for symptoms of laryngeal edema and to seek medical intervention immediately if respiratory distress occurs.
2. Instruct patients with laryngeal edema how to self-administer epinephrine.

Evaluation: Expected Outcomes

- Reports relief of pruritus with antihistamines and distraction methods.

Food Allergies

Food allergies result when the body's immune system overreacts to certain, otherwise harmless, substances. Food allergies occur in 8% of children and in 2% of adults, although the perceived prevalence is much higher because other existing adverse food reactions cause similar symptoms.

Pathophysiology and Etiology

1. Food hypersensitivity—a true food allergy is an IgE-mediated response to a food allergen (protein).
2. Food intolerance—an abnormal physical response to a food or additive; may be immunologic but not IgE-mediated.
   a. Toxicity (poisoning)—caused by toxins contained in foods, microorganisms, or parasites.
   b. Pharmacologic (chemical)—such as caffeine.
   c. Idiosyncratic—etiology unknown.
3. Common food allergens include cow's milk, eggs, shellfish, peanuts, tree nuts, soybean, and wheat.

Clinical Manifestations

1. Respiratory—rhinoconjunctivitis, sneezing, laryngeal edema, wheezing.
2. Cutaneous—urticaria, angioedema, atopic dermatitis.
3. Gastroenteritis—lip swelling, palatal itching, nausea, abdominal cramping, diarrhea, vomiting.
4. Neurologic—migraine headache in some patients.

Diagnostic Evaluation

1. Skin testing.
   a. Limited to those foods suspected of provoking symptoms based on history.
   b. Only epicutaneous testing is recommended.
   c. Intradermal testing has not been demonstrated to have a high degree of clinical correlation.
2. ImmunoCAP, RAST, or other IgE-specific antigen in vitro testing—positive result.
3. Oral challenge—the suspected food is given to the patient to identify the allergen by reproducing the symptoms caused by the initial reaction.
   a. Open—may be used if the suspected food skin test result is negative; suspected food is openly administered and the patient is monitored for a reaction.
   b. Single-blind—suspected food is disguised in capsules, liquids, or other foods and administered to the patient in increasing doses at intervals determined by history and may be interspersed with placebo. Some bias exists, however.
   c. Double-blind placebo-controlled—the "gold standard" and most definitive technique to confirm or refute food allergy. The suspected food is administered in capsules or via some other vehicle that masks its identity; it is interspersed with placebo so neither the health care provider nor the patient knows whether the suspected food or placebo is being ingested.
4. Elimination diet.
   a. To determine if the patient's symptoms will stop when certain foods are avoided.
   b. Restrict one or two foods at a time if certain foods are suspected.
   c. If no particular food is suspected, a highly restricted diet for 14 days is preferable.

Management

1. Avoidance of specific foods is the only way of effectively preventing food allergy reactions.
2. Medications:
   a. Antihistamines—may modify IgE-mediated symptoms but will not eliminate them.
   b. Corticosteroids—only used in the treatment of food allergy if associated with eosinophilic gastroenteritis or gastroenteropathy.
   c. Epinephrine—if history of anaphylaxis, patient should carry subcutaneous self-injection at all times.
3. Oral desensitization may be considered under careful observation.

Complications

Anaphylaxis.

Nursing Assessment

1. Assist with assessment for offending foods; encourage the patient to keep a food and symptom diary.
2. Auscultate lungs and document any wheezing.
3. Assess adherence with prescribed diet and relief of symptoms.

Nursing Diagnosis

- Imbalanced Nutrition: Less Than Body Requirements related to restrictive diet.

Nursing Interventions

Promoting Adequate Nutrition

1. Consult with dietitian to ensure a balanced diet that excludes identified allergens and incorporates patient's food preferences.
2. Administer dietary supplements, as needed.
3. Discuss alternative food-preparation techniques and methods of substitution (such as using extra baking powder in place of eggs).
4. Administer and teach self-administration of medications, if necessary, to reduce abdominal cramping and diarrhea, which may deter food intake.
5. Monitor weight.

Patient Education and Health Maintenance

1. Instruct the patient with history of anaphylactic reaction about self-injection technique for the administration of epinephrine.
2. Caution highly allergic patient about restaurant food; when eating out, avoid buffets and patient should request ingredient information; brochures listing ingredients of various dishes are now available in many restaurants, including fast-food establishments.
3. Explain hidden sources of foods to decrease the risk of unexpected exposure to an offending allergen. Some foods may contain allergens not as primary ingredients but as fillers or additives. Likewise, a food that has been prepared or stored in the same container or cooled on the same surface as an allergen-containing food may become contaminated with a sufficient quantity of the allergen to cause a reaction. Encourage label reading.
4. Advise patient that most young children and about one third of older children and adults lose their food sensitivity after several years of avoidance. Compliance with elimination is the key. Sensitivity to shellfish and nuts is rarely lost, however.
5. Provide resource for patient to obtain more information: The Food Allergy & Anaphylaxis Network (*www.foodallergy.org*).

Evaluation: Expected Outcomes

- Decreased frequency and severity of food allergy reactions by log; verbalizes acceptance of diet; weight stable

Latex Sensitivity

Latex sensitivity is becoming a major health concern for health care workers, patients, and others at risk by occupation. Allergic reaction may be immediate or delayed. Latex is present in approximately 40,000 medical and other products, including household products and toys. The prevalence of latex sensitivity is estimated to be 1% in the general population, 20% in nurses, and more than 60% in children with spina bifida.

Pathophysiology and Etiology

1. Natural rubber latex, manufactured from the sap of rubber trees, is highly irritating and allergenic in some people.
2. Increased use of latex, in the form of sterile and unsterile gloves, has made latex sensitivity a problem for many health care workers since the inception of Universal Precautions in the 1980s.
3. Three types of reactions to latex may occur:
   a. Irritant dermatitis—not an allergic reaction.
   b. Type IV (cell-mediated, delayed) hypersensitivity—a localized contact allergic reaction.
   c. Type I (IgE-mediated, immediate)—a systemic allergic reaction.
4. No predictable pattern exists for the progression of reactions; anaphylaxis may occur at any time. More severe reaction occurs with latex contact with mucous membrane than with intact skin.
5. Those at risk include children with spina bifida, health care workers, people with atopic allergies, people with a history of multiple surgeries, and workers in factories that produce latex products.

Clinical Manifestations

1. Irritant dermatitis—may be caused by powder or chemical residue on gloves; erythema and pruritus localized to area of contact; occurs immediately.
2. Type IV (delayed) hypersensitivity—contact allergic reaction; erythema, pruritus, urticaria; possible flushing, localized edema, rhinitis, coughing, and conjunctivitis. Symptoms occur 1 to 48 hours after contact with product.
3. Type I (immediate) hypersensitivity—urticaria, angioedema, conjunctivitis, dyspnea, pharyngeal edema, arrhythmias, and anaphylaxis. Symptoms are immediate and may be moderate to life-threatening in intensity.

Diagnostic Evaluation

1. History of symptoms gives presumptive diagnosis, but confirmation is difficult because standardized tests are not yet widely available.
2. A crude skin prick test uses a fragment of latex glove soaked in saline for 15 minutes as the solution. This is not standardized, but a positive test result is considered proof of latex sensitivity.
3. A challenge test can be done by having the patient wear a latex glove or fingertip of a glove for 15 minutes; look for a reaction. Latex-free gloves can be used as a control. Severe reactions may occur with this test.
4. Standardized skin testing will become more available pending Food and Drug Administration approval of standardized latex solution, but the threat of anaphylaxis will still exist.
5. RAST or other IgE blood testing is safe but expensive and is limited due to both false-positive and false-negative results.

Management

1. Avoidance is the key. See Box 28-1 for safety and prevention techniques in the health care workplace.
2. For irritant reactions, changing brands of gloves or changing to a powder-free glove may be sufficient.

BOX 28-1 | **Latex Safety for Patients and Health Care Workers**

- Use latex-free gloves of synthetic rubber, vinyl, nitrile, neoprene, or other material.
- Be aware that removing latex gloves with power may cause latex particles to become aerosolized for up to 5 hours and be carried to other areas on clothing and equipment.
- Do not enter OR with latex gloves or without having scrubbed after removing latex gloves in another area and remove possibly latex-laden clothing.
- Schedule latex-sensitive patients early in the day or as first surgical case.
- Post signs indicating Latex Allergy or Latex Alert.
- Encourage latex-sensitive individuals to wear identification bracelets.
- Evaluate all equipment for latex prior to use.
- A latex-free cart should accompany a latex-sensitive patient throughout the facility.
- Each facility should form a latex allergy task force with representatives from all departments.

---

3. Decreasing length of exposure time or wearing cotton liners in gloves may help, but may not solve the problem.
4. Use of latex-free gloves and products is usually necessary. Although more hospitals and medical offices are making latex-free products available, a job change may be necessary for some people.
5. A latex-free environment is necessary for treatment.
6. Topical corticosteroid creams may be used for local reactions.
7. Oral antihistamines may be used for mild to moderate reactions.
8. Epinephrine, oral or parenteral corticosteroids, and I.M. antihistamines are given for severe reactions.
9. IV fluids, oxygen, and intubation may be needed for cardiovascular and pulmonary support with severe reactions.

Complications

Unpredictable anaphylaxis and death.

Nursing Assessment

1. Assess patient for history of risk factors and pattern of suspected reactions.
2. Assess skin for erythema, swelling, vesicles, and other lesions.
3. Assess mucous membranes for conjunctivitis, rhinitis, and other lesions.
4. For suspected systemic reactions, assess vital signs for hypotension, tachycardia, arrhythmia, and respiratory distress.
5. Assess respiratory status for stridor caused by laryngeal edema and breath sounds for wheezing.
6. Assess for signs of internal edema with systemic reaction, such as nausea, vomiting, and diarrhea.

Nursing Diagnosis

- Deficient Knowledge related to sources of latex and how to avoid latex.

Nursing Interventions and Patient Education

Increasing Knowledge about Latex Avoidance

1. Educate patients about the widespread use of latex; latex-free alternatives are usually available (see Table 28-1).
2. Ensure that patients with history of type I reaction have self-injectable epinephrine and antihistamines on hand at all times to use at first sign of a reaction.
3. Encourage patients who have had immediate hypersensitivity reactions to wear a MedicAlert-type bracelet.
4. Encourage patients to notify all their health care providers, labs, and clinics before they make a visit, to facilitate the use of latex-free products. These patients should be given the first appointment of the day and all supplies that contain latex should be removed from the room or covered with a cotton cloth. Only latex-free products should be used, and staff members should be careful to avoid wearing or removing latex gloves in the hall while the patient is in the office.

Table 28-1 | Sources of Latex in Health Care Facilities and at Home

HEALTH CARE FACILITY	HOME AND COMMUNITY
Syringes	Mattresses and foam in furniture
Medication vial stoppers	Undergarments and clothing
Intravenous catheters, tubing	Bathmats and rugs
Stopcocks	Pacifiers and diapers
Tourniquet	Toys such as balls and dolls
Tape, dressings, drains	Pet toys
Elastic wraps	Bicycle helmets
Waterproof pads	Cosmetics
Blood pressure cuff	Food storage bags
Stethoscope	Drain stoppers
Reflex hammer	Spatulas
Electrocardiograph electrodes	Earphones
Oximetry sensor	Garden hose
Manual resuscitation bag	Rubber-handled tools
Oxygen canula, mask, tubing	Weather stripping
Airways, endotracheal tube	Plants—rubber, poinsettia, ficus
Urinary catheters	Scratch-off tickets and advertisements
Suction catheters	Raincoats and waterproof boots
Casting materials	Glue, envelopes, stamps

5. Support the patient who has had a severe reaction in the workplace. Remind the patient that the Americans with Disabilities Act guarantees workers reasonable modifications to the workplace to accommodate a disability. However, the area of latex sensitivity as a disability is controversial.

6. For further information, contact the American Latex Allergy Association (*www.latexallergyresources.org*) and the National Institute for Occupational Safety and Health (*www.cdc.gov/NIOSH/homepage.html*).

Evaluation: Expected Outcomes

• Verbalizes signs of reaction and appropriate treatment.

Bronchial Asthma

 Evidence Base National Heart, Lung and Blood Institute. (2007). National Asthma Education and Prevention Program Expert Panel Report 3. Guidelines for the diagnosis and management of asthma (Summary Report 2007, NIH Publication No. 08-5846). Bethesda, MD: National Institutes of Health. Available: *www.nhlbi.nih.gov/guidelines/asthma/asthsumm.pdf*.

Global Initiative for Asthma. (2011). Global strategy for asthma management and prevention. Available: *www.ginasthma.org/uploads/users/files/GINA_Report_2011.pdf*.

Asthma is a chronic inflammatory disease of the airways, characterized by airflow obstruction, which is at least partially reversible; bronchial hyperreactivity; and mucus production. The course of asthma is highly variable. In 2007, the National Asthma Education and Prevention Program Expert Panel Report 3 and in 2010, the Global Initiative for Asthma guidelines were updated. These updates are evidence-based and continue to recommend treatment that is stepwise and based on severity; however, the updates emphasize assessment of control, impairment of daily function, and risk for exacerbation at subsequent patient visits. Although severity is best established prior to the use of asthma medications, it may be determined based on the medications necessary to gain control and directs initial therapy.

Asthma therapy is characterized by periodic follow-up visits and continual reassessment. One such factor that is always assessed includes control, which can be measured at home by the patient and family and evaluated and discussed at subsequent visits. The level of control guides adjustment of medications. Nurses can use control assessment to identify patients and families who need more asthma education to gain better control of asthma.

Pharmacotherapy for asthma is now based on three age groups: ages 0 to 4 years, ages 5 to 11 (see Chapter 44), and ages 12 and older. It is comprised of six steps and has expanded to include more medications for asthma; however, inhaled corticosteroids continue as the preferred long-term control therapy for all ages.

Pathophysiology and Etiology

The basic defect appears to be an abnormality in the host, which intermittently leads to an increased constriction of smooth muscle, hypersecretion of mucus in the bronchial tree, and mucosal edema.

Neuromechanisms (Autonomic Nervous System)

1. Stimulation of the vagus nerve (which is responsible for bronchomotor tone) by viral respiratory infections, air pollutants, and other stimuli causes bronchoconstriction, increased secretion of mucus, and dilation of the pulmonary vessels.

2. Beta-adrenergic receptor cells that line the airways are also responsible for bronchomotor tone. Abnormal functioning of these cells predisposes patients to bronchoconstriction.

Antigen–Antibody Reaction

1. Susceptible individuals form abnormally large amounts of IgE when exposed to certain allergens. Most children and more than half of adults with asthma are sensitized to at least one common inhaled allergen.

2. Antigen-specific IgE fixes itself to the mast cells of the bronchial mucosa.

3. When the person is exposed to certain allergens, the resulting antigen combines with the cell-bound IgE molecules, causing the mast cell and basophil to degranulate and release chemical mediators.

4. These chemical mediators act on bronchial smooth muscle to cause bronchoconstriction, on dilated epithelium to reduce mucociliary clearance, on bronchial glands to cause mucus secretion, on blood vessels to cause vasodilation and increased permeability, and on leukocytes to cause cellular infiltration and inflammation.

5. Late-phase reactions (these occur 4 to 8 hours after the initial response) include the influx of eosinophils, neutrophils, lymphocytes, and monocytes.

Bronchial Inflammation

1. Occurs in both the immediate- and late-phase reactions caused by antigen–antibody response.

2. Factors other than allergens (such as noxious environmental stimuli) cause bronchial inflammation and hyperreactivity by mast cell activation.

Classification

Extrinsic Asthma

1. Hypersensitivity reaction to inhalant allergens (dust mites, animal allergens, cockroaches, pollen, and mold are the major ones).

2. Mediated by immunoglobulin E (IgE mediated).

Intrinsic Asthma

1. No inciting allergen.

2. Infection, typically viral.

3. Environmental stimuli (such as air pollution).

Mixed Asthma

Immediate type I reactivity appears to be combined with intrinsic factors.

Aspirin-Induced Asthma

1. Induced by ingestion of aspirin and related compounds.

2. "Samter's Triad" has been described as a combination of aspirin-induced asthma, nasal polyps, and sinusitis.

Exercise-Induced Bronchoconstriction

Symptoms vary from slight chest tightness and cough to severe wheezing and cough and shortness of breath that usually occurs after 5 to 20 minutes of sustained exercise.

Occupational Asthma

Caused by inhalation of industrial fumes, dust, allergens, and gases.

Classification by Severity

1. Asthma severity for purposes of treatment is classified as intermittent, mild persistent, moderate persistent, and severe persistent based on level of impairment and risk for exacerbation.
2. Level of impairment parameters include degree of symptoms, nighttime awakenings, need to use short-acting beta$_2$-agonist for symptom control, interference with normal activity, and lung function by spirometry.
3. Risk level is based on the number of exacerbations that required oral corticosteroids within the past year and how severe they were.
4. See details of classifying asthma severity at *www.nhlbi.nih.gov/guidelines/asthma/asthgdln.pdf.*

Clinical Manifestations

1. Episodes of coughing.
2. Wheezing.
3. Dyspnea.
4. Feeling of chest tightness.

 NURSING ALERT Do not be fooled by lack of wheezing on auscultation when the patient reports severe shortness of breath. Airflow may be so restricted that wheezing ceases.

Diagnostic Evaluation

1. Pulmonary function testing (spirometry)—more than 12% increase over baseline in forced expiratory volume in first second of exhalation (FEV$_1$) following inhalation of bronchodilator. Peak flow more than 20% variability between A.M. and P.M. measurements.
2. Bronchial challenge with airborne agent resulting in airway hyperreactivity; a positive challenge is determined by decrease in FEV$_1$ from baseline.
   a. Methacholine bronchial challenge (nebulized)—20% decrease in FEV$_1$.
   b. Mannitol (dry powder inhalation)—15% decrease in FEV$_1$.
3. Skin testing to identify causative allergens.
4. Chest x-ray to exclude other lung diseases in new onset asthma in adult.

Management

The goal is to allow the person with asthma to live a normal life. The treatment plan should be as simple as possible and individualized to the patient's lifestyle. See Figure 28-2, page 1036, for stepwise therapy for those ages 12 and older; see pages 1500 to 1501 for stepwise therapy for children younger than age 12. See Table 28-2, pages 1037 and 1038, and Table 28-3, page 1039, for medication information. For additional information on treatment and specific dosages, see "Expert Panel Report 3: Guidelines for the Diagnosis and Management of Asthma" (National Heart, Lung and Blood Institute, 2007), pages 346–352 (*www.nhlbi.nih.gov/guidelines/asthma/asthgdln.pdf*).

Long-Term Controllers

1. Inhaled corticosteroids (ICSs), such as beclomethasone, budesonide, ciclesonide, flunisolide, fluticasone, mometasone.
2. Long-acting inhaled beta-agonists (LABA) include salmeterol, formoterol. *Note:* Arformoterol is a LABA that is indicated for long-term control of chronic obstructive pulmonary disease, not asthma.
3. Combination inhalers, such as fluticasone and salmeterol, budesonide and formoterol, mometasone and formoterol.
4. Leukotriene modifiers, such as montelukast and zafirlukast.
5. Inhaled mast cell stabilizer: cromolyn sodium.
6. Long-acting oral beta-agonists, such as albuterol extended-release tablets.
7. Oral corticosteroids (maintenance dose).
8. Methylxanthines such as theophylline.
9. Muscarinic agents, namely tiropium, as adjunct therapy.
10. An IgE blocker (omalizumab) can be added to standard maintenance therapy to reduce exacerbations in moderate to severe allergic asthma.
    a. It is given by subcutaneous injection every 2 to 4 weeks.
    b. The most common adverse reactions are injection site reactions and viral infection.

 NURSING ALERT The most convenient and inexpensive method of aerosol delivery to patients is the metered-dose or dry powder inhaler; however, nebulization offers alternative delivery for those with unreliable inhaler technique.

 DRUG ALERT Beta-adrenergic blockers, such as propranolol, have the potential to cause bronchoconstriction and should not be given to patients with asthma.

Quick-Relief Medications

1. Short-acting bronchodilators by inhalation.
   a. Short-acting beta-agonists (SABAs), such as albuterol, pirbuterol, and levalbuterol.
   b. Anticholinergic agent, such as ipratropium bromide.
2. Systemic corticosteroids (short course)—prednisone, prednisolone, methylprednisolone.

DRUG ALERT Patients should be encouraged to use SABAs appropriately when needed and not to wait for severe symptoms.

Other Measures

1. Environmental control (see page 1029).
2. Immunotherapy (see page 1021).
3. Avoidance of foods that contain tartrazine (yellow dye number 5) in aspirin-sensitive patients.
4. Regular aerobic exercise should be encouraged.
5. Use of an inhaled beta-adrenergic agonist or cromolyn taken 5 to 10 minutes before exercise will decrease exercise-induced bronchoconstriction.
6. Antibiotics are prescribed only during acute exacerbations if signs and symptoms of bacterial infection are present.

Intermittent Asthma	Persistent Asthma: Daily Medication Consult with asthma specialist if step 4 care or higher is required. Consider consultation at step 3.

Step 1

Preferred:

SABA PRN

Step 2

Preferred:

Low-dose ICS

Alternative:

Cromolyn, LTRA, Nedocromil, or Theophylline

Step 3

Preferred:

Low-dose ICS + LABA
OR
Medium-dose ICS

Alternative:

Low-dose ICS + either LTRA, Theophylline, or Zileuton

Step 4

Preferred:

Medium-dose ICS + LABA

Alternative:

Medium-dose ICS + either LTRA, Theophylline, or Zileuton

Step 5

Preferred:

High-dose ICS + LABA

AND

Consider Omalizumab for patients who have allergies

Step 6

Preferred:

High-dose ICS + LABA + oral corticosteroid

AND

Consider Omalizumab for patients who have allergies

Step up if needed

(first, check adherence, environmental control, and comorbid conditions)

Assess control

Step down if possible

(and asthma is well controlled at least 3 months)

Each step: Patient education, environmental control, and management of comorbidities.

Steps 2–4:   Consider subcutaneous allergen immunotherapy for patients who have allergic asthma.

Quick-Relief Medication for All Patients

- SABA as needed for symptoms. Intensity of treatment depends on severity of symptoms: up to 3 treatments at 20-minute intervals as needed. Short course of oral systemic corticosteroids may be needed.
- Use of SABA >2 days a week for symptom relief (not prevention of EIB) generally indicates in adequate control and the need to step up treatment.

Key: **Alphabetical order is used when more than one treatment option is listed within either preferred or alternative therapy.** EIB, exercise-induced bronchospasm; ICS, inhaled corticosteroid; LABA, long-acting inhaled beta-agonist; LTRA, leukotriene receptor antagonist; SABA, inhaled short-acting beta$_2$-agonist

Figure 28-2. Stepwise approach for managing asthma in youths age 12 and older and adults.

7. Alternative and complementary therapies that include acupuncture, herbal preparations, yoga, and chiropractic treatment have been suggested for acute and chronic asthma control; however, none is a substitute for usual medical treatment. In fact, glucosamine and chondroitin have been suspected of causing asthma exacerbation in some patients.

Nursing Assessment

1. Review patient's record: ask about coughing, dyspnea, chest tightness, wheezing, exertional changes, nighttime awakenings with asthma, use of SABA, recent unscheduled or ER visits. Use an assessment tool such as the Asthma Control Test, Asthma Control Questionnaire, and Asthma Therapy Assessment Questionnaire. These tools quantify symptoms, quick-relief medication usage, effect of asthma on quality of life, and patient/family perception of control. They can be found at *www.nhlbi.nih.gov/guidelines/asthma/asthgdln.pdf.*

2. Observe the patient and assess the rate, depth, and character of respirations, especially on expiration; observe for hyperinflation. Assess peak flow.

3. Auscultate the chest for breath sounds or wheezing.

4. Assess for triggers of asthma that include the following:
   a. Allergens.
   b. Respiratory infections.
   c. Inhalation of irritating substances (dust, fumes, gases).
   d. Environmental factors (weather, air pollution, and humidity).
   e. Exercise, particularly in cold weather.
   f. Aspirin and its derivatives.
   g. Sulfite-containing agents used as food preservatives.
   h. Emotional factors.

5. After acute episode subsides, attempt to determine patient's degree of adherence with medications and management regimen.

6. Observe and correct inhalation technique and discuss care of inhaler (eg, cleaning, priming).

Nursing Diagnoses

- Ineffective Breathing Pattern related to bronchospasm.
- Anxiety related to fear of suffocating, difficulty in breathing, death.
- Risk for injury related to drug treatment and potential adverse effects.

Table 28-2	Long-Term Control Medications	
DRUG/INDICATION	**MECHANISM**	**POTENTIAL ADVERSE EFFECTS**
Inhaled Corticosteroids		
Beclomethasone, budesonide, flunisolide, ciclesonide, fluticasone, mometasone Indications: Long-term suppression of symptoms of asthma; suppression, control, and reversal of airway inflammation; reduced need for oral corticosteroids.	*Anti-inflammatory:* Block late reaction to allergen and reduce airway hyperresponsiveness; inhibit cytokine production, adhesion protein activation, and inflammatory cell migration and activation. Reverse $beta_2$-receptor downregulation. Inhibit microvascular leakage.	Cough, dysphonia, oral candidiasis. In high doses, systemic effects may occur (adrenal suppression, osteoporosis, skin thinning, easy bruising), although studies are not conclusive, and clinical significance has not been established. In low to medium doses, suppression of growth velocity has been observed in children, but this effect may be transient and the clinical significance has not been established.
Systemic Corticosteroids		
Methylprednisolone Prednisolone Prednisone Indications: Short-term burst therapy to gain control of inadequately controlled asthma; long-term prevention of symptoms in severe persistent asthma.	*Anti-inflammatory:* Block late reaction to allergen and reduce airway hyperresponsiveness; inhibit cytokine production, adhesion protein activation, and inflammatory cell migration and activation. Reverse $beta_2$-receptor downregulation. Inhibit microvascular leakage.	Short-term use: reversible abnormalities in glucose metabolism, increased appetite, fluid retention, weight gain, mood alteration, hypertension, peptic ulcer, and, rarely, aseptic necrosis. Long-term use: adrenal axis suppression, growth suppression, dermal thinning, hypertension, diabetes, Cushing's syndrome, cataracts, muscle weakness, and, rarely, impaired immune function. Consideration should be given to coexisting conditions that could be worsened by systemic corticosteroids, such as herpes virus infections, varicella, tuberculosis, hypertension, peptic ulcer, diabetes mellitus, osteoporosis, and *Strongyloides*.
Mast Cell Stabilizers		
Cromolyn sodium (nebulizer solution only) Indications: Long-term prevention of symptoms in mild persistent asthma; may modify inflammation; preventive treatment prior to exposure to exercise or known allergen.	*Anti-inflammatory:* Block early and late reaction to allergen; interfere with chloride channel function. Stabilize mast cell membranes and inhibit activation and release of mediators from eosinophils and epithelial cells. Inhibit acute response to exercise, cold dry air, and SO_2.	Cough and irritation.
Immunomodulators		
Omalizumab Indications: Long-term control and prevention of symptoms in patients (≥age 12) who have moderate or severe persistent allergic asthma inadequately controlled with ICS.	Binds to circulating IgE, preventing it from binding to high-affinity receptors on basophils and mast cells. Decreases mast cell mediator release from allergen exposure and the number of high-affinity receptors in basophils and submucosal cells.	Pain and bruising at injection sites has been reported in 45% of patients. Anaphylaxis has been reported in 0.2% of treated patients. Malignant neoplasms have been reported in 0.5% of patients compared to 0.2% of patients receiving placebo; however, relationship to drug is unlikely.
Leukotriene Modifiers		
Montelukast, zafirlukast, zileuton Indications: Long-term control and prevention of symptoms in mild persistent asthma; may be used in combination with ICS in moderate persistent asthma. Montelukast is indicated in patients >age 1; zafirlukast, >age 7; zileuton, >age 12.	*Leukotriene receptor antagonist* (montelukast and zafirlukast): Selective competitive inhibitors of CysLT1 receptor. *5-lipoxygenase inhibitor* (zileuton): Inhibits the production of leukotrienes—LTB_4 and cysteinyl leukotrienes—from arachidonic acid.	No specific adverse effects have been identified with montelukast (rare cases of Churg-Strauss have occurred, but the association is unclear). Postmarketing surveillance of zafirlukast has reported cases of reversible hepatitis and, rarely, irreversible hepatic failure resulting in liver transplantation and death. Elevation of liver enzymes has been reported with zileuton. There have been limited case reports of reversible hepatitis and hyperbilirubinemia.

(continued)

Table 28-2   Long-Term Control Medications (*continued*)

DRUG/INDICATION	MECHANISM	POTENTIAL ADVERSE EFFECTS
Long-Acting Beta₂-Agonists		
Formoterol, salmeterol, oral sustained-release albuterol *Indications:* Long-term prevention of symptoms, added to ICS; prevention of exercise-induced bronchospasm. *Note:* Not to be used to treat acute exacerbations; only used in combination with inhaled corticosteroid.	*Bronchodilation:* Smooth muscle relaxation following adenylate cyclase activation and increase in cyclic AMP, producing functional antagonism of bronchoconstriction. Compared to SABA, salmeterol (but not formoterol) has slower onset of action (15 to 30 minutes). Both salmeterol and formoterol have longer duration (>12 hours) compared to SABA.	Tachycardia, skeletal muscle tremor, hypokalemia, prolongation of QTc interval in overdose. A diminished bronchoprotective effect may occur within 1 week of chronic therapy (clinical significance has not been established). Potential risk of severe, life-threatening, or fatal exacerbation.
Methylxanthines		
Theophylline sustained-release *Indications:* Long-term control and prevention of symptoms in mild persistent asthma or as an adjunct to ICS in moderate or persistent asthma.	*Bronchodilation:* Smooth muscle relaxation from phosphodiesterase inhibition and possibly adenosine antagonism. May affect eosinophilic infiltration into bronchial mucosa as well as decreases T-lymphocyte numbers in epithelium. Increases diaphragm contractility and mucociliary clearance.	Dose-related acute toxicities include tachycardia, nausea and vomiting, tachyarrhythmias (supraventricular tachycardia), central nervous system stimulation, headache, seizures, hematemesis, hyperglycemia, and hypokalemia. Adverse effects at usual therapeutic doses include insomnia, gastric upset, aggravation of ulcer or reflux, increase in hyperactivity in some children, difficult urination in older males who have prostatism.

ICS, inhaled corticosteroid; SABA, short-acting beta-agonist.
Modified from Heart, Lung and Blood Institute, National Asthma Education and Prevention Program (2007). *Expert Panel Report 3: Guidelines for the diagnosis and management of asthma. Full report 2007* (pp. 245–246). Available: www.nhlbi.nih.gov/guidelines/asthma/asthgdln.pdf.

Nursing Interventions

Attaining Relief of Dyspneic Breathing

1. Monitor vital signs, skin color, retraction, oxygen saturation, and degree of restlessness, which may indicate hypoxia.
2. Provide medication and oxygen therapy, as prescribed.
3. Monitor airway functioning through peak flow meter or spirometry (FEV_1, FEV_1/FVC) to assess effectiveness of treatment.
4. Encourage intake of fluids to liquefy secretions.
5. Instruct patient on positioning to facilitate breathing—sitting upright (leaning forward on a table).
6. Encourage patient to use adaptive breathing techniques (eg, pursued-lip breathing) to decrease the work of breathing.

Relieving Anxiety

1. Explain rationale for interventions to gain patient's cooperation. Provide care in prompt, confident manner.
2. Help patient clarify sources of anxiety; suggest measures to reduce anxiety and to control breathing.
3. Encourage active participation and support efforts to adhere to management plan.

Preventing Adverse Effects of Drugs

1. Teach patient to rinse mouth and spit out after using ICS to prevent growth of fungi and be alert for sore throat or mouth caused by oropharyngeal candidiasis.
2. Suggest a spacer if patient is prone to candidiasis and ensure proper dosing and inhalation technique. Blood glucose testing may also be indicated to rule out hyperglycemia.
3. Monitor liver function enzymes, as directed, for patients taking zileuton and zafirlukast, and advise patient to report signs of liver dysfunction: abdominal pain, nausea, itching, jaundice.
4. Make sure patient is aware that LABAs are not used for acute symptoms or as anti-inflammatory therapy or monotherapy for asthma. Duration of protection against exercised-induced bronchospasm may decrease with regular use.
5. Monitor serum theophylline concentration periodically and maintain steady-state serum concentrations between 5 and 15 mcg/mL. Routine serum concentration monitoring is essential due to significant toxicities, narrow therapeutic range, and individual differences in metabolism. Absorption variation can produce significant changes in steady-state serum theophylline concentrations.
6. Warn patients that regular use (>2 days/week) of SABA for symptom control (not prevention of exercise-induced bronchospasm), increasing use, or lack of expected effect indicates inadequate asthma control. For patients frequently using SABA, anti-inflammatory medication should be initiated or intensified.

Community and Home Care Considerations

1. Initiate peak flow monitoring, if indicated. This may be done twice daily by the patient with persistent asthma. Provide written and verbal instruction and have the patient demonstrate the procedure.
2. The patient can buy a peak flow meter from a pharmacy or from a medical supply company.

Table 28-3   Quick Relief Medications

DRUG/INDICATION	MECHANISM	POTENTIAL ADVERSE EFFECTS
Short-Acting Beta$_2$-Agonists		
Albuterol, levalbuterol, pirbuterol *Indications:* Relief of acute symptoms; preventive treatment for exercise-induced bronchospasm prior to exercise.	*Bronchodilation:* Bind to the beta$_2$-adrenergic receptor, producing smooth muscle relaxation following adenylate cyclase activation and increase in cyclic AMP, producing functional antagonism of bronchoconstriction.	Tachycardia, skeletal muscle tremor, hypokalemia, increased lactic acid, headache, hyperglycemia. Inhaled route, in general, causes few systemic adverse effects. Patients with preexisting cardiovascular disease, especially older adults, may have adverse cardiovascular reactions with inhaled therapy.
Anticholinergic		
Ipratropium *Indications:* Acute bronchospasm; reverses only cholinergically mediated bronchospasm; does not modify reaction to antigen; does not block exercise-induced bronchospasm. Multiple doses of ipratropium in the emergency department provide additive effects to SABA. May be alternative for patients who do not tolerate SABA. Treatment of choice for bronchospasm due to beta-blocker medication.	*Bronchodilation:* Competitive inhibition of muscarinic cholinergic receptors. Reduces intrinsic vagal tone of the airways. May block reflex bronchoconstriction secondary to irritants or to reflux esophagitis. May decrease mucous gland secretion.	Drying of mouth and respiratory secretions, increased wheezing in some individuals, blurred vision if sprayed in eyes. If used in the emergency department, produces less cardiac stimulation than SABAs.
Systemic Corticosteroids		
Methylprednisolone, prednisolone, prednisone *Indications:* For moderate or severe exacerbations to prevent progression of exacerbation, reverse inflammation, speed recovery, and reduce rate of relapse.	*Anti-inflammatory:* Block late reaction to allergen and reduce airway hyper-responsiveness; inhibit cytokine production, adhesion protein activation, and inflammatory cell migration and activation. Reverse beta$_2$-receptor downregulation. Inhibit microvascular leakage.	Short-term use: reversible abnormalities in glucose metabolism, increased appetite, fluid retention, weight gain, facial flushing, mood alteration, hypertension, peptic ulcer, and, rarely, aseptic necrosis. Consideration should be given to coexisting conditions that could be worsened by systemic corticosteroids, such as herpes virus infections, varicella, tuberculosis, hypertension, peptic ulcer, diabetes mellitus, osteoporosis, and *Strongyloides*.

SABA, short-acting beta agonist.
Modified from Heart, Lung and Blood Institute, National Asthma Education and Prevention Program (2007). *Expert Panel Report 3: Guidelines for the diagnosis and management of asthma. Full report 2007* (pp. 247–248). Available: www.nhlbi.nih.gov/guidelines/asthma/asthgdln.pdf.

3. Once optimal asthma control is obtained, daily peak flow measurements in the early morning and early afternoon should be used during a 2- to 3-week period to determine the patient's personal best. The personal best peak flow measurement will be used to monitor control and to guide self-therapy in an individualized action plan.

4. Teach the patient to obtain peak flow measurement (see Patient Education Guidelines 28-2, page 1040).

5. Provide written and verbal instruction on an action plan for self-management of asthma exacerbation as outlined by the health care provider. National Asthma Education and Prevention Program Guidelines suggest the following:

   a. For symptomatic worsening of asthma or asymptomatic decrease in peak flow measurement, use initial inhalation of a short-acting beta-adrenergic agonist by metered-dose inhaler (MDI), two to four puffs for up to three treatments at 20-minute intervals, or a single nebulization treatment.

   b. After initial treatment, recheck peak flow; if it is more than 80% of personal best and no wheezing or shortness of breath, continue beta-adrenergic agonist every 3 to 4 hours for 24 to 48 hours. The patient should contact the health care provider for further instructions.

   c. If peak flow is 40% to 80% of personal best, or if the patient has persistent wheezing and shortness of breath, an oral corticosteroid should be initiated and beta-adrenergic agonist should be continued. The patient should contact the health care provider the same day for further instructions.

   d. If peak flow is less than 40% of personal best or if the patient has significant wheezing and shortness of breath, an oral corticosteroid should be started, beta-adrenergic agonist should be repeated immediately, and the patient should proceed to the emergency department.

PATIENT EDUCATION GUIDELINES 28-2

Flow Measurement

To obtain a peak flow measurement:
- Place the indicator at the base of the numbered scale.
- Stand (preferably) or sit upright.
- Take a deep breath.
- Place the meter in mouth and close lips around mouthpiece, with tongue under the mouthpiece.
- Blow out as hard and as fast as possible. Coughing or spitting will result in a falsely elevated level.
- Note the measurement that the indicator is pointing to on the number scale.
- Repeat previous steps twice more and record the highest number.

Patient Education and Health Maintenance

1. Provide information on the nature of asthma and methods of treatment.
2. Provide information regarding medications, including the difference between long-term controllers and quick-relief medications and the proper use of inhalers and spacer devices; stress avoiding overuse of inhalers and nebulizers. Ensure that patient understands that long-acting bronchodilating inhalers, such as salmeterol, are not effective for asthma exacerbations.
3. Demonstrate the use of MDIs (see Patient Education Guidelines 28-3) and nebulization equipment.
   a. Inhalers vary widely with hydrofluoroalkane (HFA) propellant and breath-actuated devices currently on the market; familiarize yourself with the manufacturer's instructions in order to help the patient.
   b. Teach patients how to clean inhalers according to manufacturer's instructions.
   c. Advise patients to count number of inhalations if the inhaler does not have an automatic counter.

 DRUG ALERT Never submerge an inhalation canister in water to determine if any medication remains. Moisture in the tip will ruin the canister.

4. Help the patient to identify what triggers asthma, warning signs of an impending attack, and strategies for preventing and treating an attack.
5. Teach adaptive-breathing techniques and breathing exercises such as pursed-lip breathing.
6. Discuss environmental control.
   a. Avoid people with respiratory infections. Get an annual flu shot.
   b. Avoid substances and situations known to precipitate bronchospasm, such as allergens, irritants, strong odors, gases, fumes, and smoke.
   c. Wear a mask if cold weather precipitates bronchospasm.
   d. Stay inside when air pollution is high.
   e. See Patient Education Guidelines 28-1, page 1029.
7. Promote optimal health practices, including nutrition, rest, and exercise.
   a. Encourage regular exercise to improve cardiorespiratory and musculoskeletal conditioning.
   b. Drink liberal amounts of fluids to keep secretions thin.
   c. Try to avoid upsetting situations.
   d. Use relaxation techniques, biofeedback management.
   e. Use community resources for smoking-cessation classes, stress management, exercises for relaxation, asthma support groups, etc.
8. Make sure that patient knows with whom to follow up and the frequency of follow-up. Discuss with patient how to overcome any barriers to follow-up, such as transportation, limited office or clinic hours, childcare, and work requirements.
9. For additional information and support, refer to American Academy of Allergy, Asthma and Immunology (*www.aaaai.org*).

Evaluation: Expected Outcomes

- Symptoms (wheezing, coughing, dyspnea, chest tightness) reduced; peak flow improved.
- Verbalizes relief of anxiety.
- No adverse reactions to drug therapy reported.

Status Asthmaticus

Status asthmaticus is a severe form of asthma in which the airway obstruction is unresponsive to usual drug therapy.

Contributing Factors

1. Infection.
2. Inhalation of air pollutants and allergens to which sensitized.
3. Noncompliance in taking medications, including overuse of bronchodilators.
4. Ingestion of aspirin or related drugs in aspirin-sensitive patient.
5. Aspiration of gastric acid.

Clinical Manifestations

1. Tachypnea, labored respirations, with increased effort on exhalation.
2. Suprasternal retractions, use of accessory muscles of respiration.
3. Diminished breath sounds, decreased ability to speak in phrases or sentences.

PATIENT EDUCATION GUIDELINES 28-3

How to Use an Inhaler and Spacer

USING AN INHALER

1. Make sure that the medication canister is attached to the plastic inhaler and shake well or, if using a dry powder inhaler system (DPI), load the medication according to the manufacturer's instructions.

2. If recommended, attach a spacer to your metered-dose inhaler (MDI) (see Using a spacer, below).

3. If using the closed-mouth method (recommended for DPI and HFA systems):

   a. Exhale fully and place the mouthpiece of the inhaler in your mouth and close lips tightly around it.

   b. While starting to inhale, use your index finger to press down firmly on the top of the canister.

   c. Continue to inhale for 3–5 seconds to obtain a full breath, then hold your breath for 5–10 seconds.

   d. Remove the inhaler from your mouth before you exhale and breathe normally.

4. If more than one inhalation of a beta$_2$-agonist is prescribed, wait 30 seconds before taking another inhalation, then repeat steps 1–5.

5. Replace the mouthpiece cap after each use.

6. Clean the inhaler according to the manufacturer's instructions.

7. Discard the canister after you have used the labeled number of inhalations. You should not use it beyond this indicated number because the correct dose amount can no longer be guaranteed.

8. For dry powdered inhalers, use a forceful, rapid inhalation with closed-mouth technique. See the instructions provided by the manufacturer of the device you use.

USING A SPACER

Unless you use your inhaler correctly, much of the medicine can end up on your tongue, on the back of your throat, or in the air. If you experience this problem, your health care

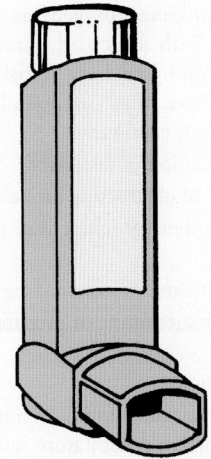

provider may recommend using a spacer. Also called a valved holding chamber, a spacer is a device that attaches to a MDI. It holds the medicine in its chamber long enough for you to inhale it in one or two slow, deep breaths, thereby enabling you to get your full dose of medicine. It also prevents you from coughing and may prevent a yeast infection in your mouth if you use a steroid inhaler. Several types of spacers are available; these devices may be purchased through your pharmacist.

1. Attach the inhaler to the spacer or holding chamber as shown in the product instructions.

2. Shake well.

3. Press the canister on the inhaler, which will put one puff of medicine into the holding chamber.

4. Place the mouthpiece of the spacer into your mouth and inhale slowly.

5. Hold your breath a few seconds, then exhale.

---

4. Anxiety, irritability, fatigue, headache, impaired mental functioning.

5. Muscle twitching, somnolence, diaphoresis—from continued carbon dioxide retention.

6. Tachycardia, elevated BP.

7. Heart failure and death from suffocation.

Management and Nursing Interventions

1. Monitor respiratory rate and oxygen saturation continuously; frequently monitor arterial blood gas levels, BP, electrocardiogram.

 NURSING ALERT In status asthmaticus, the return to normal or increasing partial pressure of carbon dioxide does not necessarily mean that the patient with asthma is improving—it may indicate a fatigue state that develops just before the patient slips into respiratory failure.

2. Administer repeated aerosol treatments with beta$_2$-agonist bronchodilators, such as albuterol or levalbuterol; add anticholinergic ipratropium, as prescribed—administer with caution until the metabolic and respiratory acidosis and hypoxemia have been corrected.

3. Monitor IV therapy.

   a. Corticosteroids are given to treat inflammation of airways; because these act slowly, their beneficial effects may not be apparent for several hours.

   b. Fluids are given to treat dehydration and loosen secretions.

4. Provide continuous humidified oxygen via nasal cannula, as prescribed. (Patients with associated chronic obstructive pulmonary disease or emphysema are at risk for depressed hypoxemic ventilatory drive, thus compounding respiratory insufficiency, so use oxygen cautiously.)

5. Initiate mechanical ventilation, if necessary.

6. Assist with mobilization of obstructing bronchial mucus.

   a. Perform chest physiotherapy (chest wall percussion and vibration).

   b. Administer expectorant and mucolytic drugs, as prescribed.

   c. Remove secretions by suctioning or prepare for bronchoscopy, if needed.

7. Provide adequate hydration.

8. Obtain portable chest x-ray and administer antibiotic, as prescribed, to treat any underlying respiratory infection.

9. Alleviate the patient's anxiety and fear by acting calmly and by reassuring the patient during an attack. Stay with the patient until the attack subsides.

SELECTED REFERENCES

Bernstein, D. I. (2012). Traffic-related pollutants and wheezing in children. *Journal of Asthma, 49*, 5–7.

Bernstein, I. L., Blessing-Moore, J., Cox, L. S., et al. (2008). Allergy diagnostic testing: An updated practice parameter. *Annals of Allergy and Asthma Immunology, 100*(3, Suppl.), S1–148.

Bozzetto, S., Carraro, S., Giordano, G., et al. (2012). Asthma, allergy and respiratory infections: The vitamin D hypothesis. *Allergy, 67*(1), 10–17.

Burks, A. W., Jones, S. M., Boyce, J. A., et al. (2011). NIAID-sponsored 2010 guidelines for managing food allergy: Applications in the pediatric population. *Pediatrics, 128*(5), 955–965.

Chipps, B. E. (2008). Adult asthma: Individualizing and optimizing care. *Medscape.* Available: *www.medscape.com/viewprogram/14649.*

Chowdhury, B. A., & Dal Pan, G. (2010). The FDA and safe use of long-acting beta-agonists in the treatment of asthma. *New England Journal of Medicine, 362*, 1169–1171.

Chu, H. W., Lloyd, C. M., Karmaus, W., et al. (2010). Developments in the field of allergy in 2009 through the eyes of *Clinical and Experimental Allergy. Clinical and Experimental Allergy, 40*(11), 1611–1631.

Cox, L. S., Nelson, H. A., Lockey, R., et al. (2010). Allergen immunotherapy: A practice parameter third update. *Journal of Allergy and Clinical Immunology, 127*(1, Suppl.), S1–S55.

de Groot, E. P., Nijkamp, A., Duiverman, E. J., et al. (2012). Allergic rhinitis is associated with poor asthma control in children with asthma. *Thorax, 67*, 582–587.

Galindo, M. J., Quirce, S., Garcia, O. L., et al. (2011). Latex allergy in primary care providers. *Journal of Investigational Allergology and Clinical Immunology, 21*(6), 459–465.

Garavello, W., Somigliana, E., Acaia, B., et al. (2010). Nasal lavage in pregnant women with seasonal allergic rhinitis: a randomized study. *International Archives of Allergy and Immunology, 151*, 137.

Global Strategy for Asthma Management and Prevention. (2010). The GINA Reports. Available: *www.ginasthma.org.*

Golden, D. B., Moffitt, J., Nicklas, R. A., et al. (2011). Stinging insect hypersensitivity: A practice parameter update 2011. *Journal of Allergy and Clinical Immunology, 127*, 852–854, e1–e23.

Hayden, M. L., Stoloff, S. W., Colice, G. L., et al. (2012). Exercise-induced bronchospasm: A case study in a nonasthmatic patient. *Journal of the American Academy of Nurse Practitioners, 24,* 19–23.

Hellings, P. W., Fokkens, W. J., Akdis, C., et al. (2013). Uncontrolled allergic rhinitis and chronic rhinosinusitis: where do we stand today? *Allergy, 68*(1), 1–7.

Herzog, R., & Cunningham-Rundles, S. (2011). Pediatric asthma: Natural history, assessment, and treatment. *Mount Sinai Journal of Medicine, 78*(5), 645–660.

Jones, S. M., & Burks, A. W. (2013). The changing CARE of patients with food allergy. *Journal of Allergy and Clinical Immunology, 131*(1), 3–11.

Kelley, K. J. (2012). Latex allergy 101: Allergy Fact Sheet. Slinger, Wisconsin: American Latex Allergy Association. Available: *www.latexallergyresources.org/allergy-fact-sheet.*

Li, H., Sha, Q., Zuo, K., et al. (2009). Nasal saline irrigation facilitates control of allergic rhinitis by topical steroid in children. *Journal of Otorhinolaryngology Related Specialties, 71*(1), 50–55.

Lieberman, P., Nicklas, R. A., Oppenheimer, J., et al. (2010). The diagnosis and management of anaphylaxis practice parameter: 2010 Update. *Journal of Allergy and Clinical Immunology, 126,* 477–522.

National Heart, Lung and Blood Institute, National Asthma Education and Prevention Program. (2007). Guidelines for the diagnosis and management of asthma. Full report 2007 (NIH Publication No. 08-4051). Bethesda, MD: National Institutes of Health. Available: *www.nhlbi.nih.gov/guidelines/asthma/asthsumm.pdf.*

National Heart, Lung and Blood Institute. (2007). National Asthma Education and Prevention Program Expert Panel Report 3. Guidelines for the diagnosis and management of asthma (Summary Report 2007, NIH Publication No. 08-5846). Bethesda, MD: National Institutes of Health. Available: *www.nhlbi.nih.gov/guidelines/asthma/asthsumm.pdf.*

Nurmatov, U., Van Schayck, C. P., Hurwitz, B., et al. (2012). House dust avoidance measure for perennial allergic rhinitis: An update. *Allergy, 67,* 158–165.

Pali-Scholl, I., Benz, H., Jensen-Jarolim, E., et al. (2009). Update on allergies in pregnancy, lactation and early childhood. *Journal of Allergy and Clinical Immunology, 123,* 1012–1021.

Peters, S. P., Kunselman, S. J., Icitovic, N., et al. (2010). Tiotropium bromide step-up therapy for adults with uncontrolled asthma. *New England Journal of Medicine, 363,* 1715–1726.

Quinto, K. B., Zuraw, B. L., Poon, K. Y., et al. (2011). The association of obesity and asthma severity and control in children. *Journal of Allergy and Clinical Immunology, 128*(5), 964–969.

Simons, F. E., & Simons, K. J. (2011). Histamine and H(1)-antihistamines: Celebrating a century of progress. *Journal of Allergy and Clinical Immunology, 128*(6), 1139–1150.

Solensky, R., Khan, D. A., Berstein, I. L., et al. (2010). Drug allergy: An updated practice parameter. *Annals of Allergy and Asthma Immunology, 105*(4), 259–273.

Szefler, S. J. (2012). Advances in pediatric asthma in 2011: Moving forward. *Journal of Allergy and Clinical Immunology, 129*(1), 60–68.

Thomas, A., Lemanske, R. F., Jackson, D. J., et al. (2011). Approaches to stepping up and stepping down care in asthmatic patients. *Journal of Allergy and Clinical Immunology, 128,* 915–924.

van den Berge, M., ten Hacken, N. H., van der Wiel, E., et al. (2013). Treatment of the bronchial tree from beginning to end: targeting small airway inflammation in asthma. *Allergy, 68*(1), 16–26.

Wallace, D. V., Dykewicz, M. S., Bernstein, D. I., et al. (2008). The diagnosis and management of rhinitis: An updated practice parameter. *Journal of Allergy and Clinical Immunology, 122,* S1–S84.

Wang, J., Godbold, J. H., Sampson, H. A., et al. (2008). Correlation of serum allergy (IgE) tests performed by different assay systems. *Journal of Allergy and Clinical Immunology, 121,* 1219–1224.

Weiler, J. M., Anderson, S. D., Randolph, C., et al. (2010). Pathogenesis, prevalence, diagnosis, and management of exercise-induced bronchoconstriction: A practice parameter. *Annals of Allergy and Asthma Immunology, 105*(6, Suppl.), S1–47.

Zeiger, R. S., Mellon, M., Chipps, B., et al. (2011). Test for respiratory and asthma control in kids (TRACK): Clinically meaningful changes in score. *Journal of Allergy and Clinical Immunology, 128,* 983–988.

29
HIV Infection and AIDS

OVERVIEW AND ASSESSMENT

Human immunodeficiency virus (HIV) is a viral infection that is transmitted from person to person. Over time, HIV overburdens the immune system's ability to coordinate an effective response against infection. This erosion of immune function takes years to occur; the eventual state of disintegrated defense against opportunistic infections is called *acquired immune deficiency syndrome (AIDS)*. Without antiretroviral treatment, HIV infection is almost universally fatal.

Since the immune deficiency syndrome associated with HIV was first described in 1981, great strides have been made in care and treatment of persons living with HIV. Nevertheless, HIV has claimed more than 25 million lives in the past 30 years and approximately 34 million persons were living with HIV in 2011 globally. In the United States, the Centers for Disease Control (CDC) estimates that more than 1.1 million persons are living with HIV.

 Evidence Base World Health Organization. (2012). WHO HIV/AIDS Fact Sheet (No. 360). Geneva: WHO. Available: *http://www.who.int/mediacentre/factsheets/fs360/en/index.html.*

Centers for Disease Control and Prevention. (2012). HIV in the United States: At a Glance. Atlanta: CDC. Available: *http://www.cdc.gov/hiv/resources/factsheets/PDF/HIV_at_a_glance.pdf.*

Transmission and Development
Etiology and Pathophysiology

1. At the beginning of this epidemic, AIDS affected men who had sex with men (MSM), persons who shared needles when using intravenous drugs, persons who received large-volume transfusions of blood or blood products, heterosexual partners of infected persons, and children of infected mothers. Today,

the majority of new HIV infections are found among MSM, and disproportionately among racial minorities and transgender persons. Others at risk include injection drug users (IDU), African Americans, those having heterosexual sex, and women. Mother-to-child transmission of HIV in the United States is reduced to <2%, owing to aggressive HIV testing, antiretroviral treatment of pregnant women, and other interventions in the intrapartum and postpartum period. Transmission from donor blood is very rare.

 NURSING ALERT Despite contemporary prevention efforts, there are approximately 50,000 new infections annually in the United States. In an effort to pierce this persistent rate of new infections, the CDC has implemented "high-impact prevention" that focuses prevention efforts on populations that are disproportionately affected by high rates of HIV transmission. Also, the CDC recommends HIV testing for all persons age 13 to 64 who access health care. The aim is to destigmatize HIV testing and provide each person with a snapshot of his or her HIV status. Earlier detection translates to earlier entry into care and treatment and provides an opportunity for each person to either avoid future infection or prevent transmission to others.

2. HIV enters the body through unprotected sexual contact or blood-to-blood transmission, then targets immune cells that carry CD4+ receptors, namely T cells and macrophages. Once inside the host cell, HIV uses the cell's components as a factory to reproduce. Eventually, reproduction of HIV within the host cell ruptures the cell membrane, releasing into the plasma more HIV virions that bind to and disable other CD4+ cells.

3. HIV infection may be viewed as a chronic condition if patients strictly adhere to treatment and care. However, some patients have difficulty managing highly structured medication and appointment regimens and need encouragement or

special interventions to support their treatment plan. Nursing care is important to tailoring a plan with the patient that optimizes her or his chances for successful and enduring treatment.

Natural History of HIV Infection

 Evidence Base U.S. Department of Health and Human Services, Health Resources and Services Administration, HIV/AIDS Bureau. (2011). Guide for HIV/AIDS clinical care. Available: *http://hab.hrsa.gov/deliverhivaidscare/clinicalguide11/*.

1. Approximately 50% to 90% of patients who become infected experience some symptom of primary HIV infection around 2 to 4 weeks after exposure to HIV. Typical symptoms include fever, adenopathy, pharyngitis, and rash. Many new HIV infections evade diagnosis because symptoms of acute HIV infection mimic other common infections. Recently, more persons who present to urgent care with these symptoms receive HIV testing and diagnosis. During this phase, the immune system is compromised by a sudden decrease in T4 helper cells and an increase in HIV viral load for a brief period before settling into a new baseline.
2. Seroconversion occurs when the person has formed enough antibodies to HIV that the serologic test is positive. This usually occurs 4 to 6 weeks after acute HIV infection.
3. The CDC provides a mechanism for staging HIV infection and defining the continuum to AIDS using clinical findings

and the CD4⁺ count (see Table 29-1). A normal CD4⁺ count is 800 to 1,000/mm³. Because HIV replication destroys CD4⁺ cells, the number of these cells diminishes slowly over time.

 NURSING ALERT The period around acute seroconversion is a time when the patient is highly infectious to others. Counsel patients to use effective prevention measures during sex and refrain from other high-risk behaviors that could transmit HIV, such as needle-sharing. Encourage and refer newly diagnosed persons into care and treatment.

4. Waning immunity in persons with untreated and treated HIV infection allows development of frequent infections, severe opportunistic infections, and malignancies. These usually appear years after exposure to HIV (see Figure 29-1).

 DRUG ALERT If a patient decides to stop taking antiretroviral (ARV) therapy, then all ARV medications must be stopped at the same time. Taking only some of the ARVs creates resistance to HIV, which could lead to loss of effective treatment options for this patient in the future. Resistance can develop within a few days to a few weeks of inadequate dosing. Special rules exist for stopping an efavirenz-containing regimen, owing to the long half-life of efavirenz. Consult the literature before a planned discontinuation of an efavirenz-containing regimen and counsel patients to contact their provider for advice before stopping an efavirenz-based regimen on their own.

Table 29-1   AIDS Surveillance Case Definition for Adolescents and Adults

CD4⁺ CELL CATEGORIES	CLINICAL CATEGORIES		
	A Asymptomatic, or PGL or Acute HIV Infection	**B** Symptomatic† (not A or C)	**C** AIDS Indicator Condition (1987)
1 ≥ 500/mm³ (≥29%)	A1	B1	C1
2 200–499 mm³ (14%–8%)	A2	B2	C2
3 200/mm³ (<14%)	A3	B3	C3

*All patients in categories A3, B3, and C1–3 are reported as acquired immunodeficiency syndrome (AIDS), based on the AIDS-indicator conditions and a CD4 cell count <200/mm³. AIDS indicator conditions include three new entries: recurrent bacterial pneumonia, invasive cervical cancer, and pulmonary tuberculosis.

†Symptomatic conditions not included in Category C that are (a) attributed to human immunodeficiency virus (HIV) infection or indicative of a defect in cell-mediated immunity or (b) considered to have a clinical course or management that is complicated by HIV infection. Examples of B conditions include, but are not limited to, bacillary angiomatosis; thrush; vulvovaginal candidiasis that is persistent, frequent, or poorly responsive to therapy; cervical dysplasia (moderate or severe); cervical carcinoma in situ; constitutional symptoms, such as fever (101.3° F [38.5° C]) or diarrhea for 1 month; oral hairy leukoplakia; herpes zoster involving two episodes or more than one dermatome; idiopathic thrombocytopenic purpura; listeriosis; pelvic inflammatory Infection (especially if complicated by a tubo-ovarian abscess); and peripheral neuropathy.

PGL, persistent generalized lymphadenopathy.

Centers for Infection Control and Prevention. (1993). AIDS surveillance case definition for adolescents and adults. *Morbidity and Mortality Weekly Report, 41(RR-17),* 2.

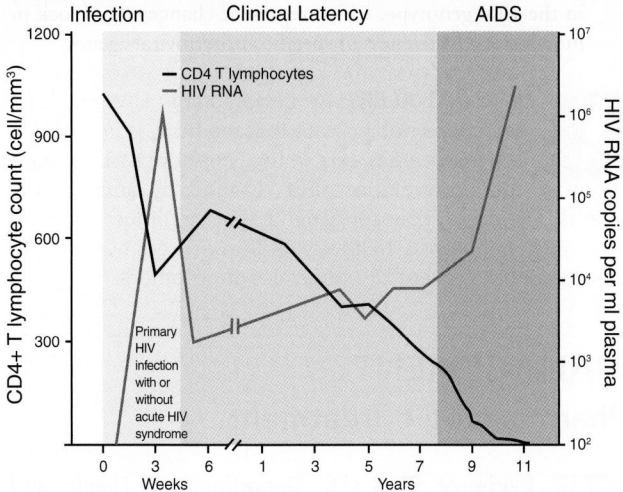

Figure 29-1. Natural history of untreated HIV Infection.

Clinical Manifestations of HIV/AIDS with Advancing Infection

1. Pulmonary manifestations.
   a. Persistent or acute cough, with or without sputum production, shortness of breath, chest pain, fever.
   b. From *Pneumocystis jiroveci* pneumonia (PCP), bacterial pneumonia (community-acquired pneumonia), *Mycobacterium* tuberculosis, disseminated *Mycobacterium avium* complex, Aspergillus, Pseudomonas, cytomegalovirus (CMV), *Histoplasma*, Kaposi's sarcoma, lung cancer, lymphoma, *Cryptococcus*, *Legionella*, or other pathogens and malignancies.
2. GI manifestations.
   a. Diarrhea, weight loss, anorexia, abdominal cramping, feeling of fullness, rectal urgency (tenesmus).
   b. From enteric pathogens or malignancies including *Salmonella*, *Shigella*, *Campylobacter*, *Entamoeba histolytica*, *C. difficile*, CMV, *M. avium* complex, herpes simplex, *Strongyloides*, *Giardia*, *Cryptosporidium*, *Isospora belli*, *Chlamydia*, lymphoma, Kaposi's sarcoma, and others.
   c. Feeling of difficulty swallowing or food feeling stuck sub-sternally upon swallowing, usually caused by *Candida* esophagitis. Also consider an esophageal ulcer caused by herpes simplex, CMV, or aphthous stomatitis.
3. Oral manifestations.
   a. Appearance of oral lesions, white plaques on oral mucosa, particularly in the posterior pharynx, and angular cheilitis from *Candida albicans* of mouth.
   b. Vesicles with ulceration from herpes simplex virus.
   c. White, thickened lesions on lateral margins of tongue from oral hairy leukoplakia.
   d. Oral warts due to human papillomavirus.
   e. Periodontitis progressing to gingival necrosis.
   f. Painful, solitary lesions with raised margins—aphthous ulcers of unclear etiology.
   g. Appearance of flat or nodular purple lesions on the hard or soft palate, buccal mucosa, posterior pharynx from Kaposi's sarcoma.
4. CNS manifestations.
   a. Cognitive, motor, and behavioral symptoms may be caused by HIV encephalopathy, AIDS dementia, acute infection, toxicity from alcohol or drugs, adverse reaction to medication, psychiatric condition, and other causes.
   b. Acute symptoms of infection with fever, malaise, headache, and/or mental status change, seizure, hemiparesis, abnormal gait or speech may be caused by toxoplasmosis, cryptococcal meningitis, herpes virus infections, CMV encephalitis, progressive multifocal leukoencephalopathy, CNS lymphoma, neuro syphilis, or other pathogens and malignancies.
   c. May also have sensory symptoms (distal symmetrical polyneuropathy)—demonstrated by numbness, tingling, and neuropathic pain of the feet or hands.
5. Ocular manifestations.
   a. Seeing floaters in the visual field, flashes of light or sudden loss of a visual field in persons with <100 CD4/mm^3 due to CMV retinitis, a sight-threatening infection that requires urgent evaluation by an ophthalmologist.
   b. Blurry vision, dry eyes, double vision, or swelling of the eyelid or conjunctiva, caused by bacterial or viral conjunctival infection, adverse reaction to medication, syphilis, Kaposi's sarcoma, or other pathogens and malignancies.
6. Malignancies.
   a. Kaposi's sarcoma (AIDS-defining cancer) (ADC).
   b. Non-Hodgkin's lymphoma (ADC) and other lymphomas (non-ADC).
   c. Cervical cancer (ADC).
   d. Liver cancer (non-ADC).
   e. Lung cancer (non-ADC).
   f. Anal cancer (non-ADC).

 Evidence Base Shiels, M. S., Pfeiffer, R. M., Gail, M. H., et al. (2011). Cancer burden in the HIV-infected population in the United States. *J Natl Cancer Inst.* 103(9):753–762.
Sigel, K., Dubrow, R., Silverberg, M., et al. (2011). Cancer screening in patients infected with HIV. *Current HIV/AIDS Reports, 8*(3), 142–152.

7. Skin manifestations.
   a. Pruritic rash with raised, erythematous papules, located on surfaces that contain hair follicles known as HIV folliculitis.
   b. Abscesses caused by methcillin-sensitive and methcillin-resistant *S. aureus* infections or other common skin pathogens.

c. Pruritic nodular rash located on any skin surface known as prurigo nodularis.

d. Purple, flat, or nodular lesions located on any skin surface including soles of feet and palms of hands—likely to be Kaposi's sarcoma and should be biopsied.

Diagnostic Evaluation

 Evidence Base Bartlett, J. G., & Gallant, J. E. (2009). *Medical management of HIV infection*. Durham, NC: Knowledge Source Solutions.

HIV Testing

Description

1. Enzyme-linked immunosorbent assay (ELISA)—serologic test for detecting antibody to HIV. Western blot test is used to confirm a positive result on ELISA.

2. Rapid test (serology or oral sample)—15- to 40-minute result; used in settings where patient is less likely to return for result such as mobile van, emergency department, urgent care center, or STD clinic.

3. Antibodies to HIV generally take 2 to 12 weeks to develop. Therefore, a negative-HIV antibody test may catch a person within this 12-week time frame to HIV seroconversion, known as the window period.

Nursing and Patient Care Considerations

1. Occasionally, an ELISA screen may yield an indeterminate result by Western blot.
   a. The cause of an indeterminate result may be early HIV seroconversion, HIV vaccine, infection with O strain or HIV-2, or a false-positive in a low-risk individual.
   b. The test should be repeated at 1, 2, and 6 months until Western blot becomes positive or there is no longer suspicion of HIV infection. If a conclusive test is needed quickly, HIV RNA viral load testing can be done.

2. The CDC recommends opt-out testing for HIV for persons age 13–64, which requires general medical consent for testing and optional prevention counseling.

Other Laboratory Tests

1. Lymphocyte panel may show decreased CD4+ count. In early infection or in long-term nonprogressors, CD4+ count may be normal.

2. A complete blood count (CBC) may show anemia, low white blood cell count, and/or decreased platelets.

3. Presence of indicator infection through microbiology or serology testing (eg, PCP, candidiasis of esophagus, herpes zoster).

4. HIV viral load testing is a measure of the amount of HIV in the blood. High viral loads (>750,000) tend to be found in acute seroconversion and late infection, but also occur in patients who have a concurrent infectious process. A viral load test result can be undetectable, meaning the amount of virus is less than the limit of the test, which may be either <400 or <50 copies/mL.

5. Resistance testing is done to determine if the patient is infected with a drug-resistant virus. The test uses genotypic assays that amplify the HIV virus and look for mutations in the viral genotype, which represent changes that block or impair the effectiveness of specific antiretroviral agents.

 NURSING ALERT An undetectable HIV viral load result does not indicate that the body is free of HIV. Latent reservoirs exist in the lymphoid tissues indefinitely. These reservoirs are not reached by antiretroviral agents. Therefore, counsel patients that they must continue with strict adherence to their medication regimen and to measures that prevent HIV transmission to others.

MANAGEMENT

Pharmacologic Treatment

 Evidence Base U.S. Department of Health and Human Services, Panel on Antiretroviral Guidelines for Adults and Adolescents. (2011). Guidelines for the use of antiretroviral agents in HIV-1-infected adults and adolescents. Available at *www.aidsinfo.nih.gov*.

Centers for Disease Control and Prevention. (2009). Guidelines for prevention and treatment of opportunistic infections in HIV-infected adults and adolescents: Recommendations from CDC, the National Institutes of Health, and the HIV Medicine Association of the Infectious Diseases Society of America. *Morbidity and Mortality Weekly Report, 58*(No. RR-4), 4–28.

1. Antiretroviral treatment (ART) has a four-part purpose: (1) to decrease HIV viral burden, increase immune function, (2) to protect against morbidity, (3) to increase quality of life and chance for survival, and (4) to prevent HIV transmission. Successful treatment requires strict adherence to medication, which means taking at least 90% of doses. Before initiating antiretrovirals, patients should be assessed for readiness to start as treatment is lifelong. However, some trepidation is expected and is not a complete bar to initiating treatment. See Table 29-2.

2. Some opportunistic infections can be prevented by prophylactic medication. All persons with CD4 <200 cells/mm³ must receive prophylaxis against PCP. Those who have CD4 < 100 cells/mm³ and are *Toxoplasma gondii* serum IgG+ must receive prophylaxis against toxoplasmosis. And those who have CD4 < 50 cells/mm³ must receive prophylaxis against *Mycobacterium avium* complex, after initial culture for *M. avium intracellulare* is negative.

3. Treatment is available for most opportunistic infections and other infections associated with AIDS. After initial treatment of an opportunistic infection, the patient may need to remain on continued suppressive therapy to prevent recurrence. This is known as secondary prophylaxis. Prophylaxis may be discontinued after a period of sustained immune reconstitution beyond the threshold of vulnerability for the particular opportunistic infection. See Table 29-3.

4. Care and treatment of HIV infection requires the expertise of many specialties including infectious infection, renal, pulmonary, gastroenterology, neurology, obstetrics and gynecology, dentistry, dermatology, cardiology, surgery, psychiatry, nursing, nutrition, and social work.

Table 29-2 Antiretroviral Therapy*

DRUG	ADVERSE REACTIONS	DRUG	ADVERSE REACTIONS
Nucleoside and Nucleotide Reverse Transcriptase Inhibitors (NRTIs)		**NRTI/NNRTI Combinations**	
Abacavir	Screen for HLA B 5701 to avoid hypersensitivity reaction. Use cautiously in cardiac Infection.	Tenofovir /Emtricitabine/Efavirenz Rilpivirine/Tenofovir/Emtricitabine	See individual agents.
Didanosine	Peripheral neuropathy, pancreatitis. Rarely used.	**Protease Inhibitors**	
Emtricitabine	Adverse reactions are rare.	Atazanavir	Most protease inhibitors are pharmacologically boosted with Ritonavir to achieve steady states of higher blood levels. This can lead to drug-induced hepatitis, hyperlipidemia, insulin resistance, and some lipodystrophy. Initial adverse effects may be nausea and diarrhea for all. (Nelfinavir and Indinavir are rarely used.)
Lamivudine	Adverse reactions are rare.	Darunavir	
Stavudine	Peripheral neuropathy, lactic acidosis.	Fosamprenavir	
Tenofovir	May make chronic renal problems worse.	Indinavir	
Zidovudine	Nausea, fatigue (first month of drug), anemia, leucopenia.	Lopinavir/Ritonavir	
		Nelfinavir	
		Ritonavir	
NRTI Combinations		Saquinavir	
Abacavir/Lamivudine	See individual agents.	Tipranavir	
Tenofovir /Emtricitabine		**Fusion Inhibitor (Entry Inhibitor)**	
Zidovudine/Lamivudine		Enfuvirtide	Twice-daily injections with possible inflammation at injection sites.
Zidovudine/Lamivudine/Abacavir		**CCR5 Antagonist (Entry Inhibitor)**	
Non-Nucleoside Reverse Transcriptase Inhibitors (NNRTIs)		Maraviroc	Screen for CCR5 tropic virus, may have a variety of adverse effects.
Delavirdine	Rarely used.	**Integrase Inhibitor and Combination**	
Efavirenz	CNS symptoms in first 14 days, rash.	Raltegravir	Adverse reactions are rare.
Ethaverine	Rash.	Emtricitabine/Tenofovir/Elvitegravir/Cobicistat	Diarrhea and rash
Nevirapine	Hepatotoxicity; should not be used in women with CD4+ > 250 or men with CD4+ > 400, rash.		
Rilpivirine			

*Monitoring for all types of ART includes complete blood count (CBC), chemistry, and HIV ribonucleic acid (RNA) viral load during the first month; CD4+, HIV RNA viral load (ultrasensitive), CBC, and chemistry panel in the second month and then every 3 months thereafter once the patient is stable and has undetectable HIV RNA viral load.

Initiating Antiretroviral Therapy in Treatment-Naive Patients

1. Antiretroviral therapy (AVRT) medications belong to six drug classifications that interfere with HIV replication at six different points in the process. The standard for ART is to use a minimum of three different drugs from at least two different drug classifications.

2. Classes of antiretroviral drugs:
   a. Nucleoside/nucleotide reverse transcriptase inhibitors (NRTI)
   b. Nonnucleoside reverse transcriptase inhibitors (NNRTI).
   c. Protease inhibitors (PIs).
   d. Entry/fusion inhibitor.
   e. Entry inhibitor/CCR5 antagonist.
   f. Integrase inhibitor.

3. Goals of antiviral therapy:
   a. Prolong life and improve quality of life.
   b. Reduce viral load to as low as possible (undetectable) for as long as possible.
   c. Increase the CD4+ count to allow immune reconstitution.

Table 29-3   Opportunistic Infections and Drug Therapies

NAME	CLINICAL MANIFESTATIONS	DIAGNOSTIC TESTS	MEDICATIONS
Pneumocystis jiroveci pneumonia	• Cough: dry or scant white sputum production • Shortness of breath • Low-grade fever	• Chest x-ray • Induced sputum specimen • Bronchoscopy	• Co-trimoxazole (may be used with corticosteroids) • Clindamycin with primaquine and possibly corticosteroids • Atovaquone • Pentamidine (IV only)
Candida esophagitis	• White coating in mouth • White coating down throat • Sensation of food getting caught in throat while swallowing	• Gross observation • Microscopy for hyphae • Endoscopy	• Nystatin • Clotrimazole • Itraconazole • Fluconazole • Amphotericin B
Mycobacterium avium complex	• Weakness • Weight loss • Diarrhea • Fever, chills	• Blood culture for acid-fast bacilli • Biopsy, if mass	• Rifabutin • Ethambutol • Azithromycin • Clarithromycin
Kaposi's sarcoma	• Pink, purple, or brown spots • Pain, edema of affected area	• Gross observation • Biopsy	• Antiviral therapy • Chemotherapy
Toxoplasmosis	• Fever • Headache • Change in mental status • Confusion • Lethargy • Frank psychosis	• CT • MRI • Serum *Toxoplasma* antibodies	• Pyrimethamine • Sulfadiazine • Folinic acid
Tuberculosis	• Cough: dry or scant frothy white or pink sputum • Shortness of breath • Fever • Lymphadenopathy	• Positive purified protein derivative (≥5 mm induration) • Interferon-gamma release assays • Chest x-ray • Sputum culture for acid-fast bacilli	• Isoniazid • Rifampin • Pyrazinamide • Ethambutol • Pyridoxine
Cryptosporidium	• Severe diarrhea • Severe abdominal cramping	• Stool culture for *Cryptosporidium*	• ART • Nitazoxanide after aggressive ART
Cryptococcal meningitis	• Headache • Confusion, memory loss • Nausea • Seizures • Change in mental status • Fever • Photophobia	• CSF culture for cryptococcosis	• Amphotericin B • Flucytosine • Fluconazole
Cytomegalovirus	• Visual changes; floaters or blindness • Difficulty swallowing • Nausea, vomiting • Abdominal cramping	• Ophthalmologic examination • Blood, urine, tissue culture for CMV	• Valganciclovir • Ganciclovir • Foscarnet • Cidofovir • Intraocular ganciclovir release device
Herpes simplex virus 1 and 2	• Lesions: mouth, lips, genitalia, rectal area • Painful vesicular rash • Ulcers	• Viral culture • Clinical observation	• Acyclovir • Famciclovir • Valacyclovir
Herpes zoster	• Painful vesicular rash on one or more dermatomes	• Viral culture • Clinical observation	• Famciclovir • Valacyclovir • Acyclovir

ART, antiretroviral therapy; CMV, cytomegalovirus; CSF, cerebrospinal fluid; CT, computed tomography; IV, intravenous; MRI, magnetic resonance imaging.

d. Maintain options for future treatment by preventing the development of treatment-resistant virus.

e. Avoid drug toxicities (see Table 29-4).

Recommendations for Starting Antiretroviral Treatment

Evidence Base U.S. Department of Health and Human Services, Panel on Antiretroviral Guidelines for Adults and Adolescents. (2011). Guidelines for the use of antiretroviral agents in HIV-1-infected adults and adolescents. Available: www.aidsinfo.nih.gov.

1. ART should be initiated in all patients with a history of an AIDS-defining illness or with a CD4 count <350 cells/mm³ (A-I*).

2. ART is also recommended for patients with CD4 counts between 350 and 500 cells/mm³ (A/B*-II).

3. ART should be initiated, regardless of CD4 count, in patients with the following conditions:
   a. HIV-associated nephropathy (A-II*).
   b. Hepatitis B virus (HBV) coinfection when treatment of HBV is indicated (A-III*).

4. A combination ARV drug regimen is also recommended for pregnant women who do not meet criteria for treatment with the goal to prevent perinatal transmission (A-I*).

5. For patients with CD4 counts >500 cells/mm³, panel members are evenly divided: 50% favor starting ART at this stage of HIV infection (B*); 50% view initiating therapy at this stage as optional (C*) (B/C-III**).

6. Patients initiating ART should be willing and able to commit to lifelong treatment and should understand the benefits and risks of therapy and the importance of adherence (A-III*). Patients may choose to postpone therapy and providers, on a case-by-case basis, may elect to defer therapy based on clinical and/or psychosocial factors.

   Note: *Rating of Recommendations: A = Strong; B = Moderate; C = Optional.

   Rating of Evidence: I = data from randomized controlled trials; II = data from well-designed nonrandomized trials or observational cohort studies with long-term clinical outcomes; III = expert opinion.

   **Panel members are divided on the strength of this recommendation: 55% voted for strong recommendation (A) and 45% voted for moderate recommendation (B).

Drug Alert For various reasons, ART may need to be interrupted or stopped by the provider or patient. Counsel patients to consult with HIV care provider before stopping a regimen. A planned discontinuation should be well thought out with the aim of reducing the risk of drug resistance and preserving treatment options for the future. Expert care or consultation should be sought when switching ART.

Complications of Treatment

Evidence Base Bartlett, J. G., & Gallant, J. E. (2012). *Medical management of HIV infection*. Durham, NC: Knowledge Source Solutions.
Bohjanen, P. R., & Boulware, D. R. (2007). Immune reconstitution inflammatory syndrome. In P. Volberding, M. A. Sande, J. Lange, et al. (Eds.), *Global HIV/AIDS medicine* (pp. 193–205). Philadelphia: Elsevier.

1. Lactic acidosis/steatohepatitis occurs with some NRTI medications; presents with nausea, vomiting, fatigue, and abdominal pain.

2. Hyperlipidemia, associated with some PI-containing regimens and some NNRTIs–containing regimens.

3. Insulin resistance leading to hyperglycemia, associated with some PI-containing regimens.

4. Lipodystrophy with fat accumulation in specific areas such as the abdomen and fat depletion in face and extremities, noted with some PI-containing regimens; lipoatrophy (depletion of fat), particularly with some NRTI medications.

5. Hepatotoxicities can occur with any class, noted especially with nevirapine and PI medications as a class. (More frequently noted in patients with chronic hepatitis B and/or hepatitis C.)

6. Immune reconstitution inflammatory syndrome (IRIS) is the emergence of acute illness in the setting of a strong response to recently started ARV therapy.

Table 29-4	HIV Treatment Considerations

CRITERIA	TREATMENT CONSIDERATIONS
History of AIDS defining illness	Treat
Asymptomatic with CD4⁺ < 350 cells/mm³	Treat
Asymptomatic with CD4⁺ 350–500 cells/mm³	Recommended
Pregnant women Where the goal is to prevent perinatal transmission	Recommended Treat
HIV-associated nephropathy	Treat, regardless of CD4⁺ count
Coinfected with HBV when treatment for HBV is indicated	Treat, regardless of CD4⁺ count

Panel on Antiretroviral Guidelines for Adults and Adolescents, U.S. Department of Health and Human Services. (2011). *Guidelines for the use of antiretroviral agents in HIV-1-infected adults and adolescents*. Available: www.aidsinfo.nih.gov.

There are two common IRIS scenarios:

   a. Unmasking of an occult opportunistic infection.

   b. Paradoxical symptomatic relapse of a prior infection despite microbiologic treatment success.

7. Treatment fatigue—emotional reaction to medication dosing and adverse effects; often needs simplified regimen and support. Drug "holidays" are not recommended, since rapid HIV replication recurs almost immediately.

Health Maintenance

Evidence Base Bartlett, J. G., & Gallant, J. E. (2012). *Medical management of HIV infection*. Durham, NC: Knowledge Source Solutions.

Prevention of Opportunistic Infections

1. PCP prophylaxis is started when the CD4+ count is 200/mm or less. The most effective medication is trimethoprim/sulfamethoxazole; others are dapsone, atovaquone, and aerosolized pentamidine.

2. *M. avium* complex prophylaxis is started when the CD4+ count is 50/mm³ or less; medications include azithromycin and clarithromycin.

3. Toxoplasmosis prophylaxis is appropriate when CD4+ count is 100/mm³ or less. Trimethoprim/sulfamethoxazole is most commonly used.

4. CMV retinitis monitoring with dilated ophthalmological exam is indicated every 6 months when the CD4+ count is ≤50/mm³.

Immunizations

1. Pneumococcal pneumonia—all patients should receive pneumococcal vaccine and it should be repeated in patients who attain a CD4+ count of ≥200/mm³.

2. Influenza—all patients should receive a flu vaccine each fall, though not the live virus formulation.

3. Tetanus booster—all patients should receive routine booster every 10 years and should be repeated when CD4+ count is >200/mm³.

4. Hepatitis A—recommended if at risk and baseline total antibody test is negative.

   a. Risk factors include MSM, IDU, and travel to endemic areas.

   b. Persons who have underlying coinfection with viral hepatitis or chronic liver infection should be vaccinated to prevent morbidity and mortality associated with acute hepatitis A infection.

5. Hepatitis B—recommended if baseline antibody test is negative.

6. Human papilloma virus—recommended for women age 13 to 26.

Supportive Care

1. Treatment of reversible illnesses.
2. Education for healthy lifestyle.

3. Assessment and management of pain.

4. Evaluation and management of psychological and social aspects of HIV infection.

5. Treatment to relieve symptoms and medication adverse effects (fatigue, nausea, diarrhea).

6. Antidepressant drugs; psychiatric interventions.

7. Substance abuse counseling and intervention.

8. All patients should be screened for tuberculosis every year with a purified protein derivative; ≥5-mm induration is considered positive.

Nursing Management of HIV Infection and AIDS

See Standard of Care Guidelines 29-1.

Evidence Base Swanson, B. (Ed.). (2010). *ANAC's core curriculum for HIV/AIDS nursing* (3rd ed.). Sudbury, MA: Jones & Bartlett.

Nursing Assessment

1. Obtain history of date of HIV diagnosis, CD4+ count at time of diagnosis, risk factors for infection, constitutional signs and symptoms, recent infections, positive blood test for HIV antibodies (confirm this if copy of original is unavailable), most recent CD4+ count, and HIV RNA viral load.

2. Review patient's present complaints, such as fever, cough, shortness of breath, diarrhea.

3. Assess patient's knowledge about HIV/AIDS, including causes, signs and symptoms, modes of transmission, methods for preventing transmission to others, infection progression, and importance of CD4+ count and HIV RNA viral load monitoring.

4. Assess the patient's adherence to medications by reviewing all prescribed drugs, the dose, and how often the patient is

---

STANDARDS OF CARE GUIDELINES 29-1
HIV/AIDS

When caring for patients with HIV infection

- Practice standard precautions.
- Protect confidentiality.
- Educate the patient about methods that prevent HIV transmission to others.
- Perform a psychosocial assessment.
- Develop adherence strategies for patients taking antiretroviral therapy.
- Provide education and interventions for HIV symptom management.

This information should serve as a general guideline only. Each patient situation presents a unique set of clinical factors and requires nursing judgment to guide care, which may include additional or alternative measures and approaches.

taking the medication. Ask the patient how many times over the last day or week he or she missed a dose. Encourage honest reporting by acknowledging that missed doses occur.

5. Evaluate nutritional and general health status by assessing weight, body mass index, anemia, or complications of drug toxicities, including hyperlipidemia, hyperglycemia, lipodystrophy.

6. Assess respiratory rate and depth and auscultate lungs for breath sounds; assess for skin color and temperature, palpable lymph nodes, and evidence of fever, night sweats.

7. Inspect mouth for lesions, especially *Candida* in the posterior pharynx; examine skin for rash, sores, and other changes. Record number, size, and locations.

8. Ask about bowel movement patterns, changes in habits, constipation, abdominal cramping, number and volume of stools, and presence of perianal pain and ulceration.

9. Note patient's orientation to time, place, and person. Note patient's affect. Ask about any problem with memory and concentration, headaches, seizures, visual changes.

10. Find out as much as possible about patient's lifestyle (assessing for ongoing risk behavior), experience and skills, social support system.

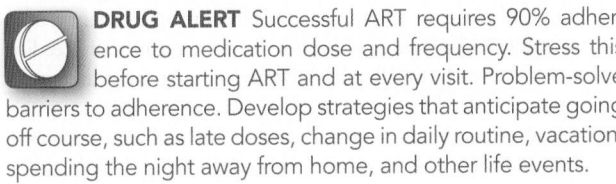 **DRUG ALERT** Successful ART requires 90% adherence to medication dose and frequency. Stress this before starting ART and at every visit. Problem-solve barriers to adherence. Develop strategies that anticipate going off course, such as late doses, change in daily routine, vacation, spending the night away from home, and other life events.

Nursing Diagnoses

- Fear of infection progression, treatment effects, isolation, and death related to having HIV/AIDS.
- Risk for infection related to immunodeficiency.
- Imbalanced Nutrition: Less Than Body Requirements related to infection or side effects to treatment.
- Impaired Oral Mucous Membranes related to opportunistic infection.
- Diarrhea related to infection and treatment side effects.
- Confusion related to infection effects and adverse effects of medicine.
- Hyperthermia related to opportunistic infection or malignancy.
- Ineffective Breathing Pattern related to opportunistic infection or malignancy.
- Ineffective Therapeutic Regimen Management related to complicated regimen of medications, treatment plans, clinical appointments, lack of social support, impaired cognitive functioning, substance use, or psychiatric illness.

Other nursing diagnoses may include:

- Fatigue related to underlying HIV infection or depression.
- Disturbed Body Image related to body changes from infection process or body changes related to adverse reaction to medication.
- Hopelessness related to chronic illness, sense of loss of control, depression, or vulnerability associated with HIV/AIDS.
- Acute and Chronic Pain related to infection, peripheral neuropathies, diarrhea, avascular necrosis, or other condition.

- Anticipatory Grieving related to awareness of implications of HIV/AIDS, changes in lifestyle, possible death.
- Disabled Family Coping related to crisis created by HIV/AIDS, guilt, fear, overwhelming caretaking responsibilities.

 NURSING ALERT Never assume the family or loved ones know that the patient is HIV-positive. Always ask the patient who knows of his or her HIV status. Confidentiality regarding HIV infection must be maintained. However, encourage the patient to share the diagnosis to decrease isolation. Offer to be with the patient when the diagnosis is shared with the family; role-playing before you meet with family or loved ones can be helpful.

Nursing Interventions

 Evidence Base Swanson, B. (Ed.). (2010). *ANAC's core curriculum for HIV/AIDS nursing* (3rd ed.). Sudbury, MA: Jones & Bartlett.

Reducing Fear

1. Maintain nonjudgmental attitude and nonprejudicial approach.

2. Anticipate that the patient may pass through a series of stages: initial crisis, transitional stage, acceptance state, and possibly preparation for death if treatment options have been exhausted.

3. Allow patient to use some degree of denial as a protective mechanism—gives some control over when and how patient will confront the diagnosis and his or her prognosis.
   a. Expect some displaced anger; avoid being personally affronted by patient's anger.
   b. Allow patient to acknowledge reality of the situation without false reassurance.

4. Explain that symptoms of anxiety and depression are common initially but generally improve with time and support. Refer patient to counseling or psychiatric care, if needed.

5. Anticipate that patients with active substance use issues may exhibit antisocial behaviors and feelings of alienation and isolation. Refer for counselling and treatment.

6. Provide careful discussion and clarification of treatment options.

7. Help patient set realistic goals and expectations.

8. Offer counseling work, especially when HIV/AIDS is initially diagnosed and if patient enters terminal phase of illness and treatment options have been exhausted.

9. Obtain social service referral for available resources such as community-based case management.

10. Help patient identify and strengthen personal resources, such as positive coping skills, relaxation techniques, strong support network, and optimistic outlook.

11. Encourage patient to join a support group—helpful in defusing stressful issues and in developing strategies to cope with the infection.

12. Observe for emerging psychiatric problems, especially in patients who are socially isolated, those with guilt about sexuality and lifestyle, and those with a history of psychiatric illness.

13. Discuss the importance of advance directives and legal guardianship of minor children. Cognitive deterioration may make it impossible for patient to act on his or her own behalf in the future.
14. If indicated, discuss hospice care and other end-of-life matters.
    a. Assure patient of palliative care, pain control, and help with anxiety and depression.
    b. Encourage patient and family participation in treatment decisions.

Preventing Infection

1. Have a high index of suspicion for infection even when clinical manifestations are subtle or absent.
2. Follow standard precautions with all patients.
3. Administer prescribed pharmacologic agents promptly and avoid medication administration delays or interruptions.
4. Administer and teach patient and family good skin care because a break in the skin is a source of secondary infection.
5. Maintain a clean environment of care.
6. Use aseptic techniques when performing invasive procedures.
7. Teach patient to make the most of his or her present immune function by minimizing the risk of infection and taking ART to reconstitute immune function.
    a. Avoid exposure to people with infections wherever possible.
    b. Encourage smoking cessation.
    c. Assist patient in finding treatment for substance abuse.
    d. Counsel patient to practice safe sex, even with an HIV-positive partner, to prevent transmission or superinfection with treatment-resistant HIV virus.
    e. Instruct visitors about handwashing before entering and leaving the inpatient room.
    f. Counsel the patient to have someone else clean a cat box or bird cage. If no one else is available, then use rubber gloves and wear a mask.
8. Ensure that the patient is up to date with immunizations.

Improving Nutritional Status

1. Monitor nutritional status by weighing patient and reviewing what patient is eating.
2. Monitor for sore throat that progresses to dysphagia or odynophagia or persistent heartburn—suggestive of esophageal candidiasis.
3. Consult with dietitian to develop strategies for optimizing patient's nutritional status.
4. Include patient in decision making regarding nutrition care.
5. Review times of drug administration in relation to meal times to optimize absorption; some medications should be taken with food and others should be taken on an empty stomach.
6. Administer or teach patient to take prescribed anti-emetic 30 minutes before meals or medication, if nausea is a problem. Use antidiarrheal medication if advised after consultation with provider.
7. For patient with oral or esophageal pain from *Candida* esophagitis or another cause:
    a. Administer prescribed antifungal and/or antiviral therapy.
    b. Avoid highly seasoned or acidic foods.
    c. Offer fluids and pureed or soft foods to minimize chewing and ease swallowing. Offer liquid nutritional supplements.
8. Discourage alcohol intake because it has immunosuppressive effect and is contraindicated if chronic hepatitis is present.
9. Make appropriate community referral if patient is unable to grocery-shop or prepare meals. Inform patient of local online grocery shopping options that are available.

Relieving Oral Discomfort

1. Ask about persistent sore throat, dysphagia, and heartburn; these symptoms are suggestive of oral and esophageal candidiasis, but may be indicative of other serious infection or malignancy.
2. Examine mouth for oral candida and other lesions and teach patient to do the same.
3. Administer antifungal treatment as indicated.

Minimizing the Effects of Diarrhea

1. Remember that diarrhea can be a complication of antibiotic therapy (ie, *C. difficile*).
2. Patients with diarrhea should have stool cultures and, if results are negative, review medication list for causative agents.
3. Counsel patient to monitor stools, reporting frequency, consistency, and presence of blood. Try to determine if bleeding is before, with, or after bowel movement to help determine source of bleeding.
4. Monitor intake and output; assess skin and mucous membranes for poor turgor and dryness, indicating dehydration.
5. Administer fluids and electrolytes, as prescribed.
6. Consider use of antidiarrheal medication.
7. Follow contact precautions and employ strict handwashing.
8. Plan regimen of skin care, including cleaning, blotting, and drying of the anal area, application of ointment or skin barrier cream.
9. Advise patient to eliminate caffeine, alcohol, dairy products, foods high in fats, and acidic juices if diarrhea persists. Drink liquids at room temperature.
10. Advise patient to avoid foods that increase motility and distention such as gas-forming fruits and vegetables.

Managing Disturbed Thought Processes

1. Remember that HIV has an affinity for the brain and is a target organ for opportunistic infections in advanced HIV infection.
2. Provide daily assessment of mental status; monitor for changes in behavior, memory, concentration ability, and motor dysfunction.
    a. Onset of dementia in advanced HIV infection is usually insidious but may be abrupt, precipitated by acute infection.
    b. Opportunistic brain infections can temporarily incapacitate mental function.
3. Reorient patient frequently; use calendar, clock, family and friends' pictures, lists, and structured care plan.
4. Provide for patient safety: bed alarm on, call signal available, articles within patient's reach. Anticipate a plan for toileting the patient.
5. Provide reassurance.

6. Assess for depressive or suicidal symptoms.

7. Anticipate necessity of guardianship, durable power of attorney for health care, and informed consent if patient has impaired cognition.

Reducing Fever

1. Assess for chills, fever, tachycardia, and tachypnea.

2. Encourage high fluid intake to replace insensible water losses incurred by fever or diaphoresis.

3. Administer or teach patient to administer antipyretics, as prescribed.

Improving Breathing Pattern

1. Provide supplemental oxygen, as ordered.

2. Watch for sudden change in respiratory function.

3. Administer or teach patient to administer prescribed opioid for postinfectious cough, a complication of PCP and viral pneumonia.

4. Encourage smoking cessation to enhance pulmonary ciliary defense.

5. Administer saline nebulization to induce sputum collection for culture and sensitivity.

   a. Wear mask and gloves during sputum collection.

   b. Instruct patient to brush tongue, buccal surfaces, teeth, and palate with water before sputum induction to remove superficial squamous epithelial cells and their adherent bacteria and foreign material.

   c. Instruct patient to gargle and rinse mouth with water.

6. Answer questions and provide support if patient has made decision for or against resuscitation and mechanical ventilation.

Improving Patient's Management of ART

1. Assess patient's adherence to medications and clinical appointments in the past; if there has been poor adherence, have patient explore what contributed to it.

2. Provide education about prescribed medications before ARVs are started and periodically thereafter; provide educational materials that can remain in the home as a resource.

3. Develop a medication schedule for the patient that incorporates his or her usual day-to-day activities; place pills in a medication box according to the schedule.

4. Encourage the involvement of a household member in the education and administration of the patient's medications.

5. Continue to monitor for medication adherence after patient has achieved an undetectable viral load.

6. Routinely ask about adverse effects. Encourage patient to call if these become a problem and offer symptom management education.

 DRUG ALERT Medication reconciliation should occur periodically, especially after hospitalizations or specialty consultations, in order to check for possible interactions and ensure that patient is taking all medications appropriately. Check with pharmacist for possible drug interactions. Some ARV medications may interact with new medications and can cause altered metabolism with increased or decreased blood levels of drug.

Community and Home Care Considerations for the End-Stage Patient

1. If patient is homebound, suggest contacting an agency that offers help specifically for HIV patients and provide home visits for services, such as hospice care and food services.

2. Assist patient, family, or significant other to locate support services in the community.

3. Assess the home for patient safety and provide durable medical goods that can enhance safety and comfort.

4. Provide latex gloves for the home for handling body fluids of the HIV-positive household member.

5. Explain that routine household cleaning of the bathroom, dishes, and laundry is sufficient to prevent HIV transmission.

6. Explain that the HIV-positive household member should never share toothbrushes or razors because they can provoke bleeding and, therefore, are a potential source of HIV transmission.

7. Establish whether there are persons in the home who will participate in the HIV-positive household member's care; engage these caregivers while attending to the patient. Assess the needs of the caregiver; acknowledge that it is important to have a break from the caregiver role. Provide information about respite services in which the patient can be cared for during the day or for days or weeks at a long-term care facility.

Patient Education and Health Maintenance

1. Indicate that patient could be a source of infection to others and should take actions to prevent transmission.

2. Encourage patient to disclose HIV status to sex partner(s) and/or needle-sharing partner(s).

3. Emphasize to HIV-infected mother that her child(ren) should be tested for HIV.

4. Discuss family planning with HIV-infected female patient. Some ARVs should not be taken by women who could become pregnant.

 DRUG ALERT Oral contraceptives interact with many protease inhibitors and NNRTI medications. Encourage the patient to discuss this with her gynecologist because she may need alternative contraception.

5. Establish both a primary care and an expert HIV provider for the patient and encourage regular follow-up care. Women should receive annual Papanicolaou (Pap) smears. Everyone should receive routine dental and eye examinations. For HIV specialty care, patients should follow up at recommended intervals, with laboratory assessment of CD4+, HIV RNA viral load, CBC with differential, and comprehensive metabolic panel.

6. Teach patient to recognize and report important symptoms such as fever or development of a new focal complaint.

7. Counsel injection drug users that continued use poses a risk of infection and may expose him or her to additional risks such as violence, missed doses of vital medications, and diversion of resources away from food, housing costs, and medication

copay fees. Provide encouragement to quit using drugs and assist him or her in finding drug treatment.

8. Encourage patient to modify sexual behaviors for safer sex. Discuss harm-reduction strategies and infection-prevention methods. Promote condom use and negotiating with partner(s) for safer sex. Refer patients to patient education materials online or in print that are appropriate to the patient's experience and literacy level.

9. Teach patient to optimize immune system function through sound dietary practices, exercise, and regular sleep; promote changes in the direction of more healthy living.

10. Ask patient if he or she uses complementary or alternative therapies, such as vitamins, herbs, and teas.

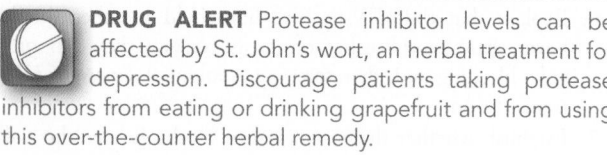

DRUG ALERT Protease inhibitor levels can be affected by St. John's wort, an herbal treatment for depression. Discourage patients taking protease inhibitors from eating or drinking grapefruit and from using this over-the-counter herbal remedy.

11. Refer patient to resources such as:

    a. Patient-oriented site with many resources including a list of hotlines for HIV infected consumers, *www.thebody .com*.

    b. Consumer-oriented magazine, which is available online and by mail, *www.poz.com*.

    c. *100 Question and Answers about HIV and AIDS*, by Joel Gallant (paperback available online and at bookstores). Excellent resource for patients in easy-to-understand language.

    d. "100 Questions and Answers about HIV and AIDS," by the New York State Health Department, *www.health. ny.gov/diseases/aids/facts/questions/index.htm* or (518) 474-3459.

12. Resources for health care professionals:

    a. U.S. Department of Health and Human Services, *www. aidsinfo.nih.gov*. Comprehensive website with links to a variety of information sources, including a list of resources for consumers.

    b. Centers for Disease Control and Prevention, *www.cdc.gov/ hiv*. General AIDS information, publications, resources, and statistics.

    c. Johns Hopkins University AIDS Service, *www.hopkins-guides.com/hopkins/ub*. Look up infections, complications, pathogens, management, and resistances.

    d. International resources, *www.unaids.org/en/*. Provides international view of AIDS epidemic with links for other international resources.

Evaluation: Expected Outcomes

• Speaks openly about HIV infection with health care providers, significant others; manages life stressors effectively.

• No signs of opportunistic infections; practicing safe sex.

• Eats three to four healthy meals per day.
• Oral mucosa without lesions.
• Reports formed stools one to three times per day.
• Responds appropriately to questions of self, time, and place; describes an accurate account of activities.
• Afebrile with normal heart rate.
• Respirations unlabored, no cough or sputum production.
• Reports medication adherence greater than 90% of doses; HIV viral load remains undetectable, CD4+ trends are upward toward normal counts and immune reconstitution.

SELECTED REFERENCES

American Academy of HIV Medicine. (2007). *AAHIVM fundamentals of HIV medicine* (2007 ed.). Washington, DC: Author.

Association of Nurses in AIDS Care. (2007). *HIV/AIDS nursing: Scope and standards of practice*. Silver Spring, MD: Author. Available: *www.nursesbooks.org*.

Bartlett, J. G., & Gallant, J. E. (2009). *Medical management of HIV infection*. Durham, NC: Knowledge Source Solutions.

Bohjanen, P. R., & Boulware, D. R. (2007). Immune reconstitution inflammatory syndrome. In P. Volberding, M. A. Sande, J. Lange, et al. (Eds.), *Global HIV/ AIDS medicine* (pp. 193–205). Philadelphia: Elsevier.

Centers for Disease Control and Prevention. (1993). AIDS surveillance case definition for adolescents and adults. *Morbidity and Mortality Weekly Report, 4*(RR-17), 2.

Centers for Disease Control and Prevention. (2006). Revised recommendations for HIV testing of adults, adolescents, and pregnant women in health care settings. *Morbidity and Mortality Weekly Report, 55*(RR-14).

Centers for Disease Control and Prevention. (2009). Guidelines for prevention and treatment of opportunistic infections in HIV-infected adults and adolescents: Recommendations from CDC, the National Institutes of Health, and the HIV Medicine Association of the Infectious Diseases Society of America. *Morbidity and Mortality Weekly Report, 58*(No. RR-4), 4–28. Available at *www.aidsinfo .nih.gov*.

Centers for Disease Control and Prevention. (2011). CDC fact sheet: Estimates of new HIV infections in the United States, 2006–2009. Available: *www.cdc.gov/ nchhstp/newsroom/docs/HIV-Infections-2006-2009.pdf*.

Cohen, M. A., & Gorman, J. M. (2008). *Comprehensive textbook of AIDS psychiatry*. New York: Oxford University Press.

Engels, E. A. (2009). Non-AIDS defining malignancies in HIV-infected persons: Etiologic puzzles, epidemiologic perils, prevention opportunities. *AIDS, 23*(8), 875–885.

Gallant, J. E. (2009). *100 questions and answers about HIV and AIDS*. Sudbury, MA: Jones & Bartlett.

Panel on Antiretroviral Guidelines for Adults and Adolescents, U.S. Department of Health and Human Services. (2011). Guidelines for the use of antiretroviral agents in HIV-1-infected adults and adolescents. Available at *www.aidsinfo .nih.gov*.

Sigel, K., Dubrow, R., Silverberg, M., et al. (2011). Cancer screening in patients infected with HIV. *Current HIV/AIDS Reports, 8*(3), 142–152.

Swanson, B. (Ed.). (2010). *ANAC's core curriculum for HIV/AIDS nursing* (3rd ed.). Sudbury, MA: Jones & Bartlett.

U.S. Department of Health and Human Services. (2010). AIDS.gov: Prevention in pregnancy and childbirth. Available: *www.aids.gov/hiv-aids-basics/prevention/ reduce-your-risk/pregnancy-and-childbirth/*

U.S. Department of Health and Human Services, Health Resources and Services Administration, HIV/AIDS Bureau. (2011). Guide for HIV/AIDS clinical care. Available: *http://hab.hrsa.gov/deliverhivaidscare/clinicalguide11/*.

World Health Organization. (2011). HIV/AIDS fact sheet (No. 360). Available: *www.who.int/mediacentre/factsheets/fs360/en/index.html*.

30
Connective Tissue Disorders

OVERVIEW AND ASSESSMENT

Connective tissue is a fibrous tissue that supports and connects internal organs, forms bones and the walls of blood vessels, attaches muscles and bones to bones (tendons and ligaments), and replaces tissue following injury (scar tissue). The long fibers of connective tissue contain a protein called *collagen*.

Connective tissue disorders are also known as *rheumatologic disorders*. They affect the integrity of the musculoskeletal system and may also affect blood vessels, the skin, and a variety of organs. They are chronic and may lead to disability; however, they can usually be controlled with medication.

Musculoskeletal and Related Assessment

Assessment for connective tissue disorders focuses on the musculoskeletal system, but also involves remote body systems. Clues to connective tissue disorders may be found in the skin, eyes, lungs, and neurologic system. Functional assessment is also important; many questionnaires and scales have been developed to assess patient function or disability related to connective tissue disorders, such as the Health Assessment Questionnaire first published in 1980, available at *www.chcr.brown.edu/pcoc/ehaqdescrscoringhaq372.pdf*.

Subjective Data

Obtain history of presenting symptoms, including duration and intensity, course of the illness, and impact of symptoms on the patient's life.

1. Musculoskeletal pain—characteristics.
   a. Joint swelling.
   b. Morning stiffness.

2. Constitutional symptoms.
   a. Fever.
   b. Weight loss, anorexia.
   c. Fatigue.
3. Involvement of other body symptoms.
   a. Skin.
   b. Ocular.
   c. Pulmonary.
   d. Neurologic.
   e. Mucous membranes.
   f. Gastrointestinal (GI).
4. Depression or psychosis.
5. Self-care activities and functional ability.
6. Social activities and roles.
7. Family history of rheumatic or autoimmune disorders.

Objective Data

1. Musculoskeletal examination:
   a. Pain on palpation or range of motion (ROM).
   b. Joint swelling, warmth, or erythema.
   c. Joint motion restriction.
   d. Pain, swelling, or warmth of soft tissues surrounding joints.
   e. Deformities.
2. Skin:
   a. Skin rash or other abnormalities such as thickening.
   b. Alopecia.
3. Oral mucosa:
   a. Ulcerations.
   b. Dryness.

1055

4. Ocular:
   a. Conjunctival inflammation.
   b. Dryness.
5. Pulmonary:
   a. Adventitious sounds.
   b. Friction rub.
6. Neurologic:
   a. Foot drop.
   b. Muscle weakness.
   c. Neurologic deficits.

Laboratory Studies

Anti–Double-Stranded DNA

Anti–double-stranded DNA (anti-dsDNA) is a highly specific marker for diagnosing systemic lupus erythematosus (SLE). This antibody is also useful for monitoring disease progression because anti-dsDNA levels fluctuate with disease activity.

Nursing and Patient Care Considerations

1. High anti-dsDNA levels are associated with the development of lupus nephritis.
2. There is a low false-positive rate (about 5%) in patients with other connective tissue disorders; in patients taking medications such as minocycline, etanercept, infliximab, and penicillamine; in first-degree relatives of patients with lupus; and in some laboratory workers.
3. There is no special preparation for this blood test.

Anticyclic Citrullinated Peptide

Anticyclic citrullinated peptide (anti-CCP) is a marker that helps diagnose rheumatoid arthritis. These autoantibodies are produced in the joint as a result of the synovial immune response of patients with rheumatoid arthritis.

Nursing and Patient Care Considerations

1. Anti-CCP is about as sensitive, but more specific (95% to 98%), than the rheumatoid factor test. Found in approximately 50% to 55% of patients with RA.
2. It may be valuable in cases of early arthritis when symptoms are mild and nonspecific and aggressive treatment is being contemplated. Anti-CCP antibody is now used with the rheumatoid factor as the gold standard in making the diagnosis of rheumatoid arthritis.
3. Some laboratories are currently doing a second generation of the test—the CCP2 assay.
4. No specific preparation is needed for this blood test, but the specimen may need to be sent out for processing, as not all labs perform this test.

Antinuclear Antibody

Antinuclear antibody (ANA) is a test for antibodies to nucleoprotein (autoantibodies or a heterogeneous group of gamma globulins); it is highly sensitive for detecting SLE, but is nonspecific (high false-positive rate).

Nursing and Patient Care Considerations

1. Be alert for drugs that may cause false-positive results.

Table 30-1	ANA Staining Patterns and Connective Tissue Disorders
ANA PATTERN	**CONNECTIVE TISSUE DISORDER**
Peripheral (rim, ring, membranous)	Active SLE, usually with renal disease
Homogenous (diffuse)	SLE, RA
Speckled	SLE, RA, scleroderma, Sjögren's syndrome, mixed connective tissue disorder
Nucleolar	Scleroderma

ANA, antinuclear antibody; RA, rheumatoid arthritis; SLE, systemic lupus erythematosus.

2. Results will be reported in a staining pattern (speckled, homogeneous, peripheral, nucleolar) if positive, which correlates to various types of connective tissue disorders and various subsets of SLE (see Table 30-1).
3. Titer will also be reported with positive ANA but does not reflect disease activity or prognosis.

Complement

1. *Complement* is a complex cascade system that activates proteins as part of the body's defense against infection.
2. Specific components include CH50 (total complement), C3, and C4; measurement helps determine immune complex formation or agammaglobulinemia.
3. Complement levels are decreased in certain autoimmune diseases, particularly SLE, because of complement consumption and because of activation of proteolytic enzymes and tissue damage. C3 and C4 are often monitored to evaluate activity in SLE.

Nursing and Patient Care Considerations

1. Obtain venous blood sample and refrigerate; send to laboratory promptly because complement deteriorates at room temperature.
2. Serial measurements may be helpful in monitoring the activity of some rheumatic diseases; decreased levels indicate increased disease activity.

C-Reactive Protein

C-reactive protein (CRP) is produced by the liver and is a nonspecific marker for infection and inflammation. It can be used to support the diagnosis for such inflammatory disorders as autoimmune disease, inflammatory bowel disease, and inflammatory arthritis.

Nursing and Patient Care Considerations

1. CRP reacts quicker to inflammatory changes than erythrocyte sedimentation rate; it rises within a few hours of an infection or inflammatory condition and then decreases quickly when inflammation resolves.
2. CRP can be used to differentiate inflammatory from noninflammatory conditions and to monitor effectiveness of treatment.
3. Normal CRP is usually below 10 mg/L; a level over 100 mg/L usually indicates infection or inflammation; however, some inflammatory conditions can raise CRP a thousandfold.

Table 30-2	Synovial Fluid Analysis				
	NORMAL COLOR	**WHITE BLOOD CELL COUNT**	**VISCOSITY**	**CRYSTALS**	
Normal	Clear, yellow	$200/\mu m^3$	Normal	None	
Osteoarthritis	Clear, slightly turbid	$200-600/\mu m^3$	Low	None	
Gout	Turbid	$2,000-75,000/\mu m^3$	Low	Monosodium urate	
Inflammatory Arthritis (Rheumatoid arthritis, systemic lupus erythematosus, Sjögren's syndrome, psoriatic)	Turbid, yellow	$2,000-75,000/\mu m^3$	Low	None	
Septic Arthritis	Pus, very turbid	Generally $80,000/\mu m^3$	Low	None	

Erythrocyte Sedimentation Rate

1. *Erythrocyte sedimentation rate (ESR)* determines the rate at which red blood cells (RBCs) fall out of unclotted blood in 1 hour.
2. The test is based on the premise that inflammatory and other disease processes create changes in blood proteins, thus causing aggregation of RBCs that makes them heavier.

Nursing and Patient Care Considerations

1. ESR is generally elevated in most rheumatic illnesses.
2. The test is sensitive for inflammatory condition, but not specific to connective tissue disorders.
   a. Result may be elevated by pregnancy, menstruation, medications (such as heparin and oral contraceptives), infection, malignancy, anemia, and advanced age.
   b. Result may be reduced by elevated blood glucose or albumin, high phospholipids, or drugs, such as corticosteroids or high-dose aspirin.
3. Most beneficial in monitoring inflammatory disease.

Rheumatoid Factor

Rheumatoid factor (RF) is a test for macroglobulin found in the blood of patients with rheumatoid arthritis (RA) and other disorders. RF has properties of an antibody and may be directed against immunoglobulin.

Nursing and Patient Care Considerations

1. It is not a highly sensitive or specific test.
2. May be positive in 50% to 75% of patients with RA, SLE, and Sjögren's syndrome. May be false-positive with endocarditis, tuberculosis, syphilis, sarcoidosis, cancer, viral infections, hepatitis C, patients with skin or renal allographs, and in some liver, lung, or kidney diseases.
3. Negative RF does not exclude the diagnosis of RA.
4. Certain disease manifestations, such as severe joint involvement and extra-articular manifestations, may be more frequent in those with high-titer RF.

Other Tests

Synovial Fluid Analysis

1. A sample of synovial (joint) fluid is analyzed for several components.

   a. Color.
   b. Clarity/turbidity.
   c. Viscosity.
   d. White blood cell (WBC) count with differential.
   e. Crystals and their identification.
2. Arthrocentesis, a sterile procedure, requires antiseptic cleaning agent, local anesthetic, a 20G needle (an 18G needle if infected fluid is suspected), and a 10- to 20-mL syringe.

Nursing and Patient Care Considerations

1. Patients are generally apprehensive about having a needle inserted into a joint. They require reassurance and explanation of the importance of information derived from test results.
2. Assist the health care provider with the test by collecting supplies, maintaining a sterile field, sending joint fluid samples for testing, and monitoring for bleeding following the procedure.
3. Results help to differentiate infection, inflammation, and crystal deposition in a painful joint (see Table 30-2).

GENERAL PROCEDURES AND TREATMENT MODALITIES

Pharmacologic Agents

 Evidence Base Singh, J. A., Furst, D. E., Bharat, A., et al. (2012). 2012 update of the 2008 American College of Rheumatology recommendations for the use of disease-modifying antirheumatic drugs and biologic agents in the treatment of rheumatoid arthritis. *Arthritis Care and Research, 64,* 625–639.

Connective tissue disorders may be treated with various drugs to relieve pain and to halt or minimize the disease process. Types of agents include nonsteroidal anti-inflammatory drugs (NSAIDs), corticosteroids, immunosuppressive agents, and a group of unrelated drugs known as disease-modifying antirheumatic drugs (DMARDs). Drug therapy may be long term and may require frequent evaluation for adverse effects (see Table 30-3). Patient education information about pharmacologic agents used to treat various disorders can be obtained from the National Institute

Table 30-3 Drug Therapy for Connective Tissue Disorders

DRUG	ACTION	ADVERSE EFFECTS
Anti-Inflammatory Agents		
Salicylates		
• Aspirin (may be buffered or enteric coated)	• Anti-inflammatory, antipyretic, and analgesic effects	• Tinnitus, gastric intolerance or GI bleeding and purpuric tendencies
Nonsteroidal Anti-Inflammatory Drugs (NSAIDs)		
• Ibuprofen • Fenoprofen • Naproxen • Tolmetin • Sulindac • Meclofenamate • Ketoprofen • Salsalate • Diclofenac • Nabumetone • Ketorolac • Oxaprozin • Flurbiprofen • Diflunisal • Piroxicam • Etodolac • Indomethacin • Trisalicylate	• Anti-inflammatory and analgesic effects • Mechanism of action may be related to inhibition of prostaglandin synthesis (prostaglandins have a role in inflammatory process, pain, and fever) • Nonsteroidal antirheumatic agents for adjunctive treatment of rheumatoid arthritis • Sometimes remarkably effective in control of articular symptoms	• GI irritation: nausea, vomiting, epigastric distress, precipitation and reactivation of peptic ulcer, hepatitis • Hematologic: bone marrow depression, anemia, leukopenia, thrombocytopenia purpura • Decrease in renal function can precipitate renal failure • Central nervous system: headache, dizziness, drowsiness, aseptic meningitis • Cardiovascular: edema, dyspnea palpitations
COX-2 Inhibitors		
• Celecoxib • Meloxicam	• Selective prostaglandin inhibition so that the inflammatory process is reduced without reducing protective prostaglandin effects on gastric mucosa	• Same adverse effects as other NSAIDs, with less risk for GI bleeding
Disease-Modifying Agents		
Antimalarial Agents		
• Hydroxychloroquine sulfate • Chloroquine phosphate	• Remission-induction agents for rheumatoid arthritis • Used also in certain forms of lupus	• Ocular toxicity (retinopathy that can result in permanent loss of vision; blurred vision, night blindness, scotoma)
Sulfonamides		
• Sulfasalazine	• Salicylate, sulfonamide	• Anorexia, rash, hemolytic anemia
Immunomodulators		
• Etanercept • Adalimumab • Golimumab • Certolizumab pegol	• Tumor necrosis factor blocker (subcutaneous)	• Infection, injection site reaction, dyspepsia, aplastic anemia, demyelinating disorders, activation of latent TB infection
• Infliximab	• IV tumor necrosis factor blocker	• Infusion reaction, headache, fatigue, optic neuritis, seizures, lupus-like syndrome, risk of severe infection
• Abatacept	• Selective co-stimulation modulator; available as IV or SC	• Risk of serious infection
• Tocilizumab	• Interleukin-receptor blocker	• Risk of severe infection, hypersensitivity reaction, gastrointestinal perforation, demyelinating disorder, malignancy

Table 30-3   Drug Therapy for Connective Tissue Disorders *(continued)*

DRUG	ACTION	ADVERSE EFFECTS
Immunosuppressives		
• Methotrexate	• Exert anti-inflammatory effect by inhibition of cellular replication	• Bone marrow suppression, hepatic and pulmonary toxicity, reduced resistance to infection
• Azathioprine	• Used in patients with inflammatory synovitis refractory to other therapy	• Bone marrow depression, GI and hepatic toxicity, carcinogenesis
• Cyclophosphamide	• Alkylating agent that interferes with the growth of rapidly dividing cells	• Possibility of a malignancy occurring many years later after initiating therapy can cause sterility, urinary bladder, fibrosis, cystitis
• Cyclosporine	• Inhibition of immunocompetent lymphocytes also inhibits lymphokine production and release	• Renal dysfunction, tremor, hypertension, gum hyperplasia
• Leflunomide	• Pyrimidine synthesis inhibitor	• Diarrhea, liver function test abnormalities, alopecia, rash, upper respiratory infection, hypertension
Corticosteroids		
• Prednisone • Prednisolone • Triamcinolone • Betamethasone • Hydrocortisone • Dexamethasone • Methylprednisolone	• Potent anti-inflammatory drugs may also reduce immune response • Usually used for short-term management of patients with severe limitations	• Osteoporosis, fractures, avascular necrosis • Gastric ulcers, infection susceptibility • Hirsutism, acne, moon facies, abnormal fat deposition, edema, emotional disorders, menstrual disorders • Hyperglycemia, hypokalemia • Hypertension, cataracts

IV, intravenous; SC, subcutaneous.

of Arthrtitis and Musculoskeletal and Skin Disease (*www.niams.nih.gov/Health_Info/default.asp*) or from the American College of Rheumatology. (ACR; *www.rheumatology.org*).

Physical and Occupational Therapy

Physical and occupational therapy provide a multimodal program to help reduce pain and to improve joint function. Many other measures can be taught to patients for home practice. Components of the program may include:

- Joint conservation.
- Energy conservation.
- Splinting (in rare instances).
- ROM exercises.
- Application of heat and cold.
- Endurance or aerobic conditioning.
- Modification of home and work environment.

Joint Conservation

Teach or reinforce the following practices:

1. Perform activities using good body mechanics.
2. Maintain ideal body weight—extra weight places undue stress on weight-bearing joints.
3. Use large joints to perform activities—spread the load over as many joints as possible.

4. Perform activities in smooth movements to avoid trauma induced by abrupt movements.

Energy Conservation

Teach or reinforce the following practices:

1. Organize materials, utensils, and tools.
2. Perform lengthy activities in a seated position.
3. Work at an even pace—avoid rushing.
4. Delegate work to others when possible.

Splinting

1. May be used for wrists and hands.
2. Ensure proper application.
3. Periodically inspect for skin irritation, neurovascular compromise, or improper fit.
4. Usually worn during acute stage of inflammation to protect joint.

Exercise

Instruct and reinforce correct method of exercise:

1. Avoid exercising inflamed joints—putting these joints through ROM exercises one to two times per day when inflamed is sufficient.

2. Perform exercises daily, as prescribed.
3. Aerobic conditioning exercises may be indicated when disease activity permits.
4. Walking, biking, swimming, and water walking for 30 minutes, three times per week. Regular exercise three times per week for at least 20 minutes for 6 months has been shown to reduce fatigue and disability in patients with RA compared to those who didn't exercise.

Other Measures

1. Reinforce correct use and application of heat and cold.
2. Obtain and teach correct use of assistive devices.

3. Reinforce use of behavior-modification and relaxation techniques as adjuncts to therapy.
4. Suggest discussion with health care provider about complementary and alternative therapies. A wide variety of herbal and nutraceutical products have been used and studied, but data remain inconclusive about efficacy (see Table 30-4).
   a. Many herbal and supplemental products are marketed for pain, inflammation, repair of cartilage, and boosting the immune system; however, scientific evidence for clear-cut treatment benefit is lacking. There is preliminary evidence for fish oil, gamma-linolenic acid, and the herb thunder god vine.

Table 30-4	Complementary and Alternative Drug Therapy for Arthritis	
DRUG AND EFFECT	**EFFECT**	**COMMENTS**
Fish oil (omega-3 fatty acid)	May reduce tenderness and stiffness; may reduce the need for NSAIDs.	May interact with blood thinners, antihypertensives. Avoid high-dose fish liver oil, which may cause vitamin A and D toxicity.
Gamma-linoleic acid (GLA) (omega-6 fatty acid, evening primrose oil, borage, black currant)	Converted into substances that reduce inflammation to relieve joint pain, stiffness, tenderness, and possibly NSAID use.	Appears to be safe but some borage oil preparations contain hepatotoxic chemicals. More research on dose and duration is needed.
Thunder god vine (*Tripterygium wilfordii*)	May fight inflammation and suppress the immune system; may relieve rheumatoid arthritis symptoms.	May cause serious side effects—diarrhea, stomach upset, hair loss, headache, skin rash, menstrual changes, male infertility; long-term use may reduce bone mineral density.
Boswellia	Anti-inflammatory and analgesic effects.	Generally safe. Lab and animal studies have been done; need clinical studies.
Ginger	Anti-inflammatory and analgesic effects.	Large doses may cause GI adverse effects; may cause bleeding if given with anticoagulant. Lab studies have been done, need clinical studies.
Green tea	Substances might be useful in rheumatoid arthritis and osteoarthritis.	More information is needed.
Turmeric (curcumin)	Animal studies show protection of joints from inflammation and damage.	Generally safe, no adverse effects; however, may cause stomach ulcers in high doses with prolonged use. Animal studies have been done, need clinical studies.
Cayenne pepper (capsicum) Thought to deplete substance P, reducing pain transmission	Applied topically to skin over joints in concentrations of 0.025%–0.25%	Takes several days to obtain pain relief; do not use with heat application.
Glucosamine and chondroitin Cartilage repair, pain relief	Glucosamine: 1,000–2,000 mg daily Chondroitin: 800–1,600 mg daily, based on weight	Bleeding risk if ASA taken with chondroitin; may be effective either alone or as combination; must be taken for several months to achieve noticeable effect. Studies showed conflicting results.

GLA, gamma-linoleic acid.

Evidence Base National Center for Complimentary and Alternative Medicine. (2010). Rheumatoid arthrits and complimentary and alternative medicine. Bethesda, MD: Author. Available: *http://nccam.nih.gov/health/RA/getthefacts.htm*.

Cameron, M., Gangier, J. J., & Chrubasik, S. (2011). Herbal therapy for treating rheumatoid arthritis. The Cochrane Library (Article No. CD002948).

   b. Reflexology, tai chi, and acupressure or acupuncture have benefited some patients with arthritis and connective tissue disorders. Assist the patient in finding certified providers in these disciplines, if desired.

 Evidence Base Han, A., Judd, M., Welch, V. et al. (2009). Tai chi for treating rheumatoid arthritis. The Cochrane Library (Article No. CD004849).

   c. Use of magnets to relieve pain has not shown effectiveness in numerous studies since the concept was introduced.
   d. For more information, refer patients to the National Center for Complimentary and Alternative Medicine at *http://nccam.nih.gov/health/RA/getthefacts.htm*.
5. Advise patient to modify home and work environments, as needed, to install safety devices, and to maintain a safe environment.
6. Advise patient to seek counseling regarding sexuality if joint pain and inflammation are barriers to performance.
7. Reinforce the chronic waxing-and-waning nature of the illness to lessen susceptibility to quackery.

DISORDERS

Rheumatoid Arthritis

Rheumatoid arthritis (RA) is a chronic inflammatory disease that affects joints and other organ systems. RA affects 0.5% to 1% of the population worldwide. 2010 criteria includes synovitis in any joint where no alternative diagnosis can explain the synovitis, and a score of 6/10 in four domains: number and site of involved joints, serologic abnormality, elevated acute phase response (markers of inflammation), and symptom duration. These criteria permit diagnosis at an earlier stage than 1987 ACR criteria, allowing for earlier treatment and less destruction of joints.

 Evidence Base Aletaha, D., Neoqi, T., Silman, A. J., et al. (2010). 2010 rheumatoid arthritis classification criteria: An American College of Rheumatology/European League Against Rheumatism Collaborative Initiative. *Annals of Rheumatic Disease, 69*(9), 1580–1588.

Pathophysiology and Etiology

1. Immunologic processes result in inflammation of synovium, producing antigens and inflammatory by-products that lead to destruction of articular cartilage, edema, and production of a granular tissue called *pannus* (see Figure 30-1).
2. Granulation tissue forms adhesions that lead to decreased joint mobility.
3. Similar adhesions can occur in supporting structures, such as ligaments and tendons, and cause contractures and ruptures that further affect joint structure and mobility.
4. The etiology is unknown but is probably a combined effect of environmental, epidemiologic, infectious, and genetic factors.
5. An infectious agent has not been identified, but many infectious processes can produce a polyarthritis similar to RA.
6. Women are affected more frequently than men.

Clinical Manifestations

1. Arthritis–2010 criteria includes synovitis in any joint, rather than symmetrical joints in the 1987 ACR criteria (see Figure 30-2, page 1062).
2. Skin manifestations.
   a. Rheumatoid nodules—elbows, occiput, sacrum.
   b. Vasculitic changes—brown, splinterlike lesions in fingers or nail folds.

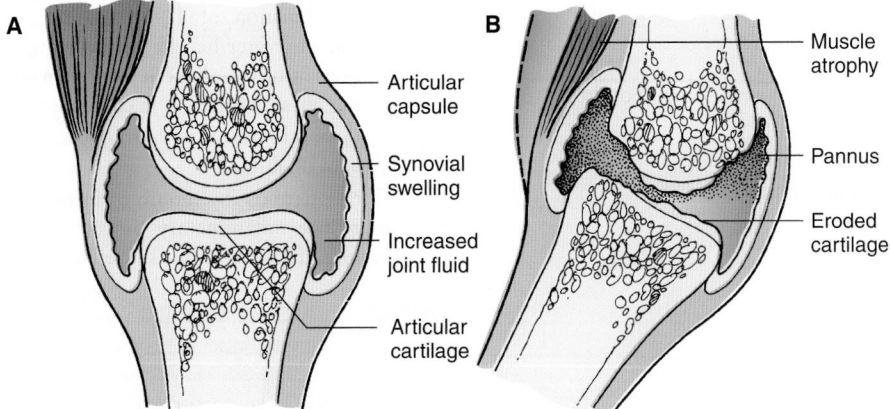

Figure 30-1. Pathophysiology of rheumatoid arthritis. (A) Joint structure with synovial swelling and fluid accumulation in joint. **(B)** Pannus, eroded articular cartilage with joint space narrowing, muscle atrophy, and ankylosis.

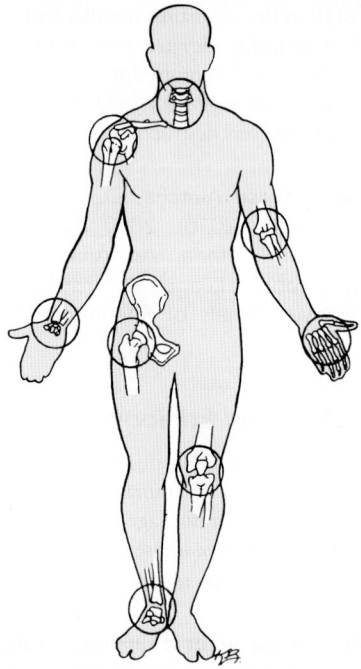

Figure 30-2. Rheumatoid arthritis characteristically involves the joints of the hands, wrist, feet, ankles, knees, elbows, and the gleno-humeral and acromioclavicular joints and the hips. The articulations of the cervical spine are also affected.

3. Cardiac manifestations.
   a. Acute pericarditis.
   b. Conduction defects.
   c. Valvular insufficiency.
   d. Coronary arteritis.
   e. Cardiac tamponade—rare.
   f. Myocardial infarction, sudden death—rare.
4. Pulmonary manifestations.
   a. Asymptomatic pulmonary disease.
   b. Pleural effusion, pleurisy.
   c. Interstitial fibrosis.
   d. Laryngeal obstruction caused by involvement of the crico-arytenoid joint—rare.
   e. Pulmonary nodules.
5. Neurologic manifestations.
   a. Mononeuritis multiplex—wrist drop, foot drop.
   b. Carpal tunnel syndrome.
   c. Compression of spinal nerve roots.
   d. Distal sensory neuropathy.
6. Other manifestations.
   a. Fever.
   b. Fatigue.
   c. Weight loss.
   d. Episcleritis.

Diagnostic Evaluation

1. Complete blood count (CBC)—normochromic, normocytic anemia of chronic disease; may also have iron-deficiency anemia (hypochromic, microcytic); platelets may be elevated with inflammation.
2. RF—positive in up to 70% to 80% of patients with RA; CCP is more specific for RA than RF testing.
3. ESR and CRP—often elevated due to active inflammation.
4. Synovial fluid analysis—see Table 30-2, page 1057.
5. X-rays—changes develop within 2 years.
   a. Hands/wrists—marginal erosions of the proximal inter-phalangeal (PIP), metacarpophalangeal, and carpal joints; generalized osteopenia.
   b. Cervical spine—erosions that produce atlantoaxial subluxation (generally after many years).
6. Magnetic resonance imaging (MRI)—detects spinal cord compression that results from C1 to C2 subluxation and compression of surrounding vascular structures. Also detects erosions earlier then x-ray.
7. Bone scan—increased uptake in the joints involved in RA.
8. Ultrasound—detects synovitis and erosion (very user dependent). Musculoskeletal ultrasound is widely used in Europe, but more sporadic use in United States.
9. Synovial biopsy.
   a. Inflammatory cells associated with RA.
   b. Excludes other causes of polyarthritis by noting the lack of other pathologic findings, such as crystals.

Management

 Evidence Base Singh, J. A., Furst, D. E., Bharat, A., et al. (2012). 2012 update of the 2008 American College of Rheumatology Recommendations for the use of disease-modifying antirheumatic drugs and biologic agents in the treatment of rheumatoid arthritis. *Arthritis Care Research, 64,* 625–639.

1. NSAIDs to relieve pain and inflammation.
2. DMARDs to reduce disease activity.
   a. Monotherapy or combination of older agent, such as methotrexate or hydroxychloroquine, with newer agent, such as tumor necrosis factor (TNF) inhibitor or other biologic agents.
   b. Combination of TNF inhibitor and methotrexate has shown greater benefit in improving signs and symptoms, preventing radiologic deterioration of the joint, and improving physical function in comparison with monotherapy.
   c. Goal is to have long-term impact on the joints and to prevent disability.
3. Corticosteroids (by mouth or intra-articular administration) to reduce inflammatory process. Generally used for short periods, due to multiple side effects.

 DRUG ALERT Do not give biologic DMARDs (immunomodulators) within 2 to 3 weeks of any live vaccine. Oral DMARDs, such as methotrexate, leflunamide, hydroxychloroquine, and sulfasalazine, may be used. Watch for signs of infection, including reactivation of viral infection, while patients are receiving these medications.

4. Local comfort measures:
   a. Application of heat and cold did not show benefit in a meta-analysis, but treatment can be individualized.
   b. Use of splints to support painful, swollen joints.
   c. Use of transcutaneous electrical nerve stimulation (TENS) unit for 15 minutes three times a week may provide some benefit.
   d. Iontophoresis—delivery of medication through the skin using direct electrical current.
   e. Parrafin wax baths with exercise may be of some benefit.

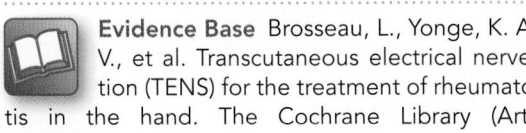 **Evidence Base** Brosseau, L., Yonge, K. A., Welch, V., et al. Transcutaneous electrical nerve stimulation (TENS) for the treatment of rheumatoid arthritis in the hand. The Cochrane Library (Article No. CD004377).
Welch, V., Brosseau, L., Casimiro, L., et al. (2009). Thermotherapy for treating rheumatoid arthritis. The Cochrane Library (Article No. CD002826).

5. Nonpharmacologic modalities:
   a. Behavior modification.
   b. Relaxation techniques.
6. Surgery:
   a. Synovectomy.
   b. Arthrodesis—joint fusion.
   c. Total joint replacement.

Complications

1. Loss of joint function because of bony adhesions and damage of supporting structures—7% of patients become disabled within 5 years of onset; 32% cannot work after 10 years.
2. Anemia of chronic disease.
3. Felty's syndrome—neutropenia, splenomegaly, and deformity; occurs in 1% of patients.

Nursing Assessment

1. Perform joint examination, if indicated, including which joints affected; ROM of each joint; presence of heat, redness, swelling; and possible joint effusion.
2. Note presence of deformities (see Figure 30-3):
   a. Swan neck—PIP joints hyperextend.
   b. Boutonniere—PIP joints flex.
   c. Ulnar deviation—fingers point toward ulna.
3. Assess pain using a pain measurement scale such as the visual analog scale (10 cm straight line scored 0 to 100; patient makes a mark indicating intensity of pain).
4. Assess functional status using the ACR revised criteria for classification for global functional status.
   a. Class I—Completely able to perform usual activities of daily living (ADLs).
   b. Class II—able to perform usual self-care and vocational activities, but limited in avocational activities.
   c. Class III—able to perform usual self-care activities, but limited in vocational and avocational activities.
   d. Class IV—limited ability to perform usual self-care, vocational, and avocational activities.
5. Assess for adherence to treatment plan, any complementary methods used, and any adverse reactions to medications.

Nursing Diagnoses

- Chronic Pain related to disease process.
- Impaired Physical Mobility related to pain and limited joint motion.
- Risk for Injury related to side effects/toxicities of DMARD therapy.
- Dressing or Grooming Self-Care Deficit related to limitations secondary to disease process.
- Ineffective Coping related to pain, physical limitations, and chronicity of RA.

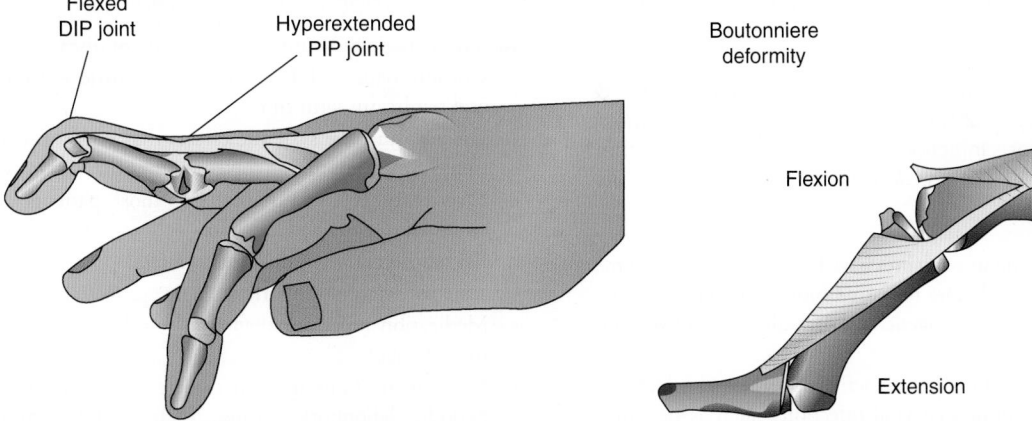

Figure 30-3. **Swan neck (A)** and boutonniere **(B)** deformities.

Nursing Interventions

Controlling Pain

1. Apply local heat or cold to affected joints for 15 to 20 minutes, three to four times per day. Avoid temperatures likely to cause skin or tissue damage by checking temperature of warm soaks or by covering cold packs with a towel.
2. Administer or teach self-administration of pharmacologic agents.
   a. Advise patient when to expect pain relief, based on mechanism of action of the drug.
3. Encourage use of adjunctive pain-control measures.
   a. Progressive muscle relaxation.
   b. TENS.
   c. Biofeedback.
   d. Meditation.
   e. Acupuncture or similar therapies.

Optimizing Mobility

1. Encourage warm bath or shower in the morning to decrease morning stiffness.
2. Encourage measures to protect affected joints.
   a. Perform gentle ROM exercises.
   b. Use splints.
   c. Assist with ADLs, if necessary.
3. Encourage exercise consistent with degree of disease activity.
4. Refer to physical therapy and occupational therapy.

Preventing Serious Adverse Reactions to Drug Therapy

1. Review drug information before administration to ensure that baseline bloodwork, such as CBC and liver function tests have been done; there are no drug interactions; and you understand reconstitution and administration information.
2. Ensure that a tuberculin test has been done prior to starting biologics. If positive, treatment for latent tuberculosis (TB) and biologic may be started simultaneously.
   a. In immunocompromised individuals, including those with auto immune diseases, greater than 5 mm reaction to tuberculin skin test is considered positive.
   b. Interferon-gamma release assays for tuberculosis screening are newer blood tests that are commonly used. These are more sensitive and specific than the purified protein derivative skin test and may be either substituted or done in conjunction with skin testing.

 Evidence Base Keystone, E. C., Papp, K. A., & Wobeser, W. (2011). Challenges in diagnosing latent tuberculosis infection in patients treated with tumor necrosis factor antagonists. *Journal of Rheumatology, 38,* 1234–1243.

3. Make sure that no live vaccines have been administered in the past 2 to 3 weeks before initiating biologic therapy because infection with vaccine agent could result. Oral DMARDs may be used safely.
4. Ensure that the patient has no active or untreated infections. Be aware that suppressed viral infections, such as hepatitis, herpes, and varicella, can result from immune therapy.
5. Administer or teach patient to administer medication subcutaneously by rotating sites of abdomen, thigh, and upper arm, as directed.
   a. Many biologics, such as etanercept, adalimumab, certolizumab, golimumab, and abatacept, are available in pre-filled syringe or pen form. Etanercept and cerolizumab are also available in powder form for reconstitution.
   b. Give IV drugs (abatacept, rituximab, infliximab, and toxilumab) by slow infusion, monitoring for fever and chills and cutaneous reaction (as per infusion protocol).

Promoting Self-Care

1. Provide pain relief before self-care activities.
2. Provide privacy and an environment conducive to performance of daily activities.
3. Schedule adequate rest periods.
4. Discuss importance of promoting the patient's self-care at an appropriate level with patient and family.
5. Help patient attain appropriate assistive devices, such as raised toilet seats, special eating utensils, and zipper pulls. Contact occupational therapist, social worker, or Arthritis Foundation for information.

Strengthening Coping Skills

1. Be aware of potential job, childcare, home maintenance, and social and family functioning problems that may result from RA.
2. Encourage patient to vocalize problems and feelings.
3. Assist with problem-solving approach to explore options and to gain control of problem areas, such as cost of drugs and medical care, limited resources at home.
   a. Patient assistance programs are available for drug therapy through the manufacturer or Partnership for Prescription Assistance (*www.ppaRx*). There are also several foundations that may be able to assist with copays and other costs.
   b. Obtain order for home care nursing or physical or occupational therapy for treatment and monitoring, as needed.
   c. Consult social worker, the Arthritis Foundation, or other community resources for additional services, as needed.
4. Reinforce effective coping mechanisms.
5. Refer to social worker or mental health counselor, as needed.

Patient Education and Health Maintenance

1. Instruct patient and family in the nature of disease.
   a. Chronic nature of RA with characteristic exacerbations and remissions with time.
   b. Disease can have systemic effects that result in constitutional symptoms and involvement of other organ systems.
   c. Severity of RA is variable, but most patients are *not* confined to bed or wheelchair.
   d. RA has no cure; avoid "miracle cures."
2. Educate patient about pharmacologic agents.
   a. Medication must be taken consistently to achieve maximum benefit.
   b. Most medications used in the treatment of RA require periodic laboratory testing, such as CBC and liver functions, to monitor for potential adverse effects.

c. Advise patient of possible adverse effects of medications and need to report adverse effects to health care provider, including fever, chills, lethargy, rash, difficulty breathing, swelling, worsening of arthritis, and severe diarrhea.

d. Advise patients to discuss the use of any complementary or alternative therapies with their health care provider.

e. Reinforce to patient the need for lifelong treatment.

3. During periods of remission, encourage patient to exercise regularly, choosing an activity that is inexpensive, convenient, enjoyable, and not dependent on the weather. Suggest dancing, mall walking, use of stationary bicycle in the home, or contacting the local YMCA about special programs for arthritis.

4. For additional information and support, refer to the Arthritis Foundation (*www.arthritis.org*) or the American College of Rheumatology (*www.rheumatology.org/public/factsheets/index.asp*).

Evaluation: Expected Outcomes

- Reports reduction in pain.
- Wears wrist splints correctly and performs ROM exercises twice per day.
- Reports no adverse reactions to drug therapy.
- Maintains independent toiletry, bathing, and feeding.
- Verbalizes concerns about cleaning and cooking; meets with occupational therapist.

Systemic Lupus Erythematosus

Systemic lupus erythematosus (SLE) is a chronic, multisystem autoimmune disease. Discoid lupus may also occur with predominant skin lesions.

Diagnostic criteria for SLE includes the presense of at least 4/17 findings, as outlined in the Systemic Lupus International Collaborating Clinics classification criteria, updating the SLICC/ACR Damage Index for SLE. Criteria include clinical manifestations and laboratory criteria.

 Evidence Base Petri, M., Orbai, A.M., Alarcon, G. S., et al. (2012). Derivation and validation of the Systemic Lupus International Collaborating Clinics classification criteria for systemic lupus erythematosus. *Arthritis and Rheumatism, 64*(8), 2677–2686.

Pathophysiology and Etiology

1. The T-lymphocyte system is affected for unknown reasons, and the failure of its regulatory system may result in an inability to slow or to halt the production of inappropriate autoantibodies.

2. B lymphocyte–stimulating factors are produced and this too may lead to production of autoantibodies.

3. Autoantibodies may combine with other elements of the immune system to activate immune complexes. These immune complexes and other immune system constituents combine to form complement, which is deposited in organs, causing inflammation and tissue necrosis.

4. More women, particularly in childbearing years, are affected than men.

Clinical Manifestations

1. Skin:
   a. Butterfly-shaped rash of the malar region of the face, characterized by erythema and edema.
   b. Discoid lesions are scarring, ring-shaped, involving the shoulders, arms, and upper back.
   c. Discoid lesions may also result in erythematous, scaly plaques on the face, scalp, external ear, and neck, resulting in alopecia.

2. Arthritis:
   a. Generally bilateral and symmetric, involving the hands, wrists, and other joints.
   b. Can resemble RA and may be mistaken for it, especially early in the course of the disease.
   c. Unlike RA, the arthritis is nonerosive; that is, no joint destruction is seen on x-ray. May (occasionally) be erosive, representing some overlap with RA.
   d. Tendon involvement is common and may lead to deformities or tendon rupture.

3. Cardiac:
   a. Pericarditis.
   b. Pleural effusion.
   c. Myocarditis.
   d. Endocarditis.
   e. Coronary artery disease.

4. Pulmonary:
   a. Pleuritis.
   b. Pleural effusion.
   c. Lupus pneumonitis.
   d. Pulmonary hemorrhage.
   e. Pulmonary embolism.

5. GI:
   a. Oral ulcers.
   b. Acute or subacute abdominal pain.
   c. Pancreatitis.
   d. Spontaneous bacterial peritonitis.
   e. Bowel infarction.

6. Renal: occurs in 50% of patients, with as many as 15% of patients developing renal failure.
   a. Nephritis.
      i. Mesangial nephritis—mild form, can be reversible, best prognosis.
      ii. Focal segmental glomerulonephritis—active necrotic or sclerosing lesions.
      iii. Proliferative—may be focal or diffuse; diffuse carries good prognosis.
      iv. Membranous nephritis—may persist for years without serious renal function decline; may present as nephrotic syndrome.
      v. Sclerosing nephritis—increase in the amount of matrix material in the glomeruli.
   b. Renal thrombosis—rare.

7. Central nervous system:
    a. Neuropsychiatric disorders.
        i. Depression.
        ii. Psychosis.
    b. Transient ischemic attacks, stroke.
    c. Seizures.
    d. Migraine headache.
    e. Myelopathy.
    f. Guillain-Barré syndrome.
    g. Chorea and other movement disorders.
    h. Poor concentration, "lupus fog"
8. Hematologic:
    a. Hemolytic anemia.
    b. Leukopenia.
    c. Thrombocytopenia.
9. Vascular:
    a. Hypertension.
    b. Raynaud's phenomenon (see Figure 30-4).
10. Constitutional:
    a. Fever.
    b. Weight loss.
    c. Fatigue.

Diagnostic Evaluation

1. CBC—leukopenia, anemia (may be hemolytic), thrombocytopenia.

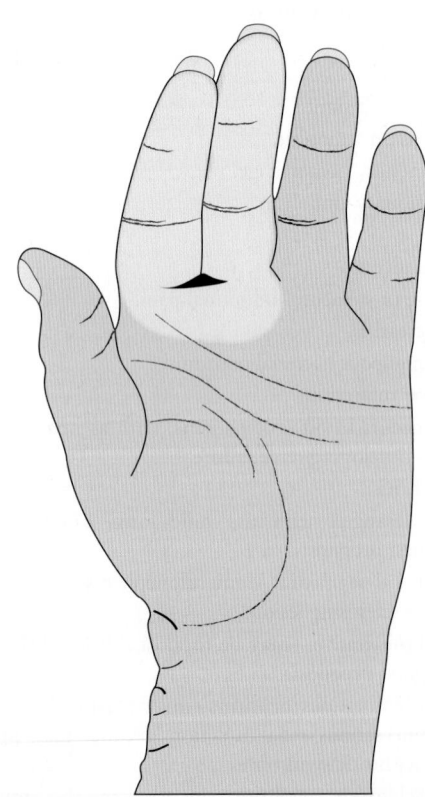

Figure 30-4. Characteristic pallor due to vasospasm in Raynaud's phenomenon.

2. ANA—positive in more than 90% of patients with SLE; predominant pattern is homogeneous.
3. Anti-dsDNA—97% specific for lupus.
4. ESR—generally elevated.
5. Complement levels—generally decreased when disease is active.
6. Urinalysis—hematuria, proteinuria, and active sediment (RBC casts).
7. Twenty-four-hour urine for protein and creatinine clearance.
8. Chest x-ray may show changes.
9. X-ray of hands and wrists—nondestructive arthritis.
10. Computed tomography (CT) or MRI may be clinically indicated.
    a. Brain—to define any neurologic manifestations.
    b. Abdomen—to rule out other abdominal processes in a patient with abdominal pain.
    c. Cerebral arteriogram—to look for evidence of cerebral vasculitis.
    d. Magnetic resonance angiography.

Management
Pharmacologic

1. NSAIDs to reduce pain and inflammation.
2. Antimalarials to decrease disease activity.
3. Corticosteroids to reduce inflammatory process.
4. Immunosuppressives to suppress immune process and to act as steroid sparing agents.
    a. Research is ongoing to develop lymphocyte-specific immunosuppressants and biologic modifiers to stop auto-antibody production.
    b. Belimumab was recently approved for intravenous infusion. This is the first new drug approved for lupus in 50 years.
    c. Belimumab is a human monoclonal antibody that neutralizes the B-cell survival factor, B-lymphocyte stimulator (BLyS).
    d. While belimumab is not effective for all lupus patients, it may serves as a model for further drug development.

 Evidence Base Stohl, W., & Hilbert, D. M. (2012). The discovery and development of belimumab: The anti BLyS–lupus connection. *Nature Biotechnology, 30*(1), 69–77.

5. Antihypertensives and diuretics to treat hypertension and fluid overload, if present due to renal disease.
6. Calcium channel blockers, angiotensin receptor blockers, or sildenafil for Raynaud's phenomenon (see page 459).

Nonpharmacologic

1. Avoid direct exposure to sunlight to reduce the chance of exacerbation. Protective clothing and sunblock with an SPF of 50 should also be used.
2. Behavior modification to prevent exacerbations and to reduce symptoms.
3. Joint protection and energy conservation.

Other Management

1. Close follow-up for evaluation of cardiac, neurologic, renal, and other body systems.
2. Referral to specialists for systemic manifestations.

Complications

1. Renal failure.
2. Permanent neurologic impairment.
3. Infection.
4. Death caused by disease process.

Nursing Assessment

1. Obtain clinical history, review systems, and perform physical examination for characteristic findings.
2. Assess for signs and symptoms of infection and other adverse effects to medications.
3. Assess patient's and family's ability to cope with impact of prolonged disease.

Nursing Diagnoses

- Chronic Pain related to inflammation of joints and juxta-articular structures.
- Powerlessness related to unpredictable course of disease.
- Risk for Impaired Skin and Oral Mucous Membrane Integrity related to skin/oral lesions.
- Fatigue related to chronic inflammatory process.
- Impaired Urinary Elimination related to renal involvement.

Nursing Interventions

Reducing Pain

1. Administer and teach self-administration of medications to reduce disease activity and of additional analgesics as ordered.
2. Suggest the use of hot or cold applications, relaxation techniques, and nonstrenuous exercise to enhance pain relief.
3. Monitor for adverse reactions to corticosteroids (see page 914).

Increasing Control Over Disease Process

1. Instruct patient to avoid factors that may exacerbate disease.
   a. Avoid exposure to sunlight and ultraviolet light.
      i. Use sunscreen with sun protection factor of 30 or greater. Avoid prolonged sun exposure.
      ii. Wear protective, lightweight clothing with long sleeves and wide-brimmed hats.
      iii. Avoid use of tanning beds.
   b. Avoid exposure to drugs and chemicals.
      i. Avoid exposure to hairspray.
      ii. Avoid exposure to hair-coloring agents.
      iii. Medications—obtain provider advice before taking any medications or supplements.
2. Teach self-administration of pharmacologic agents to reduce disease activity.
3. Encourage good nutrition, sleep habits, exercise, rest, and relaxation to improve general health and to help prevent infection.
4. Encourage expression of feelings, counseling, or referrals to social work, occupational therapy, as needed.

Maintaining Skin and Mucous Membrane Integrity

1. Apply topical corticosteroids to skin lesions, as ordered.
2. Suggest alternative hairstyles, scarves, and wigs to cover significant areas of alopecia.
3. Encourage good oral hygiene and inspect mouth for oral ulcers.
   a. Avoid hot or spicy foods that may irritate oral ulcers.
   b. Apply topical agents or analgesics to reduce pain and to promote eating.

Reducing Fatigue

1. Advise patient that fatigue level will fluctuate with disease activity.
2. Encourage patient to modify schedule to include several rest periods during the day; pace activity and exercise according to body's tolerance; use energy-conservation techniques in daily activities.
3. Teach relaxation techniques, such as deep breathing, progressive muscle relaxation, and imagery, to reduce emotional stress that causes fatigue.

Preserving Urinary Elimination

1. Assist with monitoring of urinary status as indicated by degree of renal involvement.
   a. Monitor intake and output and urine-specific gravity.
   b. Measure urine protein, microalbumin, or obtain 24-hour creatinine clearance, as ordered.
   c. Check test results of serum blood urea nitrogen and creatinine.
2. See page 785 for care of patients on dialysis.

Patient Education and Health Maintenance

1. Stress that close follow-up is essential, even in times of remission, to detect early progression of organ involvement and to alter drug therapy.
2. Advise on the use of special cosmetics to cover skin lesions.
3. Advise about reproduction.
   a. Avoid pregnancy during time of severe disease activity. Should have stable disease for 1 year before planning pregnancy.
   b. Immunomodulators may have teratogenic effects.
   c. Use of some drugs for treatment of SLE can result in sterility.
4. Stress that any complementary or alternative therapies should be discussed with the health care provider.
5. For additional information and support, refer to agencies such as the Lupus Foundation (*www.lupus.org*) or the American Occupational Therapy Association (*www.aota.org*).

Evaluation: Expected Outcomes

- Reports pain reduction.
- Verbalizes appropriate use of medications, avoidance of sun and chemicals, and need for nutrition and sleep to minimize disease process.
- Reports oral ulcers healing without interference with appetite.
- Reports resting three times per day, with adequate energy to carry out activities.
- Urine output adequate; specific gravity stable.

Systemic Sclerosis

Systemic sclerosis is a generalized disorder of connective tissue, characterized by hardening and thickening of the skin (scleroderma), blood vessels, synovium, skeletal muscles, and internal organs. Fibrotic, degenerative, and inflammatory changes result in changes in joints and several organ systems. New diagnositic criteria being evaluated and validated by the ACR and EULAR include 23 items.

 Evidence Base Johnson, S. R., Fransensen, J., Khanna, D., et al. (2012). Validation of potential classification criteria for systemic sclerosis. *Arthritis Care Research, 64*(3), 358–367.

Pathophysiology and Etiology

1. The changes seen in the skin and internal organs in systemic sclerosis are most likely caused by overproduction of collagen by fibroblasts.
2. The etiology of systemic sclerosis is unknown.
3. Systemic sclerosis affects three to four times as many women as men.
4. Major subtypes include:
   a. Diffuse scleroderma—rapidly progressive, generalized skin thickening of the proximal and distal extremities and trunk and tendency toward early internal organ involvement.
   b. Limited scleroderma—skin thickening is limited to the distal extremities and face.
   c. Localized forms of scleroderma—do not include visceral involvement.
   d. Overlap with other connective tissue disorders.

Clinical Manifestations

Skin

1. Bilateral symmetric swelling of the hands and, sometimes, the feet.
2. After the edematous phase, the skin becomes hard and thick.
3. Digits, dorsum of hand, neck, face, and trunk are involved.
4. Normal landmarks in skin are absent—no skin folds.
5. Increased or decreased skin pigmentation (salt and pepper skin).
6. Skin changes may regress after several years.
7. Telangiectasia—on/under tongue, face, fingers, and lips.
8. Areas of calcinosis—late in the course of disease.
9. Raynaud's phenomenon.
10. Decreased oral aperture.

GI

1. Esophageal dysmotility—resulting in reflux and dysphagia.
2. Distal esophageal dilation and esophagitis.
3. Barrett's metaplasia—may predispose to adenocarcinoma of the esophagus.
4. Duodenal atrophy dilatation—may cause postprandial abdominal pain, malabsorption, diarrhea, and abdominal distention.
5. Colonic hypomotility—results in constipation.

Musculoskeletal

1. Joint pain.
2. Polyarthritis—large and small joints affected.
3. Carpal tunnel syndrome.
4. Flexion contractures.
5. Inflammatory muscle atrophy.

Cardiac

1. Left ventricular dysfunction.
2. Myocardial involvement—heart failure and atrial and ventricular arrhythmias.
3. Right ventricular involvement—secondary to pulmonary disease.

Pulmonary

1. Interstitial fibrosis.
2. Restrictive lung disease.
3. Pulmonary hypertension.

Renal

Scleroderma renal crisis—rapid malignant hypertension with encephalopathy.

Localized Scleroderma

1. CREST—*c*alcinosis (calcium deposits of the subcutaneous tissue and periarticular tissue), *R*aynaud's phenomenon, *e*sophageal dysmotility, *s*clerodactyly (shiny, tight, atrophic appearance of skin of the fingers or toes), *t*elangiectasia.
2. Morphea—scattered patches may be several centimeters and may have a purple border.
3. Linear—lesions appear as streaks or bands.
4. Generally, no visceral involvement exists in localized scleroderma.

Diagnostic Evaluation

1. CBC and ESR—generally normal.
2. RF—positive in approximately 30% of patients.
3. ANA—generally positive with speckled or nucleolar patterns.
   a. Antisclerodermal antibody (Scl-70)—positive in diffuse cutaneous disease.
   b. Anticentromere antibody—highly specific for limited cutaneous disease.
4. Additional antibodies that have been identified include anti-RNA polymerase III antibody and anti-topoisomerase I antibody.
5. X-ray of hands and wrists—muscle atrophy, osteopenia, osteolysis.
6. Barium swallow—esophageal dysmotility.
7. Pulmonary function test—decreased diffusion capacity and vital capacity; CT of chest to evaluate for pulmonary fibrosis.
8. Multiple gated acquisition scan—to determine left ventricular function; echocardiogram to evaluate for pulmonary hypertension.
9. Endoscopy—to biopsy for Barrett's metaplasia.
10. Esophageal manometry—to determine contractile capacity of esophageal muscles.

Management

Pharmacologic

1. Calcium channel blockers; losartan or other angiotensin receptor blockers or sildenafil for more severe cases of Raynaud's phenomenon. Nitroglycerin ointment is sometimes used. Prazosin, an alpha-adrenergic agent, has a modest effect but may cause dizziness, headache, and lack of energy.

 Evidence Base Harding, S. E., Tingey, P. C., Pope, J., et al. (2009). Prazosin for Raynaud's phenomenon in progressive systemic sclerosis. The Cochrane Library (Article No. CD000956).
Effect of Sildenafil on the microcirculatory blood flow and endothelial progenitor cells in systemic sclerosis. (2011). Available: *www.clinicaltrials.gov*.

2. NSAIDs and or other analgesics for arthralgias, polyarthritis, and painful calcinosis.
3. Proton pump inhibitors for reflux.
4. Antibiotics for malabsorption because of bacterial overgrowth or secondarily infected skin ulcerations.
5. Antihypertensive agents, particularly a high-dose angiotensin-converting enzyme inhibitor such as enalapril.
6. Bronchodilators for pulmonary involvement; oxygen and cyclophosphamide may also be used in severe cases.
7. For Raynaud's phenomenon, topical L-arginine has been used on the hands to stimulate formation of nitric oxide, a vasodilator. Sildenafil may be helpful with symptoms. Severe symptoms may also respond to injections of botox.

 Evidence Base Botox and Raynaud's. (2012, August 2). Raynaud's & Scleroderma Association. Available: *www.raynauds.org.uk/press/botox-and-raynauds*.

 DRUG ALERT L-arginine should not be used with nitrates and antihypertensives; vasodilating effect may cause excessive drop in blood pressure.

Nonpharmacologic

1. Skin lubricants and care for ulcerations to promote healing.
2. Lifestyle modification for control of Raynaud's phenomenon:
   a. Increased environmental temperature.
   b. Appropriate dress with gloves and heavy socks.
   c. Avoidance of handling cold and frozen items without gloves.
   d. Avoidance of wind and exposure to cold weather.
   e. Use of hand and foot warmers.
   f. Smoking cessation.
3. Raynaud's attack can possibly be aborted by placing hand or foot in tepid water.
4. Biofeedback to abort or prevent Raynaud's attack.
5. Smoking cessation and immunization against pneumococcal pneumonia and influenza for pulmonary involvement.
6. Dietary modifications for GI involvement:
   a. Avoidance of caffeinated beverages.
   b. Eating smaller meals.
   c. Remaining upright after meals for at least 3 hours.
   d. Avoidance of alcohol.
   e. Elevating the head of the bed.
7. Physical therapy to help prevent contractures.

Complications

1. Skin ulcers.
2. Malabsorption.
3. Esophageal adenocarcinoma.
4. Pulmonary hypertension.
5. Renal failure.
6. Heart failure.
7. Death caused by disease process.

Nursing Assessment

1. Focus physical assessment on:
   a. Skin ulcers, thickening, subcutaneous deposits, secondary infection.
   b. Joint examination—flexion contractures.
   c. Pulmonary examination—for shortness of breath and wheezing.
   d. Blood pressure and renal status.
2. Determine nutritional intake.
3. Assess mood, support system, and coping ability.

Nursing Diagnoses

- Ineffective Peripheral Tissue Perfusion related to Raynaud's phenomenon.
- Risk for Impaired Skin Integrity related to effects of disease process.
- Imbalanced Nutrition: Less Than Body Requirements related to impaired swallowing and GI involvement.
- Disturbed Body Image related to effects of disease.

Nursing Interventions

Maintaining Tissue Perfusion

1. Teach patient to identify Raynaud's phenomenon.
   a. Characteristic color change of the fingers—white, blue, red.
   b. Coldness, pallor, numbness, pain.
2. Teach patient to reduce factors associated with precipitation or exacerbation of Raynaud's phenomenon.
   a. Dress warmly—cover head and extremities, keep trunk warm.
   b. Discontinue tobacco usage.
   c. Avoid prolonged exposure to cold.
      i. Weather.
      ii. Artificially controlled environments (eg, air conditioning).
      iii. Limit contact with cold food items, such as frozen foods, ice cube trays—use gloves or tongs.
3. Protect ulcerated digits and report signs of infection.

Preserving Skin Integrity

1. Use moisturizers on skin daily.
2. Advise patient to avoid use of drying soaps and detergents.

3. Use protective padding (eg, elbow pads) to protect the skin from friction or trauma.

4. Inspect skin daily for cracking, ulceration, and signs of infection.

5. Soak ulcerations, apply topical antibiotic, and use occlusive dressings, as directed.

Achieving Optimal Nutritional Status

1. Make sure patient is in proper position for meals to avoid aspiration (ie, in chair if possible).

2. Provide smaller, more frequent feedings of well-balanced diet.

3. Encourage patient to remain upright after meals for 45 to 60 minutes and raise head of bed during sleep to avoid reflux.

4. Administer or teach self-administration of medications to prevent nausea and reflux, as ordered.

5. Encourage good oral hygiene and frequent dental visits.

6. Advise the use of lubricating agents, if necessary, to treat dry mouth and to teach stretching exercises of mouth to maintain aperture.

7. Weigh weekly and ask patient to keep food diary.

Strengthening Body Image

1. Encourage patient to take an active role in treatment plan to feel in control of body changes.

2. Explain that changes may be gradual and slow; although not noticeable, internal organ involvement is even more important than external changes.

3. Suggest continuance of activities that patient enjoys and foster strong support network.

4. Refer for counseling, as needed.

Patient Education and Health Maintenance

1. Explain diagnostic tests and their purpose in detecting GI, pulmonary, or renal involvement.

2. Teach about drug treatment and adverse effects.

3. Advise on modifying activity and using bronchodilators and oxygen to prevent dyspnea caused by restrictive lung disease.

4. Encourage regular follow-up visits and prompt attention to worsening symptoms.

5. Refer to agencies such as United Scleroderma Foundation (*www.scleroderma.org*).

Evaluation: Expected Outcomes

- Relates factors that precipitate Raynaud's phenomenon.
- Reports no skin cracking or ulceration.
- Reports no weight loss.
- Reports participating in community and church activities and groups.

Gout

Gout is a disorder of purine metabolism, characterized by elevated uric acid levels and deposition of urate (usually in the form of crystals) in joints and other tissues. More common in men, but may affect postmenopausal women, especially those taking diuretics.

Pathophysiology and Etiology

Gout results from an overabundant accumulation and subsequent deposition of monosodium urate crystals in joints and other connective tissue. This can occur in one of two ways.

Overproduction of Uric Acid (10% of Cases)

1. Inherited enzyme defects.

2. Certain conditions:
   a. Myeloproliferative disorders.
   b. Lymphoproliferative disorders.
   c. Cancer chemotherapy.
   d. Hemolytic anemias.
   e. Psoriasis.

Underexcretion of Uric Acid (90% of Cases)

1. Renal disease.

2. Endocrine disorders.

3. Medications and chemicals:
   a. Diuretics, beta blockers, angiotensin converting enzyme inhibitors.

 Evidence Base Choi, H. K., Soriano, L. C., & Zhang, Y. (2012). Antihypertensive drugs and risk of incident gout among patients with hypertension: Population-based control study. *British Medical Journal*, 344, d8190.

   b. Ethanol (alcohol).
   c. Low-dose aspirin.
   d. Pyrazinamide—antituberculosis agent.
   e. Lead.

4. Volume depletion states—nephrogenic diabetes insipidus.

Clinical Manifestations

Acute Gouty Arthritis

1. Generally affects one joint—commonly the first metatarsophalangeal joint (called podagra); however, in women is often polyarticular.

2. Other joints can be affected, such as ankle, tarsals, knee; upper extremities are less commonly involved.

3. Pain, warmth, erythema, and swelling of tissue surrounding the affected joint.

4. Fever may occur.

5. Onset of symptoms is sudden; intensity is severe.

6. Duration of symptoms is self-limiting; lasts approximately 3 to 10 days without treatment.

Chronic Tophaceous Gout

1. Occurs if acute gout is inadequately treated or if it goes untreated.

2. Characterized by development of tophi or deposits of uric acid in and around joints, cartilage, and soft tissues.

3. Arthritis is more prolonged in nature with discrete attacks less common.

4. Arthritis can produce bone erosions and subsequent bony deformities that can resemble RA.

Hyperuricemia

1. Produces no symptoms but is characterized by persistent elevation of uric acid in the blood.
2. Renal calculi composed of uric acid may develop.
3. Deposition of uric acid in kidney tissue causing nephropathy.

Diagnostic Evaluation

1. Synovial fluid analysis.
   a. Identification of monosodium urate crystals under polarized microscopy.
   b. Synovial WBC count can range from 2,000 to 100,000/mm³.
   c. Culture of synovial fluid to rule out infection.
2. Twenty-four-hour urine for uric acid to determine overproduction of uric acid versus underexcretion.
3. ESR—elevated.
4. X-rays of affected joints may show changes consistent with diagnosis of gout.

Management

Acute Management

1. NSAIDs for acute attacks to relieve pain and swelling; considered first-line therapy.
2. Colchicine for acute treatment and prevention of attacks; considered second-line therapy.
   a. May be given orally at onset of an attack, taken b.i.d. to t.i.d. as tolerated (may cause nausea, cramping, diarrhea).
   b. Taken once daily on continuous basis to prevent attack, usually while transitioning to urate-lowering medications. May be used every other day for patients with chronic kidney disease.

 Evidence Base Schlesinger, N., Schumacher, R., Catton, M., et al. (2009). Colchicine for acute gout. The Cochrane Library (Article No. CD006190).

3. Corticosteroids.
   a. Intra-articular if attack confined to one or two joints.
   b. Oral—in short-tapering course if other treatments are contraindicated or if attack involves many joints.
4. Increase fluids (orally because usually treated as outpatient) and rest joint for 48 hours.

Chronic Management

1. Urate-lowering agents (antihyperuremic agents) are taken to prevent progressive articular damage in cases of asymptomatic hyperuricemia and chronic tophaceous gout.
   a. Allopurinol—interferes with conversion of hypoxanthine and xanthine to uric acid. May also be given to prevent renal calculi and kidney disease.
   b. Feboxustat—a xanthine oxidase inhibitor, which lowers uric acid associated with fewer drug interactions than allopurinol.
   c. Uricosuric drugs, such as probenecid—interfere with tubular reabsorption of uric acid.

2. Adverse reactions for these drugs include headache, anorexia, nausea and vomiting, allergic reaction, hemolytic anemia and other blood dyscrasias, and worsening of gout. Urinary frequency and uric acid kidney stones may occur with probenecid.
3. Rapid increase or decrease of uric acid may precipitate a gout flare, so medication usually started at a low dose and titrated up.

 DRUG ALERT Exfoliative dermatitis (sometimes fatal) and liver and biliary dysfunction may occur with use of allopurinol and feboxustat.

4. Uric acid levels and renal function are monitored during chronic therapy. A small percentage of patients develop elevated liver functions with urate-lowering treatment.

Lifestyle Modification

1. Avoidance of obesity and fluctuations in weight.
2. Avoidance of alcohol—can precipitate gout attacks through overproduction and decreased excretion of urate.
3. Low-purine diet gives only a minor decrease in serum uric acid levels.
4. Moderate coffee consumption has been linked to decreased uric acid levels.

Complications

1. Uric acid renal calculus.
2. Urate nephropathy.
3. Erosive, deforming arthritis/contractures.

Nursing Assessment

1. Obtain history for factors predisposing to gout, such as malignancy, alcoholism, renal insufficiency.
2. Perform physical examination.
   a. Inspect involved joint for pain, swelling, redness, warmth, effusion.
   b. Observe for tophi over pinna of ear, olecranon bursa, Achilles tendon, and fingertips.
3. Assess pain and pain relief pattern if attack is acute.

Nursing Diagnoses

- Acute Pain related to acute arthritis.
- Impaired Physical Mobility related to arthritis.

Nursing Interventions

Relieving Pain

1. Administer and teach self-administration of pain-relieving medications, as prescribed.
2. Encourage adequate fluid intake to assist with excretion of uric acid and to decrease likelihood of stone formation.
3. Instruct patient to take prescribed medications consistently because interruptions in therapy can precipitate acute attacks.
4. Encourage patient to follow up as directed, usually in 48 hours, then 4 to 8 weeks after acute attack to evaluate for chronic therapy.

Facilitating Mobility

1. Elevate and protect affected joint during acute attack.
2. Assist with ADLs.
3. Encourage exercise and maintenance of routine activity in chronic gout, except during acute attacks.
4. Protect draining tophi by covering and applying antibiotic ointment, as needed.

Patient Education and Health Maintenance

1. Instruct patient and family in nature of disease.
   a. Generally, acute attacks are followed by periods of remission.
   b. Once need for chronic treatment has been determined, it will generally be lifelong.
2. Encourage avoidance of alcohol.
3. Avoid rapid weight loss by fasting or crash diets because rapid weight loss results in production of chemicals that compete with uric acid for excretion from the body, resulting in increased uric acid levels.
4. Avoid medications known to increase uric acid levels, such as aspirin, diuretics, and cyclosporine.
5. Advise prompt treatment of acute attack to reduce joint damage associated with repeated attacks.
6. Instruct about signs and symptoms of allopurinol hypersensitivity syndrome and need to report promptly.
7. Advise patients to avoid foods containing purines (ie, sardines, anchovies, shellfish, organ meats) and, in general, to consume meat, seafood, and high-calorie food in moderation.

Evaluation: Expected Outcomes

- Reports relief from pain.
- Performs ADLs with minimal assistance.

Sjögren's Syndrome

Sjögren's syndrome is a chronic inflammatory autoimmune process that affects the lacrimal and salivary glands. The disease can be primary or secondary. Secondary Sjögren's syndrome is seen most commonly in RA but can be seen in SLE and some other connective tissue diseases. New diagnostic criteria involve at least two of three items (presence of antibodies, ocular staining score, lymphocytic sialadenitis).

 Evidence Base Shiboski, S. C, Shiboski, C. H., Criswell, L., et al. (2012). American College of Rheumatology classification criteria for Sjögren's syndrome: A data-driven, expert consensus approach in the Sjögren's International Collaborative Clinical Alliance cohort. *Arthritis Care and Research, 64*(4), 475–487.

Pathophysiology and Etiology

1. The etiology of the syndrome is unknown, but is thought to include several factors: genetic predisposition, immunologic, infectious, and hormonal.
2. It is thought that antibodies directed at exocrine glands are produced, leading to disturbed function of the involved tissue.

3. Lymphocytes are found infiltrating affected tissues.
4. Sjögren's syndrome occurs primarily in middle-aged women.

Clinical Manifestations

1. Ocular—xerophthalmia (dry eyes) due to decreased tear formation that leads to keratoconjunctivitis, photophobia, greater than 3 months. Positive Schermer's or positve vital dying test.
2. Oral—xerostomia (dry mouth) caused by diminished production of saliva, mucosal ulcers, stomatitis, greater than 3 months. Need for fluids to swallow food.
3. Recurrent or persistent salivary gland enlargement—unilateral or bilateral.
4. Dryness of the skin, vagina, and other tissues may also occur.
5. Extraglandular features include rash, dysphagia, Raynaud's phenomenon, arthralgias/arthritis, and myalgias.
6. Less commonly, major organ dysfunction, such as interstitial pneumonitis, glomerulonephritis, vasculitis, thyroid disease, and central and peripheral neuropathy may occur.

Diagnostic Evaluation

1. CBC—mild anemia, leukopenia present in 30% of patients.
2. ESR—elevated in 90% of patients.
3. RF—positive in 75% to 90% of patients.
4. ANA—positive in 70% of patients; speckled and nucleolar patterns are most common; titer more than 1:320.
5. Antibodies to SSA/SSB—detects antibodies to specific nuclear proteins.
   a. SSA (Ro antibody)—positive in patients with Sjögren's syndrome and SLE.
   b. SSB (La antibody)—positive in patients with Sjögren's syndrome; also in patients with SLE.
6. Organ-specific antibodies—antibodies directed against specific organ tissues have been found (eg, antithyroid antibodies).
7. Salivary scintigraphy—salivary gland function is measured by determining excretion of radioisotope dye.
8. X-rays of affected joints to rule out erosive arthritis.
9. Salivary gland biopsy—to determine lymphocytic infiltration of tissue and confirm diagnosis; usually done on one of the minor salivary glands, in the lower lip.

Management

Systemic Drugs

1. NSAIDs and hydroxychloroquine may be used to try to control symptoms.
2. Corticosteroids and immunosuppressants may be used in severe cases.
3. Antifungal agents—used for oral candidiasis.
4. Pilocarpine or cevimeline, systemic parasympathomimetic agents—used to improve salivation when there is some salivary gland function.

Topical Agents

1. Cyclosporine emulsion eyedrops to reduce ocular inflammation and increase tear production.

2. Over-the-counter products that contain salivary stimulants or substitutes.
   a. A meta-analysis of 36 randomized controlled trials showed slight benefit with oxygenated glycerol triester sprays over enzyme sprays as saliva substitutes.
   b. Integrated mouth care systems (toothpaste, gel, mouthwash) and oral reservoir devices show promising results, but more research is needed.
   c. Chewing gum is effective for people with residual salivary capacity.
3. Symptomatic relief of dryness.
   a. Artificial tears, lubricant inserts.
   b. Frequent use of nonsugared liquids, gums, and candies.
   c. Vaginal lubricants.
4. Dental care.
   a. Frequent brushing and flossing.
   b. Topical fluoride treatments.
   c. Avoidance of high-sucrose foods.
5. Avoidance of drying.
   a. Avoid windy, low-humidity environments, cigarette smoke.
   b. Avoid anticholinergic medications, such as antihistamines.
   c. Use of occlusive goggles at bedtime to prevent drying.

Complications

1. Ocular complications, such as corneal ulceration, corneal opacification, vascularization of the cornea, infection, glaucoma, cataract formation.
2. Dental caries and tooth loss.
3. Lymphoma.

Nursing Assessment

1. Obtain history of signs and symptoms, emphasizing dryness.
2. Perform complete physical examination, focusing on oral cavity, eyes, skin, lungs, GI, and neurologic systems.
3. Assess nutritional status because decreased saliva may make eating difficult.

Nursing Diagnoses

- Impaired Oral Mucous Membrane related to disease process.
- Risk for Impaired Skin Integrity related to dryness.
- Imbalanced Nutrition: Less Than Body Requirements related to disturbances in saliva production, taste, and difficulty swallowing.
- Sexual Dysfunction related to discomfort of decreased vaginal secretions.

Nursing Interventions

Maintaining Mucous Membranes

 **Evidence Base** Furness, S., Worthington, H. V., Bryan, G., et al. (2011). Interventions for the management of dry mouth: Topical therapies. The Cochrane Library (Article No. CD008934).

1. Inspect oral mucosa for oral *Candida*, ulcers, saliva pools, and dental hygiene.

2. Instruct and assist patient in proper oral hygiene.
   a. At least twice-daily brushing.
   b. Frequent rinsing with antiseptic mouthwash.
3. Encourage frequent intake of noncaffeinated, nonsugared liquids. Keep pitcher filled with cool water.
4. Promptly report any ulcers or signs of infections.

Protecting Skin Integrity

1. Instruct and assist patient with daily inspection of skin for areas of trauma or for potential breakdown.
2. Apply lubricants to skin daily.
3. Avoid shearing forces and encourage or perform frequent position changes.

Promoting Adequate Nutritional Intake

1. Increase liquid intake with meals.
2. Assist and instruct patient to avoid choosing spicy or dry foods from menu choices.
3. Suggest small, more frequent meals.
4. Weigh weekly and review diet history for deficiency in basic nutrients.

Promoting Optimal Sexual Functioning

1. Encourage patient to discuss sexual difficulty and to explain its relation to disease process.
2. Advise on proper use of water-soluble vaginal lubrication.
3. Suggest alternative positioning and practices to prevent discomfort.
4. Teach patient to report symptoms of vaginitis—discharge, irritation, itching—because infection may result from altered mucosal barrier.

Patient Education and Health Maintenance

1. Advise patient of commercially available artificial saliva preparations, artificial tears, moisturizing nasal sprays, artificial vaginal moisturizers.
2. Encourage frequent dental visits. Dental cavities are more frequent in Sjögren's syndrome.
3. Advise patient to check with health care provider before using any medications because many, such as diuretics, tricyclic antidepressants, and antihistamines, have the adverse effect of mouth dryness.
4. Advise patient to wear protective eyewear while outdoors.
5. Encourage support through Sjögren's Syndrome Foundation (*www.sjogrens.org*) or the American College of Rheumatology (*www.rheumatology.org/public/factsheets/index.asp*).

Evaluation: Expected Outcomes

- Demonstrates proper oral hygiene.
- Reports skin without cracking, scaling, or other lesions.
- Maintains weight.
- Describes correct use of water-soluble lubricants.

Fibromyalgia

Fibromyalgia is a syndrome characterized by fatigue, diffuse muscle pain and stiffness, sleep disturbance, and tender points on physical examination.

Pathophysiology and Etiology

1. Etiology is unknown.
2. It affects 3 to 6 million Americans, usually women between ages 29 to 37.
3. Fibromyalgia most likely represents a complex pain syndrome in which there is abnormality in central sensory processing, dysregulation of peripheral pain receptors, and psychoneuroendocrine dysfunction.
4. Clinical features include:
   a. Reduction in pain threshold.
   b. Increased response to painful stimuli.
   c. Mild muscle contraction or tension results in postexertion muscle pain.
   d. Decreased muscle strength and endurance, resulting in deconditioning.

Clinical Manifestations

Evidence Base Wolfe, F., Clauw, D. J., Fitzcharles, M., et al. (2010). The American College of Rheumatology preliminary diagnostic criteria for fibromyalgia and measurement of symptom severity. *Arthritis Care and Research, 62*(5), 600–610.

Wolfe, F., Smythe, H. A., Yunus, M. B., et al. (1990). The American College of Rheumatology 1990 criteria for the classification of fibromyalgia: Report of the Multicenter Criteria Committee. *Arthritis and Rheumatology, 33*, 160–172.

1. Widespread pain and tenderness on physical exam (see Figure 30-5). Diagnostic criteria proposed in 2010 include a widespread pain index, fatigue, awakening unrefreshed, and number of somatic symptoms, relying less on an absolute tender point count, which has been widely used since 1990.
2. Additional symptoms include:
   a. Chronic fatigue and easy fatigability.
   b. Sleep is poor or nonrestorative.
   c. Possible joint pain and stiffness.
   d. Additional somatic complaints such as headache, nausea, abdominal pain.

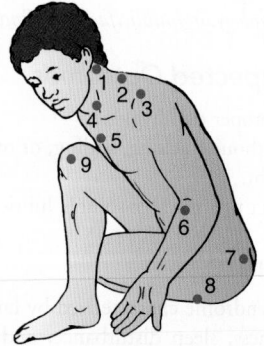

Figure 30-5. Fibromyalgia trigger points.

3. Exacerbation of symptoms occurs due to cold weather, stress, poor sleep, infection, and exertion.

Diagnostic Evaluation

1. To rule out other disorders—test results generally normal in fibromyalgia.
2. Complete history and physical examination.
   a. CBC.
   b. Blood chemistries.
   c. ESR.
   d. Thyroid-stimulating hormone.
3. Sleep study may be done to rule out organic sleep disorder causing fatigue.

Management

Treatment is aimed at symptom management and should be individualized, comprehensive, and goal-oriented.

Pharmacologic

1. Nonopioid analgesics are used to relieve pain.
   a. NSAIDs and acetaminophen are rarely effective alone.
   b. Tramadol may be effective if taken regularly at 50 to 100 mg every 4 to 6 hours.
   c. A small subgroup of patients with fibromyalgia may require and respond well to opioids.
2. Low-dose tricyclic antidepressants improve sleep quality and help control chronic pain and depression. Other antidepressants may also be used for concomitant depression.
3. Sleep medication may be used occasionally or on a regular basis in some cases.
   a. Short-acting hypnotic agents, such as zolpidem or zaleplon, are effective without causing a drug "hangover" in the morning.
   b. Ramelteon is a melatonin receptor agonist that helps to promote sleep and is indicated for treatment on a long-term basis.

DRUG ALERT Teach patients not to take ramelteon after a fatty meal due to problems with absorption. Tell patients taking sleep medication to report any unusual behavior or thoughts of suicide while taking the medication.

   c. Periodic limb movements and restless leg syndrome that interfere with sleep can be treated with such medication as ropinirole or clonazepam.
4. Gabapentin and pregabalin, anti-epileptics, may be tried for chronic pain control. Dosage is titrated and effects are seen over time for some patients.

Evidence Base Moore, R. A., Wiffen, P. J., Derry, H., et al. (2011). Gabapentin for chronic neuropathic pain and fibromyalgia in adults. The Cochrane Library (Article No. CD007938).

Moore, R. A., Straube, S., Wiffen, P. J., et al. (2010). Pregabalin for acute and chronic pain in adults. The Cochrane Library (Article No. CD007676).

DRUG ALERT There are risks for birth defects for women and men of childbearing years while taking pregabalin.

5. Duloxetine and minacipran, serotonin and norepinephrine reuptake inhibitors, are approved by the FDA for symptom relief in fibromyalgia.

Nonpharmacologic

1. Exercise is important and should be initiated at a level below the level expected for the patient and gradually increased.
   a. Overtraining is to be avoided to prevent muscle microtrauma, which increases pain.
   b. Stretching, strength training, and aerobic exercise should be included in every patient's exercise plan.
   c. Walking; water aerobics; daily activities, such as gardening; and use of exercise equipment, such as a bike or treadmill, can be part of the patient's exercise routine.
2. Relaxation training through visualization, electromyogram biofeedback, and other techniques.
3. Cognitive-behavioral therapy for feelings of depression, confusion, and irritability.
   a. Patient may learn to think non-negatively by visualizing a stop sign when negative thoughts enter the mind.
   b. Patient can be taught to control anxiety by learning to stop, become aware of his body, and take deep breaths.
4. Meditation, prayer, and other spiritual practices.

Complications

1. Deconditioning.
2. Work disability.
3. Inability to fulfill social role.
4. Unnecessary diagnostic and therapeutic maneuvers.

Nursing Assessment

1. Assess pain level because it varies during the day/week.
2. Assess functional ability.
3. Assess mood, support system, and coping mechanisms.
4. Assess lifestyle factors that may be impairing well-being—smoking, lack of exercise, poor posture.

Nursing Diagnoses

- Chronic Pain related to disease process.
- Disturbed Sleep Pattern related to disease process.
- Ineffective Role Performance related to disabling disease process.

Nursing Interventions

Controlling Pain

1. Encourage regular use of analgesics and antidepressants, as directed.
2. Encourage regular exercise routine, including stretching, aerobic activity, and muscle-strengthening exercises.
3. Suggest referrals to physical therapist or pain specialist for additional pain-control modalities, as needed.

4. Suggest referral to psychiatrist or therapist for anxiety, depression, and cognitive or behavioral impairments. Up to 80% of fibromyalgia patients have these symptoms but only 10% are referred.

Improving Sleep

1. Suggest regular nighttime ritual to promote sleep. Advise avoidance of reading, watching television, or using a computer while in bed.
2. Discourage staying up late and other erratic sleep habits.
3. Encourage relaxation periods or short naps during the day, as needed, for fatigue.
4. Advise limiting caffeine intake during the day, especially after 4:00 PM.
5. Discourage alcohol as a sleep aid; instead, advise patient to discuss sleep problems with health care provider.

Strengthening Roles

1. Encourage patient to look at fibromyalgia as a chronic condition that can be controlled.
2. Suggest a fibromyalgia support group.
3. Tell the patient that fibromyalgia is not a progressive debilitating disease and that most people gain control of their symptoms.
4. Help patient plan schedule and pace activities to accomplish routine activities.

Patient Education and Health Maintenance

1. Educate patient and family that fibromyalgia is a real disorder that causes pain and fatigue despite normal test results and lack of ill appearance.
2. Explain proper use of analgesics and potential adverse effects.
3. Encourage regular activity as much as possible and avoid physical and emotional stress.
4. Advise patient to discuss all types of alternative and complementary therapy with health care provider.
5. Encourage regular follow-up visits with primary care provider, rheumatologist, and physical therapist, as indicated.
6. Suggest further help and information from Fibromyalgia Network (*www.fmnetnews.com*) or the Arthritis Foundation (*www.arthritis.org*). Many local support groups are also available through community hospitals.

Evaluation: Expected Outcomes

- States pain at 0 to 2 level.
- Sleeping 8 hours per night with 0 to 1 short awakenings.
- Goes to work, takes care of children.

Other Rheumatologic Disorders

A number of other conditions affect the joints and periarticular tissue.

Seronegative spondyloarthropathies are inflammatory conditions with negative rheumatoid factor or other autoantibodies, but are associated with HLA-B27 antigen. NSAIDs are generally used for treatment, but DMARDs and biologic agents may also be used. Seronegative spondyloarthropathies include the following:

1. Ankylosing spondylitis—characterized by lower back stiffness and possible ocular, cardiac, and pulmonary manifestations.
2. Reiter's disease—characterized by the triad of urethritis, arthritis, and conjunctivitis.
3. Arthritis—associated with inflammatory bowel disease.
4. Psoriatic arthritis—characterized by arthritis and the skin lesions of psoriasis.
5. Polymyositis (dermatomyositis if rash around eyes is present)—an inflammatory disease of striated muscles that most commonly affects the proximal limb girdle, neck, pharynx, proximal third of the esophagus, and occasionally the heart. Corticosteroids and methotrexate are used for treatment but response is slow.
6. Calcium pyrophosphate dihydrate crystal deposition disease, also known as pseudogout—results in crystal deposition in the joint cartilage and menisci, bursae, and periarticular tissue and can present similar to gout. Treatment is similar, although urate-lowering therapies have no place in treatment.
7. Polymyalgia rheumatica—an inflammatory disease with elevated ESR that affects mostly women older than age 50 and presents with profound stiffness, usually in the shoulder girdle and hips. It responds well to low-dose corticosteroids.
8. Sarcoidosis—a chronic, granulomatous multisystem disorder that most notably affects the lungs but can mimic rheumatic disease by causing fever, arthritis, uveitis, myositis, and rash. May also be treated with steroid-sparing DMARDs and biologic agents, such as infliximab or adalimumab.

Nursing care for patients with these disorders is similar to that for RA.

SELECTED REFERENCES

Aletaha, D., Neoqi, T., Silman, A. J., et al. (2010). 2010 rheumatoid arthritis classification criteria: An American College of Rheumatology/European League Against Rheumatism Collaborative Initiative. *Annals of Rheumatic Disease, 69*(9), 1580–1588.

American College of Rheumatology. (2008) Position statement: Complementary and alternative medicine for rheumatologic disease. Atlanta, GA: Author. Available: *www.rheumatology.org/publications/position/complementary.asp.*

American College of Rheumatology. (2009). American College of Rheumatology position statement: Biologic agents for rheumatic disease. Atlanta, GA: Author. Available: *www.rheumatology.org/publications/biologics.asp.*

Aschenbrenner, D. S. (2011). New use for duloxetine. *American Journal of Nursing, 111*(3), 23.

Bernatsky, S., Kale, M., Ramsey-Goldman, R., et al. (2012). Systemic lupus and malignancies. *Current Opinion in Rheumatology, 24*(2), 177–181.

Brosseau, L., Yonge, K. A., Welch, V. et al. (2009). Transcutaneous electrical nerve stimulation (TENS) for the treatment of rheumatoid arthritis in the hand. The Cochrane Library (Article No. CD004377).

Bukhari, M. (2012). Drug induced rheumatic diseases. *Current Opinion in Rheumatology, 24*(2), 182–186.

Cameron, M., Gangier, J. J., & Chrubasik, S. (2011). Herbal therapy for treating rheumatoid arthritis. The Cochrane Library (Article No. CD002948).

Chakravarty, S. D., & Markenson, J. A. (2013). Rheumatic manifestations of endocrine disease. *Current Opinion in Rheumatology, 25*(1), 37–43.

Choi, H. K., Soriano, L. C., & Zhang, Y. (2012). Antihypertensive drugs and risk of incident gout among patients with hypertension: Population-based control study. *British Medical Journal, 344*, d8190.

Dasgupta, B., Cimmino, M. A., Kremers, H. M., et al. (2012). Provisional classification criteria for polymyalgia rheumatica: A European League Against Rheumatism/American College of Rheumatology collaborative initiative. *Arthritis and Rheumatism, 64*(4), 943–954.

Dougados, M., Khanna, D., King, C. M., et al. (2012). Multinational evidence-based recommendations for pain management by pharmacotherapy in inflammatory arthritis: Integrating systematic literature research and expert opinion of a broad panel of rheumatologists in the 3e Initiative. *Arthritis Care and Research, 64*(5), 625–639.

Fries, J. F., Spitz, P., Kraines, G., et al. (1980). Measurement of patient outcome in arthritis. *Arthritis and Rheumatism, 23*, 137–145.

Furness, S., Worthington, H. V., Bryan, G., et al. (2011). Interventions for the management of dry mouth: topical therapies. The Cochrane Library (Article No. CD008934).

Gärtner, M., Fabrizii, J. P., Koban, E., et al. (2012). Immediate access rheumatology clinic: Efficiency and outcomes. *Annals of Rheumatic Disease, 71*(3), 363–368.

Gill, D., Derry, S., Wiffen, P. J., et al. (2011). Valproic acid and sodium valproate for neuropathic pain and fibromyalgia in adults. The Cochrane Library (Article No. CD009183).

Gow, P. (2011). Treating gout in patients with comorbidities. *International Journal of Clinical Rheumatology, 6*(6), 625–633.

Guermazi, A., Roemer, F. W., Hayashi, D., et al. (2011). Imaging of osteoarthritis: Update from a radiological perspective. *Current Opinion in Rheumatology, 23*(5), 484-491.

Harding, S. E., Tingey, P. C., Pope, J., et al. (2009). Prazosin for Raynaud's phenomenon in progressive systemic sclerosis. The Cochrane Library (Article No. CD000956).

Haynes, R. B., Ackloo, E., Sahota, N., et al. (2008). Interventions for enhancing medication adherence. The Cochrane Library (Article No. CD00011).

Hochberg, M. C., Chang, R. W., Dwosh, I., et al. (1991). American College of Rheumatology–revised criteria for classification for global functional status in rheumatoid arthritis. *Arthritis and Rheumatism, 35*(5), 498–502.

Hochberg, M. C., Chang, R. W., Dwosh, I., et al. (1992). The American College of Rheumatology 1991 revised criteria for the classification of global functional status in rheumatoid arthritis. *Arthritis and Rheumatism, 35*, 498–502.

Hootman, J. M., Watson, K. B., Harris, C., et al. (2011). State-specific prevalence of no leisure-time physical activity among adults with and without doctor-diagnosed arthritis. *Morbidity and Mortality Weekly Report, 60*(48), 1641–1645.

Johnson, S. R., Fransensen, J., Khanna, D., et al. (2012). Validation of potential classification criteria for systemic sclerosis. *Arthritis Care Research, 64*(3), 358–367.

Keystone, E. C., Papp, K. A., & Wobeser W. (2011). Challenges in diagnosing latent tuberculosis infection in patients treated with tumor necrosis factor antagonists. *Journal of Rheumatology, 38*, 1234–1243.

Klippel, J. H., Stone, J. H., Crofford, L. J., et al. (2008). *Primer on the rheumatic diseases* (13th ed.). New York: Springer.

MacIsaac, A. M., Colicchia, R., Helm, J., et al. (2011). *Standards of practice: Professional nursing competencies in rheumatology.* Atlanta, GA: American College of Rheumatolgoy.

Moore, R. A., Straube, S., Wiffen, P. J., et al. (2010). Pregabalin for acute and chronic pain in adults. The Cochrane Library (Article No. CD007676).

Moore, R. A., Wiffen, P. J., Derry, H., et al. (2011). Gabapentin for chronic neuropathic pain and fibromyalgia in adults. The Cochrane Library (Article No. CD007938).

National Center for Complementary and Alternative Medicine. (2010). Rheumatoid arthritis and complementary and alternative medicine. Bethesda, MD: Author. Available: *http://nccam.nih.gov/health/RA/getthefacts.htm.*

Petri, M., Orbai, A. M., Alarcon, G. S., et al. (2012). Derivation and validation of the Systemic Lupus International Collaborating Clinics classification criteria for systemic lupus erythematosus. *Arthritis and Rheumatism, 64*(8), 2677–2686.

Richards, B. L., Whittle, S. L., & Buchbinder, R. (2011). Antidepressants for pain management in rheumatoid arthritis. The Cochrane Library (Article No. CD008920).

Richards, B. L., Whittle, S. L., & Buchbinder, R. (2012). Muscle relaxants for pain management in rheumatoid arthritis. The Cochrane Library (Article No. CD008922).

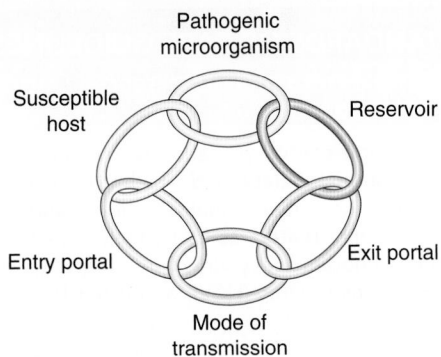

Figure 31-1. Chain of infection.

Mode of Transmission

How the pathogenic microorganism is spread to a host by an infectious source. Horizontal transmission is the spread of a pathogen from one individual to another individual or vertically from mother to offspring via transplacental transmission, contact through the birth canal, or through breastfeeding or close contact after birth. There are two main types of transmission: direct and indirect.

Direct Transmission

1. Direct contact—infected by touching the reservoir (eg, *Clostridium difficile* fecal-to-oral transmission or rubella virus crossing the placenta to the fetus).
2. Droplet transmission.
   a. Droplets of large particles more than 5 microns in size usually from respiratory secretions.
   b. Transmitted through coughing, sneezing, or talking to an infected person (eg, human metapneumovirus spread through coughing).
   c. Transmitted through aerosolizing procedures (eg, sprays of infectious agents during a nebulization treatment or a sputum induction).
3. Airborne transmission.
   a. Droplet nuclei—less than 5 microns that remains suspended in air (eg, tuberculosis and varicella [primary chickenpox]).
   b. Dust particles in the air containing the infectious agent (eg, *Aspergillus* fungi through dust).

Indirect Transmission

Touching an inanimate object or fomite that has had direct contact with the reservoir (eg, touching a tissue of a child with Influenza virus or touching a bedside table contaminated with *Clostridium difficile*).

Table 31-1	Multidrug-Resistant Organisms (MDROs)	
ORGANISM	**OVERVIEW AND TRANSMISSION**	**PREVENTION (ALL)**
Methicillin-resistant *Staphylococcus aureus* (MRSA)	Found in various body sites but especially in nares and on skin. Can produce toxins and invade body tissues. Transmitted via direct and indirect contact. Drug of choice: vancomycin.	• Hand hygiene with soap or alcohol-based hand sanitizer. • Use of gloves and gowns for patient contact. • Isolate patient in private room or cohort patients with the same organisms on contact isolation. • Use disposable equipment or disinfect reusable items after removal from room. • Utilize a system for prompt identification and isolation of patients upon readmission and for discharge planning. • Health care worker, patient and family education.
Vancomycin-resistant enterococci (VRE)	Found in GI tract and female GU tract. Relatively weak pathogen, but if infection occurs treatment options are limited. Transmitted via direct and indirect contact.	
Vancomycin intermediate- *or* vancomycin resistant-*Staphylococcus aureus* (VISA/VRSA)	Transmitted via direct and indirect contact. An epidemiologically significant organism that must be reported to the Centers for Disease Control and Prevention (CDC) and the local health department. Strictly follow contact precautions and dedicate staff for one-to-one care.	
Multidrug-resistant Gram-negative rods such as *Escherichia coli*, *Klebsiella pneumoniae*, *Acinetobacter* species, and *Pseudomonas aeruginosa*	Found in various body sites, especially sputum. Spread via direct and indirect contact.	
Emerging MDROs • Extended-spectrum metallo-beta lactamase (ESBLs) producers • Carbapenem-resistant enterobacteriaceae (CRE) • New Delhi metallo-b lactamase (NDM-1)	Produced by some Gram-negative bacteria, making them resistant to multiple antibiotics. Spread via direct and indirect contact. Limited treatment options due to resistance. Of concern worldwide.	

1. Common vehicle route (through contaminated items).
   a. Food (eg, *Salmonella* and *Campylobacter*).
   b. Water (eg, cholera and Legionellosis).
   c. Medications (eg, hepatitis C infection from contaminated multidose vials).
2. Vectorborne transmission.
   a. A living creature acts as an intermediary acquiring a pathogen from one living host and transmits the disease agent to another living organism, often an arthropod (fly, mosquito, tick).
   b. Can be mechanical (carried on the surface) or biological (host is infected with pathogen) vectors.

Susceptible Host

1. Determined by a complex interrelationship between a host and an infectious agent, by factors that influence infection or disease, such as:
   a. Pathogenicity—the ability to produce disease in a host. The organism invades a host, enters tissue, colonizes then spreads from host to host while not necessarily causing death to the host;
   b. Virulence—the wide range of damage that can occur to the host because of the toxic capabilities of the pathogen. Given that the host–pathogen relationship is fluid, the outcome can be dictated by:
      i. Number of pathogens to which the host is exposed; route and duration of exposure.
      ii. Invasiveness of the pathogen and its ability to produce toxins.
      iii. Age, genetic constitution of host, and general physical, mental, and emotional health and nutritional status of host.
      iv. Ability to bypass or overcome host defense mechanisms (immunologic response).

Collection of Specimens

 Evidence Base Garcia, L. S., et al. (Ed.-in-Chief). (2010). *Clinical microbiology procedures handbook* (3rd ed.). Washington, DC: American Society for Microbiology Press.

Proper collection and transport of specimens is important to maximize the outcome of laboratory tests for the diagnosis of infectious diseases. A variety of laboratory tests can be performed to make a presumptive or definitive diagnosis so that therapy can begin. See Standards of Care Guidelines 31-1.

Principles

1. It is imperative that specimens be collected and handled carefully if the causative agent for infection is to be identified correctly.
2. Specimens should be collected during the acute phase of infection and before the initiation of antibiotic therapy, if possible.
3. Obtain an adequate amount of the specimen necessary for all tests.

STANDARDS OF CARE GUIDELINES 31-1
Universal Precautions (Referenced OSHA 1910.1030)

These infection control precautions are mandated by the Occupational Safety and Health Administration (OSHA) and recommend that all blood and certain body fluids are treated as potentially infectious for Human Immunodeficiency Virus (HIV), Hepatitis B Virus (HBV), Hepatitis C Virus (HCV), and other bloodborne pathogens:

- Employers are required to provide appropriate personal protective equipment (PPE) and other engineering/work practice controls to eliminate or minimize employee exposure to bloodborne pathogens as mandated in OSHA regulation 1910.
- Gloves are to be worn when there is anticipation of contact with blood, other potentially infectious materials, mucous membranes, and nonintact skin.
- Gowns, aprons, or other protective body clothing are to be worn when contamination of clothing with blood or other potentially infectious materials is anticipated.
- Masks in combination with protective eyewear are to be worn when performing procedures likely to generate sprays or splashes of blood or other potentially infectious materials into the eyes, nose, or mouth.
- Hands and other skin surfaces are to be washed immediately if contaminated with blood or other potentially infectious materials.
- Utilize safety devices for needles and other sharps and do not manipulate by hand (eg, recapping, purposely bending or breaking, or removing from syringes, etc.).
- Needles and other sharps are to be placed in puncture-resistant containers for disposal.
- All specimens and items with blood or other potentially infectious materials are to be transported in containers that prevent leakage.
- Blood and body fluid spills are to be cleaned up promptly with an appropriate germicide, such as a bleach solution or phenolic.

---

4. Avoid potential contamination of the specimen by using proper collection technique.
5. Check local laboratory guidelines for the specimen collection recommendations for each test. These guidelines should include the appropriate specimen containers, sample size, as well as transport requirements (temperature, time, etc.).
6. Label the container properly according to local laboratory protocol; in general, include the patient's name, date of birth, medical record number, the source of the specimen, date and time collected, test to be performed, and any special instructions the provider may request.

7. Transport the specimen to the laboratory as soon as possible according to laboratory guidelines.

8. Be familiar with hospital policy recommending the transport of specified pathogens by staff personnel to the laboratory instead of via a pneumatic tube system.

Types of Specimen Collection

Blood Culture

1. Normally a sterile body fluid.

2. Specimens obtained by peripheral venipuncture are preferred over sampling from vascular catheters due to contamination of the catheter. Culturing hardware to determine a central line infection is not recommended in the literature.

3. Aseptic technique is essential to avoid contaminating the specimen with organisms colonizing the skin or the collector's hands.

5. Cleanse the venipuncture site with 70% alcohol followed by chlorhexidine gluconate and allow to fully dry.

6. The diaphragm tops of the culture bottles are not sterile and must be cleaned with alcohol before injection of blood.

Urine Culture

1. Normally a sterile body fluid.

2. A clean-catch, midstream urine collection provides the best method for obtaining a specimen to detect a urinary tract infection (see page 774).

3. Patients who are catheterized should have the specimen withdrawn using a sterile syringe from the catheter sampling port (see page 781).

4. Urine specimens must be transported to the laboratory promptly. If not cultured within 30 minutes of collection, urine must be refrigerated and cultured within 24 hours.

5. Other types of urine specimens may be collected, such as a straight in-and-out catheter specimen (see page 778) or suprapubic bladder drainage (see page 784).

Stool Culture

1. Obtained to culture organisms that are not part of the normal bowel flora (eg, *Salmonella* species, *Shigella* species).

2. Patient should defecate into a sterilized container or bedpan. Stool specimens should not contain urine or water from the toilet bowl.

3. Stool specimens can also be obtained directly from the rectum using a sterile swab.

Sputum Culture

1. Specimen needs to be from the lower respiratory tract, not oropharyngeal secretions. The laboratory will perform a Gram stain on all sputum specimens to determine if they are representative of pulmonary secretions and appropriately collected. A specimen containing a majority of cells from squamous epithelium may be rejected.

2. The most common method of collection is expectoration from a cooperative patient with a productive cough. Early morning is the optimal time to collect sputum specimens.

3. A sputum specimen can be collected in a sputum trap from patients who have artificial airways and require suctioning.

4. If a patient cannot produce sputum, sputum induction using an aerosol nebulizer may assist with loosening thickened secretions.

5. Bronchoscopy may be required to obtain sputum if induction fails.

Wound Culture

1. Specimens are usually cultured for aerobic and anaerobic organisms.

2. Specimens may be collected by multiple techniques, depending on the depth of the wound, including tissue samples, needle aspiration, and swabbing the surface.

3. To collect a wound culture using a sterile swab, cleanse the surface and collect as much exudate as possible from the advancing margin of the lesion. Avoid swabbing surrounding skin.

4. Place the swab immediately in appropriate transport culture tube and send to the laboratory.

5. Label with the specific anatomic site.

Throat Culture

1. Use a tongue depressor to hold the tongue down.

2. Carefully yet firmly rub swab over areas of exudate or over the tonsils and posterior pharynx, avoiding the cheeks, teeth, and gums.

3. Insert swab into packet and follow directions for handling the transport medium.

Laboratory Tests

Microbiologic Evaluation

Microscopy

1. Microscopic examination distinguishes tissue cells from microorganisms.

2. Various stains are used to highlight the structural characteristics of microorganisms (eg, Gram stain, acid-fast stains to isolate mycobacteria).

3. Classification is conducted according to physical appearance such as shape, size, or tendency to form chains or clusters and stain reactions such as Gram-positive versus Gram-negative.

4. Results of microscopy are usually available within minutes, which permits early initiation of treatment based on a presumptive diagnosis.

Culture

1. Culture is the gold standard for positive identification of most microorganisms.

2. Different culture media are used for suspected pathogens and can be selective (allow growth of only certain microorganisms) and/or differential (distinguish between different bacteria based on different characteristics).

   a. A liquid medium is used for blood specimens because lower numbers of microorganisms are detectable.

   b. A solid medium is used to isolate mixtures of organisms and grow pure cultures of each type of organism found.

3. Recovery of pathogens from culture varies depending on the microorganism type, test selected, and stage of illness.
   a. Most common pathogens, such as staphylococci, streptococci, and enterococci, are often identifiable to genus and species within 48 hours.
   b. Fungal organisms may take 10 to 14 days to grow in culture medium.
   c. Viruses may take 2 to 3 weeks to grow in culture medium.
   d. Mycobacteria may take up to 6 weeks to grow in culture medium.

Antibiotic Susceptibility Testing

1. Used to determine minimal concentration of antibiotics that will inhibit growth of an organism.
   a. Minimum inhibitory concentration is the lowest concentration of an antimicrobial drug that will inhibit organism growth and is measured by the size of the zone around the antimicrobial disk in which growth is inhibited.
   b. Based on Clinical and Laboratory Standards Institute guidelines for each organism, the size of the inhibitory zone diffusion tests are interpreted as resistant (R), sensitive (S), and intermediate (I).

Molecular Testing

1. There are technologies to detect specific genetic portions of pathogenic organisms or to identify the specific host's response to the presence of the pathogen. Examples include DNA probe testing and polymerase chain reaction.
2. These tests often yield a more rapid result than culture.

White Blood Cell Count

1. An increase in white blood cell count or "leukocytosis" may indicate infection, inflammatory response, tissue necrosis, or bone marrow failure.
2. The total number of circulating leukocytes and the differential (given as a percent of the total white blood cell [WBC] count) may change during a bacterial or viral infection.
3. During an acute bacterial infection, the WBC count often increases (greater than $11,000/mm^3$), accompanied by increased neutrophils and increased bands (immature neutrophils) in the differential. The shift (to the left) in differential reflects phagocytic activity.

Immunologic Tests

1. Pathogens that are antigenic stimulate antibodies that can be detected in the serum of patients.
2. Detection of antibodies is not necessarily diagnostic of current infection.
3. Antigen–antibody reactions must be evaluated over a period of time.
4. Immunoglobulin M (IgM) antibody production peaks during active infection and decreases during convalescence.
5. IgG antibodies peak during convalescence and persist.
6. A fourfold rise in antibody titer between the acute and convalescence samples indicates recent infection.

GENERAL PROCEDURES AND TREATMENT MODALITIES

Immunity

The human body is equipped with defense mechanisms to ward off disease. These include anatomical barriers, such as the skin, and physiological barriers, such as enzymes in saliva. The normal flora of microorganisms on and in the body also helps to prevent invasion of pathogens. If these nonspecific defense mechanisms fail, the body's specific immune response usually provides protection. Specific immunity to a particular organism implies that an individual has either generated the appropriate antibody in his or her own body or received ready-made antibodies from another source. Immunity may be natural or acquired or passive or active.

Natural active immunity occurs when antibodies are acquired following an infection. Antibodies are also acquired through natural passive immunity, such as from mother to fetus through the placenta or to infant via breast milk.

Passive artificial immunity is achieved through administration of immune globulin or antitoxin. *Active artificial immunity* occurs when antibodies are produced in response to a vaccine or toxoid (see Table 31-2).

Infection Prevention

Health-care-associated infections (HAIs) occur when a patient comes to a health care facility and acquires a new infection during their care. HAIs affect 2 million patients a year (2002) and, conservatively, 99,000 of those people die annually as a result. An intensive-care patient has a 30% chance of acquiring an HAI. In the United States, the cost for these infections is $28 to $33 billion a year.

The four most common HAIs for which hospitals perform surveillance are (1) surgical site infection; (2) central line–associated bloodstream infection; (3) ventilator-associated pneumonia; and (4) catheter-associated urinary tract infection. HAI rates are increasingly being used as indicators of quality and patient safety in health care facilities. Hospitals are reporting infection rates to the National Health Safety Network, part of the Centers for Disease Control and Prevention (CDC), and the data is being published and made available to the public.

In addition to surveillance of select HAIs, other infection prevention efforts include monitoring transmission of multidrug-resistant organisms (MDROs), hospital-wide hand hygiene compliance, antimicrobial stewardship, cleaning and disinfection, occupational health including vaccine compliance, staff education, and performance improvement initiatives to reduce HAIs.

Control and prevention of disease transmission by use of isolation precautions has a long history in health care facilities. Currently in health care facilities, those at highest risk are burn patients, neonates, those with MDROs, those with invasive lines, and anyone in intensive care units.

Fundamentals of Standard Precautions

In 1996, the CDC issued an isolation guideline for hospitals. It synthesized the major features of Universal Precautions and Body

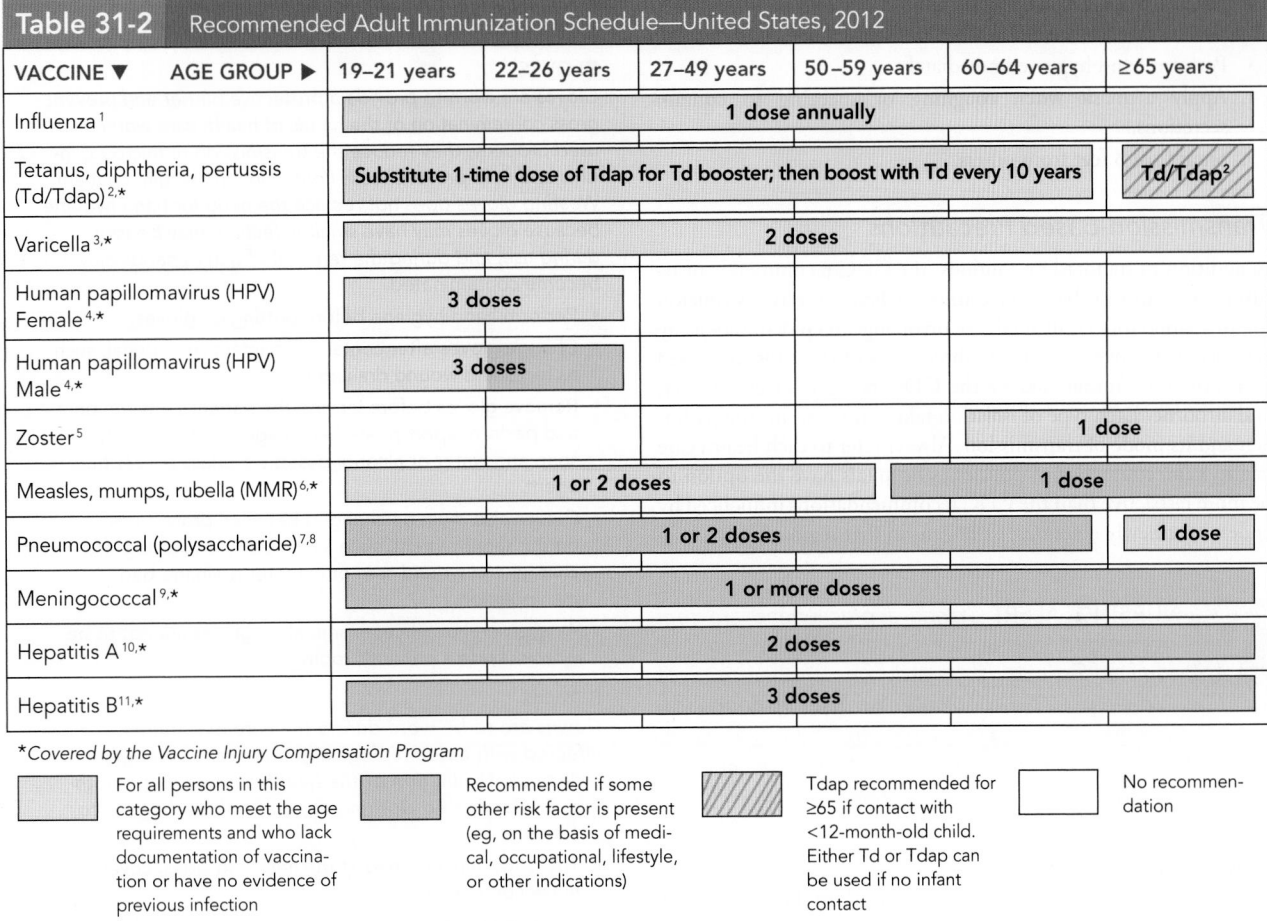

Table 31-2 Recommended Adult Immunization Schedule—United States, 2012

VACCINE ▼ AGE GROUP ▶	19–21 years	22–26 years	27–49 years	50–59 years	60–64 years	≥65 years
Influenza[1]	1 dose annually					
Tetanus, diphtheria, pertussis (Td/Tdap)[2,*]	Substitute 1-time dose of Tdap for Td booster; then boost with Td every 10 years					Td/Tdap[2]
Varicella[3,*]	2 doses					
Human papillomavirus (HPV) Female[4,*]	3 doses					
Human papillomavirus (HPV) Male[4,*]	3 doses					
Zoster[5]					1 dose	
Measles, mumps, rubella (MMR)[6,*]	1 or 2 doses				1 dose	
Pneumococcal (polysaccharide)[7,8]	1 or 2 doses					1 dose
Meningococcal[9,*]	1 or more doses					
Hepatitis A[10,*]	2 doses					
Hepatitis B[11,*]	3 doses					

Covered by the Vaccine Injury Compensation Program

- For all persons in this category who meet the age requirements and who lack documentation of vaccination or have no evidence of previous infection
- Recommended if some other risk factor is present (eg, on the basis of medical, occupational, lifestyle, or other indications)
- Tdap recommended for ≥65 if contact with <12-month-old child. Either Td or Tdap can be used if no infant contact
- No recommendation

For footnote information, see www.cdc.gov/vaccines/recs/schedules/downloads/adult/mmwr-adult-schedule.pdf.

Substance Isolation into a single set of precautions, called *standard precautions*. Standard precautions apply to (1) blood; (2) all body fluids, secretions, and excretions (except sweat), regardless of whether or not they contain visible blood; (3) nonintact skin; and (4) mucous membranes. As a common practice, standard precautions are recommended for the care of *all* patients in any environment, every time. If there is a chance of coming into contact with a potentially infectious material, a barrier is recommended to be placed between the patient and the care provider. The barrier may be a gown, glove, mask, or goggles, depending on the reason and area of contact.

Hand Hygiene

1. Hand hygiene is the single most recommended measure to reduce the risks of transmitting microorganisms.
2. Hand hygiene should be performed between patient contacts; after contact with blood, body fluids, secretions, excretions, and contaminated equipment or articles; before donning and after removing gloves is vital for infection control. It may be necessary to clean hands between tasks on the same patient to prevent cross-contamination of different body sites.
3. To perform hand hygiene, clean hands with soap and water, applying friction for 15 seconds upon all surfaces of the hands, or applying alcohol-based waterless hand sanitizer covering all surfaces of both hands until completely dry.
4. Waterless hand cleaners are recommended unless there is visible soil on the hands, before eating, after using the restroom, and when there is significant buildup of waterless hand cleaners.
5. If caring for a patient with a spore-producing pathogen such as *Clostridium difficile*–associated disease (CDAD), then use hand hygiene with soap and water applying friction for 15 seconds, as the spores this organism forms are resistant to alcohol hand gel.
6. Similarly, for other pathogens known or suspected to be resistant to alcohol waterless hand gels—such as *Norovirus*—hand hygiene with soap and water while applying friction for 15 seconds.

Respiratory Hygiene/Cough Etiquette

1. When coughing or sneezing, cover the mouth and nose with a tissue or the fabric of your sleeve.

2. Use the nearest waste receptacle to dispose of the tissue after use.
3. Perform hand hygiene immediately.
4. Apply a mask when coughing or sneezing to contain secretions.
5. Sit at least 3 feet from others.

Transmission-Based Precautions

In addition to standard precautions, the CDC recommends instituting transmission-based precautions when there is a suspicion for, or a laboratory confirmed case involving, an epidemiologically significant pathogen. There are three types of transmission-based precautions recommended by the CDC being contact, droplet, and airborne. Each type of isolation takes into account the pathogen and its mode of transmission. Always refer to each health care facility's infection control policies as hospitals have the option to be more restrictive than the CDC recommendations influenced by endemic or newly emerging pathogens in that region.

> **! NURSING ALERT** *Standard precautions are recommended for the care of each patient in all circumstances even if already on another type of isolation. When possible, dedicate the use of noncritical patient care equipment to a single patient. Thoroughly clean and disinfect reusable equipment before use on another patient.*

Contact Precautions

1. Used for patients known or suspected to be infected or colonized with epidemiologically significant microorganisms that can be transmitted by direct contact with the patient (skin-to-skin or patient's skin to staff's clothing as contact occurs when performing patient care activities that require touching the patient's skin) or indirect contact with environmental surfaces (fomites) or patient care items in the patient's environment.
2. Examples of microorganisms requiring contact precautions:
   a. Methicillin (oxacillin)–resistant *Staphylococcus aureus* (MRSA).
   b. Vancomycin-resistant *Enterococcus.*
   c. Vancomycin-intermediate or -resistant *S. aureus.*
   d. CDAD.
3. Place the patient in a private room or in a room with a patient who has the same microorganism (cohorting).
4. Personal protective equipment (PPE)—When entering a room marked as contact isolation, it is expected that everyone (including visitors) wear gloves and a gown (see Box 31-1).
5. All equipment, including intravenous poles, handles on carts, and other devices, should be cleaned, disinfected, and labeled as cleaned prior to transport in halls, elevators, or before provided to a new patient—doing so protects the environment, staff, visitors, and patients from contamination with infectious diseases.

BOX 31-1   Personal Protective Equipment

GLOVES

Gloves are worn to provide a protective barrier and prevent gross contamination of the hands of health care workers; if used properly, they reduce the transmission of microorganisms and help prevent cross-contamination within a patient. Wearing gloves does not replace the need for hand hygiene because gloves may have small defects or may be torn during use, and during the removal of gloves hands may become contaminated.

- Perform hand hygiene before putting on gloves.
- Change gloves after contact with infective material, such as feces and wound drainage.
- Remove gloves before leaving the patient's environment and perform appropriate hand hygiene immediately with soap and water or alcohol-based waterless antiseptic agent.
- Gloves also must be changed between procedures on the same patient, such as central line dressing change and wound care or catheter drainage bag manipulation.
- As a general practice, examination gloves are not to be worn outside a patient's room.

GOWNS

Gowns are to be worn during the care of patients infected with epidemiologically significant pathogens to reduce contamination of the health care worker's clothing. Contaminated clothing can transmit pathogens to patients.

- The gown must be tied at the neck and sides, covering the nurse completely.
- If the gown is too small, two gowns can be used to cover any exposed areas of the nurse.
- Water-impermeable gowns, leg coverings, boots, or shoe covers provide greater protection to the skin when large splashes of blood or body fluid are possible such as in the OR.
- Gowns must be removed and discarded prior to leaving the patient's environment, and appropriate hand hygiene must be performed.

Droplet Precautions

1. Designed for care of patients known or suspected to be infected with microorganisms transmitted by large-particle droplets generated by the patient when coughing, sneezing, talking, or during the performance of certain procedures, such as sputum induction or nebulization.
2. These large-particle droplets fall out of the air 3 to 6 feet from the patient's mouth so use of mask, eye protection, gown and gloves is mandatory.
3. Examples of illnesses requiring droplet precautions: *Neisseria meningitidis,* pneumonic plague, scarlet fever, pertussis, adenoviruses, parainfluenza viruses, influenza, respiratory syncytial virus, human metapneumovirus, rhinovirus, mumps, parvovirus B12, rubella.

4. Place the patient in a private room.

   a. When a private room is not available, place patients with the same microorganism together (cohorting).

   b. If neither of these is possible, maintain spatial separation of at least 3 feet between the infected patient and other patients and visitors.

5. Special air handling and ventilation are not necessary and the door may remain open.

6. PPE includes gowns and gloves, as well as masks, goggles, or face shields.

   a. Wear a mask when working within 3 feet (0.9 m) of the patient.

   b. In order to protect the mucous membranes of the eyes, nose, and mouth, masks and goggles or face shields are worn by health care workers during patient care to protect against splashes or sprays of blood, body fluids, or secretions.

7. Limit transport of the patient from the room for essential purposes only.

   a. If transport is necessary, minimize dispersal of droplets by masking the patient.

Airborne Precautions

1. Designed to reduce the risk of airborne transmission of infectious agents through dissemination of small-droplet nuclei less than 5 microns in size which remain suspended in the air for long periods of time.

2. Microorganisms can be dispersed widely by air currents and may become inhaled by or deposited on a susceptible host within the same room or over a longer distance from the source patient. Therefore, special air handling, filtration, and ventilation are required.

3. Examples of illnesses requiring airborne precautions: measles, varicella (including disseminated zoster), and tuberculosis.

4. PPE—gowns and gloves might be required based on the disease, so see the disease-specific hospital policy; respirators are required (N95 respirator, a high-efficiency particulate air [HEPA] filter respirator, or a powered air-purifying respirator [PAPR]).

   a. Staff members are required to be trained in the use of protective respirators and/or PAPRs annually in a program of respiratory protection that includes a "fit test." This test ensures that the respirator seals to the face of the staff member, teaches the staff member how to use the respirator, and optimizes the protection for the staff member.

   b. Persons immune to rubeola or varicella need not wear a mask but must wear gown and gloves when having exposure to lesions, to prevent carrying contaminant to a nonimmune patient outside of the room.

5. Place the patient in a private room that has:

   a. Monitored negative air pressure in relation to the surrounding areas.

   b. At least 6 but preferably 12 air changes per hour.

   c. Appropriate discharge of air outdoors or monitored high-efficiency filtration of room air before recirculation.

   d. Door that is closed at all times with the patient in the room.

6. Limit the transport of the patient from the room to essential purposes only.

   a. If transport is necessary, minimize patient dispersal of droplet nuclei by placing a surgical or procedural mask on the patient. The mask remains on the patient going to the procedure and returning from the procedure. While in the procedure room, the staff must have on appropriate PPE so the patient may remove his or hers.

   b. Transporters are not required to wear a respirator while taking the patient through the hospital. If the transporter will be assisting in the procedure room when the patient removes the mask, then appropriate PPE is expected.

   c. Notify the receiving destination about the isolation requirement of the patient so they can order the appropriate PPE and HEPA filtration to provide protection to their staff and other patients.

   d. The patient must not sit in a waiting area with other patients but go directly to the procedure and come directly back to the patient's hospital room.

Other Considerations

Limiting the Movement of Patients

1. Limiting the movement of patients with epidemiologically significant microorganisms reduces transmission. Every effort should be made to limit the movement of patients on airborne precautions.

2. When transport is necessary for a contact, droplet, or airborne patient:

   a. Patient should be in a clean hospital gown with clean linens.

   b. Appropriate barriers (such as masks and impervious dressings) are to be worn by the patient.

   c. Personnel in the area to which the patient is taken need notification with time to collect PPE, prepare a room that will meet specifications for the identified isolation, communicate with cleaning staff and ensure the patient will not sit in a waiting area with other patients, visitors, and staff.

   d. Unless transporting staff are giving care during the transport, there is no need to wear PPE. If the patient may require critical care in the hallway, consider having two transporters: one to remain without PPE to open doors, touch elevator buttons and push the patient, while the other person with PPE will only touch the patient.

3. When appropriate, patients are taught how they can assist in preventing transmission.

Attention to Equipment

1. Soiled linen should be handled, transported, and laundered in a manner that avoids transfer of microorganisms to patients, personnel, and environments. With some organisms, such as smallpox or anthrax, care must be taken to not expel the air from plastic linen bags outside of airborne patient rooms.

2. There is currently no evidence indicating a need for special precautions for dishes, glasses, cups, or eating utensils because the combination of hot water and detergents used in hospital dishwashers is sufficient for decontamination for most infectious diseases. However, appropriate hand hygiene is required when removing food trays from some isolated rooms.

3. Patient-care equipment that is soiled with blood, body fluids, secretions, and excretions must be handled in a manner that prevents skin and mucous membrane exposures, contamination of clothing, and transfer of microorganisms to other patients and environments.

    a. There must be a procedural mechanism in place labeling or otherwise identifying used equipment as not to be used on another patient.

    b. Reusable equipment must be transported in a manner to prevent contamination of the staff, the environment, and visitors until it reaches the area where it will be cleaned, disinfected, and reprocessed appropriately before use for another patient.

    c. Single-use items must be discarded properly.

4. Care must be taken to prevent injuries from needles, scalpels, and other sharp objects. Used needles must never be recapped using both hands, removed from syringes, bent, /broken, or otherwise manipulated. Used needles and sharps must have the engineered sharps injury protection activated and be disposed of immediately into an OSHA-approved puncture-resistant container. These containers should be mounted per the National Institute of Occupational Safety and Health guidelines and be located as close as is practical to the area of use.

5. Protective mouthpieces, resuscitation bags, or other ventilation devices are used instead of mouth-to-mouth resuscitation methods.

INFECTIOUS DISORDERS

Evidence Base Jarvis, W. R. (Ed.). (2007). *Bennett & Brachman's Hospital Infections* (5th ed.). New York: Lippincott Williams & Wilkins.

Infectious disorders are covered throughout the book in a variety of body system chapters. See Table 31-3, pages 1088 to 1099, for selected infectious disorders. Be aware that new data on infectious diseases are emerging daily. For the latest information on infectious diseases, contact your state public health department or the CDC at *www.cdc.gov*.

Emerging Infections

Evidence Base Centers for Disease Control and Prevention. (2008). *Emerging infectious diseases*. Atlanta, GA: Author. Available: *www.cdc.gov/ncidod/diseases/eid/*.

Hantaviral Diseases

1. Hantaviruses infect rodents worldwide.
2. In humans, hantaviruses cause either hantavirus pulmonary syndrome or hemorrhagic fever with renal syndrome.
3. Morbidity—50% of reported cases due to pulmonary syndrome.
4. Intensive care in a tertiary facility is critical in the first 24 to 48 hours.

Symptoms

1. Abrupt onset of fever, lower back pain, varying degrees of hemorrhagic manifestations and renal involvement.
2. Characterized by five, frequently overlapping, clinical phases: febrile, hypotensive, oliguric, diuretic, and convalescent.

Transmission

1. Humans become infected through direct contact with infected rodents and their droppings or by aerosolized rodent excreta.
2. No person-to-person transmission; no isolation other than standard precautions.

Implications for Nursing

1. Teach prevention through rodent control, limiting nesting sites, proper storage of food, careful wet-mop cleaning, and disinfection of rodent-contaminated areas with 10% bleach solution.

Ebola-Marburg Viral Diseases

1. Filoviruses cause severe hemorrhagic fevers, commonly accompanied by hepatic and renal damage.
2. Central nervous system (CNS) involvement and shock with multiorgan failure can occur.
3. Mortality—Marburg virus, 25%; Ebola virus, 50% to 90%.

Symptoms

1. Sudden onset of fever, myalgia, and headache; followed by pharyngitis, vomiting, diarrhea, and maculopapular rash.
2. Commonly leads to hepatic damage, renal failure, CNS involvement, and terminal shock with multiorgan dysfunction.

Transmission

1. Person to person by direct contact with infected blood, secretions, organs, or semen.
2. Risk is highest during later stages when patient is vomiting, experiencing diarrhea, and hemorrhaging.

Implications for Nursing

1. Strict adherence to standard precautions and airborne precautions and as directed by public health authorities.

2. Health-care-associated infections have occurred frequently; virtually all Ebola cases in outbreaks acquired from contaminated syringes and needles have been fatal.

West Nile Virus

1. Caused by an arbovirus.
2. First cases in United States in New York in 1999.
3. Cases have since been reported in more than 40 states.
4. Mortality is 3% to 15%, mainly in older persons.

Symptoms

Febrile illness with rash, arthritis, myalgias, weakness, lymphadenopathy, meningoencephalitis.

Transmission

1. Bite of infected mosquito that has fed on infected bird or animal; has also been transmitted through blood transfusions and transplanted organs.
2. Not transmitted person to person; no isolation other than standard precautions necessary.

Implications for Nursing

1. Teach prevention of mosquito bites by wearing proper clothing, using insect repellent, and removing sources of standing water that provide breeding grounds for mosquitoes.
2. Be alert for acute febrile illness and deteriorating condition.

Avian Flu

Evidence Base Centers for Disease Control and Prevention. (2010). *Avian influenza A virus infections of humans.* Atlanta, GA: Author. Available: www.cdc.gov/flu/avian/gen-info/facts.htm.

Avian flu refers to influenza A viruses found chiefly in birds, but it may also occur in humans—cases have been reported worldwide since 1997.

Symptoms

1. Conjunctivitis.
2. Fever, cough, sore throat, muscle aches.
3. Pneumonia, respiratory distress.
4. Nausea, vomiting.
5. Neurologic changes.

Transmission

1. Direct contact with sick or dead, infected poultry.
2. Reports of human-to-human transmission have been limited; however, because the virus has the potential to change, transmission is being monitored.

Implications for Nursing

1. Conduct a thorough travel history assessment of the patient.
2. Teach patients that for those at risk because of contact with birds or poultry, good hand hygiene and use of protective equipment is recommended.

3. For suspected contact with an infected bird, the patient should be monitored for symptoms throughout the week following exposure.
4. The CDC and World Health Organization recommend oseltamivir (as with other types of influenza A) for treatment of infection and as prophylaxis for exposure to infection.

Clostridium difficile–Associated Disease

1. Caused by the presence of toxins that are produced by certain strains of *C. difficile* in the intestinal tract.
2. This organism is a spore-forming bacteria, which makes it very resistant to disinfectants routinely used in hospital settings.
3. An especially toxic strain, NAP-1, has emerged as the leading cause of outbreaks in hospitals across the world.
4. The disease is associated with the use of almost every class of antibiotics, but the use of fluoroquinolones has become the leading class of antibiotics associated with this disease.

Symptoms

1. Although incubation rates have not been clearly established, they can range from less than 7 days to 6 months depending on the clinical picture of the patient.
2. The patient may be an asymptomatic carrier or may present with abdominal cramps, diarrhea, colitis, pseudomembranous colitis, fulminant colitis, and toxic megacolon.
3. The most common presentation is nonbloody diarrhea and cramps.
4. Recurrence of the disease is common.

Transmission

1. Contaminated environment and the contaminated hands of those who touch surfaces in that environment leads to transmission.
2. The use of alcohol hand gels is not recommended following care of a patient with CDAD. Staff and visitors should wash their hand with soap, warm water, and friction for 15 seconds to perform adequate hand hygiene.
3. The use of sodium hypochlorite at 5000-ppm, bleach diluted 1:10, or buffered commercially prepared bleach solutions or FDA-approved sporicidal disinfectant are recommended for cleaning the patient's environment and equipment.

Implications for Nursing

1. Strict contact precautions and diligent hand hygiene by all who enter the environment need to be enforced.
2. The use of dedicated patient equipment and disposable items should be considered as much as possible.
3. Close monitoring of antimicrobial use for the development of diarrhea should prompt early identification and reduced transmission.
4. Consider using a bleach-based disinfectant (or other FDA-approved sporicidal) and a highly trained environmental staff.

(Text continues on page 1100)

Table 31-3   Selected Infectious Diseases

DISEASE, INFECTIOUS AGENT, AND TRANSMISSION	CLINICAL MANIFESTATIONS	INCUBATION PERIOD	DIAGNOSTIC TESTS
Vector-Transmitted Infection			
Rocky Mountain Spotted Fever			
Rickettsia rickettsii • Transmission usually occurs via an infected tick bite with a minimum of 4–6 hours of attachment for infection to occur. May also be transmitted via contamination of breaks in the skin or mucous membranes with crushed tissues or feces of the tick. • Reservoir includes the American dog tick in the east and south, the Rocky Mountain wood tick in the northwest, and the brown dog tick. • Coinfection with other tickborne pathogens should be considered.	• Sudden onset of high fever, malaise, severe headache, chills, and conjunctival injection (red eyes). • Maculopapular rash may begin on day 3–5 on the extremities, which progresses to the soles, palms, and body trunk (in 35%–60%) into petechia and purpura on or after the 6th day. • Mortality ranges depending on the region, but occurs in 3%–5% of cases after treatment.	• 3–14 days.	• Serologic assays, although not standardized interpretations, for *R. rickettsii* antigen, including indirect immunofluorescence assay (primary diagnostic tool, considered the gold standard) and ELISA. • Specimens collected 2–3 weeks apart that show a rising IgG or IgM is essential to confirm infection. • Nucleic acid detection by PCR.
Lyme Disease			
Borrelia burgdorferi • Endemic in the Northern Hemisphere temperate regions but found worldwide. • Ixodid ticks reservoir (affecting primarily small mammals and deer). • Coinfection with other tickborne pathogens should always be considered.	• Erythema migrans occurs in 70%–80% of infected patients after a delay of 3–30 days. Appears at the site of the tick bite and gradually expands over a period of days. May be anywhere on the body. Feels warm but is rarely itchy or painful. • Flulike symptoms—malaise, fever, headache, stiff neck, myalgia, migratory arthralgias, lymphadenopathy. • Weeks to months—limb weakness, pain and swelling in the large joints, facial palsy, aseptic meningitis. • Months to years—arthritis with severe joint pain and swelling, chronic neurologic symptoms.	• 3–32 days after tick exposure (mean 7–10 days).	• IFA, ELISA, and western immunoblotting two-stage serological testing combined with supportive clinical findings. Serological tests are poorly standardized and must be interpreted with caution. • Biopsies of skin lesions yield the organism in about 80% of cases.
Viral Infections			
Influenza			
• Acute viral disease of the respiratory tract. • Spread from person to person by large-particle respiratory droplet transmission or by contact with articles recently contaminated with respiratory secretions. • Animal influenza viruses may also be spread via direct contact with infected animals.	• Usually self-limited febrile illness associated with upper and lower respiratory infection. • Characterized by sudden onset of fever, chills or rigors, headache, malaise, myalgia, and nonproductive cough, typically followed by sore throat, nasal congestion, and rhinorrhea. • Among children—otitis media, abdominal pain, and vomiting are commonly reported.	• 1–4 days (mean 2 days). • Cough may last 2 weeks or more but other symptoms generally resolve within 5–7 days.	• Isolation of virus from pharyngeal or nasal secretions or identification of viral antigens in nasopharyngeal cells by fluorescent antibody test or ELISA. • Without testing, may be clinically indistinguishable from other respiratory viruses such as rhinovirus, RSV, adenovirus, parainfluenza, human metapneumovirus.

MANAGEMENT	COMPLICATIONS	NURSING CONSIDERATIONS
• Doxycycline is the first line of treatment for adults and children of all ages: adults 100 mg b.i.d. and children under 45 kg (100 lbs): 2.2 mg/kg body weight given twice daily. • Chloramphenicol may be used for contraindications to tetracyclines. • Patients should be treated for at least 3 days after the fever subsides and until there is evidence of clinical improvement. • Considerations: The clinical presentation may resemble other tickborne diseases such as Ehrlichiosis, Lyme disease, and others.	• Damage to the endothelial cells that line the blood vessels, called "vasculitis," and bleeding or clotting in the brain or other vital organs may occur. Loss of fluid from damaged vessels can result in loss of circulation to the extremities and damaged fingers, toes, or limbs. • Amputation • Neurologic deficits • Internal organ damage	• Not communicable person to person. • Instruct patient to report reoccurrence of symptoms immediately; may be relapse. • Stress prevention through avoidance of tick-infested areas, wearing protective clothing and tick repellent, inspecting body and clothes for ticks every 3–4 hours. • Remove ticks with tweezers or forceps to avoid leaving mouth parts in skin.
• Doxycycline 100 mg b.i.d. or amoxicillin 500 mg t.i.d. P.O. for 14 to 21 days. • Ceftriaxone, cefotaxime, penicillin G IV regimens for 3–4 weeks for disseminated infection. • Single-dose antibiotic for exposure by tick bite is not recommended in most cases. • Treatment failure occurs in some cases and retreatment may be necessary.	• Meningeal irritation leading to meningitis, encephalitis • Chorea • Atrioventricular block • Chronic neurologic manifestations, such as encephalopathy, polyneuropathy • Chronic arthritis	• Not communicable person to person. • Preventive measures include: (a) avoiding tick-infested areas; (b) wearing protective clothing; (c) using insect repellent; (d) inspecting the body and clothing daily while working or playing in tick-infested areas. • Ticks should be removed from the skin with tweezers or forceps, using gentle, steady traction to avoid leaving mouth parts in the skin. Protect hands with gloves, cloth, or tissue when removing ticks.
• Aspirin or acetaminophen for control of fever. • Antivirals, oseltamivir or zanamivir, as prophylaxis for high-risk persons for influenza complications. • Agent-specific antibiotics for bacterial complications.	• Secondary bacterial pneumonia • Primary viral pneumonia • Severe illness and death may occur, primarily among older adults, the young, and the chronically ill • Acute myositis characterized by calf tenderness may develop, particularly with type B infections	• Highly infectious via aerosolization or droplets from the respiratory tract of infected persons. • Implement droplet precautions for patients for the duration of symptoms • Best means of prevention—annual influenza vaccination, particularly for high-risk groups and HCWs • Maintain bed rest for at least 48 hours after fever subsides. Encourage fluids. Report symptoms of secondary infection (purulent nasal drainage or sputum, ear pain, increase in fever) to health care provider. • Continue antibiotics prescribed for bacterial complications for defined time period (usually 7–10 days).

(continued)

Table 31-3   Selected Infectious Diseases (continued)

DISEASE, INFECTIOUS AGENT, AND TRANSMISSION	CLINICAL MANIFESTATIONS	INCUBATION PERIOD	DIAGNOSTIC TESTS
Viral Infections			
Mononucleosis			
• Epstein-Barr virus (EBV) Spread via oropharyngeal route (saliva). • Especially via kissing among young adults.	• Fever, sore throat (exudative pharyngotonsillitis), fatigue, splenomegaly, and lymphadenopathy.	• 4–6 weeks.	• Lymphocytosis >50%, with more than 10% being atypical lymphocytes, abnormalities in liver function tests, or an elevated heterophile antibody titer. Not useful diagnostic tool in children younger than age 5. If negative, EBV, IgM, and IgA tests may be performed.
Cytomegalovirus (CMV)			
Spread by intimate contact with mucous membranes, secretions, and excretions and by blood transfusion and organ transplant. A fetus may be infected in utero or at delivery.	• Ordinarily asymptomatic, especially in children. • Clinical disease in adolescents and adults resembles mononucleosis. • More extensive organ involvement in the immunosuppressed host: colitis, pneumonitis, and retinitis may occur. • GI tract disorders. • Congenital infections are serious and lead to irreversible CNS and liver damage.	• 3–8 weeks following transplant or transfusion; 3–12 weeks following delivery-produced infection.	• Virus culture. • CMV antigen detection. • CMV deoxyribonucleic acid detection by PCR. • Serologic studies for CMV-specific IgM antibody or a fourfold rise in titer.
Rabies			
Rabies virus Spread by direct contact of virus-laden saliva of a rabid animal into a bite or scratch; may also be transmitted via transplanted corneas and, possibly, other organs removed from patients dying of undiagnosed rabies.	• Initial symptoms nonspecific and consist of a sense of apprehension, malaise, fatigue, headache, and fever; possible pain or paresthesia at the site of exposure. • Usually lasts 2–6 days. • Progresses to paresis or paralysis, hydrophobia, eventually to delirium and convulsions. • Respiratory arrest usually occurs, followed by death.	• Highly variable, usually 3–8 weeks; if the bite occurs on the head rather than on an extremity, duration is shorter due to bite's proximity to the brain.	• Specific FA staining of brain tissue or by virus isolation or FA staining of frozen skin sections taken from back of neck.

MANAGEMENT	COMPLICATIONS	NURSING CONSIDERATIONS
• Supportive therapy to include aspirin or acetaminophen for sore throat and fever, bed rest. • Surgical removal of the spleen for splenic rupture. • Corticosteroids for severe neurologic complications, thrombocytopenia purpura, hemolytic anemia, or severe oropharyngeal involvement and airway encroachment.	• Splenic rupture • Thrombocytopenia purpura • Hemolytic anemia • Pericarditis, myocarditis • Aseptic meningitis, encephalitis, Guillain-Barré syndrome • Hepatitis • Orchitis	• Person-to-person spread via saliva is prolonged—can be months to a year or more after infection. • Convalescence may be as long as several months. • Patients with splenomegaly should avoid activity that may increase the risk of injury to the spleen, such as contact sports and heavy lifting. • Report any excess bruising or bleeding, jaundice, or abnormal CNS functioning.
• Supportive therapy for control of fever and sore throat. • Immune gamma globulin as a prophylactic agent for patients undergoing marrow transplantation. • Ganciclovir for retinitis in HIV-infected individuals.	• Congenital infection leads to neurologic defects (severe mental retardation, microcephaly, psychomotor retardation, hearing loss, and evidence of chronic liver disease). • Immunocompromised host—progressive pneumonitis, hemolytic anemia, hepatitis, pericarditis, and GI ulceration.	• Patients with splenomegaly should avoid activity that may increase the risk of injury to the spleen, such as contact sports and heavy lifting. • Report any excess bruising or bleeding, jaundice, or abnormal CNS functioning. • Pregnant personnel should be counseled about potential risks and urged to practice good hygiene (especially hand hygiene) and to follow standard precautions.
• Best controlled through prevention rather than treatment. • Supportive therapy to manage neurologic, respiratory, and cardiac symptoms. • Use of high-dose passive rabies immunoglobulin or vaccine after the onset of illness has not been successful.	• Almost invariably progresses to death, usually due to respiratory paralysis.	• Avoid contact with respiratory secretions, especially saliva, for duration of illness. • Preexposure prophylaxis should be offered to persons at high risk for exposure to rabies, such as veterinarians, veterinary students, wildlife personnel, park rangers, staff of kennels, and laboratory workers working with rabies. • Bites from animals, particularly dogs and cats, should be thoroughly flushed and cleaned with soap and water immediately. Wounds should not be sutured unless unavoidable. • Domestic dogs and cats should be quarantined for 10 days. • Wild animal carriers include skunks, bats, foxes, coyotes, raccoons, bobcats, wolves, jackals, and other carnivores. • Postexposure prophylaxis must include the use of human rabies immunoglobulin followed by Human Diploid Cell Vaccine (HDCV) unless preexposure prophylaxis with HDCV had been administered. HDCV requires 5 doses I.M. (fifth dose 35 days after the first).

(continued)

Table 31-3   Selected Infectious Diseases *(continued)*

DISEASE, INFECTIOUS AGENT, AND TRANSMISSION	CLINICAL MANIFESTATIONS	INCUBATION PERIOD	DIAGNOSTIC TESTS
Protozoan Infections			
Malaria			
Plasmodium vivax, P. falciparum, P. malariae, and *P. ovale* Malaria is vectorborne through the bite of a female *Anopheles* mosquito; may be congenital or transmitted by transfusions or dirty needles.	• Malarial paroxysm characterized by variations of high fever, chills, sweats, headache, rigor, cough, diarrhea, respiratory distress, nausea, vomiting, and arthralgia. • As infection becomes synchronized, fever and paroxysms are generally cyclic. • Moderate splenomegaly and tender hepatomegaly.	• 7 days to 10 months, depending on the strain.	• Diagnosis of malaria rests on the demonstration of parasites in stained peripheral blood smears. Repeated smears may be necessary. • Liver function tests reveal elevated transaminase level and increase in indirect serum bilirubin.
Amebiasis			
Entamoeba histolytica Transmitted by ingestion of fecally contaminated food or water, or sexually by oral–anal contact.	• Intestinal disease: may be asymptomatic or mild symptoms such as abdominal distention, flatulence, constipation, and, occasionally, loose stools. • Nondysenteric colitis: recurring episodes of loose stools; vague abdominal pain; hemorrhoids with occasional rectal bleeding. • Dysenteric colitis: abdominal cramps and diarrhea containing blood and mucus, alternating with periods of constipation or remission.	• Usually 2–4 weeks; however, may be as short as 3 days or as long as months or even years.	• Microscopic examination of stool, rectal secretions; positive for trophozoites or cysts of protozoan. Examination should be done on fresh specimens.
Giardiasis			
Giardia lamblia Transmitted by ingestion of fecally contaminated water or food, or sexually by anal intercourse.	• Acute: explosive, watery diarrheal stool; abdominal cramping and flatulence; nausea. • Chronic: intermittent foul-smelling diarrheal stools; increased flatulence and distention; anorexia.	• Usually 3–25 days (median 7–10 days).	• Examination of stool; positive for cysts or trophozoites of the *G. lamblia* protozoan. • Detection of *G. lamblia* antigen by enzyme immunoassay (EIA).
Hookworm			
Ancylostoma duodenale, Necator americanus Transmitted by entry into the skin of soil contaminated with feces from humans, cats, and dogs.	• Chronic, debilitating disease leading to iron deficiency and hypochromic, microcytic anemia due to intestinal blood loss to the hookworm.	• A few weeks to many months, depending on intensity of infection.	• Microscopic examination of cultured stool specimen positive for hookworm eggs; however, do not appear until 8–12 weeks after infestation.

MANAGEMENT	COMPLICATIONS	NURSING CONSIDERATIONS
<ul><li>IV fluids and electrolytes (restrict fluids in cerebral edema).</li><li>Assisted ventilation with pulmonary edema.</li><li>Dialysis in renal failure.</li><li>Transfusions in anemia.</li><li>Chemotherapy is based on infecting species, possible drug resistance, and severity of disease. Drugs used include chloroquine phosphate, quinidine gluconate, quinine dihydrochloride/sulfate plus doxycycline, tetracycline, or clindamycin.</li></ul>	<ul><li>Shock.</li><li>Acute encephalopathy.</li><li>Renal failure.</li><li>Hepatic failure.</li><li>Cerebral and pulmonary edema.</li><li>Disseminated intravascular coagulation.</li><li>Coma.</li><li>Death.</li></ul>	<ul><li>Symptoms may recur; instruct patient to report recurrence immediately.</li><li>Travelers to malaria-endemic countries should follow preventive measures:<ul><li>Proper use of mosquito netting at night.</li><li>Clothing that minimizes contact with mosquitoes.</li><li>Use of insect repellents.</li><li>Chemoprophylaxis with suppressive drugs, based on local endemicity and resistance.</li></ul></li></ul>
<ul><li>Treatment regimens depend on the severity of the illness.</li><li>Metronidazole followed by iodoquinol, paromomycin, or diloxanide furoate.</li><li>Abscess may require surgical aspiration.</li></ul>	<ul><li>Amebic granulomata of intestinal wall.</li><li>Penile lesions in active homosexuals.</li><li>Abscess of lung, brain, or pericardium.</li><li>Hepatic abscess.</li></ul>	<ul><li>Instruct patient to wash hands thoroughly after defecating to prevent transmission to others.</li><li>Household and sexual contacts should seek medical examination and treatment.</li><li>Instruct patient on safer sex practices.</li><li>Travelers to areas where the water supply is not chemically treated or protected from sewage should boil all water used for drinking and cooking.</li></ul>
<ul><li>Metronidazole is the drug of choice (5- to 7-day course).</li><li>Relapse is common in immunocompromised patients; may need prolonged therapy.</li></ul>	<ul><li>Chronic diarrhea.</li><li>Malabsorption leading to significant weight loss, failure to thrive, and anemia.</li></ul>	<ul><li>Instruct patient to wash hands thoroughly after defecating to prevent transmission to others.</li><li>Household and sexual contacts should seek medical examination and treatment.</li><li>Instruct patient on safer sex practices.</li><li>Travelers to areas where the water supply is not chemically treated or protected from sewage should boil all water used for drinking and cooking.</li></ul>
<ul><li>Albendazole, mebendazole, or pyrantel pamoate.</li><li>Iron therapy to correct anemia.</li></ul>	<ul><li>Immunosuppressed individuals—septicemia and death.</li><li>In children with heavy, long-term infection—hypoproteinemia, mental and physical retardation.</li></ul>	<ul><li>Follow-up examination of the stool 2 weeks after therapy is necessary. Repeat therapy if heavy worm burden persists.</li><li>Nutrition counseling and taking iron supplements are recommended until deficiencies are corrected.</li><li>Family members and close contacts should be examined and treated for parasites.</li><li>Educate public about dangers of soil contamination and importance of wearing shoes.</li></ul>

(continued)

Table 31-3   Selected Infectious Diseases *(continued)*

DISEASE, INFECTIOUS AGENT, AND TRANSMISSION	CLINICAL MANIFESTATIONS	INCUBATION PERIOD	DIAGNOSTIC TESTS
Protozoan Infections			
Trichinellosis, Trichinosis			
Trichinella spiralis Transmitted by ingestion of raw or insufficiently cooked meat, chiefly pork and pork products.	• Clinical disease is highly variable, from inapparent infection to a fulminating fatal disease. • During first week: abdominal discomfort, nausea, vomiting, and, possibly, diarrhea. • Early signs: sudden appearance of muscle soreness and pain accompanied by edema of upper eyelids, pain, photophobia; ocular signs may progress to subconjunctival, subungual, and retinal hemorrhages. • Remittent fever is usual, sometimes as high as 104° F (40° C).	• 5–45 days, depending on the number of worms involved; usually 8–15 days after ingestion of infected meat.	• Skeletal muscle biopsy not earlier than 10 days after exposure to infection demonstrates the *Trichinella* larvae. • Serology; complement fixation, fluorescent antibody—fourfold increase in antibody titer 3 weeks after infection. • Differential WBC count—increase in eosinophils to 70%. • Increased concentration of muscle enzymes.
Fungal Infections			
Histoplasmosis			

Histoplasma capsulatum
Transmitted by inhalation of airborne particles from soil or dust that harbor chicken or other bird droppings or bat droppings.
	• May be asymptomatic with only hypersensitivity to histoplasmin.
	• Four other clinical forms of disease:
	  • Acute benign respiratory—mild respiratory illness to temporary flu-like illness.
	  • Acute disseminated—debilitating fever, GI symptoms, bone marrow suppression, hepatosplenomegaly, and lymphadenopathy; usually fatal in infants and immunocompromised unless treated.
	  • Chronic disseminated—intermittent fever, weight loss, weakness, hepatosplenomegaly, hematologic abnormalities, and focal disease, such as endocarditis, meningitis, and mucosal ulcers; usually fatal unless treated.
	  • Chronic pulmonary disease—resembles pulmonary tuberculosis with cavitation; occurs most commonly with underlying emphysema.
		• Variable, 3–17 days after exposure.	• Complement fixation shows increase in antibodies within 3–4 weeks; fourfold increase suggests disease progression.
			• Visualization of fungus in specially stained smears of ulcer exudates, bone marrow, sputum, or blood.
			• Fungal culture or enzyme immunoassay positive for *H. capsulatum* or detection of antigen by EIA.
			• Chest x-ray—acute findings: transient parenchymal pulmonary infiltrates resembling lobar pneumonia; chronic: progressively enlarging areas of necrosis with or without cavitation.

MANAGEMENT	COMPLICATIONS	NURSING CONSIDERATIONS
• Mebendazole and albendazole. • Corticosteroids added for severe symptoms. • Supportive therapy for respiratory, neurologic, and cardiac sequelae.	• Cardiac and neurologic—third to sixth week. • Myocardial failure—first to second or fourth to eighth weeks.	• Instruct patient to thoroughly wash hands after defecation. • Proper cooking of pork to 160° F (71° C) is necessary. • Family members and close contacts of patients should be examined and treated for parasites.
• Amphotericin B, ketoconazole, and itraconazole. • Corticosteroids and diphenhydramine to minimize the adverse effects of amphotericin.	• Chronic pulmonary disease. • Pneumonitis, meningitis, lymphadenopathy, pancytopenia. • Hepatosplenomegaly. • Death.	• Investigation for the common source of infection should be done in outbreaks. • Educate public to minimize exposure to dust in chicken coops, attics, and caves—use protective masks, gloves, and disposable clothing.

(continued)

Table 31-3   Selected Infectious Diseases *(continued)*

DISEASE, INFECTIOUS AGENT, AND TRANSMISSION	CLINICAL MANIFESTATIONS	INCUBATION PERIOD	DIAGNOSTIC TESTS
Bacterial Infections			
Typhoid Fever			
Salmonella typhi Transmitted by ingestion of food and water contaminated by feces, urine, or sewage, or by direct contact with excrement.	• Systemic—insidious onset of fever, severe headache, malaise, anorexia, bradycardia, and splenomegaly. • Ulceration of the distal ileum; can progress to hemorrhage or perforation.	• Usually 8–14 days; however, may be as little as 3 days or as long as 3 months.	• Culture of urine or stool positive for *S. typhi* during second week. • Culture of blood positive for *S. typhi* during first week. • Bone marrow culture.
Botulism			
Clostridium botulinum Transmitted by ingestion of contaminated food or by contact with a contaminated wound.	• Severe intoxication characterized by visual difficulty, dysphagia, and dry mouth, followed by descending symmetrical flaccid paralysis. • Vomiting and constipation or diarrhea may be present initially.	• Usually 12–36 hours, but may be up to 8 days after eating contaminated food. • When transmitted through a wound, 4–14 days after injury.	• Culture of *C. botulinum* from stool or stomach contents. • Serum positive for botulinal toxins. • Positive wound culture.
Tetanus (Lockjaw)			
Clostridium tetani Transmitted by direct contact of soil contaminated with animal or human feces into a wound (primarily puncture wounds), burn, or laceration.	• Painful muscular contractions, primarily of the masseter and neck muscles. • Abdominal rigidity. • Generalized spasms frequently induced by sensory stimuli—opisthotonos (arching of the trunk) and risus sardonicus (distorted grin).	• Usually 3–21 days (average is 10 days); however, may range from 1 day to several months. • Shorter incubation periods generally associated with more heavily contaminated wounds, more severe disease.	• Organism rarely recovered from the site of infection. • No detectable antibody response. • Diagnosis is made clinically by excluding other possibilities.
Staphylococcal Infections			
Staphylococcus aureus, S. epidermidis, S. haemolyticus, coagulase-negative *staphylococci* Transmitted by direct contact with draining lesions or by autoinfection from colonized nares; hands are the most common vehicle of transmission.	• Skin and soft tissue infections—furuncles (boils), impetigo, carbuncles, cellulitis, abscesses, and infected lacerations. • Seeding of the bloodstream may lead to pneumonia, lung abscess, osteomyelitis, septicemia, endocarditis, pyarthrosis, meningitis, and brain abscess.	• Usually 4–10 days.	• Confirmed by isolation of the organism from culture.

MANAGEMENT	COMPLICATIONS	NURSING CONSIDERATIONS
• IV fluids and electrolytes. • Bed rest. • Avoid antispasmodics, laxatives, and salicylates. • Ampicillin, amoxicillin, cefotaxime, ceftriaxone, chloramphenicol, co-trimoxazole, or a fluoroquinolone. • Immunization is advised for travelers to areas of high endemicity.	• Endocarditis. • Meningitis. • Pneumonia. • Pyelonephritis. • Osteomyelitis. • Intestinal perforation and hemorrhage. • Septicemia. • Parotitis. • Cerebral dysfunction.	• Relapses occur in 5% to 10% of untreated cases and may be more common after antibiotic therapy. Report symptoms immediately. • Instruct patient to wash hands thoroughly after defecation and before preparing food. • Educate public—control flies, avoid raw shellfish, thoroughly rinse raw fruits and vegetables. • Family and close contacts should be examined and treated. • Typhoid is communicable as long as the infective organism is in the feces or urine, which may persist for months or, in 2% to 5% of cases, permanently.
• IV administration of trivalent botulinum antitoxin as soon as possible, obtained from CDC through state health departments. • IV fluids and electrolytes. • Intensive care to anticipate and manage respiratory failure: mechanical ventilation. • Report to health department immediately.	• Death from respiratory failure (fatality rate in the United States is 5% to 10%).	• All patient contacts known to have eaten the same food should have gastric lavage, high enemas, and cathartics and be kept under close medical supervision. • Instruct patient/patient contacts to wash hands thoroughly after defecation and before handling food. • No questionable canned food should ever be tasted.
• Tetanus immune globulin or tetanus antitoxin. • IV metronidazole. • Wound care to include cleaning, irrigation, wide debridement. • Sedatives and muscle relaxants, sometimes together with tracheostomy or intubation and mechanical ventilation. • Cardiac monitoring.	• High case fatality rate, up to 90% in infants and older adults. • Cardiac arrest. • Bacterial shock. • Autonomic disturbances.	• Refer persons with skin injuries for tetanus prophylaxis. • Remind adults to receive a tetanus booster every 10 years. • For major wounds, booster dose of vaccine should be given if none received in past 5 years.
• Penicillinase-resistant penicillins and the cephalosporins. • Vancomycin is treatment of choice for methicillin-resistant *S. aureus*. • Incision of abscesses to permit drainage of pus. • In severe systemic infection, the selection of antibiotics should be governed by results of susceptibility tests on the isolates.	• Septicemia. • Embolic skin lesions. • Toxic shock syndrome. • Death.	• Monitor patient's response to prescribed therapy. • Emphasize meticulous hand hygiene among patients and visitors. • Contain purulent drainage with a dressing. • Place soiled dressings in a paper bag before disposal.

(continued)

Table 31-3   Selected Infectious Diseases (continued)

DISEASE, INFECTIOUS AGENT, AND TRANSMISSION	CLINICAL MANIFESTATIONS	INCUBATION PERIOD	DIAGNOSTIC TESTS
Bacterial Infections			
Group A Streptococci Infections			
Streptococcus pyogenes, group A, with approximately 80 serologically distinct types Transmitted by large respiratory droplets or direct contact with secretions, or by ingestion of contaminated food and milk.	• Streptococcal pharyngitis (most common). • Wound and skin infections—impetigo, cellulitis, and erysipelas. • Scarlet fever—streptococcal sore throat with a rash that occurs if infectious agent produces erythrogenic toxin to which patient is not immune.	• Usually 1–3 days; rarely, longer.	• Identification of group A streptococcal antigen in pharyngeal secretions (rapid strep test). • Isolation of the organism by culture.
Syphilis			
Treponema pallidum, a spirochete Transmitted sexually or by direct contact with infectious exudates; transplacental infection of fetus can occur.	• Congenital: can result in spontaneous abortion or stillbirth, hydrops fetalis, prematurity, and multisystem abnormalities, including deafness. • Primary: indurated, painless, clean ulcer (chancre) with serous exudates. • Secondary: generalized macular-papular rash including palms and soles; fever; generalized lymphadenopathy, condylomata, malaise, headache, and splenomegaly. • Tertiary: aortitis, neurosyphilis; gummatous changes of skin, bone, viscera, and mucosal surfaces.	• Usually 3 weeks, but may be up to 3 months; signs of secondary syphilis develop 6 weeks to 6 months after primary syphilis.	• Nonspecific serologic tests such as RPR and VDRL; confirmed by specific antitreponemal antibody tests such as FTA-ABS and TP-RH; dark-field examination of lesion exudate for organism is definitive
Prion Disease			
Creutzfeldt-Jacob disease (CJD) and variant CJD (vCJD) Prion proteinaceous infectious particles. Transmission unknown in most cases; transmission of vCJD probably occurs through consumption of beef infected with BSE. Potential infectious organs and body fluids include the brain, spinal cord, eye, and CSF.	• Insidious onset with confusion, progressive defects in memory and personality, ataxia, rigidity, and myoclonus. • vCJD is distinguished by onset at early age, absence of EEG changes, and prolonged duration.	• 15 months to more than 30 years.	• Brain tissue biopsy. • Characteristic, periodic EEG changes.

b.i.d., twice per day; BSE, bovine spongiform encephalopathy; CDC, Centers for Disease Control and Prevention; CNS, central nervous system; CSF, cerebrospinal fluid; EEG, electroencephalography; ELISA, enzyme-linked immunosorbent assay; FA, direct fluorescent or immunofluorescent antibody test; GI, gastrointestinal; HCWs, health care workers; HIV, human immunodeficiency virus; IFA, indirect immunofluorescent antibody; IgM, immunoglobulin class M; IV, intravenous; PCR, polymerase chain reaction; P.O., by mouth; q.i.d., four times per day; t.i.d., three times per day; WBC, white blood cell.

MANAGEMENT	COMPLICATIONS	NURSING CONSIDERATIONS
• Penicillin is the drug of choice. Therapy should be continued for at least 10 days. • Erythromycin for penicillin-allergic patients. • Clindamycin or a cephalosporin may be used.	• Septicemia. • If pharyngitis is untreated, purulent complications, such as otitis media, sinusitis, abscesses, cervical adenitis, pneumonia. • Acute glomerulonephritis. • Toxic shock syndrome, necrotizing fasciitis. • Rheumatic fever, endocarditis.	• Repeated attacks of sore throat or other streptococcal disease due to different types of streptococci are relatively frequent. • Make sure the patient understands the importance of completing the course of antimicrobial therapy. • Emphasize the relationship of streptococcal infections to heart disease and glomerulonephritis. • Children should not return to school and HCWs should not return to work until at least 24 hours after appropriate antimicrobial therapy has begun.
• Primary and secondary: parenteral penicillin G; in penicillin allergy, if not pregnant, doxycycline; erythromycin is an inferior substitute in pregnant, penicillin-allergic patients but no proven alternative has been determined. • Latent syphilis of longer than 1 year or of unknown duration requires penicillin G given 1 injection per week for 3 weeks. • Tertiary syphilis requires IV penicillin for longer duration.	• Tertiary syphilis with cardiac, dermatologic, neurologic, and other systemic manifestations. • Acute syphilitic meningitis may occur in secondary or early latent syphilis. • Concurrent HIV infection may increase risk of CNS syphilis.	• Ensure that sexual activity is not resumed until treatment is complete for patient and partner. • Consider testing for HIV and other sexually transmitted diseases. • Encourage follow-up at 3 months for repeat serologic testing. • All women should be screened serologically for syphilis early in pregnancy. • All individuals, including HCWs, who have had close, unprotected contact with patient with early congenital syphilis before or during the first 24 hours of therapy should be examined for lesions in 3 weeks and again in 3 months.
• No treatment, only supportive care.	• Universally fatal degenerative disease, usually within weeks to months of symptom onset.	• Prion is extremely hardy and resistant to many disinfectants and to normal sterilization practices. • Use disposables as much as possible. • Health care facilities should have protocols in place for identification of cases and for instrument reprocessing at a higher temperature and for longer periods than typical. • Tissue from infected patients must not be used for transplants.

SELECTED REFERENCES

Centers for Disease Control and Prevention. (2002). Guideline for hand hygiene in health-care settings: Recommendations of the Healthcare Infection Control Practices Advisory Committee and the HICPAC/SHEA/APIC/IDSA Hand Hygiene Task Force. *Morbidity and Mortality Weekly Report, 51*, RR-16.

Centers for Disease Control and Prevention. (2010). *Avian influenza A virus infections of humans.* Atlanta, GA: Author. Available: *www.cdc.gov/flu/avian/gen-info/facts.htm.*

Centers for Disease Control and Prevention. (2012). CRE Toolkit—Guidance for control of carbapenem-resistant enterobacteriaceae (CRE). Atlanta: CDC. Available: *http://www.cdc.gov/hai/organisms/cre/cre-toolkit/index.html.*

Centers for Disease Control and Prevention. (2012). Healthcare associated infections. Atlanta, GA: Author. Available: *www.cdc.gov/ncidod/dhqp/pdf/isolation2007.pdf.*

Centers for Disease Control and Prevention. (2012). Recommended adult immunization schedule. *Morbidity and Mortality Weekly Report, 61*(4). Available: *www.cdc.gov/vaccines/recs/schedules/downloads/adult/mmwr-adult-schedule.pdf.*

Cohen, S. H., Gerding, D. N., Johnson, S., et al. (2010). Clinical practice guidelines for *Clostridium difficile* infection in adults: 2010 update by the Society for Healthcare Epidemiology of America (SHEA) and the Infectious Diseases Society of America (IDSA). *Infection Control and Hospital Epidemiology, 31*(5), 431–455.

Daugherty, E., Paine, L., Maragakis, L., et al. (2012). Safety Culture and Hand Hygiene: Linking Attitudes to Behavior. *Infection Control and Hospital Epidemiology, 33*(12), 1280–1282.

Drusano, G. L., & Lodise, T. P. (2013). Editorial Commentary: Saving Lives with Optimal Antimicrobial Chemotherapy. *Clin Infect Dis. 56*(2), 245–247.

Dumont, C., & Nesselrodt, D. (2012). Preventing CLABSI central line-associated bloodstream infections. *Nursing, 42*(6), 41–46.

Garcia, L.S., et al. (Eds.). (2010). *Clinical microbiology procedures handbook* (3rd ed.). Washington, DC: American Society for Microbiology Press.

Has, J. P., & Larson, E. L. (2008). Compliance with hand hygiene guidelines: Where are we in 2008? *American Journal of Nursing, 108*(8), 40–44.

Heymann, D. L. (2008). Control of communicable diseases manual (19th ed.). Washington, DC: American Public Health Association.

Jarvis, W. R. (Ed.). (2007). *Bennett & Brachman's hospital infections* (5th ed.). New York: Lippincott Williams & Wilkins.

Kelcikova, S., Skodova, Z., & Straka, S. (2012). Effectiveness of hand hygiene education in a basic nursing school curricula. *Public Health Nursing, 29*(2), 152–159.

Klevens, R. M., Edwards, J. R., Richards, C. L., et al. (2007). Estimating health care associated infections and deaths in USA 2002. *Public Health Reports, 122*(2), 160–166. Available: *www.cdc.gov/HAI/pdfs/hai/infections_deaths.pdf.*

Letto, C. (2008). An overview of sepsis. *Dimensions in Critical Care Nursing, 27*(5), 195–200.

Lora-Tamayo, J., Murillo, O., Iribarren, J. A., et al. (2013). A Large Multicenter Study of Methicillin–Susceptible and Methicillin–Resistant *Staphylococcus aureus* Prosthetic Joint Infections Managed with Implant Retention. *Clin Infect Dis. 56*(2), 182–194.

Occupational Safety & Health Administration. Standard number 1910.1030 Bloodborne Pathogens. Washington, DC: U.S. Department of Labor, OSHA. Available: *www.osha.gov/pls/oshaweb/owadisp.show_document?p_table=standards&p_id=10051.*

O'Grady, N. P., Alexander, M., Burns, L. A., et al. (2011). Guidelines for the prevention of intravascular catheter-related infections. Atlanta, GA: Centers for Disease Control and Prevention. Available: *www.cdc.gov/hicpac/pdf/guidelines/bsi-guidelines-2011.pdf.*

Rutala, W. A., Weber, D. J., and the Healthcare Infection Control Practices Advisory Committee (HICPAC). (2008). Guideline for Disinfection and Sterilization in Healthcare Facilities, 2008. Atlanta: CDC. Available: *http://www.cdc.gov/hicpac/pdf/guidelines/disinfection_nov_2008.pdf.*

Shefer, A., Atkinson, W., Friedman, C., et al. (2011). Immunization of health-care personnel recommendations of the Advisory Committee on Immunization Practices (ACIP). *Morbidity and Mortality Weekly Report, 60*(RR07), 1–45.

Siegel, J. D., Rhinehart, E., Jackson, M., et al. (2006). Management of Multidrug-Resistant Organisms in Healthcare Settings, 2006. Atlanta: CDC. Available: *http://www.cdc.gov/hicpac/pdf/guidelines/MDROGuideline2006.pdf.*

Siegel, J. D., Rhinehart, E., Jackson, M., et al. (2007). 2007 guideline for isolation precautions: Preventing transmission of infectious agents in healthcare settings. Atlanta, GA: Centers for Disease Control and Prevention. Available: *www.cdc.gov/hicpac/pdf/isolation/Isolation2007.pdf.*

Tseng, H. F., Sy, L. S., Lei, Q., et al. (2013). Safety of a Tetanus-Diphtheria-Acellular Pertussis Vaccine When Used Off-Label in an Elderly Population. *Clinical Infectious Diseases, 56*(3), 315–321.

Understanding emerging and reemerging infectious diseases: Teacher's guide. (1999). Bethesda, MD: National Institutes of Allergy and Infectious Disease. Available: *http://science.education.nih.gov/supplements/nih1/diseases/guide/understanding1.htm.*

Wormser, G. P., Dattwyler, R. J., Shapiro, E. D., et al. (2006). The clinical assessment, treatment, and prevention of Lyme disease, human granulocytic anaplasmoris, and babesiosis: Clinical practice guidelines by the IDSA. *Clinical Infectious Disease, 43*, 1089–1134.

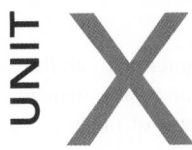
32
Musculoskeletal Disorders

OVERVIEW AND ASSESSMENT

 Evidence Base National Association for Orthopaedic Nurses. 2012. Core Curriculum for Orthopaedic Nursing. *Across the Lifespan* (3rd ed.).
Chicago: Author.
McRae, R. (2010). *Clinical orthopaedic examination*
(6th ed.). New York: Elsevier.

Subjective Data

Much can be learned about musculoskeletal disorders from
subjective data. History of injury, description of symptoms,
and associated personal health and family history can give
clues to the underlying problem and appropriate care for that
problem.

Common Manifestations of Musculoskeletal Problems

Pain
1. Where is the pain located?
   a. Joints, as in osteoarthritis (OA).
   b. Muscles or soft tissue, as in contusions, sprains, or
   strains.
   c. Bone, as in fractures or tumors.
2. Is it sharp, as in a fracture or sprain, or dull, as in a bone
   tumor?
3. Does the pain radiate?
   a. To buttocks or legs, as in lower back pain.
   b. To thigh or knee, as in hip fracture.
4. What makes the pain increase? What makes it better?
5. When was the onset of pain?

Limited Range of Motion

1. Is stiffness present? How long does it last?
   a. Present in morning for less than 30 minutes or after sitting for long period when due to OA.
   b. May persist and is associated with acute pain when due to spasm of lower back strain.
2. Is swelling present and limiting mobility?
   a. May be due to fracture.
   b. May be soft-tissue injury, such as sprain, strain, or contusion.
3. How does limited mobility affect activities of daily living (ADLs)?

Associated Symptoms

1. Any sensory or motor deficits, such as numbness, paresthesias, or weakness, indicating neurovascular compromise?
2. Any weight loss, fever, or malaise, as in bone tumors?
3. Any bony nodules or deformity, as in rheumatoid arthritis?

History

Mechanism of Injury

1. How did the injury occur? Essential for all trauma, including fractures, contusions, sprains, and strains, to help identify the extent of injury.
2. What was the progression of symptoms?
3. If not an acute injury, was there any repetitive movement or strain that may have contributed to problem, as in tendinitis?

Medical History

1. What medications are you taking (include name, dosage schedule, and last time taken—include prescription medications, vitamins, over-the-counter (OTC) medications, and herbals)?
2. Any history of corticosteroid use that predisposes to osteoporosis?
3. Is the woman postmenopausal? On estrogen replacement? If estrogen deficient, may predispose to osteoporosis.
4. Any history of prostate, breast, or lung cancer, which may metastasize to the bone?
5. What are other chronic conditions that may affect immobility imposed by casting, traction, or surgery?

Social History

1. What is the patient's occupation, which may contribute to lower back strain or OA?
2. Does the patient exercise? What type of exercise is performed, how frequently, and what is the duration of exercise? When was the last time this was performed?
3. What activities or sports does the patient participate in, such as running or tennis, which may cause tendinitis?
4. Are there risk factors for osteoporosis, such as smoking, inactivity, low calcium intake, or lack of exposure to the sun?
5. Is there a family history of osteoporosis or arthritis?
6. What cultural issues/religious beliefs contribute to this history?
7. Does the patient drink alcohol? If yes, what is the daily alcohol consumption?

Objective Data

Data on current system condition and functional abilities are secured through inspection, palpation, and measurement. Always compare with contralateral side (one side of the body to the other).

Musculoskeletal System

Skeletal Component

1. Note deviation from normal structure—bony deformities, length discrepancies, alignment, symmetry, amputations.
2. Identify abnormal motion and crepitus (grating sensation), as found with fractures.

Joint Component

1. Identify swelling that may be due to inflammation or effusion.
2. Note deformity associated with contractures or dislocations.
3. Evaluate stability, which may be altered.
4. Estimate active and passive range of motion (ROM).

Muscle Component

1. Inspect for size and contour of muscles.
2. Assess coordination of movement.
3. Palpate for muscle tone.
4. Estimate strength through cursory evaluation (ie, handshake) or scaled criteria (ie, 0 = no palpable contraction; 5 = normal ROM against gravity with full resistance).
5. Measure girth to note increases due to swelling or bleeding into muscle or decreases due to atrophy (difference of more than 1 cm is significant).
6. Identify abnormal clonus (rhythmic contraction and relaxation) or fasciculation (contraction of isolated muscle fibers).

Additional Assessment

Neurovascular Component

1. Assess circulatory status of involved extremities by noting skin color and temperature, peripheral pulses, capillary refill response, pain, and edema.
2. Assess neurologic status of involved extremities by the patient's ability to move distal muscles and description of sensation (eg, paresthesia).
3. Test reflexes of extremities.
4. Compare all to uninjured/unaffected extremity.

Skin Component

1. Inspect traumatic injuries (eg, cuts, bruises).
2. Assess chronic conditions (eg, dermatitis, stasis ulcers).
3. Note hair distribution and nail condition.
4. Inspect for Heberden's or Bouchard's nodes.
5. Assess for warmth or coolness of skin.

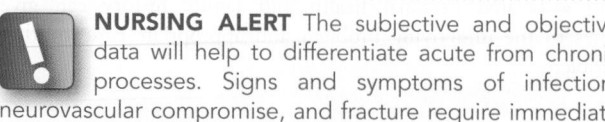 **NURSING ALERT** The subjective and objective data will help to differentiate acute from chronic processes. Signs and symptoms of infection, neurovascular compromise, and fracture require immediate diagnostic testing.

Radiologic and Imaging Studies

Many radiologic and imaging studies are helpful in evaluating musculoskeletal problems to rule out fracture or skeletal changes and to differentiate soft tissue injury.

 DRUG ALERT Many radiologic studies include injection or oral contrast. Check the patient's allergies and make sure a recent creatinine level has been obtained. Report elevated creatinine as soon as possible. Ensure that nephrotoxic drugs and metformin should be held at least 24 hours before the procedure and for 48 hours following. The patient should be well hydrated before and after the procedure.

X-rays

1. Of bone—to determine bone density, texture, integrity, erosion, changes in bone relationships.
2. Of cortex—to detect any widening, narrowing, irregularity.
3. Of medullary cavity—to detect any alteration in density.
4. Of involved joint—to show fluid, irregularity, spur formation, narrowing, changes in joint contour.
5. Tomogram—special x-ray technique for detailed view of special plane of bone.

Nursing and Patient Care Considerations

1. Tell patient that proper positioning is important to obtain a good x-ray, so cooperation is essential.
2. Advise patient to remove all jewelry, clothing with zippers or snaps, change from pockets, or other items that may interfere with x-ray.
3. Medicate for pain prior to x-ray, as needed.

Bone Scan

A *bone scan* consists of parenteral injection of bone-seeking radiopharmaceutical (such as gallium); concentration of isotope uptake revealed in primary skeletal disease (osteosarcoma), metastatic bone disease, inflammatory skeletal disease (osteomyelitis); fracture.

Nursing and Patient Care Considerations

1. There is usually no special preparation prior to the scan.
2. Injectable radionuclide is given several hours before the scan.
3. Reassure patient that the procedure will not cause pain and that scan will take 1 to 2 hours.
4. Analgesics or sedatives may be ordered for patients for whom lying immobile for any length of time is difficult.
5. Breastfeeding should be discontinued for at least 4 weeks after test to prevent radionuclide exposure to infant.
6. Inform patient that the exposure to radioactive substances is small (dose of radiation is less than a chest x-ray) and substances are excreted quickly by the body.

Bone Densitometry

Bone densitometry is a noninvasive study that yields an actual measurement of bone density and is diagnostic for osteoporosis (see page 184). It is most often performed on the lower spine and hips; however, simple portable screening tests that analyze the wrist or heel are also available.

Nursing and Patient Care Considerations

1. Calcium supplements should be avoided 24 hours prior to exam.
2. DXA scan should be avoided for 10 to 14 days if patient recently had a barium examination or has been injected with a contrast material for a computed tomography (CT) scan or radioisotope scan.
2. Have patient remove clothing and all jewelry or other metal objects.
3. Advise patient to lie still with hips flexed for about 20 minutes during test; technician will remain in the room.
4. Reassure patient that radiation exposure is minimal.

Magnetic Resonance Imaging

Magnetic resonance imaging (MRI) uses magnetic fields to demonstrate differences in hydrogen density of various tissues. Demonstrates tumors and soft tissue (muscle, ligament, tendon) abnormalities. Although it is more costly than CT scans, the cost is typically validated through the diagnostic accuracy. MRI not only clearly defines internal organs, but also is able to detect nerve damage and changes, such as edema or bruises, of bone. Bone bruises (osseous contusions) with traumatic injuries have some predictive value for future development of posttraumatic arthritis.

Nursing and Patient Care Considerations

1. Prepare patient for need to lie still for about 1 hour; repetitive clanging noise of machine will be heard; patients may feel closed in.
2. Practice relaxation techniques, such as relaxation breathing and imagery, ahead of time.
3. Some patients may need sedation; claustrophobic patients may be unable to undergo procedure or may need open MRI.
4. May be contraindicated for patients with some types of metal implants and devices. Notify the technologist or radiologist of any surgical implants, medical devices, or hardware for evaluation prior to MRI.
    a. In general, metal objects used in orthopedic surgery pose no risk during MRI. However, a recently placed artificial joint may require the use of another imaging procedure. If there is any question of their presence, an x-ray may be taken to detect the presence of and identify any metal objects.
    b. Patients who might have metal objects in certain parts of their bodies may also require an x-ray prior to an MRI. Notify the technologist or radiologist of any shrapnel, bullets, or other pieces of metal that may be present due to accidents.
    c. Dyes used in tattoos may contain iron and could heat up during MRI, but this is rarely a problem.
    d. Tooth fillings and braces usually are not affected by the magnetic field but they may distort images of the facial area or brain, so the radiologist should be aware of them.
    e. Parents who accompany children into the scanning room also need to remove metal objects and notify the technologist of any medical or electronic devices they may have.

NURSING ALERT In most cases, an MRI exam is safe for patients with metal implants, except for a few types. People with the following implants cannot be scanned and should not enter the MRI scanning area unless cleared by a radiologist:

- Internal (implanted) defibrillator or pacemaker
- Cochlear (ear) implant
- Some types of clips used on brain aneurysms
- Some types of metal coils placed within blood vessels

Other Tests

1. CT scan—narrow beam of x-ray that scans area in successive layers to evaluate disease, bone structure, joint abnormalities, and trauma (fractures).
2. Arthrogram—injection of radiopaque substance or air into joint cavity to outline soft tissue structures (eg, meniscus) and contour of joint.
3. Myelogram—injection of contrast medium into subarachnoid space at lumbar spine to determine level of disk herniation or site of tumor.
4. Diskogram—injection of small amount of contrast medium into lumbar disk abnormalities.
5. Arthrocentesis—insertion of needle into joint and aspiration of synovial fluid for purposes of examination or injection of therapeutic medications.
6. Arthroscopy—endoscopic procedure that allows direct visualization of joint structures (synovium, articular surfaces, menisci, ligaments) through a small needle incision. May be combined with arthrography.
7. Nerve studies—to differentiate nerve root compression, muscle disease (eg, dystrophy, myositis), peripheral neuropathies, central nervous system–anterior horn cell neuropathies, neuromuscular junction problems.
   a. Electromyography (EMG)—measures electrical potential generated by the muscle during relaxation and contraction.
   b. Nerve conduction velocities—measure the rate of potential generation along specific nerves (speed of impulse conduction).

GENERAL PROCEDURES AND TREATMENT MODALITIES

Evidence Base Bowden, G., McNally, M., Thomas, S., et al. (Eds.). (2011). *Oxford handbook of orthopaedics and trauma nursing*. Oxford, UK: Oxford University Press.

Crutch Walking

Crutches are artificial supports that assist patients who need aid in walking because of disease, injury, or a birth defect.

Preparation for Crutch Walking

The goals are to develop power in the shoulder girdle and upper extremities that bear the patient's weight in crutch walking and strengthen and condition the patient.

Strengthening the Muscles Needed for Ambulation

Instruct the patient as follows:

1. For quadriceps setting:
   a. Contract the quadriceps muscle while attempting to push the popliteal area against the mattress and raise the heel.
   b. Maintain the muscle contraction for a count of 5.
   c. Relax for the count of 5.
   d. Repeat this exercise 10 to 15 times hourly.
2. For gluteal setting:
   a. Contract or pinch the buttocks together for a count of 5.
   b. Relax for the count of 5.
   c. Repeat 10 to 15 times hourly.

Strengthening the Muscles of the Upper Extremities and Shoulder Girdle

Instruct the patient as follows:

1. Flex and extend arms slowly while holding traction weights; gradually increase poundage of weight and number of repetitions to increase strength and endurance.
2. Do push-ups while lying in a prone position.
3. Squeeze rubber ball—increases grasping strength.
4. Raise head and shoulders from bed; stretch hands forward as far as possible.
5. Sit up on bed or chair.
   a. Raise body from chair by pushing hands against chair seat (or mattress).
   b. Raise body out of seat. Hold. Relax.

Measuring for Crutches

1. When the patient is lying down (an approximate measurement):
   a. Measure from the anterior fold of the axilla to the sole. Then add 2 inches (5 cm).
   b. Alternatively, subtract 16 inches (40 cm) from the patient's height.
2. When the patient is standing erect:
   a. Stand the patient against the wall with feet slightly apart and away from the wall.
   b. The crutches should be fitted with large rubber suction tips.
   c. The elbow is flexed 30 degrees with the hand resting on the grip.
   d. There should be a two-finger-width insertion between the axillary fold and the underarm piece grip. A foam-rubber pad on the underarm piece will relieve pressure on the upper arm and thoracic cage.
   e. The tip of the crutch is placed 6 to 8 inches (15 to 20 cm) lateral to the forefoot.

Teaching the Crutch Stance

1. Have the patient wear well-fitting shoes with firm soles.
2. Before using the crutches, have the patient stand by a chair on the unaffected leg to achieve balance.
3. Position the patient against a wall with head in a neutral position.
4. Tripod position—basic crutch stance for balance and support.

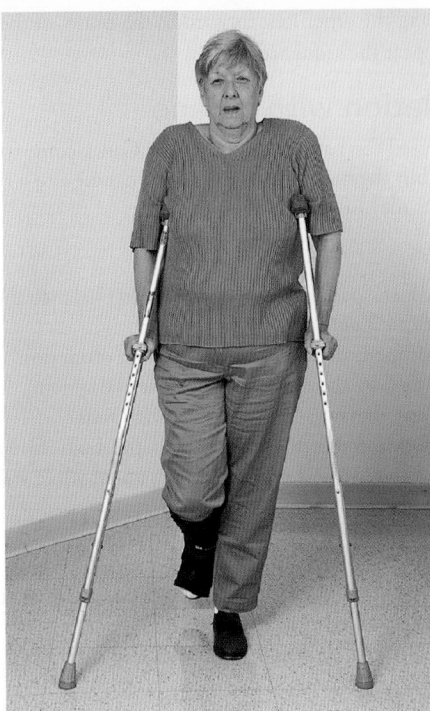

Figure 32-1. The tripod position is the basic crutch stance for balance and support.

   a. Crutches rest approximately 8 to 10 inches (20 to 25 cm) in front of and to the side of the patient's toes (see Figure 32-1).

   b. Taller patient requires a wider base, whereas shorter patient needs a narrower base.

5. Teach the patient to support weight on hands; weight borne on the axillae can damage the brachial plexus nerves and produce "crutch paralysis."

Teaching the Crutch Gait

1. Crutch walking requires balance, coordination, and a high expenditure of energy; these can be acquired with diligent and regular practice.
2. Practice balancing with crutches while leaning against the wall.
3. Practice shifting body weight in different positions while standing with crutches.
4. The selection of the crutch gait depends on the type and severity of the disability, weight-bearing status, and the patient's physical condition, arm and trunk strength, and body balance.
5. Teach the patient at least two gaits—a faster gait to be used for swiftness and a slower one to be used in crowded places.
6. Instruct the patient to change from one gait to another—relieves fatigue because a different combination of muscles is used.

Crutch Gaits

See Figure 32-2.

Four-Point Gait (Four-Point Alternate Crutch Gait)

1. Four-point gait is a slow but stable gait; the patient's weight is constantly being shifted.

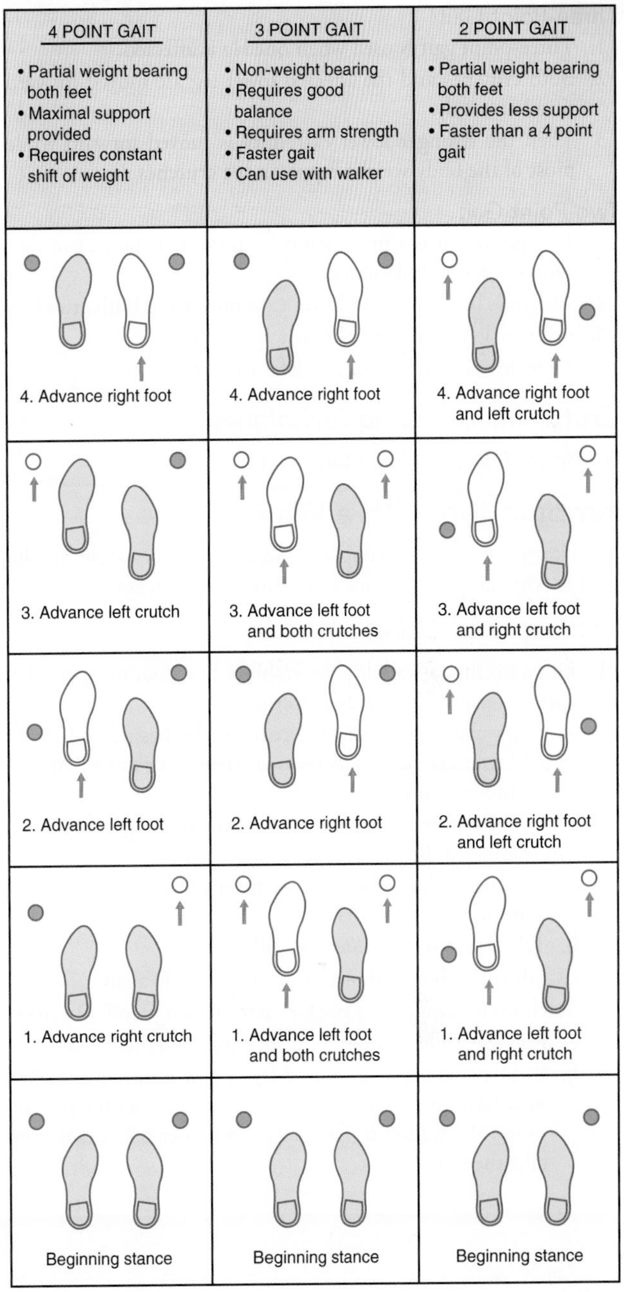

4 POINT GAIT	3 POINT GAIT	2 POINT GAIT
• Partial weight bearing both feet • Maximal support provided • Requires constant shift of weight	• Non-weight bearing • Requires good balance • Requires arm strength • Faster gait • Can use with walker	• Partial weight bearing both feet • Provides less support • Faster than a 4 point gait
4. Advance right foot	4. Advance right foot	4. Advance right foot and left crutch
3. Advance left crutch	3. Advance left foot and both crutches	3. Advance left foot and right crutch
2. Advance left foot	2. Advance right foot	2. Advance right foot and left crutch
1. Advance right crutch	1. Advance left foot and both crutches	1. Advance left foot and right crutch
Beginning stance	Beginning stance	Beginning stance

Figure 32-2. Crutch gaits. Shaded areas are weight-bearing. Arrow indicates advance of foot or crutch.

2. Four-point gait can be used only by patients who can move each leg separately and bear a considerable amount of weight on each of them.
3. Crutch-foot sequence:
   a. Right crutch.
   b. Left foot.
   c. Left crutch.
   d. Right foot.

Three-Point Gait

1. Three-point gait is used when one leg is affected.
2. Both crutches and the affected lower leg are moved forward simultaneously.
3. Then the stronger lower extremity is moved forward while most of the body weight is put on the crutches.

Two-Point Gait

1. Two-point gait is a progression from the four-point gait that allows faster ambulation.
2. Weight is borne on both lower extremities and both crutches.
3. Advance left foot and right crutch together.
4. Then advance right foot and left crutch together.

Crutch-Maneuvering Techniques

See Patient Education Guidelines 32-1.

Ambulation with a Walker

A walker provides more support than crutches or a cane for the patient who has poor balance and cannot use crutches.

Technique for Using a Walker

1. Be aware that a walker gives stability but does not permit a natural reciprocal walking pattern.
2. Rolling walkers may assist the patient who has painful joints in the lower extremities, decreased balance, or decreased cardiopulmonary function.
3. Teach the following sequence for a patient using a stationary (nonrolling) walker:
   a. Lift the walker, placing it in front of you while leaning your body slightly forward.
   b. Take a step or two into the walker.
   c. Lift the walker and place it in front of you again.
4. Teach the following sequence for a patient using a rolling walker:
   a. Roll the walker and move it forward about 12 inches.
   b. If the patient has an injured leg, a new joint, or a weaker side, step forward with that foot first. Instruct the patient to use the walker to help keep his or her balance as they take the step.

c. Bring the other foot forward to the center of the walker.
d. Repeat the sequence.

Ambulation with a Cane

A cane is used for balance and support. Canes come in a variety of shapes, but the majority have a curved handle and a rubber tip. Quad canes may offer greater support.

Purposes

1. To assist the patient to walk with greater balance and support and less fatigue.
2. To compensate for deficiencies of function normally performed by the neuromuscular skeletal system.
3. To relieve pressure on weight-bearing joints.
4. To provide forces to push or pull the body forward or to restrain the forward motion of the patient while walking.

Principles of Cane Use

1. An adjustable aluminum cane fitted with a 1½-inch (3.8-cm) rubber suction tip to provide traction while walking gives optimal stability to the patient.
2. With bilateral disease, using two canes gives better balance and weight relief.
3. To fit for a cane:
   a. Have patient flex elbow at a 30-degree angle and hold the cane 6 inches (15 cm) lateral to the base of fifth toe.
   b. Adjust the cane so the handle is approximately level with the greater trochanter.
4. Alternatively, while the patient is standing with arms at side, the handle of the cane should line up with the crease in wrist.

Technique for Walking with a Cane

1. Hold the cane in the hand opposite to the affected extremity (ie, the cane should be used on the good side)—allows partial weight-bearing relief because the cane is in contact with the floor at the same time as the affected extremity.
2. Advance the cane at the same time the affected leg is moved forward.
3. Keep the cane fairly close to the body to prevent leaning.

PATIENT EDUCATION GUIDELINES 32-1

Crutch-Maneuvering Techniques

STANDING UP

1. Move forward to the edge of the chair with the strong leg slightly under the seat.
2. Place both crutches in the hand on the side of the affected extremity.
3. Push down on the hand pieces while raising the body to a standing position.

SITTING IN A CHAIR

Grasp the crutches at the hand pieces for control and bend forward slightly while assuming a sitting position.

GOING UP STAIRS

1. Advance the stronger leg first up to the next step.
2. Advance the crutches and the weaker extremity.

GOING DOWN STAIRS

1. Place feet forward as far as possible on the step.
2. Advance crutches to the lower step. The weaker leg is advanced first and then the stronger one—the stronger extremity shares the work of raising and lowering the body weight with the patient's arms.

Note: Strong leg goes up stairs first and down stairs last.

4. If the patient cannot use the cane in the opposite hand, the cane may be carried on the same side and advanced when the affected leg is advanced.
5. To go up and down stairs:
   a. Step up on unaffected extremity.
   b. Then place cane and affected extremity on the step.
   c. Reverse this procedure for the descending steps.
   d. The strong leg goes up first and comes down last.
6. When using a quad cane, ensure that all four tips are touching the ground.

Casts

Evidence Base Bulstrode, C., Wilson-MacDonald, J., Fairbank, J., et al. (2011). *Oxford textbook of trauma and orthopaedics* (2nd ed.). Oxford, UK: Oxford University Press.

A *cast* is an immobilizing device made up of layers of plaster or fiberglass (water-activated polyurethane resin) bandages molded to the body part that it encases. See Procedure Guidelines 32-1. See also Procedure Guidelines 32-2, pages 1109 to 1110, for application and removal of a cast.

Purposes

1. To immobilize and hold bone fragments in reduction.
2. To apply uniform compression of soft tissues.
3. To permit early mobilization.
4. To correct and prevent deformities.
5. To support and stabilize weak joints.

Types of Casts

1. Short-arm cast—extends from below the elbow to the proximal palmar crease.
2. Gauntlet cast—extends from below the elbow to the proximal palmar crease, including the thumb (thumb spica).

(Text continues on page 1110)

PROCEDURE GUIDELINES 32-1

Application of a Cast

EQUIPMENT

- Plaster or synthetic bandages in desired widths
- Stockinette (tubular knitted material)*
- Cast padding (roll padding)*
- Splints (for reinforcement)

- Cotton, polyester, or polyurethane foam padding for bony prominences*
- Cast knives, scissors
- Polyethylene sheeting or newspaper—to protect floor
- Disposable gloves—to protect hands of operator

- Large, plastic-lined pail of water at room temperature—70°–75° F (21°–24° C)—or as recommended by cast material manufacturer
- Cast finishing hand cream for synthetic cast, as needed

CONSIDERATIONS

1. The application of a cast requires two to three persons: one to apply the plaster (operator), one to dip and hand the plaster bandages to the operator, and a third person to hold the extremity in correct position. (Body spicas may require additional personnel.)

2. The time required for the cast to become rigid varies with the material used—generally 2–6 minutes.
3. There should be no movement of the extremity while the cast is being applied and set.
4. In general, the joints above and below the involved bone are immobilized.

PROCEDURE

Nursing Action	Rationale
Preparatory phase	
1. Spread polyethylene sheeting or newspaper on floor.	1. Contains mess.
2. Explain to the patient that there will be a feeling of warmth as the plaster is applied.	2. Heat is produced by an endothermic reaction causing crystallization as plaster sets. The reaction of water with plaster of Paris liberates heat.

3. Apply stockinette and roll cast padding on the extremity or part to be immobilized.
 	
   a. Apply roll padding as smoothly and snugly as possible so each turn overlaps the preceding turn by one-half the width of the roll.
 	
   b. Extra pieces of padding may be placed over bony prominences: olecranon process, malleoli, patella, or ulnar protuberance.
	3. Padding is used to pad the sharp cast margins for patient comfort and to prevent pressure areas, minimize circulatory problems, and facilitate cast removal. It is applied from the distal to the proximal end of the extremity. When too much padding is used, it may shift and produce pressure areas under the cast.

(continued)

PROCEDURE GUIDELINES 32-1 *(continued)*

Application of a Cast

PROCEDURE *(continued)*

Nursing Action	Rationale
4. While keeping the thumb under the forward edge of the bandage, submerge the plaster bandage vertically in water (room temperature) for a minute or so, or until bubbles cease to rise.	4. Water that is too warm will accelerate setting time, may cause a burn, and may result in excessive plaster loss by loosening the adhesive agents that bond the plaster to the fabric.
5. Expel excess water by squeezing (not wringing) toward the center of the bandage; hand bandage to operator with free end hanging loose.	5. Cast will dry more quickly (thus will acquire maximum strength sooner) if a well-squeezed plaster bandage is used. Maximum strength is achieved by synthetic casts through chemical reaction in about 30 minutes.

Performance phase (by operator)

1. Starting at the distal end, roll the bandage gently and evenly on the extremity overlapping the preceding turn by one-half the width of the roll.	1. Roll inward toward the patient's body for ease of control.
2. Keep bandage moving and in constant contact with surface of extremity. Smooth and rub down successive layers or turns of each bandage into layers below with the thumbs and thenar eminences (mound on the palm) in circumferential and longitudinal directions.	2. Keeps the cast uniformly thick. Rubbing the plaster as it is applied will form a smooth, solid, and well-fused cast. Avoid indenting the cast with the fingertips because this may produce pressure sores on underlying skin. Handle fresh casts with palms.
3. Make tucks in the lower border of the bandage by lifting the bandage off the surface (without tension) and overlapping it in a V-shaped fashion.	3. Tucking the bandage helps to contour the cast to the changing circumference of the extremity. Do not twist or reverse the bandage to change its direction because this produces sharp cutting edges.
4. Trim the cast to size with a sharp knife. Fold stockinette over edges of cast and anchor with cast material.	4. Stockinette produces smooth, comfortable edges on cast. Do not pull too vigorously on the stockinette because this may cause pressure on bony prominences.
5. Finish synthetic cast with cast hand cream, as indicated.	5. Smoothes rough exterior surface.
6. Ask the patient if there is any discomfort or pain.	6. If a patient complains of pain, it may be due to manipulation of fracture during setting; pain should subside rapidly. If it persists, the cast and encircling dressings are split to avoid constriction, circulatory problems, and pressure sores.

Follow-up phase

1. Support the cast with the palm of the hand while moving the patient. Avoid indentations from tips of fingers.	1. Finger indentation on a fresh cast can produce pressure sores.
2. Expose the cast to warm, circulating, dry air or blow air over cast with a circulating fan to increase the evaporation of water.	2. Avoid covering the cast when it is drying because this delays drying time. Usually the plaster cast will reach its maximum temperature 5–15 minutes after it is applied and will then cool rapidly. The ultimate plaster cast strength is obtained after the cast is dry (up to 48 hours, depending on outside temperature and humidity). The synthetic cast strength is maximum within 30 minutes of application and not dependent on being dry.
3. Clean equipment and store ready for use.	

 Evidence Base National Association for Orthopaedic Nursing. (2012). *Orthopedic nursing core competencies across the lifespan*, (3rd ed.). Chicago: Author.

*Material needs to be nonabsorbent if nonplaster cast is used.

PROCEDURE GUIDELINES 32-2

Removal of a Cast

EQUIPMENT

- Cast cutter—an electric saw with circular blade that oscillates and is connected to a vacuum collector
- Cast spreader
- Plaster knife
- Scissors
- Felt-tip pen

PROCEDURE

Nursing Action	Rationale
Preparatory phase	
1. Describe to the patient how and where the cast cutter will be used and the expected sensations.	1. Reassures the patient that the cutter produces vibrations but not pain.
2. Determine whether the cast is padded.	2. An electric plaster cast cutter should not be used on unpadded casts.
3. Determine where the cut will be made. Mark the area to be cut with a felt pen.	3. The line should be in front of the lateral malleolus and behind the medial malleolus on a lower-extremity cast. An upper-extremity cast is usually split along the ulnar or flexor surface.
Performance phase	
1. Inform the patient to shield eyes.	1. Plaster dust may be irritating to the eyes.
2. Grasp the electric cutter as illustrated.	2. Correct grasp is essential for stabilizing the electric cutter.
3. Rest the thumb on the cast.	3. The thumb serves as a depth gauge and acts as a guard in front of the blade.
4. Turn on the electric cutter. Push the blade firmly and gently through the cast while holding the thumb against the cast to steady the blade while cutting through the cast.	
5. As the blade cuts through the plaster, a sudden lack of resistance is felt; plaster will "give" (or "dip") when the cut is completed.	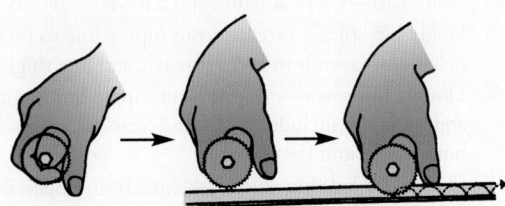
6. Lift the cutting blade up a degree (but not out of the cutting groove) and advance the blade at a slightly higher or lower level. The cast is cut by a series of alternating pressure and linear movements along the line of the cut (see accompanying figure).	*Operating a cast cutter.*
7. Avoid drawing the cutting blade along the extremity in a single motion.	7. This will cut the skin. If saw blade is in contact with padding too long, the patient will feel burning sensation on skin from rapidly oscillating blade.
8. Cut the cast on both sides. Then rock the anterior portion of the cast over the posterior portion.	8. Allows the operator to determine if the cast is completely cut.
9. Insert the blades of the cast spreader in the cut trough. Separate the two halves with the spreader at several sites along the cast split. Separate the cast with the hands.	
10. Cut through the padding and stockinette with scissors, keeping the scissor blade that is closest to the skin parallel to the skin.	10. Use bandage scissors; place the flat blade closest to the skin.
11. Lift the extremity carefully out of the posterior portion of the cast. Support the extremity so it is maintained in the same position as when in the cast.	11. When the support of the cast has been removed, stresses and strain are placed on parts that have been at rest.

(continued)

PROCEDURE GUIDELINES 32-2 *(continued)*

Removal of a Cast

PROCEDURE *(continued)*

Nursing Action	Rationale
After removal of cast	
1. Clean the skin gently with mild soap and water. Blot dry. Apply a skin cream.	1. Explain to the patient that the skin will be scaly and the extremity will appear "thin" from disuse. Reassure him or her that it will take a few weeks to regain normal appearance and function.
2. Emphasize the importance of continuing the prescribed exercises, reporting for physical therapy, and so forth.	2. Exercises are necessary to redevelop and increase strength and function. Pain and stiffness may be expected after cast removal.

 Evidence Base National Association for Orthopaedic Nursing. (2012). *Orthopedic nursing core competencies across the lifespan*, (3rd ed.). Chicago: Author.

3. Long-arm cast—extends from upper level of axillary fold to proximal palmar crease; elbow usually immobilized at right angle.
4. Short-leg cast—extends from below knee to base of toes.
5. Long-leg cast—extends from upper thigh to the base of toes; foot is at right angle in a neutral position.
6. Body cast—encircles the trunk stabilizing the spine.
7. Spica cast—incorporates the trunk and extremity.
   a. Shoulder spica cast—a body jacket that encloses trunk, shoulder, and elbow.
   b. Hip-spica cast—encloses trunk and a lower extremity.
      i. Single hip-spica—extends from nipple line to include pelvis and extends to include pelvis and one thigh.
      ii. Double hip-spica—extends from nipple line or upper abdomen to include pelvis and extends to include both thighs and lower legs.
      iii. One-and-a-half hip-spica—extends from upper abdomen, includes one entire leg and extends to the knee of the other.
8. Cast-brace—external support about a fracture that is constructed with hinges to permit early motion of joints, early mobilization, and independence.
   a. Cast bracing is based on the concept that some weight-bearing is physiologic and will promote the formation of bone and contain fluid within a tight compartment that compresses soft tissues, providing a distribution of forces across the fracture site.
   b. Cast-brace is applied after initial edema and pain have subsided and there is evidence of fracture stability.
9. Cylinder cast—Can be used for upper or lower extremity. Used for fracture or dislocation of knee (lower extremity) or elbow dislocation (upper extremity).

Complications Associated with Casts

1. Pressure of cast on neurovascular and bony structures causes necrosis, pressure sores, and nerve palsies.

2. Compartment syndrome is a condition resulting from increased progressive pressure within a confined space, thus compromising the circulation and the function of tissues within that space. This is a medical emergency and can be limb-threatening. A tight cast, trauma, fracture, prolonged compression of an extremity, bleeding, and edema put patients at risk for compartment syndrome.
3. Immobility and confinement in a cast, particularly a body cast, can result in multisystem problems.
   a. Nausea, vomiting, and abdominal distention associated with cast syndrome (superior mesenteric artery syndrome, resulting in diminished blood flow to the bowel), adynamic ileus, and possible intestinal obstruction.
   b. Acute anxiety reaction symptoms (ie, behavioral changes and autonomic responses—increased respiratory and heart rate, elevated blood pressure [BP], diaphoresis) associated with confinement in a space.
   c. Thrombophlebitis and possible pulmonary emboli associated with immobility and ineffective circulation (eg, venous stasis).
   d. Respiratory atelectasis and pneumonia associated with ineffective respiratory effort.
   e. Urinary tract infection—renal and bladder calculi associated with urinary stasis, low fluid intake, and calcium excretion associated with immobility.
   f. Anorexia and constipation associated with decreased activity.
   g. Psychological reaction (eg, depression) associated with immobility, dependence, and loss of control.

Nursing Assessment

1. Assess neurovascular status of the extremity with a cast for signs of compromise.
   a. Pain (pain out of proportion to injury is an indication for compartment syndrome).
   b. Swelling.

c. Discoloration—pale or blue.

d. Cool skin distal to injury.

e. Tingling or numbness (paresthesia).

f. Pain on passive extension (muscle stretch).

g. Slow capillary refill; diminished or absent pulse.

h. Paralysis.

2. Assess skin integrity of casted extremity. Be alert for:

a. Severe initial pain over bony prominences; this is a warning symptom of an impending pressure ulcer. Pain increases when ulceration occurs.

b. Odor.

c. Drainage on cast.

NURSING ALERT Signs and symptoms of compartment syndrome include pain, paresthesia, pallor, pulselessness, poikilothermia, and paralysis. Pain is the first sign and is usually described as deep, constant, poorly localized, and out of proportion to the injury. The pain is not relieved by analgesia and worsens with stretching of the muscle group. The other signs occur late in the course of compartment syndrome. Unrelenting pain and other signs of compartment syndrome should be reported immediately. The cast may have to be split and removed.

3. Carefully assess for positioning and potential pressure sites of the casted extremity (see Figure 32-3).

a. Lower extremity—heel, malleoli, dorsum of foot, head of fibula, anterior surface of patella.

b. Upper extremity—medial epicondyle of humerus, ulnar styloid.

c. Plaster jackets or body spica casts—sacrum, anterior and superior iliac spines, vertebral borders of scapulae.

4. Assess cardiovascular, respiratory, and GI systems for possible complications of immobility.

5. Assess psychological reaction to illness, cast, and immobility.

Nursing Diagnoses

- Risk for neurovascular injury related to swelling and constrictive bandage or cast.

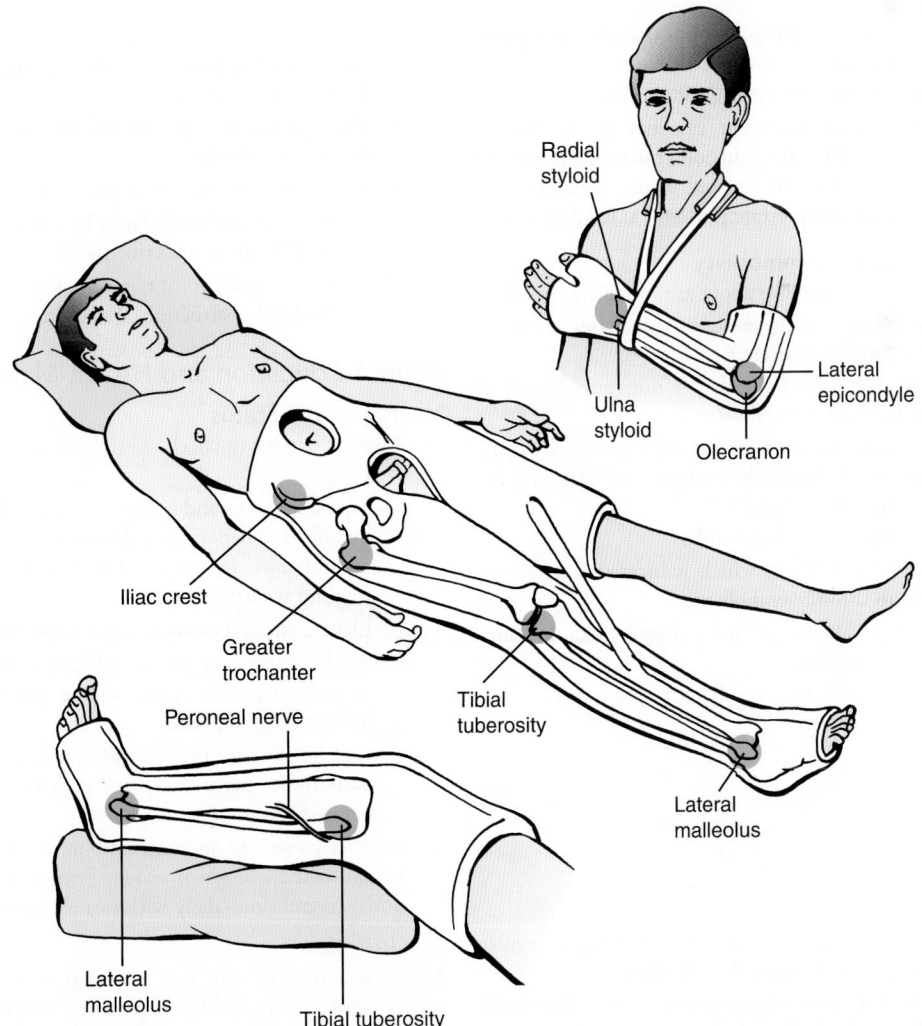

Figure 32-3. Pressure areas in different types of casts.

- Impaired Physical Mobility related to condition and casting.
- Risk for impaired gastrointestinal motility related to cast syndrome.

Nursing Interventions

Maintaining Adequate Tissue Perfusion

1. Elevate the extremity on cloth-covered pillow above the level of the heart. Keep the heel off the mattress.
2. Avoid resting cast on hard surfaces or sharp edges that can cause denting or flattening of the cast and consequent pressure sores.
3. Handle moist cast with palms of hands.
4. Turn patient every 2 hours while cast dries.
5. Instruct patient not to place objects into cast. Advise patient of alternative methods of managing itching such as blowing cool air under the cast.
6. Assess neurovascular status hourly during the first 24 hours, then less frequently as condition warrants and swelling resolves.
7. If symptoms of neurovascular compromise occur:
   a. Notify health care provider immediately.
   b. Bivalve the cast—split cast on each side over its full length into two halves.
   c. Cut the underlying padding—blood-soaked padding may shrink and cause constriction of circulation.
   d. Spread cast sufficiently to relieve constriction.
8. If symptoms of pressure area occur, cast may be "windowed" (hole cut in it) so the skin at the pain point can be examined and treated. The window must be replaced so the tissue does not swell and cause additional pressure problems at window edge.

Minimizing the Effects of Immobility

1. Encourage the patient to move about as normally as possible.
2. Encourage compliance with prescribed exercises to avoid muscle atrophy and loss of strength.
   a. Active ROM for every joint that is not immobilized at regular and frequent intervals.
   b. Isometric exercises for the muscles of the casted extremity. Instruct patient to alternately contract and relax muscles without moving affected part.
3. Reposition and turn patient frequently.
4. Avoid pressure behind knees, which reduces venous return and predisposes to thromboembolism.
5. Use anti-embolism stockings and sequential compression devices (SCDs), as indicated.
6. Administer prophylactic anticoagulants, as prescribed.

> **NURSING ALERT** People at high risk for pulmonary emboli include older adults and persons with previous thromboembolism, obesity, heart failure, or multiple trauma. These patients require prophylaxis against thromboembolism.

7. Encourage deep-breathing exercises and coughing at regular intervals to prevent atelectasis and pneumonia.
8. Encourage patient to drink liberal quantities of fluid to avoid urinary infection and calculi secondary to immobility.

9. Facilitate patient participation in care planning and activities. Encourage verbalization of feelings and concerns regarding restriction of activities.
10. Provide and encourage diversional activities.
11. Pay special attention to positioning and turning for patients in spica or body cast (see Box 32-1).

Preventing Gastrointestinal Impairment

1. Encourage balanced nutritional intake.
   a. Assess the patient's food preferences. Serve small meals.
   b. Provide natural bowel stimulants (eg, fiber) and good fluid intake.
   c. Monitor bowel movements, bowel sounds, and use a bowel program, if necessary.
2. Observe for symptoms of cast syndrome—nausea, vomiting, abdominal distention, abdominal pain, and decreased bowel sounds.

> **NURSING ALERT** Cast syndrome (superior mesenteric artery syndrome) is a rare sequela of body cast application, yet it is a potentially fatal complication. It is important to teach patients about this syndrome because this can develop as late as several weeks after cast application.

3. If symptoms of cast syndrome develop, report immediately to the health care provider.
   a. Place patient in a prone position, if tolerated, to relieve pressure symptoms.
   b. Use nasogastric suction as prescribed.
   c. Maintain electrolyte balance by intravenous (IV) replacement of fluids, as prescribed.
   d. Prepare the patient for removal of the cast or surgical relief of duodenal obstruction, if necessary.

Patient Education and Health Maintenance

Neurovascular Status

1. Instruct patient to check neurovascular status and to control swelling.
   a. Watch for signs and symptoms of circulatory disturbance, including blueness or paleness of fingernails or toenails accompanied by pain and tightness, numbness, cold or tingling sensation.
   b. Elevate affected extremity and wiggle fingers or toes.
   c. Apply ice bags, as prescribed (one third to one half full), to each side of the cast, making sure they do not make indentations in plaster.
   d. Call health care provider promptly if excessive swelling, paresthesia, persistent pain, pain on passive stretch, or paralysis occurs.
2. Instruct patient to alternate ambulation with periods of elevation to the cast when seated. Encourage the patient to lie down several times daily with cast elevated.

Skin Irritation

Advise patient to prevent skin irritation at cast edge by padding edges of cast with moleskin or "petaling" cast edges with strips of adhesive tape.

BOX 32-1   Specific Care for Patient in Spica or Body Cast

POSITIONING

1. Place a bed board under the mattress for uniform support of the body.
2. Support the curves of the cast with cloth-covered flexible pillows—prevents cracking and flat spots while cast is drying.
   a. Place three pillows crosswise on bed for body cast.
   b. Place one pillow crosswise at the waist and two pillows lengthwise for affected leg for spica cast. If both legs are involved, use two additional pillows.
3. Encourage the patient to maintain physiologic position by:
   a. Using the overhead trapeze.
   b. Placing good foot flat on bed and pushing down while lifting him-or herself up on the trapeze.
   c. Avoiding twisting motions.
   d. Avoiding positions that produce pressure on groin, back, chest, and abdomen.

TURNING

1. Move the patient to the side of the bed using a steady, even pulling motion.
2. Place pillows along the other side of the bed—one for the chest and two (lengthwise) for the legs.
3. Instruct the patient to place arms at side or above head.
4. Turn the patient as a unit. Avoid twisting the patient in the cast.
5. Turn the patient toward the leg not encased in plaster or toward the unoperated side if both legs are in plaster.
   a. One nurse stands at other side of bed to receive the patient's shoulders.

b. Second nurse supports leg in plaster while the third nurse supports the patient's back as he or she is turned.

 NURSING ALERT Do not grasp cross bar of spica cast to move the patient. The purpose of the bar is to maintain the integrity of the cast.

   c. Turn the patient in body cast to a prone position twice daily—provides postural drainage of bronchial tree; relieves pressure on back.
6. Keep the cast level by elevating the lumbar sacral area with a small pillow when the head of the bed is elevated.

OTHER CARE

1. Protect cast from soiling.
   a. Cover perineum with a towel and apply spray (lacquer-type) to perineal area of cast. Tuck 4-inch (10-cm) strips of thin polyethylene sheeting under perineal area of cast and tape to cast exterior. Replace when soiling occurs.
   b. Clean outside of soiled cast with a mild powdered cleanser and a *slightly* dampened or dry, clean cloth and pat dry completely, only when necessary.
2. Roll the patient onto fracture bedpan; use small pillow in lumbosacral area for support.
3. Inspect skin for signs of irritation around cast edge, under cast using a flashlight for illumination.
4. Reach up under cast and massage accessible skin.
5. Protect the toes from the pressure of the bedding.

Exercise

1. Instruct patient to actively exercise every joint that is not immobilized and to perform isometric exercises (contract muscles without moving joint) of those immobilized to maintain muscle strength and to prevent atrophy.
2. Tell patient to perform hourly when awake:
   a. Leg cast—push down on the popliteal space, hold it, relax, repeat. Move toes back and forth; bend toes down, then pull them back.
   b. Arm cast—make a fist, hold it, relax, repeat. Move shoulders.
3. Encourage ambulation with weight-bearing restrictions.

Cast Care

1. Advise to avoid getting cast wet, especially padding under cast—causes skin breakdown as plaster cast becomes soft.
2. Warn against covering a leg cast with plastic or rubber boots because this causes condensation and wetting of the cast.
3. Instruct to avoid weight-bearing or stress on plaster cast for 24 hours.
4. Instruct to report to health care provider if the cast cracks or breaks; instruct the patient not to try to fix it.
5. Teach how to clean the cast:
   a. Remove surface soil with slightly damp cloth.
   b. Rub soiled areas with household scouring powder.
   c. Wipe off residual moisture.

Teaching Safety Measures

To prevent falls, avoid walking on wet floors or sidewalks. To prevent pressure and injury to the skin, do not place objects inside the cast.

After Cast Removal

1. Instruct to clean skin with mild soap and water, blot dry, and apply emollient lotion to dry skin.
2. Warn against scratching the skin.
3. Advise to continue prescribed exercises. Gradually resume activities and elevate extremity to control swelling.

Evaluation: Expected Outcomes

- No pain, discoloration, or sensory or motor impairment of affected extremity; warm, with good capillary refill.
- Ambulates with assistance; performing active ROM and isometric exercises every 1 to 2 hours.
- No signs of cast syndrome.

Traction

Traction is force applied in a specific direction. To apply the force needed to overcome the natural force or pull of muscle groups, a system of ropes, pulleys, and weights is used. See Procedure Guidelines 32-3, page 1114.

PROCEDURE GUIDELINES 32-3

Application of Buck's Extension Traction

PURPOSE

Buck's extension skin traction is used as a temporary measure to provide immobility, support, and comfort until definitive treatment is accomplished.

EQUIPMENT

- Foam Buck's traction boot or traction tape and 4-inch elastic bandage
- Spreader block or metal spreader
- Pulley, nylon rope, and weights (5–7 lb [2.5–3 kg] is usual [amount of weight is prescribed, generally not more than 10 lb (4.5 kg)])
- Sheepskin pad
- Shock blocks or adjustable bed for Trendelenburg's position

PROCEDURE

Nursing Action	Rationale
Preparatory phase	
1. Bed position is flat or in Trendelenburg's position. This depends on the size of the patient and the weight applied.	1. Elevating the foot of the bed (countertraction) helps prevent the patient from sliding down toward the foot of the bed.
2. Question the patient to determine previous skin conditions (contact dermatitis). Inspect skin for evidences of atrophy, abrasions, and circulatory disturbances.	2. The skin must be in healthy condition to tolerate skin traction.
3. Make sure the skin of the extremity is clean and dry.	3. Clean, dry skin helps traction tape adherence.
4. Document the neurovascular status of the extremity, any evidence of skin problems or varicosities.	4. As baseline for future reference.
Performance phase	
1. Position the patient in center of bed in good alignment.	1. For effective line of pull.
If traction tape is used:	
2. Apply continuous traction tape to medial and lateral aspects of lower leg (below knee and loosely around foot to allow for attachment of spreader).	2. Avoid pressure over malleoli and head of fibula. Pressure sores develop rapidly over bony prominences. Pressure over the region of the fibular head and common peroneal nerve may produce peroneal palsy and footdrop.
3. Have a second person elevate and support the extremity under the ankle and knee while the elastic bandage is applied. Beginning at the ankle, wrap the elastic bandage snugly over the tape up to the tibial tubercle.	3. The elastic bandage holds tape to the skin and helps prevent slipping.
4. Attach a spreader block (or metal spreader) to the distal end of the tape. Attach a rope to the spreader block and pass it over a pulley fastened to the end of the bed and gently apply weights.	4. The spreader block prevents pressure along the side of the foot. The spreader should not be too narrow (causes pressure sores on ankle) or too wide (pulls traction tape away from the heel).
5. Place a sheepskin pad under the leg (or use a commercial heel protector).	5. Sheepskin is used to reduce friction of the heel against the bed.
If foam boot is used:	
1. Apply anti-embolism stockings, if prescribed.	1. Prophylactic measure in high-risk population.
2. Place leg in foam boot, adjusting it so the heel is in the heel of the boot.	2. Preventing sore heels is a primary concern.
3. Secure Velcro bootstraps, avoiding excessive pressure on malleoli and fibular head.	3. Pressure over bony prominences causes skin breakdown and pressure on peroneal nerve may result in footdrop.
4. Attach rope to built-in spreader plate, pass it over pulley, and apply weights gently.	4. The rope should move unobstructed and the weights should hang free of the bed and not touch the floor.

 Evidence Base National Association for Orthopaedic Nursing. (2012). *Orthopedic nursing core competencies across the lifespan*, (3rd ed.). Chicago: Author.

Purposes of Traction

1. To reduce and immobilize fracture.
2. To regain normal length and alignment of an injured extremity.
3. To lessen or eliminate muscle spasm.
4. To prevent deformity.
5. To give the patient freedom for "in-bed" activities.
6. To reduce pain.

Types of Traction

Running Traction

1. A form of traction in which the pull is exerted in one plane.
2. May use either skin or skeletal traction.
3. Buck's extension traction (see Figure 32-4) is an example of running skin traction.

Balanced Suspension Traction

1. Uses additional weights to counterbalance the traction force and floats the extremity in the traction apparatus.
2. The line of pull on the extremity remains fairly constant despite changes in the patient's position.

Application of Traction

Traction may be applied to the skin or to the skeletal system.

Skin Traction

1. Accomplished by applying a light force that pulls on tape, sponge rubber, or special device (boot, cervical halter, pelvic belt) that is in contact with the skin.
2. The pulling force is transmitted to the musculoskeletal structures.
3. Skin traction is used as a temporary measure in adults to control muscle spasm and pain.
4. It is used before surgery in the treatment of hip fracture (Buck's extension) and femoral shaft fractures (Russell's traction).
5. It may be used definitively to treat fractures in children.

Skeletal Traction

See Figure 32-5.

1. Traction applied by the orthopedic surgeon under aseptic conditions using wires, pins, or tongs placed through bones and provides a strong, steady, continuous pull.
2. Skeletal traction is used most frequently in treating fractures of the femur, humerus (supracondylar fractures), tibia, and cervical spine.

Complications

1. Infection of pin tracts in skeletal traction.
2. Skin breakdown and dermatitis under skin traction.
3. Neurovascular compromise resulting in increased pain, muscle spasms, numbness, tingling, and loss of sensation.
4. Inadequate fracture alignment resulting in posttreatment arthritis.
5. Complications of immobility include:
   a. Stasis pneumonia.
   b. Thrombophlebitis.
   c. Pressure ulcers.
   d. Urinary infection and calculi.
   e. Constipation.

Nursing Assessment

1. Assess for pain, deformity, swelling, motor and sensory function, and circulatory status of the affected extremity.
2. Assess skin condition of the affected extremity, under skin traction and around skeletal traction, as well as over bony prominences throughout the body.
3. Assess for alignment of affected body part.
4. Assess for signs and symptoms of complications.
5. Assess traction equipment for safety and effectiveness.
   a. The patient is placed on a firm mattress.
   b. The ropes and the pulleys should be in alignment.

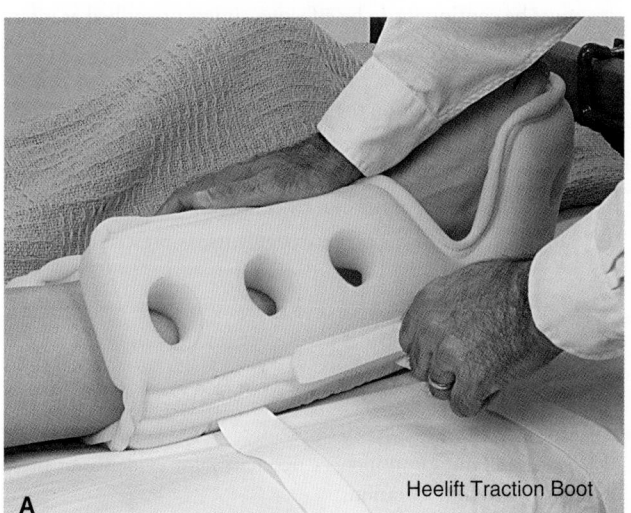
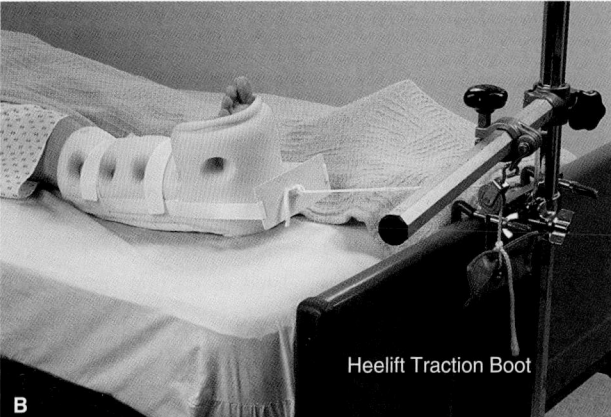

Figure 32-4. Buck's extension traction. (A) Skin traction is accomplished through a boot device in contact with the skin. **(B)** Weight is applied to exert running traction in one plane, while the body acts as a counterweight. (Courtesy DM Systems Inc., *www.dmsystems.com*.)

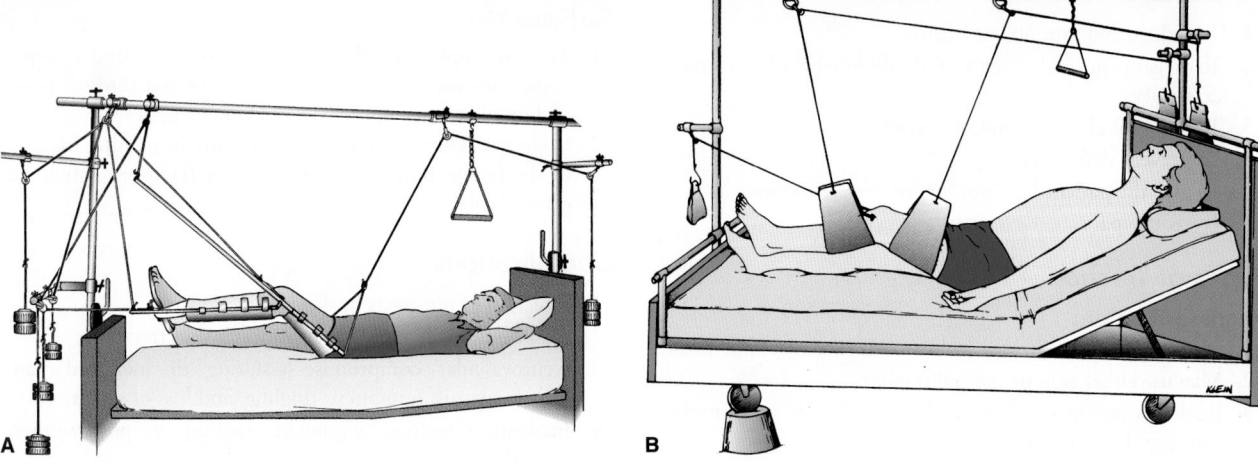

Figure 32-5. Balanced skeletal traction using (A) Thomas leg splint and Pearson attachment and **(B)** slings for support and suspension.

c. The pull should be in line with the long axis of the bone.

d. Any factor that might reduce the pull or alter its direction must be eliminated.

   i. Weights should hang freely.

   ii. Ropes should be unobstructed and not in contact with the bed or equipment.

   iii. Patient's bed should have an overhead trapeze set up to assist the patient to pull self up in bed at frequent intervals.

> **NURSING ALERT** Traction is *not* accomplished if the knot in the rope or the footplate is touching the pulley or the foot of the bed or if the weights are resting on the floor. Never remove the weights when repositioning the patient who is in skeletal traction because this will interrupt the line of pull and cause the patient considerable pain.

e. The amount of weight applied in skin traction must not exceed the tolerance of the skin. The condition of the skin must be inspected frequently.

f. Cover exposed sharp ends of skeletal pins with cork or other pin covering to protect patient and caregivers from injury.

6. Assess emotional reaction to condition and traction.

7. Assess understanding of the treatment plan.

Nursing Diagnoses

- Impaired Physical Mobility related to traction therapy and underlying pathology.
- Risk for Impaired Skin Integrity related to pressure on soft tissues.
- Risk for Infection related to bacterial invasion at skeletal traction site.
- Risk for Peripheral Neurovascular Dysfunction related to injury or traction therapy.

Nursing Interventions

Minimizing the Effects of Immobility

1. Encourage active exercise of uninvolved muscles and joints to maintain strength and function. Dorsiflex feet hourly to avoid development of footdrop and aid in venous return.

2. Encourage deep breathing hourly to facilitate expansion of lungs and movement of respiratory secretions.

3. Auscultate lung fields at least twice per day.

4. Encourage fluid intake of 2,000 to 2,500 mL daily.

5. Provide balanced high-fiber diet rich in protein; avoid excessive calcium intake.

6. Establish bowel routine through use of diet and stool softeners, laxatives, and enemas, as prescribed.

7. Prevent pressure on the calf and evaluate twice daily for the development of thrombophlebitis.

8. Check traction apparatus at repeated intervals—the traction must be continuous to be effective, unless prescribed as intermittent, as with pelvic traction.

   a. With *running traction*, the patient may not be turned without disrupting the line of pull.

   b. With *balanced suspension traction*, the patient may be elevated, turned slightly, and moved as desired.

9. Use SCDs and compression stockings, as indicated.

10. Administer prophylactic anticoagulants, as prescribed.

> **NURSING ALERT** Every complaint of the patient in traction should be investigated immediately to prevent injury.

Maintaining Skin Integrity

1. Examine bony prominences frequently for evidence of pressure or friction irritation.

2. Observe for skin irritation around the traction bandage.

3. Observe for pressure at traction–skin contact points.

4. Report complaint of burning sensation under traction.

5. Relieve pressure without disrupting traction effectiveness.
   a. Make sure that linens and clothing are wrinkle-free.
   b. Use lambs' wool pads, heel and elbow protectors, and special mattresses, as needed.
6. Special care must be given to the back every 2 hours because the patient maintains a supine position.
   a. Have patient use trapeze to pull self up and relieve back pressure.
   b. Provide backrubs.

Avoiding Infection at Pin Site

1. Monitor vital signs for fever or tachycardia.
2. Watch for signs of infection, especially around the pin tract.
   a. The pin should be immobile in the bone and the skin surrounding the wound should be dry. Small amount of serous oozing from pin site may occur.
   b. If infection is suspected, percuss gently over the tibia; this may elicit pain if infection is developing.
   c. Assess for other signs of infection: heat, redness, fever.
3. If directed, clean the pin tract with sterile applicators and prescribed solution or ointment (ie, normal saline, sterile water, chlorhexidine)—to clear drainage at the entrance of tract and around the pin because plugging at this site can predispose to bacterial invasion of the tract and bone.

Preventing Neurovascular Injury

1. Assess motor and sensory function of specific nerves that might be compromised.
   a. Peroneal nerve—have patient point great toe toward nose; check sensation on dorsum of foot; presence of footdrop.
   b. Radial nerve—have patient extend thumb; check sensation in web between thumb and index finger.
   c. Median nerve—thumb–middle finger apposition; check sensation of index finger.
2. Determine adequacy of circulation (eg, color, temperature, motion, capillary refill of peripheral fingers or toes).
   a. With Buck's traction, inspect the foot for circulatory difficulties within a few minutes and then periodically after the elastic bandage has been applied.
3. Report promptly if change in neurovascular status is identified.

Patient Education and Health Maintenance

1. Teach the patient the purpose of traction therapy.
2. Delineate limitations of activity necessary to maintain effective traction.
3. Teach use of patient aids (eg, trapeze).
4. Instruct the patient not to adjust or modify traction apparatus.
5. Instruct the patient in activities designed to minimize effects of immobility on body systems.
6. Teach the patient necessity for reporting changes in sensations, pain, movement.

Evaluation: Expected Outcomes

- Exercises as instructed; deep breaths hourly; fluid intake 2,000 to 2,500 mL/24 hours.
- No signs of skin breakdown under traction bandage or over bony prominences.
- No drainage, redness, or odor at pin site.
- No motor or sensory impairment; good capillary refill, color, and warmth of extremity.

External Fixation

External fixation is a technique of fracture immobilization in which a series of transfixing pins is inserted through bone and attached to a rigid external metal frame (see Figure 32-6). The method is used mainly in the management of open fractures with severe soft-tissue damage.

Advantages

1. Permits rigid support of severely comminuted open fractures, infected nonunions, and infected unstable joints.
2. Facilitates wound care (frequent debridements, irrigations, dressing changes) and soft tissue reconstruction (delayed wound closure, muscle flaps, skin grafts).
3. Allows early function of muscles and joints.
4. Allows early patient comfort.

Circular Fixators

Purpose

May be used for limb lengthening, correction of angulation and rotation defects, and in treatment of nonunion.

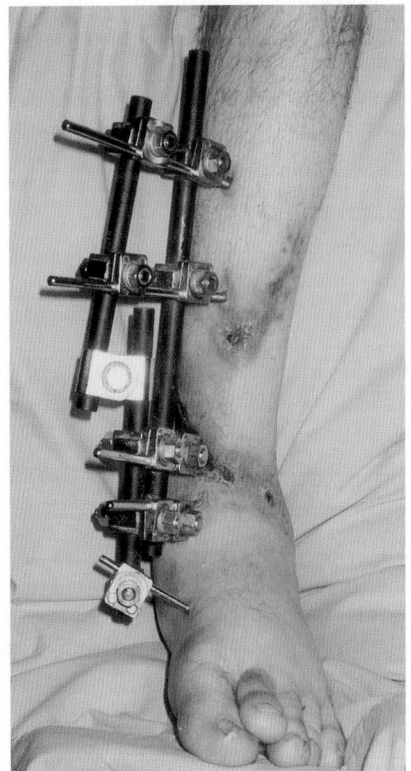

Figure 32-6. External fixation device used for reduction and immobilization of open fracture, allowing treatment of soft tissue wounds.

Components

1. This fixator apparatus consists of through-the-bone tension wires placed above and below the treatment site.
2. The wires are attached to fixator rings surrounding the limb.
3. The rings are connected to one another by telescoping rods.

Management

1. Adjustments are made daily at about 1 mm/day, stimulating callus and bone formation.
2. Patient compliance is essential.
3. Weight-bearing is encouraged.
4. When the desired length or correction is achieved, the fixator is left in place without further adjustment until bone healing occurs.

Application of External Fixator

1. Under general anesthesia, the skin is cleaned and transfixing pins are inserted into the bone through small incisions above and below the fracture.
2. After reduction of the fracture, the appliance is stabilized by adjusting and tightening the bars connecting the sets of pins.
3. The sharp pinheads are covered with plastic, cork, or rubber covers to protect the other extremity and caregivers.

Nursing Assessment

1. Determine the patient's understanding of procedure and fixation device.
2. Evaluate neurovascular status of involved body part.
3. Inspect each pin site for redness, drainage, tenderness, pain, and loosening of the pin.
4. Inspect open wounds for healing, infection, or devitalized tissue.
5. Assess functioning of other body systems affected by injury or immobilization.

Nursing Diagnoses

- Anxiety related to appearance of external fixation device and wound.
- Risk for Peripheral Neurovascular Dysfunction related to swelling, fixator, and underlying condition.
- Risk for Infection related to open injury and skeletal pin insertion.
- Impaired Physical Mobility related to presence of fixator and condition.

Nursing Interventions

Relieving Anxiety

1. If possible, before placement of the device, reassure the patient that, although the fixator appears clumsy and cumbersome, it should not hurt once it is in place.
2. Emphasize the positive aspects of this device in treating complex musculoskeletal problems.
3. Encourage the patient to verbalize reaction to the device.
4. Inform the patient that greater mobility can be achieved with an external fixation device, thereby minimizing the development of other system problems.
5. Involve the patient in care and in the management of external fixator.

Maintaining Intact Neurovascular Status

1. Assess neurovascular status frequently—every 15 minutes to 1 hour while swelling is significant and later, every 2 to 8 hours.
2. Establish baseline of functioning for comparative monitoring. Complex musculoskeletal injuries frequently result in disruption of soft tissue functioning.

 NURSING ALERT Assess neurovascular status frequently and record findings. Report abnormal findings or change in status.

3. Elevate extremity to reduce swelling.
4. Report any change in neurovascular status.

Preventing Infection

1. Provide site and fixator care.
   a. Clean pin sites and remove crusts with sterile cotton applicator, using solution as prescribed, or established standard of care.
      i. Crusts formed by serous drainage can prevent fluid from draining and can cause infection.
      ii. A small amount of serous drainage from the pin sites is normal.
   b. Note and report inflammation, swelling, tenderness, and purulent drainage at pin site.
   c. Note skin tension at pin site—tension can cause discomfort.
   d. Report loosened pins.
   e. Clean fixator with clean cloth and water, as needed.
2. Provide wound care.
   a. The open wounds at the fracture site are usually treated by daily dressing changes.
   b. Use sterile technique.
   c. Note wound appearance. Monitor healing. Report signs of infection.
3. Monitor for local and systemic indicators of infection.

Encouraging Mobility

1. Encourage the patient to participate in care activities.
2. Assure the patient that pain associated with injury will diminish as tissue reactions to injury and manipulation resolve and healing progresses.
3. Inform the patient that the external fixator maintains the fracture in a stable position and that the extremity can be moved. Adjustment of the fixator is done by the health care provider. (Patient is taught how to adjust the circular fixator.)
4. To move the extremity, grasp the frame and assist the patient to move. Reassure the patient that the fixator can withstand normal movement.
5. Teach quadriceps exercises and ROM exercises for joints; usually started on first postoperative day.
6. Teach crutch walking when soft tissue swelling has diminished; encourage weight-bearing, as prescribed.

Patient Education and Health Maintenance

1. Instruct patient to inspect around each pin site daily for signs of infection and loosening of pins. Watch for pain, soft tissue swelling, and drainage.
2. Teach patient how to clean around each pin daily, using aseptic technique. Do not touch wound with hands.
3. Advise patient to clean fixator regularly—to keep it free of dust and contamination.
4. Warn against tampering with clamps or nuts—can alter compression and misalign fracture.
5. Review weight-bearing and other restrictions associated with injury and treatment regimen.
6. Encourage the patient to follow rehabilitation regimen.

Evaluation: Expected Outcomes

- Verbalizes understanding of and comfort with fixator device.
- Swelling relieved; neurovascular status intact.
- No drainage or signs of infection at pin sites; pin tracts remain intact, no loosening of pins.
- Ambulating with ambulatory device, as directed.

Orthopedic Surgery

 Evidence Base American Academy of Orthopaedic Surgeons. (2011). *Preventing venous thromboembolic disease in patients undergoing elective hip and knee arthroplasty*. Rosemont, IL: Author.

Wiesel, S. W. (2010). *Orthopaedic surgery: Principles of diagnosis and treatment*. Philadelphia: Lippincott Williams & Wilkins.

Types of Surgery

1. Open reduction—reduction and alignment of the fracture through surgical incision.
2. Closed reduction—manipulation of bone fragments or joint dislocation without surgical incision.
3. Internal fixation—stabilization of the reduced fracture with use of metal screw, plates, nails, or pins.
4. Bone graft—placement of autologous or homologous bone tissue to replace, promote healing of, or stabilize diseased bone.
5. Arthroplasty—repair of a joint through realignment or reconstruction; may be done through arthroscope (arthroscopy) or open joint repair.
6. Joint replacement—type of arthroplasty that involves replacement of joint surfaces with metal or plastic materials.
7. Total joint replacement—replacement of both articular surfaces within a joint.
8. Meniscectomy—excision of damaged meniscus (fibrocartilage) of the knee.
9. Tendon transfer—movement of tendon insertion point to improve function.
10. Fasciotomy—cutting muscle fascia to relieve constriction or contracture.
11. Amputation—removal of a body part.
   Note: Joint replacement and amputation will be covered separately.

Preoperative Management

1. Hydration, protein, and caloric intake are assessed. The goal is to maximize healing and reduce risk of complications by providing IV fluids, vitamins, and nutritional supplements, as indicated.

 GERONTOLOGIC ALERT Many older patients are at risk for poor healing due to poor nutritional status. Suggest obtaining albumin, prealbumin, and transferrin evaluation and nutrition consult in advance of surgery.

2. Medications, including prescribed, over-the-counter, and herbals, are reviewed and patient is instructed on which medications should be held prior to surgery and for how long.
   a. Aspirin, anti-inflammatories, anticoagulants, and antiplatelet agents that may affect clotting may be held for up to a week prior to surgery.
   b. If patient has had previous corticosteroid therapy, it could contribute to current orthopedic condition (aseptic necrosis of the femoral head, osteoporosis) as well as affect the patient's response to anesthesia and the stress of surgery. The patient may need corticotropin postoperatively, so history of corticosteroid therapy must be documented.
   c. Metformin is usually held for 48 hours prior to surgery to prevent lactic acidosis, a rare complication.
   d. Antidepressants, particularly monamine oxidase inhibitors, and herbals should be explored for interaction with anesthetics.
3. Signs of infection (respiratory, dental, skin, urinary), which could contribute to development of osteomyelitis after surgery, are ruled out. It is important to determine whether preoperative antibiotics will be necessary.
4. Coughing and deep breathing, frequent vital sign and wound checks, repositioning are described to prepare patient.
5. The patient should practice voiding in bedpan or urinal in recumbent position before surgery. This helps reduce the need for postoperative catheterization.
6. The patient is acquainted with traction apparatus and the need for splint or cast, as indicated by type of surgery.
7. Type and cross match is ordered if there is a potential need for the patient to receive blood products. Autologous blood donation may be done several weeks before surgery.
8. Discharge planning is begun prior to surgery with plan for rehabilitation options post-operatively.

Postoperative Management

1. Neurovascular status is monitored and swelling caused by edema and bleeding into tissues should be assessed and controlled.
2. The affected area is immobilized and activity limited to protect the operative site and stabilize musculoskeletal structures.
3. Hemorrhage and shock, which may result from significant bleeding and poor hemostasis of muscles that occur with orthopedic surgery, are monitored.
4. Complications of immobility are prevented through aggressive and vigilant postoperative care.

Complications

1. Compartment syndrome.
2. Shock.
3. Atelectasis and pneumonia.
4. Osteomyelitis, wound infections.
5. Thromboembolism.
6. Fat embolus.
7. Anemia.

Nursing Diagnoses

- Risk for Deficient Fluid Volume related to hemorrhage.
- Ineffective Breathing Pattern related to effects of anesthesia, analgesics, and immobility.
- Risk for Peripheral Neurovascular Dysfunction related to swelling.
- Acute Pain related to surgical intervention.
- Risk for Infection related to surgical intervention.
- Impaired Physical Mobility related to immobilization therapy and pain.
- Imbalanced Nutrition: Less Than Body Requirements related to blood loss and the demands of healing and immobility.

Nursing Interventions

Monitoring for Shock and Hemorrhage

1. Evaluate BP and pulse rates frequently—rising pulse rate, widening pulse pressure, or slowly falling BP indicate persistent bleeding or development of a state of shock.
2. Monitor for hemorrhage—orthopedic wounds have a tendency to ooze more than other surgical wounds.
   a. Measure suction drainage, if used.
   b. Anticipate up to 500 mL of drainage in the first 24 hours, decreasing to less than 30 mL per 8 hours within 48 hours, depending on surgical procedure.
   c. Report increased wound drainage or steady increase in pain of operative area.
3. Administer IV fluids and blood products, as ordered.

Promoting Effective Breathing Pattern

1. Give respiratory depressant drugs cautiously. Monitor respiration depth and rate frequently. Opioid analgesic effects may be cumulative.
2. Change position every 2 hours—mobilizes secretions and helps prevent bronchial obstruction.
3. Encourage use of incentive spirometer and coughing and deep-breathing exercises every 2 hours.
4. Auscultate lungs for atelectasis and retention of secretions.

Monitoring Peripheral Neurovascular Status

1. Watch circulation distal to the part where cast, bandage, or splint has been applied.
2. Prevent constriction leading to interference with blood or nerve supply.
3. Elevate affected extremity and apply ice packs, as directed, to reduce swelling and bleeding into tissues.
4. Observe toes and fingers for healthy color and good capillary refill.
5. Check pulses of affected extremity; compare with unaffected extremity.
6. Note skin temperature and sensation.
7. Document observations.

 NURSING ALERT If neurovascular problems are identified, loosen cast or dressing at once and notify surgeon.

Relieving Pain

1. Institute comfort measures, as prescribed, as well as nursing measures, as indicated: backrubs; soft light; soft, tranquil music.
2. Be aware that muscle spasms may contribute to discomfort.
3. Use patient-controlled analgesia according to standards of care.
4. Facilitate progression from IV medications to by mouth when tolerated.
5. Prevent constipation due to opioids by obtaining order for bowel regimen.

Preventing Infection

1. Monitor vital signs for fever, tachycardia, or increased respiratory rate, which may indicate infection.
2. Examine incision for redness, increased temperature, swelling, and induration. Document findings.
3. Note and document character of drainage.
4. Evaluate complaints of recurrent or increasing discomfort.
5. Administer antibiotic therapy, as prescribed.
6. Maintain aseptic technique for dressing changes and wound care.

Minimizing the Effects of Immobility

1. Encourage patient to exercise by self with a planned program of exercise as soon as possible after surgery.
2. Have patient flex knee, extend the knee with hip still flexed, and then lower the extremity to the bed. Passive motion devices may be used to maintain range of motion.
3. Encourage patient to move fingers and toes hourly.
4. Advise patient to move joints that are not fixed by traction or appliance through their ROM as fully as possible.
5. Suggest muscle-setting exercises (quadriceps setting) if active motion is contraindicated.
6. Apply antiembolism stockings, foot pumps, or SCDs as prescribed by surgeon.
7. Give prophylactic anticoagulants as directed (eg, heparin, warfarin, aspirin, a low-molecular-weight heparin).
8. Encourage early resumption of activity.

Providing Adequate Nutrition

1. Watch for signs and symptoms of anemia, especially after fracture of long bones:
   a. Fatigue.
   b. Shortness of breath.
   c. Pallor.
   d. Tachycardia.
2. Monitor hemoglobin and hematocrit levels. Report below-normal results to health care provider.

3. Encourage a high-iron diet and administer blood products and iron supplements, as directed.
4. Provide a balanced diet and increase fluids and fiber to reduce incidence of constipation associated with immobility.
5. Maintain urinary output and prevent infection and calculi by increased fluid intake.
6. Watch for urinary retention—older men with some degree of prostatism may have difficulty voiding.

Patient Education and Health Maintenance

1. Teach patient activities that will minimize the development of complications (eg, turning, ankle pumps, anti-embolism stockings, SCDs, coughing, and deep breathing, early mobilization as able).
2. Instruct patient in dietary considerations to facilitate healing and minimize development of constipation and renal calculi.
3. Inform patient of techniques that facilitate moving while minimizing associated discomforts (eg, supporting injured area and practicing smooth, gentle position changes).
4. Encourage long-term follow-up and physical therapy (PT) exercises, as prescribed, to regain maximum functional potential.

Evaluation: Expected Outcomes

- BP stable; drainage from wound less than 30 mL.
- Respirations, deep; performing effective deep breathing and coughing every 2 hours.
- Extremity beyond operative site neurovascularly intact.
- Verbalizes decreased pain.
- Afebrile; incision without drainage.
- Ambulating as directed.
- Eats a balanced diet high in iron; hemoglobin within normal range.

Arthroplasty and Total Joint Replacement

 Evidence Base American Academy of Orthopaedic Surgeons. (2010). *The diagnosis of periprosthetic joint infections of the hip and knee.* Rosemont, IL: Author.
Brotzman, S. B., & Manske, R. C. (2011). *Clinical orthopaedic rehabilitation* (3rd ed.). New York: Mosby.

Arthroplasty is reconstructive surgery to restore joint motion and function and to relieve pain. It generally involves replacement of bony joint structure by a prosthesis. *Total joint arthroplasty* is the replacement of both articular surfaces with metal or plastic components. The most common types of joint replacement (see Figure 32-7) include:

Total hip replacement (total joint arthroplasty)—replacement of a severely damaged hip with an artificial joint. Although a large number of implants are available, most consist of a metal femoral component topped by a spherical ball fitted into a plastic acetabular socket.

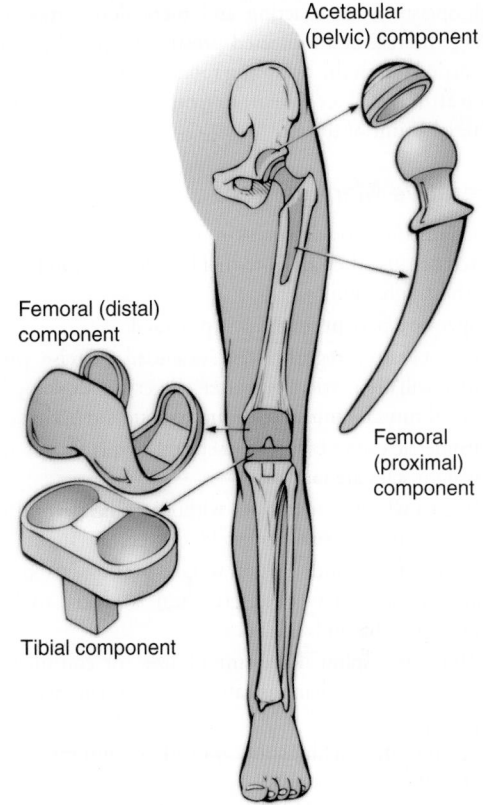

Figure 32-7. Hip and knee replacement.

Total knee arthroplasty—implant procedure in which tibial, femoral, and patellar joint surfaces are replaced because of destroyed knee joint.
Total shoulder arthroplasty—replacement of the humeral head and the glenoid surface with prostheses.

Clinical Indications

1. For patients with unremitting pain and irreversibly damaged joints:
   a. Primary OA.
   b. Rheumatoid arthritis (RA).
2. Selected fractures (eg, femoral neck fracture).
3. Failure of previous reconstructive surgery (osteotomy, cup arthroplasty, femoral neck fracture complications—nonunion, avascular necrosis).
4. Congenital hip disease.
5. Pathologic fractures from metastatic cancer.
6. Joint instability.

Considerations

1. The prostheses are of various designs and may be fixed to the remaining bone by cement, press fit, or bone ingrowth.
2. Selection of the prosthesis and fixation technique depends on patient's bone structure, joint stability, and other individual characteristics, including age, weight, and activity level.

3. Arthroplasty is an exacting and meticulous procedure. To reduce the risk of an infected prosthesis, special precautions are carried out in the operating room (impermeable operating room attire, clean air system) to reduce particulate matter and bacterial count of the air.

Preoperative Management

1. Infections (urinary, dental, skin, respiratory) are ruled out or treated because they are potential foci of infection for seeding prosthesis infection.
2. Preoperative patient teaching is provided.
   a. Postoperative regimen (eg, extended exercise program) that will be carried out after surgery is explained; atrophied muscles must be reeducated and strengthened.
   b. Isometric exercises (muscle setting) of quadriceps and gluteal muscles are taught.
   c. Bed-to-wheelchair transfer without going beyond the hip flexion limits (usually 60 to 90 degrees) is taught.
   d. Non-weight- and partial weight-bearing walking with ambulatory aid (walker, crutches) is taught to facilitate postoperative ambulation.
   e. Abduction splint, knee immobilizer, or continuous passive motion is demonstrated if equipment will be used postoperatively.
3. Antiembolism stockings are applied to minimize development of thrombophlebitis.
4. Skin preparation includes antimicrobial solution to reduce skin microorganisms, a potential source of infection.
5. Antibiotics are administered timely, as prescribed, to ensure therapeutic blood level during and immediately after surgery. Antimicrobials usually are given immediately preoperatively, intraoperatively, and postoperatively to reduce incidence of infection.
6. Cardiovascular, respiratory, renal, and hepatic function are assessed and measures are taken to maximize general health condition.
7. Discharge planning is begun, including rehabilitation options postoperatively.

Postoperative Management

Use of Appropriate Positioning
To prevent dislocation of prosthesis and facilitate healing. Numerous modifications are required in positioning these patients postoperatively.

1. After hip arthroplasty (posterior approach):
   a. The patient is usually positioned supine in bed.
   b. The affected extremity is held in slight abduction by either an abduction splint or pillow or Buck's extension traction to prevent dislocation of the prosthesis.
   c. Avoid acute flexion of the hip.

> **NURSING ALERT** The patient must not adduct the hip or flex it beyond recommended degree, as indicated by the surgeon, as this may lead to subluxation or dislocation of the hip. Signs of joint dislocation include shortened extremity, increasing discomfort, inability to move joints.

   d. When the patient is in bed immediately postoperatively, two nurses turn patient on unoperated side while supporting operated hip securely in an abducted position; the entire length of leg is supported by pillows.
      i. Use pillows to keep the leg abducted; place pillow at back for comfort.
      ii. If the bed is equipped, use overhead trapeze to assist with position changes.
   e. The bed is usually not elevated more than 45 to 60 degrees; placing patient in an upright sitting position puts a strain on the hip joint and may cause dislocation.
   f. A fracture bedpan is used. Instruct patient to flex the unoperated hip and knee and pull up on the trapeze to lift buttocks onto pan. Instruct patient *not* to bear down on the operated hip in flexion when getting off the pan.
2. After knee arthroplasty:
   a. The knee may be immobilized in extension with a firm compression dressing and an adjustable soft extension splint or long-leg plaster cast.
   b. Leg is elevated on pillows to control swelling being mindful to assure that there is nothing causing the knee to remain bent if it is not in an immobilizer.
   c. Alternatively, continuous passive motion may be started to facilitate joint healing and restoration of joint ROM.

Deterring Complications
1. Aggressive care and frequent assessment can reduce the complication rate.
2. Prevent thromboembolism by continuous use of elastic hose and sequential compression device while patient is in bed. Discontinue sequential compression device when patient is ambulatory.
3. C-reactive protein and erythrocyte sedimentation rate (ESR) can be used to quantify the risk of periprosthetic joint infection. High serum levels indicate a high risk of infection and require further diagnostic testing or biopsy.

Promoting Early Ambulation
1. Ambulation may begin on day of surgery or first postoperative day.
2. Transfers to the chair or ambulation with aids, such as walkers, are encouraged as tolerated and based on patient's condition and type of prosthesis.
3. Caution is taken in moving the patient to upright position and the patient is monitored for orthostatic hypotension.

Nursing Diagnoses
Also see "Orthopedic Surgery," page 1120.

- Impaired Physical Mobility related to prosthetic joint.

Nursing Interventions
Also see page 1120.

Promoting Mobility
After hip arthroplasty:

1. Use an abduction splint or pillows while assisting patient out of bed.
   a. Keep the hip at maximum extension.

b. Instruct patient to pivot on unoperated extremity.

c. Assess patient for orthostatic hypotension.

2. When ready to ambulate, teach patient to advance the walker and then advance the operated extremity to the walker, permitting weight-bearing, as prescribed.

3. With increased stability, assist patient to use crutches or cane, as prescribed.

4. Encourage practice of PT exercises to strengthen muscles and prevent contractures.

5. Encourage bed mobility by providing an overhead frame/trapeze.

After knee arthroplasty:

1. Assist patient with transfer out of bed into wheelchair with extension splint in place, if applicable.

2. Encourage weight-bearing, as directed by surgeon.

3. Apply continuous passive motion equipment or carry out passive ROM exercises, as prescribed.

Community and Home Care Considerations

1. Encourage patient to continue to wear elastic stockings after discharge until full activities are resumed.

2. Ensure that patient avoids excessive hip adduction, flexion, and rotation for 6 weeks after hip arthroplasty (posterior hip precautions).

a. Avoid sitting in low chair or toilet seat to avoid flexing hip more than 90 degrees.

b. Keep knees apart; do not cross legs.

c. Limit sitting to 30 minutes at a time—to minimize hip flexion and the risk of prosthetic dislocation and to prevent hip stiffness and flexion contracture.

d. Avoid internal rotation of the hip.

e. Follow weight-bearing restrictions from surgeon.

3. Encourage quadriceps setting and ROM exercises, as directed.

a. Have a daily program of stretching, exercise, and rest throughout lifetime.

b. Do not participate in any activity placing undue or sudden stress on joint (jogging, jumping, lifting heavy loads, gaining weight, excessive bending and twisting).

c. Use a cane when taking fairly long walks.

4. Suggest self-help and energy-saving devices.

a. Handrails by toilet.

b. Raised toilet seat if there is some residual hip flexion problem.

c. Bar-type stool for kitchen work.

d. Occupational therapy (OT) devices for dressing, reaching.

e. Adequate home lighting to prevent falls.

f. Removal of scatter rugs.

5. Advise patient to sleep with two pillows between legs to prevent turning over in sleep. Patient should get out of bed with nonoperative leg.

6. Tell patient to lie prone when able twice daily for 30 minutes to promote full extension of hip.

7. Monitor for late complications—deep infection, increased pain or decreased function associated with loosening of prosthetic components, implant wear, dislocation, fracture of components, avascular necrosis or dead bone caused by loss of blood supply; heterotrophic ossification (formation of bone in periprosthetic space).

8. Assess home for safety to prevent falls—long phone cords, scatter rugs, pets that run underfoot, slippery floors.

Patient Education and Health Maintenance

1. Teach patient use of supportive equipment (crutches, canes, raised toilet seat), as prescribed.

2. Advise patient to notify all health care providers about prosthetic joint because prophylactic antibiotic (to prevent implant infection) will be needed prior to other surgical procedures or any procedure known to cause bacteremia (tooth extraction, manipulation of genitourinary tract). Patients with inflammatory arthropathies, immunosuppressive therapies, and immunocompromising conditions are especially at risk.

Evidence Base American Academy of Orthopedic Surgeons. (2010). *Antibiotic prophylaxis for bacteremia in patients with joint replacements.* Rosemont, IL: Author.

3. Avoid MRI studies because of implanted metal component.

4. Advise patient that metal component in hip or knee may set off metal detectors (airports, some buildings). The patient should carry a medical identification card.

5. New hip or knee is designed for low-impact exercise, such as walking, golf, dancing. High-impact exercises, such as jogging, may cause the prosthesis to loosen.

Evaluation: Expected Outcomes

Maintains proper positioning without evidence of complications. Also see page 1121.

Amputation

Evidence Base Bulstrode, C., Wilson-MacDonald, J., Fairbank, J., et al. (2011). *Oxford textbook of trauma and orthopaedics* (2nd ed.). Oxford, UK: Oxford University Press.

Amputation is the total or partial surgical removal of an extremity. Amputation is considered a surgical reconstructive procedure.

Indications

1. Inadequate tissue perfusion caused by peripheral vascular diseases.

2. Severe trauma.

3. Malignant tumor.

4. Congenital deformity.

5. Osteomyelitis/infection.

Types of Amputation

Open (Guillotine)

1. Used with infection and for patients who are poor surgical risks.

2. Wound heals by granulation over time or secondary closure 1 week later.

Closed (Myoplastic or Flap)

1. Residual limb is covered by a flap of skin.
2. Flap of skin is sutured posteriorly.
3. Most common technique used for vascular disease.

Surgical Considerations

1. The surgeon considers possible limb-salvage techniques.
   a. Revascularization (research is focusing on angiogenesis and stem cell therapy).
   b. Hyperbaric oxygenation.
   c. Tumor resection with bone grafting.
2. Determines level for amputation based on level of maximal viable tissue for wound healing.
3. Develops a functional, nontender, pressure-tolerant residual limb.

Types of Dressings

Soft Dressing

1. Secured with elastic bandage.
2. Permits wound inspection.
3. Used with patients who should avoid early weight-bearing (eg, those with peripheral vascular disease).

Closed, Rigid Plaster Dressing

1. Applied immediately after surgery (ie, immediate postoperative prosthesis).
2. Controls edema.
3. Supports circulation, promoting healing.
4. Minimizes pain on movement.
5. Shapes residual limb.
6. Permits attachment of prosthetic extension (pylon) and early ambulation.

Preoperative Management

1. Hemodynamic evaluation is performed through testing, such as angiography, arterial blood flow, and xenon 133 scan, to determine optimal amputation level.
2. Culture and sensitivity tests of draining wounds are done to assist in control of infection preoperatively.
3. Evaluation of contralateral extremity is performed to determine functional potential postoperatively.
4. Evaluation of cardiovascular, respiratory, renal, and other body systems is necessary to determine preoperative condition of patient and reduce the risks of surgery by optimizing function.

GERONTOLOGIC ALERT Amputation of the lower extremity can be a life-threatening procedure, especially in patients older than age 60 with peripheral vascular disease. Significant morbidity accompanies above-knee amputations because of associated poor health and disease as well as the complications of sepsis and malnutrition and the physiologic insult of amputation.

5. Nutritional status is evaluated and optimized with adequate protein to enhance wound healing.

6. Exercises are taught to strengthen muscles for use of ambulatory aids (lower-limb amputee).
   a. Flex and extend arms while holding traction weights.
   b. Do push-ups from a prone position, if feasible.
   c. Do sit-ups from a seated position, if feasible.
7. Use of ambulatory aids taught to maintain mobility, prepare for postoperative status, and instill confidence in ability.
8. Phantom sensation is explained—the patient will continue to "feel" the amputated body part for some time.
9. Emotional support is given.
   a. Support concept of amputation as a surgical reconstructive procedure.
   b. Explore patient's perception of procedure and effect on lifestyle.
   c. Avoid unrealistic and misleading reassurance—management of prosthesis can be slow and painful.

Postoperative Management

1. The extremity should be in full extension and may be elevated, if possible. An extension splint/immobilizer may be indicated.
2. Complications are monitored—hemorrhage, infection, unrelieved phantom pain, nonhealing wound.
3. Rehabilitation is initiated through PT and prosthetic fitting, if indicated.
4. Optimal treatment is provided for diabetes mellitus, heart disease, infection, stroke, chronic obstructive pulmonary disease, peripheral vascular disease, and age-related deterioration, which are factors limiting rehabilitation.
5. If wound breakdown, infection, or delay in healing of residual limb occur, therapy is provided to prevent delay in rehabilitation.
6. Acceptance of body image change is promoted.

Nursing Diagnoses

- Risk for Deficient Fluid Volume related to hemorrhage from disrupted surgical homeostasis.
- Ineffective Tissue Perfusion related to edema and tissue responses to surgery and prosthesis.
- Ineffective Coping related to change in body image.
- Acute Pain related to surgical procedure.
- Impaired Physical Mobility related to amputation, muscle weakness, alteration in body weight distribution.

Nursing Interventions

NURSING ALERT Prevention of complications associated with a major operation and facilitation of early rehabilitation are essential to prevent prolonged disability. Frequent monitoring of patient's physiologic responses to anesthesia, surgery, and immobility is required.

Monitoring Fluid Balance

1. Monitor patient for systemic symptoms of excessive blood loss—hypotension, widening pulse pressure, tachycardia, diaphoresis, decreased level of consciousness.

2. Watch for excessive wound drainage.
   a. Keep tourniquet (in view) attached to end of bed to apply to residual limb (stump) if excessive bleeding occurs.
   b. Reinforce dressing, as required, using aseptic technique.
   c. Measure suction drainage.
   d. Maintain accurate record of bloody drainage on dressing and in drainage system.
3. Monitor intake and output for fluid balance.

Maintaining Adequate Tissue Perfusion

1. Control edema.
   a. Elevate residual limb to promote venous return.
   b. Use air splint, if prescribed.
2. Maintain pressure dressing.
   a. Reapply, if necessary, using sterile dressing secured with elastic bandage.
   b. Notify surgeon if rigid cast dressing comes off.

Supporting Effective Coping

1. Accept patient responses to loss of body part (ie, depression, withdrawal, denial, frustration).
2. Encourage expression of fears and concerns.
3. Recognize that modification of body image takes time.
4. Encourage participation in rehabilitation planning and self-care.
5. Assist patient to adapt to changes in self-care activities.
   a. Upper-extremity amputation—encourage independence in one-handed self-care activities using one-handed aids (eg, one-handed knife), as needed.
   b. Lower-extremity amputation—encourage mobility using transfer assistance and ambulatory aids, as needed.

Controlling Pain

1. Surgical pain.
   a. Assess patient's pain experience.
   b. Administer prescribed medications, as needed, to control postoperative pain.
   c. Use nonpharmaceutical pain-management techniques, such as progressive muscle relaxation and imagery.
   d. Recognize that increasing discomfort may indicate presence of hematoma, infection, or necrosis.
2. Phantom sensations (pain).
   a. Anticipate complaint of pain and sensation located in the missing limb ("phantom pain").
   b. The use of adjunctive pain medications may be prescribed, such as gabapentin.
   c. Use physical modalities (eg, wrapping, temperature changes) and transcutaneous electrical nerve stimulation (TENS), if prescribed, in relieving discomfort.
   d. Encourage patient activity to decrease awareness of phantom limb pain.
   e. Reassure patient that phantom limb pain will diminish over time.
   f. Patients may benefit from cognitive-behavioral therapy to assist in pain management. Virtual reality-based interventions may also be effective.

Promoting Physical Activity

1. Encourage frequent repositioning in bed.
2. Teach patient to avoid long periods in one position.
   a. Avoids dependent edema.
   b. Avoids flexion deformity.
   c. Avoids skin pressure areas.
3. Prevent deformities.
   a. Lower-extremity amputations—hip flexion contracture (avoid placing residual limb on pillow; encourage prone position twice per day) and abduction deformity (use trochanter roll; avoid pillow between legs).
   b. Upper-extremity amputations—postural abnormalities (encourage good posture).
4. Encourage active ROM and muscle-strengthening exercises when prescribed to:
   a. Minimize muscle atrophy.
   b. Increase muscle strength.
   c. Prepare residual limb for prosthesis.
5. Promote reestablishment of balance (amputation alters distribution of body weight).
   a. Transfer to chair within 48 hours after surgery.
   b. Instruct and guard lower-limb amputee during balance exercises (ie, arise from chair; stand on toes holding on to chair; bend knee holding on to chair; balance on one leg without support; hop on one foot while holding on to chair).
6. Supervise ambulation, use of wheelchair, and self-care activities.

Patient Education and Health Maintenance

1. Teach patient and family how to wrap residual limb with elastic bandage to control edema and to form a firm conical shape for prosthesis fitting (see Figures 32-8 and 32-9).
   a. Wrapping generally begins 1 to 3 days after surgery or after hard plaster dressing is removed.
   b. Use diagonal figure-eight bandaging technique.
   c. Wrap distal to proximal to maintain pressure gradient and to control edema.
   d. Begin wrapping with minimal tension and increase as wound heals and sutures are removed.
   e. Flatten skin at ends of incision to ensure conical stump shape.
   f. Rewrap residual limb a couple of times per day and as necessary to achieve a smooth, graded tension dressing.
   g. Rewrap if patient complains of more pain—dressing is probably too tight.
   h. Keep residual limb wrapped at all times except when bathing.
2. Teach patient residual limb conditioning.
   a. Push the residual limb against a soft pillow.
   b. Gradually push residual limb against harder surfaces.
   c. Massage healed residual limb to soften scar, decrease tenderness, and improve vascularity.
3. Fitting of prosthesis.
   a. Note residual limb contour.
   b. Assess for residual limb contraction.
   c. When maximum shrinkage occurs, the prosthetist measures and fits the prosthesis.
   d. Adjustments are made by the prosthetist to minimize skin problems.

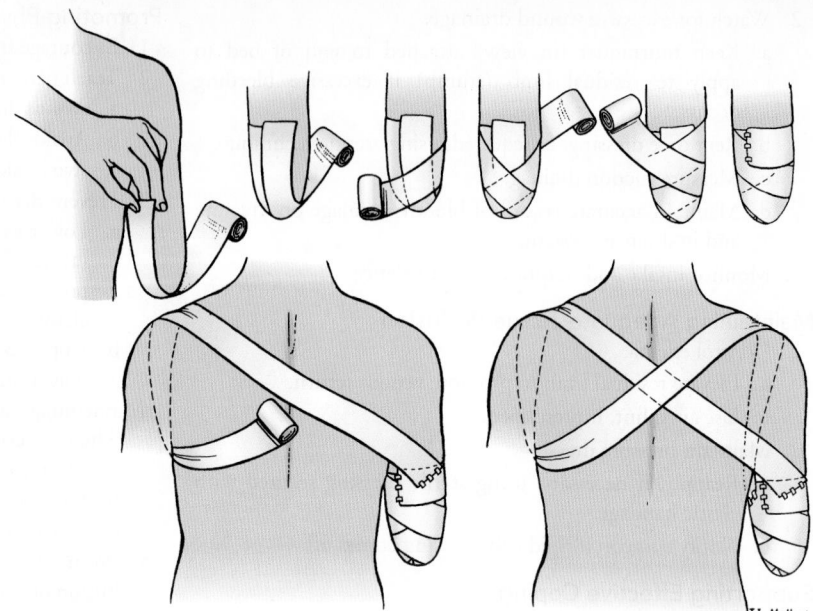

Figure 32-8. Wrapping above-elbow residual limb. Elastic bandaging reduces edema and shapes the residual limb for the prosthesis. Bandage may need to be secured by wrapping across back and shoulders.

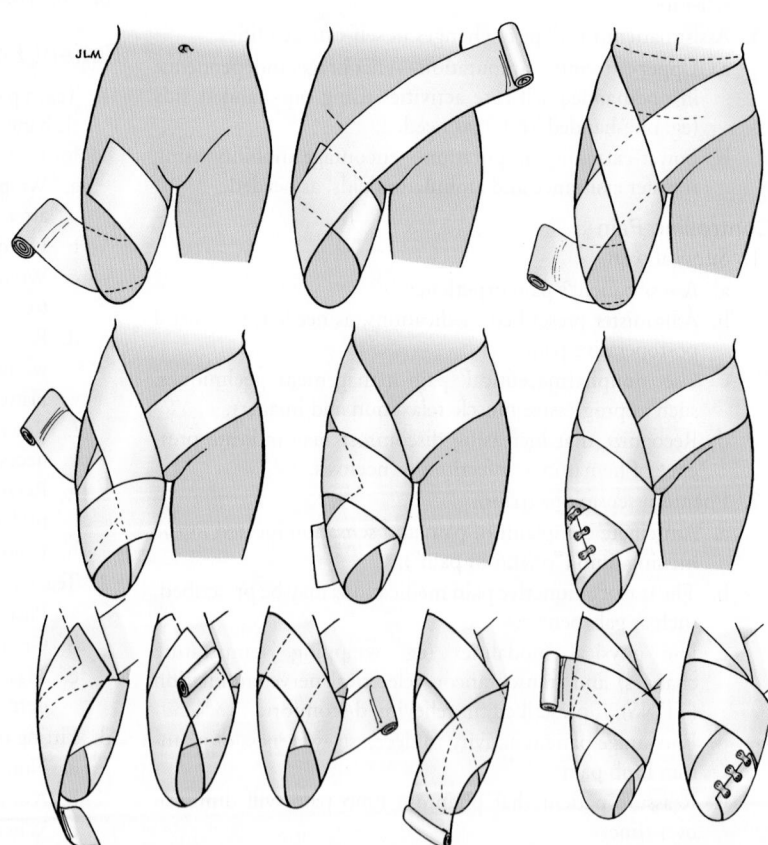

Figure 32-9. Wrapping above-knee residual limb. Elastic bandaging reduces edema and shapes the residual limb in a firm conical form for the prosthesis.

4. Continuing care of residual limb and prosthesis.
   a. Instruct patient to wash and dry limb thoroughly at least twice per day, removing all soap residue, to prevent skin irritation and infection.
   b. Avoid soaking residual limb because it results in edema.
   c. Inspect residual limb and skin under prosthesis harness daily for pressure, irritation, and actual skin breakdown.
   d. Wear residual limb sock or cotton underwear—to absorb perspiration and to avoid direct contact between prosthetic socket or harness and skin.
   e. Avoid wrinkles in residual limb sock—potential pressure areas.
   f. Wipe socket of prosthesis with a damp cloth when prosthesis is removed for evening.
   g. Have prosthesis checked periodically.
5. Teach patient to protect the remaining extremity from injury and to secure prompt treatment of problems.

Evaluation: Expected Outcomes

- Vital signs stable; dressing reinforced once in 4 hours.
- Pressure dressing intact; stump elevated without edema.
- Participates in care plan; expresses concerns about independence.
- Verbalizes relief of incisional pain; dull phantom sensation tolerable.
- Performs ROM actively; transfers to wheelchair with assistance; participates in PT and OT activities.

MUSCULOSKELETAL TRAUMA

See Standards of Care Guidelines 32-1.

Contusions, Strains, and Sprains

Evidence Base Logerstedt, D. S., Snyder-Mackler, L., Ritter, R. C., et al. (2010). Knee stability and movement coordination impairments: Knee ligament sprain. *Journal of Orthopaedic Sports and Physical Therapy, 40*(4), A1–A37.

A *contusion* is an injury to the soft tissue produced by a blunt force (blow, kick, or fall). A *strain* is a microscopic tearing of the muscle caused by excessive force, stretching, or overuse. A *sprain* is an injury to ligamentous structures surrounding a joint; it is usually caused by a wrench or twist resulting in a decrease in joint stability.

Clinical Manifestations

Contusion
1. Hemorrhage into injured part (ecchymosis)—from rupture of small blood vessels; also associated with fractures.
2. Pain, swelling, and ecchymosis.
3. Hyperkalemia may be present with extensive contusions, resulting in destruction of body tissue and loss of blood.

Strain
1. Hemorrhage into the muscle.
2. Swelling.
3. Tenderness.

STANDARDS OF CARE GUIDELINES 32-1
Caring for a Patient with Musculoskeletal Trauma, Surgery, Casting, or Immobilization

When caring for a patient with musculoskeletal trauma, surgery, casting, or immobilization, provide the following care, as indicated:

- Check neurovascular status of involved extremities.
- Palpate for intact and equal pulses bilaterally.
- Palpate for proper warmth of the skin.
- Check for brisk capillary refill.
- Test sensation to light touch and pain.
- Observe for unusual or increased swelling.
- Ensure that patient can move affected parts.
- Ensure proper positioning for comfort and alignment.
- Determine pressure points and take precautions to prevent pressure sores.
- Medicate to control pain, particularly before movement, procedures, and physical therapy.
- Provide diversional activities and emotional support during long immobilizations.
- Always document assessments and interventions meticulously, realizing that patient may be involved in workers' compensation claim or litigation due to accident and that records will be essential to patient's future well-being.

This information should serve as a general guideline only. Each patient situation presents a unique set of clinical factors and requires nursing judgment to guide care, which may include additional or alterative measures and approaches.

---

4. Pain with isometric contraction.
5. May be associated spasm.

Sprain
1. Rapid swelling—due to extravasation of blood within tissues.
2. Pain on passive movement of joint.
3. Increasing pain during first few hours due to continued swelling.

Management
1. X-ray may be done to rule out fracture.
2. Immobilize in splint, elastic wrap, or compression dressing to support painful structures and control swelling.
3. Apply ice while swelling is present.
4. Analgesics usually include nonsteroidal anti-inflammatory drugs (NSAIDs).
5. Severe sprains may require surgical repair or cast immobilization.

Nursing Interventions and Patient Education
1. Elevate the affected part to reduce swelling. Maintain splint or immobilization, as prescribed.
2. Apply cold compresses for the first several days (15 to 20 minutes at a time every few hours)—to produce vasoconstriction,

decrease edema, and reduce discomfort (do not apply ice directly to skin). Ice may be needed for up to a week to control acute swelling.

3. Assess neurovascular status of contused extremity every 1 to 4 hours as patient's condition indicates.
4. Instruct patient on use of pain medication, as prescribed.
5. Ensure correct use of crutches or other mobility aid with or without weight-bearing, as prescribed.
6. Educate on need to rest injured part for about a month to allow for healing.
7. Teach patient to resume activities gradually.
8. Teach patient to avoid excessive exercise of injured part.
9. Teach patient to avoid reinjury by "warming up" before exercise and stretching tendons and muscles before and after exercise.
10. Complementary methods, such as acupuncture, biofeedback, and imagery, may contribute to healing by reducing anxiety and pain.

> **NURSING ALERT** Teach patients to use PRICE at home for minor injuries: *Protection*—of the affected part from injury; *Rest*—to promote healing; *Ice*—to control swelling (do not use heat until acute swelling is relieved); *Compression*—with an elastic wrap or splint to control swelling and prevent stiffness, can be removed at night; *Elevation*—above the level of the heart to reduce swelling.

Tendinitis

Evidence Base American Academy of Orthopaedic Surgeons. (2010). *Optimizing the management of rotator cuff problems.* Rosemont, IL: Author.

Tendinitis is an inflammation of a tendon caused by a lack of sufficient lubrication of the tendon sheath. May be caused by acute stress on tendon structure or by chronic overuse.

Clinical Manifestations

1. Onset of pain may occur immediately after activity or delayed up to a day later. ROM and resistance testing is painful.
2. Mild swelling occurs and the tendon sheath is tender to the touch.
3. Sudden onset of sharp pain in extremity and hearing or feeling a "snap" are associated with tendon rupture, as in Achilles tendinitis due to running injuries or stop–start activities such as basketball. Also occurs in gastrocnemius and biceps.

Management

1. X-rays are not usually diagnostic.
2. Thompson's test helps with diagnosis of Achilles rupture. Patient kneels on chair or lies prone. Examiner squeezes calf of affected leg. Normal response: foot moves downward, denoting intact tendon. If foot does not move, tendon is assumed to be ruptured.
3. Initial treatment includes protection, rest, ice, compression, elevation (PRICE).

4. Splinting or casting for up to 6 weeks in functional position usually necessary.
5. Surgical intervention may be necessary if rupture is complete.
6. PT to regain strength and function.
7. Corticosteroid injection.
8. NSAIDs for pain and inflammation.

Nursing Interventions and Patient Education

1. Ensure understanding of need for proper immobilization for full time period even though fracture is not present.
2. Encourage the use of warm compresses after 24 hours to relieve pain and inflammation.
3. Advise patient not to return to full activity until strength is equal to unaffected extremity.
4. Teach proper warm-up before exercise and sports activities (stretchis of all major tendons).

Bursitis

Evidence Base Aaron, D. L., Patel, A., Kayiaros, S., et al. (2011). Four common types of bursitis: Diagnosis and management. *Journal of the American Academy of Orthopaedic Surgery, 19*(6), 359–367.

Bursitis is a painful inflammation of the bursae, fluid-filled sacs lined with synovium similar to the lining of the joint spaces. Bursae reduce friction between tendons and bones or tendons and ligaments. They are found over joints with bony prominences, such as the trochanter, patella, and olecranon. Friction between skin and musculoskeletal tissues may result in bursitis.

Clinical Manifestations

1. Pain around a joint—commonly the knee, elbow, shoulder, and hip.
2. Varying degrees of redness, warmth, and swelling may be visible.
3. There is point tenderness and limited ROM on examination.

Management and Nursing Interventions

1. Rest and immobilization of affected joint.
2. Ice for the first 48 hours; moist heat every 4 hours thereafter.
3. Nonopioid analgesics such as NSAIDs.
4. ROM exercises.
5. Corticosteroid injection into the area.
6. Surgery indicated when calcified deposits or adhesions have diminished function.

Plantar Fasciitis

Evidence Base Goff, J. D., & Crawford, R. (2011). Diagnosis and treatment of plantar fasciitis. *American Family Physician, 84*(6), 676–682.

Plantar fasciitis is inflammation of the fascia that runs along the bottom of the foot from heel to toes. As the fascia is stretched, microscopic tears develop at the point where fascia attaches to the calcaneus.

Clinical Manifestations

1. Pain along sole of foot, usually unilateral but may be bilateral.
2. Worse upon arising, long period of standing, and walking.
3. Tenderness of heel area.

Management and Nursing Interventions

1. Rest—decrease walking, running, exercise, standing.
2. NSAIDs for pain and inflammation.
3. Good supportive footwear.
4. Orthotic devices may be beneficial.
   a. Heel cup to cushion the heel (OTC).
   b. Arch support orthotics for pes planus (flat foot).
   c. Cushioning of arches for pes cavus (high arch).
5. Stretching exercises several times per day.
6. Massage of bottom of foot.
7. Steroid injection into painful area.
8. Surgery for release of fascia as last resort.

Traumatic Joint Dislocation

 Evidence Base Humbyrd, C. J., Petre, B., Chanmugam, A. S., et al. (2012). *Orthopaedic emergencies.* Oxford, UK: Oxford University Press.

Dislocation of a joint occurs when the surfaces of the bones forming the joint are no longer in anatomic contact. This is a medical emergency because of associated disruption of surrounding blood and nerve supplies. Shoulder, fingers, and elbow are the most commonly dislocated joints. Mechanism of injury can be anterior, posterior (most common), lateral, or medial force.

Clinical Manifestations

1. Pain.
2. Deformity.
3. Change in the length of the extremity.
4. Loss of normal movement.
5. X-ray confirmation of dislocation without associated fracture.

Management

1. Immobilize part while patient is transported to emergency department, x-ray department, or clinical unit.
2. Secure reduction of dislocation (bring displaced parts into normal position) as soon as possible to prevent circulatory or nerve impairments; usually performed under anesthesia.
3. Stabilize reduction until joint structures are healed to prevent permanently unstable joint or aseptic necrosis of bone.

Nursing Interventions and Patient Education

1. Assess neurovascular status of extremity before and after reduction of dislocation.
2. Administer or teach self-administration of pain medications such as NSAIDs.
3. Ensure proper use of immobilization device after reduction.
4. Review instructions for activity restrictions and need for PT and follow-up.

Knee Injuries

 Evidence Base Logerstedt, D. S., et al. (2010). Knee pain and mobility impairments: Meniscal and articular cartilage lesions. *Journal of Orthopaedic Sports and Physical Therapy, 40*(6), A1–A35.
   Work Loss Data Institute. (2010). *Knee and leg* (acute and chronic). Encinitas, CA: Author.

The knee ligaments provide stability to the knee joint. These ligaments promote rotational stability (*anterior cruciate ligament [ACL]* and *posterior cruciate ligament*) and prevent varus and valgus instability (*medial and lateral collateral ligaments*). Pieces of cartilage that stabilize the knee internally are known as the medial and lateral menisci. *ACL injuries* and *medial meniscus tears* are common due to sports injuries.

Clinical Manifestations

1. Severe stresses are applied to the knee during many sports activities (eg, soccer, skiing, running).
2. Injury to knee structures occurs during rapid position changes involving flexing and twisting of the joint.
3. Torn cartilage (meniscus) causes pain, tenderness, joint effusion, clicking sensations, and decreased ROM.
4. Knee ligaments may be torn, resulting in pain on ambulation, swelling, and joint instability. The patellar tendon may rupture.

Management

1. Special assessment techniques are done to detect ACL injury (see Table 32-1).
2. MRI shows injury to soft tissue involved.
3. Some injuries may be immobilized (splint, brace, or cast) and treated with PT.
4. ACL reconstruction frequently indicated.
   a. Arthroscopic surgery preferred; synthetic ligaments selected where ligaments failed. Graft rejection is a complication.
   b. Postoperative continuous passive motion used.
   c. Postoperative ACL rehabilitation program includes progressive ROM, bracing (not done with synthetic ligaments).
   d. Long-term bracing during sports controversial.
5. Meniscal injury—damaged cartilage removed.
   a. Arthroscopic or open meniscectomy.
   b. Rehabilitation includes progressive ROM and quadriceps strengthening.

Nursing Interventions and Patient Education

1. After arthroscopic surgery, ensure proper use of crutches, as indicated, and encourage pain control through medications, as prescribed, and RICE.
2. For open joint surgery, see care of patient undergoing orthopedic surgery, page 1119.
3. Teach patient strengthening exercises for affected extremity.
4. Teach patient to prevent fatigue through rest periods, conservation of energy.
5. Advise on prevention of injuries using proper equipment and footwear for sports.

Table 32-1	Assessment Techniques for Anterior Cruciate Ligament Injury	
TEST	**DESCRIPTION**	**POSITIVE FINDING**
Anterior drawer test	Place patient supine with knee in 90 degrees of flexion with foot flat on table. Proximal tibia is pulled forward by examiner using two hands.	Tibia subluxes (dislocates) forward on femur.
Lachman test	Place patient supine with knee in 15 to 20 degrees of flexion. Distal femur is grasped by examiner with one hand while the other hand grasps the proximal tibia and applies forward pressure.	Tibia subluxes forward on femur.
Pivot shift test (evaluates anterolateral rotational stability)	Place patient supine with knee slightly flexed. Examiner grasps patient's ankle in one hand and places palm of other hand over the lateral aspect of the knee distal to the joint. Lower leg is extended and internally rotated, applying a valgus (lateral) stress to knee.	Tibia subluxes and reduces itself ("pivots and shifts").

Fractures

Evidence Base Bucholz, R. W., Heckman, J. D., Court-Brown, C. M., et al. (Eds.). (2010). *Rockwood and Green's fractures in adults* (2nd ed.). Philadelphia: Lippincott Williams & Wilkins.

A *fracture* is a break in the continuity of bone. A fracture occurs when the stress placed on a bone is greater than the bone can absorb. Muscles, blood vessels, nerves, tendons, joints, and other organs may be injured when fracture occurs.

Types of Fractures

1. Complete—involves the entire cross section of the bone, usually displaced (abnormal position).
2. Incomplete—involves a portion of the cross section of the bone or may be longitudinal.
3. Closed (simple)—skin not broken.
4. Open (compound)—skin broken, leading directly to fracture.
   a. Grade I—minimal soft tissue injury.
   b. Grade II—laceration greater than 1 cm without extensive soft tissue flaps.
   c. Grade III—extensive soft tissue injury, including skin, muscle, neurovascular structure, with crushing.
5. Pathologic—through an area of diseased bone (osteoporosis, bone cyst, bone tumor, bony metastasis).

Patterns of Fracture

See Figure 32-10.

1. Greenstick—one side of the bone is broken and the other side is bent.
2. Transverse—straight across the bone.
3. Oblique—at an angle across the bone.
4. Spiral—twists around the shaft of the bone.
5. Comminuted—bone splintered into more than three fragments.
6. Depressed—fragments are driven inward (seen in fractures of the skull and facial bones).
7. Compression—bone collapses in on itself (seen in vertebral fractures).
8. Avulsion—fragment of bone pulled off by ligament or tendon attachment.
9. Impacted—fragment of bone wedged into other bone fragment.

GERONTOLOGIC ALERT Osteoporosis is a major risk for fractures, particularly hip and vertebral compression fractures.

10. Fracture-dislocation—fracture complicated by the bone being out of the joint.
11. Other—described according to anatomic location: epiphyseal (end of large bones containing growth plate), supracondylar (above the articular prominence of a bone), midshaft, intra-articular.

Clinical Manifestations

Physical Findings

1. Pain at site of injury.
2. Swelling.
3. Tenderness.
4. False motion and crepitus (grating sensation).
5. Deformity.
6. Loss of function.
7. Ecchymosis.
8. Paresthesia.

Altered Neurovascular Status

1. Injured muscle, blood vessels, nerves.
2. Compression of structures resulting in ischemia.
3. Findings:
   a. Progressive uncontrollable pain.
   b. Pain on passive movement.
   c. Altered sensations (paresthesia).
   d. Loss of active motion.
   e. Diminished capillary refill response, diminished distal pulse.
   f. Pallor.

Shock

1. Bone is very vascular.
2. Overt hemorrhage through open wound.

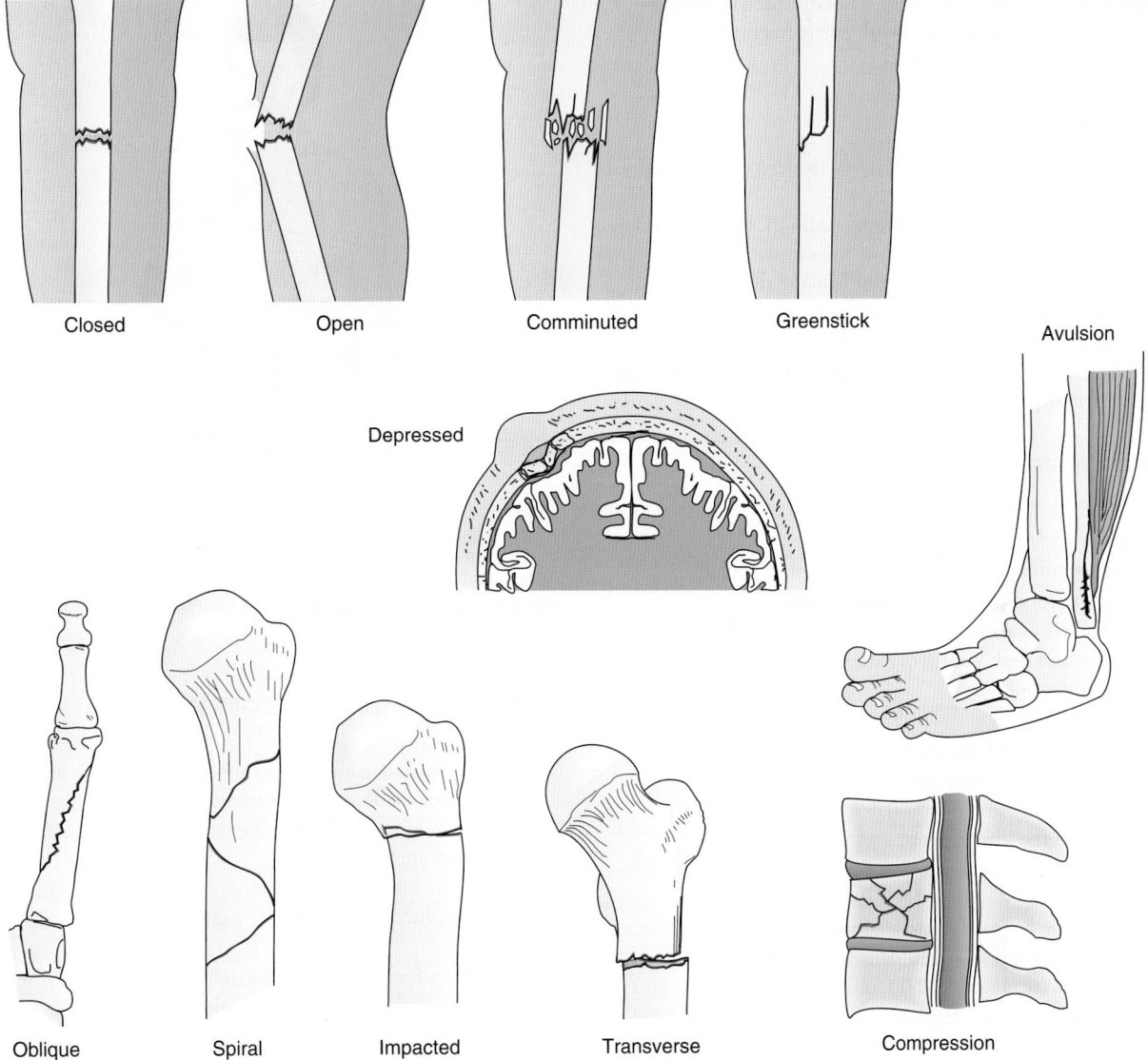

Figure 32-10. Patterns of fractures.

Avulsion—a pulling away of a fragment of bone by a ligament or tendon and its attachment.

Closed—a fracture that remains contained; does not break the skin.

Comminuted—a fracture in which bone has splintered into several fragments.

Compression—a fracture in which bone has been compressed (seen in vertebral fractures).

Depressed—a fracture in which fragments are driven inward (seen frequently in fractures of the skull and facial bones).

Epiphyseal—a fracture through the epiphysis.

Greenstick—a fracture in which one side of a bone is broken and the other side is bent.

Impacted—a fracture in which a bone fragment is driven into another bone fragment.

Oblique—a fracture occurring at an angle across the bone (less stable than transverse).

Open—a fracture in which damage also involves the skin or mucous membranes.

Pathologic—a fracture that occurs through an area of diseased bone (bone cyst, Paget's disease, bony metastasis, tumor); can occur without trauma or a fall.

Spiral—a fracture twisting around the shaft of the bone.

Transverse—a fracture that is straight across the bone.

3. Covert hemorrhage into soft tissues (especially with femoral fracture) or body cavity, as with pelvic fracture.
4. May be fatal if not detected.

Diagnostic Evaluation

1. X-ray and other imaging studies to determine integrity of bone.
2. Blood studies (complete blood count [CBC], electrolytes) with blood loss and extensive muscle damage—may show decreased hemoglobin level and hematocrit.
3. Arthroscopy to detect joint involvement.
4. Angiography if associated with blood vessel injury.
5. Nerve conduction and electromyogram studies to detect nerve injury.

Management

For emergency management, see page 1215.

Principles of Management

1. Factors influencing choice of management include:
   a. Type, location, and severity of fracture.
   b. Soft tissue damage.
   c. Age and health status of patient, including type and extent of other injuries.
2. Goals include:
   a. To regain and maintain correct position and alignment.
   b. To regain the function of the involved part.
   c. To return patient to usual activities in the shortest time and at the least expense.
3. The management process is a three-step process:
   a. Reduction—setting the bone; refers to restoration of the fracture fragments into anatomic position and alignment.
   b. Immobilization—maintains reduction until bone healing occurs (see Figures 32-11 and 32-12).
   c. Rehabilitation—regaining normal function of the affected part.

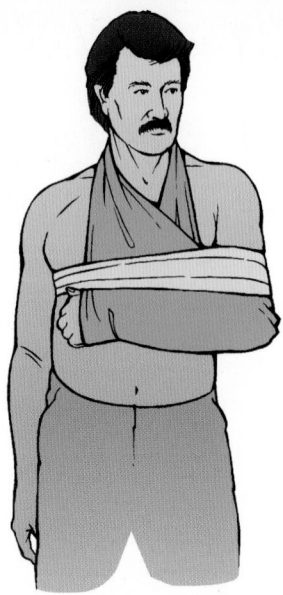

Figure 32-12. Immobilization of fracture of upper humerus can be achieved with conventional sling and swathe.

Approaches to Management

Vary by specific site of fracture (see Table 32-2, pages 1133 to 1135).

1. Closed reduction.
   a. Bony fragments are brought into apposition (ends in contact) by manipulation and manual traction restoring alignment.
   b. May be done under anesthesia for pain relief and muscle relaxation.
   c. Cast or splint applied to immobilize extremity and maintain reduction (see "Casts," page 1107).
2. Traction.
   a. Pulling force applied to accomplish and maintain reduction and alignment (see "Traction," page 1113).
   b. Used for fractures of long bones.
   c. Techniques.
      i. Skin traction—force applied to the skin using foam rubber, tape.
      ii. Skeletal traction—force applied to the bony skeleton directly, using wires, pins, or tongs placed into or through the bone.
3. Open reduction with internal fixation.
   a. Operative intervention to achieve reduction, alignment, and stabilization.
      i. Bone fragments are directly visualized.
      ii. Internal fixation devices (metal pins, wires, screws, plates, nails, rods) used to hold bone fragments in position until solid bone healing occurs (may be removed when bone is healed).
      iii. After closure of the wound, splints or casts may be used for additional stabilization and support.
4. Endoprosthetic replacement.
   a. Replacement of a fracture fragment with an implanted metal device.

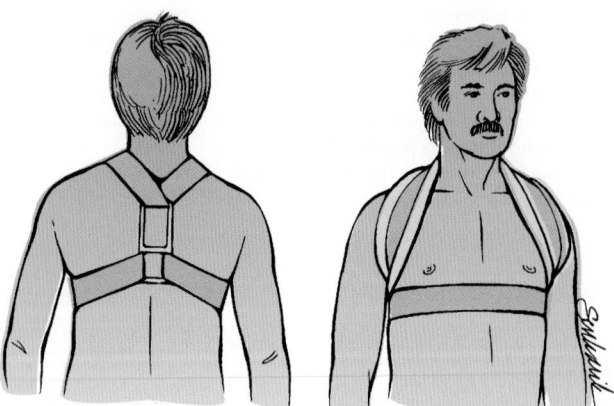

Figure 32-11. Method for immobilizing a clavicular fracture with a clavicular strap.

Table 32-2   Fractures of Specific Sites

SITE AND MECHANISM	MANAGEMENT	NURSING CONSIDERATIONS
Clavicle Fall on shoulder	• Closed reduction and immobilization with clavicular strap (see Figure 32-11) figure-eight bandage or sling. • ORIF for marked displacement, severely comminuted fracture, and extensive soft tissue injury.	• Pad axilla to prevent nerve damage from pressure of immobilizer. • Assess neurovascular status of arm. • Teach exercises of elbow, wrist, and fingers. • Teach shoulder exercises through full ROM, as prescribed.
Proximal Humerus Fall on outstretched arm; osteoporosis is predisposing factor	• Many remain in alignment and are supported by a sling and swathe or Velpeau bandage for comfort (see Figure 32-12). • If displaced, treated with reduction under x-ray control, open reduction, or replacement of humeral head with prosthesis.	• Place a soft pad under the axilla to prevent skin maceration. • Encourage shoulder ROM exercises after specified period of immobilization to prevent frozen shoulder. • Instruct patient to lean forward and allow affected arm to abduct and rotate.

Shaft of Humerus
 	
Direct fall, blow to arm, or auto injury; damage to radial nerve may occur
	• Immobilize with sling and swathe, splint, or hanging cast.
	• A hanging cast is applied for its weight to correct displaced fractures with shortening of the humeral shaft.
	• ORIF for associated vascular injury or pathologic fracture, followed by support in sling.
		• Hanging cast must remain unsupported to maintain traction.
		  • Teach patient to avoid supporting elbow in lap or arm on pillow.
		  • Patient should sleep in upright position to maintain 24-hour traction.
		• Encourage exercise of fingers immediately after application of cast.
		• Teach pendulum exercises of arm, as prescribed, to prevent frozen shoulder.

Elbow and Forearm Fall on elbow, outstretched hand, or direct blow (side-swipe injury)	• Treatment depends on specific characteristics of fracture—ORIF, arthroplasty, external fixation, casting. • Closed drainage system may be used to decrease hematoma formation and swelling.	• Assess neurovascular status of forearm and hand. • If radial pulse weakens or disappears, report immediately to prevent irreversible ischemia. • Elevate arm to control edema. • Encourage finger and shoulder exercises.

Wrist
 	
Colles' fracture is common (½–1 inch [1.2–2.5 cm] above the wrist with dorsal displacement of lower fragment); caused by fall on outstretched palm; commonly associated with osteoporosis
	• Closed reduction with splint or cast support.
	• Percutaneous pins and external fixator or plaster cast.
		• Elevate arm above level of heart for 48 hours after reduction to promote venous and lymphatic return and reduce swelling.
		• Watch for swelling of fingers and check for constricting bandages or cast.
		• Teach finger exercises to reduce swelling and stiffness.
		  • Hold hand above level of heart.
		  • Move fingers from full extension to flexion.
		  • Hold and release.
		  • Repeat at least 10 times every half hour when awake for as long as swelling occurs.
		• Encourage daily-prescribed exercises to restore full extension and supination.

(continued)

Table 32-2   Fractures of Specific Sites *(continued)*

SITE AND MECHANISM	MANAGEMENT	NURSING CONSIDERATIONS
Hand		
Caused by numerous injuries	• Splinting for undisplaced fractures of fingers. • Debridement, irrigation, and Kirchner wire fixation for open fractures. • Reconstructive surgery may be necessary for complex injuries.	• Provide aggressive care and encouragement with rehabilitation plan to regain maximal function of hand.
Hip (Proximal Femur)		

occur frequently in older adults, women with osteoporosis, and with falls
Types:
• Intracapsular—femoral neck within joint capsule.
• Extracapsular—femoral neck between greater and lesser trochanter (intertrochanteric) or of femoral shaft.
• Subtrochanteric—of femur just below level of lesser trochanter.
	• Hip fracture identified by shortening and external rotation of affected leg; pain in hip or knee; inability to move leg.
	• Immobilization with Buck's extension traction until surgery.
	• Surgery as soon as medically stable; choice depends on location, character, and patient factors.
	  • Internal fixation with nail, nail–plate combination, multiple pins, screw, or sliding nails.
	  • Femoral prosthetic replacement.
	  • Total hip replacement.
		• Provide constant monitoring and nursing care to reduce the risk of complications, such as pneumonia, thrombophlebitis, fat emboli, dislocation of prosthesis, infection, and pressure sores.
		• Administer aspirin, warfarin, subcutaneous heparin, or low-molecular-weight heparin, as ordered.
		• Use sequential compression devices, as ordered.
		• Provide meticulous skin care to prevent breakdown.
		  • Use trapeze for patient to assist with position changes.
		  • Use special bed or mattress, as indicated.
		  • Inspect heels daily and use heel protection measures.
		• Prevent UTI by increasing fluids, limiting use of indwelling catheter, and encouraging frequent voiding.
		• Keep affected leg in abduction and neutral rotation.
		• Teach quadriceps setting exercise to prevent muscle atrophy of affected leg.

Femoral Shaft		
	• Closed reduction and stabilization with skeletal traction—Thomas leg splint with Pearson attachment; followed by use of orthosis (cast-brace) to allow weight-bearing. • Open reduction with hardware or with bone grafting may be necessary. • External fixator may be used.	• Marked concealed blood loss may occur; watch for signs of shock initially and anemia later. • Examine skin under the ring of the Thomas splint for signs of pressure.
Knee		
Direct blow to knee area; involve distal shaft of femur (supracondylar), articular surfaces, or patella	• Closed reduction and immobilization through casting, traction, braces, splints. • ORIF. • Goal is to preserve knee mobility.	• Elevate extremity by raising foot gatch of bed. • Evaluate for effusion—report and loosen pressure dressing if pain is severe; prepare for joint aspiration. • Teach quadriceps setting exercises and limited weight-bearing, as prescribed.
Tibia and Fibula/Ankle		
Distal tibia or fibula, malleoli, or talus fractures generally result from forceful twisting of ankle and commonly associated with ligament disruption; also high incidence of open fractures of tibial shaft because tibia lies superficially beneath the skin	• Closed reduction and toe-to-groin cast for closed fractures, later replaced by short leg cast or orthosis. • ORIF may be necessary for some closed fractures. • External fixator for open fracture.	• Elevate lower leg to control edema. • Avoid dependent position of extremity for prolonged periods. • Prepare patient for long immobilization period, as union is slow (12–16 weeks, longer for open and comminuted fractures). • Prepare patient for stiff ankle joint following immobilization.
Foot		
Metatarsal fracture due to crush injuries of foot	• Immobilization with cast, splint, or strapping.	• Encourage partial weight-bearing, as allowed. • Elevate foot to control edema.

Table 32-2 Fractures of Specific Sites *(continued)*

SITE AND MECHANISM	MANAGEMENT	NURSING CONSIDERATIONS
Thoracic and Lumbar Spine Trauma from falls, contact sports, or auto accidents, or excessive loading may cause fracture of vertebral body, lamina, spinous and transverse processes; usually stable compression fractures	• Suspected with pain that is worsened by movement and coughing and radiates to extremities, abdomen, or intercostal muscles and presence of sensory and motor deficits. • Bed rest on firm mattress and pain relief followed by progressive ambulation and back strengthening to treat stable fractures; takes about 6 weeks to heal. • ORIF with Harrington rod, body cast, or laminectomy with spinal fusion may be necessary for unstable or displaced fractures.	• Use log roll technique to change positions. • Monitor bowel and bladder dysfunction, as paralytic ileus and bladder distention may occur with nerve root injury. • Assist patient to ambulate when pain subsides, no neurologic deficit exists, and x-rays reveal no displacement. • Teach proper body mechanics and back preservation techniques. • Encourage weight reduction. • Teach patient with osteoporosis the importance of safety measures to avoid falls.

Pelvis Sacrum, ilium, pubic, ischium, and coccyx fractures may occur from auto accidents, crush injuries, and falls; most are stable fractures that do not involve the pelvic ring and have minimal displacement	• Emergency management to treat multiple trauma, shock from intraperitoneal hemorrhage, and injury to internal organs is necessary (see pages 1215–1218).
	• Bed rest for several days followed by progressive weight-bearing for stable fracture.
	• Prolonged bed rest, external fixation, ORIF, skeletal traction, or pelvic sling are options for unstable fracture.
		• Monitor and support vital functions, as indicated.
		• Observe urine output for blood indicating genitourinary injury.
		• Do not attempt to insert urethral catheter until patency of urethra is known; incidence of urethral injury in males is high with anterior fractures.
		• Assist the patient being treated in pelvic sling.
		  • Fold sling back over buttocks to enable the patient to use bedpan.
		  • Reach under sling to give skin care; line sling with sheepskin.
		  • Loosen sling only as directed.

ORIF, open reduction with internal function; ROM, range of motion; UTI, urinary tract infection.

b. Used when fracture disrupts nutrition of the bone or treatment of choice is bony replacement.

5. External fixation device.
   a. Stabilization of complex and open fracture with use of a metal frame and pin system.
   b. Permits active treatment of injured soft tissue.
      i. Wound may be left open (delayed primary wound closure).
      ii. Repair of damage to blood vessels, soft tissue, muscles, nerves, and tendons, as indicated.
      iii. Reconstructive surgery may be necessary (see "External Fixation," page 1117).

Complications

Complications Associated with Immobility
1. Muscle atrophy, loss of muscle strength and endurance.
2. Loss of ROM due to joint contracture.
3. Pressure sores at bony prominences from immobilizing device pressing on skin.
4. Diminished respiratory, cardiovascular, GI function, resulting in possible pooling of respiratory secretions, orthostatic hypotension, ileus, anorexia, and constipation.
5. Psychosocial compromise resulting in feelings of isolation and depression.

Other Acute Complications
1. Venous stasis and thromboembolism—particularly with fractures of the hip and lower extremities.
2. Neurovascular compromise.
3. Infection, especially with open fractures.
4. Shock due to significant hemorrhage related to trauma or as a postoperative complication.
5. Pulmonary emboli.

Fat Emboli Syndrome
1. Associated with embolization of marrow or tissue fat or platelets and free fatty acids to the pulmonary capillaries, producing rapid onset of symptoms.
2. Clinical manifestations.
   a. Respiratory distress—tachypnea, hypoxemia, crackles, wheezes, acute pulmonary edema, interstitial pneumonitis.
   b. Mental disturbances—irritability, restlessness, confusion, disorientation, stupor, coma due to systemic embolization, and severe hypoxia.
   c. Fever.
   d. Petechiae in buccal membranes, hard palate, conjunctival sacs, chest, anterior axillary folds, due to occlusion of capillaries.

NURSING ALERT Restlessness, confusion, irritability, and disorientation may be the first signs of fat embolism syndrome. Confirm hypoxia with arterial blood gas (ABG) analysis. Young adults (age 20 to 30) and older adults (age 60 to 70) with multiple fractures or fractures of long bones or pelvis are particularly susceptible to development of fat emboli.

Bone Union Problems

1. Delayed union (takes longer to heal than average for type of fracture).
2. Nonunion (fractured bone fails to unite).
3. Malunion (union occurs but is faulty—misaligned).

Nursing Assessment

1. Ask patient how the fracture occurred—mechanism of injury important in determining possible associated injuries.
2. Ask patient to describe location, character, and intensity of pain to help determine possible source of discomfort.
3. Ask patient to describe sensations in injured extremity to aid in evaluation of neurovascular status.
4. Observe patient's ability to change position to assess functional mobility.
5. Note patient's emotional status and behavior—indicators of ability to cope with stress of injury.

 NURSING ALERT Change in behavior or cerebral functioning may be an early indicator of cerebral anoxia from shock or pulmonary or fat emboli.

6. Assess patient's support system; identify current and potential sources of support, assistance, and caregiving.
7. Review findings on past and present health status to aid in formulating care plan.
8. Conduct physical examination.
   a. Examine skin for lacerations, abrasions, ecchymosis, edema, and temperature.
   b. Auscultate lungs to establish baseline assessment of respiratory function.
   c. Assess pulses and BP; assess peripheral tissue perfusion, especially in injured extremity, to establish circulatory status baseline.
   d. Determine neurologic status (sensations and movement) of extremity distal to injury.
   e. Note length, alignment, and immobilization of injured extremity.
   f. Evaluate behavior and cognitive functioning of patient to determine ability to participate in care planning and patient education activities.

 GERONTOLOGIC ALERT Assessment of patient's health and functional abilities before a fracture along with available support systems facilitates development of realistic rehabilitation and discharge goals.

Nursing Diagnoses

- Risk for Deficient Fluid Volume related to hemorrhage and shock.
- Impaired Gas Exchange related to immobility and potential pulmonary emboli or fat emboli.
- Risk for Peripheral Neurovascular Dysfunction.
- Risk for vascular trauma related to thromboembolism.
- Acute Pain related to injury.
- Risk for Infection related to open fracture or surgical intervention.
- Bathing or Hygiene Self-Care Deficit related to immobility.
- Impaired Physical Mobility related to injury/treatment modality.
- Risk for Disuse Syndrome related to injury and immobilization.
- Risk for Posttrauma Syndrome related to cause of injury.

Nursing Interventions

Evaluating for Hemorrhage and Shock

1. Monitor vital signs as frequently as clinical condition indicates, observing for hypotension, elevated pulse, widening pulse pressure, cold clammy skin, restlessness, pallor.

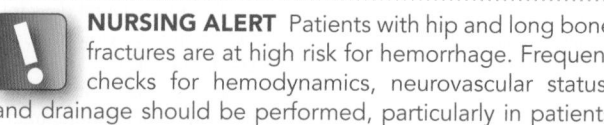 **NURSING ALERT** Patients with hip and long bone fractures are at high risk for hemorrhage. Frequent checks for hemodynamics, neurovascular status, and drainage should be performed, particularly in patients with other comorbidities who may not tolerate changes in hematocrit and hemoglobin levels.

2. Watch for evidence of hemorrhage on dressings or in drainage containers.
3. Review laboratory data; report abnormal values.
4. Administer prescribed fluids/blood to maintain circulating volume.
5. Monitor intake and output.

Monitoring for Impaired Gas Exchange

1. Evaluate changes in mental status and restlessness that may indicate hypoxia.
2. Review diagnostic evaluation data—especially ABG values and chest x-ray.
3. Position to enhance respiratory effort. Report any sudden or progressive changes in respiratory status.
4. Encourage coughing and deep breathing to promote lung expansion and diminish pooling of pulmonary secretions.
5. Monitor pulse oximetry; administer oxygen, as prescribed.
6. Maintain cervical spine precautions if spinal injury is suspected.

Preventing Neurovascular Compromise

1. Monitor neurovascular status for compression of nerve, diminished circulation, development of compartment syndrome.
   a. Pain—progressive, localized, deep throbbing, persistent, unrelieved by immobilization and medications.
   b. Pain on passive stretch.
   c. Weakness progressing to paralysis.

d. Altered sensation, hypothesia, paresthesia.

e. Poor capillary refill (>3 seconds).

f. Skin color—pale, cyanotic.

g. Elevated compartment pressure—palpable tightness of muscle compartment, elevated measured tissue pressure.

h. Pulselessness—a late sign.

 NURSING ALERT Monitoring the neurovascular integrity of the injured extremity is essential. Development of compartment syndrome (increased tissue pressure causing hypoxemia) leads to permanent loss of function in 6 to 8 hours. This situation must be identified and managed promptly.

2. Reduce swelling.

a. Elevate injured extremity (unless compartment syndrome is suspected—may contribute to vascular compromise).

b. Apply cold to injury, if prescribed.

3. Relieve pressure caused by immobilizing device, as prescribed (such as bivalving cast, rewrapping elastic bandage, or splinting device).

4. Relieve pressure on skin to prevent development of pressure sore.

a. Frequent repositioning.

b. Skin care—do not massage bony prominences.

c. Special mattresses.

Preventing Development of Thromboembolism

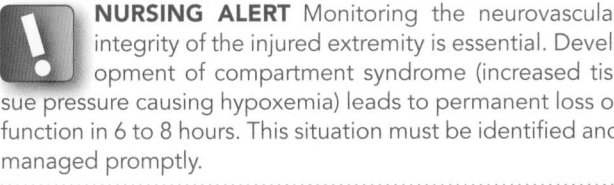 **GERONTOLOGIC ALERT** Older adults with fractures, trauma, immobility, obesity, or history of thrombophlebitis are at high risk for developing thromboembolism.

1. Encourage active and passive ankle exercises.

2. Use elastic stockings, foot pumps, or SCDs, as prescribed.

3. Elevate legs to prevent stasis, avoiding pressure on blood vessels.

4. Encourage mobility; change position frequently; encourage ambulation.

5. Administer anticoagulants, as prescribed.

6. Monitor for development of thrombophlebitis.

a. Note complaint of pain and tenderness in calf.

b. Report calf pain.

c. Report increased size and temperature of calf.

d. Homans' sign has not been proved to be an effective screen for deep vein thrombosis (DVT); therefore, it is no longer an acceptable measure for assessing DVT.

Relieving Pain

1. Perform a comprehensive pain assessment.

a. Have patient describe the pain, location, characteristics (dull, sharp, continuous, throbbing, bony, radiating, aching).

b. Ask patient what causes the pain, makes the pain worse, relieves the pain. Evaluate patient for proper body alignment, pressure from equipment (casts, traction, splints, appliances).

2. Initiate activities to prevent or modify pain.

a. Assist patient with pain-reduction techniques—cutaneous stimulation, distraction, guided imagery, TENS, biofeedback.

b. Immobilize injured part.

c. Position patient in correct alignment.

d. Support splinted fracture above and below fracture when repositioning or moving patient.

e. Reposition patient with slow and steady motion; use additional personnel, as needed.

f. Elevate painful extremity to diminish venous congestion.

g. Apply heat or cold modalities, as prescribed. Heat versus cold is controversial. One randomly controlled trial found significantly less edema with cold packs versus heat 3 to 5 days postinjury.

h. Modify environment to facilitate rest and relaxation.

3. Administer prescribed pharmaceuticals, as indicated. Encourage use of less potent drugs as severity of discomfort decreases.

 DRUG ALERT Meperidine may cause toxicity as it breaks down into the metabolite normeperidine, which has a 15- to 20-hour half-life, especially in patients with impaired renal function or older patients.

4. Establish a supportive relationship to assist patient to deal with discomfort.

5. Encourage patient to become an active participant in rehabilitative plans.

Monitoring for Development of Infection

1. Clean, debride, and irrigate open fracture wound, as prescribed, as soon as possible to minimize risk of infection.

a. All open fractures are contaminated.

b. Begin prescribed antibiotic therapy promptly after wound culture obtained.

2. Use sterile technique during dressing changes to minimize infection of wound, soft tissues, and bone.

3. Evaluate patient for elevation of temperature every 4 hours.

4. Note and report elevated white blood cell (WBC) counts.

5. Report areas of inflammation and swelling around incision or open wound.

6. Report purulent odiferous drainage.

7. Obtain specimens for culture and sensitivity to determine causative organism.

8. Administer antibiotic therapy, as prescribed.

Promoting Adequate Hygiene

1. Encourage participation in care.

2. Arrange patient area and personal items for patient convenience and to promote independence.

3. Modify activities to facilitate maximum independence within prescribed limits.

4. Allow time for patient to accomplish task.

5. Teach safe use of mobility and necessary aids.

6. Assist with ADLs, as needed.

7. Teach family how to assist patient while promoting independence in self-care.

Promoting Physical Mobility

1. Perform active and passive exercises to all nonimmobilized joints.
2. Encourage patient participation in frequent position changes, maintaining support to fracture during position changes.
3. Minimize prolonged periods of physical inactivity, encouraging ambulation when prescribed.
4. Administer prescribed analgesics judiciously to decrease pain associated with movement.

Preventing Disuse Syndrome

1. Teach and encourage isometric exercises to diminish muscle atrophy.
2. Encourage use of immobilized extremity within prescribed limits.

Minimizing the Psychological Effects of Trauma

1. Monitor patient for symptoms of posttraumatic stress disorder.
   a. Memory of event; anger, helplessness, vulnerability, mood swings, depression, cognitive impairment, sleep disturbance, increased dependency, and social withdrawal.
2. Assist patient to move through phases of posttraumatic stress (outcry, denial, intrusiveness, working through, completion).
3. Establish trusting therapeutic relationship with patient.
4. Encourage patient to express thoughts and feelings about traumatic event.
5. Encourage patient to participate in decision making to reestablish control and overcome feelings of helplessness.
6. Teach relaxation techniques to decrease anxiety.
7. Encourage development of adaptive responses and participation in support groups.
8. Refer patient to psychiatric liaison nurse or refer for psychotherapy, as needed.

Community and Home Care Considerations

1. Assist patient to actively exercise joints above and below the immobilized fracture at frequent intervals.
   a. Isometric exercises of muscles covered by cast—start exercise as soon as possible after cast application.
   b. Increase isometric exercises as fracture stabilizes.
2. After removal of immobilizing device (eg, cast, splint), have patient start isotonic exercises and continue with isometric exercises.
3. Assess the home for any fall hazards when patient ambulates.
4. Obtain PT/OT consultation for assistance with ADLs, transferring technique, gait strengthening, and conditioning after lengthy immobilization, as needed.
5. Assess orthostatic BP when patient begins to ambulate to prevent falls.

Patient Education and Health Maintenance

1. Explain basis for fracture treatment and need for patient participation in therapeutic regimen.
2. Promote adjustment of usual lifestyle and responsibilities to accommodate limitations imposed by fracture.
3. Instruct patient on exercises to strengthen upper-extremity muscles if crutch walking is planned.
4. Instruct patient in methods of safe ambulation—walker, crutches, cane.
5. Emphasize instructions concerning amount of weight-bearing that will be permitted on fractured extremity.
6. Discuss prevention of recurrent fractures—safety considerations, avoidance of fatigue, proper footwear.
7. Encourage follow-up medical supervision to monitor for union problems.
8. Teach symptoms needing attention, such as numbness, decreased function, increased pain, elevated temperature.
9. Encourage adequate balanced diet to promote bone and soft tissue healing.

Evaluation: Expected Outcomes

- Vital signs within normal parameters; urine output at least 30 mL/hour.
- Respirations unlabored; alert and oriented.
- No signs of neurovascular compromise (ie, circulation, motor, sensory intact).
- No calf pain reported.
- Reports decreased pain with elevation, ice, and analgesic.
- Afebrile; no wound drainage.
- Performing hygiene and dressing practices with minimal assistance.
- Performing active ROM correctly.
- Using affected extremity for light activity, as allowed.
- Denies acute symptoms of stress; reports working through feelings about trauma.

OTHER MUSCULOSKELETAL DISORDERS

Lower Back Pain

 Evidence Base Institute for Clinical Systems Improvement. (2011). *Adult low back pain*. Bloomington, MN: Author.

Lower back pain is characterized by an uncomfortable or acute pain in the lumbosacral area associated with severe spasm of the paraspinal muscles, usually with pain radiating to the lower extremities.

Pathophysiology and Etiology

Multiple causes:

1. Mechanical (joint, muscular, or ligamentous sprain).
2. Degenerative disk disease; acute herniation of disks.
3. Lack of physical activity and exercise; weakness of musculature of back.
4. Arthritic conditions.
5. Diseases of bone (osteoporosis, vertebral fracture, Paget's disease, metastatic carcinoma).
6. Congenital disorders.

7. Systemic diseases.
8. Infections of disk spaces or vertebrae.
9. Spinal cord tumors.
10. Referred pain from other areas.

Clinical Manifestations

1. Pain localized or radiating to buttocks or to one or both legs.
2. Paresthesias, numbness, and weakness of lower extremities.
3. Spasm in acute phase.
4. Bowel or bladder dysfunction in cauda equina syndrome.

Diagnostic Evaluation

1. X-rays of lumbar spine are usually negative.
2. CT of spine—to detect arthritic changes, degenerative disk disease, tumor, and other abnormalities.
3. Myelography—to confirm and localize disk herniation.
4. MRI—to detect pathology, disk herniation, soft tissue injury, stenosis, nerve impingement.
5. EMG of lower extremities—to detect nerve changes related to back pathology.
6. Diskogram—to evaluate herniated disk.

Management

For management of herniated disk, 566. For management of spinal cord tumors, 555.

1. Avoid activities that may strain the back until healed, but bed rest is to be avoided as well because it may significantly decrease the rate of recovery, increase pain and disability, and lengthen time spent absent from work.
   a. When in bed, sleep in a supine to semi-Fowler's position with hips and knees flexed to relieve painful muscle and ligament sprain, heal soft tissue injury, remove stress from lumbar sacral area, relieve tension on sciatic nerves, and open the posterior part of the intervertebral spaces.
   b. Acute spasm and pain should subside in 3 to 7 days if there is no nerve involvement or other serious underlying disease.
   c. Isometric exercises should be done hourly while in bed, if possible.
2. Heat or ice is used to relax muscle spasm and relieve discomfort. Follow heat with massage.
3. Medications.
   a. Oral analgesic and anti-inflammatory agent—usually NSAID is first-line agent, unless contraindicated due to history or high risk of GI bleeding, renal insufficiency, or allergy. If there is a high risk of GI bleeding, COX-2 inhibitors may be used unless the patient has a sulfa or aspirin allergy or is in the third trimester of pregnancy.
   b. Painful trigger points may be injected with hydrocortisone/Xylocaine for pain relief.
   c. Pain may be treated with opioid when severe. Opioids may be sedating.
   d. Muscle relaxant to relieve spasm and tense muscles. Muscle relaxants may be sedating.
   e. Adjunct medications to reduce chronic neuropathic pain such as amitriptyline or duloxetine.

4. Lumbosacral support may be used—provides abdominal compression and decreases load on lumbar intervertebral disks.
5. TENS may be helpful in relieving chronic pain.
6. Psychiatric intervention may be needed for patient with chronic depression, anxiety, and lower back syndrome.
   a. Psychotropic medication may be used for treatment of depression and anxiety, which potentiate pain.
   b. Focus on getting back to functional state after long disability.

 NURSING ALERT Risk factors of chronic low back pain include high severity of pain, depression, lack of positive coping skills, beliefs that the patient cannot control his or her pain, and high rate of missing work due to low back pain. Cognitive-behavioral strategies can be used to help the patient with pain management and strengthen positive coping skills. Screening tools are available to help identify risk factors and guide treatment decisions.

Complications

1. Spinal instability, infection, sensory and motor deficits.
2. Chronic pain.
3. Malingering and other psychosocial reactions.

Nursing Assessment

1. Obtain history to determine when, where, and how the pain occurs, aggravating or relieving factors, relationship of pain to specific activities, presence of numbness or paresthesia.
2. Perform physical examination of neurologic system—spots localized weakness of extremities and reflex and sensory loss.
3. Perform musculoskeletal examination for changes in strength, tone, and ROM.
4. If condition is chronic, assess coping ability of patient and family or significant others.
5. Assess effect of illness on daily living—work, school.

Nursing Diagnoses

- Acute Pain related to injury.
- Chronic Pain related to injury.
- Impaired Physical Mobility related to pain.

Nursing Interventions

Relieving Pain

1. Advise patient to stay active and avoid bed rest, in most cases.
2. Keep pillow between flexed knees while in side-lying position—minimizes strain on back muscles.
3. Apply heat (moist towels; Hydrocollator packs) or ice, as prescribed.
4. Administer or teach self-administration of pain medications and muscle relaxants, as prescribed.
   a. Give NSAIDs with meals to prevent GI upset and bleeding.
   b. Muscle relaxants and opioids may cause drowsiness.

Coping with Chronic Pain

1. Administer adjunct pain medications, as directed. Explain that medications may not completely relieve pain, but will reduce level of discomfort so that patient can increase daily activities. Encourage adherence to therapy.
2. Teach relaxation techniques such as progressive muscle relaxation and imagery (see page 28).
3. Encourage balanced diet, exercise program, and avoidance of smoking.
4. Suggest consultation with physical/occupational therapist, psychologist, or pain management clinician, as needed.

Promoting Mobility

1. Encourage ROM of all uninvolved muscle groups.
2. Suggest gradual increase of activities and alternating activities with rest in semi-Fowler's position.
3. Avoid prolonged periods of sitting, standing, or lying down.
4. Encourage patient to discuss problems that may be contributing to backache.
5. Encourage patient to do prescribed back exercises. Exercise keeps postural muscles strong, helps recondition the back and abdominal musculature, and serves as an outlet for emotional tension.

Patient Education and Health Maintenance

Instruct patient to avoid recurrences as follows:

1. Standing, sitting, lying, and lifting properly are necessary for a healthy back.
2. Alternate periods of activity with periods of rest.
   a. Avoid prolonged sitting (intradiskal pressure in lumbar spine is higher during sitting), standing, and driving.
   b. Change positions and rest at frequent intervals.
   c. Avoid assuming tense, cramped positions.
   d. Sit in a straight-back chair with the knees slightly higher than the hips. Use a footstool, if necessary.
   e. Flatten the hollow of the back by sitting with the buttocks "tucked under." Pelvic tilt (small of back is pressed against a flat surface) decreases lordosis.
   f. Avoid knee and hip extension. When driving a car, have the seat pushed forward as necessary for comfort. Place a cushion in the small of the back for support.
3. When standing for any length of time, rest one foot on a small stool or platform to relieve lumbar lordosis.
4. Avoid fatigue, which contributes to spasm of back muscles.
5. Use good body mechanics when lifting or moving about.
6. Daily exercise is important in the prevention of back problems (see Patient Education Guidelines 32-2).
   a. Do prescribed back exercises twice daily—strengthens back, leg, and abdominal muscles.
   b. Walking outdoors (progressively increasing distance and pace) is recommended.
   c. Reduce weight, if necessary—decreases strain on back muscles.

Evaluation: Expected Outcomes

- Verbalizes relief of pain with rest and medication.
- Able to participate in activities of daily living with sedation or pain >3/10.
- Performs back exercises correctly.

Osteoarthritis

 Evidence Base National Institute for Health and Clinical Excellence. (2011). *Osteoarthritis: The care and management of osteoarthritis in adults.* London: Author.
Michigan Quality Improvement Consortium. (2011). *Medical management of adults with osteoarthritis guideline.* Southfield, MI: Author.

Osteoarthritis, or degenerative joint disease, is a chronic, noninflammatory, slowly progressing disorder that causes deterioration of articular cartilage. It affects weight-bearing joints (hips and knees) as well as joints of the distal interphalangeal and proximal interphalangeal joints of the fingers.

Pathophysiology and Etiology

1. Changes in articular cartilage occur first; later, secondary soft tissue changes may occur.
2. Progressive wear and tear on cartilage leads to thinning of joint surface and ulceration into bone.
3. Leads to inflammation of the joint and increased blood flow and hypertrophy of subchondral bone.
4. New cartilage and bone formation at joint margins result in osteophytosis (bone spurs), altering the size and shape of bone.
5. Generally affects adults age 50 to 90; equal in males and females.
6. Cause is unknown, but aging and obesity are contributing factors. Previous trauma may cause secondary OA.

Clinical Manifestations

1. Pain in one or more joints, may be long-standing pain that increases with weight-bearing or use of joint; may have been a gradual, insidious onset, or may have been some history of trauma to the joint in the past.
2. Less than 30 minutes of morning stiffness.
3. Bony deformity (osteophyte) or enlargement of the joint.
4. Possible crepitation, effusion.

Diagnostic Evaluation

1. No specific laboratory examination.
2. X-rays of affected joints show joint space narrowing, osteophytes, and sclerosis.
3. Radionuclide imaging (bone scan) shows increased uptake in affected bones.
4. Analysis of synovial fluid differentiates OA from RA.

PATIENT EDUCATION GUIDELINES 32-2

Taking Care of Your Lower Back

Almost everyone has lower back pain at some time. Chronic pain will develop in some, and a few will become disabled because of it. Risk factors for chronic lower back pain include being overweight, being deconditioned (out of shape), having poor posture, and having poor abdominal muscle tone. You can relieve pain and avoid disability by adhering to the following instructions.

DO BACK EXERCISES EVERY DAY

- Lie on your back on the floor or a firm mattress. Bend one knee and bring that leg up toward your chest. Hold it against your chest a few seconds. Then repeat with the other leg. Alternate legs several times.
- Lie on your back with your knees bent and feet flat on the floor. Tighten your abdomen and buttocks and push your lower back to the floor. Hold for a few seconds, then relax. Repeat several times.
- Lie on your back with knees bent and feet flat on the floor. Do a partial sit-up by crossing your arms on your chest or behind your head and lifting your shoulders off the floor 6–12 inches (15–30.5 cm). Repeat several times.

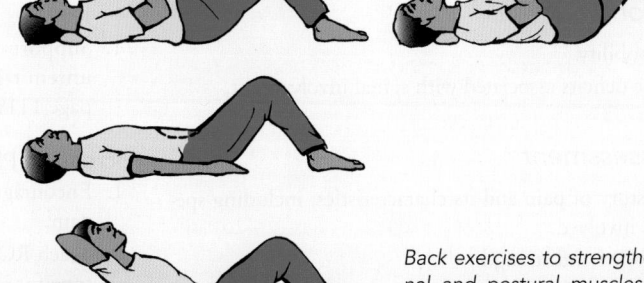

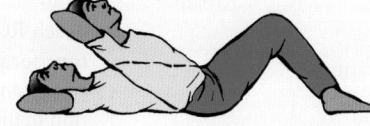

Back exercises to strengthen abdominal and postural muscles, to stretch contracted back muscles, and to maintain flexibility.

BE CAREFUL HOW YOU LIFT

- Move your body close to an object before picking it up.
- Bend at the knees, not the back, to pick up an object that is low.
- Hold the object close to your abdomen and chest.
- Bend at the knees again to put down an object.
- Avoid reaching, twisting, or turning your back as you lift or carry an object.

PROTECT YOUR BACK WHILE SITTING AND STANDING

- Avoid sitting in soft, cushioned chairs too long.
- If you sit for long periods at work, make sure your knees are level with your hips. Use a step stool, if necessary.
- If you stand for long periods, try to put one foot up on a stool, then the other. Walk around and change position periodically.

- Adjust your car seat so there is a bend in your knees. Do not stretch.
- Put a firm pillow behind your lower back if it does not feel supported while you are sitting.

STAY ACTIVE AND IN GOOD HEALTH

- Take a walk every day wearing comfortable, low-heeled shoes.
- Eat a balanced, low-fat diet with plenty of fruits and vegetables to avoid constipation.
- Get plenty of sleep on a firm mattress.
- See your health care provider promptly for worsening pain or new injury.

Management

Conservative Management

1. Includes PT and OT to maintain function while preserving the joints.
2. Pain management using nonopioid analgesics, such as acetaminophen and NSAIDs, mostly for analgesic affects and, possibly, such opioids as oxycodone, codeine, or hydrocodone (these may be used in combination with nonopioid analgesics).
3. Hyaluronate and hylan G-F 20, agents known as viscosupplements, have been approved by the Food and Drug Administration. These drugs are administered over time through intra-articular injections into the knee.
   a. They relieve pain and are most effective for people with mild to moderate knee OA.

b. After the injection, patient is instructed to avoid prolonged weight-bearing activities for 48 hours.
   c. Contraindicated for patients with joint infections and for those with allergies to hyaluronate preparations, avian proteins, and bird feathers or eggs.
4. Weight loss, if necessary, to relieve stress on joints.

> **! NURSING ALERT** The patient's body mass index can be used to determine the need for weight loss, a major factor in preventing chronic pain due to osteoarthritis. Long-term management with a primary care provider or weight-loss specialist may assist the patient in successful weight reduction.

5. Proper nutrition, sleep, and stress reduction to improve well-being.
6. OTC supplements glucosamine and chondroitin sulfate are common alternative remedies that have potential cartilage-rebuilding effects, but clinical trials in humans have been scant up to this point.

Surgical Intervention

Surgical intervention is considered when the pain becomes intolerable to patient and mobility is severely compromised. Options include osteotomy, debridement, joint fusion, arthroscopy, and arthroplasty.

Complications

1. Limited mobility.
2. Neurologic deficits associated with spinal involvement.

Nursing Assessment

1. Obtain history of pain and its characteristics, including specific joints involved.
2. Evaluate ROM and strength.
3. Assess effect on ADLs and emotional status.

Nursing Diagnoses

- Acute or Chronic Pain related to joint degeneration and muscle spasm.
- Impaired Physical Mobility related to pain and limited joint motion.
- Bathing, Hygiene, Feeding, and Toileting Self-Care Deficits related to pain and limited joint movement.

Nursing Interventions

Relieving Pain

1. Advise patient to take prescribed NSAIDs or OTC analgesics as directed to relieve inflammation and pain. May alternate with opioid analgesic, if prescribed.

GERONTOLOGIC ALERT Older patients are at greater risk for GI bleeding and renal failure associated with NSAID use. Encourage administration with meals and monitor stool for occult blood. Celecoxib is associated with less risk of GI bleeding, but may cause an increased risk of cardiovascular embolic events and deleterious effects on the kidneys.

2. Provide rest for involved joints—excessive use aggravates the symptoms and accelerates degeneration.
   a. Use splints, braces, cervical collars, traction, and lumbosacral corsets, as necessary.
   b. Have prescribed rest periods in recumbent position.
3. Advise patient to avoid activities that precipitate pain.
4. Apply heat, as prescribed—relieves muscle spasm and stiffness; avoid prolonged application of heat—may cause increased swelling and flare symptoms.

5. Teach correct posture and body mechanics—postural alterations lead to chronic muscle tension and pain.
6. Advise sleeping with a rolled terry cloth towel under the neck—for relief of cervical OA.
7. Provide crutches, braces, or cane when indicated—to reduce weight-bearing stress on hips and knees.
8. Teach use of cane in hand on side opposite involved hip or knee.
9. Advise wearing corrective shoes and metatarsal supports for foot disorders—also helps in the treatment of arthritis of the knee.
10. Encourage weight loss to decrease stress on weight-bearing joints.
11. Support patient undergoing orthopedic surgery for unremitting pain and disabling arthritis of joints (see page 1119).

Increasing Physical Mobility

1. Encourage activity as much as possible without causing pain.
2. Teach ROM exercises to maintain joint mobility and muscle tone for joint support, to prevent capsular and tendon tightening, and to prevent deformities. Avoid flexion and adduction deformities.
3. Teach isometric exercises and graded exercises to improve muscle strength around the involved joint.
4. Advise putting joints through ROM after periods of inactivity (eg, automobile ride).

Promoting Self-Care

1. Suggest performing important activities in morning, after stiffness has been abated and before fatigue and pain become a problem.
2. Advise on modifications, such as wearing looser clothing without buttons, placing bench in tub or shower for bathing, sitting at table or counter in kitchen to prepare meals.
3. Help with obtaining assistive devices, such as padded handles for utensils and grooming aids, to promote independence.
4. Refer to OT for additional assistance.

Patient Education and Health Maintenance

1. Suggest swimming or water aerobics (offered by the YMCA) as a form of nonstressful exercise to preserve mobility.
2. Encourage adequate diet and sleep to enhance general health.
3. Advise patient to discuss the use of complementary therapies, such as glucosamine and chondroitin sulfate, with health care provider.
4. For additional information and support, refer to the Arthritis Foundation (*www.arthritis.org*).

Evaluation: Expected Outcomes

- Reports reduction in pain while ambulatory.
- Performs ROM exercises.
- Dresses, bathes self, and grooms with assistive devices.

Neoplasms of the Musculoskeletal System

 Evidence Base Tobias, J., & Hochhauser, D. (2010). *Cancer and its management* (6th ed.). Somerset, NJ: Wiley-Blackwell.

Musculoskeletal neoplasms include primary *sarcomas, metastatic bone disease*, and benign tumors (*osteoma, chondroma, osteoclastoma*) of the bone. More than 60% of bone neoplasms are metastatic from other sites of cancer.

Pathophysiology and Etiology

Benign Bone Tumors

Osteoid osteoma, chondroma, and osteoclastoma (benign giant cell tumor) are examples of benign bone tumors. Malignant transformation occurs with some.

Malignant Bone Tumors

1. Chondrosarcoma and osteosarcoma are examples of primary malignant bone tumors.
   a. Tumors develop in areas of rapid growth.
   b. Risk factors include Paget's disease, previous radiation therapy to the bone, and other bone diseases.
   c. Hematogenous spread to the lung occurs.
2. Multiple myeloma is a malignant neoplasm arising from the bone marrow.

Metastatic Bone Tumors

1. Metastatic bone tumors are most frequently associated with cancers of the breast, prostate, and lung (primary malignancy site).
2. Bone metastasis most frequently occurs in the vertebrae and results in pathologic fracture.

Clinical Manifestations

1. Pain in the involved bone—from effects of tumor (destruction, erosion, and expansion of tumor).
   a. Generally mild to constant pain, which may be worse at night or with activity.
   b. Pain will be acute with fracture.
   c. Neurologic symptoms may present with nerve root compression.
2. Swelling and limitation of motion and joint effusion.
3. Physical findings.
   a. Palpable, tender, fixed bony mass.
   b. Increase in skin temperature over mass.
   c. Superficial veins dilated and prominent.

Diagnostic Evaluation

1. X-ray will usually reveal bone tumor; may show increased or decreased bone density. Tomograms may be helpful for some benign osseous lesions.
2. CT and MRI demonstrate soft tissue involvement and location of tumors.
3. Bone scan—helpful in detecting initial extent of malignancy, planning therapy, defining level of amputation, and following course of radiation or chemotherapy.

4. Ultrasound may help with identification of the lesion.
5. Serum alkaline phosphatase—usually increased.
6. Bence-Jones protein in urine with multiple myeloma.
7. Biopsy of bone—to confirm suspected diagnosis.
8. Chest x-ray and lung scan—to determine if metastasis is present.
9. Arteriography—to assess soft tissue involvement.

Management

A multidisciplinary approach in a cancer center is usually preferred. The basic objective is to halt the progression of the tumor by destroying or removing the lesion. Treatment depends on the type of tumor. Combinations of chemotherapy, surgery, and radiation may be indicated as most appropriate for specific type of tumor.

Surgery

1. Tumor curettage or resection with bone grafting may be used.
2. Limb-salvaging procedures involve resection of affected bone and surrounding normal muscle tissue and reconstruction using metallic prostheses or allografts for bone or joint replacement and skin grafting, as needed.
3. Amputation is necessary in some cases.

Chemotherapy

May be used as preoperative, adjunctive, and palliative treatment.

1. Chemotherapy may be administered before (to shrink the tumor) and after (to destroy metastasis) surgery.
2. Chemotherapy used in combination to achieve a greater patient response at a lower toxicity rate and to minimize potential problems of drug resistance and may be given in varying courses separated by rest periods.

Radiotherapy

1. Tumor irradiation may be used.
2. Prophylactic lung irradiation may be performed—to suppress metastasis.

Other Therapies

1. Immunotherapy—interferon.
2. Hormone therapy may be used with metastatic tumors of the breast and prostate.
3. If pathologic fracture occurs, the fracture is managed with open reduction and internal fixation or other fracture treatment method.

Complications

1. Lack of tumor control and metastases.
2. Pathologic fracture.
3. Hypercalcemia from bone destruction.

Nursing Assessment

1. Obtain history of progression of disease; presence of pain, fever, weight loss, malaise.
2. Examine for painless mass.
3. Review records for evidence of pathologic fracture.
4. Assess knowledge of cancer, experiences with family or others, and present coping.

Nursing Diagnoses

- Acute Pain related to effects of tumor.
- Risk for Injury related to altered bone structure.
- Ineffective Coping related to diagnosis and treatment options.

Nursing Interventions

See also "Orthopedic Surgery," page 1119, and "Amputation," page 1123.

Relieving Pain

1. Use multiple approaches to reduce discomfort.
2. Administer pain medications 30 minutes before ambulation or other uncomfortable movement.
3. Support painful extremities on pillows.

Preventing Pathologic Fractures

1. Assist patient in movement with gentleness and patience.
2. Avoid jarring patient or bed.
3. Support joints when repositioning patient.
4. Guard patient to avoid falls.
5. Create a hazard-free environment.
6. Provide patient education on safety.

Strengthening Coping Ability

1. Create a supportive environment.
2. Use psychological support services, as needed.
3. Answer questions and clear up misconceptions about treatment options.

Patient Education and Health Maintenance

1. Teach about particular treatment selected. See 146 for information on chemotherapy and 151 for radiation therapy information.
2. Encourage appropriate follow-up and diagnostic testing for recurrence.
3. Refer for additional information and support to the American Cancer Society (*www.cancer.org*).

Evaluation: Expected Outcomes

- Reports decreased pain with ambulation.
- No signs or symptoms of fractures.
- Verbalizes understanding of treatment options and strength to make decisions.

Osteomyelitis

Evidence Base Schnettler, R. (2010). *Septic bone and joint surgery.* New York: Thieme.

Osteomyelitis is a severe pyogenic infection of the bone and surrounding tissues that requires immediate treatment.

Pathophysiology and Etiology

1. Generally bacteria gain entry to the bone via three routes:
   a. Bloodstream (hematogenous spread).
   b. Adjacent soft tissue infection (contiguous focus).
   c. Direct introduction of microorganisms into the bone.
2. Bacteria lodge and multiply in bone.
3. Pressure increases as pus collects in confined rigid bone, contributing to ischemia and vascular occlusion and leading to bone necrosis.
4. *Staphylococcus aureus* is the most common infecting microorganism, although others are prevalent: *Escherichia coli, Pseudomonas, Klebsiella, Salmonella,* and *Proteus.*

Clinical Manifestations

1. Infection of long bones with acute pain and signs of sepsis.
2. Localized pain and drainage.
3. Symptoms vary in adults and children according to the site of involvement.

Diagnostic Evaluation

1. Acute osteomyelitis diagnosis made on initial clinical signs (history, physical examination, CBC, ESR).
2. Aerobic and anaerobic cultures of bone and deep tissue to identify the organism. Wound cultures are not reliable.
3. ESR elevated, WBC and hemoglobin decreased.
4. Radiographic evidence of osteomyelitis lags behind symptoms by up to 14 days.
5. Radionuclide bone scans used to diagnose early acute osteomyelitis.
6. MRI used increasingly—distinguishes between soft tissue and bone marrow.

Management

1. Acute: full recovery possible with minimal loss of function.
2. Chronic: develops with inadequate or ineffective course of antibiotics or delayed treatment.

Surgical Intervention

1. Needle aspiration or needle biopsy done initially.
2. Surgical intervention may be needed to obtain culture and sensitivity of specimen.
3. Surgical decompression considered when patient does not improve after 36 to 48 hours of antimicrobial therapy.
4. Debridement may be done, or antibiotic-impregnated beads used in wound (removed after 2 to 4 weeks and replaced with bone graft).
5. Hyperbaric oxygen therapy may be used as an adjunctive therapy.

Pharmacologic Intervention

1. Employ quickly after presentation of symptoms to avoid chronicity.
2. Parental antimicrobial therapy based on blood/wound cultures.
3. Medications depend on organism, but include:
   a. Penicillins (penicillin G, penicillin V).
   b. Semisynthetic penicillins (nafcillin, oxacillin, methicillin).
   c. Extended-spectrum penicillins (ampicillin, carbenicillin, amoxicillin).
   d. Beta-lactam agents (imipenem).
   e. Tetracyclines.
   f. Cephalosporins.
   g. Aminoglycosides.

4. Requires 6 to 8 weeks of intravenous antibiotic therapy, requiring a peripherally inserted central catheter line or other long-term access device and coordination of home care services.

Complications

1. Nonhealing wound.
2. Sepsis.
3. Immobility.
4. Amputation.

Nursing Assessment

1. Obtain detailed history of injury.
2. Assess pain and functional deficits.
3. Be aware that systemic symptoms are acute in children, but vary in intensity with adults.
4. Perform general systemic assessment because adults with long bone involvement generally have more systemic septic symptoms.

Nursing Diagnoses

- Acute Pain related to inflammatory process.
- Deficient Knowledge related to disease and medications.
- Impaired Physical Mobility related to rest of affected part.

Nursing Interventions

Relieving Pain

1. Administer opioids for acute pain; nonopioids for chronic pain.
2. Administer medications around the clock versus as necessary to establish a consistent blood level.
3. Report any increase in pain that may indicate worsening infection.

Increasing Knowledge

1. Describe the infectious process and rationale for prolonged treatment with osteomyelitis.
2. Explain IV antibiotic therapy, potential adverse effects, and reactions.
3. Explain strict adherence to infection-control practices (sterile technique, handwashing, selection of roommate) to prevent spread of infection in some cases.
4. Initiate home care nursing and infusion services referrals before discharge.

Promoting Rest without Complications

1. Support the affected extremity (splint, traction) to minimize pain.
2. If patient is on bed rest, prevent hazards of immobility (passive ROM, position changes, coughing, and deep breathing).
3. Encourage distraction activities.

Patient Education and Health Maintenance

1. Advise patient to adhere to infection-control principles—proper handwashing, disposal of wound drainage, dressings to prevent reinfection or transmission of infection at home.

2. Stress adherence to medication regimen, which may be prolonged, with frequent follow-up visits.
3. Teach care of indwelling device for medication delivery (such as Hickman catheter).
4. Educate patient on signs and symptoms of infection to monitor for and when to notify physician.

Evaluation: Expected Outcomes

- Pain managed with nonopioid analgesics.
- Infectious process minimized.
- Functional status of affected joint intact.

Paget's Disease (Osteitis Deformans)

 Evidence Base Manson, J., Chambers, S., Shipley, M., et al. (2011). *Rapid review of rheumatology and musculoskeletal disorders*. London: Manson.

Paget's disease of the bone is a skeletal disorder resulting from excessive osteoclastic activity, affecting the long bones, pelvis, lumbar vertebrae, and the skull predominantly.

Pathophysiology and Etiology

1. The cause of this disease is unknown, although there is evidence of familial tendency (25% to 40% have at least one affected relative).
2. More common in men than in women.
3. Rare before age 40 and increases as age does—12% after age 80.
4. May be caused by infection from blood-borne viruses. After acute viremia, osteoclasts become chronically infected, stimulating osteoclastic proliferation. See Figure 32-13.

Clinical Manifestations

1. Generally asymptomatic.
2. Most common symptoms are pain and predisposition to fracture.
3. Pagetic lesions can lead to OA, joint destruction, spinal deformity.
4. Decrease in hearing, tinnitus, and vertigo as a result of skull abnormality.
5. Waddling gait due to abnormality of pelvis.
6. Radiculopathy and nerve palsies due to effects from the vertebral column.
7. Rarely, heart failure and other cardiovascular effects from increased blood supply over abnormal bone.
8. Malignant bone tumors occur in 5% to 10%.

Diagnostic Evaluation

1. Elevated serum alkaline phosphatase and urine hydroxyproline.
2. Serum calcium, phosphorus, and albumin levels usually normal.
3. Generally confirmed with radiologic examinations showing characteristic abnormalities.

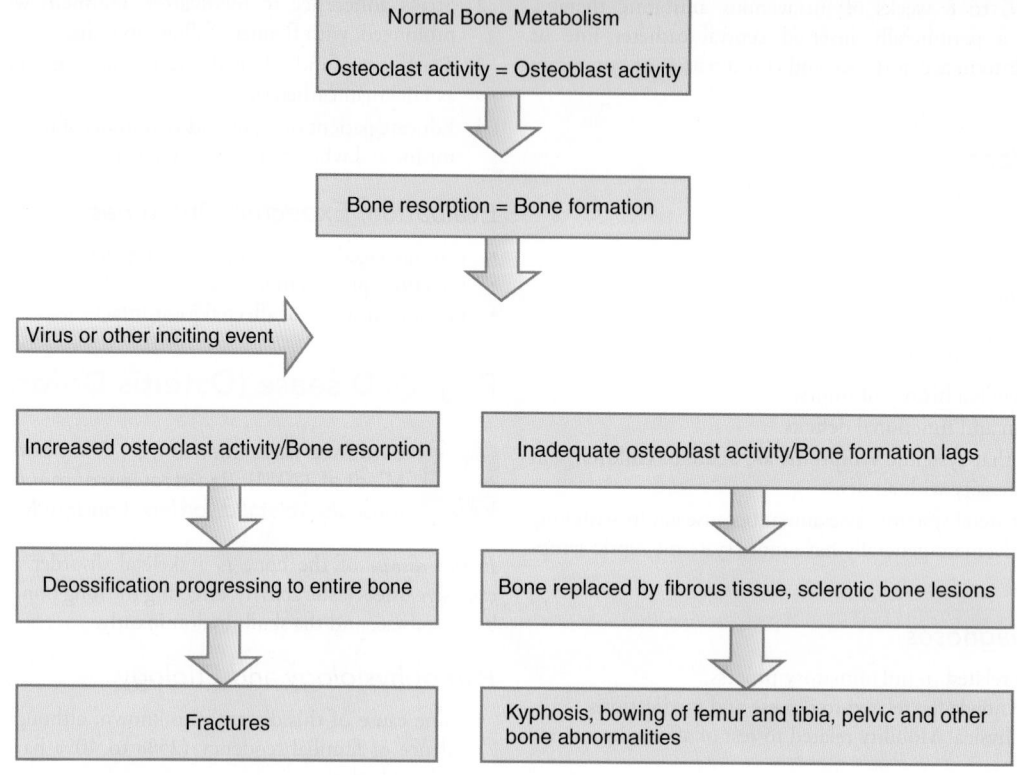

Figure 32-13. Pathophysiology of Paget's disease.

4. Bone scans can evaluate rapid bone turnover.
5. Bone biopsy to differentiate from osteomyelitis or bone tumor.

Management

1. No treatment for asymptomatic Paget's.
2. Pain management—NSAIDs, aspirin.
3. Medications—calcitonin is the main medication used to suppress bone turnover, reduce pain, and prevent progression.
4. Other medications used to block bone resorption—the bisphosphonates etidronate disodium, alendronate, pamidronate, risedronate; an antineoplastic agent, plicamycin.
5. Tibial osteotomy done to realign knees and relieve pain.

Nursing Assessment

1. Assess pain and functional ability.
2. Observe for bowing (legs) or complaint that hats feel tight.
3. Assess for cardiovascular complications.
4. Assess for auditory symptoms—tinnitus, vertigo, and hearing loss.

Nursing Diagnoses

- Chronic Pain related to pathophysiologic process.
- Risk for Injury related to falls.

Nursing Interventions

Reducing Pain

1. Administer and teach self-administration of analgesics.
2. Avoid sedation due to opioids, which may increase risk of falls.

Preventing Injury

1. Establish exercise protocols through a PT consult to maintain physical abilities and prevent falls.
2. Teach safe transferring and make sure patient can alert nurses if he or she needs help.
3. Assist patient with activities, as necessary.
4. Provide function and mobility aids such as heel lifts, walking aids, as needed, through an OT consult.

Patient Education and Health Maintenance

1. Teach safety measures in the home—removal of loose rugs and obstacles to prevent falls, good lighting.
2. Provide education about the disease process and medication treatment.
3. Make sure that patient knows how to use mobility aids.
4. Initiate home care referral, as indicated.
5. Provide information about The Paget Foundation (*www. paget.org*).
6. Encourage follow-up for periodic hearing tests and bloodwork.

Evaluation: Expected Outcomes

- Pain severity ranges 2–3/10
- No falls

Hallux Valgus

Also called *bunion*, *hallux valgus* is a deformity of the foot involving the first metatarsal and great toe. Occurs in females more frequently than males and incidence increases with age; may have a genetic predisposition. Commonly occurs with other deformities of the feet, such as hammertoe, mallet toe, and claw toe.

Clinical Manifestations

1. Pain.
2. Possible callus of skin overlying bunion and accompanying toe deformities.
3. Diminished ROM.
4. Generally associated with tight footwear.

Management and Nursing Interventions

Conservative Management

1. Wearing footwear made of soft leather with a wider toe box, rounded rather than pointed, and with low heel.
2. Special orthoses can be ordered.
3. Steroid injections to relieve pain.

Surgical Management

Surgical alignment of the great toe by osteotomy of metatarsal or proximal phalanx of the great toe or fusion of the metatarsal–metatarsophalangeal joint

Postoperative Care

1. Elevation of the foot to reduce pain.
2. Initial non-weight-bearing activity, with very gradual progress in activity.
3. Crutch walking initially, followed by wooden shoe immobilizer for several weeks.
4. NSAIDs and opioid analgesics for pain.
5. Bandages changed by surgeon initially.

SELECTED REFERENCES

Aaron, D. L., Patel, A., Kayiaros, S., et al. (2011). Four common types of bursitis: Diagnosis and management. *Journal of the American Academy of Orthopaedic Surgery, 19*(6), 359–367.

American Academy of Orthopedic Surgeons. (2010). *Antibiotic prophylaxis for bacteremia in patients with joint replacements.* Rosemont, IL: Author.

American Academy of Orthopaedic Surgeons. (2010). *The diagnosis of periprosthetic joint infections of the hip and knee.* Rosemont, IL: Author.

American Academy of Orthopaedic Surgeons. (2010). *Optimizing the management of rotator cuff problems.* Rosemont, IL: Author.

American Academy of Orthopaedic Surgeons. (2011). *Preventing venous thromboembolic disease in patients undergoing elective hip and knee arthroplasty.* Rosemont, IL: Author.

Atkins, E. (2010). *A practical approach to orthopaedic medicine: Assessment, diagnosis, treatment* (3rd ed.). New York: Elsevier.

Brotzman, S. B., & Manske, R. C. (2011). *Clinical orthopaedic rehabilitation* (3rd ed.). New York: Mosby.

Bucholz, R. W., Heckman, J. D., Court-Brown, C. M., et al. (Eds.). (2010). *Rockwood and Green's fractures in adults* (2nd ed.). Philadelphia: Lippincott, Williams & Wilkins.

Bulstrode, C., Wilson-MacDonald, J., Fairbank, J., et al. (2011). *Oxford textbook of trauma and orthopaedics* (2nd ed.). Oxford, UK: Oxford University Press.

Goff, J. D., & Crawford, R. (2011). Diagnosis and treatment of plantar fasciitis. *American Family Physician, 84*(6), 676–682.

Humbyrd, C. J., Petre, B., Chanmugam, A. S., et al. (2012). *Orthopaedic emergencies.* Oxford, UK: Oxford University Press.

Jester, R., Santy, J., & Rogers, J. (2011). *Oxford handbook of orthopaedic and trauma nursing.* Oxford, UK: Oxford University Press.

Logerstedt, D. S., Snyder-Mackler, L., Ritter, R. C., et al. (2010). Knee pain and mobility impairments: Meniscal and articular cartilage lesions. *Journal of Orthopaedic Sports and Physical Therapy, 40*(6), A1–A35.

Logerstedt, D. S., Snyder-Mackler, L., Ritter, R. C., et al. (2010). Knee stability and movement coordination impairments: knee ligament sprain. *Journal of Orthopaedic Sports Physical Therapy, 40*(4), A1–A37.

Manson, J., Chambers, S., Shipley, M., et al. (2011). *Rapid review of rheumatology and musculoskeletal disorders.* London: Manson.

McRae, R. (2010). *Clinical orthopaedic examination* (6th ed.). New York: Elsevier.

Michigan Quality Improvement Consortium. (2011). *Management of acute low back pain guideline.* Southfield, MI: Author.

Michigan Quality Improvement Consortium. (2011). *Medical management of adults with osteoarthritis guideline.* Southfield, MI: Author.

National Association for Orthopaedic Nursing. (2012). *Orthopedic nursing core competencies across the lifespan,* (3rd ed.). Chicago: Author.

National Institute for Health and Clinical Excellence, 2012. *Orthopedic nursing core competencies across the lifespan* (3rd ed.). Chicago: Author.

Schnettler, R. (2010). *Septic bone and joint surgery.* New York: Thieme.

Tobias, J., & Hochhauser, D. (2010) *Cancer and its management* (6th ed.). Somerset, NJ: Wiley-Blackwell.

Wiesel, S. W. (2010). *Orthopaedic surgery: Principles of diagnosis and treatment.* Philadelphia: Lippincott Williams & Wilkins.

Work Loss Data Institute. (2010). *Knee and leg* (acute and chronic). Encinitas, CA: Author.

33
Dermatologic Disorders

OVERVIEW AND ASSESSMENT

Description of Skin Lesions

The description of dermatologic conditions always includes the morphology of the lesions that appear on the skin (ie, their size, shape, color, pattern and distribution; see Figure 33-1).

Primary Lesions

1. Macule—flat, circumscribed discoloration of skin; may have any size or shape.
2. Papule—solid, elevated lesion less than 1 cm wide.
3. Nodule—raised, solid lesion larger than 1 cm wide.
4. Vesicle—circumscribed elevated lesion less than 0.5 cm, containing fluid.
5. Bulla—a vesicle or blister larger than 0.5 cm wide.
6. Pustule—circumscribed raised lesion that contains pus; may form as a result of purulent changes in a vesicle.
7. Wheal—elevation of the skin that lasts less than 24 hours, caused by edema of the dermis; may be surrounded by erythema or blanching.
8. Plaque—solid, elevated lesion on the skin or mucous membrane, larger than 1 cm in diameter; psoriasis is commonly manifested as plaques on the skin; leukoplakia is an example of plaques on mucous membranes.

9. Cyst—soft or firm mass in the skin, filled with semisolid or with liquid material contained in a sac.

Secondary Lesions

Secondary lesions involve changes that take place in primary lesions that modify them.

1. Scale—heaped-up, horny layer of dead epidermis; may develop as a result of inflammatory changes.
2. Crust—covering formed by the drying of serum, blood, or pus on the skin (scab).
3. Excoriation—linear scratch marks or traumatized areas of skin.
4. Fissure—linear cracks in the skin, usually from marked drying and long-standing inflammation.
5. Ulcer—lesion formed by local destruction of the epidermis and by part or all of the underlying dermis.
6. Lichenification—thickening of skin accompanied by accentuation of skin markings.
7. Scar/keloid—abnormal new formation of connective tissue that replaces the loss of substance in the dermis as a result of injury or disease. A keloid is a hypertrophic scar that is larger than the original lesion or injury.
8. Atrophy—diminution in size or in loss of skin cells that causes thinning of the skin.

Primary lesions

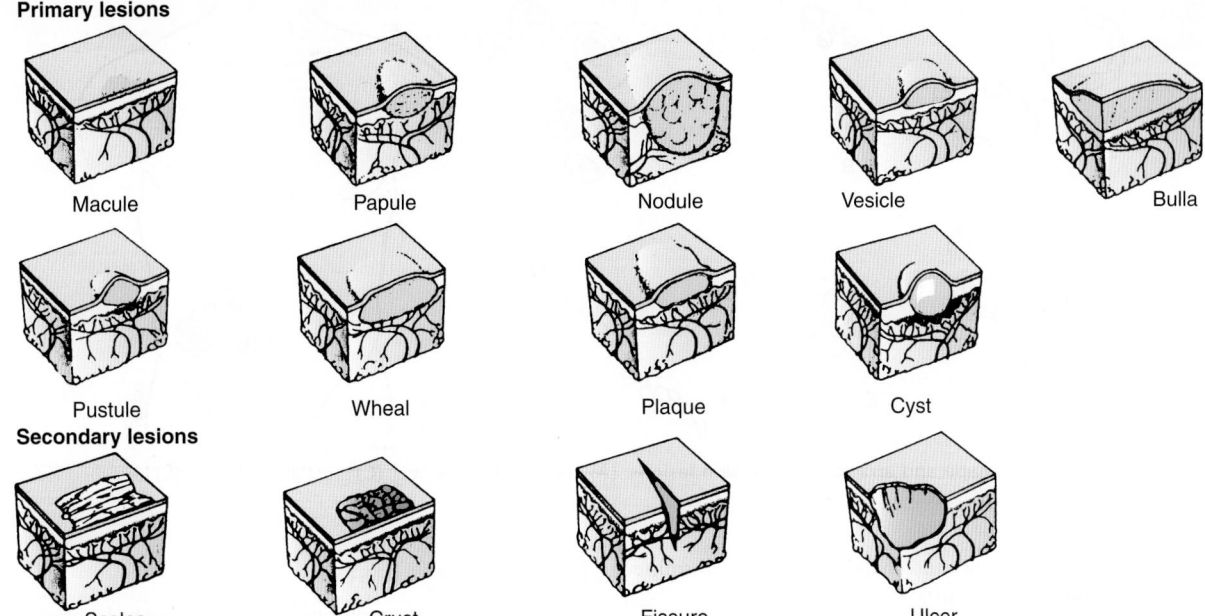

Figure 33-1. Types of skin lesions.

Other Lesions

1. Petechiae—circumscribed deposits of blood or blood pigment 1 to 2 mm wide.
2. Purpura—circumscribed deposits of blood or blood pigment greater than 0.5 cm wide.
3. Comedones—hair follicle obstructed by a sebum and keratin plug; blackheads and whiteheads.
4. Telangiectasia—small, irregular blood vessels visible in the epidermis.
5. Burrow—linear, irregular, elevated tunnel produced by parasites in the skin.

Shape and Configuration

After the type of lesion is identified, the shape, configuration or arrangement (in relation to each other), and pattern of distribution are noted (see Figure 33-2, page 1150). The following are descriptions commonly used:

1. Annular—ring-shaped.
2. Circinate—circular.
3. Confluent—lesions run together or join.
4. Discoid—disk-shaped.
5. Discrete—lesions remain separate.
6. Generalized—widespread eruption.
7. Grouped—clustering of lesions.
8. Guttate—droplike.
9. Herpetiform—grouped vesicles.
10. Iris—ring or a series of concentric circles (bull's-eye).
11. Linear—in lines.
12. Nummular—coin-shaped.
13. Polymorphous—occurring in several or many forms.
14. Reticulated—lacelike network.
15. Serpiginous—snakelike or creeping eruption.
16. Telangiectatic— a tiny red thread or line.
17. Zosteriform or dermatomal—bandlike distribution, limited to one or more dermatomes of skin.

History

Obtaining a thorough history is key to diagnosing and developing a plan of care for dermatologic conditions, as well as understanding the characteristics of the problem and its effect on the patient.

Characteristics of Rash

1. When did the rash first occur? Was the onset sudden or gradual?
2. What site was first affected? Describe the spread and its severity.
3. What was the initial color and configuration of the rash? Has it changed?
4. Is there associated itching, burning, tingling, pain, or numbness?
5. Has it been constant or intermittent?

Associated Factors

1. What makes the rash worse or better? Is it seasonal? Is it affected by stress?
2. What medications are being taken? What topical products have been used? What effect did they have?
3. What skin products are used? What chemicals have come into contact with the skin: such as laundry detergent, cleaning products, insecticides, or nickel?
4. Has there been pet contact?
5. What is the patient's occupation? Any hobbies, such as gardening or hiking, that may have contributed? Are latex gloves worn routinely? Is frequent handwashing required?

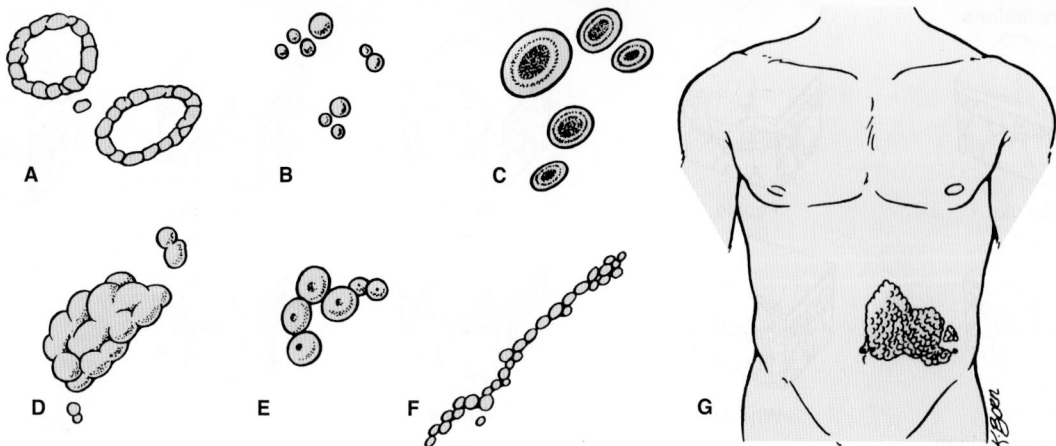

Figure 33-2. Shape and arrangement of skin lesions: (A) annular, **(B)** grouped, **(C)** iris, **(D)** confluent, **(E)** herpetiform, **(F)** linear, **(G)** zosteriform or dermatomal.

6. What is the sexual history and chance of sexually transmitted disease exposure (if relevant)?
7. Any international travel?

Medical History

1. Is there a history of hay fever, asthma, hives, eczema, or allergies?
2. Has the patient had this particular rash or other skin disorders in the past?
3. What is the family history of skin disorders?
4. Are there any long-standing medical problems? Immunosuppressive therapy?

Physical Examination

1. Focus your examination on the skin, hair, and nails. Some dermatologic conditions affect other body systems (eg, hair loss may be associated with thyroid disease or anemia); perform a general physical exam, as indicated.
2. Ask the patient to show you the area of concern and examine the skin surface under good lighting. Patients should be undressed, in a gown, and the skin of the total body should be examined, not just the area affected.
3. Note the distribution and configuration of skin lesions. Compare right and left sides of the body.
4. Note the shape, border, texture, and surface of the lesions.
5. Palpate the lesions for texture, warmth, and tenderness.
6. Use a metric ruler to determine size of lesions to serve as a baseline for comparison with subsequent measurements.
7. Examine the scalp, nails, and oral mucosa.
8. Perform diascopy—gently press a glass slide or Lucite rule over a skin lesion to detect blanching (caused by dilated blood vessels).
9. Use a Wood's light to inspect for fluorescent changes with some fungal infections. Clean skin prior to examination because some ointments, soaps, or deodorant may fluoresce.
10. For dark-skinned patients look for black, purple, or gray lesions; palpate carefully to determine if rash is present.

Laboratory Tests

Some dermatologic conditions can be evaluated by laboratory tests such as microscopy and culture.

Microscopy

1. Sample taken by scraping, swabbing, or aspirating a lesion is transferred to a glass slide for microscopic examination or staining.
   a. Direct visualization of scrapings mixed with mineral oil to detect scabies, mites, or lice nits that cling to hair.
   b. A Tzanck smear is obtained from vesicular fluid or a moist ulcer and stained to detect characteristics of herpes simplex virus, herpes zoster, and varicella. This is rarely done in the office but properly obtained specimen could be sent to the lab.
   c. Potassium hydroxide may be added to skin scrapings on a glass slide and heated to dissolve skin cells to detect hyphae and spores in fungal infections.
   d. Gram stain may be performed by the lab or dermatopathologist to tentatively identify bacteria or fungi in certain skin infections.

Nursing and Patient Care Considerations

1. To obtain the specimen for microscopy use the side of a glass slide or a scalpel held at a 45-degree angle to gently scrape the active border of a dry lesion or of an inflamed area; only mild discomfort and pinpoint bleeding should occur.
2. For moist or semi-moist ulcerations or crusted lesions, roll saline-soaked cotton or Dacron-tipped swab over the lesion; for weeping lesions, use a dry swab.
3. For intact vesicles, aspirate fluid from the edge with a 25G sterile needle; if vesicle is partially broken, gently unroof with forceps and obtain fluid on a swab.

Culture

1. Drainage from lesions may be cultured on specific media to detect causative organism and sensitivity to antimicrobial therapy; also, portions of skin, hair, and nails may be submitted for fungal culture.

2. Usually takes 24 to 48 hours for results; fungal cultures may take 4 to 5 weeks.

Nursing and Patient Care Considerations

1. Obtain specimen with cotton or Dacron-tipped swab and send to laboratory in bacterial culture container clearly labeled with the patient's name, the date, and the site where the specimen was obtained or in a viral culture container also clearly labeled. Refrigerate viral culture if laboratory pickup is delayed.

2. To obtain specimen for fungal culture, scrape or clip the affected skin, hair, or nails; then place into a dry, sterile container for transport or onto a dermatophyte test medium.

Other Tests

Patch Testing

Patch testing is an office procedure done to determine if patients are sensitive to contact materials. Materials are applied in patches to the skin and checked for reaction 48 hours after application and possibly again in 1 week. Erythema, itching, swelling, papules, and vesicles indicate an allergic contact dermatitis rather than an irritant contact dermatitis or no reaction.

See Patient Education Guidelines 33-1 and Procedure Guidelines 33-1, pages 1152 to 1153.

GENERAL PROCEDURES AND TREATMENT MODALITIES

Baths and Wet Dressings

A therapeutic bath is used to apply medication to the entire skin surface and is useful in treating widespread eruptions and general pruritus. Baths soothe, soften, and reduce inflammation and relieve itching and dryness. See Table 33-1 for types and desired effects. Wet dressings and soaks are damp compresses that contain water, normal saline solution, aluminum acetate (Burow's) solution, or magnesium sulfate solution. They may be sterile or clean, or warm or cool, depending on the skin condition and the area to which they are applied.

Therapeutic Baths

Indications

1. Vesicular disorders, eczema, atopic dermatitis.
2. Acute inflammatory conditions.
3. Erosions and exudative, crusted surfaces.

Nursing and Patient Care Considerations

1. Prepare the bath or teach patient to prepare a lukewarm bath at 90° to 100° F (32.2° to 37.8° C); with the tub half-full, add the prescribed quantity of medication and mix thoroughly to prevent sensitivity reaction. Add oatmeal products or oils to emulsifying baths.

PATIENT EDUCATION GUIDELINES 33-1

Patch Testing

Patch testing is a process used to determine what substances may be causing reactions in your skin. Your dermatologist will decide which substances to test. The goal of patch testing is to reproduce the skin rash on a small, controlled area of the skin. The patch test will identify materials, such as preservatives, fragrances, dyes, and chemicals, that cause an allergic reaction upon contact with your skin. Because patch testing does not break the skin barriers, allergies to food, inhalants, and oral medication cannot be identified by this method.

WHAT TO EXPECT

• During your initial visit, which lasts approximately 30 minutes, the nurse will apply one or more small aluminum disks or tape strips to an area on your upper back (used as the test site because the strongest responses are seen in this area). These disks, or patch test kits, contain small amounts of each suspected chemical or allergen; the substances to be tested are determined by your dermatologist or other health care provider. A visible reaction in the skin in contact with a disk indicates allergy to the substance contained in that disk. This redness or rash may itch and persist for several days to several weeks.

• You will be advised to return 48 hours later. At this time, the nurse will remove the patches, mark your skin, and do the first reading; you will be expected to remain at the office for 30 minutes so that the nurse can complete the reading.

• A final reading will be done on your next visit, which will take place 96 hours to 1 week after the disks have been removed. A copy of your test results will be provided and explained to you at this visit.

DO'S AND DON'TS

• DO wear loose or high-necked clothing throughout the day. Wear a T-shirt to bed to avoid catching the edges of the tape on the bed sheets.

• DO apply tape to the patch edges if they become loose.

• DO contact your health care provider immediately if a patch test area burns severely or if you are unable to carry out normal daily activities. *Note:* Some itching will occur if you are having a positive reaction; you do not need to call your dermatologist.

• DO NOT wet the patches during the testing period—for example, do not take showers. Sponge baths are allowed as long as care is taken to keep the patches completely dry.

• DO NOT engage in strenuous activities. Exercise may result in excess sweating, thereby causing the tape to loosen.

• DO NOT expose your back to the sun for 2 weeks before patch testing.

• DO NOT discontinue antihistamine therapy (these agents do not affect test results).

• DO NOT use nonmedicated creams and lotions on your back for at least 24 hours before testing (lotions and creams prevent patches from sticking).

PROCEDURE GUIDELINES 33-1

Patch Testing

PURPOSE
Patch testing is a sometimes useful diagnostic tool used to differentiate irritant versus allergic contact dermatitis. Patients who present with suspected allergic contact dermatitis or eczema are potential candidates for patch testing.

EQUIPMENT

- Finn chambers (strips of 10 shallow aluminum cups or chambers 3 inches [8 cm] wide) or TRUE test strip
- Allergens (2-inch [5-cm] ribbons of petrolatum-base allergen or disks with filter paper dampened with aqueous solution). Standard tray includes:
  - Benzocaine 5%
  - Mercaptobenzothiazole 1%
  - Colophony 20%

- p-Phenylenediamine 1%
- Imidazolidinyl urea 2%
- Cinnamic aldehyde 1%
- Lanolin alcohol 30%
- Carba mix 3%
- Neomycin sulfate 20%
- Thiuram mix 1%
- Formaldehyde 1%
- Ethylenediamine dihydrochloride 1%

- Epoxy resin 1%
- Quaternium-15 2%
- P-tert-Butylphenol formaldehyde resin 1%
- Mercapto mix 1%
- Black rubber mix 0.6%
- Potassium dichromate 0.25%
- Balsam of Peru
- Nickel sulfate

 DRUG ALERT Patients should not be taking oral corticosteroids at the time of the test; topical corticosteroids should be discontinued 1–2 weeks before testing to prevent a weak reaction or false-negative results. Make sure the patient has followed the health care provider's instructions.

PROCEDURE

Nursing Action	Rationale
1. Prepare Finn chambers with allergen. Aqueous allergens come in prefilled syringes that should be kept refrigerated. TRUE test is a prepackaged strip.	1. Prepackaged strips are more convenient and easier to use but may be more costly.
2. Apply strip to patient's back.	2.
a. Avoid hairy areas and areas affected by dermatitis and sunburn.	a. Should be a large area of skin unaffected by friction and free from interfering skin lesions so that results will be clear. Hair may interfere with tape adhesion.
b. Preferred area is upper back.	b. Skin on upper back is most sensitive to reaction.
3. Number the disks 1 through 10 to match the allergen placed on the disk. If the patient is having several strips applied, draw a diagram on the patient's file to record which tray is placed in which location. Optionally, take a photo.	3. Ensures that results are interpreted correctly.
4. Apply additional tape, as required, to keep patches secure.	4. Sweating and activity may reduce adherence in some people.
5. Instruct the patient to keep area dry, not to scratch or remove the patches unless they become unbearable (severe burning, stinging, or pruritus).	5. Area may become uncomfortable with positive reaction, but removal or disruption of patch will invalidate results.
6. When patient returns in 48 hours for the first reading, mark the outline of the patch strip on the patient's back, then remove the strip. A skin marker or an ultraviolet skin pen marker may be used.	6. Outline serves as a reference point to interpret results.
7. Wait 30 minutes, then do the first reading. Document based on the outcome as follows or take a picture for the patient's record:	7. The skin may be red from the application of the tape and a false reading may occur if read too soon.

1+ Weak reaction. Nonvesicular, but with erythema, induration, and possible papules.

2+ Strong reaction. Edematous and vesicular, with erythema, edema, papules, and vesicles.

PROCEDURE GUIDELINES 33-1 *(continued)*

Patch Testing

PROCEDURE *(continued)*

Nursing Action	Rationale
3+ Extreme reaction. Spreading, bullous, ulcerative IR (irritant reaction). Negative reaction. Not tested. Patches fell off.	
8. Instruct patient to keep the area dry after removal of the patches and return again in 24–72 hours (usually 48 hours) for additional reading.	8. Though the initial 48-hour reading may be negative, positive results may be seen at the 96-hour reading because of delayed reaction.
9. A final reading is done on the last visit, results are recorded, and counseling is given on negative or positive results.	
10. If the results are positive, the nurse discusses avoidance of allergens and gives the patient written information regarding the allergens to be avoided.	10. According to practice policy.

 Evidence Base Hall, J. C. (2010). *Sauer's manual of skin diseases* (10th ed.). Philadelphia: Lippincott Williams & Wilkins.

Table 33-1	Therapeutic Baths
BATH SOLUTION AND MEDICATION	**DESIRED EFFECT**
Water	• Removes crusts and relieves inflammation
Saline	• Used for widely disseminated lesions
Colloidal Oatmeal	• Antipruritic and demulcent
Sodium Bicarbonate	• Cooling
Starch	• Soothing
Tar Baths (follow package directions)	• Used for psoriasis and chronic eczematous conditions
Bath Oils	• Used for antipruritic and emollient soothing properties • Used for acute and subacute eczematous eruptions
Bleach Baths	• Reduces colonization of harmful bacteria that contribute to acute and chronic eczema

a. Bleach baths may be used for acute and chronic atopic dermatitis.

b. Add ½ cup of bleach to full tub or ¼ cup to half tub of warm water and soak limbs and torso for 5 to 10 minutes (do not submerge head), no more than twice a week.

2. Do not rub the skin. Soaking for at least 5 to 10 minutes will promote removal of loosened scales.

3. Keep the room and water at comfortable temperatures and limit bathing to 20 to 30 minutes; the bath area should be well ventilated if tars are used because they are volatile.

4. Tell patient to use a bath mat inside the tub and to use a rug outside the tub when bathing at home because medication may make the tub and other wet surfaces slippery.

5. Blot skin dry with a towel and apply emollient or topical medication to moist skin. While skin is wet, apply steroid to inflamed areas, if prescribed.

Open Wet Dressings

Indications
1. Bacterial infections that require drainage.
2. Inflammatory and pruritic conditions.
3. Oozing and crusting conditions.

Nursing and Patient Care Considerations
1. Apply dressing to affected area or teach patient to apply. Moisten to the point of slight dripping; remoisten as necessary.
2. Use warm tap water if warming is desired.

3. Application may be from 5 to 15 minutes three to four times per day, unless otherwise indicated.

4. Keep patient warm and do not treat more than one third of body at a time because open wet dressings can cause chilling and hypothermia.

5. Teach patients to prevent burns by measuring temperature of solution with a bath thermometer or by testing tap water on wrist before applying compress. Advise them not to use microwave ovens to warm dressings because uneven heating can occur.

Other Dressings

Occlusive Dressing

An *occlusive dressing* is formed by an airtight plastic or vinyl film applied over medicated areas of skin (usually with corticosteroids) to enhance absorption of medication and to promote moisture retention.

Indications

Skin conditions with thick scaling, such as psoriasis, eczema, and lichen simplex chronicus.

Nursing and Patient Care Considerations

1. Wash area and pat dry.
2. Apply medication while skin is still moist.
3. Cover with plastic wrap, vinyl gloves, or plastic bag.
4. Seal with paper tape at edges or cover with other self adhesive dressing to hold in place.

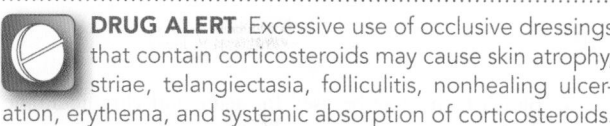

DRUG ALERT Excessive use of occlusive dressings that contain corticosteroids may cause skin atrophy, striae, telangiectasia, folliculitis, nonhealing ulceration, erythema, and systemic absorption of corticosteroids.

5. Do not apply to ulcerated or abraded skin; removal is recommended within 12 to 24 hours. High-potency steroids are for short-term use only.

Nonocclusive Dressings

Other dressing materials may be used as dry dressings to protect the skin, keep affected areas clean, absorb drainage, or to cover medication or to hold occlusive dressings in place.

Nursing and Patient Care Considerations

1. Apply dry gauze dressing using clean technique (unless sterile technique is indicated by open wounds).
2. Wrap extremities with elastic or cotton-rolled bandages or apply tape. Avoid constricting circulation.
3. Alternative dressing materials can be used for home care, such as disposable or white cotton gloves for the hands, cotton socks for the feet, sheets or towels for large areas, disposable diapers or towels folded in diaper fashion for the groin, washcloths for the axilla, cotton T-shirt or cotton pajamas for the trunk, turban or plastic shower cap for the scalp, or mask made from gauze for the face, with holes cut for the eyes, mouth, and nose.

Skin Biopsy

Removal of a piece of skin by shave, punch, or excision technique to detect malignancy or other characteristics of skin disorders.

Types of Biopsy

1. Shave biopsy—scalpel used to remove raised lesions, leaving lower layers of dermis intact.
2. Punch biopsy—special instrument used to remove round core of lesion, containing all layers of skin. Biopsy site is usually closed with sutures.
3. Excisional biopsy—scalpel and scissors used to remove entire lesion, usually with prescribed margins; suturing required.

Nursing and Patient Care Considerations

1. Position patient comfortably with the site exposed; explain that a local anesthetic will be given. Check if patient has any known allergies to local anesthetics. Ask patient what current medication he or she is taking. Aspirin, some herbal supplements, or anticoagulants may cause increased postoperative bleeding.
2. Explain the procedure.
3. Obtain written consent.
4. After the biopsy, apply hemostatic agent and pressure to the site to stop bleeding, along with an appropriate dressing. Pressure dressing may be required for larger wounds or wounds that are bleeding.
5. Place the biopsy specimen in a clearly labeled container with 10% formaldehyde and transport it to the dermatopathology lab for hematoxylin and eosin staining. It is essential that skin biopsies be sent to a specialized dermatopathology lab for examination by a dermatopathologist in order to get the best analysis and most complete information on the histology of the skin disease or lesion.

Patient Education

1. Keep the bandage on surgery site for 24 to 48 hours. During this time, keep site clean and dry.
2. After this time, remove the bandage and do the following daily:
   a. Wash the incision with soap and water.
   b. Dry the incision well.
   c. Apply petroleum- or mineral oil–based ointment, such as Vaseline or Aquaphor, one to four times per day, keeping the incision moist at all times.
3. After a few days the dressing is no longer needed, but continue to apply ointment one to four times per day to keep the site moist and help reduce scarring.
4. Do not apply makeup directly to the stitches.
5. Repeat wound care for 2 or 3 days after stitches have been removed, unless otherwise instructed.
6. Use caution when shaving around stitches on face.

DRUG ALERT Many patients are allergic to neomycin, a component of triple antibiotic ointment. Petrolatum or mineral oil–based ointments pose less risk of allergic dermatitis.

Wound Coverage: Grafts and Flaps

Wound coverage, using grafts and flaps, is a type of reconstructive (plastic) surgery performed to improve the skin's appearance and function. These are sometimes used following Mohs micrographic surgery to remove skin cancers, especially on the face, head, and neck.

Skin Graft

1. A section of skin tissue is separated from its blood supply and transferred as free tissue to a distant (recipient) site; it must obtain nourishment from capillaries at the recipient site.
2. In dermatology, skin grafting is used to repair defects that result from excision of skin tumors and to cover areas of denuded skin.
3. Definitions.
   a. Autografts—grafts done with tissue transplanted from the patient's own skin.
   b. Allografts—involve the transplant of tissue from one individual of the same species; these grafts are also called allogenic or homografts.
   c. Xenograft or heterograft—involves the transfer of tissue from another species.
4. Classification by thickness.
   a. Split thickness (thin, intermediate, or thick)—graft that is cut at varying thicknesses and is used to cover large wounds because its total potential donor area is virtually unlimited.
   b. Full thickness—graft consists of epidermis and all of the dermis without the underlying fat; used to cover wounds that are too large to close primarily. They are used frequently to cover facial defects because they provide a better contour match and less postoperative contracture.

Skin Flaps

1. A flap is a segment of tissue that has been left attached at one end (called a base or pedicle); the other end has been moved to a recipient area. It is dependent for its survival on functioning arterial and venous blood supplies and on lymphatic drainage in its pedicle or base.
   a. Free flap or free-tissue transfer—one that is completely severed from the body and is transferred to another site; receives early vascular supply from microvascular anastomosis with vessels at recipient site.
2. Flaps may consist of skin, mucosa, muscle, adipose tissue, and omentum.
3. Used for wound coverage and to provide bulk, especially when bone, tendon, blood vessels, or nerve tissue are exposed.
4. Flaps offer the best aesthetic solution because a flap retains the color, texture, and thickness match of the donor area.
5. Flaps are classified according to the method of movement, composition, location, or function.

Procedure for Skin Grafts

1. Split-thickness skin graft is obtained by razor blade, skin-grafting knife, or electric or air-powered dermatome or drum dermatome. Most commonly obtained from the inner aspect of the upper arm or outer thigh.
2. A full-thickness skin graft is primarily excised, defatted, and tailored to fit accurately over the defect area.
3. Skin is taken from the donor or host site and applied to the wound or defect site, called the recipient site or graft bed.
4. A bolster (pressure) dressing is applied to the graft to enhance the survival of the skin graft by providing stable approximation of the graft to the recipient bed.
5. The bolster dressing is left in place for 1 week. The process of revascularization and reattachment of the skin graft to the recipient bed is referred to as a take.
6. The donor site is maintained clean and dry.
   a. If Scarlet Red (a single layer dressing impregnated with epithelial growth promoter) is used on the donor site for split-thickness grafts, it is left in place for 2 to 3 weeks to allow the wound to heal.
   b. Occlusive dressings, such as Omniderm or Allevyn, may also be used to decrease pain, alleviate frequent wound care, and speed healing.
   c. Daily wound care and dressing change with an antimicrobial ointment and nonstick dressing may also be used.

 NURSING ALERT Patients usually find the donor site more painful than the graft site.

Preoperative Management and Nursing Care

1. Aspirin and nonsteroidal anti-inflammatory drugs (NSAIDs) and vitamin E are discontinued 14 days before the procedure. Coumadin should be held for several days before the procedure, and prothrombin time and International Normalized Ratio should be measured before the procedure, as ordered. Herbal supplements, such as ginkgo, ginseng, green tea, and vitamin E, can inhibit coagulation.
2. Efforts should be made to enhance wound healing several months to several weeks before the procedure, such as smoking cessation, alcohol avoidance, and proper nutrition.
3. Medical history and examination should be evaluated, particularly for latex sensitivity, cardiovascular problems requiring endocarditis antibiotic prophylaxis, bleeding problems, and high blood pressure (BP).
4. The procedure is usually done under local anesthetic, so no meals are withheld.
5. The operative site should be free from makeup.
6. The patient should have someone available to drive him or her home after surgery unless otherwise notified.

Postoperative Management and Nursing Care

Educate the patient with a skin graft on the following care:

1. Initial pressure dressing will be left in place for 24 to 48 hours.
2. If wound begins to ooze, apply firm pressure for 10 to 15 minutes (without peeking). If bleeding persists, contact surgeon.
3. Do not take aspirin or aspirin-containing medication for pain. May take one to two acetaminophen tablets every 4 to 6 hours, as needed.
4. Most skin grafts are held in place by a bolster dressing (cotton ball or foam). Do not remove the bolster dressing during the next week.
5. May clean site and apply ointment to the surrounding area of the bolster dressing.

6. Do not get the bolster dressing wet.

7. When the bolster dressing is removed, may shower, but *do not* let the water hit the graft directly.

8. Keep the graft edges moist with ointment.

9. Protect the graft from the sun. The sun will cause pigmentation changes in the graft. A sunscreen may be used in 2 to 3 weeks.

10. Skin grafts to the lower leg must be kept elevated because the new capillary connections are fragile and excess venous pressure may cause rupture. Keep leg elevated as much as possible during the next week.

11. Inspect the dressing daily. Report unusual drainage or signs of an inflammatory reaction.

12. After 2 to 3 weeks, any water-based moisturizer may be applied to the skin donor site for split-thickness skin grafts.

13. Expect some loss of sensation in the grafted area for a time.

14. Avoid strenuous exercise (jogging, lifting heavy objects). Anything that causes face flushing will raise BP, cause bleeding, and impair healing.

Aesthetic Procedures

Aesthetic procedures (cosmetic surgery) consist of reconstructive (plastic) surgery or the use of injected substances, which may be performed to reconstruct or to alter congenital or acquired defects or to restore or improve the body's appearance. Noninvasive procedures alter the skin surface through the use of light sources or chemical applications.

Types of Procedures

Rhytidectomy

1. Done through various techniques and incisions to alleviate skin folds and wrinkles to improve the appearance of the aging face (face lift).

2. The correction can last as long as 10 years, but results vary with each individual. Skin relaxes with time and the muscles may also relax, but seldom does the face revert to its preoperative condition.

3. Surgical procedures include:
   a. Operative: Standard incisions that are either temporal (hidden in hairline) or submental.
   b. Laser: Several laser modalities are now used in facial plastic surgery, including radio-frequency tissue tightening, which causes collagen shrinkage and reduction of deep wrinkles and lines.

Blepharoplasty

1. Removes loose skin, muscle, and excess fat from upper or lower eyelids. It will not remove lines at the lateral corners of the eyes ("crow's feet").

2. The procedure is generally done by either scalpel under local or general anesthetic or by carbon dioxide laser.

Dermabrasion, Chemical Peel, Laser Resurfacing, and Fillers

1. Patients with weathered skin, fine wrinkles (especially at the corners of the eyes and along the vermilion border), or acne pitting and scarring may benefit from these procedures.

2. The use of laser technology allows for a more predictable result and eliminates the porcelain appearance resulting from such chemicals as trichloroacetic acid. There is less risk of hypopigmentation than with dermabrasion.

3. Chemical peels using tretinoin cream and alpha-hydroxy acids result in the destruction of portions of the epidermis and dermis, with subsequent regeneration of new tissues.

4. New nonablative laser resurfacing is used for fine wrinkles, smoker lines, sun-damaged skin, and shallow acne scarring with minimal downtime.

5. Contraindications of laser resurfacing include:
   a. History of isotretinoin therapy 6 to 12 months prior to treatment.
   b. Status of postradiation or scleroderma.
   c. History of herpes simplex—requires perioperative treatment.

6. Hyperpigmentation can occur in persons with dark skin.

7. Purified botulinum toxin and fillers (collagen, hyaluronic acid, autologous fat) are used to correct deep wrinkles and facial hollows. Results may last 3 to 12 months.

Liposuction

1. Also called body contouring, liposuction reduces localized deposits of fat not amenable to weight loss with a cannula aided by suction or fitted to a syringe.

2. May be done on the face, neck, breasts, abdomen, flanks, hips, buttocks, and extremities.

Preoperative Management and Nursing Care

1. Local or general anesthetic will be administered. For local anesthetic, patient may eat and drink before surgery. For general anesthetic:
   a. Preoperative assessment may be necessary, depending on health status and patient's age.
   b. No eating or drinking for several hours before surgery.
   c. Patient should have escort and must be reminded not to drive home alone after surgery.

2. Review patient's allergies and medication before surgery.

3. Instruct patient to cleanse skin with antiseptic agent the night before surgery, if prescribed.

4. Make sure patient thoroughly understands the procedure and has discussed the risks and benefits with the health care provider before surgery.

5. Make sure a consent form is signed before any procedure.

6. Make sure aspirin, warfarin, and NSAIDs have been discontinued for 2 weeks before surgery, unless otherwise indicated. Herbal supplements, such as ginkgo, ginseng, green tea, and vitamin E, can inhibit coagulation.

7. If applicable, instruct the patient to stop smoking for the 2 weeks leading up to rhytidectomy and to continue cessation for 2 weeks postprocedure and permanently, if possible.

8. Be aware of signs of topical lidocaine toxicity (if used)—drowsiness, tingling of lips, metallic taste—which may lead to seizures.

Postoperative Management and Nursing Care

Rhytidectomy

1. Mild exercise can be resumed in 3 days postoperatively.

2. No strenuous exercise (that will increase the BP) for 1 month.

3. Dressings are usually removed on the first postoperative day. Elastic facial support garment is recommended for 1 to 3 weeks.

4. Eyelid sutures are removed in 3 to 5 days; facial sutures in 7 days.

5. Showering and gentle hair washing may begin on day 2 or 3.

6. The patient is to apply ointment (petroleum or a similar ointment) to all suture lines.

7. Stress to the patient not to remove crusts by "picking" at them along suture lines or scarring may result.

8. Elevate the head at night for 2 weeks after the procedure. Avoid bending and lifting, which may increase edema and provoke bleeding.

9. Expect the face or affected part to be swollen, bruised, and numb for several days to weeks.

10. Be aware that complications include bleeding and hematoma, sloughing of skin, and possible facial nerve damage. Notify surgeon if the areas become increasingly red or swollen or if they become more tender or painful.

Blepharoplasty

1. Apply iced gauze compresses to eyes for 10 minutes four to six times per day to reduce edema after surgery.

2. Head of bed should be elevated to reduce internal pressure that might cause bleeding.

3. Avoid strenuous exercise for 1 week.

4. Bruising and swelling generally resolve in 2 weeks.

5. Watch for such complications as eyelid hematomas, ocular mobility dysfunction, and postsurgical ectropion (eversion of the edge of the eyelid).

Dermabrasion and Chemical Peel

1. Instruct patients to not pick at crusts because new epithelium will be injured; soak face several times per day and apply emollient, as directed. Crusts form in 2 to 3 days and start to separate by 7 to 10 weeks. Total separation can take up to 3 weeks.

2. Keep treated areas clean and moist.

3. Avoid sun on treated areas. Apply sunscreen with sun protection factor (SPF) of 15 to 30 when outdoors.

4. Manage bruising and swelling from injectables with ice packs.

Laser Resurfacing

1. Dressings, such as hydrogel dressings (see page 185), may be applied to the affected areas immediately and left in place for 24 to 48 hours.

2. Alternately, the open technique involves using petroleum gel and daily face washes with tepid water.

Liposuction

1. After liposuction, increased fluids are required.

2. Aspirin and NSAIDs should be avoided for at least 1 week to prevent bleeding.

3. Wear compression garment, as instructed.

4. Notify the surgeon if increased swelling develops; could indicate development of a seroma.

5. Expect blood-tinged fluids from cannula injection sites for 2 to 3 days.

6. Keep sutured areas moist with ointment, as instructed.

7. Avoid jarring exercise.

8. Complications include development of seromas, lumpiness in treated areas, excessive bruising.

 NURSING ALERT Advise all postoperative patients to notify health care provider if sudden pain, swelling, or bruising develops; these suggest hematoma or abscess. Do not take aspirin for postoperative discomfort; follow surgeon's orders.

DERMATOLOGIC DISORDERS
Cellulitis

Cellulitis is a diffuse inflammation of the deep dermal and subcutaneous tissue that results from an infectious process.

Pathophysiology and Etiology

1. Caused by infection with group A beta-hemolytic streptococci, *Staphylococcus aureus*, *Haemophilus influenzae*, or other organisms.

2. Usually results from break in skin that may be as simple as athlete's foot.

3. Infection can spread rapidly through lymphatic system.

 NURSING ALERT Methicillin-resistant *S. aureus* (MRSA) is a significant problem outside of the hospital as well as within. It is resistant to previously effective antistaphylococcal antibiotics and may be fatal.

Clinical Manifestations

1. Tender, warm, erythematous, and swollen area that is poorly demarcated.

2. Tender, warm, erythematous streak that extends proximally from the area, indicating lymph vessel involvement.

3. Possible fluctuant abscesses or purulent drainage.

4. Possible fever, chills, headache, malaise.

Diagnostic Evaluation

1. Gram stain and culture of drainage.

2. Blood cultures.

Management

1. Oral antibiotics (penicillinase-resistant penicillins, cephalosporins, quinolones, or sulfa-based) may be adequate to treat small, localized areas of cellulitis of legs or trunk.

2. Parenteral antibiotics may be needed for cellulitis of the hands, face, or lymphatic or widespread involvement.

3. Surgical drainage and debridement for suppurative areas recommended for MRSA infections.

Complications

1. Tissue necrosis.

2. Septicemia.

Nursing Assessment

1. Obtain history of trauma to skin, needlestick, insect bite, or wound.

2. Observe for expanding borders and lymphatic streaking; palpate for fluctuance of abscess formation.
3. Watch for signs of antibiotic sensitivity—shortness of breath, urticaria, angioedema, maculopapular rash, or severe skin reaction, such as erythema multiforme or toxic epidermal necrolysis.
4. Assess for patient and caretaker ability to provide care at home, keep affected area clean, and adhere to medication prescribed.

Nursing Diagnoses

- Impaired Skin Integrity related to infectious process.
- Acute Pain related to inflammation of subcutaneous tissue.

Nursing Interventions

Protecting Skin Integrity

1. Administer or teach patient to administer antibiotics, as prescribed; teach dosage schedule and adverse effects. Assess ability to swallow pills. Recommend crushing or taking with food to avoid stomach irritation, if applicable.
2. Maintain intravenous (IV) infusion or venous access to administer IV antibiotics, if indicated.
3. Elevate affected extremity to promote drainage from area and reduce swelling.
4. Prepare patient for surgical drainage and debridement, if necessary.

Relieving Pain

1. Encourage comfortable position and immobilization of affected area.
2. Administer or teach patient to administer analgesics, as prescribed; monitor for adverse effects.
3. Use bed cradle to relieve pressure from bed covers.

Patient Education and Health Maintenance

1. Make sure that patient understands dosage schedule of antibiotics and the importance of complying with therapy to prevent complications.
2. Advise patient to notify health care provider immediately if condition worsens; hospitalization may be necessary.
3. Outpatient-treated cellulitis should be observed within 24 to 48 hours of starting antibiotics to determine efficacy.
4. Teach patient with impaired circulation or impaired sensation how to perform proper skin care and how to inspect skin for trauma.

Evaluation: Expected Outcomes

- Skin is normal color and temperature, nontender, nonswollen, and intact.
- Actively moves extremity; verbalizes no pain.

Necrotizing Fasciitis

Necrotizing fasciitis is a type of necrotizing infection of the soft tissue that spreads quickly along fascia. It rapidly progresses toward death if not treated quickly.

Pathophysiology and Etiology

1. Usually caused by group A *Streptococcus*, known as flesh-eating bacteria, but may also be a clostridia or polymicrobial infection. It is emerging as a complication of MRSA infection.
2. May result postoperatively or from local injury with superficial or deep infection.
3. More common in patients with diabetes, those that abuse drugs, and other immunocompromised populations.
4. Spreads along fascia, causing extensive necrosis of skin and subcutaneous tissue.

Clinical Manifestations

1. Increasing pain or pain out of proportion to local infection or injury; increasing redness, edema, and warmth.
2. Fever, rapid pulse.
3. Tissue appears darkened under skin.
4. Possible bullae or petechiae or appears hemorrhagic.
5. May be foul odor and drainage (delayed).

Diagnostic Evaluation

1. Surgical excision and debridement is diagnostic to determine extent as well as therapeutic.
2. Gram stain and culture from deep tissue to determine exact etiology.
3. Blood cultures to rule out septicemia.

Management

1. Immediate hospitalization with intensive care support.
2. Prompt and repeated surgical debridement.
3. IV antibiotic regimen using multiple agents, including clindamycin, penicillin G, erythromycin, ceftriaxone, and others.

Complications

1. Muscle gangrene—requires amputation.
2. Loss of tissue and function.
3. Death.

Nursing Assessment

1. After trauma, surgery, or with cellulitis, frequently assess for increasing pain, fever, and changes in skin appearance, which may indicate necrotizing fasciitis.

 NURSING ALERT Inform the health care provider immediately if pain is out of proportion to injury or if progressive skin changes occur. The patient should be assessed for necrotizing fasciitis.

2. Be aware of underlying conditions that may cause immunocompromise, such as diabetes, alcoholism, malnutrition, IV drug use, cancer and cancer treatment, and HIV/AIDS, which increases the risk and worsens the course of necrotizing fasciitis.
3. Monitor vital signs frequently for any change (rise or fall in BP, temperature, pulse, and respirations) that may indicate worsening condition.

4. Monitor wound dressings after debridement for amount, color, and odor of drainage. Wounds will usually be left open to heal by secondary intention.

Nursing Diagnoses

- Hyperthermia related to infectious process.
- Acute Pain related to necrosis.

Nursing Interventions

Normalizing Body Temperature

1. Administer antipyretics, as directed.
2. Encourage oral fluids and administer IV fluids, as directed.
3. Monitor intake and output to ensure adequate hydration because of fluid loss through fever and insensible loss.
4. Provide cool compresses, sponge baths, and clothing and linen changes as comfort measures.

Relieving Pain

1. Administer analgesics, as directed, and based on pain assessment; however, be alert for sedation that may mask signs of worsening condition.
2. Assist patient to position of comfort that will not place pressure on affected area.
3. Administer analgesic 30 to 60 minutes before wound care and dressing changes.

Education and Health Maintenance

1. Make sure that patient can complete wound care at home and will follow up as directed.
2. Make home care nursing referral, as necessary.
3. Teach patient signs of infection and to notify health care provider immediately if experiencing increasing pain, fever, redness, swelling, warmth, or increased and odorous drainage.
4. Advise patient to eat a balanced diet rich in protein, vitamin C, iron, and zinc for wound healing.

Evaluation: Expected Outcomes

- Core temperature 97.6° to 98.8° F (36.4° to 37.1° C).
- Patient turning in bed, verbalizing minimal pain.

Toxic Epidermal Necrolysis

Toxic epidermal necrolysis is a severe, potentially fatal skin disease associated with erythema, blistering, and epidermal sloughing. A less severe form is known as *Stevens-Johnson syndrome.*

Pathophysiology and Etiology

1. Exact mechanism is unknown, but can be induced by various drugs, including sulfonamides, anticonvulsants, NSAIDs, allopurinol.
2. Resembles second-degree burns, with sloughing of skin at epidermal or dermal junction.
3. Mortality ranges from 3.2 to 90%, based on an illness severity score with factors such as age, presence of malignancy, heart rate, and percentage of epidermal detachment.

 Evidence Base New Zealand Dermatologic Society. (2012). Stevens Johnson Syndrome and Toxic Epidermal Necrolysis. DermNet NZ. Available: *http://www .dermnetnz.org/reactions/sjs-ten.html*

Clinical Manifestations

1. Malaise, fatigue, vomiting, cough, fever, and diarrhea may be prodromal symptoms.
2. Sudden onset of urticaria and large dark-red areas; within 5 to 8 days, large, flaccid bullae appear.
3. Within hours coma may develop.
4. Bullae become confluent and slough in large sheets, leaving moist, erythematous surface.
5. Positive Nikolsky's sign (desquamation of skin on light pressure).
6. Erosions of mucosal sites, including lips, oral pharynx, or urinary tract.

Diagnostic Evaluation

1. Skin biopsy to determine level of separation.
2. Possible cultures of blood and body fluids to differentiate infection.

Management

1. Treatment in intensive-care unit or regional burn center because toxic epidermal necrolysis has similar pathophysiologic characteristics to those of extensive burns (see Chapter 34, page 1178).
2. Treatment of affected skin.
   a. Wounds are cleaned in operating room under anesthesia; loose skin and blisters are removed, necrotic areas are debrided to prevent infection.
   b. Temporary biologic dressings (porcine cutaneous xenographs, amnion, collagen-based skin substitute, or plastic semipermeable dressings) applied to prevent secondary skin infection while awaiting reepithelialization.
3. All nonessential drugs are stopped immediately.
4. Fluid replacement therapy, as necessary, and possible enteral nutrition if oral involvement.
5. Topical antimicrobial dressings to enhance reepithelialization.
6. Ophthalmologic examination and removal of corneal adhesions, as necessary.
7. Use of systemic corticosteroids is not recommended and use of human IV immunoglobulin is controversial.

Complications

1. Sepsis.
2. Pneumonia.
3. Blindness.

Nursing Assessment

1. Obtain medication and immunization history.
2. Monitor vital signs and level of consciousness closely because condition is rapidly progressive.

3. Monitor fluid and nutritional status through daily weight, vital signs, and laboratory test results (electrolytes, especially glucose, bicarbonate, blood urea nitrogen, creatinine, albumin, and total protein).

Nursing Diagnoses

- Impaired Skin Integrity related to sloughing.
- Risk for Deficient Fluid Volume related to transudation of fluid into bullae.
- Acute Pain related to exposed dermal nerve endings.
- Impaired Oral Mucous Membranes related to oral lesions.

Nursing Interventions

Restoring Skin Integrity

1. Place patient on warmed air-fluidized bed to distribute weight with minimal shearing forces.
2. Use extreme care in handling patient because skin is very fragile; obtain assistance to move patient.
3. Gently apply warm, wet compresses of prescribed antiseptic solution to reduce bacterial population of wound surface.
4. Inspect xenograft several times daily for dislodgment or purulence; these will require new xenograft.
5. Watch for new areas of toxic epidermal necrolysis; note and record progression of skin slough and chart progress.
6. Patient should be in private room on reverse isolation to prevent infection.
7. Provide nutritional supplements through enteral feeding to ensure healing.

Maintaining Fluid Balance

1. Monitor vital signs for falling BP or for rising pulse that indicates hypovolemia; use an indwelling arterial catheter to provide continuous measurement while avoiding cuff pressure on the skin.
2. Measure hourly urine output.
3. Weigh patient daily.
4. Give IV fluids, as prescribed.
5. Assess bowel sounds and give oral or enteral fluids, as tolerated.

Reducing Pain

1. If patient cannot verbalize, watch for facial expressions, guarding, or for increased pulse and respirations to indicate pain.
2. Administer analgesics, as prescribed and as required, possibly around the clock; monitor for adverse effects and document effectiveness.
3. Provide distraction through music or other measures to promote relaxation.
4. Provide emotional support and encouragement. Emotional/psychological support to patient and family are crucial.

Protecting Mucous Membranes

1. Use meticulous oral hygiene.
   a. Inspect oral cavity daily; note any changes.
   b. Rinse mouth with normal saline, diluted hydrogen peroxide, or other solution to remove debris and to cleanse ulcerations.
   c. Apply petroleum jelly or other lubricant/protectant to cracked, swollen lips.
2. Assess urethral, vaginal, and anal regions for ulcerations or bleeding.

3. Inspect eyes and remove crusts from eyelid margins using damp compresses or saline-soaked swabs; apply eyedrops, as prescribed.

Patient Education and Health Maintenance

1. Encourage follow-up appointments with plastic surgeon and other health care providers, as indicated.
2. Encourage compliance with physical therapy, as indicated, to restore function.
3. Advise patient to use sunscreen of at least SPF 15, avoid direct sunlight during the healing phase, and continue to use sunscreen.
4. Advise patient to avoid suspected medication in the future.

Evaluation: Expected Outcomes

- New epithelium noted without scarring.
- Output equals input; weight and vital signs remain stable.
- Patient verbalizes reduced pain.
- Oral mucosa intact.

Herpes Zoster

Herpes zoster (varicella zoster, shingles) is an inflammatory condition in which reactivation of the chickenpox virus produces a vesicular eruption along the distribution of the nerves from one or more dorsal root ganglia (dermatome). The prevalence increases with age. A varicella zoster vaccine is available for people older than age 60 to prevent reactivation.

Pathophysiology and Etiology

1. Caused by a varicella-zoster virus, which is a member of a group of deoxyribonucleic acid viruses.
2. Virus is identical to the causative agent of varicella (chickenpox). After the primary infection, the varicella-zoster virus may persist in a dormant state in the dorsal nerve root ganglia. The virus may emerge from this site in later years, either spontaneously or in association with immunosuppression, to cause herpes zoster.

Clinical Manifestations

1. Eruption may be accompanied or preceded by fever, malaise, headache, and pain; pain may be burning, lancinating, stabbing, or aching.
2. Inflammation is usually unilateral, involving the cranial, cervical, thoracic, lumbar, or sacral dermatome in a bandlike configuration.
3. Vesicles appear in 3 to 4 days.
   a. Characteristic patches of grouped vesicles appear on erythematous, edematous skin.
   b. Early vesicles contain serum; they later rupture and form crusts; scarring usually does not occur unless the vesicles are deep and they involve the dermis.
   c. If ophthalmic branch of the facial nerve is involved, patient may have a painful eye. (This can be a medical emergency.) Vesicles on tip of nose suggest eye involvement.
   d. In healthy host, lesions resolve in 2 to 3 weeks.
4. A susceptible person can acquire chickenpox if there is contact with the infective vesicular fluid of a zoster patient.

A person with a history of chickenpox or who has received the immunization is immune and thus is not at risk from infection after exposure to zoster patients.

 NURSING ALERT Varicella-zoster virus may be a life-threatening condition to the patient who is immunosuppressed, who is receiving cytotoxic chemotherapy, or who is a bone marrow transplant recipient.

Diagnostic Evaluation

1. Usually diagnosed by clinical presentation.
2. Culture of varicella-zoster virus from lesions or detection by fluorescent antibody techniques, including viral detection that uses monoclonal antibodies or by electron microscopy, to confirm diagnosis.

Management

1. Antiviral drugs, such as acyclovir, famciclovir, and valacyclovir, interfere with viral replication; may be used in all cases, but especially for treatment of immunosuppressed or debilitated patients. Must be started within 72 hours of onset.
2. Corticosteroids early in illness (controversial)—given for severe herpes zoster if symptomatic measures fail; given for anti-inflammatory effect and for relief of pain.
3. Pain management—aspirin, acetaminophen, NSAIDs, opioids—useful during the acute stage, but not generally effective for postherpetic neuralgia. If treated early (48 to 72 hours), may decrease risk of postherpetic neuralgia.
4. Postherpetic neuralgia may be treated with anticonvulsant agents, such as gabapentin or pregabalin, and 5% lidocaine patch.

Complications

1. Approximately 20% of patients will experience chronic pain syndrome (postherpetic neuralgia), characterized by constant aching and burning pain or by intermittent lancinating pain or hyperesthesia of affected skin after it has healed.
2. Ophthalmic complications with involvement of ophthalmic branch of trigeminal nerve with keratitis, uveitis, corneal ulceration, and possibly blindness.
3. Facial and auditory nerve involvement, resulting in hearing deficits, vertigo, and facial weakness (Ramsay Hunt syndrome).
4. Visceral dissemination—pneumonitis, esophagitis, enterocolitis, myocarditis, pancreatitis.

Nursing Diagnoses

- Acute Pain related to inflammation of cutaneous nerve endings.
- Impaired Skin Integrity related to rupture of vesicles.

Nursing Interventions

Controlling Pain

1. Assess patient's level of discomfort and medicate, as prescribed; monitor for adverse effects of pain medications.
2. Teach patient to apply wet dressings, such as aluminum acetate (Burow's) solution, for soothing effect.
3. Encourage distraction techniques such as music therapy.

4. Teach relaxation techniques, such as deep breathing, progressive muscle relaxation, and imagery, to help control pain.

Improving Skin Integrity

1. Apply wet dressings to cool and dry inflamed areas by means of evaporation.
2. Administer antiviral medication in dosage prescribed (usually high dose); warn the patient of adverse effects such as nausea.

Patient Education and Health Maintenance

1. Teach patient to use proper handwashing technique to avoid spreading herpes zoster virus.
2. Advise patient not to open the blisters to avoid secondary infection and scarring.
3. Reassure patient that shingles is a viral infection of the nerve endings; nervousness does not cause shingles.
4. A caregiver may be required to assist with dressings and meals. In older patients, the pain is more pronounced and incapacitating. Dysesthesia and skin hypersensitivity are distressing.

Evaluation: Expected Outcomes

- Verbalizes decreased pain.
- Reepithelialization of skin without scarring.

Pemphigus

Pemphigus is a serious autoimmune disease of the skin and of the mucous membranes, characterized by the appearance of flaccid blisters (bullae and vesicles) of various sizes on apparently normal skin and mucous membranes (mouth, esophagus, conjunctiva or vagina) (see Figure 33-3). Familial benign chronic pemphigus (Hailey-Hailey disease) is a familial type of pemphigus that appears in adults, particularly affecting the axillae and groin.

Pathophysiology and Etiology

1. The exact cause is unknown.
2. Certain drugs, other autoimmune diseases, and genetics may play a role in its development.
3. Many variants of pemphigus exist.

Clinical Manifestations

1. Initial lesions may appear in oral cavity; flaccid blisters (bullae) may arise on normal or erythematous skin.

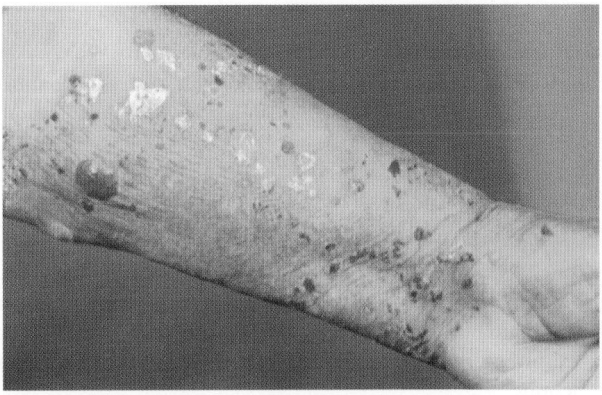

Figure 33-3. Pemphigus vulgaris blisters on the forearm.

a. The bullae enlarge and rupture, forming painful, raw, and denuded areas that eventually become crusted. These areas can become secondarily infected.

b. The eroded skin heals slowly; eventually, widespread areas of the body may become involved.

c. In the mouth, the blisters are usually multiple, of varying size and irregular shape, painful, and persistent. Oral lesions may appear initially, with lesions of the mucous membranes of the pharynx and esophagus; the conjunctivae, larynx, urethra, cervix, and rectum may become affected as well.

2. An offensive odor may emanate from the bullae due to infection.

3. Positive Nikolsky's sign—separation of epidermis when minimal pressure is applied to the skin; downward pressure on a bulla will cause it to expand laterally.

Diagnostic Evaluation

1. Skin biopsies of blisters and surrounding skin—demonstrate acantholysis (separation of epidermal cells from each other).

2. Immunofluorescence of skin cells shows antibodies that bind to the epidermis in a lacy pattern network (pemphigus antibodies).

Management

1. Corticosteroids in large doses to control the disease and keep skin free from blisters.

2. Immunosuppressive agents, such as cyclophosphamide and azathioprine, are used alone or in combination with steroids, for immunosuppressive and steroid-sparing effect.

3. Plasmapheresis—reinfusion of specially treated plasma cells; temporarily decreases serum level of antibodies.

4. Treatment of denuded skin.

Complications

1. Infections (skin, pneumonia, septicemia).

2. Adverse effects from acute and chronic corticosteroids: GI bleeding, secondary infection, psychosis, hyperglycemia, and others.

Nursing Assessment

1. Assess for odor or drainage from lesions, which may indicate infection.

2. Assess for fever and signs of systemic infection.

3. Assess for adverse effects of corticosteroids, such as abdominal pain, white patches in mouth that indicate *Candida* infection, and emotional changes.

Nursing Diagnoses

• Impaired Oral Mucous Membrane related to ruptured bullae.
• Impaired Skin Integrity related to ruptured bullae.
• Risk for Deficient Fluid Volume related to transudation of fluid into bullae.
• Disturbed Body Image related to widespread or chronic skin lesions.

Nursing Interventions

Restoring Oral Mucous Membrane Integrity

1. Inspect oral cavity daily; note and report any changes—oral lesions heal slowly.

2. Keep oral mucosa clean and allow regeneration of epithelium.

3. Give topical oral therapy, as directed.

4. Offer prescribed mouthwashes through a straw to rinse mouth of debris and to soothe ulcerative areas.

5. Teach patient to apply petrolatum to lips frequently.

6. Use cool-mist therapy to humidify environmental air.

Restoring Skin Integrity

1. Keep skin clean and eliminate debris and dead skin—the bullae will clear if epithelium at the base is clean and not infected.

2. Obtain swab of bullous fluid for cultures—most common organism is *S. aureus*.

3. Administer cool, wet dressings or baths or teach patient to administer to soothe and cleanse skin. Large areas of blistering have a characteristic odor that is lessened when secondary infection is under control.

   a. After the bath, dry and cover with talcum powder, as directed; this enables the patient to move more freely in bed. Large amounts are necessary to keep clothes and sheets from sticking.

4. The nursing management of patients with blistering or with bullous skin conditions is similar to that of the patient with a burn (see page 1191).

Restoring Fluid Balance

1. Evaluate for fluid and electrolyte imbalance—extensive denudation of the skin leads to fluid and electrolyte imbalance.

   a. Monitor serum albumin and protein levels.

   b. Monitor vital signs for hypotension or tachycardia.

   c. Weigh patient daily.

   d. Monitor intake and output.

2. Administer IV saline solutions, as directed.

3. Encourage the patient to maintain hydration; suggest cool, nonirritating fluids.

   a. Suggest soft, high-protein, high-calorie diet or liquid supplements that will not be irritating to oral mucosa but will replace lost protein.

Promoting Positive Body Image

1. Develop a trusting relationship with the patient.

2. Educate patient and family about the disease and its treatment; this reduces uncertainty and clears up misconceptions.

3. Encourage expression of anxieties, embarrassment, and discouragement.

4. Encourage patient to maintain social contacts and activities among support network.

Patient Education and Health Maintenance

Instruct the patient as follows:

1. The disease may be characterized by relapses that require continuing therapy to maintain control.

MANAGEMENT	NURSING CONSIDERATIONS
• On Wood's light examination, may fluoresce and will show hypopigmented patches. • Microscopic examination with KOH preparation of skin scraping shows characteristic "spaghetti and meatballs" appearance of hyphae and spores. • Treat with selenium sulfide shampoo (leave on for 40 minutes before showering) daily for 1 week. • Topical or systemic antifungal may be used as prescribed by health care provider.	• Common in high-temperature, high-humidity environments. • Advise patient that discoloration may persist after fungus has been eradicated; lost pigmentation will resolve with sun exposure. • Tell patient that recurrence is common after 2–12 weeks if prophylactic treatment is not given periodically.
• Identification of offending fungus by microscopic examination of shavings with KOH or by culture. • Treatment with appropriate systemic antifungal for prolonged period—usually at least 6 weeks for fingernails and at least 12 weeks for toenails. • Surgical removal of nail may be necessary.	• Encourage patient to comply with lengthy treatment, as fungal infections of the nail are difficult to treat. • Examine patient for other areas of tinea infection (feet, groin), encourage treatment, and teach patient that infection may be spread from fingernails by scratching. • After nail removal, advise patient to keep hand or foot elevated for several hours and change dressing daily by applying gauze and antibiotic ointment or other prescribed medication until nail bed is free of exudate or blood.

• Treatment for pediculosis corporis involves washing with soap and water and washing all infested clothing and linens with hot water. Alternatively, clothes may be dry-cleaned or ironed, paying close attention to the seams.
• Pediculosis capitis and pubis are treated with a topical antiparasitic preparation, such as lindane or permethrin.
• Manual removal of nits (eggs) may be performed; retreatment with topical antiparasitic in 3–7 days is recommended.
• Petroleum may be applied to eyelashes, then lice and nits removed with swab or tweezers, or pilocarpine drops can be used to paralyze the lice.
• Items that cannot be washed or dry-cleaned can be stored for 30 days without use.
	• Advise patient that pediculosis pubis is considered a sexually transmitted disease; partners must be examined and treated.
	• Teach patient the proper use of medication:
	  • Apply lotion or cream after bathing to affected hairy and adjacent areas; wash off after 8–12 hours.
	  • Alternatively, apply shampoo to affected hairy areas and lather for 4–5 minutes, rinse, and let hair dry.
	  • Use fine-tooth comb to remove nits.
	• Urge patient to wash all clothing, towels, linens, combs, and hair items by soaking in hot water for 10 minutes.
	• Advise patient not to use antiparasitic preparations more frequently than recommended.

• Parasite identified by microscopic examination of skin scraping.
• Treated with antiparasitic, such as permethrin or crotamiton, and oral treatment with Ivermectin 0.2mg/kg × 1 dose, if indicated.
• Machine wash and dry clothing and linens on hot cycle.
• Topical or systemic steroids may be needed to treat symptoms of allergic reaction to mites.
	• Teach proper use of medication:
	  • Apply thin layer from neck downward, with particular attention to hands, feet, and intertriginous areas; every inch of skin must be treated because mites are migratory. Apply to dry skin. (Wet skin allows more penetration and the possibility of toxicity.)
	  • Leave medication on for 8–12 hours—but no longer, as doing so will irritate the skin. Wash thoroughly.
	• Advise patient to avoid close contact for 24 hours after treatment to prevent transmission.
	• Encourage treatment of sexual and close contacts simultaneously.
	• Tell patient that itching may persist for days to weeks following treatment due to an allergic reaction to mites; retreatment is not necessary.

(continued)

Table 33-2   Other Dermatologic Disorders (continued)

NAME AND DESCRIPTION	CLINICAL MANIFESTATIONS

Viral Infections

Herpes Simplex

Acute vesicular eruption caused by herpes simplex virus type 1 or 2

- Prodromal pain, burning, or tingling, possible fever and malaise.
- Tiny vesicles appear on erythematous, swollen base; they rupture, forming painful ulcers and crusting; healing occurs but outbreaks are recurrent.
- Can occur anywhere, especially near mucocutaneous junctions.
- Viral shedding may occur between symptomatic periods, leading to transmission of the infection.

Other Conditions

Contact Dermatitis

Inflammatory condition caused by exposure to irritating or allergenic substances, such as plants, cosmetics, cleaning products, soaps and detergents, hair dyes, metals, and rubber

- Itching, burning, erythema, and vesiculation at point of contact.
- Progresses to weeping, crusting, drying, fissuring, and peeling.
- Lichenification (thickening of skin) and pigmentation changes may occur with chronicity.

Exfoliative Dermatitis

Chronic extensive scaling and inflammation of the skin; may be idiopathic or related to preexisting skin conditions, drug reactions, or underlying malignancy

- Starts as patchy erythema, with possible fever, chills, and malaise.
- Rapid spread until whole integument is involved.
- Skin color changes to scarlet, desquamates, and may ooze serous fluid.
- Pruritus, hair loss, and secondary infection.

Alopecia

Hair loss, may be idiopathic (alopecia areata), male-pattern, physiologic, or due to hair pulling (trichotillomania); also due to scarring from other skin or systemic disorders

- Patterned, patchy, or diffuse hair loss.
- Inflammation and scarring with some types.
- Physiologic alopecia may be associated with hormonal changes, such as childbirth, nutritional factors, or toxin exposure.

MANAGEMENT	NURSING CONSIDERATIONS
• Tzanck smear from scraping of ulcer or fluid from vesicle shows characteristic giant cells with intranuclear inclusions; also diagnosed by fluorescent antibody detection or viral culture. • Antiviral treatment with acyclovir, famciclovir, or valacyclovir for acute infection or continuous suppressive therapy to prevent or lessen recurrence. • Analgesics may be needed for widespread and genital eruptions.	• Teach patient that herpes simplex can be transmitted by close and sexual contact; good personal and hand hygiene are required for facial cases; sexual abstinence or condom use is required for genital cases. • Recurrence may be brought on by fever, illness, emotional stress, menses, pregnancy, sunlight, and other factors. • Advise patients with active herpes simplex infection to avoid contact with immunosuppressed individuals, such as those with diabetes, HIV disease, cancer (including those undergoing cancer treatment), alcoholism, and malnutrition, because herpes simplex infection can be severe in these individuals. • Tell patients that lesions usually resolve in 1–2 weeks without scarring.
• Topical or oral steroids, depending on severity. Oral steroids usually given in tapered dose—start with high dose and gradually decrease to provide greatest anti-inflammatory effect without adrenal suppression.	• Take thorough history to determine causative agent or contributing factors; have patient keep log of activities and symptoms if unsure of irritant.
• Removal or avoidance of causative agent. • Antipruritics—systemic or topical antihistamines or topical calamine preparations. • Desensitization to poison ivy and other substances may be accomplished for those who have severe reactions and cannot avoid contact.	• Teach patient to use allergen-free products, wear gloves and protective clothing, wash and rinse skin thoroughly, and wash clothing after contact with potential irritants. • Advise patient that rash—even oozing lesion of poison ivy—is not contagious; however, contaminated clothing may cause spread of poison ivy in those who are sensitive. • Advise patient to perform patch test by applying substance behind ear or on inside of wrist before trying new cosmetics, soaps, or hair products.
• Discontinuation of offending drug or treatment of underlying condition. • Systemic corticosteroids should control most cases. • Supportive treatment—bed rest, warm environment, and fluid and electrolyte replacement. • Soothing baths and topical emollients for symptomatic relief. • Possible use of immunosuppressants—azathioprine, methotrexate, and cyclophosphamide.	• Monitor fluid balance and electrolyte values. • Watch for signs of secondary infection and report; antimicrobial therapy may be necessary. • Watch for signs of heart failure caused by chronically increased cutaneous blood flow. • Teach patient how to relieve itching with oatmeal baths and emollient creams. • Tell patient to avoid environments with temperature fluctuations to avoid chilling. • Advise patient to avoid all irritants.
• Treatment of underlying causes. • Minoxidil may cause fine hair regrowth in male-pattern baldness and alopecia areata. Finasteride, an oral agent, can be used by men only, with good results. • Other methods of hair replacement—surgical grafting of hair follicles, hair weaving, or hairpieces.	• Explain that alopecia areata and physiologic hair loss are usually temporary and self-limiting. • Encourage female patient to change hairstyle or wear hairpieces or turbans until hair grows back after childbirth. • Counsel male patient on the slow, limited effects of minoxidil treatment and stress that effects reverse when treatment is stopped.

(continued)

Table 33-2   Other Dermatologic Disorders (continued)

NAME AND DESCRIPTION	CLINICAL MANIFESTATIONS
Other Conditions (continued)	
Seborrheic Dermatitis Chronic, superficial inflammatory skin disorder	• Crusted pinkish or yellow patches. • Loose scales that may be dry, moist, or greasy. • Mild itching. • Affects the scalp, eyebrows, eyelids, nasolabial creases, lips, ears, chest, axillae, umbilicus, and groin.
Hidradenitis Suppurativa Chronic follicular plugging and secondary infection of the apocrine glands of the groin and axilla	• Development of tender red nodules that enlarge, rupture, and suppurate. • Sinus tracts develop with recurrent lesions, leading to continuous inflammation and drainage.
Bullous Pemphigoid Chronic bullous disease of autoimmune etiology; occurs in older adults	• Tense vesicles and bullae arise on normal or erythematous skin, rupture, and heal without scarring. • Occurs on flexor aspects of the body, axilla, inguinal areas, abdomen, and, occasionally, on mucous membranes.
Acne Vulgaris Obstruction and inflammation of sebaceous glands and follicles	• Closed comedones (whiteheads). • Open comedones (blackheads). • Papules, pustules, nodules, cysts, or abscesses may develop. • Primary sites are face, chest, upper back, and shoulder.

MANAGEMENT	NURSING CONSIDERATIONS

- Apply selenium sulfide, tar, zinc, or resorcinol shampoo to scalp several times per week.
- Corticosteroid lotions or creams.
- For eyelid margin involvement (blepharitis), daily debridement with cotton-tipped applicator and baby shampoo and application of ophthalmic steroid ointment or lotion.
- Zinc soap or selenium lotion for washing once controlled.
- For external ear canal involvement, corticosteroid cream.

- Advise patient of chronic nature of seborrhea and that condition may be exacerbated by perspiration, neuroleptic drugs, and emotional stress; also seen more frequently in persons with Parkinson's disease, HIV disease, diabetes mellitus, malabsorption syndromes, and epilepsy.
- Teach patient to apply topical preparations, as prescribed.
- Advise using only baby shampoo and gently rubbing with swab near eyes to prevent irritation of conjunctiva in seborrheic blepharitis.

- Initially, prolonged (2 months or more) administration of an antibiotic, such as tetracycline, clindamycin, or erythromycin, as well as systemic or intralesional corticosteroids; however, progression of the condition is likely.
- Surgical treatment necessary when chronic suppuration and fistulas develop:
  - Incision and drainage or laser stripping.
  - Cauterization of sinus tracts.
  - Exteriorization with curettage and electrodesiccation.
  - Excision with possible skin grafting.
- Isotretinoin, anti-androgens, and intralesional or systematic steroid therapy may relieve exacerbations.

- Advise patient to use moisturizing soap and keep axilla and groin dry to reduce bacterial colonization of the skin.
- Teach patient the signs of bacterial infection—purulent drainage, odor, pain—that call for notification of health care provider and treatment with antibiotics.
- Encourage use of warm compresses to relieve inflammation.
  - Obesity and cigarette smoking contribute to the disease. Encourage weight loss and smoking cessation, if applicable.

- Systemic corticosteroid treatment in widespread involvement. Topical corticosteroids if limited lesions. Immunosuppressant for resistant cases.
- Condition may remit within 2–4 years even without treatment.

- Keep skin clean and dry to reduce chances of secondary infection.
- If patient is immobilized, encourage positioning to prevent undue pressure on lesions to avoid risk of premature rupture and secondary infection.
- Make sure to differentiate from early pressure sore development and treat pressure sores appropriately.
- Advise patient that lesions usually heal without scarring.

- Topical benzoyl peroxide—antibacterial and comedolytic.
- Topical retinoic acid, a comedolytic, or adapalene, a more potent synthetic retinoid.
- Topical antibiotics—suppress growth of *Propionibacterium acnes* and decrease comedones, papules, and pustules without systemic adverse effects.
- Azelaic acid, a topical agent with multiple anti-acne effects.
- Systemic antibiotics—long-term, low-dose therapy for more inflammatory and extensive causes.
- Retinoid therapy—inhibits sebum production and secretion; for severe, disfiguring cystic acne.
- Estrogen therapy—anti-androgenic effect decreases sebum production in women taking oral contraceptives. Spironolactone may be added, if needed, to increase anti-androgenic effect.
- Intralesional steroid injection—for inflamed lesions.
- Dermabrasion—surgical planing or chemical peels to smooth surface configuration of old scars. Should not be done within 6–12 months of Accutane use.

- Advise patient to wash face gently with mild soap and water one to two times per day.
- Teach proper application of topical preparation—use sparingly and decrease frequency if irritation and redness develop.
- Inform patient about adverse effects of systemic antibiotics.
- Ensure that women of childbearing potential are using contraceptives and that a negative pregnancy test has been obtained before starting isotretinoin therapy. Female patients must be on two forms of birth control. All patients must be enrolled in the Ipledge system.
- Encourage follow-up and monitoring of laboratory tests during treatment with isotretinoin for elevated liver enzymes, cholesterol, and triglycerides, and for decreased HDL.
- Advise patient taking isotretinoin to notify health care provider of persistent headache—could signal pseudotumor cerebri.
- Tell patient that initiation of therapy may worsen symptoms for several weeks, but to continue treatment.
- Advise patient not to squeeze pimples and avoid friction around face.
- Suggest use of water-based and hypoallergenic cosmetics.
- Encourage stress management, balanced diet, and avoidance of foods believed to aggravate acne.

(continued)

Table 33-2	Other Dermatologic Disorders *(continued)*

NAME AND DESCRIPTION	CLINICAL MANIFESTATIONS
Other Conditions *(continued)*	
Rosacea Erythematous, pustular eruption of the Malar cheeks, forehead, nose or around the eyes; most common in adults ages 40–60; unknown cause; may affect the eyes in 20%–50% of cases	• Diffuse redness, papules, and pustules develop over Malar cheeks, forehead, nose, or around the eyes. • Later, dilated blood vessels and flushing are seen. • Rhinophyma (hypertrophic, bulbous nose) may develop. More common in men, rare in women.

AIDS, acquired immunodeficiency syndrome; HDL, high-density lipoprotein; HIV, human immunodeficiency virus; I.M., intramuscular; INR, International Normalized Ratio; IV, intravenous; KOH, potassium hydroxide.

SELECTED REFERENCES

Gibson, L. E. (2011). What is a bleach bath? Can it treat chronic eczema symptoms? Mayo Clinic Health Information. Available: *www.mayoclinic.com/health/eczema-bleach-bath/AN02003*.

Gibbs, S., & Harvey, I. (2009). Topical treatments for cutaneous warts. The Cochrane Library (Article No. CD001781).

Gill, J. F., Yu, S. S., & Neuhaus, I. M. (2013). Tobacco smoking and dermatologic surgery. *Journal of the American Academy of Dermatology, 68*(1), 167–172.

Habif, T. P. (2010). *Clinical dermatology: A color guide to diagnosis and therapy* (5th ed.). St. Louis, MO: Mosby.

Hall, J. C. (2010). *Sauer's manual of skin diseases* (10th ed.). Philadelphia: Lippincott Williams & Wilkins.

International Programme on Chemical Safety. (1994). Environmental health criteria 160: Ultraviolet radiation. Geneva, Switzerland: World Health Organization. Available: *www.inchem.org/documents/ehc/ehc/ehc160.htm#SectionNumber:1.5*.

James, W. D., Berger, T. G., & Elston, D. M.. (2011). *Andrews' diseases of the skin clinical dermatology* (11th ed.). Philadelphia: Elsevier.

Johnson, S. R., & Taylor, M. A. (2012). Identification and management of malignant skin lesions among older adults. *Journal for Nurse Practitioners, 8*(8), 610–616.

Kwok, C. S., Holland, R., Gibbs, S., et al. (2011). Efficacy of topical treatments for cutaneous warts: A meta-analysis and pooled analysis of randomized controlled trials. *British Journal of Dermatology, 165*(2), 233–246.

New Zealand Dermatologic Society. (2012). Stevens Johnson Syndrome and Toxic Epidermal Necrolysis. DermNet NZ. Available: *http://www.dermnetnz.org/reactions/sjs-ten.html*.

Turnbull, R. (2012). Recognizing psoriasis in children. *Community Practitioner 85*(6), 39–40.

Van Lumig, P., Driessen, R., Kievit, W., et al. (2013). Results of three analytical approaches on long term efficacy of etanercept for psoriasis in daily practice. *Journal of the American Academy of Dermatolgy, 68*(1), 57–63.

Werth, V. P. (2013). The safe and appropriate use of systemic glucocorticoids in treating dermatologic disease. *Journal of the American Academy of Dermatology, 68*(1), 177–178.

Yeung, H., Wan, J., Van Voorhees, A. S., et al. (2013). Patient-reported reasons for the discontinuation of commonly used treatments for moderate to severe psoriasis. *Journal of the American Academy of Dermatology, 68*(1), 64–72.

MANAGEMENT	NURSING CONSIDERATIONS
• Topical metronidazole gel applied b.i.d. • Oral doxycycline. • Treatment necessary for 4–6 weeks and repeated if recurrence. May need long-term suppression with oral antibiotics. • Avoid exercise, stress, hot beverages, and spicy foods.	• Teach patient to avoid flushing by reducing stress, replacing strenuous exercise with low-intensity workouts, staying cool, and avoiding the sun. • Suggest contacting the National Rosacea Society (*www.rosacea.org*).

34
Burns

OVERVIEW AND ASSESSMENT

Burns are a form of traumatic injury caused by thermal, electrical, chemical, or radioactive agents.

Inhalation injury and associated pulmonary complications are a significant factor in mortality and morbidity from burn injury (50% to 60% of fire deaths are secondary to inhalation injury).

Etiology and Pathophysiology

 Evidence Base American Burn Association. (2011). *Resources: Burn incidence and treatment in the United States fact sheet.* Chicago: Author. Available: *www.ameriburn.org/resources_factsheet.php.*

Incidence

1. One million burn injuries are reported each year, resulting in 3,500 deaths as a result of fire and burns in the United States, with a survival rate of 96%. This is a significant decline from 2 million burn injuries in the early 1990s.
2. Seven hundred thousand patients visit the emergency department every year for a burn injury and 45,000 patients require admission and about one half of those patients are treated at a specialized burn center.
3. The average burn size is 14% total body surface area (TBSA).
4. Males (70%) are more commonly injured by burns than are females.
5. Flame injury (44%) is the leading cause of accidents for adults and scalding (33%) is the leading cause of accidents for children. Fires in the home, combined with smoke inhalation, account for most burn-related deaths.

Burn Injury

 Evidence Base Latenser, B. A. (2009). Critical care of the burn patient: The first 48 hours. *Critical Care Medicine, 37,* 2819–2826.
Ribbens, K. A., & DeVries, M. (2013). Burns. In B. B. Hammond & P. G. Zimmerman (Eds.), *Sheehy's manual of emergency care* (pp. 453–462). St. Louis, MO: Elsevier Mosby.

1. A burn injury usually results from energy transfer from a heat source to the body. The type of burn injury may be flame/flash, contact, scald (water, grease), chemical, electrical, inhalation, or any thermal source. Many factors alter the response of body tissues to these sources of heat.
   a. Local tissue conductivity—bone is most resistant to the heat source accumulation. Lesser resistance is seen in nerves, blood vessels, and muscle tissue.
   b. Adequacy of peripheral circulation.
   c. Skin thickness, insulating material of clothing, or dampness of the skin.
2. Physiologic reaction to a burn is a unique combination of distributive and hypovolemic shock. The release of mediators such as tumor necrosis factor-α produce a profound effect on the circulatory system. In burns greater than 20% TBSA, there is an intravascular depletion, low pulmonary artery occlusion pressures, elevated systemic vascular resistance, and depressed cardiac output.
   a. Systemic microcirculation loses its vessel wall integrity and proteins are lost into the interstitium.
   b. Protein loss causes intravascular colloid osmotic pressure to drop and allows fluid to leak from the vessels.
   c. There is an increase of fluid leaking into the interstitium, caused by decreased interstitial pressure and increased capillary permeability to protein.

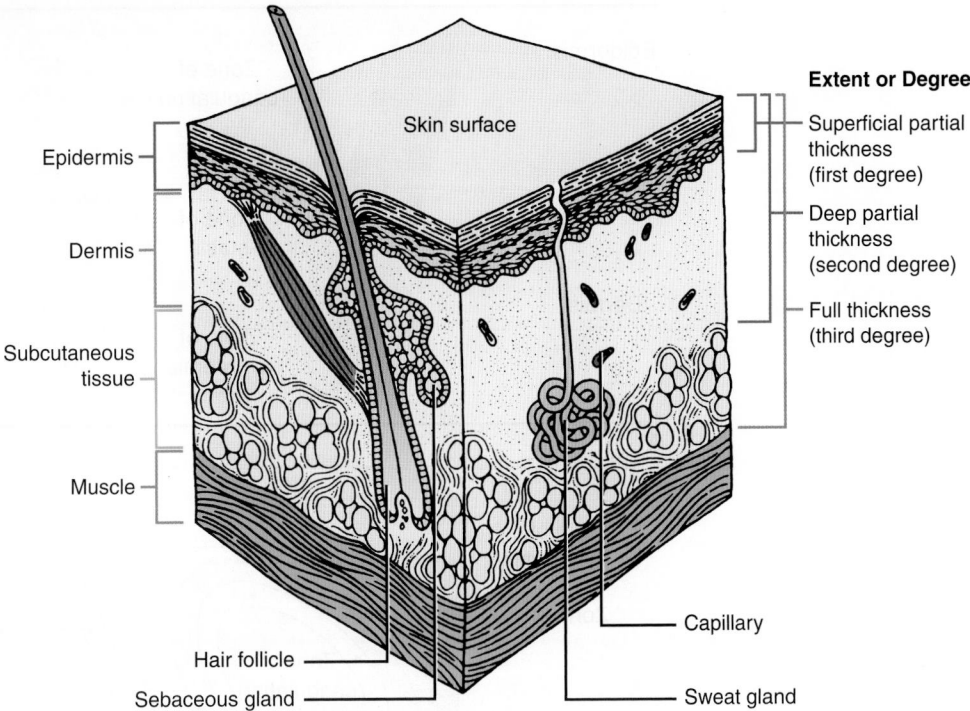

Figure 34-1. Cross-section of skin depicting blood supply, depth of burn, and relative thickness of skin grafts. (*The Burn Patient,* Ethicon.)

d. Over 24 hours, there is a loss of intravascular fluid, electrolytes, and proteins into the interstitium.

e. The resultant changes are reflected in massive edema formation, loss of circulating plasma volume, hemoconcentration, decreased urine output, and depressed cardiac function.

3. Burns may be partial (second-degree) or full (third-degree) thickness (see Figure 34-1).

   a. Superficial partial-thickness burns are commonly termed first-degree burns. Only the epidermis is involved. Local redness, blanching occurs similar to a sunburn. Healing time is 5 to 7 days.

   b. Deep partial-thickness burn injuries, commonly known as second-degree burns, involve the epidermis and upper portions of the dermis. Sweat glands, hair follicles, and nerves remain intact. The wound is moist and very painful. Some of the dermal appendages remain, from which the wound can spontaneously reepithelialize and heal on its own. A deep partial-thickness burn injury can convert to a full-thickness burn injury if patient is underresuscitated or develops an infection. Healing time is 5 to 35 days.

   c. Full-thickness injuries, commonly known as third-degree burns, involve all layers of the skin and sometimes underlying tissues are destroyed. The burn wound is dry, white, brown, or leathery in appearance. Patients typically do not have pain with full-thickness injuries due to the destruction of the nerve endings. At the core is the burn injury. There is then a zone of coagulation surrounded by a zone of stasis, surrounded by hyperemia (erythema) very similar to a bull's-eye pattern, the burn being in the center (see Figure 34-2). Grafting is usually required to close the wound.

4. Burn depth is directly related to the temperature of the burning agent and the duration of contact with body tissue.

   a. Below 112° F (44.4° C), no local damage occurs unless exposure is for a protracted period.

   b. At 120° F (48.9° C), it takes 5 minutes' exposure to create a full-thickness burn.

   c. At 125° F (51.7° C) the time requirement is 2 minutes, and at 140° F (60° C) only 6 seconds is required.

   d. At 159° F (70.6° C) it takes 1 second to create a full-thickness burn in a healthy adult—less time or temperature in children or older adults.

Inhalation Injury

 Evidence Base Colohan, S. M. (2010). Predicting prognosis in thermal burns with associated inhalational injury: A systematic review of prognostic factors in adult burn victims. *Journal of Burn Care and Research,* 31, 529–539.

Ribbens, K. A., & DeVries, M. (2013). Burns. In B. B. Hammond & P. G. Zimmerman (Eds.), *Sheehy's manual of emergency care* (pp. 453–462). St. Louis, MO: Elsevier Mosby.

1. The burn injury results in a release of mediators and an activation of neutrophils and a release of free radicals. In the lungs, free radicals are toxic and it is this injury pattern that is more significant than the thermal injury itself. Inhalation injuries combined with a large burn injury accounts for most mortality from a burn injury.

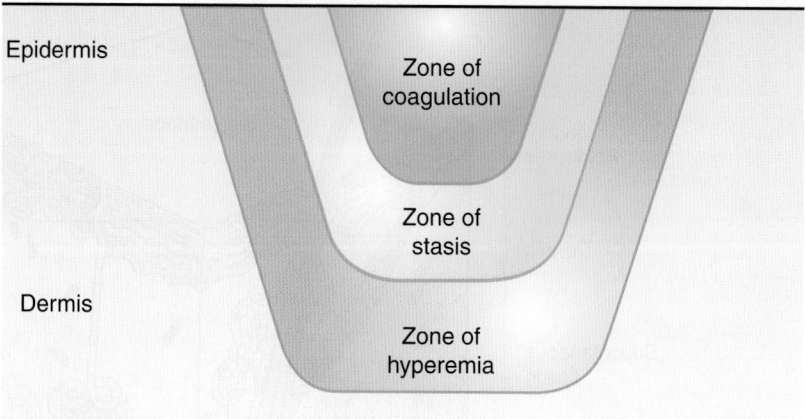

A

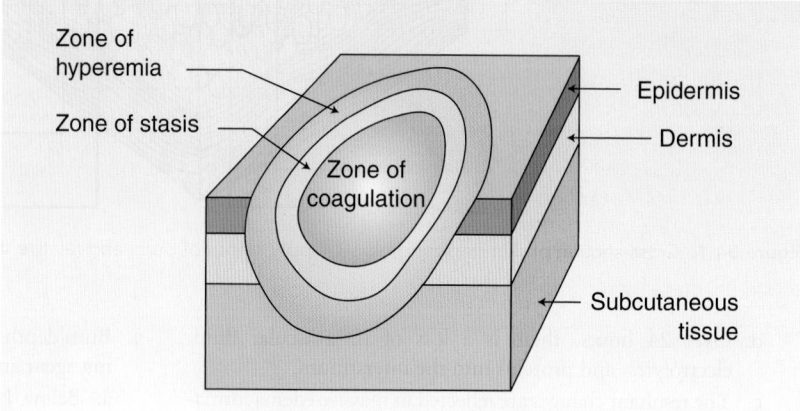

Figure 34-2. A. Shows cross-section, **B.** shows surface view and depth.

B

2. Most inhalation injuries that result in death are a result of carbon monoxide. It is a colorless, odorless, tasteless, nonirritating gas produced from incomplete combustion of carbon-containing materials.

3. Carbon monoxide's affinity for hemoglobin is 200 times greater than for oxygen.

4. Toxicity depends on concentration of carbon monoxide in inspired air and the length of time of exposure.

5. Although oxygen content of the blood is diminished, the amount of dissolved oxygen in the plasma (PaO_2) is unaffected by carbon monoxide poisoning; therefore, the arterial blood gas will appear normal.

6. Pulse oximetry only detects saturated hemoglobin and does not measure carbon monoxide; therefore, the pulse oximetry will appear normal.

7. A serum carboxyhemoglobin level must be measured in any patient with possible exposure to carbon monoxide in a fire.
   a. A carboxyhemoglobin level of less than 10% is not a cause for alarm. Normal carboxyhemoglobin in nonsmokers is less than 5% and smokers can have carboxyhemoglobin levels as high as 10%.
   b. From 10% to 20%, severe headache, flushing, and dilation of skin vessels occur.
   c. Levels of 30% to 50% can produce disorientation, nausea, irritability, dizziness, vomiting, prostration, tachypnea, and tachycardia.
   d. Levels above 50% result in coma, seizures, convulsions, and Cheyne-Stokes respirations, and death is possible.

8. Sulfur dioxide and nitrous oxide are toxic agents inhaled in soot. In the presence of water, they form corrosive acids and alkalis that are extremely toxic.

9. Toxic fumes from burning plastic are more dangerous than smoke.
   a. Noxious gases include hydrogen cyanide, hydrochloric acid, sulfuric acid, halogens, and perhaps phosgene.

10. Restrictive pulmonary complications can occur because of the tourniquet effect of edema seen with circumferential chest burns. Lung compliance and alveolar gas exchange can also be decreased because of acute respiratory distress syndrome (ARDS).

Systemic Changes in Major Burns

 Evidence Base (2010). In G. Doherty (Ed.), *Current diagnosis and treatment: Surgery.* New York: McGraw-Hill.

Major burns involving more than 25% TBSA.

Fluid Shifts

1. In addition to changes in the local burned area, there are alterations and disruptions in the vascular and other systems of the body.
2. The water-vapor barrier for the body is the outermost layer of the epidermis. When it is rendered nonfunctioning, severe systemic reactions from fluid losses can occur.
3. Fluid volume deficit is directly proportional to the extent and depth of burn injury.
4. Capillary permeability increases, permitting fluid and protein to move from vascular to interstitial spaces (edema results) for the first 24 to 36 hours, peaking at 12 hours postburn. Protein-rich fluid is lost in blebs of the burned tissues as well as by weeping of second-degree wounds and surface of full-thickness wounds. With reduced vascular volume, the patient will go into shock if untreated.
5. Capillary permeability starts to change in about 48 hours, but protein lost in interstitial spaces may remain there for 5 days to 2 weeks before returning to the vascular system.
   a. When fluid mobilizes (moves from interstitial spaces back to vascular compartment), patients with good cardiac and renal function will diurese.
   b. Patients with impaired cardiac or renal function are in danger of fluid overload and pulmonary edema at this time.
6. Red blood cell (RBC) mass is also diminished because of thrombosis, sludging, and RBC death from thermal injury; as fluid escapes from capillary walls, however, blood concentrates and the hematocrit rises, causing sluggish flow (see Figure 34-3).
7. Capillary stasis may cause ischemia and even necrosis.
8. The body attempts to compensate for losses of plasma volume.
   a. Constriction of vessels.
   b. Withdrawal of fluid from undamaged extracellular space.
   c. Patient thirst.

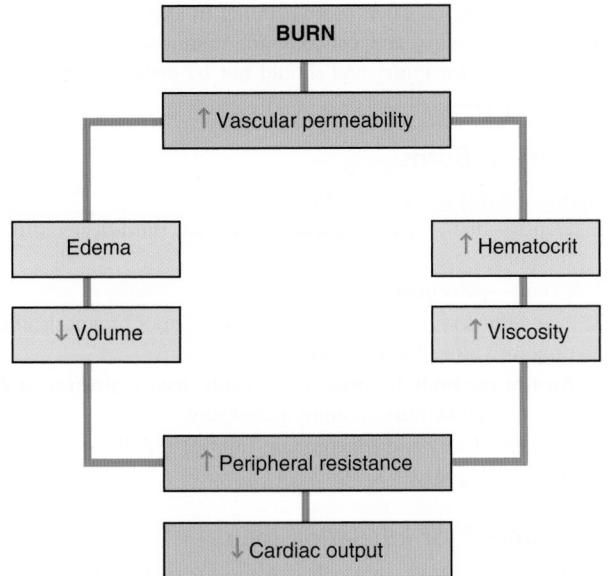

Figure 34-3. Hemodynamic changes in burn injury.

Hemodynamic Changes

1. Decreased circulating blood and plasma volume results in decreased cardiac output initially and increased pulse rate as a result of hypovolemia.
2. Afterload is increased due to a marked increase in systemic vascular resistance resulting from vasoactive mediators such as catecholamines.
3. A decrease in cardiac contractility is a predominant feature of full-thickness injuries covering more than 40% TBSA.
4. This results in inadequate tissue perfusion, which may in turn cause metabolic acidosis, renal failure, and irreversible burn shock.
5. Electrolyte imbalance may also occur.
   a. Hyponatremia usually occurs during the 3rd to 10th day due to fluid shift.
   b. The burn injury also causes hyperkalemia initially due to cell destruction, followed by hypokalemia as fluid shifts occur if potassium is not replaced.

Metabolic Demands

1. The initial metabolic response is thought to be activated by proinflammatory cytokines. The release of catecholamines, cortisol, glucagon, renin-angiotensive, antidiuretic hormone, and aldosterone is also increased. The major fuel source is stored glycogen. Major hypermetabolism and catabolism occur immediately postburn. The degree of the response is directly proportionate to the size of the burn injury.
2. Tachycardia, ranging from 100 to 120 beats per minute, is common and results from persistent elevation of catecholamine levels.
3. "Burn fever" (usually seen during the first week) is common and is dependent on depth of burn and percentage of TBSA involved. An increase of 1° F to 2° F makes it difficult to assess for infection.
4. Total body glucose stores are limited and stored liver and muscle glycogen is exhausted within the first few days postburn, hepatic glucose synthesis (gluconeogenesis) increases and patients with glucose intolerance (obese patients and older adults) usually develop hyperglycemia.
5. Increased catabolism leads to increased urea production, especially in nutritionally depleted patients.
6. Body levels of protein begin to decrease as high levels of cortisol, inflammatory cytokines continue to circulate. Skeletal and visceral protein are mobilized to meet increased nutritional demands. Ten to 15% of body protein stores can be lost within 10 days without proper nutritional supplementation. This can lead to muscular weakness, decreased wound healing, and further weakening of the immune system.
7. With adequate fluid resuscitations, the patient's weight will increase during the first few days. Fluid mobilization will result in weight loss, as will the catabolic response. Nutritional support in the form of enteral or total parenteral nutrition may be necessary. Weight loss from fluid mobilization usually starts within 3 to 4 days postresuscitation.
8. Despite all nutritional support, it is almost impossible to counteract a negative nitrogen balance; the sooner a burn wound is closed, the more rapidly a positive nitrogen balance is reached.

9. The resting metabolic expenditure increases linearly with amount of TBSA; a burn of 40% to 50% TBSA has a metabolic rate almost twice normal.
10. The adult burn patient may require 3,000 to 5,000 calories or more per day.
    a. A burn of less than 10% usually requires minimal supplementation.
    b. A high-protein, high-calorie diet is necessary for a 10% to 20% burn.
    c. Between 20% and 30%, enteral feedings are generally necessary.
    d. TBSA burns of 30% to 40% may require total parenteral nutrition. However, the current trend is to meet nutritional needs enterally, if possible.

Renal Needs

1. Glomerular filtration may be decreased in extensive injury.
2. Without resuscitation or with delay, decreased renal blood flow may lead to high output or oliguric renal failure and decreased creatinine clearance.
3. Hemoglobin and myoglobin, present in the urine of patients with deep muscle damage commonly associated with electrical injury, may cause acute tubular necrosis and call for a greater amount of initial fluid therapy and osmotic diuresis.

Pulmonary Changes

1. Hyperventilation and increased oxygen consumption are associated with major burns.
2. The majority of deaths from fire are due to smoke inhalation.
3. Overzealous fluid resuscitation and the effects of burn shock on cell membrane potential may cause pulmonary edema, contributing to decreased alveolar exchange. Therefore, with an inhalation injury, it may be necessary to keep the patient slightly less hydrated.
4. Initial respiratory alkalosis resulting from hyperventilation may change to respiratory acidosis associated with pulmonary insufficiency as a result of major burn trauma.

Hematologic Changes

1. Thrombocytopenia, abnormal platelet function, depressed fibrinogen levels, inhibition of fibrinolysis, and a deficit in several plasma clotting factors occur postburn.
2. Anemia results from the direct effect of destruction of RBCs due to burn injury, reduced life span of surviving RBCs, overt or (more commonly) occult blood loss from duodenal or gastric ulcers, and blood loss during diagnostic and therapeutic procedures.

Immunologic Activity

1. The loss of the skin barrier and presence of eschar favor bacterial growth. Methicillin-resistant *Staphylococcus aureus* (MRSA) is now being seen in the immunocompromised burn patient.
2. Polymorphonuclear chemotactic activity is suppressed, which results in decreased oxygen consumption and impaired bactericidal activity.
3. Abnormal inflammatory response after burn injury causes a decreased delivery of antibiotics, white blood cells, and oxygen to the injured area.

4. Hypoxia, acidosis, and thrombosis of vessels in the wound area impair host resistance to pathogenic bacteria.
5. Serum IgA, IgM, and IgG are depressed, reflecting depressed B cell function.
6. Depressed cellular immunity is reflected by lymphocytopenia, delayed skin sensitivity, decreased allograft rejection potential, depletion of thymus-dependent lymphoid tissue, and increased susceptibility to fungi, viruses, and Gram-negative organisms.
7. Burn wound sepsis.
   a. After colonization of the burn wound surface by bacteria, subeschar, and intrafollicular colonization develop. Intraeschar and subeschar colonization may progress to invasion of subadjacent, nonburned, previously viable tissue.
   b. A bacterial count of 10^5 per gram of tissue as determined by burn wound biopsy (quantitative culture) indicates burn wound sepsis. Usually, only a swab culture is done of the wound surface.
   c. The wound is fully colonized in 3 to 5 days.
8. Seeding of bacteria from the wound may give rise to systemic septicemia.

GI Impact

1. As a result of sympathetic nervous system response to trauma, peristalsis decreases and gastric distention, nausea, vomiting, and paralytic ileus may occur.
2. Ischemia of the gastric mucosa and other etiologic factors put the burn patient at risk for duodenal and gastric ulcers, manifested by occult bleeding and, in some cases, life-threatening hemorrhage.

Immediate Assessment

Immediate assessment of the burned patient is imperative, particulary burn size and depth, as fluid resuscitation is hallmark for initial management. As with all trauma patients, it is important to not forget the primary and secondary trauma survey, including assessment of airway, breathing, and circulation. While a major burn injury is often overwhelming in any clinical setting, mechanism of injury and concomitant traumatic injuries often accompany a burn injury and should not be missed in the early assessment phase.

Severity of Burns

Severity of burns is determined by:
1. Depth—first-, second- (partial-thickness), third-degree (full-thickness).
2. Extent—percentage of TBSA.
3. Age—the very young and very old have a poor prognosis; the prognosis alters for adults after age 45.
4. Area of the body burned—face, hands, feet, perineum, and circumferential burns require special care.
5. Medical history and concomitant injuries and illness.
6. Inhalation injury.

Assessment for Inhalation Injury

1. If victim was burned in a closed area, there should be a high index of suspicion that smoke inhalation has occurred.

Table 34-1	Signs and Symptoms of Toxicity from Carbon Monoxide
CO BLOOD LEVEL	**MANIFESTATIONS**
0%–10%	• None • Smokers may have 10% carbon monoxide level or greater
10%–20%	• Headache, vision disturbance, angina in patients with cardiovascular disease, and slowed mental function
20%–40%	• Tight feeling in head, rapid fatigue from muscular effort, decreased muscular coordination, confusion, irritability, ataxia, nausea, vomiting, increased pulse rate, decreased blood pressure, and dysrhythmias
40%–60%	• Pulmonary and cardiac dysfunction, collapse, coma, and convulsions
>60%	• Commonly fatal

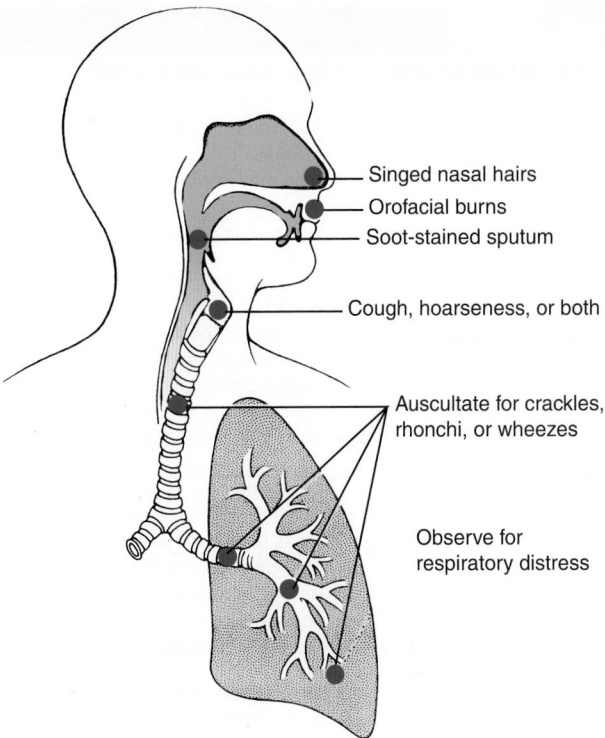

Figure 34-4. Respiratory system signs of inhalation injury.

2. Evaluate all patients in closed-space fires for symptoms of carbon monoxide poisoning—headache, visual changes, confusion, irritability, decreased judgment, nausea, ataxia, and collapse (see Table 34-1).

3. Question the patient about types of things that burned in the room—carpet, vinyl articles, and synthetics. With the increasing use of synthetics, toxicity from aldehydes, cyanide, and other substances must be considered.

4. Observe for upper-body burn erythema or blistering of lips, buccal mucosa, or pharynx; singed nasal hair; soot in oropharynx; dark gray or black sputum (see Figure 34-4).

5. Listen for hoarseness and crackles. Increasing hoarseness, stridor, and drooling are indicators of increasing need for intubation.

6. Obtain arterial blood gases (ABGs), carboxyhemoglobin levels, and spirometry.

7. Direct visualization of the vocal cords may be necessary. Further visualization may be accomplished through bronchoscopy, if necessary.

8. A chest x-ray should be obtained as a baseline.

Extent of Body Surface Burned

1. Anatomic location—burns affecting hands, feet, face, and perineum require specialized care. Circumferential burns also require special attention, possibly escharotomy.

2. Determination is based on the use of tables for this purpose, such as the "rule of nines" (see Figure 34-5), the Lund and Browder chart (see page 1772), or the rule of the palm. The patient's palm (including the fingers) is approximately 1% of the TBSA burned. The Lund and Browder chart is the most accurate. Calculation of the percentage of TBSA burned serves as a guide for fluid therapy. Full fluid resuscitation is necessary for partial- or full-thickness burns of 20% TBSA or greater.

3. Repeat assessment may be performed on the second or third day to verify demarcation of burned areas.

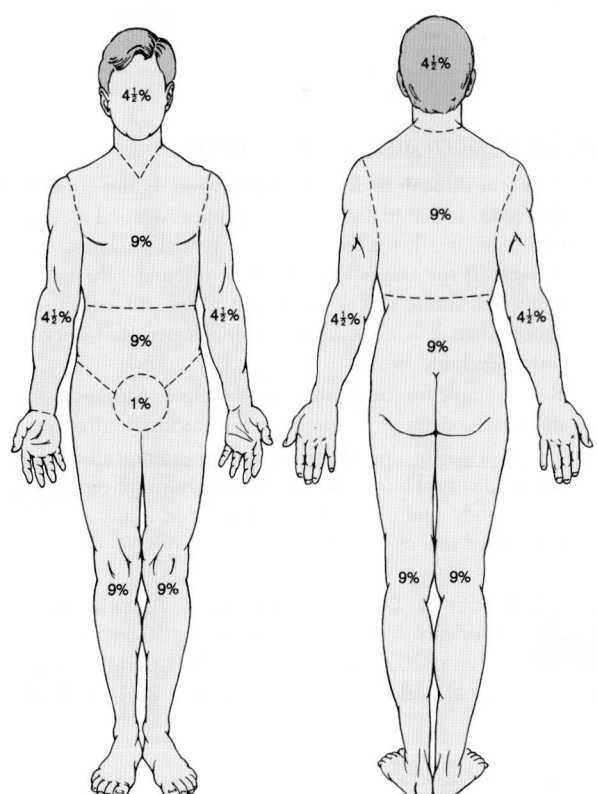

Figure 34-5. Rule of nines for calculating total burn surface area (TBSA).

Table 34-2	Assessment of Burn Injury	
EXTENT OR DEGREE	**ASSESSMENT OF EXTENT**	**REPARATIVE PROCESS**
Superficial (First degree)	• Pink to red; slight edema, which subsides quickly. • Pain may last up to 48 hours; relieved by cooling. • Sunburn is a typical example.	• In about 5 days, epidermis peels, heals spontaneously. • Itching and pink skin persist for about 1 week. • No scarring. • If burn does not become infected, heals spontaneously within 10–14 days.
Partial Thickness (Second degree)	*Superficial:* • Pink or red; blisters (vesicles) form; weeping, edematous, and elastic. • Superficial layers of skin are destroyed; wound moist and painful. • Hair does not pull out easily.	• Takes several weeks to heal. • Scarring may occur.
	Deep dermal: • Mottled white and red; edematous reddened areas blanch on pressure. • May be yellowish but soft and elastic—may or may not be sensitive to touch; sensitive to cold air. • Hair pulls out easily.	• Takes several weeks to heal. • Scarring may occur.
Full Thickness (Third degree)	• Destruction of epithelial cells—epidermis and dermis destroyed. • Reddened areas do not blanch with pressure. • Not painful; inelastic; coloration varies from waxy white to brown; leathery devitalized tissue is called eschar. • Destruction of epithelium, fat, muscles, and bone.	• Eschar must be removed. Granulation tissue forms to nearest epithelium from wound margins or support graft. • For areas larger than 1¼–2 inches (3–5 cm), grafting is required. • Expect scarring and loss of skin function. • Area requires debridement, formation of granulation tissue, and grafting.

Depth of Burn and Triage Criteria

1. It may be difficult to differentiate between second- and third-degree wounds initially. If the areas appear wet and are particularly sensate, then a second-degree (partial-thickness) injury is likely. If the area is less painful or insensate, the hairs are easily pulled out, and the area appears dry and is firm to the touch, then it is most likely a third degree (full-thickness) burn (see Table 34-2).

2. Reassess daily for the first few days because a partial-thickness burn can convert or progress to a full-thickness burn injury.

3. Deep partial-thickness burns of certain extent, full-thickness burns, chemical burns, electrical burns, burns of certain areas of the body, and any airway or inhalation injury should be transferred to a regional burn center (see Box 34-1).

 Evidence Base American Burn Association and American College of Surgeons Committee on Trauma. (2007). Guidelines for the operation of burn centers. *Journal of Burn Care and Research, 28*(1), 133–141.

MANAGEMENT

Management of the acute burn injury includes hemodynamic stabilization, metabolic support, wound debridement, use of topical antibacterial therapy, biologic dressings, and wound closure. Prevention and treatment of complications, including infection and pulmonary damage, and rehabilitation are also of major importance. The patient will also require physical and occupational therapy and psychiatric and nutritional support.

BOX 34-1	Burn Center Referral Criteria

- Partial-thickness burns of greater than 10% TBSA
- Involvement of face, hands, feet, genitalia
- Third-degree burns
- Electrical burns
- Chemical burns
- Inhalation injury
- Preexisting medical conditions that could complicate management
- Concomitant trauma where burn injury poses greatest risk
- Burned children where facilities lack qualified staff and equipment
- Patients who require special social, emotional, or rehabilitative intervention

Hemodynamic Stabilization

IV Fluid Therapy

 Evidence Base Zaletel, C. (2009). Factors affecting fluid resuscitation in the burn patient: The collaborative role of the APN. *Advanced Emergency Nursing Journal, 31,* 309–320.

The goal of fluid resuscitation is to maintain tissue perfusion and minimize complications associated with central line catheters. Overzealous fluid resuscitation has been associated with acute coronary syndrome, compartment syndrome of the extremities, ARDS, airway obstruction, and pulmonary edema. Underresuscitation may lead to inadequate organ and cellular perfusion, stress ulcer development, acute tubular necrosis, and conversion of deep partial-thickness burns to full-thickness burns.

1. The American Burn Association recommends fluid resuscitation for partial-thickness and full-thickness burns exceeding 15% TBSA.
   a. Immediate intravenous (IV) fluid resuscitation is indicated for patients with electrical injury, older patients, or those with cardiac or pulmonary disease.
   b. These patients require meticulous monitoring and may require a modification of fluid requirements.
2. Establish two large-bore peripheral IV catheters for fluid resuscitation and pain management, preferably through non-burned skin. If unable to obtain peripheral IV access, intraosseous or central line catheters may be used.
3. The goal is to give sufficient fluid to allow perfusion of vital organs without overhydrating the patient and risking later complications and circulatory overload.
4. Generally, a crystalloid (Ringer's lactate) solution is used initially. Colloid is used during the second day (5% albumin, plasma proteins, or hetastarch).
5. One of several formulas may be used to determine the amount of fluid to be given in the first 48 hours.
   a. Any formula that is utilized is only a guide. Some patients will require more or less fluid depending on their response.
   b. The Consensus formula (formerly known as the Parkland formula) is most commonly used.
6. The Consensus formula:
   a. First 24 hours: 2 to 4 mL of Ringer's lactate × weight in kg × % TBSA burned.
   b. One-half amount of fluid is given in the first 8 hours, calculated from the time of injury. If the starting of fluids is delayed, then the same amount of fluid is given over the remaining time. Remember to deduct any fluids given in the prehospital setting.
   c. The remaining half of the fluid is given over the next 16 hours. Example:
      Patient's weight: 70 kg; % TBSA burn: 80%
      4 mL × 70 kg × 80% TBSA = 22,400 mL of Ringer's lactate
      First 8 hours: 11,200 mL or 1,400 mL/hour
      Second 16 hours: 11,200 mL or 700 mL/hour
   d. Second 24 hours: 0.5 mL colloid × weight in kg × TBSA + 2,000 mL dextrose 5% in water (D_5W) run concurrently over the 24-hour period. Example:
      0.5 mL × 70 kg × 80% = 2,800 mL colloid + 2,000 mL D_5W yields 117 mL colloid/hour and 84 mL D_5W per hour

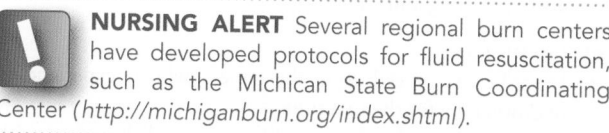 **NURSING ALERT** Several regional burn centers have developed protocols for fluid resuscitation, such as the Michican State Burn Coordinating Center (http://michiganburn.org/index.shtml).

Wound Care

Treatment of the partial-thickness burn wounds includes daily or twice-daily wound cleansing with debridement or hydrotherapy (tubbing/showering) and dressing changes. Treatment of deep partial-thickness and full-thickness burns require early surgical excision of eschar and skin grafting.

Cleansing and Debridement

1. Burn wounds must be cleansed initially and usually daily with a mild antibacterial cleansing agent and saline solution or water.
   a. May be done in the hydrotherapy tub, in the bathtub or shower, or at the bedside.
   b. See "Hydrotherapy," below.
2. Nonviable tissue (eschar) may be removed through natural, enzymatic, mechanical, and/or surgical debridement.
3. Burn eschar will begin to separate from the underlying viable tissue by a natural process of bacterial growth, which causes a lysis of protein at the viable–nonviable tissue interface.
4. Eschar can be removed through daily or twice-daily dressing changes and use of forceps and scissors at time of wound cleansing.
5. Enzymatic agents applied to the burn wound may be used for more rapid debridement of eschar.

Hydrotherapy

Hydrotherapy ("tubbing," "tanking," or "showering") is bathing of the burn patient in a tub of water or with a water shower to facilitate cleansing and debridement of the burned area. Even ventilator-dependent patients can be safely bathed when a shower table is used.

Advantages

1. Topical medications, adherent dressings, and eschar are more easily removed.
2. Provides an opportunity for the patient to practice range-of-motion (ROM) exercises.
3. Total assessment of the burn area is facilitated; total body cleansing can be achieved.

Disadvantages

1. Loss of body heat; loss of sodium.
2. Uncomfortable and at times painful for the patient.

Nursing Alert Adequately premedicating the patient with an opioid and anxiolytic allows the patient to participate and tolerate the bathing and dressing change process.

3. Maintenance of IV lines and ventilator care may be difficult during bathing and showering.

Interventions

1. Describe the procedure to the patient who is experiencing hydrotherapy for the first time.
2. Select the time for future tubbings in collaboration with the patient; administer a pain-control medication, as prescribed, before the treatment so that maximum benefit is realized. Use nursing activities to assist patient with the pain experience.
3. If the patient has an indwelling catheter, drain and plug it or maintain a closed system to avoid contamination.
4. Sterile technique is adhered to as closely as possible in preparing the patient for hydrotherapy, during hydrotherapy, and in redressing the patient's wounds after therapy.
5. During hydrotherapy, after cleansing of the wounds, debride wound, shave adjacent areas at health care provider's direction, shampoo hair, and gently wash normal skin.
6. Limit hydrotherapy to as brief a time as possible to decrease the loss of body temperature and subsequent chilling.
7. Never leave the patient unattended in the tub.
8. Respect the patient's feelings and expressions of stress, pain, cold, and fatigue.
9. After treatment, the patient may be weighed before being carefully dressed and returned to the unit.
10. Document significant data, including status of the wound.

Topical Antimicrobials

1. Topical medications are used to cover burn areas and to reduce the number of organisms. See Table 34-3. Identifying the most effective topical antimicrobial and dressing medium is an essential aspect in promoting wound closure.
2. Factors such as location of burn, burn depth, ease of application and removal, pain, frequency of dressing changes, and cost need to be considered.
3. They are applied directly to the burn area as ointments, creams, or solutions, or they may be incorporated in single-layer dressings that do not stick to the wound but permit drainage.
4. Dressings may take the form of commercial multilayered pads, standard 4 × 4 gauze pads, or several layers of stretch bandage (Kerlix type).
5. If gauze or pads are used, they may be held in place by stretch gauze or net tube dressings.
6. When wet dressings are used, that is, after a surgical procedure, then the same dressings are maintained. They are remoistened every 4 to 6 hours, as ordered. Heat loss may be prevented by limiting evaporative loss with a dry blanket and by warming the bed or using a heat cradle.

7. When wet dressings are used, 20-ply gauze will help retain solution at the proper concentration if rewet every 4 hours. A dry top layer of stockinette or a cotton bath blanket prevents evaporative heat loss.
8. Desired characteristics in a topical antimicrobial:
   a. Demonstrates action against a broad spectrum of bacteria.
   b. Has the ability to diffuse through the wound and penetrate the eschar.
   c. Nontoxic and noninjurious to body tissue.
   d. Inexpensive, pleasant to use, odorless or has pleasant odor, will not stain skin or clothing.
   e. Will not cause resistant strains of pathogenic organisms to develop.
9. Generally, all of the previously applied topical cream should be removed and the wound gently cleansed before applying new cream with each dressing change. Extremity dressings should be wrapped distally to proximally, taking care to avoid circulatory compromise when edema occurs or dressing is too tight.
10. Identifying the best evidence on dressings for superficial and partial-thickness burn injuries has produced limited results. A Cochrane Database systematic review of 26 randomized controlled trials showed some evidence that biosynthetic dressings decrease healing time and pain associated with dressing changes over silver sulphadiazene. However, methodological shortcomings of the individual studies limits usefulness of the review.

 Evidence Base Storm-Versloot, M. N., Vos, C. G., Ubbink, D. T., et al. (2010). Topical silver for preventing wound infection. *Cochrane Database of Systematic Reviews*, Issue 3 (Article No. CD006478).
Wasiak, J., Cleland, H., Campbell, F., et al. (2008). Dressings for superficial and partial thickness burns. *Cochrane Database of Systematic Reviews*, Issue 4 (Article No. CD0002106).

Surgical Management

Early excision and skin grafting is the goal to early wound closure for deep partial-thickness and full-thickness burn injuries. For types of burn wound coverings, see Table 34-4, pages 1188 to 1189.

General Considerations

1. Early surgical intervention reduces the potential for wound infection and potentially reduces the length of stay.
2. Operative excision is very stressful metabolically and incurs heavy blood loss; therefore, more conservative measures may be indicated for some patients.
3. As a general consideration, up to 190 mL of blood may be lost per 1% of burn excised in the adult patient.
4. With tangential excision, a special blade is used to slice off thin layers of damaged skin until live tissue is evidenced by capillary bleeding. Commonly used with deep partial-thickness burns and full-thickness burns and followed with immediate coverage with a biosynthetic or biologic dressing or an autograft.

Table 34-3	Topical Antimicrobial Agents for Burns		
TOPICAL AGENT	**DESCRIPTION AND INDICATIONS**	**DISADVANTAGES**	**NURSING CONSIDERATIONS**
Silver Sulfadiazine 1%	• White, crystalline, highly insoluble compound in an opaque, odorless, water-miscible cream • Exerts antimicrobial effect against Gram-negative and Gram-positive bacteria and yeasts at level of cell membrane and cell wall • Penetration of silver sulfadiazine into wound is intermediate between silver nitrate and mafenide • Systemic toxicity is rare • Most widely used agent and least common incidence of adverse effects	• May cause transient leukopenia that disappears after 2–3 days of treatment • May increase possibility of kernicterus; should not be used in pregnant women in last trimester, premature neonates, or infants younger than age 2 months • Impairment of hepatic and renal function that results in decreased excretion of drug constituents may preclude therapeutic benefits of continued silver sulfadiazine administration • Exposure to sunlight produces gray discoloration • Crystalluria and methemoglobinemia are rare toxic effects • Protracted use may be associated with emergence of sulfadiazine resistance	• Use with open treatment, or with light or occlusive dressings • Apply with sterile gloved hand directly to wound or to gauze dressing 1/16 inch (0.2 cm) thick, once or twice per day after thorough wound cleansing • Silver sulfadiazine will be discontinued if white blood cell (WBC) count is <1,500 in an adult or <2,000 in a child; WBC count usually returns to normal in 2–4 days, after which application may be resumed
Mafenide Acetate 10% cream or 5% solution	• Usually supplied in water-miscible, hydroscopic cream base • Active against most Gram-positive organisms, particularly *Clostridia* spp. • Active against common Gram-negative burn wound pathogens but has little antifungal activity • Not significantly bound by protein and wound exudate • Good penetrating power and useful for control of established invasive burn wound infection	• Painful during and for a short period following application • A potent carbonic anhydrase inhibitor resulting in metabolic acidosis, therefore not used if total body surface area is >20% • Brisk alkaline diuresis and inappropriate polyuria may result when used on patients with a large burn surface area • Compensatory hyperventilation and pulmonary failure may ensue if mafenide is not discontinued • Hemolytic anemia is a rare complication	• Cream is applied without dressing, if possible. Must be reapplied every 12 hours to maintain therapeutic effectiveness • Therapeutic solution concentration is maintained with bulky wet dressings; rewet every 2–4 hours • Application is associated with significant pain • Hypersensitivity evidenced by maculopapular rash; is treated with antihistamines or by discontinuing use • Requires careful monitoring of pulmonary status and acid-base and fluid balance
Silver Nitrate (0.5% solution)	• Clear solution with low toxicity and significant antimicrobial effect against common burn wound pathogens • Absorption is minimal due to the insolubility of its chloride and other salts • Nonallergenic and not usually painful on application • Best use is prophylaxis against infection	• Can cause electrolyte abnormalities by depleting serum sodium, chloride, potassium, and magnesium • Methemoglobinemia is a rare complication • Stains everything (including normal skin) brown or black	• Monitor electrolyte balance carefully; supplementation with sodium and potassium salts is routinely needed for patients with extensive burns • Use bulky dressings; rewet every 2–4 hours to maintain therapeutic concentration • Maintain patient warmth and minimize transcutaneous evaporative water loss with dry top layer, such as stockinette or bath blanket
Silver Sheeting	• Silver impregnated on a neutral backing	• Cannot be moistened until time of application • Moisten with sterile water only; saline deactivates the silver • Need to keep moist with sterile water every 8 hours	• Dressing change required only every 4–7 days, reducing pain • Can be used on an outpatient basis
Mupirocin	• Ointment • Active against methicillin-resistant *Staphylococcus aureus* (MRSA)	• Allergy is major contraindication • Prolonged use may result in superinfection • Apply b.i.d. to t.i.d.	• May be ordered based on culture or prophylactically

Table 34-4   Burn Wound Coverings

COVERING AND DESCRIPTION	INDICATIONS	SOURCE OR FORM	NURSING CONSIDERATIONS
Allograft/Homograft • Human cadaver skin, about 0.015-inch thick • Preferred biologic dressing	• To debride untidy wounds • To protect granulation tissue after escharotomy • To cover excised wound immediately • To serve as test graft before autograft	Fresh, cryopreserved homografts available from tissue banks throughout the United States	• Remember: Length of time dressing is left in place varies greatly. • Observe for exudate; also, watch for local and systemic signs of infection and rejection.
Xenograft Heterograft • Pigskin similar to human skin, harvested after slaughter, then cryopreserved or lyophilized for long-term storage	• Same as for homograft • To cover meshed autografts • To protect exposed tendons • To cover partial-thickness burns that are eschar-free and clean or only slightly contaminated	Available in fresh, frozen, or lyophilized form, in rolls or sheets; also available meshed and impregnated with silver sulfadiazine	• Change every 2–5 days; wound may be dressed or left open. • Observe for signs of infection.
Biobrane • Nylon fabric bonded to silicon rubber membrane, containing collagenous porcine peptides • Elastic and durable; adheres to wound surface until removed or sloughed by spontaneous reepithelialization	• To cover donor graft sites • To protect clean, superficial, partial-thickness burns and excised wounds awaiting autografts • To cover meshed autografts	Individually packaged sterile sheets of various sizes; also in glove-shaped form for hand burns	• Useful for wounds awaiting autograft because it can be left in place 3–14 days and is permeable to antimicrobials, which can be applied over it.
Duo-Derm • Hydroactive dressing that interacts with moisture on skin, creating bond that makes it adhere • Interacts with wound exudate to produce soft, moist gel, facilitating removal	• To cover small partial-thickness burns • To prevent bacterial contamination	Individual, peelable, "blister" packages containing sheets of various sizes (from 3 × 3 inches to 8 × 12 inches)	• Use size that allows dressing to extend beyond wound onto healthy skin. • Be careful to distinguish pus from liquefied material that normally remains in wound. • Used until it falls off, usually 7–10 days.
Op-Site • Thin, transparent elastic film that adheres to dry surfaces, conforms to body contours, and stretches with movement • Occlusive and waterproof; permeable to moisture, vapor, and air	• To cover clean partial-thickness burns and clean donor sites and to reduce pain from these wounds • To provide moist environment for reepithelialization	Individual, sterile, peelable packages of sheets in various sizes	• Maintain closed dressing; if exudate forms, drain aseptically with needle and syringe; seal hole with Op-Site patch. • Check for pooling of exudate in dependent areas. • Use until it falls off, usually 7–10 days.
Vigilon • Colloidal suspension on a polyethylene mesh support • Permeable to gases and water vapor; provides moist environment • Compatible with topical preparations	• To clean small partial-thickness burns	Individual sterile or nonsterile sheets in various sizes	• For occlusive use, remove one polyethylene film backing and place uncovered side on wound; for nonocclusive use, remove both backings and secure over wound with gauze or tape. Change daily.

Table 34-4 Burn Wound Coverings *(continued)*

COVERING AND DESCRIPTION	INDICATIONS	SOURCE OR FORM	NURSING CONSIDERATIONS
Integra Artificial Skin • Permanent bilayer membrane composed of a dermal portion consisting of a porous lattice of fibers of cross-linked bovine collagen and glycosaminoglycan composite and an epidermal layer of synthetic polysiloxane polymer	• To create a template for dermal regeneration by formation of a "neodermis." Provides an immediate postexcisional physiologic wound closure. Allows use of a thinner autograft.	Sterile individual sheets	• Dermal regeneration layer is very soft and fragile. No hydrotherapy immersion should occur while the silicone layer is still in place. • Change outer dressing every 4–5 days. • Removal of the silicon layer is usually done in 14–21 days.
Acticoat • Temporary covering of a nanocrystalline film of pure ionic silver	• To provide a temporary layer with optimal antimicrobial protection. May be used for immediate wound coverage as well as for postgraft site coverage. May also be used as donor site coverage.	Sterile individual sheets	• Must be moistened immediately before application. It must also be moistened with sterile water every 4–6 hours. Do not apply any topical antimicrobial over or onto the silver sheeting.
Aquacel AG	• To provide wound coverage for superficial to mid-depth partial-thickness wounds. It dries and remains on the wound until healed, at which time it will loosen and can be peeled from the wound.	Individual sterile rolls	• Do not try to wet or remove before the wound has healed.

5. With fascial (primary) excision, the skin, lymphatics, and subcutaneous tissue are removed down to fascia, with either immediate autografting or temporary coverage with biologic or biosynthetic dressings. This is repeated until all deep burn areas are removed.

Biologic Dressings

1. Biologic dressings are used to cover large surfaces of the body. Usually, they are split-thickness grafts harvested either from human cadavers or from other mammalian donors such as pigs.
2. An allograft is a graft of skin taken from a person other than the burn patient and applied to a burn wound temporarily. A cadaver is the most common source. Other sources may be live donors having a panniculectomy or other surgery.
3. A xenograft or heterograft is a segment of skin taken from an animal such as a pig. It is useful in preparing a debrided area for grafting and is really a biologic dressing.

Donor Criteria

1. Skin color is unimportant because it is only a temporary graft.
2. Donor should be an adult, free from infection. All donated skin must be tested and free from contagious diseases before it can be used for donation.

Purpose and Benefits

1. Decreases heat, fluid, and protein losses.
2. Reduces bacterial proliferation.
3. Closes wound temporarily; enhances production and protection of granulation tissue.
4. Protects exposed neurovascular and muscle tissue as well as tendons.
5. Reduces pain and facilitates patient comfort.
6. Acts as a test graft to determine when granulating wounds will accept autograft successfully.
7. Provides an effective donor-site dressing.

Clinical Procedures

1. Allograft (cadaver) skin is the most popular temporary biologic dressing.
2. Devitalized tissue is first removed surgically or enzymatically.
3. Allograft is applied directly (shiny side down) to the denuded area. Before applying, it may be dipped in saline solution. It may be trimmed to fit the wound.
4. Grafts are usually secured with adhesive strips or with staples or sutures. The graft is covered with wet non-adherent gauze (antibiotic solution or saline) and covered with stretch gauze; this is again wet down with the appropriate solution.

5. The wound remains unchanged initially for 3 to 5 days, during which time it is wet down every 4 to 6 hours. Sheet grafts do not require the wet-down procedure.

6. After the initial takedown (typically known as the first postoperative dressing removal), dressings are changed daily.

7. If allograft or xenograft is used, the wound bed may be prepared for permanent autografting.

Biosynthetic Dressings

1. Temporary biosynthetic dressings help prevent bacterial contamination.

2. Used when permanent autograft is unavailable or unnecessary (as when partial-thickness wounds will heal spontaneously over time).

3. Biobrane (Woodruff Laboratories) consists of a custom-knit nylon fabric mechanically bonded to an ultra-thin silicone rubber membrane, to which collagenous peptides of porcine skin are covalently bonded.

   a. Has a longer shelf life and lower cost than biologic dressings such as pigskin.

   b. Is widely used for coverage of shallow wounds awaiting epithelialization, excised wounds awaiting autografts, widely meshed autografts until closure of interstices, and donor sites awaiting healing.

Artificial Dermis

1. Method being studied in selected burn centers to improve survival of patients with massive burns and little donor skin available.

2. Composed of a porous collagen-chondroitin 6-sulfate fibrillar mat covered with a thin Silastic sheet.

3. Used with an epidermal graft to provide a permanent cover that is at least as satisfactory as other available grafting techniques.

4. Used with donor sites that are thinner and that heal faster; seems to result in less hypertrophic scarring than the usual grafting methods.

Wound Closure

1. Skin grafting is usually required or preferred with full-thickness burns greater than 1¼ to 2 inches (3 to 5 cm) in diameter or in deep partial-thickness wounds or in areas of function.

2. After gradual eschar removal and development of a base of granulating tissue or in the presence of viable tissue after excision, grafts of the patient's own skin (autografts) are applied.

3. Sheet grafts or meshed grafts, providing wider expansion from donor sites, may be used.

4. Blood flow is established by the 3rd or 4th day, and postgrafting, vascular continuity, and wound closure have been established by the 7th to 10th day.

5. Cultured epithelial autografts (cultured skin) may be used for patients with large burns and little available donor skin.

   a. Biopsies of unburned skin are cultured in a specialized laboratory to yield confluent sheets of epithelial cells suitable for grafting in about 3 weeks.

   b. Available donor sites can be used for coverage of the most functional or posterior surfaces, and the more delicate cultured epithelial autografts can be used to cover other large areas.

   c. Additional experience is needed to determine the long-term durability of cultured epithelial autografts, which may be life-saving treatment for the severely burned.

6. Many partial-thickness burn wounds will heal spontaneously within a few weeks, provided they are protected from infection.

7. The donor site requires meticulous care and may be covered with a synthetic dressing, Scarlet Red, silver sheeting, or an antimicrobial cream such as silver sulfadiazine 1%.

Other Interventions

Pain Management

1. Pain relief should be considered in the primary assessment of all initial burn injuries. A burn injury is one of the most feared painful injuries; all burn injuries are painful.

2. All pain medication should be given via IV line. Pain medication that is given intramuscularly may not be metabolized properly through burned tissue. Acceptable IV pain medications are morphine, hydromorphone, and fentanyl.

3. Careful administration of opioids for pediatrics, older adults, and patients with higher pain tolerances to avoid respiratory suppression or overdose.

Nutrition Support

1. Initially, institute nothing-by-mouth (NPO) status until bowel sounds return (1 to 2 days). However, small amounts (5 to 10 mL/hour) of isotonic enteral tube feedings are typically started within 24 hours to help maintain a functioning GI tract. Small amounts of erythromycin may be used to encourage GI motility.

2. Reduce metabolic stress by allaying pain, fear, and anxiety and maintaining a warm environment.

3. Nutritional management must be aggressive to combat acute nutritional deficiency and weight loss; a positive nitrogen balance should be the goal throughout postburn care.

4. When bowel sounds return, administer oral fluids and advance diet, as tolerated.

5. Offer more solid food after 2 to 3 days postburn as tolerance to food improves.

   a. Build up daily caloric intake to match daily caloric expenditure.

   b. Provide 3 gm protein/kg body weight: 20% of needed calories in the form of fats; remainder in carbohydrates.

6. Oral anabolic steroids (oxandrolone) have shown good results in helping to maintain lean muscle mass.

7. When caloric requirements cannot be met by enteral feedings, it may be necessary to initiate total parenteral nutrition (TPN) (amino acids, carbohydrates, and fat emulsions).

8. Provide potassium and vitamin and mineral supplements (zinc, iron, vitamin C).

Prevention and Treatment of Complications

Primary causes of morbidity and mortality in burn patients are those related to infection and pulmonary problems.

1. Topical antibacterial agents help to retard the proliferation of pathogenic organisms until wound closure occurs spontaneously or through surgical intervention.
2. Broad-spectrum antibiotics may be necessary to treat systemic Gram-positive and Gram-negative infections and sometimes fungal infection.
3. Critical diagnostic parameters include observing for signs of burn-wound sepsis, obtaining quantitative and qualitative wound biopsy, checking for signs of systemic septicemia, and taking blood for cultures.
4. Meticulous pulmonary care is essential because pneumonia (especially if patient remains intubated) is common.
5. Severe inhalation injury, including ARDS, can contribute significantly to mortality, even though the burn wound size may be small.

Nursing Management of the Burn Patient

Nursing Assessment

1. Obtain a thorough history, including:
   a. Causative agent—hot water, chemical, gasoline, flame, tar, radiation PUVA light, etc.
   b. Duration of exposure.
   c. Circumstances of injury, including whether in closed or open space, accidental or intentional, or self-inflicted.
   d. Initial treatment, including first aid, prefacility emergency care (including fluids, intubation, etc.), or care rendered in another facility (emergency department, etc.).
   e. Patient's age and preexisting medical problems, such as heart disease, human immunodeficiency virus, drug abuse, diabetes, ulcers, alcoholism, chronic obstructive pulmonary disease (COPD), epilepsy, psychosis, or hepatitis..
   f. Current medications—include both prescription and over the counter.
   g. Concomitant injuries (eg, from fall, explosions, assaults).
   h. Evidence of inhalation injury.
   i. Medication and food allergies, tetanus immunization status.
   j. Height and weight.
2. Perform ongoing assessment of hemodynamic and respiratory status, condition of wounds, and signs of infection.

Nursing Diagnoses

- Impaired Gas Exchange related to inhalation injury.
- Ineffective Breathing Pattern related to circumferential chest burn, upper airway obstruction, or ARDS.
- Decreased Cardiac Output related to fluid shifts and hypovolemic shock.
- Ineffective Tissue Perfusion: Peripheral related to edema and circumferential burns.
- Risk for Imbalanced Fluid Volume related to fluid resuscitation and subsequent mobilization 3 to 5 days postburn.
- Impaired Skin Integrity related to burn injury and surgical interventions (donor sites).
- Impaired Urinary Elimination related to indwelling catheter.
- Ineffective Thermoregulation related to loss of skin microcirculatory regulation and hypothalamic response.
- Risk for Infection related to loss of skin barrier and altered immune response.
- Impaired Physical Mobility related to edema, pain, skin and joint contractures.
- Imbalanced Nutrition: Less Than Body Requirements related to hypermetabolic response to burn injury.
- Risk for Bleeding related to stress response.
- Acute Pain related to burn injury.
- Ineffective Coping related to fear and anxiety.
- Disturbed Body Image related to cosmetic and functional sequelae of burn wound.
- Disturbed Sleep Pattern related to unfamiliar surroundings and pain.

Nursing Interventions

Achieving Adequate Oxygenation and Respiratory Function

1. Provide humidified 100% oxygen until carbon monoxide level is known. (*Caution:* Adjust oxygen flow rate for patient with COPD, as prescribed.) If the patient is stable, try to get the initial ABG on room air.
2. Assess for signs of hypoxemia (anxiousness, tachypnea, tachycardia) and differentiate this from pain.
3. Suspect respiratory injury if burn occurred in an enclosed space.
4. Observe for and report erythema or blistering of buccal mucosa; singed nasal hairs; burns of lips, face, or neck; increasing hoarseness.
5. Monitor respiratory rate, depth, rhythm, and cough.
6. Auscultate chest and note breath sounds.
7. Note character and amount of respiratory secretions; report carbonaceous sputum.
8. Observe for signs of inadequate ventilation and begin serial monitoring of ABG levels and oxygen saturation.
9. Provide mechanical ventilation, continuous positive airway pressure, or positive end-expiratory pressure, if requested.
10. Keep intubation equipment nearby and be alert for signs of respiratory obstruction.
11. In mild inhalation injury:
    a. Provide humidification of inspired air.
    b. Encourage coughing and deep breathing.
    c. Promote clearance of secretions through chest physical therapy (see page 234).
12. In moderate to severe inhalation injury:
    a. Initiate more frequent bronchial suctioning.
    b. Closely monitor vital signs, urine output, and ABG levels.
    c. Administer bronchodilator treatments, as ordered.
    d. For additional respiratory problems, it may be necessary to have patient intubated and placed on mechanical ventilation.

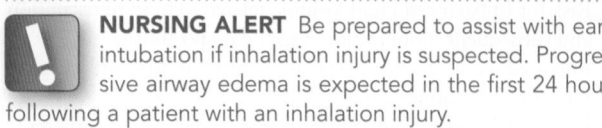 **NURSING ALERT** Be prepared to assist with early intubation if inhalation injury is suspected. Progressive airway edema is expected in the first 24 hours following a patient with an inhalation injury.

Maintaining Adequate Tidal Volume and Unrestricted Chest Movement
1. Observe rate and quality of breathing; report if progressively more rapid and shallow.
2. Assess tidal volume; report decreasing volume to health care provider.
3. Encourage deep breathing and incentive spirometry (may use sigh control on ventilator, as needed).
4. Place patient in semi-Fowler's position to permit maximal chest excursions if there are no contraindications, such as hypotension or trauma.
5. Make sure that chest dressings are not constricting.
6. Prepare the patient for escharotomy and assist, as indicated.

Supporting Cardiac Output
1. Position the patient to increase venous return.
2. Give fluids, as prescribed.
3. Monitor vital signs, including apical pulse, respirations, central venous pressure, pulmonary artery pressures, and urine output at least hourly.
4. Determine cardiac output, as requested.
5. Monitor sensorium.
6. Document all observations and particularly note trends in vital sign changes.

Promoting Peripheral Circulation
1. Remove all jewelry and clothing.
2. Elevate extremities.
3. Monitor peripheral pulses hourly; use Doppler, as necessary.
4. Prepare the patient for escharotomy if circulation is impaired.
5. Avoid tight, constrictive dressings.

Facilitating Fluid Balance
1. Titrate fluid intake, as tolerated. The initial resuscitation formula is only a base.

 GERONTOLOGIC ALERT Older patients and those with impaired renal function, cardiovascular disease, and pulmonary disease are more likely to develop fluid overload. Proceed with caution.

2. Maintain accurate intake and output records.
3. Weigh the patient daily.
4. Monitor results of serum potassium and other electrolytes.
5. Be alert to signs of fluid overload and heart failure, especially during initial fluid resuscitation and immediately afterward, when fluid mobilization is occurring.
6. Administer diuretics, as ordered.

Protecting and Reestablishing Skin Integrity
1. Cleanse wounds and change dressings twice daily. Use an antimicrobial solution or mild soap and water. Dry gently. This may be done in the hydrotherapy tank, bathtub, shower, or bedside.
2. Perform debridement of dead tissue at this time. May use gauze, scissors, or forceps as appropriate. Try to limit time to 20 to 30 minutes depending on the patient's tolerance. Additional analgesia may be necessary.
3. Apply topical bacteriostatic agents, as directed. Cream or ointment is applied 1/8-inch (3-mm) thick.
4. Dress wounds, as appropriate, using conventional burn pads, gauze rolls, or any combination. Dressings may be held in place, as necessary, with gauze rolls or netting.
5. For grafted areas, use extreme caution in removing dressings; observe for and report serous or sanguineous blebs or purulent drainage. Redress grafted areas according to facility protocol.
6. Observe all wounds daily and document wound status on the patient's record.
7. Promote healing of donor sites by:
   a. Preventing contamination of donor sites that are clean wounds.
   b. Opening to air for drying postoperatively if gauze or impregnated gauze dressing is used. If exudate occurs after the first 24 hours, swab the area for culture and apply an antimicrobial topical cream. If the culture is positive, treatment will be in accord with sensitivities.
   c. Following health care provider's or manufacturer's instructions for care of sites dressed with synthetic materials.
   d. Allowing dressing to peel off spontaneously.
   e. Cleansing healing donor site with mild soap and water when dressings are removed; lubricating site twice daily and as needed.

Preventing Urinary Infection
1. Maintain closed urinary drainage system and ensure patency. Use a catheter impregnated with an antimicrobial agent whenever possible.
2. Frequently observe color, clarity, and amount of urine.
3. Empty drainage bag per facility protocol.
4. Provide catheter care per facility protocol.
5. Encourage removal of catheter and use of urinal, bedpan, or commode as soon as frequent urine output determinations are not required.

Promoting Stable Body Temperature
1. Be efficient in care; do not expose wounds unnecessarily.
2. Maintain warm ambient temperatures.
3. Use radiant warmers, warming blankets, or adjustment of the bed temperature to keep the patient warm.
4. Obtain urine, sputum, and blood cultures for temperatures above 102° F (38.9° C) rectal or core temperature or if chills are present.
5. Provide a dry top layer for wet dressings to reduce evaporative heat loss.
6. Warm wound cleansing and dressing solutions to body temperature.
7. Use blankets in transporting patient to other areas of the hospital.
8. Administer antipyretics, as prescribed.

Avoiding Wound and Systemic Infection

1. Wash hands with antibacterial cleansing agent before and after all patient contact.
2. Use barrier garments—isolation gown or plastic apron—for all care requiring contact with the patient or the patient's bed.
3. Cover hair and wear mask when wounds are exposed or when performing a sterile procedure.
4. Use sterile examination gloves for all dressing changes and all care involving patient contact.
5. Maintain proper concentration of topical antibacterial agents used in wound care.
6. Be alert for reservoirs of infection and sources of cross-contamination in equipment, assignment of personnel.
7. Check history of tetanus immunization and provide passive or active tetanus prophylaxis as prescribed.
8. Change IV tubing and central line catheters according to Centers for Disease Control and Prevention recommendations.
9. Administer antibiotics, as prescribed, and be alert for toxic effects and incompatibilities.
10. Assess wounds daily for local signs of infection—swelling and redness around wound edges, purulent drainage, discoloration, loss of grafts.

DRUG ALERT Although pseudomonas has been and continues to be a danger to the burn patient, hospital-acquired MRSA is now another serious threat. Staple antibiotics, such as vancomycin and gentamycin, are not effective. Now, linezolid, clindamycin, sulfamethoxazole-trimethoprim, and even mupirocin ointment are being used to combat MSRA—not only in the hospital setting, but in most burn clinics as well.

11. Be alert for early signs of septicemia, including changes in mentation, tachypnea, and decreased peristalsis as well as later signs, such as increased pulse, decreased blood pressure (BP), increased or decreased urine output, facial flushing, increased and later decreased temperatures, increasing hyperglycemia, and malaise. Report to health care provider promptly.
12. Promote optimal personal hygiene for the patient, including daily cleansing of unburned areas, meticulous care of teeth and mouth, shampooing of hair every other day, shaving of hair in or near burned areas, and meticulous care of IV and urinary catheter sites.
13. Inspect skin carefully for signs of pressure and breakdown.
14. Observe for and report signs of thrombophlebitis or catheter-induced infections.
15. Prevent atelectasis and pneumonia through chest physical therapy, postural drainage, meticulous pulmonary technique, and, if indicated, tracheostomy care.

Promoting Mobility and Ability to Perform Activities of Daily Living (ADLs)

1. Ensure consultation with physical and occupational therapists, who will exercise the patient at least once or twice daily, as necessary.
2. Encourage the patient to be as active as possible and to perform active ROM exercises throughout the day.
3. Maintain splints in proper position as prescribed by occupational therapist; remove splints on regular schedule and observe for signs of skin irritation before reapplying.
4. Position the patient to decrease edema and avoid flexion of burned joints.
5. Coordinate pain management and other care to allow optimal effort during periods of physical exercise.
6. Initiate passive and active ROM and breathing exercises during early postburn period.
7. Plan with therapists for a conditioning regimen that gradually increases energy expenditure and tolerance for activity.
8. Act as advocate for the patient's need for rest by coordinating the patient's therapeutic and social activities and prioritizing interventions and visits.
9. Help the patient achieve adequate relaxation and sleep through medication and environmental measures.

Ensuring Adequate Nutrition

1. Weigh the patient daily with dressings removed.
2. Obtain consultation from dietitian for calculation of nutritional needs based on age, weight, height, and burn size. Two of the more popular formulas used to estimate nutritional needs are the Harrison-Benedict and Curari formulas.
3. Administer vitamins and mineral supplements, as prescribed. Deficiencies in zinc, copper, and selenium can occur after a burn.
4. Minimize metabolic stress by allaying fears, pain, and anxiety and by maintaining a warm environmental temperature.
5. Generally, for burns less than 10% TBSA, a well-balanced diet with emphasis on protein intake is necessary. For 10% to 20% TBSA, a high-protein, high-calorie diet is ordered. From 20% to 30% TBSA, supplementary enteral nutrition is necessary. Between 30% and 40% TBSA, TPN may be implemented.
6. When the patient is ready for oral fluids, observe tolerance. If there are no problems, advance the diet, as tolerated.
7. Provide nasogastric (NG) tube feedings, as prescribed, using caution to prevent aspiration by checking tube placement before each feeding and checking amount of gastric aspirate.
8. Administer IV hyperalimentation and fat emulsions prescribed with usual nursing precautions.
9. Keep record of caloric intake.
10. Encourage the patient to feed self.
11. Supplement meals with between-meal high-protein, high-calorie snacks, such as milkshakes or foods brought from home according to patient's preference.

Preventing Paralytic Ileus and Stress Ulcer

1. Keep on NPO status until bowel sounds resume.
2. Assess bowel sounds every 2 to 4 hours while acutely ill. (Decreased peristalsis may be an early sign of septicemia.)
3. Decompress stomach with NG tube on low intermittent suction until bowel sounds resume.
4. Recent practice now encourages small amounts of tube feedings, 5 to 10 mL/hour, immediately following the initial injury to help preserve the function of the gut and prevent paralytic ileus or stress ulcer.
5. Check amount and pH of gastric drainage or aspirate and report change.

6. Administer histamine-2 blockers and antacids, as prescribed. This will help prevent or diminish the occurrence of stress (Curling's) ulcers.

7. Heed complaints of nausea while intubated by checking for abdominal distention, tube placement, residual aspirate.

8. Provide mouth care every 4 hours while intubated.

9. Parenteral administration of vitamin A has been shown to reduce the incidence of gastric and duodenal ulcers.

Evidence Base Gaby, A. (2010). Nutritional treatment for burns. *Integrative Medicine, 9*(3), 46–51.

Reducing Pain

1. Assess for pain periodically; do not wait for complaints of pain to intervene. Common opioids used include morphine, fentanyl, hydromorphone, and propofol administered via IV line or by patient-controlled analgesia. Oral agents such as oxycodone, hydrocodone, and long-acting continuous-release agents are appropriate once the patient is tolerating P.O. food and fluids.

2. Determine previous experience with pain, the patient's response, and coping mechanisms.

3. Offer analgesics before wound care or before particularly painful treatments. Analgesia given orally should be administered 30 to 45 minutes before the procedure. Ketamine IV. is now more commonly used than before. It is also becoming more popular to use conscious sedation for dressing changes.

NURSING ALERT Check with your state board of nursing and facility policy to determine requirements for administering conscious sedation. Requirements may dictate that an anesthesiologist be in attendance or that the nurse be trained in intubation and airway management.

4. Change the patient's position when possible, supporting extremities with pillows.

5. Reduce anxiety by such approaches as sensory-oriented explanations of procedures.

6. Teach relaxation techniques, such as imagery, breathing exercises, and progressive muscle relaxation, to help the patient cope with pain.

7. Allow the patient to make choices regarding care whenever possible, thus allowing some measure of input and control in care.

8. Greater emphasis is now focusing on pain management both from an inpatient and an outpatient perspective. Mid-range analgesics are often used rather than just morphine. Medication dosages are being increased if patient is on a ventilator. It is not always possible to make a conscious patient completely pain-free, but increased comfort is the goal.

Enhancing Coping

1. Assess the patient's coping mechanisms from past history and current behavior.

2. Provide opportunities for the patient to express thoughts, feelings, fears, and anxieties regarding injury.

3. Explore with the patient alternative mechanisms for coping with the burn injury and its consequences.

4. Assure the patient of the normality of responses and the effect that time and healing will likely have on current concerns.

5. Interpret patient behavior to concerned family members and significant others.

6. Respect current coping mechanisms and discourage them only when an appropriate alternative can be provided.

7. Support family and friends' communications and visits if this is noted to help the patient.

8. Assess need for mental health consultation.

9. Offer anti-anxiety medications, as prescribed.

Preserving Positive Body Image

1. Gather data on the patient's preburn self-image and lifestyle.

2. When ready, encourage the patient to express concerns regarding changes in self-image or lifestyle that may result from burn injury.

3. Be honest, but positive, in responding to the patient and family.

4. Positively reinforce appropriate, effective coping mechanisms.

5. Arrange for the patient to see face (if burned) with appropriate supportive personnel before being placed/transferred to a room with access to a mirror.

6. Arrange for the patient to talk with other patients who have had a similar injury and are progressing satisfactorily.

7. Encourage participation in a burn survivor's group such as the Phoenix Society or other local support group.

8. Use and emphasize the concept of being a burn survivor. Survivors continue onward. Avoid the use of the term "burn victim" because it enhances the sick role.

9. Refer to psychological services, as needed. Consider other areas of the patient's traumatic experience that may require intervention as well.

Promoting Sleep

1. Assess patient's pain level at hour of sleep and administer pain medications, as needed.

2. Ensure comfort with room temperature and splints.

3. Administer sleep medications, as needed.

4. Schedule dressing changes accordingly to accommodate patient's sleep–wake cycle.

Community and Home Care Considerations

1. Demonstrate and explain wound care procedures to be continued after discharge:
   a. Wash hands.
   b. Clean small open wounds with mild soap in tub or shower.
   c. Rinse well with tap water.
   d. Pat dry with clean towel.
   e. Apply prescribed topical agent and dressing.

2. Assess for and teach patient to observe for local signs of wound infection:
   a. Increased redness of normal skin around burn area.
   b. Increased or purulent drainage.
   c. Increased pain, foul odor in burn area.
   d. Elevated body temperature.

3. Coordinate physical therapy consultation and encourage patient to develop a schedule to incorporate exercise regimen as prescribed by physical therapist.

   a. Suggest scheduling exercises immediately after wound cleansing and application of topical agent because skin may be more pliable and less sensitive to stretching then.

4. Instruct the patient in use and care of splints and pressure garments.

   a. Cleanse with mild soap and rinse well daily.

   b. Keep away from heat; dry garment by laying it flat on towels.

   c. Wear garment, as prescribed. This is usually 23 out of 24 hours/day. The garment is usually worn for 1 to 1½ years.

   d. Small open wounds should be covered with a light dressing under splints or pressure garments.

   e. Small superficial wounds smaller than ½ inch (1.5 cm) are usually treated with an antiseptic drying agent, such as merbromin 10%, twice per day.

   f. Observe for signs of skin breakdown. Reassure the patient that small blister formation is normal and generally lessens after the first year.

   g. Wear/bring splints and pressure garments to follow-up visits to be checked for proper fit.

Patient Education and Health Maintenance

Health education is closely related to rehabilitation as the burn patient prepares to return to a productive place in society. Functional and cosmetic reconstruction is accomplished and the patient attempts to integrate a new self-concept into social realities. Broadly viewed, health education focuses on biologic, psychological, and social parameters.

1. Assist the patient in transition from dependence on the health team to independence by assisting the patient to communicate needs and functional abilities to others.

2. Guide the patient in thinking positively about self. Promote ability to redirect others' attention from the scarred body to the self within.

3. Instruct the patient in measures to lubricate and enhance comfort of healing skin:

   a. After cleaning, use moisturizers such as cocoa butter or other nonperfumed hand lotion at least twice per day or more frequently, as needed.

   b. Wear clean white underwear and clothing free from irritating dyes until wounds are well healed.

   c. Take antipruritics, as prescribed.

   d. Stay in a cool environment if itching occurs.

   e. Protect skin from further trauma; use a sunscreen with a sun protection factor of 24 or higher.

   f. Discuss summer precautions, which should include a hat with a full, wide brim if there were facial or neck burns. Also limit exposure to sun because the affected areas will sunburn more easily and tan more deeply.

   g. Advise the patient that if wearing a pressure vest with or without sleeves, or tights, the Occupational Safety and Health Administration standards for work in a hot environment should be used. The patient should also be aware of the need for oral fluid replacement.

4. Review with the patient and family common emotional responses during convalescence (depression, withdrawal, grieving, dreaming, anxiety, guilt, excessive sensitivity, emotional lability, insomnia, and fear of future) and discuss usual temporary nature of these as well as effective coping mechanisms.

   a. There may be some psychological sequelae that will require long-term intervention, such as image adjustment disorders or posttraumatic stress issues. If not already in place, psychological referral is appropriate as an outpatient.

   b. Make sure that the patient has a phone number or referral to the counselor in order to make follow-up appointments, if desired.

5. Make sure that information has been given about follow-up evaluations and home health care services, as needed, in the interim.

6. For additional information and support, contact agencies such as the American Burn Association (*www.ameriburn.org*) or The Phoenix Society for Burn Survivors (*www.phoenix-society.org*). The Phoenix Society is a national foundation with local chapters whose primary function is support of other burn survivors. It has a toll-free number that burn survivors may use: (800) 888-BURN (2876).

Evaluation: Expected Outcomes

- Carboxyhemoglobin level below 10%, ABG levels within normal limits, respiratory rate 12 to 28 breaths/minute.
- Tidal volume within normal limits.
- Pulse 110 to 120 mm Hg or below, BP stable.
- Peripheral pulses strong.
- Weight stable, no edema, lungs clear.
- Wounds clean and granulating.
- Catheter patent, urine clear and quantity sufficient.
- Temperature normal to low-grade fever, no chills.
- No signs of infection.
- Normal ROM achieved and performing ADLs independently.
- Less than 5% weight loss from baseline.
- No gastric distention, aspirate and stool Hemoccult negative.
- Reports minimal pain after analgesic administration.
- Uses appropriate coping mechanisms.
- Verbalizes fears and concerns after viewing self in mirror.
- Sleeping 2- to 4-hour intervals, falls back to sleep easily.

SELECTED REFERENCES

American Burn Association. (2011). *Resources: Burn incidence and treatment in the United States fact sheet*. Chicago: Author. Available: *www.ameriburn.org/resources_factsheet.php*.

American Burn Association and American College of Surgeons Committee on Trauma. (2007). Guidelines for the operation of burn centers. *Journal of Burn Care and Research, 28*(1), 133–141.

Barkman, A. (2011). Heart failure and circulatory shock. In C. Porth (Ed.), *Essentials of pathophysiology* (pp. 486–512). Philadelphia: Lippincott Williams & Wilkins.

Colohan, S. M. (2010). Predicting prognosis in thermal burns with associated inhalational injury: A systematic review of prognostic factors in adult burn victims. *Journal of Burn Care and Research, 31*, 529–539.

Current diagnosis and treatment: Surgery. New York: McGraw-Hill.

Gaby, A. (2010). Nutritional treatment for burns. *Integrative Medicine, 9*(3), 46–51.

Goyata, S. (2009). Nursing diagnoses of burned patients and relatives' perceptions of patients' needs. *Internation Journal of Nursing Terminologies and Classifications*, *20*(1), 16–24.

Jayasekara, R. (2009). Dressings for superficial and partial thickness burns. *Journal of Advanced Nursing*, *37*, 1365–1366.

Latenser, B. A. (2009). Critical care of the burn patient: The first 48 hours. *Critical Care Medicine*, *37*, 2819–2826.

Michigan State Burn Coordinating Center. (2012). Fluid resuscitation overview: Emergency burn triage and management. Available: *www.michiganburn.org*.

Mosier, M. (2009). American Burn Association practice guidelines for prevention, diagnosis, and treatment of ventilator-associated pneumonia (VAP) in burn patients. *Journal of Burn Care & Research*, *30*, 910–928.

Pham, T., Cancio, L. C., Gibran, N. S., et al. (2008). American Burn Association practice guidelines burn shock resuscitation. *Journal of Burn Care and Research*, *29*(1), 257–266.

Ribbens, K. A., & DeVries, M. (2013). Burns. In B. B. Hammond & P. G. Zimmerman (Eds.), *Sheehy's manual of emergency care* (pp. 453–462). St. Louis, MO: Elsevier Mosby.

Singer, A. T. (2010). Thermal burns. In J. Marx (Ed.), *Rosen's emergency medicine* (pp. 758–766). Philadelphia: Mosby Elsevier.

Storm-Versloot, M. N., Vos, C. G., Ubbink, D. T., et al. (2010). Topical silver for preventing wound infection. *Cochrane Database of Systematic Reviews*, Issue 3 (Article No. CD006478).

Wasiak, J., Cleland, H., Campbell, F., et al. (2008). Dressings for superficial and partial thickness burns. *Cochrane Database of Systematic Reviews*, Issue 4 (Article No. CD0002106).

Zaletel, C. (2009). Factors affecting fluid resuscitation in the burn patient: The collaborative role of the APN. *Advanced Emergency Nursing Journal*, *31*, 309–320.

35
Emergent Conditions

OVERVIEW AND ASSESSMENT

Emergency medicine is the care, diagnosis, and treatment of unforeseen illness or injury. It is provided to patients with conditions ranging from minor to serious or life-threatening. The philosophy of emergency care includes the concept that an emergency is whatever the patient or family considers it to be. Emergency nursing is a dynamic and evolving practice that deals with unstable, undiagnosed patients usually presenting unexpectedly. See Standards of Care Guidelines 35-1, page 1198.

Emergency Assessment

When first contacting an emergency patient, it is essential that a systematic approach is used to ensure all factors are identified. Usually, the most dramatic injuries are distractors and are not immediately life-threatening. The primary and secondary surveys provide the emergency nurse with a methodical approach to help identify and prioritize patient needs.

Primary Survey

The initial, rapid ABCD (**a**irway, **b**reathing, **c**irculation, and neurologic **d**isability) assessment of the patient is meant to identify

STANDARDS OF CARE GUIDELINES 35-1
Emergency Assessment and Intervention

When a patient presents with a potentially life-threatening condition, proceed swiftly with the following:

- Call for help.
- Ensure the area is safe for you to enter, with no live electric current, hazardous materials, dangerous persons or other threats.
- Remove the patient from potential source of danger, such as live electric current, water, or fire. If hazardous materials are present, consult a MSDS book for decontamination procedures.
- Determine whether patient is conscious.
- Assess for adequate airway, breathing, and circulation in systematic manner. If any of these are absent, or inadequate, begin basic life support.
- Assess pupillary reaction and level of responsiveness to voice or touch, as indicated.
- If the patient is unconscious or has sustained a significant head injury, assume there is a spinal cord injury and maintain C-spine stabilization.
- Undress the patient to assess for wounds and skin lesions as indicated. Control any hemorrhage, as needed.
- When help arrives, assist with further assessment and transport, as needed.

This information should serve as a general guideline only. Each patient situation presents a unique set of clinical factors and requires nursing judgment to guide care, which may include additional or alternative measures and approaches.

---

life-threatening problems. If conditions are identified that present an immediate threat to life, you are required to stop and take corrective action prior to moving on to the next steps.

1. **A**—Airway: Does the patient have an open airway? Is the patient able to speak, swallow, or cry? Check for airway obstructions such as loose teeth, foreign objects, bleeding, vomitus, or other secretions. Immediately treat anything that compromises the airway. Never do a blind finger sweep of an airway.

2. **B**—Breathing: Is the patient breathing adequately? Assess for equal rise and fall of the chest (check for bilateral breath sounds), respiratory rate and pattern, skin color, use of accessory muscles, adventitious breath sounds, integrity of the chest wall, and position of the trachea. All major trauma patients require supplemental oxygen via a nonrebreather mask at 12 to 15L/min. Dress any penetrating chest injuries with occlusive dressings.

3. **C**—Circulation: Is circulation in immediate jeopardy? Can you palpate a central pulse? What is the quality (strong, weak, slow, rapid)? Is the skin warm and dry? Is the skin color normal? Obtain a blood pressure (BP; in both arms if chest trauma or dissecting aortic aneurysm is suspected). Is there any major bleeding?

4. **D**—Disability: Assess level of consciousness and pupils (a more thorough neurologic survey will be completed in the secondary survey). Assess level of consciousness using the AVPU scale:
   a. **A**—Is the patient alert? Are they looking at you and responding?
   b. **V**—Does the patient respond to voice? Do they open their eyes or respond when you call them?
   c. **P**—Does the patient respond to painful stimulus? Do they respond to sternal rub or nailbed pressure?
   d. **U**—The patient is unresponsive even to painful stimulus.

Secondary Assessment

The secondary assessment is a brief, but thorough, systematic assessment designed to identify all injuries. The steps include *Expose/environmental* control, *Full* set of vital signs, *Five* interventions, *Facilitate* family presence, and *Give* comfort measures. If your emergency department (ED) has enough staff, these interventions may be assigned to multiple staff members and performed simultaneously.

1. Expose/environmental control: It is necessary to remove all of the patient's clothing in order to identify all injuries. You must then prevent heat loss by using warm blankets, overhead warmers, and warmed intravenous (IV) fluids unless induced hypothermia is indicated. If your facility has a dedicated Trauma/Resuscitation room, keeping the temperature turned up aids in preventing heat loss.

2. Full set of vital signs:
   a. Obtain a full set of vital signs including BP, heart rate, respiratory rate, temperature, and oxygen saturation.
   b. As stated previously, obtain BP in both arms if chest trauma or dissecting aortic aneurysm is suspected.
   c. Institute continuous cardiac monitoring.
   d. Assess Glasgow Coma Scale (GCS) (see page 483) and pain scores.

3. Five interventions:
   a. Vascular access with two large-bore IV catheters, if possible.
   b. Pulse oximetry to measure the oxygen saturation; consider capnography to measure end-tidal carbon dioxide ($EtCO_2$); noninvasive ultrasonic cardiac output monitor; and 12-lead electrocardiogram (ECG).
   c. Indwelling urinary catheter (do not insert if you note blood at the meatus, blood in the scrotum, or if you suspect a pelvic fracture).
   d. Gastric tube (if there is evidence of facial fractures, insert the tube orally rather than nasally).
   e. Laboratory studies frequently include type and cross matching, complete blood count (CBC), urine drug screen, blood alcohol, electrolytes, prothrombin time and partial thromboplastin time, arterial blood gas (ABG), and pregnancy test, if applicable.

4. Facilitate family presence: Family presence is important during unexpected, potentially life-threatening events. They often have information that is critical in formulating the correct treatment plan. It is important to assess and respect the family's needs and wishes. If any member of the family wishes to be present during the resuscitation, it is imperative to assign a staff member to that person to explain what is being

done and offer support. Resuscitation rooms are often loud and appear chaotic. Assigning a staff member to any family wishing to be present can do much to alleviate their anxiety and assure them that everything is being done to help their loved one. If a family member does not wish to be present, providing them with a quiet area to wait and assigning a staff member as a contact person or liaison can be helpful.

5. Give comfort measures: These include verbal reassurances as well as pain management as appropriate. Do not forget to give comfort measures to the family as well as the patient during the resuscitation process.

History

1. Obtain prehospital information from emergency personnel, patient, family, or bystanders using the mnemonic MIVT.
   a. **M**—Mechanism of injury: It is helpful to understand the mechanism of injury to anticipate probable injuries. It is particularly helpful in motor vehicle accidents to know such information as external and internal damage to the car (or at least if the car was drivable after the accident), if the patient was ejected, if they were wearing a seat belt, if airbags were deployed, and the period of time elapsed before the patient received medical attention.
   b. **I**—Injuries sustained or suspected: Ask prehospital personnel to list any injuries that they have identified. Most prehospital providers will have completed a rapid trauma survey, including looking for DCAP/BTLS (deformities, contusions, abrasions, punctures/burns, tenderness, lacerations, and swelling)
   c. **V**—Vital signs: What were the prehospital vital signs?
   d. **T**—Treatment: What treatment did the patient receive before arriving at the hospital and what was the patient's response to those interventions?

2. If the patient is conscious, it is essential to ask him what happened. How did the accident occur? Why did it happen? A fall, for example, may not be a simple fall—perhaps the patient blacked out and then fell. If the patient is conscious and time permits, explore the chief complaint through the OPQRST mnemonic.
   O—Onset: When did they first notice symptoms? Was today the first time? Has it been ongoing? Is it getting progressively worse?
   P—Provokes, Palliates, Precipitates: What makes the symptoms better or worse?
   Q—Quality: How would they describe the discomfort? Burning, throbbing, aching, and like an electric shock are all commonly used to describe the quality of pain.
   R—Region, Radiates: Can the patient point to the pain with one finger? Does it move or shoot anywhere?
   S—Severity, associated Symptoms: How do they rate their symptom? Is it accompanied by anything else such as numbness, tingling, or nausea?
   T—Timing: Have the symptoms been constant or do they come and go? How often?

3. Obtain past medical history from the patient or a family member or friend; it may be helpful to utilize the mnemonic SAMPLE to assist in organizing history information:
   S—Signs and symptoms, including chief complaint and OPQRST.

A—Allergies to foods and medications.
M—Medications, including herbal supplements and over-the-counters.
P—Past medical and surgical history.
L—Last oral intake.
E—Events leading up to the incident.
Plus any history of alcohol or illicit drug use.

 NURSING ALERT To obtain a good descriptive history, do not ask questions that can be answered with a yes or no.

Head-to-Toe Assessment

The head-to-toe assessment begins with assessment of the patient's general appearance, including body position or any guarding or posturing. Work from the head down, systematically assessing the patient one body area at a time.

1. Head and face.
   a. Inspect for any lacerations, abrasions, contusions, avulsions, puncture wounds, impaled objects, ecchymosis, or edema. Hair can hide injuries, so take time to do a complete inspection. Scalp lacerations also tend to bleed profusely, further obscuring the area from quick inspections.
   b. Gently palpate for crepitus, crackling, or bony deformities.
   c. Inspect ears and nares for any bleeding or drainage, if present, check for Halo sign.

2. Neck (ensure proper C-spine stabilization is maintained).
   a. Inspect for any punctures, lacerations, contusions, swelling, tracheal deviation, JVD, or subcutaneous emphysema.
   b. Check for stomas or Medic Alert tags.
   c. Gently palpate for midline cervical tenderness.

3. Chest.
   a. Inspect for breathing effectiveness, paradoxical (uneven) chest wall movement, disruptions in chest wall integrity (lacerations, punctures, subcutaneous emphysema).
   b. Auscultate for bilateral breath sounds and adventitious breath sounds.
   c. Auscultate heart tones (muffled).
   d. Gently palpate for bony crepitus or deformities.

 NURSING ALERT Any penetrating chest wound has the potential to rapidly cause a life-threatening tension pneumothorax and must be treated immediately.

4. Abdomen/flanks.
   a. Inspect for lacerations, abrasions, contusions, avulsions, puncture wounds, impaled objects, ecchymosis, edema, scars, eviscerations, or distention.
   b. Auscultate for the presence of bowel sounds.
   c. Gently palpate for rigidity, guarding, masses, or areas of tenderness.

5. Pelvis/perineum.
   a. Inspect for lacerations, abrasions, contusions, avulsions, puncture wounds, impaled objects, ecchymosis, edema, or scars. Look for blood at the urinary meatus and vagina in

females. Look for priapism in males (which could indicate spinal cord injury).

   b. Gently palpate for pelvic instability or tenderness (do not rock the pelvis).

6. Neurologic/spinal (maintaining proper stabilization).

   a. Reassess mental status.

   b. Gently palpate for midline bony spinal tenderness.

   c. Check for paresthesias and determine sensory level.

   d. Check motor function and sphincter tone.

6. Extremities.

   a. Inspect skin color and temperature. Look for signs of injury and bleeding. Does the patient have movement in all four extremities? Touch the patient on a distal extremity and ask them to identify the part you are touching.

   b. Gently palpate peripheral pulses, any bony crepitus, or areas of tenderness.

   c. Check capillary refill.

   d. Gently palpate extremities for compartment firmness or signs of compartment syndrome.

 NURSING ALERT Pregnant trauma patients present a unique set of challenges. While performing assessments and interventions, a towel or roll should be placed under the right side of the backboard, tipping the patient slightly to the left and preventing fetal compression of the inferior vena cava and decreased blood return to the heart.

Focused Assessment

Any injuries that were identified during the primary and secondary surveys require a detailed assessment, which will typically include a team approach and radiographic studies.

Emergency Triage

Triage is a French verb meaning "to sort." Emergency triage is a subspecialty of emergency nursing, which requires specific, comprehensive educational preparation. The goal of an efficient triage system is to rapidly connect a patient with the proper level of care (such as fast-track or urgent care) and the correct resources in the shortest amount of time. Upon entering an ED, patients are greeted by a triage nurse, who will perform a rapid assessment, to include a general impression, chief complaint, immediate or potential life threats, and pertinent history, and then make a decision about the patient's acuity and the resources needed. These decisions can often be difficult if the patient has an altered mental status, is intoxicated, or is otherwise impaired. Thus, the primary role of the triage nurse is to make acuity and disposition decisions and set priorities while maintaining awareness for potentially violent or communicable disease situations. Secondary triage decisions involve the initiation of triage extended practices, such as the ordering of standardized labs or radiology studies. With the waiting times in EDs due to overcrowding becoming an increasing problem, the accuracy of the triage nurse in assigning acuity level is of critical importance. With extended wait times, triage is a continually ongoing process, with the triage nurse frequently reevaluating those who are waiting for changes in condition and updating their status, as needed.

Priorities of Care and Triage Categories

Standardized 5-level triage systems, such as the Australasian Triage Scale, Canadian Triage and Acuity Scale, and the Emergency Severity Index, have been developed and proven through research to possess utility, validity, reliability, and safety. All three systems utilize similar time frames and are evidence based (the Manchester Triage System is a consensus-based algorithm approach, which utilizes longer time frames).

Triage Level 1—Immediately Life-Threatening or Resuscitation

1. Conditions requiring immediate clinician assessment. Any delay in treatment is potentially life- or limb-threatening. These are the patients that are in active danger of dying if there is no immediate intervention and will require admission.

2. Includes conditions such as:

   a. Airway or severe respiratory compromise.

   b. Cardiac arrest.

   c. Severe shock.

   d. Symptomatic cervical spine injury.

   e. Multisystem trauma.

   f. Altered level of consciousness (LOC) (GCS < 10).

   g. Eclampsia.

   h. Acute mental status changes or unresponsiveness.

Triage Level 2—Imminently Life-Threatening or Emergent

1. These are conditions that are not in immediate danger, but have the potential to deteriorate rapidly if not treated.

2. Conditions include:

   a. Head injuries.

   b. Trauma.

   c. Conscious overdose.

   d. Severe allergic reaction without airway compromise.

   e. Chemical exposure to the eyes.

   f. Chest pain without hemodynamic instability.

   g. Back pain.

   h. GI bleed with unstable vital signs.

   i. Stroke with deficit.

   j. Severe asthma without airway compromise.

   l. Abdominal pain in patients older than age 50.

   m. Vomiting and diarrhea with dehydration.

   n. Fever in infants younger than age 3 months.

   o. Acute psychotic episode.

   p. Severe headache.

   q. Any pain greater than 7 on a scale of 1 to 10.

   r. Any sexual assault.

   s. Any neonate age 7 days or younger.

Triage Level 3—Potentially Life-Threatening/ Time Critical or Urgent

1. Conditions requiring urgent care–level activities with stable vital signs, but have the potential to deteriorate and utilize multiple resources.

2. Conditions include:

   a. Alert head injury with vomiting.

   b. Mild to moderate asthma.

c. Moderate trauma.

d. Abuse or neglect.

e. GI bleed with stable vital signs.

f. History of seizure, alert on arrival.

Triage Level 4—Potentially Life-Serious/Situational Urgency or Semi-urgent

1. Stable conditions that use few resources.

2. Conditions include:

a. Alert head injury without vomiting.

b. Minor trauma.

c. Vomiting and diarrhea in patient older than age 2 without evidence of dehydration.

d. Earache.

e. Minor allergic reaction.

f. Corneal foreign body.

g. Chronic back pain.

Triage Level 5—Less/Nonurgent

1. Stable conditions that utilize little to no resources.

2. Conditions include:

a. Minor trauma, not acute.

b. Sore throat.

c. Minor symptoms.

d. Chronic abdominal pain.

 NURSING ALERT When working with pediatric patients in a triage setting, it is important to remember that they can deteriorate rapidly. Pediatric patients should be triaged by those experienced in identifying the subtle clues that often precede this rapid deterioration.

Psychological Considerations

Serious illness or trauma is an insult to physiologic and psychological homeostasis; it requires physiologic and psychological healing. Both patients and families experience high levels of anxiety when being treated in the emergency department. It is important for the emergency nurse to recognize, understand, and alleviate these anxieties whenever possible.

Approach to the Patient

1. Understand and accept the basic anxieties of the acutely ill or traumatized patient. Be aware of the patient's fear of death, disablement, and isolation.

a. Personalize the situation as much as possible. Speak, react, and respond in a warm manner, reassure, but remain realistic and do not patronize the patient.

b. Give explanations on a level that the patient can grasp. An informed patient can cope with psychological/physiologic stress in a more positive manner.

c. Accept the rights of the patient and family to have and display their own feelings.

d. Maintain a calm and reassuring manner—helps the emotionally distressed patient or family to mobilize their psychological resources.

e. Include the patient's family or significant others if the patient wishes.

f. Encourage the patient or family to reach out to their support system. Often friends, other family members, or clergy can be of great comfort.

2. Understand and support the patient's feelings concerning loss of control (emotional, physical, and intellectual). If possible, giving the patient options and choices can help alleviate some of their feelings of helplessness.

3. Treat the unconscious patient as if conscious. Touch, call by name, and explain every procedure that is done. Avoid making negative comments about the patient's condition.

a. Orient the patient to person, time, and place as soon as he or she is conscious; reinforce by repeating this information.

b. Bring the patient back to reality in a calm and reassuring way.

c. Encourage the family, when possible, to touch the patient and aid in orienting the patient to reality.

4. Be prepared to handle all aspects of acute illness and trauma; know what to expect and what to do. When in doubt, stop, take a deep breath, and refocus. This alleviates the nurse's anxieties and increases the patient's confidence.

Approach to the Family

1. Inform the family where the patient is and give as much information as possible about the treatment he or she is receiving.

2. Consider allowing a family member to be present during the resuscitation. Assign a staff person to the family member to explain procedures and offer comfort.

3. Recognize the anxiety of the family and allow them to talk about their feelings. Acknowledge expressions of remorse, anger, guilt, and criticism.

4. Allow the family to relive the events, actions, and feelings preceding admission to the ED.

5. Deal with reality as gently and quickly as possible; avoid encouraging and supporting denial.

6. Assist the family to cope with sudden and unexpected death. Some helpful measures include the following:

a. Take the family to a private place.

b. Talk to all of the family together so they can mourn together.

c. Assure the family that everything possible was done; inform them of the treatment rendered.

d. Avoid using euphemisms such as "passed on." Show the family that you care by touching, offering coffee.

e. Allow family to talk about the deceased—permits ventilation of feelings of loss. Encourage family to talk about events preceding admission to the ED.

f. Encourage family to support each other and to express emotions freely—grief, loss, anger, helplessness, tears, disbelief.

g. Avoid volunteering unnecessary information (eg, patient was drinking).

h. Avoid giving sedation to family members—may mask or delay the grieving process, which is necessary to achieve emotional equilibrium and prevent prolonged depression.

i. Be cognizant of cultural and religious beliefs and needs.

j. Encourage family members to view the body if they wish—to do so helps to integrate the loss (cover mutilated areas).

   i. Prepare the family for visual images and explain any legal requirements.

   ii. Go with family to see the body.

   iii. Show acceptance of the body by touching to give family permission to touch and talk to the body.

   iv. Spend a few minutes with the family, listening to them.

   v. Allow the family some private time with the body, if appropriate.

7. Encourage the ED staff to discuss among themselves their reaction to the event to share intense feelings for review and for group support. Organize a formal debriefing session for staff if warranted by circumstances of the event.

Pain Management

Pain is an unpleasant sensory and emotional experience associated with actual or potential tissue damage and is also associated with significant morbidity. Pain inhibits immune function and has detrimental effects on cardiovascular, respiratory, GI, and other body systems. Over 60% of patients report pain on arrival at ED, making pain the most common patient complaint. It is imperative to adequately assess, monitor, and relieve pain in the ED. Despite this, significant evidence–practice gaps continue to be identified with underestimation and undertreatment of pain, as well as gaps in pain documentation, despite available clinical practice guidelines. In general, geriatric patients tend to have their pain underestimated and undertreated more frequently than younger adults do. Pain may be somatic or visceral, acute or chronic, or centrally or peripherally generated.

Primary Assessment

1. ABCD.
2. Evaluate pain using the OPQRST mnemonic.
3. Assess pain score using a pain rating tool, such as the numeric rating scale, visual analogue scale, Wong-Baker FACES pain scale (see page 1447), FLACC (faces, legs, activity, cry, and consolability) behavioral scale, verbal rating scale, or Abbey pain scale.

Primary Interventions

1. Pain is always subjective. Never doubt that a patient has pain based on how they look.
2. Establish a supportive relationship with the patient.
3. Respect the patient's response to pain and its management.
4. Educate the patient regarding methods of pain relief, preventive measures, and expectations.
5. Establish a baseline pain level, as well as a pain level the patient would consider tolerable.
6. Administer pharmaceutical and nonpharmaceutical pain control.
7. Monitor the patient's response to and effectiveness of treatment.
8. If initial interventions do not bring pain down to the tolerable level, explore other options.
9. Always reassure your patient and let them know you take their pain seriously.

NURSING ALERT Pain relief is a moral, humane, and physiologic imperative.

CARDIOPULMONARY RESUSCITATION AND AIRWAY MANAGEMENT

Evidence Base American Hearth Association. (2010). American Heart Association 2010 guidelines for CRP and ECC. *Circulation, 122*(Suppl. 3).

Nolan, J. P., Soar, J., Zideman, D. A., et al. (2010). European resuscitation council guidelines for resuscitation 2010, section 1. Executive summary. *Resuscitation, 81*, 1219–1276.

McQuillan, A. K. (2000). Inducing hypothermia after cardiac arrest. *Critical Care Nurse, 29*, 75–78.

Cardiopulmonary Resuscitation

Cardiopulmonary resuscitation (CPR) is a technique of basic life support for the purpose of oxygenating the brain and heart until appropriate, definitive medical treatment can restore normal heart and ventilatory action. Management of foreign-body airway obstruction or cricothyroidotomy may be necessary to open the airway while CPR is performed.

In 2010, there were many changes made to the CPR guidelines. The emphasis is now on performing good, high-quality chest compressions, with a minimum of interruptions, in an effort to not only preserve life but prevent anoxic brain injuries as well. The traditional "look-listen-and-feel" for breathing has been eliminated, as well as the A-B-C order for assessing the unresponsive patient. For the lay public, the focus has changed to a compressions-only resuscitation model, with no interruptions to deliver breaths. For the professional provider, airway, breathing, and circulation are all still important parts of the resuscitation effort; however, A-B-C has become C-A-B, or circulation, airway, then breathing. All efforts begin with good, high-quality chest compressions. See Procedure Guidelines 35-1.

Indications

1. Cardiac arrest.
   a. Ventricular fibrillation.
   b. Ventricular tachycardia.
   c. Asystole.
   d. Pulseless electrical activity.
2. Respiratory arrest.
   a. Drowning.
   b. Stroke.
   c. Foreign-body airway obstruction.
   d. Smoke inhalation.
   e. Drug overdose.
   f. Electrocution/injury by lightning.
   g. Suffocation.
   h. Accident/injury.
   i. Coma.
   j. Epiglottitis.

PROCEDURE GUIDELINES 35-1

Cardiopulmonary Resuscitation

EQUIPMENT

- Backboard
- Oral airway
- Bag–valve–mask (BVM) device
- Oxygen
- IV setup
- Defibrillator
- Emergency cardiac drugs
- Cardiac monitor
- Electrocardiograph machine
- Intubation equipment
- Suction

PROCEDURE

Nursing Action	Rationale
Responsiveness	
1. Determine unresponsiveness: tap or gently shake patient while shouting, "Are you okay?"	1. Prevents injury from attempted resuscitation on a person who is not unconscious.
2. Activate emergency medical service (call local emergency telephone number or 911) if outside facility.	2. Obtain help as soon as possible.
3. Place the patient supine on a firm, flat surface. Kneel at the level of the patient's shoulders. If he or she has suspected head or neck trauma, he or she should not be moved unless it is absolutely necessary (eg, at the site of an accident, fire, or other unsafe environment).	3. Enables the rescuer to perform rescue breathing and chest compression without changing position.

Circulation–Airway–Breathing

Determine if a pulse is present while checking for signs of breathing

Nursing Action	Rationale
1. Palpate the carotid or femoral pulse for no more than 10 seconds, while looking for signs the patient is attempting to breathe. If pulse is not palpable, start chest compressions.	1. Cardiac arrest is recognized by a lack of palpable pulses in the central arteries of a nonresponsive, apneic patient. For patients who are apneic but have a clearly palpable central pulse, begin rescue breathing with a BVM device or pocket mask at a rate of 1 breath every 5–6 seconds.

External Chest Compressions

Chest compressions consist of a sequence of rhythmic applications of pressure over the lower half of the sternum, which provides circulation to the vital organs

Nursing Action	Rationale
1. Kneel as close to the side of the patient's chest as possible, placing the heel of one hand on the lower half of the sternum, taking care to avoid the xiphoid process. Fingers may be interlaced or extended but care must be taken to keep them off the chest.	1. Ensure the main force of the compression is on the sternum by placing the long axis of the hand on the long axis of the sternum.
2. Keep your arms straight and your elbows locked. Ensure your shoulders are directly over your hands and quickly and forcefully depress the patient's sternum straight down to a depth of at least 2 inches.	2. Keeping your arms straight and your elbows locked allows a greater force to be delivered with each compression and aids in preventing fatigue
3. Deliver 30 compressions at a rate of *at least* 100 compressions a minute. Always allow for complete chest recoil after each compression without taking your hands off of the chest between compressions.	3. Allowing complete chest recoil gives the heart time and room to fill with blood. A partially compressed heart will eject less blood than one that is allowed to fill properly.

(continued)

PROCEDURE GUIDELINES 35-1 (continued)

Cardiopulmonary Resuscitation

PROCEDURE (continued)

Nursing Action	Rationale
4. Taking no more than 10 seconds, open the airway and deliver 2 breaths	4. Total "hands-off" time between the end of one set of 30 compressions and the start of the next needs to be less than 10 seconds to ensure adequate circulation.
a. Head-tilt/chin-lift maneuver: Place one hand on the patient's forehead and apply firm backward pressure with the palm to tilt the head back. Then, place the fingers of the other hand under the bony part of the lower jaw near the chin and lift up to bring the jaw forward and the teeth almost to occlusion.	a. In the absence of sufficient muscle tone, the tongue or epiglottis will obstruct the pharynx and larynx. This supports the jaw and helps tilt the head back.
b. If a cervical spine injury is suspected, use the jaw-thrust maneuver: Grasp the angles of the patient's lower jaw and, lifting with both hands, one on each side, displace the mandible forward while maintaining C-spine immobility.	b. The jaw-thrust technique without head tilt is the safest method for opening the airway in the presence of suspected neck injury.
c. Perform rescue breathing by using a pocket mask or other barrier device	c. Mouth to mouth is only done in extreme circumstances in the hospital setting.
d. While keeping the patient's airway open, place the pocket mask on the patient's face, making sure to maintain a good seal. Take a deep breath and ventilate the patient with two breaths of just enough volume to see chest rise (each over 1 second), taking a breath after each ventilation. If the initial ventilation attempt is unsuccessful, reposition the patient's head and repeat rescue breathing.	d. Ensuring a good seal with a pocket mask takes practice, but is essential in preventing air leakage. Full breaths are no longer required as gastric inflation can occur. Ventilate just enough to get the chest to rise.
5. When a second rescuer arrives, have them begin compressions while you take over ventilations.	5. The ratio of compressions to ventilations for the adult victim is 30:2 for one- and two- rescuer CPR.
6. While resuscitation proceeds, simultaneous efforts are made to obtain and use special resuscitation equipment to manage breathing and circulation and provide definitive care.	6. Definitive care includes defibrillation, pharmacotherapy for dysrhythmias and acid-base disturbances, and ongoing monitoring and skilled care in an intensive care unit.
7. Utilize the automated external defibrillator (AED) or, if trained, the manual defibrillator as soon as possible. Special circumstances affecting use of AEDs include:	7. The American Heart Association supports the use of AEDs in public places as well as medical centers.
a. For children <1 year of age, a manual defibrillator is preferred. If there is no manual defibrillator available, or one with pediatric dose attenuators, an adult AED may be used.	a. For children under age 8, an AED with pediatric dose attenuators is preferred. If one is not available, a normal adult AED may be used.
b. The victim should not be lying in water when using an AED. Make sure the patient's chest is dry before attaching the AED.	b. Using an AED when patients are wet or lying in water may result in burns and shocks to the rescuer.
c. Do not place the AED electrode directly over an implanted pacemaker.	c. Placing an AED pad directly over an implanted pacemaker may reduce the effectiveness of the defibrillation.
d. Remove any transdermal medication patches from the patient before using the AED.	d. Placing an AED pad over a transdermal medication patch may make the defibrillation less effective and cause a burn.
8. The four basic steps used in AED operation are:	8. The directions provided for operation of the AED were provided by the device manufacturer. Many machines will walk you through the steps for operation once the power is turned on. Be familiar with the type of device in your facility.
a. Turn the power on. Always do this first to ensure the device has power	
b. Attach the AED pads to the patient's chest, using the diagrams on the pads to show you exactly where to place them.	

PROCEDURE GUIDELINES 35-1 *(continued)*

Cardiopulmonary Resuscitation

PROCEDURE *(continued)*

Nursing Action	Rationale
c. Analyze the patient's rhythm by pushing the button on the AED labeled ANALYZE. During this time, no one should touch the patient.	c. Some AEDs will analyze automatically once the pads are connected. Touching the patient could create artifact and interfere with analysis.
d. Charge the AED and deliver the shock if indicated by the AED. Make sure that no one is touching the patient. Push the shock button; the AED will provide visual and voice prompts to tell you what to do.	d. Always call "Clear" and visually check for anyone touching the patient prior to delivering a shock. When the machine delivers a shock, anyone touching the patient will feel it.

 NURSING ALERT With two rescuers present, do not stop chest compressions to place AED pads. Pads can be correctly placed on the patient while compressions continue. Only stop compressions when instructed to do so for rhythm analysis and shock delivery.

 Evidence Base American Heart Association. (2010). American Heart Association 2010 guidelines for CPR and ECC. *Circulation, 122*(Suppl. 3).

Assessment

1. Immediate loss of consciousness.
2. Absence of palpable carotid or femoral pulse; pulselessness in large arteries.
3. Absence of breath sounds or air movement through nose or mouth.

Complications

1. Postresuscitation distress syndrome (secondary derangements in multiple organs).
2. Neurologic impairment, brain damage.

 NURSING ALERT The patient who has been resuscitated is at risk for another episode of cardiac arrest.

Induced Hypothermia Post Cardiac Arrest

In adults with persistent coma (post cardiac arrest), initiating induced hypothermia to a temperature of 89°–93° F (32° to 34° C) for 12 to 24 hours results in neuroprotection, improving neurologic function and decreasing mortality. It is also associated with beneficial hemodynamic, renal, and acid-base effects. See Procedure Guidelines 35-2, pages 1206 to 1207.

Indications

1. Persistent coma in the adult patient following cardiac arrest.
2. Return of spontaneous circulation.

 NURSING ALERT The patient who responds to verbal stimuli after cardiac arrest should not be treated with induced hypothermia.

Assessment

1. Institute continuous cardiac monitoring. Monitor for bradycardia caused by cooling or other dysrhythmias.
2. Institute continuous temperature monitoring, preferably core temperature.
3. Frequently monitor blood pressure to avoid hypotension, particularly during rewarming.
4. Monitor CBC for signs of infection, since temperature will not be an accurate sign. Monitor electrolyte panel for hypokalemia caused by hypothermia. ABGs should be analyzed at patient's actual body temperature.
5. Assess skin every 2 hours for pressure and cold injury.

Complications

1. Shivering—patient may require sedation and neuromuscular blockade to relieve shivering, which will interfere with hypothermia.
2. Seizures—continuous neuromuscular blockade may mask post–cardiac arrest seizure activity.

Commercial Cooling Devices

1. A number of commercially available cooling devices are currently available, including cooling blankets, cooling gel pads applied to the skin, and centrally inserted heat-exchange catheters.

PROCEDURE GUIDELINES 35-2

Induced Hypothermia Post Cardiac Arrest

PURPOSE

Current evidence suggests that mild induced hypothermia may reduce mortality and improve neurologic outcomes in adult post–cardiac arrest patients. Cooling should be started as soon as possible to ensure optimum effectiveness.

EQUIPMENT

- 3–6 L bag of refrigerated 39° F (4° C) lactated Ringer's solution
- Small plastic bags
- Ample supply of ice cubes

Note: *Commercially available external cooling device (may be used in addition to or instead of ice packs)

PRE PROCEDURE

Nursing Action	Rationale
1. Consider the inclusion criteria. All patients who are resuscitated from arrest but remain unconscious and are unable to respond to verbal command should be considered for immediate cooling.	1. Research has shown that an improved outcome can be attained if the patient has adequate arterial circulation and oxygenation to the brain. a. Research has shown improved outcomes in arrest patients who remain hemodynamically stable during the post-resuscitation period.

2. Consider exclusion criteria. Patients should not be considered for the following reasons:
 	
   a. Severe preexisting conditions with DNR orders.
   b. Active noncompressible bleeding.
	2. There are only two absolute contraindications for therapeutic hypothermia. All others must be considered on a case by case basis

PROCEDURE

Nursing Action	Rationale
1. Provide standard advanced life support and ongoing intensive care management. All patients must be intubated and ventilated.	1. Patient's cardiopulmonary status is unstable.
2. Perform and document thorough neurologic examination.	2. The goal of the procedure is improved neurologic outcome.

3. Measure temperature continuously, if possible, or every 15 minutes.
 	
   a. Initially, peripherally until continuous core temperature monitoring (central venous, bladder, rectal, oropharyngeal) can be instituted
   b. As rectal core temperature monitoring may be slow to change, two sites of measurement are preferred.
	3. Frequent monitoring of temperature is important to reach goal temperature quickly.
	
	   a. Central venous temperature monitoring is preferred.

4. Begin cooling as soon as possible. This should begin in the emergency department.
 	
   a. Apply ice packs to groin, axillae, sides of chest, neck; or apply cooling blanket, wrap, or pads according to manufacturer's instructions.
   b. Instill 30 mL/kg of refrigerated lactated Ringer's solution over 30 minutes through a femoral line (if patient is not in acute pulmonary edema).
	4. Internal and external cooling are required to bring down core temperature
	
	   b. One liter of cold saline infused over 15 min can drop the core temperature by 1°C.

5. Target temperature is 91.4° F (32° C). Remove ice packs once temperature is less than 91° F (33° C).	5. There is no need to bring down the temperature below 33°C, but temperature should be kept in that range for 12 to 24 hours.

PROCEDURE GUIDELINES 35-2 *(continued)*

Induced Hypothermia Post Cardiac Arrest

PROCEDURE *(continued)*

Nursing Action	Rationale
6. Replace ice packs and consider further ice-cold lactated Ringer's solution if temperature remains above 92.3° F (33.5° C).	
7. Use nondepolarizing neuromuscular blockade to prevent shivering. Provide sedation according to standard ICU protocol.	7. Shivering produces heat, which will raise core temperature.
8. Maintain patient at target temperature for a period of 12–24 hours once temperature is reached.	
9. After the targeted time has elapsed passive rewarming should occur slowly over 8–12 hours.	9. Research has shown that the best risk/benefit ratio is at 12 hours.
10. Monitor for complications:	10. Complications will compromise outcome.
a. Hyperglycemia.	
b. Ileus may occur at <93.2° F (34° C).	
c. Hypovolemia and hypotension, secondary to vasodilation, may occur during rewarming.	
d. Bleeding—this may be of increased significance in patients undergoing urgent angioplasty or thrombolytic therapy who will also receive antiplatelet agents.	
e. Infection, especially pneumonia, during and following the procedure. Fever, one of the cardinal signs of infection, will be absent in people treated with therapeutic hypothermia.	

 NURSING ALERT Do not cool below 90° F (32° C) because this increases the risk of complications.

 Evidence Base American Heart Association. (2010). American Heart Association 2010 guidelines for CPR and ECC. *Circulation, 122*(Suppl. 3)).
    Arrich, J., Holzer, M., Havel, C., et al. (2012). Hypothermia for neuroprotection in adults after cardiopulmonary resuscitation (Review). The Cochrane Library, CD004128.pub3.

2. Cooling blankets are placed under and over the patient and cool utilizing circulated chilled water. They are easy to apply; however, they can have poor surface contact, making it difficult to maintain a targeted temperature.

3. Devices utilizing adhesive gel pads are also easy to apply and provide improved surface contact to facilitate rate and maintenance of cooling. Contoured cooling garments are also available.

4. With any surface cooling method, ice packs are often used to assist in initial cooling and then removed. Maintenance is controlled by the commercial device.

5. Centrally inserted heat-exchange catheters use chilled saline passed through a coiled section of catheter.

   a. These coils provide a large surface area for blood to pass over and heat exchange to occur.

   b. Normally placed in the femoral vein, these catheters allow for rapid cooling and extremely tight control without promoting shivering.

Foreign-Body Airway Obstruction

Foreign-body obstruction of the airway may be either partial or complete. Abdominal thrusts (the Heimlich maneuver) are recommended for relieving foreign-body airway obstruction in the adult. See Procedure Guidelines 35-3, page 1208.

Assessment

1. Weak, ineffective cough.
2. High-pitched noises on inspiration.
3. Respiratory distress.

PROCEDURE GUIDELINES 35-3

Management of Foreign-Body Airway Obstruction

PROCEDURE

Nursing Action	Rationale
Airway obstruction with conscious patient sitting or standing **Abdominal thrusts**	
1. Stand behind the patient; wrap your arms around patient's waist, and proceed as follows:	1. If the patient is able to speak or cough forcefully, allow them to attempt to clear their own airway.
a. Make a fist with one hand, placing the thumb side of the fist against the patient's abdomen in the midline, slightly above the navel and well below the xiphoid process. Grasp the fist with your other hand.	
b. Press your fist into the patient's abdomen with a quick upward thrust. Each new thrust should be a separate and distinct maneuver.	b. A subdiaphragmatic abdominal thrust, by elevating the diaphragm, can force air from the lungs to create an artificial cough intended to move and expel an obstructing foreign body in the airway.
c. Continue until the obstruction is cleared, help arrives, or the patient becomes unresponsive.	
d. Should the patient become unresponsive, immediately begin CPR, checking the airway after each set of compressions and prior to attempting ventilations.	d. The obstruction may have become dislodged during chest compressions. Only attempt to remove objects you can see. Never perform a blind finger sweep.
Airway obstruction with conscious patient standing or sitting **Chest thrust**	
1. Stand behind the patient with your arms under the axillae to encircle his or her chest.	1. This technique is to be used only in advanced stages of pregnancy or in a markedly obese patient.
2. Place the thumb side of your fist on the middle of the patient's sternum, taking care to avoid the xiphoid process and rib cage margins.	2. The xiphoid process can be easily injured.
3. Grasp your fist with your other hand and perform backward thrusts until the foreign body is expelled. If the patient becomes unconscious, stop and begin CPR, as noted above.	3. The thrusting motion is intended to relieve the obstruction.

4. Inability to speak or breathe.
5. Cyanosis.
6. Hands at throat.

Cricothyroidotomy

Cricothyroidotomy is the puncture or incision of the cricothyroid membrane to establish an emergency airway in certain emergency situations when placement of an endotracheal tube or laryngeal-mask airway is not possible or is contraindicated and when adequate oxygenation cannot be maintained utilizing a bag–valve–mask device with 100% oxygen. See Procedure Guidelines 35-4, page 1209.

Indications

1. Compromised airway and inability to intubate or perform tracheostomy:
   a. Complete foreign-body airway obstruction.
   b. Trauma to head and neck.

2. Allergic reaction causing laryngeal edema.

Contraindications

1. Laryngeal fracture.
2. Tracheal rupture.
3. Tracheal transection with distal tracheal retraction into the mediastinum.

INJURIES TO THE HEAD, SPINE, AND FACE

Head Injuries

Head injuries can include fractures to the skull and face, direct injuries to the brain (as from a bullet), and indirect injuries to the brain (such as a concussion, contusion, or intracranial hemorrhage). Head injuries commonly occur from motor vehicle accidents, assaults, or falls.

PROCEDURE GUIDELINES 35-4

Cricothyroidotomy

EQUIPMENT

- Chlorhexidine or povidone iodine for site cleansing
- Cricothyrotomy catheter (if available)
- IV catheters (if commercial cricothyrotomy catheter is not available):
  16G or larger IV catheters (adult)
  16G or 18G IV catheters (children)
- 3.0 endotracheal tube connecter (bag–valve–mask connecter)
- 10 mL Luer-loc syringe with 5 mL of saline

PROCEDURE

Nursing Action	Rationale
1. Preoxygenate the patient, if possible	1. Boosts oxygen saturation during the procedure.
2. Extend the patient's neck. Place a towel roll beneath the shoulders.	2. Allows the cricothyroid membrane to be palpated readily.
3. Attach a 10-mL syringe containing 5-mL of saline to the insertion catheter	
4. Identify the prominent thyroid cartilage (Adam's apple) and allow your finger to descend in the midline to the depression between the lower border of the thyroid cartilage and the upper border of the cricoid cartilage (see accompanying figure).	4. This depression represents the cricothyroid membrane.

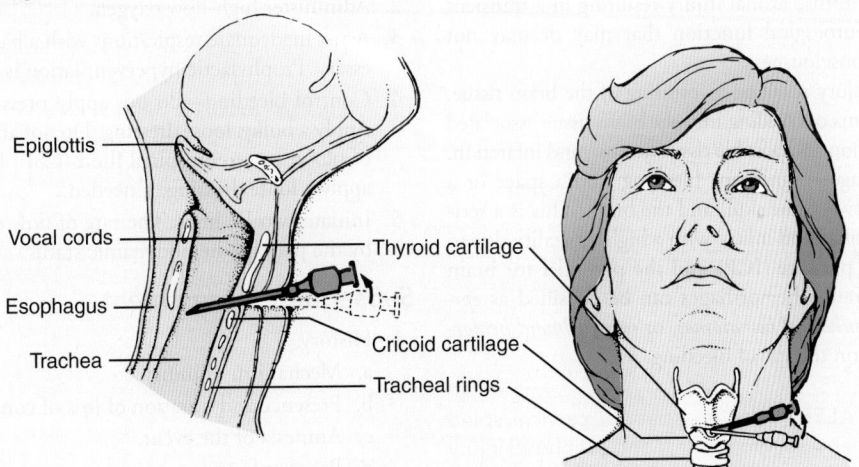

Cricothyroidotomy, or cricothyroid membrane puncture.

5. Scrub insertion site and maintain sterility throughout procedure.	5. Reduces risk of infection.
6. Provide skin tension and hold the trachea in place with the nondominant hand, using the index finger to palpate the cricothyroid membrane.	6. Attains stability and identifies the insertion site.
7. Place the catheter at the inferior margin of the cricothyroid membrane, in the midline of the neck, and direct it caudally at a 30- to 45-degree angle	7. Insertion will be in direction of airway.
8. While maintaining negative pressure on the syringe, advance the catheter through the skin and tissue until air bubbles are seen in the syringe	8. Maintaining negative pressure prevents saline from being injected into the airway.
9. Thread the catheter off of the needle until the hub rests on the skin surface and withdraw the needle.	9. Insertion needle is withdrawn; flexible catheter remains.

(continued)

PROCEDURE GUIDELINES 35-4 *(continued)*

Cricothyroidotomy

PROCEDURE *(continued)*

Nursing Action	Rationale
10. Listen for air passing back and forth through the needle synchronously with the patient's respirations.	10. Indicates correct positioning and opening of obstructed airway.
11. Secure the needle with adhesive tape or sutures.	11. Maintains stability of airway.
12. Ventilate with bag–valve–mask device, allowing for a prolonged exhalation time.	12. In cases of airway obstruction, prolonged exhalation times are necessary to prevent air trapping, or auto-PEEP.
13. Prepare for tracheostomy.	13. After the patient is stabilized, a more permanent means of ventilatory support is implemented.
14. Potential complications: bleeding, aspiration, subcutaneous emphysema.	

 Evidence Base Finucane, B., Tsui, B., & Santora, A. (2011). Surgical options in airway management. In *Principles of airway management* (pp. 569–640). New York: Springer.

Concussion—a mild diffuse axonal injury resulting in a transient disturbance of neurological function that may or may not include a loss of consciousness.

Contusion—a focal injury resulting in bruising of the brain tissue. Actual small amounts of bleeding into the brain tissue associated with edema formation and possible tissue necrosis and infarction.

Intracranial hemorrhage—significant bleeding into a space or a potential space between the skull and the brain. This is a serious complication of a head injury with a high mortality due to rising intracranial pressure (ICP) and the potential for brain herniation. Intracranial hemorrhages can be classified as *epidural hematomas, subdural hematomas,* or *subarachnoid hemorrhages,* depending on the site of bleeding.

 NURSING ALERT Always assume a cervical spine fracture for any patient with a significant head injury until proven otherwise.

Primary Assessment

1. Airway: assess for vomitus, bleeding, and foreign objects. Ensure cervical spine immobilization.
2. Breathing: assess for abnormally slow or shallow respirations. An elevated carbon dioxide partial pressure can worsen cerebral edema.
3. Circulation: assess pulse and bleeding.
4. Disability: assess the patient's neurologic status.

Primary Interventions

1. Open the airway using the jaw-thrust technique without head tilt. Oral suction equipment (to handle heavy vomitus) should be at hand. Make sure that you do not stimulate the gag reflex as this can cause increases in ICP.
2. Administer high-flow oxygen.
3. Assist inadequate respirations with a bag–valve–mask, as necessary. Prophylactic hyperventilation is not indicated.
4. Control bleeding—do not apply pressure to the injury site. Apply a bulky, loose dressing. Do not attempt to stop the flow of blood or cerebrospinal fluid (CSF) from the nose or ears; apply a loose dressing, if needed.
5. Initiate two IV lines. The rate of flow should be determined by the patient's hemodynamic status.

Subsequent Assessment

1. History.
   a. Mechanism of injury.
   b. Presence and duration of loss of consciousness.
   c. Amnesia of the event.
   d. Position found.
2. LOC.
   a. Change in mental status is the most sensitive indicator of a change in the patient's condition.
   b. GCS (see page 483).
3. Vital signs.
   a. Hypertension and bradycardia are late signs of increasing ICP.
   b. Patients with a head injury may have associated cardiac dysrhythmias, noted by an irregular or rapid pulse.
   c. Changing patterns of respiration or apnea may indicate a head injury.
   d. Elevated temperature—high temperatures may be associated with head injury.
4. Unequal or unresponsive pupils.
5. Confusion or personality changes.
6. Impaired vision.
7. One or both eyes appear sunken.

8. Seizure activity.
9. Periauricular ecchymosis—"Battle sign," a bluish discoloration behind the ears (indicates a possible basal skull fracture).
10. Rhinorrhea or otorrhea (indicative of leakage of CSF).
11. Periorbital ecchymosis (indicates anterior basilar fracture).

 **NURSING ALERT** If basilar skull fracture or severe midface fractures are suspected, a nasogastric (NG) tube is contraindicated. An orogastric tube may be considered for insertion.

General Interventions

1. Keep the neck in a neutral position with the cervical spine immobilized.
2. Establish an IV line of normal saline or lactated Ringer's solution—fluid volume should be restricted.
3. Be prepared to manage seizures—if seizures occur, they should be controlled immediately.
4. Maintain normothermia.
5. Pharmacologic interventions may include:
   a. Anticonvulsants—to control seizures.
   b. Mannitol or hypertonic saline—to reduce cerebral edema and decrease ICP.
   c. Antibiotics.
   d. Antipyretics to control hyperthermia.

Cervical Spine Injuries

Injuries to the cervical spine are serious because the crushing, stretching, and rotational shear forces exerted on the cord at the time of trauma can produce severe neurologic deficits. Edema and cord swelling contribute further to the loss of spinal cord function.

Any person with a head, neck, or back injury or fractures to the upper leg bones or to the pelvis should be suspected of having a potential spinal cord injury until proven otherwise.

Primary Assessment

1. Provide immediate immobilization of the spine and maintain immobilization throughout assessment.
2. Airway.
3. Breathing.
   a. Intercostal paralysis with diaphragmatic breathing indicates cervical spinal cord injury.
   b. In conscious patient, observe for increased respiratory rate and difficulty in speaking due to shortness of breath.
4. Circulation.
5. Disability—assess neurologic status.

Primary Interventions

1. Immobilize the cervical spine.
2. Open the airway using the jaw-thrust technique without head tilt.
3. If the patient needs to be intubated, it may be done nasally.

4. If respirations are shallow, assist with a bag–valve–mask.
5. Administer high-flow oxygen to minimize potential hypoxic spinal cord damage.

Subsequent Assessment

1. Assess the position of the patient when found; this may indicate the type of injury incurred.
2. Hypotension and bradycardia accompanied by warm, dry skin—suggests spinal shock.
3. Neck and back pain/extremity pain or burning sensation to the skin.
4. History of unconsciousness.
5. Total sensory loss and motor paralysis below level of injury.
6. Loss of bowel and bladder control; usually urinary retention and bladder distention.
7. Loss of sweating and vasomotor tone below level of cord lesion.
8. Priapism—persistent erection of penis.
9. Hypothermia—due to the inability to constrict peripheral blood vessels and conserve body heat.
10. Loss of rectal tone.

General Interventions

 NURSING ALERT A spinal cord injury can be made worse during the acute phase of injury, resulting in permanent neurologic damage. Proper handling is an immediate priority.

1. Ensure adequacy of airway, breathing, and circulation. Frequently monitor vital signs.
2. Insert an NG/OG tube.
3. Keep the patient warm.
4. Initiate IV access.
5. Insert an indwelling urinary catheter to avoid bladder distention.
6. Continue with repeated neurologic examinations to determine if there is deterioration of the spinal cord injury.
7. Be prepared to manage seizures if head injury is also suspected.
8. Pharmacologic interventions: high-dose steroids (methylprednisolone). Research has shown differing results; currently in the United States, high-dose steroids remain a treatment option but are no longer considered to be standard practice.

 NURSING ALERT Patients with spinal cord injuries can experience autonomic dysreflexia, an exaggerated sympathetic response to noxious stimuli. It has the potential to be life-threatening if signs are not immediately recognized and treated, along with the removal of the offending stimuli.

Maxillofacial Trauma

Injuries to the head frequently result in facial lacerations and fractures to the facial bones (ie, nasal fractures, orbital fractures, maxillary fractures, and mandibular fractures).

Primary Assessment

1. Maintain immobilization of the spine while performing assessment.
2. Airway—obstruction can occur due to tongue swelling, bleeding, or broken or missing teeth.
3. Breathing—have suction ready to prevent aspiration of blood or broken teeth.
4. Circulation—control bleeding; monitor vital signs for signs of instability.
5. Disability.

Primary Interventions

1. Establish and maintain an airway. This includes high-flow oxygen, inserting an oral airway in the unresponsive patient, or assisting with intubation. A nasopharyngeal airway should be used only if there is no evidence of nasal fractures or CSF leakage from the nose.
2. Control bleeding—do not apply pressure to the injury site. Apply a bulky, loose dressing. Do not attempt to stop the flow of blood or CSF from the nose or ears; apply a loose dressing, if needed.

Subsequent Assessment

1. Examine the mouth for broken or missing teeth.
2. Assess for a potential eye injury, vision loss, double vision, or pain in the eye.
3. Examine the eye for disconjugate gaze—incoordination of eye movements.
4. Paralysis of the upward gaze is indicative of an inferior orbit fracture (blowout fracture).
5. Crepitus or a crackling feeling on palpation around the nose usually indicates a nasal fracture.
6. Malocclusion of the teeth is indicative of a maxilla or mandible fracture.
7. A palpable flattening of the cheek and a loss of sensation below the orbit may indicate a zygoma (cheekbone) fracture.
8. Spasms of the jaw (trismus) and mobility of the jaw indicate a maxilla fracture.
9. Rhinorrhea or otorrhea (indicative of leakage of CSF).

General Interventions

1. Gently apply ice to areas of swelling or ecchymosis. This may reduce further swelling and pain. However, if you suspect an injury to the eye itself, do not apply ice.
2. If other injuries permit, elevate the head of the bed.
3. Possible pharmacologic interventions:
   a. Pain management.
   b. Sedation.
4. With the potential for a CSF leak, the patient should be instructed not to blow the nose because of the potential for transmitting infection to the brain or eyes.

INJURIES TO SOFT TISSUE, BONES, AND JOINTS

Soft Tissue Injuries

Soft tissue injuries involve the skin and underlying subcutaneous tissue and muscles. They can be classified as closed or open injuries. A *closed wound* is an injury to the soft tissue but without an associated break in the skin. Closed wounds include:

1. Contusion—bleeding beneath the skin into the subcutaneous tissue. Discoloration, swelling and pain may be present.
2. Hematoma—well-defined pocket of blood and fluid beneath the skin resulting from a disruption of the deeper veins and arteries. Hematomas present as an appreciable soft mass on palpation.

An *open wound* is an injury to soft tissue with an associated break in the skin. Generally, they are more serious than closed injuries due to the potential for blood loss and infection. Open wounds include:

1. Abrasion—superficial loss of skin resulting from rubbing or scraping the skin over a rough or uneven surface.
2. Laceration—a tear or cut in the skin. They can be a partial- or full-thickness cut, incisional or jagged.
3. Puncture—occurs when the skin is penetrated by a pointed object. Can be penetrating (entrance wound only) or perforating (entrance and exit wound). Generally, puncture wounds do not cause serious external bleeding, but there may be significant internal bleeding and damage to vital organs, as well as significant risk of infection.
4. Avulsion—involves a tearing off or loss of a full-thickness flap of skin.
5. Amputation—traumatic cutting or tearing off of an appendage (eg, finger, toe, arm, or leg).
6. Burn—tissue injury that results from thermal, chemical, electrical, or radiation energy.

Primary Assessment

1. Always ensure the adequacy of airway, breathing, and circulation.
2. If the bleeding from the injury has been significant, be aware of the clinical signs and symptoms of shock.
   a. Restlessness, confusion, and anxiety.
   b. Skin pale, mottled, cold, and diaphoretic.
   c. Tachycardia (rapid pulse).
   d. Tachypnea (rapid, shallow breathing).
   e. Hypotension (falling BP is a late sign of shock).
3. Assess for arterial or venous bleeding. Arterial bleeding is bright red and usually spurts from the wound. Venous bleeding is darker red and will flow steadily from a wound.

Primary Interventions

The primary goal and nursing intervention are to control severe bleeding.

 NURSING ALERT Wounds that result in severe arterial bleeding should be considered life-threatening and treatment is second only to CPR.

Direct Pressure

1. Most external bleeding can be controlled by direct pressure.
2. Cover the injury with sterile dressings.
3. Apply firm direct pressure to the site of injury.
4. While maintaining pressure, assess for distal pulses.
5. Pressure should be maintained until the bleeding stops, a pressure dressing is applied, or definitive treatment is undertaken.
6. If the dressing becomes saturated, reinforce the dressing; do not remove the dressing.
7. After bleeding has stopped, apply a pressure dressing.
   a. A pressure bandage is made by securing several gauze pads over the injury with a rolled gauze bandage.
   b. A pressure dressing allows the nurse freedom to continue assessing the patient or attend to other injuries.
   c. After applying a pressure dressing, always ensure that the patient has a pulse distal to the dressing. If no pulse is present, the dressing may be too tight.

Elevation

1. Elevating the injured area while applying direct pressure helps to control bleeding. This measure uses gravity to slow the blood flow.

2. If possible, the injured area should be elevated above the level of the heart.
3. Do not raise a limb if a fracture is suspected or if elevation causes the patient pain or discomfort.

Pressure Points

1. Pressure points are used when direct pressure and elevation cannot control bleeding alone or when direct pressure cannot be applied to a bleeding site due to a protruding bone or an embedded object.
2. Pressure points are located between the site of injury and the heart where a main artery passes over a bone or underlying muscle mass (see Figure 35-1).
3. Locate the pressure point and apply firm, steady pressure with the heel of the hand.
4. If heavy bleeding is still not controlled, the patient may exsanguinate and a tourniquet should be used or a vascular clamp can be applied to the artery.

Subsequent Assessment

1. Expose the wound; cut away clothing, if necessary. Secure any impaled objects in place.
2. Assess for the presence of concomitant injuries. The obvious wound is not necessarily the most life-threatening.

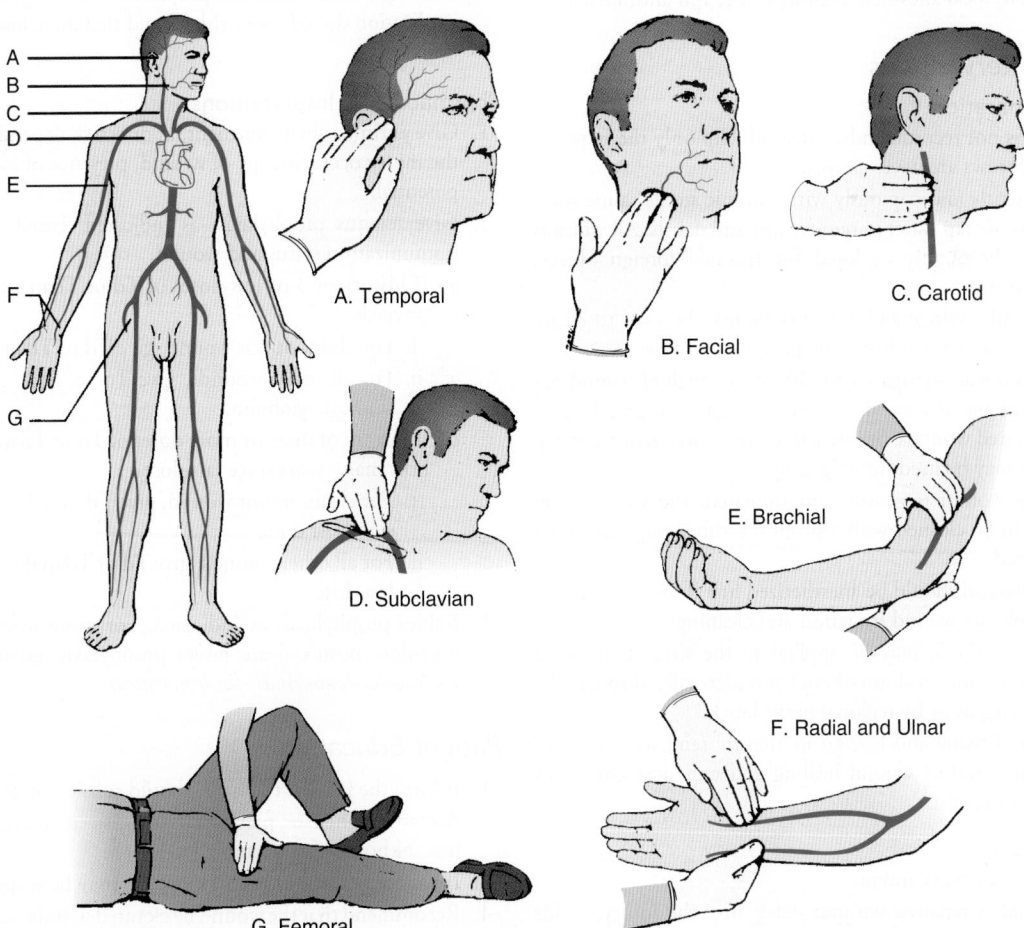

Figure 35-1. Pressure points for control of hemorrhage.

3. Assess vascular status distal to the injury and compare it to the uninjured extremity.
   a. Color of the injured extremity—pallor suggests poor arterial perfusion and cyanosis suggests venous congestion.
   b. Test capillary refill time by depressing the nailbed until it blanches and seeing how long until the nailbed returns to pink. A capillary refill time greater than 2 to 3 seconds suggests decreased capillary perfusion.
   c. Test pulses distal to the injury—generally, they should be full and strong.
4. Perform a neurologic assessment of the injured extremity to determine peripheral nerve insult, possibly caused by direct injury, compression, or edema.
   a. Sensory function—while the patient's eyes are closed, lightly touch the area distal to the injury and ask them to identify the area being touched. Have them discriminate between sharp and dull touch.
   b. Motor function—have patient move extremity distal to the injury.
5. Determine tetanus immunization status.
6. History of the injury, including when and how the wound occurred. Any wound that is more than 6 hours old is considered at high risk for infection and primary closure by suturing may not be an option.
7. Allergies to local anesthesia, epinephrine, and antibiotics.

General Interventions

Wound Preparation
1. Shaving is not recommended; instead, clip only the required area. Eyebrows are never clipped.
2. Irrigate gently and copiously with isotonic sterile saline solution or sterile tap water to remove dirt and debris. All wounds must be thoroughly explored for retained foreign objects before closure.
   a. A 10-mL syringe and 22G needle may be used to create the recommended hydraulic pressure of 13 psi.
   b. General rule—irrigate with 50 mL per inch of wound per hour of age of wound. Use more irrigant for grossly contaminated wounds. Sterile saline, sterile water, or clean tap water may be used for irrigation.
   c. If the wound is grossly contaminated, the wound may need to be cleaned with a surgical scrub sponge and then irrigated.
   d. The wound should be anesthetized first if the patient cannot tolerate wound irrigation and cleaning.
3. Topical anesthetic may be applied to the wound (prior to infiltration with local anesthetic) intradermally through the wound margins or by regional nerve block.
4. Devitalized tissue and foreign matter are removed—devitalized tissue inhibits wound healing and enhances chance of bacterial infection.

Wound Closure
1. Closure by primary intent.
   a. Wound is repaired without delay after the injury; yields the fastest healing.
   b. Primary closure may be with sutures, skin tapes, staples, or tissue adhesives. Location and size of the wound are key factors in determining closure material used.
2. Closure by secondary intent.
   a. Wound is allowed to granulate on its own without surgical closure.
   b. Wound is cleaned and covered with a sterile dressing.
3. Closure by secondary intent with delayed closure.
   a. Wound is cleaned and dressed.
   b. Patient returns in 3 to 4 days for definitive closure.

Wound Dressing
1. Dressing should be applied in three layers.
   a. The first layer is the contact layer. This should consist of a nonabsorbent hydrophilic dressing that will allow exudate to pass through to the second layer without wetting the contact layer. Examples of contact layer dressings are Adaptic, petroleum gauze, and Xeroform gauze.
   b. The second layer is the absorbent layer and is usually constructed of surgical dressing pads or 4 × 4 gauze dressings.
   c. The third layer is the outer wrap that holds the dressing in place. The outer wrap may consist of rolled gauze and tape.
2. There are many different proprietary dressings available for application directly over the wound that are constantly being updated.

Pharmacologic Interventions
1. Give antimicrobial treatment, as directed, depending on how the injury occurred, age of wound, presence of soil, infection potential.
2. Give tetanus prophylaxis, as indicated, based on patient's immunization status and wound.
   a. If history of 3 or less doses of Td or Tdap, consider prophylaxis.
      i. For clean, minor wound, give Td or Tdap.
      ii. For all other wounds, give Td or Tdap plus tetanus immune globulin.
   b. If history of three or more doses of Td or Tdap, determine how many years since last dose.
      i. For clean, minor wound, give Td or Tdap if >10 years since last dose.
      ii. For all other wounds, give Td or Tdap if >5 years since last dose.
3. Rabies prophylaxis, as indicated. For more information on four-dose postexposure rabies prophylaxis, go to *www.cdc.gov/vaccines/pubs/ACIP-list.htm#rabies*.

Patient Education
1. Inform the patient that pain should subside in 24 hours.
2. Acetaminophen or prescribed analgesic to be taken for the first 24 hours after a simple laceration.
3. If pain reappears, a wound infection may be suspected.
4. Recommend that the wound be elevated to limit accumulation of fluid in the wound's interstitial spaces.

a. Elevate extremity for first 48 hours.

b. Sleep with the head elevated if facial lacerations are present.

c. Advise that health care provider be contacted if there is sudden or persistent onset of pain, fever/chills, bleeding, rapid swelling, foul odor, purulent fluid, or redness surrounding the wound.

Injuries to Bones and Joints

Injuries to bones and joints are common. They are usually obvious injuries and may be dramatic in nature. However, rarely are these injuries life-threatening. *Fractures* may be caused by direct trauma (eg, projectiles, crush injuries) or by indirect trauma (ie, bones being pulled apart or rotational forces). In addition, bones may be fractured due to pathologic reasons. A pathologic fracture is due to a weakness in the bone secondary to a disease process such as metastatic cancer. For the classification of fractures, see page 1131.

Other injuries include:

1. Dislocation—complete displacement or separation of a bone from its normal place of articulation. It may be associated with a tearing of the ligaments. The shoulder, elbow, fingers, hips, and ankles are the joints most frequently affected.

2. Subluxation—partial disruption of the articulating surfaces.

3. Sprains—injuries in which ligaments are partially torn or stretched. These types of injuries are usually caused by a twisting of a joint beyond its normal range of motion. The severity can range from mild to severe. The more seriously injured ligaments may resemble a fracture.

4. Strains—stretching or tearing of muscle and tendon fibers. Usually caused by overexertion or overextension.

Primary Assessment

1. Always ensure the adequacy of airway, breathing, and circulation before initiating treatment.

2. Occult blood loss into a closed space from the fracture may be significant enough to produce hypovolemic shock. Death by exsanguination can occur from pelvic and femoral fractures. Estimated blood loss from closed fractures in liters:

a. Tibia—1.5 L

b. Femur—2 L

c. Pelvis—6 L

d. Humerus—2 L

3. A fractured cervical spine, pelvic fracture, or fractured femur may produce life-threatening injuries. Posterior dislocations of the hip are life- and limb-threatening emergencies due to the potential for blood loss and the disruption in blood supply to the head of the femur. Unless this dislocation is promptly reduced, the patient may develop avascular necrosis of the femoral head and subsequently may require a hip replacement.

Primary Interventions

1. Support airway, breathing, and circulation, if compromised.

2. Initiate IV line and treat for shock, if evident.

3. Assess circulation distal to the site of injury. Loss of distal pulses requires immediate intervention.

4. Protect injured part from movement or further trauma. Splinting in the position the patient was found may be helpful if circulation is not compromised.

5. Pain management is essential.

Subsequent Assessment

1. Seek information on the mechanism of injury.

a. How did the injury occur?

b. In what position was the limb after the injury?

c. Did the person fall? How many feet did the person fall? What type of surface did they land on?

d. What was the direction and amount of force? Certain musculoskeletal injuries commonly occur together.

2. Assess for the presence of concomitant injuries.

a. A fractured calcaneus as the result of a fall from a great height may also include a compression fracture of the spine.

b. A person with a fractured patella from a motor vehicle accident may also have a fractured or dislocated femur.

c. A fractured pelvis may occur with lumbosacral spine fractures and bladder injuries.

3. Perform a neurovascular assessment to include the area above and below the injury.

a. Assess for ischemia to the extremity.

i. Pallor suggests poor arterial perfusion.

ii. Cyanosis suggests venous congestion.

iii. A capillary refill time greater than 2 seconds suggests decreased arterial capillary perfusion.

b. Assess neurologic supply of the injured extremity to determine peripheral nerve insult. Damage to a peripheral nerve can be the result of a direct injury, compression, stretching, or edema.

i. Test sensory function—with the patient's eyes closed, lightly touch the area distal to the injury. Ask the patient to identify the area being touched.

ii. Test motor function—have patient move extremity distal to the injury.

iii. Numbness or paralysis indicates pressure on the nerves and may require immediate medical intervention.

4. Examine the bones and joints adjacent to the injury. If there was enough force to produce one injury, there may be other injuries.

5. Signs and symptoms of fractures:

a. Pain and tenderness over the fracture site.

b. A grating or crepitus over the fracture site.

c. Swelling, due to internal bleeding and edema.

d. Deformity, unnatural position, or movement where there is no joint.

e. Loss of use or guarding.

f. Discoloration due to bleeding into the surrounding tissue.

g. Shortening of an extremity or rotation of the extremity.

6. Signs and symptoms of dislocations:
   a. Loss of joint motion—the joint may appear "frozen."
   b. Obvious deformity—lump, ridge, or excavation.
   c. Severe pain.
7. Signs and symptoms of sprains:
   a. Pain in the joint area.
   b. Swelling.
   c. Limited use or movement.
   d. Discoloration.
8. Signs and symptoms of strains:
   a. Pain located in a muscle or its tendon, not a bone or a joint.
   b. Swelling is usually minimal.
9. Closely monitor vital signs.

General Interventions

Interventions for the Severely Injured Patient

1. Ensure adequacy of airway, breathing, and circulation. Begin frequent monitoring.
2. Initiate two IV lines and start volume replacement with lactated Ringer's solution.
3. Immobilize the injury—this will prevent further damage and will help to relieve the pain.
4. Prepare the patient for the operating room for open reduction, closed reduction, internal fixation, or wound care.
5. Antibiotics may be started.

Other Interventions

1. Elevate to prevent or limit swelling.
2. Apply ice packs or cold compresses; ice should not be placed directly on the skin.
3. Cover open fractures with a sterile dressing. If bone is protruding, do not attempt to tuck the ends under the skin. Cover with a sterile dressing.
4. Splint the extremity in as good alignment as possible until definitive care is complete. Immobilize the joint above and below the fracture.
5. Handle the part gently and as little as possible.
6. Pain management may include ice packs, simple or opioid analgesics, nonsteroidal anti-inflammatory drugs, or regional nerve blocks.
7. High-flow oxygen should be administered to patients with pelvic or femoral fractures, compartment syndrome, or signs of shock.

Assess for Compartment Syndrome

1. Increased pressure within an extremity resulting from bleeding and swelling into a closed space, causing pressure on vital structures.
2. The six P's (signs and symptoms) of compartment syndrome are:
   a. Pain—development of a different type of pain, the return of pain after treatment/splinting had caused pain relief, or pain out of proportion to the severity of the injury.
   b. Pallor—deterioration in skin color and an increase in the capillary refill time.
   c. Pulselessness.
   d. Paresthesias.
   e. Paralysis—late sign.
   f. Puffiness—late sign.

NURSING ALERT Compartment syndrome is a limb-threatening event; therefore, if suspected, do not elevate limb above the level of the heart. This may decrease perfusion to the compromised extremity. Emergent fasciotomy is often required.

NURSING ALERT Patients with long bone or pelvic fractures are at risk for developing fat emboli and should be monitored closely.

SHOCK AND INTERNAL INJURIES

Shock

Shock is the common denominator in a wide variety of disease processes that present as an immediate threat to life. Simply defined, *shock* is inadequate tissue perfusion. This inadequate tissue perfusion is the result of failure of one or more of the following: (1) the heart—pump failure, (2) blood volume, (3) arterial resistance vessels, and (4) the capacity of the venous beds. Any condition that significantly affects any of the above may precipitate a shock state. It can be classified as compensated (stable for now) or decompensated (hemodynamically unstable).

Types of shock are:

1. Hypovolemic shock—occurs when a significant amount of fluid is lost from the intravascular space. May result from hemorrhage, burns, GI losses, or fluid shifts.
2. Cardiogenic shock—occurs when the heart fails as a pump. Primary causes of this failure are myocardial infarction (MI), serious cardiac dysrhythmias, and myocardial depression. Secondary causes include mechanical restriction of cardiac function or venous obstruction, such as occurs with cardiac tamponade, vena cava obstruction, or tension pneumothorax.
3. Distributive—occurs as the result of a loss of vascular tone. It may be anaphylactic, septic, neurogenic, or due to an acute adrenal insufficiency. Septic shock may occur with or without an infection. Sepsis is characterized by a systemic inflammatory response in the presence of suspected or confirmed infection. Systemic inflammatory response syndrome (SIRS) is a clinical response to a nonspecific insult such as trauma that provokes an acute inflammatory reaction. See Table 35-1 for defining characteristics of SIRS and sepsis.

Primary Assessment and Interventions

1. Rapid recognition and prompt intervention are essential to increase the chance of survival because a downward spiral of physiologic responses culminating in multiorgan dysfunction syndrome and eventual death will occur if shock is not treated.
2. The initial priorities in the assessment are the same for all types of shock.
   a. Is the airway open?
   b. Is the patient breathing?
   c. Is there a circulation problem?
3. Initiate immediate interventions, as indicated.
   a. Resuscitate as necessary. Fluid replacement with blood products or isotonic fluids is essential.

Table 35-1	Defining Characteristics of Sepsis
SEPTIC CONDITION	**CHARACTERISTIC**
SIRS, two or more of:	Temperature > 100.4° F (38° C) or < 96.8° F (36° C)
	HR > 90 bpm
	RR > 20, arterial CO_2 < 32 mmHg or need for mechanical ventilation
	WBC > 12000/mm³ or < 4000/mm³ or more than 10% immature band forms
Sepsis	SIRS criteria
	Suspected or confirmed infection
Severe sepsis	Serum lactate level > 2 mmol/L
	Hypovolemia responsive to fluid resuscitation
	Signs of tissue hypoperfusion
Septic shock	Profound hypovolemia, hypoxia, and hypoperfusion
	Hypovolemia unresponsive to fluid resuscitation
	Multiple organ failure

bpm, beats per minute; HR, heart rate, RR, respiratory rate, SIRS, systemic inflammatory response syndrome; WBC, white blood cell.

b. Administer oxygen.
c. Start cardiac monitoring.
d. Control hemorrhage or other fluid loss, if present.
4. Pain management is essential.

Subsequent Assessment

1. Assess level of consciousness—important indicator of shock because it reflects cerebral perfusion. Changes may include:
   a. Confusion.
   b. Irritability.
   c. Anxiety.
   d. Agitation.
   e. Inability to concentrate.
2. Watch for increasing lethargy progressing to obtundation and coma, indicating progression of shock.
3. Monitor arterial BP.
   a. If the patient can compensate for the shock state, the BP may initially rise approximately 20%. A significant decrease in BP may not occur until late.
   b. Narrowing pulse pressure—early in shock, the diastolic pressure may rise due to an initial vasoconstriction produced by release of catecholamines from the sympathetic nervous system.
   c. Fall in the systolic pressure—there is no absolute value in BP that indicates a shock state. It is the deviation from

normal that is important. However, it is generally accepted that a systolic pressure below 80 mm Hg or a mean arterial pressure below 60 mm Hg is indicative of shock.
4. Assess pulse quality and rate change.
   a. The rate is usually increased.
   b. Weak, thready pulse due to decreased cardiac output and increased peripheral vascular resistance.
5. Assess urine output.
   a. A decrease in renal blood flow or pressure will result in decreased urine output.
   b. Ideally in an adult, the urine output should be 50 mL/hour. An output of less than 25 mL/hour may indicate shock in a patient without renal dysfunction.
6. Assess capillary perfusion.
   a. Pale, ashen, mottled, cold, and sweaty skin indicates potent vasoconstriction.
   b. Capillary refill greater than 2 seconds indicates vasoconstriction.
7. Also assess for:
   a. Subjective feeling of impending doom.
   b. Metabolic acidosis due to anaerobic metabolism within the cells.
   c. Excessive thirst.

General Interventions

1. Administer 100% O_2 by nonrebreather face mask to maintain the partial pressure of arterial oxygen at 90% to 100%.
2. Assist with intubation if the patient is unable to maintain airway.
3. Fluid resuscitation.
   a. Two large-bore IV lines should be established.
   b. Lactated Ringer's solution is the initial fluid choice. Normal saline is the second choice because hyperchloremic acidosis may develop if massive amount of normal saline is infused.
   c. Rate of infusion depends on severity of blood loss and clinical evidence of hypovolemia.
   d. Packed red blood cells or whole blood are infused when there is hypovolemic shock due to blood loss.
   e. Additional platelets and coagulation factors are given when large amounts of blood are needed because replacement blood is deficient in clotting factors.
   f. Warm the blood (commercial warmer)—massive blood replacement has a cooling effect that can cause cardiac dysrhythmias, paradoxical hypotension, decreased oxyhemoglobin dissociation, or cardiac arrest.
4. Insert an indwelling urinary catheter.
   a. Record urine output every 15 to 30 minutes.
   b. Urinary volume reveals adequacy of kidney and visceral perfusion.
5. Maintain patient in supine position with the legs elevated. (This position is contraindicated in patients with head injuries.)

 NURSING ALERT Trendelenburg's position is no longer recommended because of the potential for respiratory compromise caused by pressure from abdominal organs.

6. ECG monitoring—dysrhythmias may contribute to shock.

7. Maintain ongoing nursing surveillance of total patient—BP, heart rate, respiratory rate, temperature, color, central venous pressure (CVP), ABG levels, urine output, ECG, hematocrit, hemoglobin, coagulation profiles, and electrolytes—to assess patient response to treatment.

8. Immobilize fractures to minimize blood loss.

9. Maintain normothermia.
   a. Too much heat produces vasodilatation, which counteracts the body's compensatory mechanism of vasoconstriction and also increases fluid loss through perspiration.
   b. A patient who is in septic shock should be kept cool because high fever will increase the cellular metabolic effects of shock.

10. Pharmacologic interventions:
   a. Vasopressors may be necessary, but not until volume is replaced.
   b. Antibiotics—broad spectrum for septic shock.

 NURSING ALERT Rapid identification and treatment of SIRS or sepsis is essential in the treatment of septic shock. Although a source of infection may not be identified, signs include fever, tachypnea, tachycardia, and leukocytosis.

Abdominal Injuries

Abdominal injuries account for a large percentage of trauma-related injuries and deaths. The visceral organs contained within the abdomen can be classified as either hollow or solid. Damage to a hollow organ can result in acute peritonitis, leading to shock within a few hours, and damage to a solid organ can result in lethal hemorrhage. Abdominal injuries may be classified as either penetrating or blunt.

Penetrating abdominal injury—usually the result of gunshot wounds or stab wounds. The mechanism that caused the penetrating abdominal trauma may cross the diaphragm and enter the chest. The opposite can also occur.

Blunt abdominal injury—usually caused by motor vehicle accidents or falls. Trauma to the abdomen is commonly associated with extra-abdominal injuries (ie, chest, head, and extremity injuries) and severe concomitant trauma to multiple intraperitoneal organs. Blunt abdominal injury is often associated with delayed complications, especially if there is injury to the liver, spleen, or blood vessels, which can lead to substantial blood loss into the peritoneal cavity.

Primary Assessment and Interventions

1. Assess airway, breathing, and circulation.

2. Initiate resuscitation, as indicated.

3. Control bleeding and prepare to treat shock.

4. If there is an impaled object in the abdomen, leave it there. Stabilize the object in place with bulky dressings along the sides of the object.

Subsequent Assessment

1. Obtain a history of the mechanism of the injury, type of weapon, and estimated amount of blood loss.
   a. If the patient was stabbed, how long was the blade?
   b. Was the person who stabbed the patient a man or a woman?
      i. Men usually hold a knife underhand and stab/thrust upward.
      ii. Women usually will stab/thrust downward with an overhand motion.
   c. If the patient sustained a gunshot wound, attempt to ascertain the type of gun and range at which shot.
   d. Time of onset of symptoms.
   e. Passenger location (driver frequently sustains spleen/liver rupture). Were seat belts worn? Did the airbag deploy? Were there other injured parties or fatalities involved in the same accident?

2. Inspect the abdomen for obvious signs of injury (penetrating injury, bruises).

3. Evaluate for signs and symptoms of hemorrhage—usually accompanies abdominal injury, especially if the liver and spleen have been traumatized.

4. Note tenderness, rebound tenderness, guarding, rigidity, and spasm.
   a. Firmly press, with the whole hand, the area of maximal tenderness (let the patient point to the area).
   b. Remove the fingers quickly to check for rebound tenderness; pain at suspected point indicates peritoneal irritation.

5. Ask about referred pain: Kehr's sign—pain radiating to the left shoulder may be a sign of blood beneath the left diaphragm; pain in right shoulder can result from laceration of liver. The patient must be lying flat for this type of shoulder pain to occur.

6. Look for increasing abdominal distention. Measure abdominal girth at umbilical level early in your assessment—serves as a baseline from which changes can be determined. Making a mark where you measured can also assist in assuring the same place is measured each time.

7. Auscultate—a silent abdomen accompanies peritoneal irritation or ileus. The presence of bowel sounds in the chest indicates a ruptured diaphragm. Bruits over the aorta or other large arteries may indicate disrupted arterial blood flow.

8. Percuss—tympani over solid organs (liver, spleen)—indicates presence of free air; dullness over regions normally containing gas may indicate presence of blood or other fluids.

9. Look for chest injuries, which frequently accompany intra-abdominal injuries.

10. Cullen's sign, a slight bluish discoloration around the navel, is a sign of blood in the abdominal wall. Grey Turner's sign, or flank ecchymosis, is indicative of renal injuries or retroperitoneal bleeding.

11. Pain is a poor indicator of the extent of an abdominal injury. Rebound tenderness and board-like rigidity are indicative of a significant intra-abdominal injury.

12. A rectal examination and examination of the perineum should be done on all patients. The presence of blood may be indicative of trauma.

13. Continually assess vital signs, urine output, CVP readings, hematocrit values, and neurologic status. Tachypnea, tachycardia, and hypotension may be clues to intra-abdominal bleeding.

General Interventions

1. Assess adequacy of airway, breathing, and circulation. Begin frequent monitoring.
2. Goals are to control bleeding, maintain blood volume, and prevent infection.
3. Keep the patient quiet and on the stretcher because movement may fragment or dislodge a clot in a large vessel and produce massive hemorrhage.
4. Cut the clothing away from the wound. Do not cut through bullet holes or stab marks. These will be needed by law enforcement authorities as forensic evidence.
5. Count the number of wounds.
6. Look for entrance and exit wounds.
7. If the patient is comatose, immobilize the cervical spine until after cervical films are taken and cleared.
8. Apply compression to external bleeding.
9. Insert two large-bore IV lines and infuse lactated Ringer's solution. If possible, one of the lines should be in a central venous location.
10. Unless contraindicated by other injuries, insert an NG tube to decompress the abdomen. This will serve to empty the stomach, relieve gastric distention, and facilitate abdominal assessment. In addition, if blood is found, it may indicate stomach injury or esophageal injury.
11. Cover protruding abdominal viscera; do not attempt to replace the protruding organs into the abdomen. Use sterile saline dressings to protect viscera from drying.
12. Cover open wounds with dry dressings.
13. Withhold oral fluids to prevent increased peristalsis and vomiting.
14. Insert an indwelling urethral catheter to ascertain the presence of hematuria and to monitor urine output. If a fracture of the pelvis is suspected, a catheter should not be placed until the integrity of the urethra is ensured.
15. Pharmacologic interventions.
    a. Analgesics.
    b. Tetanus prophylaxis.
    c. Broad-spectrum antibiotics because bacterial contamination is a frequent complication (depending on history and nature of wound).
16. Prepare for focused ultrasound and/or peritoneal lavage when there is uncertainty about intraperitoneal bleeding. See Procedure Guidelines 35-5, page 1220. Focused assessment with sonography in trauma (FAST) is a standard for rapid bedside assessment with ultrasound performed by providers to identify free fluid in the abdomen, pericardium, or peritoneum.
17. Prepare for surgery if the patient shows evidence of unexplained shock, unstable vital signs, peritoneal irritation, bowel protrusion or evisceration, significant penetrating injury, significant GI bleeding, or peritoneal air.
18. Prepare the patient for diagnostic procedures.
    a. Catheterization and urinalysis—as a guide to possible urinary tract injury and to monitor urine output.
    b. Type and cross match and serial hemoglobin and hematocrit levels—their trend reflects presence or absence of bleeding.
    c. Complete blood count (CBC)—white blood cell count is generally elevated with trauma.
    d. Serum amylase elevation usually indicates pancreatic injury or perforations of GI tract.
    e. Computed tomography (CT) scans permit detailed evaluation of abdominal and retroperitoneal injuries.
    f. Abdominal and chest x-rays may reveal free air beneath diaphragm, indicating ruptured hollow viscus.

Multiple Injuries

The patient with multiple injuries requires rapid and definitive interventions during the first hour after the trauma to increase chance of survival; this first hour has been called the "golden hour." During this time, multiple assessments and interventions may be performed simultaneously by the health care team.

Primary Assessment and Interventions

Airway

1. Assume a cervical spine injury and open the airway using the jaw-thrust technique without head tilt.
2. Apply suction to clear the trachea and bronchial tree. Remove debris from mouth (ie, broken teeth, mucus).
3. Insert an oropharyngeal airway—to prevent occlusion by the tongue. Oropharyngeal airways are used in unconscious patients only to prevent stimulation of the gag reflex.
4. Prepare for endotracheal intubation if adequate airway cannot be maintained.
5. If upper airway trauma or edema exists, a cricothyroidotomy may be indicated.

Breathing

1. Note the character and symmetry of chest wall motion and pattern of breathing. Assess for open wounds, deformity, and flail segments.
2. Auscultate the lungs and assess for tracheal deviation. If a tension pneumothorax is present, the trachea will shift away from the injury. Tracheal deviation is a late sign.
3. Ask the conscious patient if experiencing difficulty in breathing or chest pain with breathing.
4. Administer oxygen by 100% nonrebreather mask or assist the patient's ventilations by bag–valve–mask.
5. Suspect serious intrathoracic injuries if respiratory distress continues after adequate airway has been established.
6. Assess the overall effectiveness of ventilations.

Circulation

1. Assess cardiac function and treat cardiac arrest (hypoxia, metabolic acidosis, and chest trauma may precipitate cardiac arrest).
    a. For cardiac arrest, start CPR.
2. Control hemorrhage.
    a. Apply direct pressure over bleeding points, if able.
    b. Expect significant blood loss in patients with fractures to the shaft of the femur, multiple fractures, or pelvic trauma.
    c. Use tourniquet(s) for massive arterial bleeding from extremities that cannot be halted with pressure.
    d. Prepare for immediate surgical intervention if patient is bleeding internally.

PROCEDURE GUIDELINES 35-5

PERITONEAL LAVAGE

Peritoneal lavage is a technique of irrigation of the peritoneal cavity and examination of the irrigating fluid to evaluate the effects of trauma to the abdomen. It is most often used in patients whose injuries are suspicious for internal bleeding and imaging tests are inconclusive or unavailable.

EQUIPMENT

- Peritoneal dialysis tray
- Warm sterile solution (lactated Ringer's solution)
- IV tubing; IV pole
- Peritoneal dialysis catheter (multiple perforations)
- Local skin anesthetic; sterile gloves

PROCEDURE

Nursing Action	Rationale
Preparatory phase	
1. Explain the procedure to the patient; ensure that an informed consent form has been signed.	1. Ensures understanding and cooperation.
2. Insert indwelling catheter into the bladder.	2. Prevents puncture of urinary bladder.
3. Prepare the abdomen as for surgery.	3. Minimizes or eliminates surface bacteria and decrease the possibility of wound contamination and infection.
4. Place the patient in a supine position.	4. Best position to avoid puncture of underlying organs.
5. Prime IV tubing with solution using aseptic technique.	5. Eliminates air from tubing.
Performance phase (by health care provider)	
1. The skin is infiltrated ¾–1¼ inches (2–3 cm) below the umbilicus in the midline with local anesthetic.	1. The midline area is relatively avascular. Epinephrine may be injected with local anesthetic to produce capillary constriction and prevent a false-positive tap.
2. A small vertical incision is made at the chosen site.	2. Accommodates the catheter.
3. Bleeding vessels are carefully ligated.	3. Ligation of vessels helps avoid a false-positive lavage.
4. The peritoneum is opened under direct vision and the peritoneal catheter is inserted into the peritoneal cavity, *or*	4. Open or percutaneous methods may be used to introduce the catheter into the peritoneal space.
5. A needle is passed intra-abdominally, a flexible wire is passed through the needle, and a catheter is guided over the wire.	5. Needle insertion eliminates need for incision.
6. A syringe is attached to the catheter and the peritoneal cavity is aspirated. If more than 10 mL of blood is obtained or the fluid contains bile, feces, or particulate matter, the test is considered positive and the patient is prepared for immediate laparotomy.	6. Indicates intra-abdominal bleeding and possible injury to organs.
7. If no blood (or less than 10 mL) is present, the catheter is attached to the IV tubing; 500–1,000 mL of solution is infused into the peritoneal cavity through the IV tubing attached to the dialysis catheter.	7. If not contraindicated by condition, the patient may be turned from side to side to ensure that the solution reaches all parts of the abdominal cavity.

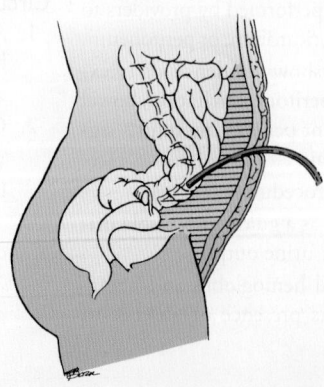

Peritoneal lavage.

PROCEDURE GUIDELINES 35-5 (continued)

PERITONEAL LAVAGE

PROCEDURE (continued)

Nursing Action	Rationale
8. After the solution is infused, the empty IV bag is removed from the pole and lowered below the abdominal level (near the floor).	8. Lowering the bag creates a siphon effect to drain the excess fluid. As much of the fluid as possible is siphoned out of the peritoneal cavity by gravity.
9. The peritoneal dialysis catheter is removed and the wound is closed (unless laparotomy is necessary).	9. Prevents infection.
10. The fluid recovered from the peritoneal cavity is examined visually and is usually sent to the laboratory for cell counts and microscopic inspection of spun-down sediment.	10. Detects occult bleeding or rupture organs such as liver or intestine.

Interpretation of lavage fluid

1. Clear fluid indicates a lack of significant intraperitoneal bleeding.	1. Indicates a negative test.
2. Criteria for positive results: • Aspiration of free blood from peritoneal cavity. • Red blood cells > 100,000 per mm³. • Presence of bile, bacteria, or fecal or food particles in lavage fluid.	2. If the test is positive, and the patient is hemodynamically unstable, a laparotomy is usually done. The hemodynamically stable patient may have injuries manageable with interventional radiology. Indeterminate or equivocal results merit monitoring and further investigation.

Follow-up phase

1. Assess the patient for complications.	1. Complications include visceral perforation, wound hematoma, perforated bowel, puncture of bladder, laceration of major vessels and infection.
2. Watch the patient closely for any signs of deterioration, such as change in vital signs, increasing pain, or altered mental status.	2. Repeated physical examinations of the abdomen should be performed when intra-abdominal injury is suspected.

3. Palpate the carotid pulse and note its rate and quality. In addition, assess the femoral and radial pulses to determine an approximate systolic pressure.
   a. If the carotid pulse is present, the systolic pressure is at least 60 mm Hg.
   b. If the femoral pulse is present, the systolic pressure is at least 70 mm Hg.
   c. If the radial pulse is present, the systolic pressure is at least 80 mm Hg.
4. Prevent and treat hypovolemic shock.
   a. Insert at least two (sometimes four) IV lines.
   b. Initiate a central venous catheter to monitor the patient's response to fluid infusion—to prevent fluid overload and as a route for fluid infusion.
   c. Fluid resuscitation—lactated Ringer's solution or normal saline is given for volume replacement until blood is available.
   d. Administer blood—massive transfusions have a cooling effect that can cause cardiac irritability and arrest; blood should be warmed.

5. Note presence or absence of pulses in fractured extremities.

Neurologic
1. Assess level of responsiveness, pupil size and reactivity, strength, and reflexes.
2. Determine a Glasgow Coma Score as a baseline (see page 483).
3. If signs of increased ICP exist, ICP monitoring may be instituted.
4. Agitation or other mental status changes are often the first sign of impending problems.

Subsequent Assessment and Interventions
1. The goals are rapid determination of the extent of the injuries and treatment prioritization.
2. Monitor ECG—to detect life-threatening dysrhythmias.
3. Insert indwelling urethral catheter and monitor urine output to aid in diagnosis of shock as well as monitor effectiveness of therapy. Do not force the catheter—the patient may have a ruptured urethra.

4. Perform an ongoing clinical evaluation to observe for improvement or deterioration, such as changes in vital signs, improvement in level of responsiveness, skin warmth, and speed of capillary filling.

5. Prepare for immediate surgical intervention if the patient does not respond to fluids or blood. Inability to restore BP and circulatory volume in the patient usually indicates major internal bleeding.

6. Splint fractures to prevent further trauma to soft tissues and blood vessels and to relieve pain.

7. Examine the patient for abdominal pain, rigidity, tenderness, rebound tenderness, diminished bowel sounds, hypotension, and shock.

8. Prepare for peritoneal lavage, FAST exam, or CT scan to assess for intraperitoneal bleeding.

9. Draw blood for laboratory studies (type and cross matching, hemoglobin, hematocrit, baseline CBC, electrolytes, blood urea nitrogen [BUN], glucose, coagulation studies).

10. Insert an NG tube to prevent vomiting and aspiration.

11. Prepare for laparotomy if the patient shows continuing signs of hemorrhage and deterioration.

12. Continue to monitor urine output every 30 minutes—reflects cardiac output and state of perfusion of vital organs.

13. Assess for hematuria and oliguria.

14. Evaluate the patient for other injuries and institute appropriate treatment, including tetanus immunization.

15. Perform a more thorough physical examination after resuscitation and management of the aforementioned priorities.

ENVIRONMENTAL EMERGENCIES

Heat Exhaustion

Heat exhaustion is the inadequacy or the collapse of peripheral circulation due to volume and electrolyte depletion. Heat exhaustion is one condition in the spectrum of heat-related illnesses, including heat rash, heat edema, heat cramps, and heat syncope. Untreated heat exhaustion may progress to heatstroke.

Primary Assessment and Interventions

1. Expect the patient to be alert without significant cardiorespiratory or neurologic compromise.

2. If vital functions are significantly impaired, suspect secondary condition, such as MI or stroke.

Subsequent Assessment

1. Obtain history of headache, fatigue, dizziness, muscle cramping, and nausea.

2. Inspect skin—usually pale, ashen, and moist.

3. The temperature may be normal, slightly elevated, or as high as 104° F (40° C).

4. Measure vital signs for hypotension, orthostatic changes, tachycardia, and tachypnea.

5. The patient will be awake but may give a history of syncope or confusion.

6. Laboratory analysis will show hemoconcentration and hyponatremia (if sodium depletion is the primary problem) or hypernatremia (if water depletion is the primary problem).

7. The ECG may show dysrhythmias without evidence of infarction.

General Interventions

1. Move the patient to a cool environment and remove all clothing.

2. Position the patient supine with feet slightly elevated.

3. If the patient complains of nausea or vomiting, do not give fluids by mouth.

4. Start an IV line with normal saline until electrolyte results are confirmed.

5. Monitor the patient for changes in the cardiac rhythm and vital signs. Vital signs should be taken at least every 15 minutes until the patient is stable.

6. Provide fans and cool sponge baths as cooling methods.

7. Provide patient education.

   a. Advise the patient to avoid immediate reexposure to high temperatures; the patient may remain hypersensitive to high temperatures for a considerable length of time.

   b. Emphasize the importance of maintaining an adequate fluid intake, wearing loose clothing, and reducing activity in hot weather.

   c. Athletes should monitor fluid losses, replace fluids, and use a gradual approach to physical conditioning, allowing sufficient time for acclimatization.

 NURSING ALERT Identify those at increased risk for heat exhaustion and heatstroke so preventive measures can be taken. Risk factors include such underlying conditions as cardiovascular disease, alcohol abuse, malnutrition, diabetes, skin diseases, and major burn scarring; very young or very old age; drugs such as anticholinergics, phenothiazines, diuretics, antihistamines, antidepressants, and beta-adrenergic blockers; and such behaviors as working outdoors, wearing inappropriate clothing, inadequate fluid intake, and living in poor environmental conditions.

Heatstroke

Heatstroke is a medical emergency that can result in significant morbidity and mortality. It is defined as the combination of hyperpyrexia greater than 104° F (40° C) and neurologic symptoms. It is caused by a shutdown or failure of the heat-regulating mechanisms of the body. It can be classified as exertional or nonexertional.

Primary Assessment and Interventions

1. Assess airway, breathing, and circulation.

2. LOC may be altered.

3. Expect to intervene immediately if cardiovascular collapse occurs.

Subsequent Assessment

1. Obtain a history from accompanying person about environmental conditions, activity, underlying health, and medications that may have contributed to heatstroke.
2. Perform a neurologic assessment.
   a. Initially, the patient may exhibit bizarre behavior or irritability. This may progress to confusion, combativeness, deliriousness, and coma.
   b. Other central nervous system (CNS) disturbances include tremors, seizures, fixed and dilated pupils, and decerebrate or decorticate posturing.
3. Assess vital signs.
   a. Temperature greater than 104° F (40° C).
   b. Hypotension.
   c. Rapid pulse; may be bounding or weak.
   d. Rapid respirations.
4. The skin may appear flushed and hot; in early heatstroke, the skin may be moist, but, as the heatstroke progresses, the skin will become dry as the body loses its ability to sweat.
5. ABGs show metabolic acidosis.

General Interventions

 NURSING ALERT When the diagnosis of heatstroke is made or suspected, it is imperative to reduce the patient's temperature.

1. Protect the airway in patients with deteriorating mental status or absent gag reflex.
2. Provide cooling measures.
   a. Reduce the core (internal) temperature to 102° F (38.9° C) as rapidly as possible.
   b. Evaporative cooling is the most efficient. Spray tepid water on the skin while electric fans are used to blow continuously over the patient to augment heat dissipation.
   c. Apply ice packs to neck, groin, axillae, and scalp (areas of maximal heat transfer).
   d. Soak sheets/towels in ice water and place on patient, using fans to accelerate evaporation/cooling rate.
   e. Immersion in cold water is contraindicated.
   f. If the temperature fails to decrease, initiate core cooling: iced saline gastric lavage, cool fluid peritoneal dialysis, cool fluid bladder irrigation, or cool fluid chest irrigation.
   g. Cooling blankets may be used after temperature is stabilized.
   h. Discontinue active cooling when the temperature reaches 102° F (38.9° C). In most cases, this will reduce the chance of overcooling because the body temperature will continue to fall after cessation of cooling.
3. Oxygenate patient to supply tissue needs that are exaggerated by the hypermetabolic condition: 100% nonrebreather mask or intubate the patient, if necessary, to support a failing cardiorespiratory system.
4. Monitor condition.
   a. Monitor and record the core temperature continually during cooling process to avoid hypothermia; also, hyperthermia may recur spontaneously within 3 to 4 hours.
   b. Monitor the vital signs continuously, including ECG, CVP, BP, pulse, and respiratory rate.
   c. Perform frequent (every 30 minutes) neurologic assessments.
   d. Monitor lab values for signs of coagulopathy, liver or renal damage.
5. Replace fluids.
   a. Start IV infusion using normal saline solution to replace fluid losses, maintain adequate circulation, and facilitate cooling.
   b. At least one IV line should be a central line.
   c. Fluid replacement is based on the patient's response and laboratory results.

 GERONTOLOGIC ALERT Vigorous fluid replacement in older adults or those with underlying cardiovascular disease may cause pulmonary edema.

6. Other measures:
   a. Dialysis for renal failure.
   b. Diuretics, such as mannitol, to promote diuresis.
   c. Anticonvulsant agents to control seizures.
   d. Potassium for hypokalemia and sodium bicarbonate to correct metabolic acidosis, depending on laboratory results.
   e. Antipyretics are not useful in treating heatstroke. They may contribute to the complications of coagulopathy and hepatic damage.
   f. Intense shivering may be controlled by diazepam. Shivering will generate heat and increase the metabolic rate.
   g. Patients with depleted clotting factors may be treated with platelets or fresh frozen plasma.
7. Insert an indwelling catheter with a urometer and measure urine output at least hourly—acute tubular necrosis is a complication of heatstroke.
8. Perform continuous ECG monitoring and frequent cardiovascular assessments for possible ischemia, infarction, and dysrhythmias.
9. Perform serial laboratory testing (coagulation studies, electrolytes, glucose, and serum enzymes).
10. The patient should be admitted to an intensive care unit (ICU); complications can occur, including heart failure, cardiovascular collapse, hepatic failure, renal failure, disseminated intravascular coagulation, and rhabdomyolysis.
11. Monitor the patient for the development of seizures and provide for a safe environment in case of seizures.

Frostbite

Frostbite is trauma due to exposure to freezing temperatures that cause actual freezing of the tissue fluids in the cell and intracellular spaces, resulting in vascular damage. The areas of the body most likely to develop frostbite are the earlobes, cheeks, nose, fingers, and toes. Frostbite may be classified as frostnip (initial response to cold, reversible), superficial frostbite, and deep frostbite.

Primary Assessment and Interventions

1. Assess airway, breathing, and circulation.
2. Deficits may indicate coexisting hypothermia or underlying condition.
3. Protect frostbitten tissue while performing other interventions.

Subsequent Assessment

Frostnip
1. History of gradual onset.
2. Skin appears pale.
3. Complaints of numbness or tingling.

Superficial Frostbite
1. Damage is limited to the skin and subcutaneous tissue.
2. The skin will appear white and waxy.
3. On palpation, the skin will feel stiff but the underlying tissue will be pliable, soft, and have its normal "bounce."
4. Sensation is absent.

Deep Frostbite
1. Skin will appear white, yellow-white, or mottled blue-white.
2. On palpation, the surface will feel frozen and the underlying tissue will feel frozen and hard.
3. The affected part is completely insensitive to touch.

General Interventions

1. Frostnip may be treated by placing a warm hand over the chilled area.
2. Leave the frostbitten area alone until definitive rewarming is undertaken. Pad the extremity to prevent damage from trauma.

 NURSING ALERT When definitive rewarming of a frostbitten extremity has started, it must not be stopped. Refreezing of a partially thawed extremity reverses ice crystal formation in tissues and increases tissue damage and loss.

3. Handle the part gently to avoid further mechanical injury.
4. Remove all constricting clothing that can impair circulation, including watchbands and rings.
5. Rewarming:
   a. Rewarm the extremity by controlled and rapid rewarming. Rewarm with a temperature of 98.6° F to 104° F (37° C to 40° C) in a fairly large, tepid water bath where the part can be fully immersed without touching the side or bottom. If clothing, socks, or gloves are frozen to the extremity, they should be left on and removed after rewarming.
   b. More warm water may be added to the container by removing some cooled water and adding warm water.
   c. Slow rewarming is less effective and may increase tissue damage.
   d. Dry heat is not recommended for rewarming.
   e. The rewarming procedure may take 20 to 30 minutes.
   f. Rewarming is complete when the area is warm to the touch and pink or flushed.
   g. Do not rub or massage a frostbitten extremity. The ice crystals in the tissue will lacerate delicate tissue.
6. Pharmacologic interventions:
   a. Opioids or nonsteroidals for pain control.
   b. Antibiotics if there is an open wound.
   c. Tetanus prophylaxis.

Post-Rewarming Care

1. Protect the thawed part from infection. Large blisters may develop in 1 hour to a few days after rewarming; these blisters should not be broken. If necessary, fluid may be aspirated from the blister with a needle.
2. Place sterile gauze or cotton between affected fingers/toes to absorb moisture.
3. Use strict sterile technique during dressing changes. Frostbite injuries make the patient susceptible to infection. Make sure any dressings are loosely applied.
4. Elevate the part to help control swelling.
5. Use a foot cradle to prevent contact with bedding if the feet are involved—prevent further tissue injury.
6. Perform a physical assessment to look for concomitant injury (soft tissue injury, dehydration, alcohol coma, fat embolism due to fracture, immobility).
7. Restore electrolyte balance; dehydration and hypovolemia are common in frostbite victims.
8. Whirlpool bath for the affected extremity—to aid circulation, debride dead tissue and help prevent infection.
9. Escharotomy (incision through the eschar)—to prevent further tissue damage, allow for normal circulation, and permit joint motion.
10. Fasciotomy (incision in fascia to release pressure on the muscles, nerves, blood vessels)—to treat compartment syndrome.
11. Encourage hourly active motion of the affected digits to promote maximum restoration of function and to prevent contractures.
12. Advise patient not to use tobacco because of the vasoconstrictive effects of nicotine, which further reduce the already deficient blood supply to injured tissues.
13. Perform serial laboratory testing (urinalysis, electrolytes and serum enzymes) to monitor for the complications of rhabdomyolysis and subsequent renal failure.

Hypothermia

Hypothermia is a condition in which the core (internal) temperature of the body is less than 95° F (35° C) as a result of exposure to cold or a loss of thermoregulation. In response to a decreased core temperature, the body will attempt to produce or conserve more heat by (1) shivering, which produces heat through muscular activity; (2) peripheral vasoconstriction, to decrease heat loss; and (3) raising the basal metabolic rate. Hypothermia may be classified as mild, moderate, or severe.

 GERONTOLOGIC ALERT Older patients are at greater risk for hypothermia due to altered compensatory mechanisms.

Primary Assessment and Interventions

 NURSING ALERT Extreme caution should be used in moving or transporting hypothermia patients because of the increased risk of cardiac arrhythmias.

1. Assess airway and breathing.
   a. Spontaneous respirations may be extremely slow and imperceptible.
   b. Assist breathing and oxygenation with supplemental oxygen at 100% or a bag–valve–mask device.
   c. If intubation is necessary, extreme caution should be used because ventricular fibrillation may be precipitated.
2. Assess circulation.
   a. If the body temperature falls below 86° F (30° C), the heart sounds may not be audible even if the heart is still beating. Tissues conduct sound poorly at low temperatures.
   b. BP readings may be extremely difficult to hear because cold tissue conducts sound waves poorly.
   c. Pupil reflexes may be blocked by a decrease in cerebral blood flow, so the pupils may appear fixed and dilated.
   d. A patient with severe hypothermia may present like a patient in cardiac arrest with fixed dilated pupils, no pulse or perfusing rhythm, and no BP. If there is any doubt about whether a pulse is present, begin CPR.

Subsequent Assessment

1. There is progressive deterioration marked by apathy, poor judgment, ataxia, dysarthria, drowsiness and, eventually, coma.
2. Speech is slow and may be slurred.
3. Shivering may be suppressed below a temperature of 90° F (32.2° C).
4. Cardiac dysrhythmias—cold disrupts the conduction system of the heart and a variety of dysrhythmias may be seen. A hypothermic heart is extremely susceptible to conduction delays. Ventricular fibrillation may occur if the temperature falls below 81° F (25° C). Patients with core temperatures below 86° F (30° C) do not respond to drugs or defibrillation.
5. The heartbeat and the BP may be so weak that the peripheral pulsations become undetectable. Always check a central pulse.
6. Urine output may increase in response to peripheral vasoconstriction—cold diuresis.
7. Initial tachypnea is usually followed by slow and shallow respirations, possibly two or three per minute in severe hypothermia.

General Interventions

The goal is to rewarm without precipitating cardiac dysrhythmias.

Supportive Measures

1. Handle the patient carefully and gently—to avoid triggering arrhythmias.
2. Continuously monitor core temperatures with a low-reading rectal thermometer.
3. Continuously monitor ECG and central pulses. Loss of a central pulse indicates a nonperfusing rhythm and the need for immediate CPR and ACLS interventions

4. Monitor the patient's condition through vital signs, CVP, urine output, ABG values, and blood chemistry determinations.
5. Maintain an arterial line for recording BP and to facilitate blood sampling—allows rapid detection of acid–base disturbances and assessment of adequacy of ventilation and oxygenation.
6. Start IV therapy with warmed normal saline. Lactated Ringer's solution is not recommended because the cold liver may not be able to metabolize the lactate.

Rewarming Techniques

The type of rewarming depends on the degree of hypothermia. Rewarming should continue until the core temperature is 93.2° F (34° C). Death in hypothermia is defined as a failure to revive after rewarming.

1. Passive external rewarming (mild hypothermia).
   a. Remove all the wet or cold clothing and replace with warm clothing.
   b. Provide insulation by wrapping the patient in several blankets.
   c. Provide warmed fluids to drink.
   d. Disadvantage: slow process.
2. Active external rewarming (moderate to severe hypothermia or hemodynamic instability).
   a. Provide external heat for the patient—warm hot water bottles to the armpits, neck, or groin. (Do not apply hot water bottles directly to the skin.)
   b. Warm water immersion.
   c. Disadvantages:
      i. Causes peripheral vasodilation, returning cool blood to the core, causing an initial lowering of the core temperature.
      ii. Acidosis due to the "washing out" of lactic acid from the peripheral tissues.
      iii. An increase in the metabolic demands before the heart is warmed to meet these needs.
      iv. A combination of active external rewarming and active core rewarming can be used to minimize rewarming shock.
3. Active core rewarming (severe hypothermia <82.4° F [<28° C]).
   a. Inhalation of warmed, humidified oxygen by mask or ventilator.
   b. Warmed IV fluids.
   c. Peritoneal dialysis with warmed standard dialysis solution.
   d. Mediastinal irrigation through open thoracotomy has been used successfully but has serious complications.
   e. Cardiopulmonary bypass.
   f. Disadvantage: invasiveness of the procedures.

TOXICOLOGIC EMERGENCIES

Toxicology is the study of the harmful effect of various substances on the body. Toxins are substances that are harmful to the body no matter how much or in what manner they enter the body. Drugs become toxic when they are taken in excess quantities or manners that are not therapeutic. Alcohol is considered a drug.

The treatment goals of toxicological emergencies are first, to support, and second, to prevent or minimize absorption; third, to provide an antidote.

Ingested Poisons

Ingested poisons can produce immediate or delayed effects. Immediate injury is caused when the poison is caustic to the body tissues (ie, a strong acid or a strong alkali). Other ingested poisons must be absorbed into the bloodstream before they become harmful. Ingested poisoning may be accidental or intentional.

Primary Assessment and Interventions

1. Maintain an open airway—some ingested substances may cause soft tissue swelling of the airway.
2. Attain control of the airway, ventilation, and oxygenation; in the absence of cerebral or renal damage, the patient's prognosis depends largely on successful management and support of vital functions.

Subsequent Assessment

1. Identify the poison.
   a. Try to determine the product taken: where, when, why, how much, who witnessed the event, time since ingestion. Histories obtained from the patient are often inaccurate and should be confirmed if at all possible.
   b. Always contact the local poison control center for assistance in identifying the toxin, if unknown; treatment recommendations; and antidote information. In the United States, local poison control centers can all be reached by calling (800) 222-1222.
2. Continue the focused assessment, observing any significant deviations from normal. Different poisons will affect the body in different ways.
3. Obtain blood and urine tests for toxicology screening. Gastric contents may also be sent for toxicology screening in serious ingestions.
4. Monitor neurologic status, including mentation; monitor the course of vital signs and neurologic status over time.
5. Monitor for fluid and electrolyte imbalance.

General Interventions
Supportive Care
1. Assess and protect the patient's airway, as needed.
2. Administer oxygen and assist ventilations, as needed.
3. Monitor and treat shock.
4. Insert two large-bore IV lines.
5. Give supportive care to maintain vital organ systems.
6. Insert an indwelling urinary catheter to monitor renal function.
7. Support the patient having seizures; many poisons excite the CNS or the patient may convulse from oxygen deprivation.
8. Monitor and treat for complications: hypotension, coma, cardiac dysrhythmias, and seizures.
9. Psychiatric evaluations should be done after the patient is stabilized.

Minimizing Absorption
1. The primary method for preventing or minimizing absorption is to administer activated charcoal. Newer super-activated charcoals can reduce absorption of a toxic substance by as much as 50%. Administering activated charcoal alone is recommended. Insertion of a large-bore orogastric tube and gastric lavage are no longer recommended. The routine use of a cathartic in combination with activated charcoal is also no longer recommended.
   a. Administration of premixed oral-activated charcoal adsorbs the poison on the surface of its particles and allows it to pass with the stool. Multiple doses may be administered.
   b. A routine NG tube may be inserted to facilitate emptying of stomach contents (without lavage) within 30 minutes of ingestion or to instill charcoal if the patient is unable to drink the mixture.

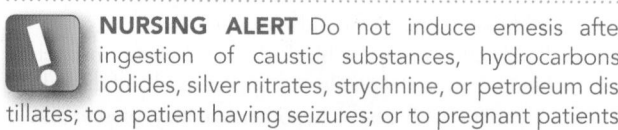

NURSING ALERT Do not induce emesis after ingestion of caustic substances, hydrocarbons, iodides, silver nitrates, strychnine, or petroleum distillates; to a patient having seizures; or to pregnant patients.

2. Gastric lavage is contraindicated due to poor outcomes and complications.
3. Procedures to enhance the removal of the ingested substance if the patient is deteriorating.
   a. Forced diuresis with urine pH alteration—to enhance renal clearance.
   b. Hemoperfusion (process of passing blood through an extracorporeal circuit and a cartridge containing an adsorbent, such as charcoal, after which the detoxified blood is returned to patient).
   c. Hemodialysis—used in selected patients to purify blood and accelerate the elimination of circulating toxins.
   d. Repeated doses of charcoal—for binding nonabsorbed drugs/toxins.

Providing an Antidote
1. An antidote is a chemical or physiologic antagonist that will neutralize the poison.
2. Administer the specific antidote as early as possible to reverse or diminish effects of the toxin.
3. Repeated antidote doses may be necessary.

Carbon Monoxide Poisoning

Carbon monoxide poisoning is an example of an inhaled poison and is the result of the inhalation of the products of incomplete hydrocarbon combustion. It may occur as an industrial or household accident or as an attempted suicide. Carbon monoxide exerts its toxic effect by binding to circulating hemoglobin to reduce the oxygen-carrying capacity of the blood. The affinity between carbon monoxide and hemoglobin is 200 to 250 times that between oxygen and hemoglobin. (Carbon monoxide combines with hemoglobin to form carboxyhemoglobin.) As a result, tissue anoxia occurs.

Primary Assessment

1. Assess airway and breathing. Assist with ventilations, as needed.
   a. Respiratory depression may be present.
   b. If the carbon monoxide poisoning is due to smoke inhalation, stridor (indicative of laryngeal edema due to thermal injury) may be present. Check for soot on the back of hard palate or pharynx if smoke inhalation is suspected.

Primary Interventions

1. Provide 100% oxygen by tight-fitting mask. (The elimination half-life of carboxyhemoglobin, in serum, for a person breathing room air is 5 hours, 20 minutes. If the patient breathes 100% oxygen, the half-life is reduced to 80 minutes; 100% oxygen in a hyperbaric chamber will reduce the half-life to 23 minutes [treatment of choice].)
2. Intubate, if necessary, to protect the airway.

Subsequent Assessment

1. A thorough history is important: determine the type and length of exposure as well as possible other fumes inhaled. An underlying anemia, cardiac disease, or pulmonary disease may place a person at higher risk.
2. Determine LOC—the patient may appear intoxicated from cerebral hypoxia; confusion may progress rapidly to coma.
3. Assess complaints of headache, muscular weakness, palpitation, dizziness.
4. Inspect skin: may be pink, cherry red, or cyanotic and pale—skin color is not a reliable sign.
5. Monitor vital signs: increased respiratory and pulse rates are generally present. Be alert for altered breathing patterns and respiratory failure.
6. Listen for rales or wheezes in the lungs (with smoke inhalation, indicates acute respiratory distress syndrome).
7. Obtain arterial blood samples for carboxyhemoglobin levels.
   a. Normal levels for a nonsmoking patient are less than 3%. For a patient who smokes one to two packs per day, 4% to 5% and two or more packs per day, 8% to 10%.
   b. Toxic concentrations are considered to be greater than 20%.

General Interventions

1. History of exposure to carbon monoxide justifies immediate treatment.
2. Goals are to reverse cerebral and myocardial hypoxia and hasten carbon monoxide elimination.
3. Give 100% oxygen at atmospheric or hyperbaric pressures to reverse hypoxia and accelerate elimination of carbon monoxide. Patients should receive hyperbaric oxygen for CNS or cardiovascular system dysfunction.
4. Use continuous ECG monitoring, treat dysrhythmias, and correct acid-base and electrolyte abnormalities.
5. Observe the patient constantly—psychoses, spastic paralysis, vision disturbances, and deterioration of personality may persist after resuscitation and may be symptoms of permanent CNS damage.

Insect Stings

Insect stings or bites are injected poisons that can produce either local or systemic reactions. Local reactions are characterized by pain, erythema, and edema at the site of injury. Systemic reactions usually begin within minutes and produce mild to severe and life-threatening reactions.

Primary Assessment and Interventions

1. Assess airway, breathing, and circulation.
2. Anaphylactic reactions may produce unconsciousness, laryngeal edema, and cardiovascular collapse.
3. Epinephrine is the drug of choice—the amount and route depend on the severity of the reaction.
4. Administer a bronchodilator to help relieve the bronchospasm.
5. Initiate an IV line with lactated Ringer's solution.
6. Prepare for CPR.

Subsequent Assessment

1. Obtain history of insect sting, previous exposure, and allergies.
2. Inspect skin for local reaction—erythema, edema, pain at site of injury—as well as generalized pruritus, urticaria, and angioedema.
3. Continue to monitor BP and respiratory status for dyspnea, wheezing, and stridor.

General Interventions

1. Apply ice packs to site to relieve pain.
2. Elevate extremity with large edematous local reaction.
3. Administer oral antihistamine for local reactions.
4. Clean the wound thoroughly with soap and water or an antiseptic solution.
5. Administer tetanus prophylaxis if not up to date.
6. Provide patient education.
   a. Always have epinephrine on hand.
   b. Wear medical emergency bracelets indicating hypersensitivity.
   c. Instructions when sting occurs:
      i. Take epinephrine immediately if stung.
      ii. Remove stinger with one quick scrape of fingernail.
      iii. Do not squeeze venom sac because this may cause additional venom to be injected.
      iv. Report to nearest health care facility for observation.
   d. Avoid exposure and become desensitized.
      i. Avoid locales with stinging insects (camp and picnic sites).
      ii. Stay away from insect feeding areas—flower beds, ripe fruit orchards, garbage, fields of clover.
      iii. Avoid going barefoot outdoors—yellow jackets may nest on ground.
      iv. Avoid perfumes, scented soaps, and bright colors—attract bees.
      v. Keep car windows closed.
      vi. Spray garbage cans with rapid-acting insecticide and keep areas meticulously clean.

Snakebites

The majority of snakes in the United States are not poisonous. The poisonous varieties are pit vipers (rattlesnakes and copperheads) and coral snakes. Bites by these snakes may result in envenomation, an injected poisoning. Other parts of the world have many snakes capable of lethal bites. Snakebites can cause neurotoxic muscle paralysis, coagulopathy, and hemolysis. Therefore, knowledge of snakes indigenous to your area is important for swift and appropriate treatment.

Primary Assessment and Interventions

1. Assess airway, breathing, and circulation.
2. Severe envenomation may lead to neurotoxicity with respiratory paralysis, shock, coma, and death.
3. Be prepared to resuscitate and provide advanced life support.

Subsequent Assessment

1. Get a description of the snake, the time of the snakebite, and the location of the bite. Bites to the head and trunk may progress more rapidly and be more severe.
   a. Pit vipers have triangular heads, vertical pupils, indentations between the eyes and nostrils, and long fangs.
   b. Coral snakes are small and brightly colored, with short fangs and teeth behind them and a series of bands of yellow, red, yellow, and black (in that order).
   c. Venom detection kits are available in some areas of the world such as Australia where venomous snakes are not uncommon. Specific antivenom may be available.
2. Assess for local reactions—burning, pain, swelling, and numbness at the site. Local reactions to coral snakebites may be delayed by several hours and may be very mild.
3. A few hours after the bite, hemorrhagic blisters may occur at the site and the entire extremity may become edematous.
4. Watch for signs of systemic reactions, including nausea, sweating, weakness, light-headedness, initial euphoria followed by drowsiness, difficulty in swallowing, paralysis of various muscle groups, signs of shock, seizures, and coma.
5. Monitor vital signs closely because tachycardia or bradycardia may develop.

> **NURSING ALERT** Patients will, on occasion, bring the snake that bit them into the Emergency Department for identification. Even dead, a snake can reflexively bite for several hours. Caution should be used to avoid becoming a second victim.

General Interventions

1. Keep the patient calm and at rest in a recumbent position with the affected extremity immobilized. Remove jewelry or other constricting items, as the area may become edematous.
2. Administer oxygen.
3. Start an IV line with normal saline or lactated Ringer's solution.
4. Administer antivenin and be alert to allergic reaction.

5. Administer vasopressors in the treatment of shock.
6. Monitor for bleeding and administer blood products for coagulopathy.

Drug Intoxication

Substance abuse includes the use of specific substances that are intended to alter mood or behavior.

Drug abuse is the use of drugs for other than legitimate medical purposes. There is a growing tendency among drug users to take a variety of drugs simultaneously (polydrug abuse), including alcohol, sedatives, hypnotics, and marijuana, which may have addictive effects. The clinical manifestations may vary with the drug used (see Table 35-2), but the underlying principles of management are essentially the same.

Overdose refers to the toxic effects that occur when a drug is taken in a larger-than-normal dose.

Primary Assessment and Interventions

1. Assess airway, breathing, and circulation.
2. Attain control of the airway, ventilation, and oxygenation.
3. Intubate and provide assisted ventilation in patients with severe respiratory depression or in patients lacking gag or cough reflexes. If possible, intubation should be held off until a trial dose of naloxone is given.
4. Begin CPR in the absence of pulse.

Subsequent Assessment

1. Do a thorough physical examination to rule out insulin shock, meningitis, head injury, stroke, or trauma.
2. If the patient is unconscious, consider all possible causes of loss of consciousness.
3. Monitor LOC continuously.
4. Monitor vital signs frequently—some drugs will cause depressed vital signs; others will elevate the vital signs.
5. Monitor the pupils: extreme miosis (pinpoint pupils) may indicate opioid overdose.
6. Look for needle marks and external evidence of trauma.
7. Perform a rapid neurologic survey: level of responsiveness, pupil size and reactivity, reflexes, and focal neurologic findings; these can all give clues for identifying the drug taken.
8. Keep in mind that many drug abusers take multiple drugs simultaneously.
9. Be aware that there is a high incidence of human immunodeficiency virus (HIV), tuberculosis, and infectious hepatitis among drug users.
10. Examine the patient's breath for characteristic odor of alcohol, acetone, and so forth.
11. Try to obtain a history of drug experiences (from the person accompanying the patient or from the patient).

General Interventions

1. Goals:
   a. Support the respiratory and cardiovascular functions.
   b. Give definitive treatment for drug overdose, such as naloxone.
   c. Prevent further absorption, enhance drug elimination, and reduce its toxicity.

Table 35-2 Specific Drug Overdose Presentations and Interventions

TYPE OF DRUG	PRESENTATION	INTERVENTIONS
CNS Stimulants • Amphetamines • Designer drugs (MDMA, Ecstasy, Ice, Eve, bath salts) • Cocaine (can be smoked in freebase or crack form, snorted, or injected)	Palpitations, feeling of impending doom, tachycardia, hypertension, dysrhythmia, myocardial ischemia or infarction, euphoria, agitation, combativeness, confusion, hallucinations, paranoia, aggressive or violent behavior, suicide attempts, hyperpyrexia, and seizures. When the drug wears off, depression, exhaustion, irritability, and sleeplessness.	• Secure airway, breathing, and circulation. • Monitor ECG and provide oxygen for ischemia. • Sedate, as necessary. • Administer anti-arrhythmics for ventricular dysrhythmia. • Administer diazepam for seizures. • Closely monitor hemodynamic status and provide IV fluids, as indicated.
Hallucinogens • Lysergic acid diethylamide (LSD) • Phencyclidine HCl (PCP) • Mescaline • Psilocybin mushrooms • Jimson weed seeds • Salvia	Marked anxiety bordering on panic, confusion, incoherence, hyperactivity, hallucinations, hazardous behavior, convulsions, coma, circulatory collapse, and death. Flashbacks may occur months to years after initial drug use.	• Reduce sensory stimuli, encourage patient to keep eyes open, and stay with patient. • Monitor for hypertensive crisis and evidence of trauma. • Sedate if hyperactivity cannot be controlled and place patient in a protected environment.
Opioids • Heroin (may be cut with other ingredients in 20:1–200:1 ratios) • Morphine and its derivatives • Codeine and its derivatives	Hypotension, respiratory depression leading to apnea, miosis, and drowsiness progressing to stupor and coma.	• Administer naloxone 0.4–2 mg via IV line or by endotracheal tube (effective in 1–2 minutes). • Maintain an open airway but defer intubation until naloxone is given, if possible. • Monitor for reappearance of symptoms and readminister naloxone. • Protect the patient from harm (may be combative on awakening).
Sedatives • Barbiturates, such as amobarbital and secobarbital • Benzodiazepines, such as diazepam and flurazepam • Other sedative/hypnotics, such as chloral hydrate and glutethimide	Incoordination, ataxia, impaired thinking and speech, lethargy to coma, early miosis; later, fixed and dilated pupils, hypoventilation, hypotension, hypothermia, and decreased reflexes.	• Administer flumazenil to reverse or diminish effects of benzodiazepines. • Administer activated charcoal. • Protect the airway. • For hypotension, infuse with lactated Ringer's solution and give vasopressors.
Alcohol Intoxication generally occurs with blood levels greater than 100 mg/dL. Levels more than 400 mg/dL are due to rapid consumption of alcohol and represent a medical emergency.	Slurred speech, incoordination, ataxia, belligerent behavior progressing to stupor and coma, odor of alcohol on breath and clothing, and respiratory depression.	• Protect the airway. • Closely monitor for CNS and respiratory depression. • Draw blood for ethanol concentration, electrolytes, glucose, and drug screen, using nonalcohol skin cleanser. • Assess for head injury and other trauma, as well as organic disease. • Administer IV fluids, magnesium sulfate (to reduce risk of seizures), thiamine (to prevent Wernicke-Korsakoff syndrome), and glucose (to treat hypoglycemia).

CNS, central nervous system; ECG, electrocardiogram.

2. Measure ABGs for hypoxia due to hypoventilation or for acid-base derangements.
3. Continuously monitor ECG.
4. Draw blood samples for testing glucose, electrolytes, BUN, creatinine, and appropriate toxicology screen.
5. Initiate IV fluids.
6. Administer oxygen.
7. Pharmacologic interventions:
    a. Give specific drug antagonist if drug is known.
    b. Naloxone for CNS depression due to opioids.
    c. Dextrose 50% IV to rule out hypoglycemic coma.

> **DRUG ALERT** Antidotes generally have a shorter half-life than the drugs they are used to treat. Repeated dosing is often necessary.

8. If the drug was taken by mouth, the primary method for preventing or minimizing absorption is to administer activated charcoal. Multiple doses may be administered. A routine NG tube may be inserted to facilitate emptying of stomach contents (without lavage) within 30 minutes of ingestion; or charcoal may be instilled if the patient is unable to drink.
9. In unconscious or semi-conscious patients who are or may be lacking gag or cough reflexes, use an NG tube only after intubation with cuffed endotracheal tube to prevent aspiration of charcoal stomach contents.
10. Take rectal temperature—extremes of thermoregulation (hyperthermia/hypothermia) must be recognized and treated.
11. Treat seizures with diazepam.
12. Assist with hemodialysis/peritoneal dialysis for potentially lethal poisoning.
13. Catheterize the patient because the drug or its metabolites are excreted in urine.
14. Do not leave the patient alone; there is a potential for the patient to harm self or ED staff.
15. Anticipate complications—sudden death from cerebral hypoxia, dysrhythmias, seizures, respiratory arrest, MI.
16. Always suspect mixtures of medications and alcohol.

> **NURSING ALERT** Many drugs will not or cannot be tested for in a standard toxicology screen. A negative drug screen does not mean an overdose is not the cause of the emergency.

Alcohol Withdrawal Delirium

Alcohol withdrawal delirium (*delirium tremens* or *alcoholic hallucinosis*) is an acute toxic state that follows a prolonged bout of steady drinking or sudden withdrawal from prolonged intake of alcohol. It may be precipitated by acute injury or infection. Symptoms can begin as early as 4 hours after a reduction of alcohol intake and usually peak at 24 to 48 hours, but may last up to 2 weeks.

> **NURSING ALERT** Alcohol withdrawal delirium is a serious complication of inadequate withdrawal management and is life-threatening.

Primary Assessment and Interventions

1. Patient may present alert, unless experiencing a seizure.
2. Ensure adequacy of airway, breathing, and circulation.

Subsequent Assessment

1. Assess for major symptoms—may occur independently or in combination.
    a. Nausea.
    b. Tremors.
    c. Paroxysmal sweating.
    d. Anxiety.
    e. Agitation.
    f. Headache.
    g. Mental status.
    h. Hallucinations (may be tactile, visual, or auditory).
2. Utilizing a standard Clinical Institute Withdrawal Assessment for Alcohol scale may assist in identifying those at risk for withdrawal problems and guide treatment. See Box 35-1.
    a. Each category is given a score and the total added. The cumulative score provides a basis for treatment. Generally a score of 8 to 10 or greater is the threshold for treatment to alleviate symptoms and prevent seizures.
    b. Reassess frequently during the first 48 hours and discontinue treatment and assessments when three subsequent determinations have been below the threshold.
3. Obtain drinking history, including the severity of past withdrawal episodes and any recent drug intake. Be aware that people tend to underestimate drinking habits.
4. Perform thorough examination for signs of autonomic hyperreactivity—tachycardia, diaphoresis, elevated temperature, dilated but reactive pupils—as well as any coexisting illnesses or injuries (head injury, pneumonia, metabolic disturbances).
5. Observe behavior for talkativeness, restlessness, agitation, or preoccupation.

General Interventions

1. Protect the patient from injury. Not all patients have hallucinations; however, if they do, the hallucinations may be visual, tactile, or auditory and are frequently frightening. Seizures may also occur.
2. Using a nonalcoholic skin preparation, draw blood for measurement of ethanol concentration, toxicology screen for other drugs of abuse, and other tests, as directed.
3. Pharmacologic interventions:
    a. Diazepam or chlordiazepoxide for sedation. Sedate the patient with sufficient dosage of medication to produce adequate relaxation and to reduce agitation, prevent exhaustion, and promote sleep without compromising airway.
    b. Diazepam or phenytoin for seizure control.
4. Monitor vital signs every 30 minutes.
5. Maintain close observation.
6. Maintain electrolyte balance and hydration through oral or IV route—fluid losses may be extreme because of profuse perspiration, vomiting, and agitation.
7. Assess respiratory, hepatic, and cardiovascular status of patient—pneumonia, liver disease, and cardiac failure are complications.

BOX 35-1   Clinical Institute of Withdrawal from Alcohol Revised (CIWA-Ar)*

NAUSEA AND VOMITING:
Ask: "Do you feel sick to your stomach? Have you vomited?"
0 = No nausea, no vomiting
1 = Mild nausea with no retching or vomiting
4 = Intermittent nausea with dry heaves
7 = Constant nausea, frequent dry heaves, and/or vomiting

TREMOR:
Arms extended and fingers spread apart.
0 = No tremor
1 = Not visible, but can be felt fingertip to fingertip
4 = Moderate with patients arm extended
7 = Severe, even with arms not extended

SWEATING:
0 = No sweat visible
1 = Barely perceptible sweating, palms moist
4 = Beads of sweat obvious on forehead
7 = Drenching sweat over face and chest

ANXIETY:
Ask, "Do you feel nervous?"
0 = No anxiety, at ease
1 = Mildly anxious
4 = Moderately anxious or guarded, so anxiety is inferred
7 = Equivalent to acute panic states, as seen in severe delirium or acute schizophrenic reaction

AGITATION:
0 = Normal activity
1 = Somewhat more than normal activity (may move legs up and down, shift position occasionally)
4 = Moderately fidgety and restless, shifting position frequently
7 = Paces back and forth or constantly thrashes about

TACTILE DISTURBANCES:
Ask, "Have you any itching, pins-and-needles sensation, burning or numbness, or do you feel bugs crawling on or under your skin?"
0 = None
1 = Very mild
2 = Mild
3 = Moderate
4 = Moderately severe hallucinations
5 = Severe hallucinations
6 = Extremely severe hallucinations
7 = Continuous hallucinations

AUDITORY DISTURBANCES:
Ask, "Are you more aware of the sounds around you? Are they harsh? Do they frighten you? Are you hearing anything disturbing? Are you hearing things you know are not there?"
0 = Not present hallucinations
1 = Very mild
2 = Mild
3 = Moderate
4 = Moderately severe
5 = severe hallucinations
6 = Extremely severe hallucinations
7 = Continuous hallucinations

VISUAL DISTURBANCES:
Ask, "Does the light appear to be too bright? Is its color different? Does it hurt your eyes? Are you seeing anything disturbing to you? Are you seeing things you know are not there?"
0 = Not present
1 = Very mild
2 = Mild
3 = Moderate
4 = Moderately severe
5 = Severe hallucinations
6 = Extremely severe hallucinations
7 = Continuous hallucinations

HEADACHE, FULLNESS IN HEAD:
Ask, "Does your head feel different? Does it feel like there is a band around your head?" Do not rate dizziness or lightheadedness. Otherwise, rate severity.
0 = Not present
1 = Very mild
2 = Mild
3 = Moderate
4 = Moderately severe
5 = Severe
6 = Very severe
7 = Extremely severe

ORIENTATION AND CLOUDING OF SENSORIUM:
Ask, "What day is this? Where are you? Who am I?"
0 = Oriented and can do serial additions
1 = Cannot do serial additions or is uncertain about date
2 = Disoriented for date by no more than 2 calendar days
3 = Disoriented for date by more than 2 calendar days
4 = Disoriented for place and/or person

*Assessment is made in each category and cumulative score is used to determine treatment (institutional protocols vary). From Sullivan, J. T., Sykora, K., Schneiderman, J., et al. (1989). Assessment of alcohol withdrawal: The revised Clinical Institute Withdrawal Assessment for Alcohol scale (CIWA-Ar). *British Journal of Addiction, 84*(11), 1373–1357.

8. Observe for hypoglycemia and treat appropriately. Hypoglycemia may accompany alcoholic withdrawal because alcohol depletes liver glycogen stores and impairs gluconeogenesis; many patients also suffer from malnutrition.

   a. Administration of thiamine is common.

BEHAVIORAL EMERGENCIES

A *behavioral emergency* is an urgent, serious disturbance of behavior, affect, or thought that makes the patient unable to cope with his or her life situation and interpersonal relationships. A patient presenting with a psychiatric emergency may be overactive or violent, depressed, or suicidal.

Violent Patients

Violent and aggressive behavior is usually episodic and is a means of expressing feelings of anger, fear, or hopelessness about a situation.

Assessment

1. Assess for overactivity, aggression, or anger out of proportion to the circumstances.
2. Determine risk factors for violence, including:
   a. Intoxicated with drugs/alcohol.
   b. Going through drug or alcohol withdrawal.
   c. Acute paranoid schizophrenic states, acute organic brain syndrome, acute psychosis, paranoia, or borderline personality.
3. Obtain psychiatric assessment.

General Interventions

1. Goals are to bring violence under control and protect patient and staff from harm.
2. Establish control.
   a. Keep room door open, and be in clear view of the staff. Always leave a clear exit pathway. Never allow the patient to be between you and safety.
   b. Help the patient bring violence under control.
      i. Give patient space; do not make sudden moves.
      ii. Avoid touching agitated patients or standing close.
      iii. Ask if the patient has a weapon; request that it be placed in a neutral area.
      iv. If the patient will not surrender weapon, leave the room and allow security personnel/police to handle the situation.
   c. Try not to leave the patient alone unless your safety is in jeopardy; this may be interpreted as rejection or the patient may try to harm self.
   d. Adopt a calm, nonconfrontational approach and remain in control of the situation. External calm and structure may help the patient gain control.
   e. Give the patient choices and options about treatments or timing of events if at all possible.
3. Provide emotional support.
   a. Talk and listen to the patient.
   b. Crisis intervention is best done with an attitude of interest in the patient's well-being and with an attempt to "tune in" to the patient while remaining firm.
   c. Acknowledge the patient's state of agitation (eg, "I want to work with you to relieve your distress").
   d. Give the patient the opportunity to ventilate anger verbally; avoid challenging the delusional state.
   e. Try to hear what the patient is saying.
   f. Convey the expectation of appropriate behavior and make the patient aware that help is available for him or her to gain control.
   g. Administer prescribed tranquilizer to reduce anxiety and hyperactivity, if verbal management techniques fail to attenuate the patient's tension.
4. Secure assistance.
   a. Allow security personnel/police to intervene if patient does not become calm.
   b. Use of a dedicated safe room is encouraged. The room should be free of cords, cables, or any object capable of being used as a weapon and be easily seen by staff. Shatterproof windows and/or cameras are encouraged. Use restraints when absolutely necessary but with minimal force.
   c. Have a specific plan and enough well-trained personnel available when applying restraints; if patient is intoxicated, restrain in a left lateral position and monitor closely for aspiration.
   d. Talk reassuringly while applying restraints; use empathic and supportive verbal interactions.
   e. Monitor patient continuously after restraints are applied; check circulation of restrained extremities.

Depression

Depression may be seen as the presenting condition at the health care facility or may be masked by the presentation of anxiety and somatic complaints.

Assessment

1. Observe for sadness, apathy, feelings of worthlessness, self-blame, suicidal thoughts, desire to escape, worsening of mood in morning, anorexia, weight loss, sleeplessness, lessening interest in sex, reduction of activity, or ceaseless activity.
2. The agitated, depressed person may exhibit motor restlessness and severe anxiety.

General Interventions

1. Listen to the patient in a calm, unhurried manner.
2. The patient will benefit from ventilation of feelings.
3. Give the patient an opportunity to talk about problems.
4. Anticipate that the patient may be suicidal.
5. Attempt to find out if the patient has thought about or attempted suicide.
   a. "Have you ever thought about taking your own life?"
   b. The patient is generally relieved because of the opportunity to discuss feelings.
6. Find out if there is an illness, perceived or real.
7. Assess whether there has been sudden worsening of depression.
8. Notify relatives about a seriously depressed patient. Do not leave the patient alone because suicide is usually an act committed in solitude.

9. Give antidepressant and anti-anxiety agents, as prescribed.

10. Point out to the patient that depression is treatable.

11. Be aware of crisis and supportive services in the community: telephone counseling and referral, suicide prevention centers, group therapy, marital and family counseling, drug/alcohol counseling, adolescent counseling, or befriending programs.

12. Refer for psychiatric consultation or to psychiatric unit.

Suicide Ideation

According to the Centers for Disease Control and Prevention (CDC), suicide is the 11th leading cause of death in the United States and the third most common cause of death in young people.

Assessment

1. Assess for risk factors:
   a. Associated psychiatric illness (affective disorders and substance abuse in adults; conduct disorders and depression in young people).
   b. Personality traits, such as aggression, impulsivity, depression, hopelessness, borderline personality disorder, or antisocial personality.
   c. Persons who have experienced early loss, decreased social support, chronic illness, or recent divorce.
   d. Genetic and familial factors: family history of suicide, certain psychiatric disorders or alcoholism, alcohol and substance abuse.

2. Determine whether patient has communicated suicidal intent, such as preoccupation with death or talking about someone else's suicide.

3. Determine whether patient has ever attempted suicide—the risk is much greater in these people.

4. Determine whether there is a specific plan for suicide and a means to carry out the plan.

General Interventions

1. Treat the consequences of the suicide attempt, if one has been made

2. After the patient has been stabilized, or if there was no active attempt made, use crisis intervention (a form of brief psychotherapy) to determine suicide potential, discover areas of depression and conflict, find out about the patient's support system, and determine whether hospitalization, psychiatric referral, and so forth is warranted.

3. Prevent further self-injury—a patient who has made a suicide gesture may do so again.

4. Admit to ICU (if condition warrants), arrange follow-up care, or admit to psychiatric unit, depending on assessment of suicide potential.

SEXUAL ASSAULT

Rape

The definition of rape has undergone several revisions during the past several years. Currently, *rape* is defined as any kind of penetration of another person, without her or his consent. This definition now includes men and women, as well as the use of objects, rather than body parts. Lack of consent is the key. *Lack of consent* can imply either force or the incapacity to make an informed judgment. Children, mentally handicapped individuals, and persons who are intoxicated are all considered unable to consent to sex.

 NURSING ALERT The management of the sexual assault is important, but immediate physical health should be ensured first. A complete primary and focused assessment should take place, being alert for signs of internal hemorrhage, shock, or respiratory distress. If the victim has suffered trauma in the form of physical assault (eg, head or abdominal trauma), the trauma should be managed in the order of established priorities.

Assessment

Initiating a Supportive Relationship

1. The manner in which the patient is received and treated in the ED is important to her or his future psychological well-being. Many areas have sexual assault nurse examiners. These nurses have specialized education and clinical experience to prepare them for forensic examination of sexual assault victims. Some metropolitan areas of the country have one facility designated for treatment of sexual assault victims. If this is true in your area, the patient should have any life-threatening injuries stabilized, then be transferred to the dedicated facility for examination.
   a. Call a rape crisis intervention counselor (if available), who will meet the patient/family in the ED.
   b. Do not leave patient alone. Accept the emotional reactions of the patient (hysteria, stoicism, overwhelmed feeling, etc.).

2. Emotional trauma may be present for weeks, months, or years. Patients may experience complex posttraumatic stress disorder or rape trauma syndrome. Patients may go through phases of psychological reactions:
   a. Acute phase (disorganization)—shock, disbelief, fear, anxiety, guilt, humiliation, suppression of feelings—may be for a few days to several weeks.
   b. Outward-adjustment phase—victim resumes what appears to be a normal life but internally faces continued turmoil, manifested as fear, flashbacks, sleep disturbances, hyperalertness, and psychosomatic reactions.
   c. Resolution phase—the rape is no longer the central focus of the victim's life and she or he is able to move on from the incident.

Interviewing the Patient

1. Consent should be obtained for the examination, the collecting of cultures/evidence, and for release of information to law-enforcement agencies.

 NURSING ALERT Most EDs have commercially prepared rape evidence collection kits as well as written protocols for treatment of injuries, legal documentation, and sexually transmitted disease (STD) and pregnancy prevention. Remember that the evidence collection kit is meant to preserve forensic evidence.

2. Record history of event in the patient's own words.

3. Ask if the patient has bathed, douched, gargled or brushed teeth, changed clothes, or urinated or defecated since attack—may alter interpretation of subsequent findings.

4. Record time of admission, time of examination, date and time of sexual assault, and the general appearance of the patient.

   a. Document any evidence of trauma—discoloration, bruises, lacerations, secretions, torn and bloody clothing.

   b. Record emotional state.

Interventions

Preparing for Physical Examination

1. Assist the patient to undress over a sheet/large piece of paper to obtain debris.

2. Place each item of clothing in a separate paper bag (plastic bags promote moisture retention, which may lead to formation of mold and mildew, which can destroy evidence).

3. Label bags appropriately; give to appropriate law-enforcement authority.

4. Advise the patient of the nature and necessity of each procedure; give the rationale for each question asked.

Physical Examination

1. Examine the patient (from head to toe) for injuries, especially to the head, neck, breasts, thighs, back, and buttocks.

2. Assess for external evidence of trauma (bruises, contusions, lacerations, stab wounds).

3. Assess for dried semen stains (appearing as crusted, flaking areas) on the patient's body.

4. Inspect fingers for broken nails and tissue and foreign materials under nails. Obtain scrapings or clippings of fingernails.

5. Assist in conducting oral examination to determine secretion status of patient compared with that of assailant. In many areas, this has been replaced with DNA testing.

   a. Obtain a saliva specimen.

   b. Take prescribed cultures of gum and tooth areas.

6. Document evidence of trauma with body diagrams or photographs.

Pelvic and Rectal Examinations

1. Examine perineum and thighs with an ultraviolet light (Wood's lamp); areas that are found to fluoresce may indicate semen stains. Urine and other stains may also fluoresce.

2. Note color and consistency of any discharge present.

3. Use water-moistened vaginal speculum for examination; do not use lubricant (contains chemicals that may interfere with later forensic testing of specimens and acid phosphatase determinations).

Obtaining Laboratory Specimens

1. Collect vaginal aspirate, which is examined for presence or absence of motile/nonmotile sperm.

2. Use sterile swab to draw from vaginal pool for acid phosphatase, blood group antigen of semen, and precipitin test against human sperm and blood.

3. Obtain separate smears from the oral, vaginal, and anal areas.

4. Obtain swabs of body orifices for gonorrhea and chlamydia testing (to determine preexisting infection or new infection if patient is not presenting immediately).

5. Comb and trim areas of pubic hair suspected of containing semen; obtain several pubic hairs with follicles; place in separate containers and identify these as patient's pubic hairs.

6. Obtain blood serum for syphilis; a sample of serum may be frozen and saved for future testing.

7. Collect foreign material (leaves, grass, dirt) and place in appropriate container.

8. Examine rectum for signs of trauma, blood, and semen stains.

9. Conduct a pregnancy test if there is a possibility that patient is pregnant.

10. Label all specimens with name of patient, date, time of collection, body area from which specimen was obtained, and names of personnel collecting specimens to preserve chain of evidence; give to designated person (eg, crime laboratory) and obtain an itemized receipt.

11. Photographs are taken by designated person.

Other Interventions

1. Treat physical trauma as with any patient.

2. Protect patient against STDs.

   a. Specimens obtained for STDs, including gonorrhea, cannot be immediately obtained (positive cultures taken in the immediate postrape period will reflect only existing disease).

   b. In addition, follow-up visits cannot be ensured, so some health care providers may treat the patient as if they have been exposed to a known case of gonorrhea or chlamydia.

   c. CDC recommendations for prophylactic treatment following a sexual assault are:

   Ceftriaxone 125 mg I.M. in a single dose

   plus

   Metronidazole 2 g by mouth (P.O.) in a single dose

   plus

   Azithromycin 1 g P.O. in a single dose

   or

   Doxycycline 100 mg P.O. twice per day for 7 days in place of azithromycin.

3. Protect patient against pregnancy.

   a. It is important to determine whether pregnancy existed before the attack.

   b. Negative pregnancy test should be obtained before administering postcoital therapy.

   c. Hormonal treatment to prevent pregnancy—morning-after pill, as indicated.

4. Allay fear of HIV or acquired immunodeficiency syndrome. Consider prophylactic treatment for HIV.

5. Possible prophylactic scabies treatment.

6. Provide the patient with cleansing facilities, including a cleansing douche, shower, and mouthwash after forensic exam is completed.

Providing for Follow-up Services

1. Make an appointment for follow-up surveillance for pregnancy, STD, and HIV counseling.

2. Inform the patient of counseling services to prevent long-term psychological effects; counseling services should also be made available to the family.

3. Encourage the patient to return to previous level of functioning as soon as possible.

4. The patient should be accompanied by a family member or friend when leaving the health care facility.

BIOLOGICAL WEAPONS AND PREPAREDNESS

Following the September 11, 2001, terrorist attacks on the United States, bioterrorism has become a real possibility. As frontline responders, emergency nurses must be aware of possible acts of bioterrorism and be familiar with their facilities' policies regarding such emergencies.

Biological Agents

Terrorism may consist of the intentional release of a chemical, biological, radiological, nuclear, or explosive device intended to cause widespread illness or death. Explosive devices tend to announce themselves rather quickly and definitively. Bioterrorism, however, can have a slow, insidious onset, leaving the population with little idea they have been the victim of an attack. The emergency nurse should be on the alert for possible signs of terrorism:

1. Large numbers of people with similar disease.
2. Cases of unexplained illness or death.
3. More severe illness than would normally be expected for a specific pathogen.
4. An illness that is resistant to usual treatment.
5. Unusual routes of exposure for a specific pathogen.
6. Disease that is unusual for an area.
7. A single case of unusual disease (smallpox, hemorrhagic fever).
8. Disease unusual for an age group.

See Table 35-3 for specific agents of bioterrorism, such as smallpox, anthrax, plague, and botulism.

For additional information regarding bioterrorism, consult the following websites:

- Association for Professionals in Infection Control and Epidemiology (*www.apic.org*)
- Centers for Disease Control and Prevention Bioterrorism and Public Health Preparedness (*www.bt.cdc.gov/bioterrorism*)

Table 35-3	Potential Biological Weapons	
AGENT AND METHOD OF TRANSMISSION	**CLINICAL MANIFESTATIONS**	**MANAGEMENT**
Smallpox Transmitted by inhalation or direct contact with the variola virus; has a 2-week incubation period.	High fever, fatigue, muscle aches, and rash that progresses to blisters after 3 days. The rash first develops on the face and around the wrists, then spreads to the trunk. Smallpox lesions progress at the same rate, unlike lesions of chickenpox, which may be seen in various stages of progression.	The patient should be isolated (preferably at home) until all of the scabs have fallen off. Management includes IV hydration. Health care providers should use masks, gowns, and gloves when caring for these patients and should receive smallpox vaccination within 2–3 days of exposure. Persons who have had contact with the patient should be isolated for 17 days.
Anthrax Transmitted through consumption of contaminated animal products, ingestion of raw meat, or inhalation of airborne spores of *Bacillus anthracis*, a Gram-positive, spore-forming bacteria. The incubation period is 1–6 days.	Fever, fatigue, cough, chest discomfort, widened mediastinum on chest x-ray, and respiratory distress.	Ensure that standard precautions are observed and that all surfaces are disinfected. Persons who have had contact with the patient should be started on the vaccine schedule and treated with ciprofloxacin or doxycycline.
Pneumonic Plague Transmitted by inhalation of *Yersinia pestis*. The incubation period is 2–6 days.	Fever, headache, weakness, and upper respiratory symptoms often including hemoptysis.	Treatment must begin within 24 hours and should include gentamicin or streptomycin drug. Isolate the patient for 48 hours after antibiotics are started. Postexposure prophylaxis consists of tetracycline or doxycycline for 7 days.
Botulism Transmitted primarily by ingestion of food contaminated with a preformed toxin produced by *Clostridium botulinum*. An inhalation form has been developed specifically as a biological agent.	Blurred or double vision, slurred speech, nausea, vomiting, diarrhea, and descending muscle weakness.	An antitoxin is effective if used early in the disease. Standard precautions are satisfactory; botulism is not contagious.

- Centers for Disease Control and Prevention Emergency Preparedness and Response (*www.bt.cdc.gov*)
- U.S. Department of Health and Human Services, Public Health Emergency (*www.ndms.dhhs.gov*)
- United States Army Medical Research Institute of Infectious Diseases (*www.usamriid.army.mil*)

SELECTED REFERENCES

American Academy of Clinical Toxicology and the European Association of Poisons Centres and Clinical Toxicologists. (2004). Position paper: Cathartics. *Journal of Toxicology, 42*(3), 243–253.

American Academy of Clinical Toxicology and the European Association of Poisons Centres and Clinical Toxicologists. (2004). Position paper: Gastric lavage. *Journal of Toxicology, 42*(7), 933–943.

American Heart Association. (2010). *ACLS provider manual 2010*. Dallas: Author.

Arrich, J., Holzer, M., Havel, C., et al. (2012). Hypothermia for neuroprotection in adults after cardiopulmonary resuscitation (Review). The Cochrane Library, CD004128.pub3.

Bernard, S. A., Gray, T. W., Buist, M. D., et al. (2002). Treatment of comatose survivors of out-of-hospital cardiac arrest with induced hypothermia. *New England Journal of Medicine, 346*(8), 557–563.

Bienvenu, O. J., Neufeld, K. J., Needham, D. M. (2012). Treatment of four psychiatric emergencies in the intensive care unit. *Critical Care Medicine, 40*(9), 2662–2670.

Bohm, K., Rosenqvist, M., Herlitz, J., et al. (2007). Survival is similar after standard treatment and chest compressions only in out of facility bystander cardiopulmonary resuscitation. *Circulation, 116*, 2908–2912.

Dellinger, R. P., Levy, M. M., Carlet, J. M., et al. (2008). Surviving Sepsis Campaign: International guidelines for management of severe sepsis and septic shock. *Critical Care Medicine, 36*, 296–327; published correction appears in *Critical Care Medicine, 36*, 1394–1396.

Emergency Nurses Association. (2007). *Emergency nursing core curriculum* (6th ed.). Philadelphia: W.B. Saunders.

Emergency Nurses Association. (2007). *Trauma nursing core course* (6th ed.). Des Plaines, IL: Author.

Fugate, J. E., Wijdicks, E. F. M., Mandraker, J., et al. (2010). Predictors of neurologic outcome in hypothermia after cardiac arrest. *Annals of Neurology, 68*(6), 907–914.

Gessner, P., Dugan, G., Janusek, L. (2012). Target temperature within 3 Hours. *AACN Advanced Critical Care, 23*(3), 246–257.

Hwang, U., Richardson, L., Harris, B., (2010). The quality of emergency department pain care for older adult patients. *Journal of the American Geriatrics Society, 58*, 2122–2128.

Hypothermia after Cardiac Arrest Study Group. (2002). Mild therapeutic hypothermia to improve the neurologic outcome after cardiac arrest. *New England Journal of Medicine, 346*(8), 549–556.

Marx, J. A. (Ed.). (2009). *Rosen's emergency medicine: Concepts and clinical practice* (7th ed.). Philadelphia: Mosby Elsevier.

McNab, A., Burns, B., Bhullar, I., et al. (2012). A prehospital shock index for trauma correlates with measures of hospital resource use and mortality. *Surgery, 152*(3), 473–476.

McQuillan, K. A., Flynn Makic, M. B., & Whalen, E. (2009). *Trauma nursing: From resuscitation through rehabilitation* (4th ed.). St. Louis, MO: Saunders Elsevier

Muntlin, A., Carlsson, M., Safwenberg, U., et al. (2011). Outcomes of a nurse-initiated intravenous analgesic protocol for abdominal pain in an emergency department: A quasi-experimental study. *International Journal of Nursing Studies, 48*, 13–23.

Nolan, J. P., Morley, P. T., Vanden Hoek, T. L., et al. (2003). Therapeutic hypothermia after cardiac arrest: An advisory statement by the Advanced Life Support Task Force of the International Liaison Committee on Resuscitation. *Circulation, 108*, 118–121.

Proehl, J. A. (2008). *Emergency nursing procedures* (4th ed.). Philadelphia: W.B. Saunders.

Sullivan, J. T., Sykora, K., Schneiderman, J., et al. (1989). Assessment of alcohol withdrawal: The revised Clinical Institute Withdrawal Assessment for Alcohol scale (CIWA-Ar). *British Journal of Addiction, 84*(11), 1373–1357.

Uray, T., Haugk, M., Sterz, F., et al. (2010). Surface cooling for rapid induction of mild hypothermia after cardiac arrest: Design determines efficacy. *Academic Emergency Medicine, 17*(4), 360–367.

Vanzant, A. M., & Schmelzer, M. (2011). Detecting and treating sepsis in the emergency department. *Journal of Emergency Nursing, 37*(1), 47–54.

SELECTED INTERNET RESOURCES

American Academy of Clinical Toxicology, *www.clintox.org*
American Association of Poison Control Centers, *www.aapc.org*
American College of Emergency Physicians, *www.acep.org*
American Heart Association, *www.americanheart.org*
Australasian College for Emergency Medicine, *www.acem.org.au*
Australian Resuscitation Council, *www.resus.org.au*
The Cochrane Collaboration, *www.cochrane.org*
College of Emergency Nursing Australasia, *www.cena.org.au*
Emergency Nurses Association, *www.ena.org*
European Resuscitation Council, *www.erc.edu*
NICS Guide to the Cochrane Library, *www.nicsl.com.au/Cochrane*
Preparing for ACLS Certification, *www.acls.net*
Society of Trauma Nurses, *www.traumanurses.org*
Surviving Sepsis Campaign, *www.survivingsepsis.org*
The Eastern Association for the Surgery of Trauma (EAST), *www.east.org/resources*

PART THREE

MATERNITY AND NEONATAL NURSING

36
Maternal and Fetal Health

INTRODUCTION TO MATERNITY NURSING

Providing care to childbearing families is aimed at the ideal of having every pregnancy result in a healthy mother, baby, and family unit. The nurse today faces many evolving and challenging issues in achieving this goal. Such advances as in vitro fertilization and embryo freezing have afforded people opportunities once thought impossible. An increasing number of high-risk pregnancies result from such factors as drug abuse, acquired immunodeficiency syndrome, late or no prenatal care, teenage pregnancies, and pregnancies in women older than age 35.

Today's childbearing families have many options. The planned birth may take place in the traditional hospital setting, a birthing center, or at home. The primary care provider may be a physician, a certified nurse-midwife, or a lay midwife. Birth-related choices commonly include the use of labor, delivery, and recovery rooms or labor, delivery, recovery, and postpartum rooms; various birthing positions and analgesic methods; alternative pain-relief strategies such as hydrotherapy; and the decision to allow children and others to be present during labor and delivery. Regionalization of obstetric services has provided childbearing families with access to the technologic advances and skilled personnel capable of managing pregnancy or neonatal complications. The combination of advancing technology, pregnancy risk factors, and changing economics due to the rising cost of health care challenges the nurse to be a highly skilled clinician and outstanding communicator.

Terminology Used in Maternity Nursing

 Evidence Base Bond, L. (2011). Physiology of pregnancy. In S. Mattson & J. E. Smith (Eds.), *Core curriculum for maternal-newborn nursing* (4th ed., pp. 80–100). St. Louis, MO: Saunders Elsevier.

1. Gestation—pregnancy or maternal condition of having a developing fetus in the body.
2. Embryo—human conceptus up to the 10th week of gestation (8th week postconception).
3. Fetus—human conceptus from 10th week of gestation (8th week postconception) until delivery.
4. Viability—capability of living, usually accepted as 24 weeks, although survival is rare.
5. Gravida (G)—woman who is or has been pregnant, regardless of pregnancy outcome.
6. Nulligravida—woman who is not now and never has been pregnant.
7. Primigravida—woman pregnant for the first time.
8. Multigravida—woman who has been pregnant more than once.
9. Para (P)—refers to past pregnancies that have reached viability.
10. Nullipara—woman who has never completed a pregnancy to the period of viability. The woman may or may not have experienced an abortion.

11. Primipara—woman who has completed one pregnancy to the period of viability regardless of the number of infants delivered and regardless of the infant being live or stillborn.

12. Multipara—woman who has completed two or more pregnancies to the stage of viability.

13. Living children—refers to the number of children a woman has delivered who are living.

A woman who is pregnant for the first time is a primigravida and is described as Gravida 1 Para 0 (or G1P0). A woman who delivered one fetus carried to the period of viability and who is pregnant again is described as Gravida 2, Para 1. A woman with two pregnancies ending in abortions and no viable children is Gravida 2, Para 0.

Obstetric History

TPAL

In some obstetric services, a woman's obstetric history is summarized by a series of four digits, such as 5-0-2-5. These digits correspond with the abbreviation TPAL.

1. **T**—represents full-term deliveries, 37 completed weeks or more.

2. **P**—represents preterm deliveries, 20 to less than 37 completed weeks.

3. **A**—represents abortions, elective or spontaneous loss (miscarriage) of a pregnancy before the period of viability.

4. **L**—represents the number of children living. If a child has died, further explanation is needed for clarification.

5. If, for example, a particular woman's history is summarized as G 7, P 5-0-2-5, then she has been pregnant seven times, had five term deliveries, zero preterm deliveries, two abortions, and five living children.

GTPALM

In some institutions a woman's obstetric history can also be summarized as GTPALM, especially when multiple gestations or births are involved.

1. **G**—represents gravida.

2. **T**—represents full-term deliveries, 37 completed weeks or more.

3. **P**—represents preterm deliveries, 20 to less than 37 completed weeks.

4. **A**—represents abortions, elective or spontaneous loss of a pregnancy before the period of viability.

5. **L**—represents the number of children living. If a child has died, further explanation is needed for clarification.

6. **M**—represents the number of multiple gestations and births (not the number of neonates delivered).

If, for example, a particular woman's history is summarized as G 5, P 5-0-0-6-1, then she has been pregnant five times, had five term deliveries, zero preterm deliveries, zero abortions, six living children, and one multiple gestation/birth.

THE EXPECTANT MOTHER
Manifestations of Pregnancy

 Evidence Base Blackburn, S. T. (2008). Physiologic changes of pregnancy. In K. Rice-Simpson & P. A. Creehan (Eds.), *AWHONN's perinatal nursing* (3rd ed., pp. 59–77). Philadelphia: Lippincott Williams & Wilkins.

Pregnancy may be determined by cessation of menses, enlargement of the uterus, and a positive result on a pregnancy test. These and the many other manifestations of pregnancy are classified into three groups: presumptive, probable, and positive.

Presumptive Signs and Symptoms

Physical signs and symptoms that suggest, but do not prove, pregnancy.

1. Abrupt cessation of menses—pregnancy is suspected if more than 10 days have elapsed since the time of the expected onset in a healthy woman who previously had predictable menstrual periods.

2. Breast changes:
   a. Breasts enlarge and become tender. Veins in breasts become increasingly visible.
   b. Nipples become larger and more pigmented. Nipple tingling may also be present.
   c. Colostrum—a thin, milky fluid—may be expressed in the second half of pregnancy.
   d. Montgomery glands—small elevations on the areolae—may appear.

3. Skin pigmentation changes:
   a. Chloasma/melasma gravidarum (the mask of pregnancy)—brownish pigmentation appearing on the face in a butterfly pattern in 50% to 70% of women. It is usually symmetric and is distributed on the forehead, cheeks, and nose. The mask of pregnancy is more common in dark-haired, brown-eyed women and is progressive throughout the pregnancy.
   b. Linea nigra—dark vertical line on the abdomen between the sternum and the symphysis pubis.
   c. Abdominal striae (striae gravidarum)—reddish or purplish linear marks sometimes appearing on the breasts, abdomen, buttocks, and thighs because of the stretching, rupture, and atrophy of the deep connective tissue of the skin.

4. Nausea with or without vomiting (morning sickness)—occurs mainly in the morning but may occur at any time of the day, lasting a few hours. Begins between 2 and 6 weeks after conception and usually disappears spontaneously near the end of the first trimester (12 weeks).

5. Frequency of urination:
   a. Caused by pressure of the expanding uterus on the bladder.

b. Decreases when the uterus rises out of the pelvis (around 12 weeks).

c. Reappears when the fetal head engages in the pelvis at the end of pregnancy.

6. Constipation—due to the decreased absorption of fluid by the gut.

7. Fatigue—characteristic of early pregnancy in response to increased hormonal levels.

Probable Signs and Symptoms

Objective findings detected by 12 to 16 weeks of gestation.

1. Enlargement of abdomen—at about 12 weeks' gestation, the uterus can be felt through the abdominal wall, just above the symphysis pubis.

2. Changes in shape, size, and consistency of the uterus:
   a. Uterus enlarges, elongates, and decreases in thickness as pregnancy progresses. The uterus changes from a pear shape to a globe shape.
   b. Hegar's sign—lower uterine segment softens 6 to 8 weeks after the onset of the last menstrual period.

3. Changes in cervix:
   a. Chadwick's sign—bluish or purplish discoloration of cervix and vaginal wall.
   b. Goodell's sign—softening of the cervix; may occur as early as 4 weeks.
   c. With inflammation and carcinoma during pregnancy, the cervix may remain firm.

4. Intermittent contractions of the uterus (Braxton-Hicks contractions)—painless, palpable contractions occurring at irregular intervals, more frequently felt after 28 weeks. They usually disappear with walking or exercise.

5. Ballottement—sinking and rebounding of the fetus in its surrounding amniotic fluid in response to a sudden tap on the uterus (occurs near midpregnancy).

6. Changes in levels of human chorionic gonadotropin (hCG) in maternal plasma and urine.

7. Leukorrhea—increase in vaginal discharge.

8. Quickening (sensations of fetal movement in the abdomen)—occurs between the 16th and 20th week after the onset of the last menses.

9. Positive hCG—laboratory (urine or serum) test for pregnancy.

Positive Signs and Symptoms
Diagnostic of Pregnancy

1. Fetal heart tones (FHTs)—usually heard between 16th and 20th week of gestation with a fetoscope or the 10th and 12th week of gestation with a Doppler stethoscope.

2. Fetal movements felt by the examiner (after about 20 weeks' gestation).

3. Outlining of the fetal body through the maternal abdomen in the second half of pregnancy.

4. Sonographic evidence (after 4 weeks' gestation) using vaginal ultrasound. Fetal cardiac motion can be detected by 6 weeks' gestation.

Maternal Physiology During Pregnancy

 Evidence Base Bond, L. (2011). Physiology of pregnancy. In S. Mattson & J. E. Smith (Eds.), *Core curriculum for maternal-newborn nursing* (4th ed., pp. 80–100). St. Louis, MO: Saunders Elsevier.

Duration of Pregnancy

1. Averages 280 days or 40 weeks (10 lunar months, 9 calendar months) from the first day of the last normal menses.

2. Duration may also be divided into three equal parts, or trimesters, of slightly more than 13 weeks or 3 calendar months each.

3. Estimated date of confinement (EDC), more commonly referred to now as estimated date of delivery (EDD), is calculated by adding 7 days to the date of the first day of the last menses and counting back 3 months (Nägele's rule). Additionally, most antenatal clinics have obstetric wheels. These devices have an outer wheel that has markings for the calendar and an inner, sliding wheel with weeks and days of gestation. These wheels facilitate the estimation of gestational age (GA) and the calculation of the EDD. The quality of these wheels varies, but in general, the larger wheels yield better results.
   a. For example, if a woman's last menstrual period (LMP) began on September 10, 1999, her EDC would be June 17, 2000. The calculation would start with September 10, 1999, plus 7 days (September 17, 1999), minus 3 months (June 17, 1999). If the date of the woman's LMP begins after March 31, an additional year must be added to give a correct EDD.
   b. Another method of calculating the EDD is McDonald's rule: after 24 weeks' gestation, the fundal height measurement will correspond to the week of gestation plus 2 to 4 weeks.
   c. EDD can also be calculated via ultrasound technology—the most accurate assessment—preferably in the first trimester. Gestational age in the first trimester is usually calculated from the fetal crown-rump length (CRL). This is the longest demonstrable length of the embryo or fetus, excluding the limbs and the yolk sac. The correlation between CRL and GA is excellent until about 12 weeks' gestation and the estimate has a 95% confidence interval of plus or minus 6 days.

Changes in the Reproductive Tract
Uterus

1. Enlargement during pregnancy involves stretching and marked hypertrophy of existing muscle cells secondary to increased estrogen and progesterone levels.

2. In addition to an increase in the size of the uterine muscle cells, there is an increase in fibrous tissue and elastic tissue. The size and number of blood vessels and lymphatics increase.

3. Enlargement and thickening of the uterine wall are most marked in the fundus.

4. By the end of the third month (12 weeks), the uterus is too large to be contained wholly within the pelvic cavity—it can now be palpated suprapubically.

5. As the uterus rises out of the pelvis, it rotates somewhat to the right because of the presence of the rectosigmoid colon on the left side of the pelvis.

6. By 20 weeks' gestation, the fundus has reached the level of the umbilicus.

7. By 36 weeks, the fundus has reached the xiphoid process.

8. By the end of the fifth month, the myometrium hypertrophy ends and the walls of the uterus become thinner, allowing palpation of the fetus.

9. During the last 3 weeks, the uterus descends slightly because of fetal descent into the pelvis.

10. Changes in contractility occur—from the first trimester, irregular painless contractions occur (Braxton-Hicks contractions). In the latter weeks of pregnancy, these contractions become stronger and more regular.

11. There is a progressive increase in uteroplacental blood flow during pregnancy.

Cervix

1. Pronounced softening and cyanosis—due to increased vascularity, edema, hypertrophy, and hyperplasia of the cervical glands.

2. Endocervical glands secrete thick mucus that forms a cervical plug and obstructs the cervical canal. This plug prevents bacteria and other substances from entering and ascending into the uterus.

3. Erosions of cervix, common during pregnancy, represent an extension of proliferating endocervical glands and columnar endocervical epithelium.

4. Evidence of Chadwick's sign, the bluish, purplish coloring of the cervix. This sign is due to the increased vascularity and hyperemia caused by increased estrogen levels.

Ovaries

1. Ovulation ceases during pregnancy; maturation of new follicles is suspended.

2. One corpus luteum functions during early pregnancy (first 10 to 12 weeks), producing mainly progesterone. However, small levels of estrogen and relaxin are also produced by the corpus luteum.

3. After 8 weeks' gestation, the corpus luteum remains the source for the hormone relaxin. However, relaxin is not required for a successful pregnancy outcome and normal delivery.

Vagina and Outlet

1. Increased vascularity, hyperemia, and softening of connective tissue in skin and muscles of the perineum and vulva.

2. Vaginal walls prepare for labor: mucosa increases in thickness, connective tissue loosens, and small-muscle cells hypertrophy. Secretions are thick, white, and acidic in nature and play a major role in the prevention of infections.

3. Vaginal secretions increase; pH is 3.5 to 6—because of increased production of lactic acid from glycogen in the vaginal epithelium by *Lactobacillus acidophilus*. (Acid pH probably aids in keeping vagina relatively free of pathogenic bacteria.)

4. Hypertrophy of the structures, along with fat deposits, causes the labia majora to close and cover the vaginal introitus (vaginal opening).

Changes in the Abdominal Wall

1. Striae gravidarum (stretch marks) may develop—reddish, slightly depressed streaks in the skin of abdomen, breast, and thighs (become glistening silvery lines after pregnancy).

2. Linea nigra may form—line of dark pigment extending from the umbilicus down the midline to the symphysis. Commonly during the first pregnancy, the linea nigra occurs at the height of the uterus. During subsequent pregnancies, the entire line may be present early in gestation.

3. Diastasis recti may occur as muscles (rectus) separate. If severe, a part of the anterior uterine wall may be covered by only a layer of skin, fascia, and peritoneum.

Breast Changes

1. Tenderness and tingling occur in early weeks of pregnancy.

2. Increase in size by second month—hypertrophy of mammary alveoli. Veins become more prominent and striae may develop as the breasts enlarge.

3. Nipples become larger, more deeply pigmented, and more erectile early in pregnancy.

4. Colostrum, a yellow secretion rich in antibodies, may be expressed by second trimester.

5. Areolae become broader and more deeply pigmented. The depth of pigmentation varies with the person's complexion.

6. Scattered through the areola are a number of small elevations (glands of Montgomery), which are hypertrophic sebaceous glands.

Metabolic Changes

Numerous and intensive changes occur in response to rapidly growing fetus and placenta.

Weight Gain Average

Twenty-five to 35 pounds (11.5 to 16 kg) (see Table 36-1).

Table 36-1	Components of Weight Gain	
AREA	**KG**	**LB**
Fetus	3.2–3.4	7–7.5
Placenta	0.5–0.7	1–1.5
Amniotic fluid	0.9	2
Uterus	1.1	2.5
Breast tissue	0.7–1.4	1.5–3
Blood volume	1.6–2.3	3.5–5
Maternal stores	1.8–4.3	4–9.5

Water Metabolism

1. The average woman retains 6 to 8 L of extra water during the pregnancy due to hormonal influence.

2. Approximately 4 to 6 L of fluid move into the extracellular spaces. This creates a physiologic increase in blood volume (hypervolemia).

3. Many pregnant women experience a normal accumulation of fluid in their legs and ankles at the end of the day. This is most common in the third trimester and is referred to as physiologic edema.

4. Sodium excretion in the normal pregnant woman is similar to the nonpregnant woman.

5. Sodium retention is usually directly proportional to the amount of water accumulated during the pregnancy. However, pregnancy lends itself toward sodium depletion, making sodium regulation more difficult.

6. Additional sodium is required during pregnancy to meet the need for increased intravascular and extracellular fluid volumes and to maintain a normal isotonic state.

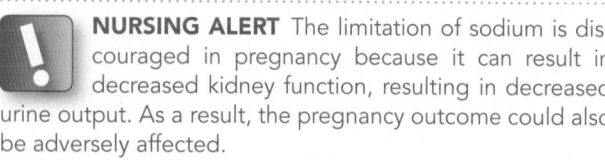

NURSING ALERT The limitation of sodium is discouraged in pregnancy because it can result in decreased kidney function, resulting in decreased urine output. As a result, the pregnancy outcome could also be adversely affected.

Protein Metabolism

1. The fetus, uterus, and maternal blood are rich in protein rather than in fat or carbohydrates.

2. At term, fetus and placenta contain approximately 500 grams of protein or approximately half of the total protein increase of pregnancy.

3. Approximately 500 grams more of protein is added to the uterus, breasts, and maternal blood in the form of hemoglobin and plasma proteins.

Carbohydrate Metabolism

1. Carbohydrate metabolism during pregnancy is controlled by glucose levels in the plasma and the metabolism of glucose in the cells.

2. The liver controls the plasma glucose level. Not only does it store glucose as glycogen, but it also converts it into glucose when the woman's blood glucose levels are low.

3. Early in pregnancy, the effects of estrogen and progesterone can induce a state of hyperinsulinemia. As pregnancy advances, there is increased tissue resistance coupled with increased hyperinsulinemia.

4. Approximately 2% to 3% of all women will develop gestational diabetes mellitus during pregnancy regardless if they have a history of carbohydrate intolerance.

5. Pregnant women with preexisting diabetes mellitus (type 1 or 2) may experience a worsening of the disease attributed to hormonal changes occurring with pregnancy.

6. During pregnancy, there is a "sparing" of glucose used by maternal tissues and a shunting of glucose to the placenta for use by the fetus.

7. Human placental lactogen (placental hormone) promotes lipolysis, increases plasma-free fatty acids, and thereby provides alternative fuel sources for the mother.

8. Human placental lactogen, estrogen, progesterone, and cortisol oppose the action of insulin during pregnancy and promote maternal lipolysis as well.

Fat Metabolism

1. Lipid metabolism during pregnancy causes an accumulation of fat stores, mostly cholesterol, phospholipids, and triglycerides.

2. This accumulation of fat stores has no negligible effect on the fetus.

3. Fat storage occurs before the 30th week of gestation. After 30 weeks' gestation, there is no further fat storage, only fat mobilization that correlates with the increased utilization of glucose and amino acids by the fetus.

4. The ratio of low-density proteins to high-density proteins is increased during pregnancy.

Nutrient Requirements

Caloric Requirements

1. Additional calories are usually not required during the first trimester due to the limited metabolic demands.

2. An additional 300 kcal/dL are required during the second and third trimester over the nonpregnant woman. However, due to the variety of women and their individualized needs, the exact caloric requirements need to be established on an individual basis.

3. Caloric expenditure varies throughout pregnancy. There is a slight increase in early pregnancy and a sharp increase near the end of the first trimester, continuing throughout pregnancy.

Protein Requirements

1. Protein is required for adequate amino acids to accommodate the normal development of the fetus, blood volume expansion, and growth of maternal breast and uterine tissue.

2. An additional requirement of 10 grams of protein per day is recommended over the nonpregnant intake.

Carbohydrate and Fat Requirements

1. As in the nonpregnant woman, carbohydrates should supply 55% to 60% of calories in the diet and should be in the form of complex carbohydrates, such as whole-grain cereal products, starchy vegetables, and legumes.

2. Fat intake should not exceed 30% of the diet. Saturated fats should not exceed 10% of the total calories.

Iron Requirements

1. Total circulating red blood cells (RBCs) increase about 20% to 30% (250 to 450 mL) during pregnancy; therefore, iron requirements are increased to 500 mg of iron needed: 270 mg by fetus; 90 mg by the placenta. This equates to 0.8 g/day in early pregnancy and 7.5 mg/day by term. This usually exceeds dietary intake.

2. Supplemental iron is valuable and necessary during pregnancy and for several weeks after pregnancy or lactation.

3. During the last half of pregnancy, iron is transferred to the fetus and stored in the fetal liver. This store lasts 3 to 6 months.

Changes in the Cardiovascular System

Heart

1. Diaphragm is progressively elevated during pregnancy; heart is displaced to the left and upward, with the apex moved laterally.
2. Heart sounds—exaggerated splitting of the first heart sound; a loud, easily heard third sound.
3. Heart murmurs—systolic murmurs are common and usually disappear after delivery.

Blood Volume Changes

1. Cardiac volume increases by 30% to 50% (1,450 to 1,750 mL), beginning as early as 6 weeks and peaking by 28 to 34 weeks' gestation, causing slight hypertrophy of the heart and increased cardiac output. Women with multiple gestation can have higher cardiac outputs, especially after 20 weeks' gestation.
2. Cardiac output increases by 30% to 50% above normal early in gestation with about one half of the increase occurring by 8 weeks' gestation. It peaks in the second trimester and plateaus until term, reaching a volume of 6 to 7 L/minute by term.
3. Position greatly influences cardiac output, especially in the third trimester. In the supine position, the large uterus compresses the venous return from the lower half of the body to the heart. This may cause arterial hypotension, referred to as *supine hypotensive syndrome*. Cardiac output increases by 25% to 30%, with an increase in uterine and renal blood flow when the woman turns from her back to lateral position (either left or right side).
4. Femoral venous pressure increases—because of slowing of blood flow from lower extremities as a result of pressure of enlarged uterus on pelvic veins and inferior vena cava.
5. Increased cutaneous blood flow dissipates excess heat caused by increased metabolism of pregnancy.
6. Plasma volume increases 40% to 60% (1,200 to 1,600 mL) by term, resulting in hemodilution, more commonly referred to as *physiologic anemia of pregnancy* or *physiologic dilutional anemia*. This "anemic" state is not a true pathologic state and does decrease the risk of thrombosis. It is due to the rapid increase in plasma volume and the later increase in RBC volume.

Blood Pressure Changes

1. Blood pressure (BP)—during the first half of pregnancy, there is a slight (5 to 10 mm Hg) decrease in systolic BP (SBP) and diastolic BP (DBP), with the lowest point occurring in the second trimester. By the third trimester, the BP gradually returns to prepregnancy levels.

> **NURSING ALERT** Hypertensive disease affects up to 22% of pregnancies and is associated with maternal and fetal death. According to the National Institutes of Health, women with hypertension in pregnancy should be referred to as having hypertensive disorders of pregnancy. Additionally the term "gestational hypertension" replaces the term "pregnancy-induced hypertension" to describe cases in which elevated BP without proteinuria occurs in a woman past 20 weeks of gestation who previously had a normal BP. Essentially, gestational hypertension is an elevated BP past 20 weeks of gestation without proteinuria.

2. Maternal position influences BP: the highest reading is obtained in the sitting position, the lowest reading is obtained in the left lateral position, and an intermediate reading is obtained in the supine position. Sitting or standing positions show minimal change in SBP readings; however, can decrease the DBP by about 10 to 15 mm Hg.
3. Maternal BP will also rise with uterine contractions and returns to the baseline level after the uterine contraction is over.

> **NURSING ALERT** Ensure that the maternal BP is not taken during uterine contractions because it may give you a false elevated BP. Blood pressure readings should be measured in the same extremity, with the woman in the same position. BP should be measured with the BP cuff at the level of the woman's heart, regardless of the position (sitting, standing, or lateral). This may mean that the BP is taken on the dependent arm (the arm the patient is lying on). If this occurs, move the dependent arm out from underneath the patient's side to ensure unobstructed vessels and take BP.

Hematologic Changes

1. Total volume of circulating RBCs increases 17% to 33%; hemoglobin concentration at term averages 12 to 16 g/dL; hematocrit concentration at term averages 37% to 47%.
2. Average leukocyte (white blood cell [WBC]) count in the third trimester is 5 to 12,000/mm^3. WBC count can be elevated as high as 30,000 or more during labor—cause unknown; probably represents the reappearance in the circulation of leukocytes previously shunted out of active circulation.
3. Pregnancy is a hypercoagulable state due to the increased levels of a number of essential coagulation factors. These factors include factor I (fibrinogen by 50%), factor V (proaccelerin or labile factor), factor VII (proconvertin or serum prothrombin conversion accelerator), factor VIII (antihemophilic factor or antihemophilic globulin), factor IX (plasma thromboplastin component or Christmas factor), factor X (Stuart or Prower factor), factor XII (Hageman or glass or contact factor) and vWF (von Willebrand factor antigen). Factor II (prothrombin) increases slightly, whereas factors XI (plasma thromboplastin antecedent) and XIII (fibrin-stabilizing factor) decrease during pregnancy.
4. There is no significant change in the number, appearance, or function of platelets. Average platelet count is 150,000 to 400,000/mm^3, which increases the risk to the pregnant woman for venous thrombosis.

Changes in the Respiratory Tract

1. Diaphragm is elevated (about 4 cm) during pregnancy—chiefly by the enlarging uterus that decreases the length of the lungs.
2. Thoracic cage expands its anteroposterior diameter (by 2 cm). The increased pressure from the uterus also widens the substernal angle by about 50%, causing slight flaring of the ribs—result of increased mobility of rib attachments.

3. Breathing is more diaphragmatic than costal.

4. Total lung volume (amount of air in lungs at maximum inspiration) decreases by about 5%. Residual volume (amount of air in lungs after maximum expiration), respiratory reserve volume (max amount of air expired during rest), and functional residual capacity (amount of air remaining in lungs at rest and allowing for gas exchange) drop by about 18% to 20%.

5. Hyperventilation occurs—that is, an increase in respiratory rate, tidal volume (amount of air inspired and expired with normal breath) increases by 30% to 40%, and minute ventilation (amount of air inspired in 1 minute) increases by 40%.

6. Increased total volume lowers partial pressure of arterial carbon dioxide ($Paco_2$), causing mild respiratory alkalosis that is compensated for by lowering of the bicarbonate concentration.

7. Increased respiratory rate and reduced $Paco_2$ are probably induced by progesterone and estrogen to a lesser degree on the respiratory center.

8. Oxygen consumption increases 15% to 20% and as much as 300% in labor. This increase leads to increased maternal alveolar and arterial oxygen partial pressure levels.

9. Partial pressure of arterial oxygen (PaO_2) elevates to 106 to 108 mm Hg in first trimester and 101 to 104 mm Hg at term. $Paco_2$ is decreased to 27 to 32 mm Hg. Bicarbonate decreases to 18 to 21 mEq/L. Normal pH during pregnancy is 7.40 to 7.45. These changes allow for removal of fetal carbon dioxide via passive diffusion in the placenta.

10. Approximately 60% to 70% of pregnant women experience shortness of breath; the cause is unknown.

11. Nasal stuffiness and epistaxis (nosebleeds) are also common during pregnancy, secondary to vascular congestion caused from the increased estrogen levels.

12. Net effect of all changes in lung volume = no change in maternal maximum breathing capacity during pregnancy.

Changes in Renal System

1. Ureters become dilated and elongated during pregnancy because of mechanical pressure and perhaps due to the effects of progesterone. When the uterus rises out of the uterine cavity, it rests on the ureters, compressing them at the pelvic brim. Dilation is greater on the right side—the left side is cushioned by the sigmoid colon.

2. Renal plasma flow (RPF) increases by 60% to 80% by the end of the first trimester due to the increases in blood volume and cardiac output and the decreases in the systemic vascular resistance (all due to the effects of progesterone).

3. Glomerular filtration rate (GFR) increases 40% to 50% by the second trimester, and the increase persists almost to term. RPF increases early in pregnancy and decreases to nonpregnant levels in the third trimester. These changes may be due to placental lactogen.

4. Glucosuria may be evident because of the increase in glomerular filtration without an increase in tubular resorptive capacity for filtered glucose.

5. Excreted protein may be increased due to the increased GFR, but is not considered abnormal until the level exceeds 250 mg/dL. Slight amounts of protein may be excreted during or just after vigorous labor.

6. Toward the end of pregnancy, pressure of the presenting part impedes drainage of blood and lymph from the bladder base, typically leaving the area edematous, easily traumatized, and more susceptible to infection.

7. Due to the increased RPF and GFR, the amount of glucose the kidneys filter increases 10- to 100-fold. The kidneys cannot always keep up with this increase; therefore, whatever glucose that is not filtered is lost in the urine, contributing to glycosuria.

8. Protein excretion is also increased to a rate not always handled by the kidneys' tubular reabsorptive capability. Therefore, protein can spill into the urine. However, protein in the urine should not be considered an abnormal finding until 24-hour urine values exceed 300 mg/dL.

Changes in GI Tract

1. Gums may become hyperemic and softened and may bleed easily.

2. A localized vascular swelling of the gums may appear—called *epulis of pregnancy*.

3. Stomach and intestines are displaced upward and laterally by the enlarging uterus. Heartburn (pyrosis) is common, caused by reflux of acid secretions in the lower esophagus.

4. Tone and motility of GI tract decrease, leading to prolongation of gastric emptying due to the large amount of progesterone produced by the placenta. Decreased motility, mechanical obstruction by the fetus, and decreased water absorption from the colon leads to constipation.

5. Hemorrhoids are common because of elevated pressure in veins below the level of the large uterus and constipation.

6. Distention and hypotonia of the gallbladder are common, which can cause stasis of bile. Additionally, there is a decrease in emptying time and thickening of bile, resulting in hypercholesterolemia and gallstone formation.

7. Liver function tests are altered. With pregnancy, bilirubin, aspartate aminotransferase, and alanine aminotransferase values are unchanged; prothrombin time may show a slight increase or be unchanged. Liver size and morphology are unchanged.

8. Peptic ulcer formation or exacerbation is uncommon during pregnancy due to decreased hydrochloric acid (caused by increased estrogen levels).

9. The appendix is pushed superiorly.

Changes in the Endocrine System

1. Anterior pituitary gland enlarges in both weight (30% increase) and volume (two-fold increase). Its shape also changes from convex to dome-shaped; posterior pituitary gland remains unchanged.

2. Thyroid is moderately enlarged because of hyperplasia of glandular tissue and increased vascularity.

a. Basal metabolic rate increases progressively during normal pregnancy (as much as 25%) because of metabolic activity of fetus.

b. Level of protein-bound iodine and thyroxine rises sharply and is maintained until after delivery because of increased circulatory estrogen and hCG.

c. Hyperthyroidism during pregnancy is rare. Although levels of thyroxine (T_4) and triiodothyronine (T_3) are elevated by as much as 40% to 100% by term, this is a result of estrogen, hCG, and increased urinary iodide secretion, resulting in "euthyroid hyperthyroxinemia."

3. Parathyroid gland size is known to increase, but there is a decrease in the parathyroid hormone (PTH) during pregnancy. This decrease is balanced by the fetus' and the placenta's increased production of PTH.

4. Adrenal secretions considerably increased—amounts of aldosterone increase as early as the 15th week to accommodate for the increased sodium excretion.

5. Pancreas—because of the fetal glucose needs for fetal growth, there are alterations in maternal insulin production and usage.

a. Estrogen, progesterone, cortisol, and human placental lactogen (hPL) decrease the maternal utilization of glucose.

b. Cortisol also increases maternal insulin production.

c. Insulinase, an enzyme produced by the placenta, deactivates maternal insulin.

d. These changes result in an increased need for insulin, and the islets of Langerhans increase their production of insulin.

Changes in Integumentary System

1. Pigment changes occur because of melanocyte-stimulating hormone (due to increased estrogen and progesterone), the level of which is elevated from the second month of pregnancy until term.

2. Striae gravidarum appear in later months of pregnancy as reddish, slightly depressed streaks in the skin of the abdomen and occasionally over the breasts and thighs and occur in as much at 50% of all pregnant women.

3. A brownish-black line of pigment is usually formed in the midline of the abdominal skin—known as *linea nigra*.

4. Brownish patches of pigment may form on the face—known as *chloasma/melasma* or "mask of pregnancy." Chloasma usually disappears after pregnancy, but can reappear with excessive exposure to the sun or with oral contraceptive treatment.

5. Angiomas (vascular spider nevis)—minute red elevations commonly on the skin of the face, neck, upper chest, legs, and arms—may develop.

6. Reddening of the palms (palmar erythema) may also occur.

7. There is also an increased warmth to the skin and increased nail growth.

Changes in the Musculoskeletal System

1. The increasing mobility of sacroiliac, sacrococcygeal, and pelvic joints during pregnancy is a result of hormonal changes, specifically the hormone relaxin.

2. The center of gravity shifts secondary to increased weight gain, fluid retention, lordosis, and mobile ligaments. This mobility and the change in the center of gravity contribute to alteration of maternal posture and to back pain.

3. Late in pregnancy, aching, numbness, and weakness in the upper extremities may occur because of lordosis and paresthesia, which ultimately produces traction on the ulnar and median nerves.

4. Separation of the rectus muscles due to pressure of the growing uterus creates what is called a diastasis recti. If this is severe, a portion of the anterior uterine wall is covered by only a layer of skin, fascia, and peritoneum.

Changes in the Neurologic System

1. Usually no system changes.

2. Mild frontal headaches are common in the first and second trimester and are usually related to tension or hormonal changes.

3. Dizziness is common and is related to vasomotor instability, postural hypotension, or hypoglycemia following long periods of standing or sitting.

4. Tingling sensations in the hands are common and are due to excessive hyperventilation, which decreases maternal $Paco_2$ levels.

 NURSING ALERT Severe headaches that occur after 20 weeks' gestation and are accompanied by visual changes, elevated BP (systolic >140 mm Hg or diastolic >90 mm Hg), and proteinuria should be evaluated immediately.

Changes in Hormonal Responses

Steroid Hormones

1. Estrogen:

a. Is secreted by the ovaries in early pregnancy, but by 7 weeks' gestation, over half of the estrogen is secreted by the placenta.

b. The three classic estrogens during pregnancy are estrone, estradiol, and estriol. More than 90% of the estrogen secreted during pregnancy is estriol.

c. Estrogens also ensure uterine growth and development, maintenance of uterine elasticity and contractility, maintenance of breast growth and its ductal structures, and enlargement of the external genitalia.

2. Progesterone:

a. Is initially secreted by the corpus luteum and later by the placenta.

b. Plays a critical role in the maintenance of the pregnancy by suppressing the maternal immunologic response to the fetus and the rejection of the trophoblasts.

c. Progesterone also helps to maintain the endometrium, inhibits uterine contractility, helps in the development of breast lobules for lactation, stimulates the maternal respiratory center, and relaxes smooth muscle.

Placental Protein Hormones

1. hCG:
   a. Secreted by the syncytiotrophoblasts and stimulates the production by the corpus luteum of progesterone and estrogen until the fully developed placenta takes over.
   b. In multiple gestations, hCG can be twice as high as in a single pregnancy.
   c. hCG levels peak around 10 weeks' gestation (50,000 to 100,000 mIU/mL) then decrease to 10,000 to 20,000 mIU/mL by 20 weeks' gestation.
2. hPL:
   a. Also referred to as *human chorionic somatomammotropin*. Produced by the syncytiotrophoblasts of the placenta; detected in maternal serum as early as 6 weeks' gestation.
   b. Serum hPL levels rise concomitantly with placental growth.
   c. hPL is an antagonist of insulin. It increases the amount of free fatty acids available to the fetus for metabolic needs and decreases the maternal metabolism of glucose allowing for protein synthesis. This action allows the fetus to have the needed nutrients when the woman is not eating.

Other Hormones

1. Prostaglandins:
   a. Exact function is still unknown.
   b. Affect smooth muscle contractility and some potent vasodilators.
   c. Essential for the cardiovascular adaptation to pregnancy, cervical ripening, and initiation of labor.
   d. Increased levels of prostaglandins may lead to vasodilation.
2. Relaxin:
   a. Secreted primarily by the corpus luteum. Can be secreted in small amounts by the decidua and the placenta.
   b. Inhibits uterine activity, decreases the strength of uterine contractions, softens the cervix, and remodels collagen.
3. Prolactin:
   a. Released from the anterior pituitary gland.
   b. Responsible for sustaining milk protein, casein, fatty acids, lactose, and the volume of milk secretion during lactation.

Structure of the Pelvis

Bones of the Pelvis

The pelvis is composed of four bones:

1. Two innominate bones (hip bones) form the sides and front.
2. Sacrum and coccyx form the back. Pelvic bones are held together by fibrocartilage of the symphysis pubis and several ligaments.

Divisions of the Pelvis

1. False pelvis—lies above an imaginary line called the *linea terminalis* or *pelvic brim* (see Figure 36-1). Function of the false pelvis is to support the enlarged uterus.
2. True pelvis lies below the pelvic brim or linea terminalis; it is the bony canal through which the fetus must pass. It is divided into three planes: the inlet, the midpelvis, and the outlet.
   a. Inlet:
      i. Upper boundary of the true pelvis—bounded by upper margin of symphysis pubis in front, linea terminalis on sides, and sacral promontory (first sacral vertebra) in back.
      ii. Largest diameter of inlet is transverse (see Figure 36-2).
      iii. Smallest diameter of inlet is anteroposterior.
      iv. Anteroposterior diameter is most important diameter of inlet: measured clinically by diagonal conjugate—distance from lower margin of symphysis to the sacral promontory (usually 5½ inches [14 cm]) (see Figure 36-3).
      v. Obstetric (true) conjugate—distance between inner surface of symphysis and sacral promontory measured by subtracting ½ to ¾ inch (1.5 to 2 cm) (thickness of symphysis) from the diagonal conjugate. Adequate diameter is usually 4½ inches (11.5 cm). This is the shortest anteroposterior diameter through which the fetus must pass.
   b. Midpelvis:
      i. Bounded by inlet above and outlet below—true bony cavity. Midpelvis contains the narrowest portion of the pelvis.
      ii. Diameters cannot be measured clinically.

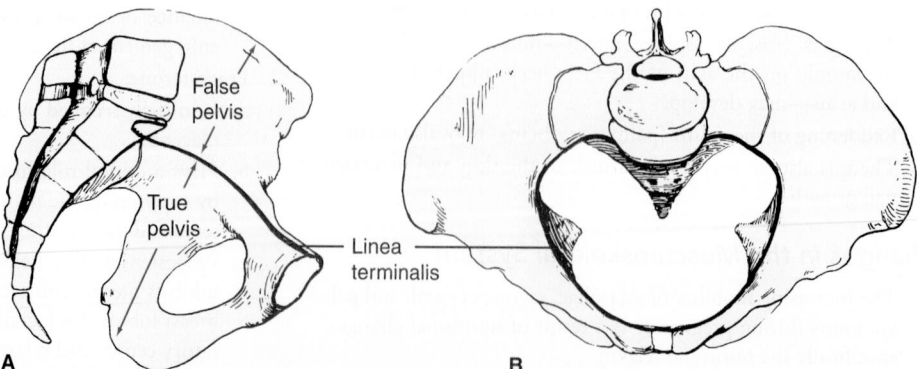

Figure 36-1. (A) Side view of the true and false pelvis. **(B)** Front view showing linea terminalis (pelvic brim).

False pelvis

True pelvis

Linea terminalis

A   B

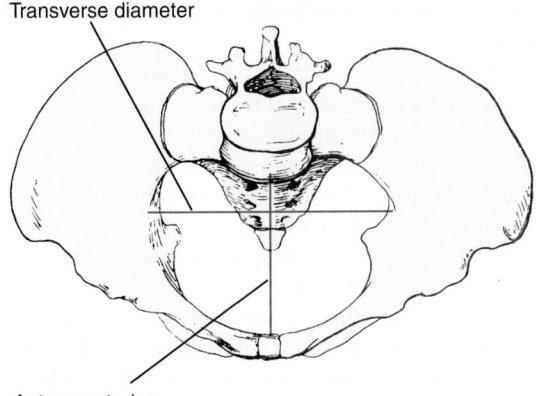

Figure 36-2. Inlet of normal female pelvis showing transverse and anteroposterior diameters.

    iii. Clinical evaluation of adequacy is made by noting the ischial spines. Prominent spines that protrude into the cavity indicate a contracted midpelvic space. The interspinous diameter is 4 inches (10 cm).
  c. Outlet:
    i. Lowest boundary of the true pelvis.
    ii. Bounded by lower margin of symphysis in front, ischial tuberosities on sides, tip of sacrum posteriorly.
    iii. Most important diameter clinically is distance between the tuberosities (>4 inches).

Shapes of the Pelvis

There are four main types of pelvic shapes (see Figure 36-4).

1. Gynecoid (normal female pelvis); optimal diameters in all three planes; 50% of all women.

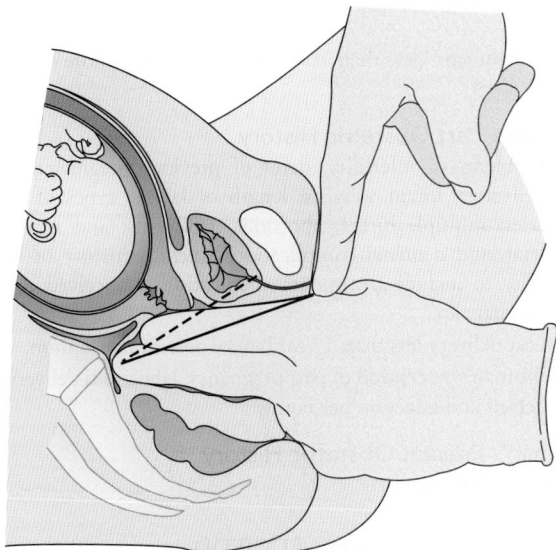

Figure 36-3. Measurement of diagonal conjugate diameter. *Straight* line shows diagonal conjugate; *dotted* line shows true conjugate.

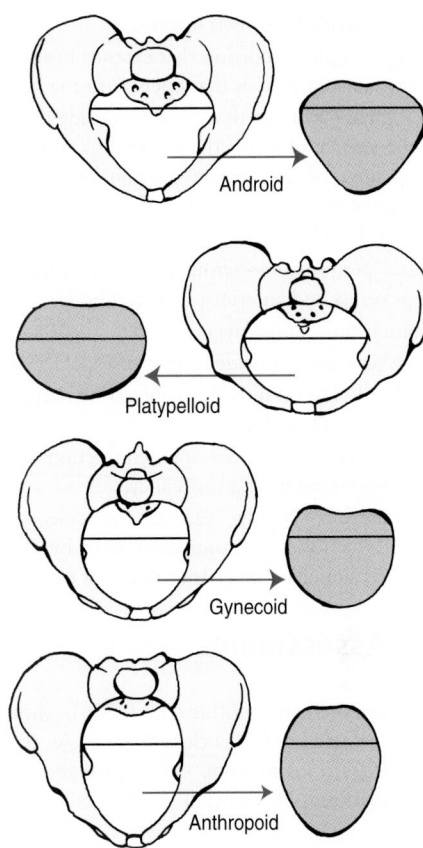

Figure 36-4. The four types of female pelvises. *Android—*male-type pelvis. *Platypelloid—*broad pelvis with shortened anteroposterior diameter and flattened, oval, transverse shape. *Gynecoid—*typical female pelvis in which inlet is round instead of oval. *Anthropoid—*pelvis in which anteroposterior diameter is equal to or greater than the transverse diameter.

2. Android (normal male pelvis); posterior segments are decreased in all three planes; deep transverse arrest of descent of the fetus and failure of rotation of the fetus are common; 20% of all women.
3. Anthropoid (apelike pelvis with long anteroposterior diameter); may allow for easy delivery of an occiput-posterior presentation of the fetus; 25% of all women.
4. Platypelloid (flat female pelvis with wide transverse diameter); arrest of fetal descent at the pelvic inlet is common; labor progress can be poor; 5% of all women.

Structure of the Uterus

1. Located behind the symphysis pubis between the bladder and the rectum.
2. Uterine size increases after childbirth.
3. Consists of four parts:
  a. Fundus—upper rounded segment that extends above the insertion of the fallopian tubes; fetal growth is measured by fundal height.
  b. Body (corpus)—main portion between cervix and fundus.
  c. Isthmus (neck)—lower uterine segment.

d. Cervix—divided into two sections:
   i. Supravaginal—portion that extends inside the uterus; contains internal os that opens into the uterine cavity.
   ii. Vaginal—portion that extends outside the uterus into the vagina; contains the external os that is the visible opening of the cervix; portion that is felt during vaginal examination in assessing cervical dilation.
4. Consists of three layers:
   a. Parietal peritoneum—serous coat; covers most of uterus except cervix and anterior portion of body.
   b. Myometrium—three layers:
      i. Outer layer—provides power to expel the fetus.
      ii. Middle layer—provides contractions after childbirth to control blood loss.
      iii. Inner layer—provides sphincter action to help keep cervix closed during pregnancy.
   c. Endometrium—highly vascular mucous membrane; responds to hormonal stimulation with hypertrophy and secretion; sloughs if pregnancy does not occur.

Prenatal Assessment

Evidence Base Gauthier, D. (2009). Maternal-fetal assessment. In A. Lyndon & L. U. Ali (Eds.), *Fetal monitoring principles and practices* (4th ed., pp. 45–64). Dubuque, IA: Kendall Hunt.

Health History

Age
1. Adolescents (younger than age 19) have an increased incidence of anemia, gestational hypertension, preterm labor (PTL), small-for-gestational-age (SGA) infants, intrauterine-growth-restricted infants, cephalopelvic disproportion, and dystocia.
2. Women of advanced maternal age (over age 35) have an increased incidence of hypertension, pregnancies complicated by underlying medical problems such as diabetes, multiple gestation, and infants with genetic abnormalities.

Family History
1. Includes maternal and paternal history.
2. Congenital disorders, hereditary diseases, multiple pregnancies, diabetes, heart disease, hypertension, mental retardation, renal disease, use of diethylstilbestrol (DES).

NURSING ALERT Daughters born to mothers who sustained their pregnancies with DES may have uterine anomalies that increase their risk of PTL or uterine tachysystole.

Woman's Medical History
1. Childhood diseases, especially rubella. Others to consider are measles and chickenpox.
2. Major illnesses, surgery (especially of the reproductive tract, spinal surgery, or appendectomy), blood transfusions.

3. Chronic medical conditions, such as epilepsy, diabetes mellitus.
4. Drug, food, and environmental sensitivities.
5. Urinary tract infections (UTIs), heart disease, hypertension, endocrine disorders, anemias.
6. Menstrual history (onset of menarche, length, amount, regularity, and pain [dysmenorrhea] of menstrual cycle). Also, assess bleeding between menses.
7. Gynecologic history (sexually transmitted diseases, contraceptive use, sexual history).
8. Use of medications (prescription and over-the-counter [OTC]), recreational drugs, alcohol, nicotine, tobacco, and caffeine.
9. History of tuberculosis, hepatitis, group B beta-hemolytic streptococcus, or human immunodeficiency virus (HIV).

Woman's Nutritional History
1. Adherence to special dietary practices (religious, social, or cultural preferences)
2. History of eating disorders (obesity, bulimia, anorexia nervosa), gastric bypass, absorption problems.
3. Eating patterns (times and frequency of eating daily), number of servings of food from the five food groups, calories, protein, vitamins, and minerals consumed daily.
4. Additional factors to be considered include where the food was eaten, quantity of food eaten, how food was prepared (ie, fried, baked), and which foods are limited and why.
5. In 2011, the Food Pyramid was changed to MyPlate. As a result, the U.S. Department of Agriculture has designed an online interactive diet program, Daily Food Plan for Moms, specifically directed to pregnant and breastfeeding women. This program gives a personalized plan for nutrition.

Evidence Base United States Department of Agriculture. (2011). Personalized food plan for pregnant and nursing mothers. Available: *www.choosemyplate.gov/mypyramidmoms*.

6. Weight gain (less than 10 lb [4.5 kg]) or loss (more than 5 lb [2.3 kg]).

Woman's Past Obstetric History
1. Problems of infertility, dates of previous pregnancies and deliveries; infant weights; length of labors; types of deliveries; multiple births; abortions; stillbirths; and maternal, fetal, and neonatal complications. Include history of infertility to include treatments, medications, conceived or lost pregnancies.
2. Last delivery less than 1 year before present conception.
3. Woman's perception of past pregnancy, labor, and delivery for herself and effect on her family.

Woman's Present Obstetric History
1. Gravidity, parity.
2. Date of last menses.
3. Estimated date of birth—EDC/EDD.
4. Signs and symptoms of pregnancy—amenorrhea, breast changes, nausea and vomiting, fetal movement, fatigue, urinary frequency, skin pigment changes. Expectations for her

present pregnancy, labor, and delivery. Expectations for her health care providers and her perception of her relationship between herself and her nurse.

5. Rest and sleep patterns—length, quality, and regularity of rest and sleep.

6. Activity and employment—exercise patterns, type and hours of employment, exposure to hazardous material (occupational hazards), plans for continued employment.

7. Sexual activity—sexual satisfaction, frequency, positions during intercourse, alternative practices used to achieve sexual satisfaction.

8. Inadequate prenatal care, intrauterine growth problems, Rh sensitization, or preterm labor.

Psychosocial History

1. Psychiatric and mental status history: history of mood or anxiety disorders; mental illness; medications or treatments for psychiatric or mental problems.

2. Self-concept or self-esteem issues.

3. Support systems available, including ones she has made contact with.

4. Stressors: personal and occupational stressors that may affect her pregnancy and the fetus; include coping strategies she may use or lack of coping skills.

5. Past history of depression, with or without an association with pregnancy.

6. Emotional changes and adjustment to pregnancy

7. The Psychosocial Screening Tool can be used to determine factors that impact a woman's physical and mental health and may interfere with her following through with prenatal care. Any positive response to the following questions deserves further investigation and intervention.

   a. Do you have any problems (job, transportation, etc.) that prevent you from keeping your health care appointments?

   b. Do you feel unsafe where you live?

   c. In the past 2 months, have you used any form of tobacco?

   d. In the past 2 months, have you used drugs or alcohol (including beer, wine, or mixed drinks)?

   e. On a scale of 1 to 5, how do you rate your current stress level?

   f. How many times have you moved in the past 12 months?

   g. If you could change the timing of this pregnancy, would you want it earlier, later, not at all, no change?

 Evidence Base American College of Obstetricians and Gynecologists. (2006/Reaffirmed 2011). *Psychosocial risk factors: Perinatal screening intervention* (Committee Opinion No. 343). Washington, DC: Author.

8. In addition to the Perinatal Screening Tool, the pregnant woman can be asked about intimate partner violence. Examples of questions for this interview are:

   a. Has your current partner ever threatened you or made you feel afraid? Threatened to hurt you or your children if you did or did not do something?

   b. Has your partner ever hit, choked, or physically hurt you? (Includes being slapped, kicked, bitten, pushed, or shoved.)

   c. Has your partner ever forced you to do something sexually that you did not want to do or refused your request to use condoms?

   d. Has your partner ever tampered with your birth control or tried to get you pregnant when you did not want to be pregnant?

   e. Has your partner prevented you from using a wheelchair, cane, respirator, or other assistive devices?

 Evidence Base American College of Obstetricians and Gynecologists. (2012). *Intimate partner violence* (Committee Opinion No. 518). Washington, DC: Author.

Laboratory Data

Urinalysis

1. Urine is tested for glucose, ketones, and protein. Urine is usually collected by way of clean-catch midstream.

2. Glucose (glucosuria) may be present in small amounts because the glomerular filtration rate is increased without the same increase in kidney tubular reabsorption. Glucosuria should be investigated to rule out diabetes.

3. Protein in the urine that exceeds 300 mg/dL/24-hour urine collection should be reported because it may be a sign of preeclampsia, renal problems, or UTI.

4. Ketones in the urine should be reported because ketonuria may be a sign of excessive weight loss, dehydration, or electrolyte imbalance. Ketonuria is commonly secondary to nausea and vomiting of pregnancy.

5. If the urine is cloudy and bacteria or leukocytes are present (more than four leukocytes per high-powered field), a urine culture is performed.

6. The presence of bilirubin is indicative of liver or gallbladder disease or breakdown of RBCs.

7. The presence of blood in the urine (hematuria) is suggestive of UTI, kidney disease, or vaginal contamination.

Blood

1. Determination of hematocrit and hemoglobin levels and description of the morphology of the RBCs are done to find evidence of anemias, such as sickle cell or Mediterranean anemia.

2. Hemoglobin levels average 12 to 16 g/dL.

3. Blood type, Rh factor, and antibody screen—if the woman is found to be Rh negative or to have a positive antibody screen, her partner is screened and a maternal antibody titer is drawn, as indicated.

   a. Coomb's test—retested at 28 weeks in the Rh-negative woman for detection of antibodies.

   b. Rh_o (D) immune globulin (RhoGAM) given at 28 weeks, as indicated. Also administered following chorionic villus sampling (CVS), percutaneous umbilical sampling, amniocentesis, trauma, or placental separation (abruptio placentae or placenta previa).

   c. Given within 72 hours of birth to a Rh_o (D) mom or Du– and without antibodies and neonate is Rh_1 (D) or Du+ with a negative Coombs' test.

4. Glucose—diabetic screening for women who are at average risk conducted at 24 to 28 weeks using a 1-hour 50-g glucose load test. According to the American Diabetes Association, average risk includes age 25 or older; obese women of any age; family history of diabetes mellitus in a first-degree relative; member of an ethnic group with a high prevalence of diabetes (Hispanic, black, Native American, Asian American); history of abnormal glucose tolerance; history of poor obstetric outcome.

5. Alpha-fetoprotein (AFP)—done at 15 to 18 weeks. High maternal levels may indicate an open neural tube defect in the fetus; low levels have been associated with Down syndrome. Inaccurate pregnancy dating is the most common cause for an abnormal AFP.

Infection

1. Venereal Disease Research Lab (VDRL) test or Fluorescent Treponemal Antibody Absorption Test for syphilis is done on the initial visit; repeat VDRL at 32 weeks, as indicated.

2. Gonorrhea—cervical cultures are usually done at the initial visit and when symptoms are present.

3. Herpes—all visible lesions are cultured and the cervix is cultured weekly beginning 4 to 8 weeks before delivery.

4. Chlamydia—done at the initial visit and when symptoms are present.

5. Rubella titer—if nonimmune, less than 1:8; immunize postpartum.

6. Hepatitis B surface antigen.

7. HIV—screen is done on high-risk women.

Other Tests

1. Toxoplasmosis—done as indicated for women at risk.

2. Tuberculin skin tests—done as indicated.

3. Papanicolaou (Pap) smear—done unless recent results available.

4. Maternal serum alpha-fetoprotein (MS-AFP)—done to detect open neural tube defects or open abdominal wall defects; offered to all women and usually drawn between 16 and 18 weeks' gestation.

5. Sickle cell screen—done to detect presence of sickle hemoglobin in at-risk women.

6. Group B beta streptococcus (cervical and pharyngeal swabs)—done to detect carriers or active group B beta streptococcus.

Physical Assessment

General Examination

1. The woman is asked to empty her bladder before the examination to enhance her comfort and to facilitate palpation of her uterus and pelvic organs during the vaginal examination.

2. Evaluation of the woman's weight and BP.

3. Examination of the eyes, ears, and nose—nasal congestion during pregnancy may occur as a result of peripheral vasodilation.

4. Examination of the mouth, teeth, throat, and thyroid—the gums may be hyperemic and softened because of increased progesterone.

5. Inspection of breasts and nipples—the breasts may be enlarged and tender; nipple and areolar pigment may be darkened.

6. Auscultation of the heart.

7. Auscultation and percussion of the lungs.

Abdominal Examination

1. Examination for scars or striations, diastasis (separation of the rectus muscle), or umbilical hernia.

2. Palpation of the abdomen for height of the fundus (palpable after 13 weeks of pregnancy); measurement recorded and used as guideline for subsequent calculations.

3. Palpation of the abdomen for fetal outline and position (Leopold's maneuvers)—third trimester.

4. Check of FHTs—FHTs are audible with a Doppler after 10 to 12 weeks and at 18 to 20 weeks with a fetoscope.

5. Record fetal position, presentation, and FHTs.

Pelvic Examination

1. The woman is placed in lithotomy position.

2. Inspection of external genitalia.

3. Vaginal examination—done to rule out abnormalities of the birth canal and to obtain cytologic smear (Pap and, if indicated, smears for gonorrhea, vaginal trichomoniasis, candidiasis, herpes, group B beta streptococcus, and chlamydia) (see Figure 36-5).

4. Examination of the cervix for position, size, mobility, and consistency. Cervix is softened and bluish (increased vascularity) during pregnancy.

5. Identification of the ovaries (size, shape, and position).

6. Rectovaginal exploration to identify hemorrhoids, fissures, herniation, or masses.

7. Evaluation of pelvic inlet—anteroposterior diameter by measuring the diagonal conjugate.

8. Evaluation of midpelvis—prominence of the ischial spines.

9. Evaluation of pelvic outlet—distance between ischial tuberosities and mobility of coccyx.

Subsequent Prenatal Assessments

1. Uterine growth and estimated fetal growth (see Figure 36-6).
   a. Fundus at symphysis pubis indicates 12 weeks' gestation.
   b. Fundus at umbilicus indicates 20 weeks' gestation.
   c. Fundal height corresponds with gestational age between 22 and 34 weeks.
   d. Fundus at lower border of rib cage indicates 36 weeks' gestation.
   e. Uterus becomes globular and drop indicates 40 weeks' gestation.

2. A greater fundal height suggests:
   a. Multiple pregnancy.
   b. Miscalculated due date.
   c. Polyhydramnios (excessive amniotic fluid).
   d. Hydatidiform mole (degeneration of villi into grapelike clusters; fetus does not usually develop).
   e. Uterine fibroids.

3. A lesser fundal height suggests:
   a. Intrauterine fetal growth restriction.
   b. Error in estimating gestation.

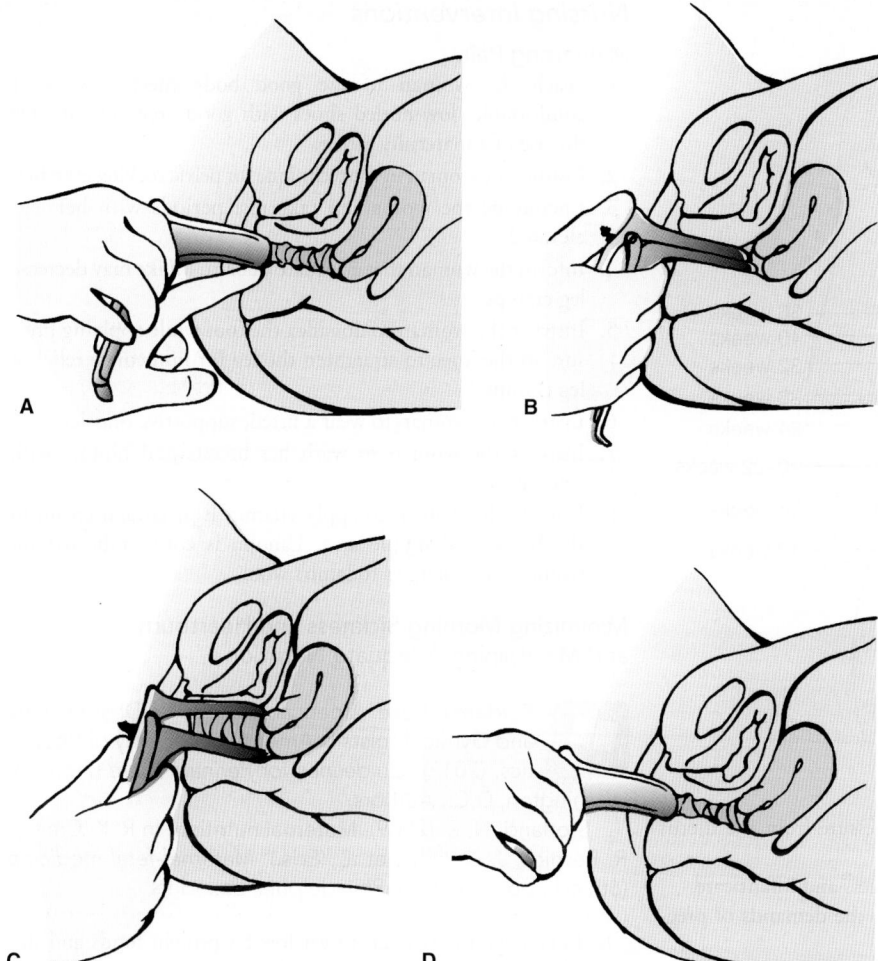

Figure 36-5. Vaginal speculum examination. (**A**) Blades held obliquely on entering the introitus. (**B**) Blades rotated to horizontal position and pushed toward cervix. (**C**) Blades separated to encircle cervix. (**D**) Blades removed with gentle pulling.

   c. Fetal or amniotic fluid abnormalities.
   d. Intrauterine fetal death.
   e. SGA.
4. FHTs—palpate abdomen for fetal position.
   a. Normal—110 to 160 beats/minute (bpm).
5. Weight—major increase in weight occurs during second half of pregnancy; usually between 0.5 lb (0.2 kg)/week and 1 lb (0.5 kg)/week. Greater weight gain may indicate fluid retention and hypertensive disorder.
6. BP—should remain near woman's prepregnant baseline.
7. Complete blood count at 28 and 32 weeks' gestation; VDRL—rechecked at 36 to 40 weeks' gestation.
8. Antibody serology screen if Rh negative at 36 weeks' gestation.
9. Culture smears for gonorrhea, chlamydia, group B beta-hemolytic streptococcus, and herpes, as indicated; usually at 36 and 40 weeks' gestation.
10. Urinalysis—for protein, glucose, blood, and nitrates.
11. AFP—done at 15 to 20 weeks.
12. Diabetic screening—done, as indicated, at 24 to 28 weeks.
13. Administer RhoGAM, as indicated, at 28 weeks.
14. Edema—check the lower legs, face, and hands.

15. Evaluate discomforts of pregnancy—fatigue, heartburn, hemorrhoids, constipation, and backache.
16. Evaluate eating and sleeping patterns, general adjustment and coping with the pregnancy.
17. Evaluate concerns of the woman and her family.
18. Evaluate preparation for labor, delivery, and parenting. See Patient Education Guidelines 36-1, page 1252.

Nursing Interventions and Patient Education

Nursing Diagnoses

- Acute Pain (backache, leg cramps, breast tenderness) related to physiologic changes of pregnancy.
- Imbalanced Nutrition: Less Than Body Requirements related to morning sickness and heartburn and lack of knowledge of requirements in pregnancy.
- Impaired Urinary Elimination (frequency) related to increased pressure from the uterus.
- Constipation related to physiologic changes of pregnancy and pressure from the uterus.

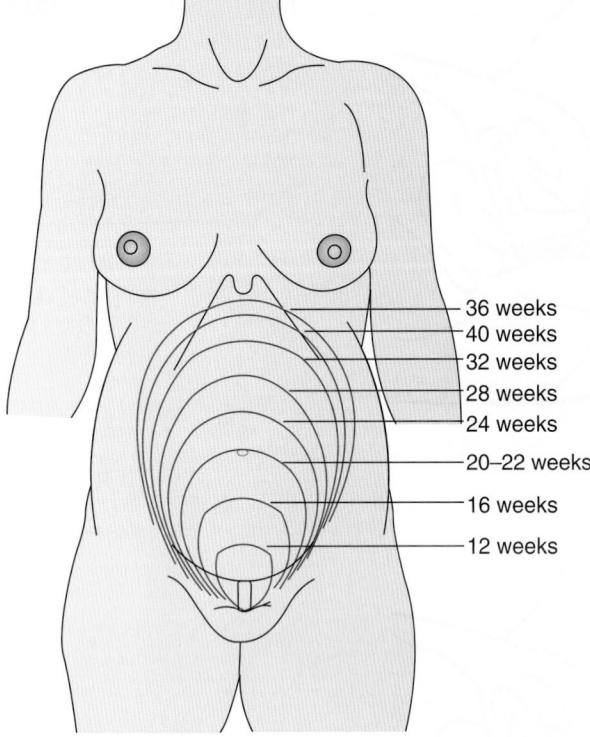

Figure 36-6. Height of fundus.

- Impaired Tissue Integrity related to pressure from the uterus and increased blood volume.
- Anxiety or Fear related to the birth process and infant care.
- Ineffective Role Performance related to the demands of pregnancy.
- Activity Intolerance related to physiologic changes of pregnancy and enlarging uterus.

Nursing Interventions

Minimizing Pain

1. Teach the woman to use good body mechanics—wear comfortable, low-heeled shoes with good arch support; try the use of a maternity girdle.
2. Instruct the woman in the technique for pelvic rocking exercises.
3. Encourage the woman to take rest periods with her legs elevated.
4. Inform the woman that adequate calcium intake may decrease leg cramps.
5. Instruct the woman to dorsiflex the foot while applying pressure to the knee to straighten the leg for immediate relief of leg cramps.
6. Instruct the woman to wear a fitted, supportive brassiere.
7. Instruct the woman to wash her breasts and nipples with water only.
8. Instruct the woman to apply vitamin E or lanolin cream to the breast and nipple area. Lanolin is contraindicated for women with allergies to lamb's wool.

Minimizing Morning Sickness and Heartburn and Maintaining Adequate Nutrition

 Evidence Base American College of Obstetricians and Gynecologists & American Academy of Pediatrics. (2012). *Guidelines for Perinatal Care* (7th ed.). Washington, D.C.: Authors.
  Stotland, N. E. (2009). Maternal nutrition. In R. K. Creasy, R. Resnick, J. D. Iams, et al. (Eds.), *Maternal-fetal medicine* (6th ed., pp. 111–124). Philadelphia: Saunders.

1. Encourage the woman to eat low-fat protein foods and dry carbohydrates, such as toast and crackers.
2. Encourage the woman to eat small, frequent meals.

PATIENT EDUCATION GUIDELINES 36-1

Prenatal Care

- It is important to keep scheduled prenatal care appointments:
  - Weeks 1–28: Every month
  - Weeks 28–36: Every 2 weeks
  - Weeks 36–delivery: Every week
- Expect the following discomforts of pregnancy, and speak with your nurse or health care provider about strategies for relief:
  - Back pain, leg cramps, breast tenderness
  - Morning sickness, heartburn
  - Frequent urination
  - Constipation
  - Swelling of legs, varicose veins
  - Fatigue
- Follow a healthy, balanced diet with three meals per day and take prenatal vitamins as directed by your health care provider.

- Get regular exercise and use proper body mechanics to avoid injury.
- Be aware of danger symptoms of pregnancy; these must be reported to your health care provider promptly:
  - Vision disturbances—blurring, spots, or double vision
  - Vaginal bleeding, new or old blood
  - Edema of the face, fingers, and sacrum
  - Headaches—frequent, severe, or continuous
  - Fluid discharge from vagina; unusual or severe abdominal pain
  - Chills, fever, or burning on urination
  - Epigastric pain (severe stomachache)
  - Muscular irritability or convulsions
  - Inability to tolerate food or liquids, leading to severe nausea and hyperemesis

3. Advise the woman to eat slowly.

4. Instruct the woman to avoid brushing her teeth soon after eating.

5. Instruct the woman to get out of bed slowly.

6. Encourage the woman to drink soups and liquids between meals to avoid stomach distention and dehydration.

7. Instruct the woman in the use of antacids; caution against the use of sodium bicarbonate because it results in the absorption of excess sodium and fluid retention.

8. Instruct the woman to avoid offensive foods or cooking odors that may trigger nausea.

9. Encourage the woman to eat a few bites of a soda cracker or dry toast before getting out of bed in the morning.

10. Teach the woman the importance of good nutrition for herself and her fetus. Review the basic food groups with appropriate daily servings for essential vitamins and nutrients.

    a. Seven servings of protein-rich foods, including one serving of a vegetable protein.

    b. Three servings of dairy products or other calcium-rich foods.

    c. Seven servings of grain products.

    d. Two or more servings of vitamin C–rich vegetable or fruit.

    e. Three servings of other fruits and vegetables.

    f. Three servings of unsaturated fats.

    g. Two or more servings of other fruits and vegetables.

11. Recommended dietary reference intakes for pregnant women can be obtained from the Food and Nutrition Board at *www.iom.edu/Reports/2006/Dietary-Reference-Intakes-Essential-Guide-Nutrient-Requirements.aspx*.

12. If the woman is a vegetarian, inform her of appropriate intake. Assess type of vegetarian and food intake.

    a. Two broad groups of vegetarians:

       i. Traditional—cultural or religious affiliation prescribes their diet.

       ii. New—adopted vegetarian dietary patterns as a personal or philosophical choice.

    b. Subgroups exist within the above two groups:

       i. Vegan—eat foods from a plant origin, eat no animal foods or anything derived from an animal (ie, eggs, milk, cream, etc.).

       ii. Lacto—eat milk/dairy products but eat no meat, poultry, fish, seafood, or eggs.

       iii. Lacto-ovo—eat milk/dairy products and eggs, but eat no meat, poultry, fish, or seafood.

       iv. Pesce—eat foods from a plant origin and fish or cheese but no meat, poultry, or eggs.

    c. Partial vegetarians may exclude a specific type of animal food, usually meat, but may consume fish and poultry.

    d. Recommend iron and folic acid supplements.

13. Inform the woman that average weight gain in pregnancy is 25 to 35 lb (11 to 16 kg). About 2 to 5 lb (0.9 to 2.3 kg) are gained in the first trimester and about 1 lb (0.5 kg) per week for the remainder of the gestation.

    a. Average weight gain for obese women is 15 lb (6.8 kg).

    b. Adolescent weight gain should be about 5 lb more than for adult women if within 2 years of starting menses.

    c. Women with a multiple pregnancy should gain between 35 and 45 lb (16 and 20 kg).

    d. Average weight gain for underweight women is 28 to 40 lb (13 to 18 kg).

    e. Assess for any cultural or religious times of fasting (eg, Lent or Ramadan).

14. Advise the woman to limit the use of caffeine.

15. Inform the woman that alcohol should be limited or eliminated during pregnancy; no safe level of intake has been established.

16. Inform the woman that smoking should be eliminated or severely reduced during pregnancy; risk of spontaneous abortion, fetal death, low birth weight, and neonatal death increases with increased levels of maternal smoking.

17. Inform the woman that ingesting any drug during pregnancy may affect fetal growth and should be discussed with her health care provider.

Minimizing Urinary Frequency and Promoting Elimination

 Evidence Base Blackburn, S. T. (2008). Physiologic changes of pregnancy. In K. Rice-Simpson & P. A. Creehan (Eds.), *AWHONN's perinatal nursing* (3rd ed., pp. 59–77). Philadelphia: Lippincott Williams & Wilkins.

Monga, M. (2009). Maternal cardiovascular, respiratory, and renal adaptation to pregnancy. In R. K. Creasy, R. Resnick, J. D. Iams, et al. (Eds.), *Maternal-fetal medicine* (6th ed., pp. 101–110). Philadelphia: Saunders.

Stotland, N. E. (2009). Maternal nutrition. In R. K. Creasy, R. Resnick, J. D. Iams, et al. (Eds.), *Maternal-fetal medicine* (6th ed., pp. 111–124). Philadelphia: Saunders.

1. Instruct the woman to limit fluid intake in the evening.

2. Instruct the woman to void before going to bed.

3. Encourage the woman to void after meals.

4. Encourage the woman to void when she feels the urge and after sexual intercourse.

5. Encourage the woman to wear loose-fitting cotton underwear.

6. Cranberry or blueberry juice may be recommended to help prevent UTIs. Caffeine should be avoided.

Avoiding Constipation

1. Instruct the woman to increase fluid intake to at least eight glasses of water per day. One to 2 quarts of fluid per day is desirable.

2. Teach the woman that foods high in fiber should be eaten daily.

3. Encourage the woman to establish regular patterns of elimination.

4. Encourage daily exercise such as walking.

5. Inform the woman that OTC laxatives should be avoided and that bulk-forming agents may be prescribed, if indicated.

Maintaining Tissue Integrity

1. Encourage the woman to take frequent rest periods with her legs elevated.
2. Instruct the woman to wear support stockings and wear loose-fitting clothing for leg varicosities.
3. Instruct the woman to rest periodically with a small pillow under the buttocks to elevate the pelvis for vulvar varicosities.
4. Instruct the woman to avoid constipation, apply cold compresses, take sitz baths, and use topical anesthetics, such as Tucks, for the relief of anal varicosities (hemorrhoids).
5. Provide reassurance that varicosities will totally or greatly resolve after delivery.

Reducing Anxiety and Fear and Promoting Preparation for Labor, Delivery, and Parenthood

1. Encourage the woman or couple to discuss their knowledge, perceptions, cultural values, and expectations of the labor and delivery process.
2. Provide information on childbirth education classes and encourage them to attend.
3. Provide information on sibling and grandparent preparation, as indicated.
4. Encourage a tour of the birth facility.
5. Discuss coping and pain-control techniques for labor and birth.
6. Inform the woman or couple of common procedures during labor and birth.
7. Provide guidelines for coming to the birth facility.
8. Encourage the woman or couple to discuss their perceptions and expectations of parenthood and their "ideal child."
9. Discuss the infant's sleeping, eating, activity, and response patterns for the first month of life.
10. Discuss physical preparations for the infant, such as a sleeping space, clothing, feeding, changing, and bathing equipment.
11. Discuss plans for returning to work and childcare arrangements.
12. Discuss the importance of planning time for themselves and each other apart from the neonate.
13. Provide information and encourage attendance at baby care, breastfeeding, and parenting classes.
14. Answer any questions the woman/couple may have.

Enhancing Role Changes

1. Encourage discussion of feelings and concerns regarding the new role of mother and father.
2. Provide emotional support to the woman/couple regarding the altered family role.
3. Discuss physiologic causes for changes in sexual relationships, such as fatigue, loss of interest, and discomfort from advancing pregnancy. Some women experience heightened sexual activity during the second trimester.
4. Teach the woman or couple that there are no contraindications to intercourse or masturbation to orgasm provided the woman's membranes are intact, there is no vaginal bleeding, and she has no current problems or history of premature labor.
5. Teach the woman or couple that female superior or side-lying positions are usually more comfortable in the latter half of pregnancy.

Minimizing Fatigue

1. Teach the woman reasons for fatigue and have her plan a schedule for adequate rest.
   a. Fatigue in the first trimester is due to increased progesterone and its effects on the sleep center.
   b. Fatigue in the third trimester is due mainly to carrying increased weight of the pregnancy.
   c. About 8 hours of rest are needed at night.
   d. Inability to sleep may be due to excessive fatigue during the day.
   e. In the latter months of pregnancy, sleeping on the side with a small pillow under the abdomen may enhance comfort.
   f. Frequent 15- to 30-minute rest periods during the day are important to avoid overfatigue.
   g. Whenever possible, the woman should work while sitting with her legs elevated.
   h. The woman should avoid standing for prolonged periods, especially during the third trimester.
   i. To promote placental perfusion, the woman should not lie flat on her back—left lateral position provides the best placental perfusion; however, either side is acceptable.
2. Help the woman plan for adequate exercise (if not contraindicated).
   a. In general, exercise during pregnancy should be in keeping with the woman's prepregnancy pattern and type of exercise.
   b. Activities or sports that have a risk of bodily harm (skiing, snowmobiling, ice skating, inline skating, horseback riding) should be avoided.
   c. During pregnancy, endurance during exercise may be decreased.
   d. Exercise classes for pregnant women that concentrate on toning and stretching have resulted in enhanced physical condition, increased self-esteem, and greater social support as a result of being in the exercise group.
   e. Relative contraindications to aerobic exercise during pregnancy: severe anemia, unevaluated maternal cardiac arrhythmia, chronic bronchitis, poorly controlled type 1 diabetes, hypertensive disorder, seizure disorder or hyperthyroidism, extreme morbid obesity, extreme underweight (eg, body mass index less than 12), history of extremely sedentary lifestyle, intrauterine growth restriction in current pregnancy, orthopedic limitations, or heavy smoker.

Evidence Base American College of Obstetricians and Gynecologists. (2002/Reaffirmed 2010). *Diagnosis and management of preeclampsia and eclampsia* (Practice Bulletin #33). Washington, DC: Author.

NURSING ALERT Absolute contraindications to aerobic exercise during pregnancy include hemodynamically significant heart disease, restrictive lung disease, incompetent cervix, cerclage, multiple gestation at risk for PTL, persistent second- or third-trimester bleeding, placenta previa after 26 weeks' gestation, ruptured membranes, PTL in current pregnancy, and preeclampsia.

Community and Home Care Instructions

1. Community and home care is prevention-oriented.
2. Case management coordinates health care management collaboratively.
3. Search out and register for prepared childbirth classes. Preferable to attend those associated with the family's intended delivery facility.
4. Social support available from Women, Infants, and Children's Special Supplemental Feeding Program, breastfeeding groups (La Leche League), and father support groups.
5. Prenatal education should focus on nutrition, sexuality, stress reduction, lifestyle behaviors, and hazards at home or work.
6. Consider cultural practices because they have important implications for the provision of nursing care.

Alternative Therapies

 Evidence Base Louik, C., Gardiner, P., Kelley, K., et al (2010). Use of herbal treatments in pregnancy. *American Journal of Obstetrics and Gynecology*, *202*(5), 439.e1–439.e10.

General Measures

1. Alternative therapies range from nutrition and lifestyle changes to mind and body programs.
2. Encourage the woman to discuss options with her health care provider and consult a credentialed naturopath, accupuncturist, or other alternative practitioner.
3. Physical activities—maintaining an active lifestyle and healthy diet. Some use macrobiotic diets and isometric exercise.
4. Attitudinal activities—maintaining a positive attitude and self-image; have fun and laugh.
5. Relational activities—maintaining social relationships—friends, pets, and family.
6. Spiritual activities—having faith, hope, prayer, and music and meditating as an active part of daily life.
7. Self-caring activities—taking care of self, balancing life, personal integrity, knowing and trusting self, and own time management.
8. Help-seeking activities—seeking assistance in health care ranging from prescribed treatments to biomedicine (self-healing touch). Help-seeking activities include ethno medicine (Chinese herbal medicine and acupuncture), structure/energy therapies (therapeutic touch and osteopathy), pharmacologic/biologic treatments (antioxidants), biofeedback, guided imagery, music therapy, meditation, and prayer.

Alternative Therapies Specific to the Prenatal Period

1. Many herbs are available to be used during pregnancy including the labor and delivery process. Herbs come in different forms—capsules, tablets, extracts, tinctures, powders, dried and prepared as teas or juices, in combinations, and as external preparations.

 DRUG ALERT It is essential that the woman and her family discuss the use of herbs with her obstetric provider before use, become familiar with manufacturers, and ask questions. Although herbs are natural, they can be harmful if misused. Herbs should be used with the same respect as medications.

2. Herbal therapies that are Food and Drug Administration–approved include:
   a. Aloe, cascara (sacred bark, bitter bark), psyllium (plantago seed), senna as a laxative.
   b. Capsicum or cayenne pepper (chili pepper; red pepper) as a topical analgesic; marketed as a cream and used topically.
   c. Slippery elm (red elm) as an oral demulcent; marketed as throat lozenges.
3. Other herbal preparations include Catnip, fennel, lobelia, papaya, spearmint, and wild yams decrease colic stomach cramps, gas, and heartburn and improve the appetite.
4. Cranberry or blueberry juice for UTI prevention.
5. Nausea is sometimes attributed to vitamin B deficiencies, but does not always improve with simple vitamin supplements. Red raspberry, peppermint, spearmint, or chamomile tea; ginger root or ginger ale may be used to alleviate the nausea. To increase the effectiveness of red raspberry tea, alfalfa may be added to the tea.
6. Certain acupressure or acupuncture points may assist with the relief of nausea.
7. Other therapies include therapeutic touch and yoga.

Evaluation: Expected Outcomes

- Verbalizes understanding of proper body mechanics and wears low-heeled shoes.
- Identifies the basic food groups and describes meals to include needed servings for pregnancy.
- Reports limited fluid intake in the evening.
- Describes foods high in fiber.
- Wears support stockings and loose-fitting clothing.
- Discusses expectations for labor, delivery, and parenthood and attends educational classes.
- Verbalizes an understanding of the physiologic causes that may change the sexual relationship.
- Reports engaging in regular exercise.

Psychosocial Adaptation of Pregnancy

 Evidence Base Coverston, C. R. (2011). Psychology of pregnancy. In S. Mattson & J. E. Smith (Eds.), *Core curriculum for maternal-newborn nursing* (4th ed., pp. 101–116). St. Louis, MO: Saunders Elsevier.

Rubin's Framework for Maternal Role Assumption

1. Attainment of motherhood role occurs with each pregnancy.

2. Involves a series of cognitive operations:
   a. Mimicry—woman begins observing and modeling her behavior after other pregnant women.
   b. Role-play—woman begins acting out behaviors of a mother (eg, rocking a baby to sleep).
   c. Searching for a role "fit"—woman has perceptions of how the motherhood role will be. She observes others' behaviors to determine how well they fit with her expectations of the motherhood role.
   d. Grief work—woman experiences a sense of loss of her "old" self as she prepares to begin her new role as a mother.
3. Maternal task—commonly divided by trimesters.
   a. First trimester (first 3 months):
      i. Acceptance of pregnancy—progressive movement from a state of conflict and ambivalence to one of acceptance of the pregnancy, the child, and the motherhood role.
      ii. Realignment of roles—expectant parents begin to realign their roles and responsibilities as they relate to the child.
      iii. Safe passage—although the mother seeks to ensure a safe passage for her fetus and self throughout her pregnancy, the main focus during this trimester is on self-safety.
   b. Second trimester (second 3 months):
      i. Safe passage—in this trimester, the mother's main focus is on appropriate nutrition and exercise.
      ii. Acceptance by others—acceptance of the child by each family member.
      iii. Binding-in to the child—maternal perception of the child as a real person.
   c. Third trimester (last 3 months):
      i. Safe passage—during this trimester, the main focus is on the safety of the fetus and is inseparable from self-safety.
      ii. Giving of oneself—the most complex task, in which the mother is learning to give to the unborn child and placing the unborn child's need in relation to her own needs.
      iii. Critical to this trimester is the preparation of the nursery because it solidifies the acceptance of the unborn child.

Rubin's Framework for Paternal Role Assumption

1. The fatherhood role can also be attained with the pregnancy.
2. Paternal tasks can also be divided by trimesters.
   a. First trimester (first 3 months):
      i. Announcement and realization of the pregnancy—father will exhibit excitement over the announcement of the pregnancy and is more interested in maternal changes. Usually, he will insist on accompanying the mother to each prenatal appointment.
      ii. Some fathers will even begin to experience the same signs and symptoms of pregnancy experienced by the mother. This is more commonly referred to as *couvadé*.

   b. Second trimester (second 3 months):
      i. Anticipation—father anticipates and adapts to the role of fatherhood.
      ii. Fantasy and exploration—along with the mother, the father begins to imagine what his child will look like and may also begin to explore the talents and attributes of the unborn child.
      iii. Adjustment of sexual expression to accommodate the pregnancy.
   c. Third trimester (last 3 months):
      i. Preparation—now, serious preparation for the forthcoming child includes preparation of the nursery and childbirth education courses to prepare for labor and delivery.
      ii. Reassurance—provided by the father to ease the anxious mother's fears regarding labor and delivery.

THE FETUS

 Evidence Base Callahan, L. (2011). Fetal and placental development and functioning. In S. Mattson & J. E. Smith (Eds.), *Core curriculum for maternal-newborn nursing* (4th ed., pp. 35–58). St. Louis, MO: Saunders Elsevier.

Fetal Growth and Development

Previously, methods used to determine how well the fetus was growing and maturing consisted of evaluating uterine growth and listening to fetal heart sounds. Advances in knowledge and technology have provided newer methods for assessing fetal well-being and maturity. Improved methods for assessment and diagnosis enable early intervention for improved outcome. See Figure 36-7 for critical periods of fetal growth.

Stages of Growth and Development

The growth and development of the fetus is typically divided into three stages.

Preembryonic Stage: Fertilization to 2 to 3 Weeks
1. Rapid cell division and differentiation.
2. Develop embryonic membranes and germ layers.

Embryonic Stage: 4 to 8 Weeks' Gestation
1. Most critical stage of physical development.
2. Organogenesis.

Fetal Stage: 9 Weeks to Birth
1. Every organ system and external structure present.
2. Refinement of fetus and organ function occurs.

Development by Month

First Lunar Month
1. Fertilization to 2 weeks of embryonic growth.
2. Implantation is complete.
3. Primary chorionic villi forming.

Age of Embryo and Fetus in weeks

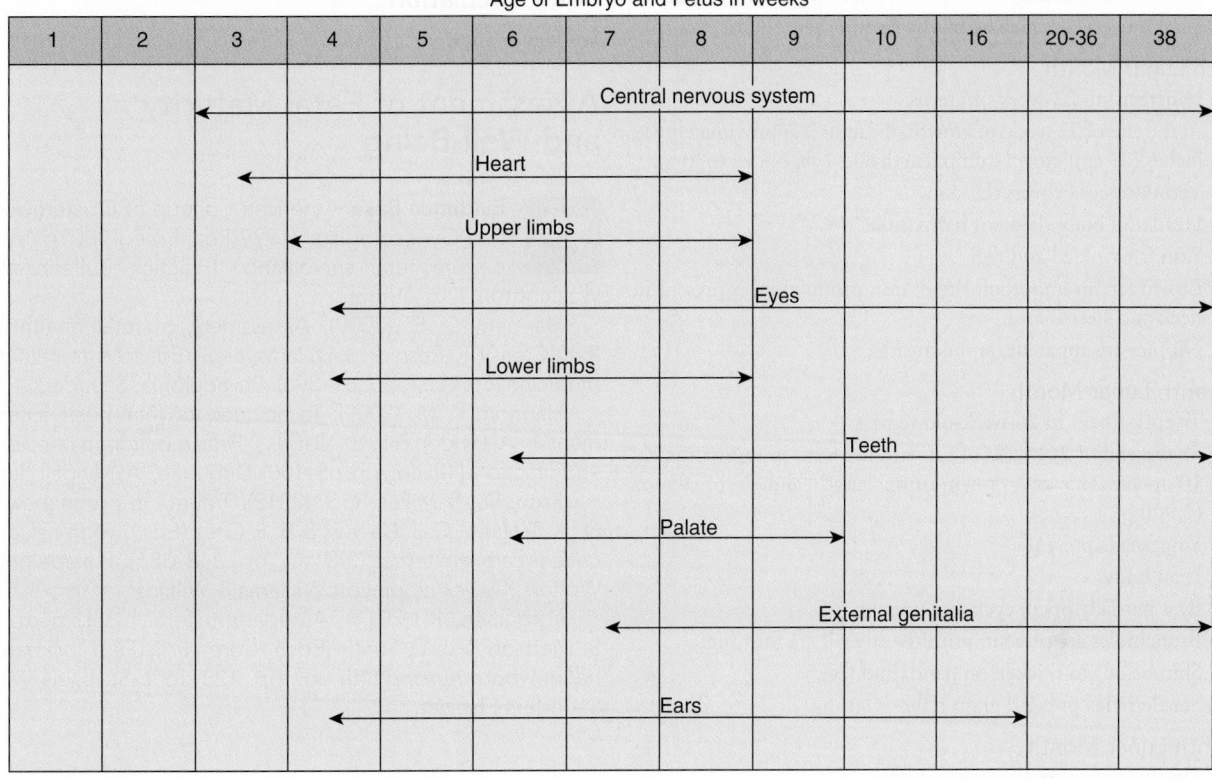

Figure 36-7. Critical periods of fetal growth. Pillitteri, A. (2003). *Maternal and child health nursing* (4th ed.). Philadelphia: Lippincott Williams & Wilkins.

4. Embryo develops into two cell layers (trophoblast and blasto-cyst).
5. Amniotic cavity appears.

Second Lunar Month
1. Three to 6 weeks of embryonic growth.
2. At the end of 6 weeks of growth, the embryo is approximately ½ inch (1.3 cm) long.
3. Arm and leg buds are visible; arm buds are more developed with finger ridges beginning to appear.
4. Rudiments of the eyes, ears, and nose appear.
5. Lung buds are developing.
6. Primitive intestinal tract is developing.
7. Primitive cardiovascular system is functioning.
8. Neural tube, which forms the brain and spinal cord, closes by the fourth week.

Third Lunar Month
1. Seven to 10 weeks of growth.
2. The middle of this period (9 weeks) marks the end of the embryonic period and the beginning of the fetal period.
3. At the end of 10 weeks of growth, the fetus is approximately 2½ inches (6.3 cm) from crown to rump and weighs ½ oz (14 g).
4. Appearance of external genitalia.

5. By the middle of this month, all major organ systems have formed.
6. The membrane over the anus has broken down.
7. The heart has formed four chambers (by 7th week).
8. The fetus assumes a human appearance.
9. Bone ossification begins.
10. Rudimentary kidney begins to secrete urine.

Fourth Lunar Month
1. Eleven- to 14-week-old fetus.
2. At the end of 14 weeks of growth, the fetus is approximately 4¾ inches (12 cm) crown–rump length and 3¾ oz (110 g).
3. Head erect; lower extremities well developed.
4. Hard palate and nasal septum have fused.
5. External genitalia of male and female can now be differentiated.
6. Eyelids are sealed.

Fifth Lunar Month
1. Fifteen- to 18-week-old fetus.
2. At the end of 18 weeks of growth, the fetus is approximately 6¼ inches (16 cm) crown–rump length and 11¼ oz (320 g).
3. Ossification of fetal skeleton can be seen on x-ray.
4. Ears stand out from head.
5. Meconium is present in the intestinal tract.

6. Fetus makes sucking motions and swallows amniotic fluid.
7. Fetal movements may be felt by the mother (end of month).

Sixth Lunar Month

1. Nineteen- to 22-week-old fetus.
2. At the end of 22 weeks of growth, the fetus is approximately 8¼ inches (21 cm) crown–rump length and 1 lb, 6¼ oz (630 g).
3. Vernix caseosa covers the skin.
4. Head and body (lanugo) hair visible.
5. Skin is wrinkled and red.
6. Brown fat, an important site of heat production, is present in neck and sternal area.
7. Nipples are apparent on the breasts.

Seventh Lunar Month

1. Twenty-three- to 26-week-old fetus.
2. At the end of 26 weeks of growth, the fetus is approximately 10 inches (25 cm) crown–rump length and 2 lb, 3¼ oz (1,000 g).
3. Fingernails present.
4. Lean body.
5. Eyes partially open; eyelashes present.
6. Bronchioles are present; primitive alveoli are forming.
7. Skin begins to thicken on hands and feet.
8. Startle reflex present; grasp reflex is strong.

Eighth Lunar Month

1. Twenty-seven- to 30-week-old fetus.
2. At the end of 30 weeks of growth, the fetus is approximately 11 inches (28 cm) crown–rump length and 3 lb, 12 oz (1,700 g).
3. Eyes open.
4. Ample hair on head; lanugo begins to fade.
5. Skin slightly wrinkled.
6. Toenails present.
7. Testes in inguinal canal, begin descent to scrotal sac.
8. Surfactant coats much of the alveolar epithelium.

Ninth Lunar Month

1. Thirty-one- to 34-week-old fetus.
2. At the end of 34 weeks of growth, the fetus is approximately 12½ inches (32 cm) crown–rump length and 5 lb, 8 oz (2,500 g).
3. Fingernails reach fingertips.
4. Skin pink and smooth.
5. Testes in scrotal sac.

Tenth Lunar Month

1. Thirty-five- to 38-week-old fetus; end of this month is also 40 weeks from onset of last menses.
2. End of 38 weeks of growth, fetus is approximately 14½ inches (37 cm) crown–rump length and 7 lb, 8 oz (3,400 g).
3. Ample subcutaneous fat.
4. Lanugo almost absent.
5. Toenails reach toe tips.
6. Testes in scrotum.
7. Vernix caseosa mainly on the back.
8. Breasts are firm.

Fetal Circulation

See Figure 36-8.

Assessment of Fetal Maturity and Well-Being

Evidence Base American College of Obstetricians and Gynecologists. (1999/Reaffirmed 2009). Antepartum fetal surveillance (Practice Bulletin #9). Washington, DC: Author.

Harman, C. R. (2009). Assessment of fetal health. In R. K. Creasy, R. Resnick, J. D. Iams, et al. (Eds.), *Maternal-fetal medicine* (6th ed., pp. 361–396). Philadelphia: Saunders.

Harmon, K. M. (2009). Techniques for fetal heart assessment. In A. Lyndon & L. U. Ali (Eds.), *Fetal monitoring principles and practices* (4th ed., pp. 65–100). Dubuque, IA: Kendall Hunt.

Ruth, D., & Miller, R. S. (2013). Trauma in pregnancy. In N. H. Troiano, C. J. Harvey, & B. F. Chez (Eds.), *High-risk and critical care obstetrics* (3rd ed., pp. 343–356). Philadelphia: Wolters Kluwer/Lippincott Williams & Wilkins.

Torgersen, K. (2011). Antepartum fetal assessment. In S. Mattson & J. E. Smith (Eds.), *Core curriculum for maternal-newborn nursing* (4th ed., pp. 128–162). St. Louis, MO: Saunders Elsevier.

Maternal History and Examination

1. The woman's family medical history, the woman's personal medical history, and her reproductive health history.
2. Comprehensive physical examination, history of current pregnancy, and identified risk factors.
3. Health during previous pregnancies.
4. Outcome of previous pregnancies.
5. Routine prenatal labs.
6. Fetal assessment after first trimester and individualized fetal surveillance, as indicated.

Fetal Heart Tones

Description

Fetal heart tones (FHTs) are representative of the fetal heart rate (FHR) and are an indicator of oxygen perfusion to the fetal brain, heart, and adrenals. The evaluation of FHTs is indicated in routine assessment of fetal well-being, in determining gestational age, and in cases of threatened abortion or other abnormalities. FHTs can be heard using techniques that amplify sound.

1. Doppler at approximately 10 to 12 weeks' fetal gestation.
2. Fetoscope (fetal stethoscope) at approximately 18 to 20 weeks' fetal gestation.
3. Electronic fetal monitoring testing is usually done when the fetus is considered viable, around 24 weeks' gestation.
4. Rate—between 110 and 160 bpm.
5. In latter months of pregnancy, fetal heart sounds found:
   a. Near the woman's midline in fetal occipitoanterior positions.
   b. Lateral to midline in fetal occipitotransverse positions.
   c. In the woman's flank in fetal occipitoposterior positions.

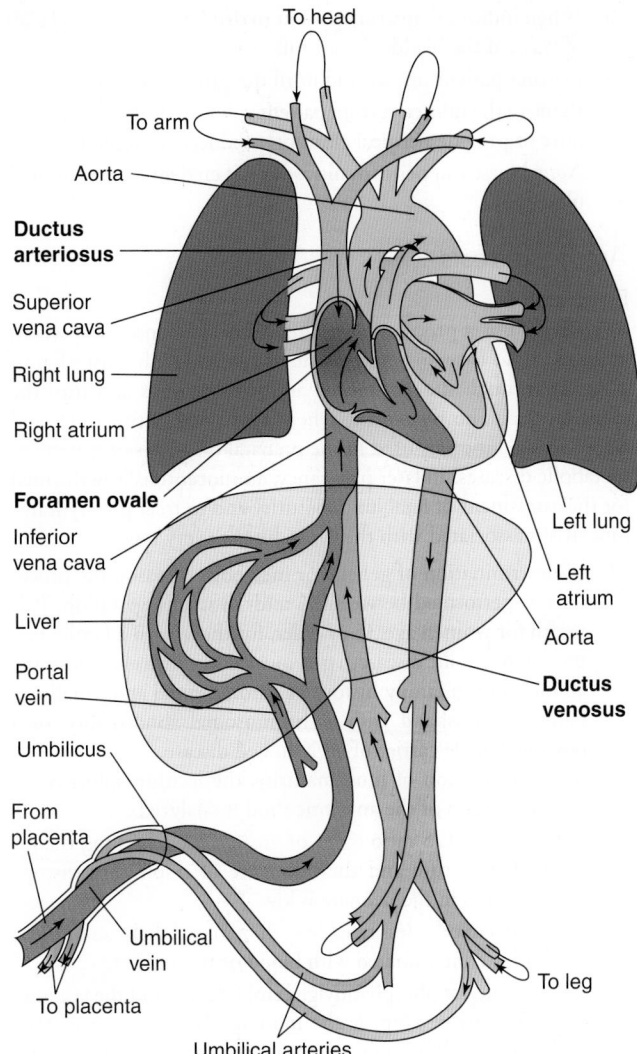

To head

To arm

Aorta

Ductus arteriosus

Superior vena cava

Right lung

Right atrium

Foramen ovale

Inferior vena cava

Liver

Portal vein

Umbilicus

From placenta

Umbilical vein

To placenta

Umbilical arteries

Left lung

Left atrium

Aorta

Ductus venosus

To leg

Figure 36-8. Diagram of the fetal circulation shortly before birth. Arrows indicate course of blood.

d. Below the woman's umbilicus in cephalic presentations.

e. At or above the woman's umbilicus in breech presentations.

6. Failure to hear FHTs at the expected time may be due to maternal obesity, polyhydramnios, error in date calculation, or fetal death.

Nursing and Patient Care Considerations

1. Explain equipment, purpose, and procedure to patient.

2. Assist patient to a side-lying or semi-Fowler's position. Position may affect the ability to clearly hear the heart tones. Perform Leopold's maneuvers.

3. Document findings on patient's chart and monitor strip along with date, time, activity level, medications, and other information per your health care facility's guidelines.

4. Discontinue electronic fetal monitoring, as indicated, according to facility guidelines.

5. Communicate appropriate information to patient and other personnel.

NURSING ALERT Monitor tracings become part of the neonate's and mother's chart and are legal documents. They may be used in litigation if certain health problems develop in years to come.

Fetal Movement

Description

Fetal movements or "kick counts" may be evaluated daily by the pregnant woman to provide reassurance of fetal well-being. Several methods have been proposed; however, neither the ideal number of kicks nor the ideal interval for movement counting has been defined. Although there are two methods defined in the literature, Cardiff Count-to-Ten and the Sadowsky, it is critical for the facility policy to be standardized and the instructions to the patient consistently the same. Testing can be as short as 5 minutes or as long as 2 hours.

Nursing and Patient Care Considerations

1. Instruct patient to lie on her side in a quiet place with no distractions. Have her place her hands on the largest part of her abdomen and concentrate on fetal movement.

2. Instruct patient to use a clock and record the movements felt. Once the tenth movement is felt, the testing is stopped. If fewer than 10 movements are felt in 2 hours or if the time it takes to get the 10 movements takes longer to achieve than earlier testing, she should contact her primary care provider.

3. Instruct patient that fetal movements are best assessed after meals, after or with light abdominal massage, or after short walks, and if she has not smoked for the last 2 hours.

4. Instruct patient that the fetus can sleep for up to 40 minutes.

5. Request patient to explain the procedure so her understanding is ensured.

Maternal Serum Alpha-Fetoprotein

Description

MS-AFP levels are analyzed at 15 to 20 weeks' gestation to identify certain birth defects and chromosomal abnormalities during pregnancy. AFP is a major protein produced in the fetal yolk sac during the first trimester and in the fetal liver during late term.

1. Elevated AFP levels are associated with birth defects and chromosomal abnormalities, such as open neural tube defects, open abdominal defects, and congenital nephrosis. Also associated with Rh isoimmunization, multiple gestation, maternal diabetes mellitus, and fetoplacental dysfunction.

2. Decreased levels are associated with Down syndrome and other chromosome anomalies (eg, gestational trophoblastic disease).

3. Follow-up for abnormal high or low levels includes ultrasound examination and amniocentesis.

Nursing and Patient Care Considerations

1. Obtain health and pregnancy history, including the date of patient's last menses and risk factors. Accurate dating of the pregnancy is crucial to interpret the results of the serum levels.

2. Explain the purpose and procedure for the test.

3. Discuss patient's concerns.

Ultrasound and Doppler Studies

Description

Ultrasonography is a noninvasive, safe technique that uses reflected sound waves as they travel in tissue to produce a picture. In the abdominal approach, a clear gel is applied to the woman's abdomen or to the transducer and the transducer is moved along the abdomen by the examiner. Images are produced onto a screen. During the early weeks of gestation, when the uterus remains a pelvic organ, a full bladder may be necessary to facilitate visualization. In the endovaginal approach, a lubricated transducer probe is inserted (either by the woman or by the examiner) into the vagina. No full bladder is necessary and this technique is especially useful during the early weeks of pregnancy or when cervical evaluation is important (ie, for assessment of preterm labor). Three-dimensional ultrasonography is a newer technology that is believed to offer improved assessment of fetal growth and weight parameters.

1. Uses in the first trimester of pregnancy include:
   a. Early confirmation of pregnancy and determination of the estimated date of confinement.
   b. Diagnosis of an ectopic pregnancy.
   c. Detection of an intrauterine device.
   d. Evaluation of placental location.
   e. Diagnosis of a multiple gestation.
   f. Guidance for CVS.
2. Uses in the second and third trimester include:
   a. Evaluation of fetal growth, weight, and gestational age.
   b. Evaluation of the placenta for placenta previa or separation associated with vaginal bleeding.
   c. Evaluation of fetal presentation and position.
   d. Evaluation of fetal abnormalities.
   e. Evaluation of fetal viability.
   f. Determination of the Biophysical Profile (BPP) Score.
   g. Evaluation of amniotic fluid volume.
   h. Guidance for amniocentesis or fetal blood sampling.
   i. Secondary survey for pregnant trauma patient.
3. Doppler flow study, also known as Doppler velocimetry, is a noninvasive way to analyze uteroplacental blood flow within the umbilical, uterine, and cerebral arteries. The use of this technology primarily focuses on placental analysis to identify patients at risk for increased perinatal mortality. Systolic and diastolic ratios are measured within the arteries. If the ratios rise above normal, it means that blood flow to the placenta is decreased.
4. Three- and four-dimensional (3-D and 4-D) ultrasonography evaluates major and superficial vessels of the placenta, including the cord; fetal physiologic development; and fetal behavior. There are a number of advantages to 3-D and 4-D ultrasonography over Doppler velocimetry, such as decreased time of fetal exposure to ultrasound beam (2 to 5 minutes for 3-D versus 15 to 30 minutes for velocimetry), off-line image processing, and identification of placental anastomoses, to mention a few.

Nursing and Patient Care Considerations

1. Explain the purpose and procedure to patient, emphasizing the need to remain still.
2. Inform patient of the need for a full bladder, if indicated, before the procedure.
3. When indicated, instruct patient to drink three to four glasses of water if the bladder is not full.
4. Instruct patient not to void until the procedure is over.
5. Remove the lubricant from patient's abdomen after the procedure or provide perineal cleaning products, as needed.
   Note: Nurse can perform ultrasound if credentialed in limited ultrasound.

Amniocentesis

Description

Amniocentesis is a procedure needing informed consent, in which amniotic fluid is removed from the uterine cavity by insertion of a needle through the abdominal and uterine walls and into the amniotic sac. The procedure, when performed between 15 and 20 weeks' gestation, is used in the prenatal diagnosis of genetic or metabolic diseases. In later pregnancy, amniocentesis is performed for the assessment of fetal lung maturity and to treat polyhydramnios. Risks associated with the procedure are very low.

1. In determination of genetic or metabolic diseases, the procedure is performed between 16 and 18 weeks' gestation. It is useful for women age 35 or older, for those with a family history of metabolic disease, a previous child with a chromosomal abnormality, a family history of chromosomal abnormality, a patient or husband with a chromosomal abnormality, or a possible female carrier of an X-linked disease.
2. In determination of lung maturity, the lecithin/sphingomyelin (L/S) ratio of the amniotic fluid is analyzed.
   a. When the L/S ratio is 2:1 or greater, the fetal lung is considered mature and the incidence of respiratory distress syndrome in the neonate is low.
   b. Results may be less reliable with maternal diabetes or if the fluid is contaminated with blood or meconium.
3. The presence of phosphatidylglycerol (PG), one of the last lung surfactants to develop, is the most reliable indicator of fetal lung maturity. PG is not present until 36 weeks' gestation and is measured as being present or absent. Unlike the L/S ratio, PG is not affected by hypoglycemia, hypoxia, or hypothermia.
4. A Triple Marker Screening (TMS) can also be used for the evaluation of trisomy 18 and 21 and neural tube defects. This test is costly when compared to MS-AFP, thus it is limited in its use. The TMS evaluates unconjugated estriol and hCG: Down syndrome shows increased hCG and decreased estriol levels; trisomy 18 shows decreased hCG and decreased estriol levels. The quadruple screen, which includes a measurement of the substance Dimeric Inhibin-A, provides a more sensitive and accurate detection of trisomy 21.
5. In the treatment of polyhydramnios (2,000 mL amniotic fluid or >25 cm amniotic fluid index [AFI]), amniocentesis may be performed to drain excess fluid and relieve pressure. Polyhydramnios can be associated with specific fetal abnormalities, such as trisomy 18, anencephaly, spina bifida, and esophageal atresia or tracheoesophageal fistula.

Nursing and Patient Care Considerations

1. Reduce anxiety related to the procedure.
   a. Reduce the parents' anxiety by determining their understanding of the procedure and the meaning it holds for them.

b. Reexplain the procedure before it begins, and answer any questions they have. Ensure informed consent is signed.

c. Provide explanations during the procedure, correct misinformation they may have, and make sure they know when the results will be available and how they may obtain the results as soon as possible.

2. Reduce pain and discomfort related to the procedure.

a. Reduce discomfort by having patient lie comfortably on her back with her hands and a pillow under her head. Relaxation breathing may help.

b. Ensure adequate time between infiltration of local anesthetic and introduction of needle into the amniotic sac.

c. Start intravenous (IV) administration of fluids in accordance with facility policy. Administer terbutaline subcutaneously or IV per your facility's policy.

3. Reduce potential for traumatic injury to fetus, placenta, or maternal structures.

a. Have patient empty her bladder if the fetus is more than 20 weeks' gestation to avoid injury to patient's bladder. If the fetus is less than 20 weeks' gestation, patient's full bladder will hold the uterus steady and out of the pelvis. The placenta is localized with the use of ultrasound.

b. Obtain maternal vital signs and a 20-minute FHR tracing to serve as a baseline to evaluate possible complications.

c. Monitor patient during and after the procedure for signs of premature labor or bleeding.

d. Tell patient to report signs of bleeding, unusual fetal activity or abdominal pain, cramping, or fever while at home after the procedure.

Chorionic Villus Sampling

Description

Chorionic villus sampling (CVS) involves obtaining samples of chorionic villus (placental tissue [fetal origin]) to test for chromosomal (via deoxyribonucleic acid [DNA]) and enzymatic disorders of the fetus. CVS is ideally performed between 10 and 11½ weeks' gestation.

1. Using an ultrasound picture, a catheter is passed vaginally into the woman's uterus, where a specimen of chorionic villus tissue is snipped off or obtained by suction.

2. Results from CVS are available in 4 days.

3. Complications include rupture of membranes, intrauterine infection, spontaneous abortion, hematoma, fetal trauma, or maternal tissue contamination.

4. Incidence of fetal loss is about 2% to 5%.

Nursing and Patient Care Considerations

1. Obtain maternal vital signs.

2. Instruct patient to void.

3. Reduce patient's anxiety as related to the procedure.

4. Inform patient that a small amount of spotting is normal, but heavy bleeding or passing clots or tissue should be reported.

5. Instruct patient to rest at home for a few hours after the procedure.

Percutaneous Umbilical Blood Sampling

Description

Percutaneous umbilical blood sampling (PUBS), or *cordocentesis*, involves a puncture of the umbilical cord (vein) for aspiration of fetal blood under ultrasound guidance.

1. It is used in the diagnosis of fetal blood disorders, infections, Rh isoimmunization, metabolic disorders, and karyotyping.

2. Transfusion to the fetus may be conducted with this procedure.

3. Using ultrasound picture, the provider inserts a needle (guided by ultrasound) into one of the umbilical vessels. A small amount of blood is withdrawn.

4. Can also be used for fetal therapies, such as RBC and platelet transfusion.

Nursing and Patient Care Considerations

1. Explain the procedure to patient.

2. Provide support to patient during the procedure.

3. Monitor patient after the procedure for uterine contractions and the FHR for distress.

Biochemical Markers

 Evidence Base Adeza Biomedical. (2005). *Fetal fibronectin enzyme immunoassay and rapid fFN for the TLi™ system: Information for health care providers.* Sunnyvale, CA: Author.

American College of Obstetricians and Gynecologists. (2011). *Screening and diagnosis of gestational diabetes mellitus* (Committee Opinion No. 504). Washington, DC: Author.

Description

1. *Fetal fibronectin (fFN)* is a protein that is secreted by the trophoblast of the implanted egg. It can be detected by the use of a monoclonal antibody known as FDC-6. The exact function is unknown; however, this protein is thought to play a key role in placental–uterine attachment. It is considered to be a better marker of women who will *not* go into PTL than those who *will* go into PTL.

a. Normally present in cervical or vaginal fluid before 20 weeks' gestation.

b. After 20 weeks' gestation, the presence of fFN can indicate a detachment of the fetal membranes and should be evaluated as an early marker for preterm birth.

c. Specimen is collected no earlier than 24 weeks and no later than 34 weeks and 6 days.

2. Delta OD 450 is used to determine the amount of bilirubin in the fetus. It reflects the increasing optical density, at a wavelength of 450 nanometers, of the amniotic fluid when it contains increasing amounts of bilirubin.

a. The value obtained is plotted on a gestational age–based nomogram, either the 1961 Liley curve or the newer Queenan curve.

b. With the advancement in technology and the use of Doppler velocity flow studies, the use of the invasive testing using the Delta OD-450 has begun to be replaced in the management of Rh-alloimmunized pregnancies.

Nursing and Patient Care Considerations

1. Explain the procedure to patient.
2. Collect specimen with a Dacron swab placed in the posterior fornix of the vagina and rotated for 10 seconds. Sexual activity within 24 hours of sample collection, recent cervical examination, and vaginal bleeding may result in a false-positive test.
3. Provide support to patient during the procedure.

Nonstress Test

Description

The *nonstress test (NST)* is used to evaluate FHR accelerations that normally occur in response to fetal activity in a fetus in good condition. Accelerations are indicative of an intact central and autonomic nervous system and are a sign of fetal well-being. Absence of FHR accelerations in response to fetal movements may be associated with hypoxia, acidosis, drugs (analgesics, barbiturates), fetal sleep, and some fetal anomalies.

1. Maternal indications include postdates, Rh sensitization, maternal age 35 or older, chronic renal disease, hypertension, collagen disease, sickle cell disease, diabetes, premature rupture of membranes, history of stillbirth, trauma, vaginal bleeding in the second and third trimesters.
2. There are no contraindications or known adverse effects associated with the NST.
3. Fetal indications include decreased fetal movement, intrauterine growth restriction, fetal evaluation after an amniocentesis, oligohydramnios or polyhydramnios.
   a. Criteria for a reactive NST include two accelerations within 20 minutes, each lasting at least 15 seconds with an FHR increased by 15 bpm above baseline in response to fetal activity. The quality of the tracing is an important factor in the test interpretation.
   b. Criteria for a reactive NST in a preterm fetus (<32 completed weeks' gestation) include two accelerations within 20 minutes, each lasting at least 10 seconds with an FHR increased by 10 bpm above baseline in response to fetal activity.
   c. Testing time for the term NST can be as long as 40 minutes. Testing time for the preterm NST can be as long as 60 to 90 minutes.
   d. In a nonreactive NST, the above criteria are not met.

Significance/Management

1. Reactive NST—suggests less than 1% chance of fetal death within 1 week of the NST.
2. Nonreactive NST—suggests fetus may be compromised and there needs to be further follow-up with a BPP, modified BPP, Contraction Stress Test (CST), or Oxytocin Challenge Test (OCT).

Nursing and Patient Care Considerations

1. Explain the procedure and equipment to patient. Make sure patient has had adequate nutrition and fluid intake and, if a smoker, has not been smoking within the past 2 hours.

2. Assist patient to a semi-Fowler's position in bed. Perform Leopold's maneuvers and apply the external fetal and uterine monitors.
3. Event markers do not need to be used unless the fetal movement is not observed on the fetal monitor. If fetal movement not observed, instruct patient to make a mark on the monitor strip each time fetal movement is felt. The nurse will do this if patient cannot.
4. Evaluate the response of the FHR immediately after fetal activity.
5. Monitor patient's BP and uterine activity for deviations during the procedure.

Fetal Acoustic Stimulation Test and Vibroacoustic Stimulation Test

Description

Acoustic (sound) and vibroacoustic stimulation (sound plus vibration) involve the use of handheld battery-operated devices (usually a laryngeal stimulator) placed over the mother's abdomen near the fetal head. This technique produces a low-frequency vibration and a buzzing tone intended to induce fetal movement along with associated FHR accelerations. The sound stimulus should last for up to 3 seconds. The *fetal acoustic stimulation test (FAST)* and *vibroacoustic stimulation test (VST)* are used as an adjunct following a nonreactive NST; these tests may also be used with fetuses that exhibit decreased FHR variability during labor. If no FHR accelerations occur in response to the stimulus, it is repeated at 1-minute intervals up to three times (total of 6 seconds). If the FHR pattern remains nonreactive, further evaluation with BPP or CST is indicated. In the light of advanced ultrasound technology, this test is being used less frequently than several years ago. However, there are still facilities that do not have the ultrasound capabilities of large facilities; therefore, this testing is quite appropriate.

1. It is not known whether the fetus responds more to the sound or to the vibration.
2. Both methods of testing are noninvasive, easy to perform, and yield rapid results.
3. Interpretation depends on individualized institutional guidelines. Usually:
   a. Reactive—two accelerations meeting 15 × 15 criteria (preterm 10 × 10 criteria).
   b. Nonreactive—no accelerations.
4. Tachycardic rate may result from stimulus and may last >1 hour. If this occurs, observe FHR for normal baseline characteristics, other than the tachycardia, until the FHR returns to the prestimulus rate.

Nursing and Patient Care Considerations

1. Explain procedure, equipment, and purpose to patient.
2. Assist patient to a semi-Fowler's position in bed.
3. Apply external fetal monitors to patient.
4. Demonstrate how the stimulus may feel on patient's forearm or leg.
5. Observe for reactivity.

Oxytocin Challenge Test or Contraction Stress Test

Description

Oxytocin challenge test or the *contraction stress test* is used to evaluate the ability of the fetus to withstand the stress of uterine contractions as would occur during labor.

1. The test is generally used when a woman has a nonreactive NST or FAST/VST, although in many areas, the CST has been replaced by the BPP.
2. The test is contraindicated in women with third-trimester bleeding, multiple gestation, incompetent cervix, placenta previa, previous classic uterine incision, hydramnios, history of PTL, or premature rupture of membranes.
3. Contractions may occur spontaneously (unusual) or they may be induced.
4. The CST utilizes endogenously produced oxytocin by way of nipple or breast stimulation.
5. The OCT utilizes exogenous oxytocin, which is administered by way of titrated IV infusion.

Nursing and Patient Care Considerations

1. Obtain maternal vital signs, especially BP.
2. Instruct patient to void.
3. Assist patient to a semi-Fowler's or side-lying position in bed.
4. Obtain a 20-minute strip of the FHR and uterine activity for baseline data.
5. For CST:
   a. Apply warm packs to the breasts for 10 minutes before the CST.
   b. Instruct patient on nipple stimulation. Instruct patient to brush or roll the nipple, using the palmar surface of the index finger and thumb. The patient can do this through her clothes or skin-to-skin. If using skin-to-skin, provide the patient with some mineral oil to use on her fingers to ease stimulation. Stimulation occurs in 4 cycles of 2 minutes *on* and 2 to 5 minutes off *(for ease of memory: 1 cycle = 2 minutes on and 2 minutes off)*. The nipple is stimulated until contractions begin *or* 2 minutes have passed.
   c. If contractions occur during stimulation, instruct the patient to stop the stimulation; she can begin the stimulation again when the contraction is over. If no contractions after four cycles, two different methods can be used:
      i. Let the patient rest for 5 to 10 minutes, then begin bilateral continuous stimulation for 5 to 10 minutes, stopping when contractions begin (have the patient resume stimulation when contraction ends).
      ii. Let the patient rest for 5 to 10 minutes, then begin stimulation again, alternating nipples, stopping when contractions begin (have the patient resume stimulation when contraction ends).
   d. Stop the stimulation if:
      i. Three or more contractions occur within 10 minutes that last more than or equal to 40 seconds.
      ii. Tetanic uterine contractions or tachysystole occurs.
      iii. Unsuccessful nipple stimulation (two rounds of four cycles without contractions). Notify health care provider and prepare for OCT, BPP, or modified BPP.
6. For OCT: follow 1 through 4 above. In addition:
   a. Administer diluted oxytocin through an IV infusion pump, as indicated, until three contractions occur within 10 minutes and last ≥40 seconds. Maintain mainline IV fluids in accordance with facility policy.
   b. Discontinue the infusion when:
      i. Criteria are met.
      ii. Maximum dose of 16 milliunits per minute has been achieved.
      iii. Tachysystole or tetanic contractions occurs.
      iv. Prolonged deceleration or bradycardia occurs.
      v. Late decelerations are present.

Interpretation of CST/OCT

1. Negative (normal)—three uterine contractions in 10 minutes without late or significant variable decelerations.
2. Positive (abnormal)—late decelerations with more than 50% of uterine contractions even if frequency is less than three contractions in 10 minutes; usually associated with absent or minimal variability.
3. Equivocal-suspicious—intermittent late decelerations (<50% of uterine contractions) or significant variables (usually >1 minute in duration × 60 to 70 seconds).
4. Equivocal-"hyperstimulatory"—uterine contractions more frequent than every 2 minutes or lasting more than 90 seconds with accompanying late, significant variable, or prolonged decelerations.
5. Unsatisfactory—quality of tracing inadequate to assess or less than three contractions in 10 minutes or contractions <40 seconds in duration.

Significance/Management of CST/OCT

1. Negative—reassuring.
2. Positive—nonreassuring.
3. Equivocal-suspicious—repeat in 24 hours unless post-term, indication for delivery is present, or follow immediately with further antenatal assessment (eg, BPP).
4. Equivocal-"hyperstimulatory"—stop testing; repeat in 2 to 24 hours depending on clinical presentation, provider preference, or hyperstimulatory pattern is resolved.
5. Unsatisfactory—repeat in 24 hours or use alternative antenatal assessment (ie, BPP).
6. Regardless of the result, if variable decelerations are present, further testing should be done to look for oligohydramnios.
7. If test remains equivocal after 3 consecutive days, NSTs may be used in place of CSTs.

Biophysical Profile

Description

The *biophysical profile (BPP)* uses ultrasonography and NST to assess five biophysical variables in determining fetal well-being. A BPP is performed during a 30-minute time frame by someone credentialed in ultrasonography.

1. NST—assessing for FHR acceleration (fetal reactivity) in relation to fetal movements.
2. AFI volume—assessing for one or more pockets of amniotic fluid measuring ¾ inch (2 cm) or more in two perpendicular planes.
3. Fetal breathing movements—one or more episodes lasting at least 30 seconds.
4. Gross fetal body movements—three or more body or limb movements, to include rolling, in 30 minutes.
5. Fetal muscle tone—one or more episodes of active extension with return to flexion of spine, hand, or limbs.

For each variable, if the criteria are met, a score of 2 is given. For an abnormal observation, a score of 0 is given. A score of 8 to 10 is considered normal, 6 is equivocal, and 4 or less is abnormal.

Nursing and Patient Care Considerations

1. Explain the purpose and procedure to patient; provide emotional support.
2. Instruct patient to empty her bladder.
3. Assist patient onto the examination table and help her to assume a position of comfort.
4. Remove the lubricant from patient's abdomen after the procedure.
5. Assist patient in rising from the examination table.

Modified BPP

Description

The modified BPP is more common today than the BPP. It consists of an NST and an AFI check. The modified BPP performed twice per week provides the same predictive results as the weekly CST. Interpretation of the modified BPP is either normal or abnormal. Normal is a reactive NST with an AFI greater than 5 cm. A normal AFI is 9 to 25 cm with a borderline "normal" being 5 to 8 cm. Oligohydramnios is when there is less than 5 cm of amniotic fluid. If abnormal, a full ultrasound evaluation is required and the fetus is evaluated for functioning renal tissue. If renal function is abnormal = delivery.

Nursing and Patient Care Considerations

1. Explain NST and AFI check in accordance with previously stated guidelines, as noted in this chapter.
2. Document findings in patient's prenatal record.

SELECTED REFERENCES

Adeza Biomedical. (2005). *Fetal fibronectin enzyme immunoassay and rapid fFN for the TLi™ system: Information for health care providers.* Sunnyvale, CA: Author.

American Academy of Pediatrics (AAP) & American College of Obstetricians and Gynecologists (ACOG). (2007). *Guidelines for perinatal care* (6th ed.). Washington, DC: ACOG.

American College of Obstetricians and Gynecologists. (2001/Reaffirmed 2010). *Gestational diabetes* (Practice Bulletin No. 30). Washington, DC: Author.

American College of Obstetricians and Gynecologists. (2002/Reaffirmed 2010). *Diagnosis and management of preeclampsia and eclampsia* (Practice Bulletin #33). Washington, DC: Author.

American College of Obstetricians and Gynecologists. (2005). *Intrapartum fetal heart rate monitoring* (Practice Bulletin #70). Washington, DC: Author.

American College of Obstetricians and Gynecologists. (2006/Reaffirmed 2011). *Psychosocial risk factors: Perinatal screening and intervention* (Committee Opinion #343). Washington, DC: Author.

American College of Obstetricians and Gynecologists. (2008). *Planning your pregnancy and birth* (3rd ed.). Washington, DC: Author.

American College of Obstetricians and Gynecologists. (2011). Screening and diagnosis of gestational diabetes mellitus (Committee Opinion No. 504). Washington, DC: Author.

American College of Obstetricians and Gynecologists. (2012). *Intimate partner violence* (Committee Opinion No. 518). Washington, DC: Author.

Association of Women's Health, Obstetric, and Neonatal Nurses. (2009). *Standards and guidelines* (7th ed.). Washington, DC: Author.

Barron, M. L. (2008). *Nursing assessment of the pregnant woman: Antepartal screening and laboratory evaluation* (Nursing Module). White Plains, NY: March of Dimes Birth Defects Foundation.

Benirschke, K. (2009). Normal early development. In R. K. Creasy, R. Resnick, J. D. Iams, et al. (Eds.), *Maternal-fetal medicine* (6th ed., pp. 37–46). Philadelphia: Saunders.

Blackburn, S. T. (2008). Physiologic changes of pregnancy. In K. Rice-Simpson & P. A. Creehan (Eds.), *AWHONN's perinatal nursing* (3rd ed., pp. 59–77). Philadelphia: Lippincott Williams & Wilkins.

Bond, L. (2011). Physiology of pregnancy. In S. Mattson & J. E. Smith (Eds.), *Core curriculum for maternal-newborn nursing* (4th ed., pp. 80–100). St. Louis, MO: Saunders Elsevier.

Callahan, L. (2011). Fetal and placental development and functioning. In S. Mattson & J. E. Smith (Eds.), *Core curriculum for maternal-newborn nursing* (4th ed., pp. 35–58). St. Louis, MO: Saunders Elsevier.

Clark, S., Sabey, P., & Jolley, K. (1989). Nonstress testing with acoustic stimulation and amniotic volume assessment: 5,973 tests without unexpected fetal death. *American Journal of Obstetrics and Gynecology, 160,* 694–697.

Coverston, C. R. (2011). Psychology of pregnancy. In S. Mattson & J. E. Smith (Eds.), *Core curriculum for maternal-newborn nursing* (4th ed., pp. 101–116). St. Louis, MO: Saunders Elsevier.

Felton, M. B. (2011). Normal childbirth. In S. Mattson & J. E. Smith (Eds.), *Core curriculum for maternal-newborn nursing* (4th ed., pp. 225–247). St. Louis, MO: Saunders Elsevier.

Foyouzi, N., Frisbaek, Y., & Norwitz, E. R. (2004). Pituitary gland and pregnancy. *Obstetrics and Gynecology Clinics of North America, 31,* 873–892.

Gauthier, D. (2009). Maternal-fetal assessment. In A. Lyndon & L. U. Ali (Eds.), *Fetal monitoring principles and practices* (4th ed., pp. 45–64). Dubuque, IA: Kendall Hunt.

Harman, C. R. (2009). Assessment of fetal health. In R. K. Creasy, R. Resnick, J. D. Iams, et al. (Eds.), *Maternal-fetal medicine* (6th ed., pp. 361–396). Philadelphia: Saunders.

Harmon, K. M. (2009). Techniques for fetal heart assessment. In A. Lyndon & L. U. Ali (Eds.), *Fetal monitoring principles and practices* (4th ed., pp. 65–100). Dubuque, IA: Kendall Hunt.

Iams, J. D., Romero, R., & Creasy, R. K. (2009). Preterm labor and birth. In R. K. Creasy, R. Resnick, J. D. Iams, et al. (Eds.) *Maternal-fetal medicine* (6th ed., pp. 545–582). Philadelphia: Saunders.

Liu, J. H. (2009). Endocrinology of pregnancy. In R. K. Creasy, R. Resnick, J. D. Iams, et al. (Eds.), *Maternal-fetal medicine* (6th ed., pp. 111–124). Philadelphia: Saunders.

Louik, C., Gardiner, P., Kelley, K., et al (2010). Use of herbal treatments in pregnancy. *American Journal of Obstetrics and Gynecology, 202*(5), 439.e1–439.e10.

Moise, K. J. (2009). Hemolytic disease of the fetus and newborn. In R. K. Creasy, R. Resnick, J. D. Iams, et al. (Eds.), *Creasey & Resnick's maternal-fetal medicine: Principles and practice* (6th ed., pp 477–503). Philadelphia: Saunders.

Monga, M. (2009). Maternal cardiovascular, respiratory, and renal adaptation to pregnancy. In R. K. Creasy, R. Resnick, J. D. Iams, et al. (Eds.), *Maternal-fetal medicine* (6th ed., pp. 101–110). Philadelphia: Saunders.

Mongelli, M., Gardosi, J., Trupin, S. R., et al. (2010). Evaluation of gestation. Available: *http://emedicine.medscape.com/article/25926.*

National Institutes of Health. (2000). National high blood pressure education program working group on high blood pressure in pregnancy (NIH Publication #00-3029). Bethesda, MD: Author.

Norwitz, E. R., & Lye, S. J. (2009). Biology of parturition. In R. K. Creasy, R. Resnick, J. D. Iams, et al. (Eds.) *Maternal-fetal medicine* (6th ed., pp. 69–86). Philadelphia: Saunders.

Records, K. (2011). Intimate partner violence. In S. Mattson & J. E. Smith (Eds.), *Core curriculum for maternal-newborn nursing* (4th ed., pp. 417–431). St. Louis, MO: Saunders Elsevier.

Richardson, B. S., & Gagnon, R. (2009). Behavioral state activity and fetal health and development. In R. K. Creasy, R. Resnick, J. D. Iams, et al. (Eds.) *Maternal-fetal medicine* (6th ed., pp. 171–180). Philadelphia: Saunders.

Ruth, D., & Miller, R. S. (2013). Trauma in pregnancy. In N. H. Troiano, C. J. Harvey, & B. F. Chez (Eds.), *High-risk and critical care obstetrics* (3rd ed., pp. 343–356). Philadelphia: Wolters Kluwer/Lippincott Williams & Wilkins.

Stotland, N. E. (2009). Maternal nutrition. In R. K. Creasy, R. Resnick, J. D. Iams, et al. (Eds.), *Maternal-fetal medicine* (6th ed., pp. 111–124). Philadelphia: Saunders.

Torgersen, K. (2011). In S. Mattson & J. E. Smith (Eds.), *Core curriculum for maternal-newborn nursing* (4th ed., pp. 128-162). St. Louis, MO: Saunders Elsevier.

Yonkers, K. A. (2009). Management of depression and psychoses in pregnancy and the puerperium. In R. K. Creasy, R. Resnick, J. D. Iams, et al. (Eds.), *Maternal-fetal medicine* (6th ed., pp. 1113–1122). Philadelphia: Saunders.

SELECTED INTERNET RESOURCES

American Association of Acupuncture and Oriental Medicine, *www.aaaomonline.org*

Bradley Method of Natural Childbirth, *www.bradleybirth.com*

Lamaze International: *www.lamaze.org*

Multilingual Facts for Prenatal Health, *www.safemotherhood.org*

National Women's Health Resource Center Inc., *www.healthywomen.org*

Personalized Food Pyramid, *www.choosemyplate.gov/mypyramidmoms*

Pregnancy and Childbirth Prenatal Care, *www.makewayforbaby.com/babies/prenatal-care.html*

Pregnancy and Exercise, *www.familydoctor.org/handouts/305.html*

37

Nursing Management During Labor and Delivery

THE LABOR PROCESS

The phases of pregnancy, labor, and birth are normal physiologic processes. A pregnant woman typically approaches the birth process with possible concerns of personal well-being, that of her unborn child, and fear of labor pain. Addressing these concerns, minimizing her discomfort, and optimizing patient safety should be of paramount importance to all participants involved in the care of the mother and her fetus during the intrapartum period.

General Considerations

Evidence Base Lowdermilk, D., & Perry, S. (2012). *Maternity and women's health care* (10th ed.). St. Louis, MO: Elsevier.
  Mattson, S., & Smith, J. E. (2011). *Core curriculum for maternal-newborn nursing* (4th ed.). St. Louis, MO: Elsevier.

Prepared Childbirth

Historically, the term *natural childbirth* has evolved to mean (1) delivery outside in nature, (2) home birth, (3) nonhospital birth (birthing center), (4) facility birth—no medical intervention (ie, no intravenous [IV] medications), and, most recently, (5) facility birth without analgesia or anesthesia. Preparation through education and training prior to labor gives the pregnant woman a method of coping with the discomforts of labor and delivery. This method is known as *prepared childbirth* and incorporates analgesia and anesthesia into the process. The latter method dominates

current culture in the United States. Variances in prepared childbirth are outlined.

Psychoprophylactic or Lamaze Method

1. Psychoprophylactic childbirth has a rationale based on Pavlov's concept of pain perception and his theory of conditioned reflexes (the substitution of favorable conditioned reflexes for unfavorable ones). The Lamaze method is an example of this technique.
2. The woman is taught to replace responses of restlessness, fear, and loss of control with more controlled measures, which can excite the cerebral cortex efficiently to inhibit other stimuli such as pain in labor.
3. The mother-to-be is taught exercises that strengthen the abdominal muscles and relax the perineum.
4. Various breathing techniques to help the process of labor are practiced.
5. The woman is conditioned to respond with respiratory measures and disassociation or relaxation of the uninvolved muscles, while controlling her perception of the stimuli associated with labor.

The Bradley Method of Delivery

1. Commonly referred to as "husband-coached childbirth." A coach may be *any* significant other such as a friend, mother, sister, boyfriend, aunt, grandmother, or husband.
2. Involves the concepts of leading, guiding, supporting, caring, and fostering specific skills and confidence.
3. Coaches attend classes and learn to help the woman prior to initiation of labor.

4. The coach serves as a conditioned stimulus using the sound of his or her voice, use of particular words, and repetition of practice.

5. Medications are not encouraged for pain relief. Relaxation is the core component. Increased tolerance to pain is accomplished by decreased mental anxiety and fear, which ultimately decreases the awareness of the pain stimulus. This occurs through cognitive and physical rehearsal.

Home Delivery

1. Motivations for home delivery:
   a. Increases patient choices and flexibility during the birth process while decreasing patient separation and fear of intrusive intervention.
   b. Desire to avoid such practices as routine cesarean delivery for breech presentation, episiotomy, forceps delivery, oxytocin stimulation, routine monitoring of the fetal heart tones, and other practices associated with facilities.
   c. Risk of in-hospital infections; belief that infant is immune to own-home bacteria.
   d. Rising costs of hospitalization.
2. Contraindications:
   a. High-risk pregnancy.
   b. History of premature or postdate delivery in previous or current pregnancy or previous cesarean delivery, pre-eclampsia, gestational diabetes.
   c. Woman with medical, surgical, or emotional complications.
   d. Fetal complications: cardiac anomalies, placental abnormalities, and so on.
3. Alternatives to home delivery:
   a. Family-centered hospital setting.
   b. Birthing centers with adequate facilities for emergency care for low-risk women.

Initiation of Labor

Evidence Base Cunningham, F. G., Leveno, K., Bloom, S., et al. (2010). *Williams obstetrics* (23rd ed.). New York: McGraw-Hill.

Parturition is a multifactorial physiologic process involving both maternal and fetal influences. The exact mechanism initiating labor is unknown. The following four phases outline the labor process:

1. Phase 0, *Quiescence* (inhibition)—inhibition of labor is maintained by a constant release of progesterone and other uterotonic inhibitors (ie, PgI_2, relaxin, nitric oxide, and parathyroid hormone).
2. Phase 1, *Activation* (preparation)—levels of uterotonic inhibitors decrease while myometrial preparatory processes evolve (ie, gap junction development, oxytocin receptors, prostaglandin [PG] receptors, and calcium channels). This phase leads to uterine contractility, cervical ripening, and stimulation of fetal membranes.

3. Phase 2, *Stimulation* (contractions)—initiation of coordinated and rhythmic contractions by two uterotonics, primarily oxytocin and PG.
4. Phase 3, *Involution* (restitution)—oxytocin initiates resolution of the uterus to its prepregnant state.

Factors Affecting Labor

Evidence Base Davidson, M. W., London, M. L., & Ladeweig, P. W. (2012). *Olds' maternal-newborn nursing and women's health across the lifespan* (9th ed.). Upper Saddle River, NJ: Pearson Education.

The success of labor and delivery depends on three concepts: *passage*, adequacy of maternal pelvic dimensions; *passenger*, fetal dimensions and presentation; and *power*, uterine contractions.

Passage: Pelvic Dimensions
1. Pelvic inlet (anteroposterior diameter): The obstetric conjugate anterior–posterior measurement is typically more than 10 cm. Over 50% of women have a gynecoid-shaped pelvis to accommodate proper descent.
2. Midpelvis (ischial spines): Intraspinous diameter is typically more than 10 cm; protrusion of the spines into the birthing canal may complicate descent.
3. Pelvic outlet (intertuberous diameter + suprapubic arch): Dimensions are estimated as the anterior–posterior diameter from the coccyx to the symphysis pubis. This is typically 13 centimeters in length, but again one must subtract 1.5 to 2 cm from the calculation due to the thickness of the symphysis. A prominent coccyx may impede descent.

Passenger: Fetal Dimensions
1. Size—assessed via palpation using Leopold's maneuvers or ultrasound. Excessive size may lead to inadequate or asynclitic descent, labor dystocia, shoulder dystocia, or postpartum hemorrhage.

Evidence Base American College of Obstetricians and Gynecologists. (2003/Reaffirmed 2011). *Dystocia and augmentation of labor* (Practice Bulletin #49). Washington, DC: Author.

2. Posture—typically, the fetal head and extremities are flexed while the back is rounded. Flexion of the head allows for the smallest diameter (occiput) to present and pass through the birth canal with ease (see Figure 37-1). Nonflexed presentations may increase risk of asynclitic conditions.
3. Lie—constitutes the comparison of the fetal long axis to the long axis of the mother. Variances include transverse, longitudinal, or oblique; 99% of fetuses present as a longitudinal lie parallel to the mother's spine. This improves ease of access into the birth canal.
4. Presentation—the fetal body part presenting into the birth canal first and is felt on vaginal exam (see Figure 37-2).
   a. Cephalic (head)—occiput, sinciput, brow, face, or chin (mentum).
   b. Breech (feet)—frank, complete, or footling (single or double).

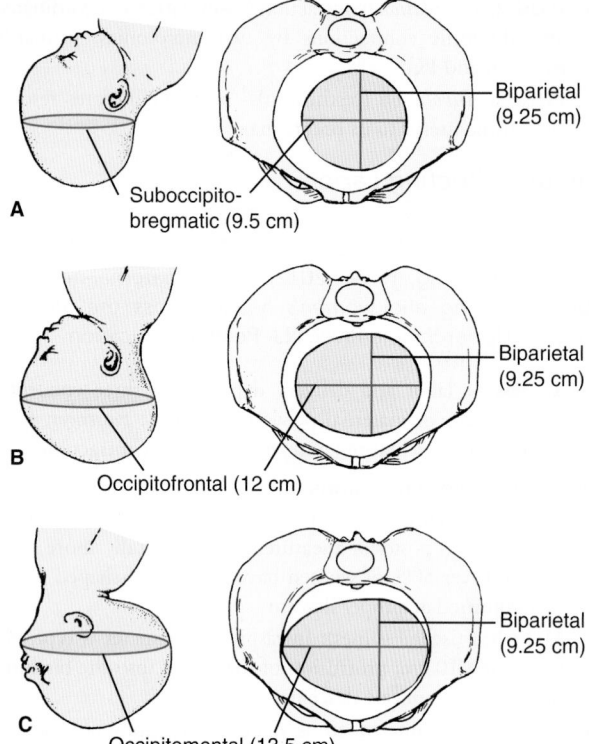

A Suboccipito-bregmatic (9.5 cm) — Biparietal (9.25 cm)

B Occipitofrontal (12 cm) — Biparietal (9.25 cm)

C Occipitomental (13.5 cm) — Biparietal (9.25 cm)

Figure 37-1. (A) Complete flexion allows smallest diameter of head to enter pelvis. **(B)** Moderate extension causes larger diameter to enter pelvis. **(C)** Marked extension forces largest diameter against pelvic brim, but head is too large to enter pelvis.

c. Shoulder (transverse).

d. Compound—two or more parts presenting at same time.

5. Position—Specific landmark of fetal presenting part (occiput, mentum, sacrum, scapula) in comparison to the anterior, posterior, or transverse portion of the woman's pelvis and the maternal left or right side; designated by a three-letter abbreviation.

a. The first letter L or R represents the side (right or left) in the maternal pelvis the presenting part is facing.

b. The second letter represents the landmark that is presenting: O for occiput, M for mentum (chin), S for sacrum, Sc for scapula or shoulder.

c. The third letter represents the direction (anterior [A], posterior [P], or transverse [T]) the presenting part is facing in the pelvis.

d. For example, the fetus with the head presenting and facing toward the maternal right anterior pelvis is ROA.

Passenger: Fetal Head (Vertex)

In approximately 95% of all births, the fetal head (vertex) presents first. Sutures and fontanelles provide important landmarks for determining fetal position during a vaginal examination (see Figure 37-3).

1. Bones of the fetal skull:

a. One occipital bone posteriorly.

b. Two parietal bones bilaterally.

c. Two temporal bones bilaterally.

d. Two frontal bones anteriorly.

2. Sutures of the fetal skull—membranous spaces between the bones of the fetal skull:

a. Frontal—between the two frontal bones.

b. Sagittal—between the two parietal bones.

c. Coronal—between the frontal and parietal bones.

d. Lambdoidal—between the back of the parietal bones and the margin of the occipital bone.

3. Fontanelles of the fetal skull—irregular spaces formed where two or more sutures meet. Sutures and fontanelles allow fetal skull bones to overlap in order to pass through the maternal pelvis.

a. Anterior—largest fontanelle; junction of the sagittal, frontal, and coronal sutures; closes by age 18 to 24 months; "diamond" shaped.

b. Posterior—located where the sagittal suture meets the lambdoidal suture (smaller than anterior); closes by 1 year; "triangle" shaped.

Power: Uterine Contractions

Successful labor depends on regular uterine contractions of adequate intensity that lead to cervical advancement and facilitate fetal descent. The following are characteristics of labor contractions:

1. Uterine contractions typically increase in intensity, frequency, and duration as labor progresses.

2. Uterine contractions may cause vasoconstriction of the umbilical cord leading to potential alterations in the fetal heart rate (ie, variable decelerations).

3. The active upper portion of the uterus (fundus) stimulates activation of contractions during labor (referred to as fundal dominance).

4. At the completion of a contraction, the upper uterine segment retains its shortened, thickened cell size and, with each succeeding contraction, becomes thicker and shorter. As a result, the upper uterine segment never totally relaxes during labor. Cells of the lower uterine segment become thinner and longer with each contraction. This mechanism is greatly responsible for the progress of the fetus through the birth canal.

5. The differentiation point between the upper and lower uterine segment is known as the "physiologic retraction ring."

Preparatory Events to Labor

1. Lightening (the settling of the fetus in the lower uterine segment) occurs 2 to 3 weeks before term in the primigravida and typically later, during labor, in the multigravida.

a. Breathing becomes easier as the fetus falls away from the diaphragm.

b. Lordosis of the spine is increased as the fetus enters the pelvis and falls forward. Walking may become more difficult; leg cramping may increase.

c. Urinary frequency may occur due to pressure on the adjacent bladder.

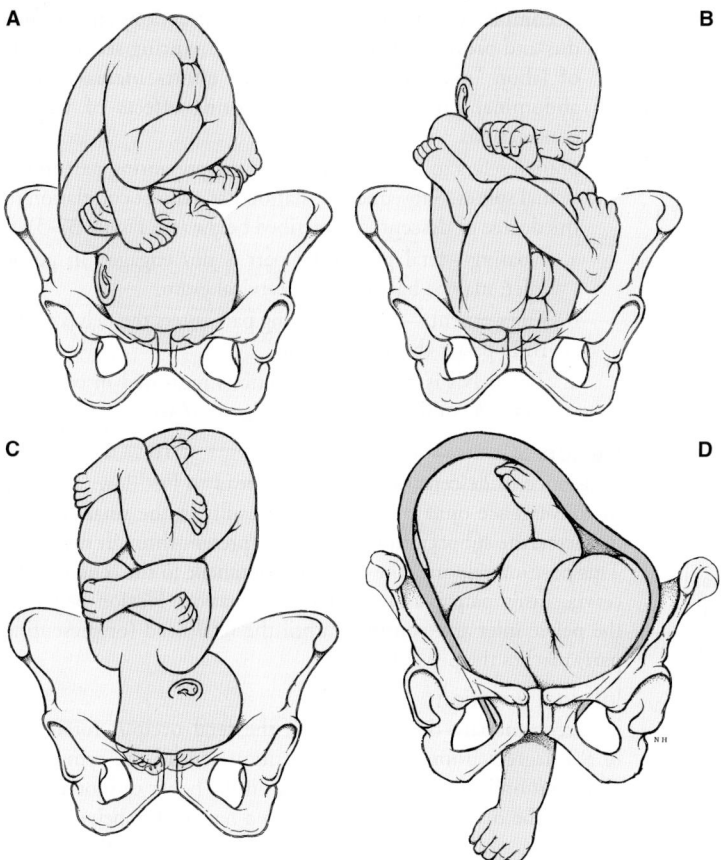

Figure 37-2. Fetal presentations. (A) Cephalic; **(B)** breech; **(C)**; face; **(D)** transverse.

2. Vaginal secretions may increase due to hormonal changes.
3. Mucus plug is discharged from the cervix along with a small amount of blood from surrounding capillaries—referred to as "bloody show."
4. Cervix becomes soft, effaces (shortens), and gradually moves from a posterior to an anterior position.
5. Membranes may rupture spontaneously.
6. False labor contractions may occur (see Table 37-1) in preparation for true labor.
7. Backaches may occur due to fetal size and lightening.

8. GI alterations (ie, diarrhea) may occur.
9. Weight loss of 1 to 3 lb (0.5 to 1.5 kg) with advanced pregnancy.
10. Energy may increase (referred to as "nesting") or decrease in the last few weeks.

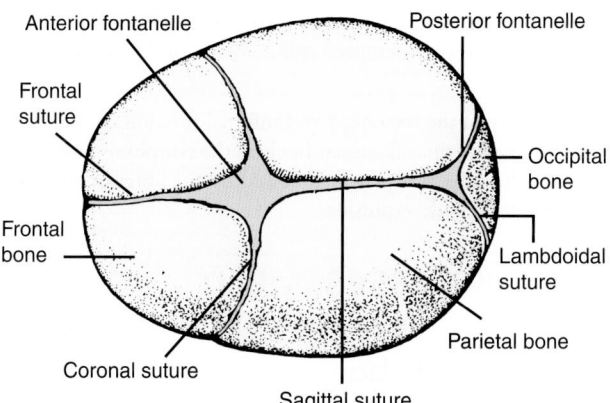

Figure 37-3. Fetal head.

Table 37-1	True and False Labor Contractions
TRUE LABOR CONTRACTIONS	**FALSE LABOR CONTRACTIONS**
Result in progressive cervical dilation and effacement	Do not result in progressive cervical dilation and effacement
Occur at regular intervals	Occur at irregular intervals
Interval between contractions decreases	Interval between contractions remains the same or increases
Frequency, duration, and intensity increase	Intensity decreases or remains the same
Located mainly in back and abdomen	Located mainly in lower abdomen and groin
Generally intensified by walking	Generally unaffected by walking
Not easily disrupted by medications	Generally relieved by mild sedation

Stages of Labor

First Stage of Labor (Cervical Completion, Dilation, and Effacement)

1. Begins with regular and rhythmic true labor contractions and ends with complete effacement (100%) and dilation of the cervix (10 cm).
2. The length of the first stage varies and is almost double in a primiparous patient; this stage of labor consists of two phases:
   a. Latent phase (early):
      i. Dilation from 0 to 3 cm; effacement tends to precede dilation in the primiparous patient.
      ii. At the end of the phase, contractions typically occur regularly every 5 minutes on average and are mild via palpation.
   b. Active phase:
      i. Dilation from 4 to 7 cm; completion of effacement evolves over this period in multiparous patients.
      ii. Contractions are more frequent at every 2 to 5 minutes, lasting 40 to 60 seconds and of moderate to strong intensity (60 to 80 mm Hg) via palpation.
      iii. Dilation averages 1.2 cm/hour in the nullipara and 1.5 cm/hour in the multipara.
   c. Transition (final segment of active phase): Dilation from 8 to 10 cm with contractions occurring every 2 to 3 minutes, lasting 50 to 60 seconds and of moderate to strong intensity (<90 mm Hg and typically nonindentable by palpation). Some contractions may last up to (but not exceed) 120 seconds.

Second Stage of Labor (Fetal Expulsion)

1. Begins with complete effacement and dilation ending with delivery of the fetus.
2. The second stage may last from 1 to 4 hours in the nullipara and typically less than 1 hour in the multipara. Variance in time depends on maternal pushing efforts, contraction pattern, anesthesia, and fetal descent.

Third Stage of Labor (Placental Expulsion)

1. Begins with delivery of the fetus and ends with delivery of the placenta.
2. The third stage may last from a few minutes to 30 minutes (typical). Prolonged periods may be attributable to abnormal placentation (ie, placenta accreta).

Fourth Stage (Immediate Postpartum)

This period lasts from delivery of the placenta until the postpartum condition of the woman has become stabilized (typically 1 to 2 hours after delivery).

Seven Cardinal Fetal Movements of Labor

When the biparietal diameter (BPD) of the fetal head has passed through the pelvic inlet, engagement occurs. Once the fetus enters the pelvis, seven "cardinal movements" are performed to assist in proper passage through the maternal pelvis during labor and birth (see Figure 37-4).

Descent

1. The downward movement of the fetus through the birth canal.

2. Accomplished by force of uterine contractions in the fundus and pressure of the amniotic fluid; during second stage of labor, "maternal bearing down" efforts increase intra-abdominal pressure, thus augmenting effects of uterine contractions.
3. *Station* refers to the relationship of the presenting part to the ischial spines. Subsequently, station has a direct correlation to the degree of descent, as described below (see Figure 37-5):
   a. Floating—fetal presenting part is not engaged in pelvic inlet; may be ballotable via cervical exam.
   b. Engagement—fetal presenting part enters the pelvis as the BPD passes through the inlet.
   c. The pelvis is divided into sections measured in centimeters; a 5 cm scale is used (see Figure 37-6).

Flexion

Resistance to descent causes the fetal head to flex down, leading to convergence onto the chest. This results in the smallest head diameter, the suboccipitobregmatic, to present through the canal. This position relocates the posterior fontanelle to the center of the cervix, easily palpable on vaginal examination. Flexion begins at the pelvic inlet and continues until the fetal head (or presenting part) reaches the pelvic floor.

Internal Rotation

To accommodate the birth canal, the fetal occiput rotates 45 or 90 degrees from its original position toward the symphysis. The rotation is usually anteriorly, but if the pelvis cannot accommodate the occiput anteriorly due to a narrow forepelvis, it will rotate posteriorly, resulting in an occipitoposterior (OP) position of the fetus. This movement results from the shape of the fetal head and maternal pelvis, as well as the contour of the perineal muscles. The ischial spines project into the midpelvis, causing the fetal head to rotate anteriorly to accommodate the available space.

Extension

As the fetal head meets the pelvic floor, it meets resistance from the perineal muscles and is forced to extend up and outward. The fetal head becomes visible at the vulvovaginal ring; its largest diameter is encircled (crowning) and later emerges from the vagina.

External Rotation

Initial phase is called *restitution*. Once the fetal head realigns with the shoulders, restitution is complete. After restitution, the second phase of external rotation occurs as the body rotates so that the shoulders are in the anteroposterior diameter of the pelvis.

Expulsion

After delivery of the fetal head and internal rotation of the shoulders, the anterior shoulder resets beneath the symphysis pubis. The posterior shoulder is expelled, followed by the anterior shoulder, leading to total body expulsion.

NURSING ASSESSMENT AND INTERVENTIONS

Initiation of Labor

Nursing responsibilities begin with an initial assessment once a patient presents in labor.

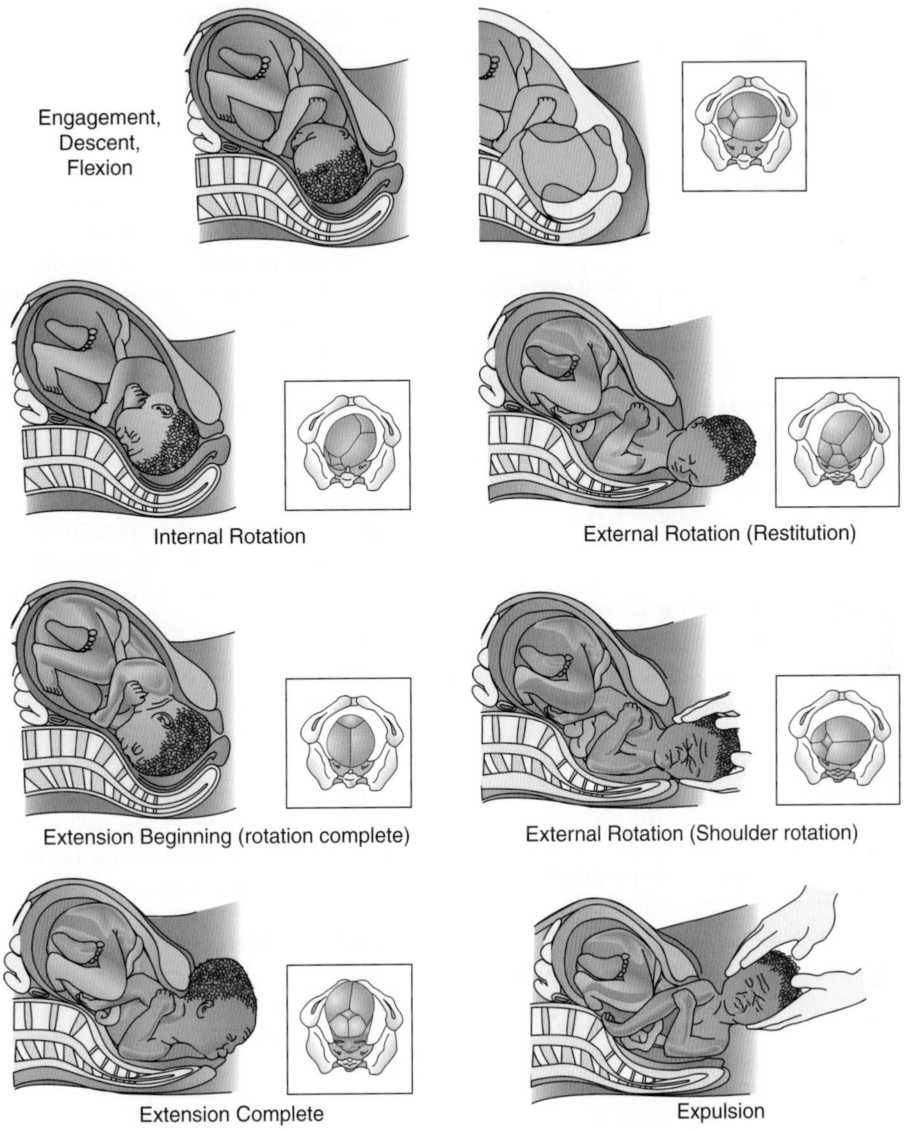

Engagement,
Descent,
Flexion

Internal Rotation

External Rotation (Restitution)

Extension Beginning (rotation complete)

External Rotation (Shoulder rotation)

Extension Complete

Expulsion

Figure 37-4. Seven fetal cardinal movements of labor (vertex presentation).

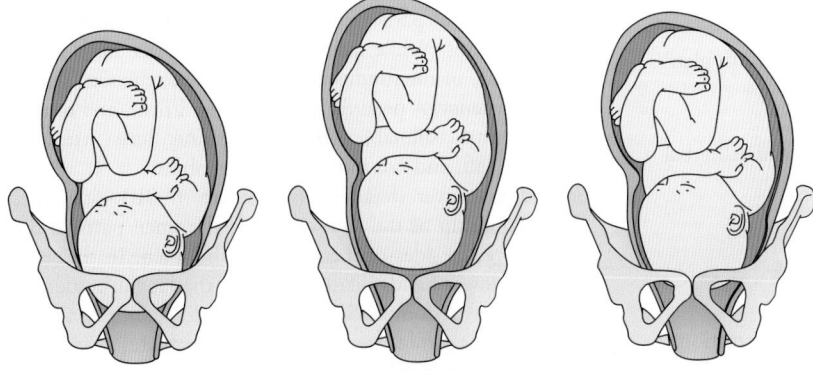

Figure 37-5. Engagement, floating, and dipping.

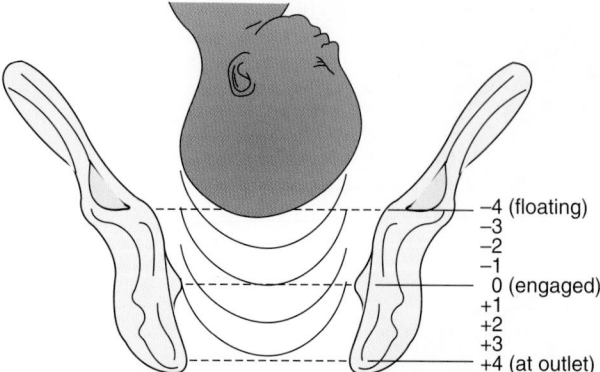

Figure 37-6. Stations of presenting part. The location of the presenting part in relation to the level of the ischial spines is designated station and indicates the degree of advancement of the presenting part through the pelvis. Stations are expressed in centimeters above (minus) or below (plus) the level of the ischial spines (zero).

Collection of History and Baseline Data

 Evidence Base Lowdermilk, D., & Perry, S. (2012). *Maternity and women's health care* (10th ed.). St. Louis, MO: Elsevier.
Mattson, S., & Smith, J. E. (2011). *Core curriculum for maternal-newborn nursing* (4th ed.). St. Louis, MO: Elsevier.

1. Introduce yourself; maintain eye contact; ask for name of woman's health care provider, inquire if the provider has been notified that the woman was coming to the facility or birth center; ask about presenting complaints/concerns.
2. Establish baseline obstetric, medical, and surgical information.
   a. Inquire and validate patient information with the prenatal care record, if available. Complete brief review of past medical, surgical, and obstetric history. Obtain a history of the current pregnancy: Gravidity? Parity? Expected date of delivery or confinement? Complications? Fetal growth? Antepartal testing results?
   b. Inquire about obstetric course and validate uterine contraction data with palpation: When did contractions begin? Frequency? Intensity? Duration? Bloody show? Have the membranes ruptured? Time of rupture? Color? Consistency? Amount of fluid? Odor?
   c. Assess patient's pain tolerance? Does she have a birth plan? Has she participated in Lamaze classes?
   d. Last meal/drink? What type of food/drink?
   e. Medications—nonprescription/prescription/illicit/herbal preparations or supplements?
   f. Support system?
3. Obtain baseline maternal and fetal vital signs.
   a. Temperature—elevation more than 100.0° F (37.8° C) suggests a possible infection or dehydration.
   b. Pulse—elevated over the resting rate during contractions; may be elevated between contractions due to medications, bleeding, or drug use; goal: 60 to 100 bpm.
   c. Respirations—increases as labor progresses; goal: 12 to 24 breaths/minute.
   d. Blood pressure (BP).
      i. A slight elevation over baseline may be attributed to anxiety.
      ii. BP more than 140 diastolic or 90 systolic (mm Hg) may be suggestive of hypertensive disorder of pregnancy and requires further evaluation and notification to primary care provider. A BP of more than 160/110 needs immediate attention and notification of the primary health care provider due to potential for stroke or seizure. Goal: Systolic more than 90 and less than 140 mm Hg; diastolic more than 60 and less than 90 mm Hg; mean arterial pressure (MAP) less than 100.

 Evidence Base American College of Obstetricians and Gynecologists. (2002/Reaffirmed 2010). *Diagnosis and management of preeclampsia and eclampsia* (Practice Bulletin #33). Washington, DC: Author.

   e. Complete fetal heart rate assessment; if a fetal monitor is to be used, run a 20- to 30-minute strip for baseline data and assessment of fetal well-being.
   f. Physical assessment—complete review of systems on admission to include heart and lung sounds, as well as peripheral deep tendon reflexes.
4. Obtain a urine specimen—test urine at bedside or send to lab for interpretation; assess results for dehydration, infection, blood, protein, or glucose.

Methods for Determining Fetal Presentation

 Evidence Base Curran, C., & Torgersen, K. (2012). *abcdEFM TEXTBook: Electronic fetal monitoring* (2nd ed.). Virginia Beach, VA: Clinical Specialists Consulting.

Leopold's Maneuvers

This involves manual manipulation of the maternal abdomen to determine fetal placement in relation to maternal structures (see Figure 37-7).

1. First maneuver (fundal contents) (see Figure 37-7A)—determines fetal parts (fetal head or breech) located in the uterine fundus. While facing the woman, place both hands on each side of the fundus and palpate; note the size, shape, and consistency. A head feels smooth, hard/firm, and round, mobile, and ballotable. Breech position feels irregular, rounded, soft, and not independently mobile.
2. Second maneuver (fetal lie) (see Figure 37-7B)—identifies the relationship of the fetal back and the small parts to the front, back, or sides of the maternal abdomen. In the same position, lower hands bilaterally along the lateral borders of the maternal abdomen. Select one hand to stabilize one side of the uterus while the opposite hand palpates downward over the opposite side. Repeat on the opposing side. Determine fetal anatomy by palpated contents: firm, smooth, and

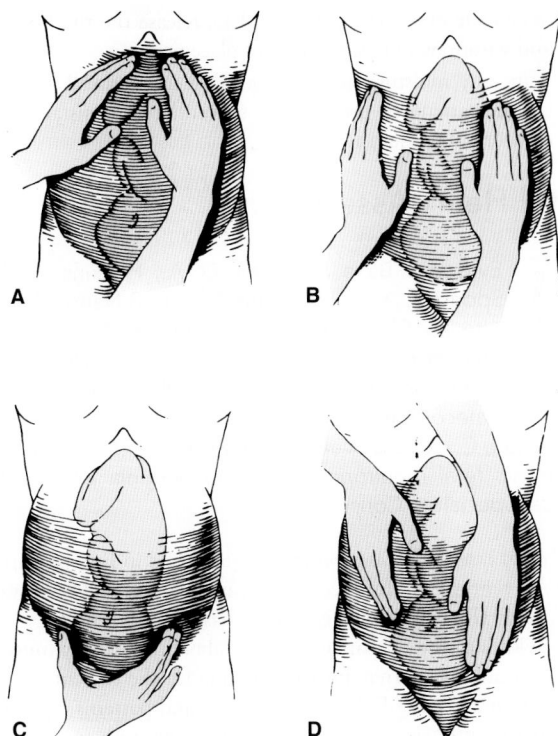

Figure 37-7. Leopold's maneuvers.

a hard continuous structure = fetal back; if small, knobby, irregular, protruding, and moving = fetal extremities.

3. Third maneuver (fetal presentation) (see Figure 37-7C)—determines the portion of the fetus that is presenting into the pelvic inlet. Grasp the part of the fetal presenting part situated in the lower uterine segment between the thumb and middle finger of one hand. Assess contents as described in the first maneuver; findings should be opposite of information found in the fundus. This maneuver is also known as Pallach's maneuver or grip.

4. Fourth maneuver (fetal attitude and engagement) (see Figure 37-7D)—determines flexion or attitude of the fetal vertex or the greatest prominence of the fetal head over the pelvic brim. In this maneuver, the examiner faces the woman's feet. The examiner places their hands on each side of the uterus, below the umbilicus and pointing toward the symphysis pubis. The examiner presses deeply with the fingertips, toward the symphysis pubis, locating the cephalic prominence. If the cephalic prominence is felt on the same side as the small parts: sinciput (fetus' forehead), fetus vertex is flexed. If the cephalic prominence is felt on the same side as the back: occiput (or crown), fetal vertex slightly extended. If the cephalic prominence is felt equally on both sides: military position (common in posterior position), or nonflexed. As hands move toward the pelvic brim, assess for the following: if the hands converge (come together) around the presenting part, it is floating; if the hands diverge (move apart), the presenting part is either dipping or engaged in the pelvis.

Ultrasonography
See page 1260.

Vaginal Examination
See Figure 37-8.

1. Explain the procedure to the woman and assist her to a lithotomy position.
2. Conduct examination gently, under sterile conditions.
3. Perineum—visually assess perineum for lesions, ulcerations, bruising, discharge, odor, rupture of membranes, or bleeding. If contagious condition is suspected (ie, syphilis or genital herpes) or active bleeding exists, stop the examination and notify the primary care provider.
4. Perform manual examination with dominant hand (may use nondominant hand over fundus to stabilize fetal presenting part against the cervix):
   a. Cervical assessment.
      i. Location? Posterior, mid, or anterior (facing the introitus and aligned parallel to the vagina).

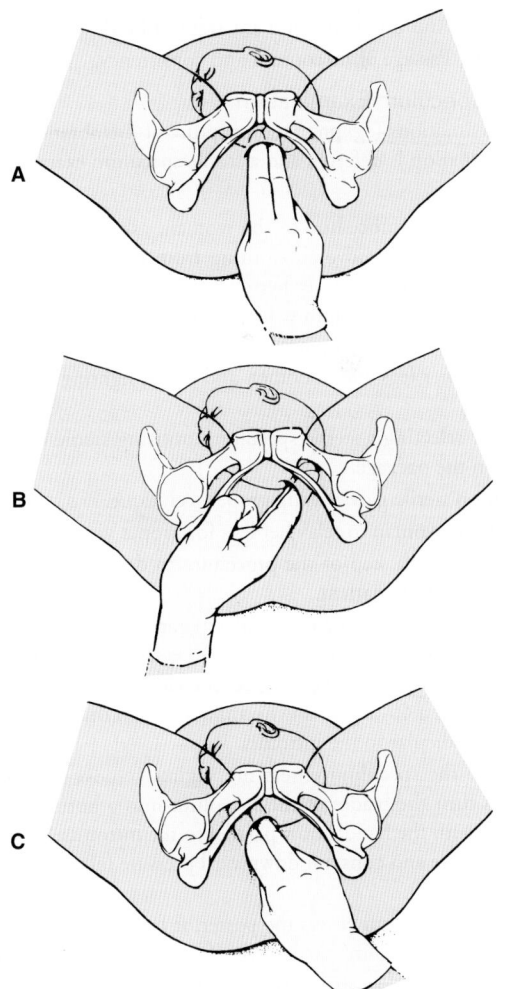

Figure 37-8. Vaginal examination. (A) Determining the station and palpating the sagittal suture. **(B)** Identifying the posterior fontanelle. **(C)** Identifying the anterior fontanelle.

ii. Hard or soft? Cervix softens during latent phase of labor.

iii. Long or short? As effacement occurs, the cervix shortens and thins. Measured in percentages from 0% to 100%.

iv. Open or closed? Measure degree of dilation in centimeters from 1 to 10 cm (complete).

b. Presentation.

i. Breech, cephalic/vertex (head), face, shoulder, transverse, or compound.

ii. Caput succedaneum (edema occurring in and under fetal scalp) present (mild, moderate, severe) or absent.

iii. Station identified: signifies descent in relation to maternal pelvis (–5 to +5).

c. Position.

i. Cephalic presentation (in relation to maternal pelvis anterior, posterior, transverse).

ii. Location of fontanelles.

d. Membranes—intact or ruptured.

i. Amount, color, and any odor of fluid.

ii. Passage of meconium and consistency.

Sterile Speculum Examination

In some situations (eg, premature rupture of membranes), a vaginal examination is deferred and a sterile speculum examination is completed.

1. Explain the procedure to the woman, ask her to empty her bladder and remove all clothing from the waist down, and give her a sheet to cover herself.

2. Assist the patient into a lithotomy position (place hip roll under one hip to displace the uterus).

3. Drape her legs and abdomen and adjust lighting at the perineum.

4. After selecting a sterile speculum, utilizing sterile technique, open the package.

5. Put on sterile gloves using proper technique.

6. Ask the woman to relax her legs for proper visualization.

7. Explain each step of the procedure to decrease anticipatory anxiety of the patient.

8. With the nondominant hand separate the labia, place two fingers just inside the introitus, and gently press down on the base of the vagina. Next, insert the closed speculum past the fingers at a 45-degree downward angle such that the handle is perpendicular to the introitus.

9. Once the speculum enters the vagina, remove your fingers and turn the blades of the speculum into a horizontal position with the handle now parallel to the introitus; maintain a moderate and constant downward pressure (alleviates pain to the urethra).

10. As the speculum enters the posterior fornix, gently open the blades to visualize the cervix. If you still cannot visualize, close the blades, withdraw the speculum slightly, and move the blades toward the back of the vagina and try again. Once the cervix is in view, tighten the thumbscrew to maintain the blades in an open position. Complete a visual cervical assessment and obtain any samples necessary.

11. When the examination is complete, release the thumbscrew and withdraw in reverse order of placement.

12. Wipe any moisture or discharge from the perineal area and tell the patient the procedure is over; offer her assistance to a comfortable position.

Fetal Heart Assessment

Evidence Base Macones, G. A., Hankins, G. D., Spong, C. Y., et al. (2008). The 2008 National Institute of Child Health and Human Development workshop report on electronic fetal monitoring: Update on definitions, interpretation, and research guidelines. *Obstetrics and Gynecology, 112,* 661–666.

Curran, C., & Torgersen, K. (2012). *abcdEFM TEXTbook: Electronic fetal monitoring* (2nd ed.). Virginia Beach, VA: Clinical Specialists Consulting.

Fetal heart rate (FHR) assessment was established in Europe during the 17th century and fostered in the United States by Dr. Edward Hon. As FHR analysis evolved, so too has its purpose.

Providers caring for patients during labor and delivery must be skilled in utilizing correct instrumentation for the current clinical scenario, interpreting FHR characteristics and patterns, applying appropriate interventions, and communicating both routine and critical data to the perinatal team as the patient's (mother, fetus, or both) condition warrants.

Maternal Risk Factors, Fetal/Neonatal Risks, and Fetal Heart Rate Implications

One cannot sufficiently interpret FHR variances without considering the impact of maternal physiology and pathophysiology during gestation. Maternal conditions that may negatively impact oxygenation and perfusion of the mother may lead to oxygen deprivation and hypoxemia in the fetus. The large majority of maternal and fetal couplets tolerate physiologic challenges of pregnancy, labor, and birth without consequence. Under extreme conditions (ie, asthma attack, seizure, hemorrhage), the maternal patient diverts blood and oxygen away from the nonvital uterus to vital organs at the expense of the fetus. Several maternal conditions outlined below explain risk factors to the fetus and subsequent FHR changes possibly witnessed during the intrapartum period.

1. Cardiac—acquired or congenital cardiac disease, anemia, or hypertensive disorders.

a. *Fetal/neonatal secondary risks*: small for gestational age (SGA), intrauterine growth restriction (IUGR), hydrops fetalis, hypoxemia, decreased amniotic fluid volume (AFV), preterm labor (PTL)/birth, placental abruption.

b. *Potential FHR alterations*: tachycardia, bradycardia, minimal or absent variability, absent accelerations, late decelerations, variable decelerations, prolonged decelerations, or sinusoidal patterns.

2. Respiratory—*chronic disease:* asthma, sickle cell, smoking; *acute disease:* status asthmaticus, acute respiratory distress syndrome, pulmonary embolus, amniotic fluid embolus, or infections.

a. *Fetal/neonatal secondary risks*: SGA, IUGR, hypoxemia, PTL/birth, presence of meconium.

b. *Potential FHR alterations*: tachycardia, bradycardia, minimal or absent variability, absent accelerations, late decelerations or prolonged decelerations.

3. Neurologic—*chronic disease*: epilepsy, underlying; *acute disease*: stroke, eclampsia.

   a. *Fetal/neonatal secondary risks*: hypoxemia, PTL/birth.

   b. *Potential FHR alterations*: bradycardia, minimal or absent variability, absent accelerations, late decelerations, or prolonged decelerations.

4. Renal—*chronic disease*: dialysis, transplant; *acute disease*: acute tubular necrosis, acute renal failure, development of calculi, fluid/electrolyte imbalance, infection.

   a. *Fetal/neonatal secondary risks*: SGA, IUGR, hypoxemia, decreased AFV, decreased/reversed umbilical blood flow, PTL/birth. (*Note*: Altered electrolytes may adversely affect fetus if prolonged.)

   b. *Potential FHR alterations*: tachycardia, bradycardia, minimal or absent variability, absent accelerations, variable decelerations, late decelerations, or prolonged decelerations.

5. Psychosocial and other risk factors—lack of prenatal care, medications, malnutrition/inadequate weight gain, excessive stress, domestic violence, substance abuse (eg, alcohol, illicit drug use).

   a. *Fetal/neonatal secondary risks*: SGA, IUGR, congenital anomalies, placental anomalies, hypoxemia, decreased AFV, or PTL/birth.

   b. *Potential FHR alterations*: tachycardia, bradycardia, minimal or absent or marked variability, absent accelerations, variable decelerations, late decelerations, or prolonged decelerations.

Fetal Heart Monitoring Instrumentation: External Options

Uterine Contraction Assessment by Palpation

1. Uterine palpation is performed periodically throughout labor to validate labor adequacy and progression; if applicable, palpation is also utilized to validate information received from internal equipment (ie, intrauterine pressure catheter).

2. Intensity may be described as follows (this may be taught to patient and labor coach):

   a. Uterus easily indented: feels like the tip of the nose (mild intensity).

   b. Able to slightly indent uterus: feels like the chin (moderate intensity).

   c. Unable to indent uterus: feels like the forehead (strong intensity).

3. Uterine contraction data include:

   a. Frequency: beginning of one contraction to the beginning of the next.

   b. Duration: beginning of one contraction to the end of the same contraction.

   c. Intensity: peak pressure of a contraction.

   d. Resting tone: pressure of uterus at rest or between contractions.

4. Benefits:

   a. Noninvasive; increases provider–patient interaction; direct assessment; easy to use/teach.

   b. Provides information regarding relative frequency, duration, strength, and resting tone.

   c. Allows freedom of movement and ambulation for woman.

5. Limitations:

   a. Subjective information that leads to potential practitioner variance.

   b. No permanent record for visual comparison analysis or collaboration.

   c. Clinical conditions that may limit or alter data collection: overextended uterus (ie, multiple gestation, polyhydramnios, macrosomia) or maternal obesity.

6. Procedure:

   a. Position patient in semi-Fowler's or lateral position; place hip roll on one side to displace the uterus; explain the procedure to the patient.

   b. Place the pads of your fingers on the patient's abdomen in the area of the fundus and at the point of maximum intensity (this is not always midline).

   c. Assess uterine contraction frequency, duration, intensity, and resting tone.

      i. Normal findings/intrapartum active phase: frequency: less than or equal to five contractions in 10 minutes, averaged over a 30-minute period; duration: <90 to 120 seconds; intensity: <80 mm Hg; resting tone: <20 to 25 mm Hg.

      ii. Abnormal findings—tachysystole: more than five contractions in 10 minutes; hypertonus: intensity > 80 mm Hg, resting tone > 20 to 25 mm Hg or Montevideo units (MVUs) > 400.

Uterine Contraction Assessment by Tocodynamometer (Tocotransducer)

1. A *tocodynamometer* detects changes in tension or muscular tone over the fundus on the outside layer of the maternal abdomen. The electronic data are then converted into a number and printed on the lower half of the electronic fetal monitor (EFM) paper. However, proper placement is key for accuracy:

   a. If patient is at term—place over the point of maximum intensity in the fundal region of the maternal abdomen.

   b. If patient is preterm—place over the lower uterine segment below the umbilicus, typically beside the ultrasound device if the fetus is vertex.

2. Benefits:

   a. Noninvasive, easy to use.

   b. Detects relative uterine resting tone, frequency, intensity, and duration of uterine contraction.

   c. Does not require ruptured amniotic membranes.

   d. Generates a tracing for future assessment and permanent record keeping.

3. Limitations:

   a. Nonspecific data gathered, particularly intensity and resting tone.

   b. Difficult to obtain data in patients with the following conditions: obesity, polyhydramnios, macrosomia, PTL, maternal vomiting, maternal bearing-down efforts/pushing during second stage or during procedures.

c. Location sensitive; placement may result in false or inadequate information.

d. Sensitive to maternal and fetal movement—may be superimposed on contraction waveform.

e. Limits maternal movement and ambulation during labor.

4. Procedure:

a. Position patient in a semi-Fowler's or lateral position; place hip roll on one side to displace the uterus; explain the procedure to the patient and support persons.

b. Palpate the point of maximum intensity over the fundus and secure belt.

c. Press the uterine activity (UA) reference button on the EFM between contractions to set the resting tone between 5 and 15 mm Hg.

d. Palpate the fundus and compare printed data.

e. Reposition the device periodically, as needed, for patient comfort and during labor as the fetus descends.

f. Interpret data and document and communicate findings.

Fetal Heart Rate Assessment by Auscultation

1. *Auscultation* is a FHR counting technique accompanied by a listening device (ie, fetoscope or Doppler). The examiner counts the FHR over a specified time frame (see Table 37-2).

2. Interpretation of data includes: FHR baseline rate, rhythm, and general increases and decreases.

3. Devices for interpretation may include: fetoscope, Leffscope or Pinard stethoscope (rarely used today), and Doptone/Doppler.

4. Capabilities of a fetoscope—detects:

a. Differentiation of fetal and maternal heart rates—eliminates error due to fetal demise and EFM with nonelectrical device (ie, fetoscope).

b. Verification of FHR dysrhythmias visualized on EFM tracing.

c. Clarification of halving or doubling (may occur due to dysrhythmia) on the EFM tracing.

5. Benefits:

a. Neonatal outcomes comparable to the use of EFM, in low-risk populations and with 1:1 nurse–patient ratios.

b. Noninvasive, easy to use, and most methods require no electricity.

c. Patient has increased freedom of movement and ambulation.

d. Patient can be monitored if submerged in water (eg, water/Jacuzzi births).

6. Limitations:

a. Subjective data collection; variances between practitioners may exist.

b. Conditions may limit the practitioner's ability to assess the FHR (obesity, increased fetal movement or amniotic fluid).

c. Cannot assess FHR variability or periodic/episodic decelerations or accelerations.

d. Lack of continuous recording from monitor for visual comparative analysis.

e. Requires education, practice, skill in auditory assessment.

f. Requires a 1:1 nurse–patient ratio during intrapartum; therefore, may create need to increase or realign labor and delivery staff.

7. Procedure:

a. Position patient in a semi-Fowler's or lateral position; place hip roll on one side to displace the uterus; explain the procedure to the patient and her support persons.

b. Palpate the maternal abdomen to locate the fetal back by using Leopold's maneuvers (see page 1272). Figure 37-9 outlines FHR locations and corresponding fetal positions.

Table 37-2	Frequency of Auscultation: Recommended Assessment and Documentation		
ORGANIZATION	**LATENT PHASE**	**ACTIVE PHASE**	**SECOND STAGE**
ACOG			
Low risk	—	q 30 minutes	q 15 minutes
High risk	—	q 15 minutes	q 5 minutes
AWHONN			
Low risk	—	q 30 minutes	q 15 minutes
High risk	—	q 15 minutes	q 5 minutes
SOGC	Regularly after rupture of membranes or clinically significant change	q 15 minutes	q 5 minutes when pushing is initiated

ACOG, American College of Obstetrics and Gynecologists; AWHONN, Association of Women's Health, Obstetric and Neonatal Nurses; SOGC, Society of Obstetrics and Gynecology of Canada.

Assess fetal heart rate (FHR) before initiation of labor-enhancing procedures, ambulation, administration of medications, administration or initiation of analgesia or anesthesia, and transfer or discharge of patient.

Assess FHR after admission of patient, artificial or spontaneous rupture of membranes, ambulation, recognition of abnormal uterine activity patterns, and administration of medications.

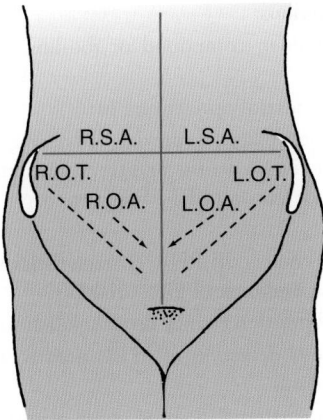

Figure 37-9. Fetal heart tone locations on the abdominal wall indicating possible corresponding fetal positions and the effects of the internal rotation of the fetus.

   c. If using Doppler device, apply conduction gel to underside of device.

   d. Position the bell of the fetoscope or Doppler on the area of the abdomen where maximum fetal heart sounds can be heard, usually over the back or chest of fetus. If using a fetoscope, use firm pressure. If using Doppler device, avoid friction noises caused by fingers on the abdominal surface area.

   e. Assess and compare maternal heart rate (radial pulse) against the FHR; confirm differentiation.

   f. Palpate uterine contractions simultaneously and compare with FHR data.

   g. Differentiate between fetal heart rate/tone and other abdominal sounds.

     i. FHR—a rapid crisp ticking or galloping sound.

     ii. Uterine bruit—a soft murmur, caused by the passage of blood through dilated uterine vessels; synchronous with maternal pulse.

     iii. Funic souffle (uterine souffle)—a hissing sound produced by passage of blood through the umbilical arteries; synchronous with the FHR.

   h. Count the FHR between contractions for at least 30 to 60 seconds (60 seconds per Society of Obstetricians and Gynaecologists of Canada).

   i. Interpret findings to include FHR baseline rate, rhythm, increases or decreases; further evaluation via EFM is indicated if:

     i. Baseline FHR less than 110 or more than 160, irregular rhythm, abrupt or gradual decreases in FHR during, immediately after, or 30 seconds after a contraction.

   j. Document and communicate findings with woman and her support persons.

   k. Communicate abnormal findings to primary practitioner immediately.

8. Troubleshooting interventions:

   a. Verify placement; utilize Leopold's maneuvers to verify fetal position.

   b. Assess all four quadrants of the maternal abdomen slowly; fetal malpresentation or demise may exist.

   c. Repositioning the patient may reposition the fetus.

   d. Reaffirm and compare data to the maternal pulse.

   e. Use alternative equipment options (eg, EFM) if unable to assess.

   f. Consult with other members of the perinatal team (patient care team) and notify the practitioner as warranted.

   g. Multiple gestations require a keen sense of auscultation; each FHR should be documented by location. For example, baby A/#1 = left lower quadrant, 150 beats/minute; baby B/#2 = right upper quadrant, 120 beats/minute. Ultrasound may be warranted to discern two separate FHRs.

Fetal Heart Rate Assessment by Ultrasound Transducer

Monitoring the FHR via ultrasound transducer allows detection of the FHR baseline rate, variability, accelerations, and decelerations.

1. Benefits:
   a. Noninvasive.
   b. Rupture of membranes not required.
   c. Provides permanent record for review and collaboration.

2. Limitations:
   a. Signal transmission may be influenced by maternal obesity, polyhydramnios, or anterior placental placement providing a weak, absent, or false signal.
   b. Restricts maternal mobility.
   c. Episodic maternal and fetal movement may interfere with continuous recording.
   d. Half- or double-counting of FHR may occur, especially with fetal tachycardia or bradycardia.
   e. May document maternal pulse with undiagnosed intrauterine fetal demise; always validate and compare data to maternal pulse.

3. Procedure:
   a. Gather equipment, explain procedure to patient, and perform Leopold's maneuvers to locate the fetal back or chest (point of maximum intensity [PMI]).
   b. Lubricate the face of the transducer with a thin layer of ultrasonic gel to aid in the transmission of sounds. Place the transducer over the PMI.
   c. Readjust the device periodically to maximize signal quality. Maintain a constant strip of FHR data as diligently as possible during course of labor.

Fetal Heart Monitoring Instrumentation: Internal Options

Uterine Contraction Assessment by Intrauterine Pressure Catheter

An *intrauterine pressure catheter (IUPC)* is the most objective technique to evaluate all uterine contraction characteristics and patterns. The device may be utilized for amniotic fluid testing and to perform an intrapartum amnioinfusion. IUPCs are either fluid-filled or solid-tipped catheters. Currently, there is no absolute indication for use of the IUPC in labor. Although not required, many practitioners utilize this device during labor of a woman with a previous uterine scar (eg, vaginal birth after cesarean). IUPCs are typically placed by the primary practitioner.

1. Benefits (fluid-filled and solid-tipped catheters):
   a. Utilized to calculate MVUs.
   b. Assists in the interpretation of the FHR (ie, comparison of a variable vs. late deceleration).
   c. Tracing generated as a permanent part of the medical record.
   d. Offers a portal for amniotic fluid sampling and amnioinfusion.
   e. Solid-tipped—easy, quick setup with decreased pressure artifact.
   f. Fluid-filled—least expensive; most accurate readings if correctly installed.

2. Limitations (fluid-filled and solid-tipped catheters):
   a. Rupture of membranes (ROM) and adequate cervical dilation are required for insertion.
   b. Invasive procedure.
   c. Increased risk of uterine infection.
   d. Improper insertion can lead to maternal or fetal trauma (ie, uterine perforation, uterine cord prolapse, extraovular placement).
   e. Limits the potential for maternal ambulation during labor.
   f. May be contraindicated in presence of vaginal bleeding and infection where ROM is discouraged to prevent maternal–fetal transmissions (eg, human immunodeficiency virus [HIV], herpes, group B-strep).
   g. Differences may occur in readings between fluid-filled and sensor-tipped catheters.
   h. Solid-tipped—pressure readings higher than fluid-filled catheters.
   i. Fluid-filled—lengthy setup; may be difficult to maintain with maternal repositioning; may become compressed between the uterine wall and fetus, distorting the waveform.

3. Contraindications:
   a. Placenta previa, active vaginal or cervical herpes, active hepatitis, or HIV infection; active vaginal bleeding.
   b. Presence of Category III FHR pattern requiring immediate delivery.

> **NURSING ALERT** If internal monitoring with an IUPC is used, uterine activity (UA) (frequency, duration, intensity, and resting tone) can be calculated and documented using mm Hg and MVUs. MVUs are derived by subtracting the resting tone of the uterus from the peak pressure of the contraction (in mm Hg) for each contraction occurring in a 10-minute period. These numbers are then added together for the total number of MVUs during that 10-minute period. IUPC data should also be periodically checked against manual palpation until delivery.

Fetal Heart Assessment by Fetal Spiral Electrode

The use of the *fetal spiral electrode (FSE)* to monitor the FHR allows for detection of FHR baseline rate, variability, accelerations, decelerations, and FHR dysrhythmias. Indications for use during labor include FHR not detected or abnormal findings via an external device.

1. Contraindications:
   a. Face, shoulder, compound or footling breech presentations.
   b. Unable to identify presenting part.
   c. Presence of placenta previa, active vaginal or cervical herpes, active hepatitis, or HIV infection; active vaginal bleeding or Category III FHR pattern.

2. Benefits:
   a. Ability to detect all FHR characteristics to include dysrhythmias and direct FHR variability.
   b. Maternal position change does not alter quality of tracing.
   c. Continuous detection of FHR; permanent recording in health record.
   d. Enhanced maternal comfort with removal of abdominal belt from external device.

3. Limitations:
   a. Invasive procedure; requires ROM, cervical dilation, and accessible/appropriate fetal presenting part.
   b. Potentially small risk of fetal hemorrhage, injury, or infection.
   c. May record maternal heart rate in the presence of fetal demise.
   d. Fetal arrhythmias may be missed (not detected) if EFM logic or electrocardiogram activation switch is turned on.
   e. A moist environment is necessary for FHR detection.
   f. Electronic interference and artifact may occur (ie, may become twisted in fetal hair).

4. Procedure:
   a. Gather equipment and explain procedure to patient.
   b. Perform EFM test if turning on EFM for the first time.
   c. Open FSE package utilizing sterile technique and place sterile glove on dominant hand.
   d. Following completion of a cervical exam, secure hand inside the cervix with second and third fingers pressed against presenting part, avoiding face, genitalia, and fontanels.
   e. Press catheter against presenting part and turn clockwise one full turn, pinch locking device at end, remove introducer, and attach to the EFM while securing to maternal abdomen or inner thigh.
   f. Interpret and document data.

Interpretation of Fetal Heart Rate

 Evidence Base Curran, C., & Torgersen, K. (2012). *abcdEFM TEXTbook: Electronic fetal monitoring* (2nd ed.). Virginia Beach, VA: Clinical Specialists Consulting.

American College of Obstetricians and Gynecologists. (2009). *Intrapartum fetal heart rate monitoring: Nomenclature, interpretation, and general management principles* (Practice Bulletin #106). Washington, DC: Author.

American College of Obstetricians and Gynecologists. (2010). *Management of intrapartum fetal heart rate tracings* (Practice Bulletin #116). Washington, DC: Author.

The following FHR interpretation criteria meets the current National Institute of Child Health and Human Development (NICHD) terminology and update and guidelines adopted by American College of Obstetricians and Gynecologists and Association of Women's Health, Obstetric and Neonatal Nurses in 2005, as well as management updates by ACOG in 2009 and 2010.

Fetal Heart Rate Baseline

1. *Fetal heart rate baseline (FHRB)* is the approximate mean FHR rounded to increments of 5 beats/minute during a 10-minute segment and excluding periodic/episodic changes, periods of marked FHR variability, segments of the baseline that differ by more than 25 beats/minute; interpretation between contractions is recommended but not required.
2. Documented as a single number.
3. Normal FHRB: 110 to 160 beats/minute; tachycardia: more than 160 beats/minute for 10 minutes or greater; bradycardia: less than 110 beats/minute for 10 minutes or greater.
4. In any 10-minute window, the minimum baseline duration must be at least 2 minutes or the baseline for that period is indeterminate. In this case, one may need to refer to the previous 10-minute segment for determination of the baseline. Two consecutive minutes are recommended but not required.
5. FHRB is calculated by determining the range of FHRV first then calculating the mean in increments of 5 (if FHRV equals 10 [ie, 140 to 150], mean FHRB = 145; if FHRV equals 15 [ie, 120 to 135], mean = 7.5, round up to FHRB of 130).
6. Variations from the normal baseline rate are tachycardia, bradycardia, and sinusoidal patterns.

Tachycardia

1. Etiology—maternal causes:
   a. Maternal fever.
   b. Maternal infection.
   c. Dehydration.
   d. Hyperthyroidism.
   e. Endogenous adrenaline or anxiety.
   f. Medications.
      i. Beta-sympathomimetics (terbutaline, ritodrine).
      ii. Ketamine, atropine, and phenothiazines.
      iii. Hydroxyzine.
      iv. Parasympathomimetics (epinephrine).
      v. Selected positive inotropic agents (dobutamine and positive chronotropic drugs).
      vi. Over-the-counter medications (decongestants, appetite suppressants, and stimulants or caffeine).
      vii. Illicit drugs (cocaine, amphetamines).
      viii. Nicotine, if inhaled (if inhaled, nicotine may increase FHR; if absorbed through a nicotine patch, it may decrease FHR).
      ix. Labor enhancement agents (ie, oxytocin, misoprostol), leading to persistent abnormal uterine contraction patterns.
2. Etiology—fetal causes:
   a. Infection.
   b. Fetal activity or stimulation.
   c. Compensatory response to acute hypoxemia.

d. Chronic hypoxemia.
e. Fetal hyperthyroidism.
f. Fetal tachyarrhythmias (supraventricular tachycardia).
g. Prematurity.
h. Congenital anomalies.
i. Cardiac abnormalities or heart failure.
j. Anemia.

3. Interventions:
   a. Monitor vital signs: maternal temperature and pulse; compare to FHR data.
   b. Assess maternal hydration (initiate or increase IV fluids, as needed).
   c. Decrease maternal temperature, if elevated, via an antipyretic, as ordered.
   d. Decrease maternal anxiety, give explanations for treatment measures, provide comfort measures, and assist with breathing/relaxation techniques.
   e. Assess additional FHR characteristics: if decelerations exist, consider the need to:
      i. Change patient to a lateral position.
      ii. Administer oxygen via face mask (8 to 10 L/minute); prolonged use discouraged.
      iii. Assess medication history and use.
      iv. Assess for tachydysrhythmia.
      v. If auscultating, apply EFM, as needed.
      vi. Notify the primary health care provider and perinatal team.

Bradycardia

Bradycardia in the fetus may result from maternal or fetal conditions. Severe bradycardia is defined as FHR less than 60 beats per minute. Sudden and sustained bradycardia accompanied by absent FHR variability (FHRV) has the highest risk of fetal and neonatal morbidity or mortality.

1. Etiology—maternal causes:
   a. Adrenergic-receptor blocking drugs (propranolol).
   b. Connective tissue disease (systemic lupus erythema).
   c. Prolonged maternal hypoglycemia.
   d. Maternal hypotension or hypothermia.
   e. Anesthetics (epidural, spinal, pudendal, or paracervical).
   f. Conditions that may cause acute maternal cardiopulmonary compromise (ie, amniotic fluid embolus, pulmonary embolus, cerebral vascular ischemia, hemorrhage, uterine rupture, trauma).
2. Etiology—fetal causes:
   a. Congenital heart block, typically secondary to maternal Lupus.
   b. Mature parasympathetic nervous system.
   c. Acute hypoxia.
   d. Cardiac structural defect.
   e. Umbilical cord occlusion.
   f. Maternal or fetal sentinel event precipitating hypoxia.
3. Hypoxic causes: umbilical cord prolapse or compression, uterine rupture, maternal hemorrhage, prolonged maternal hypoglycemia, placental abruption, maternal trauma, and persistent

abnormal uterine contraction patterns (ie, tachysystole). A FHR category III pattern of lengthy and severe bradycardia accompanied by absent FHR variability may lead to permanent central nervous system (CNS) injury or death in the fetus or neonate.

4. Interventions:
   a. Validate maternal heart rate versus FHR; validate if fetus has complete heart block.
   b. Perform vaginal examination to assess for umbilical cord prolapse.
   c. Assess maternal vital signs to rule out hypotension (pulse and BP); increase fluids, as necessary, to alleviate unstable vital signs.
   d. Assess FHR variability and other FHR characteristics—consider:
      i. Maternal lateral position change.
      ii. Discontinue oxytocin administration or augmentation agents.
      iii. Modify maternal pushing techniques or stop pushing during second stage of labor until FHR resolves.
      iv. Administer oxygen via face mask (8 to 10 L/minute) as necessary; prolonged use discouraged.
   e. If auscultating, apply EFM to assess FHR variability.
   f. Notify the primary health care provider and perinatal team.

Sinusoidal

1. This pattern differs from variability in that it has a smooth, sine wave-like pattern (equal deflections above and below the FHRB) of regular frequency and amplitude and is excluded in the definition of variability; described as *sinusoidal* or *pseudosinusoidal (medication induced)*.
2. Etiology:
   a. Chronic fetal anemia: Rh isoimmunization.
   b. Fetal–maternal hemorrhage.
   c. Severe fetal acidosis.
   d. Maternal opioid administration; leads to pseudosinusoidal pattern.
3. Interventions:
   a. Lateral positioning.
   b. Administer IV hydration.
   c. Administer oxygen via face mask (8 to 10 L/minute); prolonged use discouraged.
   d. Analyze patient for causes of hemorrhage and treat accordingly.
   e. Notify the primary health care provider and perinatal team.
   f. If etiology necessitates, consider:
      i. Kleihauer-Betke test to assess for fetal red cells in maternal blood due to hemorrhage.
      ii. Expeditious delivery.

Fetal Heart Rate Variability

1. *Fetal heart rate variability (FHRV)* is the result of electrical impulses received by the cardiac muscle from the brain stem's medulla oblongata. The medulla oblongata receives information from both the parasympathetic (slow) and the sympathetic (fast) nervous systems; the combined effect leads to a cyclic push and pull of the heart rate over time (heart rates are never static unless permanent CNS damage has occurred). Oxygenation must remain constant for communication to occur between the CNS and cardiac muscle.

2. At the time of observation, variability indicates adequate oxygenation of the fetal CNS.
3. FHRV is defined as fluctuations in the baseline FHR. These fluctuations are irregular in amplitude and frequency and are visually quantified as the *amplitude of the peak-to-trough range* in beats per minute as follows:
   a. Absent FHRV—undetectable.
   b. Minimal FHRV—more than undetectable but less than or equal to 5 beats/minute.
   c. Moderate FHRV—6 to 25 beats/minute.
   d. Marked FHRV—more than 25 beats/minute.
4. Calculation of FHRV range is determined by the mean peak-to-trough range rounded to increments 5 beats per minute (ie, 120 to 135, 115 to 130, 150 to 155); the mean is reported as the FHRB.
5. Absent or minimal variability may be due to preterm gestation (less than 28 to 32 weeks), alteration in nervous system function, medications, abnormal uterine contraction patterns, or inadequate oxygenation.
6. Normal sleep and wake states, medications, alcohol, and illicit drugs that cause fetal neurologic damage; morphine; methadone; anomalies; and previous insults that have damaged the fetal brain can affect the baseline variability.
7. Moderate FHRV, even in the presence of decelerations, is strongly associated (98%) with an umbilical pH more than 7.15 (nonacidemic) or newborn vigor (Apgar score ≥ 7 at 5 minutes).
8. Abnormal findings: prolonged periods of absent, minimal, or marked FHRV; if absent FHRV is accompanied by recurrent decelerations (late, variable, or prolonged), fetal or neonatal morbidity or mortality may result.
9. Interventions for Category III pattern: recurrent late, variable or prolonged decelerations accompanied by absent FHRV (caused by CNS dysfunction, hypoxia, asphyxia):
   a. Notification to primary practitioner and perinatal team for expeditious delivery.
   b. Prepare for expeditious and immediate delivery; route dependent on clinical conditions.
   c. Discontinue oxytocin administration, if applicable.
   d. Assess maternal vital signs (initiate/increase intravenous infusion (IVF), as needed).
   e. Administer oxygen via face mask (8 to 10 L/minute); prolonged use discouraged.
   f. Change maternal lateral position.
10. Interventions for minimal FHRV (caused by sleep state, medications, hypoxia, CNS dysfunction, dysrhythmias):
    a. Rule out nonhypoxic causes: sleep state, medications?
    b. If minimal FHRV is accompanied by recurrent late, variable, or prolonged decelerations, extended time to complete all interventions outlined in 9 a–f (previous paragraph) is afforded. If pattern does not resolve within 60 to 90 minutes, delivery via the most expeditious route is recommended.
11. Interventions for marked FHRV (possibly caused by cord entanglement, excessive release of fetal catecholamines, asphyxia): same as for minimal FHRV.

Periodic/Episodic Fetal Heart Rate Patterns

Periodic or episodic changes are visually apparent increases or decreases in the FHRB in the form of an acceleration or deceleration. Their duration is greater than 15 seconds and less than 2 minutes. After 2 minutes, they are considered prolonged. If duration exceeds 10 minutes, a baseline rate change has occurred. *Periodic* patterns occur simultaneously with contractions and *episodic* patterns occur in the absence of contractions. Periodic and episodic patterns are distinguished on the basis of waveforms, currently accepted as "abrupt" (onset to peak or nadir [lowest point] is less than 30 seconds) or "gradual" (onset to nadir is equal to or greater than 30 seconds). Decelerations are defined as recurrent if they appear with 50% or greater of uterine contractions in any 20-minute period, or intermittent, if they occur with less than 50% of uterine contractions, in any 20-minute period.

1. Acceleration: visually apparent, abrupt increase in the FHR above the baseline rate; calculated from the most recently determined FHRB.
   a. The following criteria reflect gestational age implications:
      i. Term (greater than or equal to 32 weeks): peak of acceleration is 15 or more beats per minute (bpm) above the FHR baseline and 15 seconds or more in duration but less than 2 minutes.
      ii. Preterm (less than 32 weeks): peak of acceleration is at least 10 bpm above the FHR baseline and at least 10 seconds in duration but less than 2 minutes.
      iii. Prolonged: duration 2 minutes or longer but less than 10 minutes.
   b. Etiology: fetal movement, uterine contraction, partial umbilical cord occlusion, breech presentation, occiput posterior position of the fetal vertex, vaginal examination, fetal scalp stimulation, following application of vibro-acoustic stimulator, application of FSE.
   c. Accelerations are associated with a nonhypoxic fetus and normal fetal pH at time of observation.
   d. Interventions—none required.
2. Early deceleration— Visually apparent usually symmetrical gradual decrease and return of the FHR associated with a uterine contraction; calculated from the most recently determined portion of the FHR baseline. It is coincident in timing, with the nadir of the deceleration occurring with the peak of a contraction. In most cases, the onset, nadir, and recovery of the deceleration occur with the beginning, peak, and end of the contraction, respectively.
   a. Physiology—head compression causing a vagal response. It is a benign pattern and not associated with fetal hypoxemia; may evolve into variable decelerations.
   b. Interventions—none required.
3. Late decelerations—visually apparent, usually symmetrical gradual decrease and return of the FHR associated with a uterine contraction. The decrease in FHR is calculated from the onset to the nadir of the deceleration. The deceleration is delayed in timing, with the nadir of the deceleration occurring after the peak of the contraction. In most cases, the onset, nadir, and recovery of the deceleration occur after the beginning, peak, and ending of the contraction, respectively.

a. Physiology.
   i. Reflex—chemoreceptor stimulation leading to the transient decrease in FHR accompanied by normal FHRB and moderate variability. Prolonged supine positioning may precipitate reflex late decelerations; repositioning patient laterally often resolves pattern.
   ii. Myocardial depression—decreased oxygen transfer at the placental interface may lead to uteroplacental insufficiency (UPI). Prolonged periods of UPI may lead to progressive fetal hypoxia and metabolic acidosis. Metabolic acidosis can directly influence electrical conduction and performance of the fetal heart, causing direct myocardial depression. These late decelerations are "myocardial mediated" and may be accompanied by a change in the fetal heart baseline (tachycardia or bradycardia), absent or minimal variability, and the absence of accelerations; usually indicative of a fetus in metabolic acidemia. A category III FHR pattern of recurrent late decelerations accompanied by absent FHRV requires immediate delivery via the most expeditious route.
b. Maternal factors that may promote UPI:
   i. Hypotension (may also be associated with reflex late decelerations).
   ii. Severe hypertension.
   iii. Placental changes that may affect uteroplacental gas exchange (ie, postmaturity, premature placental aging, calcification, placental abruption, placenta previa, or placental malformations).
   iv. Physiologic conditions that may be associated with decreased maternal oxygen saturation or hemoglobin levels (ie, asthma attack, cardiopulmonary disease, or trauma).
   v. Persistent abnormal uterine contraction patterns (ie, tachysystole, tetany, or hypertonus).
c. Interventions—aimed at increasing uteroplacental perfusion by correcting cause.
   i. Alter maternal position: lateral position (right or left) or knee chest.
   ii. Correct maternal hypotension with hydration and/or medication.
   iii. Discontinue labor stimulation or cervical ripening agents.
   iv. Administer oxygen by face mask at 8 to 10 L/minute via a nonrebreather mask; prolonged use discouraged.
   v. If category III FHR pattern of recurrent late decelerations accompanied by absent FHRV, immediate delivery is warranted by the most expeditious route. Notification of the primary practitioner and perinatal team is indicated. Preparations for emergent delivery are warranted.
4. Variable deceleration—visually apparent abrupt decrease in FHR from the onset of the deceleration to the beginning of the FHR nadir is less than 30 seconds. When variable decelerations are associated with uterine contractions, their onset, depth, and duration commonly vary with successive uterine

contractions. It is important to note that variable decelerations vary in shape, timing, and return to baseline. Severe variable decelerations last more than 60 seconds yet less than 2 minutes and fall more than 70 beats below the FHRB. Therefore, deceleration depth correlates with the degree of acidemia.

a. Physiology—decreased umbilical cord perfusion, resulting from compression or stretch. Compression may result from maternal positioning, prolapsed cord, cord entanglement, second-stage labor, short cord, and a true knot in the cord.

b. Interventions.

i. Change maternal position, which may dislodge an occluded cord.

ii. Perform a vaginal examination to assess for cord prolapse or imminent delivery.

iii. If prolapse, elevate presenting part off the cord while palpating for an umbilical pulse, FHR.

iv. Amnioinfusion, if appropriate.

v. Decrease or discontinue oxytocin, if appropriate.

vi. Provide oxygen by face mask at 8 to 10 L/minute; prolonged use discouraged.

vii. Discontinue or alter second-stage pushing technique if repetitive, severe variables occur in second stage.

viii. If category III FHR pattern of recurrent variable decelerations accompanied by absent FHRV, immediate delivery is warranted by the most expeditious route. Notification of the primary practitioner and perinatal team is indicated. Preparations for emergent delivery are warranted.

5. Prolonged deceleration—visually apparent decrease of FHR of at least 15 beats per minute or more below the baseline and lasting more than 2 minutes but less than 10.

a. Physiology—causes may reflect similar pathophysiology of late or variable deceleration

b. Interventions—if more than 4 to 5 minutes and causes unknown or unresolved, perinatal team should prepare for an emergent delivery.

6. Document all findings and classify patterns as normal (category I FHR), indeterminate (category II FHR), or abnormal (category III FHR) per NICHD guidelines (refer to Table 37-3).

First Stage of Labor—Latent Phase (0 to 3 cm)

Nursing Diagnoses

- Deficient Fluid Volume related to decreased oral intake, dietary restrictions, and energy requirement of labor.
- Anxiety related to concern for self and fetus.
- Acute Pain related to uterine contractions, position of fetus, advancement of labor.

Nursing Interventions

Maintaining Nutrition and Hydration

1. Provide clear liquids and ice chips, as allowed.
2. Evaluate urine for ketones and glucose.
3. Administer IV fluids, as indicated and ordered.

Table 37-3	Three-Tier Fetal Heart Rate Interpretation System
CATEGORY	**FHR PATTERNS**
Category I: normal patterns	Baseline rate: 110 to 160 beats per minute Baseline FHR variability: moderate Late or variable decelerations: absent Early decelerations: present or absent Accelerations: present or absent
Category II: indeterminate patterns (includes all tracings not categorized in Categories I or III)	Bradycardia not accompanied by absent baseline variability Tachycardia Minimal variability Absent variability not accompanied by recurrent decelerations Marked variability Absence of induced accelerations after fetal stimulation Recurrent variable decelerations accompanied by minimal or moderate variability Prolonged decelerations Recurrent late decelerations with moderate variability Variable decelerations with other characteristics, such as slow return to baseline, overshoots, or "shoulders"
Category III: abnormal patterns	Absent variability plus any of the following: Recurrent late or variable decelerations Bradycardia Sinusoidal pattern

Relieving Anxiety

1. Establish a relationship with the woman/support persons.
2. Inform the woman/support persons of maternal status, fetal status, and labor progress periodically during the labor process.
3. Explain all procedures and equipment used during labor; answer questions and offer support.
4. Review birth plan and make appropriate revisions, if applicable.
5. Monitor maternal vital signs as the patient's condition warrants.

a. Temperature every 2 to 4 hours, unless elevated or membranes ruptured, then every 1 to 2 hours.

b. Pulse and respirations, as indicated by facility policy, medical condition, or medication administration (eg, oxytocin or MgSO$_4$).

c. BP typically every hour unless hypertension or hypotension exists or woman has received pain medication or anesthesia; then evaluate more frequently based on findings or as indicated.

6. Monitor FHR periodically (refer to Table 37-2, page 1276).

Controlling Pain

1. Encourage ambulation and frequent repositioning, as tolerated.
2. Encourage diversional activities, such as reading, talking, watching TV, playing cards, listening to music.
3. Review, evaluate, and teach proper breathing techniques:
   a. Slow chest breathing (slow paced/Lamaze)—relax, take one deep cleansing breath, and exhale slowly and completely. Breathe deeply, slowly, rhythmically throughout the contraction. Average 10 to 12 breaths per minute. Breathe slowly and deeply in through the nose and out through nose or slightly pursed lips.
   b. Modified-paced breathing—used when slow chest breathing no longer effective, typically as labor progresses. Take one deep breath and exhale slowly and completely. As contractions intensify, breathe with more frequent shallow breaths during a contraction. At conclusion of contraction, take a deep breath and exhale slowly. Maintain a pace not to exceed twice the woman's average respiratory rate or less than 24 breaths/minute.
   c. Patterned-paced breathing (pant-blow breathing/Lamaze)—utilized in later stages of labor as contractions intensify and deep long breaths are not obtainable. Concentrate on breathing in controlled manner. Take a deep breath and exhale slowly and completely. Then take four shallow breaths through the mouth, making a "hee" or "heh" sound; maintain steady rhythm. Finish with a deep cleansing breath at end of contraction. This breathing pattern is most commonly used during transition prior to active pushing.
4. Teach effleurage—light touch and massage over maternal skin, typically the abdomen, with fingertips; can be used with slow chest and modified-paced breathing. Start at pubic bone and move hands slowly up sides of abdomen in wide circular sweep; during exhalation, move fingertips down center of abdomen. Usually performed by laboring mother, but can be done with one hand if side-lying or coach assisted (see Figure 37-10).
5. Encourage a warm shower or whirlpool, if approved by primary practitioner.
6. Provide comfort measures.
   a. Give back or foot rubs.
   b. Assist the woman to change position. Walking, squatting, semi-sitting, hands and knees, kneeling, standing, side-lying, or sitting on the toilet assist fetal descent and alleviate pain. Side-lying position or hands and knees position will assist to rotate a persistent OP position to an anterior position.

Alternative Therapies

Birthing Balls

Sturdy inflatable vinyl balls approximately 2½ feet (0.8 m) in diameter used by the laboring woman. The laboring woman can sit on the ball and sway from side to side, or she may kneel and lean forward resting on the birthing ball to assist in fetal descent.

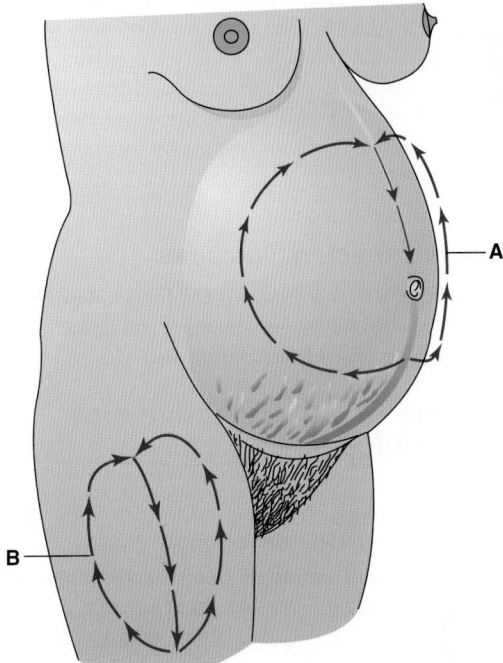

FIGURE 37-10 Effleurage. (**A**) During uterine contractions, a woman creates the pattern on her bare abdomen with her fingers. (**B**) If electronic fetal monitoring is being used, effleurage may be performed on the thigh.

Self-Hypnosis

Women are trained to rehearse the birth mentally and to control physical reactions to labor, such as BP, pulse, or pain. The American Psychotherapy and Medical Hypnosis Association (*www.apmha.com*) can provide referrals.

Acupuncture

Although there are no current U.S. studies on acupuncture, the practice is active in this country and is said to relieve as much as 90% of the pain in early labor and 60% of the pain during transition. Referrals can be made to the American Academy of Medical Acupuncture (*www.medicalacupuncture.org*).

Herbal Therapies

 Evidence Base Skidmore-Roth, L. (2009). *Mosby's handbook on herbs and natural supplements* (4th ed.). St. Louis, MO: Mosby.

Although many of the herbs used are not approved by the Food and Drug Administration, they have been researched and found to be effective in laboring women and are documented in myriad medical and nursing references.

1. Evening primrose oil—rubbed on abdomen in prelabor to stimulate uterine activity.
2. Corn silk—stimulates sluggish labor.
3. Nutmeg—enhances uterine contractions; if added, cayenne and bayberry help to reduce bleeding after delivery.
4. Nutmeg with yarrow, mistletoe, and corn silk—utilized as a treatment for postpartum hemorrhage.

DRUG ALERT Although red raspberry is effective when used to expel retained placenta, it should only be used during the immediate postpartum period—not during labor. Avoid licorice, mistletoe, thyme, and slippery elm during labor because they can significantly increase uterine tone.

Evaluation: Expected Outcomes

- Tolerates fluids well and urine negative for ketones and glucose.
- Verbalizes positive statements about self and fetus.
- Reports pain decreased from comfort strategies.

First Stage of Labor: Active and Transition Phase (4 to 10 cm)

 Evidence Base Davidson, M. W., London, M. L., & Ladewig, P. W. (2011). *Olds' maternal-newborn nursing and women's health across the lifespan* (9th ed.). Upper Saddle River, NJ: Prentice Hall.

Nursing Diagnoses

- Anxiety related to concern for self and fetus.
- Acute Pain related to uterine contractions, nausea, and vomiting.
- Impaired Urinary Elimination related to epidural anesthesia or from pressure of the fetus.
- Ineffective Coping related to discomfort.
- Risk for Infection related to rupture of the membranes and prolonged labor.
- Impaired Physical Mobility related to medical interventions and discomfort.
- Ineffective Breathing Pattern related to pain and fatigue.

Nursing Interventions

Relieving Anxiety

1. Monitor maternal vital signs every hour if low-risk pregnancy or every 30 minutes if high-risk pregnancy; assess FHR as outlined in Table 37-2, page 1276.
2. Provide encouragement and support and involve the patient and significant other(s) in the maternal–fetal plan of care.

Minimizing Pain

1. Encourage frequent position changes for comfort.
2. Assist the woman with breathing and relaxation techniques, as needed.
3. Provide back, leg, and shoulder massage, as needed.
4. Evaluate cervical status periodically for labor progression (typically every 2 hours and periodically prior to labor enhancement medication dose adjustments).
5. Assist with preparation for analgesia and anesthesia following patient request (see Table 37-4).
   a. Confirm known allergies.
   b. Assess and document baseline temperature, BP, pulse, and respiratory rate. Monitor FHR during anesthetic procedures and before and after intramuscular (I.M.) or IV administration of medication.
   c. Review maternal health information, laboratory results, labor status, and current obstetric complications with anesthesia and obstetric care.
   d. Administer IV fluid bolus of lactated Ringer's solution (500 to 1,000 mL), if not contraindicated (ie, severe pre-eclampsia, pulmonary edema).
   e. Assist anesthesia care provider; position and hold patient for catheter insertion (lateral decubitus or sitting with feet supported, head flexed forward, elbows resting on knees with feet supported on a stool).
   f. Monitor FHR during procedure, continuous or intermittent.

 DRUG ALERT A licensed, credentialed anesthesia care provider should be readily available to manage anesthesia-related obstetrical emergencies. The American Society of Anesthesiologists guidelines require that the administrator of anesthesia/analgesia remain with the patient for the first 20 minutes after regional anesthesia administration.

6. Monitor the woman following administration of analgesia/anesthesia.
   a. Monitor maternal BP, pulse, and respiratory rate after initiation or rebolus of regional block per facility protocol; typically every 5 minutes for the first 15 minutes.
   b. Support patient to lateral or Semi-Fowler's position with uterine displacement.
   c. Intervene for maternal hypotension with lateral positioning; additional IV fluids, as ordered; and administration of ephedrine per facility protocol.
   d. Monitor for adverse reactions from IV injection of local anesthetic: maternal tachycardia or bradycardia, hypertension, dizziness, tinnitus, metallic taste in mouth, loss of consciousness, or cardiopulmonary collapse.
   e. Monitor for adverse effects of opioids or anesthetics:
      i. Pruritus (itching on chest, face, and arms), especially during first hour after medication administration (usually begins within 30 to 60 minutes and decreases during the next hour).
      ii. Nausea/emesis—can occur in up to 50% of women; administer medications to help with nausea/emesis, as directed by provider.
      iii. Headache: (1) pain in the frontal/occipital regions or radiating to neck; (2) stiff neck; (3) pain increases in upright position and may decrease in horizontal position; (4) relieved by abdominal compression; (5) accompanied by nausea/vomiting, ocular symptoms (photophobia, diplopia, difficulty in accommodation), and auditory symptoms (hearing loss, hyperacusis, tinnitus).
      iv. Urine retention—observe for bladder distention; may utilize straight catheter to empty bladder if patient loses ability to sense fullness.

Table 37-4   Obstetric Analgesia and Anesthesia

DRUG	COMMENTS
Analgesics/Parenteral Opioids	
Meperidine Butorphanol Nalbuphine Fentanyl	Decreases fear and anxiety, promotes physical relaxation and rest between contractions; may cause nausea and vomiting; respiratory depression is the main adverse effect and is seen primarily in the neonate. Most commonly given via IV line or I.M. every 3–4 hours.
Tranquilizers	
Promethazine Hydroxyzine Propiomazine	May be used in combination with opioids; potentiates opioids; may be used as an antiemetic. Used in latent and first stage of labor to relieve anxiety, increase sedation and rest, and decrease nausea and vomiting.
Sedatives	
Sodium pentobarbital Sodium phenobarbital	Produces sedation and hypnosis. Used for latent stage of labor to decrease anxiety, inhibit uterine contractions, and allow for rest. Does not relieve pain. Given orally or I.M.
Epidural Anesthesia/Analgesia	
Epidural opioids	Used with a local anesthetic to provide pain relief with a decreased motor block in labor. Used postoperatively to promote long-acting analgesia.
Epidural block	Used for labor to provide a sensory block up to the T10–T12 level. Medication is given through the epidural catheter. Used for cesarean delivery and postpartum tubal ligation by increasing the level of anesthesia up to T4–T6.
Subarachnoid block (spinal/intrathecal)	Used for such surgical procedures as a cesarean delivery and postpartum tubal ligation. The procedure is quicker and easier to perform. There is no catheter left in place for the procedure. Medication lasts for a finite period.
Local anesthesia	Used for pain control of the perineal area for an episiotomy or repair during a vaginal delivery.
Pudendal block	Used during the second stage of labor just before delivery to numb the lower vaginal canal, vulva, and the perineum for delivery. May also be used to provide pain relief for a forceps delivery if the woman does not have an epidural and for perineal repair.
General anesthesia	Used for emergency delivery involving cesarean delivery; if the woman refuses regional anesthesia; if regional anesthesia cannot be performed.

DRUG ALERT Nembutal and promethazine can cause the following fetal or neonatal complications: fetal tachycardia, minimal or absent variability, absent short-term variability, hypotonia, hypothermia, generalized drowsiness, and a reluctance to feed in the first days of life. Meperidine, fentanyl, morphine, nalbuphine, and butorphanol can cause subtle effects on neonatal behavior in the first 24 hours secondary to these drugs crossing the placenta.

f. Assess EFM data before, during, and after initiation or rebolus of anesthesia or analgesia, including patient-controlled epidural analgesia.

g. Periodically evaluate and document maternal pain level on continuum using pain assessment tools in accordance with facility policy.

h. Evaluate labor progress; anesthetics may slow labor progression; augmentation agents may be necessary.

7. Following delivery, assess neonate for effects of analgesia or anesthesia (neurobehavioral change, such as decreased motor tone and decreased respiratory rate). Initiate neonatal resuscitation, as indicated, in accordance with established guidelines.

Encouraging Bladder Emptying

1. Encourage the woman to void every 2 hours at least 100 mL, if possible.

2. Palpate the lower abdomen, evaluate for a distended bladder periodically throughout labor.

3. Provide privacy to the patient to complete task. Running water or providing a perineal bottle of warm water for the woman to squirt against her perineum may assist success.

4. Catheterize patient if unable to void voluntarily.

5. Monitor intake and output per facility policy, particularly for certain medical conditions or following medication administration of IV oxytocin or $MgSO_4$.

Strengthening Coping with Active Labor and Transition

1. Assist the woman with breathing and relaxation techniques.
2. Encourage the labor coach to assist with coping strategies.
3. Provide comfort measures, which may include:
   a. Effleurage, back rubs, and leg stroking.
   b. Cool cloth to face, neck, abdomen, or back.
   c. Ice chips to moisten mouth.
   d. Clean pads and linens, as needed.
   e. Quiet, calm environment.
   f. Repositioning frequently for comfort with pillow and blanket.
4. Assist patient to pace herself and to encourage her to deal with one contraction at a time.
5. Provide information on the contraction's ascent, peak, and descent; encourage resting between contractions. Anticipatory guidance helps to assist with the patient's ability to tolerate labor.
6. Encourage the woman not to push with feelings of rectal pressure until complete cervical dilation has occurred. Short panting breaths may assist to divert bearing-down sensation.

Preventing Intrauterine Infection

1. Assess temperature every 2 hours if membranes are not ruptured. If ruptured, assess temperature every hour.
2. Periodically change pads and linens when wet or soiled.
3. Provide perineal care after voiding and as needed.
4. Discourage the use of perineal pads or folded towels against the perineum because they create a warm, moist environment for bacteria.
5. Minimize vaginal examinations.
6. Observe for fetal tachycardia and warmth of maternal skin as signs of infection.
7. Assess complete blood count, as indicated and available.

Maintaining Mobility

1. Provide information regarding limitations and opportunities for movement with EFM.
2. Encourage ambulation or sitting in a chair while being monitored, if appropriate.
3. Encourage frequent upright or lateral position changes.

Encouraging Effective Breathing Techniques

1. Assist the woman to alter her breathing and utilize relaxation techniques, as needed, to maintain pain control.
2. Inform the woman that the urge to push is common during transition and occurs as the fetal presenting part meets the perineal floor muscles. Pushing with feelings of rectal pressure before complete cervical dilation should be avoided due to risks of increasing cervical edema and lacerations.
3. Assist the woman to avoid pushing prematurely by:
   a. Maintaining close eye contact during breathing and keeping patient focused.
   b. Breathing with the woman, having her blow out strong, short breaths.

Evaluation: Expected Outcomes

- Verbalizes positive statements about self and fetus.
- Reports pain decreased from comfort strategies and medical interventions.
- Bladder remains nondistended.
- Directs strategies for decreasing discomfort.
- Absence of fever and signs of infection.
- Changes position during labor.
- Utilizes patterned breathing techniques during contractions.

Second Stage of Labor

The second stage of labor is typically the most challenging for both the mother and fetus. As contractions become more frequent and increase in intensity, perineal pressure is heightened as the fetus completes the last few cardinal movements through the birth canal. Breathing techniques and positioning may either help or hinder descent and oxygenation. It is important for each practitioner to assist the maternal–fetal couplet with strategies to optimize oxygenation, encouragement, descent, and patient safety.

Positioning

It is most beneficial for practitioners who offer labor support to encourage the patient to utilize upright positions in order to facilitate fetal descent. Research supports that the most successful position is the squat; additional options exist (ie, standing, upright kneeling, leaning against a wall). Advanced imaging techniques have verified an increase in the pelvic outlet during squat positioning of approximately 1 to 2 centimeters. Subsequent findings also conclude that a squat position is accompanied by a shorter second stage, higher Apgar scores, reduced pain, decreased perineal trauma, and decreased need for neonatal resuscitation intervention. With advancements in anesthesia preparations and dosing, patients have increased mobility during anesthetic infusions. Therefore, encouraging and assisting the epidural-induced patient into a squat position is achievable. Additional positions are available to encourage fetal rotation and descent: side-lying, knee-chest, hands-and-knees, and forward lean accompanied by a pelvic tilt or pelvic rocking. Supine positioning is inappropriate during labor—at all stages—as it promotes maternal vena caval compression with subsequent deoxygenation and perfusion of the mother and fetus.

Pushing Techniques

For optimum success, pushing techniques should be initiated once the cervix is fully dilated, fetal presenting part is on the pelvic floor (+1, +2, or > station), and the patient has a sense to push/bear down (Ferguson's reflex). Due to the expanded use and effects of anesthetics during labor and birth, some women lose sensitivity to perineal pressure, requiring guidance and instruction with pushing efforts. Two methods of pushing exist: passive pushing or laboring down and active pushing.

1. Passive pushing ("laboring down"/"rest and descend")—this technique offers no active participation by the patient or practitioner to facilitate descent; strength of second-stage labor contractions moves the fetus down the birth canal. Reasons that may necessitate the need for this method include the following:
   a. Due to epidural anesthesia/analgesia, the woman does not feel the urge to push.
   b. Maternal clinical conditions such as cardiac disease, respiratory distress, or trauma.

c. Fetal clinical conditions such as category III FHR or persistent abnormal UA data.

d. Maternal exhaustion; need for periods of rest during prolonged second stage.

e. Lack of nursing personnel to provide 1:1 support.

f. Absence or unavailability of primary practitioner to assist with delivery.

2. Active pushing—this technique involves active participation (breathing techniques and positioning) by the patient and practitioner to assist in fetal descent. Closed-glottis (ie, breath holding) is no longer recommended during second stage as it limits oxygenation and encourages CO_2 retention. If prolonged, this technique may negatively impact the fetus and potentially lead to abnormal FHR patterns. Strategies that promote oxygen exchange in the mother include:

a. Open-glottis pushing—this technique allows the woman to maintain a patent airway for gas exchange while enhancing bearing-down efforts with several short, quick breaths over the duration of a contraction (60 to 90 seconds). The method includes several short, quick breaths of 4 to 6 seconds accompanied by bearing-down efforts that utilize muscles in the upper abdomen; improves maternal–fetal oxygenation.

b. Tug-of-war—utilization of a gown or short sheet tied in a knot at both ends. When the mother has the urge to push, she grabs one end of the gown or sheet and pulls as much as she can while the coach or nurse provides resistance by holding the other end (alternative way is to tie knot in one end and tie other end to squat bar of labor bed); relaxes the perineum and has been found to decrease the second stage of labor by as much as 20 minutes.

c. Birthing aids—birthing balls, squat bars, birthing stools, and cushions may also be utilized to support the woman and her fetus.

Nursing Diagnoses

- Fear or Anxiety related to impending delivery.
- Acute Pain related to descent of the fetus.
- Risk for Infection related to episiotomy and tissue trauma.

Nursing Interventions

Minimizing Fear and Anxiety

1. Monitor maternal vital signs per facility policy.

2. Assess FHR and UA data every 15 minutes in low-risk women and every 5 minutes in high-risk women.

3. Explain procedures, breathing technique, and equipment during the delivery process.

4. Periodically inform the woman or couple of their progress and alterations in care plan.

5. Provide frequent, positive encouragement and utilize a mirror to assist the woman to see her progress.

6. Assist with positioning and pushing, as outlined above.

Promoting Comfort

1. Change positions frequently to increase comfort and promote fetal descent.

2. Evaluate bladder fullness and encourage voiding or catheterize, as needed.

3. Evaluate effectiveness of analgesia or anesthesia, as indicated; notify if alterations in dosing are needed to facilitate progression while maintaining pain control.

Preventing Infection and Promoting Safety

1. Prepare the birthing room or delivery room using sterile technique, allowing ample time for setup before delivery.

2. Prepare the infant resuscitation area; notify pediatric personnel, if appropriate, per facility policy; if category III pattern, have two practitioners available to administer neonatal resuscitation, as indicated.

3. Notify necessary obstetric personnel and primary practitioner to prepare for delivery. Because it is often difficult to predict delivery time, err on the side of safety and call early in order to limit deliveries without a primary provider.

4. If delivery room is to be used, safely transfer the patient to the delivery room bed once the fetal head is crowning.

5. If delivering in LDR (Labor, Delivery, Recovery) or LDRP (Labor, Delivery, Recovery, Postpartum) room, prepare labor bed for delivery in accordance with manufacturer's instructions. Prepare infant warmer and remain in the room for delivery.

6. Position the woman for vaginal birth in a semi-Fowler's position supported by a large cushion for her head, back, and shoulders. Padded stirrups or footrests may be used for foot support. Gently place both legs in the stirrups at the same time to avoid ligament strain, backache, or injury.

7. Clean the vulva and perineal areas.

a. Cleanse from the lower abdomen to the mons.

b. Next, clean the groin to the inner thigh on each side and then clean labia.

c. Finally, clean the introitus.

8. Support and guide the woman step by step during the delivery process.

a. When the fetal head is encircled by the vulvovaginal ring, an episiotomy may be performed by the primary practitioner. Episiotomies are no longer recommended as research shows advanced tearing may progress once an incision has been made.

b. Once the head is delivered, the mother is instructed to stop pushing. Mucus is wiped from the infant's face and the mouth and nose are aspirated with a bulb syringe. Neonatal resuscitator guidelines no longer recommend suctioning of any kind on the perineum for the presence of meconium. However, if positive pressure ventilation is required, the airway should be cleared prior to bag and mask ventilation.

 Evidence Base American Academy of Pediatrics & American Heart Association. (2011). *Textbook of neonatal resuscitation* (6th ed.). Elk Grove, IL: American Academy of Pediatrics.

c. Nuchal cord intervention—loops of umbilical cord found around the neonate's neck are loosened and slipped over the head, if possible. If the cord cannot be slipped over the head, it is clamped with two clamps and a cut is made between the two clamps.

d. Next, the woman is instructed to give a gentle push to assist with delivery of the remainder of the neonate's body.

e. Cord clamping—once the entire newborn has delivered, two cord clamps are placed on the umbilical cord and a cut is made between the two clamps. The infant is then presented to the mother or shown to the mother and passed to the neonatal team for immediate care, if indicated. If color and tone are adequate and accompanied by a vigorous cry, basic neonatal care can be delayed to support immediate skin-to-skin contact with mother and family bonding.

9. Practice standard universal precautions during labor and delivery.

Evaluation: Expected Outcomes

- Verbalizes positive statements about delivery outcome.
- Reports decreased pain from proper positioning.
- Absence of infection noted.

Third Stage of Labor: Delivery of the Placenta

 Evidence Base Davidson, M. W., London, M. L., & Ladewig, P. W. (2011). *Olds maternal-newborn nursing and women's health across the lifespan* (9th ed.). Upper Saddle River, NJ: Prentice Hall.

Nursing Diagnoses

- Impaired Tissue Integrity related to placental separation.
- Risk for Bleeding related to complications of delivery.

Nursing Interventions

Promoting Tissue Integrity

1. Delivery of the placenta typically occurs within the first 5 to 10 minutes, but may persist past 30 minutes, particularly in preterm gestations. Once signs of placental separation are

noted, the woman may assist delivery of the placenta with gentle bearing-down efforts. Observe for signs of placental separation (see Figure 37-11):

a. Uterus rises upward in the abdomen.

b. Umbilical cord lengthens.

c. Small amount of blood appears.

d. The uterus becomes globular in shape.

2. Evaluate the placenta for size, shape, implantation site of cord, and intact cotyledons. Umbilical cord should be inspected for true knots, clots, length, and number of vessels. Abnormalities in the placenta, cord, or both should be confirmed by an additional practitioner and documented in the labor record. Occasionally, the primary practitioner may request the placenta be sent to pathology for evaluation.

Preventing Hemorrhage

1. Maintain accurate measurement of intake and output throughout labor and delivery.

2. Immediately after delivery of the placenta, administer oxytocin as directed by facility policy and provider. At high doses or rapid administration, oxytocin administration may cause hypotension. Titration of the medication to uterine response is indicated (ie, if uterus is firm, decrease infusion; if boggy, increase infusion). Oxytocin should never be administered via IV push, as it can cause cardiac dysrhythmia and death.

3. Immediately after delivery of the placenta, gently massage uterine fundus periodically to promote firmness and extract placental clots. Uterine massage is performed with a bimanual technique. The nondominant hand is anchored over the lower uterine segment above the symphysis pubis to inhibit uterine inversion while the dominant hand gently massages the fundus. Visual inspection of the perineum should occur simultaneously to assess results of lochia.

4. Assess for possible causes of hemorrhage, including undiagnosed lacerations, or retained placental fragments or membranes. Placental evaluation should include visual assessment of intact cotyledons; the presence of even one cotyledon remaining intact within the uterus may stimulate a hemorrhagic state.

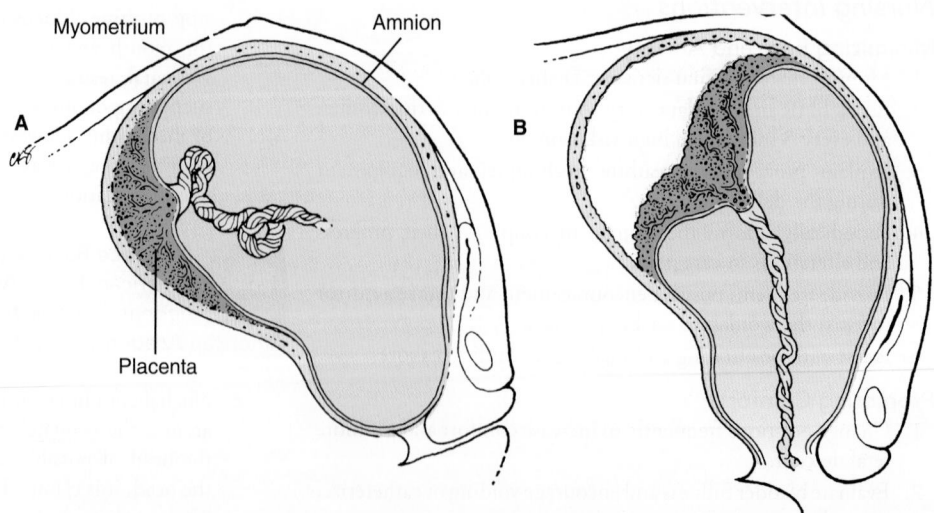

Figure 37-11. Placental separation. (A) Placenta attached to uterine wall. **(B)** Placenta separated from uterine wall.

Enlarged clots and retained amniotic membranes may stimulate bleeding. Periodic expression of clots should be performed during the immediate postpartum period.

5. Evaluate actual blood loss (ABL) versus estimated blood loss during periods of excessive bleeding. Weight machines may be used to assess for ABL of blood-saturated items; 1cc = 1gm = 1ml. Patient vital signs offer clinical triggers of deterioration during periods of hypovolemia; patient may be stable or unstable based on these parameters and uterine response.

    a. Stable: The uterus should remain firm between assessments or quickly firms after fundal massage. Moderate amount of lochia for 1 hour, should reduce to small or trace amounts over the next 2 to 4 hours postpartum.

    b. Unstable: An MAP less than 60, a systolic blood pressure less than 80, or a 15% drop from normal are clinical triggers of hemorrhage. Severe tachycardia ($\geq$ 110), severe tachypnea (>24/minute), or BP < 80/50 are signs of impending compromise. Increasing IV fluids (lactated Ringer's [LR] solution of choice) improve circulating volume; replacement should occur at a rate of 3cc of LR per each 1 cc of blood loss. A second IV may be warranted as clinical conditions evolve. Continuous vaginal bleeding and a boggy (soft) uterine tone are signs of uterine atony.

NURSING ALERT Hypotension is a late sign of hypovolemia; increased pulse rate is the first indicator.

6. Anticipate the need for medication to treat postpartum hemorrhage:

    a. Methergine I.M. 0.2 mg every 2 to 4 hours.

    b. Prostaglandin F_2 alpha I.M. 0.25 mg every 15 to 90 minutes up to eight doses.

    c. Dinoprostone 20 mg per rectum (PR).

    d. Misoprostol 200 to 400 for a maximum dose of 1,000 mcg PR.

DRUG ALERT Methergine is contraindicated in women with hypertension. If the woman had ephedrine in the past 2 hours, the woman can experience a hypertensive crisis with or without a history of hypertension. Hemabate is contraindicated in women with asthma, active cardiac disease, active renal disease, or active hepatic disease. Prostin is contraindicated in women with hypotension.

7. If bleeding continues and uterus is firm, notify health care provider for evaluation of lacerations or retained placental fragments. Inspection and repair of lacerations of the vagina and cervix are made by the health care provider.

8. If abnormal vaginal bleeding continues, notify health care provider and prepare patient for possible surgery (dilation and curettage, B-lynch suture, pelvic pressure packing, and selective arterial embolization). Autotransfusion (transfusion with one's own blood) is a viable treatment option and approved for use by Jehovah's Witnesses.

Evaluation: Expected Outcomes

- Delivery of an intact placenta.
- Blood loss controlled and hemorrhage prevented.

Immediate Care of the Neonate

Evidence Base Lowdermilk, D., & Perry, S. (2012). *Maternity and women's health care* (10th ed.). St. Louis, MO: Elsevier.

American Academy of Pediatrics & American Heart Association. (2011). *Textbook of neonatal resuscitation* (6th ed.). Elk Grove Village, IL: American Academy of Pediatrics.

Nursing Diagnoses

- Ineffective Airway Clearance related to nasal and oral secretions from delivery.
- Ineffective Thermoregulation related to environment and immature ability for adaptation.
- Risk for Infection related to immature defenses of the neonate.

Nursing Interventions

Promoting Airway Clearance and Transitioning of the Neonate

1. Over 90% of newborns complete intrauterine to extrauterine transition without compromise or assistance. Close observation of all neonates is recommended for a minimum of 4 to 6 hours after birth.

2. Clean mucus from the face, mouth, and nose. Aspirate with a bulb syringe, as necessary.

    a. Neonatal resuscitator protocols no longer require suctioning on the perineum if meconium is present in the amniotic fluid.

    b. If a neonate is born vigorous (strong respiratory efforts, good muscle tone, and heart rate greater than 100), bulb suction of mouth and nose only are required. If meconium-stained amniotic fluid is present and baby is not vigorous (depressed respirations, depressed muscle tone, and/or heart rate less than 100 bpm), direct suctioning of the mouth and trachea are necessary to prevent aspiration.

3. Clamp the umbilical cord approximately 1 inch (2.5 cm) from the abdominal wall with a cord clamp.

    a. Count the number of vessels in the cord—fewer than three vessels is associated with renal and cardiac anomalies, which may or may not result in a normal outcome.

4. Assess neonate's condition by utilization of the Apgar scoring system (see Table 37-5) at 1 and 5 minutes after birth. When the 5-minute score is <7, scoring continues every 5 minutes or until transition to neonatal special or intensive care unit. An Apgar score of 0 to 3 at 20 minutes is associated with neonatal encephalopathy and cerebral palsy.

Promoting Thermoregulation

1. Dry the neonate immediately after delivery, remove wet towels, and place skin-to-skin on mother and cover with a blanket if stable and vigorous. If nonvigorous newborn, place under a prewarmed radiant warmer bed. A wet, small neonate

SIGN	0	1	2
Heart rate	Absent	Slow (<100)	>100
Respiratory effort	Absent	Slow, irregular	Good, crying
Muscle tone	Flaccid	Some flexion of extremities	Active motion
Reflex irritability	No response	Cry	Vigorous cry
Color	Blue, pale	Body pink, extremities blue	Completely pink

Table 37-5 — Apgar Scoring Chart

looses up to 200 cal/kg/minute through evaporation, convection, conduction, and radiation.

2. Cover the neonate's head with a cotton stocking cap to prevent heat loss.

3. Wrap the neonate in several warm blankets and return to mother, if stable.

4. Provide a warm, draft-free environment for the neonate.

5. Assess neonate's axillary temperature—a normal temperature is between 97.5° and 99° F (36.4° and 37.2° C).

Preventing Infection

1. Administer prophylactic treatment against ophthalmia neonatorum (gonorrheal or chlamydial).
   a. Treatment may be with ½- to ¾-inch (1- to 2-cm) ribbon of sterile ointment of tetracycline (1%) or erythromycin (0.5%) ophthalmic ointment or ophthalmic solution of povidone-iodine (2.5%).
   b. This treatment can be delayed up to 1 hour after birth and usually delayed until after the first breastfeeding episode.

 DRUG ALERT Excessive ophthalmic ointment should be wiped away with a sterile pad or cotton ball at least 1 minute after installation.

   c. If the mother has a positive gonococcal or chlamydial culture, the neonate will require further treatment.
   d. Treatment is mandatory in all states.

2. Administer a single parental prophylactic injection of vitamin K.
   a. This is done to prevent a vitamin K–dependent hemorrhagic disease of the neonate.
   b. If the parents do not want vitamin K administered, inform the parents that circumcision may not be performed. However, inform parents that vitamin K levels will reach their peak (without neonatal injection) at 8 days after birth.

3. While in the delivery room (DR), place identical identification bracelets on the mother and the neonate. The nurse in the DR should be responsible for preparing and securely fastening the bands on the neonate. Security devices may also be secured at this time to prevent infant abduction.

   a. Information on bands may include mother's name, hospital/admission number, neonate's sex, race, primary practitioner, and date and time of birth and other information specified in the facility's policy.
   b. The father or significant other may also wear an identical bracelet matching the mother's.
   c. Footprinting and fingerprinting the neonate are not adequate methods of patient identification and may or may not be performed.
   d. Complete all identification procedures before the infant is taken from the DR.
   e. Many hospitals have security systems and small infant locators are attached to the umbilical cord or cord clamp prior to leaving labor and delivery.

4. Weigh and measure the infant shortly after birth.
   a. Normal neonate weight is 6 to 9 lb (2,700 to 4,000 g).
   b. Normal neonate length is 19 to 21 inches (48 to 53 cm).

5. After birth, nursery/mother-baby personnel should evaluate the neonate's status and assess risks.

6. Administer hepatitis B vaccine according to your facility's policy.
   a. Vaccination of all infants born in the United States is recommended regardless of mother's hepatitis status. If the mother's hepatitis B surface antigen (HBsAg) status is negative, the vaccine is given within 12 hours of birth to age 2 months and then again at 1 to 2 months after the initial dose with the final vaccine (#3) given at 6 to 18 months. The vaccine is given for the prevention of acute and chronic hepatitis B infection.
   b. If mother is hepatitis B positive, infant will receive hepatitis B immunoglobulin (HBIG) and the HBV vaccine at birth to within 12 hours. Additionally, infants of hepatitis-positive mothers will receive HBV at ages 1 to 2 months and age 6 months.
   c. Neonates born to nonscreened mothers will receive the HBV at birth within 12 hours of birth. If the mother later proves to be hepatitis B positive, the neonate will also receive HBIG (0.5 mL) I.M. as soon as possible, but no later than 1 week after birth. The infant will also receive HBV at 1 to 2 months and another injection at 6 to 18 months.

Community and Home Care Considerations

1. Issues regarding promoting airway clearance, transitioning, and thermoregulation promotion are essentially unchanged for home births; Apgar scores are not always given at home deliveries.

2. Eye prophylaxis remains necessary; parents may choose not to use prophylaxis.

3. Vitamin K administration is not a requirement for home deliveries. Vitamin K levels naturally increase at 8 days of life. If infant is a boy and parents desire circumcision, the procedure is withheld until after day 8.

4. Make sure attendants are familiar with neonatal resuscitation and that emergency numbers and procedures are readily available.

5. Identification procedures are not required for home births, although required state paperwork must be completed by the health care provider.

Evaluation: Expected Outcomes

- Neonate transitions appropriately, as evidenced by Apgar score between 7 and 10.
- Temperature remains between 97.5° F to 99° F (36.4° C and 37.2° C).
- Proper identification bracelets are placed on neonate and initial neonate care complete.

Fourth Stage of Labor

 Evidence Base American College of Obstetricians and Gynecologists. (2006/Reaffirmed 2011). *Postpartum hemorrhage* (Practice Bulletin #76). Washington, DC: Author.

Nursing Diagnoses

- Risk for Bleeding related to uterine atony and hemorrhage.
- Deficient Fluid Volume related to decreased oral intake, bleeding, and diaphoresis.
- Acute Pain related to tissue trauma and birth process, intensified by fatigue.
- Impaired Urinary Elimination related to epidural or spinal anesthesia and tissue trauma.
- Risk for Injury related to disturbed sensation of lower extremitie after regional anesthesia.
- Risk for Impaired Parenting related to inexperience or birth trauma.

Nursing Interventions

Promoting Normal Involution and Controlled Bleeding

1. Monitor BP, pulse, and respirations every 15 minutes for 1 hour, then every half to 1 hour until stable or transferred to the postpartum unit. Vital signs are assessed as the patient's condition warrants, increased frequency during periods of instability are necessary.
2. Take temperature every 4 hours unless elevated or additional signs of infection present.
3. Evaluate the following clinical parameters with vital signs per facility's policy:
   a. Uterine fundal tone, height, and position. The uterus should be firm at or around the level of the umbilicus and midline. If deviated to the side (usually the right side), it is indicative of a full bladder. Assist the mother to void spontaneously or utilize a straight catheter to empty her bladder if anesthesia effects remain.
   b. Assess vaginal bleeding (lochia):
      i. Scant—blood only on tissue when wiped or less than 1-inch (2.5-cm) stain on perineal pad.
      ii. Small/light—less than 4-inch (10.2-cm) stain on perineal pad.
      iii. Moderate—less than 6-inch (15.2-cm) stain on perineal pad.
      iv. Heavy—saturated perineal pad.
      v. Clots—note size and frequency; weigh for ABL.

   c. Assess perineum for edema, discoloration, bleeding, odor, or hematoma formation.
   d. Assess episiotomy for approximation, drainage, bleeding, or infection.

Maintaining Fluid Volume

1. Maintain IV fluids as orders dictate and clinical condition warrants.
2. Provide oral fluids and a snack or meal, as tolerated, if vital signs are stable and bleeding is controlled.

Relieving Discomfort and Fatigue

1. Apply a covered ice pack to the perineum periodically during the first 24 hours for an episiotomy, perineal laceration, or edema.

 NURSING ALERT Excessive perineal pain unrelieved by medications suggests hematoma formation and mandates careful examination of vulva, vagina, and rectum.

2. Administer analgesics, as indicated.
3. Ensure that epidural catheter has been removed, if appropriate.
4. Assist the woman in finding comfortable positions.
5. Assist the woman with a partial bath and perineal care. Periodically change linens and pads, as necessary.
6. Allow for privacy and rest periods between postpartum checks.
7. Provide warm blankets and reassure the woman that tremors are common during this period due to intravascular fluid shifts.

Encouraging Bladder Emptying

1. Evaluate the bladder for distention.
2. Encourage the woman to void periodically.
   a. Provide adequate time and privacy.
   b. The sound of running water may stimulate voiding.
   c. Gently squirting tepid water against the perineum may facilitate voiding.
3. Catheterize the woman if the bladder is full and she is unable to void.
   a. Birth trauma, anesthesia, and pain from lacerations and episiotomy may reduce or alter the voiding reflex.
   b. Bladder distention may displace the uterus upward and to the right side.

Preventing Injury Pending Return of Sensation

1. Evaluate mobility and sensation of the lower extremities.
2. Evaluate vital signs.
3. Remain with the woman, and assist her out of bed for the first time. Evaluate her ability to support her weight and ambulate.

Promoting Parenting

1. Once stable, bring neonate to the mother and support person immediately after birth.
2. Encourage the parents to hold infant as soon as possible.

3. Teach parents to hold the neonate close to their faces, about 8 to 12 inches (20.5 to 30.5 cm) to engage neonate.

4. Assist parents to inspect the infant's body to familiarize themselves with their child.

5. Assist with breastfeeding as soon as possible once both mother and newborn are stable. This is typically a period of quiet alert time for the neonate often optimizing successful breastfeeding.

6. Document appropriate and inappropriate bonding; notify primary practitioner and social services if suspect lack of or inappropriate response in mother, father, or any other potential caregiver.

Evaluation: Expected Outcomes

- Vital signs remain stable, vaginal bleeding remains light to moderate, and uterus remains firm at the midline below umbilicus.
- Tolerates fluids and food well after delivery.
- Verbalizes decreased perineal pain and feels more rested.
- Voids within 2 hours of delivery.
- Ambulates without assistance.
- Interacts with the neonate.

SPECIAL CONSIDERATIONS
Neonatal Resuscitation

 Evidence Base American Academy of Pediatrics & American Heart Association. (2011). *Textbook of neonatal resuscitation* (6th ed.). Elk Grove, IL: American Academy of Pediatrics.

Neonatal resuscitation is most effective with an organized and efficient team. At every delivery there should be at least one person whose primary responsibility is the neonate and who is capable of initiating neonatal resuscitation. Any high-risk delivery (requiring more advanced neonatal resuscitation) requires at least two people to be present to manage the resuscitation—one with complete resuscitation skills (intubation and umbilical catheter placement) and one to assist.

Causes

Perinatal asphyxia is the main cause for neonatal resuscitation. When the infant is deprived of oxygen, an initial period of rapid respirations occurs followed by apnea, decreased heart rate, and decreased neuromuscular tone. This is a period of primary apnea.

Primary Apnea

1. Intrauterine asphyxia may result in passage of meconium, fetal tachycardia, absent variability, recurrent late or variable decelerations, or prolonged bradycardia.

2. Infants born with primary apnea will need sensory stimuli (tactile or positive-pressure ventilation) to initiate respirations.

3. May occur in utero or after birth.

Secondary Apnea

1. Secondary apnea occurs when primary apnea is unresolved. The heart rate continues to drop lower (begins to drop about the same time the infant enters into primary apnea), the BP drops, the infant becomes flaccid, and spontaneous gasps occur.

2. May occur in utero or after birth.

3. At birth, these infants are pale, flaccid, and bradycardic.

 NURSING ALERT When the infant is apneic at birth, it is difficult to distinguish between primary and secondary apnea; therefore, one must assume secondary apnea and resuscitation must begin immediately.

4. Anticipation and preparation of neonatal resuscitation should occur at every birth.

Initial Steps in Neonatal Resuscitation

1. A: Airway
2. B: Breathing
3. C: Circulation

How to Achieve Initial Steps

Performing the initial steps should take no more than 30 seconds.

1. Call for assistance, if needed.
2. Place infant on a warm, dry radiant warmer.
3. Dry infant thoroughly with warmed towels, dispose of wet towels, and stimulate infant by rubbing back or slapping soles of feet, if necessary.
4. Assess respirations (rise and fall of chest, air moving in the lungs) and pulse (heart rate more than 100 bpm).
5. If apnea or the heart rate is less than 100 bpm, begin positive-pressure ventilation (PPV; bag and mask ventilation) and SpO$_2$ monitoring. Breaths are administered at a rate of 40 to 60 per minute. Oxygen is to be delivered with a compressed air source an oxygen blender. Titration of oxygen delivery is based on preductal oximetry values during the first 10 minutes of birth. Resuscitation starts with room air (21%) and increases are made to the concentration of oxygen demonstrated by an uncompromised term neonate.

   a. Observe chest movement and auscultate for air movement in all lung fields.

   b. To prevent air filling the stomach during PPV, an orogastric tube can be inserted orally.

6. If heart rate is less than 60 bpm, administer chest compressions and provide PPV simultaneously. Once cycle of events consists of three compressions plus one ventilation, resulting in 120 "events" per 60 seconds or 90 compressions plus 30 breaths. If the heart rate increases to above 60 bpm, cease chest compressions and maintain PPV at a rate of 40 to 60 breaths per minute. Once the heart rate exceeds 100 and spontaneous breathing resumes, gradually decrease rate of PPV.

7. Assist with endotracheal intubation, if needed.

8. Assist with insertion of an umbilical catheter for administration of medications and fluids, if needed. If heart rate remains below 60 bpm for over 60 seconds of PPV and chest compressions, intensive care medications (eg, epinephrine) should be considered and administered intravenously via an umbilical catheter.

9. Continue to assess neonate periodically once stabilization is reestablished and transport accordingly.

Precipitous Delivery or Delivery in Absence of Health Care Provider (Nurse-Assisted)

A precipitous delivery is an emergent event. During this event, consider the woman and infant as a unit. Coordination to prevent maternal and fetal infection, injury, and hemorrhage is key.

Interventions

1. Provide reassurance and instruct the woman in a calm, controlled manner. Sustain eye contact and assist the mother to utilize pant-blow breathing until told to push. Do not break down the birthing bed. The lower half of the bed will be utilized as a table and promotes fetal safety.

2. Instruct the woman to assume a lateral Sims' position; this will help to slow her labor down, prevent lacerations, and improve visualization.

3. Wash hands, put on gloves, and clean the perineum as time permits.

4. Exert gentle pressure against the head of the fetus, using pads of thumb, index finger, and middle fingers or cupped palm of hand, to control progress and prevent precipitous (fast) delivery; this prevents undue stretching of the perineum and sudden expulsion through the vulva with subsequent infant and maternal complications.

5. Encourage the woman to pant at this time to prevent bearing down.

6. Rupture the membranes by tearing at the nape of the infant's neck. This is done if membranes have not ruptured by the time the head is delivered.

7. Wipe the infant's face and mouth with a clean towel. Suction the mouth and nose with a bulb syringe, if available.

8. Check for nuchal cord and reduce, if possible. If the cord is too tight to permit slipping over the infant's head, it must be clamped in two places and cut between the clamps before the rest of the body is delivered.

9. Allow head to restitute. Place one hand over each ear bilaterally to support the infant's head; gently exert downward pressure toward the floor, thus slipping the anterior shoulder under the symphysis pubis.

10. As soon as the anterior shoulder is delivered, provide upward, outward traction to the head to deliver the posterior shoulder.

11. Support the infant's body and head in the lower hand. As the body is delivered, slide the upper hand down the back to grasp the infant's feet.

12. Hold the infant with the head down to help drain mucus; wipe away excess mucus from the mouth and nose. Gentle rubbing of the back may stimulate breathing.

13. Place the infant skin-to-skin with the mother and cover both with a blanket.

14. Avoid pulling on the cord, which might break and cause hemorrhage.

15. Watch for signs of placental separation (gush of dark blood from introitus, lengthening of umbilical cord, change in uterine contour).

16. Check fundal contractions; massage, if indicated. Putting the baby to breast may assist fundal contraction.

17. Place identification bands on both the mother and infant.

18. Offer the patient fluids (IV or by mouth).

19. Teach the woman to massage her fundus.

20. Record the time and date of birth, as well as:
    a. Notifications and preparations for the birth.
    b. Fetal presentation and position.
    c. Presence of nuchal or body cord.
    d. Rupture of membranes: character, color, odor, amount of amniotic fluid.
    e. Time of placental expulsion.
    f. Placental appearance.
    g. Maternal condition.
    h. Unusual occurrences during birth (ie, shoulder dystocia).

21. Assist and transport as necessary.

SELECTED REFERENCES

American College of Obstetricians and Gynecologists. (2002/Reaffirmed 2010). *Diagnosis and management of preeclampsia and eclampsia* (Practice Bulletin #33). Washington, DC: Author.

American College of Obstetricians and Gynecologists. (2003/Reaffirmed 2011). *Dystocia aids augmentation of labor* (Practice Bulletin #49). Washington, DC: Author.

American College of Obstetricians and Gynecologists. (2005). *Intrapartum fetal heart rate monitoring* (Practice Bulletin #62). Washington, DC: Author.

American College of Obstetricians and Gynecologists. (2006/Reaffirmed 2011). *Postpartum hemorrhage* (Practice Bulletin #76). Washington, DC: Author.

American College of Obstetricians and Gynecologists. (2009). *Intrapartum fetal heart rate monitoring: Nomenclature, interpretation, and general management principles* (Practice Bulletin #106). Washington, DC: Author.

American College of Obstetricians and Gynecologists. (2010). Management of intrapartum fetal heart rate tracings (Practice Bulletin #116). Washington, DC: Author.

American Academy of Pediatrics & American College of Obstetricians and Gynecologists. (2007). *Guidelines for perinatal care* (6th ed.). Elk Grove Village, IL: Authors.

American Academy of Pediatrics & American Heart Association. (2011). *Textbook of neonatal resuscitation* (6th ed.). Elk Grove Village, IL: American Academy of Pediatrics.

American Society of Anesthesiologists Task Force on Obstetric Anesthesia. (2007). Practice guidelines for obstetric anesthesia: An updated report by the American Society of Anesthesiologists Task Force on Obstetric Anesthesia. *Anesthesiology, 106*(4), 843–863.

Association of Women's Health, Obstetric and Neonatal Nurses. (2003). *Standards for professional nursing practice in the care of women and newborns* (6th ed.). Washington, DC: Author.

Association of Women's Health, Obstetric and Neonatal Nurses. (Ed.). (2009). *Fetal heart monitoring principles and practices* (4th ed.). Dubuque, IA: Kendall-Hunt Publishing Co.

Berlit, S., Welzel, G., Tuschy, B., et al. (2012). Emergency caesarean section: Risk factors for adverse neonatal outcome. *Arch Gynecol Obstet.* 2012 Dec 16 [Epub ahead of print].

Blackburn, S. (2007). *Maternal, fetal and neonatal physiology: A clinical perspective* (3rd ed.). St. Louis, MO: Elsevier.

Bradbury, C. L., Singh, S. I., Badder, S. R., et al. (2012). Prevention of post-dural puncture headache in parturients: A systematic review and meta-analysis. *Acta Anaesthesiol Scand.* Dec 28. [Epub ahead of print]

Carlton, T., Callister, L. C., Christiaens, G., et al. (2009). Labor and delivery nurses' perceptions of caring for childbearing women in nurse-managed birthing units. *MCN: The American Journal of Maternal/Child Nursing, 34*(1), 50–56.

Cunningham, F. G., Leveno, K., Bloom, S., et al. (2010). *Williams obstetrics* (23rd ed.). New York: McGraw-Hill.

Curran, C., & Torgersen, K. (2013). *abcdEFM TEXTbook: Electronic fetal monitoring* (2nd ed.). Virginia Beach, VA: Clinical Specialists Consulting.

Davidson, M. W., London, M. L., & Ladewig, P. W. (2012). *Olds' maternal-newborn nursing and women's health across the lifespan* (9th ed.). Upper Saddle River, NJ: Pearson Education.

Feinstein, N. F., Sprague, A., & Trepanier, M.-J. (2009). *Fetal heart rate auscultation* (2nd ed.). Washington, DC: Association of Women's Health, Obstetric and Neonatal Nurses.

Fleming, S. E., Smart, D., & Eide, P. (2011). Grand multiparous women's perceptions of birthing, nursing care, and childbirth technology. *Journal of Perinatal Education, 20*(2), 108–117.

Freeman, R. K., Garite, T. J., & Nageotte, M. P. (2003). *Fetal heart rate monitoring* (3rd ed.). Philadelphia: Lippincott Williams & Wilkins.

Gabbe, S. G., Niebyl, J. R., Simpson, J. L., et al. (2007). *Obstetrics: Normal and problem pregnancies* (5th ed.). New York: Churchill Livingstone.

Gallo, A. (2003). The fifth vital sign: Implementation of the neonatal infant pain scale. *Journal of Obstetric, Gynecologic, and Neonatal Nursing, 32*(2), 199–206.

Goldbort, J., Knepp, A., Mueller, C., et al. (2011). Intrapartum nurses' lived experience in a traumatic birthing process. *MCN: The American Journal of Maternal/Child Nursing, 36*(6), 373–380.

Grassley, J. S., & Sauls, D. J. (in press). Evaluation of the supportive needs of adolescents during childbirth intrapartum nursing intervention on adolescents' childbirth satisfaction and breastfeeding rates. *Journal of Obstetric, Gynecologic and Neonatal Nursing.*

Grivell, R. M., Alfirevic, Z., Gyte, G. M., et al. (2012). Antenatal cardiotocography for fetal assessment. *Cochrane Database Syst Rev.* Article CD007863.

Hwang, M., Shrestha, A., Yazzie, S., et al. (2013). Preterm Birth Among American Indian/Alaskan Natives in Washington and Montana: Comparison with Non-Hispanic Whites. *Matern Child Health J.* 2013 Jan 4 [Epub ahead of print].

Jones, L., Othman, M., Dowswell, T., et al. (2012). Pain management for women in labour: An overview of systematic reviews. *Cochrane Database of systematic reviews*, 2012(3). Article No. CD009234.

Kolkman, D. G., Verhoeven, C. J., Brinkhorst, S. J., et al. (2013). The Bishop Score as a Predictor of Labor Induction Success: A Systematic Review. *American Journal of Perinatology.* 2013 Jan 2 [Epub ahead of print].

Koyanagi, A., Zhang, J., Dagvadorj, A., et al. (2013). Macrosomia in 23 developing countries: An analysis of a multicountry, facility-based, cross-sectional survey. *Lancet.* Jan 3 [Epub ahead of print].

Lowdermilk, D., & Perry, S. (2012). *Maternity and women's health care* (10th ed.). St. Louis, MO: Mosby.

Macones, G. A., Hankins, G. D., Spong, C. Y., et al. (2008). The 2008 National Institute of Child Health and Human Development workshop report on electronic fetal monitoring: Update on definitions, interpretation, and research guidelines. *Obstetrics and Gynecology, 112*, 661–666.

Mattson, S., & Smith, J. E. (2011). *Core curriculum for maternal-newborn nursing* (4th ed.). St. Louis, MO: W.B. Saunders.

Mori, R., Tokumasu, H., Pledge, D., et al. (2011). High dose versus low dose oxytocin for augmentation of delayed labour. *Cochrane Database of Systematic Reviews,* Issue 5 (Article No. CD007201).

National Institutes of Health. (1979). *Antenatal diagnosis. Report of a consensus development conference* (NIH Publication No. 79–1973). Bethesda, MD: Author.

NICHD Research Planning Workshop. (1997). Electronic fetal heart rate monitoring: Research guidelines for interpretation. *Journal of Obstetric, Gynecologic and Neonatal Nursing, 26*(6), 635–640.

Parer, J., King, T., Flanders, S., et al. (2006). Fetal acidemia and electronic fetal heart rate patterns: Is there evidence of an association? *Journal of Maternal-Fetal and Neonatal Medicine, 19*(5), 289–294.

Poole, J. (2001). *Epidural analgesia/anesthesia evidence-based clinical guideline* (2nd ed.). Washington, DC: Association of Women's Health, Obstetric and Neonatal Nurses.

Poole, J. (2003). Analgesia and anesthesia during labor and birth: Implications for mother and fetus. *Journal of Obstetric, Gynecologic and Neonatal Nursing, 32*(6), 780–793.

Simpson, K. R., and Knox, G. E. (2009). Communication of fetal heart monitoring information. In Feinstein, N., et al. (eds.). *Fetal heart monitoring principles and practices* (4th ed.). Dubuque, Iowa: Kendall-Hunt Publications. Chapter 8, pp. 177–209.

Skidmore-Roth, L. (2009). *Mosby's handbook on herbs and natural supplements* (4th ed.). St. Louis, MO: Mosby.

Society of Obstetricians and Gynaecologists of Canada (SOGC). (2002). SOGC Policy statement: Fetal health surveillance in labour (SOGC Clinical Practice Guidelines No. 112). *Journal of Obstetrics and Gynaecology in Canada, 112*, 1–13.

Todd, S., Malinoski, D., Muller, P., et al. (2007). Lactated Ringer's is superior to normal saline in the resuscitation of uncontrolled hemorrhagic shock. *Journal of Trauma, 62*(3), 636–639.

Tranquilli, A. L. (2012). Fetal heart rate in the second stage of labor: recording, reading, interpreting and acting. *J Matern Fetal Neonatal Med., 25*(12):2551–2554.

38

Care of Mother and Neonate During the Postpartum Period

NURSING CARE OF THE MOTHER

The Puerperium

The *puerperium* is the period beginning after delivery and ending when the woman's body has returned as closely as possible to its prepregnant state. The period lasts approximately 6 weeks. (See Standards of Care Guidelines 38-1, page 1296.)

Physiologic Changes of the Puerperium

 Evidence Base Cunningham, F. G., Leveno, K. J., Bloom, S. L. et al. (2010). The puerperium. In *Williams obstetrics* (23rd ed., pp. 646–660). New York: McGraw-Hill.
   Whitmer, T. (2011). Physical and psychologic changes. In S. Mattson & J. E. Smith (Eds.), *Core curriculum for maternal-newborn nursing* (4th ed., pp. 301–314). St. Louis, MO: Saunders Elsevier.

1. Uterine changes.
   a. Immediately after delivery, the fundus is palpable halfway between the umbilicus and symphysis pubis. At 1 hour postpartum, the fundus is usually level with or slightly below the level of the umbilicus. The fundus is usually midline. Within 12 hours of delivery, the fundus may be ½ inch (1.3 cm) above the umbilicus and by 24 hours, ¼ inch (1 cm) below the umbilicus. After this, the level of the fundus descends approximately 1 fingerbreadth (or ½ inch) each day, until by the 10th to the 14th day, it has descended into the pelvic cavity and can no longer be palpated (see Figure 38-1).
   b. After delivery, *lochia*—a vaginal discharge that consists of fatty epithelial cells, shreds of membrane, decidua, and blood—is red or dark brown with clots (lochia rubra) for approximately 1 to 3 days. It then progresses to a paler pink or more brown-tinged color of serosanguineous consistency (lochia serosa) for 3 to 10 days, followed by a whitish or yellowish color (lochia alba) in the 10th to 14th day. Lochia usually ceases by 3 weeks and the placental site is completely healed by the 6th week.
   c. The amount of lochial flow can be scant (less than 2.5 cm stain [1 inch]/hour), light (less than 10 cm stain [4 inches]/hour), moderate (less than 15.2 cm stain [6 inches]/hour), or heavy (one pad saturated within 1 hour). Lochial flow is considered to be "excessive" if the perineal pad becomes saturated in less than 15 minutes (see Figure 38-2).
   d. Immediately after delivery of the placenta, the cervix has little tone or resemblance to the prepregnant state. In approximately 2 to 3 days, it appears more like the prepregnant state and is dilated to 2 to 3 cm. By the end

1295

STANDARDS OF CARE GUIDELINES 38-1
Postpartum Care

- Perform assessment regularly for BUBBLERS—breasts, uterus size and consistency, bladder distention, bowel elimination, lochia, episiotomy, emotional response, and Homans' sign.
- Notify health care provider immediately if abnormalities are present:
  - Increased respiration and pulse, decreased blood pressure, and orthostatic changes may indicate hemorrhage.
  - Excessive vaginal bleeding (saturation of peripad within 1 hour for 2 or more hours), expulsion of large clots, or steady increase in vaginal bleeding, which indicates hemorrhage.
  - Boggy uterine fundus that does not become firm and remain firm with massage, indicating uterine atony.
  - Inability to void and bladder distention, which may displace uterus, leading to uterine atony.
  - Decreased urine output, which may indicate hemorrhage.
  - Elevated temperature, increased pain, swelling, and redness from incisions, indicating infection.
  - Calf tenderness, swelling, redness, or warmth, which may indicate a blood clot.
  - Excessive irritability, crying, moodiness, withdrawal, insomnia, and loss of interest in activities, which may indicate postpartum depression.
- Encourage rest, nutrition, and bonding with the infant.
- Provide education on feeding, bathing, changing, safety measures, signs of illness, and when to call infant's pediatric care provider with questions.

This information should serve as a general guideline only. Each patient situation presents a unique set of clinical factors and requires nursing judgment to guide care, which may include additional or alternative measures and approaches.

of the first postpartum week, it is approximately 1 cm in diameter. The cervical opening is more slitlike than the prepregnant dimple and remains that way. The cervical opening does not return to the prepregnant dimple following delivery unless the cervix has never been dilated.

2. The vaginal walls, uterine ligaments, and muscles of the pelvic floor and abdominal wall regain most of their tone during the puerperium. Immediately after delivery, the vaginal walls are smooth and swollen because the vaginal rugae are absent. Rugae reappears approximately 3 weeks postpartum. At approximately 6 weeks postpartum, involution of the vagina is complete.

3. Postpartum diuresis begins within 12 hours after birth and continues for 2 to 5 days postpartum, as extracellular water accumulated during pregnancy is excreted. Diuresis may also occur shortly after delivery if urine output was obstructed because of the pressure of the presenting part, or if IV fluids were given during labor.

4. Breasts.
   a. With loss of the placenta, circulating levels of estrogen and progesterone decrease and levels of prolactin increase, thus initiating lactation in the postpartum woman.
   b. *Colostrum*—a thick, yellowish fluid that contains more minerals and protein but less sugar and fat than mature breast milk and has a laxative effect on the infant—is secreted for the first 2 days postpartum.
   c. Mature milk secretion is usually present by the third postpartum day, but may be present earlier if a woman breast-feeds immediately after delivery. Usually by the end of the second postpartum week mature breast milk is present.
   d. Breast engorgement with milk, venous and lymphatic stasis, and swollen, tense, and tender breast tissue may occur between day 3 and day 5 postpartum.

5. Endocrine/metabolic function.
   a. Human chorionic gonadotropin declines rapidly and is nonexistent by the end of the first postpartum week.
   b. Thyroid levels are normal by 4 to 6 weeks postpartum.
   c. Glucose levels are low secondary to decreased human placental lactogen, decreased cortisol, decreased estrogen,

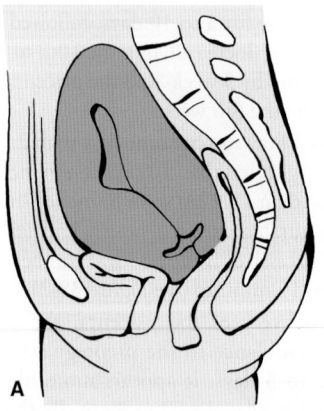 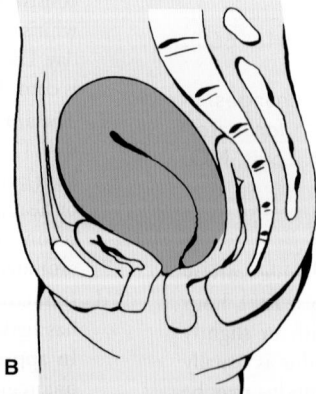 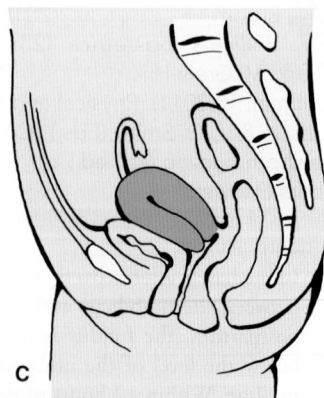

Figure 38-1. Changes in uterine size and shape following delivery. (A) Uterus after delivery. **(B)** Uterus at 6th day. **(C)** Nongravid uterus.

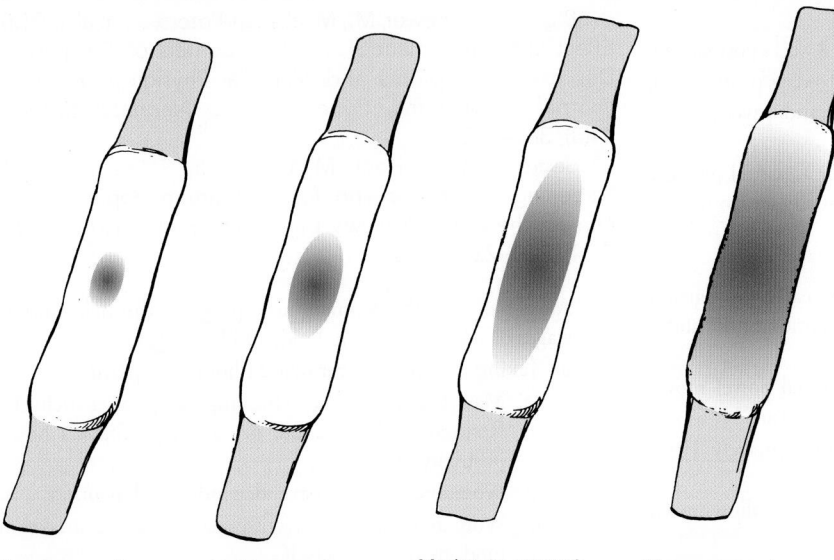

Scant amount
Blood only on tissue when wiped or less than 1-inch (2.5 cm) stain on peripad.

Light amount
Less than 4-inch (10-cm) stain on peripad.

Moderate amount
Less than 6-inch (15.2-cm) stain on peripad.

Heavy amount
Saturated peripad within 1 hour.

Figure 38-2. Assessing the volume of lochia by peripad saturation.

and decreased growth hormone. Blood glucose levels of women with gestational (type 2) diabetes may return to normal limits shortly after birth.

6. Ovarian function.
   a. Estrogen and progesterone levels decrease rapidly after delivery of the placenta and are usually their lowest by the seventh postpartum day.
   b. Estrogen reaches the follicular phase by 3 weeks after birth, as long as the woman is not lactating.
   c. Ovulation may occur as early as 27 days after delivery. The average time is 70 to 75 days postdelivery and 190 days postdelivery if breastfeeding.
   d. The start of menses after delivery is individualized. Usually, the first menses occurs approximately 7 to 9 weeks after delivery in non-nursing mothers, although breastfeeding women may not start their first menses until as late as 18 months.

7. Kidneys and bladder function.
   a. Mild proteinuria (+1 on urine dipstick) is common for 1 to 2 days after delivery in 40% to 50% of postpartum women.
   b. Spontaneous voiding should return by 6 to 8 hours postpartum. Bladder tone returns between 5 and 7 days postpartum.
   c. The catabolic process of involution can cause an increase in blood urea nitrogen levels during the postpartum period.
   d. Stress incontinence is common during the first 6 weeks postpartum.

 **NURSING ALERT** Hematuria immediately after normal spontaneous vaginal birth is usually indicative of bladder trauma. If hematuria occurs after the first 24 hours, it is indicative of urinary tract infection (UTI).

8. Neurologic function.
   a. Discomfort and fatigue are common.
   b. Afterpains and discomfort from the delivery, lacerations, episiotomy, and muscle aches are common for the first 2 to 3 days postdelivery.
   c. Frontal and bilateral headaches are common and are caused by fluid shifts in the first week postpartum.
   d. Non-rapid-eye-movement (REM) sleep is absent after birth and increases during the next 2 weeks. REM sleep decreases as non-REM sleep increases.
   e. Carpal tunnel syndrome (resulting from physiologic edema causing pressure on the median nerve) is usually relieved by postpartum diuresis.

NURSING ALERT Postpartum eclamptic seizures can begin more than 48 hours and less than 4 weeks postdelivery. They are commonly preceded by severe headache or vision disturbances (spots before the eyes, double vision, etc.). Extra care is taken to observe for these symptoms, especially in women with prenatal diagnosis of preeclampsia or hypertension.

9. Cardiovascular function.
   a. Most dramatic changes occur in this system and can take between 6 and 12 weeks to return to the prepregnant state.
   b. Cardiac output peaks to about 80% immediately after birth (10 to 15 minutes) then decreases rapidly, reaching prelabor values by about 1 hour postpartum. However, it can remain elevated for as much as 48 hours postpartum. Cardiac output values return to normal by 2 to 3 weeks postpartum.
   c. Hematocrit increases and increased red blood cell (RBC) production stops.
   d. Leukocytosis with increased white blood cells (WBCs) common during the first postpartum week.

10. Respiratory function.
    a. Returns to normal by approximately 6 to 8 weeks postpartum.
    b. Basal metabolic rate increases for 7 to 14 days postpartum, secondary to mild anemia, lactation, and psychological changes.
    c. Partial pressure of arterial oxygen (PaO_2), partial pressure of carbon dioxide ($PaCO_2$), and pH usually return to normal by 3 weeks postpartum.
11. GI/hepatic function.
    a. GI tone and motility decreases in the early postpartum period, commonly causing gaseous distention of the abdomen and constipation.
    b. Normal bowel function, including normal bowel movements, returns at about 2 to 3 days postpartum.
    c. Liver function returns to normal approximately 10 to 14 days postpartum.
    d. Gallbladder contractility increases to normal, allowing for expulsion of small gallstones.
12. Musculoskeletal function.
    a. Generalized fatigue and weakness is common.
    b. Decreased abdominal tone is common.
    c. Diastasis recti heals and resolves by the 4th to 6th week postpartum. Until healing is complete, usually 1 to 2 weeks postpartum, abdominal exercises are contraindicated.
    d. Joint instability returns to normal between 6 and 8 weeks postpartum.

 NURSING ALERT A positive Homans' sign may indicate thrombophlebitis and should be reported to the primary care provider. The woman should be instructed not to massage her legs.

13. Integumentary function.
    a. Striae lighten and melasma is usually gone by 6 weeks postpartum.
    b. Hair loss can increase for the first 4 to 20 weeks postpartum and then regrowth will occur, although the hair may not be as thick as it was before pregnancy.
14. A good method to remember how to check the postpartum changes is the use of the acronym BUBBLERS:
    a. **B**—Breast.
    b. **U**—Uterus.
    c. **B**—Bladder.
    d. **B**—Bowel.
    e. **L**—Lochia.
    f. **E**—Episiotomy.
    g. **R**—Emotional response.
    h. **S**—Homans' sign.

Emotional and Behavioral (Psychosocial) Status

 Evidence Base American College of Obstetricians and Gynecologists. (2008/Reaffirmed 2009). *Use of psychiatric medications during pregnancy and lactation* (Practice Bulletin #92). Washington, DC: Author.

Bigelow, A., Power, M., MacLellan-Peters, J., et al. (2012). Effect of Mother/Infant Skin-to-Skin Contact on Postpartum Depressive Symptoms and Maternal Physiological Stress. *Journal of Obstetric, Gynecologic, & Neonatal Nursing, 41*(3), 369–382.

Segre, L. S., O'Hara, M. W., Amdt, S., et al. (2011). Screening and counseling for postpartum depression by nurses: The women's views, part 2. *Maternal Child Nursing, 35*(4), 220–225.

1. After delivery, the woman may progress through Rubin's stages of taking in, taking hold, and letting go.
   a. Taking in (extends over first 24 hours postpartum:
      i. May begin with a refreshing sleep after delivery. Restorative sleep should occur within first 24 hours postdelivery.
      ii. Woman exhibits passive, dependent behavior.
      iii. Woman is concerned with sleep and the intake of food, mainly for herself.
   b. Taking hold (if not in first 24 hours postpartum then between days 2 and 4 postpartum):
      i. Woman begins to initiate action and to function more independently. First sign mother is in this phase is alert interest in her infant.
      ii. Woman may require more explanation and reassurance that she is functioning well, especially in caring for her infant.
      iii. Openness to teaching on care of self and neonate.
      iv. Today, with early hospital discharge, this phase may occur earlier, or it may occur after discharge.
   c. Letting go:
      i. Begins near the end of the first week; no specific end time noted.
      ii. Is influenced by cultural beliefs.
      iii. Reestablishment of couple relationship.
      iv. As the woman meets success in caring for the neonate, her concern extends to other family members and to their activities.
2. Some women may experience euphoria in the first few days after delivery and set unrealistic goals for activities after discharge from the birthing place.
3. Many women may experience temporary mood swings during this period because of the discomfort, fatigue, and exhaustion following labor and delivery and because of hormonal changes after delivery.
4. Up to 50% to 75% of mothers may experience postpartum (or maternity) blues. They can last for a few hours to 1 to 2 weeks and usually peak at approximately the 5th postpartum day. Women may exhibit irritability, poor appetite, insomnia, tearfulness, or crying. This is a normal reaction to the physiologic shifts that occur postdelivery and is a temporary situation.
5. Postpartum depression is a more serious problem. Research shows that women feel a loss of control of all aspects of life and go through a four-stage process that includes: encountering terror, dying of self, struggling to survive, and regaining control.

6. Nursing research findings indicate that new mothers commonly identify postpartum needs such as coping with:
   a. The physical changes and discomforts of the puerperium, including a need to regain their prepregnancy figure.
   b. Changing family relationships and meeting the needs of family members, including the infant.
   c. Fatigue, emotional stress, feelings of isolation, and being tied down.
   d. A lack of time for personal needs and interests.

Nursing Assessment

Evidence Base Cunningham, F. G., Leveno, K. J., Bloom, S. L., et al. (2010). The puerperium. In *Williams obstetrics* (23rd ed., pp. 646–660). New York: McGraw-Hill.

Intermountain Utah Valley Regional Medical Mother/Baby Unit. (2010). *Assessment of the new mother & baby* [DVD/CD]. Salt Lake City, UT: Concept Media.

Immediate Postpartum Assessment

The first hour after delivery of the placenta (fourth stage of labor) is a critical period; postpartum hemorrhage is most likely to occur at this time (see page 1364).

Subsequent Postpartum Assessment

1. Check firmness of the fundus at regular intervals. Perform fundal massage if the uterus is boggy (not firm) (see Figure 38-3).

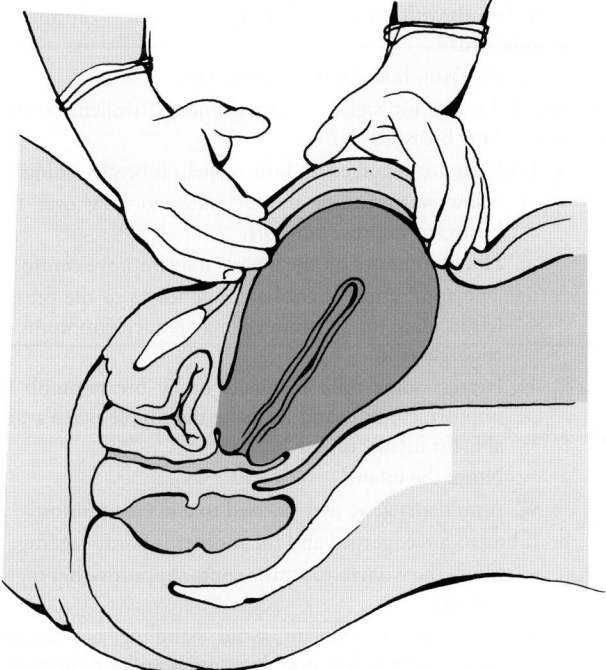

Figure 38-3. Fundal massage. With hands correctly positioned, gentle fundal massage stimulates the uterine muscles to contract, helping to restore normal tone and control bleeding.

2. Inspect the perineum regularly for frank bleeding.
   a. Note color, amount, and odor of the lochia.
   b. Count the number of perineal pads that are saturated in each 8-hour period.
3. Assess vital signs at least twice daily and more frequently, if indicated.
4. Assess bowel and bladder elimination.
5. Evaluate interaction and care skills of the mother and family with infant.
6. Assess for breast engorgement and condition of the nipples if breastfeeding.
7. Inspect legs for signs of thromboembolism and assess Homans' sign.
8. Assess incisions for signs of infection and healing.
9. A good method to remember how to evaluate the episiotomy is the use of the acronym REEDA:
   a. **R**—Redness.
   b. **E**—Edema.
   c. **E**—Ecchymosis (purplish patch of blood flow).
   d. **D**—Discharge.
   e. **A**—Approximation, or the closeness of the skin edges.

REEDA is based on a 3-point scale. A score of 3 indicates an assessment of very poor wound healing. On the first postpartum day, the REEDA score may range from 0 to 3; by the second postpartum week, the score should be 0 to 1.

10. If the patient is Rh negative, evaluate her need for Rho(D) immune globulin (RhoGAM). If indicated, administer the RhoGAM within 72 hours of delivery.
11. If the woman is not rubella immune, a rubella vaccination may be given and pregnancy must be avoided for at least 3 months.

Nursing Management

Evidence Base Bond, L. (2011). Physiology of pregnancy. In S. Mattson & J. E. Smith (Eds.), *Core curriculum for maternal-newborn nursing* (4th ed., pp. 80–100). St. Louis, MO: Saunders Elsevier.

Rhode, M. A. (2011). Postpartum complications. In S. Mattson & J. E. Smith (Eds.), *core curriculum for maternal neonatal nursing* (4th ed., pp. 650–666). St. Louis, MO: Saunders Elsevier.

Nursing Diagnoses

- Risk for Deficient Fluid Volume related to blood loss and effects from anesthesia.
- Impaired Urinary Elimination related to birth trauma.
- Constipation related to physiologic changes from birth.
- Risk for Infection related to birth process.
- Fatigue related to labor.
- Acute Pain related to perineal discomfort from birth trauma, hemorrhoids, and physiologic changes from birth.
- Readiness for Enhanced Self-health Management pertaining to postpartum care.
- Readiness for enhanced parenting related to neonatal care.
- Ineffective Breast-feeding related to lack of knowledge and inexperience.

Nursing Interventions

Monitoring for Hypotension and Bleeding

1. Monitor vital signs every 4 hours during the first 24 hours, then every 8 to 12 hours or as delineated by facility policy. Observe for the following:
   a. Decreased respiratory rate below 14 to 16 breaths/minute may occur after receiving epidural opioids or opioid analgesics.
   b. Increased respiratory rate greater than 24 breaths/minute may be caused by increased blood loss, pulmonary edema, or a pulmonary embolus.
   c. Increased pulse rate greater than 100 beats/minute (bpm) may be present with increased blood loss, fever, or pain.
   d. Decrease in blood pressure (BP) 15 to 20 mm Hg below baseline pressures may indicate decreased fluid volume or increased blood loss.
2. Assess the woman for light-headedness and dizziness when sitting upright or before walking.
   a. Evaluate orthostatic BP.
   b. Have the woman lie in bed if symptoms exist.
   c. Emphasize the importance of asking for assistance before ambulating the first time.
3. Assess vaginal discharge for clots and amount.
4. Evaluate lower-extremity sensory function and motor function before ambulation if the woman had regional anesthesia.
5. Encourage food and drink, as tolerated.
6. Maintain IV line, as indicated.
7. Monitor postpartum hemoglobin levels and hematocrit.

Promoting Urinary Elimination

1. Observe for the woman's first void within 6 to 8 hours after delivery.
2. Palpate the abdomen for bladder distention if the woman cannot void or if she complains of fullness after voiding.
   a. Uterine displacement from the midline suggests bladder distention.
   b. Frequent voidings of small amounts of urine suggest urine retention with overflow.
3. Catheterize the woman (in and out), if indicated.
4. Instruct the woman to void every several hours and after meals to keep her bladder empty. An undistended bladder may help decrease uterine cramping.

Promoting Proper Bowel Function

1. Teach the woman that bowel activity is sluggish because of decreased abdominal muscle tone, anesthetic effects, effects of progesterone, decreased solid food intake during labor, and prelabor diarrhea.
2. Inform the woman that pain from hemorrhoids, lacerations, and episiotomies may cause her to delay her first bowel movement.
3. Review the woman's dietary intake with her.
4. Encourage adequate amounts of fresh fruit, vegetables, fiber, and at least eight glasses of water daily.
5. Encourage frequent ambulation.
6. Administer stool softeners, as indicated.

Preventing Infection

1. Observe for elevated temperature above 100.4° F (38° C).
2. Evaluate episiotomy/perineum for REEDA.
3. Assess for pain, burning, and frequency on urination.
4. Administer antibiotics as ordered.

Reducing Fatigue

1. Provide a quiet and minimally disturbed environment.
2. Organize nursing care to keep interruptions to a minimum.
3. Encourage the woman to minimize visitors and phone calls.
4. Encourage the woman to sleep while the baby is sleeping and specifically to nap or lie down and get off her feet at least 30 minutes per day.

Minimizing Pain

1. Instruct the woman to apply ice packs to her perineal area for the first 24 hours for perineal trauma or edema, then to apply heat to the area.
   a. Take breaks between applications to prevent tissue damage.
   b. Commercial or handmade packs of ice chips in a glove may be used.
   c. Place a thin barrier between the ice pack and her skin.
2. Initiate the use of sitz baths for perineal discomfort after the first 24 hours.
   a. Use three times per day for 15 to 20 minutes.
3. Instruct the woman to contract her buttocks before sitting to reduce perineal discomfort.
4. Assist the woman in the use of positioning cushions and pillows while sitting or lying.
5. Teach the woman to use a perineal bottle and squirt warm water against her perineum while voiding.
6. Provide pads with witch hazel or topical creams or ointments, as indicated.
7. Administer pain medication, as indicated.
8. Check breasts for signs of engorgement (swollen, tender, tense, shiny breast tissue).
   a. If breasts are engorged and the woman is breastfeeding:
      i. Allow warm-to-hot shower water to flow over the breasts to improve comfort.
      ii. Hot compresses on the breasts may improve comfort.
      iii. The application of cool cabbage leaves to the breast, left in place for 20 minutes, may reduce symptoms of engorgement.
      iv. Express some milk manually or by breast pump to improve comfort and to make the nipple more available for infant feeding.
      v. Nurse the infant.
      vi. A mild analgesic may be used to enhance comfort.
   b. If breasts are engorged and the mother is bottle-feeding:
      i. Teach the woman to wear a snug, supportive bra night and day.
      ii. Teach the woman to avoid handling her breasts because this action stimulates more milk production.
      iii. Teach the woman to avoid letting warm water fall on her breasts during showers because the heat stimulates milk production.

iv. Suggest the application of ice bags to the breasts to provide comfort.

v. Moderately strong analgesics may be needed to provide comfort.

Promoting Postpartum Health Maintenance

1. Teach the woman to perform perineal care—warm water over the perineum after each voiding and after each bowel movement several times per day to promote comfort, cleanliness, and healing.

2. Promote sitz baths for the same purpose.

3. Teach the woman to apply perineal pads by touching the outside only, thus keeping clean the portion that will touch her perineum.

4. Assess the condition of the woman's breasts and nipples. Inspect nipples for reddening, erosions, or fissures. Reddened areas may be improved with vitamin A & D ointment, a lanolin cream (always remove before breastfeeding), and air-drying for 15 minutes, several times per day. She may also be instructed to squeeze a small amount of breast milk onto her nipples for lubrication.

5. Teach the woman to wash her breasts with warm water *without* soap, which prevents the removal of the protective skin oils.

6. Teach the woman to wear a bra that provides good support night and day.

7. Instruct the breastfeeding woman to add between 500 and 750 additional calories daily for milk production. Inform her that she also needs 2 to 3 quarts (2 to 3 L) of liquid per day; 20 g more protein than before pregnancy; additional calcium, phosphorus, and vitamins D, A, C, E, B, and B_2; and additional niacin, zinc, and iodine.

8. Instruct the woman in postpartum exercises for the immediate and later postpartum period.

   a. Immediate postpartum exercises can be performed in bed.

      i. Toe stretch (tightens calf muscles)—while lying on your back, keep your legs straight and point your toes away from you, then pull your legs toward you and point your toes toward your chest. Repeat 10 times.

      ii. Pelvic floor exercise (tightens perineal muscles)—contract your buttocks for a count of 5 and relax. Contract your buttocks and press thighs together for a count of 7 and relax. Contract buttocks, press thighs together, and draw in anus for a count of 10 and relax.

      iii. Kegel exercises (tightens vaginal muscles)—contract vaginal muscles as if stopping stream of urine. Do 15 per day, increasing 5 more each week to a maximum of 40 per day. When conditioned, patient can do 4 or 5 Kegels per day for maintenance.

      iv. Abdominal breathing—lie on back, knees bent, hands on belly, feet flat. Suck in your belly, trying to pull your navel toward your spine. Hold 5 seconds; release. When you can do 10 (this can take a week), add a head lift. Suck in your belly, then hold it as you lift head toward chest, counting slowly to 4. Lower head for 4 slow counts; release belly. Muscles are working if fingers move down when you suck in belly, not up. Work up to 10 repetitions.

      v. Arm circles—stand with feet approximately 12 inches (30.5 cm) apart, arms at sides. Keeping arms at sides, draw large circles with your shoulders by moving them forward, up, and back, and finish with a press down. Do 10 to 20 repetitions. Next, extend both arms as you reach forward, up, back, and down. Move slowly, breathe deeply for 5 to 10 repetitions.

      vi. Short walks—start with 5 minutes at first, then increase 5 minutes per day as desired.

      vii. Shoulder-side roll—lying on back, fold left arm across chest. Lift right arm and cross it over to left side. Feel as if your right arm is pulling you over so your right shoulder lifts and you roll to left. Continue to spiral movement as rib cage turns, then hips. Use left arm to take pressure off breasts, which may feel full. Lying on your left side, roll hips back toward right, followed by ribs, then shoulders until you are on your back. Repeat, other side. Perform five slow repetitions each side.

   b. Exercises for the later postpartum period can be done after the first postpartum visit (1 to 2 weeks postpartum).

      i. Bicycle (tightens thighs, stomach, and waist)—lie on your back on the floor, arms at sides, palms down. Begin rotating your legs as if you were riding a bicycle, bringing the knees all the way in toward the chest and stretching the legs out as long and as straight as possible. Breathe deeply and evenly. Do the exercises at a moderate speed and do not tire yourself.

      ii. Buttocks exercise (tightens buttocks)—lie on your stomach and keep your legs straight. Raise your left leg in the air, then repeat with your right leg (feel the contraction in your buttocks). Keep your hips on the floor. Repeat 10 times.

      iii. Twist (tightens waist)—stand with legs wide apart. Hold your arms at your sides, shoulder level, palms down. Twist your body from side to front and back again. Feel the twist in your waist.

      iv. Back bridge—begin by doing a pelvic tilt while lying on your back and flattening the lower back against the floor. Then continue to push your hips forward, lifting them off the floor. Hold the pelvic tilt for 4 seconds so that your back is flat, supporting your weight with your upper back. Lower your body slowly for 4 seconds so that upper back touches floor first, then waist touches, then pelvis.

      v. All fours—begin on your hands and knees. First do a pelvic tilt, tucking in your buttocks and sucking in your belly. Do not allow your back to arch. Next, keeping your pelvic tilt, lift your left leg out behind you and extend your right arm in front of you. Slowly lower arm and leg. At first, you will have to work hard to keep your balance.

      vi. Lift and laugh—this is a fun exercise to do with your baby. Sit with legs crossed, back straight, belly sucked in. Cradle your baby in your folded arms and lift until your elbows are at shoulder height. Laugh and cuddle as you hold for 2 seconds. Slowly lower your baby, keeping shoulders even, if possible. Do 5 to 10 repetitions.

NURSING ALERT Advise the mother to listen to her body. Avoid pain and fatigue. If pain or fatigue occurs, instruct the mother to stop her exercises. She may consult her obstetric provider, if desired.

Promoting Health Maintenance of the Neonate

Evidence Base Cheffer, N. D., & Rannalli, D. A. (2011). Transitional care of the newborn. In S. Mattson & J. E. Smith (Eds.), *Core curriculum for maternal-newborn nursing* (4th ed., pp. 345–361). St. Louis, MO: Saunders Elsevier.

1. Encourage the parents to participate in the daily care of the infant.
2. Advise the parents to attend parenting and baby care classes offered during their stay at the birth facility.
3. Teach the parents to bathe and diaper the infant, perform circumcision care, and initiate either breast- or bottle-feeding.
4. Foster bonding by encouraging skin-to-skin contact with the infant ("kangaroo care"), eye contact, and talking to and touching the infant.
5. Instruct the parents to contact the infant's health care provider for the following:
   a. Fever above 100° F (37.8° C).
   b. Loss of appetite for two consecutive feedings.
   c. Inability to awaken the baby to his or her usual activity state.
   d. Vomiting all or part of two feedings.
   e. Diarrhea—three watery stools.
   f. Extreme irritability or inconsolable crying.
6. Inform the parents that by law, infants and young children in cars are required to be in a car safety seat that is located in the back seat and that faces the back of the seat. Demonstrate and review the proper technique for use of the car seat.
7. Provide positive reinforcement and reassurance to the parents.
8. Provide written instructions and educational material on discharge.

Promoting Breastfeeding

Evidence Base Orr, S. S. (2011). Breastfeeding. In S. Mattson & J. E. Smith (Eds.), *Core curriculum for maternal-newborn nursing* (4th ed., pp. 315–334). St. Louis, MO: Saunders Elsevier.

1. Assist the woman and infant in the breastfeeding process.
   a. Have the mother wash her hands before feeding to help prevent infection.
   b. Encourage the mother to assume a comfortable position, such as sitting upright in the bed or in a chair or lying on her side.
   c. Have the woman hold the baby so that she is facing the mother. Common positions for holding the baby are the cradle hold, with the baby's head and body supported against the mother's arm, with buttocks resting in her hand; the football hold, in which the baby's legs are supported under the mother's arm, and the head is at the breast, resting in the mother's hand; and lying on the side with the baby lying on his or her side facing the mother.
   d. Teach the woman to bring the baby close to her to prevent back, shoulder, and arm strain.
   e. Have the woman cup the breast in her hand in a C position, with bottom of the breast in the palm of her hand and the thumb on top; or the U position, with the fingers and the thumb to the sides of the breast and the breast resting in the palm of the hand.
   f. Have the woman place her nipple against the side of the baby's mouth, and when the mouth opens, guide the nipple and the areola into the mouth. The baby should latch on so that as much of the areola as possible is in his or her mouth. If the baby has latched on to the nipple only, take the baby off the breast by putting the tip of the mother's finger in the corner of the baby's mouth to break the suction, and then reposition on the breast to prevent nipple pain and trauma.
   g. Encourage the woman to alternate the breast with which she begins feeding at each feeding to ensure emptying of both breasts and stimulation for maintaining milk supply.
   h. Advise the mother to use each breast at each feeding. Begin with approximately 10 minutes at each breast, then increase the time at each breast, allowing the infant to suck until he or she stops sucking actively. Pinning a safety pin to the bra as a reminder of which breast to start with at the next feeding is helpful.
   i. Have the mother breast-feed frequently (8 to 12 times/ 24 hours) to help maintain the milk supply. Although there is no time limit on each breastfeeding session, it is recommended to last at least 10 to 15 minutes on each breast.
   j. Have the mother air-dry her nipples for approximately 15 to 20 minutes after feeding to help prevent nipple trauma.
   k. Have the mother burp the infant at the end of the feeding to help release the air in the stomach and to make the infant less fretful.
2. Alert the mother that uterine cramping may occur, especially in multiparous women, because of the release of oxytocin, which can be worse in women with lessened uterine tone. Commonly referred to as afterpains.
3. Teach the mother to provide for adequate rest and to avoid tension, fatigue, and a stressful environment, which can inhibit the letdown reflex and make breast milk less available at feeding.
4. Advise the woman to avoid taking medications and drugs without health care provider approval because many substances pass into the breast milk and may affect milk production or the infant.

Evaluation: Expected Outcomes

- Vital signs within normal limits; decreasing color and amount of lochia.
- Voids freely and without discomfort.
- Lack of constipation; eats high-fiber foods and uses stool softeners.

- Afebrile, no abnormal redness of perineum, no purulent discharge or foul odor of lochia.
- Verbalizes feeling rested.
- Verbalizes decreased pain.
- Incorporates postpartum care into activities of daily living.
- Demonstrates confidence in performing infant care; shows signs of maternal–child bonding.
- Demonstrates successful breastfeeding; breasts and nipples intact and without redness or cracks.

Postpartum Patient Education

1. Advise the woman that healing occurs within 2 to 4 weeks; however, evaluation by the health care provider during the follow-up visit is necessary.

2. Inform the woman that intercourse may be resumed when perineal and uterine wounds have healed and when vaginal bleeding has stopped. Inform the woman that normal vaginal secretions may not occur for up to 6 months. Also inform the mother that for the first 3 months following delivery, her sexual arousal and desire may be diminished due to infant needs and fatigue. Review methods of contraception. Sexual arousal may cause milk to leak from her breasts. Breastfeeding is not a reliable method of contraception.

3. Inform the woman that menstruation usually returns within 4 to 8 weeks if bottle-feeding; if breastfeeding, menstruation usually returns within 4 months, but may return between 2 and 18 months postpartum. Nursing mothers may ovulate even if they are experiencing amenorrhea. Thus, a form of contraception should be used if pregnancy is to be avoided.

4. Counsel the woman to rest for at least 30 minutes after she arrives home from the birthing facility and to rest several times during the day for the first few weeks.

5. Advise the woman to confine her activities to one floor if possible and to avoid stair climbing as much as possible for the first several days at home.

6. Counsel the woman to provide quiet times for herself at home and to help her establish realistic goals for resuming her own interests and activities.

7. Encourage the couple to provide times to reestablish their own relationship and to renew their social interests and relationships.

NURSING CARE OF THE NEONATE
Physiology of the Neonate

Evidence Base Cheffer, N. D., & Rannalli, D. A. (2011). Transitional care of the newborn. In S. Mattson & J. E. Smith (Eds.), *Core curriculum for maternal-newborn nursing* (4th ed., pp. 345361). St. Louis, MO: Saunders Elsevier.

Verklan, M. T., & Walden, M. (Eds.). (2010). *Core curriculum for neonatal intensive care nursing* (4th ed.). St. Louis, MO: Saunders Elsevier.

The first 24 hours of life constitute a highly vulnerable time, during which the infant must make major physiologic adjustments to extrauterine life. Most neonates transition without difficulty during the first 6 to 10 hours of life.

Transitional Stages

During the period of postnatal transition, six overlapping stages have been identified:

- Stage 1. Receives stimulation (during labor) from the pressure of the uterine contractions and from changes in pressure when the membranes rupture.
- Stage 2. Encounters various foreign stimuli—light, cold, gravity, and sound.
- Stage 3. Initiates breathing.
- Stage 4. Changes from fetal circulation to neonatal circulation.
- Stage 5. Undergoes alteration in metabolic processes, with activation of liver and GI tract for passage of meconium.
- Stage 6. Achieves a steady level of equilibrium in metabolic processes (production of enzymes, increased blood oxygen saturation, decrease in acidosis associated with birth, and recovery of the neurologic tissues from the trauma of labor and delivery).

Respiratory Changes

Factors Initiating Respiration

1. Mechanical—pressure changes (eg, compression of the fetal chest with delivery) from intrauterine life to extrauterine life produce stimulation to initiate respirations.

2. Chemical—changes in the blood, as a result of transitory asphyxia, include:
   a. Cessation of placental blood flow.
   b. Lowered oxygen level.
   c. Increased carbon dioxide level.
   d. Lowered pH—if asphyxia is prolonged, depression of the respiratory center (rather than stimulation) occurs and resuscitation is necessary.

3. Sensory—light (visual), sound (auditory), olfactory, and tactile stimulation, beginning in utero with uterine contraction and when the infant is touched and dried, contribute to the initiation of respiration by stimulating the neonate's respiratory center in the brain.

4. Thermal—a drop in environmental temperature from 98.6° F (37° C) to 70° to 75° F (21° to 23.9° C) produced by sudden chilling of the moist infant stimulates the respiratory center in the brain.

5. First breath—maximum effort is required to expand the lungs and to fill the collapsed alveoli.
   a. Surface tension in the respiratory tract and resistance in lung tissue, thorax, diaphragm, and respiratory muscles must be overcome.
   b. First active inspiration comes from a strong contraction of the diaphragm, which creates a high negative intrathoracic pressure, causing a marked retraction of the ribs and distention of the alveolar space. (Any remaining fluid is reabsorbed rapidly if the pulmonary capillary blood flow is adequate because the fluid is hypotonic and passes easily into the capillaries.)

6. Contributing factors, such as pulmonary blood flow, sur-factant production, and respiratory musculature, also increase the respiratory effort of the neonate.

Character of Normal Respirations

1. First period of reactivity occurs immediately after birth. Vigorous, diffuse, purposeless movements alternate with peri-ods of relative immobility/inactivity.
2. Respirations are rapid, as frequent as 80 breaths/minute, accompanied by tachycardia, 140 to 180 breaths/minute.
3. Relaxation occurs and the infant usually sleeps; he or she then awakes to a second period of activity. Oral mucus may be a major problem during this period.
4. Respirations are reduced to 30 to 60 breaths/minute and become quiet and shallow; respiration is carried out by the diaphragm and abdominal muscles.
5. Period of dyspnea and cyanosis may occur suddenly in an infant who is breathing normally; this may indicate an anom-aly or a pathologic condition.
6. Pauses in respirations of less than 20 seconds are normal in the neonatal period.

Circulatory Changes

1. Cord clamping causes increased systemic vascular resistance (SVR), an increase in blood pressure, and increased pressures in the left side of the heart.
2. Removal of the placenta = functional closure of the ductus venosus shunt and anatomic closure the first week of life (see page 1258).
3. With the neonate's first breath, the foramen ovale shunt closes. Permanent closure occurs by 3 months of age.
4. Increased SVR, falling pulmonary VR, and increased sensi-tivity to rising arterial oxygen concentrations in the blood = closure of ductus arteriosus shunt. The shunt is completely closed in all infants by 96 hours of age with permanent clo-sure within 3 weeks to 3 months of age.
5. Blood volume can be as high as 300 mL/kg immediately after birth, then decrease to 80 to 85 mL/kg shortly after birth. Factors that influence blood volume:
   a. Maternal blood volume (affected by maternal diseases and iron intake).
   b. Placental function.
   c. Uterine contractions during labor.
   d. Amount of blood loss associated with delivery.
   e. Placental transfusion at birth—increase in blood volume of 60% if cord is clamped and cut after pulsation ceases.
6. Residual cyanosis in hands and feet (acrocyanosis) is present for 1 to 2 hours after birth because of sluggish circulation.
7. Normal apical pulse rate 110 to 160 bpm; may rise to 180 bpm when the infant is crying or drop to 80 to 110 bpm dur-ing deep sleep.
8. BP is 65 to 95/30 to 60 mm Hg at birth (slightly higher in legs).
9. BP measurement is best accomplished with a Doppler device while the infant is at rest.

 NURSING ALERT A systolic BP in the upper extremities that is 20 mm Hg greater than in the lower extremities strongly suggests coarctation of the aorta.

10. Coagulability is temporarily diminished because of lack of bacteria in the intestinal tract that contributes to the synthesis of vitamin K.
    a. Coagulation time is 5 to 8 minutes (glass tubes), 5 to 15 minutes (room temperature), or 30 minutes (silicone tube).
    b. Bleeding time is 2 to 4 minutes.
    c. Prothrombin 50%, decreasing to 20% to 30% (approxi-mately 13 to 18 seconds).
11. Values for blood components in the neonate:
    a. Hemoglobin, 14.5 to 22 g/dL.
    b. Hematocrit, 14% to 72%.
    c. Reticulocytes, 4% to 6%.
    d. Leukocytes, 9,000 to 34,000/mm^3.

Temperature Regulation

1. Mechanism not fully developed; heat production low.
2. Infant responds readily to environmental heat and cold stimuli.
3. Heat loss of 35.6° F to 37.4° F (2° C to 3° C) may occur at birth by radiation, convection, and evaporation.
   a. Radiation—transfer of heat from neonate to cooler object not in direct contact with the infant.
   b. Convection—transfer of heat when flow of cool air passes over infant's skin.
   c. Evaporation—loss of heat when water on infant's skin is converted to vapor.
   d. Conduction—transfer of heat when neonate comes into direct contact with cooler surface/object.
4. Decreased adipose tissue, thinner skin, blood vessels closer to the skin results in increased heat loss.
5. Infant develops mechanisms to counterbalance heat loss.
   a. Vasoconstriction—blood directed away from skin surfaces.
   b. Insulation—from subcutaneous adipose tissue.
   c. Heat production—by nonshivering thermogenesis (brown fat metabolism) elicited by the sympathetic nervous sys-tem's response to decreased temperatures; activated by adrenaline.
   d. Fetal position—by assuming a flexed position.

Basal Metabolism

1. Surface area of infant, especially the head, is large in compari-son to weight.
2. Basal metabolism per kilogram of body weight is higher than that of an adult.
3. Calorie requirements are high—117 calories per kilogram of body weight per day.

Renal Function

Neonatal kidneys have functional deficiency in concentrating urine and coping with fluid and electrolyte fluctuations. Low arterial BP and increased renal vascular resistance lead to the following effects:

1. Decreased ability to concentrate urine because of low tubular resorption rate and low levels of antidiuretic hormone.
2. Limited ability to maintain water balance by excretion of excess water or retention of needed water.
3. Decreased ability to maintain acid-base mechanism; slower excretion of electrolytes, especially sodium and hydrogen ions, results in accumulation of these substances, which predisposes the infant to dehydration, acidosis, and hyperkalemia.
4. Excretion of large amount of uric acid during neonatal period—appears as brick dust stain on diaper.

Hepatic Function

Function limited because of lack of GI tract activity, deficiency in forming plasma proteins, and limited blood supply; consequences include the following:

1. Decreased ability to conjugate bilirubin (rationale for physiologic jaundice).
2. Decreased ability to regulate blood glucose concentration (less glycogen stores) (rationale for neonatal hypoglycemia).
3. Deficient production of prothrombin and other coagulation factors that depend on vitamin K for synthesis (rationale for neonate's predisposition to hemorrhage).

Endocrine Function

Endocrine glands are better organized than other systems: disturbances are most commonly related to maternally provided hormones. This can cause the following:

1. Vaginal discharge (or bleeding [pseudomenstruation]) in female infants.
2. Enlargement of mammary glands (breast engorgement) in both sexes—related to increased estrogen, luteal, and prolactin activity. Milky secretions may be present (witch's milk).
3. Disturbances related to maternal endocrine pathology (eg, mother with diabetes or mother with inadequate iodine intake).

GI Changes

The neonate's intestinal tract is proportionately longer than the adult's; however, elastic tissue and musculature are not fully developed and neurologic control is variable and inadequate.

1. Most digestive enzymes are present, with the exception of pancreatic amylase and lipase. Protein and carbohydrates are easily absorbed, but fat absorption is poor.
2. Limitations relate primarily to anatomic structures and neutrality of the gastric contents.
3. Limited production of pancreatic amylase leads to inadequate utilization of complex carbohydrates.
4. Imperfect control of the cardiac and pyloric sphincters and immaturity of neurologic control cause mild regurgitation or slight vomiting.
5. Irregularities in peristaltic motility slow stomach emptying.
6. Peristalsis increases in the lower ileum, resulting in stool frequency—one to six stools per day. No stools within 48 hours after birth is indicative of intestinal obstruction.

Neurologic Changes

Neurologic mechanisms are immature; they are not fully developed anatomically or physiologically. As a result, uncoordinated movements, labile temperature regulation, and poor control over musculature are characteristic of the infant. Reflexes are important indicators of infant neural development (see page 1310).

Nursing Assessment

 Evidence Base Hockenberry, M. J., & Wilson, D. (Eds.). (2010). *Wong's nursing care of infants and children* (9th ed.). St. Louis, MO: Elsevier Mosby.

Delivery of effective neonatal care is enhanced by communication of pertinent information about the mother and her infant to the pediatrician or other health care provider. It is important that the obstetric staff record the following information on the medical record that accompanies the neonate during any transfer of care.

Pertinent Maternal History

1. Mother's age, socioeconomic status, ethnic or cultural group, educational level, marital status.
2. Mother's/family's past medical history.
3. Mother's past obstetric history.
4. Mother's prenatal history with this pregnancy includes rubella status, hepatitis B testing, history of psychiatric disease, domestic violence, or history of previous child abuse or neglect. Also includes other maternal test results relevant to neonatal care (ie, human immunodeficiency virus test results and colonization with group B-hemolytic streptococci).
5. Labor and delivery. (Includes intrapartum maternal antibiotic therapy, along with type and dosage of antibiotics.)

Physical Assessment Findings and Physiologic Functioning

 Evidence Base Cheffer, N. D., & Rannalli, D. A. (2011). Transitional care of the newborn. In S. Mattson & J. E. Smith (Eds.), *Core curriculum for maternal-newborn nursing* (4th ed., pp. 345–361). St. Louis, MO: Saunders Elsevier.
  Verklan, M. T., & Walden, M. (Eds.). (2010). *Core curriculum for neonatal intensive care nursing* (4th ed.). St. Louis, MO: Saunders Elsevier.
  Hockenberry, M. J., & Wilson, D. (Eds.). (2010). *Wong's nursing care of infants and children* (9th ed.). St. Louis, MO: Elsevier Mosby.

Posture
1. Full-term neonate assumes symmetric posture; face turned to side; flexed extremities; hands tightly fisted with thumb covered by fingers.
2. Asymmetric posture may be caused by fractures of clavicle or humerus or by nerve injuries commonly of the brachial plexus.
3. Infants born in breech position may keep knees and legs straightened or in frog position, depending on the type of breech birth.

Length

Average length of full-term neonate is 20 inches (51 cm); range, 18 to 22 inches (46 to 56 cm).

Weight

Average weight of male neonates is 7½ lb (3,400 g); female neonates, 7 lb (3,200 g). Weight range of 80% of full-term neonates is 6 lb, 5 oz to 9 lb, 2 oz (2,900 to 4,100 g).

Skin

Examine under natural light for:

1. Hair distribution—term infant will have some lanugo over back; most of the lanugo will have disappeared on extremities and other areas of the body.
2. Turgor—term infant should have good skin turgor (ie, after gently pinching small portion of skin and releasing it, the skin should return to its original position).
3. Color.
   a. Cyanosis—acrocyanosis, bluish color in palms of hands and soles of feet, is common because of immature peripheral circulation. This condition is exacerbated by cold temperatures.
   b. Pallor—may indicate cold, stress, anemia, or cardiac failure.
   c. Plethora—reddish (ruddy) coloration may be caused by a high level of RBCs to total blood volume from intrauterine intravascular transfusion (twins), cardiac disease, or diabetes in the mother.
   d. Jaundice—physiologic jaundice caused by immaturity of liver is common beginning on day 2, peaking at 1 week, and disappearing by the 2nd week. It first appears in skin over the face or upper body, then progresses over a larger area; it can also be seen in conjunctivae of eyes.
   e. Meconium staining—staining of skin, fingernails, and umbilical cord indicates passage of meconium in utero (possibly caused by fetal hypoxia in utero).
4. Dryness/peeling—marked scaling and desquamation are signs of postmaturity.
5. Vernix—in full-term infants, most vernix is found in skin folds under the arms and in the groin under the scrotum (in males) and in the labia (in females).
6. Nails—should reach end of fingertips and be well developed in the full-term infant. There should be no evidence of pits, ridges, aplasia, or hypertrophy.
7. Edema—some edema may occur over buttocks, back, and occiput if the infant has been supine; pitting edema may be caused by erythroblastosis, heart failure, and electrolyte imbalance.
8. Ecchymosis—may appear over the presenting part in a difficult delivery; may also indicate infection or a bleeding problem.
9. Petechiae—pinpoint hemorrhages on skin caused by increased intravascular pressure, infection, or thrombocytopenia; regresses within 48 hours.
10. Erythema toxicum (newborn rash)—small white, yellow, or pink to red papular rash that appears on trunk, face, and extremities; regresses within 48 hours.
11. Hemangiomas—vascular lesions present at birth; some may fade, but others may be permanent.
    a. Strawberry (nevus vasculosus)—bright red, raised, lobulated tumor that occurs on the head, neck, trunk, or extremities; soft, palpable, with sharp demarcated margins; increases in size for approximately 6 months, then regresses after several years.
    b. Cavernous—larger, more mature vascular elements; involves dermis and subcutaneous tissues; soft, palpable, with poorly defined margins; increases in size the first 6 to 12 months, then involutes spontaneously.
12. Telangiectatic nevi (stork bites)—flat red or purple lesions most commonly found on the back of the neck, lower occiput, upper eyelid, and bridge of the nose; regress by age 2, although the ones on the neck may persist through adulthood.
13. Milia—enlarged sebaceous glands found on nose, chin, cheeks, brow, and forehead; regress in several days to a few weeks. They appear as multiple yellow or pearly white papules, approximately 1 mm in diameter. When found in the mouth, they are referred to as Epstein pearls.
14. Mongolian spots—blue-green or gray pigmentation on the lower back, sacrum, and buttocks; common in blacks (90%), Asians, and infants of southern European heritage; regress by age 4. May be mistaken for signs of child abuse.
15. Café-au-lait spots—tan or light brown macules or patches. When less than 1¼ inches (3 cm) in length and less than six in number, there is no pathologic significance; if greater than 1¼ inches or more than six in number, may indicate cutaneous neurofibromatosis.
16. Harlequin color change—when on side, dependent half turns red, upper half pale; caused by gravity and vasomotor instability.
17. Abrasions or lacerations can result from internal monitoring and instruments used at birth.
18. Cutis marmorata—bluish mottling or marbling of skin in response to chilling, stress, or overstimulation.
19. Port-wine nevus (nevus flammeus)—flat pink or reddish purple lesion consisting of dilated, congested capillaries directly beneath the epidermis; does not blanch.

Head

1. Examine head and face for symmetry, paralysis, shape, swelling, movement.
   a. Caput succedaneum—swelling of soft tissues of the scalp because of pressure; swelling crosses suture lines. Associated with vacuum-assisted birth.
   b. Cephalohematoma—subperiosteal hemorrhage with collection of blood between periosteum and bone; swelling does not cross suture lines. May result from vacuum-assisted birth (use of the vacuum extractor).
   c. Molding—overlapping of skull bones, caused by compression during labor and delivery (disappears in a few days).
   d. Examine symmetry of facial movements.
   e. Forceps marks—U-shaped bruising usually on cheeks following forceps delivery.
2. Measure head circumference—13 to 14 inches (33 to 36 cm), approximately ¾ inch (2 cm) larger than chest. Measure just above the eyebrows and over the occiput.

3. Fontanelles—area where more than two skull bones meet; covered with strong band of connective tissue; also called the soft spot.
   a. Enlarged or bulging—may indicate increased intracranial pressure (ICP).
   b. Sunken—commonly indicates dehydration.
   c. Size—posterior may be obliterated because of molding; generally closes in 2 to 3 months. Anterior is palpable; generally closes in 12 to 18 months.
4. Sutures—junctions of adjoining skull bones.
   a. Overriding—caused by molding during labor and delivery.
   b. Separation—extensive separation may be found in malnourished infants and with increased ICP.

Face

1. Eyes—examine the following:
   a. Color—sclera in most full-term infants are white; blue sclera is indicative of osteogenesis imperfecta. Eye color usually slate-gray, brown, or dark blue; final eye color is evident by 6 to 12 months.
   b. Hemorrhagic areas—subconjunctival hemorrhages may appear as a red band from pressure during delivery; regress within 2 weeks.
   c. Edema—edema of the eyelids may be caused by pressure on the head and face during labor and delivery.
   d. Conjunctivitis or discharge—may be caused by instillation of silver nitrate (if still used) or infections from organisms, such as staphylococcus, chlamydia trachomatis, or gonococcus. Tear formation does not usually begin until age 2 to 3 months.
   e. Jaundice—may be seen in sclera because of physiologic jaundice or, if severe, blood-group incompatibility.
   f. Pupils—equal in size and should constrict equally in bright light.
   g. Infant can see and discriminate patterns; limited by imperfect oculomotor coordination and inability to accommodate for varying distances.
   h. Red reflex—red-orange color seen when light from an ophthalmoscope is reflected from the retina. No red reflex indicates cataracts.
   i. Brushfield's spots—white or yellow pinpoint areas on iris that may indicate trisomy 21 or even a normal variant.
   j. Abnormal placement of eyes or small eye openings can signify a syndrome or chromosomal anomaly.
   k. Strabismus—cross-eyed appearance that is common; nystagmus (constant, rapid, involuntary movement of the eye) is also common and disappears by age 4 months.
2. Nose—examine the following:
   a. Patency—necessary because infants breathe through the nose, not the mouth.
   b. Nasal flaring—abnormal and may indicate respiratory distress. Check for appropriate size and shape of the nose; should be placed vertically midline in face.
   c. Discharge—stuffiness is normal unless chronic nasal discharge is present; may be caused by possible infection.

d. Sense of smell—infants will turn toward familiar odors and away from noxious odors.
e. Septum should be midline; low nasal bridge with broad base may be associated with Down syndrome.
f. Periodic sneezing is common.
3. Ears—examine the following:
   a. Formation—large, flabby ears that slant forward may indicate abnormalities of the kidney or other parts of the urinary tract.
   b. Position in relation to the eye—helix (top of ear) on the same plane as eye; low-set ears may indicate chromosomal or renal abnormalities.
   c. Cartilage—full-term infant has sufficient cartilage to make the ear feel firm.
   d. Hearing—auditory canals may be congested for a day or two after birth; the infant should hear well in a few days.
   e. Observe for skin tags; preauricular sinus located in front of the ear may be normal or may be associated with genetic disorders.
4. Mouth—examine the following:
   a. Size—small mouth found in trisomy 18 and 21; corners of mouth turn down (fish mouth) in fetal alcohol syndrome. Mucous membranes should be pink.
   b. Palate—examine hard and soft palate for closure.
   c. Size of tongue in relation to mouth—normally does not extend much past the margin of gums. Excessively large tongue seen in congenital anomalies, such as cretinism and trisomy 21.
   d. Teeth—predeciduous teeth are found on rare occasions; if they interfere with feeding, they may be removed.
   e. Epstein's pearls—small white nodules found on sides of hard palate (commonly mistaken for teeth); regress in a few weeks.
   f. Frenulum linguae—thin ridge of tissue running from base of tongue along undersurface to tip of tongue, formerly believed to cause tongue-tie; no treatment necessary. True congenital ankyloglossia (tongue-tie) is rare.
   g. Sucking blisters (labial tuberales)—thickened areas on midline of upper lip that may be filled with fluid or callous; no treatment necessary.
   h. Infections—thrush, caused by *Candida albicans*, may appear as white patches on tongue and/or insides of cheeks that do not wash away with fluids; treated with nystatin suspension.

Neck

Examine the following:
1. Mobility—infant can move head from side to side; palpate for lymph nodes; palpate clavicle for fractures, especially after a difficult delivery.
2. Torticollis—appears as a spasmodic, one-sided contraction of neck muscles; generally from hematoma of sternocleidomastoid muscle; usually no treatment required.
3. Excessive skin folds may be associated with congenital abnormalities such as trisomy 21.
4. Stiffness and hyperextension may be caused by trauma or infection.

5. Clavicle—for intactness.
6. Observe for masses such as cystic hygroma—soft and usually seen laterally or over the clavicle.

Chest

1. Circumference and symmetry—average circumference is 12 to 13 inches (30 to 33 cm), approximately ¾ inch (2 cm) smaller than head circumference.
2. Breast.
   a. Engorgement—may occur at day 3 because of withdrawal of maternal hormones, especially estrogen; no treatment required. Regresses in 2 weeks.
   b. Nipples and areolae—less formed and pronounced in preterm infants.

Respiratory System

1. Rate—normally between 30 to 60 breaths/minute; influenced by sleep–wake status, when last fed, drugs taken by mother, and room temperature.
2. Rhythm—respirations may be shallow with irregular rhythm.
   a. Respiratory movements are symmetric and mainly diaphragmatic because of weak thoracic muscles. For example, the lower thorax pulls in and the abdomen bulges with each respiration.
   b. Periodic breathing—resumption of respiration after 5- to 15-second period without respiration; decreases with time; more common in preterm infants. Substernal retractions, if accompanied by gasps or stridor, are indicative of upper airway obstruction.
   c. Observe for abnormal respiratory signs.
3. Breath sounds—determined by auscultation.
   a. Bronchial sounds are heard over most of the chest.
   b. Crackles may be heard immediately after birth.
   c. Expiratory grunting is indicative of respiratory distress syndrome (RDS).

Cardiovascular System

1. Rate—normal between 110 and 160 bpm (80 to 110 normal with deep sleep); influenced by behavioral state, environmental temperature, medication; take apical count for 1 minute.
2. Rhythm—common to find periods of deceleration followed by periods of acceleration.
3. Heart sounds—second sound higher in pitch and sharper than first; third and fourth sounds rarely heard; murmurs common, majority are transitory and benign.
4. Pulses—examine equality and strength of brachial, radial, pedal, and femoral pulses; lack of femoral pulses indicative of inadequate aortic blood flow.
5. Cyanosis—examine for cyanosis. Acrocyanosis of distal extremities is common; record location of any cyanosis, color changes with time, and when crying.
6. BP—neonates who weigh more than 3 kg (6½ lbs) have systolic BP between 65 and 95 mm Hg; diastolic, between 30 and 60 mm Hg. BP is usually higher in the lower extremities than in the upper extremities. BP assessment may not be conducted routinely on healthy neonates. Measurement of BP is essential for infants who show signs of distress, are premature, or are suspected of having a cardiac anomaly.

Abdomen

1. Shape—cylindrical, protrudes slightly, moves synchronously with chest in respiration.
2. Distention may be caused by bowel obstruction, organ enlargement, or infection.
3. Palpate abdomen for masses; gap between rectus muscles is common; palpate liver and spleen.
   a. Liver has decreased ability to conjugate bilirubin (rationale for physiologic jaundice).
   b. Liver has decreased production of prothrombin and factors that depend on vitamin K for synthesis (rationale for neonate's predisposition to hemorrhage).
4. Auscultate abdomen in all four quadrants for bowel sounds; usually bowel sounds occur 1 hour after delivery.
5. Kidneys—palpate kidneys for size and shape.
   a. Infant has decreased ability of kidney to concentrate urine, excrete a solute load, maintain water and electrolyte balance.
   b. Urine may contain uric acid crystals, which appear on diaper as reddish blotches; uric acid crystals may yield false-positive result when the infant's urine is tested for protein.
6. Umbilical cord.
   a. Normally contains two arteries, one vein; single artery sometimes associated with renal and other congenital abnormalities.
   b. Signs of infection around insertion into abdominal wall—redness, discharge.
   c. Meconium staining—associated with intrauterine compromise or postmaturity.
   d. By 24 hours, becomes yellowish brown; dries and falls off in approximately 10 to 14 days.
   e. Umbilical hernia—defect in abdominal wall.
7. Genitalia.
   a. Female:
      i. Labia majora cover labia minora and clitoris in full-term female infants.
      ii. Hymenal tag (tissue) may protrude from vagina—regresses within several weeks.
      iii. Vaginal discharge—white mucus discharge common; pink-tinged mucus discharge (pseudomenstruation) may be present because of the drop in maternal hormones; no treatment necessary.
   b. Male:
      i. Full-term—testes in scrotal sac; scrotal sac appears markedly wrinkled due to rugae.
      ii. Edema may be present in scrotal sac if the infant was born in breech presentation; a frank collection of fluid in the scrotal sac is a hydrocele—regresses in approximately a month.
      iii. Examine glans penis for urethral opening—normally central; opening ventral (hypospadias); opening dorsally (epispadias); abnormally adherent foreskin (phimosis).

c. Check for patent anus—infant should stool within 24 hours after delivery. If passed meconium in utero, patent anus has been established.

Back

1. Examine spinal column for normal curvature, closure, and pilonidal dimple or sinus; also for tufts of hair or skin disruptions that would indicate possible spina bifida.
2. Examine anal area for anal opening, response of anal sphincter, fissures.

Musculoskeletal System

1. Examine extremities for fractures, paralysis, range of motion, irregular position.
2. Examine fingers and toes for number and separation: extra digits, polydactyly; fused digits, syndactyly.
3. Examine hips for dislocation—with the infant in supine position, flex knees and abduct hips to side and down to table surface; clicking sound indicates dislocation (Ortolani's sign).
4. Asymmetrical gluteal folds also indicate congenital hip dislocation.
5. Examine feet for structural and positional deformities, that is, club foot (talipes equinovarus) or metatarsus adductus (inward turning of the foot).

Neurologic System

1. Neurologic mechanisms are immature anatomically and physiologically; as a result, uncoordinated movements, labile temperature regulation, and lack of control over musculature are characteristic of the infant.
2. Examine muscle tone, head control, and reflexes.
3. Two types of reflexes are present in the neonate:
   a. Protective in nature (blink, cough, sneeze, gag)—remain throughout life.
   b. Primitive in nature (rooting/sucking, Moro, startle, tonic neck, stepping, and palmar/plantar grasp)—either disappear within months or become highly developed and voluntary (sucking and grasping) (see Figure 38-4, page 1310).

Behavioral Assessment

Response to Stimulation

1. Neonates exhibit predictable, directed responses in social interactions with nurturing adults or in response to attractive auditory or visual stimuli.
2. Neonate responses are influenced by states of consciousness, such as:
   a. Quiet, deep sleep (sleep state)—no spontaneous activity, eyes closed, respirations regular, with delayed response to external stimuli.
   b. Light, active sleep (sleep state)—random startles, eyes closed, REMs, frequent change of state with response to stimulation.
   c. Drowsy awake (transitional state)—eyes open or closed, appearing dull and heavy lidded, eyelids flutter, variable activity level, mild startles periodically, delayed response to stimulation.

d. Quiet alert (awake state)—eyes open, little motor activity, focuses on source of stimulation. Interacts most with environment; respirations regular.
   e. Alert active (awake state)—eyes open, less bright and attentive, much motor activity, increase in startles in response to stimulation.
   f. Crying (awake state)—intense crying that is difficult to interrupt with stimulation; increased motor activity and color changes.

Sleeping Pattern

1. Length of sleep cycles (REM, active and quiet sleep) changes with maturation of the central nervous system (CNS).
2. Quiet sleep should increase with time in relation to REM sleep.
3. Neonates usually sleep 20 hours per day.

Feeding Pattern

1. Most neonates eat 10 to 12 times per day with 2 to 4 hours between feedings; establish fairly regular feeding patterns in approximately 2 weeks.
2. Caloric requirements are high—110 to 130 calories/kg of body weight daily.
3. Most digestive enzymes are present at birth.
4. Imperfect control of cardiac and pyloric sphincters; immaturity results in regurgitation.

Pattern of Elimination

1. Stools.
   a. Meconium is usually passed in 24 to 48 hours.
   b. Passage of meconium (tarry green-black stools) continues for about 72 hours, followed by transitional stools (greenish brown to yellowish brown; thin; may contain milk curds). Milk stools (for breast-fed, yellow to golden; pasty; odor like sour milk; for formula-fed, pale yellow to light brown; firmer; more offensive odor) are passed by day 4 to 5.
   c. Neonate has up to six stools per day in the first weeks after birth.
2. Voiding.
   a. Neonate voids within first 24 hours.
   b. After first few days, infant voids from 10 to 20 times per day.

Temperature Regulation

1. Infant's body responds readily to changes in environmental temperature.
2. Heat loss at birth may occur through evaporation, convection, conduction, and radiation.
3. Physiologic mechanisms to avoid heat loss include:
   a. Vasoconstriction.
   b. Nonshivering thermogenesis elicited by sympathetic nervous system in response to decreased temperature.
   c. Adipose tissue and brown fat—the latter contains many small blood vessels, fat vacuoles, and mitochondria and is a site of heat production. Brown fat is found between scapulae, around neck and thorax, behind sternum, and around kidneys and adrenals.
   d. Flexed position of full-term neonate.

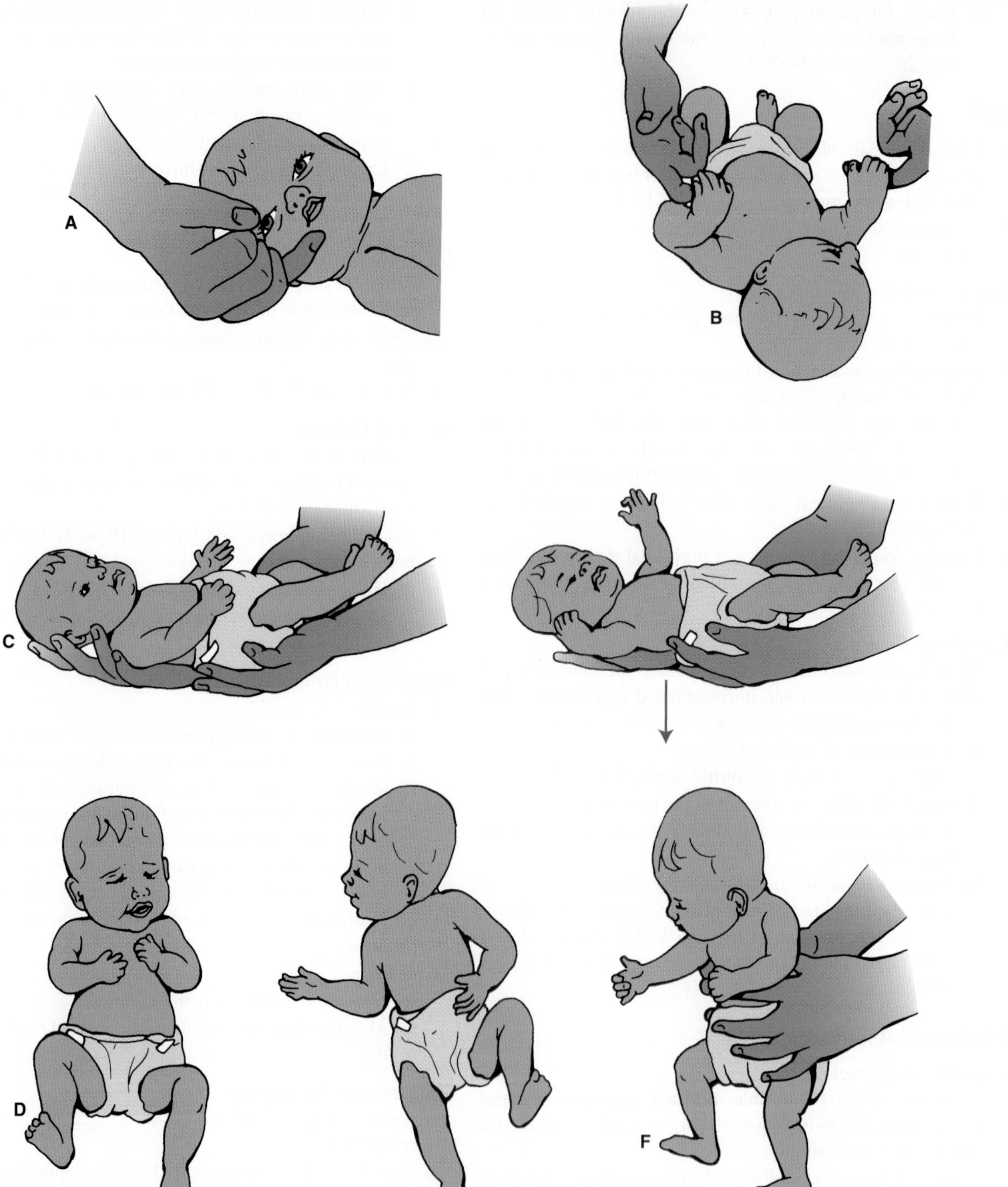

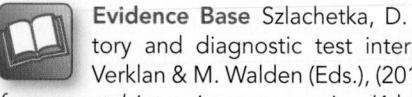

Figure 38-4. Newborn reflexes. (A) Rooting. **(B)** Grasp. **(C)** Moro. **(D)** Startle. **(E)** Tonic neck. **(F)** Stepping.

Metabolic Screening Tests

📖 **Evidence Base** Szlachetka, D. M. (2010). Laboratory and diagnostic test interpretation. In M. T. Verklan & M. Walden (Eds.), (2010). *Core curriculum for neonatal intensive care nursing* (4th ed., pp. 252–269). St. Louis, MO: Saunders Elsevier.

1. Phenylketonuria—inability of the infant to metabolize phenylalanine; scheduled after 48 hours of protein feedings.
2. Galactosemia—inborn error of carbohydrate metabolism, in which galactose and lactose cannot be converted to glucose.
3. Hypothyroidism—thyroid hormone deficiency.
4. Maple sugar urine disease—inability to metabolize leucine, isoleucine, and valine.

5. Homocystinuria—inborn error of sulfur amino acid metabolism.

6. Sickle cell anemia—abnormally shaped RBCs with lower oxygen solubility.

Community and Home Care Considerations

1. The American Academy of Pediatrics (AAP) and the American College of Obstetricians and Gynecologists have established guidelines and have suggested criteria for discharging childbearing women before 48 hours after birth.

 Evidence Base American Academy of Pediatrics. (2010). Policy statement: Hospital stay for healthy term newborns. *Pediatrics, 125*(2), 403–409.

   a. Singleton birth between 38 and 42 weeks' gestation.

   b. Mother with uncomplicated vaginal birth and mother and neonate with uncomplicated, antepartum, intrapartum, and postpartum course.

   c. Pertinent laboratory data within normal limits for mother and neonate.

   d. Neonate has spontaneously passed at least one stool and urinated at least once.

   e. Neonate stable, maintaining thermal homeostasis, and feeding well (eg, completed at least two successful feedings with coordinated sucking, swallowing, and breathing).

   f. If circumcised, no excessive bleeding from circumcision site for 2 hours postprocedure.

   g. All necessary vaccines have been administered (eg, hepatitis B) according to current AAP immunization schedules.

   h. Hearing screening has been completed per facility protocol.

   i. Cord or infant blood type and direct Coombs results (if required) have been reviewed.

   j. Family members and support persons are available at home for next several days.

   k. Mother aware of complications for self and neonate.

   l. Facility has in place mechanisms to address patient questions after discharge.

   m. Continuing medical care is planned, usually within 48 hours after discharge and especially for neonates discharged prior to 48 hours after birth.

2. The first visit at home by the perinatal home care personnel is the longest because a complete physical of mother and the neonate is conducted. Subsequent visits are shorter.

3. Listening is important. The approach for care is a collaborative one.

4. Nurse needs to have a thorough knowledge base in:

   a. Normal postpartum and neonatal care.

   b. Potential complications in the postpartum and neonatal periods.

   c. Nursing interventions for postpartum and neonatal complications.

5. Personal safety is also a concern. There should be a mechanism in place to locate home care personnel, if needed. Staff should also be trained in actions to take when encountering potentially unsafe situations. It is recommended that home care personnel leave their purse and other pertinent information in their vehicle or at home. Do not carry it on your person should quick escape be necessary.

Nursing Management

 Evidence Base Cheffer, N. D., & Rannalli, D. A. (2011). Transitional care of the newborn. In S. Mattson & J. E. Smith (Eds.), *Core curriculum for maternal-newborn nursing* (4th ed., pp. 345–361). St. Louis, MO: Saunders Elsevier.

   Hockenberry, M. J., & Wilson, D. (Eds.). (2010). *Wong's nursing care of infants and children* (9th ed.). St. Louis, MO: Elsevier Mosby.

See Procedure Guidelines 38-1, page 1312.

In caring for the neonate, the nurse establishes an ongoing care plan for the infant and the family until discharge. The nurse's assessment of the neonate includes observing and recording vital signs, daily weight gain or loss, bowel and bladder function, activity and sleep patterns, and thermoregulation. Observation for potential problems in the neonate, ensuring safety, and the prevention of infection are the main goals of nursing care.

Another main component of caring for the neonate is to assist with establishing a healthy family unit. Because so much of the baby's time is spent with parents, the nurse has the opportunity to assist them with promoting health maintenance by teaching feeding methods and by demonstrating baby care techniques, such as diapering, bathing, and circumcision care. The nurse provides health counseling and education and answers questions to enable the parents to gain confidence, control, and satisfaction in caring for their child at home.

PROBLEMS OF THE NEWBORN
Premature Infant

 Evidence Base American College of Obstetricians and Gynecologists. (2008/Reaffirmed 2011). *Late-preterm infants* (Committee Opinion #404). Washington, DC: Author.

   Verklan, M. T., Askin, D. F., Hill, C., et al. (2010). *Assessment and care of late preterm infant guideline*. Washington, DC: Association of Women's Health, Obstetric and Neonatal Nurses.

The *premature neonate* is a neonate born before the completion of 37 weeks' gestation. Other classifications include moderately preterm (32 to 36 weeks), late preterm (34 to 36-6/7 weeks), and very preterm birth (less than 32 weeks).

A low-birth-weight (weight at birth) neonate is one whose birth weight is less than 5 lb, 8 oz (2,500 g), regardless of gestational age.

A very-low-birth-weight neonate is one whose birth weight is below 3 lb, 5 oz (1,500 g), regardless of gestational age.

PROCEDURE GUIDELINES 38-1

Newborn Care

EQUIPMENT

- Cotton balls or disposable washcloths
- Neutral soap (varies with facility, but examples include Castile, Dove, and Neutrogena)
- 70% alcohol
- Petrolatum gauze
- Protective ointment

PROCEDURE

Nursing Action	Rationale
Weight, temperature, and blood pressure	
1. Weigh infant and record weight.	1. Newborn may lose 5%–10% of birth weight because of minimal intake of nutrients and fluid and loss of excess fluid.
2. Take axillary temperature by placing thermometer in axilla and pressing infant's arm gently but firmly against it for 10 minutes. Prevent undue exposure; provide warm environment (75°–80° F [24°–27° C]).	2. Use of rectal thermometer predisposes to irritation of rectal mucosa.
3. Take blood pressure, if indicated.	3. Hypotension may be present and require remedial action.
Bathing technique	
1. Use cotton balls or soft, disposable washcloths to wipe eyes, face, and outer ears. Eyes are wiped from inside corner outward.	1. Moves secretions from cleanest to most soiled area.
2. Use a neutral soap—check pH. Clear water may be used if infant's skin is dry (bath water temperature 98° F–100° F [37° C–38° C]).	2. Prevents irritation of skin. The use of hexachlorophene to prevent staphylococcal infection is controversial. Hexachlorophene may cause brain damage if a sufficient quantity is absorbed through the skin.
3. Wash infant's head, using gentle circular motions.	3. Prevents cradle cap from forming, especially over the frontal areas.
4. Tilt head back to cleanse neck.	4. Exposes neck folds for more thorough cleansing.
5. Bathe torso and extremities quickly.	5. Prevents unnecessary exposure and chilling.
6. Carefully dry each area after washing.	6. Prevents heat loss and maintains thermoregulation.
7. Inspect umbilical cord. Check area for bleeding or foul odor. A drying agent, such as 70% alcohol or merthiolate, may be applied several times daily (according to your facility's policy). Do not cover with diaper. Dressings are not used.	7. Minimizes colonization by bacteria.
8. Cleanse genital area of male infants.	8.
a. Cleanse penis without retracting foreskin.	a. Edema and constriction of the penis may result if foreskin is retracted.
b. Circumcision care—keep area clean. Place sterile petrolatum gauze over area for first 24 hours; change after voiding. Observe hourly for bleeding. Position infant and diaper to avoid friction.	b. Prevents infection and promotes healing. Bleeding can be controlled by pressure or by application of adrenaline solution. Prevents discomfort.
9. Cleanse genital area of female infants.	
a. Wash vulva from front to back.	a. Removes vernix and other discharge.
b. Wipe vulva with cotton ball, using one stroke in a front-to-back direction.	b. Front-to-back cleansing prevents contamination of vagina.
10. Bathe buttocks, using a gentle, patting motion. Keep area clean and dry to prevent diaper rash. If rash does occur, protective ointment (zinc oxide or vitamin A & D) may be used. Exposure of buttocks to air or heat lamp is helpful.	10. Area is susceptible to skin breakdown because of acid reaction of urine and feces.

PROCEDURE GUIDELINES 38-1 *(continued)*

Newborn Care

PROCEDURE *(continued)*

Nursing Action	Rationale
Stool observation	
1. Observe stool pattern—meconium during first 2 to 3 days.	1. Material composed of epithelial and epidermal cells, lanugo, and bile pigments.
2. Transitional stools—change from tarry black to greenish black, to greenish brown to brownish yellow to greenish yellow.	2. Changes reflect intake of milk—stools are composed of meconium and milk stools.
3. Number, color, and consistency are recorded daily.	3. For early identification of abnormalities.
	a. No stools within 48 hours indicates an intestinal obstruction.
	b. Passage of meconium only (without other stools) suggests obstruction in the ileum.
	c. Thick, puttylike meconium may indicate cystic fibrosis.
	d. Diarrhea may be caused by overfeeding or by gastroenteritis.
	e. Blood in the stools is an indication of intestinal bleeding.
Nutritional considerations	
1. Provide for nutritional intake.	1. Newborn infants vary in their readiness to feed.
2. Promote feeding method of choice.	2. Although recommendations may be made, family decisions should be respected and continuity of care provided.
3. Test blood glucose using enzymatic strip test (according to your facility's policy).	3. Newborn may be hypoglycemic and require feeding sooner than the usual 4- to 6-hour wait.
4. Instruct the parent in technique of bottle-feeding.	4.
a. Hold infant in semi-upright position.	a. Gravity assists flow of milk into stomach.
b. Position bottle so that neck of bottle is filled.	b. Prevents the infant from swallowing air.
c. Insert nipple into infant's mouth so that his or her tongue is under nipple.	c. Sucking and swallowing reflexes are used in feeding.
d. Burp during feeding by holding infant upright.	d. Allows air to escape from stomach, preventing distention or milk regurgitation.
Community and home care considerations	
1. Preparation for home care: instruction is given concerning infant bathing and care, preparation of formula, and infant feeding. Written formula with instructions for preparation is provided to parents.	1. Instruction for newborn care is a combined responsibility of the medical and nursing staffs.
2. Provide ample opportunity for parent contact and care of infant while nursing support is available. Take every opportunity to teach.	2. Early attachment results in improved parent–child relationships.
3. Arrange home visits, as necessary.	

A extremely-low-birth-weight neonate is one whose birth weight is below 2 lb, 2 oz (1,000 g), regardless of gestational age.

Pathophysiology and Etiology

1. A wide range of maternal factors is associated with prematurity.
2. Possible risk factors associated with prematurity include, but are not limited to:

a. Chronic health problems, such as hypertension, obesity, or diabetes.

b. Behavioral and environmental risks, such as late or no prenatal care, smoking, illicit drug use, alcohol, domestic violence, stress, or lack of social support.

c. Demographic risks, such as non-Hispanic black race, younger than age 17, older than age 35, or low socioeconomic status.

d. Genetics.

e. Assisted reproductive technologies.

f. Medical risks in current pregnancy, such as preeclampsia or gestational hypertension, bleeding, placenta previa or abruptio placentae, uterine or cervical anomalies (incompetent cervix), premature rupture of membranes, preterm premature rupture of membranes, polyhydramnios or oligohydramnios, infection, or periodontal disease.

g. Changes in delivery practices, concern about postmaturity complications, or risk of stillbirth (late preterm).

3. Fetal factors associated with prematurity include:

a. Chromosomal abnormalities.

b. Anatomic abnormalities, such as tracheoesophageal atresia or fistula and intestinal obstruction.

c. Fetoplacental unit dysfunction.

4. The premature infant has altered physiology because of immature and typically poorly developed systems. The severity of any problem that occurs depends somewhat on the gestational age of the infant. Systems and situations that are most likely to cause problems in the premature infant include:

a. Respiratory system.

b. Digestive system.

c. Thermoregulation.

d. Immune system.

e. Neurologic system.

Nursing Assessment and Interventions

1. Notice physical characteristics of the premature neonate:

a. Hair—lanugo, fluffy.

b. Poor ear cartilage.

c. Skin—thin; capillaries are visible (may be red and wrinkled).

d. Lack of subcutaneous fat.

e. Sole of foot is smooth.

  i. 36 weeks' gestation—anterior $^1/_3$ of foot is creased.

  ii. 38 weeks' gestation— $^2/_3$ of foot is creased.

f. Breast buds 5 mm.

  i. 36 weeks' gestation—none.

  ii. 38 weeks' gestation—1¼ inches (3 cm).

g. Testes—undescended.

h. Labia majora—undeveloped.

i. Rugae of scrotum—fine.

j. Fingernails—soft.

k. Abdomen—relatively large.

l. Thorax—relatively small.

m. Head—appears disproportionately large.

n. Muscle tone poor, possibly weak reflexes.

2. Obtain accurate body measurements.

a. Head circumference—frontal–occipital circumference one finger above eyebrows, using parallel lines of tape around head.

b. Abdominal girth—one finger above umbilicus, mark location.

c. Heel to crown.

d. Shoulder to umbilicus—used to calculate proper length of catheter for umbilical arterial catheter placement.

e. Weight in grams.

3. Assess gestational age (see Figure 38-5) using a tool such as the Ballard scoring system (recommended by Committee of Fetus and Newborn of AAP):

a. Observation of physical and neurologic characteristics that change predictably with growth and maturation. Ideally done in the first 12 to 24 hours of life.

	0	1	2	3	4	5
SKIN	gelatinous red, transparent	smooth pink, visible veins	superficial peeling &/or rash, few veins	cracking pale area, rare veins	parchment, deep cracking, no vessels	leathery, cracked, wrinkled
LANUGO	none	abundant	thinning	bald areas	mostly bald	
PLANTAR CREASES	no crease	faint red marks	anterior transverse crease only	creases ant. 2/3	creases cover entire sole	
BREAST	barely percept.	flat areola, no bud	stippled areola, 1–2 mm bud	raised areola, 3–4 mm bud	full areola, 5–10 mm bud	
EAR	pinna flat, stays folded	sl. curved pinna, soft with slow recoil	well-curv. pinna, soft but ready recoil	formed & firm with instant recoil	thick cartilage, ear stiff	
GENITALS Male	scrotum empty, no rugae		testes descending, few rugae	testes down, good rugae	testes pendulous, deep rugae	
GENITALS Female	prominent clitoris & labia minora		majora & minora equally prominent	majora large, minora small	clitoris & minora completely covered	

	0	1	2	3	4	5
Posture						
Square Window (Wrist)	90°	60°	45°	30°	0°	
Arm Recoil	180°		100°–180°	90°–100°	<90°	
Popliteal Angle	180°	160°	130°	110°	90°	<90°
Scarf Sign						
Heel to Ear						

Score	Wks
5	26
10	28
15	30
20	32
25	34
30	36
35	38
40	40
45	42
50	44

Figure 38-5. Ballard assessment of gestational age criteria. (Ballard, J. L., Khoury, J. C., Wedig, K., et al. [1991]. New Ballard score, expanded to include extremely premature infants. *Journal of Pediatrics, 119,* 417–423.)

b. Later, adjusted, or corrected age will be determined once the neonate reaches term (40 weeks after conception). Chronological age is adjusted for prematurity by taking gestational age – 40 + chronologic age = developmental or corrected age. This is the age the neonate would have been if he or she had been born at 40 weeks' gestation.

4. Assist with laboratory testing, as indicated, for blood gases, blood glucose, complete blood count or hemoglobin and hematocrit, electrolytes, calcium, bilirubin.

5. Monitor closely for respiratory or cardiac complications.

   a. Respirations above 60/minute may indicate respiratory difficulty.

   b. Expiratory grunting, retractions, chest lag, or nasal flaring should be reported immediately.

   c. Watch for cyanosis (other than acrocyanosis—coldness and cyanosis of hands and feet) and other signs of respiratory distress.

   d. Increased (>180 bpm) or irregular heart rate may indicate cardiac or circulatory difficulties.

   e. Muscle tone and activity should be evaluated.

   f. Hypotension, indicated by BP measurement, may be caused by hypovolemia.

   g. Hypoglycemia may result from inadequate glycogen stores, respiratory distress, and cold stress.

6. Institute cardiac monitoring and care for infant in isolette or radiant heater. Omit bath until infant's temperature has stabilized. Temperature instability is a risk factor for hypoglycemia.

7. Observe for early signs of jaundice and check maternal history for any blood incompatibilities. Also be aware of maternal factors that can lead to additional complications, such as drug use, diabetes, and infection.

8. Once the infant is admitted to the nursery, be aware that the first 24 to 48 hours after birth is a critical time, usually requiring constant observation and intensive care management. Make the following observations:

   a. Note bleeding from the umbilical cord—apply pressure and notify health care provider.

   b. Note first voiding—may occur up to 36 hours after birth; after first voiding, report any 4- to 6-hour period when voiding does not occur.

   c. Note stools—abdominal distention and lack of stools may indicate intestinal obstruction or other intestinal tract anomalies. Measure abdominal girth at regular intervals.

   d. Note activity and behavior—look for sucking movement and hand-to-mouth maneuver, which can help to determine oral feeding initiation.

   e. Observe for a tense and bulging fontanelle; feel suture lines, noting separation or overriding—may indicate intracranial hemorrhage. Be alert to twitching and seizures.

   f. Note color of skin for cyanosis and jaundice, rashes, paleness, ruddiness.

   g. Carefully monitor, record, and report vital signs.

9. Have available resuscitative equipment, oxygen, and suction apparatus.

   a. A rubber ear bulb syringe is usually all that is necessary for clearing the mouth.

   b. Frequent suctioning of the pharynx may not be necessary.

10. Position neonate to allow for easy ventilation, paying careful attention to maintaining body alignment and facilitating hand-to-mouth positioning.

    a. Elevate head and trunk to decrease pressure on diaphragm from abdominal organs.

    b. Change position from side to side.

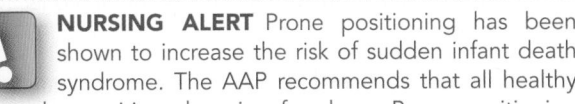

NURSING ALERT Prone positioning has been shown to increase the risk of sudden infant death syndrome. The AAP recommends that all healthy infants be positioned supine for sleep. Prone positioning offers some advantage for oxygenation in preterm neonate with respiratory compromise. During the initial phase of illness, these infants are cared for with cardiorespiratory monitoring and may be placed prone according to your facility's policy. Before discharge, these neonates should become accustomed to sleeping supine and supine positioning should be reinforced with the neonate's care providers.

11. Provide oxygen therapy with moisture in the percentage necessary to maintain appropriate blood gas values.

    a. Monitor oxygen with analyzer continuously to ensure consistency in percentage used.

    b. Pulse oximeter correlates well with oxygen (O_2) saturation of arterial hemoglobin of the blood.

12. Monitor for apnea (pauses more than 20 seconds) versus periodic breathing (regular repetition of breathing pauses of less than 15 seconds, alternating with breaths of regularly increasing then decreasing amplitude for 10 to 15 seconds). Theophylline may be given to reduce apneic episodes.

13. Protect the infant from infection by following scrupulous handwashing policy, minimizing neonate's contact with unsterile equipment, and minimizing the number of people who come in contact with the neonate.

14. Provide good skin care using water for bathing, an approved emollient for the skin, avoiding adhesives, and providing adequate hydration.

15. Avoid cranial deformity by using gel head pillow, frequent turning, and upright position.

16. Protect the neonate's eyes from bright lights.

17. Continue to provide IV and oral feedings according to neonate's needs. Assist the mother with breast pumping, as needed, and encourage both parents to hold and feed infant.

18. Continue to monitor for complications, such as hypoglycemia, hyperglycemia, RDS (see page 1505), apnea, infection, hypocalcemia, cardiac abnormalities, necrotizing enterocolitis, intracranial hemorrhage, and hyperbilirubinemia. Long-term complications may include retinopathy of prematurity, chronic lung disease, hearing loss, and learning disabilities.

19. Do not neglect the needs of the parents. Instead, make every effort to include them in the infant's care and update them frequently on the infant's condition.

Postmature Infant

Evidence Base Kattwinkle, J. (2011). Endotracheal intubation and laryngeal mask airway insertion. In American Academy of Pediatrics & American Heart Association, *Textbook of neonatal resuscitation* (6th ed., pp. 159–210). Chicago: American Academy of Pediatrics.

McGrath, J. M., & Hardy, W. (2011). The infant at risk. In S. Mattson & J. E. Smith (Eds.), *Core curriculum for maternal-newborn nursing* (4th ed., pp. 362–416). St. Louis, MO: Saunders Elsevier.

The postmature newborn infant is one whose gestation is 42 weeks or longer and who may show signs of weight loss with placental insufficiency.

Pathophysiology and Etiology

1. Cause is not known in many cases. Maternal factors associated with postmaturity include primigravida and high-parity mother at any given age and prolonged gestation in preceding pregnancies.
2. The postmature infant appears to have suffered from intrauterine malnutrition and hypoxia. Before the termination of the pregnancy, but at the point when the birth should have occurred, the placental function begins to diminish, resulting in impaired oxygen exchange and inadequate nutrient transfer to the fetus.
3. There are stages of postmaturity—severity of associated problems is determined by length of gestation (ie, the longer the gestation, the more severe the problems).

Nursing Assessment and Interventions

1. Be alert for the physical appearance of a postmature neonate. The following characteristics are most commonly seen in a neonate of 42 weeks' gestation or more:
   a. Reduced subcutaneous tissue—loose skin, especially of buttocks and thighs.
   b. Long, curved fingernails and toenails.
   c. Reduced amount of vernix caseosa.
   d. Abundant scalp hair.
   e. Wrinkled, macerated skin; possibly pale, cracked, parchment-like skin.
   f. Having the alert appearance of a 2- to 3-week-old neonate after delivery.
   g. Greenish yellow staining of skin, fingernails, or cord, indicating fetal distress.
2. Determine gestational age by physical examination. Measure weight, length, and head circumference and plot on Colorado intrauterine growth chart. Compare percentiles.
3. Determine blood sugar; below 40 mg/100 mL indicates hypoglycemia.
4. Assess for asphyxia neonatorum by Apgar score and blood gas analysis.
5. Be alert for meconium aspiration; signs include:
   a. Thick meconium in amniotic fluid at delivery.
   b. Tachypnea, increasing signs of cyanosis; difficulty breathing, with need for ventilation.
   c. Tachycardia.
   d. Inspiratory nasal flaring and retraction of chest.
   e. Expiratory grunting.
   f. Increased anteroposterior diameter of the chest.
   g. Palpable liver.
   h. Crackles and rhonchi on chest auscultation.
   i. Concomitant cerebral irritation—jitteriness, hypotonia, seizures.
   j. X-ray—classic coarse, patchy, irregular pulmonary infiltrates ranging in severity.
   k. Additional signs: metabolic acidosis, hypotension, hypoglycemia, hypocalcemia.
6. Provide supportive treatment for meconium aspiration. The consistency of the meconium in the amniotic fluid (thin vs. thick) is no longer used to determine the need for tracheal suctioning. The indication for *selective* intubation and tracheal suctioning of an infant born through meconium aspiration syndrome includes any infant who is nonvigorous. The Neonatal Resuscitation Program (NRP) defines a nonvigorous infant as an infant who meets one or more of the following conditions: depressed respirations, depressed muscle tone, or heart rate below 100 beats/minute.
   a. Warmth—maintain thermally neutral environment so the infant uses fewer calories and less oxygen.
   b. Adequate oxygenation and humidification to maintain PaO_2 at 50 to 70 mm Hg.
   c. Respiratory support with ventilator; extracorporeal membrane oxygenation may be needed if persistent pulmonary hypertension of the neonate develops.
   d. Adequate administration of calories and fluid.
   e. Accurate monitoring of intake and output—assess possible alteration in kidney function caused by hypoxia.
   f. Administration of antibiotics prophylactically.

NURSING ALERT A contraindication to *selective* intubation and tracheal suctioning is apparent vigor. The NRP defines a vigorous infant as one with all of the following: strong respiratory effort, good muscle tone, or heart rate above 100 beats/minute.

7. Provide oral feeding or IV glucose soon after birth to treat or prevent hypoglycemia. If oral feedings are not contraindicated, they can begin 1 to 2 hours after birth. Monitor blood sugar every hour until condition stabilizes.
8. Be alert for persistent pulmonary hypertension of the newborn (PPHN)—physiologic disorder characterized by severe, labile cyanosis arising from persistent or return to suprasystemic pulmonary vascular resistance and pressure normally found in the fetus.
   a. Cyanosis, pronounced respiratory distress, murmur, and heart failure.
   b. Treatment is aggressive respiratory support in a tertiary care nursery.
9. Provide psychological support to the parents. Long-term sequelae common in the postmature infant are CNS problems.

Infant of Mother Who Has Diabetes

A mother may have overt diabetes or gestational diabetes. The severity of neonatal problems depends on the severity of the maternal diabetes. Also known as infant of diabetic mother (IDM).

Pathophysiology and Etiology

Hyperinsulinemia in utero, secondary to elevated maternal glucose levels, results in the following in the neonate:

1. Macrosomia/large for gestational age (LGA)—increased amount of body fat, not edema.
   a. Total body water is somewhat reduced at birth.
   b. High urine output during first 2 days of life, probably from freeing of intracellular water.
2. Hypoglycemia (defined as serum glucose < 40 mg/dL).
   a. Occurs within first ½ to 12 hours of life; may occur within minutes after birth.
   b. The neonate's response to glucose is excessive (ie, insulin blood level has a slight elevation, will drop and then peak within 1 hour). This response is probably caused by maternal hyperglycemia.
   c. The neonate's cord insulin levels may not be higher than in a normal infant unless a large amount of glucose is given.
   d. Neonate may be symptomatic, with blood sugars less than 20 mg/100 mL.
   e. When present, symptoms may include the following: lethargy; jitteriness; poor feeding; vomiting; pallor; apnea; irregular respirations; hypotonia; tremors; seizure activity; high-pitched cry.
3. Hypocalcemia (<7 mg/dL).
   a. Associated with prematurity, difficult labor and delivery, asphyxia at birth, and decreased functioning of parathyroid glands.
   b. Generally occurs during the first 24 to 72 hours of life.
   c. Tremors constitute the clinical sign and may be secondary to prematurity or the stress of a difficult pregnancy, labor, and birth.
   d. Can also have hypomagnesemia (<1.4 mg/dL) resulting from functional hypoparathyroidism due to maternal magnesium loss.
4. Polycythemia and hyperbilirubinemia.
   a. Most likely to occur within 48 to 72 hours after birth.
   b. Immature liver results in inability to conjugate bilirubin.
   c. Hematocrit is higher on the third day after birth and extracellular volume is decreased.
   d. Because of large size, birth trauma may increase risk of enclosed hemorrhage.
   e. Prematurity.
   f. May be premature or small for gestational age when associated with placental insufficiency in some cases.
   g. Respiratory function is similar to that of other premature neonates. Thus, neonate is prone to RDS.
5. Polycythemia.
   a. Venous hematocrit greater than 65% or venous hemoglobin 22 g/100 mL.
   b. Polycythemia increases the risks of occurrence of renal vein thrombosis, respiratory distress, hypoglycemia, and hypocalcemia.
6. Congenital anomalies.
   a. Increased incidence of congenital anomalies may be caused by:
      i. Divergent gene pattern.
      ii. Glucose homeostasis in utero.
      iii. Episodes of ketoacidosis in early pregnancy.
   b. Common anomalies are renal and CNS anomalies, caudal regression syndrome, facial clefts, patent ductus arteriosus, transposition of the great vessels, ventricular septal defect, and small colon syndrome.
7. Infection.
   a. Prematurity and lowered passive immunity.
   b. Possible maternal UTI and bacteria crossing the placenta.

Nursing Assessment and Interventions

1. Be alert for typical appearance of IDM—macrosomia, cardiomegaly, hepatomegaly, large umbilical cord and placenta, plethora, full-face, tendency to be large for gestational age (some may be normal weight or small for gestational age), abundant fat, abundant hair, liberally coated with vernix caseosa, and hypertrichosis pinnae (excessive hair growth on the external ear).
2. Assist with diagnostic evaluation of the infant.
   a. Maternal history of diabetes.
   b. Physical assessment of neonate and determination of gestational age.
   c. Laboratory tests—serum glucose, calcium, phosphorus, magnesium, electrolytes, bilirubin, arterial blood gas analysis, blood hemoglobin, and hematocrit.
3. Monitor for hypoglycemia.
   a. Monitor serum glucose levels every 30 to 60 minutes beginning immediately after birth for 24 hours, then every 4 to 8 hours until stabilized.
   b. May be asymptomatic or may show signs of jitteriness, tremors, convulsions, sweating, cyanosis, weak or high-pitched cry, refusal to eat, hypotonia, apnea, temperature instability.
   c. Hypoglycemia may be prevented or treated by early feedings of 10% glucose or formula by nipple or gavage, if plasma glucose less than 36 mg/dL. If less than 25 mg/dL, will require an IV solution with appropriate glucose concentration. Maintain glucose levels above 45 mg/dL. In neonates with profound, recurrent, or persistent hyperinsulinemic hypoglycemia, serum glucose levels should remain above 60 mg/dL.
4. Monitor neonate closely for changes in acid-base status, respiratory distress, temperature instability, hypocalcemia, and sepsis.
5. Observe for hyperbilirubinemia.
   a. Neonates of mothers with diabetes have a higher incidence of hyperbilirubinemia. Levels will be elevated 48 to 72 hours after birth.
   b. The neonate may need an exchange transfusion at relatively lower bilirubin levels (as in the premature infant) to

prevent kernicterus. Phototherapy may need to be initiated early.

6. Monitor intake and output, ensure adequate fluid intake, and assess for dehydration.

7. Observe for possible cardiac anomalies and secondary heart failure.

8. Observe for other complications, including RDS, renal vein thrombosis, infection, hypermagnesemia or hypomagnesemia, birth injuries (encephalohematomas, facial nerve paralysis, fractured clavicles, brachial nerve plexus injuries), prematurity, asphyxia neonatorum, and organomegaly.

9. Support the family, especially the mother, who may feel guilty about being responsible for the neonate's problems.

Jaundice in the Newborn (Hyperbilirubinemia)

 Evidence Base American College of Obstetricians and Gynecologists. (2008/Reaffirmed 2011). Late-preterm infants (Committee Opinion #404). Washington, DC: Author.

Hyperbilirubinemia (jaundice) in the neonate is an accumulation of serum bilirubin above normal levels. Onset of clinical jaundice is seen when serum bilirubin levels are 5 to 7 mg/100 dL. Jaundice appears first on the face and progresses and serum bilirubin levels increase. *Kernicterus* is a yellow discoloration of specific areas of brain tissue by unconjugated bilirubin; can be confirmed only by death and autopsy. Bilirubin encephalopathy best describes the occurrence of the syndrome and the accompanying neurologic sequela in neonates.

Pathophysiology and Etiology

Causes

1. Increased bilirubin load.
   a. Hemolytic disease—Rh and ABO incompatibility.
   b. Morphologic abnormalities of RBCs.
   c. RBC enzyme defects.
   d. Physiologic jaundice.
   e. Sepsis.
2. Extravascular blood.
   a. Cephalohematoma.
   b. Pulmonary or cerebral hemorrhage.
   c. Any enclosed occult blood.
3. Decrease or inhibition of bilirubin conjugation.
   a. Inherited bilirubin conjugation defect: Crigler-Najjar syndrome (deficiency of glucuronyl transferase).
   b. Acquired bilirubin conjugation defect: breast-milk jaundice, Lucey-Driscoll syndrome, IDM, asphyxiated infant with respiratory distress.
4. Increased extrahepatic circulation.
   a. Intestinal obstruction.
5. Polycythemia.
   a. Twin–twin transfusion.
   b. Maternal–fetal transfusion.

c. IDM.
d. Infant small for gestational age.

6. Hypothyroidism.
7. Familial, transient—associated with inhibiting factor in plasma.
8. Unknown.
9. Obstructive disorders.
10. Intrauterine infection.

Physiologic Jaundice

1. Increased load of bilirubin on liver cells.
   a. Increased bilirubin production—more rapid hemolysis because of higher level of circulating RBCs per kg of body weight and a shorter RBC life span.
   b. Enterohepatic circulation—reabsorption of unconjugated bilirubin.
2. Decreased clearance of bilirubin from plasma.
   a. Predominant bilirubin-binding protein in liver cells may be deficient in the first days of life.
   b. Glucuronyl transferase enzyme activity may be decreased, resulting in impaired conjugation of bilirubin.
   c. Liver may show decreased ability to excrete large amounts of conjugated bilirubin.
   d. Poor portal blood supply may decrease the liver's capacity to act effectively.
3. Physiologic jaundice occurs 3 to 5 days after birth.
   a. Increase in unconjugated bilirubin levels; levels must not exceed 5 mg/100 dL per day.
   b. Full-term peak levels are reached 48 to 72 hours after birth; clinical jaundice declines in 1 week.
   c. Premature peak levels are reached by 5 to 6 days of age; clinical jaundice declines in 2 weeks.
   d. Jaundice progresses in head-to-toe fashion. A yellow hue can be seen on the face and on the abdomen with levels of 15 mg/dL and on the soles of the feet with levels of more than or equal to 20 mg/dL.
4. Pathologic unconjugated hyperbilirubinemia.
   a. Jaundice usually appears in first 24 hours of life.
   b. Total serum bilirubin usually increases >5 mg/dL/day; total serum bilirubin > 12.9 mg/dL in term infant or 15 mg/dL in preterm infant.
   c. Direct serum bilirubin usually exceeds 1 to 2 mg/dL.

Erythrocyte Destruction

1. Erythroblastosis fetalis (isoimmunization caused by Rh factor or ABO incompatibility).
   a. Immune hemolysis or Rh/ABO blood group incompatibility; the mother's and fetus's blood are different. Rh factor; different ABO blood groups (see Coombs' test, page 1249).
   b. Mother produces antibodies against the antigen of the fetus's blood. Fetal cells frequently cross the placenta.
   c. Antibodies of the mother's blood are in the infant's blood at birth, causing hemolysis of the neonate's red blood cells, leading to a rising level of indirect bilirubin.

2. Glucose-6-phosphate dehydrogenase deficiency—nonimmune hemolytic disease (erythrocyte biochemical factor).
   a. Deficiency results in reduced stability to oxidative destruction from substances that act as oxidizing agents (ie, vitamin K, naphthalene, salicylates).
   b. X-linked recessive disease that affects primarily black and Mediterranean-Asian groups.
   c. Screen maternal blood for carrier state and screen neonatal blood in high-risk groups.
3. Other conditions associated with increased erythrocyte destruction:
   a. Infection—bacterial, viral, or protozoan.
   b. Structural abnormal erythrocyte.
   c. Sequestered blood (ie, cephalohematoma, ecchymoses).

Nursing Assessment and Interventions

1. Be alert for signs and symptoms of jaundice:
   a. Sclerae appears yellow before skin appears yellow.
   b. Skin appears light to bright yellow or orange.
   c. Lethargy.
   d. Dark amber, concentrated urine.
   e. Poor feeding.
   f. Dark stools.
2. Make observations in daylight, sunlight, or white fluorescent light.
   a. Blanch the skin during the observation to clear away capillary coloration: forehead, cheeks, and clavicle sites allow for clear view.
   b. Be alert to the neonate's age in connection with the appearance of jaundice.
   c. With dark-skinned neonates, observing the color of the sclera and buccal mucosa is useful.
3. Assist with treatment.
   a. Fluids—ensure adequate hydration.
   b. Exchange transfusion—mechanically remove bilirubin.
   c. Phototherapy—allow for utilization of alternative pathways for bilirubin excretion.
   d. Enzyme induction agent—reduce bilirubin levels by inducing hepatic enzyme system involved in bilirubin clearance (ie, phenobarbital).
4. Provide nursing care related to phototherapy.
   a. Photoisomerization of tissue bilirubin occurs when the neonate is exposed to 420 to 460 nm of light.
   b. Check light intensity for therapeutic range daily. Use commercial Bili light.
   c. Have the neonate completely undressed so entire skin surface is exposed to light.
   d. Keep the neonate's eyes covered, unless using a Bili blanket, to protect from constant exposure to high-intensity light, which may cause retinal injury.
   e. Shield gonads.
   f. Develop a systematic schedule of turning neonate so all body surfaces are exposed (ie, every 2 hours).
   g. Maintain thermo-neutrality—light affects the ambient temperature.
   h. Shield the neonate (by Plexiglas) from direct exposure to lights.
   i. Obtain bilirubin levels, as directed. The diminishing icterus (ie, the lowering of unconjugated bilirubin from cutaneous tissue) does not reflect the serum bilirubin concentration. Lights should be turned off when blood is being collected to eliminate false-low bilirubin levels.
   j. If possible, remove the neonate from under the lights, remove eye covers, and encourage parents to hold the neonate for feedings.
   k. A fiber-optic blanket, which delivers continuous phototherapy by wrapping light around the neonate's torso, may be used. This method allows the neonate to remain in the mother's room in an open crib. Encourage the mother to remove the infant from the bili blanket, remove eye covers, and hold for feedings.

 NURSING ALERT If priapism (abnormally persistent erection of the penis) occurs during phototherapy, turn the neonate on his abdomen for short periods of time and this will cease.

Septicemia Neonatorum

Septicemia neonatorum (sepsis of the neonate) is a generalized infection that is characterized by the proliferation of bacteria in the bloodstream and commonly involves the meninges (as distinguished from simple bacteremia, congenital infection, septicemia after major diseases or surgery, or major congenital anomalies). High mortality.

Pathophysiology and Etiology

1. The distribution of etiologic agents varies from year to year and from facility to facility.
   a. Gram-negative organisms include *Escherichia coli*, *Klebsiella* (Enterobacteriaceae), *Pseudomonas*, *Proteus*, *Salmonella*, *Hemophilus influenzae*.
   b. Gram-positive organisms include group B beta-hemolytic *Streptococcus*, *Listeria monocytogenes*, *Staphylococcus aureus* (coagulase-negative and coagulase-positive), *Staphylococcus epidermidis*, *Streptococcus pneumoniae*, *Streptococcus faecalis*.
2. Fungal infections from the organism *Candida albicans* are increasing in incidence, especially in the low-birth-weight neonate.
3. Predisposing factors include a wide range of maternal perinatal complications; iatrogenic factors, such as use of catheters, oxygen, and resuscitative equipment; and infant complications, such as prematurity, congenital anomalies, RDS, skin infections, and asphyxia.
4. Infection occurs because of a temporary breakdown or depression of the neonate's defense mechanism for an unknown reason.
5. Risk factors for bacterial infection: prematurity, premature rupture of membranes (≥ 12 hours), foul-smelling amniotic fluid, maternal temperature; urinary tract infection with group B *Streptococci*, low socioeconomic status, no or limited prenatal care, or antenatal or intrapartum asphyxia.

Nursing Assessment and Interventions

1. Be alert for early signs of sepsis, which are usually vague and subtle.
   a. Poor feeding; gastric retention; weak sucking.
   b. Lethargy, limpness; weak crying, irritability.
   c. Temperature alteration—generally hypothermia, but infant may have hyperthermia or temperature instability.
   d. Hypoglycemia or hyperglycemia.
   e. Tachycardia (due to inability to change contractility of heart).
   f. Decreased perfusion and pulses.
2. Assist with diagnostic tests.
   a. Cultures from the blood, urine, spinal fluid, skin lesions, nose, throat, rectum, gastric fluid.
   b. WBC and differential, hemoglobin, hematocrit. Be alert for neutrophils < 5000 cells/mm³ or >25,000 cells/mm³; absolute neutrophil count < 1800 cells mm³; immature/total neutrophils > 0.2; platelets < 150,000.
   c. Blood chemistries—glucose, calcium, pH, electrolytes.
   d. C-reactive protein and erythrocyte sedimentation rate.
   e. Acid-base studies (acidosis).
   f. Bilirubin.
   g. TORCH (toxoplasmosis–rubella–cytomegalic inclusion virus–herpes–other) detects antibodies against common intrauterine-infective agents.
   h. Arterial blood gases.
   i. Chest x-ray—may demonstrate pulmonary infection.
   j. Urinalysis.
   k. CSF: look for protein 150 to 200 mg/L term and 300 mg/L preterm; Glucose: 50% to 60% or more of blood glucose level.
3. Assist with treatment.
   a. Before the specific organism is identified and after cultures have been obtained, the antibacterial therapy is based on the more common causative agents and their anticipated susceptibilities.
   b. Supportive therapy includes observation, isolation, hydration, nutrition, oxygen, regulation of thermal environment, blood transfusion to correct anemia and shock, and protection from further infection.
4. Observe for complications, such as meningitis (very common), shock, adrenal hemorrhage, disseminated intravascular coagulation, PPHN, metabolic derangements, seizures, pneumonia, UTI, and heart failure.

Infant of Substance-Abusing Mother

Maternal abuse of such substances as drugs, alcohol, and tobacco may have an impact on the growth, development, and well-being of her fetus or neonate. Working mechanisms include direct toxic effects on fetal circulation and CNS (heroin/cocaine), indirect toxic effects affecting placental circulation (alcohol and marijuana), and both direct or indirect toxic effects (polydrug use).

Pathophysiology and Etiology

1. Drugs and alcohol cross the placental barrier and enter the fetal circulation. The supply to the neonate is abruptly terminated at delivery, causing withdrawal symptoms.
2. Fetal alcohol syndrome is direct ethanol toxicity to the developing fetus. Additional effects on the fetus come from maternal malnutrition, maternal hypoglycemia, smoking, and alcohol-induced illness (ie, gastric hemorrhage, cirrhosis of liver).
3. Cocaine is a CNS stimulant that results in increased norepinephrine levels, which leads to vasoconstriction, tachycardia, hypertension, and uterine contractions; may lead to cerebral hemorrhage. This can result in fetal complications such as decreased uterine blood flow, increased fetal mean arterial pressure, increased FHR, decreased fetal oxygen, and damage to fetal brain transmitters.
4. The long-term biologic effects on the neonate of a drug-dependent mother are not fully known.
5. These children may have:
   a. Abnormal psychomotor development associated with intrauterine growth restriction due to the decreased perfusion/blood flow.
   b. Behavioral disturbances, such as hyperactivity, brief attention spans, temper tantrums, and seizures, due to exposure to large doses of the drug.
   c. Fetal anoxia (due to decrease perfusion) and meconium aspiration, prematurity (due to uterine hypertension and hyperirritability), and a wide variety of complications to include but not limited to limb reduction defects, uterine tract anomalies such as urethral obstruction malformation, prune belly syndrome, or hydronephrosis.
   d. Neurodevelopmental abnormalities due to damage to the fetal brain neurotransmitters; this may be permanent.
6. Infants and children with fetal alcohol syndrome may develop intellectual impairment, poor fine motor control, difficulty feeding, hyperactivity, delay of gross motor skills, and brain dysfunction.
7. Complications of cocaine abuse include spontaneous abortion, premature labor, abruptio placentae, uterine rupture, meconium staining, congenital anomalies, and neonatal death.

Nursing Assessment and Interventions

1. Obtain maternal history of drug, dosage, time of last dose. Be alert for onset of symptoms of opioid withdrawal.
   a. Heroin—several hours after birth to 3 to 4 days of life.
   b. Methadone—7 to 10 days after birth to several weeks of life.
   c. Cardinal signs of neonatal opioid withdrawal include coarse, flapping tremors; irritability; hyperactivity; hypertonicity; persistent high-pitched cry; restlessness; sleepiness.
2. Be alert for fetal alcohol syndrome.
   a. Difficulty establishing respirations.
   b. Metabolic problems.
   c. Irritability.

d. Increased muscle tone, tremulousness.

e. Lethargy.

f. Opisthotonos.

g. Poor sucking reflex.

h. Abdominal distention.

i. Seizure activity.

j. Facial abnormalities.

3. Be alert for neonate born to mother of cocaine abuse—does not appear to experience classic neonatal abstinence syndrome. Instead, may exhibit:

a. Mild tremulousness.

b. Increased irritability and startle response.

c. Muscular rigidity.

d. Difficulty in being consoled.

e. Pronounced state of lability.

f. Tachycardia and tachypnea.

g. Poor tolerance for oral feedings, diarrhea.

h. Disturbed sleep pattern.

4. Collect urine for toxicology screen within 24 hours after birth. Obtain blood gases, blood glucose, and other laboratory tests, as indicated, including meconium stools sent for toxicology screen.

5. Administer medications, as directed.

a. Opioid antagonist such as naloxone for opioid-induced respiratory depression at birth. There has been a report of seizures secondary to acute opioid withdrawal after administration to a baby born to an opioid user, so use with caution.

b. Drug therapy for alleviation of signs of opioid withdrawal. Duration of therapy using decreasing dosages may be from 4 to 40 days.

    i. Paregoric (camphorated tincture of opium) orally.

    ii. Phenobarbital orally.

    iii. Chlorpromazine orally.

    iv. Diazepam I.M.

    v. Methadone.

6. Provide nursing care to support infant and to relieve symptoms.

a. Irritability and restlessness, high-pitched crying.

    i. Loosely swaddle (may increase infant's temperature).

    ii. Minimize handling.

    iii. Decrease environmental stimuli (ie, light, noise).

    iv. Organize care to allow for periods of uninterrupted sleep.

    v. Prone positioning may help the infant organize motor movements.

    vi. Give medications with meals unless patient vomits; then 30 minutes before.

b. Floppy tremors—protect skin from irritation and abrasions.

    i. Change position frequently.

    ii. Give good, frequent skin care—keep the neonate clean and dry.

c. Frantic sucking—give pacifier between feedings; protect the neonate's hands from excoriation.

d. Poor feeding—give small, frequent feedings; maintain caloric and fluid intake requirement for the neonate's desired weight.

e. Vomiting/diarrhea—position the neonate to prevent aspiration; provide good skin care to areas exposed to vomitus or stools.

f. Muscle rigidity, hypertonicity.

    i. Change position frequently to minimize development of pressure areas.

    ii. Use sheepskin and provide good skin care.

g. Increased salivation and nasal stuffiness.

    i. Aspirate nasopharynx; suction tracheal mucus.

    ii. Provide frequent nose and mouth care.

    iii. Note respiration rate and characteristics and infant's color.

h. Tachypnea.

    i. Note onset and severity of accompanying signs of respiratory distress; place the infant on respiratory monitor.

    ii. Position the infant for easier ventilation—semi-Fowler's position; tilt head back slightly.

    iii. Minimize handling.

    iv. Have resuscitative equipment available.

i. Tachycardia and hypertension—monitor vital signs closely; cardiopulmonary monitor may be indicated.

7. Assist mother in learning to care for neonate, in efforts to promote bonding, and in her own alcohol or drug rehabilitation efforts.

8. Obtain further information and resources from March of Dimes Birth Defects Foundation (*www.modimes.org*).

SELECTED REFERENCES

American Academy of Pediatrics. (2010). Policy statement: Hospital stay for healthy term newborns. Elk Grove Village, IL: Author.

American Academy of Pediatrics. (2010). Policy statement: Hospital stay for healthy term newborns. *Pediatrics, 125*(2), 403–409.

American Academy of Pediatrics & American College of Obstetricians and Gynecologists. (2007). *Guidelines for perinatal care* (6th ed.). Elk Grove Village, IL: Authors.

American Academy of Pediatrics, Newborn Screening Task Force. (2000). Newborn screening: A blueprint for the future. *Pediatrics, 106*(2), 389–427.

American Academy of Pediatrics, Task Force on Sudden Infant Death Syndrome and Other Sleep-Related Infant Deaths. (2005). The changing concepts of sudden infant death syndrome: Diagnostic coding shifts, controversies regarding the sleeping environment and new variables to consider risk. *Pediatrics, 116*(5), 1245–1255

American Academy of Pediatrics, Task Force on Sudden Infant Death Syndrome and Other Sleep-Related Infant Deaths (2011). Expansion of recommendations for a safe infant sleeping environment. *Pediatrics, 128*(5), 1341–1367.

American College of Obstetricians and Gynecologists. (2007/Reaffirmed 2011). *Breastfeeding: Maternal and infant aspects* (Committee Opinion No. 361). Washington, DC: Author.

American College of Obstetricians and Gynecologists. (2008/Reaffirmed 2009). *Use of psychiatric medications during pregnancy and lactation* (Practice Bulletin #92). Washington, DC: Author.

American College of Obstetricians and Gynecologists. (2008/Reaffirmed 2011). Late-preterm infants (Committee Opinion #404). Washington, DC: Author.

American College of Obstetricians and Gynecologists. (2008). *Planning your pregnancy and birth* (3rd ed.). Washington, DC: Author.

American College of Obstetricians and Gynecologists & American Academy of Pediatrics. (2007). Neonatal complications. In *Guidelines for perinatal care* (pp. 251–301). Washington, DC: Authors.

Armentrout, D. (2010). Glucose management. In M. T. Verklan & M. Walden (Eds.), *Core curriculum for neonatal intensive care nursing* (4th ed., pp. 172–181). St. Louis, MO: Saunders Elsevier.

Askin, D. F. (2003). Chest and lungs assessment. In E. P. Tappero & M. E. Honeyfield (Eds.), *Physical assessment of the newborn* (3rd ed., pp. 69–80. Santa Rosa, CA: NICU Ink.

Association of Women's Health, Obstetrics, and Neonatal Nurses. (2006). *Compendium of postpartum care* (2nd ed.). New Brunswick, NJ: Johnson & Johnson Pediatric Institute.

Ballard, J. L., Khoury, J. C., Wedig, K., et al. (1991). New Ballard score, expanded to include extremely premature infants. *Journal of Pediatrics, 119*, 417–423.

Beck, C. T. (1993). Teetering on the edge: A substantive theory of postpartum depression. *Nursing Research, 44*, 293–304.

Bigelow, A., Power, M., MacLellan-Peters, J., et al. (2012). Effect of Mother/Infant Skin-to-Skin Contact on Postpartum Depressive Symptoms and Maternal Physiological Stress. *Journal of Obstetric, Gynecologic, & Neonatal Nursing, 41*(3), 369–382.

Bond, L. (2011). Physiology of pregnancy. In S. Mattson & J. E. Smith (Eds.), *Core curriculum for maternal-newborn nursing* (4th ed., pp. 80–100). St. Louis, MO: Saunders Elsevier.

Bradshaw, W. T. (2010). Gastrointestinal disorders. In M. T. Verklan & M. Walden (Eds.), *Core curriculum for neonatal intensive care nursing* (4th ed., pp. 589–637). St. Louis, MO: Saunders Elsevier.

Brooten, D., Youngblut, J. M., Golembeski, S., et al. (2012). Perceived weight gain, risk, and nutrition in pregnancy in five racial groups. *Journal of the American Academy of Nurse Practitioners, 24*(1), 32–42.

Cary, B. E. (2003). Neurologic assessment. In E. P. Tappero & M. E. Honeyfield (Eds.), *Physical assessment of the newborn* (3rd ed., pp. 149–172). Santa Rosa, CA: NICU Ink.

Cavaliere, T. A. (2003). Genitourinary assessment. In E. P. Tappero & M. E. Honeyfield (Eds.), *Physical assessment of the newborn* (3rd ed., pp. 107–124). Santa Rosa, CA: NICU Ink.

Charsa, D. S. (2010). Care of the extremely low birth weight infant. In M. T. Verklan & M. Walden (Eds.), *Core curriculum for neonatal intensive care nursing* (4th ed., pp. 434–446). St. Louis, MO: Saunders Elsevier.

Cheffer, N. D., & Rannalli, D. A. (2011). Transitional care of the newborn. In S. Mattson & J. E. Smith (Eds.), *Core curriculum for maternal-newborn nursing* (4th ed.), pp. 345–361). St. Louis, MO: Saunders Elsevier.

Cunningham, F. G., Leveno, K. J., Bloom, S. L., et al. (2010). Postterm pregnancy. In *Williams obstetrics* (23rd ed., pp. 832–841). New York: McGraw-Hill.

Cunningham, F. G., Leveno, K. J., Bloom, S. L., et al. (2010). Puerperal infection. In *Williams obstetrics* (23rd ed., pp. 661–672). New York: McGraw-Hill.

Cunningham, F. G., Leveno, K. J., Bloom, S. L., et al. (2010). The puerperium. In *Williams obstetrics* (23rd ed., pp. 646–660). New York: McGraw-Hill.

Furdon, S. A., & Benjamin, K. (2010). Physical assessment. In M. T. Verklan & M. Walden (Eds.), *Core curriculum for neonatal intensive care nursing* (4th ed., pp. 135–172). St. Louis, MO: Saunders Elsevier.

Goodwin, M. (2003). Abdomen assessment. In E. P. Tappero & M. E. Honeyfield (Eds.), *Physical assessment of the newborn* (3rd ed., pp. 97–106). Santa Rosa, CA: NICU Ink.

Greenberg, J. M., Narendran, V., Schibler, K. R., et al. (2009). Neonatal morbidities of prenatal and perinatal origin. In R. K. Creasy, R. Resnick, J. D. Iams, et al. (Eds.), *Maternal-fetal medicine* (6th ed., pp. 1197–1228). Philadelphia: Saunders.

Hockenberry, M. J. (2010). Communication and physical assessment of the child. In M. J. Hockenberry & D. Wilson (Eds.), *Wong's nursing care of infants and children* (9th ed., pp. 1117–1178). St. Louis, MO: Elsevier Mosby.

Hockenberry, M. J. (2010). Family influence on child health promotion. In M. J. Hockenberry & D. Wilson (Eds.), *Wong's nursing care of infants and children* (9th ed., pp. 46–67). St. Louis, MO: Elsevier Mosby.

Hummel, P. (2010). Discharge planning and transition to home care. In M. T. Verklan & M. Walden (Eds.), *Core curriculum for neonatal intensive care nursing* (4th ed., pp. 383–398). St. Louis, MO: Saunders Elsevier.

Hudak, M., & Tan, R. C. (1998/Reaffirmed 2012). American Academy of Pediatrics (APP), Committee on Drugs and Committee on Fetus and Newborn. Elk Grove Village, IL: American Academy of Pediatrics.

Iams, J. D., Romero, R., & Creasy, R. K. (2009). Preterm labor and birth. In R. K. Creasy, R. Resnick, J. D. Iams, et al. (Eds.), *Maternal-fetal medicine* (6th ed., pp. 545–582). Philadelphia: Saunders Co.

Intermountain Utah Valley Regional Medical Mother/Baby Unit. (2010). Assessment of the new mother & baby [DVD/CD]. Salt Lake City, UT: Concept Media.

Jacob, E. (2010). Pain assessment and management in children. In M. J. Hockenberry & D. Wilson (Eds.), *Wong's nursing care of infants and children* (9th ed., pp. 179–226). St. Louis, MO: Elsevier Mosby.

Johnson, C. B. (2003). Head, eyes, ears, nose, mouth, and neck assessment. In E. P. Tappero & M. E. Honeyfield (Eds.), *Physical assessment of the newborn* (3rd ed., pp. 55–68). Santa Rosa, CA: NICU Ink.

Kattwinkle, J. (2011). Endotracheal intubation and laryngeal mask airway insertion. In American Academy of Pediatrics & American Heart Association (Eds.), *Textbook of neonatal resuscitation* (6th ed., pp. 159–210). Chicago: American Academy of Pediatrics.

Landry, N., & Shviraga, B. (2010). Antepartum, intrapartum and transition to extrauterine life. In M. T. Verklan & M. Walden (Eds.), *Core curriculum for neonatal intensive care nursing* (4th ed., pp. 1–19). St. Louis, MO: Saunders Elsevier.

Lott, J. W. (2010). Immunology and infectious diseases. In M. T. Verklan & M. Walden (Eds.), *Core curriculum for neonatal intensive care nursing* (4th ed., pp. 694–723). St. Louis, MO: Saunders Elsevier.

McGrath, J. M., & Hardy, W. (2011). The infant at risk. In S. Mattson & J. E. Smith (Eds.), *Core curriculum for maternal-newborn nursing* (4th ed., pp. 362–414). St. Louis, MO: Saunders Elsevier.

Moore, T. R., & Catalano, P. (2009). Diabetes in pregnancy. In R. K. Creasy, R. Resnick, J. D. Iams, et al. (Eds.), *Maternal-fetal medicine* (6th ed., pp. 953–994). Philadelphia: Saunders.

Moran, B. A. (2010). Substance abuse in pregnancy. In S. Mattson & J. E. Smith (Eds.), *Core Curriculum for maternal-newborn nursing* (4th ed., pp. 573–586). St. Louis, MO: Saunders Elsevier.

Orr, S. S. (2011). Breastfeeding. In S. Mattson & J. E. Smith (Eds.), *Core curriculum for maternal neonatal nursing* (4th ed., pp. 315–334). St. Louis, MO: Saunders Elsevier.

Pappas, B. E., & Walker, B. (2010). Care of the late preterm infant. Hospital stay for healthy term newborns. In M. T. Verklan & M. Walden (Eds.), *Core curriculum for neonatal intensive care nursing* (4th ed., pp. 447–452). St. Louis, MO: Saunders Elsevier.

Pappas, B. E., & Walker, B. (2010). Neonatal delivery room resuscitation. In M. T. Verklan & M. Walden (Eds.), *Core curriculum for neonatal intensive care nursing* (4th ed., pp. 91–109). St. Louis, MO: Saunders Elsevier.

Pitts, K. (2010). Perinatal substance abuse. In M. T. Verklan & M. Walden (Eds.), *Core curriculum for neonatal intensive care nursing* (4th ed., pp. 41–71). St. Louis, MO: Saunders Elsevier.

Resnick, J. L., & Resnick, R. (2009). Post-term pregnancy. In R. K. Creasy, R. Resnick, J. D. Iams, et al. (Eds.) *Maternal-fetal medicine* (6th ed., pp. 613–618). Philadelphia: Saunders.

Rhode, M. A. (2011). Postpartum complications. In S. Mattson & J. E. Smith (Eds.), *Core curriculum for maternal-newborn nursing* (4th ed., pp. 650–666). St. Louis, MO: Saunders Elsevier.

Rubin, R. (1984). *Maternal identity and the maternal experience.* New York: Springer.

Schefelbien, J. (2010). Genetics: From bench to bedside. In M. T. Verklan & M. Walden (Eds.), *Core curriculum for neonatal intensive care nursing* (4th ed., pp. 399–414). St. Louis, MO: Saunders Elsevier.

Segre, L. S., O'Hara, M. W., Amdt, S., et al. (2010). Nursing care of postpartum depression, part 1: Do nurses think they should offer both screening and counseling? *Maternal Child Nursing, 35*(5), 280–285.

Segre, L. S., O'Hara, M. W., Amdt, S., et al. (2011). Screening and counseling for postpartum depression by nurses: The women's views, part 2. *Maternal Child Nursing, 35*(4), 220–225.

Sterk, L. (2010). Congenital anomalies. In M. T. Verklan & M. Walden (Eds.), *Core curriculum for neonatal intensive care nursing* (4th ed., pp. 782–812). St. Louis, MO: Saunders Elsevier.

Promoting Comfort

1. Instruct patient on the cause of pain to decrease anxiety.
2. Instruct and encourage the use of relaxation techniques to augment analgesics.
3. Administer pain medications, as needed and prescribed.

Community and Home Care Considerations

1. Review symptoms of hemorrhage if a threatened abortion is suspected.
2. Discuss an emergency access care plan with patient and support personnel.
3. Instruct the patient to collect any expelled specimen and to bring to facility with her for evaluation.

Patient Education and Health Maintenance

1. Provide the names of local support groups; Resolve Through Sharing groups may be available through a local hospital.
2. Discuss with the patient methods of contraception to be used.
3. Explain the need to wait 2 to 4 months before attempting another pregnancy.
4. Teach the woman to observe for signs of infection (fever, pelvic pain, change in character and amount of vaginal discharge) and advise to report to provider immediately.
5. Provide information regarding genetic testing of the products of conception, if indicated; send the specimen according to facility policy.

Evaluation: Expected Outcomes

- Vital signs remain normal; minimal blood loss.
- Expresses feelings regarding the loss of the pregnancy by demonstrating normal signs of grief.
- No signs of infection, temperature normal, performs perineal care.
- Verbalizes relief of pain.

Hyperemesis Gravidarum

 Evidence Base American College of Obstetricians and Gynecologists. (2004/Reaffirmed 2011). *Nausea and vomiting in pregnancy* (Practice Bulletin #52). Washington, DC: Author.

Hyperemesis gravidarum is exaggerated and persistent nausea and vomiting that occurs during pregnancy. It is a clinical diagnosis of exclusion based on a typical presentation in the absence of other diseases that could explain the findings, such as GI conditions, metabolic disease, neurologic disorders, drug use, or acute fatty liver or preeclampsia during pregnancy.

Pathophysiology and Etiology

1. Typically occurs during the first 16 weeks' gestation but may last into the third trimester in severe cases. Etiology is unknown, but two theories prevail: psychosomatic or hormonal stimulus (high levels of β-hCG or estrogen).
2. Accompanied by appetite disturbances that are intractable in nature.
3. Psychological factors, including neurosis or altered self-concept, may be contributory.
4. Seen in molar pregnancies, multiple gestation, and history of hyperemesis in previous pregnancies.
5. Decreased gastric motility often accompanies the condition.
6. Persistent vomiting may result in fluid and electrolyte imbalances, dehydration, jaundice, and elevation of serum transaminase.

Clinical Manifestations

1. Persistent vomiting; inability to tolerate anything by mouth.
2. Dehydration—fever, dry skin, decreased urine output, large ketonuria.
3. Weight loss (up to 5% to 10% of body weight).
4. Severity of symptoms commonly increases as the condition progresses.

Diagnostic Evaluation

1. Tests may be done to rule out other conditions causing vomiting (cholecystitis, appendicitis, pancreatitis, thyroid disease, or hepatitis).
2. Liver function studies—alanine aminotransferase (ALT) and aspartate transaminase (AST) are elevated four times normal in severe cases.
3. Prothrombin time (PT), partial thromboplastin time (PTT) usually normal.
4. Blood urea nitrogen (BUN) and creatinine—may be slightly elevated.
5. Serum electrolytes—may result in hypokalemia, hyponatremia, or hypernatremia; loss of hydrogen and chloride.
6. Ketones in blood and urine.

Management

1. Try withholding food and fluid for 24 to 48 hours or until vomiting stops and appetite returns; then restart small meals.
2. Control of vomiting may require anti-emetics (benefits to therapy may outweigh the risks of drugs), such as:
   a. Phenothiazines—prochlorperazine (injectable or rectal suppository); promethazine; or chlorpromazine.
   b. Droperidol.
   c. Metoclopramide—do not give in combination with phenothiazines.
   d. Meclizine.
   e. Methylprednisolone (recently found to be more helpful than promethazine; 16 mg three times per day for 3 days then tapered over 2 weeks).
3. Treat dehydration with IV fluids—typically 1 to 3 L of dextrose solution with electrolytes and vitamins, as needed.
4. Most women respond quickly to restricting oral intake and giving IV fluids, but repeated episodes may occur.
5. Total parenteral nutrition rarely needed.
6. Complications of hepatic or renal failure or coma could result from disease progression but rare.

Complications

1. Hypovolemia and renal insufficiency.
2. Electrolyte imbalance.
3. Malnutrition.

Nursing Assessment

1. Evaluate weight loss pattern; compare to prepregnant weight.
2. Evaluate 24- or 48-hour dietary recall.
3. Evaluate environmental factors that may affect the woman's appetite. Determine if woman is ingesting nonfood substances (pica), such as starch, clay, or toothpaste.
4. Monitor vital signs for tachycardia, hypotension, and fever due to dehydration.
5. Assess skin turgor and mucous membranes for signs of dehydration.

Nursing Diagnoses

- Risk for Deficient Fluid Volume related to prolonged vomiting.
- Imbalanced Nutrition: Less Than Body Requirements related to prolonged vomiting.
- Ineffective Coping related to stress of pregnancy and illness.
- Fear related to concerns for fetal well-being.

Nursing Interventions

Maintaining Fluid Volume

1. Establish an IV line and administer IV fluids, as prescribed.
2. Monitor serum electrolytes and report abnormalities.
3. Medicate with anti-emetics, as prescribed.
4. Maintain nothing-by-mouth status until vomiting has stopped; introduce ice chips slowly and add clear fluids once tolerated; solid food introduced later.
5. Assess intake and output, urine specific gravity and ketones, vital signs, skin turgor, and fetal heart rate (FHR), as indicated by condition.

Encouraging Adequate Nutrition

1. Advise the woman that oral intake can be restarted once emesis ceases and appetite returns.
2. Begin small bland meals (ie, rice and chicken). Avoid greasy, gassy, and spicy foods.

3. Suggest or provide an environment conducive to eating.
4. Administer parenteral calorie replacement if multiple anti-emetic treatments and enteral tube feeding have been unsuccessful.
5. Consult with a dietitian, as indicated.

Strengthening Coping Mechanisms

1. Allow patient to verbalize feelings regarding this pregnancy and associated stressors.
2. Refer the patient to social service and counseling services, as needed.

Allaying Fears

1. Explain the effects of all medications and procedures on maternal as well as fetal health.
2. Once confirmed, accentuate the positive signs of fetal well-being.
3. Praise and support patient for attempts at following nutritious diet and healthy lifestyle.

Patient Education and Health Maintenance

1. Educate the woman about proper diet, nutrition, and healthy weight gain.
2. Educate the woman on the need to take anti-emetics continuously during the nausea phase to alleviate vomiting episodes.

Evaluation: Expected Outcomes

- Demonstrates signs of normal hydration with no ketosis; urine output adequate; urine-specific gravity within normal limits; blood pressure (BP) stable.
- Tolerates clear liquids then small, bland diet without vomiting.
- Verbalizes concerns and stresses related to pregnancy.
- Expresses confidence in fetal well-being.

Placenta Previa

Placenta previa is the abnormal implantation of the placenta in the lower uterine segment, partially or completely covering the internal cervical os (Figure 39-2). Classification may change over

Figure 39-2. Degrees of placenta previa. (A) Low implantation. **(B)** Partial placenta previa. **(C)** Total placenta previa.

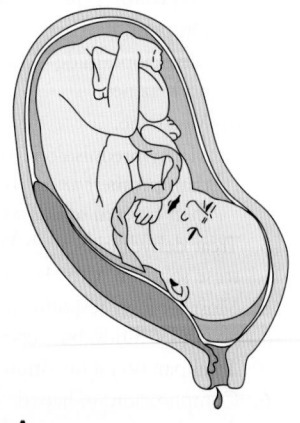
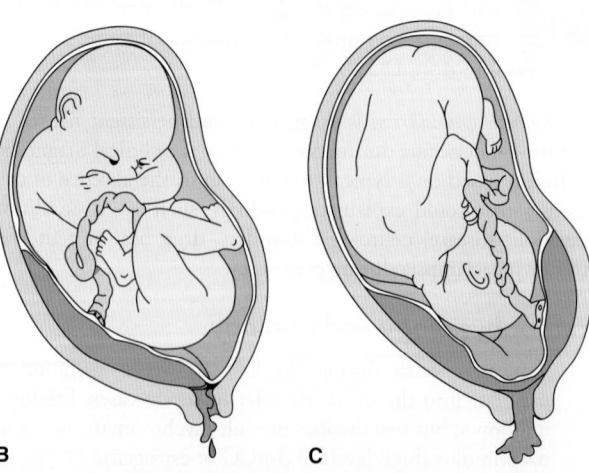

A   B   C

the course of the pregnancy or during labor as the cervix dilates. Placenta previa occurs in 1 in 200 live births and is associated with intrauterine growth restriction (IUGR).

Pathophysiology and Etiology

1. *Classifications* of placenta previa:
   a. Complete: placenta covers the cervical os completely.
   b. Partial: placenta partially covers the cervical os.
   c. Marginal: placenta lies at the margin of the internal os, but does not cover it.
   d. Low-lying placenta: placental implantation in the lower uterine segment next to the cervical os; the placenta may migrate and be pulled upward as the uterus stretches and grows during the course of the pregnancy.
2. *Causation* is unknown, but risk factors include:
   a. Previous myomectomy.
   b. Endometritis.
   c. Scarred uterus to include vaginal birth after cesarean delivery (VBAC).
   d. Induced or spontaneous abortions involving suction curettage.
   e. Advanced maternal age, multiparity, cigarette smoking.
   f. Fetal hydrops fetalis.
   g. Previous placenta previa.

Clinical Manifestations

1. Cardinal sign is sudden onset of painless vaginal bleeding during the second or third trimester; some women may not exhibit bleeding until labor starts.
2. Initial episode is rarely fatal and usually stops spontaneously.
3. With a complete placenta previa, bleeding typically occurs earlier in the pregnancy.

Diagnostic Evaluation

1. Ultrasound (transabdominal, transvaginal, or translabial) is the method of choice to show location of placental implantation.

Management

1. Conservative management is usually possible with nonviable pregnancy and maternal stability.
2. Once viable and fetal lung maturity is established, delivery may be attempted based on maternal–fetal status.
3. If bleeding is heavy, IV access should be established immediately, along with CBC, type, and crossmatching for blood component therapy, as indicated.
4. Typically in the medical facility setting, continuous maternal and fetal monitoring is necessary.
5. Cesarean delivery is usually indicated if maternal–fetal status unstable or complete previa.
6. Vaginal delivery may be attempted in a marginal or low-lying placenta without active bleeding. Operating room personnel should be available.
7. Notify neonatal team.

Complications

1. Placenta accreta (abnormally adherent placenta difficult to expel); increased incidence if placenta previa exists with maternal history of uterine surgery.
2. Immediate hemorrhage, possible shock, and maternal death.
3. Postpartum hemorrhage.
4. Prematurity.

Nursing Assessment

1. Estimate current episode of blood loss; review history of bleeding throughout current pregnancy.
2. Assess pain in association with the bleeding.
3. Assess maternal and fetal vital signs through electronic fetal monitoring (EFM).
4. Assess for symptoms of labor: preterm or term.
5. Evaluate laboratory data to assess signs of hemorrhage: hemoglobin and hematocrit.

 NURSING ALERT   Withhold vaginal examinations in patients with active vaginal bleeding until placenta previa (or other cause) has been ruled out; an examination may aggravate the condition.

Nursing Diagnoses

- Ineffective Tissue Perfusion: Placental related to excessive bleeding causing fetal compromise.
- Deficient Fluid Volume related to excessive bleeding.
- Risk for Infection Related to operative intervention or delivery.
- Anxiety related to excessive bleeding, procedures, and possible maternal–fetal complications.

Nursing Interventions

Promoting Tissue Perfusion

1. Monitor both the mother and fetus frequently; pulse, respirations, and BP should be taken as the patient's condition warrants; continuous EFM if fetus viable.
2. Administer IV fluids, as prescribed.
3. Prepare for emergency delivery and neonatal resuscitation, as needed.

Maintaining Fluid Volume

1. Establish and maintain one or two large-bore IV lines, as needed; obtain CBC, type and screen/cross for blood replacement, platelets, PT/PTT, fibrinogen. Repeat periodically as patient's condition warrants.
2. Assess bleeding periodically to note changes in frequency and volume.
3. Maintain strict bed rest during any bleeding episode in a lateral supine position.
4. If bleeding is profuse and delivery cannot be delayed, prepare for a cesarean delivery.
5. Administer blood component therapy, as necessary.

Preventing Infection

1. Use sterile technique when providing care.
2. Evaluate temperature and pulse periodically; if ruptured membranes, hypothermia, or hyperthermia, evaluate more frequently.

3. Evaluate white blood cell (WBC) and differential count.
4. Teach perineal care and handwashing techniques.
5. Assess for perineal odor after vaginal bleeding episodes.

Decreasing Anxiety

1. Explain all treatments and procedures; answer related questions to patient satisfaction.
2. Provide information on a cesarean delivery and prepare patient emotionally, if applicable.

Community and Home Care Considerations

1. Home care for patients with placenta previa and other antenatal bleeding disorders can occur if the following criteria are met:
   a. No active bleeding.
   b. No signs and symptoms of preterm labor (PTL).
   c. Home close to medical facility.
   d. Emergency support readily available.
2. Teach the woman signs and symptoms of hemorrhage; patient report to labor and delivery immediately if bleeding occurs.
3. Monitor vaginal discharge and bleeding after each urination and bowel movement.
4. Instruct the woman on home uterine activity monitoring, if ordered; use of palpation and electronic telemetry units included.
5. Instruct the woman on performing daily fetal movement counts (kick counts).
6. Antepartum testing may be increased, as indicated periodically.
7. Instruct the woman to have support persons readily available.
8. Instruct patient of the need for vaginal and sexual abstinence; discuss options.

Patient Education and Health Maintenance

1. Educate the woman and her family about the diagnosis, etiology, and treatment of placenta previa.
2. Educate the woman who is discharged from the hospital with placenta previa to avoid intercourse or inserting anything into her vagina, limit physical activity, have an accessible person in the event of an emergency, and report to the hospital immediately if repeat bleeding, more than six uterine contractions per hour, or decreased fetal movement.

Evaluation: Expected Outcomes

- Fetal condition stable.
- Absence of shock, stable vital signs, absence of bleeding.
- Absence of signs or symptoms of infection.
- Verbalizes concerns and understanding of procedures and treatments.

Abruptio Placentae

Abruptio placentae results from the premature separation of a normally implanted placenta before the birth of the fetus; typically occurs after 20 weeks' gestation. Classifications include partial, complete, or marginal (Figure 39-3). Hemorrhage can be concealed (occult/hidden) or revealed (exposed). During an occult hemorrhage, the placenta detaches from the center, leaving the edges attached; this offers a concealed area for blood to pool behind the placenta. Even though bleeding is not evident at the perineum, concealed hemorrhage is accompanied by constant cramping or general abdominal pain. Prompt intervention is warranted.

Pathophysiology and Etiology

1. Typically, the etiology is unknown, but risks include:
   a. History of abdominal trauma, prior cesarean birth, uterine anomalies (fibroids, septum).
   b. Maternal hypertension: 50% of placental abruptions are associated with some form of hypertension.
   c. Cigarette smoking, cocaine or amphetamine abuse.
   d. Thrombophilias, such as Factor V Leiden or antiphospholipid antibody.
   e. Previous history of abruptio placentae or partial abruption in current pregnancy.
   f. Rapid decompression of the uterus (reduction of fluid with polyhydramnios).
   g. Preterm premature rupture of membranes: less than 34 weeks.
2. Hemorrhage occurs into the decidua basalis behind the placenta and forms a hematoma. This hematoma will expand as

Figure 39-3. Abruptio placentae—premature separation of the placenta.

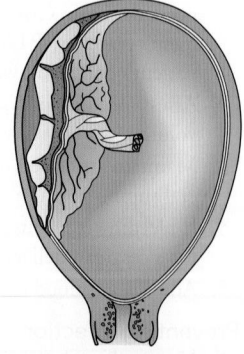
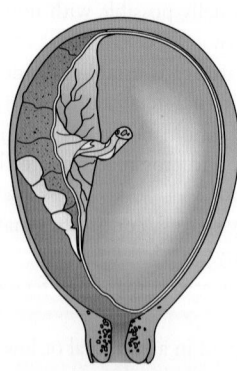
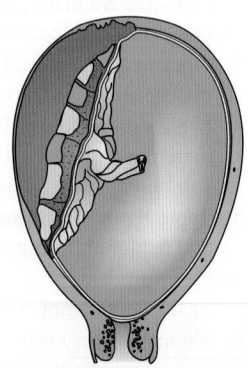

Partial Separation
(Concealed Hemorrhage)

Partial Separation
(Apparent Hemorrhage)

Complete Separation
(Concealed Hemorrhage)

bleeding increases; enlargement further detaches the placenta from the uterine wall.

Clinical Manifestations

1. Sudden-onset, intense, constant, generalized abdominal pain/tenderness with (revealed) or without (concealed) vaginal bleeding; approximately 10% of women present with concealed hemorrhage.
2. Uterine contractions are typically low amplitude and high frequency. Uterine baseline resting tone may be elevated over course of evolving abruption.
3. Changes in the FHR may commonly be the first sign of maternal hemodynamic imbalance. Category II or III patterns may evolve to include tachycardia or bradycardia, recurrent late decelerations with minimal or absent variability. Fetal response depends on amount of blood loss and extent of uteroplacental insufficiency present.
4. Patient may exhibit signs and symptoms of rapid labor progress and delivery.

Diagnostic Evaluation

1. Based on woman's history, physical examination, laboratory studies, EFM data, and signs and symptoms to include vaginal bleeding, abdominal pain, uterine contractions, uterine tenderness, and/or maternal–fetal distress. Presentations vary per patient.
2. Ultrasound is performed to exclude placenta previa, but may not be sensitive enough to diagnose or rule out abruptio placentae; EFM is frequently more accurate.
3. Kleihauer-Betke lab test may be ordered to determine maternal–fetal hemorrhage by assessing maternal blood for the presence of fetal RBCs.

Management

1. Management depends on maternal and fetal status and degree of bleeding. Any viable fetus and patient with suspected abruptio placentae should be admitted immediately and continuous EFM applied.
2. In fetal compromise, severe hemorrhage, coagulopathy, or increasing uterine activity dysfunction, emergent cesarean delivery is highly recommended.
3. If the mother is hemodynamically stable and the fetus is stable (normal FHR/UA data) or has an intrauterine fetal demise, vaginal delivery may be recommended.
4. If mother is hemodynamically unstable, she may need stabilization with IV/blood/blood products replacement to maintain urine output and appropriate hematocrit levels. With rapid infusion of fluids, monitor woman for signs/symptoms of pulmonary edema.
5. A neonatal specialty team is necessary at delivery due to prematurity and neonatal complications.

Complications

1. Maternal shock, DIC.
2. Anaphylactoid syndrome of pregnancy (formerly amniotic fluid embolism).
3. Postpartum hemorrhage.
4. Acute respiratory distress syndrome.
5. Sheehan's syndrome (postpartum pituitary necrosis).
6. Renal tubular necrosis.
7. Precipitous labor and delivery.
8. Prematurity.
9. Maternal or fetal death.

Nursing Assessment

See Table 39-2.

1. Determine the amount and type of bleeding along with the presence or absence of pain; labor pain is episodic whereas placental abruption pain is constant.
2. Monitor maternal and fetal vital signs, especially maternal BP, pulse, FHR, FHR characteristics, and uterine activity data.

Table 39-2	Characteristics of Abruptio Placentae and Placenta Previa	
CHARACTERISTIC	**ABRUPTIO PLACENTAE**	**PLACENTA PREVIA**
Onset	Third trimester	Third trimester (commonly at 32–36 weeks)
Bleeding	May be concealed, external dark hemorrhage, or bloody amniotic fluid	Mostly external, small to profuse in amount, bright red
Pain and uterine tenderness	Usually present; irritable uterus, progresses to boardlike consistency	Usually absent; uterus soft
Fetal heart tone	May be irregular or absent	Usually normal
Presenting part	May be engaged	Usually not engaged
Shock	Moderate to severe depending on extent of concealed and external hemorrhage	Usually not present unless bleeding is excessive
Delivery	Immediate delivery, usually cesarean delivery	Delivery may be delayed, depending on size of fetus and amount of bleeding

3. Palpate the abdomen.
   a. Note presence of contractions and note relaxation between each subsequent contraction.
   b. If contractions are not present, assess abdominal firmness (relaxed or tight).
4. Measure and record fundal height periodically to evaluate accumulation of concealed bleeding.
5. Prepare for possible delivery.

Nursing Diagnoses

- Ineffective Tissue Perfusion: Placental related to excessive bleeding, hypotension, and decreased cardiac output, causing maternal–fetal compromise.
- Deficient Fluid Volume related to excessive bleeding.
- Fear related to excessive bleeding, procedures, and unknown outcome.

Nursing Interventions

Maintaining Tissue Perfusion

1. Evaluate amount of bleeding by weight of pads (actual blood loss) and direct visualization, rather than estimated blood loss, particularly if moderate to severe. Monitor CBC results and vital signs.
2. Position in the left lateral position, with head elevated.
3. Administer oxygen via face mask at 8 to 10 L/minute. Maintain oxygen saturation level above 90% to 95%. Limit prolonged use, particularly if delivery is imminent.
4. Evaluate fetal status with continuous external fetal monitoring.
5. Encourage relaxation techniques.
6. Prepare for possible cesarean delivery if maternal or fetal compromise is evident.

Maintaining Fluid Volume

1. Establish and maintain one to two large-bore IV lines for fluids and blood component therapy, as prescribed.
2. Evaluate coagulation studies and intake and output totals.
3. Monitor maternal vital signs and uterine activity.
4. Monitor vaginal bleeding and evaluate fundal height to detect an increase in bleeding.

Decreasing Fear

1. Inform the woman and her family about maternal–fetal status frequently.
2. Explain all procedures in advance when possible or as they are performed.
3. Answer questions in a calm manner, using simple terms.
4. Encourage the presence of a support person.

Patient Education and Health Maintenance

1. Provide information regarding etiology and treatment for abruptio placentae.
2. Encourage involvement from the neonatal team regarding education related to fetal/neonatal outcome.
3. Teach high-risk women the signs and symptoms of placental abruption.
4. Instruct woman to report to labor and delivery immediately should excessive bleeding or constant pain occur at home.

5. Instruct woman to have emergency plan in place for transport to medical facility. It is important to have support persons aware of procedures as well.

Evaluation: Expected Outcomes

- FHR remains as Category I or II with minimal fetal deterioration noted.
- Absence of shock, demonstrated by stable maternal vital signs after initiation of treatment.
- Verbalizes concerns; asks questions.

Hypertensive Disorders of Pregnancy

Evidence Base American College of Obstetricians and Gynecologists. (2002/Reaffirmed 2010). *Diagnosis and management of preeclampsia and eclampsia* (Practice Bulletin #33). Washington, DC: Author.

American College of Obstetricians and Gynecologists. (2011). *Emergent therapy for acute-onset severe hypertension with preeclampsia and eclampsia* (Committee Opinion # 514). Washington, DC: Author.

Hypertensive disorders of pregnancy are considered the most common medical complications of pregnancy, affecting 12% to 22% of all pregnancies and responsible for 17.6% of maternal deaths in the United States. Classification varies from prepregnancy disease and beyond 12 weeks postpartum.

Classification

Chronic Hypertension

Hypertension is defined as mild—systolic BP ≥ 140 mm Hg *or* diastolic BP ≥ 90 mm Hg; or severe—systolic BP ≥ 180 mm Hg *or* diastolic BP ≥ 110 mm Hg. The condition may be observable before pregnancy, diagnosed before the 20th week of gestation, or persisting beyond 12 weeks postpartum. Condition increases risk of placental abruption.

Gestational Hypertension

1. New onset of hypertension (systolic BP ≥ 140 mm Hg *or* diastolic BP ≥ 90 mm Hg), generally after 20 weeks' gestation in the absence of gestational proteinuria; replaces the term *pregnancy-induced hypertension.*
2. BP typically normalizes to prepregnancy values by 12 weeks postpartum; if it remains elevated past 12 weeks, then a diagnosis of chronic hypertension is confirmed.

Preeclampsia and Eclampsia

1. Preeclampsia—elevated BP accompanied by proteinuria (without evidence of urinary tract infection [UTI]); both must be present for a diagnosis.
   a. Mild: systolic BP ≥ 140 mm Hg *or* diastolic BP ≥ 90 mm Hg on more than two occasions; gestational proteinuria >300 mg on random specimen or >1+ on dipstick; urinary excretion ≥ 0.3 g protein in a 24-hour specimen (24-hour specimens are recommended for diagnosis).
   b. Severe: diagnosis considered if preeclampsia evident and at least one of the following present: systolic BP ≥ 160 mm Hg; diastolic BP ≥ 110 mm Hg; proteinuria

BOX 39-1   HELLP Syndrome

HELLP syndrome—consisting of **H**emolysis of RBCs, **E**levated **L**iver enzymes, and **L**ow **P**latelets (<100,000 mm³)—is a severe complication with or without preeclampsia.

- These findings are commonly associated with disseminated intravascular coagulation (DIC) and, in fact, may be diagnosed as DIC.
- The hemolysis of erythrocytes is seen in the abnormal morphology of the cells.
- The elevated liver enzyme measurement is associated with decreased blood flow to the liver as a result of fibrin thrombi.
- The low platelet count is related to vasospasm and platelet adhesions.
- Treatment is similar to treatment for preeclampsia with close monitoring of liver function and bleeding.
- These women are at increased risk for postpartum hemorrhage.
- Complaints range from malaise, epigastric pain, and nausea and vomiting to nonspecific viral syndrome-like symptoms.

5 g or >/24-hour specimen or 3+ on two or more random urine specimens; oliguria of <500 mL/24 hours, cerebral or visual disturbances, pulmonary edema or cyanosis, epigastric or right upper quadrant pain, impaired liver function, thrombocytopenia (<100,000/mm³ platelets), or fetal growth restriction.

2. HELLP syndrome—acronym stands for **H**emolysis: microangiopathic hemolytic anemia, **E**levated **L**iver **E**nzymes, and **L**ow **P**latelets; form of severe preeclampsia (refer to Box 39-1).

3. Eclampsia—new onset of seizure activity or coma in a preeclamptic patient that cannot be attributed to any underlying neurologic condition or preexisting disease.

Preeclampsia/Eclampsia Superimposed on Chronic Hypertension

1. Diagnosis based on presence of one or more of the following in woman with hypertension and proteinuria prior to 20 weeks' gestation:
   a. New onset of proteinuria.
   b. Sudden increase in proteinuria.
   c. Sudden increase in hypertension.
   d. Development of HELLP syndrome.

Pathophysiology and Etiology

1. Etiologic theories include primary or excessive exposure to chorionic villi, as well as immunologic, genetic, and endocrine factors. These factors lead to endothelial dysfunction, systemic inflammatory response, and subsequent increased capillary permeability resulting in multisystem organ dysfunction. New research incorporates an allergic response from the mother against the fetus, similar to rejection of a transplanted organ. Hemoconcentration occurs due to vasoconstriction, increased vascular permeability, or both. Physiologic anemia

results as a symptom due to decreased intravascular plasma volume.

2. The disease is more commonly seen in primigravidas.

3. Risk factors—chronic hypertension, hydatidiform mole, multiple gestation, polyhydramnios, preexisting vascular disease, obesity, and diabetes mellitus may predispose a patient to preeclampsia. Adolescents (younger than age 17) and women older than age 35 are at higher risk.

 NURSING ALERT The risk of preeclampsia is increased for multigravida women if they have a new partner (father of the baby different from previous children) due to new paternal genetic makeup of the fetus.

Diagnostic Evaluation

1. Evaluate BP with appropriate auditory sounds (Korotkoff Phase I–systolic and V–diastolic), cuff size (1.5 times circumference of upper arm), placement (arm resting at level of heart), and proper maternal position (sitting or semi-Fowler's).

2. A 24-hour urine test is recommended for absolute diagnosis of preeclampsia.

3. Serum BUN, serum creatinine, and serum uric acid levels evaluate renal function and glomerular filtration capability, signaling advanced disease.

4. Liver function tests (AST, ALT); elevations indicative of organ dysfunction and disease.

5. Coagulation studies, specifically platelets, antithrombin III, and factor VIII levels.

6. Ultrasound assesses fetal growth, amniotic fluid volume, and placental implantation and function.

7. Periodic antepartum testing may be required to assess advanced or evolving disease and maternal–fetal tolerance: nonstress test (NST), oxytocin challenge test (OCT), biophysical profile (BPP).

8. Deep tendon reflexes and clonus evaluation assesses evolving disease and level of medications administered to treat disease.

Management

Treatment for hypertensive disorders of pregnancy focus on stabilization of the mother and pregnancy prolongation while observing for fetal intolerance. Delivery may be necessary for maternal indications, fetal indications, or both.

Expectant Management

Expectant management can be considered if the following maternal and fetal factors are present:

1. Maternal factors:
   a. Controlled hypertension.
   b. Urinary protein not severe; organ function adequate.
   c. Oliguria (<0.5 mL/kg/hour) that resolves with hydration.
   d. Liver enzymes not excessive, organ function adequate.

2. Fetal factors:
   a. BPP > 6.
   b. Amniotic fluid index (AFI) > 2 cm.
   c. Ultrasound fetal weight > 5th percentile.

Delivery

Delivery may be considered if any of the following occur:

1. Maternal factors:
   a. Uncontrolled hypertension: persistent > 160 systolic or 110 diastolic.
   b. Eclampsia unresolved or controlled.
   c. Thrombocytopenia: platelet count < 100,000/mm^3.
   d. Compromised liver function.
   e. Pulmonary edema.
   f. Compromised renal function.
   g. Abruptio placentae.
   h. Persistent and unresolved severe headache or visual changes.
   i. Evidence of hemorrhagic stroke or coma.
2. Fetal factors:
   a. Evolving Category II patterns or Category III FHR patterns (see page 1282).
   b. BPP < 4 on two occasions, 4 hours apart.
   c. AFI < 2 cm.
   d. Ultrasound fetal weight less than 5th percentile.
   e. Reverse umbilical artery diastolic flow.
   f. Evidence of acute placental abruption.

Pharmacologic Therapies

1. Magnesium sulfate (MgSO$_4$) is the primary medication for prophylactic treatment of seizure activity precipitated by hypertensive distress; may be given either via IV line or I.M., yet IV route is preferred; I.M. administration is reserved for eclamptic patients without IV access.
   a. A 4-g loading dose of 50% MgSO$_4$ is usually given via IV line over 15 to 30 minutes followed by a maintenance dose (secondary infusion) of 2 g/hour.
   b. The therapeutic level for MgSO$_4$ is a serum level of 4 to 7 mEq/dL. Periodic laboratory analysis of serum levels is required.
   c. Actions: decreases neuromuscular irritability and blocks release of acetylcholine at the neuromuscular junction; depresses vasomotor center; depresses central nervous system (CNS) irritability.
2. Phenytoin, although proposed for eclampsia prophylaxis, is considered second-line therapy in the United States; preferred for patients with kidney dysfunction.
3. If seizures develop and the patient is not on MgSO$_4$, 2 g may be given via IV line every 15 minutes to a maximum of 6 g or stabilization of patient. If patient has an existing MgSO$_4$ infusion, give 1 to 2 g IV piggyback. Continue to check magnesium levels periodically to assess toxicity/therapeutic levels.
4. If seizures continue, paralytic agents may be necessary and the patient may require mechanical ventilation.
5. Calcium gluconate is maintained bedside (but must remain secure) as a reversal agent for magnesium toxicity; dosage is 1 g (10 mL of 10% solution) by slow IV push.

 NURSING ALERT Signs of MgSO$_4$ toxicity include loss of deep tendon reflexes, including knee-jerk reflex, respiratory depression, oliguria, respiratory arrest, and cardiac arrest.

Antihypertensive Drug Therapy

Acute and persistent (>15 minutes) onset of severe preeclampsia, systolic >160 or diastolic >110, is considered a hypertensive emergency warranting prompt medical management. A clinical relationship between severe systolic hypertension and risk of hemorrhagic stroke has been observed in pregnant and nonpregnant adults. Therefore, a systolic BP of 160 mm Hg or greater is widely adopted as the definition of severe hypertension in pregnant or postpartum women. The goal of antihypertensive therapy is not to achieve normotension but to reduce risk of stroke and coma. Blood pressure is maintained with a margin of safety (<100 mm Hg) without compromising adequate uterine perfusion.

1. Hydralazine—relaxes vascular arterioles and stimulates cardiac output via direct peripheral vasodilation.
   a. Dosage: 5 to 10 mg IV push every 15 to 20 minutes to a maximum dose of 20 mg; dose cautiously and avoid hypotension.
   b. Onset of action can occur in 10 to 20 minutes, with peak action in 20 minutes; duration of the drug can last 3 to 8 hours.
   c. Monitor BP and pulse closely.
   d. If desired response is not obtained after 20 mg, change agents or consider hemodynamic monitoring.
   e. Adverse effects: flushing, headache, maternal and fetal tachycardia, palpitations, uteroplacental insufficiency with subsequent fetal tachycardia, late decelerations, and worsening hypertension (if due to elevated cardiac output). Rebound hypotension is possible if drug is given too rapidly.
2. Labetalol—alpha/beta-adrenergic blocker that decreases systemic vascular resistance without reflex tachycardia; it slows the maternal heart rate.
   a. Contraindicated in women with asthma, heart failure, and/or second- or third-degree heart block.
   b. Cardiac monitoring is required.
   c. Administered as 20 mg IV bolus dose, followed by 40 mg if no effect is seen in 10 minutes, then 80 mg every 10 minutes to a maximum dose of 220 mg.
   d. Onset of action is 1 to 2 minutes, with peak of action at 10 minutes; duration of drug effect lasts 6 to 16 hours.
   e. Adverse effects: transient fetal and neonatal hypotension, bradycardia, and hypoglycemia. Small doses excreted in breast milk.

Complications

Complications of preeclampsia affect many organ systems to include cardiovascular, renal, hematologic, neurologic, hepatic, and uteroplacental.

1. Abruptio placentae.
2. DIC.
3. HELLP syndrome (see page 1335).
4. Maternal or fetal death.
5. Hypertensive crisis, hemorrhagic stroke, or coma.
6. Pulmonary edema; cerebral edema.
7. Oliguria; acute renal dysfunction or failure.
8. Thrombocytopenia; acute liver dysfunction or failure.

9. Postpartum hemorrhage.
10. Blindness; retinal detachment.
11. Fetal intolerance of labor; evolving Category II or Category III patterns.
12. Hypoglycemia.
13. Hepatocellular dysfunction; hepatic rupture.
14. Prematurity.
15. Growth restriction and placental dysfunction.

Nursing Assessment

1. Evaluate BP with appropriate auditory sounds (Korotkoff Phase I–systolic and V–diastolic), cuff size (1.5 times circumference of upper arm), placement (arm resting at level of heart), and proper maternal position (sitting or semi-Fowler's). Utilizing wrong size cuff may inadvertently increase or decrease BP.
2. Assess urine protein at the bedside and initiate a 24-hour urine specimen, as ordered.
3. Evaluate DTRs and clonus on admission and periodically throughout therapy.
4. Evaluate fetal status with NST, fetal movement (kick) counts, BPP, contraction stress test (CST) via nipple stimulation or OCT, and continuous EFM, as directed.
5. Evaluate uterine activity for high-frequency, low-intensity uterine contractions; possible signs and symptoms of PTL or placental abruption.
6. Periodically observe for signs and symptoms of advancing disease.
7. Monitor for signs of $MgSO_4$ toxicity—absent knee-jerk reflex, respiratory depression, oliguria, absent FHR variability; if evident discontinue $MgSO_4$ and notify health care provider immediately.
8. Monitor serum magnesium serum level every 24 hours or per facility's policy.

Nursing Diagnoses

- Risk for Fluid Excess Volume related to pathophysiologic aspects of disease leading to fluid overload.
- Risk for Decreased Cardiac/Ineffective Cerebral Tissue Perfusion related to altered vascular perfusion caused by vasospasm and thrombosis formation.
- Risk for Injury related to seizures, prolonged bed rest, or other therapeutic regimens.
- Anxiety related to diagnosis and concern for self and fetus.
- Deficient Diversional Activity related to prolonged bed rest.
- Decreased Cardiac Output related to antihypertensive therapy.

Nursing Interventions

Maintaining Fluid Balance

1. Strict intake and output—control IV fluid intake using a continuous infusion pump. Utilize Foley catheter with urometer for adequate assessment of output. Notify health care provider if urine output is less than 25 mL/hour.
2. Monitor hematocrit levels to evaluate intravascular fluid status.

3. Monitor vital signs periodically as the patient's condition warrants.
4. Auscultate breath sounds at admission and periodically; report signs of pulmonary edema (ie, wheezing, crackles, shortness of breath, increased pulse rate, increased respiratory rate, or reduced SpO_2 saturation).

Promoting Adequate Tissue Perfusion

1. Position laterally to optimize maternal and placental perfusion.
2. Monitor fetal activity.
3. Evaluate NST and continuous EFM, if applicable, to determine fetal status.

Preventing Injury

1. Instruct patient on importance of reporting signs of advancing disease: headaches, visual changes, dizziness, respiratory distress, and/or epigastric pain.
2. Keep the environment quiet and calm as possible.
3. Hospitalized patients should have side rails remain up to prevent injury if seizure occurs.
4. Hospitalized patients should have oxygen, suction, and emergency medications immediately available for seizure management.
5. Assess DTRs and clonus periodically; increase frequency as patient's condition warrants.

 DRUG ALERT Keep calcium gluconate at bedside as a reversal agent for magnesium toxicity. Dosage is 1 g (10 mL of a 10% solution) slow IV push. Be cautious with concurrent administration of opioids, CNS depressants, calcium channel blockers, and beta-adrenergic blockers.

Decreasing Anxiety and Increasing Knowledge

1. Explain disease process and care plan including signs and symptoms of evolving disease.
2. Discuss the effects of all medications on mother and fetus.
3. Allow time to ask questions and discuss feelings regarding the diagnosis and treatment plan.

Promoting Diversional Activities

1. Explain need for bed rest to the woman and her support persons.
2. Explore woman's hobbies/diversional activities if prolonged hospitalization necessary.
3. Instruct family to arrange for community support (eg, church, women's groups).

Maintaining Cardiac Output

1. Strict intake and output—control IV fluid intake using a continuous infusion pump. Utilize Foley catheter with urimeter for adequate assessment of output. Notify health care provider if urine output is less than 25 mL/hour.
2. Monitor maternal vital signs, especially mean BP, pulse, and respirations.
3. Assess formation of edema: peripheral and pulmonary. Report pitting edema of +2 or less or evidence of pulmonary edema to primary care provider immediately.
4. Monitor oxygenation saturation levels with pulse oximetry. Report rate of less than 95% to primary care provider.

Community and Home Care Considerations

1. Mild preeclampsia, if stable, may be considered for home care at the discretion of the primary practitioner.
2. Ensure patient has daily phone access to primary care provider.
3. Periodic home visits by nursing personnel may be warranted.
4. Teach woman signs and symptoms of evolving disease.
5. At-home BP monitoring requires use of same arm and same physical position (eg, on left side, on right side) during each assessment.
6. Assess urine protein status daily on the first voided urine or obtain 24-hour urine each week, as ordered.
7. Teach woman to assess daily fetal movement (kick) counts; arrange for weekly NST, if indicated.

Patient Education and Health Maintenance

1. Teach the woman the importance of bed rest.
2. Encourage support of family and friends; suggest diversional activities on bed rest.
3. Include support of the neonatal team for discussion of fetal prognosis with the woman and her family.

Evaluation: Expected Outcomes

- BP and other vital parameters stable.
- Absence of evolving Category II or Category III FHR patterns.
- No seizure activity.
- Expresses concern for self and fetus.
- Maintains bed rest and pursues diversional activities.
- No evidence of pulmonary edema; urine output adequate.

Polyhydramnios

Polyhydramnios or *hydramnios* is excess amniotic fluid; volume typically exceeds 1.5 to 2 L between 32 and 36 weeks' gestation. About 50% of cases result in good outcomes.

Pathophysiology and Etiology

1. Amniotic fluid is 98% to 99% water, with the remainder consisting of proteins, carbohydrates, fats, electrolytes, enzymes, hormones, urinary by-products, fetal cells, lanugo, and vernix.
   a. Volume facilitates normal lung and neuromuscular maturity.
   b. At 36 weeks' gestation, approximately 1 L of fluid is present with subsequent decreases over the duration of gestation.
   c. The amount of amniotic fluid present is controlled in part by fetal urination and swallowing.
2. Polyhydramnios is idiopathic in 60% of women, but is associated with multiple gestation, immune and nonimmune hydrops fetalis, chromosomal anomalies such as Down syndrome, and fetal GI–cardiac–neural tube abnormalities.

Clinical Manifestations

1. Excessive weight gain, dyspnea.
2. Abdomen may be tense and shiny.
3. Edema of the vulva, legs, and lower extremities may be evident.
4. Increased uterine size for gestational age; usually accompanied by difficulty in palpating fetal parts or auscultation of the FHR.
5. Possible evolving Category II or Category III FHR patterns.

Diagnostic Evaluation

1. Ultrasound evaluation: AFI > 20 cm or single vertical depth pocket > 8 cm or total volume > 1.5 to 2L.
2. Difficult to palpate fetus or auscultate FHR.
3. Fundal height (FH) greater than age of gestation.

Management

1. Treatment is based on severity and underlying conditions; may include direct fetal therapy, serial amniocentesis, or administration of prostaglandin inhibitors such as indomethacin.
2. Indomethacin may be administered to increase fetal lung absorption, decrease fetal urine production, and increase fluid movement across the membranes of the mother.
3. Serial amniocentesis:
   a. Fluid is slowly removed under ultrasound-guided needle aspiration; rapid removal can result in a premature separation of the placenta.
   b. Usually 500 to 1,000 mL of fluid is removed during one procedure.

Complications

1. Potential for dysfunctional labor with increased risk for cesarean delivery.
2. Postpartum hemorrhage due to uterine atony from prolonged gross distention of the uterus.
3. Acute fetal hypoxia secondary to prolapsed cord or trauma.
4. Potential for preterm delivery.

Nursing Assessment

1. Evaluate maternal respiratory status; dyspnea may be present as hydramnios increases.
2. Evaluate EFM, continuously if viable, to assess fetal status.
3. Inspect abdomen and evaluate uterine height and compare with previous findings.
4. Evaluate for abdominal pain, edema, varicosities of lower extremities and vulva.

Nursing Diagnoses

- Ineffective Breathing Pattern related to pressure on the diaphragm.
- Impaired Physical Mobility related to edema and discomfort from the enlarged uterus.
- Anxiety related to fetal outcome.
- Risk for Bleeding at delivery related to prolonged overdistention of the uterus.

Nursing Interventions

Promoting Effective Breathing

1. Position to promote chest expansion with head elevated.
2. Provide oxygen (8 to 10 L/minute) by face mask, if indicated; prolonged use prior to delivery is not recommended.
3. Limit activities and plan for frequent rest periods.
4. Maintain adequate intake and output.

Promoting Mobility

1. Assist the woman with position changes and ambulation, as needed.
2. Advise on alternating activity with rest periods to promote circulation.
3. Instruct the woman to wear loose-fitting clothing and low-heeled shoes with good support.

Decreasing Anxiety

1. Explain probable causes of polyhydramnios, if known.
2. Encourage the patient and family to ask questions and express feelings regarding any treatment or procedure.
3. Prepare patient for mode of delivery that is anticipated and for the expected findings at the time of delivery.
4. Encourage presence and participation of support person in plan of care.

Preventing Hemorrhage during Labor

1. Notify primary care provider of inadequate or abnormal labor curve.
2. Place peripheral IV and maintain throughout labor with normal saline or dextrose (5%) in lactated Ringer's solution (D$_5$LR).
3. Administer medications (ie, oxytocin, misoprostol) to decrease postpartum bleeding, as necessary.
4. Observe for alterations in vital signs indicating excessive blood loss, such as decreasing BP and increasing pulse.
5. Medications for the prevention of postpartum hemorrhage should be immediately available following delivery (eg, oxytocin, misoprostol).

Patient Education and Health Maintenance

1. Instruct the woman to notify her health care provider if she experiences respiratory distress.
2. Teach the woman signs of PTL and importance to report them to health care provider.

Evaluation: Expected Outcomes

- Respirations: normal rate of 18 to 24 and unlabored.
- Verbalizes improved comfort; moves freely.
- Discusses pregnancy outcome realistically; asks questions regarding treatment for self and fetus.
- Labor progresses and involution occurs without hemorrhage.

Oligohydramnios

Oligohydramnios is the marked decrease of amniotic fluid of less than 500mL in the amniotic sac. It is rarer than polyhydramnios and is associated with amnion abnormalities, placental insufficiency, premature rupture of membranes, and fetal urinary anomalies.

Pathophysiology and Etiology

1. Commonly related to fetal problems, such as obstruction in the urinary tract, renal agenesis, and IUGR (any condition that prevents the formation of urine or the entry of urine into the amniotic sac usually results in oligohydramnios).
2. Commonly seen in postdate pregnancies

3. May be due to placental insufficiency
4. Associated with premature rupture of membranes (PROM) and severe preeclampsia
5. The fetus may suffer from pulmonary hypoplasia (especially if associated with Potter's syndrome) due to compression of the fetal chest and body by the uterine wall.
6. Skeletal abnormalities may also occur due to a lack of fluid in the terminal air sacs if oligohydramnios occurs in the first or second trimester.

Clinical Manifestations

1. Prominent fetal parts on palpation of the abdomen.
2. Small-for-date uterine size.
3. FHR variable decelerations or repetitive late decelerations may present on EFM tracing.

Diagnostic Evaluation

1. Ultrasound evaluation of the AFI—decrease of amniotic fluid in all four vertical plane quadrants of the uterus of less than 500 mL, single vertical depth pocket: < 2 cm, or AFI < 5 cm at term.

Management

1. Frequent evaluation of fetal status through NST, BPP, CST, or OCT, as indicated.
2. Periodic ultrasound evaluations performed to evaluate fetal renal dysfunction and abnormal fetal growth.
3. Amnioinfusion (the installation of fluid into the amniotic cavity to replace depleted volumes of amniotic fluid) during labor is optional to decrease occurrence and severity of FHR variable decelerations.

 NURSING ALERT Contraindications to amnioinfusion include suspected or diagnosed abruptio placentae, acute fetal compromise, fetal head that is engaged and tightly applied to the cervix, or the inability to measure intrauterine pressures.

4. Delivery may be indicated for such conditions as IUGR or fetal compromise.

Complications

1. Preterm labor.
2. Umbilical cord compression.
3. Passage of meconium.
4. Fetal/neonatal death.
5. Neonatal respiratory distress due to pulmonary hypoplasia.

Nursing Interventions and Patient Education

1. Evaluate fetal status via EFM.
2. Evaluate maternal vital signs periodically; note signs of infection, especially if oligohydramnios is secondary to PROM.
3. Assist with an amnioinfusion, as indicated.
4. Inform health care provider of fetal intolerance to labor and treat, as indicated.

Multiple Gestation

Multiple gestation or *multifetal pregnancy* results when two or more fetuses are present in the uterus at the same time. Since 1980, there has been a 65% increase in the frequency of twins and a 500% rise in triplet and high-order multiples due to advanced maternal age and infertility treatment. Multiple gestation is not a complication of pregnancy; rather, it is a condition that presents an increased risk of morbidity and mortality for mother and neonates. One fifth of triplet pregnancies and one half of quadruplet pregnancies result in at least one child with a major long-term handicap, such as cerebral palsy.

 Evidence Base American College of Obstetricians and Gynecologists. (2004/Reaffirmed 2010). *Multiple gestation: Complicated twin, triplet, and high-order multifetal pregnancy* (Practice Bulletin #56). Washington, DC: Author.

Pathophysiology and Etiology

1. Types of twinning (Figure 39-4): The degree to which structures are shared (amnion, chorion, placenta) is related to the time of zygotic division after conception (within 72 hours).
   a. Monozygotic (identical)—one ovum fertilizes with one sperm, later dividing early in gestation resulting in two embryos. Each embryo has identical genetic makeup and sexual identity but may vary in size due to unequal splitting of the cytoplasm; etiology unclear; rarest type of twinning with increased risk of twin-to-twin transfusion syndrome.
   b. Dizygotic, trizygotic (fraternal, nonidentical)—two or more ova are fertilized by two or more separate sperm. The twins do not always share same genetic makeup or sexual identity.

2. Artificially induced ovulation, as well as in vitro fertilization with multiple embryos transferred into the uterus, increase risk of multiple gestation.
3. Increasing maternal age and parity increase odds of twinning.
4. Other terminology:
   a. Monochorionic—one chorionic membrane.
   b. Monoamniotic—one amniotic sac.
   c. Dichorionic—two chorionic membranes.
   d. Diamniotic—two amniotic sacs.

Clinical Manifestations

1. Uterine size is large for gestational age. Fundal height is typically 2 cm larger than normal.
2. Auscultation of two or more distinct and separate fetal hearts may occur with a Doppler late in the first trimester or with a fetoscope after 20 weeks' gestation.
3. Ultrasound is the primary diagnostic tool; used for 95% to 100% of cases. Gestation sacs identified as early as 6 to 8 weeks.
4. High initial quantitative β-hCG is one of the earliest indicators. However, due to the possibility of false-positive results, ultrasound should be used to confirm the diagnosis in the presence of elevated β-hCG levels.

Complications

1. Cardiopulmonary.
   a. Pulmonary edema.
   b. Complications from tocolysis.
   c. Hypertension or preeclampsia.
   d. Venal caval hypotension syndrome.
   e. Peripartum cardiomyopathy.
2. GI.
   a. Acute fatty liver of pregnancy.
   b. Cholestasis of pregnancy.

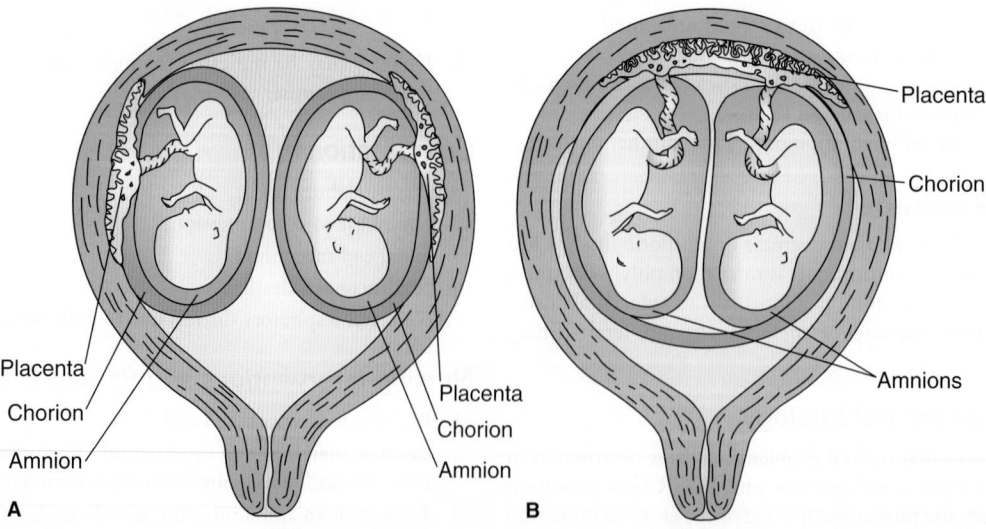

Figure 39-4. Multiple gestations. (A) Dizygotic twins showing two placentas, two chorions, and two amnions. **(B)** Monozygotic twins with one placenta, one chorion, and two amnions.

3. Hematologic—anemia.
4. Obstetric.
   a. PTL or birth.
   b. Incompetent cervix.
   c. Increased incidence of cesarean delivery.
   d. Increased use of tocolysis.
   e. Antepartum and postpartum hemorrhage.
   f. Abruptio placentae.
   g. Uterine rupture.
   h. Gestational diabetes.
   i. Polyhydramnios; oligohydramnios common with twins.
   j. Spontaneous abortion.
   k. IUGR.
   l. Umbilical cord problems, such as entanglement, cord prolapse, or vasa previa.
5. Fetal risks—structural abnormalities, such as congenital heart defects, intestinal tract anomalies, neural tube defects, hydrocephaly, craniofacial defects, skeletal defects, anencephaly, encephalocele, or acardia (ie, absence of the heart).
6. Conjoined twins.
7. Twin-to-twin transfusion syndrome leads to anastomoses of placental vessels; increased risk with one placenta.

Management and Nursing Interventions

1. Nutrition counseling—increased caloric and protein intake as well as vitamin supplements are needed to meet demands of multiple fetuses.
2. Fetal evaluation—serial sonograms during the pregnancy evaluate growth and development to growth inconsistencies. NST, BPP, and amniocentesis are utilized for detection of fetal lung maturity and fetal tolerance. Percutaneous umbilical cord sampling may be used to establish fetal well-being if twin-to-twin transfusion is suspected.
3. PTL prevention—hospitalization may be necessary for signs and symptoms of PTL.
   a. Encourage bed rest and hydration.
   b. Institute fetal monitoring and assist with tocolytic therapy, if ordered.
4. Mode of delivery—dependent on the presentation of the twins, maternal and fetal status, and gestational age. Cesarean delivery is commonly used for multiples other than twins; however, vaginal birth of triplets may be indicated in the presence of noncontracted pelvis, unscarred uterus, and onset of labor at more than 32 to 34 completed weeks of gestation.
5. Intrapartum management.
   a. Establish IV access for fluid resuscitation and for anticipation of potential cesarean delivery.
   b. Provide for EFM for each fetus with multiple monitors; triplets and high-order multiples may need serial ultrasounds during labor or preoperatively.
   c. Double setup (vaginal delivery attempted in operating room suite) is recommended for delivery, if appropriate. Guidelines for vaginal birth of twins:
      i. Multiple neonatal teams to care for each newborn.
      ii. IV access with large bore catheter.
      iii. Surgical suite immediately available.
      iv. An obstetrician and assistant experienced in vaginal births of twins at delivery.
      v. Anesthesia of choice: epidural, although alternatives exist; consult with anesthesiologist. Anesthesia provider capable of administering general anesthesia should be immediately available.
   d. Pitocin induction/augmentation may be required secondary to hypotonic labor.
   e. An increased risk of postpartum hemorrhage exists; prepare accordingly.
6. Emotional support—encourage family to discuss feelings about multiple births and identify ways in which they will need assistance. Refer to resources such as National Organization of Mothers of Twins Clubs (*www.nomotc.org*).

Community and Home Care Considerations

1. Discuss the warning signs of PTL.
2. Teach uterine self-palpation. Patient should evaluate uterine activity twice daily.
3. Home care may include nursing visits and fetal assessments.
4. Offer provider phone contact information for notification of complications.

INTRAPARTUM COMPLICATIONS OF LABOR

Preterm Labor

Preterm labor (PTL) is defined as regular contractions associated with cervical change between 20 and 37 completed weeks of gestation. PTL is second, only to birth defects, as a leading cause of neonatal mortality. It occurs in up to 12% of all pregnancies and is one of the most frustrating clinical dilemmas in obstetrics. However, neonatal intensive care and technology has advanced to meet the various needs of extrauterine transition of the preterm fetus.

It is important to differentiate PTL from other sequelae to avoid misdiagnosis. For example, uterine irritability without cervical change is not PTL. Likewise, preterm birth (PTB) and low birth weight (LBW) are not synonymous; preterm birth is any birth that occurs before 37 completed weeks of pregnancy, whereas LBW refers to birth weight alone (<2,500 g [5½ lb]), regardless of gestational age.

Pathophysiology and Etiology

1. The exact etiology for PTL remains unknown, but may include:
   a. Decidual hemorrhage (placental abruption).
   b. Mechanical factors such as uterine overdistention or cervical incompetence.
   c. Hormonal changes.
   d. Infectious etiology (eg, bacterial vaginosis, Group B beta strep).
2. Physiologic alterations occur with onset of spontaneous labor.
   a. Cervical changes occurs: softening, shortening, and location.
   b. Oxytocin receptors present in the myometrium respond to circulating levels.
   c. Prostaglandin levels in the amniotic fluid rise.

Risk Factors for PTL

1. Medical/obstetric complications (predating the current pregnancy):
   a. Prior PTB triples risk in current pregnancy.
   b. Multiple abortions.
   c. Low prepregnancy weight for height.
   d. Uterine/cervical abnormalities.
   e. Parity (0 or >4).
   f. Hypertension.
   g. Diabetes.
2. Current pregnancy complications:
   a. Anemia.
   b. Multiple gestation.
   c. Placenta previa.
   d. Abruptio placentae.
   e. Fetal anomaly.
   f. Hydramnios (polyhydramnios, oligohydramnios).
   g. Abdominal surgery.
   h. Infection.
   i. Bleeding in first trimester.
   j. Short interpregnancy interval.
   k. PROM.
   l. Cervical incompetence.
   m. UTIs/pyelonephritis.
3. Demographic data:
   a. Maternal age younger than 17 or older than 35.
   b. African American (doubles the risk).
   c. Low socioeconomic status.
4. Behavioral and environmental:
   a. DES exposure.
   b. Smoking (especially if more than 11 cigarettes/day).
   c. Poor nutrition or excessive stress.
   d. Alcohol or other substance use.
   e. Late or no prenatal care.
   f. Domestic violence.

Clinical Manifestations

1. Uterine cramps (menstrual-like, intermittent, or constant).
2. Uterine contractions occurring at intervals of 10 minutes or less.
3. Low abdominal pain or pressure (pelvic pressure).
4. Dull low backache (intermittent or constant).
5. Increase or change in vaginal discharge.
6. Feeling that baby is "pushing down" or that "something" is in the vagina.

Diagnostic Evaluation

1. Transvaginal cervical ultrasound can predict cervical length and direct internal changes.
2. Fetal fibronectin (fFN): protein produced by fetal membranes and functions as an adhesive to hold membranes against the uterine myometrium. It is normally absent in cervical secretions after 16 to 20 weeks and reappears after 34 weeks. Therefore, a midtrimester assay with positive fFN is an indicator of PTL/PTB and possible infection.

Management

Management of PTL is focused on early education, prevention, and limiting neonatal morbidity.

Preconception Care

1. Baseline assessment of health and risks; advise patient to decrease risks attributable to PTL/PTB.
2. Pregnancy planning and identification of barriers to care.
3. Adjustment of prescribed and over-the-counter medications that may pose a threat to the developing fetus.
4. Nutritional counseling, as needed.
5. Genetic counseling, as indicated.

Antepartum Treatment

1. Educate mother regarding signs/symptoms of PTL.
2. Instruct mother and provide resources for lifestyle modifications:
   a. If applicable, encourage smoking-cessation classes.
   b. Discuss aspects of a healthy diet and adequate maternal weight gain during pregnancy.
3. Early therapy options include bed rest, hydration, and abstention from intercourse and orgasm; effectiveness of each method is uncertain.

Tocolytic Therapy

If antepartum therapy is not successful, tocolytic therapy may be instituted. These drugs should be used only when the potential benefit to the fetus outweighs the potential risk. If tocolytic drugs are used, the choice of drug should be individualized and based on maternal condition, potential drug side effects, and gestational age.

1. Betamimetic—terbutaline: acts on β_2 receptor cells located in smooth muscle, inhibiting uterine contractions. Injectable terbutaline should not be used in pregnant women for prevention or prolonged treatment (beyond 48 to 72 hours) of preterm labor in either the hospital or outpatient setting because of the potential for serious maternal heart problems and death. In addition, oral terbutaline should not be used for prevention or any treatment of preterm labor because it has not been shown to be effective and has similar safety concerns.
   a. Withhold medication for a maternal pulse >120.
   b. Contraindications: cardiac arrhythmias.
   c. Potential maternal adverse effects: tachycardia, cardiac arrhythmias, pulmonary edema, myocardial ischemia, hypotension, death.
   d. Potential fetal adverse effects: tachycardia, hyperinsulinemia, hyperglycemia, myocardial or septal hypertrophy, myocardial ischemia.
2. $MgSO_4$—interferes with smooth-muscle contractility, although its exact mechanism of action is unknown.
   a. Dosage: 4 to 6 g IV piggyback bolus over 20 minutes, then 2 to 3 g maintenance dose via continuous IV drip.
   b. Contraindications: myasthenia gravis, renal disease.
   c. Potential maternal adverse effects: flushing, lethargy, headache, muscle weakness, diplopia, dry mouth, pulmonary edema, cardiac arrest.
   d. Potential fetal adverse effects: lethargy, hypotonia, respiratory depression, demineralization with prolonged use.
   e. Antidote: calcium gluconate.

3. Prostaglandin inhibitors—Indomethacin: inhibits prostaglandin stimulation of contractions; however, after 34 weeks' gestation, indomethacin may cause premature closure of the fetal ductus arteriosus, increasing the risk of fetal pulmonary hypertension.
   a. Dosage: loading dose of 50 mg rectally or 50 to 100 mg orally, then 25 to 50 mg orally every 6 hours for 48 hours.
   b. Contraindications: significant renal or hepatic impairment.
   c. Potential maternal adverse effects: nausea, heartburn, postpartum hemorrhage.
   d. Potential fetal adverse effects: constriction of the ductus arteriosus, pulmonary hypertension, reversible decreased renal function with oligohydramnios, intraventricular hemorrhage, hyperbilirubinemia, necrotizing enterocolitis (NEC).
4. Calcium channel blocker—nifedipine: relaxes smooth muscle by inhibiting the transport of calcium negating contraction formation.
   a. Dosage: 30 mg loading dose, then 10 to 20 mg every 4 to 6 hours.
   b. Contraindications: cardiac disease, use caution with renal disease, maternal hypotension (<90/50 mm Hg), avoid concomitant use with $MgSO_4$.
   c. Potential maternal adverse effects: flushing, dizziness, headache, nausea, transient hypotension.
   d. Potential fetal adverse effects: none currently known.
5. Antibiotic therapy: several regimens exist for intrapartum antimicrobial prophylaxis for perinatal group B streptococcal (GBS) disease prevention. Even if unable to arrest PTL, treatment is indicated if the mother tests positive.

General Contraindications to Tocolytic Therapy
1. Category III FHR patterns.
2. Intra-amniotic infection.
3. Eclampsia or severe preeclampsia.
4. Fetal demise.
5. Fetal maturity.
6. Maternal hemodynamic instability.
7. Severe bleeding of any cause.
8. Fetal anomaly incompatible with life.
9. Severe IUGR.
10. Cervix dilated more than 5 cm.

Acceleration of Fetal Lung Maturity
1. Corticosteroid administration—betamethasone or dexamethasone.
   a. Given to potential PTL patients between 24 and 34 weeks' gestation.
   b. Betamethasone is given I.M. in two doses of 12 mg each, 24 hours apart.
   c. Dexamethasone is given I.M. in four doses of 6 mg each, every 12 hours.
      i. Decreases intraventricular hemorrhage (IVH), NEC, and respiratory distress syndrome (RDS), mortality that may be a result of prematurity.
   d. Timely administration is essential; given before delivery to mother; postponing delivery for administration is an option.
   e. Serial administration of the agents is no longer recommended.
2. Artificial surfactant therapy.
   a. Decreases need for ventilatory support in the neonate with RDS.
   b. Administered via endotracheal tube directly into the neonate's lungs after delivery.

Complications
1. Prematurity and associated neonatal complications include:
   a. IVH.
   b. RDS due to lung immaturity.
   c. Patent ductus arteriosus.
   d. NEC.

Nursing Assessment
During tocolytic therapy, assess the following:
1. Fetal status and UA data by EFM.
2. Respiratory status (pulmonary edema is a common adverse effect).
3. Muscular tremors.
4. Palpitations.
5. Dizziness/light-headedness.
6. Urine output.
7. Patient education to signs and symptoms of PTL.
8. Patient education to signs and symptoms of infection.

Nursing Diagnoses
- Anxiety related to medication and fear of outcome of pregnancy.
- Risk for Injury to fetus secondary to prematurity.
- Risk for Shock related to tocolytic therapy.
- Compromised Family Coping secondary to hospitalization.

Nursing Interventions
Decreasing Anxiety
1. Know the contraindications and potential complications of tocolytic therapy.
2. Explain the purpose and common adverse effects of tocolytic therapy.
3. Provide accurate information on the status of the fetus and progressive labor.
4. Allow the woman and her support person to verbalize their feelings.
5. Encourage relationship with other patients who are also experiencing PTL.

Minimizing Injury to Fetus
1. Encourage the woman to assume lateral positions that will enhance placental perfusion.
2. Monitor fetal status and labor progress.
3. Assist with delivery of infant, as needed.
4. Notify provider of signs of advancing labor.

Minimizing Risk of Drug-Related Injury

1. Maintain accurate intake and output at least periodically based on tocolytic agent and dosing.
2. Assess maternal vital signs in accordance with facility policy. Notify the primary health care provider if maternal pulse greater than 120 beats/minute.
3. Assess for signs and symptoms of pulmonary edema.
4. Periodically assess deep tendon reflexes to note signs of hyporeflexia due to $MgSO_4$ infusion; excessive dosage or poor renal clearance may lead to magnesium toxicity.
5. Discontinue infusion if adverse effects occur; notify primary health care provider.
6. Educate the woman on tocolytic therapy, explaining the purpose and common adverse effects.

Promoting Maternal-Family Coping

1. Encourage private time for woman and partner.
2. Allow visitation with other children, as tolerated by woman.
3. Encourage patient to participate in other family activities such as helping with homework. This will assist in maintaining the family unit.

Community and Home Care Considerations

1. Ensure that woman meets following criteria for home management of PTL:
   a. No evidence of active PTL.
   b. No evidence of intra-amniotic infection.
   c. Cervical dilatation less than 3 cm.
2. Ensure that protocols or orders are in place for each of the following:
   a. Warning signs for PTL.
   b. Demonstration of uterine self-palpation by woman.
   c. Monitoring vaginal discharge; signs of spontaneous rupture of membranes.
   d. Assessment of urinary frequency, signs and symptoms for UTI, diarrhea, pelvic heaviness/pressure, maternal temperature, uterine cramping/tenderness.
   e. Frequent home visits; NST, FHR assessment, and vaginal examination evaluation necessary.
   f. Close health care provider contact.

Patient Education and Health Maintenance

1. Educate the patient about the importance of continuing the pregnancy until term or fetal lung maturity.
2. Encourage the need for compliance with a decreased activity level or bed rest, as indicated.
3. Teach the patient the importance of proper nutrition and need for adequate hydration.
4. Instruct the woman not to engage in sexual activity if diagnosed with PTL.
5. Teach the woman signs and symptoms of infection and to report them immediately.

Evaluation: Expected Outcomes

- Demonstrates concern about treatment and pregnancy outcome.
- No fetal compromise or complications; term delivery.
- Adequate fluid intake and output.
- Family focused on woman's well-being.

Premature Rupture of Membranes

Premature rupture of membranes (PROM) is defined as rupture of the membranes before the onset of labor. PROM is independent of gestational age; when it occurs prior to term it is referred to as preterm PROM. This condition occurs in approximately one-third of preterm births and 8% of term pregnancies. This condition increases risk of FHR variable decelerations.

Pathophysiology and Etiology

1. Rupture of membranes occurs during the normal course of labor. The exact etiology of PROM is not clearly understood, although nonpathologic causes, such as the combination of stretching of the membranes and biochemical changes, are suspected to contribute; infection has commonly been found to be a primary cause.
2. PROM is manifested by a gush of amniotic fluid or leaking of fluid through the vagina, which usually persists; flow may decrease in the sitting or supine position.

Diagnostic Evaluation

1. Patient history and physical exam.
2. Sterile speculum examination for identification of "pooling" of fluid in the vagina, cervicitis, umbilical or fetal prolapse, and cervical advancement. Collect cultures as appropriate.
3. Nitrazine test—amniotic fluid changes pH paper from yellow-green to blue.
4. Fern test—swab of the posterior vaginal fornix is taken to obtain amniotic fluid. Positive test will reveal arborization or "ferning" (visually appears as a fern leaf) on a slide viewed under a microscope.
5. Ultrasound to assess amniotic fluid volume.
6. Amniocentesis to inject indigo carmine or Evans blue dye. Watch for vaginal leakage of blue fluid to assess for ruptured membranes.

Management (>34 weeks)

1. When PROM is confirmed, the patient is admitted to the hospital and usually remains there until delivery. Gestational age, fetal presentation, and well-being should be determined.
2. At any gestational age, a patient with evident intrauterine infection, placental abruption, or evidence of Category III FHR pattern is best cared for by expeditious delivery.
3. If immediate delivery is not indicated, cultures of the cervix should be obtained to identify best antibiotic management (chlamydia, gonorrhea, and group B beta-hemolytic streptococcus, if appropriate).
4. Expectant management: offer adequate time for the latent phase of labor to progress (may be as long as hours to days or at the discretion of the primary practitioner) and EFM.
   a. Vaginal examinations are kept to a minimum to prevent infection.
   b. Once the decision to deliver is made, GBS prophylaxis should be initiated based on prior culture results or risk factors.

5. Active management:
    a. Oxytocin induction may be initiated at the time of presentation to reduce:
        i. Risk of chorioamnionitis.
        ii. Postpartum febrile morbidity.
        iii. Neonatal antibiotic treatments.

Complications

1. Maternal infection—intrapartum and postpartum.
2. Potential increased rates of cesarean delivery.
3. Fetal or neonatal infection or compromise.

Nursing Assessment

1. Evaluate maternal BP, respirations, pulse, and temperature periodically. If temperature or pulse is elevated, continue monitoring more frequently.
2. Monitor the amount and type of amniotic fluid that is leaking. Observe for purulent, foul-smelling discharge and report immediately.
3. Assess patient periodically for diffuse abdominal pain or pain on palpation, signs of increased infection.
4. Evaluate periodic CBC with differentials results; any shift to the left (ie, increase of immature forms of neutrophils/WBCs) signals infection.
5. Communicate any findings related to signs of infection to the primary practitioner and perinatal team.
6. Evaluate fetal status periodically depending on stages of labor; maternal infection is the primary cause of fetal tachycardia.

Nursing Diagnosis

- Risk for Infection related to ascending bacteria.

Nursing Interventions

Preventing Infection

1. Evaluate amount and odor of amniotic fluid leakage.
2. Limit vaginal examinations.
3. Place patient on disposable pads to collect leaking fluid and change pads every 1 to 2 hours or more frequently, as needed.
4. Review the need for good handwashing technique and hygiene after urination and defecation.
5. Monitor FHR and fetal activity periodically, as indicated.
6. Monitor maternal temperature, pulse respirations, BP, and uterine tenderness frequently, as indicated.
7. Administer GBS therapy or antibiotics, as indicated.

Evaluation: Expected Outcomes

- No signs of infection.

Preterm Premature Rupture of Membranes

Preterm premature rupture of membranes (PPROM) is defined as rupture of membranes before 37 completed weeks' gestation without the onset of spontaneous labor. Regardless of management or clinical presentation, delivery within 1 week is the most likely outcome. However, approximately 3% to 13% of patients can anticipate cessation of fluid leakage and possible restoration of normal amniotic fluid volume over remaining course of gestation.

PPROM patients are at high risk for infection during the intrapartum and postpartum phases. Secondary complications include fetal malpresentation, placental abruption, and prematurity.

Pathophysiology and Etiology

1. Although the exact cause is unknown, PPROM is likely to be either a pathologic intrinsic weakness or related to an extrinsic factor that causes the membranes to rupture prematurely.
2. The primary cause of PPROM is infection, particularly in earlier gestations (amnionitis; group B beta-hemolytic *Streptococcus*).
3. Other causes:
    a. History of PROM/PTB.
    b. Low body mass index (<19.8).
    c. Nutritional deficiencies.
    d. Connective tissue disorders.
    e. Maternal smoking.
    f. Cervical conization or cerclage.
    g. Pulmonary disease.
    h. Uterine overdistention.
    i. Amniocentesis.

Diagnostic Evaluation

1. Same as PROM.

Management

1. When PPROM is confirmed, the patient is admitted to the facility and usually remains there until delivery. Gestational age, fetal presentation, and well-being should be determined.
2. At any gestational age, a patient with evident intrauterine infection, placental abruption, or evidence of a nonreassuring fetal status is best cared for by expeditious delivery.
3. If immediate delivery is not indicated, cultures of the cervix should be obtained (chlamydia, gonorrhea, and GBS, if appropriate).
4. Expectant management (24 to 37 weeks): once labor, fetal compromise, and infection are ruled out, expectant management is maintained with EFM to assess fetal and uterine data accompanied by periodic antepartum testing, as indicated.
    a. Vaginal examinations are kept to a minimum to prevent infection.
    b. GBS prophylaxis is recommended.
    c. Corticosteroid therapy—single course.
    d. Tocolytic therapy- may or may not be beneficial.
    e. Antibiotics are recommended if there are no contraindications.
5. Expectant management (less than 24 weeks) or induction of labor:
    a. Patient counseling.
    b. Vaginal examinations are kept to a minimum to prevent infection.

c. GBS prophylaxis—start antibiotics for latency and obtain GBS culture, if labor initiates or GBS positive prophylaxis is indicated; if culture negative, repeat culture at 35 to 37 weeks.

d. Corticosteroid therapy—data does not support use in <24 weeks' gestation.

e. Antibiotics—there are incomplete data on use in prolonging latency in the absence of a positive GBS culture.

Complications

1. Maternal.
    a. Increased risk of intrauterine infection.
    b. Postpartum endometritis.
    c. Placental abruption.
2. Fetal—infection.
3. Neonatal—RDS, infection, death.

Nursing Assessment

1. Evaluate maternal vital signs periodically to assess for infection and include fetal assessment. If temperature or pulse is elevated, notify practitioner and assess more frequently.
2. Monitor for fetal infection: tachycardia, minimal or absent FHR variability, or variable decelerations due to decreased amniotic fluid.
3. Monitor for maternal chorioamnionitis (purulent, foul-smelling vaginal discharge, increased temperature, increased uterine activity).
4. Minimize infection with decreased or no vaginal examinations, sterile technique, and appropriate perineal cleansing.
5. Strict bed rest with or without bathroom privileges, as ordered.
6. Evaluate daily CBC with differentials, noting any shift to the left, and communicate findings to primary practitioner.
7. Communicate any findings of infection or maternal–fetal intolerance to the perinatal team promptly.
8. Offer supportive care for woman and her family.
9. Organize a neonatal consult for anticipatory guidance, as indicated.

Nursing Diagnosis

• Risk for Infection related to ascending bacteria.
• Also see "Preterm labor," page 1341.

Nursing Interventions

Preventing Infection

1. Evaluate amount and odor of amniotic fluid leakage.
2. Do not perform vaginal examinations without consulting the primary health care provider.
3. Place patient on disposable pads to collect leaking fluid and change pads approximately every 2 hours or more frequently, as needed.
4. Review the need for good handwashing technique and hygiene after urination and defecation.
5. Monitor FHR and fetal activity periodically, as indicated.

6. Monitor maternal temperature, pulse respirations, BP, and uterine tenderness periodically as the patient's condition warrants.
7. Administer antibiotics, GBS, or corticosteroid therapy, as prescribed.

Evaluation: Expected Outcomes

• No signs of infection.

Induction and Augmentation of Labor

 Evidence Base Troiano, N., Harvey, C., & Chez, B. (Eds.). (2013). High-risk and critical care obstetrics (3rd ed.). Philadelphia: Lippincott Williams & Wilkins.

Induction of labor refers to utilization of exogenous labor enhancement agents or procedures resulting in rhythmic contractions and spontaneous onset of labor. Cervical ripening utilizes medications and procedures to effecting the physical properties (softening and dilation) of the cervix in preparation for labor and delivery. Benefits of induction must outweigh the risks to the maternal–fetal unit. Inductions may be medically indicated or elective. Elective procedures prior to 39 completed weeks of gestation are contraindicated.

Augmentation refers to the administration of uterine stimulants once labor dystocia (dysfunction) ensues. Dysfunctional labor may result for several reasons (outlined in the next section) and remains the number one cause for primary cesarean deliveries. Similar medications are utilized for induction, augmentation, and sometimes cervical ripening.

Indications for Induction

Medically Indicated

1. Abruptio placentae.
2. Chorioamnionitis (intra-amniotic infection).
3. Fetal demise.
4. Hypertensive disorders: chronic, gestational, preeclampsia, or eclampsia.
5. PROM.
6. Postterm pregnancy.
7. Maternal medical conditions: diabetes mellitus, renal disease, chronic pulmonary disease, or underlying cardiac disease
8. Fetal conditions: severe fetal growth restriction, anomalies, isoimmunization, evolving Category II FHR pattern, or Category III FHR pattern.

Elective

1. Patient or physician request.
2. Logistic reasons: risk of rapid labor, distance from hospital.
3. Psychosocial indications.
4. In addition to the other reasons for elective induction, there must also be fetal lung maturity or 39 or more weeks' gestational age determined by one of the following criteria:
    a. Fetal heart tones documented from 20 weeks onward by nonelectronic fetoscope or for at least 30 weeks by Doppler.

b. Thirty-six weeks or more since a positive serum or urine hCG pregnancy test from a reliable laboratory.

c. An ultrasound measurement of the crown to rump length obtained at 6 to 12 weeks, which supports a gestational age of at least 39 weeks.

d. An ultrasound examination between 13 and 20 weeks, confirming at least 39 weeks' gestation as determined by clinical history and physical exam.

Contraindications for Induction

1. Vaginal bleeding, known placenta previa or vasa previa.
2. Abnormal presentation: transverse or funic (cord).
3. Previous transfundal/"classic" uterine incision or extensive myomectomy.
4. Pelvic structural deformities.
5. Active or culture-proven genital herpes infection.
6. Invasive cervical carcinoma.
7. Umbilical cord prolapse.
8. Fetal presenting part above pelvic inlet.
9. Category III FHR pattern.

Indications for Augmentation

1. Uterine hypocontractility.
2. Dystocia (slow, abnormal progression of labor).
3. Augmentation should be considered in the absence of cervical change if the frequency of contractions is less than 3 over 10 minutes or the intensity of contractions is less than 25 mm Hg above baseline or both.

Contraindications for Augmentation

1. Same as induction.

Management

Cervical Ripening

Cervical ripening is performed if induction is indicated and the cervix is unfavorable. Typically the cervix is evaluated according to the Bishop pelvic scoring system; if the score is 6 or more, the probability of vaginal delivery after labor induction is similar to that of spontaneous labor.

1. Methods:
   a. Manual stripping of the membranes.
   b. Mechanical cervical dilators.
      i. Laminaria digitata—a seaweed preparation that is inserted directly into and dilates the cervix by absorption of water.
      ii. Indwelling urinary catheter tip is inserted through the cervix, balloon is inflated, and gentle traction is applied to dilate the cervix.
   c. Prostaglandin E$_1$ (PGE$_1$): misoprostol—small tablet inserted directly into posterior fornix of vagina for direct absorption.
   d. Prostaglandin E$_2$ (PGE$_2$): dinoprostone—prefilled or time-released medication administration devices administered into the posterior fornix of vagina for direct absorption.

Stripping the Membranes

1. Following a cervical exam, the procedure entails separating the membranes from the lower uterine segment without rupturing the membranes.
2. Outpatient or inpatient option.
3. Complications include maternal/fetal infection, PPROM, umbilical cord prolapse, precipitous labor and birth, and personal discomfort.

Prostaglandin E$_1$

1. Misoprostol is a tablet containing prostaglandins. Misoprostol is not FDA-approved but has off-label use for cervical ripening or labor induction.
   a. Various dosing regimens are available; however, lower doses are associated with less uterine tachysystole; typical intravaginal dose is 25 mcg every 4 hours. Oral dosing is less successful.
   b. Redosing is withheld if more than five contractions occur in 10 minutes, adequate cervical ripening is achieved (cervix 80% effaced and 3 cm dilated), the patient is in active labor, or FHR Category III pattern.
   c. Patient should be observed for up to 2 hours after spontaneous rupture of membranes. If cervix remains unfavorable, uterine activity minimal, absence of Category III FHR pattern, and at least 3 hours since last dose, redosing is acceptable.
   d. Oxytocin can be given after 4 hours after last dose.
   e. Misoprostol should be administered at or near the labor and delivery/birthing suite to allow continuous monitoring of fetal and uterine status.

 DRUG ALERT Adverse effects of misoprostol include shivering, backache, vomiting, diarrhea, shortness of breath, uterine hypertonus, or uterine rupture. Misoprostol is not recommended for women with a history of prior cesarean delivery or other uterine scarring.

Prostaglandin E$_2$

1. PGE$_2$ is primarily used before induction of labor for cervical ripening, administered intracervically or vaginally.
2. If labor results from administration of PGE$_2$, it is similar to spontaneous labor.
3. Uterine tachysystole is a complication.
4. PGE$_2$ gel is given via catheter or diaphragm in doses ranging from 0.5 to 5 mg.
   a. Unstable at room temperature; store in refrigerator; bring to room temperature just before administration (do not use microwave; warm water, or any other heating method to speed the warming process as the gel is sensitive to heat and may be inactivated).
   b. Patient should stay recumbent for at least 30 minutes. If no response, additional doses may be administered every 6 hours.
   c. Oxytocin should be delayed for 6 to 12 hours after last dose of gel.
   d. Should be administered at or near labor and delivery/birthing suite (to monitor fetal and uterine status—continue monitoring for 30 minutes to 2 hours after administration).

5. Dinoprostone is a solid, time-released suppository placed into the vagina. The suppository contains 10 mg that releases 0.3 mg/hour. Requires continuous fetal monitoring as evidenced by manufacturer and research guidelines.

   a. Keep frozen until immediately before use; unstable at room temperature; stable up to 3 years when frozen.

   b. Patient is to remain supine for 2 hours after insertion; may ambulate after 2 hours.

   c. Removal after 12 hours or at onset of labor; oxytocin may be delayed at least 30 to 60 minutes after removal. Removal may be required if evidence of uterine hyperstimulatory response or fetal intolerance (evolving FHR Category II or Category III pattern).

   d. Should be administered at or near labor and delivery/birthing suite with continuous EFM to monitor fetal and uterine status and for at least 15 minutes after removal.

Amniotomy (Artificial Rupture of Membranes [AROM])

1. Perform cervical exam.

2. Insert amniohook through cervix and perform a slight twisting motion to catch a small area of the membranes. Fluid should be clear or cloudy without odor.

3. Data shows when amniotomy is used alone it has unpredictable results with often long intervals before the onset of labor; increasing risk of infection.

4. Utilized with oxytocin at onset, induction-to-delivery is shorter than with amniotomy alone.

5. Monitor UA and FHR data at periodic intervals.

6. Complications include umbilical cord prolapse or compression and possible maternal or fetal infection.

Oxytocin Infusion

Oxytocin, an octapeptide, is one of the most common drugs utilized in the United States. Patient sensitivity varies. Based on pharmacokinetic studies, uterine response begins within 3 to 5 minutes of infusion and reaches a steady state in 40 minutes. Cervical dilation, parity, and gestational age predict the dose response of oxytocin.

1. Oxytocin is mixed as an IV piggyback solution that is infused into the primary IV at the port of entry nearest the skin insertion. Solution concentrations vary and may be mixed by pharmacy or on labor and delivery by a staff registered nurse.

2. Oxytocin is only given via infusion pump accompanied by constant monitoring of maternal and fetal status in the inpatient setting.

3. Dosing requirements adequate for labor vary as low- and high-dose options.

   a. Typical starting doses vary from 0.5 to 2 milliunits (mU) and increase 1 to 2 mU every 15 to 40 minutes; pharmacodynamics recommend dosing intervals of 45 to 60 minutes to limit risk of oxytocin resistance over intrapartum period.

   b. The goal is to establish regular uterine contractions leading to cervical advancement and fetal descent. Cervical dilation of 1.5 to 2 cm/hour in the active phase of labor—contractions occurring every 2 to 5 minutes lasting 50 to 70 seconds and an intensity of 50 to 70 mm Hg (moderate) or greater than 180 Montevideo units but less than 400.

   c. Be aware that cervical dilation, effacement, and subsequent fetal descent are the true indicators of adequate labor progression, not uterine activity.

4. If oxytocin is discontinued for 20 to 30 minutes, it may be restarted at one half the previous dose once reassuring UA and FHR data are established. However, if the oxytocin has been discontinued for over 30 to 40 minutes, it must be restarted at the initial dose.

5. Complications:

   a. Uterine tachysystole (more than 5 contractions in 10 minutes).

   b. Uterine hypertonus (resting tone > 20 to 25 mm Hg, depending on the type of intrauterine pressure catheter; intensity > 80 mm Hg).

   c. Contractions longer than 2 minutes in duration.

   d. Increased incidence of cesarean delivery.

   e. Hypotension with rapid infusion.

6. Uterine tachysystole accompanied by fetal bradycardia may be treated with tocolytics prior to emergent delivery, if indicated.

 DRUG ALERT Administration of oxytocin requires close monitoring of intake and output, especially IV fluid monitoring. A major adverse effect of oxytocin is water intoxication, which can lead to heart failure. Symptoms of water intoxification include headache, nausea and vomiting, mental confusion, decreased urine output, hypotension, tachycardia, and cardiac arrhythmia.

Active Management of Labor

1. Augmentation high-dose oxytocin protocol directed toward reducing cesarean deliveries due to dystocia in nulliparous woman; reduction of cesarean delivery with active management has not been confirmed in research.

2. Goal is vaginal birth within 12 hours after admission.

3. Criteria for active management of labor:

   a. Nulliparity; multiparous is optional.

   b. Greater than 37 weeks' gestation.

   c. Singleton pregnancy with cephalic presentation.

   d. Active or true labor defined as contractions with bloody show, spontaneous rupture of membranes, or complete (100%) cervical effacement.

   e. Artificial rupture of membranes within 1 hour after labor has been diagnosed.

   f. If no cervical change of at least 1 cm/hour, oxytocin augmentation is initiated.

   g. Dosage is 6 µU/minute; increase by 6 milliunits/minute every 15 minutes until adequate labor is achieved or to a maximum of 40 µU/minute.

   h. One-to-one nurse-to-patient ratio is recommended; this is difficult to maintain in many facilities nationwide.

Complications

1. Hyperstimulatory effects (eg, tachysystole or hypertonus).

2. Evolving Category II or Category III FHR pattern.

3. Uterine rupture.

Nursing Assessment

 NURSING ALERT Make sure that patient is aware of the procedures to be used, questions have been answered, and informed consent obtained prior to initiation of procedure.

Prior to Induction
1. Obtain an NST to assess fetal well-being.
2. Evaluate maternal vital signs, especially BP.
3. Place an IV and evaluate patency prior to initiation.

Following Administration of Oxytocin
1. Monitor FHR and uterine activity periodically, typically every 15 minutes.
2. Assess maternal vital signs in accordance with your facility's policy; BP and pulse should be assessed at each dose interval.
3. Limit vaginal examinations, especially after the membranes have ruptured.
4. Maintain intake and output records and watch for signs of water intoxication—dizziness, headache, confusion, nausea and vomiting, hypotension, tachycardia, decreased urine output.

Nursing Diagnoses
- Anxiety related to planned childbirth and outcome.
- Risk for Injury related to hyperstimulatory uterine response.
- Acute Pain related to uterine activity and evolution of labor and birth process.

Nursing Interventions

Decreasing Anxiety
1. Teach or review the use of relaxation and distraction techniques.
2. Prior to induction or augmentation, explain the procedure to the woman and her support person.
3. Answer questions and offer support.

Preventing Injury through Ureteroplacental Oxygenation
1. Assess fetal status and uterine contractions periodically. Assess for signs of uteroplacental insufficiency (minimal-absent variability, abnormal baseline FHR, recurrent or repetitive late or variable decelerations).
2. Place patient in lateral position and assess vital signs; increase IV fluids if hypotension evolves.
3. Administer prescribed oxygen (8 to 10 L/minute by face mask) if nonreassuring FHR characteristics develop (evolving Category II or Category III FHR pattern) and notify provider.
4. If any persistent hyperstimulatory uterine response (eg, tachysystole or hypertonus) develops, discontinue the augmentation or induction agent, if possible; induce intrauterine resuscitation techniques; and notify health care provider immediately. Administer tocolytics, as ordered, and prepare for emergent cesarean delivery.

Pain Control
1. Encourage use of breathing techniques, distraction, and non-pharmacologic comfort measures.
2. Administer analgesia/anesthesia as requested and prescribed.
3. Maintain positive outlook and support as labor progresses.

Evaluation: Expected Outcomes
- Verbalizes understanding of the induction process.
- No evidence of hyperstimulatory uterine response or Category III FHR pattern.
- Labor progressing and pain controlled.

Dystocia

Dystocia is characterized by slow, abnormal labor progression typically resulting from abnormal uterine activity patterns or maternal expulsive forces. Dystocia is the leading indication for augmentation and primary cesarean delivery. Causes include power (contractions), passageway (pelvis), or passenger (fetus) abnormalities.

Pathophysiology and Etiology

Power Abnormalities
1. Inadequate contractions result in poor labor progression and slow fetal descent. Common causes include increased uterine tone, abnormal contraction pressure, hypotonic labor (prolonged latent phase, protracted or arrested active phase, or prolonged second stage of labor), and abnormal contraction pressure.
2. Problems with the force of labor result in ineffective contractions or bearing-down efforts (pushing) during the second stage of labor.
3. Etiology of abnormalities in the force of labor includes:
   a. Early or excessive use of analgesia.
   b. Overdistention of the uterus.
   c. Excessive cervical rigidity.
   d. Grand multiparity (>6).

Passageway Abnormalities
1. Abnormalities in the passageway may be the result of pelvic or soft tissue anomalies.
2. Pelvic abnormalities that interfere with the engagement, descent, and expulsion of the fetus include:
   a. Size and shape of the pelvis.
   b. Obstruction that may result from soft tissue problems, such as a uterine or ovarian fibromyoma.
3. Contractions of the inlet are noted when the anteroposterior diameter is less than 10 cm or the greatest transverse diameter is less than 12 cm. Contracted inlets may be of genetic origin or a result of rickets.
4. Cephalopelvic disproportion (CPD) is a disparity between the size of the maternal pelvis and fetal head that prevents or precludes fetal descent and subsequent vaginal birth; cesarean birth is indicated if unresolved.

Passenger Abnormalities
1. Breech presentations occur in approximately 3% of all deliveries.

a. This presentation is more common in multiple gestations, increased parity, hydramnios, congenital dislocated hip, placenta previa, and preterm neonates.

b. Usually the method of choice for delivery is a cesarean delivery.

2. Shoulder presentation (transverse lie) occurs when the infant lies perpendicular to the maternal spine and cervical os. The infant is delivered by cesarean delivery if external cephalic version (ECV) is unsuccessful.

3. A large fetus increases the risk of trauma, both maternal and fetal; CPD may result.

Diagnostic Evaluation

1. Inadequate progress of cervical effacement, dilation, or descent of the presenting part as determined by vaginal examination.

2. Comparison of serial evaluations of labor progress using Friedman's curve criteria, if available.

   a. A prolonged latent phase in the primigravida is >20 hours and >14 hours in the multigravida.

   b. During the active phase, the cervix of a primigravida will normally dilate at a rate of 1.2 cm/hour and a multigravida 1.5 cm/hour. In addition, the fetus should descend at a typical rate of 1 cm/hour in a primigravida and 2 cm/hour for a multigravida.

Management

1. Treatment for contraction abnormalities involves stimulation of labor through the use of labor enhancement medications such as oxytocin; an intrauterine pressure catheter may be utilized for direct assessment of uterine contraction data.

2. Management for maternal passageway or fetal passenger problems involves delivery in the safest manner for the mother and fetus.

   a. If the problem is related to the inlet or midpelvis, a cesarean delivery is indicated.

   b. If the problem is related to the pelvic outlet, an operative vaginal delivery with forceps or vacuum extraction may be performed.

Complications

1. Maternal exhaustion.
2. Infection.
3. Postpartum hemorrhage.
4. Fetal intolerance: evolving Category II or Category III FHR patterns.
5. Fetal or maternal trauma from operative vaginal delivery.

Nursing Assessment

1. Perform Leopold's maneuvers and evaluate fetal presentation, position, and size.
2. Using Friedman's labor curve, periodically evaluate progress of labor.
3. Monitor FHR and contraction status periodically per facility policy.

Nursing Diagnoses

• Acute Pain related to physical and psychological factors of difficult labor.
• Anxiety related to threat of possible operative delivery.

Nursing Interventions

Promoting Comfort

1. Review relaxation techniques.
2. Encourage use of breathing techniques learned in prenatal classes.
3. Encourage frequent change of position.
4. Encourage voiding periodically throughout labor.
5. Provide back rubs and sacral pressure, as needed.
6. Offer ice chips, as needed, to combat a dry mouth, if permitted.
7. Provide frequent encouragement to the woman and her support person.
8. Administer pain medication as ordered.
9. Assist with the administration of anesthesia, as requested and indicated.

Decreasing Anxiety

1. Provide anticipatory guidance regarding the use of medication, equipment, and procedures.
2. Educate the woman regarding augmentation agents: oxytocin.
3. Prepare the family for cesarean delivery, if necessary.

Evaluation: Expected Outcomes

• Verbalizes increased comfort.
• Verbalizes understanding of procedures.

Shoulder Dystocia

Shoulder dystocia is the dysfunctional descent and expulsion of the fetal shoulders, resulting in impaction of the anterior shoulder behind the maternal pubis symphysis or posterior shoulder on the sacral promontory during the second stage of labor. This condition is often relieved with gentle manipulation but may turn into an obstetrical emergency within minutes. Approximately 50% of shoulder dystocia incidents have no risk factors.

Pathophysiology and Etiology

1. Antepartum risk factors:
   a. Fetal macrosomia.
   b. Maternal diabetes.
   c. Fetal macrosomia more than 5,000 g or more than 4,500 g with maternal diabetes (collaborative risks have highest rate of shoulder dystocia).
   d. Postterm gestation.
   e. Previous history of shoulder dystocia, macrosomia, or postterm pregnancy.

2. Intrapartum factors:
   a. Labor induction.
   b. Epidural anesthesia.
   c. Protraction or arrest of labor.
   d. Prolonged second stage.
   e. Operative vaginal delivery.

3. None of the risk factors noted above individually, or collectively, can predict shoulder dystocia. Anticipatory preparations should be made at every delivery.

Management

1. Compare labor progression to Friedman labor graph per facility policy and communicate dysfunctional patterns early and prepare accordingly.
2. Prevention is the key because shoulder dystocia is difficult to predict.
   a. Early identification and treatment of gestational diabetes mellitus.
   b. Antepartum control of insulin-dependent diabetes mellitus.
   c. Periodic estimated fetal weight measurements; third-trimester ultrasound measurements are significantly inaccurate.
   d. Avoid postdated deliveries.
   e. Prevent abnormal progression of labor or treat early.
   f. Promote adequate maternal weight gain.
3. Once shoulder dystocia is identified, the following interventions may be indicated based on individual clinical conditions:
   a. Document the time shoulder dystocia diagnosed.
   b. Avoid fundal pressure.
   c. Perform appropriate nursing maneuvers, as indicated (see below).
   d. Assist with appropriate medical maneuvers, if applicable (see below).
   e. Call for assistance to support maneuvers and to treat immediate postpartum complications.
   f. Notify neonatal team.
   g. Document delivery time and calculate total time frame of shoulder dystocia incident. List all maneuvers performed during incident, time of application, and individual(s) who performed the intervention(s). Record Apgar scores and neonatal resuscitative interventions, if applicable. Lastly, manage and document any postpartum complications.
4. Nursing maneuvers; begin with least invasive; no particular order is recommended:
   a. McRoberts' maneuver—exaggerated flexion of the mother's legs, simulating a supine squat position. The squat position increases pelvic diameter by 1 to 3 cm.
   b. Suprapubic pressure—place the heel or palm of one hand over the suprapubic area and press down and to the left or right, as directed by the primary practitioner, to assist in dislodging the anterior shoulder under the maternal pubic bone.
   c. Gaskin's maneuver—Hands-and-knees position; assist the patient onto her hands and knees in an "all-fours" position; it is suspected the anterior shoulder drops posteriorly in this position, releasing the dystocia and resulting in delivery. This may be difficult but obtainable in the patient with epidural anesthesia.
5. Medical maneuvers:
   a. Episiotomy.
   b. Rotation of the anterior shoulder to oblique position.

   c. Barnum maneuver- delivery of posterior arm across fetal chest.
   d. Rubin's maneuver—displacement of the posterior shoulder anteriorly, with respect to fetus.
   e. Wood's screw maneuver—rotation of the shoulders to an oblique position.
   f. Zavanelli maneuver—replacement of the head by reverse cardinal movements into the vagina and delivery by cesarean.

Complications
Fetal
1. Fetal hypoxia and asphyxia; neonatal hypoxic ischemic encephalopathy.
2. Brachial plexus injury.
3. Fractured clavicle or humerus.
4. Facial nerve paralysis.
5. Neuropsychiatric dysfunction or death.

Maternal
1. Postpartum hemorrhage (11%).
2. Vaginal lacerations (fourth degree: 3.8%).
3. Cervical lacerations.

Nursing Assessment

1. Continuously evaluate labor curve for signs of dystocia.
2. Maintain EFM until delivery is successful.
3. Notify all perinatal team members of delivery time frame.

Nursing Diagnoses

- Fear and Anxiety related to inability of fetus to deliver.
- Acute Pain associated with operative and instrumented procedures or uterine manipulation.
- Risk for Injury to fetus or mother secondary to instrumented delivery or manual maneuvers.

Nursing Interventions

Reducing Fear and Anxiety
1. Inform patient of complication and offer support.
2. Limit family members in the delivery room should shoulder dystocia occur, as additional health care personnel may be required.
3. Keep voice calm and controlled during delivery process.

Decreasing Pain
1. Maintain appropriate anesthesia/analgesia for pain relief during maneuvers.
2. Offer additional anesthesia/analgesia after delivery, as needed or indicated.

Reducing and Identifying Trauma
1. Monitor labor curve and notify primary care provider if abnormalities exist.
2. Performing fundal pressure may further impact the shoulder; utilize other maneuvers to dislodge shoulder.
3. Perform critical assessment of neonate after delivery, particularly face and upper limbs.

NURSING ALERT Fundal pressure is not utilized for the treatment of shoulder dystocia. It can lead to further impaction of the anterior shoulder, irreversible brachial plexus injury, fetal neurologic injury secondary to hypoxia, and even fetal death.

Evaluation: Expected Outcomes

- Verbalizes understanding of situation and is cooperative with plan.
- Verbalizes control of pain.
- No maternal or neonatal injury.

Uterine Rupture

 Evidence Base American College of Obstetricians and Gynecologists. (2010). *Vaginal birth after cesarean* (Practice Bulletin #115). Washington, DC: Author.

Uterine rupture is a spontaneous or traumatic tear exposing the internal uterine compartment to the peritoneal cavity; extrusion of the umbilical cord, fetus, or fetal parts may occur. *Uterine dehiscence* occurs due to partial separation of an old scar prior to full rupture. Uterine rupture is a catastrophic event with significant risk of maternal, fetal, and neonatal morbidity and mortality.

Pathophysiology and Etiology

Risk factors:

1. Number of prior cesarean births and scar type.
2. Interpregnancy interval (time frame of the end of one gestation to the beginning of the subsequent gestation).
3. Trial of labor after cesarean.
4. Uterine closure technique: single-layer closure has higher risk over double-layer closure.
5. Trauma.
6. Obstetric maneuvers.
7. Uterine abnormalities.

Clinical Manifestations

Clinical manifestations depend on location, size, and duration of rupture. Clinical conditions may evolve acutely (minutes) or chronically (hours) during the intrapartum period.

Signs and Symptoms

May be absent or present individually or collectively.

1. Constant abdominal pain and tenderness (may be dulled by anesthesia or analgesia).
2. Uterine contractions will usually continue but may diminish in intensity and tone.
3. Vaginal or abdominal bleeding into the peritoneal cavity.
4. Nausea/vomiting.
5. Syncope.
6. Vital sign instability: early—tachycardia, tachypnea, hypertension; late—signs of shock: rapid, weak pulse; hypotension; cold, clammy skin; pale color.

7. Uteroplacental insufficiency as evidenced by evolving Category II or Category III FHR patterns.
8. Clinical signs of placental abruption or cord prolapse (sudden onset of FHR variable decelerations).

Management

1. Immediate stabilization of maternal hemodynamics followed by emergent cesarean delivery. Anticipatory preparations may require intraoperative blood component therapy.
2. Fetus is delivered expeditiously and neonatal resuscitation is performed, as indicated. The uterus is repaired, if possible, otherwise a hysterectomy may be indicated.
3. Adequate fluid replacement is maintained.
4. Antibiotic therapy.

Complications

Maternal

1. Urologic injury.
2. Hysterectomy.
3. Concurrent complete or partial abruptio placentae; hemorrhage.
4. Hypovolemic shock.
5. Severe blood loss or anemia, with possibility of transfusion.
6. Bowel laceration, with possibility of peritonitis.
7. Infection.
8. Death.

Fetal

1. Hypoxia leading to fetal acidosis and perinatal asphyxia (occurs 39% to 91%).
2. Hypoxic-ischemic encephalopathy; neonatal brain injury.
3. Death.

Nursing Assessment

1. Continuously evaluate maternal vital signs for clinical triggers of decompensation.
2. Observe for signs and symptoms of impending rupture periodically during labor progression, particularly during VBAC delivery or a history of uterine surgery (see Box 39-2).
3. Assess fetal status by continuous monitoring.
4. Speak with family and debrief them on event following stabilization of mother and newborn.

Nursing Diagnoses

- Deficient Fluid Volume related to active fluid loss secondary to hemorrhage.
- Risk for Decreased Cardiac Tissue Perfusion: Maternal and Fetal, related to hypovolemia.
- Fear related to outcome for fetus and mother.

Nursing Interventions

Maintaining Fluid Volume

1. Maintain primary IV line and start a secondary line, as indicated by the patient's condition; if patient is unstable, place a second line with a 16G needle in the antecubital fossa with lactated Ringer's solution with rapid infusion.

BOX 39-2 Vaginal Birth after Cesarean

- Selection criteria to identify women eligible for vaginal birth after cesarean (VBAC):
  - One or two low-transverse cesarean births
  - Clinically adequate pelvis
  - No other uterine scars or previous rupture
  - Physician (capable of monitoring labor and performing an emergent cesarean delivery) is immediately available throughout active labor
  - Anesthesia and surgical team available for emergent cesarean delivery
- Contraindications for VBAC (due to high risk of uterine rupture):
  - Prior classic or T-shaped incision or other transfundal uterine surgery
  - Contracted pelvis
  - Medical or obstetric complication that prevents/precludes vaginal delivery
  - Inability to perform emergency cesarean delivery because of unavailability of surgeon, anesthesia provider, sufficient personnel, physician capable of performing cesarean delivery, or sufficient facility

2. Monitor vital signs frequently to observe for maternal decompensation.
3. Assist with and maintain central venous pressure and arterial lines, as indicated, for hemodynamic monitoring.
4. Maintain bed rest to decrease metabolic demands.
5. Place indwelling urinary catheter and monitor urine output hourly or as indicated.
6. Obtain and administer blood component therapy, as ordered.
7. Monitor for signs of DIC—spontaneous bleeding from IV sites, oral mucous membranes, and vagina; bruising.

Maintaining Maternal Vital Organ and Fetal Tissue Perfusion

1. Administer oxygen using a face mask at 8 to 10 L/minute or as indicated; prolonged use prior to delivery is not recommended unless clinical conditions dictate.
2. Apply pulse oximeter and monitor oxygen saturation, as indicated. Pulse oximeter is unreliable during episodes of severe hemorrhage, therefore, monitor patient closely.
3. Monitor arterial blood gas levels and serum electrolyte levels, as indicated, to assess respiratory status, observing for hypoxemia and electrolyte imbalance.
4. Continually monitor maternal vital signs and FHR and UA data on EFM for clinical triggers of decompensation; rapid deterioration may indicate shock.
5. Evaluate actual blood loss as determined by weight periodically.

Reducing Fear

1. Offer explanation of events and procedures to the patient and her support person.
2. Answer questions.
3. Maintain a quiet and calm atmosphere to enhance relaxation.

4. Remain with the patient during anesthesia administration; offer support, as needed.
5. Update family members on the current situation, while the woman is in surgery, and then again postoperatively. Debrief family on expected outcomes of mother and newborn.

Patient Education and Health Maintenance

1. Provide information and support regarding the possibility for future pregnancies.
2. Encourage the support of family and friends.
3. Offer dietary options high in iron to improve secondary anemia.
4. Inform patient to limit activity during postpartum period to aid in recovery process.

Evaluation: Expected Outcomes

- Vital signs stable; no evidence of shock.
- Hemoglobin and hematocrit stable.
- Verbalizes concerns about self and her fetus.

Amniotic Fluid Embolism

Amniotic fluid embolism (AFE), also known as *anaphylactic syndrome of pregnancy*, occurs once amniotic fluid filled with fetal cells and debris enters the maternal circulation. Deposits of fluid or debris into the pulmonary arterioles results in rapid onset of respiratory distress, shock, and possible development of DIC. The mortality for this condition is 60% to 90%. Incidence is 1 per 8,000 to 20,000 births in the United States.

Pathophysiology and Etiology

1. The exact mechanism or portal of entry is uncertain yet many researchers have postulated the following theories:
   a. Fluid and debris may enter through small endocervical tears, vessels of the lower uterine segment, or cervical veins.
   b. Diffusion across amniotic membranes.
   c. Once fluid and debris enter the maternal vasculature, the maternal system may stimulate an immunologic (allergic) response to the foreign entity similar to rejection of a transplanted organ or infusion of the wrong blood type; this often stimulates the coagulation system, resulting in DIC (see Figure 39-5).
   d. Debris may be large enough to block the perfusion through the pulmonary artery, leading to pulmonary hypertension and right-sided heart failure; over a short time subsequent left-sided heart failure ensues, accompanied by hypoxia and acidosis.
2. If prolonged, DIC, shock, and cardiopulmonary collapse may occur.
3. It can occur in the intrapartum or postpartum period.
4. Risk factors include:
   a. Intrapartum period (70%).
   b. Multiparous (75%).
   c. Abruptio placentae.
   d. History of allergy or atopy (41%).
   e. Male fetal gender (controversial).
   f. Multiple gestations.
   g. Genetic influences.

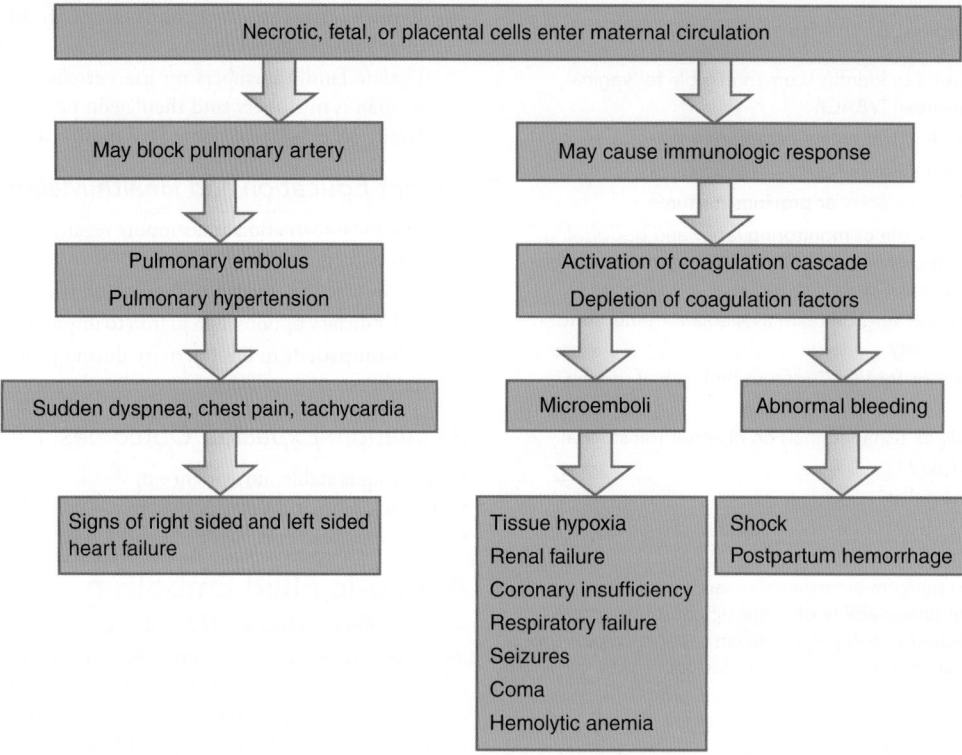

Figure 39-5. Pathogenesis of disseminated intravascular coagulation from amniotic fluid embolism.

Clinical Manifestations

1. Sudden dyspnea and chest pain.
2. Cyanosis, tachycardia.
3. Pulmonary edema.
4. Seizures.
5. Increasing restlessness and anxiety.
6. Feeling of impending doom.
7. DIC.
8. Cardiac dysrhythmias.
9. Cardiopulmonary collapse.

Diagnostic Evaluation

1. Clinical picture of sudden onset of respiratory collapse, shock, and cardiopulmonary arrest.
2. DIC confirmed by coagulation studies (prolonged thrombin time, PT, and PPT; decreased factor V, VIII, X; decreased platelets; increased fibrin split products).
3. Pulmonary aspirate evaluation for fetal cells.
4. Autopsy evaluation to confirm fetal cells and debris intravascularly.

Management

1. Respiratory support with oxygen therapy and intubation, as necessary.
2. Administration of IV crystalloid fluids in the treatment of shock.
3. Administration of blood component therapy to combat hemorrhage, shock, and DIC.
4. Establishment of a pulmonary artery catheter, if appropriate.
5. Cardiopulmonary resuscitation in a wedge position or abdominal displacement.
6. Perimortem cesarean delivery within 5 minutes of cardiopulmonary collapse.

Nursing Assessment and Interventions

See pages 998–999 for additional nursing care.

1. Be alert and suspicious to signs and symptoms of potential AFE and patients at risk (see above risk factors).
2. Monitor maternal vital signs to assess for signs of shock.
3. Monitor FHR for signs of intolerance.
4. Administer oxygen to assist respiratory status.
5. Alert medical staff immediately and assist with emergency procedures, such as delivery and cardiopulmonary resuscitation, as needed.
6. Provide information and comfort to the family or support persons. If unable to do this personally due to the emergent needs of the woman, delegate another member of the staff to stay with the family or support persons.

Umbilical Cord Prolapse

If the umbilical cord precedes the presenting part of the fetus or lies adjacent to the primary presenting part, prolapse has occurred. Types of cord prolapse include:

Complete—the cord completely and significantly precedes the primary fetal presenting part; may be in the vagina or visible outside the introitus.

Occult—the cord is beside or just in front of the presenting part of the fetus.

Funic—the cord can be felt on vaginal examination through intact membranes preceding the fetal presenting part.

Pathophysiology and Etiology

Predisposing factors include:

1. Rupture of membranes before the presenting part is engaged in the pelvis.
2. More common in abnormal fetal positions, such as shoulder and foot presentations.
3. Prematurity.
4. Polyhydramnios.
5. Multifetal gestation.
6. Cephalopelvic disproportion (CPD).
7. Abnormally long umbilical cord.
8. Result of interventions or maneuvers (ie, ECV or amniotomy).

Clinical Manifestations

1. Cord may be seen protruding from vagina or palpated in the vagina or through the cervix.
2. Compression of the cord may cause variable decelerations; prolonged decelerations or bradycardia may develop over time.

 NURSING ALERT Prolapsed cord should be suspected with FHR prolonged deceleration or bradycardia resulting immediately after spontaneous or artificial rupture of membranes.

Management

1. Deliver fetus as soon as possible via the most expeditious route.
2. With an occult prolapse, relieve pressure off the umbilical cord by positioning the cord between your two examination fingers and pushing the fetal presenting part up and off the cord; palpate the cord for the FHR simultaneously.
3. Change maternal positions to potentially alleviate compression (typically knee-chest position or side-lying is adequate).
4. Prepare for emergent delivery.

Complications

Maternal

1. Infection.
2. Risk of increased perineal trauma from emergency operative delivery.

Fetal

1. Prematurity.
2. Hypoxia and perinatal asphyxia.
3. Meconium aspiration.
4. Fetal death if delayed or undiagnosed.

Nursing Assessment and Interventions

1. Observe for prolonged FHR deceleration or bradycardia following spontaneous or artificial rupture of membranes.
2. Perform vaginal exam; if cord is palpated, call for assistance and prepare for emergent delivery. Push the presenting part up and off the cord while palpating a pulse. Do not remove hand from vagina (see Figure 39-6). Extreme conditions may include lack of additional staff to assist; if so, remove hand and place patient in a reverse Trendelenburg position or up on all four extremities so that she is supported by knees and elbows to alleviate pressure on the cord while preparing for emergent delivery.
3. Palpate FHR between your fingers and notify team of results. A cord exposed to room air may exhibit a reflex constriction of the umbilical blood vessels. These conditions may further restrict oxygen and blood flow to the fetus. Place warm blankets over the patient's legs while transporting to the operating room.

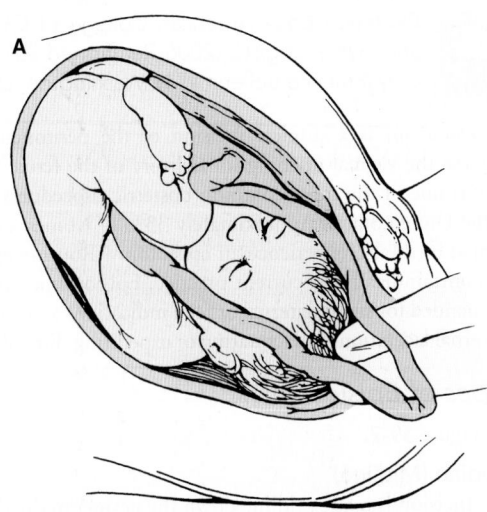
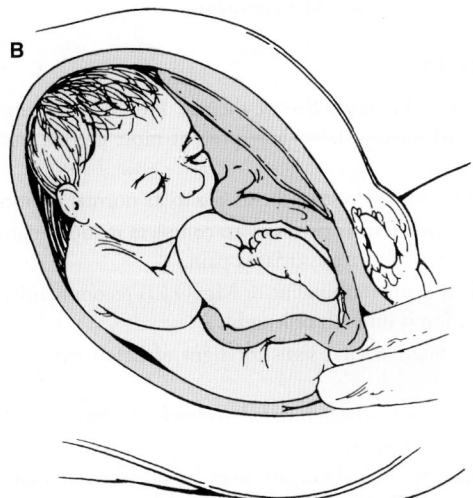

Figure 39-6. Prolapsed cord. Reduction of cord compression using gloved examiner's hand in vagina to elevate presenting part. (**A**) Vertex. (**B**) Breech.

4. Do not pinch or squeeze the umbilical cord as this may cause the cord to spasm, decreasing umbilical blood flow and oxygen to the fetus.
5. Explain procedures as much as possible to the woman during this emergent situation.
6. Administer oxygen at 8 to 10 L/minute.

Uterine Inversion

Uterine inversion is a potentially life-threatening complication in which the uterus turns inside out during the third stage of delivery. Uterine inversions may be classified as:

Complete—fundus inverts and passes through the cervical os into the vagina and may prolapse through the introitus.

Partial—fundus of uterus partially inverts but not beyond the cervical os.

Pathophysiology and Etiology

1. Excessive traction on the cord while the placenta is still attached.
2. Fundal pressure.
3. Lax or thin uterine wall.
4. Spontaneous inversion.
5. Abnormally short umbilical cord.
6. Uterine atony.
7. Uterine anomalies.
8. Fundal placentation.
9. Abnormally adherent placental tissue (placenta accreta or increta).
10. Fetal macrosomia.

Clinical Manifestations

1. Maternal instability accompanied by hemorrhage and sudden, severe pelvic pain (anesthesia may dull pain sensation).
2. Inability to palpate fundus in association with clinical manifestations.
3. Confirmed with bimanual examination.

Management

1. Prevention is the most effective therapy. Proper management of the third stage of labor may prevent most uterine inversions.
2. Goal is to manually restore the uterus to its normal position.
3. Typically, anesthesia is necessary to complete manual manipulation and to alleviate associated pain.
4. Tocolytic therapy (terbutaline or $MgSO_4$) is recommended if manipulation is difficult or lengthy.
5. Monitor maternal vital signs for signs of deterioration and shock.
6. After the uterus has been restored, oxytocin is administered to alleviate uterine atony.
7. Abdominal or vaginal surgery may be necessary if manual replacement fails.
8. Postprocedure, a broad-spectrum antibiotic is ordered.

Complications

1. Infection.
2. Anemia.
3. Hysterectomy.
4. Hemorrhagic shock.
5. Death.

Nursing Assessment and Interventions

See page 1216 for additional nursing care.

Before Correction of the Inversion

1. Check maternal vital signs and evaluate blood loss.
2. Assist practitioner, as needed, for manual replacement.
3. Administer oxygen, as warranted.
4. Maintain primary IV line and establish a second line with a 16G or 18G catheter for administration of fluids, blood products, and/or medications.
5. Apply a pulse oximeter to determine oxygen saturation.
6. If replacement of the uterus is unsuccessful, prepare the woman and her support persons for emergency surgery.

After Correction of the Inversion

1. Check maternal vital signs, and monitor CBC for signs of bleeding and infection.
2. Administer oxytocin and other uterine tonics, as ordered.
3. Measure and record accurate intake and output.
4. Evaluate uterine fundus carefully for position and firmness.
5. Evaluate lochia for amount of blood loss.
6. Evaluate for transfusion reactions (ie, itching, wheezing, anaphylaxis).
7. Administer antibiotics, as ordered, to minimize risk of infection.
8. Provide support to the woman and encourage her to express her feelings.

OPERATIVE OBSTETRICS
Episiotomy

Evidence Base American College of Obstetricians and Gynecologists. (2006/Reaffirmed 2011). *Episiotomy* (Practice Bulletin #71). Washington, DC: Author.

An *episiotomy* is a surgical incision of the peritoneum used to increase the vaginal opening for delivery of the fetus. An episiotomy is one of the most common obstetric procedures performed in the United States. Approximately 33% of women experiencing vaginal birth also experience an episiotomy. Routine episiotomies are contraindicated in current practice. Episiotomies are only recommended for such maternal or fetal indications as avoiding severe maternal lacerations or facilitating or expediting difficult deliveries.

Types of Episiotomies

See Figure 39-7.

Median (Midline)

1. Incision is made midline down the perineum directed toward the rectum.

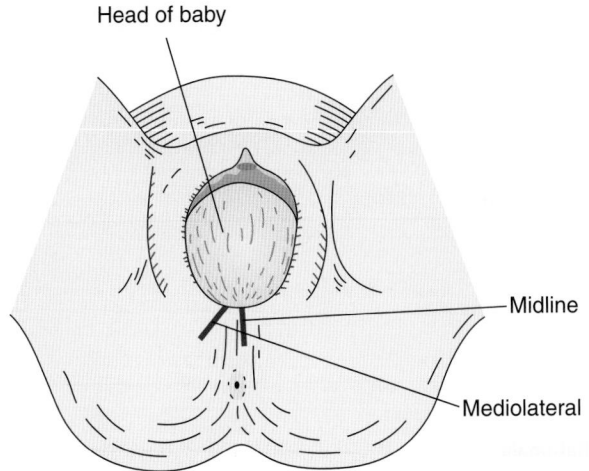

Figure 39-7. Position of episiotomy incision in a woman during second stage of labor. Baby's head is presenting to vaginal outlet (crowning).

2. This method is believed to heal with few complications, is more comfortable for the woman during healing, is easy to repair, and is associated with minimal blood loss.
3. Increases risk of third- and fourth-degree lacerations.
4. Decreased postpartum dyspareunia.
5. Most commonly performed in the United States.

Mediolateral
1. Incision 45 degrees or more from the midline.
2. This method avoids the anal sphincter if an extension is needed.
3. Women find it extremely uncomfortable during healing.
4. Difficult to repair.
5. Associated with increased blood loss.
6. Necessitates longer wound healing time.

Management
1. Pain relief.
   a. The stretching of the perineum and pressure from the fetal head may provide a natural numbing effect.
   b. Local perineal infiltration with lidocaine provides anesthesia for performing and repairing the episiotomy.
   c. A pudendal block provides anesthesia to the lower two thirds of the perineum and vagina using lidocaine injection into the vaginal walls.
   d. Epidural anesthesia provides anesthesia from the level of the umbilicus to the midthigh area.
2. The episiotomy is performed once the fetal head is 3 to 4 cm visible with a contraction.
3. The repair of the episiotomy usually begins after the delivery of the placenta.

Complications
1. Infection.
2. Bleeding.

3. Third- and fourth-degree lacerations.
4. Pain.
5. Hematoma.
6. Dyspareunia (painful intercourse).

Nursing Assessment
During the recovery period, the episiotomy should be evaluated periodically after delivery.
1. Describe and document the degree of healing.
2. Assess for infection; signs and symptoms include edema, redness, purulent drainage at the site, and/or increased temperature.
3. Notify health care provider of signs of infection or excessive bleeding at site, other than slight oozing.
4. Monitor for hematoma formation.
5. Apply ice packs periodically to limit edema and pain.

Nursing Diagnoses
- Risk for Infection related to traumatized tissue.
- Acute Pain related to surgical procedure.

Nursing Interventions
Preventing Infection
1. Instruct the woman to clean the perineum from front to back.
2. Provide instructions on perineal care.
   a. Provide a peri bottle; teach patient to squirt the water gently on her perineum after voiding.
3. Instruct patient to change the perineal pad each time after urination and defecation; dispose of in proper receptacle.
4. Explain the importance of proper handwashing before and after perineal care.
5. Explain that perineal care should be performed after urination and defecation and periodically throughout the day.
6. Encourage a diet that is high in protein and vitamin C and encourage hydration.

Promoting Comfort
1. Apply ice packs to the perineal area for the first 24 hours after delivery. The ice packs should not remain in place longer than 30 minutes at a time to get the maximum benefit from the treatment.
2. Encourage sitz baths with either warm or cool water. The warm water is soothing, whereas the cool water helps to decrease pain sensation and edema. See Procedure Guidelines 39-1, page 1358.
3. Administer pain medication and topical anesthetics, as ordered.
4. Instruct the woman to tighten her buttocks and perineal muscles before sitting in a chair and to release the muscles once seated.
5. Abstain from sexual intercourse until healing is complete, typically 4 to 6 weeks.

Evaluation: Expected Outcomes
- No evidence of infection; afebrile.
- Demonstrates increase in comfort.

PROCEDURE GUIDELINES 39-1

Sitz Bath

PURPOSE

A sitz bath aids the healing of the perineum through application of moist heat.

EQUIPMENT

- Sitz bath basin, bag, and tubing
- Towel
- Perineal pad

PROCEDURE

Nursing Action	Rationale
1. Assess patient's condition, pain level, and ability to ambulate to bathroom.	1. Effects of childbirth, pain medication, and lost sleep may make patient light-headed, fatigued, or drowsy, impairing her ability to ambulate and tolerate sitting on toilet without support.
2. Wash hands.	2. Prevents spread of germs onto clean equipment.
3. Fill sitz bath basin with warm water and place on toilet bowl (with toilet seat up). Fill bag with warm water at a temperature of 105° to 110° F (40.6° to 43.3° C) and attach tubing to basin.	3. Warm water is soothing and results in vasodilation to enhance healing, but should not create thermal injury.
4. Hang bag overhead so a steady stream of water will flow from the bag, through the tubing, into the basin.	4. Flow of water in the basin continuously replenishes warm water and enhances cleansing and circulation of the perineum, reducing inflammation and enhancing healing.

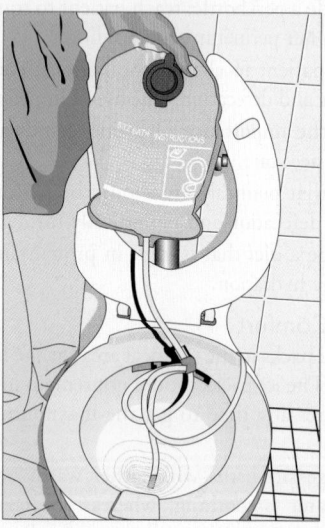

Nursing Action	Rationale
5. Assist patient with removal of peripad from front to back and positioning on sitz basin.	5. Removal of peripad from front to back prevents rectal contamination of incision.
6. Instruct patient to use clamp on tubing to control water flow. Make sure that she has robe or blanket to prevent chilling and that she can call for assistance, if necessary.	6. Adequate circulation of water enhances comfort and healing, but too brisk a flow will drain water too quickly to achieve benefit. Privacy should be protected.
7. Allow patient to sit for 20 minutes, then assist her with drying and applying a clean peripad (avoid touching front of pad).	7. Beneficial effects of heat are lost after 20 minutes due to vasoconstriction. Contamination of front of peripad might result in infection of healing tissue.
8. Assist patient back to bed, noting tolerance of the procedure.	8. Use of warm water and prolonged sitting in one position may result in light-headedness on arising.
9. Document tolerance of procedure, pain, and appearance of the perineal area.	9. Decreased swelling, redness, and drainage and complete healing are the goals.

Table 39-3   Representative Types of Forceps*

MAJOR CLASSIFICATIONS	USE
Simpson—separated shanks (eg, DeLee forceps)	Extract fetus with elongated, molded head; commonly used with nulliparas who have long labors
Elliot—overlapping shanks (eg, Tucker-McLean)	Extract fetus with unmolded, rounder heads; commonly used with multiparas who have briefer labors
Specialized Types	
Piper	Deliver aftercoming head in a breech presentation
Kielland	Rotate head from transverse or posterior position to an anterior position; used with women with anthropoid pelves
Barton	Rotate head from transverse to an anterior position; designed for use in women with flat pelves

*There are more than 600 types of forceps.

Forceps Delivery

Obstetric forceps (see Table 39-3) are designed for rotating or extracting the fetus. Most forceps are placed on each side of the fetal vertex and others are utilized for special considerations (Pipers: breech extraction). Forceps consist of two pieces: a right blade, which is slipped into the right side of the mother's pelvis, and a left blade, which is slipped into the left side. Unfortunately, forceps increase the diameter of the presenting part, which may hinder delivery. Special training and skill are required.

Types of Forceps Deliveries

American College of Obstetricians and Gynecologists definitions for obstetric forceps:

Outlet Forceps
1. Scalp is visible at the introitus without separating labia.
2. Fetal skull has reached pelvic floor.
3. Sagittal suture in anteroposterior diameter or right or left occiput anterior or posterior position.
4. Fetal head is at or on perineum.
5. Rotation does not exceed 45 degrees.

Low Forceps
1. Leading point of fetal skull is at station +2 cm or above and not on the pelvic floor.
   a. Rotation is less than 45 degrees (left or right occiput anterior to occiput anterior or left or right occiput posterior to occiput posterior).
   b. Rotation is greater than 45 degrees.

Indications for Forceps Delivery
1. No absolute indication exists. The fetal head must be engaged and the cervix fully dilated.
2. Prolonged second-stage labor.
   a. Nulliparous women: lack of continuing progress for 3 hours with regional anesthesia or 2 hours without regional anesthesia.
   b. Multiparous women: lack of continuing progress for 2 hours with regional anesthesia or 1 hour without regional anesthesia.
3. Category III FHR pattern.
4. Cardiac or neurologic disease.

Contraindications
1. Malpresentations: face or brow presentation.
2. Incomplete dilation of the cervix.
3. Unengaged fetal head.
4. Gestational age <34 weeks.
5. Live fetus with bone demineralization.
6. Fetal coagulopathies.
7. Inexperience of practitioner or unavailable operative personnel.

Management
1. The woman is placed in lithotomy position.
2. The bladder is usually emptied by catheterization.
3. Regional anesthesia is most frequently used; pudendal block is optional.
4. The neonatal staff is in attendance at delivery.
5. An episiotomy may be performed prior to manipulation.
6. Each blade is placed bilaterally over the fetal ear, avoiding the face.
7. Gentle traction is administered in a downward motion.

Complications
Maternal
1. Perineal trauma: lacerations of the vulva, cervix, vagina, and rectum; coccyx fracture.
2. Extensions of an episiotomy into the rectum: fourth-degree laceration.
3. Bladder trauma, uterine rupture.
4. Postpartum infection, postpartum hemorrhage secondary to uterine atony.
5. Anemia secondary to uterine atony/hemorrhage.
6. Urinary or fecal incontinence; fistula formation.

Fetal

1. Bruising.
2. Cephalohematoma.
3. Facial paralysis or brachial palsy.
4. Skull fracture.
5. Ocular trauma.
6. Intracranial hemorrhage.
7. Hypoxic-ischemic encephalopathy.
8. Shoulder dystocia.

Nursing Assessment

1. After application of forceps, the FHR should be evaluated at least every 5 minutes until delivery.
2. Evaluate bladder fullness—bladder should be empty before the application of the forceps.
3. Ensure sterile technique is maintained.

Nursing Diagnoses

- Anxiety related to fetal outcome.
- Acute Pain related to procedures.

Nursing Interventions

Decreasing Anxiety

1. Explain how forceps are applied.
2. Explain that a sensation of pressure will be felt.
3. Answer any questions.
4. Stay with the woman and provide guidance during the delivery process.

Promoting Comfort

1. Encourage use of breathing and relaxation techniques.
2. Make sure bladder is completely empty.
3. Encourage relaxation between contractions and use of abdominal muscles and pushing with the contractions.
4. Use blankets and pillows for support when positioning the woman for delivery.

Evaluation: Expected Outcomes

- Verbalizes concerns regarding forceps; responds to instructions.
- Demonstrates increased level of comfort.

Vacuum Extraction

Vacuum extraction applies suction to the fetal vertex to assist in delivery without increasing the diameter of the presenting part. Advantages include ease of application and ability; therefore, the procedure is gaining favor in the United States. It is also associated with less maternal trauma and less need for general or regional anesthesia.

Indications

1. Same as forceps.

Contraindications

1. Same as forceps.

Management

1. Fetus is in vertex presentation.
2. The woman is in the lithotomy position.
3. The bladder is emptied by catheterization.
4. Pressure is applied during contractions and released between contractions. Fetal descent should occur with each contraction.
5. Anesthesia may be indicated.
6. Unsuccessful extraction is followed by a cesarean delivery.
7. Neonatal staff is in attendance at delivery.

Complications

Complications are usually less frequent and less severe with vacuum extraction than with forceps.

Maternal

1. Lacerations of the cervix or vagina.

Fetal

1. Cephalohematoma.
2. Caput succedaneum (swelling of the scalp) from the vacuum.
3. Intracranial hemorrhage.
4. Retinal hemorrhage.
5. Abrasions.
6. Subgaleal hemorrhage.

Nursing Assessment

1. After application of the vacuum extractor, the FHR should be evaluated at least every 5 minutes until delivery.
2. Evaluate maternal sensation.
3. Evaluate bladder fullness—bladder should be empty before the application of the vacuum extractor.
4. Make sure sterile technique is maintained.
5. Monitor the vacuum pressure of the equipment according to your facility's protocol and document maternal–fetal response during procedure.
6. Monitor "pop-offs" (vacuum extractor cup pops off the fetal head); if three pop-offs have occurred of greater than 5 minutes have passed, other options (forceps, cesarean) should be considered.

Nursing Interventions

Same as for forceps delivery.

Cesarean Delivery

Cesarean delivery is the surgical removal of the infant from the uterus through an abdominal incision. Cesarean births are on the rise, up to 30% in 2005 from 29% in 2004. Maternal request for this procedure is a popular option.

Types of Cesarean Delivery

Uterine Incisions

Incision choice is based on the clinical scenario and future fertility.

1. Low transverse—transverse incision made across the lower uterine segment.
   a. Incision is made across the thickest section and away from uterine activity (fundus); minimizes blood loss and

improves the integrity of the scar, decreasing risk of future dehiscence or rupture.

  b. Postoperative convalescence is more comfortable.

  c. Incidence of postoperative adhesions and danger of intestinal obstruction are reduced.

  d. First-line choice of incision in most clinical scenarios.

2. Classic—vertical incision from the fundus down the body of the uterus to the lower uterine segment; may be utilized for emergent or preterm deliveries.

  a. Useful when bladder and lower segment are involved in extensive adhesions.

  b. Surgery of choice with a diagnosed anterior placenta previa, which inhibits the use of the low transverse incision.

  c. Increased blood loss versus low transverse.

  d. Increased risk of uterine rupture in subsequent deliveries.

3. T-extension (low transverse with midline vertical incision extending upward from the middle of the horizontal incision).

  a. Utilized to enlarge incision to complete the delivery.

  b. Commonly used with preterm deliveries.

Abdominal Incisions

1. Pfannenstiel—a horizontal incision across the suprapubic area.

  a. Cosmetic advantage; incision is hidden by clothing and often pubic hair.

  b. Decreased chance of dehiscence or hernia formation.

  c. Most common.

2. Vertical—a midline vertical incision from below the umbilicus to the symphysis pubis.

  a. Quicker to perform.

  b. Provides better uterine visualization.

  c. Cosmetically less appealing.

  d. Greater chance of wound dehiscence and hernia formation.

Indications for Cesarean Delivery

1. Any maternal medical complications, such as asthma, chronic hypertension, cardiac disease.

2. Labor complications: dystocia, malpresentation, CPD, Category III FHR pattern, prolonged or arrest of first or second stage of labor, early labor induction prior to cervical ripening.

3. Obstetric complications: placenta previa, breech, elective induction of nulliparous (50% higher risk than spontaneous labor).

4. Possible indications for cesarean hysterectomy:

  a. Ruptured uterus.

  b. Intrauterine infection.

  c. Postpartum hemorrhage: unresponsive to conservative management options.

  d. Laceration of major uterine vessel.

  e. Severe dysplasia or carcinoma in situ of the cervix.

  f. Placenta accreta.

  g. Gross multiple fibromyomas.

  h. Uterine inversion unresponsive to manual replacement.

Management

Preoperative

1. Assess patient's last intake of food, surgery should be delayed for 6 to 8 hours following last meal; consult anesthesia.

2. A blood sample should be typed and screened and available to be cross matched, if needed; a CBC is obtained.

3. Anesthesia, regional or general, depends on indication for surgery.

4. Consents signed and witnessed.

5. A large-bore IV is established with D_5LR or normal saline infusion.

6. Insert indwelling urinary catheter; may wait until after anesthesia placement to minimize discomfort.

7. Administer an antacid; reduces gastric acidity, limiting complications should aspiration occur.

8. Antibiotics may be given prophylactically.

Intraoperative

1. Patient is moved onto and secured to the operating table.

2. Abdominal preparation is completed with Betadine and air-dried.

3. Grounding pad for electrocautery unit is applied to patient's upper thigh.

4. Perform instrument, needle/knife, and lap pad counts periodically: before, during, and after surgery.

5. Assist with anesthesia, as needed.

6. Assist personnel with gowning and gloving.

7. Receive newborn and perform neonatal assessment.

8. Maintain sterile integrity.

9. Remove drapes and assist with application of dressing.

10. Assist patient to stretcher.

Postoperative

1. Assist patient to postoperative recovery room.

2. Complete care or give report to postoperative care provider.

3. Assist with patient stabilization as warranted by patient's condition.

Complications

1. Hemorrhage.

2. Endometritis.

3. Paralytic ileus (intestinal obstruction).

4. Pulmonary embolism.

5. Thrombophlebitis.

6. Anesthesia complications.

7. Bowel or bladder injury.

8. Respiratory depression of the infant from anesthetic drugs.

9. Possible delay in mother-infant bonding.

Nursing Assessment

Before Delivery

1. Assess knowledge of procedure.

2. Perform admission assessment.

3. Obtain 20- to 30-minute fetal tracing strip to assess fetal and uterine status.

4. Identify drug allergies; identify other allergies (eg, latex, iodine, tape).
5. Refer to interventions outlined above under "Management."

After Delivery

1. Assess maternal vital signs every 15 minutes the first hour or more frequently as the patient's condition warrants.
   a. Assess respiratory status: airway patency, oxygen needs, rate/quality/depth of respirations, auscultation of breath sounds, oxygen saturation readings.
   b. Circulation: BP, pulse, electrocardiogram monitoring for assessing dysrhythmias, color; assess dressing for drainage.
   c. LOC: orientation and response to verbal/tactile/painful stimulation.
2. Assess postpartum status (same intervals for assessment): fundal position and contractions, condition of incision and abdominal dressing, maternal–neonatal attachment, lochia (color, amount), neonate condition (if applicable), feeding preferences.
3. Assess hourly intake and output and reestablishment of bowel sounds.
4. Perform pain assessment: evaluate level of anesthesia, medications given (amount/time/results).

Nursing Diagnoses

- Anxiety related to surgical procedure.
- Acute Pain related to surgical procedure.
- Risk for Infection related to open abdominal cavity.
- Risk for Ineffective Parent/Infant Attachment related to interruption in bonding process.

Nursing Interventions

Relieving Anxiety

1. Explain the reason for the cesarean delivery.
2. Answer any questions.
3. Allow the support person to attend the birth, if appropriate.
4. Explain sensations of pressure that may be felt during the procedure; pain should be reported.
5. Explain procedures prior to initiation.
6. Inform patient and significant other of procedural progress.

Promoting Comfort

1. Encourage use of relaxation techniques after medication has been given for pain.

 DRUG ALERT Do not administer parenteral opioids if patient is receiving epidural opioids unless ordered by anesthesiologist or nurse anesthetist.

2. Monitor for respiratory depression up to 24 hours after epidural opioid administration.
3. Monitor and instruct patient on use of patient-controlled anesthesia pump, as applicable.
4. Use a back rub and a quiet environment to promote the effectiveness of the medication.
5. Support and splint the abdominal incision when moving or coughing and deep breathing.

6. Encourage frequent rest periods.
7. To reduce pain caused by gas, encourage ambulation or use of rocking chair.

Preventing Infection

1. Perform shaving or clipping of pubic hair per facility guidelines.
2. Maintain sterile technique during surgery and use sterile technique when changing dressings postoperatively.
3. Provide perineal care along with vital signs every 4 hours or as needed.
4. Provide routine postoperative care measures to prevent urinary or pulmonary infection.

Promoting Effective Bonding

1. Encourage mother–child bonding as soon as possible.
2. Emphasize that adjustments to parenting under any circumstances are necessary and normal.

Patient Education and Health Maintenance

1. Teach and assist the woman with the "football hold" for breastfeeding; alleviates pressure on the abdominal incision.
2. Teach the woman to observe for signs of infection (foul-smelling lochia, elevated temperature, increased pain, redness and edema at the incision site) and to report them immediately through 12 weeks' postpartum.
3. Assist the woman in planning for the assistance of friends, family, or hired help at home during the period immediately after discharge.

Evaluation: Expected Outcomes

- Verbalizes an understanding of the cesarean delivery procedure and postdelivery care.
- Reports relief of pain.
- No signs of infection.
- Participates in care of self and infant.

POSTPARTUM COMPLICATIONS

Postpartum Infection

Postpartum (puerperal) infection should be suspected if the patient's temperature exceeds 100° F (37.8° C) on two occasions at least 6 hours apart during the first 10 days postpartum. Postpartum endometritis occurs in 1% to 3% of postpartum women. The infection may remain localized or extend to various parts of the body such as connective tissue by lymphatic dissemination (parametritis). The broad ligament is the main pathway for systemic infection.

 NURSING ALERT The most effective method of prevention is handwashing.

Pathophysiology and Etiology

The most common cause is polymicrobial ascent to the uterus from the lower genital tract. Hematogenous bacterial spread may also occur.

1. Types of infection include:
   a. Endometritis: inflammation of the endometrium.

b. Endomyometritis: inflammation of the endometrium and myometrium.

c. Parametritis: inflammation of the endometrium and parametrial tissue.

2. Other infections include:

a. Wound or UTIs.

b. Pneumonia.

c. Mastitis.

d. Pelvic thrombophlebitis.

e. Necrotizing fasciitis.

3. Risk factors:

a. Operative birth.

b. Prolonged labor or rupture of membranes.

c. Use of invasive procedures (ie, internal monitoring, amnioinfusion, fetal scalp sampling).

d. Multiple pelvic examinations.

e. Excessive blood loss.

f. Pyelonephritis or diabetes.

g. Socioeconomic and nutritional factors compromising host defense mechanisms.

h. Anemia and systemic illness.

i. Smoking.

j. Mastitis-specific risk factors: infrequent breastfeeding, incomplete breast emptying, plugged milk duct, cracked or bleeding nipples (may be secondary to improper latch-on and removal).

Clinical Manifestations

Endometritis Postpartum

1. Fever occurring around third day postpartum is the most important finding.

2. Uterus usually larger than expected for postdelivery day and tender.

3. Lochia may be profuse, bloody, and foul-smelling.

4. Chills, malaise, and fever occur if lochial discharge is obstructed by clots.

5. WBC greater than 20,000/mm³ with increased neutrophils.

6. Infection may spread to myometrium (endomyometritis), parametrium, fallopian tubes, peritoneum, and blood.

Parametritis (Pelvic Cellulitis)

1. Chills, fever (102° to 104° F [38.9° to 40° C]), tachycardia.

2. Severe unilateral or bilateral pain in lower abdomen.

3. Enlarged and tender uterus.

4. Uterine position may become fixed as it is displaced by the exudate along the broad ligament.

5. Commonly the result of an infected wound in the cervix, vagina, perineum, or lower uterine segment.

Diagnostic Evaluation and Management

1. Obtain urinalysis and urine culture to rule out UTI.

2. Obtain blood sample for CBC and report results; assess for leukocytosis more than 20,000/mm³.

3. Antibiotic therapy: obtain cultures to identify causative agent. Broad-spectrum antibiotics are the treatment of choice including penicillins, cephalosporins (cefoxitin, cefazolin), clindamycin, and aminoglycosides (gentamicin, tobramycin). Antibiotics are given

until the woman is afebrile for 48 hours (maternal response usually occurs within 48 to 72 hours) and may include home therapy.

4. Increase daily fluid intake.

5. Encourage intake of 1,800 to 2,000 calories if lactating; diet should include a variety of foods, usually high in protein and vitamin C (promotes wound healing).

6. Ensure adequate urine output (30 mL/hour).

7. Supportive therapy is used to control pain and to maintain hydration and nutritional status.

8. Drainage is indicated for abscess development.

9. Instruct woman to discontinue breastfeeding, yet continue to pump (and dump) milk until infection clears.

 DRUG ALERT Clindamycin/gentamycin treatment is successful in only 75% to 92% of cases and is associated with renal toxicity. It is not effective against enterococci—ampicillin is the drug of choice in this instance.

Complications

1. Thrombophlebitis may result from postpartum infection spread along the veins or immobility.

a. Femoral thrombophlebitis—appears 10 to 20 days after delivery as pain in calf, fever, edema; affected leg circumference is 2 cm greater than unaffected leg.

b. Pelvic thrombophlebitis—infection of the veins of uterine wall and broad ligament usually caused by anaerobic streptococci; presents 14 days after delivery with severe chills and wide range of temperature changes.

c. Treatment includes strict bed rest, anticoagulants, and antibiotics.

2. Pulmonary embolus may occur—respiratory distress and chest pain.

3. Peritonitis—spread of infection through lymphatic channels.

Nursing Assessment

1. Perform postpartum assessment: note uterine tenderness on palpation and the color, amount, and odor of lochia; assess for proper breastfeeding techniques.

2. Monitor vital signs periodically for signs of infection.

3. Assess knowledge and skill of perineal and breast hygiene to prevent infection.

Nursing Diagnoses

- Hyperthermia related to infection.
- Risk for impaired attachment due to management of infection

Nursing Interventions

Restoring Normothermia

Teach proper technique and assist, if necessary.

1. Provide for adequate rest periods.

2. Increase fluid intake to make up for insensible loss.

3. Position in high-Fowler's position to promote drainage.

4. Administer antibiotics and analgesics, as ordered.

5. Explain the benefit of perineal washing or sitz baths; assist, as needed.

6. Explain importance of good handwashing technique; proper cleaning (front to back) during voiding or defecation.

7. Assist with perineal pads and medications; encourage changing pads with each voiding, bowel movement, and periodically throughout the day.

8. Observe for signs of septic shock: severe tachycardia, hypotension, tachypnea, changes in sensorium, and decreased urine output.

9. If pulmonary embolism is in question, elevate the head of the bed, provide oxygen, and notify rapid response team and primary practitioner.

Promoting Infant Attachment

1. Encourage minimal separation from the infant and continuation of breastfeeding, as able.

2. Promote good handwashing technique for the mother before contact with the infant.

3. Encourage father/family participation in care of mother/baby unit.

Evaluation

- Afebrile, tolerating antibiotics well, using good hand hygiene.
- Infant bonding time uninterrupted.

Postpartum Hemorrhage

 Evidence Base American College of Obstetricians and Gynecologists. (2006/Reaffirmed 2011). *Postpartum hemorrhage* (Practice Bulletin #76). Washington, DC: Author.

Postpartum hemorrhage reflects a blood loss in excess of 1,000 mL or greater regardless of mode of delivery. Hemorrhage is the single most significant cause of maternal death worldwide. Early postpartum hemorrhage occurs in the first 24 hours and may be considered late after 24 hours up until 12 weeks after birth. The greatest risk is during the first hour following delivery. Hemorrhage may also be defined as a decrease in hematocrit of at least 10%, but determinations of hemoglobin and hematocrit concentrations may not reflect current hematologic status. Worldwide, a woman dies of postpartum hemorrhage every 4 minutes.

Pathophysiology and Etiology

Excessive bleeding from a point between the uterus and perineum. Visual estimates are frequently imprecise and inaccurate, delaying diagnosis and treatment. See Figure 39-8.

Primary: Early Postpartum Hemorrhage (First Hour after Birth)

1. Occurs in 4% to 6% of pregnancies. Main cause: uterine atony (80%)—relaxation of the uterus secondary to:
   a. Overdistention of uterus secondary to multiple pregnancy, polyhydramnios, or macrosomia.
   b. High parity (more than six pregnancies).
   c. Prolonged labor.
   d. Medications—oxytocin, $MgSO_4$, tocolytics, anesthetics (halothane).
   e. Fibroids—prevents uterus from contracting.

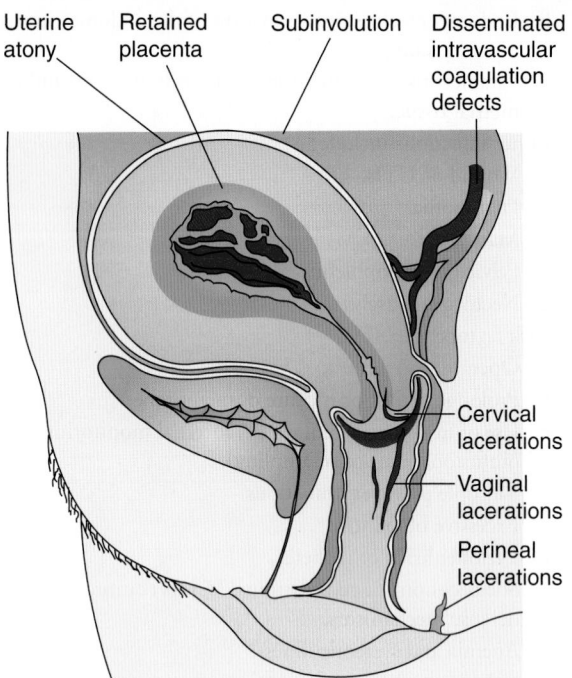

Figure 39-8. Common causes of postpartum hemorrhage.

   f. Retained placental fragments—result from manual removal of placenta, succenturiate (additional) lobe, abnormal adherent placenta (placenta accreta), or spontaneous Schultze placenta (periphery detaches first instead of central [Duncan] detachment).

2. Uterine inversion.

3. Bleeding disorders such as DIC.

4. Trauma, laceration, or hematomas of the vagina, cervix, or perineum secondary to:
   a. Forceps delivery, especially rotation forceps.
   b. Large infant.
   c. Multiple gestation.

5. Difficult third stage of labor (aggressive fundal manipulation or cord traction).

6. Sepsis.

7. Uterine rupture; uterine inversion.

8. Other risk factors include augmented or induced labor, rapid labor, history of postpartum hemorrhage, preeclampsia, Asian or Hispanic ethnicity.

Secondary: Late Postpartum Hemorrhage (Birth to 12 Weeks Postpartum)

1. Main cause is retained placental fragments.

2. Infection.

3. Subinvolution (delayed healing) of placental site.

Clinical Manifestations

Early Postpartum Hemorrhage

1. With uterine atony, uterus is soft or boggy, usually difficult to palpate, and will not remain contracted; excessive vaginal bleeding occurs.

2. Lacerations of the vagina, cervix, or perineum cause bright red, continuous bleeding even when the fundus is firm.

3. Tachycardia, hypotension, dizziness, pallor, and decreased urine output occur after loss of 10% total blood volume.

Late Postpartum Hemorrhage

1. Uterus is soft or boggy.
2. Slow, reddish oozing or heavy bleeding (first 6 weeks postdelivery).
3. Low persistent backache.
4. Abdominal pain or tenderness.
5. Fatigue.
6. Loss of appetite.

 NURSING ALERT For each 450 to 500 mL of blood loss, there will be a decrease in the hematocrit of 2% to 4% and a decrease in the hemoglobin of 1 to 1.5 g/dL.

Management

Goal is to stop hemorrhage by alleviating cause, correct hypovolemia, and return maternal hemostasis. These goals are accomplished through identification of risk factors and early identification and treatment of the underlying cause.

1. Maintain IV access with Lactated Ringers infusion and add a secondary line with 16G catheter for severe loss.
2. Notify blood bank, as indicated; order 4 to 6 units, as needed.
3. Prompt notification and communication to the perinatal team, which includes anesthesia, primary care provider, nursing and operating personnel, as indicated by the patient's condition.
4. Administer medications, as ordered: for uterine atony—IV administration of oxytocin, I.M. administration of methylergonovine, or prostaglandins (such as carboprost tromethamine, prostaglandins F2 alpha) administered I.M. or directly into myometrium during cesarean delivery, or misoprostel 200 to 1000 mcg rectally.
5. Bimanual massage of the uterus.
6. Pain medication may be needed to counter uterine contractions.
7. If placental fragments have been retained, curettage of the uterus may be indicated.
8. Assess for undiagnosed lacerations and repair.
9. Emergency hysterectomy may be necessary.

Complications

1. Hypovolemic shock.
2. Hysterectomy.
3. Death.

Nursing Assessment

1. Assess maternal history for risk factors; plan accordingly and communicate to the perinatal team.

2. Perform ongoing cumulative assessment of blood loss during the entire postpartum period. As the patient changes hands between practitioners and departments, blood loss is commonly estimated only by what one practitioner visualizes over his or her own shift, not taking into consideration what has transpired over the course of the entire postpartum period. Therefore, documentation and communication should reflect a cumulative total and any acute changes relative to the changes in the patient's immediate status.

3. Evaluate for presence of clots expelled or passed during voiding; note number of pads saturated in 1 hour or shorter time frame, if applicable. Weigh pads, as necessary, to determine loss (1 g = 1 mL).

4. Assess vital signs periodically and increase assessments if the patient shows signs of instability—tachycardia, hypotension, pallor, diaphoresis, altered LOC, tachypnea, nausea and vomiting, feelings of impending doom—all of which may indicate hypovolemic shock.

 NURSING ALERT Normal vital signs are not an indication that the woman is *not* in shock. Traditional signs of hypovolemic shock are not evident until approximately 15% to 20% of total maternal blood volume is lost. Continuous BP monitor readings may falsely lower diastolic and raise systolic readings. Assessments more frequent than 2 minutes apart may not allow for vessels within the extremity to reperfuse between assessments.

5. Assess pulse pressure (calculated from subtracting diastolic from systolic BP); recordings consistently less than 30 bpm are consistent with hypotensive crisis.

6. Assess intake and output (maintain >25 mL/hour); make sure intake includes a cumulative total to include all labor and delivery infusions as well as any fluids administered during surgery, such as with cesarean delivery.

7. Assess location and firmness of uterine fundus.

8. Percuss and palpate for bladder distention, which may interfere with contracting of the uterus.

9. Inspect for intactness of any perineal repair.

10. Due to rapid infusion of fluid during fluid resuscitation, periodically assess breath sounds for signs of pulmonary edema.

11. Abdominal girth assessments may be indicated if intra-abdominal bleeding is suspected, particularly after cesarean delivery. Use measuring tape under and around abdomen at level of umbilicus and mark the skin; assess every 30 minutes to 1 hour for any changes (increase in size), which may indicate internal bleeding and abdominal pooling.

12. Assist with surgical techniques for blood control, as indicated.

 NURSING ALERT In cases of postpartum hemorrhage, remember the acronym ORDER:
- Oxygen
- Restore circulation
- Drugs to alleviate bleeding
- Evaluate interventions
- Remedy underlying cause

Nursing Diagnoses

- Anxiety related to unexpected blood loss and uncertainty of outcome.
- Deficient Fluid Volume related to blood loss.
- Risk for Infection related to blood loss and vaginal examinations.

Nursing Interventions

Decreasing Anxiety

1. Maintain a quiet and calm atmosphere; provide emotional support.
2. Provide information about the current clinical situation; answer questions.
3. Encourage the presence of a support person.
4. Explain changes to care plan.

Maintaining Fluid Volume

1. Maintain primary IV access and place a second large-bore 16G catheter infusing normal saline or volume expanders, as indicated.
2. Monitor and maintain accurate intake and output; use of indwelling urinary catheter provides accurate output measurements.
3. Make sure that cross-matched blood is available; administer per facility protocol when necessary.
4. Provide supplemental oxygen by face mask; monitor oxygen saturation with pulse oximetry.
5. Administer medications, as ordered.
6. Change patient positions to facilitate perfusion to vital organs: elevate legs 20 to 30 degrees.
7. Use proper technique (two hands, gentle fundal pressure) during uterine massage; document findings.
8. Monitor CBC for anemia.
9. Dilatation and curettage may be needed for late postpartum hemorrhage.

> **NURSING ALERT** Avoid Trendelenburg's position for treatment of shock as it interferes with the cardiac and respiratory function by increasing pressure on the chemoreceptor and baroreceptors while decreasing lung expansion. The most effective position is to elevate the legs 20 to 30 degrees.

Preventing Infection

1. Maintain sterile technique.
2. Evaluate for symptoms of infection: chills, elevated temperature, increased WBCs, uterine tenderness, and odor of lochia.
3. Administer antibiotics, as prescribed.
4. Maintain adequate rest and proper nutrition.

Patient Education and Health Maintenance

1. Educate the woman about the cause of hemorrhage.
2. Teach the woman the importance of eating a balanced diet high in iron-rich options and taking vitamin supplements.
3. Advise the woman she may feel tired and fatigued and to schedule daily rest periods.
4. Teach woman and family signs and symptoms of hemorrhage for home care.
5. Ensure woman has emergency procedures and numbers readily available.
6. Advise the woman to notify her health care provider of increased bleeding or other changes in her status.

Evaluation: Expected Outcomes

- Verbalizes concerns about her well-being.
- Vital signs stable, urine output adequate, hematocrit stable.
- Remains afebrile, WBC count within normal limits.

Postpartum Hematomas

Postpartum hematomas are localized collections of blood in loose connective tissue beneath the skin covering external genitalia, beneath the vaginal mucosa, or in the broad ligaments. Usually occurs without laceration of the overlying tissue.

Pathophysiology and Etiology

1. Trauma during spontaneous labor or operative vaginal delivery.
2. Inadequate suturing of an episiotomy.
3. Delayed homeostasis or difficult or prolonged second stage of labor, or both.

Clinical Manifestations

1. Complaints of pressure and pain; pain may be verbalized as excruciating.
2. Discolored skin that is tight, full feeling, and painful to the touch.
3. Possible decrease in BP, tachycardia.
4. Decrease or absence of lochia flow if the vagina is impeded.

Management

1. Small hematomas (<3 cm) are left to resolve on their own— ice packs may be applied.
2. Large hematomas (>3 cm) may require evacuation of the blood and ligation of the bleeding vessel.
3. Analgesics and broad-spectrum antibiotics may be ordered (due to increased chance of infection).

Complications

1. Hypovolemia and shock from extreme blood loss.
2. Anemia, infection.
3. Increased length of postpartum recovery period.
4. Sepsis.
5. Calcification and scar tissue.
6. Dyspareunia (painful intercourse).

Nursing Interventions and Patient Education

1. Inspect perineal and vulvar area for signs of a hematoma periodically postpartum.
2. Inspect vaginal area for signs of a hematoma if woman is unable to void.

3. Monitor vital signs periodically and evaluate for signs of shock.

4. Relieve pain of a hematoma by applying an ice bag to perineal area, medicating with mild analgesics, and positioning for comfort to decrease pressure on the affected area.

5. Help relieve voiding problems by assisting to bathroom if able to ambulate. If patient is unable to ambulate, then assist her on to a bedpan with legs hanging over side of bed. Provide privacy and run water while the woman is attempting to void.

6. Catheterize patient if unable to void.

7. Teach the woman the importance of eating a balanced diet and to include food high in iron.

8. Encourage the woman to take vitamin supplements and to take medications, as ordered.

9. Instruct the woman in the use of a sitz bath to provide perineal comfort after the first 24 hours and at home.

Postpartum Depression

 Evidence Base American College of Obstetricians and Gynecologists. (2010). *Screening for depression during and after pregnancy* (Committee Opinion #453). Washington, DC: Author.

There is no consensus regarding the classification of postpartum depression. The most common conditions are typically identified as:

1. Maternity blues; postpartum blues; baby blues; mother's blues; or 3rd-, 4th-, or 10th-day blues.

2. Postpartum or postnatal depression.

3. Postpartum or puerperal psychosis.

4. Postpartum panic disorder.

5. Postpartum obsessive–compulsive disorder.

Pathophysiology and Etiology

Social, cultural, physiologic, and psychological factors may contribute to postpartum depression. Predisposing factors include:

1. Stressful life events during pregnancy or the postpartum period.
   a. Loss of loved one (fetus, neonate, partner, or other child).
   b. Illness of loved one.
   c. Financial difficulties.
   d. Loss of job.
   e. Move to new area, home, or job.

2. Poor interpersonal relationships.

3. Inadequate support.

4. Poor psychological history before or after pregnancy.

5. History of sexual abuse or domestic violence.

6. High levels of anxiety, neurotic behavior, and depression or emotional distress.

7. Personal or family history of psychopathology, especially depression.

Clinical Manifestations

1. Confusion.

2. Exaggerated and prolonged periods of irritability, moodiness, hostility, fatigue.

3. Ineffective coping.

4. Withdrawal and inappropriate response to the infant or family.

5. Loss of interest in activities.

6. Insomnia or sleep disturbances.

7. Headache.

8. Constipation or other GI difficulty.

9. Hair loss.

10. Dysmenorrhea.

11. Difficulties with lactation.

12. Decreased sexual responsiveness.

Evaluation and Management

Signs and symptoms may be overlooked, making the diagnosis of depression difficult. Several assessment tools, designed to screen for women who may need further evaluation for postpartum depression, are available. The psychosocial screening tool recommended by the American College of Obstetricians and Gynecologists can be used by the nurse or health care provider as a means of communication. Questions should be worded empathically and nonjudgmentally to stimulate an honest response from the mother.

Counseling with a mental health professional, medication, and continuous support from family and friends may be helpful in managing the depressed patient. If untreated, the woman may possibly harm the infant, herself, or others.

 DRUG ALERT The use of psychotropic medications during breastfeeding remains a controversial issue. All of the major classes of psychotropic drugs are expressed in breast milk.

 NURSING ALERT Any indication of suicide or harm to infant requires immediate referral to mental health professional.

Nursing Interventions and Patient Education

1. Listen to the woman regarding her adjustment to role of mother and observe for any clinical manifestations suggesting depression.

2. Ask the woman about the infant's behavior. Negative statements about the infant may suggest that the woman is having difficulty coping. Notify the woman's obstetric or primary care provider.

3. Consult or refer woman to health care provider and other resources skilled in postpartum depression, as indicated. Refer patients to Postpartum Support International (*www.postpartum.net* or 631-422-2255).

4. Provide support and encourage family and friends to support and assist with the infant and mother. Physical support as well as emotional support may be indicated.

5. Educate the woman that treatment may help alleviate her symptoms and allow her to better care for herself and her infant.

6. Encourage the woman to engage in activities that enhance attachment: rooming-in, breastfeeding, becoming involved in the medical examination of the neonate.

7. Realize that effective attachment behaviors differ from culture to culture and do not necessarily indicate maladaptive parenting behaviors.

SELECTED REFERENCES

American College of Obstetricians and Gynecologists. (2002/Reaffirmed 2008). *Shoulder dystocia* (Practice Bulletin # 40). Washington, DC: Author.

American College of Obstetricians and Gynecologists. (2002/Reaffirmed 2010). *Diagnosis and management of preeclampsia and eclampsia* (Practice Bulletin #33). Washington, DC: Author.

American College of Obstetricians and Gynecologists. (2003/Reaffirmed 2011). *Dystocia and augmentation of labor* (Practice Bulletin #10). Washington, DC: Author.

American College of Obstetricians and Gynecologists. (2003/Reaffirmed 2011). *Management of preterm labor* (Practice Bulletin #43). Washington, DC: Author.

American College of Obstetricians and Gynecologists. (2004/Reaffirmed 2008). *Diagnosis and treatment of gestational trophoblastic disease* (Practice Bulletin #53). Washington, DC: Author.

American College of Obstetricians and Gynecologists. (2004/Reaffirmed 2010). *Multiple gestation: Complicated twin, triplet, and high-order multifetal pregnancy* (Practice Bulletin #56). Washington, DC: Author.

American College of Obstetricians and Gynecologists. (2004/Reaffirmed 2011). *Nausea and vomiting of pregnancy* (Practice Bulletin #52). Washington, DC: Author.

American College of Obstetricians and Gynecologists. (2005/Reaffirmed 2011). *Medical management of abortion* (Practice Bulletin #67). Washington, DC: Author.

American College of Obstetricians and Gynecologists. (2006/Reaffirmed 2011). *Episiotomy* (Practice Bulletin #71). Washington, DC: Author.

American College of Obstetricians and Gynecologists. (2006/Reaffirmed 2011). *Postpartum hemorrhage* (Practice Bulletin #76). Washington, DC: Author.

American College of Obstetricians and Gynecologists. (2007/Reaffirmed 2009). *Premature rupture of membranes* (Practice Bulletin #80). Washington, DC: Author.

American College of Obstetricians and Gynecologists. (2010). *Screening for depression during and after pregnancy* (Committee Opinion #453). Washington, DC: Author.

American College of Obstetricians and Gynecologists. (2010). *Vaginal birth after cesarean* (Practice Bulletin #115). Washington, DC: Author.

American College of Obstetricians and Gynecologists. (2011). *Emergent therapy for acute-onset severe hypertension with preeclampsia and eclampsia* (Committee Opinion # 514). Washington, DC: Author.

American Academy of Pediatrics & American College of Obstetricians and Gynecologists. (2007). *Guidelines for perinatal care.* Elk Grove Village, IL: Authors.

Barron, M. L. (2008). Antenatal care. In K. Rice-Simpson & P. A. Creehan (Eds.), *AWHONN perinatal nursing* (3rd ed.). Philadelphia: Lippincott Williams & Wilkins, pp. 88–124.

Bishop, E. H. (1964). Pelvic scoring for elective induction. *Obstetrics and Gynecology, 24,* 267.

Blackburn, S. (2007). *Maternal, fetal and neonatal physiology: A clinical perspective* (3rd ed.). Philadelphia: W.B. Saunders.

Blackburn, S. T. (2008). Physiologic changes of pregnancy. In K. Rice-Simpson & P. A. Creehan (Eds.), *AWHONN perinatal nursing* (3rd ed.). Philadelphia: Lippincott Williams & Wilkins, pp. 59–77.

Bowers, N. A., et al. (2008). High risk pregnancy. In K. Rice-Simpson & P. A. Creehan (Eds.), *AWHONN perinatal nursing* (3rd ed.). Philadelphia: Lippincott Williams & Wilkins, pp. 125–299.

Calì, G., Giambanco, L., Puccio, G., et al. (2013). Morbidly adherent placenta: An evaluation of ultrasound diagnostic criteria and an attempt to differentiate placenta accreta from percreta. *Ultrasound Obstet Gynecol.*, Jan 3. [Epub ahead of print].

Carolan, M. (2012). Maternal age ≥45 years and maternal and perinatal outcomes: A review of the evidence. *Midwifery.* Nov. 15. [Epub ahead of print].

Clark, S., Simpson, K. R., Knox, E., et al. (2009). Oxytocin: New perspective on an old drug. *American Journal of Obstetrics and Gynecology, 200,* 35e1–35e6.

Clemmens, D., Driscoll, J. W., & Beck, C. T. (2004). Postpartum depression as profiled through the postpartum depression screening scale. *MCN: The American Journal of Maternal/Child Nursing, 29*(3), 181–185.

Creasy, R., Resnick, R., Iams, J., et al. (2009). *Creasy & Resnick's maternal-fetal medicine principles and practice* (6th ed.). Philadelphia: Saunders Elsevier.

Davidson, M. W., London, M. L., & Ladewig, P. W. (2011). *Olds' maternal-newborn nursing and women's health across the lifespan* (9th ed.). Upper Saddle River, NJ: Prentice Hall.

Gabbe, S., Neebyl, J., & Simpson, J. (2007). *Obstetrics: Normal and problem pregnancies* (5th ed.). Philadelphia: Elsevier

Gennaro, S. (2007). The evidence supporting nursing management of labor. *Journal of Obstetric, Gynecologic, and Neonatal Nursing, 36*(6), 598–604.

Hartmann, K. E., Andrews, J. C., Jerome, R. N., et al. (2012). Strategies to Reduce Cesarean Birth in Low-Risk Women (Report No. 12(13)-EHC 128-EF). Rockville, MD: Agency for Healthcare Research and Quality (US).

James, D. (2008). Postpartum care. In K. Rice-Simpson & P. A. Creehan (Eds.), *AWHONN perinatal nursing* (3rd ed.). Philadelphia: Lippincott Williams & Wilkins, pp. 473–526.

Kohari, K., Rebarber, A. (2013). Natural history of placenta previa in twins. *Obstet Gynecol., 121*(1), 190.

Kramer, J., Bowen, A., Stewart, N., et al. (2013). Nausea and Vomiting of Pregnancy: Prevalence, Severity and Relation to Psychosocial Health. *MCN Am J Matern Child Nurs., 38*(1), 21–27.

Kidner, M. G., & Flanders-Stepans, M. B. (2004). A model for the HELLP syndrome: The maternal experience. *Journal of Obstetric, Gynecologic, and Neonatal Nursing, 33*(1), 44–53.

Mattson, S., & Smith, J. (2011). *Core curriculum for maternal-neonate nursing* (4th ed.). Philadelphia: W.B. Saunders.

National High Blood Pressure Education Program. (2000). *Working group report on high blood pressure in pregnancy* (NIH Publication No. 00-3029). Bethesda, MD: National Institutes of Health, National Heart, Lung, and Blood Institute, National High Blood Pressure Education Program.

Phillips, F. (2012). Obesity in pregnancy. Part 1: prevalence and risks. *Pract Midwife., 15*(9), 20, 22–23.

Power, M. L., Schulkin, J. (2012). Maternal obesity, metabolic disease, and allostatic load. *Physiol Behav., 106*(1), 22–28.

Pri-Paz, S., Khalek, N., Fuchs, K. M., et al. (2012). Maximal amniotic fluid index as a prognostic factor in pregnancies complicated by polyhydramnios. *Ultrasound Obstet Gynecol., 39*(6), 648–653.

Rice-Simpson, K. (2008). Labor and birth. In K. Rice-Simpson & P. A. Creehan (Eds.), *AWHONN perinatal nursing* (3rd ed.). Philadelphia: Lippincott Williams & Wilkins, pp. 300–398.

Romano, A. M., & Lothian, J. A. (2008). Promoting, protecting, and supporting normal birth: A look at the evidence. *Journal of Obstetric, Gynecologic, and Neonatal Nursing, 37*(1), 94–105.

Sehgal, N. N. (1980). Early detection of abnormal labor using the Friedman labor graph. *Postgraduate Medicine, 68*(3), 189–196.

Simpson, K. S. (2008). *AWHONN cervical ripening and induction and augmentation of labor* (3rd ed.). Washington, DC: Association of Women's Health, Obstetric and Neonatal Nurses.

Stringer, M., Miesnik, S. R., Brown, L., et al. (2004). Nursing care of the patient with preterm premature rupture of membranes. *MCN: The American Journal of Maternal/Child Nursing, 29*(3), 144–150.

Troiano, N., Harvey, C., & Chez, B. (Eds.). (2013). *High-risk and critical care obstetrics* (3rd ed.). Philadelphia: Lippincott Williams & Wilkins.

U.S. Food and Drug Administration. (2011). FDA Drug Safety Communication: New warnings against use of terbutaline to treat preterm labor. Available: *www.fda.gov/drugs/drugsafety/ucm243539.htm.*

PART FOUR

PEDIATRIC NURSING

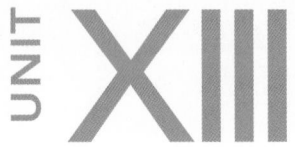
40

Pediatric Growth and Development

GROWTH AND DEVELOPMENT

Infant to Adolescent Growth and Development

Growth and development begin with birth. As infants and children grow and mature, they pass through predictable stages of development. Knowledge and assessment of growth and development help the nurse provide screening for physical and emotional problems; offer anticipatory guidance to parents and caregivers; develop a rapport with the child to enhance the provision of health care; and provide education to the family to build a healthy lifestyle for the future. For assessment of the neonate, see Chapter 38, page 1305. This chapter covers the beginning of infancy (age 1 month) to adolescence (ages 12 to 14). See Table 40-1.

Developmental Screening

Assessment tools have been created to determine the overall developmental age of a child or to detect specific areas of development that are lacking. The most widely used developmental screening tool is the Denver II Developmental Screening Test (Denver II). This tool provides for a quick overview of development in children from birth to age 6 years and identifies areas of strength and weakness relative to age norms. Denver II test forms and an instruction manual can be obtained from *www.denverii.com*. This test has been criticized for a lack of sensitivity in detecting children with more subtle developmental delays. The American Academy of Pediatrics recommends that developmental surveillance be conducted at all well-child exams and screening tests administered at the 9-, 18-, and 30-month visits; however, they do not recommend a specific test.

Another method for developmental screening involves interviewing the parent or caregiver about attainment of developmental milestones. Persistent deficits or deficits in multiple areas indicate a more serious problem than deficits in a single area. See Table 40-2, pages 1382 and 1383.

Table 40-1 Infant to Adolescent Growth and Development

AGE AND PHYSICAL CHARACTERISTICS	BEHAVIOR PATTERNS	NURSING CONSIDERATIONS
Birth–4 Weeks (1 Month) • Significant neurologic disorganization. • Strong Moro reflex. • Sleep cycle disorganized. • GI system too immature for solid foods.	**Motor development** • Momentary visual fixation on objects and adult face. • Eyes follow bright moving objects. • Lies awake on back. • Immediately drops objects placed in hands. • Responds to sounds of bell and other similar noises. • Keeps hands fisted. **Socialization and vocalization** • Mews and makes throaty noises. • Shows interest in human face. **Cognitive and emotional development** • Reflexive. • External stimuli are meaningless. • Responses are generally limited to tension states or discomfort. • Gains satisfaction from feeding and being held, rocked, fondled, and cuddled. • Has an intense need for sucking pleasure. • Quiets when picked up.	**Play stimulation** • Use human face—smile and talk. • Dangle bright moving object (eg, mobile) in field of vision. • Hold, touch, caress, fondle, kiss. • Rock, pat, change position. • Play soft music or have infant listen to ticking clock, sing. • Talk to infant, call by name. **Parental guidance** • Begin to expose infant to different household sounds. • Change crib location in room. • Use brightly colored clothing and linens. • Put infant to sleep on back until old enough to roll. • Keep infant nearby. • Play with infant when awake. • Hold during feeding. **NURSING ALERT** Educate parents about infant sleep stages and putting infant to sleep on back.
4–8 Weeks (2 Months) • Crossed extensor reflex disappears. • Tonic neck reflex begins to fade.	**Motor development** • Reflexive behavior is slowly being replaced by voluntary movements. • Turns from side to back. • Begins to lift head momentarily from prone position. • Shows eye coordination to light and objects. • If bell is sounded nearby, infant will stop activity and listen. • Eyes follow better, both vertically and horizontally. Focuses well. **Socialization and vocalization** • Begins vocalization—coos, especially to a voice. • Crying becomes differentiated. • Visually looks for sounds. • May squeal with delight when stimulated by touching, talking, or singing. • Begins to smile socially. • Eyes follow person or object more intently. **Cognitive and emotional development** • Recognizes familiar face. • Becomes more aware and interested in environment. • Anticipates being fed when in feeding position. • Enjoys sucking—puts hand in mouth.	**Play stimulation** • Arrange mobile over crib so infant's movement will set it in motion. • Hang wind chimes near infant. • Hang brightly colored pictures on wall. • Use cradle gym and infant seat. • Use rattles. • Hold infant and walk around room. • Allow freedom of kicking with clothes off. **Parental guidance** • Talk to infant and smile; get excited when infant coos. • Place infant seat on a secure surface (eg, floor, center of a table—never near edge of table) near mother's activities. • Put infant in prone position in bed or on floor. • Expose infant to different textures. • Exercise infant's arms and legs. • Sing to infant. • Provide tactile experience during bathing, diapering, and feeding.
8–12 Weeks (2–3 Months) • Landau reflex appears at 3–4 months. • Positive support reflex disappears.	**Motor development** • When prone, will rest on forearms and keep head in midline—makes crawling movements with legs, arches back, and holds head high; may get chest off surface.	**Play stimulation** • Encourage socialization, smiling, and laughing. • Place on mat on floor. • Continue to introduce new sounds.

(continued)

Table 40-1   Infant to Adolescent Growth and Development (*continued*)

AGE AND PHYSICAL CHARACTERISTICS	BEHAVIOR PATTERNS	NURSING CONSIDERATIONS
8–12 Weeks (2–3 Months) (*continued*) • Posterior fontanelle closes. • Increase in body fluids—real tears appear, drooling and GI juices increase.	***Motor development (continued)*** • Indicates preference for prone or supine. • Discovers hands—bats objects with hands. • Holds objects in hands and brings to mouth. • Has fairly good head control. ***Socialization and vocalization*** • Smiles more readily, babbles, and coos. • Stops crying when mother enters room or when caressed. • Enjoys playing during feeding. • Stays awake longer without crying. • Turns head to follow familiar person. ***Cognitive and emotional development*** • Shows active interest in environment. • Recognizes familiar faces and objects. • Focuses and follows objects. • Shows repetitiveness in play activity. • Is aware of strange situations. • Derives pleasure from sucking—purposefully gets hand to mouth. • Begins to establish routine preceding sleep.	***Parental guidance*** • Take outdoors with proper clothing (similar warmth as that of adults), hat, and PABA-free sunscreen. • Bounce on bed. • Play with infant during feeding. • Rattles can be used effectively for visual following and for hand play. • Encourage older siblings to "make faces," sing, and talk to infant. **NURSING ALERT** Children of all ages should avoid intense sun exposure, particularly during the middle of the day. PABA-free sunscreen with a sun protection factor of at least 15 should be used on children of all ages, particularly if sun exposure is longer than 30 minutes.
12–16 Weeks (3–4 Months) • Moro reflex fades. • Stepping reflex disappears. • Rooting reflex disappears. • By 4–5 months infant's weight approximately doubles birth weight. • Average weekly weight gain, 4–7 ounces (113.5–198.5 g). • Average monthly height gain, 1 inch (2.5 cm). • Pulse rate slows to 100–140 beats/minute. • Respirations, 20–40 breaths/minute. • Grasp becomes voluntary. • Sucking becomes voluntary.	***Motor development*** • Eyes focus on small objects, may pick a dangling ring. • Holds head up (when being pulled to sitting position). • Becomes more interested in environment. • Hand comes to meet rattle. • Listens—turns head to familiar sound. • Sits with minimal support. • Intentional rolling over, back to side. • Reaches for offered objects. • Grasps objects with both hands and everything goes into mouth. ***Socialization and vocalization*** • Laughs and chuckles socially. • Demands social attention by fussing. • Recognizes mother. • Begins to respond to "No, no." • Enjoys being propped in sitting position. ***Cognitive and emotional development*** • Actively interested in environment. • Enjoys attention; becomes bored when alone for long periods. • Recognizes bottle. • More interested in mother. • Indicates increasing trust and security. • Sleeps through night; has defined nap time.	***Play stimulation*** • Encourage mirror play. • Provide soft squeeze toys in vivid colors of varying textures. • Allow infant to splash in bath. • Infant still enjoys holding and playing with rattles. • Enjoys old-fashioned clothespins and playing pat-a-cake and peek-a-boo. ***Parental guidance*** • Be certain button eyes on toys and other small objects cannot be pulled off. • Hold rattle and let infant reach and grasp it. • When infant is in high chair, strap in. • Move mobile out of reach—infant may grab it and cause injury. • Repeat child's sounds. • Talk in varying degrees of loudness. • Begin looking at and naming pictures in book. • Begin roughhousing play by both parents. • Give space in playpen or on sheet on floor to practice rolling over. • Place on abdomen for part of playtime.
16–26 Weeks (4–7 Months) • By 5–6 months, tonic neck reflex disappears. • By 6–7 months, palmar grasp disappears.	***Motor development*** • Shows momentary sitting with hand support. • Bounces and bears some weight when held in standing position. • Transfers and mouths objects in one hand.	***Play stimulation*** • Enjoys social games, hide-and-seek with adult, toys, and large blocks. • Likes to bang objects. • Plays in bounce chair and walker.

Table 40-1 Infant to Adolescent Growth and Development (*continued*)

AGE AND PHYSICAL CHARACTERISTICS	BEHAVIOR PATTERNS	NURSING CONSIDERATIONS
16–26 Weeks (4–7 Months) (*continued*) • Two central lower incisors erupt. • Spine "C-shaped"—lacks lordotic and lumbar curves. • Eustachian tube short and horizontal, which may be a factor in ear infections. • GI system mature enough for solid foods.	***Motor development (continued)*** • Discovers feet. • Bangs objects together. • Rolls over well. • May begin some form of mobility. ***Socialization and vocalization*** • Discriminates between strangers and familiar people. • Crows and squeals. • Starts to say "Ma," "Da." • Play is self-contained. • Laughs out loud. • Makes "talking" sounds in response to others' talking. ***Cognitive and emotional development*** • Secures objects by pulling on string. • Searches for lost objects that are out of sight. • Inspects objects; localizes sounds. • Likes to sit in high chair. • Drops and picks up objects. • Displays exploratory behavior with food. • Exhibits beginning fear of strangers. • Becomes fretful when mother leaves. • Shows much mouthing and biting.	***Play stimulation (continued)*** • Enjoys large nesting toys (round rather than square). • Likes to drop and retrieve things. • Likes metal cups, wooden spoons, and things to bang with. • Loves crumpled paper. • Enjoys squeeze toys in bath. • Likes peek-a-boo, bye-bye, and pat-a-cake. ***Parental guidance*** • Will play as long as you can. • Tie toys to chair with short string. • Let play with extra spoon at feeding. • Give soft finger foods. • Because infant puts everything in mouth, use safety precautions. • Keep small items away from infant; could choke on them. • Show excitement at achievements. • Supply safe kitchen items for toys.
26–40 Weeks (7–10 Months) • By 7–9 months, develops eye-to-eye contact while talking; engages in social games. • Four upper incisors erupt around 7–9 months. • By 9–12 months, plantar reflex disappears. • By 9–12 months, neck-righting reflex disappears. **6–12 months** • Average weekly weight gain, 3–5 ounces (85–141.7 g). • Average monthly height gain, ½ inch (1.25 cm).	***Motor development*** • Sits without support. • Recovers balance. • Manipulates objects with hands. • Unwraps objects. • Creeps. • Pulls self upright at crib rails. • Uses index finger and thumb to hold objects. • Rings a bell. • Can feed self a cracker and can hold a bottle. Chewing reflex develops. • Can control lips around cup. • Does not like supine position. • Can hold index finger and thumb in opposition. ***Socialization and vocalization*** • Claps hands on request. • Responds to own name. • Is very aware of social environment. • Imitates gestures, facial expressions, and sounds. • Smiles at image in mirror. • Offers toy to adult, but does not release it. • Begins to test parental reaction during feeding and at bedtime. • Will entertain self for long periods. • Begins fear of strangers, 8½–10 months. ***Cognitive and emotional development*** • Begins to imitate. • Shows more interest in picture books. • Enjoys achievements. • Has strong urge toward independence—locomotion, feeding, dressing.	***Play stimulation*** • Encourage use of motion toys—rocking horse and stroller. • Water play. • Imitate animal sounds. • Allow exploration outdoors. • Provide for learning by imitation. • Offer new objects (blocks). • Child likes freedom of creeping and walking, but closeness of family is important. • Good toys: plastic milk carton; bean bag for tossing; fabric books; things to move around, fill up, empty out; pile-up and knock-down toys. ***Parental guidance*** • Protect from dangerous objects—cover electrical outlets, block stairs, remove breakable objects from tables. • Have child with family at mealtime. • Offer cup. • Talk and sing to infant.

(continued)

Table 40-1   Infant to Adolescent Growth and Development (*continued*)

AGE AND PHYSICAL CHARACTERISTICS	BEHAVIOR PATTERNS	NURSING CONSIDERATIONS

10–12 Months (1 Year)
 	
• Develops lordotic and lumbar curves to make walking possible.
• Weight should approximately triple birth weight.
• Two lower lateral incisors appear.
• Four first molars appear by 14 months.
 	
Child development theories
• Freudian: Behavior
  • birth–1 year—Oral Stage
• Eriksonian: Emotion/Personality
  • birth–1 year—Sense of Trust vs. Mistrust
• Piagetian: Intellectual Activity (Thought Process)
  • birth–2 years—Sensori-motor Period
	Motor development
	• Cruises around furniture.
	• Beginning to stand alone and toddle.
	• Turns pages in book.
	• Tries tossing object.
	• Shows hand dominance.
	• Navigates stairs; climbs on chairs.
	• Builds a tower of two blocks.
	• Puts balls in box.
	• May use spoon.
	• Can release objects at will.
	• Has regular bowel movements.
	
	Socialization and vocalization
	• Uses jargon.
	• Points to indicate wants.
	• Loves give-and-take game.
	• Responds to music.
	• Enjoys being center of attention and will repeat laughed-at activities.
	
	Cognitive and emotional development
	• Shows fear, anger, affection, jealousy, anxiety, and sympathy.
	• Experiments to reach new goals.
	• Displays intense determination to remove barriers to action.
	• Begins to develop concepts of space, time, and causality.
	• Has increased attention span.
		Play stimulation
		• Ball play.
		• Cloth doll.
		• Motion objects and toys.
		• Transporting objects.
		• Name and point to body parts.
		• "Put-in" and "take-out" toys.
		• Sand box with spoons and other simple objects.
		• Blocks.
		• Music.
		
		Parental guidance
		• Allow self-directed play rather than adult-directed play.
		• Continue to expose to foods of different texture, taste, smell, and substance.
		• Offer cup.
		• Show affection and encourage child to return affection.
		• Safety teaching: Child gets into everything within reach. Place medications in safe, locked place. Create a safe environment for child. Use stair guards, faucet protectors, and drawer locks. Have Poison Control Center phone number readily available.

12–18 Months • *Note:* Between ages 1 and 3 years the child is called a "toddler." • By 12–24 months, Landau reflex disappears. • Anterior fontanelle closes. • Abdomen protrudes, arms and legs lengthen. • Big muscles become well developed. • Four cuspids appear by 18 months. • Fine muscle coordination begins to develop. • Average yearly weight gain, 4½–6½ lb (2–3 kg). • Average height gain during second year, 4¾ inch (12 cm).	***Motor development*** • Walks up stairs with help, creeps downstairs. • Walks without support and with balance. • Falls less frequently. • Throws ball. • Stoops to pick up toys, look at bug. • Turns pages of book. • Holds and lifts cup. • Builds three-block tower. • Picks up and places small beads in container. • Begins to use spoon. ***Cognitive and emotional development*** • Has vocabulary of 10 words that have meanings. • Uses phrases, imitates words. • Points to objects named by adult. • Follows directions and requests. • Imitates adult behavior. • Retrieves toy from several hiding places. ***Psychosocial development*** • Develops new awareness of strangers. • Wants to explore everything in reach. • Plays alone, but near others. • Is dependent on parents, but begins to reach out for autonomy. • Finds security in a blanket, toy, or thumbsucking.	***Play stimulation*** • Allow unrestricted motor activity (within safety limits). • Offer push–pull toys. • Child selects favorite toy. • Child likes blocks, pyramid toys, teddy bears, dolls, pots and pans, cloth picture books with large colorful pictures, telephone, musical top, and nested blocks. ***Parental guidance*** • Begin to teach toothbrushing to establish good dental habits; however, continue to brush child's teeth. • Establish limits to give toddler sense of security, but encourage exploration. • Reinforce safety teaching.

Table 40-1   Infant to Adolescent Growth and Development (*continued*)

AGE AND PHYSICAL CHARACTERISTICS	BEHAVIOR PATTERNS	NURSING CONSIDERATIONS
1½–2 Years • Protruding abdomen less noticeable. • During first 2 years, 14 inches (35 cm) are added to height. • Slight bowing of legs with a wide-based walk. • Handedness may become apparent.	**Motor development** • Walks up and down stairs. • Opens doors; turns knobs. • Has steady gait. • Holds drinking cup well with one hand. • Uses spoon without spilling food (may prefer fingers). • Kicks a ball in front of him or her without support. • Builds a tower of four to six blocks. • Scribbles. • Rides tricycle or kiddie car (without pedals). **Cognitive development** • Has 200–300 words in vocabulary. • Begins to use short sentences. • Refers to self by pronoun. • Obeys simple commands. • Does not know right from wrong. • Begins to learn about time sequences. **Psychosocial development** • Uses word "mine" constantly. • Is possessive with toys. • Displays negativism—uses "no" as assertion of self. • Routine and rituals are important. • May begin cooperation in toilet training. • Resists restrictions on freedom. • Has fear of parents leaving. • Shows parallel play. • Dawdles. • Resists bedtime—uses transitional objects (blanket, toy). • Vacillates between dependence and independence.	**Play stimulation** • Shows parallel play, although enjoys having other children around. • Has very short attention span. • Enjoys same toys as child of 18 months. • Likes doll play and balls. • Imitates parents in domestic activities. • Likes swing, hammering, paper, and large crayons. **Parental guidance** • Has need for peer companionship, although displays immaturity by inability to share and take turns. • A decrease in appetite normally occurs at this stage. • Toilet training should be started (each child follows own pattern). • Begin to have child eat meals with family if not already doing so. • Begin to read to child; child likes storybooks with large pictures.

2–3 Years
• Height approximates one half adult height.
• Legs are about 34% of body length.
• Begins 5 lb (2.3 kg) or more weight gain per year until age 5 years.
• At 2½ years has full set (20) of baby teeth.
• Four second molars appear by 2½ years.
• Height gain, 2⅜–3¼ inches (6–8 cm).
• Lordosis and protuberant abdomen of toddler disappear.
 	
Child development theories
• Freudian:
  • 1–3 years—Anal Stage
• Eriksonian:
  • 1–3 years—Sense of Autonomy vs. Shame and Doubt
	Motor development
	• Throws objects overhead.
	• Pedals tricycle.
	• Walks backward.
	• Washes and dries hands.
	• Begins to use scissors.
	• Can string large beads.
	• Can undress him- or herself.
	• Feeds himself well.
	• Tries to dance.
	• Jumps in place.
	• Builds tower of eight blocks.
	• Balances on one foot.
	• Swings and climbs.
	• Can eat an ice cream cone.
	• Drinks from a straw.
	• Chews gum without swallowing it.
	
	Cognitive development
	• Shows increased attention span.
	• Gives first and last name.
	• Begins to ask "why."
	• Is egocentric in thought and behavior.
	• Beginning ability to reflect on own behavior.
	• Talks in short sentences.
		Play stimulation
		• Plays simple games with other children.
		• Enjoys storytelling and dress-up play.
		• Plays "house."
		• Colors.
		• Uses scissors and paper.
		• Rides tricycle.
		• Read simple books to child.
		• Will assist in developing memory skills, visual discrimination skills, and language.
		
		Parental guidance
		• From 2–3 years, the child develops a seeming maturity; do not expect more than child is able to do.
		• Arrange first visit to the dentist to have teeth checked.
		• Be aware that negativistic and ritualistic behavior is normal.
		• Be consistent in discipline.
		• Control temper tantrums.
		• Begin to teach traffic safety.
		• Supervise outdoor play.

Table 40-1   Infant to Adolescent Growth and Development (*continued*)

AGE AND PHYSICAL CHARACTERISTICS	BEHAVIOR PATTERNS	NURSING CONSIDERATIONS
2–3 Years (*continued*) • Piagetian: • 2–7 years—Preoperational Period; shows egocentrism and centering	**Cognitive development (*continued*)** • Uses plurals. • May attempt to sing simple songs. • Has vocabulary of 900 words. • Begins fantasy. • Begins to understand what it means to take turns. • Can repeat three numbers. • Shows interest in colors. **Psychosocial development** • Negativism grows out of child's sense of developing independence—says "no" to every command. • Ritualism is important to toddler for security (follows certain pattern, especially at bedtime). • Temper tantrums may result from toddler's frustration in wanting to do everything for self. • Shows parallel play as well as beginning interaction with others. • Engages in associative play. • Fears become pronounced. • Continues to react to separation from parents but shows increasing ability to handle short periods of separation. • Has daytime bladder control and is beginning to develop nighttime bladder control. • Becomes more independent. • Begins to identify sex (gender) roles. • Explores environment outside the home. • Can create different ways of getting desired outcome.	
3–4 Years • *Note:* Between ages 3 and 5 years, the child is called a "preschooler." • May appear "knock-kneed."	**Motor development** • Drawings have form and meaning, not detail. • Copies a circle and a cross. • Buttons front and side of clothes. • Laces shoes. • Bathes self, but needs direction. • Brushes teeth. • Shows continuous movement going up and down stairs. • Climbs and jumps well. • Attempts to print letters. **Cognitive development** • Awareness of body is more stable; child becomes more aware of own vulnerability. • Is less negativistic. • Learns some number concepts. • Begins naming colors. • Can identify longer of two lines. • Has vocabulary of 1,500 words. • Uses mild profanities and name-calling. • Uses language aggressively. • Asks many questions. • May not be abstract enough to understand body parts that cannot be seen or felt. • Can be given simple explanation as to cause and effect. • Thinks very concretely; demonstrates irreversibility of thought.	**Play stimulation** • Plays and interacts with other children. • Shows creativity. • Likes ring-around-the-rosy. • "Helps" adults. • Likes costumes and enjoys dramatic play. • Toys and games: record player, nursery rhymes, housekeeping toys, transportation toys (tricycle, trucks, cars, wagon), blocks, hammer and peg bench, floor trains, blackboard and chalk, easel and brushes, clay, crayon and finger paints, outside toys (sandbox, swing, small slide), books (short stories, action stories), drum, scrapbook. **Parental guidance** • Base your expectations within child's limitations. • Provide limited frustrations from environment to assist in coping. • Give small tasks to do around the house (putting silverware on table, drying a dish). • Expand child's world with trips to the zoo, to the supermarket, to restaurant, etc. • Prevent accidents. • Provide for brief nonthreatening separation from parents and home. • Reinforce correct use of language. • Use opportunities for simple sexual education as child's needs arise.

Table 40-1 Infant to Adolescent Growth and Development (*continued*)

AGE AND PHYSICAL CHARACTERISTICS	BEHAVIOR PATTERNS	NURSING CONSIDERATIONS
3–4 Years (*continued*)	**Cognitive development (continued)** • Immature concept of death—believes it is reversible. • Has beginning understanding of past and future. • Is egocentric in thought. **Psychosocial development** • Is more active with peers and engages in cooperative play. • Performs simple tasks. • Frequently has imaginary companion. • Dramatizes experiences. • Is proud of accomplishments. • Exaggerates, boasts, and tattles on others. • Can tolerate separation from mother longer without feeling anxiety. • Is keen observer. • Has good sense of "mine" and "yours." • Behavior still frequently ritualistic. • Becomes curious about life and sex. Often indulges in masturbation.	**Parental guidance (continued)** • Accept masturbation as a normal phenomenon to be discouraged in public. • Provide consistent discipline, motivated by love rather than anger. • Consider nursery school.

4–5 Years
• By 2–5 years adds 9½ inches (25 cm) to height.
• At age 4, legs comprise about 44% of body length.
 	
Child development theories
• Freudian:
  • 3–6 years—Phallic Stage
• Eriksonian:
  • 3–6 years—Sense of Initiative vs. Guilt
• Piagetian:
  • 2–7 years—Preoperational Period; shows egocentrism and centering
	Motor development
	• Hops two or more times.
	• Dresses without supervision.
	• Has good motor control—climbs and jumps well.
	• Walks up stairs without grasping handrail.
	• Walks backward.
	• Washes self without wetting clothes.
	• Prints first name and other words.
	• Adds three or more details in drawings.
	• Draws a square.
	
	Cognitive development
	• Has 2,100-word vocabulary.
	• Talks constantly.
	• Uses adult speech forms.
	• Participates in conversations.
	• Asks for definitions.
	• Knows age and residence.
	• Identifies heavier of two objects.
	• Knows weeks as time units.
	• Names days of week.
	• Begins to understand kinship.
	• Knows primary colors.
	• Can count to 10.
	• Can copy a triangle.
	• Has high degree of imagination.
	• Questioning is at a peak.
	• Begins to develop power of reasoning.
	
	Psychosocial development
	• May have an imaginary companion.
	• Has a sense of order (likes to finish what was started).
	• Is obedient and reliable.
	• Is protective toward younger children.
	• Begins to develop an elementary conscience with some influence in governing behavior.
	• Has increased self-confidence.
		Play stimulation
		• Demonstrates gross motor activity—likes to jump rope, skip, climb on jungle gym, etc.
		• Prefers group play and cooperates in projects.
		• Plays simple letter, number, form, and picture games.
		• Plays with cars and trucks.
		• Still likes being read to.
		• Continues to enjoy fantasy play.
		
		Parental guidance
		• Child no longer takes an afternoon nap.
		• Prepare child for kindergarten.
		• Tell him or her stories.
		• Provide opportunities and reassurance for group play; have his or her friends visit for lunch and an afternoon of playing.
		• Prevent accidents.
		• Encourage child's participation in household activities.

(continued)

Table 40-1   Infant to Adolescent Growth and Development (continued)

AGE AND PHYSICAL CHARACTERISTICS	BEHAVIOR PATTERNS	NURSING CONSIDERATIONS
4–5 Years (continued)	**Psychosocial development (continued)** • Accepts responsibility for acts. • Is less rebellious. • Has dreams and nightmares. • Is cooperative and sympathetic. • Shows generosity with toys. • Begins to question parents' thinking. • Identifies strongly with parent of same sex.	

Middle Childhood (5–9 Years)
• Growth rate is slow and steady.
• Gains an average of 7 lb (3.2 kg) per year. Height increases approximately 2½ inch (6.3 cm) per year.
• Among children there is considerable variation in height and weight.
• Appears taller and slimmer.
• Early lordosis disappears.
• Begins to lose baby teeth; permanent teeth appear at a rate of about 4 teeth per year from 7–14 years.
• Neuromuscular and skeletal development allows improved coordination.
• Eyes become fully developed; vision approaches 20/20.
• Handedness should be well developed.
 	
Child development theories
• Freudian:
  • 5–9 years—Beginning of Latency Period
• Eriksonian:
  • 5–9 years—Industry vs. Inferiority
• Piagetian:
  • 5–9 years—Enters Stage of Concrete Operations
	Motor development
	6 years
	• Is active and impulsive.
	• Balance improves.
	• Uses hands as manipulative tools in cutting, pasting, hammering.
	• Can draw large letters or figures.
	7 years
	• Has lower activity level.
	• Capable of fine hand movements; can print sentences.
	• Nervous habits, such as nail biting, are common.
	• Muscular skills, such as ball throwing, have improved.
	8 years
	• Moves with less restlessness.
	• Has developed grace and balance, even in active sports.
	• Has developed coordination of fine muscles, allowing child to write in script.
	9 years
	• Uses both hands independently.
	• Has become skillful in manual activities because of improved eye–hand coordination.
	
	Cognitive development
	6 years
	• Begins to learn to read. Defines objects in terms of use. Time sense is as much in past as present.
	• Is interested in relationship between home and neighborhood; knows some streets.
	• Uses sentences well; uses language to share others' experiences; may swear or use slang.
	• Distinguishes morning from afternoon.
	7 years
	• More reflective and has deeper understanding of meanings.
	• Interested in conclusions and logical endings. Begins to have scientific interests in cause and effect.
	• More responsible in relation to time, more punctual. Sense of space is more realistic; child wants some space of own.
	• Knows value of coins.
	• Concept of death maturing—includes idea of irreversibility.
	8 years
	• Thinking is less animistic. Is aware of impersonal forces of nature. Begins to understand logical reasoning, conclusions, and implications.
		Parental guidance
		• Family atmosphere continues to have an impact on the child's emotional development and future response within the family.
		• The child needs ongoing guidance in an open, inviting atmosphere. Limits should be set with conviction. Deal with only one incident at a time. When punishment is necessary, the child should not be humiliated. Child should know that it was the act that the adult found undesirable, not the child.
		• Needs assistance in adjusting to new experiences and demands of school. Should be able to share experiences with family. Parents need to have communication with the teacher to work together for the health of the child.
		• Convey love and caring in communication. The child understands language directed at feelings better than at intellect. Get down to eye level with the child.
		• Focus attention on child's abilities and accomplishments rather than shortcomings and limitations.
		• The child is sex-conscious and should be able to discuss questions at home rather than with friends. Requires simple, honest answers to questions.
		• Common problems include teasing, quarreling, nail biting, enuresis, whining, poor manners, swearing, lying, cheating, and stealing. These are usually fleeting phases and should not be handled negatively. The causes for such behavior should be investigated and dealt with constructively.
		• The child needs order and consistency to help in coping with doubts, fears, unacceptable impulses, and unfamiliar experiences.
		• Encourage peer activities as well as home responsibilities and give recognition to child's accomplishments and unique talents.
		• Television may stimulate learning in several spheres, but should be monitored.
		• Accidents are a major cause of disability and death. Safety practices should be continued. (Refer to section on safety, page 1415.)
		• Exercise is essential to promote motor and psychosocial development. The child should have a safe place to play and simple pieces of equipment.

Table 40-1 Infant to Adolescent Growth and Development (continued)

AGE AND PHYSICAL CHARACTERISTICS	BEHAVIOR PATTERNS	NURSING CONSIDERATIONS
Middle Childhood (5–9 Years) (continued)	**Cognitive development** (continued) • Less self-centered in thinking. Personal space is expanding; goes places on own. Aware of time; plans events of day. Understands right from left. *9 years* • Intellectually energetic and curious. Realistic; reasonable in thinking. Able to plan in advance. Breaks complex activities into steps. • Focuses on detail. • Sense of space includes the entire earth. • Participates in family discussions. • Likes to have secrets. **Psychosocial development** *5–9 years* • Still requires parental support, but pulls away from overt signs of affection. • Peer groups provide companionship in widening circle of persons outside the home. Child learns more about self as he or she learns about others. • "Chum" stage occurs at about age 9 or 10. Child chooses a special friend of same sex and age in whom to confide. This is usually child's first love relationship outside of home, when someone becomes as important to him or her as oneself. • Play teaches the child new ideas and independence. Child progressively uses tools of competition, compromise, cooperation, and beginning collaboration. • Body image and self-concept are fluid because of rapid physical, emotional, and social changes. • Latency-stage sexual drive is controlled and repressed. Emphasis is on the development of skills and talent. **Patterns of play** *6–7 years* • Child acts out ideas of family and occupational groups with which he or she has contact. • Painting, pasting, reading, simple games, watching television, digging, running games, skating, riding bicycle, and swimming are all enjoyed activities. *8 years* • Child enjoys collections; loosely formed, short-lived clubs; table games; card games; books; television; and music.	**Parental guidance** (continued) • A school health program should be available and concerned with the child's physical, emotional, mental, and social health. This should be augmented by information and example at home. • Medical supervision should continue with yearly examination to detect developmental delay and disease. Appropriate immunizations should be administered. • The child frequently has "quiet days"— periods of shyness, which should be tolerated as part of growing up and deciding who he or she is. • The child may be subject to nightmares, a situation that requires reassurance and understanding. • Parents, teachers, and health professionals should be available and able to provide information and answer questions about the physical changes that occur.
Late Childhood (9–12 Years) • Vital signs approach adult values. • Loses childish appearance of face and takes on features that will characterize individual as an adult.	**Motor development** • Energetic, restless, active movements such as finger-drumming or foot-tapping appear. • Has skillful manipulative movements nearly equal to those of adults. • Works hard to perfect physical skills.	**Parental guidance** • Continue appropriate interventions related to early childhood. • Continue sex education and preparation for adolescent body changes. • Understanding is important.

(continued)

Table 40-1   Infant to Adolescent Growth and Development (*continued*)

AGE AND PHYSICAL CHARACTERISTICS	BEHAVIOR PATTERNS	NURSING CONSIDERATIONS

Late Childhood (9–12 Years) (*continued*)
 	
• Growth spurt occurs and some secondary sex characteristics appear: in girls, between ages 10 and 12 years; in boys, between ages 12 and 14 years.
 	
Physical changes of puberty:
• Increased height and weight, increased perspiration and activity of sebaceous glands; vasomotor instability; increased fat deposition.
 	
Physical changes in girls:
• Pelvis increases in transverse diameter; hips broaden; tenderness in developing breast tissue; enlargement of areola diameter; appearance of pubic hair.
 	
Physical changes in boys:
• Size of testes increases; scrotum color changes; breasts enlarge, temporarily; height and shoulder breadth increase.
• Appearance of lightly pigmented hair at base of penis.
• Increase in length and width of penis.
 	
Child development theories
• Freudian:
  • 9–12 years—Latency Period continues
• Eriksonian:
  • 9–12 years—Industry vs. Inferiority continues
• Piagetian:
  • 9–12 years—Stage of Concrete Operations continues
	Cognitive development
	10 years
	• Likes to reason, enjoys learning.
	• Thinking is concrete, matter of fact.
	• Wants to measure up to challenge.
	• Likes to memorize, identify facts.
	• Attention span may be short. Space is rather specific (ie, where things are).
	• Can write for relatively long time with speed.
	• Likes action in learning.
	• Concentrates well when working competitively.
	• Can understand relational terms, such as weight and size.
	• Perceives space as nothingness that goes on forever.
	• Can discuss problems.
	• Can conceptualize symbolically enough to understand body parts.
	• Can describe some abstract terms.
	
	12 years
	• Enjoys learning.
	• Considers all aspects of a situation.
	• Motivated more by inner drive than by competition.
	• Able to classify, arrange, and generalize.
	• Likes to discuss and debate.
	• Begins conceptual thinking.
	• Verbal, formal reasoning now possible.
	• Can recognize moral of a story.
	• Defines time as duration; likes to plan ahead.
	• Understands that space is abstract.
	• Can be critical of own work.
	
	Psychosocial development
	• Gang becomes important and gang code takes precedence over nearly everything. Gang codes are typically characterized by collective action against the mores of the adult world. Here, children begin to work out their own social patterns without adult interference. Early gangs may include both sexes; later gangs are separated by sex.
	• May strive for unreasonable independence from adult control.
	• Usually interested in religion and morality.
	• Has increased interest in sexuality.
	• May reach puberty; resurgence of sexual drives causes recapitulation of Oedipal struggle.
	
	Patterns of play
	• Continues to enjoy reading, TV, and table games.
	• More interested in active sports as a means to improve skills.
	• Creative talents may appear; may enjoy drawing and modeling clay. By age 10, sex differences in play become profound.
	• Occasional privacy is important.
	• Begins to have vocational aspirations.
		Parental guidance (continued)
		• Encourage participation in organized clubs and youth groups.
		• Democratic guidance is essential as child works through a conflict between dependence (on parents) and independence. The child needs realistic limits set.
		• Needs help channeling energy in proper direction—work and sports.
		• Requires adequate explanation of body changes. Special understanding is required for the child who lags in physical development.
		• Continue consistent disciplinary style.

Table 40-1 Infant to Adolescent Growth and Development (*continued*)

AGE AND PHYSICAL CHARACTERISTICS	BEHAVIOR PATTERNS	NURSING CONSIDERATIONS

Early Adolescence (12–14 Years)
 	
 • Phase of development begins when reproductive organs become functionally operative; phase ends when physical growth is completed.
 • Skeletal system grows faster than supporting muscles.
 • Hands and feet grow proportionately faster than rest of body.
 • Large muscles develop more quickly than small muscles.
 	
 Girls:
 • Physical changes include beginning of menarche; growth of axillary and perineal hair; deepened voice; ovulation; further development of breasts.
 • Nutritional need for iron and calcium increase dramatically.
 	
 Boys:
 • Physical changes include growth of axillary, perineal, facial, chest hair; deepening of voice; production of spermatozoa; nocturnal emissions.
 	
 Child development theories
 • Freudian:
    • 12–14 years—Begins Stage of Sexuality
 • Eriksonian:
    • 12–14 years—Identity vs. Role Diffusion
 • Piagetian:
    • 12–14 years—Begins Stage of Formal Operations
	Motor development
	 • Usually uncoordinated; has poor posture.
	 • Tires easily.
	
	 Cognitive development
	 • Mind has great ability to acquire and use knowledge.
	 • Abstract thinking is sufficient to learn multivariable ideas such as the influence of hormones on emotions.
	 • Categorizes thoughts into usable forms.
	 • May project thinking into the future.
	 • Is capable of highly imaginative thinking.
	
	 Psychosocial development
	 • Interest in opposite sex increases.
	 • Often revolts from adult authority to conform to peer-group standards.
	 • Continues to rework feelings for parent of opposite sex and unravel the ambivalence toward parent of same sex.
	 • Affection may turn temporarily to an adult outside of the family (eg, crush on family friend, neighbor, or teacher).
	 • Uses peer-group dialect—highly informal language or specially coined terminology.
	 • Peer groups are especially important and help adolescent to define own identity, to adapt to changing body image, to establish more mature relationships with others, and to deal with heightened sexual feelings. Cliques may develop.
	 • Dating generally progresses from groups of couples to double dates and finally single couples.
	 • Teenage "hangouts" become important centers of activity.
	 • Begins questioning existing moral values.
		Parental guidance
		 • Stresses frequently result from conflicting value systems between generations. The parents may need help to see that the adolescent is a product of the times and that actions reflect what is happening around the youngster.
		 • The parents' limits and rules should be realistic and consistent. They should convey the parent's love and concern and should be a source of comfort and reassurance, protecting the child from activities for which he or she is not ready.
		 • The home should be an accepting, emotionally stable environment.
		 • Continue sex education, including discussion of ovulation, fertilization, menstruation, pregnancy, contraception, masturbation, nocturnal emissions, and hygiene.
		 • Adolescents have an increased need for rest and sleep because they are expending large amounts of energy and are functioning with an inadequate oxygen supply.
		 • Recreational interests should be fostered. Favorite activities include sports, dating, dancing, reading, hobbies, and television. Socializing via telephone or computer and listening to music are favorite pastimes.
		 • Adolescent health problems that require preventive education are accidents, obesity, acne, pregnancy, sexually transmitted disease, and drug abuse.
		 • Allow the adolescent to handle his or her own affairs as much as possible, but be aware of physical and psychosocial problems that may require help. Encourage independence but allow the child to lean on the parents for support when frightened or unable to attain goals.
		 • Adolescents with special problems should have access to specialists, such as adolescent clinics and psychologists.
		 • Requires reassurance and help in accepting a changing body image. Parents should make the most of the child's positive qualities.
		 • Give gentle encouragement and guidance regarding dating. Avoid strong pressures in either direction.
		 • Understand conflicts as the child attempts to deal with social, moral, and intellectual issues.

Table 40-2   Developmental Milestones

AGE	GROSS MOTOR	VISUAL-MOTOR/ PROBLEM SOLVING	LANGUAGE	SOCIAL/ADAPTIVE
1 month	Raises head slightly from prone, makes crawling movements	*Birth:* visually fixes *1 month:* has tight grasp, follows to midline	Alerts to sound	Regards face
2 months	Holds head in midline, lifts chest off table	No longer clenches fist tightly, follows object past midline	Smiles socially (after being stroked or talked to)	Recognizes parent
3 months	Supports on forearms in prone, holds head up steadily	Holds hands open at rest, follows in circular fashion, responds to visual threat	Coos (produces long vowel sounds in musical fashion)	Reaches for familiar people or objects, anticipates feeding
4 months	Rolls front to back, supports on wrists and shifts weight	Reaches with arms in unison, brings hands to midline	Laughs, orients to voice	Enjoys looking around environment
5 months	Rolls back to front, sits supported	Transfers objects	Says "ah-goo," blows raspberries, orients to bell (localizes laterally)	—
6 months	Sits unsupported, puts feet in mouth in supine position	Unilateral reach, uses raking grasp	Babbles	Recognizes strangers
7 months	Creeps	—	Orients to bell (localized indirectly)	—
8 months	Comes to sit, crawls	Inspects objects	"Dada" indiscriminately	Finger-feeds
9 months	Pivots when sitting, pulls to stand, cruises	Uses pincer grasp, probes with forefinger, holds bottle, throws objects	"Mama" indiscriminately, gestures, waves bye-bye, inhibits to "no"	Starts to explore environment; plays gesture games (eg, pat-a-cake)
10 months	Walks when led with both hands held	—	"Dada/mama" discriminately; orients to bell (directly)	—
11 months	Walks when led with one hand held	—	One word other than "dada/mama," follows one-step command with gesture	—
12 months	Walks alone	Uses mature pincer grasp, releases voluntarily, marks paper with pencil	Uses two words other than "dada/mama," immature jargoning (runs several unintelligible syllables together)	Imitates actions, comes when called, cooperates with dressing
13 months	—	—	Uses three words	—
14 months	—	—	Follows one-step command without gesture	—
15 months	Creeps up stairs, walks backward	Scribbles in imitation, builds tower of two blocks in imitation	Uses four to six words	*15–18 months:* uses spoon, uses cup independently
17 months	—	—	Uses seven to 20 words, points to five body parts, uses mature jargoning (includes intelligible words in jargoning)	—

Table 40-2 Developmental Milestones (*continued*)

AGE	GROSS MOTOR	VISUAL-MOTOR/ PROBLEM SOLVING	LANGUAGE	SOCIAL/ADAPTIVE
18 months	Runs, throws objects from standing without falling	Scribbles spontaneously, builds tower of three blocks, turns two to three pages at a time	Uses two-word combinations	Copies parent in tasks (sweeping, dusting), plays in company of other children
19 months	—	—	Knows 8 body parts	—
21 months	Squats in play, goes up steps	Builds tower of five blocks	Uses 50 words, two-word sentences	Asks to have food and to go to toilet
24 months	Walks up and down steps without help	Imitates stroke with pencil, builds tower of seven blocks, turns pages one at a time, removes shoes, pants, etc.	Uses pronouns (*I, you, me*) inappropriately, follows two-step commands	Parallel play
30 months	Jumps with both feet off floor, throws ball overhand	Holds pencil in adult fashion, performs horizontal and vertical strokes, unbuttons	Uses pronouns appropriately, understands concept of "1," repeats two digits forward	Tells first and last names when asked; gets self drink without help
3 years	Can alternate feet when going up steps, pedals tricycle	Copies a circle, undresses completely, dresses partially, dries hands if reminded	Uses minimum 250 words, three-word sentences; uses plurals, past tense; knows all pronouns; understands concept of "2"	Group play, shares toys, takes turns, plays well with others, knows full name, age, sex
4 years	Hops, skips, alternates feet going down steps	Copies a square, buttons clothing, dresses self completely, catches ball	Knows colors, says song or poem from memory, asks questions	Tells "tall tales," plays cooperatively with a group of children
5 years	Skips alternating feet, jumps over low obstacles	Copies triangle, ties shoes, spreads with knife	Prints first name, asks what a word means	Plays competitive games, abides by rules, likes to help in household tasks

SELECTED REFERENCES

American Academy of Pediatrics. (2006). Identifying infants and young children with developmental disorders in the medical home: An algorithm for developmental surveillance and screening. *Pediatrics, 118*(1), 405–420. Available: *http:// aappolicy.aappublications.org/cgi/content/abstract/pediatrics;118/1/405.*

Augustyn, M. C., Zuckerman, B. S., & Caronna, E. B. (2010). *The Zuckerman Parker handbook of developmental and behavioral pediatrics: A handbook for primary care* (3rd ed.). Philadelphia: Lippincott Williams & Wilkins.

Burns, C., Dunn, A., Brady, M., & Starr, N. (2013). *Pediatric Primary Care.* (5th ed.). Philadelphia: Saunders.

Dixon, S., & Stein, M. (2005). *Encounters with children: Pediatric behavior and development* (4th ed.). St. Louis, MO: Mosby

Johns Hopkins Hospital, Arkara, K., & Tschudy, M. (Eds.). (2012.) *The Harriet Lane handbook* (19th ed.). Philadelphia: Elsevier Mosby.

Kyle, T. (Ed.). (2012). *Essentials of pediatric nursing.* Philadelphia: Wolters Kluwer Health.

McKinney, E., James, S., Murray, S., et al. (2013). *Maternal-Child Nursing.* (4th ed.). St. Louis, MO: Saunders.

National Institute of Child Health and Human Development. (2012). SIDS: Back to Sleep Public Education Campaign. Available: *www.nichd.nih.gov/sids/.*

Pillitteri, A. (2009). *Maternal and child health nursing: Care of the childbearing and childrearing family.* (6th ed.). Philadelphia: Lippincott Williams & Wilkins.

41

Pediatric Physical Assessment

HISTORY

Obtaining a History

A history of the child is obtained to establish a relationship with the child and family; to assess what a family understands about the child's health; to formulate an individual care plan; and to correct misinformation the family may have.

Focus on specific topics in the history, depending on the child's age, including:

- Infant—prenatal and postnatal history, nutrition, development.
- Toddler—home environment, safety issues, development, parent's response.
- School-age—school, friends, reaction to previous hospitalizations.
- Adolescent—alcohol, drugs, friends, sexual history, relationships with parents, identity.

Identifying Information

Type of Information Needed

1. Date and time.
2. Health care provider's name and telephone number, if known.
3. Insurance data.
4. Patient's name, address, telephone number, birth date.
5. Referring health care source (eg, school, other health care provider, clinic).

   Note: Permission from the legal guardian must be obtained to treat a child.

Method of Collecting Data

1. Identify the care person in charge of the patient by name and relationship to the patient; obtain a relative's or care person's address and home and work telephone numbers, if different from those of the patient.
2. To make the informant feel more at ease, the questions should begin in a friendly, nonthreatening manner. Questions addressed to the parent should be phrased appropriately.
3. Casual, friendly responses or remarks on the part of the interviewer may also help break the ice, such as:
   a. "Whoever takes care of this baby certainly does a good job."
   b. "That is a lovely outfit the baby is wearing." (Remember that families will usually put good clothes on a baby for a visit to a health care agency.)
4. Sometimes repeat the information to verify data. This will give you a better judgment of the care person's cooperation and reliability.
5. If age appropriate, get some data directly from the child.

Chief Complaint

Method of Recording

1. Write an exact description of the complaint.
2. Use quotation marks to clearly indicate that the informant's words are being used. It is helpful to explain:
   a. "I will write it down so there will be no mistake."
   b. "Let me read this back to you to make sure it is correct."

3. Quotation of the care person's exact words may give an indication of how he feels about the symptoms; it may reflect fear, guilt, defensiveness.

Method of Collecting Information

1. Begin with a helpful, open-ended question. That is the first overture made to this patient:
   a. "How have things been going?"
   b. "Please tell me the reason for your coming here today."
   c. "Do you have any particular worries or concerns about the baby?"
2. Then proceed to more specific questions.

Duration of Complaint

1. The information obtained may indicate the natural history of the disease, if one is present, and its gradual evolution. Pursue the information with a series of probing questions.
   a. "How long has the baby (child) had this problem?"
   b. If the informant cannot remember, try another route: "When did he (or she) last act well?"; "Do you remember last Christmas? Did the baby have the trouble then?"
2. Write down the responses; try to assess, as more questions are asked, how accurate the informant's answers may be.

History of Present Illness

Type of Information Needed

When the patient is an infant or a preverbal child, information will consist mainly of what the informant has been able to observe. Having established what the chief complaint is, identify further problems, if any. Obtain the following information for each problem:

1. Body location—of pain, itching, weakness.
2. Quality and quantity of complaint—both type (a burning pain) and severity (knifelike, comes and goes).
3. Degree of symptom—(eg, pain, how severe; cough, day and night; eye drainage, amount).
4. Chronology—indicate time sequence and whether the problem is episodic (lasts for a while and then clears up completely).
5. Environment or setting—where and when the symptoms occur.
6. Aggravating and alleviating factors—what makes the pain worse or better.
7. Associated manifestations or symptoms—accompanied by vomiting, blurred vision.

Importance of Detail

1. Typically, a carefully written description of a symptom will be the source of a future diagnosis and will serve all who are involved in helping the patient.
2. Do not worry about how many notes you have to take at first.
3. You will be able to recheck this information when you do the review of systems.

Family History

1. Family members—mother's age and state of health, father's age and health, siblings—who is at home with you?
2. Family health history:
   a. Eyes, ears, nose, throat—nosebleeds, sinus problems, glaucoma, cataracts, myopia, strabismus, other problems of eyes, ears, nose, throat.
   b. Cardiorespiratory—tuberculosis, asthma, hay fever, hypertension, heart murmurs, heart attacks, strokes, rheumatic fever, pneumonia, emphysema, other problems.
   c. Gastrointestinal—ulcers, colitis, vomiting, diarrhea, other problems.
   d. Genitourinary—kidney infections, bladder problems, congenital abnormalities.
   e. Musculoskeletal—congenital hip or foot problems, muscular dystrophy, arthritis, other problems.
   f. Neurologic—seizures, epilepsy, nervous disorder, mental retardation, emotional problems, comas, headaches, others.
   g. Chronic disease—diabetes, liver disease, cancer, tumors, anemia, thyroid problems, congenital disorder.
   h. Special senses—anyone deaf or blind.
   i. Miscellaneous—other medical problem not mentioned.
3. Family social history:
   a. Residence—apartment or house and size. Yard, stairs, proximity to transportation, shopping, playground, school, safe neighborhood? City or well water?
   b. Financial situation—who works, where employed, occupation, welfare, food stamps.
   c. Primary care person—babysitters, day-care center.
   d. Family interrelationships—happy, cooperative, antagonistic, chaotic, multiproblem, violent.

Past History

Prenatal

1. Pregnancy—planned or not; source of care; approximate date of seeking care; birth order of this pregnancy, including miscarriages. This area of the history may be one of great sensitivity. Try to make the questions gentle and supportive:
   a. "Did you plan a baby around this time?"
   b. "When did you manage to get your first checkup for the pregnancy?"
   c. "Were there any unusual problems related to your pregnancy or delivery?"
2. Maternal health—includes illnesses and dates, abnormal symptoms (eg, fever, rash, vaginal bleeding, edema, hypertension, urine abnormalities, sexually transmitted disease). Avoid technical words, if possible.
   a. "Were the doctors or nurses worried about your health?"
   b. "Were your rings tight?"
   c. "Do you know if your blood pressure went up?"
   d. "Did you have trouble with your urine?"
3. Weight gain—validate by trying to get a figure for nonpregnant weight and weight at delivery.
4. Medications taken—eg, vitamins, iron, calcium, aspirin, cold preparations, tranquilizers ("nerve medicine"), antibiotics; use of ointments, hormones, injections during pregnancy; special or unusual diet; radiation exposure; sonography; and amniocentesis.
5. Quality of the fetal movements—when felt?
6. Use of alcohol, tobacco, or drugs during pregnancy.

Natal

1. Expected date of delivery and approximate duration of pregnancy.

2. Place of delivery and name of person who conducted the delivery.
3. Labor—spontaneous or induced, duration, and intensity.
4. Analgesia or anesthesia.
5. Type of delivery—vaginal (breech or vertex presentation); cesarean delivery; forceps delivery.
6. Complications (eg, need for blood transfusion or delay in delivery).

Neonatal
1. Condition of infant.
2. Color (if seen) at delivery.
3. Activity of infant.
4. Type of crying heard.
5. Breathing abnormality.
6. Birth weight and length.
7. Problems that occurred immediately at birth.

Postnatal
1. Duration of hospitalization of the mother and infant.
2. Problems with baby's breathing or feeding.
3. Need of supportive care (eg, oxygen, incubator, special care nursery, isolation, medications).
4. Weight changes, weight at discharge, if known.
5. Color—cyanosis or jaundice.
6. Bowel movements—when.
7. Problems—seizures, deformities identified, consultation required.
8. Hearing—was a hearing screen conducted in the nursery? The United States Preventative Services Task Force recommends universal screening for all newborns using otoacoustic emissions and/or auditory brain stem response testing. The guideline is available online at *www.guideline.gov/content. aspx?id=12640.*
9. Mother's contact with the baby and her first impression:
   a. "What was it like when you first saw your baby?"
   b. "What did the baby do when you were first together?"

Nutrition
1. Breast- or bottle-fed? What formula? How prepared?
2. Amounts offered and consumed.
3. Frequency of feeding—weight gain.
4. Addition of juice or solid foods.
5. Food preferences or allergies.
6. Feeding problems—variations in appetite.
7. Age of weaning.
8. Vitamins—type, amount, regularity.
9. Pattern of weight gain.
10. Current diet—frequency and content of meals.

Growth and Development
1. Past weights and lengths, if available.
2. Milestones—sat alone unsupported; walked alone; used words, then sentences.
3. Teeth—eruption, difficulty, cavities, brushing, flossing.
4. Toilet training.
5. Current motor, social, and language skills.
6. Sexual development.

a. Infant—swollen breast tissue, vaginal discharge, hypertrophy of the labia.
b. Toddler or school-age child—early development of breasts or pubic hair.
c. Prepubertal or pubertal child—in girls, time of development of breasts and pubic hair and onset of menstruation. In boys, time of enlargement of testes and penis, development of pubic and facial hair, and voice changes.

Health Maintenance
1. Immunizations—rubella, rubeola, mumps, polio, diphtheria, pertussis, tetanus toxoid, varicella, pneumococcal, bacille Calmette-Guérin, influenza, *Haemophilus influenzae* type b, hepatitis A and B, meningococcal conjugate, human papillomavirus, and rotavirus. Indicate number and dates. Recommended immunization schedules are available online at *www. cdc.gov/vaccines/recs/schedules/.*
2. Screening procedures—hematocrit or hemoglobin level, urinalysis, tuberculin testing, visual and auditory acuity, color vision, lead testing, cholesterol screening, syphilis testing, HIV testing, gonorrhea and chlamydia screening.
3. Dental care—source and frequency of care, dental hygienist visits, fillings, extractions, last checkup.

Acute Infectious Diseases
Rubella, rubeola, mumps, chickenpox, group A beta-hemolytic pharyngitis, parvovirus B19 (Fifth disease), hepatitis, infectious mononucleosis, sexually transmitted disease, tuberculosis, influenza. Recent exposure to a communicable disease.

Hospitalizations and Surgeries
1. Dates, hospital, health care provider.
2. Indications, diagnosis, procedures.
3. Complications.
4. Reactions to previous hospitalizations.

Injuries
1. Emergency department visits—frequency and diagnosis.
2. Fractures—location and treatment.
3. Trauma, burns, bruises.
4. Ingestions.
5. Ask the parents about provision of a safe environment; for example, cleaning supplies out of reach, electrical outlets with appropriate covers, guns in the house unloaded and kept in a locked room or cabinet, water safety education. Ask about use of safety equipment, such as seat belts, bike helmets, childproof safety caps on medications.

Medications
1. For general use, such as vitamins, antihistamines, laxatives.
2. Special or fad diets.
3. Recent antibiotics.
4. Routine use of aspirin.
5. Hormonal contraceptives—types, dose, duration.
6. Drugs, opioids, marijuana, hallucinogens, mood elevators, tranquilizers, alcohol.
7. Determine when last dose of medication was taken; is the medication with the patient? How does the child take the medication?
8. Allergy to medication?

School History

Type of Information Needed

1. Present and past schooling, grade, and performance.
2. Favored and least-favored subjects.
3. School-related behavior—anxious to go, anxious to stay home.
4. General attitude toward school and career plans; attitude toward peer groups.
5. Gang dress or behavior.

Method of Collecting Data

1. Straightforward questions to a child (eg, "What grade are you in?"; "Who are your friends?").
2. Three wishes offered to the child:
   a. "If your birthday were here, what would you ask for?"
   b. "If you could be anyone, who would it be?"
   c. "What would be the best thing that could happen to you?"
3. "Who is your best friend?"
4. Questions to parents: "How does that seem to you?"
5. Adolescents—Interviews with older children and teens may start with the parents present but the child should also be provided with some private time away from the parents to discuss concerns. The parents should also be allowed a brief time away from their child to voice any concerns.
6. Emphasize the positive (eg, "What is your best subject?")

Social History

Type of Information Needed

1. Environment—rural, urban.
2. Housing—type, location, heating, sewage, water supply, family pets, other animal exposure.
3. Parents' occupations (employment) and marital status.
4. Number of individuals living in home, sleeping arrangements.
5. Religious affiliations.
6. Previous utilization of social agencies.
7. Health insurance and usual source of care.
8. After assuring older children of the confidentiality of their answers, inquire about risk-taking behaviors, such as cigarette smoking, alcohol and drug use, drinking and driving, and sexual history.

Method of Collecting Data

Parents are proud, so use tact and diplomacy when asking some questions. Ask permission.

1. "Can you tell me a little bit about your home?"
2. "I need to know more about how you live to help you with your child's problem."

Personal History

Type of Information Needed

1. Hygiene.
2. Exercise.
3. Sleep habits.
4. Elimination habits.
5. Activities, hobbies, special talents.
6. Friends, teacher relationships.
7. Sibling and parent relationships.
8. Expression of emotions.
   a. Blows up easily.
   b. Quiet.
9. Idiosyncratic behavior and habits (eg, thumb-sucking, nail-biting, temper tantrums, head-banging, pica, breath-holding, rituals, tics).
10. Emotional issues, such as school avoidance, somatic complaints.

Review of Systems

Type of Information Needed

1. General—activity, appetite, affect, sleep patterns, weight changes, edema, fever, behavior.
2. Allergy—eczema, hay fever, asthma, hives, food or drug allergy, sinus disorders.
3. Skin—rash or eruption, nodules, pigmentation or texture change, sweating or dryness, infection, hair growth, itching.
4. Head—headache, head trauma, dizziness.
5. Eyes—visual acuity, corrective lenses, strabismus, lacrimation, discharge, itching, redness, photophobia.
6. Ears—auditory acuity, earaches (frequency, ages, response to specific medications), infection, drainage.
7. Nose—colds and runny nose (frequency), infection, drainage.
8. Teeth—hygiene practices, frequency of brushing, general condition, cavities, malocclusions.
9. Throat—sore throat, tonsillitis, difficulty swallowing.
10. Speech—peculiarity of or change in voice, hoarseness, clarity, enunciation, stuttering, development of articulation, vocabulary, use of sentences.
11. Respiratory—difficulty breathing, shortness of breath, chest pain, cough, wheezing, croup, pneumonia, tuberculosis or exposure.
12. Cardiovascular—cyanosis, fainting, exercise intolerance, palpitations, murmurs.
13. Hematologic—pallor, anemia, tendency to bruise or bleed.
14. Gastrointestinal—appetite (amount, frequency, cravings), nausea, vomiting, abdominal pain, abnormal size, bowel habits and nature of stools, parasites, encopresis (incontinence of feces), colic.
15. Genitourinary—age of toilet training, frequency of urination, straining, dysuria, hematuria (or unusual color or odor of infant's soiled diaper), previous urinary tract infection, enuresis (age of onset; day or nighttime), urethral or vaginal discharge. Girls and young women: age at menarche, last menses, cramps, changes in interval and duration.
16. Musculoskeletal—deformities, fractures, sprains, joint pains or swelling, limited motion, abnormality of nails.
17. Neurologic—weakness or clumsiness, coordination, balance, gait, dominance, fatigability, tone, tremor, seizures or paroxysmal behavior, personality changes.

PHYSICAL EXAMINATION

General Principles

1. Establish the order of all data collection according to the needs of the patient. For example:
   a. An exhausted parent with a screaming baby will not give a careful, comprehensive history.
   b. Alternative care may not be available for preschoolers when the neonate comes in for his or her first checkup.
2. If the parent has come in with more than one child, try to organize some supervision of the other children so that you can have a little time alone with the parent.
3. Remember that the safest place for a young child is on the parent's knee. Privacy may not be possible when other children are present.
4. Attempt to develop rapport with the young patient from the moment you first see or meet him or her.
5. Explain to the school-age child or teenager what you are looking for as you proceed with the examination and provide feedback.

APPROACH TO THE PATIENT

1. Offer the young child a choice of being examined on the parent's lap or on your "special table."
2. To evaluate the chest properly, you need to listen through 10 heartbeats when the child is not screaming; therefore, the chest is a good place to begin the examination.
3. The part to be examined should be completely exposed, but if an apprehensive child objects to having clothes removed, slip your stethoscope under the shirt.
4. After listening to the heart, begin with parts of the body that are already exposed.
5. Start with either the head or the toes and work thoroughly and systematically toward the other end.
6. Gradually remove the child's clothes (may best be done by usual caregiver); look for asymmetry very carefully in the bodies of all children.
7. Develop a pattern appropriate to the patient's age.
   a. With infants it may be wise to leave the diaper area until last.
   b. Adolescents and school-age children are usually embarrassed at the genital examination—you may want to leave this until last.
8. Using a cold stethoscope may result in a frightened and screaming child, so warm the stethoscope before bringing it into contact with the child.
9. Some children are less frightened if allowed to hold the examination equipment first.
10. Show the child the procedure by demonstrating on the parent first.
11. Many young children enjoy listening to their own hearts.
12. Toddlers and preschoolers enjoy blowing your otoscope light out.

Pediatric Physical Assessment

Technique	Findings

VITAL SIGNS

1. Obtain temperature, pulse rate, respiratory rate, and blood pressure as often as necessary, based on the child's condition.
2. Measure core temperature, whenever possible, via rectal or ear route. A mercury thermometer must remain in place 3–5 minutes. Alternately, use an electronic thermometer. Avoid taking temperature via oral route following fluid or food intake.
3. Obtain apical pulse rate on an infant or small child; radial, temporal, or carotid pulse may be measured on an older child. Pulse may be counted for 30 seconds and multiplied by 2.
4. Count respirations on an infant for 1 full minute; observe the chest as well as the abdomen. Respirations may be counted for 30 seconds and multiplied by 2 in an older child.
5. Obtain blood pressure by auscultatory method, rather than palpation method, whenever possible. Make sure the cuff covers no less than ½ and no more than ⅔ the length of the upper arm or leg.

Temperature

Oral	Rectal	Axillary
97.6° F–99.3° F	97° F–100° F	96.6° F–98° F
(36.4° C–37.4° C)	(36.1° C–37.8° C)	(35.9° C–36.7° C)

Pulse and respiratory rates

Age	Pulse	Respirations
Neonate	70–170	30–50
11 months	80–160	26–40
2 years	80–130	20–30
4 years	80–120	20–30
6 years	75–115	20–26
8 years	70–110	18–24
10 years	70–110	18–24
Adolescent	60–110	12–20

Blood pressure
Varies with age, height, and weight of child.

Pediatric Physical Assessment (continued)

Technique	Findings

STANDING HEIGHT, HEAD CIRCUMFERENCE, AND CHEST CIRCUMFERENCE

1. Use a tape measure to obtain accurate head circumference. Measure the widest part of head.

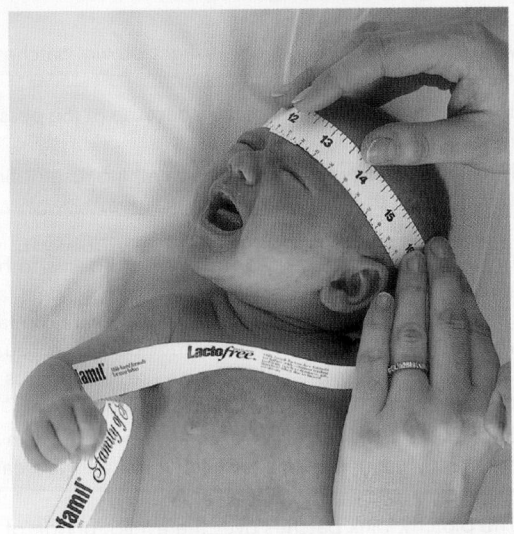

2. Measure the chest at the level of the nipples.

3. Record height and weight at each visit. Plot on growth chart.

   3. A variety of clinical growth charts on which to record length, head, circumference, BMI, and weight can be downloaded from *www.cdc.gov/growthcharts/*. Trends in growth are as important as the basic measurements.

4. Calculate body mass index (BMI) and plot on appropriate chart.

   4. BMI is calculated by following the formula on page 743, or for online pediatric BMI calculator, *http://apps.mccd .cdc.gov/dnpabmi*.

GENERAL APPEARANCE

1. Begin your observations with the first contact with the patient, taking into account that there are at least two people to observe (child and parent).

   1. If the child is easily distracted or sleepy, it may be naptime.

2. The patient's interaction with the caretaker, whether it be the mother, father, a babysitter, an older sibling, or a friend of the family, is vital in the assessment of the child. As you observe for race, sex, general physical development, nutritional state, mental alertness, evidence of pain, restlessness, body position, clothes, apparent age, hygiene, and grooming, remember that many of these things are a measure of the parent's caretaking.

   2. Careful observation of the general state of the child will provide many clues about the child's relationship with the family and its response to the child.

SKIN AND LYMPHATICS

Examine as you move through each body region (include hair and skin).

Inspection

Inspection of the skin is the same as for the adult.

1. Observe for skin color, pigmentation, lesions, jaundice, cyanosis, scars, superficial vascularity, moisture, edema, color of mucous membranes, hair distribution.

   1. In young infants, the skin is soft, smooth, and velvety in texture.

(continued)

Pediatric Physical Assessment *(continued)*

Technique	Findings

SKIN AND LYMPHATICS *(continued)*

Inspection *(continued)*

2. Describe any variation in color, particularly in children with increased pigmentation. No pigment, or vitiligo, in darker children can be noted.

3. Birthmarks of any type are recorded. (May change as child grows older.)

4. Bruises or unusual marks, wounds or insect bites, scratch marks, or scars may have particular significance.

5. Draw a picture of anything unusual such as a scar and measure the dimensions of the lesion when recording the findings.

6. To ascertain suspected jaundice, take the child to the window to get a true picture of the color of the skin. (A room with yellow walls and artificial lighting may create a wrong impression when jaundice is suspected.)

7. The skin of neonates will still be covered with vernix caseosa, the oily material that covers the fetus's body while in utero.

8. Postmature infants may have scaliness that persists for several weeks after birth, particularly around the feet. The color of the skin may change as the child gets a little older.

9. Note striae.

10. Dark-skinned children may have Mongolian spots at the base of spine or elsewhere.

Palpation

1. Use the tips of your fingers to palpate—fingertips are more sensitive.

2. Check the tension of the skin by pinching up a fold of skin—normal skin quickly falls back, but dehydrated skin remains in pinched position.

2. Pigmentations vary in children, depending on race, and will change as the child gets older.

3. A suntan, freckles, and small, light-brown patches or café-au-lait spots may occur.

4. Bruises are particularly important because of the possibility of child abuse.

5. If you have difficulty describing something, use ordinary words rather than inaccurate technical terms.

6. Carotenemia, which causes the nose and palms to have a yellowish tinge, may lead the parents to suspect jaundice; however, carotenemia is caused by eating a large amount of yellow vegetables (sweet potatoes, squash, carrots). In carotenemia, the sclerae are clear; this is not the case in jaundice.

7. Swollen sebaceous glands over the nose and chin are commonly seen immediately after birth and are called *milia.*

8. The blotchy, pink patches over the eyelid, bridge of the nose, and the back of the neck may persist until the child is almost age 2.

9. May indicate rapid weight gain.

10. Important to distinguish from child abuse.

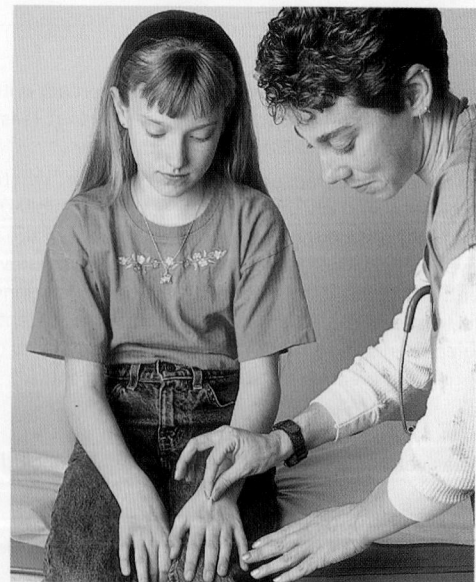

3. Feel the skin for texture, moisture, temperature, turgor, elasticity, masses, tenderness.

3. Skin that is rough and dry in texture may actually have a discrete rash that can be felt but not seen.

Pediatric Physical Assessment *(continued)*

Technique	Findings

SKIN AND LYMPHATICS *(continued)*

Palpation *(continued)*

Lymph

1. Observe and palpate for lymph node enlargement in lymph chain areas.
   a. Neck.
   b. Axilla.
   c. Inguinal.
   d. Epitrochlear.
2. Note tenderness, size, and consistency.

1. May be large or readily palpable, but should be non-tender, mobile, and slightly spongy.

Nails

1. Observe for color, shape, irregularities in surface, and general nail care; cleanliness, evidence of biting.
2. Palpate the skin around the fingernails for firmness. Palpate any part that appears inflamed.

1. Nail beds should be pink, nails convex.
2. General care of the child is frequently reflected in good care of nails.

Hair

1. Observe for color and distribution.
   a. Note according to the age of the child and race.
   b. Be aware that tufts of hair over the spine or sacral area may mark an underlying abnormality.
2. Note changes in pigmentation.
3. Palpate the hair for texture and thickness.
4. Examine to see if there are patches on the head where hair is missing.

5. Separate thick hair on the head to get a good view of the scalp. Check for dandruff or scaliness in older children.
6. Check scalp for signs of lice infestation.

7. Inspect in the axillae and over the pubis and the extremities for hair and its quantity, to gauge the development and level of puberty.

1. *Neonate:* Normally varies from no hair to a thick bush. Infant: lanugo, a soft, downy covering commonly seen over the shoulders, back, arms, face, and sacral area, especially in dark-skinned children; lanugo is present for the first 1–2 months, after which it disappears.
2. Remember, children may experiment with hair dye or rinse.
3. Texture may be thick or thin, coarse or fine, straight or curly.
4. May denote underlying skin infection; however, some children pull their hair out; sometimes the hair is braided so tightly that it falls out. Infants who sleep consistently on their backs may have thinning or absent hair in the occiput.
5. Look carefully for broken hairs, for scaliness on the scalp, or cradle cap in infants.
6. Nits (louse eggs) appear on the hair as little white dots. Lice may be seen on the scalp; they move quickly and may jump.
7. The child does not need to be totally undressed; a prepubertal child will usually be embarrassed if all clothes are removed.

HEAD AND NECK

1. Unless specifically requested, examine the eyes and ears last, especially in the younger child.
2. Also, examine the throat toward the end of the examination, unless the child exhibits concern about the "throat stick." It is then best to examine the throat right away to "get it over with." If a child cries you may be able to avoid using a tongue blade.
3. To avoid frightening the child when palpating the head, make a game out of it—ask, "Where is your nose?" "Where are your eyes?"

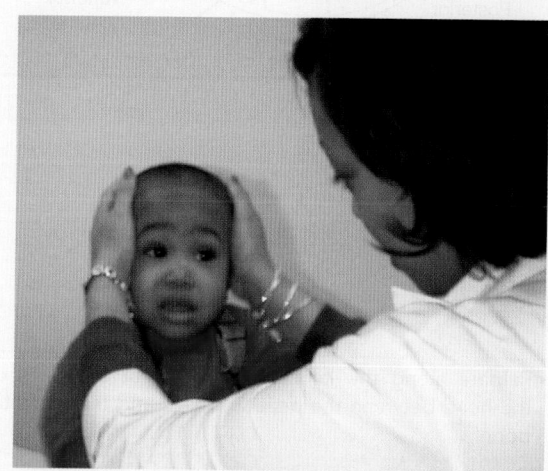

(continued)

Pediatric Physical Assessment *(continued)*

Technique	Findings

HEAD AND NECK *(continued)*

Inspection

1. Observe the face and skull for asymmetry, deformity, and abnormal or limited movements.

2. Closely observe facial expressions and blinking, if the child is not crying. This may be one of your few moments to see the child when he or she is not crying. If you are examining a crying infant, watch particularly for asymmetry of the face.

3. Observe the movement of the head on the neck as the infant looks around. When turning an infant over, observe the head for control, position, and movement.

4. Because an infant's neck is typically short and there are usually several folds of skin under the chin, it is necessary to lift the chin a little to observe the skin completely—to see that it is clear and free from perspiration rash or irritation.

Palpation

1. Palpate the skull for the suture lines. Feel the face for masses, noting size, consistency, surface, temperature, and tenderness.

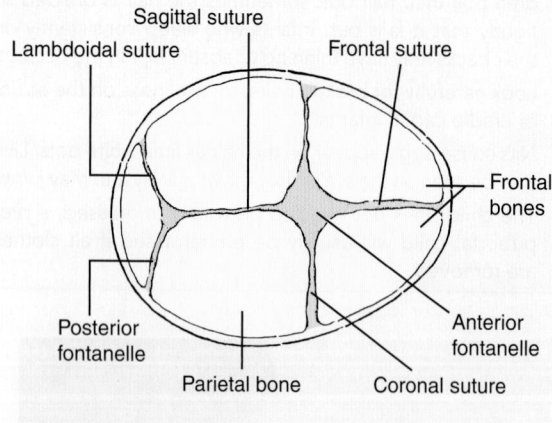

2. Palpate the anterior and posterior fontanelles.

3. Palpate along the lambdoidal suture at the back of the head between the parietal bones and the occipital bone.

Findings column:

1. An infant's head may be asymmetrical because of pressure during pregnancy and delivery. The rounded head of an infant born by breech delivery contrasts with the long, pointed head of an infant who is a firstborn and whose head was molded during a prolonged labor.

2. In an infant born by forceps delivery, there may be signs of weakness of the facial nerve caused by pressure of the forceps over the front of the ear where the facial nerve emerges. When the infant cries, the involved side will show weakness and downturning of the mouth.

3. There should be very little head lag after age 3 months.

4. In the back, the neck should be free of webbing or extra folds of skin extending from just beneath the ear toward the shoulder.

1. The suture lines of the skull may be felt to override as a result of the pressure applied when contractions occurred during labor. This is usually most marked between the frontal and the parietal bone, where the coronal suture is located.

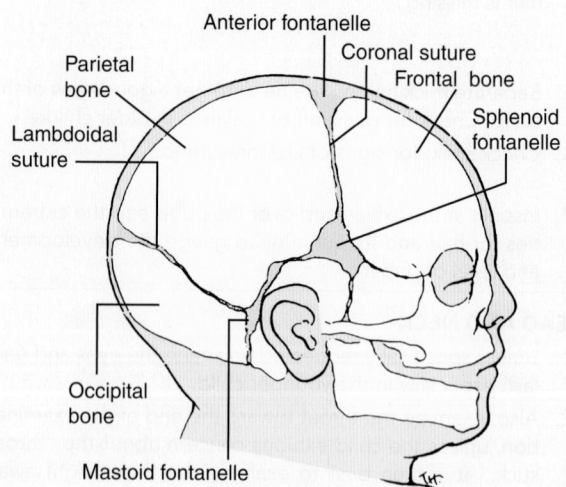

2. The fontanelles are soft and flat when the child is quiet. Tense or bulging fontanelles may indicate hydrocephalus. Depressed fontanelles are often a sign of dehydration. The posterior fontanelle usually closes by 1–2 months; anterior fontanelle by 18 months.

Pediatric Physical Assessment *(continued)*

Technique	Findings

HEAD AND NECK *(continued)*

Palpation *(continued)*

4. Palpate the neck for swollen lymph nodes, noting tenderness, mobility, location, and consistency.

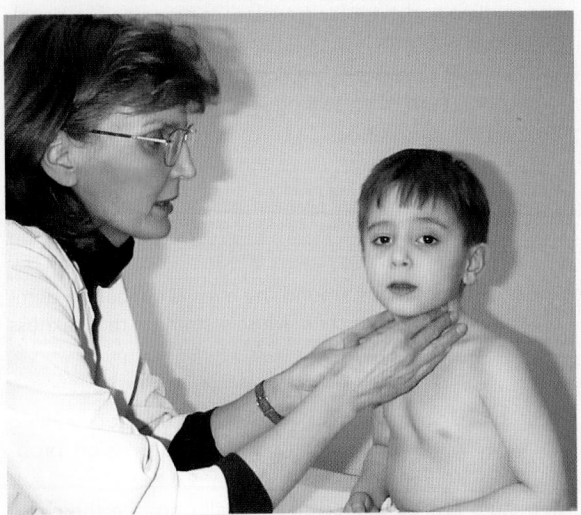

4. Palpation of the lymph nodes may reveal slightly enlarged nodes in the anterior cervical chain secondary to sore throat.

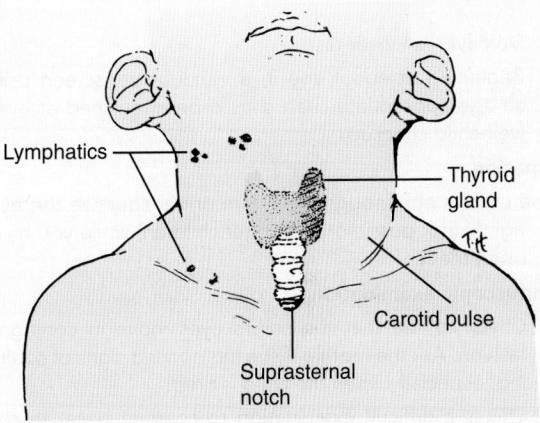

5. Note that there are other nodes, which are normally not palpable.

5. These include the preauricular and postauricular, the posterior cervical (behind the sternomastoid), the submental and submandibular (under the jaw), the supraclavicular, and the occipital nodes (along the prominence of the occiput).

6. Feel the pulses in the neck for location, strength, and equality.
7. Check the thyroid for enlargement, position, texture, and tenderness.
8. Locate the trachea in the suprasternal notch for position in the center of the neck.
9. Palpate the sternocleidomastoids, making sure they are equal in size.

Percussion

1. Percussion of the face may elicit tenderness over the sinuses.
2. Percuss over the head and neck directly with the fingertips, usually the middle finger of the right hand.

3. Percuss over the forehead for tenderness in the sinuses and across the zygoma, or cheekbone.

1. Tenderness may be caused by a tooth cavity or by a sinus infection.
2. Gentle tapping over the skull elicits a typical sound when the sutures are open and elicits a different sound when the sutures are closed.

3. Determines underlying tenderness in the frontal or maxillary sinus.

Auscultation

Auscultate the skull and carotid arteries in the neck.

To determine bruits.

EYES AND VISION

Inspection

Similar to adult examination; see pages 52–55.

1. Pay particular attention to the lacrimal duct and excessive tearing.

1. Discharge from the eyes along the lower lid or from the lacrimal duct can occur as a result of infection or reaction to silver nitrate administered to the neonate.

(continued)

Pediatric Physical Assessment *(continued)*

Technique	Findings

EYES AND VISION *(continued)*

Inspection *(continued)*

2. Note the distance between the eyes and the distribution of the eyebrows.

3. Test the eyes for light perception.

4. Do cover–uncover test.

5. Beginning at about age 3, a visual acuity screen using an age-appropriate chart should be attempted at every well-child checkup.

2. Hypertelorism denotes a wider than normal area between the eyes. Excessively long and full eyebrows that meet in the midline and extra-long eyelashes may signify a developmental abnormality.

3. It is difficult to prevent children from blinking their eyes or closing them when testing light response.

4. To discover strabismus.

Palpation

If the child is old enough, have him or her squeeze the eyes tightly (not possible in younger children) while you try to open them.

Weakness of the muscles around the eyes is difficult to demonstrate in the young child. Muscle strength or weakness can be evaluated when the child cries.

Funduscopic examination

1. Check to see that the child's eyes move in conjugate fashion. Ask the mother if she has noticed signs of squinting, especially when the child is tired.

2. This is a difficult examination to conduct because children tend to watch the light and stare directly at you, which constricts their pupils. If the child cannot cooperate, it may be necessary to dilate the pupil to see the fundus and this is only infrequently necessary.

3. Start your examination at about 1 foot (0.3 m) from the patient. Look for the red reflex, which should be readily observable.

4. Look for opacities and then slowly approach the patient, turning the ophthalmoscope dial to the smaller plus (+) numbers. Start originally at +8 to +10.

1. Loss of vision can occur if the eyes are not working together properly. Squinting can indicate vision problems.

2. A picture can be pinned to the wall opposite the child, who is then instructed to look at the picture during the examination. If the child is examined while lying down, a picture can be placed on the ceiling.

3. The corneal light reflex and red reflex should be symmetrical.

4. The red reflex is diminished if there is something obstructing your view. A cataract or opacity in the retina can cause this, as would a tumor filling the posterior chamber. If there is any paleness in the red reflex or difficulty in identifying it, a consultation should be sought immediately.

5. To help guide your gaze, put your hand on top of the child's head or at the side, with your thumb at the corner of the eye at the outer edge. If you lose the fundus, you can return to your thumb and get your bearings by directing your gaze medial to the tip of your thumbnail.

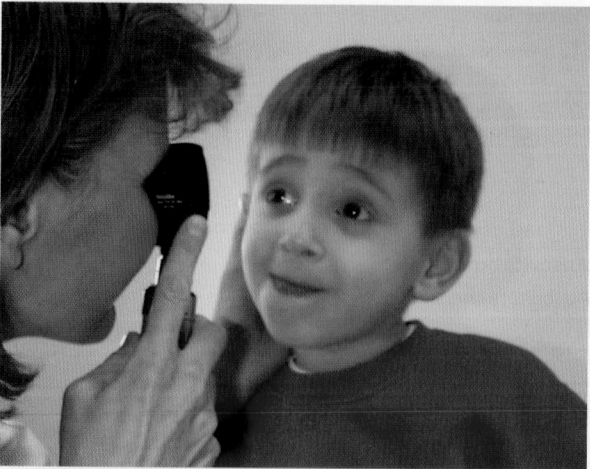

Pediatric Physical Assessment *(continued)*

Technique	Findings

EARS AND HEARING

Equipment
- Otoscope with insufflator (pneumatic bulb and tubing)
- Varying sizes of ear speculum
- Fresh batteries to ensure a bright light

Inspection

1. When examining the external ear, the auricle, or the pinna, be sure to note the position of the ear.

1. The top of the ear should cross an imaginary line drawn between the edge of the eye and the back of the occiput. If the ear is positioned more obliquely or is low-set, some underlying abnormality, particularly of the genitourinary system, may be present.

2. If you cannot get the child to cooperate by offering an explanation or by playing a game, the child will need to be restrained. Many children will enjoy watching the light on their legs or seeing the red glow of their fingers with the light shining through or blowing the light out. If restraint is needed:

2. If the child is in a supine position, be sure to remove the child's shoes because some children will kick when frightened.

   a. The child can be seated on the parent's knee, facing the parent, with arms and legs wrapped around the parent. The parent can then use one hand to hold the child's head firmly against the parent's chest and the other hand to hold the child's back.

   a. This allows a good secure hold and provides the child with the security of a "hug."

   b. An older child may be held in a supine position, with the parent controlling the head by holding the child's arms above his head.

Inspection with otoscope

1. Attach the insufflator, a small bulb and tube device, to the otoscope. Hold the otoscope gently with the handle between the thumb and forefinger. This will enable you to control the head of the otoscope while keeping your hand steady on the child's head.

1. Small children will jerk about, so be careful not to push the speculum into the eardrum. The insufflator allows assessment of mobility of the tympanic membrane.

2. With your free hand, pull the pinna back and slightly upward to straighten the canal. Examine the canal.

2. Cerumen or wax may interfere with your view of the eardrum. You may need to remove the wax with an ear curette or hydrogen peroxide instillation.

3. Use the insufflator to inspect the eardrum and test for mobility. Do not use an insufflator if there is any suspicion of a perforated eardrum.

3. The normal eardrum moves slightly when air is introduced into the ear canal.

Palpation
Palpate behind the ear over the mastoid process.

Tenderness behind the ear may denote infection. Sometimes a lymph node can be felt in this area.

Special testing

1. Most children will be able to respond to a test of gross hearing.

1. A small bell, such as that found in the Denver kit, can be used to determine hearing ability by noting if the child stops moving when the bell is rung and turns his or her head toward the sound.

2. More specific tests using an electric screening device are used before school age.

(continued)

Pediatric Physical Assessment (*continued*)

Technique	Findings

NOSE AND SINUSES

Equipment

- Nasoscope
- Small speculum

Inspection

1. Observe for general deformity.

2. With a nasoscope, examine the nasal septum, mucous membranes and turbinates, and observe for discharge and nasal obstruction (see "Adult Physical Examination," page 57).

3. Check for the presence of a foreign body. Always remember that a foul odor may indicate a foreign body in the nose, ear, or any other body orifice including the anus or the vagina.

4. Observe for nasal flaring.

Palpation

Palpate the sinuses, remembering the order of development.

2. Dry mucous membranes may bleed and cause clots of blood to form in the nares. Scratches may also occur if the child picks at his or her nose or scratches when itching occurs.

3. A foreign body in the nose will cause a foul odor, purulent discharge, and possibly cause bleeding.

4. Indicates respiratory distress.

Sinuses develop in a set order; the ethmoid and maxillary sinuses are present at birth. The frontal sinuses begin to develop at about 7 years and are fully formed by adolescence. The sphenoid sinuses develop after puberty.

MOUTH AND THROAT

Equipment

- Penlight
- Tongue blade

Inspection

Note: The child may gag when the tongue blade is placed on the tongue. To avoid this unpleasant occurrence, encourage the child to stick out tongue, breathe deeply, and say "ah." This may allow for easy visualization of the palate and uvula without need for the "stick."

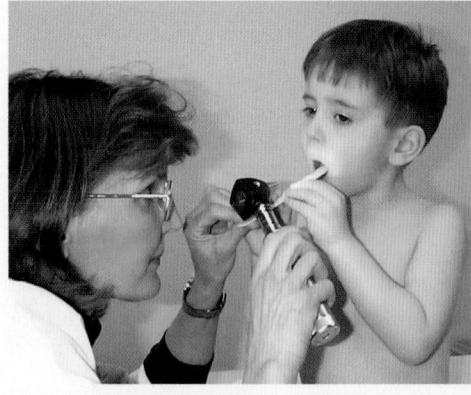

A child may also be allowed to place the tongue blade directly on own tongue while you guide with your hand.

1. Observe the lips, noting the color. (Remember that cyanosis is difficult to detect in a black child.)

2. Count the teeth (see page 1397) and note any extra or missing teeth and any evidence of caries, staining, tartar, and malocclusion.

3. Check the gums for swelling and signs of easy bleeding. Also note mouth odor.

4. Check the tongue for movement, color, and taste buds on the surface. Check to see that the frenulum under the tongue is the proper length.

5. As the gag reflex is elicited, note how the palate moves upward and the uvula springs into view.

1. *Infants:* There may be a protuberance on the upper lip, the so-called "sucking blister."

   Children: May have dry lips and redness around the lips caused by allergy.

4. If the frenulum is too short, the child may be tongue-tied (meaning that he or she cannot advance the tip of the tongue beyond the lips), which may interfere with sucking or speech.

5. It should be midline and single, although occasionally it will be divided or bifurcated.

Pediatric Physical Assessment *(continued)*

Technique	Findings

MOUTH AND THROAT *(continued)*

Inspection *(continued)*

6. Examine the roof of the mouth.

7. Inspect the height of the arch of the palate.

8. Note the tonsils on each side of the uvula and immediately posterior to it for position, surface, size, equality, and color.

9. As the child cries, note the odor of the breath and any hoarseness of the voice; note difficulty on inspiration, as in croup, or wheezing on expiration.

Palpation

1. Palpate the lips and cheeks manually using a finger cot or glove.

2. Note evidence of swelling.

3. Palpate for submucous cleft.

6. Whitish lesions, called Epstein's pearls, may be noted on the roof of the mouth at the junction of the hard and soft palate and persist through infancy.

7. With experience, an unusually high arch is easily recognizable.

8. Any coating with pus or ulcers or a pocket or cryptic appearance should be recorded.

9. These signs may indicate throat and chest disturbances.

1. By comparing one side with the other, differences caused by abnormality can be detected.

3. Submucous cleft may indicate a genetic disposition toward cleft palate.

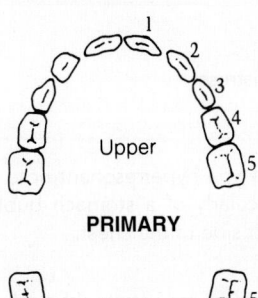

Upper

PRIMARY

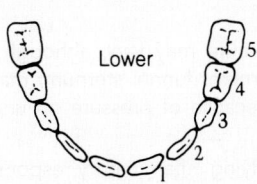

Lower

	(Upper)	(Lower)
1 Central incisor	8 to 12 months	5 to 9 months
2 Lateral incisor	8 to 12 months	12 to 18 months
3 Cuspid	18 to 24 months	18 to 24 months
4 First molar	12 to 18 months	12 to 18 months
5 Second molar	24 to 30 months	24 to 30 months

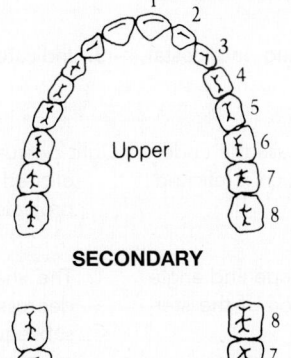

Upper

SECONDARY

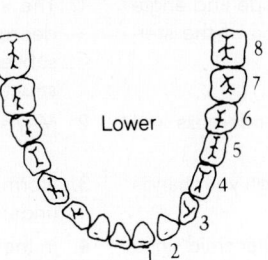

Lower

	(Upper)	(Lower)
1 Central incisor	6 to 7 years	7 to 8 years
2 Lateral incisor	7 to 8 years	8 to 9 years
3 Cuspid	9 to 10 years	11 to 12 years
4 First bicuspid	10 to 11 years	10 to 11 years
5 Second bicuspid	11 to 12 years	10 to 12 years
6 First molar	6 to 7 years	6 to 7 years
7 Second molar	11 to 13 years	12 to 13 years
8 Third molar	17 years	17 to 18 years

BREAST

1. Realize that a child may be resistant to examination because of not wanting to remove clothes.

2. The following approaches may help overcome this problem:

   a. Distract the child by having him or her listen to a few heartbeats.

   b. Have the parent (while the child is sitting on parent's knee) remove the underclothing while you stand by.

   c. For an older child entering puberty, provide an examination sheet or gown.

1. Resistance may be due to modesty or fear of being exposed.

(continued)

Pediatric Physical Assessment (*continued*)

Technique	Findings

BREAST (*continued*)

Inspection

1. Check to see if there are any small extra nipples present.

2. In the neonate, the nipples appear a little darker than normal and breast tissue underneath may form a small knot with occasional leakage of fluid.

3. In the child, a lump may be found under or near one or both nipples in either males or females, causing parents to worry about cancer.

4. Occasionally, the breasts begin to develop earlier than normal, at about age 5 or 6 years.

1. These would appear along a line extending from the anterior axillary line through the normal nipple down toward the symphysis pubis.

2. This leakage is a secondary effect of the hormone level in the mother; instruct the mother not to try to express the fluid because of the danger of infection.

3. Such lumps are almost always secondary to hormone stimulation and occur toward puberty or during the neonatal period.

4. This may indicate the need for referral to an endocrinologist.

THORAX

Inspection

1. Observe the entire thorax as the child breathes; note symmetry and equal expansion of both sides as the lungs inflate.

2. Confirm the respiratory rate as you observe the child with shirt off.

3. Observe for substernal, suprasternal, and intercostal retractions.

1. Diaphragm excursion is more marked than intercostal expansion in infants (especially an infant lying on the parent's knee) and young children. Thus, the abdomen goes up and down more than the chest expands.

3. Indicates respiratory distress.

Percussion

Percussion of the child's chest is difficult. Because the underlying structures are crowded, not too much is elicited. The heart edge is difficult to outline.

Light percussion is necessary; a hyperresonant note may be elicited over air, particularly of a stomach bubble that projects up into the left side of the chest.

Palpation

1. Use warmed hands as you palpate the shape and angle of the sternum. Note if there is depression of the sternum.

2. Palpate the costochondral junctions for tenderness and enlargement.

3. As you palpate, vibration may be felt through your hands as the child cries.

4. Vocal fremitus is difficult to elicit in the smaller child since it is difficult to have him or her make repetitive sounds on command.

1. The shape of the sternum may vary, although a large depression of the sternum (funnel sternum) may cause subsequent trouble because of pressure on underlying structures.

2. May suggest an underlying inflammatory response.

3. Normal inspiration and expiration do not give a sensation under the fingers, except for the expansion of the chest.

4. In the older child, it is worth trying to obtain transmission of sound through the lung tissue (see page 63).

Auscultation

1. Try to examine the child before crying begins.

2. Warm the stethoscope before using by rubbing it between your hands.

3. Be aware that breathing is louder in younger children with slightly increased length of inspiration, almost to the point of bronchovesicular breathing in the adult.

4. Crackles (discontinuous; interrupted, explosive sounds) may be heard more easily in children.

5. Wheezes.

1. Note, however, that crying increases lung expansion.

2. A cold stethoscope will startle the child.

3. Bronchial breathing with equal inspiration and expiration is very loud and easy to hear in children with respiratory tract infections.

4. Added coarse-quality sounds in the chest are commonly associated with mucus in the trachea or in the back of the nose and usually clear with cough.

5. Recurrent wheeze is an important finding in children.

Pediatric Physical Assessment *(continued)*

Technique	Findings

HEART

Inspection

In thin children, the apical beat or the point of maximal impulse can easily be seen, particularly if you look obliquely across the chest wall.

Measurement and documentation of the distance from the midline and the exact rib space are worth noting.

Palpation

The apical beat may be felt in the 6th intercostal space about 2 inches (5 cm) from the midline in the school-age child. It is more difficult to feel in the infant, particularly a plump child, and would not be so far out toward the anterior axillary line.

The apical beat will be deviated to the left with cardiac enlargement or a collapsed lung on that side. The apical pulse could be pushed toward the right by a tumor or a collapsed lung on the right. Pneumothorax under tension will push the heart away from the side of the increased pressure.

Auscultation

1. Identify the first heart sound (S_1) (occurs during systole).

    a. Locate the apical beat (closing of the mitral valve) by placing the stethoscope over the maximum impulse area, concentrating on the first heart sound. (As the ventricle on the left contracts, pushing the blood up into the aorta, the sound of the mitral valve closing is heard.)

    b. That sound can be identified by placing the thumb on the carotid pulse of the neck, which will coincide very closely with the heart sounds.

2. Identify the second heart sound (S_2).

    a. Move the stethoscope up toward the sternum and to the left.

    b. At the base of the heart, both over the aortic and pulmonic areas, S_2 is louder than S_1.

3. Move the stethoscope in small jumps from the apical area medially toward the sternum. Go up to the left side of the sternum, listening at each interspace next to the sternum.

4. Move next to the child's right second intercostal space—again next to the sternum.

5. Listen to only one sound; concentrate on that to the exclusion of all others. Can you identify this sound? Is it clear? Compare it with your own heart sound or that of the parent.

6. If there is question of a heart murmur or added sounds, refer to the health care provider.

7. As you listen to the heart sounds, you are also listening to the rhythm to confirm your findings on pulse.

    a. If the child breathes in and out deeply, a sinus arrhythmia will be obvious.

    b. If the child holds his or her breath, the sinus arrhythmia will disappear.

8. Be sure to note a rapid heart rate that is present even when the child is at rest and quiet.

9. In the infant, heart sounds are just a series of taps; they occur so fast that it may be very difficult to determine which sound is S_1.

1. Consists of the "lub" portion of the "lub-dub" heart sound.

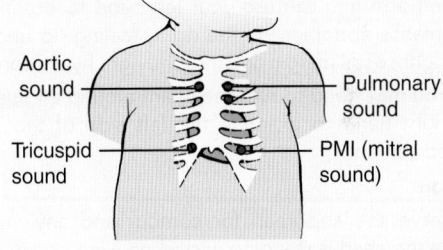

2. Represents the "dub" portion of the "lub-dub" heart sound.

    b. In a child, S_2 can be heard as two heart sounds because the two valves in the aorta and pulmonary vessels do not close at the same time. This split will increase with inspiration and decrease with expiration.

3. Represents the area of maximum intensity of sound of the pulmonary vessels.

4. It is at this area that you will hear the aortic sound best.

5. The child will enjoy this comparison if allowed to listen.

7. The typical rhythm of a child is called *sinus arrhythmia*. As the heart speeds up, the child is breathing in; the heart slows down on expiration.

8. This may be indicative of a tachycardia that requires further investigation.

9. In the infant, the S_1 and S_2 are equal in intensity.

(continued)

Pediatric Physical Assessment *(continued)*

Technique	Findings

ABDOMEN

1. For examination of the abdomen, the child should be lying down, relaxed, and not crying. Placing a small child, particularly those between ages 1 and 3, on a high table on cold paper can be frightening; as a result, his or her abdomen will not be relaxed.

2. Infants up to age 1 do not seem to be perturbed and will usually lie down and play nicely as long as they can see the parent, who should be stationed at the head of the child while you examine the abdomen.

3. Having the child lie across the parent's knees with the legs dangling on one side and the head cradled in his or her arms will enable you to feel the abdomen quite well.

   a. You may find that with the infant's head in the parent's left arm you can use your left hand to examine the infant's abdomen on the right, feeling up under the right costal margin and into the right hypochondrium.

   b. You may need to turn the infant around and use your right hand to examine the left side of the infant's abdomen.

1. The abdomen needs to be relaxed to palpate abnormal masses or enlarged liver or spleen as well as to auscultate for abnormal sounds.

Inspection

1. Observe the abdomen for contour and any markings while the child is standing and when lying down. As you inspect, you may see some abdominal movement with respiration. (Remember that the diaphragm, as it goes up and down, will move the contents of the abdomen.)

2. Check for early signs of puberty as evidenced by pubic hair over the symphysis pubis.

3. Carefully inspect the umbilicus for cleanliness and the presence of scar tissue.

1. Sometimes superficial veins are seen on the abdomen, particularly in a very blond infant. Striae are commonly noticed on the flank following rapid loss or gain of weight.

2. Early pubic hair in younger children (ages 8 to 10 years) may appear long and silky. This will ultimately become curly toward the onset of puberty.

3. A deep umbilicus may be difficult to keep clean. Immediately after the cord has dropped off, a granuloma may occur.

Auscultation

1. Because percussion and palpation will stimulate the small bowel and increase bowel sounds, auscultation should precede these two techniques.

2. To obtain the child's cooperation, you can conduct a running commentary as you listen, saying such things as, "I can hear the Cheerios in there."

1. Bowel sounds are heard as tinkling, irregular sounds that indicate that fluid is moving from one section of the bowel to the next.

2. In a quiet infant who has just eaten, not many bowel sounds will be heard. In a hungry child, noisy bowel sounds can be heard, even without a stethoscope.

Percussion

1. On the right side, percuss for the liver. Confirm on palpation.

2. Percuss over the left upper quadrant (LUQ).

3. Percuss the lower abdomen, particularly above the symphysis pubis.

1. Liver dullness can frequently be outlined to determine size of the liver.

2. Percussion over a gas-filled bowel or stomach results in a high-pitched, hollow sound.

3. Above the symphysis pubis, a filled bladder can produce a duller sound, as does a pregnant uterus. (A mass in the abdomen of a girl over age 10 may be a fetus.)

   a. The liver is frequently felt about ⅜ inch (1 cm) below the right costal margin and in some instances as low as ¾ inch (2 cm). This is a common finding in the neonate and through the early school-age years.

Pediatric Physical Assessment *(continued)*

Technique	Findings

ABDOMEN *(continued)*

Palpation

1. Divide the abdomen into imaginary quadrants, palpating each with the fingertips.
2. In the right upper quadrant, palpate for the liver edge.
   a. Although the liver is easily palpable in many children, you may have to press quite firmly.

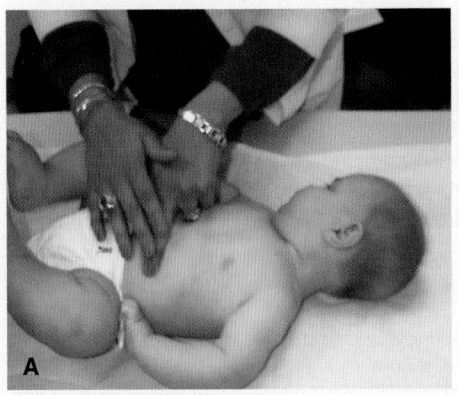 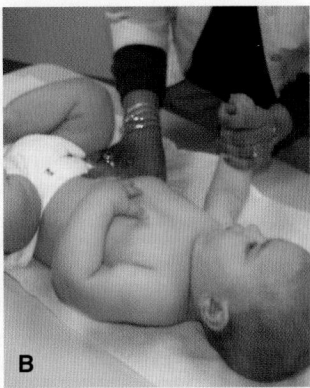

3. In the LUQ, palpate for the spleen. Less resistance is encountered as you feel up under the left costal margin.

3. Typically, only the tip of the spleen can be felt in the outer LUQ in the early months of life and in very thin children of preschool age.

4. In the upper quadrants also try to palpate for the kidneys. Deep palpation for both kidneys should routinely be a part of the examination to make sure there is no enlargement of the kidney. Normally, the kidney is not palpable.

4. Kidney palpation is difficult, but during the neonatal period, the lower pole of the right kidney may be felt and sometimes the left as well. (This applies to the period immediately after delivery, when the neonate's abdomen is relaxed and the bowel is not distended.)

5. In the iliac fossa or the left lower quadrant, palpate for the descending bowel.

5. The descending colon can be felt, particularly if it's filled with firm stool and the child is quiet. It may be slightly tender, but it should not cause severe pain on gentle palpation.

6. Palpate on the right lower quadrant (RLQ) where the appendix is located.

6. In the RLQ, usually the only sensation is that of gas-filled bowel. Tenderness in this area could be related to an inflamed appendix.

7. If the child has pain in any area or has pointed to the umbilicus when asked to show where the pain is, avoid the area demonstrated and leave it until last. Note whether the pain is with pressure or rebound.

7. If the painful area is palpated first, the child may tense up when the other areas of the abdomen are examined.

8. Palpate around the umbilicus for any masses that may indicate a hernia, especially in preterm and black children. As you press over the protruding hernia, you can feel the sensation of gurgling under your fingers as the bowel returns to the abdomen.

8. Most of these hernias heal naturally by age 6. A hernia above the umbilicus can be revealed by asking the child to lift his or her head from the table. (Widening of the muscles above the umbilicus is called *diastasis recti*.)

RECTUM AND ANUS

1. Rectal examinations are rarely necessary in infants and young children.
2. If the child will be examined by a another health care provider, it is not necessary to duplicate this part of the examination.
3. Rectal examinations are embarrassing and uncomfortable for most children. Explain the procedure before performing the examination.

(continued)

Pediatric Physical Assessment *(continued)*

Technique	Findings

RECTUM AND ANUS *(continued)*

4. Positioning for a rectal examination:
   a. Infants can be placed on their abdomens, sides, or backs with their legs raised to their chests.
   b. Young children and teenagers can be positioned on their sides.

Inspection

1. When examining an infant or toddler, place the child on a flat surface so that the weight is evenly distributed on the front of the pelvis. As the infant moves about on the abdomen, observe the entire back, the lower back, the upper thigh, and the tightening of the buttocks.

2. Check particularly the lower part of the back for hairiness or a mass.

3. As the child moves away, part the buttocks and look at the cleft between them.

4. Pay careful attention to the outer appearance of the anus and the perineum, the underside of the scrotum in the male, and the labia majora in the female.

1. If one buttock is larger than the other, you will see that side projected above the other. Weakness of one side will be obvious as the infant moves around, although a child in the early stages of crawling will tend to use one knee as a predominant leader, dragging the other.

2. This may indicate an underlying abnormality of the vertebrae in spina bifida.

3. A pilonidal dimple or sinus may be seen over the lower back. This is a common finding, but parents should be told about it for cleaning purposes. Make sure there is no drainage.

4. The anus is inspected for blood, fissures, or splitting in the external tissue; redness; swelling; or pads of extra flesh. On occasion, small white pinworms may be seen adhering to the anal skin.

Palpation

1. Consider the child's age and feelings; ask the mother to assist, if necessary. This part of the examination is not always needed.

2. Start by parting the buttocks with the left hand and introducing a well-lubricated finger (with finger cot) into the anus.

3. Gently apply pressure on the anal sphincter to allow the muscles to relax and the fingertip to slide into the rectum.

4. Gently palpate the inner ring, feeling for areas of thickening and tenderness and simultaneously judging the sphincter tone.

5. If the rectum is full of stool, it will be impossible to feel any other mass.

6. Palpate the walls of the rectum.

7. In the male, gently turn your finger through 180 degrees and feel the posterior surface of the prostate. Note size, consistency, tenderness, and contour.

8. In the female, perform a bimanual examination and palpate the cervix.

2. When an infant is being examined, the small finger should be used.

3. Apply pressure with pulp of the finger rather than jab at the anus with the fingertip.

4. As the perianal area is pressed on from the inside, tenderness will be elicited if a deep fissure exists or if an infection has occurred around a fissure.

5. In a young child, particularly an infant, dilatation provided by the finger may result in a bowel movement. In an older child, a suppository or even an enema may be required.

6. The mucosal walls should be smooth and deep palpation should elicit mild tenderness and no acute pain.

EXAMINING MALE GENITALIA

1. This part of the examination requires a direct, matter-of-fact approach. Acknowledge that it is normal to feel embarrassed during an examination of the genitals. Explain what you are looking for as you proceed through the examination with a teenager.

2. Reassure the child after the examination that his genitals are normal. This decreases anxiety.

Pediatric Physical Assessment (continued)

Technique	Findings

EXAMINING MALE GENITALIA (*continued*)

3. When examining the testes in a young boy, you may need to block the canals to prevent them from retracting into the abdomen.

Scrotum and testes

Inspection

1. Before touching the child, determine by observation of the testes whether they are in the scrotum.

2. Observe the skin over the scrotum for color and surface appearance, noting the presence of wrinkles, or rugae.

1. Retraction of the testes into the abdomen occurs frequently in young children; the development of the scrotum depends on the presence of the testes.

2. The skin over the scrotum varies in color, being a darker brown to black in the more pigmented races and reddish in children with light complexions. The wrinkles, or rugae, are more developed as the child grows older.

Palpation

1. Check the scrotum wall for swelling or sensitivity. Gently feel the testes, palpating across the upper pole and feeling for the epididymis. (Remember the scrotum is extremely sensitive to pressure.)

2. Estimate the size of the testes and identify the spermatic cord, tracing it from the testis up toward the groin.

3. Make a special effort to locate the testis in a young child whose testes may be retracted into the abdomen via a hyperactive cremasteric reflex. You may need to have the child in a sitting or standing position. Occasionally, you may need to ask a parent to check at home with the child sitting in a warm bathtub.
   a. If the testes cannot be felt in the scrotum, gently run the skin of the upper scrotum between your fingers, moving superiorly and approaching the external inguinal ring.
   b. Try to milk the testis down toward the scrotum from above with your hand.
   c. If this fails, have the child sit cross-legged to abolish the reflex of the cremaster muscle.

4. When examining a boy in the early stages of puberty, it is important to note the size of the testis as well as the greater number of rugae on the scrotum and the appearance of pubic hair around the penis.

1. The epididymis is a ridge of soft, bumpy tissue extending from the superior pole and running down and behind the testis.

2. The spermatic cord, with the vas deferens, feels firm and is accompanied by softer nerves, arteries, veins, and a few muscle fibers.

3. Ascertaining the presence of the testes in the scrotum is vital in older infant or toddler. Nondescent of the testes requires further evaluation.

   a. During this period the testis is about ½–¾ inch (1.5–2 cm) in length. In the quiescent period before puberty, the male genitalia remain fairly infantile.

4. In early puberty, the testes start to grow. Onset of puberty varies, occurring between the ages of 10 and 14 years. In most teenagers, the findings are similar to those in adults.

Penis

1. Evaluate the penis on all sides by lifting up the shaft.

2. If the child is not circumcised, partially retract the foreskin to observe the glans and meatus.

3. Observe the position of the meatus and evert the lips of the meatus to reveal an adequate orifice.

4. In the older child, inspect the penis for ulcers, sores, or discharge from the meatus.

1. The shaft of the penis contains the urethra on the under, or ventral, surface and is easily palpable.

2. The foreskin may adhere to the glans for the first few years of life. It is not necessary for the parent to "stretch" the foreskin by retraction.

   Whitish discharge around the glans under the foreskin is normal and not a sign of infection. The foreskin should completely encircle the glans.

3. The meatus may be positioned off center. If the meatus is located on the dorsal or ventral surface of the shaft, the child should be evaluated by a pediatric urologist.

4. Consider sexually transmitted diseases in children of all ages; the possibility of sexual abuse must be considered.

(continued)

Pediatric Physical Assessment *(continued)*

Technique	Findings

EXAMINING MALE GENITALIA *(continued)*

Inguinal area

Palpation

1. Palpate for a hernia over the external inguinal ring. Have the child cough to enhance your observation.

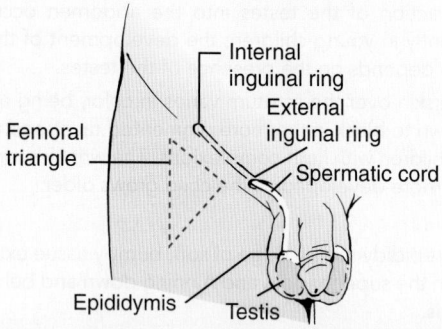

Labels: Internal inguinal ring · External inguinal ring · Spermatic cord · Femoral triangle · Epididymis · Testis

2. An increased cough reflex or swelling in the area should be checked by carefully placing a finger on the scrotal skin and invaginating the skin over your fingers toward the external ring. You are trying to follow the course of a hernia that would descend into the scrotum while you feel the external ring from below. A hernia in the inguinal region presents as a bulge that can be either seen or felt from below by placing the finger in the scrotum pointing up toward the external inguinal ring.

3. Also palpate for the inguinal lymph nodes.

1. Having the child stand either with the parent holding him or placing him against the parent's knee will help you in locating a hernia in the inguinal area.

3. The inguinal lymph nodes in an infant are palpable as small and "shotty." Anything more than this should alert you to possible infection because the perianal area drains into the superficial inguinal lymph nodes. For example, diaper rash may explain enlargement of the lymph nodes, which should be noted and reported.

Femoral area

Palpation

Palpate the femoral triangle carefully for a hernia and for lymph nodes.

In the femoral area, a swelling that can be reduced with a gurgling sound is an unusual finding.

Auscultation

If you are trying to reduce a mass, listen over the scrotum to determine if there is a gurgling sound.

This will locate the bowel and confirm a hernia.

Transillumination

1. To locate the testis, darken the room and shine a bright light from behind the scrotum. In a normal child, the testis will stand out as a darker area.

2. Transilluminate any suspicious mass to help locate a hernia.

1. A scrotal sac that is swollen by fluid (hydrocele) will transilluminate. Fluid around the testes or cord must be differentiated from a hernia.

2. Any mass in this area must be reported to a health care provider immediately.

EXAMINING FEMALE GENITALIA

1. If the child will be examined by a health care provider, it is not necessary to duplicate this part of the examination.

2. Place the infant or toddler on the table or on her parent's knee while the parent holds the child's knees in an abducted and flexed position.

Pediatric Physical Assessment *(continued)*

Technique	Findings

EXAMINING FEMALE GENITALIA *(continued)*

3. A preschool child can be allowed to lean over her parent's knee. However, remember that the structures are being visualized upside down.

4. The older child or teenager should be draped as an adult would and should be placed in a lithotomy position with the aid of stirrups.

Equipment

- Disposable gloves   • Speculum   • Light source

1. Carefully inspect the perineal area for cleanliness, inflammation, and abnormality.

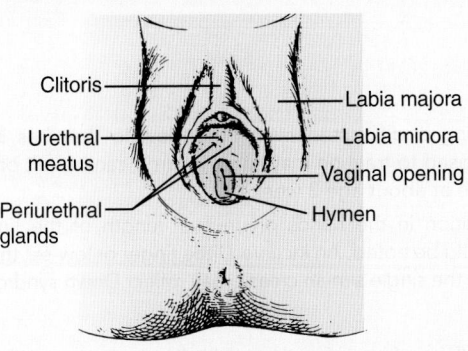

2. If the mother of a neonate has noted a bloody discharge from the infant's vagina during the first few days of life, reassure her that this is not an uncommon occurrence; the discharge will disappear, as will swelling of the labia majora and clitoris and enlargement of the infant's breasts.

3. Note the vaginal opening, which may vary in size because of the presence of a thin membrane, the hymen. The hymen varies in appearance according to the child's age.

4. In the young child it is usually unnecessary to examine inside the vagina. If a young child requires an extensive vaginal exam, it is frequently done under sedation.

1. This includes the mons pubis, clitoris, labia, urethra, and perineum. The labia minora are seen as two slender folds of tissue inside the labia majora. In some instances, adhesions of the labia minora occur because of the lack of natural hormones.

2. Hormone stimulation from the mother's body accounts for this occurrence. The discharge usually stops after the hormones are excreted. The bloody appearance on the diaper may be confused with the presence of urates, which are also orange-red and appear normally in urine.

3. The lack of an opening into the vagina may result in the retention of menstrual fluid when the child reaches puberty. In the sexually active adolescent, vestigial remains on the hymen may appear as small particles (caruncles) at the fringe of the vagina.

   The possibility of sexual abuse should always be considered and, if necessary, the child referred to a specialist in sexual abuse.

4. A foreign body or sexually transmitted infection may be suspected if there is a vaginal discharge, bleeding, or odor.

MUSCULOSKELETAL SYSTEM

1. Evaluation of the musculoskeletal system can be done both in an informal manner, while watching the child at rest and at play, and in a formal manner as specific findings are methodically checked.

2. In the neonate, observe the position of the extremities during sleep and the quality of movement when the child is awake.

(continued)

Pediatric Physical Assessment (continued)

Technique	Findings

MUSCULOSKELETAL SYSTEM (continued)

3. Various aspects of size, shape, and movement are evaluated as the child is observed pushing up on his or her arms and turning his or her head toward the mother.

4. A child in the early stages of walking offers many opportunities for evaluation of muscle strength and movement.

5. At the same time, rapport with the mother can be reinforced by your admiring the child's ability and by inquiring if she is concerned about the manner in which the child is walking.

6. A more mobile child can be evaluated as you watch him or her play and explore the room.

7. Having the older child reach for crayons, run after a ball, or walk around the room enables you to evaluate the musculoskeletal system and the child's sense of balance.

Upper extremities

1. In the infant, evaluate the status of the clavicles when examining the skull and neck.

2. Carefully examine the hands to note the shape of the hand, shape and length of the fingers, changes in the nails, and creases on the palms.

Findings for Upper extremities:

1. During a difficult delivery, the clavicle that has been exposed to traction may snap. A lump can be felt on the bone at about age 3 weeks.

2. Variation in the hands or unusual length of the fingers should be noted. An incurved little finger or low-set thumb with the single simian crease may reflect Down syndrome.

Lower extremities

1. Examine the appearance of the infant's foot, noting arch formation.

2. Inspect the angle of the foot and lower leg and then manipulate the ankle to evaluate the range of motion.

3. Place the legs together and see how far the ankles and knees are separated.

4. Evaluate the child's ability to walk, noting the appearance of his or her legs and foot placement. Remember to look at the child's shoes and see which side of the sole is worn down.

Findings for Lower extremities:

1. The foot of an infant is usually flat and appears broad because the arch on the inside of the foot is covered by a fat pad. Parents may need reassurance about this.

2. Full flexibility of the foot (plantar flexion) rules out underlying abnormality. The foot should return to the neutral position after manipulation. Typically, the foot will turn in, or adduct. Such a finding should be recorded.

3. Toddlers typically have external hip rotation and internal knee rotation, which results in a "bowed" appearance. The preschooler has a normally knock-kneed walk, but with knees touching, ankles should be no more than two fingerbreadths apart.

4. Infants commonly appear to be bow-legged when they first start to walk because the feet are kept wide apart and turn slightly in. The ankles appear curved when viewed from behind.

Hip

When examining children under age 1, check for signs of hip dislocation. See page 1759.

Spine

1. Check the spine for signs of abnormal curvature.

2. Observe the child from the side and back in the standing position to see forward curving of the shoulders.

3. Have the child bend forward with the arms hanging down. A unilateral rib prominence will be seen in children with scoliosis.

Findings for Spine:

1. The normal young child has a curve inward at the lumbar region (lordosis), but this should not be exaggerated. It is normally more exaggerated in black children.

2. These appear most commonly during school-age years and adolescence.

Pediatric Physical Assessment (continued)

Technique   **Findings**

MUSCULOSKELETAL SYSTEM (continued)

Spine (continued)

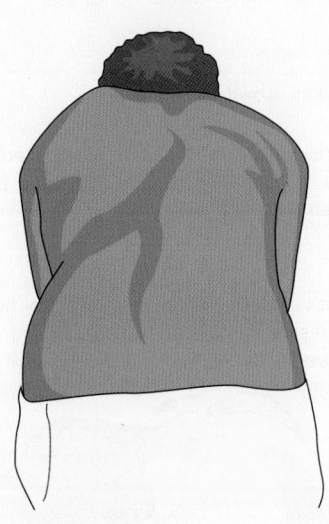

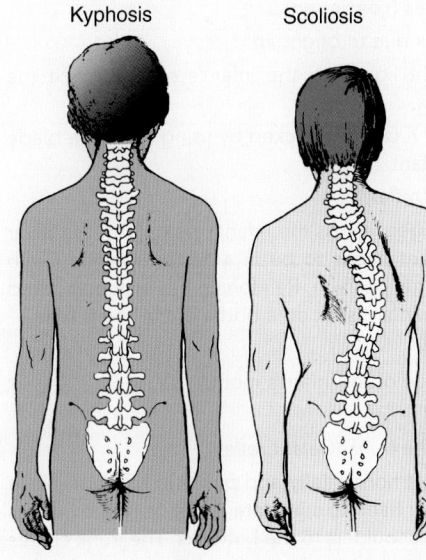

Kyphosis   Scoliosis

Kyphosis: Forward curvature of the shoulders.

Scoliosis: Side-to-side curvature of the spine.

NEUROLOGIC EXAMINATION

1. The neurologic system at birth is different from that in an infant age 3 months. There is an even greater contrast between the infant and children and adults.
2. The central nervous system at birth is underdeveloped and the functions tested are below the level of the cortex.

Equipment

- Flashlight
- Ophthalmoscope
- Tuning fork
- Noisemaker
- Tongue depressor

Procedure for the neonate and young infant

1. Observe the neonate for general appearance, positioning, activity, crying, and alertness. Take note of the posture—including head, neck, and extremities.
2. Note the pitch, volume, and character of his or her cry.
3. Observe the infant's facial expression and the symmetry of his or her face when crying or sucking.
4. Most of the cranial nerves are difficult to check at this early age.

Automatic reflexes

1. *Blinking reflex due to loud noise*

   Clap your hands or produce a loud clicking noise. Be careful not to clap near the infant to prevent a wave of air from causing a blinking of the eyes.

1. Stiffness of the neck or marked extension of the head will cause a position of opisthotonos and necessitates referral.
2. The high-pitched cry of the infant who has intracranial irritation is distinctive.
3. Poor sucking, with dribbling, is abnormal. Transient weakness of the mouth caused by cranial nerve VII paralysis is commonly seen as a result of a forceps delivery in which the forceps is pressed on the facial nerve where it emerges from the ear.

1. Lack of a blink in response to a loud noise may indicate deafness.

(continued)

Pediatric Physical Assessment *(continued)*

Technique	Findings

NEUROLOGIC EXAMINATION *(continued)*
Procedure for the neonate and young infant *(continued)*
Automatic reflexes *(continued)*

2. *Blinking reflex due to bright light*

   Shine a bright light into the infant's eyes to elicit the blinking reflex.

3. Cranial nerve X can be checked by using a tongue blade to gag the infant.

4. *Palmar grasp reflex*

   Place your fingers across the infant's palm from the ulnar side. The infant needs to be in a relaxed position with head in a central position. Reinforcement may be offered by having the infant suck on a bottle at the same time.

5. *Rooting reflex*

   Touch the edge of the infant's mouth.

6. *Incurving of the trunk (Galant reflex)*

   Hold the infant horizontally and prone in one arm while using the other hand to stimulate one side of the infant's back from the shoulders to the buttocks. The trunk curves toward the stimulated side as the shoulders and pelvis move toward the stroking hand (persists until the infant is about age 2 months).

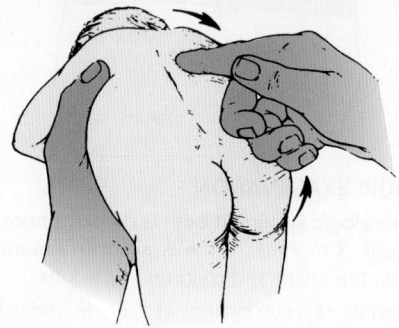

7. *Vertical suspension position*

   Place your hands under the infant's axillae with thumbs supporting the back of the head and hold the infant upright.

8. *Stepping response*

   Hold the infant under its axillae with thumbs supporting the back of the head. Allow the infant's foot to touch a firm surface.

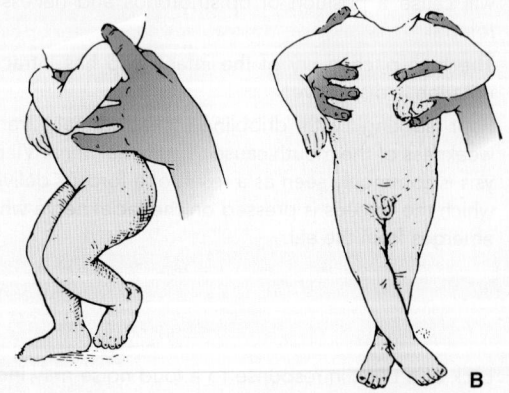

A   B

---

2. Failure to blink may indicate blindness.

3. Palate moves upward.

4. Both hands will flex and can be compared for strength. Weakness on one side may be indicated by a failure to grasp when the palm is stimulated.

5. The infant's mouth will open and the head will turn toward the side stimulated. This reflex is marked during the early weeks of life.

7. The legs flex at the hips and knees (persists for about 4 months).

8. Normally, the infant responds by lifting one knee and hip into a flexed position and moving the opposite leg forward—making a series of stepping movements (see 8A).

   a. Difficulty with the stepping reflex and stiffness or spasticity connected with crossing of the feet and scissoring (see 8B) is indicative of spastic paraplegia or diplegia.

   b. It should be noted that the stepping response may be affected by breech delivery. (It may also be affected by weakness.)

   c. The stepping response is evident toward the end of the first week after birth and persists for a variable time.

Pediatric Physical Assessment *(continued)*

Technique	Findings

NEUROLOGIC EXAMINATION *(continued)*

Procedure for the neonate and young infant (*continued*)

Automatic reflexes *(continued)*

9. Tonic neck reflex

   Hold the infant in a supine position with the head turned to one side and the jaw held in place over the shoulder.

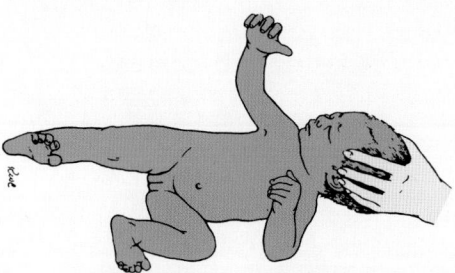

9.

   a. The arm and leg on the side to which the head is turned will extend, whereas those on the other side will flex (the so-called "fencing reflex").

   b. This reflex persists for about 5–6 months; it may be present at birth or delayed until the infant is age 6 or 8 weeks.

   c. Persistence beyond 6 months suggests major cerebral damage.

10. *Mass reflexes* (Moro or startle reflex)

    Hold the infant along your arm with the other hand below the lower legs. Lower the feet and body in a sudden motion.

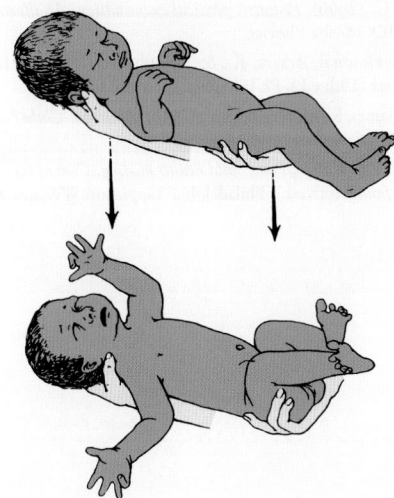

10. The arms will spring up and out, abducting and extending; the fingers are also extended. The arms then return forward over the body with a clasping motion. At the same time, the legs flex slightly and the hips abduct.

    a. The Moro reflex is present at birth and disappears at approximately the end of the third month. Persistence beyond 6 months is significant.

    b. Asymmetrical response may be caused by paralysis of the arm after difficult delivery, tension and injury to the brachial plexus, or a fracture of the clavicle or humerus. A dislocated hip would produce an asymmetrical response in the lower extremities.

11. *Perez reflex*

    Hold the infant in a prone position along your arm; place the thumb of the other hand on the sacrum and move it firmly toward the head, along the entire length of the spine.

11. The head and spine will extend and the knees will flex upward.

Summary

1. Some of the jerking and shaking movements seen in neonates are normal, but they should be rechecked frequently during the first few weeks of life.

2. Variants in the findings caused by the infant's sleepiness or hunger should be taken into account and reevaluations should be carried out under different conditions.

3. Severe neurologic damage may be completely asymptomatic and impossible to detect during the first few weeks of life.

(continued)

Pediatric Physical Assessment *(continued)*

Technique	Findings

NEUROLOGIC EXAMINATION *(continued)*

Procedure for the toddler and early school-age child

1. The neurologic examination for the toddler and the early school-age child is similar to that for the adult (see page 78).

2. The Draw-A-Person Test and the Denver Developmental Assessment are both well-accepted methods for testing areas in the development of the child.

3. Beyond the neonatal period, specific gross and fine motor coordination testing, accompanied by appropriate evaluation of the Denver test, will assist in assessing the child's level of development.

4. These tests also assess social and language development and are important screening devices.

5. Interview techniques can also be useful in assessing development in the preschool child.

2. See *www.denverii.com* for instructions and findings of the Denver Development Assessment.

SELECTED REFERENCES

American Academy of Pediatrics. (2008). *Bright futures: Guidelines for health supervision of infants, children, and adolescents* (3rd ed.). Elk Grove Village, IL: Author.

American Academy of Pediatrics. (2011). *Bright futures: Nutrition* (3rd ed.). Elk Grove Village, IL: Author.

Bickley, L. S. (2008). *Bates' guide to physical examination and history taking* (10th ed.). Philadelphia: Lippincott Williams & Wilkins.

Burns, C., Dunn, A., Brady, M., & Starr, N. (2013). *Pediatric Primary Care* (5th ed.). Philadephia: Saunders.

Centers for Disease Control and Prevention. (2010). Growth charts. Atlanta, GA: Author. Available: *www.cdc.gov/growthcharts/*.

Duderstadt K. G. (2006). *Pediatric physical examination: An illustrated handbook*. St. Louis, MO: Mosby Elsevier.

Johns Hopkins Hospital, Arkara, K., & Tschudy, M. (Eds.). (2012). *The Harriet Lane handbook* (19th ed.). Philadelphia: Elsevier Mosby.

McKinney, E., James, S., Murray, S., et al. (2013). *Maternal-Child Nursing*. (4th ed.). St. Louis, MO: Saunders.

Pillitteri, A. (2009). *Maternal and child health nursing: Care of the childbearing and childrearing family* (6th ed.). Philadelphia: Lippincott Williams & Wilkins.

42

Pediatric Primary Care

HEALTH MAINTENANCE

Pediatric primary care includes health promotion and disease prevention interventions that will positively affect the well-being of children and their families. The goal of pediatric primary care is to achieve physical, emotional, and developmental health for all children. Primary prevention—through immunizations, proper nutrition, and safety counseling—are essential components of pediatric health care.

Immunizations

Disease prevention through immunizations has significantly reduced childhood morbidity and mortality from infectious diseases. However, despite effective immunization availability, vaccine-preventable diseases are still present in the United States and continue to pose significant public health problems. The rate of immunization in the United States exceeds 90% for children ages 19 to 35 months for poliovirus vaccine; measles, mumps, rubella; Hepatitis B, and varicella vaccine. However, rates vary by state and decrease after this age. Rate of immunization for routine vaccines for adolescents ages 13 to 17 range from 26.7% (human papillomavirus vaccine) to 55.6% (Tdap vaccine).

 Evidence Base Centers for Control Disease and Prevention. (2011). National and state vaccination coverage among children aged 19–35 months— United States, 2010. *Morbidity and Mortality Weekly Report, 60*(34), 1157–1163.
 Niederhauser, V., & Baker, D. (2011). What's new in child and adolescent immunizations? *The Nurse Practitioner, 36*(10), 39–44.

Nurses are in a vital position to promote child health by assessing, recommending, and administering immunizations. Also, nurses are frequently asked to provide documentation (to parents or caregivers) of the immunizations that have been administered in order to facilitate children's enrollment in day care, school programs, and summer camp participation. A review of immunizations and administration of needed vaccines should be done at every health care visit.

Barriers to Vaccination

 Evidence Base Connors, J., Arushanyan, E., Bellanca, G., et al. (2012). A description of barriers and facilitators to childhood vaccinations in the military health system. *Journal of the American Academy of Nurse Practitioners, 24*(12), 716–725.
 Murphy, P., Frazee, S., Cantlin, J. P., et al. (2012). Pharmacy provision of influenza vaccinations in medically underserved communities. *Journal of the American Pharmacists Association, 52*(1), 67–70.

There are many reasons that parents or caregivers may give to refuse vaccination for their children.

1. Safety concerns, such as concerns that the child may develop learning disabilities. Information about vaccine safety can be obtained from the Centers for Disease Control and Prevention (CDC) at *www.cdc.gov/vaccinesafety/Concerns/Index.html*.
2. Concern for the pain inflicted on the child.
3. Because the vaccine programs have been successful for many years, many parents have no memory or knowledge of the serious vaccine-preventable illnesses that have been near eradicated.
4. Unfortunately many parents may be influenced by high-impact negative media information regarding vaccinations despite the fact that most is not supported by evidence.

NURSING ALERT Nurses can be instrumental in assisting caregivers in discerning factual information from myths and erroneous information that may be presented in the media.

General Considerations

Requirements of National Childhood Vaccine Injury Act (Effective 1988)

1. This act mandated providers to notify all patients and parents about the risks and benefits associated with vaccines.
2. The patient, parent, or legal guardian should be informed about the benefits and risks of immunizations. They must be provided with the current Vaccine Information Statement (VIS), developed by the CDC, before the administration of the vaccine. Health care providers must record the name of the VIS publication (eg, polio), date of VIS publication, and the date the VIS was given to the patient or his or her family on the child's medical record.
3. Federal law mandates that all health care providers must record the following information in the patient's permanent medical record: month, day, and year of administration; vaccine or other biologic administered; manufacturer, lot number, and expiration date; and name, address, and title of the health care provider administering the vaccine.
4. In addition, the site and route of administration should be documented in the patient's record.
5. Health care providers are required to report selected events occurring after vaccination to the Vaccine Adverse Events Reporting System, part of the CDC Immunization Safety Office, which monitors and investigates possible vaccine adverse effects.

Routine Vaccinations for Children in the United States

The Advisory Committee on Immunization Practices (ACIP) annually develops written recommendations for the CDC regarding the routine administration of vaccines, along with schedules detailing the appropriate timing, dosage, and contraindications for children and adults in the civilian population in the United States. The most recent recommendations are reviewed below, but complete immunization schedules can be found at *www.cdc.gov/vaccines*.

Childhood-recommended vaccines (ages 0 to 6 years) include diphtheria, tetanus toxoid, acellular pertussis (DTaP); inactivated poliovirus vaccine (IPV); measles, mumps, rubella (MMR); *Haemophilus influenzae* type b (Hib) vaccine; hepatitis B vaccine (HBV); *Varicella*; pneumococcal conjugate vaccine (PCV7 and PCV13); rotavirus (Rota); hepatitis A (HepA); and meningococcal vaccine (MCV4). An influenza vaccine is recommended to be given annually for healthy children ages 6 months to 19 years old.

The recommended immunization schedule for persons ages 7 to 18 years includes tetanus toxoid, diphtheria, and acellular pertussis (Tdap); human papillomavirus vaccine (HPV); MCV4; pneumococcal polysaccharide vaccine (PPV)—to certain groups at high risk; annual influenza vaccine (live attenuated influenza vaccine [LAIV] or trivalent inactivated influenza vaccine [TIV]); HepA—for certain groups of children; HBV; MMR; *Varicella*; and IPV, if necessary, to equal a total of four doses.

Immunization Schedules

1. Routine immunizations are started in infancy. However, if a child is not immunized in infancy, immunizations may be started at any age and a slightly different schedule may be followed, depending on the child's age and the prevalence of specific diseases at that time.
2. An interrupted primary series of immunizations does not need to be restarted; rather, the original series should be resumed regardless of the length of time that has elapsed.
3. The immunoresponse is limited in a significant proportion of infants and the recommended booster doses are designed to ensure and maintain immunity.
4. Current recommended immunization schedules can be found at *www.cdc.gov/vaccines/*.
5. When using a combination vaccine, if there is a contraindication to any of the components, do not vaccinate.

Contraindications and Precautions

It is important to read the manufacturer's insert for each vaccine before administration.

1. Contraindications to all vaccines:
   a. Anaphylactic reaction to a vaccine or a vaccine constituent.
   b. Moderate or severe illnesses with or without a fever. Children with moderate or severe illnesses, with or without fever, can be vaccinated as soon as they are recovering and no longer acutely ill.
2. All live virus vaccines (live oral poliovirus vaccine [OPV], MMR, *Varicella*) are contraindicated in pregnancy, immunosuppression or immunodeficiency, and household or close contact with those who are immunosuppressed or immunodeficient.
   a. MMR vaccine should be considered for all symptomatic human immunodeficiency virus (HIV)–infected persons who do not have evidence of severe immunosuppression or evidence of measles immunity.
   b. *Varicella* vaccine should be considered for asymptomatic or mildly symptomatic HIV-infected children.
3. Diphtheria, tetanus, and pertussis (DTP)/DTaP—encephalopathy within 7 days of administration of previous dose of DTP/DTaP.
   a. Infants and children with stable neurologic conditions, including well-controlled seizures, may be vaccinated; however, such vaccination should be decided on an individual basis.
4. IPV—anaphylactic reaction to neomycin, streptomycin, or polymyxin B.
5. MMR and *Varicella*—anaphylactic reactions to neomycin or gelatin.
6. Influenza—anaphylactic reaction to eggs or egg protein. Persons with asthma, reactive airway disease, or other chronic pulmonary or cardiovascular disorders should not receive LAIV.
7. HBV—anaphylactic reaction to baker's yeast.
8. Meningococcal vaccines—can be given to pregnant women; should not be administered with other vaccines for children with sickle cell disease or those without a functioning spleen.

Misconceptions Concerning Vaccine Contraindications

1. Some health care providers and parents inappropriately consider certain conditions or circumstances to be contraindications to vaccination. Conditions most commonly regarded as such include:
   a. Mild acute illness with low-grade fever or mild diarrheal illness in an otherwise well child.
   b. Current antimicrobial therapy or the convalescent phase of illness.
   c. Reaction to a previous DTaP dose that involved only soreness, redness, swelling in the immediate vicinity of the vaccination site, or temperature of less than 105° F (40.5° C).
   d. Prematurity.
   e. Person using aerosolized steroids, short course of oral steroids (less than 14 days), or topical steroids.
   f. Pregnancy of mother or other household contact.
   g. Recent exposure to an infectious disease.
   h. Breastfeeding.
   i. History of nonspecific allergies or relatives with allergies.
   j. Allergies to penicillin or other antibiotic, except anaphylactic reactions to neomycin or streptomycin.
   k. Allergies to duck meat or duck feathers.
   l. Family history of seizures in people considered for pertussis or measles vaccination.
   m. Family history of sudden infant death syndrome in children considered for DTaP vaccination.
   n. Family history of an adverse event, unrelated to immunosuppression, after vaccination.
   o. Malnutrition.
2. In most cases, children with the above conditions can still be immunized.

Vaccine Administration Considerations

1. Strict adherence to the manufacturer's storage and handling recommendation is vital. Failure to observe these precautions and recommendations may reduce the potency and effectiveness of vaccines.
2. Health care personnel administering vaccines should be immunized against measles, mumps, rubella, hepatitis B, influenza, tetanus, pertussis, and diphtheria. *Varicella* vaccine is recommended for health care providers with no serologic proof of immunity, prior vaccination, or previous disease. Gloves should be worn when administering vaccines. Good handwashing technique is mandatory before and after vaccine administration.
3. Sterile, disposable needles and syringes should be discarded promptly in appropriate biohazard containers. Do not recap needles.
4. Parenteral vaccines should be administered in the anterolateral aspect of the upper thigh in infants and in the deltoid area of the upper arm in older children and adolescents. Recommended routes of administration are included in the package inserts of vaccines.
5. Before administering a subsequent dose of any vaccine, question patients and parents about adverse effects and possible reactions from previous doses.

6. Routine vaccines can be safely and effectively administered simultaneously in most healthy children.

Specific Immunizations

DTaP

1. Administered I.M.
2. A time lapse of 8 weeks is recommended between the first three DTaP injections for desirable maximum effects.
3. Administration of acetaminophen at the time of immunization and at 4 and 8 hours after immunization decreases the incidence of febrile and local reactions.
4. Tdap is recommended for children over age 7 years. In 2006, vaccination guidelines for pertussis included recommendations that Tdap be routinely used in adolescents 11 to 18 years of age and single doses for adults 19 to 64 years of age in attempts to control recent pertussis outbreaks.
5. For contaminated wounds, a booster dose of tetanus should be given if more than 5 years have elapsed since the last dose.
6. For infant pertussis protection, ACIP has recommended that Tdap be given during each pregnancy between 27 and 36 weeks gestation to maximize the maternal antibody response and passive antibody transfer to the infant.

Tuberculin Skin Test

1. It is recommended that, if indicated, the tuberculin test be given before or at the time of the MMR vaccine. The measles vaccine may temporarily suppress tuberculin reactivity for 4 to 6 weeks, so result many not be accurate during that time frame.
2. The frequency of repeated tuberculin testing depends on the following:
   a. Risk of tuberculosis exposure to the child.
   b. Prevalence of tuberculosis in the population group.
   c. Presence of underlying host factors in the child (immunosuppressive conditions or HIV infection).
3. Children who have immigrated or been adopted from another country may have received an immunization for tuberculosis (BCG vaccine). It is not recommended in the United States due to low effectiveness.
   a. BCG may cause a false-positive tuberculosis (TB) skin test; however, screening for tuberculosis should still occur.
   b. Interferon-gamma release assays (IGRAs) are the preferred method of testing for tuberculosis in those immunized with BCG. An IGRA measures how strong a person's immune system reacts to TB bacteria by testing the person's blood in a laboratory.
   c. Chest x-ray confirms pulmonary disease.

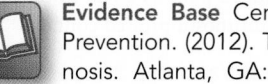

Evidence Base Centers for Disease Control and Prevention. (2012). Tuberculosis: Testing and diagnosis. Atlanta, GA: Author. Available: *www.cdc.gov/tb/topic/testing/default.htm#bcg.*

Measles Vaccine

1. Usually given between ages 12 and 15 months, but should be given at 12 months in high-risk areas. Second dose is recommended between ages 4 and 6 years.

2. Administered subcutaneously.

3. During an outbreak, infants as young as age 6 months can be immunized. A second dose should be given between ages 12 and 15 months and again at school entry.

4. Mild postimmunization symptoms include transient skin rashes and fever up to 2 weeks after vaccination.

5. Immunoglobulin preparations will interfere with the serologic response to measles vaccine; therefore, wait the specified time after administration for vaccination.

Meningococcal Vaccine

1. Usually given between the ages of 11 and 12 years, with a booster dose at age 16 years for healthy children. Is administered earlier (minimum age of 9 months) for some children with underlying conditions or children who are resident or travel to countries with epidemic disease.

2. Administer the MPSV4 vaccine subcutaneously into the fat of the arm. The MCV4 vaccines are given I.M.

3. Mild postimmunization symptoms such as local discomfort may occur. A small percentage of those who receive the vaccine may develop a fever. Severe reactions (such as an allergic reaction) are very rare.

Mumps Vaccine

1. Usually administered in combination with measles and rubella vaccine between ages 12 and 15 months.

2. Second dose administered as MMR is important because a substantial number of cases have occurred in people with previous immunizations.

3. Important to immunize susceptible children approaching puberty, adolescents, and adults.

Rubella Vaccine

1. Two doses of rubella vaccine are recommended to avoid consequences such as congenital rubella syndrome; usually administered in combination with mumps and measles.

2. Important to immunize postpubertal individuals, especially college students and military recruits.

3. Women should avoid pregnancy within 3 months of vaccine due to the theoretical risk to the fetus.

Polio Vaccine

1. Two types of trivalent vaccine have been developed—OPV and IPV (given I.M. or subcutaneously). Both are effective in preventing poliomyelitis; however, as of 2000, both the ACIP and CDC recommend exclusive use of IPV for infants and children in the United States, in order to reduce the risk of vaccine-induced polio from OPV.

2. Since live OPV is excreted in the stool for up to 1 month after vaccination, vaccine-induced polio is a risk to both the nonimmune child and any immunosuppressed contact.

Haemophilus Influenzae Type B Vaccine

1. Incidence of invasive disease caused by Hib has declined dramatically since the introduction of the conjugate vaccine.

2. Several different types of Hib vaccines are available. Different vaccines have different schedules.

3. Minimal adverse reactions (pain, redness, or swelling at immunization site for less than 24 hours).

Hepatitis B Vaccine

1. There are two schedules for this vaccine. Infants born to hepatitis B surface antigen (HBsAg)–negative mothers should receive the routine schedule. Infants born to HBsAg-positive mothers should be on an accelerated vaccination schedule

2. Recommended for all infants born to HBsAg-negative mothers. Three-dose schedule is initiated in neonatal period or by age 2 months; the second dose is given 1 to 2 months later; the third dose, 6 to 18 months later.

3. All infants born to HBsAg-positive mothers, including premature neonates, should receive hepatitis B immunoglobulin and HBV within 12 hours after birth. The second dose is given between ages 1 and 2 months; the third dose at age 6 months.

4. Preterm neonates weighing less than 2,000 g may have lower seroconversion rates. Initiation of HBV should be delayed until just before hospital discharge if the infant weighs 2,000 g or more or until about age 2 months when other routine immunizations are given.

5. All children and adolescents who have not had HBV should be immunized.

6. Administered I.M.

Pneumococcal Vaccines

1. There are two types of pneumococcal vaccines:
   a. PCV7/Prevnar (must be administered I.M.).
   b. 23-valent PPV/Pneumovax (may be given I.M. or subcutaneously).

2. Since 2000, the pneumococcal has been included in the recommended childhood vaccines for all children ages 2 to 23 months and for certain children ages 2 to 5 years.

3. Efficacy for the vaccine is 97% and the adverse effects are mild (fever and localized tenderness and redness at the injection site).

4. PPV is recommended for children ages 2 to 5 years in certain high-risk groups (sickle cell disease, functional or anatomic asplenia, nephrotic syndrome, chronic renal failure, immunosuppressive disorders, HIV infection, and cerebrospinal fluid leak).

Influenza Vaccine

1. The influenza vaccine known as TIV or LAIV contains three virus strains and is changed yearly, based on predictions of predominate strains expected to circulate in the upcoming influenza season. LAIV was approved for use in those ages 2 through 49 years in the United States in 2003 and is administered intranasally. TIV is available in both pediatric and adult formulations and is administered I.M.

2. The influenza vaccine should be given annually to children ages 6 months through 18 years. The "Recommended Immunization Schedule" provides more specifics.

3. This vaccine is given annually, before flu season, usually in October, November, or December.

4. In children ages 8 years and younger, the first time influenza vaccine is administered, two doses should be given 1 month apart. In subsequent years, only one dose is needed.

5. TIV should be used for children with asthma, children 2 to 4 years who had wheezing in the past 12 months, or children who have any other underlying medical contraindications to the LAIV.

Rotavirus Vaccine

1. In 2006, a live, oral vaccine—Rotateq—was licensed. In the United States, routine vaccination of infants—with three doses of rotavirus vaccine administered at 2, 4, and 6 months—is recommended.

Varicella Virus Vaccine

1. Varicella virus vaccine contains live, attenuated virus; approved for children 12 months and older and for adults.
2. Administered subcutaneously at 12 to 15 months; second dose at 4 to 6 years (or at least 3 months after first dose).
3. May be given to older children and adults who do not have immunity. In those older than age 13, the second dose may be delayed only 4 weeks following first dose.

 NURSING ALERT Millions of children travel overseas every year, risking exposure to infectious diseases not covered by routine immunizations. Refer families to their local public health department or retail travel clinic for special immunizations and malaria prophylaxis.

Nutrition in Children

The nutritional status of the child is an important aspect of health maintenance. A balanced diet influences child growth and psychosocial development. Feeding provides emotional and psychological benefits in addition to nutritional needs. In the United States, obesity in childhood has become a major problem and in developing countries, undernutrition—due to scarcity of nutrient-rich foods—leads to malnutrition and illness. In addition, anorexia, bulimia, and other dietary restrictions may place children and adolescents at risk for serious health consequences. Good eating habits, nutrient-rich foods, and physical activity introduced early in life can help foster good nutrition practices into adulthood. Nurses can be instrumental in providing factual information to both parents and children on typical nutritional needs and those required for specific sport participation. Table 42-1 presents nutritional guidelines based on age and developmental maturation.

Breastfeeding

1. Breastfeeding is the natural and ideal nourishment that will supply an infant with adequate nutrition as well as immunologic and anti-infection properties. With breast milk being at the proper temperature, it may prevent other GI disturbances as well. The development of allergies is reduced in breastfed babies.
2. Breastfeeding is recommended solely for infants to 6 months of age. As the infant grows and develops, the breast milk properties change in respect to amounts of fat, carbohydrates, and protein as well as physical properties such as pH needed for the respective age of the infant.

 Evidence Base American Academy of Pediatrics. (2012). Breastfeeding and the use of human milk. *Pediatrics, 129*(3), e827–e841.

3. Breastfeeding provides psychological and emotional satisfaction for the infant and mother and can promote bonding.

The physical closeness may also provide comfort after a frightening or painful procedure.

4. Breastfeeding can be continued through most illnesses and hospitalizations of the infant. In times of stress, the infant may cope with breastfeeding better than bottle-feeding. Because breast milk is more easily and quickly digested, shorter periods without food preoperatively and postoperatively may be necessary. Attempts should be made to maintain the breastfeeding bond and routines of the child and mother.
   a. Supplemental artificial formula can be given to the infant if the mother is not available.
   b. The mother can pump her breasts so that milk can be given to the infant by way of bottle when she is not available.
   c. Breast milk can be frozen for up to 6 months (check the facility's specific policy).
   d. Thaw frozen breast milk for use in tepid water. Do not use a microwave, which may destroy vitamins and nutritional properties as well as result in extreme overheating of portions of the breast milk.
5. Stress of new motherhood or illness in the infant or mother may decrease the mother's milk supply and inhibit her "let-down" reflex, as well as increase or decrease the infant's desire to suckle. Pumping may be initiated to help stimulate the mother's milk supply. An electronic pump may be necessary if prolonged pumping is expected or if manual pumping is not successful.
6. Education and encouragement should be offered to all new mothers and those having difficulty or concerns about breastfeeding (see Patient Education Guidelines 42-1, page 1420).

Bottle-Feeding

1. Bottle-feeding is a method of supplying nutrition to the infant by oral feedings, using a bottle and nipple setup.
2. Bottle-feeding can supplement breastfeeding with formula or water, or can be the sole means of nutritional intake for the infant.
3. Bottle-feeding can also provide intermittent feedings of expressed breast milk when the mother cannot be present at the time of the feeding.
4. Bottle-feeding can be a time of bonding between the mother and infant. The father or other capable members of the family should be taught bottle-feeding technique as well (see Procedure Guidelines 42-1, pages 1421 and 1422).
5. Some mothers may have chosen bottle-feeding for a variety of reasons, ranging from poor milk production, discomfort (psychological or physical) with breastfeeding, or drug treatment not compatible with breastfeeding. It is important that health care providers offer mothers information on all methods but not be judgmental when the mother choses one method over another.

Safety

Safety is an important aspect of child health and well-being. Injuries are the leading cause of death for children in the United States. Additionally, injury is a significant cause of childhood morbidity. Although childhood deaths from other causes have decreased, deaths from injuries remain constant.

(Text continues on page 1420)

Table 42-1   Nutrition in Children

AGE AND DEVELOPMENTAL INFLUENCE ON NUTRITIONAL REQUIREMENTS AND FEEDING PATTERNS	FEEDING PATTERN AND DIET	NURSING CONSIDERATIONS AND PARENTAL GUIDANCE

Neonate
 	
Birth–4 weeks
• Neonate's rapid growth makes infant especially vulnerable to dietary inadequacies, dehydration, and iron-deficiency anemia.
• Feeding process is basis for infant's first human relationship, formation of trust. Feeding reinforces mother's sense of "motherliness."
• Neonates require more fluid relative to their size than adults.
• Sucking ability is influenced by individual neuromuscular maturity.
 	
Infant
 	
1–3 months
• Infants consume more formula or breast milk with each feeding and sleep for longer periods.
• Infants have increased interaction during feeding due to cooing and development of a social milestone.
• Bowel movements become less frequent. Breast-fed infants may not have a bowel movement after each feeding.
	• Breast milk or formula is generally given in 6–8 feedings per day, spaced 2–4 hours apart.
	• Feeding schedules should be individualized according to infant's needs.
	• Breast-fed infant up to 6 months will not need supplemental vitamins or minerals.
	• Bottle-fed infant may benefit from supplements.
		• Provide information to help parents make decision concerning breast- or bottle-feeding.
		• Support parents in their decision.
		
		Breast-fed infant:
		• Help mother assume comfortable and satisfying position for self and baby.
		• Help mother to determine schedule, timing, and when infant is satisfied.
		• Provide specific information about:
		  • Feeding technique: position, "bubbling."
		  • Care of breasts.
		  • Manual expression of milk from breast.
		  • Maternal diet.
		
		Bottle-fed infant:
		• Provide specific information about:
		  • Type of formula.
		  • Preparation of formula: measuring and sterilization.
		  • Equipment—types of bottles and nipples.
		  • Sterilization of equipment.
		  • Technique of feeding: position, "bubbling."
		• Help mother to determine when infant is satisfied; develop schedule for feeding.
		• Provide information about normal characteristics of stools, signs of dehydration, constipation, colic, milk allergy.
		• Discuss need for prescribed supplements and how to administer (by dropper).
		• Discuss need for additional fluids during periods of hot weather and with fever, diarrhea, and vomiting.
		• Observe for evidence of common problems and intervene accordingly:
		  • Overfeeding.
		  • Underfeeding.
		  • Difficulty digesting formula because of its composition.
		  • Improper feeding technique; holes in nipples too large or too small; formula too hot or too cold; uncomfortable feeding position; failure to "bubble"; improper sterilization; bottle propping.
		  • Bottles should never be given to infants to take to bed.

Infant **3 months–1 year overview** • Increased neuromuscular development allows infant to make transition from a totally liquid diet to a diet of milk and solid foods as well as to more active participation in the feeding process. **3–6 months** • Sucking reflex becomes voluntary and chewing action begins; infant can approximate lips to rim and cup and may begin drinking from cup at 6 months.	• Number of feedings per day decreases through the first year. • By ages 4–6 months, generally ready to begin strained foods. The usual sequence of foods is cereal followed by fruits and vegetables. Meats may be started between 8 and 9 months. Sequence may vary according to preferences of the family and health care provider.	• The person feeding should be calm, gentle, relaxed, and patient in approach. • When first offered puréed foods with a spoon, the child expects and wants to suck. The protrusion of the tongue, which is needed in sucking, makes it appear as if the child is pushing the food out of the mouth. This response should not be interpreted as dislike for the food; it is a result of immature muscle coordination and surprise at the taste and feel of the new food. • The baby foods selected should be high in nutrients without providing excessive calories. Personal and cultural preferences should be considered. Iron-fortified formulas and cereals are needed to prevent physiologic anemia. • New foods should be offered one at a time and early in the feeding while the infant is still hungry. Allow 3–5 days between new foods.

Table 42-1   Nutrition in Children (*continued*)

AGE AND DEVELOPMENTAL INFLUENCE ON NUTRITIONAL REQUIREMENTS AND FEEDING PATTERNS	FEEDING PATTERN AND DIET	NURSING CONSIDERATIONS AND PARENTAL GUIDANCE
Infant (*continued*)		

6–12 months
• Loses maternal iron stores at 6 months; first tooth erupts between ages 6 and 9 months; eyes and hands can work together; infant can sit without support and has developed grasp; can feed self a biscuit; bangs objects on table; able to hold own bottle between ages 9 and 12 months; can "pincer" grasp food; able to be weaned from bottle as child becomes developmentally able to take sufficient fluids from the cup.
• Food provides the infant with a variety of learning experiences; motor control and coordination in self-feeding; recognition of shape, texture, color; stimulation of speech movement through use of mouth muscles.
• Mealtime allows the infant to continue development of trust in a consistent, loving atmosphere. The infant is forming lifetime eating habits; it is therefore important to make mealtime a positive experience.
	• Mashed table foods or junior foods are generally started between ages 6 and 8 months, when infant begins chewing action.
	• Infant begins to enjoy finger foods between ages 10 and 12 months.
	• The transition from iron-fortified formula or breast milk to cow's milk is usually advised at about age 12 months.
	• By age 1 year, most infants are satisfied with three meals and additional fluids throughout the day.
		• Infants should be observed for allergic reactions when new foods are added. Common allergies are to citrus juices, egg whites, cow's milk, and peanut butter. These foods should be avoided until age 12 months. Also avoid honey until age 12 months due to the risk of infantile botulism.
		• Finger foods should be selected for their nutritional value. Good choices include teething biscuits, cooked vegetables, bananas, cheese sticks, and enriched cereals. Avoid nuts, raisins, and raw vegetables, which can cause choking.
		• Parents can be taught to prepare their own strained or junior foods using a commercial baby food grinder or blender.
		• Weaning is a gradual process.
		  • Assist parents to recognize indications of readiness.
		  • Do not expect the infant to completely drop old pattern of behavior while learning a new one; allow overlap of old and new techniques.
		  • Evening feedings are usually the most difficult to eliminate because the infant is tired and in need of sucking comfort.
		  • During illness or household disorganization, the infant may regress and return to sucking to relieve his or her discomfort and frustration.

		 **NURSING ALERT** Obtain a thorough nursing history for the hospitalized infant that includes feeding pattern and schedule; types of foods that have been introduced; likes and dislikes; breast- or bottle-fed; type of bottle; temperature at which infant prefers foods and fluids.

Toddler		

1–3 years
• Growth slows at the end of the first year. The slower growth rate is reflected in a decreased appetite.
• The toddler has a total of 14–16 teeth, making him or her more able to chew foods.
• Increased self-awareness causes the toddler to want to do more for self. Refusal of food or of assistance in feedings are common ways in which the toddler asserts him- or herself.
• Because body tissues, especially muscles, continue to grow quite rapidly, protein needs are high.
	• Transition from a bottle to a cup at age 1 is recommended to prevent tooth decay.
	• Appetite is sporadic; specific foods may be favored exclusively or refused from time to time.
	• Child may be ritualistic concerning food preferences, schedule, and manner of eating.
	• Diet should include a full range of foods: milk, meat, fruits, vegetables, breads, and cereals. Iron-fortified dry cereals (rice, barley) are an excellent source of iron during the second year of life.
		• Provide foods with a variety of colors, textures, and flavors. Toddlers need to experience the feel of foods.
		• Offer small portions. It is fun for the child to ask for more. It is more effective to give small helpings than to insist that he or she eat a specific amount.
		• Maintain a regular mealtime schedule.
		• Provide appropriate mealtime equipment:
		  • Silverware scaled to size.
		  • Dishes—colorful, unbreakable; shallow, round bowls are preferable to flat plates.
		  • Plastic bibs, placemats, and floor coverings permit a relaxed attitude toward child's self-feeding attempts.
		  • Comfortable seating at good height and distance from table.
		• Adults who help toddlers at mealtime should be calm and relaxed. Avoid bribes or force-feeding because this reinforces negative behavior and may lead to a dislike for mealtime. Encourage independence, but provide assistance when necessary. Do not be concerned about table manners.
		• Avoid the use of soda or "sweets" as rewards or between-meal snacks. Instead, substitute fruit, juice, or cereal.

(continued)

Table 42-1   Nutrition in Children (continued)

AGE AND DEVELOPMENTAL INFLUENCE ON NUTRITIONAL REQUIREMENTS AND FEEDING PATTERNS	FEEDING PATTERN AND DIET	NURSING CONSIDERATIONS AND PARENTAL GUIDANCE
Toddler *(continued)*	• Older toddler can be expected to consume about one half the amount of food than an adult consumes. • Whole milk is recommended up to age 2 years.	• Toddlers who show little interest in eggs, meat, or vegetables should not be permitted to appease their appetite with carbohydrates or milk because this may lead to iron-deficiency anemia. Milk should be limited to approximately 16 ounces/day. **NURSING ALERT** Nursing history for the hospitalized toddler should include feeding pattern and schedule; food likes and dislikes; food allergies; special eating equipment and utensils; whether child is weaned; what child is fed when ill.

Preschooler
3–5 years
• Increased manual dexterity enables child to have complete independence at mealtime.
• Psychosocially, this is a period of increased imitation and sex identification. The preschooler identifies with parents at the table and will enjoy what parents enjoy.
• Additional nutritional habits are developed that become part of the child's lifetime practices.
• Slower growth rate and increased interest in exploring his or her environment may decrease the preschooler's interest in eating.
• Eating assumes increasing social significance. Mealtime promotes socialization and provides the preschooler with opportunities to learn appropriate mealtime behavior, language skills, and understanding of family rituals.

 **NURSING ALERT** Consider cultural differences. Allow parents to bring in favorite foods or eating utensils from home for the hospitalized preschooler. Encourage family members to be present at mealtime.
	• Appetite tends to be sporadic.
	• Child requires the same basic four food groups as the adult, but in smaller quantities.
	• Generally likes to eat one food from plate at a time.
	• Likes vegetables that are crisp, raw, and cut into finger-sized pieces. Often dislikes strong-tasting foods.
		• Emphasis should be placed on the quality rather than the amount of food ingested.
		• Foods should be attractively served, mildly flavored, plain, as well as being separated and distinctly identifiable in flavor and appearance.
		• Nutritional foods (eg, crackers and cheese, yogurt, fruit) should be offered as snacks.
		• Desserts should be nutritious and a natural part of the meal, not used as a reward for finishing the meal or omitted as punishment.
		• Unless they persist, periods of overeating or not wanting to eat certain foods should not cause concern. The overall eating pattern from month to month is more pertinent to assess.
		• Frequent causes of insufficient eating:
		  • Unhappy atmosphere at mealtime.
		  • Overeating between meals.
		  • Parental example.
		  • Attention-seeking.
		  • Excessive parental expectations.
		  • Inadequate variety or quantity of foods.
		  • Tooth decay.
		  • Physical illness.
		  • Fatigue.
		  • Emotional disturbance.
		• Measures to increase food intake:
		  • Allow child to help with preparations, planning menu, setting table, and other simple chores.
		  • Maintain calm environment with no distractions.
		  • Avoid between-meal snacks.
		  • Provide rest period before meal.
		  • Avoid coaxing, bribing, threatening.
		• Place children in small groups, preferably at tables during mealtime. Use nursing history to determine likes and provide simple foods in small portions. Peanut butter and jelly sandwiches are often favorites. Allow and encourage children to feed themselves. Do not punish children who refuse to eat. Offer alternative foods.

Table 42-1 Nutrition in Children *(continued)*

AGE AND DEVELOPMENTAL INFLUENCE ON NUTRITIONAL REQUIREMENTS AND FEEDING PATTERNS	FEEDING PATTERN AND DIET	NURSING CONSIDERATIONS AND PARENTAL GUIDANCE
School-age Child • Slowed growth rate during middle childhood results in gradual decline in food requirements per unit of body weight. • The preadolescent growth spurt occurs about age 10 in girls and about age 12 in boys. At this time, energy needs increase and approach those of the adult. Intake is particularly important because reserves are laid down for the demands of adolescence. • The child becomes dependent on peers for approval and makes food choices accordingly. • The child experiences increased socialization and independence through opportunities to eat away from home (eg, at school and homes of peers).	• By this time, food practices are generally well established, a product of the eating experiences of the toddler and preschool period. • Many children are too busy with other affairs to take time out to eat. Play readily takes priority unless a firm understanding is reached and mealtime is relaxed and enjoyable.	• Nutrition education should help the child to select foods wisely and to begin to plan and prepare meals. • Parental attitudes continue to be important as the child copies parental behavior (eg, skipping breakfast, not eating certain foods, consuming fast foods frequently). • Most children require a nutritious breakfast to avoid lassitude in late morning. • Mealtime should continue to be relaxed and enjoyable. Diversions, such as television, should be avoided. • Calcium and vitamin D intake warrant special consideration. They must be adequate to support the rapid enlargement of bones. • Parents and health care professionals should be alert to signs of developing obesity. Intake should be altered accordingly. • Table manners should not be overemphasized. The young child typically stuffs mouth, spills food, and chatters incessantly while eating. Time and experience will improve habits. • Provide some companionship and conversation at the child's level during meals. Peers should be invited occasionally for meals. **NURSING ALERT** Nursing history of the hospitalized child should include food preferences; mealtime patterns and snacks; food allergies; food preferences when ill. Provide opportunities for children to eat in small groups at tables. Consider cultural differences. Allow parents to bring in favorite foods from home. Allow child to order his or her own meal.

Adolescent
 	
11–17 years
• Dietary requirements vary according to stage of sexual maturation, rate of physical growth, and extent of athletic and social activity.
• When rapid growth of puberty appears, there is a corresponding increase in energy requirements and appetite.
• Menstruating teen is particularly susceptible to iron-deficiency anemia.
	• Previously learned dietary patterns are difficult to change.
	• Food choices and eating habits may be quite unusual and are related to the adolescent's psychological and social milieu.
	• Generally, a significant percentage of the daily caloric intake of the adolescent comes from snacking.
		• Continue nutrition education, with emphasis on:
		  • Selecting nutritious foods high in iron.
		  • Nutritional needs related to growth.
		  • Preparing favorite "adolescent foods."
		  • Foods and physical fitness.
		• Informal sessions are generally more effective than lectures on nutrition.
		• Special problems requiring intervention:
		  • Obesity.
		  • Excessive dieting.
		  • Extreme fads—eccentric and grossly restricted diets.
		  • Anorexia nervosa and bulimia.
		  • Adolescent pregnancy.
		  • Iron-deficiency anemia.
		• Provide nutritious foods relevant to the adolescent's lifestyle.
		• Discourage cigarette smoking, which may contribute to poor nutritional status by decreasing appetite and increasing the body's metabolic rate.
		
		 NURSING ALERT Allow hospitalized adolescent to choose own foods, especially if on a special diet. Provide a refrigerator in the recreation room for snacks or utilize a snack cart. Serve foods that appeal to adolescents. Use a nursing history similar to that for the school-age child.

PATIENT EDUCATION GUIDELINES 42-1

Breastfeeding

Breastfeeding is the best possible source of nutrition for your infant. It provides an immunologic boost for the infant, protects against breast cancer, hastens postpartum healing, and serves as a wonderful bond between the infant and mother.

1. You should begin breastfeeding in a quiet, comfortable place that is free from interruption. You may need a pillow to help support the infant and a footstool to use to elevate your leg.

2. Make sure the infant is awake and dry before the feeding is started. If awake and comfortable, the infant will settle down and feed better. The infant should also be hungry.

3. Dress the infant appropriately so that the infant is not too warm or too cool during the feeding. If too warm, the infant may fall asleep after the first few sucks of milk. A sleepy infant will not nurse well. If too cool, the infant may be fussy and restless.

4. Position infant at the breast by placing the infant in a semi-sitting position with face close to the breast and supported by one of your arms and hand. A pillow may be used under the infant for support. You may need to support your breast with your other hand. Proper positioning will provide the infant with comfort and security and make it easier for the infant to suck and swallow. This makes the nipple more easily accessible to the infant's mouth and prevents obstruction of nasal breathing.

5. When the feeding is to start, let the breast touch the infant's cheek. Do not hold the cheek, but try to help the infant find the nipple. The rooting reflex will take over and the infant will turn head toward breast with mouth open. If you touch the cheek, the infant will become confused, perhaps turning toward your hand.

6. The infant's lips should be out over the areola and not just around the nipple before beginning to suck. Because the nipple is so small, suction cannot be achieved merely by grasping it. The areola must be in the infant's mouth to establish suction and make the suck effective.

7. You may notice the "let-down" reflex during the nursing period. Milk flowing from the other breast during nursing is quite normal.

8. The length of feeding time may vary from 5 to 30 minutes. Let the infant nurse until satisfied. When the infant is satisfied and has nursed well, the infant is relaxed and usually falls asleep. The infant will stop sucking.

9. Burp the infant during and at the end of the feeding to prevent abdominal distention or regurgitation from air swallowed during the feeding.

10. One or both breasts may be used at each feeding. It makes no difference as long as the infant is satisfied at the end of the feeding and one breast is completely emptied at the feeding. If both breasts were used, the second breast is not usually emptied and should be used first at the next feeding. Regular and complete emptying of the breast is the only stimulation for the production of milk.

11. When the infant has stopped sucking, the infant typically likes to cling to the breast. To break this suction, insert a finger to the corner of the infant's mouth and gently pull.

12. When the infant has finished feeding, change the diaper if it is wet or soiled. Position the infant on the right side in bed. Note whether the infant appears satisfied or still seems to be hungry.

13. To continue successful breastfeeding, get adequate rest and nutrition.

14. For information and support, contact La Leche League International, 957 N. Plum Grove Rd., Schaumburg, IL 60173, (800) 525-3243, *www: illi.org*; or read their publication *The Womanly Art of Breast-feeding* (8th ed.).

Role of the Nurse

1. Identify environmental hazards and act to reduce or eliminate them.

2. Identify behavioral characteristics of individual children that may be related to accidental liability and caution parents accordingly. Pay particular attention to children who show the following:
   a. Characteristics that increase exposure to hazards, such as excessive curiosity, inability to delay gratification, hyperactivity, and daringness.
   b. Characteristics that reduce the child's ability to cope with hazards, such as aggressiveness, stubbornness, poor concentration, low frustration threshold, and lack of self-control.

3. Provide anticipatory guidance about child development as it relates to accidents. Direct preventive teaching toward the intended audience, be it individuals or groups, children or adults.

4. Participate in policy-setting for accident prevention with great emphasis on effective public health measures.

Principles of Safety

1. The type of accident likely to occur is influenced by the child's age and developmental level. Parents who have knowledge of their own child's typical behavior patterns may foresee potential accident situations.

2. Children are naturally curious, impulsive, and impatient. The young child needs to touch, feel, and investigate. Consistent adult supervision will enable children to learn in a safe environment.

3. Children copy the behavior of their parents and absorb parental attitudes. Parents and other adults should be a role model for using proper and safe methods.

PROCEDURE GUIDELINES 42-1

Bottle Feeding

EQUIPMENT
- Sterile nipple and bottle (can be washed in dishwasher or in hot soapy water and rinsed well)
- Formula or breast milk (prepared according to manufacturer's directions)

PROCEDURE

Nursing Action	Rationale
Preparatory phase	
1. Infant should be awake and hungry. Change wet or soiled diaper.	1. A sleepy infant will not feed well. A dry diaper will provide comfort so that the infant will settle down and feed more easily.
2. If using new bottle and nipple, boil for 5 minutes immersed in a covered pan. Remove bottle and nipple and place upside down on a clean towel to cool and dry. Commercial sterilizers may also be used.	2. Prevent possible contamination by bacteria or other particles.
3. Check formula for proper type and amount. Prepare according to manufacturer instructions.	3.
a. For babies up to 6 months, mix concentrated or powdered formula with water that has been boiled (unless commercially prepared water is marked as sterile).	a. Boiling water kills bacteria in the event of contaminated water supply.
b. If using tap water, run the faucet for 2 minutes to flush out any lead or other impurities before boiling.	b. Running the tap removes impurities that standing water may pick up from the plumbing.
c. Boil water vigorously for 1–2 minutes, let cool, and add to formula.	
4. Use cold formula, if tolerated, but some infants prefer warmed formula.	4. Infants may prefer cold formula if started on it from the beginning.
a. Warm bottle by holding it under very warm running water for a few minutes or putting the bottle in a pan of warm water (away from the heat source). Commercial bottle warmers may be used. Shake bottle vigorously after warming.	a. Overheating must be avoided to prevent burns to the infant's sensitive mouth. Shaking will distribute fluid temperature evenly.
b. Test formula temperature by squirting some on your inner wrist before feeding.	b. The inside of the wrist is more sensitive to test temperature than other areas of the skin.
5. Sit in a comfortable chair. Cradle the infant with one hand and arm, while supporting the infant against your body or lap.	5. Proper position will provide the infant with comfort and security and will make it easier to suck and swallow. Holding the infant will enhance bonding and provide sensory stimulation.
Performance phase	
1. Let the infant root for the nipple by touching the corner of the infant's mouth with the nipple.	1.
a. When the infant's mouth opens, insert the nipple.	a. Rooting is a natural reflex.
b. Position the nipple on top of the tongue and far enough into the mouth so suction can be created.	b. Suction will be created when the infant sucks if the nipple is positioned properly in the mouth.
2. Hold the bottle at an angle to completely fill the nipple with fluid.	2. Prevents the infant from sucking and swallowing excessive air.
3. Never prop the bottle or leave the infant unattended during feeding.	3. This is unsafe. Should vomiting occur, aspiration is more likely.
4. Handle the bottle carefully so as not to contaminate the nipple or fluid.	4. Contamination will increase the risk of GI disturbances.
5. Feed until the infant stops sucking; varies from 10 to 25 minutes.	5. Feeding time is individual, based on age, size, how vigorously the infant sucks.

(continued)

PROCEDURE GUIDELINES 42-1 *(continued)*

Bottle Feeding

PROCEDURE *(continued)*

Nursing Action	Rationale
6. Burp the infant after every 2–3 ounces during the feeding and at the end of the feeding. a. Place the infant in a sitting position in your lap, tilt slightly forward, and gently rub or pat the back. b. Place the infant in a prone position on your shoulder or in your lap and gently pat or rub the back.	6. Most infants swallow some air with feeding. These positions aid in expelling air and thus prevent abdominal distention, discomfort, and regurgitation. Vigorous handling or patting may result in the infant spitting up or regurgitating fluid.

Follow-up phase

Nursing Action	Rationale
1. After final burping, keep the infant in an upright position for 10–15 minutes (longer if the infant has reflux). If restless, burp the infant. Note if any spitting up occurs.	1. Prevents regurgitation, but it is not abnormal to bring up small amounts of formula.
2. Throw away any leftover formula in the bottle after the feeding. a. Discard any formula that has been left out unrefrigerated for 2 hours. b. Refrigerate extra bottles after mixing formula; discard if not used in 24 hours. c. Do not reuse the bottle for a subsequent feeding (refill and reuse) without properly cleaning.	2. Avoids bacterial contamination.

 NURSING ALERT When feeding a premature infant, the infant will tire more easily and fall asleep. Allow frequent rest periods and use a soft nipple so that less energy is needed to suck. To stimulate the premature infant to suck, the nurse can brush the infant's cheek with her or his finger, place the thumb or finger under the infant's chin, or move the nipple slowly back and forth in the infant's mouth. Feeding time should not exceed 30 minutes. Keep the infant warm during feeding.

 Evidence Base Infant Nutrition Council. (2013). *Safe Preparation, Storage and Handling of Powdered Infant Formulas*. Available: *http://infantnutritioncouncil.com/safe-prep-and-handling/.*

---

4. Children become less careful and less willing to listen to warnings and to observe routine safety precautions when they are tired or hungry.
5. An estimated 90% of all accidents are preventable.

General Areas of Adult Responsibility for Child Safety

Motor Vehicle

 Evidence Base American Academy of Pediatrics. (2012). *Car safety seats: A guide for families.* Available: *www.healthychildren.org/English/safety-prevention/on-the-go/Pages/Car-Safety-Seats-Information-for-Families.aspx.*

1. Automobiles should be in good mechanical condition.
2. Use properly fitted and installed car seats and seat belts. Be aware of the guidelines for restraints based on the child's age, weight, and height.
   a. Rear-facing car seat until age 2, or if child has outgrown the manufacturer's recommendation for maximum height and weight.
   b. Front-facing car seat from age 2 until the child has outgrown the manufacturer's recommendation for maximum height and weight.
   c. Belt-positioning booster seat until the vehicle seat belt fits properly, typically when the child has reached 4 feet, 9 inches in height, between 8 and 12 years of age.
3. All children younger than 13 years should be restrained in the rear seats of vehicles (when the vehicle has a rear seat with lap

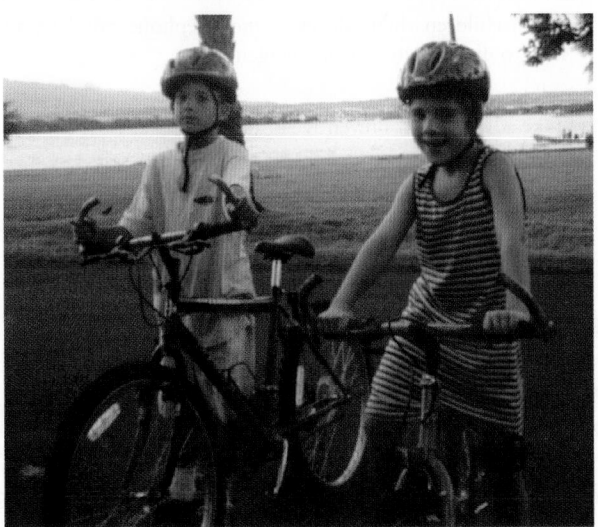

Figure 42-1. Use of bike helmets by all children for safety.

and shoulder belts) for optimal protection. The center rear seat is the safest seat for a child.

4. The driver should look carefully in front and back of the car before getting into the car.
5. Lock all car doors.
6. Never leave young children in a car alone.
7. Do not place heavy or sharp objects on the same seat with a child.

Sports and Recreation

1. Keep equipment in good condition and proper working order.
2. Ensure that children are aware of the correct use of sports equipment.
3. Encourage the routine use of bike helmets (see Figure 42-1).
4. Wear appropriate clothing and safety equipment for the activity (see Figure 42-2).

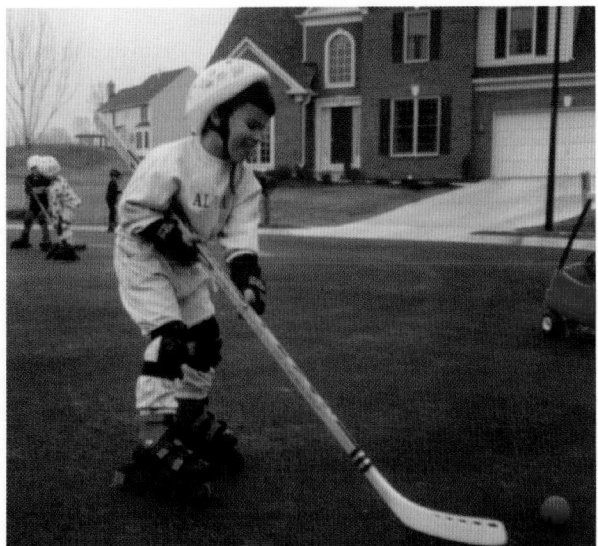

Figure 42-2. Use of appropriate pads and helmets for safety.

5. Do not attempt activities beyond one's physical endurance.
6. Keep firearms and ammunition locked up.

Electrical and Mechanical Equipment

1. Only underwriter-approved devices should be installed; they should be inspected periodically.
2. Dry hands before touching appliances. Keep radios, transportable heaters, and hair dryers out of the bathroom.
3. Disconnect appliances after each use and before attempting minor repairs.
4. Keep garden equipment and machinery in a restricted area. Teach proper use of the equipment as soon as the child is old enough.
5. Avoid overloading electrical circuits.
6. Discourage children from playing with or being in area where appliances or power tools (eg, washing machine, clothes dryer, saw, lawnmower) are in operation.

Prevention of Falls

1. Keep stairs well lighted and free from clutter.
2. Use gates at tops and bottoms of stairways where toddlers have access.
3. Provide sturdy railings.
4. Anchor small rugs securely.
5. Use rubber mats in the bathtub and shower.
6. Use only sturdy ladders for climbing.
7. The American Academy of Pediatrics and the National Association of Children's Hospitals and Related Institutions have recommended that baby walkers be banned as most injuries using these walkers will occur even when adults are present (rolling down stairs, burns, drowning, reaching unsafe objects due to greater stability provided by walkers).

Poisonings and Ingestions

1. Do not mix bleaches with ammonia, vinegar, and other household cleaners.
2. See section on ingested poisons and pediatric poisoning (see page 1428).
3. Become familiar with the telephone number for poison control centers where available.
4. Label poisonous household materials and keep them out of child's reach.
5. Post local poison control phone number in easily accessible location (eg, refrigerator door).

Fire

1. Maintain an adequate fire escape plan and routinely conduct home fire drills. Teach children escape routes as soon as they are old enough.
2. Keep a pressure-type, handheld fire extinguisher on each floor. Regularly check expiration or necessary inspection dates. Consider additional units in areas where there are higher risk of fires (kitchen, laundry room, garage). Instruct all family members who are old enough in its use.
3. Fit fireplaces with snug fireplace screens.
4. Store gasoline and other flammable fluids in tightly covered containers that are clearly labeled and away from heat and sparks.

5. Dispose of paint- and oil-soaked cloths promptly.
6. Use flame-retardant sleepwear.
7. Mark children's rooms so they are obvious to firefighters.
8. Teach children about the danger of smoke inhalation.
9. Teach children to stop, drop, and roll if their clothing catches fire.
10. Maintain smoke detectors in working order.
11. Keep lighters and matches out of the reach of children.
12. Keep children away from heated oven, stovetop, and outdoor grill.

Swimming Pools

1. Completely enclose pool with a fence that complies with local regulations. The gate should be self-closing and have a lock.
2. Indicate water depth with numbers on the edge of the pool. Place a safety float line where the bottom of the slope begins to deepen.
3. Install at least one ladder at each end of the pool. Ladders should have handrails on both sides and the diameter of the rails should be small enough for a child to grasp.
4. Use nonslip materials on ladders, deck, and diving boards.
5. If the pool is used at night, install underwater lighting as well as outdoor lights.
6. Install a ground fault circuit interrupter on the pool circuit to cut off electrical power and thus prevent electrocutions should electrical fault occur.
7. Instruct children about safety rules, such as not swimming alone, need for adult supervision, not running around the pool, and not pushing others. Avoid using radios or other electrical appliances around the pool.
8. Warn children not to attempt to walk on any remaining pool water after the season—frozen water or pool-covering equipment.
9. Keep essential rescue devices and first-aid equipment close to the pool.

Emergency Precautions

1. Record emergency telephone numbers in an obvious and easily accessible place.
2. Keep a well-stocked first-aid kit immediately available for emergencies. It is helpful to also carry a small first-aid kit in family vehicles.
3. Give instruction in principles of first aid to all family members who are old enough.
   a. Responsible adults should enroll in first-aid courses offered by the American Red Cross and adult education programs.
   b. Be aware of first-aid procedure for the following conditions: burns, electric shock, poisoning, bites and stings, wounds, near drowning, fractures, cardiopulmonary arrest.
   c. Teach children safety precautions concerning bicycles, answering the telephone or door, strangers outside the home, street safety.
4. Know the location of gas, water, and electrical switches and how to turn them off in an emergency.

5. Teach children their addresses and telephone numbers and how to dial 911 in case of emergency.

Miscellaneous

1. Take advantage of preventive health care.
   a. Obtain recommended immunizations.
   b. Have regular physical and dental examinations.
2. Seek immediate treatment of all diseases and health problems.
3. Balance periods of work, rest, and exercise in daily living.

PEDIATRIC CARE TECHNIQUES

Nursing Management of the Child with Fever

 Evidence Base van den Anker, J. (2013). Optimising the management of fever and pain in children. *International Journal of Clinical Practice, 67* (supplement 178), 26–32.

Fever is an abnormal elevation of body temperature. Prolonged elevation of temperature above 104° F (40° C) may produce dehydration and harmful effects on the central nervous system (CNS).

General Considerations

1. Consider basic principles related to temperature regulation in pediatric patients.
   a. Usually an infant's temperature does not stabilize before age 1 week. A neonate's temperature varies with the temperature of the environment.
   b. The degree of fever does not always reflect the severity of the disease. A child may have a serious illness with a normal or subnormal temperature.
   c. Febrile seizures may occur in some children when the temperature rises rapidly.
   d. The range for normal temperature varies widely in children. A common explanation for "fever" is misinterpretation of a normal temperature reading.
   e. A child's temperature is influenced by activity and by the time of day; temperatures are highest in late afternoon.
2. Temperature interpretation depends on accurate temperature measurement in a child. The mode should be appropriate for the child's age and condition and the thermometer should be left in place for the required time period. Parents or caregivers should be taught the appropriate assessment of temperature as the child grows.

Causes of Fever in Children

1. Infection.
2. Inflammatory disease.
3. Dehydration.
4. Tumors.
5. Disturbance of temperature-regulating center.
6. Extravasation of blood into the tissues.
7. Drugs or toxins.

Nursing Assessment

1. Assess history of present illness for source of fever.
   a. Age of the child.
   b. Pattern of the fever.
   c. Length of the illness.
   d. Change in normal patterns of eating, elimination, and recreation.
   e. Other symptoms—poor feeding, cough, earache, diarrhea, vomiting, and rash.
   f. Exposure to any illness.
   g. Recent immunizations or drugs.
   h. Treatment of fever and effectiveness of treatment.
   i. Previous experiences with fever and its control.
2. Assess the general appearance of the child.
3. Perform a systematic physical assessment.
   a. Inspection of the skin for rashes, sores, flushed appearance.
   b. Inspection of eyes, ears, nose, and throat for redness and drainage.
   c. Auscultation of lungs for abnormal sounds.
   d. Neurologic observation for changes in state of consciousness, pupillary reaction, strength of grip, abnormal muscle movement, or lack of movement.
   e. Inspection of external genitals for redness and drainage.
   f. Presence of abdominal or flank tenderness.
4. Assist with laboratory tests, as indicated. Initial tests typically include complete blood count; urinalysis; cultures of the throat, nasopharynx, urine, blood, and spinal fluid; and chest x-ray.
5. Attempt to identify the pattern of the fever. Take the child's temperature by the same method every hour until stable, then every 2 hours until normal, then every 4 hours for 24 hours.

Nursing Measures to Reduce Fever

Fever does not necessarily require treatment. The presence of fever should not be obscured by the indiscriminate use of antipyretic measures. However, if the child is uncomfortable or appears toxic because of fever, an attempt should be made to reduce it by any of the following nursing measures or by a combination of these measures:

1. Increase the child's fluid intake to prevent dehydration.
2. Expose the skin to the air by leaving the child lightly dressed in absorbent material. Avoid warm, binding clothing and blankets.
3. Administer antipyretic drugs, as prescribed. Avoid aspirin/acetyl salicylic acid as its use is known to result in Reye's syndrome (encephalopathy, fatty degeneration of the liver with associated hypoglycemia) in some children. Children ages 4 to 12 years with a viral illness are at greatest risk.
4. Use a tub bath or a hypothermia blanket. Do not allow the child to shiver, as that may increase the body temperature.

Administering Medications to Children

Administration of medication is usually traumatic for children. The proper approach to administration can facilitate the process and enhance the child's understanding of the importance of taking medications.

Important Considerations

1. The manner of approach should indicate that the nurse firmly expects the child to take the medication. This manner usually convinces the child of the necessity of the procedure.
2. Establishing a positive relationship with the child will allow expression of feelings, concerns, and fantasies regarding medications.
3. Explanation about medication should appeal to the child's level of understanding (ie, through play or comparison to something familiar).
4. The nurse must mask her or his own feelings regarding the medication.
5. Always be truthful when the child asks, "Does it taste bad?" or "Will it hurt?" Respond by saying, "The medication does not taste good, but I will give you some juice as soon as you swallow it," or "It will hurt for just a minute."
6. It is typically necessary to mix distasteful medications or crushed pills with a small amount of carbonated drink, cherry syrup, ice cream, or applesauce. After mixing, monitor to ensure that the child finishes the preparation.
7. Never threaten a child with an injection when refusing oral medication.
8. Do not mix medications with large quantities of food or with any food that is taken regularly (eg, milk).
9. Avoid giving medications to a child at mealtime unless specifically prescribed.
10. For each medication administered, the nurse should know the common use, safe dosage based on the child's weight, contraindications, adverse effects, and toxic effects.
11. The child must be accurately identified before medication is given.
12. When preparing I.M. injections, draw 0.2 cc of air into the syringe, in addition to the correct amount of medication. This clears the medication from the needle on injection and prevents backflow and the depositing of medication in subcutaneous fat when the needle is withdrawn.
13. Physical intervention (through swaddling, side or stomach position, shushing, swinging, sucking) and oral sucrose administration have been shown through research to reduce pain reactions in infants ages 2 months and 4 months during vaccine injections.

 Evidence Base Harrison, D., Beggs, S., & Stevens, B. (2012). Sucrose for Procedural Pain Management in Infants. *Pediatrics*, *130*(5), 918–925.
Harrington, J. W., Logan, S., Harwell, C., et al. (2012). Effective analgesia using physical interventions for infant immunizations. *Pediatrics*, *129*, 815–822.

Calculating the Pediatric Dosage

General Principles

1. The nurse is responsible for knowing the safe dosage range for the medication she administers.
2. Factors determining the amount of drug prescribed include:

a. Action, absorption, detoxification, and excretion of the drug are related to the maturity and metabolic rate of the child.

b. Neonates and premature neonates require a reduced dosage because of:

   i. Deficient or absent detoxifying enzymes.

   ii. Decreased effective renal function.

   iii. Altered blood–brain barrier and protein-binding capacity.

c. Dosage recommendations based on age-groups are not satisfactory because a child may be much smaller or larger than the average child in the age-group.

d. Dosages based on child's weight are more accurate; however, these calculations have limitations.

3. Be alert to a prescription that would be inappropriate for a child.

4. Consult drug literature for recommended dosage and other information.

Calculating by Body Surface Area

The following formulas are used to estimate the pediatric dosage based on the child's body surface area (BSA). BSA calculations are generally preferred because many physiologic processes in the child (eg, blood volume, glomerular filtration) are related to BSA.

1. Surface area in square meters × Dose per square meter = Approximate child dose.

2. Surface area of child/surface area of adult × Dose of adult = Approximate child dose.

3. Surface area of child in square meters/1.75 × Adult dose = Child dose.

Calculating by Clark's Rule

Clark's rule may be used as an estimate of the pediatric dosage based on the child's weight in respect to the adult dose of the drug:

Child's weight in pounds/150 × Adult dose = Approximate dose for child

 NURSING ALERT Ensure proper identification of all patients via the identification bracelet before administration of medication.

Oral Medications

Infants

1. Draw up medication in a plastic dropper or disposable syringe.

2. Elevate infant's head and shoulders; depress chin with thumb to open mouth.

3. Place dropper or syringe on the middle of the tongue and slowly drop the medication on the tongue.

4. Release thumb and allow the child to swallow.

5. When the correct amount of medication has been measured, it can be placed in a nipple and the infant can suck the medication through the nipple.

6. If the nurse feels comfortable managing the infant in her or his lap, it is acceptable to hold the infant for medication administration.

Toddlers

1. Draw up liquid medications in a syringe or measure into medicine cup. Medications may be placed in a medicine cup or spoon after being measured accurately in a syringe.

2. Elevate the child's head and shoulders.

3. Squeeze the cup and put it to the child's lips or place the syringe (without needle) in the child's mouth, positioning the syringe tip in the space between the cheek mucosa and gum, and slowly expel the medicine. Child may prefer using a familiar teaspoon.

4. Allow the child time to swallow.

5. Allow the child to hold the medicine cup if able and to drink it at his or her own pace. (This may be a more agreeable method.) Offer a favorite drink as a "chaser," if not contraindicated.

6. The small, safe medicine cups can be given to the child for play.

School-Age Children

1. When a child is old enough to take medicine in pill or capsule form, teach the child to place the pill near the back of the tongue and immediately swallow fluid such as water or fruit juice. If swallowing of the fluid is emphasized, the child will no longer think about the pill.

2. Always give praise after a child takes medication.

3. If the child finds it particularly difficult to take oral medications, express understanding and offer help.

Subcutaneous and Intramuscular Medications

General Considerations

1. After the medication to be given I.M. is drawn from the vial, draw up an additional 0.2 to 0.3 cc of air into the syringe, thus clearing the needle of medication and preventing medication seepage from the injection site.

2. When injecting less than 1 mL of medication, use a tuberculin syringe for accuracy.

3. Clean site thoroughly, using friction with an antiseptic solution; let site dry.

4. Establish anatomic landmarks and prepare to position the needle at a 45-degree angle for subcutaneous (S.C.) injection and a 90-degree angle for I.M. injection (see Figure 42-3). Alternate injection sites and keep record at bedside or on medication card.

5. With I.M. injections, after penetrating site, aspirate to check for blood vessel puncture. If this occurs, withdraw the needle, discard the medicine, and start again.

6. After injection, massage site (unless contraindicated). When multiple injections are being administered, such complications as fibrosis and contracture of the muscle can be diminished by massage, warm soaks, and range-of-motion exercises to disrupt and stretch immature scar tissue.

Infants

1. Acceptable sites for I.M. injections include the rectus femoris (anterior thigh, middle third), vastus lateralis (lateral thigh, middle third), or ventrogluteal, as these sites are relatively free from major nerves and blood vessels. The gluteus maximus and deltoid muscles are underdeveloped in the infant and use of these sites can result in nerve damage.

2. Rectus femoris injection.

   a. Place the child in a secure position to prevent movement of the extremity.

   b. Do not use a needle longer than 1 inch.

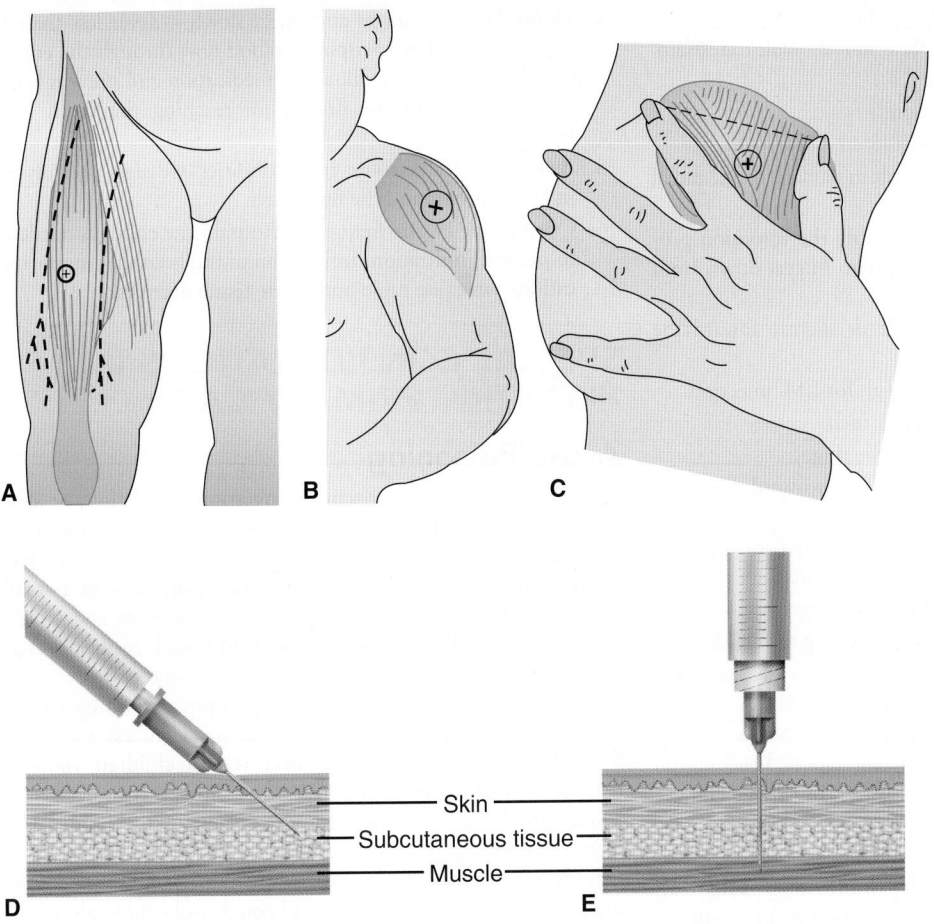

Skin

Subcutaneous tissue

Muscle

Figure 42-3. I.M. and subcutaneous injections in children. Sites for I.M. injections: (A) rectus femoris, **(B)** deltoid, **(C)** ventrogluteal. **(D)** Subcutaneous injection. **(E)** I.M. injection.

c. Bunch the muscle between your thumb and forefinger.

d. Insert needle at 90-degree angle or slightly toward the knee.

3. Vastus lateralis injection.

a. Place the child in a prone or supine position.

b. Area is a narrow strip of muscle extending along a line from the greater trochanter to lateral femoral condyle below.

c. Insert needle at 90-degree angle, ¾ to 1½ inches (2 to 4 cm) deep.

4. Ventrogluteal injection.

a. This site provides a dense muscle mass that is relatively free from the danger of injuring the nervous and vascular systems.

b. The disadvantage is that the injection site is visible to the child.

c. Administration.

i. Position the child supine.

ii. Place the index finger on the anterosuperior spine.

iii. With the middle finger moving dorsally, locate the iliac crest; drop finger below the crest. The triangle formed by the iliac crest, index finger, and middle finger is the injection site.

iv. Inject needle perpendicular to the surface on which the child is lying.

5. After administration of medication, hold and cuddle the infant.

6. Administer subcutaneous injection in the fatty tissue over the anterolateral thigh.

Toddlers and School-Age Children

1. Posterogluteal injection—upper outer quadrant for I.M. injection.

a. Gluteal muscles do not develop until a child begins to walk; they should be used only when the child has been walking for 1 year or more. Complications include sciatic nerve injury or subcutaneous injury (due to medication being injected) and poor absorption.

b. Upper outer quadrant of the young child's buttock is smaller in diameter than that of an adult; thus accuracy in determining the area comprising the upper outer quadrant is essential.

c. Administration.

i. Do not use a needle longer than 1 inch.

ii. Position the child in a prone position.

iii. Place thumb on the trochanter.

iv. Place middle finger on the iliac crest.

v. Let index finger drop at a point midway between the thumb and middle finger to the upper outer quadrant of the buttock. This is the injection site.

vi. Insert needle perpendicular to the surface on which the child is lying, not to the skin.

2. Ventrogluteal injection for I.M. injection.
   a. May be used for the older child who is difficult to restrain.
   b. See description given above.
3. Deltoid injection for I.M. injection.
   a. May be used for older, larger children.
   b. Inaccurate site injection can result in damage to the radial nerve or brachial artery.
   c. Determine injection site by palpating the acromion process of the shoulder and placing two fingers down from the acromion process.
   d. Inject needle at 90-degree angle or slightly toward the shoulder.
4. Lateral and anterior aspect of the thigh for I.M. injection.
   a. Do not use a needle longer than 1 inch.
   b. Use the upper outer quadrant of the thigh.
   c. Insert needle at 45-degree angle in a downward direction, toward the knee.
5. Administer subcutaneous injection in the fatty tissue over the anterolateral thigh or outer aspect of upper arm.
6. Nursing support of toddlers and older children.
   a. Prepare all equipment before approaching the child.
   b. Explain to the child where you are going to give the injection (site) and why you are giving it.
   c. Allow the child to express fears.
   d. Carry out the procedure quickly and gently. Have needle and syringe completely prepared and ready before contact with the child.
   e. Numb the site of injection by rubbing the skin firmly with cleaning swab or with ice (older children may assist with this). Minimize pain of an I.M. injection by injecting the needle into the muscle with a quick, darting motion.
   f. Always secure the assistance of a second nurse to help immobilize the child and divert his or her attention as well as to offer support and comfort.
   g. Praise the child for behavior after the injection. Allowing the child to assist with applying an elastic bandage will give some feeling of comfort.
   h. Also encourage activity that will use the muscle site of the injection—promotes dispersal of medication and decreases soreness. This can also be done by firmly massaging the muscle after injection, unless contraindicated.
   i. Accurately record the injection site to ensure proper site rotation.

Intravenous Medications

1. Intravenous (IV) administration of medications may be done through a variety of techniques, including piggyback or through a heparin lock, volume control set, or implantable port. See pages 84–94 for information on these techniques.
2. Prepare mixtures aseptically (laminar-flow hood) and use sterile technique when accessing the IV line. (Sepsis is a constant threat when a child is receiving IV medications.)
3. Be aware that an exaggerated pharmacologic effect may exist with IV medications. As with any medication, know the use, adverse effects, and toxic effects of the drug as well as the pharmacologic effect on the body.

4. Dilute IV medications and inject slowly—never less than 1 minute (this allows peripheral blood flow through the entire circulating system to dilute the medication and prevent high concentrations of the drug from reaching the brain and heart).
5. Be knowledgeable about compatibilities of drugs, electrolytes in IV solutions, and the fluid itself.
6. Observe the IV site frequently. Restrain the child, as needed, to prevent infiltration. Infiltration of fluids containing medications can cause rapid and severe tissue necrosis.

SPECIAL CONSIDERATIONS IN PEDIATRIC PRIMARY CARE

Acute Poisoning

Exposure to poisons can occur by ingestion, inhalation, or skin or mucous membrane contact. This section focuses on the most common poisoning, toxic ingestions. Poisoning by ingestion refers to the oral intake of a harmful substance that, even in a small amount, can damage tissues, disturb body functions and, possibly, cause death. The substances may include such medications as acetaminophen and iron, household products, and plants.

Children are at risk for acute poisoning. According to the American Association of Poison Control Centers, in 2010, 50.5% of poisoning exposures occurred in children younger than age 6, and the majority (37.7%) of these were under age 3. More than 89% of poison exposures occur in the home. The most common agents ingested by children younger than age 6 include cosmetics and personal care products; however, cleaning products, analgesics, plants, and cough and cold medications also pose risk.

 Evidence Base Bronstein, A. C., Spyker, D. A., Cantilena, L. R., et al. (2011). 2010 annual report of the American Association of Poison Control Centers' National Poison Data System (NPDS): 28th annual report. *Clinical Toxicology, 49*, 910–949.

Pathophysiology and Etiology

1. Improper or dangerous storage of potentially toxic substances.
2. Poor lighting—causes errors in reading.
3. Human factors:
   a. Failure to read label properly.
   b. Failure to return poisons to their proper place.
   c. Failure to recognize the material as poisonous.
   d. Lack of supervision of the child.
   e. Purposeful use of poison.
4. Toxin is ingested and may have limited local effects or continue to a stage of absorption and interference with metabolic processes and organ function.
5. Typically occurs in children younger than age 6, with a peak incidence between 12 and 24 months.
6. Acute poisoning may result in arrhythmias or permanent multiorgan damage due to initial loss of airway, breathing, and circulation (ABCs) and specific organ toxicity.

Poisoning with Acetaminophen

Acetaminophen is a common drug-poisoning agent in children due to its replacement of salicylates and the pleasant taste of the preparations developed to facilitate administration. Ingestion by adolescents is frequently intentional. Acetaminophen is toxic to the liver, resulting in cell necrosis and, possibly, cell death.

Clinical Manifestations

Phase I (first 24 hours after ingestion):

1. May be asymptomatic.
2. Anorexia.
3. Nausea and vomiting.
4. Diaphoresis.
5. Malaise.
6. Pallor.

Phase II (24 to 48 hours after ingestion):

1. Symptoms of phase I diminish or disappear.
2. Right upper quadrant pain due to liver damage.
3. Liver enlargement with elevated bilirubin and hepatic enzymes and prolonged prothrombin time.
4. Oliguria.

Phase III (days 3 to 5 after ingestion):

1. Signs of hepatic failure, such as jaundice, hypoglycemia, coagulopathy, and encephalopathy.
2. Peak liver function abnormalities.
3. Anorexia, nausea, vomiting, and malaise may reappear.
4. Renal failure and cardiomyopathy may occur.

Phase IV:

1. Associated with recovery or progression to complete liver failure and death.

Diagnostic Evaluation

1. Serum acetaminophen level 4 hours after ingestion.
2. Serial liver function tests.
3. Urine and serum chemistry studies for renal function.

Management

1. Activated charcoal should be given if treatment is instituted within 6 to 8 hours after ingestion; if treatment is begun after this time frame, activated charcoal is not used unless another toxic substance was ingested.
2. N-Acetylcysteine as an antidote given orally or via IV line. This is the most extensively studied regimen for acetaminophen overdose.
3. As with all poisons, ABCs and treatment of shock are always the priority in management.

Iron Poisoning

Iron poisoning occurs frequently in childhood due to the prevalence of iron-containing preparations. The severity of iron poisoning is related to the amount of elemental iron absorbed. The range of potential toxicity is between 50 and 60 mg/kg.

Clinical Manifestations

1. Thirty minutes to 2 hours after ingestion:
   a. Local necrosis and hemorrhage of GI tract.
   b. Nausea and vomiting, including hematemesis.
   c. Abdominal pain.
   d. Diarrhea, usually bloody.
   e. Severe hypotension.
   f. Symptoms subside after 6 to 12 hours.
2. Six to 24 hours—period of apparent recovery.
3. Twenty-four to 40 hours:
   a. Systemic toxicity with cardiovascular collapse, shock, hepatic and renal failure, seizures, coma, and, possibly, death.
   b. Metabolic acidosis.
4. Two to 4 weeks after ingestion:
   a. Pyloric and duodenal stenosis.
   b. Hepatic cirrhosis.

Diagnostic Evaluation

1. Measurement of serum-free iron.
   a. Total serum iron.
   b. Total serum iron-binding capacity.
2. Abdominal x-ray to visualize iron tablets; limited use for visualizing liquid toxins.

Management

1. Gastric lavage may be of some benefit because iron is not absorbed by activated charcoal; however, wide lumen must be used, which may not be possible in small children.
2. Whole-bowel irrigation reduces the absorption of iron and sustained-release drugs.
3. Administration of deferoxamine for severe cases—iron-chelating agent that binds with iron and is excreted in urine (urine will be bright red).

Primary Assessment in Acute Poisoning

1. Initial assessment should include evaluation of ABCs, level of consciousness, vital signs, and neurologic assessment.

 NURSING ALERT It may be necessary to initiate emergency respiratory and circulatory support at this time. If needed, obtain venous access, maintain safety during seizure activity, and treat shock. Otherwise, continue with assessment.

2. Assess for symptomatic effects of poisoning by systems.
   a. GI—common in metallic acid, alkali, and bacterial poisoning. These may include nausea and vomiting, diarrhea, abdominal pain or cramping, and anorexia.
   b. CNS—may include seizures (especially with CNS depressants, such as alcohol, chloral hydrate, barbiturates) and behavioral changes. Dilated or pinpoint pupils may be noted.
   c. Skin—rashes; burns to the mouth, esophagus, and stomach; eye inflammation; skin irritations; stains around the mouth; lesions of the mucous membranes. Cyanosis may be visible, especially with cyanide and strychnine.
   d. Cardiopulmonary—dyspnea (especially with aspiration of hydrocarbons) and cardiopulmonary depression or arrest.
   e. Other—odor around the mouth.
3. Identify the poison when possible.
   a. Determine the nature of the ingested substance from the child's history or by reading the label on the container.

Nursing intervention may need to be implemented immediately after this assessment.

b. Call the nearest poison control center or toxicology section of the medical examiner's office to identify the toxic ingredient and obtain recommendations for emergency treatment. The United States toll-free number is (800) 222-1222.

c. Save vomitus, stool, and urine for analysis when the child reaches the hospital.

Primary Interventions

Assisting the Family by Telephone Management

1. Calmly obtain and record the following information:
   a. Name, address, and telephone number of caller.
   b. Evaluation of the severity of the ingestion.
   c. Age, weight, and signs and symptoms of the child, including neurologic status.
   d. Route of exposure.
   e. Name of the ingested product, approximate amount ingested, and time of ingestion.
   f. Brief past medical history.
   g. Caller's relationship to victim.
2. Instruct the caller about appropriate emergency actions or refer to (800) 222-1222.
3. Direct the patient to the nearest emergency department. Dispatch an ambulance, if necessary.
4. Instruct the caller to clear the child's mouth of any unswallowed poison.
5. Identify what treatments have already been initiated.
6. Instruct the parents to save vomitus, unswallowed liquid or pills, and the container and to bring them to the hospital as aids in identifying the poison.
7. Identify whether other children were involved in the poisoning to initiate treatment for them also.

Intervention Related to the Patient's Condition

Support ABCs, as needed.

Removing the Poison from the Body

1. If the poison is nonpharmaceutical, have the child drink 100 to 200 mL of water. If a medication was ingested, do not dilute with water, as this may speed absorption.
2. For skin or eye contact, remove contaminated clothing and flush with water for 15 to 20 minutes.
3. For inhalation poisons, remove from the exposed site.

DRUG ALERT Do not administer household neutralizing foods or products (unless recommended by poison control specialist) because the heat generated by the chemical reaction could result in a burn (or exacerbation of an existing burn).

4. Administer gastric lavage if the toxin is not bound by charcoal (most effective within 50 minutes after ingestion).
5. Follow lavage with a cathartic and activated charcoal to hasten removal of the poison from the GI tract. Use cautiously with young children.

6. Be aware of the dangers associated with lavage.
   a. Esophageal perforation—may occur in corrosive poisoning.
   b. Gastric hemorrhage.
   c. Impaired pulmonary function resulting from aspiration.
   d. Cardiac arrest.
   e. Seizures—may result from stimulation in strychnine ingestion.
7. Follow lavage (if performed) with activated charcoal (preferably within 1 hour after ingestion) to hasten removal of the poison from the GI tract.
   a. Charcoal poorly absorbs most electrolytes, iron, lithium, mineral acids and bases, alcohols, cyanide, most solvents, and hydrocarbons.
   b. Administer 30 to 50 g for an adolescent, in 6 to 8 ounces (180 to 240 mL) of water with sweetener.
   c. It is sometimes easier to administer in an opaque beverage container as some children are hesitant to drink the charcoal because of its unusual dark color.

Reducing the Effect of the Poison by Administering an Antidote

1. An antidote may either react with the poison to prevent its absorption or counteract the effects of the poison after its absorption.
2. Not all poisons have specific antidotes.
3. Information about appropriate antidotes for specific poisons is available through all poison control centers. Antidotes for the most common poisons should be listed in the emergency department of the hospital.
4. Effectiveness of the antidote usually depends on the amount of time that elapses between ingestion of the poison and administration of the antidote.

Eliminating the Absorbed Poison

1. Force diuresis.
   a. Administer large quantities of fluid either orally or via IV line.
   b. Carefully monitor intake and output.
2. Assist with kidney dialysis, which may be necessary if the child's kidneys are not functioning effectively.
3. Assist with exchange transfusion if this method is indicated for removing the poison.

Providing Emotional Support

1. Remain calm and efficient while working rapidly.
2. Reassure the child and his or her family that therapeutic measures are being taken immediately.
3. Discourage anxious parents from holding, caressing, and overstimulating the child.

Subsequent Nursing Assessment and Interventions

Observing the Child for Progression of Symptoms

1. CNS involvement.
   a. Observe for restlessness, confusion, delirium, seizures, lethargy, stupor, or coma.

b. Administer sedation with caution—to avoid CNS depression and masking of symptoms.

c. Avoid excessive manipulation of the child.

d. See nursing care of the child with seizures, page 1569.

e. See nursing care of the unconscious patient, Chapter 15.

2. Respiratory involvement.

a. Observe for respiratory depression, obstruction, pulmonary edema, pneumonia, or tachypnea.

b. Have artificial airway and tracheostomy set available.

c. Be prepared to administer oxygen and provide artificial respiration.

d. Other nursing concerns:

i. Nursing care for mechanical ventilation, see page 1479.

ii. Procedures for administration of oxygen, see pages 1480.

iii. Procedure for cardiopulmonary resuscitation, see page 1474.

3. Cardiovascular involvement.

a. Observe for peripheral circulatory collapse, disturbances of heart rate and rhythm, or heart failure.

b. Maintain IV therapy, as directed, to prevent shock. Assess for complications of overhydration.

c. Be prepared for cardiac arrest.

4. GI involvement.

a. Observe for nausea, pain, abdominal distention, and difficulty swallowing.

b. Maintain IV therapy to replace water and electrolyte losses.

c. Offer a diet that is easily swallowed and digested.

i. Begin with clear liquids.

ii. Progress to full liquids, soft foods, and then a regular diet as the child's condition improves.

5. Kidney involvement.

a. Observe the child for decreased urine output. Record oral and IV intake and urine output exactly.

b. Observe for hypertension.

c. Insert indwelling catheter, if necessary, for urinary retention.

d. Administer appropriate amounts of fluids and electrolytes.

e. See nursing care of child with renal failure, page 1651.

f. Correct and monitor acid-base balance.

Providing Supportive Care

1. Maintain adequate caloric, fluid, and vitamin intake. Oral fluids are preferable if they can be retained.

2. Avoid hypothermia or hyperthermia. (Control of body temperature is impaired in many types of poisoning.) Monitor the child's temperature frequently.

3. Observe closely for inflammation and tissue irritation.

a. This is especially important in ingestion of kerosene or other hydrocarbons, which cause chemical pneumonitis.

b. Isolate the patient from other children, especially those with respiratory infections.

c. Administer antibiotics, as prescribed by the physician.

4. Counsel parents who typically feel guilty about the accident.

a. Encourage parents to talk about the poisoning.

b. Emphasize how their quick action in getting treatment for the child has helped.

c. Discuss ways that they can be supportive to their child during the hospitalization.

d. Do not allow prolonged periods of self-incrimination to continue. Refer parents to a psychologist for assistance in resolving these feelings, if necessary.

5. Involve the young child in therapeutic play to determine how he or she views the situation.

a. The child commonly sees nursing measures as punishments for misdeed involving the poisoning.

b. Explain treatment and correct misinterpretations in a manner appropriate for child's age.

6. Initiate a community health nursing referral for any childhood poisoning incident. A home assessment should be made to identify any potential or actual problems and provide proper poisoning prevention interventions and education.

Family Education and Health Maintenance

Stressing Prevention

1. Information concerning poison prevention should be available on every hospital pediatric unit and during every child health care visit.

a. Many free booklets and home safety checklists are available from such sources as insurance companies and drug companies.

b. Teaching may be done with any parent regardless of the reason for the child's hospitalization or office visit.

2. Teach the following precautions:

a. Keep medicines and poisons out of the reach of children.

b. Provide locked storage for highly toxic substances; select cabinet that is higher than child can reach or climb.

c. Do not store poisons in the same areas as foods.

d. Make sure all containers are properly marked and labeled. Keep medicines, drugs, and household chemicals in their original containers.

e. Do not discard poisonous substances in receptacles where children can reach them; however, do discard used containers of poisonous substances.

f. Teach children not to taste or eat unfamiliar substances.

g. Clean out medicine cabinets periodically.

h. Keep medications in childproof containers that are securely closed.

i. Read all labels carefully before each use.

j. Do not give medicines prescribed for one child to another.

k. Never refer to drugs as candy or bribe children with such inducements.

l. Never give or take medications in the dark.

m. Encourage parents not to take medication in front of young children because children role-play adult behavior.

n. Suggest that mothers avoid keeping medications in their purses or on the kitchen table.

o. Keep baby creams and ointments away from young children.

p. Never puncture or heat aerosol containers.

q. Store lawn and garden pesticides in a separate place under lock and key outside of the house; do not store large quantities of cleaning products or pesticides.

3. Advise parents to dispose of syrup of ipecac if they keep it in the household. According to the American Academy of Pediatrics, there is no evidence supporting improved outcomes of poisonings with the use of ipecac. In addition, there is potential for abuse of ipecac with bulimic or anorexic teenagers; therefore, the recommendation for keeping ipecac on hand to induce vomiting has been rescinded.

4. Tell family to keep a list of emergency telephone numbers including the poison control center, health care provider's number, nearest hospital, and ambulance service.

5. Reinforce the need for vigilance and consistent supervision of infants and young children due to their increased mobility, increased curiosity, and increased dexterity.

Teaching Emergency Actions

1. Suspect poisoning with the occurrence of sudden, bizarre symptoms or peculiar behavior in toddlers and preschoolers.

2. Read label on the ingested product or call the health care provider, hospital, or poison control center for instructions about treatment for the poisoning. Give all relevant information about the child, condition, and substance ingested.

3. Maintain an adequate airway in a child who is convulsing or who is not fully conscious.

4. Dilute the poison with 100 to 200 mL of water, if advised.

5. Transport the child promptly to the nearest medical facility.

a. Wrap the child in a blanket to prevent chilling.

b. Bring the container and any vomitus or urine to the hospital with the child.

6. Avoid excessive manipulation of the child.

7. Act promptly but calmly.

8. Do not assume the child is safe simply because the emesis shows no trace of the poison or because the child appears well. The poison may have produced a delayed reaction or may have reached the small intestine where it is still being absorbed.

Lead Poisoning

There are approximately 250,000 children with elevated blood lead levels (> 10 mg/dL) in the United States. Lead poisoning, referred to as *plumbism*, results from some form of lead consumption. Blood lead levels even lower than the prior accepted level of 10 mg/dL can affect intellectual functioning in children.

Millions of children live in housing built before 1950, which contains the highest surface soil level and internal household dust contaminated with lead. Normal hand-to-mouth activities of children may introduce leaded household dust, soil, and nonfood items into their GI tract. Pica (eating nonfood substances, particularly leaded paint chips) is generally associated with more severe degrees of poisoning.

Pathophysiology and Etiology

Etiologic Factors

1. Multiple episodes of chewing on, sucking, or ingestion of nonfood substances.

a. Toys, furniture, windowsills, household fixtures, and plaster painted with lead-containing paint.

 NURSING ALERT Legislation stipulates that toys, children's furniture, and the interior of homes be painted with lead-free paint; however, the problem arises when deeper layers of paint and plaster on older products are contaminated with lead. One paint chip contains much more lead than is considered safe.

b. Cigarette butts and ashes.

c. Acidic juices or foods served in lead-based earthenware pottery made with lead glazes.

d. Colored paints used in newspapers, magazines, children's books, matches, playing cards, and food wrappers.

e. Water from lead pipes.

f. Fruit treated with insecticides.

g. Dirt containing lead fallout from automobile exhaust.

h. Antique pewter, especially when used to serve acidic juices or foods.

i. Lead weights (curtain weights, fishing sinkers).

j. Continuous proximity to lead-processing center.

k. Occupations or hobbies that use lead.

l. Imported folk remedies, cosmetics, food, or cookware that contain lead.

2. Inhalation of fumes containing lead (less common cause in children).

a. Leaded gasoline.

b. Burning storage batteries.

c. Dust containing lead salts.

d. Dust in the air at shooting galleries and in enclosed firing ranges with poor ventilation.

e. Cigarette smoke.

3. Highest incidence in children between ages 1 and 6 years, especially those between ages 1 and 3 years.

a. High incidence in individuals living in old homes or deteriorated housing conditions.

b. No significant difference in incidence by sex.

c. High incidence among siblings.

4. Symptomatic lead poisoning occurs most frequently in summer months.

Systemic Effects

1. Lead absorption from GI tract is affected by age, diet, and nutritional deficiency. Young children absorb 40% to 50% and retain 20% to 25% of dietary lead.

2. It takes the body twice as long to excrete lead as it does to absorb lead.

3. Lead is stored in two places in the body:

a. Bone.

b. Soft tissue.

4. Principal toxic effects occur in nervous system, bone marrow, and kidneys.
5. Nervous system.
   a. Brain—increased capillary permeability results in edema, increased intracranial pressure, and vascular damage; destruction of brain cells causes seizures, mental retardation, paralysis, blindness, and learning disabilities.
   b. Neurologic damage cannot be reversed.
   c. CNS of young children and fetuses is most sensitive to lead.
6. Bone marrow.
   a. Lead attaches to red blood cells (RBCs).
   b. Inhibition of a number of steps in the biosynthesis of heme, thus reducing the number of RBCs, increasing fragility, and reducing half-life.
   c. The decreased production of hemoglobin results in anemia and respiratory distress.
7. Kidneys—injury to the cells of the proximal tubules, causing increased excretion of amino acids, protein, glucose, and phosphate.
8. Recurrence rate is high, especially if the lead is not removed from the home environment.

Clinical Manifestations

Symptoms in young children may develop insidiously and may abate spontaneously.

1. GI—anorexia, sporadic vomiting, intermittent abdominal pain (colic), constipation.
2. CNS—hyperirritability; decreased activity; personality changes; loss of recently acquired developmental skills; falling, clumsiness, loss of coordination (ataxia); local paralysis; peripheral nerve palsies.
3. Hematologic—anemia, pallor.
4. Cardiovascular—hypertension, bradycardia.

Diagnostic Evaluation

1. Detailed history with emphasis on the presence or absence of clinical symptoms; evidence of pica; family history of lead poisoning; possible source of exposure to lead; recent change in behavior, developmental delay, or behavior problems; recent change of address; or recent renovations in the home.
2. Assess serum lead level and repeat confirmatory, preferably by way of venipuncture. Recent changes in screening recommendations have been made to include targeted screening of all Medacaid-enrolled and Medicaid-eligible children. Additionally, all children born outside the United States should be screened.

 **NURSING ALERT** Venous sampling is the best method for assessing the level of lead in the blood as it limits cutaneous contamination. If a finger-stick sample is being used, careful collection should include a free flowing specimen.

a. For levels under 10 µg/dL, no action is required.
b. For levels between 10 and 14 µg/dL, level should be confirmed and repeated in 3 months. Education on decreasing exposure and limiting absorption of lead should be done on all levels greater than 10 µg/dL.
c. Levels between 15 and 19 µg/dL should be repeated within 2 months, while an environmental history additionally is reviewed.
d. Levels between 20 and 44 µg/dL should be repeated within 2 days and referred to local health department plus a thorough medical history and physical examination added to education as noted above.
e. Levels between 45 and 69 µg/dL should be confirmed immediately, referred to the local health department, and should be considered for chelation therapy in consultation with an expert.
f. Immediate hospitalization is required for levels >70 µg/dL.

 Evidence Base: Warniment, C., Tsang, K., & Galezka, S. (2010). Lead poisoning in children. *American Family Physician, 81*(6), 751-757.
Levin, R., Brown, M. J., Kashtock, M. E., et al. (2008). Lead exposures in U.S. children, 2008: implications for prevention. *Environ Health Perspect., 116*(10), 1285–1293.

3. Hematologic evaluation for iron-deficiency anemia.
4. Flat plate of abdomen—may reveal radiopaque material if lead has been ingested during the preceding 24 to 36 hours.
5. Erythrocyte protoporphyrin level—not sensitive enough for identifying lead levels below 25 mg/dL. Can be used to follow levels after medical and environmental interventions for poisoned children have occurred. A progressive decline in erythrocyte protoporphyrin levels indicates that management is successful.
6. 24-hour urine—more accurate than a single voided specimen in determining elevated urinary components that correspond with elevated blood lead levels.
7. Radiologic examination of long bones—unreliable for diagnosis of acute lead poisoning; may provide some indication of past lead poisoning or length of time poisoning has occurred.
8. Edetate calcium disodium provocation chelation test—used only in selected medical centers treating large numbers of lead-poisoned children; demonstrates increased lead levels in urine over an 8-hour period after injection of edetate disodium.

Management
Removal of Lead from the Environment
1. Remove leaded paint and paint chips or objects containing lead from the child's environment.
2. Remove child from environment during lead abatement process.

Nutritional Considerations
1. Consume adequate amounts of iron. Iron supplementation may be indicated to correct anemia.

2. Reduced-fat diet and small, frequent meals will reduce the GI absorption of lead.

3. Encourage foods high in vitamin C (such as fruits and juices) and calcium (such as milk, yogurt, and ice cream).

Chelation Therapy

According to the CDC, although chelation therapy is considered a mainstay in the medical management of children with blood lead levels > 45 µg/dL, it should be used with caution. Indeed, an expert in the management of lead chemotherapy should be consulted prior to using chelation agents. State lead poisoning programs, local poison control centers, or the Lead Poisoning Prevention Branch at the CDC can be used as resources to identify accessible experts.

 Evidence Base Centers for Disease Control and Prevention. (2008). Childhood lead poisoning prevention program; managing elevated lead levels among young children: Recommendations from the Advisory Committee on Childhood Lead Poisoning Prevention. Available: *www.cdc.gov/nceh/lead/*.

(*Note*: ACLPP draft report, January 2012, has not been adopted at the time of publication.)

Complications

1. Severe and usually permanent mental, emotional, and physical impairment.
2. Neurologic deficits.
   a. Learning disabilities.
   b. Mental retardation.
   c. Seizures.
   d. Encephalopathy.

Nursing Assessment

1. Partake in primary prevention through screening for lead poisoning—should target high-risk groups. This includes children:
   a. Who live in homes built before 1950.
   b. With iron-deficiency anemia.
   c. Who are exposed to contaminated dust or soil.
   d. Who have developmental delays.
   e. Who are victims of abuse or neglect.
   f. Whose parents are exposed to lead through occupational hazards or hobbies.
   g. Who live in low-income families.
2. Screening should also be targeted at children who live in communities with more than 27% of houses built before 1950 or in populations where 12% or more of the children have elevated lead levels.
3. Assess all children for signs of lead toxicity, including hyperactivity, developmental delay, constipation, anorexia, colicky abdominal pain, clumsiness, and pallor.
4. Inquire about presence of pica behavior in children younger than age 6 years.
5. Assess the child's level of development. The Denver Developmental Screening Test II may be useful for this purpose and will help detect delays possibly caused by lead poisoning.

Nursing Diagnoses

- Risk for Injury related to seizures and encephalopathy.
- Acute Pain related to chelation therapy injections.
- Delayed Growth and Development related to the effects of chronic lead exposure.
- Compromised Family Coping related to guilt and concern for child.

Nursing Interventions

Protecting the Child with Seizures and Encephalopathy

1. Maintain seizure precautions.
   a. Crib or bed rails elevated and padded.
   b. Tongue blade (if indicated per institutional guidelines) and suction equipment at bedside.
2. Be aware that encephalopathy may occur 4 to 6 weeks after first symptoms:
   a. Sudden onset of persistent vomiting.
   b. Severe ataxia.
   c. Altered state of consciousness.
   d. Coma.
   e. Seizures.
   f. Massive cerebral edema in younger children.
3. Observe for signs of increased intracranial pressure (ICP) in the child with encephalopathy:
   a. Rising blood pressure.
   b. Papilledema.
   c. Slow pulse.
   d. Seizures.
   e. Unconsciousness.
4. Provide supportive care to maintain vital functions.

Reducing Pain Associated with Chelation Therapy

1. Plan appropriate play activities to prepare the child for the injections and as an outlet for the pain and anger the child feels.
2. Implement measures to decrease pain at injection site.
   a. Rotate injection sites.
   b. Apply warm packs to the site to decrease pain.
   c. Move painful areas slowly.
3. Provide diversion activities, fluids, and meals between injections.
4. Monitor intake and output and blood studies, such as electrolytes and liver and renal function tests, as directed.

Promoting Growth and Development

1. Provide and encourage activities that will help the child to learn and progress from his or her present developmental state to meet the next appropriate milestone.
2. Initiate appropriate referrals in cases of obvious developmental delays or learning difficulties. The referrals may be to such professionals as psychologists, psychiatrists, and specialists in early child education.
3. Share the results of developmental testing with the parents and discuss ways to provide stimulation for the child at home.

Strengthening Family Coping

1. Use sensitivity in interviewing and teaching to avoid causing or increasing guilt feelings about the poisoning and to

establish a positive, trusting relationship between the family and the health care facility.

2. Explain the treatment and its purpose because parents are commonly faced with putting an asymptomatic child through painful treatments.

3. Encourage frequent visits by parents and siblings and facilitate family involvement.

Community and Home Care Considerations

1. Carry out lead screening in the community. It is recommended that all high-risk children be screened for high lead levels between ages 9 and 12 months and, if feasible, again at 24 months. Screening policies, universal or targeted, are determined by local departments of health, based on the prevalence of risk factors in the community.

2. Coordinate community care efforts to return the child to a safe home. Communicate with community outreach workers so that environmental case management is conducted. Lead abatement must be conducted by experts, not untrained parents, property owners, or contractors.

3. Suggest periodic, focused household cleaning to remove the lead dust; use a wet mop.

4. Encourage handwashing before meals and at bedtime to eliminate lead consumption from normal hand-to-mouth activity.

5. Observe the child and other children in the home for pica.
   a. Observe and record the child's eating habits and food preferences.
   b. Report any attempted eating of nonfood substances.
   c. Encourage caregivers to provide regular meals and make mealtime a pleasurable time for the child.
   d. Teach caregivers to discourage oral activity and to substitute activity that contributes to play, social skills, and ego development.
   e. Refer the family for additional social or psychiatric casework, if indicated, to reduce economic and other factors that result in pica in the child.

6. Screen siblings and playmates of known cases immediately.

7. Make sure that the family is able to provide close supervision of the child or assist them to make arrangements to ensure that the child is adequately supervised at home.

Family Education and Health Maintenance

Ensuring Long-Term Follow-Up

1. Teach the parents why long-term follow-up is important. Tell them that residual lead is liberated gradually after treatment and:
   a. May result in the renewal of symptoms.
   b. May increase serum lead to a dangerous level.
   c. May cause additional damage to the CNS, which may not become apparent for several months.

2. Stress that acute infections must be recognized and treated promptly because these may reactivate the disease.

3. Teach that iron supplementation may be continued to treat anemia. Advise the parents about medication administration and adverse effects and periodic complete blood count monitoring.

Preventing Reexposure of the Child to Lead

1. Advise the parents that the single most important factor in managing childhood lead poisoning is reducing the child's reexposure to lead.

 NURSING ALERT Children should not return home until their home environment is lead free.

2. Instruct the parents about the seriousness of repeated lead exposure.

3. Initiate referrals to home health nursing and community agencies, as indicated.

Providing Community Education

1. Initiate and support educational campaigns through schools, day care centers, and news media to alert parents and children to hazards and symptoms of lead poisoning.

2. Provide literature in clinics, waiting rooms, and other appropriate settings that stresses the hazards of lead, sources of lead, and signs of lead intoxication.

3. Support legislation to study the nature and extent of the lead poisoning problem and to eliminate the causes of lead poisoning.

4. Include the topic of pica and lead poisoning in nutritional teaching.

5. For additional information, contact the state or local health department or CDC (*www.cdc.gov*).

Evaluation: Expected Outcomes

- Seizure precautions maintained; no signs of increased ICP.
- Tolerates chelation therapy injections; expresses anger through doll play.
- Parents provide appropriate play and stimulation for development.
- Family involved in care; provides support to the child.

Communicable Diseases

With the dramatic success of immunizations, many childhood diseases have decreased in frequency. However, a number of communicable diseases still cause significant morbidity in children (see Table 42-2). Many other infections that occur in childhood are covered elsewhere in the book such as Chapter 31, Infectious diseases, or the chapters of each body system.

Child Abuse and Neglect

 Evidence Base Raman, S., Holdgate, A., & Torrens, R. (2012). Are our frontline clinicians equipped with the ability and confidence to address child abuse and neglect? *Child Abuse Review, 21*(2), 114–130.

Child abuse is any type of maltreatment of children or adolescents by their parents, guardians, or caretakers. It is considered a major problem worldwide, with most countries tracking the problem and allocating some resources toward services to prevent and treat child abuse. Child abuse includes physical or emotional abuse, injury, trauma, neglect, or sexual abuse of a child that is intentional and nonaccidental. Abuse includes:

(Text continues on page 1440)

Table 42-2   Communicable Diseases

DISEASE, AGENT, MODE OF TRANSMISSION, AGE WHEN MOST COMMON	INCUBATION AND COMMUNICABILITY PERIODS	SYMPTOMS
Chickenpox ***Varicella-zoster virus*** • Highly communicable; acquired in direct contact, droplet spread, and airborne transmission. • 2–9 years; January to May. *Diagnostic tests:* Tzanck smear shows multinucleated giant cells; a culture may be done for confirmation.	*Incubation (I):* 11–21 days after exposure. *Communicability (C):* Onset of fever (1–2 days before first lesion) until last vesicle is dried (5–7 days).	• General malaise, low-grade fever, and anorexia for 24 hours. • Rash—macules to papules and vesicles to crusts within several hours. • Pruritus of lesions may be severe and scratching may cause scarring. • *Rash characteristics:* Rash appears first on the head and mucous membranes, then becomes concentrated on body and sparse on extremities, papulovesicular eruption.
Rubella (German 3-day Measles) ***Rubella virus; RNA toga virus*** • Oral droplet or transplacentally. • School age, young adults; spring, winter. *Diagnostic tests:* Tissue culture of throat, blood, or urine; latex agglutination, enzyme immunoassay, passive hemagglutination, fluorescent immunoassay tests. *Passive immunity:* Birth to age 6 months from maternal antibodies.	*I:* 14–21 days after exposure. *C:* Virus can be passed from 7 days before to 5 days after rash appears.	• Enlarged lymph nodes in postauricular, auricular, suboccipital, and cervical areas 24 hours before rash develops. • Enanthem: discrete rose spots on soft palate. • Exanthem: variable; begins on face, spreads quickly over entire body; usually maculopapular; clears by third day.
Roseola Infantum (Exanthem subitum) ***Human herpes virus–6*** • Direct contact or droplet. • 6–24 months; late fall to early spring.	*I:* 5–15 days. *C:* Not known—believed not to be highly contagious.	• Fever of 103°–106° F (39.4°–41.1° C), either intermittent or sustained 3–4 days with no clinical findings. • Fever suddenly drops and macular or maculopapular rash develops on trunk, spreading to arms and neck; mild involvement of face and legs; rash fades quickly.
Rubeola (Hard, Red, 7-day Measles) ***Measles virus, RNA-containing paramyxovirus*** • Direct contact with droplets from infected persons, respiratory route. *Diagnostic tests:* Serologic procedures not routinely done. *Passive immunity:* Birth to between ages 4 and 6 months if mother is immune before pregnancy. • 5–10 years, adolescents; spring.	*I:* 10–12 days. *C:* 5th day of incubation to 4th day of rash.	• Fever, lethargy, cough, coryza, and conjunctivitis. • 2–3 days later; Koplik's spots on buccal pharyngeal mucosa (grayish white spots with reddish areolae), which disappear within 12–18 hours. • 2 days later: maculopapular rash appears at hairline and spreads to feet in 1 day; rash begins to clear after 3–4 days.
Mumps ***Mumps virus, paramyxovirus*** • Direct contact, through families, airborne droplets, saliva, and possibly urine. • School age; all seasons but slightly more frequent in late winter and early spring. *Diagnostic tests:* Serologic testing and viral culture from throat swab. *Passive immunity:* Birth to age 6 months if mother is immune before pregnancy.	*I:* 16–18 days. *C:* 3 days before to 9 days after swelling appears; virus in saliva greatest just before and after parotitis onset.	• Headache, anorexia, generalized malaise; fever 1 day before glandular swelling; fever lasts 1–6 days. • Glandular swelling usually of parotid—one side or bilaterally. • Enlargement and reddening of Wharton's duct and Stensen's duct. • Subclinical infection may occur.

TREATMENT	COMPLICATIONS	NURSING CONSIDERATIONS
• Symptomatic: Shorten fingernails to prevent scratching. • Daily antiseptic baths. • Oral antihistamines to decrease pruritus. • Treatment of itching: Baking soda (sodium bicarbonate) or oatmeal baths, Calamine lotion to lesions. • Isolation until all lesions have crusted. • Acyclovir by mouth (P.O.) within first 24 hours. • Avoid salicylates.	• Complications are rare in otherwise healthy children. • Secondary bacterial infection of lesions. • Hemorrhagic varicella, pneumonia, encephalitis, and thrombocytopenia are not common but they can occur. • Reye's syndrome.	• Severe in neonate and pregnant women. • Varicella zoster immune globulin is available for high-risk susceptible children who have been exposed to varicella zoster. • Prevention through immunization is the best practice.
• Symptomatic—isolation.	• In adolescent females: arthritis; arthralgias. • Encephalitis. • Thrombocytopenia.	• Exposure of nonimmune pregnant women in the first trimester results in a high percentage of affected fetuses and infants born with various birth defects: cataracts, deafness, growth retardation, congenital heart disease, mental retardation. • Prevention is the best practice.
• Symptomatic—antipyretic.	• Seizures due to high fever. • Encephalitis (rare).	• Reassure family that this is a self-limiting illness.

• Symptomatic:
  • Sedatives.
  • Antipyretic.
  • Bed rest in humid, comfortably warm room.
  • Dark room for photophobia.
  • Adequate fluids.
	• Otitis media.
	• Pneumonia, laryngitis.
	• Mastoiditis, encephalitis.
	• Appendicitis.
		• Provide symptomatic care and respiratory isolation.
		• Prevention through immunization is the best practice.

• Isolation until swelling has subsided.
• Symptomatic:
  • Analgesics.
  • Hydration.
  • Alimentation.
  • Antipyretics.
  • Rest.
	• Meningoencephalitis.
	• Orchitis, epididymitis.
	• Auditory nerve involvement, resulting in unilateral deafness.
		• Provide symptomatic care.
		• Prevention through immunization is the best practice.

(continued)

Table 42-2   Communicable Diseases (continued)

DISEASE, AGENT, MODE OF TRANSMISSION, AGE WHEN MOST COMMON	INCUBATION AND COMMUNICABILITY PERIODS	SYMPTOMS
Diphtheria		
Corynebacterium diphtheriae • Acquired through secretions of carrier or infected individual by direct contact with contaminated articles and environment. • Unimmunized children under 15 years old; incidence increased in autumn and winter. *Diagnostic tests:* Cultures of nose and throat.	*I:* 2–4 days. *C:* 2–4 weeks untreated; 1–2 days with antibiotic treatment.	***Nasal diphtheria*** • Coryza with increasing viscosity, possibly epistaxis, low-grade fever. • Whitish gray membrane may appear over nasal septum. ***Pharyngeal and tonsillar diphtheria*** • General malaise, low-grade fever, anorexia. • 1–2 days later, whitish gray membranous patch on tonsils, soft palate, and uvula. • Lymph node swelling, fever, rapid pulse, "bull neck." ***Laryngeal diphtheria*** • Usually spread from pharynx to larynx. • Fever, harsh voice, stridor, barking cough; respiratory difficulty with inspiratory retraction. ***Nonrespiratory diphtheria*** • Affects eye, ear, genitals, or, rarely, skin.
Pertussis (Whooping Cough)		
Bordetella pertussis • Direct contact or respiratory droplet spread. • Infants and young children; females more than males. *Diagnostic tests:* Culture of nasopharyngeal mucus.	*I:* 3–12 days; mean of 7 days. *C:* 7 days after exposure (greatest just before catarrhal stage) to 3 weeks after onset of paroxysms or until cough has ceased.	***Stage I (catarrhal stage)*** • Lasts 1–2 weeks. • Rhinorrhea, conjunctival injection, lacrimation, mild cough, and low-grade fever. ***Stage II (paroxysmal stage)*** • Lasts 2–4 weeks or longer. • Frequent severe, violent coughing attacks occurring in clusters, leading to vomiting, cyanosis, and exhaustion. ***Stage III (convalescent stage)*** • Lasts 2 weeks to several months. • Coughing attacks decrease, but may return with each respiratory infection. • Duration: 9 months to 2 years.
Staphylococcal Scalded Skin Syndrome (Ritter's Disease)		

Group II phage-type Staphylococcus aureus
• Disseminated from a primary infection site (usually nose or around eyes).
• Infants and children under 10 years old.
Diagnostic tests: Cultures of skin, conjunctiva, nasopharynx, stools, and blood. Biopsy of exfoliated epidermis.
	I: Few days.
	C: Onset of rash until after antibiotics initiated.
		• Malaise, fever, irritability, or asymptomatic.
		• Rash develops in three phases:
		  • Erythematous—macular involving face, neck, axilla, and groin.
		  • Exfoliative—upper layer of epidermis becomes wrinkled and can be removed by light stroking (Nikolsky sign); crusting around eyes, mouth, and nose produce characteristic "sunburst," radial pattern; irritable due to extreme tenderness of skin.
		  • Desquamative—epidermis peels away, leaving moist areas that dry quickly and heal in 10–14 days.

Erythema Infectiosum (Fifth Disease or Slapped Cheek)		

Parvovirus B 19
• Respiratory route.
• School-age children.
Diagnostic tests: Not widely available; IgM antibody test, polymerase chain reaction detection test.
	I: 6–14 days.
	C: Until rash develops.
		• Mild fever, chills, fatigue, or nonpruritic rash develops in three stages:
		  • Sudden appearance of bright erythema on cheeks.
		  • Erythematous, maculopapular rash on trunk and extremities.
		  • Rash on body fades with central clearing, giving a lacy or reticulated appearance.
		• Rash lasts 2–39 days; frequently pruritic without desquamation.
		• Occasional joint arthropathy.

TREATMENT	COMPLICATIONS	NURSING CONSIDERATIONS

• Diphtheria antitoxin via IV line or I.M.
• Antibiotic therapy (penicillin, erythromycin).
• Supportive treatment:
  • Respiratory support and cardiac monitoring.
  • Isolation until three cultures are negative after antibiotic therapy is completed.
  • Bed rest for 2–3 weeks.
  • Hydration.
  • Immunization with diphtheria toxoid after recovery.
	• Myocarditis.
	• Neuritis.
	• Paralysis.
	• Toxic neurosis and hyaline degeneration of heart, liver, adrenal glands, and kidneys.
	• Gastritis, hepatitis.
	• Nephritis.
		• Identify close contacts and monitor for illness; culture nose, throat, and cutaneous lesions and administer prophylactic antimicrobial therapy.
		• Prevention through immunization is the best practice.

• Specific:
  • Erythromycin estolate.
  • Azithromycin.
  • Clarithromycin.
• Supportive:
  • Antipyretics.
  • Bed rest.
  • Quiet environment to reduce coughing.
  • Gentle suctioning.
  • Increase fluid intake.
  • Oxygen.
	• Respiratory: pneumonia, atelectasis, emphysema, aspiration pneumonia, pneumothorax.
	• CNS: convulsions, encephalopathy, coma.
	• Death may occur among the unvaccinated.
		• Erythromycin should be given to all close and household contacts for 14 days.
		• Neither immunization nor natural disease confers complete or lifelong immunity.

• Specific:
  • Therapy with penicillinase-resistant penicillin P.O., I.M., or via IV line
• Symptomatic:
  • Gentle cleaning of skin with compresses.
	• Excessive fluid loss, electrolyte imbalance, pneumonia, septicemia, cellulitis.	• Provide symptomatic care.

• Symptomatic treatment. • Immunoglobulin for immunocompromised patients.	• Complications are rare among otherwise healthy children. • Children with abnormal red blood cells (sickle cell disease, hereditary spherocytosis, and thalassemia) can develop transient aplastic anemia and may require multiple transfusions. • Immunocompromised patients may develop severe, chronic anemia.	• Avoid contact of child with pregnant female (< 5% of exposed unborn children will have severe anemia; rare chance of miscarriage).

(continued)

Table 42-2   Communicable Diseases *(continued)*

DISEASE, AGENT, MODE OF TRANSMISSION, AGE WHEN MOST COMMON	INCUBATION AND COMMUNICABILITY PERIODS	SYMPTOMS
Rotavirus		
Reoviridae group A • Most common agent responsible for infantile diarrhea. • Fecal-oral route. • Ages 6 months to 2 years; most common in winter in temperate climates. *Diagnostic tests:* Enzyme-linked immunosorbent assay.	*I:* 1–3 days. *C:* Until 2–5 days after diarrhea.	• Fever. • Vomiting. • Profuse, watery, non-foul-smelling diarrhea.
Hand, Foot, Mouth Disease		
Coxsackie virus A16 or other enteroviruses • Moderately contagious by direct contact with nose and throat secretions, fluid from blisters, and stool. • Most common in children under age 10 during summer and fall. *Diagnostic tests:* Throat swab or stool culture for virus; rarely indicated.	*I:* 3–7 days. *C:* 1st week of illness.	• Mild fever, poor appetite, malaise, and sore throat. • Painful sores develop in the mouth 1–2 days after fever begins (usually on the tongue, gums, and buccal mucosa). A nonpruritic rash follows on the palms and soles, occasionally on the buttocks.

• Battering—physical injury.
• Drug abuse—intentional administration of harmful drugs, especially during pregnancy.
• Sexual abuse.
• Sexual assault or molestation (non-family member).
• Incest (family offender).
• Emotional abuse—scapegoating, belittling, humiliating, lack of mothering.

Neglect is the omission of certain appropriate behaviors, with such omission having detrimental physical or psychological effects on development. Neglect includes:
• Child abandonment.
• Lack of provision of the basic needs of survival, including shelter, clothing, stimulation, medical care, food, love, supervision, education, attention, emotional nurturing, and safety.

Etiology and Incidence

 Evidence Base U.S. Department of Health and Human Services, Administration for Children and Families. (2012). *Child Maltreatment 2011.* Washington, DC: Author.

The cause of child abuse and maltreatment is multidimensional. The abuse may be related to the combined presence of three factors: special kind of child, special kind of parent or caretaker, special circumstances of crisis. Abuse occurs in all ethnic, geographic, religious, educational, occupational, and socioeconomic groups.

1. In 2010, there were 695,000 reported victims of child abuse and neglect in the United States. Furthermore, 1,537 reported fatalities occurred.

2. Maltreatment occurred approximately 80% of the time at the hands of one or both parents.

3. The most common type of abuse is neglect (78.3% of cases), followed by physical abuse (17.6%), sexual abuse (9.2%), emotional maltreatment (5.1%), and medical neglect (2.4%).

Contributing Factors

1. Incidents of child abuse may develop as a result of disciplinary action taken by the abuser who responds in uncontrolled anger to real or perceived misconduct of the child. The parents may confuse punishment with discipline. "Good parenting" may be equated with physical contact to eradicate child behavior. The abuser may be a stern, authoritarian disciplinarian.

2. Incidents of child abuse may develop out of a quarrel between caretakers. The child may come to the aid of one parent and may be entered into the midst of the quarrel; marital discord is common.

3. The abuser may be under a great deal of stress because of life circumstances (debt, poverty, illness) and may thus resort to child abuse. Crisis and stress may be ongoing. The abuser may have a low frustration-tolerance level and may not have a well-developed means of coping with stress in general.

4. The abuser may be intoxicated with alcohol or drugs at the time of the abuse; only 10% of abusers have a history of mental illness.

5. Child abuse may occur by a surrogate caregiver, such as a babysitter or boyfriend.

6. Lack of effective parenting, inappropriate parent–child bonding, and punitive treatment as a child may contribute to the parent becoming an abuser.

TREATMENT	COMPLICATIONS	NURSING CONSIDERATIONS
• Oral fluid and electrohydrate solution.	• Isotonic dehydration with acidosis. • Malnourished infants may develop malabsorption dehydration and die.	• Excellent hygiene (handwashing) is necessary to avoid spreading disease. • Current vaccine will prevent 74% of all cases, 98% of severe cases.
• Symptomatic for fever, aches, and mouth lesions.	• Rare, asymptomatic meningitis.	• Provide pain relief and monitor fluid intake to prevent dehydration from not eating.

7. Specific characteristics evident in many abusing parents include:
   a. Low self-esteem—a sense of incompetence in role, unworthiness, unimportance, have difficulty controlling aggressive impulses; commonly live in social isolation.
   b. Unrealistic attitudes and expectations of the child, little regard for the child's own needs and age-appropriate abilities, lack of knowledge related to parenting skills.
   c. Fear of rejection—a deep need to feel wanted and loved, but a feeling of rejection when love is not obvious; a crying infant may elicit a feeling of rejection.
   d. Inability to accept help—isolation from the community, loneliness.
   e. Unhappiness due to unsatisfactory relationships; may look to child for satisfaction of own emotional needs.
   f. Child abusers are commonly the children of abuse or victims of spousal abuse.
8. Incidents of child abuse may develop from a general attitude or resentment or rejection on the part of the abuser toward the child.
9. Atypical child behavior (eg, hyperactivity or a technology-dependent child who needs additional care) may unintentionally provoke the abuser.
10. The degree of the family crisis is not usually in proportion to the degree of abuse.

Clinical Manifestations

Characteristics of the Child that Should Raise Suspicion

1. The child is usually younger than age 3 years. School-age children and adolescents are also subject to abuse. The average age of a sexually abused child is 9 years.
2. General health of the child indicates neglect (diaper rash, poor hygiene, malnutrition, unattended physical problem).
3. Characteristic distribution of fractures (scattered over many parts of body).
4. Disproportionate amount of soft tissue injury.
5. Evidence that injuries occurred at different times (healed and new fractures, resolving and fresh bruises).
6. Cause of recent trauma in question.
7. History of similar episodes in the past.
8. No new lesions during the child's stay in the hospital.
9. May show a wide range of reactions—may be either very withdrawn or overactive. The child may be anxious, tense, or nervous or show regressive behavior.
10. The child may show unusual affection for strangers or may be overly fearful of adults and avoid any physical contact with them.
11. For sexual abuse: the child may fear no one will believe him or her; may experience self-blame; most know their abusers.
12. Children may not "tell" about abuse from parents, fearing a loss of security; "a bad parent is better than no parent at all."
13. Behavior problems, depression, acting-out behaviors, and aggression toward younger children may result.
14. For abuse that occurs in school or day care, the child may exhibit fear of the teacher, have nightmares, decrease school attendance, or develop psychosomatic illnesses.

Injuries or Types of Abuse that May Occur

1. Bruises, welts (linear or looplike).
2. Abrasions, contusions, lacerations (most common).
3. Wounds, cuts, punctures.

4. Burns (cigarette, radiator), scalding—stocking or glove distribution.
5. Bone fractures.
6. Sprains, dislocations.
7. Subdural hemorrhage or hematoma; "shaken baby syndrome."
8. Brain damage.
9. Internal injuries.
10. Drug intoxication.
11. Malnutrition (deliberately inflicted).
12. Freezing, exposure.
13. Whiplash-type injury.
14. Eye injuries, periorbital injuries, ear bruises.
15. Dirty, infected wounds or rashes.
16. Unexplained coma in infant.
17. Failure to thrive—developmental delay; malnutrition with decreased muscle mass; decreased interaction with environment and with others; dental caries; listlessness; behavior problems.
18. Sexually transmitted diseases—genital trauma, recurrent urinary tract infection, pregnancy.

NURSING ALERT Munchausen syndrome by proxy is a condition in which symptoms are induced in a child by the actions of a parent or caregiver. A wide range of methods have been noted as the basis for the fabricated illness, with most falling into one of four general categories: poisoning, bleeding, infections, and injuries. Many of the conditions cannot be observed by a health care provider nor can diagnosis be confirmed by further evaluation. Munchausen syndrome by proxy is a serious form of child abuse and is associated with a high rate of morbidity and mortality. It is important for nurses to obtain thorough histories of any illness or injury and be observant in any unusual cases.

Management

1. The goal of treatment is to ensure the physical and emotional safety of the child. Therefore, treatment is inclusive of other family members and caretakers and is often focused on the parents. A team approach is employed to determine the most effective use of community resources to protect the child and help the parents.
2. It is estimated that 80% to 90% of abusing parents can be rehabilitated. The ideal approach is to return the child to the biological parents after treatment concludes.
3. Counseling is offered to help parents do the following:
   a. Understand and redirect their anger.
   b. Develop an adequate parent–child relationship.
   c. See their child as an individual with his or her own needs and differences.
   d. Understand child development and normal behaviors of developing children.
   e. Learn about effective discipline techniques.
   f. Enjoy the child.
   g. Develop realistic expectations of their child.
   h. Decrease their use of criticism.
   i. Increase parents' self-esteem and confidence.
   j. Establish supportive relationships with others.
   k. Improve their economic situation (if appropriate).
   l. Show progress toward the physical, emotional, and intellectual development of their child.

Nursing Assessment

1. Identify family or child at risk.
   a. Alcohol or drug abuser.
   b. Adolescent parent.
   c. Low-income, single-parent family.
   d. Multiple births.
   e. Unwanted child.
   f. Sickly and more demanding child.
   g. Premature child with long separation from mother at birth.
2. Inspect for evidence of possible abuse.
   a. Describe completely on the medical record all bruises, lacerations, and similar lesions as to location and state of healing. Look carefully at areas generally covered with clothing (ie, buttocks, underarms, behind knees, bottom of feet).
   b. Ask how injuries occurred and record descriptions of the injury, including the date, time, and place of the event.
3. Collect necessary specimens for identification of organisms, sperm, or semen.
4. Take color photographs, as indicated.
5. Assess developmental level of the child.
6. Observe for behaviors common in abusing or neglecting parents. Be aware that not all abusing parents exhibit these behaviors but be alert for the parent who:
   a. Anxiously volunteers information or withholds information related to an injury.
   b. Gives explanation of the injury that does not fit the condition or gets story confused concerning the injury.
   c. Shows inappropriate reaction or concern to severity of injury.
   d. Becomes irritable about questions being asked.
   e. Seldom touches or speaks to the child; does not respond to child. May be critical or indicate unreal expectations of child (or may be oversolicitous to the child).
   f. Delays seeking medical help; refuses to sign permit for diagnostic studies; frequently changes hospitals or health care providers.
   g. Shows no involvement in the care of the hospitalized child; does not inquire about the child.
   h. Obtains little or no prenatal care and shows inappropriate response to the neonate; acts disinterested or unhappy with the child.
7. Assess the parent–child relationship in the areas of appropriate involvement in care, show of affection, reaction to arrival and leaving, expectations, role portrayal.

8. Assess for signs of sexual abuse. Sexual abuse should be suspected when the young, prepubertal child presents with:
   a. Genital trauma not readily explained.
   b. Gonorrhea, syphilis, or other sexually transmitted organisms.
   c. Blood in urine or stool.
   d. Painful urination or defecation.
   e. Penile or vaginal infection or itch.
   f. Penile or vaginal discharge.
   g. Report of increased, excessive masturbation.
   h. Report of increased, unusual fears.
   i. Trauma to genitalia, inner thigh, breast.
9. Establish a relationship with the child based on mutual respect, empathy, and sensitivity to facilitate further investigation.
   a. Consideration of the child's emotions in conjunction with a good relationship may encourage the child to express feelings either verbally or through drawings or play.
   b. Prepare the child physically and psychologically for the necessary physical and pelvic examination.
   c. Talk with the child without the presence of the parents, especially when incest is possible.

 NURSING ALERT If the alleged sexual abuse occurred within 72 hours of the health care visit, or if trauma or bleeding is present, an immediate physical examination should be done. Assessment and evidence collection is very important and every attempt should be made to enlist the assistance of a health care provider experienced in this task. Many emergency departments have SANE-P (Sexual Abuse Nurse Examiners–Pediatric) who have had extensive training on the acute management of sexual abuse but also managing the long-term needs of the abused child. If more than 72 hours have passed since the alleged sexual abuse, the physical examination might be delayed. After child abuse has been reported, additional children in the family may be examined as well.

10. Report suspicion of child abuse based on your assessment. All states (as well as the District of Columbia) have mandatory reporting laws based on Public Law 94-247 (Child Abuse and Neglect Act, 1973). All states provide statutory immunity for those who report real or suspected child abuse. There is no immunity from civil or criminal liability for failure to report such. Notify the appropriate officials.

 NURSING ALERT Every nurse is morally and legally responsible to report and provide protective services for the abused child. Become familiar with laws, procedures, and protective services in your community and state.

Nursing Diagnoses

- Fear related to experiences with abuse.
- Impaired Parenting related to abusive treatment of a child.

Nursing Interventions

Relieving Fear and Fostering Trust

1. Be aware that some of these children have never learned how to trust an adult; they are fearful of giving affection for fear of rejection.
2. Assign one nurse to care for the child over a period of time.
3. Make no threatening moves toward the child. The child will indicate readiness and awareness of the environment by verbal or facial expressions.
4. Touch the child gently.
5. Provide nonthreatening physical contact (hold and frequently cuddle the child). Pick up and carry child around; encourage any exploration of your face and hair.
6. Provide appropriate opportunities for play.
7. Set limits for the child.
8. Provide therapeutic play to allow the child to express fears and anger in a nonverbal manner; be nonjudgmental and supportive with expression of feelings; correct misconceptions.
9. Provide additional help in these areas:
   a. Having ambivalent feelings toward the parents or any adult caretaker.
   b. Overcoming low self-image and the fear that something is wrong with him or her.
   c. Fearing future abuse upon his or her return home or for misbehavior in the hospital.

Providing Support in Parenting

1. Assume a nonjudgmental attitude that is neither punitive nor threatening. Convey a desire to help the parents through the healing process.
2. Refrain from questioning them about the incident of abuse. The health care provider, social worker, and investigative authority will interview the suspected abuser.
3. Include the parents in the hospital experience (ie, orient them to the unit and to any procedure to be done to the child). Serve as a role model in the management of the child's behavior as well as their own. Try to give the parents as much information as possible about the care of their child. Listen to what they are saying.
4. Refrain from challenging all the information they may give.
5. Express appropriate concern and kindness. Remain objective, yet empathic. This will help foster the parents' self-respect and improve their self-image and dignity.
6. Discuss the reporting to the authorities with them because of the widespread nature of the problem and the need for education and assistance.
7. Support the parents who may have feelings of guilt, anger, and helplessness. Explain to them the extent of trauma and educate them. Allow them to express their feelings. Support their parental role in handling the child (eg, allow the child to talk about or play out the incident, but do not force it).
8. Build a relationship by working with the parents' strengths rather than their weaknesses. Use compliments as positive reinforcement.

9. Assist the parents to learn safe and appropriate parenting skills.

   a. Remember that many of these parents were abused as children and have no role models or personal experience with nurturing behaviors.

   b. Foster attachment between child and parents, not between child and nurse, when the parents are present; the latter would increase their feelings of incompetence in the parenting role.

   c. Correct erroneous expectations as to what is appropriate behavior for a particular age group.

   d. Encourage the parents to take time out from caring for their children to meet their own needs; assist them in identifying safe and appropriate resources for their child's care.

10. Provide the parents with psychological support and reinforcement for appropriate parenting behaviors.

11. Work with the parents in planning for the child's future care.

12. Determine in what areas the parents need help. Does the infant cry often? How does this make the parents feel? How do the parents comfort the child? Is there someone the parents can call for help?

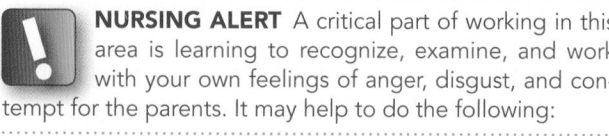 **NURSING ALERT** A critical part of working in this area is learning to recognize, examine, and work with your own feelings of anger, disgust, and contempt for the parents. It may help to do the following:

1. Realize that most abusing parents do love their children and want the best for them despite their ambivalent feelings for the children.

2. Understand the dynamics of child abuse and neglect. This crisis is due to stress, with which the parents are unable to cope, and to deprivations they have themselves suffered in the past.

Community and Home Care Considerations

Nurses typically provide home care visits as part of a multidisciplinary team engaging in extensive community follow-up. Education and continued assessment are the focus.

1. Teach the parents about normal growth and development (see Chapter 40).

   a. Give specific information about and examples of the types of behavior to expect at the various stages of development. Point out in a nonthreatening way normal behavior exhibited by their child.

   b. Provide specific strategies for dealing with whatever behavior the child exhibits.

   c. Serve as a role model and teacher; minimize intensity when the parents become threatened.

2. Teach the parents how to use discipline without resorting to physical force.

   a. Discipline must be consistent. Offer suggestions for alternative ways of handling undesirable behavior (eg, time-out).

   b. Suggest using a reward system for acceptable behavior (eg, a trip to the zoo, staying up later than usual for a special television show, a special treat).

   c. Instruct the parents to withhold rewards for unacceptable behavior.

3. Teach children how to avoid being the victims of abuse.

   a. Teach them about "good touch" and "bad touch."

   b. Emphasize that they can say no to anyone who wants to touch their body.

   c. Provide names or places where they can go if they feel they are being abused.

   d. Assist them in dealing with their fears that their parents will be sent to jail or that they will be removed from the home.

4. Be alert for signs of abuse in the school. If a teacher is suspected of being the abuser, the child may:

   a. Display increased fear of the teacher.

   b. Decrease school attendance.

   c. Develop psychosomatic symptoms during school days.

   d. Develop nightmares.

   e. Worry excessively over school performance.

Family Education and Health Maintenance

1. Teach the parents and child (if age is appropriate) any specific instructions relative to injury and follow-up care.

2. Ensure that the family knows where and when to follow up.

3. Review schedule for well-child visits and immunizations so the family can keep up with routine care.

4. Make known to the parents your continued concern and your availability as a source of help. Help them to use resources in the community, including the home health nurse, social worker, and therapists.

5. Refer those interested in learning more about abuse to the following agencies: Prevent Child Abuse America (*www.preventchildabuse.org*, 1-800-CHILDREN) and Child Welfare Information Gateway (*www.childwelfare.gov*).

Evaluation: Expected Outcomes

- Exhibits appropriate developmental behavior.
- Both parents participate in feeding and playing with child.

SELECTED REFERENCES

Acara, K., & Tschudy, M. (Eds.). (2012). *The Harriet Lane Handbook* (19th ed.). Philadelphia: Elsevier.

American Academy of Pediatrics Advisory Committee on Childhood Lead Poisoning Policy Statement. (2007). Lead exposure in children: Prevention, detection, and management. *Pediatrics, 116*(4), 1036–1046.

American Academy of Pediatrics. (2012). Breastfeeding and the use of human milk. *Pediatrics, 129*(3), e827–e841.

Blosser, C., Brady, M., & Royal, R. (2013) Infectious Diseases and Immunizations. In C. Burns, A. Dunn, M. Brady, et al. (Eds.), *Pediatric primary care* (pp. 427–493). Philadelphia: Elsevier.

Bronstein, A. C., Spyker, D. A., Cantilena, L. R., et al. (2011). 2010 annual report of the American Association of Poison Control Centers' National Poison Data System (NPDS): 28th annual report. *Clinical Toxicology, 49*, 910–949.

Centers for Disease Control and Prevention. (2008). Childhood lead poisoning prevention program; managing elevated lead levels among young children: Recommendations from the Advisory Committee on Childhood Lead Poisoning Prevention. Available: *www.cdc.gov/nceh/lead/*.

Centers for Disease Control and Prevention. (2009). Recommendations for blood lead screening of Medicaid-eligible children aged 1–5 years: An updated approach to targeting a group at high risk. *Morbidity and Mortality Weekly Report, 58*(RR09), 1–11.

Centers for Disease Control and Prevention. (2011). National and state vaccination coverage among children aged 19–35 months—United States, 2010. *Morbidity and Mortality Weekly Report, 60*(34), 1157–1163.

Centers for Disease Control and Prevention. (2012). Tuberculosis: Testing and diagnosis. Atlanta, GA: Author. Available: *www.cdc.gov/tb/topic/testing/default.htm#bcg.*

Centers for Disease Control and Prevention. (2013). Recommended immunization schedules for persons aged 0 through 18 years. Available: *www.cdc.gov/vaccines/recs/acip.*

Centers for Disease Control and Prevention. (2013). Tdap for pregnant women: Information for providers. Available: *www.cdc.gov/vaccines/vpd-vac/pertussis/tdap-pregnancy-hcp.htm.*

Chantry, C. J., & Howard, C. R. (2013). Clinical protocols for management of breastfeeding. *Pediatric Clinics of North America, 60*(1), 75–113.

Connors, J., Arushanyan, E., Bellanca, G., et al. (2012). A description of barriers and facilitators to childhood vaccinations in the military health system. *Journal of the American Academy of Nurse Practitioners, 24*(12), 716–725.

Criddle, L. (2010). Monsters in the closet: Munchausen syndrome by proxy. *Critical Care Nurse, 30*(6), 46–55.

Dieterich, C. M., Felice, J. P., O'Sullivan, E., et al. (2013). Breastfeeding and health outcomes for the mother-infant dyad. *Pediatric Clinics of North America, 60*(1), 31–48.

Fadda, G. (2012). Tuberculosis: novel approaches to an old disease. *Journal of Infection in Developing Countries, 6*(1), 4–5.

Feldman-Winter, L. (2013). Evidence-based interventions to support breastfeeding. *Pediatric Clinics of North America, 60*(1), 169–187.

Harrington, J. W., Logan, S., Harwell, C., et al. (2012). Effective analgesia using physical interventions for infant immunizations. *Pediatrics, 129*, 815–822.

Harrison, D., Beggs, S., & Stevens, B. (2012). Sucrose for procedural pain management in infants. *Pediatrics, 130*(5), 918–925.

Institute of Medicine. (2004). *Immunization safety review: Vaccines and autism.* Washington, DC: National Academies Press.

Infant Nutrition Council. (2013). Safe preparation, storage and handling of powdered infant formulas. Available: *http://infantnutritioncouncil.com/safe-prep-and-handling/.*

Levin, R., Brown, M. J., Kashtock, M. E., et al. (2008). Lead exposures in U.S. children, 2008: Implications for prevention. *Environ Health Perspect., 116*(10), 1285–1293.

Meifert, M., & Bunik, M. (2013). Overcoming clinical barriers to exclusive breastfeeding. *Pediatric Clinics of North America, 60*(1), 115–145.

Murphy, P., Frazee, S., Cantlin, J. P., et al. (2012). Pharmacy provision of influenza vaccinations in medically underserved communities. *Journal of the American Pharmacists Association, 52*(1), 67–70.

National Network for Immunization Information. (2009). Vaccines and autism. Galveston, TX: Author. Available: *www.immunizationinfo.org/issues/thimerosal-mercury/vaccines-and-autism-2009.*

Niederhauser, V., & Baker, D. (2011). What's new in child and adolescent immunizations? *The Nurse Practitioner, 36*(10), 39–44.

Pickering, L. K., Kimberlin, D. W, Long, S., et al. (Eds.). (2012). *Red Book: 2012 Reports of the Committee on Infectious Disease*s (29th ed.). Elk Grove Village, IL: American Academy of Pediatrics.

Raman, S., Holdgate, A., & Torrens, R. (2012). Are our frontline clinicians equipped with the ability and confidence to address child abuse and neglect? *Child Abuse Review, 21*(2), 114–130.

Rosenman, J., & Fischer, P. (2011). Travel clinics in pediatric and adolescent travel. *Pediatric Annals, 40*(7), 371–375.

Spratling, R., & Carmon, M. (2010). Pertussis: An overview of the disease, immunizations, and trends for nurses. *Pediatric Nursing, 36*(5), 238–243.

Taddio, A., Appleton, M., Bortolussi, R., et al. (2010). Reducing the pain of childhood vaccination: An evidence-based clinical practice guideline (summary). *Canadian Medical Association Journal, 182*(18), 1989–1895.

U.S. Department of Health and Human Services, Administration for Children and Families. (2012). *Child maltreatment 2011.* Washington, DC: Author.

van den Anker, J. (2013). Optimising the management of fever and pain in children. *International Journal of Clinical Practice, 67* (supplement 178), 26–32.

Warniment, C., Tsang, K., & Galezka, S. (2010). Lead poisoning in children. *American Family Physician, 81*(6), 751–757.

43
Care of the Sick or Hospitalized Child

GENERAL PRINCIPLES

Hospitalization of a child brings about a range of emotions in the child and his or her family. In order to care for the hospitalized child, one must take into consideration the child's development and family coping skills. Being hospitalized versus receiving care at home affects the child's response to his or her illness. In addition, family presence is often an integral part of pediatric patient care. Facilitating family-centered care allows the family to fully support the child during his or her hospitalization. Knowledge of these aspects will assist the registered nurse in providing appropriate pediatric patient care.

Pain Management

 Evidence Base Habich, M., Wilson, D., Thielk, D., et al. (2012). Evaluating the effectiveness of pediatric pain management guidelines. *Journal of Pediatric Nursing—Nursing Care of Children & Families, 27*(4), 336–345.

Accurate assessment and timely management of pain in children is an important and challenging nursing responsibility because infants and young children cannot express their pain, as adults can.

General Considerations

1. Pain experienced by infants and children is not effectively identified or managed in many cases.
2. There are still misunderstandings about the ways pain is experienced and expressed by infants and children.
3. Behavioral and physiologic cues are used to assess pain in infants. Special rating tools are available to involve children in assessing the intensity of their pain, including the Pain Experience Inventory, CRIES Neonatal Postoperative Pain Measurement Scale, Oucher Pain Rating Scale, Numerical or Visual Analog Scale, FLACC Behavioral Pain Assessment Scale, and the Wong-Baker FACES Pain Rating Scale (see Figure 43-1).
4. Pain caused by a condition is not always proportional to the seriousness of the illness or injury. For example, a relatively minor illness, such as an earache, is a very painful experience, whereas an enlarging tumor may not cause pain in early stages.
5. It is important to consider pain when a child is noncommunicative, has decreased consciousness, is intubated, or whose chosen language is not understood by the health caregivers.
6. It is equally important to consider pain when a child requires an injection, blood test, or noninvasive or invasive diagnostic test.

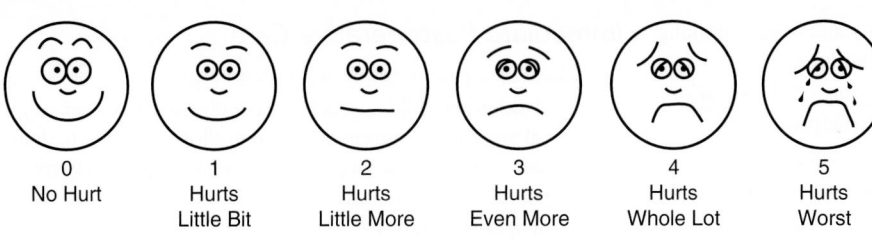

Figure 43-1. Wong-Baker FACES Pain Rating Scale. (Hockenberry, M. J., & Wilson, D. (2012). Wong's essentials of pediatric nursing (9th ed.). Philadelphia: Elsevier.)

7. Consider parents when assessing and managing the pain of their child. It is well documented that parents are important influences on their children.
   a. Consider the way in which the parents view the situation experienced by the child and work with them to intervene effectively.
   b. Presence of the parents during a procedure can be very positive, especially when the family has been prepared.
   c. At other times, it is recommended that the parents mutually agree to wait in a nearby area.
   d. Arbitrary rules against parental presence are often designed to meet the needs of staff, not the needs of the child and his or her parents.

Nursing Interventions

1. Anticipate pain and intervene early.
2. Use a rating scale that the child can understand and use it consistently with that child for initial pain assessment and to determine the effectiveness of interventions. Attempt to introduce the pain rating scale to the child prior to the surgery or procedure.
3. Use self as therapeutic presence to help ease pain.
4. Teach self-regulation and self-control techniques.
5. Utilize distraction by sounds, music, audio images, and movies.
6. Allow self-soothing maneuvers (thumbsucking, clinging to blanket, rocking).
7. Reposition patient, as needed.
8. Decrease environmental light and noise when possible.
9. Consider referral for self-hypnosis and conscious relaxation techniques.
10. Utilize medication delivered by way of noninvasive routes where possible.
11. Administer premedication—anesthetizing, anti-anxiety, and anti-emetic medications, as indicated.
12. Assist with conscious sedation when indicated, following standards of practice related to assessment, staffing, care, and documentation.
13. Reassess the patient's response to the intervention and document appropriately. This is important to evaluate effectiveness and identify possible new pain issues.

The Child Undergoing Surgery

 Evidence Base Vincent, C., Chiappetta, M., Beach, A., et al. (2012). Parents' management of children's pain at home after surgery. *Journal for Specialists in Pediatric Nursing*, 17(2), 108–120.

Physical and emotional preparation for surgery will minimize stress and will help the child and family cope effectively with surgery. Also see Chapter 7, Perioperative Nursing.

Psychological Preparation and Support

1. Potential threats for the hospitalized child anticipating surgery are:
   a. Physical harm—bodily injury, pain, mutilation, death.
   b. Separation from parents; peers for the older child or adolescent.
   c. The strange and unknown—possibility of surprise.
   d. Confusion and uncertainty about limits and expected behavior.
   e. Relative loss of control of their world, loss of autonomy.
   f. Fear of anesthesia.
   g. Fear of the surgical procedure itself.
   h. Misinterpretation of medical jargon (eg, *dye/die*).
2. The attitudes of the parents toward hospitalization and surgery largely determine the attitudes of their child.
   a. The experience may be emotionally distressing.
   b. Parents may have feelings of fear or guilt.
   c. The preparation and support should be integrated for parent, child, and family unit.
   d. Give individual attention to parents; explore and clarify their feelings and thoughts; provide accurate information and appropriate reassurance.
   e. Stress parents' importance to the child. Help parents understand how they can care for their child.

Preoperative Teaching

1. All preparation and support must be based on the child's age, developmental stage, and level; personality; past history and experience with health professionals and hospitals; background including religion, socioeconomic circumstances, culture, and family attitudes and dynamics. Anxiety level and coping skills should be taken into consideration.
2. Inquire as to what information the child has already received.
3. Determine what the child knows or expects; identify family myths and possible misunderstandings.
4. Additional guidelines in preparation include:
   a. Use illustration or model of a child's body, concrete examples, and simple terms (not medical jargon).
   b. Identify changes that may occur as a result of the procedure, both in body and daily routine.
   c. Give explanations slowly and clearly, saving anxiety-producing aspects until the end. Repeat as needed.

d. Make use of the child's creative ability and logical thinking powers to aid in preparation for procedures.

e. Involve parents, as indicated, depending on the situation.

f. Allow and encourage the child to participate as able.

g. Suggest ways for the child to cope—crying is okay.

h. Offer constant reassurance; speak in a calm manner.

i. Evaluate the child's understanding of your teaching. Repeat and correct information, as necessary.

5. Orient the patient and family to the unit, room, location of playroom, operating room and recovery room (if applicable) and introduce them to appropriate personnel. Make arrangements for the child to meet the anesthesiologist as well as the operating room nurse and recovery room nurse.

6. Allow and encourage questions. Give honest answers.

a. Such questions will give the nurse a better understanding of the child's fears and perceptions of what is happening.

b. Infants and young children need to form a trusting relationship with those who care for them.

c. The older the child, the more reassuring information can be.

7. Provide opportunity for the child and parents to work out concerns and feelings (play, talk). Such supportive care should result in less upset behavior and more cooperation.

8. Prepare the child for what to expect postoperatively (ie, equipment to be used or attached to child, where the child will wake up, how the child will feel, what the child will be expected to do, diet, any physical restrictions). Be honest about what pain they may experience.

9. Educate parents regarding the option to be with their child, if available at the facility, during induction of anesthesia to reduce separation anxiety and fear.

Physical Preparation

1. Assist with necessary laboratory studies. Explain to the child what is going to happen before the procedure and how he or she may respond. Give continual support during the procedure.

2. See that the patient has nothing by mouth (NPO). Explain to the child and his or her parents what NPO means and the importance of it. Place signs on the patient's hospital door indicating the NPO status to ensure that non-family members and non-staff members do not give the patient food.

3. Assist with fever reduction.

a. Fever can result from some surgical problems (eg, intestinal obstruction).

b. Fever increases risk of anesthesia and need for fluids and calories.

4. Administer appropriate medications, as prescribed. Sedatives and drugs to dry the secretions are often given on the unit preoperatively.

5. Establish good hydration. Parental therapy may be necessary to hydrate the child, especially if the child is NPO, vomiting, or febrile.

6. With the parents in attendance, assist the surgeon with marking the patient's intended surgical site, as recommended by The Joint Commission as part of the National Safety Goals.

7. Allow the child to carry a toy or other comfort item to the preoperative area.

Immediate Postoperative Care

1. Maintain a patent airway and prevent aspiration.

a. Position the child as ordered depending on his or her surgical procedure; position as needed to allow secretions to drain and to prevent the tongue from obstructing the pharynx.

b. Suction any secretions present. Avoid causing a gag reflex or spasm during suctioning.

2. Make frequent observations of general condition and vital signs. Postoperative protocols may vary per procedure and facility.

a. Take vital signs every 15 minutes until the child is awake and his or her condition is stable.

b. Note temperature, respiratory rate and quality, pulse rate and quality, blood pressure, skin color.

c. Watch for signs of shock.

i. Children in shock may have signs of pallor, coldness, increased pulse, and irregular respiration.

ii. Older children have decreased blood pressure and respiration.

d. Change in vital signs may indicate airway obstruction or compromise, hemorrhage, atelectasis, altered hemodynamics.

e. Restlessness may indicate pain or hypoxia. Medication for pain is not usually given until anesthesia has worn off. Give analgesics and sedatives per the pain management team orders.

f. Check dressings for drainage, constriction, and pressure. Perform dressing changes per protocol.

3. See that all drainage tubes are connected and functioning properly. Gastric decompression relieves abdominal distention and decreases the possibility of respiratory compromise. Chest tubes evacuate pleural air and fluid. Ensure all tubes are secure to prevent accidental removal.

4. Monitor parenteral fluids, as prescribed.

5. Be physically near as the child awakens to offer soothing words and a gentle touch. Reunite the parents and child as soon as possible after the child recovers from anesthesia. If a language barrier exists, the parents should be with the child during recovery from anesthesia and an interpreter should be present when medical explanations are being given to the parents or child.

After Recovery from Anesthesia

After undergoing simple surgery and receiving a small amount of anesthesia, the child may be ready to play and eat in a few hours. More complicated and extensive surgery debilitates the child for a longer period of time.

1. Continue to make frequent and astute observations in regard to behavior, comfort level and pain control, vital signs, dressings or operative site, and special apparatus (intravenous [IV] lines, chest tubes, oxygen, nasogastric tubes).

a. Note signs of dehydration—dry skin and membranes; sunken eyes; poor skin turgor; sunken fontanelle in an infant; poor urine output.

b. Record any passage of flatus or stool and bowel sounds. Observe for intestinal ileus because crying children swallow air, which may cause gastric distention.

c. Record vomiting time, amount, and characteristics.

2. Assess behavior for signs of pain and medicate appropriately.

3. Record intake and output accurately.
   a. Parenteral fluids and oral intake.
   b. Drainage from gastric tubes or chest tubes, colostomy, wound, and urinary output.
   c. Parenteral fluid is evaluated and prescribed by considering output and intake. It is usually maintained until the child is taking adequate oral fluids.
4. Advance diet as tolerated, according to the child's age and the health care provider's directions.
   a. First feedings are usually clear fluids; if tolerated, advance slowly to full diet for age. Note any vomiting or abdominal distention.
   b. Because anorexia may occur, offer what the child likes in small amounts and in an attractive manner.
5. Prevent infection.
   a. Keep the child away from other children or personnel with respiratory or other infections.
   b. Change the child's position every 2 to 4 hours; support infant with a blanket roll.
   c. Encourage the child to cough and breathe deeply; let the infant cry for short periods of time, unless contraindicated. Offer older children incentive spirometry every hour while awake.
   d. Keep operative site clean—change dressing, as ordered; in infant, keep the diaper away from the wound.
   e. Enforce diligent handwashing by family members and staff before any contact with the patient.
   f. Do not cohort surgical patients with patients with a proven or presumptive infection.
   g. Administer prophylactic antibiotics, as ordered.
6. Provide good general hygiene and opportunities for exercise and diversional activity; encourage sleep and rest.
7. Provide emotional support and psychological security. Reassure the child that things are going well; if there are complications, offer honest information based on the patient's health and developmental level and the parents' willingness to share this information with their child. Talk about going home, if appropriate.
8. Begin early to prepare for discharge: teach special procedures, provide written instructions, and arrange for community nurse referral.

The Dying Child

The nursing role is to assist the child and family to cope with the experience in such a way that it will promote growth rather than destroy family integrity and emotional well-being.

Recognize the Stages of Dying

Evidence Base Kubler-Ross, E. (1997). *On death and dying.* New York: Scribner.
Nielson, D. (2012). Discussing death with pediatric patients: Implications for nurses. *Journal of Pediatric Nursing, 27*(5), e59–64.

See Table 43-1.

1. Be aware that dying children, their families, and the staff will all progress through these stages, not necessarily at the same time.
2. Children experience the stages with much variation. They tend to pass more quickly through the stages and may merge some of these stages.
3. The nursing goal is to accept the child and his or her family at whatever stage they are experiencing, not to push them through the stages.

Table 43-1	Stages of Dying as Identified by Dr. Elizabeth Kübler-Ross
STAGE	**NURSING CONSIDERATIONS**
I. Denial, shock, disbelief	• Accept denial, but function within a reality sphere. Do not tear down the child's (or family's) defenses. • Be aware that denial usually breaks down in the early morning when it may be dark and lonely. • Be certain that it is the child or family who is using denial, not the staff.
II. Anger, rage, hostility	• Accept anger and help the child express it through positive channels. • Be aware that anger may be expressed toward other family members, nursing staff, physicians, and other persons involved. • Help families recognize that it is normal for children to express anger for what they are losing.
III. Bargaining (from "No, not me," to "Yes, me, but ...")	• Recognize this period as a time for the child and family to regain strength. • Encourage the family to finish any unfinished business with the child. This is the time to do things such as take a promised trip or buy a promised toy.
IV. Depression (The child and/or family experiences silent grief and mourns past and future losses.)	• Recognize this as a normal reaction and expression of strength. • Help families to accept the child who does not want to talk and excludes help. This is the usual pattern of behavior. • Reassure the child that you can understand his or her feelings.
V. Acceptance	• Assist families to provide significant loving human contact with their child and one another.

Table 43-2	Stages in the Development of a Child's Concept of Death
AGE OF CHILD	**STAGE OF DEVELOPMENT**
Child up to age 3	• At this stage, the child cannot comprehend the relationship of life to death because the child has not developed the concept of infinite time. • The child fears separation from protecting and comforting adults. • The child perceives death as a reversible act.
Preschool child	• At this age, the child has no real understanding of the meaning of death; the child feels safe and secure with parents. • The child may view death as something that happens to others. • The child may interpret the separation that occurs with hospitalization as punishment; the painful tests and procedures that the child is subjected to support this idea. • The child may become depressed because of not being able to correct these wrongdoings and regain the grace of adults. • The concept may be connected with magical thoughts of mystery.
School-age child	• The child at this age sees death as the cessation of life; child understands that he or she is alive and can become "not alive"; child fears dying. • The child differentiates death from sleep. Unlike sleep, the horror of death is in pain, progressive mutilation, and mystery. • The child is vulnerable to guilt feelings related to death because of difficulty in differentiating death wishes and the actual event. • The child believes death may be caused by angry feelings or bad thoughts. • The child learns the meaning of death from own personal experiences, such as the death of pets, family members, and public figures. • Television and movies have contributed to the concept of death and understanding of the meaning of illness. There may be more knowledge in the meaning of the diagnosis and an awareness that death may occur violently.
Adolescent	• The adolescent comprehends the permanence of death as the adult does, although the adolescent may not comprehend death as an event occurring to persons close to self. • The adolescent wants to live—sees death as thwarting pursuit of goals: independence, success, achievement, physical improvement, and self-image. • The adolescent fears death before fulfillment. • The adolescent may become depressed and resentful because of bodily changes that may occur, dependency, and the loss of social environment. • The adolescent may feel isolated and rejected because adolescent friends may withdraw when faced with impending death of a friend. • The adolescent may express rage, bitterness, and resentment; especially resents the fact that fate is to die.

4. Understand the meaning of illness and death at various stages of growth and development (see Table 43-2).
5. Be aware of other factors that influence a child's personal concept of death. Of particular importance are:
   a. The amount and type of direct exposure a child has had to death.
   b. Cultural values, beliefs, and patterns of bereavement.
   c. Religious beliefs about death and an afterlife.
6. Meet with the parents separately from the child and discuss their wishes regarding dissemination of information to their child.

Communicate with the Child about Death

Research indicates that children generally can cope with more than adults will allow and that children appreciate the opportunity to know and understand what is happening to them. It is important that the child's questions be answered simply but truthfully. The answers should be based on the child's particular level of understanding. The following responses have been suggested by Easson

in *The Dying Child: The Management of the Child or Adolescent Who Is Dying* and may be useful as a guide:

Preschool-Age Child

1. When the child at this age is comfortable enough to ask questions about illness, questions should be answered. When death is anticipated at some future time and the child asks "Am I going to die?", a response might be, "We will all die someday, but you are not going to die today or tomorrow."
2. When death is imminent and the child asks "Am I going to die?", the response might be, "Yes, you are going to die, but we will take care of you and stay with you."
3. When the child asks "Will it hurt?", the response should be truthful and factual.
4. Death should never be described as a form of sleep. Some children may fear sleep as the result of this type of explanation. Anesthesia is sometimes called a "special sleep" so it is not currently recommended to refer to death as "sleep."

5. Parents can express to the child the fact that they do not want the child to go and that they will miss the child very much; they feel sad, too, that they are going to be separated.

School-Age Child

1. Responses to the school-age child's questions about death should be answered truthfully. The child looks for support from those he or she trusts.
2. The school-age child should be given a simple explanation of his or her diagnosis and its meaning; the child should also receive an explanation of all treatments and procedures.
3. The child should be given no specific time in terms of days or months because each individual and each illness is different.
4. When the school-age child asks "Am I going to die?" and death is inevitable, the child should be told the truth. The school-age child has the emotional ability to look to parents and those he or she trusts for comfort and support.
5. The school-age child believes in his or her parents. The child should be allowed to die in the comfort and security of his or her family.
6. The school-age child knows death means final separation and knows what will be missed. The child must be allowed to mourn this loss. The dying child may be sad and bitter and demonstrate aggressive behavior. The child must be allowed the opportunity to verbalize this if able to do so.

Adolescent

1. The adolescent should be given an explanation of his or her illness and all necessary treatments and procedures.
2. The adolescent feels deprived and reasonably resentful regarding his or her illness because he or she wants to live and reach fulfillment.
3. As death approaches, the adolescent becomes emotionally closer to his family.
4. The adolescent should be allowed to maintain emotional defenses—including absolute denial. The adolescent will indicate by questions what types of answers are desired.
5. If the adolescent states, "I am not going to die," he or she is pleading for support. Be truthful and state, "No, you are not going to die right now."
6. The adolescent may ask, "How long do I have to live?" Adolescents are able to face reality more directly and can tolerate more direct answers. No absolute time should be given because that blocks all hope. If an adolescent has what is felt to be a prognosis of approximately 3 months, the response might be, "People with an illness like yours may die in 3 to 6 months, but some may live much longer."

Support Parents' Adaptation to Child's Death

1. Develop a care plan that includes this approach:
   a. The primary responsibility for communicating with the parents should be designated to one nurse.
   b. Information regarding the parents' concerns should be communicated to all staff members and should be included in the patient's care plan.
2. Accept parental feelings about the child's anticipated death and help parents deal with these feelings.

a. It is not unusual for parents to reach the point of wishing the child dead and to experience guilt and self-blame because of this thought.
   b. The parents may withdraw emotional attachments to the child if the process of dying is lengthy. This occurs because the parents complete most of the mourning process before the child reaches biologic death. They may relate to the child as if he or she were already dead.
3. Provide anticipatory guidance regarding the child's actual death and immediate decisions and responsibilities afterward.
   a. Describe what the death will probably be like and how to know when it is imminent. This is necessary to dispel the horrifying fantasies that many parents have. Reassure the parents that all measures will be taken to keep the child comfortable at the time of death. (*Note:* Certain diseases, despite appropriate medical interventions, may cause an uncomfortable or painful death. Parents should be promised complete comfort for their child only if this expectation is realistic.)
   b. Clarify the parents' wishes about being present at the child's death and respect their desires. See if they want to hold the child—before, during, or after the death.
   c. If appropriate, allow the parents to discuss their feelings about issues such as autopsy and organ donation in order that they may make appropriate decisions. Do not make them feel guilty if they do not consent.
   d. If necessary, assist the parents to think about funeral arrangements.
4. Be aware of factors that affect the family's capacity to cope with fatal illness, especially social and cultural features of the family system, previous experiences with death, present stage of family development, and resources available to them.
5. Contact the appropriate clergy if the family desires. Contact other extended family members for support if they wish.
6. During final hours, do not leave the family alone, unless they request it.
7. Encourage parents and siblings to share their thoughts with the dying child.
8. Provide information on bereavement support groups, usually available through hospital or church.

PEDIATRIC PROCEDURES
Restraints

 Evidence Base Crellin, D., Babl, F., Sullivan, T., et al. (2011). Procedural restraint use in preverbal and early-verbal children. *Pediatric Emergency Care, 27*(7), 622–627.

Protective measures to limit movement may be necessary for restraining children in the health care setting (see Figure 43-2). They can be a short-term restraint to facilitate examination and minimize the child's discomfort during special tests, procedures, and specimen collections. Restraints can also be used for a longer period of time to maintain the child's safety and protection from injury.

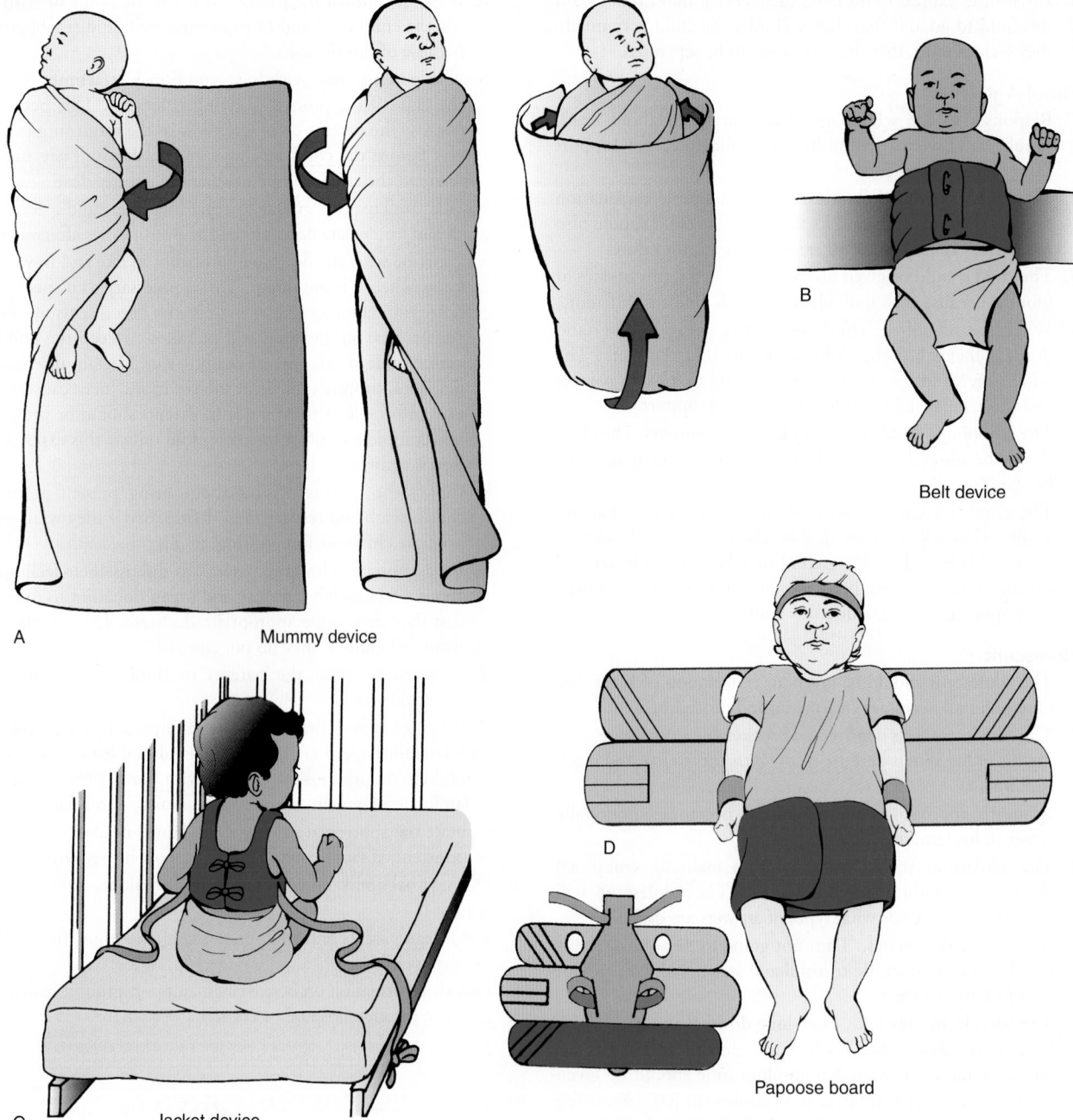

Figure 43-2. Types of restraints.

General Considerations

1. Protective devices should be used only when necessary and after all other considerations are exhausted, never as a substitute for careful observation of the child.

2. Protective devices cannot be used on a continuous basis without an order. Continuous use requires justification and full documentation of the type of restraint used, reason for use, and the effectiveness of the restraint used. Ongoing monitoring, documentation, and renewal of the order, with the length of time the restraint will be in place, are required.

3. The reason for using the protective device should be explained to the child and parents to prevent misinterpretation and to ensure their cooperation with the procedure. Children often interpret restraints as punishment.

4. Teach the child and family about specific devices they may be using in the hospital (ie, side rails) and after discharge (ie, mitts, elbow restraints).

5. Any protective device should be checked frequently to make sure it is effective and is not causing any ill side effects. It should be removed periodically to prevent skin irritation or

circulation impairment. Provide range of motion and skin care routinely.

6. Do not cover an IV site with a restraint when possible.

7. Protective devices should always be applied in a manner that maintains proper body alignment and ensures the child's comfort.

8. Any protective device that requires attachment to the child's bed should be secured to the bed springs or frame, never the mattress or side rails. This allows the side rails to be adjusted without removing the restraint or injuring the child's extremity.

9. Any required knots should be tied in a manner that permits their quick release. This is a safety precaution.

10. When a child must be immobilized, an attempt should be made to replace the lost activity with another form of motion. For example, although restrained, a child can be moved in a stroller, wheelchair, or in bed. When arms are restrained, the child may be allowed to play kicking games. Water play, mirrors, body games, and blowing bubbles are helpful replacements.

11. Restraints should be removed as soon as the child is no longer considered a danger to self or others or when medical devices are no longer in place.

 NURSING ALERT An order from a health care provider is needed to initiate continuous restraints. Proper documentation is required when restraints are in use. Do not secure restraints to bed rails or mattresses. Hourly assessment of the restrained extremity is needed to ensure there has been no impairment of circulation and constriction or respiratory compromise with chest restraints.

Mummy Device

The *mummy device* involves securing a sheet or blanket around the child's body in such a way that the arms are held to the sides and leg movements are restricted (see Figure 43-2). This short-term type of restraint is used on infants and small children during treatments and examinations involving the head and neck.

Equipment
Small sheet or blanket.

Nursing Action
1. Place the blanket or sheet flat on the bed.
2. Fold over one corner of the blanket.
3. Place the child on the blanket with shoulder at the edge of the fold.
4. Pull the right side of the blanket firmly over the child's right shoulder.
5. Tuck the remainder of the right side of the blanket under the left side of the child's body.
6. Repeat the procedure with the left side of the blanket.
7. Separate the corners of the bottom portion of the sheet and fold it up toward the child's neck.
8. Tuck both sides of the sheet under the child's body.
9. Secure by crossing one side over the other in the back and tucking in the excess, or by pinning or taping the blanket in place.

Special Precautions
Make certain the child's extremities are in a comfortable position during this procedure. Make sure that the restraint is not obstructing the child's airway.

Jacket Device

The *jacket device* is a piece of material that fits the child like a jacket or halter. Long tapes are attached to the sides of the jacket (see Figure 43-2). Jacket device restraints are used to keep the child in a wheelchair, high chair, or crib.

Nursing Action
1. Put the jacket on the child so the opening is in the back.
2. Tie the strings securely with a knot that can be easily released, if necessary.
3. Position the child in a wheelchair, high chair, or crib.
4. Secure the long tapes appropriately:
   a. Under the arm supports of a chair.
   b. Around the back of the wheelchair or high chair.
   c. To the springs or frame of a crib.

Special Precautions
Children in cribs must be observed frequently to make certain they do not become entangled in the long tapes of the jacket device. Release, reposition, and perform range of motion exercises as per hospital policy.

Belt Device

The *belt device* is exactly like the jacket method of restraining, except that the material fits the child like a wide belt and buckles in the back (see Figure 43-2).

Elbow Device

The *elbow device* is a plastic device that fits around the arm at the elbow bend and is secured with a Velcro strap. This type of restraint prevents flexion of the elbow. It is especially useful for pediatric patients receiving IV therapy, those with eczema or other skin rashes, and those following a cleft lip repair, eye surgery, or any other type of procedure or surgery in which touching the upper extremities, head, or neck should be prevented.

Equipment
1. Elbow device.
2. Skin protective material for under the device (long-sleeved shirt or gauze).

Nursing Action
1. Cover the elbow with a long-sleeved shirt or gauze if irritation or sweating is expected.
2. Place the child's arm in the center of the appropriately sized elbow restraint.
3. Wrap the restraint around the child's arm.
4. Secure with Velcro.

Special Precautions
1. The child's fingers should be observed frequently for coldness or discoloration and the skin under the device should be checked for signs of irritation.

2. The device should be removed periodically according to facility policy or standards of care to provide skin care and range of motion.

Devices to Limit Movement of the Extremities

Many different kinds of devices are available to limit motion of one or more extremities. One commercial variety consists of a piece of material with tapes on both ends to be secured to the frame of the bed. The material also has two small flaps sewn to it for securing the child's ankles or wrists. Similar devices are available that use sheepskin flaps. These should be used when the device will be necessary over a prolonged period or for children with sensitive skin. This restraining device may be used to restrain infants and young children for procedures, such as IV therapies and urine collection.

Equipment
1. Extremity restraint of appropriate size for the child (small, medium, or large).

Nursing Action
1. Secure the device to the crib or bed frame.
2. Velcro the small flaps securely around the child's ankles or wrists.

Special Precautions
1. The child's fingers or toes should be observed frequently for coldness or discoloration and the skin under the device should be checked for signs of irritation.
2. The device should be removed periodically according to policy or standards of care to provide skin care and range of motion exercises and documentation should be completed.

Abdominal Device

The *abdominal device* is used for restraining a small child in a crib. It operates exactly like the method described for limiting the movements of extremities. However, the strip of material is wider and has only one wide flap sewn in the center for fastening around the child's abdomen.

Mitts

Mitts are used to prevent a child from injuring self with his or her hands and from removing tubes or IV lines. They are especially useful for children with dermatologic conditions such as eczema or burns and for those with nasogastric or nasojejunal feeding tubes. Mitts can be purchased commercially or made by wrapping the child's hands in Kling gauze or by covering the child's hands with a pair of clean socks and securing them to the wrist with tape.

 NURSING ALERT Mitts should be removed at least every 4 hours to permit skin care and to allow the child to exercise fingers.

Crib Top Device

A *crib top device* is used to prevent an infant or small child from climbing over the crib sides. Several types of commercial devices are available, including nets, plastic tops, and domes. A crib top device should be applied to the crib of a child capable of climbing over the crib sides (usually between ages 1 and 4).

 NURSING ALERT In all instances, it is essential to be certain that the crib sides are kept all of the way up and latched securely.

Papoose Board

A *papoose board* is the most cumbersome restraint device that may be used for procedures of the head, chest, and abdomen. Straps restrain the child or infant at the forehead, lower arms, and thighs (see Figure 43-2, page 1452).

Specimen Collection

Evaluation of specimens such as blood, urine, and stool is important in determining the status of the child. The nurse should be adept in the techniques for obtaining specimens, as well as meticulous in labeling and recording them.

For blood collection, see Procedure Guidelines 43-1.

For urine specimen collection, see Procedure Guidelines 43-2, pages 1457 to 1458.

For catheterization of the urinary bladder, refer to Chapter 21. For infants and children, the catheter size is 6 to 10 F, depending on the size of the child.

For stool collection, see Procedure Guidelines 43-3, page 1459.

Feeding and Nutrition

 Evidence Base Heyland, D., Cahill, N., Dhaliwal, R., et al. (2010). Impact of enteral feeding protocols on enteral nutrition delivery: Results of a multicenter observational study. *Journal of Parenteral and Enteral Nutrition, 34*(6), 675–684.

Nutritional requirements may increase while infant or child is ill, but the ability to feed naturally may be impaired by illness or the child's response to illness. If existing feeding patterns cannot be maintained, alternate methods may be necessary. The ability to feed enterally is preferred over parenteral nutrition due to decreased risk of complications as well as improved physiological response.

Gavage Feeding

See Procedure Guidelines 43-4, pages 1460 to 1462.
1. *Gavage feeding* is a means of providing food by way of a catheter passed through the nares or mouth, past the pharynx, down the esophagus, and into the stomach, slightly beyond the cardiac sphincter. Feedings may be continuous or intermittent.
2. Gavage feedings can provide a method of feeding or administering medications that require minimal patient effort when the child is unable to suck or swallow adequately.
3. Gavage feedings can be used to administer supplemental calories to a patient who is unable to meet their caloric needs by mouth. They also can be used to provide full calories to those unable to tolerate oral intake.
4. Gavage feedings can prevent fatigue or cyanosis that can occur from bottle-feeding in susceptible infants. They can provide supplements for an infant who is a poor bottle-feeder.

(Text continues on page 1456)

PROCEDURE GUIDELINES 43-1

Assisting with Blood Collection

EQUIPMENT

- 23- to 19-gauge short needle or scalp vein needle
- Smaller volume or micro blood-collecting tubes
- Antiseptic wipes (alcohol)
- Warm compresses
- Smaller tourniquet (rubber band may be used with infant)
- Gloves per standard precautions
- Band-aid or pressure dressing

PROCEDURE

Nursing Action	Rationale
Preparatory phase	
1. Perform hand hygiene.	1. Standard precautions.
2. Immobilize the child by placing in a mummy restraint, if necessary or use distraction techniques.	2. Allows easier access to the venipuncture site and protects child from injury.
3. Position the patient.	3. These positions allow for optimal visualization and stabilization of the patient.
a. *Femoral venipuncture:* Place child on back with legs in froglike position. Place your hands on the child's knees.	a. Cover perineum to protect site in case child voids.

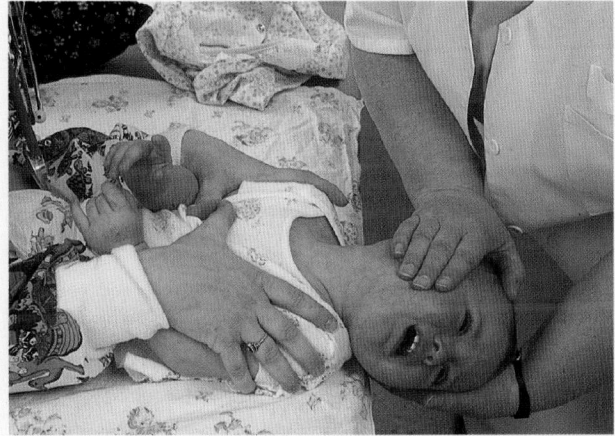

Assisting with jugular venipuncture.

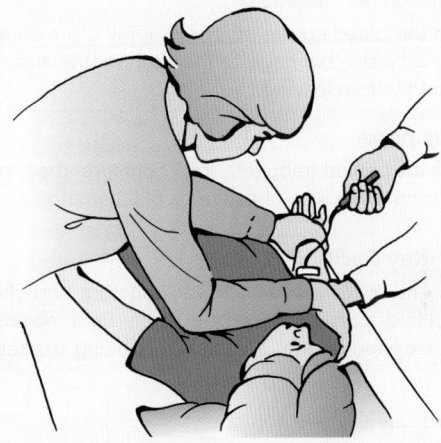

Assisting with antecubital fossa venipuncture.

b. *External jugular venipuncture:* Place the child in mummy restraint and lower head over the side of the bed or table. Turn head to side and stabilize. (See accompanying figure.)	b. Crying will make external jugular vein visible and causes blood to flow more readily.
c. *Antecubital fossa venipuncture:* Place the child in a supine position. The nurse stands on the side opposite the site to be used (across from the person drawing the specimen). The nurse positions her right arm across the upper part of the child's chest and grasps the shoulder at the axilla position. The nurse's left arm is placed across the lower part of the child's chest and is used to extend the child's arm at the wrist (see accompanying figure). If possible, allow child to sit upright while being held by parent to decrease stress of child and parent.	c. The nurse's hands are used to straighten and hold the child's arm still; arms are used to maintain stability of child's upper body.
d. *Infant—heel, toe, or digital puncture:* Warm area with warm compress for 5–10 minutes.	d. This dilates vessels, allowing blood to flow more freely, and reduces bruising.

PROCEDURE GUIDELINES 43-1 (continued)

Assisting with Blood Collection

PROCEDURE (continued)

Nursing Action	Rationale
Performance phase	
1. *Capillary:* Clean area with antiseptic and dry with sterile 2″ × 2″ gauze. Hold heel firmly and with free hand quickly puncture with microlancet or sterile 21-gauge needle on most medial or lateral part of plantar surface. Puncture deeply enough to get free-flowing blood—never deeper than 2 mm. Discard first drop of blood; rapidly collect specimen in proper capillary tube.	1. Standard precautions. Both persons holding the infant and drawing the blood should wear gloves. Gowns, masks, and goggles may be used if splattering is anticipated.
2. After the specimen is collected and the needle is removed, apply pressure to the site with dry gauze for 3–5 minutes.	2. The femoral and jugular veins are large vessels. Because intravascular pressure is great, bleeding, oozing, and hematoma formation may result. External pressure prevents this from happening.
a. *Jugular venipuncture:* While applying pressure to the site, place the patient in an upright sitting position. Do not apply excessive pressure that may compromise circulation or respiration.	a. Upright position will reduce pressure in jugular vein.
3. When the bleeding has stopped, apply a pressure dressing or adhesive bandage to the site. Soothe and comfort the child before leaving.	3. Crying and thrashing about may initiate bleeding.

Follow-up phase

1. Check the patient frequently for 1 hour after the procedure for oozing, bleeding, or evidence of a hematoma.

Key Decision Point

Anticipate bleeding if venipuncture was difficult. Hold pressure over the area until oozing has stopped (longer if the child is being treated with aspirin or an anticoagulant). Assess frequently and reapply pressure, if needed; report continued oozing or hematoma formation.

2. Record carefully and accurately:
   a. Site of venipuncture
   b. How the patient tolerated procedure
   c. Bleeding stopped or continued and for how long
   d. Test for which the specimen was collected as well as the place to which it was sent for analysis and the time at which it was sent
   e. Amount of blood loss

2. For continuity of care.

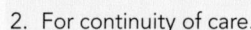

Evidence Base Bowden, V. R., & Greenberg, C. S. (2011). *Pediatric nursing procedures* (3rd ed.). Philadelphia: Lippincott Williams & Wilkins.

5. Gavage feedings can provide a safe method of feeding patients with hypotonia, patients experiencing respiratory distress, patients with uncoordinated suck and swallow, patients that are intubated, patients with a debilitation, and patients with anomalies of the digestive tract.

Gastrostomy Feeding

See Procedure Guidelines 43-5, pages 1463 and 1465.

1. Gastrostomy feeding is a means of providing nourishment and fluids by way of a tube that is surgically inserted through an

PROCEDURE GUIDELINES 43-2

Collecting a Urine Specimen from the Infant or Young Child

EQUIPMENT

- Collecting device—plastic, disposable urine bag or collector (Hollister, U-Bag, double chamber)
- Cleansing agent
- Wiping material—4" × 4" gauze pads or cotton balls
- Sterile water
- Containers for solutions
- Specimen container
- Gloves
- Chemical adhesive (tincture of benzoin)

PROCEDURE

Nursing Action	Rationale
Preparatory phase	
1. Prior to obtaining urine sample, consult facility policy or laboratory manual for type of specimen container and amount of urine to be collected.	1. Amount of urine and type of container may vary by test ordered.
2. Offer the young child a choice of fluids to drink 30–60 minutes before the procedure, if no contraindications.	2. Increases urine production.
3. Position the patient so genitalia are exposed by placing child on back with legs in a froglike position. Assistance may be needed to hold the legs of the young child in proper position.	3. Proper positioning will facilitate cleansing and allow for proper placement of collection device.
4. When small samples of urine are needed for tests to be done by the nurse, such as dipstick tests, urine can be extracted from the diaper using a syringe or dropper.	4. Several mL of urine may be collected by dropper.
Performance phase	
1. Perform hand hygiene; wear gloves.	1. Standard precautions.
2. Cleanse genital area.	2. This method of cleansing the female will prevent contamination of the genitalia from the anus and will prevent contamination of the urine specimen obtained. During the cleansing, be gentle to avoid any injury or possible stimulation of urination.
a. *Female:* Using cotton balls, dip into cleansing agent, wipe labia majora from top to bottom (clitoris to anus) only once with each cotton ball. Repeat this once more. Wipe again with sterile water. Then spread labia apart with one hand while wiping the labia minora in the same manner with other hand. Wipe area dry.	
b. *Male:* Wipe tip of penis in circular motion down toward the scrotum. Be certain to retract foreskin, if present. Wipe first with cleansing agent two to three times, then sterile water. Dry the area.	
3. Apply a chemical adhesive.	3. Helps to provide a better seal between bag and child's skin.
4. Apply collecting bag firmly so the opening is exposed to receive urine.	4. If collecting bag is properly and securely placed, it is less likely that the procedure will have to be repeated.
a. *Female:* Stretch perineum taut during application. Attach bag to perineum first, then proceed up to symphysis.	a. This should ensure leakproof contact.
b. *Male (small boys):* Place penis inside bag.	
5. Apply diaper and comfort patient; possibly give additional clear fluids.	
6. Elevate head of bed or place the child in an infant seat, if appropriate.	6. Aids flow of urine by gravity.
7. Check the patient every 5–10 minutes to see whether he or she has voided. When the patient has voided, and after gloves are on, gently remove the bag. Cleanse area and reapply diaper to the child. If the child has not voided within 45 minutes, procedure must be repeated.	7. The adhesive on the collecting bag may tend to be sticky. Careful removal of the bag will prevent skin injury on and around genitalia. Also avoid spilling urine out of the bag during removal. Reapplication of the bag will decrease the possibility of unreliable test results.

PROCEDURE GUIDELINES 43-2 *(continued)*

Collecting a Urine Specimen from the Infant or Young Child

PROCEDURE *(continued)*

Nursing Action	Rationale

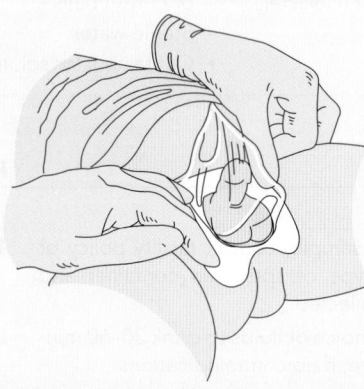

Urine collector for male infants.

Follow-up phase

Nursing Action	Rationale
1. Pour specimen into proper collecting container. Send specimen to the laboratory within 30 minutes or refrigerate.	1. Prompt delivery of specimen to the laboratory will prevent growth of organisms in an uncontrolled environment and distortion of the test results.
2. Accurately chart and describe the following in the nurse's notes:	2. For continuity of care.
a. Time specimen collection was started and ended	
b. Amount of urine voided	
c. Color of urine (cloudy, clear, any sediment)	
d. Type of test to be done	
e. Condition of skin in perianal area	

Note: If 24-hour urine collection is needed, use a collection bag that has a long tube attachment to facilitate frequent emptying of urine every 1–2 hours. Place urine in a labeled receptacle in refrigerator. Adherence of bag to skin can be improved by applying a thin coating of tincture of benzoin to skin and allowing this to dry before attaching the collection bag.

---

incision made through the abdominal wall into the stomach. A gastrostomy tube may also be placed surgically or by endoscopy using interventional radiology. Gastrostomy placement is the method of choice for those requiring tube feedings for an extended period of time (usually longer than 4 to 6 months).

2. Gastrostomy feedings provide a safe method of feeding a hypotonic or debilitated patient or one who cannot tolerate alternative methods. Prolonged feeding problems occur frequently in those with physical disabilities, prematurity, and chronic disease. Gastrostomy feedings may provide a route that allows adequate calorie or fluid intake in a child with chronic lung disease or in one who does not have continuity of the GI tract, such as in esophageal atresia, chronic reflux, or aspiration processes.

3. Gastrostomy tubes can also allow better decompression of the stomach due to larger tube size.

Community and Home Care Considerations

Gastrostomy feedings are commonly maintained for an extended period of time. If a child is receiving these tube feedings at home, nursing responsibilities include the following:

1. Teach the child (if age appropriate) and caregivers about the gastrostomy tube and feeding regimen.
   a. Anatomy of tube placement.
   b. Type of gastrostomy tube (button or tube).
   c. Amount and timing of feedings.
   d. Signs and symptoms of problems—tube obstruction or displacement, distended stomach, infection.
   e. Appropriate actions to be taken if problems occur—call home care nurse or health care provider.
2. Teach use of equipment: syringes, feeding bag, feeding tubing.

PROCEDURE GUIDELINES 43-3

Collecting a Stool Specimen

EQUIPMENT

- Diaper
- Cellophane or plastic liner (used when stool is loose or watery)
- Specimen container
- Tongue blade
- Gloves

Note: Collecting a stool specimen from an older child who is toilet-trained is the same as collecting a specimen from an adult.

PROCEDURE

Nursing Action	Rationale
Preparatory phase	
1. If a specimen is needed from a patient whose stools are loose or watery enough to be absorbed in the diaper, line the diaper with a piece of cellophane or plastic, or use urine bag to collect stool. Place liner between the diaper and the skin. Then apply diaper to the child and position so head is slightly elevated. If stools are soft or formed, apply only diaper.	1. The liner and position will allow the loose stool specimen to collect in the liner and not be absorbed by the diaper.
Performance phase	
1. Wear gloves.	1. Standard precautions.
2. Check the child frequently to see if a bowel movement has occurred.	2. A fresh specimen should be obtained so test results will not be distorted by time lapse. This will also decrease the chance of contamination of the stool with urine and will prevent skin irritation from the stool.
3. Remove soiled diaper from the child. Clean perineal area, apply clean diaper, and leave the child comfortable.	
4. Remove small amount of stool from diaper with the tongue blade and place it in the clean specimen container.	
5. Send labeled specimen to the laboratory promptly.	5. Prompt delivery to the laboratory will prevent changes from occurring in the specimen that could alter the test results.
Follow-up phase	

1. Accurately describe and record the following:
  a. Time specimen was collected
  b. Color, amount, and consistency of stool (note any foul smell or blood-tinged stool)
  c. Type of specimen collected
  d. Nature of test for which the specimen was collected
  e. Condition of the perineal and anal areas.
	1. For continuity of care.

---

3. Teach the use of feeding pump (for continuous feedings or slow boluses).
4. Teach care of the gastrostomy tube—how to clamp, observe for leakage, determine amount of water in the balloon, and change a gastrostomy tube at home if site is mature and family is willing to learn.
5. Teach stoma care—clean area with soap and water, observe for breakdown, apply skin barrier cream or powder, as appropriate.

6. Instruct about formula—proper mixing if not reconstituted; need to refrigerate if opened; discard any unused and nonrefrigerated formula after 4 hours.
7. Teach measures to take in an emergency.
   a. Procedure to follow if the tube falls out—replace tube (gastrostomy or Foley catheter), secure and cover site with gauze dressing, and call health care provider or proceed to emergency room if the tube has been in place less than 6 weeks. If tube has been in place for longer than

(Text continues on page 1465)

PROCEDURE GUIDELINES 43-4

Infant Gavage Feeding

EQUIPMENT

- Sterile rubber or plastic catheter, rounded-tip, size 5–12 French (Argyle feeding tubes)
- Clear, calibrated reservoir for feeding fluid

- 5–10 mL syringe
- Stethoscope
- Sterile water or normal saline

- Tape—hypoallergenic
- Feeding fluid, room temperature
- Pacifier

PROCEDURE

Nursing Action	Rationale
Preparatory phase	
1. Perform hand hygiene.	1. Standard precautions.
2. Position child on side or back with a rolled diaper placed under shoulders. A mummy restraint may be necessary to help maintain this position (see page 1452).	2. Allows for easy passage of the catheter, facilitates observation, and helps avoid obstruction of the airway.
3. Measure the distance from the tip of the patient's nose to earlobe to xiphoid process of sternum and mark the length on the feeding tube with tape.	3. Premeasuring the catheter provides a guideline as to how far to insert the catheter.
4. Have suction apparatus readily available.	4. Suctioning clears the airway and prevents aspiration if regurgitation occurs.
Performance phase	
1. Lubricate catheter with sterile water, normal saline solution, or water-soluble lubricant.	1. Do not use oil because of danger of aspiration.
2. Stabilize the patient's head with one hand; use the other hand to insert catheter.	2.
a. *Insertion through nares:* Slip the catheter into the patient's nostril and direct it toward the occiput in a horizontal plane along the floor of the nasal cavity. Do not direct the catheter upward. Observe for respiratory distress.	a. This direction will follow the nares' passageway into the pharynx. Positioning in nares may cause partial airway obstruction. Avoid this route if there is critical airway compromise.
b. *Insertion through the mouth:* Pass the catheter through the patient's mouth toward the back of the throat, with his or her head tilted slightly forward.	b. Facilitates passage into the esophagus
3. If the patient swallows, passage of the catheter may be synchronized with the swallowing. Do not push against resistance. Gently try rotating the tube if resistance is met.	3. Swallowing motions will cause esophageal peristalsis, which opens the cardiac sphincter and facilitates passage of the catheter. Perforation can occur with very little pressure. Prevents trauma to tissue.
4. If there is no swallowing, insert the catheter smoothly and quickly. Avoid inserting the catheter into the infant's trachea.	4. Because of cardiac sphincter spasm, resistance may be met at this point. Pause a few seconds, then proceed. An infant's anatomy makes it relatively difficult to enter the trachea because the esophagus is behind the trachea, but it may occur.

Key Decision Point

If improper placement occurs and the catheter enters the trachea, the patient may cough, fight, and become cyanotic. Remove the catheter immediately and allow the patient to rest before attempting to insert the tube again.

5. In the infant especially, observe for vagal stimulation (ie, bradycardia and apnea).	5. Stimulation of vagal nerve branches with the catheter will slow the heart rate.

PROCEDURE GUIDELINES 43-4 (continued)

Infant Gavage Feeding

PROCEDURE (continued)

Nursing Action	Rationale

Key Decision Point

If bradycardia occurs, remove tube and allow the patient to relax. If the child appears to be in distress, follow basic life support protocols and contact the health care provider. When the patient's vital signs normalize, attempt tube replacement.

6. When the catheter has been inserted to the premeasured length, tape the catheter to the patient's face (see accompanying figure).

6. Prevents movement of the catheter from the premeasured, preestablished correct position. Alternative method: Loop narrow cloth tape around the tube just below the nostril, then secure it above lip or nose with tape. Some movement of the tube may be seen with swallowing. Avoid upward pressure of the nares in order to prevent ulceration.

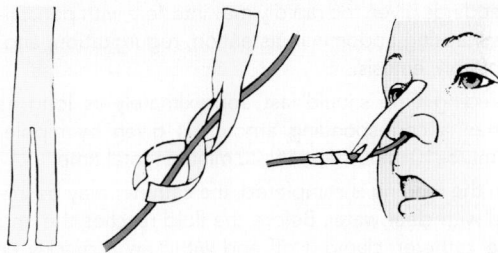

Steps in preparing adhesive tape to retain gavage tube.

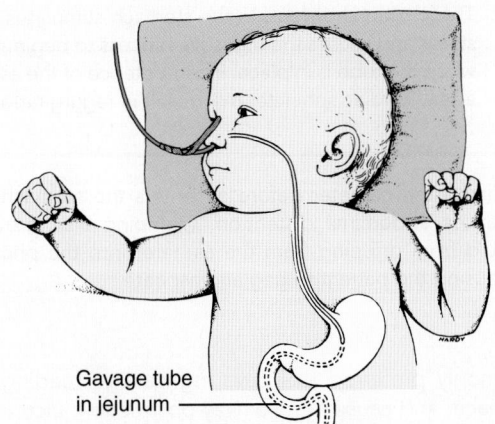

Gavage tube
in jejunum

Gavage tube in jejunum.

7. Test for correct position of the catheter in the stomach, according to institution policy. Radiographic assessment is most reliable but may subject the patient to multiple x-rays and increased exposure to radiation. Injection of air into the catheter while auscultating over the stomach is a procedure used by some; however, the preferred method is to aspirate a small amount of stomach content and test for acidity.

   If unsure of placement at any time, obtain an abdominal x-ray.

7. X-ray is the most reliable method to verify placement, but another method may be used.

   Injection of air may cause abdominal distention.

   Failure to obtain aspirate does not indicate improper placement; there may not be any stomach content or the catheter may not be in contact with the fluid.

8. Further secure the tube to the patient's cheek by using tape or Opsite. Avoid using paper tape, which loosens if exposed to secretions or formula.

8. Adhesive should not loosen easily and should be washable because it may be exposed to secretions.

9. The feeding position should be right side-lying or supine, with head and chest elevated 30 degrees. Attach the reservoir to catheter and fill with feeding fluid. Encourage the infant to suck on a pacifier during feeding. Hold the infant when possible.

9. This position allows the flow of fluid to be aided by gravity. The use of the pacifier will relax the infant, allowing for easier flow of fluid as well as provide for normal sucking needs. Sucking will help develop muscles and provide a positive association between sucking and relief of hunger.

10. Aspirate the tube before feeding begins to assess for residual contents and to remove any air.

10. This is done to monitor for appropriate fluid intake, digestion time, and overfeeding that can cause distention. Notify the health care provider of a large residual. Document any residual amount after each aspiration

(continued)

PROCEDURE GUIDELINES 43-4 (continued)

Infant Gavage Feeding

PROCEDURE (continued)

Nursing Action	Rationale
a. If over one half of the previous feeding is obtained by aspiration, withhold the next feeding. Do not return aspirate to the stomach. Notify the health care provider of the large residual volume.	a. Indicates slow gastric emptying. Overfeeding will result in distention.
b. If a small residual of formula is obtained, return it to the stomach and subtract that amount from the total amount of formula to be given. Document any residual contents.	b. Residual of less than 25% of the feeding is considered small and should be tolerated if refed. Recheck residual in 30–60 minutes and notify health care provider if it is over half.
11. The flow of the feeding should be slow. Do not apply pressure. Elevate the reservoir 6–8 inches (15–20 cm) above the patient's head.	11. The rate of flow is controlled by the size of the feeding catheter; the smaller the size, the slower the flow. If the reservoir is too high, the pressure of the fluid itself increases the rate of flow.
a. Feedings given too rapidly may interfere with peristalsis, causing abdominal distention, regurgitation, and, possibly, emesis.	a. The presence of food in the stomach stimulates peristalsis and causes the digestive process to begin. Also, when the tube is in place, incompetence of the esophageal–cardiac sphincter may result in regurgitation.
b. Feeding time should last approximately as long as when a corresponding amount is given by nipple, 5 mL/5–10 minutes or 15–20 minutes total time.	
12. When the feeding is completed, the catheter may be irrigated with clear water. Before the fluid reaches the end of the catheter, clamp it off and withdraw it quickly or keep in place for the next feeding.	12. Clamp the catheter before air enters the stomach and causes abdominal distention. Clamping also prevents fluid from dripping from the catheter into the pharynx, causing the patient to gag and aspirate.
13. Discard the feeding tube and any leftover solution.	

> **! NURSING ALERT** Intermittent gavage feeding is commonly preferred to indwelling gavage feeding. An indwelling catheter may coil and knot, perforate the stomach, and cause nasal airway obstruction, ulceration, irritation of the mucous membranes, incompetence of esophageal–cardiac sphincter, and epistaxis. However, if intermittent placement is not well tolerated and the indwelling method is used, the catheter should be clamped to prevent loss of feeding or entry of air. Some new catheters can remain in place for up to 30 days. (Use alternate sides of the nares with each tube change.) Constant alertness to the above problems should be stressed. Indwelling method may be preferred with an older infant or child.

Follow-up phase

1. Burp the patient. (The patient may not burp if air was aspirated from the tube following the feeding.)	1. Adequate expulsion of air swallowed or ingested during feeding will decrease abdominal distention and allow for better tolerance of the feeding.
2. Place the patient on right side for at least 1 hour.	2. Facilitates gastric emptying and minimize regurgitation and aspiration.
3. Observe the patient's condition after feeding; bradycardia and apnea may still occur.	3. Because of vagal stimulation, as mentioned above.
4. Note vomiting or abdominal distention.	4. Due to overfeeding or too-rapid feeding. Regurgitation of 1–2 mL may occur in the premature infant as the musculature of the sphincter of the GI tract is relaxed and allows for easy reflex.
5. Note the infant's activity.	5. Fatigue or peaceful sleep offers insight as to tolerance of the feeding.

PROCEDURE GUIDELINES 43-4 *(continued)*

Infant Gavage Feeding

PROCEDURE *(continued)*

Nursing Action	Rationale
6. Accurately describe and record procedure, including type and size of tube used, verification of placement, time of feeding, type of gavage tube feeding, type and amount of feeding fluid given, amount retained or vomited, how the patient tolerated feeding, and activity before, during, and after feeding.	6. Continuity of care. Observe for readiness of the infant to feed by nipple—note sucking activity and sleep–wake cycle in relation to feeding.

 Evidence Base Simons, S., & Abdallah, L. M. (2012). Bedside assessment of enteral tube placement: Aligning practice with evidence. *American Journal of Nursing, 112*(2), 40–48.

PROCEDURE GUIDELINES 43-5

Gastrostomy Feeding

EQUIPMENT

- Appropriately prepared feeding fluid
- Pacifier
- Reservoir syringe or feeding bag
- Syringe for aspirating

PROCEDURE

Nursing Action	Rationale
Preparatory phase	
1. Gastrostomy tube may be in one of three positions between feedings:	1.
a. Lowered and open for drainage.	a. Constant decompression.
b. Open, connected to reservoir (funnel, syringe) that is elevated 4–6 inches (10–15 cm).	b. Serves as safety valve outlet to prevent esophageal reflux and increased stomach pressure.
c. Clamped.	c. Most "normal" physiologic setup.
2. Perform hand hygiene.	2. Universal precautions.
3. The nurse may be directed to check residual stomach contents before any feeding.	3. This is done to monitor for appropriate fluid intake, digestion time, and overfeeding, which can cause distention.
a. Attach syringe and aspirate stomach contents.	
b. Measure volume.	
c. Residual fluid may be returned to stomach or discarded, depending on the amount, as per order.	c. Residual may be returned to the stomach or discarded, depending on the amount as per order. Large-volume residual may indicate reduced gastric emptying and cause abdominal distention.
d. Assess the skin around the tube for excoriation, redness, drainage.	d. May indicate infection.
4. A Y-tube that is connected at the point where reservoir and gastrostomy tube join may be used during feeding.	4. Provides simultaneous decompression (venting) during feeding.

(continued)

PROCEDURE GUIDELINES 43-5 *(continued)*

Gastrostomy Feeding

PROCEDURE *(continued)*

Nursing Action	Rationale
5. When feeding is about to begin, the patient should be placed in a comfortable position in bed—with head slightly elevated. If condition permits, the nurse or family member should hold the patient. A pacifier can be given.	5. When the patient is comfortable and relaxed, feeding fluid will flow more easily into stomach. Pacifier will satisfy normal sucking activity, provide exercise for jaw muscles, and relax musculature as well as provide pleasure normally associated with feeding.

Note: The child may have a gastrostomy button in place. In this case, insert the appropriate extension set into the button and follow the feeding procedure in the performance phase.

Performance phase

1. Attach reservoir syringe or primed feeding bag to the tube or extension set (if not already open to continuous venting) and fill reservoir syringe with feeding fluid. Unclamp the tube.	1. Prevents air from entering tube (and then stomach), which may cause distention.
2. If providing bolus feed via syringe, elevate tube and reservoir to 4–4¾ inches (10–12 cm) above the abdominal wall. Do not apply pressure to start flow. If providing continuous feedings or bolus feed via pump, program pump as prescribed and start feed via pump.	2. This elevation level will allow for slow, gravity-induced flow. Pressure may cause a backflow of fluid into the esophagus.
3. Feed slowly, taking 20–45 minutes. Fill reservoir with remaining fluid before it is empty to avoid instillation of air.	3. Too rapid a feeding will interfere with normal peristalsis and will cause abdominal distention and backflow into reservoir or esophagus.
4. Continue to provide the infant with pleasant feelings associated with feeding (ie, pacifier).	

5. When feeding is completed either:
  a. Instill clear water (0.3–1 ounce [10–30 mL]) if the tube is to be clamped. Apply clamp before water level reaches end of reservoir.
<div align="center">or</div> b. Leave tube unclamped and open to continuous elevation.
	5.
	  a. This rinses tubing and will prevent clogging.
	
	  b. Feeding fluid is allowed to return to the reservoir if the infant cries or changes position, and thus decreases pressure in the stomach.

> **Key Decision Point**
>
> If the gastrostomy tube becomes dislodged and if it is newly placed (less than 6 weeks), replace tube (if allowed in scope of practice) with gastrostomy tube or Foley catheter and secure tube. Frequently a smaller size must be used if stoma is closing. Notify health care provider before using the tube and accurately record events.
>
> If gastrostomy tube is established (more than 6 weeks) and dislodged, replace with a Foley catheter or comparable-sized gastrostomy tube and aspirate the tube for gastric contents. If gastric contents are obtained, feeds may be resumed. If there is difficulty verifying placement, notify the health care provider.

6. Commonly, when oral feedings are started, they are given simultaneously with gastrostomy feedings.	6. Allows the infant to learn or reestablish the sucking–swallowing process as well as to build up tolerance to eating without compromising nutritional intake.

Follow-up phase

1. Check dressing and skin around point of tube entry for wetness. Clean skin and apply skin barrier, if ordered. Ensure that there is no pull on the tube.	1. Skin breakdown is caused by continued exposure to stomach contents that may be leaking out around the tube, causing excoriation and infection. Constant pulling on the tube can cause widening of skin opening and subsequent leakage.

PROCEDURE GUIDELINES 43-5 (continued)

Gastrostomy Feeding

PROCEDURE (continued)

Nursing Action	Rationale
2. Leave the patient dry and comfortable. If unable to hold the patient during feeding, this may be a good time to hold and provide warmth and love. Place on right side or in Fowler's position.	2. Promotes relaxation and improved digestion of feeding.
3. Accurately describe and record procedure, including time of feeding, type and amount of feeding fluid given, amount and characteristics of residual (if any) and what was done with it, how the patient tolerated the feeding, any abdominal distention, and activity after feeding.	3. Continuity of care.

6 weeks, the tube may be replaced by the family or home care nurse
  b. Troubleshooting for nonfunctioning equipment—ensure that the pump is plugged in and turned on, tubing is unclamped, not kinked; abdomen is not distended.
  c. Proper phone numbers available to have as a resource or to obtain assistance.
8. Perform regular home visits as prescribed to assess nutritional and hydration status of the child, check tube placement and stoma site, and modify the care plan, as needed.
	1. Nasojejunal (NJ) or nasoduodenal (ND) feedings are means of providing full enteral feedings by way of a catheter passed through the nares, past the pharynx, down the esophagus, through the stomach, through the pylorus into the duodenum or jejunum.
	2. Duodenal or jejunal feedings may decrease the risk of aspiration and can minimize regurgitation and gastric distention because the feeding bypasses the stomach and pylorus.
	3. ND and NJ feedings provide a route that allows for adequate calorie or fluid intake (a full enteral feeding) by way of continuous drip.
	4. ND or NJ feedings may also provide a route for administration of enteral medications.

Nasojejunal and Nasoduodenal Feedings

See Procedure Guidelines 43-6.

PROCEDURE GUIDELINES 43-6

Nasojejunal and Nasoduodenal Feedings

EQUIPMENT

- Sterile radiopaque silicone or polyvinyl nasojejunal (NJ) or nasoduodenal (ND) tube, 36 inches (91 cm) (appropriate size for child); may have weighted tip
- Tape
- pH paper or pH probe
- Reservoir (syringe or bag) for feeding
- Appropriate feeding pump
- Three-way stopcock
- Syringe–0.5 mL normal saline solution or sterile water
- Equipment for nasogastric (NG) tube insertion; introducer catheter
- Cardiac monitoring equipment

PROCEDURE

Nursing Action	Rationale
Preparatory phase	
1. Perform hand hygiene.	1. Standard precautions.
2. Apply cardiac monitoring leads.	2. Allows for continuous monitoring of heart rate and rhythm in the event that the vagus nerve is stimulated as the catheter is passed, causing bradycardia.
3. Flush tube with 5 mL of water.	3. Confirms tube's patency and functionality.

(continued)

PROCEDURE GUIDELINES 43-6 *(continued)*

Nasojejunal and Nasoduodenal Feedings

PROCEDURE *(continued)*

Nursing Action	Rationale
4. Tube is generally inserted by a health care provider (with or without fluoroscopy).	4.
a. Measure from the tip of the patient's nose to the ear lobe then down to between the xiphoid process and the umbilicus. Add 8–10 inches and mark the tube at this measurement.	a. Equals distance to stomach.
b. Measure and mark the remaining length of tubing and record.	b. Serves as a double-check to ensure that the tube has not advanced farther than intended.
5. Place patient on right side with his or her hips slightly elevated. Gentle restraint or soft mittens may have to be applied.	5. Facilitates passage of the tube. Restraints prevent the patient from pulling out the tube before the tip passes the pylorus. Do not place on left side.
6. The tube is inserted by threading the NJ or ND through the nostril into the stomach and through the pylorus.	6. Oral insertion may cause increased salivation, air swallowing, and regurgitation.
7. Check intestinal aspirate for pH every 1–2 hours. The infant may be positioned on right side, back, or abdomen. When the tube is past the pylorus, abdominal posteroanterior and lateral x-rays are taken to confirm that the tip of the catheter is at the ligament of Treitz. Remove the guidewire. If the pH results are inconclusive or the NJ is difficult to place, it may be placed under fluoroscopy.	7. When aspiration fluid reaches a pH of 6–8 or bile-colored fluid is obtained, the tip of the tube may have passed the pylorus and duodenum into the jejunum.
8. A small NG feeding tube may be passed through the other nostril at this time and left indwelling. This is used to check stomach for residual fluid and regurgitation through the pylorus.	8. If gastric residual is significant, it will interfere with prescribed feeding. Notify the health care provider (4 mL/kg reflux in stomach is usually tolerated). Do not remove NG tube because it will adhere to NJ tube during withdrawal and also pull out the NJ tube.

Performance phase

1. NJ feedings are generally given by continuous slow drip.	1. Commonly preferred method to minimize the satiety–hunger cycle and large-volume instillation to prevent dumping syndrome.
a. Fill reservoir as needed, with no more than 4 hours' worth of feeding fluid	a. Ensures a constant flow and minimizes overinfusion directly into the jejunum or duodenum.
b. Feeding is given at room temperature. Avoid cold fluid,	b. Cold fluid may cause infant discomfort.
c. If breast milk is used, gently knead the reservoir periodically to mix settled-out fat content.	c. Breast milk may separate, providing uneven infusion of nutrients.
2. Reservoir chamber and tubing should be changed every 4 hours in the hospital and daily at home.	2. Prevents growth of bacteria.
3. Many medications may be given by way of ND and NJ tubes, if prescribed.	3.
a. A three-way stopcock will have to be placed at the connection of the NJ tube and the line from the feeding fluid.	a. Provides access port for medications without disconnecting the line each time a medication is to be administered.
b. Flush tubing with small amounts of sterile water after medication is administered. Pills should be crushed finely.	b. Ensures that the infant receives entire dosage prescribed, prevents any sediment from remaining in the tubing, and prevents tube clogging.
c. Alternative method for administering oral medications is by passing an oral–gastric or NG feeding tube	c. The stomach and process of digestion and absorption are not bypassed.

PROCEDURE GUIDELINES 43-6 (continued)

Nasojejunal and Nasoduodenal Feedings

PROCEDURE (continued)

Nursing Action	Rationale

Follow-up phase

1. Be constantly alert for mechanical problems:
   a. Tube clogging—check external tube measurement.

   b. Check for abdominal distention by palpating abdomen, measuring abdominal girth every 3–8 hours, and checking residual formula in the stomach every 3–8 hours.
   c. Check external tube measurement.
2. Discard or refeed residual formula, as prescribed.
3. Check stools for occult blood and blood glucose as ordered.

a. Due to inadequate flushing or tube advancing too far into jejunum.

b. Resulting from the patient's inability to handle ingested amount of fluid.

c. May indicate dislodgement of tube.
2. Increasing residual may cause aspiration.
3. Determines tolerance of feeding fluid.

 Key Decision Point

If abdominal pain, distention, diarrhea, or vomiting occur, stop feeds and check emesis and stools for gross blood and report to health care provider immediately—this may be a sign of necrotizing enterocolitis.

4. Stop feeding and flush tube with warm water every 4–6 hours.
5. Hold and give positive stimulation to the patient, if conditions permit.
6. Accurately document condition of the patient and the procedure, including type and amount of feeding given, amount of residual and characteristics, and any signs of impending patient distress or problems.

4. Maintains patency of tube.
5. This procedure limits the normal pleasures associated with feeding. The patient needs attention to oromotor needs.
6. Continuity of care.

---

5. ND or NJ feedings can provide a method of feeding that requires minimal patient effort when the child or infant is unable to tolerate alternative feeding methods (low birth weight, increased respiratory effort, and intubated patient).
6. ND or NJ feeding tubes may be placed under fluoroscopy, endoscopically, or at the bedside.

Fluid and Electrolyte Balance

Basic Principles

1. Infants and small children have different proportions of body water (see Table 43-3) and body fat than adults.

Table 43-3	Body Fluids Expressed as Percentage of Body Weight		
FLUID	**ADULT**		**Infant (%)**
	Male (%)	Female (%)	
Total body fluids	60	54	75
Intracellular	40	36	35
Extracellular	20	18	40

a. The body water of a neonate is approximately 75% of body weight compared with that of an average adult man, which is approximately 60%.
b. The normal neonate demonstrates a rapid physiologic decline in the ratio of body weight to body water during the immediate postpartum period.
c. Proportion of body water declines more slowly throughout infancy and reaches the characteristic value for adults by about age 2.
2. Compared with adults, a greater percentage of the body water of infants and small children is contained in the extracellular compartment.
   a. Infants—approximately one half of the body water is extracellular.
   b. Adults—approximately one third of the body water is extracellular.
3. Compared with adults, the water turnover rate per unit of body weight is three or more times greater in infants and small children.
   a. The child has more body surface in relation to weight.
   b. The immaturity of kidney function in infants may impair their ability to conserve water.
4. Electrolyte balance depends on fluid balance and cardiovascular, renal, adrenal, pituitary, parathyroid, and pulmonary regulatory mechanisms (see Table 43-4).

Table 43-4 Common Abnormalities of Fluid and Electrolyte Metabolism

SUBSTANCE AND MAJOR FUNCTION	ABNORMALITY	CAUSE	CLINICAL MANIFESTATION	LABORATORY DATA
Water				
Medium of body fluids, chemical changes, body temperature, lubricant	Volume deficit	• Primary—inadequate water intake • Secondary—loss following vomiting, diarrhea, and GI obstruction	Oliguria, weight loss, signs of dehydration including dry skin and mucous membranes, lassitude, sunken fontanelles, lack of tear formation, increased pulse rate, decreased blood pressure	Concentrated urine; azotemia; elevated hematocrit, hemoglobin level, erythrocyte count, and sodium level
	Volume excess	• Failure to excrete water in the presence of normal intake, such as in cardiac disease or failure or renal disease • Water intake in excess of output	Weight gain, peripheral edema, signs of pulmonary congestion	Variable urine volume, low specific gravity of urine, decreased hematocrit
Potassium				
Intracellular fluid balance, regular heart rhythm, muscle and nerve irritability	Potassium deficit	• Excessive loss of potassium due to vomiting, diarrhea, prolonged cortisone, corticotropin or diuretic therapy, diabetic acidosis • Shift of potassium into the cells, such as occurs with the healing phase of burns, recovery from diabetic acidosis	Signs and symptoms variable, including weakness, lethargy, irritability, abdominal distention, and, eventually, cardiac arrhythmias	Low plasma potassium level (<3.5 mEq/L) may be normal in some situations; hypochloremic alkalosis; ECG changes
	Potassium excess	• Excessive administration of potassium-containing solutions, excessive release of potassium due to burns, severe kidney disease, adrenal insufficiency • Beta-blocker therapy	Variable, including listlessness, confusion, heaviness of the legs, nausea, diarrhea, abdominal cramping, ECG changes, and, ultimately, paralysis and cardiac arrest	Elevated potassium plasma level; decreased arterial pH; ECG abnormalities
Sodium				
Osmotic pressure, muscle and nerve irritability	Sodium deficit	• Water intake in excess of excretory capacity, replacement of fluid loss without sufficient sodium; excessive sodium losses	Headache, nausea, abdominal cramps, confusion alternating with stupor, diarrhea, lacrimation, salivation, later hypotension; early polyuria, later oliguria	Sodium plasma level may be normal or low (<135 mEq/L)
	Sodium excess	• Inadequate water intake especially in the presence of fever or sweating; increased intake without increased output; decreased output	Thirst, oliguria, weakness, muscular pain, excitement, dry mucous membranes, hypotension, tachycardia, fever, agitation	Elevated sodium plasma level (>148 mEq/L), high plasma volume
Bicarbonate				
Acid-base balance	Primary bicarbonate deficit	• Diarrhea (especially in infants), diabetes mellitus, starvation, infectious disease, shock or cardiac failure producing tissue anoxia and renal failure	Progressively increasing rate and depth of respiration—ultimately becoming Kussmaul respiration; flushed, warm skin; weakness; disorientation progressive to coma	• Urine pH usually <6.0 • Plasma bicarbonate < 20 mEq/L • Plasma pH < 7.35
	Primary bicarbonate excess	• Loss of chloride through vomiting, gastric suction, or the use of excessive diuretics; excessive ingestion of alkali	Depressed respiration, muscle hypertonicity, hyperactive reflexes, tingling of fingers and toes, tetany, and, sometimes, convulsions.	Urine pH usually >7, plasma bicarbonate > 26 mEq/L (30 mEq/L in adults), plasma pH > 7.45

ECG, electrocardiographic.

5. Infants and children are more vulnerable to dehydration than adults.
   a. The basic principles relating to fluid balance in children make the magnitude of fluid losses considerably greater in children than in adults.
   b. Children are prone to severe disturbances of the GI tract that result in diarrhea and vomiting.
   c. Young children cannot independently respond to increased losses by increased intake. They depend on others to provide them with adequate fluid.

Common Fluid and Electrolyte Therapy

1. Repair of preexisting deficits that may occur with prolonged or severe diarrhea or vomiting.
   a. Deficits are estimated and corrected as soon and as safely as possible.
   b. Initial therapy is aimed at restoring intravascular and intracellular fluid volume to relieve or prevent shock and restore renal function.
   c. Intracellular deficits are replaced slowly over an 8- to 12-hour period after the circulatory status is improved.
2. Provision of maintenance requirements.
   a. Maintenance requirements occur as a result of normal expenditures of water and electrolytes due to metabolism.
   b. Maintenance requirements bear a close relationship to metabolic rate and are ideally formulated in terms of caloric expenditure.
3. Correction of concurrent losses that may occur by way of the GI tract as a result of vomiting, diarrhea, or drainage of secretions.
4. Replacement should be similar in type and amount to the fluid being lost.
5. Replacement is usually formulated as milliliters of fluid and milliequivalents of electrolytes lost.

Intravenous Fluid Therapy

IV therapy refers to the infusion of fluids directly into the venous system. This may be accomplished through the use of a needle or by venous cutdown and insertion of a small catheter directly into the vein (see Figure 43-3). IV therapy is used to restore and maintain the child's fluid and electrolyte balance and body homeostasis when oral intake is inadequate to serve this purpose (see Procedure Guidelines 43-7, pages 1470 to 1473).

1. Infusion pumps are often used in pediatrics to provide a controlled, constant rate of infusion.
2. Because infants and children are vulnerable to fluid shifts, the rates need to be monitored carefully.
3. During an IV infusion, every hour, check:
   a. Rate of infusion.
   b. Volume delivered.
   c. IV site for infiltration, because many pumps will continue to infuse solution even if infiltration has occurred.

See Standards of Care Guidelines 42-1, page 1473.

Cardiac and Respiratory Monitoring

Cardiac and respiratory monitoring refers to electrical surveillance of heart and respiratory rates and patterns. It is indicated for patients whose conditions are unstable, patients with cardiac or respiratory disorders, and patients receiving anesthesia or conscious sedation.

Nursing Management

1. Select a monitor that is appropriate for the child's needs. This will depend on the child's age and ability to cooperate, purpose for monitoring, information desired, and equipment available.
2. Stabilize the device to reduce the amount of mechanical noise and for safety considerations. Ensure the equipment is functioning well and there are no frayed cords. Plug into an emergency power outlet.
3. Reduce the child's anxiety:
   a. Provide age-appropriate explanations of the equipment.
   b. When possible, involve the child in care, including change of electrodes.

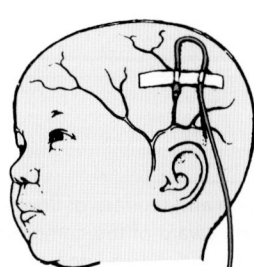

Venipuncture of scalp vein

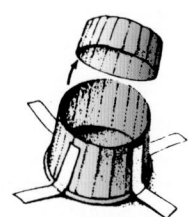

Paper cup taped over venipuncture site for protection. A clear plastic cup may also be used.

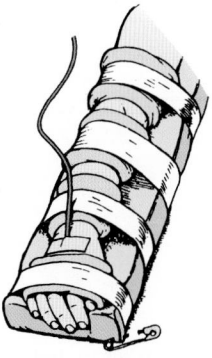

Restraint of arm when hand is site of infusion

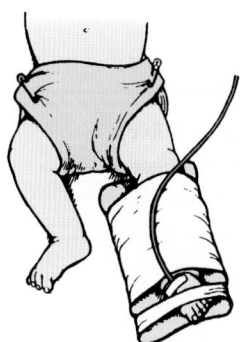

Infant's leg taped to sandbag for immobilization (I.V. site should be visible)

Figure 43-3. IV fluid therapy.

(Text continues on page 1474)

PROCEDURE GUIDELINES 43-7

Intravenous Fluid Therapy

EQUIPMENT

Needle method

- IV solution
  - The kind of solution is specified by the health care provider.
  - For small children, 250-mL bottles should be used for purposes of safety.
- IV pole, pump device
- IV administration set, pump tubing
- Micropore filter
- Syringe, 3 mL—with normal saline solution
- Butterfly needle or catheter of appropriate gauge
  - The size of the needle depends on the age and size of the child, the size and location of the vascular access, and the type of fluid to be administered
- Alcohol pads, dry pads
- Betadine or other antibacterial cleansing solution
- Normal saline solution
- Small tourniquet or rubber band
- 5-0 black silk suture with a straight-eye needle
- 1%–2% procaine
- Normal saline solution
- Tourniquet
- Sterile gloves
- Restraining devices
- Hypoallergenic (silk or cloth) tape, ½ inch, 1 inch, 2 inches
- Padded armboard
- Gauze bandage for securing the extremity to the armboard
- Restraining devices—bath blanket, extremity restraint, covered sandbags (the type of restraint depends on the child's age, level of cooperation, and the location of the IV line to be started)
- Safety razor (if scalp vein is to be used)

Cutdown method

- IV solution, IV pole, IV administration set
- Alcohol wipes
- Hypoallergenic (silk or cloth) tape, ½ inch, 1 inch, 2 inches
- Padded armboard
- Dry wipes
- Gauze bandage
- Sterile cutdown tray
  - The tray should include the following equipment: medicine cups, sterile treatment towels, wound towel, syringes, 25-gauge ⅝-inch needle and catheter, 20-gauge 1-inch needle, knife handle and #15 blade, forceps, scissors, gauze sponges, 4-0 black silk suture, needle holder
- Assorted sizes of sterile polyethylene tubing and Luer adapters
- 5-0 black silk suture with a straight-eye needle
- 1%–2% procaine
- Normal saline solution
- Tourniquet
- Sterile gloves
- Restraining devices

PROCEDURE

Nursing Action	Rationale
Inserting an IV line	
Preparatory phase	
1. Perform hand hygiene.	1. Standard precautions.
2. Obtain the IV solution.	2. Although the type of solution and the rate of flow are prescribed, the nurse should be aware of the composition of common parenteral solutions and should know how to calculate maintenance therapy.
3. Check the IV fluid for sediment or contaminant by holding the container up to the light. Ensure light-sensitive IV fluids are properly contained and covered.	3. Contaminant is most easily identified with the container in this position. If sediment is observed, the solution should be discarded.
4. Check the container for cracks.	4. If a flash of light can be seen through the bottle, it has a razor-thin crack and should be discarded.

PROCEDURE GUIDELINES 43-7 *(continued)*

Intravenous Fluid Therapy

PROCEDURE *(continued)*

Nursing Action	Rationale
5. Attach a micropore filter to the end of the infusion tubing that attaches to the catheter hub. Use aseptic technique.	5. A 0.45-μm filter prevents entry into the vein of larger particles, air emboli, and most bacterial and fungal organisms except some *Pseudomonas* organisms. A 0.22-μm filter prevents entry of any organisms but requires the use of an IV pump.
6. Remove the seal from the IV container without touching the rubber top.	6. Do not use the solution if the seal has been broken. It is not necessary to cleanse the sterile, rubber top with alcohol unless it has been accidentally contaminated.
7. Following product information, insert the end of the administration set into the container's opening. Fill the tubing with solution.	
8. Label the IV fluid and tubing with the date, time, and initials.	8. Serves as a reminder of when tubing and fluid should be changed.
9. Perform the procedure in the treatment room unless another location is requested by the patient or his or her family.	9. Although it is usually best to move the child to a different room for the procedure, some children will be less fearful if the procedure is performed in the familiar surroundings of their own rooms.
10. Promote the cooperation of the child. The family may be present, if desired. a. *Infant:* Provide with a pacifier. b. *Young child:* Avoid placing IV into the dominant extremity (ie, the hand used to suck the thumb). c. *Older child:* Explain the procedure and its purpose. d. *Adolescent:* Give choice as to the location of the IV, if possible.	10. The procedure will be less traumatic if the child is cooperative and does not resist.
11. Position the child for comfort.	
12. Restrain the child, as necessary.	12. Protective devices may be necessary to prevent the child from dislodging the IV needle or catheter. The type and size of such devices should be appropriate for the child's age and the position of the IV.
a. *Infant or young child:* Restraints may include mummy wrappings, jacket or elbow restraints, or small sandbags. b. *Older child:* The extremity to be used should be comfortably restrained on the armboard. Free extremities may also require light restraints to remind the child not to move.	b. Toes and fingers should be visible to avoid compromising blood flow. The restraint board must be padded and the main pressure points (heel, palm) padded with gauze. Before strapping an extremity to the armboard, back the adhesive with tape or gauze wherever it touches the skin.

Performance phase

1. The persons starting the IV and holding the infant should wear gloves and other protective equipment (gown, mask, and goggles) if blood splattering is anticipated.	1. Standard precautions.
2. Assist, as necessary.	2. The nurse may insert the IV, based on facility policy.
3. Check the restraints at intervals and adjust them, as necessary.	3. The restraints may become loose after a period of time and must be secured to ensure the child's safety. They may also become too tight and require loosening to maintain adequate circulation.
4. Connect and start IV fluids, as prescribed.	

(continued)

PROCEDURE GUIDELINES 43-7 (continued)

Intravenous Fluid Therapy

PROCEDURE (continued)

Nursing Action	Rationale
Follow-up phase	
1. Comfort and reassure the child.	1. The procedure is usually disturbing for the child. This should be acknowledged. If crying and upset, the child should be reassured that this behavior is acceptable.
2. Regulate the IV rate by way of a pump	2. Pump infusion devices should always be used in IV rate regulation of infants and children.
3. Record: • Type of solution being used • Reading on the container or reservoir • Rate of flow • Time that the infusion began • Name of the physician or nurse who started the IV • Site of administration • Reaction of the child to the procedure.	3. Continuity of care.
Irrigating an IV line	
1. Perform hand hygiene. Then, irrigate the IV, as necessary, if an occlusion or infiltration is suspected. Irrigate intermittent infusion devices every 8 hours.	1. Irrigation may be required to dislodge small clots in the catheter or to maintain the infusion rate of a sluggish IV.
2. Gather equipment: • Syringe with 1–3 mL normal saline solution or heparinized saline • Several alcohol wipes	
3. Clamp off the IV solution.	
4. Disconnect the IV tubing at the catheter insertion site. Keep it sterile by covering the tip with a cap.	4. Tubing can be reinserted and infusion restarted if sterility is maintained.
5. Remove the needle from the syringe.	5. Just the syringe is needed for irrigation.
6. Connect the syringe to the tubing at the catheter insertion site or stopcock.	
7. Slowly inject the normal saline solution or heparinized saline. If the catheter cannot be flushed, it may be occluded or infiltrated and removal may be necessary.	7. Great force of injector should be avoided because this may cause the vein to rupture or the catheter to become dislodged from the vein.
8. Disconnect the syringe and reconnect the IV tubing to the needle insertion site.	
9. Unclamp the IV and regulate the flow of the solution.	
10. Check frequently to make certain that the IV is functioning properly and there is no apparent infiltration.	10. Manipulation of the catheter increases risk of infiltration.
Removing an IV line	
1. Perform hand hygiene. Gather equipment: • Scissors, gloves • 2" × 2" gauze square • Adhesive bandage	
2. Stop the IV infusion when prescribed or if it has obviously infiltrated.	
3. Explain the procedure to the child (depending on the child's age).	3. Enlists cooperation.
4. Apply gloves.	4. Standard precautions.

PROCEDURE GUIDELINES 43-7 *(continued)*

Intravenous Fluid Therapy

PROCEDURE *(continued)*

Nursing Action	Rationale
5. Remove the tape and armboard from the extremity.	5. Provides open access to IV site.
6. Loosen the tape around the catheter, holding it firmly in position so it does not slip out.	6. Careless dislodgment of the catheter may cause bleeding and bruising.
7. Hold the 2″ × 2″ gauze lightly over the insertion site and remove the needle quickly and carefully.	7. Alcohol wipes should not be used for removing IV catheters because the stinging of alcohol on the puncture site causes unnecessary discomfort. If the intracath or plastic needle is not intact, notify the health care provider.
8. Apply pressure to the site immediately and hold until bleeding stops.	8. Aids clotting.
9. Apply adhesive bandage.	9. The bandage should not be applied until all bleeding has stopped to minimize the possibility of prolonged or unnoticed bleeding.
10. Comfort the child as required.	
11. Note the fluid level on the container or reservoir and complete recordings.	11. Documentation for continuity of care.
12. Record that the IV was discontinued.	

For additional information relating to IV therapy, including criteria for selecting a suitable vein for venipuncture, guidelines for administering an infusion using the antecubital fossa, and complications of IV therapy, refer to Chapter 6, Intravenous therapy.

STANDARDS OF CARE GUIDELINES 43-1
Pediatric IV Therapy

When caring for a child undergoing IV therapy:

- Check IV site hourly, noting skin color and evidence of swelling. Compare to the opposite extremity or look for asymmetry. Feel area for sponginess. Observe for leakage.
- Check the IV tubing and equipment hourly. Stop the infusion if any cracks are noted in the tubing or there is discoloration of the IV fluid.
- Record the reading on the container or reservoir, amount of fluid absorbed in the hour, flow rate.
- Check for blood return in the tube by stopping IV fluid flow. It may be normal not to see blood return due to small catheter size.
- Check function of pump rate set versus amount infused.
- Maintain accurate intake and output record and 24-hour totals.
- Describe consistency and approximate volume of all stools and vomitus.

- Weigh child at regular intervals, using the same scale each time. An increase or decrease of 5% body weight in a relatively brief time period is usually significant.
- Monitor electrolytes (see Table 43-4, page 1468).
- Report evidence of electrolyte imbalances: decreased skin turgor, marked increase or decrease in urination, fever, sunken or bulging fontanelles, sudden change in vital signs, diarrhea, weakness, lethargy, apathy, pyrogenic reactions, and arrhythmias.
- If the child is experiencing severe reactions, the IV should be discontinued and the solution saved for possible analysis.
- Change the IV container and tubing every 24 hours or as per facility policy.
- If infiltration occurs, remove the IV, raise the affected extremity, apply heat to the site, and restart the IV at an alternative site. Notify the health care provider if irritation develops or toxic medication has infiltrated.

This information should serve as a general guideline only. Each patient situation presents a unique set of clinical factors and requires nursing judgment to guide care, which may include additional or alternative measures and approaches.

4. Select lead placement sites according to equipment specifications:
   a. Cardiac monitors frequently use three leads located at:
      i. Right upper chest wall below the clavicle.
      ii. Left lower chest wall in the anterior axillary line.
      iii. Left upper chest wall below the clavicle.
   b. Respiratory monitors frequently use three electrodes located:
      i. On either side of the chest (anterior axillary line in fourth or fifth intercostal space).
      ii. A reference electrode placed on the manubrium or other suitable distal point.
5. Apply electrodes by:
   a. Cleaning the appropriate areas on the chest with soap and water.
   b. Placing pregelled, disposable electrodes to dry skin.
6. Plug the leads into the lead cable at appropriate insertion points.
7. Make sure that the monitor alarms are in the "on" position. High and low alarm limits should be set according to the child's age and condition so that apnea, tachypnea, bradycardia, and tachycardia can be readily detected.
8. Avoid skin breakdown by changing lead placement sites, as needed. Clean and dry old sites and expose them to air.
9. Check integrity of the entire system at least once per shift.
   a. Carefully inspect lead wires and cable for breaks and proper attachment.
   b. If malfunction is suspected, change equipment and notify the engineering department or manufacturer immediately.
10. Continue to count respiratory and apical rates at least once per shift.
   a. Compare with monitor rates to verify accuracy of equipment.
   b. It must be remembered that monitors cannot substitute for close observation and nursing assessments of the child.

Cardiopulmonary Resuscitation

Evidence Base American Heart Association. (2010). *BLS for the healthcare provider: Student manual.* Dallas, TX: Author.

Cardiopulmonary resuscitation (CPR) involves measures instituted to provide effective ventilation and circulation when the patient's heart and lungs have ceased to function. In children, the most common initial cause is respiratory distress.

Underlying Considerations

Cardiac Arrest
1. Signs—absence of heartbeat and absence of carotid and femoral pulses.
2. Causes—asystole, ventricular fibrillation, cardiovascular collapse, shock, or progression of respiratory failure.

Respiratory Arrest
1. Signs—apnea and cyanosis.
2. Causes—obstructed airway, depression of the central nervous system, neuromuscular paralysis.

Emergency Preparation
1. Every hospital should have a well-defined and organized plan to be carried out in the event of cardiac or respiratory arrest.
2. Emergency carts should be placed in strategic locations in the hospital and checked daily to ensure that all equipment is available.
3. Personnel should be trained in up-to-date CPR maneuvers and be certified in Basic Life Support at least every 2 years.

Equipment
1. Emergency cart—assembled and ready for use.
2. Positive-pressure breathing bag with nonrebreathing valve and universal 15-mm adapter.
3. Mask (premature neonate, child, adult sizes).
4. Oropharyngeal airway tubes, sizes 0 to 4.
5. Laryngoscope with blades of various sizes.
6. Extra batteries and light bulbs for laryngoscope.
7. Endotracheal tubes with connectors (complete sterile set, 2.5- to 8-mm inner diameter).
8. Portable suction equipment and sterile catheters of various sizes.
9. Bulb syringe, DeLee trap.
10. Oxygen source—portable supply, gauge, and tubing.
11. Cardiac board (30 × 50 cm).
12. Emergency drugs:
    a. Sodium bicarbonate.
    b. Epinephrine.
    c. Isoproterenol.
    d. Normal saline solution (for dilution).
    e. Diphenhydramine.
    f. Diazepam.
    g. Hydrocortisone sodium succinate.
    h. Digoxin.
    i. Naloxone.
    j. Calcium gluconate.
    k. Calcium chloride 10%.
    l. Dextrose 50%.
    m. Lidocaine.
    n. Atropine.
    o. Phenytoin.
    p. Insulin.
    q. Procainamide.
    r. Propranolol.
    s. Dopamine.
    t. Bretylium tosylate.
    u. Volume expanders (lactated Ringer's solution, normal saline solution).
    v. Vasopressin.
    w. Amiodarone.
    x. Magnesium sulfate.
    y. Vecuronium.
13. Intracardiac needles, 20 and 22G, 2 to 3 inches long.
14. IV equipment, including infusion set, IV fluids.
15. Tourniquet, armboards, tape.
16. Scalp vein needles of various sizes.

17. Gloves, mask, gown, other protective barriers.
18. Nasogastric tubes of various sizes.
19. Syringes and syringe needles of various sizes.
20. Intraosseous needles.
21. Longdwell catheters of various sizes.
22. Three-way stopcock.
23. Cutdown set.
24. Alcohol wipes.
25. Tongue blades.
26. Sterile 4″ × 4″ gauze pads.
27. Sterile hemostat.
28. Sterile scissors.
29. Blood specimen tubes.
30. Electrocardiograph (ECG) monitor, lead wires.
31. Defibrillator and paddles (pediatric and adult), lubricating jelly.
32. Arrest documentation record and patient-specific labels.

Artificial Ventilation

Mouth-to-Mouth Technique

1. Infants:
   a. Slightly extend neck by gently pulling chin up and forward and the head back by pressing forehead into a neutral position (known as head tilt–chin lift; use jaw thrust if cervical trauma is suspected). Place a rolled towel or diaper under the infant's shoulder or use one hand to support the neck in an extended position. Do not hyperextend the neck because this narrows the airway.
   b. Check the mouth and throat, and clear mucus or vomitus with finger or suction, if visible.
   c. Take a breath.
   d. Make a tight seal with your mouth over the infant's mouth and nose.
   e. Gently blow air from the cheeks and observe for chest rise. Give a total of two slow breaths.
   f. Remove your mouth from infant's mouth and nose and allow the infant to exhale.
   g. If spontaneous respiration does not return, continue breathing at a rate and volume appropriate for the size of the infant (usually 12 to 20 times/minute or 1 breath every 3 to 5 seconds).
2. Children older than age 1 year:
   a. Clear mouth of mucus or vomitus with fingers or suction.
   b. Extend neck with one hand or a rolled towel (head tilt, chin lift, or jaw thrust, if cervical trauma is suspected).
   c. Clamp the nostrils with the fingers of one hand, which also continues to exert pressure on the forehead to maintain the neck extension.
   d. Take a deep breath.
   e. Make a tight seal with your mouth over the child's mouth.
   f. Force air into the lungs until the chest expansion is observed.
   g. Release your mouth from the child's mouth and release nostrils to allow the child to exhale passively. Give a total of two slow breaths.
   h. Repeat approximately 10 to 12 times/minute or 1 breath every 5 to 6 seconds if spontaneous breathing does not occur.

Hand-Operated Ventilation Devices

1. Remove secretions from mouth and throat and move chin forward.
2. Appropriately extend the neck with one hand or place a diaper roll behind the neck.
3. Select an appropriate-sized mask to obtain an adequate seal and connect mask to bag.
4. Hold the mask snugly over the mouth and nose, holding the chin forward and the neck in extension.
5. Squeeze the bag, noting inflation of the lungs by chest expansion. If there is no chest expansion, realign the patient's head and adjust the mask; retry.
6. Release the bag, which will expand spontaneously. The child will exhale and the chest will fall.
7. Repeat 12 to 20 times/minute (depending on the size of the child).
8. Because this technique is commonly difficult to master, it should be practiced in advance, under supervision.

Indications of Effective Technique

1. Victim's chest rises and falls.
2. Rescuer can feel in his or her own airway the resistance and compliance of the victim's lungs as they expand.
3. Rescuer can hear and feel the air escape during exhalation.
4. Victim's color improves.

Management of Complications

1. Gastric distention (occurs frequently if excessive pressure is used for inflation).
   a. Turn victim's head and shoulders to one side.
   b. Exert moderate pressure over the epigastrium between the umbilicus and the rib cage.
   c. A nasogastric tube may be used to decompress the stomach.
2. Vomiting.
   a. Turn patient on side for drainage.
   b. Clear the airway with finger or suction.
   c. Resume ventilations after the airway is clear and patent.

Artificial Circulation

General Principles Related to Artificial Circulation

See Table 43-5, page 1476. See also Figure 43-4, page 1477.

1. A backward tilt of the head lifts the back in infants and small children. A firm support beneath the back is therefore essential if external cardiac compression is to be effective.
2. A supine position on a firm surface is mandatory. Only in this position can chest compression squeeze the heart against the immobile spine enough to force blood into the systemic circulation.
   Because most infant/child cardiac arrests are the result of respiratory failure or shock, there is a decrease in the oxygen levels in the blood prior to the arrest. Thus, chest compressions alone are not an effective method for delivering oxygen to the heart and brain.
   a. This is different from cardiac arrest in an adult, in which the blood usually has a high level of oxygen and compressions alone are an effective way to deliver oxygen to the heart and brain.

Table 43-5	Technique of Artificial Circulation			
SIZE OF CHILD	PREPARATORY PHASE	ACTION PHASE	COMPRESSION	RATE
Neonate, premature, or otherwise small infant	1. Place in supine position. 2. Encircle the chest with the hands, with thumbs over the midsternum. *or* Use method for a larger infant.	1. Compress midsternum with both thumbs, gently but firmly.	⅓ the depth of the chest (approximately 1½ inches)	At least 100/min
Larger infant	1. Place on a firm, flat surface. 2. Support the back with one hand or use a small blanket under the shoulders. 3. Place the tips of the index and middle fingers of one hand over the midsternum, just below the nipple line.	1. Compress the midsternum with the tips of the index and middle fingers.	⅓ the depth of the chest (approximately 1½–2 inches)	At least 100/min
Small child	1. Place on a firm, flat surface. 2. Support the back by slipping one hand beneath it, or use a small blanket. 3. Place the heel of one hand over the midsternum, parallel with the long axis of the body (at the nipple line).	1. Apply a rapid downward thrust to the midsternum, keeping the elbow straight. 3. Instantly and completely release the pressure so the chest wall can recoil. 4. Do not remove the heel of the hand from the chest.	⅓ the depth of the chest (approximately 2 inches)	At least 100/min
Larger child, adolescent	1. Place on a flat, firm surface, or place a board under the thorax. 2. Place the heel of one hand on the lower half of the sternum, about 1–1½ inches (2.5–3.8 cm) from the tip of the xiphoid process and parallel with the long axis of the body. 3. Place the other hand on top of the first one (may interlock fingers). 4. Place shoulders directly over child's sternum, in order to use own weight in application of pressure.	1. Exert pressure vertically downward to depress lower sternum, keeping elbows straight. 3. Instantly and completely release the pressure so the chest wall can recoil. 4. Do not remove the hands from the chest.	2 inches (5 cm)	At least 100/min

3. Compressions must be regular, smooth, and uninterrupted. Avoid sudden or jerking movements. Push hard and push fast. Compressions should be done at a rate of at least 100 compressions/minute.

4. The chest must recoil (return to normal position) fully after each compression.

5. Between compressions, the fingers or heel of the hand must completely release their pressure but should remain in constant contact with the chest. This allows for complete recoil of the chest while minimizing interruptions to the compressions.

6. Fingers should not rest on the patient's ribs during compression. Pressure with fingers on the ribs or lateral pressure increases the possibility of fractured ribs and costochondral separation.

7. Never compress the xiphoid process at the tip of the sternum. Pressure on it may cause laceration of the liver.

8. Indications of effective technique include:
   a. A palpable femoral or carotid pulse.
   b. Decrease in size of pupils.
   c. Improvement in the patient's color.

Nursing Management

1. Recognize cardiac and respiratory arrest.

2. Send for assistance and note time.

3. Initiate CPR:
   a. Check for responsiveness and breathing; if the patient is unresponsive and not breathing, palpate a pulse. Checking for a pulse should not take more than 10 seconds.
   b. If no pulse is felt, institute artificial circulation using appropriate technique.
   c. For an infant or child, each cycle contains a ratio of 30 compressions to two breaths, starting with compressions.
   d. Continue repeating this cycle until help arrives.
   e. If alone, perform CPR as previously described for five cycles or 2 minutes of CPR, then call for help. After call, resume CPR until help arrives.

4. When help arrives:
   a. One rescuer performs mouth-to-mouth resuscitation or institutes bag breathing.
   b. Another rescuer performs cardiac compressions.
   c. A ratio of 15 compressions to two breaths is maintained for both infants and children.
   d. Cardiac compression should not be stopped for respiration. Breaths should be interposed on the upstroke of each fifth cardiac compression.

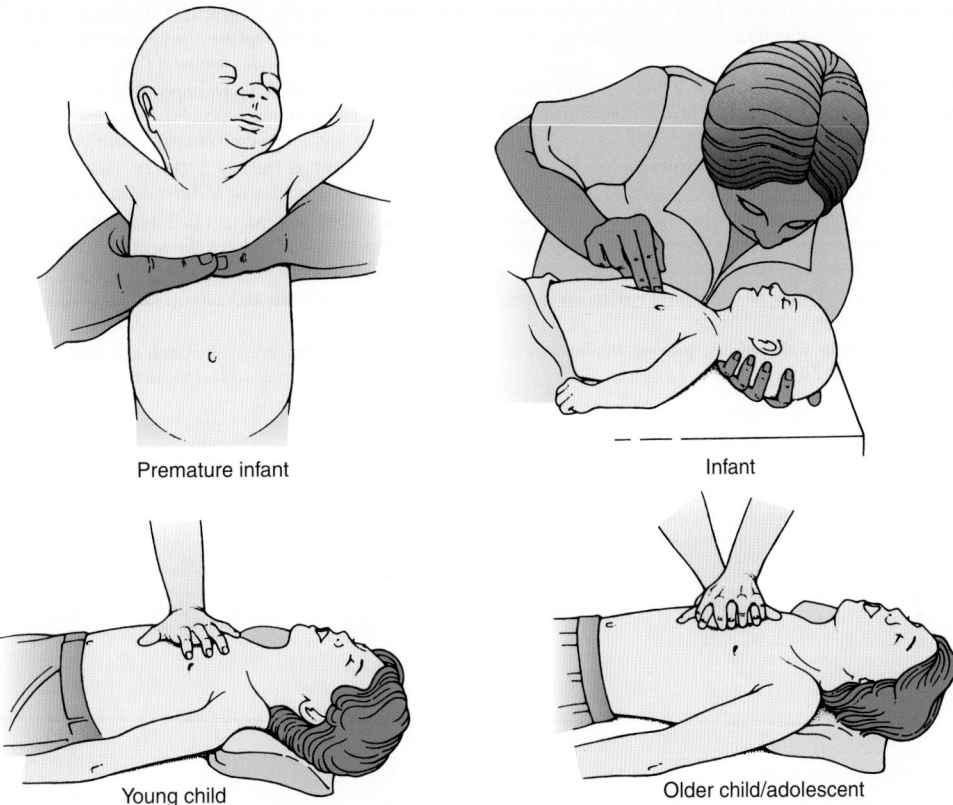

Premature infant

Infant

Young child

Older child/adolescent

Figure 43-4. Cardiopulmonary resuscitation in children. In the young child, the heel of the hand is placed over the lower sternum at the nipple line. In older children and adolescents, both hands are used.

5. Anticipate and assist with emergency procedures.
   a. Assist with intubation, monitoring, placement of intravascular access, administration of IV fluids, defibrillation, and other definitive measures.
   b. Prepare and administer emergency medications, as prescribed. Record dose and time.
   c. Notify family of current management and CPR.
6. After resuscitation:
   a. Care for the child, as required.
   b. Determine if family members have been notified and are being cared for.
   c. Record all events.
   d. Restock emergency cart.

SELECTED REFERENCES

Acara, K., & Tschudy, M. (Eds.). (2011). *The Harriet Lane handbook* (19th ed.). Philadelphia: Elsevier.

American Heart Association. (2011). *BLS for the healthcare provider: Student manual.* Dallas, TX: Author.

Arbour, R., & Kirk, A. (2012). Patient safety: Restraint reduction, restraint elimination, and best practice. *Critical Care Nurse,* 2012 Apr; *32*(2): e54–5.

Arif-Rah, M., Fisher, D., Matsuda, Y. (2012). Biobehavioral measures for pain in the pediatric patient. *Pain Management Nursing, 13*(3), 157–168.

Bowden, V. R., & Greenberg, C. S. (2011). *Pediatric nursing procedures* (3rd ed.). Philadelphia: Lippincott Williams & Wilkins.

Braegger, C., Decsi, T., Dias, J. A., et al. (2010). Practical approach to paediatric enteral nutrition: A comment by the ESPGHAN committee on nutrition. *Journal of Pediatric Gastroenterology and Nutrition, 51*(1), 110–122.

Burton-Shepard, A. (2012). Nutritional management of children who follow therapeutic diets for medical reasons. *Primary Health Care, 22*(9), 32–39.

Chorney, J., & Kain, Z. (2010). Family-centered pediatric perioperative care. *Anesthesiology, 112*(3), 751–755.

Fergusson, D. M., Boden, J. M., Horwood, L. J. (2013). Nine-year follow-up of a home visitation program: A randomized trial. *Pediatrics, 131*(2), 297–303.

Field, J. M., Hazinski, M., Sayre, M., et al. (2010). Part 1: Executive summary: 2010 American Heart Association guidelines for cardiopulmonary resuscitation and emergency cardiovascular care. *Circulation, 122*(18, Suppl. 3), S640–S656.

Goldberg, E., Barton, S., Xanthopoulos, M., et al. (2010). A descriptive study of complications of gastrostomy tubes in children. *Journal of Pediatric Nursing, 25*(2), 72–80.

Habich, M., Wilson, D., Thielk, D., et al. (2012). Evaluating the effectiveness of pediatric pain management guidelines. *Journal of Pediatric Nursing–Nursing Care of Children & Families, 27*(4), 336–345.

Herr, K., Coyne, P. J., McCaffery, M., et al. (2011). Pain assessment in the patient unable to self-report: Position statement with clinical practice recommendations. *Pain Management Nursing, 12*(4), 230–250.

Heyland, D., Cahill, N., Dhaliwal, R., et al. (2010). Impact of enteral feeding protocols on enteral nutrition delivery: Results of a multicenter observational study. *Journal of Parenteral and Enteral Nutrition, 34*(6), 675–684.

Hockenberry, M. J., & Wilson, D. (2010). *Wong's essentials of pediatric nursing* (9th ed.). Philadelphia: Elsevier.

Johnston, C., Rennick, J. E., Filion, F., et al. (2012). Maternal touch and talk for invasive procedures in infants and toddlers in the pediatric intensive care unit. *Journal of Pediatric Nursing, 27*(2), 144–153.

Kars, M. C., Grypdonck, M. H. F., & van Delden, J. J. M. (2011). Being a parent of a child with cancer throughout the end-of-life course. *Oncology Nursing Forum, 38*(4), E260–E271.

Kozlowski, L. J., Kost-Byerly, S., Colantuoni, E. (in press). Pain prevalence, intensity, assessment, and management in a hospitalized pediatric population. *Pain Management Nursing.* (posted online June 2012).

Kubler-Ross, E. (1997). *On death and dying.* New York: Scribner.

Landier, W., & Tse, A. (2010). Use of complementary and alternative medical interventions for the management of procedure-related pain, anxiety, and distress in pediatric oncology: An integrative review. *Journal of Pediatric Nursing, 25*(6), 566–579.

Longo, M. (2011). Best evidence: Nasogastric tube placement verification. *Journal of Pediatric Nursing, 26*(4), 373–376.

Nielson, D. (2012). Discussing death with pediatric patients: Implications for nurses. *Journal of Pediatric Nursing, 27*(5), e59–64.

Pagé, M., Katz, J., Stinson, J., et al. (2012). Validation of the numerical rating scale for pain intensity and unpleasantness in pediatric acute postoperative pain: Sensitivity to change over time. *Journal of Pain, 13*(4), 359–369.

Peterson, K. A., Phillips, A. L., Truemper, E., et al. (2012). Does the use of an assistive device by nurses impact peripheral intravenous catheter insertion success in children? *Journal of Pediatric Nursing, 27*(2), 134–143.

Rhoda, K., Porter, M., & Quintini, C. (2011). Fluid and electrolyte management: Putting a plan in motion. *Journal of Parenteral and Enteral Nutrition, 35*(6), 675–685.

Simons, S., & Abdallah, L. M. (2012). Bedside assessment of enteral tube placement: Aligning practice with evidence. *American Journal of Nursing, 112*(2), 40–48.

Vincent, C., Chiappetta, M., Beach, A., et al. (2012). Parents' management of children's pain at home after surgery. *Journal for Specialists in Pediatric Nursing, 17*(2), 108–120.

Woods, W. (2012). Pediatric resuscitation and cardiac arrest. *Emergency Medicine Clinics of North America, 30*(1), 153–168.

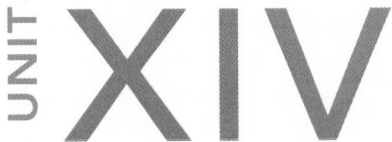

44

Pediatric Respiratory Disorders

PEDIATRIC RESPIRATORY PROCEDURES

Oxygen Therapy

Children with respiratory problems may receive oxygen therapy via nasal cannula, mask, face tent, endotracheal tube, or tracheostomy device. An Isolette or oxygen hood may also be used for infants and young children. See Procedure Guidelines 44-1, pages 1480 to 1482.

Mechanical Ventilation

Infants and children requiring mechanical ventilation need specialized care. These patients are typically treated in facilities that focus on providing a safe environment for technology-dependent children, with care provided by highly skilled nurses, respiratory therapists, and pediatricians. Specific nursing procedures and interventions and management of technology-dependent infants and children are beyond the scope of this text. General considerations are as follows.

Maintenance of a Patent Airway

1. Artificial airway options include nasotracheal, orotracheal, and tracheostomy. Endotracheal (ET) and tracheostomy tubes are available in several sizes, cuffed and uncuffed, for the pediatric population.

a. Several methods are available to determine the appropriate size, such as: ET tube size = age in years + 16 divided by 4 (consult facility policy).

2. The patient should be closely monitored for hypoxia and bradycardia during intubation.

a. Only experienced and highly trained and skilled practitioners should perform intubation.

b. Resuscitation and reintubation equipment, access to oxygen and suction equipment must always be readily available.

c. An appropriate-size self-inflating bag with reservoir for oxygenation and mask should remain with the patient.

3. Action should be taken to prevent dislodgement of the artificial airway (especially during movement of the child) and obstruction of the airway.

a. Pediatric ET tubes have small diameters and are easily obstructed by thick secretions.

b. Adequate humidification will loosen secretions and suctioning will prevent airway obstruction.

c. Frequent vital signs and respiratory assessments are necessary. Cardiorespiratory monitors, pulse oximeter, end-tidal carbon dioxide, or transcutaneous carbon dioxide monitors are also necessary.

PROCEDURE GUIDELINES 44-1

Oxygen Therapy for Children

PROCEDURE

Nursing Action	Rationale
1. Explain the procedure to the child and allow the child to feel the equipment and the oxygen flowing through the tube and mask.	1. The child will be reassured if he or she understands the procedure and knows what to expect.
2. Maintain a clear airway by suctioning, if necessary.	2. The delivery of oxygen requires a clear airway.
3. Provide a source of humidification.	3. Oxygen is a dry gas and requires the addition of moisture to prevent drying of the tracheobronchial tree and thickening and consolidating secretions.

4. Measure oxygen concentrations every 1–2 hours when a child is receiving oxygen through incubator hood.
    a. Measure when the oxygen environment is closed.
    b. Measure the concentration close to the child's airway.
    c. Record oxygen concentrations and simultaneous measurements of the pulse and respirations.
	4. It is desirable to keep the oxygen concentration as low as possible while still providing for physiologic requirements. This minimizes the child's risk of developing retinopathy of prematurity. (Desired oxygen concentrations are determined by the arterial oxygen tension measurement.) The oxygen analyzer should be calibrated daily on both room air and 100% oxygen. The concentration of oxygen within the space is determined by litre flow, efficiency of the equipment, and frequency with which it is opened to the external environment.

5. Observe the child's response to oxygen.	5. Desired response includes:
	    a. Decreased restlessness.
	    b. Decreased respiratory distress.
	    c. Improved color.
	    d. Improved vital sign values.

6. Organize nursing care so interruption of therapy is minimal.	6. Interruption of therapy may result in the return of anoxia and defeats the goals of therapy.
7. Periodically check all equipment during each span of duty.	7. For optimal functioning, the equipment should be clean, undamaged, and in good working order.
8. Clean equipment daily and change it at least once per week. (Tubing and nebulizer jars should be changed daily.)	8. Unclean equipment may be a source of contamination.

9. Keep combustible materials and potential sources of fire away from oxygen equipment.
    a. Avoid using oil or grease around oxygen connections.
    b. Avoid the use of wool blankets and those made from some synthetic fibers.
    c. Prohibit smoking in areas where oxygen is being used.
    d. Have a fire extinguisher available.
    e. Avoid lengthy oxygen tubing in any young child that is not being constantly supervised.
	9. Oxygen supports combustion.
	
	    a. Are easily combustible.
	    b. May cause injury due to static electricity.
	
	    c. Limits the risk of fire.
	
	    e. May be at risk for injury including strangulation in active children.

10. Terminate oxygen therapy gradually.
    a. Slowly reduce litre flow.
    b. Open air vents in incubators.
	10. Allows the child to adjust to normal atmospheric oxygen concentrations.

11. Continually monitor the child's response during weaning. Observe for restlessness, increased pulse rate, respiratory distress, and cyanosis.	11. These are indications that the child is unable to tolerate reduced oxygen concentration.

Oxygen by nasal cannula or catheter

1. Refer to Procedure Guidelines 10-12, page 239.	
2. Nasal cannulas are available in a variety of sizes for neonates, infants, and children.	
3. Low-flow meters are available to titrate oxygen at levels under 1 L/minute.	3. Lower flow rate may be necessary for infants.

PROCEDURE GUIDELINES 44-1 *(continued)*

Oxygen Therapy for Children

PROCEDURE *(continued)*

Nursing Action	Rationale

Oxygen by mask

1. Choose an appropriate-size mask that covers the mouth and nose of the child but not the eyes.
2. Use a mask that is capable of delivering the desired oxygen concentration.
3. Place the mask over the child's mouth and nose so it fits securely. Secure the mask with an elastic head grip.
4. Remove the oxygen mask at hourly intervals; wash and dry the face.
5. Do not use masks for comatose infants or children.

6. For additional information, refer to Procedure Guidelines 10-14, page 242, and Procedure Guidelines 10–13, page 240.

1. Extra space under mask and around face is added dead space and decreases effectiveness of the therapy.
2. Venturi masks for pediatric use deliver low to moderate concentrations of oxygen: 24%, 28%, 31%, 35%, or 40%.
3. Make sure the mask is adjusted properly over the mouth and nose. Do not allow the oxygen to blow in the child's eyes.
4. Makes the patient feel more comfortable.
5. Such children are more likely to vomit. The risk of aspiration may be increased with mask therapy because of obstruction of the flow of vomitus.

Face tent

1. Face tents are available in adult size only. They can be used effectively in pediatric patients if inverted to create a smaller reservoir and better fit.
2. A flow of 8–10 L/minute should be used to flush the system and provide a stable oxygen concentration.

1. Face tents combine the positive qualities of aerosol masks and mist tents. The child is accessible and may continue to play without feeling confined.
2. Larger children will require higher flows.

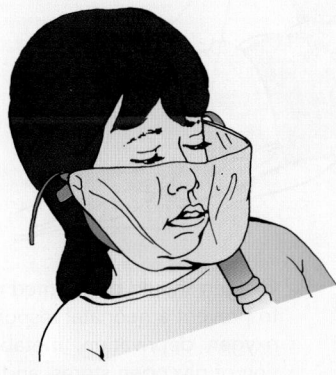

A child receiving humidity and oxygen by way of an aerosol face tent.

T-Bars and tracheostomy masks

1. These devices are used to deliver oxygen to intubated patients.
2. The flow rate must be set to meet the minute volume requirements of the child and to provide a 100% source of gas.

2. T-bars require a short, flexible tube on the distal end to act as a reservoir and prevent room-air entrapment.

Closed incubator and Isolettes

1. The incubator is used to provide a controlled environment for the neonate.
2. Adjust the oxygen flow to achieve the desired oxygen concentration.
   a. An oxygen limiter prevents the oxygen concentration inside the incubator from exceeding 40%.
   b. Higher concentrations (up to 85%) may be obtained by placing the red reminder flag in the vertical position.

1. The unit is able to provide precise environmental control of temperature, oxygen, humidity, and isolation.
2. Follow manufacturer's instructions for each make of incubator.
   a. This is desirable because it reduces the hazard of the child's developing retinopathy of prematurity.
   b. This operates by reducing the air intake.

(continued)

PROCEDURE GUIDELINES 44-1 *(continued)*

Oxygen Therapy for Children

PROCEDURE *(continued)*

Nursing Action	Rationale
3. Secure a nebulizer to the inside wall of the incubator if mist therapy is desired.	3. This should be cleaned and autoclaved daily. Sterile solutions are used to keep the bacteria count at a minimum.
4. Keep sleeves of incubator closed to prevent loss of oxygen.	4. When the incubator or sleeves are opened, supply supplemental oxygen with oxygen mask to face and nose.
5. Periodically analyze the incubator atmosphere.	5. Be certain the child is receiving the desired concentration of oxygen.
6. Drain and fill reservoirs with sterile water at least every 24 hours.	6. Decreases risk of *Pseudomonas* contamination.

Oxygen hood/box

1. Warmed, humidified oxygen is supplied through a plastic container that fits over the child's head. This method is more suitable for a child under 1 year of age.	1. This is especially useful when high concentrations of oxygen are desired. The hood may be used in an incubator or with a warming unit.
	Oxygen should not be allowed to blow directly into the infant's face.

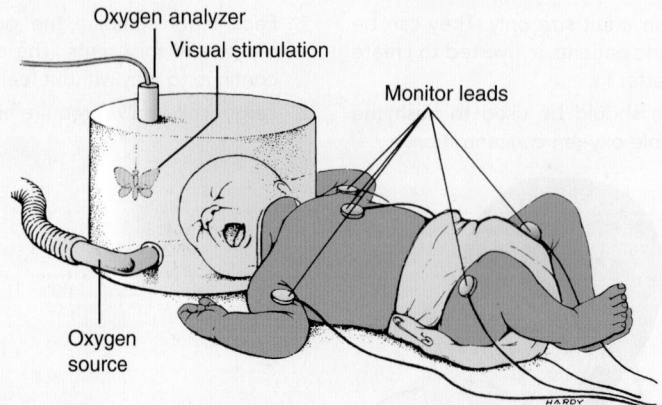

Oxygen analyzer
Visual stimulation
Monitor leads
Oxygen source

2. Continuously monitor the oxygen concentration, temperature, and humidity inside the hood.	2. Oxygen should be warmed to 87.8°–93.2° F (31°–34° C) to prevent a neonatal response to cold stress, including oxygen deprivation, metabolic acidosis, rapid depletion of glycogen stores, and reduction of blood glucose levels.
3. Open the hood or remove the baby from it as infrequently as possible.	3. Prevents fluctuations of heat and oxygen, which may further debilitate the young infant.
4. Several different designs are available for use. The manufacturer's directions should be carefully followed.	4. This is a safety consideration.

 Evidence Base Ghuman, A. K., Newth, C. J. L., & Khemani, R. G. (2010). Respiratory support in children. *Paediatrics and Child Health, 21,* 4.

4. Nursing care should continue to address issues of hydration, nutrition, sedation, skin integrity, tissue perfusion, infection control, communication, safety, and parental support and education.

5. Available ventilators for pediatric use have a wide range of capabilities, versatility, and clinical application. Some are more suitable for use with infants, others with older children.

   a. Nurses must be well acquainted with the characteristics of the particular machine being used and the meaning of the settings and alarms on the machine.

Nursing Management

See Procedure Guidelines 10-19, page 254. In addition, the nurse who is caring for a pediatric patient should remember the following.

Setting Controls

In setting controls, inspiratory flow rate will be less and the respiratory rate will be greater than in the adult patient. These depend on the patient's size and condition and are determined by the health care provider or respiratory therapist.

Humidification

During ventilation of an infant in an incubator, the amount of ventilator tubing outside the incubator should be kept to a minimum. The warm temperature inside the incubator helps decrease the amount of condensation in the tubing and thus provides higher water content in the inspired gas.

Oxygen Concentration

1. In infants, inspired concentrations of oxygen should always be kept as low as possible (while still providing for physiologic requirements) to prevent the development of retinopathy of prematurity or pulmonary oxygen toxicity.

2. The oxygen concentration should be checked periodically with an analyzer.

Blood Gases

1. Blood gas analysis to monitor oxygenation, via arteriopuncture or umbilical or arterial lines.

2. The arterialized capillary sample method is inaccurate for infants in respiratory distress because the constricted peripheral circulation may not reflect the ABG (arterial blood gases) levels accurately.

Sterile Precautions

The neonate has only those antibodies transferred across the placenta from the mother. Therefore, sterile precautions are essential.

1. Ventilator tubing should be changed every 24 hours.

2. Routine cultures should be taken after intubation; there should be daily Gram staining of secretions.

3. Suctioning requires aseptic technique.

Tubing Support

1. Special frames are available to support ventilator tubing; this helps to prevent accidental decannulation in infants and small children.

2. Infants may require support or padding on either side and at the top of their heads to decrease mobility and take up space between the head and the frame.

Monitoring the Ventilator

1. Pressure gauges should be checked at frequent intervals because this gives an indication of changing compliance or increased airway resistance.

2. Volume measurements are difficult to obtain in infants because most spirometers incorporated into ventilators and meters do not read accurately at low volumes and flows. However, they are helpful with older children.

3. Measure respiratory rates of the machine and the patient at least every hour and record.

DISORDERS
Common Pediatric Respiratory Infections

Respiratory tract infection is a frequent cause of acute illness in infants and children. Many pediatric infections are seasonal. The child's response to the infection will vary based on the age of the child, causative organism, general health of the child, existence of chronic medical conditions, and degree of contact with other children. Information about specific respiratory infections, including bacterial pneumonia, viral pneumonia, *Pneumocystis* pneumonia, *Mycoplasma* pneumonia, bronchiolitis, croup, and epiglottitis, may be found in Figure 44-1 and Table 44-1, pages 1484 to 1492.

Nursing Assessment

Determine the severity of the respiratory distress that the child is experiencing. Make an initial nursing assessment.

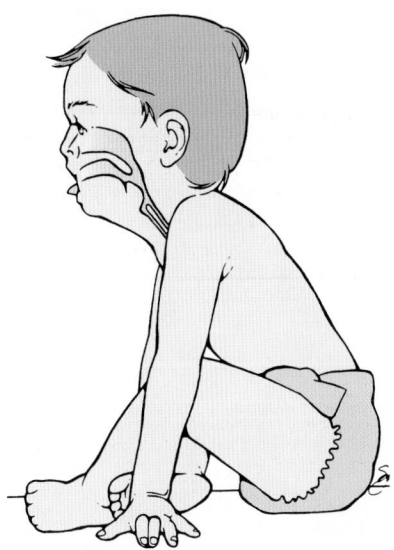

Figure 44-1. Characteristic posture of a child with acute epiglottitis: leaning forward on hands, in the "tripod" position; mouth open, tongue out, head forward and tilted up in a sniffing position in an effort to relieve the acute airway obstruction secondary to swollen epiglottis.

(*Text continues on page 1492*)

Table 44-1   Common Pediatric Respiratory Infections

CONDITION AND CAUSATIVE AGENT	AGE AND INCIDENCE	CLINICAL MANIFESTATIONS
Bacterial Pneumonia Bacterial infection of the lung parenchyma. General considerations: In the normal child, bacterial pneumonias are not common. A viral respiratory infection commonly occurs before bacterial pneumonia. The initial viral infection alters the lungs' defense mechanisms.		
Pneumococcal pneumonia • The most common causative agent is *Streptococcus pneumoniae*. **NURSING ALERT** Pneumococcal polysaccharide vaccine provides protection from 23 types of *Streptococcus pneumoniae*. It is recommended for children age 2 years and older with sickle cell disease, functional or anatomic asplenia, nephrotic syndrome, human immunodeficiency virus (HIV) infection, and Hodgkin's disease before beginning cytoreduction therapy.	• Responsible for the majority of bacterial pneumonias in ages 1 month through 6 years. However, it is seen in all age groups. • The incidence has declined due to the use of the vaccine. • Most common in winter and spring.	• *Infants:* Mild URI of several days' duration, poor feeding, decreased appetite. • Abrupt onset of fever 102.2° F (39° C) or higher; restlessness, respiratory distress, air hunger, pallor, cyanosis (common), nasal flaring, retractions, grunting, tachypnea, tachycardia, irritability; may see abdominal distention due to swallowed air or ileus. • *Older child:* Mild URI, followed by fever up to 104.9° F (40.5° C), shaking chills, headache, decreased appetite, abdominal pain, vomiting, drowsiness, restlessness, irritability, lethargy, rhonchi, fine crackles, dry hacking cough, increased respirations, anxiety, occasionally circumoral cyanosis, pleuritic pain, diminished breath sounds, may develop a pleural effusion, empyema.
Streptococcal pneumonia • Beta-hemolytic Streptococcus group A	• Ages 3–5 years. Uncommon, serious. • An endemic influenza predisposes to streptococcal pneumonia and tracheobronchitis.	• Sudden onset, high fever, chills, worsening cough, pleuritic pain, respiratory distress, grunting, retractions, altered mental status, signs of shock, decreased capillary refill, tachycardia. • May be insidious, mildly ill, low-grade fever. • Severe infections—toxic shock syndrome with erythematous rash, desquamation, hypotension, hepatic dysfunction, renal involvement, vomiting and diarrhea, hematologic abnormalities, acute respiratory distress syndrome.
Staphylococcal pneumonia • Staphylococcus aureus, Gram-positive	Most common in children ages 6 months to 1 year. October–May (rare)	• Predisposing factors: cystic fibrosis, maternal infection, immunodeficiency. • Usually preceded by a viral URI. Changes abruptly to high fever, cough, respiratory distress, tachypnea, grunting, nasal flaring, cyanosis, retractions. • Anxiety, lethargic, occasionally vomiting, diarrhea, anorexia, abdominal distention, toxic appearance.

DIAGNOSTIC EVALUATION	TREATMENT	NURSING CONSIDERATIONS	COMPLICATIONS
• Chest x-ray: Commonly does not correspond to clinical findings. • *Infants:* Patchy, diffuse areas follow a bronchial distribution, many limited areas of consolidation around smaller airways. • *Young and older child:* Lobar or segmental consolidation; pleural fluid may be present. • WBC count elevated, ABG analysis indicates hypoxemia. • *Cultures:* Sputum, nasopharyngeal secretions, pleural fluid, blood.	• Oxygen. • Penicillin G; penicillin allergy: erythromycin, trimethoprim-sulfamethoxazole, alternately amoxicillin, ampicillin, cefuroxime, cefotaxime, ceftriaxone, clindamycin, chloramphenicol. • Due to the increased incidence of penicillinase-resistant pneumococci, all pneumococcal isolates should be tested for resistance. Vancomycin has been recommended for penicillin-resistant strains. • Bronchodilators.	• Bed rest, monitor fluids, intake and output. Give oral fluids cautiously to avoid aspiration. Do not give oral fluids to a child in respiratory distress. • Administer oxygen with humidification. Perform frequent, thorough respiratory assessment. • Administer antipyretics as prescribed. • Change position frequently. Isolation procedures, as ordered or per facility policy.	• Rare, but include bacteremia, empyema, pleural effusion, otitis media, sinusitis, meningitis, hemolytic uremic syndrome, lung abscess, necrotizing pneumonia.
• Initial chest x-ray may be normal or slightly abnormal. Within 24 hours, chest x-ray worsens. • Unilateral lobar disease, bilateral diffuse infiltrates with severe disease. • Blood cultures, nasopharyngeal secretions cultured, throat swab, culture pleural fluid and lung aspirate. • Leukocytosis, sedimentation rate increased, elevated serum ASO titer.	• Penicillin G	• Administer antipyretics. • Provide humidified oxygen, as needed. Rest. Monitor intake and output.	• Empyema, toxic shock syndrome, severe respiratory compromise, pneumatoceles. Can be life-threatening.
• *Older infant/child:* Elevated WBC count, especially polymorphonuclear cells. • *Young infant:* WBC count may be normal, mild to moderate anemia. • Cultures—pleural fluid, lung aspirate, sputum, gastric aspirate, blood. • If pulmonary fluid is purulent and of a large amount, closed chest drainage may be utilized. • Chest x-ray: Patchy infiltrate, may involve entire lobe or hemithorax. Right lung involvement common; bilateral involvement is also seen. Pleural effusion, empyema, pyopneumothorax, pneumatoceles, pneumothorax, lung abscesses.	• Thoracentesis • Nafcillin, oxacillin, methicillin, cefazolin, clindamycin, vancomycin. MRSA exists, especially in long-term care facilities or in patients with a prolonged hospital stay.	• Isolation per policy, check for MRSA, prevent nosocomial infection. • Rapid treatment is important. Administer antibiotics as soon as possible. Monitor for signs of tension pneumothorax. Monitor fluid status closely. • Strict handwashing. • Staphylococcal pneumonia is rare and must be treated aggressively due to rapid onset and deterioration.	• Empyema, tension pneumothorax, abscess, fibrothorax, bronchiectasis, osteomyelitis, staphylococcal pericarditis. Consider screening infants for cystic fibrosis and immunodeficiency.

(continued)

Table 44-1   Common Pediatric Respiratory Infections (*continued*)

CONDITION AND CAUSATIVE AGENT	AGE AND INCIDENCE	CLINICAL MANIFESTATIONS
Bacterial Pneumonia (*continued*)		
***Haemophilus influenzae*, type B**	• Majority of children younger than age 4 years. • Infants and children who are not immunized. • Winter and spring.	• Usually preceded by URI. Associated with otitis media, epiglottitis, and meningitis; appears toxic. • Insidious onset; cough, febrile, tachypneic, nasal flaring, retractions.
Viral Pneumonia		
• Respiratory syncytial virus (RSV); para-influenza virus types 1, 2, 3; Adenoviruses types 1, 2, 5, 6 and types 3, 7, 11, 21; Influenza A and B.	• Peak age for bronchiolitis is within the first year of life. Peak age for viral pneumonia is age 2.3 years. • Typically seen in the winter months.	• Usually preceded by URI with symptoms of cough, rhinitis, and mild fever. Progressing to tachypnea, poor feeding in infants and retractions (suprasternal, intercostal, subcostal and substernal), leading to nasal flaring. Along with use of accessory muscles, wheezing, severe cough, cyanosis, and respiratory fatigue. • Viral pneumonia may present concurrently with bacterial pneumonia. Adenovirus types 3, 7, 11, and 21 may cause severe necrotizing pneumonia in infants.
• RSV subgroup A (more virulent, associated with more severe disease); RSV subgroup B	• In infants, RSV is the most common cause of pneumonia, bronchiolitis, and hospitalizations. • Severity of RSV infection decreases with age and subsequent infections. • Peak age is 2–7 months, October–April.	• Typically begins with URI, rhinorrhea, fever usually less than 102° F (38.9° C), otitis media, and conjunctivitis. • Progressing to coughing, wheezing, tachypnea (greater than 70 breaths/minute), intercostal and subcostal retractions, poor air exchange, hypoxia, decreased breath sounds, cyanosis, lethargy, listless apneic episodes, and irritability. Infants will present with poor feeding, inability to suck and breathe.

DIAGNOSTIC EVALUATION	TREATMENT	NURSING CONSIDERATIONS	COMPLICATIONS

• Chest x-ray: Usually lobar infiltrates; however, segmental, single, or multiple lobe infiltrates are also seen. Pleural effusion, pneumatocele. CBC: elevated WBC, lymphopenia.
• Cultures: blood, pleural fluid, lung aspirates, and nasal secretions. In the absence of a positive culture, a positive urine latex agglutination can confirm diagnosis.
• If atelectasis is present, bronchoscopy to rule out foreign body.
	• Patients may present receiving antibiotics for otitis media.
	• Ceftriaxone and other cephalosporins, ampicillin, chloramphenicol, azithromycin.
		• Administer antibiotics on time.
		• Ensure adequate hydration. Monitor for signs of upper respiratory impairment, drooling, stridor, and dusky color.
		• Respiratory isolation until 24 hours after appropriate antibiotic therapy is initiated.
		• Rifampin prophylaxis should be considered for close household contacts if there are:
		  • Incomplete or unvaccinated members younger than age 2 years.
		  • Immunocompromised child.
		  • Daycare setting with two or more cases of invasive disease within 2 months and incompletely vaccinated children in attendance.
		• Not recommended for pregnant women.
			• Frequently in young infants, bacteremia, pericarditis, cellulitis, empyema, meningitis, pyarthrosis.

• Chest x-ray shows patchy infiltrates, transient lobal infiltration, and hyperinflation. • CBC: slightly elevated WBC count. • Cultures: blood and nasopharyngeal secretions. • Viral antigens for rapid diagnosis.	• If bacterial pneumonia is suspected, administer antibiotics. • Supportive measures: IV fluids, antipyretics, humidified oxygen, assisted ventilation. • Avoid aspirin due to risk of Reye's syndrome. • Oseltamivir or zanamivir for influenza infection.	• Monitor closely for signs of respiratory fatigue or distress. • Monitor oxygen saturation levels and response to oxygen therapy if hypoxic. • Close cardiac monitoring may be indicated. • Monitor for adequate hydration and nutritional status. Elevate infants up to an angle of 10–30 degrees to ease breathing. Infants and children who require mechanical ventilation require close supervision and frequent monitoring. Institute contact precautions with strict handwashing. • Prevention: influenza vaccine.	• Influenza: severe fulminant pneumonia with hemorrhagic exudate. Death may result. Severe disease may be seen in children with cardiopulmonary disease, cystic fibrosis, bronchopulmonary dysplasia, and neurovascular disease. • Type B—myositis.
• Nasopharyngeal secretions for rapid antibody or assay for RSV antigen detection. • Chest x-ray: chest hyperexpanded, air trapping, multiple lobe infiltrates, atelectasis. • ABG analysis. • Pulse oximetry.	• Supportive measures, such as oxygen, respiratory support, hydration. • Bronchodilators should not be used routinely. • Racemic epinephrine can be effective in bronchiolitis. • Glucocorticoids and ribavirin are not supported in the literature. • Antibiotics only if a secondary bacterial infection is suspected.	• Prevent nosocomial spread. Institute contact isolation. Strict handwashing. • RSV-positive patients should not be in contact with other high-risk patients, such as those with chronic cardiac or respiratory illness or immunocompromised patients. • Assess frequently for signs of respiratory failure. • Use noninvasive oxygen monitoring.	• RSV can be fatal, especially in children with chronic cardiac and respiratory diseases, premature infants, and those with underlying neuromuscular or immunologic diseases. • Respiratory failure, intubation, and mechanical ventilation. • In older children with asthma, RSV can cause an acute asthmatic episode.

(continued)

Table 44-1   Common Pediatric Respiratory Infections (*continued*)

CONDITION AND CAUSATIVE AGENT	AGE AND INCIDENCE	CLINICAL MANIFESTATIONS
Viral pneumonia (*continued*)		
Respiratory syncytial virus (continued)		
***Pneumocystis Carinii* Pneumonia** • *P. carinii*, also known as *P. jiroveci*, is a fungus with similarities to a protozoa. The organism exists in three forms in the tissues: trophozoite, sporozoite, and cyst.	• Most healthy humans are infected before age 4 years and are asymptomatic. • Life-threatening pneumonia is seen in the immunosuppressed host. PCP in severely immunocompromised children with acquired or congenital immunodeficiency disorders, malignancies, organ transplant recipients, and debilitated, malnourished, and premature infants. In HIV-infected children it most commonly occurs between ages 3 and 6 months. PCP can occur during remission or relapse in patients with leukemia or lymphoma.	• Slow onset, tachypnea, retractions, and nasal flaring cyanosis. • Sporadic form in immunocompromised patients. Signs may vary; onset may be acute or fulminant. • Fever, tachypnea, dyspnea, cough, nasal flaring, cyanosis, subacute, diffuse pneumonitis with dyspnea at rest, tachypnea and decreasing oxygen saturation. Extrapulmonary sites rarely occur and usually produce no symptoms.
Mycoplasma Pneumonia • *Mycoplasma pneumoniae*, microorganisms with properties between bacteria and viruses.	• Fall and winter. • Crowded living conditions. Seen frequently in school age children and adolescents.	• Slow onset; 2- to 3-week incubation period. Coryza, malaise, headache, anorexia, normal temp or low-grade fever, sore throat, muscle pain, vomiting, subacute tracheobronchitis, shortness of breath, dry cough that progresses to mucopurulent cough, mild chest pain, wheezing. May present with maculopapular rash.
Bronchiolitis • Inflammation of the bronchioles. Causative agents: RSV, adenovirus, parainfluenza type 1 or 3, influenza virus, and *M. pneumoniae*.	• Winter and spring. • Most common in infants younger than 6 months old, may occur up to age 2 years. • Greater incidence in males than females. • Increased in daycare centers.	• Gradual onset after exposure to an individual with URI. Coryza, tachypnea, respiratory rate greater than 50 bpm, retractions, wheezing, paroxysmal cough, fever, cyanosis, dehydration, poor feeding, vomiting, tachycardia, irritability, dyspnea. • Apnea may be first sign in infants with RSV. Decreased breath sounds with prolonged expiratory phase. Hypoxemia may persist for 4–6 weeks.

DIAGNOSTIC EVALUATION	TREATMENT	NURSING CONSIDERATIONS	COMPLICATIONS
	• Early detection is important in hospitalized patients. Institute contact precautions with strict handwashing. RSV Immune Globulin (RSV-IGIV) and palivizumab may be given to prevent infection in select patient populations. Consult AAP Guidelines for specific information.	• In tachypneic patients and those in respiratory distress, oral fluids are contraindicated due to risk of aspiration.	
• Chest x-ray: Bilateral, diffuse, alveolar disease with a granular pattern, initially perihilar densities, which progress to peripheral and apical areas. • Organism cannot be cultured from routine specimens. • Open lung biopsy is the most reliable method. • Bronchoalveolar lavage is also utilized to obtain samples. Needle aspiration of the lung. IgM-ELISA: elevated. CBC: mild leukocytosis, moderate eosinophilia.	• PCP mortality is 5%–40% in immunocompromised patients; if untreated, 100%. • Trimethoprim-sulfamethoxazole; rate of adverse reactions is high in HIV-infected patients. • Pentamidine, parenterally or aerosolized. IV form associated with increased risk of adverse reactions. Aerosolized for children ages 5 and older. • Corticosteroids recommended for children older than age 13, may be used in younger children.	• Close monitoring of respiratory status, hydration, and nutrition. • Monitor for adverse reactions to therapy: vomiting, nausea, rash. • Respiratory isolation should be instituted for 48 hours after initiation of therapy. • PCP prophylaxis (see page 1717). **NURSING ALERT** Pentamidine is associated with a high incidence of adverse reactions: pancreatitis, renal dysfunction, hypoglycemia, hyperglycemia, hypotension, fever, and neutropenia. Pentamidine should not be used with didanosine, which also causes pancreatitis, and in patients with hepatic dysfunction.	—
• Chest x-ray: bronchopneumonic, diffuse bilateral infiltrates. • Complement fixation test: increased. Cold agglutinins: increased. Immunofluorescent and enzyme immunoassay tests. • Positive sputum culture.	• Erythromycin, azithromycin, clarithromycin, tetracycline, and doxycycline may be used in children ages 8 and older.	• Children should be on secretion precautions. • Monitor fever. • Assess need for cough suppressants.	• May be fatal if infection becomes systemic or if the child has a preexisting chronic lung disease, sickle cell anemia, immunodeficiencies, or cardiac disease. Those with Down syndrome can develop severe pneumonia. • Pleural effusions.
• Chest x-ray: patchy or peribronchial infiltrates, hyperinflation of lungs with flattening of diaphragms. Some will present with a normal chest x-ray. • Nasopharyngeal viral cultures. • Serologic studies for specific organisms. ABG analysis for children with respiratory distress.	• Humidified oxygen, ventilatory assistance as needed. (Note treatment for RSV above regarding bronchodilators, glucocorticoids, antibiotics.) • Antipyretics for fever. • Continuous cardiac monitoring for apnea or bradycardia. • Pulse oximetry.	• Avoid high-density humidity; may cause bronchospasm. • Monitor fluid and electrolyte balance closely. Place infant on apnea monitor. • Keep nasal passages free of secretions; infants are obligate nose breathers. • Position patient upright to facilitate breathing. Monitor closely for signs of impending respiratory failure. • There is a high risk of cross-contamination to noninfected children. Institute contact precautions and respiratory isolation. • Monitor oxygenation levels with noninvasive monitoring.	• Increasing respiratory distress resulting in the need for mechanical ventilation. • Secondary bacterial infection. • Pneumothorax and pneumomediastinum. Apneic episodes, may be life-threatening in children with chronic respiratory or cardiac disease. • Some infants demonstrate abnormal lung functions months after infection.

(continued)

Table 44-1   Common Pediatric Respiratory Infections (*continued*)

CONDITION AND CAUSATIVE AGENT	AGE AND INCIDENCE	CLINICAL MANIFESTATIONS
Croup Syndromes Croup syndromes refer to infections of the supraglottis, glottis, subglottis, and trachea.		
Acute laryngotracheobronchitis (subglottic croup) • Parainfluenza types 1, 2, 3; RSV; influenza A and B; adenovirus; measles.	• Ages 3 months to 5 years. Peak ages 1–2 years. • Greater incidence in males than females. • Late autumn, early winter.	• Usually a preceding URI is seen. Initially, a mild brassy or barking cough, hoarse, intermittent stridor, progresses to continuous stridor. • Nasal flaring, suprasternal, infrasternal, intercostals, retractions. • Breathing labored, prolonged expiratory phase. Temperature slightly elevated. • Crying and agitation aggravate signs. • Child prefers to be held upright or sit up in bed. Symptoms are worse at night. • Severe croup: restlessness, air hunger, decreased breath sounds, hypoxemia, hypercapnia, anxiety, cyanosis, tachycardia, and cessation of breathing.

 NURSING ALERT If ABG analysis is done, a normal partial pressure of arterial carbon dioxide may not indicate decreased severity. By the time hypercapnia is seen, intubation will be required.

Spasmodic croup and acute spasmodic laryngitis • No infectious agents seen. Thought to be related to spasm of laryngeal muscle. • Cause may be viral in a few cases, allergic or psychological.	• Ages 1–6 years. • Peak incidence 7–36 months.	• Similar to acute laryngotracheobronchitis. Symptoms are sudden, in the evening. • Afebrile, barking, brassy cough, hoarse, stridor. Child may be anxious and frightened. • Breathing is noisy on inspiration, slow, and labored; respiratory distresses. • Tachycardia. Skin cool, moist. Dyspnea is worse with excitement. • Cyanosis is rare; severity decreases over time. Patient appears well in the morning, may cough or sound hoarse. The symptoms may recur for subsequent nights; however, they will be less severe.
Bacterial tracheitis (pseudomembranous croup) • Tracheal inflammation in the subglottic region. • *S. aureus, H. influenzae*, streptococci groups A and B, *Escherichia coli, Klebsiella, Moraxella catarrhalis*, Pseudomonas, *Chlamydia trachomatis*, and *Corynebacterium diphtheriae* should be considered in the nonvaccinated patient.	• No season variation. • Age is variable, 1 month to 6 years; however, most are younger than age 3 years.	• Usually follows a viral illness. Slow or sudden deterioration, child appears toxic. • High fever, stridor, hoarse, respiratory distress. Thick, purulent, copious airway secretions. • Mucosal necrosis, brassy or barking cough. Epiglottitis may coexist. May cause life-threatening airway obstruction.
Acute epiglottitis • Supraglottitis, inflammation of the epiglottis and edema of the arytenoepiglottic folds. • *H. influenzae* type B, most common. *S. pneumoniae, S. aureus*, group A. *Beta-hemolytic streptococcus, Streptococcus pyogenes, Moraxella catarrhalis*, and *Candida albicans* (in the immunocompromised).	• Range ages 2–7 years; peak ages 3–5 years. • Autumn and winter. • Incidence significantly decreased due to the routine use of the *H. influenzae* vaccine.	• Sudden fulminating course, high fever, toxic appearance, sore throat, drooling, dysphagia, aphonia, retractions, air hunger, anxiety, tachycardia, hoarseness, irritability, restlessness, rapid progression to respiratory distress. • Sitting forward, neck hyperextended, mouth open, tongue protruding. Older child will sit in tripod position. Drooling, agitation, and absence of spontaneous cough are predictive of epiglottitis. • Absence of croupy cough.

DIAGNOSTIC EVALUATION	TREATMENT	NURSING CONSIDERATIONS	COMPLICATIONS
• Diagnosis is made by clinical evaluation and careful history. A croup score may be assigned to grade severity. Lateral neck x-ray: subglottic edema, narrowing with normal supraglottic structures. Anterior/posterior neck film: steeple sign. • Lower airway involvement.	• Racemic epinephrine nebulized with oxygen. Monitor pulse and cardiac rhythm. • Severe airway edema may require intubation. • Corticosteroid therapy. • Antibiotic therapy.	• Maintain a calm environment, avoid agitating the child, and disturb as little as possible. Monitor oxygenation with noninvasive pulse oximeter. Monitor respiratory status closely and frequently. Closely observe response to racemic epinephrine. Have intubation equipment at bedside and available during transport. Increasing tachypnea may be first sign of hypoxia. If severe distress does not respond to initial treatment, ABG analysis should be obtained. In a hypoxic, pale, cyanotic, or obtunded patient, do not manipulate larynx and do not examine with a tongue blade; it may lead to sudden cardiopulmonary arrest.	• Dehydration, intubation, airway obstruction, death.
• CBC is normal, x-ray: subglottic narrowing. • Endoscopic exam: inflammation of the arytenoids cartilage, epithelium intact, pale mucosa.	• Corticosteroid therapy. • Racemic epinephrine, nebulized.	• Same as for acute laryngotracheobronchitis (above). • Allow the parent to hold the child, remain in upright position. • Use racemic epinephrine with caution and provide cardiac monitoring, due to possible tachycardia.	
• Neck x-ray: subglottic narrowing, large epiglottis, thick arytenoepiglottic folds, pseudomembrane in trachea. • Tracheal culture. Laryngoscopy, CBC, leukocytosis, bandemia.	• Humidified oxygen as required, mist, antibiotic therapy, cephalosporin, antipyretics. • Admit to the intensive care unit (ICU), intubation, and frequent suctioning. • Racemic epinephrine ineffective.	• Monitor closely for airway obstruction.	• Airway obstruction, death, tracheostomy, pneumothorax, toxic shock syndrome.
• Clinical evaluation and history, determining the onset of symptoms. • Monitor oxygen saturation level. • Lateral neck films: while sitting in parent's lap with portable radiology, swollen epiglottis.	• Medical emergency. • Establish a stable artificial airway first. Approach child in a calm manner; emotional upset and agitation may result in complete airway obstruction.	• Allow the parents to remain with and hold the child. Before transport to the operating room, observe closely for signs of airway obstruction. Allow the child to maintain a position of comfort (not supine).	• Airway obstruction, death, tracheostomy, pneumothorax, toxic shock syndrome. **NURSING ALERT** Do not attempt to visualize the epiglottis with a tongue blade or take a throat culture. May cause laryngospasm and airway obstruction.

(continued)

Table 44-1   Common Pediatric Respiratory Infections (*continued*)

CONDITION AND CAUSATIVE AGENT	AGE AND INCIDENCE	CLINICAL MANIFESTATIONS
Croup Syndromes (*continued*) ***Acute epiglottitis*** (*continued*)		• Complete fatal airway obstruction and death may occur within hours if not treated. In group A beta-hemolytic streptococcus and *H. influenzae*, patient will present with acute respiratory distress. • Stridor and breath sounds decrease as child begins to tire. • A brief episode of air hunger with restlessness and agitation may rapidly progress into increasing cyanosis, coma, and death.

ABG, arterial blood gas; ASO, antistreptolysin; CBC, complete blood count; HIV, human immunodeficiency virus; ICU, intensive care unit; MRSA: Methicillin-resistant S. aureus; PCP, Pneumocystis carinii pneumonia; RSV, respiratory syncytial virus; URI, upper respiratory infection.

1. Observe the respiratory rate and pattern. Count the respirations for 1 full minute, document and note level of activity, such as awake or asleep. Determine if the rate is appropriate for age (see page 1388).
2. Observe respiratory rhythm and depth. Rhythm is described as regular, irregular, or periodic. Depth is normal, hypopnea or too shallow, hyperpnea or too deep.
3. Auscultate breath sounds for a full cycle of inspiration and expiration over all lung fields. Note airflow and presence of adventitious sounds such as crackles, wheeze, or stridor.
4. Observe degree of respiratory effort—normal, difficult, or labored. Normal breathing is effortless and easy.
5. Document character of dyspnea or labored breathing; continuous, intermittent, worsening, or sudden onset. Note relation to activity, such as rest, exertion, crying, feeding, and association with pain, positioning, or orthopnea.
6. Note presence of additional signs of respiratory distress: nasal flaring, grunting, and retractions. Note location of retractions (see Figure 44-2) and character (mild, moderate, or severe).
7. Observe for head bobbing, usually noted in a sleeping or exhausted infant. The infant is held by caregiver with head supported on the caregiver's arm at the suboccipital area. The head bobs forward with each inspiration.

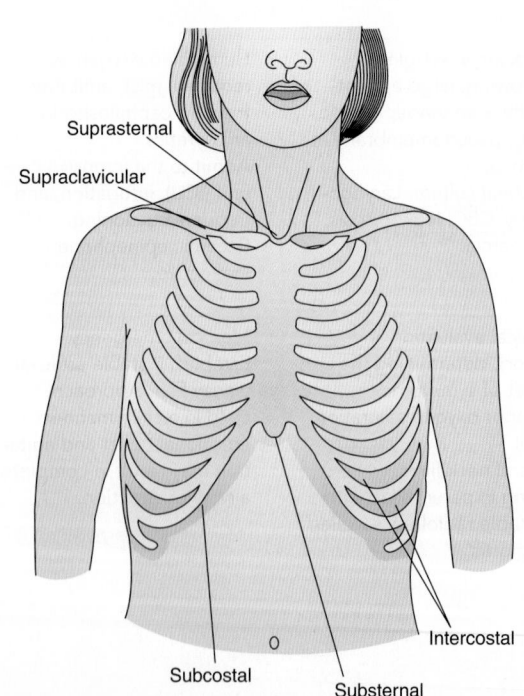

Figure 44-2. Sites of respiratory retractions.

DIAGNOSTIC EVALUATION	TREATMENT	NURSING CONSIDERATIONS	COMPLICATIONS
• Direct exam or laryngoscopy: large, swollen cherry-red epiglottis, edema of arytenoepiglottic folds. CBC, cultures, IV catheters must be done after intubation.	• Proceed to the operating room or ICU with personnel skilled and equipped to intubate or perform a percutaneous tracheostomy. • Lateral neck films should be done in the operating room or ICU after airway is established. • Antibiotics: intravenous cefotaxime, ceftriaxone, ampicillin with sulbactam. • Supplemental humidified oxygen; mechanical ventilation, if necessary. • If epiglottitis is strongly suspected, examination of the throat is contraindicated; due to reflex laryngospasm, acute airway obstruction, aspiration, and cardiopulmonary arrest during or immediately after examination of the pharynx with a tongue blade. Do not attempt throat culture.	• Equipment for intubation and tracheostomy must remain with the patient at all times. A practitioner skilled in intubation and tracheostomy procedures must accompany the child to the operating room or ICU. After intubation, the child should remain in the ICU with frequent assessment of oxygenation levels and need for mechanical ventilation. Prevent self-extubation; use arm boards or restraints to prevent arm movements, extubation, and death. After intubation, administer sedation, as needed. When the decision is made to extubate the child, emergency tracheostomy and intubation equipment must be at bedside.	

8. Observe the child's color. Note the presence and location of cyanosis—peripheral, perioral, facial, and trunk. Note degree of color changes, duration, and association with activity such as crying, feeding, and sleeping.

9. Observe the presence of cough, noting type and duration, such as dry, barking, paroxysmal, or productive. Note any pattern, such as time of day or night, association with activity, physical exertion, or feeding. Severity of croup may be determined by cough and signs of respiratory effort.
   a. Mild croup—occasional barking cough, no audible stridor at rest, and either mild or no suprasternal or intercostal retractions.
   b. Moderate croup—frequent barking cough, easily audible stridor at rest, and suprasternal and sternal retractions at rest, but little or no agitation.
   c. Severe croup—frequent barking cough, prominent inspiratory and occasional expiratory stridor, marked sternal retractions, and agitation and distress.
   d. Impending respiratory failure—barking cough (often not prominent), audible stridor at rest (may be hard to hear), sternal retractions (may be marked), lethargy or decreased level of consciousness, and often dusky appearance in the absence of supplemental oxygen.

 Evidence Base Ledoux, M., Perkin, R., Sharieff, G. (2012). Upper airway obstruction in pediatrics. *Pediatric Emergency Medicine Reports, 17*(1), 1–11.

10. Note the presence of sputum, including color, amount, consistency, and frequency.
11. Observe the child's fingernails and toenails for cyanosis and the presence and degree of clubbing, which indicate underlying chronic respiratory disease.
12. Evaluate the child's degree of restlessness, apprehension, and muscle tone.
13. Note the presence or complaint of chest pain and its location, whether it is local or generalized, dull or sharp, and associated with respiration or grunting.
14. Assess for signs of infection, such as elevated temperature; enlarged cervical lymph glands; purulent discharge from nose or ears; sputum; or inflamed mucous membranes.

Nursing Diagnoses

- Ineffective Airway Clearance related to inflammation, obstruction, secretions, or pain.
- Ineffective Breathing Pattern related to inflammatory process or pain.

- Deficient Fluid Volume related to fever, decreased appetite, and vomiting.
- Fatigue related to increased work of breathing.
- Anxiety related to respiratory distress and hospitalization.
- Parental Role Conflict related to hospitalization of the child.

Nursing Interventions

Promoting Effective Airway Clearance

1. Provide a humidified environment enriched with oxygen to combat hypoxia and to liquify secretions (see Procedure Guidelines 44-1, pages 1480 to 1482).
2. Advise the parents to use a jet or ultrasonic nebulizer at home and encourage fluids, as tolerated.
3. Keep nasal passages free of secretions. Infants are obligate nose breathers. Use a bulb syringe to clear nares and oropharynx.

Improving Breathing Pattern

1. Place the child in a comfortable position to promote easier ventilation.
   a. Semi-Fowler's—use infant seat or elevate head of bed.
   b. Occasional side or abdominal position will aid drainage of liquefied secretions. Do not place infant in prone position.
   c. Do not position the child in severe respiratory distress in a supine position. Allow the child to assume a position of comfort.

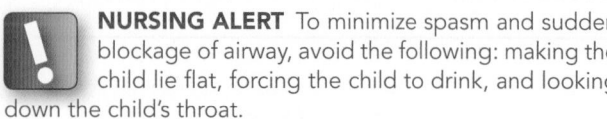 **NURSING ALERT** To minimize spasm and sudden blockage of airway, avoid the following: making the child lie flat, forcing the child to drink, and looking down the child's throat.

2. Provide measures to improve ventilation of the affected portion of the lung.
   a. Change position frequently.
   b. Provide postural drainage, if prescribed.
   c. Relieve nasal obstruction that contributes to breathing difficulty. Instill normal saline solution or prescribed nose drops and apply nasal suctioning.
   d. Quiet prolonged crying, which can irritate the airway, by soothing the child; however, crying may be an effective way to inflate the lungs.
   e. Realize that coughing is a normal tracheobronchial cleansing procedure, but temporarily relieve coughing by allowing the child to sip water; use extreme caution to prevent aspiration.
   f. Insert a nasogastric tube, as ordered, to relieve abdominal distention, which can limit diaphragmatic excursion.
3. Ensure that the child's oxygen input is not compromised.
   a. Monitor oxygen saturations, as indicated; pulse oximetry should be performed if hypoxia is suspected.
   b. If compressed air or oxygen is administered, use a head box to avoid excess carbon dioxide concentrations and increased respiratory rate.
4. Administer appropriate antibiotic or antiviral therapy.
   a. Observe for drug sensitivity.
   b. Observe the child's response to therapy.

5. Administer specific treatment for respiratory syncytial virus (RSV), if ordered.
   a. There is presently no evidence that supports the use of ribavirin or inhaled corticosteroids in acute bronchiolitis; however, some health care providers do consider these options in the management of RSV.

 Evidence Base Kelsall-Knight, L. (2012). Clinical assessment of a child with bronchiolitis. *Nursing Children & Young People*, Oct; *24*(8), 29–34.

6. If the decision is made to initiate ribavirin therapy, appropriate precautions should be implemented to protect personnel and caregivers.
   a. Information should be provided about the potential but unknown risk of exposure to ribavirin.
   b. Pregnant women should be advised to refrain from providing direct care to patients who are receiving ribavirin therapy.
   c. Methods to reduce environmental exposure to ribavirin should be employed:
      i. Stop aerosol administration before opening hood or tent.
      ii. Use room with adequate ventilation of at least six air exchanges per hour.
      iii. Consider the use of scavenger devices to help decrease the escape of ribavirin into the air.
      iv. Staff should wear aprons and face masks for the duration of the time the nebulizer is in use.
7. For cases of severe respiratory distress, assist with intubation or tracheostomy and mechanical ventilation.
   a. Tracheostomy and endotracheal tubes are generally not cuffed for infants and small children because the tube itself is big enough relative to the size of the trachea to act as its own sealer.
   b. Position the infant with a tracheostomy with the neck extended by placing a small roll under the shoulders to prevent occlusion of the tube by the chin. Support his or her head and neck carefully when moving the infant to prevent dislodgement of the tube.
   c. When feeding, cover the tracheostomy with a moist piece of gauze, or use a bib for older infants or young children.
   d. See page 1479 in this chapter as well as Chapter 10 for care of the patient on mechanical ventilation.

 NURSING ALERT Infants with a history of very low birth weight and bronchopulmonary dysplasia have chronic compensated carbon dioxide retention. Careful attention must be given to oxygen administration to avoid respiratory depression by suppressing their hypoxic drive.

Promoting Adequate Hydration

1. Administer fluids via intravenous (IV) route at the prescribed rate.
2. To prevent aspiration, withhold oral food and fluids if the child is in severe respiratory distress.

3. Offer the child small sips of clear fluid when respiratory status improves.
   a. Note any vomiting or abdominal distention after the oral fluid is given.
   b. As the child begins to take more fluid by mouth, notify the health care provider and modify the IV fluid rate to prevent fluid overload.
   c. Do not force the child to take fluids orally because this may cause increased distress and possibly vomiting. Anorexia will subside as the condition improves.
4. Assist in the control of fever to reduce respiratory rate and fluid loss.
   a. Give antipyretics, as prescribed.
5. Record the child's intake and output and monitor urine-specific gravity.
6. Provide mouth care or offer mouth rinse if child is able to perform this safely.

Promoting Adequate Rest
1. Disturb the child as little as possible by organizing nursing care, and protect the child from unnecessary interruptions.
2. Be aware of the age of the child and be familiar with the level of growth and development as it applies to hospitalization.
3. Encourage the parents to stay with the child as much as possible to provide comfort and security.
4. Provide opportunities for quiet play as the child's condition improves.

Reducing Anxiety
1. Explain procedures and hospital routine to the child as appropriate for age.
2. Provide a quiet, stress-free environment.
3. Observe the child's response to the oxygen therapy environment and provide reassurance.
   a. The child may experience fear of confinement or suffocation.
   b. Vision is distorted through the plastic.
   c. The environment is noisy and damp.
   d. Physical and diversional activities are restricted.
   e. Parental contact is decreased.
   f. The environment is often uncomfortable.
4. Avoid the use of sedatives and opiates, which may obscure restlessness. Restlessness is a sign of increasing respiratory distress or obstruction.
5. Allow the child to assume a position of comfort.

Strengthening the Parents' Role
1. Help the parents understand the purpose of the oxygen therapy/humidifier and how to work with it.
2. Discuss their fears and concerns about the child's therapy.
3. Include the parents in planning for the child's care. Promote their participation in caring for the child.
4. Recognize that the parents will need rest periods. Encourage them to take breaks and eat on a regular basis.

Family Education and Health Maintenance
1. Teach the importance of good hygiene. Include information on handwashing and appropriate ways to handle respiratory secretions at home.

2. Teach the family when it is appropriate to keep the child home from school (any fever, coughing up secretions, and significant runny nose in toddler or younger child).
3. Teach methods to keep the ill child well hydrated.
   a. Provide small amounts of fluids frequently.
   b. Offer clear liquids and prepared electrolyte preparations.
   c. Offer frozen juice pops.
   d. Avoid juices with a high sugar content.
4. Teach ways to assess the child's hydration status at home.
   a. Decreased number of wet diapers or number of times the child urinates per day.
   b. Decreased activity level.
   c. Dry lips and mucous membranes.
   d. No tears when the child cries.
5. Teach the parents when to contact their health care provider—signs of respiratory distress, recurrent fever, decreased appetite and activity, and signs of dehydration.
6. Teach about medications and follow-up.
7. If a tracheostomy was required, teach care of the tracheostomy, use of equipment, safety, and referral for home nursing care before discharge.

Evaluation: Expected Outcomes
- Breath sounds clear and equal.
- Easy, regular, unlabored respirations on room air (or back to baseline if the child is on oxygen).
- Mucous membranes moist; urine output adequate.
- Bathing and feeding tolerated well.
- Child calm and interacts appropriately with family and staff.
- Parents participate in the child's care.

Disorders Requiring Surgery of the Tonsils and Adenoids

 Evidence Base Scottish Intercollegiate Guidelines Network. (2010). *Management of sore throat and indications for tonsillectomy—A national clinical guideline.* Edinburgh: NHS Quality Improvement Scotland.

Tonsillectomy and *adenoidectomy* are the surgical removal of the adenoidal and tonsillar structures, part of the lymphoid tissue that encircles the pharynx. These are one of the most frequently performed surgical procedures in the child. The most common disease processes that require tonsillectomy and adenoidectomy are obstructive sleep apnea; chronic, persistent tonsillitis or adenoiditis; and chronic persistent otitis media.

Pathophysiology and Etiology

Function of Tonsils and Adenoids
1. They are a first line of defense against respiratory infections.
2. Because the growth of the tonsils and adenoids in the first 10 years of life exceeds general somatic growth, these structures appear especially large in the child.
3. The natural process of involution of tonsillar and adenoidal lymphoid tissue in the prepubertal years is associated with decreased frequency of throat and ear infections.

Obstructive Sleep Apnea

1. Adenotonsillar hypertrophy causes airway obstruction during sleep, leading to persistent hypoventilation during sleep.
2. Peak incidence in children is between ages 3 and 6 years.
3. Incidence is increased in children with Down syndrome.

Tonsillitis and Adenoiditis

1. In tonsillitis and adenoiditis, structures that are already large become inflamed due to an infectious agent and cause airway obstruction, decreased appetite, and pain.
2. Infection is caused by bacterial or viral organisms, with viral organisms most commonly implicated.
3. Group A beta-hemolytic *Streptococcus* is the most common bacterial cause.
4. Enlarged adenoids may block nasal passages, resulting in persistent mouth breathing.
5. Chronic adenoiditis without tonsillitis is typically seen in children younger than age 4 years.

Otitis Media

1. Bacterial infection caused most commonly by *Streptococcus pneumoniae* or *Haemophilus influenzae*.
2. Chronic infection may be associated with enlarged adenoids that block drainage from the eustachian tubes.

Clinical Manifestations

Obstructive Sleep Apnea

1. Loud snoring or noisy breathing in sleep.
2. Excessive daytime sleepiness.
3. Mouth breathing.

Chronic Infection of Tonsils and Adenoids

1. Mouth breathing or difficulty breathing.
2. Frequent sore throat.
3. Anorexia, decreased growth velocity.
4. Fever.
5. Obstruction to swallowing or breathing.
6. Nasal, muffled voice.
7. Night cough.
8. Offensive breath.

Chronic Otitis Media

1. Ear pain or general irritability in young children.
2. Alterations in hearing.
3. Fever.
4. Enlarged lymph nodes.
5. Anorexia.

Diagnostic Evaluation

1. Thorough ear, nose, and throat examination and appropriate cultures to determine presence and source of infection.
2. Preoperative blood studies to determine risk of bleeding—clotting time, smear for platelets, prothrombin time, and partial thromboplastin time.

Management

Appropriate antibiotics are given and the decision is made to perform surgery. Tonsillectomy and adenoidectomy may be performed together or separately. Debate continues over indications for and benefits of surgery.

Indications for Tonsillectomy

1. Conservative.
   a. Recurrent or persistent tonsillitis. The widely accepted criteria for surgery is seven episodes of tonsillitis in the previous 12 months or five episodes in each of the preceding 2 years.
   b. Marked hypertrophy of tonsils, which distorts speech, causes swallowing difficulties, and causes subsequent weight loss.
   c. Tonsillar malignancy.
   d. Diphtheria carrier.
   e. Cor pulmonale due to obstruction.
2. Controversial.
   a. Peritonsillar abscess or retrotonsillar abscess.
   b. Suppurative cervical adenitis with tonsillar focus.
   c. Persistent hyperemia of anterior pillars.
   d. Enlarged cervical lymph nodes.

Indications for Adenoidectomy

1. Conservative.
   a. Adenoid hypertrophy resulting in obstruction of airway, leading to hypoxia, pulmonary hypertension, and cor pulmonale.
   b. Hypertrophy with nasal obstruction accompanied by breathing difficulty and severe speech distortion.
   c. Hypertrophy associated with chronic suppurative or serous otitis media and sensorineural or conductive hearing loss, chronic mastoiditis, or cholesteatoma.
   d. Mouth breathing due to hypertrophied adenoids.
2. Controversial.
   a. Enlarged adenoids.
   b. Chronic otitis media and no evidence of complications.
   c. Child younger than age 4 years, unless life-threatening situation.

Contraindications to Surgery

1. Bleeding or coagulation disorders.
2. Uncontrolled systemic disorders (eg, diabetes, rheumatic fever, cardiac or renal disease).
3. Presence of upper respiratory infection in the child or immediate family.
4. Specific for adenoidectomy—certain palate abnormalities (ie, cleft palate or submucous cleft palate).

Complications

1. If untreated, obstructive sleep apnea in the child may result in pulmonary hypertension, cor pulmonale, failure to thrive, respiratory failure, attention-deficit disorders, and cardiac arrhythmias.
2. Untreated chronic tonsillitis may result in failure to thrive, peritonsillar or retropharyngeal abscess, difficulty swallowing, and poor eating.
3. Untreated chronic otitis media may result in hearing loss, scarring of the eardrum (tympanosclerosis), mastoiditis, and meningitis.
4. Complications of surgery include hemorrhage, reactions to anesthesia, otitis media, and bacteremia.

Nursing Assessment

Preoperative Assessment

1. Assess the child's developmental level.
2. Assess the parents' and child's understanding of the surgical procedure.
3. Assess psychological preparation of the child for hospitalization and surgery.
   a. Does the child understand what will happen?
   b. Do the parents know the importance of telling the child the truth, and do they have a good understanding of the procedure?
   c. Does the child have preconceived ideas from peers that may pose a threat?

 NURSING ALERT The preschool child is especially vulnerable to psychological trauma as a result of surgical procedures or hospitalization.

4. Obtain thorough nursing history from the child and parents to gather any pertinent information that would impact the child's care.
   a. Has the child had a recent infection? It is desirable for the child to be free of respiratory infection for at least 2 weeks.
   b. Has the child recently been exposed to any communicable diseases?
   c. Does the child have any loose teeth that may pose the threat of aspiration?
   d. Are there any bleeding tendencies in the child or family?
   e. Are there any family members with a history of adverse reactions to anesthesia?
5. Obtain the child's baseline vital signs along with his or her height and weight.
6. Assess the child's hydration status.

Postoperative Assessment

1. Assess respiratory status and pain often.
2. Assess frequently for signs of postoperative bleeding; monitor vital signs, as warranted.
3. Assess oral intake.
4. Assess for indications of negative psychological sequelae related to the surgery and hospitalization.

Nursing Diagnoses

- Fear related to painful procedure, unfamiliar environment.
- Anxiety of the parents related to concept of surgery.
- Risk for Deficient Fluid Volume related to reduced intake postoperatively and blood loss.
- Ineffective Airway Clearance related to pain and effects of anesthesia.
- Acute Pain related to surgical incision.

Nursing Interventions

Reducing Fear

1. Prepare the child and parents by encouraging participation in hospital tours and preadmission programs specifically for children.
2. Share information with the child, commensurate with their development stage and cognitive ability, as well as the family.
3. Prepare the child specifically for what to expect postoperatively, using techniques appropriate to the child's developmental level (books, dolls, drawings). Include the following:
   a. Where the child will wake up.
   b. Temporary sore throat, emesis of blood, position, and foul taste and smell in mouth.
   c. Medications.
   d. Fluid regimen and possible intravenous infusion.
4. Talk to the child about the new things to be seen in the operating room and clear up any misconceptions. Whenever possible, allow the child to see, touch, and examine equipment, such as thermometers, beds, tubings, and suction equipment.
5. Where available, involve the play specialist in the preparation.

Relieving Parental Anxiety

1. Help the parents prepare the child by talking at first in general terms about surgery and progressing to more specific information.
2. Reassure the parents that complication rates are low and that recovery is usually swift.
3. Encourage the parents to stay with the child and help provide care.

Maintaining Adequate Fluid Volume

1. Assess the child frequently for postoperative bleeding. Check all secretions and emesis for the presence of fresh blood. These are indications of hemorrhage:
   a. Increased pulse.
   b. Frequent swallowing while awake and asleep.
   c. Pallor.
   d. Restlessness.
   e. Clearing of throat and vomiting of blood.
   f. Continuous slight oozing of blood over a number of hours.
   g. Oozing of blood in back of throat.

 NURSING ALERT Notify the surgeon immediately if bleeding is suspected.

2. Have suction equipment, oxygen, and packing material readily available in case of emergency.
3. Provide adequate fluid intake.
   a. Give ice cubes 1 to 2 hours after awakening from anesthesia.
   b. When vomiting has ceased, cautiously advance to clear liquids.
   c. Offer cool fruit juices without pulp at first because they are best tolerated; then offer ice pops and cool water for the first 12 to 24 hours. Avoid red and brown fluids.
   d. There is some debate regarding the intake of milk and ice cream the evening of surgery. It can be soothing and can reduce swelling; however, it coats the mouth and throat, causing the child to clear the throat more often, which may initiate bleeding.

Promoting Effective Airway Clearance

1. Assist the child in maintaining a patent airway by draining secretions and preventing aspiration of vomitus.
2. Assess the child for signs and symptoms of airway obstruction and respiratory distress (stridor, drooling, restlessness, agitation, tachypnea, and cyanosis), which may result from edema or the accumulation of secretions.
   a. Place the child prone or semi-prone with his or her head turned to side while still under the effects of anesthesia.
   b. Allow the child to assume a position of comfort when alert. (The parent may hold the child.)
   c. The child may vomit old blood initially. If suctioning is necessary, avoid trauma to the oropharynx.
   d. Remind the child not to cough, clear throat, or blow nose.

Improving Comfort

1. Give analgesics, as ordered, parenteral or rectally.
2. Rinse the child's mouth with cool water or alkaline solution.
3. Keep the child and environment free from blood-tinged drainage to help decrease anxiety.
4. Encourage the parents to be with the child when the child awakens. This is the most important comfort measure the nurse can provide for the child.
5. When the parents must leave, reassure the child that they will return.

Family Education and Health Maintenance

1. Explain and write instructions concerning the care of the child at home after discharge.
   a. Diet should still consist of large amounts of fluids and soft, cool, nonirritating foods. (Supply a list of suggestions for the family.)
   b. Eating helps promote healing because it increases the blood supply to the tissues.
   c. Bed rest should be maintained for 1 to 2 days and then daily rest periods for about 1 week. Resume normal eating and activities within 2 weeks after surgery.
   d. Avoid contact with people with infections.
   e. Discourage the child from blowing nose and frequent coughing and clearing of his or her throat.
   f. Avoid gargling. Mouth odor may be present for a few days after surgery; only mouth rinsing is acceptable.
   g. Discourage use of red dye enhanced foods or analgesics if possible—can be difficult to differentiate from bleeding.
2. Advise the parents to call the health care provider if the following occur. (Ensure that the parents have the phone numbers of the health care provider and hospital emergency department.)
   a. Earache accompanied by fever.
   b. Any bleeding, often indicated only by frequent swallowing; most common between the 5th and 10th postoperative days when membrane sloughs from surgical site.
3. Teach about medications prescribed or suggested for pain relief.
4. Discuss with the parents what results they can expect from the surgery.
   a. Decreased number of sore throats.
   b. Lessened evidence of obstructive symptoms.
   c. Decreased incidence of cervical lymphadenitis.
   d. Improvement in nutritional status.
   e. No improvement in nasal allergies.
   f. No improvement in secretory otitis media.
5. Guide the parents in helping the child think of the experience as a positive one after the surgery is over, to make subsequent health care experiences easier.
   a. Talk about what happened and the positive outcomes.
   b. Let the child play out his or her feelings.

Evaluation: Expected Outcomes

- Acts out surgery with dolls, asks questions.
- Parents interact with the child, ask appropriate questions.
- Takes fluids well; no signs of bleeding.
- No vomiting; breathing without difficulty.
- Verbalizes reduced pain.

Asthma

Asthma is a chronic, inflammatory disease of the airways, characterized by airflow obstruction, bronchial hyperreactivity, and mucus production. The course of asthma is highly variable. Many cells and mediators play a role, including mast cells, eosinophils, neutrophils, and epithelial cells. Classic signs and symptoms include cough, wheezing, shortness of breath/dyspnea, and chest tightness. Children may also claim that their stomach aches when they are experiencing asthma. The Global Initiative for Asthma (GINA) guidelines (2011), published by the World Health Organization, and the National Asthma Education and Prevention Program of the National Institutes of Health provide evidence-based categorization, treatment, and ongoing control information.

Assessment of Asthma Control

1. Although severity is best evaluated prior to the use of asthma medications, it can be established based on the medications necessary to gain control and directs initial therapy.
2. Two domains of asthma control are assessed at each encounter: risk and impairment.
   a. Risk is measured by exacerbations.
   b. Impairment is determined both on initial diagnosis and ongoing assessment.
3. Factors that affect impairment include:
   a. Day and nighttime asthma symptoms.
   b. Usage of quick-relief medication.
   c. Pulmonary function tests/peak flow measurements if the child is capable.
   d. Limitations of daily activities.
   e. Adverse effects of medications.
   f. Progression of lung disease.
4. Several validated tools are available for patients age 12 years and older to complete, including the Asthma Control Test, Asthma Control Questionnaire, and Asthma Therapy Assessment Questionnaire.
   a. These tools quantify symptoms, quick-relief medication usage, effect of asthma on quality of life, and patient/family perception of control.
   b. To assist in the diagnosis of asthma, particularly in very small children who cannot perform lung function tests, an asthma predictive index can help identify children likely to have asthma.

NURSING ALERT Level of control guides adjustment of medications, and nurses can use such assessment to identify patients/families who need more asthma education to better gain control of asthma.

 Evidence Base Castro-Rodriguez, J. A. (2010). The asthma predictive index: A very useful tool for predicting asthma in young children. *Journal of Allergy and Clinical Immunology, 126,* 212–216.

Variations of Asthma

Cough Variant Asthma

Cough variant asthma is typically seen in children, where cough (especially at night) is the principal symptom. The child may never wheeze. Although the symptoms are chronic and commonly mild in many children, severe exacerbations (attacks) may arise, even resulting in respiratory failure and death.

Exercise-Induced Bronchospasm

Exercise-induced bronchospasm refers to symptoms of cough, shortness of breath, chest pain, tightness, wheezing, and endurance problems during or after vigorous activity. Typically, symptoms begin during exercise and peak 5 to 10 minutes after stopping; they may resolve spontaneously within 20 to 30 minutes. Diagnosis is confirmed by documenting a decrease in peak expiratory flow (PEF) or forced expiratory volume in 1 second (FEV_1), before and after exercise and at 5-minute intervals for 20 to 30 minutes. This condition may occur without chronic asthma and has a different pathophysiology from asthma that is triggered by exercise. The preferred treatment consists of short-acting beta-2 agonists, taken 15 minutes prior to exercise. Cromolyn sodium, available only for a nebulizer, is an alternative, although less effective.

Factors that Increase Risk of Asthma Death

 Evidence Base Sala, K. A., Carroll, C. L., Yang, Y. S., et al. (2011). Factors associated with the development of severe asthma exacerbations in children. *Journal of Asthma, 48,* 558–564.
Global Initiative for Asthma. (2011). Pocket Guide for Asthma Managment and Prevention. Available: *www.ginasthma.org.*

1. Previous severe exacerbation (intubation or intensive care admission).
2. Hospitalization two or more times within the year, three or more emergency department (ED) visits in the last year.
3. Use of more than two canisters per month of short-acting beta-adrenergic (SABA).
4. Difficulty perceiving airway obstruction or the severity of worsening asthma.
5. Low socioeconomic status or inner-city residence.
6. Illicit drug use.
7. Major psychological problems or psychiatric disease.
8. Comorbidity, such as cardiovascular disease or other chronic lung disease.
9. Other factors, lack of asthma action plan, sensitivity to *Alternaria.*

Management

The Stepwise Approach to Managing Asthma, developed by the EPR 3, identifies classifications of asthma according to symptoms and suggests pharmacologic options for the control of asthma. Medications may be "stepped up or down" depending on the patient's response to therapy. See Table 44-2, page 1500, and Table 44-3, page 1501, for the recommended management of asthma for infants and children age 0 to 4 and 5 to 12 years. See page 1036 for the management of older children with asthma.

For additional information on treatment and specific dosages, see Expert Panel Report 3: Guidelines for the Diagnosis and Management of Asthma, National Heart, Lung and Blood Institute, National Asthma Education and Prevention Program, Full Report, NIH Publication No. 08-4051, 2007, pages 346–352. Available: *www.nhlbi.nih.gov/guidelines/asthma/asthgdln.pdf.*

Acute Exacerbation

1. Be alert for severe asthma exacerbation. Exacerbations are usually associated with viral respiratory infections
2. In a severe exacerbation, the child is short of breath, may be audibly wheezing with a prolonged expiratory phase, restless, apprehensive, anxious, and diaphoretic, tachycardic; color may be pale or flushed and lips may be dark red or cyanotic.

 NURSING ALERT Cyanosis of the lips and nail beds is an ominous sign.

   a. There are signs of respiratory distress, such as nasal flaring, use of accessory muscles, retractions, one- to two-word dyspnea (speaking in short phrases), tachypnea, hypoxemia, and respiratory alkalosis progressing to respiratory acidosis.
   b. Breath sounds may be decreased and there may be decreased level of consciousness.
   c. A young child will assume tripod position; an older child will sit upright with shoulders hunched.
3. Signs of respiratory distress in infants include use of accessory muscles, inspiratory and expiratory wheezing, paradoxical breathing, cyanosis, respiratory rate greater than 60, and oxygen saturation less than 90%. These infants are at greater risk of respiratory failure.

 NURSING ALERT Absence of wheezing with decreased breath sounds and inability to blow a PEF indicates minimal air exchange. This situation requires immediate, swift attention to prevent respiratory failure. Respiratory failure tends to progress quickly and is difficult to reverse.

4. The goals of emergency management are to quickly reverse airflow obstruction, to correct hypoxemia, and to reduce the likelihood of recurrence.
5. Assess PEF rate or FEV_1 upon arrival; assess degree of respiratory distress or fatigue.
6. Obtain an oxygen saturation level by pulse oximetry.
7. Obtain arterial or capillary blood gas levels in infants with an oxygen saturation of 90% or less and in a child with moderate to severe respiratory distress.

(*Text continues on page 1502*)

Table 44-2   Stepwise Approach for Managing Asthma in Children 0–4 Years of Age

Intermittent Asthma	Persistent Asthma: Daily Medication Consult with asthma specialist if step 3 care or higher is required. Consider consultation at step 2.

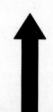

Step 1

Preferred:

SABA PRN

Step 2

Preferred:

Low-dose ICS

Alternative:

Cromolyn or Montelukast

Step 3

Preferred:

Medium-dose ICS

Step 4

Preferred:

Medium-dose ICS + either LABA or Montelukast

Step 5

Preferred:

High-dose ICS + either LABA or Montelukast

Step 6

Preferred:

High-dose ICS + either LABA or Montelukast

Oral systemic corticosteroids

Step up if needed

(first, check adherence, inhaler technique, and environmental control)

Assess control

Step down if possible

(and asthma is well controlled at least 3 months)

Patient Education and Environmental Control at Each Step

Quick-Relief Medication for All Patients

- SABA as needed for symptoms. Intensity of treatment depends on severity of symptoms.
- With viral respiratory infection: SABA q 4–6 hours up to 24 hours (longer with physician consult). Consider short course of oral systemic corticosteroids if exacerbation is severe or patient has history of previous severe exacerbations.
- Caution: Frequent use of SABA may indicate the need to step up treatment. See text for recommendations on initiating daily long-term-control therapy.

Key: Alphabetical order is used when more than one treatment option is listed within either preferred or alternative therapy. ICS, inhaled corticosteroid; LABA, inhaled long-acting beta2-agonist; SABA, inhaled short-acting beta2-agonist

Notes:

- The stepwise approach is meant to assist, not replace, the clinical decisionmaking required to meet individual patient needs.

- If alternative treatment is used and response is inadequate, discontinue it and use the preferred treatment before stepping up.

- If clear benefit is not observed within 4-6 weeks and patient/family medication technique and adherence are satisfactory, consider adjusting therapy or alternative diagnosis.

- Studies on children 0-4 years of age are limited. Step 2 preferred therapy is based on Evidence A. All other recommendations are based on expert opinion and extrapolation from studies in older children.

National Heart, Lung and Blood Institute, National Asthma Education and Prevention Program. (2007). Expert panel report 3: Guidelines for the diagnosis and management of asthma. p. 305. Available: www.nhlbi.nih.gov/guidelines/asthma/asthgdln.pdf.

Table 44-3   Stepwise Approach for Managing Asthma in Children 5–11 Years of Age

Intermittent Asthma	Persistent Asthma: Daily Medication Consult with asthma specialist if step 4 care or higher is required. Consider consultation at step 3.

Step 1
Preferred:
SABA PRN

Step 2
Preferred:
Low-dose ICS
Alternative:
Cromolyn, LTRA, Nedocromil, or Theophylline

Step 3
Preferred:
EITHER:
Low-dose ICS + either LABA, LTRA, or Theophylline
OR
Medium-dose ICS

Step 4
Preferred:
Medium-dose ICS + LABA
Alternative:
Medium-dose ICS + either LTRA or Theophylline

Step 5
Preferred:
High-dose ICS + LABA
Alternative:
High-dose ICS + either LTRA or Theophylline

Step 6
Preferred:
High-dose ICS + LABA + oral systemic corticosteroid
Alternative:
High-dose ICS + either LTRA or Theophylline + oral systemic corticosteroid

Step up if needed (first, check adherence, inhaler technique, environmental control, and comorbid conditions)

Assess control

Step down if possible (and asthma is well controlled at least 3 months)

Each step: Patient education, environmental control, and management of comorbidities.

Steps 2-4: Consider subcutaneous allergen immunotherapy for patients who have allergic asthma (see notes).

Quick-Relief Medication for All Patients

• SABA as needed for symptoms. Intensity of treatment depends on severity of symptoms: up to 3 treatments at 20-minute intervals as needed. Short course of oral systemic corticosteroids may be needed.

• Caution: Increasing use of SABA or use >2 days a week for symptom relief (not prevention of EIB) generally indicates inadequate control and the need to step up treatment.

Key: Alphabetical order is used when more than one treatment option is listed within either preferred or alternative therapy. ICS, inhaled corticosteroid; LABA, inhaled long-acting beta2-agonist, LTRA, leukotriene receptor antagonist; SABA, inhaled short-acting beta2-agonist

Notes:

■ The stepwise approach is meant to assist, not replace, the clinical decision making required to meet individual patient needs.

■ If alternative treatment is used and response is inadequate, discontinue it and use the preferred treatment before stepping up.

■ Theophylline is a less desirable alternative due to the need to monitor serum concentration levels.

■ Step 1 and step 2 medications are based on Evidence A. Step 3 ICS + adjunctive therapy and ICS are based on Evidence B for efficacy of each treatment and extrapolation from comparator trials in older children and adults—comparator trials are not available for this age group; steps 4-6 are based on expert opinion and extrapolation from studies in older children and adults.

■ Immunotherapy for steps 2-4 is based on Evidence B for house-dust mites, animal danders, and pollens; evidence is weak or lacking for molds and cockroaches. Evidence is strongest for immunotherapy with single allergens. The role of allergy in asthma is greater in children than in adults. Clinicians who administer immunotherapy should be prepared and equipped to identify and treat anaphylaxis that may occur.

National Heart, Lung and Blood Institute, National Asthma Education and Prevention Program. (2007). Expert panel report 3: Guidelines for the diagnosis and management of asthma. p. 306. Available: www.nhlbi.nih.gov/guidelines/asthma/asthgdln.pdf.

8. Deliver humidified oxygen via nasal cannula, hood, or face mask. Maintain oxygen tension greater than 64 mm Hg but less than 100 mm Hg to prevent oxygen narcosis.

9. Obtain a brief history and physical and focus on prior treatment and possible triggers of the episode, such as respiratory infection or lack of medication.

10. Administer emergency treatment, as indicated.

    a. SABA with ipratropium, either by nebulization or by MDI with spacer (with face mask in young child).

    b. Systemic corticosteroids should be administered early in treatment.

    c. Adjunctive treatments include IV leukotriene modifiers, heliox, and magnesium sulfate.

    d. Antibiotics are generally not used unless there is evidence of bacterial infection.

11. Hospitalized patients will need frequent assessment, repeat or continuous SABA treatments, corticosteroids, and treatment of any comorbid condition, such as sinusitis.

12. Discharge planning for patients with exacerbations should include an action plan for medications, recognition and treatment of acute asthma, and plans for follow-up.

13. Children in severe status asthmaticus unresponsive to the above therapy may require:

    a. Intubation and mechanical ventilation with 100% oxygen for impending or actual respiratory distress, decreased mental alertness, increased fatigue, or partial pressure of arterial carbon dioxide ($Paco_2$) greater than or equal to 42 mm Hg.

    b. Nebulized beta-2 agonist, hourly or continuously.

    c. Anticholinergic such as ipratropium, although generally limited to the emergency department.

    d. IV corticosteroid therapy.

    e. Admission to ICU.

    f. Pharmacologic paralysis to ventilate effectively.

    g. Cardiopulmonary monitoring of the child's response to treatment.

    h. Placement of an arterial line for blood monitoring.

14. Therapies not recommended for treating an exacerbation, based on the 2007 National Heart, Lung, and Blood Institute Expert Panel Report:

    a. Subcutaneous beta-2 agonist provides no advantage over inhaled medication.

    b. Theophylline or aminophylline therapy is not recommended in the ED. It does not provide additional benefit to short-acting beta-2 agonists; it may produce adverse effects.

    c. Chest physiotherapy (CPT) and mucolytics.

    d. Antibiotics are not recommended for asthma treatment. However, antibiotics may be needed in patients with fever, purulent sputum, and evidence of bacterial pneumonia.

    e. Anxiolytic and hypnotic drugs are contraindicated.

    f. Aggressive hydration is not recommended in older children. Assess fluid status; make corrections, as needed, for infants and young children to decrease risk of dehydration.

Long-Term Management

1. As the child becomes stabilized, begin to develop a home and school management plan. Components of the plan should include:

    a. The use of quick-relief medications (SABA); expected effect and side effects.

    b. The use of long-term controllers, which include corticosteroids, leukotriene modifiers, mast cell stabilizers, and long-acting beta agonists (LABA). See page 1037 for mechanism and adverse reactions. Note: LABA should only be prescribed if poor control with other medications due to increeasd risk of asthma-related deaths.

    c. Inhalation technique with nebulizer or multidose inhaler with spacer (see Figure 44-3).

    d. Peak flow and symptom monitoring.

    e. Use of PEF zone system, if indicated (see below).

    f. Identification of triggers (eg, exercise, weather change, infection, allergen exposure [pollen, mold, dust mite, animals, cockroach, mouse]).

    g. Environmental control by removal of suspected stimuli.

    h. Hydration, nutrition, rest, and exercise regimens.

    i. Emergency action plans.

2. Plan a team conference involving the child, parents, school nurse, and teacher, if possible. Ideally, the plan should be clear and easy for the child and family to follow, adapted to their lifestyle, and using the least amount of medications necessary to control and prevent the child's asthma symptoms. A written action plan should be submitted to the school, including information on medications (possible self-medication by the adolescent), identified triggers, steps in an emergency plan, and emergency contact information. Emergency action plans may need to include multiple family caregivers, and residences. A copy of this form can be found in *Guidelines for the Diagnosis and Management of Asthma*, available at *www.nhlbi. nih.gov/guidelines/asthma/*.

3. Stress that, without exception, no smoking should be permitted in the home or car of a child with asthma. Even if the

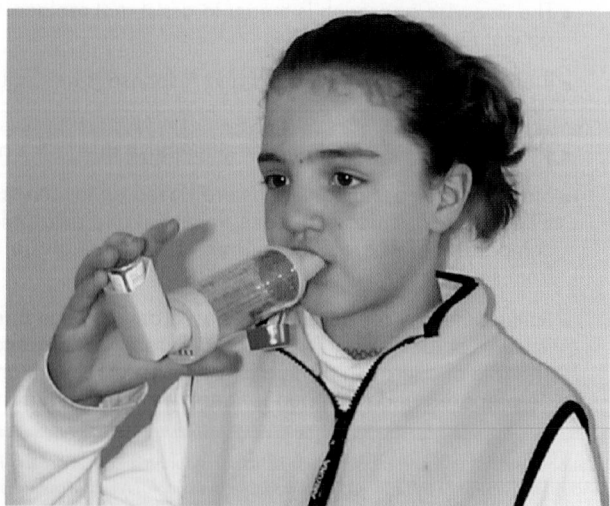

Figure 44-3. Multidose inhaler use with spacers. Aero Chamber.

child is out of the home, the residual odor will cause symptoms. Opening windows or using sprays and air cleaners are not acceptable alternatives.

4. Encourage the parents to pay particular attention to environmental control in the child's bedroom, including elimination of dust, not allowing any pets, and avoidance of any strong smells or sprays. If using wood stoves in the home, find out if there is an alternative source of heat.

5. Obtain more information from the National Asthma Education Program (*www.nhlbi.nih.gov/about/naepp/*), the American Academy of Allergy, Asthma and Immunology (*www.aaaai. org*), or the American Lung Association (*www.lungusa.org*).

Peak Expiratory Flow Monitoring and the Zone System

1. Teach the family and child about PEF monitoring at home as well as other important indicators, as directed (see Figure 44-4).
   a. PEF monitoring is not emphasized as much in current guidelines as in the past.
   b. Other indicators of severity include symptom assessment, need for medication, and measures of control such as the asthma control questionnaire.

2. A PEF meter measures the PEF rate that can be produced during a forced expiration. It measures airflow through the large airways; the result is effort dependent. PEF measurements can be initiated in children as young as age 5. Given time and practice, consistent readings will be produced. (See page xxxx for directions on use of PEF meter.)

3. A table of predicted PEF values should be included in the packaging of the home PEF meter. These values are based on age and height. A few patients may find their readings above or below the published values. Therefore, each child should establish a personal best PEF value. Ideally, this should be implemented during a time when the child is symptom-free. If PEF readings are consistently below predicted values, the health care provider should be contacted and additional medications may be necessary.

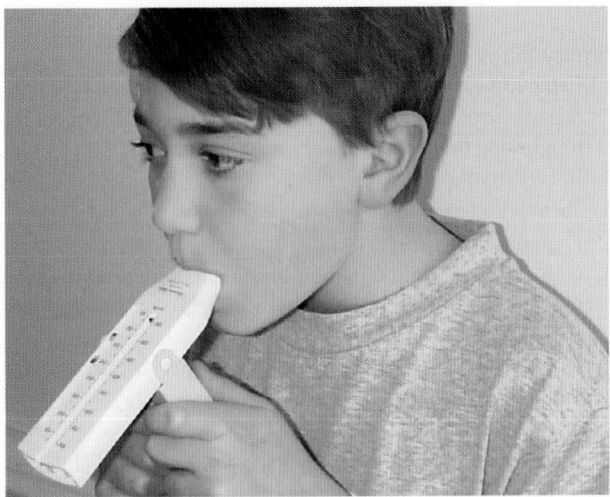

Figure 44-4. Peak flow monitoring.

4. Use of the PEF zone system along with a home asthma management plan can assist families in the proper use of medications, and assists in decision making regarding the degree of airflow obstruction. After the personal best PEF value is identified, teach the patient that subsequent PEF measurements can be classified into three zones that will dictate a home management plan.
   a. Green Zone = 80% to 100% of personal best. No asthma symptoms are present. Continue usual medications.
   b. Yellow Zone = 50% to less than 79% of personal best. Signals caution. May be experiencing an asthma episode or day-to-day control is suboptimal. Need to use short-acting inhaled beta-2 agonist, follow emergency plan, and contact health care provider for further instructions.
   c. Red Zone = less than 50% of personal best value. This zone signals danger. Must take a short-acting inhaled beta-2 agonist immediately and, if PEF does not return to yellow or green zone, contact health care provider or proceed to the ED immediately.

Respiratory Distress Syndrome (Hyaline Membrane Disease)

Respiratory distress syndrome (RDS), formerly known as hyaline membrane disease, is a syndrome of premature neonates that is characterized by progressive and usually fatal respiratory failure resulting from atelectasis and immaturity of the lungs. RDS occurs most commonly in premature neonates (primarily weighing between 1,000 and 1,500 g) and between 28 and 37 weeks' gestation. In neonates 26 to 28 weeks' gestation, the incidence is 50% to 70% and increases with degree of prematurity. RDS can be fatal; those who survive are at risk for chronic respiratory and neurologic complications.

Pathophysiology and Etiology

1. Adequate pulmonary function at birth depends on:
   a. An adequate amount of surfactant (a lipoprotein mixture) lining the alveolar cells, which allows for alveolar stability and prevents alveolar collapse at the end of expiration.
   b. An adequate surface area in air spaces to allow for gas exchange (ie, sufficient pulmonary capillary bed in contact with this alveolar surface area).

2. RDS is ultimately the result of decreased pulmonary surfactant, incomplete structural development of lung, and a highly compliant chest wall.

3. Contributing factors are any factor that decreases surfactant, such as:
   a. Prematurity and immature alveolar lining cells.
   b. Acidosis.
   c. Hypothermia.
   d. Hypoxia.
   e. Hypovolemia.
   f. Diabetes.
   g. Elective cesarean delivery.
   h. Fetal or intrapartum stress that compromises blood supply to fetal lungs: vaginal bleeding, maternal hypertension, difficult resuscitation associated with birth asphyxia.

(Some situations, such as steroid therapy or a heroin-addicted mother, result in the acceleration of surfactant.)

i. RDS due to nonpulmonary factors such as cardiac defects, sepsis, airway obstruction, intraventricular hemorrhage, hypoglycemia, and acute blood loss.

4. Surfactant production is deficient by type II alveolar cells. (Although some surfactant may be present at birth, it may not be regenerated at an adequate rate.) Surfactant production may be reduced due to:

a. Extreme immaturity of alveolar lining cells.

b. Diminished or impaired production rate resulting from fetal or early neonatal stress.

c. Impairment of release mechanism for phospholipid from type II alveolar cells.

d. Death of many of these cells responsible for decreased surfactant production.

5. Intra-alveolar surface tension is increased and alveoli are unstable and collapse at the end of expiration. Functional reserve capacity—the amount of air left in the lungs after expiration—is decreased; thus, the next breath requires almost as much effort as the first breath after birth.

6. More oxygen and energy are required to expand the alveoli with each breath, causing fatigue.

7. The number of alveoli that expand progressively decreases, leading to alveolar instability and atelectasis.

8. Pulmonary vascular resistance increases, causing hypoperfusion of lung.

9. Persistence of fetal circulation right-to-left shunt results, leading to hypoxemia and hypercapnia, which lead to respiratory and metabolic acidosis.

10. Hypoxemia and pulmonary vascular pressure cause ischemia in the alveoli, leading to transudate in the alveoli and formation of a membranous layer (see Figure 44-5).

11. Gas exchange becomes inhibited. Lungs become stiff (decreased compliance), requiring more pressure to expand them.

12. Airway obstruction leads to increased hypoxia and vasoconstriction, and the cycle continues.

13. RDS is usually a self-limiting disease and symptoms peak in about 3 to 4 days, at which time surfactant synthesis begins to accelerate and pulmonary function and clinical appearance begin to improve.

a. Moderately ill infants or those who do not require assisted ventilation usually show slow improvement by about 48 hours and rapid recovery over 3 to 4 days with few complications.

b. Severely ill and very immature infants who require some ventilatory assistance usually demonstrate rapid deterioration, such as decreased cardiac inflow, decreased arterial pressure, apneic episodes, cyanosis, pallor, and flaccid, unresponsive shocklike state. Ventilatory assistance may be required for several days and chronic lung disease and other complications are common.

Clinical Manifestations

Symptoms are usually observed soon after birth and may include those listed here and increase in severity over the first 2 days of life.

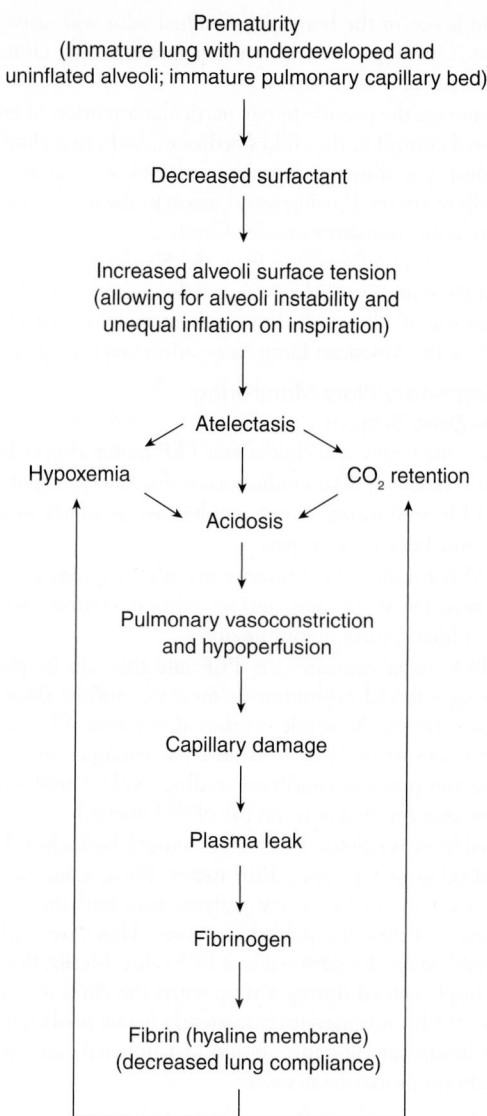

Figure 44-5. Schematic outline of respiratory distress syndrome.

Primary Signs and Symptoms

1. Expiratory grunting or whining (when the infant is not crying).

2. Sternal, suprasternal, substernal, and intercostal retractions progressing to paradoxical seesaw respirations.

3. Inspiratory nasal flaring.

4. Tachypnea less than 60 breaths per minute.

5. Hypothermia.

6. Cyanosis when child is in room air (infants with severe disease may be cyanotic even when given oxygen), increasing need for oxygen.

7. Decreased breath sounds and dry "sandpaper" breath sounds.

8. Pulmonary edema.

9. As the disease progresses:

a. Seesaw retractions become marked with marked abdominal protrusion on expiration.

b. Peripheral edema increases.

c. Muscle tone decreases.

d. Cyanosis increases.

e. Body temperature drops.

f. Short periods of apnea occur.

g. Bradycardia may occur.

h. Changes in distribution of blood throughout the body result in pale gray skin color.

i. Diminished breath sounds.

Secondary Signs and Symptoms

1. Hypotension.
2. Edema of the hands and feet.
3. Absent bowel sounds early in the illness.
4. Decreased urine output.

Diagnostic Evaluation

1. Prenatal diagnosis: Evaluation of amniotic fluids to assess fetal lung maturity.
   a. Lecithin/sphingomyelin ratio—tests of surfactant phospholipids in amniotic fluid.
   b. Phosphatidylcholine and phosphatidylglycerol (PG)—phospholipids that stabilize surfactant.
   c. Fetal maturity assay—determines PG levels in amniotic fluid or neonatal tracheal aspirates.
   d. Lamellar bodies test—measures a storage form of surfactant in amniotic fluids.
2. Laboratory tests:
   a. $PaCO_2$—elevated.
   b. Partial pressure of arterial oxygen (PaO_2)—low.
   c. Blood pH—low due to metabolic acidosis.
   d. Calcium—low.
   e. Serum glucose—low.
3. Chest x-ray—diffuse, fine granularity; "whiteout," very heavy, uniform granularity reflecting fluid-filled alveoli and atelectasis of some alveoli, surrounded by hyperdistended bronchioles; "ground glass" appearance with prominent air bronchogram extending into periphery of lung fields. Pulmonary interstitial emphysema is observed in premature neonates with RDS due to overdistension of distal airways.
4. Pulmonary function studies—stiff lung with a reduced effective pulmonary blood flow.

Management

Evidence Base Engle, W. A., & American Academy of Pediatrics. (2008). Surfactant replacement therapy for respiratory distress in the preterm neonate. *Pediatrics, 121*(2), 419–432.

Early recognition is imperative so that treatment may be initiated to halt the progression of RDS. In fact, treatment should begin prior to birth if the mother is at risk for delivering the baby preterm. Transportation to a facility providing specialized care is desirable, when possible.

Supportive

1. Maintenance of oxygenation—PaO_2 at 60 to 80 mm Hg to prevent hypoxia; frequent arterial pH and blood gas measurements and use of a pulse oximeter.

2. Maintenance of respiration with ventilatory support, if necessary.
   a. Intermittent mandatory ventilations delivered via ET tube. Allows the infant to breathe spontaneously at his or her own rate while the ventilator provides a preset cycle of respirations and pressure.
   b. Positive end-expiratory pressure (PEEP) via ET tube. The ventilator is pressure or volume limited. Provides increased PEEP during expiration to prevent alveolar collapse; residual airway pressure is maintained.
   c. Continuous positive airway pressure (CPAP) delivered via mask or nasal prongs. Used in spontaneous respiration to improve oxygenation by preventing collapse of the alveoli and increasing diffusion time.
   d. Synchronized intermittent mandatory ventilation allows the infant to breathe spontaneously between mechanical breaths. In assist or control mode, mechanical breaths are delivered at a regular rate if spontaneous breaths are not detected.
3. Maintenance of normal body temperature.
4. Maintenance of fluid, electrolyte, and acid-base balance—metabolic acidosis buffered with sodium bicarbonate.
5. Maintenance of nutrition—IV fluids, as prescribed.
6. Antibiotics, as needed, to treat infection.
7. Constant observation for complications—pneumothorax, disseminated intravascular coagulation (DIC), patent ductus arteriosus (PDA) with heart failure, chronic lung disease.
8. Care appropriate for a small, premature neonate.
9. Prevent hypotension.
10. Maintain a hematocrit of 40% to 45%.

Aggressive (Offered in Tertiary Care Centers)

1. Administration of exogenous surfactant into lungs early in the disease.
   a. Especially beneficial in the very low birth weight (VLBW) infant.
   b. May be given preventively to VLBW infants at birth.
   c. Available preparations are natural (derived from animal lungs) and synthetic (protein-free): bovine and synthetic surfactant.
   d. Administered into the ET tube.
2. Surfactant replacement therapy.
   a. Prophylactic surfactant therapy: infants at increased risk for RDS, infants of less than 27 weeks' gestational age, infants with a birth weight of less than 1,250 g.
   b. Treatment initiated after infant is stabilized in the delivery room or within 15 minutes of life.
   c. Rescue surfactant therapy: infants with moderate to severe RDS, requiring ventilatory assistance, with an oxygen requirement greater than 40%.
   d. Benefits of surfactant: decreases oxygen requirement and mean airway pressure; decreases pulmonary leaks.
   e. Complications observed in surfactant administration: pulmonary hemorrhage, PDA, mucus plugging.
   f. Nursing assessment with surfactant administration: suctioning delayed for 1 hour or as indicated by protocol. Assist with delivery of surfactant, collection and monitoring of

ABG studies, meticulous monitoring of oxygenation status with pulse oximeter or transcutaneous monitor ($Tcpco_2$).

   g. Assess the infant's tolerance of the procedure: increase in respiratory compliance, which will require adjustments of the ventilator.

3. High-frequency ventilation—mechanical ventilation that uses rapid rates (can be greater than 900 breaths per minute) and tidal volumes near and, commonly, less than anatomical dead spaces.
   a. Jet ventilator delivers short burst of gases at high flow.
      i. Exhalation is passive.
      ii. Necrotizing tracheitis is a significant complication, along with hypotension and pneumopericardium.
   b. Oscillator ventilator delivers gases by vibrating columns of air.
      i. Exhalation is active.
      ii. The child appears to shake on the bed, which may be frightening for the parents.

4. Extracorporeal membrane oxygenation (ECMO)—indicated in infants with reversible cardiac or respiratory failure. ECMO is a modified heart–lung bypass machine used to allow gas exchange outside the body.
   a. Blood is removed from the venous system by a catheter placed in the internal jugular vein or right atrium.
   b. Oxygen is added and carbon dioxide removed with a membrane oxygenator.
   c. Oxygenated blood is returned by way of the right common carotid (in venoarterial ECMO) or the femoral vein (in venovenous ECMO).
   d. The infant must be heparinized for the procedure, increasing the risk of intraventricular hemorrhage. For this reason, VLBW infants or infants of decreased gestational age are usually not candidates for the procedure.
   e. One nurse and one perfusionist must be present at the bedside at all times to monitor the patient and equipment. The patient will receive paralytic agents as well as analgesia and sedation; therefore, diligent continuous monitoring is required.
   f. Cannula dislodgement or tubing separation will result in immediate hemorrhage. Tubing and cannula must be secured and visible.
   g. Administration of dopamine or dobutamine may be required to support alteration in cardiac output and blood pressure.
   h. Blood transfusions may be indicated due to blood loss from frequent sampling or anemia of prematurity.

5. Ventilatory support modalities for RDS currently under study: nitric oxide, liquid ventilation (tidal or partial), and perfluorocarbon assisted gas exchange.

Complications

1. Complications related to respiratory therapy:
   a. Air leak: pneumothorax, pneumomediastinum, pneumopericardium, and pneumoperitoneum.
   b. Pneumonia, especially Gram-negative organisms.
   c. Pulmonary interstitial emphysema.

2. PDA or heart failure.
3. Hypotension.
4. Intraventricular hemorrhage—typically seen in infants weighing less than 1,500 g.
5. DIC.
6. Chronic problems associated with long-term use of oxygen:
   a. Bronchopulmonary dysplasia (BPD)—cystic-appearing lungs with hyperinfiltration, obstructive bronchiolitis, dysplastic changes, and pulmonary fibrosis.
   b. Chronic respiratory infections.
7. Necrotizing enterocolitis.
8. Tracheal stenosis.
9. Retinopathy of prematurity (retrolental fibroplasia).
10. Other complications related to prematurity.

Nursing Assessment

1. Review the birth history.
   a. Apgar scores 1 and 5 minutes after birth.
   b. Type of resuscitation required.
   c. Treatments or medications administered.
   d. Medications or anesthesia administered to the mother during labor.
   e. Estimated gestational age.
   f. Maternal history—contributing factors or complications.
2. Carefully assess the infant's respiratory status to determine the degree of respiratory distress.
   a. Determine the degree and severity of retractions.
   b. Count the respiratory rate for 1 full minute, note level of activity, and determine if they are regular or irregular.
   c. Identify periods of apnea, length, and type of stimulation necessary.
   d. Listen for expiratory grunting or whining sounds from the infant when quiet. This indicates an attempt to maintain PEEP and prevent alveoli from collapse.
   e. Note nasal flaring.
   f. Note cyanosis—location, improvement with oxygen.
   g. Auscultate chest for diminished breath sounds and presence of crackles.
3. Determine the infant's cardiac rate and rhythm.
   a. Count the apical pulse for 1 full minute.
   b. Note irregularities in the rate or bounding pulses.
4. Observe the infant's general activity.
   a. Lethargic or listless.
   b. Active and responds to stimuli.
   c. Infant's cry.
5. Assess the skin for cyanosis, jaundice, mottling, paleness or grayness, and edema.

Nursing Diagnoses

• Impaired Gas Exchange related to disease process.
• Imbalanced Nutrition: Less than Body Requirements related to prematurity and increased energy expenditure on breathing.
• Ineffective Thermoregulation related to immaturity.
• Impaired Parenting related to separation from the neonate due to hospitalization.

Nursing Interventions

Promoting Adequate Gas Exchange

1. Have emergency equipment readily available for use in the event of cardiac or respiratory arrest.
2. Institute cardiorespiratory monitoring to continuously monitor heart and respiratory rates.
3. Administer supplemental oxygen.
   a. Incubator with oxygen at prescribed concentration.
   b. Plastic hood with oxygen at prescribed concentration when using radiant warmer.
   c. CPAP, if indicated, using nasal prongs or ET tube.
4. Assist with ET intubation and maintain mechanical ventilation, as indicated.
5. Measure oxygen concentration every hour and record.
6. Monitor ABG levels, as appropriate. Obtain sample of blood through indwelling umbilical line, arterial puncture, or capillary puncture. (Capillary gas analysis for monitoring $PaCO_2$ and pH but not PaO_2.)
7. Institute pulse oximetry, if available, for continuous monitoring of the blood's arterial oxygen saturation (SaO_2).
   a. Avoid using adhesive to secure the sensor when the infant is active. Wrap it snugly enough to reduce sensitivity to movement but not tight enough to constrict blood flow.
   b. If transcutaneous PaO_2 monitor is used, reposition the probe every 3 to 4 hours to avoid burns caused by heating the probe to achieve sufficient arterialization.
8. Observe the infant's response to oxygen.
   a. Observe for improvement in color, respiratory rate and pattern, and nasal flaring.
   b. Note response by improvement in arterial or capillary blood gas levels.
   c. Observe closely for apnea.
9. Stimulate infant if apnea occurs. If unable to produce spontaneous respiration with stimulation within 15 to 30 seconds, initiate resuscitation.
10. Position the infant to allow for maximal lung expansion.
    a. Prone position provides for a larger lung volume because of the position of the diaphragm, decreases energy expenditure, and increases the time spent in quiet sleep; however, it may be contraindicated due to placement of the umbilical catheter. The risk for sudden infant death syndrome (SIDS) is increased, but the infant is continuously monitored.
    b. Change position frequently.
11. Suction, as needed, because the gag reflex is weak and cough is ineffective.
12. Try to minimize time spent on procedures and interventions and monitor effects on respiratory status. (Infants undergoing multiple procedures lasting 45 minutes to 1 hour have shown a moderate decrease in PaO_2.)
13. The decision to suction should be based on assessment of the infant, such as auscultation of chest, decrease in oxygenation, excessive moisture in the ET tube, and irritability.
    a. Nasopharyngeal, tracheal, or ET tube suctioning should be done gently, quickly, 5 seconds or less, with intermittent suction applied as the catheter is withdrawn.
   b. To prevent hypoxemia, observe oximeter before, during, and after the procedure.
   c. Suctioning of the ET tube is done to maintain a patent airway. The practice of inducing a catheter into the tube until resistance is met and then withdrawn has been shown to cause trauma to the tracheal wall. Instead, the suction catheter should be premeasured according to the size of the infant's ET tube length and documented. When suctioning, do not insert the catheter beyond this predetermined length. This will prevent damage to the mucosa.
14. Observe for complications of suctioning: bronchospasm, vagal nerve stimulation, bradycardia, hypoxia, increased intracranial pressure, trauma to airway, infection, and pneumothoraces.
15. VLBW and extremely low birth weight neonates cannot tolerate percussion and vibration. Trendelenburg's position is contraindicated in premature neonates and may result in increased intracranial pressure.
16. Record all nursing observations.

 NURSING ALERT Prone position may present several problems: Turning head to side can compromise upper airway and increase airflow resistance; observation of chest is obstructed, making retractions difficult to detect; and abdominal distention is more difficult to recognize.

Promoting Adequate Nutrition and Hydration

1. Administer IV fluids or enteral feeding, as ordered, and observe infusion rate closely to prevent fluid overload.
2. Observe IV sites for infiltration or infection; use meticulous technique to prevent sepsis.
3. If umbilical artery catheter is in place, observe for bleeding.
4. Provide adequate caloric intake (80 to 120 kcal/kg/24 hours) through the following:
   a. Nasojejunal tube (best tolerated by VLBW neonates).
   b. Nasogastric tube.
   c. Parenteral nutrition—$D_{10}W$ or hyperalimentation fluid usually required, especially in the acute phase of illness.
5. Monitor for hypoglycemia, which is especially common during stress. Maintain serum glucose greater than 45 mg/dL.
6. Monitor intake and output closely.
   a. Include amount of blood drawn (small infants can become anemic due to frequent blood sampling).
   b. Apply urine collection bag to obtain sample of urine and measure specific gravity periodically.
7. Weigh the infant daily and record.

Maintaining Thermoregulation

1. Provide a neutral thermal environment to maintain the infant's abdominal skin temperature between 97° and 98° F (36.1° and 36.7° C) to prevent hypothermia, which may result in vasoconstriction and acidosis.
2. Adjust incubator or radiant warmer to obtain desired skin temperature. For the infant weighing less than 1,250 g, the radiant warmer should be used with caution because of increased water loss and potential for hypoglycemia.

3. Prevent frequent opening of incubator.
4. Ensure that oxygen is warmed to a temperature between 87.6° and 93.2° F (30.9° and 34° C) with 60% to 80% humidity.

Encouraging Parental Attachment

1. Identify factors that may prohibit the parents' visitation and communication: geographic distance, lack of transportation, care of siblings, employment restrictions, economic issues, lack of telephone in the home, fear. Refer to social services for assistance and intervention, if required.
2. If the neonate was transported to a tertiary care center immediately after birth, send the mother a photograph of the neonate.
3. Call the parents daily to update them on the infant's condition until they are able to visit the child. Emphasize positive aspects of the infant's status.
4. Refer to the child by his or her first name when speaking with the parents.
5. Prepare the parents for the neonatal intensive care unit (NICU) environment and how their child will appear before their first visit.
6. Assist the parents to participate in the child's care, as appropriate.
7. Demonstrate for the parents how they can touch and speak to the child while the child is in an Isolette/incubator.
8. Allow the parents to hold the infant as soon as possible.
9. If the mother plans to breastfeed, assist her with expressing her milk and use the breast milk to feed the infant when enteral feedings are initiated.
10. If the infant has siblings, provide the parents with information on how to discuss the infant's illness with them.
11. If unit policies allow and the situation is appropriate, encourage sibling visitation with adequate preparation.
12. Provide the parents with information concerning the disease process, expected outcomes, and usual course of the NICU stay. Encourage the parents to ask questions and participate in the care plan.
13. Help parents work through their distress at the birth of a premature child.
14. Assess parents' support mechanisms (eg, grandparents, friends).

Family Education and Health Management

1. Prepare the family for long-term follow-up, as appropriate. Infants with BPD may eventually go home on oxygen therapy.
2. Stress the importance of regular health care, periodic eye examinations, and developmental follow-up with the parents.
3. Ensure that the family receives information on routine well-baby care.
4. Before discharge, parents should feel comfortable in their abilities to care for the infant. Referrals for home nursing visits should be completed and a physician identified for follow-up care.

Evaluation: Expected Outcomes

- Respiratory rate within normal range for age; pattern regular and unlabored.
- Tolerates enteral feedings well; weight gain noted.

- Maintains temperature within normal limits.
- Parents interact with infant, participate in care, and ask appropriate questions.

Cystic Fibrosis

 Evidence Base Royal Brompton Hospital Paediatric Cystic Fibrosis Team. (2011). *Clinical guidelines: Care of children with cystic fibrosis* (5th ed.). London: Royal Brompton & Harefield NHS Foundation Trust. Available: www.rbht.nhs.uk/chldrencf.

Cantine, M., & Lomas, P. (2012) Cystic fibrosis patients: Step-up to better breathing. *The Journal for Respiratory Care Practitioners, 25*(11), 14–17.

Cystic fibrosis (CF) is an autosomal recessive disorder affecting the exocrine glands, causing abnormal viscosity of secretions. It primarily affects the pulmonary and GI systems. Approximately 4% to 5% of Caucasians are symptomless carriers of the CF gene. Slightly more males than females are affected. Incidence is estimated at approximately 1 in 3,500 live Caucasian births. CF is found in all racial groups. There are approximately 30,000 people living with CF in the United States, 45% of whom are age 18 or older. Presently the predicted survival age extends to the late 40s, compared with a life expectancy of less than 1 year in the 1950s.

Pathophysiology and Etiology

1. CF is caused by a genetic defect in a single gene located on the long arm of chromosome 7 that encodes the cystic fibrosis transmembrane conductance regulator (CFTR).
2. The variations in the onset of the disease, symptomatology, and clinical presentation within the CF population are attributed to the over 1,000 mutations of the CF gene. CFTR is responsible for the fluid balance across epithelial cells.
3. The malfunction of CFTR results in:
   a. Decreased chloride secretion into the airway lumen.
   b. Increased sodium reabsorption, which leads to decreased airway surface liquid volume.
   c. Thickened mucus, impaired mucociliary clearance, chronic infection, plugged bronchi.
   d. Chronic inflammation, airway damage, atelectasis, and hyperinflation of lungs.
   e. Progressive bronchiectasis, irreversible fibrotic changes in lungs.
4. GI and pancreatic involvement includes:
   a. Acini and ducts of pancreas become filled with thick mucus and are obstructed.
   b. Trypsin, chymotrypsin, lipase, and amylase do not reach the small intestine.
   c. Digestion is impaired. Interruption of the enterohepatic circulation of bile acids probably results in interference with normal pancreatic lipolysis and fat absorption through the intestinal wall.
   d. Stools are abnormal and indicate malabsorption syndrome.
   e. Meconium ileus often occurs in infants, indicating that bowel is obstructed by thick intestinal secretions.

f. Biliary cirrhosis occurs because the intrahepatic biliary tract is obstructed by thick secretions.

g. In 30% of CF patients, the gallbladder is small, with suboptimal function. Gallstones develop in up to 10% of patients.

5. Sweat gland involvement includes:

a. Secretions contain excessive amount of sodium and chloride, leading to excessive loss, especially with hot weather, fever, or exertion.

b. Saliva also contains an excess of sodium and chloride.

Clinical Manifestations

Presentation usually occurs younger than age 6 months but may occur at any age. Signs and symptoms and severity of the disease vary and change over time as the disease progresses.

Respiratory Manifestations

1. Recurrent pulmonary infections—*H. influenza, S. aureus, P. aeruginosa.*

2. Cough, dry to productive. Chronic clearing of throat may indicate increased mucus production.

3. Wheezing, crackles on auscultation are indicative of respiratory exacerbation.

4. Dyspnea.

5. Barrel-shaped chest (increased anteroposterior chest diameter).

6. Cyanosis.

7. Clubbing of fingers and toes.

8. Nasal polyps and pansinusitis.

9. Progressive chronic obstructive pulmonary disease (COPD). A 10% drop in FEV_1 is a sign of an acute exacerbation or worsening lung disease.

a. Mild form of CF—slightly decreased FEV_1 (70% to 90%).

b. Moderate CF—FEV_1 of 40% to 69%.

c. Severe forms of CF—life-threatening pulmonary disease with FEV_1 of less than 40%.

GI Manifestations

1. Meconium ileus found in neonates.

2. Failure to thrive and failure to gain weight in the presence of a good appetite.

3. Abdominal distention.

4. Vomiting, dehydration, and electrolyte imbalance.

5. Maldigestion, steatorrhea (fatty stools, loss of fat-soluble vitamins).

6. Rectal prolapse.

7. Distal intestinal obstructive syndrome.

8. Biliary cirrhosis, obstructive jaundice.

9. Pancreatitis.

Other Manifestations

1. Thin extremities, sallow skin, wasted buttocks.

2. Hyperglycemia, glucosuria, polyuria, weight loss.

3. Salty taste when parents kiss skin.

4. Sterility in males.

5. Hypoproteinemia and anemia.

6. Bleeding diathesis.

7. Hyponatremia and heat prostration.

8. Kyphosis.

Diagnostic Evaluation

1. Quantitative sweat chloride test; pilocarpine iontophoresis, performed at a CF Foundation accredited center by skilled personnel. Measures sodium and chloride content in sweat.

a. Chloride level greater than 60 mEq/L is virtually diagnostic.

b. Chloride of 40 to 60 mEq/L is borderline and should be repeated, followed by genotype for the most frequent CFTR mutations.

c. Sodium level greater than 60 mEq/L is diagnostic.

2. Measurement of trypsin concentration in duodenal secretions; absence of normal concentration virtually diagnostic.

3. Analysis of digestive enzymes (trypsin and chymotrypsin) in stool—reduced, used for initial screening for CF.

4. Chest x-ray—may be normal initially; later shows areas of infection, overinflation, bronchial thickening and plugging, atelectasis, fibrosis, and emphysema.

5. Sinus radiograph or computed tomography shows mucus plugging.

6. Analysis of stool for steatorrhea.

7. Meconium strip test for stool includes lactose and protein content; used for screening.

8. Sputum or throat cultures to rule out infection.

9. Pulmonary function studies (after age 4).

a. Decreased vital capacity and flow rates.

b. Increased residual volume or increased total lung capacity.

10. Diagnosis made when a positive sweat test is seen in conjunction with one or more of the following:

a. Positive family history for CF.

b. Typical COPD.

c. Documented exocrine pancreatic insufficiency.

d. Failure to thrive.

e. History of frequent respiratory infections.

11. Prenatal diagnostic tests—prenatal genetic screening for families affected with CF:

a. Chorionic villus sampling at approximately 12 weeks' gestation.

b. Deoxyribonucleic acid (DNA) probes.

c. Microvillar enzymes.

12. Neonatal screening: immunoreactive trypsinogen; if elevated, DNA assay for single and multiple CFTR mutations.

Management

Goals of treatment are to prevent and minimize pulmonary complications, ensure adequate nutrition for growth, and assist the family and child to adapt to chronic disease.

Pulmonary Interventions

1. Antimicrobial therapy, as indicated, for pulmonary infection.

a. Oral antibiotics may be given prophylactically or when symptomatic.

b. IV antibiotics are given when the child fails to respond to oral antibiotics; this may be inpatient or at-home therapy.

c. Inhaled antibiotics such as tobramycin. Colistin may be used for severe lung disease or colonization of organisms. Recently, some practitioners advocate using nebulized antibiotics earlier in therapy.

d. Patients with CF metabolize antibiotics rapidly; if drug dosage is higher than normal, monitor for signs of toxicity.

2. Bronchodilators to increase the airway size and assist with mucociliary clearance. Many CF patients also have airway hyperreactivity.

a. Long-term clinical improvement with inhaled broncho-dilators has not been well supported in the literature. Sal-meterol, a long-acting bronchodilator, has demonstrated improvements in pulmonary function and is effective in decreasing nocturnal hypoxia.

b. Inhaled steroids for treatment of airway hyperreactivity.

3. Aerosols, expectorants, and mucolytic agents to decrease viscosity of secretions.

a. Recombinate human DNase administered via nebulizer improves pulmonary function and decreases sputum viscosity and pulmonary exacerbations.

b. Hypertonic saline solution 3% to 7%.

c. Improves airway clearance and lung function, although it is not as effective as recombinant human DNase.

d. Acetylcysteine solution is not recommended due to irritant effect on airways.

4. CPT for bronchial drainage, especially during acute exacerbations.

a. Postural drainage (see Figure 44-6, and Procedure Guidelines 44-2, pages 1512 and 1513).

b. Some patients use a vibrating vest that utilizes a shaking motion rather than manual postural drainage.

c. Coughing and deep-breathing exercises; huffing helps move secretions from smaller airways.

d. Increase physical activity—aerobic activity.

e. Active cycle of breathing, a new technique, improves lung function without decreasing oxygenation. Consists of breathing control, thoracic expansion, forced expiratory technique, and huffing. An assistant is not required.

f. Autogenic drainage—breathing at various lung volumes to move and evacuate mucus. Oxygenation should not be affected during procedure.

g. Positive expiratory pressure (PEP) and flutter. PEP airway technique is utilized by those with severe disease. It reduces airway collapse due to bronchiectasis. Available as low-pressure PEP, high-pressure PEP, and oscillating PEP with a flutter or acapella device.

h. High-frequency chest compressions—externally applied device provides oscillation to the chest, resulting in release of mucus from the airway wall.

Evidence Base Flume, P. A., Robinson, K. A., & O'Sullivan, B. P. (2009). Cystic fibrosis guidelines: Airway clearance therapies. *Respiratory Care, 54*(4), 522–537.

5. Bronchopulmonary lavage—treatment of atelectasis and mucoid impaction using large volumes of saline (used in some institutions in the United States).

6. Lobectomy—resection of symptomatic lobar bronchiectasis to retard progression of lesion to total lung involvement.

GI Interventions

1. Pancreatic enzyme supplementation is provided with each feeding.

a. Favored preparation is pancrelipase.

b. Occasionally, antacid is helpful to improve tolerance of enzymes.

c. Favorable response to enzymes is based on tolerance of fatty foods, decreased stool frequency, absence of steatorrhea, improved appetite, and lack of abdominal pain.

2. Provide a high-energy diet by increasing carbohydrates, protein, and fat (possibly as high as 40%). Increases in dietary intake should consider growth and repair, infection, the work of breathing and energy expenditure for coughing, malabsorption, and physical activity.

3. Provide zinc and iron supplements and water-soluble and fat-soluble vitamins.

4. Ensure adequate fluid and salt intake.

Controversial and Experimental Treatments

1. Heart–lung, double-lung, or single-lung transplantation for end-stage lung disease.

a. This treatment is limited by availability of donor organs.

b. Long-term survival at 5 years is approximately 50%.

c. Bilateral lobar transplantation using a new method, called bipartitioning of a single-donor lung, is under study. This method could result in increased availability of donor organs.

2. Liver transplant.

3. Gene therapy.

a. This treatment is at present only being undertaken by a small number of centers due to its complexity.

b. Therapy is based on somatic gene correction; an attempt to correct the defect in the cells of the individual is made by adding the correct gene sequence to the cells.

c. One trial method will use a virus carrying DNA with the appropriate gene sequence, which will be introduced into the affected lung cells by nebulization.

d. A second method being investigated is the introduction into the lungs of DNA by nebulization with the appropriate gene sequence suspended in liposomes.

e. It is thought that the treatment will need to be repeated at regular intervals.

4. *Pseudomonas aeruginosa* genome is complete, which should lead to the development of new medications to combat this common lung infection in CF.

Complications

1. Pulmonary infections:

a. Most frequently caused by *P. aeruginosa, S. aureus, H. influenzae,* and *Burkholderia cepacia. Pseudomonas* is the most difficult organism to treat.

b. Bronchiectasis and bronchiolitis.

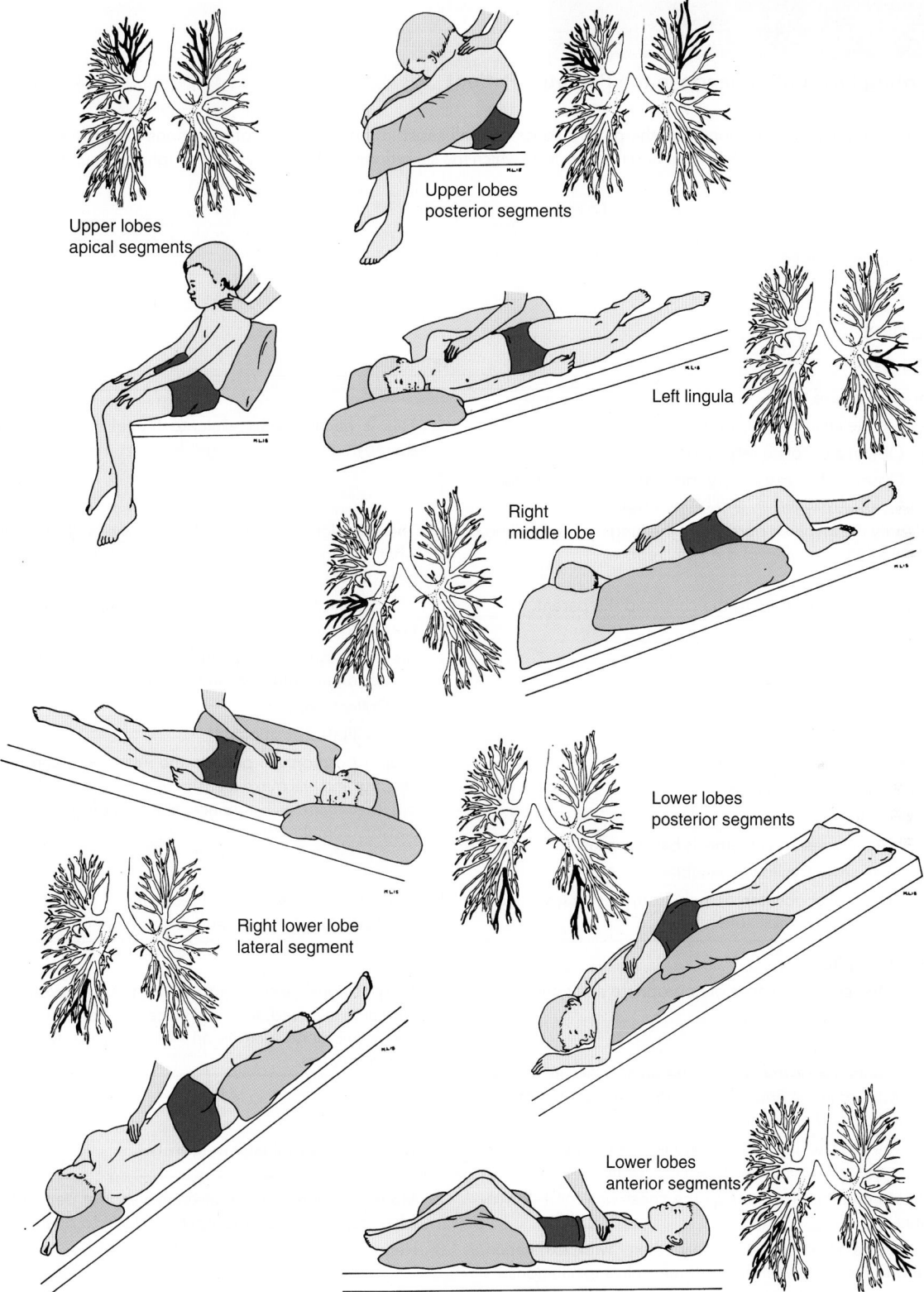

Upper lobes
apical segments

Upper lobes
posterior segments

Left lingula

Right
middle lobe

Right lower lobe
lateral segment

Lower lobes
posterior segments

Lower lobes
anterior segments

Figure 44-6. Positions for postural drainage.

PROCEDURE GUIDELINES 44-2

Promoting Postural Drainage in the Pediatric Patient

Postural drainage is the positioning of the patient so gravity will assist in the movement of secretions from the smaller bronchial airways to the main bronchus and trachea, from which the secretions can be removed by coughing or suctioning.

 NURSING ALERT Percussion, vibration, and squeezing of the chest are contraindicated in children with pulmonary hemorrhage, pulmonary embolism, end-stage renal disease, increased intracranial pressure, osteogenesis imperfecta, and minimum cardiac reserve.

PROCEDURE

Nursing Action	Rationale
Preparatory phase	
1. Assess the child's respiratory status.	1. This is necessary to evaluate the effectiveness of the therapy.
a. Obtain a baseline respiratory rate.	
b. Observe for respiratory distress, retractions, nasal flaring, hypoxemia, and bronchospasm.	
2. Identify the involved portions of the lung by auscultation, percussion, or review of the x-ray report.	2. The positions selected for drainage will depend on what portion of the lung is involved (see Figure 44-6, page 1511).
3. Explain the procedure to the child and the parent.	3. Allays anxiety and helps to secure the child's cooperation.
	a. Assists in relaxing and decreasing strain on the abdominal muscles during coughing.
	b. Collects mucus.
	c. Facilitates positioning.
4. Make the child comfortable.	4. Proper position will provide the infant with comfort and security and will make it easier to suck and swallow. Holding the infant will enhance trust-building and provide sensory stimulation.
a. Remove constricting clothes.	
b. Flex the child's knees and hips.	
c. Have tissues and an emesis basin available.	
d. Have several pillows available.	
5. Provide bronchodilator or nebulization therapy before the procedure, if indicated.	5. It is easier to raise mucus mechanically after the bronchi are dilated and the secretions are thinned.
Performance phase	
1. Place the child in a series of appropriate positions.	1. The positions are selected and modified according to the lung area involved, the child's age and general condition, and equipment such as an IV tracheostomy, monitors, and ventilators.
a. Infants are positioned on the nurse's lap, in the Isolette, or in the crib; older children may be treated on a tilt board or in bed.	
b. The area to be drained should be elevated and its respective bronchus placed in a vertical position.	b. Facilitates drainage by gravity.
2. Unless contraindicated, cup the chest wall for 1–2 minutes.	2. More secretions can be raised in a shorter period of time when cupping and vibration are added to posturing.
3. Have the child inhale deeply; then, with exhalation, vibrate the chest wall during three to five exhalations.	3. Helps open airways and mobilize secretions.
4. Encourage the child to cough. Infants and young children may require suctioning.	4. Facilitates movement of secretions.

PROCEDURE GUIDELINES 44-2 *(continued)*

Promoting Postural Drainage in the Pediatric Patient

PROCEDURE *(continued)*

Nursing Action	Rationale
5. Allow the child to rest for a minute, then repeat cupping, vibration, and coughing until no more mucus is produced or the child's condition indicates that the procedure should be stopped.	5. Procedure may be tiring, so rest will be necessary.

Total treatment time should generally not exceed 20–30 minutes.

a. In acute conditions such as atelectasis, postural drainage may be done for 5 minutes of every hour.

b. In chronic conditions such as cystic fibrosis, postural drainage may be done two to five times per day for 15–30 minutes.

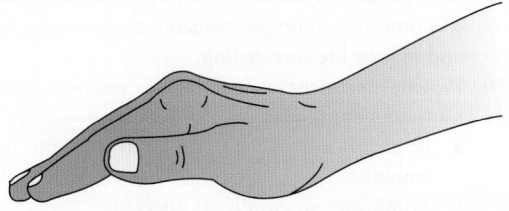

Cupping the chest.

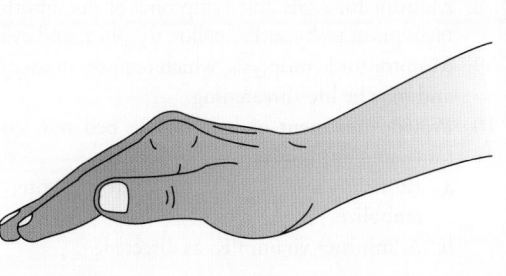

To assist with percussing an infant or small child, an alternative percussion device may be used, such as a mask from a manual resuscitation bag.

6. Stay with the child during the procedure, especially when in a head-down position.

6. Provides for patient safety.

 NURSING ALERT Postural drainage should not be done immediately after meals because it may induce vomiting.

 Evidence Base Flume, P. A., Robinson, K. A., O'Sullivan, B. P., et al. (2009). Cystic fibrosis guidelines: Airway clearance therapies. *Respiratory Care, 54*(4), 522–537.

NURSING ALERT *B. cepacia* affects approximately 5% of CF patients, is associated with a rapid decline in pulmonary function, and is multiple antibiotic-resistant. Twenty percent of colonized patients develop fulminant septicemia and necrotizing pneumonia, leading to death.

2. Other pulmonary complications—emphysema, atelectasis, pneumothorax, hemoptysis (primarily seen in adolescents), and pulmonary hypertension.

3. Biliary cirrhosis, leading to portal hypertension, esophageal varices, and splenomegaly.

4. Pancreatic fibrosis with islets of Langerhans involvement, resulting in glucose intolerance and CF-related diabetes.

5. Cor pulmonale.
6. Chronic sinusitis.
7. Rectal polyps (3 months to 3 years).
8. Rectal prolapse.
9. Intussusception (younger than 2 years).
10. Pancreatitis.
11. Hypertrophic pulmonary osteoarthropathy—arthritis, clubbing, periosteitis; the long tubular bones are most commonly involved.
12. Bone thinning and demineralization.
13. Depression.
14. Heat prostration.
15. Fibrosis of epididymis and vas deferens in male; aspermia.
16. Growth retardation.
17. Gastroesophageal reflux.
18. Allergic bronchopulmonary aspergillosis.
19. Respiratory failure and death.

Nursing Assessment

1. Check for family history of CF, failure to thrive, and unexplained infant death; check the child's history and physical condition. Carefully listen for subtle information that may suggest CF.
2. Assess respiratory status—respiratory rate, presence of tachypnea, wheeze, cough, character of sputum, and oxygen saturation level.
   a. Increased work of breathing.
   b. Quality of breath sounds by auscultation.
   c. Child's perception of respiratory status.
   d. Ability to participate in activities of daily living, exercise tolerance, quality of sleep.
   e. Assess for oxygen desaturation with sleep.
3. Assess nutritional status and characteristics of stool.

Nursing Diagnoses

- Ineffective Airway Clearance related to thick pulmonary secretions.
- Risk for Infection related to thick, tenacious secretions.
- Imbalanced Nutrition: Less than Body Requirements related to decreased appetite or inadequate absorption.
- Disturbed Body Image related to chronic disease process.
- Interrupted Family Processes related to the child with a chronic disease.

Nursing Interventions

Promoting Airway Clearance

1. Use intermittent nebulizer therapy three to four times per day when child is symptomatic.
   a. Use pretreatment postural drainage.
   b. Administer bronchodilators and other medications, diluted in normal saline, in aerosol form to penetrate respiratory tract. Proper technique is necessary to deliver the correct dose of medication. If using a face mask, it should fit snugly; movement of the mask by ¾ inch (2 cm) could decrease the delivery of medication by 85%.

 NURSING ALERT Mist therapy is no longer recommended because water droplets may cause bronchospasm in some patients and the equipment required to deliver the therapy is frequently contaminated with opportunistic organisms.

2. Perform CPT three to four times per day after nebulizer therapy; perform more frequently if infection is present.
   a. Perform prior to meals or 1 hour after eating to prevent vomiting or discomfort.
   b. Place the child in a position that gives the greatest access to the affected lobes of the lung and facilitates gravity drainage of mucus from specific lung areas.
   c. Children with gastro-esophageal reflux should not use the head-down position during CPT.
3. Help the child to relax to cough more easily after postural drainage.
4. Suction the infant or young child when necessary if he or she is unable to cough.
5. Teach child breathing exercises using pursed lips to increase duration of exhalation.
6. Monitor child's oxygen saturation levels during procedures.
7. Maintain cautious oxygen therapy due to chronic carbon dioxide retention.
8. Monitor for signs and symptoms of pneumothorax, such as tachypnea, tachycardia, pallor, dyspnea, and cyanosis.
9. Monitor for hemoptysis, which requires immediate treatment and may be life-threatening.
10. Provide treatment of hemoptysis: bed rest, cough suppressants, and antibiotics.
    a. Bronchoscopy is used to locate the site, cauterize, or embolize.
    b. Administer vitamin K, as directed.

Preventing Infection

Adherence to infection control procedures must be enforced to prevent the spread of nosocomial infections.

1. Provide frequent mouth care to reduce the chance of infection because mucus is present.
2. Restrict contact with people with respiratory infections.

 NURSING ALERT To decrease the risk of transmission of *B. cepacia* within the hospital setting, children who test positive for the pathogen are placed on room isolation.

3. Administer antibiotics, as prescribed, to treat specific organisms when the child is symptomatic.
4. Monitor closely for deteriorating respiratory status.
5. Provide good skin care and position changes to prevent skin breakdown of malnourished child.
6. Change diapers promptly to prevent diaper rash and superimposed infection.

Promoting Adequate Nutrition

1. Refer to dietitian for dietary assessment.
2. Encourage diet composed of foods high in calories and protein and moderate to high in fat because absorption of food is

incomplete. Provide 120% to 150% of recommended dietary allowances because only 80% to 85% of intake is absorbed.

3. Administer fat-soluble vitamins in water-miscible solution in two to three times the normal dose, as prescribed, to counteract malabsorption.

   a. Give vitamins A, D, and E on a daily basis.

   b. Give vitamin K when the child has an infection or is being treated with antibiotics.

4. Administer pancreatic enzymes with each meal and snack. Dose is based on the child's weight, weight gain, growth, food intake, and number and character of bowel movements.

   a. Mix capsule, granules, or powder with small portion of food for infant or small child; do not mix with formula, which may not be finished.

   b. Offer the older child capsules or tablets.

   c. Withhold enzymes, as ordered, if the child is taking only clear liquid diet or enteral feedings.

   d. Beads should not be chewed or crushed.

   e. The CF Foundation discourages the use of generic enzymes.

5. Increase salt intake during hot weather, fever, or excessive exercise to prevent sodium depletion and cardiovascular compromise.

6. To prevent vomiting, allow ample time for feeding, especially if irritable because of not feeling well and coughing.

7. Check weights at least weekly to assess nutritional interventions. Document and plot height and weight every 3 months.

8. Infants who are breastfed will need enzyme supplementation. If supplementation with formula is necessary, choose a high-calorie preparation.

9. Administer supplemental parenteral or enteral feedings, as required.

10. Constipation, due to malabsorption, decreased gastric motility; viscous intestinal secretions may be treated with laxatives, stool softeners, or rectal administration of x-ray contrast material.

Enhancing Self-Esteem and Body Image

1. Explain each procedure, medication, and treatment to the child as appropriate for age.

2. Allow the child to show frustrations, fears, and feelings by talking, complaining, or crying.

3. Support and comfort the child by talking to and holding him or her.

4. Provide diversional activities related to the child's interests and praise the child for his or her accomplishments.

5. Encourage older child to take an active role in his or her self-management and be involved in the care plan.

6. Help the child to identify strengths and limitations and to feel good about self.

7. If the child resists CPT due to anger, fear, or frustration, help to redirect those feelings.

8. Encourage regular exercise and activity to foster a sense of accomplishment and independence and improve pulmonary function. Consent from health care provider is necessary prior to the initiation of an exercise program. Oxygenation status during exercise should be assessed.

Enhancing Family Processes

1. Provide opportunities for the parents to learn all aspects of care for the child.

2. Provide education and support during hospitalization to make home care easier.

3. Encourage maintenance of family activities and involvement with other children.

4. Initiate social work referral, as needed.

5. Encourage information sharing about CF with friends, teachers, and relatives. Explain that one of the most important things people can do to help a child with CF is to treat him or her just as they would any other child.

6. Help family share and interpret feelings about CF and its impact on all of their lives.

7. Encourage families to foster the older child's independence when the time comes.

Family Education and Health Maintenance

1. Teach parents to have a thorough understanding of the dietary regimen and special need for calories, fat, and vitamins. Consultation with a registered dietitian is recommended.

2. Discuss the child's need for salt replacement and free access to salt as well as the increased need for salt during hot weather or in the presence of fever, vomiting, or diarrhea.

3. Help the parents to become skilled at CPT and other pulmonary treatments. Demonstrate and explain procedures and evaluate their return demonstration.

4. Help the family to schedule care for the child within the framework of family life.

   a. CPT should be done at least 1 hour after meals.

   b. Nebulizer treatments should be done before CPT.

   c. Mild exercise and activity are beneficial to the child.

   d. Vacations and major family outings can be planned for remissions of the child's symptoms.

5. Help the parents to provide emotional support to their child. The child needs love, understanding, and security, not overprotection.

6. Stress the importance of regular medical care.

   a. Routine immunizations.

   b. Prompt attention to infection.

   c. Continued evaluation and supervision in home management.

   d. Attention to developments through research that may change therapy.

   e. Prevention or early detection of complications.

7. Stress the importance of following up with regular health care provider for routine follow-up according to Cystic Fibrosis Foundation.

   a. Outpatient visits, four per year.

   b. Pulmonary function tests, two or more per year.

   c. Respiratory cultures, at least one per year.

   d. Creatinine level, every year.

   e. Glucose level, every year if older than age 13.

   f. Liver enzymes, every year.

8. Discuss with parents the limitations and expectations for the child.
   a. With proper care, the child will most likely live to adulthood but may be smaller and shorter than peers.
   b. Play and school participation depends on severity of illness.
   c. Involve teachers and school nurses in planning of the child's day.
9. Suggest parents and child meet other CF families. Investigate location and participation in summer camps for children with CF.
10. Investigate home care options for families, especially respite services for caregivers.
11. After the diagnosis is confirmed, refer the parents to genetic counseling. It is important for the parents to realize that the affected child inherits the defective gene from both parents. Each pregnancy will result in a 25% chance that the infant will have CF, a 50% chance that it will be a carrier of the CF gene and *not* have CF, and a 25% chance that the infant will neither be a carrier of the CF gene nor have CF.
12. Refer families for additional information and support to agencies such as Cystic Fibrosis Foundation (*www.cff.org*). Most areas have local chapters of the organization.
13. The pediatric health care team should discuss with the patient and parents the concept of eventual transitioning of care from a pediatric CF center to an adult CF center as early as possible—an important issue that should not be left until adolescence. Facilitate a planned, efficient, and smooth transition by:
   a. Encouraging the child to gradually assume responsibility for health care.
   b. Encouraging the parents to foster the adolescent's independence.
   c. Providing patient and family time to adjust and educate themselves about the transitioning process.
   d. Identifying and introducing the child and his or her family to members of the adult care team.
   e. Advocating for the patient in regard to any restrictions superimposed by the patient's health insurance plan.
14. Sadly, at some point, it will become apparent to the health care team that the time has arrived to discuss end-of-life issues. Use a family-centered approach to provide care for the child and family facing a life-threatening illness or death. Discuss hospice care and other available services with the family (see page 1449).

 Evidence Base Sands, D., Reppetto, T., Dupont, L. J., et al. (2011). End of life care for patients with cystic fibrosis. *Journal of Cystic Fibrosis, 10*(2), 37–44.

Evaluation: Expected Outcomes

- Tolerates CPT four times per day for 30 minutes with stable oxygen saturation.
- No signs of respiratory infection.
- Eats well with no vomiting; weight stable.
- Plays, interacts appropriately.
- Parents ask questions; meet, as necessary, with a social worker; and take part in care of their child.

Apnea of Infancy and Apparent Life-Threatening Event

Apnea of infancy (AOI) is defined as an unexplained episode of cessation of breathing for 20 seconds or longer or a shorter respiratory pause associated with bradycardia, cyanosis, pallor, and marked hypotonia in an infant of 37 weeks' gestation or more at the onset of apnea.

Apnea of prematurity (AOP) is defined as sudden cessation of breathing that lasts for 20 seconds and may or may not be accompanied by bradycardia and cyanosis in an infant younger than 37 weeks' gestation.

An *apparent life-threatening event (ALTE)* is defined as an episode that is frightening to the observer and is characterized by some combination of apnea (central or obstructive), color change, cyanosis, pallor or plethora, marked change in muscle tone, extreme limpness, choking, or gagging.

Pathophysiology and Etiology

1. Cause is often unknown—may result from many different pathologic processes; may be idiopathic.
2. Apnea may be related to organic disorders, such as seizure disorders, sepsis, severe infection, hypoglycemia, and impaired regulation of breathing while sleeping or feeding, gastroesophageal reflux, upper airway abnormalities, metabolic disorders, or abuse.
3. Abnormal properties of surfactant have been reported in some children with recurrent ALTE.
4. A diagnosis of AOI is made when no identifiable cause of ALTE is found.
5. AOP is related to immature neurologic and respiratory control mechanisms.

Clinical Manifestations

1. The infant may be found by parents or caretaker to be limp, cyanotic, and pale with no respiration. Skin is cool to the touch.
2. Some form of resuscitation may be required.
3. The infant usually exhibits symptoms when asleep, although the syndrome may occur during waking hours.
4. Types of AOP:
   a. Central or diaphragmatic—chest movement ceases, absence of airflow.
   b. Obstructive—chest and diaphragm move, but there is no air exchange.
   c. Mixed—cessation of airflow and chest movement, followed by respiratory effort without airflow.

Diagnostic Evaluation

Complete history, physical examination, and diagnostic tests are aimed at ruling out other medical problems that could result in respiratory failure as a secondary cause.

1. Complete blood count with differential, serum glucose, electrolytes, calcium, phosphate, magnesium, and ABG levels, as indicated.
2. Chest x-ray.

3. Electrocardiogram.

4. Electroencephalogram (may not be routine) and neurologic examination.

5. Respiratory studies—a 12- to 24-hour pneumogram recording of small changes in electrical resistance with each breath or respiratory pattern; multichannel sleep test with continuous printout, monitoring heart rate, chest impedance, nasal airflow, and oxygen saturation.

6. Continuous cardiac and apnea monitoring for recurrence of event, prolonged apnea, or bradycardia.

7. Barium swallow for GER.

8. Because of hypoxemia that may have occurred, the child should be assessed for learning difficulties, discrete neurologic impairments, impaired hearing or vision, and personality disorders.

9. Polysomnograph—records brain waves, eye movements, esophageal manometry, and end tidal carbon dioxide.

Management

1. Cardiopulmonary monitoring is critical; hospitalization if ALTE has occurred.

2. Specific treatment of the underlying cause, if identified.

3. Theophylline may be used to decrease apneic episodes (therapeutic levels of 6 to 13 mcg/mL). Caffeine, which also acts as a central nervous system stimulant for breathing, may be given to maintain a trough level of 5 to 20 mcg/mL.

4. Long-term follow-up for physiologic and neurologic behavioral functions.

5. Prevention of SIDS: the most effective method of prevention is public education to avoid prone sleeping. More education is needed, with an emphasis on poor, underserved areas (see Box 44-1).

 NURSING ALERT Infants who have experienced apnea may be at risk for recurrent apnea, hypoxia, and sudden death and should be monitored closely. Research has shown that SIDS is more likely in infants sleeping prone. It is now recommended that all infants be put to sleep on their backs or sides.

Nursing Assessment

1. Obtain a nursing history, including the parents' description of the events that preceded the hospitalization, and their understanding of prolonged apnea.
   a. This information may provide clues for factors to observe during hospitalization and provides data for the development of a teaching plan.
   b. It allows for the correction of misinformation and misconceptions.

2. Have the parents describe sleep patterns, feeding habits, prior health problems, immunizations, and medications; this may provide data regarding possible influencing factors or causes of the condition.

3. Have the parents describe a typical day in the life of the infant and the family unit. This provides important data on how

---

BOX 44-1 Sudden Infant Death Syndrome

 Evidence Base American Academy of Pediatrics, Task Force on Sudden Infant Death Syndrome. (2005). The changing concept of sudden infant death syndrome: Diagnostic coding shifts, controversies regarding the sleeping environment, and new variables to consider in reducing risk. *Pediatrics, 116*(5), 1245–1255. (Reaffirmed 2007.)

Sudden infant death syndrome (SIDS) is sudden death of an infant under the age of 1 year, which remains unexplained after a thorough case investigation, including performance of a complete autopsy, examination of the death scene, and review of clinical history.

The peak incidence occurs between 2 and 3 months of age. In addition, it has been found that there is a higher rate of incidence, two to three times the national average, in children who are black or American Indian or of Alaskan origin. Additional infant risk factors include male gender, prematurity, preterm birth or low birth weight, low Apgar scores, prone sleeping position, overheating, sleeping on soft surfaces, and twin victim of SIDS. Maternal risk factors include young maternal age, late or no prenatal care, smoking or exposure to smoking during pregnancy, history of sexually transmitted disease or urinary tract infection, anemia, and poverty.

There has generally been a reduction in death rate, with 1.2 deaths per 1,000 live births reported in 1992 and 0.5% deaths per 1,000 live births in 2002. However, since 2001, there has been a slightly higher proportion of deaths occurring in the neonatal period and after 6 months of age, possibly due to classification.

Current theories on the cause of SIDS focus on abnormalities of the brain stem and its network. Recent autopsy results from victims of SIDS have indicated deficits in serotonin receptors in this network, which are responsible for breathing, body temperature, blood pressure, and arousal.

The American Academy of Pediatric's Task Force on Sudden Infant Death Syndrome introduced a policy statement in November 2005 that put forth a number of recommendations that were developed to reduce the risk of SIDS.

The recommendations are:

- Infants should be placed in the supine position for sleep.

- A firm sleep surface should be used. For example, soft items, such as quilts or pillows, should not be placed under the infant.

- Soft objects and loose bedding should not be part of the infant's sleeping environment.

- Smoking and exposure to passive smoke during pregnancy should be avoided.

- Infants should not share the same bed as adults.

- Overheating should be avoided.

- Using a pacifier, when placing the infant down to sleep, should be considered.

- Home monitors should not be used as a strategy to reduce the risk of SIDS as there is no evidence that proves their effectiveness for this purpose. This is only suggested for infants who have had an apparent life-threatening event.

home monitoring may affect family life and contributes to the effective development of home management and family teaching plans; it also provides a basis for continuity of care for the infant.

Nursing Diagnoses

- Ineffective Breathing Pattern related to periods of apnea.
- Anxiety of the parents related to life-threatening event.
- Deficient Knowledge regarding home monitoring.

Nursing Interventions

Maintaining Breathing Pattern

1. Be prepared for the infant's admission and have all equipment, including apnea monitor, ready for use. Continuous cardiac monitoring is also recommended.
   a. Select a room that is clearly visible from the nursing station; the room should be quiet to reduce sensory stimulation, which may reduce the likelihood of a recurring episode.
   b. Be aware that the family has just experienced the extreme stress of feeling that their infant has almost died. Reassure them with empathy and efficiency at the time of admission.
2. Continuously monitor respirations. Document apnea along with state of consciousness; sleep state; color; position of infant; muscle tone; respiratory effort before, during, and after event; relationship to activity (eg, feeding); and intervention necessary (nothing, gentle stimulation, vigorous stimulation, resuscitation).
3. Administer theophylline, if prescribed. Observe for signs of toxicity: apical rate above 200, vomiting, and agitation. Concentration of theophylline for apnea is lower than the concentration for bronchospasm.
4. Continue the infant's normal activities whenever possible (eg, holding him or her for feedings, playing with him or her, disconnecting from monitor for bathing); allow for continuation of usual eating or sleeping patterns. Simulating the home environment as much as possible will encourage deep-sleep patterns, which may stimulate apnea and provide valuable diagnostic information.

Minimizing Anxiety

1. Encourage the parents to continue involvement in infant care during hospitalization.
2. Clarify any misconceptions about apnea and SIDS.
3. Allow ventilation of feelings and concerns.
4. Assess family dynamics for any conflicts or maladapted responses; intervene or refer, as appropriate.
5. Use anticipatory guidance in preparing the parents for emotional responses to home monitoring.
   a. Increased anxiety or tension.
   b. Constant worry about the alarm even when it does not go off.
   c. Fatigue.
   d. Financial and emotional burdens encountered by the family.
   e. Perceived loss of "normal, healthy child"; parents may grieve when given the diagnosis.

Increasing Confidence in Home Monitoring

1. Demonstrate operation and maintenance of the monitor. Reinforce teaching by equipment supplier. Provide information on contacting a monitor technician. Teach parents proper electrode and belt placement and skin care.
   a. Do not adjust monitor to eliminate false alarms.
   b. Maintain an unobstructed view of the monitor. Plug power cord directly into outlet—do not use extension cords. Check battery and charger. Place monitor on firm surface.
   c. Monitored infant should not share his or her bed.
2. Identify the presence of a telephone in the home and, if not, an alternative plan in the event of an emergency situation.
3. Describe how to record apnea in relation to activity and position and when to report apnea to health care provider.
4. Teach methods of responding to alarms; what to observe and document in diary (eg, color, presence or absence of breathing) and how to respond (gentle vs. vigorous stimulation, cardiopulmonary resuscitation [CPR]). Never vigorously shake the child.
5. Discuss the necessary adjustments in daily living and anticipated changes.
   a. Emphasize that responsibility must be shared by family members.
   b. Discuss the possible impact on siblings.
   c. Advise the parents to eliminate noises that would interfere with their ability to hear the alarm (eg, showering, vacuuming). Someone must always be available to hear and respond to the alarm. Be aware of electrical interference from appliances or cellular phones and in public places such as airports.
   d. Avoid traveling long distances alone with the infant.
   e. Encourage the parents to enlist the assistance of a third person who is willing to learn CPR and to help care for the infant and provide the parents with an opportunity for respite time.
6. Emphasize the healthy aspects of the infant. Encourage the parents to continue as many usual routines as possible. Provide specific things parents can do to encourage normal development and a healthy parent–child relationship.
7. Encourage the parents to provide total care for their infant 24 hours before discharge so they regain confidence in caring for their child.

Family Education and Health Maintenance

1. Advise the family to keep emergency numbers near the telephone or set on speed dial.
2. Educate about feeding precautions: frequent burping, no bottle in bed, upright position after feeding, positioning the infant on his or her back or side, not abdomen. Avoid soft, moldable sleeping surfaces and pillows; toys and stuffed animals should be removed from the crib.
3. Have parents contact local emergency service to inform them about their infant and to be certain that they have infant resuscitation equipment. Arrange for notification of the utility company in order to plan for the event of a power outage.

4. Instruct the parents in the administration of any new medications.

5. Teach CPR to all those involved in providing care for the infant.

6. Refer the family to a home care agency for home nursing visits, additional teaching, and support.

Evaluation: Expected Outcomes

• Monitoring maintained; respirations regular without apnea.
• Parents verbalize concern over infant's well-being.
• Parents demonstrate correct operation of respiratory monitor and response to alarms.

SELECTED REFERENCES

Alberta Medical Association. (2008). *Guidelines for the diagnosis and management of croup.* Edmonton, Alberta, Canada: Alberta Medical Association.

Al-Yakeem, N. (2012). Child to adult: Transitional care for young adults with cystic fibrosis. *British Journal of Nursing, 21*, 850–854.

American Academy of Pediatrics, Task Force on Sudden Infant Death Syndrome. (2005). The changing concept of sudden infant death syndrome: Diagnostic coding shifts, controversies regarding the sleeping environment, and new variables to consider in reducing risk. *Pediatrics, 116*(5), 1245–1255.

Avnita, A., Oragui, E., Khan, W., et al. (2010). Psychosocial consideration os perioperative care in children, with a focus on effective management strategies. *Journal of Perioperative Practice, 20*(6), 198–202.

Balfour-Lynn, I. M. (2008). Newborn screening for cystic fibrosis: Evidence for benefit. *Archives of Disease in Childhood, 93*(1), 7–10.

Bissett, L. (2010). Skincare as a tool in the prevention of health care-associated infection. *British Journal of Community Nursing, 15*(5), 226–231.

Bradley, J. S., Byington, C. L., Shah, S. S., et al. (2011). The management of community-acquired pneumonia in infants and children older than 3 months of age: Clinical practice guidelines by the Pediatric Infectious Disease Society and the Infectious Disease Society of America. *Clinical Infectious Diseases, 53*, 617–630.

Burton, M. J., & Glaszouu, P. (2009). Tonsillectomy or adeno-tonsillectomy versus non-surgical treatment for chronic/recurrent acute tonsillitis. *The Cochrane Library*, Issue 1.

Cantine, M., & Lomas, P. (2012). Cystic fibrosis patients: Step-up to better breathing. *The Journal for Respiratory Care Practitioners, 25*(11), 14–17.

Castro-Rodriguez, J. A. (2010). The asthma predictive index: A very useful tool for predicting asthma in young children. *Journal of Allergy and Clinical Immunology, 126*, 212–216.

Flume, P. A., Mogayzel, P. J., Robinson, K. A., et al. (2010). Cystic fibrosis pulmonary guidelines: Pulmonary complications: Hemoptysis and pneumothorax. *American Journal of Respiratory and Critical Care Medicine, 182*, 298–306.

Flume, P. A., Robinson, K. A., O'Sullivan, B. P., et al. (2009). Cystic fibrosis guidelines: Airway clearance therapies. *Respiratory Care, 54*(4), 522–537.

Garibaldi, B. T., Illei, P., Danoff, S. K. (2012). *Bronchiolitis. Immunology & Allergy Clinics of North America, 32*(4), 601–619.

Glasscoe, C. A., & Quittners, A. L. (2009). Psychological interventions for people with cystic fibrosis and their families. *Cochrane Database of Systematic Reviews*, Issue 3 (Article No. CD003148).

Ghuman, A. K., Newth, C. J. L., & Khemani, R. G. (2010). Respiratory support in children. *Paediatrics and Child Health, 21*, 4.

Global Initiative for Asthma Report. (2011). Global strategy for asthma management and prevention. Available: *www.ginasthma.com.*

Hockenberry, M., & Wilson, D. (2011). *Wong's nursing care of infants and children* (9th ed.). St. Louis, MO: Mosby.

Illes, N., & Lowton, K. (2010). What is the perceived nature of parental care and support for young people with cystic fibrosis as they enter adult health services? *Health and Social Care in the Community, 18*(1), 21–29.

Kliegman, R. M., Stanton, B., St. Geme, J., et al. (2011). *Nelson textbook of pediatrics* (19th ed.). Philadelphia: Elsevier

Lenny, W., Boner, A. L., Bont, L., et al. (2009). Medicines used in respiratory diseases only seen in children. *European Respiratory Journal, 34*(3), 531–551.

Lock, C., Wilson, J., Steen, N., et al. (2010). North of England and Scotland Study of Tonsillectomy and Adeno-tonsillectomy in Children (NESSTAC): A pragmatic randomized controlled trial with a parallel non-randomised preference study. *Health Technology Assessment, 14*(13).

Marlais, M., Evans, J., & Abrahamson, E. (2011). Clinical predictors of admission in infants with acute bronchiolitis. *Archives of Disease in Childhood, 96*(7), 648–652.

McDougall, P. (2011). Caring for bronchiolitic infant's needing continuous positive airway pressure. *Paediatric Nursing, 23*(1), 30–35.

Mcllwaine, M. (2007). Chest physical therapy, breathing techniques and exercise in children with CF. *Paediatric Respiratory Reviews, 8*(1), 8–16.

National Heart, Lung and Blood Institute, National Asthma Education and Prevention Program. (2007). Guidelines for the diagnosis and management of asthma. Full report (NIH Publication No. 08-4051). Available: *www.nhlbi.nih.gov/guidelines/asthma/asthgdln.htm.*

National Heart, Lung and Blood Institute, National Asthma Education and Prevention Program. (2007). Guidelines for the diagnosis and management of asthma. Summary report (NIH Publication No. 08-5846). Available: *www.nhlbi.nih.gov/guidelines/asthma/asthsumm.htm.*

Paranjape, S. M., Barnes, L. A., Carson, A. C., et al. (2012). Exercise improves lung function and habitual activity in children with cystic fibrosis. *Journal of Cystic Fibrosis, 11*, 18–23.

Paul, S. (2011). Treating lower respiratory tract ailments in children and infants. *Emergency Nurse, 19*(80), 21–25.

Paul, S. P., O'Callaghan, C., & McKee, N. (2011) Effective management of lower respiratory tract infections in childhood. *Nursing Children and Young People, 23*(9), 27–34.

Royal Brompton Hospital Paediatric Cystic Fibrosis Team. (2011). *Clinical guidelines: Care of children with cystic fibrosis* (5th ed.). London: Royal Brompton & Harefield NHS Foundation Trust. Available: *www.rbht.nhs.uk/chldrencf.*

Sala, K. A., Carroll, C. L., Yang, Y. S., et al. (2011). Factors associated with the development of severe asthma exacerbations in children. *Journal of Asthma, 48*, 558–564.

Sands, D., Reppetto, T., Dupont, L. J., et al. (2011). End of life care for patients with cystic fibrosis. *Journal of Cystic Fibrosis, 10*(2), 37–44.

Scottish Intercollegiate Guidelines Network. (2010). *Management of sore throat and indications for tonsillectomy—A national clinical guideline.* Edinburgh: NHS Quality Improvement Scotland.

Singh, N., Hawley, K. L., & Viswanathan K. (2011). Efficacy of porcine versus bovine surfactants for preterm newborns with respiratory distress syndrome: Systematic review and meta-analysis. *Pediatrics, 128*(6), 1588–1595.

Stapleton, J., Howard-Thompson, A., George, C., et al. (2011). Smoking and asthma. *Journal of the American Board of Family Medicine, 24*(3), 313–322.

Szefler, S. J. (2012). Advances in pediatric asthma in 2011: Moving forward. *Journal of Allergy and Clinical Immunology, 129*, 60–68.

Verger, J. T., Verger, E. E. (2012). Respiratory syncytial virus bronchiolitis in children. *Clinical Care Nursing Clinics of North America, 24*(4), 555–572.

Zemek, R., Plint, A., Osmond, M. H., et al. (2012). Triage nurse initiation of corticosteroids in pediatric asthma is associated with improved emergency department efficiency. *Pediatrics, 129*(4), 671–680.

Zentz, S. E. (2011). Care of infants and children with bronchiolitis: A systematic review. *Journal of Pediatric Nursing, 26*, 519–529.

Zorc, J. J., & Breese Hall, C. (2010). Bronchiolitis: Recent evidence on diagnosis and management. *Pediatrics, 125*(2), 342–349.

45

Pediatric Cardiovascular Disorders

CARDIAC PROCEDURES

Cardiac Catheterization

Cardiac catheterization is an invasive procedure used to identify cardiac anatomy; measure intracardiac pressures, shunts, and oxygen saturations; and calculate systemic and pulmonary vascular resistance.

Procedure

1. Catheter insertion sites include femoral vein or artery, umbilical vein or artery, brachial vein, or internal jugular vein.
2. Under fluoroscopy, catheters are guided through the heart, collecting pressure measurements and oxygen saturations.
3. Contrast dye is injected through the catheters to visualize blood flow patterns and structural abnormalities.
4. Cardiac catheterization is usually an outpatient procedure for children who undergo an elective procedure. After interventional procedures, some children are observed in the hospital for 12 to 24 hours.

Indications

1. To confirm or establish the diagnosis.
2. To measure cardiac output.
3. To measure pressures and oxygen saturations.
4. To calculate intracardiac shunting and pulmonary and systemic vascular resistance.
5. To visualize coronary arteries.

6. To assess for myocarditis or rejection following heart transplantation.
7. To intervene in congenital heart disease (see Box 45-1 for definitions of abbreviations):
   a. Balloon atrial septostomy (Rashkind) for restrictive atrial septum.
   b. Balloon valvuloplasty (arterial stenosis [AS], pulmonary stenosis [PS]) and angioplasty (recurrent coarctation of the aorta [CoA]).
   c. Endomyocardial biopsy.
   d. To occlude vessels (coil embolization) or defects (atrial septal defect [ASD], ventricular septal defect [VSD], or patent ductus arteriosus [PDA] closure devices).
   e. To stent vessels open (branch pulmonary artery [PA] stenosis, recurrent CoA).
   f. To dilate stenotic valves (mitral valve, pulmonary valve, tricuspid valve).

Complications

1. Arrhythmias (usually catheter induced).
2. Infection.
3. Bleeding at catheter insertion site; large hematoma.
4. Allergic reaction to contrast material.
5. Loss of pulse in the extremity used for cannulation.
6. Perforation of heart or vessels.
7. Stroke.
8. Dislodgment of coils, closure devices, or stents.
9. Death.

BOX 45-1	Abbreviations Used for Congenital Heart Disease
ASD	Atrial septal defect
AV	Atrioventricular
CoA	Coarctation of the aorta
HLHS	Hypoplastic left heart syndrome
IAA	Interrupted aortic arch
IVC	Inferior vena cava
LVOTO	Left ventricular outflow tract obstruction
PA	Pulmonary artery
PAPVR	Partial anomalous pulmonary venous return
PDA	Patent ductus arteriosus
PFO	Patent foramen ovale
PS	Pulmonary stenosis
PVR	Pulmonary vascular resistance
SVC	Superior vena cava
TA	Tricuspid atresia
TAPVR	Total anomalous pulmonary venous return
TGA	Transposition of great arteries
TOF	Tetralogy of Fallot
VSD	Ventricular septal defect

Nursing Diagnoses

Preoperative
- Fear related to surgical procedure.
- Deficient Knowledge regarding surgical procedure and associated nursing care.

Postoperative
- Risk for Injury related to complications of cardiac catheterization.

Nursing Interventions

Reducing Fear in Child and Parents
1. Provide specific instructions in nonthreatening manner:
   a. Day and time of the procedure.
   b. Nothing-by-mouth (NPO) guidelines.
   c. Sedation versus general anesthesia.
   d. Site of the planned arterial and venous puncture.
   e. Routine postprocedure care.
2. Provide appropriate teaching geared toward the child's age and level of cognitive development. Use diagrams and models, as appropriate.
3. Provide parents an opportunity, without the child present, to discuss the procedure, risks, benefits, and alternative choices.
4. Give child opportunity to express fears and ask questions.
5. Provide tour of the cardiac catheterization laboratory, if appropriate.

Explaining and Providing Nursing Care
1. Obtain baseline set of vital signs: heart rate, BP, respiratory rate, and oxygen saturation.
2. Measure and record child's height and weight.
3. Note time of last oral intake: solids and liquids.
4. Identify known allergies.
5. List current medications and note time last taken.
6. Help child change into a hospital gown.
7. Start peripheral IV, as needed.
8. Administer sedation, as prescribed.
9. Assess and mark the location of pulses (dorsalis pedis, posterior tibial).

Observe for and Prevent Complications
1. Monitor and record routine vital signs (q 15 min × 4, q 30 min × 2, then q 1 hr); extremity temperature, color, and pulse check with vital signs.
2. Notify health care provider for:
   a. Heart rate, respiratory rate, or BP outside normal parameters for age.
   b. Bleeding or increasing hematoma at puncture site.
   c. Change in oxygen saturations.
   d. Fever.
   e. Cool, pulseless extremity.
3. Observe puncture site for redness, pain, swelling, or induration.
4. Maintain the child in a reclining position for 4 to 6 hours after the procedure.
5. Offer fluids as soon as the child is ready.

Family Education and Health Maintenance
1. Provide discharge information:
   a. Care of incision or puncture site (keep dry for 48 hours).
   b. Activity restrictions (usually for 48 hours, but may be up to 2 weeks following placement of closure devices).
   c. Observe for and report late complications: redness, swelling, drainage from puncture site.
   d. Follow-up medical care.
   e. Reinforce infective endocarditis precautions.
2. If cardiac catheterization was a preoperative procedure, use the recovery time to teach the child and family about upcoming hospital stay.

Evaluation: Expected Outcomes
- Child describes procedure in own words; parents and child discuss procedure and ask appropriate questions.
- Child cooperative with preoperative nursing care.
- Insertion site intact without drainage, redness, or hematoma.

Cardiac Surgery

The ultimate goal of treatment of cardiovascular disease in children is to restore normal heart structure and function. Most types of CHDs can be palliated or definitively repaired.

Procedures

Closed-Heart Surgery

1. Surgical approach: lateral thoracotomy or mediastinal incision.
2. Indications:
   a. PDA ligation.
   b. PA banding.
   c. CoA repair.
   d. Vascular ring repair.
   e. Blalock-Taussig shunt (BT shunt) placement.
   f. Occasionally, Glenn and Fontan procedures.

Open-Heart Surgery

1. Surgery is done through a mediastinal incision.
2. With the use of cardiopulmonary bypass, the surgeon can stop the heart and operate inside to repair the defects.
3. Deep hypothermia with circulatory arrest allows the surgeon to safely stop cardiopulmonary bypass and remove arterial or venous cannulas to better visualize and repair the defects.
4. Indications:
   a. ASD, VSD, atrioventricular (AV) canal defect.
   b. Aortic stenosis, pulmonary stenosis.
   c. Tetralogy of Fallot (TOF).
   d. Transposition of great arteries (TGA).
   e. Tricuspid atresia.
   f. Total anomalous pulmonary venous return (TAPVR) or partial APVR.
   g. Truncus arteriosus.
   h. Hypoplastic left heart syndrome (HLHS).
   i. Complex single ventricle.

Potential Complications of Specific Surgeries

1. PDA ligation: laryngeal nerve damage, phrenic nerve damage, diaphragm paralysis, thoracic duct injury.
2. CoA: rebound hypertension, mesenteric arteritis (abdominal pain), coarctation restenosis.
3. Aorta-pulmonary shunt (BT shunt): shunt occlusion, PA distortion, pulmonary overcirculation.
4. ASD: atrial arrhythmias, sinoatrial node dysfunction.
5. VSD: transient or permanent heart block, residual VSD, ventricular dysfunction.
6. TOF: low cardiac output, residual right ventricular outflow tract obstruction (RVOTO) or VSD, ectopic junctional tachycardia or arrhythmias, thoracic duct injury.
7. TGA: arterial switch operation—coronary artery injury, ventricular dysfunction, suprapulmonary stenosis.
8. TGA: atrial switch operation—baffle obstruction, RV failure, atrial arrhythmias.
9. Valvotomy (for valve stenosis): valve insufficiency.
10. Bidirectional Glenn shunt: superior vena cava (SVC) syndrome, low cardiac output, hypoxia, pleural effusions.
11. Fontan completion: low cardiac output, pleural effusions, ventricular dysfunction, thrombus formation, arrhythmias, hepatic dysfunction.

Cardiac Transplant Surgery

Cardiac transplantation is a treatment option for children with progressive congestive heart failure (CHF) or certain cardiac diseases not amenable to conventional medical-surgical therapy. Children who cannot grow and meet developmental milestones or who have unacceptable quality-of-life issues may benefit from cardiac transplant surgery. However, approximately one in four children die while waiting for an organ donor. Those children who receive a donor heart must take lifelong immunosuppression medications to prevent organ rejection.

Indications for Cardiac Transplantation

1. End-stage cardiomyopathy.
2. Untreatable complex CHD.
3. Malignant arrhythmia.
4. Retransplant for cardiac graft failure.

Immunosuppressive Medications

 Evidence Base Denfield, S. W. (2010). Strategies to prevent cellular rejection in pediatric heart transplant recipients. *Paediatric Drugs, 12*(6), 391–403.

Immunosuppressive therapy is divided into two phases, induction and maintenance. Induction therapies reduce early rejection and may help to reduce the child's overall exposure to corticosteroids. Combination therapy is usually used in the maintenance phase to ensure ongoing protection against rejection.

1. Phase I: Induction.
   a. Polyclonal antibodies.
      i. Rabbit or equine antithymocyte globulin.
      ii. Interlukin-2 receptor antibodies.
         1) Daclizumab.
         2) Basiliximab.
2. Phase II: Maintenance therapies.
   a. Calcineurin inhibitors.
      i. Ciclosporin (cyclosporine).
      ii. Tacrolimus.
   b. Antiproliferative agent.
      i. Azathioprine.
      ii. Mycophenolate mofetil.
   c. Mammalian target of rapamycin inhibitors.
      i. Sirolimus.
      ii. Everolimus.
   d. Corticosteroids.
      i. Prednisone.

Complications

1. Organ rejection: routine surveillance endomyocardial biopsies are performed to assess for rejection.
   a. With mild to moderate rejection, children may initially be asymptomatic.
   b. With severe rejection, children are usually symptomatic with hemodynamic instability.
2. Infection.

3. Adverse effects of immunosuppressive agents.
   a. Polyclonal antibodies—fever, chills, rash, headaches, abdominal pain, leukopenia, and thrombocytopenia
   b. Calcineurin inhibitors.
      i. Ciclosporin—nephrotoxicity, hypertension, diabetes mellitus, hirsutism, gingival hyperplasia, tremor.
      ii. Tacrolimus—nephrotoxicity, diabetes mellitus, hypertension, hyperkalemia, hypomagnesemia, tremor.
   c. Antiproliferative agent.
      i. Azathioprine—leukopenia, thrombocytopenia, nausea, vomiting.
      ii. Mycophenolate mofetil—leukopenia, nausea, vomiting, diarrhea, anorexia.
   d. Mammalian target of rapamycin inhibitors—hyperlipidemia, thrombocytopenia, anemia, leukopenia.
   e. Prednisone—hypertension, Cushing syndrome, growth retardation.
4. Accelerated diffuse coronary artery disease.
5. Posttransplant lymphoproliferative disease.

Routine Follow-Up

1. Routine well-child care visits to primary care provider.
   a. Transplant children should not receive any live virus immunizations (oral polio, measles–mumps–rubella, varicella). Monitor for adverse effects of chronic steroids and immunosuppressive medications.
2. Routine cardiology clinic visits.
   a. Laboratory studies: chemistry, hematology, therapeutic drug levels.
   b. Vital signs.
   c. Electrocardiogram (ECG).
   d. Echocardiography.
3. Serial cardiac catheterizations and endomyocardial biopsies.
4. Yearly coronary angiography or dobutamine stress echocardiography.

Nursing Assessment

Baseline Assessment on Day of Surgery

1. Measure and record height and weight.
2. Document vital signs: heart rate, respiratory rate, BP, and oxygen saturation.
3. Assess for preoperative infection: fever, signs of upper respiratory infection (cough, runny nose, crackles), vomiting, or diarrhea might necessitate delaying surgery.
4. Document last oral intake.
5. Void on call to the operating room.

Nursing Diagnoses

Preoperative

• Fear related to surgical procedure.

Postoperative

• Risk for Injury related to complications of surgery.
• Impaired Adjustment related to postsurgery care.

Nursing Interventions

Preparing the Child and Family and Reducing Fear

1. Be honest and use nonthreatening language the child can understand.
2. The following are frequently asked questions from parents. Address them with the parents:
   a. What to tell the child.
   b. When to tell the child.
   c. What to bring to the hospital.
   d. Anticipated hospital course: how long in the operating room; how many days in the intensive care unit (ICU); how many days on the general care unit; visiting policy, rooming-in accommodations.
3. Review preoperative instructions.
   a. NPO guidelines.
   b. Where to report on the day of the surgery.
   c. Time to arrive at the hospital; time of surgery.
   d. Preoperative medications (injection, liquid, inhalation).
   e. What the operating room looks like; what the people wear in the operating room (hats, gowns, and masks).
4. Explain the preoperative period.
   a. Change into a hospital gown.
   b. Parents stay with the child.
   c. Transportation to the operating room (walking, wheelchair, or stretcher).
5. Explain the operative period.
   a. Operating room waiting room.
   b. Updates during the surgery will come from the surgical scrub nurses.
   c. Surgeon will meet the family after surgery to review the surgical findings and to describe the operation.
6. Explain the postoperative period. Use models and diagrams.
   a. Pediatric ICU routines and procedures.
   b. Monitoring lines and equipment.
   c. Ventilators, oxygen therapy.
   d. Protective restraints.
7. Offer medical equipment to handle and play with (ECG leads, face mask, BP cuff), age-appropriate books about surgery and hospital stays, and tour of ICU and surgical area, as available.
8. Prehospital tour of the pediatric ICU and general pediatric care unit.
9. Allow an opportunity for the child and family to ask questions, express their concern, or to ask for more detail.

Observing for and Preventing Complications

1. Assess respiratory status and maintain respiratory support.
   a. Maintain ventilatory support, as needed.
   b. Maintain patent airway with routine endotracheal suctioning.
   c. Auscultate breath sounds frequently. Decreased breath sounds may indicate pleural effusions, atelectasis, pneumothorax, hemothorax.

d. Report results of routine chest x-ray.

e. Perform frequent position changes: side–back–side.

f. Monitor arterial blood gas levels and oxygen saturations.

g. Assess chest tube drainage.

h. Extubate when hemodynamically stable and when patient meets extubation criteria.

i. Administer oxygen therapy, as needed, after extubation.

2. Assess cardiac status.

a. Monitor vital signs and oxygen saturations.

b. Maintain continuous ECG monitoring.

    i. Daily 12-lead ECG to assess rhythm.

    ii. Temporary epicardial pacemaker wires available for pacing, as needed.

c. Continuous BP monitoring (arterial line).

d. Monitor intracardiac pressures (central venous pressure [CVP], left atrial [LA], PA).

e. Monitor peripheral perfusion, capillary refill, toe temperature.

f. Titrate vasopressors (dopamine, dobutamine, milrinone), as prescribed.

3. Assess fluid status.

a. Record hourly intake (IV fluids, blood products, fluid boluses).

b. Record hourly output (urine, chest tube drainage, nasogastric drainage).

c. Perform daily weights.

d. Administer diuretics, as prescribed.

4. Assess neurologic status.

a. Monitor level of responsiveness, response to verbal commands, and response to pain.

b. Check pupil size and reactivity to light.

c. Document movement of all extremities.

d. Monitor all invasive lines for air bubbles and potential air embolism.

e. Observe for signs of neurologic injury related to hypoperfusion or embolism.

5. Monitor for potential specific complications related to particular surgery for CHD.

6. Assess for postoperative pain.

a. Monitor level of responsiveness, agitation.

b. Implement pediatric pain scale rating to assist the child in identifying the severity of pain.

c. Administer pain medication, as prescribed: continuous IV infusion and IV boluses, as necessary.

d. Utilize patient-controlled analgesia continuous pump, as appropriate.

7. Assess serum electrolyte balance. Obtain blood tests and report results. Treat deficits with supplements.

8. Assess packed cell volume, platelet count, and coagulation studies.

a. Low hematocrit (less than 30): consider directed donor transfusion or blood bank transfusion.

b. Low platelet count: continue to monitor; if bleeding persists, transfuse platelets.

c. Prolonged coagulation studies: continue to monitor; if bleeding or oozing persists, give protamine, fresh frozen plasma.

Enhancing Adjustment Postoperatively

1. Provide continuity of care (primary nursing and consistent medical team).

2. Explain all procedures and routines to the child and parents to minimize fear.

3. Explain to the parents a child's typical reactions to stressful events.

a. Regression—temporary loss of developmental milestones.

b. Fear of any medical personnel (white coat anxiety).

c. Sibling jealousy that one child is receiving a lot of attention.

d. Withdrawal—related to stimulation overload and lack of undisturbed sleep.

e. Nightmares.

f. Increased dependency; clinging behavior.

4. Suggest parent and patient support groups, Child Life Therapy, community resources, and counseling, as needed.

Family Education and Health Maintenance

1. Provide the child and family with oral and written discharge instructions and recommendations.

a. Medications.

b. Activity restrictions.

    i. No strenuous activity or contact sports for 6 to 8 weeks after surgery.

    ii. Most children are ready to return to school at least part time about 2 weeks after surgery.

    iii. If child needs prolonged recovery time at home, may need to consider home tutoring.

    iv. No gym class until full recovery.

c. Care of the incision.

d. Dietary recommendations.

e. Bathing or showering guidelines.

2. Provide the child and family with a list of potential signs of complications and instructions to notify the health care provider.

a. Fever greater than or equal to 101.5° F (38.6° C).

b. Any redness, swelling, or drainage from chest incision.

c. Partial opening of the chest incision.

d. Poor appetite, nausea, vomiting.

e. Breathing difficulties, shortness of breath.

3. Provide the family with the names and phone numbers of people to call for questions and emergencies.

4. Make follow-up appointments for the child to be seen by his or her primary care provider 2 to 3 days after discharge from the hospital and 10 to 14 days to be seen by their pediatric cardiologist.

5. Review American Heart Association's recommendations for infective endocarditis prophylaxis: standard general prophylaxis for children at risk: amoxicillin 50 mg/kg (maximum dose = 2 g) given orally 1 hour before the procedure.

Community and Home Care Considerations

1. Arrange skilled home nursing visits, as needed, to:

a. Review medications.

b. Assess wound healing.

c. Monitor vital signs and oxygen saturations.

d. Assess oral intake; nutritional supplements.

e. Resource for family.

2. Make referral to community agencies, as needed (infant and toddler program).

3. Arrange for home medical equipment (oxygen, feeding pump, and supplies), as needed.

4. Review safety precautions in the home:

    a. Childproof medication bottles.

    b. Poison control phone number for accidental medication overdose.

    c. Infant and child CPR techniques.

    d. Bleeding precautions for children on anticoagulation therapy. No aspirin or ibuprofen products. Be sure to read the labels on over-the-counter cold and cough syrups. Avoid activities with high risk of injury. All head injuries need to be evaluated by a physician. Signs of bleeding:

        i. Blood in the urine.

        ii. Black tarry stools.

        iii. Prolonged nosebleeds.

        iv. Bleeding gums.

        v. Bruising for no known trauma.

        vi. Spitting or coughing up blood.

        vii. Any unusual swelling or pain.

    e. MedicAlert bracelet or tags.

5. Discuss developmental issues with the family.

    a. A child on diuretics may have difficulty with toilet training.

    b. Disciplining, establishing behavioral expectations, and setting limits in a child with CHD should be similar to those for a child without CHD.

6. Discuss the need for home schooling or tutoring during recovery time. Return to the classroom as soon as the child is ready.

7. Discuss infants with CHD in daycare situations—address each case individually. Daycare programs usually have increased risk of URIs and other communicable diseases.

8. Encourage routine dental visits to prevent dental caries (dental caries predispose to bacteremia and endocarditis).

9. Encourage heart-healthy eating and exercise routines.

10. Encourage age-appropriate activities. A few children will need exercise restrictions. Children with CHD should be allowed to participate in activities with rest periods, as needed. Children with pacemakers and children on anticoagulation therapy should refrain from contact sports.

11. Maintain standard childhood immunization schedule. Delay vaccines around the perioperative time until fully recovered from surgery (no immunizations for 6 weeks postoperatively).

12. Encourage yearly influenza vaccine for children with unrepaired or complex CHD.

13. Encourage respiratory syncytial virus (RSV) immunization for children younger than age 2 with complex CHD and those at risk of CHF or pulmonary hypertension.

Evaluation: Expected Outcomes

- Child describes procedure without fear; parents and child discuss procedure and ask appropriate questions.
- Vital signs stable, no signs of infection.
- Parents offer support to child.

CONGENITAL HEART DISEASE

Evidence Base Dolbec, K., & Mick, N. W. (2011). Congenital heart disease. *Emergency Medical Clinics of North America, 29*(4), 811–827.

Congenital heart disease (or *defects*) *(CHD)* is one of the most common forms of congenital anomalies. It involves the chambers, valves, and vessels arising from the heart (see Figure 45-1, page 1526).

In most cases, the cause of CHD is not known. Some infants and children with CHD may appear perfectly healthy, whereas others may be critically ill. Most infants and children with CHD can be successfully managed with medications and surgeries.

Etiology and Incidence

1. CHD affects 8 to 12 of every 1,000 neonates.

2. Exact cause of CHD is unknown in 90% of cases.

3. The heart begins as a single cell and develops into a four-chambered pumping system during the 3rd to 8th weeks of gestation.

4. Associated factors for CHD include:

    a. Fetal or maternal infection during the first trimester (rubella).

    b. Chromosomal abnormalities (trisomy 21, 18, 13).

    c. Maternal insulin-dependent diabetes.

    d. Systemic lupus erythematosus.

    e. Teratogenic effects of drugs and alcohol.

        i. Lithium—Ebstein anomaly.

        ii. Phenytoin—aortic and pulmonic stenosis.

        iii. Alcohol—ASD and VSD.

DRUG ALERT Teratogenic drugs also include amphetamines, estrogen, progesterone, retinoic acid, selective serotonin reuptake inhibitors, trimethadione, valproic acid.

5. Syndromes that include CHD:

    a. Marfan's syndrome—mitral valve prolapse (MVP), dilated aortic root.

    b. Turner's syndrome—aortic valve stenosis (AVS), CoA.

    c. Noonan's syndrome—dysplastic pulmonary valve.

    d. William's syndrome—supravalvular PS.

    e. DiGeorge syndrome—interrupted aortic arch (IAA), truncus arteriosus, TGA, TOF.

    f. Down syndrome (trisomy 21)—AV canal defect, VSD. About 50% of children with Down syndrome have a CHD.

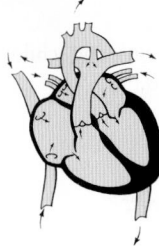

Patent Ductus Arteriosus

Patent ductus arteriosus (PDA) is a vascular connection that, during fetal life, shunts blood from the pulmonary artery to the aorta. Functional closure of the ductus normally occurs soon after birth. If the ductus remains patent after birth, the direction of blood flow in the ductus is reversed from aorta to pulmonary circuit by the higher pressure in the aorta.

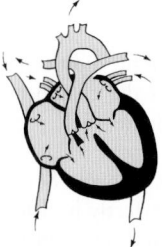

Ventricular Septal Defect

Ventricular septal defect (VSD) is an abnormal opening between the right and left ventricle. VSDs vary in size and may occur in either the membranous or muscular portion of the ventricular septum. Due to the higher pressure in the left ventricle, a shunting of blood from the left to right ventricle occurs during systole. If pulmonary hypertension or obstruction to pulmonary flow exists, the shunt of blood is then reversed from the right to the left ventricle, with cyanosis resulting.

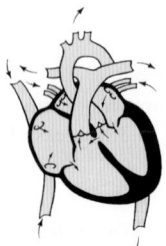

Pulmonary Stenosis

Pulmonary stenosis refers to any lesion that obstructs the blood flow from the right ventricle to the pulmonary artery. This obstruction may cause right ventricular hypertrophy and eventual right-sided heart failure.

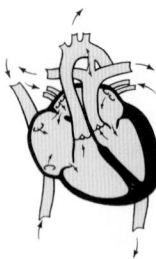

Aortic Stenosis

Aortic stenosis may be at the subvalvular, valvular (with thickening or fusion of the cusps), or supravalvular level. Subaortic stenosis is caused by a fibrous ring below the aortic valve in the outflow tract of the left ventricle. At times, valvular and subaortic stenosis exist in combination. The obstruction presents an increased workload for the normal output of the left ventricular blood and results in left ventricular enlargement.

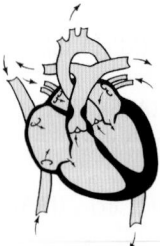

Coarctation of the Aorta

Coarctation of the aorta is characterized by a narrowed aortic lumen. It normally occurs in the juxtaductal position. Coarctations exist with great variation in anatomic features. The lesion produces an obstruction to the flow of blood through the aorta, causing increased left ventricular pressure and workload.

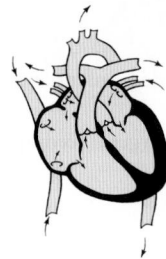

Tetralogy of Fallot

Tetralogy of Fallot is characterized by the combination of four defects: (1) pulmonary stenosis, (2) ventricular septal defects, (3) overriding aorta, (4) hypertrophy of right ventricle. It is the most common defect causing cyanosis in patients surviving past age 2. The severity of symptoms depends on the degree of pulmonary stenosis, the size of the VSD, and the degree to which the aorta overrides the ventricular septal defect.

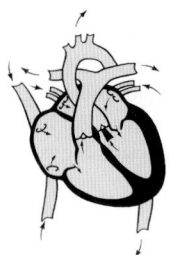

Complete Transposition of Great Vessels

The aorta originates from the right ventricle and the pulmonary artery from the left ventricle. An abnormal communication between the two circulations (atrial septal defect [ASD] or VSD) must be present to sustain life.

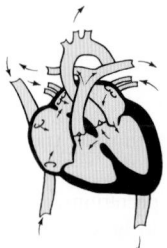

Atrial Septal Defect

An atrial septal defect (ASD) is an abnormal opening between the right and left atria. Basically, three types of abnormalities result from incorrect development of the atrial septum: (1) sinus venosus at the top of the atrial septum, (2) ostium secundum at the middle of the atrial septum, (3) ostium primum at the bottom of the atrial septum. In general, left-to-right shunting of blood occurs in all ASDs.

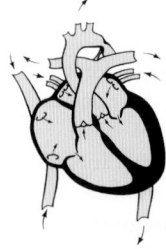

Tricuspid Atresia

Tricuspid valvular atresia is characterized by absence of the tricuspid valve, a small right ventricle, and usually diminished pulmonary circulation. Cyanosis is present because blood from the right atrium passes through an ASD into the left atrium, mixes with oxygenated blood returning from the lungs, flows into the left ventricle, and is propelled into the systemic circulation. The lungs may receive blood through one of three routes: (1) VSD, (2) PDA, and (3) collateral aortopulmonary vessels.

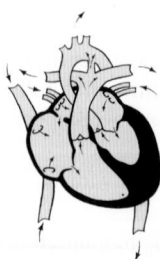

Hypoplastic Left Heart Syndrome

A collection of complex congenital heat lesions results in the abnormal development of the left side of the heart. These lesions include: (1) mitral stenosis/atresia, (2) aortic stenosis or atresia, (3) aortic arch hypoplasia, and (4) hypoplastic left ventricle. The right ventricle pumps blood through the pulmonary and systemic circulations. A patent foramen ovale allows a left-to-right shunt and blood is shunted from left atrium back to right atrium. A PDA is often the sole supply of blood to the systemic circulation.

Figure 45-1 Congenital heart abnormalities.

Common Congenital Heart Malformations

Congenital heart defects can be classified into three categories: obstruction to blood flow, increased pulmonary blood flow (acyanotic lesions), and decreased pulmonary blood flow (cyanotic lesions).

1. Obstructive lesions:
    a. AS—valvular, subvalvular, or supravalvular.
    b. CoA.
    c. PS—valvular, subvalvular, or supravalvular.
    d. IAA.
2. Increased pulmonary blood flow (acyanotic):
    a. PDA.
    b. ASD.
    c. VSD.
    d. AV canal.
    e. PAPVR.
3. Decreased pulmonary blood flow (cyanotic):
    a. TOF.
    b. TA.
    c. TAPVR.
    d. TGA.
    e. Truncus arteriosus.
    f. HLHS.
    g. DORV.

Aortic Stenosis

Evidence Base Loscalzo, M. L. (2010). Left outflow tract anomalies in children. *Current Opinion in Pediatrics, 22*(5), 593–597.

Schnieder, D. J., & Moore, J. W. (2013). Aortic stenosis. In H. D. Allen, D. J. Driscoll, R. E. Shaddy, & T. F. Feltes, (Eds.), *Moss and Adams' heart disease in infants, children, and adolescents* (8th ed.), (pp. 1023–1043). Philadelphia: Lippincott Williams & Wilkins.

Congenital *aortic stenosis (AS)* may be caused by a bicuspid aortic valve with fused commissures that does not open completely, by a hypoplastic aortic valve annulus, or by stenosis above or below the aortic valve (subvalvular or supravalvular stenosis). The result is turbulent blood flow across the aortic valve and into the ascending aorta. Patients with AS must be evaluated for additional left heart lesions that include CoA, mitral valve stenosis, hypertrophic cardiomyopathy, and hypoplastic left heart. AS is the most common form of left ventricular outflow tract obstruction (LVOTO). It accounts for 3% to 6% of CHDs. AS may occur at any age, and it occurs more commonly in boys than in girls (4:1 ratio). In most children, it is a progressive lesion that creates LVOTO.

Pathophysiology and Etiology

1. Blood flows at an increased velocity across the obstructive valve or stenotic area and into the aorta.
2. During systole, left ventricular pressure rises dramatically to overcome the increased resistance at the aortic valve.
3. Myocardial ischemia may occur because of an imbalance between the increased oxygen requirements related to the hypertrophied left ventricle (LV) and the amount of oxygen that can be supplied.
4. Left-sided heart failure results in an increased LV end diastolic pressure that is reflected back to the left atrium and pulmonary veins.

Clinical Manifestations

Neonate

1. Severe CHF.
2. Metabolic acidosis.
3. Tachypnea.
4. Faint peripheral pulses, poor perfusion, poor capillary refill, cool skin.
5. Poor feeding and feeding intolerance.

Child and Adolescent

1. Chest pain on exertion, decreased exercise tolerance.
2. Dyspnea, fatigue, shortness of breath.
3. Syncope, light-headedness.
4. Palpitations.
5. Sudden death.

Diagnostic Evaluation

1. Auscultation.
    a. Systolic ejection murmur heard best at right upper sternal border, radiates to neck.
    b. Ejection click. May be absent with severe stenosis.
    c. S_2 splits normally or narrowly.
2. Four-limb blood pressure.
    a. Systolic blood pressure normally 5 to 10 mm higher in lower extremities.
    b. Systolic blood pressure in lower limbs the same as or lower than that in the arms seen in coarctation of the aorta.
3. Palpation.
    a. Thrill may be palpable in right upper sternal border.
4. ECG: left ventricular hypertrophy (LVH) with a strain pattern may be seen in severe cases.
5. Chest x-ray: increased cardiac silhouette, increased pulmonary vascular markings. A prominent aortic knob may be seen occasionally from poststenotic dilatation with valvular AS.
6. Echocardiogram: two-dimensional echocardiogram with Doppler study and color flow mapping to visualize the anatomy and to estimate the gradient across the valve and through the aorta.

Management

Neonate

1. Stabilize with prostaglandin E_1 (PGE$_1$) infusion to maintain cardiac output through the PDA.
2. Inotropic support, as needed.
3. Intubation and ventilation, as needed.
4. Infective endocarditis prophylaxis (lifelong).
5. Cardiac catheterization: aortic balloon valvuloplasty or aortic balloon angioplasty.
6. Surgical valvotomy, commissurotomy, or myectomy/myotomy.

Child and Adolescent

1. Medical management with close follow-up to monitor increasing gradient across the aortic valve or through the aorta.
2. Restrict strenuous exercise and anaerobic exercise (eg, weight lifting).
3. Restrict participation in competitive sports.
4. Aortic balloon valvuloplasty or aortic balloon angioplasty.
5. Infective endocarditis prophylaxis (lifelong).
6. Surgical intervention.
    a. Surgical valvotomy, commissurotomy, or myectomy/myotomy.
    b. Aortic valve replacement.
        i. Mechanical prosthesis (St. Jude valve).
        ii. Ross procedure (pulmonary autograft).

Complications

1. CHF and pulmonary edema.
2. Dizziness, light-headedness, and syncope.
3. Palpitations, arrhythmias.
4. Infective endocarditis.
5. Sudden death.

Coarctation of the Aorta

Evidence Base Beekerman, R. H. (2013). Coarctation of the Aorta. In H. D. Allen, D. J. Driscoll, R. E. Shaddy, & T. F. Feltes, (Eds.), *Moss and Adams' heart disease in infants, children, and adolescents* (8th ed.). Philadelphia: Lippincott Williams & Wilkins.
Kenny, D., & Hijazi, Z. M. (2011). Coarctation of the aorta: From fetal life to adulthood. Cardiology Journal, 18(5), 487–495.

Coarctation of the aorta (CoA) is a discrete narrowing or a long segment hypoplasia of the aortic arch, usually in the juxtaductal position. It accounts for 8% to 10% of CHDs and is two to five times more common in males. Thirty percent of infants with Turner syndrome have CoA. Commonly associated defects include VSD, mitral valve stenosis, and bicuspid aortic valve.

Pathophysiology and Etiology

1. The discrete narrowing or hypoplastic segment of the aorta increases the workload of the left ventricle (increased LV systolic pressure).
2. In a neonate with critical CoA, lower-body blood flow occurs through the PDA (right-to-left shunting).
3. In the older child, collateral vessels grow and bypass the coarctation to perfuse the lower body.

Clinical Manifestations

1. The neonate with critical CoA (ductal dependent lesion):
    a. Asymptomatic until the PDA begins to close.
    b. After PDA closure: severe CHF, poor lower body perfusion, tachypnea, acidosis, progressive circulatory shock, absent femoral and pedal pulses.

2. The child or adolescent with CoA:
    a. Usually asymptomatic—normal growth and development.
    b. Hypertension in the upper extremities, with absent or weak femoral pulses.
    c. Nosebleeds, headaches, leg cramps.

Diagnostic Evaluation

1. Auscultation—varies; nonspecific systolic ejection murmur. Murmur may be heard over the back or spinous processes. Single S_2 loud S_3 gallop is usually present.
2. Four-limb blood pressure.
    a. Systolic blood pressure normally 5 to 10 mm higher in lower extremities
    b. Systolic blood pressure in lower limbs the same as or lower than that in the arms seen in CoA.
3. Chest x-ray—cardiomegaly and pulmonary edema or pulmonary venous congestion.
4. ECG—varies; normal or right ventricular hypertrophy (RVH) in infants and LVH in older children.
5. Two-dimensional echocardiography with Doppler and color flow mapping identifies area of aortic arch narrowing and associated lesions (bicuspid aortic valve, VSD, PDA).
6. Invasive studies (cardiac catheterization) usually not needed to make the initial diagnosis; may need aortic angiography to identify collateral vessels before surgery.
7. Cardiac magnetic resonance imaging may be done to noninvasively assess the location and degree of narrowing and identify collateral vessels.

Management

Critical Coarctation in the Neonate

1. Medical management:
    a. Resuscitation and stabilization with PGE_1 infusion: monitor for complications related to PGE_1 therapy (fever, apnea).
    b. Intubation and ventilation, as needed.
    c. Infective endocarditis prophylaxis (lifelong).
    d. Anticongestive therapy (digoxin and Lasix) and inotropic support, as needed.
    e. Assessment of renal, hepatic, and neurologic function.
2. Balloon angioplasty may be indicated for infants who are at high surgical risk.
3. Surgical intervention: usually performed as soon as the diagnosis is made.
    a. Subclavian flap repair (Waldhausen procedure).
    b. End-to-end anastomosis.
    c. Dacron patch repair.
    d. Stent implantation.

Coarctation in the Child or Adolescent

1. Surgical intervention.
    a. End-to-end anastomosis.
    b. Dacron patch.
    c. Stent implantation.

2. Medical management for hypertension (beta-adrenergic blockers).

3. Infective endocarditis prophylaxis (lifelong).

Recurrent Coarctation in the Neonate or Child

1. Balloon angioplasty in the cardiac catheterization laboratory.
2. Redo surgical intervention.

Complications

1. Systemic hypertension.
2. CHF—occurs in 20% to 30% of all infants with CoA by age 3 months.
3. Cerebral hemorrhage.
4. Infective endocarditis.
5. Left ventricular failure.
6. Aortic aneurysm.

Pulmonary Stenosis

Evidence Base Prieto, L. R., & Latson, L. A. (2013). Pulmonary stenosis. In H. D. Allen, D. J. Driscoll, R. E. Shaddy, & T. F. Feltes, (Eds.), *Moss and Adams' heart disease in infants, children, and adolescents* (8th ed.). (pp. 913–938). Philadelphia: Lippincott Williams & Wilkins.

The pulmonary valve opens during systole to let blood flow from the right ventricle into the main PA. Obstruction to flow can occur at three levels: subvalvular, valvular, or supravalvular. The most common cause of RV outflow tract obstruction is pulmonary valve stenosis (PS). PS accounts for 8% to 12% of CHDs.

Pathophysiology and Etiology

1. Critical PS in the neonate: blood flows into the right atrium, across a patent foramen ovale (PFO) into the left side of heart; pulmonary blood flow comes from a left-to-right shunt through a PDA.
2. Right ventricular pressure increases to pump blood across the obstructive pulmonary valve.
3. RVH develops in response to the increased pressure gradient across the pulmonary valve.
4. Signs of right-sided heart failure include hepatic congestion, neck vein distention, elevated CVP.

Clinical Manifestations

Critical PS in the Neonate

1. Hypoxia.
2. Tachypnea.
3. RV failure.

Mild to Moderate PS in the Child and Adolescent

1. Asymptomatic.
2. Decreased exercise tolerance, fatigue, dyspnea.
3. Chest pain.

Diagnostic Evaluation

1. Auscultation: systolic ejection murmur heard best at the left upper sternal border; ejection click.
2. ECG: varies; normal in mild cases and RVH in moderate to severe cases.
3. Chest x-ray: varies; may show right ventricular enlargement; poststenotic dilatation of PA.
4. Two-dimensional echocardiography with Doppler study and color flow mapping to visualize the sites of obstruction, observe the degree of RVH, and estimate the pressure gradient across the valve.
5. Cardiac catheterization is usually not needed for the initial diagnosis.

Management

Neonate with Critical PS

1. Medical management:
   a. Stabilize and improve oxygen saturations with PGE_1 infusion.
   b. Intubation and ventilation, as needed.
   c. Inotropic support, as needed.
   d. Infective endocarditis prophylaxis (lifelong).
2. Balloon pulmonary valvuloplasty.
3. Blalock-Taussig shunt (Gore-Tex graft between the subclavian artery and the PA to supply pulmonary blood flow).

Child and Adolescent with PS

1. Medical management:
   a. Close follow-up to monitor and record RV to PA gradient and assess RV function.
   b. Restrict strenuous exercise and participation in competitive sports.
   c. Infective endocarditis prophylaxis (lifelong).
   d. Refer for intervention when RV pressure is greater than two thirds of the systemic pressure.
2. Balloon pulmonary valvuloplasty in the cardiac catheterization laboratory.
3. Surgical intervention:
   a. Valvotomy or valvectomy for dysplastic pulmonary valve.
   b. Patch repair of the right ventricular outflow tract.
   c. Placement of an RV-to-PA conduit.

Complications

1. Cyanosis (critical PS in the neonate).
2. Arrhythmia; sudden death.
3. Infective endocarditis.
4. Right ventricular failure.

Patent Ductus Arteriosus

Evidence Base Barrett, A. (2012). PDA—an overview. *Synergy: Imaging & Therapy Practice*, July: 4–9.
Hoffman, T. M., & Welty, S. E. (2013). Physiology of the preterm and term infant. In H. D. Allen, D. J. Driscoll, R. E. Shaddy, & T. F. Feltes, (Eds.), *Moss and Adams' heart disease in infants, children, and adolescents* (8th ed.). (pp. 473–482). Philadelphia: Lippincott Williams & Wilkins.

The *ductus arteriosus* is a normal fetal connection between the left PA and the descending aorta. During fetal life, blood flow is shunted away from the lungs through the ductus arteriosus and directly into the systemic circulation. PDAs occur in up to 60% of premature neonates who weigh less than 1,000 g. In term infants, PDAs account for 5% to 10% of CHDs; the male to female ratio is 1:3.

Pathophysiology and Etiology

1. During fetal life, the ductus arteriosus allows blood to bypass the pulmonary circulation (fetus receives oxygen from the placenta) and flow directly into the systemic circulation.
2. After birth, the ductus arteriosus is no longer needed. Functional closure usually occurs within 48 hours after birth. Anatomic closure is completed by age 2 to 3 weeks.
3. When the ductus arteriosus fails to close, blood from the aorta (high pressure) flows into the low-pressure PA, resulting in pulmonary overcirculation.
4. Increased pulmonary blood flow leads to a volume-loaded LV.

Clinical Presentation

Small- to Moderate-Sized PDA
Usually asymptomatic.

Large PDA
1. CHF, tachypnea, frequent respiratory tract infections.
2. Poor weight gain, failure to thrive.
3. Feeding difficulties.
4. Decreased exercise tolerance.
5. Infective endocarditis.

Diagnostic Evaluation

1. Auscultation: continuous murmur heard best at left upper sternal border. Hyperactive precordium with large PDAs.
2. Wide pulse pressure; bounding pulses.
3. Chest x-ray: varies; normal or cardiomegaly with increased pulmonary vascular markings.
4. ECG: varies; normal, LVH or RVH.
5. Two-dimensional echocardiogram with Doppler study and color flow mapping to visualize the PDA with left-to-right blood flow.
6. Elevated levels of N-terminal pro-B-type natriuretic peptide and cardiac troponin T.
7. Cardiac catheterization is not needed for the initial diagnosis.

Management

1. In the symptomatic premature neonate—indomethacin or ibuprofen given via IV line. These drugs are not effective in term infants.
2. Medical management:
   a. Monitor growth and development.
   b. Reassess for spontaneous PDA closure.
   c. Increase caloric intake as needed for normal weight gain.
   d. Infective endocarditis prophylaxis for 6 months after surgery or coil occlusion.

3. Cardiac catheterization:
   a. For small PDAs, coil occlusion.
   b. For larger PDAs, a closure device may be used.
4. Surgical management through PDA ligation.

Complications

1. CHF, pulmonary edema.
2. Infective endocarditis.
3. Pulmonary hypertension/pulmonary vascular occlusive disease.
4. Recurrent pneumonia.

Atrial Septal Defect

 Evidence Base Sachdeva, R. (2013). Atrial septal defect. In H. D. Allen, D. J. Driscoll, R. E. Shaddy, & T. F. Feltes, (Eds.), *Moss and Adams' heart disease in infants, children, and adolescents* (8th ed.). (pp. 672–690). Philadelphia: Lippincott Williams & Wilkins.
Webb, G. D., et al. (2011). Congenital heart disease. In L. Libby (Ed.), *Braunwald's heart disease: A textbook of cardiovascular medicine* (9th ed.). (pp. 1412–1426). St. Louis, MO: Elsevier.

Atrial septal defect (ASD) is an abnormal communication between the left and right atria. ASDs account for 6% to 10% of CHDs. Thirty-five percent of children with ASD also have Down syndrome. There are four types:

1. Ostium secundum ASD: most common type of ASD (accounts for 50%–70%); abnormal opening in the middle of the atrial septum.
2. Ostium primum ASD (accounts for 30%): abnormal opening at the bottom of the atrial septum; increased association with cleft mitral valve and atrioventricular defects.
3. Sinus venosus ASD (accounts for 10%): abnormal opening at the top of the atrial septum; increased association with partial anomalous pulmonary venous return.
4. Coronary sinus defect (rare): abnormal opening between coronary sinus and left atrium.

Pathophysiology and Etiology

1. Blood flows from the higher-pressure left atrium across the ASD into the lower-pressure right atrium (left-to-right shunt).
2. Increased blood return to the right side of the heart leads to right ventricular volume overload and right ventricular dilation.
3. Increased pulmonary blood flow leads to elevated pulmonary artery pressures.

Clinical Manifestations

1. Usually asymptomatic.
2. Clinical symptoms vary depending on type of associated defects:
   a. CHF (usually not until the third or fourth decade of life).
   b. Frequent upper respiratory infections (URIs).
   c. Poor weight gain.
   d. Decreased exercise tolerance.
   e. Dyspnea and fatigue.

Diagnostic Evaluation

1. Auscultation: soft systolic ejection murmur heard best at the left upper sternal border; widely split, fixed second heart sound.
2. Prominent systolic impulse.
3. Chest x-ray: varies; normal to right atrial and ventricular dilation, increased pulmonary markings.
4. ECG: varies; right axis deviation and mild RVH or right bundle-branch block. Alterations are present only when the shunt is large and the pulmonary resistance to systemic resistance ratio is greater than 1.5:1 (Qp:Qs > 1.5:1).
5. Two-dimensional echocardiogram with Doppler study and color flow mapping to identify the site of the ASD and associated lesions and document left-to-right flow across the atrial septum.
6. Cardiac catheterization usually not needed for initial diagnosis; performed if defect can be closed using an atrial occlusion device (device can be used only in ostium secundum defects).

Management

1. Medical management:
   a. Monitor and reassess (spontaneous closure rate is small but may occur up to age 2).
   b. Treatment with anticongestive therapy (digoxin and furosemide) may be necessary if signs of CHF are present (usually not until third to fourth decade of life if ASD unrepaired).
   c. Infective endocarditis prophylaxis for 6 months after surgery or atrial occlusion device is used.
2. Cardiac catheterization for placement of an atrial occlusion device for ostium secundum defects.
3. Surgical intervention:
   a. Primary repair: suture closure of the ASD.
   b. Patch repair of the ASD.

Complications

1. CHF (rare).
2. Infective endocarditis.
3. Embolic stroke.
4. Pulmonary hypertension.
5. Atrial arrhythmias.

Ventricular Septal Defect

 Evidence Base Rubio, A., & Lewin, M. (2013). Ventricular septal defects. In H. D. Allen, D. J. Driscoll, R. E. Shaddy, & T. F. Feltes, (Eds.), *Moss and Adams' heart disease in infants, children, and adolescents* (8th ed.). (pp. 713–721). Philadelphia: Lippincott Williams & Wilkins.
Pedra, C. A., Pedra, S. R., Chaccur, P., et al. (2010). Perventricular device closure of congenital muscular ventricular septal defects. *Expert Review of Cardiovascular Therapy, 8*(5), 663–674.

A *ventricular septal defect (VSD)* is an abnormal communication between the right and left ventricles. It is the most common type of CHD, accounting for approximately 20% to 25% of all CHDs. VSD is slightly more common in females and is the most common lesion found in chromosomal syndromes (Trisomy 13, 18, 21). However, 95% of VSDs are not associated with such syndromes. VSDs vary in size (small and restrictive to large and nonrestrictive), number (single vs. multiple), and type (perimembranous or muscular).

Pathophysiology and Etiology

1. Blood flows from the high-pressure left ventricle across the VSD into the low-pressure right ventricle and into the PA, resulting in pulmonary overcirculation. The size of the defect determines the physiologic effect on the infant.
2. A left-to-right shunt because of a VSD results in increased right ventricular pressure and increased PA pressure.
3. The increased pulmonary venous return to the left side of the heart results in left atrial dilation.
4. Long-standing pulmonary overcirculation causes a change in the pulmonary arterial bed, leading to increased pulmonary vascular resistance. High pulmonary vascular resistance (PVR) can reverse the blood flow pattern that leads to a right-to-left shunt across the VSD (Eisenmenger's syndrome), resulting in cyanosis. Once this develops, the child is no longer a candidate for surgical repair.

Clinical Manifestations

1. Small VSDs—usually asymptomatic; high spontaneous closure rate during the first year of life. Ongoing risk of endocarditis.
2. Large VSDs.
   a. CHF: tachypnea, tachycardia, excessive sweating associated with feeding, hepatomegaly.
   b. Frequent URIs.
   c. Poor weight gain, failure to thrive presenting at age 2 to 3 months.
   d. Feeding difficulties.
   e. Decreased exercise tolerance.

Diagnostic Evaluation

1. Auscultation: harsh systolic regurgitant murmur heard best at the lower left sternal border (LLSB); systolic thrill felt at LLSB, narrowly split S_2. The murmur may radiate toward the head along the left parasternal border or to the right of the sternum.
2. Chest x-ray: varies; normal or cardiomegaly and increased pulmonary vascular markings. Pulmonary vascular markings are directly proportionate to the amount of left-to-right shunting.
3. ECG: varies; normal to biventricular hypertrophy.
4. Two-dimensional echocardiogram with Doppler study and color flow mapping to identify the size, number, and sites of the defects; estimate pulmonary artery pressure; and identify associated lesions.
5. Cardiac catheterization usually not needed for initial diagnosis; may be needed to calculate the size of the shunt or to assess PVR. May be performed if defect can be closed using a ventricular occlusion device (device can be used only in muscular defects).

Management

Small VSD

1. Medical management:
   a. Usually no anticongestive therapy is needed.
   b. Infective endocarditis prophylaxis for 6 months after surgical implantation of a ventricular occlusion device.
2. Cardiac catheterization for placement of a ventricular occlusion device for muscular defects (for Qp:Qs > 1.5:1).
3. Surgical intervention is usually not necessary.

Moderate to Large VSD

1. Medical management:
   a. CHF management: digoxin and diuretics such as furosemide and spironolactone and afterload reduction enalapril.
   b. Avoid oxygen; oxygen is a potent pulmonary vasodilator and will increase blood flow into the PA.
   c. Increase caloric intake: fortify formula or breast milk to make 24 to 30 cal/oz formula; supplemental nasogastric feeds, as needed.
   d. Infective endocarditis prophylaxis for 6 months after surgery/ventricular device occluder.
2. Cardiac catheterization for placement of a ventricular occlusion device for muscular defects (for Qp:Qs > 1.5:1).
3. Refer for surgical intervention.
   a. Usually repaired before age 1.
   b. One-stage approach: preferred surgical plan; patch closure of VSD.
   c. Two-stage approach: first surgery is to band the PA to restrict pulmonary blood flow; second surgery is to patch close the VSD and remove the PA band.

Long-Term Follow-Up

1. Monitor ventricular function.
2. Monitor for subaortic membrane and double-chamber RV.

Complications

1. CHF.
2. Frequent URIs.
3. Failure to thrive; poor weight gain.
4. Infective endocarditis.
5. Eisenmenger's syndrome.
6. Pulmonary hypertension.
7. Aortic insufficiency.

Tetralogy of Fallot

Evidence Base Bailliard, F., & Anderson, R. H. (2009). Tetralogy of Fallot. *Orphanet Journal of Rare Diseases, 13*(4), 2.
Roche, S. L., Greenway, S., & Redington, A. (2013). Tetralogy of Fallot with Pulmonary Stenosis and Tetralogy of Fallot with Absent Pulmonary Valve. In H. D. Allen, D. J. Driscoll, R. E. Shaddy, & T. F. Feltes, (Eds.), *Moss and Adams' heart disease in infants, children, and adolescents* (8th ed.). Philadelphia: Lippincott Williams & Wilkins.
Webb, G. D., et al. (2011). Congenital heart disease. In L. Libby, (Ed.), *Braunwald's heart disease: A textbook of cardiovascular medicine* (9th ed.). St. Louis, MO: Elsevier.

Tetralogy of Fallot (TOF) is the most common complex CHD; it accounts for 6% to 10% of all CHDs. The four abnormalities of TOF include:

1. A large, nonrestrictive VSD.
2. Aortic override.
3. Pulmonary stenosis (right ventricular outflow tract obstruction).
4. Right ventricular hypertrophy.

Pathophysiology and Etiology

1. Degree of cyanosis depends on the size of the VSD and the degree of RVOTO.
2. Obstruction of blood flow from the right ventricle to the PA results in deoxygenated blood being shunted across the VSD and into the aorta (right-to-left shunt causes cyanosis).
3. RVOTO can occur at any or all of three levels: pulmonary valve stenosis, infundibular stenosis, or supravalvular stenosis.
4. The right ventricle becomes hypertrophied as a result of the increased gradient across the RVOT.
5. Minimal RVOTO results in a pink TOF variant, with the physiology behaving more like a large, nonrestrictive VSD.

Clinical Manifestations

1. Clinical manifestations are variable and depend on the size of the VSD and the degree of RVOTO.
2. Cyanosis.
   a. Neonate may have normal oxygen saturations; as the infant grows, the RVOTO increases and the oxygen saturation falls.
   b. Neonate with unacceptably low oxygen saturation needs PGE$_1$ infusion to maintain ductal patency and adequate oxygen saturation.
   c. Cyanosis may initially be observed only with crying and with exertion.
3. Loud second heart sound with a harsh systolic ejection murmur.
4. Polycythemia.
5. Decreased exercise tolerance.
6. A common clinical manifestation years ago was squatting, a posture characteristically assumed by older children to increase systemic vascular resistance and to encourage increased pulmonary blood flow. Squatting is rarely seen currently, however, because TOF is now surgically repaired during the first year of life.
7. Hypercyanotic spells (formerly known as Tet spells): life-threatening hypoxic event with a dramatic decrease in oxygen saturations; mechanism is usually infundibular spasm, which further obstructs pulmonary blood flow and increases right-to-left flow across the VSD.
   a. Typical hypoxic spells occur in the morning soon after awakening; during or after a crying episode; during or after a feeding; during painful procedures such as blood draws.
   b. Typical scenario includes tachypnea, irritability, and increasing cyanosis, followed by flaccidity and loss of consciousness.
   c. Home treatment for the caregiver: soothe the infant and place him or her in a knee–chest position; notify the health care provider immediately.

d. Hospital treatment includes knee–chest position, sedation (morphine), oxygen, beta-adrenergic blockers (propranolol, esmolol) to relax the infundibulum, and administration of medications to increase systemic vascular resistance (phenylephrine).

e. Hypercyanotic spells usually prompt the cardiologist to refer for surgical intervention.

Diagnostic Evaluation

1. Auscultation: harsh systolic ejection murmur heard best at the upper left sternal border (RVOT murmur); single loud second heart sound; aortic ejection click. Murmur is caused by pulmonary stenosis—in mild stenosis, the murmur is louder and longer than when stenosis is more severe; during a hypercyanotic spell, the murmur disappears.

2. Palpation: systolic thrill palpable along left lower and left middle sternal border (50% of cases). RV tap at left sternal border.

3. Chest x-ray: varies; normal or decreased pulmonary vascular markings. The heart may appear "boot shaped" because of a concave main PA with an upturned apex resulting from RVH.

4. ECG: varies; normal or RVH.

5. Two-dimensional echocardiogram with Doppler study and color flow mapping to identify the structural abnormalities, estimate the degree of RVOTO, and assess the coronary artery pattern.

6. Cardiac catheterization is usually not needed for the initial diagnosis. May be performed before surgical intervention to identify the location and number of VSDs, the PVR, the degree of RVOTO, and the presence of any coronary abnormalities.

Management

1. Medical management:
   a. Monitor oxygen saturation level.
   b. Monitor growth and development.
   c. Monitor for hypercyanotic spells (many spells go unnoticed by parents).
   d. Infective endocarditis prophylaxis (lifelong).
   e. Restrict strenuous activity and participation in competitive sports.

2. Balloon pulmonary angioplasty (rarely).

3. Infants with severe pulmonary stenosis may require PGE$_1$ to maintain ductal patency.

4. Surgical intervention: palliative versus definitive repair.
   a. Many centers prefer definitive, one-stage repair.
   b. Potential obstacles for one-stage repair: abnormal coronary artery distribution (left anterior descending arises from right coronary artery and crosses RVOT); multiple VSDs; hypoplastic branch pulmonary arteries; small infant weighing less than 5.5 lb (2.5 kg).
   c. Palliative surgery: modified BT shunt; tube Gore-Tex graft between the left subclavian artery and the PA; increased

pulmonary blood flow results in higher oxygen saturations.

   d. Definitive surgery: patch closure of VSD, relief of right ventricular outflow tract obstruction; with or without transannular patch across the pulmonary valve.

Long-Term Follow-Up

1. Assess RV outflow tract, monitor degree of pulmonary insufficiency.
2. Monitor RV function and exercise tolerance.
3. Monitor for arrhythmias.

Complications

1. Hypoxia.
2. Hypercyanotic spells.
3. Polycythemia.
4. CHF: rare; associated with pink TOF.
5. Right ventricular dysfunction.
6. Ventricular arrhythmias.
7. Infective endocarditis.

Transposition of the Great Arteries

 Evidence Base Park, M. (2008). *Pediatric cardiology for practitioners* (5th ed.). St. Louis, MO: Mosby. Wernovsky, G. (2013). Transposition of the great arteries. In H. D. Allen, D. J. Driscoll, R. E. Shaddy, & T. F. Feltes, (Eds.), *Moss and Adams' heart disease in infants, children, and adolescents* (8th ed.). Philadelphia: Lippincott Williams & Wilkins.

Transposition of the great arteries (TGA) occurs when the PA arises off the left ventricle and the aorta arises off the right ventricle. It accounts for 5% to 8% of CHDs with a male-to-female ratio of 1.5 to 3:1. Associated lesions occur in 50% of cases and include VSD (30% to 40%), ASD, PDA, PS, and CoA. Ten percent of infants with TGA also have noncardiac malformations.

Pathophysiology and Etiology

1. This defect results in two parallel circulations:
   a. The right atrium receives deoxygenated blood from the inferior vena cava (IVC) and SVC; blood flow continues through the tricuspid valve into the right ventricle and is pumped back to the aorta.
   b. The left atrium receives richly oxygenated blood from the pulmonary veins; blood flow continues through the mitral valve into the left ventricle and is pumped back into the PA.

2. To sustain life, there must be an accompanying defect that allows mixing of deoxygenated blood and oxygenated blood between the two circuits, such as PDA, ASD, PFO, or VSD.

3. Neonates born with TGA with an intact ventricular system are usually more cyanotic and sicker than neonates born with TGA with a VSD.

Clinical Manifestations

Symptoms evident soon after birth; clinical scenario is influenced by the extent of intercirculatory mixing.

1. Cyanosis.
2. Tachypnea.
3. Metabolic acidosis.
4. CHF.
5. Feeding difficulties.

Diagnostic Evaluation

1. Auscultation: varies; no murmur or a murmur related to an associated defect, single loud S_2.
2. Chest x-ray: varies; neonate chest x-ray usually normal; cardiomegaly with a narrow mediastinum (egg-shaped cardiac silhouette) and increased pulmonary markings; or decreased pulmonary markings with pulmonary stenosis.
3. ECG: RVH or biventricular hypertrophy.
4. Two-dimensional echocardiogram with Doppler study and color flow mapping identifies the structural abnormalities: transposed vessels, coronary artery pattern, and degree of mixing across the atrial septum plus associated lesions.

Management

Medical Management

1. Stabilize with PGE_1 infusion.
2. Correct metabolic acidosis.
3. Provide oxygen to decrease PVR.
4. Treat pulmonary overcirculation with digoxin and diuretics, as needed.
5. Intubate and ventilate, as needed.
6. Inotropic support, as needed.
7. Infective endocarditis prophylaxis (lifelong).

Cardiac Catheterization

1. Balloon atrial septostomy (Rashkind) is indicated for severe hypoxia to create or improve atrial level mixing.

Surgical Management

1. Arterial switch operation (Jatene)—procedure of choice:
   a. Ideally performed during the first week of life.
   b. The aorta and PA are switched back to their anatomically correct ventricle above the level of the valve.
   c. Coronary arteries are transferred to the new aorta.
   d. Associated lesions are also repaired at this time.
2. Rastelli operation—performed for TGA, VSD, and PS.
   a. Repaired during the first year of life.
   b. VSD patch repaired to include LV to aortic outflow continuity with pulmonary blood flow provided via an RV to PA homograft.
3. Atrial switch operation—Mustard or Senning procedure:
   a. Rerouting of atrial blood flow: RA → mitral valve → LV → PA and LA → tricuspid valve → RV → Ao.
   b. Restores oxygenated blood into the systemic system and deoxygenated blood guided to the pulmonary system.
   c. Disadvantages:
      i. RV is left as the systemic ventricle—will develop RV dysfunction.
      ii. Increased incidence of atrial dysrhythmias and baffle obstruction.

Complications

1. Severe hypoxia.
2. Multiorgan ischemia.
3. Arrhythmias.
4. RV dysfunction.
5. Coronary artery obstruction leading to myocardial ischemia or death.

Tricuspid Atresia

 Evidence Base Epstein, M. L. (2013). Tricuspid atresia, stenosis, regurgitation, and Uhl's Anomaly. In H. D. Allen, D. J. Driscoll, R. E. Shaddy, & T. F. Feltes, (Eds.), *Moss and Adams' heart disease in infants, children, and adolescents* (8th ed.). (pp. 877–888). Philadelphia: Lippincott Williams & Wilkins.

Webb, G. D., et al. (2011). Congenital heart disease. In L. Libby (Ed.), *Braunwald's heart disease: A textbook of cardiovascular medicine* (9th ed.). (pp. 1412–1426). St. Louis, MO: Elsevier.

Tricuspid atresia involves the absence of the tricuspid valve and hypoplasia of the right ventricle. Such associated defects as ASD, VSD, or PDA are necessary for survival. Tricuspid atresia accounts for 1% to 3% of CHDs.

Pathophysiology and Etiology

1. With tricuspid atresia, systemic venous return enters the right atrium and cannot continue into the RV; blood flows across an atrial septal opening into the left atrium.
2. Pulmonary blood flow occurs through a PDA or VSD.

Clinical Manifestations

1. Cyanosis.
2. Tachypnea.
3. Feeding difficulties.

Diagnostic Evaluation

1. Auscultation: murmurs vary depending on the associated lesions; single S_2.
2. Palpation: if a restrictive VSD is present, a thrill may be palpated.
3. Chest x-ray: pulmonary vascular markings related to the amount of pulmonary blood flow (usually decreased); normal to slightly increased cardiac silhouette.
4. ECG: superior axis; right and left atrial hypertrophy; LVH.
5. Two-dimensional echocardiogram identifies the atretic tricuspid valve and hypoplastic RV; Doppler study and color flow mapping documents the right-to-left atrial shunt and the size of the PDA or VSD.
6. Cardiac catheterization may be necessary to delineate anatomy.

Management

Medical Management

1. Stabilize with PGE_1 infusion.
2. Maintain oxygen saturation at greater than 75%.
3. Intubate and ventilate, as needed.
4. Inotropic support, as needed.
5. Infective endocarditis prophylaxis (lifelong).

Surgical Management

1. First surgery—neonate:
   a. BT shunt—indicated if pulmonary blood flow is insufficient.
   b. Pulmonary artery band—indicated if pulmonary blood flow is excessive.
   c. No treatment is required if pulmonary blood flow is balanced.
2. Second surgery—ages 6 to 9 months:
   a. Bidirectional Glenn shunt: end-to-side anastomosis of the SVC to the right PA.
3. Third surgery—ages 18 months to 3 years:
   a. Fontan completion: IVC to PA connection (extracardiac conduit or intracardiac baffle).

Complications

1. CHF.
2. Persistent pleural effusion (especially after stage II and stage III repairs).
3. Thrombus formation in the systemic venous system.
4. Infective endocarditis.
5. Rarely, heart block.

Hypoplastic Left Heart Syndrome

Evidence Base Feinstein, J. A., Benson, D. W., Dubin, A. M., et al. (2012). Hypoplastic left heart syndrome: current considerations and expectations. *Journal of the American College of Cardiology*, 59(1, Suppl.), S1–S42.

Treddell, J. S., et al. (2013). Hypoplastic left heart syndrome. In H. D. Allen, D. J. Driscoll, R. E. Shaddy, & T. F. Feltes, (Eds.), *Moss and Adams' heart disease in infants, children, and adolescents* (8th ed.). (pp. 1061–1096). Philadelphia: Lippincott Williams & Wilkins.

Webb, G. D., et al. (2011). Congenital heart disease. In L. Libby (Ed.), *Braunwald's heart disease: A textbook of cardiovascular medicine* (9th ed.). (pp. 1412–1426). St. Louis, MO: Elsevier.

Hypoplasic left heart syndrome (HLHS) is a constellation of left-sided heart abnormalities that include:

1. Critical mitral stenosis or atresia.
2. Hypoplastic LV.
3. Critical aortic stenosis or atresia.
4. Hypoplastic ascending aorta with severe coarctation of the aorta.
5. Associated anomalies include CoA (75%), ASD (15%), and VSD (10%).

HLHS accounts for 1% of all CHDs. It is the most common cause of death from cardiac defects in the first month of life.

Pathophysiology and Etiology

1. The left side of the heart is underdeveloped and essentially nonfunctional.
2. The right ventricle supports the pulmonary and systemic circulations.
3. An ASD allows blood to flow from the left atrium into the right heart.
4. Blood flows right to left across the PDA and into the descending aorta to deliver oxygen and nutrients to the body.

Clinical Manifestations

1. Neonate may appear completely well initially, but becomes critically ill when the PDA closes.
2. Once the PDA begins to close:
   a. Tachypnea due to CHF.
   b. Decreased urine output.
   c. Poor feeding and feeding intolerance.
   d. Lethargic; change in level of alertness.
   e. Pallor; gray.
   f. Weak peripheral pulses.
   g. Cyanosis.
   h. Metabolic acidosis.

Diagnostic Evaluation

1. Auscultation: single S_2; usually no heart murmur is present, but occasionally a soft systolic ejection murmur may be heard. As CHF develops, gallop rhythm may be heard.
2. Chest x-ray: cardiac silhouette varies (normal to increased size); increased pulmonary markings and pulmonary edema.
3. ECG: RV hypertrophy; decreased electrical forces in V_5 and V_6.
4. Two-dimensional echocardiogram with Doppler study and color flow mapping identifies the structural abnormalities and the altered blood flow patterns.
5. A cardiac catheterization is usually not needed for initial diagnosis. It may be performed if a balloon atrial septostomy is needed to improve oxygenation.

Management

Medical Management

1. Resuscitation and stabilization with PGE_1 infusion.
2. Inotropic support, as needed (dopamine, dobutamine).
3. Intubate and ventilate, as needed.
4. Correct metabolic acidosis.
5. Assess hepatic, renal, and neurologic function.
6. Infective endocarditis prophylaxis (lifelong).
7. Refer for surgical intervention.

Cardiac Catheterization

1. May need balloon atrial septostomy to allow unrestrictive LA to RA blood flow.

Surgical Management

1. Palliative, staged repair:
   a. Stage I Norwood (neonate): reconstruction of the hypoplastic aorta using the PA and an aortic or pulmonary allograft, an atrial septectomy, repair of the coarctation and placement of a BT shunt.
   b. Stage II bidirectional Glenn shunt (ages 6 to 9 months): transect the SVC off the right atrium and directly suture end to side to right PA; ligate BT shunt.
   c. Stage III Fontan (ages 12 to 18 months): IVC to PA connection (extracardiac conduit or intracardiac baffle).
2. Cardiac transplantation.

Complications

1. Cyanosis.
2. Metabolic acidosis.
3. Persistent pleural effusion (especially after stage II and stage III repairs).
4. Thrombus formation in the systemic venous system.
5. Infective endocarditis.
6. Cardiovascular collapse.
7. Multisystem failure.
8. Death.

Nursing Care of the Child with Congenital Heart Disease

 Evidence Base Frank, J. E., & Jacobe, K. M. (2011). Evaluation and management of heart murmurs in children. *American Family Physician, 84*(7), 793–800.

Thangaratinam, S., Brown, K., Zamora, J., Khan, K., & Ewer, A. (2012). Pulse oximetry screening for critical congenital heart defects in asymptomatic newborn babies: A systematic review and meta-analysis. *Lancet, 379*(9835), 2459–2464.

Smith, M., Newey, C., Jones, M., & Martin, J. (2011). Congenital heart disease and its effects on children and their families. *Paediatric Nursing, 23*(2), 30–35.

Nursing Assessment

1. Obtain a thorough nursing history.
2. Discuss the care plan with the health care team (cardiologist, cardiac surgeon, nursing case manager, social worker, and nutritionist). Discuss the care plan with the patient, parents, and other caregivers.
3. Measure and record height and weight and plot on a growth chart.
4. Record vital signs and oxygen saturations.
   a. Measure vital signs at a time when the infant/child is quiet.
   b. Choose appropriate-size blood pressure (BP) cuff.
   c. Check four extremity BP × 1.
5. Assess and record:
   a. Skin color: pink, cyanotic, mottled.
   b. Mucous membranes: moist, dry, cyanotic.
   c. Extremities: check peripheral pulses for quality and symmetry; dependent edema; capillary refill; color and temperature.
6. Assess for clubbing (cyanotic heart disease).
7. Assess chest wall for deformities; prominent precordial activity.
8. Assess respiratory pattern.
   a. Before disturbing the child, stand back and count the respiratory rate.
   b. Loosen or remove clothing to directly observe chest movement.
   c. Assess for signs of respiratory distress: increased respiratory rate, grunting, retractions, nasal flaring.
   d. Auscultate for crackles, wheezing, congestion, stridor.
9. Assess heart sounds.
   a. Determine rate (bradycardia, tachycardia, or normal for age) and rhythm (regular or irregular).
   b. Identify murmur (type, location, and grade).
10. Assess fluid status.
    a. Daily weights.
    b. Strict intake and output (number of wet diapers; urine output).
11. Assess and record the child's level of activity.
    a. Observe the infant while feeding. Does the infant need frequent breaks or does he or she fall asleep during feeding? Assess for sweating, color change, or respiratory distress while feeding.
    b. Observe the child at play. Is play interrupted to rest? Ask the parent if the child keeps up with peers while at play.
    c. Assess and record findings relevant to the child's developmental level: age-appropriate behavior, cognitive skills, gross and fine motor skills.

Nursing Diagnoses

- Impaired Gas Exchange related to altered pulmonary blood flow or pulmonary congestion.
- Decreased Cardiac Output related to decreased myocardial function.
- Activity Intolerance related to hypoxia or decreased myocardial function.
- Imbalanced Nutrition: Less Than Body Requirements related to excessive energy demands required by increased cardiac workload.
- Risk for Infection related to chronic illness.
- Fear and Anxiety related to life-threatening illness.

Nursing Interventions

Relieving Respiratory Distress

1. Position the child in a reclining, semi-upright position.
2. Suction oral and nasal secretions, as needed.
3. Identify target oxygen saturations and administer oxygen, as prescribed.
4. Administer prescribed medications and document response to medications (improved, no change, or worsening respiratory status).

Table 45-1 Common Cardiac Drugs

DRUG CLASSIFICATION	MECHANISM OF ACTION	EXAMPLES
Beta-adrenergic blockers	Antagonize epinephrine receptors resulting in decreased cardiac contractility and decreased heart rate	Propranolol, esmolol, atenolol
Angiotensin-converting enzyme (ACE) inhibitor	Lowers blood pressure by decreasing blood vessel tone	Captopril, enalapril
Angiotensin II receptor blockers	Decrease blood pressure by causing dilation of blood vessels	Losartan, valsartan
Calcium-channel blockers	Decrease intracellular calcium leading to reduced cardiac and vascular smooth muscle contraction and lower blood pressure	Amlodipine, diltiazem, felodipine, isradipine, intravenous nicardipine, nifedipine, and verapamil
Vasopressors	Increase cardiac contractility and vascular muscle tone resulting in increased blood pressure	Dopamine, dobutamine, milrinone, epinephrine
Diuretics	Reduce blood volume by increasing urinary output. Used to treat high blood pressure and congestive heart failure	Furosemide, spironolactone
Anti-arrhythmics	Various classifications used to treat cardiac dysrhythmias	Lidocaine, amiodarone, disopyramide adenosine
Cardiac glycosides	Strengthens cardiac contractility and decreases heart rate. Used to treat congestive heart failure	Digoxin

a. Diuretics.
b. Bronchodilators.
5. May need to change oral feedings to nasogastric feedings because of increased risk of aspiration with respiratory distress.

Improving Cardiac Output

See Table 45-1.
1. Organize nursing care and medication schedule to provide periods of uninterrupted rest.
2. Provide play or educational activities that can be done in bed with minimal exertion.
3. Maintain normothermia.
4. Administer diuretics (furosemide, spironolactone), as prescribed.
   a. Give the medication at the same time each day. For older children, do not give a dose right before bedtime.
   b. Monitor the effectiveness of the dose: measure and record urine output.
5. Administer digoxin, as prescribed.
   a. Check heart rate for 1 minute. Withhold the dose and notify the physician for bradycardia (heart rate less than 90 beats/minute).
   b. Lead II rhythm strip may be ordered for PR interval monitoring. Prolonged PR interval indicates first-degree heart block (dose of digoxin may be withheld).
   c. Give medication at the same time each day. For infants and children, digoxin is usually divided and given twice per day.
   d. Monitor serum electrolytes. Increased incidence of digoxin toxicity associated with hypokalemia.

6. Administer afterload-reducing medications (captopril, enalapril), as prescribed.
   a. When initiating medication for the first time: check BP immediately before and 1 hour after dose.
   b. Monitor for signs of hypotension: syncope, light-headedness, faint pulses.
   c. Withhold medication and notify the physician according to ordered parameters.

Improving Oxygenation and Activity Tolerance

1. Place pulse oximeter probe (continuous monitoring or measure with vital signs) on finger, earlobe, or toe. Pre- and postductal saturation monitoring provides the most comprehensive information about oxygenation.
2. Administer oxygen, as needed.
3. Titrate amount of oxygen to reach target oxygen saturations.
4. Assess response to oxygen therapy: increase in baseline oxygen saturations, improved work of breathing, and change in patient comfort.
5. Explain to the child how oxygen will help. If possible, give the child the choice for face mask oxygen or nasal cannula oxygen.

Providing Adequate Nutrition

1. For the infant:
   a. Small, frequent feedings.
   b. Fortified formula or breast milk (up to 30 cal/oz).
   c. Limit oral feeding time to 15 to 20 minutes.
   d. Supplement oral feeds with nasogastric feedings, as needed, to provide weight gain (ie, continuous nasogastric feedings at night with ad-lib by-mouth feeds during the day).

2. For the child:
   a. Small, frequent meals.
   b. High-calorie, nutritional supplements.
   c. Determine child's likes and dislikes and plan meals accordingly.
   d. Allow the parents to bring the child's favorite foods to the hospital.
3. Report feeding intolerance: nausea, vomiting, diarrhea.
4. Document daily weight (same time of day, same scale, same clothing).
5. Record accurate intake and output; assess for fluid retention.
6. Fluid restriction not usually needed for children; manage excess fluid with diuretics.

Preventing Infection
1. Maintain routine childhood immunization schedule. With the exception of RSV and influenza, immunizations should not be given for 6 weeks after cardiovascular surgery.
2. Administer yearly influenza vaccine.
3. Administer RSV immunization for children younger than age 2 with complex CHD and those at risk for CHF or pulmonary hypertension.
4. Prevent exposure to communicable diseases.
5. Good handwashing.
6. Report fevers.
7. Report signs of URI: runny nose, cough, increase in nasal secretions.
8. Report signs of GI illness: diarrhea, abdominal pain, irritability.

Reducing Fear and Anxiety
1. Educate the patient and family.
2. Provide the family with contact phone numbers: how to schedule a follow-up visit; how to reach a cardiologist during the work week, evenings, weekends, and holidays.

Family Education and Health Maintenance
1. Instruct the family in necessary measures to maintain the child's health:
   a. Complete immunization.
   b. Adequate diet and rest.
   c. Prevention and control of infections.
   d. Regular medical and dental checkups. The child should be protected against infective endocarditis when undergoing certain dental procedures.
   e. Regular cardiac checkups.
2. Teach the family about the defect and its treatment.
   a. Provide patients and families with written and verbal information regarding the CHD. Offer appropriate Internet resources for information about CHD and medical and surgical treatment options.
   b. Signs and symptoms of CHF (see page 1539).
   c. Signs of hypercyanotic spells associated with cyanotic defects and need to place child in knee–chest position.
   d. Need to prevent dehydration, which increases risk of thrombotic complications.

   e. Emergency precautions related to hypercyanotic spells, pulmonary edema, cardiac arrest (if appropriate).
   f. Special home care equipment, monitors, oxygen.
3. Encourage the parents and other people (teachers, peers) to treat the child in as normal a manner as possible.
   a. Avoid overprotection and overindulgence.
   b. Avoid rejection.
   c. Promote growth and development with modifications. Facilitate performance of the usual developmental tasks within the limits of the child's physiologic state.
   d. Prevent adults from projecting their fears and anxieties onto the child.
   e. Help family deal with anger, guilt, and concerns related to the disabled child.
4. Initiate a community health nursing referral, if indicated.
5. Stress the need for follow-up care.
6. Encourage attendance in support groups for patients and families.

Evaluation: Expected Outcomes
- Improved oxygenation evidenced by easy, comfortable respirations.
- Improved cardiac output demonstrated by stable vital signs, adequate peripheral perfusion, and adequate urine output.
- Increased activity level.
- Maximal nutritional status demonstrated by weight gain and increase in growth curve percentile.
- No signs or symptoms of infection.
- Parents discuss diagnosis and treatment together and with child.

Congestive Heart Failure

Evidence Base Kantor, P. F., & Mertens, L. L. (2010). Clinical practice: Heart failure in children. Part I: Clinical evaluation, diagnostic testing, and initial medical management. *European Journal of Pediatrics*, *169*(3), 269–279.

Kantor, P. F., & Mertens, L. L. (2010). Clinical practice: Heart failure in children. Part II: Current maintenance therapy and new therapeutic approaches. European Journal of Pediatrics, *169*(4), 403–410.

Congestive heart failure (CHF) occurs when cardiac output cannot meet the metabolic demands of the body.

Pathophysiology and Etiology
1. May result from:
   a. CHDs with a volume or pressure overload (moderate to large left-to-right shunt [PDA, VSD], AV valve insufficiency or outflow obstruction [HLHS, CoA]).
   b. Acquired heart disease: myocarditis, cardiomyopathy, acute rheumatic fever.
   c. Chronic pulmonary disease: cor pulmonale, bronchopulmonary dysplasia.

d. Arrhythmias: prolonged SVT, complete heart block.

e. Anemia.

f. Iatrogenic fluid overload.

2. In an attempt to meet the metabolic needs of the body, the heart rate increases to increase cardiac output.

   a. Cardiac output = heart rate × stroke volume.

   b. Stroke volume is the amount of blood (mL) ejected from the heart with each heartbeat; it depends on preload and vascular resistance.

3. Preload (CVP) increases as the failing heart contracts poorly.

4. With decreased cardiac output, the systemic vascular resistance increases to maintain BP. This increase in afterload limits cardiac output.

5. With decreased blood flow to the kidneys, the glomerular filtration rate decreases as tubular reabsorption increases sodium and water retention, resulting in decreased urine output.

6. Long term, these compensatory mechanisms are detrimental to the failing myocardium. The chronic increase in preload and afterload contributes to chamber dilation and myocardial hypertrophy, leading to progressive CHF.

Clinical Manifestations

1. Impaired myocardial function.

   a. Tachycardia, S_3 gallop.

   b. Poor peripheral perfusion: weak peripheral pulses, cool extremities, delayed capillary refill.

   c. Pallor.

   d. Exercise or activity intolerance.

2. Pulmonary congestion.

   a. Tachypnea.

   b. Cyanosis.

   c. Retractions, nasal flaring, grunting.

   d. Cough.

3. Systemic venous congestion.

   a. Hepatomegaly.

   b. Peripheral edema: scrotal and orbital.

   c. Water weight gain.

   d. Decreased urine output.

Diagnostic Evaluation

1. Characteristic physical examination findings.

2. Chest x-ray shows cardiomegaly and pulmonary congestion.

Management

1. Diuretics to reduce intravascular volume (furosemide, spironolactone).

2. Digoxin to increase myocardial contractility.

3. Afterload reduction to decrease the workload of the ailing myocardium (angiotensin-converting enzyme inhibitors—captopril, enalapril, lisinopril).

4. Beta-adrenergic blockers to counteract increased sympathetic activity and reduce systemic vascular resistance (metoprolol, carvedilol).

5. Inotropic support, as needed.

Complications

1. Pulmonary edema.

2. Metabolic acidosis.

3. Failure to thrive.

4. URIs.

5. Arrhythmia.

6. Death.

Nursing Assessment

1. Assess response to medical treatment plan.

2. Document vital signs and oxygen saturations.

3. Observe infant or child during feeding or activity. Assess for diaphoresis, need for frequent rest periods, and inability to keep up with peers.

4. Follow growth curve.

Nursing Diagnoses

- Decreased Cardiac Output related to myocardial dysfunction.

- Excess Fluid Volume related to decreased cardiac contractility and decreased excretion from the kidney.

- Impaired Gas Exchange related to pulmonary venous congestion.

- Activity Intolerance related to myocardial dysfunction and pulmonary congestion.

- Risk for Infection related to pulmonary congestion.

- Imbalanced Nutrition: Less Than Body Requirements related to increased metabolic demands with decreased caloric intake.

- Anxiety related to diagnosis and prognosis.

Nursing Interventions

Improving Myocardial Efficiency

1. Administer digoxin, as prescribed.

   a. Measure heart rate. Hold medication and notify health care provider for heart rate less than 90 beats/minute.

   b. Check most recent potassium level. Hold medication and notify health care provider for potassium less than 3.5 mEg/L.

   c. Run lead II ECG, if ordered, to monitor PR interval. If first-degree AV block occurs, notify health care provider and hold medication, as directed.

   d. Report signs of possible digoxin toxicity: vomiting, nausea, visual changes, bradycardia.

   e. Double-check dose of digoxin with another nurse before administering the dose. Make sure the digoxin order has two signatures.

2. Administer afterload reduction medications, as prescribed.

   a. Measure BP before and after giving the patient the medication. Hold the medication and notify the health care provider for low BP (greater than a 15-mm Hg drop from baseline).

   b. Observe for other signs of hypotension: dizziness, lightheadedness, syncope.

Maintaining Fluid and Electrolyte Balance

1. Administer diuretics, as prescribed.

   a. Obtain daily weights.

   b. Keep strict intake and output record.

   c. Monitor serum electrolytes. Provide potassium supplements, as needed.

2. Sodium restriction: not usually needed in children; provide dietary assistance, as needed.
3. Fluid restriction: not usually needed in children.

Relieving Respiratory Distress

1. Administer oxygen therapy, as prescribed.
2. Elevate head of bed; infants may be more comfortable in an upright infant seat.

Promoting Activity Tolerance

1. Organize nursing care to provide periods of uninterrupted sleep/rest.
2. Avoid unnecessary activities.
3. Respond efficiently to a crying infant. Provide comfort and treat the source of distress: wet or dirty diaper, hunger.
4. Provide diversional activities that require limited expenditure of energy.
5. Provide small, frequent feedings.

Decreasing Risk of Infection

1. Ensure good handwashing by everyone.
2. Avoid exposure to ill children or caretakers.
3. Monitor signs of infection: fever, cough, runny nose, diarrhea, vomiting.

Providing Adequate Nutrition

1. For the older child: provide nutritious foods that the child likes, along with supplemental high-calorie snacks (milkshake, pudding).
2. For the infant:
   a. High-calorie formula (24 to 30 cal/oz).
   b. Supplement oral intake with nasogastric feedings. Allow ad-lib oral intake through the day with continuous nasogastric feedings at night.

Reducing Anxiety and Fear

1. Communicate the care plan to the child and family.
2. Educate the family about CHF and provide home care nursing referral to reinforce teaching after discharge.
3. Encourage questions; answer questions as able or refer to another member of the health care team.

Family Education and Health Maintenance

1. Teach the signs and symptoms of CHF.
2. Teach medications: brand name and generic name, expected effects, adverse effects, dose.
3. Demonstrate medication administration.
4. With the family, design a medication administration time schedule.
5. Provide guidelines for when to seek medical help.
6. Teach infant and child cardiopulmonary resuscitation (CPR), as needed.
7. Reinforce dietary guidelines; provide a recipe to the parent on how to make high-calorie formula.
8. Reinforce ways to prevent infection.
9. Make sure that follow-up visit with health care providers is scheduled.

10. Educate the patient and family on infective endocarditis guidelines and provide them with written materials. Standard general prophylaxis for children at risk: amoxicillin 50 mg/kg (maximum dose = 2 g) given orally 1 hour before the procedure.

Evaluation: Expected Outcomes

- Heart rate within normal range for age; adequate urine output.
- No unexpected weight gain.
- Clear lungs; normal respiratory rate and effort.
- Participates in quiet diversional activities.
- No signs or symptoms of infection.
- Adequate intake of small, frequent feedings.
- Parents express understanding of disease process and treatment.

ACQUIRED HEART DISEASE

Note: Kawasaki disease is discussed in Chapter 53.

Acute Rheumatic Fever

Evidence Base Marijon, E., Mirabel, M., Celermajer, D. S., et al. (2012). Rheumatic heart disease. *Lancet, 379*, 953–964.

Acute rheumatic fever (ARF) is an acute autoimmune disease that occurs as a sequelae of group A beta-hemolytic streptococcal infection. It is characterized by inflammatory lesions of connective tissue and endothelial tissue, primarily affecting the joints and heart.

Pathophysiology and Etiology

1. Most initial attacks of ARF occur 1 to 5 weeks (average 3 weeks) after a streptococcal infection of the throat or of the upper respiratory tract.
2. Peak incidence occurs in children ages 5 to 14. Incidence after a mild streptococcal pharyngeal infection is 0.3%; after a severe streptococcal infection, 1% to 3%.
3. Family history of rheumatic fever is usually positive.
4. Streptococcal infection abates with or without treatment; however, autoantibodies attack the myocardium, pericardium, and cardiac valves.
   a. Aschoff's bodies (fibrin deposits) develop on the valves, possibly leading to permanent valve dysfunction, especially of the mitral and aortic valves.
   b. Severe myocarditis may cause dilation of the heart and CHF.
5. Inflammation of the large joints causes painful arthritis that may last 6 to 8 weeks.
6. Involvement of the nervous system causes chorea (sudden involuntary movements).

Clinical Manifestations

Documented or undocumented group A beta-hemolytic streptococcal infection is usually followed (within several weeks) by fever, malaise, and anorexia. Major symptoms of ARF may appear several weeks to several months after initial infection.

Major Manifestations

1. Carditis—manifested by sinus tachycardia, a soft blowing pansystolic murmur, prolonged PR and QT intervals on ECG, and possibly by signs of CHF (see page 1539).
2. Polyarthritis—pain and limited movement of two or more joints; joints are swollen, red, warm, and tender.
3. Chorea—purposeless, involuntary, rapid movements commonly associated with muscle weakness, involuntary facial grimaces, speech disturbance, and emotional lability.
4. Erythema marginatum—nonpruritic pink, macular rash mostly of the trunk with pale central areas; migratory.
5. Subcutaneous nodules—firm, painless nodules over the scalp, extensor surface of joints, such as wrists, elbows, knees, and vertebral column.

Minor Manifestations

1. History of previous rheumatic fever or evidence of preexisting rheumatic heart disease.
2. Arthralgia—pain in one or more joints without evidence of inflammation, tenderness, or limited movement.
3. Fever—temperature greater than 100.4° F (38° C).
4. Laboratory abnormalities—elevated erythrocyte sedimentation rate, positive C-reactive protein, elevated white blood cell count.
5. ECG changes—prolonged PR interval.

Diagnostic Evaluation

1. Diagnosed clinically through use of the Jones criteria from the American Heart Association—presence of two major manifestations or one major and two minor manifestations (as listed above), with supporting evidence of a recent streptococcal infection.
2. ECG to evaluate PR interval and other changes.
3. Laboratory tests listed above. In addition, group A streptococcal culture and/or antistreptolysin-O titer to detect streptococcal antibodies from recent infection.
4. Chest x-ray for cardiomegaly, pulmonary congestion, or edema.

Management

1. Course of antibiotic therapy to completely eradicate streptococcal infection (may be given despite previous treatment).
   a. Usually benzathine penicillin is given I.M. in a single dose or a 10-day course of oral penicillin V.
   b. Oral erythromycin may be used for children who are allergic to penicillin.
2. Nonsteroidal anti-inflammatory drugs (naproxen sodium) usually used to control pain and inflammation of arthritis.
3. Corticosteroids may be used in severe cases to try to control cardiac inflammation, however, there is limited evidence to support their use.
4. Phenobarbital, diazepam, or other neurologic agent to control chorea.
5. Bed rest during the acute phase to rest the heart. Gradual return to activities is recommended once acute symptoms resolve.

6. Mitral valve replacement may be necessary in some cases.
7. Secondary prevention of recurrent ARF:
   a. Risk of recurrence greatest within first 5 years, with multiple episodes of ARF, and with rheumatic heart disease. Prophylactic antibiotic treatment may be lifelong.
   b. For those at low risk for recurrence, antibiotic prophylaxis may be continued for 5 years or longer.
   c. Antibiotic regimens may include:
      i. Benzathine penicillin I.M. every 28 days.
      ii. Penicillin V or erythromycin 250 mg twice per day.
      iii. Sulfisoxazole 0.5 to 1 g (dosage calculated according to patient's weight) once per day.

Complications

1. CHF.
2. Pericarditis, pericardial effusion.
3. Permanent damage to the aortic or mitral valve, possibly requiring valve replacement.

Nursing Assessment

1. Assess for signs of cardiac involvement by auscultation of the heart for murmur and cardiac monitoring for prolonged PR interval.
2. Monitor pulse for 1 full minute to determine heart rate.
3. Assess temperature for elevation.
4. Observe for involuntary movements: stick out tongue or smile; garbled or hesitant speech when asked to recite numbers or the ABCs; hyperextension of the wrists and fingers when trying to extend arms.
5. Assess child's ability to feed self, dress, and do other activities if chorea or arthritis present.
6. Assess pain level using scale appropriate for child's age.
7. Assess parents' ability to cope with illness and care for child.
8. Assess need for home schooling while patient is on bed rest.

Nursing Diagnoses

- Decreased Cardiac Output related to carditis.
- Acute and Chronic Pain related to arthritis.
- Risk for Injury related to chorea.

Nursing Interventions

Improving Cardiac Output

1. Explain to the child and family the need for bed rest during the acute phase and as long as CHF is present. In milder cases, light indoor activity is allowed.
2. In severe cases, organize care to minimize exertion and provide uninterrupted rest.
3. Maintain cardiac monitoring, if indicated.
4. Administer course of antibiotics, as directed. Be alert to adverse effects, such as nausea, vomiting, and GI distress.
5. Administer medications for CHF, as directed. Monitor BP, intake and output, and heart rate.

Relieving Pain

1. Administer anti-inflammatory medication, analgesics, and antipyretics, as directed.
   a. Monitor for side effects of corticosteroid use—GI distress, acne, weight gain, emotional disturbances—or long-term effects, such as rounded face, ulcer formation, and decreased resistance to infection.
   b. Administer all anti-inflammatory medications with food to reduce GI injury.
   c. Be aware that anti-inflammatories may not alter the course of myocardial injury.
2. Teach family the importance of maintaining dosage schedule, continuing medication until all signs and symptoms of the ARF have gone, and tapering the dose, as directed by health care provider.
3. Assist child with positioning for comfort and protecting inflamed joints.
4. Suggest diversional activities that do not require use of painful joints.

Protecting the Child with Chorea

1. Use padded side rails if chorea is severe.
2. Assist with feeding and other fine-motor activities, as needed.
3. Assist with ambulation if weak.
4. Avoid the use of straws and sharp utensils if chorea involves the face.
5. Make sure that child consumes nutritious diet with recommended vitamins, protein, and calories.
6. Be patient if speech is affected and offer emotional support.
7. Protect the child from stress.
8. Administer phenobarbital or other medication for chorea, as directed. Observe for drowsiness.

Family Education and Health Maintenance

1. Teach the appropriate administration of all medications, including prophylactic antibiotic.
2. Encourage all family and household members to be screened for streptococcus and receive the appropriate treatment.
3. Instruct on additional prophylaxis for endocarditis with dental procedures and surgery, as indicated.
4. Encourage following activity restrictions, resuming activity gradually, and resting whenever tired.
5. Encourage keeping appointments for follow-up evaluation by cardiologist and other health care providers.
6. Advise the parents that child cannot return to school until health care provider assesses that all disease activity is gone. Parents may need to discuss with teachers how the child can catch up with schoolwork.
7. Instruct on follow-up with usual health care provider for immunizations, well-child evaluations, hearing and vision screening, and other health maintenance needs.
8. Provide general health education about early identification and treatment seeking for any possible streptococcal infection (fever, sore throat). Compliance with 10 to 14 days of antibiotics can greatly reduce the risk of ARF and other post-streptococcal sequelae.

Evaluation: Expected Outcomes

- Heart rate and PR interval within normal range for age; no signs of CHF.
- Compliant with anti-inflammatory therapy; reports pain as 1 to 2 on scale of 1 to 10.
- Feeds self, washes face and hands, and ambulates to bathroom without injury.

Cardiomyopathy

 Evidence Base Durani, Y., Giordano, K., & Goudie, B. W. (2010). Myocarditis and pericarditis in children. *Pediatric Clinics of North America, 57*(6), 1281–1303.
Williams, G. D., & Hammer, G. B. (2011). Cardiomyopathy in childhood. *Current Opinion in Anesthesiology, 24*(3), 289–300.

According to the type of myocardial changes, *cardiomyopathy* can be classified into three categories: dilated, hypertrophic, and restrictive. The most common type in children is dilated cardiomyopathy. Hypertrophic cardiomyopathy is a leading cause of death in young athletes.

Pathophysiology and Etiology

1. Familial (family history, genetic predisposition) tendency.
2. Idiopathic in most cases.
3. May be related to:
   a. Nutritional deficiency (carnitine or selenium).
   b. Viral infection (myocarditis), human immunodeficiency virus.
   c. Collagen vascular disease (systemic lupus erythematosus).
   d. Cardiotoxic drugs (doxorubicin).
   e. Cocaine abuse.
   f. Infants of diabetic mothers
   g. Sustained tachycardia (ectopic atrial tachycardia).
   h. Catecholamine surge; hyperthyroidism.
4. Dilated cardiomyopathy involves dilatation of one or both ventricles associated with normal septal and LV free wall thickness.
5. Decreased systolic function (contractility) results in CHF.
6. Increasing end-systolic dimension results in AV valve insufficiency, further worsening CHF.

Clinical Manifestations

1. Signs of CHF—tachycardia, tachypnea, dyspnea, crackles, hepatosplenomegaly.
2. Decreased exercise tolerance, fatigue, sweating.
3. Poor weight gain, nausea, abdominal tenderness.
4. Ventricular arrhythmia.
5. Chest pain.
6. Syncope.

Diagnostic Evaluation

1. Auscultation: systolic regurgitant murmur (if mitral or tricuspid insufficiency is present), S_2 is normal or narrowly split, prominent S_3 gallop.
2. ECG: tachycardia, abnormal ST segments, arrhythmia, ectopic atrial tachycardia, deep Q waves, LVH.
3. Chest x-ray: cardiomegaly, pulmonary congestion.
4. Two-dimensional echocardiogram: increased wall thickness, poor ventricular systolic function, dilated heart chambers; AV valve insufficiency.
5. Cardiac MRI will provide useful information on cardiac function and may demonstrate ventricular hypertrophy or fibrosis.
6. Cardiac catheterization: not needed for initial diagnosis; endomyocardial biopsy (to rule out myocarditis); assess PVR.

Management

General Measures

1. Identify and treat the underlying cause.
2. Maximize caloric intake: fortify formula; supplemental nasogastric feedings.
3. Supplemental oxygen, as needed.
4. Activity restriction (usually self-imposed by the younger child and infant). Restrict participation in strenuous and competitive sports.

Treatment of Systolic Dysfunction with Dilated Cardiomyopathy

1. Diuretics: furosemide, spironolactone.
2. Inotropics: digoxin.
3. Afterload reduction: captopril, enalapril, lisinopril.
4. Anticoagulation: warfarin, low-molecular-weight heparin (enoxaparin).
5. Anti-arrhythmics.
6. Placement of an automatic implantable cardioverter-defibrillator.
7. Biventricular pacing.
8. Cardiac transplant.

Treatment of Diastolic Dysfunction with Hypertrophic Cardiomyopathy

1. Beta-adrenergic blockers: propranolol.
2. Calcium channel blockers: verapamil.
3. AV sequential pacing.
4. Myomectomy or myotomy.

Treatment of Diastolic Dysfunction with Restrictive Cardiomyopathy

1. Diuretics.
2. Anticoagulation.
3. Permanent pacemaker for advanced heart block.

Complications

1. Severe CHF.
2. Increased pulmonary vascular resistance.
3. Intracardiac thrombus.
4. Embolus.
5. Malignant arrhythmias.
6. Sudden death.

Nursing Assessment

Perform a thorough nursing assessment as for CHD (see page 1536).

Nursing Diagnoses

- Decreased Cardiac Output related to impaired systolic or diastolic ventricular function.
- Imbalanced Nutrition: Less Than Body Requirements related to increased metabolic demands and poor feeding from dyspnea, fatigue, and poor appetite.
- Ineffective Family Coping related to chronic illness.

Nursing Interventions

Maximizing Cardiac Output

1. Monitor vital signs; notify physician for hypotension, tachycardia, arrhythmia; increasing tachypnea.
2. Administer oxygen therapy, as prescribed.
3. Administer medications, as prescribed.
   a. Maintain bleeding precautions for anticoagulated patients.
   b. Document response to diuretics; monitor intake and output.
4. Monitor electrolytes.
5. Restrict level of activity.

Providing Maximal Nutritional Support

1. Encourage frequent, small meals. Provide foods the child likes.
2. Provide high-calorie supplements (milkshakes, pudding).
3. Administer supplemental tube feedings if nutritional needs are not being met.
4. Administer parenteral hyperalimentation and intralipids, as directed (rarely needed).

Promoting Effective Coping and Control within the Family

1. Organize a family meeting with various members of the health care team to review the child's medical condition and to explain the treatment plan.
2. Allow the child and family to express their questions, fears, and concerns.
3. Identify support systems and services for the child and family: extended family members, clergy, support groups, community resources.

Family Education and Health Maintenance

1. Teach child and family medication administration: purpose of the drug, drug dosage, drug schedule, and adverse effects.
2. Help family design a realistic medication schedule.
   a. Identify usual wake-up time and bedtime. Schedule medications accordingly.
   b. Do not give a diuretic right before bedtime or nap time.
   c. If possible, avoid having to give medications at school.

3. Teach bleeding precautions if the child is on anticoagulation agents (coumadin).
   a. Monitor prothrombin International Normalized Ratio regularly.
   b. Observe for signs of bleeding.
   c. Counsel regarding menses and pregnancy.
   d. Instruct on foods and medications that interfere with coumadin.
4. Give guidelines for notifying the physician.
   a. Worsening shortness of breath.
   b. Irregular pulse; palpitations.
   c. Syncope, dizziness, or light-headedness.
   d. Increasing fatigue, exercise intolerance.
5. Teach infant and child CPR to family members and other caregivers.

Evaluation: Expected Outcomes

- Stable vital signs.
- Maximal nutritional status, as evidenced by weight gain and growth.
- Compliance with the treatment plan and follow-up visits.

SELECTED REFERENCES

Andrews, R. E., Fenton, M. J., Ridout, D. A., et al. (2008). New-onset heart failure due to heart muscle disease in childhood: A prospective study in the United Kingdom and Ireland. *Circulation, 117*(1), 79–84.

Bailliard, F., & Anderson, R. H. (2009). Tetralogy of Fallot. *Orphanet Journal of Rare Diseases, 13*(4), 1–10.

Beekman, R. H. (2008). Coarctation of the aorta. In R. E. Shaddy & T. F. Feltes, (Eds.), *Moss and Adams' heart disease in infants, children, and adolescents* (7th ed.). Philadelphia: Lippincott Williams & Wilkins.

Benitz, W. E. (2011). Learning to live with patency of the ductus arteriosus in preterm infants. *Journal of Perinatology, 31*(Suppl. 1), S42–S48.

Davidson, D. J., & Bonow, R. O. (2011). Cardiac catheterization. In L. Libby (Ed.), *Braunwald's heart disease: A textbook of cardiovascular medicine* (9th ed.) pp. 383–405. St. Louis, MO: Elsevier.

Denfield, S. W. (2010). Strategies to prevent cellular rejection in pediatric heart transplant recipients. *Paediatric Drugs, 12*(6), 391–403.

Dolbec, K., & Mick, N. W. (2011). Congenital heart disease. *Emergency Medical Clinics of North America, 29*(4), 811–827.

Durani, Y., Giordano, K., & Goudie, B. W. (2010). Myocarditis and pericarditis in children. *Pediatric Clinics of North America, 57*(6), 1281–1303.

Epstein, M. L. (2013). Tricuspid atresia, stenosis, regurgitation, and Uhl's Anomaly. In H. D. Allen, D. J. Driscoll, R. E. Shaddy, & T. F. Feltes, (Eds.), *Moss and Adams' heart disease in infants, children, and adolescents* (8th ed.). pp. 877–888. Philadelphia: Lippincott Williams & Wilkins.

Feinstein, J. A., Benson, D. W., Dubin, A. M., et al. (2012). Hypoplastic left heart syndrome: current considerations and expectations. *Journal of the American College of Cardiology, 59*(1, Suppl.), S1–S42.

Feltes, T. F., et al. (2011). Indications for cardiac catheterization and intervention in pediatric cardiac disease: A scientific statement from the American Heart Association. *Circulation 123* (22):2607–2652.

Frank, J. E., & Jacobe, K. M. (2011). Evaluation and management of heart murmurs in children. *American Family Physician, 84*(7), 793–800.

Hartas, G. A., Tsounias, E., & Gupta-Malhotra, M. (2009). Approach to diagnosing congenital cardiac disorders. *Critical Care Nursing Clinics of North America, 21*(1), 27–36.

Hoffman, T. M., & Welty, S. E. (2013). Physiology of the preterm and term Infant. In H. D. Allen, D. J. Driscoll, R. E. Shaddy, & T. F. Feltes, (Eds.), *Moss and Adams' heart disease in infants, children, and adolescents* (8th ed.) pp. 473–482. Philadelphia: Lippincott Williams & Wilkins.

Kantor, P. F., & Mertens, L. L. (2010). Clinical practice: Heart failure in children. Part I: Clinical evaluation, diagnostic testing, and initial medical management. *European Journal of Pediatrics, 169*(3), 269–279.

Kantor, P. F., & Mertens, L. L.(2010). Clinical practice: Heart failure in children. Part II: Current maintenance therapy and new therapeutic approaches. *European Journal of Pediatrics, 169*(4), 403–410.

Kenny, D., & Hijazi, Z. M. (2011). Coarctation of the aorta: From fetal life to adulthood. *Cardiology Journal, 18*(5), 487–495.

Lawrence, K., Stilley, C. S., Pollock, S. A., et al. (2011). A family-centered educational program to promote indpendence in pediatric heart transplant recipients. *Progress in Trasnplantation, 21*(1): 61–66.

Loscalzo, M. L. (2010). Left outflow tract anomalies in children. *Current Opinion in Pediatrics, 22*(5), 593–597.

Marijon, E., Mirabel, M., Celermajer, D. S., et al. (2012). Rheumatic heart disease. *Lancet, 379*, 953–964.

Martins, P., & Castela, E. (2008). Transposition of the great arteries. *Orphanet Journal of Rare Diseases, 3*(27), 1–10.

Park, M. (2008). *Pediatric cardiology for practitioners* (5th ed.). St. Louis, MO: Mosby.

Pedra, C. A., Pedra, S. R., Chaccur, P., et al. (2010). Perventricular device closure of congenital muscular ventricular septal defects. *Expert Review of Cardiovascular Therapy, 8*(5), 663–674.

Prieto, L. R., & Latson, L. A. (2013). Pulmonary stenosis. In H. D. Allen, D. J. Driscoll, R. E. Shaddy, & T. F. Feltes, (Eds.), *Moss and Adams' heart disease in infants, children, and adolescents* (8th ed.), pp. 913–938. Philadelphia: Lippincott Williams & Wilkins.

Roche, S. L., Greenway, S., & Redington, A. (2013). Tetralogy of Fallot with Pulmonary Stenosis and Tetralogy of Fallot with Absent Pulmonary Valve. In H. D. Allen, D. J. Driscoll, R. E. Shaddy, & T. F. Feltes, (Eds.), *Moss and Adams' heart disease in infants, children, and adolescents* (8th ed.). Philadelphia: Lippincott Williams & Wilkins.

Rubio, A., & Lewin, M. (2013). Ventricular septal defects. In H. D. Allen, D. J. Driscoll, R. E. Shaddy, & T. F. Feltes, (Eds.), *Moss and Adams' heart disease in infants, children, and adolescents* (8th ed.) pp. 713–721. Philadelphia: Lippincott Williams & Wilkins.

Sachdeva, R. (2013). Atrial Septal Defects. In H. D. Allen, D. J. Driscoll, R. E. Shaddy, & T. F. Feltes, (Eds.), *Moss and Adams' heart disease in infants, children, and adolescents* (8th ed.), pp. 672–690. Philadelphia: Lippincott Williams & Wilkins.

Sadowski, S. L. (2009). Congenital cardiac disease in the newborn infant: Past, present, and future. *Critical Care Nursing Clinics of North America, 21*(1), 37–48.

Schnieder, D. J., & Moore, J. W. (2013). Aortic stenosis. In H. D. Allen, D. J. Driscoll, R. E. Shaddy, & T. F. Feltes, (Eds.), *Moss and Adams' heart disease in infants, children, and adolescents* (8th ed.), pp.1023–1043. Philadelphia: Lippincott Williams & Wilkins.

Smith, M., Newey, C., Jones, M., & Martin, J. (2011). Congenital heart disease and its effects on children and their families. *Paediatric Nursing, 23*(2), 30–35.

Taggart, N., & Cabalka, A. (2013). Cardiac catheterization and Angiography. In H. D. Allen, D. J. Driscoll, R. E. Shaddy, & T. F. Feltes, (Eds.), *Moss and Adams' heart disease in infants, children, and adolescents* (8th ed.), pp. 258–287. Philadelphia: Lippincott Williams & Wilkins.

Thangaratinam, S., Brown, K., Zamora, J., et al. (2012). Pulse oximetry screening for critical congenital heart defects in asymptomatic newborn babies: A systematic review and meta-analysis. *Lancet, 379*(9835), 2459–2464.

Treddell, J. S., Hoffman, G., et al. (2013). Hypoplastic left heart syndrome. In H. D. Allen, D. J. Driscoll, R. E. Shaddy, & T. F. Feltes, (Eds.), *Moss and Adams' heart disease in infants, children, and adolescents* (8th ed.), pp. 1061–1096. Philadelphia: Lippincott Williams & Wilkins.

Webb, G. D., Smallhorn, J., et al. (2011). Congenital heart disease. In L. Libby (Ed.), *Braunwald's heart disease: A textbook of cardiovascular medicine* (9th ed.), pp. 1412–1426. St. Louis, MO: Elsevier.

Wernovsky, G. (2013). Transposition of the Great Arteries. In H. D. Allen, D. J. Driscoll, R. E. Shaddy, & T. F. Feltes, (Eds.), *Moss and Adams' heart disease in infants, children, and adolescents* (8th ed.), pp. 1097–1146. Philadelphia: Lippincott Williams & Wilkins.

Williams, G. D., & Hammer, G. B. (2011). Cardiomyopathy in childhood. *Current Opinion in Anesthesiology, 24*(3), 289–300.

46
Pediatric Neurologic Disorders

NEUROLOGIC AND NEUROSURGICAL DISORDERS

It is essential to have strong knowledge of growth and development and use physical assessment skills while caring for a child with a neurological or neurosurgical condition. Young children often cannot either speak or express how they feel, so a good ongoing physical assessment is essential. Parents and caregivers are also a valuable information source as to differences in their child's physical condition and should always be included in the assessment. It is also important to remember that children are not little adults. They have their own unique physiology, which is important to consider when assessing and understanding the manifestation of neurological conditions in children. The plasticity of the infant brain can make for greater recovery than that of an adolescent.

Cerebral Palsy

Cerebral palsy (CP) is a nonprogressive disorder of posture and movement. It is a result of a fixed lesion or anomaly of the brain that occurred in the early stages of brain development. The incidence of CP is 2 to 2.5 per 1,000 live births. The rate of CP in premature infants continues to rise as survival rates have increased in such infants.

Pathophysiology and Etiology

Antenatal Causes (80% of all cases)

1. Vascular occlusion.
2. Cortical migration disorders.
3. Structural maldevelopment during gestation—gene deletions.
4. Genetic syndromes.
5. Congenital infection.

Natal Causes (10% of all cases)

1. Hypoxic ischemic injury at birth.

Postnatal Causes (10% of all cases)

1. Preterm infants vulnerable to brain damage from periventricular leukomalacia secondary to ischemia and/or severe intraventricular hemorrhage.
2. Meningitis, encephalitis, encephalopathy, head trauma (accidental and nonaccidental).
3. Symptomatic hypoglycemia, hydrocephalus, hyperbilirubinemia.

Types of Cerebral Palsy

CP can be classified into three categories.

1. Neuropathic—motor dysfunction.
   a. Spastic: hyperreflexia, hypertonicity, clonus, Babinski sign.
   b. Athetoid: involuntary movements, dystonia, no joint contractures.
   c. Ataxic: lack of balance and coordination, wide-based gait.
   d. Mixed: spastic and athetoid signs, total body usually involved.
   e. Hypotonic: rare in the first 2 to 3 years, evolves into athetoid.
2. Anatomic—region of involvement.
   a. Monoplegia: one limb involved, usually spastic.
   b. Hemiplegia: spastic ipsilateral limbs.
   c. Paraplegia: lower limbs only, familial type.
   d. Diplegia: lower limbs more involved than upper limbs, spastic.
   e. Triplegia: three limbs involved.
   f. Quadriplegia—all four limbs involved including head, neck, and trunk.

3. Functional.
   a. Independent community ambulators.
   b. Dependent community ambulators.
   c. Wheelchair bound.

Clinical Manifestations

1. The types of CP mentioned above correlate with clinical presentation.
2. Early clinical signs include:
   a. Abnormal tone and limb and/or trunk posture in infancy with delay in achieving motor milestones, with or without slowing of head growth.
   b. Difficulty or slow feeding, gagging and vomiting, oromotor incoordination.
   c. Abnormal gait once child is walking.
   d. Asymmetric hand function before age 12 months.
3. Persistence of primitive reflexes.
4. Common associated findings include:
   a. Seizures.
   b. Hearing impairment.
   c. Visual impairment.
   d. Mental retardation.
   e. Speech and language disorders.
   f. Growth disorders, developmental delays.
   g. Gastroesophageal reflux, nutritional deficiencies (due to poor feeding, reflux, aspiration).
   h. Behavioral/emotional problems.

Diagnostic Evaluation

Diagnosis is based on clinical examination and history. Various testing also helps determine cause or evaluate for associated problems.

1. Neuroimaging—magnetic resonance imaging (MRI) and computed tomography (CT).
   a. Recommended when cause has not been identified.
   b. MRI is preferred over CT as it has a higher yield for suggesting the cause and timing of the insult.
2. Metabolic and genetic testing.
   a. Not routinely required.
   b. Should be considered in cases when the clinical history or findings on neuroimaging do not identify a specific structural abnormality or if additional and atypical features in the history or clinical examination are identified.
3. Consider completing testing for coagulation disorders, particularly in children with a hemiplegic CP as the incidence of cerebral infarction is very high in these children.
4. Associated conditions.
   a. Electroencephalography (EEG) should not be obtained for the purpose of determining cause, but should be obtained when there is evidence on history and examination suggesting epilepsy or epileptic syndrome.
   b. Initial assessment should include screening for mental retardation, ophthalmologic and hearing impairments, speech and language disorders, and oral-motor dysfunction, as many children with CP have these associated deficits.

Management

1. Spasticity should be treated first to improve function, reduce pain, and provide ease in caregiving. It requires an organized approach and begins with thorough assessment.
   a. Focal spasticity.
      i. Botulinum injections help reduce spasticity and improve gait; may be given in upper or lower limbs. Botulinum toxin type A is an effective and generally safe treatment.
      ii. Serial casting may be done with or without Botulinum injections.
   b. Generalized spasticity.
      i. Diazepam is usually used for short-term treatment of generalized spasticity; tizanidine may also be used.
      ii. Currently there is insufficient evidence to support the use of dantrolene, oral baclofen, or continuous intrathecal baclofen.

 Evidence Base Delgado, M. R., Hirtz, D., Aisen, M., et al. (2010). Practice parameter: Pharmacologic treatment of spasticity in children and adolescents with cerebral palsy (an evidence-based review). *Neurology, 74*, 336–343.

 DRUG ALERT Intrathecal baclofen lowers the seizure threshold. Children may develop severe withdrawal syndrome characterized by fever, hypertension, tachycardia, agitation, and hallucinations. May occur in situations of pump malfunction, catheter breakage, or improper filling of pump.

      iii. Selective dorsal rhizotomy—25% to 60% of dorsal nerve rootlets are cut from L4 to S1 through a L1–S1 laminectomy (guided by the response to intraoperative electromyogram).
2. Monitor for and treat scoliosis and hip subluxation.
   a. Scoliosis is very common and increases with age and severity of CP; highest risk is among the nonambulatory.
      i. Curve progression occurs most quickly during a growth spurt but, unlike idiopathic scoliosis, may continue to progress after skeletal maturity.
      ii. Early detection is critical to slow progression. Interventions, such as external bracing, customized seating and seating inserts, and maintenance of good seating posture by correcting hip and pelvic deformities, is essential in preventing or delaying the need for corrective spine surgery.
   b. Hip subluxation and dislocation results from spasticity in hip adductors and iliopsoas muscles; if left untreated, it may result in acetabular dysplasia and degenerative joint disease.
      i. Routine hip radiographs are important to monitor hip condition.
      ii. Stretching and positioning are essential in preventing hip subluxation.

iii. Tendon releases are required when stretching and positioning are ineffective.

iv. Botulinum toxin injections into hip adductors have been found to limit progression.

3. Growth and nutritional problems are common among children with moderate to severe CP, resulting in poor health, increase in use of health resources, and decreased participation in school and community activities; may require gastrostomy tube feeding.

4. Drooling results from impaired swallowing or poor lip closure.

   a. Anticholinergic medications, such as glycopyrolate and hydroxyzine, are used but have significant side effects.

   b. It has recently been reported that injecting Botulinum toxin into the parotid glands decreased salivary flow without the side effects seen with anticholinergic therapy.

   c. Surgery to treat sialorrhea (excessive saliva secretion) may be of benefit.

5. Treatment of involuntary movements.

   a. Dystonia—levodopa is used as an initial medication; trihexyphenidyl may also be used.

   b. Chorea—benzodiazepines, such as clonazepam, and dopamine-depleting medications, such as haloperidol, are used.

6. Treatment of hemisyndromes.

   a. Balance training improves symmetry of gait.

   b. Constraint-induced movement therapy—affected arm/hand is restrained for a prolonged period of time, which results in increased use of the affected hand; well tolerated in children.

7. Treatment of osteopenia.

   a. Encourage weight-bearing activities (use of stander, rolator walker).

   b. Provide vitamin D and calcium supplements.

   c. Bisphosphonates may be considered for those children with low bone mineral density and those who are at particular risk for fragility fractures.

   d. Risk for fracture is assessed through bone density scanning and other tests and is reported as the Z score. It is not valid in children less than 5 years old.

 Evidence Base Fehlings, D., Switzer, L., Agarwal, P., et al. (2012). Informing evidence-based clinical practice guidelines for children with cerebral palsy at risk of osteoporosis: A systematic review. *Developmental Medicine and Child Neurology, 54*, 106–116.

Complications

1. Contractures.
2. Hip subluxation/dislocation.
3. Malnutrition.
4. Scoliosis.
5. Osteopenia/fractures.
6. Gastroesophageal reflux.
7. Constipation.
8. Seizures.
9. Spasticity.
10. Pain.

Nursing Assessment

1. Perform a functional assessment; determine ability to perform activities of daily living (ADLs).

2. Perform a developmental assessment; use Denver II developmental or other screening tools.

3. Evaluate ability to protect airway—gag reflex, swallowing.

4. Assess nutritional status—growth, signs of deficiency, risk of aspiration.

5. Assess neuromuscular function and mobility—range of motion (ROM), spasticity, coordination.

6. Assess speech, hearing, vision.

7. Evaluate parent–child interaction.

8. Determine parents' understanding of and compliance with treatment plan.

9. Assess skin for pressure sores, especially in areas of friction (splints).

10. Assess for presence of pain (chronic or acute due to hip subluxation, dislocation).

Nursing Diagnoses

- Impaired Physical Mobility related to altered neuromuscular functioning.
- Delayed Growth and Development related to the nature and extent of the disorder.
- Interrupted Family Processes related to nature of disorder, role disturbances, and uncertain future.
- Risk for Injury related to deficit in motor activity and coordination.

Nursing Interventions

Increasing Mobility and Minimizing Deformity

1. Teach the parents to carry out appropriate exercises under the direction of the physical therapist and occupational therapist.

2. Use splints and braces to facilitate muscle control and improve body functioning.

   a. Apply, as directed.

   b. Remove for recommended time.

   c. Inspect underlying skin for redness, irritation, skin breakdown, and signs of improper application or fit of splints or orthoses.

   d. Regularly inspect orthoses for cracks, loose screws, or broken Velcro straps.

   e. Use splint as directed for constraint-induced therapy in children with unilateral CP.

3. Use assistive devices, such as adapted grooming tools, writing implements, and utensils, to enhance independence. Handles of toothbrushes, spoons, and forks can be built up with sponges or specially curved to make holding easier.

4. Encourage self-dressing with easy pull-on pants, large sweatshirts, Velcro closures, and other loose clothing.

5. Use play, such as board games, ball games, pegboards, and puzzles, to improve coordination.
6. Maintain good body alignment to prevent contractures.
7. Provide adequate rest periods.
   a. Avoid exciting events before rest or bedtime.
   b. Administer or teach parents about side effects of medications and how to administer medications, as prescribed.

Maximizing Growth and Development

1. Evaluate the child's developmental level and then assist with age-appropriate tasks.
2. Provide for continuity of care at home, daycare, therapy centers, and the hospital.
   a. Obtain a thorough history from the parents regarding the child's usual home routines, weaknesses and strengths, and likes and dislikes.
   b. Communicate with representatives from all disciplines involved in the child's care to ensure that the specific needs of the child are identified.
   c. Formulate a consistent care plan that incorporates the goals of all related disciplines and meets the needs of the child and family. Include in the care plan guidelines for the following:
      i. Feeding.
      ii. Sleeping.
      iii. Physical therapy.
      iv. Play.
      v. Other ways to foster growth and development.
      vi. Medications.
      vii. Psychosocial needs.
      viii. Family needs.
      ix. Pain assessment/management.
3. During feeding, maintain a pleasant, distraction-free environment.
   a. Provide a comfortable chair.
   b. Serve the child alone, initially. After the child begins to master the task of eating, encourage the child to eat with other children.
   c. Do not attempt feedings if the child is very fatigued.
   d. Find the eating position in which the child can be most self-sufficient.
   e. Allow the child to hold the spoon even if self-feeding is minimal.
   f. Stand behind and reach over the child's shoulder to guide the spoon from the plate to the child's mouth.
   g. Serve foods that stick to the spoon, such as thick applesauce or mashed potatoes.
   h. Encourage finger foods that the child can handle alone.
   i. Provide appropriate assistive devices for independent feeding, such as spoon and fork with special handles, plate and glass holders, and special feeding chair.
   j. Disregard "messy" eating; use a large plastic bib, smock, or towel to protect the child's clothes.
4. If the child must be fed, do so slowly and carefully. Be aware of difficulty sucking and swallowing caused by poor muscle control. Cut large pieces of food into small pieces.

5. Be alert for associated sensory deficits that delay development and could be corrected.
   a. Hearing, speech, vision.
   b. Squinting, failure to follow objects, or bringing objects very close to the face.

Strengthening Family Processes

1. Assess parental coping and provide anticipatory guidance, emotional support, and contact with social worker, as needed.
2. Help the parents to recognize immediate needs and identify short-term goals that can be integrated into the long-term plan.
3. Assess for caregiver burden due to the numerous challenges of daily care and link with appropriate resources (eg, home care, respite, funding) and provide access to social work for assistance in obtaining such support.
4. Provide positive feedback for effective parenting skills and positive approaches to caring for the child.
5. Assist the parents to deal with siblings' responses to the disabled child.
   a. Encourage parents to find time to spend with each sibling separately.
   b. Encourage family to maintain contact with friends and community and engage in outside activities as much as possible.
   c. Suggest family counseling.
6. Assist parents to find local resources to help in the child's care.
   a. Contact hospital social worker or discharge planner for information about local CP organizations, chapters, funding sources, community supports, or charities.
   b. Use the Internet to identify national and regional programs that may have local chapters.

Protecting the Child from Injury

1. Evaluate the child's need for specific safety measures, such as suction machine, safety helmet, or seizure precautions, and modify the environment as appropriate to ensure the child's safety.
2. Provide for frequent position changes and adequate fit on orthotics, wheelchairs, and walking or standing devices to prevent skin breakdown. Assess skin integrity daily.

Community and Home Care Considerations

1. Assess the home environment for safety. Stairs should be gated and paths should be cleared for walking with assistive devices or for adequate passage of wheelchairs, walkers, etc.
2. Assist parents in arranging for equipment that may be required in the home (eg, wheelchair, pump for intermittent G-tube feedings, walkers).
3. Check all adaptive equipment, braces, and walkers for correct fit. Arrange for replacement, as needed.

Family Education and Health Maintenance

1. Instruct the parents in all areas of the child's physical care.
2. Encourage regular medical and dental evaluations.
3. Advise parents that the child needs discipline to feel secure.

4. Refer parents to such agencies as the United Cerebral Palsy Association of America (*www.ucp.org*).

5. Connect families with other families who have a child with CP so that they may provide a supportive network.

6. Encourage maintenance of good nutritional status.

Evaluation: Expected Outcomes

- Dresses and feeds self as independently as possible; minimal contractures noted.
- Consistent growth curve maintained; sequential developmental milestones consistent with condition achieved.
- Family participates in usual school and community activities; uses respite care when available.
- Safety equipment used; no injury reported.

Hydrocephalus

Hydrocephalus is characterized by an increased volume of cerebrospinal fluid (CSF), which is associated with progressive ventricular dilatation. There are two main categories of hydrocephalus: communicating and noncommunicating. Hydrocephalus occurs with such conditions as tumors, infections, congenital malformations, and hemorrhage. The incidence of hydrocephalus is 0.5 to 4 per 1,000 live births.

Pathophysiology and Etiology

1. Noncommunicating hydrocephalus—obstruction of CSF flow within the ventricular system or blockage of CSF flow from the ventricular system to the subarachnoid space.
   a. May be partial, intermittent, or complete.
   b. More common than communicating type.
   c. Congenital causes.
      i. Aqueductal stenosis.
      ii. Congenital lesions (vein of Galen malformation, congenital tumors).
      iii. Arachnoid cyst.
      iv. Chiari malformations (with or without myelomeningocele).
      v. X-linked hydrocephalus.
      vi. Dandy-Walker malformation.
   d. Acquired causes.
      i. Aqueductal gliosis (posthemorrhagic or postinfectious).
      ii. Space-occupying lesions (tumors or cysts).
      iii. Head injuries.
2. Communicating hydrocephalus—CSF circulates through the ventricular system into the subarachnoid space with no obstruction.
   a. Congenital causes.
      i. Achondroplasia.
      ii. Arachnoid cyst.
      iii. Craniofacial syndromes.
   b. Acquired causes.
      i. Posthemorrhagic (intraventricular or subarachnoid)
      ii. Choroid plexus papilloma or choroid plexus carcinoma

---

BOX 46-1 | **Signs and Symptoms of Increased Intracranial Pressure in Infants and Children**

- Vomiting
- Restlessness and irritability
- High-pitched, shrill cry (infants)
- Rapid increase in head circumference (infants)
- Tense, bulging fontanelle (infants)
- Changes in vital signs:
  - Increased systolic blood pressure
  - Decreased pulse
  - Decreased and irregular respirations
  - Increased temperature
- Pupillary changes
- Papilledema
- Possible seizures
- Lethargy, stupor, coma
- Older children may also experience:
  - Headache, especially on awakening
  - Lethargy, fatigue, apathy
  - Personality changes
  - Separation of cranial sutures (may be seen in children up to age 10)
  - Visual changes such as double vision

---

iii. Venous obstruction (eg, superior vena cava syndrome)
iv. Postinfectious

Clinical Manifestations

May be rapid, slow and steadily advancing, or intermittent. Clinical signs depend on the age of the child, whether the anterior fontanelle has closed, whether the cranial sutures have fused, and the type and duration of hydrocephalus.

Infants

1. Excessive head growth (may be seen up to age 3).
2. Delayed closure of the anterior fontanelle.
3. Fontanelle tense and elevated above the surface of the skull.
4. Signs of increased intracranial pressure (ICP) (see Box 46-1).
5. Alteration of muscle tone of the extremities, including clonus or spasticity.
6. Later physical signs:
   a. Forehead becomes prominent ("bossing").
   b. Scalp appears shiny with prominent scalp veins.
   c. Eyebrows and eyelids may be drawn upward, exposing the sclera above the iris.
   d. Infant cannot gaze upward, causing "sunset eyes."
   e. Strabismus, nystagmus, and optic atrophy may occur.
   f. Infant has difficulty holding head up.
   g. Child may experience physical or mental developmental lag.
7. Pseudobulbar palsy (difficulty sucking, feeding, and phonation, which leads to regurgitation, drooling, and aspiration).

> **! NURSING ALERT** It is important to measure head circumference because the infant's skull is highly elastic and can accommodate an increase in ventricular size. Ventriculomegaly may progress without obvious signs of increased ICP.

Older Children

Older children have closed sutures and present with signs of increased ICP.

Diagnostic Evaluation

1. Percussion of the infant's skull may produce a typical "cracked pot" sound (MacEwen's sign).
2. Ophthalmoscopy may reveal papilledema.
3. MRI is the diagnostic tool of choice.
4. CT is also used for diagnosis in cases where sedation poses added risk due to need for general anesthetic or in situations in which MRI is not available.
5. Ultrasonography is also used.

Management

Hydrocephalus can be treated through a variety of surgical procedures, including direct operation on the lesion causing the obstruction, such as a tumor; intracranial shunts for selected cases of noncommunicating hydrocephalus to divert fluid from the obstructed segment of the ventricular system to the subarachnoid space; and extracranial shunts (most common) to divert fluid from the ventricular system to an extracranial compartment, frequently the peritoneum or right atrium. CSF production may also be reduced by medication or surgical intervention.

Extracranial Shunt Procedures

1. Ventriculoperitoneal (VP) shunt (see Figure 46-1):
   a. Diverts CSF from a lateral ventricle or the spinal subarachnoid space to the peritoneal cavity.
   b. A tube is passed from the lateral ventricle through an occipital burr hole subcutaneously through the posterior aspect of neck and paraspinal region to the peritoneal cavity through a small incision in the right lower quadrant.
   c. A ventricular access device is an implanted reservoir and catheter used for premature neonates less than 2,000 g in lieu of a shunt. The catheter drains fluid from the ventricles into the reservoir, which can then be emptied using aseptic technique. When infant weight exceeds 2,000 g, a shunt can be placed.
2. Ventriculoatrial (VA) shunt:
   a. A tube is passed from the dilated lateral ventricle through a burr hole in the parietal region of the skull.
   b. It then is passed under the skin behind the ear and into a vein down to a point where it discharges into the right atrium or superior vena cava.
   c. A one-way pressure-sensitive valve will close to prevent reflux of blood into the ventricle and open as ventricular pressure rises, allowing fluid to pass from the ventricle into the bloodstream.

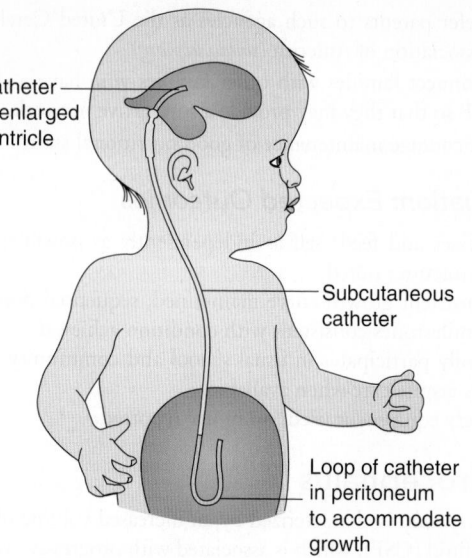

Figure 46-1. A ventriculoperitoneal shunt removes excessive cerebrospinal fluid from the ventricles and shunts it to the peritoneum. A one-way valve is present in the tubing behind the ear.

3. Ventriculopleural shunt:
   a. Diverts CSF to the pleural cavity.
   b. Indicated when the VP or VA route cannot be used.
4. Ventricle–gall bladder shunt:
   a. Diverts CSF to the common bile duct.
   b. Used when all other routes are unavailable.
5. Most shunts have the following components:
   a. Ventricular tubing.
   b. A one-way or unidirectional pressure-sensitive flow valve.
   c. A pumping chamber.
   d. Distal tubing.
6. Programmable shunts are available. These can be programmed to a certain flow pressure and pressure settings can be readjusted based on patient response. A magnetic device is used to adjust the pressure setting of the shunt valve. The use of a programmable shunt eliminates the need for multiple surgeries or hospital visits to adjust shunt pressure.

Shunt Complications

1. Need for shunt revision frequently occurs because of occlusion, infection, or malfunction, especially in the first year of life.
2. Shunt revision may be necessary because of growth of the child. Newer models, however, include coiled tubing to allow the shunt to grow with the child.
3. Shunt dependency frequently occurs. The child rapidly manifests symptoms of increased ICP if the shunt does not function optimally. Onset may be sudden or insidious.
4. Children with VA shunts may experience endocardial contusions and clotting, leading to bacterial endocarditis, bacteremia, and ventriculitis or thromboembolism and cor pulmonale.
5. Children with VA shunts require biannual or annual chest x-ray to check length of tubing. Chest x-ray is also done

during growth spurts, especially during puberty. When tubing is short or close to being out of the right atrium, shunt replacement needs to be scheduled.

Prognosis

1. Prognosis depends on early diagnosis and prompt therapy and the underlying etiology.
2. With improved diagnostic and management techniques, the prognosis is becoming considerably better.
   a. Many children experience normal motor and intellectual development.
   b. The severity of neurologic deficits is directly proportional to the interval between onset of hydrocephalus and the time of diagnosis.
3. Approximately two thirds of patients will die at an early age if they do not receive surgical treatment.
4. Surgery reduces mortality and decreases morbidity, with a survival rate of greater than 90%.

Complications

1. Seizures, headaches.
2. Herniation of the brain.
3. Spontaneous arrest due to natural compensatory mechanisms, persistent increased ICP, and brain herniation.
4. Developmental delays.
5. Depression in adolescents is common.
6. Shunt malfunctions.

Nursing Assessment

Infants

1. Assess head circumference.
   a. Measure at the occipitofrontal circumference—point of largest measurement.
   b. Measure the head at approximately the same time each day.
   c. Use a centimeter measure for greatest accuracy.
2. Palpate fontanelle for firmness and bulging.
3. Assess pupillary response.
4. Assess level of consciousness (LOC).
5. Evaluate breathing patterns and effectiveness.
6. Assess feeding patterns and patterns of emesis.
7. Assess motor function.
8. Assess developmental milestones.

Older Children

1. Measure vital signs for signs of increased ICP.
2. Assess patterns of headache, emesis.
3. Determine pupillary response.
4. Evaluate LOC using the Glasgow Coma Scale.
5. Assess motor function.
6. Evaluate attainment of milestones, school performance.
7. Assess for behavioral changes.

Nursing Diagnoses

- Ineffective Cerebral Tissue Perfusion related to increased ICP before surgery.
- Imbalanced Nutrition: Less Than Body Requirements related to reduced oral intake and vomiting.
- Risk for Impaired Skin Integrity related to alterations in LOC and enlarged head.
- Anxiety of parents related to child undergoing surgery.
- Risk for Injury related to malfunctioning shunt.
- Risk for Deficient Fluid Volume related to CSF drainage, decreased intake postoperatively.
- Risk for Infection related to bacterial infiltration of the shunt.
- Ineffective Family Coping related to diagnosis and surgery.

Nursing Interventions

Maintaining Cerebral Perfusion

1. Observe for evidence of increased ICP and report immediately.

 NURSING ALERT Brain stem herniation can occur with increased ICP and is manifested by opisthotonic positioning (flexion of head and feet backward). This is a grave sign and may be followed by respiratory arrest. Prepare for emergency resuscitation and corrective measures, as directed.

2. Assist with diagnostic procedures to determine cause of hydrocephalus and indication for surgical intervention.
   a. Explain the procedure to the child and parents at their levels of comprehension.
   b. Administer prescribed sedatives 30 minutes before the procedure to ensure their effectiveness.
   c. Organize activities so that the child is permitted to rest after administration of the sedative.

 DRUG ALERT Sedatives are contraindicated in many cases because increased ICP predisposes the child to hypoventilation or respiratory arrest. If they are administered, the child should be observed very closely for evidence of respiratory depression.

   d. Observe closely after ventriculography for the following:
      i. Leaking CSF from the sites of subdural or ventricular taps. These tap holes should be covered with a small piece of gauze or other dressing per institutional policy.
      ii. Reactions to the sedative, especially respiratory depression.
      iii. Changes in vital signs indicative of shock.
      iv. Signs of increased ICP, which may occur if air has been injected into the ventricles.

Providing Adequate Nutrition

1. Be aware that feeding is frequently difficult because the child may be listless, have a diminished appetite, and be prone to vomiting.
2. Complete nursing care and treatments before feeding so that the child will not be disturbed after feeding.
3. Hold the infant in a semi-sitting position with head well supported during feeding. Allow ample time for bubbling.
4. Offer small, frequent feedings.
5. Place the child on side with head elevated after feeding to prevent aspiration.

Maintaining Skin Integrity

1. Prevent pressure sores (pressure sores of the head are a frequent problem) by placing the child on a sponge rubber or lamb's wool pad or an alternating-pressure or egg-crate mattress to keep weight evenly distributed. Be mindful of latex allergies and the type of padding used.
2. Keep the scalp clean and dry.
3. Turn the child's head frequently; change position at least every 2 hours.
   a. When turning the child, rotate head and body together to prevent strain on the neck.
   b. A firm pillow may be placed under the child's head and shoulders for further support when lifting the child.
   c. Keep weight off incision during immediate postoperative period.
4. Provide meticulous skin care to all parts of the body and observe skin for signs of breakdown or pressure.
5. Give passive ROM exercises to the extremities, especially the legs.
6. Keep the eyes moistened with artificial tears if the child is unable to close the eyelids normally. This prevents corneal ulcerations and infections.

Reducing Anxiety

1. Prepare the parents for their child's surgery by answering questions, describing what nursing care will take place postoperatively, and explaining how the shunt will work.
2. Encourage the parents to discuss all the risks and benefits with the surgeon. Help them to understand the prognosis and what to expect of the child's neurologic and cognitive development.
3. Prepare the child for surgery by using dolls or other forms of play to describe what interventions will occur.

Improving Cerebral Tissue Perfusion Postoperatively

1. Monitor the child's temperature, pulse, respiration, blood pressure (BP), and pupillary size and reaction every 15 minutes until stable; then monitor every 1 to 2 hours or as indicated by child's condition and institutional policy.
2. Maintain normothermia.
   a. Provide appropriate blankets or covers, an Isolette or infant warmer, or hypothermia blanket.
   b. Administer a tepid sponge bath or antipyretic medication for temperature elevation.
3. Aspirate mucus from the nose and throat, as necessary, to prevent respiratory difficulty.
4. Turn the child frequently.
5. Promote optimal drainage of CSF through the shunt by pumping the shunt and positioning the child, as directed.
   a. If pumping is prescribed, carefully compress the valve the specified number of times at regularly scheduled intervals.
   b. Report any difficulties in pumping the shunt.
   c. Gradually elevate the head of child's bed to 30 to 45 degrees, as ordered. Initially, the child will be positioned flat to prevent excessive CSF drainage.
6. Assess for excessive drainage of CSF.
   a. Sunken fontanelle, agitation, restlessness (infant).
   b. Decreased LOC (older child).

7. Assess closely for increased ICP, indicating shunt malfunction.
   a. Note especially change in LOC, change in vital signs (increased systolic BP, decreased pulse rate, decreased or irregular respirations), vomiting, pupillary changes.
   b. Report these changes immediately to prevent cerebral hypoxia and possible brain herniation.
8. Prevent excessive pressure on skin overlying shunt by placing cotton behind and over the ears under the head dressing and avoiding positioning the child on the area of the valve or the incision until the wound is healed.

Maintaining Fluid Balance

1. Accurately measure and record total fluid intake and output.
2. Administer intravenous (IV) fluids, as prescribed; carefully monitor infusion rate to prevent fluid overload.
3. Use a nasogastric tube, if necessary, for abdominal distention. This is most frequently used when a VP shunt has been performed.
   a. Measure the drainage and record the amount and color.
   b. Monitor for return of bowel sounds after nasogastric suction has been disconnected for at least 30 minutes.
4. Give frequent mouth care while the child is to have nothing by mouth.
5. Begin oral feedings when the child is fully recovered from the anesthetic and displays interest.
   a. Begin with small amounts of dextrose 5% in water.
   b. Gradually introduce formula.
   c. Introduce solid foods suitable to the child's age and tolerance.
   d. Encourage a high-protein diet.
   e. Observe for and report any decrease in urine output, increased urine-specific gravity, diminished skin turgor, dryness of mucous membranes, or lethargy, indicating dehydration.

Preventing Infection

1. Assess for fever (temperature normally fluctuates during the first 24 hours after surgery), purulent drainage from the incision, or swelling, redness, and tenderness along the shunt tract.
2. Administer prescribed prophylactic antibiotics.

 NURSING ALERT All children who have had surgery require pain assessments. Although pain management is institution specific, acetaminophen is often the medication of choice. Also use alternative modes of pain management, such as distraction and relaxation techniques and ensure a quiet environment.

Strengthening Family Coping

1. Begin discharge planning early, including specific techniques for care of the shunt and suggested methods for providing daily care.
   a. Turning, holding, and positioning.
   b. Skin care over shunt.
   c. Exercises to strengthen muscles—incorporated with play.
   d. Feeding techniques and schedule.
   e. Pumping the shunt.

2. Accompany all instructions with reassurance necessary to prevent the parents from becoming anxious or fearful about assuming the care of the child.

3. Help the parents to assist siblings to understand hydrocephalus and the child's special needs. Encourage parents to spend individual time with siblings and not to neglect their needs as well. Suggest family counseling, if needed.

4. Assist parents in locating additional resources.
   a. Social worker, discharge planner, or department of social services.
   b. Visiting or home health nurses or aides.
   c. Parent groups.
   d. Community agencies.
   e. Special programs at school.

Community and Home Care Considerations

1. Follow the community and home care considerations listed under "Cerebral Palsy" on page 1548. Check shunt functioning regularly and reinforce parental performance of shunt checks and assessment for shunt malfunction and increased ICP.

2. Perform total physical assessment regularly, looking for signs of trauma or skin breakdown.

3. Patient should wear a medical alert bracelet when he or she starts to attend school or daycare.

4. Make sure that parents or caregivers are certified in cardiopulmonary resuscitation (CPR).

Family Education and Health Maintenance

1. Stress the importance of recognizing symptoms of increased ICP and reporting them immediately.

2. Advise parents to report shunt malfunction or infection immediately to prevent increased ICP.

3. Teach parents that illnesses that cause vomiting and diarrhea or illnesses that prevent an adequate fluid intake are a great threat to the child who has had a shunt procedure. Advise parents to consult with the child's health care provider about immediate treatment of fever, control of vomiting and diarrhea, and replacement of fluids.

4. Tell the parents that few restrictions are required for children with shunts and to consult with the health care provider about specific concerns.

5. Alert parents that additional information and support are available from the Hydrocephalus Association (*www.hydroassoc.org*).

Evaluation: Expected Outcomes

- No changes in vital signs, LOC, or head size; no vomiting; pupils equal and responsive.
- Feeds every 4 hours without vomiting; no significant weight loss.
- No erythema, blanching, or skin breakdown; wound healing evident.
- Parents verbalizing purpose and type of operative procedure, risks, and benefits.
- Shunt pumping without resistance; stable LOC and vital signs.
- Urine output equal to intake; skin turgor normal; electrolytes within normal limits.
- Afebrile; no drainage from shunt site.
- Parents actively seeking resources.

Spina Bifida

Spina bifida, also called *spinal dysraphia*, is a malformation of the spine in which the posterior portion of the laminae of the vertebrae fails to close. It occurs in approximately 1 per 1,000 live births in the United States and is the most common developmental defect of the central nervous system (CNS). It is more common in Caucasians than in other races. The incidence of spina bifida defects has been declining in the United States and United Kingdom due to antenatal screening and changes in environmental factors such as the consumption of folic acid in early pregnancy.

Several types of spina bifida are recognized, of which the following three are most common (see Figure 46-2).

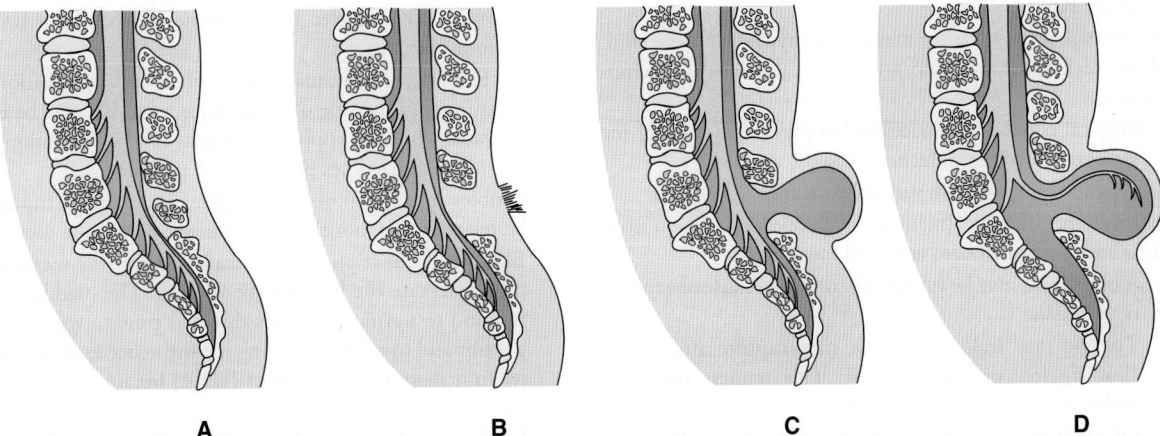

Figure 46-2. Spina bifida. (A) Normal spine. **(B)** Spina bifida occulta. **(C)** Spina bifida with meningocele. **(D)** Spina bifida with myelomeningocele.

Spina Bifida Occulta

Spina bifida occulta is seen in 10% of the United States population. It is a result of the posterior verteberal arches failing to fuse. A fat pad, dermal sinus, hairy tuft, or dimple in the lower back/lumbosacral region is often seen.

Meningocele

Meningocele is a herniation of the meninges through the defective posterior arches. The sac does not contain neural elements.

Myelomeningocele (or Meningomyelocele)

The spinal nerve roots and cord membranes protrude through the defect in the laminae of the vertebral column. Myelomeningoceles are covered by a thin membrane.

Pathophysiology and Etiology

1. Unknown etiology, but generally thought to result from genetic predisposition triggered by something in the environment.
   a. Certain drugs, including valproic acid, have been known to cause neural tube defects if administered during pregnancy.
   b. Women who have spina bifida and parents who have one affected child have an increased risk of producing children with neural tube defects.
2. Involves an arrest in the orderly formation of the vertebral arches and spinal cord that occurs between the 4th and 6th weeks of embryogenesis.
3. Theories of causation include:
   a. Incomplete closure of the neural tube during the 4th week of embryonic life.
   b. The neural tube forms adequately, then ruptures.

 DRUG ALERT Maternal periconceptional use of folic acid supplementation reduces by 50% or more the incidence of neural tube defects in pregnancies at risk.

4. In spina bifida occulta, the bony defect may range from a very thin slit separating one lamina from the spinous process to a complete absence of the spine and laminae.
   a. A thin, fibrous membrane sometimes covers the defect.
   b. The spinal cord and its meninges may be connected with a fistulous tract extending to and opening onto the surface of the skin.
5. In meningocele, the defect may occur anywhere on the cord. Higher defects (from thorax and upward) are usually meningoceles.
   a. Surgical correction is necessary to prevent rupture of the sac and subsequent infection.
   b. Prognosis is good with surgical correction.
6. In myelomeningocele (meningomyelocele), the lesion contains both the spinal cord and cord membranes.
   a. A bluish area may be evident on the top because of exposed neural tissue.
   b. The sac may leak in utero or may rupture after birth, allowing free drainage of CSF. This renders the child highly susceptible to meningitis.
   c. Of all defects known as spina bifida cystica, 95% are myelomeningoceles and 5% are meningoceles.

Clinical Manifestations

Spina Bifida Occulta

1. Most patients have no symptoms.
   a. They may have a dimple in the skin or a growth of hair over the malformed vertebra.
   b. There is no externally visible sac.
2. With growth, the child may develop foot weakness or bowel and bladder sphincter disturbances.
3. This condition is occasionally associated with more significant developmental abnormalities of the spinal cord, including syringomyelia and tethered cord.

Meningocele

1. An external cystic defect can be seen in the spinal cord, usually in the midline.
   a. The sac is composed only of meninges and is filled with CSF.
   b. The cord and nerve roots are usually normal.
2. There is seldom evidence of weakness of the legs or lack of sphincter control.

Myelomeningocele

1. A round, raised, and poorly epithelialized area may be noted at any level of the spinal column. However, the highest incidence of the lesion occurs in the lumbosacral area.
2. Hydrocephalus occurs in approximately 90% of children with myelomeningocele due to associated Arnold-Chiari malformation, which causes a block in the flow of CSF through the ventricles.
3. Loss of motor control and sensation below the level of the lesion can occur. These conditions are highly variable and depend on the size of the lesion and its position on the cord.
   a. A low thoracic lesion may cause total flaccid paralysis below the waist.
   b. A small sacral lesion may cause only patchy spots of decreased sensation in the feet.
4. Contractures may occur in the ankles, knees, or hips. Hips may become dislocated.
   a. Nature and degree of involvement depend on size and location of lesion.
   b. This occurs because some fibers of innervation get through. One side of a hip, knee, or ankle may be innervated while the opposing side may not be. The unopposed side then becomes pulled out of position.
5. Clubfeet are a common accompanying anomaly; thought to be related to the position of paraplegic feet in the uterus.
6. Bladder dysfunction occurs because of how the sacral nerves that innervate the bladder are affected. The bladder fails to respond to normal messages that it is time to void and simply fills and overflows, causing incontinence and susceptibility to urinary tract infections (UTIs) because of incomplete emptying.
7. Fecal incontinence and constipation are caused by poor innervation of the anal sphincter and bowel musculature.

8. Most children have average intellectual ability despite hydrocephalus. Developmental disabilities include the following:
   a. Gross motor development—children will need assistance in gaining and maintaining mobility.
   b. Most children are able to learn in a "mainstream" school environment, provided they are able to overcome other barriers (architectural and attitudinal).

Diagnostic Evaluation

1. Prenatal detection is done through prenatal ultrasound and fetal MRI. This testing should be offered to all women at risk (women who are affected or who have had other affected children).
2. Diagnosis is primarily based on clinical manifestations.
3. CT scan and MRI may be performed to further evaluate the brain and spinal cord.

Management

Surgical Intervention

1. Procedure: laminectomy and closure of the open lesion or removal of the sac usually can be done soon after birth.
2. Purpose:
   a. To prevent further deterioration of neural function.
   b. To minimize the danger of rupture and infection, especially meningitis.
   c. To improve cosmetic effect.
   d. To facilitate handling of the infant.

Multidisciplinary Follow-Up for Associated Problems

1. A coordinated team approach will help maximize the physical and intellectual potential of each affected child.
2. The team may include a neurologist, neurosurgeon, orthopedic surgeon, urologist, primary care provider, social worker, physical therapist, occupational therapist, a variety of community-based and hospital staff nurses, and the child and family.
3. Numerous neurosurgical, orthopedic, and urologic procedures may be necessary to help the child achieve maximum function.

Prognosis

1. Influenced by the site of the lesion and the presence and degree of associated hydrocephalus. Generally, the higher the defect, the greater the extent of neurologic deficit and the greater the likelihood of hydrocephalus.
2. In the absence of treatment, most infants with meningomyelocele die early in infancy.
3. Surgical intervention is most effective if it is done early in the neonatal period, preferably within the first few days of life.
4. Even with surgical intervention, infants can be expected to manifest associated neurosurgical, orthopedic, or urologic problems.
5. New techniques of treatment, intensive research, and improved services have increased life expectancy and have greatly enhanced the quality of life for most children who receive treatment.

Complications

1. Hydrocephalus associated with meningocele; may be aggravated by surgical repair.
2. Scoliosis, contractures, and joint dislocation.
3. Skin breakdown in sensory denervated areas and under braces.

Nursing Assessment

1. Assess sensory and motor response of lower extremities.
2. Assess ability to void spontaneously, retention of urine, symptoms of UTI.
3. Assess usual stooling patterns, need for medications to facilitate elimination.
4. Assess mobility and use of orthoses, casts, and other special equipment.

Nursing Diagnoses

Neonates (Preoperative)

- Risk for Impaired Skin Integrity related to impaired motor and sensory function.
- Risk for Infection related to contamination of the myelomeningocele site.
- Impaired Urinary Elimination related to neurologic deficits.
- Ineffective Tissue Perfusion: Cerebral related to potential hydrocephalus.
- Fear (parents) related to neonate with neurologic disorder and to surgery.

Infants and Children (Postoperative)

- Ineffective Thermoregulation following surgery.
- Impaired Urinary Elimination related to sacral denervation.
- Bowel Incontinence or Constipation related to impaired innervation of anal sphincter and bowel musculature.
- Disturbed Body Image related to the child's appearance, difficulties with locomotion, and lack of control over excretory functions.

Nursing Interventions

Protecting Skin Integrity

1. Avoid positioning on the infant's back to prevent pressure on the sac. Check position at least once every hour.
2. Do not place a diaper or other covering directly over the sac.
3. Observe the sac frequently for evidence of irritation or leakage of CSF.
4. Use prone positioning and prevent hip flexion to decrease tension on the sac.
5. Place a foam rubber pad covered with a soft cloth between the infant's legs to maintain the hips in abduction and to prevent or counteract subluxation. A diaper roll or small pillow may be used in place of the foam rubber pad.
6. Allow the infant's feet to hang freely over the pads or mattress edge to prevent aggravation of foot deformities.
7. Provide meticulous skin care to all areas of the body, especially ankles, knees, tip of nose, cheeks, and chin.

8. Provide passive ROM exercises for muscles and joints that the infant does not use spontaneously. Avoid hip exercises because of common hip dislocation, unless otherwise recommended.
9. Use a foam or fleece pad to reduce pressure of the mattress against the infant's skin.
10. Avoid pressure on the infant's back during feeding by holding the infant with your elbow rotated to avoid touching the sac, or feeding while infant is lying on side or prone on your lap. Encourage the parents to use these positions to provide infant stimulation and bonding.

Preventing Infection

1. Be aware that infection of the sac is most commonly caused by contamination by urine and feces.
2. Keep the infant's buttocks and genitalia scrupulously clean.
   a. Do not diaper the infant if the defect is in the lower portion of the spine.
   b. Use a small plastic drape taped between the defect and the anus to help prevent contamination.
3. Apply a sterile gauze pad or towel or a sterile, moistened dressing over the sac, as directed.
   a. When the sterile covering is used, it should be changed frequently to keep the area free from exudate and to maintain sterility.
   b. Care must be taken to prevent the covering from adhering to and damaging the sac.
4. Monitor and report immediately any signs of infection.
   a. Oozing of fluid or pus from the sac.
   b. Fever.
   c. Irritability or listlessness.
   d. Seizure.

Promoting Urinary Elimination

1. Use Crede's method for emptying the bladder (unless contraindicated by vesicoureteral reflux) and teach parents the technique.
   a. Apply firm, gentle pressure to the abdomen, beginning in the umbilical area and progressing toward the symphysis pubis.
   b. Continue the procedure as long as urine can be manually expressed.
2. Ensure fluid intake to dilute the urine.
3. Administer prescribed prophylactic antibiotics.
4. Monitor and report concentrated or foul-smelling urine.

Maintaining Cerebral Tissue Perfusion

1. Monitor for signs of hydrocephalus and report immediately.
   a. Irritability.
   b. Feeding difficulty, vomiting, decreased appetite.
   c. Temperature fluctuation.
   d. Decreased alertness.
   e. Tense fontanelle.
   f. Increased head circumference.

Reducing Fear

1. Encourage parents to express feelings of guilt, fear, lack of control, or helplessness.

2. Provide accurate information about spina bifida and what to expect postoperatively.
3. Include the parents in all of infant's care and encourage private bonding time.

Maintaining Thermoregulation and Preventing Complications

1. Frequently monitor temperature, pulse, respirations, color, and level of responsiveness postoperatively, based on the infant's stability.
2. Use an Isolette or infant warmer to prevent temperature fluctuation.
3. Prevent respiratory complications.
   a. Periodically reposition the infant to promote lung expansion.
   b. Watch for abdominal distention, which could interfere with breathing.
   c. Have oxygen available.
4. Maintain hydration and nutritional intake.
   a. Administer IV fluids, as ordered; keep accurate intake and output log.
   b. Administer gavage feedings, as ordered.
   c. Begin bottle-feeding when infant is responsive and tolerating feedings. Give small, frequent feedings slowly so air can be expelled naturally without bubbling.
5. Keep the surgical dressing clean and dry and observe for drainage. Avoid pressure to the area and diapers that cover the incision until healed.
6. Monitor for and teach parents to recognize signs of hydrocephalus. Report immediately.
7. Limit or prevent direct contact of the child to products routinely used that contain latex, due to risk of latex allergy and severe reaction. Latex products include BP cuffs, tourniquets, tape, indwelling catheters, gloves, and IV tubing injection ports. Develop protocols specifying modification of care for children at risk for latex allergy.

 NURSING ALERT Be aware that children with spina bifida have a far greater risk of latex allergy than the general population. It is estimated that up to 20% of spina bifida patients have a latex allergy. Symptoms include hives, itching, wheezing, and anaphylaxis. Incidence increases with time and may be related to repeated exposure to products containing latex.

Achieving Continence

1. Teach parents that continence can usually be achieved with clean, intermittent self-catheterization.
   a. Children can generally be taught to catheterize themselves by age 6 or 7.
   b. Parents can catheterize younger children.
2. Teach the following procedure:
   a. Gather equipment: catheter, water-soluble lubricant, soap and water, urine collection container.
   b. Wash hands.
   c. Position patient.

d. Clean the area around the urethral meatus.

e. Lubricate the catheter tip.

f. Insert the catheter until urine starts to flow. Have urine collection container or diaper available.

g. Remove catheter when urine is drained from bladder.

h. Clean any lubricant off the child.

i. Dispose of urine.

j. Wash hands.

3. Teach about the action of medications, such as imipramine and ephedrine, if prescribed, which are used to help children retain urine rather than dribbling. When used with self-catheterization, many children can stay dry for 3 to 4 hours at a time.

4. Teach the signs of UTI (concentrated, foul-smelling urine; irritability; pain or burning; and fever) and the proper administration of antibiotics either prophylactically or when prescribed for infection.

5. For children who cannot achieve urinary continence through intermittent catheterization, provide information about options, such as surgically implanted mechanical urinary sphincters and bladder pacemakers, indwelling catheters, external collecting devices, and urinary diversion (may be necessary in some cases).

Achieving Regular Bowel Elimination

1. Assist with bowel training program to compensate for decreased sacral sensation.

a. Children are placed on a toileting schedule and are taught to push.

b. Medications, such as stool softeners, suppositories, or enemas, may be used initially to help determine scheduling.

2. To prevent constipation and enhance bowel control, encourage intake of high-fiber, high-fluid diet. Such medications as psyllium may be used to increase bulk or soften stool.

Fostering Positive Body Image

1. Emphasize rehabilitation that makes use of the child's strengths and minimizes disabilities.

2. Continually reassess functional abilities and offer suggestions to increase independence. Periodically consult with physical or occupational therapists to help maximize function.

3. Encourage the use of braces and specialized equipment to enhance ambulation while minimizing the appearance of the equipment. For example, wear pants instead of dresses or shorts to cover leg braces; choose a compact wheelchair that can be decorated or personalized for the child.

4. Encourage participation with peer group and in activities that build on strengths, such as cognitive abilities, interest in music or art.

5. Periodically reassess bowel and bladder programs. The ability to stay dry for reasonable time intervals is one of the greatest factors in enhancing self-esteem and positive body image.

Community and Home Care Considerations

1. Follow the community and home care considerations listed under "Cerebral Palsy" on page 1548.

2. Survey the home environment for latex and substitute products obtained, if possible. Toys and equipment for children, such as nipples, pacifiers, and elastic on the legs of disposable diapers, also contain latex. Teach the parents how to recognize latex allergy and to notify the child's health care provider.

 NURSING ALERT Ensure there is an emergency epinephrine injection available in case of inadvertent latex exposure.

3. Teach the family how to clean and reuse urinary catheters. The catheter should be washed in warm, soapy water and rinsed well in warm water. The catheter should be air-dried and, when completely dried, placed in a clean jar or plastic bag. A catheter should be replaced when it becomes dry, cracked, stiff, or if the child develops a UTI.

4. Instruct the parents to notify the health care provider for signs of associated problems, such as hydrocephalus, meningitis, UTI, and latex sensitivity.

Family Education and Health Maintenance

1. Prepare the parents to feed, hold, and stimulate their infant as naturally as possible.

2. Teach the parents the special techniques that may be required for holding and positioning, feeding, caring for the incision, emptying the bladder, and exercising muscles.

3. Alert the parents to safety needs of the child with decreased sensation, such as protection from prolonged pressure, the risk of burns due to bath water that is too warm, and avoidance of trauma from contact with sharp objects.

4. Urge continued follow-up and health maintenance, including immunizations and evaluation of growth and development.

5. Advise parents that children with paralysis are at risk for becoming overweight due to inactivity, so they should provide a low-fat, balanced diet; control snacking; and encourage as much activity as possible.

6. For additional resources, refer families to agencies such as the Spina Bifida Association of America (*www.sbaa.org*).

Evaluation: Expected Outcomes

- No signs of meningeal sac or skin breakdown.
- Afebrile, alert, and active.
- Clear urine without odor; adequate elimination; no infection.
- Fontanelle soft; head circumference stable.
- Parents asking questions about surgery, showing affection for infant.
- Vital signs stable; incisional dressing dry and intact.
- Parents or child demonstrate proper catheterization technique.
- Passes stool once per day; adequate elimination; no constipation.
- Verbalizes participation in school and other social activities.

Muscular Dystrophy

Muscular dystrophy (MD) refers to a group of genetically determined, progressive, degenerative myopathies affecting a variety of muscle groups—most patients are children. The common muscular dystrophies include Duchenne's MD, affecting 1 in 3,500 live-born males, and Becker's MD, affecting 1 in 30,000 live-born males. Most with Duchenne's MD rarely survive beyond ages 20 to 25.

Pathophysiology and Etiology

1. Inherited; may be X-linked, autosomal dominant, or recessive.
2. Genetic coding defect causes abnormal muscle development and function—mutations in the dystrophin gene.
3. Loss of skeletal muscle fibers, but no associated structural abnormalities in peripheral nerves or spinal cord.
4. Marked reduction of dystrophin, a protein vital to muscle function. The amount of dystrophin levels vary with the type of MD.

Clinical Manifestations

1. Progressive muscular weakness (see Table 46-1).
2. Gower's sign is a hallmark feature of Duchenne's MD, characterized by a child's difficulty rising from the floor. The child must take the following steps to assume a standing position:
   a. Roll onto hands and knees.
   b. Bear weight with legs by creating a wide base of support, while using hands on floor to support some weight.
   c. Use arms to climb up legs.
   d. Push torso to an upright stance with legs remaining wide apart.
3. Heart muscle weakens and tachycardia develops.
4. Respiratory muscles weaken, causing ineffective cough and frequent infections.

Diagnostic Evaluation

1. Nerve conduction test and electromyography show abnormalities.
2. Serum creatinine kinase—elevated.
3. Deoxyribonucleic acid (DNA) analysis of blood.
4. Muscle biopsy may provide definitive diagnosis.

Management

1. Goals of treatment are directed toward maintaining mobility, quality of life, and prevention of complications.
2. Medications to control symptoms, such as anti-arrhythmics and bronchodilators.
3. Promotion of ambulation with appropriate aid after loss of ability to walk.
4. Provision of spinal orthotic supports.
5. Surgical tendon releasing to treat contractures.
6. Physical therapy, such as passive stretching, to preserve function.
7. Vigorous respiratory therapy, such as chest percussion, inspirometry, and assisted cough.
8. Pulmonary function monitoring.
9. Carrier detection and genetic counseling to explain implications of MD to parents and detect sibling carriers.
10. Corticosteroids are used to delay the progression of muscle weakness; often, need for early surgical intervention to correct scoliosis.
11. Nutritional management to prevent obesity is necessary as this may affect quality of life, life expectancy, and burden of care.
12. Frequent surveillance of cardiac function.

Table 46-1 Clinical Manifestations of Muscular Dystrophies

TYPE	ONSET	CLINICAL MANIFESTATIONS	OTHER INFORMATION
Duchenne	Age 2–6 years	Muscle atrophy and weakness over time affecting pelvis, thighs, upper arms, and eventually all voluntary muscles; waddling gait, need for wheelchair by age 12; pulmonary and cardiac abnormalities; survival beyond age 20 is rare.	Affects only males. Most common type of MD in children.
Becker	Age 2–16 years	Similar to Duchenne, but less severe, very mild in some cases; slower progression. Survival into middle age.	Affects only males.
Limb-girdle	Late teen to adult	Progressive weakness of the pelvic and shoulder girdles, then arms and legs. Walking becomes difficult over 20-year period. Survival may be to late adulthood.	Affects males and females. Most common type overall.
Facioscapulohumeral	Teen to early adult	Weakness of fascial muscles, wasting of shoulders and upper arms; slow progression with short periods of rapid deterioration. Causes problems with chewing, swallowing, speaking; characteristic "Popeye" arms and scapular winging. Survival well into adulthood.	Affects males and females. Severity varies widely.
Congenital	At birth	General muscle weakness; possible joint deformities due to contractures; slow progression. Seizures and other brain abnormalities with Fukuyama type. Shortened life span.	Affects males and females. Several types have been identified.
Emery-Dreifuss	Childhood to early teen	Slowly progressive weakness and atrophy of shoulder, upper arm, and lower leg muscles; joint deformities; possible cardiac problems causing sudden death. Cardiac problems may affect carriers (including women).	Affects males only. Rare form.

Complications

1. Infections (pulmonary, urinary, systemic).
2. Cardiac dysrhythmias.
3. Respiratory insufficiency and failure secondary to weakness of diaphragm and chest muscles.
4. Aspiration pneumonia due to oropharyngeal dysfunction.
5. Depression.
6. Orthopedic deformities—contractures, lordosis, scoliosis.
7. Learning and behavioral disorders.
8. Malignant hyperthermia—may develop in small number of children with mild or nonapparent muscle disease.
9. Osteopenia related to immobility.

Nursing Assessment

1. Assess muscle strength, atrophy, gait, age-related motor development, progressive loss of function.
2. Evaluate respiratory and cardiac status—breath sounds, heart sounds, pulse rate and rhythm, BP, and peripheral perfusion.
3. Evaluate ADLs.
4. Identify psychosocial issues, such as altered self-concept, decreased socialization, and family discord.

Nursing Diagnoses

- Ineffective Breathing Pattern related to muscle weakness.
- Impaired Physical Mobility related to disease process.
- Decreased Cardiac Output related to cardiac muscle involvement.
- Impaired Swallowing related to muscle weakness.
- Deficient Diversional Activity related to weakness.

Nursing Interventions

Maintaining Breathing Pattern

1. Encourage upright positioning to provide for maximum chest excursion.
2. Encourage energy-conservation techniques and avoidance of exertion.
3. Teach deep-breathing exercises to strengthen respiratory muscles.
4. Assess rate, depth, and pattern of respirations; listen to breath sounds; and report any change in condition.
5. Note results of arterial blood gas levels, sputum cultures, and chest x-rays.
6. Encourage coughing and deep breathing or perform chest physiotherapy, as indicated.

Preserving Optimal Motor Function

1. Refer to physical therapy for stretching and strengthening exercises to optimize remaining motor function.
2. Perform ROM exercises to preserve mobility and prevent atrophy.
3. Schedule activity with consideration to energy highs throughout the day.
4. Consult with occupational therapist for assistive devices to maintain independence.
5. Apply braces and splints to prevent contractures.

Improving Cardiac Output

1. Monitor vital signs, cardiac rhythm, and signs of heart failure, such as edema, adventitious breath sounds, and weight gain.
2. Monitor intake and output and maintain IV or oral fluid intake, as ordered.

Monitoring Swallowing Function

1. Assess cranial nerve function for swallowing (gag reflex) and chewing.
2. Provide a diet that the patient can handle; a pureed diet may be necessary.
3. Diet should be high protein and controlled calories to provide optimal nutritional value.
4. Encourage eating in upright position without talking and encourage consumption of smaller, frequent meals.
5. Administer alternative enteral feeding if gag reflex is diminished.

Encouraging Diversional Activities

1. Encourage diversional activities that prevent overexertion and frustration, but discourage long periods of bed rest and inactivity such as TV watching.
2. If upper extremities are mostly affected, suggest walking or riding a stationary bike; if lower extremities are mostly affected, encourage use of a wheelchair to promote mobility and performing simple crafts.
3. Discuss patient's interests and assist with preferred activities.
4. Investigate with the patient various methods of stress management to deal with frustration.
5. Administer analgesics and antidepressants, as ordered, to facilitate participation in activities.

Community and Home Care Considerations

1. Follow the community and home care considerations listed under "Cerebral Palsy" on page 1548.
2. Obtain services and devices that will promote maximal functioning, such as wheelchair ramp, wheelchair van for transportation, assistive devices.
3. Explore physical and recreational activities with family such as Special Olympics.
4. Assess child's educational progress and ability to attend school versus home schooling.
5. Collaborate with patient and family to establish daily plan of activities that incorporates patient's interests, ability, and need for rest periods.

Family Education and Health Maintenance

1. Offer genetic counseling, if indicated, to determine options of family planning.
2. Instruct the patient and family in ROM exercises, pulmonary care, and methods of transfer and locomotion.
3. Refer to community respite and counseling services.
4. Stress the importance of fluids to decrease risk of urinary/pulmonary infection and minimize constipation.
5. Advise patient or family to report signs of respiratory infection immediately to obtain treatment and prevent heart failure.
6. Refer patient and family to agencies such as the Muscular Dystrophy Association (*www.mdausa.org*).

Evaluation: Expected Outcomes

- Deep, unlabored respirations with clear breath sounds.
- Ambulates unassisted, no contractures noted.
- Vital signs stable, no edema.
- Tolerates small pureed feeds without aspiration.
- Out of bed most of day, engages in diversional and social activities.

Bacterial Meningitis

Bacterial meningitis is an inflammation of the meninges that follows the invasion of the spinal fluid by a bacterial agent. Most cases are seen in children younger than age 5.

Pathophysiology and Etiology

1. The proportion of cases due to a specific organism varies from year to year; there is also considerable geographic difference. The organisms most commonly causing bacterial meningitis in different age groups include:
   a. Birth to age 3 months—*Escherichia coli, Streptococcus* group B, *Listeria monocytogenes, Pseudomonas aeruginosa, Staphylococcus* species.
   b. Ages 3 months to 6 years—*Streptococcus pneumoniae, Neisseria meningitidis* (meningococcal meningitis), *Haemophilus influenzae.*
   c. Ages 6 to 16—*S. pneumoniae, N. meningitidis, Mycobacterium tuberculosis.*
2. Bacterial meningitis is frequently preceded by an upper respiratory infection, which is complicated by bacteremia. Bacteria in the circulating blood then invade the CSF.
   a. Less commonly, bacterial meningitis may occur as an extension of a local bacterial infection, such as otitis media, mastoiditis, or sinusitis.
   b. Bacteria may also gain direct entry through a penetrating wound, spinal tap, surgery, or anatomic abnormality.
3. The infective process results in inflammation, exudation, and varying degrees of tissue damage in the brain.

Clinical Manifestations

1. Signs and symptoms are variable, depending on the patient's age, the etiologic agent, and the duration of the illness when diagnosed. Onset may be insidious or fulminant.
2. Infants younger than age 2 months usually display irritability, lethargy, vomiting, lack of appetite, seizures, high-pitched cry, fever, or hypothermia.
3. Infants up to age 2 manifest symptoms similar to those of the young infant and may have altered sleep patterns, fever, tenseness of the fontanelle, nuchal rigidity, positive Kernig's or Brudzinski's signs (see page 514).
4. Children older than age 2 initially have vomiting, headache, fever, mental confusion, lethargy, and photophobia. Later symptoms include nuchal rigidity within 12 to 24 hours after onset, positive Kernig's or Brudzinski's sign, seizures, and progressive decline in responsiveness.
5. Petechiae or purpura may develop.
   a. Characteristic skin lesions are most commonly observed in cases of meningococcal or *Pseudomonas* infection.
   b. Hemorrhagic rashes may occur in any child with overwhelming bacterial sepsis because of disseminated intravascular coagulation (DIC).
6. Septic arthritis suggests either meningococcal or *H. influenzae* infection.

Diagnostic Evaluation

1. Diagnosis is usually established through lumbar puncture and examination of CSF.
   a. Cloudy or turbid appearance.
   b. Elevated CSF pressure.
   c. High cell count with mostly polymorphonuclear cells.
   d. Low glucose level.
   e. Elevated protein level (also may be normal).
   f. Positive Gram stain and cultures (identifies the causative organism).
2. Additional laboratory studies include:
   a. Complete blood count (CBC)—total white blood cell count usually increased, with a preponderance of young neutrophils in the differential blood count (known as "shift to the left").
   b. Blood, urine, and nasopharyngeal cultures to look for source of infection.
   c. Platelet count, serum electrolytes, glucose, blood urea nitrogen and creatinine, and urinalysis usually done to monitor critically ill patient.

Management

1. IV administration of the appropriate antimicrobial agents to promote rapid destruction of the bacteria and to suppress the emergence of resistant strains. The first dose of antibiotics should be administered as soon as possible (cultures should be taken before an antibiotic is given).
2. Recognition and treatment of hyponatremia caused by syndrome of inappropriate antidiuretic hormone (SIADH).
3. Supportive management of the comatose child or the child with seizures including neuroprotective measures.
4. Appropriate prophylactic treatment provided for contacts when indicated.

Complications

1. Acute—seizures, cerebral edema and increased ICP, shock, SIADH.
2. Long-term—sensorineural hearing loss, hydrocephalus, blindness, learning disabilities or developmental delays.
3. DIC.

Nursing Assessment

1. Obtain a history from the parents about recent upper respiratory or other infection.

2. Assess LOC and neurologic status.
   a. Evaluate for *Kernig's sign*—with the child in the supine position and knees flexed, flex the leg at the hip so the thigh is brought to a position perpendicular to the trunk. Attempt to extend the knee. If meningeal irritation is present, this cannot be done, and attempts to extend the knee result in pain.
   b. Evaluate for *Brudzinski's sign*—flex the patient's neck. Spontaneous flexion of the lower extremities indicates meningeal irritation.
3. Monitor breathing pattern and circulatory status.

Nursing Diagnoses

- Ineffective Tissue Perfusion: Cerebral related to endotoxin release into the CSF.
- Hyperthermia related to infectious process.
- Acute Pain related to neurologic effects from the disease process.
- Anxiety related to infection transmission precautions.
- Ineffective Tissue Perfusion: Cerebral related to complications of infectious process.
- Anxiety of parents related to severity of illness and hospitalization.

Nursing Interventions

See Standards of Care Guidelines 46-1.

Maintaining Cerebral Tissue Perfusion

1. Administer antimicrobial agents at specified time intervals to obtain optimal serum levels. Obtain blood studies for peak and trough levels, as ordered.
2. Maintain patent IV line for medication administration; observe for signs of infiltration and phlebitis.
3. Monitor closely for signs of complications affecting cerebral perfusion.
   a. Monitor vital signs, LOC, and neurologic status at frequent intervals.
   b. Monitor intake and output, weight, and head circumference daily to assess for hydrocephalus.
   c. Be especially alert for lethargy or subtle changes in condition, which may indicate cerebral edema.
   d. Accurately chart child's behavior and clinical signs.

Reducing Fever

1. Administer antipyretics, tepid sponge baths, and hypothermia blanket, as ordered, to reduce fever. Fever increases metabolic rate and energy requirements by the brain; this may lead to hypoxemia and brain damage in the child with cerebral vascular compromise.
2. Monitor for seizures and use seizure precautions in the febrile child.
   a. There is an increased potential for seizures in the febrile child.
   b. Ensure safety by using padded bed or crib rails and having airway and suction equipment on hand.

STANDARDS OF CARE GUIDELINES 46-1
Caring for a Child with Neurologic Dysfunction

- Monitor vital signs, level of consciousness, pupillary reaction, and behavior, as indicated, and observe for signs of increased intracranial pressure; report significant changes immediately.
- Make sure that the patient receives all seizure medications and antibiotics, as directed, and that any deviation from dosage schedule or change in therapeutic serum drug levels is reported immediately.
- Assess for adequate elimination: ability for the child to urinate, or caregiver or child to do catheterization. Report deviation from normal pattern and take measures to prevent constipation and stool impaction.
- Assess for signs of secondary infection: postoperative incision infection; shunt malfunction and infection; pneumonia; skin breakdown. Report abnormality in timely fashion.
- Monitor for seizures and maintain safety. Document and report all seizures, including type, time of onset, duration, and behavior afterward. Administer medications, as needed, and as directed.
- Make sure that any assistive devices fit adequately to avoid tissue breakdown. Check more frequently if child is restless.
- Observe and assist with ambulation for safety.
- Train all caregivers in standards of home safety, including cardiopulmonary resuscitation, seizure control, and accident prevention.
- Make sure that the patient and family are aware of all community resources, including respite and support groups, educational assistance, and social services.
- Teach caregivers to do range of motion exercises to prevent contractures. Utilize physical and occupational therapy, as needed.
- Encourage regular health maintenance visits to monitor growth, development, and general health.

This information should serve as a general guideline only. Each patient situation presents a unique set of clinical factors and requires nursing judgment to guide care, which may include additional or alternative measures and approaches.

Relieving Pain and Irritability

1. Reduce the general noise level around the child and prevent sudden loud noises.
2. Organize nursing care to provide for periods of uninterrupted rest.
3. Keep general handling of the child at a minimum. When necessary, approach the child slowly and gently.
4. Maintain subdued lighting as much as possible.
5. Speak in a low, well-modulated tone of voice.
6. Medicate for pain, as ordered, avoiding opioids that cause CNS and respiratory depression.

Preventing Transmission of Infection Without Anxiety

1. Use infection control precautions at all times to prevent transmission of infection.
2. Practice careful handwashing technique.
3. Explain use of all protective equipment and procedures to child and family to allay anxiety.
4. Make sure that personnel with colds or other infections avoid contact with infants with meningitis and wear a mask when it is necessary to enter the nursery.
5. Teach parents and other visitors proper handwashing and gown techniques.
6. Maintain sterile technique for procedures, when indicated.
7. Identify close contacts of the child with meningitis caused by *H. influenzae* or *N. meningitidis* who might benefit from prophylactic treatment.

Avoiding Complications

1. Monitor for and report any of the following:
   a. Decreased respirations, decreased pulse rate, increased systolic BP, pupillary changes, or decreased responsiveness, which may indicate increased ICP.
   b. Decreased urine volume and increased body weight, which may indicate SIADH.
   c. Sudden appearance of a skin rash and bleeding from other sites, which may indicate DIC.
   d. Persistent or recurring fever, bulging fontanelle, signs of increased ICP, focal neurologic signs, seizures, or increased head circumference, which may indicate subdural effusion.
   e. Hearing disturbances and apparent deafness, indicating cranial nerve involvement.
2. Observe for episodes of apnea and initiate measures to stimulate respiration.
   a. Institute respiratory monitoring.
   b. Stimulate the infant when apnea does occur.
      i. Pinch feet and provide more vigorous stimulation, if necessary.
      ii. When spontaneous respiration does not occur within 15 to 20 seconds, provide bag or mask ventilation.
   c. Report any periods of apnea.
   d. Record length of apneic episode and response to stimulation.

Allaying Parental Anxiety

1. Encourage the parents to engage in quiet activities with their child, such as reading or listening to soft music.
2. Provide the parents with an opportunity to express their concerns and answer questions they may have regarding the child's progress and care.
3. Engage the parents in the supportive care of the child so they may feel some control over the situation.

Family Education and Health Maintenance

1. Provide parents with appropriate information if they and other family members are to receive antibiotic prophylaxis.
2. Discuss symptoms for which the parents should watch as signs of possible latent complications, especially hydrocephalus.
3. Give specific instructions about medications to be administered at home.
4. Encourage regular health maintenance visits to chart growth and development and assess for any delays.
5. Parents can obtain more information about meningitis at *www.aboutkidshealth.ca/En/HealthAZ/ConditionsandDiseases/InfectiousDiseases/Pages/Meningitis.aspx*.

Evaluation: Expected Outcomes

- Alert without signs of increased ICP.
- Fever below 101° F (38.3° C), no subsequent infection.
- Resting comfortably, verbalizing reduced pain.
- Child expresses understanding of infection precautions.
- Vital signs stable; breathing pattern regular without apnea.
- Parents participate in child's care, ask questions.

Seizure Disorders (Convulsive Disorders, Epilepsy)

Seizure disorder is a term used to encompass a number of varieties of episodic disturbances of brain function. Seizures should not be regarded as one specific disorder, but as a symptom of an underlying disorder. They are relatively common in children, being more prevalent during the first 2 years of life than at any other time. Incidence of epilepsy is estimated at 15 cases per 100,000 people. Of individuals with seizure disorders, 90% are diagnosed before age 20. *Epilepsy* is defined as the occurrence of two or more unprovoked seizures. Seizures result from an abnormal and excessive discharge of neurons along with behavioral or sensorimoter symptoms. Of children under age 16, approximately 0.5% to 1% experience seizures. Of 326,000 children under age 15 with epilepsy, approximately 90,000 have seizures not completely controlled by treatment. Seizures are the most common pediatric neurologic problem.

Pathophysiology and Etiology

Etiologic Factors

Seizure disorders are idiopathic or related to a variety of contributing factors.

1. Genetic (inherited)—channelopathies, chromosomal abnormalities, mitochondrial DNA disorders, metabolic disorders, hereditary neurocutaneous disorders.
2. Congenital (inherited or acquired)—developmental cortical malformations, cerebral tumors, vascular malformations, prenatal injury.
3. Acquired—trauma, neurosurgery, infection, vascular disease, hippocampal sclerosis, tumors, neurodegenerative disorders, metabolic disorders, toxic disorders.
4. Causes in newborns—brain malformations, infections, metabolic disorders (pyridoxine deficiency, hypoglycemia, hyponatremia, hypocalcemia), urea cycle disorders, hypoxic ischemic encephalopathy, intracranial hemorrhage, familial neonatal convulsions.
5. Causes in children—inherited metabolic or developmental diseases, idiopathic/genetic syndromes, infections, cortical dysplasias, degenerative disorders.
6. Causes in adolescents—mesial temporal sclerosis, degenerative diseases, trauma, tumors.

Altered Physiology

1. The basic mechanism for all seizures appears to be prolonged depolarization and other chemical changes, causing neurons to discharge in an uncontrolled manner.
2. This paroxysmal burst of electrical energy spreads to adjacent areas of the brain or may jump to distant areas of the CNS, resulting in a seizure.
3. Some seizures appear to occur under the influence of a triggering factor.
   a. Hormonal factors, such as those related to the menstrual period, menarche, and menopause.
   b. Nonsensory factors, such as hyperthermia, hyperventilation, metabolic disorders, sleep deprivation, emotional disturbances, and physical stress.
   c. Sensory factors, such as those related to vision, hearing, touch, the startle reaction, and those that are self-induced.

Clinical Manifestations: Types of Seizures

Epileptic seizures are classified according to the International League Against Epilepsy classification system and are either partial or generalized.

Generalized seizures may be myoclonic, tonic, tonic-clonic, astatic, or clonic. Generalized seizures are characterized by global synchronized activation of neurons, resulting in impaired consciousness, bilateral motor changes, and ECG abnormalities.

Partial seizures are either simple (no impairment of consciousness) or complex (impairment of consciousness). Obtaining a thorough history and physical examination is crucial because the diagnosis of epilepsy is primarily based on clinical features.

Partial Seizures Simple-Partial Seizures

1. Caused by abnormal activation of a limited number of neurons resulting in symptoms that allow for localization of the epileptic focus.
   a. Motor: jerking of extremities.
   b. Somatosensory or special sensory: tingling or numbness, simple visual phenomena, rising epigastric sensation.
   c. Autonomic: changes in skin color, BP, heart rate, pupil size, piloerection.
   d. Psychic: dysphasia or aphasia, flashbacks, déjà vu, jamais vu, panoramic experiences, dreamy state, sensations of unreality or depersonalization, fear, depression, anger, irritability, illusions of perception (size [macro or micropsia], shape, weight, distance, sound), hallucinations (visual, auditory, gustatory, olfactory).

Complex-Partial Seizures

1. Often preceded by aura or accompanied by various types of automatisms.
2. May begin with simple-partial onset but lead to impairment of consciousness (secondary generalization).
3. May have impairment of consciousness at onset of seizure.
4. Features may include mouth movements (ie, chewing, lip-smacking), hand movements (ie, picking at clothing, "pill-rolling," grasping at objects), rubbing genitalia, eye-blinking, head-turning, raising of arm, or autonomic symptoms such as vomiting, retching, and drooling.

Generalized Seizures Typical Absence Seizures

1. Frequent, brief, abrupt loss of consciousness, often accompanied by eyelid-flickering and ending abruptly with resumption of normal activity; usually last less than 10 seconds, occur in clusters, with no postictal phase.
2. May be induced by hyperventilation or photic stimulation.
3. Idiopathic in nature.

Atypical Absence Seizures

1. Frequently associated with symptomatic epilepsies.
2. Partial impairment of consciousness, usually lasting several minutes. Postictal confusion, headache, and emotional disturbance are common.
3. Often associated with mixed seizure disorders; may have aura or automatisms.

Myoclonic Seizures

1. Consist of brief, involuntary contractions of only one muscle group or several muscle groups; caused by a cortical discharge.
2. May be triggered by action, noise, being startled, photic stimulation, or percussion.

Clonic Seizures

1. Consist of jerking that is often asymmetric and irregular.
2. Occur more frequently in neonates, infants, or young children.

Tonic Seizures

1. Consist of sustained muscle contraction with no clonic phase.
2. Can occur at any age.
3. Frequently associated with diffuse cerebral damage and are seen in children with Lennox-Gastaut syndrome.

Tonic-Clonic Seizures

1. Consist of a tonic phase, clonic phase, and postictal phase.
2. Tonic phase lasts for 10 to 30 seconds.
3. The seizure progresses to a clonic phase that lasts 30 to 60 seconds.
4. The postictal period consists of confusion or fatigue that may last for 2 to 30 minutes.

Infantile Spasms (Myoclonic Seizures, Massive Myoclonic Spasms)

1. These seizures occur in infants; they are second in incidence only to generalized seizures in this age group.
2. Peak incidence is in children between ages 4 and 8 months; onset after age 2 is rare.
3. Clinical signs include the following:
   a. Sudden, forceful, myoclonic contractions involving the musculature of the trunk, neck, and extremities.
      i. Flexor type—infant adducts and flexes the extremities, drops the head, and doubles on him- or herself.
      ii. Extensor type—infant extends neck, spreads out arms, and bends body backward in a position described as "spread eagle."
      iii. Mixed—combination of the above two types, occurring in clusters or volleys of each.
   b. A cry or grunt may accompany severe attacks.
   c. The infant may grimace, laugh, or appear fearful during or after the attack.

4. Duration is momentary (usually less than 1 minute).
5. Frequency varies from a few attacks per day to hundreds per day.
6. Almost always associated with cerebral abnormalities. Mental retardation usually accompanies this disorder in 95% of cases.
7. Usually, this type of seizure disappears spontaneously by the time the child reaches age 4. Subsequent generalized or other types of seizures usually develop.

 NURSING ALERT Occurrence of infantile spasms is a pediatric emergency. Delay in treatment could lead to permanent cognitive impairment and developmental delay.

Status Epilepticus

1. A prolonged seizure or repeated seizures lasting longer than 30 minutes with no interictal recovery.
2. Most common pediatric neurologic emergency, possibly resulting in permanent neurologic sequelae.
3. May be overt seizure activity (convulsive) or subclinical (nonconvulsive).
4. Generalized tonic-clonic status epilepticus is life-threatening.
5. Causes include new acute illness, progressive neurologic disease, loss of seizure control in an epileptic, or a febrile seizure in a child who is otherwise in good health.
6. Recurrence occurs more often in children who have other neurologic abnormalities; recurrence is rare in children who experience febrile seizures.
7. Absence and complex-partial status epilepticus are often difficult to identify and children often appear to be in a mildly confused state.

Psychogenic Nonepileptic Seizures

1. Previously known as "hysterical" or "pseudoseizures" and are usually a method of seeking attention and secondary gain.
2. Occur most frequently in adolescents and more often in girls than boys (3:1).
3. History of sexual abuse is common in women with nonepileptic seizures.
4. May occur in people with true seizures that have come under control.
5. Difficult to distinguish by observation alone.
6. Often include three broad patterns:
   a. Unilateral or bilateral motor activity that may include tonic posturing or tremulousness—movements are thrashing or jerking, rather than tonic-clonic, and often different movements occur simultaneously.
   b. Behavioral or emotional changes—distress or discomfort, followed by semi-purposeless—but not stereotyped—behaviors and may include walking or fumbling with objects.
   c. Periods of unresponsiveness with precipitation or cessation of the attack occurring after suggestion—no self-harm occurs, with no associated incontinence during these episodes.

Diagnostic Evaluation

Electroencephalogram

1. Used to confirm the clinical diagnosis, classify type of epilepsy, localize the area of epileptic focus, and determine when it is safe to discontinue treatment.
2. A normal EEG does not preclude the diagnosis of epilepsy. Indeed, about 10% to 20% of children who have epilepsy have a normal EEG.

Brain Imaging

1. CT scan and MRI—provide an anatomic picture of the brain; essential in ruling out the presence of a lesion. MRI is the gold standard in evaluation of epilepsy, although CT scan is used when MRI is not available.
2. Single-photon emission computed tomography, positron emission tomography, and functional MRI—brain imaging techniques that measure local vascular or metabolic changes associated with neuronal activity; they can also map cortical function when resective surgery is being planned.
3. Magnetoencephalography—noninvasive technology that helps map the sensory and language cortex when resective surgery is being planned.

Neuropsychological Evaluation

1. Used to evaluate the specific learning needs of children with epilepsy because many have learning difficulties.
2. Part of the presurgical workup is to determine cognitive deficits and predict long-term consequences of epilepsy, particularly when surgery is performed in an eloquent area.
3. WADA testing (named after its inventor, Juhn Wada) evaluates hemisphere dominance for language and memory when resective surgery is being planned.
   a. Involves the intracarotid administration of amobarbital to anesthetize each hemisphere of the brain separately.
   b. The patient is then shown objects to name and recall over a short period of time.

Laboratory Studies

1. Serum electrolytes, magnesium, calcium, and fasting blood sugar to rule out metabolic causes.
2. Toxicology screen—drug overdoses may cause seizures.
3. Blood cultures—fever and CNS infections may cause seizures.
4. Lumbar puncture may be done if fever is present.
5. Serum levels of seizure medications should follow therapy.
6. Metabolic workup in infants or children with developmental delay.
7. Genetic testing to determine underlying epilepsy syndrome.

Management

Pharmacologic Management

1. Selection of the most effective drug depends on correct identification of the clinical seizure type (see Table 46-2, page 1565).
2. A desirable drug level is one that will prevent seizures without producing undesirable adverse effects.
3. Dosages are adjusted according to blood level, clinical signs, and the child's weight.

(Text continues on page 1568)

Table 46-2   Drugs Used to Treat Seizures in Children

DRUGS AND DOSAGE	ADVANTAGES	ADVERSE EFFECTS	NURSING CONSIDERATIONS
Phenobarbital *Maintenance dosage:* 3–5 mg/kg given q.i.d. or b.i.d. *Status epilepticus:* 10–20 mg/kg, may repeat to maximum 40 mg/kg	Relatively safe and inexpensive	Excitement, hyperactivity, rash, GI distress, dizziness, ataxia, worsening of psychomotor seizures, drowsiness; toxicity causing respiratory depression, circulatory collapse, and renal impairment	• Contraindicated in hepatic or renal dysfunction, hypersensitivity. • I.M. or IV loading dose can be given. • IV rate should not exceed 1 mg/kg/minute.
Phenytoin *Loading dose:* 20 mg/kg *Maintenance:* 3–9 mg/kg given q.i.d. or b.i.d.	Safest drug for psycho-motor seizures; does not cause drowsiness	Hypertrophy of gums, hirsutism, rickets, nystagmus, ataxia, rash; may accentuate absence seizures; toxicity may cause blood dyscrasias and liver damage	• May interact with a wide variety of drugs due to extensive protein binding. • Daily gum massage may prevent gum disease. • Avoid I.M. administration. • If given IV, do not exceed rate of 0.5 mg/kg/minute. • Dilute with normal saline to prevent formation of precipitant.
Ethosuximide *Maintenance:* 20–40 mg/kg given q.i.d. by oral route only	Used for absence seizures	Drowsiness, GI distress, lethargy, euphoria; may aggravate generalized seizures; toxicity causes blood dyscrasias and psychiatric symptoms	• This is contraindicated in hepatic or renal disease. • Dosage should not be increased more frequently than every 4–7 days.
Primidone *Children younger than age 8 years:* 10–25 mg/kg given t.i.d. *Children older than age 8 years:* 750–1,500 mg t.i.d. or q.i.d. by oral route only	May control generalized seizures not responsive to treatment by other drugs	Ataxia, vertigo, GI symptoms; megaloblastic anemia is a rare idiosyncratic reaction; drowsiness in breastfed infants of treated mothers; Stevens-Johnson syndrome, gum hypertrophy, night terrors	• Contraindicated in those hypersensitive to phenobarbital and those with porphyria. • Commonly used with other drugs for mixed seizures. • Dosage increases are usually done weekly until effect is seen.
Diazepam *IV dosage:* 0.04–0.2 mg/kg to maximum of 10 mg if age 5 years or older; maximum of 5 mg if younger than age 5 years *Rectal dosage:* 0.5 mg/kg	Given IV, I.M., or rectally for status epilepticus or as adjunct therapy	Ataxia, drowsiness, fatigue, venous thrombosis or phlebitis at injection site, confusion, depression, headache; tonic status epilepticus when given IV for absence seizures; toxicity may cause somnolence, confusion, diminished reflexes, hypotension, coma, apnea, cardiac arrest	• If administered IV, give no faster than 1 mg/minute. Drug used cautiously in children with limited pulmonary reserve. • Monitor respiratory status closely.
Carbamazepine 20–30 mg/kg t.i.d. or q.i.d. *Maximum dose:* 1,000 mg/day if older than age 12 years; 100 mg b.i.d. if ages 6–12 years; 20 mg/kg/day if younger than age 6 years	Especially useful for major motor and psychomotor seizures	Most likely to occur during initiation of therapy: dizziness, drowsiness, nausea and vomiting; toxicity may cause bone marrow depression (fever, sore throat, oral ulcers, easy bruising)	• Administration with phenytoin reduces half-life of phenytoin; higher dose of phenytoin may be needed. • Contraindicated in previous bone marrow depression and is used cautiously in patients with cardiac, hepatic, or renal problems. • Erythromycin increases plasma levels. • Give with food.

(continued)

Table 46-2 Drugs Used to Treat Seizures in Children *(continued)*

DRUGS AND DOSAGE	ADVANTAGES	ADVERSE EFFECTS	NURSING CONSIDERATIONS
Lorazepam 0.05 to 0.1 mg/kg q 10–15 minutes *Maximum dose:* 4 mg	Given IV or rectally for status epilepticus; longer acting; may cause less respiratory depression	Sedation, dizziness, respiratory depression, hypotension, ataxia, weakness	• Use with caution in patients with hepatic or renal dysfunction. • Monitor respiratory status closely.
Valproic Acid *Loading dose:* 10 mg/kg/day *Maximum dose:* 30–60 mg/kg t.i.d. or q.i.d.	Adjunct for poor seizure control; some success with behavioral problems	Nausea, vomiting, anorexia, amenorrhea, sedation tremor, weight gain, alopecia, hepatotoxicity	• Use caution with hepatic dysfunction. Increases serum levels of phenytoin, phenobarbital, and primidone.
Gabapentin *Loading dose:* 10–15 mg/kg/day in three divided doses *Maximum dose:* 25–40 mg/kg/day in three divided doses	Recommended for add-on therapy in children over age 3 with refractory partial seizures	May interfere with the action of other drugs, including cimetidine; nausea/dizziness	• Must exercise caution in patients with renal impairment.
Topiramate *Loading dose:* 25 mg/day at bedtime for the first week *Maximum dose:* 200–400 mg/day in two divided doses	Recommended for patients ages 2–16 with partial-onset seizures and those seizures related to Lennox-Gastaut syndrome	Most commonly associated with fatigue, dizziness, sleepiness	• Must exercise caution in patients with renal impairment. • Interacts with other anticonvulsants, altering drug concentrations; may interfere with effectiveness of hormonal contraceptives.
Oxcarbazepine *Loading dose:* 8–10 mg/kg/day in two divided doses *Maximum dose:* 900–1,800 mg/day based on weight	Adjunctive therapy in children ages 4–16	Fatigue, abnormal gait, sedation, difficulty in concentration, and memory impairment	• Need to monitor serum sodium. • May interfere with other anticonvulsants by increasing serum concentration; decreases the effectiveness of hormonal contraceptives.
Zonisamide *Loading dose:* 2–4 mg/kg/day *Maximum dose:* 12 mg/kg/day in two to three divided doses	Adjunctive therapy in children older than age 16; especially effective in refractive seizures, such as absence, Lennox-Gastaut syndrome, or infantile spasms	Drowsiness, ataxia, loss of appetite, GI upset, and slowing of mental activity	• Must exercise caution in patients with renal impairment and patients with sensitivity to sulfonamides.
Lacosamide *Adolescents ≥17 years, initial dose:* 50 mg b.i.d.; *maintenance dose:* 200–400 mg/day	Adjunctive therapy in the treatment of partial-onset seizures	Dizziness, ataxia, lightheadedness, excessive drowsiness, headaches, nausea, vomiting, tremors, change in vision or multi-organ sensitivity reactions. Report signs of suicide ideation or depression.	• Carbamazepine, fosphenytoin, phenobarbital, and phenytoin may decrease lacosamide serum concentration. • May prolong PR interval (patients with conduction problems or severe cardiac disease should have ECG tracing prior to/during treatment).

Table 46-2   Drugs Used to Treat Seizures in Children (continued)

DRUGS AND DOSAGE	ADVANTAGES	ADVERSE EFFECTS	NURSING CONSIDERATIONS
Clobazam Lennox-Gastaut (adjunctive), U.S. labeling: *Children ≥2 years:* refer to adult dosing. Epilepsy (adjunctive): Canadian labeling (not in U.S. labeling), oral: *Children <2 years, initial dose:* 0.5–1 mg/kg/day *Children 2–16 years, initial dose:* 5 mg/day; *maximum:* 40 mg/day	Adjunctive treatment of seizures associated with Lennox-Gastaut syndrome (FDA approved in ages ≥2 years and adults); has also been used as monotherapy and adjunctive treatment for other forms of epilepsy	Somnolence, fever, lethargy, upper respiratory tract infection, GI issues, muscle weakness, paradoxical reactions including hyperactive or aggressive behavior, anterograde amnesia, suicidal ideation.	• May be administered with or without food. • Tablets can be crushed and mixed in applesauce. • Tolerance and loss of seizure control have been reported with chronic administration. • Rebound or withdrawal symptoms may occur following abrupt discontinuation or large decreases in dose. • Use caution, adjust dose in patients with hepatic impairment, respiratory disease, and preexisting muscle weakness (Canadian labeling contraindicates use in myasthenia gravis).
Rufinamide, Oral Lennox-Gastaut syndrome: *Children ≥4 years, initial dose:* 10 mg/kg/day in two equally divided doses; *target dose:* 45 mg/kg/day; *maximum dose:* 3,200 mg/day)	Adjunctive therapy of seizures associated with Lennox-Gastaut syndrome (FDA approved in ages ≥4 years and adults)	Cardiovascular: QT shortening (46%–65%; may be dose-related), headache, somnolence, dizziness, fatigue, aggression, anxiety, ataxia/gait disturbance, vertigo, tremor, attention disturbance, back pain, hyperactivity, seizures, status epilepticus, suicidal thinking, pruritus, rash, frequent urination, anemia, leucopenia; visual, respiratory or GI disturbances	• Contraindicated in patients with familial short QT syndrome. • Administer with food. • Monitor for signs and symptoms of anxiety, depression, unusual mood or behavior changes, suicide ideation.
Vigabatrin Adjunctive treatment of seizures (Canadian labeling; not in U.S. labeling): *Children, oral, initial dose:* 40 mg/kg/day in two divided doses, maintenance dosages based on patient weight Infantile spasms: *children 1 month to 2 years, initial dose:* 50 mg/kg/day in two divided doses; *maximum dose:* 150 mg/kg/day	Treatment of infantile spasms; refractory complex partial seizures not controlled by usual treatments Canadian labeling: Additional uses (not in U.S. labeling): Active management of partial or secondary generalized seizures not controlled by usual treatments	Anemia, somnolence, headache, fatigue, irritability, sedation, nystagmus, tremor, insomnia, GI issues, weight gain, edema, peripheral neuropathy, neurotoxicity, suicidal ideation, vision loss, abnormal MRI changes have been reported in some infants	• May be administered without regard to meals. • Assess vision prior to initiating therapy or within 4 weeks from start, at least every 3 months during therapy and at 3–6 months after therapy has been discontinued. • Assess for CNS depression, changes in behavior, and suicidal tendencies.

(continued)

Table 46-2 Drugs Used to Treat Seizures in Children (continued)

DRUGS AND DOSAGE	ADVANTAGES	ADVERSE EFFECTS	NURSING CONSIDERATIONS
Levetiracetam			
Partial-onset seizures: *Children 1 to <6 months, initial dose:* 7 mg/kg b.i.d.; *maximum dose:* 21 mg/kg b.i.d. *Children 6 months to <4 years, initial dose:* 10 mg/kg b.i.d.; *maximum dose:* 25 mg/kg b.i.d. *Children 4 to <16 years, initial dose:* 10 mg/kg/day b.i.d.; *maximum dose:* 30 mg/kg/day b.i.d. (*maximum daily dose:* 3,000 mg/day) Tonic-clonic seizures: *Children 6 to <16 years, initial dose:* 10 mg/kg b.i.d.; *recommended dose:* 30 mg/kg twice daily.	Adjunctive therapy in the treatment of partial onset, myoclonic, and/or primary generalized tonic-clonic seizures	Behavioral/psychiatric symptoms, agitation, amnesia, anxiety, somnolence, fatigue, anorexia and other GI symptoms, ataxia and coordination problems, hypertension	• Be aware of neuropsychiatric adverse events as incidence of behavioral abnormalities and psychiatric symptoms may be increased in children • Use with caution and decrease dose in patients with renal dysfunction. • May be administered without regard to meals.
Stiripentol			
Children ≥3 years and adults, in conjunction with clobazam and valproic acid: increased over 3 days to a final dose of 50 mg/kg/day in 2–3 divided doses with food	Treatment of refractory generalized tonic-clonic seizures in conjunction with clobazam and valproic acid in patients with severe myoclonic epilepsy in infancy (Dravet's syndrome) whose seizures are not adequately controlled with clobazam and valproic acid alone	Clobazam concentrations have increased 2- to 3-fold when given with stiripentol; a clobazam dosage reduction of 25% per week may be required in the presence of clobazam toxicity (drowsiness, hypotonia, and irritability)	• Product available in various countries; not currently available in the United States. • Should be given with food, excluding fruit juice, dairy, or caffeinated or carbonated products.

b.i.d., twice a day; CNS, central nervous system; ECG, electrocardiogram; FDA, Food and Drug Administration; GI, gastrointestinal; I.M., intramuscular; IV, intravenous; q.i.d., four times a day; t.i.d., three times a day.

4. Accurate timing is essential to prevent seizures. This is especially true when the child tends to have seizures at a certain time each day.
5. Enteric-coated tablets, which have a delayed effect, should be used for children who are prone to attacks during sleep.
6. Most anticonvulsants are available in liquid form and in capsules or tablets. Some drugs are less well absorbed in liquid form.
7. It may take several months to find the best combination of medications and the best dosages of each to control the child's seizures. Monotherapy is attempted initially. If this is not successful, a second drug may be tried or added on.
8. Symptoms may not be controlled 100% in every patient.
9. Dosage adjustments may be required from time to time because of the child's growth.
10. Blood counts, urinalysis, therapeutic drug levels, and liver function studies are done at regular intervals in children receiving certain anticonvulsants.

11. Medication is commonly not discontinued until 2 to 3 years after the last attack and if the EEG is normal.
12. Weaning from medication should always be gradual, with stepwise reduction of dosage and withdrawal of one drug at a time.
13. There is some evidence to suggest that long-term use of some anti-epileptic agents may cause intellectual impairment in children with epilepsy.
14. Monitor bone health and provide calcium supplementation if inadequate calcium intake.

Surgical Management

1. If a cerebral lesion, such as a tumor, is found, surgical removal is the treatment of choice.
2. Surgical treatment, such as hemispherectomy, resection of localized seizure focus/epileptogenic zone, or corpus callostomy may be performed in children with severe, medically intractable seizure disorders.

Ketogenic Diet Therapy

1. The ketogenic diet is a high-fat, adequate protein, and low-carbohydrate diet that is used for control of seizures that are refractory to medications. The diet consists of precisely calculated portions of protein, fat, and carbohydrates. The diet causes the child to become ketotic because fats are used for fuel rather than carbohydrates. It is thought that ketones may inhibit seizures, although the mechanism of action is not known.
2. Children on this diet should not be given IV fluids with dextrose.
3. All medications should be in sugar-free and carbohydrate-free suspensions, tablets, or capsules.
4. The child will be on strict fluid restriction.
5. This diet must be carefully monitored by a dietitian.
6. There is some evidence that this diet may put the child at increased risk for developing kidney stones. The risk may be increased when the child receives concomitant therapy with topiramate.
7. Another form of the ketogenic diet is the medium-chain triglyceride (MCT) diet. The MCT diet allows for consumption of more carbohydrates than the classic ketogenic diet, causing lower side effects of vomiting and lack of energy.

Evidence Base Jung da, E., Kang, H. C., Lee, L. S., et al. (2012). Safety and role of ketogenic parenteral nutrition for intractable childhood epilepsy. *Brain & Development, 34*(8), 620–624.

8. Valproic acid must be weaned off prior to commencing treatment with the MCT ketogenic diet to prevent hepatic toxicity.

Modified Atkins Diet

1. Emerging as another form of diet therapy for seizure control.
2. Carbohydrates are restricted to 10 to 20 g per day, with no restriction of protein, fluid, or calories.
3. Hospital admission is not required to initiate the diet. The diet is often self-administered.

Vagal Nerve Stimulation

The vagal nerve stimulator is a pacemaker-like device that is surgically implanted into the chest and attached to coiled electrodes, which are tunneled to the left cervical vagus nerve. The generator emits a programmed stimulus to stop seizures of long duration (usually 1 minute or longer) and children/families may activate the generator to allow for additional stimulus at times of seizure activity. Vagal nerve stimulation is an adjunctive treatment for intractable epilepsy—the mechanism of action is unknown.

Evidence Base Chen, C. Y., Lee, H. T., Chen, C. C., et al. (2012). Short-term results of vagus nerve stimulation in pediatric patients with refractory epilepsy. *Pediatrics and Neonatology, 53*(3), 184–187.

Behavioral Management

1. Psychiatric disorders, especially attention-deficit hyperactivity disorder, depression, and anxiety, are common in children and adolescents who have epilepsy. They are more prevalent in this population than in children and adolescents in the general population or children who have other chronic conditions. Psychosis occurs infrequently.
2. It is important to monitor children with epilepsy for these disorders to ensure early recognition and treatment to minimize lifelong negative sequelae.
3. Further studies are needed to identify the most effective treatments.

General Prognosis

1. General prognosis depends on type and severity of seizure disorder, coexisting mental retardation, organic disorders, and the type of medical management.
2. Medically treated seizures—spontaneous cessation of seizures may occur. Drugs may be gradually discontinued when the child has been free from attacks for an extensive period and the EEG pattern has reverted to normal.
3. Untreated epilepsy—seizures tend to become more numerous.

Complications

1. Apnea/hypoventilation.
2. Hypoglycemia in status epilepticus.
3. Injuries sustained during a seizure.
4. Sudden unexpected death in epilepsy (SUDEP).
5. Osteopenia—due to restrictions in physical activity as a result of seizures or other conditions, such as CP, or treatment with anti-epileptic medications, such as valproic acid and carbamazepine.

Nursing Assessment

1. During a seizure, assess the following:
   a. Indications of difficulties with airway or breathing.
   b. Significant preseizure events, such as noise, excitement, lethargy.
   c. Behavior before the seizure, aura.
   d. Types of movements observed.
   e. Time seizure began and ended.
   f. Site where twitching or contraction began.
   g. Areas of the body involved.
   h. Movements of the eyes and changes in pupil size.
   i. Incontinence.
   j. Color change—pallor, cyanosis, flushing.
   k. Mouth—teeth clenched, abnormal movements, tongue bitten.
   l. Degree of consciousness during the seizure.
2. After a seizure, assess the following:
   a. Degree of memory for recent events.
   b. Types of speech.
   c. Coordination, paralysis, or weakness.
   d. Length of time the child is postictal.
   e. Pupillary reaction.

Nursing Diagnoses

- Risk for Injury related to seizure activity.
- Ineffective Breathing Pattern related to spasms of respiratory musculature.

- Social Isolation related to the child's feelings about seizures or public fears and misconceptions.
- Chronic Low Self-Esteem related to lack of control over seizures.

Nursing Interventions

Ensuring Safety during a Seizure

1. Remove hard toys from the bed.
2. Pad the sides of the crib or side rails of the bed.
3. Assess level of consciousness.
4. Make sure the child can be readily observed.
5. During a seizure, monitor vital signs and assess neurologic status frequently.
6. After a seizure, check the child frequently and report the following:
   a. Behavior changes.
   b. Irritability.
   c. Restlessness.
   d. Listlessness.
   e. Neurologic signs.

Preventing Respiratory Arrest and Aspiration

1. During a seizure, take the following emergency actions:
   a. Clear the area around the child.
   b. Do not restrain the child.
   c. Loosen the clothing around the neck.
   d. Turn the child on side so saliva can flow out of the mouth.
   e. Place a small, folded blanket under the head to prevent trauma if the seizure occurs when the child is on the floor.
2. Do not give anything by mouth or attempt to place anything in the mouth.
3. After the seizure, place the child in a side-lying position.

Promoting Socialization

1. Advise the parents that the child should be in an environment that is as normal as possible.
2. Encourage regular attendance at school after the school nurse and teachers have been notified and emergency treatment of seizures is understood.
3. Encourage the child to participate in organizations and outside activities with limited restrictions.
   a. Each child must be treated individually; the kind of activity depends on the degree of seizure control.
   b. Generally, children with seizure disorders should not be allowed to climb in high places or to swim alone.
   c. Responsible adults should be made aware of the child's disorder.
   d. Children with seizures should wear a MedicAlert bracelet at all times.

Strengthening Self-Esteem

1. Offer reassurance and praise to the parents and child for coping effectively with seizures.
2. Observe parent–child interactions for evidence of rejection or overprotection.
   a. Tell the parents that the child should not be made to feel that he or she can never be left alone.

   b. Advise the parents that the child needs to be disciplined as any other child and should not gain attention directly or indirectly by having seizures.
3. Help the child gain more control by providing education about seizure disorders.
   a. Include the child in treatment planning.
   b. Allow the opportunity to ask questions and answer them honestly.
   c. Make sure the child is aware of restrictions and can deal with them.
   d. Encourage parents gradually to give the child responsibility for taking medications.
4. Help the older child or adolescent to achieve independence.
   a. Encourage the parents to give the older child the opportunity for privacy to discuss concerns with the physician.
   b. Encourage parents to allow the older child to use his or her own judgment in making decisions.
   c. Help the older child to develop realistic educational and career goals.
5. Help parents deal with a noncompliant child. Refusal to take medications requires prompt intervention. Children need to be reassured that they are not abnormal, but that they do require medication to control seizures. Children need to be taught that they are normal and can have normal lives. This is most commonly seen during adolescence. Family counseling may be necessary.
6. Teach the parents and child seizure safety.

Community and Home Care Considerations

1. Follow community and home care considerations listed under "Cerebral Palsy" on page 1548.
2. Make sure that the home environment is safe, especially where the child sleeps and plays. Remove toys with sharp edges or parts or small pieces the child could choke on if they are put in the mouth and cover very hard surfaces, such as the floor, against which the child could fall.
3. Reinforce parents' knowledge and ability to dispense seizure medications.
4. Help the family acquire a medical alert tag that the child should wear at all times, especially when attending daycare or school.
5. Make sure that parents and caregivers know the seizure type, name of all medications, when to call the health care provider, and when to call 911.
   a. The health care provider should be notified of an increased frequency of seizures or new onset of symptoms.
   b. Emergency response should be activated when the child has been seizing for longer than 5 minutes or is unresponsive after a seizure.
6. Make sure that parents and caregivers are trained in CPR and seizure management.

Family Education and Health Maintenance

1. Describe completely any examinations, evaluations, and treatments that the child is receiving.

2. Provide information regarding the disorder itself.
   a. Epilepsy is not contagious, is seldom dangerous, and does not indicate insanity or mental retardation.
   b. Most children with epilepsy have infrequent seizures and with medications can completely control their convulsions.
   c. The child may have normal intelligence and can live a useful and productive life.
3. Prepare the parents for the fact that it may take several months of regulating drug dosages before adequate control is obtained.
4. Encourage parents and older children to obtain genetic counseling.
   a. There is no proof that epilepsy is hereditary. However, there is a genetic predisposition with certain types of seizures, such as absence, febrile, and juvenile myoclonic seizures.
   b. It is impossible to predict accurately the possibility of the seizure disorder appearing in siblings or offspring of the affected child.
5. Teach the parents and child factors that may precipitate a seizure.
   a. The child should be kept in optimal physical condition with routine immunizations, medical care, dental care, and eye care and should receive prompt evaluation and treatment of infections.
   b. Excessive fatigue, dehydration, and sleep deprivation should be avoided.
   c. Irregular, fluctuating schedules are detrimental. Advise the parents to maintain a daily routine.
   d. Fever or illness of any kind can trigger seizures in children diagnosed with epilepsy even though their seizures may otherwise be under control.
6. For additional resources, refer families to *www.aboutkidshealth .ca/En/ResourceCentres/Epilepsy/Pages/default.aspx*.

Evaluation: Expected Outcomes

- Padded bed rails in place.
- Breathing unlabored after seizure, with lungs clear.
- Parents and child verbalize understanding of child's ability to participate in activities.
- Child participates in treatment plan, takes medications as ordered without reminders; serum drug levels are therapeutic.

Febrile Seizures

Febrile seizures occur in childhood after 1 month of age and are associated with a febrile illness that is not caused by an infection of the central nervous system. There is no history of a previous neonatal seizure or a previous unprovoked seizure and the child does not have an acute symptomatic seizure. Most febrile seizures occur between 6 and 36 months of age, with the peak incidence at 18 months. In North America, 3% to 4% of all children will have at least one febrile seizure before age 5 years.

Febrile seizures may be simple or complex:

- Simple febrile seizures—brief, last less than 10 minutes; tonic-clonic convulsion occurs once in 24 hours; absence of focal features; resolve spontaneously; 70% to 75% of febrile seizures are simple.

- Complex febrile seizures—prolonged, last more than 10 to 15 minutes; focal in nature; may recur within the same febrile illness over 24 hours; 9% to 35% of febrile seizures are complex.

Pathophysiology and Etiology

1. Febrile seizures are associated with first- or second-degree relatives with a history of febrile seizure, day care attendance, developmental delay, influenza A viral infection, herpes virus–6 infection, metapneumovirus, and iron-deficiency anemia.
2. Seizures accompany intercurrent infections, especially viral illness, tonsillitis, pharyngitis, and otitis.
3. They appear to occur in a familial pattern, although exact pattern of inheritance is not completely understood. Children with a positive family history of febrile seizures have a greater risk of recurrent febrile seizures.
4. It is unclear whether the seizure is triggered by a rapid rise in temperature or the actual temperature attained.
5. Most febrile seizures consist of generalized tonic-clonic seizures (see above).

Clinical Manifestations

1. Fever is usually more than 101.8° F (38.8° C) rectally.
2. Seizures usually occur near the onset of fever rather than after prolonged fever.

Diagnostic Evaluation

Measures are directed toward delineating the cause of any seizure as precisely as possible so its implications and prognosis may be discussed with the parents. Diagnostic methods may include the following:

1. Careful history-taking and physical examination.
2. CSF examination to detect CNS infection—strongly recommended in children experiencing their first febrile seizure, especially in children less than age 18 months.
3. CBC and urinalysis to detect signs of infection.
4. Cultures of nasopharynx, blood, or urine, as appropriate, to determine cause of fever.
5. Blood glucose, calcium, and electrolyte levels to detect abnormalities that may cause seizures.
6. EEG (for atypical seizures or for a child at risk for epilepsy).
   a. Demonstrates mild, postictal slowing soon after the attack.
   b. Pattern is generally normal after a few days.

Management

The goals of treatment are to control seizures and decrease temperature.

1. Administration of antipyretics and other cooling measures.
2. Prevention of febrile seizures with anticonvulsants is not common practice. Prompt control of fevers is the desired course of action.
3. Rectal diazepam gel is the preferred method of acute seizure management for prolonged seizures greater than 5 minutes or for someone who is at risk for status epilepticus. It is used only in extreme cases.
   a. Intermittent therapy with phenobarbital during febrile episodes is apparently of no value because of the length of time required to achieve therapeutic serum levels of the drug.

4. Airway management, as required.
5. Prognosis—likelihood of recurrence is about 33% in those who have had two febrile seizures. The younger the child is at the time of the first seizure, the greater the risk for additional febrile seizures.
6. The risk of development of nonfebrile seizures is relatively low (about 5%). At risk are children who demonstrate the following characteristics:
   a. Prolonged or complex febrile seizures.
   b. Abnormal or suspected abnormal development before the first seizure.
   c. Family history of nonfebrile seizures.
   d. Persistent EEG abnormalities.

Complications

Injury may occur during seizure.

Nursing Assessment and Interventions

Nursing assessment and interventions are the same as for seizure disorders, pages 1569–1570.

Family Education and Health Maintenance

1. Reinforce realistic, reassuring information, such as the following:
   a. A seizure does not necessarily imply that the underlying disease is serious.
   b. Febrile seizures are relatively common in children.
   c. The prognosis depends on the cause of the seizure.
      i. A single febrile seizure does not indicate later chronic epilepsy.
      ii. Children usually outgrow the tendency to develop febrile seizures by age 4 or 5.
      iii. Occasional or brief seizures are thought to not have any effect on the child's overall development, although this is controversial.
2. Discuss and demonstrate emergency management of seizures.
   a. The child should be positioned on the side, on a flat surface from which he or she cannot fall.
   b. The surface should be padded, if possible, to prevent injury.
   c. An adult should stay with the child to monitor the airway and breathing until the seizure is complete.
   d. If the child vomits, immediately clear the mouth of all foreign material.
3. Stress that medical evaluation is indicated as soon as the child develops a fever.
   a. Review technique of temperature measurement.
   b. Prompt administration of antipyretic measures is necessary when the child is febrile but may not prevent a febrile seizure.
4. Review administration schedule, adverse reactions, and appropriate follow-up regarding anticonvulsant therapy.
5. Let the family know that when a child is diagnosed with febrile seizures, future events can be adequately managed at home and do not require emergency transport if less than 5 minutes in duration. However, parents should notify pediatrician of febrile illness and seizure occurrence.

Subdural Hematoma

Subdural hematoma refers to an accumulation of fluid, blood, and its degradation products within the potential space between the dura and arachnoid (subdural space). Subdural hematomas are classified as acute or chronic, depending on the time between injury and the onset of symptoms.

Also see Chapter 15 for care of unconscious patient, ICP monitoring, and other neurologic care.

Pathophysiology and Etiology

Causes

1. Direct or indirect trauma to the head:
   a. Birth trauma.
   b. Accidental causes.
   c. Purposeful violence, as in cases of child abuse.
2. Meningitis.

Classification

1. Acute syndrome—presents as an acute problem, closely related to the time of presumed injury.
2. Chronic:
   a. Signs and symptoms are nonlocalizing and subacute.
   b. This is the most common type of subdural hematoma in children.
   c. It is usually difficult to delineate the exact time and type of injury because the precipitating episode may appear relatively insignificant.

Altered Physiology

1. Trauma to the head causes tearing of the delicate subdural veins, resulting in small hemorrhages into the subdural space. (Bleeding may be of arterial origin in cases of acute subdural hematoma.)
2. As the blood breaks down, there is an increased capillary permeability and effusion of blood cells and protein into the subdural space.
3. The breakdown products of blood stimulate the growth of connective tissue and capillaries largely from the dura.
4. A membrane is formed that usually extends frontally and laterally over the hemispheres, surrounding the clot.
5. Fluid accumulates within the membrane and increases the width of the subdural space.
6. Further hemorrhages occur.
7. The lesion enlarges, compressing the brain and expanding the skull, and, if unrelieved, ultimately causes cerebral atrophy or death from compression and herniation.
8. The lesion may arrest spontaneously at any point.
9. Further bleeding may occur into an already existing sac and may increase symptoms.
10. In long-standing subdural hematoma, the fluid may disappear, leaving a constricting membrane that prevents normal brain growth.

Clinical Manifestations

Acute

1. Typically present with continuous unconsciousness from the time of injury, but child may present with a lucid interval.
2. Ensuing manifestations include deterioration of LOC, progressive hemiplegia, focal seizures, and signs of brain stem involvement and herniation (pupillary enlargement, changes in vital signs, decerebrate posturing, and respiratory failure; see Figure 46-3).

Chronic

This has a slow, gradual onset; symptoms are variable and are related to the age of the child.

1. Infants—early signs:
   a. Anorexia, difficulty feeding, vomiting.
   b. Irritability.
   c. Low-grade fever.
   d. Retinal hemorrhages.
   e. Failure to gain weight.
2. Infants—later signs:
   a. Enlargement of the head.
   b. Bulging and pulsation of the anterior fontanelle.
   c. Tight, glossy scalp with dilated scalp veins.
   d. Strabismus, pupillary inequality, ocular palsies (rare).
   e. Hyperactive reflexes.
   f. Seizures.
   g. Retarded motor development.
3. Older children—early signs:
   a. Lethargy, anorexia.
   b. Symptoms of increased ICP (vomiting, irritability, headache).
4. Older children—later signs (may also occur immediately if bleeding takes place rapidly):
   a. Seizures.
   b. Coma.

Diagnostic Evaluation

1. Clinical features.
   a. In infants who are irritable, have failed to gain weight, and have developed an enlarged and tense fontanelle, chronic subdural hematoma should be suspected.
   b. Biparietal bulge of the head.
2. Imaging.
   a. Diagnosis and size of hematoma is confirmed by CT and, if necessary, by MRI.

Management

Acute Subdural Hematoma

This requires evacuation of the clot through a burr hole or craniotomy.

Chronic Subdural Hematoma

1. Repeated subdural taps are done to remove the collecting fluid.
   a. In infants, the needle can be inserted through the fontanelle or suture line.
   b. In older children, burr holes into the skull are necessary before the needle can be inserted.
   c. Subdural taps may be the only treatment required if the fluid disappears entirely and symptoms do not recur.
   d. Concurrently, treatment is instituted to correct anemia, electrolyte imbalance, and malnutrition.
2. Shunting procedure may be indicated if repeated taps fail to significantly reduce the volume or protein content of the subdural collections. Shunting is usually to the peritoneal cavity.

Prognosis

1. Treatment is usually successful when the diagnosis is made before cerebral atrophy and a fixed neurologic deficit have occurred. In such cases, subsequent development is normal.
2. Prognosis depends on the effect of the initial trauma on the brain and the effect of continued fluid collection.
3. Mortality in massive, acute subdural bleeding is very high, even if promptly diagnosed.

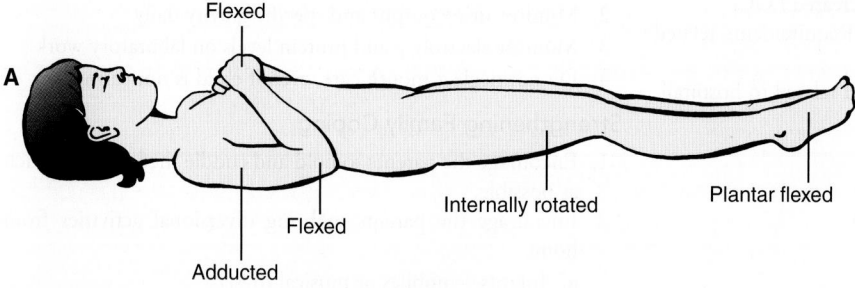

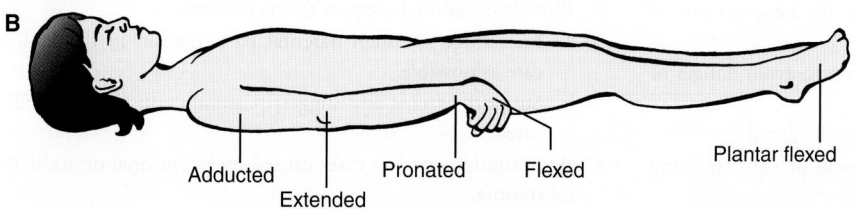

Figure 46-3. Primitive posturing in unconscious states due to loss of motor control. (A) Decorticate posturing occurs when cortical loss is present. **(B)** Decerebrate posturing occurs when the midbrain is involved.

Complications

1. Mental retardation.
2. Ocular abnormalities.
3. Seizures.
4. Spasticity, paralysis.
5. Brain stem herniation and death.
6. Neurologic impairment (cognitive or physical).

Nursing Assessment

Assess the child's neurologic status to evaluate the effectiveness of treatment or to identify disease progress.

1. Observe general behavior, especially irritability, lethargy, and evidence of personality changes. It is important to obtain a thorough history from the parents regarding normal behavior and level of functioning so abnormalities can be more easily recognized.
2. Evaluate appetite and feeding difficulties, including vomiting.
3. Assess vital signs for signs of increased ICP—be alert for the following:
   a. Increased systolic BP.
   b. Widened pulse pressure.
   c. Decreased pulse or irregularities.
   d. Changes in respiratory rate or difficulty breathing.
4. Assess LOC; describe response explicitly, including what type of stimulus was required to elicit a response.
5. Assess pupillary and visual changes, especially dilated pupil, double vision, lack of response to light, alterations in visual acuity, and nonsymmetric or abnormal eye movements.
6. Monitor for seizures.
7. Evaluate motor function, including ability to move all extremities. The ability to grasp should be checked and compared bilaterally.
8. Inspect for drainage of CSF from the nose or ears, indicating fractured skull with CSF leak.

Nursing Diagnoses

- Ineffective Tissue Perfusion: Cerebral related to disease process.
- Impaired Physical Mobility related to decreased LOC.
- Imbalanced Nutrition: Less Than Body Requirements related to decreased LOC.
- Ineffective Family Coping: Compromised related to hospitalization of child.

Nursing Interventions

Maintaining Cerebral Tissue Perfusion

1. Avoid additional increase in ICP.
   a. Maintain a quiet environment.
   b. Avoid sudden changes in position.
   c. Organize nursing activities to allow for long periods of uninterrupted rest.
   d. Carefully regulate fluid administration to avoid danger of fluid overload.
   e. Measure urine output and record specific gravity.
   f. Administer laxatives or suppositories to prevent straining during a bowel movement.

2. Assist with subdural taps.
   a. Protect and restrain the child, as needed (see page 1542).
   b. Hold the child securely to avoid injury caused by sudden movement.
   c. Apply firm pressure over the puncture site for a few minutes after the tap has been completed to prevent fluid leakage along the needle tract.
   d. Observe the child frequently after the procedure for shock or drainage from the site of the tap.
   e. Note whether there is serous drainage or frank blood.
   f. Reinforce the dressing, as needed, to prevent contamination of the wound.
   g. Monitor temperature frequently and monitor for signs of developing infection.
   h. Report purulent drainage from the site of the subdural tap.
3. Avoid discussing the child's condition near the bed. Even though comatose, the child may be able to hear.
4. Have emergency equipment available for resuscitation.

Preventing Complications of Immobility

1. Change the child's position frequently and provide meticulous skin care to prevent hypostatic pneumonia and decubitus ulcers.
2. Prevent contractures.
   a. Apply passive ROM exercises to all extremities.
   b. Place pillows appropriately to support the child's body in good alignment.
   c. Use splints designed by physical therapy, as instructed.
3. Suction the child as necessary to remove secretions in the mouth and nasopharynx.
4. Observe for signs of respiratory or urinary infection related to stasis.
5. Keep the child's eyes well lubricated to prevent corneal damage.

Maintaining Nutritional Status

1. Provide nutrition and fluids through nasogastric feedings, as ordered. Observe for gastric distention.
2. Monitor urine output and specific gravity daily.
3. Monitor electrolyte and protein levels on laboratory work.
4. Do not neglect mouth care, even if child is not eating.

Strengthening Family Coping

1. Encourage the parents to hold and cuddle the infant as much as possible.
2. Encourage the parents to bring diversional activities from home.
   a. Infants—mobiles or musical toys.
   b. Older children—quiet games, books, dolls.
3. Provide emotional support to the parents.
   a. Encourage as much parental participation in the child's care as possible.
   b. Support parents and suggest pastoral counseling, as indicated.
4. Be nonjudgmental in cases caused by intentional or accidental trauma.

5. Make sure that cases of suspected child abuse have been reported to the appropriate agency and that parents have been referred for counseling.

6. Encourage visitation by siblings.

Community and Home Care Considerations

1. Follow community and home care considerations listed under "Cerebral Palsy" on page 1548.

2. Perform periodic developmental assessments and reinforce the need to report any signs of developmental delay to the health care provider.

3. Discuss return-to-activity/play as the child progresses, as directed by health care provider.

Family Education and Health Maintenance

1. Reinforce explanations in the following areas:
   a. Condition.
   b. Causes of the child's specific symptoms.
   c. Need and rationale for treatment.
   d. Postoperative and recovery expectations.

2. Encourage parents to keep all follow-up appointments for medical evaluation and physical and occupational therapy.

3. Teach parents safety measures to prevent injuries in the future.

4. Assist parents in seeking additional support and resources through social work department, church groups, community agencies, or private counseling.

Evaluation: Expected Outcomes

- Drowsy but responsive to verbal stimuli; pupils equal and reactive to light; vital signs stable; ventricular tap site without drainage.
- Skin without signs of erythema or breakdown; full ROM of all joints; functional position maintained.
- Tolerates nasogastric feedings without distention; urine output sufficient.
- Parents participate in child's care, hold and read to child; parents receive counseling.

SELECTED REFERENCES

Benini, R., & Shevell, M. (2012). Updates in the treatment of spasticity associated with cerebral palsy. *Current Treatments in Neurology, 14*(6), 650–659.

Bialer, M. (2012). Why are antiepileptic drugs used for nonepileptic conditions? *Epilepsia, 53* (Suppl. 7), 26–33.

Blevins, J. Y. (2011). Oral health care for hospitalized children. *Pediatric Nursing, 37*(5), 229–235.

Cervasio, K. (2011). Lower extremity orthoses in children with spastic quadriplegic cerebral palsy implications for nurses, parents, and caregivers. *Orthopaedic Nursing, 30*(1), 155–159.

Chen, C. Y., Lee, H. T., Chen, C. C., et al. (2012). Short-term results of vagus nerve stimulation in pediatric patients with refractory epilepsy. *Pediatrics and Neonatology, 53*(3), 184–187.

Chiron, C., & Dulac, O. (2011). The pharmacologic treatment of dravet syndrome. *Epilepsia, 52*(Suppl. 2), 72–75.

Chu-Shore, C. J., & Thiele, E. A. (2010). New drugs for pediatric epilepsy. *Seminars in Pediatric Neurology, 17*, 214–223.

Collins, S. (2011). The psychosocial effect of epilepsy on adolescents and young adults. *Nursing Standard, 25*(43), 48–56.

De Los Angeles Beytia, M., Vry, J., & Kirschner, J. (2012). Drug treatment of Duchenne muscular dystrophy: Available evidence and perspectives. *Acta Myologica,* XXXI: 4–8.

Delanty, N., Jones, J., & Tonner, F. (2012). Adjunctive levetiracetam in children, adolescents, and adults with primary generalized seizures: Open-label, noncomparative, multicenter, long-term follow-up study. *Epilepsia, 53*(1), 111–119.

Delgado, M. R., Hirtz, D., Aisen, M., et al. (2010). Practice parameter: Pharmacologic treatment of spasticity in children and adolescents with cerebral palsy (an evidence-based review). *Neurology, 74*, 336–343.

Ducruet, A. F., Grobelny, B.T., & Zacharia, B. E., et al. (2012). The surgical management of chronic subdural hematoma. *Neurosurgical Review, 35*(2), 155–169.

Duffy, L. V. (2011). Parental coping and childhood epilepsy: the need for future research. *Journal of Neuroscience Nurses, 43*(1), 29–35.

Fehlings, D., Switzer, L., Agarwal, P., et al. (2012). Informing evidence-based clinical practice guidelines for children with cerebral palsy at risk of osteoporosis: A systematic review. *Developmental Medicine and Child Neurology, 54*, 106–116.

Foster, H., Popplewell, L., & Dickson, G. (2012). Genetic therapeutic approaches for Duchenne muscular dystrophy. *Human Genetic Therapy, 23*(7), 676–687.

Frimberger, D., & Kropp, B. P. (2012). The current management of the neurogenic bladder in children with spina bifida. *Pediatric Clinics of North America, 59*(4), 757–767.

Go, C. Y., MacKay, M. T., Weiss, S. K., et al. (2012). Evidence-based guideline update: Medical treatment of infantile spasms: Report of the Guideline Development Subcommittee of the American Academy of Neurology and the Practice Committee of the Child Neurology Society. *Neurology, 78*, 1974–1980.

Gordon, A. M. (2011). To constrain or not to constrain, and other stories of intensive upper extremity training for children with unilateral cerebral palsy. *Developmental Medicine and Child Neurology, 53*(Suppl. 4), 56–61.

Jung da, E., Kang, H. C., Lee, L. S., et al. (2012). Safety and role of ketogenic parenteral nutrition for intractable childhood epilepsy. *Brain & Development, 34*(8), 620–624.

Kulkarni, A. (2010). Quality of life in childhood hydrocephalus: a review. *Childs Nervous System, 26*, 737–743.

Lipson-Aisen, M., Kerkovich, D., Mast, J., et al. (2011). Cerebral palsy: Clinical care and neurological rehabilitation. *Lancet Neurology, 10*, 844–852.

Liu, Y. M. (2008). Medium-chain triglyceride (mct) ketogenic therapy. *Epilepsia, 49*(Suppl. 8), 33–36.

Narayanan, U. G. (2012). Management of children with ambulatory cerebral palsy: An evidence-based review. *Journal of Pediatric Orthopedics, 32* (Suppl. 2), S172–181.

Oskoui, M. (2012). Growing up with cerebral palsy: Contemporary challenges of healthcare transition. *Canadian Journal of Neurological Sciences, 39*, 23–25.

Paul, S. P., Blaikley, S., & Chinthapalli, R. (2012). Clinical update: Febrile convulsion in childhood. *Community Practice, 85*(7), 36–38.

Pellock, J. M., Hrachovy, R., Shinnar, S., et al. (2010). Infantile spasms: A US concensus report. *Epilepsia, 51*(10), 2175–2189.

Resnick, T., Arzimanoglou, A., Brown, L. W., et al. (2011). Rufinamide from clinical trials to clinical practice in the United States and Europe. *Epileptic Disorders, 13* (Suppl. 1), S 27–S 43.

Sergott, R. C. (2010). Recommendations for visual evaluations of patients treated with vigabatrin. *Current Opinion in Ophthalmology, 21*, 442–446.

Shorvon, S., & Tomson, T. (2011). Sudden unexpected death in epilepsy. *Lancet, 378*, 2028–2038.

Stafstrom, C. E., Arnason, B. G. W., Baram, T. Z., et al. (2011). Treatment of infantile spasms: Emerging insights from clinical and basic science perspectives. *Journal of Child Neurology, 26*(11), 1141–1421.

Walshe, M., Smith, M., & Pennington, L. (2012). Interventions for drooling in children with cerebral palsy. *Cochrane Database Systematic Review, 15, 2* CD008624.

Wheless, J. W., Gibson, P. A., Rosbeck, L. L., et al. (2012). Infantile spasms (West Syndrome): Update and resources for pediatricians and providers to share with parents. *BMC Pediatrics, 12*(108).

47

Pediatric Eye and Ear Problems

CONDITIONS OF THE EYE

Also see Chapter 16 for additional information on eye problems.

Infectious Processes

Infectious processes of the eye include conjunctivitis, periorbital or orbital cellulitis, and hordeolum (stye). They are characterized by inflammation, infectious exudate, and tissue damage caused by microbes, such as bacteria, viruses, or *Chlamydia trachomatis*. Conjunctivitis is a common problem, affecting almost all children at some time or another.

Pathophysiology and Etiology

1. Microbes are usually introduced into the eye or surrounding tissues including eyelids, eyebrow, and cheeks by direct contact with infected objects. Orbital infections occur secondary to microbial spread from an adjacent sinus, direct inoculation from trauma (insect bites or eyelid injury), surrounding skin infection, or postoperative contamination or, in the case of sepsis or dental infection, from hematogenous spread.
2. This initiates an inflammatory response that includes dilation of blood vessels, swelling, antibody production, and destruction of the offending agent by white blood cells.
3. Common bacterial agents include nontypeable *Haemophilus influenzae, Streptococcus pneumoniae, Moraxella catarrhalis*, and *Staphylococcus aureus*. Viral infections are common and are usually caused by adenovirus. Less commonly, herpesvirus may occur.
4. The infecting agents can be contagious and easily spread from person to person or from infected objects (fomites). Therefore, conjunctivitis may occur in outbreaks in which several children in the same family, classroom, or community are affected.

5. Allergic reaction from pollen can be a major contributor to conjunctivitis.

Clinical Manifestations

Redness of the eye is a common ophthalmic symptom. The problem causing this redness could arise from within or outside the globe. These range from cases of simple inflammation following minor trauma to severe cases, such as orbital cellulitis and tumor. Such diverse causes of redness must be differentiated from the red eye of noninfectious processes (see Table 47-1).

Conjunctivitis
1. Inflammation of palpebral and bulbar conjunctival layer of eyes that leads to dilation of the blood vessels.
2. Eyelid and conjunctiva edema.
3. Excessive tearing or exudate.
4. Gritty feeling in the eye and itching.
5. Photophobia.
6. Fluctuating blurring and cloudy vision.

Periorbital Cellulitis
1. Inflammation of the eyelids and surrounding tissues that does not involve eyeball or internal structures.
2. No significant fever.
3. No pain on eye movement.
4. No impaired vision.
5. Age less than 5 years.

Orbital Cellulitis
1. Red, swollen eyelid with swelling and inflammation of soft tissues surrounding the eye.
2. Tenderness, pain.
3. Proptosis (forward displacement of the eye) and, sometimes, chemosis (edema of conjunctiva).

Table 47-1   Common Causes of Eye Redness in Children

CAUSE	ASSOCIATED SYMPTOMS	MANAGEMENT
Conjunctivitis		
Viral	Commonly associated with other symptoms of generalized viral illness Commonly known as "pink eye," with adenovirus and epidemic keroconjunctivitis being the most infectious	Hygiene (see page 1578), rest
Bacterial	Yellow, green, or white discharge, photophobia	Antibiotic eyedrops or ointment, hygiene
Chlamydial	Cough, history of maternal infection	Systemic antibiotic
Herpetic	Pain, photophobia, skin lesions	Evaluation by specialist, antiviral agents
Allergic	Itching, seasonal onset of symptoms, other allergic symptoms, watery discharge	Topical mast cell stabilizer eyedrops, histamine-1 antagonist eyedrops, avoidance of allergens
Chemical	Watery discharge, onset of symptoms when exposed to cigarettes or other irritants	Avoidance of irritating substances
Trauma	Pain, photophobia, increased tear production	May require eye patch, referral to specialist
Congenital glaucoma	Increased tear production, cloudiness of cornea	Referral to specialist

4. Restrictive eye movement and orbital tension.
5. Increased temperature of affected areas.
6. Reduced visual acuity.
7. Elevated fever.
8. Age over 5 years.

Hordeolum

1. Inflammation of lubricating glands of eyelids and eyelashes.
2. Unilateral.
3. Pustule in area of eyelash follicle.
4. Tenderness, pain.
5. Localized eyelid swelling and erythema.
6. "Lump under the eyelid."

Diagnostic Evaluation

1. Due to the cost of and the delay in results, laboratory testing is limited to cases which fail to respond to treatment. Appropriate laboratory media must be used to transport a swab of eye exudate for bacterial culture, viral culture, and antigen testing. Swabs should be obtained immediately, but treatment not delayed, especially in the cases of suspected *N. gonorrhoea* or *C. trachomatis.*
2. Screening vision exam may be done; a thorough visual and ocular exam may be done if vision is impaired or if internal involvement is suspected.
3. A dendritic ulcer caused by herpesvirus can be visualized by instilling fluorescein dye and examining the cornea with a cobalt-filtered blue light, looking for the dendrite lesion.
4. Clinical evaluation and computed tomography scan are the best methods to distinguish periorbital from orbital cellulitis.

 NURSING ALERT A child who has a painful red eye should be referred immediately for medical evaluation because this could indicate an infectious process, exposure to a chemical or foreign body, or other traumatic etiology.

Management

1. Allergic conjunctivitis may respond to removal of the underlying allergen. Treatment may include systemic or topical agents (depending on severity), including antihistamine, mast cell stabilizer, and corticosteroid.

 DRUG ALERT Topical corticosteroids should only be prescribed by an ophthalmologist because they may aggravate a herpetic infection.

2. Antibiotic eyedrops or ointment—such as erythromycin, trimethoprim sulfate and polymyxin B, sulfacetamide, ciprofloxacin, tobramycin, azithromycin, or doxycycline—will shorten the course of bacterial conjunctivitis and make the child more comfortable.
3. Hordeolum will usually resolve without antibiotic treatment. Warm compresses applied four times daily are recommended. Lid washes of diluted baby shampoo in water aid with drainage. Incision and drainage may be necessary to promote healing.
4. Systemic antibiotic treatment is indicated for orbital cellulitis. These children may be admitted to the hospital for close observation and aggressive management. A multidisciplinary approach, including an ophthalmologist, pediatrician, otolaryngologist, and, possibly, a neurosurgeon may be indicated.

Complications

1. Permanent scarring of the cornea and visual impairment with herpetic infection, *N. gonorrhoeae*, and *C. trachomatis*.
2. Spread of orbital cellulitis to the central nervous system, with optic nerve damage and vision loss.
3. Eyelid deformity.
4. Septicemia.
5. Ptosis and strabismus after resolution of orbital cellulitis.

Nursing Assessment

1. Assess nature and extent of symptoms and their effect on child's activities.
2. Assess visual acuity.
3. Determine resources available to family for treatment and rehabilitation.

Nursing Diagnoses

- Risk for Infection (spread, secondary, transmission to others) related to hand-to-hand or hand-to-object contact.
- Acute Pain and discomfort related to tissue swelling, inflammation, and light sensitivity.

Nursing Interventions

Preventing Spread of Infection

1. Perform or teach proper cleansing of drainage.
   a. Use warm water or saline and a disposable applicator, such as cotton balls or gauze.
   b. Use a separate applicator for each eye.
   c. Wipe from inner to outer canthus to avoid contamination of the other eye.
2. Teach self-care measures to prevent spread to others.
   a. Observe good handwashing practices.
   b. Wipe eyes and nose with tissues and dispose promptly. Do not wipe the nose, then eyes with same tissue.
   c. Avoid rubbing eyes to prevent spread to other eye.
3. Administer and teach proper instillation of eyedrops or ointment (see page 576).
4. Administer oral or IV antibiotics, as prescribed.
5. Advise parents to only use eye drops prescribed or recommended by a health care provider and dispose of leftover medication at end of treatment period.

Minimizing Pain

1. Apply warm compresses to affected area.
2. Suggest darkened room and sunglasses for patients with photophobia.
3. Administer an analgesic, as prescribed.
4. Administer lubricating eyedrops and ointment, as needed.
5. Minimize environmental stimulation.

Family Education and Health Maintenance

1. Advise of ways to prevent transmission to others.
   a. Handwashing is the most important factor in infection control.
   b. Do not share washcloths or towels or handkerchief.
   c. Change pillowcases frequently.
   d. Avoid swimming until infection is resolved.
   e. Return child to school only after having received antibiotic treatment for 24 hours.
   f. Dispose of contaminated items in proper receptacles.
   g. Discontinue use of contact lenses until infection is cleared.
2. Advise parents of indications for reevaluation by health care provider.
   a. Lack of response to antibiotic treatment.
   b. Increased swelling and tenderness; eye pain.
   c. Worsening of visual acuity.
   d. Identification of dry eye.
   e. Development of additional symptoms such as fever.
3. Encourage routine follow-up visits and vision evaluation.
4. Advise about proper detection and early treatment of sinus, dental, and other infection.
5. Recommend updated immunization, including the *Haemophilus influenzae* type B vaccine in children.

Evaluation: Expected Outcomes

- Parents perform treatment correctly; hygiene procedures followed.
- Patient verbalizes less pain; tolerates bright light.

Congenital Problems

Congenital problems of the eye include structural defects present at birth or developing soon thereafter. These are usually genetically transmitted and include cataract, dacryostenosis, glaucoma, ptosis, and strabismus. See Table 47-2 for pathophysiology, clinical manifestations, and management of each.

Nursing Assessment

1. Assess for red light reflex, especially in neonates and infants. Absence or asymmetry of the red light reflex may indicate congenital cataract or an intraocular tumor or other eye disease.
2. Inspect the eyes for redness of conjunctiva, cloudiness of the cornea, excessive tearing, drooping eyelids that partially occlude the pupil, or obvious misalignment, which provide clues to congenital eye problems.
3. Assess visual acuity routinely in infants and children. Changes in acuity may be the first manifestation of a problem or indication of effectiveness of treatment. Prompt referral to a specialist is necessary.
4. Perform pupillary light reflex test using a penlight or "muscle light" or use a distant light source to help detect strabismus.
   a. Hirschberg's test for symmetry of the pupillary light reflexes—normally, the light reflexes are in the same position in each pupil when a light is shone on the bridge of the nose, but asymmetrical reflection will occur with strabismus (positive Hirschberg's test).
   b. Krimsky test—prism is used to center the light reflex in each eye. It is said to be more accurate than the Hirschberg method.
5. Perform the cover–uncover test to detect latent strabismus caused by weak eye muscles. When the patient is fixated on

Table 47-2 Congenital Eye Problems

CONDITION AND DESCRIPTION	CLINICAL MANIFESTATIONS	MANAGEMENT
Congenital Cataract Opacity of the lens. Possible causes include abnormal embryonic development, intrauterine infection, metabolic disorders, retinopathy of prematurity. Incidence is 1 in 250 neonates.	• Absence of red reflex • Visible clouding of lens • Varying impairment of vision, depending on size, location, and density of cataract • May result in amblyopia	• Surgical removal within first 3 months to promote visual stimulation. • Postoperative care: sedation for first 24 hours to prevent crying, vomiting, and increased IOP; dilating eyedrops; antibiotic and steroid ointments to prevent infection; eye patch and shield for several days. • Aggressive optical therapy and patching of nonoperative eye; monitoring for IOP.
Dacryostenosis Relatively common obstruction of the nasolacrimal duct caused by incomplete duct development and persistence of membrane at lower end of duct. Tears cannot exit via the duct into the nasal cavity and continuously spill over onto the cheek. May be unilateral or bilateral.	• Excessive tearing and spilling onto cheek • Crusted eyelashes and lids • Excoriated cheek • Normal-appearing eye structures and vision • Possible episodes of secondary conjunctivitis and lacrimal duct infection • Increased risk of dacryocystitis	• Resolves spontaneously in 90% of infants in first year of life. • Some recommend gentle massage of lacrimal duct, but effectiveness has not been documented. • Topical antibiotics for secondary infection. • Surgical probing of duct if persists beyond age 12 months; more complex surgery if probing unsuccessful.
Glaucoma Rare, congenital or acquired abnormality in which the balance between aqueous fluid production and outflow is disrupted. Increased pressure of fluid in anterior chamber causes damage to the retina, cornea, and other structures.	• Corneal enlargement • Haziness of the cornea • Photophobia and intolerance to ordinary light • Excessive tearing • Decreased visual acuity (symptoms present in 35% at birth) • Amblyopia and permanent loss may result without treatment	• Early diagnosis is essential. • Monitoring of IOP by tonometry and central corneal thickness by pachymetry and funduscopy. • Medical therapy. • Surgical intervention is first-line treatment. • Postoperatively, a patch and shield may be worn for several days to protect sutures. • Lifetime follow-up.
Ptosis Drooping of the upper eyelid caused by weakness of levator palpebrae or, less frequently, Möller's muscle. May be congenital or acquired. Affects either the muscle or the nerve that innervates it. Particularly challenging to treat if amblyopia is also present.	• Drooping is visible on inspection • Vision may be impaired if eyelid covers the pupil • May be unilateral or bilateral • If unilateral, amblyopia may result without treatment	• Surgical correction to raise the eyelid and increase visual field. • Patching not necessary postoperatively. • Nonsurgical modalities, such as the use of "crutch" glasses to support the eyelid.
Strabismus Malalignment of the eyes caused by muscle imbalance or by paralysis, which prevents both eyes from focusing correctly on the same image. Affects 2% to 5% of the preschool population. Can cause visual and psychological disability.	• Asymmetric pupillary light reflexes • Asymmetric extraocular movements • Diplopia, impaired depth • Tendency to close one eye or tilt head during vision testing • Amblyopia may result without treatment	• Early and rigorous amblyopic occlusion therapy (patching of the stronger eye for a prescribed period each day may correct latent strabismus by exercising the muscles of the weaker eye). • Correction of refractive error. • Surgical repositioning of the extraocular muscles for severe or fixed cases. • Postoperatively: antibiotic ointment, no eye patch.

IOP, intraocular pressure.

an object approximately 12 inches (30.5 cm) away, cover one eye. The eye with weak muscles will drift when covered and will snap back when uncovered. An eye with normal muscles will remain straight.

Nursing Diagnoses

- Disturbed Sensory Perception (Visual) related to reduction in visual acuity or no visual stimulation.
- Disturbed Body Image related to the need for patch or glasses.
- Risk for Injury related to reduced visual acuity and modified depth perception.
- Delayed Growth and Development related to altered visual stimulation and possible overprotective behavior of parents.

Nursing Interventions

Minimizing Effects of Vision Loss

1. Participate in visual acuity problem identification and encourage prompt treatment to minimize functional impairment. Accurate assessment of (corrected) monocular visual acuity is the single most important element in an examination.
   a. Effective newborn screening in the nursery helps to detect congenital eye problems.
   b. All children should be screened for visual acuity and strabismus. In young children, this is accomplished by physical examination and assessment of developmental milestones (ie, looks at mother's face, smiles responsively, reaches for objects). Special assessment tools are available to assess preverbal children. By age 3 to 5 years, most children can cooperate for performance of accurate visual acuity screening tests.
2. Encourage and assist parents in obtaining corrective lenses for the child.
3. Advise and encourage parents to adhere to the postoperative treatment plan, such as occlusion therapy following cataract surgery or proper use of eyedrops after glaucoma surgery.
4. Encourage and assist parents in providing normal experiences for child to achieve maximum potential:
   a. Assist parents in locating and accessing resources, such as financial assistance, special education in Braille, or parent support groups.
   b. Remind parents of their child's right to an education.

Minimizing Body Image Disturbance

1. Encourage parents to focus on normalization rather than on overprotection. Place expectations on the child's abilities rather than disabilities, provide opportunities for interaction with peers, and make the child's life as normal as possible.
2. Encourage acceptance of appearance and emphasize the positive aspects of treatment.

Preventing Injury

1. Encourage the family to be aware of safety in the home, school, and community.
   a. Suggest the use of impact-resistant polycarbonate eyeglasses and devices to keep eyeglasses from falling off.
   b. Advise the family to maintain a consistent and uncluttered furniture arrangement; notify child of planned changes.

c. Instruct child in the use of a cane or other assistive device, if warranted.
   d. Teach traffic safety and personal security measures.
2. Orient visually impaired children to their immediate environment.
   a. Orient child to food placement on meal trays.
   b. Assist child with ambulation and use side rails on bed or crib to prevent falls.

Promoting Normal Growth and Development

1. Encourage parents to provide many sensory opportunities, such as manipulating objects, hearing various sounds, noting the smells in the environment, and tasting an assortment of substances.
2. Allow child to perform activities of daily living (ADLs) as independently as possible.

Family Education and Health Maintenance

Postoperative Teaching

1. In the interest of hygiene and safety, the patient (if older) and parent should be taught correct handwashing technique before and after instilling eye medication, particularly eyedrops. This must be reinforced before discharge.
2. Teach about instillation of medications and use of eye shield to prevent injury to the operative eye after surgery.
3. Teach about activity restrictions after glaucoma surgery.
   a. Bed rest may be required immediately postoperatively.
   b. Older children should not engage in strenuous activity or contact sports for 2 weeks.
4. Advise that activity is not usually restricted after repair of ptosis.
5. Following strabismus repair, strenuous activity, contact sports, and swimming are restricted for 2 to 4 weeks.
6. After cataract surgery due to inflammatory reaction, encourage behaviors to reduce the risk of damage to sutures from increased intraocular pressure (IOP):
   a. Prevent vomiting.
   b. Minimize crying.
   c. Encourage intense occlusion therapy and use of optical correction with glasses or contact lenses as advised.
7. Encourage parents to remove eye discharge or crusts on lashes regularly by wiping the eyes with warm water. Separate washcloths should be used for each eye and each child. Moistened cotton balls may be used.
8. Advise and encourage about the importance of keeping postoperative follow-up appointments.
9. Advise of indications that would require reevaluation by health care provider:
   a. Worsening of visual acuity.
   b. Evidence of inflammation and infection, such as pain, redness, swelling, drainage, and increased temperature.
10. Refer family to Prevent Blindness America (*www.preventblindness.org*) for information on eye disease and safety measures. For cataract and glaucoma patients, refer to the Pediatric Glaucoma and Cataract Family Association (*www.pgcfa.org*). Lighthouse International (*www.lighthouse.org*) aids with rehabilitation of visual impairment.

Evaluation: Expected Outcomes

- Child wears glasses or contact lens, as prescribed; good visual outcome with adequate optical rehabilitation.
- Parents and child report involvement in activities, satisfactory school performance, and positive peer interactions.
- No injuries reported.
- Achieves age-appropriate developmental milestones.

Eye Trauma

 Evidence Base Gerstenblith, A. T., & Rabinowitz, M. P. (2012). *The Wills eye manual: Office and emergency room diagnosis and treatment of eye disease* (6th ed.). Philadelphia: Lippincott Williams & Wilkins.

Eye trauma causes structural damage to the eye and is produced by mechanical force or contact with a corrosive chemical. Some common types of eye trauma are corneal abrasions, blunt trauma, perforating injuries, and chemical injuries. Eye injuries are common among children and are usually related to their involvement in vigorous play activities.

Pathophysiology and Etiology

Corneal Abrasion

1. Injury to corneal epithelium.
2. This may happen when a foreign object becomes lodged in the eye (eg, flying dust particle; contact lens rubbing against the eye because of inadequate tear production; injury from a fingernail, tree branch, or other sharp object entering the eye and scraping the cornea).
3. May occur from the effects of general anesthetic, which cause decreased tear production, decreased eyelid reflexes, decreased perception of pain, and failure of the eye to close properly.
4. May result from corneal exposure with such conditions as ptosis or pressure on the globe, especially in the presence of dry eyes.
5. May result from contact with household or industrial chemicals.

Blunt Trauma

1. Occurs when the eye or surrounding tissues are struck by a blunt object such as a ball, a hockey puck, a bat, or a stick.
2. The resulting injury depends on the size, hardness, and velocity of the blunt object and the force imparted. Injury may include tissue swelling and seepage of blood into the surrounding tissues.
3. The bony structures surrounding the eye may be fractured.
4. Subconjunctival hemorrhage, lens dislocation, hyphema (blood in the anterior chamber of the eye), and a retinal detachment may occur.

Perforating Injury

1. When an object penetrates the eyeball, there may be loss of vitreous material and/or damage to the internal structures of the eye—vitreous hemorrhage, choroidal rupture, retinal tears, retinal detachment, and ruptured globe.
2. Bacteria may also be introduced into the interior of the eye, causing infection.

Chemical Injury

1. Corrosive chemicals burn the delicate tissues of the cornea and may penetrate into deeper layers of the eye.

 NURSING ALERT A chemical injury is a medical emergency.

2. Healing may occur with scarring.

Clinical Manifestations

1. Pain or sensation of a foreign body in the affected eye—because of the high concentration of nerve endings in the cornea from the ciliary body.

 NURSING ALERT At times, pain may be useful in distinguishing a serious eye problem from a self-limiting condition.

2. Increased tear production—one of the eye's defenses against injury or irritation.
3. Injection of the blood vessels of the cornea—increase of blood flow to the cornea is another protective mechanism; most likely seen with foreign bodies, abrasions, or chemical burns that affect the cornea.
4. Impaired visual acuity caused by:
   a. Swelling of the cornea, reducing its clarity.
   b. Swelling of the soft tissues surrounding the eye, causing the eye to partially or completely close.
   c. Excessive tear production, impairing vision.
   d. Damage to internal structures of the eye, altering or obstructing visual pathways.
5. Visible signs of injury—bruising, swelling, or a foreign object visible in the eye.

Diagnostic Evaluation

1. Thorough inspection of the eye, including eversion of the upper lid to inspect for a foreign object.
2. A slit-lamp examination to determine the extent of the corneal abrasion.
3. Funduscopic examination may detect abnormalities, such as a dislodged lens, retinal hemorrhage, retinal detachment, or papilledema with increased IOP.
4. Staining with fluorescein dye reveals lesions of the cornea such as abrasions.
5. Assessment of eye function, including near and far acuity, extraocular movements, and visual field testing.

Management

Most childhood injuries will resolve spontaneously with no adverse long-term consequences. Early detection and prompt intervention may help reduce the incidence of ocular morbidity.

Corneal Abrasion

1. Removal of the offending foreign body, such as contact lens.
2. Antibiotic drops or ointment for superficial abrasion.

3. For infected or inflamed abrasion, antibiotic eyedrops or ointment to prevent infection and anti-inflammatory drops to decrease inflammation.

4. Follow up for any recurrent symptoms because recurrent corneal erosion can occur months or years following injury because of spontaneous disruption of corneal epithelium that occurs near the site of the corneal abrasion.

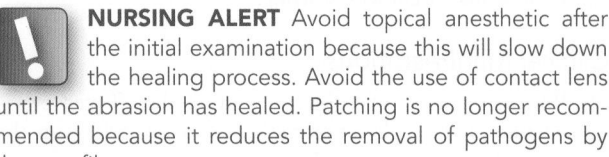 **NURSING ALERT** Avoid topical anesthetic after the initial examination because this will slow down the healing process. Avoid the use of contact lens until the abrasion has healed. Patching is no longer recommended because it reduces the removal of pathogens by the tear film.

Blunt Trauma

1. Application of cold compresses may help control pain and swelling.
2. The head should be elevated 30 degrees to facilitate settling of hyphema, if present.
3. Surgery may be required because of damage to underlying bones or eye structures.

Perforating Injury

1. Surgery is usually necessary to remove the object and reconstruct damaged tissues.
2. The head should be elevated 30 degrees to facilitate settling of hyphema.
3. The child should be kept on nothing-by-mouth status in preparation for surgery.

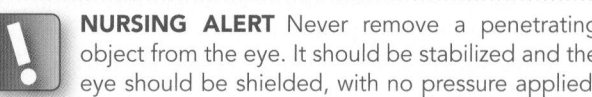 **NURSING ALERT** Never remove a penetrating object from the eye. It should be stabilized and the eye should be shielded, with no pressure applied. In an emergency, use a foam cup with part of the bottom cut off, if necessary, to support the object. Patch the unaffected eye during transport to the hospital.

Chemical Injury

1. Continuous, gentle flushing of the affected eyes with any available water until able to change to normal saline solution for at least 30 minutes (see page 580). This will help remove the offending chemical. This should be done from the inner aspect of eye to the outer aspect to prevent contaminated water from flowing into the other eye.
2. Further management depends on the nature and extent of the injury.

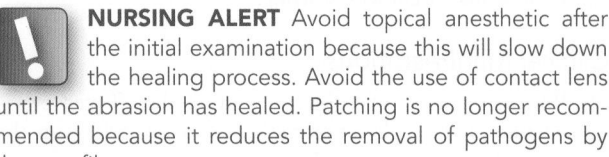 **NURSING ALERT** Acid chemicals coagulate the conjunctival protein, leaving the blood vessels undamaged. Alkaline chemicals rapidly permeate the eye's structure, thus causing more damage.

Complications

1. Infection.
2. Bleeding.

3. Refractive problems due to corneal scar, cataract, glaucoma, shrinkage of the affected eye, and inflammation of the unaffected eye; may result in vision impairment or loss of vision.
4. Disfigurement may result from severe or extensive tissue damage.

Nursing Assessment

1. Obtain history of injury, including the child's account of how the injury occurred, and a description of symptoms experienced.
2. Inspect for location and extent of swelling and bruising, asymmetry, or abnormality in appearance of any part of the eye.
3. Obtain visual history preinjury. Assess visual acuity. This should include near and far acuity in each eye. If the patient cannot see well enough to read a Snellen chart, assess ability to count fingers or perceive light. Compare findings with preinjury visual history.

Nursing Diagnoses

• Acute Pain related to inflammation, photophobia, or trauma to eye tissue.
• Risk for Injury related to impaired vision and adverse effects of pain medications.
• Feeding, Dressing, and Grooming Self-Care Deficit related to impaired vision and adverse effects of pain medications.

Nursing Interventions

Minimizing Pain

1. Apply cold compresses to the affected area to help reduce swelling and discomfort.
2. Keep the child's room as dark as possible to help reduce pain for photophobic patients.
3. Administer analgesics, as prescribed.
4. Encourage quiet activities to act as a distraction to pain.

Preventing Injury

1. Enforce safety measures:
   a. Use of bed side rails.
   b. Assistance with ambulation.
   c. Close observation.

Maintaining ADLs

1. Provide assistance with eating, bathing, toileting, and other ADLs, as needed.
2. Teach child location of self-care items and positioning of food on tray to promote independence.
3. Encourage child to attempt self-care and offer praise even if unsuccessful.

Family Education and Health Maintenance

1. Teach indications for reevaluation by health care provider.
   a. Increase in swelling, tenderness, discoloration, or pain.
   b. Worsening of visual acuity.
   c. Development of additional symptoms, such as fever, alteration in sensorium, or other indications of neurologic injury.

2. Provide safety education to all families to prevent common causes of injury. Encourage families to use protective eyewear when participating in sports or other activities; proper use of infant car seat, booster seat, and seat belt; proper storage of household chemicals.

3. Provide families with information and support as they cope with having a visually impaired child in the home. The American Academy of Ophthalmology has patient information and a list of helpful resources at its website (*www.aao.org/aao/news/eyenet/*).

Evaluation: Expected Outcomes

- Demonstrates decreased pain.
- No injuries reported.
- Dressing and feeding self with minimal assistance.

Functional Problems

Functional problems of the eye involve vision impairment because of refractive errors or disuse of visual pathways. Such problems frequently result in amblyopia—impaired vision in one or both eyes due to poor visual stimulation rather than an organic problem. Abnormal vision screening with referral occurs in 1.2% of 5-year-old patients and increases to 9.1% by the time the child reaches age 13. Amblyopia affects 1% to 3% of the population.

Pathophysiology and Etiology

1. Refractive errors are usually caused by a genetic predisposition to shortened or elongated eyeballs or by individual variations in growth.
   a. In an elongated or shortened eyeball, the visual image is focused either in front of or behind the retina, resulting in unclear images.
   b. The nearsighted (myopic) child can see near objects, such as print in schoolbooks, but cannot focus clearly on far objects such as writing on the blackboard.
   c. The farsighted (hyperopic) child can see far objects clearly but has difficulty seeing near objects.
   d. The problem may be unilateral or bilateral.
2. Amblyopia may result from any condition that causes the two retinas to receive different images. Etiology may include:
   a. Diplopia caused by strabismus.
   b. Significant difference in acuity of the two eyes.
   c. Cataract.
   d. Unilateral severe ptosis.
3. When a discrepancy exists between images received on the two retinas, the more unclear image is suppressed.
   a. Over time, a young child will become permanently unable to use the visual pathways of the suppressed eye.
   b. Although the visual pathways are structurally normal, the child is visually impaired in that eye due to poor visual stimulation.

Clinical Manifestations

Children usually do not complain that they cannot see well, but may exhibit other signs of vision problems, including:

1. Poor academic performance or behavioral problems in school.
2. Dislike for reading.
3. Head tilting.
4. Squinting.
5. Sitting close to the television or holding reading materials close to the face.
6. Refusal or resistance to covering one eye during vision screening.

Diagnostic Evaluation

1. Standardized vision screening tests, such as the Snellen chart, the Titmus test, or the H:O:T:V matching symbol test, may be used for distance acuity screening.
   a. Tests can be administered to children as young as age 3.
   b. Each eye should be tested separately.
2. Near vision may be tested by having the child read or by the Titmus test. Each eye should be tested separately.
3. Muscle balance can be tested using the cross cover test and the Titmus test.

Management

1. Most visual acuity problems can be treated by the use of corrective lenses or refractive surgery.
2. Amblyopia management focuses on prevention through early identification and treatment of conditions that caused it.
   a. Strabismus is treated with patching the stronger eye to strengthen the weaker eye. Glasses may also be prescribed to improve the vision. In some cases, however, surgery may be required.
   b. Topical miotic drops may be used if the child is not able to tolerate the daily patching required to correct amblyopia.

 Evidence Base Matta, N., Singman, E., & Silbert, D. (2010). Evidenced-Based Medicine: Treatment for Amblyopia. *American Orthoptic Journal, 60,* 17–22.

   c. Surgery may also be required to correct ptosis.
   d. Acuity problems due to refractive error are usually managed with the use of corrective lenses.
3. Optimal outcome is accomplished when treatment is begun early in life, while visual pathways are still developing. However, some visual function may be recovered even if the problem is treated in adolescence or adulthood. Ideally, the problem can be prevented by early identification and treatment of factors that may cause it.

Complications

Injuries caused by visual impairment.

Nursing Assessment

1. Begin visual acuity screening early, in the preschool years and whenever a child displays behaviors suggestive of acuity problems.

2. Assess Hirschberg's test for symmetry of the pupillary light reflexes routinely, beginning at birth.
3. Perform the cover–uncover test as part of routine eye assessment.
4. Assess the effect of the functional deficit on the child's overall function, including academic progress, self-esteem, and safety.

Nursing Diagnoses

- Disturbed Sensory Perception (Visual) related to reduced acuity or inability to use one eye.
- Risk for Injury related to impaired visual acuity or lack of depth perception.
- Chronic Low Self-Esteem related to lowered performance caused by poor vision.

Nursing Interventions

Minimizing Effects of Sensory Deficits

1. Encourage the consistent use of corrective lenses, as prescribed.
2. Teach the parents ways to help develop the child's skills in interpreting information through the senses of hearing, smell, and touch.
   a. Familiarize the child with common sounds and smells in the environment. Also, orient the child to traffic sounds and sounds associated with danger, such as animals and speeding vehicles, and instruct the child how to respond.
   b. Use voice or touch, rather than facial expressions or gestures, to express emotion.
   c. Speak to the child before touching to reduce startling.
   d. Allow the child to touch and handle unfamiliar objects to learn about them.
   e. Have the child practice such things as retelling stories and giving the home telephone number and address.
   f. Explain unfamiliar sounds and smells to the hospitalized child.

Preventing Injury

1. Recommend the use of shatterproof eyeglasses with flexible frames.
2. Recommend the use of eye protection on a routine basis because eye trauma can occur unexpectedly. This is especially important for children who rely on only one eye.
3. Suggest extra protection, such as shatterproof goggles or shields, when participating in contact or ball sports and activities.
4. Maintain a stable arrangement of furniture in the home, adequate lighting, and an uncluttered environment to minimize falls.
5. Orient hospitalized children to the hospital room and offer assistance when walking.

Promoting a Positive Sense of Self-Esteem

1. Provide opportunities for mastery of developmentally appropriate activities.
2. Encourage interactions with sighted children to decrease feelings of isolation. Also, suggest interactions with children with similar alterations in vision.

3. Encourage the child to discuss feelings and strategies for coping with negative peer reactions such as teasing.
4. Encourage independence in self-care activities to promote autonomy, such as dressing, feeding, and use of bathroom.
5. Assist the patient and family with effective coping mechanisms to promote family stability.

Community and Home Care Considerations

1. Perform a safety inspection of the home environment and make changes as necessary to help prevent falls and other injuries.
2. Assist family access to financial and social resources, as needed.
3. Make sure that the child is receiving specialized educational resources, as needed.

Family Education and Health Maintenance

1. Teach the importance of patching for amblyopia and the wearing of corrective lenses, as prescribed, and their proper care.
2. Refer families of blind children to community resources that can help their child learn special skills, such as reading Braille, using a cane, or developing self-care skills. Information can be obtained from agencies such as the American Foundation for the Blind (*www.afb.org*).

Evaluation: Expected Outcomes

- Identifies common sounds.
- No injury reported; wears protective eyeglasses.
- Reports good school performance and participation in extracurricular activities; can eat and dress independently.

CONDITIONS OF THE EAR

Also see Chapter 17 for additional information on ear, nose, and throat problems.

Eustachian Tube Dysfunction

Eustachian tube dysfunction (ETD) is an umbrella term describing disorders that arise from closure of the eustachian tube, which ventilates the middle ear to equalize pressure on both sides of the tympanic membrane. ETD may be associated with otitis media with effusion (OME), also known as serous otitis; acute otitis media (AOM); and recurrent otitis media. Approximately 90% of children experience one or more episodes of middle ear effusion by age 2.

Pathophysiology and Etiology

1. Inflammation of the eustachian tube lining is caused by an acute upper respiratory infection or an allergic response.
   a. Infected secretions may pass through the tube from the nasal area into the middle ear.
   b. When inflammation and swelling causes the eustachian tube to close, the passage of air into and out of the middle ear is prevented.

BOX 47-1 Risk Factors for Eustachean Tube Dysfunction

- Frequent episodes of upper respiratory infections in younger children.
- Nasal allergies.
- Genetic predisposition to floppy eustachian tube.
- Native American or Eskimo heritage.
- Craniofacial abnormalities.
- Down syndrome.
- Lower socioeconomic status.
- Exposure to cigarette smoke.
- Bottle-feeding.
- Male gender.
- Daycare attendance with greater than six attendees.
- Pacifier use after 2 years of age.
- Immune deficiencies.

c. The air in the middle ear is absorbed into the middle ear lining and a vacuum is created.

d. The vacuum is filled by serous fluid that seeps out of the middle ear lining.

e. The warm, moist environment of the middle ear and nutrients in the serous fluid are conducive to the growth of viruses or bacteria that may be present in the middle ear cavity.

2. Children between ages 6 and 24 months are predisposed to the development of AOM because their short, relatively straight eustachian tubes more easily allow the passage of infected nasal secretions into the middle ear cavity. See Box 47-1 for additional risk factors.

Evidence Base Armengol, C. E., Hendley, J. O., & Winter, B. (2011). Occurrence of acute otitis media during colds in children younger than four years. *Pediatric Infectious Disease Journal, 30*(6), 518–520.

Gould, J. M., & Matz, P. S. (2010). Otitis media. *Pediatrics in Review, 31*(3), 102–116.

3. Viruses account for 48% of AOM cases. In 33% of AOM cases there is no identifiable bacterial pathogen. The most common bacterial agents include:

a. *S. pneumoniae.*

b. Nontypeable *H. influenzae.*

c. *Moraxella catarrhalis.*

Evidence Base Tahtinen, P., Laine, M., Ruuskanen, O., & Ruohola, A. (2012). Delayed versus immediate antimicrobial treatment for otitis media. *Pediatric Infectious Disease Journal, 31*(12), 1227–1232.

4. Barotrauma, caused by rapid changes in atmospheric pressure, may also lead to closure of the eustachian tube and to the development of serous otitis. This is less likely to involve introduction of microorganisms through infected nasal secretions; development of AOM is less common.

Clinical Manifestations

1. Decreased hearing—temporary conductive hearing loss; usually resolves when tympanic membrane mobility is restored.
2. Sensation of fullness in the affected ears.
3. Popping sensations in the affected ears may be experienced as the eustachian tube begins to open and admits air into the middle ear cavity.
4. Ear pain.
5. Signs of infection—fever, irritability, or decreased appetite.

Diagnostic Evaluation

1. Otoscopic examination.
   a. OME—yellowish effusion, prominent bony landmarks, a diffuse light reflex, and decreased mobility of tympanic membrane.
   b. AOM—inflamed tympanic membrane with decreased or absent mobility; bulging of the tympanic membrane may obscure the bony landmarks and light reflex.
2. Tympanometry—quick and simple way to assess tympanic membrane mobility (see Figure 47-1).
   a. A probe occludes the ear canal while pressure is varied and a test sound is emitted. The test produces a graphic display that shows the mobility of the tympanic membrane at various air pressures.
   b. A normal reading has a distinct peak in the middle of the graph (see Figure 47-1A).
   c. A flat tympanogram (no peak) indicates lack of mobility of the tympanic membrane, usually caused by serous otitis or AOM (see Figure 47-1B).
   d. A peak to the left of the center indicates negative pressure in the middle ear (see Figure 47-1C).
3. Acoustic reflectometry—useful in infants older than age 3 months.
   a. A probe held at the opening of the ear canal measures reflected sound waves from the middle ear.
   b. Reduction in reflected sound is an indication of middle ear effusion.

Management

Evidence Base McConnochie, K. (2012). Development of an algorithm for the diagnosis of otitis media. *Academic Pediatrics*, May-Jun; *12*(3), 159–160.

Otitis Media with Effusion

1. Usually resolves spontaneously.
2. Treatment of underlying predisposing factors (eg, allergies) may provide some relief.
3. Placement of ventilating tubes may be considered for effusions that persist for 3 or more months with bilateral hearing loss of 20 or more decibels.
4. Some children may benefit from adenoidectomy.

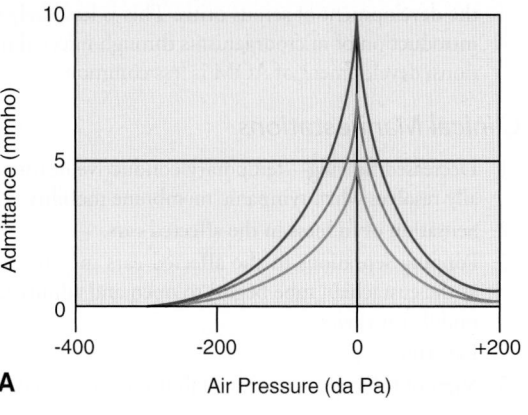

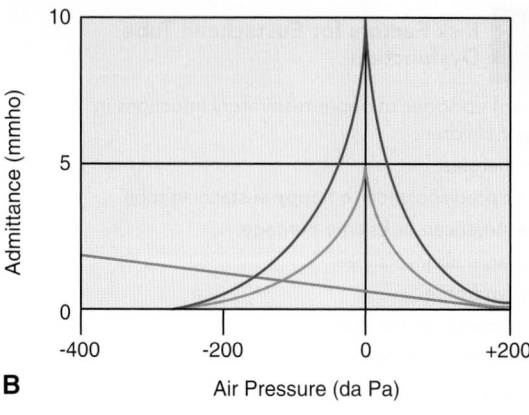

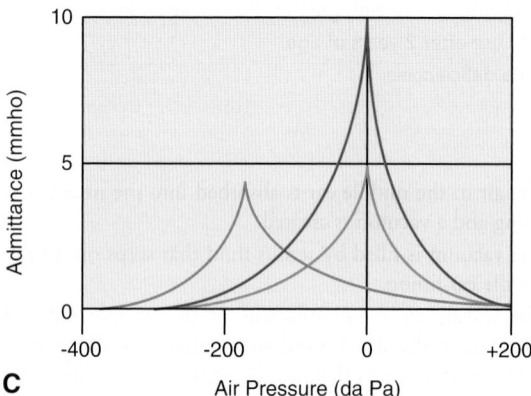

Figure 47-1. **(A)** Type A tympanogram: This is the normal pattern showing mobility of the tympanic membrane with a peak mobility at the 0 point (the point at which there is neither positive nor negative pressure in the external ear canal). **(B)** Type B tympanogram: This pattern shows a low level of mobility with no peak. It is characteristic of impaired mobility due to the presence of fluid in the middle ear. **(C)** Type C tympanogram: This pattern shows a distinct peak in the mobility level of the tympanic membrane, but the peak occurs when there is negative pressure in the external ear canal. This indicates eustachian tube dysfunction causing negative pressure in the middle ear cavity. Negative pressure in the external ear canal equalizes pressure on both sides of the tympanic membrane and allows for maximum mobility.

Acute Otitis Media

1. All infants under age 6 months with presumed or certain AOM should be treated.
2. Children ages 6 to 24 months with certain AOM should be treated, whereas those with presumed AOM may be monitored.
3. For children over age 2 years, observation may be considered for those with certain AOM, but who do not have severe illness—defined as acute onset and significant pain with or without fever.
4. If not treating, the clinician should ensure an adult caregiver is able to observe the child, recognize signs of serious illness, and be able to provide prompt access to medical care if improvement does not occur. If there is worsening of illness or no improvement in 48 to 72 hours, antibacterial therapy should be considered.
5. Amoxicillin remains the drug of choice, although higher doses are now given (80 to 90 mg/kg divided into b.i.d. doses) because of growing prevalence of resistant bacteria (*S. pneumoniae*). Children under the age of 5 and those with severe disease should be treated for 10 days.
6. Those at risk for resistance include children younger than age 2, those treated with antibiotics within the past 2 months, and those who attend daycare.
7. Alternative antibiotics for treatment failures include amoxicillin-clavulanate or one of the cephalosporins.

Recurrent Otitis Media

1. Placement of ventilating tubes by myringotomy (incision into the tympanic membrane) may be considered for children who experience three or more episodes in 6 months or four or more episodes per year (see Figure 47-2).
2. Antibiotic prophylaxis is no longer recommended because it may contribute to the problem of antibiotic-resistant bacteria.

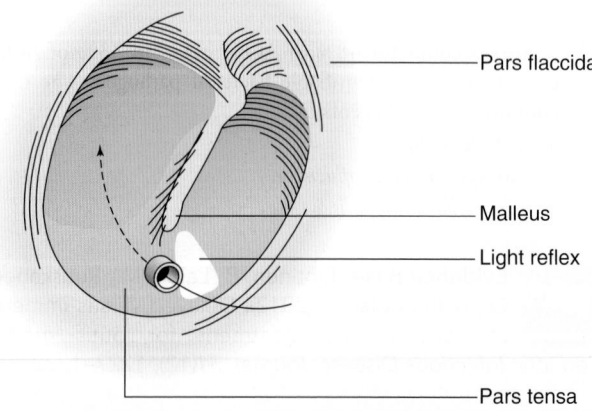

Figure 47-2. A ventilating (myringotomy) tube provides air to the middle ear to prevent otitis media.

Complications

1. Perforations of the tympanic membrane, scarring because of healed perforations, or damage to the ossicles of the middle ear may occur; permanent hearing loss is a rare complication.
2. Delayed speech and language development.
3. Mastoiditis, meningitis, lateral sinus thrombosis, or intracranial abscess; spread of bacterial infection may occur, although all are uncommon.

Nursing Assessment

1. Assess for etiologic factors that contribute to eustachian tube dysfunction.
2. Assess for symptoms of serous otitis and AOM to identify and to document the nature and severity of the illness.
3. Assess hearing after the middle ear effusion is resolved. Promptly identify any hearing loss that may have social and educational consequences.
4. Assess speech and language development in children who experience recurrent or prolonged infections to determine deficits.

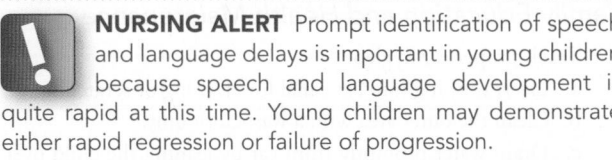 **NURSING ALERT** Prompt identification of speech and language delays is important in young children because speech and language development is quite rapid at this time. Young children may demonstrate either rapid regression or failure of progression.

5. Assess for effects of illness on family, such as sleep deprivation of parents caused by staying up with child at night or decreased attendance at work caused by keeping child out of school.

Nursing Diagnoses

- Acute Pain related to increased pressure in the middle ear.
- Impaired Verbal Communication caused by conductive hearing loss.

Nursing Interventions

Minimizing Discomfort

1. Administer and teach parents to administer antibiotics. Provide instruction in:
   a. Measurement of correct dosage.
   b. Time of doses.
   c. Importance of administering all doses.
   d. Proper storage and disposal of unused medication.
   e. Adverse effects.
2. Administer acetaminophen or ibuprofen, as directed, for pain or fever.
3. Apply warm compresses to the external ear.
4. Administer analgesic otic drops, if prescribed; only indicated if no perforation of the tympanic membrane exists.
5. Advise elevation of head to facilitate drainage of fluid from the middle ear into the pharynx.
6. Teach older children to stimulate opening of their eustachian tubes by yawning or performing Valsalva's maneuver.

Facilitating Verbal Communication

1. Assess hearing, speech, and language development regularly.
2. Alert parents to report signs of hearing difficulty or delayed speech immediately to ensure early intervention.
3. Refer to a specialist for evaluation and treatment, if necessary.

Family Education and Health Maintenance

1. Teach parents that episodes of otitis may be minimized by:
   a. Breastfeeding.
   b. Placing older, bottle-fed infants in a sitting position during feeding.
   c. Identifying and eliminating allergens, such as particular foods, molds, and dust.
   d. Not exposing the child to cigarette smoke.
   e. Immunization with pneumococcal and influenza vaccines.

 Evidence Base Principi, N., Baggi, E., & Esposito, S. (2012). Prevention of acute otitis media using currently available vaccines. *Future Microbiology*, 7(4), 457–465.

2. Teach the importance of taking antibiotics at prescribed times for the indicated length of therapy to prevent partial treatment and the development of resistance.
3. Teach all parents the difference between viral and bacterial infections, emphasizing that overuse of antibiotics for viral infections contributes to the development of resistant bacteria.
4. If ventilating tubes are placed, instruct parents to do the following.
   a. Prevent water or other fluids from entering the ear canal. Encourage use of earplugs when the child is bathing or swimming.
   b. Discourage instillation of eardrops or other medications in the external ear unless they have been prescribed by the health care provider.
   c. Tubes will fall out of the ear spontaneously, usually in 6 to 12 months.

Evaluation: Expected Outcomes

- Demonstrates improved comfort; family states proper treatment regimen.
- Speech and language development appropriate for age; reports regular assessment; receives therapy from specialist, if indicated.

External Otitis

Acute *otitis externa* is inflammation in the external ear canal. It is frequently unilateral but may be bilateral. Commonly known as "swimmer's ear."

Pathophysiology and Etiology

1. Caused by bacteria or fungi. Common pathogens include:
   a. *Pseudomonas aeruginosa.*
   b. *Staphylococcus aureus.*

c. *Proteus mirabilis.*

d. *Streptococcus pyogenes.*

e. Fungi *(Candida, Aspergillus).*

2. Risk factors include:

a. Frequent swimming.

b. Insertion of objects, such as cotton swabs, into the ear canals.

c. AOM with perforation of the tympanic membrane.

d. Ventilation tubes with drainage.

e. Poorly fitting ear plugs.

3. When water remains in the external ear canal, a warm, moist environment is created.

4. Skin lining the canal is irritated, causing breakdown of its protective barrier.

5. Bacteria or fungi overgrow in the conducive environment and cause symptoms of inflammation and infection in 1 to 2 days.

6. Breakdown of protective barrier and introduction and proliferation of infectious organisms can also occur through trauma to the ear canal, such as cleaning the ear with an inappropriate object or using an improper technique.

Clinical Manifestations

1. Intense ear pain, itching, and white, yellow, or greenish drainage.

2. Inflammation of the external ear canal and structures.

3. Pain when the ear pinna is manipulated.

Diagnostic Evaluation

1. Otoscopic examination may be difficult because of severe pain and swelling; redness, swelling, and drainage in external canal is noted while tympanic membrane appears normal.

2. Ear pain may be severe.

3. Cellulitis of the surrounding structures can result in displacement of the external ear out and away from the head.

4. Cultures are usually not necessary.

Management

1. Ear pain may be severe and appropriate analgesia should be provided.

2. Effective topical treatments include acetic and boric acid solutions, which dry and modify the pH of the ear canal.

3. Topical antibiotic solution, possibly combined with a steroid to reduce significant discomfort and swelling.

4. Ear canal may be gently cleansed with curette, cotton swab, mild suctioning, or irrigation to remove drainage.

5. An ear wick may be used to aid in medication getting to the lining of the deeper ear canal.

6. Oral antibiotics may be used in addition to topical medications in severe cases or if cellulitis extends beyond the external canal.

Nursing Assessment

1. Assess severity of symptoms and need for pain relief.

2. Assess ear hygiene and the need for earplugs.

Nursing Diagnosis

• Acute Pain related to inflammation and irritation of drainage.

Nursing Interventions

Relieving Pain

1. Administer eardrops or teach parents administration, as prescribed.

a. Have child lie on side with affected ear upward.

b. Instill drops, using caution not to contaminate dropper, and press gently on tragus.

c. Have child maintain position for 5 minutes to facilitate penetration of medication into ear canal.

d. Repeat on other side, if ordered.

2. Administer analgesics, such as acetaminophen or ibuprofen, as directed.

3. Suggest application of warm or cold compresses to outer ear to relieve discomfort.

4. Frequently clean drainage from area surrounding opening of ear canal to relieve irritation.

Family Education and Health Maintenance

1. Teach proper ear hygiene.

a. Insert nothing into ear canal for cleaning or scratching.

b. Clean the outer area with a washcloth only.

c. Drain water promptly from ear by leaning the child over and pulling auricle slightly downward and outward.

2. Instruct in the use of well-fitting earplugs, if necessary.

3. Instruct in the use of routine acetic acid solution instillation after water activity, if prescribed.

Evaluation: Expected Outcomes

• Reports pain relieved; uses compresses and analgesics, if necessary.

Functional Hearing Disorders

Functional hearing disorders arise from problems in the function of the ear. In a quiet environment, the healthy child can hear tones between 0 and 25 decibels. Categories of hearing impairment include slight, 15 to 25 decibels; mild, 25 to 40 decibels; moderate, 40 to 65 decibels; severe, 65 to 95 decibels; and profound, 95 or more decibels. In the United States, moderate to profound bilateral sensorineural hearing loss occurs in 0.5 to 1.0 per 1,000 live births each year. Factors that place an infant at high risk for hearing loss include low birth weight, craniofacial anomalies, family history of hereditary childhood hearing loss, and certain infections, such as rubella or bacterial meningitis.

Pathophysiology and Etiology

1. Hearing loss may be conductive, sensorineural, or mixed.

2. Conductive loss may uncommonly result from a congenital ear deformity. More commonly, conductive loss is acquired and occurs when sound transmission through the outer

and/or middle ear is impaired, caused by impaction of cerumen in the external ear canal, fluid in the middle ear cavity, or scarring of the tympanic membrane.

a. A mechanical obstruction, such as cerumen or a foreign object blocking the external ear canal, may block the passage of sound waves to the tympanic membrane.

b. With otitis media or OME, fluid in the middle ear cavity does not transmit sound as well as air.

c. A scarred or perforated tympanic membrane has lost its normal mobility and does not transmit sound as well as a normal one.

d. Most cases of conductive hearing loss in children are reversible and produce no permanent effect.

3. Sensorineural hearing loss results from damage to the cochlea or auditory nerve and congenital defects of the cochlea. Examples include damage caused by ototoxic drugs, damage resulting from prenatal infections, and damage caused by prolonged exposure to loud noise.

a. Damage to the auditory nerve prevents transmission of sound impulses to the brain for interpretation.

b. Damage to hair cells of the cochlea may be caused by prolonged exposure to loud noise, resulting in hearing loss, especially pronounced for high-pitched sounds.

c. Sensorineural problems are usually irreversible.

Clinical Manifestations

1. Infants may be noted to be unresponsive to sound. Response to sound, however, is not sufficiently reliable as a screening method, especially for high-risk infants.

2. Children usually do not complain that they cannot hear well. They may exhibit other signs of hearing problems, including:

a. Poor academic performance or behavior problems in school.

b. Lack of response to sounds.

c. Delayed language development.

d. Listening to the television or radio at a loud volume.

e. Speaking loudly.

Diagnostic Evaluation

 Evidence Base Buz Harlor, Jr., A. D., & Bower, C., Committee on Practice and Ambulatory Medicine, et al. (2009). Hearing assessment in infants and children: Recommendation beyond neonatal screening. *Pediatrics, 124*, 1252–1263.

Eichwald, J. (2010). CDC expert commentary: Identifying hearing loss in newborns. Available: *www.cdc.gov/ncbddd/hearingloss/hcp.html*.

1. Universal newborn hearing screening using a two-stage process is advocated by the American Academy of Pediatrics and the Agency for Healthcare Research and Quality and is widely accepted as the standard of care for infants in the United States. This is accomplished by an initial automated transient evoked otoacoustic emission (OAE) before discharge from the hospital newborn nursery. If indicated, an automated auditory brain response test is used to confirm a positive OAE screen.

2. Infants who fail their initial screening need a follow-up evaluation at 1 month of age. Any infants with a second abnormal result should be evaluated by an audiologist as soon as possible. Infants with risk factors such as sepsis at birth requiring antibiotics require a repeat hearing evaluation at 3 months of age.

3. Infants with documented hearing loss need referral to specialists (otolaryngology and ophthalmology) by 3 months of age. Referral to other subspecialists (genetics, nephrology, neurology, etc.) may be necessary. The infant should be enrolled in Early Intervention Services (Part C) through the local school system in the United States no later than 6 months of age, which will supply physical therapy, occupational therapy, speech therapy, and visual intervention, as indicated.

4. Infants whose initial hearing screen is normal should be routinely assessed for their response to sound and achievement of developmental speech language milestones.

5. Routine audiometric screening should be done beginning as soon as the child can cooperate and follow instructions (between ages 3 and 5). It is important that the child be screened and hearing deficits addressed before entry into school.

Management

1. Treatment of the underlying problem, such as impacted cerumen or otitis media.

2. Hearing aids may be helpful for both conductive and sensorineural hearing loss.

3. Cochlear implants help some children with sensorineural hearing loss.

a. Consists of an external microphone and speech processor, which sends radio signals to an internal electrode array implanted in the cochlea.

b. Most effective in the young child who has had shorter hearing deprivation, but requires a long period of rehabilitation.

4. If the problem cannot be corrected, the focus of treatment is on development of adaptive skills through special education, sign language or other communication alternatives, and/or technical devices for the hearing impaired.

Complications

1. Speech and language delays.

2. Inadequate social development.

Nursing Assessment

1. Periodically assess hearing in the child with an identified hearing impairment to follow up promptly on changes in ability to hear.

2. Assess speech and language development frequently so that children may obtain special assistance, as indicated.

3. Assess social development and academic progress periodically so that counseling and intervention can be instituted.

Nursing Diagnoses

- Disturbed Sensory Perception (Auditory) related to limited ability to hear.
- Impaired Verbal Communication related to inability to hear and imitate speech sounds.
- Risk for Injury related to inability to hear warning sounds of impending danger.
- Chronic Low Self-Esteem related to social and academic difficulties.

Nursing Interventions

Minimizing Effects of Hearing Loss

1. Face the child, use appropriate facial expressions, and make sure the child can see your face clearly when communicating.
2. Approach the child so that you can be seen; touch the deaf child on the shoulder to get attention.
3. Assist the child in utilizing hearing aid, as prescribed.

Promoting Effective Communication

1. Determine usual method of communication: ability to write, using verbal cues, or reading lips. Do not depend on gestures to communicate with child or with a third party who does not know sign language.
2. Obtain an interpreter, when necessary, for children who communicate using sign language. Adequate communication is especially important when providing health education or when treating children who may have been abused.
3. Help the parents of a young child to stimulate and communicate with him or her.
   a. Teach them to use gestures, mime, and nonverbal communication.
   b. Teach them to help the infant to develop watching behavior by giving rewards of pleasure and praise.
   c. Teach them to talk to the child while looking directly into his or her eyes and using appropriate facial expressions.

Preventing Injury

1. Advise parents that home safety devices, such as smoke detectors, may require visual or tactile alarms (flashing lights or vibration) rather than auditory alarms.
2. Encourage the use of other senses to compensate for inability to hear. For example, the child should be especially careful to look in all directions when crossing the street.
3. Do not leave the child alone in an unfamiliar environment without means of communication.
4. Provide close surveillance and frequent visual contact for the hospitalized child.

Increasing Self-Esteem

1. Inform families of the child's right to a public education in the least restrictive setting and promote use of augmented communication devices.
2. Encourage interaction with hearing and nonhearing children to promote integration.
3. Encourage mastery of developmental milestones and skills through self-care activities and play.
4. Help parents understand that the child may not be able to express anxiety or frustration and may act out instead.

5. Teach them to be consistent in their use of discipline and to provide alternative ways for the child to gain attention or to relieve stress.
6. Praise the child for accomplishments and attempts at social interaction.

Family Education and Health Maintenance

1. Encourage families to learn sign language and alternative methods of communication with the child.
2. Advise on proper hearing aid cleaning and maintenance.
3. Encourage attention to health maintenance needs, such as immunizations and well-child visits.
4. For additional support and information, refer to agencies such as the American Speech-Hearing Association (*www.asha.org*).

Evaluation: Expected Outcomes

- Responds appropriately to environmental stimuli.
- Communicates effectively through sign language, interpreter, and visual cues.
- Reports no injuries.
- Reports adequate progress in school and participation in extracurricular activities.

SELECTED REFERENCES

American Academy of Family Physicians, American Academy of Otolaryngology-Head and Neck Surgery, & American Academy of Pediatrics Subcommittee on Otitis Media with Effusion. (2004). Otitis media with effusion. *Pediatrics, 113*(5), 1412–1429.

American Academy of Pediatrics, Joint Commission on Infant Hearing. (2007). Year 2007 Position Statement: Principles and guidelines for early hearing detection and intervention programs. *Pediatrics, 120*(4), 898–921.

American Academy of Pediatrics, Section on Ophthalmology and Strabismus, American Academy of Ophthalmology, & American Academy of Certified Orthoptists. (2008). Red reflex examination in neonates, infants, and children. *Pediatrics, 122*(6), 1401–1404.

Armengol, C. E., Hendley, J. O., & Winter, B. (2011). Occurrence of acute otitis media during colds in children younger than four years. *Pediatric Infectious Disease Journal, 30*(6), 518–520.

Buz Harlor, Jr., A. D., Bower, C., Committee on Practice and Ambulatory Medicine, et al. (2009). Hearing assessment in infants and children: Recommendation beyond neonatal screening. *Pediatrics, 124*, 1252–1263.

Coco, A., Vernacchio, L., Horst, M., et al. (2010). Management of acute otitis media after publication of the 2004 AAP and AAFP clinical practice guideline. *Pediatrics, 125*(2), 214–220.

Committee on Practice and Ambulatory Medicine, Section on Ophthalmology; American Association of Certified Orthoptists; American Association for Pediatric Ophthalmology and Strabismus; & American Academy of Ophthalmology. (2003). Eye examination in infants, children, and young adults by pediatricians. *Pediatrics, 111*(4, Part 1), 902–907.

Cronau, H., Kankanala, R. R., & Mauger, T. (2010). Diagnosis and management of red eye in primary care. *American Family Physician, 81*(2), 137–144.

Eichwald, J. (2010). CDC Expert Commentary: Identifying hearing loss in newborns. Available: *www.cdc.gov/ncbddd/hearingloss/hcp.html*.

Gerstenblith, A. T., & Rabinowitz, M. P. (2012). *The Wills eye manual: Office and emergency room diagnosis and treatment of eye disease* (6th ed.). Philadelphia: Lippincott Williams & Wilkins.

Goss, L. K. (2011). A close up view of pneumococcal disease. *Nurse Practitioner, 36*(12), 41–45.

Gould, J. M., & Matz, P. S. (2010). Otitis media. *Pediatrics in Review, 31*(3), 102–116.

Hoberman, A., Paradise, J. L., Rockette, H. E., et al. (2011). Treatment of acute otitis media in children under 2 years of age. *New England Journal of Medicine, 364*(2), 105–115.

Matta, N., Singman, E., & Silbert, D. (2010). Evidenced-Based Medicine: Treatment for Amblyopia. *American Orthoptic Journal, 60,* 17–22.

McConnochie, K. (2012). Development of an algorithm for the diagnosis of otitis media. *Academic Pediatrics, 12*(3), 159–160.

Morris, P. S., & Leach, A. J. (2009). Acute and chronic otitis media. *Pediatric Clinics of North America, 56*(6), 1383–1399.

Pelton, S., & Leibovitz, E. (2009). Recent advances in otitis media. *Pediatric Infectious Disease Journal, 28*(Suppl. 10), S113–S137.

Pettigrew, M. M., Gent, J. F., Pyles, R. B., et al. (2011). Viral–bacterial interactions and risk of acute otitis media complicating upper respiratory infection. *Journal of Clinical Microbiology, 49*(11), 3750–3755.

Principi, N., Baggi, E., & Esposito, S. (2012). Prevention of acute otitis media using currently available vaccines. *Future Microbiology, 7*(4), 457–465.

Repka, M. X. (2008). How much amblyopia treatment is enough? *Archives of Ophthalmology, 126*(7), 990–991.

Sethuraman, U., & Kamat, D. (2009). The red eye: Evaluation and management. *Clinical Pediatrics, 48*(6), 588–600.

Sethuraman, U., & Kamat, D. (2012). Eye infection: Cures for a common ailment, part 2. *Consultant for Pediatricians, 11*(12), 405–409.

Spering, K. A. (2011, August). Therapeutic strategies for bacterial conjunctivitis. *The Clinical Advisor, pp.* 31–39.

Tahtinen, P. A., Laine, M. K., Huovinen, P., et al. (2011). A placebo-controlled trial of antimicrobial treatment for acute otitis media. *New England Journal of Medicine, 364*(2), 116–126.

Tahtinen, P., Laine, M., Ruuskanen, O., & Ruohola, A. (2012). Delayed versus immediate antimicrobial treatment for otitis media. *Pediatric Infectious Disease Journal, 31*(12), 1227–1232.

Thornton, K., Parrish, F., & Swords, C. (2011). Topical vs. systemic treatment for acute otitis media. *Pediatric Nursing, 37*(5), 263–267.

Todman, M. S., & Enzer, Y. R. (2011). Medical management vs. surgical intervention of pediatric orbital cellulitis: The importance of subperiosteal abscess volume as a new criterion. *Ophthalmic Plastic and Reconstructive Surgery, 27*(4), 255–259.

Wallace, D. K., Kraker, R. T., Beck, R. W., et al. (2011). Randomized trial to evaluate combined patching and atropine for residual amblyopia. *Archives of Ophthalmology, 129*(7), 960–962.

Wicker, A. M., & Mohundro, B. L. (2011). Management of pediatric otitis media. *U.S. Pharmacist, 35*(3), 44–49.

COMMON PEDIATRIC GASTROINTESTINAL DISORDERS

Cleft Lip and Palate

Cleft lip and palate are congenital anomalies, known as *oral-facial clefts*, resulting in structural facial malformation. These defects are usually present in early fetal development, are one of the most common birth defects in the United States, and associated with any of more than 400 syndromes. The lip, or the lip and palate, fail to close in approximately 1 in every 1,000 neonates. This equals approximately 7,000 infants born each year in the United States. Infants born with both cleft lip and palate number 4,437 per year.

Cleft lip and palate is most prevalent among Native Americans. Cleft lip (with or without cleft palate) occurs more frequently in males and isolated cleft palate is more frequent in females. The chance of having a child with an oral-facial cleft increases if one or both parents have a defect and if there is a sibling born with a defect.

 Evidence Base Parker, S. E., Mai, C. T., Canfield, M. A., et al. (2010). Updated national birth prevalence estimates for selected birth defects in the United States, 2004–2006. *Birth Defects Research, Part A: Clinical and Molecular Teratology, 88*(12), 1008–1016.

Pathophysiology and Etiology

 **Evidence Base** Kohli, S. S., & Kohli, V. S. (2012). A comprehensive review of the genetic basis of cleft lip and palate. *Journal of Oral and Maxillofacial Pathology, 16,* 64–72.

1. A failure of fusion of lip/palate tissue between 5 and 7 weeks of gestation, resulting in defect in morphogenesis. It involves patterns of DNA signaling, gene and biochemical organizers, nuclear and cellular differentiation, proliferation, and migration. A major impact is at the level of the neural crest cell.

2. Although the syndrome is not well understood, genetic/hereditary factors may play a role; a fetus with an affected parent or sibling has a 3% to 5% risk of being affected.

3. In 2004, a gene variant was identified as being a major contributor to oral-facial clefts. This gene variant may triple the risk of developing the defect in signaling and transcription proteins that are involved in development and differentiation. There is a 50% risk in monozygotic twins.

 Evidence Base Grosen, D., Bille, C., Petersen, I., et al. (2011). Risks of oral clefts in twins. *Epidemiology, 22*(3), 313–319.

4. Environmental factors may include:
    a. Vitamin B and folic acid deficiency. Some studies have shown that consumption of multivitamins with folic acid prior to conception and during the first trimester may lower the incidence of cleft lip and palate. A 2007 study by the National Institute of Environmental Health Sciences suggests taking a multivitamin containing 400 mcg of folic acid.

 Evidence Base Jia, Z. L., Shi, B., Chen, C. H., et al. (2011). Maternal malnutrition, environmental exposure during pregnancy and the risk of nonsyndromic orofacial clefts. *Oral Diseases, 17*(6), 584–589.

b. Medications taken during pregnancy, including antiseizure drugs and corticosteroids.

c. Maternal alcohol and smoking.

d. Infections.

e. Diabetes.

Types of Defects

1. Cleft lip—prealveolar cleft (see Figure 48-1):
   a. Varies from a notch in the lip to complete separation of the lip into the nose.
   b. May be unilateral or bilateral.
   c. Failure of maxillary process to fuse with nasal elevations on frontal prominence; normally occurs during 5th and 6th weeks of gestation.
   d. Merging of upper lip at midline complete between 7th and 8th weeks of gestation.

2. Isolated cleft palate—postalveolar cleft:
   a. Cleft of uvula.
   b. Cleft of soft palate.
   c. Cleft of both soft and hard palate through roof of mouth.
   d. Unilateral or bilateral.
   e. Failure of mesodermal masses of lateral palatine process to meet and fuse; normally occurs between 7th and 12th weeks of gestation.

3. Submucous cleft:
   a. Muscles of soft palate not joined.
   b. Not recognized until child talks; cannot be seen at birth.

4. Pierre Robin syndrome—cleft palate, glossoptosis (tongue lays back on pharynx), and micrognathia (underdeveloped mandible):
   a. This causes feeding difficulties, potential airway obstruction by tongue, slow weight gain, and ear infections.

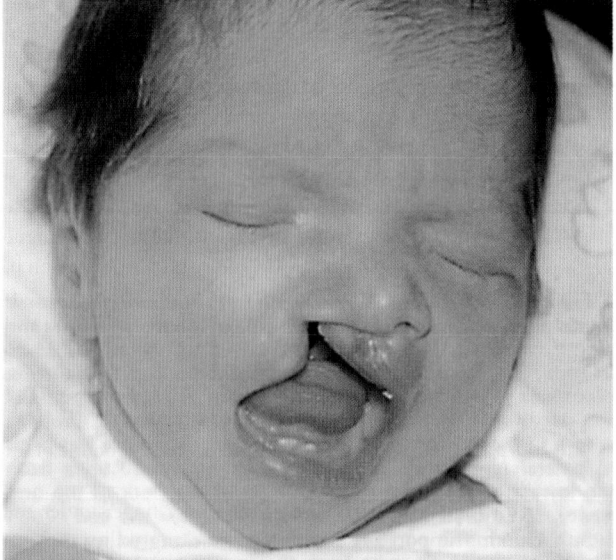

Figure 48-1. Cleft lip.

b. By age 3 to 4 months, the mandible has grown enough to accommodate the tongue and respiratory difficulty is greatly diminished.

Clinical Manifestations

1. Physical appearance of cleft lip or palate:
   a. Incompletely formed lip—varies from slight notch in vermilion to complete separation of lip.
   b. Opening in roof of mouth felt with examiner's finger on palate.
2. Eating difficulty:
   a. Suction cannot be created for effective sucking.
   b. Food returns through the nose.
3. Nasal speech.
4. Increased incidence of otitis media, which may lead to mild to moderate hearing loss.
5. Speech delay secondary to lip defect as well as related to chronic otitis media.
6. Dental problems.

Diagnostic Evaluation

 Evidence Base Aras, I., Olmez, S., & Dogan, S. (2012). Comparative evaluation of nasopharyngeal airways of unilateral cleft lip and palate patients using three-dimensional and two-dimensional methods. *Cleft Palate Craniofacial Journal, 49*(6), e75–81.

1. Prenatal ultrasonography to detect cleft lips and some cleft palates in utero.
2. Magnetic resonance imaging (MRI) and three-dimensional computed tomography to evaluate extent of abnormality before treatment.
3. Photography to document the abnormality.
4. Serial x-rays before and after treatment.
5. Dental impressions for expansion prosthesis.
6. Genetic evaluation to determine recurrence risk.

Management

 Evidence Base McGrattan, K. E., & Ellis, C. (2013). Team oriented care for orofacial clefts: A review of the literature. *Cleft Palate Craniofacial Journal 50*(1), 13–18.

Interdisciplinary approach begins early and continues into late adolescence. Craniofacial team consists of a plastic surgeon, otolaryngologist, pediatric dentist, prosthodontist, orthodontist, feeding specialist, speech pathologist, audiologist, geneticist, psychologist, and community health nurse. Each team member has a role at some point in the child's care.

1. General management is focused on proper growth and nutrition, closure of the clefts, prevention of complications, oral-motor rehabilitation, and facilitation of normal growth and development of the child.

2. Patients with isolated cleft lips have a greater chance of overcoming feeding difficulties than those with combined defects.

3. The cleft lip is repaired before the palate defect, generally around age 3 months.

   a. Techniques performed include the Millard repair, which results in a zigzag scar on the lip, or placement of sutures where the line of the columella would have been.

   b. The surgical goals are adherence and the most cosmetically pleasing and naturally appearing lip.

4. Cleft palate repair may be done any time between ages 6 and 18 months. Surgery and timing is based on degree of deformity, width of oropharynx, neuromuscular function of palate and pharynx, and surgeon's preference. Some children may require more than one reconstructive surgery.

   a. Palatoplasty is the reconstruction of the palatal musculature.

   b. The surgical goal is adherence, development of normal speech pattern, and safe/appropriate eating skills. Additionally, it should decrease the incidence of otitis media.

   c. Surgery may be performed by craniofacial or plastic surgeon in conjunction with other specialists, including oral surgeon and dentist.

Complications

1. Respiratory distress.
2. Infection.
3. Palatal fistulas.
4. Dehydration and electrolyte imbalance.
5. Bleeding.

Nursing Assessment

1. If the newborn has a cleft lip, assess for cleft palate by direct visualization and palpation with finger.
2. Obtain family history of cleft lip or palate.
3. Evaluate feeding abilities.
   a. Effectiveness of suck and swallow.
   b. Amount taken.
   c. Vomiting, regurgitation, or formula coming from nose.
4. Observe for other syndromic features, such as small jaw, abnormal facies, micro/macrocephaly, heart murmur, anal–rectal defects.

Nursing Diagnoses

- Ineffective Infant Feeding Pattern related to defect.
- Risk for Infection related to open wound created by malformation, ear infections.
- Risk for Impaired Attachment related to malformation and special care needs of the infant.
- Risk for Aspiration related to tongue and palate deformities in Pierre Robin syndrome.
- Deficient Knowledge related to home management of infant with cleft malformation.

- Fear related to surgery.
- Deficient Knowledge related to postoperative care.

Nursing Interventions

 Evidence Base Cleft Palate Foundation. (2012). Neonatal cleft lip and palate protocol: Instructions for hospital nurseries. Chapel Hill, NC: Author. Available: *www.cleftline.org/healthcare-professionals/tips for-hospital-nurseries.*

Maintaining Adequate Nutrition

1. Facilitate nutrition and speech therapy for all infants.
2. Encourage the mother to begin feeding the infant as soon as possible to enhance bonding and to strengthen the oral structures needed for mastication and speech production.
3. If sucking is permitted:
   a. Encourage breastfeeding.
   b. Encourage and demonstrate breast pump.
   c. Use a soft nipple with crosscut to facilitate feeding.
4. If sucking is ineffective due to inability to create a vacuum, try alternate oral feeding methods.
   a. Feeding devices include preemie nipple, crosscut nipple, NUK nipple, Ross Cleft Palate Nurser, Mead Johnson Cleft Palate Nurser, Pidgeon nipple bottle system, Haberman Feeder, or palatal obturator.
   b. Avoid enlarging nipple holes due to infant's inability to control flow of milk, which will result in choking. Crosscut nipples allow milk to flow only when infant squeezes the crosscut open.
   c. Using a squeezable bottle (eg, Mead Johnson Cleft Palate Nurser) or plastic liner can be helpful by applying rhythmic pressure along with the infant's normal sucking and swallowing.
   d. Rubber-tipped asepto syringe or dropper; the rubber extension should be long enough to extend back into the mouth to prevent regurgitation through the nose. Direct tip to side of mouth and feed slowly.
5. Feed infant in an upright, sitting position or the upright side-lying position if airway support is needed. This decreases possibility of fluid being aspirated or returned through the nose or back to the auditory canal.
   a. Feeding is usually easier if the nipple is angled to the side of the mouth away from the cleft so the infant's tongue can press the nipple against the upper gum or dental arch.
   b. Feed slowly over approximately 18 to 30 minutes. Feedings longer than 45 minutes expend too many calories and tire infant.
   c. Smaller but more frequent feedings may be necessary if the infant tires or requires extended time to eat.
   d. Burp frequently during feeding to decrease amount of air swallowed.
   e. If micrognathia exists, use of the pinky finger under the chin for support aids in improved sucking ability.
   f. Feed infant before he or she becomes too hungry. If the infant is too agitated, feeding becomes a problem.

6. Administer enteral tube feedings if nipple feeding is to be delayed.

7. Advance diet as appropriate for age and needs of infant. Eating usually improves when solids are introduced because they are easier for the infant to manipulate.

8. Assess and calculate adequate nutritional intake.

Preventing Infection

1. Protect child from infection so that surgery will not be delayed.
   a. Use and teach good handwashing practice.
   b. Avoid patient contact with anyone who has an infection.
   c. Provide frequent assessment for otitis media.

2. Clean the cleft after each feeding with water and a cotton-tipped applicator.

3. Observe for fever, irritability, redness, or drainage around cleft and report promptly.

4. Monitor vital signs; report temperature greater than 101° F (38.3° C).

Promoting Acceptance and Adjustment

1. Show acceptance of the infant; maintain composure and do not show negative emotion when handling the infant. The manner in which the nurse handles the infant can make a lasting impression on the parents.

2. Support parents when showing a neonate for the first time. Demonstrate acceptance of the infant's and the parents' feelings. Parents may be grieving about the infant's cosmetic imperfections and may harbor ambivalent feelings.

3. Offer information and answer any questions in a simple, matter-of-fact manner. The better informed the family, the easier it will be for them to see the infant as a normal child with a physical difference that will require surgery, dental work, and possibly speech therapy.

4. Be aware that the normal sequence of parental responses may include shock, disbelief, worry, grief, and anger and then proceed to a state of equilibrium and reorganization.

5. Encourage parental involvement in infant's care: frequent holding, cuddling, and playing.

Preventing Aspiration and Airway Obstruction

1. Prevent respiratory obstruction by the tongue, especially on inspiration and when the infant is quiet.
   a. Positioning: elevated and side-lying.
   b. Tilt head back as tolerated by the infant, and elevate upper trunk slightly.
   c. Tongue/lip suture may be placed by otolaryngologist to prevent the tongue from interfering with airway. Assess for slippage, infection, pain, interference with eating.
   d. Suction nasopharynx, as needed.

2. Infants with Pierre Robin syndrome are at greater risk for airway compromise, especially when feeding.
   a. Feeding can be done with a nursing bottle (feeding techniques similar to those used for cleft palate).
   b. Generally use orthopneic position—vertical and slightly forward; this allows infant to push jaw forward to suck and allows the feeder a clear view of the infant.
   c. Use gentle finger pressure at mandibular attachment to bring the jaw forward.

Preparing for Home Management

1. Prepare family for home feedings by providing several days to practice feeding and to become familiar with the infant's feeding pattern.

2. Alert caregiver to difficulties with feeding and how to manage them.
   a. Nasal regurgitation: feed in more upright position or stop feeding and allow the infant to cough and clear the airway; then continue with smaller feedings.
   b. Respiratory distress: feed slowly, give smaller feedings. Observe for signs of aspiration, such as coughing, color changes, increased respiration, fever, and/or formula coming from nose.
   c. Prolonged feeding: if oral feedings take longer than 20 to 30 minutes, energy expenditure increases. Smaller, more frequent feedings are indicated or enteral tube feeding supplements may be warranted.

3. Suggest that about 1 week before scheduled admission for surgery the mother begin using feeding techniques preferred by multidisciplinary team. Infants who feed well prior to surgery may do better postoperatively than poor feeders.

4. Encourage the parents to prepare siblings at home for the arrival of the infant. Suggest they show a picture of the new infant.

5. Offer parents available resources regarding children with cleft lip and palate.

6. Encourage parental involvement with local self-help groups that provide information and parent-to-parent contact.

7. Initiate referrals, as indicated, for additional support and financial assistance and early intervention programs.

8. Describe and reinforce surgical treatment plans to the parents to promote communication and hope.

9. Stress compliance with follow-up care with the pediatrician, plastic surgeon, dentist, orthodontist, psychologist, and speech therapist to prevent chronic otitis media, hearing loss, speech impairment, and emotional problems.

10. Initiate a community nurse referral to continue emotional support and teaching progress at home.

Providing Preoperative Care and Allaying Fear in the Child Undergoing Surgery

1. Prepare the infant or toddler for the postoperative experience to decrease fear and increase cooperation.
   a. Practice the feeding measure that will be used postoperatively—cup, side of spoon, or syringe.
   b. Use elbow immobilizers for short periods; allow the child to play with them and the caregiver to use them. Check your facility's policy regarding the use of immobilizers because this is considered a form of restraint, but may be deemed medically necessary.
   c. Demonstrate and practice mouth irrigation because it will be done postoperatively for cleft palate repair; allow the child to assist if age appropriate.

2. Prepare the parents emotionally for the postoperative appearance of the child.
   a. Explain the use of the Logan bow (a curved metal wire that prevents stress on the suture line for cleft lip repair) and restraints.

b. Encourage a parent to be with the child, especially when awakening from anesthesia, to offer security and comfort.

3. Address and explain pain management, collaborating with the parents as to what comforts their child.

Providing Postoperative Care

1. Protect surgical site:
   a. Apply elbow immobilizers to prevent hands from reaching the mouth while still allowing some freedom of movement; follow your institution's policy regarding medical restraints.
      i. Assess the patient's skin and/or intravenous (IV) line every 2 hours while the immobilizer is in place.
      ii. Remove the immobilizer to exercise the arms.
      iii. Do not allow anything in the child's mouth, such as straw, eating utensils, or fingers.
2. Maintain adherence device: check that Logan bow or other device is intact and maintaining adherence of lip repair.
   a. Prevent wetting tape or it will loosen.
   b. Observe for and report bleeding or dislodgement of Logan bow.
3. Prevent the child from stressing the suture site—not crying, blowing, sucking, talking, or laughing.
4. Assess and manage pain.
   a. Consult institution's pain management team, if necessary.
   b. Use pain medications appropriate for age, weight, and condition.
   c. Use pain assessment tools appropriate for age (see page 1446).
   d. Recognize signs of pain, such as crying, agitation, poor feeding, increased vital signs.
   e. Discourage pacifiers until cleared by surgeon.
   f. Encourage the mother to hold the infant, swaddle, use security/comfort items from home.
5. Positioning—elevated head of bed and side-lying.
   a. An infant seat may be useful for variation of position, comfort, entertainment, and to prevent interference with suture line.
   b. Provide for appropriate diversional activity, hanging toys, and mobiles.
   c. If only cleft palate was repaired, child may lie on abdomen.
6. Monitor respiratory effort after cleft palate repair.
   a. Be aware that breathing with a closed palate is different from the child's customary way of breathing; the child must also contend with increased mucus production.
   b. Provide humidified air, if needed, to provide moisture to mucous membranes that may become dry from mouth breathing.
7. Prevent infection.
   a. Clean suture line after every feeding.
   b. Gently wipe lip incision with cotton-tipped applicator and solution of choice, such as water, saline, or diluted hydrogen peroxide. Gently pat dry and apply antibiotic ointment or petroleum jelly, if ordered.
   c. Rinse the mouth with water or offer a drink of water after each feeding.
   d. Irrigate the mouth with normal saline solution or water after cleft palate repair. Technique may vary based on

preference of surgeon. You can direct a gentle stream over the suture line using an ear bulb syringe with the child in a sitting position with head forward.

8. Avoid tension on the suture line during feeding for several days after lip repair.
   a. Use dropper or syringe with a rubber tip and insert from the side to avoid suture line or to avoid stimulating sucking.
   b. Use side of spoon. Never put spoon into the mouth.
   c. Perform enteral tube feedings, if prescribed; usually this is last treatment of choice.
   d. Advance slowly to nipple feeding, as directed. The infant should be able to suck more efficiently after the lip is repaired.
   e. After palate repair, feed the child in the manner used preoperatively (cup, side of spoon, or rubber-tipped syringe). Never use straw, nipple, or plain syringe.
   f. Consult with speech/occupational therapy if feeding/swallowing continues to be difficult.
9. Facilitate adequate nutrition.
   a. Obtain nutrition consult, if indicated.
   b. Diet progresses from clear liquids to full liquids to soft foods.
   c. Soft foods are usually continued for about 1 month after surgery, at which time a regular diet is started, but excludes hard food.
   d. Ensure that child is receiving adequate calories.
   e. Weigh daily and plot on growth charts (*www.cdc.gov/growthcharts/*).
   f. Early feeding intervention relates to appropriate growth.
10. Administer an antibiotic, if prescribed, to prevent infection as the mouth and skin contain bacteria.

Community and Home Care Considerations

1. As the patient's advocate, alert members of the craniofacial team when a family is overwhelmed by too many appointments and interventions. Act as liaison to case manager, social worker, and home care agency.
2. Continue to assess weight gain, feeding behavior, overall development, parent–child bonding and interactions.
3. Advise the parents to discuss the child's problem with teachers and other responsible adults in close contact with the child.
   a. Aesthetic touch-up and bone graft surgery performed later may interfere with schooling.
   b. Speech differences require early identification and intervention.
   c. Monitor for reading and learning problems related to speech and language delays.
   d. Hypernasality may develop at ages 10 to 14 due to normal shrinkage of adenoid tissue occurring at this time.
4. Assess the child's self-perception and coping skills. Assess the family's support systems and coping mechanisms.

 Evidence Base Nelson, P., Glenny, A.-M., Kirk, S., et al. (2012), Parents' experiences of caring for a child with a cleft lip and/or palate: A review of the literature. *Child: Care, Health and Development, 38(1)*, 6–20.

5. Help school-age children deal with teasing (as a result of being "different" from their peers) by allowing them to express their feelings and guiding their response: ignoring the remark, responding with a joke or good-natured tease, or educating the teaser.

6. The school nurse can also help by performing frequent hearing evaluations, communicating with staff, and educating the school community on the child's condition and individual needs.

Family Education and Health Maintenance

1. Instruct on continued protection of the mouth after surgery. Child cannot put anything in mouth, including lollipops.

2. Demonstrate how to rinse mouth after eating.

3. Advise parents on the introduction of solid foods; semi-upright position or upright position; avoid spicy or acidic foods, which may irritate the oral and nasal cavities; avoid hard, sharp-edged foods, such as raw carrots or potato chips.

4. Advise on increased risk of ear infections and need to seek medical attention for colds, ear pain, fever, or other signs and symptoms. Frequent hearing screens and tympanometry should be done to monitor the effects of middle ear pathology. *Note*: Hearing should be monitored at least every 6 months during the first year of life and then annually to prevent hearing impairment.

5. Encourage modeling "good speech" by providing a stimulating language environment, and encourage spontaneous imitations of sounds at home.

6. Stress the importance of speech therapy and practicing exercises as directed by the speech therapist.

7. Encourage thorough brushing of teeth, regular dental examinations, and fluoride treatment as indicated due to risk of tooth decay related to defective enamel and abnormally positioned teeth with clefts.

8. Advise the parents on current therapies available: bone grafting providing permanent teeth support, dental implants to replace missing teeth, speech prosthesis for incomplete velopharyngeal closure.

9. Help the parents realize that, although rehabilitation is extensive, their child can live a normal life.

10. For additional information and support, refer patients and family to the Cleft Palate Foundation (*www.cleftline.org*) and Velo-Cardio-Facial Syndrome Educational Foundation (*www.vcfsef.org*).

11. Refer families to companies that manufacture bottles for cleft palate: Enfamil (Mead Johnson) Cleft Palate Nurser, 1-800-222-9123; Medela Haberman Feeder, 1-800-435-8316; Pigeon Bottle (Children's Medical Ventures), 1-888-766-8443.

Evaluation: Expected Outcomes

- Infant feeds with appropriate feeding device in small amounts every 2 to 3 hours.
- No signs of infection.
- Parents involved with care; demonstrate contact with infant as seen by holding and talking to infant.
- Proper positioning maintained, no signs of aspiration.

- Parents demonstrate proper feeding technique as evidenced by adequate nutrition and weight gain.
- Parents and child prepared for surgery.
- Parents express understanding of postoperative home care procedures and identify supportive resources.

Esophageal Atresia with Tracheoesophageal Fistula

 Evidence Base Alberti, D., Boroni, G., Corasaniti, L., et al. (2011). Esophageal atresia: Pre and postoperative management. *Journal of Maternal-Fetal and Neonatal Medicine, 24*(Suppl. 1), 4–6.

Pinheiro, P., Simoes e Silva, A., & Pereira, R. (2012). Current knowledge on esophageal atresia. *World Journal of Gastroenterology, 18*(28), 3662–3672.

Esophageal atresia (EA) is failure of the esophagus to form a continuous passage from the pharynx to the stomach during embryonic development. EA can occur with *tracheoesophageal fistula (TEF)*, which is an abnormal connection between the trachea and esophagus. EA/TEF occurs in approximately 1 in 3,500 births.

Clinically, EA/TEF is divided equally into isolated EA and syndromic EA. Additional defects vary in severity, with cardiac anomalies as the most common (14.7% to 28%) and life-threatening. Currently, an overall survival of 85% to 90% has been reported from developed countries. In developing countries, however, several factors contribute to higher mortality rates. Such factors include prematurity, delay in diagnosis with an increased incidence of aspiration pneumonia, and a shortage of qualified nurses.

Pathophysiology and Etiology

1. Cause is unknown in most cases and likely multifactorial. Possible influences include:
   a. Low evidence for inheritable genetic factor
   b. Six to 10% due to chromosomal (structural) abnormalities, including trisomies (12, 18, 21), and partial deletions such as 13q13-qter, 22q11.2.

 Evidence Base Genevieve, D., de Pontual, L., Amiel, J., et al. (2011). Genetic factors in isolated and syndromic esophageal atresia. *Journal of Pediatric Gastroenterology and Nutrition, 52*(Suppl. 1), S6–S8.

   c. Teratogenic stimuli, such as the anticancer drug adriamycin and diethylstilbestrol (DES).

2. Failure of proper separation of the embryonic channel into the esophagus and trachea occurring during the 4th and 5th weeks of gestation.

3. Esophageal atresia can be classified as (see Figure 48-2):
   a. *Type I* (Type A): proximal and distal segments of esophagus are blind; there is no connection to trachea; accounts for approximately 7% of cases; second most common.
   b. *Type II* (Type B): proximal segment of esophagus opens into trachea by a fistula; distal segment is blind; rare, 0.8% of cases.

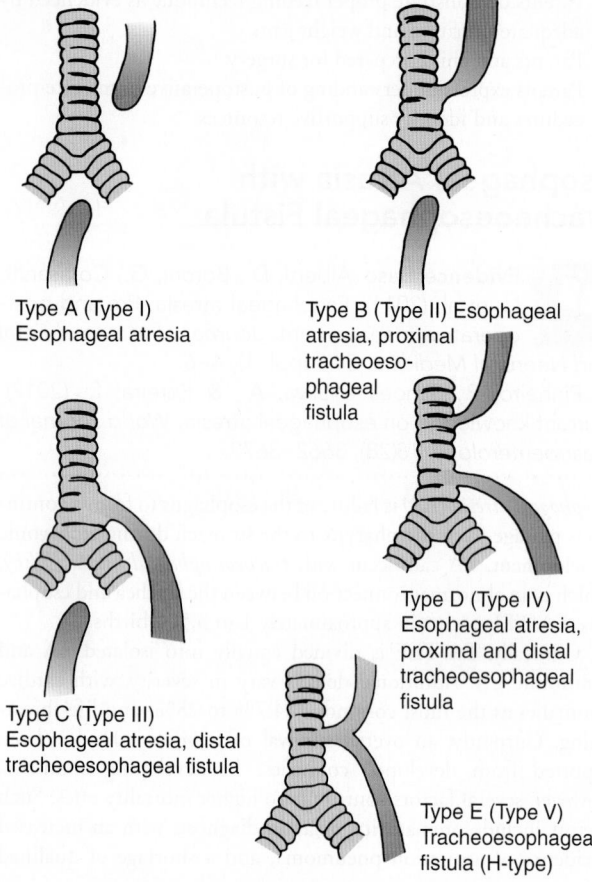

Figure 48-2. Types of esophageal atresia: esophageal atresia and tracheoesophageal fistula.

Type A (Type I)
Esophageal atresia

Type B (Type II) Esophageal atresia, proximal tracheoeso-phageal fistula

Type C (Type III) Esophageal atresia, distal tracheoesophageal fistula

Type D (Type IV) Esophageal atresia, proximal and distal tracheoesophageal fistula

Type E (Type V) Tracheoesophageal fistula (H-type)

c. *Type III* (Type C): proximal segment of esophagus has blind end; distal segment of esophagus connects into trachea by a fistula; most common, with 86% of cases. (Discussion is limited to this type.)

d. *Type IV* (Type D): esophageal atresia with fistula between proximal and distal ends of trachea and esophagus (rare, 0.7% of cases).

e. *Type V* (Type E): proximal and distal segments of esophagus open into trachea by a fistula; no esophageal atresia but sometimes referred to as an H-type fistula; occurs in 4.2% of cases; not usually diagnosed at birth.

4. Associations:
   a. Down syndrome.
   b. VACTERL syndrome (vertebral defects, anal atresia, cardiac anomaly, TEF fistula with EA, renal defects, and radial limb dysplasia).
   c. Feingold syndrome.

Clinical Manifestations

These appear soon after birth.

1. Excessive secretions.
   a. Constant drooling.
   b. Large amount of secretions from nose.
   c. Saliva or formula accumulates in upper esophageal pouch and is aspirated into airway.
2. Intermittent, unexplained cyanosis and laryngospasm.
   a. Caused by aspiration of accumulated saliva in blind pouch.
   b. Gastric acid is regurgitated through distal fistula.
3. Abdominal distention.
   a. Occurs as a result of air entering the lower esophagus through the fistula and passing into the stomach, especially when the child is crying.
4. Violent response after first or second swallow of feeding.
   a. Infant coughs and chokes.
   b. Fluid returns through nose and mouth.
   c. Cyanosis occurs.
   d. Infant struggles.
5. Poor feeding.
6. Inability to pass catheter through nose or mouth into stomach; tip of catheter stops at blind pouch, or atresia. *Note*: Be aware of coiling of catheter; coiling may make catheter appear to be descending into stomach.
7. Infant can be premature and pregnancy complicated by polyhydramnios. Look for other birth anomalies.

Diagnostic Evaluation

1. Ultrasound scanning techniques enable TEF to be identified in utero for some infants.
2. Failure to pass a 10F catheter (smaller catheters may coil) into the stomach through nose or mouth. Catheter is left in situ while an x-ray confirms the diagnosis.
3. pH of tracheal secretions is acidic.
4. Flat-plate x-ray of abdomen and chest may reveal presence of gas in stomach and catheter coiled in the blind pouch. Barium x-ray may be used in some cases.
5. Electrocardiogram and echocardiogram are performed because there is a high association with cardiac anomalies.

Management

Immediate Treatment

1. Propping infant at 30-degree angle, supine or side-lying, to prevent reflux of gastric contents.
2. Nasogastric (NG) tube remains in the esophagus and is aspirated frequently to prevent aspiration until continuous low suction is applied.
3. Pouch is washed out with normal saline to prevent thick mucus from blocking the tube.
4. Gastrostomy to decompress stomach and prevent aspiration; later used for feedings.
5. Nothing by mouth (NPO); IV fluids.
6. Comorbidities, such as pneumonitis and heart failure, are treated.
7. Supportive therapy includes meeting nutritional requirements, IV fluids, antibiotics, respiratory support, and maintaining thermally neutral environment.

Surgery

1. Prompt primary repair: fistula found by bronchoscopy is divided, followed by esophageal anastomosis of proximal and distal segments if infant weight permits and is without pneumonia.
2. Short-term delay: subsequent primary repair is used to stabilize infant and prevent deterioration when the patient's condition contraindicates immediate surgery.
3. Staging: initially, fistula division and gastrostomy are performed with later secondary esophageal anastomosis or colonic transposition performed approximately 1 year later to effect total repair. Approach may be used with a very small, premature infant or a very sick neonate or when severe congenital anomalies exist.
4. Circular esophagomyotomy may be performed on proximal pouch to gain length and allow for primary anastomosis at initial surgery.
5. Cervical esophagostomy: when ends of esophagus are too widely separated, esophageal replacement with segment of intestine (colonic transposition) is done at ages 18 to 24 months.
6. Fiberoptic tracheoscopy-assisted repair of tracheoesophageal fistula can expedite and facilitate surgery on ventilated patients.
7. Staged repair resulted in least amount of GI dysmotility postoperatively.

 Evidence Base Lacher, M., Froehlich, S., von Schweinitz, D., et al. (2009) Early and long term outcome in children with esophageal atresia treated over the last 22 years. *Surgery, 145*(6), 675–681.

Complications

Note: Higher rates of complications occur in patients with cardiac anomalies and low birth weight.

1. Death from asphyxia.
2. Pneumonitis/pneumonia secondary to salivary aspiration and/or gastric acid reflux.
3. Leak at anastomosis site: most common and dangerous complication (15–20%).
4. Recurrent fistulas.
5. Esophageal strictures (30–40%).
6. Abnormal function of distal esophagus sphincter (gastroesophageal reflux can be found in approximately 50% of these infants).
7. Esophagitis.
8. Tracheomalacia (10–20% of these patients).
9. GERD (40–65%).
10. Feeding problems with older children due to esophageal dysmotility (95%).

Nursing Assessment

Assessment begins immediately after birth.

1. Be alert for risk factors of polyhydramnios and prematurity.
2. Suspect in infant with the following:

   a. Excessive amount of mucus.
   b. Difficulty with secretions.
   c. Cyanotic episodes (unexplained).
3. Report suspicion to health care provider immediately.

Nursing Diagnoses

Preoperative

- Risk for Aspiration related to structural abnormality.
- Risk for Deficient Fluid Volume related to inability to take oral fluids.
- Anxiety of parents related to critical situation of neonate.

Postoperative

- Ineffective Airway Clearance related to surgical intervention.
- Ineffective Infant Feeding Pattern related to defect.
- Acute Pain related to surgical procedure.
- Impaired Tissue Integrity related to postoperative drainage.
- Risk for Injury related to complex surgery.
- Risk for Impaired Attachment related to prolonged hospitalization.

Nursing Interventions

Preventing Aspiration

1. Position the infant supine with head and chest elevated 20 to 30 degrees to prevent or decrease reflux of gastric juices into the tracheobronchial tree.

   a. This position may also ease respiratory effort by dropping the distended intestines away from the diaphragm.
   b. Side-lying position can be used if the risk of aspiration from being supine is greater than the risk of sudden infant death syndrome (SIDS); supine positioning is preferred to reduce the risk of SIDS.
   c. Turn frequently to prevent atelectasis and pneumonia.
2. Perform intermittent nasopharyngeal suctioning or maintain indwelling Sump tube with constant suction to remove secretions from esophageal blind pouch.

   a. Tip of tube is placed in the blind pouch.
   b. Sump tube allows air to be drawn in through a second lumen and prevents tube obstruction by mucous membrane of pouch.
   c. Maintain indwelling tube patency by irrigating with 1 mL normal saline solution frequently.
3. Place the infant in an Isolette or under a radiant warmer with high humidity to aid in liquefying secretions and thick mucus. Maintain the infant's temperature in thermoneutral zone and ensure environmental isolation to prevent infection by using Isolette.
4. Administer oxygen, as needed.
5. Suction mouth to keep it clear of secretions and prevent aspiration. Provide mouth care.
6. Be alert for indications of respiratory distress.

   a. Retractions.
   b. Circumoral cyanosis.
   c. Restlessness.
   d. Nasal flaring.
   e. Increased respiration and heart rate.

7. Maintain NPO status.

8. Administer antibiotics, as ordered, to prevent or treat associated pneumonitis.

9. Observe infant carefully for any change in condition; report changes immediately.
   a. Check vital signs, color and amount of secretions, abdominal distention, and respiratory distress.
   b. Evaluate for complications that can occur in any neonate or premature infant.

10. Be available and recognize need for emergency care or resuscitation.
    a. Have resuscitation equipment on hand.
    b. Accompany the infant to other departments and the operating room in Isolette with portable oxygen and suction equipment.

11. Monitor for signs or symptoms that may indicate additional congenital anomalies or complications.

12. Gastrostomy tube (GT) may be placed before definitive surgery to aid in gastric decompression, prevention of reflux, or nutrition.

Preventing Dehydration

1. Administer parenteral fluids and electrolytes as prescribed.

2. Monitor vital signs frequently for changes in blood pressure (BP) and pulse, which may indicate dehydration or fluid volume overload.

3. Record intake and output, including gastric drainage (if GT for decompression is present) and weight of diapers.

Reducing Parental Anxiety

1. Explain procedures and necessary events to parents as soon as possible.

2. Orient parents to hospital and intensive care nursery environment.

3. Allow family to hold and assist in caring for infant.

4. Offer reassurance and encouragement to family frequently. Provide for additional support by social worker, clergy, and counselor, as needed.

Maintaining Patent Airway

1. Keep endotracheal (ET) tube patent by frequent lavage and suction. *Note*: Reintubation could damage the anastomosis.

2. Suction frequently; every 5 to 10 minutes may be necessary, but at least every 1 to 2 hours.

3. Observe for signs of obstructed airway. Ventilatory support is continued until clinically stable (usually 24 to 48 hours).

4. Request that the surgeon mark a suction catheter, indicating how far the catheter can be safely inserted without disturbing the anastomosis (usually 2 to 3 cm).

5. Administer chest physiotherapy, as prescribed.
   a. Change the infant's position by turning; stimulate crying to promote full expansion of lungs.
   b. Elevate head and shoulders 20 to 30 degrees.
   c. Use mechanical vibrator 2 to 3 days postoperatively (to minimize trauma to anastomosis), followed by more vigorous physical therapy after the third day.

 NURSING ALERT Care should be taken not to hyperextend the neck, causing stress to the operative site.

6. Continue use of Isolette or radiant warmer with humidity.

7. Be prepared for an emergency: have emergency equipment available, including suction machine, catheter, oxygen, laryngoscope, ET tubes in varying sizes.

Providing Adequate Nutrition

Feedings may be given by mouth, by gastrostomy, or (rarely) by a feeding tube into the esophagus, depending on the type of operation performed and the infant's condition.

1. The gastrostomy is generally attached to gravity drainage postoperatively, then elevated and left open to allow for air to escape and gastric secretions to pass into the duodenum before feedings are begun.

2. Practice patterns differ regarding when to start feedings but generally minimal enteral nutrition is beneficial in promoting gut motility, decreasing bacterial overgrowth, and decreasing the stress on the liver; these "trickle" feedings are given at a rate of 5 to 20 mL/kg per day.

3. Give the infant a pacifier to suck during feedings, unless contraindicated.

4. Use care to prevent air from entering the stomach, thereby causing gastric distention and possible reflux.

5. Continue gastrostomy feedings until the infant can tolerate full feedings orally.

Providing Comfort Measures

1. Position comfortably.

2. Avoid restraints when possible.

3. Administer mouth care frequently.

4. Offer pacifier frequently.

5. Assess for pain and administer analgesics, as ordered (see page 1446).

6. Caress and speak or sing to infant frequently. Handling should be kept to a gentle minimum.

Maintaining Chest Drainage

1. Assess type of chest drainage present (determined by surgical approach). Report saliva or hemorrhage.
   a. Retropleural—small tube in posterior mediastinum; may be left open for drainage.
   b. Transthoracic—chest tube placed in pleural space and connected to suction.

2. Keep tubing patent: free from clots, unkinked, and without tension.

3. If a break occurs in the closed drainage system, immediately clamp tubing close to the infant to prevent pneumothorax.

Observing for Complications

1. Inspect for leak at the anastomosis, causing mediastinitis, pneumothorax, and saliva in chest tube: hypothermia or hyperthermia, severe respiratory distress, cyanosis, restlessness, weak pulses.

2. Continue to monitor for complications during the recovery process.

a. Stricture at the anastomosis: difficulty in swallowing, vomiting, or spitting-up of ingested fluid; refusing to eat; fever secondary to aspiration and pneumonia.

b. Recurrent fistula: coughing, choking, and cyanosis associated with feeding; excessive salivation; difficulty in swallowing associated with abnormal distention; repeated episodes of pneumonitis; general poor physical condition (no weight gain).

c. Atelectasis or pneumonitis: aspiration, respiratory distress.

3. Provide meticulous care for cervical esophagostomy—artificial opening in the neck that allows for drainage of the upper esophagus.

a. Keep the area clean of saliva.

b. Wash with clear water.

c. Place an absorbent pad over the area.

4. As soon as possible, allow the infant to suck a few milliliters of milk at the same time gastrostomy feeding is being done. Advance the infant to solid foods, as appropriate, if esophagostomy is maintained for a few months.

a. Encourage sucking and swallowing.

b. Familiarize the infant with food so that when able to eat orally, infant will be used to it.

5. Begin oral feedings 10 to 14 days postoperatively after anastomosis, as directed.

a. Feed slowly to allow the infant time to swallow.

b. Use upright sitting position to avoid risk of regurgitation.

c. Burp frequently or vent GT.

d. Do not allow the infant to become overtired at feeding time. Note heart rate.

e. Try to make each feeding a pleasant experience for the infant. Use a consistent approach and patience. Encourage parental involvement.

Stimulating Parent–Infant Attachment

1. Gently hold and cuddle the infant for feedings and after feedings.

2. Encourage parents to cuddle and talk to the infant.

3. Provide for visual, auditory, and tactile stimulation, as appropriate, for the infant's physical condition and age.

4. Provide opportunities for the parents to learn all aspects of care of their infant.

5. Encourage the parents to talk about their feelings, fears, and concerns.

6. Help to develop a healthy parent–child relationship through flexible visiting, frequent phone calls, and encouraging physical contact between child and parents.

Community and Home Care Considerations

Evidence Base Delacourt, C., Hadchouel, A., Toelen, J., et al. (2012). Long term respiratory outcomes of congenital diaphragmatic hernia, esophageal atresia and cardiovascular anomalies. *Seminars in Fetal Neonatal Medicine, 17*(2), 105–111.

1. Teach carefully and thoroughly all procedures to be done at home. Show the parents how to do them and then watch return demonstration of the following procedures:

a. Gastrostomy feedings and care.

b. Esophagostomy care with feeding technique.

c. Suctioning.

d. Identifying signs of respiratory distress.

2. Advise parents that esophageal motility will be affected for many years, due to the narrowed abnormal esophagus emptying slowly and tension on the stomach from the anastomosis.

3. Reflux may increase after surgery, thus should be maximally treated due to the risk of developing esophageal strictures.

4. Monitor weight gain and developmental progress.

5. Observe parental feeding technique.

6. Encourage parents to discuss child's condition with daycare workers, teachers, school nurse, or other responsible adults in close contact with the child so that they will be able to recognize possible problems and reinforce good eating habits.

7. To compensate for altered motility, encourage cutting food into small pieces, chewing food well, swallowing food with fluid, and sitting upright while eating.

8. Observe parent–child interaction to assess for overprotection and appropriate coping skills.

Family Education and Health Maintenance

1. Help the parents understand the psychological needs of the infant for sucking, warmth, comfort, stimulation, and affection. Suggest that activity be appropriate for age.

2. Encourage the parents to continue close medical follow-up and help them learn to recognize possible problems.

a. Eating problems may occur, especially when solids are introduced.

b. Repeated respiratory tract infection should be reported.

c. Occurrence of stricture at site of anastomosis weeks to months later may be recognized by difficulty in swallowing, spitting of ingested fluid, and fever. Continue all reflux medications until advised otherwise. Medications should be adjusted by weight as infant grows.

d. Dilatation of esophagus may be necessary to treat stricture at the site of the anastomosis.

e. Signs of fistula leakage are dusky color or choking with feeding.

3. Help the parents understand the need for good nutrition and the need to follow the diet regimen suggested by the health care provider.

4. Reassure parents that an infant's raspy cough is normal and will gradually diminish as the infant's trachea becomes stronger over 6 to 24 months (most infants have some tracheomalacia).

5. Teach parents to guard against the child swallowing foreign objects.

6. Help and support can be given by introducing the parents to other parents of children with TEF.

7. For additional information and support, refer parents to EA/TEF Family Support Connection (*www.eatef.org*), TEF Vater (*www.tefvater.org*), Birth Defect Research for Children (*www.birthdefects.org*), International Foundation for Functional Gastrointestinal Disorders (*www.aboutkidsgi.org*), Boston Children's Hospital (*www.childrenshospital.org*), or the March of Dimes Foundation (*www.modimes.org*).

Evaluation: Expected Outcomes

- No cyanosis or respiratory distress.
- Hydrated; urine output adequate.
- Parents hold and talk to infant; express concerns.
- Postoperatively, tolerates gastrostomy feedings without distention or regurgitation.
- Infant thrives, with adequate weight gain.
- Infant sleeps and rests without irritability or pain.
- Chest tube in place with minimal drainage.
- Feeds without regurgitation 12 days postoperatively.
- Parents caring for infant postoperatively and assisting with feedings.

Gastroesophageal Reflux (GER) and Gastroesophageal Reflux Disease (GERD)

 Evidence Base Vandenplas, Y., Rudolph, D., Di Lorenzo, C., et al. (2009). Joint Recommendations of the North American Society for Pediatric Gastroenterology, Hepatology, and Nutrition and the European Society for Pediatric Gastroenterology, Hepatology, and Nutrition. *Journal of Pediatric Gastroenterology and Nutrition, 49*(4), 498–547.

Gastroesophageal reflux (GER) is the passage of gastric contents into the esophagus. The barrier between the stomach and esophagus is controlled primarily by pressure at the lower esophageal sphincter (LES). GER is a normal physiologic process and occurs in all healthy infants and children, usually several times a day, without symptoms or sequelae. Of all infants with GER, 50% will be symptomatic (vomiting) during the first 3 months of life; 67% of infants ages 4 to 9 months will have symptoms; and 5% of ages 10 to 12 months will have symptoms. Symptomatic GER often self-resolves by 12 to 14 months of age.

Gastroesophageal reflux disease (GERD) is defined as the symptom complex that results as a complication of GER. GERD is used to describe a condition when this reflux process causes bothersome symptoms and complications, such as significant discomfort and altered feeding and sleeping patterns. Clinical manifestations include vomiting, dysphagia, food refusal, poor weight gain, failure to thrive (FTT), esophagitis, irritability, abdominal pain, substernal pain, respiratory disorders, asthma, and apparent life-threatening events (ALTE) or apnea.

The North American Society for Pediatric Gastroenterology, Hepatology, and Nutrition has formulated guidelines for the diagnosis and management of GER and GERD in infants and children; however, these guidelines are not intended for the management of neonates less than 72 hours old, premature neonates, or infants/children with neurologic or anatomic abnormalities of the upper GI tract. The American Academy of Pediatrics has also endorsed these guidelines.

Supportive care by nurses and other health care staff regarding feeding techniques and nutrition is often sufficient for patients with GER. GERD may require additional interventions such as changes to feeding regimen or medication therapy.

Pathophysiology and Etiology

GER

1. The LES is a physiologic, rather than an anatomic, segment that forms an antireflux barrier.
   a. Two to 5 cm in length.
   b. Characterized by a pressure greater than that found proximally in the esophagus or distally in the stomach.
   c. Constitutes an effective barrier to protect the esophageal mucosa and airway passages from damage by gastric contents (acid, pepsin, bile salts, food).
   d. Neuromuscular connection is weak in infants, GER peaks at age 6 months and usually resolves by 12 months.

GERD

1. Episodes of GERD with aspiration of refluxed material are more likely to occur during the nocturnal period—when the esophagus and stomach are leveled and the swallowing response to reflux and airway protection mechanisms are blunted by sleep.
2. Cause is undetermined in most patients; however, possible causes include:
   a. Delayed neuromuscular development.
   b. Cerebral defects.
   c. Obstruction at or just below the pylorus (eg, pyloric stenosis, malrotation).
   d. Physiologic immaturity.
   e. Increased abdominal pressure.
   f. Obesity.
   g. Cystic fibrosis.
   h. Congenital esophageal disease.
3. Associated conditions that contribute to reflux include:
   a. Chronic lung disease—there is a higher incidence of reflux in infants with this condition. It appears to be related to the duration of the episode and how proximal the reflux occurs, possibly contributing to poor clearance.
   b. Trauma/mechanical causes that affect the LES.
      i. Indwelling orogastric/NG enteric feeding tube.
      ii. Surgery on the esophagus or stomach.
      iii. Mechanical ventilation.
      iv. Extreme changes in position, lying completely flat, seating devices for infants greater than a 30% incline (increases intra-abdominal pressure).
      v. Hiatal hernia.
   c. Studies show a reduced incidence of reflux in the prone position versus the supine position; however, the American Academy of Pediatrics' "Back to Sleep" program discourages prone positioning due to increased incidence of SIDS.
   d. Protein allergy: increased inflammation in the mucosa of the esophagus and stomach, altering motility.
   e. Medications/drugs that affect LES and increase gastric acidity, such as bronchodilators, antihypertensives, diazepam, meperidine, morphine, prostaglandins, calcium channel blockers, nitrate heart medications, anticholinergics, adrenergic drugs, caffeine, alcohol, and nicotine.
   f. Cystic fibrosis, cardiac disease, and other chronic illnesses.

Clinical Manifestations of GERD

Infants

1. Vomiting or regurgitation of formula or breast milk.
2. Irritability, excessive crying with or without association with vomiting.
3. Sleep disturbances.
4. Arching, stiffening.
5. It is recommended that the infant be referred to a pediatric gastroenterologist if the following manifestations occur:
   a. Refusal to eat.
   b. Weight loss or failure to gain weight.
   c. Dehydration.
   d. Recurrent respiratory symptoms, such as cough, wheezing, stridor, pneumonia, otitis media, bronchitis.
   e. ALTE: blue spell, decreased responsiveness, limp, apnea, bradycardia. (*Note*: The exact relationship between GER and ALTE is not clear despite continued investigation. Indeed, both apnea and reflux are common in premature neonates.)
   f. Eructation (belching).
   g. Sandifer's syndrome (rare)—dystonic posturing caused by reflux.
   h. Anemia (from chronic esophagitis).
   i. Hematemesis (vomitus with blood).
   j. Occult blood in stool.
   k. Hypoproteinemia: low albumin due to severe inflammation and protein losses in the GI tract; can be seen with or without malnutrition and FTT.

Older Children

1. Intermittent vomiting.
2. Chronic heartburn or regurgitation.
3. Upper abdominal discomfort; pressure or "squeezing" feeling.
4. Chronic respiratory/airway symptoms, such as cough, stridor, otitis media, bronchitis, asthma.
5. Food refusal.
6. Dysphagia: difficulty swallowing.
7. Odynophagia: painful swallowing.
8. Anemia (from chronic esophagitis).
9. Hematemesis.
10. Hypoproteinemia.
11. Occult blood in stool.

Diagnostic Evaluation

1. History of infant's or child's feeding habits.
2. Multiple intraluminal impedance and esophageal pH monitoring can be performed on all ages; no sedation necessary.
   a. Considered gold standard for reflux and is performed over 24 hours, but does not indicate whether aspiration is occurring.
   b. Used as an index of esophageal acid exposure; however, esophageal impedance studies have been found to be more accurate, especially in the neurologically impaired child.
   c. The child must be off acid-suppressing medications for 48 to 72 hours so that acid pH can be detected.
   d. Gastric motility medications may or may not be held depending on the reason for performing the study.
   e. Most centers allow the patient to go home and return 24 hours later. Exceptions include the fragile child, premature infant, infant with active respiratory symptoms, or the child with significant symptoms who requires close observation because reflux may exacerbate while off reflux medications.
   f. Not indicated in the infant/child who is vomiting, unable to tolerate bolus feedings, or acutely ill. Because the probe is inserted in a nares, infant/children with oxygen requirements may not tolerate the study.
3. Endoscopy and biopsy allow for visualization of esophageal, gastric, and duodenal mucosa.
   a. Indicated for severe GERD or failure of medical management.
   b. Biopsy can determine cause: allergy (eosinophilic), inflammation, chemical injury, or Barrett's esophagus.
   c. Mechanical problems such as strictures, webs, and duplication/cysts will be visualized.
   d. For this procedure, sedation and anesthesia are necessary.
   e. Reflux medications do not have to be discontinued for the study.
   f. Can be done on the child who is not tolerating feedings. However, severity of illness may prevent study from being performed due to risk associated with procedure, such as with anesthesia, infection, bleeding, cardiac.
4. Technetium scintigraphy (milk/emptying scan) to assess gastric emptying and associated aspiration. This is not a reliable test for determining GERD.
   a. Sedation is not necessary and the study can be performed on children of all ages.
   b. Involves drinking/eating food with radionuclide, followed by dynamic sequenced imaging.
   c. Not indicated in the infant/child who is vomiting, unable to tolerate bolus feedings, or acutely ill.
   d. Acid suppression medications do not interfere with the study.
5. Modified barium swallow—also called *videofluoroscopy*.
   a. Assesses oral pharyngeal function and potential for aspiration from oral intake using several consistencies of feedings. This is not a reliable test for determining GERD.
   b. Sedation is not necessary for this procedure, but does require cooperation with eating.
   c. Should not be performed on the infant/child with acute respiratory symptoms or one identified by speech therapy or occupational therapy as being at risk for aspiration.
   d. Reflux medications do not have to be discontinued for the study.
   e. Speech therapist can be present for the exam to offer detailed assessment of oral-motor skills and swallowing.
6. Esophageal manometry to measure pressure inside the LES.
   a. It is a cooperative, nonsedated procedure and can only be used on an older child.
   b. Reflux medications generally do not have to be discontinued for the study.

7. Intraluminal esophageal impedance to detect the flow of liquids and gas through the esophagus may be used in combination with manometry.
8. Polysomnography may be used for evaluation of infant apnea and sleep apnea.

Complications

Complications result from frequent and sustained reflux of gastric contents into lower esophagus.

1. Recurrent pulmonary disease.
2. Chronic esophagitis.
3. FTT.
4. Anemia.
5. ALTE, although evidence is not strong.
6. Esophageal stricture from scarring.
7. Barrett's esophagus: the replacement of distal esophageal mucosa with a potentially malignant metaplastic epithelium caused by chronic exposure to acid.
8. Chronic sinusitis/otitis media.
9. There is an unclear relationship between GERD and dental erosion/caries.

Management

Goal of treatment is to alleviate and relieve symptoms and prevent complications. May be treated medically through careful positioning, feeding techniques, and medication or surgically.

Positioning for GER

1. Esophageal monitoring has demonstrated that infants have significantly fewer episodes of GER when prone. Several studies support less incidence of reflux episodes in the prone and left-side sleeping position; however, the North American Society for Pediatric Gastroenterology, Hepatology and Nutrition, along with the American Academy of Pediatrics, endorses the following recommendations:
   a. Place infant up over shoulder after feedings, avoid sitting on lap to burp, which increases intra-abdominal pressure.
   b. Handle the infant gently, with minimal movement during and after feeding.

Feeding for GER

1. Two- to 4-week trial of hypoallergenic formula in the formula-fed infant. Continuance of breastfeeding with the mother eliminating milk and soy products is encouraged, as allergen sensitivity can contribute to GER. No studies support the need for dietary restriction in mothers who breastfeed, but in anecdotal reports, infants appear to improve when dairy products are reduced. Trial of partially hydrolyzed formula and/or hydrolyzed formula is useful for refractory symptoms or for those infants/children with signs of allergy, anemia, constipation, occult positive stools, vomiting.
2. Thickened feedings with dry rice cereal (1 tbsp per ounce of formula) or commercial thickening agent may be used. Thickening does not decrease episodes of reflux but does decrease episodes of vomiting. Commercial formulas thickened with rice starch are now available, but no studies regarding their efficacy have been published; they require an acidic environment to work and, therefore, necessitate the discontinuation of acid suppression medications. Thickening of breast milk may be necessary in infants with poor weight gain.
3. Pectin liquid partially decreases GER, as measured by esophageal pH monitoring, and might improve vomiting and respiratory symptoms in children with cerebral palsy.
4. Small, frequent feedings followed by upright positioning with infant held over the shoulder.
5. Concentrating formula is a method of increasing calories for the volume-sensitive infant.
6. Avoid constant feeding (grazing), which reduces appetite and, ultimately, caloric intake.
7. Comfort the infant to reduce crying before and after meals, which increases intra-abdominal pressure and swallowing of air, increasing the likelihood of reflux.
8. Use a pacifier for nonnutritive sucking after eating to avoid overeating.

Feeding for GERD

1. Transgastric (transpyloric) enteric feeding tube used for infants when reflux medical management fails and symptoms persist; can reduce number of reflux episodes, but has not been shown to significantly reduce episodes of apnea.
   a. There are concerns regarding using these feeding tubes in neonates; however, the rate of complications does not appear to be statistically significant in recent reports.
   b. The procedure should be performed by a skilled pediatric radiologist or neonatal intensive care nurse, using a small-caliber soft polyurethane nonweighted feeding tube.
   c. Considered a temporary feeding method (to help infant/child gain weight and improve respiratory symptoms) until further options can be explored, such as surgery—Nissen fundoplication or jejunostomy.
   d. To prevent clogging, tubes should be flushed at least four to six times per day and before and after medication administration. If the tube clogs or dislodges, the family must return to a qualified center for reinsertion.
   e. If feeding difficulty persists, consult dietitian and speech and/or occupational therapist.
2. Older child:
   a. Nothing to eat 2 hours before bedtime.
   b. Avoid spicy and acidic foods (onions, citrus products, apple juice, tomatoes), esophageal irritants (chocolate, caffeinated beverages, peppermint, and secondhand smoke), and carbonated beverages.
   c. Chew gum (stimulates parotid secretions, which augment esophageal clearance and provide a buffering effect).

Other Lifestyle Changes for GERD

1. Prevent obesity.
2. Avoid tight or constrictive clothing.
3. Avoid nonsteroidal anti-inflammatory drugs, especially at bedtime.

Drug Therapy for GERD

1. Often used in combination with lifestyle changes. Prescribed for a 12-week trial and can be tapered and discontinued if symptoms resolve.

2. Antacids—buffer existing acids and also increase serum gastrin levels, leading to increase in LES pressure (symptomatic relief). Chronic antacid therapy is generally not recommended unless ordered by a gastroenterologist.

3. Histamine-2 (H_2) receptor antagonists—act by reducing hydrochloric acid and pepsinogen secretion by blocking histamine receptors on the parietal cells.
   a. Cimetidine, ranitidine, famotidine, nizatidine.
   b. Oral dosing of t.i.d. versus b.i.d. has demonstrated improved duration of acid suppression in study of infants (44% vs. 90%).
   c. Tolerance to IV dosing within 6 weeks of usage has been observed.

4. PPIs—block all gastric acid secretion by binding and deactivating the H^+/K^+ ATPase enzyme pumps. To be activated, PPIs require acid in the parietal cell canaliculus; therefore, they are most effective when the parietal cells are stimulated by a meal following a fast.
   a. Omeprazole, lansoprazole, pantoprazole, esomeprazole, rabeprazole.
   b. Generally given 15 to 30 minutes before a meal, one to two times per day.
   c. Generally not recommended in combination with H_2-antagonists due to interference with absorption (H_2 reduces the acid necessary for PPI to work).
   d. Reserved for infants and children resistant to H_2-antagonist therapy. Gastroenterology specialist should be involved. Data on the pharmacology in infants and children are limited.
   e. Dominant regurgitation in neonates and infants responds poorly to PPIs.

 DRUG ALERT All acid-altering medications may affect the efficacy of pH-dependent medications. Additionally, PPIs are metabolized to varying degrees by the hepatic cytochrome P450 enzymatic system and may alter drug metabolism by induction or inhibition of the cytochrome P enzymes.

5. Prokinetic agents—the rationale for prokinetic therapy is based on the evidence that it enhances esophageal peristalsis and accelerates gastric emptying.
   a. Metoclopramide most commonly used—an antidopaminergic agent whose efficacy is not well observed in clinical trials. Adverse effects include parkinsonian reactions, tardive dyskinesia, irritability, sleeplessness, and lowered seizure threshold.
   b. Erythromycin at low dose: motility receptor agonist. Can be associated with dysrhythmia and increased incidence of hypertrophic pyloric stenosis. Contraindicated in some patients with preexisting cardiac conditions.

6. A surface agent sucralfate may be used—an aluminum complex that acts by adhering to mucosal lesions, reducing symptoms, and promoting healing.
   a. May be used as an adjunct to an H_2 blocker or PPI, and usually for a period of several weeks or less.

   b. If used for esophagitis, should be made into a liquid preparation.
   c. If used for ulcer or gastritis, it is inhibited by H_2 blockers and PPIs due to the need for an acidic environment.

 DRUG ALERT The potential adverse effects of aluminum in infants and children should be considered before administering sucralfate; data on its efficacy and safety in children are inadequate.

Surgical Management for GERD

1. Nissen fundoplication is the most commonly used surgical method to treat moderate to severe GERD that is unresponsive to medication therapy. Decisions concerning appropriate long-term feeding access must be individualized.
   a. Involves wrapping of the fundus around the LES (see Figure 48-3).
   b. Overall complication rate ranges from 2.2% to 45%.
   c. Other surgical approaches include ventral (Thal) or dorsal (Toupet) semifundoplication.
   d. In some studies, recurrence of reflux in the neurodisabled child is as high as 46%.
   e. Simultaneous gastrostomy is usually performed for feeding purposes or as a temporary measure to decompress the stomach.
   f. The most commonly reported complications of surgery include breakdown of the wrap, small bowel obstruction, gas bloat syndrome, infection, perforation, leaking at the anastomosis site, persistent esophageal stricture, esophageal obstruction, dumping syndrome, incisional hernia, and gastroparesis.
   g. Reoperation rates range from 3% to 18%.
   h. The greater the complexity of the infant or child's health status, the greater the chance of complications.

2. Jejunostomy feeding tubes can be placed but are usually restricted to severe cases of recurrent GERD and/or failed Nissen procedure.
   a. Most surgeons use either a standard GT or a low-profile tube (button).
   b. Complications include intestinal obstruction and leaking.

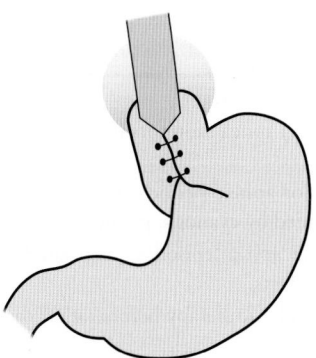

View of stomach after the surgery

Figure 48-3. Nissen fundoplication for gastroesophageal reflux disease.

Other Treatments Under Investigation

Investigation is underway to identify pathways and mechanisms that interfere or control the transient relaxation of the LES. Future understanding of this mechanism will aid in the development of lifestyle changes and medical management, which will assist in inhibiting transient relaxations. Reduction of gastric mechano-receptor signaling to the brain has emerged as one of the likely sites of action for new reflux inhibitor drugs. The most promising among these appear to be the $GABA_B$ receptor agonists and metabotropic glutamate receptor 5 (mGluR5).

Nursing Assessment

1. Obtain history of infant's or child's eating habits, including formula history, food allergies, volume tolerated at each meal.
2. Obtain history of complications from GER (ie, recurrent respiratory infections, asthma, poor weight gain).
3. Observe infant's or child's feeding behaviors. (Does child eat with a bottle, spoon, fingers? Can child feed self?)
4. Assess general appearance, skin integrity, and growth and development.

Nursing Diagnoses

- Risk for Aspiration related to reflux of gastric contents.
- Imbalanced Nutrition: Less Than Body Requirements related to decreased oral intake.
- Risk for Deficient Fluid Volume related to frequent vomiting.
- Fear of eating related to distress.

Nursing Interventions

Preventing Aspiration

1. Administer medications via IV line until tolerating enteral feedings.
   a. Administer prokinetics (motility agents) and acid suppressants 30 minutes before meals when bolus feeding schedule is instituted. Monitor for adverse effects.
   b. Unless abnormal gastric dysmotility prior to surgery, most prokinetics are discontinued after Nissen fundoplication.
2. Maintain positioning, as stated above.

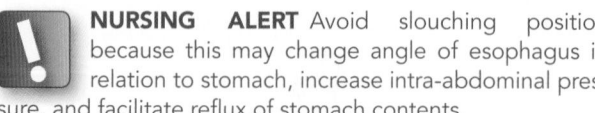 **NURSING ALERT** Avoid slouching position because this may change angle of esophagus in relation to stomach, increase intra-abdominal pressure, and facilitate reflux of stomach contents.

3. Use cardiac and apnea monitors for infants and children with severe reflux.
   a. Observe for apneic periods of more than 20 seconds or accompanied by cyanosis, pallor, or bradycardia.
   b. Document apnea episodes, associated symptoms, and recovery efforts.
4. Provide chest physiotherapy before rather than after meals, if ordered.

Maintaining Adequate Nutrition

See also section on feeding, page 1604.

1. Provide concentrated formula if volume cannot be tolerated.

2. Seek nutrition consult if patient continues to have difficulty feeding.
3. Monitor for fatigue during feeding; increased effort to suck requires higher energy expenditures. If noted, referral to occupational/speech therapy and possible modified barium swallow study are advised.
4. Monitor weight on the same scale.
5. Accurately record activity of infant.
   a. Amount of feeding taken; whether retained.
   b. Any change in behavior as a result of feeding technique.
6. Explain to the breastfeeding mother that feeding modifications may need to be made, especially in infants with poor weight gain. Assist her to express milk, quantitate volume, thicken with cereal, and fortify breast milk with formula, as needed.
7. Follow postoperative instructions on initiation of feedings.
8. If the child has a GT:
   a. Usually elevated and vented until return of bowel function.
   b. Monitor drainage, avoid kinking, and follow orders for positioning for straight drainage, elevation, or clamping.

Maintaining Fluid and Electrolyte Balance

1. Monitor vital signs and assess skin turgor for signs of dehydration.
2. Observe and record accurately urine output.
   a. Weigh diapers.
   b. Measure amount, frequency, color, and concentration of voided urine.
   c. Check specific gravity, if possible.
3. Monitor IV therapy, if ordered.
4. Monitor serum electrolytes, magnesium, phosphorus, and calcium. Replace, as ordered. Particular close monitoring is warranted if infant/child has draining gastrostomy.

 NURSING ALERT If patient is malnourished, monitor for refeeding syndrome until laboratory studies are stable. Refeeding syndrome can cause intracellular shifting of electrolytes, calcium, magnesium, and phosphorus, resulting in death. Laboratory studies should be monitored daily or more frequently if abnormal.

5. Promote good skin care to prevent lesions of dry and delicate tissues.
   a. Change position frequently.
   b. Change soiled diapers promptly.
   c. Apply lotion and gently massage any reddened areas.

Reducing Fear of Eating

1. Provide thickened feedings to increase satisfaction for the infant.
2. Identify and attempt to reduce stress, especially around mealtime.
3. Feed the child in a quiet, calm environment.
4. Children like routines; feed at routine intervals by the person with whom the child is familiar and comfortable.
5. For the older child, encourage participation in family dinnertime so the child observes eating as a pleasurable experience.
6. Advise parents that clinical specialists in feeding disorders are available.

Community and Home Care Considerations

1. Recognize that home health care referral is appropriate for the following situations:
   a. FTT: medication teaching and monitoring, teaching of formula preparation, positioning, weight.
   b. Respiratory complications/ALTE: medication teaching and monitoring, assessment of respiratory status, teaching of monitor/cardiopulmonary resuscitation (CPR), use of nebulizer.
   c. Nissen fundoplication (with GT): medication teaching and monitoring; wound assessment; monitoring of bloating; dumping syndrome; formula intolerance; GT teaching, including pump teaching, venting, medication administration, tube changing.
2. Recommend careful feeding and behavioral diary to monitor symptoms and improvements.
3. Recognize that school and community activities may affect compliance for older children; work with the family to devise individualized management strategies.
4. Assist parents to discuss medication and lunchtime behaviors with teacher and school nurse so consistency can be maintained.
5. Assess need for community services, such as respite care, especially for single parent.

Family Education and Health Maintenance

1. Plan a program of intensive parental teaching on how to handle and care for the infant. Explain rationale to parents. Make sure that they have proper equipment for propping the infant. Help the parents understand that it is not necessary to keep infant in infant seat or propped up at all times.
   a. Bathe or play with the infant before feeding.
   b. Change position about 1 hour after feeding.
   c. During the night after feeding, the infant can sleep in a semi-reclining (30 degrees) position.
   d. Expect occasional small amounts of vomiting.
2. Offer clear, concise instructions. Focus on parental fears. Discuss techniques to promote development of infants while facilitating bonding and normal parental behavior.
3. If infant or child is not demonstrating complication of GER (ie, GERD), assist parents in understanding that GER is self-limited; symptoms usually disappear within 12 months.
4. If complications exist (GERD), referral to pediatric gastroenterology and nutrition specialists is recommended.
5. If Nissen fundoplication has been performed:
   a. Teach gastrostomy care, if applicable (see page 1463). Make sure that the parents know how to use, clear, vent, assess, and replace the tube. Help them to understand the purpose of GT placement (feedings, venting, medications) and the need for surgical or gastroenterology follow-up care.
   b. Explain about potential complications and when to call the health care provider. Such complications include gagging, retching, bloating, abdominal distention, fever, vomiting, diaphoresis, lethargy, diarrhea, weight loss. Generally, the

family should contact the surgeon within the first 6 weeks postoperatively, whereas eventual follow-up is with the gastroenterologist.
   c. It usually takes 12 weeks to heal; if the GT becomes dislodged in this period, the patient should be taken to the emergency department immediately.
   d. Complications of a dislodged GT in the early postoperative period include peritonitis and bacteremia.
6. Help the parents understand the importance of follow-up for assessment of weight gain and development.
7. Assist with community resource planning (eg, education, advocacy, and financial assistance). Identify support groups.
8. Instruct parents and caregivers in CPR training before discharge of infant, if indicated.
9. Provide written and verbal instructions for medications and adverse effects.
10. Advise parents on when to call their health care provider in regard to their child's symptoms. Danger signs of dehydration include a decrease in wet diapers, listlessness, lethargy, reduced appetite, sunken fontanelle; those for aspiration include respiratory distress and cyanotic spells, fever.
11. Encourage family to contact their health care provider immediately with treatment concerns or problems.
12. For additional information and support, contact the North American Society of Pediatric Gastroenterology, Hepatology and Nutrition (*www.naspghan.org*), the United Ostomy Association (*www.uao.org*), or the Pediatric/Adolescent Gastroesophageal Reflux Association (*www.reflux.org*).

Evaluation: Expected Outcomes

- Mild regurgitation immediately after feeding; no apnea or cyanosis noted.
- Takes regular feedings without significant symptoms; weight gain noted.
- Urine output adequate.
- Exhibits pleasure in eating.

Failure to Thrive

 Evidence Base World Health Organization, United Nations Children's Fund. (2009). *WHO child growth standards and the identification of severe acute malnutrition in infants and children*. Geneva: World Health Organization.

Jaffe, A. C. (2012). Failure to thrive: Current clinical concepts. *Pediatrics in Review, 32*, 100.

Failure to thrive (FTT) is the inadequate physical development of an infant or child manifested as a deceleration in weight gain, a low weight/height ratio, or a low weight/height/head circumference ratio. The exact prevalence is unknown, although research suggests FTT accounts for 3% to 5% of pediatric hospital admissions. Children with FTT are at risk for adverse outcomes, such as short stature, behavior problems, and developmental delay. The Agency for Healthcare Research and Quality has an evidenced-based practice program on which clinical guidelines can be developed. The primary causative factors of FTT are insufficient nutrition availability, inadequate absorption and/or utilization of nutrients, and added metabolic requirements.

Most practitioners diagnose FTT when a child's weight for age falls below the fifth percentile of the standard National Center for Health Statistics growth chart or if it crosses two major percentile lines. Recent research has validated that the weight-for-age approach is the simplest and most reasonable marker for FTT.

About 25% of normal infants will shift to a lower growth percentile in the first 2 years of life and then follow that percentile; this should not be diagnosed as FTT (see Standards of Care Guidelines 48-1).

Pathophysiology and Etiology

1. FTT is a nutritional disorder having organic and nonorganic components.
   a. Organic FTT implies a major illness or organ system dysfunction as the etiology of the growth failure. It occurs equally in all populations and accounts for approximately 25% of FTT cases.
   b. Nonorganic FTT is the result of multiple psychosocial factors, including disturbances in parent–child interaction. This type accounts for 50% of cases of FTT and is most common among the psychosocially and economically deprived.
   c. The remaining 25% of cases represent mixed etiology.

STANDARDS OF CARE GUIDELINES 48-1
Care of a Child with a GI or Nutritional Disorder

When caring for a child with a GI or nutritional disorder:

- Monitor weight.
- Monitor urinary and bowel elimination.
- Monitor intake and output.
- Assess developmental milestone attainment.
- Provide and teach appropriate feeding products and techniques.
- Use most efficient position for feeding.
- Facilitate a calm, pleasant environment for feeding.
- Avoid foods that may inhibit absorption of nutrients or cause such symptoms as gas.
- Encourage and support parental involvement in care and feeding of the child.
- Encourage and support normal play and other activities for the child as condition allows.
- Identify and respond to signs and symptoms that may indicate lack of adequate nutrition or sign of complications.

This information should serve as a general guideline only. Each patient situation presents a unique set of clinical factors and requires nursing judgment to guide care, which may include additional or alternative measures and approaches.

---

2. Organic FTT has a pathophysiologic cause that reduces the availability of nutrients for maintenance and growth and is best divided into three categories:
   a. Insufficient nutrition because of the child's inability to feed properly, which may be a result of severe neurologic dysfunction, GER, or cleft palate/lip.
   b. Nutrition is adequate but poorly absorbed and/or utilized (malabsorption syndromes), which may result from chronic ileocecal intussusception, GER, milk protein allergy, malrotation of the colon, hypoplastic stomach, short bowel syndrome (anatomic and functional), pancreatic insufficiency (including cystic fibrosis), pyloric stenosis, inflammatory bowel disease, and acquired immunodeficiency syndrome.
   c. Associated disorders include asthma, cardiac failure, thyroiditis, congenital heart disease, neurologic lesions, hydronephrosis, adrenal hyperplasia, diabetes insipidus, cystic fibrosis, chronic or recurrent urinary tract infection (UTI), hypothyroidism, autoimmune disorders, immunodeficiency.
3. Nonorganic FTT occurs in the absence of GI, endocrine, congenital, or chronic diseases. It is usually associated with psychological deprivation but can also be related to behavioral or economic problems. Multiple features of the parents, child, and environment interact over time, resulting in parent–child interaction that ultimately leads to undernutrition and undernurturance of the child.

Clinical Manifestations

Organic FTT

1. Retarded growth accompanied by manifestations of the underlying disease.
2. Weight loss in early stages. If poor intake continues, linear growth slows down or ceases. In latent stage, head circumference growth is retarded, indicating compromised brain development.
3. Developmental delays.
4. Infant stress—irritability, fussiness, jitteriness.
5. Feeding disorders—ineffective sucking, difficulty chewing, difficulty swallowing.
6. Clinical symptoms can include vomiting, hypothermia, lethargy, muscle wasting, decreased subcutaneous tissue, hypoalbuminemia, eczema, hair loss, diarrhea.

Nonorganic FTT

1. Retarded growth.
2. Infant stress—irritability, fussiness, jitteriness.
3. Feeding disorders—ineffective sucking, difficulty chewing, difficulty swallowing.
4. Reduced energy level.
5. Difficult temperament.
6. Fitful sleep.
7. Reduced responsiveness and interaction with the environment.
8. Social isolation, lack of vocalization.
9. Spasticity or rigidity when touched.
10. Inability to make eye contact or smile.

11. Refusal to eat; rejection of foods.
12. Spits up, gags, coughs with feeding, rumination.

Parental Characteristics
1. Characteristics associated with parents of nonorganic FTT include lack of social and financial support, maladaptive relationships, alcohol or drug abuse, history of anxiety or depression, lack of parenting skills, family stress and crisis, absent father.
2. Postnatal depression corresponds to a higher association of FTT, but on its own depression does not contribute to a higher incidence of FTT.

Diagnostic Evaluation

Comprehensive Assessment
1. FTT suggested if a child is falling off a previously established growth curve or falls below the 5th percentile. If FTT is of recent onset, weight but not height will fall below accepted standards. Depression of weight and height indicates chronic malnutrition.
2. Technique for evaluating growth—look at growth percentage of the median for that age. Divide the actual value of height or weight by median value for that age. For example, 12-month-old female weighs 15 lb (6.8 kg); the median for age is 21 1/2 lb (9.8 kg). Child is 70% of median for age.

 NURSING ALERT Children whose weight is less than 60% of the median value for age or less than 70% for height are in acute danger of severe morbidity and malnutrition.

3. Complete health and dietary history—feeding, eating patterns, 3-day calorie count.
4. Physical examination for evidence of organic causes, with particular attention to ears, facial structure, mouth, heart, lungs, abdomen, and neurologic system.
5. Assessment of prenatal, perinatal, and postnatal infections.
6. Developmental assessment.
7. Family assessment—family short stature syndrome, family dynamics.
   a. With the assistance of endocrinologist and dietitian, calculate the midparental height:

   {(Father's height in cm + mother's height in cm) + 13 cm} divided by 2

Note: Subtract 13 cm for girls and add 13 cm for boys. For example, if the father is 180 cm and the mother is 167 cm, the daughter's equation would be {(180 + 167) − 13} ÷ 2.

Tests to Rule Out Organic Conditions
1. Complete blood count (CBC) with differential and indices, sedimentation rate to rule out anemia or hematologic or inflammatory cause.
2. Blood cultures if fever present.
3. Urinalysis and urine culture as baseline for bladder and renal function.
4. Thyroid-stimulating hormone and free thyroxine to rule out hypothyroidism.
5. Blood chemistry: provide data on electrolyte balance, renal function, and skeletal disorders.

6. Neonate screening tests, TORCH studies.
7. Stool screening tests:
   a. Infection: culture, ova and parasite, *Clostridium difficile*, white blood cell (WBC) count (may have false-negative results if recently on antibiotics).
   b. Protein malabsorption: alpha-one antitrypsin (may have false-negative results if not fed during collection).
   c. Carbohydrate malabsorption: pH, reducing substances (time sensitive, need to be fresh stool; may have false-negative results if not fed during collection).
   d. Fat malabsorption: random qualitative fecal fat (one-time sample); if needed, a 72-hour quantitative fecal fat should be collected. Results are more accurate when sample is collected while patient is receiving adequate nutrition.
   e. Pancreatic sufficiency: stool pancreatic elastase, stool chymotrypsin and serum trypsin to detect primary or secondary pancreatic insufficiency.
8. Radiologic studies including upper GI series, barium swallow, reflux workup, upper endoscopy, sweat test.

 NURSING ALERT One of the best tests to determine organic from nonorganic FTT is through observed feedings or enteral tube feedings to assess weight gain and caloric intake.

Management
1. Immediate treatment is directed at reversing malnutrition.
2. All children with FTT need additional calories for catch-up growth (typically 150% of the caloric requirement for their expected, not actual, weight).
3. Nutritional treatment is aimed at providing sufficient calories to support "catch-up" growth to restore deficits in weight and height. Protein and energy requirements for normal and FTT children are outlined in Table 48-1.
   a. This may require NG tube feedings for safe refeeding.
   b. If fat malabsorption present, may need formula with high level of medium-chain triglycerides for direct absorption of fat.
4. Multivitamin supplementation containing zinc and iron is usually recommended, fat-soluble vitamins (A, D, E, K) if fat malabsorption is present.

Table 48-1	Protein and Energy Requirements			
	NORMAL CHILDREN		**FTT CHILDREN**	
AGE (YEARS)	**Protein (g/kg)**	**Energy (kcal/kg)**	**Protein (g/kg)**	**Energy (kcal/kg)**
0–0.5	2.2	.08	3.2	150–250
0.5–1	1.6	98	3.2	150–250
1–3	1.2	102	2.5	150–250
4–6	1.1	90	2.5	150–250
7–10	1.0	70	2.5	150–250

5. If cause is organic, the underlying disease entity is treated or managed.

6. In nonorganic FTT, hospitalization is avoided (unless the child is in imminent danger) because it further disrupts the parent–child relationship. Therefore, frequent home or clinic visits are necessary. Referral to feeding disorder clinic or rehabilitation center may be necessary.

7. Developmental interventions through occupational and physical therapy are instituted, if necessary, to prevent further delay.

8. Support, education, and financial assistance are offered to the family.

9. Nutrition, occupational therapy, and physical therapy consults are indicated.

Complications

Studies are inconsistent regarding the long-term complications of FTT.

1. Anemia, fatigue, hypothermia.
2. Vulnerability to infection.
3. Delayed healing.
4. Behavior problems, poor academic performance.
5. Developmental, speech, and language delays.
6. Perceptual difficulties.

Nursing Assessment

1. Obtain accurate anthropometric measurements.
   a. Weight of children younger than age 3 should be done unclothed in a supine position using a calibrated beam scale. Children older than age 3 should be done standing on a standard scale wearing same clothing each time. Effort should be made to use the same scale each time.
   b. Height should be recumbent up to age 2. All children should be measured without shoes.
   c. Head circumference is measured each visit until age 2 with a nonstretchable tape placed firmly from maximal occipital prominence to just above the eyebrow.
   d. All measurements need to be corrected for prematurity up to the second birthday by subtracting the number of weeks premature from the chronological age.
   e. Measurements should be plotted on growth chart using a straight edge or plot grid. Birth measurements should be obtained and entered for comparison.

2. Obtain nutritional history regarding eating patterns; nutritional beliefs for food allocation; 24-hour recall; who normally feeds the child; the type, amount, and frequency of feedings; the amount of time and effort required for meals; the child's reactions (physiologic and psychological) to feedings; food likes and dislikes; and environmental factors.

3. Observe parent–child interactions, such as sensitivity to child's needs, eye-to-eye contact, if and how the infant is held, and how the parent speaks to the child.

4. If possible, observe the parent feeding the child. Assess child's overall tone, sucking pattern, oral sensitivity (gag reflex), lip and tongue function, and swallowing ability. A videotape of the child eating in the home can be reviewed later to reduce the chance of observer distraction.

5. Assess neurologic and cardiovascular status for alertness, attentiveness, developmental delays, cardiac arrhythmias or murmurs.

6. Assess skin, hair, and musculoskeletal system.

7. Assess developmental status using a Denver II developmental tool, as indicated.

Nursing Diagnoses

• Imbalanced Nutrition: Less Than Body Requirements related to FTT process.
• Delayed Growth and Development related to malnutrition.
• Impaired Parenting related to inability to meet the needs of the FTT child.

Nursing Interventions

Promoting Adequate Nutrition

1. Facilitate nutritional consultation.

2. If hospitalized, provide a primary core of staff to feed the child. Ask the parents to do so when present in a nonthreatening manner.

3. Develop individualized teaching plan to instruct parents of child's dietary needs. Specify type of diet, essential nutrients, serving sizes, and method of preparation.

4. Provide a quiet, nonstimulating environment for eating.

5. Demonstrate proper feeding techniques including details on how to hold and how long to feed the child.

6. Administer multivitamin supplements, as prescribed.

7. Encourage nutritious, high-calorie, and fortified fluids to increase nutrient density. For infants, use 24 to 30 cal/oz rather than 20 cal/oz. For older children, suggest fruit smoothies using whole milk and ice cream.

8. Refeed the malnourished child with caution, monitoring electrolytes, calcium, magnesium, and phosphorus daily or more frequently, if abnormal.

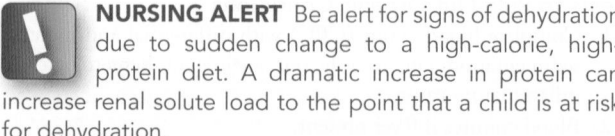 **NURSING ALERT** If patient is malnourished, monitor for refeeding syndrome until laboratory studies are stable. Refeeding syndrome can cause intracellular shifting of electrolytes, calcium, magnesium, and phosphorus, resulting in death. Laboratory studies should be monitored daily or more frequently, if abnormal.

   a. Gradually increase nutrients and use small, frequent feedings with adequate fluids to ensure hydration.

NURSING ALERT Be alert for signs of dehydration due to sudden change to a high-calorie, high-protein diet. A dramatic increase in protein can increase renal solute load to the point that a child is at risk for dehydration.

   b. Monitor intake and output.

9. Maintain high-nutrient diet until weight is appropriate for height (usually age 4 to 9 months).

10. Advise family that some nutritional intervention will be continued until appropriate height for age is reached.

Promoting Adequate Growth and Development

1. Obtain accurate weight at every visit or every day, if hospitalized.
2. Assess child's growth by using age- and gender-appropriate growth charts. Extremely low-birth-weight infants born with major anomalies have nearly twice the risk of neurodevelopmental impairment and increased risk of poor growth.

 Evidence Base Bocca-Tjeertes, I. F., Kerstjens, J. M., Reijneveld, S. A., et al. (2011). Growth and predictors of growth restraint in moderately preterm children aged 0 to 4 years. *Pediatrics, 128*(5), e1187–1194.

3. Assess child's development by interviewing the parent or caregiver or using developmental screening tests, such as the Denver II (Denver Developmental Materials, Inc., *http://denverii.com/denverii/*).
4. Observe interactions between parents and child and among family members, including eye contact, communication patterns, coping ability.
5. Provide the infant with visual and auditory stimulation by exposing to bright colors, shapes, and music. Provide the older child with age-appropriate stimulation, such as books, games, and toys. Place the infant prone, while awake, on the floor to encourage trunk control.
6. Encourage periods of scheduled rest and sleep.

Promoting Effective Parenting

1. Teach the parents (especially the mother) normal parenting skills by demonstrating proper holding, stroking, feeding, and communication using age-appropriate words and gestures.
2. If hospitalized, encourage and facilitate the parents to spend as much time as possible with the child.
3. Educate the parents to recognize and respond to the child's distress and hunger calls.
4. Help the parents to develop organizational skills—write down daily schedule with mealtimes, time for shopping, and so forth.
5. Refer for counseling, if necessary, to help parents overcome feelings of mistrust or neglect resulting from adverse personal childhood experiences.
6. Refer to social services to help resolve any social and financial difficulties that might interfere with providing a nurturing environment.
7. Monitor parents' progress and provide positive reinforcement.

Community and Home Care Considerations

 Evidence Base Didenbahi, N., Kelly, K., Austin, L., et al. (2011). Role of parental stress on pediatric feeding disorders. *Children's Health Care, 40*(2), 85–100.
Dido, O. F., Wakili, T. A., & Asekun-Olarinmove, E. O. (2011). Enhancing recovery of malnourished children: Mothers' counseling and participation ensures intervention effectiveness. *West African Journal of Nursing, 22*(1), 85–90.)

Early intervention home visiting has been shown to reduce the long-term complications associated with FTT. This may be due to promotion of maternal sensitivity and helping children build strong work habits that enables them to flourish at school.

1. Make regular home visits to:
   a. Observe for continued parent–child interaction.
   b. Encourage continued developmentally appropriate play.
   c. Monitor feeding status and assess intake amount.
   d. Determine frequency of voiding and stooling.
   e. Assess child's weight, height, and head circumference.
   f. Monitor vital signs and watch for signs of dehydration.
   g. Auscultate bowel sounds.
   h. Assess muscle tone and vigor of activity.
   i. Assess family dynamics and use of support systems.
2. Inform parents of community resources, such as Women in Crisis program, food banks, parenting groups.
3. Make sure that daycare providers can meet child's special needs in terms of diet, feeding, and developmentally appropriate play. Daycare may be beneficial in the presence of family dysfunction by providing structure.
4. Make referrals to social work and occupational or physical therapy, as needed.

Family Education and Health Maintenance

1. Reinforce the need for a quiet, nonthreatening, nurturing environment.
2. Encourage the parents to be consistent with feedings. Although forced feeding is avoided, strict adherence to appropriate feeding is essential for growth.
3. Advise the parents to introduce new foods slowly and follow the child's rhythm of feeding.
4. Review the importance of providing a routine rest schedule in an environment that is conducive to sleep.
5. Review development, stressing need for visual, auditory, and tactile stimulation and age-appropriate toys for continued development.
6. Reinforce the need for follow-up care, well-child visits, and immunizations.

Evaluation: Expected Outcomes

- Increases weight steadily.
- Attains developmental milestones at appropriate age.
- Parents participating in child's care, using appropriate feeding technique.

Hypertrophic Pyloric Stenosis

 Evidence Base Pandya, S., & Heiss K. (2012). Pyloric stenosis in pediatric surgery: An evidence-base review. *Surgery Clinics of North America, 92*(3), 527–539.

Hypertrophic pyloric stenosis is an acquired condition in which the circumferential muscle of the pyloric sphincter becomes thickened, causing a high-grade gastric outlet obstruction that results in dilation, hypertrophy, and hyperperistalsis of the stomach. It is the second most common condition (after inguinal hernia) requiring surgery, which rarely occurs before age 2 weeks or later than age 5 months. Incidence is 1 in 250 live births and is predominant in males (5:1) and more common in first-born males. Incidence peaks in spring and fall. It is more likely to affect a full-term infant than a premature infant.

Pathophysiology and Etiology

1. Unknown cause, although new research has identified several genetic markers associated with the condition. Multiple theories of etiology exist, including immature or degenerated pyloric neural elements, variations in infant feeding regimens, excessive production of gastrin (maternal or infant), dyscoordination between gastric peristalsis and pyloric relaxation, deficiency of nitric acid, abnormalities in enteric nervous system, and abnormalities in neurotransmitters.

 Evidence Base Feenstra, B., Geller, F., Krogh, C., et al. (2012). Common variants near MBNL1 and NKX2-5 are associated with infantile hypertrophic pyloric stenosis. *Nature Genetics, 44*(3), 334–337.

2. Current studies of combined imaging (pressure recordings, MRI, ultrasound, and fluid-mechanical analysis) have offered new understanding of the role of the pylorus in gastric emptying and digestion. Other studies have shown that persistent duodenal hyperacidity can lead to increased incidence of pyloric stenosis. This is associated with repeated contractions of the pylorus.

3. The use of erythromycin to treat reflux and gastric dysmotility has led to research regarding the association with pyloric stenosis. The published evidence has concluded that young infants exposed to erythromycin in the first few weeks of life are at greater risk for developing hypertrophic pyloric stenosis. The highest risk seems to be in the first 2 weeks of life in term or near-term infants, with a course of more than 14 days.

 DRUG ALERT Erythromycin should only be used in young infants (<4 weeks) when the therapeutic benefits outweigh the risks and no alternative agent is available.

4. Increase in size of the circular musculature of the pylorus with thickening (size and shape of an olive). The pylorus muscle becomes elongated and thickened and is enlarged to about twice the usual size. On clinical exam, palpation of an "olive" is diagnostic.
5. Hypertrophy of the pylorus musculature occurs with narrowing of the pyloric lumen.
6. Constriction of the lumen of the pyloric canal (at the distal end of the stomach) causes the stomach to become dilated.
7. Gastric emptying is delayed.

Clinical Manifestations

Onset usually occurs between ages 3 and 12 weeks.

1. Cardinal sign is projectile, nonbilious vomiting.
   a. Initially, occasional regurgitation (similar to GER) may be present, but eventually vomiting increases in frequency and intensity.
   b. Vomitus contains milk and gastric juices; however, it may be blood-streaked or have a "coffee ground" appearance.
   c. Emesis occurs just after or near the end of a feeding.
2. Constipation or decreased quantity of stools.
3. Loss of weight or failure to gain weight.
4. Epigastric distention.
5. Visible gastric peristaltic waves, left to right, seen just after infant vomits.
6. Excessive hunger—willingness to eat immediately after vomiting.
7. Dehydration—electrolyte disturbance with alkalosis, hypoglycemia, hypochloremia.
8. Decreased urine output.
9. Palpable pyloric mass in upper right quadrant of abdomen, to the right of the umbilicus and best felt during feeding or immediately after vomiting.
10. Jaundice.

Diagnostic Evaluation

1. Palpation of pyloric mass ("olive") in conjunction with persistent, projectile vomiting is pathognomonic.
2. Ultrasound evaluation—broadly used, noninvasive method to evaluate the length and diameter of the pyloric muscle.
   a. Criteria for a positive diagnosis: pyloric muscle thickness (PMT) ≥ 3 mm and pyloric muscle length (PML) ≥ 17 mm.
   b. Sensitivity and specificity of PMT, 91% and 85%, respectively; for PML, 76% and 85%, respectively.
   c. No significant correlation among age, weight, or prematurity and a sonographic diagnosis of infantile hypertrophic pyloric stenosis; therefore, the same ultrasound criteria should apply irrespective of prematurity, age, or weight. Borderline PMT and PML measurements necessitate repeat ultrasound or alternative imaging.

 Evidence Base Cogley, J. R., O'Connor, S. C., Houshyar, R., et al. (2012). Emergent pediatric US: What every radiologist should know. *Radiographics, 32*(3), 651–665.

3. Barium upper GI series—indicated if ultrasound is inconclusive.
4. Flat film of abdomen—dilated, air-filled stomach; nondilated pyloric canal.
5. Tests for metabolic alkalosis (seen in less than 10% due to more prompt diagnosis over the past 20 years).
6. Urinalysis—urine alkaline and concentrated.
7. Blood hemoglobin and hematocrit—elevated due to hemoconcentration.

Management

 Evidence Base Siddiqui, S., Heidel, R. E., Angel, C. A., et al. (2012). Pyloromyotomy: Randomized controlled trial of open vs laparoscopic technique. *Journal of Pediatric Surgery, 47*(1), 93–98.

1. Considered a medical emergency due to dehydration and electrolyte imbalance, with initial treatment to rehydrate to correct electrolytes and alkalosis.

2. Surgical treatment is corrective and takes place when electrolytes are stable—Rammstedt pyloromyotomy is procedure of choice, performed through a short transverse incision in the right upper quadrant over the rectus muscle at or above the liver edge. Laparoscopic pyloromyotomy may also be done but the open procedure continues to be the most performed technique.

   a. Hypertrophy of the pyloric muscle regresses to normal size about 12 weeks postoperatively.

   b. Some postoperative vomiting is expected but should decrease over 48 hours. If persistent vomiting continues, a contrast study should be completed to rule out gastric leak, fluid collection obstructing the gastric outlet, or other causes of obstruction. If these are ruled out, incomplete pyloromyotomy should be considered.

   c. Postoperative complications include duodenal perforation, gastric leak, wound infection, small bowel obstruction, and postoperative vomiting.

3. Good outcomes following surgery appear to be strongly related to the qualifications of the pediatric surgeon, the use of pediatric certified anesthesiologists, qualified pediatric nurses, adequate correction of fluids and electrolytes preoperatively.

Complications

1. Starvation.
2. Dehydration.
3. Severe electrolyte imbalance.
4. Hematemesis.

Nursing Assessment

1. Obtain a thorough history of infant's feeding behaviors and history of vomiting.
2. Assess hydration status and for signs and symptoms of electrolyte imbalance.
3. Assess and chart growth and development parameters.

Nursing Diagnoses

Preoperative

- Deficient Fluid Volume related to frequent vomiting.
- Imbalanced Nutrition: Less Than Body Requirements related to vomiting.
- Acute Pain related to gastric distention.
- Anxiety of parents related to illness, hospitalization, and impending surgery of child.

Postoperative

- Risk for Injury related to postoperative complications.
- Risk for Deficient Fluid Volume after surgery.
- Impaired Tissue Integrity related to surgical incision.

Nursing Interventions

Maintaining Fluid and Electrolyte Balance

1. Administer IV therapy, as ordered, to treat dehydration, metabolic alkalosis, and electrolyte deficiency.

2. Carefully monitor output, including amount and characteristics of urine (check specific gravity), vomiting, and stools.
3. Accurately measure daily weight as a guide for calculating need for parenteral fluid.
4. Monitor laboratory data for serum electrolytes.
5. Position infants to prevent interference with fluid therapy.
6. Provide pacifier for infants who are NPO.
7. Monitor vital signs, as indicated by condition. Watch for tachycardia, hypotension, change in respirations.

 NURSING ALERT Irregular respiratory rate with apnea is a sign of severe alkalosis.

Maintaining Nutrition

1. Emphasize rehydration, electrolyte balance, and replacement of body fat and protein stores. This depends on severity of depletion and may require total parenteral nutrition for several days or weeks before surgery to reduce surgical risk.
2. Maintain NPO status with indwelling NG tube (inserted to remove any residual barium and retained formula), as ordered. Ensure placement, position, and patency. Record drainage type, color, and amount.
3. If oral feedings are to be continued, do the following:

   a. Provide small, frequent feedings, given slowly.
   b. Burp frequently before, during, and after feeding.
   c. Allow breastfeeding, as tolerated.

4. Prop the patient in 30-degree upright position (see Figure 48-4).
5. Handle gently and minimally after feeding.

Providing Comfort

1. Provide mouth care and wet lips frequently if NPO.
2. Let the infant suck on a pacifier.
3. Provide for physical contact or nearness without excessive stimulation.
4. Provide for audio and visual stimulation that may be soothing.
5. Do not palpate pyloric "olive" to decrease risk of postoperative wound infection from bruising abdominal wall and excoriating tissue in operative site.
6. Administer analgesics, as ordered.

Alleviating Parental Anxiety

1. Assess understanding of diagnosis and care plan.
2. Help minimize guilt feelings by providing adequate, specific information and clarifying any misconceptions.
3. Prepare the parents for the surgery of their child.

   a. Be honest with them.
   b. Prepare them for the expected postoperative appearance of the infant.
   c. Show them where the operating room and recovery room are located and where to wait during surgery.

4. Allow them to hold the infant to maintain bonding.
5. Encourage them to rest to care better for the infant postoperatively.

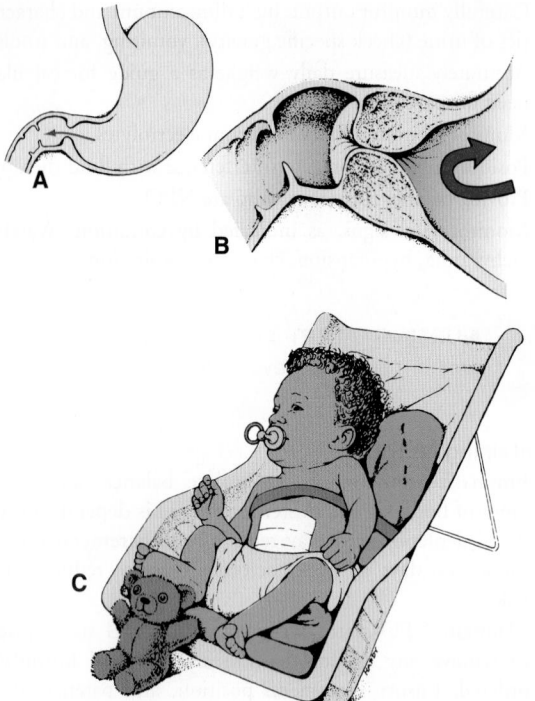

Figure 48-4. Pyloric stenosis. (A) Normal passage through pyloric sphincter. **(B)** Stoppage of flow due to stenotic sphincter. **(C)** Post-operative treatment: child propped upright, slightly on right side, aids in gastric emptying.

6. Accept and explore negative displays of emotion, which may be due to fatigue and frustration because of the extensive care given to the child before hospitalization.
7. Reassure them that surgery is considered curative and normal feeding should resume shortly afterward.

Preventing Complications

1. Assess vital signs to evaluate for fluid and electrolyte imbalances.
2. Assess skin and mucous membranes for hydration status.
3. Weigh daily to assess gain or loss.
4. Elevate head slightly.
5. If placed intraoperatively, maintain patent NG tube to prevent gastric distention. Record losses.
6. Monitor blood glucose levels to prevent hypoglycemia.

Maintaining Hydration

1. Administer IV fluids until adequate intake has been established.
2. Resume oral feeding 2 to 8 hours (standard is 6 hours) after surgery when infant is alert or as ordered.
3. After surgery, infants may progress to ad-lib feedings within 12 to 16 hours provided they did not have a prolonged preoperative course.
4. Start with small, frequent feedings of glucose water and slowly advance to full-strength (FS) formula and regular diet,

as tolerated. An example of a postoperative feeding schedule includes:
   a. NPO for 6 hours.
   b. Sugar water solution orally 30 mL every 2 hours for two feedings.
   c. Then half-strength formula 30 mL every 2 hours for two feedings.
   d. Then FS formula 45 mL every 2 hours for two feedings.
   e. Then FS formula 60 mL every 3 hours for two feedings.
   f. Then formula ad lib every 4 hours.
5. Report any vomiting—amount and characteristics. Feeding schedule may be withheld 2 hours and then reinitiated.
6. Feed slowly and burp frequently.
7. Note how feeding is taken and if it is retained.
8. Increase the amount of feeding as the time interval between feedings is lengthened.
9. Allow breastfeeding to resume, as tolerated, if permitted by the operating surgeon, beginning with limited nursing of 5 to 8 minutes and gradually increase.
10. Continue to elevate the infant's head and shoulders after feeding for 45 to 60 minutes for several feedings after surgery. Place on right side to aid gastric emptying.
11. Expect that regurgitation may continue for a short period after surgery.

Promoting Healing

1. Provide analgesia and comfort measures, such as a pacifier, rocking, and other soothing stimulation to keep infant quiet and prevent tension on incision.
2. Involve parents in care of infant postoperatively to prepare them for care of wound after discharge.
3. Observe for drainage or signs of inflammation at incision site and provide care to incision, as ordered.
4. Note that poor nutritional status may delay wound healing.

Community and Home Care Considerations

1. Teach proper care of the operative site.
   a. Check for signs and symptoms of inflammation.
   b. Observe for drainage.
   c. Provide specific care of site, as ordered by provider.
2. Monitor weight and feeding behavior. Encourage close follow-up for growth and development.

 Evidence Base Walker, K., Halliday, R., Holland, A. J., et al. (2010). Early developmental outcome of infants with infantile hypertrophic pyloric stenosis *Journal of Pediatric Surgery, 45*(12), 2369–2372.

3. Observe for signs of delayed gastric emptying or GER.
4. Assess parent–infant interaction and parental coping.

Family Education and Health Maintenance

1. Teach feeding technique to be continued at home; length of feeding technique varies depending on wound healing, nutritional status, and growth.

2. Provide written and verbal instructions as to infant's care and follow-up schedule.

3. Review with family when medical attention is needed and appropriate resources:
   a. Signs of infection.
   b. Frequent vomiting, vomiting longer than 5 days, or poor feeding with signs of dehydration.
   c. Abdominal distention.

Evaluation: Expected Outcomes

- Vital signs stable; urine output adequate.
- Tolerates 1- to 2-oz feedings in upright position without vomiting.
- Rests quietly with pacifier.
- Parents verbalize understanding of surgery and postoperative care.
- Vital signs stable; blood glucose within normal limits.
- No signs of dehydration.
- Incision healing without signs of infection.

Celiac Disease

 Evidence Base Husby, S., Koletzko, S., Korponay-Szabó, I. R., et al. (2012). European Society for Pediatric Gastroenterology, Hepatology and Nutrition guidelines for the diagnosis of celiac disease. *Journal of Pediatric Gastroenterology and Nutrition, 54,* 136–160.

Milito, T., Muri, M., Oakes, J., et al. (2012). Celiac disease: Early diagnosis leads to the best possible outcome. *JAAPA, 25*(11), 43–47.

Celiac disease (CD), or *gluten-sensitive enteropathy*, is a complex autoimmune genetic disorder with multiple contributing genes. CD affects the small intestine and is characterized by a permanent inability to tolerate dietary gluten; however, it can have systemic manifestations as well. Gluten is a protein found in wheat, rye, and barley (see Figure 48-5). The disease process is reversible with strict adherence to a gluten-free diet.

CD occurs more frequently in Caucasians; however, it is found in all ethnic groups. In the United States and Europe, the prevalence of CD in the pediatric population is between 1 in 300 and 1 in 80, respectively. It is thought to be grossly underdiagnosed.

Pathophysiology and Etiology

1. CD is an immune-mediated disease. The two necessary components of the disease are exposure to gluten and a genetic predisposition resulting in immune activation to gluten. Linkage studies have identified several genomic regions that probably contain CD-susceptibility genes.
   a. The genes implicated in celiac disease are HLA-DQ2 and HLA DQ8. However, these genes can be found in 30% of the normal population as well.
   b. A familial connection is found in 5% to 15% of celiac patients, with an 83% to 86% concordance rate among monozygotic twins.

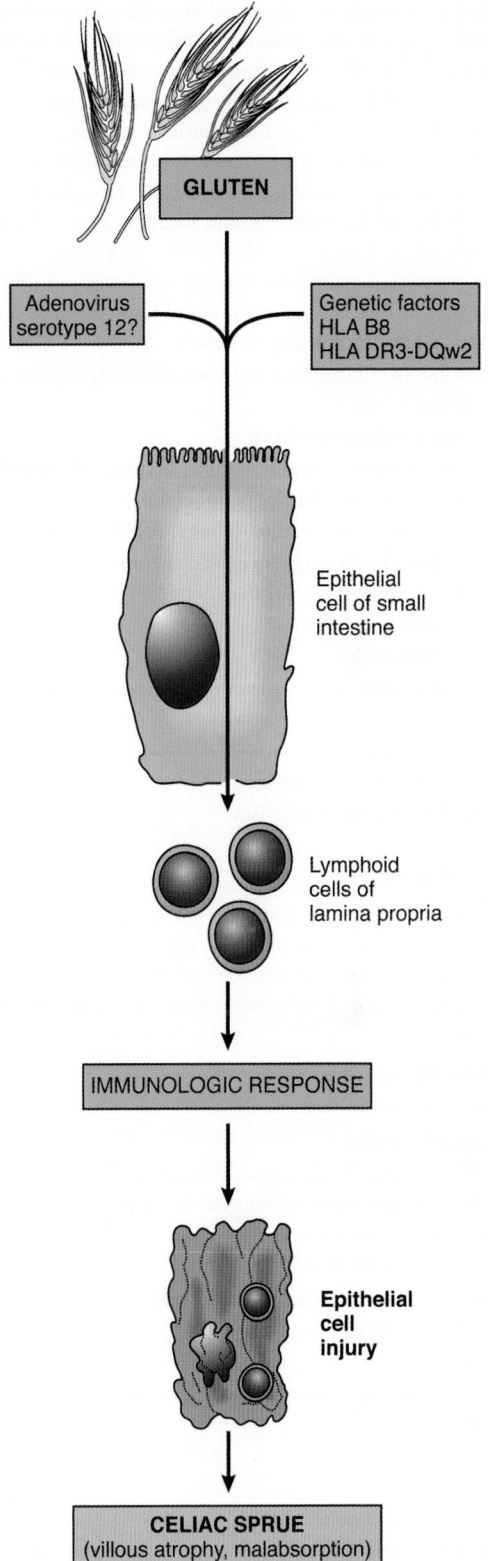

Figure 48-5. Mechanisms in the pathogenesis of celiac disease.

2. The disease results in inflammation in the mucosa of the small bowel, especially the duodenum and jejunum. This results in damage to the villi, which can be shortened or totally lost.

3. The mucosal damage results in deficiency of enzymes on the mucosal surface, such as disaccharidase and peptidase. This, along with a reduced surface area, leads to malabsorption.

4. The body may be unable to absorb fats, fat-soluble vitamins (A, D, E, and K), minerals, and some protein and carbohydrates.

5. The severity of symptoms depends on the extent of affected intestine. If involvement is focal and limited to the proximal bowel, GI symptoms may be absent.

6. A number of conditions may be associated with celiac disease, including:
   a. Type 1 diabetes mellitus.
   b. Mucocutaneous manifestations, dermatitis herpetiformis.
   c. Cystic fibrosis, seizures, peripheral neuropathy.
   d. Autoimmune thyroiditis, adrenal insufficiency.
   e. Systemic lupus erythematosus, rheumatoid arthritis, and other connective tissue disorders.
   f. Sclerosing cholangitis.
   g. Trisomy 21.
   h. Unexplained folate or iron deficiency, refractory to treatment.
   i. Alopecia areata.
   j. Dental enamel hypoplasia.
   k. Risk of thromboembolism.

Clinical Manifestations

The age and mode of presenting signs and symptoms are extremely variable. Diagnosis may be made by ages 6 to 24 months when infants are introduced to cereal; however, more subtle gastrointestinal and extraintestinal symptoms often lead to diagnosis much later in life.

Ages 6 to 18 months
Presentation may include:

1. Impaired growth.
   a. Normal growth during early months of life.
   b. Slackening of weight followed by weight loss.
2. Diarrhea—more frequent, pale, soft, bulky, greasy (steatorrhea) with offensive odor.
3. Recalcitrant constipation (occasionally).
4. Abdominal distention.
5. Anorexia.
6. Muscle wasting—most obvious in buttocks and proximal parts of extremities.
7. Vomiting.
8. Seizures.
9. Loss of tooth enamel.
10. Painful/pruritic skin rash called "dermatitis herpetiformis."

Older Children
1. Complications of malabsorption:
   a. Anemia, vitamin deficiency.
   b. Hypoproteinemia (hypoalbuminemia) with edema.
   c. Hypocalcemia, hypokalemia, hypomagnesemia.
   d. Hypoprothrombinemia resulting from impaired vitamin K absorption.
   e. Disaccharide intolerance—with acid sugar-containing stools (secondary to the altered small-bowel mucosa).
   f. Low bone density, osteoporosis secondary to decreased calcium absorption.
2. Diarrhea or constipation.
3. Overweight status.

Evidence Base Reilly, N. R., Aguilar, K., Hassid, B. G., et al. (2011). Celiac disease in normal-weight and overweight children: Clinical features and growth outcomes following a gluten-free diet. *Journal of Pediatric Gastroenterology, Hepatology and Nutrition, 53*(5), 528–531.

4. Linear growth delay.
5. Abdominal pain.
6. Fatigue.

Diagnostic Evaluation

Evidence Base Alessio, M., Tonutti, E., Brusca, I., et al. (2011). Correlation between IgA tissue transglutaminase antibody ratio and histological finding in celiac disease: A multicentre study. *Journal of Pediatric Gastroenterology and Nutrition, 55*(1), 44–49.

Dogan, Y., Yildirmaz, S., & Ozercan, I. H. (2012). Prevalence of celiac disease among first-degree relatives of patients with celiac disease. *Journal of Pediatric Gastroenterology and Nutrition, 55*(2), 205–208.

1. Thorough history, including family history of autoimmune disorders, diabetes, dietary history, growth history, and general status of the child.
2. Serologic testing is done to screen the individual at risk. It has been recommended that all short-stature children be screened irrespective of GI symptoms. Assays detect immunoglobulin (Ig) A antibody to endomysium or tissue transglutaminase. These antibodies have a very high sensitivity and specificity for CD; however, they may be falsely low in a child with IgA deficiency. Therefore, the total IgA level must also be checked.
3. An upper endoscopy is the gold-standard test to confirm the diagnosis and must be done in all individuals whose serologic screening is positive. It might show infiltration of the mucosa with lymphocytes and variable degrees of flattened villi.
4. Videocapsule endoscopy shows good sensitivity and excellent specificity for the detection of villous atrophy in patients with suspected CD, but is not often practical in the pediatric population; the gold standard of diagnosis remains the small intestinal biopsy.

NURSING ALERT Ages 3–6 months is too early to be able to detect celiac disease with testing because of the length of time of gluten exposure.

Management

1. Lifelong gluten-free diet.
   a. Avoid all foods containing wheat, rye, and barley and their derivatives because even a small amount, such as a trace contaminant, may cause a pathologic response. Oats are naturally gluten-free; however, they are often cross-contaminated during the manufacturing process, so their exclusion may be recommended.
   b. The small intestinal mucosa will always respond abnormally to dietary gluten, although clinical signs may not be immediately evident.
   c. Biopsy and serologic screening revert to normal with appropriate diet.
   d. Clinical signs of improvement are often seen days to weeks after proper diet is initiated, but can take up to 1 year in the case of more insidious symptoms such as delayed linear growth.
2. Adequate caloric and nutrient intake.
3. Supplemental vitamins and minerals may be used when clinically indicated, although there is currently no standard for use.
   a. Folic acid if low level is suspected or detected.
   b. Vitamins A and D.
   c. Iron up to 3 months if anemic.
   d. Vitamin K if evidence of hypoprothrombinemia and bleeding.
   e. Calcium if milk is restricted.
4. Temporary restriction of lactose and sucrose (disaccharidases) from diet for 6 to 8 weeks may be indicated in some cases, if these products are shown to worsen symptoms.
5. Enzyme therapy that protects the mucosal lining from gluten exposure is being investigated in clinical trials.

Complications

1. Nutritional deficiencies (most important short-term risks, which can lead to anemia, osteoporosis, and growth failure).
2. Long-term risks of untreated CD include increased risk of lymphoma and adenocarcinoma of small intestine.
3. Refractory CD.
4. Seizures related to inadequate absorption of folic acid and buildup of calcium deposits on the brain.

Nursing Assessment

1. Obtain family dietary history as it relates to onset of symptoms.
2. Assess child's nutritional status.
3. Check for signs of infection.
4. Assess growth and developmental parameters.

Nursing Diagnoses

- Imbalanced Nutrition: Less Than Body Requirements related to malabsorption of nutrients, diarrhea, and vomiting.
- Impaired Parenting related to inability to control behavioral problems.

Nursing Interventions

Provide Adequate Nutrition and Dietary Restrictions

1. Provide gluten-free diet, being careful to avoid accidental exposure via cross-contamination while food is prepared and/or cooked.
2. An initial diet high in protein, relatively low in fat, low in lactose and free from gluten may be necessary if the newly diagnosed child exhibits severe malabsorption.
   a. Initiate a referral with a dietitian for precise diet recommendations.
   b. Soy milk or lactaid drops may be indicated if the patient is exhibiting signs of lactose intolerance.
   c. Watch for fat intolerance in infants and young children.
3. Maintain NPO status during the initial treatment of celiac crisis or during diagnostic testing. Take special precautions to ensure proper restriction if the child is ambulatory.
4. Encourage small, frequent, appetizing meals, but do not force eating if the child has anorexia.
5. Note the child's reaction to food. Close observation of the child's responses to food may reveal other intolerances. Note and record:
   a. Foods taken and refused.
   b. Appetite.
   c. Change in behavior after eating.
   d. Characteristics and frequency of stools.
   e. General disposition—behavior improvement commonly seen within 2 to 3 days after diet control is initiated.
6. Be prepared to temporarily eliminate new food introduced if symptoms increase.
7. A gluten-challenged diet is not routinely indicated.
8. Provide the family with assistance to obtain a variety of gluten-free foods. Studies demonstrate that poor availability and expense of gluten-free foods lead to dietary noncompliance.

 Evidence Base Errichielleo, S., (2010). Celiac disease: Predictors of compliance with a gluten-free diet in adolescents and young adults. *Journal of Pediatric Gastroenterology and Nutrition, 50*(1), 54–60.

Promoting Effective Parenting

1. Teach the parents to develop an awareness of the child's behavior; recognize changes and care for child accordingly.
2. Explain that diet and eating have a direct effect on behavior and that behavior may indicate how the child is feeling.
3. Help the parents recognize and understand mood swings, from having temper tantrums to being very timid, nervous, or unstable.
4. Advise the parents to allow the child to express feelings freely through safe and age-appropriate media.
5. Encourage parents to define limits of behavior for the child and convey them to all family members.
6. Encourage patience, routines, and consistency.
7. Advise parents to record changes in behavior, especially in relation to eating and diet, to document effectiveness of therapy.

8. Help the parents to maintain a balance between the child with celiac disease, the other family members, and additional roles and responsibilities.

9. If the child is withdrawn, advise providing opportunity for play with other children, especially when the child begins to feel better.

10. Explain that the toddler may cling to infantile habits for security. Allow this behavior; it may disappear as physical condition improves.

11. Suggest offering the child other sensory stimulation to compensate for lack of eating pleasure.

12. Help the parents to understand that, after initial rapid weight gain, further improvement may be slow.

13. Provide emotional support for the child and parents.

14. Refer for counseling, if indicated.

Family Education and Health Maintenance

 Evidence Base Hogen Esch, C. E., Wolters, V. M., Gerritsen, S. A., et al. (2011). Specific celiac disease antibodies in children on gluten-free diet. *Pediatrics, 128*(3), 547–552.

Ryan, M., & Grossman, S. (2011). Celiac disease: Implications for management. *Gastroenterology Nursing, 34*(3), 225–228.

1. Teach parents about celiac disease and how it is controlled by diet. Help them to understand that severe, long-term damage to the intestinal lining has occurred and must be controlled to allow for normal growth and development.

2. Long-term follow-up with a qualified dietitian has been shown to improve compliance based on symptoms and follow-up serological testing.

3. Provide a specific list of restricted and acceptable foods to get the family started; because there is much variation among brands of packaged foods, it is best for the family to check with the manufacturers.

4. Teach the parents how to read labels on foods to identify those containing wheat, rye, and barley glutens, thus avoiding them.
   a. Advise that any ingredient of unknown or unspecified grain origin should be assumed to contain gluten, unless the manufacturer confirms that it is gluten-free.
   b. Advise that medications should also be checked; filler and excipients, such as alcohol in cough medication, may be wheat based.
   c. Advise parents that gluten is found in many manufactured products as a filler or thickener, such as gravy powder.

5. Provide substitutes for wheat, rye, and barley such as corn, rice, potato, soybean flour, and gluten-free starch.

6. Help the parents become comfortable in situation problem solving (eg, supplying gluten-free cupcakes for birthday party to which child has been invited).

7. Initiate referral to dietitian to ensure that nutrient and energy requirements are being met. There is no standardized vitamin regimen.

8. Discuss the importance of continued adherence to gluten-free diet, even though the child is feeling well, eating well, and has normal stools. Encourage child to become involved in diet.

9. Adolescent compliance may be variable. Encourage support and understanding.

10. Alteration in diet may have significant cultural, ethnic, and religious implications. Help parents identify how adjustments can be made.

11. Advise parents on eating out—check ahead of time with fast-food chains and restaurant chefs or management to determine if they can ensure gluten-free items. (Be aware that even a gluten-free hamburger cooked on a grill with a breaded chicken breast cannot be considered gluten-free).
    a. Many gluten-free menus at chain restaurants can be found on the Internet by searching keyword "gluten-free."
    b. Inform friends before visiting and bring gluten-free products, if necessary.
    c. Discuss dietary restrictions with the child's school and other parents.

12. Advise parents to investigate support groups, Internet companies, natural food stores, and major food brands that offer information and sell gluten-free products.

13. Tell parents that common problems with long-term gluten-free diet are constipation due to low dietary fiber intake and weight gain due to now normal absorption; therefore, encourage regular physical activity and avoidance of high-calorie foods.

14. Impress on the parents the importance of regular medical follow-up.

15. Encourage the parents to practice good hygiene to prevent infection because the child may be especially prone to infection if malnutrition and/or anemia are present.

16. Advise the family that patients with CD have a predisposition to nonresponse of the hepatitis B vaccine; therefore, titers should be considered.

17. Help the parents to understand that the emotional climate in the home and around the child is vitally important in maintaining the child's medical and physical stability. Stress the importance of not making the child feel abnormal or a nuisance to the family. Family support is invaluable in facilitating acceptance of the diet.

18. Stress that the disorder is lifelong; however, changes in the mucosal lining of the intestine and the general clinical condition of the child are reversible when dietary gluten is avoided.

19. Advise screening for all first-degree relatives, due to heredity nature of the disease.

20. For additional information and support, refer to Celiac Sprue Association (*www.csaceliacs.org*), Canadian Celiac Association (*www.celiac.ca*), or Celiac Disease Foundation (*www.celiac.org*).

Evaluation: Expected Outcomes

- Tolerates gluten-free diet well, Poor growth is not the symptom for every child, therefore gaining weight is not an appropriate expected outcome for each child.
- Parents setting limits with child and documenting behavior in relation to meals.

Diarrhea

Diarrhea is the rapid movement of fecal matter through the intestine, resulting in an excessive loss of water and electrolytes and producing more frequent loose, unformed, or watery stools. It is a symptom of many conditions and may be caused by many diseases (see Table 48-2). Commonly, the cause is difficult to determine; occasionally, it is unknown. Worldwide, approximately 1.8 million children die from diarrhea annually. Studies show that approximately 40% of cases of diarrhea have no direct cause, although some viruses have yet to be identified.

Pathophysiology and Etiology

Evidence Base Zella, G. C., & Israel, E. J. (2012). Chronic diarrhea in children. *Pediatrics in Review, 33*(5), 207–217.
  Ammoury, R. F., & Croffie, J. M. (2010). Malabsorptive disorders of childhood. *Pediatrics in Review, 31*(10), 407–416.

Mechanisms of Diarrhea

1. Secretory—decreased absorption, increased secretion
2. Osmotic—maldigestion, transport defects, ingestion of unabsorbable solute
3. Intestinal dysmotility—intact absorption with decreased intestinal transit time
4. Inflammatory—malabsorption; can be caused by infectious or noninfectious agents.

Physiologic Effects of Diarrhea

1. Dehydration (extracellular fluid [ECF] loss).
   a. Large loss of fluid and electrolytes in watery stools.
   b. May be compounded by vomiting, decreased fluid intake, and increased insensible loss due to fever and rapid respirations.
2. Electrolyte imbalance.
   a. Potassium—may be hyper or hypokalemic.
   b. Sodium and chloride are directly related and may be increased or decreased.
      i. Hypernatremic hyperchloremic (hypertonic) dehydration occurs with acute diarrhea.
      ii. Hyponatremic hypochloremic (hypotonic) hypervolemia occurs with too rapid fluid replacement.
3. Acid-base imbalance—metabolic acidosis.
   a. From large losses of potassium, sodium, and bicarbonate in stools.
   b. From impaired renal function.
4. Monosaccharide intolerance and protein hypersensitivity.

Table 48-2	Differential Diagnosis of Diarrhea		
	INFANT	**CHILD**	**ADOLESCENT**
Acute			
Common	• Gastroenteritis • Systemic infection • Antibiotic associated • Overfeeding	• Gastroenteritis • Food poisoning • Systemic infection • Antibiotic associated	• Gastroenteritis • Food poisoning • Antibiotic associated
Rare	• Primary disaccharidase deficiency • Hirschsprung's toxic colitis • Adrenogenital syndrome	• Toxic ingestion	• Hyperthyroidism
Chronic			
Common	• Postinfectious secondary lactase deficiency • Cow's milk or soy protein intolerance • Chronic nonspecific diarrhea of infancy • Celiac disease • Cystic fibrosis • AIDS enteropathy	• Postinfectious secondary lactase deficiency • Irritable bowel syndrome • Celiac disease • Lactose intolerance • Giardiasis • Inflammatory bowel disease • AIDS enteropathy	• Irritable bowel syndrome • Inflammatory bowel disease • Lactose intolerance • Giardiasis • Laxative abuse (anorexia nervosa)
Rare	• Primary immune defects • Familial villous atrophy • Secretory tumors • Acrodermatitis enteropathica • Lymphangiectasia • Abetalipoproteinemia • Eosinophilic gastroenteritis • Short-bowel syndrome • Intractable diarrhea syndrome • Autoimmune enteropathy	• Acquired immune defects • Secretory tumors • Pseudo-obstruction	• Secretory tumor • Primary bowel tumor • Anal intercourse (inflammation confined to the rectum) • Kaposi sarcoma–associated diarrhea

AIDS, acquired immunodeficiency syndrome.

Pathogenic Etiology

1. Bacteria—*Escherichia coli* O157:H7, *Salmonella, Shigella, Yersinia enterocolitica, Campylobacter jejuni, Clostridium difficile*, dysentery, cholera.
2. Antibiotic-associated diarrhea, such as *C. difficile* diarrhea, is a leading cause of nosocomial outbreaks.
3. Viral—rotavirus (most common; peaks during winter months), enteroviruses (echovirus), adenoviruses, human reovirus-like agent, Norwalk virus.
4. Fungal—*Candida enteritis*.
5. Parasitic—*Giardia lamblia, Cryptosporidium parvum*.
6. Protozoal.

Noninfectious Etiologic Factors

1. Malabsorption—lactase deficiency, cow's milk protein allergy, food protein-induced enteropathy, celiac disease, cystic fibrosis, microvillus inclusion disease.
2. Inflammatory bowel disease—ulcerative colitis, Crohn's disease, rare in infants.
3. Immune deficiency—severe combined immunodeficiency, IgA deficiency.
4. Infant exposed to overeating.
5. Direct irritation of GI tract by foods, medications, chemicals, radiation.
6. Inappropriate use of laxatives and purgatives.
7. Mechanical disorders—malrotation, incomplete small-bowel obstruction, intermittent volvulus.
8. Congenital anomalies (eg, Hirschsprung's disease-related enterocolitis).
9. Drug consumption—increases the risk of colitis, especially in predisposed persons; some agents may just exacerbate underlying colitis.
10. Functional—diagnosis of exclusion, although etiology may be a virus that has not been identified. For example, child exposed to excessive stress, emotional excitement, and fatigue.

Acute Diarrhea

1. Sudden increase in frequency of stools.
2. Usually self-limited, but can result in dehydration.

Chronic or Persistent Diarrhea

1. Defined as three loose or liquid bowel movements a day for at least 2 to 4 weeks and a stool weight >200 g/day.
2. Associated with disorders of malabsorption, anatomic defects, abnormal bowel motility, hypersensitivity reaction, or a long-term inflammatory response.
3. May be due to behaviors that continue to expose children to pathogens as well as increased resistance of bacteria to commonly used antibacterial agents.

> **NURSING ALERT** Infants and young children in daycare centers may be at increased risk for diarrhea due to *Shigella, Salmonella*, rotavirus, endopathogenic *E. coli*, and giardiasis. Handwashing is the major preventive measure. These infections are usually reportable to the health department. Bloody diarrhea should be immediately referred for medical evaluation.

Risk Factors for Diarrhea

1. Age—the younger the child, the greater the susceptibility and severity.
   a. ECF volume is proportionately larger in the infant and young child.
   b. Nutritional reserves are relatively smaller in the young child.
2. Impaired health—susceptibility is increased in the malnourished or debilitated child.
3. Climate—susceptibility is increased in warm weather.
4. Environment—frequency is increased where there is overcrowding, poor sanitation, inadequate refrigeration of food, and inadequate health care and education.
5. Virulence of a potential pathogen affects severity.
6. Internationally adopted child.

Clinical Manifestations

Symptoms vary with severity, specific cause, and type of onset (insidious vs. acute).

1. Low-grade fever to 100° F (37.8° C).
2. Anorexia.
3. Vomiting (can precede diarrhea by several days); mild and intermittent to severe.
4. Stools—appearance of diarrhea from a few hours to 3 days.
   a. Loose and fluid consistency.
   b. Greenish or yellow-green, although can be any color.
   c. May contain mucus, pus, or blood.
   d. Frequency varies from 3 to 20 per day.
   e. Expelled with force; may be preceded by pain.
5. Behavioral changes.
   a. Irritability and restlessness.
   b. Weakness.
   c. Extreme prostration.
   d. Stupor and convulsions.
   e. Flaccidity.
6. Physical changes.
   a. Little to extreme loss of subcutaneous fat.
   b. Up to 50% total body weight loss.
   c. Poor skin turgor; capillary refill longer than 2 seconds.
   d. Dry mucous membranes and dry, cracked lips.
   e. Pallor.
   f. Sunken fontanelles and eyes.
   g. Petechiae may be seen with bacterial infections.
   h. Excoriated buttocks and perineum.
   i. Urine with blood.
7. Vital sign and urine output changes (signal imminent cardiovascular collapse).
   a. Low BP.
   b. High pulse rate.
   c. Respirations rapid and hyperpneic.
   d. Decreased or absent urine output.

Diagnostic Evaluation

Studies to Evaluate Condition

1. Thorough history and physical examination to determine hydration status.

NURSING ALERT A postural change in heart rate and blood pressure is a useful clue in assessing the fluid state of a toddler (or any child). An increase greater than 20 beats/minute when moving from lying to standing is an indicator of hypovolemia. A decrease of at least 20mmHg in systolic BP or a decrease of at least 10 mmHg in diastolic BP when moving from lying to standing is considered orthostatic and likely indicates hypovolemia.

2. Electrolyte and kidney function tests—serum sodium, chloride, potassium, and blood urea nitrogen variable.
3. Acid-base balance—serum carbon dioxide; arterial pH and carbon dioxide possibly abnormal.
4. CBC to determine plasma volume by hematocrit; infection by WBC count and differential.
5. Sedimentation rate—elevated in infection and inflammation.

Studies to Determine Cause

1. Thorough history to determine recent contact or exposure, contact with potentially contaminated water (swimming in lakes and ponds, well water), travel to at-risk countries, antibiotic therapy, and possible immunosuppression.
2. Enzyme immunoassay tests such as Rotazyme to test stool for rotavirus.
3. Multiple stool and rectal swab for bacterial cultures, ova and parasites, and *C. difficile*. Some labs require the sample specify for *Giardia* profile, *Cryptosporidium*, and *E. coli* O157:H7 serotyping. If immunosuppressed, add *Microsporidian*, *Cryptosporidium*, and *G. lamblia* antigen 65.

4. Stool for WBC count to screen for colitis that may be of a bacterial or inflammatory nature.
5. Stool pH, reducing substances—decreased pH may indicate various noninfectious causes; acid stool containing sugar is characteristic of disaccharide intolerance, abnormality of bile salt reabsorption.
6. Blood cultures can rule out septicemia.
7. Serologic studies can detect viral pathogens.
8. Breath hydrogen test can determine carbohydrate malabsorption and bacterial overgrowth.
9. Urinalysis can exclude UTI as cause of nonspecific diarrhea and screen for blood, which may be part of hemolytic uremic syndrome associated with *E. coli* O157:H7 infection.

Management

 Evidence Base Fox, J., Richards, S., Jenkins, H., et al. (2012). Management of gastroenteritis over 10 years: Changing culture and maintaining the change. *Archives of Disease in Childhood, 97*(5), 415–417.

Treatment is based on the degree of dehydration; mild (loss of less than 5% of body weight), moderate (5% to 10% loss), and severe (greater than 10% loss) (see Table 48-3).

1. Goal is to prevent spread of disease; communicable disease is suspected until proved otherwise; enteric precautions are followed.
2. Bowel rest may be required based on degree of diarrhea and vomiting, if blood present, or electrolyte abnormalities.

Table 48-3	Assessment for Dehydration in Children		
CLINICAL SIGNS	**DEGREE OF DEHYDRATION**		
	Mild	**Moderate**	**Severe**
General			
Infant's behavior	Thirsty, alert, restless	Restless or lethargic; irritable to touch	Limp, drowsy; cyanotic extremities
Child's behavior	Thirsty, alert, restless	Thirsty, alert; postural hypotension	Usually conscious; cyanotic extremities
Respirations	Slightly increased	Increased	Deep and rapid
Pulse	Slightly increased	Increased	Rapid
Blood pressure	Normal	Decreased	May be unrecordable
Capillary refill	2 seconds	2–3 seconds	3 seconds
Skin turgor	Normal	Slightly reduced	Reduced
Skin color	Pale	Gray	Mottled
Weight loss	Up to 5%	Up to 10%	Up to 15%
Mucous membrane	Tacky	Tacky/dry	Parched
Anterior fontanelle	Flat	Slightly depressed	Sunken
Urine volume	Small	Oliguria	Oliguria/anuria
Specific gravity	1.020	1.030	1.035

3. For mild to moderate dehydration, oral rehydration solution is given to maintain fluid and electrolyte balance (WHO solution, Pedialyte, Infalyte). BRAT (banana, rice, apple, tea) diet is no longer recommended, as it is nutritionally suboptimal.

   a. For oral rehydration, 100 mL/kg over 4 hours, with additional fluids after each liquid bowel movement.

   b. Candidates for oral rehydration include mild to moderate dehydration, older than age 4 months, no persistent vomiting, and probable gastroenteritis.

4. For moderate to severe dehydration, IV fluid and electrolyte replacement is given slowly, as ordered (usually 20 mL/kg), usually over 2 days to prevent hypotonic hypervolemia (water intoxication). Administration of larger amounts of IV dextrose is associated with reduced return visits in children with gastroenteritis and dehydration.

5. Supportive care is given: monitoring oral and IV fluid intake, output from all sources, and patient's response to treatment.

6. Specific antimicrobial therapy may be given in some cases such as immunosuppression, bacteremia, documented *C. difficile*, and traveler's diarrhea.

   a. Metronidazole 30 mg/kg/day in divided doses orally or via IV line may be used to treat *C. difficile* infection, although IV dosing may be less efficacious.

   b. Vancomycin P.O. for resistant *C. difficile*.

   c. Rifampin has been shown to be effective in traveler's diarrhea without associated side effects.

DRUG ALERT Fidaxomicin was recently approved by the FDA for treatment of *C. difficile*–associated diarrhea in adults, but has not yet been studied in children.

7. Probiotics (*Saccharomyces boulardii*, *Lactobacillus rhamnosus* GG, and probiotic mixtures) significantly reduced the development of antibiotic-associated diarrhea. *S. boulardii* was effective for *C. difficile* infection.

Evidence Base Ringel-Kulka, T. (2012). Evidence base for probiotic products for the pediatric population. *Journal of Pediatric Gastroenterology and Nutrition, 54*(5), 578–579.

8. The World Health Organization and the American Academy of Pediatrics discourage the use of antidiarrheal agents in children. In children who are younger than age 3 years, malnourished, moderately or severely dehydrated, systemically ill, or who have bloody diarrhea, adverse events outweigh benefits. In children who are older than age 3 years, with no/minimal dehydration, loperamide may be a useful adjunct to oral rehydration and early refeeding.

Complications

1. Severe dehydration and acid-base derangements with acidosis.
2. Shock.

Nursing Assessment

1. Obtain accurate history of signs and symptoms: nature and frequency of stools, type of onset, length of illness, associated symptoms.
2. Assess degree of dehydration (see Table 48-3).
3. Monitor intake and output including oral and IV fluids, fluid loss from diarrhea, urine output, and vomitus; monitor weight.
4. Note color and consistency of stool and vomitus.
5. Successful rehydration (at 4 hours) is defined as resolution of moderate dehydration, production of urine, weight gain, and the absence of severe emesis (≥ 5 mL/kg).

NURSING ALERT Assess child's behavior to determine comfort level. Crying or legs drawn up to abdomen usually indicates pain.

Nursing Diagnoses

- Deficient Fluid Volume related to diarrhea and ECF loss.
- Risk for Infection and transmission to others related to infectious diarrhea.
- Risk for Impaired Skin Integrity related to irritation by frequent stools.
- Imbalanced Nutrition: Less Than Body Requirements related to malabsorption.
- Anxiety and Fear related to hospitalization and illness.

Nursing Interventions

Restoring Fluid Balance

1. Monitor amount and rate of IV fluid therapy, which have been calculated by the health care provider. Fluid needs are based on fluid deficit, ongoing losses, and body weight.
2. Prevent overload of circulatory system.

   a. Check flow rate and amount absorbed hourly and totally.

   b. Adhere to prescribed volume carefully when oral feedings are given in conjunction with IV fluid.

   c. Never administer IV fluids to pediatric patient without safeguard of a volume-control infusion device or pump.

   d. Observe for signs of fluid overload: edema, increased BP, bounding pulse, labored respirations, and crackles in lung fields.

3. Check IV site for infiltration or improper flow so site can be changed as necessary.
4. Use appropriate protective devices to prevent the child from injuring involved extremity or causing IV to malfunction.
5. Weigh the patient daily as a guide for fluid needs and patient status.
6. Monitor urine output and keep accurate intake and output record, including vomitus and liquid stools.
7. If NPO, provide frequent mouth care and nonnutritive sucking with a pacifier. Continue to burp infant to expel air swallowed while crying or sucking.
8. If oral rehydration solution is used, reassess hydration status every 2 to 4 hours; once rehydrated, continue for 8 to

12 hours, then resume breastfeeding with increased frequency of feedings or formula at full strength or increased frequency if half strength.

Note: Unless vomiting is severe, do not deprive the patient of nutrition for longer than 1or 2 days. If adequate nutrition cannot be provided, parenteral nutrition should be instituted.

 NURSING ALERT Diluted fruit juices and soft drinks are not recommended. High disaccharide content aggravates diarrhea by osmotic effect.

Preventing Spread of Infection

1. Ensure adherence to good handwashing and gown technique protocols for all people having contact with infant or child.
2. Follow your facility's policy on care of diapers.
3. Handle specimens collected using universal precautions and transport to laboratories in appropriate containers per policy. Collect stool sample for culture before instituting antibiotic therapy.
4. Teach good hygiene measures to older children.

Preventing Skin Impairment

1. Protect infant's diaper area from becoming excoriated by making frequent diaper changes.
2. Expose to air and light as much as possible.
3. Avoid commercial baby wipes, which contain alcohol and may sting inflamed or excoriated diaper area. Use mild soap and water, place infant in tub of water or baking soda bath (soothing and neutralizing) for cleaning.
4. Prevent scratching or rubbing of irritated area. Holding infant on parent's protected lap may provide comfort and stimulation for parent and infant.
5. Use protective barrier creams, such as zinc oxide; if excoriated, soak off cream and pat dry—do not rub. Not all cream barrier has to be removed because this can denude skin.
6. Leave diaper area open to air until thoroughly dried.

Resuming Adequate Nutritional Intake

1. After rehydration, advance slowly from clear liquids to half-strength formula, to regular diet.
   a. If chronic diarrhea, bloody diarrhea, or secretory diarrhea, limit milk products containing lactose.
   b. In older infants and children, offer nonlactose, bland, carbohydrate-rich foods shortly after successful rehydration.
2. As diet is advanced, note any vomiting or increase in stools and report it immediately. Oral feedings should not be resumed too early or advanced too rapidly because diarrhea may recur.

Reducing Fear and Anxiety

1. Acknowledge that hospitalization is frightening, especially when it is sudden, as with diarrhea.
2. Many treatments and procedures may be painful. Give reassurance to the child before, during, and after treatment.
   a. Explain treatment in age-appropriate language.
   b. Include family in care and treatments when possible.

3. Explain to family that intermittent abdominal cramps may be painful and provide support.
4. Provide some means of pleasant stimulation, entertainment, or diversion, especially while child remains in bed.
   a. Infant—mobile, musical toy.
   b. Young child—books, tapes.
   c. Older child—television, videos.
5. Provide physical closeness to provide comfort, if child displays interest.
   a. Petting, stroking.
   b. Holding, rocking.

Community and Home Care Considerations

1. Infants and young children in daycare centers may be at increased risk for diarrhea due to *Shigella*, *Salmonella*, rotavirus, *E. coli*, *Cryptosporidium*, *Campylobacter*, *C. difficile*, and *Giardia*. Good handwashing is the major preventive measure. This is especially important with rotavirus because it can be excreted for as long as 57 days in some cases.
2. If infectious agent is identified, it should be reported because other children may be at risk.
   a. Encourage parents to contact the child daycare center and report.
   b. A child with diarrhea containing blood or mucus should be excluded from daycare and medically evaluated. Exclusion from daycare should occur until the diarrhea resolves.
   c. Stool cultures positive for *E. coli* O157:H7 or *Shigella* are reportable to the county health department and the child should be excluded until the diarrhea resolves and two cultures, from two different stools, are negative for these organisms.
3. Assess sanitation and hygiene practices in the home or daycare center for overcrowding, number of working toilets in the home for number of people, availability of working sinks with soap and towels in the bathrooms and their proximity to food preparation areas, disposal of diapers, and handwashing practices of caregivers and children.
4. Because most treatment for diarrhea is done on an outpatient basis, nurses in the community need to be available to answer questions.

Family Education and Health Maintenance

1. After the cause of the diarrhea is determined, it may be necessary to teach proper hygiene, formula or food preparation, handling, and storage.
   a. Use handwashing before bottle and food preparation.
   b. Use disposable bottles or sterilize or use dishwasher for reusable bottles.
   c. Refrigerate reconstituted formula and all other fluids between uses. Milk may become contaminated within 1 hour if left out at room temperature; juice becomes contaminated within several hours.
   d. Discard small amounts of food or fluid from containers already used.

2. Explain the fecal–oral mode of transmission of infectious diarrheal illnesses.

3. Explain the early symptoms of a diarrheal illness and of dehydration, which requires notification of the health care provider.

4. Discourage the use of anti-emetics and antidiarrheal medications for infants and children with gastroenteritis; they have little effect on infantile diarrhea, may cause toxicity, and can mask signs and symptoms of more serious illness.

DRUG ALERT Bismuth subsalicylate, an over-the-counter drug that is readily available, has shown only modest beneficial effects in children and may increase the risk of Reye's syndrome due to salicylate absorption.

5. Advise parents when traveling internationally with their children to eat and drink only boiled, bottled, or carbonated water, be aware of drinks with ice cubes, food rinsed with water, and make sure all food is well cooked.

6. Help parents understand the importance of medical care and general good hygiene.

7. For additional information and support, refer to National Institute of Diabetes and Digestive and Kidney Diseases (*www.niddk.nih.gov*).

Evaluation: Expected Outcomes

- Vital signs stable; urine output adequate.
- Family, staff members handwashing properly and frequently.
- No redness or excoriation of diaper area.
- Tolerates small feedings of clear liquids without diarrhea or vomiting.
- No signs or symptoms of pain or discomfort.

Hirschsprung's Disease

Hirschsprung's disease (congenital aganglionic megacolon) is a form of chronic intestinal obstruction affecting primarily full-term infants.

It occurs due to the congenital absence of the parasympathetic ganglion nerve cells from within the muscle wall of the intestinal tract, usually at the distal end of the colon. Ganglion cells are located throughout the intestinal tract from the mouth down to the rectum. It occurs in 1 in 5,000 (ranges 1:4,400 to 1:7,000) live births with no racial predilection.

The male:female ratio is reported as 4:1, except in long segment disease, in which it is closer to 1:1, possibly favoring females. Strong evidence supports a genetic component and the association of other congenital anomalies such as Down syndrome, small/large intestinal atresias, trisomy 18, and other rare disorders.

Pathophysiology and Etiology

1. An arrest in embryologic development affecting the migration of parasympathetic nerve innervation of the intestine.
   a. Normally, the nerve cells migrate to the upper end of the alimentary tract and then proceed in the caudal direction, with migration to the distal colon complete by 12 weeks.
   b. Migration occurs first in the intermuscular layer, called *Auerbach's plexus*, and then moves into the submucosal plexus, moving along the GI tract in a descending manner.

2. The process of aganglionosis is almost always continuous within the affected segment, ending in proximal segment with ganglion cells. Intermittent ganglion cells in the colon have been reported, but this is extremely unusual.
   a. Most commonly affected site is the rectosigmoid colon (referred to as short-segment disease) (80%).
   b. Long-segment disease extends to the upper descending colon and transverse colon (10%) and occasionally throughout the entire colon, involving the small bowel (5%).
   c. Total angiogliosis of the bowel, involving the entire small and large bowel, is rare.

3. No peristalsis occurs in the affected portion of intestine (ie, spastic and contracted). This section is usually narrow; therefore, no fecal material passes through it.

4. Proximal to the narrow affected section, the colon is dilated (see Figure 48-6).
   a. Filled with fecal material and gas.
   b. Hypertrophy of muscular coating.
   c. Ulceration of mucosa may be seen in neonate.

5. The internal rectal sphincter fails to relax and evacuation of fecal material and gas is prevented. Abdominal distention and constipation result.

Clinical Manifestations

Clinical manifestations vary depending on degree of involved bowel.

1. Neonate—symptoms appearing at birth or within first weeks of life.
   a. No meconium passed in the first 48 hours of life.
   b. Vomiting—bile-stained or fecal.
   c. Abdominal distention.
   d. Constipation—occurs in 100% of patients.
   e. Overflow-type diarrhea.
   f. Dehydration; failure to thrive.
   g. Temporary relief of symptoms with enema.
   h. Bowel perforation—uncommon presentation.

2. Older child—symptoms not prominent at birth. Short-segment disease commonly presents later.
   a. History of obstipation at birth.
   b. Progressive abdominal distention.
   c. Peristaltic activity observable over abdomen.
   d. Absence of retentive posturing (ability to contract the internal and external sphincter to purposefully avoid defecation).
   e. Constipation—unresponsive to conventional remedies.
   f. Presence of encopresis.
   g. Ribbonlike, fluidlike, or pellet stools.
   h. Failure to grow—loss of subcutaneous fat; appears malnourished, stunted growth.
   i. Presentation insidious or catastrophic as with enterocolitis.

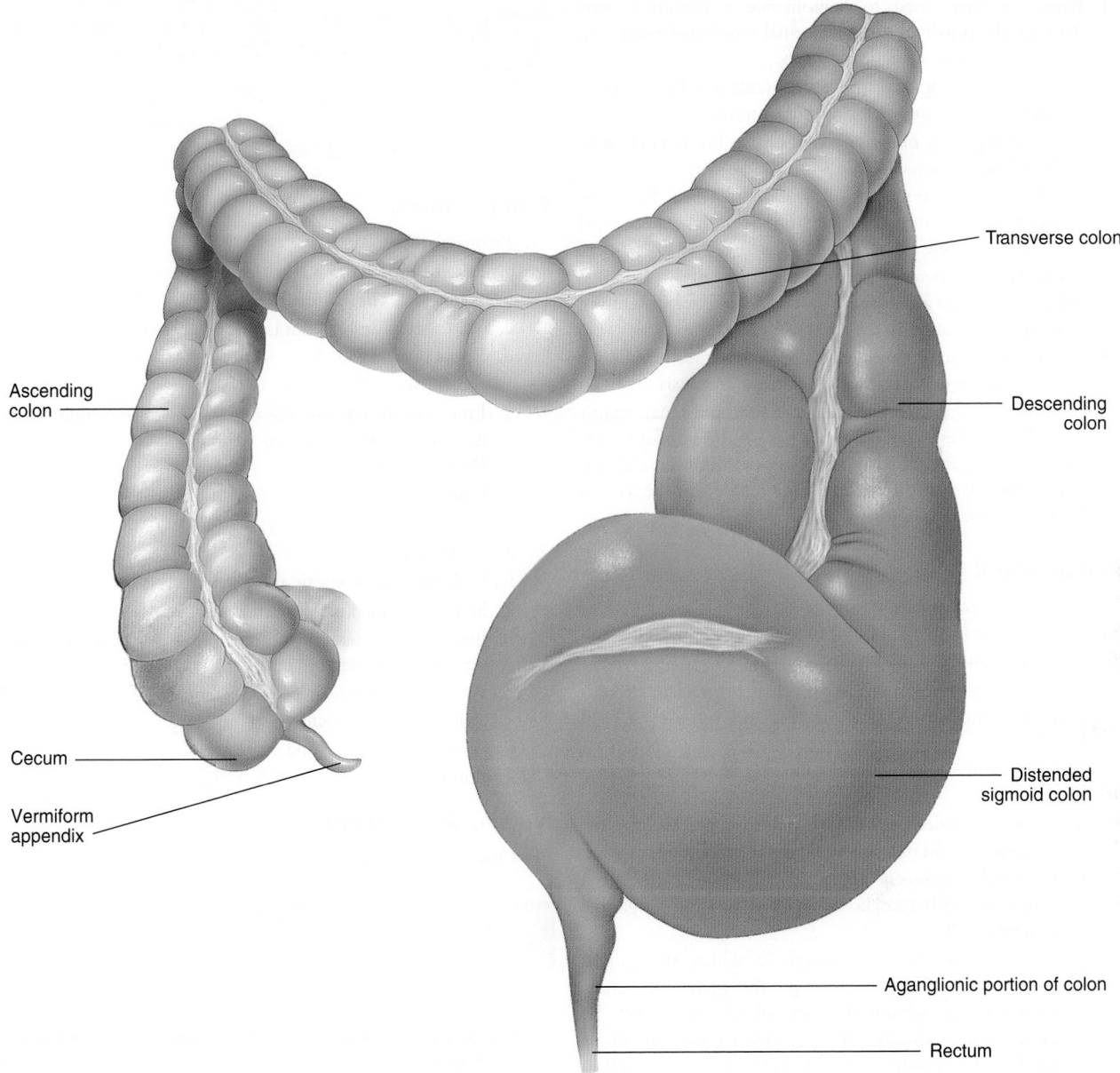

Figure 48-6. Bowel dilation in Hirschsprung's disease.

3. Enterocolitis—consists of severe toxemia and a proliferation of bacteria in the colonic lumen.
   a. Abdominal distention.
   b. Explosive diarrhea.
   c. Vomiting.
   d. Fever.
   e. Lethargy.
   f. Rectal bleeding.
   g. Shock.

Diagnostic Evaluation

1. Supportive findings on history and physical examination indicate Hirschsprung's disease.
2. Digital rectal examination—reveals a tight anal sphincter and a rectum that is narrow and empty of stool (in long-segment disease). In short-segment disease, rectal impaction may be present; removal of finger may be associated with a rush of stool as the obstruction is relieved.
3. Plain films—show severe gaseous distention of the bowel, with absence of air in the rectum.

4. Barium enema—used to demonstrate a transition zone between the proximal dilated, normal innervated colon and the distal, narrow, aganglionic colon.
   a. May be nondiagnostic in young infants who have not had sufficient time to develop a transition zone.
   b. Delayed passage of barium is suggestive, but not definitive for Hirschsprung's disease.
   c. Must be an unprepped study, as results may be falsely negative if laxatives or rectal stimulation have been used to facilitate defecation.
5. Anorectal manometry—demonstrates failure of the intestinal sphincter to relax in response to transient rectal distention. Requires cooperation of the child.
6. Full thickness or suction rectal biopsy—absence or reduced number of ganglion nerve cells; definitive diagnosis.
7. Radiopaque markers, ingested, measure intestinal transit time. Use of these markers is not part of the standard diagnostic workup for Hirschsprung's disease; however, children with short-segment disease retain the markers in the rectum for long periods.

Management

Definitive treatment is removal of the aganglionic, nonfunctioning, dilated segment of the bowel, followed by anastomosis and improved functioning of internal rectal sphincter.

1. Initially, a colostomy or ileostomy is performed to decompress intestine, divert fecal stream, and rest the normal bowel.
2. Definitive surgery includes the following reconstructive procedures:
   a. Swenson—abdominoperineal pull-through leaving the smallest amount of aganglionic bowel remaining.
   b. Duhamel—retrorectal transanal pull-through creating a neorectum with aganglionic anterior wall and ganglionic posterior wall.
   c. Soave—endorectal pull-through in which the ganglionic segment is pulled through the aganglionic muscular cuff, preserving the internal sphincter; may be done laparoscopically. May be delayed until infant is age 9 to 12 months or until weight reaches 15 to 20 lb (6.5 to 9 kg).
3. Many surgeons are now performing the endorectal pull-through without colostomy in neonates. This depends on the degree of defect, degree of dilatation of the colon, and the clinical status of the infant.
4. In older child whose symptoms are chronic but not severe, treatment may consist of isotonic enemas, stool softeners, and low-residue diet until surgery is performed.
5. Treatment of enterocolitis.
   a. Broad-spectrum IV antibiotics.
   b. Colonic irrigation and decompression with saline solution is initial emergency treatment. Hypertonic phosphate enemas are contraindicated because they may be retained, leading to electrolyte abnormalities.
   c. Surgical decompression colostomy.
   d. At least 1 month after, abdominal perineal pull-through.

 NURSING ALERT Enterocolitis is a potentially life-threatening event. Notify health care provider immediately if change in abdominal distention occurs in an infant or child with Hirschsprung's disease (whether preoperatively or postoperatively), especially if accompanied by fever, diarrhea, vomiting, or lethargy.

Complications

1. Preoperative.
   a. Enterocolitis—a major cause of death.
   b. Hydroureter or hydronephrosis.
   c. Water intoxication from tap water enemas.
   d. Bowel perforation.
2. Postoperative.
   a. Enterocolitis: remains the major cause of morbidity and mortality (mortality 6% to 30%).
   b. Diarrhea (69%).
   c. Vomiting (51%).
   d. Fever (34%).
   e. Lethargy (27%).
   f. Leaking of anastomosis and pelvic abscess.
   g. Stenosis, sudden inability to evacuate colon.
   h. Intestinal obstruction from adhesions, volvulus, or intussusception can develop late.
   i. Fecal incontinence is common but can improve with a proper bowel regimen.
   j. Adverse reaction to foods.
   k. Enuresis.

Nursing Assessment

1. Observe neonate for constipation.

 NURSING ALERT Diagnosis of Hirschsprung's should be suspected in any infant who fails to pass meconium within the first 24 hours and requires repeated rectal stimulation to induce bowel movements.

2. Obtain parents' history, especially on infant's bowel and feeding habits.
   a. Onset of constipation.
   b. Character of stools (ribbonlike or fluid-filled).
   c. Frequency of bowel movements.
   d. Enemas needed.
   e. Suppositories or laxatives needed.
3. Observe for irritability, feeding difficulty, distended abdomen, and signs of malnutrition (pallor, muscle weakness, thin extremities, fatigue).

Nursing Diagnoses

Preoperative
- Ineffective Breathing Pattern related to abdominal distention.
- Acute Pain related to intestinal obstruction.
- Imbalanced Nutrition: Less Than Body Requirements related to poor intake.
- Constipation due to pathophysiologic process.

Postoperative

- Impaired tissue integrity related to postoperative intervention.
- Risk for Infection of surgical incision.
- Risk for Dysfunctional Gastrointestinal Motility related to decreased peristalsis postoperatively.
- Ineffective Family Coping related to care of child with colostomy.

Nursing Interventions

Improving Breathing Pattern

1. Monitor for respiratory compromise that may result from abdominal distention; watch for rapid, shallow respirations; cyanosis; sternal retractions.
2. Elevate infant's head and chest by tilting the mattress to facilitate an open airway
3. Administer oxygen, as ordered, to support respiratory status.

Relieving Pain

1. Note degree of abdominal tenderness.
   a. Infant's legs drawn up.
   b. Chest breathing.
2. Note color of abdomen and presence of gastric waves; take sequential measurements of abdominal girth for evidence of changes.
3. Assist in emptying the bowel by giving repeated colonic irrigations.
   a. Procedure for irrigation in an infant is similar to that in an older child, except that less fluid and pressure are used.
   b. Physiologic saline solution (warmed) should be used for irrigations. Tap water may result in large quantities of water being absorbed and in water intoxication.
4. Administer medications (antibiotics), as ordered, to reduce the bacterial flora of the bowel.
5. Note any change in degree of distention before and after irrigation. Record if location of distention changes (ie, upper or lower abdomen).
6. Record all intake and output of irrigant and drainage. Report marked discrepancies in retention or loss of fluid.
7. Insert rectal tube for escape of accumulated fluid and gas, as ordered.
8. If abdominal distention is not relieved by irrigation and decompression and discomfort is significant, insert an NG tube, as ordered.
   a. Note drainage from NG tube and chart characteristics.
   b. Check for patency; saline irrigations may be requested. Carefully record intake and output.
   c. Perform frequent mouth care.
   d. Alternate nares when changing NG tube, and use minimal amount of tape to prevent skin irritation.
9. Offer pacifier for non-nutritive sucking if NPO, on parenteral fluids.
10. Encourage parents to hold and rock infant.
11. Maintain position of comfort with head elevated. Offer soothing stimulation (eg, music, touch, play therapy).

Providing Adequate Nutrition

1. Obtain a dietary history regarding food and eating habits.
   a. Discuss history with dietitian to facilitate potential dietary alterations.
   b. Explain to parents that eating problems are common with Hirschsprung's disease.
2. Monitor IV fluids appropriately; measure all output.
3. Offer small, frequent feedings.
   a. Feed child slowly.
   b. Provide as comfortable a position as possible for child during feedings.
4. Inform parents that defect can be corrected, but it may take some time for the child's physical status and feeding habits to improve.
   a. Feeding may cause additional discomfort because of distention and nausea.
   b. Parenteral nutrition may be necessary.

Controlling Constipation in the Older Child

1. Note and record frequency and characteristics of stools (constipation is likely to occur).
2. Provide demonstration and written and verbal instructions to family for saline enema administration and use of stool softeners.
3. Obtain dietary consultation for teaching of dietary alterations.

Preventing Complications Related to Colostomy

1. Monitor vital signs and respiratory status closely.

 NURSING ALERT Prevent injury to rectal mucosa by taking axillary or external ear temperature.

2. Monitor for proper functioning of colostomy, if present.
   a. Note drainage from colostomy: characteristics, frequency, fecal material, or liquid drainage.
   b. Record stoma color, size, and return of function.
   c. Note abdominal distention.
   d. Measure fluid loss from colostomy because the amount will affect fluid replacement.
3. Report signs of obstruction from peritonitis, paralytic ileus, handling bowel during surgery, or swelling.
   a. No output from colostomy.
   b. Increased tenderness.
   c. Irritability.
   d. Vomiting.
   e. Increased temperature.
4. Place child in a lateral position on a flat or only slightly elevated bed. When head of bed is elevated, the residual carbon dioxide in the child's abdominal cavity may cause referred pain in neck and shoulder.
5. Differentiate type and cause of pain to determine appropriate pain management interventions. Proper positioning, patent catheters and tubes, and timely administration of analgesics are key to ensuring patient comfort.

6. "Nothing per rectum" sign should be placed at head of bed so no rectal temperatures, rectal medications, or digital rectal examinations are done.

 NURSING ALERT Any rectal examination or procedure has the potential to cause serious harm to the patient and surgical site.

Preventing Postoperative Infections

1. Change wound dressing using sterile technique. If done laparoscopically, wound is minimal.
2. Prevent contamination from diaper.
   a. Apply diaper below dressing.
   b. Change diaper frequently.
3. Be aware that 7 to 10 stools per day may be passed postoperatively via ostomy bag. When cleared by surgery, prevent perianal and anal excoriation by thorough cleansing sitz baths and application of zinc oxide paste after soiling.
4. If skin is denuded and moist, apply a skin barrier and provide specific instruction to the family to prevent further damage to skin with aggressive removal.
5. Use careful handwashing technique.
6. Report wound redness, swelling or drainage, evisceration, or dehiscence immediately.
7. Suction secretions frequently to prevent infection of the tracheobronchial tree and lungs.
8. Encourage frequent coughing and deep breathing to maintain respiratory status.
9. Allow the infant to cry for short periods to prevent atelectasis.
10. Change the infant's position frequently to increase circulation and allow for aeration of all lung areas.

Preventing Abdominal Distention

1. Maintain patency of NG tube immediately postoperatively.
   a. NG suction, as ordered, for 24 to 48 hours or until adequate bowel sounds, gas from rectum or gas from ostomy.
   b. Watch for increasing abdominal distention; measure abdominal girth.
   c. Measure fluid loss because amount will affect fluid replacement.
2. Maintain NPO status until bowel sounds return and the bowel is ready for feedings as determined by provider.
3. Administer fluids to maintain hydration and replace lost electrolytes.
4. Maintain Foley catheter for 24 to 48 hours, as ordered.
5. Provide frequent oral hygiene while NPO.
6. Begin oral feedings, as ordered.
   a. Avoid overfeeding.
   b. Burp frequently during feeding.
   c. Turn head to side or elevate after feeding to prevent aspiration.

Supporting the Parents

1. Acknowledge that even a temporary colostomy can be a difficult procedure to accept and learn to manage.
   a. Initiate ostomy referral.
   b. Support the parents when teaching them to care for the colostomy.
   c. Include the parents in dressing changes and any other appropriate activities soon after surgery.
   d. Assist and encourage the parents to treat the infant or child as normally as possible.
   e. Reassure parents that colostomy will not cause delay in the child's normal development.
2. Encourage the parents to talk about their fears and anxieties. Anticipating future surgery for resection may be confusing and frightening.
3. Initiate community-nurse referral to help the parents care for the child at home away from the comforting situation of the hospital and obtain necessary equipment.
4. Initiate a genetic counseling referral, especially if the parents plan to have more children.

Ostomy Care in Children

Care of the colostomy and ileostomy in the infant and young child is based on the same principles and is essentially the same as that for an adult (see Chapter 18), with the following exceptions:

1. Colostomy irrigation is not part of management in small children. Irrigation is primarily for the purpose of regulating the colostomy to empty at regular intervals. Because children have bowel movements at more frequent intervals, this type of control is not feasible. Irrigation may be done only in preparation for tests or surgery and occasionally for the treatment of constipation.
2. Dehydration occurs quickly in the infant or small child; therefore, it is particularly important to observe drainage for amount and characteristics. Drainage should be measured to provide an accurate basis for computation of fluid replacement.
3. Prevention and treatment of skin excoriation around the stoma are of primary concern. With the advent of better skin shields and equipment designed especially for the pediatric patient, keeping an ostomy appliance in place is now less difficult. Through careful application and trying different types of pouches until a proper fit is obtained, most children can be kept clean and dry for at least 24 hours between changes. This is a significant factor in preventing skin breakdown and subsequent infections in the peristomal area. Remember, however, that infant dressings must be checked frequently.
   a. Check ostomy bag for leakage every 2 hours and change bag as soon as leakage is suspected.
   b. Teach the parents the importance of emptying the bag when it is one-quarter to one-third full.
   c. Skin breakdown is more frequent. Reinforce to parents to treat breakdown with method and products recommended by ostomy nurse.
   d. Be aware that infant elimination is more frequent than in the older child.
4. For older children with ostomies:
   a. "Potty training" may be achieved for colostomy pouch emptying. This will not be possible for a child with an ileostomy.
   b. Pouching optimizes socialization and developmental activities.

c. Encourage a matter-of-fact and accepting attitude to help build child's self-confidence.

d. Encourage the child to participate in ostomy care.

e. Encourage child to join age-appropriate ostomy support group.

5. Additional information and support can be obtained from the United Ostomy Associations of America (*www.ostomy.org*).

Community and Home Care Considerations

1. Begin early teaching about the colostomy (preoperatively, before discharge, and at home), including how it works and how to care for it and the child. Explanations should be thorough and in accordance with family readiness. Encourage care of the ostomy as part of normal activities of daily living.

2. Arrange frequent home visits to carry out comprehensive teaching plan. Consult with ostomy nurse, as needed, for any skin breakdown or other ostomy problems.

3. Involve the entire family in teaching colostomy care to enhance acceptance of body change of the child. An older child should become totally responsible for own colostomy care.

4. Assess family's self-care of the ostomy, including such procedures as preparation of skin, application of collecting appliance, care of appliance, and control of odor.

5. Observe for and teach family about signs of stomal complications, including ribbonlike stool, diarrhea, failure of evacuation of stool or flatus, and bleeding.

6. Assess hydration status and teach increased fluid intake because colon absorption is decreased or may be absent if an ileostomy is present.

7. Review GT feeding techniques, if ordered.

8. Assist family to discuss the child's needs with daycare workers, teachers, and school nurse, as applicable. Review care of ostomy with child's care providers.

9. Assist with preoperative preparation for colostomy closure when the time comes.

Family Education and Health Maintenance

1. Instruct the parents to serve small, frequent meals to the child and be alert for and eliminate foods that cause gas and diarrhea, such as cabbage, spicy foods, beans, brussels sprouts, fruits, and fruit juices.

2. Advise parents that colds or viruses may cause loose stools, which increases risk of dehydration, especially in long-segment disease, so to increase fluids in these situations.

3. Alert parents of common postoperative problems, including bacterial overgrowth, colitis or enterocolitis, and lactose intolerance. Advise parents to contact their health care provider if persistent diarrhea, abdominal distention, abdominal pain, fever, vomiting, or constipation occur.

4. Encourage parents to practice all procedures long before the infant is to be discharged.

5. Emphasize the importance of treating the child as normally as possible to prevent behavior problems later.

6. Teach the basics of good nutrition and diet. Involve the dietitian, as necessary.

7. Encourage close medical follow-up and general good health and hygiene.
   a. Safety.
   b. General growth and development.
   c. Immunizations.

8. Advise older children without colostomies that fecal staining may occur, but this will improve with time.

Evaluation: Expected Outcomes

- Respirations unlabored; no cyanosis.
- Abdominal girth decreased; resting comfortably.
- Tolerates 1- to 2-oz feedings every hour, depending on the age of the child.
- Passes stool at least every 2 days spontaneously or after enema.
- Vital signs within normal limits, afebrile, no abdominal distention.
- Stoma pink without drainage, redness, warmth, and tenderness.
- Bowel sounds present, NG tube discontinued.
- Parents listen, ask questions about care of child, and demonstrate adequate care/technique for device care/maintenance.

Intussusception

Intussusception is the invagination or telescoping of a portion of the intestine into an adjacent, more distal section of the intestine, which creates a mechanical obstruction. Intussusception is one of the most common causes of intestinal obstruction in infancy. It can occur at any time in life but most commonly occurs in children younger than age 3, with the greatest incidence between ages 5 and 10 months. It is twice as common in male infants as in female infants. Incidence in the United States is 1.5 to 4 cases per 1,000 births. Intussusception should be high on the differential list when a child younger than age 1 presents with sudden onset of abdominal pain.

Pathophysiology and Etiology

1. The cause can fall into one of three categories: idiopathic, lead point, or postoperative.

   a. Idiopathic: this is the most common type, with no identifiable cause. It is not unusual, however, to obtain a history of a recent upper respiratory or GI virus. It is hypothesized that hypertrophy of Peyer's patches create a thickened segment. It's most common in infants.

   b. Lead point: an identifiable change in the intestinal mucosa can be discovered, usually during surgical treatment, and is most common in children ages 2 to 3. Malformations include polyps, cysts, tumors, Meckel's diverticulum, and hematomas (seen in Henoch-Schönlein purpura). Children with cystic fibrosis are at risk for lead point intussusception due to mucus and thick stool.

   c. Postoperative: uncommon but can occur after surgery of the abdomen and even the chest. It may be due to interrupted motility from anesthesia or direct handling of the intestine. It can also occur from placing long tubes into the bowel.

2. Invagination results in complete intestinal obstruction.
   a. Mesentery/lymphatics/blood vessels pulled into intestine when invagination occurs.
   b. Intestine becomes curved, sausagelike; blood supply is cut off.
   c. Bowel begins to swell; hemorrhage may occur.
   d. Necrosis of involved segment occurs.
   e. If not recognized and treated, bowel death occurs, possibly resulting in significant loss of intestine, shock, and death.
3. Classification of location:
   a. Ileocecal (most common): when ileum and the attached mesentery, lymphatic tissue, and blood vessels invaginate into the cecum (see Figure 48-7).
   b. Ileocolic: ileum invaginates into colon.
   c. Colocolic: colon invaginates into colon.
   d. Ileo-ileo (enteroenteric): small bowel invaginates into small bowel.
4. There was a recent increase in cases of intussusception noted after the introduction of the first rotavirus vaccine (Rota-Shield), so this vaccine was taken off the market. The second generation of rotavirus vaccines (RotaTeq and Rotarix) do not carry the same risk of intussusception.

 Evidence Base Eng, P. M., Mast, T. C., Loughlin, J., et al. (2012). Incidence of intussusception among infants in a large commercially insured population in the United States. *Pediatric Infectious Disease Journal*, *31*(3), 287–291.

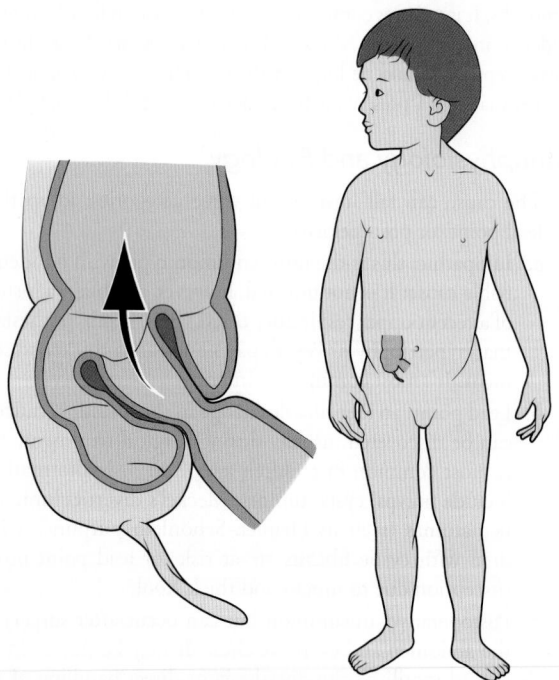

Figure 48-7. Intussusception. A portion of the ileum has been pushed into the lumen of the adjoining cecum.

Clinical Manifestations

1. Classic four signs of intussusception—vomiting, abdominal pain, bloody/red currant jelly–like stool, and abdominal mass—only occur in about 45% of children.
2. Pain is usually paroxysmal.
   a. "Attacks of pain" that awaken child from sleep; inconsolable, drawing up legs, colicky.
   b. Cyclic repetition of symptoms at approximately 5- to 30-minute intervals.
   c. Between episodes, child may act normal.
3. Stool may be like currant jelly—sloughed mucosa of dark red color with a mucoid consistency.

 **NURSING ALERT** Currant jelly–like stool indicates damage to the intestine and can be a late sign. *Any* gross blood in the stool should raise suspicion of intussusception, especially when associated with abdominal pain; one should not wait for currant jelly–like stool to report.

4. Vomiting may begin with decreased appetite and progress to bilious vomiting.
5. Bowel sounds vary:
   a. During a crisis of pain, bowel sounds may be hyperperistaltic rushes (borborygmi).
   b. Ileus/peritonitis: bowel sounds are diminished or absent.
6. Decreasing frequency of bowel movements.
7. Increasing abdominal distention and tenderness.
8. Sausagelike mass palpable in abdomen. This is pathognomonic and is known as *Dance's sign*—elongated mass in the right upper quadrant of the abdomen with absence of bowel sounds in the right lower quadrant.
9. Unusual-looking anus; may look like rectal prolapse.
10. Dehydration, fever, lethargy; shocklike state with rapid pulse, pallor, marked sweating.
11. Hematochezia (maroon-colored stools)—not always present.
    a. Rectal examination is significant if bloody mucus on examiner's finger.
    b. Occult or gross blood on rectal exam in 60% to 90% of patients.
12. The groin should be inspected for incarcerated hernia or torsion of testicle or ovary as differential diagnosis.

Diagnostic Evaluation

1. X-ray examination.
   a. Supine and upright abdomen film. Early course may be normal, but as it progresses absence of gas in the colon is found. Can also have finding of right upper quadrant mass and/or the meniscus/crescent sign.
   b. If no intraperitoneal air found on abdominal film, an air or barium enema is attempted.
   c. Commonly, a concave filling defect is seen in the transverse colon that can be reduced to the cecum.

NURSING ALERT Enemas are contraindicated in cases involving clinical findings of peritonitis, shock, or signs of perforation on abdominal x-ray.

2. Ultrasonogram to locate area of telescoped bowel and color Doppler sonography used to determine whether reducible or not. Absence of blood flow (color) indicates ischemia and, therefore, enema reduction should be avoided. Ultrasound will usually be obtained prior to contrast enema due to the low risk and excellent accuracy.

Management

 Evidence Base Niramis, R., Watanatittan, S., Krua-trachue, A., et al. (2010). Management of recurrent intussusception: Nonoperative or operative reduction? *Journal of Pediatric Surgery, 45*(11), 2175–2180.

1. Air or barium enema—both for diagnosis and treatment (hydrostatic reduction) in reducing intussusception.
   a. A surgeon should be present during the barium enema due to risk of perforation.
   b. A noninflatable tube is passed into rectum; contrast enters by gravity under fluoroscopic guidance. If air is used, it is delivered under constant pressure.
   c. As the intussusception is reduced, the contrast or air should reflux freely into the small intestine; this radiographic evidence is needed to confirm a successful reduction.
   d. Success ranges from 70% to 90%. Recurrence is the most common complication, but perforation can also occur.
   e. Nonoperative reduction using air enema or other hydrostatic reduction methods has been the standard treatment in most cases. The success rate can be as high as 84%. However, if nonoperative method is not indicated or fails, open surgery is still necessary.
2. Surgical reduction of intussusception may be necessary when radiologic reduction is unsuccessful, a pathologic lead point or peritonitis is suspected, or with multiple recurrences. Factors associated with increased risk of intestinal resection include abdominal distension (32%), bowel obstruction on abdominal x-ray (27%), and hypovolemic shock (40%).

 Evidence Base Weihmiller, S. N., Buonomo, C., & Bachur, R. (2011). Risk stratification of children being evaluated for intussusception. *Pediatrics, 127*(2), e296–e303.

3. Surgery involves a laparotomy—manual milking-out of the intussuscepted segment from the distal to proximal end, followed by resection of the nonviable bowel and, commonly, an incidental appendectomy. Up to 86% successful in reduction.
4. Recurrence is 5% to 7% regardless of the type of treatment undertaken.

Complications

1. Perforation.
2. Peritonitis.
3. Shock.
4. Loss of bowel resulting in short bowel syndrome.

Nursing Assessment

1. Obtain careful history of infant's or child's physical and behavioral symptoms, including any recent or chronic illness.

 NURSING ALERT Report of episodic, severe, colicky abdominal pain combined with vomiting suggests intussusception.

2. Perform physical examination, which may reveal a well-developed, well-nourished, afebrile infant with abdominal tenderness and distention.
3. Observe for dehydration; may be mild or severe. Poor capillary refill, decreased mental status, and decreased urine output are reliable indicators of shock in children.

Nursing Diagnoses

Preoperative

- Acute Pain related to paroxysmal abdominal pain, fever, and treatments.
- Risk for Decreased Fluid Volume related to vomiting.
- Ineffective Breathing Pattern related to abdominal distention.
- Anxiety related to hospitalization, knowledge deficit of illness, surgery, and treatments.

Postoperative

- Risk for Infection and other complications related to postoperative course.

Nursing Interventions

Minimizing Pain

1. Observe behavior as indicator of pain; the infant may be irritable and very sensitive to handling or lethargic or unresponsive. Handle very gently.
2. Encourage family to participate in comfort measures. Explain cause of pain and reassure parents as to purpose of diagnostic tests and treatments.
3. Administer medications, as prescribed.

Maintaining Fluid and Electrolyte Balance

1. Monitor fluids and maintain NPO status.
2. Restrain infant, as necessary, for IV therapy.
3. Monitor intake and output.

Promoting Effective Breathing

1. Be alert for respiratory distress because of abdominal distention. Watch for grunting or shallow and rapid respirations if in shocklike state.
2. Insert NG tube, if ordered, to decompress stomach.
   a. Irrigate, as ordered.
   b. Note drainage and return from irrigation.
3. Maintain NPO status, as ordered.
   a. Wet lips and perform mouth care.
   b. Give infant pacifier to suck.

4. Continually reassess condition because disordered breathing or respiratory distress may indicate progression of disease process.

 NURSING ALERT Passage of one normal brown stool may occur, clearing the colon distal to the intussusception. Passage of more than one normal brown stool may indicate that the intussusception has reduced itself. Report any stools immediately to the physician.

Preparing for Surgery

1. Offer support to the parents during time of crisis and fear.
2. Offer specific teaching to parents.
   a. Compare intussusception to a collapsible telescope or antenna or by drawing a picture.
   b. Visual aids, such as a rubber glove with one finger into itself, may be helpful. Reduction can be demonstrated by filling glove with water until inverted finger resumes its normal position.
3. Children need brief, simple explanations in age-appropriate language.

Preventing Infection and Other Postoperative Complications

1. Monitor vital signs and general condition, notify health care provider of any change or unexpected trend.
2. Assess temperature and administer antipyretics and other cooling measures. Fever may be present from the translocation of bacteria into the bloodstream through the damaged intestinal wall.
3. Assess for abdominal tenderness, bowel sounds, and distention of abdomen. Maintain NG suction, as ordered.
4. Assess pain and level of consciousness.
5. When able to take fluids, assess tolerance carefully and advance intake slowly.

Family Education and Health Maintenance

1. Explain that recurrences may occur, and usually occur within 36 hours after reduction. Review signs and symptoms with parents.
2. Review activity restrictions with parents (eg, positioning on back or side, quiet play, and avoidance of water sports until wound heals).
3. Encourage follow-up care.
4. Provide anticipatory guidance for developmental age of child.
5. Encourage awareness of symptoms that require prompt medical attention among daycare centers and other childcare providers (eg, paroxysmal abdominal pain, blood or mucus in stool).

Evaluation: Expected Outcomes

- Decreased irritability/pain.
- Urine output adequate.
- Respirations unlabored; abdominal distention relieved.
- Parents verbalize understanding of condition and surgery.
- Postoperative vital signs stable; audible bowel sounds; passes stool postoperatively.

Anorectal Malformations

The term *anorectal malformation* encompasses multiple congenital anomalies of the rectum, urinary tract, and reproductive system. Incidence is 1 in 2,500 to 1 in 4,000 live births, with a slight male predominance. Complexity varies from isolated imperforate anus to the extremely rare cloacal exstrophy (occurs in males and females 1 in every 250,000 births).

Pathophysiology and Etiology

 Evidence Base Warne, S. A., Hiorns, M. P., Curry, J., et al. (2011). Understanding cloacal anomalies. *Archives of Disease in Childhood, 96*, 1072–1076.
Zwink, N., Jenetzky, E., & Brenner, H. (2011). Parental risk factors and anorectal malformations: Systematic review and meta-analysis. *Orphanet Journal of Rare Diseases, 6*(25), 1–16.

1. An arrest in embryologic development of the anus, lower rectum, and urogenital tract at the 6th week of embryonic life; however, cause is unknown.
2. Approximately 40% of infants with anorectal malformations have associated major anomalies, including:
   a. Down syndrome.
   b. VACTERL syndrome (vertebral defects, anal atresia, cardiac anomaly, TEF with EA, renal defects, and radial limb dysplasia).
   c. Congenital heart disease.
   d. Renal abnormalities.
   e. Cryptorchidism.
   f. Esophageal atresia.
   g. Malformation of the spine.
   h. Variant of infantile hemangioma occurring in the extremity.
3. Abnormal development of the terminal hindgut ranges from mild anal stenosis, corrected by simple dilatation, to complex deformities, such as rectal atresia and fistula, with varying degrees of fecal and urinary incontinence.
4. BMP4 and Hox genes may play a role.

Types

See Figure 48-8.

1. Imperforate anal membrane—infant fails to pass meconium; greenish, bulging membrane is seen; bowel and sphincter return to normal after excision.
2. Rectoperineal fistula—rectum opens into the perineum; excellent function.
3. Anal atresia and stenosis—complete obstruction (atresia) or stenosis (decrease in caliber) is present approximately 2 cm above the anal opening.
4. Imperforate anus without fistula (anal agenesis)—rectum is completely blind, ending 2 cm from perineum; intestinal obstruction occurs if no associated fistula.
5. Anorectal malformation with rectourinary fistula in males (present in 80% of males with anorectal malformations).
   a. Rectourethral bulbar fistula.
   b. Rectourethral prostatic fistula.
   c. Rectobladder neck fistula.

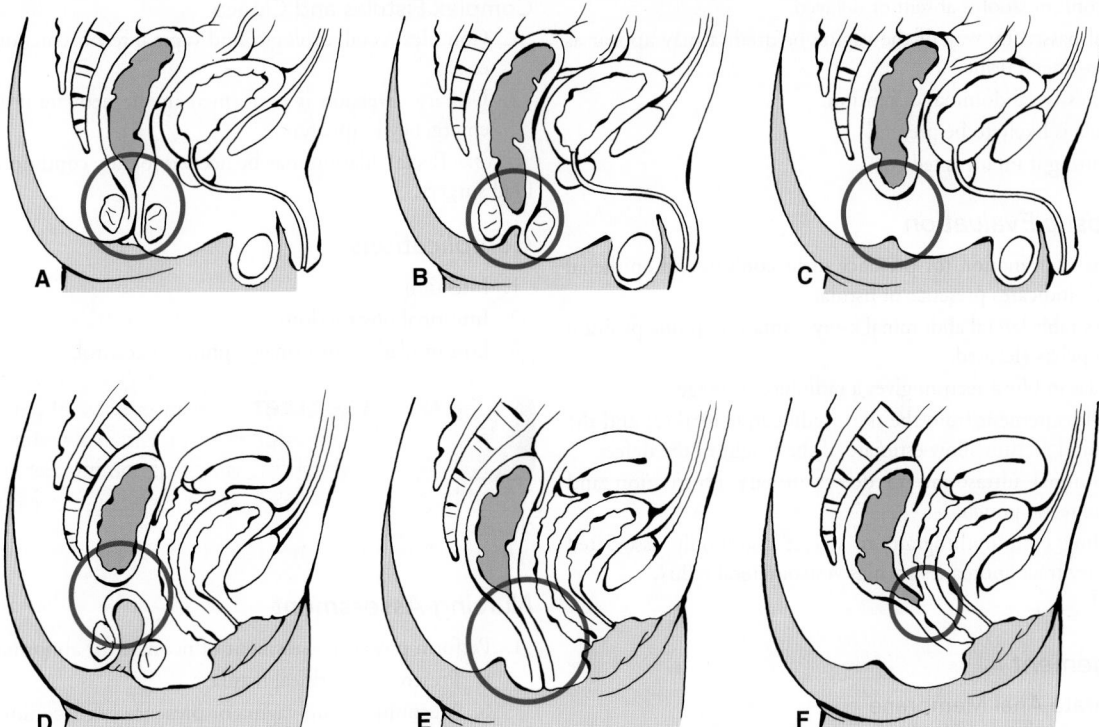

Figure 48-8. Anorectal malformations. (A) Anal stenosis. **(B)** Imperforate anal membrane. **(C)** Anal agenesis. **(D)** Rectal agenesis. **(E)** Rectoperineal fistula. **(F)** Small orifice located in the perineum. (Adapted with permission from Wong, D. L. [1995]. *Whaley and Wong's nursing care of infants and children* [5th ed.]. St. Louis, MO: Mosby.)

6. Anorectal malformation with fistula and cloaca in females.
   a. Vestibular fistula—rectum opens through an abnormal narrow orifice located in the vestibule of the genitalia outside the hymen; most common defect in females.
   b. Vagina fistula—rectum opens via fistula into vagina; exceptionally rare malformation.
   c. Persistent cloaca—complex defect in which the rectum, vagina, and urinary tract are fused together into one common channel ending in a single perineal orifice at the site of the urethra; requires colostomy, urinary diversion, or vaginal diversion.
7. Cloacal exstrophy—complex anorectal anomaly that includes omphalocele, two exstrophied hemibladders with cecum between them, imperforate anus, and abnormalities of sexual structures; rare; occurs in males and females.
8. Ectopic anus—mild displacement of the anus, which causes constipation. It is not a true anorectal malformation but may require dilatations or surgery. The anal position can be measured using the anal position index, which is the ratio of anus–fourchette distance in girls and anus–scrotum distance in boys to the distance between coccyx and fourchette/scrotum.

 Evidence Base Feldkamp, M. L., Botto, L. D., Amar, E., et al. (2011), Cloacal exstrophy: An epidemiologic study from the International Clearinghouse for Birth Defects Surveillance and Research. *American Journal of Medical Genetics, 157,* 333–343.

Degree of Incontinence

1. It may be difficult to absolutely predict what pediatric patients will obtain bowel and bladder continence for those with congenital GI/GU abnormalities or those who have suffered an injury to the area.
2. Bowel and bladder incontinence can be caused by damage to the nerves that control the sphincter muscles that control the outflow or damage to the muscle wall itself.
3. Complications may also occur from extensive surgical repairs required for surgery of the gastrointestinal or urologic system.
4. Gender and the type of abnormality will impact the likelihood of continence.
5. Some disorders; such as perineal fistula, rectal atresia, and rectal stenosis frequently result in 100% of patients having neither bowel nor bladder control.
6. Disorders such as rectobladder neck fistulas usually cause incontinence of urine but allow for bowel control.

Clinical Manifestations

1. Absence of anal opening; stimulation of perineum leads to puckering.
2. Displaced anal opening.
3. Anal opening near vaginal opening in female.
4. Thermometer, small finger, or rectal tube cannot be inserted into the rectum.

5. Meconium stool is absent or delayed.
6. Stool passed by way of the vagina or urethra may appear as green-tinged urine.
7. Progressive abdominal distention.
8. Fistula is likely to be present.
9. Vomiting if infant is fed.

Diagnostic Evaluation

1. Urine examination for presence of meconium and epithelial debris indicates presence of fistula.
2. Cross-table lateral abdominal x-ray—infant in prone position with pelvis elevated.
   a. Gas in blind rectum gives a radiolucent image.
   b. Measurement from the skin (radiopaque marker) and the blind rectum allow estimate of the height of the defect.
3. Abdominal ultrasound to detect urinary obstruction and locate rectal pouch.
4. Voiding cystourethrogram to detect commonly associated urinary tract anomalies such as vesicoureteral reflux.
5. MRI.

Management

Imperforate Anal Membrane

1. Internal and external sphincters are intact, so usually requires only a membrane excision from the anal opening.
2. Repaired at birth; no colostomy required.

Anal Stenosis

1. Internal and external sphincters are intact, so usually treated with anal dilation.
2. Occasionally requires myotomy (cutting of anal muscle).
3. Treated at birth; no colostomy required.

Imperforate Anus (Anal Agenesis)

1. Low lesion.
   a. Can usually be repaired with perineal anoplasty, which creates an anal opening for passage of stool.
   b. Usually accompanied by fistulas that need to be closed at the same time.
   c. Repaired at birth; colostomy usually not needed unless a fistula is present or more time for healing is needed.
2. High lesion.
   a. Requires more extensive surgery due to missing innervation.
   b. Usually requires a two-stage procedure, occasionally three-stage if complex defect is present.
   c. First step is a colostomy.
   d. Second step is anal repair, colon/rectum anastomosis, possible colostomy closure.
      i. Posterior sagittal anorectoplasty, also known as the *Pena procedure* (after the surgeon who developed it). The rectum is "pulled down" and sewn into a newly made anal opening in the perineum.
      ii. Most surgeons wait 4 to 6 months to complete it to allow for growth.
   e. Third step is colostomy closure if defect is complex and more healing time is needed.

Complex Fistulas and Cloaca

1. Complex rectal, urologic, and vaginal reconstruction are necessary.
2. Urinary diversion is performed in the neonate if a urologic emergency is apparent.

   Note: Rectal dilation may be needed for any condition after the final surgery.

Complications

1. Infection.
2. Intestinal obstruction.
3. Loss of bladder or urinary sphincter control.

 NURSING ALERT Condition is usually discovered immediately after birth or within several hours. A delay in diagnosis is not uncommon and can significantly increase the risk of serious early complications and death.

Nursing Assessment

1. Perform physical assessment of neonate for abnormalities.
   a. Presence of perineal fistula.
   b. Meconium from vagina or presence of meconium-stained urine.
   c. No anal opening or inability to pass thermometer into rectum.
2. Perform thorough examination for other congenital anomalies.

 NURSING ALERT A neonate who does not pass a stool in the first 24 hours after birth requires further assessment.

3. Assess parents' level of understanding of condition and ability to cope with infant's surgery.

Nursing Diagnoses

Preoperative

• Risk for Activity Intolerance related to instability before surgery.

Postoperative

• Risk for Infection related to surgical incision of anoplasty.
• Risk for Impaired Skin Integrity related to ostomy and anoplasty.
• Risk for Decreased Fluid Volume related to restricted intake.
• Readiness for Enhanced Family Processes related to increased needs of infant.
• Delayed Surgical Recovery related to definitive repair surgery.

Nursing Interventions

Maintaining Stability Before Surgery

1. Maintain NPO status. Note any vomiting: color and amount.
2. Minimize energy expenditure due to altered nutritional status.
3. Maintain NG tube passed to decompress the stomach, as ordered. Measure abdominal girth.

4. Observe the patient carefully for any signs of distress and report. Check vital signs frequently.

5. Use an Isolette or radiant warmer to maintain temperature stability.

6. Minimal handling; cluster procedures together to encourage rest and sleep.

7. Keep fistula area clean to prevent urinary tract infection.

8. Administer good oral care.

Preventing Infection of Suture Line

1. Following anoplasty, do not put anything in the rectum.
   a. Position the infant for easy access to perineum for cleansing and minimal irritation to site (ie, place the infant on his or her abdomen, possibly with hips elevated, to prevent pressure on perineal surfaces; turn side-to-side).
   b. Expose the perineum to air.
   c. Observe incision site for redness, drainage, poor healing.
   d. Apply antibiotic ointment to perineum, as directed.
2. Following colostomy, observe wound and stoma for redness, drainage, poor healing.
3. Administer IV antibiotics, as directed (usually 2 to 3 days).

Preventing Skin Breakdown

See "Ostomy care in children," page 1628.

Maintaining Fluid and Electrolyte Balance

1. Monitor for return of peristalsis; NG tube may be discontinued by the health care provider when bowel sounds present.
2. Start oral feedings, as ordered.
   a. Anoplasty: usually within hours.
   b. Colostomy: when bowel sounds present and colostomy has output.
3. Monitor parenteral fluids and discontinue when oral intake is sustained.
4. Report vomiting.
5. Describe stool frequency, consistency, and character. Report blood in stool or lack of stool output.
6. Monitor urine output, particularly important with urethral defects (including cloaca).

Strengthening Coping

1. Assure the parents that colostomy is temporary (unless complex surgery performed).
2. Encourage the parents to participate in care of the child and to provide emotional security for the child.
3. Provide thorough teaching program for special care needed at home.
   a. Colostomy care.
   b. Anal dilatation to prevent a stricture at site of anastomosis from scar tissue (after instructions by health care provider).
4. Initiate referral to community nurse, especially if the parents are particularly anxious about caring for the child at home.
5. Encourage the parents to talk about their concerns.
6. Enlist help of enterostomal nurse specialist before the child leaves the hospital and for continued home care needs.
7. Assist breastfeeding mother to maintain milk supply through frequent pumping.

Maximizing Recovery Following Definitive Pull-Through Surgery

1. Maintain GT or NG tube decompression until peristalsis returns.
2. If a bladder catheter is used, provide care, as directed, and measure urine output accurately.
3. Observe carefully for abdominal distention, bleeding from perineum, and respiratory compromise. Report immediately.
4. Carry out perineal care.

Family Education and Health Maintenance

1. Review special care and procedures to be continued at home. Involve parents and other caregivers in teaching. Advise parents to make daycare providers, teachers, and school nurse aware of child's needs.
2. It is important that the family understands the rationale and technique for anal dilation as indicated by the surgeon. Provide written instructions and assess their understanding of the procedure.
3. Help the parents to understand situations that may be encountered as a result of anorectal malformation repair as the infant gets older.
   a. Fecal impaction due to lack of sensation to defecate.
   b. Future surgery if primary repair was not done or defect complicated.
   c. Toilet training—may be delayed, especially after a pull-through procedure.
   d. Inability to control fecal seepage from rectum.
4. Offer practical guidelines to help parents cope.
   a. Fecal control may not be achieved until age 10; however, about 85% of children achieve normal or socially acceptable continence if defect limited to imperforate anus.
   b. If incontinence occurs, anorectal manometric evaluation in postoperative period can give more realistic information about future incontinence.
   c. Encourage bowel habit training or patterning of defecation (eg, after breakfast).
   d. Promote diet modifications; teach foods that produce laxative effect (plums, prunes, chocolate, nuts, corn) and foods that have binding effect (peanut butter, hot cereal, cheese).
   e. Stool softeners or antidiarrheal medications, such as loperamide, may be effective, according to the child's needs.

 DRUG ALERT Antidiarrheal medications should be used with caution in children.

   f. Rectal inertia may cause fecal impaction in rectosigmoid colon with soiling from fluid overflow. Bisacodyl suppository or cleansing enema provides assistance in management.
5. Antegrade continence enema procedures may allow for continence in children without anal sphincter function.

6. Encourage mutual support from other families who have a child with an anorectal malformation.

7. For additional information and support, refer the parents to the National Organization for Rare Disorders (*www.rarediseases.org*) or the United Ostomy Associations of America (*www.ostomy.org*).

Evaluation: Expected Outcomes

- Vital signs stable, abdominal girth stable.
- No signs of infection of suture line.
- Skin intact surrounding ostomy.
- Bowel sounds present; oral feeding tolerated without vomiting; NG tube discontinued.
- Family discusses plans for home care with enterostomal therapist.

SELECTED REFERENCES

Alberti, D., Boroni, G., Corasaniti, L., et al. (2011). Esophageal atresia: Pre and post-operative management. *Journal of Maternal-Fetal and Neonatal Medicine, 24*(Suppl. 1), 4–6.

Alessio, M., Tonutti, E., Brusca, I., et al. (2011). Correlation between IgA tissue transglutaminase antibody ratio and histological finding in celiac disease: A multicentre study. *Journal of Pediatric Gastroenterology and Nutrition, 55*(1), 44–49.

American Gastroenterological Association, Bharucha, A. E., Dorn, S. D., et al. (2013). American Gastroenterological Association Medical Position Statement on Constipation. *Gastroenterology, 144*(1), 211–217.

Ammoury, R. F., & Croffie, J. M. (2010). Malabsorptive disorders of childhood. *Pediatrics in Review, 31*(10), 407–416.

Aras, I., Olmez, S., & Dogan, S. (2012). Comparative evaluation of nasopharyngeal airways of unilateral cleft lip and palate patients using three-dimensional and two-dimensional methods. *Cleft Palate Craniofacial Journal, 49*(6), e75–81.

Bocca-Tjeertes, I. F., Kerstjens, J. M., Reijneveld, S. A., et al. (2011). Growth and predictors of growth restraint in moderately preterm children aged 0 to 4 years. *Pediatrics, 128*(5), e1187–1194.

Chumpitazi, B. P., & Nurko, S. (2011). Defecation disorders in children after surgery for Hirschsprung disease. *Journal of Pediatric Gastroenterology and Nutrition, 53*, 74–79.

Cleft Palate Foundation. (2012). *Neonatal cleft lip and palate protocol: Tips for hospital nurseries.* Chapel Hill, NC: Author. Retrieved from: *www.cleftline.org/healthcare-professionals/tips-for-hospital-nurseries.*

Cogley, J. R., O'Connor, S. C., Houshyar, R., et al. (2012). Emergent pediatric US: What every radiologist should know. *Radiographics, 32*(3), 651–665.

Delacourt, C., Hadchouel, A., Toelen, J., et al. (2012). Long term respiratory outcomes of congenital diaphragmatic hernia, esophageal atresia and cardiovascular anomalies. *Seminars in Fetal Neonatal Medicine, 17*(2), 105–111.

Dido, O. F., Wakili, T. A., & Asekun-Olarinmowe, E. O. (2011). Enhancing recovery of malnourished children: Mothers' counseling and participation ensures intervention effectiveness. *West African Journal of Nursing, 22*(1), 85–90.

Dogan, Y., Yildirmaz, S., & Ozercan, I. H. (2012). Prevalence of celiac disease among first-degree relatives of patients with celiac disease. *Journal of Pediatric Gastroenterology and Nutrition, 55*(2), 205–208.

Eng, P. M., Mast, T. C., Loughlin, J., et al. (2012). Incidence of intussusception among infants in a large commercially insured population in the United States. *Pediatric Infectious Disease Journal, 31*(3), 287–291.

Errichielleo, S., Esposito, O., Di Mase, R., et al. (2010). Celiac disease: Predictors of compliance with a gluten-free diet in adolescents and young adults. *Journal of Pediatric Gastroenterology and Nutrition, 50*(1), 54–60.

Feenstra, B., Geller, F., Krogh, C., et al. (2012). Common variants near MBNL1 and NKX2-5 are associated with infantile hypertrophic pyloric stenosis. *Nature Genetics, 44*(3), 334–337.

Feldkamp, M. L., Botto, L. D., Amar, E., et al. (2011), Cloacal exstrophy: An epidemiologic study from the International Clearinghouse for Birth Defects Surveillance and Research. *American Journal of Medical Genetics, 157*, 333–343.

Fox, J., Richards, S., Jenkins, H., et al. (2012). Management of gastroenteritis over 10 years: Changing culture and maintaining the change. *Archives of Disease in Childhood, 97*(5), 415–417.

Genevieve, D., de Pontual, L., Amiel, J., et al. (2011). Genetic factors in isolated and syndromic esophageal atresia. *Journal of Pediatric Gastroenterology and Nutrition, 52*(Suppl. 1), S6–S8.

Grosen, D., Bille, C., Petersen, I., et al. (2011). Risks of oral clefts in twins. *Epidemiology, 22*(3), 313–319.

Gunnarsdottir, A., Sandblom, G., Arnbjornsson, E., et al. (2010). Quality of life in adults operated on for Hirschsprung disease in childhood. *Journal of Pediatric Gastroenterology, Hepatology and Nutrition, 51*(2), 160–166.

Hartman, E. E., Oort, F. J., Aronson, D. C., et al. (2011). Quality of life and disease-specific functioning of patients with anorectal malformations or Hirschsprung's disease: A review. *Archives of Disease in Childhood, 96*, 398–406.

Hogen Esch, C. E., Wolters, V. M., Gerritsen, S. A., et al. (2011). Specific celiac disease antibodies in children on gluten-free diet. *Pediatrics, 128*(3), 547–552.

Husby, S., Koletzko, S., Korponay-Szabó, I. R., et al. (2012). European Society for Pediatric Gastroenterology, Hepatology and Nutrition guidelines for the diagnosis of celiac disease. *Journal of Pediatric Gastroenterology and Nutrition, 54*, 136–160.

Jaffe, A. C. (2012). Failure to thrive: Current clinical concepts. *Pediatrics in Review, 32*, 100.

Jia, Z. L., Shi, B., Chen, C. H., et al. (2011). Maternal malnutrition, environmental exposure during pregnancy and the risk of non-syndromic orofacial clefts. *Oral Diseases, 17*(6), 584–589.

Johnston, B. C., Goldenberg, J. Z., Vandvik, P. O., et al. (2011). Probiotics for the prevention of pediatric antibiotic-associated diarrhea. *Cochrane Database of Systematic Reviews*, Issue 11 (Article No. CD004827).

Joint Recommendations of the North American Society for Pediatric Gastroenterology, Hepatology, and Nutrition and the European Society for Pediatric Gastroenterology, Hepatology, and Nutrition. (2009). *Journal of Pediatric Gastroenterology and Nutrition, 49*, 498–547.

Kohli, S. S., & Kohli, V. S. (2012). A comprehensive review of the genetic basis of cleft lip and palate. (2012). *Journal of Oral and Maxillofacial Pathology, 16*, 64–72.

Lacher, M., Froehlich, S., von Schweinitz, D., et al. (2009) Early and long term outcome in children with esophageal atresia treated over the last 22 years. *Surgery, 145*(6), 675–681.

McGrattan, K. E., & Ellis, C. (2013). Team oriented care for orofacial clefts: A review of the literature. *Cleft Palate Craniofacial Journal, 50*(1), 13–18

Mossey, P., & Modell, B. (2012). Epidemiology of Oral Clefts 2012: An International Perspective. *Frontiers of Oral Biology, (16)*, 1–18.

Mueller, A. A., Zschokke, I., Brand, S., et al. (2012). One-stage cleft repair outcome at age 6- to 18-years—a comparison to the Eurocleft study data. *British Journal of Oral Maxillofacial Surgery, 50*(8), 762–768.

Nelson, P., Glenny, A. M., Kirk, S., et al. (2012), Parents' experiences of caring for a child with a cleft lip and/or palate: a review of the literature. *Child: Care, Health and Development, 38*, 6–20.

Niramis, R., Watanatittan, S., Kruatrachue, A., et al. (2010). Management of recurrent intussusception: Nonoperative or operative reduction? *Journal of Pediatric Surgery, 45*(11), 2175–2180.

Pandya, S., & Heiss, K. (2012). Pyloric stenosis in pediatric surgery: An evidence-base review. *Surgery Clinics of North America, 92*(3), 527–539.

Parker, S. E., Mai, C. T., Canfield, M. A., et al. (2010). Updated national birth prevalence estimates for selected birth defects in the United States, 2004–2006. *Birth Defects Research, Part A: Clinical and Molecular Teratology, 88*(12), 1008–1016.

Pinheiro, P., Simoes e Silva, A., & Pereira, R. (2012). Current knowledge on esophageal atresia. *World Journal of Gastroenterology, 18*(28), 3662–3672.

Reilly, N. R., Aguilar, K., Hassid, B. G., et al. (2011). Celiac disease in normal-weight and overweight children: Clinical features and growth outcomes following a gluten-free diet. *Journal of Pediatric Gastroenterology, Hepatology and Nutrition, 53*(5), 528–531.

Ryan, M., & Grossman, S. (2011). Celiac disease: Implications for management. *Gastroenterology Nursing, 34*(3), 225–228.

Scott, D. A. (2009). Esophageal atresia/tracheoesophageal fistula overview. In R. A. Pagon, T. D. Bird, C. R. Dolan, et al. (Eds.), *GeneReviews™*. Seattle: University of Washington. Available: *www.ncbi.nlm.nih.gov/books/NBK5192/*.

Sharp, W. G., Jaquess, D. L., Morton, J. F., et al. (2010). Pediatric feeding disorders: A quantitative synthesis of treatment outcomes. *Clinical Child and Family Psychology Review, 13*(4), 348–365.

Sharma, M., Rai, P., Thawrani, A. (2013). GI bleed in an infant. *Gastroenterology, 144*(1), e15–e16.

Siddiqui, A. A., Fishman, S. J., Bauer, S. B., et al. (2011). Long-term follow-up of patients after antegrade continence enema procedure. *Journal of Pediatric Gastroenterology and Nutrition, 52*(5), 574–580.

Siddiqui, S., Heidel, R. E., Angel, C. A., et al. (2012). Pyloromyotomy: randomized controlled trial of open vs laparoscopic technique. *Journal of Pediatric Surgery, 47*(1), 93–98.

Soares-Weiser, K., MacLehose, H., Bergman, H., et al. (2012). Vaccines for preventing rotavirus diarrhea: Vaccines in use. *Cochrane Database of Systematic Reviews*, Issue 2 (Article No. CD008521).

Venugopal, A. A., & Johnson, S. (2012). Fidaxomicin: A novel macrocyclic antibiotic approved for treatment of clostridium difficile infection. *Clinical Infectious Diseases, 54*(4), 568–574.

Walker, K., Halliday, R., Holland, A. J., et al. (2010). Early developmental outcome of infants with infantile hypertrophic pyloric stenosis *Journal of Pediatric Surgery, 45*(12), 2369–2372.

Warne, S. A., Hiorns, M. P., Curry, J., et al. (2011). Understanding cloacal anomalies. *Archives of Disease in Childhood, 96*, 1072–1076.

Weihmiller, S. N., Buonomo, C., & Bachur, R. (2011). Risk stratification of children being evaluated for intussusception. *Pediatrics, 127*(2), e296–e303.

Williams, J. (2012). The recognition and management of isolated cleft palate. *Community Practitioner, 85*(10), 28–31.

World Health Organization, United Nations Children's Fund. (2009). WHO child growth standards and the identification of severe acute malnutrition in infants and children. Geneva: Author. Available at: *www.who.int/nutrition/publications/severemalnutrition/9789241598163/en/*.

Zella, G. C., & Israel, E. J. (2012). Chronic diarrhea in children. *Pediatrics in Review, 33*(5), 207–217.

Zwink, N., Jenetzky, E., & Brenner, H. (2011). Parental risk factors and anorectal malformations: Systematic review and meta-analysis. *Orphanet Journal of Rare Diseases, 6*(25), 1–16.

49

Pediatric Renal and Genitourinary Disorders

ACUTE DISORDERS

Acute Glomerulonephritis

Acute glomerulonephritis is a broad term used to describe several disease processes that result in glomerular injury. The glomerular injury is the result of antigen–antibody deposits within the glomeruli. It occurs most frequently in school-age children, is rare in children younger than age 2, and occurs more frequently in males than in females (2:1).

Pathophysiology and Etiology

1. Presumed cause—antigen–antibody reaction secondary to an infection elsewhere in the body (see Figure 49-1).
2. The initial infection is usually either an upper respiratory infection (URI) or a skin infection.
3. Most frequent causative agent—nephritogenic strains of group A beta-hemolytic streptococcus.
4. It is speculated that the streptococcal infection is followed by the release of a membrane-like material from the organism into the circulation.
5. Antibodies produced to fight the invading organism also react against the glomerular tissue, thus forming immune complexes.
6. The immune complexes become trapped in the glomerular loop and cause an inflammatory reaction in the affected glomeruli.
7. Changes in the glomerular capillaries reduce the amount of the glomerular filtrate, allow passage of blood cells and protein into the filtrate, and reduce the amount of sodium and water that is passed to the tubules for reabsorption.

8. General vascular disturbances, including loss of capillary integrity and spasm of arterioles, are secondary.

Clinical Manifestations

Onset
1. Usually 7 to 15 days after acute pharyngitis. In streptococcal skin infections, the latency period may be as long as 4 to 6 weeks.
2. May be abrupt and severe or mild and detected only by laboratory measures.

Signs and Symptoms
1. Urinary symptoms:
   a. Decreased urine output.
   b. Bloody or brown-colored urine.
2. Edema.
   a. Present in most patients.
   b. Usually mild.
   c. Commonly manifested by periorbital edema in the morning.
   d. May appear only as rapid weight gain.
   e. May be generalized and influenced by posture.
3. Hypertension.
   a. Present in up to 70% of those hospitalized with glomerulonephritis.
   b. Usually mild.
   c. Rise in blood pressure (BP) may be sudden.
   d. Usually appears during the first 4 to 5 days of the illness.

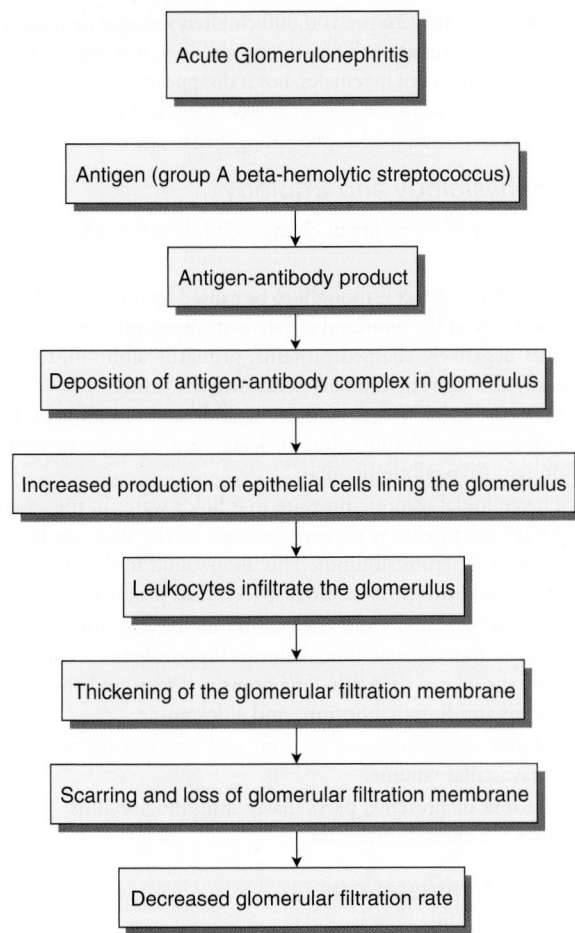

Figure 49-1. Sequence of events in acute glomerulonephritis.

4. Pallor.
5. Malaise, lethargy.
6. Low-grade fever.
7. Mild headache.
8. GI disturbances, especially anorexia and vomiting.

Diagnostic Evaluation

1. Urinalysis:
   a. Decreased output (oliguria)—may approach anuria.
   b. Microscopic or gross hematuria (noted in 30% to 70% of all cases).
   c. Specific gravity—moderately elevated.
   d. Proteinuria may be mild to severe.
   e. Microscopic—red blood cells, leukocytes, epithelial cells, and casts.
   f. Low urinary sodium may be noted.
2. Blood urea nitrogen (BUN) and creatinine—usually mildly to moderately elevated; however, normal in 50% of cases.
3. Antistreptolysin-O titer—elevated initially.
4. Anti-DNase B titer—elevated.
5. Erythrocyte sedimentation rate—elevated.

6. Complement C3 and complement C4—depressed.
7. If indicated chest x-ray—may show pulmonary congestion, cardiac enlargement during the edematous phase.

Management

1. Antibiotic therapy may be initiated if there is any concern that streptococci or other organisms are still present.
2. Other management is mostly symptomatic; in most patients, spontaneous recovery is expected. Hospitalization is usually not necessary.
3. Salt and fluid intake should be restricted during the acute phase of the disease.
4. Diuretics should be administered if significant edema or hypertension develops.
5. A renal biopsy may be indicated if the child does not recover from apparent acute poststreptococcal glomerulonephritis.

Complications

The following complications occur infrequently.

1. Circulatory congestion—if severe can lead to pulmonary edema.
2. Hypertensive encephalopathy.
3. Acute renal failure.
4. Anemia.

Nursing Assessment

1. Obtain history regarding recent streptococcal infection.
2. Obtain appropriate cultures and assess for current infection.
3. Measure urine output and degree of hematuria and proteinuria.
4. Weigh child and document areas and extent of edema.
5. Obtain baseline BP reading to assess for hypertension.

Nursing Diagnoses

- Impaired Urinary Elimination related to glomerular dysfunction.
- Excess Fluid Volume related to impaired renal function.
- Deficient Diversional Activity related to prolonged illness and restrictions.
- Deficient Knowledge regarding acute glomerulonephritis and its management.

Nursing Interventions

Promoting Normal Urine Output

1. Monitor daily intake and output.
2. Test and record urine for hematuria and proteinuria, as directed. Note color of urine.
3. Monitor daily weight.

Reducing Excess Fluid Volume

1. Provide a no-salt-added diet during the acute phase of the illness. Other restrictions may be indicated if renal function is impaired. Protein intake is not usually restricted because of the possible risk of malnutrition.
2. Restrict fluids in children with hypertension, edema, heart failure, or renal failure.
3. Place a sign that indicates dietary restrictions on the child's bed so that staff and visitors will be aware of special needs.

4. With fluid restrictions, offer small amounts of fluids spaced at regular intervals throughout the day and evening. Use an appropriate-size cup for the amount of fluid being offered.

5. Check BP, as ordered or needed, and observe for signs of hypertension. Administer antihypertensive and diuretic drugs, as ordered by health care provider.

Promoting Diversional Activity

1. Explain fluid restriction at an age-appropriate level and direct the child's focus away from restrictions.
2. Provide the child with diversional activity and play therapy.
3. Encourage activity, as tolerated.

Providing Information

1. Explain all aspects of the diagnostic tests and treatment in terms the family can understand.
2. Explain the purpose of all medications and the restricted diet, including a review of high-sodium foods to avoid and sample menus.
3. Encourage family participation in the child's care.
4. Help the family plan for adaptation of the child's nursing care to the home environment.
5. Arrange for appointments for continued medical supervision and initiate referrals when appropriate.

Family Education and Health Maintenance

1. Reinforce medical explanation of the disease process.
   a. Emphasize the need for medical evaluation and culture of all sore throats for all family members.
   b. Alert the family to signs and symptoms of disease recurrence.
   c. Be aware that microscopic hematuria may persist up to 2 years.
2. Reinforce activity recommendation; usually not restricted.
3. Advise that tonsillectomy or other oral surgery is not recommended for several months after the acute phase of glomerulonephritis.
   a. If this type of surgery is necessary, penicillin may be recommended before and after the procedure to prevent bacterial infection.
   b. Obtain information regarding drug allergies before administering penicillin.

Evaluation: Expected Outcomes

- Output remains adequate.
- Weight returns to baseline.
- Child does age-appropriate activities, as tolerated, and does not complain of thirst.
- Parents and child can state rationale for treatment.

Nephrotic Syndrome

Nephrotic syndrome is characterized by heavy proteinuria, hypoalbuminemia, and edema. The syndrome can be subdivided into congenital, primary (idiopathic), and secondary types. Approximately 85% to 95% of primary cases in preadolescents are classified as minimal-change nephrotic syndrome (MCNS) and are associated with minimal histologic change in the glomeruli. Nephrotic syndrome afflicts approximately 16 per 100,000 children younger than age 16 in the United States annually; in young children, it is slightly more common in males than in females, but it disappears in teenagers and adults. The most common age for presentation is 2 years and 70% to 80% of cases occur in children younger than age 6.

Pathophysiology and Etiology

Primary (idiopathic, minimal change, childhood) nephrotic syndrome.

1. Underlying defect is thought to be caused by the loss of charge selectivity of the glomerular basement membrane, which permits negatively charged proteins, primarily albumin, to pass easily through the capillary walls into the urine.
2. Excessive urinary loss of protein and catabolization by the kidney of circulating albumin leads to a decrease in serum protein (hypoalbuminemia).
3. The colloidal osmotic pressure that holds water in the vascular compartments is reduced because of the decrease in the amount of serum albumin. This allows fluid to flow from the capillaries into the interstitial spaces, thus producing edema.
4. The shift of fluid from the plasma to the interstitial spaces reduces the vascular fluid volume (hypovolemia), which in turn stimulates the renin–angiotensin system and the secretion of antidiuretic hormone and aldosterone.
5. Tubular reabsorption of sodium and water is increased for intravascular volume.
6. The loss of proteins, particularly immunoglobulins, predisposes the child to infection.

Clinical Manifestations

1. Onset is insidious—thought to be caused by immune system disturbances because it commonly occurs after a mild URI.
2. Edema is typically the presenting symptom.
   a. Edema may be minimal or massive.
   b. Edema is usually first apparent around the eyes.
   c. Dependent edema occurs in areas of the body such as the hands, ankles, feet, and genitalia.
   d. Fluid that accumulates in the body spaces may give rise to ascites and pleural effusions.
   e. Striae may appear on the skin from overstretching.
3. Profound weight gain caused by edema; the child may actually double normal weight.
4. Decreased urine output during the edematous phase—urine appears concentrated and frothy.
5. Pallor, irritability, lethargy, and fatigue.
6. GI disturbances, including vomiting, diarrhea, abdominal pain, and anorexia caused by edema of intestinal mucosa.

Diagnostic Evaluation

1. Urinalysis:
   a. Proteinuria (tests for albumin)—2+ (>1.0 g/L) on urine dipstick; should be sent for urine protein to creatinine ratio (first voided or random spot urine) to confirm. Considered nephrotic range if >200 to 250 mg/mmol.
   b. Blood—gross hematuria is not present but microscopic hematuria may be found in about 20% of patients.

2. Twenty-four-hour urine collection is the gold standard for quantification of urine protein—nephrotic range >40 mg/m²/hour.

3. Blood tests.
   a. Total protein—reduced.
   b. Albumin—less than 2.5 g/dL.
   c. Complete blood count may show decreased hematocrit due to hemodilution.
   d. BUN may be elevated, indicating general renal function.
   e. Creatinine—usually normal but may be increased if intravascularly depleted.
   f. Electrolytes—may be sodium, potassium, CO_2, and calcium imbalances.
   g. Increased serum cholesterol and triglycerides—due to reactive protein synthesis by the liver in response to hypoproteinemia.

4. Renal biopsy is indicated to look for other cause of renal dysfunction if patient has persistent proteinuria after 4 to 8 weeks of steroid therapy (median time to remission is 10 days—negative or trace proteinuria for 3 consecutive days). Biopsy also indicated if atypical presentation such as persistent renal failure, age less than 1 year or greater than 10 years, use of nephrotoxic drugs, or persistent hematuria.

Management

Steroid Therapy

1. Corticosteroid therapy—prednisone or prednisolone are drugs of choice due to lower cost and are less likely to induce salt retention and potassium loss.

2. No standard program of therapy exists; however, the 2012 Kidney Disease: Improving Global Outcomes guidelines recommend:
   a. Corticosteroid therapy be given for at least 12 weeks.
   b. Oral prednisone be administered as a single daily dose starting at 60 mg/m²/day or 2 mg/kg/day to a maximum 60 mg/day.
   c. Daily oral prednisone be given for 4 to 6 weeks followed by alternate-day medication as a single daily dose starting at 40mg/m² or 1.5mg/kg (maximum 40mg on alternate days) and continued for 2 to 5 months with tapering of the dose.

 Evidence Base Kidney Disease: Improving Global Outcomes (KDIGO) Work Group. (2012). Clinical Practice Guideline for the Evaluation and Management of Chronic Kidney Disease. *Kidney International, 3*(1). 1–150.

3. Corticosteroid therapy should be discontinued slowly to avoid complications of steroid withdrawal, particularly benign intracranial hypertension.

4. Children with nephrotic syndrome may respond to steroid therapy in several ways:
   a. Steroid sensitive: achieving remission within 28 days of the start of corticosteroid therapy.
   b. Steroid-dependent: relapses on alternate-day dosing or relapses within 14 days of corticosteroid discontinuation.
   c. Steroid resistant: persistent proteinuria after 8 weeks of corticosteroid therapy.

5. Children with steroid-responsive MCNS have a favorable long-term prognosis.

Alternative Drug Therapies

1. Should be considered when children relapse frequently (greater than four relapses in 1 year or two relapses in 6 months), become steroid resistant or steroid dependent, or demonstrate unacceptable adverse effects of steroid therapy (steroid toxicity). The decision to use alternative therapy in conjunction with steroids should be made by an experienced pediatric nephrologist.

2. Immunosuppressants.
   a. Cyclophosphamide.
   b. Cyclosporin A.
   c. Tacrolimus.
   d. Mycophenolate mofetil.
   e. Rituximab.

Intravenous (IV) Albumin 25%

1. To shift fluid from interstitial space into the vascular system.

2. Only a temporary treatment to relieve edema but may be used in severe cases of edema that cause respiratory distress or severe discomfort.

3. Diuretic therapy is used in combination with IV albumin to help relieve edema. In cases of hypovolemia, diuretics may not be indicated.

Complications

1. Infections:
   a. Peritonitis, most commonly caused by *Streptococcus pneumoniae*, but may also be caused by *Escherichia coli* and *Haemophilus influenzae*.
   b. Gram-negative septicemia.
   c. Staphylococcal cellulitis.

2. Thromboembolic events.

3. Hypertension.

4. Hyperlipidemia.

5. Pulmonary edema.

6. Bone disease secondary to corticosteroid therapy.

7. Acute renal failure.

Nursing Assessment

1. Obtain history of onset of illness and symptoms.
   a. Precipitating events.
   b. Recent immunizations.
   c. Recent URIs.
   d. Flulike symptoms.
   e. Time of onset and location of edema.
   f. Urinary pattern changes.

2. Perform physical examination focusing on vital signs; auscultation of breath sounds to determine adventitious sounds; areas and extent of edema, especially periorbital region, extremities, genitalia, abdomen; and peripheral perfusion, including pulses, color, warmth of extremities.

Nursing Diagnoses

- Excess Fluid Volume related to fluid accumulation in tissues.
- Risk for Infection related to urinary loss of proteins and chronic steroid use.
- Imbalanced Nutrition: Less Than Body Requirements related to loss of proteins through urine and anorexia.
- Interrupted Family Processes related to childhood illness.

Nursing Interventions

Relieving Excess Fluid

1. Administer corticosteroids, as directed.
   a. Observe for adverse effects and complications of therapy such as Cushing's syndrome—increased body hair (hirsutism), rounding of the face ("moon face"), abdominal distention, striae, increased appetite with weight gain, cataracts, and aggravation of adolescent acne.
   b. Stress that these physical changes are not harmful or permanent and that they will disappear after the steroid treatment is stopped.
   c. Observe for serious adverse effects and uncommon complications of corticosteroids (see page 914).

 NURSING ALERT No live vaccinations or immunizations should be given during active episodes of nephrosis or while the child receives immunosuppressive therapy.

2. Administer immunosuppressive drugs, as prescribed.
   a. Make sure that patient and parents understand the desired and adverse effects of therapy.
   b. Observe for complications of therapy, such as decreased white blood cell (WBC) count, increased susceptibility to infection, hair loss or increased hair growth (hirsutism), gingival hyperplasia, hemorrhagic cystitis.

 DRUG ALERT Administer cyclophosphamide in the morning, with large volumes of fluid, to prevent concentration of the drug in the urine and increased susceptibility to cystitis.

3. Administer diuretics, as prescribed.
   a. Be aware of those diuretics that may cause potassium depletion.
   b. Offer foods high in potassium, such as orange juice, bananas, and dried fruits (eg, raisins, apricots).
   c. Administer supplemental potassium chloride, as ordered, and if the urine output is adequate.
4. Encourage activity, as tolerated.
5. Restrict fluids as ordered (usually only during the extreme edematous phases).
   a. Restriction is carefully calculated at frequent intervals, based on the urine output of the previous day plus estimated insensible losses.
   b. Offer small amounts of fluids spaced at regular intervals throughout the day and evening. Use a cup of appropriate size for the amount of fluid being offered.

   c. Measure fluids accurately in graduated containers. Do not estimate fluid intake or output.
   d. Place a sign on the child's bed to make sure that no urine is accidentally discarded and that all intake is recorded.
   e. Determine total intake and output every 8 hours. In children who are not toilet trained, a fairly accurate record of output can be obtained by weighing diapers before and after voiding.
   f. Record other causes of fluid loss, such as the number of stools per day, perspiration.
6. Assist with abdominal paracentesis; this may be required because of marked ascites. During the procedure, fluid is withdrawn from the peritoneal cavity to relieve pressure symptoms and respiratory distress.
7. Restrict sodium, as ordered (usually done while the child is on corticosteroid therapy). A starting point is 1.5 to 2 g/day.
   a. Use a low-sodium menu when ordering meals from the hospital.
   b. Assist family in making food choices that are low in sodium.
   c. Foods that should be limited include cured, salted, canned, or smoked meats; processed cheese; regular canned or frozen soups and bouillon cubes; salted crackers and other snack foods.

Preventing Infection

1. Monitor complete blood count for decreased WBC count and neutropenia.
2. Closely observe the child who takes corticosteroids for signs of infection. Be aware that fever and other symptoms may be masked.
3. Provide meticulous skin care to edematous areas of the body.
   a. Bathe the child frequently and apply powder. Areas of concern are moist parts of the body and edematous male genitalia. Support the scrotum with a cotton pad held in place by a T-binder, if necessary, for the child's comfort.
   b. Position the child so that edematous skin surfaces are not in contact. Place a pillow between the child's legs when lying on side.
   c. Elevate the child's head to reduce edema.
4. If possible, avoid invasive procedures, such as femoral venipunctures and I.M. injections, to decrease the chance of introducing pathogens. Venipuncture of the lower extremities may also predispose the child to thromboembolism because of hypovolemia, stasis, and increased plasma concentration of clotting factors.
5. Educate parents regarding signs and symptoms of possible infections.

Enhancing Nutritional Status

1. Assess nutritional intake, growth, and development as appropriate for age.
2. Provide a diet low in sodium, fat, and sugar. Place a sign on the child's bed that indicates dietary restrictions so that everyone will be aware of special needs.
3. Provide food choices that appeal to the child and that are easy to eat according to stage of development.
4. Provide nutritional supplements, as needed.

Providing Emotional Support

1. Encourage frequent visiting and allow as much parental participation in the child's care as possible. Hospitalization, if necessary, is usually brief.
2. Allow the child as much activity as tolerated.
   a. Balance periods of rest, recreation, and quiet activities during the convalescent phase.
   b. Allow the child to eat meals with family or other children.
3. Encourage the child and family to verbalize fears, frustrations, and questions.
   a. Be aware that young children frequently fear abandonment by their parents.
   b. Allow parents to express frustrations regarding the uncertainties associated with the cause of the disease, the clinical course, and the prognosis.
   c. Explain the difference between nephritis and nephrosis if parents have questions.
4. Help the child adjust to changes in body image, such as cushingoid appearance, by explaining changes ahead of time.
5. Discuss the problems of discipline with the parents. Encourage them to set consistent limits and reasonable expectations of their child's behavior.
6. Suggest parents get involved with a support group for families of children with chronic illnesses, as needed.

Family Education and Health Maintenance

1. Prepare the family for home management of the child's care plan.
   a. Have the dietitian discuss special diets with the parents.
   b. Teach the parents about the child's medication—the desired effects and the potential adverse effects.
   c. Demonstrate urine testing for protein.
   d. Initiate a community health nursing referral, if necessary, for reassessment and reinforcement of teaching.
2. Encourage continued medical follow-up visits.
3. Emphasize the necessity of taking medication according to the prescribed schedule and for an extended time. Discuss complications encountered with steroid therapy.
4. Teach prevention and recognition of signs and symptoms of infection.
5. Advise family on necessary activity restrictions.
6. Teach signs and symptoms of relapse (proteinuria on urine dipstick at home, increased edema, decreased urine output) and whom and when to call with questions.
7. Teach signs and symptoms of fluid imbalances (excess or dehydration).

Evaluation: Expected Outcomes

- Decreased edema and ascites; adequate urine output.
- Exhibits no signs of infection.
- Family verbalizes and follows dietary restrictions as demonstrated by appropriate weight gain/loss.
- Family verbalizes concerns regarding child's illness as demonstrated by open communication with staff and other family members.

Urinary Tract Infection

 Evidence Base American Academy of Pediatrics. (2011). Urinary tract infection: Clinical practice guideline for the diagnosis and management of the initial UTI in febrile infants and children 2 to 24 months. Subcommittee on Urinary Tract Infection. Steering Committee on Quality Improvement and Management. *Pediatrics, 128*, 595–610.

Koyle, M., & Shifrin, D. (2012). Issues in febrile urinary tract infection management. *Pediatric Clinics of North America, 59*(4), 909–922.

Urinary tract infection (UTI) is defined as bacteria that exists anywhere between the renal cortex and the urethral meatus. Because it is usually difficult to determine the exact location of the infection, the term UTI is used to explain microorganisms anywhere within the urinary tract. UTIs are categorized as cystitis or urethritis (located in the bladder or urethra), upper tract (located in the ureters or collecting system), and pyelonephritis (renal parenchyma). The greatest incidence of UTI in males occurs in the first year of life (most common in uncircumcized males), after which it rapidly declines, remaining low through childhood and adolescence. Incidence in females is also highest in the first year of life and steadily declines through adolescence, but remains higher than the incidence for males at a rate of 10:1.

Pathophysiology and Etiology

1. Causative organisms—*E. coli* (80%), *Klebsiella pneumoniae*, *Proteus mirabilis*, *Staphlyococcus*, *Enterococcus*.
2. Route of entry:
   a. Ascent from the urethra (most common).
   b. Circulating blood (rare).
3. Contributing causes:
   a. Female specific.
      i. Perineal location of urethral orifice and shorter urethra.
      ii. Sexual intercourse (mechanics of vaginal penetration).
      iii. Vaginal voiding—reflux of urine into the vagina while voiding, with subsequent dribbling of urine.
   b. Male specific—foreskin (prepuce can be a reservoir for bacteria).
   c. Abnormal bladder or voiding with or without incontinence.
      i. High pressures in the bladder.
      ii. Incomplete bladder emptying, infrequent voiding.
      iii. Difficulty relaxing pelvic floor.
   d. Constipation.
   e. Congenital urinary tract anomalies—vesicoureteral reflux, posterior urethral valves, prune belly syndrome, hydronephrosis, bladder exstrophy.
   f. Neurogenic bladder (spina bifida, spinal injury).
   g. Catheterization, urinary drains/tubes.
   h. Bacterial colonization.
4. Pathophysiology—inflammatory changes occur in the affected portions of the urinary tract, including kidneys, ureters, or bladder and urethra.
   a. Clumps of bacteria may be present.
   b. Inflammation results in urine retention and stasis of urine in the bladder.

c. Backflow of urine into the kidneys may occur through the ureters; this is called *vesicoureteral reflux* (VUR).

d. Inflammatory changes in the renal pelvis, and throughout the kidney, occur when the kidney is involved.

e. Scarring of the kidney parenchyma occurs in chronic infection and interferes with kidney function, particularly with the ability to concentrate urine.

f. If left untreated, the kidney may become small, tissue may be destroyed, and renal function could fail.

Clinical Manifestations

1. Onset may be abrupt or gradual; may be asymptomatic.
2. Failure to thrive in infancy.
3. Young children: may be nonspecific (vomiting, irritability, poor feeding, diarrhea); fever is often the only presenting complaint.
4. Older children and adolescents: urinary frequency, urgency or voiding hesitancy, dysuria, suprapubic tenderness, dribbling, and nocturnal enuresis (more common in lower UTI).
5. Hematuria: often occurs with viral cystitis.
6. Fever.
   a. May be moderate or severe.
   b. May fluctuate rapidly.
   c. May be accompanied by chills or convulsions.
7. Anorexia and general malaise.
8. Foul odor or change in the appearance of urine.
9. Abdominal or suprapubic pain (more common in upper-tract disease).
10. Tenderness over one or both kidneys.
11. Systemic symptoms: flank pain, fever, chills, nausea, vomiting may occur with pyelonephritis.

Diagnostic Evaluation

1. Urine culture:
   a. Documentation of pathogenic organisms in the urine is the only means of definitive diagnosis.
   b. A urine culture demonstrating more than 100,000 bacteria per mL indicates significant bacteriuria.
   c. A catheterized urine specimen, with growth greater than 10,000 colonies of bacteria per mL, is considered significant.
2. Urinalysis:
   a. Leukocytes, nitrites suggestive but not indicative.
   b. Casts, especially WBC casts, may be present and are indicative of intrarenal infection.
   c. Hematuria—occurs occasionally.
   d. Decreased specific gravity due to decreased renal concentrating ability.
4. Urologic and radiologic studies to identify anatomic abnormalities or renal changes that stem from recurrent infections—renal ultrasound, voiding cystourethrogram (VCUG).
   a. Dimercaptosuccinic acid scan—evaluates renal function and scarring.

Management

See Table 49-1.

1. Treatment depends on child's age, severity of infection, and antimicrobial resistance rates in the community.
2. Oral antibiotic therapy for uncomplicated UTI. Usually 10- to 14-day antibiotic therapy for febrile UTIs.
3. IV antibiotics for complicated UTI—infections that do not respond to oral therapy or that develop into pyelonephritis or those that appear septic or dehydrated.

Table 49-1	Antimicrobial Agents Commonly Used in the Management of Childhood Urinary Tract Infection	
DRUG	**ADVERSE EFFECTS**	**NURSING CONSIDERATIONS**
Amoxicillin	• Occasional nausea, vomiting, diarrhea • Hypersensitivity reactions of skin	• Readily absorbed. • May be taken with food.
Ampicillin	• Diarrhea, urticaria • Anaphylactic reaction	• Contraindicated in penicillin-sensitive children. Package insert should be consulted regarding reconstitution, administration, and storage of I.M. and IV preparations. Absorption of oral preparations may be decreased with food. Dose must be repeated q6h to ensure therapeutic blood levels.
Cephalexin	• Diarrhea, nausea, vomiting	• May be taken with food. Dose should be reduced if renal function is impaired.
Gentamicin	• Renal and auditory toxicity; respiratory paralysis	• Toxic effects can be minimized by slow IV infusion (over 1 hour).
Nitrofurantoin	• Fever, nausea, vomiting, peripheral neuropathy	• Recommended for prolonged use. Give with food or milk to decrease GI adverse effects. May cause urine to be amber or brown in color. Contraindicated in renal failure and in infants younger than 3 months old.
Co-trimoxazole	• Nausea, vomiting, fever, rash, photosensitivity	• Commonly used if bacterial resistance is anticipated or the child fails to respond to initial therapy.

4. Repeat culture following therapy if still symptomatic, has chronic renal disease, or has known colonization of bacteria.

Complications

1. A tendency for recurrent infection exists.
2. Children with obstructive lesions of the urinary tract and those with severe VUR are at highest risk for kidney damage. These patients may need prophylactic oral antibacterial therapy.

Nursing Assessment

1. Obtain history to determine if UTI is initial or recurrent and to determine if there may be other disease processes contributing to this infection.
2. Focus assessment on identifying clinical manifestations and determining location of infection, such as presence and appearance of urethral discharge, high-grade fever (more common with upper UTI), or low-grade fever (more common with lower UTI).
3. Determine urinary pattern (ie, amount and frequency) and associated discomfort.
4. Determine bowel pattern and possibility of constipation.

Nursing Diagnoses

- Impaired Urinary Elimination related to infection.
- Acute Pain related to inflammatory changes and fever.
- Anxiety related to exposure and manipulation of the genitourinary tract.

Nursing Interventions

Promoting Urinary Elimination

1. Obtain a clean urine specimen for urinalysis or culture (see page 1457).
   a. Obtain freshly voided early morning specimen, if possible (most accurate). This urine is usually acidic and concentrated, which tends to preserve the formed elements.
   b. Provide fluids to help the child void.
   c. Perform catheterization, if necessary, to obtain a sterile specimen; however, this procedure may cause emotional trauma and the accidental introduction of additional bacteria.
   d. Send urine to the laboratory immediately or refrigerate to avoid a falsely high bacterial count.
2. Administer antibiotics, as ordered by the health care provider (after specimen has been obtained for culture).
   a. Antibiotic therapy is generally determined by the results of the urine cultures and sensitivities and by the child's response to therapy; however, empirical therapy may be started before culture results are back.
   b. Become familiar with toxic effects of antimicrobial agents and assess the child regularly for any signs and symptoms.

Maintaining Comfort and Providing Symptomatic Relief

1. Administer analgesics and antipyretics, as ordered.
2. Maintain child on bed rest while febrile.
3. Encourage fluids to reduce the fever and dilute the concentration of the urine. (Water is the best clear fluid.)
4. Administer IV fluids, if necessary.

Promoting Self-Esteem

1. Reinforce medical explanations of the disease and its therapy.
2. Explain all diagnostic tests and procedures to the child, allowing time for questions and answers.
3. Encourage verbalizing. Correct any misconceptions and particularly address concerns about the functioning of the urinary tract and sexual function. Reassure the child that he or she did not cause the problem.
4. Maintain privacy for the child as much as possible.
5. Provide an environment that is as close to normal as possible during hospitalization. Include opportunities for the child to play.
6. Prepare the child and family for discharge and begin discussions of rest, fluids, and medications.

Family Education and Health Maintenance

1. Review long-term antibiotic therapy, if prescribed, to prevent recurrence of UTI. Schedules for prolonged therapy vary from several months to continuous prophylaxis.
2. Encourage scheduled follow-up visits because of the possibility of disease recurrence.
   a. Emphasize that even though this disease may have few symptoms, it can lead to serious, permanent disability.
   b. Advise family that subsequent suspected UTIs should be assessed and followed by health care provider.
3. Teach measures of prevention:
   a. Minimize spread of bacteria from the anal and vaginal areas to the urethra in female children by cleansing the perianal area from the urethra back toward the anus.
   b. Encourage adequate fluid intake, especially water.
   c. Avoid carbonated and caffeinated beverages because of their irritative effect on bladder mucosa.
   d. Encourage the child to void frequently and to empty the bladder completely with each voiding (double voiding).
   e. Encourage a high-fiber diet to avoid constipation.

Evaluation: Expected Outcomes

- Voids regularly in adequate amounts.
- No complaints of pain during or after voiding; afebrile.
- Shows less anxiety about hospitalization; appears more relaxed about appearance, body image, tests.

ABNORMALITIES OF THE GENITOURINARY TRACT THAT REQUIRE SURGERY

Exstrophy of the Bladder

Bladder exstrophy is an abnormality present at birth in which the bladder and associated structures are improperly formed. Rather than being its normal round shape, the bladder is flattened. The skin, muscle, and pelvic bones joining the lower part of the abdomen did not form properly so the inside of the bladder is exposed outside the abdomen. There are also associated deficiencies of the abdominal muscles and pelvic bones. These occur in approximately 1 in 30,000 to 50,000 deliveries, with the male-to-female

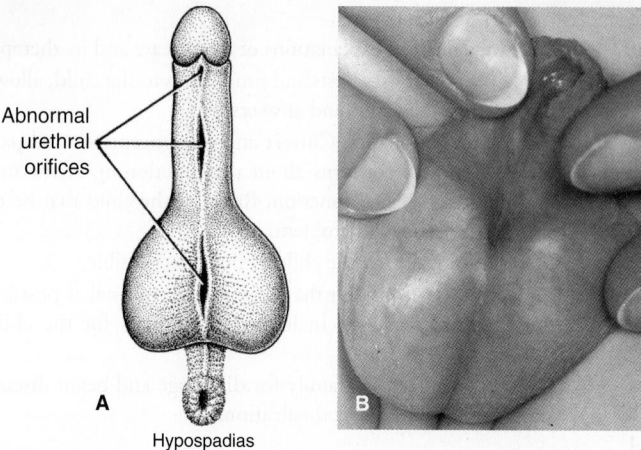

Abnormal urethral orifices

A

Hypospadias

B

Mucosa of urinary bladder

Ureteric opening

Urethra

C

Figure 49-2. (A) Hypospadias showing the various locations of abnormal urethral orifices. **(B)** Patient with hypospadias. The urethra is open on the ventral surface of the penis. **(C)** Epispadias combined with exstrophy of the bladder. Bladder mucosa is exposed. (A and C courtesy of Dr. R. J. Gorlin, Department of Oral Pathology and Genetics, University of Minnesota.)

ratio at 3:1. Recent published evidence suggests that the risk of bladder exstrophy in children born as a result of assisted fertility techniques is seven times greater than in children conceived naturally without assistance.

Hypospadias is an anomaly of the urethra only and is discussed separately (see Figure 49-2).

Pathophysiology and Etiology

1. Results from failure of the abdominal wall and its underlying structures to fuse in utero during the 3rd to 4th week of gestation.
2. In classic exstrophy (about 60% of bladder anomalies), the posterior bladder wall is externalized and lies open on the lower part of the abdomen with an epispadial urethra, allowing constant passage of urine to the outside.
3. Epispadias may occur without exstrophy (about 30% of bladder anomalies); the bladder remains an internal organ, but the urethra is laid open, possibly with a split glans penis and the meatus located proximally.
4. Cloacal anomalies (about 10% of bladder anomalies) involve externalization of the bladder and portions of the GI tract.

Clinical Manifestations

1. Urine dribbles constantly.
2. Infection and ulceration of the bladder mucosa may occur.
3. Genitalia may be ambiguous.
4. Affected children may walk with a waddling or an unsteady gait due to diastasis (separation) of pelvic bones.

Diagnostic Evaluation

1. Inspection is the most important tool in evaluation. The obvious anomaly may involve multiple systems.
2. Diagnostic procedures, such as radiography, ultrasound, magnetic resonance imaging, and urodynamic testing, determine extent of the anomaly.

Management

Evidence Base Stec, A. A., Baradaran, N., Schaeffer, A., et al. (2012). The modern staged repair of classic bladder exstrophy: A detailed postoperative management strategy for primary bladder closure. *Journal of Pediatric Urology, 8*(5), 549–555.

1. Surgical closure of bladder within first 24 to 48 hours of life by means of primary complete bladder closure and epispadias repair. This approach allows for maximal continence postrepair.
2. Urinary diversion should be rare.

Complications

1. Skin excoriation, infection.
2. Trauma to bladder mucosa.

Nursing Assessment

1. Assess for growth and development milestones during reconstruction.
2. Assess the family for coping ability.

Nursing Diagnoses

- Impaired Urinary Elimination related to anatomical defect.
- Risk for Infection as a complication of surgery.

Nursing Interventions

Facilitating Urine Output Preoperatively

1. Protect the bladder area from trauma and infection.
   a. Apply gauze soaked in normal saline solution, then cover with silastic or smooth plastic (common kitchen plastic wrap may be used).
   b. Position on back or side.
   c. Ensure umbilical cord is sutured and not clamped.

2. Observe the infant closely for signs of infection.

3. Involve other members of the health care team for parental support because of the psychosocial implications of a child who has special needs.

4. Assist the parents in dealing with their emotional reactions regarding the child's defect.

5. Prepare child and parents for the proposed surgery (see page 1649).

Providing Postoperative Care to Prevent Infection

1. Provide care for the ureteral and urethral catheters. Observe and record the amount of urinary drainage, catheter positions, and bladder spasms.

2. Care for the child in a traction system (see page 1745).

3. Provide care and instruction for an ileal conduit, as necessary (see page 792).

4. Observe for complications.
   a. Urinary or incisional infections.
   b. Fistulae in the suprapubic or penile incisions.

5. Recommend long-term support for children and families to help them deal with such fears as appearance of genitalia, potential inability to reproduce, rejection by peers, and sexual function. Ongoing discussion groups for parents and children may be helpful.

6. Teach the parents how to care for the child at home and make appropriate referrals.

Family Education and Health Maintenance

1. Provide community nursing referral, as needed, to support family and make sure that family understands the importance of follow-up with the various specialists.

2. Act as a liaison, as necessary, to coordinate care.

3. For more information and support, refer families to the following resources:
   a. Association for the Bladder Exstrophy Community (ABC) (*www.bladderexstrophy.com*).
   b. Book—*Living with Bladder Exstrophy: A Book for Families* (Murrey and Schremmer, 1996). Available through ABC.
   c. Book—*A Story About You … and the Boo-Boo on Your Bladder* (Brehm, 2002). Available through ABC.

Evaluation: Expected Outcomes

- No skin breakdown or infection.
- Incision healing well without infection or fistula; eventually, voiding without difficulty.

Vesicoureteral Reflux

 Evidence Base Routh, J. C., Bogaert, G. A., Kaefer, M., et al. (2012) Vesicoureteral reflux: Current trends in diagnosis, screening, and treatment. *European Urology, 61*(4), 773–882.

Vesicoureteral reflux (VUR) is the abnormal retrograde flow of urine from the bladder into the upper urinary tract. In the absence of bacterial infection, VUR is not considered to be critical. In the presence of bacteria, however, VUR is a risk factor for the development of UTIs and pyelonephritis, which can lead to renal damage and scarring. With linear growth, spontaneous resolution of VUR occurs in most children.

Pathophysiology and Etiology

VUR occurs as a result of congenital deficiency in the formation of the ureterovesical junction, resulting in a laterally displaced ureteral orifice.

Clinical Manifestations

1. UTI.
2. Unexplained febrile illnesses.
3. Associated urogenital anomalies (bladder exstrophy, posterior urethral valves, neurogenic bladder).
4. Prenatal diagnosis (hydronephrosis detected on prenatal screening ultrasounds).

Diagnostic Evaluation

1. VCUG—to establish diagnosis of VUR.
2. Renal ultrasound—to assess for renal damage, associated hydronephrosis.

Management

1. The goals of medical and/or surgical management are to prevent pyelonephritis, recurrent UTIs, and formation of renal cortical scarring.
2. Prophylactic antibiotic therapy should be initiated and continued until VUR resolves spontaneously or is surgically corrected.
3. Surgical intervention is indicated when medical therapy is unsuccessful.

Complications

1. Recurrent UTI can lead to renal damage and failure.
2. Recurrence of VUR following surgical intervention.

For nursing assessment, diagnoses, and interventions, see "Care of the Child Who Undergoes Urologic Surgery," page 1649.

Obstructive Lesions of the Lower Urinary Tract

Obstruction of the lower urinary tract may be caused by structural lesions, such as posterior or anterior urethral valves, bladder neck obstruction, meatal stricture, and urolithiasis (stones), or by functional lesions, such as neuromuscular dysfunction. The effect of obstruction on ureteral and renal function depends on the degree and duration of obstruction, on the rate of urine formation, and whether infection exists.

Pathophysiology and Etiology

Types of Obstruction

1. Urethral valves—filamentous valves that obstruct urine flow.
2. Congenital narrowing of the urethra.
3. Bladder neck obstruction—most common site of lower urinary tract obstruction.
4. Meatal stricture.
5. Neuromuscular dysfunction.

6. Severe phimosis (rare).
7. Inflammatory processes.
8. Neoplasia.
9. Urolithiasis.
10. Trauma.

Effects of Obstruction

1. Urinary tract becomes distended, proximal to the point of obstruction.
2. The bladder dilates and hypertrophies.
3. Stasis of urine occurs.
4. The ureters become elongated, dilated, and tortuous.
5. Hydronephrosis and destruction of kidney tissue inevitably result if left untreated.

Clinical Manifestations

1. Abnormal urination.
   a. Dysuria, frequency.
   b. Enuresis, dribbling.
   c. Reduced force of urine stream.
   d. Difficulty starting urine stream.
   e. Straining during urination.
   f. Abrupt cessation during urination.
2. Signs of infection—fever, pain, irritability, and, occasionally, hematuria.

Diagnostic Evaluation

1. Physical examination may reveal abdominal mass.
2. Laboratory findings depend on the degree that renal function is compromised.
3. Renal ultrasound may show hydronephrosis.
4. Radionuclide scanning.
5. Endoscopic examination.
6. Ureteroscopy.
7. Urodynamic examination.

Management

1. Prevention or eradication of infection with antibiotics.
2. Dilation of urethral stenosis or stricture.
3. Urinary diversion may be necessary.
4. Surgical relief of the obstruction.

Complications

1. Urinary stasis and recurrent UTI could lead to renal failure.
2. Severe and recurrent UTI.
3. Recurrence of the obstruction.

For nursing assessment, diagnoses, and interventions, see "Care of the Child Who Undergoes Urologic Surgery."

Obstructive Lesions of the Upper Urinary Tract

Obstructive lesions of the upper urinary tract include ureteropelvic junction obstruction, ureterovesical junction obstruction, ureteral stricture, congenital absence or duplication of a ureter, and urolithiasis. These obstructive lesions are primarily congenital.

Pathophysiology and Etiology

1. Congenital anomalies develop in the upper urinary tract.
   a. Ureteropelvic junction obstruction.
   b. Ureterovesical junction obstruction.
   c. Stricture of a ureter.
   d. Congenital absence of one ureter.
   e. Duplication of the ureter of one kidney.
2. Urolithiasis (renal calculi) is rare in children but may be associated with metabolic disease, such as cystinosis or oxalosis.

Clinical Manifestations

1. Hydronephrosis may present as an abdominal mass.
2. Commonly asymptomatic (seldom any problem with voiding).
3. Vague signs, such as failure to thrive, may be present.
4. UTIs may be frequent.
5. Hypertension may occur.

Diagnostic Evaluation

1. Laboratory tests to determine renal function.
2. Renal ultrasound, radionuclide imaging, and ureteroscopy to determine the extent of the lesion.

Management

1. Prevention or eradication of infection.
2. Surgical correction of the obstruction.

Complications

Renal failure.

For nursing assessment, diagnoses, and interventions, see "Care of the Child Who Undergoes Urologic Surgery."

Hypospadias

Hypospadias is a congenital defect of the penis, resulting in the incomplete development of the anterior urethra, corpora cavernosa, and foreskin. Hypospadias is also associated with penile curvature (chordee) and may result in infertility secondary to difficulty in semen delivery. Hypospadias is a common birth defect, occurring in one out of every 150 to 300 boys.

Pathophysiology and Etiology

1. At 1 month gestation, the male and female genitalia are indistinguishable. However, under the influence of testosterone, the male genitalia become masculinized. By the end of the first trimester, the penile urethra and foreskin are completely formed. Abnormalities in this development, such as subsequent, decreased testosterone production, can lead to hypospadias.
2. Classification is determined by the location of the urethral meatus.
3. Majority of cases have no known etiology, but may show genetic inheritability—14% incidence in siblings; 8% incidence in offspring.
4. Undescended testicle, hydrocele, or inguinal hernia may be associated.

Clinical Manifestations

1. Inability to void with penis in normal elevated position.
2. Spraying of urine when voiding.

Diagnostic Evaluation

1. Usually not difficult to diagnose because of visual anomaly. Assess glans penis for possible hypospadias before circumcision.
2. Severe cases require genotypic/phenotypic sex determination, chromosomal, and hormonal studies.

Treatment

Surgical reconstruction between ages 6 and 18 months, if possible (to minimize psychological issues surrounding toileting and genital awareness), and before circumcision because foreskin is essential for most repairs.

Complications

1. Fistula, meatal stenosis.
2. Urethral diverticulum.
3. Wound infection.

For nursing assessment, diagnoses, and interventions, see "Care of the Child Who Undergoes Urologic Surgery."

Cryptorchidism

Cryptorchidism refers to the failure of one or both testes to descend through the inguinal canal to the normal position in the scrotum. It is more common in premature infants and is the most common surgical problem in pediatric urology.

Pathophysiology and Etiology

1. Possibly caused by delayed descent, prevention of descent by mechanical lesion, or endocrine disorder (rare).
2. Testicular and ductal development are abnormal. It is unclear whether this is because of congenital dysplasia or because of underdevelopment.
3. Degeneration of the sperm-forming cells occurs after puberty because of the higher temperatures of the abdomen, compared with normal location in the scrotum.

Clinical Manifestations

Testicle nonpalpable within the scrotum.

Diagnostic Evaluation

1. Ultrasonography may reveal undescended testicle, but not as reliable as physical examination.
2. Serum testosterone measurements may be decreased.

Management

1. Orchiopexy surgery to achieve permanent fixation of the testis in the scrotum. Surgery should be performed between ages 6 and 15 months to prevent damage to the tissues and to lessen emotional concerns related to body image.
2. Surgical placement of testicular prosthesis, if testicle(s) absent.

3. Administration of human chorionic gonadotropin has produced descent of the testicles in some children. Testicles may have descended spontaneously in many of these cases.

Complications

1. Testicular torsion.
2. Associated hernias.
3. Emotional disturbances.
4. Significant increase in sterility and malignancy later in life.

For nursing assessment, diagnoses, and interventions, see "Care of the Child Who Undergoes Urologic Surgery."

Care of the Child Who Undergoes Urologic Surgery

Also see Chapter 21, page 787, for a discussion of kidney surgery and urinary diversion.

Nursing Assessment

1. Obtain history from prenatal and birth record, family, and child.
2. Assess feeding and crying patterns, indicating potential obstruction or abdominal pain.
3. Assess urinary elimination pattern to determine degree of disorder.
4. Assess for associated congenital defects.
5. Assess for failure to thrive.
6. Determine family's response to body image changes. Expect anxieties regarding sterility and gender identity and perceptions of the child as defective or inadequate.
7. Measure and record vital signs, height, weight, abdominal girth, and compare with previous measurements, if available. Renal insufficiency may alter growth. Fever may be indicative of infection.
8. Visually and manually inspect genitalia and record abnormalities (eg, if bladder mucosa is visible, describe signs of irritation).
9. Palpate abdomen; note masses.
10. Obtain urine for culture and sensitivity. Note color, amount, odor, degree of cloudiness.
11. Review results of all laboratory and diagnostic procedures.

Nursing Diagnoses

- Deficient Knowledge related to surgery.
- Impaired Urinary Elimination related to surgical intervention.
- Disturbed Body Image related to appearance of genitalia.
- Risk for Infection related to surgical incision and drainage tubes.
- Risk for Deficient Fluid Volume related to surgical losses.
- Acute Pain related to surgical incision and drainage tubes.

Nursing Interventions

Promoting Understanding of Surgical Treatment

1. Determine the child's expectation regarding illness and hospitalization through discussion and play therapy.
2. Explain the anatomy and physiology of the urinary system in terms the child can understand.
   a. Use a body outline appropriate for the age of the child.
   b. Explain how the child differs from the normal. Relate defect to symptoms whenever possible.

3. Explain all diagnostic tests before their occurrence. These may include urinalysis, 24-hour urine collections, IV, retrograde pyelography, ultrasound, and/or VCUG. Descriptions should include such information as:
   a. Preparation required—fasting, enemas, catheterization.
   b. Location of the test—operating room, radiology department.
   c. Appearance and attire of personnel.
   d. Positioning.
   e. Anesthesia.
   f. Pain or discomfort.
   g. Expectations after the procedure—diet, rest, urine collections.
4. Determine the child's understanding of the procedure.
   a. Ask simple, direct questions.
   b. Allow child to perform the procedure on a doll or to demonstrate it on a diagram.
5. Explain the surgical procedure, including the following:
   a. Preparation required—fasting, enemas.
   b. Description of the operating room, including the appearance of the personnel.
   c. Anesthesia.
   d. Postoperative appearance—urinary drainage tubing and collection devices, appearance of urine, sutures, bandages, IV infusion.
6. Reassess the child's understanding of the surgery and reinforce teaching when necessary.
7. Emphasize additional points:
   a. The child is in no way to blame for illness.
   b. No other part of the body will be operated on.

Promoting Normal Urine Output

1. Monitor daily intake and output.
2. Encourage adequate fluids and monitor daily weight.
3. Care for all catheters and urinary tubes according to facility policy. Maintain appropriate position of tubes.
4. Observe and record amount and appearance of urinary drainage, occurrence of bladder spasms, symptoms of urinary or incisional infection.

Providing Emotional Support Regarding Body Image

1. Continue reassurance about appearance of genitalia.
2. Maintain discussions regarding reactions. This may need to be done with patient and family alone as well as the family unit.
3. If additional surgical intervention is required, discuss plans for interim period from initial surgery until secondary or reconstructive procedures can be performed.
4. Initiate independence of care.
5. Focus on activities the child can perform and accomplish.

Preventing Infection

1. Administer antibiotics and IV fluids, as ordered.
2. Maintain patency of catheters. Provide catheter care, as directed.
3. Administer wound care using aseptic technique. Inspect incision for drainage or signs of infection.

Maintaining Fluid Volume

1. Administer fluids, as ordered.
2. Monitor vital signs for hypotension or tachycardia.
3. Assess patient's skin turgor and mucous membranes for signs of dehydration.
4. Measure and record accurate intake and output.

Promoting Comfort

1. Administer analgesics, as ordered and according to assessment of complaints of pain, restlessness, crying, or withdrawal.
2. Administer antispasmodics, as ordered, for bladder spasm.
3. Provide distraction and comfort measures.

Family Education and Health Maintenance

1. Advise the family about follow-up appointments, additional surgeries, or procedures.
2. Teach care of incision, signs of infection.
3. Advise on avoidance of straddle toys for 6 weeks to promote healing.
4. Encourage good nutrition to promote healing and to prevent infection.

Evaluation: Expected Outcomes

- Child and family verbalize understanding of surgery.
- Clear urine draining via catheter.
- Child and family verbalize relief that defects can be surgically repaired and reconstructed.
- Incision without drainage or signs of infection.
- Vital signs stable; urine output adequate.
- Decreased crying and increased restful periods and sleep noted.

RENAL FAILURE AND DIALYSIS
Acute Renal Failure

Acute renal failure is a sudden, usually reversible deterioration in normal renal function. This results in fluid and electrolyte imbalance and accumulation of metabolic toxins. Nursing care of children with acute renal failure is generally the same as that of adults (see page 795), although there are special considerations for pediatric patients.

Pathophysiology and Etiology

1. Causes are divided into *prerenal* (problem occurs in blood supply to the kidneys), *intrarenal* (problem is within the kidney or kidneys), and *postrenal* (problem occurs in urinary system after the kidneys).
   a. Prerenal causes: conditions causing hypovolemia (dehydration, shock, trauma, or burns) cause decreased blood flow to the kidneys. The nephrons, however, are structurally and functionally intact.
   b. Intrarenal causes: conditions causing a reduction in glomerular filtration rate (GFR), renal ischemia, and tubular damage. May be due to vascular diseases (hemolytic uremic syndrome, thrombosis), tubular nephropathies (myoglobinuria, hemoglobinuria, toxins), or interstitial

nephritis (penicillins, allergies). These are the largest group to require extended medical management.

c. Postrenal causes: conditions causing obstruction to urine flow. Uncommon, except for obstructive uropathies in the first year of life. Renal function is restored with relief of the obstruction.

2. The exact pathophysiology of acute renal failure is not always known. Three phases of acute renal failure are recognized in children:

a. Initiating phase: begins when kidney is injured and lasts from hours to days. Signs and symptoms of renal impairment are present.

b. Oliguric phase: usually lasts 5 to 15 days but can persist for weeks; shorter in infants and young children (3 to 5 days) and longer in older children and adolescents (10 to 14 days). Not all patients have an oliguric phase.

c. Diuretic phase: highly variable, from mild and lasting only a few days to profound.

3. Trauma, burns, and nephrotoxic agents may cause acute tubular necrosis and temporary cessation of renal function. Myoglobin (a protein released from muscle when injury occurs) and hemoglobin are released, causing renal toxicity, ischemia, or both.

4. Severe transfusion reactions may result in hemoglobin that filters through the kidney glomeruli. This becomes concentrated in the kidney tubules. Resulting precipitation interferes with the excretion of urine.

5. Nonsteroidal anti-inflammatory drugs (NSAIDs) interfere with prostaglandins that normally protect renal blood flow, decreasing GFR.

 DRUG ALERT Nephrotoxic agents include aminoglycosides, penicillins, cephalosporins, sulfonamides, calcineurin inhibitor immunosuppressives, NSAIDs and certain antineoplastic drugs. Large doses of vitamin A, chemicals that contain arsenic, and mercury are also nephrotoxic.

Clinical Manifestations

1. Nausea and vomiting.
2. Diarrhea.
3. Decreased tissue turgor.
4. Dry mucous membranes.
5. Lethargy.
6. Difficulty in voiding; changes in urine flow; decreased urine output.
7. Steady rise in serum creatinine.
8. Fever.
9. Edema—periorbital, pitting lower leg edema, ascites.
10. Changes in mental status or mood.
11. Headaches and blurry vision due to hypertension.
12. Seizures.

Diagnostic Evaluation

1. Serum creatinine level—the most reliable measure of the GFR, found to be rising.

2. Radionuclide studies—evaluate GFR and renal blood flow and distribution.
3. Urinalysis—reveals proteinuria, hematuria, casts.
4. Ultrasonography—determines anatomic abnormalities.

Management

1. Seventy-five percent of children with acute renal failure attain complete recovery.
2. Treatment is directed toward the underlying cause.
3. Correction of any reversible cause of acute renal failure (ie, surgical relief of obstruction).
4. Correction and control of fluid and electrolyte imbalances.
5. Restoration and maintenance of stable vital signs.
6. Maintenance of nutrition with low-sodium, low-potassium, low-phosphate, low-protein diet.
7. Initiation of dialysis (hemodialysis, peritoneal dialysis, or continuous venovenous hemofiltration) for patients with life-threatening complications.

Complications

1. Fluid and electrolyte imbalance, especially hyperkalemia—when GFR is reduced, patient cannot excrete potassium.
2. Metabolic acidosis, caused by decreased acid excretion and reduced bicarbonate reabsorption (see Box 49-1).
3. Insufficient nutritional intake because of metabolic abnormalities and symptoms, such as nausea and vomiting.

BOX 49-1	**Clinical Manifestations of Metabolic Acidosis**

GI
- Anorexia
- Nausea and vomiting
- Abdominal pain

NEUROLOGIC
- Lethargy
- Stupor
- Coma

CARDIOVASCULAR
- Decreased heart rate
- Cardiac dysrhythmias
- Peripheral vasodilation

OTHER MANIFESTATIONS
- Warm and flushed skin
- Weakness and malaise
- Bone resorption (with chronic acidosis)
- Increased rate and depth of respirations (Kussmaul breathing due to compensation)

LABORATORY FINDINGS
- Decreased pH
- Decreased HCO_3^- (initially)
- Decreased PCO_2 (compensatory)
- Hyperkalemia
- Acidic urine (compensatory)

Nursing Assessment

1. Obtain history of all medications, recent and past illnesses or injuries, allergies, and potential exposure to toxic substances.
2. Measure intake and output. Insert indwelling urinary catheter, as indicated.
3. Monitor vital signs, especially blood pressure. Institute cardiac monitoring, as indicated.
4. Assess for edema and fluid overload (cardiac and respiratory assessment).
5. Monitor urine-specific gravity, as directed. Fixed specific gravity of 1.010 indicates the kidneys' inability to concentrate or dilute urine.

Nursing Diagnoses

- Risk for Imbalanced Fluid Volume related to inability of the kidneys to maintain fluid balance.
- Risk for electrolyte imbalance: hyperkalemia.

Nursing Interventions

Maintaining Fluid Volume

1. Administer IV fluids slowly to prevent heart failure.
2. Maintain fluid restriction, as ordered.
3. Keep strict intake and output records.
4. Weigh child daily.
5. Promptly report signs of heart failure—edema, bounding pulse, third heart sound, shortness of breath, and adventitious breath sounds.

Preventing Severe Electrolyte Disturbance

1. Monitor blood test results (creatinine, BUN, electrolytes, calcium) and notify health care provider promptly of abnormal levels.
2. Watch for signs of hyperkalemia—weak, irregular pulse, abdominal cramps, muscle weakness.
3. Do not administer IV fluids with potassium while renal function is impaired.
4. Maintain low-protein, low-potassium, low-sodium, and high-carbohydrate diet.
5. Administer treatments for hyperkalemia, as ordered, such as IV sodium bicarbonate and IV glucose and insulin (requires careful glucose monitoring), both of which drive potassium into cells and temporarily out of the bloodstream.
6. Administer cation exchange enemas to reduce potassium, as ordered.
7. Watch for signs of hypocalcemia—muscle twitching and tetany.

Family Education and Health Maintenance

1. Explain all steps of the diagnostic and treatment process to the family.
2. Teach about dialysis if this becomes necessary.
3. Explain that as kidney function resumes, diuresis may occur to eliminate excess fluid the body was storing.
4. Educate about prompt medical attention for illnesses that may cause dehydration to prevent renal injury in the future.

Evaluation: Expected Outcomes

- No signs of heart failure.
- Potassium remains within upper range of normal; kidney function returns to baseline.

Chronic Renal Failure

Chronic renal failure (CRF) is irreversible destruction of nephrons so that they are no longer capable of maintaining normal fluid and electrolyte balance. *Chronic kidney disease (CKD)* refers to kidney damage with a decreased GFR of <60mL/min/1.73m² for 3 months or greater. Nursing care of children with CRF is similar to that of adults (see page 798). The following considerations are important for pediatric patients.

Pathophysiology and Etiology

1. Congenital renal and urinary tract abnormalities are the most common causes in children younger than age 5 (eg, polycystic kidney disease, congenital nephrotic syndrome, hyperoxaluria).
2. Most common causes in ages 5 to 15:
   a. Glomerular disease (eg, glomerulonephritis).
   b. Urologic abnormalities.
   c. Cystic kidney disease.
3. Similar progression regardless of cause.
   a. Nephron damage that results in hypertrophy and hyperplasia of remaining nephrons.
   b. Overload results in decreased ability for nephrons to excrete effectively.
   c. Results in azotemia and clinical uremia.
   d. Inability of kidney to excrete phosphate causes hypocalcemia, which results in osteodystrophy.
   e. Kidneys cannot synthesize vitamin D, thus impairing calcium absorption. Bones may become so calcium depleted that growth halts and bones become brittle (renal rickets).
   f. Kidneys cannot synthesize erythropoietin, thus resulting in anemia.
   g. Excretion of nitrogenous waste through sweat causes pruritus.
   h. Overload of fluid results in edema and hypertension.
4. Severity of CRF is indicated by GFR. The lower the GFR, the greater the loss of renal function.

Clinical Manifestations

Variable and not chronological.
1. Nausea and vomiting, decreased appetite and energy level.
2. Initial polyuria caused by kidneys' inability to concentrate urine; later oliguria and anuria.
3. Bone or joint pain.
4. Dryness and itching of skin.
5. Poor growth.
6. Fatigue, lethargy due to anemia.

Diagnostic Evaluation

1. Serum studies:
   a. Anemia and iron studies: decreased hemoglobin, hematocrit, iron levels

b. Decreased Na+, Ca++, and CO_2 (metabolic acidosis), increased K+ and phosphorus.

c. As renal function declines, BUN, uric acid, and creatinine values continue to climb.

d. Elevated PTH.

2. Urine studies:

a. Specific gravity—increased or decreased.

b. Twenty-four-hour urine for creatinine clearance is decreased (increased creatinine in urine), thus reflecting decreased GFR.

c. Changes in total output (may initially be polyuric due to difficulty concentrating urine, then oliguric).

d. Proteinuria.

3. Many other tests may be ordered to evaluate other systems and extent of disease (eg, chest x-ray, echocardiogram, bone age).

Management

1. Correction of calcium–phosphorus imbalance. Initiate low-phosphorus diet. Administer activated vitamin D to increase calcium absorption and phosphate binders with meals to bind phosphate in the GI tract.

2. Correction of acidosis with buffers, such as sodium bicarbonate tablets.

3. Correction of hyperkalemia through low-potassium diet or administration of potassium-lowering agents such as sodium polystyrene.

4. Diets should meet caloric needs of the child and contain adequate protein for development (0.9 to 1.5 g/kg per day).

5. Correction of anemia through the use of oral iron and erythropoietin administered subcutaneously at home.

6. BP should be managed with appropriate antihypertensive medications (angiotensin-converting enzyme inhibitors, angiotensin receptor blockers, calcium channel blockers, or diuretics).

7. Growth retardation should be evaluated for possible use of growth hormone. Consult dietitian to ensure optimal nutrition for use of growth hormone.

8. Renal replacement options for end-stage renal disease include hemodialysis, peritoneal dialysis, transplantation, or no treatment.

9. Dialysis, while renal transplant workup is in progress.

Complications

1. Growth retardation.

2. Delayed or absent sexual maturation.

3. Severe anemia—kidneys cannot stimulate erythropoietin; uremic toxins deplete erythrocytes; nutritional deficiencies.

4. Hypertension—renal ischemia stimulates renin–angiotensin system.

5. Cardiovascular disease (left ventricular hypertrophy, heart failure).

6. Renal osteodystrophy due to vitamin D deficiency and secondary hyperparathyroidism.

7. Azotemia/uremia—nitrogen waste products accumulate in blood. Toxic levels manifest themselves in many ways, such as coma, headache, GI disturbances, neuromuscular disturbances.

8. Neurodevelopmental delay due to uremic effects.

9. Metabolic acidosis, which may cause poor growth, confusion, dull headache, and lethargy.

10. Electrolyte imbalance—hypocalcemia, hyperkalemia.

Nursing Assessment

1. Perform a comprehensive, multisystem assessment to help in planning care.

2. Assess nutrition, growth, and developmental status.

3. Assess coping, support systems, and other resources.

Nursing Diagnoses

Children with CRF are in multisystem physiologic crises. The nursing diagnoses throughout the chapter are applicable, but focus may be:

- Risk for electrolyte imbalance: hypocalcemia, hyperkalemia.
- Risk for Imbalanced Fluid Volume related to renal failure and dialysis.
- Imbalanced Nutrition: Less Than Body Requirements related to GI disturbances, diet restrictions, and protein loss.
- Activity Intolerance related to fatigue and anemia.
- Ineffective Coping related to changes in lifestyle and body image on dialysis.

Nursing Interventions

Ensuring Safety

1. Protect the child from the effects of decreased level of consciousness and involuntary movements by maintaining crib or bed side rails up and padded, as necessary.

2. Monitor for seizure activity and have airway or tongue blade and suction equipment on hand.

3. Monitor BUN, creatinine, electrolyte, and calcium levels and report abnormalities promptly.

Promoting Fluid Balance

See "Acute renal failure," page 1650.

Ensuring Adequate Nutrition

1. Ensure adequate protein in diet. Obtain consultation from a registered dietitian.

2. Encourage appropriate fluid intake between meals.

3. Consult with dietitian regarding appropriate milk intake and alternatives because of high phosphate, sodium, and potassium content. Instead, administer feedings high in calories and low in wastes, as directed.

Increasing Activity Tolerance

1. Plan activities when child is rested.

2. Encourage activity as tolerated, but excessive exercise should be avoided to reduce nitrogenous waste from metabolism.

3. Administer blood transfusions or IV iron therapy, as ordered (if patient is resistant to erythropoietin therapy and unable to tolerate oral iron supplementation).

Enhancing Coping

Because numerous issues may interfere with the child's psychological and social development and education, help the child and family to cope with:

1. Uncertainty regarding the course of the disease and ultimate prognosis.
2. Abnormal lifestyle necessitated by dialysis (including interference with school).
3. Burden of dialysis and continuous administration of medications.
4. Problems of adjustment related to growth failure.
5. Fear of death, present in most children, adolescents, and family members.
6. Possible kidney transplantation, involving major surgery and prolonged hospitalization, followed by altered body image that is caused by high-dose steroids and potential for rejection, which may threaten survival.

Family Education and Health Maintenance

1. Teach child to avoid high-sodium foods, such as chips, pretzels, and popcorn; luncheon meats; canned foods; and fast foods, if sodium is restricted.
2. Encourage follow-up as advised by kidney specialist and primary health care provider.
3. Encourage family to keep up with regular dental care, immunizations, and health assessments to help prevent infections, problems with growth, and more severe childhood diseases.
4. Teach about medications and support child who may be taking multiple medications—calcium, phosphate binder, acid neutralizer, recombinant erythropoietin, antihypertensives, and others.
5. Teach about maintaining good hygiene and peritoneal dialysis catheter care.
6. Advise the family about support services and media resources available—for example, *It's Just a Part of My Life—A Kid's View of Dialysis*, by the National Kidney Foundation (*www.kidney.org*).

Evaluation: Expected Outcomes

- Side rails up with airway and suction at bedside.
- Fluid restriction maintained, weight stable, no signs of heart failure.
- Taking 100% of renal diet.
- Engaging in play without shortness of breath.
- Parents asking questions and discussing treatment with child.

The Child Who Undergoes Dialysis

Dialysis is the passage of a solute through a semipermeable membrane. The purpose of dialysis is to preserve life by replacing some of the normal kidney functions. See page 785 for a complete description of different types of dialysis.

General Considerations

The following principles should be considered by the nurse who works with pediatric patients:
1. Peritoneal dialysis:
   a. This mode of dialysis continues to be the favored mode in young children.
   b. Because of the child's small size, the volume of dialysate is 1,100 to 1,400 mL/m².

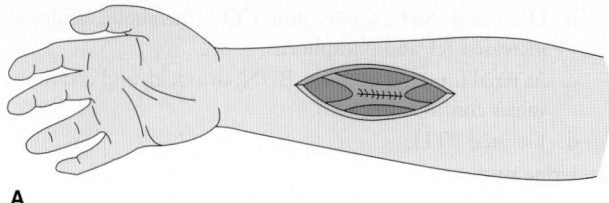

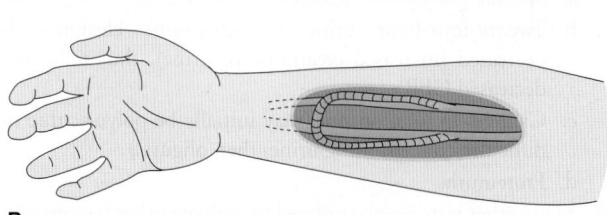

Figure 49-3. Vascular access devices for hemodialysis. (**A**) An internal arteriovenous fistula. (**B**) An internal arteriovenous graft.

   c. The child can be expected to participate at a developmentally appropriate level with his or her own care.
2. Hemodialysis:
   a. When possible, subcutaneous or I.M. injections are avoided because the child is anticoagulated with heparin.
   b. BP cuff and tourniquets should not be applied to a limb with a fistula and peripheral IVs should not be placed in a limb with a graft or fistula.
3. Specific care for the child during dialysis is generally provided by specially trained personnel in a dialysis unit. However, the following considerations should be noted:
   a. Choice for vascular access depends on patient size and availability of peripheral blood vessels of suitable size (see Figure 49-3). A central venous catheter may also be used.
   b. Extracorporeal blood volume (blood outside of the body at any given time) should be as small as possible. It should not exceed 8% to 10% of the child's total blood volume.
   c. Efficiency or adequacy of the dialyzer, relative to the child's weight, should be noted and blood pump speed adjusted accordingly.
   d. External catheter should be secured to make sure catheter is not traumatized.

Nursing Care of the Child Who Undergoes Dialysis

1. Prepare the child for the procedure. Dialysis is threatening to most children and may evoke fears of pain, mutilation, immobilization, helplessness, and dependency. Many children have fears of losing all of their blood during hemodialysis. A child who is well prepared will be less frightened and better able to cooperate during the procedure.
   a. Explain the procedure in terms that the child can understand.
   b. Allow the child to handle equipment similar to that which will be used during dialysis.
   c. Encourage the child to express fears so that misinterpretations can be corrected.

d. Provide simple pictures and diagrams, if appropriate.

e. Allow the child to talk with peers who have undergone dialysis.

2. Explain the procedure to family members and answer questions so that they will be in the best position to support the child.

3. Protect the child from infection.

a. Keep the dressings and area around the catheter (if used) clean and dry.

b. Use aseptic technique throughout the dialysis procedure.

c. Provide supplemental vitamins because diet may be low in vitamins.

d. Provide meticulous daily hygiene.

4. Maintain appropriate nutritional and fluid modifications. Because anorexia is commonly seen in CRF, provide small frequent meals.

5. Restrict fluids and sodium to prevent fluid overload in children who are hypertensive or who have minimal urine output. Potassium is limited (more so in hemodialysis patients) to prevent complications related to hyperkalemia. The child may see dietary restrictions as a punishment and must be helped to realize the purpose of restrictions.

6. Do not restrict protein, which is vital to allow for normal growth and development. Peritoneal dialysis is a continual treatment and therefore can constantly dialyze metabolic waste and fluids off.

7. Maintain careful records of intake and output, vital signs, BP, and daily weight. These provide valuable information about the effectiveness of the therapy.

8. Support the child during the dialysis procedure.

a. Provide symptomatic relief of nausea, vomiting, malaise, muscle cramping, or headache. Notify the health care provider if these symptoms are severe.

b. Involve the child in diversional activities, such as play therapy, crafts, television, and books.

c. Encourage the family to bring in articles that will make the child's room appear more homelike (eg, pictures, posters).

d. Encourage the child to be as independent as possible in daily care.

9. Help the child to keep up with schoolwork by initiating a referral to a tutor and providing study times.

Community and Home Care Considerations

1. Be aware that although life is preserved, it is by no means normal during the time on dialysis or between dialysis treatments. These measures may increase the child's feeling of self-esteem and diminish regression and social isolation. By serving as role models, health professionals may encourage parents to recognize and foster the normal, healthy aspects of the child's daily life.

2. Offer appropriate support to the family.

a. Provide opportunity for family members to discuss their feelings, fears, and frustrations and to ask questions.

b. Allow family members to become involved in the child's care.

c. Provide for continuity of personnel.

d. Initiate appropriate referrals and provide resources. These may include referrals to a social worker, psychiatrist, dietitian, community health agency, or other families who are coping with dialysis.

3. Be aware that families usually need extensive support from many health professionals to cope with the physical, psychological, financial, and logistical aspects of renal failure and dialysis. Attention must be focused on siblings and parents because sibling relationships are usually strained and difficult.

4. Teach the child and family about all of the important aspects of renal failure and dialysis, including the following:

a. Protection from infection.

b. Dietary restrictions and recommendations; ways of incorporating the special diet into the family meal plan.

c. Dialysis schedule.

d. Medications.

e. Emergency procedures.

f. Reintegration into the community and school.

5. Empower the family to care for the child at home. Learning about the child's care also helps restore some sense of control in a frightening situation.

Renal Transplantation

Renal (kidney) transplantation is the optimal therapeutic modality for end-stage renal disease in the pediatric age group. With successful transplantation, there is a greater likelihood of optimum rehabilitation than with any other form of dialytic therapy. The potential for normal growth and pubertal development is significantly increased after transplantation. However, it should be noted that posttransplant growth is affected by many variables: age of onset of chronic renal disease, caloric intake, corticosteroid dosage, bone age at transplantation, transplant function, and rejection episodes. Requirements of preoperative management and nursing care of children or teens for renal transplantation are similar to that of adults (see page 788). However, they are also more exhaustive because the recipient as well as the parents must be included. The emotional, psychological, and financial needs of the recipient and the family must be evaluated. An appropriate care plan must then be designed to address identified needs; this care plan must be appropriate for the developmental age of the recipient.

Evaluation of Recipient

The major issues that must be evaluated when considering renal transplantation in children are:

1. Patient age and size.
2. Primary renal disease.
3. Psychological status.
4. Live versus deceased donor allograft.
5. Optimal immunosuppressive regimen.
6. Maximization of growth and pubertal development.

Donor Selection (by Priority)

A tissue-compatible transplantation from a relative is 90% successful.

1. Identical twin sibling.
2. Siblings cannot be used as donors until they are of legal age to give consent for removal of a kidney.
3. Parent.

4. Other relative.
5. Unrelated live donor such as a family friend.
6. Deceased donor.

Operative Procedure

A child who weighs more than 22 pounds (10 kg) usually receives the kidney of an adult. In a very small child, the kidney transplant is placed within the abdomen, with vessel anastomosis to the aorta and superior vena cava.

Potential Emotional Concerns of Children with Transplants

1. The concept of a foreign body, especially a cadaver kidney, inside one's own body may be disturbing.
2. Fear that the kidney may wear out sooner if it is from an older person.
3. Altered body image because of growth failure and the effects of steroid therapy.
4. Guilt feelings if a live donor transplant fails, especially that of a family donor.

Nursing Interventions

Also see "After kidney transplantation," page 789.

1. Support the child and family through the preoperative phase, including diagnostic testing and blood transfusions.
2. After surgery, maintain strict infection precautions.
3. Administer immunosuppressants and other medications, as directed.
4. Continue support through dialysis, if necessary.
5. Monitor urine output, bloodwork results, and urine-specific gravity.
6. Watch for signs of rejection—fever, oliguria, proteinuria, weight gain, hypertension, and tenderness over transplanted kidney. Acute rejection usually occurs in the first 3 months after transplant. Chronic rejection may develop at any time. It occurs slowly over months to years and leads to progressive loss of renal function.
7. Watch for signs of infection: fever, leukopenia, neutropenia.
8. Infection can be bacterial (most common are pneumonia and UTIs) or viral (cytomegalovirus and Epstein-Barr virus are the most common infections).

Community and Home Care Considerations

The practice of discharging patients from an in-hospital setting as quickly as possible is also true for the pediatric transplant recipient. Community and home care nurses must have:

1. The knowledge to care for a child who receives IV and immunosuppressive medications.
2. The ability to access and heparinize central venous lines and peripheral IV catheters.
3. The ability to aid in reinforcing discharge teaching, aid in BP monitoring, and assess medication adherence.

Family Education and Health Maintenance

1. Teach families about the signs of rejection and infection.
2. Encourage close follow-up for proper dosing of immunosuppressants.
3. Education, communication, and employ strategies to promote medication adherence.
4. Advise family that close medical surveillance will always be necessary because the incidence of malignant disease is six times more likely in transplant recipients than in the general population.
5. Teach parents not to overprotect the child. When the child has healed from surgery, regular activity can be resumed. This includes returning to school; however, the school needs to be aware of the patient's immunosuppressive status.
6. Teach families and patients the importance of good handwashing.
7. Encourage patient to wear a MedicAlert bracelet or necklace, and inform the community emergency services of transplant status.
8. Advise parents that no live vaccine should be given to the child who is immunosuppressed.
9. Advise the family about resources available.

SELECTED REFERENCES

American Academy of Pediatrics Subcommittee on Urinary Tract Infection, Steering Committee on Quality Improvement and Management. (2011). Urinary tract infection: Clinical practice guideline for the diagnosis and management of the initial UTI in febrile infants and children 2 to 24 months. *Pediatrics, 128,* 595–610.

Atkinson, M., & Furth, S. (2011). Anemia in children with chronic kidney disease. *Nature Reviews Nephrology, 7,* 635–649.

Dolan, N., Borzych-Duzalka, D., Suarez, A., et al. (2013). Ventriculoperitoneal shunts in children on peritoneal dialysis: A survey of the International Pediatric Peritoneal Dialysis Network. *Pediatric Nephrology, 28*(2), 315–319.

Kidney Disease: Improving Global Outcomes (KDIGO) Work Group. (2012). Clinical Practice Guideline for the Evaluation and Management of Chronic Kidney Disease. *Kidney International, 3*(1), 1–150.

Koyle, M., & Shifrin, D. (2012). Issues in febrile urinary tract infection management. *Pediatric Clinics of North America, 59*(4), 909–922.

Mattoo, T. K. (2011). Vesicoureteral reflux and reflux nephropathy. *Advanced Chronic Kidney Disease, 18*(5), 348–354.

Rees, L., & Mak, R. (2011). Nutrition and growth in children with chronic kidney disease. *Nature Reviews Nephrology, 7,* 615–623.

Routh, J. C., Bogaert, G. A., Kaefer, M., et al. (2012) Vesicoureteral reflux: Current trends in diagnosis, screening, and treatment. *European Urology, 61*(4), 773–882.

Schaefer, F., & Warady, B. (2011). Peritoneal dialysis in children with end-stage renal disease. *Nature Reviews Nephrology, 7,* 659–668.

Schmitt, C., & Mehls, O. (2011), Mineral and bone disorders in children with chronic kidney disease. *Nature Reviews Nephrology, 7,* 624–634.

Stec, A. A., Baradaran, N., Schaeffer, A., et al. (2012). The modern staged repair of classic bladder exstrophy: A detailed postoperative management strategy for primary bladder closure. *Journal of Pediatric Urology, 8*(5), 549–555.

50
Pediatric Metabolic and Endocrine Disorders

OVERVIEW AND ASSESSMENT

Common Nursing Assessment for Growth and Development

Endocrine dysfunction in children frequently leads to altered growth and development. Accurate nursing assessment can help detect variations in growth and developmental patterns, identify such factors as diet and medications that may have an impact on growth and development, and obtain information about compliance and understanding of treatment.

Evaluation of Growth Patterns

1. Perform frequent and accurate measurements of height and weight.
2. Accurately plot measurements on growth curve for absolute chronologic age.
3. Assess growth pattern for any deviation from the child's percentile or from the parallel of the growth curve for age (includes both an upward as well as a downward deviation).
4. Calculate growth velocity—take the difference of current height from previous height and divide by the time period. Growth rate for a prepubertal child should be 2 to 3 inches (5 to 7 cm) on an annual basis.
5. Report any child whose pattern deviates from the expected pattern for age to health care provider.

General Health History

1. Dietary history—what is the child's meal frequency, volume, and food preferences? Be vigilant while obtaining the history of a child when anorexia may be possible—growth velocity will usually be low, in addition to poor weight gain.
2. History of major illnesses or surgeries that have altered the child's growth and development.
3. Family history—is there a family history of growth or developmental issues? Is there a family history of delayed puberty? Are family members unusually short or tall in stature, or is there obvious dysmorphology?
4. Clothing—outgrowing clothing and shoes?
5. Social history relative to friendships.
6. Academic and school performance—recent changes?
7. Activity—activities the child participates in? Intensity and type of exercise?

Medication History and Compliance

1. Is child on any steroid medications (such as prednisone) that would suppress growth? Inquire about over-the-counter medications or herbal supplementation.
2. When pubertal signs are present on physical examination, does child have access to any gonadal steroids (ie, birth control pills, anabolic steroids)?
3. Do child and family understand treatment medication indication and usage instructions?
4. Are child and family compliant with medications according to dose, frequency, and route? Is medication stored properly?
5. If taking oral medication, is it being taken with food, if indicated? If pills are being chewed, are teeth being brushed soon after, which could be rinsing out the medications?
6. If injectable, are injection sites being rotated appropriately? Review technique.

Physical Examination Relative to Development

1. Dental development—eruption of teeth and presence of permanent teeth (see page 1397).
2. Pubertal development—Tanner staging of pubic hair and gonadal development (see Table 50-1).
3. Presence of genetic dysmorphology—such as short-limbed dwarfism and various atypical stigmata.

Causes of Disorders of Growth and Stature

It is important to realize that growth and stature problems are caused by a wide variety of factors. Thorough history, physical examination, and diagnostic testing can help reveal the underlying cause. Many of the disorders are associated with other anomalies, such as mental retardation, cardiac problems, metabolic issues, and secondary sex characteristic abnormalities. The cause may be treatable to resolve the growth problem, be amenable to growth hormone supplementation, or may be untreatable due to genetic cause.

Short Stature and Growth Failure

Genetic Causes

1. Familial short stature—short target height relative to U.S. standards; however, growth rate is normal.
2. Constitutional delay—short stature with retarded linear growth beginning in the first 3 years of life followed by short stature relative to peers; however, final height normal upon completion of pubertal development. Puberty is usually delayed.
3. Genetic disorders:
   a. Dwarfism—multiple types and causes relative to chondrodysplasias.
   b. Turner syndrome—occurs in about 1 in 2,500 female births. Characterized by short stature, ovarian dysgenesis (underdeveloped, degenerate ovaries), and, in some cases, unusual physical appearance (see page 1799).
   c. Russell-Silver syndrome—characterized by unilateral poor growth, short stature, characteristic facies, mental delays. Whenever unilateral change in growth is present, abdominal tumor needs to be ruled out.
   d. Prader-Willi syndrome—rare syndrome characterized by below-normal intelligence, small stature, hypogonadism (see page 37), failure to thrive in infancy followed by obesity and insatiable appetite, bizarre binge-type eating behaviors.
   e. Down syndrome—occurs in 1 in 700 live births; characterized by growth retardation and mental retardation (see page 1796).
   f. Cystic fibrosis—occurs in 1 in 2,000 live births. In addition to respiratory and GI symptoms, growth retardation occurs (see page 1508).

Endocrine Disorders

1. Hypothyroidism.
2. Growth hormone (GH) deficiency.
3. Glucocorticoid excess—Cushing syndrome.

Nonendocrine Disorders

1. Glucocorticoid (prednisone) therapy for asthma, prevention of transplant rejection, adjunct medication in cancer chemotherapy.
2. Nutritional deficiency.
3. Psychosocial issues.
4. Chronic diseases—cardiovascular, renal, hematologic, pulmonary, malabsorptive disorders, inborn errors of metabolism.
5. Medical interventions—surgical tumor resection, radiation for brain tumors.

Tall Stature and Excessive Growth

Genetic Causes

1. Familial tall stature—tall stature relative to U.S. standards; however, normal for family. Growth rate is usually normal.
2. Genetic disorders:
   a. Marfan syndrome—tall, long extremities, long fingers and toes; cardiac and other anomalies.
   b. Klinefelter's syndrome—tall, slim, underweight, gynecomastia, small testicles, infertile.

Endocrine Disorders

1. Congenital adrenal hyperplasia.
2. Precocious puberty (see page 1670).
3. Hyperthyroidism (see page 1664).
4. Acromegaly—overproduction of GH usually related to pituitary tumors; very rare in children.

Nonendocrine Disorders

1. Exogenous use of androgens (ie, testosterone injections):
   a. Although stature and growth will initially be above the normal expected for age, ultimate height will be decreased due to undue advance of bone maturation at growth plate.
   b. The child will ultimately end up shorter than genetically determined.
2. Sotos syndrome (cerebral gigantism)—usually large at birth with rapid growth in first year of life, intellectual impairment. Hypothesized to be a hypothalamic defect; normal endocrine function.

DISORDERS OF THE ANTERIOR PITUITARY

The anterior pituitary is under the control of the hypothalamus and secretes six specific hormones: GH, thyroid-stimulating hormone (TSH), adrenocorticotropic hormone (ACTH), luteinizing hormone (LH), follicle-stimulating hormone (FSH), and prolactin. GH is the only hormone that does not have a target gland to induce further hormonal secretion. Hypopituitarism is a deficiency of one, some, or all of the hormones secreted by the pituitary gland. With the exception of GH, decreased secretion results in hypofunction of the consequential target gland.

TSH deficiency, ACTH deficiency, and LH/FSH deficiency are discussed under disorders of the thyroid gland, disorders of the adrenal glands, and disorders of gonadal function, respectively.

Table 50-1   Tanner Staging of Puberty

BOYS' GENITAL DEVELOPMENT	GIRLS' BREAST DEVELOPMENT	BOTH SEXES: PUBIC HAIR
Stage I Preadolescent. Testes, scrotum, and penis are of about the same size and proportion as in early childhood. 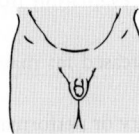	Preadolescent. Elevation of papilla only. 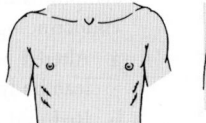	Preadolescent. The vellus over the pubis is not further developed than that over the abdominal wall (ie, no pubic hair). 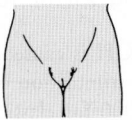 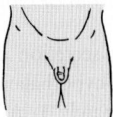
Stage 2 Enlargement of scrotum and testes. Skin of scrotum reddens and changes in texture. Little or no enlargement of penis at this time. 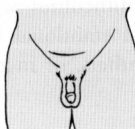	Breast bud stage. Elevation of breast and papilla as small mound. Enlargement of areola diameter. 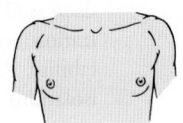 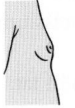	Sparse growth of long, slightly pigmented downy hair. Straight or slightly curled at base of penis or along labia. 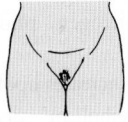 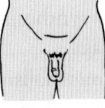
Stage 3 Enlargement of penis that occurs at first mainly in length. Further growth of testes and scrotum. 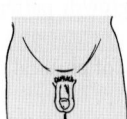	Further enlargement and elevation of breast and areola with no separation of their contours. 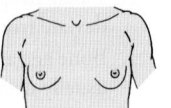	Considerably darker, coarser, and more curled. The hair spreads sparsely over the symphysis pubis. 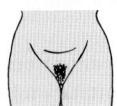 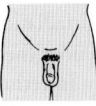
Stage 4 Increased size of penis with growth in breadth and development of glans. Testes and scrotum larger; scrotal skin darkened. 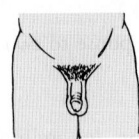	Projection of areola and papilla to form a secondary mound above level of the breast. 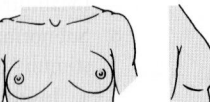 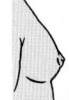	Hair now adult in type, but area covered is still considerably smaller than in adult. No spread to medial surface of thighs. 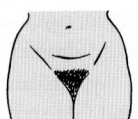 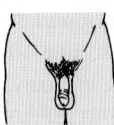
Stage 5 Genitalia adult in size and shape. 	Mature stage: projection of papilla only, due to recession of the areola to the general contour of the breast. 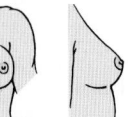	Adult in quantity and type; distribution of the horizontal (or classically "feminine") pattern. Spread to medial surface of thighs or above base of the inverse triangle occurs late (stage 6). 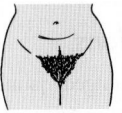 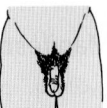

Adapted from Tanner, J. M. (1975). Growth and endocrinology of the adolescent. In L. Gardner (Ed.), Endocrine and genetic diseases of childhood and adolescence (2nd ed.). Philadelphia: W.B. Saunders.

Growth Hormone Deficiency

Evidence Base Cook, D. M., & Rose, S. R. (2012). A review of guidelines for use of growth hormone in pediatric and transition patients. *Pituitary, 15*(3), 301–310.

Acerini, C., Albanese, F., Casey, A., et al. (2012). Initiating growth hormone therapy for children and adolescents. *British Journal of Nursing, 21*(18), 1091–1097.

Insufficient secretion of GH is caused by lack of pituitary production or hypothalamic stimulation on the pituitary. Incidence is approximately 1 in 4,000 for classic GH insufficiency and is unknown for varying degrees of insufficiency.

Pathophysiology and Etiology

1. The lack of GH impairs the body's ability to perform the following functions:
   a. Protein metabolism—growth through increased protein synthesis; nitrogen, phosphorus, and potassium storage.
   b. Fat metabolism—increases lipolysis and oxidation of fat.
   c. Carbohydrate metabolism—decreases conversion of glucose to fat in adipose tissue.
2. Organic etiology:
   a. Intracranial cyst.
   b. Central nervous system (CNS) tumor (hypothalamic-pituitary structural lesions).
   c. CNS irradiation.
   d. Exogenous (head trauma from various causes such as birth injury, infection, pituitary infarction, or aneurysm).
   e. Histiocytosis X.
   f. Septo-optic dysplasia (abnormal forebrain development).
3. Idiopathic causes:
   a. Isolated GH deficiency; aplasia.
   b. Traumatic birth or breech delivery.
   c. Genetic (GH gene deletion).
   d. Nutritional deprivation; psychosocial issues.
4. Genetic cause—Turner syndrome:
   a. The pituitary and hypothalamus are not abnormal in Turner syndrome and GH secretion measurement is usually normal; however, GH is bioinactive due to binding problems.
   b. Hypothyroidism is common with Turner syndrome.
   c. Growth rate usually declines within the first year of life.
   d. Treatment with GH is a commonly accepted therapy to restore growth.

Clinical Manifestations

1. Hypoglycemia, prolonged jaundice, microphallus (small penis); usually in the neonate.
2. Growth velocity usually less than the 5th percentile for chronologic age.

3. Delayed skeletal maturation—bone age at least 1 year delayed from chronologic age.
4. "Pudgy" when the weight age (50% for weight) exceeds the height age (50% for height).
5. Frequently delayed eruption of primary and secondary teeth (not as severe as in hypothyroidism).
6. Delayed or lack of sexual development.
7. In young adulthood after epiphyseal fusion, the following symptoms may develop, requiring evaluation from an adult endocrinologist:
   a. Altered body composition (increased fat mass, decreased lean body mass).
   b. Reduced aerobic exercise capacity or performance.
   c. Decreased muscle strength.
   d. Abnormal blood lipid (fat and cholesterol) concentrations.
   e. Decreased bone mineral density or content.
   f. Impaired cardiac function.
   g. Impaired health-related quality of life (low energy level, decreased physical mobility, difficulties with concentration and memory, increased emotional lability, irritability, difficulty relating to others, or increased social isolation).

Diagnostic Evaluation

1. Rule out organic, nonendocrine causes of short stature (ie, chronic illness, nutritional deficiencies, genetic disorders, psychosocial factors).
2. Calculate growth velocity. (Does growth pattern parallel or deviate from the growth curve?)
3. Bone age assessment—ascertain age of physical development; usually delayed.
4. General physical examination—physical development that of a younger-appearing child, microphallus in the neonate.
5. Chromosome testing of females (rule out Turner syndrome).
6. Thyroid function tests to rule out hypothyroidism.
7. GH secretion laboratory indicators: IGF-1 (insulin-like growth factor 1), IGF-binding protein 3 are decreased. (Malnutrition can cause low IGF-1.)
8. Subnormal secretion of GH in response to two provocative stimuli:
   a. Insulin-induced hypoglycemia.
   b. Abnormal stimulatory response to arginine infusion, L-dopa, clonidine, or glucagon—all of which have specific actions resulting in GH secretion from pituitary. Pharmacologic agent is given, followed by blood sampling for GH response; GH levels less than 10 ng/mL are abnormal.
9. In the neonate with hypoglycemia, GH release is reduced at time of documented hypoglycemia (concomitant GH level relative to documented hypoglycemia is abnormally low).
10. GH has been associated with reduction in serum levels of free T4. Patients starting on GH should have their thyroid function monitored in the first 6 months of treatment.

NURSING ALERT In the neonate with hypoglycemia, always draw blood for cortisol and GH *before* initiating corrective action for the hypoglycemia. Early detection and diagnosis will protect child from future episodes if related to hypopituitarism.

11. Magnetic resonance imaging (MRI) of head to rule out tumor (MRI is gold standard).

Management

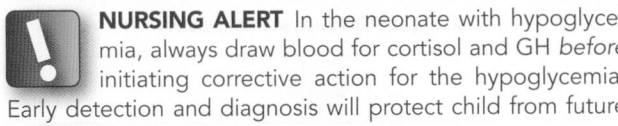 **Evidence Base** National Institute for Health and Clinical Excellence. (2010). *Human growth hormone (somatropin) for the treatment of growth failure in children.* London: Author.

1. Goal of treatment is to restore normal growth and development as well as to maximize growth potential and prevent hypoglycemia.
2. Replacement of deficiency uses recombinant deoxyribonucleic acid–derived GH given as subcutaneous injection.
3. Typical dose is 0.2 to 0.3 mg/kg per week divided in six or seven doses weekly until final height is achieved. In treatment of Turner syndrome, dose is generally 0.375 mg/kg per week divided in doses as above. *Note*: Administration three times per week is not as effective as six to seven times per week.
4. Therapy is being recommended for adult replacement. Depending on the degree of insufficiency, continued treatment into adulthood may be useful. Dosing recommendations range from less than 0.006 mg/kg/day to as high as 0.0125 mg/kg/day after epiphyseal fusion has occurred.

Complications

1. Altered carbohydrate, protein, and fat metabolism.
2. Hypoglycemia—seizures/death in neonates.
3. Adverse effects of therapy.
   a. Leukemia.
   b. Recurrence of CNS tumors.
   c. Pseudotumor cerebri.
   d. Slipped capital femoral epiphysis.
   e. Glucose intolerance/diabetes.

Nursing Assessment

1. See "Common nursing assessment for growth and development," page 1657.
2. Obtain family history related to parental heights and ages of pubertal maturation.

Nursing Diagnoses

- Delayed Growth and Development related to lack of GH.
- Impaired Social Interaction related to short stature and peer acceptance.
- Chronic Low Self-Esteem related to discordant expectations by peers and adults.

Nursing Interventions

Providing Education and Evaluation

1. Teach method of injecting GH through written and verbal instructions. Give demonstration and encourage return demonstration.
2. Encourage rotation of sites in the subcutaneous tissue of the upper arms or thighs to prevent skin irritation and hypertrophy.
3. Document growth every 3 to 6 months while on therapy.
4. If poor growth response, evaluate for appropriate dose, compliance, and injection technique. There may be initial "catch-up" growth that will be exhibited by a growth velocity above normal.
5. Instruct patient and family to report adverse effects: severe headache, hip and knee pain, limp, increased thirst and urination.

Encouraging Social Interaction

1. Encourage the child to verbalize feelings regarding short stature.
2. Have the child describe what he or she likes about certain people to help the child understand that friendships and social value are based on personality traits rather than absolute height.
3. Suggest involvement in activities that do not use height as an advantage, such as music, art, and gymnastics.
4. Ask the child to identify behaviors that may deter socialization (may or may not be related to short stature) and find ways to change behavior.

Strengthening Self-Esteem

1. Help child and parents to identify age-appropriate behaviors and develop a plan for maintaining consistent behaviors in the home and socially.
2. Make sure parents have realistic expectations of child.
3. Encourage the use of positive feedback rather than punishment.

Community and Home Care Considerations

1. Become familiar with the GH preparation being used and develop a teaching plan for home injection (mixing and injection technique). Provide periodic evaluation and ongoing support.
2. If home injections are difficult relative to family learning or parental availability, attempt to include school nurse in administering daily injections.
3. Review storage and stability of GH product relative to manufacturer's specifications for the home as well as use in travel.

Family Education and Health Maintenance

1. Tell child and family that short stature is not a "disease."
   a. Growth often catches up with peers usually when peers have stopped growing.
   b. After initial startup of treatment, growth rate should be 4 to 5 inches (10 to 12 cm)/year in year 1 and 2¾ to 3½ inches (7 to 9 cm)/year thereafter.
   c. Treatment is not to make child tall; rather, its purpose is to optimize final height potential.

2. Review medication dosage and injection technique periodically.
3. Tell family to think of GH as a replacement that is essential rather than a medication; therefore, it should always be given regardless of illness or other medication therapies.
4. Encourage regular follow-up for growth evaluation and maintenance of therapy.
5. Discuss potential lifelong therapy, which may be necessary depending on the degree of deficiency. Many hypopituitary patients require lifelong replacement therapy.
6. Recommend counseling about probable infertility for female with Turner syndrome. This should be done with a genetic counselor, if available.

Evaluation: Expected Outcomes

- Growth rate in initial 2 years of therapy should be two to four times pretreatment growth velocity with final gain of one to two standard deviations in height.
- Child reports interest in school activities and playing with friends.
- Parents report more positive behavior relative to self-esteem.

DISORDERS OF THE POSTERIOR PITUITARY

The posterior pituitary is under the control of the hypothalamus and secretes two hormones, vasopressin (antidiuretic hormone [ADH]) and oxytocin. Abnormality of ADH function is the most common disorder seen in children. The function of ADH is to conserve water at the distal tubules and collecting ducts of the kidney and to act on smooth muscle to increase blood pressure (BP).

Diabetes insipidus

 Evidence Base Di Iorgi, N., Napoli, F., Allegri, A., et al. (2012). Diabetes insipidus—diagnosis and treatment. *Hormone Research in Paediatrics, 77*(2), 69–84.

Diabetes insipidus (DI) is failure of the body to conserve water due to a deficiency of ADH, decreased renal sensitivity to ADH, or suppression of ADH secondary to excessive ingestion of fluids (primary polydipsia).

Pathophysiology and Etiology

1. The function of water metabolism in the body is to maintain a constant plasma osmolality near the mean level of 287 mOsm/kg.
2. Intake and output of water are governed by the centers in the hypothalamus to control thirst and synthesis of ADH.
3. Thirst ensures adequate intake of water and ADH prevents water loss through the kidney.
4. Patients with DI are unable to produce appropriate levels or action of ADH, leading to polyuria, increased plasma osmolality, and increased thirst (see Figure 50-1).
5. Classified as central or nephrogenic DI:

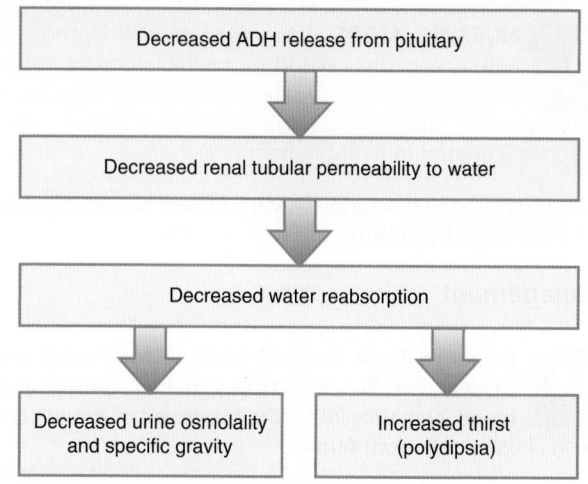

Figure 50-1. Mechanism of antidiuretic hormone (ADH) deficiency in diabetes insipidus.

a. Central DI—low levels of ADH; may be congenital or acquired.
   i. Congenital causes—CNS defects, hereditary.
   ii. Acquired causes—CNS tumors, head trauma (orbital trauma), infections, vascular disorders, idiopathic.
b. Nephrogenic DI—renal unresponsiveness to vasopressin; usually caused by chronic renal disease.
c. Acquired causes—dietary abnormalities such as primary polydipsia, decreased sodium chloride intake, severe protein restriction or depletion, sickle cell disease, drugs (alcohol, lithium, diuretics, medications such as tetracycline).

Clinical Manifestations

1. Sudden onset of excessive thirst and polyuria.
2. In infants:
   a. Excessive crying—quieted with water more than milk feeding.
   b. Rapid weight loss—caloric loss due to water preference over feedings.
   c. Constipation.
   d. Growth failure—weight loss, failure to thrive.
   e. Dehydration—sunken fontanelle, rapid heart rate, headache, fever, low blood pressure.
3. In children:
   a. More abrupt onset, excessive thirst and drinking, preference for ice water.
   b. Polyuria (usually more than 2 L/day) with nocturia and enuresis.
   c. Pale, dry skin with reduced sweating.
   d. Lethargy.

Diagnostic Evaluation

Tests document inability to produce ADH in the face of hyperosmolality of plasma.

1. Urine-specific gravity, sodium, and osmolality are decreased.
2. Serum osmolality and sodium are elevated.
3. Serum measurement of ADH is low in conjunction with high plasma osmolality.
4. Water deprivation test (potentially dangerous):
   a. Fluids are restricted and the urinary volumes and concentrations are monitored hourly along with the child's weight.
   b. Test is terminated if child loses more than 3% to 5% of body weight. Serum sodium and osmolality are measured at completion of test and are high; urine osmolality remains lower.
   c. Test is completed by giving the child a dose of ADH, which should stop the abnormal diuresis. If it does not, child may have nephrogenic DI.
5. Assess for underlying cause:
   a. MRI of hypothalamic–pituitary region.
   b. High incidence of associated anterior pituitary disorders.

Management

1. Daily replacement of ADH using desmopressin (DDAVP), a synthetic analogue.
2. Available as a metered nasal spray, measured insufflation (nasal) tube, or tablets. In children with cleft lip and palate, sublingual administration has been shown to be effective.
3. Thiazide diuretics in nephrogenic DI.

Complications

1. Dehydration.
2. Hypernatremia.
3. Adverse reactions to DDAVP therapy—hyponatremia and hypertension.

Nursing Assessment

1. Assess children with complaints or behaviors of polyuria and polydipsia for dehydration.
2. Obtain a thorough history of symptoms and behaviors—specific attention to changes in sleep patterns (may be caused by enuresis) and choices of fluids, including sources of water (eg, does child drink from toilet bowls or dog dishes?).
3. Evaluate height and weight—assess for weight loss related to possible decrease in calories due to excessive drinking, which decreases appetite.
4. For the child on treatment, assess for hydration status. Obtain history of fluid intake and output from the parents to assess appropriate dosage, frequency, and administration of medication.

Nursing Diagnoses

- Deficient Fluid Volume related to disease process.
- Imbalanced Nutrition: Less Than Body Requirements due to fluid preference over food.
- Disturbed Sleep Pattern related to nocturia and enuresis.

Nursing Interventions

Regaining Fluid Balance

1. Assess for and teach parents assessment of dehydration—dry mucous membranes, weight loss, increased pulse, listlessness or irritability, sunken fontanelle in infants, fever, poor skin turgor.
2. Administer fluid via intravenous (IV) route, as ordered, if acutely dehydrated.
3. Monitor intake and output and teach parents to maintain record of fluid intake and output in child. Reduced output may require restriction of fluids to prevent hyponatremia if overdosage of DDAVP is suspected.
4. Keep record of daily weight.

 NURSING ALERT Watch for and report signs of water intoxication due to excess free water and hyponatremia—drowsiness, listlessness, headache, confusion, anuria, weight gain. Hold DDAVP to prevent seizures, coma, and death.

5. Family education of DDAVP administration includes nurse demonstration and family administration. Proper management should eliminate symptoms.
6. Teach parents to provide free access to fluid (water) sources at all times. However, caution parents that child is unprotected from water excess.
7. Calculate rough estimated total daily (24-hour) fluid requirements based on body size to assess fluid replacement versus excess: 100 mL/kg for first 10 kg of body weight, 50 mL/kg for second 10 kg of body weight, 20 mL/kg for each additional kilogram.

Maintaining Adequate Nutrition

1. Make sure that adequate formula is ingested between plain water bottles.
2. For older child, provide liquid nutritional supplements.
3. Stress to parents or caregivers the importance of providing nutritional requirements with fluids to ensure meeting caloric demands for growth.
4. Consult with dietitian about need for vitamin or other supplements.
5. Monitor length and weight and developmental milestones at regular intervals.

Normalizing Sleep Pattern

1. Ensure adequate evening administration of DDAVP to prevent nighttime water craving and enuresis.
2. Suggest the use of diapers at night and plastic padding on bed to make controlling bedwetting easier until optimum management of condition is attained.
3. Encourage easy access to fluids and toilet or commode for older child during night.

Family Education and Health Maintenance

1. Teach family insufflation method (for infants and young children):
   a. Correct dose is measured and drawn up into catheter.
   b. Catheter is inserted into patient's nostril.
   c. Parent or patient inserts other end of catheter into mouth and gently blows.
   d. Older children may be able to inhale the solution.

2. Advise that nostrils should be as clear as possible before administration of dose.

3. Advise that, if dose is thought to be swallowed, do not readminister due to potential overdosage. Split the dose into both nares if swallowing is occurring.

4. Tell family to store drug away from heat and direct light and moisture (not in bathroom).

5. Advise parents that children should wear MedicAlert bracelet for DI.

6. Tell parents that school personnel should be aware of condition and symptoms needing attention (water intoxication).

7. Advise routine follow-up; treatment may be temporary or lifelong, depending on cause.

Evaluation: Expected Outcomes

- No signs of dehydration; intake equals output.
- No weight loss, growth curve maintained.
- Child sleeping through night.

DISORDERS OF THE THYROID GLAND

Under hypothalamic–pituitary regulation, the thyroid gland secretes thyroxine (T_4) and triiodothyronine (T_3). The action of these hormones promotes cellular growth and differentiation, protein synthesis, and lipid metabolism (cholesterol turnover). Lack of adequate thyroid hormones can affect mental development and sexual maturity. Function of the thyroid gland is controlled by a negative feedback mechanism utilizing TSH released from the pituitary gland (see Figure 50-2). Disorders of the thyroid gland are broadly classified as hypothyroidism and hyperthyroidism.

Hypothyroidism

Hypothyroidism is low circulating level of T_4. Congenital hypothyroidism occurs in 1 in 4,000 live births.

Pathophysiology and Etiology

1. Circulating levels of T_4 are dependent on hypothalamic–pituitary stimulation (TRH [thyrotropin-releasing hormone]/TSH) of the thyroid gland.

2. Low levels of T_4 cause an increase in TSH level.

3. Absent or decreased levels of T_4 result in abnormal development of the CNS of the neonate.

4. In older children, hypothyroidism results in a decrease in metabolism, growth, and physical maturation.

5. Congenital causes:
   a. Thyroid agenesis or dysgenesis.
   b. Hormone synthesis defect.
   c. Maternal thyroid antibodies crossing placenta.
   d. Iodine deficiency.
   e. Drug-induced destruction (thioamides for treatment of hyperthyroidism, iodide excess).
   f. Peripheral T_4 resistance.

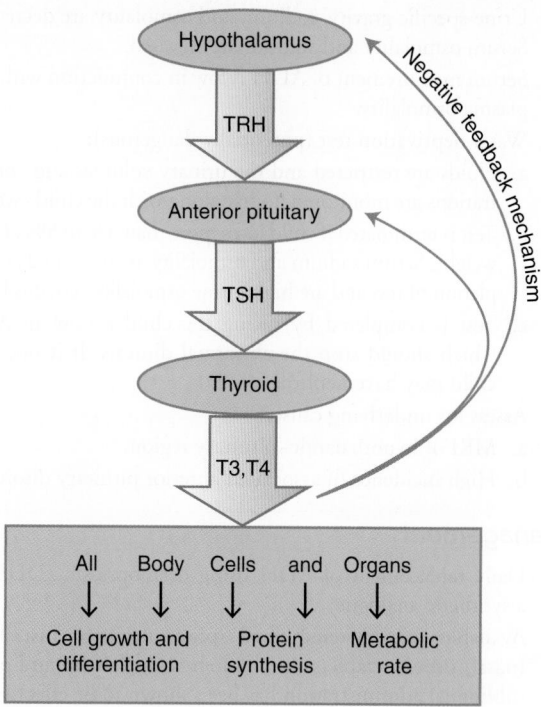

Figure 50-2. Normal thyroid hormone function.

6. Acquired (postnatal) causes:
   a. Autoimmune thyroiditis (Hashimoto's disease or chronic lymphocytic thyroiditis).
   b. Radiation.
   c. Surgical ablation (thyroidectomy).
   d. Antithyroid drugs.
   e. Iodine deficiency.
   f. Central hypothyroidism (TRH/TSH deficiency).

Clinical Manifestations

Neonates

1. Very subtle physical signs, if any.
2. Markedly open posterior fontanelle.
3. Prolonged physiologic jaundice.
4. Feeding difficulties.
5. Skin cool to touch, mottled.
6. Poor muscle tone—hypotonia, umbilical hernia.

After Age 6 Months

1. Growth failure.
2. Large, protruding tongue.
3. Coarse facial features.
4. Poor feeding and constipation.

Acquired Cases

1. Growth retardation—slow growth rate, increased weight gain.
2. Lethargy—obedient, nonaggressive, somnolent.
3. Cold intolerance.
4. Possible poor school performance.
5. Constipation.

Diagnostic Evaluation

1. Neonatal screening of TSH with backup T_4; elevation of TSH or a low T_4 may indicate congenital hypothyroidism.
   a. Testing is ideally done at 2 to 4 days of life or immediately before the neonate is discharged from the hospital. TSH levels in the first 24 to 28 hours of life may be falsely elevated.
   b. Abnormal screening test should be confirmed and treatment begun within 2 weeks after birth.

Evidence Base U.S. Preventive Services Task Force. (2008). Screening for congenital hypothyroidism (CH): U.S. Preventive Services Task Force reaffirmation recommendation statement. *Annals of Family Medicine, 6*(2), 166.

2. Thyroid nuclear scan—reduced uptake.
3. Abnormal growth rate.
4. Bone age x-ray; delayed.
5. Blood studies:
   a. Free T_4 decreased; TSH elevated.
   b. Thyroid antibodies—elevated in autoimmune thyroiditis.

Management

1. Replacement of thyroid hormone: levothyroxine.
2. Treatment must not be delayed.
3. Therapy goal is to maintain normalcy of thyroid function tests (free T_4, T_4, and T_3 concentrations) in the upper half of normal range.

Complications

1. Mental retardation in neonate who is undiagnosed or untreated.
2. Short stature, growth failure, and delayed physical maturation and development in the older child.

Nursing Assessment

1. Assess neonate for clinical manifestations listed above.
2. Perform behavioral assessment to include sleeping, eating, bowel patterns, level of alertness, and school performance.
3. Assess growth patterns: growth velocity (rate of growth over time), weight gain, and head circumference.

Nursing Diagnoses

- Delayed Growth and Development related to effects of hypothyroidism.
- Deficient Knowledge regarding hypothyroidism and its treatment.

Interventions

Evidence Base Allen, P. J., & Fomenko, S. D. (2011). Congenital hypothyroidism. *Pediatric Nursing, 37*(6), 324–326.

Promoting Growth and Development

1. Administer or teach parents to administer thyroid hormone replacement daily.
2. Discourage mixing thyroid medication with liquid in bottle that may not be completely finished during a feeding; instead, mix with small amount of fluid and give with dropper or syringe or crush tablet and place in teaspoon of infant food. Do not mix with soy formula.
3. If thyroid pill is being chewed rather than swallowed, have patient avoid brushing teeth immediately after to protect against rinsing away dose.
4. Monitor growth and developmental milestones at regular intervals.

Increasing Knowledge

1. Encourage the parents to verbalize feelings about child and the condition.
2. Educate the parents as to the importance of the therapy so child will grow and develop normally.
3. Stress that with replacement therapy, the child can participate in all usual activities.

Family Education and Health Maintenance

1. Encourage follow-up by a primary care provider or pediatric endocrinologist for blood studies to assess and monitor thyroid levels and evaluation of neurologic development to ensure adequate treatment and optimal cognitive development.
2. Make sure the family understands that therapy is usually lifelong. May do a 6-week trial off medication after age 3 under health care provider's supervision.
3. Support the parents and refer child for special testing and therapy if mental retardation is suspected.
4. Teach family the importance of avoiding overdosage of levothyroxine and of being alert for signs of overdosage (weight loss, restlessness, heat intolerance, fatigue, muscle weakness, tachycardia).

Evaluation: Expected Outcomes

- Growth curve and developmental milestones appropriate for age.
- Parents verbalize understanding and acceptance of therapy.

Hyperthyroidism

Hyperthyroidism is a disorder of the thyroid gland in which a high circulating level of T_4 results in abnormally increased body metabolism (thyrotoxicosis).

Pathophysiology and Etiology

1. May be caused by autoimmune process—thyrotropin receptor antibodies of a stimulating nature are produced.
   a. Graves' disease—most common cause of hyperthyroidism in children, affecting 1% to 2% of school-age children.
   b. Chronic thyroiditis—Hashimoto's disease; usually short-term hyperthyroidism before developing hypothyroidism.
2. Autoantibodies stimulate thyroid gland to produce and secrete T_4.

3. Elevated circulating thyroid hormone increases the body's metabolic rate, causing an increase in excitability of the neuromuscular, cardiovascular, and sympathetic nervous systems.
4. May also be caused by ingestion or overdosage of thyroid medication (iatrogenic) or pituitary adenoma (TSH initiated).

Clinical Manifestations

1. Thyromegaly—enlargement of the thyroid, possibly with a bruit.
2. Polyphagia with weight loss.
3. Exophthalmos, proptosis, lid retraction.
4. Hyperactivity—restlessness, nervousness, hand tremors, perspiration, sleeping disturbances, emotional lability; inability to concentrate, decreased school performance.
5. Heat intolerance, excessive diaphoresis.
6. Fatigue (proximal), muscle weakness.
7. Tachycardia, palpitations, wide pulse pressure.
8. Tall stature, underweight for height.

Diagnostic Evaluation

1. Serum thyroid function tests—elevated T_4, T_3 resin uptake with a suppressed TSH.
2. Microsomal antibodies—positive.
3. Thyroid radionuclide scan of goiter—rules out cold nodules that could indicate thyroid carcinoma.

Management

1. Propranolol, a beta-adrenergic blocking agent, for cardiac effects, antipyretics, and anxiolytics.
2. Inorganic iodide preparation, such as propylthiouracil or methimazole, to block release of thyroid hormone. Adverse effects include headache, nausea, diarrhea, skin rash, itching, liver disease, jaundice, arthralgia, and, rarely, agranulocytosis (severe leukopenia).
3. Radioactive ablation of thyroid gland using radioiodine—preferred over thyroidectomy. This is chosen when medical management is ineffective. Results in permanent hypothyroidism that requires treatment.

Complications

1. Development of a goiter (glandular enlargement due to overstimulation).
2. Cardiac problems of tachycardia and hypertension.
3. Exophthalmos—abnormal protrusion of the eyeball.

Nursing Assessment

1. Perform physical assessment to include temperature, heart rate, BP, height, and weight.
2. Obtain history of symptoms specific to onset and subsequent development of symptoms.
3. Elicit history of any changes in behavior, school performance, emotions, or sleep patterns.
4. Assess for presence of goiter—pain with swallowing or talking, palpation of thyroid.

Nursing Diagnoses

- Activity Intolerance related to effects of excessive metabolic activity.
- Imbalanced Nutrition: Less Than Body Requirements due to increased metabolic demand.
- Disturbed Sleep Pattern related to high metabolic rate.
- Fear related to radioiodine ablation of gland if therapy choice.

Nursing Interventions
Improving Activity Tolerance

1. Administer and teach parents to administer medications and comply with treatment to gradually lower the metabolic rate and improve activity tolerance.
2. Assess activity tolerance periodically. Ascertain if fatigue is present at rest, with activities of daily living, or with exercise. Promote relaxation and rest between activities.
3. Avoid overactivity.

Ensuring Adequate Diet

1. Encourage high-calorie, nutritious diet until thyroid hormone levels are stabilized to try to maintain weight.
2. Advise parents that effective treatment will lower metabolic rate and facilitate appropriate weight gain.
3. Periodically assess growth and development parameters.

Normalizing Sleep Pattern

1. Assess sleep pattern, including naps and sleeping through the night.
2. Adjust schedule to allow maximum amount of rest until sleeping through the night.
3. Allow short naps, as needed.

Reducing Fear

1. Encourage parents and child to verbalize fears related to the thyroid ablation.
2. Teach them about the procedure and clear up misconceptions.
   a. Ablation is accomplished through radioactive destruction of thyroid tissue by administration of a radioactive iodine pill.
   b. The thyroid gland is the only tissue in the body that absorbs iodine; therefore, the radiation only destroys thyroid tissue.
   c. Radiation will be eliminated through the child's urine and feces; precautions for disposal must be followed according to nuclear medicine department policies.
3. Tell them that the resultant effect will most likely be hypothyroidism, which can be managed with lifelong treatment of T_4 replacement.

Family Education and Health Maintenance

1. Review prescribed medications and their functions. Stress the importance of compliance.
2. Advise about periodic blood testing and monitoring for adverse effects of antithyroid medication.

DRUG ALERT Antihyperthyroid medications may cause agranulocytosis (severe leukopenia), thrombocytopenia, and aplastic anemia. Periodic blood testing is necessary to monitor blood counts. Agranulocytosis may present with sore throat and fever. Drug should be discontinued immediately and health care provider notified.

3. Educate family about possibility of oversuppression, from which hypothyroidism could develop.
4. If midday dose of medication is necessary, have family contact school nurse to coordinate dosing.
5. If gland is radioactively ablated, be certain family and other caregivers are appropriately instructed on storage and disposal of human waste after ablative therapy.
6. Encourage follow-up to monitor treatment through blood tests, growth and development evaluation, and size of thyroid gland.

Evaluation: Expected Outcomes
- The child can play normally without early fatigue.
- No weight loss noted.
- The child displays normal sleep patterns through the night as well as during naps.
- Parents and child verbalize understanding of radiation procedure and its rationale.

DISORDERS OF THE ADRENAL GLANDS

The adrenal glands are responsible for the life-sustaining production of mineralocorticoids (aldosterone) for sodium retention, glucocorticoids (cortisol) for blood glucose regulation, and androgens (Dehydroepiandrosterone [DHEA], androstenedione) for phallic and secondary sex characteristic development (adrenarche).

Adrenocortical insufficiency is the inability of the adrenal gland to produce aldosterone and cortisol due to adrenal failure or lack of adrenal stimulation. With the exception of congenital adrenal hyperplasia (discussed below), pediatric adrenocortical insufficiency is similar in adults (see page 934).

Hyperadrenalism, although rare in children, does occur, causing tissue to be exposed to excessive glucocorticoids (cortisol). This is commonly called *Cushing's syndrome*. Additionally, hyperfunction of the adrenal medulla, in which epinephrine, norepinephrine, and other catecholamines are secreted, is commonly seen in the disorder of pheochromocytoma. See pages 931 and 935 for a discussion of these conditions.

Congenital Adrenal Hyperplasia

Congenital adrenal hyperplasia (CAH) is the most common type of adrenocortical insufficiency in children. Adrenal dysfunction is a result of an enzyme deficiency in the steroid pathway converting cholesterol to cortisol, resulting in overproduction of androgens (sex hormones). The most common form of the condition is life-threatening and requires diagnosis and treatment soon after birth.

Pathophysiology and Etiology
1. Production of adrenal mineralocorticoids and glucocorticoids is blocked by an enzyme deficiency in the steroid pathway. "Blocks" may be severe or partial.
   a. Deficiency of 21-hydroxylase (90% to 95% of CAH cases)—insufficiency in cortisol and usually aldosterone production.
   b. Deficiency of 11-β-hydroxylase (5% to 8%)—insufficiency of cortisol and aldosterone; however, precursor block to aldosterone is a potent mineralocorticoid.
   c. Deficiency of 3-β-hydroxysteroid dehydrogenase (5%)—insufficiency in cortisol, aldosterone, and androgen production.
2. Due to lack of feedback suppression, ACTH and renin are secreted to stimulate adrenal gland production, causing hyperplasia of the gland.
3. Aldosterone insufficiency results in fluid and electrolyte imbalance.
   a. Loss of sodium at the kidney results in loss of fluid and an increase in serum potassium (cation exchange).
   b. Depletion of extracellular fluid leads to decreased BP.
   c. Low BP stimulates renin in the kidney to activate the adrenal aldosterone pathway.
4. Cortisol insufficiency results in diminished hepatic gluconeogenesis and tissue glucose uptake.
   a. Diminished production/secretion results in low blood sugar levels—more pronounced in times of stress.
   b. Low blood sugar, stress, or low cortisol stimulates feedback to hypothalamic–pituitary axis to release ACTH to stimulate adrenal activity, which also stimulates the release of melanocyte-stimulating hormone (MSH).
   c. Constant ACTH stimulation of gland causes overproduction and "backup" of blocked steroid pathways, resulting in "spillover" production of adrenal androgens.
5. Depending on etiology, overproduction of androgens will virilize female external genitalia or underproduction of androgens will block virilization of male external genitalia.

Clinical Manifestations
1. Ambiguous female genitalia—varying degrees of virilization due to exposure of androgens during development in utero:
   a. Clitoromegaly (may be penile shaped).
   b. Labial fusion (partial or complete).
   c. Rugated labia-appearing scrotal.
   d. Vagina may be incomplete, ending in a blind pouch.
2. Ambiguous male genitalia (3-β-dehydrogenase)—incomplete virilization development of external genitalia:
   a. Small phallic development.
   b. Incomplete scrotal fusion.
3. Hyperpigmentation (due to MSH secretion).
4. Dehydration.
5. Vomiting/poor feeding.
6. Shock.

7. Latent signs—basal cortisol levels are normal due to compensated chronic ACTH stimulation:
   a. Weakness, fatigue.
   b. Anorexia, nausea, diarrhea.
   c. Weight loss (failure to thrive).
   d. Hyperpigmentation.
   e. Hypotension/postural dizziness.
   f. Rapid growth rate—adrenal androgen effect.
   g. Premature adrenarche—pubic hair, axillary hair, acne, body odor.

Diagnostic Evaluation

Neonates

1. Pelvic ultrasound for identification of uterus, ovaries, or testes to determine true sex (internal development of gender-specific organs depends on presence or absence of Y chromosomal activity; external genital development depends on the presence or absence of androgens).
2. Karyotyping.
3. Serum electrolytes—sodium depletion.
4. Serum glucose levels—hypoglycemia.
5. Serum 17-hydroxyprogesterone (most common precursor to 21-hydroxylase)—elevated.

Latent Diagnosis

1. Rapid growth velocity, premature adrenarche.
2. Advanced bone age x-ray for chronologic age.
3. Elevated serum 17-hydroxyprogesterone.
4. Elevated plasma renin activity—compensated prevention of salt loss.

Management

1. Glucocorticoid replacement—physiologic production of cortisol is 15 to 20 mg/m² per day. Doses are individually dependent. Replacement is with hydrocortisone twice or three times per day or prednisone once per day when final growth has been achieved.
2. Mineralocorticoid replacement—aldosterone is replaced with fludrocortisone tablets at 0.05 to 0.20 mg daily.

 DRUG ALERT Overdosage of chronic corticosteroid use will result in growth failure. If child fails to grow and exhibits excessive hunger, corticosteroid dosing should be reviewed.

3. Added salt to the diet of neonates if salt loss is severe.
4. Surgical correction of ambiguous genitalia—can require multiple corrections over time.

Complications

1. Aldosterone insufficiency:
   a. Hyponatremia, hyperkalemia.
   b. Hypotension.
   c. Shock.
   d. Hypertension in 11-β-hydroxylase insufficiency in which aldosterone precursor is potent mineralocorticoid.
2. Cortisol insufficiency—hypoglycemia.

Nursing Assessment

Neonates

1. Assess genitalia for ambiguity.

 NURSING ALERT In male-appearing genitals, at least one testis must be palpated; if not, assumption must be that child is female with severe virilization. Notify health care provider so diagnostic evaluation can be initiated.

2. Assess for signs of hypoglycemia, hyponatremia, and hyperkalemia (see Box 50-1).
3. Assess feeding pattern of neonate.
4. Look for hyperpigmentation—may be subjective.

Latent Diagnosis of Child on Treatment

1. Assess growth and development.
2. Monitor vital signs; include sitting and recumbent BP for orthostatic changes.
3. Assess skin for hyperpigmentation.
4. Obtain history to include level of activity/fatigue, dietary history, salt craving, behavior, and school performance.

Nursing Diagnoses

- Fatigue related to hypoglycemia and electrolytic imbalances.
- Risk for Deficient Fluid Volume related to aldosterone deficiency.
- Deficient Knowledge related to risk of acute insufficiency.
- Anxiety of parents related to gender, sexual ambiguity, and chronic illness.

Nursing Interventions

Minimizing Fatigue

1. Administer glucocorticoids and emphasize compliance to increase energy level.
2. Encourage frequent rest periods and prevent overactivity.

BOX 50-1   Manifestations of Hyponatremia and Hyperkalemia

HYPONATREMIA
- Caused by dilution of sodium (Na⁺) when water intake exceeds output. Signs and symptoms occur when Na⁺ level falls below 120 mEq/L.
- Gradual fall: anorexia, apathy, mild nausea and vomiting
- Rapid fall: headache, mental confusion, muscular irritability, delirium, convulsions

HYPERKALEMIA
- Caused by a shift of potassium out of cells to compensate for decreased Na⁺ caused by an oliguric state. Usually asymptomatic, except for electrocardiogram (ECG) changes.
- ECG characteristics: (progressive) shortened QT interval; tall, peaked T waves; ventricular arrhythmias; degeneration of QRS complex; ventricular asystole or fibrillation.

3. Assess activity tolerance to determine adequacy of replacement therapy.

4. Tell family that child's activity level as well as growth rate should be normalized on therapy.
   a. If growth rate is too high, review corticosteroid dose and compliance with family.
   b. If growth rate is too low, overdosage of corticosteroid should be suspected.
   c. Review dosing with family.

Maintaining Fluid Balance

1. Assess fluid status and review history of fluid intake and output for appropriate volumes. Assess hydration status of child.

2. If child is vomiting and unable to take oral fluids and mineralocorticoids, administer IV fluids. Start with 5% dextrose in normal saline and monitor serum sodium level.

 NURSING ALERT No less than 0.5% normal saline should be infused in the child who is aldosterone deficient, due to the inability to retain mineralocorticoid replacement.

3. Emphasize compliance with mineralocorticoid replacement.

Preventing Acute Adrenocortical Insufficiency

1. Identify times of stress, such as acute infections, surgical procedures, or extreme emotional stress, which require increased corticosteroid replacement.

2. Teach the parents how to use and give intramuscular (I.M.) injections of hydrocortisone for stress management when oral supplementation is not possible due to vomiting.

3. Make sure that child is evaluated by the primary care provider and treated for the cause of stress.

Reducing Anxiety

1. Encourage parents to verbalize feelings regarding diagnosis, gender decisions or changes, and treatment plans.

2. Explain to the parents that the ambiguity is a result of the development process not being completed, rather than being a "mistake."

Family Education and Health Maintenance

1. Stress and reinforce the function of and need for constant replacement of adrenal steroid therapy to maintain normal daily activities.

2. Encourage parents to obtain a MedicAlert bracelet, which indicates steroid dependency, for the child.

3. Facilitate instructions to school nurse to notify parents and health care provider of signs of illness and for emergency injection of hydrocortisone should it become necessary.

4. Explain to parents and child why pubic hair may be developing and encourage discussion with teachers and school officials to prevent embarrassment of child in the locker room and other situations.

Evaluation: Expected Outcomes

- Parents report child is more active.
- No signs of dehydration.

- Parents verbalize understanding when to call health care provider or when to use emergency hydrocortisone injection; parents also demonstrate correct technique for hydrocortisone injection.
- Parents verbalize understanding of disorder and need for reconstructive surgery.

DISORDERS OF GONADAL FUNCTION

Proper gonadal function is necessary for developing sexual maturation (puberty). The process involves the hypothalamic release of gonadotropin-releasing hormone (GnRH), which in turn stimulates the pituitary to release LH and FSH. In turn, these stimulate the gonads to produce and release the gonadal steroid testosterone from the testes in males or estrogen from the ovaries in females. The actions of these steroids lead to the development of secondary sexual characteristics and maturation.

Delayed Sexual Development

 Evidence Base Palmert, M., & Dunkel, L. (2012). Delayed puberty. *New England Journal of Medicine*, 355(5), 443–453.

Delayed sexual development is the lack of pubertal development or progression.

Pathophysiology and Etiology

1. Lack of production or secretion of gonadal steroids from the testes (testosterone) or ovaries (estrogen), due either to the lack of pituitary stimulation (secondary delayed sexual development) or to gonad dysfunction (primary delayed sexual development).

2. Primary delayed sexual development—absence or dysfunction of the gonads.
   a. 45 XO Turner syndrome (chromosomal variants).
   b. Sporadic gonadal dysgenesis.
   c. Bilateral gonadal failure due to radiation, chemotherapy, infection, defect in gonadal steroid synthesis, trauma.

3. Secondary delayed sexual development—lack of hypothalamic–pituitary stimulation to gonads.
   a. Hypothalamic lesions due to infections, trauma, irradiation, or isolated deficiency of GnRH (Kallmann's syndrome).
   b. Pituitary lesions due to infection, trauma, or irradiation; also hypopituitarism or isolated LH and FSH deficiencies.

4. Failure of end organs to respond to circulating gonadal steroid—androgen insensitivity.

5. Other causes include chronic illness, anorexia nervosa, and autoimmune atrophy.

6. Resultant effect is failure to achieve sexual maturity.

Clinical Manifestations

1. Females—lack of breast development by age 13 or failure to progress through puberty.

2. Males—lack of testicular enlargement by age 14 or failure to progress through puberty.
3. Emotional lability.

Diagnostic Evaluation

1. Bone age x-ray to determine physical age—pubertal delay is not consistent with bone age.
2. Laboratory measurement of sex steroids (testosterone and estrogen) and gonadotropins (LH, FSH).
   a. Gonadal failure will show elevated LH and FSH with low estrogen.
   b. No good test is available to distinguish isolated gonadotropin deficiency (LH or FSH).
3. End organ insensitivity (lack of gonadal steroid receptor)—sex steroid and gonadotropins will be elevated. Hypothalamic receptors for feedback inhibition are the same as the end organ receptors; therefore, there is no hypothalamic "shut-off."
4. Abdominal ultrasound to view internal organ structure and development.

Management

1. Replacement of gonadal steroid—should be as close to the physiologic level as possible; however, maximal adult height may be compromised due to potential adverse effect of acceleration of skeletal maturation.
   a. Males—testosterone supplement; 50 to 100 mg monthly by injection until final height is achieved, then 200 mg monthly.
   b. Females—conjugated estrogen 0.3 to 0.625 mg daily by oral tablet. When appropriate, a progestational agent is added to the therapy for normal periods to occur. An alternative is the use of birth control pills that have the combination of estrogen and progesterone.
2. There is no pituitary or hypothalamic agent for use in secondary gonadal failure.

Complications

1. Sterility.
2. Ambiguity—in androgen insensitivity, male genital development does not respond to circulating level of testosterone from testes; may result in mistaken gender assignment.
3. Potential for dysfunctional dormant gonad to become malignant.

Nursing Assessment

1. Assess growth and development, particularly height.
2. Assess sexual development at regular intervals.

Nursing Diagnoses

• Delayed Growth and Development related to lack of sexual development.
• Disturbed Body Image related to delayed sexual maturation.
• Chronic Low Self-Esteem related to delayed sexual maturation.

Nursing Interventions

Promoting Sexual Development

1. Administer or teach self-administration of medication, as prescribed.
2. Teach technique for I.M. injections of testosterone enanthate. Watch return demonstration.
3. Stress compliance with prescribed dose and not to exceed recommended dose. Excessive use of testosterone will stunt potential statural growth.

Improving Body Image

1. Discuss strategies for assisting the child to become more comfortable with appearance and ways that may minimize appearance of physical delay in sex characteristics.
2. Stress the importance of cautious therapy to prevent loss of potential height, therefore making sexual development a slow process.

Improving Self-Esteem

1. Encourage child to discuss self-concept; list positive and negative characteristics.
2. Explore ways to strengthen and add to positive characteristics.
3. Encourage participation in age-appropriate activities and social functions.

Family Education and Health Maintenance

1. Teach the patient about adverse effects of testosterone replacement—possible behavioral changes (aggressiveness, moodiness) and an increase in acne.
   a. Suggest over-the-counter acne products or referral to dermatologist if indicated.
   b. Alert family to report behavioral changes to the health care provider.
2. Teach the patient taking estrogen replacement the importance of daily compliance. Missed doses could result in breakthrough bleeding or spotting due to drop in circulatory estrogen levels. Alert patient to notify health care provider if spotting does occur with estrogen replacement.
3. In both treatments, stress to child not to exceed prescribed dose to prevent loss of final adult height.

Evaluation: Expected Outcomes

• At follow-up visit, there is an increase in height and progression of sexual development.
• Child verbalizes improved feelings of body image.
• Child lists more positive concepts of self.

Advanced Sexual Development and Precocious Puberty

Advanced sexual development is secondary sexual development earlier than the normal timing for a child's maturation. There is abnormal early production and secretion of the gonadal steroids or adrenal androgens. Normal pubertal development occurs abnormally early. Skeletal maturation is also advanced under presence of sex steroids and adrenal androgens.

Pathophysiology and Etiology

Central Precocious Puberty

1. Central precocious puberty (CPP)—early activation of the hypothalamic–pituitary gonadotropin axis.
2. May be idiopathic or caused by:
   a. Tumors of hypothalamus/pituitary.
   b. Cranial irradiation.
   c. Trauma.
   d. Infection—meningitis.
   e. Hydrocephalus.
3. Most common form of precocious puberty.

Peripheral Precocious Puberty

1. Peripheral precocious puberty (PPP)—sex hormone production at the glandular level independent of central stimulation.
2. Ovarian PPP caused by estrogen-producing tumors or cysts.
3. Testicular PPP caused by androgen- and estrogen-producing tumors or autonomous production of testosterone.
4. Adrenal PPP caused by enzyme defects (CAH) or androgen- and estrogen-producing tumors.

Other Causes

1. Hypothyroidism.
2. Exogenous estrogen or androgen exposure.

Clinical Manifestations

1. Males:
   a. Testicular enlargement (4 mL): younger than age 9½.
   b. Tanner stage II pubic hair: younger than age 9.
   c. Tanner stage III pubic hair: younger than age 10.
2. Females:
   a. Breast bud (stage II): younger than age 8.
   b. Tanner stage III pubic hair: younger than age 8½.
   c. Menarche: younger than age 9½.
3. In both sexes, rapid growth (increased growth velocity) evident.

Diagnostic Evaluation

1. Physical assessment—Tanner staging:
   a. If adrenarche is present without thelarche (breast development) or testicular enlargement, adrenal cause is likely.
   b. In females, if only thelarche is present, ovarian or exogenous estrogen involvement is likely.
   c. If adrenarche and pubarche (gonadal signs) are present, central cause is likely.
2. Skeletal x-ray for bone age—usually advanced. Pubertal stage development is usually commensurate with bone age maturation.
3. Laboratory analysis:
   a. Gonadal steroid levels—may be elevated; however, secretion is diurnal early in development.
   b. Elevated gonadotropins to GnRH stimulation if CPP. Basal levels are frequently unreliable. Lack of elevation of gonadotropins may indicate peripheral source.
   c. Thyroid function to rule out hypothyroidism.
4. MRI of head to rule out central etiology.
5. Ultrasound of abdomen, pelvis, testes for presence of cysts or tumors.

Management

For CPP, most common form of advanced sexual development in children.

1. Goal is to inhibit puberty to preserve psychosocial well-being and to delay epiphyseal closure to maximize adult height.
2. GnRH agonist—down-regulates GnRH receptors of the pituitary against endogenous GnRH.
   a. Nafarelin—intranasal spray, twice daily.
   b. Leuprolide—daily subcutaneous injection.
   c. Depot-leuprolide —monthly I.M. injection.
   d. Histrelin—subcutaneous daily injection.

 DRUG ALERT I.M. injections of leuprolide have, rarely, been linked to sterile abscesses. The site should not be reused and the health care provider should be notified immediately if abscess occurs.

3. Progestins.
   a. Medroxyprogesterone injections—biweekly I.M. injections.
   b. Medroxyprogesterone tablets—oral daily dosing.

Complications

1. Complications of underlying tumor.
2. Behavioral problems.
3. Short stature for final height due to early epiphyseal closure.

Nursing Assessment

1. Assess sexual development using Tanner scale.
2. Obtain history of when signs and symptoms began with specific attention to chronology of events.
3. Perform psychosocial assessment relative to peer relations.
4. While child is on treatment, perform ongoing assessment of height and sexual characteristics.

Nursing Diagnoses

- Disturbed Body Image related to early presence of secondary sexual characteristics.
- Deficient Knowledge regarding maturing body and sexuality.
- Disturbed Personal Identity due to societal height expectations versus appropriate age-related expectations.

Nursing Interventions

Fostering Positive Body Image

1. Encourage the child to verbalize concerns regarding body development changes.
2. Stress to child that the changes are normal events that peers will go through; however, they are occurring early.
3. Teach the child that therapy will halt the process and soon peers will catch up.

Teaching about the Effects of Treatment

1. Assist and encourage parents to teach the child about sexual development to reduce fear of the unknown.
2. Encourage proper hygiene practices for body odor, hair growth, and menses.

3. Teach administration techniques for medication treatment, including intranasal, I.M., or subcutaneous administration, as indicated.

4. In GnRH-agonist treatment in females, instruct child and parents that it takes 10 to 12 days to fully down-regulate the pituitary receptors. The suppression results in a fall of estrogen and may cause breakthrough bleeding or even a period to occur. This will happen only once if child remains suppressed on therapy.

Promoting Sense of Identity

1. Encourage the child and parents to discuss normal age-related behaviors and identify inappropriate behaviors that are associated with society's expectations of advanced height and development.

2. Encourage the child to wear age-appropriate clothing, participate in age-appropriate activities, and socialize with peers.

3. Suggest counseling, as needed.

Family Education and Health Maintenance

1. Encourage follow-up at regular intervals while on treatment and, if condition is not treated, to monitor progress and address behavioral issues.

2. Discuss with parents that child may act out relative to advancing pubertal development. (This may include masturbation.) This behavior needs to be dealt in an understanding way, not necessarily through punishment.

3. Encourage parents to meet with school personnel regarding potential embarrassment in a locker room situation; alternatives to changing clothes in front of peers may be necessary.

4. Prepare family for the start of menstruation if puberty is advanced. The school nurse may need to assist with feminine hygiene during the cycle. Parents may need to meet with the nurse to plan for assistance during school days.

5. Teach family to inspect injection sites and notify health care provider immediately upon noticing a hard, painful, reddened area, which may be a sterile abscess from Lupron injections and require treatment.

6. Teach family to maintain strict adherence to hormonal therapy. Failure to maintain suppression of gonadotropins can result in relative rise in estrogen. Subsequent suppression may cause breakthrough bleeding.

Evaluation: Expected Outcomes

- Child accepts body changes through verbalization at follow-up visits.
- Parents or child give adequate return demonstration of I.M. injection; verbalizes understanding of sexual development.
- Child participates in school activities and socializes with peers of same age.

DISORDERS OF THE PANCREAS

The pancreas manufactures powerful enzymes for digestion as well as the hormones insulin and glucagon. These hormones are manufactured and secreted from cell clusters called the islets of Langerhans. Glucagon and insulin regulate the amount of sugar that is present in the bloodstream. Glucagon is a potent counter-regulatory hormone that raises the blood sugar by foster-ing the release of glucose from stores in the liver. Insulin stimulates glucose uptake by peripheral tissues, inhibits lipolysis, and inhibits hepatic glucose production.

Type 1 Diabetes Mellitus

Evidence Base American Diabetes Association. (2013). Clinical practice recommendations: Standards of medical care in diabetes. *Diabetes Care, 36*(suppl. 1), s11–66.

American Association of Clinical Endocrinologists. (2011). Medical guidelines for clinical practice for developing a diabetes mellitus comprehensive care plan. *Endocrine Practice, 17*(Suppl. 2), 1–53.

Diabetes mellitus (DM) is a disorder of glucose intolerance caused by deficiency in insulin production and action, resulting in hyperglycemia and abnormal carbohydrate, protein, and fat metabolism. In younger and school-age children, most cases are type 1, formerly called juvenile-onset or insulin-dependent DM. Type 1 DM affects as many as 1 in 500 children.

Type 2 DM (formerly called adult-onset or noninsulin-dependent DM) traditionally was found in only about 2% of cases of diabetes in children and adolescents. This is rapidly changing, and type 2 diabetes now accounts for up to 40% of cases of diabetes diagnosed in adolescents. Etiology suggests morbid obesity, sedentary lifestyle, high caloric intake, and family history of diabetes. There is also an increased risk in black, Hispanic, and Native American populations. The onset of pubertal development and the insulin resistance that is characteristic of puberty may be a factor in the onset of type 2 diabetes in susceptible adolescents. Type 2 DM is discussed in Chapter 25.

Pathophysiology and Etiology

1. Etiology for type 1 DM suggests genetic and environmental or acquired factors, association with certain human leukocyte antigen types, and abnormal immune responses, including autoimmune reactions.

2. Autoimmune destruction of the islets of Langerhans in the pancreas which secrete insulin, resulting in insulin deficiency.

3. Because insulin facilitates glucose transport into cells, glucose builds up in the bloodstream, causing hyperglycemia.

4. As the kidneys attempt to lower blood glucose levels, glycosuria and polyuria result, with electrolyte excretion.

5. Because the body cells are unable to use glucose for energy, protein and fat are broken down.

6. Fat metabolism results in a buildup of ketones and acidosis.

7. Diabetic ketoacidosis (DKA) occurs in 20% to 40% of patients at the time of diagnosis. Also, DKA at diagnosis is more common in children under 5 years of age and in children who have limited or no access to medical care. It is a potentially fatal condition characterized by hyperglycemia, ketonemia, ketonuria, and metabolic acidosis (pH less than 7.3, bicarbonate less than 15 mEq/L) and caused by insulin deficiency. In children with established T1DM, there is an increased incidence of DKA in those individuals with poor metabolic control, children who omit insulin doses or when caregivers omit doses of their child's insulin, children with

psychiatric or eating disorders, peripubertal or adolescent girls, and interruption or failure of insulin pump therapy.

Clinical Manifestations

Onset is rapid (usually over a period of a few weeks).

Major Symptoms

1. Increased thirst.
2. Increased urination, enuresis.
3. Increased food ingestion.
4. Weight loss.
5. Fatigue.

Minor Symptoms

1. Skin infections.
2. Dry skin, poor wound healing.
3. Monilial vaginitis in adolescent females.

Diabetic Ketoacidosis

1. Hyperglycemia, polyuria, and polydipsia.
2. Dehydration, decreased skin turgor.
3. Nausea, vomiting, generalized malaise, weakness.
4. Kussmaul respirations (rapid, deep, sighing), fruity or acetone breath odor, altered level of consciousness (LOC), confusion.

Diagnostic Evaluation

1. Criteria for diagnosis of type 1 and type 2 DM are the same: fasting blood glucose of more than 126 mg/dL on two occasions (different day); random blood glucose of more than 200 in the presence of symptoms (polydipsia, polyphagia, polyuria); glucose >200 following 2 hour oral glucose tolerance test; random hemoglobin A1C ≥6.5% (less sensitive and has not been validated in children).

 Evidence Base Kapadia, C. (2013). Are the ADA hemoglobin A criteria relevant for the diagnosis of type 2 diabetes in youth? *Current Diabetes Reports*, 13(1), 51–55.

2. Glycosuria or ketonuria on routine examination may arouse suspicion of diabetes.
3. Evaluation for metabolic acidosis with acute presentation (pH less than 7.3 and bicarbonate less than 14 mEq/L).
4. Hemoglobin A1c testing every 3 months to determine long-term plasma glucose control is dependent on age. Children, especially young children, are at high risk for hypoglycemia and are at low risk for complications prior to puberty. Goals are age-dependent.
   a. Toddlers, children <6 years: <8.5% (<8% if hypoglycemia is avoided).
   b. Children ages 6 to 12: less than 8%.
   c. Adolescents ages 13 to 19: less than 7.5%. (A lower goal may be reasonable if excessive hypoglycemia does not result.)
5. Screening for celiac disease should be done at the time of diagnosis and if disease is detected, child should be referred to a pediatric gastroenterologist. A gluten-free diet is recommended for children with celiac disease.
6. Thyroid function is also recommended at the time of diagnosis.

Management

1. Insulin therapy (see Table 50-2).
   a. New insulin analogs provide more options for insulin duration and frequency of administration. Basal insulins, such as glargine and detemir, provide a duration of up to 24 hours without a pronounced peak of action. Rapid-acting insulins, such as lispro, glulisine, and aspart, offer rapid onset with shorter duration.
   b. Dosage needs are based on the child's weight, diet, and level of activity. Dosages are adjusted through daily monitoring of blood glucose levels.
   c. Insulin pump therapy, consisting of a continuous subcutaneous infusion of insulin that can be programmed to give bolus and basal rates, may be used by some children.
2. Treatment of DKA (see Box 50-2).
   a. I.V. fluid therapy to increase perfusion and glucose uptake in the periphery which will reduce hyperglycemia; also increases glomerular filtration and reverses acidosis.
   b. Regular I.V. insulin administration at a rate of 0.1U/kg/hour after initial fluid replacement. Provide I.V. dextrose solution as plasma glucose decreases, titrate rate of insulin infusion to achieve a rate of glucose decline of 50 to 150mg/dL per hour.
   c. Bicarbonate is not indicated; acidosis will correct with adequate insulin infusion.
   d. Close monitoring of vital signs, electrocardiogram, mental status, and neurologic system.
   e. Replacement of electrolytes--sodium, potassium, ionized calcium.

 Evidence Base Rosenbloom, A. L. (2010). The management of diabetic ketoacidosis in children. *Diabetes Therapy*, 1(2), 103–120.

3. Balanced diet with controlled carbohydrates and adequate protein and fat to meet energy and growth requirements.

Table 50-2	Types of Insulin and Their Effects		
TYPE OF INSULIN	**ONSET (MINUTES)**	**MAXIMAL ACTIVITY (HOURS)**	**DURATION (HOURS)**
Aspart	10–20	1–3	3–5
Glulisine	2–5	1	2
Lispro	<15	0.5–1.5	6–8
Regular	30–60	2–4	6–8
Semilente	30–60	2–4	10–12
NPH	120	4–12	24
Lente	120	8–10	24
Ultralente	4–8 hours	14–20	36
Detemir	Slow	3–6	6–11
Glargine	≥60	N/A	≥24

N/A, not applicable.

BOX 50-2   Treatment of Diabetic Ketoacidosis

INITIATE IV FLUIDS

- Start with 0.9% normal saline (NS) solution.
- Estimate fluid deficit by amount of weight loss (2.2 lb [1 kg] equals 1 L of fluid). Infuse fluids to replace one half of estimated loss plus maintenance needs (10 to 20 mL/kg) over first 8 to 12 hours; second half plus maintenance needs over next 16 to 36 hours.
- When blood glucose falls below 250 mg/dL, change to 5% glucose in 0.45% NS solution.
- Closely monitor vital signs, electrocardiogram (ECG), and intake and output, and obtain laboratory values, including urine and blood glucose, electrolytes, blood urea nitrogen and creatinine, serum osmolarity, arterial or venous pH, serum and urine ketones, calcium, and phosphorus every 1 to 4 hours as condition warrants.

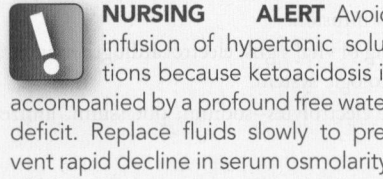 **NURSING ALERT** Avoid infusion of hypertonic solutions because ketoacidosis is accompanied by a profound free water deficit. Replace fluids slowly to prevent rapid decline in serum osmolarity, which may precipitate cerebral edema.

ADMINISTER INSULIN

- Give IV bolus of 0.1 unit/kg of regular insulin if no intermediate-acting insulin has been given in the past 6 to 8 hours.
- Provide continuous IV drip of regular insulin at rate of 0.1 unit/kg/hour.
- Continue IV insulin until metabolic acidosis is corrected (pH greater than 7.3 and bicarbonate greater than 13 to 15) and bowel sounds have returned and can take oral fluids.
- When meals are tolerated, begin subcutaneous short-acting or rapid-acting insulin at least 30 minutes before discontinuing IV insulin.
- When stabilized, return to previous insulin regimen or begin therapy using conventional dosing (intermediate-acting insulin with short-acting insulin) or basal-bolus therapy (basal insulin with rapid-acting insulin)

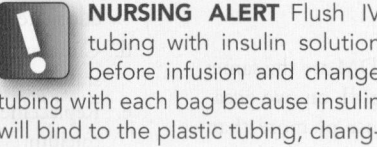 **NURSING ALERT** Flush IV tubing with insulin solution before infusion and change tubing with each bag because insulin will bind to the plastic tubing, changing concentration.

POTASSIUM AND BICARBONATE REPLACEMENT

- Initial serum K levels will be normal or high even though intracellular levels are low. Serum levels will fall as insulin therapy drives K into the cells.
- Begin replacement of K when urine output and renal function have been established.
- Add KCl 20 to 40 mEq to each liter of fluid.
- Monitor T waves on ECG for peaking (hyperkalemia) or flattening (hypokalemia).
- Bicarbonate administration is controversial in correcting acidosis but may be indicated for respiratory depression, decreased myocardial contractility, or refractory, severe acidosis.

Complications

Acute

1. Usually reversible.
2. DKA accounting for 70% of diabetes-related deaths in children younger than age 10.
3. Cerebral edema—related to treatment of DKA; thought to be due to a rapid decline in blood glucose causing a fluid shift in the brain.
4. Hyperglycemia (untreated or undertreated).
5. Hypoglycemia (insulin reaction).

Subacute

Develops over a short period.
1. Lipohypertrophy (localized tissue buildup from giving injections in the same site)—repeated injections in the same area; can cause abnormal absorption.
2. Skeletal and joint abnormalities—limited joint mobility.
3. Growth failure and delayed sexual maturation due to underinsulinization.

Chronic

Very rarely seen in children, but develop after years to decades with inadequate treatment.

1. Retinopathy/cataracts—may cause blindness.
2. Neuropathy—peripheral and autonomic.
3. Nephropathy—proteinuria/renal failure.
4. Cardiopathy—heart failure.

Nursing Assessment

1. When child first presents with suspected DM:
   a. Obtain history of onset of signs and symptoms of clinical manifestations.
   b. Assess for levels of dehydration and weight loss with level of appetite.
   c. Check for sores that are slow to heal.
   d. Identify any fruity smell to breath—acetone breath due to ketosis.
   e. Assess abdominal pain—may mimic appendicitis.
2. For child with DKA:
   a. Assess for potential cerebral edema (diminished LOC) on presentation and when fluid replacement is initiated. Fluid replacements precede and are then concurrent with insulin therapy.
   b. Assess cardiac function—tachycardia with dehydration, arrhythmias related to potassium imbalances.

c. Assess renal function—urine output with intake and output, ketonuria, glycosuria.

d. Watch for hypoglycemia—overtreatment of insulin; glucose level correction should be slow. IV replacements frequently contain glucose to prevent large osmotic fluid shifts leading to cerebral edema.

3. During treatment/routine follow-up:

a. Assess growth parameters—excessive weight gain may indicate overtreatment of insulin (child eats due to constant hunger). Loss or lack of weight gain may indicate underinsulinization (losing calories that are not metabolized).

b. Review blood glucose diaries and glucose monitor for level of control and need for insulin adjustments. (Check for appropriate adjustments of insulin made by parents.) Glucose should be checked before meals (preprandial) and at bedtime. Optimal levels are age related.

   i. Toddlers and children under age 6: 100 to 180 mg/dL preprandial; 110 to 200 mg/dL at bedtime.

   ii. Children ages 6 to 12: 90 to 180 mg/dL preprandial; 100 to 180 mg/dL at bedtime.

   iii. Adolescents ages 13 to 19: 90 to 130 mg/dL preprandial; 90 to 150 mg/dL at bedtime.

c. Obtain history of any hypoglycemic reactions—be specific to time of day, dietary record, and exercise and activity.

d. Assess injection sites—look for signs of lipohypertrophy.

e. Assess for signs of hyperglycemia—polyuria, polydipsia. Does child need to get up during the night to go to the bathroom?

Nursing Diagnoses

- Deficient Fluid Volume related to osmotic diuresis and vomiting.
- Imbalanced Nutrition: Less Than Body Requirements due to metabolic catabolism due to lack of insulin.
- Deficient Knowledge related to insulin management.
- Deficient Knowledge related to blood glucose monitoring.
- Risk for Unstable Blood Glucose.
- Fear/Anxiety of child and family related to diagnosis, treatment, and management procedures.

Nursing Interventions

Restoring Fluid Balance

1. Administer IV fluids, as ordered.
2. Monitor intake and output, BP, serum electrolyte results, and daily weight.
3. Report abnormal sodium and potassium results promptly.
4. Assess for signs of dehydration—dry skin and mucous membranes, constipation.
5. Encourage oral fluids when able.

Meeting Nutritional Requirements

1. Provide an adequate diet for the child and teach the family about the diet.

a. The most common meal plan is one based on carbohydrate counting. This type of meal plan offers flexibility and a wide variety of choices. Total carbohydrate requirements will be calculated, then labels can be read and charts consulted to determine grams of carbohydrate per serving of food eaten. Insulin dosage is based on the total amount of carbohydrates eaten; for example, 1 unit of short- or rapid-acting insulin for every 15 g of carbohydrate.

b. Occasionally, a more rigid, strictly controlled diet is necessary.

c. The diet should be composed of approximately 55% carbohydrate, 30% fat, and 15% protein.

   i. Some diets are restricted in carbohydrates, saturated fats, and cholesterol and may be based on the exchange method as recommended by the American Diabetes Association.

   ii. Approximately 70% of the carbohydrate content should be derived from complex carbohydrates such as starch.

   iii. Foods with high fiber content should be encouraged.

   iv. All diets must supply sufficient caloric intake for activity and growth, sufficient protein for growth, and the required vitamins and minerals.

d. Foods are distributed throughout the day to accommodate varying peak action of insulin. Distribution may be adjusted for increased or decreased amounts of exercise.

e. Include fluids containing sugar (sodas, juices, milk) in carbohydrate count.

2. Determine the child's usual dietary habits so that adherence to the controlled diet will be easier.

3. Include the child and parents in meal planning as soon as possible.

4. Allow the child normal activity while hospitalized so that the observed result of the dietary control will be valid. Because the child's activity level usually decreases during the hospital stay, the child and family must understand that the insulin and dietary needs will alter on discharge.

5. Allow the child to eat with other children.

6. Make certain that the child adheres to the prescribed diet and understands the rationale for it.

7. Refer family to a dietitian for additional planning and education.

Increasing Knowledge About Insulin Administration

1. Insulin should be given, as directed. Rapid-acting insulin analogues lispro and aspart begin to work immediately and should be given right before the meal. If taking regular insulin, the child should not eat until 20 to 30 minutes after injection is given.

2. Be aware of the major types of insulin and their effects.

3. Develop a systematic plan for injections that emphasizes rotation of sites (Figure 50-3, page 1676).

a. The upper arms and thighs are the most acceptable sites for injection in children, but the outer areas of the abdomen or hips may also be used.

b. Subsequent injections are given about 1 inch (2.5 cm) apart.

c. Guidelines for site location:

   i. Arms—begin below the deltoid muscle and end one handbreadth above the elbow. Begin at the midline and progress outward laterally, using the external surface only.

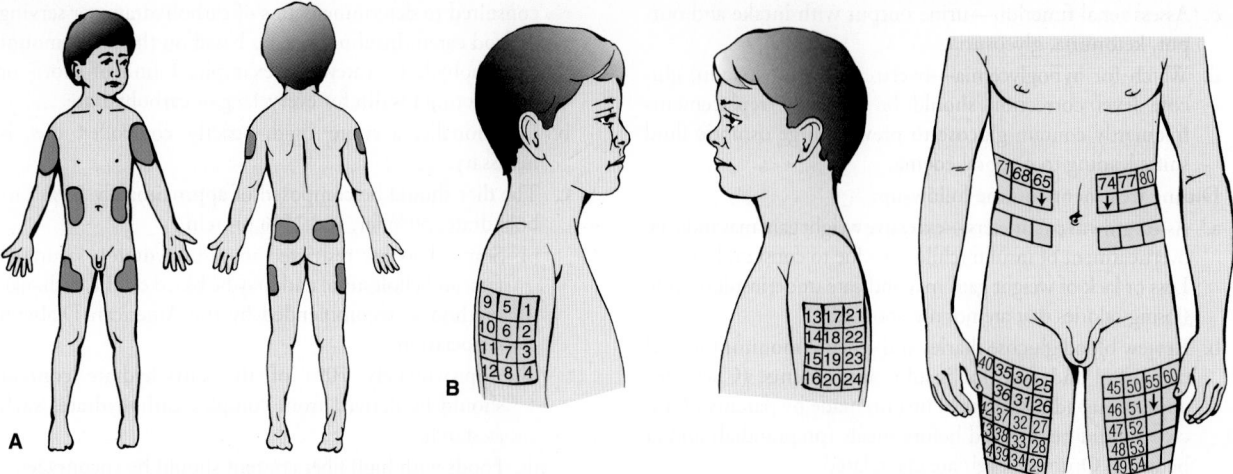

Figure 50-3. (A) Insulin injection sites are the upper outer portions of the arms, the thighs, and the abdominal area. **(B)** Injection sites are rotated, with subsequent injections given about 1 inch (2.5 cm) apart.

ii. Thighs (see Figure 50-4, page 1676)—begin one handbreadth below the hip and end one handbreadth above the knee. Begin at the midline and progress outward laterally, using only the outer, anterior surface.

iii. Abdomen—avoid the beltline and 1 inch (2.5 cm) around the umbilicus.

iv. Buttocks—use the upper outer quadrant of the buttocks.

4. Be certain that the measuring scale of the syringe matches the unit strength on the bottle of insulin. U-100 insulin is preferred because it allows the smallest possible amount to be given. Other concentrations of insulin are rarely used.

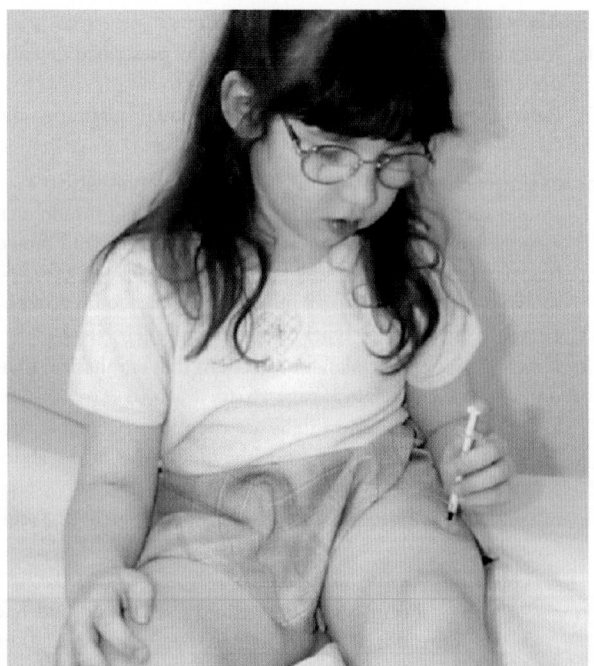

Figure 50-4. Insulin injection by a child.

5. Opened bottles of insulin may be stored at room temperature or in the refrigerator. Open bottles should be discarded after 28 days. Use insulin that is at room temperature.

a. The bottle in use may be kept at room temperature for approximately 1 month without losing appreciable strength.

b. Extra bottles should be stored in the refrigerator.

6. Insulin pens (either prefilled or using insulin cartridges) are increasing in popularity. Pens are generally kept at room temperature once opened and discarded after 28 days; check the manufacturer's directions. All insulin pens require an "air shot" (clearing air from pen) prior to giving *each* dose.

7. Mix insulin solutions, such as NPH and Ultralente, thoroughly by shaking the bottle (rolling may not be effective).

8. Administer insulin subcutaneously. Do not aspirate.

9. Observe the skin closely for signs of irritation. Avoid the injection site for several weeks if signs of local irritation are observed.

10. Observe the skin for a rash indicating an allergic reaction to the insulin (rare with newer preparations). Notify the health care provider immediately if there is an allergic reaction.

11. Be aware of factors that vary the need for and utilization of insulin, particularly exercise and infection.

a. Exercise tends to lower the blood sugar level. Encourage normal activity, regulated in amount and time.

b. Infection or illness increases the child's insulin requirement (insulin is still administered during illness). Be alert for signs of infection and dehydration.

12. Encourage the child to express feelings about the injections. The child may be helped to master fear of injections by gaining control of the situation through play and active participation in the procedure.

 DRUG ALERT None of the basal insulins (detemir, glargine, or glusiline) have been approved by the Food and Drug Administration for mixing with any other insulin.

Providing Information About Blood Glucose Monitoring

1. Teach child and parents the chosen method for blood glucose monitoring.
2. The procedure requires a drop of blood (obtained by fingerstick), a reagent strip, and a glucometer.
3. Specific instructions for performing the procedure vary with the equipment being used and must be followed explicitly.
4. Blood glucose measurements are usually made four times per day—before meals and at bedtime.
5. Additional blood tests are helpful during episodes of hypoglycemic symptoms or other problem situations.
6. Urine tests for ketones should be performed if the child is ill or if blood glucose level is greater than 240 mg/100 dL.
7. Record the results of blood glucose testing accurately.
   a. Use a standard form for recording so that the information will be clear and readily available.
   b. Help the child to understand how the disease is controlled by teaching the child to test his or her own blood, record results, and report information to health care personnel or parents.

Identifying and Controlling Hypoglycemia

1. Have glucagon available for injection if a hypoglycemic reaction occurs and the child is unconscious, has a seizure or is unable to swallow liquids safely, or is combative. Administer 0.5 to 1 mg I.M. or subcutaneously and assess response.
2. Teach family the causes, signs and symptoms, and treatment for hypoglycemia.
   a. Common causes:
      i. Overdose of insulin.
      ii. Reduction in diet or increased exercise without sufficient caloric coverage.
   b. Symptoms:
      i. Trembling, shaking, dizziness.
      ii. Sweating, apprehension.
      iii. Tachycardia.
      iv. Hunger, weakness.
      v. Drowsiness, unusual behavior.
      vi. Mental confusion.
      vii. Seizures, coma.
   c. Be prepared to give glucose tablets, orange juice, sugar cubes, or another food containing readily available simple sugars.
3. Watch for a pattern of activity or time of day that precedes hypoglycemic reactions and work with family to alter behavior to prevent reactions.
4. If prescribed, teach the child and family how to use an emergency glucagon injection kit.
5. If glucagon is not available and the child is unresponsive, activate the emergency response system (911).

Reducing Fear and Anxiety

1. Explain the need and purpose of every test to child and parents. Allow child to vent feelings and cry if fearful. When appropriate, demonstrate procedures on yourself first (eg, fingersticks for glucose testing, allowing parent to give saline injection for practice of insulin injection).
2. Teach family the pathophysiology of diabetes. Understanding the disease process aids in understanding the treatment and signs and symptoms. Assess knowledge level of teaching by having family verbalize knowledge of disease management.
3. Allow parents to verbalize feelings related to the expectations of their performance. Stress that the learning is through the actual "hands-on" management. Assist the parents in performing the needed tasks (fingersticks, insulin injections) to build their confidence. Give the parents clear objectives and directions for home management.
4. Stress that the child's condition is now the family's condition as well. Only foods appropriate for the child should be in the home. Stress that child does not need "special foods" different from the rest of the family.
5. Caution the parents that the focus on the child may cause sibling rivalry. Encourage involvement by all family members in making the home a healthy one and urge the parents to give individual attention to nondiabetic children as well.
6. Explain to child that he or she did not cause the disease to occur—young children usually blame themselves for "bad" things that happen to them. Help the child understand that good management is the key to participating in all usual activities. The perspective should be that he or she is a "child with diabetes," not a "diabetic child."

Community and Home Care Considerations

1. Perform home assessment for adequate nutritional resources.
2. Reteach and assess family's adherence to insulin administration and blood glucose monitoring.
3. Reteach and assess family's ability to respond to hypoglycemia.
4. Make sure that school is able to follow through with management plan for insulin administration, planned exercise and mealtimes, and responding to hypoglycemia.
5. When child is ill, evaluate for dehydration, hyperglycemia, and ketonuria. Teach family how to monitor condition, maintain insulin coverage, and notify the health care provider. (See "Diabetes sick-day guidelines," page 966).

Family Education and Health Maintenance

Patient or parental education is one of the most important aspects in the nursing care of the child with diabetes. Thorough instruction is essential in the following areas:

1. Influence of exercise, emotional stress, and other illnesses on insulin and diet needs.
2. Recognition of the symptoms of insulin shock and diabetic acidosis and knowledge of related emergency management.
3. Prevention of infection:
   a. Attend to regular body hygiene, with special attention to foot care.
   b. Report any breaks in the skin. Treat them promptly.
   c. Use only properly fitted shoes; do not wear vinyl or plastic, which do not permit ventilation. Avoid calluses and blisters. Teach child not to walk barefoot.
   d. Dress the child appropriately for the weather.
   e. See that the child receives regular dental checkups and maintenance every 6 months.
   f. Follow routine immunizations according to the recommended schedule; receive yearly flu vaccination.

4. Precautionary measures:
   a. Have the child carry an identifying card that states that he or she has diabetes and includes name, address, telephone number, and health care provider's name and telephone number.
   b. Suggest a simple, convenient source of sugar that can be carried easily by the child or parents in a pocket, purse, or backpack to have available for hypoglycemic symptoms. A good example is glucose tablets, glucose gel, five sugar cubes, or cake decorating gel that comes in a tube.
   c. Help the family discuss the child's disease with the school nurse and other responsible adults who are in close contact with the child (eg, teachers, scout leaders).
   d. Advise parents that vials of insulin should be kept on one's person when traveling because baggage may be subjected to extreme temperatures and pressures incompatible with the stability of insulin. If necessary, a thermos can be used to keep the insulin at the appropriate temperature.

5. Follow up with primary care provider or pediatrician for immunizations, all regular health checkups, and growth and development evaluations.

6. For additional information and support, refer to agencies, such as American Diabetes Association, ATTN: National Call Center, 1701 N. Beauregard Street, Alexandria, VA 22311, 800-DIABETES, *www.diabetes.org*; and Juvenile Diabetes Research Foundation International, 26 Broadway, New York, NY 10004; 800-JDF-CURE, *www.jdrf.org*.

Evaluation: Expected Outcomes

- No signs of dehydration.
- Parents and child describe consistent meal plan.
- Child and parents demonstrate correct insulin administration technique.
- Child and parents demonstrate correct glucose monitoring technique.
- Child and parents verbalize causes, signs and symptoms, and treatment for hypoglycemia.
- Child and parents speak openly about diabetes, ask appropriate questions, display no crying.

SELECTED REFERENCES

Abduljabbar, M., & Afifi, A. (2012). Congenital hypothyroidism. *Journal of Pediatric Endocrinology & Metabolism, 25*(1-2), 13–29.

Acerini, C., Albanese, F., Casey, A., et al. (2012). Initiating growth hormone therapy for children and adolescents. *British Journal of Nursing, 21*(18), 1091–1097.

Allen, P. J., & Fomenko, S. D. (2011). Congenital hypothyroidism. *Pediatric Nursing, 37*(6), 324–326.

Amer, K. S. (2005). Advances in assessment, diagnosis, and treatment of hyperthyroidism in children. *Journal of Pediatric Nursing, 20*(2), 119–126.

American Association of Clinical Endocrinologists Growth Hormone Task Force. (2003). Medical guidelines for clinical practice for growth hormone use in adults and children. *Endocrine Practice, 9*(1), 64–76.

American Diabetes Association. (2013). Clinical practice recommendations: Diabetes care in the school and daycare setting. *Diabetes Care, 36*(suppl. 1), s75–s79.

American Diabetes Association. (2013). Clinical practice recommendations: Standards of medical care in diabetes. *Diabetes Care, 36*(suppl. 1), s11–s66.

American Diabetes Association. (2013). Third-party reimbursement for diabetes care, self management education, and supplies. *Diabetes Care, 36*(suppl. 1), s98–99.

Bondy, C. A. (2007). Care of girls and women with Turner syndrome: A guideline of the Turner syndrome study group. *Journal of Clinical Endocrinology and Metabolism, 92*(1), 10–25.

Cook, D. M., & Rose, S. R. (2012). A review of guidelines for use of growth hormone in pediatric and transition patients. *Pituitary, 15*(3), 301–310.

Copeland, K., Silverstein, J., Moore, K., et al. (2013). Clinical Practice Guideline: Management of Newly Diagnosed Type 2 Diabetes Mellitus (T2DM) in Children and Adolescents. Pediatrics (published online January 28, 2013). Available: *http://pediatrics.aappublications.org/content/early/2013/01/23/peds.2012-3493*.

Copland, W., Shanahan, L., Miller, S., et al. (2010. Outcomes of early pubertal timing in young women: A prospective population based study. *American Journal of Psychiatry, 167*(10), 1218–1225.

Crocker, M. K., & Kaplowitz, P. (2010). Treatment of pediatric hyperthyroidism but not hypothyroidism has a significant effect on weight. *Clinical Endocrinology, 73*(6), 752–759.

D'Adamo, E., & Caprio, S. (2011). Type 2 diabetes in youth: Epidemiology and pathophysiology. *Diabetes Care, 34*(Suppl. 2), S161–S165.

Demirbilek, H., Kandemir, N., Gonc, E. N., et al. (2009). Assessment of thyroid function during the long course of Hashimoto's thyroiditis in children and adolescents. *Clinical Endocrinology, 71*, 451–454.

Di Iorgi, N., Napoli, F., Allegri, A., et al. (2012). Diabetes insipidus—diagnosis and treatment. *Hormone Research in Paediatrics, 77*(2), 69–84.

Endocrine Society. (2006). *Evaluation and treatment of adult growth hormone deficiency: An Endocrine Society clinical practice guideline.* Chevy Chase, MD: Author.

Fuhrman, B., & Zimmerman, J. (2011). *Pediatric critical care.* Philadelphia: Elsevier.

Garvey, K., Wolpert, H., Rhodes, E., et al. (2012). Health care transition with patients with Type 1 Diabetes: Young adult experiences and relationship to glycemic control. *Diabetes Care, 35*(8), 1716–1722.

Global International Diabetes Federation/International Society of Pediatric and Adolescent Diabetes. (2011). Guideline for diabetes in childhood and adolescence. Available: *www.ispad.org/NewsFiles/IDF-ISPAD_Diabetes_in_Childhood_and%20Adolescence_Guidelines_2011.pdf*.

Kapadia, C. (2013). Are the ADA hemoglobin A criteria relevant for the diagnosis of type 2 diabetes in youth? *Current Diabetes Reports, 13*(1), 51–55.

Kaplowitz, P. B. (2010). Subclinical hypothyroidism in children: Normal variation or sign of failing thyroid gland? *International Journal of Pediatric Endocrinology.* Available: *www.ijpeonline.com/content/2010/1/281453*.

Kester, L., Hey, H., Hannon, T. (2012). Using Hemoglobin A1c for prediabetes and diabetes diagnosis in adolescents: Can adult recommendations be upheld for pediatric use? *Journal of Adolescent Health, 50*(4), 321–323.

Kirk, J. (2012). Indications for growth hormone therapy in children. *Archives of Disease in Childhood, 97*(1), 63–68.

Rosenbloom, A. L. (2010). The management of diabetic ketoacidosis in children. *Diabetes Therapy, 1*(2), 103–120.

U.S. Preventive Services Task Force. (2008). Screening for congenital hypothyroidism in newborns: Clinical summary of U.S. preventive services task force recommendation (AHRQ Publication No. 08-05109-EF-3). Rockville, MD: Agency for Healthcare Research and Quality. Available: *www.ahrq.gov/clinic/uspstf08/conhyposum.htm*.

51
Pediatric Oncology

PEDIATRIC ONCOLOGIC DISORDERS

 Evidence Base National Cancer Institute. (2011). A snapshot of pediatric cancer. Bethesda, MD: Author. Available: *www.cancer.gov/aboutnci/servingpeople/snapshots/pediatric.pdf.*

Cancer is the leading cause of death from disease in children ages 1 to 14. It affects approximately 1 to 2 out of 10,000 children annually in the United States. The incidence of specific cancers is related to age, gender, and ethnic background.

Common types of cancer in children (in order of frequency) include leukemia, central nervous system (CNS) cancers, lymphoma, neuroblastoma, rhabdomyosarcoma, Wilms' tumor, bone cancer, and retinoblastoma. Treatment modalities include surgery, radiation and chemotherapy, blood and marrow transplant, immunotherapy, and gene therapy (see Chapter 8, page 134). See Chapter 43 for general nursing care of the sick or hospitalized child.

Acute Lymphocytic Leukemia

 Evidence Base Meenaghan, T., Dowling, M., & Kelly, M. (2012). Acute leukemia: making sense of a complex blood disorder. *British Journal of Nursing, 21*(2), 76–83.

Acute lymphocytic leukemia (ALL) is a primary disorder of the bone marrow in which the normal marrow elements are replaced by immature or undifferentiated blast cells. When the quantity of normal marrow is depleted below the level necessary to maintain peripheral blood elements within normal ranges, anemia, neutropenia, and thrombocytopenia occur. ALL is the most common malignancy in children, occurring in 3 to 4 out of 100,000 children younger than age 15. It is more common among white and Hispanic children and is more common in boys than in girls.

Pathophysiology and Etiology

1. The exact cause of ALL is unknown.
2. Environmental factors, including viral agents, as well as genetic factors and chromosomal abnormalities are suspected in some cases.
3. ALL results from the growth of an abnormal type of non-granular, fragile leukocyte in the blood-forming tissues, particularly in the bone marrow, spleen, and lymph nodes.
4. The abnormal lymphoblast has little cytoplasm and a round, homogeneous nucleus (see Figure 51-1, page 1680).
5. ALL is classified according to the cell type involved: T lymphoblasic leukemia or B lymphoblastic leukemia.
6. Normal bone marrow elements may be displaced or replaced in this type of leukemia.
7. The changes in the blood and bone marrow result from the accumulation of leukemic cells and from the deficiency of normal cells.
   a. Red blood cell (RBC) precursors and megakaryocytes from which platelets are formed are decreased, causing anemia, prolonged and unusual bleeding, tendency to bruise easily, and petechiae.
   b. Normal white blood cells (WBCs) are significantly decreased, predisposing the child to infection.
   c. The bone marrow is hyperplastic, with a uniform appearance caused by leukemic cells.
8. Leukemic cells may infiltrate into lymph nodes, spleen, and liver, causing diffuse adenopathy and hepatosplenomegaly.
9. Expansion of marrow or infiltration of leukemic cells into bone causes bone and joint pain.
10. Invasion of the CNS by leukemic cells may cause headache, vomiting, cranial nerve palsies, convulsions, coma, papilledema, and blurred or double vision.
11. Weight loss, muscle wasting, and fatigue may occur when the body cells are deprived of nutrients because of the immense metabolic needs of the proliferating leukemic cells.

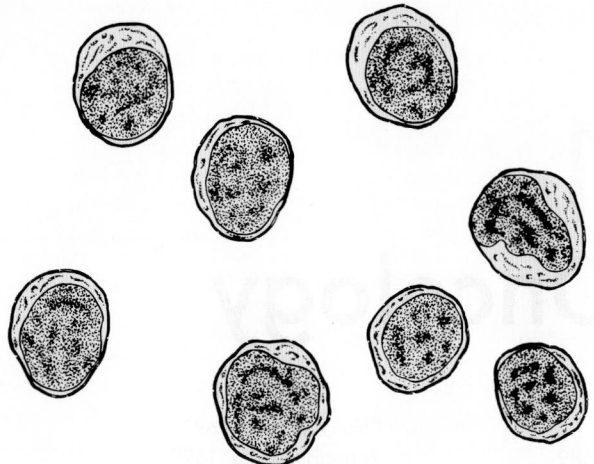

Figure 51-1. Abnormal lymphoblast in acute lymphocytic leukemia.

Clinical Manifestations

1. Manifestations depend on the degree to which the bone marrow has been compromised and the location and extent of extramedullary infiltration.
2. Presenting symptoms:
   a. Fatigability.
   b. General malaise, listlessness.
   c. Persistent fever of unknown cause.
   d. Recurrent infection.
   e. Petechiae, purpura, and ecchymoses after minor trauma.
   f. Pallor.
   g. Generalized lymphadenopathy.
   h. Abdominal pain caused by organomegaly.
   i. Bone and joint pain.
   j. Headache and vomiting (with CNS involvement).
3. Presenting symptoms may be isolated or in any combination or sequence.

Diagnostic Evaluation

1. May have altered peripheral blood counts. Blood studies may show the following:
   a. Low hemoglobin level, RBC count, hematocrit, and platelet count.
   b. Decreased, elevated, or normal WBC count.
2. Bone marrow examination and stained peripheral smear examination show large numbers of lymphoblasts and lymphocytes.
3. Lumbar puncture to assess for lymphoblasts in CNS to determine CNS involvement.
4. Renal and liver function studies determine contraindications or precautions for chemotherapy.
5. Chest x-ray determines whether a mediastinal mass or pneumonia is present.
6. Varicella and cytomegalovirus titer determine risk of infection.
7. The CNS and testes are sites of "sanctuary"; CNS treatment and surveillance is standard and testes are evaluated with physical examinations.

Management

1. Supportive therapy is indicated to control such disease complications as hyperuricemia, electrolyte imbalance, infection, anemia, bleeding, pain, nausea/vomiting, and fatigue.
2. Specific therapy is warranted to eradicate malignant cells and to restore normal marrow function.
3. Chemotherapy is used to achieve complete remission, with restoration of normal peripheral blood and physical findings; it is administered through an indwelling central catheter or implantable port. See Table 51-1.
4. Although no universally accepted standard therapy for the treatment of children with ALL exists, most facilities have similar protocols that use a combination of drugs.
5. Components of therapy:
   a. Induction, the initial course of therapy designed to achieve complete remission, usually includes a combination of vincristine, L-asparaginase, and corticosteroids. A fourth drug, such as daunorubicin, doxorubicin, or cytosine arabinoside, may be added.

Table 51-1	Commonly Used Chemotherapeutic Agents to Treat Acute Lymphocytic Leukemia
CHEMOTHERAPEUTIC AGENT	**COMMON SIDE EFFECTS**
Asparaginase	Pain at injection site Allergic reaction Increased plasma ammonia level Clotting factor abnormalities Fatigue, weakness Diarrhea
Cytarabine	Nausea, vomiting Fever Headache
Methotrexate	Nausea, vomiting Headache Elevated liver enzymes
Vincristine	Hair loss Neuropathy Constipation
Daunorubicin	Nausea, vomiting Hair loss Red urine Bone marrow suppression Cardiac dysfunction
Cytoxan	Nausea, vomiting Hair loss Loss of appetite Gonadal dysfunction Bone marrow suppression
Mercaptopurine	Bone marrow suppression
Thioguanine	Bone marrow suppression

b. CNS prophylaxis generally consists of intrathecal administration of methotrexate alone or in combination with hydrocortisone and cytarabine. Craniospinal irradiation may also be used to treat CNS disease.

c. Consolidation treatment, a period of intensified treatment immediately after remission induction, attempts total eradication of leukemic cells. It usually includes a combination of methotrexate, 6-mercaptopurine, etoposide, cytosine arabinoside, cyclophosphamide, prednisone, vincristine, L-asparaginase, and doxorubicin or daunorubicin.

d. Maintenance or continuation therapy prevents reappearance of the disease (usually continued for approximately 2½ to 3 years; boys require longer maintenance therapy to prevent testicular relapse). It usually includes daily oral administration of 6-mercaptopurine and weekly oral or I.M. administration of methotrexate with intermittent administration of other drugs, such as vincristine, corticosteroids, cyclophosphamide, cytosine arabinoside, or daunorubicin.

e. Reinduction therapy induces remission if relapse occurs and usually includes the same initial drugs. Sometimes, however, additional agents may be added.

f. If testicular relapse occurs, radiation therapy to the testicles is administered.

6. Current standards of treatment are designed on risk-based criteria; patients with worse prognostic indicators receive more intensive therapy.

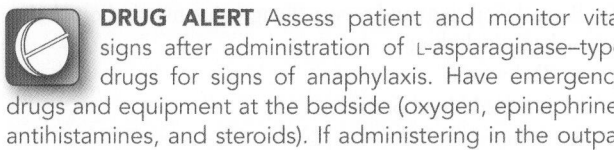

DRUG ALERT Assess patient and monitor vital signs after administration of L-asparaginase–type drugs for signs of anaphylaxis. Have emergency drugs and equipment at the bedside (oxygen, epinephrine, antihistamines, and steroids). If administering in the outpatient setting, observe patients for at least 1 hour.

7. Blood and marrow transplantation has been used successfully to treat children who fail to respond to conventional treatment.

Prognosis

1. At least 98% of children with ALL can be expected to achieve an initial remission if treated in a specialized facility.
2. Overall 5-year survival is 90%.
3. The prognosis becomes poorer with each relapse the child experiences.
4. Relapse is rare after 7 years from diagnosis.
5. Factors associated with prognosis:
   a. Initial WBC count (WBC count >50,000 has worse prognosis).
   b. Age (younger than age 2 and older than age 10 have poorer prognosis, and infants younger than age 1 have even worse prognosis).
   c. Extramedullary involvement (poorer prognosis).
   d. Type of leukemia cytogenetic factors and immunophenotype (DNA index, karyotype).

Complications

1. Infection—most frequently occurs in the blood, lungs, GI tract, or skin. Patients with central lines are at increased risk.
2. Hemorrhage—usually caused by thrombocytopenia.
3. CNS involvement.
4. Bony involvement.
5. Testicular involvement.
6. Urate nephropathy (rarely seen except in induction).
7. Acute complications of treatment (eg, cardiomyopathy).
8. Late effects of treatment (treatment-specific). Most frequent long-term complication is neurocognitive dysfunction causing school difficulty.

Nursing Assessment

1. Obtain a history.
   a. When taking the history, focus on symptoms that led to the diagnosis and previous symptoms for the past 2 weeks. For example, inquire about fatigue, headache, nausea, vomiting, pallor, bleeding, pain, or fever.
   b. Ask about past history of varicella zoster infection (chickenpox), which could lead to disseminated infection if acquired during immunosuppression. Also ask about recent exposures, including sibling exposures.
2. Perform a physical examination, including:
   a. Examination of skin for petechiae, purpura, and ecchymoses.
   b. Palpation of lymph nodes for enlargement, tenderness, and mobility.
   c. Palpation of spleen and liver for enlargement.
   d. Examination of fundi to detect papilledema with CNS disease.
   e. Inspection of skin for areas of infection, including indwelling catheter sites.
   f. Auscultation of lungs for crackles or rhonchi, indicative of pneumonia.
   g. Temperature for fever.
3. Assess family coping mechanisms and use of resources such as support systems.

NURSING ALERT Report changes in behavior or personality, persistent nausea, vomiting, headache, lethargy, irritability, dizziness, ataxia, convulsions, or alterations in state of consciousness. These may be signs of CNS disease or relapse. CNS relapse is usually caught on routine screening.

Nursing Diagnoses

- Anxiety of parents related to learning of diagnosis.
- Risk for Infection and hemorrhage related to bone marrow suppression caused by chemotherapy and disease.
- Disturbed Body Image related to alopecia associated with chemotherapy.
- Imbalanced Nutrition: Less than Body Requirements related to anemia, anorexia, nausea, vomiting, and mucosal ulceration secondary to chemotherapy or radiation.

- Acute Pain related to diagnostic procedures, progression of the disease, and adverse effects of treatment.
- Activity Intolerance related to fatigue that results from the disease and treatment.
- Anxiety of child related to hospitalization and diagnostic and treatment procedures.

Nursing Interventions

Decreasing Parental Anxiety

1. Be available to the parents when they want to discuss their feelings.
2. Offer kindness, concern, consideration, and sincerity toward the child and parents; be a source of consolation.
3. Contact the family's clergyman or the hospital chaplain.
4. Obtain the services of a social worker, as appropriate, to help the family use appropriate community resources.
5. Offer hope that therapy will be effective and will prolong life.
6. Have parents speak with parents of a child currently on therapy.
7. Encourage parents to participate in activities of daily living to help them feel a part of their child's care.
8. Assess family dynamics and coping mechanisms and plan interventions accordingly.
9. Help the parents to deal with anticipatory grief.
10. Help the parents to deal with other family members and friends.
11. Encourage the parents to discuss concerns about limiting their child's activities, protecting child from infection, disciplining child, and having anxieties about the illness.
12. Facilitate communication with the clinic nurse or clinical specialist who may interact with the child during the entire course of illness.
13. Encourage parents to continue established family patterns, including school attendance, social life, and family activities, as medically indicated.

Preventing Infection and Hemorrhage

 Evidence Base Alexander, S., Nieder, M., Zerr, D., et al. (2012). Prevention of bacterial infection in pediatric oncology: What do we know, what can we learn? *Pediatric Blood & Cancer, 59*(1), pp. 16–20.

1. Monitor complete blood count (CBC), as ordered.
2. Provide adequate hydration.
   a. Maintain parenteral fluid administration.
   b. Offer small amounts of oral fluids, if tolerated.
3. Observe renal function carefully.
   a. Measure and record urine output.
   b. Check specific gravity.
   c. Observe the urine for evidence of gross bleeding.
   d. Use labsticks to determine if occult urinary bleeding is present.
4. Protect the child from infection sources.
   a. Never use a rectal thermometer, suppositories, or enemas when caring for a neutropenic patient.

b. Family, friends, personnel, and other patients who have infections should not visit or care for the child. Discuss care of siblings while child is on therapy.
c. Private rooms are preferred, but if it is necessary to share, do not place a child with an infection in the same room with a child with leukemia.
d. Good handwashing is the most important way to control infection.

5. Observe the child closely and be alert for signs of impending infection.
   a. Observe broken skin or mucous membrane for signs of infection.
   b. Report fever of more than 101° F (38.3° C).
   c. Assess central line site for redness or tenderness.

 NURSING ALERT Patients with low WBC count may not respond to infection with usual signs and symptoms (ie, fever and purulent drainage from infected wound).

6. Administer growth factors, such as granulocyte colony-stimulating factor, to stimulate the production of neutrophils and to decrease the incidence of severe infections in the child after high-dose chemotherapy.
7. Administer IV antibiotics, as ordered.
8. Administer PCP prophylaxis, such as co-trimoxazole, if ordered, twice daily three times per week to prevent infection with *Pneumocystis carinii*. (Dapsone and pentamidine are also given for patients unable to take co-trimoxazole.)
9. Record vital signs and report changes that may indicate hemorrhage, including:
   a. Tachycardia.
   b. Lowered blood pressure.
   c. Pallor.
   d. Diaphoresis.
   e. Increasing anxiety and restlessness.
10. Observe for GI bleeding and Hematest all emesis and stool.
11. Move and turn the child gently because hemarthrosis may occur and may cause pain.
    a. Handle the child in a gentle manner.
    b. Turn the child frequently to prevent pressure ulcers.
    c. Place the child in proper body alignment in a comfortable position.
    d. Allow the child to be out of bed in a chair if this position is more comfortable.
    e. Encourage the child to ambulate, if possible.
12. Avoid I.M. injections, if possible; if not possible, ensure platelet count has been obtained prior to injection and hold pressure to the area for at least 5 minutes.
13. Handle catheters and drainage and suction tubes carefully to prevent mucosal bleeding.
14. Protect the child from injury by monitoring activities and exposure to environmental hazards, such as slippery floors or uneven surfaces.

15. Be aware of emergency procedures for control of bleeding:
    a. Apply local pressure carefully so as not to interfere with clot formation.
    b. Administer leukocyte-poor, irradiated, packed RBCs and platelets, as ordered.

Promoting Acceptance of Body Changes

1. Prepare patient for potential changes in body image (alopecia, weight loss, muscle wasting) and help child cope with related feelings.
2. Engage Child Life therapist for medical play and support.
3. Contact the school nurse and teacher to help them prepare for the child's return to school. Discuss the bodily changes that have occurred and that may happen in the future.

Promoting Optimal Nutrition

Evidence Base Bauer, J., Jurgens, H., & Fruhwald, M. C. (2011). Important aspects of nutrition in children with cancer. *Advances in Nutrition, 2*(2), 67–77.

1. Provide a highly nutritious diet as tolerated by the child.
    a. Determine the child's food likes and dislikes.
    b. Offer frequent, small meals.
    c. Offer high-calorie, high-protein supplemental feedings.
    d. Encourage the parents to assist at mealtime.
    e. Allow the child to eat with a group at a table if his or her condition allows.
    f. Avoid foods high in salt while child is taking steroids.
    g. Administer enteral and parenteral feeds, as ordered.
2. Give careful oral hygiene; the gums and mucous membranes of the mouth may bleed easily.
    a. Use a soft toothbrush.
    b. If the child's mouth is bleeding or painful, clean the teeth and mouth with a moistened cotton swab or sponge-tipped swab.
    c. Use a nonirritating rinse for the mouth (no alcohol-containing mouthwash or sodium bicarbonate).
    d. Apply petroleum to dry, cracked lips.
    e. Assess for mucositis and provide appropriate mouth rinse.
3. Be alert for nausea and vomiting.
    a. Administer anti-emetic drugs on a round-the-clock, regular schedule (eg, serotonin antagonist, dexamethasone).
    b. Become knowledgeable about chemotherapeutic agents and adjust anti-emetic therapy for those drugs with delayed nausea and vomiting.
    c. Monitor strict intake and output.
    d. Maintain parenteral fluid administration and assess for signs of dehydration or overhydration.
    e. Administer anti-emetic drugs for patients who receive radiation to the chest, abdomen, pelvis, or craniospinal axis.
    f. Suggest relaxation techniques or guided imagery for patients who experience anticipatory nausea and vomiting.

Relieving Pain

Evidence Base Van de Wetering, M. D., & Schouten-van Meeteren, N. Y. N. (2011). Supportive care for children with cancer. *Seminars in Oncology, 38*(3), 374–379.

1. Position the child for comfort.
2. Assess the child's pain using a developmentally appropriate pain scale at regular intervals.
3. Administer drugs on a preventive schedule before pain becomes intense. Continuous infusion pumps for opioid administration are commonly used.
4. Manipulate the environment, as necessary, to increase the child's comfort and to minimize unnecessary exertion.
5. Prepare the child for treatment and diagnostic procedures.
    a. Use knowledge of growth and development to prepare the child for such procedures as bone marrow aspirations, spinal taps, blood transfusions, and chemotherapy.
    b. Provide a means for talking about the experience. Play, storytelling, or role-playing may be helpful.
    c. Convey to the child an acceptance of fears and anger.
    d. Use anesthetic cream at spinal tap, injection, and bone marrow sites to decrease pain.
    e. Administer conscious sedation before procedures and monitor pulse, BP, respirations, and pulse oximetry during and after procedures.
6. Consider implementing complementary and alternative medicine (CAM) interventions for pain control as well as for management of nausea, vomiting, and anxiety. CAM strategies to consider include:
    a. Hypnosis/self-hypnosis.
    b. Imagery.
    c. Distraction/relaxation techniques.
    d. Cognitive-behavioral therapy.
    e. Music therapy.
    f. Massage.

Conserving Energy

1. Assess the child's energy level and space needed activities accordingly. Allow the child to rest, if necessary.
2. Encourage the child to limit strenuous activity after such diagnostic procedures as bone marrow aspirations and spinal taps.

Reducing the Child's Anxiety

1. Provide for continuity of care.
2. Encourage family-centered care.
3. Facilitate play activities for the child and use opportunities to communicate through play.
4. Maintain some discipline, placing calm limitations on unacceptable behavior.
5. Provide appropriate diversional activities.
6. Encourage independence and provide opportunities that allow the child to control his or her environment.
7. Explain the diagnosis and treatment in age-appropriate terms.

Community and Home Care Considerations

Evidence Base Carter, B., Coad, J., Bray, L., et al. (2012). Home-based care for special healthcare needs: Community children's nursing services. *Nursing Research, 61*(4), 260–268.

1. Begin to develop a home care plan before the child leaves the hospital.
2. Communicate with health care provider, hospital nurses, family, and others familiar with the case to gather information about the child's illness, treatment plan, and specific needs in the home.
3. Arrange schedule for blood draws and how results will be managed.
4. Contact the child's school and arrange a meeting with the school nurse, principal, and appropriate teachers to explain child's diagnosis, treatment, and potential time away from school.
5. Discuss with patient the possibility of making a visit to the classroom; explain about cancer and the adverse effects of chemotherapy to facilitate school reentry.
6. Collaborate with primary care provider regarding immunization schedule and the contraindication for children on immunosuppressive therapy.
7. Make sure that parents or caregivers can demonstrate the proper technique for care of venous access, such as dressing changes, flushing, and assessing for infection.
8. Ensure parents or caregivers receive education for home medications, including medication schedule, side effects, and indications for scheduled and PRN medications.

Family Education and Health Maintenance

1. Teach parents about normal CBC values and expected variations caused by therapy.
2. Instruct parents about leukemia and adverse effects of chemotherapy.
3. Tell parents to call the health care provider if child has a fever of more than 101° F (38.3° C), which may indicate overwhelming infection and impending septic shock, bleeding, and signs of infection. Parents should also immediately report if the child has been exposed to chickenpox. Immunosuppressed children are in danger of developing disseminated varicella and may be treated prophylactically with varicella immune globulin.
4. Teach preventive measures, such as handwashing and isolation from children with communicable diseases.
5. Reinforce that parents are *never* to use a rectal thermometer.
6. Refer parents to such agencies as Candlelighters (*www .candlelighters.org*) or the Leukemia and Lymphoma Society (*www.leukemia-lymphoma.org*).

Evaluation: Expected Outcomes

- Parents discuss their feelings about the child's diagnosis and treatment.
- Remains afebrile, no signs of localized infection or bleeding.
- Maintains a positive body image.
- Eats enough calories to maintain weight.
- Experiences relief from pain (no crying or expression of pain).
- Rests at intervals.
- Acts out feelings in play; participates in age-appropriate activities.

Brain Tumors in Children

Evidence Base Flemming, A. J., & Chi, S. N. (2012). Brain tumors in children. *Current Problems in Pediatric and Adolescent Health Care, 42*(2), 80–103.

Brain tumors are expanding lesions within the skull. Approximately 25% of the malignant tumors that occur in children are brain tumors, with an incidence rate of 4.84 per 100,000 children age 0 to 19. Four main types of brain tumors appear in children. Glial cell tumors, including *astrocytoma* and *diffuse pontine glioma*, can grow at any location in the brain and account for approximately 30% to 40% of all pediatric brain tumors. *Medulloblastoma* is a type of embryonal tumor, which is highly malignant and rapidly growing, usually found in the cerebellum. Embryonal tumors are the most common tumors of the CNS in children. *Ependymoma* is a tumor derived from the ependyma, or lining of the central canal of the spinal cord and cerebral ventricles. It frequently arises on the floor of the fourth ventricle, causing obstruction of the flow of cerebrospinal fluid (CSF). Ependymomas represent approximately 5% to 10% of all primary childhood CNS tumors. *Germ cell tumors* are midline tumors typically diagnosed in children age 6 to 14 with a higher incidence in parts of Asia, specifically Japan.

Pathophysiology and Etiology

1. The etiology of brain tumors is unknown. Symptoms are associated with the location of the tumor and rate of growth.
2. Astrocytomas typically present in the infratentorial region, producing increased intracranial pressure (ICP). It is classified according to its malignancy, from grade I (least malignant) to grade IV (most malignant). Surgery and radiation are the primary therapies.
3. Medulloblastoma grows rapidly and produces evidence of increased ICP progressing during several weeks. It is classified as standard risk or high risk depending on tumor histology. Combination therapy of surgery, radiation, and chemotherapy is usually required.
4. Germ cell tumors grow in the midline of the brain and the majority present in the supraseller or pineal regions. The growth rate varies, but frequently symptoms precede diagnosis by several months.
5. Ependymomas grow with varying speed. Because of location, tumors can invade the cardiorespiratory center, cerebellum, and spinal cord. They are graded according to degree of differentiation.

Clinical Manifestations

Glial Cell Tumors

Onset and growth is related to stage of tumor.

1. Evidence of increased ICP—especially ataxia, vomiting, or headache.

2. Cerebellar signs—ataxia, dysmetria (inability to control the range of muscular movement), nystagmus.
3. Behavioral changes.
4. Seizures.
5. Precocious puberty.

Medulloblastoma

Fast growing, malignant, and invasive.

1. The child may present with unsteady gait, anorexia, vomiting, and early morning headache.
2. May later develop ataxia, nystagmus, papilledema, drowsiness, increased head circumference, head tilt, and cranial nerve palsies. May develop obstructive hydrocephalus.

Germ Cell Tumor

Signs of midline shifts.

1. Visual disturbances.
2. Personality and sleep pattern alterations.
3. Dramatic weight loss.
4. Hydrocephalus.
5. Endocrinopathies.
6. Seizures.

Ependymoma of the Fourth Ventricle

1. Signs of increased ICP.
   a. Nausea or vomiting.
   b. Headache.
2. Unsteady gait or ataxia; dysmetria.
3. Focal motor weakness, vision disturbances, seizures.

Diagnostic Evaluation

Determined by the type of tumor that is suspected; usually includes many or all of the following procedures to localize and determine extent of the tumor:

1. Computed tomography (CT).
2. Magnetic resonance imaging (MRI).
3. Fluid attenuated inversion recovery imaging.
4. Positron emission tomography (PET).
5. Lumbar puncture with CSF cytologic evaluation.
6. Angiography (occasional).

Management

1. Surgery is performed to determine the type of tumor, to assess the extent of invasiveness, and to excise as much of the lesion as possible.
2. Radiation therapy is usually initiated as soon as the diagnosis is established and the surgical wound is healed.
3. Chemotherapy is used to treat chemoresponsive tumors and is particularly important in children who are too young to receive radiation therapy.
4. A ventriculoperitoneal shunt is usually necessary for children who develop hydrocephalus.
5. The use of immunotherapy is being investigated for potential for future treatment.

6. Prognosis is improved in cases that involve early diagnosis and adequate therapy. Five-year survivors are increasing, especially in children with low-grade astrocytomas or ependymomas. However, there are still tumors such as diffuse intrinsic pontine glioma that have no known cure.

Complications

1. Brain stem herniation.
2. Hydrocephalus.

Nursing Assessment

Assess the child's neurologic status to help locate the site of the tumor and the extent of involvement as well as to identify signs of disease progression.

1. Obtain a thorough nursing history from the child and parents, particularly data related to normal behavioral patterns and presenting symptoms.
2. Perform portions of the neurologic examination, as appropriate. Assess muscle strength, coordination, gait, and posture.
3. Observe for the appearance or disappearance of the clinical manifestations previously described. Report these to the health care provider and record each of the following in detail:
   a. Headache—duration, location, severity.
   b. Vomiting—time of occurrence, projectile, blood.
   c. Seizures—activity before seizure, type of seizure, areas of body involved, behavior during and after seizure.
4. Monitor vital signs frequently, including BP and pupillary reaction.
5. Monitor ocular signs. Check pupils for size, equality, reaction to light, and accommodation.
6. Observe for signs of brain stem herniation—should be considered a neurosurgical emergency.
   a. Attacks of opisthotonos (see Figure 51-2).
   b. Tilting of the head; neck stiffness.
   c. Poorly reactive pupils.
   d. Increased BP; widened pulse pressure.
   e. Change in respiratory rate and nature of respirations
   f. Irregularity of pulse or lowered pulse rate.
   g. Alterations of body temperature.

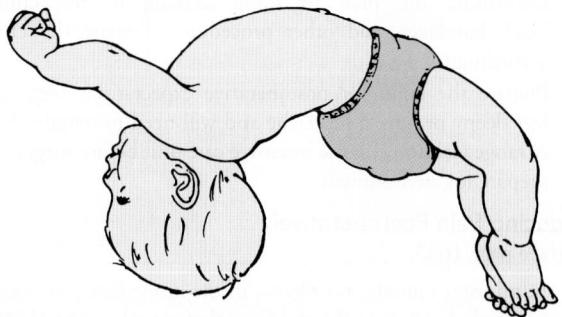

Figure 51-2. Opisthotonos, a sign of brain stem herniation.

NURSING ALERT Signs of brain stem herniation, especially opisthotonos, are ominous. The health care provider should be called immediately and the child should be prepared for ventricular tap to relieve pressure. Have resuscitation equipment on hand.

Nursing Diagnoses

- Anxiety of parents related to the nature of the diagnosis and the need for surgery.
- Fear of child related to hospitalization and to diagnostic and treatment procedures.
- Acute Pain related to increased ICP and surgery.
- Imbalanced Nutrition: Less than Body Requirements related to nausea and vomiting associated with increased ICP, chemotherapy, and radiation.
- Risk for Infection postoperatively.
- Disturbed Body Image related to appearance of the incision, shaved head, or changes caused by radiation, chemotherapy, and steroids.

Nursing Interventions

Reducing Parents' Anxiety
See also page 1682.

1. Encourage the parents to ask questions and to understand fully the risks and benefits of surgery.
2. Prepare the parents for the postoperative appearance of their child and for the fact that the child might be comatose immediately after surgery.
3. Continue supporting the parents during the postoperative period. They may be frightened and upset by the appearance of their child and by necessary emergency procedures.
4. Facilitate the return of normal parent–child relationships.
   a. The parents may be overprotective.
   b. Help the parents to see the child's increasing capabilities and encourage them to foster independence.

Reducing the Child's Fear
See also page 1683.

1. Prepare the child for surgery in realistic terms, but at the appropriate developmental level. Involve the Child Life therapist.
2. Determine the plan regarding shaving of the child's head, bandages, and other procedures. Prepare the child accordingly.
3. Prepare the child for postoperative expectations (eg, may feel sleepy or have a headache and will need to remain flat). Arrange visit to pediatric intensive care unit before surgery to prepare for environment.

Reducing Pain Postoperatively
Also see page 1683.

1. Administer opioids, as ordered, in the immediate postoperative period, assessing the child's level of consciousness (LOC) before administration.
2. Keep the child as comfortable as possible by repositioning.

Maintaining Nutritional Status

1. Feed the child after vomiting. (Vomiting is not usually associated with nausea.)
2. Allow the child to participate in the selection of foods.
3. Maintain IV hydration or hyperalimentation and intralipids, if indicated.
4. Encourage the child to eat progressively larger meals as he or she recovers.
5. If the child cannot eat, provide tube feedings. A gastrostomy tube may be inserted.
6. Be aware that children taking steroids to decrease swelling may have increased appetite.

Preventing Infection and Other Complications Postoperatively

1. Position the child according to surgeon's request—usually on unaffected side with head level with body.
   a. Raising the foot of the bed may increase ICP and bleeding.
   b. Post a sign above the bed, noting the exact position of the head.
2. Check the dressing for bleeding and for drainage of CSF.
3. Monitor the child's temperature closely.
   a. A significant rise in temperature may be caused by trauma, disturbance of the heat-regulating center, or intracranial edema.
   b. If hyperthermia occurs, administer antipyretics and use cooling techniques, as ordered. Temperature should not be reduced too rapidly.
4. Observe child closely for signs of shock, increased ICP, and alterations in LOC.
5. Assess the child for edema of the head, face, and neck.
6. Carefully regulate fluid administration to prevent increased cerebral edema.
7. Change the child's position frequently and provide meticulous skin care to prevent hypostatic pneumonia and pressure ulcers.
   a. Move the child carefully and slowly, being certain to move the head in line with the body.
   b. Support paralyzed or spastic extremities with pillows, rolls, or other means.
8. Have equipment readily available for cardiopulmonary resuscitation, respiratory assistance, oxygen inhalation, blood transfusion, ventricular tap, and other potential emergency situations.
9. Report fever or sign of infection.
10. If the child is receiving chemotherapy or radiation, assess for fever greater than 101° F (38.3° C) or nausea and vomiting unrelated to chemotherapy.

Promoting Acceptance of Body Changes

1. Encourage the child to express feelings regarding the threat to body image.
2. Reassure the child that a wig or a hat can be worn after recovery. Refer parents to *www.locksoflove.org* or *www.wigsforkids.org*.
3. If the child's hair has not been totally shaved, comb it so that the area of baldness is not evident.

4. Reassure the child that hair will grow back after surgery and chemotherapy (hair does not grow back at site of radiation therapy).

5. Prepare child and family for cushingoid changes (moon face, edema) if long-term steroids are required.

Family Education and Health Maintenance

1. Provide parents with written information regarding the child's needs—medications, activity, care of the incision, and follow-up appointments.

2. Teach the parents about radiation and chemotherapy and their adverse effects.

3. If a child has a ventriculoperitoneal shunt, teach parents to report fever, nausea, vomiting, irritability, or a bulging anterior fontanelle.

4. Initiate a referral to a home health nurse to provide care and teaching at home and to maintain therapeutic support for the family.

5. Encourage parents to contact the child's teacher and the school nurse before the child returns to school so that they can prepare classmates for child's return and help them to deal with their feelings.

6. Provide the parents with the phone number of the clinic or nursing unit so that they may call if questions occur to them after discharge.

7. For additional resources, refer family to such agencies as the American Brain Tumor Association (*www.abta.org*) or Candlelighters (*www.candlelighters.org*).

Evaluation: Expected Outcomes

- Parents discuss feelings about the child's diagnosis and surgery.
- Demonstrates lessened fear and anxiety through verbalization, play, or other age-appropriate activities.
- Verbalizes relief from pain.
- Maintains weight through adequate intake.
- Afebrile, lungs clear, vital signs stable.
- Verbalizes acceptance of appearance with hat, desire to visit with friends.

Neuroblastoma

Evidence Base Wylie, L., & Philpott, A. (2012). Neuroblastoma progress on many fronts: The neuroblastoma research symposium. *Pediatric Blood and Cancer, 58,* 649–451.

Mazur, K. A. (2010). Neuroblastoma: What the nurse practitioner should know. *Journal of the American Academy of Nurse Practitioners, 22,* 236–245.

Neuroblastoma refers to a malignant tumor that arises from the sympathetic nervous system. It is the most common extracranial solid tumor of childhood, with a prevalence of 1 in 7,000 children or 800 new cases per year in the United States. It primarily affects infants and young children and occurs slightly more frequently in boys.

Pathophysiology and Etiology

1. Etiology is unknown.
2. Tumors arise from embryonic neural crest cells anywhere along the craniospinal axis. A type of small, round, blue cell tumor.

3. Histologic picture varies greatly from tumor to tumor and even within the same tumor.

4. Tumors are staged primarily by extent of disease; International Neuroblastoma Staging System:
   a. Stage 1 (tumor confined to the organ or structure of origin with complete surgical resection) to stage 4 (remote disease involving the skeleton, parenchymal organs, soft tissue, distant lymph nodes, or bone marrow).
   b. Stage 4S refers to cases that would otherwise be stage 1 or 2 but that have dissemination limited to the liver, skin, or bone marrow in a patient <1 year of age.

5. Neuroblastoma is one of the few tumors that may demonstrate spontaneous remission.

Clinical Manifestations

1. Symptoms depend on the location of the tumor and the stage of the disease.

2. Most tumors are located within the abdomen and present as firm, nontender, irregular masses that may or may not cross the midline.

3. Other common signs:
   a. Bowel or bladder dysfunction that results from compression by a paraspinal or pelvic tumor.
   b. Neurologic symptoms because of compression by the tumor on nerve roots or because of tumor extension.
   c. Supraorbital ecchymosis, periorbital edema, and exophthalmos that results from metastases to the skull bones and retrobulbar soft tissue.
   d. Lymphadenopathy, especially in the cervical area.
   e. Bone pain with skeletal involvement.
   f. Swelling of the neck or face, wheezing, dyspnea, and cough with thoracic masses.
   g. Symptoms of bone marrow failure, such as anemia, bleeding, or infection.
   h. General symptoms of pallor, anorexia, weight loss, and weakness with widespread metastasis.

Diagnostic Evaluation

Workup done to document the extent of the disease throughout the body:

1. Chest and skeletal x-rays.
2. Bone scan.
3. Bone marrow aspiration and biopsy.
4. CBC, platelet count, ferritin.
5. Twenty-four-hour urine collection—elevated excretion of homovanillic acid (HVA) and vanillylmandelic acid (VMA).
6. Liver and kidney function tests.
7. Histologic confirmation.
8. Additional studies:
   a. CT of primary site and chest.
   b. MRI—areas above diaphragm.
   c. Ultrasound examination.
   d. Liver and spleen scan.
   e. Meta-iodo (131)-benzylguanidine scan.

9. Genetic indicators of poor prognosis include n-Myc onco-gene amplification, hyperdiploid karyotype, and chromosome deletion.

Management

1. Surgery—role is diagnostic and therapeutic. Either primary (before chemotherapy or radiation) or delayed/secondary (after therapy).
2. When complete surgical resection of a stage I tumor is possible, this may be the only treatment required.
3. Children with other than stage I disease generally receive a combination of surgery, radiation therapy, and chemotherapy. Drugs of choice include vincristine, topotecan, irinotecan, cyclophosphamide, doxorubicin, cisplatin, carboplatin, ifosfamide, and etoposide. See Table 51-2.
4. Survival rate for early stages is as high as 95%; advanced stages, 40%.

Table 51-2	Commonly Used Chemotherapeutic Agents to Treat Neuroblastoma
CHEMOTHERAPEUTIC AGENT	**COMMON SIDE EFFECTS**
Carboplatin	Nausea, vomiting Bone marrow suppression Electrolyte imbalance
Cytoxan	Nausea, vomiting Hair loss Loss of appetite Gonadal dysfunction Bone marrow suppression
Doxorubicin	Nausea, vomiting Hair loss Red urine Bone marrow suppression Cardiac dysfunction
Etoposide	Nausea, vomiting Hair loss Weakness Bone marrow suppression
Irinotecan	Diarrhea, abdominal cramping, runny nose, tearing, salivation, sweating, photophobia Nausea, vomiting Loss of appetite Bone marrow suppression Fever Weakness Elevated liver enzymes Elevated eosinophils
Temozolomide	Bone marrow suppression Nausea, vomiting Constipation Loss of appetite

5. Influencing factors for prognosis:
   a. Stage of disease—the earlier the stage, the better the prognosis.
   b. Age—infants younger than age 1 demonstrate the best survival.
   c. Site of primary tumor—children with tumors above the diaphragm appear to do better than children with abdominal tumors.
   d. Pattern of metastasis—children with metastasis to the bone marrow, liver, and skin have better prognosis than those with radiographic bone involvement.
   e. Genetic and histologic factors.
6. The use of autologous stem cell transplantation, newer chemotherapy drugs, and immunotherapy are under investigation in the hope of improving survival rates for these children.

Complications

1. Metastasis to the liver, soft tissue, bones, lymph nodes, bone marrow, and skin.
2. Neurologic deficits due to nerve compression.

Nursing Assessment

 Evidence Base Kline, N. (Ed.). (2009). *Essentials of pediatric oncology nursing: A core curriculum* (3rd ed.). Glenview, IL: Association of Pediatric Hematology/Oncology Nurses.

1. Obtain a history.
   a. Inquire about when symptoms began. Focus on decrease in appetite, weakness, pain, abdominal distention, or change in bowel and bladder function.
   b. Symptoms exhibited depend on the location of the primary tumor.
2. Perform a physical examination, including:
   a. Examination of skin for signs of increased bruising or petechiae.
   b. Palpation of liver and spleen for enlargement.
   c. Palpation of abdominal mass or other primary site of tumor.
   d. Auscultation of lungs.
   e. Palpation of lymph nodes.
   f. BP for detection of hypertension.
   g. Temperature for fever caused by infection or disease.
   h. Assessment of bones and joints for pain or swelling.
   i. Neurologic examination for signs of compression by tumor. Nerves involved depend on location of tumor.
3. Assess coping mechanisms of family.

Nursing Diagnoses

- Anxiety of parents related to learning of diagnosis.
- Fear of child related to diagnostic procedures and surgery or biopsy.
- Activity Intolerance related to fatigue from tumor growth and bone marrow suppression.

- Constipation or Bowel and Bladder Incontinence related to pressure of tumor.
- Risk for Infection related to bone marrow suppression from chemotherapy and radiation.
- Acute Pain related to tumor, surgery, or progression of disease.
- Disturbed Body Image related to hair loss.

Nursing Interventions

Reducing Parents' Anxiety
See page 1682.

Reducing Child's Anxiety and Fear
See page 1683.

Increasing Activity Tolerance
See page 1683.

Regaining Normal Bowel and Bladder Function
1. Assess normal elimination patterns the child had before the illness began.
2. Keep careful intake and output records.
3. Assess for urinary overflow incontinence and loss of bowel function, depending on the child's age.
4. Notify health care provider if these should occur.

Preventing Infection
See page 1683.

Observe the surgical incision for erythema, drainage, or separation of the incision. Report these changes.

Relieving Pain
See page 1683.

Monitor for increasing or new location of pain, indicating progression of disease (eg, fracture due to bone involvement).

Promoting Acceptance of Body Changes
See page 1683.

Family Education and Health Maintenance

1. Teach parents about the laboratory tests and imaging studies needed at diagnosis and periodically throughout therapy.
2. Instruct parents about chemotherapy drugs used and their potential adverse effects.
3. Inform parents about potential treatment methods, such as radiation therapy and bone marrow transplantation.
4. Advise parents to use good handwashing technique and to prevent exposure to children with communicable diseases.
5. Refer families to resources such as Candlelighters (*www.candlelighters.org*).

Evaluation: Expected Outcomes

- Parents and child discuss their feelings about diagnosis and treatment.
- Participates in play and expresses feelings through play.
- Maintains normal activity level.
- Resumes normal voiding and stooling pattern.
- Remains afebrile, lungs clear, no signs of localized infections.
- Rests without crying or guarding of surgical incision; good pain control according to developmentally appropriate scale.
- Interacts with others, seems comfortable with self.

Rhabdomyosarcoma

 Evidence Base Dasgupta, R., & Rodeberg, D. A. (2012). Update on rhabdomyosarcoma. *Seminars in Pediatric Surgery, 21*, 68–78.

Rhabdomyosarcoma is a highly malignant soft-tissue tumor that arises from the immature mesenchymal cells that form striated muscle. The incidence is approximately 4.5 per 1 million children in the United States and rhabdomyosarcoma accounts for 3.5% of all malignant disease in children younger than age 14. It has bimodal distribution with a peak between 2 and 6 years old and again between 10 and 18 years old. The most common sites are the head and neck, genitourinary (GU) tract, and extremities.

Pathophysiology and Etiology

1. Etiology is unknown in most cases.
2. Certain genetic and environmental factors have been associated with its development.
3. Two major variants are embryonal and alveolar, with embryonal more common in young children and alveolar more common in adolescents.
4. Tumor spreads either by local extension or by metastasis via the venous and lymphatic system.
5. The lung is the most common site of metastasis.
6. Tumor staging is based on the extent of the disease:
   a. Stage/Group I: localized tumor, completely resected.
   b. Stage/Group II: local tumor resected, microscopic residual disease.
   c. Stage/Group III: localized disease, with gross residual disease after resection.
   d. Stage/Group IV: metastatic disease at diagnosis.

Clinical Manifestations

1. Commonly presents as an asymptomatic lump noted by patient or parent.
2. Signs and symptoms are variable and reflect the location of the tumor and metastasis.
   a. Orbit—ptosis, ocular paralysis, exophthalmos.
   b. Nasopharynx—epistaxis, pain, dysphagia, nasal voice, airway obstruction.
   c. Sinuses—swelling, pain, discharge, sinusitis.
   d. Middle ear—pain, chronic otitis, facial nerve palsy.
   e. Neck—hoarseness, dysphagia.
   f. Trunk, extremities, testicular areas—enlarging soft tissue masses.
   g. Prostate, bladder—urinary tract symptoms.
   h. Retroperitoneal tumors—GI and urinary tract obstruction, weakness, paresthesia, pain.
   i. Vaginal—abnormal vaginal bleeding or mass.

Diagnostic Evaluation

To document the extent of the disease and to provide objective criteria for measuring response to therapy:

1. Open biopsy of the primary tumor—definitive diagnostic procedure.

2. CT of the chest and primary lesion.
3. MRI.
4. Bone marrow aspiration and biopsy.
5. Bone scan or skeletal survey.
6. Ultrasonography.
7. Chest x-ray.
8. PET.
9. CBC, liver and renal function tests, electrolytes, serum calcium and phosphorus, uric acid.
10. Monoclonal antibody assays.
11. Urinalysis.
12. Lumbar puncture—for children with cranial lesions.

Management

1. Surgery—to biopsy the lesion, determine the stage of the disease, and completely remove or reduce the primary tumor. Increasingly, chemotherapy and radiation therapy are used before surgery to avoid the disability associated with radical surgery for selected anatomic sites (head, neck, and pelvis).
2. Radiation—high-dose radiation is generally recommended for the primary tumor and metastasis.
3. Chemotherapy:
   a. Used for all patients, usually in combination with irradiation (see Table 51-3).
   b. Commonly used drugs include dactinomycin, vincristine, cyclophosphamide, doxorubicin, cisplatin, etoposide, ifosfamide, irinotecan, melphalan topotecan, paclitaxel, and docetaxel.
4. Survival rates have improved considerably in recent years and overall survival is approximately 70%. Survival for stage I, with favorable histology, is greater than 85%; stage IV, less than 30%.
5. Prognosis is related to the stage of the disease at diagnosis, the location of the primary tumor, and the age at diagnosis.

Complications

1. Direct tumor extension to CNS with cranial nerve palsy, brain stem compromise with bradypnea and bradycardia.
2. Metastasis to bone, bone marrow, lung.

Table 51-3	Commonly Used Chemotherapeutic Agents to Treat Rhabdomyosarcoma	
CHEMOTHERAPEUTIC AGENT	**COMMON SIDE EFFECTS**
Cytoxan	Nausea, vomiting Hair loss Loss of appetite Gonadal dysfunction Bone marrow suppression
Dactinomycin	Nausea, vomiting Bone marrow suppression
Vincristine	Hair loss Neuropathy Constipation

Nursing Assessment

1. Obtain a history.
   a. Ask about recent illness history and when the child became symptomatic.
   b. Obtain review of systems to help identify the primary tumor and metastasis present.
2. Perform physical examination, including:
   a. Palpation of lymph nodes for enlargement, tenderness, and mobility.
   b. Palpation of the liver and spleen to detect hepatosplenomegaly.
   c. Palpation of primary site of tumor and suspected areas of metastasis.
   d. Auscultation of lungs to assess breath sounds or abnormality caused by the spread of the tumor.
3. Assess family coping, resources, and emotional state of child and parents.

Nursing Diagnoses

- Anxiety of parents related to learning of diagnosis.
- Fear of child related to diagnostic procedures and surgery or biopsy.
- Imbalanced Nutrition: Less than Body Requirements related to anemia, anorexia, nausea, vomiting, and mucosal ulceration secondary to chemotherapy or radiation.
- Acute Pain related to surgery or possible progression of disease.
- Disturbed Body Image related to alopecia associated with chemotherapy.
- Risk for Infection related to bone marrow suppression from chemotherapy or radiation.

Nursing Interventions

Reducing Parents' Anxiety
See page 1682.

Reducing the Child's Fear and Anxiety
See page 1683.

Promoting Optimal Nutrition
See page 1683.

Relieving Pain
See page 1683.

Promoting Acceptance of Body Changes
See page 1683.

Preventing Infection
See page 1683.

Family Education and Health Maintenance

1. Teach parents about laboratory diagnostic tests that will be done periodically to follow the child's condition.
2. Instruct parents about treatment methods, including chemotherapy and radiation protocols postoperatively, and their adverse effects.
3. Stress the importance of follow-up so that recurrence can be detected early and appropriate treatment can be instituted.
4. Refer families to such resources as Candlelighters (*www.candlelighters.org*).

Evaluation: Expected Outcomes

- Parents verbalize understanding of diagnosis.
- Plays, interacts with others, and asks questions.
- Eats sufficient calories to maintain weight.
- Verbalizes reduced pain.
- Verbalizes acceptance of self; looks in mirror.
- Remains afebrile, no signs of localized infection.

Wilms' Tumor

 Evidence Base Hamilton, T. E., & Shamberger, R. C. (2012). Wilms tumor: Recent advances in clinical care and biology. *Seminars in Pediatric Surgery, 21,* 15–20.

National Cancer Institute. (2012). Wilm's tumor PDQ. Available: *www.cancer.gov/cancertopics/pdq/treatment/wilms/HealthProfessional/page1.*

Wilms' tumor is a malignant renal tumor and is the most common renal neoplasm in children. It constitutes approximately 6% of all childhood tumors. Incidence is 7.6 cases per million for children younger than age 15, which means about 500 cases are diagnosed each year in the United States; 75% of cases occur before the child is age 5. Most commonly a unilateral disease, but in 5% to 10%, both kidneys are involved.

Pathophysiology and Etiology

1. The etiology is not known.
2. Genetic inheritance has been documented in 1% to 2% of cases.
3. Children with Wilms' tumor may have associated anomalies.
4. Wilms' tumor has a capacity for rapid growth and usually grows to a large size before it is diagnosed.
5. The effect of the tumor on the kidney depends on the site of the tumor.
6. In most cases, the tumor expands the renal parenchyma and the capsule of the kidney becomes stretched over the surface of the tumor, which is encapsulated at the time of surgery.
7. Wilms' tumors present various histologic patterns and are grouped into two general categories; favorable histology and unfavorable histology.
8. The neoplasms metastasize either by direct extension or by way of the bloodstream. They may invade perirenal tissues, lymph nodes, the liver, the diaphragm, abdominal muscles, and the lungs. Invasions of bone and brain are less common.
9. Staging of Wilms' tumor is done based on clinical and anatomic findings. It ranges from stage I (tumor is limited to the kidney and is completely resected) to stage IV (metastasis is present in the liver, lung, bone, or brain). Stage V includes those cases that include bilateral involvement, either initially or subsequently.

Clinical Manifestations

1. A firm, nontender upper quadrant abdominal mass is usually the presenting sign; it may be on either side. (It is usually first observed by the parents.)
2. Abdominal pain, which is related to rapid growth of the tumor, may occur. As the tumor enlarges, pressure may cause constipation, vomiting, abdominal distress, anorexia, weight loss, and dyspnea.
3. Less common are hypertension, fever, hematuria, and anemia.
4. Associated anomalies:
   a. Hemihypertrophy.
   b. Aniridia (without the iris).
   c. GU anomalies.
   d. Overgrowth syndromes (ie, Beckwith-Wiedemann syndrome).

Diagnostic Evaluation

1. Abdominal ultrasound to show the tumor and assess the status of the opposite kidney.
2. Radiography of chest to identify metastases.
3. CBC and peripheral smear to determine baseline data.
4. Urinalysis to detect for hematuria.
5. Blood chemistries, especially serum electrolytes, uric acid, renal function tests (blood urea nitrogen and creatinine), and liver function tests (bilirubin, alanine aminotransferase, aspartate aminotransferase, lactate dehydrogenase [LD], total protein, albumin, and alkaline phosphatase) may show abnormalities.
6. Urinary VMA and HVA to distinguish from neuroblastoma.
7. MRI or CT of the abdomen to evaluate local spread to lymph nodes or adjacent organs.
8. Real-time ultrasonography.

Management

1. Surgical removal of primary tumor remains the cornerstone of therapy. Accurate staging and assessment of tumor spread is also done.
2. Radiation or chemotherapy may be administered preoperatively to patients with advanced tumors or risky intravascular extension to reduce tumor burden.
3. Radiation therapy may be given to the tumor bed postoperatively to render nonviable all cells that have escaped locally from the excised tumor. Children who have stage III and IV Wilms' tumor, or who have an unfavorable histology, usually receive this treatment.
4. Whole-lung radiation is used to treat stage IV tumors with lung metastasis.
5. Late effects of radiation therapy to the abdomen include scoliosis and underdevelopment of soft tissues and possible organ dysfunction in radiation field.
6. Chemotherapy is initiated postoperatively to achieve complete eradication of tumor cells (see Table 51-4).
7. Overall survival rates for Wilms' tumor are among the highest for all childhood cancers—greater than 90% survival at 4 years.
8. Prognosis is based on histologic tumor features, lymph node involvement, age, tumor size, and possible chromosomal factors.

Table 51-4	Commonly Used Chemotherapeutic Agents to Treat Wilms' Tumor
CHEMOTHERAPEUTIC AGENT	**COMMON SIDE EFFECTS**
Vincristine	Hair loss Neuropathy Constipation
Dactinomycin	Nausea, vomiting Bone marrow suppression
Doxorubicin	Nausea, vomiting Hair loss Red urine Bone marrow suppression Cardiac dysfunction

Complications

1. Metastasis to the lungs, lymph nodes, liver, bone, and brain.
2. Complications from radiation therapy include bowel obstruction, hepatic damage, nephritis, sterility in girls, interstitial pneumonia, scoliosis.
3. Cumulative incidence of second malignancy is 1.6% after 15 years, with radiation being the greatest risk factor.

Nursing Assessment

1. Obtain a history.
   a. Ask how tumor was first discovered.
   b. Ask whether the child has history of other GU anomalies or whether there is a family history of cancer.
   c. Determine whether the child has had hematuria, dysuria, constipation, abdominal pain, decreased appetite, or fever before hospitalization and ask how these were treated.
2. Perform a physical examination that includes:
   a. Assessment for associated anomalies: aniridia, hemihypertrophy of the spine, or cryptorchidism.
   b. Palpation of lymph nodes for enlargement, tenderness, and mobility.
   c. Palpation of the liver and spleen for enlargement.
   d. Palpation of the abdomen to determine the size and location of the tumor.
   e. Auscultation of the lungs to assess breath sounds or abnormality because of spread of tumor.
3. Assess coping, resources, and emotional state of the family.

 NURSING ALERT Avoid indiscriminate manipulation of the abdomen preoperatively and postoperatively to decrease the danger of metastasis. Because the tumor is soft and highly vascular, seeding may occur with excessive palpation or handling of the child's abdomen.

Nursing Diagnoses

- Anxiety of parents related to learning of diagnosis.
- Fear of child related to surgery and diagnostic tests.

- Risk for Deficient Fluid Volume postoperatively.
- Acute Pain related to surgery and possible progression of the disease.
- Imbalanced Nutrition: Less than Body Requirements related to anemia, anorexia, nausea, vomiting, and mucosal ulceration secondary to chemotherapy or radiation.
- Disturbed Body Image related to alopecia associated with chemotherapy.
- Activity Intolerance related to fatigue that results from the size of the tumor and treatment.
- Risk for Infection and hemorrhage related to bone marrow suppression caused by chemotherapy.

Nursing Interventions

Reducing Parents' Anxiety
See page 1682.

Reducing the Child's Fear and Anxiety
See page 1683.

Preventing Fluid Volume Deficit and Other Complications

1. Insert a nasogastric tube, as ordered. Many children require gastric suction postoperatively to prevent distention or vomiting.
2. Monitor gastric output accurately and replace it with the appropriate IV fluids, as ordered.
3. When bowel sounds have returned, begin with small amounts of clear fluids.
4. Keep accurate intake and output record.
5. Monitor vital signs as the child's condition warrants and check the surgical dressing frequently for drainage.

Relieving Pain
See page 1683.

Promoting Optimal Nutrition
See page 1683.

Promoting Acceptance of Body Changes
See page 1683.

Increasing Activity Tolerance
See page 1683.

Preventing Infection
See page 1683.

Family Education and Health Maintenance

1. Teach parents of children with one kidney the signs and symptoms of kidney disease.
2. Advise parents to call health care provider if child has a fever of more than 101° F (38.3° C), bleeding, signs of infections or has been exposed to chickenpox.
3. Teach measures to prevent infection, such as handwashing and isolation from children with communicable disease.
4. Refer families to resources such as Candlelighters (*www.candlelighters.org*).

Evaluation: Expected Outcomes

- Parents discuss their feelings about diagnosis and treatment.

- Expresses feelings during play and participates in playroom activities.
- Has no abdominal distention or vomiting, vital signs stable.
- Verbalizes relief from pain.
- Eats adequate calories to maintain weight, nausea relieved by anti-emetics.
- Plays with others without notice to alopecia.
- Participates in all normal daily activities without fatigue.
- Remains afebrile, no signs of local infection.

Osteosarcoma

 Evidence Base Bölling, T., Hardes, J., Dirksen, U., (2013). Management of bone tumours in paediatric oncology. *Journal of Clinical Oncology, 25*(1),19–26.

Osteosarcoma is a malignant tumor of the bone. It is the most common malignant bone cancer in children, with approximately 8.7 cases per million adolescents. It is the most common secondary malignancy in survivors of retinoblastoma. Osteosarcoma occurs most often at the peak of the adolescent growth spurt, with the majority of cases occurring between the ages of 8 and 25. It is somewhat more likely to affect males than females.

Pathophysiology and Etiology

1. Etiology is unknown.
2. Presumably arises from bone-forming mesenchyme tissue.
3. Produces malignant spindle-cell stroma, which gives rise to malignant osteoid tissue.
4. Common sites of occurrence—distal femur, proximal tibia, and proximal humerus. Less common sites include the pelvis, phalanges, and jaw.
5. Most commonly metastasizes to lungs and other bones.

Clinical Manifestations

1. Pain in the affected site, frequently causing limp or limitation of motion.
2. Palpable, tender, fixed bony mass.
3. Additional symptoms related to site of metastasis, if present.

Diagnostic Evaluation

1. Radiographic examination of lesion—to visualize the tumor.
2. Biopsy of lesion—to confirm the diagnosis and to provide histologic date for the selection of a treatment plan.
3. CT and MRI—to determine local tumor extent before surgery.
4. Bone scan—helpful in detecting initial extent of malignancy, planning therapy, and evaluating effects of treatment.
5. Renal and liver function tests; serum LD will be elevated.
6. Arteriography—possibility if limb salvage procedure is a consideration.

Management

1. Surgery—procedures fall into two categories:
   a. Limb salvage procedure is priority—greater than 80% of tumors can be treated with limb salvage surgery.

Table 51-5	Commonly Used Chemotherapeutic Agents to Treat Osteosarcoma
CHEMOTHERAPY	**COMMON SIDE EFFECTS**
Doxorubicin	Nausea, vomiting Hair loss Red urine Bone marrow suppression Cardiac dysfunction
Cisplatin	Nausea, vomiting Bone marrow suppression Hypomagnesemia Loss of appetite Hearing loss Renal dysfunction
Methotrexate	Elevated liver enzymes
Etoposide	Nausea, vomiting Hair loss Weakness Bone marrow suppression
Ifosfamide	Nausea, vomiting Hair loss Bone marrow suppression Gonadal dysfunction Renal dysfunction

   b. Radical amputation of the affected extremity and, commonly, the joint proximal to the involved area.
2. The type of surgery performed depends on tumor location, size, extramedullary extent, distant metastasis, age, skeletal development, and lifestyle preference.
3. Chemotherapy is necessary following surgery. It is also used preoperatively for patients who undergo resection surgery and for the treatment of metastatic disease (see Table 51-5).
4. Survival has greatly improved with the aggressive use of multimodal therapy.
5. Approximately 70% of patients who have localized tumors and undergo surgery followed by chemotherapy can expect to be disease-free after 10 years. Metastasis at diagnosis—decreased prognosis to 25% at 10 years.
6. Important prognostic factors are extent of disease at diagnosis, age, gender, serum LD, and amount of tumor necrosis at the time of surgery. Osteosarcomas arising in previously irradiated areas have a worse prognosis.
7. Limb salvage surgery has improved the quality of life for many survivors.
8. Patients with relapse to lung may still be curable with surgical excision.

Complications

1. Metastasis to lung and bones.
2. Later metastasis to CNS and lymph nodes.

Nursing Assessment

1. Obtain a history.
   a. Inquire about how symptoms first presented and the duration of symptoms.
   b. Determine whether the child has pain or limitation of motion in the affected area.
2. Perform a physical examination, including:
   a. Palpation of the mass to determine the size and location. (Determine whether the mass is tender or is fixed to the bone.)
   b. Palpation of other bones to check for metastasis.
   c. Auscultation of the lungs to assess breath sounds or other abnormalities caused by spread of tumor.
3. Assess family coping, resources such as support systems, and emotional state of patient and parents.
4. Assess degree of mobility, especially for lower extremity tumors.

Nursing Diagnoses

- Anxiety of parents related to learning of diagnosis.
- Fear of child or adolescent related to surgery, diagnostic tests, and treatment.
- Disturbed Body Image related to surgery and possible amputation and alopecia associated with chemotherapy.
- Acute Pain related to surgery and possible progression of the disease.
- Imbalanced Nutrition: Less than Body Requirements related to anemia, anorexia, nausea, vomiting, and mucosal ulceration caused by chemotherapy.
- Risk for Infection related to surgery or bone marrow suppression secondary to chemotherapy.
- Impaired Mobility due to surgery or disease.

Nursing Interventions

Reducing Parents' Anxiety
See page 1682.

Reducing the Adolescent's Fear and Anxiety

1. Incorporate the adolescent's developmental level and develop a teaching program to include diagnostic tests and postoperative care.
2. Support and prepare the child for routine surgical care or care of the amputated limb. Involve the parents in the teaching plan and make sure they know what to expect before going to surgery.
3. If an amputation will be done, teach the child about the need for physical therapy for exercises and to learn crutch walking and the need for a prosthesis.
4. If limb salvage surgery will be done, reinforce the importance of physical therapy exercises following surgery in order to restore as much function as possible to the affected bone and/or joint.
5. Nursing care of the adolescent with osteosarcoma is the same as care of the adult (see page 1143).

Promoting Acceptance of New Self-Image

1. Understand that adolescents need time and support to accept the diagnosis and the surgery and to grieve for their lost body part if an amputation is done.
2. Try to introduce the adolescent to another adolescent with the same diagnosis who has undergone similar treatment.
3. Suggest the selection of clothing that will camouflage the prosthesis and that is fashionable and appealing.
4. Suggest wigs, scarves, or hats for adolescents who experience hair loss because of chemotherapy.
5. Encourage visits by peers and help the child to deal with questions and reactions from peers.

Relieving Pain
See page 1683.

Promoting Optimal Nutrition
See page 1683.

Preventing Infection and Hemorrhage
See page 1683.

Community and Home Care Considerations

1. Assess the home for accessibility of adolescent who has had an amputation.
2. Educate parents about changes they may need to make in the home.
3. Encourage the parents to contact the school system to arrange for a tutor for a student who needs to remain out of school for a lengthy period.
4. Assist the parents in contacting the school nurse to facilitate reentry into the classroom.

Family Education and Health Maintenance

1. Teach adolescent and parents about infection control measures, such as good handwashing and preventing exposure to children with communicable diseases, because chemotherapy is usually long term.
2. Parents and adolescents should be instructed about chemotherapy medications used and their potential adverse effects.
3. Teach parents and adolescents about the radiation procedure and effects.
4. Advise the adolescent to protect a leg that has received radiation treatment by avoiding excessive pressure on the leg through sports. Consult orthopedic specialist for appropriate activity limitations.
5. Refer families to resources such as Candlelighters (*www.candlelighters.org*).

Evaluation: Expected Outcomes

- Parents discuss feelings about surgery and chemotherapy treatments.
- Verbalizes feelings about surgery and asks questions.
- Looks in mirror, touches amputation site.
- Verbalizes relief from pain.

- Eating pattern adequate, nausea relieved by antiemetics.
- Remains afebrile, vital signs stable, no signs of bleeding.
- Maintains skin integrity.

Retinoblastoma

 Evidence Base National Cancer Institute. (2012). Retinoblastoma PDQ. Available: *www.cancer.gov/ cancertopics/pdq/treatment/retinoblastoma/ HealthProfessional/page1.*
　Dimaras, H., Kimani, K., Dimba, E. A., et al. (2012). Retinoblastoma. *Lancet, 379,* 1436–1446.

Retinoblastoma is a malignant, congenital tumor, arising in the retina of one or both eyes. It affects 9,000 children each year, or approximately 1 in 18,000 live births; this rate of diagnosis is consistent worldwide. Median age of diagnosis is age 2 and it is rarely diagnosed after age 6.

Pathophysiology and Etiology

1. Most cases appear sporadically and have been associated with advanced paternal age; there is also an inherited form of the disease.
   a. Nonhereditary somatic mutations account for approximately 60% of all retinoblastomas; always demonstrate unilateral involvement.
   b. All bilateral cases are heritable.
      i. Mode of inheritance is autosomal dominant.
      ii. Fifty percent chance that children of patient with retinoblastoma will inherit the disease.
2. Can be associated with chromosomal aberrations.
3. Usually arise in multiple foci rather than a single tumor from any of the nucleated retinal layers.
4. Some tumors (endophytic type) arise in the internal nuclear layers of the retina and grow forward into the vitreous cavity.
5. Some tumors (exophytic type) arise in the external nuclear layer and grow into the subretinal space, with detachment of the retina.
6. Most tumors have a combination of endophytic and exophytic growth.
7. Extension of the tumor may occur into the choroid, sclera, and optic nerve.
8. "Trilateral retinoblastoma" is the presence of bilateral retinoblastoma in addition to an intracranial midline neuroblastic tumor.
9. Hematogenous spread of the tumor may occur to the bone marrow, skeleton, lymph nodes, and liver.
10. Tumor staging reflects the extent of the disease and the probability of preserving useful vision in the affected eye, from group I (very favorable) to group V (very unfavorable).

Clinical Manifestations

1. Signs and symptoms of an intraocular tumor depend on its size and position.
2. "Cat's-eye reflex"—whitish appearance of the pupil (leukocoria) represents visualization of the tumor through the lens as light falls on the tumor mass—most common sign. Also characterized by the absence of red reflex on photographs.
3. Strabismus—second most common presenting sign.
4. Other occasional presenting signs:
   a. Orbital inflammation.
   b. Hyphema.
   c. Fixed pupil.
   d. Heterochromia iridis—different colors of each iris or in the same iris.
5. Vision loss is not a symptom because young children do not complain of unilaterally decreased vision.
6. Symptoms of distant metastasis—anorexia, weight loss, vomiting, headache, bone pain.

Diagnostic Evaluation

1. Bilateral indirect ophthalmoscopy under general anesthesia.
2. Ultrasonography and CT or MRI of head and eyes to visualize tumor.
3. Bone marrow aspiration and lumbar puncture under anesthesia to determine metastasis.

Management

1. Depends on the stage of the disease at the time of diagnosis.
2. Unilateral tumors in stages I, II, or III are usually treated with intraocular and systemic chemotherapy.
   a. Goal of treatment is to eradicate the tumors and to preserve useful vision.
   b. Most common chemotherapies are carboplatin, etoposide, and vincristine (see Table 51-6).
3. Surgery (enucleation) is the treatment of choice for advanced tumor growth, especially with optic nerve involvement when no hope exists for useful vision.
4. Bilateral disease usually requires enucleation of the severely diseased eye and treatment of the least affected eye.
   a. Every attempt is made to salvage whatever vision there may be.
   b. Bilateral enucleation is indicated with extensive bilateral retinoblastoma when no hope of vision exists.
5. Focal lasar treatment, light coagulation, and cryotherapy are sometimes used to treat small, localized tumors.
6. Overall survival rate is high (90%).

Table 51-6	Commonly Used Chemotherapeutic Agents to Treat Retinoblastoma
CHEMOTHERAPEUTIC AGENT	**COMMON SIDE EFFECTS**
Carboplatin	Nausea, vomiting Bone marrow suppression Electrolyte imbalance
Vincristine	Hair loss Neuropathy Constipation

7. Heritable retinoblastoma and bilateral retinoblastoma are associated with a high incidence of spontaneous and radiation-related new tumors, particularly sarcomas.

Complications

1. Spread to brain and other eye.
2. Metastasis to bone, bone marrow, liver, and lymph nodes.

Nursing Assessment

1. Obtain a history.
   a. Ask about a family history that is positive for retinoblastoma or other types of cancer.
   b. Inquire about when symptoms began and strabismus, cat's-eye reflex, orbital inflammation, vomiting, or headache.
2. Perform a physical examination.
   a. Assess pupils for reactivity of light, size, and leukocoria.
   b. Evaluate strabismus when checking muscle balance.
   c. Assess eyes for associated signs, such as erythema, inflammation of the orbit, hyphema, and heterochromia iridis.
3. Assess family's ability to cope, to use support systems, and to communicate feelings.

Nursing Diagnoses

- Anxiety of parents related to the diagnosis, treatment, and genetic implications of the diagnosis.
- Impaired Tissue Integrity related to skin changes, loss of lashes, fat atrophy, impaired bone growth, and dryness caused by radiation.
- Fear of child related to hospitalization and to diagnostic and treatment procedures.
- Disturbed Body Image and Ineffective Coping related to enucleation and need for an eye prosthesis.
- Impaired Sensory Perception (Visual) related to disease process or enucleation.

Nursing Interventions

Decreasing Parental Anxiety and Guilt

1. Listen to the parental feelings of guilt about transmitting the disease to the child or because they did not notice symptoms earlier.
2. Discuss the benefit of consultation about the probability of having another affected child.
   a. Risk ranges from approximately 1% to 10%, depending on family history and whether the affected child had unilateral or bilateral disease.
   b. The reportedly high lifelong cancer burden among retinoblastoma patients may also be important to parents in making informed decisions.
   c. Refer for genetic counseling and support parental decisions regarding future pregnancies.
3. Encourage the parents to seek genetic counseling for the affected child when he or she reaches puberty.
   a. The risk to offspring is from 1% to 50%, depending on family history and whether disease was unilateral or bilateral.

b. Among affected offspring, there is a high probability (greater than 50%) of bilateral disease.

Preserving Tissue Integrity

1. Administer sedatives or assist with anesthesia for intraocular chemotherapy, if necessary.
   a. Administer the medication in a timely manner so that sedation is adequate for positioning of the child.
2. Observe for possible adverse effects of chemotherapy and prepare the parents for their occurrence.
   a. Swelling and edema surrounding the intraocular chemotherapy site.
   b. Nausea and vomiting with systemic chemotherapy.

Reducing the Child's Anxiety and Fear
See also page 1693.

1. Encourage the parents to room-in and participate in the child's care to minimize separation anxiety.
2. Prepare the child and parents for all diagnostic procedures.
3. Describe the surgery and anticipated postoperative appearance of the child. Draw pictures or use a doll, if one is available.
   a. A surgically implanted sphere maintains the shape of the eyeball.
   b. The child's face may be edematous and ecchymotic.
4. Offer the family the opportunity to talk with another parent who has gone through the experience or to see pictures of another child with an artificial eye.
5. See "Nursing management of eye enucleation," page 587.

Promoting Acceptance of Prosthesis

1. Explain to child the changes in terms of losing diseased eye, having a bandaged orbit until it heals after surgery, and receiving a prosthetic eye.
2. Explain that the prosthesis will be made for him or her and will look like the removed eye.
3. Tell parents to expect the child to grieve the loss and to help him or her by talking about it, but to treat the child as the same person.

Minimizing Effects of Vision Loss

1. Maintain a safe, uncluttered environment for the child.
2. Hold the child frequently and stand close, within child's field of vision, while speaking or providing care.
3. Encourage the use of touch and other senses for exploring.
4. Set environmental limits so the child feels safe and can obtain help easily.

Family Education and Health Maintenance

1. Teach care of the orbit.
2. Teach care of the prosthesis—initial instructions are provided by the ocularist and should be reinforced by the nurse.
3. Advise protection of the remaining eye from accidental injury, such as wearing safety glass for sports, not putting sharp objects near eye, treating eye infections promptly.
4. Encourage maintenance of routine checkups for eye and medical care.

5. Stress need to have subsequent children carefully evaluated for retinoblastoma.
    a. An ophthalmologic examination under anesthesia is usually recommended at approximately age 2 months.
    b. The child should receive frequent examinations thereafter until judged safe from developing retinoblastoma, usually approximately age 3.
6. Refer families to resources such as Candlelighters (*www.candlelighters.org*).

Evaluation: Expected Outcomes

- Parents discuss feelings openly, show affection to the child.
- Parents describe possible adverse effects of radiation and how to care for skin around eyes.
- Demonstrates lessened anxiety by participating in age-appropriate activities.
- Shows acceptance of the prosthesis and not inhibited in behavior.
- Moves about environment with ease.

SELECTED REFERENCES

Aburn, G., & Gott, M. (2011). Education given to parents newly diagnosed with ALL: A narrative review. *Journal of Pediatric Oncology Nursing, 28*(5), 300–305.

Alexander, S., Nieder, M., Zerr, D., et al. (2012). Prevention of bacterial infection in pediatric oncology: What do we know, what can we learn? *Pediatric Blood & Cancer, 59*(1), pp. 16–20.

Bartlett, F., Kortmann, R., Saran, F. (2013). Medulloblastoma. *Journal of Clinical Oncology, 25*(1), 36–45.

Bölling, T., Hardes, J., Dirksen, U. (2013). Management of bone tumours in paediatric oncology. *Journal of Clinical Oncology, 25*(1), 19–26.

Carter, B., Coad, J., Bray, L., et al. (2012). Home-based care for special healthcare needs: Community children's nursing services. *Nursing Research, 61*(4), 260–268.

Dasgupta, R., & Rodeberg, D. A. (2012). Update on rhabdomyosarcoma. *Seminars in Pediatric Surgery, 21,* 68–78.

Dimaras, H., Kimani, K., Dimba, E. A., et al. (2012). Retinoblastoma. *Lancet, 379,* 1436–1446.

Dores G. M., Devesa S. S., Curtis R. E., et al. (2012). Acute leukemia incidence and patient survival among children and adults in the United States, 2001–2007. *Blood, 119*(1), 34–43.

Hunger, S. P., Lu, X., Devidas, M., et al. (2012). Improved survival for children and adolescents with acute lymphoblastic leukemia between 1990 and 2005: A report from the Children's Oncology Group. *Journal of Clinical Oncology, 30*(14), 1663–1669.

Kim, H. J., Chalmers, P. N., & Morris, C. D. (2010). Pediatric osteogenic sarcoma. *Current Opinion in Pediatrics, 22,* 61–66.

Kwaan, H. C., & Huych, T. (2010). Thromboembolic and bleeding complications in acute leukemia. *Expert Reviews in Hematology, 3*(6), 719–730.

Nagaswara Rao, Amulya A., Scafidi, J., Wells, E. M., & Packer, R. J. (2012). Biologically targeted therapies in pediatric brain tumors. *Pediatric Neurology, 46,* 203–211.

National Cancer Institute. (2013). Childhood Acute Lymphoblastic Leukemia Treatment. *www.cancer.gov/cancertopics/pdq/treatment/child/all/healthprofessional.*

National Cancer Institute. (2011). *A snapshot of pediatric cancer.* Bethesda, MD: Author. Available: *www.cancer.gov/aboutnci/servingpeople/snapshots/pediatric.pdf.*

Terezakis, S., Wharam, M. (2013). Radiotherapy for rhabdomyosarcoma: Indications and outcome. *Journal of Clinical Oncology, 25*(1), 27–35.

Thorp, N. (2013). Basic principles of paediatric radiotherapy. *Journal of Clinical Oncology, 25*(1), 3–10.

Van Cleve, L., Munoz, C., Riggs, M., et al. (2012). Pain experience in children with advanced cancer. *Journal of Pediatric Oncology Nursing, 29*(1), 28–36.

Zimmerman, K., Ammann, R., Cuehni, C., et al. (2012). Malnutrition in paediatric patients with cancer at diagnosis and throughout therapy: A multicenter cohort study. *Paediatric Blood and Cancer*, ePub ahead of print.

52
Pediatric Hematologic Disorders

PEDIATRIC HEMATOLOGIC DISORDERS

Anemia

 Evidence Base Janus, J., & Moerschel, S. K. (2010). Evaluation of anemia in children. *American Family Physician, 81*(12), 1462–1471.

Anemia refers to a deficit of red blood cells (RBCs) or hemoglobin (Hb) in the blood, resulting in decreased oxygen-carrying capacity. It is the most frequent hematologic disorder encountered in children.

Pathophysiology and Etiology

1. RBCs and Hb are normally formed at the same rate at which they are destroyed. Whenever formation of RBCs or Hb is decreased or their destruction is increased, anemia results. The ability of Hb to carry oxygen to the tissues and remove carbon dioxide for excretion by the lungs is decreased.
2. May be caused by blood loss related to:
   a. Trauma and ulceration.
   b. Decreased production of platelets.
   c. Increased destruction of platelets.
   d. Decreased number of clotting factors.
3. May be caused by impairment of RBC production caused by nutritional deficiency.
   a. Iron deficiency—most common type of anemia in ages 6 months to 3 years; approximately 3% of all children.
   b. Folic acid deficiency—causes formation of large RBCs with abnormal nuclear maturation (megaloblastic anemia).
   c. Vitamin B_{12} deficiency—causes megaloblastic anemia; called *pernicious anemia* if due to lack of intrinsic factor for absorption of vitamin B_{12}.
   d. Vitamin B_6 deficiency.
   e. Lead poisoning—lead absorbed by the bone marrow attaches to newly formed RBCs and inhibits synthesis of heme.
4. May be caused by decreased erythrocyte production.
   a. Pure RBC anemia.
   b. Secondary hemolytic anemias associated with chronic infection, renal disease, and drugs. In anemia of chronic infection and inflammation, the life span of the RBC is moderately decreased and the ability of the bone marrow to produce RBCs is significantly decreased.
   c. Bone marrow depression—leukemia, aplastic anemias, transient erythrocytopenia of childhood.
5. May be caused by increased erythrocyte destruction.
   a. Extrinsic factors:
      i. Drugs and chemicals.
      ii. Infections—transient erythroblastopenia of childhood caused by parvovirus (fifth disease), usually between ages 6 months and 4 years.
      iii. Antibody reactions—passively acquired antibodies against Rh, A, or B isoimmunization, autoimmune hemolytic anemia, burns, poisons (including lead poisoning).
   b. Intrinsic factors:
      i. Abnormalities of the RBC membrane.
      ii. Enzymatic defects—glucose-6-phosphate dehydrogenase deficiency.
      iii. Abnormal Hb synthesis—sickle cell disease, thalassemia syndromes.

c. In hemolytic anemias, the RBCs are destroyed at abnormally high rates, primarily by the spleen.

  i. The activity of the bone marrow increases to compensate for the shortened survival time of the RBCs.

  ii. Bone marrow hypertrophies and occupies a larger than normal share of the inner structure of bones.

  iii. Products of RBC breakdown increase with hemolysis.

  iv. Jaundice results when the liver cannot clear the blood of the pigment that results from the breakdown of Hb from destroyed RBCs.

  v. Iron builds up (hemosiderosis) and may deposit on body tissues.

6. May result from chronic illness such as rheumatoid arthritis and other inflammatory disorders (anemia of chronic disease).

7. "Physiologic anemia" occurs in term infants at ages 8 to 12 weeks; hematocrit (Hct) should not fall below 30%.

Clinical Manifestations

1. Condition may be acute or chronic. The more slowly the onset of anemia, the less likely patient will be symptomatic.

2. Early symptoms:
   a. Listlessness.
   b. Fatigability.
   c. Anorexia related to decreased energy.

3. Late symptoms:
   a. Pallor.
   b. Weakness.
   c. Tachycardia.
   d. Palpitations.
   e. Tachypnea; shortness of breath on exertion.
   f. Jaundice (with hemolytic anemias).

Diagnostic Evaluation

1. Complete blood count (CBC) with indices and reticulocytes—vary with types of anemia (see Table 52-1).

2. Serum iron and total iron-binding capacity—ratio of less than 0.2.

3. Serum ferritin—less than 12 g/dL.

4. Lead—greater than 20 g/dL.

5. Free erythrocyte protoporphyrin—greater than 35 g/dL.

6. B_{12}, B_6, folate levels—may be decreased.

7. Hb electrophoresis—may show Hb S or other abnormality.

8. Parvovirus B19 titer—may be elevated in transient erythroblastopenia.

9. Coombs test.

Management

Iron-Deficiency Anemia

1. Oral iron at a dose of 3 to 6 mg elemental iron/kg per day given between meals. Reticulocyte count should increase in 7 to 10 days; Hct increases in approximately 4 weeks.

2. Dietary: decrease milk intake to 16 oz per day; include iron-fortified cereals and bread products; increase consumption of red meat; include foods rich in vitamin C.

3. Currently, iron is rarely administered via intramuscular (I.M.) or intravenous (IV) route because of high incidence of allergic reactions. If administered, monitor the child closely.

Anemia of Chronic Lead Poisoning

See page 1432.

1. Early detection of high lead levels through screening questionnaires and blood tests.

2. Maintenance of a well-balanced diet, high in calcium and vitamin D.

3. Administration of chelating agents such as edetate disodium calcium, dimercaprol, or succimer according to recommendations of the Centers for Disease Control and Prevention.

4. Use of lead-free paints, gasoline.

5. Testing of house and soil.

6. Removal of individuals from unsafe environment.

Megaloblastic Anemia

1. Folate deficiency—administration of folic acid orally.

2. B_{12} deficiency—administration of B_{12} (cyanocobalamin) I.M.

Hemoglobinopathies

1. Sickle cell anemia (see page 1701).

2. Thalassemia (see page 1708).

Table 52-1	Blood Tests in Anemia by Cause				
	MCV	MCHC	RETICULOCYTE	FERRITIN	FEP
Iron Deficiency	Low	Low	Low	Low	High
Lead Poisoning	Low	Low	Low	Normal	High
ß-Thalassemia	Low	Low	Low	Normal	Normal
Folate Deficiency	High	Normal	Low	Normal	Normal
B_{12} Deficiency	High	Normal	Low	Normal	Normal
Sickle Cell Disease	Normal	Normal	High	Normal	Normal

FEP, free erythrocyte protoporphyrin; MCHC, mean corpuscular hemoglobin concentration; MCV, mean corpuscular volume.

Transient Erythroblastopenia of Childhood

1. Spontaneous recovery in 4 to 8 weeks.
2. For Hb levels of less than 5 g/dL or cardiac failure, transfuse packed RBCs.
3. Usually, unless cardiac failure occurs, supportive care, not therapy, is provided.

Anemia from Blood Loss or Bone Marrow Suppression

Packed RBC transfusions may be necessary (see page 1004).

Complications

1. Mental sluggishness, as a result of decreased oxygen and energy for normal neural activity; usually associated with a decreased attention span, decreased intelligence, and lethargy.
2. Growth retardation related to anorexia and decreased cellular metabolism.
3. Delayed puberty related to growth retardation.
4. Cardiac enlargement related to muscle hypertrophy because of increased strain on the heart, attempting to compensate for increased oxygen demand by the tissues; eventually results in heart failure.
5. Death from cardiac failure related to circulatory collapse and shock.

Nursing Assessment

1. Obtain history of potential causes.
   a. Dietary history, including the amount of milk and meat consumed; medications.
   b. Family history for genetic causes.
   c. Persistent infection, fever, or chronic disease.
   d. Exposure to drugs, poisons.
   e. Pica—craving and consuming nonfood items (eg, paint chips, paper).
2. Obtain a baseline assessment.
   a. Observe skin and mucous membranes for pallor.
   b. Obtain height and weight and plot on growth curve.
   c. Measure vital signs, including blood pressure (BP).
   d. Assess child's functional level—level of exercise tolerance, mental functioning.
   e. Assess attainment of developmental milestones.
3. Observe for fatigue, listlessness, irritability.
4. Observe for blood loss: bruising, bleeding, hematuria, or hematochezia (blood in stool). Assess for excessive menstrual bleeding in adolescent females.

 NURSING ALERT Be alert for children at risk for iron-deficiency anemia—children in rapid growth stages (toddlers and adolescents) and pregnant or lactating adolescents.

Nursing Diagnoses

- Fatigue related to decreased ability of blood to transport oxygen to the tissues.
- Imbalanced Nutrition: Less than Body Requirements of recommended daily dietary allowances.

- Risk for Infection related to debilitated state.
- Anxiety related to hospitalization and painful diagnostic procedures (venipunctures, fingersticks).
- Delayed Growth and Development related to decreased energy.

Nursing Interventions

Minimizing Fatigue

1. Plan nursing care to allow for lengthy periods when the child is not disturbed by hospital routines, procedures, treatments; set priorities.
2. Observe for early signs of fatigue, such as irritability, hyperactivity, listlessness.
3. Encourage sedentary rather than active projects.
4. Administer oxygen and position upright if dyspnea present.
5. Do not always encourage self-care.
6. Provide finger foods that are easy to chew to conserve energy.
7. Transfuse packed RBCs, as directed.

 NURSING ALERT Monitor transfusion for signs and symptoms of reaction: headache, anxiety, chills, dyspnea, chest pain, hypotension, flank pain, rash, hives, bronchospasm, pruritus, hypertension, more than 1 degree increase in baseline temperature.

Providing Adequate Nutritional Intake

1. Be aware of the child's food preferences and plan diet accordingly.
2. Offer small amounts of food at frequent intervals.
3. Reward the child for positive attempts to eat.
4. Allow the child to participate in selection of foods.
5. Avoid tiring activities and unpleasant procedures at mealtime.
6. Make mealtime as pleasurable as possible.
7. Provide iron-rich food and vitamins when necessary.
8. If iron is ordered, give between meals and with orange juice (iron is absorbed best in an acidic environment).
9. Limit milk and milk products to 16 to 24 oz per day. Milk products inhibit the absorption of oral iron.
10. Administer liquid iron with a dropper or straw or dilute with water or fruit juice to prevent staining the teeth.
    a. If administered by dropper, make sure that liquid iron is deposited in the back of the mouth.
    b. Dental stains can be removed by brushing the teeth with sodium bicarbonate or hydrogen peroxide and then rinsing with water after each administration.
11. Be alert for adverse effects of iron supplements—gastric distress, colicky pain, diarrhea, or constipation; may call for decreased dose.
12. Advise family that child's stool may turn dark green or black.
13. Stress the importance of continuing iron therapy according to health care provider's directions, even though the child may not appear to be ill.
14. Inform parents that iron overdoses can be harmful or fatal.

Preventing Infection

1. Teach and assist with good hygiene practices, such as handwashing and mouth care.
2. Avoid exposure to others with colds, infections.

3. Make sure that staff, family, and visitors always wash hands thoroughly.
4. Report temperature elevation or other signs of infection.

Reducing Anxiety

1. Allow the child to handle equipment used for tests and procedures (tourniquets, syringes).
2. Explain all procedures and the treatment plan to the child in a way that the child can understand.
3. Allow the older child to look through a microscope at a blood smear, if interested and if appropriate for child's age.
4. Permit the child to cleanse the area for a venipuncture or a fingerstick and to choose the finger.

Promoting Normal Growth and Development

1. Make sure that nutrition is adequate for age and activity level.
2. Encourage participation in age-related activities.
3. Encourage doing homework and tutored activities.
4. Encourage peer socialization.
5. Promote age-appropriate play and therapeutic play.
6. Perform periodic growth chart evaluation and developmental testing.
   a. Share results with parents and explain the association between diet/anemia and growth and development.
   b. Notify health care provider and make referrals, as indicated.

Family Education and Health Maintenance

1. Stress to the parents the importance of continuing the iron therapy according to the provider's directions even though the child may not appear ill.

 DRUG ALERT Much variation exists in the elemental iron content of commercially available liquid preparations that contain iron. To avoid confusion, the dosage should be expressed in terms of elemental iron and then converted to the proper amount of the therapeutic agent selected.

2. Initiate and reinforce good dietary habits.
   a. Foods rich in iron include dark green leafy vegetables, fortified cereals, dried fruits, nuts, and red meats.
   b. Do not allow the child to drink excessive quantities of milk to the exclusion of other foods that contain more iron. Limit milk intake to 16 to 24 oz per day.
   c. Provide vitamin supplements, if necessary. Vitamin C appears to enhance the absorption of iron.
   d. Explain the reasons for diet change to parents in language they can understand. Visual aids and pictures may be helpful.
   e. Assist the parents to select iron-rich foods that are acceptable to the child, within the family's food budget, and culturally acceptable.
3. Initiate a nutritional consultation, as indicated.
4. Discuss with parents any of the social, economic, and environmental problems that may contribute to the child's disease.

5. Emphasize to the parents the benefits of a referral to a community health nurse if it appears that the family will need support in dealing with the child's chronic disease.
6. Discuss general health measures, including adequate rest, diet, sunshine, and fresh-air activity.
7. Encourage regular medical and dental evaluations. Emphasize the need for appropriate follow-up visits.
8. Explain that infection may be prevented by dressing the child according to the weather and by keeping the child away from people with colds, sore throats, and other infections.
9. Teach the parents how to administer medication.
10. Alert the parents to signs of disease progression—increased fatigue, pallor, weakness, developmental delays, and poor performance in school and activities.
11. Prepare for possible adverse GI effects, including constipation and change in stool color.

Evaluation: Expected Outcomes

- Increasing activity noted.
- Eats frequent small feedings of cereal, bread, red meat, vegetables; tolerates iron supplement without adverse effects.
- Remains free from infection; normal temperature.
- Cooperates with frequent blood sampling.
- Maintains growth curve; manages age-appropriate developmental activities.

Sickle Cell Disease (Sickle Cell Anemia)

 Evidence Base McCavit, T. L. (2011). Sickle cell disease. *Pediatrics in Review, 33*, 195–206.

Sickle cell disease is a severe, chronic, hemolytic anemia occurring in people who possess two copies of the sickle gene (homozygous). The clinical course is characterized by episodes of pain caused by the occlusion of small blood vessels by sickled RBCs. Persons heterozygous (with one copy) for the sickling gene are said to possess the sickle cell trait, which is associated with a benign clinical course. Sickle cell disease is found almost entirely in blacks and people of Arabic or northern Mediterranean ancestry. Approximately 8% of blacks have the sickle cell trait. Approximately 1 of every 500 blacks and 1 of every 1,000 to 1,400 Hispanic American infants born in the United States has sickle cell anemia. Approximately 90,000 people in the United States are affected.

Pathophysiology and Etiology

1. Genetically determined, inherited disease—autosomal recessive.
2. Each person inherits one gene from each parent, which governs the synthesis of Hb (see Table 52-2).
3. Normally, each Hb molecule consists of four molecules of heme folded into one molecule of globin. Each globin molecule consists of two alpha chains and two beta chains.
4. The amino acid sequence on the chain is altered in sickle cell Hb—valine is substituted for glutamic acid in the sixth position of the 574 amino acids that make up the globin fraction of Hb.

Table 52-2	Transmission of Sickle Cell Disease		
GENOTYPE OF PARENTS	PROBABILITY OF ABNORMAL HEMOGLOBIN IN OFFSPRING		
	Normal	Trait	Disease
One parent with trait	50%	50%	0
Both parents with trait	25%	50%	25%
One parent with trait; One parent with disease	0	50%	50%
Both parents with disease	0	0	100%

5. Sickle cell Hb aggregates into elongated crystals under conditions of low oxygen concentration, acidosis, and dehydration.
6. This distorts the membrane of the RBC, causing it to assume a crescent or sickle shape. The cells easily become entangled and enmeshed, leading to increased blood viscosity, vessel occlusion, and tissue necrosis.
7. Sickled RBCs are fragile and are rapidly destroyed in the circulation; they live 6 to 20 days versus 120 days for normal RBCs.
8. Anemia results when the rate of destruction of RBCs is greater than the rate of production.
9. Increased sequestration of RBCs occurs in the spleen.

Clinical Manifestations

Children are rarely symptomatic until late in the first year of life, related to increased amounts of fetal hemoglobin (Hb F). Clinical manifestations are sporadic; the child may be asymptomatic for several months. Periods of crisis occur at variable intervals.

Signs of Anemia

May last 1 to 2 weeks and subside spontaneously.

1. Hb level—6 to 9 g/dL.
2. Loss of appetite.
3. Paleness.
4. Weakness.
5. Fever.
6. Irritability.
7. Jaundice; increased hemolysis results in hemosiderosis (increased iron storage in the liver).

Precipitating Factors of Crisis

1. Dehydration.
2. Infection.
3. Trauma.
4. Strenuous physical exertion.
5. Extreme fatigue.
6. Cold exposure.
7. Hypoxia.
8. Acidosis.
9. Surgery.
10. Pregnancy.

Sickle Cell (Vaso-occlusive) Crisis

Most common form of crisis.

1. Small blood vessels are occluded by the sickle-shaped cells, causing distal ischemia and infarction (see Figure 52-1).
2. Extremities:
   a. Bony destruction—related to erythroid hyperplasia of marrow, leading to osteoporosis or ischemic necrosis.
   b. Bone pain; painful and swollen large joints.
   c. Dactylitis ("hand-foot" syndrome)—aseptic infarction of metacarpals and metatarsals, causing symmetrical swelling and pain; commonly first vaso-occlusive event seen in infants and toddlers.
3. Spleen:
   a. Abdominal pain.
   b. Splenomegaly—initially enlarges because of increased activity at site of RBC hemolysis; increased size results in discomfort.
   c. After multiple episodes of splenic vaso-occlusion, the spleen becomes fibrotic and atrophied.
   d. Decreased splenic function increases the risk of infection, especially by encapsulated organisms such as *Streptococcus pneumoniae*.
4. Cerebral occlusion:
   a. Stroke.
   b. Hemiplegia.
   c. Retinal damage, leading to blindness.
   d. Seizures.

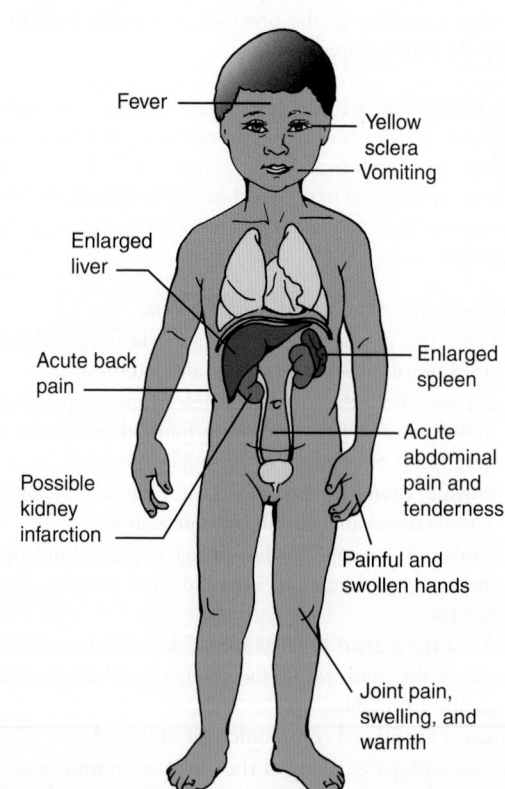

Fever

Yellow sclera

Vomiting

Enlarged liver

Acute back pain

Possible kidney infarction

Enlarged spleen

Acute abdominal pain and tenderness

Painful and swollen hands

Joint pain, swelling, and warmth

Figure 52-1. Sickle cell crisis signs and symptoms.

5. Pulmonary infarction.
6. Altered renal function: enuresis, hematuria.
7. Impaired liver function.
8. Priapism—abnormal, recurrent, prolonged, painful penile erection.

Splenic Sequestration Crisis

1. Large amounts of blood become pooled in the spleen.
2. Spleen becomes massively enlarged.
3. Great decrease in RBC mass occurs within hours.
4. Signs of circulatory collapse (eg, shock and hypotension) develop rapidly.
5. Frequent cause of death in infants with sickle cell disease.
6. Exchange blood transfusion may be required.

Aplastic Crisis

1. Bone marrow ceases production of RBCs only.
2. Results in low reticulocyte counts.

Chronic Symptoms

Chronic organ damage results in organ dysfunction.

1. Jaundice.
2. Gallstones.
3. Progressive impairment of kidney function.
4. Fibrotic spleen, resulting in high susceptibility to *Haemophilus influenzae* and *S. pneumoniae* infections, osteomyelitis, and pneumococcal septicemia.
5. Growth retardation of the long bones and spine deformities.
6. Delayed growth and puberty.
7. Cardiac decompensation related to chronic anemia (may develop heart failure).
8. Chronic, painful leg ulcers related to decreased peripheral circulation and unrelated to injury; may take months to heal or may not heal without intense therapy, including blood transfusions and grafting.
9. Decreased life span.
10. Altered bony structures—aseptic necrosis of the bones, especially the femoral and humoral heads.

Diagnostic Evaluation

1. Sickle cell prep (sickling test):
   a. Done by finger or heelstick.
   b. Oxygen is removed from a drop of blood.
   c. The blood is observed under the microscope for sickle-shaped cells.
   d. Test does not distinguish between people with sickle cell trait and disease or other sickle hemoglobinopathies.
   e. Routinely done on infants shortly after birth.
2. Sickledex:
   a. Done by fingerstick.
   b. A small amount of blood is placed in a solution containing a chemical-reducing agent.
   c. Sickle hemoglobin is indicated if the solution turns cloudy.
   d. Test also does not distinguish between people with sickle cell trait and disease or other sickle hemoglobinopathies.

3. Hemoglobin electrophoresis:
   a. Requires venipuncture.
   b. Hb is subjected to an electric current that separates the various types and determines the amounts present.
   c. Test is used to diagnose both sickle cell trait and sickle cell disease if two types of Hb are demonstrated in approximately equal amounts.
   d. A person is diagnosed as having sickle cell anemia if most Hb is sickle hemoglobin (Hb S). This may also diagnose other sickle hemoglobinopathies, including sickle C, sickle-ß-thalassemia, or other Hb variants.
4. Antenatal diagnosis is available to the high-risk group through amniocentesis and gene mapping (important if both parents have the trait).

Management

Preventing Sickling

1. Promote adequate oxygenation and hemodilution.
   a. Encourage increased intake of fluids—150 mL/kg per day or 2,250 mL/m² per day.
   b. Avoid high altitudes and other low-oxygen environments.
   c. Avoid strenuous physical exertion.
   d. Administer oxygen for pulse oximetry of 90% or less.
   e. Avoid extreme heat or cold.
   f. Routine blood transfusions (increase number of normal RBCs) (see page 1004).

Acute Management

Supportive and symptomatic care depend on type of crisis.

1. Aplastic episode—usually requires a blood transfusion starting at 10 mL/kg.
2. Splenic sequestration—usually requires a blood transfusion to release trapped RBCs in severe cases. Plasma volume expanders may also be used to correct hypovolemia. One or more episodes may require splenectomy.
3. Hemolytic episode—usually requires only hydration. May occur with splenic sequestration, aplastic, and painful episodes, which are then treated accordingly. Transfusions are required if a significant drop in Hb occurs.
4. Vaso-occlusive or painful episode—must be individualized; must determine if the painful event is a manifestation of an underlying illness (infection) or of an inflammatory condition. Most commonly caused by increased sickling, resulting from hypoxia and acidosis.
   a. Hydration—to reverse dehydration that may have been caused by decreased fluid intake, increased insensible loss, hyposthenuria, and hyperthermia (fever). This is accomplished by increased oral and parenteral fluid intake of up to two times fluid maintenance needs.
   b. Electrolyte and pH balance must be closely monitored.
   c. Analgesics—administered on fixed schedule, not to extend beyond the duration of the pharmacologic effect. IV opioids, such as morphine, are preferred for severe pain, either as a continuous infusion or on a patient-controlled analgesia pump to reach desired effects. Other agents, such as nonsteroidal anti-inflammatory drugs (NSAIDs) and

acetaminophen, are used for milder pain or to increase the analgesic effects of opioids.

   d. Alternative pain management techniques—behavior modification programs, relaxation therapy, hypnosis, music therapy, massage, and transcutaneous electrical nerve stimulation (TENS).

   e. Those with chronic or severe vaso-occlusive crises may benefit from monthly blood transfusions, which will improve anemia and decrease total amount of sickle hemoglobin; however, iron overload is a possible complication.

   f. There is ongoing research into hydroxyurea, which increases Hb F and prevents sickling.

   g. The only known cure for SCD, hematopoietic stem cell transplantation, is also under investigation; it is currently reserved for the most aggressive cases of SCD because of associated morbidity and mortality.

5. Infection—major cause of morbidity and mortality.

   a. Most serious include *S. pneumoniae, H. influenzae, Neisseria meningitidis, Salmonella* species, *Mycoplasma pneumoniae, Staphylococcus aureus, Escherichia coli,* and *S. pyogenes.*

   b. Infection of any type is more difficult to eradicate in patients with sickle cell and commonly exacerbates crises such as aplastic episodes caused by parvovirus (fifth disease), increases the rate of hemolysis, and precipitates vaso-occlusive episodes.

   c. Not at increased risk for viral or fungal infections, but these may precipitate a crisis.

   d. Prevention is most important—give usual primary immunizations as well as pneumococcal, *Haemophilus* b conjugate, hepatitis, meningococcal, and trivalent influenza vaccines.

   e. Antibiotic prophylaxis—prevents bacteremia and reduces nasopharyngeal colonization.

   f. Fever of 102° F (38.9° C), with minimal clinical signs, should be treated with broad-spectrum antibiotics to prevent septicemia. The choice of subsequent antibiotics can be guided by results of cultures and clinical course.

6. Stroke prevention—starting at age 2; routine transcranial ultrasound (TCD) to monitor blood flow to brain. Children with abnormal TCD have better outcomes if transfusion therapy is initiated.

Complications

1. Chronic hemolytic anemia.
2. Greatest risk of death is in children younger than age 5, mainly from overwhelming sepsis or sequestration.
3. Episodes of splenic sequestration, hemolysis, aplasia, vaso-occlusion.
4. Life expectancy is variable; however, it is improving with new forms of treatment. Survival through fourth decade of life is possible.

Nursing Assessment

1. Obtain history for possible dehydration, hypoxia, infection, or other precipitating event.
2. Observe for pallor and jaundice, changes in vital signs (elevated temperature, tachycardia, hypotension, tachypnea),

change in mental status, swelling of extremities, ulcers or skin lesions, or signs of dehydration (decreased elasticity of skin, dry mucous membranes, decreased urine output, increased urine concentration and specific gravity).

3. Examine for enlarged liver and spleen, tenderness of hands or feet.
4. Evaluate growth and development.

Nursing Diagnoses

- Acute Pain related to tissue anoxia from disease process.
- Ineffective Tissue Perfusion related to increased blood viscosity.
- Risk for Infection related to fibrotic changes in the spleen.
- Impaired Gas Exchange related to effects of opioids, anesthesia, and blood loss of surgery.
- Activity Intolerance related to anemia.
- Interrupted Family Processes related to frequent medical care, hospitalization, and chronic illness.

Nursing Interventions

 Evidence Base Vijenthira, A., Stinson, J., Friedman, J., et al. (2012). Benchmarking pain outcomes for children with sickle cell disease hospitalized in a tertiary referral pediatric hospital. *Pain Research & Management: The Journal of the Canadian Pain Society, 13*(7), 656–665.
   McClain, B., & Suresh, S. (2011). Sickle cell pain, in *Handbook of Pediatric Chronic Pain: Current Science and Integrative Practice,* pp. 177–192. New York: Springer.

Also see Nursing Care Plan 52-1.

Relieving Pain

1. Identify and use effective measures to alleviate pain, such as:
   a. Carefully position and support painful areas.
   b. Hold or rock the infant; handle gently.
   c. Distract the child by singing, reading stories, providing appropriate play activities, or television or videos.
   d. Provide familiar objects; encourage visits by familiar people.
   e. Bathe the child in warm water, applying local heat or massage.
   f. Give prescribed medications. Do not give aspirin because it enhances acidosis.
   g. Maintain bed rest during crisis.
2. Share effective methods of reducing pain with other staff members and family.
3. Patients with chronic pain may not display typical pain behavior; remember, "pain is what the patient says it is."
4. Assess effectiveness of intervention.

Increasing Tissue Perfusion

1. Administer blood for severe anemia and vaso-occlusion.
2. Administer oxygen via tent, face mask, or nasal cannula, depending on age.

Reducing Infection

1. Administer antibiotics, as prescribed.
2. Give meticulous care to leg ulcers and other open wounds.
3. Use good handwashing and meticulous technique in all procedures.

NURSING CARE PLAN 52-1

Painful Vaso-Occlusive Crisis

You are assigned Danielle, a 6-year-old with sickle cell anemia, who has been admitted with a fever of 102° F (38.9° C), chest pain, bilateral leg pain, and an oxygen saturation of 90%.

Subjective Data: Danielle complains of bilateral leg pain, states that it hurts to breathe, and says that she has the chills. She felt tired and had much pain yesterday and was unable to go to school. Her mother was giving her some pain medication at home, but when Danielle spiked a fever, she was brought to the emergency room and was admitted to your unit.

Objective Data: Vital signs—temperature of 100.7° F (38.2° C), pulse 120, BP 90/52, and respirations of 34. You notice that her legs are warm and swollen, tender to touch. Respiratory evaluation reveals bilateral crackles at the lung bases, labored respirations with oxygen mask on, and pallor.

Laboratory data:

- CBC—WBC, 15.4×10^9/L; HB, 6.5 g/dl; HCT, 20.1%; and platelets, 636,000 mm^3
- Pulse oximetry—90%
- Chest x-ray—bilateral lower lobe pneumonia
- Electrolytes—Na, 131 mEq/L; Cl, 110 mEq/L; K, 4.8 mEq/L
- Blood, urine, and throat cultures are pending

You know that hypoxia, dehydration, and acidosis may have been caused by the underlying respiratory infection and can all precipitate vaso-occlusive crisis. You develop your care plan to focus on resolution of these factors and to support the patient through crisis.

NURSING DIAGNOSIS

Impaired Gas Exchange related to pneumonia.

EXPECTED OUTCOME/GOAL

Oxygenation will be enhanced and respiratory acidosis will be prevented.

Nursing Interventions	Rationale	Actual Outcomes (Evaluation)

1. Administer oxygen via face mask to relieve dyspnea and promote oxygenation.
  a. Obtain pulse oximetry reading frequently and correlate with arterial blood gas (ABG) level results.
  b. Assess respiratory rate, use of accessory muscles, and depth of respirations.
	1. Secretion-filled alveoli impair gas exchange, leading to hypoxemia.
	  a. Pulse oximetry serves as guide to improving or worsening oxygenation. ABG levels should be done for correlation and to evaluate acid-base status.
	  b. Increasing rate, decreasing depth, and increased effort of breathing may lead to respiratory failure.
		1. On face mask, respirations 34, shallow, and with sternal retractions. Pulse oximetry 88%. Health care provider contacted and changed to Venturi mask at 40%.

2. Administer bronchodilator nebulization treatments every 4 hours, followed by coughing and deep-breathing exercises. Auscultate lungs hourly.	2. Will promote opening of airways and expectoration of secretions. Frequent auscultation of lungs will help evaluate effectiveness of therapy and determine the need for corticosteroids to reduce inflammation and open the airways further.	2. Lungs clearer following nebulization and coughing.
3. Administer IV antibiotics, as ordered.	3. Resolves pneumonia.	3. Antibiotic infusing via peripheral line.

NURSING DIAGNOSIS

Pain related to tissue anoxia caused by abnormal hemoglobin and clumping of sickled cells within the small vessels

---

EXPECTED OUTCOME/GOAL

Pain will be relieved.

Nursing Interventions	Rationale	Actual Outcomes (Evaluation)
1. Use nonpharmacologic strategies to help manage pain: distraction, relaxation, guided imagery, positive self-talk, cutaneous stimulation (warm soaks, massage), behavioral contracting.	1. Will limit the amount of analgesia, which may depress respirations.	1. Child uses blowing, looks at magic wand, listens to relaxation tapes and videos; states that they help.

(continued)

NURSING CARE PLAN 52-1 (continued)

Painful Vaso-Occlusive Crisis

Nursing Interventions	Rationale	Actual Outcomes (Evaluation)
2. a. Involve parent and child in selecting strategies. b. Institute and teach selected strategies before pain becomes severe.	2. a. Child will be more receptive to own choices and allows participation in care. b. If pain is severe, child may not be able to concentrate on these strategies if not practiced.	
3. Administer prescribed analgesia around the clock. Avoid as-needed orders when pain is predictable and continuous.	3. Maintains a steady state of analgesia and prevents clock-watching.	3. Receives medication every 4 hours without breakthrough pain reported.

> ! **NURSING ALERT** Avoid I.M. analgesia, if possible because children associate great deal of pain with shots and may deny pain to avoid getting a shot.

Nursing Interventions	Rationale	Actual Outcomes (Evaluation)
4. Assess pain relief using a developmentally appropriate scale and increase or decrease dose or time interval of medication for adequate control. a. Avoid placebo. b. Assess for respiratory depression, hypotension, and drowsiness with opioids.	4. Maximizes analgesia with minimal adverse effects. a. If expected effect is not received by placebo, child may lose trust in caretakers. b. Opioids may cause central nervous system depression, shallow respirations, and hypotension in large or frequent dosing.	4. No breakthrough pain with increased time interval (6 hours) between doses. b. Alert, respirations 24 and deep, BP 96/56.

NURSING DIAGNOSIS
Deficient Fluid Volume related to fever, insensible loss through mouth breathing and increased respiratory rate, and increased blood viscosity.

EXPECTED OUTCOME/GOAL
Hydration will be optimized.

Nursing Interventions	Rationale	Actual Outcomes (Evaluation)
1. Administer IV fluids, as ordered, based on calculation of recommended daily fluid intake requirements plus estimated loss.	1. Child should consume approximately 1,500 mL/m². Loss may be established by decrease in body weight (1 kg equals 1 L of fluid).	1. D_5NS infusing via peripheral IV volumetric pump.
2. Encourage child to drink by providing preferred fluids.	2. Intake will be enhanced by using preferences.	2. Sipping juices at intervals.
3. Monitor intake and output. Monitor urine-specific gravity.	3. Determines fluid balance and hydration status.	3. Intake and output equal; urine-specific gravity 1.020.
4. Administer acetaminophen for fever over 100.4° F (38° C).	4. Reduces fluid loss through perspiration due to fever.	4. Temperature 99.5° F (37.5° C).

Preventing Hypoxia

1. Monitor for and prevent respiratory depression caused by opioids.
   a. Check respiratory rate and depth frequently.
   b. Encourage coughing and deep breathing.
   c. Use incentive spirometry.
   d. Obtain pulse oximetry reading, as indicated.
   e. Raise side rails and supervise ambulation if drowsiness occurs.
2. Help reduce the risks of anesthesia and blood loss during surgery.
   a. Administer preoperative blood transfusions, as prescribed, to suppress the formation of new sickle cells and to reduce the threat of anoxia.
   b. Maintain adequate hydration before and after surgery.
   c. Observe the child closely for signs of infection, especially of the respiratory tract.
   d. Inform anesthesia department of child's disease status.
   e. Monitor vital signs frequently and obtain pulse oximetry readings.

Improving Activity Tolerance

1. Maintain bed rest during crisis, then increase activity gradually to increase endurance.
2. Encourage rest periods, alternating with activity.
3. Encourage good eating habits, sleep, and relaxation.

Normalizing Family Processes

1. Encourage parents to talk about their child, the illness, and how they feel about it.
2. Expect such feelings as guilt, shock, frustration, depression, and resentment.
3. Accept negative feelings, but try to build on positive coping mechanisms.
4. Provide factual information to child and parents about their concerns.
5. Encourage role-playing and play activities to identify fears.
6. Assure adolescents that although sexual development is delayed, they will eventually catch up with their peers.
7. Stress the normalcy of the child despite sickle cell disease.
   a. Sickle cell disease does not affect intelligence; the child should go to school and keep up with classwork while stable.
   b. Between periods of crisis the child can usually participate in peer group activities, with the exception of some strenuous sports.
   c. The child needs the same discipline as other children in family.

Community and Home Care Considerations

Home care nurses and school nurses can be instrumental in the care of patients with sickle cell anemia by ensuring that their primary health care needs are met.

1. Because of the child's predisposition to infections, be sure that the following are carried out routinely:
   a. Ophthalmology examinations every 1 to 2 years after age 10.
   b. Hearing tests yearly after age 3.
   c. A tuberculin skin test every 2 to 3 years (every year in at-risk populations). Any positive findings should be followed up promptly.
   d. All routine childhood immunizations, as well as the hepatitis B series, pneumococcal, meningococcal, *H. influenzae* type B, and yearly trivalent influenza.
   e. Dental checkups and teeth cleaning every 6 months.
2. Educate parents, teachers, and daycare providers involved in the care of children with sickle cell disease about their common problems and special needs:
   a. Frequent absences because of pain and illness.
   b. Fatigue and inattention, caused by anemia or ischemia of central nervous system tissue.
   c. Inability to concentrate urine, requiring frequent restroom breaks.
   d. Permanent learning disabilities or delays, requiring individualized teaching plans.
   e. Need for a controlled environment to prevent sickling, avoiding temperature extremes, dehydration, and excessive stress.
   f. Need for moderate physical exercise, with avoidance of rough contact sports and activities.
   g. Desire to feel "normal" and have opportunities and environmental stimulation similar to other children their age.
3. Assess the child's home environment for protection from infection and injury, adequate nutritional resources, transportation to medical appointments, and emotional support. Initiate social service and other referrals, as needed.
4. Consider/explore possible complementary and alternative therapies.

Family Education and Health Maintenance

1. Discuss the genetic implications of sickle cell disease and offer genetic counseling to the family.
2. Instruct the parents in ways that they can help their child to avoid sickling episodes.
   a. Do not allow the child to become chilled or to wear tight clothing that might impede circulation.
   b. Provide adequate fluids and notify health care provider if excessive fluids are lost through vomiting, diarrhea, fever, excessive sweating.
3. Instruct parents how to recognize signs of dehydration (dry skin and mucous membranes, decreased urine output; irritability or listlessness in the infant).
4. Encourage parents to seek prompt treatment of cuts, sores, and mosquito bites and to notify the health care provider if the child is exposed to a communicable disease.
5. Encourage good dental hygiene and frequent dental checkups to avoid dental infections.
6. Instruct on preventive care, including all the recommended childhood immunizations and screening tests.
7. Encourage a calm, emotionally stable environment.
8. Warn against trips to the mountains or against trips in unpressurized airplanes that will decrease oxygen concentration.
9. Provide sexually active adolescents with information on contraception and sexually transmitted disease.

10. Teach signs of a mild crisis:
    a. Fever.
    b. Decreased appetite.
    c. Irritability.
    d. Pain or swelling in abdomen, extremities, back.
    e. Teach parents to palpate spleen.
11. Instruct on home management of mild crisis.
    a. Encourage fluids.
    b. Administer antipyretic medications, as directed by health care provider familiar with condition.
    c. Encourage rest.
    d. Keep the child warm.
    e. Apply warm compresses to the painful area.
    f. Hospitalization may be required for the child if pain becomes severe or if IV hydration is required.
12. Teach the signs of severe crisis and whom to notify:
    a. Pallor.
    b. Lethargy and listlessness.
    c. Difficulty in awakening.
    d. Irritability.
    e. Severe pain.
    f. Fever of 102° F (38.9° C)—report immediately.
13. Instruct the parents to have emergency information available to those involved in the child's care (school nurse, teacher, babysitter, family members).
    a. Name and phone number of health care provider or clinic.
    b. Closest emergency facility and ambulance phone number.
    c. Child's blood type, allergies, medications, and medical records number.
    d. Name of informed neighbor or relative to be notified in an emergency.
14. Stress the benefit of wearing a MedicAlert bracelet.
15. For additional information and support, refer to Sickle Cell Foundation (*www.scdfc.org*).

Evaluation: Expected Outcomes

- Appears more comfortable and does not cry or complain of pain.
- Less pallor noted with oxygen use.
- Afebrile with no signs of infection.
- No change in respirations; uses incentive spirometer hourly.
- Ambulates 20 minutes four or five times per day.
- Parents verbalize concerns about chronic illness.

Thalassemia Major (Cooley's Anemia)

 Evidence Base Peters, M., Heijboer, H., Smiers, F., et al. (2012). Diagnosis and management of thalassaemia. *BMJ, 344*(7841), 40–44.

Thalassemia major is the most severe of the beta-thalassemia syndromes and represents the homozygous form of the disease. Beta-thalassemia (ß-thalassemia) refers to an inherited hemolytic anemia, characterized by a reduction or absence of the ß-globulin chain in Hb synthesis. This RBC has a decreased amount of Hb, resulting in a fragile RBC with a short life span. It is most prevalent in the Mediterranean basin, Middle East, Southeast Asia, and Africa. In the United States, it is most common in children of Italian, Greek, and Southeastern Asian ancestry. About 1,400 people in the United States are affected.

Pathophysiology and Etiology

1. Genetically determined, inherited disease—autosomal recessive pattern of inheritance.
2. Insufficient ß-globin chain synthesis allows large amounts of unstable chains to accumulate.
3. The precipitates of beta chains that form cause RBCs to be rigid and easily destroyed, leading to severe hemolytic anemia and resultant chronic hypoxia.
4. Erythroid activity is significantly increased in an attempt to overcome the increased rate of destruction, resulting in enormous expansion of bone marrow, thinning of bony cortex leading to:
    a. Skeletal deformities: frontal and maxillary bossing.
    b. Growth retardation.
    c. Pathologic fractures.
5. Rapid destruction of defective RBCs, decreased production of Hb, and increased absorption of dietary iron caused by the body's response to anemia result in an excess supply of available iron (hemosiderosis), which deposits iron on organ tissues, resulting in decreased function (especially cardiac).
6. In response to the low level of adult Hb, large concentrations of Hb F, which does not contain alpha chains, are produced; Hb F does not hold oxygen well.

Clinical Manifestations

1. Onset is usually insidious, with symptoms noted between ages 3 and 6 months when Hb F is diminished.
2. Symptoms are primarily related to the progressive anemia, expansion of the marrow cavities of the bone, and the development of hemosiderosis.
3. Early symptoms commonly include progressive pallor, poor feeding, and lethargy.
4. Further signs of progressive anemia include headache, bone pain, exercise intolerance, jaundice, and protuberant abdomen caused by hepatosplenomegaly.

Diagnostic Evaluation

1. Hb level—decreased.
2. RBCs—increased number.
3. Low mean corpuscular volume and mean corpuscular Hb concentration—microcytosis and hypochromia.
4. Peripheral blood smear—many anisopoikilocytes, nucleated RBCs.
5. Reticulocyte count—low, usually less than 10%.
6. Hb electrophoresis—elevated levels of HbF and HbA$_2$; limited amount of HbA.

Management

1. Frequent and regular blood transfusions of packed RBCs to maintain Hb levels above 9.5 g/dL.
    a. Washed, packed RBCs are usually used to minimize the possibility of transfusion reactions. If unavailable, leuko-filtered cells can be substituted.

b. The frequency and amount of transfusions depend on the size of the child, usually 10 to 15 mL packed RBCs per kg body weight every 2 to 3 weeks.

2. Iron chelation therapy with deferasirox or deferoxamine reduces the toxic adverse effects of excess iron; increases iron excretion through urine and feces.

   a. Deferoxamine: IV infusion of 100 to 150 mg/kg per day given in hospital during blood transfusion or for child with high ferritin level and poor compliance with home chelation therapy or subcutaneous infusion of 50 mg/kg per day usually infused 12 hours during night for home therapy.

   b. Deferasirox: 20mg/kg/day by mouth.

3. Splenectomy.

4. Supportive management of complications.

5. Hematopoietic stem cell transplants is the only known cure. Young patients with few complications are the best candidates.

6. Prognosis is poor; commonly fatal in late adolescence or early adulthood.

Complications

1. Splenomegaly—usually requires splenectomy; overwhelming postsplenectomy infection rate seen in 25% of these patients.

2. Growth retardation in second decade.

3. Endocrine abnormalities:

   a. Delayed development of secondary sex characteristics—most boys fail to undergo puberty; most girls experience alteration in menstruation.

   b. Diabetes mellitus is commonly seen in older patients, related to iron deposits on the pancreas.

   c. Hypermetabolic rate results in increased temperature and lethargy.

4. Skeletal complications—become less common because of early transfusion therapy and maintenance of Hb levels above 10 g/dL:

   a. Frontal and parietal bossing (enlarging).

   b. Maxillary hypertrophy, leading to malocclusion.

   c. Pathologic fractures.

   d. Premature fusion of epiphyses of long bones.

   e. Generalized skeletal osteoporosis.

   f. Pathologic fractures of the long bones and vertebral collapse.

5. Cardiac complications:

   a. Fibrosis and hypertrophy.

   b. Pericarditis.

   c. Heart failure—usual cause of death.

6. Liver enlargement—fibrosis, coagulation abnormalities, and eventually cirrhosis.

7. Gallbladder disease—gallstones are common by late adolescence; may require cholecystectomy.

8. Megaloblastic anemia—caused by sporadic folic acid deficiency from increased use by hyperplastic marrow.

9. Skin—bronze pigmentation caused by iron deposits in the dermis; jaundice.

10. Leg ulcers.

Nursing Assessment

1. Obtain family history of thalassemia or unexplained anemia or heart failure.

2. Perform whole-body examination to assess for anemia and systemic complications of thalassemia.

3. Measure growth and development parameters.

Nursing Diagnoses

- Ineffective Tissue Perfusion related to abnormal Hb.
- Chronic Pain related to progression of disease in bone.
- Activity Intolerance related to bone pain, cardiac dysfunction, and anemia.
- Risk for Infection related to progressive anemia and splenectomy.
- Deficient Knowledge related to iron chelation therapy.
- Disturbed Body Image related to endocrine and skeletal abnormalities.
- Ineffective Family Coping related to poor prognosis.

Nursing Interventions

Maximizing Tissue Perfusion

1. Administer blood transfusions, as ordered.

   a. Observe for signs of transfusion reaction (increased chance caused by frequency) including allergic, febrile, septic, circulatory overload, and hemolytic reactions.

   b. Allergic reactions usually occur within 15 to 20 minutes of start of the transfusion, although delayed reactions may occur up to several months later.

2. Monitor cardiovascular status for complications.

   a. Monitor apical pulse, BP, and respirations.

   b. Assess for edema.

   c. Auscultate heart sounds for gallop and lungs for rales.

   d. Assess extremities for ulcer formation.

3. Refer to "Care of the child with heart failure," page 1539.

Relieving Bone Pain

1. Monitor CBC, as ordered, and report Hb levels of less than 10 g/dL.

2. Elevate lower extremities.

3. Provide warm baths or soaks.

4. Administer or teach proper administration of NSAIDs, such as ibuprofen or naproxen. Use carefully and monitor liver enzymes in patients with liver complications.

Minimizing Activity Intolerance

1. Encourage participation in activities that do not require significant strenuous activity. Full participation in some activities, especially with peers, will increase self-esteem.

2. Facilitate physical and occupational therapy consultation to develop an acceptable exercise plan.

3. Assist the parents in contacting the child's school and develop a plan of gym activities, classes, and rest periods that allow the greatest level of participation and slowly develop endurance. Advise parents that during the week of the scheduled transfusion, the fatigue will be greatest, so gym and other exertional activities should be modified.

4. Suggest that driving the child to school and providing adequate rest at home will provide child with more energy for school activities.

5. Discourage participation in contact or other sports that increase the child's risk of a fracture (skateboarding, football, soccer).

Preventing Infection

1. Explain to parents that after splenectomy, child has increased susceptibility to infection and should be maintained on oral penicillin prophylaxis.
2. Make sure that child has been vaccinated against *H. influenzae*, pneumococcal, and meningococcal infections before splenectomy and encourage yearly trivalent influenza vaccination.
3. Encourage prompt medical attention for fever or signs of infection. Fever of 102° F (38.9° C) should be reported immediately and IV broad-spectrum antibiotics, such as ceftriaxone, started.

Promoting Understanding and Compliance

1. Explain to family the importance of chelating (binding) agents to decrease iron deposits in tissues and to increase iron excretion through urine and feces.
2. Administer IV deferoxamine, as ordered.
   a. Infuse slowly, during 8 to 24 hours, through peripheral line or implanted infusion device, via volumetric pump.
   b. Have emergency resuscitation equipment nearby in case a severe allergic reaction occurs.
3. Teach administration of oral deferasirox at home and encourage adherence to the medication schedule.
4. Be alert for visual and hearing deficits associated with use of deferoxamine and encourage follow-up visits for periodic visual and audiometric testing.

 NURSING ALERT Because of the excess iron deposition in children with thalassemia, dietary iron should be decreased as much as possible.

Improving Body Image

1. Explore the child's feelings of being different from other children.
2. Encourage the child to express feelings through the use of play: art, role playing.
3. Give positive reinforcement regarding appearance.
4. Encourage socialization and peer interaction.
5. Suggest endocrine consultation for delayed growth and puberty and craniofacial specialist for bony abnormalities.
6. Encourage the use of makeup, clothing, and hairstyles with adolescent, as indicated.
7. Suggest support group or individual counseling, as needed.

Improving Family Coping Strategies

1. Alleviate the child's anxieties about illness by providing explanation in a way the child can understand.
2. Use role-playing and play activities to identify concerns.
3. Assist parents in strengthening coping mechanisms, such as support network, problem solving, and planning ahead.
4. Help identify resources for financial support, medical supplies, respite care, etc.
5. Encourage parents to continue education of child and obtain vocational planning, if realistic.

6. Encourage parents to set limits and to provide discipline for child that is consistent with that for other children in family.
7. Provide supportive care to the dying child.
8. Encourage bereavement support for parents, siblings, and family.

Family Education and Health Maintenance

1. Discuss the genetic implications of thalassemia and refer for genetic counseling.
2. Provide detailed instruction about:
   a. Prevention and prompt treatment of infections.
   b. Medications.
   c. Home chelation therapy.
   d. Dietary modifications to limit iron intake.
   e. Activity restrictions, including avoidance of activities that increase the risk of fractures.
   f. Signs of complications.
3. Encourage parents to provide information about the child's condition to significant adults who are involved with the child (teacher, school nurse, babysitter, scout leader).
4. For additional information and support, refer to Cooley's Anemia Foundation (*www.thalassemia.org*).

Evaluation: Expected Outcomes

- BP stable; no edema; no leg ulcers.
- Rates pain as less than 4 out of 10 on developmentally appropriate scale.
- Reports increased participation in activity, less fatigue.
- Afebrile; immunizations current.
- Parents verbalize purpose of chelation therapy, treatment of allergic reaction, how to treat site; demonstrate correct technique for infusion.
- Verbalizes interest in appearance and positive statements about self.
- Parents seek help from support group and social worker; discuss illness with child and siblings.

Hemophilia

 Evidence Base Fijnvandraat, K., Cnossen, M. H., Leebeek, F. W. G., et al. (2012). Diagnosis and management of haemophilia. *British Medical Journal*, *334*, e2707.

Hemophilia is usually an inherited, congenital bleeding disorder characterized by a lack of blood clotting factors, especially factors VIII and IX. It is an X-linked disorder primarily affecting males; females act as carriers. The disease occurs in 1 in 5,000 males. There is no racial predilection, and hemophilia is found in all ethnic groups. It affects 18,000 people in the United States.

- 80% to 85% have factor VIII deficiency or hemophilia A (classic hemophilia).
- 15% to 20% have factor IX deficiency or hemophilia B (Christmas disease).
- Few have factor XI deficiency or hemophilia C.

Von Willebrand disease (pseudohemophilia) is a bleeding disorder caused by deficiency or abnormality in von Willebrand protein.

It is the most common inherited bleeding disorder (1 in 100 people have some form of the disease), and most forms of the disease are mild, presenting in later childhood or adulthood (see page 999).

Pathophysiology and Etiology

1. Hereditary (approximately 80% of patients).
   a. Sex-linked, recessive trait—caused by a gene carried on the X chromosome.
   b. Transmitted by asymptomatic females (see Table 52-3).
   c. Appears in males who have the hemophilic gene on their X chromosome.
   d. Affected males pass the gene to female offspring, making them carriers.
   e. May appear in females if a female carrier bears offspring with a male hemophiliac, although this is rare.
2. Spontaneous mutations may cause the condition when the family history is negative for the disease (about 30% of patients).
3. The basic defect is in the intrinsic phase of the coagulation cascade. The blood clotting factors are necessary for the formation of prothrombin activator, which acts as a catalyst in the conversion of prothrombin to thrombin.
   a. The rate of formation of thrombin from prothrombin is almost directly proportional to the amount of prothrombin activator available.
   b. The rapidity of the clotting process is proportional to the amount of thrombin formed.
4. The result is an unstable fibrin clot.
5. Platelet number and function are normal; therefore, small lacerations and minor hemorrhages are usually not a problem.

Clinical Manifestations

1. Seldom diagnosed in infancy unless excessive bleeding is observed from the umbilical cord or after circumcision.
2. Usually diagnosed after the child becomes active.
3. Varies in severity, depending on the plasma level of the coagulation factor involved.
   a. Level of less than 1% of normal—severe hemophilia; commonly severe clinical bleeding, with a tendency for spontaneous bleeds (factor level less than 0.01 µ/mL).
   b. Level of 1% to 5% of normal—moderately afflicted; may be free from spontaneous bleeding and may not manifest severe bleeding until trauma occurs (factor level less than 0.02 to 0.05 µ/mL).
   c. Level of 6% to 40% of normal—mildly afflicted; patients usually lead normal lives and bleed only with severe injury or surgery (factor level greater than 0.05 µ/mL).
   d. Degree of severity tends to be constant within a given family. Within an individual, severity does not vary over time unless inhibitor (autoantibody to infused factor) develops.
4. Signs and symptoms of abnormal bleeding include:
   a. History of prolonged bleeding episodes such as after circumcision.
   b. Easily bruised.
   c. Prolonged bleeding from the mucous membranes of the nose and mouth from lacerations.
   d. Spontaneous soft tissue hematomas.
   e. Hemorrhages into the joints (hemarthrosis)—especially elbows, knees, and ankles, causing pain, swelling, limitation of movement.
   f. Spontaneous hematuria.
   g. GI bleeding.
   h. Cyclic bleeding episodes may occur with periods of little bleeding, followed by periods of severe bleeding.
   i. Head trauma, resulting in intracranial hemorrhage.

Diagnostic Evaluation

1. Prothrombin time and bleeding time—normal.
2. Partial thromboplastin time—prolonged.
3. Prothrombin consumption—decreased.
4. Thromboplastin—increased.
5. Assays for specific clotting factors—abnormal.
6. Gene analysis—to detect carrier state, for prenatal diagnosis.

Management

1. Prompt, early, appropriate treatment is the key to preventing most complications.
2. Must replace missing coagulation factor (VIII or IX) through the administration of type-specific coagulation concentrates during bleeding episodes.
   a. *Factor VIII*—made from cryoprecipitate that has been viral inactivated, monoclonal, or solvent detergent purified. The monoclonal concentrates are the cleanest because most viruses and extraneous proteins have been removed. Since 1993, recombinant factor VIII concentrates are available for use. The factor VIII molecule has been sequenced and placed in a mammalian cell culture to produce recombinant factor VIII, which is free from all viruses.

Table 52-3 Transmission of Hemophilia

GENOTYPE OF PARENTS	PROBABILITY OF ABNORMALITY IN OFFSPRING				
	Female			Male	
	Normal	Carrier	Hemophiliac	Normal	Hemophiliac
Female carrier/normal male	50%	50%	0	50%	50%
Noncarrier female/hemophiliac male	0	100%	0	100%	0
Female carrier/hemophiliac male	0	50%	50%	50%	50%

b. *Factor IX*—made from fresh frozen plasma that has been viral inactivated by solvent detergent; monoclonal, heptane vapor; or affinity chromatography. The purest factor IX products are those that have gone through the monoclonal process or the affinity chromatography process, which removes most viruses and any other extraneous proteins and other factors. These are known as factor IX coagulation concentrates.

3. No viral inactivated concentrate exists for hemophilia C; fresh frozen plasma is given to supply factor XI.

4. Mild and moderate factor VIII–deficient hemophiliacs may respond to desmopressin, which causes the release of factor VIII from the endothelial stores. It is given in a dose of 0.3 mcg/kg per dose, usually every 24 hours.

5. Antifibrinolytics, such as aminocaproic acid and tranexamic acid, are given as adjunctive therapy for mucosal bleeding to prevent clot breakdown by salivary proteins.

6. Activated prothrombin complex concentrates that have activated factors VII, IX, and X are used when inhibitors (autoantibodies) have developed to bypass factor VIII or IX. In the case of factor VIII inhibitors, porcine factor VIII may also be given.

7. Supportive therapies:
   a. NSAIDs are used to decrease inflammation and arthritic-like pain associated with chronic hemarthroses. They must be used with caution because some types and higher doses interfere with platelet adhesion.
   b. Physical therapy to prevent contractures and muscle atrophy. This includes exercise, whirlpool, and icing.
   c. Orthotics to prevent injury to affected joint and to help resolve hemorrhages.

8. Synovectomy—orthopedic surgical intervention to remove damaged synovium in chronically involved joints.
   a. Open procedure provides direct visualization of joint and removal of damaged tissue.
   b. Arthroscopic—visualization and removal of the joint synovium through the use of an arthroscope.
   c. Radionucleotide—instillation of 32P, which removes damaged synovium; usually done through a needle.

9. Research into gene therapy—genetic copies of sequenced factor VIII and IX molecules are inserted into the body via some type of vector cell to find their way into the human host genetic machinery and begin to produce either factor VIII or factor IX in deficient patients.

Complications

1. Airway obstruction caused by hemorrhage into the neck and pharynx.
2. Repeated hemorrhages may produce degenerative joint changes with osteoporosis and muscle atrophy.
3. Intestinal obstruction caused by bleeding into intestinal walls or peritoneum.
4. Compression of nerves with paralysis caused by hemorrhaging into deep tissues; known as *compartment syndrome*.
5. Intracranial bleeding, resulting in serious neurologic impairments.
6. Death may result from exsanguination after any serious hemorrhage, such as intracranial, airway, or other highly vascular areas.

7. Contaminated cryoprecipitate, fresh frozen plasma, and concentrates have resulted in chronic active hepatitis and secondary cirrhosis.

8. Acquired immunodeficiency syndrome (AIDS) and human immunodeficiency virus (HIV)–related infections in patients receiving transfusions before 1985 with untested IV-contaminated blood products; 90% of patients who received products between 1979 and 1984 are HIV positive.

9. Uncertain life span for many hemophiliacs as a result of complications from hemorrhage or blood-borne viruses (hepatitis, AIDS). However, as a result of advances in therapy, viral inactivation of human plasma–derived factor concentrates and the new recombinant factor VIII concentrate, a normal life span is now possible.

10. It has been estimated that 20% of patients with hemophilia will develop an inhibitor or an autoantibody to the infused factor replacement. This results in decreased control of hemorrhages; these patients require massive doses of factor or activated prothrombin complex to overcome or bypass the inhibitor.

Nursing Assessment

1. Obtain history of and observe for unusual bleeding—ecchymosis, prolonged bleeding from mucous membranes and lacerations, hematomas, hemarthroses, hematuria, rectal and GI bleeding.
2. Assess joints for swelling, warmth, tenderness, range of motion (ROM), contractures, and surrounding muscle atrophy.
3. Assess family resources and coping skills.

Nursing Diagnoses

- Risk for Deficient Fluid Volume related to hemorrhage.
- Risk for bleeding related to inability of blood to clot.
- Impaired Physical Mobility related to repeated hemarthroses.
- Acute Pain related to bleeding into joints and muscles.
- Ineffective Family Coping related to disabling and life-threatening disease.

Nursing Interventions

Preventing Hypovolemia Through Control of Bleeding

1. Provide emergency care for bleeding.
   a. Apply pressure and cold on the area for 10 to 15 minutes to allow clot formation. This should be done especially after venipuncture or injection.
   b. Place fibrin foam or absorbable gelatin foam in the wound.
   c. Suturing and cauterization should be avoided.
2. Immobilize the affected part and elevate above the level of the heart.
3. Administer recombinant factor VIII or factor IX coagulation concentrate.
   a. Avoid rapid administration to minimize the possibility of transfusion reaction; usually 2 to 3 mL/minute; consult package inserts.
   b. In the case of head trauma, administer factor replacement prior to obtaining imaging—waiting to administer factor can have serious neurologic effects.
   c. Cryoprecipitate and fresh frozen plasma are not recommended because of their lack of viral inactivation treatment.

d. Stop the transfusion if hives, headaches, tingling, chills, flushing, or fever occurs.

4. Apply fibrinolytic agents to wound for oral bleeding.

5. Keep child quiet during treatment to decrease pulse and rate of bleeding.

6. Monitor vital signs and treat for shock if child becomes hypotensive.

Providing Protection Against Bleeding

1. For patients with severe hemophilia, administer prophylactic Factor IX or XIII two to three times weekly to prevent spontaneous bleeds.

2. Avoid obtaining rectal temperatures; insert thermometer probe gently and use axillary, oral (if age appropriate), or external ear route.

3. Avoid injections, if possible.
   a. Administer medications orally whenever possible.
   b. Subcutaneous route is preferred over I.M.
   c. Apply pressure to injection site for 10 to 15 minutes. Then apply a pressure dressing with self-adhesive gauze.

 DRUG ALERT Children with hemophilia should not receive aspirin or compounds containing aspirin because these medications affect platelet function and prolong bleeding time.

4. Maintain a safe environment and teach parents safety measures.
   a. Pad crib or bed rails.
   b. Inspect toys for sharp or rough edges.
   c. Offer finger foods and fluids in plastic or paper containers.
   d. Supervise small children when they are ambulatory.
   e. Use protective devices that the child brings from home. (Many children wear helmets and knee and elbow pads.)
   f. Continually assess environment for potential hazards.
   g. No straws or sharp eating utensils.
   h. No hard candy, suckers, or candy canes.

Preserving Mobility

1. Treat hemarthrosis or muscle bleed as soon as possible.
2. Provide supportive care for hemarthrosis.
   a. Immobilize the joint in a position of slight flexion.
   b. Elevate the affected part above the level of the heart.
   c. Apply ice packs. Later, after active bleeding has stopped, apply heat to promote absorption of blood.
3. For severe hemarthroses, continue immobilization through casting, if necessary, and prevent weight-bearing on the affected limb.
4. For less severe hemarthroses, begin gentle, passive exercise 48 hours after the acute phase to prevent joint stiffness and fibrosis. Progress to active exercises.
5. Administer short course of corticosteroids, as ordered, to relieve inflammation.
6. Refer for physical therapy if persistent deformity or if crutches, braces, splints, or specialized treatments are needed.

Relieving Pain

1. Be aware that increased pain usually means that bleeding continues and further replacement therapy may be needed.

2. Assess for further swelling of joints and limitation of movement.
3. Administer or teach administration of acetaminophen during acute phase. NSAIDs may be used for chronic pain, but cautiously, to prevent interference with platelet function.
4. Administer opioids sparingly, as ordered, for severe, acute pain.
5. For chronic pain, consider such alternatives as hypnosis, biofeedback, relaxation techniques, and TENS.

Enhancing Family Coping

1. Help parents understand that no one is to blame.
2. Allow the child and other family members to handle equipment used in care.
3. Use play to help the young child and siblings adjust to illness by "transfusing" teddy bear.
4. Encourage the parents to allow the child to participate in as many normal activities as possible within the realm of safety.
5. Encourage the child's continuing education. Parents fear sending the child to school, but safety issues can be addressed through discussions with the school nurse, teachers, and principal. Home or hospital tutoring should be continued while child is away from school.
6. Refer to social worker for counseling and identification of resources for financial concerns.
7. Encourage avoidance of overprotection—this can be more disabling than the disease itself.
   a. Promote a sense of independence and self-care within patient's limitations.
   b. Encourage healthful activity and reasonably aggressive pursuits. Reinforce self-judgment of child or teenager in selection of safe physical activities.
   c. Participate in as many age-appropriate activities as possible.
   d. Help parents understand the importance of vocational guidance for their child—emphasis should be given to occupations using intellect or skills rather than physical effort.
   e. Encourage older children to learn self-care and independent management.
8. Encourage involvement in support group.

Community and Home Care Considerations

1. Perform a home safety survey to identify potential hazards to the hemophiliac child, such as cluttered furniture the child may bump into, sharp edges on furniture or other objects, loose rugs that promote falls, slippery tub or floor surfaces, rocks or holes in backyard, or concrete play areas.
2. Provide teaching and referrals to initiate an infusion therapy program at home when hemorrhage begins. Assist with teaching the following:
   a. How to assess the child to determine if and what treatment is needed.
   b. Storage and preparation of replacement factors.
   c. Venipuncture technique.
   d. Transfusion management.
   e. Record-keeping.
   f. Awareness of signs of transfusion reaction and its management.
   g. Recognition of indications of need for subsequent transfusions.

3. Make sure that primary health care needs are being met by facilitating the following:

    a. Regular visits to primary care provider for preventive health maintenance to address growth and development, behavior, and psychosocial issues.

    b. Dental examinations and teeth cleaning every 6 months.

    c. All the recommended childhood immunizations, plus hepatitis A, to prevent infection from blood-borne pathogens.

4. Provide education to family and all caregivers about recognizing and treating bleeds appropriately.

5. Provide emotional support through the provision of educational materials, information about support groups, and a list of resources within the community.

6. Educate teachers and other school faculty about the child's special needs.

    a. These children can have permanent mental or physical disabilities from old hemorrhages, necessitating individualized plans.

    b. They must avoid rough or contact sports and activities; they do better with individual or calm group activities.

    c. All injuries must be taken seriously. The school nurse should be notified so that proper first aid and treatment can be initiated.

    d. Although they have a chronic illness, these children have a strong desire to be "normal," with the same opportunities and environmental stimulation as other children.

Family Education and Health Maintenance

1. Review safety measures to prevent or minimize trauma.

2. Encourage education by parents to teachers, babysitters, and others involved in child's care so that they can be responsive in an emergency.

3. Advise wearing a MedicAlert bracelet.

4. Remind parents not to administer aspirin to the child.

5. Teach emergency treatment for hemorrhage.

    a. Immobilize the part with splints or an elastic compression bandage. (These materials should be immediately available in the home.)

    b. Apply ice packs. Parents should keep two or three plastic bags of ice immediately available in the freezer.

    c. Consult the child's health care provider and initiate additional recommended therapy.

6. Encourage regular medical and dental supervision.

    a. Preventive dental care is important. Soft-bristled or sponge-tipped toothbrushes should be used to prevent bleeding. Factor replacement therapy is necessary for extensive dental work and extractions.

    b. Hepatitis B vaccine is necessary to protect against the rare occurrence of hepatitis B from blood transfusions, but does not guard against hepatitis C.

7. Teach healthy diet to avoid obesity, which places additional strain on the child's weight-bearing joints and predisposes to hemarthroses. Also teach the child to avoid sharp utensils, hard candy, suckers, and other foods with sharp edges that may cause mucosal lacerations.

8. Assist the parents in teaching the child to understand the exact nature of the illness as early as possible. Special attention should be given to the signs of hemorrhage and the child should be told of the need to report even the slightest bleeding to an adult immediately.

9. Advise families that genetic counseling and family planning are available for parents and adolescent patients.

10. Educate regarding hepatitis B and C and HIV disease as well as risks of treatment.

11. For additional information and support, refer to National Hemophilia Foundation (*www.hemophilia.org*).

Evaluation: Expected Outcomes

- Bleeding controlled; BP stable.
- Needlesticks avoided; staff and parents observe safety precautions.
- Performs passive ROM without pain.
- Rates pain at less than 4 out of 10 on a developmentally appropriate scale.
- Parents participate in care, play with child.

SELECTED REFERENCES

Black, M. M., Quigg, A. M., Hurley, K. M., et al. (2011). Iron deficiency and iron deficiency anemia in the first two years of life: Strategies to prevent loss of developmental potential. *Nutrition Reviews, 69,* 564–570.

DeBaun, M., & Telfair, J. (2012). Transition and sickle cell disease. *Pediatrics, 130*(5), 926–935.

Emiliani, F., Bertocchi, S., Poti, S., & Palareti, L. (2011). Process of normalization in families with children affected by hemophilia. *Qualitative Health Research, 21*(12), 1667–1678.

Fijnvandraat, K., Cnossen, M. H., Leebeek, F. W. G., et al. (2012). Diagnosis and management of haemophilia. *British Medical Journal, 334,* e2707.

Higgs, D. R., Engel, J. D., & Stamatoyannopoulos, G. (2012). Thalassemia. *Lancet, 379,* 373–383.

Janus, J., & Moerschel, S. K. (2010). Evaluation of anemia in children. *American Family Physician, 81*(12), 1462–1471.

Livesay, S., & Ruppert, S. D. (2012). Acute chest syndrome of sickle cell disease. *Critical Care Nursing Quarterly, 35*(2), 183–195.

Maguire, J. L., Lebovic, G., Kandasamy, et al. (2013). The relationship between cow's milk and stores of vitamin D and iron in early childhood. *Pediatrics, 131*(1), e144–e151.

McClain, B., & Suresh, S. (2011). Sickle cell pain, in *Handbook of Pediatric Chronic Pain: Current Science and Integrative Practice,* pp. 177–192. New York: Springer.

McCavit, T. L. (2011). Sickle cell disease. *Pediatrics in Review, 33,* 195–206.

Musumadi, L., Westerdale, N., & Appleby, H. (2012). An overview of the effects of sickle cell disease in adolescents. *Nursing Standard, 26*(26), 35–40.

Peters. M., Heijboer, H., Smiers, F., et al. (2012). Diagnosis and management of thalassaemia. *BMJ, 344*(7841), 40–44.

Pitrolo, M. M., Pinto, L., Sanfillippo, N., et al. (2011). Detection of early cardiac dysfunction in patients with beta thalassemia major by tissue doplar echocardiography. *Echocardiography, 28*(2), 175–180.

Rice, H. E., Crary, S. E., Langer, J. C., et al. (2012). Comparative effectiveness of different types of splenectomy for children with congential hemolytic anemias. *Journal of Pediatrics, 160*(4), 684–689.

Vijenthira, A., Stinson, J., Friedman, J., et al. (2012). Benchmarking pain outcomes for children with sickle cell disease hospitalized in a tertiary referral pediatric hospital. *Pain Research & Management: The Journal of the Canadian Pain Society, 13*(7), 656–665.

53
Pediatric Immunologic Disorders

IMMUNOLOGIC DISORDERS

Pediatric Human Immunodeficiency Virus/Acquired Immunodeficiency Syndrome

Human immunodeficiency virus (HIV) infection for infants, children, and adolescents is represented by a continuum of immunologic and clinical classifications ranging from no to severe immunologic suppression and asymptomatic to severely symptomatic. *Acquired immunodeficiency syndrome (AIDS)* is the end-stage of the continuum. Also see Chapter 29, HIV disease and AIDS, page 1043.

Epidemiology

 Evidence Base Joint United Nations Programme on HIV/AIDS. (2012). UNAIDS report on global AIDS epidemic 2012. Available: *http://www.unaids .org/en/resources/campaigns/20121120_globalreport2012/ globalreport/*.
  Centers for Disease Control and Prevention. (2012). HIV surveillance report, diagnosis of HIV infection and AIDS in the United States and dependent areas 2010. Atlanta, GA: Author. Available: *www.cdc.gov/hiv/topics/surveillance/ resources/reports/*.

1. HIV is a pandemic, affecting people all over the world; the World Health Organization estimated 34 million people living with HIV in 2011.
2. Children under age 15 account for 3.3 million infected with HIV worldwide; in North America, there are 4,500 cases.
3. In North America, UNAIDS reported there were more than 1.4 million people living with the virus in 2011.

4. In the United States it is estimated that youth aged 13–24 represent the second highest rate of newly acquired HIV.

 Evidence Base Centers for Disease Control and Prevention. (2012). Diagnoses of HIV infection and AIDS among adolescents and young adults in the United States and 5 U.S. dependent areas, 2006–2009. *HIV Surveillance Supplemental Report, 17*(2). Available: *www .cdc.gov/hiv/topics/surveillance/resources/reports/*.

5. HIV is transmitted through sexual contact with an infected person; through exposure to infected blood and blood components (sharing needles via IV drug use, tattooing, piercing, and unsterilized medical equipment); or from an HIV-infected mother to her baby before or during birth or through breastfeeding.
6. Numerous studies have indicated that a majority of HIV-infected males and females continue to be sexually active and the incidence of sexually acquired HIV infection among adolescents, in particular, has increased.
7. The availability of highly active antiretroviral therapy (HAART) and effective perinatal transmission prevention approaches has resulted in an increased number of HIV-infected females who choose to become pregnant.
8. In the United States, perinatally acquired HIV infection has dramatically decreased from about 25% to less than 2% (although the number of new cases worldwide continues to rise).
   a. This decrease reflects concerted efforts to provide voluntary HIV testing for pregnant women, along with the use of combination antiretroviral regimens during pregnancy, additional IV zidovudine during labor (ideally more than 4 hours before delivery), and zidovudine to the HIV-exposed

infant for the first 6 weeks of life, along with the avoidance of breastfeeding.

b. The use of cesarean birth in the mother whose viral load is greater than 1,000 copies/mL may also be indicated to reduce vertical transmission.

Evidence Base Panel on Treatment of HIV-Infected Pregnant Women and Prevention of Perinatal Transmission. (2012). Recommendations for use of antiretroviral drugs in pregnant HIV-1-infected women for maternal health and interventions to reduce perinatal HIV transmission in the United States. Available: *http://aidsinfo .nih.gov/contentfiles/lvguidelines/PerinatalGL.pdf.*

9. An HIV-infected mother can have a child who is infected and subsequent children who are not infected. Likewise, one infant in a multiple birth can be infected, whereas the other infants are not.

10. Children born to mothers with high HIV RNA viral load, low CD4+ lymphocyte counts, and severely symptomatic HIV disease are at greater risk for infection.

a. Infants born to such mothers and who become infected appear to be at increased risk for more rapid disease progression.

b. Infants born to mothers who seroconvert during pregnancy are at an increased risk for becoming infected.

11. With the advent of HAART, the morbidity and mortality in HIV-infected children has decreased significantly. Thus, in those who have access to medication and who are adherent to therapy, HIV has become a chronic, manageable illness.

Pathophysiology and Etiology

Evidence Base American Academy of Pediatrics. (2012). Section 3: Summaries of Infectious Diseases. In: Pickering, L. K., Baker, C. J., Kimberlin, D. W., Long, S. S., (eds). *Red Book: 2012 Report of the Committee on Infectious Diseases* (29th ed.) Elk Grove Village, IL: American Academy of Pediatrics (418–439).

1. The causative agent is a retrovirus that damages the immune system by infecting and depleting the CD4+ lymphocytes (T4-helper cells). These CD4+ lymphocytes play a central role in the regulation of the immune system.

2. There are also abnormalities in the function of cellular and humoral immunity (B cells, CD8+ cells, natural killer cells, monocytes, macrophages, and specific antibodies).

3. Progressive destruction of the immune system leads to:

a. Increased incidence of serious bacterial infections, such as bacteremias, bacterial pneumonias, and osteomyelitis.

b. Opportunistic infections, which commonly include *Pneumocystis jirovecii* pneumonia (PCP), esophageal candidiasis, and *Mycobacterium avium* infection.

c. More aggressive forms of viral infections, such as severe varicella, disseminated zoster, and cytomegalovirus pneumonitis.

d. Cancers, especially lymphomas.

e. Wasting syndromes and encephalopathy.

4. Multisystem organ involvement results in cardiomyopathies, nephropathies, neurologic impairment, GI dysfunction, endocrine disorders, dermatologic manifestations, musculoskeletal abnormalities, ocular impairments, ear, nose, and throat problems, and hematologic disorders.

5. An AIDS diagnosis occurs when a child presents as severely symptomatic (Category C) or with lymphoid interstitial pneumonitis (LIP from Category B) along with severe immune suppression (see Tables 53-1 and 53-2).

6. Once an AIDS diagnosis is made, it is not reversed even with reconstitution of the immune system and recovery from the opportunistic infection.

Clinical Manifestations

1. Generalized lymphadenopathy, especially in less common sites, such as epitrochlear and axillary areas.

2. Persistent, recurrent oral candidiasis.

3. Failure to thrive.

4. Developmental delays or loss of previously acquired milestones.

5. Hepatomegaly.

6. Splenomegaly.

7. Persistent diarrhea.

Table 53-1	Pediatric HIV Classification*			
IMMUNOLOGIC CATEGORIES	**CLINICAL CATEGORIES**			
	N: No Signs/Symptoms	**A: Mild Signs/Symptoms**	**B: + Moderate Signs/Symptoms**	**C: + Severe Signs/Symptoms**
1: No evidence of suppression	N1	A1	B1	C1
2: Evidence of moderate suppression	N2	A2	B2	C2
3: Severe suppression	N3	A3	B3	C3

*Children whose HIV infection status is not confirmed are classified by using the above grid with a letter E (for perinatally exposed) placed before the appropriate classification code (eg, EN2)

+Category C and lymphoid interstitial pneumonitis in Category B are reportable to state and local health departments as acquired immunodeficiency syndrome.

Centers for Disease Control and Prevention. (1994). 1994 revised classification system for human immunodeficiency virus infection in children less than 13 years of age. Morbidity and Mortality Weekly Report, 43(RR-12), 1–10. Available: www.cdc.gov/mmwr/preview/mmwrhtml/00032890.htm.

Table 53-2	Immunologic Categories Based on Age-specific CD4+ T-lymphocyte Counts and Percentage of Total Lymphocytes						
IMMUNOLOGIC CATEGORY	**AGE OF CHILD**						
	Younger than Age 12 Months		Ages 1–5		Ages 6–12		
	mm³	(%)	mm³	(%)	mm³	(%)	
1: No evidence of suppression	≥1,500	(≥25)	≥1,000	(≥25)	≥500	(≥25)	
2: Evidence of moderate suppression	750–1,499	(15–24)	500–999	(15–24)	200–499	(15–24)	
3: Severe suppression	<750	(<15)	<500	(<15)	<200	(<15)	

Centers for Disease Control and Prevention. 1994 revised classification system for human immunodeficiency virus infection in children less than 13 years of age. Morbidity and Mortality Weekly Report, 43(RR-12), 1–10. Available: www.cdc.gov/mmwr/preview/mmwrhtml/00032890.htm.

8. Hypergammaglobulinemia or hypogammaglobulinemia (elevated or diminished levels of immunoglobulin [Ig] G, IgM, IgA).

9. Parotitis.

10. Unexplained anemias, thrombocytopenia.

11. Unexplained cardiac or kidney disease.

12. Recurrent mild or serious bacterial infections.

Diagnostic Evaluation

1. All pregnant women in the United States should be tested for HIV before delivery. Neonatal testing with enzyme-linked immunoassay (ELISA) is an indication of the presence of circulating maternal antibodies to HIV and is not an indication of the child's infection status.

2. Polymerase chain reaction (PCR) assay is the most sensitive, specific, and preferred method for detecting HIV infection in a child younger than 18 months. The 2011 Centers for Disease Prevention and Control (CDC) guidelines recommend testing for infants using PCR at ages 14 to 21 days, 1 to 2 months, and 4 to 6 months.

3. After age 18 months, HIV antibody assays can be used for testing because maternal antibodies should not be present by this age. As with adults, a reactive ELISA must be followed by a confirmatory Western blot test.

4. Additional laboratory studies important to follow on the HIV-exposed infant include complete blood count (CBC) with differential to monitor for anemia and neutropenia and lymphocyte subsets (CD4+ counts).

5. For a known infected child, CBC with differential, platelet counts, serum chemistries, serial CD4+ counts, and HIV PCR (viral load) should be done every 3 to 6 months (depending on previous results and the stage of disease). In addition, a baseline echocardiogram and chest x-ray should be done and repeated yearly.

6. In known infected children or at-risk infants (those born to an HIV-infected mother but whose own status is still indeterminate), computed tomography scanning or magnetic resonance imaging of the head may be indicated if there is evidence of neurologic impairment, falling rate of head growth, or developmental delays or regression.

Management

1. Initiation of PCP prophylaxis is indicated when low CD4+ counts occur, with the exception that all infants born to HIV-infected women should be started on PCP prophylaxis at age 4 to 6 weeks, regardless of their CD4+ count (see Table 53-3).
   a. The first drug of choice is cotrimoxazole.

Table 53-3	Recommendations for PCP Prophylaxis and CD4+ Monitoring for HIV-Exposed Infants and HIV-Infected Children, by Age and HIV-Infection Status	
AGE/HIV-INFECTION STATUS	**PCP PROPHYLAXIS**	**CD4+ MONITORING**
Birth to ages 4–6 weeks, HIV exposed	No prophylaxis	1 month
Ages 4–6 weeks to 4 months, HIV exposed	Prophylaxis	3 months
Ages 4–12 months, HIV infected or indeterminate	Prophylaxis	6, 9, and 12 months
Under ages 4–12 months, HIV infection reasonably excluded	No prophylaxis	None
Ages 1–5, HIV infected	Prophylaxis if: CD4+ count is <500 cells/L or CD4+ percentage is <15%	Every 3–4 months
Ages 6–12, HIV infected	Prophylaxis if: CD4+ count is <200 cells/L or CD4+ percentage is <15%	Every 3–4 months

Adapted from Centers for Disease Control and Prevention. (1995). 1995 revised guidelines for prophylaxis against Pneumocystis carinii pneumonia for children infected with or perinatally exposed to human immunodeficiency virus. Morbidity and Mortality Weekly Report, 44(RR-4), 1–11. Available: www.cdc.gov/mmwr/preview/mmwrhtml/00037275.htm.

b. Pentamidine, atovaquone, and dapsone are alternative choices.

c. PCP prophylaxis should be discontinued in infants whose infection has been reasonably excluded on the basis of two or more negative viral diagnostic tests performed at >4 weeks and >8 weeks of age. Some experts may choose not to prophylaxis infants in whom antenatal and peripartum management has been appropriate and in whom the risk of infection is very low.

2. The choice to start therapy early while an individual is still asymptomatic versus delaying therapy until clinical or immunologic symptoms appear continues to generate considerable controversy among pediatric and adult HIV experts. Antiretroviral therapy is recommended for all HIV-infected children <1 year of age and in older children who have clinical symptoms of HIV or evidence of immune suppression regardless of the age of the child or HIV PCR level (viral load).

a. Clinical trial data from both adults and children have demonstrated that antiretroviral therapy in symptomatic patients slows clinical and immunologic disease progression and reduces mortality.

b. Seven classes of antiretrovirals (ARVs) have been approved for use in children: nucleoside reverse transcriptase inhibitors (NRTIs), non-nucleoside reverse transcriptase inhibitors (NNRTIs), protease inhibitors (PIs), integrase inhibitor, CCR5 antagonist, and fusion inhibitor.

c. Combination therapy is now standard care; using at least three ARVs from at least two drug classes. Special emphasis on adherence is essential to prevent viral resistance; particularly, NNRTI resistance develops rapidly with even slight fluctuations in drug levels.

 DRUG ALERT Test for the presence of ARV drug-resistant virus in both experienced and naive patients before initiating ARV combination therapy, thus ensuring the most effective regime.

 DRUG ALERT Lack of adherence to prescribed antiretroviral regimens and subtherapeutic drug levels increase the possibility that resistant virus will develop. Strict adherence (more than 95%) to combination regimens is critical in ensuring sustained response to treatment.

3. Adherence is the basis for successful viral suppression; strategies should be developed to encourage adherence.

4. Historically, use of IV immune globulin has been and continues to be common. It is still recommended for HIV-infected children who have had two or more serious bacterial infections within 1 year and for the treatment of HIV-related thrombocytopenia or immunoglobulin deficiency.

5. Use of antifungal drugs, such as nystatin, ketoconazole, fluconazole, itraconazole, and clotrimazole, for persistent or recurrent oral candidiasis.

6. Use of antivirals, such as acyclovir, valacyclovir, ganciclovir, and cidofovir, for suppression or treatment of recurrent viral infections.

7. Aggressive, prompt assessment and treatment of febrile illnesses.

8. Nutritional support.

9. Evaluation and treatment of developmental delays and regression.

10. Adequate pain management in advanced or end-stage disease.

11. Support and interventions for the child and family (including all caregivers) with issues of bereavement, disclosure, parental guilt, and long-term care.

 NURSING ALERT Families can find out about clinical treatment trials available for their child by calling (800) TRIALS-A or visiting www.clinicaltrials.gov.

Complications

1. Untreated or inadequately treated HIV:

a. Repeated, overwhelming infections and certain cancers, particularly lymphomas.

b. Hearing loss, tooth and gum disease, acute and chronic ear, nose, and throat infections.

c. Opportunistic infections.

d. Reactive airway disease.

e. Cardiomyopathy.

f. Failure to thrive, malabsorption, wasting.

g. Chronic atopic dermatitis and other skin reactions.

h. Nephropathy.

i. Neuropathy, myopathy.

j. Anemia, thrombocytopenia, neutropenia.

k. Loss of treatment options related to the development of drug resistance.

l. Developmental delay.

m. Learning disabilities.

n. Psychological challenges for children and caregivers, including multiple losses, issues of disclosure, fear, discrimination, stigmatization, and isolation.

o. Death.

2. HIV treatment:

a. NRTIs—anemia, neutropenia, lactic acidosis, pancreatitis, abacavir hypersensitivity reaction, peripheral neuropathy, lipodystrophy/lipoatrophy, renal dysfunction, osteopenia, headache, nausea, potential for vascular dysfunction.

b. NNRTIs—psychological changes, sleep disturbances/nightmares, neural tube defects (fetal exposure), hepatitis, rash.

c. PIs—dyslipidemia, GI upset, diarrhea.

d. Fusion inhibitors—injection site reactions.

 DRUG ALERT Because some liquid preparations are unpalatable, nonadherence to the drug regimen is common. Suggestions to overcome this would include using popsicle just before ingestion to numb the taste buds, followed by a teaspoon of chocolate/strawberry syrup, jam, or peanut butter immediately after. Speak to pharmacist about other ways to mask the taste.

Nursing Assessment

1. Review maternal records to identify infants who may be at risk for HIV disease. Infected infants are not easily identifiable by outward appearance.
2. Review records of at-risk or known infected children to determine nutritional status, growth and development, frequency of serious bacterial infections, presence or risk of opportunistic infections, laboratory values, and immunization status.
3. Assess growth, development, lymph nodes, hepatomegaly, splenomegaly, and oropharynx for presence of oral candidiasis and dental caries.
4. Assess the family's understanding of the child's condition, care needs, prognosis, and medical care plan.
5. Assess the family's coping mechanisms, comfort with disclosure issues, and long-term plans for care including transition plans for the child to an adult care program.
6. Assess the health of primary caregiver and discuss long-term care plans for respite and permanent alternative caregivers (including guardianship issues), as appropriate.

 NURSING ALERT Always discuss with the primary caregiver how much the child knows about own HIV status or about other family members' status. Never assume anyone knows the child's diagnosis; not friends, family members, loved ones, school contacts, or daycare providers, not even the child may know.

7. Assess the child's understanding of health condition and medications.
8. In children with advanced or end-stage disease, assess the level of pain and discomfort.
9. Assess the child's coping and response to the frequent painful and invasive procedures experienced as part of the ongoing diagnosis and management of the disease.
10. Assess for animal contact.
11. Take a thorough travel history to evaluate risk of coinfections, such as tuberculosis (TB), malaria, or other parasitic infections. Also evaluate potential travel plans, particularly to developing countries.
12. In the adolescent, assess increased at-risk behaviors, such as substance use, piercing, or sexual activity. Also determine methods of birth control, as appropriate.

 DRUG ALERT Some medications interact with the effect of birth control pills. Efavirenz during pregnancy may cause harmful effects to the developing fetus.

Nursing Diagnoses

- Risk for Infection related to immunodeficiency, neutropenia.
- Ineffective Therapeutic Regimen Management related to insufficient knowledge of HIV, noncompliance, and limited resources.
- Imbalanced Nutrition: Less than Body Requirements related to malabsorption, anorexia, or pain.
- Impaired Oral Mucous Membranes related to candidiasis and herpes stomatitis.
- Diarrhea related to enteric pathogens, disease process, and medications.

- Hyperthermia related to HIV infection and secondary infection.
- Delayed Growth and Development related to HIV Central Nervous System (CNS) infection.
- Ineffective Family Coping related to parental guilt and nature of disease.
- Ineffective Coping by child related to unresolved issues around disclosure, hospitalization, and losses.
- Pain related to advanced or end-stage HIV disease.
- Fear related to frequent invasive procedures, diagnosis, stagmatization.

Nursing Interventions

Preventing Infection

 Evidence Base Centers for Disease Control and Prevention. (2013). Recommended immunization schedules for persons aged 0 through 18 years. Available: www.cdc.gov/vaccines/recs/acip.

1. Have a high index of suspicion for secondary infection even when clinical manifestations are subtle or absent.
2. Administer or teach caregiver to administer prescribed pharmacologic agents that may help prevent serious bacterial infections, prevent opportunistic infections, and treat infections that occur.
   a. Educate caregiver or patient about the importance of more than 95% compliance with prescribed HAART regimen to maximize viral reduction, which, in turn, will maximize immune reconstitution.
3. Monitor viral load and total white blood cell (WBC) count. The absolute neutrophil counts may drop significantly as an adverse effect of antiretroviral drugs.
4. Maintain cleanliness of the environment and teach family members the essentials of environmental sanitation.
5. Use aseptic techniques when performing invasive procedures.
6. Administer and teach the family the importance of proper oral hygiene to prevent dental caries, which is a source of secondary infection.
7. Administer and teach the family good skin care—a break in the skin is a source of secondary infection.
8. Teach the family the importance of safe food preparation, including use of safe water, to avoid introducing pathogens through contaminated or undercooked food.
9. Monitor immunization status and advise families of the need to complete all recommended childhood immunizations (see Table 53-4, page 1720). In general, live virus vaccines should be used with caution. Also see page 1411 for routine pediatric immunization information based on the CDC. In general, live vaccines should be used with caution in children with HIV infections.
   a. The measles, mumps, rubella (MMR) and varicella vaccines are recommended for HIV-infected children who are not severely immunocompromised.
   b. Oral polio vaccine should be avoided because there is an alternative injectable inactivated polio vaccine available.
   c. Yellow fever vaccine should be avoided unless the risk of exposure is extremely high; consultation with an expert is recommended.

Table 53-4	Vaccination of Individuals with HIV Based on the Canadian Immunization Guide

INACTIVATED/COMPONENT VACCINES

VACCINE	HIV/AIDS
Dtap, Tdap, Td	Routine use*
IPV	Routine use
Hib	Routine use
Influenza	Recommended
Pneumococcal	Recommended
Meningococcal	Routine use
Hep A	Recommended (MSM, IDU)
Hep B	Recommended/Routine use†
Human papilloma virus	Recommended

*Routine vaccination schedules should be followed with age-appropriate booster doses.
†Hep B vaccine (HB) is now recommended for all infants.

LIVE VACCINES

VACCINE	HIV/AIDS
MMR	Routine use‡ (if no significant compromise)
Varicella	Consider in asymptomatic and mild symptomatic disease
OPV	Contraindicated (alternate available)
Oral typhoid	Contraindicated (alternate available)
BCG	Contraindicated
Yellow fever	Contraindicated**
Oral cholera	Contraindicated

‡Most HIV-positive children can receive the first MMR vaccine without significant risk. Administration of the second MMR dose (particularly in adults) must be evaluated on a case-by-case basis.
**Unless the risk of exposure is extremely high, consultation with an expert is recommended.
Modified from Public Health Agency of Canada and National Advisory Committee on Immunization. (2006). Canadian immunization guide. Immunization of immunocompromised persons. Available: www.phac-aspc.gc.ca/publicat/cig-gci/p03-07-eng.php.

d. In the United States, the bacille Calmette-Guérin vaccine is also not recommended.
e. Yearly influenza vaccine and a 3- to 5-year pneumococcal vaccine are also recommended in addition to the standard childhood immunization schedule.
f. An annual TB skin test should also be administered.

 DRUG ALERT Noninfected children living with HIV-infected parents or siblings should not receive the oral polio vaccine, but rather the injectable inactivated polio vaccine. This is due to the prolonged shedding of the virus from the live oral vaccine, which may prove to be hazardous for immunocompromised individuals.

10. Provide appropriate chemoprophylaxis following exposure to communicable diseases.
11. Educate families on the potential risks associated with pet ownership. In particular, cats may transmit *Toxoplasmosis* or *Bartonella* infections; birds may transmit *Cryptococcus neoformans* or *M. avium*; reptiles may cause salmonellosis. Good handwashing with soap and water is recommended after handling animals; contact with animal feces should be avoided.
12. Encourage families to meet with an expert in travel medicine before traveling—particularly to developing countries—to minimize the risk of acquiring opportunistic pathogens.
13. Educate teens about the use and importance of using condoms to prevent spread of HIV and to protect them from getting secondary sexually transmitted diseases such as syphilis or chlamydia.

Maximizing Adherence to HAART

 Evidence Base Panel on Antiretroviral Therapy and Medical Management of HIV-Infected Children. (2012). Guidelines for the use of antiretroviral agents in pediatric HIV infection. Available: *http://aidsinfo.nih.gov/ContentFiles/PediatricGuidelines.pdf.*

1. Develop a trusting relationship with patient by maintaining a nonjudgemental attitude to maintain open communication and assist in assessing barriers to adherence.
2. Assess drug readiness and strategies to maximize adherence before initiating therapy.
3. Provide the simplest regimen possible; for example, least number of pills (combination therapies), least often (once daily), based on viral resistance.
4. Stress the need for adherence at every visit.
5. Use several strategies for evaluating adherence (eg, viral load, pill count, self reporting, pharmacy refill checks).
6. Collaborate with patient to determine what reminder tools may work the best (pill box, calendar, stickers, alarm, associating pill-taking with daily routine).

Maintaining Adequate Nutrition

1. Carefully monitor growth parameters (height, weight, head circumference).
2. Consult with a dietitian to develop strategies for nutritional care, including additional calories, nutritional supplements while reducing cholesterol.
3. Teach the family to prepare high-calorie, nutritious meals that are pleasing and acceptable to children.
4. As age-appropriate, involve the child in meal planning.
5. Encourage small, frequent meals if the child is experiencing absorption problems.

Maintaining Oral Mucosa and Dental Integrity

1. Include regular examinations of the oral mucosa and teeth in the physical assessment of the child.
2. Administer prescribed antifungal and antiviral therapy.
3. Offer fluids and pureed foods to minimize chewing and facilitate swallowing; avoid highly seasoned or acidic foods.
4. Encourage regular dental hygiene and dental visits.

Minimizing Effects of Diarrhea

1. Monitor for the presence or development of diarrhea.
2. Monitor daily weight when diarrhea is present.
3. Monitor intake and output and assess skin and mucous membranes for turgor and dryness.
4. Use enteric precautions.
5. Avoid foods that increase intestinal motility.
6. Administer IV hydration, as indicated.
7. Plan a regimen of skin care, including cleansing/blot drying of the anal area and application of ointment or skin barrier cream.
8. Teach the family safe food preparation techniques to minimize contamination of food.
9. Administer medications, as directed, for relief of severe diarrhea and enteric infections.

Detecting and Controlling Fever

1. Monitor for fever and report any core temperature over 101° F (38.3° C).
2. Institute comfort measures, such as sponge baths, dry clothing and linens, and antipyretics, as ordered.
3. Teach the family how to accurately monitor the child's rectal temperature.
4. Teach the family to promptly report any febrile episode over 101° F rectally.
5. Administer antipyretics.

Promoting Developmental Goals

1. Assess the child's developmental status on a regular basis.
2. Report regression or delay in achieving developmental milestones.
3. Make appropriate referrals for more in-depth developmental evaluation when delays and regression are noted.
4. Teach the family appropriate developmental stimulation activities for their child.
5. Implement recommendations for developmental stimulation (including school-based programs) and assist the family in doing likewise.
6. Facilitate successful transition to adult care (see Box 53-1).

BOX 53-1 **Transition to Adult Care**

Transition is the purposeful, planned movement of adolescents and young adults with chronic illness/disabilities from child-centered to adult-oriented systems. With the advent of highly active antiretroviral therapy, children with human immunodeficiency virus (HIV) are surviving and living well into adulthood. As they become adults, they are graduating from pediatric health care programs—with parents the child's advocate—to adult programs where individual care becomes the focus, with the young adult becoming his or her own advocate.

It is imperative for the pediatric health care team to prepare children and families for the changes and challenges of adolescence, with a focus on increased autonomy and self-reliance and independence.

The transition into adolescence is a normal part of growth and development; however, special considerations need to be addressed when caring for a teenager with a chronic illness.

KEY ELEMENTS OF TRANSITION:
- Focus the orientation on the future and keep it proactive and flexible.
- Start as early as possible.
- Build on knowledge about HIV and issues of confidentiality and disclosure.
- Make sure your approach fosters personal and medical interdependence and creative problem solving.
- Provide opportunities for own consultations during clinic visit.
- Have open, honest, age-appropriate sexual health discussions.
- Develop a written transition policy—agreed upon by all members of the multidisciplinary team and target adult services—posted for families and young adults to see.

- Discuss different care models and possible settings in which the young adult can access care as an adult.
- Provide liaison personnel in both pediatric and adult health care centers.
- Coordinate an initial meeting for teen to meet adult care provider and staff.
- Ensure a flexible policy on the timing of events, with anticipation of change.
- Provide an education program for young people and their families that addresses medical, psychosocial, and educational/vocational aspects of care.
- Develop an individualized health-care transition plan by age 14, in collaboration with the young adult and his or her family, and continuously update, as needed.
- Identify a network of relevant community agencies and adult primary and subspecialty care providers.
- Implement a training program for pediatric and adult providers on transition and adolescent issues.
- Provide for appropriate primary preventive care.
- Ensure affordable continuous health and medication insurance coverage.

 Evidence Base Boudreau, M., & Fisher, C. (2012). Providing effective medical and case management services to HIV-infected youth preparing to transition to adult care. *Journal of the Association of Nurses in AIDS Care, 23*(4), 318–328.

Evidence Base Childrens HIV Association (CHIVA). (2010). CHIVA guidance on transition for adolescents living with HIV. London: Author. Available: www.chiva.org.uk/professionals/health/guidelines/youngpeople/transition.html.

Promoting Effective Family Coping

1. Practice within a framework of family-centered care.
2. Assess the family's coping mechanisms, strengths, and weaknesses.
3. Provide emotional support to the family.
4. Refer the family to appropriate community resources for grief counseling and legal assistance (eg, wills, custody issues).
5. Help the family set realistic goals and expectations for the child.
6. Maintain a nonjudgmental attitude and nonprejudicial approach.
7. Allow the family to use denial as a protective mechanism because this gives them some sense of control.
8. Explain all care and treatment plans to the family.
9. Involve the family in planning for the care and management of their child.
10. Give strategies and guidance to families regarding *partial truth telling* so they can answer child's questions as honestly as possible.
11. Provide support to new mothers who grieve the loss of not being able to breastfeed. Provide strategies on how to deflect questions about the choice not to breastfeed.
12. Encourage parent to allow adolescent to start taking increased responsibility for own health care, including individual time alone with health care provider and self-advocacy.
13. Provide family and disclosed patient with hopeful information about the future, such as continuing education or, possibly, getting married and having a family.
14. Refer the family to community resources for home care, daycare of other siblings, transportation services, school-based services, respite care, and hospice.

Strengthening Coping Skills of the Child

Evidence Base Saunders, C. (2012). Disclosing HIV status to HIV positive children before adolescence. *British Journal of Nursing, 21*(11), 663–669.

1. Introduce the subject of disclosure of diagnosis to the child with the family. Offer the family guidelines as to age-appropriate approaches.
2. Accept that some families may not be able to disclose the nature of the disease to their child, even after much support and guidance.
   a. Explore with families how they want you to address questions the child may present to you.
   b. The illness and its impact can be effectively handled without actually telling the child about the HIV disease or AIDS status, if the family refuses to disclose it.

3. Answer the child's questions as honestly as possible within parental constraints that may be present.
4. Actively involve the child in as much of the care as possible, such as by having the child decide where to place the IV line, cleaning off skin for needle insertion, and so forth.
5. Use therapeutic play techniques (age-appropriate), such as drawing, playing with dolls, playing with medical equipment, and storytelling, to allow the child to express him- or herself in less verbal ways.
6. Refer the child and family for counseling if the child's coping skills do not progress or there appears to be regression in handling the issue of illness and chronic health care needs. Signs indicating possible need for additional in-depth interventions include more acting out by the child, withdrawn behavior, and difficulty in school (either behaviorally or academically).
7. Recommend and facilitate peer support groups.

Minimizing Discomfort

1. Assess for signs of pain in the child. In the infant or nonverbal child, such signs include restlessness, crying, withdrawn behavior, and changes in vital signs.
2. Discuss concerns over pain issues with the primary health care provider and team providing care for the child. Initiate or request referral to a pain management team if the child does not experience relief.
3. Stress to the parent or guardian the need for adequate pain management in children; many people do not acknowledge that infants or children suffer from pain and that this needs to be alleviated.
4. Use appropriate techniques to assess the level of pain or discomfort a child is experiencing.

Minimizing Fear

1. Make sure that all painful and invasive procedures are done in a location other than the child's bed in the hospital.
2. Monitor central line if used for venous access. Central line access may be less traumatic over time than repeated peripheral access attempts. Some children with HIV will need long-term, probably lifelong, IV therapies and blood monitoring, and a central line greatly eliminates the pain and anxiety associated with these procedures.
3. Make sure that the parent/caregiver realizes that most clinic visits will involve blood tests so that they do not falsely reassure the child that "no needlesticks" will occur.
4. Use diversionary techniques, such as bubble-blowing, for distraction during painful procedures. Practice first with the child and tell him or her this is an activity that you will help with during the procedure. Children can also be taught other relaxation techniques.
5. Offer small rewards (such as stickers, small toy items) after painful procedures to reduce anxiety. Such rewards should be given regardless of how the child reacted. The reward is not for "not crying" but acknowledges difficulty in going through painful and invasive procedures on a regular basis.
6. Involve the child in the procedure as much as possible (age-appropriate). Such involvement can include selecting a possible site for accessing or receiving IV medications, cleaning

the site, selecting a special bandage for after the procedure. Use topical anesthetic.

Community and Home Care Considerations

1. Assess home environment for resources, such as nutritious foods and safe food preparation; adequate water, heat, electricity, and space; developmentally appropriate toys; and supplies needed for care and hygiene.
2. Assess caregiver's correct administration of medications.
3. Draw blood samples using universal precautions and careful transport of blood and used equipment.
4. Perform developmental assessment periodically.
5. Act as liaison among family, specialists, school officials, and other team members.

Family Education and Health Maintenance

1. Teach families and other caregivers of the child universal precautions. In caring for HIV-infected infants and children, gloves are recommended when handling potentially contaminated body fluids (such as blood) but are not considered necessary for routine diaper-changing unless bloody diarrhea or hematuria exists.
2. Facilitate supply of adequate numbers of latex (or nonlatex, if necessary) gloves to families to use, as indicated.
3. Facilitate education as well as a supply of latex condoms and other forms of birth control for teens who are sexually active or about to become sexually active.
4. Offer guidance as to how to initiate discussion of their child's HIV status with schools and daycare settings. The "need to know" principle serves as a guideline when deciding to whom disclosure should be made (generally the principal, school nurse, and classroom teacher). It is not currently required that schools and daycare centers be advised, but is generally encouraged because this alerts the school to notify the parent promptly in the event of an outbreak of infectious disease that could pose a threat to the HIV-infected child (such as varicella).
5. Offer guidance to teens about how to initiate disclosure of HIV status to sexual partners or peers. Provide support during the process and offer to help facilitate the disclosure in the clinical setting.
6. Give families concrete guidelines as to when to notify health care provider about their child's condition. Signs and symptoms of illness require prompt notification, all fevers over 101° F (38.3° C) should be reported, and any adverse experiences or suspected adverse experiences with medications need prompt reporting.
7. Assess whether the parents are receiving care for themselves. Typically, parents will neglect their own care to provide for their child. As a result, the parents' immune status may become more quickly compromised.
8. Refer families to a social worker or social services agency. Children with HIV may qualify for certain entitlement programs that help with their health care and the family's financial situation. Many states have initiated case management programs for people with HIV.
9. Provide guidance using a childhood chronic illness model that addresses such psychosocial issues as disclosure and parental guilt as well as such medical issues as multiorgan involvement and likelihood of exacerbations of a variety of related conditions (eg, infections and nutritional deficiencies).
10. Assist parents in obtaining the latest information regarding treatment protocols of pediatric HIV. Such information can be obtained through (800) TRIALS-A or *www.aidsinfor.nih.gov*.

Evaluation: Expected Outcomes

- Absolute neutrophil count within normal limits; aseptic technique maintained.
- Maintains medication regimen, keeps follow-up appointments; achieves an undetectable viral load (less than 40 copies/mL).
- Nutritional intake adequate to meet body requirements; growth curve maintained.
- Oral mucous membranes without ulceration, good dentition.
- Two to three loose stools per day; perianal skin without irritation.
- Afebrile; parent or caregiver demonstrates accurate monitoring of temperature.
- Achieves normal growth patterns as evidenced by height, weight, and developmental tasks.
- Parents discuss their feelings about the diagnosis of HIV; family seeks help through community resources.
- Child participates in care, asks questions; adolescent successfully transitions to an adult care program without disruption in care.
- Reports increase in comfort level.
- Practices distraction techniques during procedures; reports reduced fear.

Primary Immunodeficiencies

Primary immunodeficiencies (PID) encompass more than 150 types of disorders that affect distinct components of the innate and adaptive immune systems. More than 120 genes have been identified to account for the known forms of PID. The overall incidence of PID is estimated to be 1:10,000. However, the exact incidence and prevalence of PID is unknown. The most common presentation of an immunodeficiency is increased frequency of infections or infections that are unusual or difficult to treat. PID diseases are often undiagnosed or have a significant delay in diagnosis, which can lead to significant end-organ damage from recurrent infections.

 Evidence Base Gray, P., Namasivayam, M., Ziegler, J. (2012). Recurrent infection in children: When and how to investigate for primary immunodeficiency. *Journal of Paediatrics and Child Health, 48*(3), 202–209.

Pathophysiology and Etiology

 Evidence Base Reid, B. (2012) Immunodeficiencies. In K. Reuter-Rice & B. Bolick (Eds.), *Pediatric acute care: A guide for interprofessional practice*, 679–690. Burlington, VT: Jones & Bartlett.

1. PID diseases are due to genetic alterations in the immune system. Inheritance may be X-linked, autosomal recessive, or autosomal dominant depending on the PID disease. The genetic mutation may be de novo with no prior family history.
2. About three quarters of PID diseases are caused by humoral or combined humoral and cellular abnormalities, with the remainder being defects in phagocytic or complement components of the immune system.
3. Risk factors for PID diseases include a family history of immunodeficiency, early infant deaths, parental consanguinity, autoimmunity, and increased incidence of lymphoid malignancy in family members.

Clinical Manifestations

1. Hallmark of PID diseases is susceptibility to infection, including recurrent pneumonia, sinusitis, otitis, sepsis, meningitis, recurrent or resistant candidiasis, or infection with an opportunistic organism. Course of infection may be unusual with a need for intravenous antibiotics and/or hospitalization to clear infections. See Table 53-5.
2. Chronic diarrhea.
3. Nonhealing wounds.
4. Extensive skin lesions.
5. Failure to gain weight or grow normally (failure to thrive).
6. Complications from a live viral vaccine.
7. Unexplained autoimmunity or fevers.
8. Absence or enlargement of lymphoid tissue, including tonsils, spleen, and liver.

Diagnostic Evaluation

Specific Evaluation for Immunodeficiency

1. Complete blood count with differential to look for decreased numbers of lymphocytes and evidence of abnormalities in other cell lines, such as decreased platelets, neutrophils, or hemoglobin.
2. Immunoglobulin levels (IgG, IgA, IgM, and IgE) include total protein and albumin to rule out protein loss.
3. Antibody titres to previously administered vaccines to evaluate the ability to produce functional specific antibodies to infectious agents. Measurement of isoagglutinins (isoantibodies to blood groups) in children older than 2 years.
4. Measurement of the classical (CH50) and alternate pathway (AH50) of the complement system to rule out a complement deficiency.
5. Lymphocyte subset analysis by flowcytometry including CD3 (total T cells), CD4 (T helper), CD8 (T cytotoxic), CD19 or CD20 (B cells), and CD16/56 (natural killer cells) for suspected T cell, B cell, or combined immunodeficiency.
6. Lymphoproliferative assays to assess the cellular immune system.
7. Measurement of phagocytic oxidative responses (neutrophil oxidative burst index [NOBI] by flowcytometry) if a phagocytic disorder is suggested, such as chronic granulomatous disease.
8. Genetic testing for suspected cause of immunodeficiency.

Other Tests

1. Evaluation for infection, including inflammatory markers (C-reactive protein, sedimentation rate), appropriate cultures, radiological image of the site of suspected infections.

Table 53-5	Infections Associated with Subtypes of PID Diseases		
TYPE	**TYPES OF INFECTIONS**	**ORGANISMS**	**OTHER FEATURES**
Humoral (B cell)	Sinopulmonary, otitis media, gastrointestinal, cellulitis, meningitis, osteomyelitis	Encapsulated bacteria: *Haemophilus*, pneumococci, streptococci Parasites: *Giardia lamblia*, *Cryptosporidium* Virus: *Enterovirus*	Autoimmunity GI problems including malabsorption
Cellular (T cell or combined T and B cell)	Pulmonary, gastrointestinal, skin	Fungal: *Candida* species, *Pneumocystis jiroveci* Viral: CMV*, EBV**, RSV, parainfluenza, adenovirus, viral GI disease mycobacterium species	Failure to thrive Oral thrush Skin: rashes, dermatitis Postvaccination disease from live viral vaccines
Phagocytic disorders	Severe skin and visceral infections by common pathogens	Bacteria: *Staphylococcus aureus*, *Pseudomonas* species, *Serratia* species, *Klebsiella* species Fungi: *Candida*, *Nocardia*, *Aspergillus*	Granuloma formation, including granulomatous enteritis Poor wound healing Abscesses Oral cavity infections Anorectal infections
Complement disorders	Meningitis Septicemia	*Neiserria* infections: meningococcal, pneumococcal	Rheumatoid disorders: lupus-like syndrome Angioedema

CMV, cytomegalovirus; EBV, Ebstein-Barr virus.

2. Electrolytes, glucose, urea, creatinine, arterial blood gases, if indicated.

3. HIV testing by PCR (patient may not produce antibodies) as clinical presentation of congenital HIV and severe combined immune deficiency are similar.

Management

1. Prompt recognition and treatment of infections. Empiric antibiotic therapy pending culture results should be instituted.

2. May consider preventive antibiotic treatment for some PID diseases.

3. Avoidance of live viral vaccines, as they may be disease-causing in immunodeficient patients.

4. Postexposure infectious prophylaxis may be necessary following exposure to varicella.

5. For suspected T-cell immunodeficiency, blood products must be irradiated to eliminate leukocytes and screened for cytomegalovirus.

6. Pneumocystis jiroveci prophylaxis for T-cell immunodeficiencies.

7. Antibody replacement therapy with intravenous or subcutaneous gammaglobulin for antibody deficiencies (X-linked agammaglobulinemia, common variable immune deficiency, CD40 ligand or CD40 deficiency, or selective antibody deficiency).

8. Bone marrow transplant (BMT) to replace the defective immune system in severe PID diseases (severe combined immune deficiency, combined immunodeficiencies, Wiscott Aldrich syndrome, and chronic granulomatous disease). Indications for BMT in PID diseases are constantly expanding as new genes are identified.

9. Gene therapy is an experimental option for some PID diseases (adenosine deaminase deficiency [a type of severe combined immune deficiency] and chronic granulomatous disease).

Complications

1. Organ damage from infection, particularly lungs, gastrointestinal tract, and joints.

2. Chronic lung disease (bronchiectasis).

3. Granulomatous lesions in the skin, liver, spleen, and lungs (common variable immune deficiency and chronic granulomatous disease).

4. Gastrointestinal malabsorption due to infection or from bacterial overgrowth.

5. Autoimmunity.

6. Early death (less than 1 year of age for severe combined immune deficiency).

7. Malignancy (especially lymphoma and leukemia).

8. Psychological and social reactions to chronic disease.

Nursing Assessment

1. Focus history on infections including age of onset, sites, number, frequency, types, duration, and response to treatment.

2. Detailed family history including focus on unexplained infant deaths, recurrent miscarriages, consanguinity, malignancies, and autoimmunity in other members.

3. Review of immunization record and history to determine complications from vaccines and to ensure that immunizations are given at proper intervals.

4. Focus physical examination on the site of infections, such as lung air entry, as well as vital signs, growth and development, presence or absence of lymphoid tissue, examination of skin for evidence of candidiasis or other skin abnormalities.

5. Assess the family and child's understanding of the condition, care needs, prognosis, and medical plan of care.

6. Assess the family's coping mechanisms and resources, particularly for patients that may require bone marrow transplant or lifelong treatment with immunoglobulins.

Nursing Diagnoses

- Risk for Infection related to immunodeficiency.
- Imbalanced Nutrition: Less than Body Requirements related to infections, malabsorption, or autoimmune gastrointestinal diseases.
- Impaired Oral Mucous Membranes related to candidiasis or other infections.
- Ineffective Therapeutic Regimen Management related to insufficient knowledge, nonadherence, and limited resources.
- Delayed Growth and Development related to infection or specific PID disease.
- Ineffective Family Coping related to diagnosis of immunodeficiency.
- Impaired Family Processes due to chronic diseases.

Nursing Interventions

Preventing Infection

1. Educate families about signs and symptoms of infection that specific PID disease is susceptible to and when to seek health care advice.

2. Administer or teach caregiver to administer prescribed pharmacologic agents including treatment protocols for gammaglobulin therapy, if indicated.

3. Maintain reverse isolation for protection of severe T-cell immunodeficiencies when hospitalized.

4. Avoid administration of live viral vaccines for suspected PID (oral polio, measles, mumps, rubella, varicella, yellow fever, rotavirus, inhaled influenza, and bacilli Calmette-Guerin (BCG) vaccine.

5. Encourage yearly influenza vaccine for patients and family members unless patient is antibody deficient.

6. Administer and teach family good skin care techniques to avoid infection.

Maintaining Adequate Nutrition

1. Carefully monitor growth parameters including height, weight, and head circumference.

2. Consult with a dietician to develop nutritional plan of care, including adequate caloric intake and parental teaching.

3. Administer and teach families to administer supplemental feeds via NG or G-tube if indicated.

Maintaining Oral Mucosa

1. Include assessment of oral mucosa in routine physical assessments.
2. Administer and teach families to administer prescribed antifungal or antiviral medications.
3. Promote good dental hygiene and dental care.

Promoting therapeutic regime management

1. Teach patients and families about prescribed medications and treatments. Review teaching periodically.
2. For patients on gammaglobulin treatment, doses should be adjusted to reflect increased weight, so as to ensure adequate replacement of antibodies. For patients on subcutaneous gammaglobulin, periodically assess patient adherence to infusion protocol and reeducate, as necessary.

Promoting Growth and Development

1. Assess for normal growth and development.
2. Make appropriate referrals for more in-depth developmental assessments and adhere to treatment programs instituted (important for prolonged admissions, such as bone marrow transplant).
3. Teach the family appropriate developmental activities for their child.
4. Facilitate successful transition to adult care.

Promote Effective Family Coping

Evidence Base Burton, J., Murphy, E., & Riley, P. (2010). Primary immunodeficiency disease: A model for case management of chronic diseases. *Professional Case Management, 15*(1), 5–14.

1. Assess family coping skills including strengths and weaknesses.
2. Provide emotional support and counseling, as necessary.
3. Refer the family for genetic counseling, as diagnosis may impact other family members or future pregnancies.
4. Encourage families to allow children to take increased responsibility for their care as they mature.
5. Provide continuous teaching about disease process and treatment. It is particularly important for children diagnosed at very young ages to learn as they grow—lifelong diseases.

Normalizing family processes

1. Refer to community resources and support groups.
2. Encourage family and child to verbalize feelings about diagnosis and treatment.
3. Encourage attendance at school, participation in activities, and socialization with peers as much as possible.
4. Encourage parents to spend time with siblings and each other, as well as affected child.

Community and Home Care Considerations

1. Assess home environment for resources, such as nutritious foods, developmentally appropriate toys, and supplies needed for care and hygiene.

2. Assess caregivers' correct administration of medications.
3. For PID patient requiring gammaglobulin treatment, assess ability of parents to adhere to infusion regime for IVIG treatment. For SCIG treatment, assess home for adequate storage of gammaglobulin products and supplies.
4. Provide education to school nurses so that individual educational plans are implemented and maintained.

Family Education and Health Maintenance

1. Give families guidelines as to when to notify health care provider about their child's condition. Signs and symptoms of illness require prompt notification, all fevers over 101°F (38.3°C) should be reported, and any adverse experiences or suspected adverse events to medications require prompt reporting.
2. Assess family coping and refer to social worker or social services, as required.
3. Refer families to immunodeficiency patient support agencies so as to provide ongoing PID disease–specific education to patients and families.

Evaluation and Expected Outcomes

- Reduced incidence of infections.
- Adequate intake for child's age and developmental stage.
- No oral lesions, denies oral discomfort.
- Adherence to treatment regimes.
- Achieves normal growth, as evidenced by height, weight, and developmental tasks.
- Child and family seek appropriate support and resources, as required.
- Child and parents verbalize feelings about the illness; include siblings in activities.

CONNECTIVE TISSUE DISORDERS

Juvenile Idiopathic Arthritis

Evidence Base Gowdie, P., & Tse, S. (2012). Juvenile idiopathic arthritis. *Pediatric Clinics of North America, 59*(2), 301–327.

Juvenile idiopathic arthritis (JIA) has replaced the terms "juvenile chronic arthritis" and "juvenile rheumatoid arthritis" as the commonly agreed-upon terminology to describe arthritis in children. JIA is defined as persistent arthritis for longer than 6 weeks in children ≤16 years of age. The disease is a heterogeneous disease that has been further classified into seven subtypes with similar presentation, clinical features, disease course, and outcomes.

JIA is a chronic disease affecting approximately 1 in 1,000 children, often persisting into the adult years. There are epidemiological differences between sexes and age of onset that are specific to subtype.

Pathophysiology and Etiology

 Evidence Base Cassidy J. T., Laxer R. M., Petty R. E., et al. (Eds.). (2011). *Textbook of pediatric rheumatology* (6th ed.). Philadelphia: Saunders Elsevier.

1. The cause of JIA is unknown. It is likely multifactorial and variable between subtypes. Hypotheses suggest that environmental stimuli trigger disease in genetically susceptible children during a time of susceptibility.
   a. Genetic risk factors—associations with specific human leukocyte antigen (HLA) Class I (B27) and Class II genes, protein tyrosine phosphatase N22 gene, and interleukin-2 receptor alpha gene have been well established.
   b. Immune dysregulation of the adaptive and innate immune system. Autoantibodies including antinuclear antibody (ANA); rheumatoid factor (RF); t-lymphocytes and cytokines, commonly tissue necrosis factor (TNF) of adaptive immunity as well as neutrophils and interleukin (IL)-1, IL-6 of innate immunity are present in sera and synovial fluids.
   c. Infection as a trigger to immune dysregulation is suspected but has not been clearly established.
   d. Hormonal factors.
2. Arthritis is inflammation of one or more synovial joints. Immune complexes trigger the inflammatory response, causing:
   a. The synovium to become thickened from congestion and edema.
   b. Increased production of intra-articular fluid exhibited as a joint effusion. It is not uncommon for synovial cysts to develop (Baker's cyst).
   c. Development of periarticular soft tissue edema.
   d. Extension of the inflammatory process to the tendons, tendon sheaths, and entheses results in inflammatory changes similar to the synovial tissues.
   e. Weakness and atrophy of muscle surrounding affected joints leads to flexion contractures.
   f. Growth centers in long bones may undergo either premature epiphyseal closure or accelerated epiphyseal growth. The result is overgrowth or shortening of the affected limb.
3. Long-term disease activity can result in joint destruction and eventual joint failure, necessitating joint replacement.
   a. Degrading enzymes released during synovial inflammation result in chondrolysis and osteolysis; erosion of the articular cartilage and bone.
   b. Following destruction the overgrowth of granulation tissue may result in the formulation of new cartilage and bone, leading to ankylosis.
   c. Joint destruction is characterized by joint-space narrowing, erosions, deformities, subluxation, and ankylosis.
   d. Generalized osteopenia is common, increasing the risk for fracture.

Clinical Manifestations

Clinical manifestations include joint and extra-articular features that vary among subtypes (see Table 53-6, page 1728).

1. The inflamed joint is characterized by four of the five cardinal signs of inflammation: swelling, pain, heat, loss of function. Erythema occurs in some cases.
   a. Joint stiffness in the morning or after prolonged inactivity (gelling) is common.
   b. Pain may not be expressed verbally; the child may alter activities to protect the painful joint.
2. Extra-articular features include fever, rash, fatigue, weight loss, altered growth, subcutaneous nodules, and uveitis.
   a. Fevers occur in systemic JIA and occasionally at the onset of polyarticular JIA. In systemic JIA fevers are daily, usually above 102.2° F (39° C), following a quotidian pattern of one or two spikes with a rapid return to baseline and accompanied by a classic salmon pink rash.
   b. Altered growth includes localized growth abnormalities and poor linear growth.
      i. Overgrowth or undergrowth of bones in sites affected by arthritis result in leg length discrepancies, shortened limbs, and micronathia (receding chin) with arthritis of the temporomandibular joint (TMJ).
      ii. Poor linear growth is attributed to the inhibitory affects chronic inflammation and circulating cytokines have on growth.
   c. Uveitis is commonly asymptomatic at onset requiring frequent examinations by an eye specialist. An exception is the patient with subtype, enthesitis-related arthritis (ERA), who present with redness, pain, photophobia, headache, and decreased visual acuity.

Diagnostic Evaluation

1. Laboratory studies cannot confirm diagnosis. They are used to support diagnosis; measure disease activity; predict prognoses; and monitor toxicity of therapy.
   a. Elevated erythrocyte sedimentation rate (ESR).
   b. Leukocytosis, thrombocytosis, anemia.
   c. Elevated serum immunoglobulins.
   d. Elevated C-reactive protein.
   e. Presence of ANA, RF, and anticyclic citrullinated peptide (anti-CCP) antibodies. ANA is associated with high incidence of uveitis. Anti-CCP is an early predictor of erosive disease in polyarticular JIA.
2. Radiographic studies.
   a. Early x-ray changes include soft tissue swelling, osteopenia, and effusions.
   b. Late x-ray changes include erosions, joint space narrowing, boutonniere or swan neck deformity of the fingers, early maturation of cartilage, subluxations.
   c. Ultrasound for detection of tenosynovitis.
   d. Magnetic resonance imaging (MRI) is most sensitive to detect specific joint disease, including TMJ and sacroiliac.
3. Ophthalmologic examination.
   a. Slit lamp examination to monitor for uveitis is required within 1 month of diagnosis and every 3 to 12 months, depending on age, presence of ANA, and duration of illness.

Table 53-6	Characteristics of Juvenile Idiopathic Arthritis		
ILAR SUBTYPE	**OLIGOARTICULAR** • **PERSISTENT** • **EXTENDED**	**POLYARTICULAR (RF NEGATIVE)**	**POLYARTICULAR (RF POSITIVE)**
% Total JIA patients	40%–50%	20%–25%	5%
Age of Onset	Early childhood; 1–3 years	2 peaks: 2–4 years and 6–12 years	Early adolescence
Sex	F>M	F>M	F>M
Typical Joint Involvement	≤4 joints in first 6 months Large joints: knees, ankles, wrist Extended disease: involves >4 joints after first 6 months	≥5 joints Symmetric distribution Knees, wrists, ankles TMJ can be affected	≥5 joints Small and large joints Symmetric C-spine and TMJ affected Erosive joint disease
Laboratory Tests	ANA 60%–80% positive	ANA 50% positive	ANA 75% positive RF positive
Occurrence of Uveitis	Common (30%) Usually asymptomatic	Common (15%)	Rare (<1%)
Other Features	Leg length discrepancies Contractures	Fatigue	Rheumatoid nodules Fever and constitutional signs at onset of disease

Abbreviations: ILAR: International League for Associations of Rheumatology; F: female; M: male; ANA: antinuclear antibody; HLA: human leukocyte antigen; RF: rheumatoid factor
Adapted from: Gowdie, P. and Tse, S. "Juvenile idiopathic arthritis," Pediatric Clinics of North America, 59(2), 301–327, 2012.

Management

1. There is no cure for JIA.
2. Management of JIA should be provided by a multidisciplinary team in a family-centered approach.
3. The primary goal of treatment is to facilitate disease remission.
4. In the process of working toward remission, other goals of therapy include:
   a. To control pain.
   b. To maintain range of motion, muscle strength, and function.
   c. To promote normal growth.
   d. To support normal psychological and social development.
5. Goal attainment requires nonpharmacological and pharmacological approaches.
6. Nonpharmacological approaches to treatment include:
   a. Occupational and physical therapies utilize strength and stretching exercises, splinting, serial casting, orthotics, and thermal modalities to reduce stiffness or pain and to protect function.
   b. Strengthening and aerobic-based exercise are safe in children with JIA. Studies have demonstrated improved physical function and quality of life.

 Evidence Base Tarakci, E., Yeldan, I., Baydogan, S., et al. (2012). Efficacy of a land-based home exercise programme for patients with juvenile idiopathic arthritis: A randomized, controlled, single-blind study. *Journal of Rehabilitation Medicine*, 44(11), 962–967.

   c. Nutritional and vitamin supplementation are required to promote growth, maintain bone mineralization, and prevent toxicity from medication. Vitamin D, calcium, iron, and folic acid may be prescribed.
   d. Orthopedic surgeries to manage joint complications; tendon lengthening for severe contractures; tenosynovectomy to treat trigger finger; total joint replacements, particularly hips and knees.
7. Pharmacological therapies are introduced in a systematic stepwise approach targeted to the specific subtypes of JIA. Refer to Table 53-7. Recently, a more aggressive progression through the steps is advocated, as evidence suggests rapid control of inflammation may positively influence prognosis.
   a. Nonsteroidal anti-inflammatory drugs are the first line of therapy aimed at symptom relief.
   b. Disease-modifying antirheumatic drugs (DMARD) are second-line immunosuppressive agents that can achieve disease control and influence the course of disease.

SYSTEMIC	ENTHESITIS RELATED ARTHRITIS	PSORIATIC ARTHRITIS	UNDIFFERENTIATED
5%–10%	5%–10%	5%–10%	10%
Throughout childhood	Late childhood and adolescence	2 peaks: 2–4 years and 9–11 years	
F=M	M>F	F>M	
Oligoarticular or Polyarticular distribution Progressive and destructive arthritis	Weight bearing joints: hip, feet Axial and sacroiliac joint involvement Enthesitis	Asymmetric or Symmetric small or large joints Dactylitis Enthesitis	
ANA 5–10% positive	HLA–B27 positive		
Rare (<1%)	Symptomatic; acute onset, painful red eye Unilateral	Common (10%)	
Daily quotidian fever ≥2 week Evanescent rash Lymphadenopathy Hepatosplenomegaly Serositis Macrophage Activation Syndrome is life threatening complication	Association with inflammatory bowel disease	Nail pits, onycholysis Psoriasis	Does not fulfill criteria for any of the other categories or fulfills criteria for >1 category

c. Newer biologic agents are selected when DMARDs fail. They target very specific immune responses responsible for inflammation. Biologics offer treatment options for children with refractory arthritis.

d. Corticosteroids are potent anti-inflammatories used mainly as a bridging therapy until other treatments begin to take effect. Steroids have not been shown to be disease-modifying. They can be administered by oral, intramuscular, intravenous, intra-articular, or intraocular route and should be administered at the lowest effective dose. With the exception of intra-articular steroid injections, which are well tolerated, steroids can lead to serious toxic side effects including weight gain, edema, acne, fatigue, growth suppression, decreased bone density, hypertension, hyperglycemia, glaucoma, and cataracts.

8. Children receiving the immunosuppressive therapies used to treat arthritis require special considerations.

a. Close monitoring for signs of infection.

b. Screening for tuberculosis prior to initiation of corticosteroid or biologic therapy. Testing should be repeated annually for those taking biologics. Steroids can alter the result of tuberculin skin testing. Biologic therapy can reactivate latent tuberculosis.

c. Children receiving DMARDs, corticosteroids, or biologics should not receive live vaccines (varicella, measles, mumps, rubella). When considering treatment with methotrexate, varicella immunization may be recommended prior to starting therapy in susceptible children. In such circumstances, methotrexate cannot be started for 28 days postimmunization.

d. Regular blood monitoring for toxicity.

e. Regular clinical examinations to assess for adverse effects. In 2008, the FDA reported several cases of malignancies in children receiving biologic therapy. Recent studies have both supported and refuted possible links between cancer and biologic therapy.

Evidence Base Simard, J. F., Neovius, M., Hagelberg, S., et al. (2012). Juvenile idiopathic arthritis and risk of cancer: A nationwide cohort study. *Arthritis and Rheumatism, 62*(12), 3776–3782.

Diak, P., Siegel, J., La Grenade, L., et al. (2010). Tumor necrosis factor alpha blockers and malignancy in children: Forty-eight cases reported to the Food and Drug Administration. *Arthritis and Rheumatism, 62*(8), 2517–2524.

Table 53-7	Pharmacologic Treatment for Juvenile Idiopathic Arthritis		
	MEDICATION	**INDICATION**	**DOSING**
NSAIDs	COX-1, COX-2 inhibitors, naproxen, ibuprofen, indomethacin, celecoxib	First-line therapy for all subtypes of JIA; symptom management	P.O. Variable dose frequency
DMRADs	Methotrexate	Second-line therapy for all sub-types except systemic JIA	P.O. or sc once weekly 15 mg/m²/dose (maximum 25 mg) Therapeutic effect in 6–12 weeks
	Sulfasalazine	Oligoarticular JIA; polyarticular JIA; ERA	P.O. 50 mg/kg/day divided b.i.d. Therapeutic effect in 6–12 weeks
	Leflunomide	Oligoarticular; polyarticular	P.O. once daily 10–20 mg/day Therapeutic effect in 6–12 weeks
Glucocorticoids	Methylprednisolone, prednisone, prednisolone, triamcinolone, hexacetonide	Used for quick anti-inflammatory effect or bridging agent for all subtypes of JIA	IV, I.M., P.O., intra-articular, topical, intraocular for uveitis Dose/frequency depends on route and severity of inflammation
Biologics	TNF inhibitors: Entanercept Infliximab Adalimumab Golimumab	Used when fail second-line agents Effective to treat uveitis	sc (Entanercept, Adalimumab) IV (Infliximab) Dose/frequency variable Therapeutic effect reported after three doses
	IL Inhibitors: Anakinra (IL-1) Canakinumab (IL-1β) Tocilizumab (IL-6)	Systemic JIA Tocilizumab under study for other forms of JIA	Anakinra sc once/day Canakinumab sc q 4 weeks Tocilizumab IV q 2 weeks
	t-cell costimulatory modulators: Abatacept	JIA except systemic subtype	IV 10 mg/kg/dose Give at 0, 2 weeks then q 4 weeks Therapeutic effect reported as early as second infusion

I.M., intramuscular; IV, intravenous; JIA, juvenile idiopathic arthritis; P.O., oral; SC, subcutaneous.

9. The course and outcome of JIA has changed dramatically with early intervention and more successful therapies. However, active disease continues into adulthood in 50% to 70 % of children with polyarticular and systemic JIA; 40% to 50% of oligoarticular JIA.

Complications

1. Bone and growth changes:
   a. Growth disturbance, short stature.
   b. Osteopenia, osteoporosis.
   c. Cervical spine and temporomandibular joint problems (micrognathia—receding chin).
   d. Leg length discrepancies.
   e. Joint contractures.
2. Psychological and social reactions to illness.
3. Cataracts, glaucoma, or blindness secondary to uncontrolled, chronic uveitis.
4. Pericarditis.
5. Macrophage activation syndrome—a life-threatening complication of systemic JIA characterized by massive activation of T cells and macrophages; features include sustained fever, hepatosplenomegaly, anemia, liver function abnormalities, coagulopathy, encephalophathy, sudden drop in ESR, extreme elevation of ferritin, marked elevation of d-dimers.

ADVERSE EFFECTS	MONITORING	CONSIDERATIONS
Gastritis; pseudoporphyria; hepatotoxicity; renal toxicity	CBC, liver enzymes, creatinine at baseline then q 6 months	Pseudoporphyria most commonly seen in fair-skinned children
GI upset; mouth ulcers; hepatotoxicity; teratogenicity	CBC, liver enzymes at baseline, 1 month then q 3–4 months on stable dose	Provide folate supplement Avoid live vaccines Give VZIG within 96 hours for chicken pox exposure Avoid alcohol Avoid pregnancy Interaction with the antibiotics sulfamethoxazole and trimethopim (bone marrow suppression)
GI upset; rash; bone marrow suppression; hepatotoxicity; allergy	CBC, liver enzymes at baseline, then q 4–12 weeks	Inquire about sulfa allergies Avoid live vaccines Beware of additive hepatotoxicity in combination with methotrexate
GI upset; rash; hepatotoxicity; teratogenicity	CBC, liver enzymes at baseline, then q 4 to 12 weeks	Use when methotrexate not tolerated Cholestyramine used to enhance elimination Avoid pregnancy Avoid alcohol Avoid live vaccines
Increased appetite; GI upset; mood changes; hypertension; acne; straie; Cushing syndrome; growth suppression; osteoporosis; hyperglycemia; cataracts; glaucoma	Dependent on route of administration and length of treatment	Monitor BP; urine for glycosuria Annual bone mineral density Delay immunization schedule Give VZIG within 96 hours for chicken pox exposure
Allergic reaction; infection; demyelinating disease; possible risk for malignancy	CBC, liver enzymes, creatinine at baseline then q 3–6 months Tuberculosis screen prior to start then yearly	Assess for family history of multiple sclerosis; if positive then MRI prior to start
Injection site or infusion reactions; infection	Tuberculosis screen prior to start then yearly	Monitor for infection Avoid live vaccines
Infection	Tuberculosis screen prior to start then yearly	Monitor for infection Avoid live vaccines Monitor for infection Avoid live vaccines Avoid pregnancy

Nursing Assessment

1. History should include a thorough musculoskeletal inquiry including location, onset, duration of joint pain and stiffness; alleviating and exacerbating factors; activity limitations; medication and other nonpharmacological treatments used; review of systems to look for associated symptoms, complications of JIA and side effects of medication; most recent ophthalmology examination; immunizations and tuberculosis screening.

2. Physical examination focused on the clinical manifestations of the different subtypes of JIA including joint and gait assessment; vital signs; growth parameters; a pain assessment using a developmentally appropriate tool.

3. Gather data for psychosocial assessment including inquiry into the impact of this chronic, painful disease on the child's self-esteem and coping and the family's coping.

Nursing Diagnoses

- Acute and Chronic Pain related to joint inflammation.
- Impaired Physical Mobility related to joint inflammation and pain.
- Delayed Growth and Development related to chronic inflammation and side effects of medication.

- Impaired Family Processes related to caring for a child with a chronic, painful illness.
- Risk for Impaired Liver Function related to side effect of medications.

Other Nursing Diagnoses may include:

- Disturbed Sleep Pattern related to pain.
- Fatigue related to inflammation.
- Disturbed Body Image related to short stature; leg length discrepancy; side effects of prednisone (stretch marks, weight gain, acne); microagnathia.
- Risk for Chronic Low Self-Esteem related to changes in body image and physical capabilities.
- Impaired Nutrition: Less Than Body Requirements related to increased metabolic activity associated with inflammation.
- Risk for Imbalanced Nutrition: More Than Body Requirements related to side effect of medication.
- Deficient Knowledge related to potential adverse effects of medications.

Nursing Interventions

Minimizing Discomfort

1. Administer or teach parents to administer medications to reduce inflammation and control pain. When inflammation and pain are controlled, a child is more willing and able to do exercises to improve joint strength and prevent loss of movement.
2. Encourage a warm bath or shower to relieve morning stiffness. Use other thermal modalities such as soaking or warm, moist pads or ice packs to soothe inflamed joints. Some children respond to heat and some to cold.
3. Use assistive devices to make mobility and activities of daily living (ADLs) easier. Examples include splints; orthotics; special adaptors for pencils, doorknobs, utensils; velcro or zipper pulls.

Preserving Joint Mobility

1. Encourage compliance with physical therapy regimen to strengthen muscles and mobilize joints. Assist with range of motion (ROM) exercises, as indicated.
2. Splint joints to maintain proper position (joint extension) and decrease pain and deformity.
3. Encourage prone position with a thin pillow or no pillow and firm mattress.
4. Encourage therapeutic play (swimming, throwing, bike riding).
5. Encourage child to do own ADLs to maintain joint mobility. Refer to occupational therapy for provision of adaptation devices to facilitate completion of daily activities (velcro closures, utensils and self-care implements with enlarged handles).
6. Schedule rest periods to maximize energy; discourage complete immobilization or lengthy inactivity because they increase stiffness.

Promote Normal Growth and Development

1. Identify developmental tasks appropriate to age of child. Educate parents and work with child and family to set goals with necessary adaptations to promote successful achievement.

2. Encourage attendance in school, participation in activities, and socialization with peers as much as possible.
3. Encourage compliance with treatment plan to prevent complications related to prolonged inflammation.
4. Promote healthy diet; obtain diet history; make referral to dietician, as necessary.

Normalizing Family Processes

1. Refer to community resources and support groups.
2. Encourage child and family to verbalize feelings.
3. Remind parents to devote time to other children, themselves, and each other because the disease affects the whole family.

Family Education and Health Maintenance

1. Educate and motivate parents and child to continue program of treatment at home. This is a chronic disease with an unpredictable course; however, compliance with prescribed treatment is important to improve functional outcome and to allow the child to grow and develop to his or her full potential.
2. Encourage medication compliance by helping to create a medication calendar; suggesting weekly pill boxes; strategies to reduce side effects such as taking NSAIDS with food or taking methotrexate on the weekends before bed.
3. Encourage open communication with school authorities. Child should receive accommodations such as use of school elevator, two sets of textbooks so child does not need to carry heavy backpack to and from school, use of a computer for difficulties with writing, allowance to move around during prolonged periods of sitting.
4. Educate the family about the importance of a daily exercise routine to maintain ROM, muscle strength, and function. Periodically reevaluate need for physical and occupational therapy.
5. Provide nutritional counseling to promote a balanced diet with special attention given to the intake of calcium, vitamin D, folic acid, and iron. Portion control and healthy snacks should be encouraged to prevent obesity.
6. Stress the need for routine follow-up care and ophthalmologic evaluation.
7. Educate families about the special considerations required when their child is receiving immunosuppressive medications: seek prompt medical attention for fever and other signs of infection; child and family members should receive annual influenza vaccine; live vaccinations need to be postponed until child is no longer receiving immunosuppression.
8. Refer family to agencies such as the Arthritis Foundation (*www.arthritis.org*).

Evaluation: Expected Outcomes

- Reports decreased pain.
- ROM, muscle strength, and joint function is preserved.
- Growth and development parameters, including psychological and social, are appropriate for age.
- Parents seek additional resources.

Systemic Lupus Erythematosus

Systemic lupus erythematosus (SLE) is a systemic multisystem autoimmune disease that has the potential to affect any organ or organ system. Different types of lupus can occur, including discoid lupus (rare in pediatrics and primarily affecting only the skin), subacute cutaneous lupus erythematosus (skin and mild systemic manifestations), neonatal lupus erythematosus (NLE), and drug-induced lupus (lupus-like syndrome that may resolve when drug is discontinued).

The incidence is higher in females than in males (1:2 to 1:5), higher in Hispanic, black, North American First Nations, Southeast and South Asian, and is most common during the childbearing period (ages 15 to 44). However, it can affect neonates (1 in 20,000 live births) and children ages 5 to 15.

Pathophysiology and Etiology

1. Cause is unknown. Etiologic factors include:
   a. Immune-system dysregulation.
   b. Genetic susceptibility—associations with certain HLA types, complement deficiencies and TNF polymorphisms have been made.
   c. Environmental factors.
   d. Hormonal factors.
2. Possible factors that trigger or unmask initial symptoms:
   a. Photosensitivity (ultraviolet B light).
   b. Viral infection.
   c. Stress, extreme fatigue.
   d. Radiation therapy.
   e. Vaccination.
   f. Antioxidants.
   g. Chemical exposure.
3. SLE is characterized by the production of autoantibodies and the deposition of immune complexes in tissues and organs throughout the body.
   a. Spontaneous hyperactivity of B lymphocytes leads to increased antibody production. Additionally, the life of the B lymphocytes is abnormally prolonged, enhancing antibody production.
   b. These antibodies combine with antigen to form immune complexes, which deposit in tissue.
   c. The immune complexes activate the complement cascade, leading to inflammation (recruitment of inflammatory cells and production of oxidants, proteases, prostaglandins, and cytokines).
   d. Long-term inflammation can lead to irreversible cell destruction and tissue and organ damage.
4. Antiphospholipid syndrome (APS) produces a variety of antibodies against phospholipids and may occur singularly or in association with other diseases, commonly lupus. The primary event resulting from APS is thrombolytic in nature.
5. Neonate born to a known SLE (anti-SSA/Ro or anti-SSB/La) mother.
   a. Autoantibodies are transmitted transplacentally.
   b. Infant may or may not develop clinical symptoms.
   c. The most common clinical manifestations of NLE are cardiac, dermatologic, hematologic, and hepatic.
   d. The most serious manifestation is congenital heart block (CHB), requiring pacemaker insertion as an infant or child.
   e. The skin, liver, and hematologic symptoms gradually resolve over time, with few long-term effects.

Clinical Manifestations

1. Onset may be gradual with vague symptoms or acute with significant manifestations.
2. General characteristic signs and symptoms may include:
   a. Malar erythema (butterfly rash), which usually spreads over bridge of nose; rash may vary from a faint blush to scaly erythematous papules and may be photosensitive. Rash may spread from face and scalp to neck, chest, and extremities. There is nasiolabial sparing of the rash.
   b. Acute polyarthritis, arthralgia.
   c. Fatigue, malaise.
   d Fever, oral ulcers.
   e. Anorexia, weight loss.
   f. Hair loss.
   g. Renal (proteinuria), neurologic (seizures in the absence of known metabolic disorders or drug-associated causes), hematologic (hemolytic anemia, lymphopenia, or thrombocytopenia) and immunologic.
3. Cutaneous lesions in NLE can occur shortly after birth; most commonly develops from 6 weeks to 6 months of age. The rash resolves without scarring.
4. Cardiac involvement—CHB in neonates due to AV node absence or degeneration. The node is replaced by fibrosis, fatty tissue, or calcification. There can be pericarditis, myocarditis, and valvulitis. Risk for heart block increases significantly for siblings born after an infant with CHB or cutaneous neonatal lupus.
5. Nephritis—at onset or during course of disease. Clinically evident nephritis occurs in at least 20% to 80% of patients and is more frequent and of greater severity in children than in adults. It usually develops within 2 years of diagnosis.
   a. Routine monitoring of urine is essential in management of children with SLE.
   b. Hematuria, proteinuria, hypertension may be evident.
6. CNS involvement during course of disease—neuropsychiatric disease manifested by psychosis (visual and/or auditory hallucinations), depression, headache (severe, unremitting), cerebrovascular disease (stroke), cognitive impairment (worsening school performance), and seizures.
7. Splenomegaly, hepatomegaly, lymphadenopathy.
8. Anemia, leukopenia, thrombocytopenia, hypoglobulinemia.
9. Raynaud's phenomenon (15% to 20% of patients)
10. Pulmonary involvement with pleural effusion and lupus pneumonitis.

Diagnostic Evaluation

1. Diagnosis is made largely by clinical manifestations (see Box 53-2).
2. Antibody studies:
   a. ANA—nonspecific but positive in 90% of people with SLE.
   b. Other antibodies such as anti-dsDNA, anti-ssDNA, anti-RNP, anti-Ro, and anti-La.
3. ESR—elevated.
4. Serum complements studies—decreased.

BOX 53-2	Criteria for Diagnosis of Systemic Lupus Erythematosus

According to the American College of Rheumatology, the presence of four or more criteria must be documented to diagnose SLE.

- Malar (butterfly) rash
- Discoid lupus rash
- Photosensitivity
- Oral or nasal mucocutaneous ulcerations
- Nonerosive arthritis
- Nephritis*
  - Proteinuria >0.5 g/day
  - Cellular casts
- Encephalopathy*
  - Seizures
  - Psychosis
- Pleuritis or pericarditis
- Hemolytic anemia, leukopenia, thrombocytopenia
- Positive immunoserology*
  - Antibodies to double-stranded DNA
  - Antibodies to Sm nuclear antigen
  - Positive finding of antiphospholipid antibodies based on immunoglobulin (Ig) G or IgM anticardiolipin antibodies, lupus anticoagulant, or confirmed false-positive serologic test for syphilis for at least 6 months
- Positive antinuclear antibody

*Any one item satisfies this criterion.

5. CBC—leukopenia and mild to moderate anemia; can be hemolytic anemia, thrombocytopenia.

6. Tests for APS (antiphospholipid syndrome)—elevated prothrombin time, partial thromboplastin time; false-positive syphilis tests such as VDRL; elevated anticardiolipin antibodies; and elevated dilute Russell's viper venom time. The presence of one or more suggests APS and the need for aspirin or Coumadin therapy to prevent thrombosis.

7. Serum chemistry and urine studies to detect kidney and other body system involvement.

8. Renal biopsy—verifies lupus nephritis and classification.

9. Electrocardiogram and other cardiac testing.

Management

1. Course is unpredictable, usually progressive, and may terminate in death, if untreated. Therapy is based on the extent and severity of disease. To simplify therapy, SLE is classified as:
   a. Mild (fever, arthritis, rash).
   b. Moderate (clinically significant but non-life-threatening involvement of kidneys or other major organs)
   c. Severe (substantial renal, pulmonary, hematological, or neurologic disease).

2. Goal of medication therapy is to control symptoms and decrease inflammation.

3. NSAIDs are used to relieve joint symptoms, fever, fatigue, and pain.

4. Methotrexate may be used for joint/skin symptoms. Also used as a steroid-sparing agent.

5. Antimalarials, such as hydroxychloroquine and chloroquine, are used to:
   a. Relieve joint symptoms and skin rash.
   b. Renal—protective when renal function is stabilized.
   c. Maintain remission.

6. Corticosteroids are required for almost all children with SLE and are administered either orally as prednisone or via IV line as methylprednisilone.
   a. Low-dose oral steroids are usually used to control arthritis, fever, dermatitis, or serositis.
   b. High-dose oral or IV steroids are used to treat moderate or severe SLE, especially in the presence of CNS involvement, pulmonary disease, hemolytic anemia, and nephritis.

 DRUG ALERT IV glucocorticoid "pulse" therapy has been known to cause hypertension or hypotension, tachycardia, blurring of vision, flushing, sweating, and metallic taste in mouth. Close monitoring of temperature, pulse rate, respiratory rate, and blood pressure (BP) is indicated.

7. Immunosuppressive agents, such as azathioprine, cyclophosphamide, cyclosporine, mycophenolate mofetil, and rituximab—used in severe disease including nephritis and neuropsychiatric disease

8. Dialysis and renal transplantation as adjunctive therapy for severe lupus nephritis.

9. Supportive therapy:
   a. Rest.
   b. Adequate nutrition; aim to avoid large increases in weight.
   c. Treatment of existing complications with antibiotics, antihypertensives, and anticonvulsants.
   d. Early identification and treatment of opportunistic infection.
   e. Topical corticosteroid preparations—may help suppress cutaneous lesions (discoid lupus is rare in children).

10. Pacemaker may be necessary in neonates.

Complications

1. Infection—primarily resulting from steroid and immunosuppressive therapy.

2. Renal—hypertension, renal failure.

3. Cardiac—atherosclerosis, myocardial infarction, and valvular disease.

4. Growth impairment and weight gain related to steroid therapy.

5. Musculoskeletal—osteopenia/osteoporosis, avascular necrosis, and compression fractures (resulting from steroid therapy).

6. Ocular—cataracts, glaucoma (resulting from steroid and/or hydroxychloroquine therapy).

Nursing Assessment

1. Obtain a review of systems to determine involvement of different body systems.
2. Perform a complete physical examination, focusing on vital signs that might indicate renal or cardiac involvement, auscultation of the chest for heart and lung involvement, abdominal examination, and evaluation of the skin and extremities for vascular or cutaneous lesions.
3. Assess psychosocial status to evaluate child's and family's coping with chronic illness, school performance, and socialization. Assess adherence to medication regime, especially with adolescents.

Nursing Diagnoses

- Fatigue related to disease process.
- Acute and Chronic Pain related to arthritis.
- Hyperthermia related to disease process.
- Risk for Injury related to CNS involvement (seizures).
- Risk for Injury related to IV glucocorticoid therapy.
- Impaired Urinary Elimination related to kidney involvement.
- Imbalanced Nutrition: Less than Body Requirements related to anorexia and oral ulcers.
- Disturbed Body Image related to manifestations of disease or drugs.

Nursing Interventions

Minimizing Fatigue

1. Intersperse periods of rest between activities.
2. Caution to resume school activities slowly. Parents should contact the school to make arrangements to minimize fatigue (ie, second set of textbooks to be kept at home). Consider half days at school until fatigue is diminished. The child may also be a candidate for homeschooling.
3. Maintain good sleep hygiene.

Promoting Comfort

1. Administer or teach parents to administer analgesics, NSAIDs, steroids, and other medications, as prescribed. Review medication side effects with family. Provide written medication aids.
2. For child on steroids, monitor for glycosuria and check blood test results for hyperglycemia, hypokalemia, and hyperlipidemia.
3. Provide diversional activities appropriate for age.

Controlling Fever

1. Monitor temperature every 4 hours and document pattern.
2. Administer or teach parents to administer antipyretics, as prescribed; note results.
3. Encourage increased fluids by mouth when feverish. Dress in lightweight clothing.

Protecting from Injury Due to Seizures

1. Institute seizure precautions, if indicated.
2. Monitor condition during seizure and behavior after seizure.

Protecting from Adverse Reactions

1. While administering IV glucocorticoid therapy, monitor pulse and BP every 15 minutes for 1 hour, then every 30 minutes for 1 hour.
2. Slow the rate or discontinue infusion if there are significant changes in BP or pulse.
3. Notify the health care provider and continue to monitor vital signs frequently until they return to normal.

Maintaining Urinary Elimination

1. Monitor laboratory work for signs of renal abnormalities (blood urea nitrogen [BUN], creatinine, urine-specific gravity, hematuria, and proteinuria).
2. Monitor intake and output.
3. Monitor BP; watch for development of edema.

Promoting Appropriate Nutritional Intake

1. Allow child to help in selecting and preparing foods. Family members should set an example for healthy diet and consider complying with the same diet plan as has been recommended for the child.
2. Apply topical medication to oral ulcers or give analgesics before meals.
3. Monitor food intake and weight. Consider consultation with a dietician to assist with healthy food choices.
4. Low-sodium diet for those with nephritis and those on high-dose steroid therapy.
5. Encourage food high in calcium or use of calcium and vitamin D supplements to decrease risk of low bone density.

Improving Self-Image

1. Encourage contact with peers and family.
2. Allow child to vent feelings about bodily changes and chronic illness.
3. Allow child to be involved in planning care and making decisions.
4. Consider a referral for counseling for adolescents to help with the development of coping strategies, if required.

Family Education and Health Maintenance

1. Teach ways to prevent exacerbations and complications of the disease. Teaching points include:
   a. Get enough rest; try not to overexert.
   b. Minimize stress and anxiety.
   c. Follow treatment plan and medication schedule; understand adverse medication effects (especially with corticosteroids and other immunosuppressive drugs).
   d. Follow medication regime, as prescribed. Check with health care provider prior to using over-the-counter drugs or therapies found on the Internet.
   e. Avoid contact with people with infectious diseases; get pneumococcal and flu vaccine and keep routine immunizations up to date.
   f. Follow prescribed diet, especially when receiving steroids.
   g. Seek medical attention at times of illness or stress.
   h. Minimize sun exposure.
   i. Recognize warning signs of exacerbation such as fatigue, weight loss, joint pain, hair loss, new rashes, mouth sores, headaches, trouble with concentration, seizures, shortness of breath, chest pain, abdominal pain, fever, urinary changes.

j. Remember sun protection (hats, sunscreen, and long-sleeve shirts).

2. Teach parents about normal growth and development, emphasizing normal issues such as adolescent body image and peer relationships and how chronic illness can affect the child and the family.

3. Teach the importance of continual medical follow-up.

   a. Disease management requires frequent reevaluation; drug therapy and laboratory results need frequent monitoring to prevent complications.

   b. Prognosis varies widely depending on the organ involvement and the intensity of the inflammatory reaction. Some children have milder SLE with little organ involvement. Prolonged spontaneous remission is unusual in children. The 5-year survival rate is close to 100%; 10 years is 85%.

5. Advise family that all children with SLE need annual ophthalmologic exams. Those taking hydroxychloroquine require more frequent ophthalmologic evaluation to prevent blindness due to corneal and retinal changes.

6. Refer to agencies such as the Lupus Foundation of America (*www.lupus.org*).

Evaluation: Expected Outcomes

- Participates in activities with peers without fatigue; attends school full time.
- Reports reduced level of pain.
- Remains afebrile, knows what to do if febrile.
- Seizure precautions maintained.
- No changes in vital signs during glucocorticoid infusion.
- Urine output adequate.
- Appropriate dietary intake, weight stable.
- Compliant with medication regime.

Henoch-Schönlein Purpura

Henoch-Schönlein purpura (HSP) is an immune-mediated vasculitis with IgA deposition and subsequent inflammatory reaction around capillaries and arterioles. It is considered a small-vessel vasculitis. HSP can affect the skin, intestines, joints, kidneys, and nervous system. Incidence is higher in males than in females (2:1). Onset generally is between ages 3 and 15; it is seen most commonly in winter and can occur in clusters. Higher rate has been noted in those children diagnosed with familial Mediterranean fever.

Pathophysiology and Etiology

1. Cause is unknown; however, theories include an immunologic reaction to a variety of antigenic stimuli, such as infection (eg, streptococci), dietary allergens, insect bites, and drugs.

2. Acute vasculitis develops.

   a. Swelling and edema of capillaries, small venules, and arterioles.

   b. Fibrin is deposited in the glomeruli of the kidney.

3. Vasculitis results in skin manifestations (nonthrombocytopenic palpable purpura), arthritis, GI (abdominal pain, GI bleeding), and renal symptoms.

Clinical Manifestations

1. Rash—sudden onset may precede or follow other manifestations.

   a. Typical rash begins with maculopapular erythematous or urticarial rash.

   b. These lesions become less raised and purpuric in character and do not fade with pressure. They blanch initially, then progress to ecchymotic areas until they fade.

   c. Several stages of the rash may be present at one time.

   d. Rash appears primarily on buttocks, lower back, and extensor aspects of arms, legs, and face, then disappears.

   e. Localized subcutaneous edema in dependent and periorbital area is common.

2. Arthritis occurs in 50% to 80% of patients, primarily affecting the knee and ankle joints; the wrists, elbows, and finger joints may also be affected, although this is rare.

   a. The arthritis is moderately severe, with painful swelling due to periarticular edema and limitation of motion.

   b. The arthritis is self-limited and does not cause permanent sequelae.

3. Orchitis in 2% to 35% of male children.

4. Colicky abdominal pain—from submucosal and subserosal hemorrhage and edema.

5. Nausea, vomiting, malaise, low-grade fever.

6. Proteinuria.

7. Microscopic hematuria.

8. Rarely, CNS involvement, such as headache, seizure, or cerebral hemorrhage.

9. Symptoms may appear acutely or gradually and vary in intensity and duration.

Diagnostic Evaluation

1. Blood studies (not diagnostic, but support clinical evidence):

   a. IgA may be elevated (more than 50% of cases).

   b. Coagulation studies and platelet count are typically normal in presence of purpura.

   c. ESR and WBC count may be elevated.

   d. Anemia is possible.

   e. Elevated BUN and creatinine with severe kidney involvement.

2. Urine studies show proteinuria, microscopic hematuria, and casts.

3. Stools may show occult or gross blood.

4. Abdominal ultrasound or x-rays may help confirm bowel involvement.

Management

Treatment is primarily symptomatic and supportive. Hydration, rest, and adequate pain relief are the goals of treatment.

1. Bed rest until the child is able to ambulate and can do so without increasing edema of lower extremities, genital area, and buttocks.

2. Antibiotic therapy if acute episode was preceded by infection, especially streptococcal.

3. Management of complicating abdominal or renal involvement and arthritis.
   a. Steroid use is controversial. Suggested for use if symptoms prevent adequate oral intake or if the child has challenges with ambulation or performing ADL.
   b. Immunosuppressive therapy, such as azathioprine or cyclophosphamide, may be given to stabilize persistent renal involvement (rare).
   c. High-dose immune globulin has been recommended for severe cases.
4. Provide comfort measures and analgesics, such as acetaminophen or NSAIDS.

Complications

1. Acute nephritis or nephrosis that may lead to chronic nephritis. Ninety percent of children who develop renal involvement will do so within 2 months of diagnosis.
2. Intussusception (approximately 5% incidence).
3. Significant GI bleeding may require a transfusion (rare).
4. Neurologic vasculitis with headaches, seizures, and neuropathies.

 NURSING ALERT Be alert for signs of intussusception—sudden onset of paroxysmal, colicky abdominal pain, blood in stools, vomiting, and increasing abdominal distention and tenderness—report immediately.

Nursing Assessment

1. Obtain a complete history. There is some suggestion of allergy to insect bites or medications as a basis for development of the disease. Also controversial is association with streptococci, viruses, and vaccination.
2. Perform physical assessment of renal, integumentary, musculoskeletal, and GI systems.
3. Determine impact of illness on the psychosocial well-being of the child and family.

Nursing Diagnoses

- Acute Pain related to arthritis and abdominal pain.
- Activity Intolerance related to fatigue and pain.
- Risk for Impaired Skin Integrity related to rash and itching.
- Impaired Urinary Elimination related to renal involvement.
- Fear related to discomfort, hospitalization, and lack of knowledge.

Nursing Interventions

Reducing Discomfort

1. Monitor pain level and location. Use appropriate developmental pain scales to determine level of pain.
2. Administer or teach parents to administer pain medications, as prescribed, and monitor child's response.
3. Apply warm or cool compresses to joints or abdomen for 30-minute periods to help soothe painful areas.
4. Provide diversional activities in accordance with the child's age.

Increasing Participation in Activities

1. Monitor completion of daily and diversional activities; offer choice.
2. Alternate activities with rest periods.

Maintaining Skin Integrity

1. Assess skin condition and turgor.
2. Maintain adequate fluids.
3. Provide loose, comfortable clothing.
4. Administer or teach parents to administer antipruritics, if necessary.
5. Avoid soap, scratching, or dry skin that may exacerbate rash.

Maintaining Urinary Output

1. Record intake and output, vital signs, weight, urine-specific gravity, and level of edema.
2. Check urine for protein, hematuria, and color; monitor creatinine
3. Report or teach parents to report changes promptly.

Alleviating Fear

1. Allow child and family to verbalize feelings about hospitalization and illness.
2. Monitor anxiety level of child and family. Ensure information is given at the child's level of understanding.
3. Offer realistic encouragement. The long-term outlook is good when renal involvement is minimal.
4. Encourage the family and peers to visit the hospitalized child and bring in familiar items from home.
5. Allow child to make age-appropriate decisions and become involved in planning care.

Family Education and Health Maintenance

1. Reassure the parents that symptoms are usually self-limiting.
2. Make sure that parents and child understand the disease and the need to report changes in urine or signs of intussusception.
3. Educate the parents about the importance of continued care. Long-term follow-up of urinalysis will be necessary to evaluate renal function.

Evaluation: Expected Outcomes

- Reports relief from pain.
- Participates in activity for longer period each day.
- Rash resolved, skin intact.
- Urine output adequate, negative protein.
- Child verbalizes feelings about illness.

Kawasaki Disease

Kawasaki disease (KD) is a common vasculitis of childhood affecting medium and small blood vessels. Coronary arteries are the most common site of damage, giving KD the potential to cause severe morbidity and even death without early diagnosis and treatment. It is characterized by multisystem inflammation including fever, conjunctivitis, lymphadenopathy, and changes in blood vessels. It is the leading cause of acquired heart disease in children in the United States.

Pathophysiology and Etiology

 Evidence Base Yeung, R. S. M. (2011). Vasculitis: Kawasaki disease. In A. Y. Elzouki, H. A. Harfi, H. Nazer, et al. (Eds.), *Textbook of clinical pediatrics* (2nd ed., pp. 1675–1684). New York: Springer.

1. KD is a disease of early childhood with 85% of affected children under 5 years of age. It occurs in children of all origins, although those of Asian descent have the highest incidence.

2. Etiology is unknown, although most investigators believe the disease is related to an infectious or environmental trigger in a genetically susceptible host. The result is a prolonged immune response targeted at vessel walls of medium and small arteries.

3. Infection as a trigger is supported by the fact that KD is endemic with seasonal fluctuations (winter and early spring). It is further hypothesized that superantigens, proteins present in certain organisms (*Staphylococci, Streptococci, Mycobacterium, Mycoplasma,* Epstein-Barr virus), are responsible for the prolonged inflammation through stimulation of large numbers of T cells.

4. Genetic predisposition to KD is evident in the observations that siblings have 10-fold higher risk of developing the disease and the children of parents who had KD have a two-fold increase in risk than the general population.

5. Researchers have not found associations between exposure to drugs, environmental toxins, pesticides, chemicals, or heavy metals and KD.

6. KD is a generalized systemic vasculitis involving blood vessels throughout the body. The full extent of the inflammatory process leading to aneurysm formation is not understood. Marked elevation in the cytokine TNF is thought to activate matrix metalloproteinase enzymes capable of breaking down elastin in arterial vessel walls. This breakdown leads to loss of integrity and ballooning and aneurysm formation.

7. Aneurysms, the result of prolonged inflammation, usually develop in the second to eighth week of the illness. The most common site for development is the coronary artery although other sites such as celiac, mesenteric, femoral, iliac, renal, and axillary may be affected. Early treatment following the recommended protocol of Intravenous gamma globulin (IVIG) and aspirin has reduced aneurysm development by 85%.

 Evidence Base Sundel, R., & Petty R. (2011). Kawasaki disease. In J. T. Cassidy, R. M. Laxer, R. E. Petty, et al. (Eds.), *Textbook of Pediatric Rheumatology* (6th ed., pp. 505–520). Philadelphia: Saunders Elsevier.

Clinical Manifestations

Kawasaki disease is divided into three phases, each with distinct clinical features. See Figure 53-1.

Acute Phase (First 10 to 14 Days of Illness)

1. During the acute phase the children exhibit classic signs of inflammation (redness, swelling, heat) presented as multisystem changes. They appear ill and irritable.

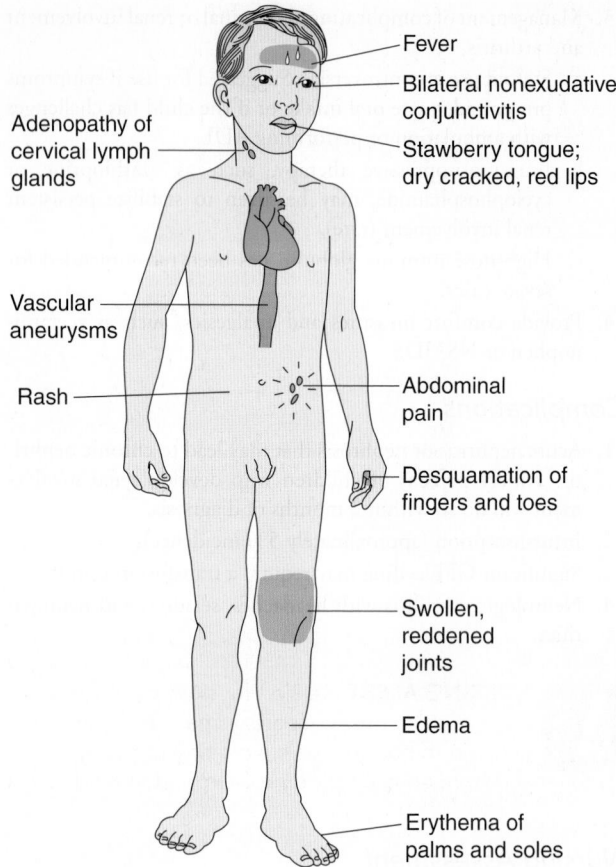

Figure 53-1. Clinical manifestations of acute Kawasaki disease.

2. The diagnostic criteria of Kawasaki disease occur during the acute phase. See Box 53-3. Fever, in addition to four out of five of the other features, is required for diagnosis; not all features occur at a single point in time.

 Evidence Base Kuo, H., Kang, K., Chang, W., et al. (2012). Kawasaki disease: An update on diagnosis and treatment. *Pediatrics and Neonatology, 53*(1), 4–11.

3. Other associated findings:
   a. Cardiovascular—early tachycardia, myocarditis, pericarditis, S3 gallop; with the reduced contractibility may progress to signs of heart failure
   b. Aseptic meningitis; anterior uveitis—children extremely irritable; photophobic
   c. Arthritis—painful; usually large joints; short duration with rapid response to standard treatment for KD.
   d. Gastrointestinal—diarrhea, vomiting, abdominal pain, hepatomegaly, hydrops of the gallbladder.

Subacute Phase (11 to 25 Days After Onset of Illness)

1. The classic inflammatory features of the acute phase resolve and the temperature returns to normal. If treated, many children are asymptomatic. If untreated or unresponsive to treatment, then fever, oral changes, and conjunctivitis

---

BOX 53-3	American Heart Association Diagnostic Features for Kawasaki Disease

Fever for at least 5 days plus at least four out of the following five features.
- Fever is high (generally >102.2° F [39 ° C]) and persistent; usually unresponsive to antipyretics

Bilateral nonexudative conjunctivitis

Oral-mucosal changes
- Swollen, red, cracked lips
- Strawberry tongue
- Erythema of the oral and pharyngeal mucosa

Cervical lymphadenopathy; at least one node >1.5 cm; usually unilateral

Rash; usually nonspecific, maculopapular involving trunk, extremities, and perineal region

Extremity changes
- Swelling of the hands and/or feet
- Erythema of the palms and/or soles
- (Subacute phase) periungual peeling of the fingers and/or toes

---

may be present until third or fourth week. Arthritis may be present.
2. Desquamation of toes and fingers in classic distribution starting in periungal region.
3. Coronary artery aneurysm is detected.
4. Thrombocytosis peaks at about 14 days.

Convalescent Phase
1. The acute phase reactants (ESR and platelets) return to normal.
2. The child appears well.
3. Transverse grooves present on fingernails and toenails (Beau's lines).
4. Vessels undergo healing, remodeling, fibrosis, and scarring. Preexisting small aneurysms may resolve and large aneurysms may develop thrombosis, leading to complications including myocardial infarction, dysrhythmias, or death.

Diagnostic Evaluation
1. There are no specific diagnostic tests for Kawasaki disease. The diagnosis is based on the clinical manifestations occurring in phases. There is a subset of children, usually the very young or old, who do not meet the diagnostic criteria for KD, yet present with prolonged fever and two or three of the features. They are a challenge to diagnose and are the group who has the highest risk for developing coronary aneurysms.
2. Although there are no specific laboratory tests, the following may help support diagnosis or rule out other diseases:
   a. CBC—leukocytosis; mild normochromic, normocytic anemia.
   b. Platelet count (from 500,000 to 1 million/mm³)—increased during second to fourth week of illness.
   c. ESR (usually >40 mm/hour).

d. C-reactive protein (usually >3.0 mg/dL).
   e. Albumin—low levels associated with more severe and prolonged disease.
   f. Liver enzymes (AST, ALT)—moderately elevated.
   g. Serum lipids—reduced high-density lipoprotein levels; elevated triglyceride and low-density lipoprotein levels during the subacute phase.
3. Lumbar puncture often performed because of the degree of child's irritability demonstrates aseptic meningitis; cerebral spinal fluid analysis shows elevated white blood cell count; normal protein; normal glucose.
4. Echocardiogram—should be performed as soon as the diagnosis is suspected and at 2 weeks and at 6 to 8 weeks after diagnosis. More frequent assessment may be required for complicated cases.
5. Cardiac catheterization and angiocardiography may be required for more complex cardiac abnormalities.

Management

 Evidence Base Daniels, L., Gordon, J., Burns, J. (2012). Kawasaki disease: Late cardiovascular sequelae. *Current Opinion in Cardiology, 27*(6), 572–577.

1. The goal of treatment is to prevent the long-term sequelae associated with KD by controlling inflammation.
2. The American Heart Association recommends that children with KD should be treated with IVIG and aspirin within 10 days of illness to reduce aneurysm formation. Treatment before day 5 has not shown any effect on coronary outcome and may increase the requirement for a second treatment.
   a. IVIG should be given as a single infusion at a dose of 2g/kg. Most infusion protocols run very slow with stepwise increases in rate for a total infusion time of 8 to 12 hours.
   b. Ten to 20% of children will have persistent fever or recurrence of fever within the first 36 hours after treatment with IVIG. Experts agree that these children should be retreated with a single infusion of 2g/kg.

 DRUG ALERT Inflammation of the child's heart may compromise the heart's ability to handle the fluid challenge associated with IVIG. The infusion may need to be of longer duration.

   c. Aspirin therapy—the anti-inflammatory dose of 80 to 100 mg/kg/day divided into four doses is recommended during the acute phase. The length of treatment varies from 24 to 72 hours after fever resolves to 2 weeks. The aspirin is then reduced to antiplatelet dosing of 3 to 5 mg/kg/day, which is continued until laboratory measures of inflammation have returned to normal and the echocardiogram at 6 to 8 weeks shows no sign of coronary aneurysm. Children with aneurysms will continue aspirin for life.

DRUG ALERT Risk of Reye's syndrome exists for children on aspirin therapy if they develop varicella or influenza. For children who are not immune to chickenpox, aspirin may need to be withheld after an exposure. Families should be instructed to receive annual influenza vaccines to minimize the risk for influenza.

3. In more complicated aneurysms, other anticoagulant and thrombolytic medications may be required.
4. Rarely, coronary artery bypass surgery or cardiac catheterization techniques are indicated.
5. Supportive measures:
    a. Maintain fluid and electrolyte balance.
    b. Give nutritional support.
    c. Provide comfort.
6. Follow-up by pediatric cardiologist with serial echocardiograms is necessary to monitor aneurysms.

Complications

1. Coronary aneurysm.
2. Aspirin toxicity.
3. Mortality is less than 0.3%.

Nursing Assessment

1. A thorough history to document data that support the diagnosis of Kawasaki disease; features of KD do not always present simultaneously.
2. Perform physical examination focusing on clinical features; hydration; cardiovascular status. Document vital signs including accurate temperature, BP, heart rate, rhythm, heart sounds, respiratory rate.
3. Perform pain assessment using age-appropriate pain scale.

Nursing Diagnoses

- Acute Pain related to conjunctival inflammation; swollen, cracked lips; and joint inflammation.
- Risk for Decreased Cardiac Tissue Perfusion related to inflammation of coronary blood vessels.
- Impaired Oral Mucous Membrane related to oral vessel inflammation.
- Risk for Impaired Skin Integrity related to edema, dehydration, and desquamation of digits.
- Deficient Fluid Volume related to hyperthermia, anorexia, and oral changes.
- Fear of parents and child related to severity of illness and hospitalization.

Other Nursing Diagnoses may include:

- Hyperthermia related to inflammatory pathology of disease.
- Risk for Ineffective Peripheral Tissue Perfusion related to inflammation of blood vessels.
- Imbalanced Nutrition: Less Than Body Requirements related to anorexia, oral changes, increased metabolic requirements of inflammatory state.

Nursing Interventions

Reducing Discomfort

1. Offer pain medication on a scheduled basis rather than as needed during acute phase. Monitor pain level and child's response to analgesics.
2. Conjunctivitis and associated uveitis can cause photosensitivity; darken the room; offer sunglasses; apply cool compresses.
3. Use age-appropriate diversional techniques such as relaxation breathing, guided imagery, and distraction.

Maintaining Cardiac Output

1. Implement continual cardiac monitoring during acute phase hospitalization.
2. Assess the child for signs of myocarditis and heart failure (tachycardia, gallop rhythm, chest pain, dyspnea, nasal flaring, grunting, retractions, cyanosis, orthopnea, crackles, moist respirations, distended neck veins, edema).
3. Closely monitor intake and output. Calculate fluid balance. Administer oral and IV fluids, as ordered.
4. If administering IVIG, give premedication, as directed, and monitor closely for adverse effects.

 DRUG ALERT Infusion of IVIG has been known to cause a precipitous drop in BP mimicking anaphylaxis. Monitor BP and heart rate at the start of infusion, after 15 minutes, 30 minutes, and then hourly until infusion is complete. Slow the infusion and have patient evaluated for any drop in BP. Give premedication as prescribed to help prevent adverse effects. Make sure medications to treat anaphylaxis are readily available.

Preserving Oral Mucous Membranes

1. Offer and encourage frequent cool liquids (ice chips and ice pops). Avoid acidic, sugary, or carbonated beverages; progress to soft, bland foods.
2. Give mouth care every 1 to 4 hours; use soft toothbrush.
3. Apply petroleum to dry, cracked lips.
4. Observe the mouth frequently for signs of infection.
5. Monitor food and fluid intake for nutrition appropriate for age.

Improving Skin Integrity

1. Avoid the use of soap to prevent drying; apply emollients to skin, as ordered.
2. Elevate edematous extremities.
3. Use sheepskin, convoluted foam mattress, and smooth sheets.
4. Encourage soft flannel or terry cloth loose-fitting clothing; change damp garments and linens frequently when febrile.
5. Protect peeling skin; observe for signs of infection.

Maintaining Fluid Balance

1. Offer fluids at least every hour when child is awake; monitor and document fluid intake and output.
2. Monitor hydration status by checking skin turgor, daily weight, urine output, presence of tears and moist mucous membranes, and urine-specific gravity.

3. Pay attention to insensible loss during febrile stage. Monitor temperature every 4 to 8 hours and administer antipyretics, as directed. Maintain temperature graph chart.

Reducing Fear

1. Use play therapy (passive and active) to help the child express feelings. Consult a Child Life therapist, as needed.
2. Explain all procedures and treatment plans to the child and family. Encourage the parents and child to verbalize their concerns, fears, and questions.
3. Provide respite for parents during irritable stage of illness when child may be inconsolable. Provide emotional support, as necessary.
4. Keep family informed of progress and reinforce information about stages and prognosis.

Family Education and Health Maintenance

1. Advise parents to take child's temperature daily for 2 weeks postdischarge. Call health practitioner for temperatures over 101° F (38.3° C).
2. Ensure family is aware of plan for follow-up. Emphasize the need for long-term care. Complications can occur during the convalescent period months after the acute illness.
3. Advise parents that IVIG is pooled immunoglobulin. Immunizations, although not harmful, may not mount a protective response after IVIG administration. Live vaccinations are not recommended for 6 months posttreatment. Catch-up vaccinations may be needed.
4. Advocate for compliance with the prescribed level of physical activity. Activity will be restricted if child is receiving anticoagulant therapy or if child has cardiac complications identified on stress testing.
5. Encourage family members to learn cardiopulmonary resuscitation.
6. Teach parents to report the possible development of salicylate toxicity—tinnitus, nausea and vomiting, GI distress, blood in stool, increased respirations.
7. For children without physical activity limitations, educate parents that children may be fatigued for several weeks. They may require naps, shorter school days, special accommodations by school.
8. Provide anticipatory guidance about child's behavior.
   a. Do not overprotect the child. Discuss with parents the grief process of denial, anger, bargaining, depression, and acceptance they may be going through because of the illness.
   b. Discuss regression that often occurs during stresses such as hospitalization and illness.
9. Refer to community organizations such as the American Heart Association (*www.heart.org*).

Evaluation: Expected Outcomes

- Reports improved comfort level.
- Vital signs stable, no signs of reduced cardiac output.
- Eating and drinking without difficulty, reports no oral discomfort.
- No pain or signs of infection with desquamation.
- Child expresses feelings about illness, parents report confidence in ability to manage care.

SELECTED REFERENCES

American Academy of Pediatrics. (2012). Section 3: Summaries of Infectious Diseases. In: Pickering, L. K., Baker, C. J., Kimberlin, D. W., Long, S. S., (eds). *Red Book: 2012 Report of the Committee on Infectious Diseases* (29th ed.). Elk Grove Village, IL: *American Academy of Pediatrics*, (418–439).

Anderson, V. L. (2006). Uncovering a pediatric immunodeficiency, Part 1. *Journal for Nurse Practitioners, 2*(3), 186–192.

Anderson, V. L. (2006). Uncovering a pediatric immunodeficiency, Part 2. *Journal for Nurse Practitioners, 2*(4), 237–246.

Bertsias, G., Ioannidis, J., Boletis, J., et al. (2008). EULAR recommendations for the management of systemic lupus erythematosus. Report of a Task Force of the EULAR Standing Committee for International Clinical Studies Including Therapeutics. *Ann Rheum Dis. 67*(2), 195–205.

Beukelman T., Patkar N. M., Saag K. G., et al. (2011). 2011 American College of Rheumatology recommendations for the treatment of juvenile idiopathic arthritis: Initiation and safety monitoring of therapeutic agents for the treatment of arthritis and systemic features. *Arthritis Care and Research, 63*(4), 465–482.

Boudreau, M., & Fisher, C. (2012). Providing effective medical and case management services to HIV-infected youth preparing to transition to adult care. *Journal of the Association of Nurses in AIDS Care, 23*(4), 318–328.

Brogan, P., & Bagga, A. (2011). Leukocytoclastic vasculitis. In J. T. Cassidy, R. M. Laxer, R. E. Petty (Eds.), *Textbook of pediatric rheumatology* (6th ed.). Philadelphia: Elsevier, 483–490.

Brucato A., Cimaz, R., Caporali, R., et al. (2011). Pregnancy outcomes in patients with autoimmune diseases and anti-Ro/SSA antibodies. *Clinical Reviews in Allergy and Immunology, 40*(1), 27.

Burton, J., Murphy, E., & Riley, P. (2010). Primary immunodeficiency disease: A model for case management of chronic diseases. *Professional Case Management, 15*(1), 5–14.

Cassidy J. T., Laxer R. M., Petty R. E., et al. (Eds.). (2011). *Textbook of pediatric rheumatology* (6th ed.). Philadelphia: Saunders Elsevier.

Cassidy J., Kilvlin C., Lindsley C., et al. (2006). Ophthalmologic examinations in children with juvenile rheumatoid arthritis. *Pediatrics, 117*(5), 1843–1845.

Centers for Disease Control and Prevention. (2012). *HIV Surveillance Report,* Available: *http://www.cdc.gov/hiv/topics/surveillance/incidence.htm.*

Centers for Disease Control and Prevention. (2013). Recommended immunization schedules for persons aged 0 through 18 years. Available: *www.cdc.gov/vaccines/recs/acip.*

Chang, J. (2012). Juvenile idiopathic arthritis. In K. Reuter-Rice & B. Nachtsheim Bolick (Eds.), *Pediatric acute care: A guide for interprofessional practice* (pp. 691–700). Chicago: Jones & Bartlett.

Chartapisak, W., Opastiraku, S., Willis, N., et al. (2009). Prevention and treatment of renal disease in Henoch-Schonlein purpura: A systematic review. *Archives of Disease in Childhood, 94*(2), 132–137.

Children's HIV Association of the UK and Ireland. (2005). Guidance on transition and long term follow up services for adolescents with HIV infection acquired in infancy. Available: *www.chiva.org.uk/publications/index.html.*

Childrens HIV Association (CHIVA). (2010). CHIVA guidance on transition for adolescents living with HIV. London: Author. Available: *www.chiva.org.uk/professionals/health/guidelines/youngpeople/transition.html.*

Council on Cardiovascular Disease in the Young, Committee on Rheumatic Fever Endocarditis and Kawasaki Disease, & American Heart Association. (2001). AHA scientific statement: Diagnostic guidelines for Kawasaki disease. *Circulation, 103*, 335–336.

Daniels, L., Gordon, J., Burns, J. (2012). Kawasaki disease: Late cardiovascular sequelae. *Current Opinion in Cardiology, 27*(6), 572–577.

Diak, P., Siegel, J., La Grenade, L., et al. (2010). Tumor necrosis factor alpha blockers and malignancy in children: Forty-eight cases reported to the Food and Drug Administration. *Arthritis and Rheumatism, 62*(8), 2517–2524.

Geha, R., Notarangelo, L. D., Casanova, J. L., et al. et al (2008). Primary immunodeficiency diseases: An update from the International Union of Immunological Societies Primary Immunodeficiency Diseases Classification Committee. *Journal of Allergy and Clinical Immunology, 120*(4), 776–794.

Gowdie, P., & Tse, S. (2012). Juvenile idiopathic arthritis. *Pediatric Clinics of North America, 59*(2), 301–327.

Gray, P., Namasivayam, M., Ziegler, J. (2012). Recurrent infection in children: When and how to investigate for primary immunodeficiency. *Journal of Paediatrics and Child Health, 48*(3), 202–209.

Hahn, B., McMahon, M., Wilkinson, A., et al. (2012). American College of Rheumatology guidelines for screening, treatment and management of lupus nephritis. *Arthritis Care and Research, 64,* 797–808.

HIV Transitional Care Working Group. (2011). Transitioning HIV-infected adolescents into adult care. New York State Department of Health, AIDS Institute. Available: *www.hivguidelines.org.*

Holman R. C., Curns A. T., Belay E. D., et al. (2003) Kawasaki syndrome hospitalizations in the United States, 1997 and 2000. *Pediatrics, 112*(3), 495–501.

Jeffrey Modell Foundation. (2009). *10 warning signs of immunodeficiency.* Available: *www.infoforpi.org/aboutpi.*

Joint United Nations Programme on HIV/AIDS. (2012). UNAIDS report on global AIDS epidemic 2010. Available: *http://www.unaids.org/en/resources/campaigns/20121120_globalreport2012/globalreport/.*

Kuo, H., Yang, K., Chang, W., et al. (2012). Kawasaki disease: An update on diagnosis and treatment. *Pediatrics and Neonatology, 53*(1), 4–11.

Lim, D. C. E., Cheng, L. N. C., & Wong, F. W. S. (2009). Could it be henochschönlein purpura? *Australian Family Physician, 38*(5), 321–324.

McLellan, M. C., & Baker, A. L. (2011). At the heart of the fever: Kawasaki disease. *American Journal of Nursing, 111*(6), 57–63.

Muscal, E., Nadeem, T., Li, X., et al. (2010). Evaluation and treatment of acute psychosis in children with systemic lupus erythematosus (SLE): Consultation-liaison service experiences at a tertiary-care pediatric institution. *Psychosomatics, 51*(6), 508–514.

Newburger, J. W., Takahashi, M., Gerber, M. A., et al. (n.d.). Diagnosis, treatment and long-term management of Kawasaki disease: A statement for health professionals from the Committee on Rheumatic Fever, Endocarditis and Kawasaki Disease, Council on Cardiovascular Disease in the Young, & American Heart Association. *Circulation, 110,* 2747–2771.

Panel on Antiretroviral Therapy and Medical Management of HIV-Infected Children. (2012). Guidelines for the use of antiretroviral agents in pediatric HIV infection. Available: *http://aidsinfo.nih.gov/ContentFiles/PediatricGuidelines.pdf.*

Panel on Treatment of HIV-Infected Pregnant Women and Prevention of Perinatal Transmission. (2012). Recommendations for use of antiretroviral drugs in pregnant HIV-1-infected women for maternal health and interventions to reduce perinatal HIV transmission in the United States. Available: *http://aidsinfo.nih.gov/contentfi les/lvguidelines/PerinatalGL.pdf.*

Petty, R. E., Southwood, T. R., Manners, P., et al. (2004). International League of Associations for Rheumatology classification of juvenile idiopathic arthritis: second revision. *Journal of Rheumatology, 31*(2), 390–392.

Public Health Agency of Canada and National Advisory Committee on Immunization. (2006). Vaccination of individuals with immunodeficiency. Available: *www.phac-aspc.gc.ca/publicat/cig-gci/p03-07-eng.php.*

Reid, B. (2012). Immunodeficiencies. In K. Reuter-Rice & B. Bolick (Eds.), *Pediatric acute care: A guide for interprofessional practice,* 679–690. Burlington, VT: Jones & Bartlett.

Saunders, C. (2012). Disclosing HIV status to HIV positive children before adolescence. *British Journal of Nursing, 21*(11), 663–669.

Silverman, E., & Eddy, A. (2011). Systemic lupus erythematosus. In J. T. Cassidy, R. M. Laxer, R. E. Petty, et al. (Eds.), *Textbook of pediatric rheumatology* (6th ed., pp. 315–343). Philadelphia: Saunders Elsevier.

Simard, J. F., Neovius, M., Hagelberg, S., et al. (2012). Juvenile idiopathic arthritis and risk of cancer: A nationwide cohort study. *Arthritis and Rheumatism, 62*(12), 3776–3782.

Singh-Grewal D., Schneiderman-Walker J., Wright V., et al. (2007). The effects of vigorous exercise training on physical function in children with arthritis: a randomized, controlled, single-blinded trial. *Arthritis and Rheumatism, 57*(7), 1202–1210.

Sundel, R., & Petty R. (2011). Kawasaki disease. In J. T. Cassidy, R. M. Laxer, R. E. Petty, et al. (Eds.), *Textbook of pediatric rheumatology* (6th ed., pp. 505–520). Philadelphia: Saunders Elsevier.

Tarakci, E., Yeldan, I., Baydogan, S., et al. (2012). Efficacy of a land-based home exercise programme for patients with juvenile idiopathic arthritis: A randomized, controlled, single-blind study. *Journal of Rehabilitation Medicine, 44*(11), 962–967.

United States Public Health Service Task Force. (2007). Recommendations for use of antiretroviral drugs in pregnant HIV-infected women for maternal health and interventions to reduce perinatal transmission in the United States. Available: *http://aidsinfo.nih.gov/contentfiles/PerinatalGL.pdf.*

UNAIDS Report on Global AIDS Epidemic 2010. Available: *www.unaids.org/globalreport/Epi_slides.htm.*

Wheeler, T. (2010). Systemic lupus erythematosis: The basics of nursing care. *British Journal of Nursing, 19*(4), 249–253.

Yeung, R. S. M. (2011). Vasculitis: Kawasaki disease. In A. Y. Elzouki, H. A. Harfi, H. Nazer, et al. (Eds.), *Textbook of clinical pediatrics* (2nd ed., pp. 1675–1684). New York: Springer.

INTERNET RESOURCES

The Body: The Complete HIV/AIDS Resource (*www.thebody.com/index/whatis/children.html*).

Canadian AIDS Treatment Information Exchange (*www.catie.ca*).

CHIVA: Children's HIV Association of UK and Ireland (*www.chiva.org.uk*).

Francis-Xavier Bagnoud Center (Resources/Clinical Information/Patient Education Resources) (*http://fxbcenter.org*).

U.S. Department of Health and Human Services, AIDS Information (*www.aidsinfo.nih.gov*).

Transitioning HIV-Infected Adolescents into Adult Care (*www.hivguidelines.rg/clinical-guidelines/adolescents/*).

54
Pediatric Orthopedic Problems

ORTHOPEDIC PROCEDURES

Immobilization: Casts, Braces, and Splints

 Evidence Base Reed, C., Carroll, L., Baccari, S., et al. (2011). Spica cast care: A collaborative staff-led education initiative for improved patient care. *Orthopaedic Nursing, 30*(6), 353–358.
Young, S., Fevang, J. M., Gullaksen, G., et al. (2010) Deformity and functional outcome after treatment for supracondylar humerus fractures in children: A 5- to 10-year follow-up of 139 supracondylar humerus fractures treated by plaster cast, skeletal traction or crossed wire fixation. *Journal of Child Orthopedics, 4*, 445–453.

Casting, bracing, and splinting are all means of immobilizing an injured or diseased body part. The length of time can vary from a few days to several months, depending on the nature of the problem. The management of children who are immobilized differs little from that of the adult; however, age-appropriate changes must be considered. See Procedure Guidelines 54-1, pages 1744 to 1745.

Complications of Immobilization

1. Peripheral neurovascular compromise.
2. Alteration in skin integrity due to pressure or friction.
3. Loss of efficient use of affected extremity due to noncompliance.

Traction

Traction is the application of a pulling force to an injured or diseased part of the body or an extremity while a counter traction pulls in the opposite direction. Traction may be used to reduce fractures or dislocations, maintain alignment and correct deformities, decrease muscle spasms and relieve pain, promote rest of a diseased or injured body part, and promote exercise. Advances in nailing and rodding, especially external fixators for fractures and spinal curvatures, have reduced the use of traction in many centers. See Procedure Guidelines 54-2, pages 1745 to 1751.

Types of Traction

1. Manual—direct pulling on the extremity or body part. Usually used to reduce fractures before treatment or immobilization.
2. Skin—force is applied directly to the skin by means of traction strips or tapes secured by elastic bandages or by means of traction boots. Usually of short-term duration and commonly used in children in whom small amounts of force are required.
3. Skeletal—force is applied to the body part through fixation directly into or through bone by means of a traction pin or screw. Allows for greater force over longer periods or used when skin traction is not feasible, as in soft tissue injury or damage.
4. Continuous or intermittent—traction forces should be disrupted only in accordance with the health care provider's orders.

PROCEDURE GUIDELINES 54-1

Care of the Child with a Cast, Splint, or Brace

EQUIPMENT

- Casting materials or immobilization device
- Cotton padding material, plastic padding

PROCEDURE

Nursing Action	Rationale
1. Prepare child for the procedure by showing materials to be used and describing procedure in age-appropriate terms.	1. Reduces fear and enlists cooperation.
2. Assess the need for pain medication, sedation, distraction techniques, or restraint and administer, as ordered.	2. Manipulation of the affected part may be painful, so pharmacologic preparation is usually necessary.
3. Obtain baseline neurovascular assessment, including discoloration or cyanosis, impaired movement, loss of sensation, edema, absent pulses, and pain disproportionate to injury or not relieved by analgesics.	3. Will serve as a baseline to compare subsequent assessments after immobilization.
4. Assist with application of the immobilization device.	

5. Help facilitate drying of a cast or splint.
  a. Keep the child and affected part still until dry.
  b. Support the curves of the cast with pillows.
  c. Avoid excessive handling of the cast, and use palms when handling it.
	5. About 24 to 48 hours are required for drying a plaster cast. Dries from the outside inward, so may appear dry but is still moldable with movement or pressure.

6. Assess the skin around edges of the device daily for signs of skin irritation. Teach child or parents to look for and report redness, skin breakdown, localized pain, foul odor that may indicate open wounds under device.	6. Pressure or friction may disrupt skin integrity. May be readily visible or occur under the device and not detected until advanced. Braces can be altered if skin irritation becomes apparent.
7. Try to prevent skin breakdown by padding edges of device and telling child to avoid placing anything inside the device.	7. Avoids friction or pressure damage to skin and underlying tissue.
8. Assess neurovascular status frequently after application of device, then daily to detect compromise.	8. Initial swelling from the injury may contribute to vascular insufficiency or nerve compression.

9. If child is in hip-spica cast, prevent skin breakdown from frequent soiling around perineum.
  a. Line cast edges around the perineum with a plastic covering to prevent soiling of cast.
  b. Use a fracture bedpan or urinal to facilitate toileting.
  c. If not toilet trained, use a small diaper or perineal pad tucked under the edges of the cast, covered by a larger diaper, and change diapers as soon as soiled.
  d. Wash the perineum frequently and dry thoroughly.
  e. If the cast is synthetic and becomes soiled, clean it with a damp cloth and small amount of detergent.
	9. Soiled edges of the cast may contribute to skin irritation or begin to disintegrate.
	
	  e. Plaster casts cannot be washed because they absorb water and soften.

Cast removal

1. Prepare the child for cast removal by describing the sensation (warmth, vibration) and demonstrating the cast cutter by touching it lightly to your palm.	1. Children are frightened by the loud noise and believe that the cast cutter will cut through their skin or extremity.

PROCEDURE GUIDELINES 54-1 (continued)

Care of the Child with a Cast, Splint, or Brace

PROCEDURE (continued)

Nursing Action	Rationale
2. Provide and teach care of skin after cast, brace, or splint removal.	2. An accumulation of dead skin and sebaceous secretions causes the skin to appear brown and flaky.
a. Wash with soapy warm water.	
b. Soak the area daily with warm water to facilitate removal of desquamated skin and secretions.	
c. Advise child to avoid scratching; instead apply lotion or oil to relieve itching.	c. Excessive rubbing may cause trauma.
d. Encourage exercise as prescribed to regain strength and function.	d. May initially be weak and stiff due to lack of use.

PROCEDURE GUIDELINES 54-2

Care of a Child in Traction

EQUIPMENT

- Traction tapes
- Elastic bandages
- Spreader blocks, ropes, weights, pulleys
- Adhesive tape
- Tincture of benzoin/other adhesive agent
- Traction bars, slings

PROCEDURE

Nursing Action	Rationale
1. Explain the procedure to the child and parents.	1. If the traction is to be effective, it is essential that the parents and child understand traction.
2. Maintain even, constant traction.	2. Traction must be kept constant to achieve the desired results.
a. Do not add or remove weights unless ordered.	
b. Allow the weights to hang free at all times.	
c. Be certain that the ropes are in the wheel grooves of the pulleys.	c. Maintains proper alignment.
d. Keep the weights out of the child's reach.	d. Prevents loosening or undoing of traction knots.
e. Wrap knotted areas of the ropes with adhesive tape to prevent slipping.	
f. Do not elevate the head or foot of the bed without consulting health care provider.	f. May disrupt traction forces.
g. Supervise the child's position so that the purpose of the traction is accomplished.	
3. Check for disturbance of circulation by observing:	3. Compares the affected extremity with the unaffected one.
a. Skin color—for redness, pallor, cyanosis.	a. May indicate neurovascular compromise.
b. Joint motion restriction.	
c. Skin temperature—warmth.	
d. Tingling, numbness.	
e. Swelling, edema.	

(continued)

PROCEDURE GUIDELINES 54-2 (continued)

Care of a Child in Traction

PROCEDURE (continued)

Nursing Action	Rationale
4. Provide skin care.	4. Immobilized children readily develop areas of pressure unless meticulous skin care is provided.
a. Pad bony prominences (ankles) with cotton padding before wrapping with elastic bandages.	a. Protects skin from injury.
b. Wash and dry all exposed areas thoroughly.	
c. Massage the child's back and sacral area frequently, using lotion.	c. Stimulates microcirculation and acts as a lubricant.
d. Inspect the heels, ankles, popliteal space, and top of the foot for signs of pressure from elastic bandages.	d. These are the areas most prone to breakdown.
e. Keep the linen free from wrinkles and food crumbs.	e. Prevents undue pressure areas.
f. Do not allow the traction cords to dig into child's skin.	f. This is a safety measure.
g. Use a fracture bedpan.	g. This is less awkward and more comfortable for the child.
5. Plan for short periods of muscle exercise every day.	5. Disuse of muscles can result in atrophy, contractures, and deformities.
a. Encourage use of unaffected extremity.	
b. Assist the child to exercise unaffected joints.	
c. Provide for diversionary activities that require movement of unaffected joints and muscles.	
6. Encourage deep-breathing exercises.	6. Prevents respiratory complications of prolonged immobilization.
7. Record intake and output.	7. Prolonged immobilization renders the child prone to urine retention and renal calculi.
8. Encourage a diet high in fiber and fluids.	8. Helps to prevent constipation and urinary calculi.
9. Provide daily diversion and encourage visitation from family and friends.	9. Helps prevent boredom and assists the child to cope with immobilization.
a. Suspend or place favorite toys within easy reach of child.	
b. Provide for continuing education for school-age children.	b. Length of immobilization in traction may be considerable.
c. Encourage activities that will allow for diversion: drawing, coloring, video games.	c. Activities that can be done while remaining in traction.
d. Immobilized patients should be roomed together, if possible.	d. Encourages peer support.
10. If not contraindicated, provide the child with an overhead trapeze.	10. This will assist with movement and self-help.
11. Document the following:	11. Proper documentation facilitates communication between health care providers.
a. Color, temperature, and appearance of the affected limb.	
b. Skin condition.	
c. Body alignment.	c. Proper alignment facilitates proper extremity positioning and maintains proper traction force.
d. Functioning of traction system.	
e. Response of child to treatment.	
12. Make sure countertraction is provided.	12. The child's body is the usual counterweight.
a. Foot of bed may need to be raised or placed on "shock blocks" to prevent child from being pulled to foot of bed.	a. Frequently the child's weight is insufficient to maintain proper alignment of the extremity.

PROCEDURE GUIDELINES 54-2 *(continued)*

Care of a Child in Traction

PROCEDURE *(continued)*

Nursing Action	Rationale
13. Do not alter the traction system.	13. Notify the health care provider if adjustment is indicated.
14. Avoid sudden movement or jarring of bed.	14. This can cause pain to the child and disturb alignment.
15. Do not allow weights to hang over the child's bed.	15. This is a safety precaution.

Skin traction

1. Do not apply over an open wound or over damaged skin.	1. The skin must be intact for the pull of the traction to be effective. Prevents contamination of the wound and further skin breakdown.
2. Prepare the skin with an adhesive agent before application of traction tapes.	2. Adhesive agents allow the traction tapes to adhere better, preventing friction on the skin surface.

Skeletal traction

1. Treat all entry sites as surgical wounds.	1. Reduces the chance of infection along the pin or screw tract.
a. Clean entry site according to your facility's policy or guidelines. This should be done at least once per shift.	a. Policies vary. Cleaning the pin site prevents infection, promotes comfort by preventing skin from adhering to pin.
b. Assess the entry site every shift for indications of infection or slippage.	b. Notify health care provider if either of these conditions exists.
2. Protect the exposed ends of skeletal traction pins.	2. Protects the health care provider as well as the child from injury.

Specific traction types

Bryant's traction

Indications

1. To reduce fractures of the femur in children younger than age 2 or weighing less than 30 lb (14 kg).
2. Also used to stabilize the hip joint when casting is not indicated.
3. Preoperatively to attempt reduction of a developmentally dislocated hip in the same age group.

Mechanism of action

Involves the bilateral vertical extension of the child's legs. The child's weight serves as the countertraction. Skin traction is applied to both limbs to minimize potential trauma and maintain stability and alignment of child.

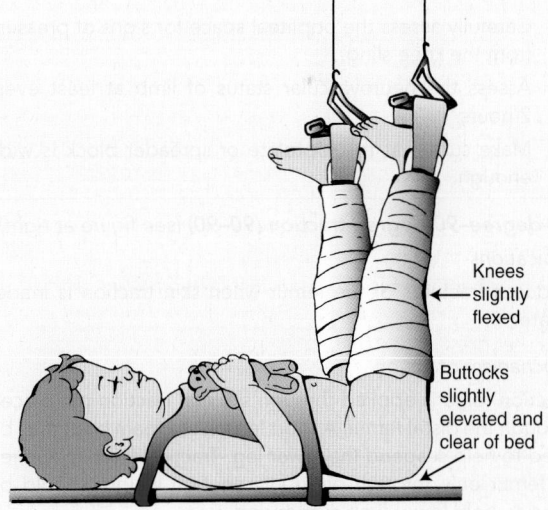

Knees slightly flexed

Buttocks slightly elevated and clear of bed

Bryant's traction.

1. Maintain appropriate position:	1. Proper positioning is needed to achieve desired results.
a. The legs are extended at right angles to the body.	
b. The hips are elevated slightly from the bed.	
c. The buttocks are elevated slightly from the bed.	c. Ensures proper traction pull.
d. The heels and ankles are free from pressure.	d. Prevents skin breakdown.
2. Check condition and position of elastic bandages every shift. Rewrap, as indicated and permitted by the health care provider.	2. Elastic bandages can cause compression and compromise circulation. In addition, force across skin surfaces needs to be constant and free from constriction to prevent skin breakdown and ensure adequate traction force.

(continued)

PROCEDURE GUIDELINES 54-2 (continued)

Care of a Child in Traction

PROCEDURE (continued)

Nursing Action	Rationale

Russel's traction (see figure at right)

Indications

1. Reduces fractures of the femur or hip.
2. Treatment of specific types of knee injuries or contractures.

Mechanism of action

Traction force is applied to the limb through application of skin traction. This can be accomplished with traction tapes or a traction boot in older individuals.

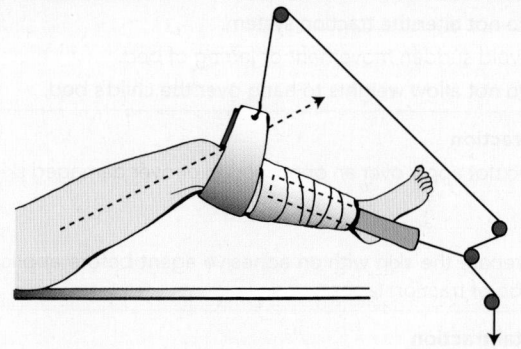

Russel's traction.

Nursing Action	Rationale

1. Application of elastic bandages:
   a. Wrap bandages from ankle to thigh on patients younger than age 2.
   b. Older patients should have bandages wrapped from ankle to the knee.
	1. Proper application of the tapes prevents neurovascular compromise and ensures proper and adequate pull on the extremity.

2. Place foot support against both feet.	2. Prevents footdrop.
3. Keep the heel free from the bed.	3. Prevents pressure sores and ensures continuous traction pull.
4. Carefully assess the popliteal space for signs of pressure from the knee sling.	4. Prevents pressure sores or neurovascular compression.
5. Assess the neurovascular status of limb at least every 2 hours.	5. Early detection can prevent injury to patient.
6. Make sure that the footplate or spreader block is wide enough.	6. Prevents pressure sores and circulatory compromise.

90-degree–90-degree traction (90–90) (see figure at right)

Indications

Reduces fractures of the femur when skin traction is inadequate.

Mechanism of action

Traction force is applied through skeletal traction pin placed through the distal femur. A short leg cast or foam boot may be used to help suspend the lower leg. Traction force is applied to femur only through pin. Only enough weight should be used to hold lower limb suspended.

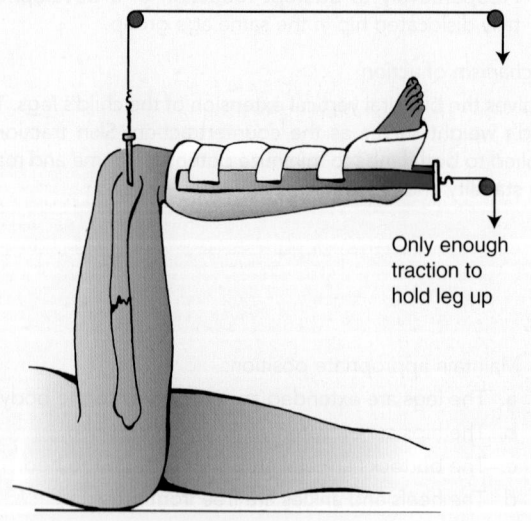

Only enough traction to hold leg up

90–90 traction.

PROCEDURE GUIDELINES 54-2 *(continued)*

Care of a Child in Traction

PROCEDURE *(continued)*

Nursing Action	Rationale

4. Be alert for symptoms of injury to spinal cord:
  a. Weakness, numbness in legs.
  b. Loss of bladder function.
  c. Upturning or downturning of toes.
  d. Clonus of ankles or knees.
	4. These complaints may indicate lower spinal nerve root or cauda equina damage and should be reported promptly.

5. Be alert for symptoms of brachial plexus injuries:
  a. Difficulty in moving hand, shoulder, or arm.
  b. Numbness or weakness in hand.
	5. These complaints or findings may be caused by impingement on spinal nerves.

6. Assess all pin sites for loosening every shift.	6. Loose pins can cause harm to the child as well as prevent proper traction pull. Halo-gravity traction, using the child's body and gravity as counterweights, may be used instead of pins.
7. Keep the torque wrench for the halo pins at the bedside at all times.	7. The halo or pins may have to be removed or adjusted in an emergency or to ensure proper tension on the pins.

Complications of Traction

1. Neurovascular compromise to extremity.
2. Skin and soft tissue injury.
3. Pin or screw tract infection, osteomyelitis (with skeletal traction).

COMMON ORTHOPEDIC DISORDERS IN CHILDREN

Fractures

A *fracture* is a break or disruption in the continuity of bone. Fractures in children differ from those in adults due to the differences in anatomy, biomechanics, and physiology of the child's skeleton compared to that of an adult. Involvement of the epiphysis or metaphysis can disrupt the epiphyseal plate, interfering with growth (see Figure 54-1). Fractures are extremely common in children, with an estimated 42% of boys and 27% of girls sustaining fractures during childhood.

> **Evidence Base** Abzug, J., & Zlotolow, D. (2012). Pediatric hand and wrist fractures. *Current Orthopaedic Practice, 23*(4), 327–330.
> Sponsellar, P. (2011). *Handbook of pediatric orthopedics.* New York: Thieme.

Pathophysiology and Etiology

1. Most fractures in children are a result of low-velocity trauma such as a fall.
   a. Up to age 2, most fractures are sustained as a result of the child being injured by another person.
   b. Fractures in neonates and infants are commonly the result of child maltreatment. Child maltreatment should be suspected when treating fractures in this age group.
2. A bone fractures when the force applied to it exceeds the amount the bone can absorb.
   a. Children's long bones are more resilient than those of adults. They are able to withstand greater deflection without fracturing.
   b. Children's bones also have thick periosteum.

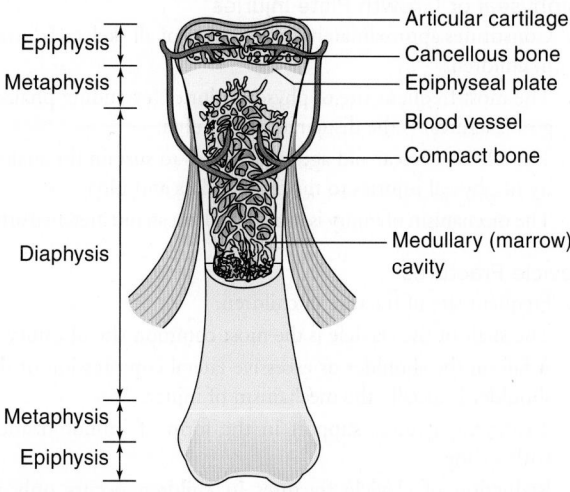

Figure 54-1. Structure of a bone.

3. The involvement of growth plates (epiphyseal plate) is unique to fractures in children. Cartilaginous growth plates are present at each end of the long bones and at one end of metacarpals and metatarsals. The plate is weaker than surrounding ligaments, tendons, and joint capsules and is disrupted before these tissues are injured.

   a. Damage to the growth plate may result in cessation of or a disturbance in bone growth (depending on the extent of damage sustained at the growth plate).

   b. On the other hand, acceleration in bone growth commonly occurs after a fracture in the long bones of children.

4. Children's fractures heal more rapidly than adult fractures. The younger the child, the more rapidly bone heals.

5. Children's fractures remodel more completely and actively than adult fractures and usually result in less disability and deformity.

Sites of Fractures in Children

Evidence Base Gourde, J., & Damian, F. (2012). ED fracture pain management in children. *Journal of Emergency Nursing, 38*(1), 91–97.

Woratanarat, P., Angsanuntsukh, C., Rattanasiri, S., et al.. (2012). Meta-analysis of pinning in supracondylar fracture of the humerus in children. *Journal of Orthopedic Trauma, 26*, 48–53.

As children grow, the fracture rate increases, with the peak incidence occurring in early adolescence. Forearm fractures are the most common injury.

Forearm and Wrist Fractures

1. Most common site of fracture in children, with most occurring in children older than age 5.
2. Major categories of classification include fracture dislocations, midshaft fractures, and distal fractures.
3. Most common cause is from a fall on an outstretched arm.

Epiphyseal or Growth Plate Injuries

1. Constitutes approximately 15% to 25% of all skeletal injuries in children.
2. The most frequent site of physeal injuries (excluding phalangeal fractures) is the distal radius and ulna.
3. The 11- to 15-year-old age group tends to sustain the majority of physeal injuries to the distal radius and ulna.
4. The mechanism of injury is usually a fall on an outstretched arm.

Clavicle Fractures

1. Frequent site of fracture in children.
2. The shaft of the clavicle is the most common site of injury.
3. A fall on the shoulder or excessive lateral compression of the shoulder is usually the mechanism of injury.
4. Treatment involves support in the form of immobilization with a sling.
5. Reduction of clavicle fractures in children occurs only in instances of extreme displacement.

Humerus Fractures

1. The mechanism of injury for the majority of humeral fractures is a fall onto an outstretched arm or hand.
2. Supracondylar fractures are the most common fractures of the humerus; they may be associated with acute vascular injury.
3. Approximately 10% of all humeral fractures occur at the shaft of the humerus; they are usually a result of twisting injuries in infants and toddlers. Direct trauma to the humeral shaft is the most common mechanism of injury in older children.
4. Distal humeral fractures occur more often in the lateral epicondyle than the medial epicondyle.
5. Less than 1% of fractures occur at the proximal humerus.

Spinal Fractures

1. Rare in children.
2. Mechanism of injury is due to significant trauma, such as a motor vehicle accident, fall from a significant height, athletic activities, beatings, or pedestrian–motor vehicle accident.
3. Most spinal fractures involve the cervical spine.

Pelvic Fractures

1. Pelvic fractures are uncommon in children and adolescents; they are commonly the result of high-energy trauma or a crush-type injury.
2. Associated injuries are present in approximately 75% of children with pelvic fractures and include hemorrhage and damage to the abdominal wall and pelvic organs.

Hip Fractures

1. Hip fractures in children are uncommon, but may occur from motor vehicle accidents, bicycle accidents, falls from significant heights, or child maltreatment (in children under age 3).
2. Hip fractures can result in avascular necrosis of the femoral head and damage to the physis resulting in growth arrest, malunion, and nonunion.
3. Pelvic avulsion fractures are more common, especially in boys ages 12 to 14.

Femur Fractures

1. Common in children. Peak incidence occurs in two age groups—children ages 2 to 3 and adolescents.
2. Femoral shaft (diaphysis) fractures are the most common location.
3. Usually the result of high-energy trauma, such as a motor vehicle accident or fall from a significant height; most common cause in children younger than age 1 is child maltreatment.

Tibial Fractures

1. The most common lower extremity fracture in children occurs in the tibial and fibular shaft—constitutes 10% to 15% of all pediatric fractures.
2. Most diaphyseal tibia fractures in children ages 5 to 6 are nondisplaced or minimally displaced spiral or oblique fractures. A rotational mechanism of injury to the lower leg is the most common cause of tibial fractures in children under age 3 (toddler's fracture or CAST [childhood accidental spiral tibial]).
3. Greater force is required to injure the tibia in older children; motor vehicle accidents and sports injuries are the most common causes of tibial fractures in children and adolescents.

Ankle Fractures

1. Common in children and adolescents—approximately 5% of all pediatric fractures.
2. Involve the growth plate in approximately every one of six injuries.
3. Greatest incidence is in males ages 10 to 15.
4. Usually the result of direct trauma.
5. Mortise view as well as anteroposterior (AP) and lateral x-rays should be obtained.

Foot Fractures

1. Foot fractures account for approximately 6% of all fractures in children and 50% of foot fractures occur at the metatarsals.
2. Most metatarsal and phalangeal fractures are nondisplaced.
3. Mechanism of injury is usually a direct or indirect trauma, such as from falls, jumping from heights, object falling on foot, and twisting injuries.

Classification of Fractures

1. Open fractures: underlying fracture in bone communicates with an external wound; usually the result of high-energy trauma or penetrating wounds.
2. Closed fractures: underlying fracture with no open wound.
3. Plastic deformation: a bending of the bone in such a manner as to cause a microscopic fracture line that does not cross the bone. When the force is removed, the bone remains bent. Unique to children and most common in the ulna (see Figure 54-2A).
4. Buckle (torus) fractures: fracture on the tension side of the bone near the softer metaphyseal bone; crosses the bone and buckles the harder diaphyseal bone on the opposite side, causing a bulge (see Figure 54-2B).

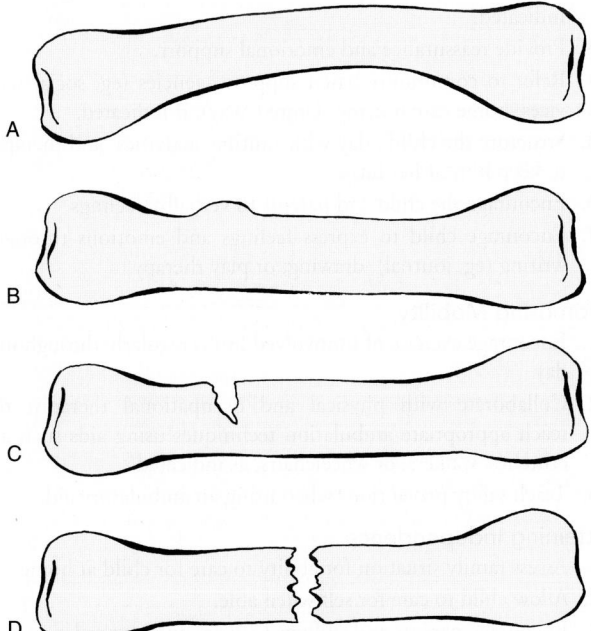

Figure 54-2. Common fractures in children. (A) Plastic deformation (bend). **(B)** Buckle (torus). **(C)** Greenstick. **(D)** Complete.

5. Greenstick fracture: bone is bent and the fracture begins but does not entirely cross through the bone (see Figure 54-2C).
6. Complete fractures (see Figure 54-2D):
   a. Spiral—from a rotational force.
   b. Oblique—diagonally across the diaphysis.
   c. Transverse—usually diaphyseal.
   d. Epiphyseal—through the physis.

Clinical Manifestations

1. Inability to stand, walk, or use injured part.
2. Limb deformity (visible or palpable).
3. Ecchymosis.
4. Pain.
5. History of injury or trauma (may not be the case with pathologic fractures).
6. Spontaneous onset of pain (usually seen with pathologic fractures).
7. Local swelling and marked tenderness.
8. Movement between bone fragments.
9. Crepitus or grating.
10. Muscle spasm.

Diagnostic Evaluation

1. X-rays of suspected limb fractures should include the joint above and below the injury.
   a. Should always include a minimum of two views at 90-degree angles to each other (AP and lateral).
   b. Comparison views of the opposite extremity are frequently needed. They help to distinguish the fracture line from the growth plate.
   c. In some situations, oblique x-rays are warranted in order to help identify a fracture that is difficult to detect.
2. Further radiologic studies may be indicated in certain instances to evaluate a fracture: ultrasound, tomography, computed tomography (CT) scan, magnetic resonance imaging (MRI), bone scan, fluoroscopy.
3. Vascular assessment may include the use of:
   a. Doppler studies.
   b. Compartment pressure monitoring.
   c. Angiography.

Management

Treatment is dependent upon the type of fracture, its location, and the age of the child.

1. Treatment may consist of:
   a. Immobilization by cast, splint, or brace.
   b. Closed reduction followed by a period of immobilization in a cast or splint.
   c. Open reduction with or without internal fixation and usually followed by a period of immobilization in a cast or splint.
   d. Closed reduction and percutaneous pinning followed by a period of immobilization.

e. Closed or open reduction and application of an external fixator.

f. Traction (skin, skeletal) followed by a period of immobilization.

2. Most children's fractures heal in 12 weeks or less. Simple fractures that are closed and nondisplaced can heal enough to be free from immobilization within 3 weeks.

Complications

1. Infection, avascular necrosis.
2. Delayed union, nonunion, malunion.
3. Shortening—epiphyseal arrest (deformities in angulation or limb length).
4. Vascular injuries.
5. Nerve injuries—palsies.
6. Visceral injuries.
7. Tendon and joint injuries.
8. Fat embolism.
9. Compartment syndrome (orthopedic emergency).
10. Osteoarthritis (occurs later).
11. Reflex sympathetic dystrophy.

Nursing Assessment

1. Follow the basic assessment for the trauma victim (see page 1197).
2. Obtain history from child, parents, and others to include accident or trauma details, noting the position of the extremity at impact.
3. Perform physical examination for location of deformity, swelling, ecchymosis, and pain; vital signs; and neurovascular assessment.
4. Assess child's support mechanisms/social situation with consideration of discharge needs.

Nursing Diagnoses

- Acute Pain related to tissue trauma and reflex muscle spasms secondary to fracture.
- Ineffective Peripheral Tissue Perfusion related to swelling and immobilization.
- Impaired Skin Integrity related to mechanical trauma (eg, fixation device, traction, casts, other orthopedic devices).
- Ineffective Coping related to separation from family and home.
- Impaired Physical Mobility related to fracture and external immobilization device (eg, cast, splint, external fixator).
- Bathing/Dressing/Feeding/Toileting Self-Care Deficit related to external devices (eg, cast, splint).
- Risk for Infection related to trauma (fracture) and surgery.
- Risk for Peripheral Neurovascular Dysfunction related to restrictive envelope secondary to cast or splint.

Nursing Interventions

Also see page 1119 for orthopedic surgery.

Promoting Comfort

1. Monitor and assess pain level using an age-appropriate pain scale (eg, Oucher or FACES scale).

2. Properly position, align, and support affected body part.
3. Administer analgesics, as indicated, and monitor effectiveness of analgesia.
4. Use nontraditional methods of pain relief—music therapy, diversionary activities, relaxation techniques, therapeutic touch, play therapy.

Maintaining Tissue Perfusion

1. Frequently assess perfusion of limb by checking temperature, color, sensation, and pulses.
2. Elevate extremity above heart level to prevent edema.
3. Encourage movement of digits on affected limb.
4. Remove compressive bandages (eg, elastic bandages, splints) that restrict flow of circulation.

Maintaining Skin Integrity

1. Assess for and relieve pressure caused by tight bandages, casts, and splints.
2. Provide periodic cleaning, thorough drying, and lubrication to pressure points if in traction.
3. Encourage frequent position changes as allowed.
4. Assess skin condition on a regular basis.
5. Massage healthy skin around affected area to stimulate circulation.
6. Protect skin at risk with special dressings or products (eg, barrier cream, moisture-permeable dressing).
7. Discourage the use of sticks, pens or pencils, or small toys or other objects to scratch itchy skin.
8. Promote a diet high in protein, carbohydrates, and calcium.

Promoting Effective Coping

1. Assess the child's and parents' response to events.
2. Explain condition, treatment, and rehabilitation goals, as indicated.
3. Provide reassurance and emotional support.
4. Refer to community-based support agencies (eg, social services, home care nursing, United Way), if indicated.
5. Structure the child's day with routine, activities, and therapy to keep him or her busy.
6. Encourage the child and parents to verbalize feelings.
7. Encourage child to express feelings and emotions through writing (eg, journal), drawing, or play therapy.

Promoting Mobility

1. Encourage exercise of uninvolved limbs regularly throughout day.
2. Collaborate with physical and occupational therapist to teach appropriate ambulation techniques using aids such as crutches, walkers, or wheelchairs, as indicated.
3. Teach safety precautions when using an ambulatory aid.

Attaining Independence

1. Assess family situation for ability to care for child at home.
2. Allow child to care for self when able.
3. Encourage parents and siblings to assist only as needed.
4. Encourage child to participate in care as much as possible.
5. Evaluate child's ability to participate in self-care activities.

Preventing Infection

 Evidence Base Timms, A., & Pugh, H. (2012). Pin site care: Guidance and key recommendations. *Nursing Standard, 27*(1), 50–55.

Walker, J. (2012). Pin site infection in orthopaedic external fixation devices. *British Journal of Nursing, 21*(3), 148–151.

1. Assess wounds, including pin sites, frequently for warmth, erythema, swelling, tenderness, or purulent drainage.
2. Pin site care is indicated by the orthopedist or institution. A cleansing ritual with chlorhexidine or other antiseptic is beneficial, which includes gentle massage to remove superficial drainage. The use of dressings is determined by institution.
3. Report signs of infection.
4. Provide appropriate wound care for open injuries and surgical wounds.
5. Administer antibiotics, as ordered.
6. Encourage child to eat and maintain good caloric and protein intake to promote healing.
7. Teach good handwashing technique to child and parents.

Preventing Peripheral Neurovascular Dysfunction

1. Assess the neurovascular status of affected limb every hour for the first 24 hours (or as indicated by hospital protocol)—compare with unaffected limb.
2. Assess for nerve injury (eg, abduct all fingers, touch thumb to small finger, plantar flexion, dorsiflexion).
3. Assess for presence of numbness, tingling, "pins and needles," excessive pain (disproportionate to injury and analgesia administered).
4. Encourage range of motion (ROM) exercises in fingers, toes, and unaffected limbs.
5. Teach child and parents signs and symptoms of neurovascular compromise and advise them to contact the health care provider immediately if signs of compromise occur.

Community and Home Care Considerations

A home care visit may be necessary in the initial postoperative stage to make sure that the family is coping with the care of their immobilized child. Usually, reinforcement is needed to help reassure the parents that they are able to care for their child. Make sure that the family has a way of contacting a nurse after home care visits have been discontinued.

1. Assess coping ability of family members.
2. Assess skin of child for signs of breakdown.
3. Assess condition of the hip-spica cast, especially around perineal area.
4. Assess neurovascular status of affected limb.
5. Assess child's coping ability—participation in self-care.
6. Assess traction device to make sure it is intact and maintained.
7. Assess child's nutritional status.
8. Assess child's bowel and bladder routine.
9. Answer questions parents may have about care of their immobilized child.
10. Teach patient and family about care of their child's external fixation device (pin site care and adjustment of screws).
11. Have the family do a return demonstration so as to assess their skill and ability to care for their child's pin sites.
12. Teach the child and family about signs and symptoms of infection and whom to contact should an infection occur.

Family Education and Health Maintenance

1. Teach proper care of casts, splints, and immobilization devices (see Patient Education Guidelines 54-1).
2. Teach safety measures and prevention of further injuries.
    a. Advise use of bicycle helmets and knee, elbow, and wrist pads.
    b. Emphasize importance of supervising young children while playing.
    c. Teach safety measures, such as placing gates at stairs and installing top-opening windows on second floors.
3. Teach family and child the natural history of fracture healing (eg, presence of fracture bump, gradual recovery of ROM, predicted time frame for healing).

Evaluation: Expected Outcomes

- Reports acceptable level of comfort.
- Extremity warm with good color sensation, pulses, and capillary refill.

PATIENT EDUCATION GUIDELINES 54-1

Cast Care

- Keep the casted body part elevated on a pillow for the first few days to decrease swelling.
- Avoid touching the cast until it is fully dry to avoid denting it.
- Watch the body part below the cast for swelling or bluish discoloration of the skin.
- Move the body part below the cast at least every 4 hours for the first 24 hours.
- Avoid strenuous activity such as roughhousing or sports while the cast is in place.
- Do not put anything inside the cast.
- Keep the cast dry; cover with plastic bag to shower; do not swim or submerge cast in water.
- If itching occurs under the cast, blow some cool air into it from a hair dryer.
- Develop a plan for carrying out usual activity, such as dressing, walking up and down steps, and carrying books.
- Call your health care provider if there is pain, blueness, swelling, or inability to move the body part.
- Be sure to keep follow-up appointments.

- No skin breakdown noted.
- Parents comfort child; child responds appropriately.
- Uses ambulatory aids and ambulates independently.
- Bathes and feeds self with minimal assistance.
- No signs of infection surrounding wound.
- Denies numbness and tingling.

Osteomyelitis

Osteomyelitis is a pyogenic infection of the bone and surrounding soft tissues. It occurs mostly in children between ages 3 and 12 and is primarily a disease of growing bones. Long bones are frequently involved and the characteristic site of involvement is the metaphyseal region. Males are afflicted two times as frequently as females.

Pathophysiology and Etiology

Etiologic Agents and Risk Factors

1. Microorganisms that cause osteomyelitis vary and are related to the age of the child.
   a. The most commonly identified pathogenic organism in acute osteoarticular infections is *Staphylococcus aureus*, causing up to 90% of cases among those having an identified etiologic agent; methicillin-resistant *S. aureus* infections have risen in the last several years.
   b. Group B streptococcus, *Escherichia coli*, and *Streptococcus pneumoniae* are other etiologic agents.
   c. Vertebral infections are increasingly a result of Gram-negative microorganisms.
2. Classification based on pathogen's mode of entry:
   a. Hematogenous osteomyelitis (through the bloodstream)—occurs primarily in children.
   b. Contiguous osteomyelitis—caused by pathogenic spread from outside the body or by progressive spread of infection from tissue adjacent to bone.
3. Risk factors include:
   a. Infected lesions of varicella.
   b. Impetigo.
   c. Furunculosis.
   d. Direct trauma to area adjacent to site of osteomyelitis.
   e. Infected burns.
   f. Prolonged use of an intravenous (IV) line.
   g. Immunization with bacille Calmette Guérin.
   h. Drug addiction.
   i. Sickle cell disease.

Pathophysiologic Changes

1. When the site is inoculated, the invading pathogen provokes the following responses:
   a. Inflammatory response.
   b. Pus formation.
   c. Edema.
   d. Vascular congestion.
   e. Leukocyte activity.
   f. Abscess formation.
2. Small terminal vessels thrombose and exudate bone's canaliculi.

   a. Inflammatory exudate extends into the metaphyseal and marrow cavity and through small metaphyseal openings into the cortex.
3. Exudate reaches outer surface of cortex, forming abscesses that lift periosteum off underlying bone, disrupting blood vessels and entering bone through periosteum, thereby causing deprivation of blood supply to the bone. This leads to necrosis and death of the infected bone.
4. Sequestrum or devitalized bone is produced.
5. Intense osteoblastic response is stimulated upon lifting of the periosteum.
6. New bone is lain down by osteoblasts that partially or completely surround infected bone.
7. New bone, also known as *involucrum*, is formed.
8. Exudate escapes into surrounding soft tissue through openings in the involucrum, from which it escapes though the skin via sinus tracts.
9. Acute osteomyelitis is an abrupt onset of inflammation. Failure to halt acute osteomyelitis can lead to chronic osteomyelitis.
10. Chronic osteomyelitis:
    a. Signs and symptoms are usually vague.
    b. Infection is silent between exacerbations.
    c. Small abscesses or fragments containing microorganisms produce occasional flare-ups of acute osteomyelitis.
    d. Inadequate or inappropriate therapy and drug-resistant microorganisms can result in progression of acute osteomyelitis to chronic osteomyelitis.

Clinical Manifestations

1. Infants—involvement of multiple sites within same bone or in multiple bones.
   a. Acute illness characterized by fever and failure to move affected limb.
2. Children—usually affects long bones but can affect pelvis and spine.
   a. Abrupt onset of fever and systemic signs of toxicity.
   b. Swelling, redness, and discrete tenderness over affected area.
   c. Decreased ability to bear weight as well as decreased ROM of affected limb.
3. Adolescents (less affected)—affects long bones but may involve vertebrae.
   a. Back pain.
   b. Signs and symptoms described above for children.

Diagnostic Evaluation

1. Blood cultures (positive in 30% to 40% of cases) should be obtained before initiation of antibiotic therapy to help identify the causative pathogen.
2. Needle aspiration of soft tissue should be done to identify the causative agent.
   a. Gram stain, culture, and sensitivity of specimen once obtained.
   b. Negative aspirate does not always rule out infection.
3. Complete blood count—marked leukocytosis, low hemoglobin.

4. Erythrocyte sedimentation rate (ESR) and C-reactive protein (CRP)—elevated.
5. X-ray:
   a. Detects deep soft tissue swelling and loss of normal fat planes.
   b. Detects presence of bone resorption and periosteal new bone formation.
   c. Comparison films of one limb with another should be done.
6. Bone scan in children younger than age 1 is required to determine multisite involvement.
   a. Localizes area of skeleton with altered physiology but does not identify the cause.
7. CT scan—used to detect focal areas of bone destruction and to delineate soft tissue abscesses associated with the bone infection.
   a. Unable to detect early changes in marrow in early stages of osteomyelitis.
8. MRI—useful in showing anatomic detail in many planes as well as detecting pathologic changes within marrow and soft tissues.
   a. MRI is not necessary to diagnose osteomyelitis but is helpful is cases of uncertainty.
9. Ultrasound—overall limited value because it does not detect changes within bone, but may be useful in guiding aspiration as the ultrasound detects soft tissue changes in periosteum and surrounding soft tissue.

Management

1. Aspiration is necessary to confirm the diagnosis of osteomyelitis and to identify the responsible microorganism in order to treat with the appropriate antibiotic. Aspiration is also needed to determine if surgical debridement is required.
   a. Aspirated fluid is sent for culture and Gram stain.
2. IV antibiotics:
   a. Broad-spectrum antibiotics until organism sensitivity obtained.
   b. IV antibiotics for 3 to 6 weeks, based on symptoms and CRP level (there are no established guidelines for duration of therapy).
   c. May require placement of a central intermittent infusion catheter (eg, midline or peripherally inserted central catheter [PICC] line).
   d. After course of IV antibiotics, switch to oral antibiotic is made.
3. Surgical debridement—helps to stop further tissue destruction, thereby allowing a shorter course of antibiotic therapy.
4. Bed rest and immobilization to help with pain management.

Complications

Evidence Base Belthur, M. V., Birchansky, S. B., Verdugo, A. A., et al. (2012). Pathologic fractures in children with staphylococcus aureus osteomyelitis. *Journal of Bone and Joint Surgery, 94,* 34–42.

1. Chronic osteomyelitis.
2. Fracture.
3. Growth arrest.
4. Osteonecrosis.
5. Recurrence of infection.
6. Septic arthritis.
7. Systemic infection—life-threatening if unrecognized and untreated.

Nursing Assessment

1. Obtain a detailed history, including recent infections (ear, tonsils, chest, urinary tract), trauma, and onset of symptoms.
2. Obtain history of current or recent antibiotic therapy and its effect.
3. Perform physical assessment for signs of primary infection as well as osteomyelitis.
4. Assess coping mechanisms and resources of family.

Nursing Diagnoses

- Acute Pain related to swelling, hyperthermia, and infectious process of bone.
- Hyperthermia related to inflammatory response secondary to osteomyelitis.
- Impaired Physical Mobility related to pain in affected limb secondary to inflammatory response or surgical treatment.
- Readiness for Enhanced Self-Health Management related to IV drug therapy.

Nursing Interventions

Maintaining Comfort

1. Assess pain characteristics and use age-appropriate pain-measurement tools.
2. Maintain rest and immobilization of affected part.
3. Administer analgesics, as indicated, and monitor their effectiveness.

Reducing Temperature

1. Assess temperature every 4 hours.
2. Increase fluid intake to prevent dehydration.
3. Administer antipyretics, as indicated.

Preventing Complications of Immobility

1. Instruct on allowable activities—generally no weight bearing on affected limb and remain on bed rest during acute phase.
2. Encourage use and exercise of unaffected limbs and joints through play.
3. Provide ambulatory aids if indicated (eg, crutches, walker) and instruct on safe and proper use.

Promoting Compliance with Therapeutic Regimen

1. Instruct patient and family on need for maintaining serum levels of antibiotics after discharge, even after signs and symptoms of infection improve.
2. Initiate appropriate home care referrals for administration and monitoring of IV therapy and wound care.
3. Evaluate response to treatment through periodic laboratory tests (ESR, CRP, serum drug levels) and follow-up.

4. Teach family about proper maintenance and care of vascular access device (eg, midline, PICC line).
5. Teach family and patient about oral antibiotic and importance of compliance with therapy.

Community and Home Care Considerations

Many visits may be necessary to make sure parents are comfortable with medication administration through a vascular access device and maintenance of the device. Parents may also need coaching about wound care.

1. Teach parents and child (if appropriate) about signs and symptoms of an infection.
2. Teach parents how to prepare the antibiotic for IV administration.
3. Teach parents how to administer the IV antibiotic.
4. Teach parents about the antibiotic being administered.
5. Teach parents and child about maintenance of the vascular access device.
6. Teach parents and child how to care for the child's wound.
7. Assess parents' and patient's coping abilities.
8. Reinforce teaching to parents on a frequent basis. Employ the use of return demonstrations to assess parental ability to administer IV antibiotics and care for their child's wound.
9. Provide the family with the phone number of a nurse whom they may contact for advice or if they have concerns.

Family Education and Health Maintenance

1. Instruct the family on the signs and symptoms of recurrent or chronic infection.
2. Stress the importance of compliance with treatment.
3. Encourage parents to seek early medical intervention for subsequent infections.

Evaluation: Expected Outcomes

- Reports reduced pain or no pain.
- Remains afebrile.
- Exercises unaffected limbs.
- Surgical wounds without signs of infection; child and parents demonstrate proper techniques for care of IV access device and infusion.

Developmental Dysplasia of the Hip

Developmental dysplasia of the hip (DDH) is now the accepted term used to describe abnormalities of the developing hip, including subluxation, dislocation, and dysplasia of the hip joint. DDH may be associated with other congenital anomalies; its incidence is 1.5 to 20 per 1,000 live births in whites and less frequently affects blacks. Bilateral involvement occurs in more than 50% of cases and the left hip is more frequently involved than the right hip. Females are afflicted four to eight times more frequently than males.

Pathophysiology and Etiology

1. Risk factors include breech birth, first born, large infants, oligohydramnios, female gender, positive family history of DDH, ethnic background (Native American, extreme

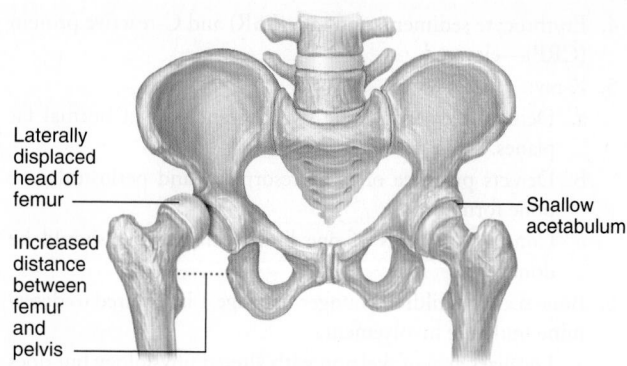

Figure 54-3. Developmental dysplasia of the hip.

northern Europe), lower limb deformity, torticollis, metatarsus adductus, hip asymmetry, and other congenital musculoskeletal abnormalities.

2. Subluxed hip—maintains contact with the acetabulum but not fully located within the hip joint.
3. Dislocated hip—no contact between the femoral head and acetabulum; sometimes located but may be dislocated easily.
4. Dysplasia—acetabulum is shallow or sloping instead of cup shaped (see Figure 54-3).

Clinical Manifestations

Physical findings change as the child ages; the presence of one or more of the following should be noted (see Figure 54-4).

1. Thigh asymmetry or thigh gluteal folds (present in 10% of normal infants).
2. Limited hip abduction.
3. Positive Barlow's test (dislocation).
4. Positive Ortolani's test (reduction).
5. Shortening of affected femur (Galeazzi's sign).
6. Abnormal gait patterns—Trendelenburg gait (downward tilt of pelvis on affected side).
7. Pain in older children.

Diagnostic Evaluation

Evidence Base Roposch, A., Liu, L. Q., Hefti, F., et al. (2011). Standardized diagnostic criteria for developmental dysplasia of the hip in early infancy. *Clinical Orthopaedics and Related Research, 469,* 3451–3461.

1. X-rays—cartilaginous femoral head is difficult to visualize in the newborn. As the child ages, the ossification center can be better viewed and the efficiency of this examination increases, usually after age 6 months. It can be useful in ruling out other pelvic, spinal, and femoral anomalies.
2. Ultrasound examination (with a skilled technician)—yields a high degree of accuracy in diagnosing DDH in children younger than age 6 months.
   a. Enables visualization of the femoral head and outer lip of the acetabulum.

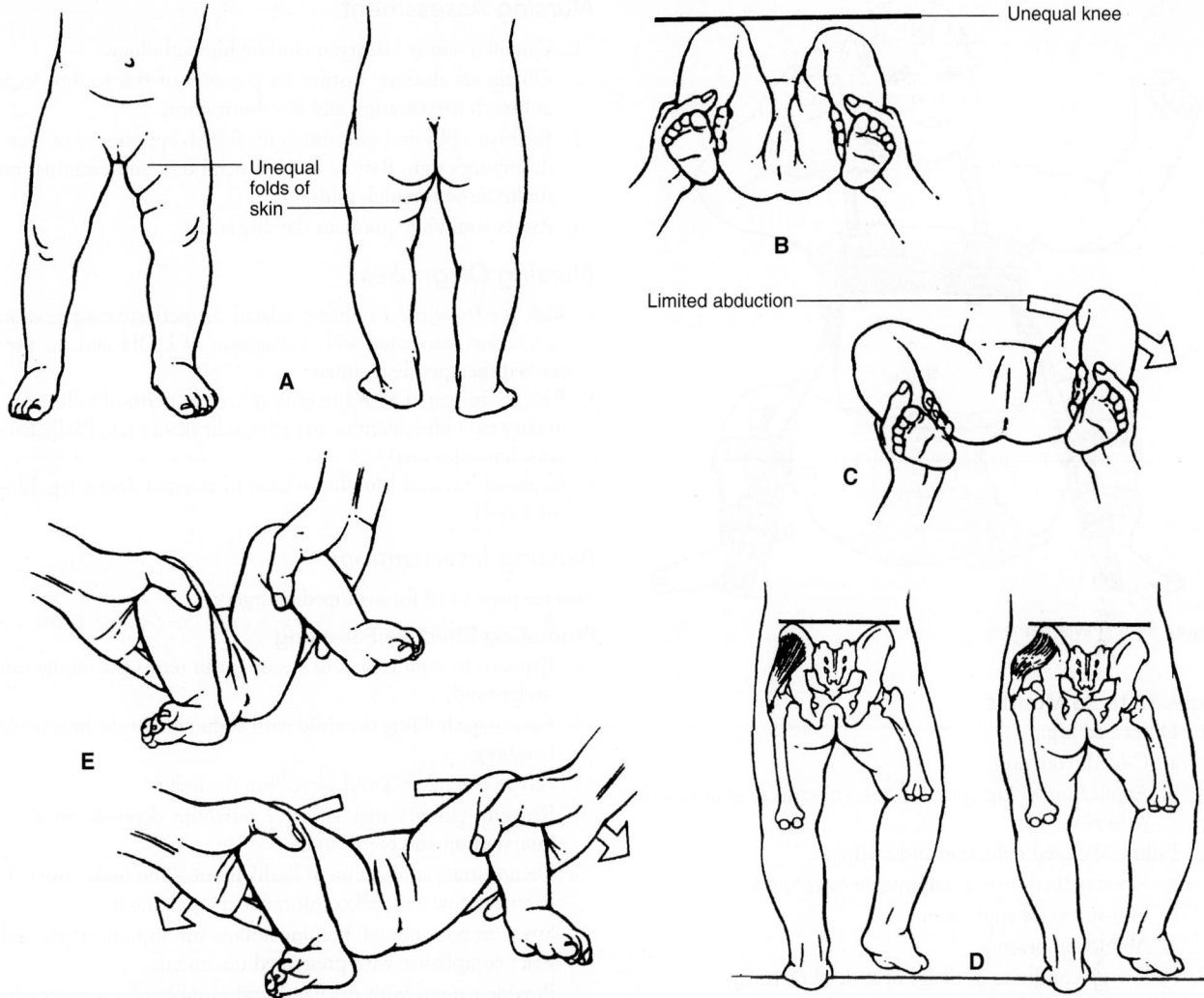

Figure 54-4. Signs of developmental dysplasia of the hip. (A) Unequal thigh folds; **(B)** apparent short femur (Galeazzi's sign); **(C)** limited abduction of affected hip; **(D)** downward tilt of pelvis on affected side (Trendelenberg's sign); and **(E)** adduction and depression of the femur dislocates hip (Barlow's test) and a "click" is felt when dislocated hip is abducted and relocated (Ortolani's sign).

Management

To restore as closely as possible the anatomic alignment of the hip. Methodology depends on the age of the child at presentation. More than 80% of clinically unstable hips at birth have been shown to resolve spontaneously.

Birth to Age 6 Months

1. Subluxable hips:
   a. Observe for 3 weeks.
   b. If persistent, treat in Pavlik harness (see Figure 54-5, page 1760).
2. Dislocated or dislocatable hips:
   a. Pavlik harness—frequent follow-up is needed to check position, make strap adjustments, and determine hip stability.
   b. Ultrasound to determine if hip was reduced.

c. Infant will wear harness on a full-time basis until clinical and ultrasound examinations are normal.

Ages 6 to 18 Months

1. Hip subluxation and dislocation in children between ages 6 and 9 months:
   a. Pavlik harness—followed on a frequent basis.
   b. Treatment in the Pavlik harness may continue for 4 months or until the child is able to stand in the harness.
   c. When the child is standing, the harness is exchanged for an abduction brace until the hip is normal.
   d. Closed reduction and hip spica application if harness treatment is unsuccessful.
2. Hip subluxation and dislocation in children ages 9 to 18 months—follow-up continues until age of skeletal maturity.

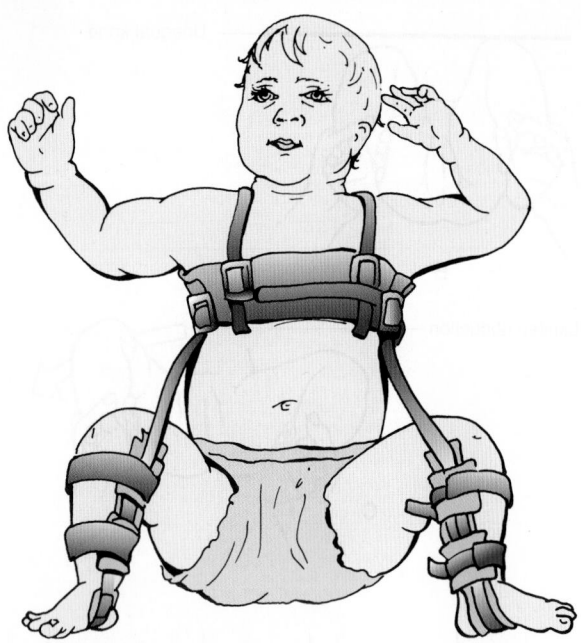

Figure 54-5. Pavlik harness.

Ages 18 to 36 Months
1. Dislocated hip:
   a. Closed reduction.
   b. Application of hip-spica cast for 3 months to maintain the reduction.
2. Failure of closed reduction and casting:
   a. Open reduction and innominate osteotomy.
   b. Hip-spica cast application.
   c. Abduction bracing.
3. Follow-up continues until age of skeletal maturity.

Age 3 and Older
1. Subluxation or dislocation of hip—treated surgically by open reduction.
2. Follow-up continues until age of skeletal maturity.

Adolescents
1. Acetabular dysplasia:
   a. Use of nonsteroidal anti-inflammatory drugs and an ambulation device (eg, crutches, cane) to limit weight-bearing on the affected limb.
   b. Usually need surgical correction.

Complications
1. Avascular necrosis.
2. Redislocation or subluxation.
3. Loss of ROM.
4. Leg length discrepancy.
5. Early osteoarthritis.
6. Recurrent dislocation or unstable hip.
7. Femoral nerve palsy.
8. Iatrogenic hip dislocation.

Nursing Assessment
1. Obtain a family history, including hip pathology.
2. Obtain an obstetric history for presence of risk factors, such as breech presentation and first-born status.
3. Perform a physical assessment for ROM, appearance of Trendelenburg's sign, Barlow test, Ortolani test, and examination for asymmetric thigh folds.
4. Assess family's response to the diagnosis.

Nursing Diagnoses
- Risk for Impaired Parenting related to ineffective adaptation to stressors associated with a diagnosis of DDH and the prescribed therapeutic regimen.
- Risk for Impaired Skin Integrity related to perineal soiling secondary to confinement in an orthopedic device (eg, Pavlik harness, hip-spica cast).
- Impaired Physical Mobility related to external device (eg, hip-spica cast).

Nursing Interventions
Also see page 1119 for orthopedic surgery.

Promoting Effective Parenting
1. Explain the condition and treatment in terms the family can understand.
2. Encourage holding the child with abduction of the hips while handling.
3. Advise parents to avoid swaddling the infant.
4. Reassure parents that effective outcome depends on early intervention and compliance.
5. Demonstrate application of Pavlik harness and make sure that parents know and feel comfortable in applying it.
6. Stress importance of keeping follow-up appointments and strict compliance with prescribed treatment.
7. Provide parents with the name and number of a contact person if they have concerns about their child's care.

Maintaining Skin Integrity
See page 1754.

Preventing Complications of Immobility
1. Stimulate the child with games and activities to exercise upper body and feet as able.
2. Turn the child frequently and encourage ambulation as able. Support the head and legs to reposition.
3. Encourage deep-breathing exercises at intervals to prevent atelectasis and hypostatic pneumonia. Children can blow bubbles, party favors, and cotton balls across the table as appropriate.
4. Encourage fluids and a high-fiber diet to prevent constipation.

Community and Home Care Considerations
1. An initial home care visit may be required to assess the child in a Pavlik harness.
2. For children in a hip-spica cast, see the "Community and Home Care Considerations," section under "Fractures," page 1755.
3. Carefully assess parental role development and educate them on normal care of infant as well as special care needed by their child, such as safety measures and positioning.

Family Education and Health Maintenance

1. If the child is to be treated with an abduction splint, explain its purpose and demonstrate its application and removal to the parents.
   a. Instruct the parents as to if and when the device can be removed.
   b. Instruct the parents to check fit of abduction splint at every diaper change.
   c. Allow the parents to demonstrate their ability to properly place the device on the child.
   d. Provide the parents with written instructions whenever possible.
2. Instruct the parents on skin care and reporting any skin breakdown or disruption of the cast, brace, or splint.
3. Encourage regular follow-up evaluations and regular health maintenance visits.

Evaluation: Expected Outcomes

- Parents hold child and participate in care (eg, applying Pavlik harness).
- No perineal skin breakdown.
- Lungs clear with good aeration bilaterally.

Congenital Clubfoot (Talipes Equinovarus)

Clubfoot is a congenital anomaly characterized by a three-part deformity of the foot, consisting of inversion of the heel (hindfoot varus), adduction and supination of the forefoot, and ankle equinus. Clubfoot typically points down and twists inward. Bone, muscle, ligaments, nerves, and blood vessels below the knee may all be displaced. Other congenital disorders of the foot and ankle occur but are less common. Incidence of clubfoot is 1 to 3 in 1,000 live births. It is bilateral in 30% to 50% of afflicted children and the ratio of occurrence in males to females is 2.5:1.

Pathophysiology and Etiology

1. Equinovarus type (forefoot adduction, about 95% of cases)—foot is plantar flexed (talipes equines) and inverted (talipes varus). See Figure 54-6.
2. Calcaneovalgus type (reverse club foot, about 5% of cases)—foot is dorsiflexed and everted (talipes valgus).
3. Exact etiology is unknown. Suggested theories point to vascular, viral, genetic, anatomic, and environmental factors; may also result from position in utero.

Clinical Manifestations

1. Deformity usually is obvious at birth with varying degrees of rigidity and ability to correct position. May range from a mild postural clubfoot to severe neuromuscular clubfoot that coexists with various diagnoses such as arthrogryposis and spina bifida.
2. Deformity becomes fixed if untreated, which can lead to:
   a. Child bearing weight on lateral border of foot.
   b. Awkward gait.
   c. Development of callosities and bursae over the lateral side of the foot.

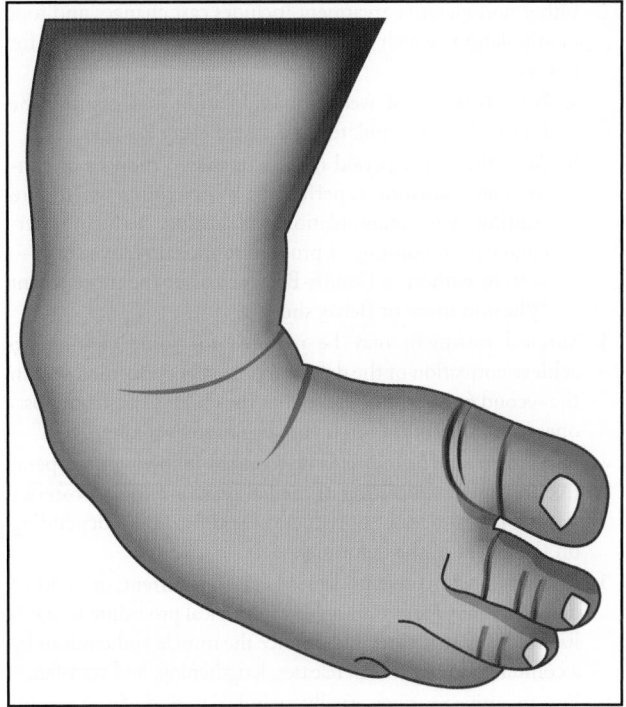

Figure 54-6. Equinovarus-type clubfoot.

Diagnostic Evaluation

1. Clinical presentation and physical examination.
2. X-rays determine bony anatomy and assess treatment efficiency.

Management

 Evidence Base Carroll, N. C. (2012) Clubfoot in the twentieth century: Where we were and where we may be going in the twenty-first century. *Journal of Pediatric Orthopaedics, 21*, 1–6.
   Gray, K., Pacey, V., Gibbons, P., et al. (2012). Interventions for congenital talipes equinovarus (clubfoot). Cochrane Database of Systematic Reviews, 4:CD008602.

Management should begin as soon after birth as possible, with the goal to establish a functional, pain-free foot that can be fit with standard footwear. Despite management, however, child will always have a small calf and foot on the affected side. Nonoperative management, including manipulation, stretching, and serial casting, is becoming the treatment of choice.

1. The Ponsetti method is the initial method of choice for treatment and incorporates gentle stretching and manipulation, followed by cast immobilization to promote relaxation and softening of tissues and remodeling of abnormal joint surfaces.
   a. Consists of weekly casting for approximately 6 weeks, followed by an Achilles tenotomy performed under local anesthetic and subsequent wearing of orthotic boots for 23 to 24 hours per day for 3 to 4 months.
   b. Treatment is completed with daytime ankle-foot orthoses (AFOs) and nighttime boots situated on a bar for 2 years.

2. Other nonoperative treatment includes cast changes and foot manipulation, which is usually done on a weekly basis for 6 weeks.

   a. After 6 weeks of weekly manipulation and casting, the foot is then manipulated and casted every 2 weeks.

   b. After the initial period (approximately 3 months of casting), an evaluation is performed to determine whether to continue with manipulation and casting, perform a percutaneous tenotomy, or proceed to use corrective shoes—with or without a Dennis-Browne bar or the more recent Wheaton brace or Bebax shoe.

3. Surgical treatment may be required for some children to achieve correction of the deformity; usually performed within the second 6 months of life so that the child is free from postoperative immobilization before beginning walking.

4. Surgical treatment may also be required following nonoperative treatment; consisting of medial plantar release, posterior release, lateral release, or reduction and fixation—depending on the extent of the deformity.

5. The child who presents late or has a recurrent or residual deformity may require an aggressive surgical procedure to stabilize the bony structures and balance the muscle and tendons by a combination of fusions, releases, lengthening, and transfers.

6. Postoperative routines usually include a period of cast immobilization of up to 12 weeks, followed by a brace (AFO) or corrective shoe for a period of 2 to 4 years.

Complications

1. "Rocker bottom" deformity from excessive dorsiflexion and "breaking through" the midtarsal bones.

2. Disturbances in epiphyseal plates from overaggressive manipulation.

3. Recurrent or residual deformity.

Nursing Assessment

1. Obtain a family history of foot deformities.

2. Obtain an obstetric history for risk factors.

3. Perform a physical assessment for presence of other anomalies and classic foot position and ROM. If late presentation, perform a thorough neurologic examination to rule out causative factors.

4. Assess family coping and resources available for lengthy treatment.

Nursing Diagnoses

• Risk for Impaired Parenting related to ineffective adaptation to stressors associated with a diagnosis of clubfoot and the intense therapeutic regimen.

• Risk for Impaired Skin Integrity related to serial casting.

• Ineffective Peripheral Tissue Perfusion related to postoperative edema or casting.

• Acute Pain related to tissue and muscle trauma secondary to surgery.

Nursing Interventions

Also see page 1119 for orthopedic surgery.

Promoting Effective Parenting

1. Provide an accurate description of deformity and the importance of treatment in terms the parents can understand.

2. Provide opportunity for parents to verbalize questions and concerns.

3. Reinforce causative factors and the fact that it was not anyone's fault that the child has clubfoot.

4. Encourage parents to hold and play with child and participate in care.

5. Provide parents with a contact family that has been through the treatment process for support.

Protecting Skin Integrity

1. Assess fit of cast, splint, orthotic device, or special shoes. Advise parents that due to rapid growth rate of infant, the cast or splint may need to be replaced to prevent skin breakdown.

2. Assess and teach assessment of excessive pressure on skin—redness, excoriation, foul odor from underneath cast, or pain.

Preserving Tissue Perfusion

1. Perform frequent neurovascular assessments after tenotomy and surgery, including color, warmth, sensation, capillary refill, pulses, and presence of pain.

2. Elevate the extremity to prevent edema in the postoperative period.

3. Protect and assess foot for injury.

Relieving Pain

1. Assess for signs of discomfort, such as irritability, crying, poor feeding and sleeping, tachycardia, and increased blood pressure.

2. Administer analgesics regularly for 24 to 48 hours after surgery.

3. Provide comfort measures, such as soft music, pacifier, teething ring, and rocking and cuddling with parent.

4. Encourage parents to administer analgesics after discharge from hospital (when needed). Discuss dosage and administration and dispel misconceptions about addiction.

Family Education and Health Maintenance

1. Teach parents to remove cast at home before weekly manipulation and recasting by soaking in water and vinegar mixture.

2. Teach the parents when orthotic devices may be removed—usually for bathing. Stress that devices must be worn as prescribed.

3. Advise parents that infant's sleep may be disturbed initially due to wearing brace at night and that he or she may be irritable while awake due to fatigue.

4. Instruct parents on providing a safe environment for the ambulatory child.

5. Discuss the importance of long-term and frequent follow-up and assist parents with special needs such as transportation, flexible appointment times, and financing orthotic equipment.

6. Teach parents to check color, warmth, capillary refill, movement of toes, and position of cast (make sure cast does not slip to hide toes).

7. Encourage parents to comply with treatment regimen to achieve the best possible outcome.

Evaluation: Expected Outcomes

- Parents hold infant, participating in care.
- No signs of skin breakdown.
- Neurovascular status of affected foot intact.
- Rests and feeds well.

Legg-Calvé-Perthes Disease

Legg-Calvé-Perthes (LCP) disease is a self-limiting condition of the proximal femur characterized by a temporary loss of blood supply, which leads to avascular necrosis of the femoral head. The incidence of LCP is 2 per 100,000 in the general population. It occurs most commonly in children between ages 4 and 8. Ratio of occurrence in males to females is 5:1 and it is frequently found in whites and Asians. It is bilateral in 10% to 20% of cases. There is a 30% to 40% familial occurrence rate.

Evidence Base Perry, D. C., Machin, D. M. G., Pope, D., et al. (2012). Racial and geographic factors in the incidence of Legg-Calve-Perthes' disease: A systematic review. *American Journal of Epidemiology, 175*(3), 159–166.

Pathophysiology and Etiology

General Information

1. Etiology is unknown. May be due to factors such as second-hand smoke, poverty, hyperactivity, delayed bone age, short stature, mechanical dysfunction, and metabolic disorders.
2. Interruption of the vascular supply to the femoral head leads to the death of bone. Deformity can occur with loss of the spherical nature of the femoral head during the disease process. The disease progresses through four identifiable stages.

Stage I (Avascularity)

1. Spontaneous interruption of the blood supply to the upper femoral epiphysis.
2. Bone-forming cells in the epiphysis die and bone ceases to grow.
3. Slight widening of the joint space.
4. Swelling of the soft tissues around the hip.
5. The first stage lasts only a few weeks.

Stage II (Revascularization or Fragmentation)

1. The femoral head is flattened and fragmented. Growth of new vessels supplies the area of necrosis; bone resorption and deposition take place.
2. The new bone lacks strength and pathologic fractures may occur.
3. Abnormal forces on the weakened epiphysis may produce progressive deformity.
4. This stage lasts several months to 1 year.

Stage III (Reossification)

1. The head of the femur gradually reforms.
2. Nucleus of the epiphysis breaks up into a number of fragments with cystlike spaces between them.
3. New bone starts to develop at the medial and lateral edges of the epiphysis, which becomes widened.

4. Dead bone is removed and is replaced with new bone, which gradually spreads to heal the lesion.
5. This stage lasts 2 to 4 years.

Stage IV (Healing)

1. Without treatment:
   a. Head of the femur flattens and becomes mushroom shaped.
   b. Incongruity between the head of the femur and the acetabulum persists and worsens.
2. With treatment:
   a. Head of femur remains near spherical.
   b. Acetabulum appears normal.
   c. Width of the neck of the femur is normal.

Clinical Manifestations

1. Child presents with limp or pain in the hip; may be intermittent initially or may last for several months.
2. Referred pain to knee, inner thigh, and groin—usually with activity and often resolved with rest.
3. Limited abduction and internal rotation of the hip.
4. Mild to moderate muscle spasm on rotation of the hip in extension, limited internal rotation flexion and abduction.
5. Trendelenburg gait—dip on the opposite side of the pelvis when weight-bearing on the affected limb.
6. History of related trauma.

Diagnostic Evaluation

1. X-rays (AP and frog leg lateral) allow assessment of the extent of epiphyseal involvement and stage of disease—early findings may be normal.
2. MRI has been useful in detecting infarction but is not accurate in showing the stages of healing.
3. Bone scan is used to help diagnose LCP in the early stage of the disease, where the diagnosis is questionable.
4. Ultrasound may show early joint effusion.
5. Arthrograms may be useful in evaluating sphericity of the femoral head.

Management

Evidence Base Joseph, B., & Price, C.T. (2012). Principles of containment treatment aimed at preventing femoral head deformation in Perthes disease. *Orthopedic Clinics of North America, 42,* 317–327.

Kim, H. K. (2012). Pathophysiology and new strategies for the treatment of Legg-Calve-Perthes disease. *Journal of Bone and Joint Surgery, 94*(7), 659–669.

The goal of management is to preserve and restore the femoral head and to relieve pain.

1. Restore motion—initial relief of synovitis, muscle spasm, and pain in the joint:
   a. Salicylates (with caution), anti-inflammatory medications.
   b. Limitation of activities, bed rest with or without activity modification.

2. Monitor progress of the disease and make sure the hip remains congruent through serial x-rays.
3. Surgical intervention, now rarely done, may vary, but generally involves varus osteotomy, innominate osteotomy, osteotomy of the proximal femur or pelvis, or a combination of these, if the femoral head becomes subluxed or incongruent with the acetabulum before the reparative process.
4. Treatment outcome depends on age of the child, extent of necrosis, stage of disease at time of treatment, and congruence of joint with skeletal maturity.

Complications

1. Early degenerative joint disease.
2. Residual deformity.
3. Loss of motion or function of involved hip.
4. Persistent pain and gait disturbance.

Nursing Assessment

1. Obtain a detailed history, including onset of symptoms and characteristics of pain.
2. Perform a physical assessment to include evaluation of gait, ROM, and presence of any contractures.

Nursing Diagnoses

- Acute Pain secondary to disease process.
- Impaired Physical Mobility related to pain on ambulation.

Nursing Interventions

Also see page 1119 for orthopedic surgery.

Promoting Comfort
1. Monitor and assess pain level using age-appropriate pain measurement tool.
2. Instruct child and parents as to which activities can be continued and which to avoid (eg, contact sports or high-impact sports).
3. Administer analgesics, as indicated, and monitor effectiveness.

Promoting Mobility
1. Encourage activities to maintain ROM (eg, swimming, bicycle riding).
2. Encourage parents to allow activities that involve unaffected body parts within restriction guidelines.
3. Provide equipment to assist with mobility (eg, wheelchair, walker).

Family Education and Health Maintenance

1. Teach proper care of assistive ambulatory aids and the need to remain compliant with usage.
2. Stress need to remain active within restrictions and to promote positive body image.
3. Reinforce to child that he or she is only temporarily restricted. Stress remaining positive aspects of activity.
4. Explain the disease process to parents and child, emphasizing the importance of compliance with treatment.

5. Allow child to voice concerns and ask questions about his or her treatment.
6. Encourage attendance at regular follow-up appointments.

Evaluation: Expected Outcomes

- Pain is adequately managed.
- ROM and function maintained.

Structural Scoliosis

Scoliosis is lateral curvature of the spine. The different types of scoliosis vary by age of onset and structure of the spine.

Pathophysiology and Etiology

1. Idiopathic scoliosis—exact etiology is unknown. Possible causes include genetic factors, vertebral growth abnormality, or central nervous system abnormality. Classified into three groups (based on age at time of diagnosis):
   a. Infantile—birth to age 3.
   b. Juvenile—presentation between ages 4 and 10 or before onset of adolescence.
   c. Adolescent—presentation between ages 11 and 17:
      i. Partially familial.
      ii. Diagnosed when curve is greater than 10 degrees and occurs in 2% to 3% of children. Boys and girls equally affected.
      iii. Prevalence for curves greater than 30 degrees is less common—1½ to 3 per 1,000; severe curvatures are rare.
      iv. Progressive curves are more prevalent in females than in males (7:1 females to males for curves greater than 25 degrees). Progression is greatest during adolescent growth spurt, just prior to onset of menses.
2. Congenital scoliosis—exact etiology unknown; represented as malformation of one or more vertebral bodies that results in asymmetric growth.
   a. Type I—failure of vertebral body formation (eg, isolated hemivertebra, wedged vertebra, multiple wedged vertebrae, multiple hemivertebrae).
   b. Type II—failure of segmentation (eg, unilateral unsegmented bar, bilateral block vertebra).
   c. Commonly associated with other congenital anomalies (eg, Klippel-Feil syndrome, 25%; genitourinary tract abnormalities, 30%; cardiac abnormalities, 12%; cervical spine anomalies, 15%; and intraspinal anomalies, 15%). Thoracic insufficiency syndrome, which includes rib fusion and the chest's inability to support normal breathing or lung growth, may also accompany congenital scoliosis.
3. Neuromuscular scoliosis—child has a definite neuromuscular condition that directly contributes to the deformity:
   a. Most severe in nonambulatory patients.
   b. Occurs in children with cerebral palsy, muscular dystrophy, spinal muscle atrophy, spina bifida, syringomyelia, spinocerebellar degeneration, Charcot-Marie-Tooth syndrome.
4. Additional, but less common causes of scoliosis, include osteopathic conditions, such as fractures, bone disease, arthritic conditions, and infections.

5. Miscellaneous factors that can cause scoliosis include spinal irradiation, endocrine disorders, post-thoracotomy, and nerve root irritation.
6. In all types of scoliosis, the vertebral column develops lateral curvature.
   a. The vertebrae rotate to the convex side of the curve, which rotates the spinous processes toward the concavity.
   b. Vertebrae become wedge-shaped.
   c. Disk shape is altered, as are the neural canal and posterior arch of the vertebral body.
7. As the deformity progresses, changes in the thoracic cage increase. Respiratory and cardiovascular compromise can occur in cases of severe progression.
   a. Changes in the thoracic cage, ribs, and sternum lead to further characteristic deformities such as the "rib hump."
   b. Neurologic compromise in idiopathic scoliosis is rare.

Clinical Manifestations

1. Physical characteristics (see Figure 54-7).
   a. Poor posture.
   b. Increased or decreased thoracic kyphosis or lumbar lordosis.
   c. Leg length discrepancy.
   d. Shoulder asymmetry.
   e. Scapular prominence.
   f. Truncal imbalance (relationship of trunk over pelvis).
   g. Lump (rib hump) on back.
   h. Uneven waistline.
   i. Uneven breast size.
2. Back pain may be present but is not a routine finding in idiopathic scoliosis. (The adolescent who presents with back pain and scoliosis warrants close consideration to rule out a distinct pathologic condition, such as a tumor, disk disease, or intraspinal anomalies.)

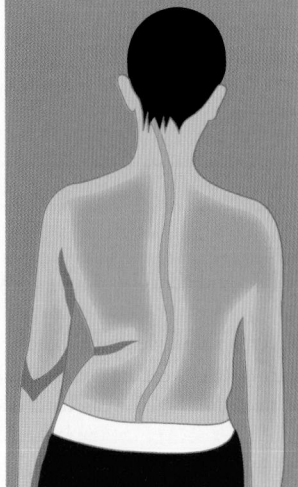
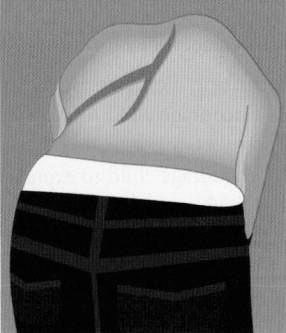

Figure 54-7. Characteristic truncal imbalance and scapular prominence with scoliosis.

Diagnostic Evaluation

Evidence Base American Academy of Orthopedic Surgeons. (2010). Idiopathic scoliosis in children and adolescents. Available: *http://orthoinfo.aaos. org/topic.cfm?topic=A00353*.
    Linker, B. (2012). A dangerous curve: The role of history in scoliosis screening programs. *American Journal of Public Health, 102*(4), 606–616.

1. Thorough history should include onset of menses, recent growth spurt, and family history of scoliosis.
2. Physical examination—Adams forward bending test to screen for scoliosis.
3. Thorough neurologic evaluation:
   a. Evaluate balance, motor strength, sensation, and reflexes (including abdominal).
   b. Skin examination for café au lait spots, axillary freckles to rule out neurofibromatosis.
   c. Examination for presence of a hairy patch in the lumbosacral area, which is suggestive of an underlying spinal dysraphism.
   d. Examination for limb length difference that could cause the appearance of scoliosis.
4. Radiologic assessment of the spine in the upright position, preferably posterior–anterior and lateral views on one long (36-inch [91-cm]) plate—shows characteristic curvature.
5. MRI may be used to determine presence of neural elements of spine; CT scan, with or without three-dimensional reconstruction, may be indicated for children with severe curvatures who have a known or suspected spinal column anomaly before management decisions are made (infantile, juvenile, and congenital).
6. Pulmonary function tests for those with compromised respiratory status.
7. Clinical photographs to assist with documenting the appearance of the spine over time.
8. Workup for associated renal abnormalities with a congenital scoliosis due to a high correlation between the two.

Management

Goal of management is to stop progression of the existing curve by nonoperative means. When this fails, the goal of operative management should be to correct the scoliosis as much as possible and balance and stabilize the spine by fusion to prevent further progression.

Medical Management

1. Observation—periodic (usually every 6 months) physical and radiographic examinations to detect curve progression.
   a. Child is not skeletally mature.
   b. Curves less than 25 degrees.
2. Brace management—goal is to prevent progression of the curve.
   a. Requires faithful compliance on the part of the child for success.
   b. Some curves progress despite brace wear.
   c. Recommended wearing time is 23 hours per day.
   d. Bracing is for skeletally immature children with curves that are about 25 to 40 degrees.

3. Types of braces include:
   a. Boston orthosis for low thoracic and thoracolumbar curves. This is an underarm molded orthosis.
   b. Milwaukee brace for thoracic or double major curves. Standard brace has neck ring with chin rest.
   c. Charleston bending brace has been tried for nighttime usage in selected patients. Results have been positive in some centers, but widespread acceptance has not occurred.
4. Exercise therapy has been promoted to help maintain flexibility in the spine and prevent muscle atrophy during prolonged bracing by strengthening back muscles.

Surgical Correction

 Evidence Base Kepler, C. K., Meredith, D. S., Green, D. W., et al. (2012). Long term outcomes after posterior spine fusion for adolescent idiopathic scoliosis. *Current Opinion in Pediatrics, 24*(1), 68–75.
Erickson, M. A., & Baulesh, D. M. (2011). Pathways that distinguish simple from complex scoliosis repair and their outcomes. *Current Opinions in Pediatrics, 23*, 339–345.

1. Stabilization of the spinal column is the goal. This is usually accomplished with a spinal fusion and one of several methods of instrumentation.
2. Indications for surgical correction vary, but generally accepted principles include:
   a. Progression of the curve over a short period in a curve greater than 45 degrees despite bracing.
   b. Management with a brace is not possible.
   c. Cosmesis.
3. Surgical approach and techniques may be anterior or posterior with various instrumentation methods.
4. Strategies have evolved from body cast fixation to nonsegmental rods, such as the Harrington; to segmental wire fixation, such as the Dwyer, Luque, or Unit Rod; to segmental hook fixation, such as the Texas Scottish Rite Hospital system, Cotrel-Dubousset instrumentation, or USS system; to current techniques, such as segmental screw fixation.
5. Segmental fixation systems provide a three-dimensional correction of coronal, sagittal, and rotational deformities.
   a. Posterior fusion is the standard approach, which allows correction and instrumentation of the majority of curves and levels.
   b. Stainless or titanium rods with segmental hooks (see Figure 54-8) and pedicle screw fixation are currently the instrumentation systems of choice.
   c. A reduction in the number of vertebrae requiring fusion may be achieved with anterior fusion.
   d. Combined anterior and posterior fusion may be used to correct severe curves.
   e. Perioperative halo-gravity traction may be used in rare cases when risk of neurologic compromise from rapid correction exists.
   f. Vertical, expandable prosthetic titanium ribs may be used to lengthen and expand a constricted hemithorax and allow for growth of thoracic spine and rib cage in thoracic

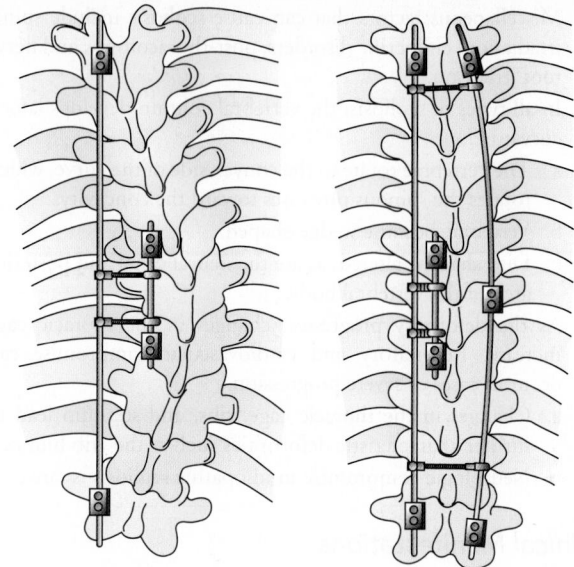

Figure 54-8. Cotrel-Dubousset rods to correct scoliosis. A short distraction rod is linked to a longer one to correct the major curve.

insufficiency. Once the child's lungs have fully developed, a spinal instrumentation and fusion can be performed.

Nursing Assessment

1. Assess respiratory, cardiovascular, and neurologic systems.
2. Perform a physical examination in the upright and forward-bending positions and observe physical characteristics, such as leg lengths, gait, hips, shoulders, and overall development.

Nursing Diagnoses

- Disturbed Body Image related to negative feelings about spinal deformity and appearance in brace.
- Risk for Impaired Skin Integrity related to mechanical irritation of brace.
- Risk for Injury related to postoperative complications.
- Ineffective Therapeutic Regimen (Family) related to chronicity and complexity of treatment regimen.

Nursing Interventions

Also see page 1119 for orthopedic surgery.

Promoting Positive Body Image

1. Encourage child to express feelings and concerns about body image.
2. Encourage child to express concerns about wearing a brace.
3. Discuss options for brace-wearing (eg, wear baggy clothes) and disclosing condition and need for brace wear to classmates.
4. Encourage child to discuss scoliosis with peers, including disease process and treatment.
5. Provide a peer support person when possible so the child can associate positive outcomes and expressions from others.

Preserving Skin Integrity

1. Assess skin integrity and fit of brace at every follow-up appointment.
2. Assess for proper fit of brace or cast.
3. Teach proper skin care to patient and family.
4. Instruct patient to wear cotton shirt under brace to avoid rubbing.

Preventing Postoperative Complications

1. Prepare patient for surgery by teaching deep-breathing and coughing exercises, explaining positioning, and explaining patient-controlled analgesia or another method of pain control.
2. Following surgery, encourage frequent log-rolling side to side to prevent skin breakdown and respiratory complications. Medicate for pain prior to repositioning and ambulation.
3. Perform frequent neurovascular assessments and monitor vital signs frequently.
4. Monitor drainage or bleeding from incision site.
5. Maintain indwelling catheter for first couple of days. Monitor intake and output.
6. Encourage patient to be out of bed as allowed and assist as necessary to avoid orthostatic hypotension from position change.
7. Assessment of active bowel sounds should be done before diet is advanced. If constipation occurs (from lack of mobility and opioid use), provide patients with a bowel regimen consisting of stool softener, stimulant suppository, or laxative, as needed.

Promoting Compliance with Treatment

1. Explain scoliosis and the treatment options to the child in language she or he can understand.
2. Explain the importance of complying with treatment and possible outcomes with noncompliance.
3. Encourage the child and family to discuss concerns and questions they may have about scoliosis and the prescribed treatment.
4. Assist with social service referral for financial, transportation, and other needs.

Family Education and Health Maintenance

1. Provide adequate information on condition and treatment.
2. Instruct parents to examine brace daily for fit or breakage. Also instruct them to contact orthotist when repairs or adjustments are needed.
3. Teach family to inspect skin for irritation under brace.
4. Suggest to family to discuss child's treatment with teachers and school officials so child can receive tutoring or home schooling in order to keep up with grade requirements if out for surgery.

Evaluation: Expected Outcomes

- Child makes positive comments about self.
- Skin without signs of breakdown.
- Neurovascular status intact; no bleeding noted; bowel sounds present; pain is adequately managed.
- Wears brace as prescribed, following up as directed.

Slipped Capital Femoral Epiphysis

 Evidence Base Gordon, E., Herrera-Soto, J., Loder, R., et al. (2012). Slipped capital femoral epiphysis: Controversies and current treatment options. *Orthopedics Today, 32*(10), 34–38.

Slipped capital femoral epiphysis (SCFE) is the most common hip disorder in adolescents, which occurs in puberty just before the physis (growth plate) closes. It is characterized by a slipping of the epiphysis and metaphysis due to weakening of the perichondral ring of the physis. The epiphysis slips downward and backward. Incidence is 10 per 100,000 and it is three times more common in males than in females. Approximately 20% of patients present with bilateral slips at time of presentation and 20% to 30% will develop a contralateral slip within 12 to 18 months of initial slip.

Pathophysiology and Etiology

1. Skeletally immature and obese adolescents are at greatest risk.
2. Left hip is most frequently affected.
3. Exact etiology is unknown; possible risk factors include:
   a. Sedentary lifestyle.
   b. Rapid growth spurt.
   c. Overweight and obesity.
   d. African American ethnicity.
4. Femoral neck slips off the proximal femoral epiphysis and is contained within the acetabulum.
5. Classified by duration of symptoms:
   a. Acute—sudden onset; symptoms for less than 3 weeks.
   b. Chronic—symptoms lasting more than 3 weeks.
6. Approximately 85% of children have stable slips.

Clinical Manifestations

1. Pain in groin, medial thigh, or knee (referred pain).
2. Decreased ROM in affected hip.
3. Sudden onset of pain (acute SCFE).
4. Inability to bear weight (acute SCFE).
5. Limp when walking (usually found in chronic cases).
6. Intermittent pain.
7. Trendelenburg gait.
8. External rotation of the lower limb; involved limb may be shortened.

Diagnostic Evaluation

1. X-rays confirm diagnosis—AP and frog leg lateral views.
2. Bone scan—rules out presence of avascular necrosis.
3. CT scan—helps to define extent of slip.

Management

1. Goal is to prevent progressive slippage and minimize deformity while avoiding necrosis of cartilage (chondrolysis) and avascular necrosis.
2. Treatment is surgical—in situ pinning with one or two screws is usually done within 24 to 48 hours.

Complications

1. Chondrolysis over femoral head resulting in permanent loss of ROM.
2. Avascular necrosis of femoral head.
3. Osteoarthritis.

Nursing Assessment

1. Obtain a detailed history, including onset of symptoms and characteristics of pain.
2. Perform a physical assessment and include evaluation of gait and ROM in hips.

Nursing Diagnoses

- Acute and Chronic Pain related to disease process.
- Impaired Physical Mobility related to disease process.
- Deficient Diversional Activity related to activity restriction.

Nursing Interventions

Also see page 1119 for orthopedic surgery.

Promoting Comfort

1. Monitor and assess pain level using age-appropriate pain-measurement tools.
2. Instruct child and parents as to which activities can be continued and which to avoid (eg, contact sports, high-impact activities).
3. Administer analgesics, as indicated, and monitor effectiveness.

Promoting Mobility

1. Facilitate bed rest or other activity restriction, as directed.
2. Provide equipment to assist with mobility (eg, wheelchair, crutches).

Promoting Diversional Activities

1. Be alert to the needs of adolescents to socialize with peers. Encourage visitation and communication with friends and family.
2. Encourage family to provide books, magazines, games, and electronics for the adolescent to use.
3. Provide support for the family and reinforce the importance of following activity restrictions to prevent permanent damage to femur.

Family Education and Health Maintenance

1. Teach proper use of mobility devices (eg, crutches).
2. Stress need to maintain activity within restrictions and to promote positive body image.
3. Encourage follow-up during active treatment and following surgery. About 25% of children later develop the same condition in the opposite hip, so careful attention must be paid to both legs at follow-up.

Evaluation: Expected Outcomes

- Child reports feeling little or no pain.
- Child follows activity restriction.
- Child maintains socialization with friends and partakes of hobbies in room.

SELECTED REFERENCES

American Academy of Orthopedic Surgeons (2010). Idiopathic scoliosis in children and adolescents. Available: *http://orthoinfo.aaos.org/topic.cfm?topic=A00353.*

Belthur, M. V., Birchansky, S. B., Verdugo, A. A., et al. (2012). Pathologic fractures in children with staphylococcus aureus osteomyelitis. *Journal of Bone and Joint Surgery, 94,* 34–42.

Benson, M., Fixsen, J., Macnicol, M., et al. (2011). *Children's upper and lower limb fractures.* New York: Springer.

Carroll, N. C. (2012). Clubfoot in the twentieth century: Where we were and where we may be going in the twenty-first century. *Journal of Pediatric Orthopaedics, 21,* 1–6.

Clarke, N., & Castaneda, P. (2012). Strategies to improve nonoperative childhood management. *Orthopedic Clinics of North America, 43*(3), 281–289.

Ellis, H. B., Ho, C. A., Podeszwa, D. A., et al. (2011). A comparison of locked versus nonlocked Enders rods for length unstable pediatric femoral shaft fractures. *Journal of Pediatric Orthopedics, 31*(8), 825–833.

Erickson, M. A., & Baulesh, D. M. (2011). Pathways that distinguish simple from complex scoliosis repair and their outcomes. *Current Opinions in Pediatrics, 23,* 339–345.

Gordon, E., Herrera-Soto, J., Loder, R., et al. (2012). Slipped capital femoral epiphysis: Controversies and current treatment options. *Orthopedics Today, 32*(10), 34–38.

Gourde, J., & Damian, F. (2012). ED fracture pain management in children. *Journal of Emergency Nursing, 38*(1), 91–97.

Gray, K., Pacey, V., Gibbons, P., et al. (2012). Interventions for congenital talipes equinovarus (clubfoot). *Cochrane Database of Systematic Reviews, 4:*CD008602.

Harris, G. D., & Lavernia, G. J. (2010). Legg-Calve-Perthes disease. *Medscape.* Available: *http://emedicine.medscape.com/article/1248267-overview.*

Hart, E. S., Turner, A., Albright, M., et al. (2011). Common pediatric elbow fractures. *Orthopedic Nursing, 30*(1), 11–17.

Hatzenbeuhler, J., & Pulling, T. J. (2011). The diagnosis and management of osteomyelitis. *American Family Physician, 84*(9), 1027–1033.

Joseph, B., & Price, C. T. (2012) Principles of containment treatment aimed at preventing femoral head deformation in Perthes disease. *Orthopedic Clinics of North America, 42,* 317–327.

Jowett, C. R., Morcuende, J. A., & Ramachandran. M. (2011). Management of congenital talipes equinovarus using the Ponseti method: A systematic review. *Journal of Bone and Joint Surgery, 93*(9), 1160–1164.

Kepler, C. K., Meredith, D. S., Green, D. W., & Widmann, R. F. (2012). Long term outcomes after posterior spine fusion for adolescent idiopathic scoliosis. *Current Opinion in Pediatrics, 24*(1), 68–75.

Kim, H. K. (2012). Pathophysiology and new strategies for the treatment of Legg-Calve-Perthes disease. *Journal of Bone and Joint Surgery, 94*(7), 659–669.

Laine, J. C., Kaiser, S. P., & Diab, M. (2010). High risk pediatric orthopedic pitfalls. *Emergency Medical Clinics of North America, 28,* 85–102.

Linker, B. (2012). A dangerous curve: The role of history in scoliosis screening programs. *American Journal of Public Health, 102*(4), 606–616.

Mehrpour, S., Aghamirsalim, M., Motamedi, S., et al. (2013). A supplemental video teaching tool enhances splinting skills. *Clinical Orthopaedics & Related Research, 471*(2), 649–654.

Peck, D. (2010). Slipped capital femoral epiphysis: Diagnosis and management. *American Family Physician, 82*(3), 258–262.

Pediatric Orthopaedic Society of North America. (2010). Growth plate fractures. Available: *http://orthoinfo.aaos.org/topic.cfm?topic=A00040.*

Perry, D. C., Machin, D. M. G., Pope, D., et al. (2012). Racial and geographic factor in the incidence of Legg-Calvé-Perthes' disease: A systematic review. *American Journal of Epidemiology, 175*(3), 159–166.

Pillitterri, A. (2012) Nursing care of the child with a musculoskeletal disorder. In A. Pilliterri (Ed.), *Maternal-child health nursing: Care of the childbearing and child rearing family,* 216–220. Philadelphia: Lippincott, Williams and Wilkins.

Ramseier, L. E., Janicki, J. A., Weir, S., et al. (2010). Femoral fractures in adolescents: A comparison of four methods of fixation. *Journal of Bone and Joint Surgery, 92,* 1122–1129.

Reed, C., Carroll, L., Baccari, S., et al. (2011). Spica cast care: A collaborative staff-led education initiative for improved patient care. *Orthopedic Nursing, 30*(6), 353–358.

Roposch, A., Liu, L. Q., Hefti, F., et al. (2011). Standardized diagnostic criteria for developmental dysplasia of the hip in early infancy. *Clinical Orthopaedics and Related Research, 469*, 3451–3461.

Santy, J. (2010). A review of pin site wound infection assessment criteria. *International Journal of Orthopaedic and Trauma Nursing, 14*(3), 125–131.

Seel, E. H., Noble, S., Clarke, N. M. P., et al. (2011). Outcome of distal fibial injuries. *Journal of Pediatric Orthopedics, 20*, 242–248.

Sponsellar, P. (2011). *Handbook of pediatric orthopedics.* New York: Thieme.

Timms, A., & Pugh, H. (2012). Pin site care: Guidance and key recommendations. *Nursing Standard, 27*(1), 50–55.

Valerio, G., Galle, F., Mancusi, C., et al. (2010). Patterns of fractures across pediatric age groups: Analysis of individual and lifestyle factors. *BMC Public Health, 10*, 2–9.

VonKries, R., Ihme, N., Altenhofen, L., et al. (2012). General ultrasound screening reduces the rate of first operative procedures for developmental dysplasia of the hip: A case-control study. *Journal of Pediatrics, 160*(2), 272–275.

Walker, J. (2012). Pin site infection in orthopaedic external fixation devices. *British Journal of Nursing, 21*(3), 148–151.

Woratanarat, P., Angsanuntsukh, C., Rattanasiri, S., et al. (2012). Meta-analysis of pinning in supracondylar fracture of the humerus in children. *Journal of Orthopedic Trauma, 26*, 48–53.

Wu, G. S., & Pollock, A. N. (2011). Slipped capital femoral epiphysis. *Pediatric Emergency Care, 27*(11), 1095–1096.

Young, S., Fevang, J. M., Gullaksen, G., et al. (2010). Deformity and functional outcome after treatment for supracondylar humerus fractures in children: A 5-to 10-year follow-up of 139 supracondylar humerus fractures treated by plaster cast, skeletal traction or crossed wire fixation. *Journal of Child Orthopedics, 4*, 445–453.

Zhang, H., Wang, Y., Guo, C., et al. (2011). Posterior-only surgery with strong halo-femoral traction for the treatment of adolescent idiopathic scoliotic curves more than 100°. *International Orthopedics, 35*, 1037–1042.

55

Pediatric Integumentary Disorders

BURNS

Management of Burns in Children

Burns are common childhood injuries. They may be caused by heat, electrical energy, or chemicals. Long-term surgical and psychological sequela often follow a burn injury and may include reconstruction and issues related to posttraumatic stress disorder. Very serious burns may include:

1. Partial-thickness (second-degree) burns of 12% to 15% or more of body surface area and full-thickness burns.
2. Burns of face, hands, feet, perineum, or joint surfaces.
3. Electrical burns.
4. Burns in the presence of other injuries.
5. Any burn that cannot be cared for adequately at home.

Epidemiology

1. Burns are the third leading cause of accidental deaths in childhood, with the highest incidence of burns occurring in children younger than age 5.
2. Children at high risk are of lower socioeconomic status and of single parents. However, any child, supervised or unsupervised, is at risk for a burn injury.
3. Scalds are the leading cause of injury in children, followed by flame burns.
4. Burns from a hot liquid are most common in children younger than age 3.
   a. Tap water temperature above 120° F (48.9° C) (at 130° F [54.4° C]) takes only 30 seconds to produce a full-thickness injury in adult skin—less time in the very young; at 155° F (68.3° C), tap water will cause a full-thickness injury in a child in 1 second.
   b. Child left unsupervised in tub turns on hot water tap.
   c. Child placed in tub of hot water that has not been tested.
   d. Spilling of hot liquid, such as coffee or tea, on child. Spilling occurs especially when pot handles stick out on top of stove, when hot liquids and foods are removed from microwave oven, and when child grabs or pulls items from surfaces.
   e. Ingestion and aspiration of hot foods and liquids from microwave oven as well as scald burns to skin and palate from hot formula.

5. Burns from open flames:
   a. House fires.
   b. Child climbing on stove, resulting in ignited clothing.
   c. Children playing with lighters, especially 3- to 10-year-olds.
   d. Playing or working with gasoline.
   e. Automobile accidents with subsequent fire.
   f. Juvenile fire-setters.

6. Electrical burns are most common in toddlers and adolescents and may be caused by:
   a. Child playing with electrical outlets or appliances.
   b. Child playing with extension cords; children commonly bite through the cord.
   c. Child playing on railroad tracks; climbing trees and touching high-tension wires; lightning.

7. Other causes:
   a. Caustic acid or alkali burns, often of the mouth and esophagus.
   b. Chemical burns of the skin—child playing with gasoline or chemical cleaning agents.
   c. Burns inflicted on the child as a result of neglect or abuse (immersion and contact burns most common).
   d. Smoke inhalation and inhalation from products of combustion of synthetics, such as plastics and rayon; may yield cyanide, formaldehyde.

e. Radiation burns—sunburn most common, may be secondary to cancer radiation therapy.

f. Contact burns from touching hot surfaces, such as radiators, wood-burning stoves, fireplaces, or open ovens.

g. Fireworks burns, typically as a result of misuse and lack of adult supervision; may be combined with explosive hand injuries.

h. Friction burns such as those seen with exercise treadmills in the home.

 NURSING ALERT With combined injury, management of trauma takes precedence over the burn.

Pathophysiology and Etiology

See "Burns in Adults," page 1178.

Clinical Manifestations

Characteristics of Burn Wounds

1. See page 1184 for characteristics of superficial, partial-thickness, and full-thickness burns.
2. Electrical burns:
   a. Especially of the mouth in child younger than age 2; may chew or suck on live wire.
   b. Are progressive and may take up to 3 weeks to fully manifest the extent of injury.

Symptoms of Shock

Symptoms of hypovolemic shock are dependent upon the size and thickness of the burn. Hypovolemic shock may develop in large surface size burns within the first 1 to 2 hours of the injury.

1. Rapid pulse, low blood pressure.
2. Subnormal temperature.
3. Pallor, cyanosis, prostration.
4. Failure to recognize parents or other familiar people.
5. Poor muscle tone; flaccid extremities.

Symptoms of Toxemia

Symptoms may develop 1 to 2 days after burn.

1. Prostration, fever, rapid pulse.

 **NURSING ALERT** The fever of toxemia is not to be confused with expected "burn fever," which may be as high as 103° F (39.4° C) because of the hypermetabolic state.

2. Glucosuria, decreased urine output.
3. Vomiting, edema.
4. These symptoms may progress to coma or death.

Upper Respiratory Tract Injury

Causes inflammation or edema of the glottis, vocal cords, and upper trachea and is characterized by symptoms of upper airway obstruction and immediate attention to securing and maintaining the airway takes precedence over the burn injury. Signs of inhalation are:

1. Dyspnea, tachypnea, hoarseness.
2. Stridor, substernal and intercostal retractions, nasal flaring.

3. Restlessness, drooling, cough, increasing hoarseness.
4. Carbonaceous sputum.
5. Facial burns and/or edematous lips.
6. Black nasal or oral secretions.
7. Hypoxemia.
8. History of burn within a closed space.

 NURSING ALERT Increasing hoarseness, drooling, and stridor are leading indicators for immediate intubation.

Smoke Inhalation

Smoke inhalation may cause no initial symptoms other than mild bronchial obstruction during the initial phase after the burn. Within 6 to 48 hours, the child may develop sudden onset of the following conditions:

1. Bronchiolitis.
2. Pulmonary edema (acute respiratory distress syndrome)—of noncardiac origin.
3. Severe airway obstruction.
4. Delayed damage: up to 7 days after the burn injury.

Suspicious Burns in Children

Mechanism of injury is an important assessment when a burn injury involves a child. If the mechanism of injury seems out of proportion to the injuries of the child, notification to law enforcement is mandated by all nursing practice acts. Be alert for the following characteristics that may require further investigation by law enforcement:

1. Burns in a pattern.
2. History and physical findings inconsistent with the burn injury.
3. Burn injuries incompatible with child's developmental level.
4. Burn to buttocks, perineum, or genitals.
5. Burns involving immersion into hot water. Typical findings reveal the back of the knees will be spared of burn injury, with entire feet and lower legs burned.
6. Multiple and new and old burns in different stages of healing.
7. Burns that are circular in nature, likely due to cigarette burns.
8. Presence of other nonburn injuries such as bruises, scrapes, or previous fractures.

Diagnostic Evaluation

Calculation of the Burn Area

1. Rule of Nines (used in assessment of extent of burns in adults) has not proven to be exact when applied to young children; it may be acceptable to use in child older than age 10. It is not recommended for hospital use; the Lund and Browder chart is recommended. Total body surface area (TBSA) is based on age, thus compensating for changes in body surface area that change during growth (see Figure 55-1).
   a. During infancy and early childhood, the relative surface area of different parts of the body varies with age.
   b. The younger the child, the greater the proportion of the surface area is constituted by the head and the lesser the proportion of the surface area is constituted by the legs.

AREA OF BODY	RELATIVE PERCENTAGE OF BODY SURFACE (VARIES BY AGE)					ESTIMATED PERCENTAGE OF BODY AREA WITH:	
	0–1 Years	1–4 Years	5–9 Years	10–15 Years	Adult	2nd-degree burns	3rd- and 4th-degree burns
Head	19	17	13	10	7		
Neck	2	2	2	2	2		
Anterior trunk	13	13	13	13	13		
Posterior trunk	13	13	13	13	13		
Right buttock	2	2	2	2	2		
Left buttock	2	2	2	2	2		
Genitalia	1	1	1	1	1		
Right upper arm	4	4	4	4	4		
Left upper arm	4	4	4	4	4		
Right lower arm	3	3	3	3	3		
Left lower arm	3	3	3	3	3		
Right hand	2	2	2	2	2		
Left hand	2	2	2	2	2		
Right thigh	5	6	8	8	9		
Left thigh	5	6	8	8	9		
Right lower leg	5	5	5	6	7		
Left lower leg	5	5	5	6	7		
Right foot	3	3	3	3	3		
Left foot	3	3	3	3	3		
					TOTAL:	+	=

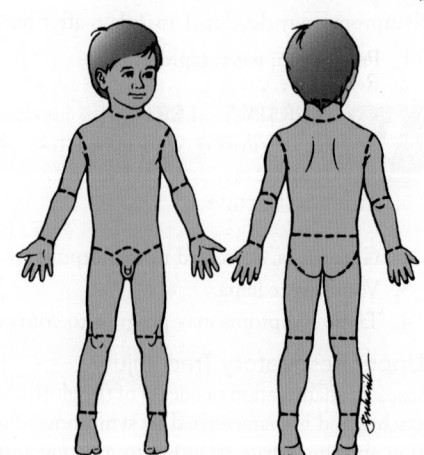

Figure 55-1. The Lund and Browder chart is used to determine the extent of burns in children because it is based on age, thus compensating for changes based on growth.

2. A rough estimate can be obtained by using the child's hand (palm, with fingers extended), which is equal to 1%.

Categorization of Severity of Burn

1. Total area injured, depth of injury, location of injury.
2. Age of child.
3. Condition of patient (ie, level of consciousness). Confusion is the hallmark of an anoxic brain.
4. Medical history (ie, comorbidities, chronic disease).
5. Additional injuries.

Schematic Classification of Burn Severity

1. Minor burn—10% TBSA or less; first- and second-degree burn
2. Moderate burn:
   a. 10% to 20% TBSA; second-degree burn.
   b. 2% to 5% TBSA; third-degree burn not involving eyes, ears, face, genitals, hands, or feet or circumferential burns.
3. Major burn:
   a. 20% TBSA or greater; second-degree burn.
   b. All third-degree burns greater than 10%; depending on age of child, 5% is sometimes used.
   c. All burns involving hands, face, eyes, ears, feet, or genitals.
   d. All electrical burns.
   e. Complicated burn injuries involving fracture or other major trauma.
   f. All poor-risk patients (ie, head injury, cancer, lung disease, diabetes).

Management

Fluid Resuscitation: Intravenous (IV) Fluid Replacement

Note: Controversy exists regarding fluid resuscitation solution and amount. Not all pediatric patients require fluid resuscitation. Children with burns 15% TBSA or less may be treated with oral rehydration therapies and supplemental maintance IV fluids.

1. Fluid loss from transcapillary leakage is greatest during the first 12 hours after injury and diminishes to almost zero 12 to 24 hours after injury. Fluid loss after 48 hours is due to vaporization of water from the wound.
2. Replacement usually consists of lactated Ringer's solution, an isotonic electrolyte solution. Lactated Ringer's solution has a much lower sodium content than 0.9% saline (130 mEq/L vs. 154 mEq/L), has a much higher pH (6.5 vs. 6.0), and has 28 mmol/L of lactate, which is used as a buffering agent.
3. The Consensus formula is commonly used to determine the fluid needed for resuscitation for burns greater than 15% TBSA (see page 1185). Children age 6 months to 5 years should receive a maintenance containing formula with dextrose to prevent hypoglycemia (5% dextrose or D5LR).
   a. One half of the requirements are given during the first 8 hours.
   b. The remainder is given over the next 24 hours
   c. In children, the second day's crystalloid consists of the maintenance requirements; 5% dextrose and 0.45% normal saline or 5% dextrose and 0.2% normal saline is used instead of 5% dextrose solution. Colloid is per Consensus formula.

Burn Treatment

1. Burns are most commonly treated by the closed method. However, dependent on the location of the burn a combination technique using both open and closed methods may be necessary.
2. Using the closed method is preferred as it allows children to be more mobile when a burn injury is covered and because they experience less pain.
3. Hydrotherapy is the treatment of choice for cleaning wounds. Isotonic saline rather than water may be needed for large wounds and small children. A large stainless steel tub, commonly with a one-use-only tub liner, is used to ensure a clean environment during the treatment. During a tub treatment, children should be encouraged to participate with washing off cream whenever possible. A gentle soap or shampoo can be used to wash the burned and nonburned parts of the body and hair. Tub or shower treatments are usually done daily unless a longer-acting dressing is in place between hydrotherapy sessions.
4. The use of a hand-held shower to facilitate the loosening and removal of sloughing tissue, eschar, exudate, and topical medications is gaining popularity. The shower—water about 90° F (32.2° C)—flows over the child; debridement is then performed.
5. Use pharmaceutical and psychological interventions, unique to each child and appropriate for their developmental stage and comfort needs, to ensure appropriate pain and anxiety management.
6. See page 1184 for wound cleaning and debridement, hydrotherapy, topical antimicrobials, surgical management, and burn wound grafting. It is important to use bacitracin ophthalmic ointment on a child's face because touching or rubbing the face may get ointment into the eyes. Topical bacitracin will cause conjunctivitis if it gets into the eyes.

Complications

Vary according to severity of burn injury; commonly occur, especially with severe burn injury.

Acute

1. Infection; burn wound sepsis, pneumonia, urinary tract infection (UTI), phlebitis, toxic shock syndrome.
2. Curling's (stress) ulcer, GI hemorrhage; rarely seen now that histamine-2 (H_2) blockers are commonly used prophylactically, especially in burns greater than 20% TBSA.
3. Acute gastric dilation, paralytic ileus; occurs especially in child younger than age 2 with greater than 20% injury and develops early in postburn period, lasting 2 to 3 days.
4. Renal failure.
5. Respiratory failure; severe inhalation injury is the insult most likely to cause death.
6. Postburn seizures.
7. Hypertension.
8. Central nervous system dysfunction.
9. Vascular ischemia.
10. Anxiety and complex pain (acute to chronic presentations).
11. Anemia and malnutrition; may resolve when the burn area is covered.

12. Constipation and fecal impaction.
13. Labile moods secondary to hospitalization, repeated procedures, and changing body image.

Long Term
1. Growth and development delays secondary to malnutrition, hospitalization, complexities of injury and recovery.
2. Developmental regression.
3. Scarring, disfigurement, and contractures.
4. Impact of psychological trauma.

Nursing Assessment

1. Initially, perform emergency assessment of the burn patient to determine priorities of care.
   a. Airway, breathing, and circulation: airway may be compromised with inhalation injury.
   b. Extent of burn injury.
   c. Additional injuries. (Although establishing a patent airway always comes first, trauma takes precedence over the burn.).
2. Obtain a history of the injury—for example, when the injury occurred; what first aid was given; location of the child; if smoke was present, if child was in a closed space; who was supervising the child; what the specific mechanism of injury was; what other factors need to be considered in terms of the context of the injury; consider if additional injuries may exist.
3. Obtain a complete medical history, including childhood diseases, immunizations (especially tetanus status), current medications, allergies, recent infections, general health and developmental status.
4. Assess level of pain and emotional status; provide pain relief and reassurance while performing assessment and determining priorities.
5. Subsequently, focus assessment on fluid volume balance, condition of the burn wounds, and signs of infection (burn wound, pulmonary, urinary).
6. Remain vigilant for signs of sepsis. The American Burn Association 2007 consensus guidelines provide clear definitions for sepsis and common infections in burn patients, but it's not perfect. Additional markers such as procalcitonin, C-reactive protein, and erythrocyte sedimentation rate can be used. Sepsis occurs in children when at least three of the following occur:
   a. Temperature above 102.2° F (39° C) or below 97.7° F (36.5° C).
   b. Progressive tachycardia more than 2 standard deviations (SD) above age-specific norms.
   c. Progressive tachypnea more than 2 SD above age-specific norms.
   d. Thrombocytopenia (not applicable until 3 days after initial recuscitation) less than 2 SD below age-specific norms.
   e. Hyperglycemia (in the absence of preexisting diabetes mellitus).
      i. Untreated plasma glucose greater than 200 mg/dL.
      ii. Insulin resistance.
   f. Inability to continue enteral feedings for more than 24 hours.
      i. Abdominal distention.
      ii. Enteral feeding intolerance.
      iii. Uncontrollable diarrhea.
7. In addition, it is required that infection be documented by positive culture, pathologic tissue source identified, or clinical response to antimicrobials observed.

 Evidence Base Greenhalgh, D. G., Saffle, J. R., Holmes, J. H. IV, et al. (2007). American Burn Association Consensus Conference to define sepsis and infection in burn. *Journal of Burn Care and Rehabilitation, 28*(6), 776–790.
    Hogan, B. K., Wolf, S. E., Hospenthal, D. R., et al. (2012). Correlation of American Burn Association sepsis criteria with the presence of bacteremia in burned patients admitted to the intensive care unit. *Journal of Burn Care and Rehabilitation, 33*(3), 371–378.

Nursing Diagnoses

- Decreased Cardiac Output related to fluid shifts and hypovolemic shock.
- Risk for Infection related to altered skin integrity, decreased circulation, and immobility.
- Impaired Gas Exchange related to inhalation injury, pain, and immobility.
- Imbalanced Nutrition: Less Than Body Requirements related to hypermetabolic response to burn injury.
- Dysfunctional gastrointestinal motility related to paralytic ileus and stress.
- Ineffective Peripheral Tissue Perfusion related to edema and circumferential burns.
- Risk for Imbalanced Fluid Volume related to fluid resuscitation and subsequent mobilization 3 to 5 days postburn.
- Impaired Skin Integrity related to burn injury and surgical interventions (donor sites).
- Impaired Urinary Elimination related to indwelling catheter.
- Ineffective Thermoregulation related to loss of skin microcirculatory regulation and hypothalamic response.
- Impaired Physical Mobility related to edema, pain, dressings and splints.
- Acute Pain related to burn wound and associated treatments.
- Disturbed Body Image related to cosmetic and functional sequelae of burn wound.
- Fear and Anxiety related to pain, treatments, procedures, and hospitalization.
- Impaired Parenting related to crisis situation, prolonged hospitalization, and disfigurement.
- Disturbed Sleep Pattern related to unfamiliar surroundings and pain.

Nursing Interventions

Supporting Cardiac Output
1. Be alert to the symptoms of shock that occur shortly after a severe burn—tachycardia, hypothermia, hypotension, pallor, prostration, shallow respirations, anuria.

2. Monitor the administration of IV fluids because major burns are followed by a reduction in blood volume due to outflow of plasma into the tissues.

3. Maintain and record intake and output to provide an accurate measure of volume.
   a. Record time and amount of all fluids given.
   b. Measure urine output every hour and report diminished output, as ordered (0.5 mL/kg/hour is considered minimally acceptable urine output; however, 1 mL/kg/hour is preferable).
   c. Check urine-specific gravity to determine concentration or dilution.

4. With severe burn injuries, insert an indwelling catheter.

5. Weigh patient daily to help evaluate fluid balance.

6. Monitor sensorium, pulse, pulse pressure, capillary refill, and blood gas values.

7. Provide a rich oxygen environment to combat hypoxia, as necessary.

8. Monitor electrolyte and hematocrit results as a guide to fluid replacement.

9. Maintain a warm, humidified ambient environment (especially with burns of 20% TBSA) to maintain body temperature and decrease fluid needs.

Preventing Infection

1. Wash hands with antibacterial cleansing agent before and after all patient contact and use appropriate precautions.
   a. Use barrier garments—isolation gown or plastic apron—for all care requiring contact with the patient or the patient's bed.
   b. Cover hair and wear mask when wounds are exposed or when performing a sterile procedure.
   c. Use sterile examination gloves for all dressing changes and all care involving patient contact.

2. Be alert for reservoirs of infection and sources of cross-contamination in equipment, assignment of personnel.

3. Observe burn wounds with each dressing change: assess drainage for color, odor, and amount; necrosis; increase in pain; and surrounding erythema, warmth, swelling, and tenderness, which may indicate infection.

4. Administer topical antimicrobials and systemic antibiotics, as ordered.

5. Provide meticulous skin care to prevent infection and promote healing.

6. Be alert for early signs of septicemia, including changes in mentation, tachypnea, and decreased peristalsis as well as later signs, such as increased pulse, decreased blood pressure (BP), increased or decreased urine output, facial flushing, increased and later decreased temperatures, increasing hyperglycemia, and malaise. Report to health care provider promptly.

7. Obtain serial cultures, as ordered.
   a. Obtain urine, sputum, and blood cultures for two or more consecutive temperatures of 103° F (39.4° C) or a single temperature of 104° F (40° C).
   b. Pan culturing (urine, wound, blood, and sputum) may be ordered.

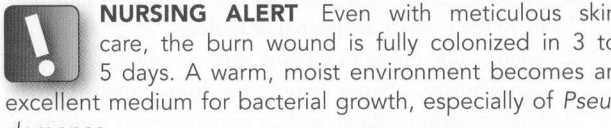

NURSING ALERT Even with meticulous skin care, the burn wound is fully colonized in 3 to 5 days. A warm, moist environment becomes an excellent medium for bacterial growth, especially of *Pseudomonas*.

8. Promote optimal personal hygiene for the patient, including daily cleansing of unburned areas, meticulous care of teeth and mouth, shampooing of hair every other day, and meticulous care of IV and urinary catheter sites.

9. Prevent the child from scratching by administering antipruritics and applying protective devices to his or her hands.

10. Be alert for the development of pneumonia or UTI related to immobility and invasive procedures. Encourage coughing, turning, deep breathing, ambulation, and early discontinuation of indwelling catheter to minimize complications.

11. Ensure that appropriate nutrition and enteral feeding are in place within 6 to 8 hours of injury to prevent translocation of bacteria in the gut.

12. Administer tetanus prophylaxis based on immunization history.
   a. If primary series complete (or at least three doses of tetanus toxoid obtained) and last injection within past 5 years, it is not necessary.
   b. If at least three doses obtained and last injection more than 5 years, give tetanus toxoid.
   c. If two or fewer doses obtained, give tetanus immunoglobulin and tetanus toxoid.

Optimizing Gas Exchange

1. Be alert for and report symptoms of respiratory distress—dyspnea, stridor, tachypnea, restlessness, cyanosis, coughing, increasing hoarseness, drooling.

2. Administer supplemental humidified oxygen.

3. Monitor arterial blood gas (ABG) levels as necessary.

4. Evaluate the carboxyhemoglobin on ABG results (due to inhalation of carbon monoxide, a product of combustion) and be prepared to support ventilation if signs of hypoxemia and respiratory failure develop.

5. Assist with pulmonary function and bronchoscopy, as indicated.

6. Have intubation supplies readily available. If unable to intubate the child, then tracheostomy may be necessary. If unable to extubate in 14 to 21 days, then may be converted to tracheostomy for continuous pulmonary management. The current trend is to use the earlier time frame.

7. Prevent atelectasis and pneumonia through chest physical therapy, postural drainage, meticulous pulmonary technique, and, if indicated, tracheostomy care.

Ensuring Adequate Nutrition for Healing and Growth Needs

1. Be aware that hypernutrition is important because of the extreme hypermetabolism related to large burn injuries.
   a. Twice the predicted basal metabolic rate in calories, based on ideal weight, may be necessary. Caloric recommendation is 1,800 kcal/m² total body surface for maintenance, plus 2,000 kcal/m² of burned surface area.

b. Hypermetabolic state generally subsides when the majority of the wounds are grafted or healed.

c. High caloric intake to support hypermetabolic state; protein synthesis; calories should come from carbohydrates.

d. High-protein intake to replace protein lost by exudation; support synthesis of immunoglobulins and structural protein; prevent negative nitrogen balance.

e. Vitamin and mineral supplement needed, particularly vitamins B and C, iron, and zinc.

2. Maintain ambient temperature at 82.4° F to 90° F (28° C to 32.2° C) to minimize metabolic expenditure by maintaining core temperature.

3. Minimize anorexia to increase caloric intake.

a. Offer small amounts of food, perhaps four to five feedings rather than three per day.

b. Give choice of foods; determine favorites.

c. Provide high-calorie, high-protein oral or nasogastric (NG) supplementation, as necessary.

d. Consider long-term use of G-tube or NJ-tube for supplemental nutrition.

e. Make meals a pleasant time, unassociated with treatments or unpleasant interruptions. Maintain oral intake as much as possible.

4. Monitor dietary compliance with dietary goals and adjust, as needed.

5. Administer total parenteral nutrition, if necessary.

6. Administer serum albumin or fresh frozen plasma to combat hypoalbuminemia when burn area exceeds 20% TBSA.

7. Monitor nutritional status through weight gain, wound healing, serum transferrin, and serum albumin.

Relieving Gastric Dilation and Preventing Stress Ulcer

1. Be alert for the development of gastric distention, especially with burns greater than 20% TBSA, associated injury, or tachypnea.

2. Maintain nothing-by-mouth status if distention or decreased bowel sounds develop.

3. Insert NG tube, as indicated, to prevent vomiting, aspiration, and paralytic ileus.

4. Monitor the return of bowel sounds after NG extubation and before reinstituting oral feeding.

5. Administer H_2-blockers such as cimetidine to prevent Curling's ulcer development.

Promoting Peripheral Perfusion

1. Remove all jewelry and clothing.

2. Elevate extremities.

3. Monitor peripheral pulses hourly. Use Doppler, as necessary.

4. Prepare the patient for escharotomy if circulation is impaired.

5. Avoid tight constrictive dressings.

6. Observe for and report signs of thrombophlebitis or catheter-induced infections.

Facilitating Fluid Balance

1. Titrate fluid intake as tolerated. The initial resuscitation formula is only a guide.

2. Maintain accurate intake and output records.

3. Weigh the patient daily.

4. Monitor results of serum potassium and other electrolytes.

5. Be alert to signs of fluid overload, especially during initial fluid resuscitation and immediately afterward, when fluid mobilization is occurring.

6. Administer diuretics, as ordered.

Protecting and Reestablishing Skin Integrity

1. Cleanse wounds and change dressings twice daily. Use an antimicrobial solution or mild soap and water. Dry gently. This may be done in the hydrotherapy tank, bathtub, shower, or at the bedside.

2. Perform debridement of dead tissue at this time. May use gauze, scissors, or forceps, as appropriate. Try to limit time to 20 to 30 minutes depending on the patient's tolerance. Additional analgesia may be necessary.

3. Apply topical bacteriostatic agents, as directed. Cream or ointment is applied 1⅛-inch (3-mm) thick.

4. Dress wounds, as appropriate, using conventional burn pads, gauze rolls, or any combination. Dressings may be held in place, as necessary, with gauze rolls or netting.

5. For grafted areas, use extreme caution in removing dressings; observe for and report serous or sanguineous blebs or purulent drainage. Redress grafted areas according to facility protocol.

6. Observe all wounds daily and document wound status on the patient's record.

7. Promote healing of donor sites by:

a. Preventing contamination of donor sites that are clean wounds.

b. Opening to air for drying postoperatively if gauze or impregnated gauze dressing is used. If exudate occurs after the first 24 hours, swab the area for culture and apply an antimicrobial topical cream. If the culture is positive, treatment will be in accord with sensitivities.

c. Following health care provider's or manufacturer's instructions for care of sites dressed with synthetic materials.

d. Allowing dressing to peel off spontaneously.

e. Cleansing healing donor site with mild soap and water when dressings are removed; lubricating site twice daily and as needed.

8. Inspect unburned skin carefully for signs of pressure and breakdown.

Preventing Urinary Infection

1. Maintain closed urinary drainage system and ensure patency. Use a catheter impregnated with an antimicrobial agent whenever possible.

2. Frequently observe color, clarity, and amount of urine.

3. Empty drainage bag per facility protocol.

4. Provide catheter care per facility protocol.

5. Encourage removal of catheter and use of urinal, bedpan, or commode as soon as frequent urine output determinations are not required.

Promoting Stable Body Temperature

1. Be efficient in care; do not expose wounds unnecessarily.

2. Maintain warm ambient temperatures.

3. Use radiant warmers, warming blankets, or adjustment of the bed temperature to keep the patient warm.

4. Obtain urine, sputum, and blood cultures for temperatures above 102° F (38.9° C) rectal or core temperature or if chills are present.

5. Provide a dry top layer for wet dressings to reduce evaporative heat loss.

6. Warm wound cleansing and dressing solutions to body temperature.

7. Use blankets in transporting patient to other areas of the hospital.

8. Administer antipyretics, as prescribed.

Preserving Mobility

1. Make sure that physical and occupational therapy are begun early to facilitate rehabilitation.

2. Child Life professionals can also assist in making therapy and routines child-friendly, thereby increasing the child's participation and ultimately preserving and improving mobility.

3. Encourage range-of-motion exercises, ambulation, and position changes to minimize joint and skin complications.

4. Position joint in opposite direction of expected contracture. Reassess positioning regularly, reconfigure patient room or positioning of bed or television to encourage different positions if patient is bedridden.

5. Apply splints to aid joint positioning and decrease skin contractures and hypertrophy.

6. Apply pressure garments to aid circulation, protect newly healed skin, and prevent and treat hypertrophic scar formation by promoting dermal collagen fiber growth in parallel direction. Encourage the use of pressure garments for as long as 12 to 18 months after injury, until the healed skin has matured.

7. Medicate for pain before therapy or exercise to minimize discomfort.

8. Use play opportunities to help the child accept the therapy program (eg, tricycle riding may be used as form of exercise).

Controlling Pain

 Evidence Base World Health Organization. (2012). WHO's pain ladder. Geneva: Author. Available: *www.who.int/cancer/palliative/painladder/en.*

1. Assess for signs of pain, such as irritability, crying, increased BP, tachycardia, decreased mobility, and inability to sleep using reliable and valid assessment measures.

2. Use principles of the WHO analgesic ladder using combinations of analgesic where one type is ineffective alone until pain relief is achieved.
   a. Step 1: Nonopioids
   b. Step 2: Mild opioids
   c. Step 3: Strong opioids

3. Acetaminophen has been shown to safely manage background pain in pediatric burns and is considered the first step in managing such pain.

4. Regular nonsteroidal anti-inflammatory drugs should also be prescribed unless contraindicated.

5. Opioid analgesia is the gold standard for burn pain and should be dosed for each individual with concurrent laxative treatment provided. Strong (morphine) versus mild (codeine) opioids should be considered for severe pain.

6. In severe burns, analgesia should be given via IV line because of lack of absorption of I.M. injections during the emergency phase. Emphasis is on maintaining an alert, reasonably comfortable child. Monitor child closely when using IV opioids and sedatives.

7. Other adjunctive medications, such as anti-emetics and sedatives, should be considered to increase comfort and decrease distress.

8. Use a therapeutic surface to relieve pressure and provide comfort.

9. Maintain warmth and prevent chilling.

10. Provide diversional activities appropriate for age to distract from focus on pain.

11. Teach simple relaxation techniques, such as relaxation breathing and guided imagery.

12. Recognize that fear may exacerbate discomfort; assess anxiety and child temperament. Provide reassurance and empathy. Develop a plan to minimize anxiety and fear. Collaborate with other health care professional, such as a Child Life therapist.

13. Ensure an adequate sleep routine and establish good sleep hygiene as possible to minimize sleep disturbances.

Addressing Body Image Disturbance

1. Encourage the child to talk about the way he or she feels and looks; let the child set the pace for discussions.
   a. The child may feel guilty and think that the burn is punishment for some wrong deed.
   b. Small children may be fearful of the appearance of bandages, scars, or pressure garments; offer reassurance.
   c. Encourage the use of play with dolls or puppets, role-playing, or picture drawing to help the child express feelings and fears.

2. Treat the child with warmth and affection and encourage parents to continually express their love and provide physical and emotional comfort.

3. Support child in viewing self in mirror when ready and encourage the presence of family members.

4. Encourage early contact with other children. Maintain connections with siblings, friends, and community where possible.

5. Suggest psychiatric consultation and work with psychosocial resources for anticipatory guidance and ongoing adjustment and adaptation to burn injury. Specific requests may be related to heightened anxiety, alterations in mood, or problems manifesting as:
   a. Refusal to eat.
   b. Developmental regression.
   c. Resistance to procedures.
   d. Aggressive behaviors, excessive sadness or withdrawal.
   e. Increasing isolation or resisting socialization.

6. Advise parents that returning to home and community routines and separation from the hospital environment, caregivers,

and other patients can produce excessive anxiety or disruption in the child's coping. Consider a plan to develop a graduated discharge process with time-limited home passes (overnight, weekend), as well as plan for aftercare to support the transition home.

7. If the child is school age, help prepare for school reentry; contact teacher or discuss with parents the need to prepare peers for what to expect.

8. Discuss and plan for issues of social reentry, such as responding to questions and stares from strangers and perceived rejection by friends.
   a. Ensure enrollment in an aftercare (follow-up) program, ideally one that is targeted at both child and family adjustment.
   b. Refer to a support group or peer mentor where possible.
   c. Refer to a burn camp—usually this may be the first opportunity for the child to wear a swimsuit after the injury.

9. Initiate family consultation with a plastic surgeon about future scar revision.

10. Encourage the older child to engage in long-term follow-up to address issues of concern as they arise at various developmental stages. Some children and teens may wish to experiment with clothing and consult with a burn cosmetic specialist to enhance appearance and body image.

Reducing Fear and Anxiety

1. Explain procedures, surgeries, and treatments to the child according to age and level of understanding.

2. Allow the child to express fears through puppets, dolls, water play, clay, and drawings.

3. Expect regression due to the physical pain and psychological trauma the child is experiencing.

4. Encourage parents to stay with a young child as much as possible.

5. Teach parents how to engage their child to foster development of coping skills.

6. Encourage involvement with treatment plan and self-care activities.

Promoting Effective Parenting

1. Be alert to signs of depression or stress syndromes in parents and encourage counseling for them to promote a healthier family.

2. Encourage parents to assess the effects on siblings at home; they may have needs that are unrecognized or neglected as a result of this crisis.

3. Attempt to have parents become actively involved in the child's care when they are ready to do so.
   a. Provide training for parents to effectively participate in treatments and respect their wishes not to participate if the situation is too distressful—the focus for parents is on their ability to comfort their child.
   b. Advise parents that their visits and involvement can have a positive effect on the child's survival and recovery.
   c. If the parents are unable to visit, telephone calls and family photographs are helpful. New technologies like video conferencing can also be helpful to maintain connections with family and community supports.

4. Give the parents the opportunity to discuss their feelings.
   a. Parents commonly express guilt regarding their lack of supervision when the accident occurred.
   b. Typically, burn injury is associated with actual or perceived parental neglect. Remember that this type of injury is sudden and acute, placing the family in a state of crisis.

5. Keep the parents informed of the child's progress.
   a. Begin initial teaching at admission with supportive words and limited technical information.
   b. Education and orientation to the facility and the burn injury will decrease some anxiety and begin to build rapport on which future support can be based.
   c. Encourage meetings with other parents who have coped with trauma.
   d. Refer families for aftercare programs intended to support adjustment over time.

Sleep Pattern Disturbance

1. Allow a parent to stay with the patient.

2. Provide a structured environment. Perform dressing changes, therapy, and meals at the same time everyday.

3. Combine interventions so that child can get longest possible intervals of uninterrupted sleep.

4. Minimize noise and lights within room.

5. Ensure adequate pain relief and comfort measures at bedtime or naptime.

Community and Home Care Considerations

1. Make routine home visits to perform, teach, and supervise burn wound care and rehabilitation program.

2. Inspect the wounds for signs of infection at every visit.

3. Assess coping ability of child and family to care for child and provide psychological support and counseling referrals, as needed.

4. Make sure that parents can:
   a. Discuss and demonstrate treatments, procedures, and dressing changes.
   b. Obtain equipment necessary to perform treatment at home.
   c. Understand reason for and adverse effects of medications as well as dietary requirements.
   d. Follow up at appropriate intervals with the designated health care provider.

5. Encourage the use of smoke alarms on every floor in the home, a fire extinguisher, and an emergency fire escape plan. Assist parents to review strategies for childhood safety.

Family Education and Health Maintenance

1. Teach the family that special skin care is necessary after burn injury.
   a. Avoid exposure to sunlight; use sunscreen with sun protective factor 24 or higher and apply frequently.
   b. Use pressure garments to prevent hypertrophic scar formation—worn 23 of 24 hours each day for effectiveness for 1 to 2 years depending on the maturation of the scar.
   c. Use lotions and creams to prevent skin from drying, cracking, and itching; topical or oral antihistamines or antipruritics may be necessary to reduce itching.

    d. Burn area has decreased sensation to touch, heat, and pressure; take precautions to prevent injury to area.

2. Advise the family that adjustment after burn is usually prolonged and painful. Adjustment can ebb and flow with developmental stages. Encourage ongoing family and individual psychological and social support.

3. Encourage continued physical therapy to prevent and minimize contractures and preserve function.

4. Monitor outcomes over time in keeping with the Health Outcomes Burn Questionnaire for Infants and Children 5 years of Age and Younger; burn size and visible scarring are not predictive of psychological adaptation.

5. Initiate home health, psychiatric referral, physical and occupational therapy, financial assistance, and other referrals, as necessary.

6. Teach parents and children the prevention of burn injury as well as other safety measures (see page 1422).

7. Teach first-aid emergency care for burn injury (ie, cool burned area with cool water, remove clothing, seek medical assistance).

8. Teach children how to stop, drop, and roll if their clothes catch on fire and how to crawl to safety if a fire occurs in the house.

Evaluation: Expected Outcomes

- Absence of shock: stabilization of vital signs, normal serum and electrolyte values.
- Absence of infection: normal laboratory values, clean wound, and normal temperature.
- No respiratory distress: stable vital signs, respiratory status, and ABG levels.
- Adequate nutritional status: weight gain and wound healing.
- No GI complications: normal bowel sounds and ability to tolerate oral feeding.
- Tissue perfusion.
- No signs of fluid overload, weight stable.
- Donor site and burn wounds healing without signs of infection.
- Urine output adequate via catheter.
- Temperature remains below 102° F (38.9° C).
- Improved mobility: involved in play and other activities.
- Minimal discomfort: stable vital signs, verbalization, and involved in play.
- Positive body image: verbalization, socialization, and ability to look in mirror.
- Relief of fear: able to play, participates in care.
- Effective parenting: involved in child's care, accurate discussion of child's progress and treatment plan.
- Sleeping between treatments through the night and napping for 1-hour intervals during the day.

DERMATOLOGIC DISORDERS

Atopic Dermatitis (Infantile and Childhood Eczema)

Atopic dermatitis, the most common cause of eczema in childhood, is a highly pruritic chronic inflammatory skin disorder affecting 15% to 25% of the pediatric population. Peak prevalence is age 6 months to 8 to 10 years. Ninety-five percent of children with atopic dermatitis have asthma or allergic rhinitis. It is an abnormal immune response to environmental allergens in a genetically susceptible individual. These individuals tend to have dry skin and a lower threshold for itching. Itching leads to scratching, which causes lichenification or skin thickening, creating increased sensitivity to renewed itching. Many children with atopic dermatitis have a personal or family history of disorders in the atopic triad (allergic rhinitis, asthma, and atopic dermatitis). During the past three decades, the incidence of atopic dermatitis has increased, especially in industrialized nations. Possible causes include urban migration, increased antibiotic use, and decreased incidence of early childhood infections.

Atopic dermatitis has a typical age-related morphology and distribution and a chronic or chronically relapsing nature. By age 5, 90% of patients who will develop atopic dermatitis have already manifested the disease. The appearance and location of the lesions change with age in a characteristic manner. Atopic dermatitis usually improves or resolves by adolescence but can persist in some form throughout adulthood. Hand dermatitis is a common finding in adults with a history of atopic dermatitis.

Pathophysiology and Etiology

1. Although it has both immunologic and genetic components, the etiology of atopic dermatitis is unknown. Approximately 80% of children with atopic dermatitis have elevated immunoglobulin (Ig) E levels and increased rates of sensitization to common allergens. Histamine release from basophils is increased, and hyperreactive cutaneous T cells, which secrete proinflammatory cytokines, cause increased Th2 and decreased Th1 cytokine responses. There is also a hereditary component. When both parents have a history of atopic dermatitis, there is an 80% chance a child will be affected. When only one parent is affected, the prevalence drops to 50%. A number of genes have been tentatively linked to atopic dermatitis.

2. Atopic dermatitis causes breakdown of the statum corneum, which allows allergens and bacteria to penetrate deeper layers, causing inflammation and possible infection.

3. Atopic dermatitis is known as the "itch that rashes." The skin is dry and becomes pruritic when exposed to common environmental allergens, such as wool; occlusive synthetic fabrics, soaps, and detergents; perspiration; extremes of temperature and humidity; and emotional stress.

4. Food allergies contribute to atopic dermatitis in up to 30% of infants and very young children with moderate to severe disease. Eggs, milk, peanut, soy, wheat, tree nuts, fish, and shellfish account for more than 90% of the reactions. The most common offender is eggs.

5. One third to one half of children with atopic dermatitis are allergic to house dust mites, animal dander, weeds, and molds.

6. Children with atopic dermatitis are at increased risk for developing allergic rhinitis or asthma, known as the "atopic march" or "atopic triad."

Clinical Manifestations

Age and Distribution of Lesions

Atopic dermatitis is divided into three phases based on the age of the patient and the distribution of the lesions. These are referred to as the infant, childhood, and adult phases.

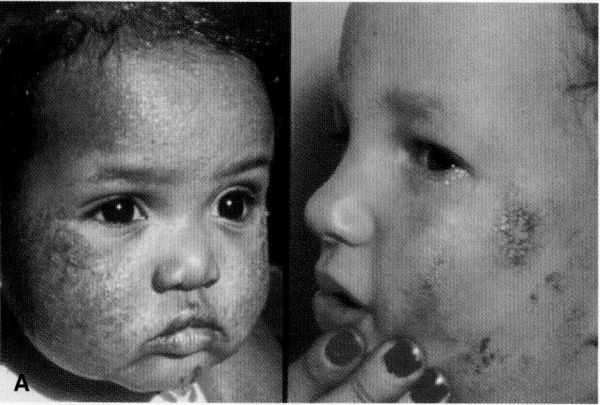
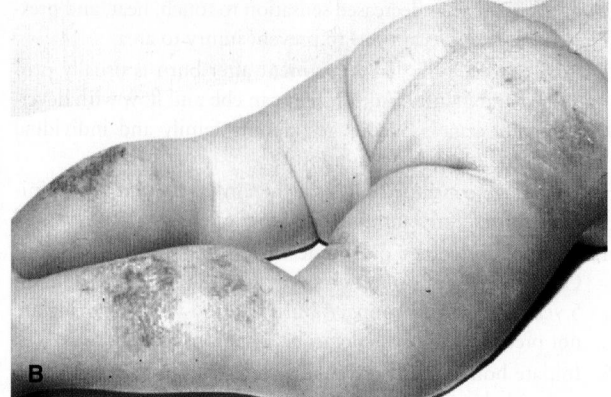

Figure 55-2. Characteristic rash of infant atopic dermatitis of the head **(A)** and of the limbs **(B)**. (Courtesy of Schering.)

1. Infant (age 2 months to 3 years):
   a. The onset is between ages 2 and 6 months. One half of affected infants have spontaneous resolution by age 2 or 3.
   b. Characterized by intense itching, erythema, papules, vesicles, oozing, and crusting (see Figure 55-2).
   c. The rash usually begins on the cheeks, forehead, or scalp and then extends to the trunk or extremities in scattered, commonly symmetric patches. The perioral, paranasal, and diaper areas are usually spared (see Figure 55-3).
2. Childhood (ages 4 to 10):
   a. Affected people in this age group are less likely to have exudative and crusted lesions. Eruptions are characteristically more dry and papular and commonly occur as circumscribed scaly patches. There is a greater tendency toward chronicity and lichenification.

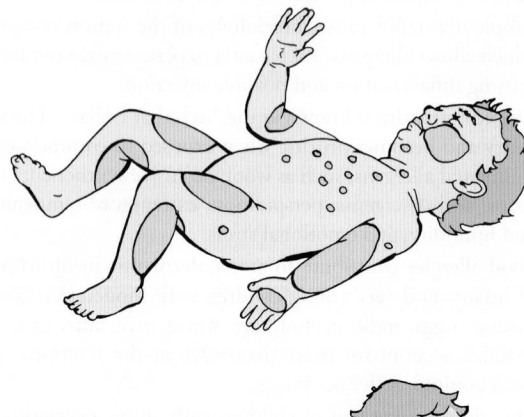

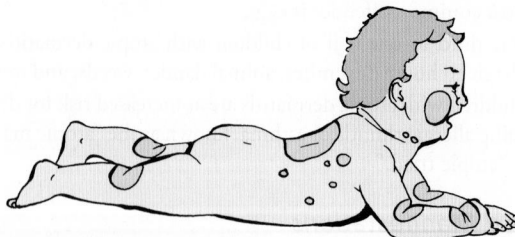

Figure 55-3. Distribution of infant atopic dermatitis occurs primarily on the face but may develop on symmetrical areas of the body. Diaper areas are usually clear.

b. The typical areas of involvement are the face, including the perioral and paranasal areas, neck, antecubital and popliteal fossae, wrists, and ankles. May have severe pruritus.
3. Adult (puberty to old age):
   a. Predominant areas of involvement include the flexor folds, face, neck, upper arms, back, dorsa of the hands and feet, fingers, and toes.
   b. The eruption appears as thick, dry lesions, confluent papules, and large lichenified plaques. Weeping, crusting, and exudation can occur, but they are usually the result of superimposed external irritation or infection.

Clinical Appearance

Atopic dermatitis is also divided into three stages based on the clinical appearance of the lesions. The acute, subacute, and chronic stages can occur in infants, children, and adults.

1. Acute (see Figure 55-4A)—moderate to intense erythema, vesicles, a wet surface, and severe itching.
2. Subacute:
   a. Erythema and scaling are present in various patterns with indistinct borders. The redness may be faint or intense. The surface is dry. There are varying degrees of pruritus.
   b. The subacute stage may be an initial stage or may follow an acute inflammation or exacerbation of a chronic stage. Irritation, allergy, or infection can convert a subacute process into an acute one.
3. Chronic (see Figure 55-4B)—the inflamed area thickens and the surface skin markings become more prominent. Thick plaques with deep parallel skin markings are called *lichenified*. Lichenification is the hallmark of chronic eczema. The surface of the skin is dry and the border of the lesion well defined. There is moderate to intense itching. There may be post-inflammatory hypopigmentation.

Diagnostic Evaluation

1. There is no single clinical, laboratory, or histologic marker that will definitively diagnose atopic dermatitis. It is a clinical diagnosis based on the evaluation of the aggregate of signs, symptoms, stigmata, course, and associated familial findings. The presence of pruritus, recurring symptoms, and age-specific

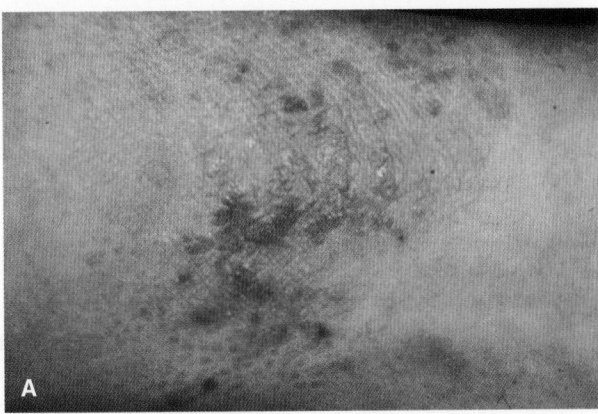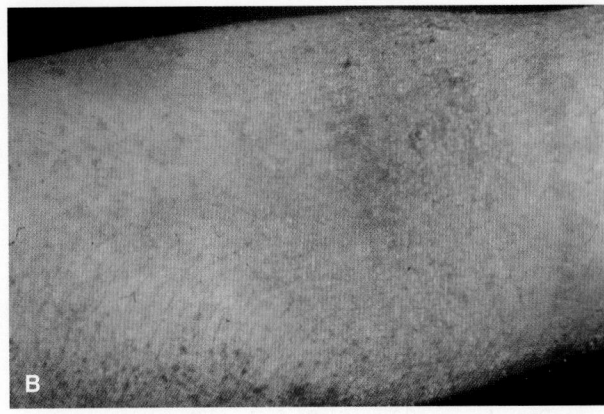

Figure 55-4. **(A)** Acute atopic dermatitis. **(B)** Chronic atopic dermatitis. (Courtesy of Schering.)

morphology and distribution are the most important diagnostic features. Several sets of clinical diagnostic criteria have been established. See Box 55-1.

2. Although not diagnostic for atopic dermatitis, prick skin testing, patch testing, and radioallergosorbent test may be helpful in the identification of food and aeroallergen triggers in infants and young children with moderate to severe disease. Negative skin prick sensitivity tests eliminate the possibility of IgE-mediated food allergy. Positive tests, which predict 30% to 50% of food allergies, may be useful. To avoid unnecessary dietary restrictions, positive tests should be confirmed by controlled food challenges, elimination diets, or atopy patches.

Treatment

 Evidence Base Nicol, N. H. (2011). Efficacy and safety considerations in topical treatment for atopic dermatitis. *Pediatric Nursing, 37*(6), 295–301.

Daily skin care is the cornerstone of prevention and treatment, including proper cleansing, moisturizing, and protection from triggers.

Acute

1. Open, wet dressings, such as Burrows solution, for 1 to 3 days.
2. Avoidance of known allergen or trigger. Atopic dermatitis patients have decreased threshold to irritants.
3. Management of secondary infection.
4. Topical corticosteroids:
   a. Topical corticosteroids are the mainstay of drug therapy. These agents are ranked into seven groups according to potency. Group 1 contains the most potent topical steroids and group 7 the least potent agents. The concentration listed on the medication does not correlate with its potency or safety, but is merely a statement of its specific chemical formulation. Adverse effects are related to the potency rating of the compound, the duration of use, and the thickness of the skin to which it is applied.
   b. Group 1 topical corticosteroids are avoided in children younger than age 12 because of greater skin absorption.

 DRUG ALERT Topical corticosteroids of adequate strength should be used two to four times per day for a specific length of time, such as 7 to 21 days, in order to achieve control and avoid adverse effects. Long-term use of topical corticosteroids can cause striae, cutaneous atrophy, telangiectasia, acne, growth retardation, adrenal suppression, Cushing's syndrome, and cataracts.

BOX 55-1 | **Clinical Criteria for Atopic Dermatitis**

MAJOR FEATURES: THREE OR MORE
- Pruritus
- Eczematous changes
- Typical and age-specific morphology and location
- Face, neck, and extensor surfaces in infants/children
- Flexural lesions in older children/adults
- Chronicity or chronically relapsing
- Personal or family history of atopy (allergic rhinitis, asthma, atopic dermatitis)

MINOR FEATURES: THREE OR MORE
- Early age of onset
- Elevated serum immunoglobulin E
- Itching with sweating
- Intolerance to wool and lipid solvents
- Immediate (type 1) skin test reactivity
- Tendency toward skin infections
- Facial pallor or erythema
- Food intolerance
- Xerosis (very dry skin)
- Ichthyosis/palmar hyperlinearity/keratosis pilaris
- Hand or foot dermatitis
- Pityriasis alba (white patches on face)
- Conjunctivitis
- Severity of symptoms influenced by environmental or emotional factors

5. Oral medications to relieve itching—hydroxyzine, diphenhydramine, or promethazine. Diphenhydramine and promethazine cause more sedation than hydroxyzine. Mild sedation may be desirable to allow sleep.

Subacute and Chronic

1. Prevention of dry skin:
   a. Diminish the frequency and duration of bathing.
   b. Use mild soap or hydrophilic cleanser.
   c. Lubricate the skin with emollients. Apply within 3 minutes after exiting bath. Apply over, not under, topical corticosteroids. Newer barrier repair moisturizers contain the skin lipid ceramide and help rebuild/repair skin. (Some over-the-counter products are CeraVe, Cetaphil Restoderm, and Eucerin Professional Repair.)
   d. Maintain environmental humidity above 40% during winter months.
   e. Tar preparations may be added to bath water; however, they are rarely used due to odor and staining.
2. Avoidance of known allergens or triggers.
3. Management of secondary infection.
4. Topical corticosteroids as described above. Apply the least potent topical corticosteroid that provides adequate control. Topical corticosteroids may be applied under occlusion, which is under plastic wrap to increase absorption, for short-term therapy.
5. Topical immunomodulators, also called *calcineurin inhibitors*, are approved for the short-term and intermittent long-term treatment of subacute and chronic atopic dermatitis for patients age 2 and older when conventional therapies are inadvisable, ineffective, or not tolerated.
   a. Tacrolimus 0.03% ointment and pimecrolimus 1% cream.
   b. These agents do not cause skin atrophy (which corticosteroids may cause) and can be used on the face and neck. However, they are expensive and their long-term safety is unknown.
   c. Active viral, bacterial, or fungal skin infections must be cleared before use.
   d. Topical immunomodulators should be discontinued if lymphadenopathy of unknown etiology develops.

 DRUG ALERT The U.S. Food and Drug Administration issued a black-box warning for *calcineurin inhibitors* stating long-term safety has not been established. Although causal relationship has not been proven, rare cases of malignancy (skin and lymphoma) have been reported. Drugs should be used for short-term, second-line therapy for patients over 2 years of age.

Complications

1. Increased risk of secondary infection by bacterial, viral, or fungal agents. Bacterial infections are typically caused by *Staphylococcus aureus*. Rate of infection with methicillin-resistant *S. aureus* is increasing. Infections secondary to papilloma viruses (warts), molluscum contagiosum, herpes simplex, tinea, and candida are more common.

2. Adverse effects from topical corticosteroids (folliculitis, skin atrophy) or topical immunomodulators (local reactions, acne).

Nursing Assessment

1. Take a nursing history focusing on clinical manifestations:
   a. Onset and duration of rash.
   b. Location, course, and distribution of lesions.
   c. Change in morphology of lesions.
   d. Previous episodes of rashes.
   e. Local and systemic symptoms, especially itching.
   f. Exposure to possible allergens or triggers, especially wool, occlusive synthetic fabrics, soaps, detergents, perspiration, extremes of temperature and humidity, emotional stress, and certain foods in infants and toddlers.
   g. Personal history of allergies, asthma, or allergic rhinitis.
   h. Family history of eczema, asthma, or allergic rhinitis.
   i. Medications, treatments tried, and their effect.
   j. Diet for possible triggers.
2. Perform a physical assessment.
   a. Examine the entire skin in an orderly fashion with specific attention to the type of lesion (ie, macule, papule, or vesicle), its appearance (shape, border, color, texture, and surface), and its distribution (areas of the body involved).
   b. Note associated symptoms, such as scratching, fever, or drainage.
   c. Assess patient for signs of other atopic disorders, including nasal congestion, mouth breathing, cough, or wheezing.
   d. Palpate for lymphadenopathy.
3. Document findings:
   a. Describe skin findings using dermatologic terminology.
   b. Draw pictures to facilitate communication.
   c. Document presence or absence of associated signs or symptoms.

Nursing Diagnoses

- Impaired Skin Integrity or Risk for Impaired Skin Integrity related to skin pathology and scratching.
- Deficient Knowledge related to identification and elimination of triggers.
- Impaired Comfort related to itching.
- Risk for Infection related to increased bacterial colonization of skin and possible break in defensive barrier.

Nursing Interventions

The nurse may perform the following interventions or teach patient or family to do them.

Improving Skin Integrity

1. Reduce inflammation during the acute stage with the topical application of open wet dressings.
   a. Use a soft, lightweight cloth, such as a handkerchief, a thin cloth diaper, or strips of bed sheeting. Do not use gauze (adheres to skin), washcloths, or towels (too heavy). Warm moist pajamas layered under dry pajamas are effective and soothing.

b. Open wet dressings should be clean. In certain situations, they should be sterile to prevent contamination.

c. Solutions should be lukewarm or at body temperature to soothe the skin and prevent chilling.

d. Compresses should be moderately wet, not dripping, and removed after 20 minutes, unless otherwise directed. They should be reapplied three to four times per day.

e. After the compress, a topical corticosteroid may be applied to further reduce itching and inflammation.

f. Observe the skin for changes in response to therapy.

2. Prevent dry skin during the subacute and chronic stages.

a. Decrease the frequency and duration of bathing. Long, hot tub baths should be avoided.

b. Avoid hot water and harsh soaps. Patients should bathe in lukewarm water using mild soap with a neutral pH (eg, Dove, Neutrogena); avoid bubble baths; rinse well and pat skin dry with towel.

c. If bath water stings, add 1 cup of table salt.

d. Apply unscented emollients (eg, Eucerin, Keri, Aquaphor, and Lubriderm) within 3 minutes of bathing, when the skin is still slightly moist. Apply over topical medications. This traps water in the skin. Creams and ointments are more effective than lotions because they are better at preventing evaporation of water from the skin.

e. Some patients may benefit from soaking in a tar bath for 15 to 20 minutes daily, preferably in the evening. Add to bath water as directed. Instructions must include the ability to stain the skin and clothing and cause sunlight sensitivity.

f. For patients with extremely dry skin, clean with a hydrophilic cleanser (eg, Cetaphil). Apply without water until light foam occurs. Remove by wiping with soft cotton cloth or cleansing tissue.

g. Keep environmental humidity above 40% during winter months. Use a humidifier.

h. Observe the skin for changes in response to therapy.

 NURSING ALERT Apply unscented emollients to the skin within 3 minutes of bathing when the skin has been patted dry but is still moist to maintain a high level of hydration to the epidermis.

Identifying and Eliminating Triggering Factors

1. Employ these interventions to prevent food allergies.

a. Follow the American Academy of Pediatrics guidelines of delaying the introduction of solid foods until age 5 to 7 months and dairy products until age 12 months. Eggs should be delayed until age 24 months, and the most allergenic foods—peanuts, tree nuts, and seafood—until age 36 months.

 Evidence Base Burks, A. W., Tang, M., Sicherer, S., et al. (2012). ICON: Food allergy. *Journal of Allergy and Clinical Immunology, 129*(4), 906–920.

b. Encourage breastfeeding during the first 6 months. For infants not breastfed, extensively or partially hydrolyzed formulas (Nutramigen, Alimentum) are preferable to cow's-milk formula.

2. Eliminate trigger foods for infants and toddlers with known or suspected food allergies.

a. Observe skin for flare-ups after exposure to potential allergens.

b. Suggest referral to allergy specialist for infants and young children with moderate to severe atopic dermatitis.

c. Be aware of the results of skin prick sensitivity, patch testing, or blood testing.

d. Record known allergens on chart and care plan.

e. Notify dietary department, caregivers, school personnel of food allergies.

f. Consult with dietitian to ensure a balanced diet that excludes identified allergens.

g. Check food for known allergens before feedings.

h. Prevent accidental ingestion by informing visitors of food allergies and keeping offending foods from patient.

i. Teach parents and caregivers to read food labels for the elimination of offending food proteins.

j. Assess compliance with prescribed diet and relief of symptoms.

3. Be aware of environmental triggers.

a. Maintain a warm climate with moderate humidity.

b. Dress child in soft, lightweight cotton clothing. Avoid wool and occlusive synthetic fabrics. A new type of non-irritating, antimicrobial fabric impregnated with silver is useful as a sleep garment.

c. Avoid harsh soap and hot water. Avoid fabric softeners. Use fragrance-free and dye-free detergents.

d. Prevent excessive sweating.

e. Discourage smoking in child's presence.

4. Try to alleviate stress.

a. Encourage parents to stay with young child as much as possible.

b. Involve child in age-appropriate diversional activities.

Controlling Pruritus

1. Apply topical corticosteroids.

a. Apply a thin layer of topical corticosteroids to the affected skin two to four times per day, as directed. Use only for the duration prescribed. Apply under emollients.

b. Observe for possible adverse effects from long-term use of topical corticosteroids (ie, striae, cutaneous atrophy, telangiectasia, acne, and growth retardation).

c. Note scratching and intervene, as necessary.

2. Apply topical immunomodulators.

a. Assess skin for active viral, bacterial, or fungal infection before use.

b. Apply a thin layer of topical calcineurin inhibitors to the affected dry skin twice per day, as directed.

c. Do not apply to wet or occluded skin.

d. Observe patient for possible adverse effects including burning, itching, and erythema. Check for lymphadenopathy.

e. Instruct family to have child use sunscreen to decrease exposure to ultraviolet light and sunlight.

f. Note scratching and apply age-appropriate interventions.

3. Administer oral antipruritic medications.

a. Give medications exactly as prescribed.

b. Note the degree of sedation and presence of scratching.

Preventing Infection

1. Assess and treat secondary infection.

a. Observe the skin for signs of bacterial, viral, or fungal infection (discharge, oozing, crusts, increased redness, fever). Report any positive findings.

b. Administer medications, as prescribed.

c. Loosen exudate and crusts with water or wet dressings, unless otherwise specified.

d. Note changes in the skin in response to therapy.

Family Education and Health Maintenance

1. Teach patient and family to avoid potential precipitants, including:

a. Exposure to excessive heat and cold or extremes of humidity.

b. Contact with wool and occlusive synthetic fabrics. Soft, lightweight cotton fabrics are preferred. Infants should not be allowed to crawl on wool carpeting.

c. Participation in strenuous athletic activities that promote sweating. Activities should be modified according to the needs of the child. Swimming is recommended in chlorinated pools, although bromine in pool water may be irritating. The child should shower afterward and apply a lubricant or other topical medication.

 NURSING ALERT   Advise family that fresh water (pond, lake, river) should be avoided if child has breaks in skin integrity, due to risk of infection.

d. Use of irritating soaps, perfumes, detergents, and chemicals.

Table 55-1	Common Pediatric Skin Problems

DISORDER/ORGANISM	CLINICAL MANIFESTATIONS

Impetigo
 	
Bacterial infectious disease affecting the superficial layers of the skin and characterized by the formation of vesicles, honey-colored crusts, or bullae.
Etiology and incidence:
• Caused by *Staphylococcus aureus* and *Streptococcus pyogenes*. Occurs most commonly when personal hygiene is poor.
• Common in children younger than age 10.
• Spread by close contact—easily conveyed from person to person via hands, nasal discharge, shared towels, toys; plastic wading pools in summer—when water is not replaced and no disinfectant is used; highly contagious.
• An abrasion of skin may serve as a portal of entry.
Diagnosis:
• Usually clinical.
• Rarely, a culture of the lesion's exudate is indicated to confirm the diagnosis.
	• Incubation period is 1–10 days.
	• Lesion first appears as pink-red macules that quickly change to vesicles, which, in turn, rupture, develop crusts, and leave a temporary superficial erythematous area.
	  • Bullous (neonate and older child)—large, thin-roofed blisters break to form thin, light-brown crusts. Lesions may occur anywhere on the body but are more common on the face, axillae, and groin.
	  • Crusted (preschool age—seen more commonly in summer on exposed body parts)—lesions appear with thick, yellow crusts; skin around crusts is red and weeping with satellite lesions.
	• Regional lymphadenopathy is common with secondary infection of insect bites, eczema, poison ivy, and scabies.
	• Autoinoculation is major cause of spreading.
	• Pruritus may occur.

Ringworm of the Scalp (Tinea Capitis)
 	
(See page 1168 for ringworm of the body [Tinea corporis]) A fungal infection of the scalp and hair follicles
Etiology and incidence:
• Most ringworm of the scalp is caused by *Trichophyton tonsurans*. *Microsporum canis* and *Microsporum audouinii* are also causative agents.
• Is seen primarily in children before puberty (usually ages 3–10).
• May be spread through child-to-child contact as well as through the common use of towels, pillows, combs, brushes, and hats. Cats and dogs may also be the source of the infection.
	• The lesions appear on the scalp in a variety of ways:
	  • One or more patchy areas of dandruff like scaling with little or extensive alopecia (hair loss).
	  • One or more discrete areas of alopecia with tiny broken hairs.
	  • Numerous discrete pustules or excoriations with little alopecia.
	  • A kerion or boggy, tender, inflammatory mass that produces edema and pustules.
	• Pruritus usually occurs in the involved area.

e. Avoidance of stressful situations, when possible.

f. Foods that are associated with skin reactions (see "Food Allergies," page 1031).

g. Identified other allergens such as pets, live Christmas trees, cigarette smoke, stuffed animals, and objects that harbor dust.

2. Encourage mothers to breast-feed and follow a hypoallergenic diet to decrease the risk of atopic dermatitis.

3. Advise parents and caregivers to follow the American Academy of Pediatrics guidelines of delaying the introduction of solid foods until age 6 months and dairy products until age 12 months for infants at risk for food allergies.

4. Make sure that the family knows the common triggers to avoid, how to prevent dry skin, signs of flares or secondary infection, when to apply topical medications, and the need for routine follow-up appointments.

5. Recommend consultation with dermatology specialist for children with severe or persistent atopic dermatitis.

6. Suggest locating additional information from the following websites:

a. American Academy of Dermatology (*www.aad.org*)

b. American Academy of Pediatrics (*www.aap.org*)

c. National Eczema Society (*www.eczema.org*)

7. Stress the importance of regular health maintenance examinations, immunizations, and preventive practices.

Evaluation: Expected Outcomes

- Skin intact with minimal erythema and lichenification.
- Names common triggers and avoidance measures.
- Verbalizes less itching; less scratching observed.
- No signs of secondary infection.

Other Dermatologic Disorders

See Table 55-1.

TREATMENT/PREVENTION	NURSING CONSIDERATIONS

Based on etiology and type of infection.
- Gently wash affected area with soap and water three times per day.
- Crusts and debris can be removed from the affected area by gentle soaking or wet compresses. Use tap water, normal saline, or 1:20 Burrow's solution.
* If indicated, obtain lipid drainage or debris for culture before antibiotics are provided.
- Apply topical antibacterial medication, such as bacitracin or mupirocin ointment or retapamulin.
- Systemic antibiotics (cephalosporins, erythromycin, or dicloxacillin) if widespread or recurrent.
- Methicillin-resistant *S. aureus* infection is common.
- Prevention—close contact with other children should be avoided until 24 hours after treatment is initiated.
	- Assess the child's skin condition and document the location and appearance of lesions. Note new lesions.
	- Initiate and teach measures to prevent the spread of infection.
	  - Engage in frequent hand washing. Use separate towels.
	  - Daily bathing with soap and water. Regular laundering for contaminated bed linens, towels, and clothing.
	  - Observe drainage and secretion precautions for 24 hours after the start of therapy.
	  - Isolate the child from direct contact with other children (school or day care) until 24 hours after treatment has started.
	  - Trim fingernails and toenails. Apply small amount of bacitracin or mupirocin ointment under the fingernails to prevent the spread of infection.
	  - Engage the child in diversional activities to discourage scratching.
	- Be aware that the patient with streptococcal impetigo has an increased risk of acute glomerulonephritis.

- Micronized griseofulvin—an antifungal antibiotic that is administered orally, 15–20 mg/kg/day (maximum 1 g) in a single dose with a high-fat food for 4–12 weeks. Some children may require higher doses or micronized griseofulvin 20–25 mg/kg/day or ultra-micronized griseofulvin 5–10 mg/kg/day (maximum 750 mg). - Topical antifungal medicines are not effective. Selenium sulfide lotion 2.5% used twice per week decreases fungal shedding and may curb the spread of infection. - Treatment should be continued for 2 weeks after clinical resolution.	- Assess the scalp for characteristic lesions. - Administer or teach the patient and family to administer medications as prescribed. - Be aware of adverse effects, such as headache, heartburn, nausea, epigastric discomfort, diarrhea, urticaria, photosensitivity, and possible granulocytopenia caused by griseofulvin. - Griseofulvin is absorbed more efficiently with a fatty meal. Children can be given the medicine once per day with ice cream or peanut butter. - Liver function monitoring may be required for prolonged treatment (greater than 6 months) or for children with baseline abnormal liver functiion.

(continued)

Table 55-1   Common Pediatric Skin Problems (*continued*)

DISORDER/ORGANISM	CLINICAL MANIFESTATIONS
Ringworm of the Scalp (Tinea Capitis) (*continued*) *Diagnosis:* • Hair or skin scrapings for microscopic evaluation or fungal culture, obtained by rubbing a swab or toothbrush over the affected area. *Differential diagnosis:* • Tinea amiantacea, lichen planopilaris, and perifolliculitis capitis abscendens et suffodiens must be ruled out clinically or histologically. Woods lamp inspection has limited benefit.	

Pediculosis
 	
Infestation of humans by lice.
Etiology:
• Three types of lice affect human beings:
  • *Pediculosis capitis* (head lice)—commonly infests school-age children.
  • *Pediculosis corporis* (body lice)—rare in the United States.
  • *Pediculosis pubis* (pubic or crab lice)—common in sexually active adolescents or adults—can be found on pubic hair, chest hair, axillary hair, eyebrows, eyelashes, and beards.
• Each type of louse generally remains in the area designated by its name.
• Lice are transmitted by personal contact with people harboring them or through contact with articles that temporarily harbor them (clothing or bed linens).
• Head and pubic lice are not health hazards or signs of uncleanliness. Only body lice can transmit disease.
Diagnosis:
• Identification of lice or their eggs with the naked eye confirmed by using a hand lens or microscope.
• In active infection of head or pubic lice, nits and eggs are found on the hair shaft within 1 cm of the skin and are difficult to remove.
• Body lice and their eggs are found in the seams of undergarments.
	• Itching in the area affected is the primary symptom of pediculosis. Scratch marks may be evident in these areas. However, not all affected people itch.
	• Other signs of infestation are pillows or clothing that look unusually dirty.
	• Infested scalp areas may become secondarily infected from scratching.
	• Crusts, lice, nits, eggs, and dirt may combine to cause a foul odor and matted hair.
	• Body lice may produce minute red lesions.

TREATMENT/PREVENTION	NURSING CONSIDERATIONS

• Treatment with oral itraconazole, oral terbinafine, or oral fluconazole is effective, but only terbinafine has been approved by the Food and Drug Administration for this disorder.	• Teach the child and family methods to prevent further episodes.
	  • Teach general hygiene measures—regular shampooing and bathing.
	  • Advise them to avoid sharing hats, combs, brushes, pillows.
	  • Routine cleaning of heavily contaminated articles, such as pillowcases, sheets, towels, hats, bike helmets, combs, brushes.
	  • All family members and close contacts should be screened for tinea infections. The child's school should be notified to facilitate the screening of classmates.
	• Hair loss is usually temporary, except in some cases with a kerion, when the hair follicles may have been destroyed.
	• Child may attend school after treatment has been initiated. Hats are not necessary.

• Pediculosis capitis and Pediculosis pubis may be treated with over-the-counter agents, such as permethrin or natural pyrethrin-based products. Lindane 1% (Rx) is indicated for second-line therapy only. Natural pyrethrin-based products and lindane may be reapplied 7–10 days later. Lindane should be avoided in children younger than age 2, people with known seizures, and pregnant or lactating women.
• For infestation of eyelashes by crab lice, petroleum jelly applied twice daily to the eyelashes for 8 to 10 days is effective.
• Pediculicides are not necessary for the treatment of Pediculosis corporis. Washing infested clothing and linens, where the lice harbor, in hot water and machine drying (on hot cycle) is adequate.
• Because pediculicides kill lice shortly after application, the detection of living lice on scalp inspection 24 hours or more after treatment suggests incorrect use, reinfection, or resistance. Immediate retreatment with a different pediculicide followed by a second application 7 days later is recommended.
• A suffocation-based pediculicide (DSP) lotion applied and then blown dry with a hair dryer weekly for up to 3 weeks effectively treats 95% of head lice. The hair can be shampooed 8 hours after application. The lotion is not visible and the hair can be styled.
• Studies of the efficacy of suffocation of lice by the application of occlusive agents, such as petroleum jelly, olive oil, or mayonnaise, have not been performed. Cotrimoxazole and ivermectin have been shown to be effective, but neither is approved by the FDA as a pediculicide.
• "No nit" policies requiring children to be free from nits for the return to school do not reduce transmission and are not recommended.
• Shaving head is not necessary.
	• Administer or teach administration of antiparasitic as directed. Natural pyrethrin-based products work best on dry hair. Avoid shampoo, cream rinses, and conditioners before application.
	• Although both pyrethrins and permethrin are quite safe, limit exposure to the skin by rinsing the hair in a sink rather than the shower and use cool water to minimize absorption from vasodilation.
	• Removal of nits with a fine-tooth comb may be attempted for aesthetic reasons or to decrease diagnostic confusion. However, mechanical removal of nits after treatment does not prevent spread.
	• Inspect the scalp (or have the family inspect the scalp) 24–48 hours after treatment to see what lice remain. The presence of large lice may mean that the treatment was ineffective or that the lice are resistant.
	• Provide appropriate teaching for the family to prevent recurrences.
	  • Wash clothing, bed linens, and towels in hot water and machine dry (on hot cycle). Temperature above 128.3° F (53.5° C) for 5 minutes will kill lice and eggs. Dry cleaning or simply storing contaminated articles in a well-sealed plastic bag for 10 days is also effective.
	  • Teach children not to share combs, brushes, head gear or hats. Combs and brushes can be disinfected by soaking in hot water for 10 minutes or washing with a pediculicide shampoo.
	  • Environmental insecticide sprays are not helpful. Vacuuming carpets and car seats is a safe alternative.
	  • Household, other close contacts, and classmates of the child with head lice should be screened for parasites and treated if affected. Prophylactic treatment of head lice is unnecessary and may increase resistance. Notify the child's school or day care so classmates can be screened.
	  • Children should be allowed back to school or day care the morning after their first treatment. "No nit" policies for the return to school are unnecessary.
	  • Prophylactic treatment of all sexual contacts of adolescents and adults with pubic lice is warranted because of the high co-infection rate.

(continued)

Table 55-1	Common Pediatric Skin Problems (*continued*)
DISORDER/ORGANISM	**CLINICAL MANIFESTATIONS**

Scabies

A disease of the skin produced by the burrowing action of a parasitic mite in the epidermis, resulting in irritation and the formation of burrows, vesicles, or pustules
Etiology:
- The mite, *Sarcoptes scabiei*, is the cause of this disorder.
- Occurs in people of all socioeconomic levels, regardless of personal hygiene standards.
- Is transmitted by direct skin contact with infected people or by indirect contact through soiled bed linens, clothing.

Diagnosis:
- Identification of a mite, ova, or feces from skin scrapings.
- Often based on clinical presentation.

- Itching, particularly at night, is the primary symptom. The onset of itching is usually insidious.
- Secondary skin infection is common and may confuse the diagnosis.
- Systemic manifestations are absent, unless they result from the secondary infection.
- The burrow, a gray or white, tortuous, threadlike line, is seen most commonly in older children and adults between the fingers, in the wrists, in the axillary and buttock folds, along the belt-line, on the male genitalia, on the female breasts, and on the knees, elbows, and ankles.
- In infants and small children, the lesions may occur on any part of the body and are usually widespread. Vesicles on the palms and soles are characteristic.
- Incubation period in children without previous exposure is 4–6 weeks.

Oral Candidiasis (Thrush)

Oral candidiasis is a mycotic stomatitis characterized by the appearance of white plaques on the oral mucous membranes, gums, and tongue. (Chronic mucocutaneous candidiasis may be associated with endocrine diseases or immunodeficiency disorders or use of systemic antibiotic or inhaled corticosteroids.)
Etiology:
- Caused by *Candida albicans*.
- Maternal vulvovaginitis is the primary source of neonatal thrush. Evaluate for endocrine diseases or immunodeficiency disorders if thrush occurs after 6 months of life or is chronic.
- Nipples, pacifiers may be reservoirs.

- The infant develops small plaques on the oral mucous membranes, tongue, or gums. These plaques look like curds of milk but cannot be wiped out of the mouth.
- Most infants with thrush appear to have little pain or discomfort, unless the case is severe and there is erosion and ulceration of the mucosa.
- The mouth may be dry.
- Occasionally, the infant may appear to have some difficulty swallowing or may eat less vigorously.
- Enteric infection is usually associated with oral thrush.

Diaper Dermatitis

Candidal diaper dermatitis—a rash characterized by bright red, sharply circumscribed but moist patches with pustular satellite lesions
Etiology:
- 80% of diaper rashes present for 3 or more days are caused by *Candida albicans*.
- Most commonly seen in infants and toddlers who wear diapers.
- May be associated with oral candidiasis.

- Buttock rash consisting of erythematous maculopapular eruption with perianal distribution.
- Generally causes discomfort, especially with wetting and cleanings. Lesions last approximately 2 weeks, desquamate, and resolve without scarring.

TREATMENT/PREVENTION	NURSING CONSIDERATIONS
<ul><li>Application of a scabicide to the skin:<ul><li>The drug of choice is 5% permethrin. Alternative drugs are lindane 1% and crotamiton. Permethrin should be removed after 8–14 hours by bathing, lindane after 8–12 hours, and crotamiton after 48 hours.</li><li>Lindane can cause neurotoxicity from absorption through the skin. It should be avoided in children younger than age 2, people with known seizures, pregnant and lactating women, and people with extensive dermatitis.</li><li>Infected children and adults should apply the scabicidal lotion or cream on the entire body from the neck down. The entire head, neck, and body of infants and young children should be treated. Bathing immediately before treatment should be avoided.</li><li>Oral ivermectin at 200 mcg/kg/dose is not FDA-approved, but has been shown to be effective.</li></ul></li></ul>	<ul><li>People caring for affected children should wear gloves.</li><li>Contagion is unlikely 24 hours after treatment. Children may return to school or day care.</li><li>Teach the patient and family to launder all clothing, bed linens, and towels used by the patient during the 4 days prior to therapy with hot water and hot drying cycle to kill mites. Clothing that cannot be laundered can be stored in a plastic bag for 1 week. Further environmental disinfection is rarely necessary.</li><li>Itching may continue 2–3 weeks after successful therapy due to a hypersensitivity reaction to the mites. The use of oral antihistamines and topical corticosteroids can help relieve symptoms.</li><li>All household and close contacts should be treated prophylactically and at the same time to prevent reinfection. Caretakers with prolonged skin-to-skin contact with infected patients may also benefit from prophylactic treatment. Manifestations of scabies can occur as late as 2 months after exposure.</li></ul>
<ul><li>Topical administration of nystatin in suspension three to four times daily is the treatment of choice. Apply ½ doses to each side of the mouth after feeding.</li><li>Retain in mouth as long as possible before swallowing. Allow the child to swallow any medication to treat any lesions along the GI tract.</li><li>Clotrimazole troches can be used in children older than age 3.</li><li>Amphotericin B, clotrimazole, ketoconazole, fluconazole, and newer antifungal agents are used for candidiasis resistant to nystatin. Not all of these drugs are approved for use in infants and children.</li></ul>	<ul><li>Recognize the appearance of thrush.</li><li>Be aware of the infant or child who is particularly susceptible to the development of this condition, especially normal infants younger than age 6 months, low-birth-weight infants, immunocompromised or debilitated hosts, and people on prolonged, broad-spectrum antibiotics.</li><li>Teach parents to inspect the child's mouth before every feeding for presence of thrush and report the appearance of thrush.</li></ul>
<ul><li>Keep the affected area clean and dry by frequent diaper changes.</li><li>Clean the skin with water-based, alcohol-free baby wipes with a pH of 5.5 or with water.</li><li>Use disposable diapers with sodium polyacrylate polymers in the diaper core that form a gel when hydrated to keep liquid away from the skin or a breathable diaper.</li><li>Topical application of nystatin, clotrimazole, or miconazole cream or ointment after gentle cleaning of the affected area. If no improvement in 2 days, consider nonadherence, failure to relieve aggravating factors, or need for a different drug.</li><li>Nystatin may be given orally if rash is persistent.</li><li>Burrow's solution compresses for severe inflammation or vesiculation.</li><li>Low-potency topical corticosteroids for short-term use may be added.</li></ul>	<ul><li>Teach parents the general principles of prevention.<ul><li>Change diaper as soon as possible after wetting or soiling. Prolonged contact of feces with the skin promotes the development of candidal diaper dermatitis. Check diaper frequently (every 3–4 hours). Encourage use of disposable diapers.</li><li>Wash entire diaper area with warm water or use water-based, alcohol-free baby wipes.</li><li>If using cloth diapers, use a second hot rinse when washing diapers to neutralize ammonia produced when infant urinates; use vinegar, Borax, or Diaparene in wash.</li><li>Avoid powder and oil, which tend to clog pores and cake on skin, retaining bacteria.</li><li>Avoid occlusive plastic coverings, and tightly pinned or double diapers, all of which tend to increase production and retention of body heat and moisture.</li></ul></li><li>Allow the infant to go without a diaper for short periods to leave area open to air.</li><li>Diaper rashes present for 3 or more days should be evaluated by a health care provider.</li></ul>

SELECTED REFERENCES

Burks, A. E., Tang, M., Sicherer, S., et al. (2012). ICON: Food allergy. *Journal of Allergy and Clinical Immunology, 129*(4), 906–920.

Colohan, S. M. (2010). Predicting prognosis in thermal burns with associated inhalational injury: A systematic review of prognostic factors in adult burn victims. *Journal of Burn Care and Research, 31*(4), 529–539.

Demling, R. (2010). Burns and other thermal injuries. In G. Doherty (Ed.), *Current diagnosis and treatment: Surgery,* 210–223. New York: McGraw-Hill.

Dempster, J., Jani, B., & Daly, T. (2011). Managing eczema in children—a treatment update. *Journal of Family Practice, 60*(11), 660–668.

DeYoung, A. C., Kenardy, J. A., Cobham, V. E., et al. (2012). Prevalence, comorbidity and course of trauma reactions in young burn-injured children. *Journal of Child Psychology and Psychiatry, 53*(1), 56–63.

Diamantis, M. L., Ortega-Loayza, A. G., & Morell, D. S. (2011). Update on the characterization of *Staphylococcus aureus* skin infections in a pediatric dermatology tertiary health care outpatient facility: Antibiotic susceptibility patterns and decreased methicillin resistance. *Journal of the American Academy of Dermatology, 64*(2), 440–441.

Fiocchi, A., Assa'ad, A., Bahan, S., et al. (2006). Food allergy and the introduction of solid foods to infants: A consensus document. *Annals of Allergy, Asthma, and Immunology, 97*(1), 10–21.

Friedstat, J., Moore, M., Weber, J., et al. (2013). Selection of appropriate empiric gram-negative coverage in a multinational pediatric burn hospital. *Journal of Burn Care & Research, 34*(1), 203–210.

Greenhalgh, D. G., Saffle, J. R., Holmes, J. H. IV, et al. (2007). American Burn Association Consensus Conference to define sepsis and infection in burn. *Journal of Burn Care and Rehabilitation, 28*(6), 776–790.

Haisley-Royster, C. (2011). Cutaneous infestations and infections. *Adolescent Medicine: State of the Art Reviews, 22*(1), 129–145.

Hall, B. J., & Hall, J. C. (2010). *Sauer's manual of skin diseases* (10th ed.). Philadelphia: Lippincott Williams & Wilkins.

Hogan, B., Wolf, S. E., Hospenthal, D. R., et al. (2012). Correlation of American Burn Association sepsis criteria with the presence of bacteremia in burned patients admitted to the intensive care unit. *Journal of Burn Care and Rehabilitation, 33*(3), 371–378.

James, W. D., Berger, T., & Elston, D. M. (2011). *Andrews' diseases of the skin clinical dermatology* (11th ed.). Philadelphia: W.B. Saunders.

Kapdia, N. (2011). Dermatology. In M. M. Tschudy (Ed.), *The Harriet Lane handbook* (19th ed.), 201–225. Philadelphia: Elsevier Mosby.

Kazis, L. E. (2002). The development, validations and testing of a Health Outcomes Burn Questionnaire for infants and children 5 years of age and younger: American Burn Association/Shriners Hospitals for Children. *Journal of Burn Care and Rehabilitation, 23*(3), 196–206.

Latenser, B. A. (2009). Critical care of the burn patient: The first 48 hours. *Critical Care Medicine, 37*(10), 2819–2826.

Liu, C., Bayer, A., Cosgrove, S. E., et al. (2011). Clinical practice guidelines by the Infectious Diseases Society of America for the treatment of methicillin-resistant *Staphylococcus aureus* infections in adults and children. *Clinical Infectious Disease, 52*, 1–38.

Martin-Herz, S. P., Thurber, C. A., & Patterson, D. R. (2000). Psychological principles of burn wound pain in children. II: Treatment applications. *Journal of Burn Care and Rehabilitation, 21*(5), 458–472.

Michigan State Burn Coordinating Center. (2012). Fluid resuscitation overview: Emergency Burn Triage and Management. Available: *www.michiganburn.org.*

National Collaborating Centre for Women's and Children's Health. (2007). *Atopic eczema in children. Management of atopic eczema in children from birth up to the age of 12 years* (Clinical Guideline No. 57). London: National Institute for Health and Clinical Excellence.

Nicol, N. H. (2011). Efficacy and safety considerations in topical treatments for atopic dermatitis. *Pediatric Nursing, 37*(6), 295–301.

Paller, A. S., & Mancini, A. J. (2011). *Hurwitz clinical pediatric dermatology* (4th ed.). Philadelphia: Elsevier.

Ribbens, K. A., & DeVries, M. (2013). Burns. In B. B. Hammond & P. G. Zimmerman (Eds.), *Sheehy's manual of emergency care* (pp. 453–462). St. Louis, MO: Elsevier Mosby.

Royal Children's Hospital. (2012). Clinical practice guideline on eczema. Available: *www.rch.org.au/clinicalguide/index.cfm.*

U.S. Food and Drug Administration. (2009). FDA approves updated labeling with boxed warning and medication guide for two eczema drugs, Elidel and Protopic. *FDA News.* Available: *www.fda.gov/bbs/topics/news/2006/new01299.html.*

Watson, W., & Kapur, S. (2011) Atopic dermatitis. *Allergy, Asthma, and Clinical Immunology, 7*(Suppl. 1), S4

Weinberg, J. M., & Tyring, S. K. (2010). Retapamulin: An antibacterial with a novel mode of action in an age of emerging resistance to Staphylococcus aureus. *Journal of Drugs in Dermatology, 9*(10), 1198–1204.

Willebrand, M. S., Sveen, J., Ramklint, M. D., et al. (2011). Psychological problems in children with burn—parents' reports on the Strengths and Difficulties Questionnaire. *Burns, 37*(8), 1309–1316.

World Health Organization. (2012). WHO's pain ladder. Geneva: Author. Available: *www.who.int/cancer/palliative/painladder/en.*

56
Developmental Disabilities

OVERVIEW AND ASSESSMENT

The spectrum of developmental disabilities is a group of interrelated chronic neurodevelopmental disorders. It includes cerebral palsy, mental retardation, autism, learning disabilities, communication disorders, anxiety disorders, and attention-deficit disorders. These conditions are suspected or noticed at varying stages during childhood. Some conditions, such as Down syndrome, can be recognized prenatally or at birth; other conditions, such as cerebral palsy or autism, may not present themselves until the child fails to meet typical developmental milestones. This phenomenon makes the nurse's role in developmental assessment crucial. The pediatric nurse who understands that the development of the child occurs in an orderly, predictable manner and who knows what the milestones should be may be the first person to recognize the deviation and raise the suspicion to the parent or pediatrician. Because there are many confusing and overlapping characteristics for many of these conditions, it is important for the health care provider and family to refer to clinicians who are experienced and knowledgeable in typical and atypical child development to arrive at an accurate diagnosis and coordinate an appropriate care plan. Nurses can play a significant role in supporting the family in navigating the complex needs of many of these disorders.

When a known condition exists, the nurse should be aware of the predisposing health issues associated with the condition and the resources available to promote optimal growth and development of the child within the family.

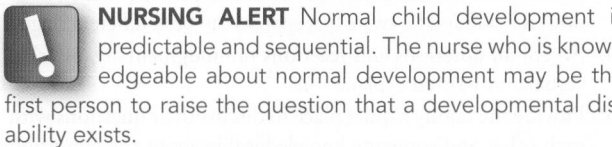

NURSING ALERT Normal child development is predictable and sequential. The nurse who is knowledgeable about normal development may be the first person to raise the question that a developmental disability exists.

Signs of Developmental Delay
Criteria for Referral
Communication and Feeding

1. Feeding difficulties—weak sucking or poor coordination of suck–swallowing to sustain normal weight gain.
2. No social smile by age 4 months.
3. No babbling (*ga-ga*, *da-da*) by age 9 months.
4. No *mama*, *dada* (specific) by age 14 months.
5. No name of object (one word) by age 14 months.
6. At least 10 words by age 18 months (not just repeating).
7. Combines words (eg, *me outside*, *more milk*) and uses pronouns by age 24 months.
8. Regression in language or social responses at any age.
9. Unresponsive to name.

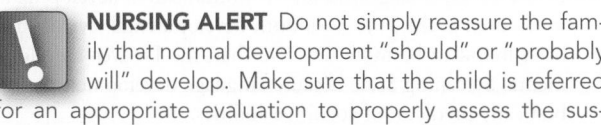

NURSING ALERT Do not simply reassure the family that normal development "should" or "probably will" develop. Make sure that the child is referred for an appropriate evaluation to properly assess the suspected delay and establish a diagnosis, if possible. In the presence of a developmental delay, a comprehensive vision and hearing evaluation should also be included.

Motor Delay

1. Assymmetrical movements and poor tone are noted.
2. Not rolling over by age 6 months.
3. Not sitting by age 9 months.
4. Not walking by age 15 months.
5. Not stair-climbing by age 2 years.

See Chapter 40 for normal pediatric growth and development.

Care of the Child with a Developmental Disability

Nursing Assessment

1. Review the child's record including the prenatal and birth history to determine existing health problems that may cause or affect the developmental disability. Always rule out a vision or hearing impairment.
2. Review the family history, if available, to determine if there are any family members with a history of developmental disabilities. If possible, assess when parents and siblings of the patient reached specified developmental milestones.
3. Assess the family's understanding of the diagnosis and its ramifications. The parents' experiences, cultural beliefs, attitudes toward disabilities, cognitive ability, stage of grief, and their own health affect their ability to assimilate information provided. It will be necessary to repeat the information. (For example, a woman who has just given birth to a child with Down syndrome may have difficulty processing much information shortly after birth.) If possible, provide the family with written information that reinforces verbal information given at the visit. Provide resources with careful consideration of information overload. Additional information and resources may be better introduced at subsequent visits.
4. Determine the developmental age of the child. The pediatric nurse should be familiar with normal developmental milestones (see Chapter 40, page 1370), noting the child's strengths and areas presenting challenges, for example, the communication skills are at a 12-month level and the gross motor skills are at a 36-month level. Children who are found to be functioning at one half or less of their chronological age have a moderate to severe developmental delay.

 NURSING ALERT Be aware of the diversity of cultural norms that may impact developmental milestones.

5. Administer a developmental tool such as the Clinical Adaptive Test–Clinical Linguistic Auditory Milestone Scales (CAT-CLAMS). It is a reliable tool that nurses can be trained to use to assess cognitive and communicative development in children at the 1- to 36-month developmental level. It has been found to be more sensitive than the Denver Developmental Screening Scale because language development is the best early predictor of cognitive abilities.

 Evidence Base Honigfield, L., Chandhok, L., Spiegelman, K. (2012). Engaging pediatricians in developmental screening: The effectiveness of academic detailing. *Journal of Autism & Developmental Disorders,* 42(6), 1175–1182.
Bricker, D., Macy, M., Squires, J., Marks, K. (2013). *Developmental Screening in Your Community: An Integrated Approach for Connecting Children with Services.* Baltimore: Brookes.

6. Assess the functional level of the child. The WeeFIM is a tool used to track functional independence in children. It has had multiple revisions and is reliable and valid. It uses the following categories to describe function: completely dependent, needs some physical assistance, can physically perform the task but needs verbal cues and coaching, and completely independent. Functional areas to assess include:
   a. Feeding.
   b. Grooming and bathing.
   c. Dressing.
   d. Mobility.
   e. Problem solving.
   f. Communication.

 Evidence Base DeVeney, S., Hoffman, L., Cress, C. (2012). Communication-based assessment of developmental age for young children with developmental disabilities. *Journal of Speech, Language & Hearing Research,* 55(3), 695–709.

7. Assess parents' perception of the child's development level and the appropriateness of parental expectations. Use such questions as, "Do you have any concerns regarding things your child is doing or should be doing?" "Is your child progressing like your other children have?"
8. Assess parent–child interaction. Observe and explore bonding and attachment, ability to set appropriate limits, management of behavioral problems, and methods of discipline.
9. Assess the need for additional resources, such as financial aid, transportation, and counseling, for long-term support of child and family.

Nursing Diagnoses

- Impaired Parenting related to birth and diagnosis of developmentally disabled child.
- Interrupted Family Processes related to multiple needs of child and difficult bonding.
- Ineffective Infant Feeding Pattern related to protruding tongue, poor muscle tone, and weak sucking.
- Delayed Growth and Development related to impaired cognitive and motor functioning.
- Social Isolation related to developmental differences from other children.
- Risk for Injury related to neurologic impairment and developmental delay.

Nursing Interventions

Promoting Adjustment

1. Allow the parents access to the infant at all possible times to promote bonding when parents appear ready.
2. Focus on the positive aspects of the infant and serve as a role model for handling and stimulating.
3. Be cognizant of the grieving process (loss of the anticipated and planned-for "normal child") that families experience when a diagnosis is made and be aware that spouses can be at different stages.
4. Accept all questions and reactions nonjudgmentally, offering verbal and written explanations.
5. Provide the family a quiet place to discuss their questions with each other and someone knowledgeable about the condition (primary care provider, clinical nurse specialist) to support their concerns.

6. Offer the family the option to take advantage of counseling. A social worker or psychologist can help families deal with immediate reactions. Many parents benefit from continuous or periodic support of counseling professionals.

 NURSING ALERT Children with developmental disabilities and chronic illness are at greater risk for experiencing divorce, child abuse, and neglect than the general population.

Strengthening the Role of the Family

1. Help the family to realize what strengths they have in caring for their child. The role of the parents is critical; a nurturing, loving environment gives the child the best chance at maximizing potential. An individual who grows up at home has markedly higher adaptive abilities and an increased life span compared with those raised in residential care facilities.
2. Enlist the help of family and siblings, who can offer valuable support to the parents and child and assist with stimulation activities. Including siblings in the care can help them feel needed and involved, thus strengthening the family.
3. If sibling issues arise, suggest family counseling to address the needs of all family members.
4. Identify resources available to the family, such as parent support groups, early intervention programs, specialty clinics, pediatrician or primary health care provider, respite care, financial support programs, and advocacy groups for individuals with developmental disabilities.
5. For those parents concerned with their ability to care for the child, explore with them their options of foster care, adoption, and residential placement in a nonjudgmental manner.
6. Ensure that the family has adequate respite services to prevent exhaustion and mental fatigue.

Establishing Effective Feeding Techniques

 Evidence Base Cloud, H. (2012). Developmental disabilities. In P. Q. Samour & K. King, *Pediatric nutrition* (4th ed.), 219–236. Sudbury, MA: Jones & Bartlett.

1. Be aware that the presence of hypotonia, as in children with many genetic syndromes and metabolic disorders, or hypertonia, as in children with cerebral palsy, can interfere with feeding by compromising sucking and swallowing.
2. Demonstrate proper feeding positioning, with the infant's head elevated, and encourage the parents to always hold the infant during feedings with his or her head elevated and supported in arms.
3. Try different nipples and bottles to find the easiest for the infant to use without leakage or danger of aspiration.
4. Allow adequate time for feeding and increase frequency of feedings if infant tires easily.
5. Offer support and guidance for breastfeeding. Refer to lactation consultant, if needed.
6. Consider referral for a feeding evaluation to a speech therapist or to an occupational therapist who has experience working with children and families.
7. Be aware of and anticipate the need for initiation of tube feeding (nasogastric or gastrostomy) so that early referral and education of the parents about feeding options can be discussed

8. Assess for signs of feeding intolerance and gastroesophageal reflux disease, which is common in children with hypotonia; implement management strategies to optimize feeding and minimize risk of aspiration, such as upright position after feedings.
9. Frequently assess growth (length or height, weight, and head circumference) to ensure adequate dietary intake and be aware that growth in children with neurologic impairment and genetic syndromes may be slower or limited in relation to the general pediatric population and standard growth charts.
10. Monitor bowel and elimination patterns of children with neurologic impairment, especially those with generalized hypotonia, as they are at risk for poor gastric motility and constipation. Dietary measures, such as increased fiber and fluid intake, or pharmacologic agents to promote adequate elimination may be needed.

Promoting Optimum Growth and Development

1. Refer parents to the Early Intervention Program administered by their county so that they can take advantage of the educational and support services available for children from birth to age 3.
2. If the condition is identified after age 3 years, refer parents to the school district in which they reside.
3. Help the parents to understand the concept of developmental age and identify the functional level of the child.
4. Determine whether there is consistency between the developmental age of the child and degree of independence. Cognitive and physical limitations may interfere with emerging independence; however, parents may "baby" or overindulge a child who has a disability.
5. Work with parents to set reasonable expectations and to break down tasks into simple, achievable steps. Care should be taken not to address too many areas at one time so as not to overwhelm the family.
6. Use appropriate discipline and behavior-modification techniques, such as extinction, time-out, and reward, to achieve cooperation and success.
7. Demonstrate and encourage play with the child at the appropriate level to provide stimulation and work toward achieving developmental milestones.
8. Provide parents with information and links to community, regional, or national associations for children with special needs and refer to parent support groups. These resources are frequently found online and can be easily accessed to provide an ongoing source of information and support to families.
9. Ensure that the child's physical well-being is optimized to promote optimal development and self-esteem. Any congenital defects should be repaired (ie, orthopedic, cardiac, craniofacial, etc), and attention should be paid to dental health and restorative orthodontic procedures that can improve facial appearance.

Providing Opportunities to Develop Social and Self-Care Skills

1. Be aware that feeding, toileting, dressing, and grooming are important aspects of socialization and development of self-esteem. These tasks should be taught in a developmentally appropriate manner to children with a focus on maximizing independence. Many adaptive devices are available and

an occupational therapist can guide families in effective techniques to help children with developmental disabilities master these important self-care skills.

2. Make parents aware that recreational and leisure-time experiences are valuable in building social skills and self-esteem. Rehearse and role-play desirable social behaviors—such as waving goodbye, saying "hello," taking turns, saying "please" and "thank you," and responding to their name—will help build social confidence and acceptance within the child's peer group.

3. Offer suggestions that will be enjoyable and developmentally appropriate for the child. Interaction with developmentally delayed and nondevelopmentally delayed peers is desirable. The Special Olympics is one example of an adaptive program. Local programs are also available in many areas.

4. Praise the child for participation in activities, regardless of whether the child succeeds.

Maintaining Safety

1. When handling the infant, provide adequate support with a firm grasp because the infant may be floppy due to poor muscle tone.

2. If hypotonia is accompanied by poor head control and neck strength, position the infant to prevent aspiration should vomiting occur.
   a. Support the infant with a diaper roll, if needed, to maintain position.
   b. Change the infant's position frequently.
   c. Continuously check the environment for the safety needs of the child.

3. Be aware that hypotonia can also lead to increased heat loss as more surface area is exposed; therefore, infants may need close attention paid to swaddling and environmental control to maintain thermoregulation.

 NURSING ALERT Teach caregivers to base safety needs on the developmental, not the chronological, age of the child.

4. Advise the parents to:
   a. Maintain appropriate surveillance of the child when cooking or exposing him or her to other potential hazards that he or she may be able to get into but not understand.
   b. Help the child to read words, such as *danger* and *stop*.
   c. Teach the child how to call and ask for help.
   d. Teach the child to say no to strangers.
   e. Teach the child appropriate and socially acceptable sexual behaviors to prevent exploitation.
   f. Teach sex education, with practical information about anatomy, physical development, and contraception, in a way the child and adolescent can understand.

5. Ensure that parents and caregivers have the knowledge and resources to transport their child safely.

Family Education and Health Maintenance

1. Remind the parents to recognize the child's routine health care needs and maintain regular follow-up with a primary care provider.
   a. Immunizations.

b. Regular dental checkups.
   c. Vision and hearing examinations.
   d. Anticipatory guidance related to developmental stages, safety, behavior, and transition planning.

2. Provide guidance and support to parents with their child's multidimensional treatment plan. Make sure parents know whom to contact when problems arise. Encourage parents to develop and maintain a notebook with a calendar to keep track of agencies, subspecialists, and professionals who will be involved with their child. It should include such information as business cards, names, addresses, phone numbers, appointment dates, health providers' orders, and insurance information.

3. Teach parents the benefits of a therapeutic home environment.
   a. Develop optimum sleeping, eating, working, and playing routines.
   b. Ensure adequate nutrition.
   c. Divide tasks and expectations into small, manageable parts. Give only one or two instructions at a time.
   d. Set firm but reasonable limits on behavior and carry through with consistent discipline.
   e. Avoid situations that cause excessive excitement, stimulation, or fatigue.
   f. Provide an energy outlet through physical activity and outdoor play, as well as vocal outlet.
   g. Channel the need for movement into safe, appropriate activities.

4. Discuss preparation for independent living, when appropriate.
   a. Help the parents identify areas of home responsibilities that may be delegated to the cognitively impaired child.
   b. Guide development of social skills that will be an asset to later vocational life.
   c. Help the child to develop a set of attitudes and behaviors that will increase motivation.
   d. Refer for vocational assistance to ARC (formerly Association of Retarded Citizens) or other rehabilitative agencies.
   e. Begin planning for transition from pediatric care providers to adult providers well in advance of when eligibility for services will run out to ensure appropriate provider(s) can be established in a timely way and to avoid gaps in health care.

 Evidence Base Wang, G., McGrath, B., & Watts, C. (2010). Health care transitions among youth with disabilities or special health needs: An ecological approach. *Journal of Pediatric Nursing, 25*(6), 505–550.
Richmond, N., Tran, T., Berry, S. (2012). Can the medical home eliminate racial and ethnic disparities for transition services among youth with special health care needs? *Maternal & Child Health Journal, 16*(4), 824–833.

5. Refer for genetic consultation for information about genetics of the disorder, risk in subsequent pregnancies (parents) or risk to offspring (patient), or risk to other relatives as it is warranted by the diagnosis.

Evaluation: Expected Outcomes

• Parents hold infant frequently and seek information from health care provider.

- Family members feed, assist with care, and bond with child.
- Parents and health care providers monitor nutrition, growth, and development closely, with ongoing assessment of most effective feeding techniques and management of any feeding-related problems.
- Parents describe developmental level of child and have realistic goals for attainment of next milestones in collaboration with their health care team and occupational, speech, and physical therapists.
- Parents seek out support and resources that enable them to share their experience in raising a child with special needs and gain information needed to optimize the child's developmental and health outcomes throughout childhood.
- Child remains safe through careful handling and appropriate supervision.

DEVELOPMENTAL DISABILITIES

Cognitive Developmental Delay

Cognitive developmental delay, also known as *intellectual disabilities*, refers to the most severe, general lack of cognitive and problem-solving skills. The American Association on Intellectual and Developmental Disabilities defines intellectual disabilities as a disability characterized by significant limitations both in intellectual functioning and in adaptive behavior, which covers many everyday social and practical skills. This disability originates before the age of 18 years. There are many causes and a wide range of impairments. Approximately 3% of the United States population—6.6 million people—are considered mentally retarded. Of every 1,000 infants born, 30 will be classified as mentally retarded before they reach age 18 years.

Pathophysiology and Etiology

1. No identifiable organic or biologic cause can be found for 50% of children with cognitive delays.
2. Identifiable causes include:
   a. Genetic causes, such as Down syndrome, fragile X syndrome, Angelman's syndrome, and inborn errors of metabolism such as phenylketonuria (PKU).
   b. Congenital anomalies, including brain malformations, hydrocephalus, and microcephaly.
   c. Intrauterine influences, such as alcohol and drug exposure, congenital infections, and teratogens.
   d. Perinatal trauma—birth hypoxia, intracranial hemorrhage.
   e. Postnatal trauma—acquired brain injury from falls, automobile accidents, near drownings, child abuse (shaken baby syndrome).
   f. Postnatal infections and diseases (meningitis, encephalitis, sepsis, hypoxia, brain tumors).
   g. Environmental exposure to toxins such as lead; environmental deprivation; neglect.
3. The malfunctioning brain is poorly understood in most cases, but physiologic alterations identified in some cases include:
   a. Congenital brain malformations, brain tissue damage, or underdevelopment of the brain as shown by normal results of computed tomography (CT) scan or magnetic resonance imaging (MRI).
   b. Biochemical errors or errors of metabolism, in which an absence of an enzyme or hormone produces abnormal brain function or formation, as in PKU or hypothyroidism.
4. IQ is 75 or below; classification has been recently changed to mild and severe and includes both cognitive and functional ability.
   a. The more severe types of intellectual developmental disability tend to be diagnosed in early infancy, especially when they coexist with an identifiable syndrome or congenital anomaly.
   b. Milder forms of intellectual developmental disability tend to be diagnosed in the preschool years, when language and behavioral concerns call attention to slower development.
5. Limitations in adaptive ability occur in communication, self-care, home living, social skills, community use, self-direction, health and safety, functional academics, leisure, and work.

Clinical Manifestations

Developmental delays (failure to achieve age-appropriate skills) are evident to some degree in almost all areas.

Infancy

1. "Poor feeder"—a weak or uncoordinated suck results in poor breast- or bottle-feeding, leading to poor weight gain.
2. Delayed or decreased visual alertness and curiosity with poor visual tracking of face or objects.
3. Decreased or lack of auditory response.
4. Decreased spontaneous activity or asymmetric activity.
5. Delayed head and trunk control.
6. Floppy (hypotonic) or spastic (hypertonic) muscle tone.

 NURSING ALERT Although 75% of individuals with intellectual developmental disabilities have no physical signs, they typically achieve motor milestones at a slower rate.

Toddler

1. Delayed independent sitting, crawling, pulling to stand, and independent ambulation.
2. Delayed communication—failure to develop receptive and expressive language milestones. Almost 50% of children with intellectual developmental disability are identified after age 3 years, when speech delays manifest themselves.
3. Failure of the child to make progress or show interest in the area of independence in self-feeding, dressing, and toilet training may reflect cognitive impairment.
4. Short attention span and distractibility.
5. Behavioral disturbances.
6. Decreased muscle coordination.

Diagnostic Evaluation

Federal law (PL 94-142—Education for All Handicapped Children and PL 101-476—Individuals with Disabilities

Education Act [IDEA]) ensures that each child with a delay or suspected of having a delay has a comprehensive evaluation by a multidisciplinary team. Part C of PL 105-17 calls for the creation of statewide, coordinated, multidisciplinary interagency programs for the provision of early intervention services. Each state has its own definitions and organizational framework to provide these services. No single test can diagnose intellectual developmental disabilities. The multidisciplinary evaluation should be individually tailored to the child.

1. Rule out sensory deficits by assessment of vision and hearing, even if neonate hearing screen was normal.
2. Medical evaluation should include prenatal history, developmental history, sequential developmental assessments, family history including genetic assessment, and physical examination. The positive findings determine the direction of the individual evaluation and any diagnostic testing.
   a. Unusual appearance (dysmorphic features) warrants evaluation by a genetic specialist.
   b. History consistent with loss of developmental milestones and positive family history warrants workup for presence of an inborn error of metabolism (diagnosed by blood, urine, or DNA analysis) or lead poisoning.
   c. Children with macrocephaly, microcephaly, or neurologic abnormalities may require imaging studies, such as CT scan or MRI.
   d. EEG is indicated for children with seizures.
3. Psychological testing (appropriate tests selected by a child psychologist):
   a. The Bayley Scales are used to assess children ages 2 months to 3 years. This test is weighted on nonlanguage items and is used to assess fine motor, gross motor, language skills, and visual problem solving.
   b. The McCarthy Scale offers a "general cognitive index" that is roughly equivalent to an IQ score.
   c. The Stanford–Binet Intelligence Scale is used to test the mental abilities of children age 2 and older.
   d. The Wechsler Preschool and Primary Scale of Intelligence—Third Edition (WPPSI-3) measures mental age of 3 to 7 years.
   e. The Wechsler Intelligence Scale for Children—Fourth Edition (WISC-IV) tests children whose functional age is above a 6-year level.
   f. The Vineland Scale tests social-adaptive abilities—self-help skills, self-control, interaction with others, cooperation; the Adaptive Behavior Scale is similar to Vineland but also measures adjustment.

Complications and Associated Findings

1. Seizures.
2. Cerebral palsy.
3. Sensory deficits.
4. Communication disorders (speech and language).
5. Neurodevelopmental disorders.
6. Psychiatric illness.
7. Specific learning disabilities.
8. Emotional and behavioral problems (self-injury, hyperactivity, aggression).

Management

1. An interdisciplinary team evaluation by a developmental pediatrician, clinical psychologist, and counselor is usually the initial step in the management of mental retardation. This type of evaluation can be obtained through a state or private diagnostic and evaluation center, public school, or university-affiliated program.
2. Associated medical problems, such as seizures, feeding difficulties and poor nutrition, sensory deficits, or dental problems, must be treated to allow the child to maximize his or her potential.
3. If a treatable cause is identified, such as an inborn error of metabolism, a therapeutic diet can be instituted. Hypothyroidism can be treated with thyroid hormone.
4. A family assessment is essential to address:
   a. Financial stressors—financial aid may be available through Social Security, Medicaid, or state and local programs to help families with children with developmental delays.
   b. Family functioning and coping abilities.
   c. Support for parents, siblings, and extended family.
   d. Respite services.
   e. Support groups.
   f. Recreational programs, such as the Special Olympics and summer camps.
   g. Identification of other affected or at-risk people and the need for genetic counseling for recurrence risk.
5. The initial evaluation usually leads to recommendations for more targeted evaluations, such as physical therapy, occupational therapy, and social work assessment.

See "Care of the Child with a Developmental Disability," page 1792.

Down Syndrome

Evidence Base American Academy of Pediatrics. (2011). Health supervision for children with Down syndrome. *Pediatrics, 128*(2), 393–406.

Down syndrome was first described in 1866. It is the most common genetic cause of intellectual disability and is also referred to as trisomy 21. According to the National Down Syndrome Society, the incidence of this error in cell division is 1 in 733 live births. Each child with Down syndrome has a unique set of genes, besides the effects of the extra genes on chromosome 21, and the child will need individualized evaluation. The most common life experience of a child with Down syndrome is to live with the family, participate in infant stimulation and preschool programs, and attend school while receiving support from special education services. Adults with Down syndrome can function in supported employment programs and live in small residential group homes. Life expectancy depends on the presence of medical complications; when there are no complications, life expectancy is slightly shorter than average.

Pathophysiology and Etiology

See Chapter 4, page 35.

Clinical Manifestations and Associated Problems

1. Characteristic facies—brachycephaly; oblique palpebral fissures; epicanthal folds; flat nasal bridge; protruding tongue; small, low-set ears; simian crease of palms (see Figure 56-1).
2. Congenital heart defects (seen in approximately 40% of infants with Down syndrome), most commonly ventricular septal defects and patent ductus arteriosus.
3. Mental retardation.
4. Hypotonia.
5. Growth retardation.
6. Dry, scaly skin.
7. Table 56-1, pages 1788 and 1789, provides a comprehensive list of potential problems that occur with Down syndrome. Some are identified at birth; others arise and cause difficulties later in the life cycle. Percentages are listed that represent occurrence within the Down syndrome population.

Diagnosis and Management

1. See "Care of the Child with a Developmental Disability," page 1792, for a general approach to assessment.

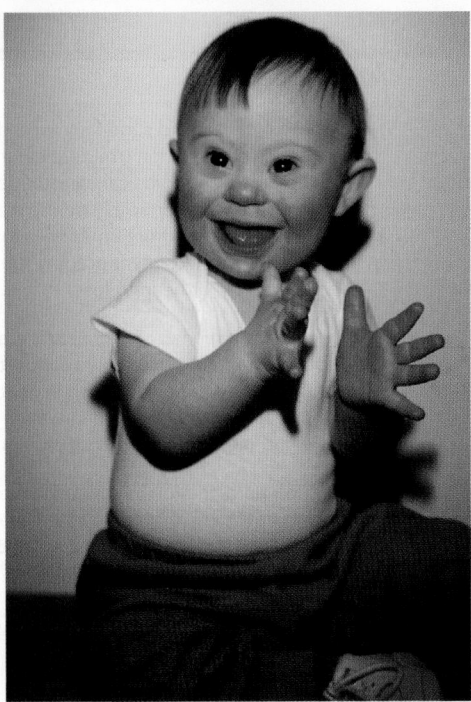

FIGURE 56-1. One-year-old with Down syndrome, recently diagnosed with hypothyroidism.

Table 56-1	Down Syndrome (DS)	
POTENTIAL PROBLEMS	**EVALUATION**	**MANAGEMENT**
Congenital heart malformations (ie, AV canal, VSD, PDA, and tetralogy of Fallot) (40%)	• Observe for color changes, pulse, and respiratory rate at rest and with stress. Assess tolerance of feeding for early tiring or frequent interruptions in feeding. Echocardiogram usually done during neonatal period on all infants with DS.	• Early identification and treatment can prevent heart failure and decompensation or poor growth. Medical or surgical intervention correction has minimized mortality from simple cardiac defects.
Congenital GI malformations (12%) • Pyloric stenosis • Duodenal atresia, tracheoesophageal fistula	• Observe for coughing or vomiting, especially with feeding: bile-stained vomitus suggests lower-tract abnormalities; partially digested contents suggest upper-tract problem. Observe bowel movements and for abdominal distention. • Radiographic studies are done.	• GI reflux (spillage of material from esophagus into the trachea) can cause arching during feedings, poor weight gain, chronic respiratory problems, allergy and asthma symptomatology, pneumonia, and aspiration. Medication management and, if needed, surgical intervention can occur in the early neonatal period.
Hypothyroidism (10%–20%)	• Monitor for weight gain, hair loss, lethargy, short stature, voice changes, and depression (can develop at any time over life cycle). Neonatal screening includes T_3, TSH, T_4 biannually.	• Thyroid hormone replacement.
Visual defects • Refractive errors (70%) • Strabismus (50%) • Nystagmus (35%) • Cataracts (3%)	• Observe for indication of vision problems, such as head tilt or poor visual tracking. Use Teller activity as a visual screen tool for those who cannot cooperate with Snellen chart. • Positive findings in first year of life warrant immediate referral to ophthalmologist. All individuals should be seen by a pediatric ophthalmologist (or one who is skilled in evaluating children) at age 1, and vision evaluations should continue throughout life.	• Undetected visual deficits can cause failure to achieve developmental milestones and cause permanent loss of vision.

(continued)

Table 56-1   Down Syndrome (DS) (continued)

POTENTIAL PROBLEMS	EVALUATION	MANAGEMENT
Hearing defects (60%–90%): • Mild to moderate conductive hearing loss • Enlarged adenoids • Sleep apnea	• Assess for curiosity and response to sounds of varying quality. Auditory brain stem response assesses hearing in infants. Sound field testing for children older than age 1. • Tympanometry to assess middle ear function.	• Narrow ear canals and subtle immune deficiencies can cause chronic middle ear infections. Enlarged adenoids can cause upper airway obstruction, especially during sleep. • Treatment can range from antibiotics for simple otitis media to myringotomy tubes, adenoidectomy, or hearing loss.
Hypotonia of infants (100%)	• Observe for floppiness, poor head control, poor oral motor function. Infant should be placed on abdomen periodically while being observed and monitored for potential for suffocation.	• Physical, occupational, and speech therapy. Adaptive equipment gives extra support to head and neck when handling neonate. Always keep head elevated for at least 1 hour after meals. Change position regularly.
Atlanto-occipital and atlanto-axial subluxation (dislocation of the upper spine due to joint laxity) (15%)	• Assess for head tilt; increasing clumsiness, limping, or refusal to walk; weakness of arms. X-ray of cervical spine to evaluate for atlanto-axial dislocation at age 2 and then every 5 years during childhood. Precise measurements are taken to document alignment of the skull and vertebrae. Shifting of the two can cause compression and neurologic damage. Participation in Special Olympics and other activities that may require neck flexion should warrant a baseline evaluation.	• If present, participation in contact sports and gymnastics is contraindicated. In severe cases, surgery to fuse the vertebrae and occiput and stabilize spinal column.
Gait abnormalities (15%)	• Monitor for onset of limp, leg length discrepancy. Hip x-rays can document dislocation or subluxation.	• Physical therapy and, sometimes, orthopedic surgery are necessary.
Failure to thrive	• Monitor growth on DS growth chart. Monitor feedings for length of feeding, feeding schedule, loss of feeding by vomiting or poor seal on nipple. Monitor type of formula and caloric content.	• Nutritionist can advise on formula adjustments. Therapists can help with positioning and types of nipples used to counteract effects of weak sucking reflex and large, protruding tongue.
Short stature (100%)	• Plot growth on DS growth chart. Monitor stages of puberty. Delayed puberty may warrant further investigation.	• Use of human growth hormone may be considered; this is still controversial.
Obesity (50%)	• Monitor thyroid hormone levels. Serial monitoring of weight. Monitor for amount of exercise, caloric intake.	• Overindulgence by adults or use of food in behavior management increases risk of overeating. Lack of social involvement leads to decreased activity. Behavior modification is necessary.
Malocclusions (60%–100%)	• Assess for malocclusions, periodontal disease, delayed eruption of teeth. Regular dental checkups begin at age 1 year of age or when teeth erupt.	• Encourage good oral hygiene with proper toothbrushing.
Mental retardation with varying degrees from mild to moderate (100%)	• Routine developmental assessment using standardized tools of measurement.	• Special education and training.
Alzheimer's disease after age 40 (15%–30%)	• Assess for decreased cognitive function and loss of memory. MRI or CT scan shows areas of plaque.	• Increased supervision is needed.
Seizures (6%)	• Onset of seizures is seen primarily during adolescence and middle age.	• Neurologic evaluation and appropriate antiseizure medications.
Other problems • Communication disorders • Alopecia (10%) • Leukemia (1%)		

VSD, ventricular septal defect; AV, atrioventricular; GI, gastrointestinal; PDA, patent ductus arteriosus; T3, triiodothyronine; TSH, thyroid-stimulating hormone; T_4, levothyroxine; MRI, magnetic resonance imaging; CT, computed tomography.

2. See Table 56-1, pages 1797 to 1798, for specific conditions requiring medical management related to Down syndrome, such as otolaryngologic, endocrine, orthopedic, gastrointestinal, and cardiac problems.

3. Alternative therapies—nutritional and supplemental vitamin therapy for Down syndrome remains controversial and effects have not been medically proven.

Considerations for Adult Patients with Down Syndrome

 Evidence Base Heavey, E., & Peterson-Sweeney, K. (2010, June). Caring for an adult with Down syndrome. *Nursing*, pp. 53–56.

Infants born with Down syndrome today are expected to live well into their 50s. Adults with Down syndrome experience accelerated aging and have a higher incidence of dementia. Other medical problems more prevalent in this population include spinal and neck problems, pulmonary hypertension, hypothyroidism, testicular cancer, sleep apnea, and dermatologic problems. Mental health disorders can include depression and obsessive–compulsive disorder. Annual health exams are crucial and every attempt should be made to find a health care provider that is comfortable with these patients and knowledgeable of the specific health maintenance concerns.

Fragile X Syndrome

Fragile X syndrome is the second most common identifiable cause of intellectual developmental disability as well as the most common inherited cause. It is responsible for about 40% of X-linked intellectual disabilities. The fragile X phenotype is nonspecific and commonly becomes more apparent with age, therefore, diagnosis usually is not made until mid-childhood or later. This syndrome can cause a wide range of cognitive and behavioral characteristics, ranging from mild to severe. Chromosome analysis reveals that the long arm of the X chromosome is constricted and appears fragile, but this cannot be detected in all cases; thus, deoxyribonucleic acid (DNA) analysis is preferred for diagnosis. Fragile X is more common in males, occurring in 1 in 4,000 boys and 1 in 8,000 girls. Genetic counseling and testing of family members is necessary to evaluate recurrence risks.

Pathophysiology and Etiology

See Chapter 4, page 36.

Clinical Manifestations and Associated Problems

1. Mild to moderate mental retardation (IQ range 41 to 88).
2. Elongated face, prominent ears, macrocephaly, high-arched palate, dental crowding, epicanthal folds (fold of skin on either side of nose), hypertelorism (increased distance between eyes), flattened nasal bridge.
3. Macro-orchidism (enlarged testicles) after puberty.
4. Delay in both expressive and receptive language, perseverative or repetitive speech
5. Delay in adaptive behavior skills.
6. Autistic-like communication disorders.

7. Attention deficit, hyperactivity.
8. Self-stimulating and self-injurious behaviors such as hand biting.
9. Associated problems, including mitral valve prolapse, seizures, joint laxity or hyperextensibility, and feeding problems.
10. Adult patients may develop tremors and ataxia.
11. Women are at risk for premature ovarian failure and early menopause.

Diagnosis and Management

1. See "Care of the Child with a Developmental Disability," page 1792, for a general approach to management.
2. See Table 56-2, page 1800 for specific medical issues related to fragile X syndrome.

Turner Syndrome

Turner syndrome is a genetic disorder found in females. The incidence of this syndrome is approximately 1 in 2,000 female live births. The most severe phenotype occurs in approximately 50% of females with the absence of an X chromosome. There are typically mosaic variations seen with Turner syndrome and the clinical effects can vary between individuals. It is important to note that most girls will present with short stature and/or ovarian failure but the other syndrome characteristics may not be present or may be present in mild form, causing a delay in diagnosis. The cognitive impairments and phenotype can be nonspecific in early childhood and a diagnosis is commonly not made until failure of pubertal development is noted.

Pathophysiology and Etiology

See Chapter 4, page 36.

Clinical Manifestations and Associated Problems

1. The most prevalent characteristics of Turner syndrome include:
   a. Short stature, webbed neck, low posterior hairline, edema of the hands and feet (see Figure 56-2).
   b. Congenital cardiac defects.
   c. Broad chest with inverted or underdeveloped nipples.
   d. Immature reproductive organs, delayed puberty, primary amenorrhea.
   e. Hypothyroidism, obesity, type II diabetes, osteoporosis and fractures in adulthood.
   f. Learning disabilities.
2. Associated problems include:
   a. Coarctation of the aorta, idiopathic hypertension.
   b. Hearing loss—conductive or sensorineural.
   c. Obesity, glucose intolerance.
   d. Feeding problems.
   e. Renal anomalies.

Diagnosis and Management

1. See "Care of the Child with a Developmental Disability," page 1792, for a general approach to assessment.

Table 56-2   Fragile X Syndrome

POTENTIAL PROBLEMS	EVALUATION	MANAGEMENT
Hypotonia of infancy	• Assess ability to control head and assume upright posture. • Assess feeding for efficient suck and coordination of suck/swallow.	Physical therapy, stimulation program, feeding adaptations.
Seizures (20% of cases)	• Assess for muscle tremors, deviation of eyes to one side, rhythmic jerking of the body, and loss of consciousness.	Referral to neurologist for diagnosis and anticonvulsants to treat seizures.
Mitral valve prolapse (80% of males)	• Assess dyspnea, cyanosis, murmur. Echocardiogram to evaluate valve function.	Antibiotics for prophylaxis before invasive procedures to prevent endocarditis. Treatment of heart failure; surgical repair may be necessary.
Self-stimulating behavior	• Rule out source of pain (ie, otitis media, tooth pain) that may be causing behavior. Rule out sensory deficits.	Behavior management techniques: Focus on replacing undesirable behaviors with purposeful, meaningful ones, with emphasis on positive reinforcement and extinguishing negative reinforcement.
Hyperactivity, attention deficits	• Assess activity of attention span within the context of the developmental age of the child.	Behavior management and special educational techniques.
Discipline problems	• Assess social skills.	Males tend to do best in self-contained classrooms for children with similar degrees of mental retardation.
Communication disorders	• Assess language development (usually weakest area of development).	Speech-language therapy can be beneficial.
Poor auditory memory; auditory reception	• Assess how child lets needs be known: cries, gestures, single words, or sentences.	Speech therapy, behavior modification.
Cognitive dysfunction • Short-term memory deficits • Poor problem-solving skills • Functional limitations in self-care	• Assess for appropriateness of educational placement and child's reaction to situation.	Specialized training and education, assisted living.

2. See Table 56-3, for specific medical issues related to Turner syndrome.
3. Diagnosis may occur prenatally through an amniocentesis, with genetic testing, or any time after birth. A preliminary diagnosis may be made based on physical characteristics. This should then be confirmed by genetic testing. A diagnosis is often not made until there is a failure to begin menstruation.

Fetal Alcohol Spectrum Disorder

Fetal alcohol spectrum disorder (FASD) is a significant problem. Children with FASD have a wide range of physical, mental, behavioral, and/or learning disabilities that put them at risk. FASD is the leading known preventable cause of intellectual developmental disabilities in developed countries.

Pathophysiology and Etiology

1. The incidence is approximately 0.3 to 1.5 per 1,000 children. Approximately 40,000 children are diagnosed each year in the United States.
2. Caused by use or abuse of alcohol during pregnancy. The alcohol ingested by the mother passes easily across the placenta to the fetus.
   a. There is no "safe" level of alcohol use during pregnancy and a pregnant woman who drinks any amount of alcohol is at risk.
   b. Larger amounts of alcohol and binge drinking appear to cause more significant risk to the fetus.
   c. Alcohol use in the first trimester is more problematic.

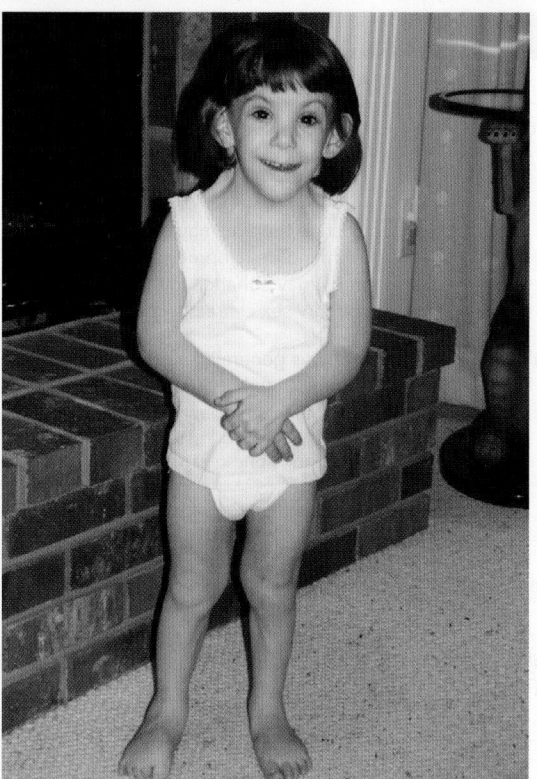

FIGURE 56-2. Three-year-old with Turner syndrome. Note the webbed neck.

Clinical Manifestations and Associated Problems

Evidence Base Defendi, G. (2010). Fetal alcohol spectrum disorder: How to recognize the various manifestations. *Consultant for Pediatricians, 9*(10). Available: *www.pediatricsconsultant360.com/content/fetal-alcohol-spectrum-disorder-how-recognize-various-manifestations.*

1. Intrauterine growth delay.
2. Decreased muscle tone and poor coordination.
3. Delayed development and problems in three or more major areas: cognitive, speech, motor, or social skills.
4. Hyperactivity and attention deficits.
5. Vision or hearing problems.
6. Heart defects such as ventricular septal defect or atrial septal defect.
7. Craniofacial abnormalities including narrow, small eyes with large epicanthal folds; small head; small upper jaw; smooth groove in upper lip; smooth and thin upper lip.
8. The average IQ is 65 with a range from 20 to 120, with many of these children qualifying for special education services.
9. Many will go on to have disrupted school progress, criminal offenses, and alcohol- and drug-related problems.

Table 56-3	Turner Syndrome	
POTENTIAL PROBLEMS	**EVALUATION**	**MANAGEMENT**
Congenital heart malformations: • Increased incidence of left-sided heart anomalies • Aortic valve anomalies • Coarctation of aorta	Observe for color changes, pulse, and respiratory rate at rest and with stress. Monitor blood pressure. Assess tolerance of feeding for early tiring or frequent interruptions in feeding. An electrocardiogram should be done in the neonatal period. A yearly echocardiogram or magnetic resonance imaging should also be done.	Early identification and treatment can prevent secondary problems. If needed, prophylactic antibiotic for subacute bacterial endocarditis. Referral to a cardiologist.
Renal and renovascular anomalies: • Horseshoe kidney • Duplicated renal pelvis • Vascular anomalies	Renal sonogram should be done to rule out anomalies. Routine urinalysis and culture to screen for urinary tract infection, glycosuria.	Referral to a nephrologist if a renal anomaly is present. Monitor for the development of diabetes mellitus.
Edema in the hands and feet	Edema may persist for months or may recur; if recurrence, monitor for renal or cardiac causes.	—
Dysmorphic features: webbed neck, face, ears	Parents may elect plastic surgery to minimize the visible defects.	Enhances the socialization of females with Turner syndrome in school. May need additional support or therapy.
Nutrition: failure to thrive in the infant period and obesity in childhood	Infants may have inefficient sucking and swallowing reflexes. Monitor growth utilizing a Turner syndrome growth chart.	Nutrition counseling and encouragement of exercise to maintain appropriate weight.

(continued)

Table 56-3   Turner Syndrome *(continued)*

POTENTIAL PROBLEMS	EVALUATION	MANAGEMENT
Hearing loss	Hearing loss may be conductive or sensorineural. Routine screening should be performed.	Otitis media should be treated aggressively to minimize potential hearing loss.
Short stature and failure to develop secondary sex characteristics	—	Endocrine therapy may be indicated for growth and development. Hormonal therapy may enhance the development of secondary sex characteristics.
Infertility	Ovaries are not developed. Usually no need for testing.	Infertility is generally expected in Turner syndrome. Infertility techniques may be able to assist with childbearing.
Hypothyroidism	Periodic laboratory testing.	Thyroid hormone replacement therapy.
Behavioral problems, learning disabilities	—	Behavioral management. Special education.
Strabismus	If detected, referral to an ophthalmologist is recommended.	Patching or surgical repair.
Cognitive function	Average to slightly below-average intelligence. Problem areas include spatial perception and math functions.	Special education.

Diagnosis and Management

1. Diagnosis is usually made with history and clinical presentation. Ultrasounds during pregnancy may demonstrate physical features. Brain imaging studies (CT and MRI) may be performed later to document neuroabnormalities.
2. Management includes evaluation and regular monitoring of growth and nutrition. Ongoing management of symptoms related to other medical issues is a priority.
3. Nurses should be knowledgeable of educational and community resources that may be necessary for the child to reach his or her maximum potential. See "Care of the Child with a Developmental Disability," page 1792.

PERVASIVE DEVELOPMENTAL DISORDER OR AUTISM SPECTRUM DISORDER

Autism spectrum disorders refer to a group of pervasive developmental disorders including autism, Asperger's disorder (AD), and disorders noted as pervasive developmental disorder not otherwise specified. These disorders impact 1 in 150 children.

Autism

Evidence Base Lee, C., Walter, G., Cleary, M. (2012). Communicating with children with autism spectrum disorder and their families: A practical introduction. *Journal of Psychosocial Nursing & Mental Health Services, 50*(8), 40–44.

Autism is a complex neurobiological developmental disorder that most typically appears during the first 2 years of life. The diagnosis of autism is based on the display of at least six out of 12 symptoms in three categories. Autism is a lifelong disorder defined by the individual's interactive difficulties, which can range from mild to severely impaired. It is four to five times more common in males than in females, but affected females tend to be more severely impaired.

Approximately 75% of people with autism are cognitively impaired, with a wide range of potential IQs. Autism is seen in approximately 60 to 70 per 10,000 live births.

Pathophysiology and Etiology

1. A clear cause has not been identified; however, evidence suggests a genetic predisposition, but no specific mutation has been identified.
2. Studies have shown that measles, mumps, and rubella vaccine do *not* cause autism. Likewise, thimerosal, a preservative found in many vaccines, does *not* cause autism.
3. Before diagnosis, parents may be initially concerned about their infant's social interactions, delayed or unusual speech development, and reactions to various stimuli (ie, tactile defensiveness).
4. Individuals with ASD have neuroanatomical differences, including small neuron cell size, increased cell packing, relative macrocephaly, and large third ventricles.

Clinical Manifestations

1. In general, the features present with the diagnosis include problems with social interactions, communication, and language skills.

2. Patients with autism have abnormalities in relating to people, objects, and events. They have abnormal responses to sensory stimuli, usually sound.

3. The stereotypical behaviors of autism are restricted and repetitive, like the commonly known symptom of echolalic speech.

Diagnosis and Management

 **Evidence Base** Webb, P. (2011). Screening for autism spectrum disorders during well-child visits in a primary care setting. *Journal for Nurse Practitioners, 7*(3), 229–235.

Scarpinato, N., Bradley, J., Kurbjun, K., et al. (2010). Caring for the child with an autism spectrum disorder in the acute care setting. *Journal of Specialists in Pediatric Nursing, 15*(3), 244–254.

1. Early diagnosis leads to earlier interventions, resulting in improved outcomes for these children.

2. The two major diagnostic challenges in the evaluation of ASD include making the differential diagnosis and searching for the etiologic disorder associated with ASD (ie, 3% to 5% of children with ASD will also have a diagnosis of fragile X syndrome).

3. Comprehensive standardized assessment tools specific for ASD usually require specialized training; these tools include Childhood Autism Rating Scale (CARS), Diagnostic Interview of Social and Communication Disorders (DISCO), Autism Diagnostic Interview (ADI), Autism Diagnostic Interview Schedule (ADIS), and CHAT (Checklist for Autism in Toddlers).

4. Alternative treatments such as nutrition and vitamin therapy are being investigated, but no definitive research has been conclusive to date.

5. Many children with ASD also have psychiatric comorbidities with such conditions as obsessive–compulsive disorder, attention-deficit/hyperactivity disorder (ADHD), depression, mood disorders, and Tourette syndrome. These conditions can be challenging to diagnose as it may be difficult to assess the child with communication and behavioral problems. Indeed, health care providers need to be vigilant in screening and monitoring for these comorbidities to ensure optimal functioning of the child with ASD.

6. Treatment is focused on management of symptoms. Medications may be helpful in treating some of the more disruptive behavioral symptoms. The most commonly used medications include select serotonin reuptake inhibitors, atypical antipsychotic/neuroleptics, stimulants, and alpha agonists.

7. Medical comorbidities are also common in children with ASD, including seizure disorders, sleep disturbances, GI disorders, and dental problems. As with psychiatric comorbidities, health care providers need to be vigilant in their assessment, as it can improve behavior and functioning of the child with ASD.

8. A multidisciplinary team—including primary care provider; medical subspecialists; occupational, speech, and physical therapists; and educational specialist—is essential for optimal care. See "Care of the Child with a Developmental Disability," page 1792.

Childhood Disintegrative Disorder

Childhood disintegrative disorder follows a period of normal development. This normal developmental period may last from ages 2 to 10 years, with the most common age of onset being 3 and 4 years of age. The child begins to experience a significant loss of previously acquired skills. Areas that may be affected include expressive and receptive language, social skills or adaptive behavior, bowel and bladder control, and motor skills. The loss of these skills generally reaches a point at which they do not disintegrate further. At such point, some limited improvements may be seen.

Pathophysiology and Etiology

Etiology is unknown. Childhood disintegrative disorder appears to be more common in males. The incidence of this disorder is rare.

Diagnosis and Management

See "Care of the Child with a Developmental Disability," page 1792, for a general approach to assessment.

Asperger's Disorder

Asperger's disorder is considered a milder form of autism and is characterized by poor peer relationships, lack of empathy, and the tendency to be overfocused on certain topics.

Asperger's disorder is one of several developmental disabilities associated with normal intelligence. Academic and functional underachievement in the preschool and school-age child with normal intelligence is the common picture. Proper diagnosis, utilizing a cooperative team effort from several individuals, is imperative to develop an individualized treatment plan.

Pathophysiology and Etiology

The etiology is unknown. Asperger's disorder is commonly not diagnosed until the child reaches school age. One study showed the prevalence of Asperger's disorder to be approximately 3 per 1,000 children. The male-to-female ratio is 4:1.

Clinical Manifestations

1. Child does not seek spontaneous interpersonal interactions.

2. Average to above-average intelligence and development of normal language skills with regard to vocabulary and grammar.

3. No significant delays in the areas of cognitive development, development of age-appropriate self-help skills, adaptive behavior, and curiosity about the environment.

4. Limited range of interests, strict adherence to routines and rituals, and repetitive motor movements or sequences.

5. May have obsessional interests and appear "eccentric" to others.

Diagnosis and Management

1. Complete medical review, family history, and physical examination, including vision and hearing assessment and neurologic evaluation, to rule out other disorders.

2. Genetic evaluation and counseling to identify the presence of recurrence risks.

3. Psychological testing to determine the exact nature of cognitive and perceptual dysfunctions.

4. Behavioral and social assessment.

5. Assessment of academic performance.

6. MRI and other testing to determine underlying neurologic abnormality, if appropriate.

7. Occupational and physical therapy, speech and language evaluations, as necessary.

8. School evaluation—involves IQ testing and achievement testing (teacher's input is also essential).

    a. The focus of a school evaluation is to determine eligibility for services. Most school systems will provide services only when moderate to severe problems exist.

    b. It may be necessary for the family to provide remediation for problems considered mild or outside of the educational setting.

9. Because the disorder may include health manifestations as well as behavioral and educational implications, the school nurse should be prepared to provide guidance on complex management.

 Evidence Base Minchella, L., & Preti, L. (2011). Autism spectrum disorder: Clinical considerations for the school nurse. *NASN School Nurse, 26*(3), 143–145.

Pervasive Developmental Disorder, Not Otherwise Specified

Pervasive developmental disorder, not otherwise specified (PDD-NOS) is used when the child meets some but not all criteria for the diagnosis of autism. For example, a young child may not meet all of the diagnostic criteria for an autistic disorder, but the diagnosis may be made later due to the appearance of additional manifestations. The American Psychiatric Association's *Diagnostic and Statistical Manual of Mental Disorders, Fourth Edition* added the criteria that for a diagnosis of PDD-NOS, at least one criteria from the domain of Social Interaction is required. The recognition of PDD-NOS suggests that ASD, Asperger disorder, and other PDDs represent a spectrum of developmental disorders with common features, which may range widely in severity and represent a range of genetically influenced impairments.

ATTENTION DISORDERS AND LEARNING DISABILITIES

Attention disorders and learning disabilities are separate but overlapping problems and may need specific approaches based on the nature of the disability. An estimated 5% to 10% of children (ranging up to 30%) have attention-deficit disorder (ADD); learning disabilities are reportedly present in 12.6% of children by the end of the second grade. Learning disabilities and ADD commonly occur together.

Pathophysiology and Etiology

1. Multiple hypotheses exist because the exact causes are unknown and may be genetic.

    a. A family trait—other members of the family have similar difficulties.

    b. Characteristic of inborn errors of metabolism.

    c. Sex chromosome abnormalities commonly exhibit these traits.

2. Not shown to be associated with a history of birth trauma or brain damage.

3. Exposure to prenatal and postnatal factors that might adversely affect brain development and function—lead, alcohol, cocaine, central nervous system (CNS) infections, low birth weight, and prematurity.

4. May coexist with other disabling conditions, such as spina bifida, cerebral palsy, or seizure disorders.

5. May have biomedical, emotional, social, and environmental components.

6. ADD is an alteration in the response-inhibition mechanisms of the brain controlled by the frontal cortex and reticular activating system; alteration in neurotransmitter.

7. Learning disabilities—authorities are investigating abnormalities in the parietal lobe of the brain and in the central visual pathways located in the occipital lobe.

8. Although emotional and environmental factors play a role, serotonin deficiency may serve as a physiologic basis for these disorders.

Attention Disorders

 Evidence Base Goodman, D., Lasser, R., Babcock, T., et al. (2011). Managing ADHD across the lifespan in the primary care setting. *Postgraduate Medicine, 123*(5), 4–26.

Attention disorders are characterized by a cluster of symptoms, including developmentally inappropriate short attention span, impulsivity, and distractibility. The classification system identifies three subtypes of attention disorders: predominantly inattentive, predominantly hyperactive–impulsive, and combined. Attention disorders are more common in boys than in girls by a ratio of 3 to 1. Females are much more likely to have inattentive type, showing more symptoms of attention deficit rather than hyperactivity.

There is no specific laboratory test or radiographical test that can diagnose attention disorders. The best way to diagnose attention disorders is through careful history from parents, child, and teachers; use of standardized questionnaires or rating scales; and observation. There are a number of behavior rating scales that are used to establish the diagnosis of ADD and ADHD. Examples of rating scales include the Connors Rating Scale, the Brown Attention Deficit Disorder Scale for Children and Adolescents, and the Vanderbilt ADHD Rating Scale.

Clinical Manifestations and Diagnostic Evaluation

General Behavior

 Evidence Base Burns, C. (2013). Genetic disorders. In C. Burns, A. Dunn, M. Brady, et al. (Eds.), *Pediatric primary care* (pp. 1032–1054). Philadelphia: Elsevier.

Behavior varies slightly based on the child's age. Some impairments across the lifespan can include:

1. Childhood: Needs for special education, grade retention, classroom behavior management issues, behavioral difficulties at home and other settings.
2. Adolescence: School failure and dropout, social difficulties with peer relationships, substance abuse (in untreated), high comorbidity with other psychiatric disorders, involvement in juvenile criminal activities.
3. Adult: Fewer employment possibilities and frequent job hopping; high risk of tobacco, drug, and alcohol use; high risk of motor vehicle accidents; marital problems and higher divorce rates; increased incidence of criminal activity.

Diagnostic Criteria for ADHD

Diagnostic criteria are outlined in the *Diagnostic and Statistical Manual of Mental Disorders, Fourth Edition*, Text Revision (DSM-IV-TR) criteria for attention-deficit/hyperactivity disorder. Examples of questions include:

1. Does the child often fidget with hands or feet or squirm in seat?
2. Does the child have difficulty remaining seated when required to do so?
3. Is the child easily distracted by extraneous stimuli?
4. Does the child have difficulty awaiting his or her turn in games or group situations?
5. Does the child often blurt out answers to questions before they have been completed?
6. Does the child often have difficulty following instructions from others?
7. Does the child have difficulty sustaining attention in tasks or play activities?
8. Does the child often shift from one uncompleted activity to another?
9. Does the child have difficulty playing quietly?
10. Does the child often talk excessively?
11. Does the child often interrupt or intrude on others?
12. Does the child often not seem to listen to what is being said to him or her?
13. Does the child often lose things necessary for tasks or activities at school or at home?
14. Does the child often engage in physically dangerous activities without considering possible consequences?

Management

Multidisciplinary Approach

A multidisciplinary approach, including environmental and behavioral approaches, is the treatment of choice.

Pharmacologic Treatment

1. CNS stimulants are effective for 70% to 75% of children with attention disorders.
   a. Effective in decreasing motor activities and increasing attention span and concentration, thereby allowing the child to be more available to learn.
   b. Medications generally include stimulant medications but nonstimulant medications may also be effective, especially in adults. Examples include methylphenidate, dextroamphetamine, amphetamine, lisdexamfetamine, and atomoxetine.
2. Adverse effects:
   a. Insomnia may result from increased dosage or if administered too late in the day.
   b. Anorexia, weight loss, hair loss, and temporary growth retardation.
   c. Increased pulse and respiratory rates, nervousness, nausea, and stomachache.
   d. Altered effects of many antiseizure drugs and tricyclic antidepressants.
   e. Do not cause euphoric effect or addiction in children.

Nursing Responsibilities and Family Education

1. Administer the drug before breakfast and lunch (sustained-release forms may not require a second dose).
2. Work with school system to make sure that the lunch dose is given.
3. Consider "drug holidays" during vacations and on weekends to monitor effectiveness and the need for a dosage change; this is especially recommended at the start of each academic school year.
4. Frequently a cardiac evaluation is done prior to administration of long-term stimulant use to rule out conduction disorders.
5. Stimulant drugs are not usually given to children younger than age 6.
6. The child is usually started on a small dose, which is gradually increased until the desired response is achieved.
7. Evaluate the child's response to the drug by direct observation and consultation with others, such as parents and teachers.

 DRUG ALERT Stimulant drugs for attention disorders should be used in conjunction with a comprehensive therapeutic regimen and not as the sole method of treatment. Stimulant drugs require monitoring and feedback from the parents and teachers who directly observe the effects.

Learning Disability

Difficulties with academic achievement fall under a broad category of learning problems. The cause or influencing factors can be biomedical, developmental, behavioral, emotional, social, environmental, and family issues. The problem may be in the area of reading, math, written expression, motor skills, and communication disorders. Attention deficit, anxiety, and behavioral disorders must be ruled out.

Clinical Manifestations

1. Signs of learning disabilities include:
   a. School achievement significantly lower than potential.
   b. Perceptual-motor impairments.
   c. Emotional lability.
   d. Speech and language disorders.
   e. Coordination deficits.
2. There can be a wide range of cognitive ability from mild retardation to above-average intelligence.

Areas of Learning Disabilities

Auditory Perception

Auditory perception is characterized by difficulty distinguishing between similar sounds or words. This includes the inability to process the sounds into words that have a meaning at a rapid enough rate to be able to follow conversations.

Visual Perception

Visual perception difficulties involve problems interpreting what is seen. This may include problems recognizing shapes and positions of letters or words. Depth perception may pose a problem to some children with visual perception disorders.

Integrative Processing

Integrative processing disabilities encompass, to varying degrees, the inability to sequence events or facts; comprehend abstract ideas or implied meanings; and organize learned information and apply it to what has been previously acquired.

Memory

Disabilities generally affect short-term memory, which stores information that has just been perceived for a brief period before it is either discarded or stored in long-term memory.

Expressive Language

An *expressive language* disorder affects the child's verbal communication. Characteristics depend on the child's age and the severity of the disorder. Language skills in terms of vocabulary, grammatical content, fluency, and language formulation can be affected.

Motor

Motor disabilities can affect either gross motor or fine motor muscle groups. A disability affecting the gross motor development can cause children to be "clumsy." These children have a tendency to fall or bump into things and have difficulty running and playing sports. Fine motor disabilities affect muscles for detailed tasks, such as writing, using scissors, and painting.

Management and Special Teaching Strategies

1. For visual perceptual deficit—present material verbally; use hands-on experience; tape-record teaching sessions.
2. For auditory perceptual deficit—provide materials in written form; use pictures; provide tactile learning.
3. For integrative deficit—use multisensory approaches; print directions while you verbalize them; use calendars and lists to organize tasks and activities.
4. For motor and expressive deficits—break down skills and projects into their multiple component parts; verbally describe the component parts; provide extra time to perform; allow the child to type work rather than use cursive writing.
5. For highly distractible child—provide a structured environment; have child sit in the front of the class; place child away from doors or windows; decrease clutter on his or her desk.

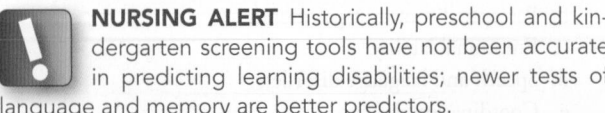

NURSING ALERT Historically, preschool and kindergarten screening tools have not been accurate in predicting learning disabilities; newer tests of language and memory are better predictors.

RESOURCES AND SUPPORT GROUPS

Agencies that may provide information, support, and additional resources include:

The ARC of the United States (formerly Association for Retarded Citizens of the United States)
1825 K Street NW, Suite 1200
Washington, DC 20006
(800) 433-5255
www.thearc.org

Autism Society
4340 East-West Hwy, Suite 350
Bethesda, MD 20814
www.autism-society.org

Children and Adults with Attention Deficit/Hyperactivity Disorder (CHADD)
8181 Professional Place, Suite 150
Landover, MD 20785
(301) 306-7070
www.chadd.org

Council for Learning Disabilities
11184 Antioch Road
P.O. Box 405
Overland Park, KS 66210
(913) 491-1011
www.cldinternational.org

The Joseph P. Kennedy, Jr. Foundation
1133 19th Street NW
Washington, DC 20005
(202) 393-1250
www.jpkf.org

Learning Disabilities Association of America
4156 Library Road
Pittsburgh, PA 15234-1349
(412) 341-1515
www.ldanatl.org

National Dissemination Center for Children with Disabilities (NICHCY)
1825 Connecticut Avenue NW, Suite 700
Washington, DC 20009
(800) 695-0285
www.nichcy.org

National Down Syndrome Congress
30 Mansell Court, Suite 108
Roswell, GA 30076
(800) 232-NDSC
www.ndsccenter.org

National Down Syndrome Society
666 Broadway
New York, NY 10012
(800) 221-4602
www.ndss.org

National Fragile X Foundation
1615 Bonanza Street, Suite 202
P.O. Box 37
Walnut Creek, CA 94597
(800) 688-8765
www.nfxf.org

SELECTED REFERENCES

American Psychiatric Association. (2000). *Diagnostic and statistical manual of mental disorders* (4th ed., Text rev.). Washington, DC: Author.

Bellando, J., & Lopez, M. (2009). The school nurse's role in treatment of the student with autism spectrum disorders. *Journal of Specialists in Pediatric Nursing, 14*(3), 173–182.

Bricker, D., Macy, M., Squires, J., Marks, K. (2013). *Developmental Screening in Your Community: An Integrated Approach for Connecting Children with Services.* Baltimore: Brookes.

Bull, M. (2011). Health supervision for children with Down syndrome. *Pediatrics, 128*(2), 393–406.

Burns, C. (2013). Genetic disorders. In C. Burns, A. Dunn, M. Brady, et al. (Eds.), *Pediatric primary care* (pp. 1032–1054). Philadelphia: Elsevier.

Butter, E., & Mulick, J. (2009). Autism. In T. McInerny, H. Adam, & D. Campbell (Eds.), *American Academy of Pediatrics textbook of pediatric care.* Elk Grove Village, IL: American Academy of Pediatrics.

Caley, L., Kramer, C., & Robinson, L. (2005). Fetal alcohol spectrum disorder. *Journal of School Nursing, 21*(3), 139–146.

Cloud, H. (2012). Developmental disabilities. In P. Samour & K. King, *Pediatric nutrition* (4th ed., pp. 219–236). Sudbury, MA: Jones & Bartlett.

Defendi, G. (2010). Fetal alcohol spectrum disorder: How to recognize the various manifestations. *Consultant for Pediatricians, 9*(10). Available: *www.pediatricsconsultant360.com/content/fetal-alcohol-spectrum-disorder-how-recognize-various-manifestations.*

DeVeney, S., Hoffman, L., Cress, C. (2012). Communication-based assessment of developmental age for young children with developmental disabilities. *Journal of Speech, Language & Hearing Research, 55*(3), 695–709.

Elder, J., & D'Alessandro, T. (2009). Supporting families of children with autism spectrum disorders: Questions parents ask and what nurses need to know. *Pediatric Nursing, 35*(4), 240–253.

Goodman, D., Lasser, R., Babcock, T., et al. (2011). Managing ADHD across the lifespan in the primary care setting. *Postgraduate Medicine, 123*(5), 4–26.

Heavey, E., & Peterson-Sweeney, K. (2010, June). Caring for an adult with Down syndrome. *Nursing,* pp. 53–56.

Heslam, S. (2011). Health issues for adults with Down's syndrome. *Learning Disability Practice, 14*(6), 26–27.

Hockenberry, M. J. (2011). *Wong's nursing care of infants and children* (9th ed.). St. Louis, MO: Elsevier Mosby.

Honigfeld, L., Chandhok, L., Spiegelman, K. (2012). Engaging pediatricians in developmental screening: The effectiveness of academic detailing. *Journal of Autism & Developmental Disorders, 42*(6), 1175–1182.

Hoon, A. H., Jr., Pulsifer, M. B., Gopalan, R., et al. (1993). Clinical Adaptive Test/Clinical Linguistic Auditory Milestone Scale in early cognitive assessment. *Journal of Pediatrics, 123*(1), S1–S8.

Laver-Bradbury, C. (2012). The treatment of ADHD in children and young people. *British Journal of School Nursing, 7*(2), 71–75.

Lee, C., Walter, G., Cleary, M. (2012). Communicating with children with autism spectrum disorder and their families: A practical introduction. *Journal of Psychosocial Nursing & Mental Health Services, 50*(8), 40–44.

Leenaars, L., Denys, K., Henneveld, D., et al. (2012). The impact of fetal alcohol spectrum disorders on families: Evaluation of a family intervention program. *Community Mental Health Journal, 48*(4), 431–435.

Lovette, B. (2008). Safe transportation for children with special needs. *Journal of Pediatric Health Care, 22*, 323–328.

McConkie-Rosell, A., Finucane, B., Cronister, A., et al. (2005). Genetic counseling for fragile X syndrome: Updated recommendations of the National Society of Genetic Counselors. *Journal of Genetic Counseling, 14*(4), 249–270.

Minchella, L., & Preti, L. (2011). Autism spectrum disorder: Clinical considerations for the school nurse. *NASN School Nurse, 26*(3), 143–145.

Msall, M. E., DiGaudio, K., Duffy, L. C., et al. (1994). WeeFIM. Normative sample of an instrument for tracking functional independence in children. *Clinical Pediatrics, 33*(7), 431–438.

Nehring, W. M. (2007). Cultural considerations for children with intellectual and developmental disabilities. *Journal of Pediatric Nursing, 22*(2), 93–102.

Niewczyk, P., & Granger, C. (2010). Measuring functions in young children with impairments. *Pediatric Physical Therapy, 22*(1), 42–50.

Pasco, G. (2011). The diagnosis and epidemiology of autism. *Tizard Learning Disability Review, 16*(4), 5–19.

Pati, A. (2011). Early assessment and diagnosis for children with hyperactivity disorder. *Nursing Children & Young People, 23*(7), 5–15.

Ranweiler, R. (2009). Assessment and care of the newborn with Down syndrome. *Advances in Neonatal Care, 9*(1), 17–24.

Richmond, N., Tran, T., Berry, S. (2012). Can the medical home eliminate racial and ethnic disparities for transition services among youth with special health care needs? *Maternal & Child Health Journal, 16*(4), 824–833.

Scales, R., & Weber, C. (2010). Turner syndrome: Do not miss this diagnosis. *Journal of Pediatric Nursing, 25*, 66–68.

Scarpinato, N., Bradley, J., Kurbjun, K., et al. (2010). Caring for the child with an autism spectrum disorder in the acute care setting. *Journal of Specialists in Pediatric Nursing, 15*(3), 244–254.

Shevell, M., Ashwal, S., Donley, D., et al. (2003). Practice parameter: Evaluation of the child with global developmental delay: Report of the Quality Standards Subcommittee of the American Academy of Neurology and the Practice Committee of the Child Neurology Society. *Neurology, 60*(3), 367–380.

Subcommittee on Attention-Deficit/Hyperactivity Disorder. (2011). ADHD: Clinical practice guideline for the diagnosis, evaluation, and treatment of attention-deficit/hyperactivity disorder in children and adolescents. *Pediatrics, 128*(5), 1007–1022.

Tsai, A., Pickler, L., Tartaglia, N., et al. (2009). Chromosomal disorders and fragile x syndrome. In W. Carey, A. Crocker, W. Coleman, et al. (Eds.), *Developmental-behavioral pediatrics* (4th ed., pp. 224–234). Philadelphia: Saunders.

U.S. Preventive Services Task Force. (2012). *Screening for speech and language delay in preschool children: Recommendation statement.* Rockville, MD: Agency for Healthcare Research and Quality.

Wang, G., McGrath, B., & Watts, C. (2010). Health care transitions among youth with disabilities or special health needs: An ecological approach. *Journal of Pediatric Nursing, 25*(6), 505–550.

Webb, P. (2011). Screening for autism spectrum disorders during well-child visits in a primary care setting. *Journal for Nurse Practitioners, 7*(3), 229–235.

PART FIVE

PSYCHIATRIC
NURSING

57
Problems of Mental Health

ANXIETY-RELATED DISORDERS
Anxiety and Dissociative Disorders

 Evidence Base American Psychiatric Association. (2000). *Diagnostic and statistical manual of mental disorders* (4th ed., text rev.). Washington, DC: Author.

Anxiety disorders are the most common of all psychiatric disorders. An individual with one of these disorders experiences physiologic, cognitive, and behavioral symptoms of anxiety. The physiologic manifestations are related to the "fight-or-flight" response and result in cardiovascular, respiratory, neuromuscular, and GI stimulation. The cognitive symptoms include subjective feelings of apprehension, uneasiness, uncertainty, or dread. Behavioral manifestations include irritability, restlessness, pacing, crying and sighing, and complaints of tension and nervousness. The common theme among anxiety disorders is that the individual experiences a level of anxiety that interferes with functioning in personal, occupational, and social areas.

Anxiety experienced in response to a traumatic event may interrupt the formation of memories related to the event and disrupt learning processes resulting in dissociation. Disassociation can be initially viewed as an adaptive defense against painful memories or feelings of helplessness. When aspects of disassociation interfere with the ability of the individual to function socially, vocationally, or interpersonally, then such dissociative aspects may be considered a disorder.

In most situations of disassociation, the response to a traumatic event is not consciously connected to memories of the event. Such dissociative disorders are characterized by an alteration in conscious awareness, which includes forgetfulness and memory loss for past stressful events. Other dissociate methods of withdrawing from anxiety-producing stimuli are depersonalization (a feeling of disconnection from one's self) and derealization (a feeling of being disconnected from the surrounding environment). The individual may also develop what appear to be distinctly different personalities.

Classification

Anxiety-related disorders, as defined by the *Diagnostic and Statistical Manual of Mental Disorders*, Fourth Edition, Text Revision (DSM-IV-TR), include those listed here.

Anxiety Disorders
1. Panic disorder without agoraphobia.
2. Panic disorder with agoraphobia.
3. Agoraphobia without history of panic disorder.
4. Specific phobia.
5. Social phobia.
6. Obsessive–compulsive disorder (OCD).
7. Posttraumatic stress disorder (PTSD).
8. Acute stress disorder.
9. Generalized anxiety disorder.
10. Anxiety disorder due to a general medical condition.
11. Substance-induced anxiety disorder.
12. Anxiety disorder not otherwise specified.

Dissociative Disorders
1. Dissociative amnesia.
2. Dissociative fugue.
3. Dissociative identity disorder.
4. Depersonalization disorder.
5. Dissociative disorder not otherwise specified.

Pathophysiology and Etiology

The underlying etiology of anxiety disorders as well as any of the psychiatric disorders, is complex, having multiple factors that interact. Therefore, it is essential to examine the biochemical, genetic, psychosocial, and sociocultural factors.

Biochemical Factors

1. The limbic system, which is called the *emotional brain*, regulates emotional responses. Anxiety disorders are associated with abnormalities within this system (including the frontal cortex, hypothalamus, amygdala, hippocampus, brain stem, and the autonomic nervous system).
2. Neurotransmitters and their specific receptor sites function to transmit inhibiting or stimulating messages across the synapses between nerve cells in the brain. Abnormalities in the neurotransmitters or the receptor sites have been associated with multiple psychiatric disorders, including anxiety disorders.
3. Gamma-aminobutyric acid (GABA) is an inhibitory neurotransmitter that normally acts to decrease anxiety responses. An individual that genetically produces lower amounts of GABA may have an increased likelihood of developing anxiety or stress-related disorders (eg, PTSD).
4. Norepinephrine is a stimulating neurotransmitter, which is released as part of the fight-or-flight response and is associated with the cardiovascular and respiratory effects of anxiety. Serotonin is a neurotransmitter that regulates multiple responses, including sleep and alertness and sensations of hunger and satiation. Genetic variation resulting in a decrease in the number of select serotonin receptors (particularly 1A) may be associated with the development of panic disorder.
5. Panic disorders may be related to the reception of a false signal from the brain that there is a shortage of oxygen or an increase in carbon dioxide (suffocation alarm theory). Those who have panic attacks have also been reported to have higher levels of norepinephrine.
6. Suppression of cortisol through administration of dexamethasone has been associated with PTSD, suggesting heightened glucocorticoid feedback sensitivity.
7. Positron-emission tomography (PET) and computed tomography (CT) scanning have shown abnormalities in glucose metabolism in the frontal and prefrontal cortex and the basal ganglia of the brains of individuals with panic disorder. PET scans have also demonstrated increased blood flow and cerebral metabolism in the basal ganglia and frontal cortex of individuals with OCD.
8. OCD has been associated with increased serotonin responsiveness as well as striatum dysfunction. The striatum controls voluntary movement and it is hypothesized that individuals with OCD may be doing repetitive rituals to "self-medicate" for serotonin deficiencies.
9. Dissociative symptoms have been related to shrinkage of the hippocampus. Studies of physically, sexually, and psychologically abused children found increased electroencapholography (ECG) abnormalities in the frontal and temporal lobes.

Genetic Factors

1. First-degree relatives of individuals with panic disorder have a four to seven times greater chance of developing this disorder. Twin studies demonstrate a higher concordance rate for monozygotic than dizygotic twins.
2. Approximately 20% of first-degree relatives of people with agoraphobia also have agoraphobia.
3. Approximately 3% to 7% of people with OCD have first-degree relatives with the same disorder.
4. Approximately 25% of first-degree relatives with generalized anxiety disorder are also affected by generalized anxiety disorder.
5. Environmental influences may interact with genetic predispositions in the pathogenesis of dissociative and other trauma-related disorders. Variations in regions of the serotonin transporter gene, among others, which regulates an enzyme that degrades several neurotransmitters (catechol-O-methyl transferase), have been found to be associated with adverse life events in individuals with dissociation. It has been speculated that the nature of this variation may be associated with development of anxiety or depression depending on the stressor.

Psychosocial Factors

1. Psychodynamic theory describes unconscious conflicts having early childhood origin and resulting from repressed wishes and drives. These conflicts cause guilt and shame, which lead to anxiety and associated symptoms.
2. Interpersonal theory implicates early relationships, which directly affect development of self-concept and self-esteem. Individuals with poor self-concept and decreased self-esteem have increased susceptibility to anxiety-related disorders.
3. Behavioral theory describes anxiety and associated symptoms as a conditioned response to internal and external stressors.
4. Cognitive theory describes faulty thinking patterns that lead to an individual's misperceiving events affecting self, the future, and the world. These faulty thinking patterns contribute to the subjective experience of anxiety.
5. Dissociative disorders are generally associated with traumatic events. An individual responds to severe trauma (especially in early childhood) by "splitting off" or dissociating the self from the memory of the trauma. Severe physical, sexual, and psychological abuse in early childhood is associated with dissociative identity disorder.

Sociocultural Factors

1. Anxiety disorders and ritualistic behaviors are commonly seen in high-technology societies.
2. There is a higher incidence of anxiety disorders in urban communities than in rural communities.
3. Women are diagnosed more commonly with anxiety disorders except with OCD, which affects men and women equally. It is thought that this may represent a sociocultural rather than a genetic factor.

Clinical Manifestations

Acute Stress and Posttraumatic Stress Disorder

1. Acute and posttraumatic stress disorder share several symptoms, with the major difference between the two conditions being the time frame in which symptoms develop.

2. For acute stress, symptoms develop within 1 month of the traumatic event, and last for 2 days to 3 weeks whereas for posttraumatic stress disorder, the symptoms are more enduring and have lasted for a least 1 month at the time of diagnosis.

3. During the initial traumatic event, the individual needs to have displayed an initial response of horror, accompanied by intense feelings of helplessness in order to meet criteria for each of these disorders.

4. Both disorders share a cluster of dissociative symptoms with attempts to avoid stimuli associated with the original trauma while also reexperiencing intrusive memories and recollections of the traumatic event.

5. An examination and history would elicit findings that would include three or more of the following: a sense of numbness, a lack of emotional responses, feelings of depersonalization or derealization, a feeling of confusion, and a loss of memory for aspects of the original event.

6. There will also be increased sympathetic activation, hypervigilance and a pattern of reexperiencing the event through intrusive dreams, flashbacks or increased anxiety when presented with stimuli associated with the traumatic event. Increased sympathetic activation associated with anxiety is demonstrated through insomnia, difficulty concentrating, feelings of restlessness, and hypervigilance.

Generalized Anxiety Disorder

1. A pattern of worrying or anxiety that results in increased autonomic activity persisting for a period of at least 6 months.

2. An examination and history would reveal symptoms from three of four categories:
   a. Motor (eg, trembling, restlessness, inability to relax, and fatigue).
   b. Autonomic hyperactivity (eg, sweating, palpitations, cold clammy hands, urinary frequency, lump in throat, pallor or flushing, increased pulse, and rapid respirations).
   c. Apprehensiveness (eg, worry, dread, fear, rumination, insomnia, and inability to concentrate).
   d. Hypervigilance (eg, feeling edgy, scanning the environment, and distractibility).

   Obsessive–Compulsive Disorder
1. A preoccupation with persistent intrusive thoughts (obsessions), repeated performance of rituals designed to prevent some event (compulsions), or both.
2. Anxiety occurs if obsessions or compulsions are resisted and from feeling powerless to resist the thoughts or rituals.

Panic Disorder

1. The presence of recurrent unexpected anxiety attacks for at least 1 month with a sudden onset of feelings of intense apprehension and dread.

2. These feelings result in sympathetic activation that manifests through the appearance of at least four of the following symptoms: chest discomfort or pain, dyspnea, palpitations, syncope, diaphoresis, trembling, hot or cold flashes, and dizziness.

Phobias

1. A phobia is a persistent irrational fear of an object or situation that the person may recognize as being unreasonable.

2. Exposure to the feared object or situation may result in a panic attack.

3. An example is agoraphobia, which is a fear of being alone in open or public places where escape might be difficult.

Dissociative Disorders

Dissociative disorders are conditions in which the anxiety associated with a stressful or traumatic event induces a subjective feeling of being not connected to one's body or to reality. These conditions are viewed as defense mechanisms that result in a disorder when the ability to function in social or work environments is significantly impaired due to feelings of dissociation.

1. Depersonalization disorder—a persistent or recurrent experience of feeling detached from oneself. A common sensation is of being an outside observer of one's body. This experience can cause significant impairment in daily function.

2. Dissociative amnesia—one or more episodes of inability to recall important information, usually of a traumatic or stressful nature

3. Dissociative fugue—state manifested by sudden, unexpected travel away from home or one's place of work with inability to remember the past. There may be confusion about personal identity or the assumption of a new identity.

4. Dissociative identity disorder—previously known as multiple personality disorder, this disorder is evidenced by the presence of two or more distinct identities, each with its own patterns of relating, perceiving, and thinking. At least two of these identities take control of the person's behavior.

Diagnostic Evaluation

1. Measurement tools for anxiety:
   a. Hamilton Rating Scale for Anxiety
   b. State–Trait Anxiety Inventory
2. Measurement tools for OCDs:
   a. Yale-Brown Obsessive–Compulsive Scale
   b. Florida Obsessive–Compulsive Inventory (FOCI)
3. Measurement tools for panic disorders:
   a. Acute Panic Inventory
   b. Sheehan Client-Rated Anxiety Scale
4. Sodium lactate infusion or carbon dioxide inhalation will likely produce a panic attack in a person with panic disorder.
5. Increased arousal may be measured through studies of autonomic functioning (ie, heart rate, electromyography, sweat gland activity) in a person with PTSD.
6. Dexamethasone suppression test (DST) may be used to demonstrate heightened glucocorticoid feedback in individuals with PTSD.
7. Measurement tools for dissociation:
   a. Dissociation Impulsivity Scale (DIS)
   b. Dissociative Experiences Scale (DES)
   c. Dissociative Disorders Interview Schedule (DDIS)

Management

Evidence Base Koen, N., & Stein, D. J. (2011). Pharmacotherapy of anxiety disorders: a critical review. *Dialogues in Clinical Neuroscience, 13,* 423–437.

Wampold, B. E., Budge, S. L., Laska, K. M., et al. (2011). Evidence-based treatments for depression and anxiety versus treatment-as-usual: A meta-analysis of direct comparisons. *Clinical Psychology Review, 31,* 1304–1312.

1. Various levels and sites of care can be provided: psychiatric inpatient, outpatient, or home care. Most care is provided on an outpatient basis. Site of care is based on many factors, including degree of disability of affected individual, community services available, and insurance and managed care considerations. Generally, the recommended treatment is a combination of drugs and psychotherapy, along with education of the individual and family.

2. Psychoeducational strategies:
   a. Relaxation techniques.
   b. Progressive muscle relaxation.
   c. Guided imagery or visualization exercises.
   d. Stress management.
   e. Assertiveness training.

3. Psychotherapy:
   a. Psychodynamic—assists people in understanding their experiences by identifying unconscious conflicts and developing effective coping behaviors.
   b. Behavioral—focuses on the individual problematic behavior and works to modify or extinguish the behavior. One form of behavioral therapy effective in management of phobic disorders is systematic desensitization.
   c. Cognitive—assists patient to question faulty thought patterns (reframing) and examine alternatives. In treatment of PTSD and dissociative disorders, reframing is used to help the patient view self as a survivor rather than a victim.
   d. Hypnotherapy—can be used as part of therapy for those suffering dissociative disorders.
   e. Support group therapy—useful in providing a supportive and psychoeducational approach for patients with anxiety or dissociative disorders.

4. Somatic therapies:
   a. Biofeedback—relaxation through biofeedback is achieved when a person learns to control physiologic mechanisms that are not ordinarily within one's awareness. Awareness and control are accomplished by monitoring body processes, including muscle tone, heart rate, and brain waves.
   b. Psychopharmacologic—traditionally, drugs used to treat anxiety-related disorders were those that would increase GABA (benzodiazepines), regulate serotonin levels (antidepressants), or reduce physiologic effects of anxiety by causing peripheral beta-adrenergic blockade (beta-adrenergic blockers). Currently, selective serotonin reuptake inhibitors are prescribed as first-line treatment for managing several anxiety-related disorders due to their safety and tolerability. See Table 57-1, page 1814.
   c. Narcotherapy—sodium amobarbital or IV sodium thiopental may assist the therapist in gaining access to a patient's repressed memories and buried conflicts. In a person experiencing dissociative amnesia or dissociative fugue, the therapist may explore dissociated events. If the person is diagnosed with dissociative identity disorder, this type of interview may facilitate the access of other personalities.

Complications

1. Undiagnosed medical reasons for anxiety could lead to physical deterioration and a delay in obtaining appropriate medical care. It is important to screen for coexisting medical illness.
2. If panic and phobic disorders are left untreated, they can lead to increasing social withdrawal and isolation, which may severely impair the person's social and work life.
3. Untreated OCD can lead to aggressive behavior toward self or others as well as depression. It can also lead to injuries from compulsive behavior such as skin breakdown from repeated handwashing.
4. Undiagnosed or untreated PTSD or acute stress disorder can lead to substance abuse or dependence, aggressive or violent behavior and, possibly, suicide.
5. If a person with a dissociative disorder goes untreated, aggressive behavior may develop toward self or others. Such behaviors may include assaults, depression, PTSD, psychoactive substance abuse disorder, rape, self-mutilation, and suicide attempts.

Nursing Assessment

1. Assess psychological, cognitive, and behavioral symptoms.
   a. Defense mechanisms or coping measures used.
   b. Mood.
   c. Suicide potential.
   d. Thought content and process.
   e. Severity of subjective experience of anxiety.
   f. Understanding of specific disorder.
2. Explore social functioning.
   a. Ability to function in social and work situations.
   b. Impact of symptoms on patient's relationships, especially work and family relationships.
   c. Diversional and recreational behavior.
   d. Identification of stressors related to self-concept, role performance, life values, social status, and support systems.
   e. Benefits (primary and secondary gains) and risks of the presenting symptoms.

Nursing Diagnoses

- Anxiety related to unexpected panic attacks or related to reexperiencing traumatic events.
- Acute Confusion related to severe anxiety.

Table 57-1   Dosage and Adverse Reactions of Anti-Anxiety Drugs

DRUG: CLASS/GENERIC/TRADE NAME	ADULT THERAPEUTIC DOSAGE RANGE (MG/DAY)	ADVERSE REACTIONS
Benzodiazepines		*For all benzodiazepines:*
Alprazolam	0.75–1 mg	• Drowsiness, sedation, and dizziness.
Chlordiazepoxide	15–75 mg	• Possibility of dependence.
Clonazepam	0.5–2 mg	
Clorazepate	15–60 mg	
Diazepam	4–40 mg	
Lorazepam	2–6 mg	
Oxazepam	30–120 mg	
Tetracyclic Agent		
Mirtazapine	15–45 mg	• Somnolence, increased appetite, weight gain, dry mouth, constipation
Selective Serotonin Reuptake Inhibitors (SSRIs)		
Citalopram	20–60 mg	• Nausea, dry mouth, diarrhea, fatigue, drowsiness, ejaculatory delay, impotence
Duloxetene	40–60 mg	• Nausea, dry mouth, dizziness, constipation, diarrhea, fatigue, increased sweating
Escitalopram	10–20 mg	• Nausea, ejaculatory delay, impotence
Fluoxetine	20–80 mg	• Delayed orgasm, headache, nervousness, insomnia, anxiety, tremor, dizziness, nausea, diarrhea, anorexia, dry mouth
Fluvoxamine	50–300 mg	• Nausea, vomiting, drowsiness, anorexia, constipation, tremor, insomnia
Paroxetine	10–50 mg	• Nausea, dry mouth, headache, somnolence, insomnia, diarrhea, constipation, tremor

- Impaired Social Interaction related to avoidance behavior or related to embarrassment and shame associated with symptoms.
- Ineffective Role Performance related to inability to function in usual social and occupational situations secondary to anxiety-related symptoms.
- Disturbed Personal Identity related to a traumatic event.
- Risk for Injury related to compulsive behaviors.

Nursing Interventions

Reducing Symptoms of Anxiety

1. Help patient identify anxiety-producing situations and plan for such events.
2. Assist patient to develop assertiveness and communication skills.
3. Practice stress-reduction techniques with patient.
4. Teach patient to monitor for objective and subjective manifestations of anxiety.
   a. Tachycardia, tachypnea.
   b. Signs and symptoms associated with autonomic stimulation—perspiration, difficulty concentrating, insomnia.

5. Promote use of stress-reduction techniques in managing symptoms of anxiety.
6. Encourage patient to verbalize feelings of anxiety.
7. Administer prescribed anxiolytics to decrease anxiety level.

 DRUG ALERT Benzodiazepines are associated with tolerance and dependence and are appropriate for short-term use. Withdrawal symptoms may occur when drug is abruptly discontinued. Gradual dosage reduction is necessary. Overdose or taking benzodiazepines with alcohol or other central nervous system (CNS) depressants can cause respiratory depression requiring emergency intervention.

Improving Concentration

1. Use short, simple sentences when communicating with patient.
2. Maintain a calm, serene manner.
3. Use adjuncts to verbal communication, such as visual aids and role-playing, to stimulate memory and retention of information.
4. Teach relaxation techniques to diminish distress that interferes with concentration ability.

Increasing Social Interaction

1. Encourage discussion of reasons for and feelings about social isolation.
2. Help patient identify specific causes and situations that produce anxiety that inhibits social interaction.
3. Recommend participation in programs directed at specific conflict areas or skill deficiencies. Such programs may focus on assertiveness skills, body awareness, managing multiple role responsibilities, and stress management.

Encouraging Independence

1. Identify secondary benefits, such as decreased responsibility and increased dependency, that inhibit patient's move to independence.
2. Provide experiences in which patient can be successful.
3. Explore alternative methods of meeting dependency needs.
4. Explore beliefs that support a helpless or dependent mode of behavior.
5. Teach and role-play assertive behaviors in specific situations.
6. Provide instruction in decision-making skills, allowing opportunities for practice and rehearsal of techniques in role-play situations.
7. Assist patient to improve skills based on performance.
8. Encourage family members to avoid fostering dependency.

Strengthening Identity

1. Develop an honest, nonjudgmental relationship with patient.
2. Try to establish open communication.
3. Do not overwhelm patient.
4. Teach patient containment techniques to assist in coping with the painful memories becoming conscious (eg, visualizing a safe environment, recall of past successes in dealing with anxiety, focusing on slowing of physiologic responses).

Reducing Harm from Behavior

1. Encourage patient to set limits on ritualistic behavior as part of established treatment plan.
2. Assist patient in listing all objects and places that trigger anxiety as part of exposure-response prevention program.
3. Use cognitive strategies, such as reframing, to assist patient in placing thoughts and feelings in a different perspective.
4. Participate as member of treatment team in establishing program for systematic desensitization.
5. Intervene as needed and obtain emergency assistance when patient is in immediate danger.

Community and Home Care Considerations

1. Patients with anxiety-related disorders are generally treated in an outpatient setting. Many of these patients may not see a mental health professional but will be treated by their family health care provider, utilizing pharmacologic therapy. Nurses who encounter patients taking prescribed drugs for anxiety should assess effectiveness and patient knowledge base regarding safe use of these drugs. Patients should be encouraged to utilize anxiety-reduction techniques.
2. Because anxiety disorders will affect family functioning, the nurse should provide support for the family, including teaching family members about the disorder and treatment measures.
3. Patients may elect to utilize alternative and complementary therapies in order to obtain relief from symptoms. Advise patients not to use nutritional supplement or "natural" remedy, such as St. John's wort or kava kava, without discussing it with a health care provider; many drug interactions exist.
4. Several community support groups are available to provide patient with continued support. Patient may also be able to learn further techniques for the management of anxiety through participation in these programs. Such programs may also provide patient with an opportunity to practice previously learned skills in a supportive environment.

Family Education and Health Maintenance

1. Teach patient and family members about anxiety.
   a. Define anxiety and differentiate it from fear.
   b. Explain causes of anxiety.
   c. Identify events that can trigger anxiety.
   d. Identify relevant signs and symptoms of anxiety.
2. Describe the drug regimen, including significant action, adverse effects, dosage considerations, and any food or drug interactions.
3. Identify, describe, and practice deep-muscle relaxation techniques, relaxation breathing, imagery, and other relaxation therapies (see page 30).
4. Teach family to give positive reinforcement for use of healthy behaviors.
5. Teach family not to assume responsibilities or roles normally assigned to patient.
6. Teach family to give attention to patient, not patient's symptoms.
7. Teach alternative ways to perform activities of daily living (ADLs) if physical or emotional disability inhibits function and performance.
8. For additional information and support, refer to such agencies as the Anxiety Disorders Association of America (*www.adaa.org*).
9. Many websites provide support for individuals and family members. Some examples include Agoraphobics Building Independent Lives, *www.anxietysupport.org* (for sufferers from anxiety disorders), and for panic and anxiety disorders, *www.anxietynetwork.com/pdhome.html*.

Evaluation: Expected Outcomes

- Identifies stressors and demonstrates normal heart rate, respirations, sleep pattern, and subjective feelings of anxiety.
- Demonstrates improved concentration and thought processes through improved ability to focus, think, and solve problems.
- Reports increased participation and enjoyment in family- and community-related events
- Reports going to work, keeps appointments.
- Uses coping strategies in situations that are anxiety provoking.
- Does not injure self or others.

Somatoform Disorders

Evidence Base American Psychiatric Association. (2000). *Diagnostic and statistical manual of mental disorders* (4th ed., text rev.). Washington, DC: Author.

de C Williams, A. C., & Cella, M. (2012). Medically unexplained symptoms and pain: Misunderstanding and myth. *Current Opinion in Supportive and Palliative Care, 6*(2), 201–206.

Somatoform disorders are characterized by physical symptoms that cannot be explained by known physical mechanisms. These disorders have in common the belief that physical symptoms are real despite evidence to the contrary. The affected individual experiences changes or loss in physical function. The physical symptoms are not under the individual's voluntary control. Significant impairment occurs in social or occupational functioning. For these reasons, it has been argued that these conditions should be located under the Axis III category of medical disorders rather than as primary psychiatric diagnoses.

Classification

1. Somatization disorder.
2. Undifferentiated somatoform disorder.
3. Conversion disorder.
4. Pain disorder.
5. Hypochondriasis.
6. Body dysmorphic disorder.
7. Somatoform disorder not otherwise specified.

Pathophysiology and Etiology

The underlying etiology of somatoform disorders is difficult to define. The following factors may interact in the individual with these disorders.

Biochemical Factors

1. An individual with a somatoform disorder may experience high levels of physiologic arousal (increased awareness of somatic sensations).
2. The phenomenon of alexithymia, or deficient communication between brain hemispheres, may result in difficulty expressing emotions directly, and therefore distress may be expressed as physical symptoms.
3. The concept of somatosensory amplification, in which there is the tendency to experience somatic sensation as intense, noxious, and disturbing, may be related to the development of somatoform disorders.

Genetic Factors

1. Somatization disorder has been found to have a 10% to 20% frequency in first-degree female biological relatives of women with this disorder.
2. Twin studies have validated some increased risk in conversion disorder in monozygotic twins.
3. The genetic basis for other somatoform disorders is not well established.

Psychosocial Factors

1. Psychodynamic theory—the psychological source of ego conflict is denied and finds expression through displacement of anxiety onto physical symptoms. Both primary gain (anxiety relief) and secondary gains (increased dependence and relief from normal responsibilities) are common to these disorders.
2. Behavioral theory—the child learns from parent to express anxiety through somatization; secondary gains reinforce symptoms.
3. Cognitive theory—the individual has cognitive distortions in which benign symptoms are magnified and interpreted as serious disease.
4. Family theory—a family system that is overly enmeshed may utilize dysfunction in one person as a means to handle anxiety. In such families, the individual may not see self as a separate and distinct person; instead, the person may view him- or herself as an extension of the family.

Sociocultural Factors

1. Incidence of somatoform disorders is highest in rural populations and in low socioeconomic groups.
2. Somatic symptoms are more common in cultures that view direct expression of emotions as unacceptable.
3. Women may experience certain chronic pain conditions more commonly than men (this may have more of a cultural than a genetic basis).

Clinical Manifestations

Somatoform disorders are psychiatric conditions that manifest in the appearance of symptoms that reflect medical illnesses or injuries. For the diagnosis of these conditions to be made, other physical health issues must be ruled out. As with other mental health conditions, these problems lead to problems with the ability to perform necessary activities of daily living.

Body Dysmorphic Disorder

1. This disorder is characterized by a preoccupation with some imagined defect in appearance in an otherwise normal-appearing person (or excessive concern, if the defect is present).
2. The preoccupation causes significant impairment in social or occupational functioning or cause marked distress.

Conversion Disorder

1. With this condition, the individual develops symptoms compatible with a neurological disorder.
2. Examples include loss of vision, deafness, peripheral neuropathy, or bladder and bowel dysfunction. Some patients may exhibit paralysis or seizure activity.
3. These symptoms cannot be associated with a physical illness for the diagnosis of this disorder.

Hypochondriasis

1. A fixed preoccupation the individual has a serious medical condition.
2. This belief often persists in spite of medical tests or procedures that do not find any physical condition.
3. This preoccupation often leads to significant problems with daily function.

Pain Disorder

1. Characterized by the presence of acute or chronic pain, which may be associated with a physical injury or have a psychological cause.
2. When associated with a physical cause, the pain appears to be more intense or disabling than expected.
3. Pain is generally found in more than one place on the body.

Somatization Disorder

1. A chronic condition characterized by the presence of numerous physical complaints prior to age 30, with at least 6 months' duration at time of diagnosis.
2. Physical examination and history elicits reports of pain in at least four bodily locations, gastrointestinal dysfunction, reproductive concerns or dysfunction, and at least one symptom reflecting a neurologic disorder.
3. An undifferentiated form of the disorder exists, with fewer presenting symptoms primarily consisting of fatigue, gastrointestinal symptoms, and pain.

Diagnostic Evaluation

1. Individuals with somatoform disorders will present in the medical rather than the psychiatric setting because of their belief that the problems are medical.
2. The individual should receive a thorough medical evaluation (if possible, avoiding repeating tests that have already had negative results).
3. The diagnosis of somatoform disorder will be made after a thorough medical evaluation in which no organic basis for the symptoms is found.

Management

1. Level and setting of care to be provided is determined. In general, the individual will be treated on an outpatient basis, unless underlying mood disorder is present leading to risk for self-harm.
2. Referral to psychiatric treatment is generally rejected by the individual with a somatoform disorder; therefore, the goal of management is to maintain a long-term relationship with a specific health care provider to prevent patient from seeking multiple providers with multiple recommendations for testing, treatments, and drugs.
3. Psychotherapy:
   a. Psychodynamic—assist the individual to express conflicts and emotions verbally rather than displacing them onto physical symptoms.
   b. Behavioral—establish a program whereby adaptive behavior is reinforced and illness behaviors do not receive secondary gains.
   c. Cognitive—restructure belief system that perpetuates illness-related behaviors.
   d. Family therapy—assist family members to define appropriate boundaries and support patient in increasing self-responsibility.
4. Somatic therapies: somatoform disorders are usually not treated with psychopharmacologic drugs because these patients are susceptible to dependency on drugs used.
5. Mood disorders, especially depression, are a common comorbid problem in individuals with somatoform disorders. Antidepressant drugs may be used to treat the mood disorder.

Complications

1. A patient with a known history of a somatoform disorder may have a coexisting medical condition that could go undiagnosed. Careful screening is essential to rule out medical problems.
2. Increased risk of suicide and substance abuse and dependence disorders is possible in patient with an untreated somatoform disorder.

Nursing Assessment

1. Assess physical complaints.
   a. Current and past history as well as duration of problems.
   b. Diagnostic testing completed.
   c. Number of health care providers consulted.
   d. Types and amounts of drugs as well as whether self-medicating (over-the-counter) or prescribed.
2. Assess psychological processes.
   a. Perception of illness and current stressors.
   b. Self-concept and body image.
   c. Secondary gains from physical symptoms.
   d. Mood.
   e. Suicide potential.
3. Explore social functioning.

Refer to section on anxiety disorders, page 1813, for assessment data.

Nursing Diagnoses

- Anxiety related to multiple physical symptoms and belief that serious disease exists.
- Ineffective Coping related to preoccupation with physical symptoms.

Other nursing diagnoses and nursing interventions under anxiety disorders may apply.

Nursing Interventions

Encouraging Recognition of Anxiety

1. Discuss current life stressors in the areas of social, occupational, and family functioning.
2. Assist patient to identify anxiety-producing situations and plan coping strategies.
3. Avoid focus on physical symptoms (after appropriate screening to rule out physical etiology).
4. Maintain focus on feelings and emotional responses rather than on somatic symptoms.

Improving Coping

1. Teach and reinforce problem-solving approach to stressors.
2. Practice use of stress-reduction techniques with patient.
3. Encourage use of support groups.
4. Set limits on manipulative behaviors in a matter-of-fact manner.

5. Decrease reinforcement of secondary gains for physical symptoms.
6. Help patient identify and use positive means to meet emotional needs.

Community and Home Care Considerations

1. Encourage patient to cooperate with referrals for psychiatric or psychotherapy treatments.
2. Promote patient attendance and participation at community support groups.
3. Teach patient and family the importance of remaining with one health care provider to ensure continuity of care.
4. Nurses who encounter patients with somatoform disorders in the community should maintain a matter-of-fact attitude in order to decrease emphasis on dramatic symptoms. Any approach to patient should include a focus on patient's strengths and capabilities rather than on disability.

Family Education and Health Maintenance

1. Teach patient and family about the relationship between stressors, anxiety, and physical symptoms.
2. Family should expect person to function despite physical symptoms; doing things and making decisions for patient will increase dependent behaviors.
3. Encourage family therapy, which may be helpful in order to clarify roles, communication, and expectations.

Evaluation: Expected Outcomes

- Verbalizes anxiety about specific problems rather than expressing anxiety with physical symptoms.
- Makes decisions on own; demonstrates less dependence on family and friends.

MOOD DISTURBANCES
Depressive Disorders

Depressive disorders are considered mood disorders. A mood is a sustained emotion that, when extreme, affects the person's view of the world. Mood disorders are characterized by disturbances in feelings, thinking, and behavior. These disorders may occur on a continuum ranging from severe depression to severe mania (hyperactivity). A depressive illness is painful and can be psychophysiologically debilitating. Depression is much more than just sadness; it affects the way one feels about the future and can alter basic attitudes about the self. A depressed person can become so despairing as to express hopelessness. When moods become severe or prolonged or interfere with a person's interpersonal or occupational functioning, this may signal a mood disorder.

Pathophysiology and Etiology

The exact causes for depressive disorders have not been established. These disorders are thought to result from complex interactions among various factors.

Biochemical Factors

1. Biogenic amine theory proposes that there is a norepinephrine and serotonin deficiency in individuals with a depressive disorder. Changes in quantity and sensitivity of receptor sites for these neurotransmitters may also be important.
2. Kindling theory describes a process whereby external environmental stressors activate internal physiologic stress responses, which trigger the first depressive episode. Subsequent episodes can occur with less stress in response to the electrophysiologic sensitivity that was established in the brain from the initial episode.
3. Neuroendocrine dysfunction:
   a. Hypothalamic–pituitary–adrenal axis dysfunction may be present in some individuals. Abnormalities include increased cortisol levels, resistance of cortisol to suppression by dexamethasone, and blunted adrenocorticotropin hormone response to corticotropin-releasing factor.
   b. Subclinical hypothyroidism has been associated with depression, especially in women.
   c. Dysfunction of circadian rhythms has been theorized to be related to depression. Abnormal sleep EEGs have been demonstrated in many individuals. Increased early morning awakening is common, as are multiple nighttime awakenings.

Genetic Factors

1. Risk of developing a mood disorder is 1½ to 3 times greater in individuals with a first-degree relative with a mood disorder.
2. Twin studies reveal a higher rate of concordance in monozygotic twins than in dizygotic twins.
3. Mood states are associated with activation of several neuroendocrine pathways within the central and peripheral nervous systems. These pathways involve a number of neurochemical processes that involve activation of a particular binding protein identified as cyclic amp response binding protein 1 (CREB-1). Genetic profiles of individuals with depression have found evidence that genes involved in the cellular signaling pathways utilizing CREB-1 are associated with major depression. There then may be alleles (coding genes) that are related to the development of mood disorder.
4. Genetic variation in a certain region of the serotonin transporter gene (5-HTT) has been found to interact with the perception of stressful events (possibly through neuroendocrine pathways) to produce higher levels of depression and suicidality than in individuals without this variation.
5. While genetic evidence has supported conceptualizations of neurochemical and biologic alteration in the development of mood and other psychiatric disorders, no one single gene or factor has appeared to emerge as the main culprit. Most likely, a number of different genes and disposing factors are involved. Possible genes include 5-HTT, brain-derived neurotrophic growth factor, and the monoamine oxidase A gene.

Medical Factors

1. Many drugs have the adverse effect of depression, including hormones, cardiovascular drugs, psychotropic drugs, and anti-inflammatory and anti-ulcer drugs.
2. Clinically significant depressive symptoms are detected in approximately 12% to 36% of individuals with a nonpsychiatric general medical condition.

Psychosocial Factors

1. Psychodynamic theory describes the occurrence of a significant loss (object loss) that is associated with anger and aggression, which is turned inward and leads to negative feelings about self. The negative feelings about the self, including shame and guilt, then lead to depression.
2. Life events and environmental stress, such as loss of a family member through death, divorce, or separation; lack of social support; and significant health problems, have all been associated with the onset of depression.
3. Cognitive theory describes how faulty thought patterns, including negative distortions of life experiences, produce negative self-evaluation, pessimistic thinking, and hopelessness.
4. Learned helplessness theory posits that a person who internalizes the belief that an unwanted event is his or her own fault and that nothing can be done to avoid or change it is prone to developing depression.

Clinical Manifestations

 Evidence Base American Psychiatric Association. (2000). *Diagnostic and statistical manual of mental disorders* (4th ed., text rev.). Washington, DC: APA.

Depression

1. A major depressive episode reflects a level of depression that persists over a 2-week period.
2. Certain qualifying terms can be used that indicate whether the depression is associated with a change in the seasons (seasonal affective disorder) or follows the birth of an infant (postpartum).
3. Should delusions or hallucinations exist, the depression would be said to have psychotic features.
4. Major depression results in a significant change in ability to work or participate in social activities.
5. Physical examination and history findings should reveal at least five or more symptoms that include:
   a. Depressed mood, fatigue.
   b. Insomnia or an increased need for sleep.
   c. Lack of interest in pleasurable activities (anhedonia).
   d. Recent gain or loss of weight that represents at least 5% of body weight.
   e. Feelings of worthlessness.
   f. Inability to concentrate or make a decision.
   g. Suicidal ideation.

Dysthymic Disorder

1. A chronic, less intense level of depressed mood characterized by the same symptoms as seen in major depression and that lasts for at least 2 years in adults, at least 1 year in children and adolescents.
2. A major distinguishing feature is that dysthymia does not alter the ability to participate in social or work-related functions to the extent of major depression.

Diagnostic Evaluation

1. Rating scales of depression—to determine presence and severity of the problem:
   a. Zung Depression Scale
   b. Raskin Depression Rating Scale
   c. Hamilton Rating Scale for Depression
   d. Beck Depression Inventory
2. Laboratory studies:
   a. Thyroid function tests and thyrotropin-releasing hormone stimulation test—to detect underlying hypothyroidism, which may cause depression.
   b. DST—to evaluate depression that may be responsive to antidepressant or electroconvulsive therapy (ECT).
   c. Twenty-four-hour urinary 3-methoxy-4-hydroxyphenylglycol (MHPG)—may show slightly lower level in unipolar depression than in bipolar depression.
3. Polysomnography—an increase in the overall amount of rapid-eye-movement (REM) sleep and shortened REM latency period in patients with major depression.
4. Additional diagnostic tests to evaluate physical conditions, such as CT scan or magnetic resonance imaging (MRI), complete blood count (CBC), chemistry panel, rapid plasma reagin (RPR), human immunodeficiency virus (HIV) test, EEG, vitamin B_{12} and folate levels, and toxicology studies.

Management

1. Patients may receive treatment in acute inpatient psychiatric hospitals or in the community in an outpatient program. Decision about treatment setting is made according to the severity of patient's illness, with primary concern being the risk of self-harm (suicide) as well as the presence of symptoms that are severely disabling.
2. Inpatient treatment is directed toward drug management and supportive psychotherapy using milieu management.
3. Somatic therapies:
   a. Psychopharmacologic: drugs used to treat depression are those that will increase serotonin and norepinephrine (see Table 57-2, pages 1820 to 1821). A selective norepinephrine reuptake inhibitor (reboxetine) has seen used in Europe, but is not yet approved for use in the United States.

 DRUG ALERT Several drug classes interact with these medications, posing a risk of development of serotonin syndrome.

   b. ECT may be used to treat severe depression that is unresponsive to antidepressant drugs.
   c. Ultraviolet light therapy may be recommended for depression that occurs during fall and winter months (seasonal affective disorder).
4. Patient may select complementary and alternative treatments. The use of herbal supplements, especially St. John's wort, is a popular alternative for antidepressant drugs. However, use of nutritional or herbal supplements should be discussed with the health care provider because of the potential for drug interactions.

Table 57-2   Dosage and Adverse Reactions of Antidepressant Drugs

DRUG: CLASS/GENERIC/ TRADE NAME	ADULT THERAPEUTIC DOSAGE RANGE (MG/DAY)	ADVERSE REACTIONS
Tricyclic Agents		
Amitriptyline (Elavil, Endep)	50–300 mg	*For all tricyclic and tetracyclic agents:*
Clomipramine (Anafranil)	25–250 mg	• Possibility of triggering a manic episode in bipolar patients
Desipramine	75–300 mg	• Anticholinergic effects. Dry mouth, constipation, blurred vision, urine retention.
Doxepin	75–300 mg	• Sedative effects
Imipramine	75–300 mg	• Autonomic effects: orthostatic hypotension, sweating, palpitations, and increased blood pressure
Nortriptyline	25–150 mg	• Cardiac effects: tachycardia, T-wave flattening, prolonged QT interval
Protriptyline	15–60 mg	• Twitch, extrapyramidal movement effects
Trimipramine	75–200 mg	
Tetracyclic Agent		*See tricyclic agents:*
Mirtazapine	15–45 mg	• Somnolence, increased appetite, weight gain, dry mouth, constipation
Bicyclic Agent		
Venlafaxine	75–375 mg	• Nervousness, weight loss, dizziness, hypertension
Desvenlafaxine	50–100 mg	• Nausea, headache, dry mouth, insomnia, fatigue, dizziness
Selective Serotonin Reuptake Inhibitors (SSRIs)		
Citalopram	20–60 mg	• Nausea, dry mouth, diarrhea, fatigue, drowsiness, ejaculatory delay, impotence
Duloxetene	40–60 mg	• Nausea, dry mouth, dizziness, constipation, diarrhea, fatigue, increased sweating
Escitalopram	10–20 mg	• Nausea, ejaculatory delay, impotence
Fluoxetine	20–80 mg	• Delayed orgasm, headache, nervousness, insomnia, anxiety, tremor, dizziness, nausea, diarrhea, anorexia, dry mouth
Fluvoxamine	50–300 mg	• Nausea, vomiting, drowsiness, anorexia, constipation, tremor, insomnia
Paroxetine	10–50 mg	• Nausea, dry mouth, headache, somnolence, insomnia, diarrhea, constipation, tremor
Sertraline	50–150 mg	• Insomnia, diarrhea, nausea, weight loss
Vilazodone	40 mg	• Nausea, vomiting, insomnia, diarrhea
Monoamine Oxidase Inhibitors (MAOIs)		
Isocarboxazid	30–50 mg	*For all MAOIs:*
Phenelzine	45–90 mg	• Orthostatic hypotension, weight gain, edema, insomnia, sexual dysfunction, myoclonus, muscle pains, paresthesia, anticholinergic effects
Tranylcypromine	20–60 mg	• Food and beverages containing tyramine in combination with MAOIs as well as combining sympathetic drugs with an MAOI can cause hypertensive crisis
Selegiline	10 mg	
Dibenzoxazepine Agent		
Amoxapine	100–600 mg	• Dizziness, orthostatic hypotension, reflex tachycardia, extrapyramidal movement disorders
Unicyclic Agent		
Bupropion	225–450 mg	• Dry mouth, constipation, headache, insomnia, restlessness, agitation, menstrual irregularities, increased seizure risk

Table 57-2 Dosage and Adverse Reactions of Antidepressant Drugs (*continued*)

DRUG: CLASS/GENERIC/ TRADE NAME	ADULT THERAPEUTIC DOSAGE RANGE (MG/DAY)	ADVERSE REACTIONS
Triazolopyridine Agent		
Trazodone	150–600 mg	• Sedation, orthostatic hypotension, dizziness, headache, nausea, priapism
Phenylpiperazine Agent	200–600 mg	• Orthostatic hypotension, anxiety, nervous tremor, agitation
Nefazodone		
Combination Therapies		
Amitriptyline and chlordiazepoxide	2.5–5 mg/10–25 mg	• Blurred vision, dizziness, drowsiness, fatigue, tremor
Fluoxetine and olanzapine	3–12 mg/ 25–50 mg	• Dry mouth, fatigue, somnolence, increased appetite and increased weight
Perphenazine and amitriptyline	2–4 mg/10–25 mg	• Extrapyramidal reactions are possible due to the presence of perphenazine

 DRUG ALERT Antidepressant therapy takes 2 to 4 weeks before beneficial effects occur. Antidepressant drugs cannot be combined due to additive serotonergic effects leading to serotonin syndrome, a state of excessive serotonin in the synaptic cleft. Symptoms include insomnia, confusion, agitation, hyperreflexia, involuntary movements, and hypotension. Hypertensive crisis can occur if patients take a monoamine oxidase inhibitor antidepressant in combination with a sympathomimetic drug or eat foods high in tyramine.

5. Psychotherapy:
   a. *Psychodynamic therapy* helps patient to become aware of unconscious anger directed toward object loss and "work through" these feelings to alleviate depression.
   b. *Cognitive therapy* is the recommended psychotherapeutic approach for depression. This approach includes identifying and challenging the accuracy of patient's negative thought patterns and encouraging behaviors designed to counteract depressive symptoms.
   c. *Family therapy* assists patient and family members in developing a sense of self that is separate from that of the family as a whole. Patient is then encouraged to take responsibility for his or her own actions.

Complications

1. An undiagnosed medical condition causing depressive symptoms could lead to physical deterioration and delay in obtaining appropriate treatments.
2. Untreated depressive illness can lead to suicide.
3. Use of alcohol or drugs to "feel better" or numb dysphoric feelings.

NURSING ALERT During the first 60 days of antidepressant therapy, young adults and children (those under age 24) are considered to be at increased risk for suicidal thinking and behavior. The Food and Drug Administration has issued black box warnings of this risk for most antidepressants. Those taking these medications require additional monitoring and supervision during this period. The evidence does not support the need for this type of monitoring in those over age 24.

 Evidence Base Adegbite-Adeniyi, C., Gron, B., Rowles, B. M., et al. (2012). An update on antidepressant use and suicidality in pediatric depression. *Expert Opinion on Pharmacotherapy, 13,* 2119–2030.

Nursing Assessment

1. Assess posture and affect for:
   a. Poor or slumped posture.
   b. Appearance of being older than stated age.
   c. Facial expression of sadness, dejection.
   d. Episodes of weeping.
   e. Anhedonia—inability to experience pleasure.
2. Assess thought processes:
   a. Identify the presence of suicidal thoughts.
   b. Poor judgment, indecisiveness.
   c. Impaired problem solving, poor concentration.
   d. Negative thoughts.
3. Explore feelings for:
   a. Anger and irritability.
   b. Anxiety, guilt.
   c. Worthlessness.
   d. Helplessness, hopelessness.
4. Assess physical behavior for:
   a. Psychomotor agitation or retardation.
   b. Vegetative signs of depression.
      i. Change in eating patterns.
      ii. Change in sleeping patterns.
      iii. Change in elimination patterns.

    iv. Change in level of interest in sex.

    v. Change in personal hygiene.

5. Assess for evidence of "masked depression":

  a. Hypochondriasis.

  b. Psychosomatic disorders.

  c. Compulsive gambling.

  d. Compulsive overwork.

  e. Accident proneness.

  f. Eating disorders.

  g. Addictive illnesses.

6. Assess for risk of suicide.

 NURSING ALERT All mentally ill individuals, especially those who are depressed, should be assessed for suicide risk and referred for crisis intervention if they are deemed at risk.

Nursing Diagnoses

- Hopelessness related to depressive thoughts.
- Risk for Injury related to hopelessness and impaired problem solving.
- Bathing and Dressing Self-Care Deficit related to lack of motivation and poor concentration.
- Disturbed Sleep Pattern related to insomnia.

Nursing Interventions

Strengthening Coping and Sense of Hope

1. Initiate interaction with patient at a regularly scheduled time.
2. Be clear and honest about your own feelings related to patient's behavior.
3. Encourage verbal expression of feelings.
4. Validate feelings that are appropriate to the situation.
5. Explore with patient what is producing and maintaining the feeling of depression.
6. Encourage patient to identify events that cause unpleasant emotional responses.
7. Assess significant losses patient has experienced.
8. Identify cultural and social factors that may contribute to how patient copes with loss and feelings.
9. Assess patient's support network.

Maintaining Safety

1. Assess current suicide risk.
2. Implement appropriate level of observation based on a focused suicide assessment (eg, constant observation or 15-minute checks).
3. Explain observation precautions to patient.
4. Remove harmful objects from patient's possession and assess environmental safety of patient's room and unit.
5. Encourage patient to negotiate a "no-self-harm and no-suicide" agreement with the staff.
6. Monitor need to revise level of observation.
7. Provide additional structure by keeping patient involved in therapeutic and psychorehabilitative activities.

Encouraging Participation in ADLs

1. Collaborate with occupational and physical therapists to determine patient's functional capacity to accomplish ADLs.
2. If patient cannot accomplish ADLs independently, provide hygiene activities in collaboration with patient.
3. Acknowledge and reinforce patient's efforts to maintain appearance; do not rush patient when self-care is slow.
4. Reinforce what patient can do rather than what patient cannot do without assistance.
5. Remain with patient during mealtimes to determine the level of need for assistance or cueing in the ability to eat.

Facilitating Sleep

1. Determine patient's past and current sleep patterns and sleep hygiene.
2. Ask what strategies patient has already used to improve sleep and elicit which ones have been successful.
3. Consider decreasing the amount of daytime sleep by encouraging participation in an activity.
4. Discuss alternative methods for facilitating sleep:

  a. Avoid caffeine and nicotine.

  b. Avoid emotionally charged or upsetting discussions before bedtime.

  c. Avoid exercise 30 minutes to 1 hour before bed.

  d. Increase physical activity within functional limits.

  e. Use relaxation techniques.

  f. Try a warm bath or warm milk.

5. Administer prescribed drugs that cause sleepiness at bedtime; avoid giving drugs that cause insomnia at night.

Community and Home Care Considerations

1. Mood disorders tend to be chronic, with acute episodes that may require inpatient treatment. In the home or community setting, patient will require ongoing monitoring regarding the use of drugs as well as support and education in terms of the disorder.
2. Community health care providers, including nurses, must be aware of the need for primary and secondary prevention programs directed at education as well as early case finding and prompt treatment.

Family Education and Health Maintenance

1. Instruct patient and family members about symptoms of depression.
2. Instruct patient and family members about purpose of antidepressant drugs, effects, adverse effects and their management, and how to recognize early signs and symptoms of relapse.
3. Instruct patient and family members about the effect of a depressive disorder on the family system.
4. Provide patient and family members with written material on coping with depression.
5. Provide patient and family members with information about appropriate community-based programs and support groups. Contact the National Foundation for Depressive Illness (*www.depression.org*).

Evaluation: Expected Outcomes

- Reports improvement in mood and increased interest in daily living.
- Remains free from self-harm.
- Accomplishes ADLs in an independent manner.
- Obtains a minimum of 5 hours of uninterrupted sleep.

Bipolar Disorders

Bipolar disorders, also considered *mood disorders*, include the occurrence of depressive episodes and one or more elated mood episodes. An elated mood can include a range of affect, from normal mood to hypomania to mania. In the most intense presentation, the person with bipolar disorder experiences altered thought processes, which can produce bizarre delusions.

Pathophysiology and Etiology

Genetic Factors

1. Twin studies reveal a concordance rate of 65% in monozygotic twins for bipolar disorder.
2. Risk of developing bipolar disorder is increased 4% to 24% in first-degree relatives of people with bipolar disorder.
3. Current research indicates that defective genes located within chromosomes 18 and 21 may be related to bipolar disorder.

Biochemical Factors

1. Patients with bipolar disorders may have lower plasma norepinephrine, urinary MHPG, and platelet serotonin uptake and higher red blood cell/plasma lithium rates than do unipolar populations.
2. Pathology of the limbic system, basal ganglia, and hypothalamus is proposed to contribute to the development of mood disorders.

Psychosocial Factors

1. Psychosocial stressors appear to have an important role early in the illness, in concert with the electrical kindling and behavioral sensitization models.
2. Mania and hypomania have been viewed by psychoanalytic theorists as a defense against depression.

Clinical Manifestations

Evidence Base American Psychiatric Association. (2000). *Diagnostic and statistical manual of mental disorders* (4th ed., text rev.). Washington, DC: Author.

Mood disorders are often characterized by varying degrees of mania that can alternate with periods of depression. The distinguishing characteristic between forms of bipolar disorder is the degree of mania, with or without the signs of depression. Mania is an elevation of mood that persists for at least 1 week.

Bipolar Disorder I

1. Physical examination and history findings for bipolar I disorder are the presence of a single manic episode generally without the individual also meeting the criteria for a major depressive episode.

2. A mixed episode refers to the symptoms of mania and depression coexisting across the course of 1 week.
3. Mania is characterized by a cluster of at least three symptoms across the course of at least 1 week that result in a disruption in daily function. These behaviors can include:
   a. Excessive or pressured speech.
   b. Difficulty in maintaining concentration or focus.
   c. A reduced need for sleep and an increase in either goal-directed or pleasure-seeking behaviors.

Bipolar Disorder II

1. In bipolar II disorder, there has been an episode of hypomania along with an episode of major depression.
2. Hypomania is a less intense form of mania (increased energy does not result in significant changes in functional ability) with duration of at least 4 days, but less than a week.

Cyclothymic Disorder

1. A chronic alteration in mood that persists over a 2-year period of time during which there are several episodes of hypomania and depressed mood, but no episodes of major depression.
2. In children and adolescents, a 1-year time frame is used.
3. During the course of the 2 years, symptoms cannot have abated for more than 2 months.

Diagnostic Evaluation

1. Rating scale assessment tools:
   a. Young Mania Rating Scale
   b. Manic State Rating Scale
2. There appear to be no laboratory features that distinguish major depressive episodes found in major depressive disorder from those in bipolar I or bipolar II disorder.
3. Complete psychophysiologic examination.
4. Complete assessment to rule out medical conditions.

Management

Evidence Base Stoffers, J. M., Völlm, B. A., Rücker, G., et al. (2012). Psychological therapies for people with borderline personality disorder. *Cochrane Database Systematic Review, 15*(8), CD005652.

1. Patients may receive treatment in acute inpatient psychiatric hospitals or in the community in an outpatient program. The decision about treatment setting is made according to severity of patient's illness, including degree of mania or depression as well as risk of self-harm or harm to others.
2. Inpatient treatment is directed toward drug management as well as supportive psychotherapy in order to alleviate the acute manic symptoms.
3. Pharmacologic treatment for acute mania and bipolar disorder consists of:
   a. Lithium.
   b. Anticonvulsants, such as carbamazepine and valproate, for mood-stabilizing properties.
   c. Neuroleptic agents, such as risperidone, for acute psychotic thinking.

d. Benzodiazepines, such as clonazepam or lorazepam, for acute agitation.

e. Combination therapies, often incorporating an antipsychotic (perphenazine or olanzapine) along with an antidepressant (amitriptyline or fluoxetine). Another approach involves combining a benzodiazine (chlordiazepoxide) with an antidepressant (amitriptyline) to combat comorbid depression and anxiety.

 DRUG ALERT Patients taking lithium can develop toxicity related to elevated levels in the blood; therefore, lithium blood levels must be monitored periodically. Initial therapy requires daily monitoring until a safe, therapeutic level is attained; weekly and then monthly monitoring is then recommended. Lithium toxicity is related to decreased serum sodium levels and inadequate hydration. Therefore, patients taking lithium must have normal sodium intake and drink at least 2 to 3 qt (2 to 3 L) of water daily.

4. Psychotherapy is used as described above in the section related to depression.
5. Psychiatric home care nursing to facilitate compliance with drugs and therapeutic interventions.
6. Community-based support group participation.

Complications

1. Untreated bipolar disorder can lead to physical exhaustion.
2. Poor judgment and risk-taking behavior can lead to financial problems.
3. Alcohol and drug abuse problems can develop and cause disruption in the family.
4. Concurrent medical conditions may be exacerbated.

Nursing Assessment

1. Assess mood for stability; range of affect, from elation to irritability to severe agitation; laughing, joking, and talking continuously; uninhibited familiarity with interviewer.
2. Assess behavior for constant activity, starting many projects but finishing few, mild to severe hyperactivity, spending large sums of money, increased appetite, indiscriminate sexual behavior, minimal to no sleeping, outlandish or bizarre dress, poor concentration.
3. Assess thought processes for flight of ideas; pressured speech, usually with content that is sexually explicit; clang associations (sound of word, rather than its meaning, directs subsequent associations); delusions; hallucinations.

Nursing Diagnoses

• Ineffective Impulse Control related to biological changes as demonstrated by agitation, hyperactivity, and inability to concentrate.
• Disturbed Sleep Pattern related to hyperactivity and perceived lack of need for sleep.
• Compromised Family Processes related to role changes, economic strain, and lack of knowledge about patient's illness.

• Imbalanced Nutrition: Less than Body Requirements related to hyperactivity.

Nursing Interventions

Improving Impulse Control and Decreasing Disturbed Thoughts

1. Assess patient's degree of distorted thinking.
2. Redirect patient when you are unable to follow thought processes.
3. Use brief explanations.
4. Remain consistent in approach and expectations.
5. Frequently orient patient to reality; speak in a clear, simple manner.
6. Provide patient with a relaxing area with decreased environmental stimulation.
7. Assist patient with a gradual and progressive integration into the social environment while observing for behavioral changes that indicate readiness for participation in further activities.

Improving Sleep Pattern

1. Establish a distraction-free environment at bedtime.
2. Help patient avoid the intake of caffeine and nicotine.
3. Administer prescribed drugs, as ordered, and monitor patient's response.

Improving the Effect of Bipolar Illness on Family

1. Assess family's external support network and encourage participation in family therapy and support groups.
2. Assess communication and boundaries within family.
3. Observe and assess interaction patterns within family and discuss their influence on patient and family functioning.
4. Provide patient and family with information about bipolar disorder and the treatment plan, prognosis, and aftercare plan.

Ensuring Adequate Nutrition

1. Maintain accurate documentation of food and fluid intake.
2. Offer small, frequent meals of high-calorie foods. Include foods that patient likes and that can be eaten "on the move."
3. Serve patient meals in a low-stimulus environment.
4. Monitor patient's serum electrolyte and albumin levels and weigh patient every other day.
5. Monitor patient's vital signs.

Family Education and Health Maintenance

1. Instruct patient and family about bipolar illness, including symptoms of relapse.
2. Instruct patient and family members about psychopharmacologic treatment, including its purpose, effects, adverse effects, and management.
3. Advise patient and family members about community-based support groups or health care agencies that are relevant to his or her care.
4. For additional information, refer them to such organizations as the National Association on Mental Illness (*www.nami.org*).

Evaluation: Expected Outcomes

- Improved thought processes demonstrated by clear sentences with no evidence of flight of ideas and completion of simple tasks.
- Sleeps for at least 5 hours at night.
- Family members verbalize realistic, goal-directed thinking related to patient's abilities, recovery, and control of condition.
- No weight loss noted.

THOUGHT DISTURBANCES (PSYCHOTIC DISORDERS)

Schizophrenia, Schizophreniform, and Delusional Disorders

Schizophrenia, schizophreniform, and delusional disorders included in this section have defining features of psychotic symptoms. Psychotic symptoms are produced by a loss of ego boundaries or a gross impairment in reality testing, which includes prominent hallucinations and delusions, disorganized speech, and grossly disorganized or catatonic behavior. Schizophrenia can be classified as positive or negative type, although most patients have a mixture of these symptoms. The positive symptoms include hallucinations, delusions, loose associations, and bizarre or disorganized behavior. The negative symptoms include restricted emotion (flat affect), anhedonia (lack of interest in pleasurable activities), avolition (lack of motivation or initiative), alogia (lack of speech or content), and social withdrawal.

Pathophysiology and Etiology

The exact cause of these disorders remains unclear. The current consensus is that they result from complex interactions among various factors.

Schizophrenia, Schizophreniform Disorder

1. Genetic factors:
   a. Studies of monozygotic twins reveal a 50% concordance rate with a 15% rate with dizygotic twins.
   b. If one parent is affected with schizophrenia, a 12% rate is demonstrated in the children, while having two parents with the disorder increases the risk to 35% to 39%.
   c. Research is focused on a number of different genes that may be related to the development of schizophrenia. An increased risk of schizophrenia is seen in individuals with genetic variation in the catechol-O-methyltransferase gene, which is involved in the manufacture of an enzyme that metabolizes neurotransmitters. Other current candidate genes include GRM3, DISC1, dysbindin, and neuregulin.
2. Biochemical and structural brain factors:
   a. Dopamine hypothesis—hyperactivity in the dopaminergic system, possibly due to receptor neurons that are functionally hyperactive.
   b. Norepinephrine, serotonin, glutamate, and GABA may also play a role in modulating the symptoms of schizophrenia.
   c. Endogenous dysfunction of N-methyl-D-aspartate receptor-mediated neurotransmission could lead to the development of schizophrenia.
   d. Neuroanatomic studies—cerebral ventricular enlargement; sulcal enlargement; cerebellar atrophy; decreased cranial, cerebral, and frontal size; abnormalities in basal ganglia; structural abnormalities at the cellular level, particularly in the limbic and periventricular regions.
   e. Functional and metabolic studies—regional cerebral blood flow studies demonstrated hypofrontality: schizophrenic patients were unable to increase blood flow to their frontal lobes during a task thought to increase frontal lobe functions; PET studies also consistently found evidence for a relative hypofrontality.
   f. Electrophysiologic studies—EEG findings in schizophrenic patients demonstrated decreased alpha and increased delta activity; changes in evoked potential studies and amplitude reduction may occur in responses reflecting selective attention and stimulus evaluation. P300 response (reduced amplitude to unexpected stimuli using auditory and visual parameters) is the most pronounced and is prolonged. This defect leads to information or sensory overload and an inability to "screen out" irrelevant stimuli.
   g. Research evidence supports speculation that schizophrenia is a neurodevelopmental disorder that may result from brain injury occurring early in life and interfering with normal developmental events.
3. Psychosocial factors:
   a. Psychodynamic theory proposes that the essential feature of schizophrenia is a defect in interpersonal relationships due to a withdrawal of the libido into the self.
   b. Interpersonal theory proposes that the lack of a warm, nurturing relationship in the early years of life contributes to the lack of self-identity, reality misperception, and relationship withdrawal that is apparent in the disorder.
   c. Family theory related to the role of the family in the development of schizophrenia has not been validated by research. An area of family functioning that has been implicated is increased relapse risks in families characterized by high expressed emotion. This characteristic is described as emotional overinvolvement along with hostile and critical feedback.

Delusional Disorder

1. Little has been established about the etiology of delusional disorder.
2. There is no demonstrated genetic linkage.
3. It is possible that psychosocial stressors have a role in the etiology of delusional disorder in some people. This is illustrated in some of the rarer conditions such as shared psychotic disorder.

Clinical Manifestations

Evidence Base American Psychiatric Association. (2000). *Diagnostic and statistical manual of mental disorders* (4th ed., text rev.). Washington, DC: Author.

Thought disorders are characterized by the appearance of positive and negative symptomatology. Positive symptomatology refers to the presence of delusions or hallucinations, while negative is the lack of personality traits that should normally be present. A lack of affect, interest in daily activities, and an inability to attend to daily hygiene or self-care reflect negative symptomatology. Distinguishing between the various thought disorders requires careful attention to the presence and duration of positive and negative symptomatology. As with other psychiatric disorders, the symptoms must be severe enough to alter daily function.

Schizophrenia

There are five primary forms of schizophrenia (paranoid, disorganized, undifferentiated, catatonic, and residual), in which certain clusters of symptoms are noted over a period of between 1 and 6 months.

1. Paranoid—primarily characterized by the presence of delusions and/or hallucinations that can result in feelings of persecution or grandiosity.
2. Disorganized—characterized by patterns of behavior and speech that are often unfocused and lack organization usually in connection with flat or labile affect. Positive symptoms may accompany these behaviors but are not the main feature.
3. Undifferentiated—characterized by the presence of positive symptoms and unusual behavior that does not fit into the symptom clusters seen with other forms of schizophrenia (paranoid, disorganized, or catatonic).
4. Catatonic—characterized by a marked lack of responsiveness to external stimuli. Increased or decreased motor activity may be present, with the copying of the speech patterns (echolalia) or behaviors (echopraxia) of others.
5. Residual—positive symptoms are not present, but select negative symptoms remain.
   a. Examples include social isolation, a lack of energy, a lack of interest in activities of daily living, restricted or flat affect.
   b. These symptoms often cause difficulty in daily function.

Schizophreniform Disorder

1. The primary difference between schizophreniform disorder and schizophrenia is a period of symptom duration of less than 6 months but more than 1 month.
2. Those with this disorder can appear schizophrenic with the presence of positive and/or negative symptomatology.
3. Diagnostic criteria includes delusions, hallucinations, and patterns of disorganized behavior or speech along with negative symptoms.

Schizoaffective Disorder

1. A psychiatric condition in which there is a comorbid thought and mood disorder.
2. Those with this disorder may display signs and symptoms of depression or mania along with the positive and negative symptoms of schizophrenia.

Other Psychotic Disorders

1. Delusional disorders encompass nonbizarre delusions of at least 1 month's duration, but no positive or negative symptoms of schizophrenia present.

2. Psychotic disorder due to a general medical disorder contains prominent hallucinations that may last longer than the course of the underlying disorder.
3. Brief psychotic disorders contain one or more of the following: delusions, disorganized speech, grossly disorganized or catatonic behavior, hallucinations. Duration is at least 1 day and less than 1 month, then return to previous level of functioning.
4. Shared psychotic disorder occurs in an individual with an already established delusion who develops another delusion similar to another's in the context of a close relationship with that person.
5. Substance-induced psychotic disorder contains prominent hallucinations and delusions associated with substance intoxication or withdrawal, but not exclusively during the course of underlying drug use.

Diagnostic Evaluation

1. Clinical diagnosis is developed on historical information and thorough mental status examination.
2. No laboratory findings have been identified that are diagnostic of schizophrenia.
3. Routine battery of laboratory tests may be useful in ruling out possible organic etiologies, including CBC, urinalysis, liver function tests, thyroid function tests, RPR, HIV test, serum ceruloplasmin (rules out an inherited disease, Wilson's disease, in which the body retains excessive amounts of copper), PET scan, CT scan, and MRI.
4. Rating scale assessment:
   a. Scale for the Assessment of Negative Symptoms
   b. Scale for the Assessment of Positive Symptoms
   c. Brief Psychiatric Rating Scale

Management

Evidence Base Barnes, T. R. (2011). Evidence-based guidelines for the pharmacological treatment of schizophrenia: Recommendations from the British Association for Psychopharmacology. *Journal of Psychopharmacology, 25,* 567–620.

Schizophrenia and Schizophreniform Disorder

1. Patients may receive treatment in inpatient settings or in community-based outpatient programs or psychiatric home care. The level of care depends on the severity of symptoms and the risk of harm to self and others.
2. These disorders generally require long-term treatment; therefore, a case management approach is important in order to coordinate multiple services.
3. Pharmacologic therapy with either the typical or atypical neuroleptics (antipsychotics) is the mainstay of treatment (see Table 57-3).
   a. The typical neuroleptics have multiple adverse effects that require careful management (see Table 57-4, page 1828).
   b. The atypical neuroleptics have fewer adverse effects and may also be more effective in decreasing the negative symptoms of schizophrenia.

Table 57-3 Dosage and Adverse Reactions of Antipsychotic Drugs

DRUG: CLASS/GENERIC/ TRADE NAME	ADULT THERAPEUTIC DOSAGE RANGE (MG/DAY)	ADVERSE REACTIONS
Butyrophenone		
Haloperidol	2–40 mg	Extrapyramidal adverse effects are common. Decreased incidence of orthostatic hypotension as compared with phenothiazines
Aliphatic Phenothiazine		
Chlorpromazine	30–800 mg	Orthostatic hypotension, sedation, dry mouth, extrapyramidal adverse effects, agranulocytosis, ocular changes
Piperidine Phenothiazine		
Thioridazine	200–800 mg	Sedation, orthostatic hypotension, fewer extrapyramidal symptoms than other phenothiazines
Piperazine Phenothiazine		
Fluphenazine	2.5–40 mg	Extrapyramidal symptoms and lower incidence of orthostatic hypotension than with other phenothiazines
Perphenazine	8–64 mg	
Trifluoperazine	15–40 mg	
Dibenzoxipine		
Loxapine	60–250 mg	Extrapyramidal adverse effects, hypotension, dizziness
Thioxanthene		
Thiothixene	20–60 mg	Extrapyramidal adverse effects, hypotension, tachycardia, insomnia
Atypical Antipsychotics		Extrapyramidal adverse effects can occur with the use of any of the atypical antipsychotics, although the incidence of occurrence usually is less than that seen with other classes of antipsychotic medications
Aripiprazole	10–30 mg	Headache, anxiety, insomnia, nausea, vomiting, dizziness, and drowsiness
Asenapine	10–20 mg	Extrapyramidal adverse effects, drowsiness, oral hypoesthesia, weight gain
Clozapine	150–600 mg (requires careful titration)	Seizure, agranulocytosis (obtain weekly white blood cell count), hypotension, tachycardia, cardiac dysrhythmia, drowsiness, sedation, increased salivation
Iloperidone	12–24 mg	Extrapyramidal adverse effects, orthostatic hypotension, weight gain
Lurasidone	40–160 mg	Extrapyramidal adverse effects primarily akathisia and pseudoparkinsonism, nausea, somnolence
Olanzapine	5–20 mg	Orthostatic hypotension, tachycardia, drowsiness, agitation, akathisia, constipation
Paliperidone	3–6 mg	Extrapyramidal adverse effects, tremor, muscle stiffness
Pimozide	1–10 mg	Orthostatic hypotension, tachycardia, drowsiness, sedation, akathisia, akinesia
Quetiapine	200–800 mg	Orthostatic hypotension, tachycardia, drowsiness, dizziness, dry mouth
Risperidone	4–16 mg	Orthostatic hypotension, tachycardia, drowsiness, dizziness, dry mouth
Ziprasidone	20–80 mg	Dysrhythmia, drowsiness, dizziness, nausea, restlessness, constipation

Table 57-4	Management of Adverse Effects of Neuroleptic Drugs
SYMPTOM	**MANAGEMENT**
Orthostatic Hypotension	Assess for orthostatic blood pressure changes and dizziness and teach the patient: • When rising from bed or chair, get up slowly. • Sit at side of bed for a few minutes, dangling legs. • Do ankle pumps before standing. • Once standing, move slowly. • Do not twist or turn quickly. • Use assistive devices, hand rails, canes, walkers when necessary for functional deficits. • Do not drive or operate machinery when dizzy.
Peripheral Anticholinergic Effects Dry mouth and nose, blurred vision, constipation, urine retention	*Dry mouth:* • Brush teeth after each meal with a fluoridated toothpaste. • Rinse mouth frequently. • Limit caffeinated or alcoholic drinks because they can be dehydrating. • Stop smoking due to the irritation of oral mucosa. • Suck on sugarless candy or gum; avoid sugared candy to decrease the risk of fungal infections and dental caries. • Avoid dry or spicy foods. • Drink fluids between meals unless on a specific fluid restriction. • Avoid acidic beverages due to potential irritation. • Use dressing, juices, or sauces (if allowed) to moisten food. *Constipation:* • Drink fluids (within prescribed limits set by health care provider). • Eat roughage: fruits, vegetables (raw leafy types) to increase bulk and help soften stool. • Eat dried fruits, such as prunes or dates, for laxative effect. • Maintain activity level within functional limits. • Consult with health care provider to determine appropriate use of over-the-counter laxatives or prescribed stool softeners. *Urine retention:* • Void at regular intervals. • Ensure privacy.
Extrapyramidal Adverse Effects ***Short term*** Akathisia: restless legs, jitters, nervous energy, motor agitation	• Reassure patient. • Differentiate between agitation and akathisia. • Consider reducing dosage. • Consider switching patient to another class of antipsychotic.
Akinesia: weakness (hypotonia), fatigue, painful muscles, anergy (lack of energy), absence of movement	• Assess functional ability. • Dose reduction or cessation should improve movement if problems are due to akinesia versus psychotic symptoms.
Dystonias, dyskinesias: grimacing, torticollis, intermittent spasms, opisthotonos, oculogyric crises, head-neck stiffness, myoclonic twitches, laryngeal-pharyngeal dystonia	• Consider prophylaxis with anticholinergic medications. • Treat with I.M. or IV anticholinergics, as prescribed.
Parkinsonian effects: muscle stiffness, cog wheel rigidity, shuffling gait, stooped posture, drooling	• Treat with anticholinergics, as prescribed. • Stop the antipsychotic, as directed.
Long term *Tardive dyskinesia:* a delayed effect of neuroleptic drugs usually occurring after 6 months of treatment involving abnormal, involuntary, irregular, and choreoathetoid movements of the muscles of the head, limbs, and trunk	• Complete regular objective rating/assessment of the movement disorder. • Reduce or stop neuroleptic, as directed. • Consider clozapine or risperidone. • Comprehensive medical psychiatric assessment necessary with close monitoring of movement disorder.

c. Pharmacologic therapy with both the typical and atypical neuroleptics can include the use of long-lasting, or depot, injections. The use of such injections is increasing. Five drugs are currently available in depot formulations, haloperidol, fluphenazine, olanzapine, paliperidone, and risperidone.

4. Psychosocial treatments (social skills training, ADL instruction).
5. Supportive therapy that is reality oriented and pragmatic.
6. Family therapy.
7. Psychoeducational individual, group, and family support.
8. Support groups in the community.
9. Community-based partial hospitalization programs.
10. Psychiatric home care nursing.
11. Vocational and social skills education.

Delusional Disorder

1. Neuroleptic drugs have demonstrated some success in reducing the intensity of the delusion.
2. Individual psychotherapy.
3. Hospitalization for comprehensive assessment for diagnostic purposes or if suicidal or homicidal.

Complications

1. If left undiagnosed, untreated, or ineffectively treated, schizophrenia can lead to profound inability to function and contributes to the problem of homelessness in our society.
2. Neglect of other medical conditions; therefore, complications due to untreated medical illness are common.
3. Depression and suicide.
4. Substance use, abuse, or dependency.

Nursing Assessment

Assess for positive symptoms of schizophrenia. These symptoms reflect aberrant mental activity and are usually present early in the first phase of the schizophrenic illness.

Alterations in Thinking

1. Delusion—false, fixed belief that is not amenable to change by reasoning. The most frequent elicited delusions include:
   a. Ideas of reference.
   b. Delusions of grandeur.
   c. Delusions of jealousy.
   d. Delusions of persecution.
   e. Somatic delusions.
2. Loose associations—the thought process becomes illogical and confused.
3. Neologisms—made-up words that have a special meaning to the delusional person.
4. Concrete thinking—an overemphasis on small or specific details and an impaired ability to abstract.
5. Echolalia—pathologic repeating of another's words.
6. Clang associations—the meaningless rhyming of a word in a forceful way.
7. Word salad—a mixture of words that is meaningless to the listener.

Alterations in Perceiving

1. Hallucinations—sensory perceptions that have no external stimulus. The most common are auditory, visual, gustatory, olfactory, and tactile.
2. Loss of ego boundaries—lack a sense of their body and how they relate to the environment.
   a. Depersonalization is a nonspecific feeling or sense that a person has lost his or her identity or is unreal.
   b. Derealization is the perception by a person that the environment has changed.

Alterations in Behavioral Responses

1. Bizarre behavioral patterns.
   a. Motor agitation and restlessness.
   b. Automatic obedience or robotlike movement.
   c. Negativism.
   d. Stereotyped behaviors.
   e. Stupor.
   f. Waxy flexibility (allowing another person to reposition extremities).
2. Agitated or impulsive behavior.
3. Negative symptoms of schizophrenia that reflect a deficiency of mental functioning.
   a. Alogia—lack of speech.
   b. Anergia—inability to react.
   c. Anhedonia—inability to experience pleasure.
   d. Avolition—lack of motivation or initiation.
   e. Poor social functioning.
   f. Poverty of speech.
   g. Social withdrawal.
   h. Thought blocking.
4. Associated symptoms of schizophrenia.
   a. Substance use, abuse, or dependence.
   b. Depression.
   c. Fantasy.
   d. Violent or aggressive behavior.
   e. Water intoxication.
   f. Withdrawal.

Nursing Diagnoses

- Acute Confusion related to perceptual and cognitive distortions, as demonstrated by suspiciousness, defensive behavior, and disruptions in thought.
- Social Isolation related to an inability to trust.
- Activity Intolerance related to adverse reactions to psychopharmacologic drugs.
- Ineffective Coping related to misinterpretation of environment and impaired communication ability.
- Risk for Self-directed or Other-directed Violence related to delusional thinking and hallucinatory experiences.

Nursing Interventions

Strengthening Differentiation Between Delusions and Reality

1. Provide patient with honest and consistent feedback in a nonthreatening manner.

2. Avoid challenging the content of patient's behaviors.

3. Focus interactions on patient's behaviors.

4. Administer drugs, as prescribed, while monitoring and documenting patient's response to the drug regimen.

5. Use simple and clear language when speaking with patient.

6. Explain all procedures, tests, and activities to patient before starting them and provide written or video material for learning purposes.

Promoting Socialization

1. Encourage patient to talk about feelings in the context of a trusting, supportive relationship.

2. Allow patient time to reveal delusions to you without engaging in a power struggle over the content or the reality of the delusions.

3. Use a supportive, empathic approach to focus on patient's feelings about troubling events or conflicts.

4. Provide opportunities for socialization and encourage participation in group activities.

5. Be aware of patient's personal space and use touch judiciously.

6. Help patient to identify behaviors that alienate significant others and family members.

Improving Activity Tolerance

1. Assess patient's response to prescribed antipsychotic drug.

2. Collaborate with patient and occupational and physical therapy specialists to assess patient's ability to perform ADLs.

3. Collaborate with patient to establish a daily, achievable routine within physical limitations.

4. Teach strategies to manage adverse effects of antipsychotic drug that affect patient's functional status, including:

   a. Change positions slowly.

   b. Gradually increase physical activities.

   c. Limit overdoing it in hot, sunny weather.

   d. Use sun precautions.

   e. Use caution in activities if extrapyramidal symptoms develop.

Improving Coping with Thoughts and Feelings

1. Encourage patient to express feelings.

2. Focus on patient's feelings and behavior.

3. Provide honest perceptions of reality and feedback about symptoms and behaviors.

4. Encourage patient to explore adaptive behaviors that increase abilities and success in socializing and accomplishing ADLs.

5. Decrease environmental stimuli.

Ensuring Safety

1. Monitor patient for behaviors that indicate increased anxiety and agitation.

2. Collaborate with patient to identify anxious behaviors as well as the causes.

3. Tell patient that you will help with maintaining behavioral control.

4. Establish consistent limits on patient's behaviors and clearly communicate these limits to patient, family members, and health care providers.

5. Secure all potential weapons and articles from patient's room and the unit environment that could be used to inflict an injury.

6. To prepare for possible continued escalation, form a psychiatric emergency assist team and designate a leader to facilitate an effective and safe aggression-management process.

7. Determine the need for external control, including seclusion or restraints. Communicate the decision to patient and put plan into action.

8. Frequently monitor patient within the guidelines of facility's policy on restrictive devices and assess patient's level of agitation.

9. When patient's level of agitation begins to decrease and self-control is regained, establish a behavioral agreement that identifies specific behaviors that indicate self-control against a reescalation of agitation.

Community and Home Care Considerations

1. Patients with these disorders may be in supportive housing, such as transitional living halfway houses, foster homes, and board and care homes. Supervision and drug management are important areas of concern for the nurse working in the community.

2. Psychosocial rehabilitation approach may be used in the community setting, where skills necessary for independent living are taught. Patient who has been symptomatic since early adulthood may not have learned these skills. The nurse working in the community setting may work as a member of the treatment team using this approach.

Family Education and Health Maintenance

1. Instruct patient and family members in disease process and how to recognize and cope with relapse symptoms.

2. Instruct patient and family members about the uses, actions, and adverse effects of prescribed drugs.

3. Provide instruction on when to notify primary care provider regarding adverse drug effects or increased disease symptomatology.

4. Instruct patient and family about community resources, support groups, and possible use of psychiatric home care nursing.

5. For additional information and support, refer patient and family to such agencies as the Brain and Behavior Research Foundation (*www.bbrfoundation.org*) or Schizophrenia.com, an informative and supportive website run by volunteers (*www.schizophrenia.com*).

Evaluation: Expected Outcomes

• Exhibits improved reality orientation, concentration, and attention span, as demonstrated through speech and behavior.

• Communicates with family and staff in a clear manner without evidence of loose, dissociated thinking.

• Independently maintains personal hygiene without fatigue.

• Attends group activities.

• Remains free from harm or violent acts.

COGNITIVE IMPAIRMENT DISTURBANCES

Delirium, Dementia, and Amnesic Disorder

Cognitive impairment disturbances encompass specific disorders that produce either temporary or permanent neuronal damage, resulting in psychological or behavioral dysfunction. Cognitive impairment disorders described in DSM-IV-TR include delirium, dementia, and amnesic disorder.

Delirium is an acute disturbance of consciousness and a change in cognition that develops over a brief period. *Dementia* is a chronic disturbance involving multiple cognitive deficits, including memory impairment. *Amnesic disorder* is characterized by memory impairment in the absence of other significant cognitive impairments.

Pathophysiology and Etiology

Delirium

Can be caused by numerous pathophysiologic conditions. Some of the major possibilities include:

1. CNS pathology: head trauma, hypertensive cerebral changes, seizures, tumors.
2. Endocrinopathies: thyroidism, parathyroidism.
3. Hypoxemia.
4. Hypothermia or hyperthermia.
5. Substance intoxication or abstinence and withdrawal states.
6. Exposure to certain metals, toxins, or drugs.
7. Metabolic: diabetic acidosis, hypoglycemia, acid-base imbalances.
8. Hepatic encephalopathy.
9. Thiamine deficiency.
10. Postoperative states.
11. Psychosocial stressors: relocation stress, sensory deprivation or overload, sleep deprivation, immobilization.

Primary Dementia

Primary dementias are degenerative disorders that are progressive, irreversible, and not due to any other condition. Specific disorders are dementia of the Alzheimer's type (DAT) and vascular dementia (formerly multi-infarct dementia). DAT demonstrates progression of symptoms from the initial stage, which is characterized by mild cognitive deficits in the area of short-term memory and accomplishment of goal-directed activity, to the final stage in which profound impairment occurs in the areas of cognition and self-care abilities. Research is ongoing; however, DAT is thought to have multiple causative factors. (See page 188 for Alzheimer's disease.)

1. Genetic factors:
   a. Familial Alzheimer's disease is associated with abnormal genes on chromosomes 1, 14, and 21, particularly with genes located on these chromosomes (1 and 14) that encode for amyloid precursor protein, which leads to accumulation of the amyloid beta-peptide in plaques.
   b. A specific cholesterol-bearing protein, apolipoprotein E4 (Apo E4), is found on chromosome 19 twice as often in people with DAT as in the general population.

2. Biochemical and brain structural factors:
   a. The neurotransmitter acetylcholine has been implicated in terms of relative deficit or receptor abnormalities as related to Alzheimer's disease.
   b. Autopsy findings reveal presence of brain changes, that is, the presence of amyloid plaques and neurofibrillary tangles associated with nerve cell destruction.
   c. Additional areas of investigation include:
      i. Slow viral infection.
      ii. Autoimmune processes.
      iii. Head trauma.

Secondary Dementias

Occur as a result of another pathologic process.

1. Infection-related dementias.
   a. Acquired immunodeficiency syndrome.
   b. Chronic meningitis.
   c. Creutzfeldt-Jakob disease.
   d. Progressive multifocal leukoencephalopathy.
   e. Postencephalitic dementia syndrome.
   f. Syphilis.
   g. Subacute sclerosing panencephalitis.
   h. Tuberculosis.
2. Subcortical degenerative disorders.
   a. Huntington's disease.
   b. Parkinson's disease.
   c. Wilson's disease.
   d. Thalamic dementia.
3. Hydrocephalic dementias.
4. Vascular dementias.
5. Traumatic conditions, such as posttraumatic encephalopathy and subdural hematoma.
6. Neoplastic dementias.
   a. Glioma.
   b. Meningioma.
   c. Meningeal carcinomatosis.
   d. Metastatic deposits.
7. Inflammatory conditions, such as sarcoidosis, systemic lupus erythematosus, and temporal arteritis.
8. Toxic conditions, such as alcohol-related syndrome and iatrogenic dementias (anticonvulsant, anticholinergic, antihypertensive, psychotropic drugs).
9. Metabolic disorders.
   a. Anemias.
   b. Deficiency states (minerals and vitamins).
   c. Cardiac or pulmonary failure.
   d. Hepatic encephalopathy.
   e. Porphyria (deficiency in enzymes involved in heme synthesis).
   f. Uremia.

Amnesic Disorder

1. Posttraumatic amnesia: head trauma is the most common cause of amnesia.
2. Poststroke amnesia: damage to the fornix or hippocampus.
3. Neoplasms.

4. Anoxic states.
5. Herpes simplex encephalitis.
6. Hypoglycemic states.
7. Epileptic seizures.
8. ECT.
9. Substance-induced.

Clinical Manifestations

See Table 57-5.

Diagnostic Evaluation

Various diagnostic tests may be done to determine the cause. A comprehensive neuropsychiatric evaluation must be completed to make an accurate diagnosis.

1. Basic laboratory examination, including CBC with differential, chemistry panel (including blood urea nitrogen, creatine, and ammonia), arterial blood gas values, chest x-ray, toxicology screen (comprehensive), thyroid function tests, and serologic tests for syphilis.

Table 57-5	Clinical Manifestations of Cognitive Impairment Disorders
DISORDER	**CLINICAL MANIFESTATIONS**
Delirium (severe impairment in functioning)	• Fluctuating levels of awareness • Clouding of consciousness (confused and disoriented) • Perceptual disturbances (illusions and hallucinations) • Memory, especially recent memory, is disturbed • Alteration in sleep–wake cycle • EEG changes • Abrupt onset may last about 1 week • Reversible when underlying cause has been treated
Dementia (severe impairment in functioning)	• Slow, insidious onset • Impaired long- and short-term memory • Deterioration of cognitive abilities—judgment, abstract thinking • Often irreversible if untreated • Personality changes • No or slow EEG changes
Amnesic syndrome (moderate to severe impairment in functioning)	• Impairment in short- and long-term memory • Inability to learn new material • Remote memory better than that of recent events • Confabulation • Apathy, lack of initiative • Emotionally bland

2. Additional tests may include CT scan, MRI, additional blood chemistries (heavy metals, thiamine, folate, antinuclear antibody, and urinary porphobilinogen), lumbar puncture, PET/single-photon emission computed tomography scans.
3. Complete mental status examination.
4. Comprehensive physical examination.

Management

 Evidence Base Ballard, C., Khan, Z., Clack, H., et al. (2011). Nonpharmacological treatment of Alzheimer disease. *Canadian Journal of Psychiatry*, 56(10), 589–595.

Delirium

1. Treatment generally occurs in acute hospital-based setting where the goal is diagnosis to identify specific reversible causes of the delirium so that treatment is focused on ameliorating the causative factors.
2. Pharmacologic therapy is dependent on underlying causes. Additional drugs may be used that are directed toward the reduction of the acute symptoms of delirium. These include:
   a. Benzodiazepines, such as lorazepam, for substance withdrawal states.
   b. Neuroleptics, such as risperidone and haloperidol, for agitation.
   c. Combined administration of haloperidol and lorazepam for agitated and psychotic symptomatology.
3. Environmental management:
   a. Safe, structured environment.
   b. Orientation facilitated by accurate clocks and calendars.
4. Family teaching about the nature of the disorder.
5. Family participation in the treatment plan in order to assist in the management of behavior.

Dementia

1. Treatment is generally community focused; the goal of treatment is to maintain the quality of life as long as possible despite the progressive nature of the disease. Effective treatment is based on:
   a. Diagnosis of primary illness and concurrent psychiatric disorders.
   b. Assessment of auditory and visual impairment.
   c. Measurement of the degree, nature, and progression of cognitive deficits.
   d. Assessment of functional capacity and ability for self-care.
   e. Family and social system assessment.
2. Environmental strategies in order to assist in maintaining the safety and functional abilities of patient as long as possible.
3. Pharmacologic therapy used for the person with DAT is directed toward the use of anticholinesterase drugs to slow the progression of the disorder by increasing the relative amount of acetylcholine. Available drugs include donepezil, galantamine, rivastigmine, and tacrine. An NMDA-receptor antagonist memantine may be provided in an attempt to improve cognition. (see Table 57-6). Other drugs may be used for behavioral control and symptom reduction.

Table 57-6 Dosage and Adverse Reactions of Drugs used in the Treatment of Dementia

DRUG: CLASS/GENERIC/TRADE NAME	ADULT THERAPEUTIC DOSAGE RANGE (MG/DAY)	ADVERSE REACTIONS
Cholinesterase Inhibitors		
Donepezil	10–23 mg	Nausea, diarrhea, anorexia, fatigue.
Galantamine	8–24 mg	Nausea, diarrhea, dizziness, fatigue.
Rivastigmine	6–12 mg	Nausea, vomiting, anorexia, dizziness.
Tacrine	40–160 mg	Nausea, vomiting, agitation, rash, anorexia.
NMDA Receptor Antagonist Memantine	2–6 mg	Fatigue, dizziness, headache.

a. Agitation management: neuroleptic drugs.
b. Psychosis: neuroleptic drugs.
c. Depression: select antidepressants such as citalopram, duloxetene, escitalopram, fluoxetine, fluvoxamine, paroxetine, and mirtazapine; ECT.
4. Hypertension management in vascular dementia is important in reducing the severity of symptoms.
5. Family education is a treatment strategy because statistics indicate that family caregivers provide care for patients with DAT in 7 out of 10 cases. The family and the treatment team collaborate in the delivery of care.

Complications

1. Without accurate diagnosis and treatment, secondary dementias may become permanent.
2. Falls with serious orthopedic or cerebral injuries.
3. Self-inflicted injuries.
4. Aggression or violence toward self, others, or property.
5. Wandering events, in which the person can get lost and potentially suffer exposure, hypothermia, injury, and even death.
6. Serious depression is demonstrated in caregivers who receive inadequate support.
7. Caregiver stress and burden may result in patient neglect or abuse.

Nursing Assessment

See Table 57-7.

1. Assess the onset and characteristics of symptoms (determine type and stage of disorder).
2. Establish cognitive status using standard measurement tools.
3. Determine self-care abilities.
4. Assess threats to physical safety (eg, wandering, poor reality testing).
5. Assess affect and emotional responsiveness.
6. Assess ability and level of support available to caregivers.

Table 57-7 Nursing Assessment for Delirium, Dementia, and Amnesic Disorder

	DELIRIUM	DEMENTIA	AMNESTIC DISORDER
Onset	Acute	Slow, insidious	Sudden
Course	Usually brief	Progresses over years	Transient or chronic
Mood	Fearfulness, anxiety, irritability	Mood labile, personality traits accentuated	Apathy, agitation, emotional blandness, shallow range of affective expression
Perception	Auditory, visual, tactile hallucinations; illusions	Hallucinations not a prominent feature	No hallucinatory experiences
Memory	Short-term memory impaired	Short-term memory damage followed by long-term memory damage	Impaired ability to learn new information; unable to recall previously learned information or past events
Communication	Slurred speech; confabulation	Normal—early stage: progressive aphasia and confabulation	Confabulation

Nursing Diagnoses

- Impaired Verbal Communication related to cerebral impairment as demonstrated by altered memory, judgment, and word finding.
- Bathing and Dressing Self-Care Deficit related to cognitive impairment as demonstrated by inattention and inability to complete ADLs.
- Risk for Injury related to cognitive impairment and wandering behavior.
- Impaired Social Interaction related to cognitive impairment.
- Risk for Violence: Self-directed or Other-directed related to suspicion and inability to recognize people or places.

Nursing Interventions

Improving Communication

1. Speak slowly and use short, simple words and phrases.
2. Consistently identify yourself and address the person by name at each meeting.
3. Focus on one piece of information at a time. Review what has been discussed with patient.
4. If patient has vision or hearing disturbances, have him or her wear prescription eyeglasses or a hearing device.
5. Keep environment well lit.
6. Use clocks, calendars, and familiar personal effects in patient's view.
7. If patient becomes verbally aggressive, identify and acknowledge feelings.
8. If patient becomes aggressive, shift the topic to a safer, more familiar one.
9. If patient becomes delusional, acknowledge feelings and reinforce reality. Do not attempt to challenge the content of the delusion.

Promoting Independence in Self-Care

1. Assess and monitor patient's ability to perform ADLs.
2. Encourage decision making regarding ADLs as much as possible.
3. Label clothes with patient's name, address, and telephone number.
4. Use clothing with elastic and velcro for fastenings rather than buttons or zippers, which may be too difficult for patient to manipulate.
5. Monitor food and fluid intake.
6. Weigh patient weekly.
7. Provide food that patient can eat while moving.
8. Sit with patient during meals and assist by cueing.
9. Initiate a bowel and bladder program early in the disease process to maintain continence and prevent constipation or urine retention.

Ensuring Safety

1. Discuss restriction of driving when recommended.
2. Assess patient's home for safety: remove throw rugs, label rooms, and keep the house well lit.
3. Assess community for safety.
4. Alert neighbors about patient's wandering behavior.
5. Alert police and have current pictures taken.
6. Provide patient with a MedicAlert bracelet.
7. Install complex safety locks on doors to outside or basement.
8. Install safety bars in bathroom.
9. Closely observe patient while he or she is smoking.
10. Encourage physical activity during the daytime.
11. Give patient a card with simple instructions (address and phone number) in case he or she gets lost.
12. Use nightlights.
13. Install alarm and sensor devices on doors.

Improving Socialization

1. Provide magazines with pictures as reading and language abilities diminish.
2. Encourage participation in simple, familiar group activities, such as singing, reminiscing, doing puzzles, and painting.
3. Encourage participation in simple activities that promote the exercise of large muscle groups.

Preventing Violence and Aggression

1. Respond calmly and do not raise your voice.
2. Remove objects that might be used to harm self or others.
3. Identify stressors that increase agitation.
4. Distract patient when an upsetting situation develops.

Community and Home Care Considerations

1. Multidisciplinary team approach is important, along with collaboration among professionals in nursing, medicine, psychiatry, nutrition, social work, pharmacy, and rehabilitative specialties.
2. Nurses involved in community care need to utilize case-finding approach as well as provide long-term support for family members involved in caregiving.
3. Adult day care and respite care may be utilized in order to provide the level of care needed by patient as well as allow the family to continue to maintain normal functioning.

Family Education and Health Maintenance

1. Instruct family about the process of the disorder, whether delirium, dementia, or amnesic disorder.
2. Instruct family about safety measures, environmental supports, and effective interventions for common symptoms in order to provide care in the home.
3. Instruct about and refer family members to community-based groups (adult day care centers, senior assessment centers, home care, respite care, and family support groups).
4. For additional information and support, refer to Alzheimer's Association (*www.alz.org*) or National Institutes of Health, National Institute on Aging, Alzheimer's Disease Education and Referral Center (800-438-4380; *www.nia.nih.gov/alzheimers*). For information on caregiving tips and advice with referral to local community groups, consult Caregiver.com at *www.caregiver.com* or Alzheimer's Caregiver Support Online (800-677-1116; *http://alzonline.phhp.ufl.edu*).

Evaluation: Expected Outcomes

- Demonstrates decreased anxiety and increased feelings of security in supportive environment.

- Maintains maximum degree of orientation and self-care within level of ability.
- Safety precautions and close surveillance maintained; no injury.
- Attends group activities; sings, exercises with group.
- Decreased occurrence of acting-out behaviors.

SUBSTANCE-RELATED DISORDERS

Substance Abuse and Dependence

The abuse of alcohol and other psychoactive substances has become an endemic problem throughout all levels of society. In terms of substance abuse or dependence, a substance can be defined as a prescribed drug, an illegal drug, or a substance used in an unintended manner to produce mood or mind-altering effect (eg, inhalants, glues, or steroids). Substance abuse may arise unintentionally from the initial use of a substance for its approved purpose. The individual commonly faces not only the psychological ramifications of a substance-related disorder but also physiologic consequences resulting from substance use or abuse.

Substance abuse and dependence share certain criteria and can be difficult to distinguish from one another. With substance abuse, the pattern of use has led to the development of one or more life problems. In dependence, these problems can coexist with a pattern of tolerance and physiologic or psychological dependence. Withdrawal and tolerance are significant criteria related to substance dependence; however, dependence can exist without either of these criteria being met. Dependence has been characterized as loss of control over the use of a substance. Dual diagnosis is defined as the presence of a substance-related diagnosis along with another psychiatric disorder.

Classification

 Evidence Base American Psychiatric Association. (2000). *Diagnostic and statistical manual of mental disorders* (4th ed., text rev.). Washington, DC: Author.

Substance abuse and dependence disorders are defined according to criteria found in DSM-IV-TR. Substance-related disorders include abuse of, and dependence on, a particular substance (eg, cocaine, alcohol). According to DSM-IV-TR, a diagnosis of substance abuse cannot be applied to caffeine or nicotine use.

- Substance (Specify) Abuse
- Substance (Specify) Dependence
- Substance (Specify) Intoxication
- Polydrug Dependence

A number of disorders can be induced through the use of a particular substance; in such cases, the symptoms cannot be explained by another condition or disorder and are related to substance use. Such substance-induced disorders include:

- Substance-Induced Anxiety Disorder
- Substance-Induced Mood Disorder
- Substance-Abuse Intoxication
- Substance-Induced Sexual Disorder
- Substance-Induced Sleep Disorder

- Substance Withdrawal
- Substance Withdrawal Delirium

Pathophysiology and Etiology

As with the development of other psychiatric conditions and disorders, the development of substance-related disorders reflects a complex interaction of biological, genetic, sociologic, and psychological factors. Several theoretical approaches have been developed to describe the process of abuse and dependence.

Biochemical Factors

1. Dopamine is one of the primary neurotransmitters within the CNS and is known to be involved in the integration of environmental stimuli with physiologic responses. Cannabis, cocaine, and alcohol increase the dopamine level, thereby producing a strong association between physiologic effects and behavior.
2. Dopamine is also involved in CNS pathways that mediate feelings of pleasure. Opioids indirectly increase dopamine activity by modulation of the mesolimbic system, leading to reinforcement of substance use.
3. Neurons in the mesolimbic system can become sensitized to the presence of amphetamine and cocaine. Such sensitization is the reverse of tolerance, with the development of an enhanced neuronal response upon repeated exposure. These responses appear to be associated with the development of substance dependence.

Genetic Factors

1. Alcoholism is strongly associated with a familial history of alcoholism. In these individuals, a genetic disposition (attention-deficit/hyperactivity disorder [ADHD] allele) to alcoholism combines with a learning environment in which patient develops certain beliefs about the use of a substance and its effects. The presence of genetic disposition, in the absence of parental alcoholism, does not result in a significantly higher risk of alcoholism than in those individuals without such disposition. These findings provide support for models focusing on genetic and environmental interaction in the etiology of substance abuse.
2. Genetic variation in gene regulation resulting in lower levels of serotonin in the CNS may be associated with the development of alcoholism.

Psychosocial Factors

1. An individual learns to use substances in certain situations with certain expectations as to the effects of the substance (eg, relaxation, disinhibition). As the individual experiences the desired effects, this may reinforce the desire to use the substance.
2. Use may begin with an attempt to fit in with a larger peer group as a means of boosting self-esteem.
3. Substances may be used to relieve anxiety or as a means of coping with other traumatic events (self-medication).

Sociocultural Factors

1. Societies around the world use psychoactive substances for a number of reasons. The individual learns the approved use of the substance within the societal or familial structure and may consider such use to be appropriate.

2. The society in which an individual resides may consider dependence on certain substances to be a minor issue, thereby providing a justification for continued use.

Clinical Manifestations

 Evidence Base American Psychiatric Association. (2000). *Diagnostic and statistical manual of mental disorders* (4th ed., text rev.). Washington, DC: Author.

Overview

1. Substance abuse and dependence are characterized by a loss of control over substance use.
2. For either abuse or dependence, a pattern of substance use must be sustained over a period of 12 months and impair activities of daily living.
3. Whether the pattern is one of steady or binge drinking, activities related to substance use must interfere with daily functioning, in terms of time off work or curtailing of social activities to provide more time to participate in, or recover from, substance use.
4. A differentiating factor between abuse and dependence is that dependence is characterized by the development of tolerance with the appearance of substance-specific withdrawal symptomatology in the absence of use.

Substance Abuse

Physical examination and history findings compatible with substance abuse includes at least one of the following:

1. Continued use even in the face of an inability to meet major life obligations,
2. Use in situations that pose a danger of harm to self or others (ie, driving while intoxicated).
3. Continued use regardless of legal issues associated with use (ie, continued driving while intoxicated after suspension of a license) or continued use after the development of problems in social relationships (ie, an impending divorce brought about by substance use).

Substance Dependence

Physical examination and history findings include meeting at least three diagnostic criteria, which include:

1. Tolerance to substance-related effects.
2. Withdrawal in the absence of the substance.
3. Unsuccessful attempts to reduce or halt use.
4. Cutting down or avoiding social obligations or work responsibilities to spend time in substance-related activity (eg, obtaining, using, recovering from).
5. Continued use despite the development of significant life problems (ie, loss of job).

Diagnostic Evaluation

A number of tools have been designed to assess for the presence of substance-related disorders in specific populations (eg, adolescents, pregnancy). The tool used should be specific to patient being assessed.

1. Measurement tools for alcohol abuse or dependence:
   a. CAGE
   b. Michigan Alcohol Screening Test (MAST)
   c. Alcohol Use Disorders Identification Test (AUDIT)
2. Measurement tools for other substance abuse and dependence:
   a. CAGE-AID
   b. Drug Abuse Screening Tool (DAST)
3. Laboratory testing of blood, saliva, sweat, and hair for the presence of a substance or metabolite. The period of effective measurement varies based on the procedure and the substance.
4. States of drug intoxication or withdrawal can be identified through the presence of physiologic and behavioral symptoms associated with the use of a particular substance.
5. Additional screening and testing is recommended for the presence of other disease conditions or illnesses (HIV, hepatitis) that may have resulted from risk-taking behavior while under the influence of substances or may have resulted from the physiologic effects of the substance (as in cardiac dysrhythmia in the case of cocaine use).

Management

For the treatment of substance overdose and alcohol-related delirium, see Chapter 35, pages 1228–1232.

1. The management of substance abuse and dependence includes outpatient and inpatient treatment modalities. Inpatient modalities include programs of detoxification and therapy sessions designed to aid in the recognition of a substance-related disorder. Outpatient therapies include support groups, continued therapy sessions, and the use of pharmacologic drugs to aid in the maintenance of sobriety.
2. Initial detoxification is typically provided through inpatient hospitalization. Detoxification protocols are unique to each substance. Benzodiazepine taper is utilized during detoxification from alcohol. The treatment of cocaine withdrawal may include administration of prescribed drugs that can reduce craving, such as amantadine or bromocriptine. The treatment of heroin withdrawal generally involves transdermal clonidine along with oral administration, as necessary.
3. Drugs may also be used in the treatment of alcohol abuse.
   a. Disulfiram is used as aversion therapy. It leads to accumulation of acetaldehyde in the blood system, causing flushing, tachycardia, vomiting, nausea, and chest pain if alcohol is consumed.
   b. A nonaversion therapy, acamprosate sodium, may be used in attempts to ensure abstinence fron alcohol. It interacts with the GABA neurotransmitter system to restore balance between neuronal excitation and inhibition.
   c. Topiramate, an anticonvulsant, may reduce craving for alcohol. Clinical trials have demonstrated that ondansetron may aid in reducing drinking.
4. Drug therapy in the treatment of opiate withdrawal includes several classes.
   a. Administration of an opioid antagonist, such as naloxone and naltrexone, reverses the effects of opioids. Injectable

sustained-release formulations of naltrexone may also be used.

   b. Outpatient detoxification is typically focused on the administration of the opioid agonist, methadone, or levo-alpha-acetylmethadol, a longer-lasting formulation, to substitute for the illicit drug.

   c. Another opioid agonist, buprenorphine, is available in the outpatient treatment of opiod addiction. An injectable form is used in the treatment of chronic pain. It is also available in sublingual and transdermal formulations and often blended with naloxone to prevent euphoria from intravenous injection of oral formulations.

5. Psychosocial support through the use of 12-step or other treatment programs (Rational Recovery).

6. Psychoeducational therapy to understand triggers of substance use and prevention of relapse.

7. Family support and educational groups.

Complications

1. The physiologic complications of substance-related disorders are specific to the substance involved. Physiologic complications can also result from exposure to other substances (eg, talcum powder, strychnine) that are mixed with cocaine or heroin.

2. Psychological complications include increased potential for risk-taking and suicidal behavior.

3. Individuals under the influence of substances are more likely to experience automobile or other accidents.

4. Suicide rates increase in the presence of substance use and abuse. This includes accidental overdose related to the substance.

5. The physiologic complications or consequences associated with alcohol abuse involve each organ system and include the development of GI ulcers, liver disease, malnutrition, anemia, and dehydration.

6. Complications associated with the use of cocaine or amphetamines include cardiac dysrhythmia, seizures, dehydration, and acute renal failure. Mood lability and psychosis are commonly associated with the use of amphetamines and cocaine.

7. Heroin use can result in respiratory complications and the development of infectious disease through the sharing of needles. Endocarditis, skin abscesses, and other infectious sequelae may result.

8. The use of 3-4 methylenedioxymethamphetamine (Ecstasy) can have complications similar to those associated with amphetamine use. Research has also demonstrated effects on short- and long-term memory through neurotoxic effects on serotonergic pathways, with possible additional effects on dopamine pathways in the CNS.

Nursing Assessment

1. Assess physiologic stability.
   a. Elevated or decreased blood pressure.
   b. Cardiac abnormalities.
   c. Confusion, memory deficits, ataxia, nystagmus (Wernicke's encephalopathy, a thiamine deficiency).
   d. Lasting memory deficits (Korsakoff's amnesic disorder).
   e. Lung congestion or diminished breath sounds.
   f. Fever.
   g. Mood lability.

2. Assess for evidence of medical complications.
   a. Hepatic disease.
   b. Renal disease.
   c. Anemia.
   d. Sexually transmitted disease.
   e. Chronic obstructive pulmonary disease.
   f. Anxiety.
   g. Depression.

3. Identify risk-taking behaviors.
   a. Participation in criminal activities.
   b. Sexual activity and behaviors, including use of protective devices.
   c. Motor vehicle violations.
   d. Participation in hazardous sports or activities.

4. Gather information regarding substance use.
   a. Substances used and amounts.
   b. Method of use (eg, injection, inhalation).
   c. Previous attempts to reduce or stop use.
   d. Prior history of withdrawal symptoms.
   e. Longest previous period of sobriety.
   f. Prior treatment programs attended.
   g. Familial history of substance abuse.
   h. Precipitating events to substance use.

5. Examine coping mechanisms and behaviors.
   a. Denies presence of a substance-related problem.
   b. Does not recognize the presence of physical or emotional health problems.
   c. Blames others for the presence of problems.
   d. Uses substance in stress-provoking situations.
   e. Justifies use of substance.
   f. Prior psychiatric history.

6. Monitor for withdrawal symptoms.
   a. Agitation, mood lability, paranoia, or mania (cocaine, amphetamines).
   b. Dehydration, nutritional deficiencies, hallucinations, seizures, GI disturbances (alcohol and other substances).
   c. Nausea, vomiting, flulike symptoms, diarrhea, and muscle pain (opioids).

Nursing Diagnoses

The following is a partial list of nursing diagnoses that may be appropriate in working with an individual with a substance-related disorder.

- Ineffective Denial related to substance use.
- Compromised Family Coping related to roles and relationships.
- Risk for Injury related to effects of the substance.
- Readiness for Enhanced Coping related to life stressors.

Other nursing diagnoses may apply depending on the particular substance involved and may include the following:

- Risk for Self-directed or Other-directed Violence.
- Powerlessness.
- Self-Care Deficit.
- Imbalanced Nutrition: Less than Body Requirements.

Nursing Interventions

Facilitate Recognition of Substance-Related Disorder
1. Approach patient in a direct, nonjudgmental manner.
2. Assess patient's level of knowledge about substance.
3. Have patient identify situations preceding substance use.
4. Discuss consequences of substance use.
5. Reinforce desire for change.

Encourage Participation of Family and Significant Others
1. Provide support to family and significant others while acknowledging substance-related disorder of patient.
2. Encourage family to attend supportive and educational group meetings.
3. Have family members identify effects of substance use on family functioning.
4. Discuss role relationships with family that may be related to substance-seeking behavior.

Ensuring Safety
1. Monitor patient for symptoms of substance withdrawal.
2. Provide prescribed medications, as indicated, for the treatment of withdrawal symptomatology.
3. Educate patient on relationship between symptoms and substance use.
4. Monitor hydration and nutritional status.
5. Reduce level of stimulation, as appropriate.
6. Assess for presence of agitation or mood lability.

Enhancing Coping Strategies
1. Aid in identifying triggers to use.
2. Have patient develop a list of personal strengths.
3. Help patient develop an understanding of dependence as an illness.
4. Assist patient in developing alternative coping strategies through participation in role-playing activities and groups.
5. Identify alternative methods of participating in social situations without resorting to use of substance.
6. Reinforce need for ongoing attendance of support group meetings.

Community and Home Care Considerations
1. Assist in resource finding for inpatient or outpatient program. Provide referral and information about community-based programs and activities that can aid in the maintenance of sobriety. The individual may benefit from placement in a residential treatment program or halfway house that provides supportive services and continued programs of treatment in a community setting.
2. Assist in educating and encouraging adherence to drug therapy regimen. Provide information about medication therapy, as appropriate, including known adverse effects and means of obtaining prescribed drugs, as necessary (eg, methadone).

Family Education and Health Maintenance
1. Instruct patient and family about adverse physiologic and psychological effects of substance use.
2. Discuss health maintenance practices to minimize potential effects of substance use (eg, vitamin use, proper diet).
3. Explain the potential for injury from risk-taking behaviors.
4. Reinforce the need for aftercare groups and activities.
5. For general information and support, consult such agencies as the National Institute on Drug Abuse, National Institutes of Health (*www.drugabuse.gov*) or National Institute on Alcohol Abuse and Alcoholism, National Institutes of Health (*www.niaaa.nih.gov*). General information can also be obtained from Substance Abuse & Mental Health Services Administration, Room 12-105 Parklawn Building, 5600 Fishers Lane, Rockville, MD 20857 or Alcoholics Anonymous (*www.aa.org*).

Evaluation: Expected Outcomes
- Acknowledges the presence of a substance-related disorder.
- Identifies negative effects of substance use or abuse on family, work, and other relationships.
- Describes negative effects of substance use or abuse on physical and emotional health.
- Continues to attend treatment programs; refrains from substance use.

CHILD AND ADOLESCENT PROBLEMS

Children and adolescents are capable of developing the same psychiatric disorders seen in adult populations, such as major depression, bipolar disorder, and substance-related disorders. In addition, children and adolescents face a number of developmental and age-specific mental health issues. A child faced with a traumatic situation may engage in a pattern of destructive or deviant behavior. Working with such a child can be frustrating to both health care personnel and parents. The intent of this section is to provide a brief overview of a select group of mental health issues specific to pediatric populations. For further information, the reader is strongly encouraged to seek out texts and materials dedicated to pediatric mental health and child development.

Classification

 Evidence Base American Psychiatric Association. (2000). *Diagnostic and statistical manual of mental disorders* (4th ed., text rev.). Washington, DC: Author.

Psychiatric disorders specific to child populations, as defined by the *DSM-IV-TR*, include:

1. Attentional and developmental disorders (see Chapter 56, page 1804).
2. Behavioral disorders.
   a. Conduct disorder.
   b. Oppositional defiant disorder.

3. Elimination disorders.
   a. Encopresis—incontinence of feces not caused by organic process.
   b. Enuresis—involuntary voiding during sleep; may be physiologic during early childhood.

Other psychiatric disorders already discussed in this chapter may appear in childhood and adolescence and persist into adulthood. Eating disorders (anorexia and bulimia) commonly begin during the adolescent years and continue well into adulthood (see Chapter 20, page 758).

Behavioral Disorders

Conduct disorder and oppositional defiant disorder may arise in children of all ages. The most significant difference between the two is that in conduct disorder, the child or adolescent is violating societal norms and rules. With oppositional defiant disorder, the child or adolescent is displaying disruptive and negative behavior primarily toward authority figures, without violation of societal norms.

Pathophysiology and Etiology

The development of a psychiatric disorder commonly reflects a complex interaction of several etiologic factors.

1. Twin studies have provided some evidence that conduct disorder may have a genetic predisposition.
2. Other genetic studies have indicated that regions located on chromosomes 2 and 19 may be associated with the development of conduct disorder.
3. These predisposing genetic factors most likely interact with environmental influences, such as household violence, neglect, and other situational variables, in contributing to the development of behavioral or attentional disorders.

Clinical Manifestations

1. Conduct disorder is a pattern of persistent behavior during which the individual violates either the rights of another person or accepted societal norms. Behavioral criteria incorporates four possible domains, across which three or more behaviors must be observed within a 12-month period:
   a. Aggression toward people or animals (threatening behaviors, physical cruelty, initiating of physical confrontations, or weapon use).
   b. Aggression toward property (intentional fire-setting or destruction of property).
   c. Theft or deceitfulness (breaking into property of others, stealing of items).
   d. Violation of rules (before age 13, staying out late at night, regardless of parental instruction; running away from home, absence from school).
2. If the individual does not violate societal norms but engages in a pattern of hostile, defiant, and negative behavior toward authority figures or adults in general, oppositional defiant disorder may be considered. This pattern of behavior must endure for at least 6 months, during which time at least four of the following behaviors are exhibited:
   a. Frequently loses temper.
   b. Often argues with adults.
   c. Often refuses to comply with, or actually defies, rules.
   d. Often blames others for behavior or mistakes.
   e. Intentionally provokes others on a frequent basis.
   f. Often appears easily annoyed or irritated by others.
   g. Often appears angry or resentful toward others.
   h. Frequently engages in spiteful and vindictive behavior.
3. The behavioral disorders have been found to have a significant degree of comorbidity. These disorders may also coexist with attention deficits such as ADHD.

Diagnostic Evaluation

1. The evaluation of a child and adolescent ideally incorporates information from patient, parents, other family members, and teachers.
2. Evaluation should also include a detailed physical and nutritional assessment.
3. Depending on patient's age, play activities may be incorporated into the interview to facilitate trust and patient expression. Younger children may be more capable of depicting family dynamics and their own feelings through play or art.

Management

1. Care of the individual with a behavioral disorder may initially involve treatment in a structured inpatient program that incorporates many behavioral modification techniques, including a level system, a token economy, and close monitoring.
2. Residential or partial hospitalization treatment programs may also be employed.
3. Treatment of a behavioral disorder includes family therapy, parental and patient education, and, ideally, teacher interaction. Family counseling and education are essential aspects of any treatment modality.
4. Drugs may be employed in the treatment program, based on the presence of comorbidities and behavioral severity.

Nursing Diagnoses

Any of the following may be individualized to the child or adolescent:

- Chronic Low Self-Esteem.
- Compromised Family Coping.
- Impaired Parenting.
- Risk for Injury.
- Risk for Suicide.
- Readiness for Enhanced Coping.
- Readiness for Enhanced Parenting.
- Readiness for Enhanced Self-Concept.

Nursing Interventions

Interventions should be selected that encourage the verbal expression of feelings and provide alternatives to destructive behavior. Interventions should also be included that address parental education. Interventions to be considered include:

- Aid patient in identifying events that trigger inappropriate behavioral responses.
- Assist patient in developing communication skills.
- Teach alternative behaviors and methods of expression.
- Provide consistent limits and consequences for inappropriate behaviors.
- Provide positive feedback for appropriate behaviors.
- Monitor behavior for violence directed toward self or others.
- Utilize role-play to practice alternative behavioral responses.
- Teach parenting skills to parents or primary caregivers.
- Teach parents appropriate limit-setting and emphasize need to clearly state expectations.

Evaluation: Expected Outcomes

- Reduction in frequency and intensity of outbursts while interacting with others.
- Uses alternative coping strategies in situations in which he or she would previously have been angered or engaged in destructive behavior.
- Attends school on consistent basis.
- Does not injure self or others.

SELECTED REFERENCES

Abbass, A., Town, J., & Driessen, E. (2012). Intensive short-term dynamic psychotherapy: A systematic review and meta-analysis of outcome research. *Harvard Review of Psychiatry, 20*(2), 97–108.

Adegbite-Adeniyi, C., Gron, B., Rowles, B. M., et al. (2012). An update on antidepressant use and suicidality in pediatric depression. *Expert Opinion on Pharmacotherapy, 13,* 2119–2030.

American Psychiatric Association. (2000). *Diagnostic and statistical manual of mental disorders* (4th ed., text rev.). Washington, DC: Author.

Ardizzone, I., Nardecchia, F., Marconi, A., et al. (2010). Antipsychotic medication in adolescents suffering from schizophrenia: A meta-analysis of randomized controlled trials. *Psychopharmacology Bulletin, 43*(2), 45–66.

Baldassano, C. F., Hosey, A., & Coello, J. (2011). Bipolar depression: An evidence-based approach. *Current Psychiatry Reports, 13*(6), 483–487.

Baldwin, D., Woods, R., Lawson, R., et al. (2011). Efficacy of drug treatments for generalised anxiety disorder: systematic review and meta-analysis. *British Medical Journal, 342,* d1199.

Ballard, C., Khan, Z., Clack, H., et al. (2011). Nonpharmacological treatment of Alzheimer disease. *Canadian Journal of Psychiatry, 56*(10), 589–595.

Barnes, T. R. (2011). Evidence-based guidelines for the pharmacological treatment of schizophrenia: Recommendations from the British Association for Psychopharmacology. *Journal of Psychopharmacology, 25*(5), 567–620.

Bishop, J. R., & Bishop, D. L. (2010). Iloperidone for the treatment of schizophrenia. *Drugs Today, 46*(8), 567–579.

Carlat, D. (2012). Evidence-based somatic treatment of depression in adults. *Psychiatric Clinics of North America, 35*(1), 131–142.

Chan, M. K., Guest, P. C., Levin, Y., et al. (2011). Converging evidence of blood-based biomarkers for schizophrenia: An update. *International Review of Neurobiology, 101,* 95–144.

Correll, C. U., Kishimoto, T., Nielsen, J., et al. (2011). Quantifying clinical relevance in the treatment of schizophrenia. *Clinical Therapeutics, 33*(12), B16–39.

Cox, G. R., Callahan P., Churchill R., et al. (2012). Psychological therapies versus antidepressant medication, alone and in combination for depression in children and adolescents. *Cochrane Database Systematic Review, 11,* CD008324.

D'Angelo, E. J., & Augenstein, T. M. (2012). Developmentally informed evaluation of depression: Evidence-based instruments. *Child and Adolescent Psychiatric Clinics of North America, 21*(2), 279–298.

Davis, T. E., III, May, A., & Whiting, S. E. (2011). Evidence-based treatment of anxiety and phobia in children and adolescents: Current status and effects on the emotional response. *Clinical Psychology Review, 31*(4), 592–602.

de C Williams, A. C., & Cella, M. (2012). Medically unexplained symptoms and pain: Misunderstanding and myth. *Current Opinion in Supportive and Palliative Care, 6*(2), 201–206.

Dellava, J. E., Kendler, K. S., & Neale, M. C. (2011). Generalized anxiety disorder and anorexia nervosa: Evidence of shared genetic variation. *Depression and Anxiety, 28*(8), 728–733.

Depp, C. A., Mausbach, B. T., Harmell, A. L., et al. (2012). Meta-analysis of the association between cognitive abilities and everyday functioning in bipolar disorder. *Bipolar Disorder, 14*(3), 217–226.

Divr, Y., & Smallwood, P. (2008). Serotonin syndrome: A complex but easily avoidable condition. *General Hospital Psychiatry, 3,* 284–287.

Figueira, M. L., & Brissos, S. (2011). Measuring psychosocial outcomes in schizophrenia patients. *Current Opinion in Psychiatry, 24*(2), 91–99.

Gili, M., Comas, A., Garcia-Garcia, M., et al. (2010). Comorbidity between common mental disorders and chronic somatic diseases in primary care patients. *General Hospital Psychiatry, 32*(3), 240–245.

Huntley, A. L., Araya, R., & Salisbury, C. (2012). Group psychological therapies for depression in the community: Systematic review and meta-analysis. *British Journal of Psychiatry, 200*(3), 184–190.

Kelly, T. M., Daley, D. C., & Douaihy, A. B. (2012). Treatment of substance abusing patients with comorbid psychiatric disorders. *Addictive Behaviors, 37*(1), 11–24.

Kiosses, D. N., Leon, A. C., & Arean, P. A. (2011). Psychosocial interventions for late-life major depression: Evidence-based treatments, predictors of treatment outcomes, and moderators of treatment effects. *Psychiatric Clinics of North America, 34*(2), 377–401, viii.

Kircanski, K., Craske, M. G., Epstein, A. M., et al. (2009). Subtypes of panic attacks: A critical review of the empirical literature. *Depression and Anxiety, 26*(10), 878–887.

Koen, N., & Stein, D. J. (2011). Pharmacotherapy of anxiety disorders: A critical review. *Dialogues in Clinical Neuroscience, 13*(4), 423–437.

Lowe, B., Mundt, C., Herzog, W., et al. (2008). Validity of current somatoform disorder diagnoses: Perspectives for classification in DSM-V and ICD-11. *Psychopathology, 41*(1), 4–9.

Moore, T. A. (2011). Schizophrenia treatment guidelines in the United States. *Clinical Schizophrenia and Related Psychoses, 5*(1), 40–49.

Morlino, M., Calento, A., Pannone, G., et al. (2009). Systematic reviews to support evidence-based psychiatry: What about schizophrenia? *Journal of Evaluation in Clinical Practice, 15*(6), 1025–1028.

Nelson, J. C., & Devanand, D. P. (2011). A systematic review and meta-analysis of placebo-controlled antidepressant studies in people with depression and dementia. *Journal of the American Geriatrics Society, 59*(4), 577–585.

Oertel-Knochel, V., Bittner, R. A., Knochel, C., et al. (2011). Discovery and development of integrative biological markers for schizophrenia. *Progress in Neurobiology, 95*(4), 686–702.

Plassman, B. L., Williams, J. W., Jr., Burke, J. R., et al. (2010). Systematic review: Factors associated with risk for and possible prevention of cognitive decline in later life. *Annals of Internal Medicine, 153*(3), 182–193.

Ripoll, L. H., Triebwasser, J., & Siever, L. J. (2011). Evidence-based pharmacotherapy for personality disorders. *International Journal of Neuropsychopharmacology, 14*(9), 1257–1288.

Rynn, M., Puliafico, A., Heleniak, C., et al. (2011). Advances in pharmacotherapy for pediatric anxiety disorders. *Depression and Anxiety, 28*(1), 76–87.

Seitz, D. P., Adunuri, N., Gill, S. S., et al. (2011). Antidepressants for agitation and psychosis in dementia. *Cochrane Database of Systematic Reviews,* Issue 2 (Article No. CD008191).

Stoffers, J. M., Völlm, B. A., Rücker, G., et al. (2012). Psychological therapies for people with borderline personality disorder. *Cochrane Database Systematic Review, 15*(8), CD005652.

Thaler, K., Delivuk, M., Chapman, A., et al. (2011). Second-generation antidepressants for seasonal affective disorder. *Cochrane Database of Systematic Reviews,* Issue 12 (Article No. CD008591).

Zhang, J. P., & Malhotra, A. K. (2011). Pharmacogenetics and antipsychotics: Therapeutic efficacy and side effects prediction. *Expert Opinion on Drug Metabolism and Toxicology, 7*(1), 9–37.

APPENDICES
AND INDEX

APPENDIX A
Diagnostic Studies and Interpretation

BOX A-1	Selected Abbreviations Used in Appendices

CONVENTIONAL UNITS

kg = kilogram	mM = millimole	
g = gram	nM = nanomole	
mg = milligram	mOsm = milliosmole	
µg = microgram	mm = millimeter	
µµg = micromicrogram	µm = micron or micrometer	
ng = nanogram	mm Hg = millimeters of mercury	
pg = picogram	U = unit	
dL = 100 milliliters	mU = milliunit	
mL = milliliter	µU = microunit	
mm^3 = cubic millimeter	mEq = milliequivalent	
fL = femtoliter	IU = International Unit	
	mIU = milliInternational Unit	

SI UNITS

g = gram
L = liter
mol = mole
mmol = millimole
µmol = micromole
nmol = nanomole
pmol = picomole

Table A-1	Reference Ranges—Hematology and Coagulation	

LABORATORY TEST	NORMAL ADULT REFERENCE RANGE		CLINICAL SIGNIFICANCE
	Conventional Units	SI Units	
Bleeding Time	3–10 minutes	3–10 minutes	• Prolonged in thrombocytopenia, defective platelet function, and aspirin therapy
D-dimer	<250 mg/mL	<0.25 mg/L	• Increased in disseminated intravascular coagulation, malignancy, and arterial and venous thrombosis
Erythrocyte Count Males	4,600,000– 6,200,000/mm^3	4.6–6.2 × 10^{12}/L	• Increased in severe diarrhea and dehydration, polycythemia, acute poisoning, and pulmonary fibrosis
Females	4,200,000– 5,400,000/mm^3	4.2–5.4 × 10^{12}/L	• Decreased in all anemias in leukemia and after hemorrhage, when blood volume has been restored

Table A-1   Reference Ranges—Hematology and Coagulation (continued)

LABORATORY TEST	NORMAL ADULT REFERENCE RANGE		CLINICAL SIGNIFICANCE
	Conventional Units	SI Units	
Erythrocyte Indices			• Increased in macrocytic anemia; decreased in microcytic anemia
Mean corpuscular volume (MCV)	84–96 μm³	84–96 fL	
Mean corpuscular hemoglobin (MCH)	28–34 μμg/cell	28–34 pg	• Increased in macrocytic anemia; decreased in microcytic anemia
Mean corpuscular hemoglobin concentration (MCHC)	32%–36%	Concentration fraction: 0.32–0.36	• Decreased in severe hypochromic anemia
Erythrocyte Sedimentation Rate (ESR)—Westergren Method			• Increased in tissue destruction, whether inflammatory or degenerative; during menstruation and pregnancy; and in acute febrile diseases
Males younger than age 50	<15 mm/hour	<15 mm/hour	
Males older than age 50	<20 mm/hour	<20 mm/hour	
Females younger than 50	<20 mm/hour	<20 mm/hour	
Females older than age 50	<30 mm/hour	<30 mm/hour	
Fibrinogen	200–400 mg/dL	2–4 g/dL	• Increased in pregnancy, cancer, inflammation, and nephrosis • Decreased in severe liver disease and abruptio placentae
Fibrin Split (Degradation) Products	<10 mg/L	<10 mg/L	• Increased in disseminated intravascular coagulation, myocardial infarction, and pulmonary embolism
Fibrinolysis (Whole Blood Clot Lysis Time)	No lysis in 24 hours	—	• Increased activity associated with massive hemorrhage, extensive surgery, transfusion reactions, and liver disease
Hematocrit			• Decreased in severe anemia, anemia of pregnancy, and acute massive blood loss • Increased in erythrocytosis of any cause and in dehydration or hemoconcentration associated with shock
Males	42%–52%	Volume fraction: 0.42–0.52	
Females	37%–47%	Volume fraction: 0.37–0.47	
Hemoglobin			• Decreased in various anemias, pregnancy, severe or prolonged hemorrhage, and with excessive fluid intake • Increased in polycythemia, chronic obstructive pulmonary disease, failure of oxygenation due to heart failure, and normally in people living at high altitudes
Males	13–18 g/dL	2.02–2.79 mmol/L	
Females	12–16 g/dL	1.86–2.48 mmol/L	
International Normalized Ratio (INR)	1.0	—	• INR used to standardize the prothrombin time and anticoagulation therapy
	2–3 for therapy in atrial fibrillation, deep vein thrombosis, and pulmonary embolism		
	2.5–3.5 for therapy in prosthetic heart valves		

(continued)

Table A-1   Reference Ranges—Hematology and Coagulation (continued)

LABORATORY TEST	NORMAL ADULT REFERENCE RANGE		CLINICAL SIGNIFICANCE
	Conventional Units	SI Units	
Leukocyte Count			• Total is elevated in acute infectious diseases, predominantly in the neutrophilic fraction with bacterial diseases, and in the lymphocytic and monocytic fractions in viral diseases
Total	5,000–10,000/mm³	5–10 × 10⁹/L	
Basophils	0%–0.5%	Number fraction: 0.6–0.7	
Eosinophils	1%–4%	Number fraction: 0.01–0.04	• Elevated in acute leukemia, following menstruation, and following surgery or trauma • Eosinophils elevated in collagen disease, allergy, and intestinal parasitosis
Lymphocytes	20%–30%	Number fraction: 0.00–0.05	• Depressed in aplastic anemia, agranulocytosis, and by toxic chemotherapeutic agents used in treating malignancy
Monocytes	2%–6%	Number fraction: 0.2–0.3	
Neutrophils	60%–70%	Number fraction: 0.02–0.06	
Partial Thromboplastin Time (Activated)	20–35 seconds	—	• Prolonged in deficiency of fibrinogen, factors II, V, VIII, IX, X, XI, and XII, and in heparin therapy
Platelet Count	140,000–400,000/mm³	0.14–0.4 × 10¹²/L	• Increased in malignancy, myeloproliferative disease, rheumatoid arthritis, and postoperatively; about 50% of patients with unexpected increase of platelet count will be found to have a malignancy • Decreased in thrombocytopenic purpura, acute leukemia, aplastic anemia, and during cancer chemotherapy
Prothrombin Time	9.5–12 seconds	—	• Prolonged by deficiency of factors I, II, V, VII, and X, for malabsorption, severe liver disease, and coumarin anticoagulant therapy
Reticulocytes	0.5%–1.5% of red blood cells	Number fraction: 0.005–0.015	• Increased with any condition stimulating increase in bone marrow activity (infection, blood loss [acute and chronically following iron therapy in iron-deficiency anemia], and polycythemia vera) • Decreased with any condition depressing bone marrow activity, acute leukemia, and late stage of severe anemias

Laboratory values may vary according to the techniques used in different laboratories.

Table A-2   Reference Ranges—Serum, Plasma, and Whole Blood Chemistries

LABORATORY TEST	NORMAL ADULT REFERENCE RANGE		CLINICAL SIGNIFICANCE	
	Conventional Units	SI Units	Increased	Decreased
Alkaline Phosphatase			• Conditions reflecting increased osteoblastic activity of bone • Rickets • Hyperparathyroidism • Hepatic disease	• Malnutrition • Cretinism • Severe anemia • Celiac disease
Adults	40–150 IU/L	40–150 IU/L		

(continued)

Table A-2   Reference Ranges—Serum, Plasma, and Whole Blood Chemistries (*continued*)

LABORATORY TEST	NORMAL ADULT REFERENCE RANGE		CLINICAL SIGNIFICANCE	
	Conventional Units	SI Units	Increased	Decreased
Alanine Aminotransferase (ALT)	5–40 IU/L	5–40 IU/L	• Liver disease • Muscle trauma • MI	• Azotemia • Chronic dialysis
Aspartate Aminotransferase (AST)	5–40 IU/L	5–40 IU/L	• Same as ALT	—
Bilirubin				—
Total	0.1–1.2 mg/dL	2–20 µmol/L	• Hemolytic anemia (indirect) • Biliary obstruction and disease • Hepatocellular damage (hepatitis) • Pernicious anemia • Hemolytic disease of the newborn	
Direct (conjugated)	0.1–0.2 mg/dL	0–4 µmol/L		
Indirect (unconjugated)	0.1–1 mg/dL	1.7–17.1 µmol/L		
Calcium	8.6–10.3 mg/dL	2.15–2.57 mmol/L	• Tumor or hyperplasia of parathyroid • Hypervitaminosis D • Multiple myeloma • Nephritis with uremia • Malignant tumors • Sarcoidosis • Hyperthyroidism • Skeletal immobilization • Excess calcium intake: milk alkali syndrome	• Hypoparathyroidism • Diarrhea • Celiac disease • Vitamin D deficiency • Acute pancreatitis • Nephrosis • After parathyroidectomy
Carbon Dioxide, Venous			• Respiratory acidosis (CO_2 retention) • Metabolic alkalosis (vomiting)	• Respiratory alkalosis (hyperventilation) • Metabolic acidosis (diabetic ketoacidosis)
Adults	22–30 mEq/L	22–30 mmol/L		
Infants	18–24 mEq/L	18–24 mmol/L		
Chloride	98–106 mEq/L	98–106 mmol/L	• Nephrosis • Nephritis • Urinary obstruction • Cardiac decompensation • Anemia	• Diabetes • Diarrhea • Vomiting • Pneumonia • Heavy metal poisoning • Cushing's syndrome • Intestinal obstruction • Febrile conditions
Creatinine	0.7–1.4 mg/dL	62–124 µmol/L	• Renal insufficiency, muscle disease • Chronic renal disease	• Advanced liver disease
Glucose			• Diabetes • Cushing's disease • *Note:* 100–126 is impaired fasting glucose; >126 fasting is diagnostic for diabetes	• Hyperinsulinism/insulinemia • Addison's disease • Insulin therapy
Fasting	60–99 mg/dL	3.3–6.05 mmol/L		
Postprandial (2 hours)	65–140 mg/dL	3.58–7.7 mmol/L		
Potassium (K)	3.5–5 mEq/L	3.5–5 mmol/L	• Renal failure • Acidosis • Cell lysis • Tissue breakdown or hemolysis	• GI losses • Diuretic administration

(continued)

Table A-2   Reference Ranges—Serum, Plasma, and Whole Blood Chemistries (*continued*)

LABORATORY TEST	NORMAL ADULT REFERENCE RANGE		CLINICAL SIGNIFICANCE	
	Conventional Units	SI Units	Increased	Decreased
Protein, Total	6–8 g/dL	60–80 g/L	• Hemoconcentration • Shock • Multiple myeloma (globulin fraction) • Chronic infections (globulin function) • Liver disease (globulin)	• Malnutrition • Hemorrhage • Loss of plasma from burns • Proteinuria
Albumin	3.5–5 g/dL	35–50 g/L		
Globulin	1.5–3 g/dL	15–30 g/L		
Sodium	135–145 mEq/L	135–145 mmol/L	• Hemoconcentration • Diabetes insipidus	• Diuretic therapy • Water intoxication
Urea Nitrogen, Blood (BUN)	10–20 mg/dL	3.6–7.2 mmol/L	• Acute glomerulonephritis • Obstructive uropathy • Mercury poisoning • Nephrotic syndrome	• Severe hepatic failure • Pregnancy

APPENDIX B
Conversion Tables

Metric Units and Symbols, 1847
Celsius (Centigrade) and Fahrenheit Temperatures, 1848

Metric and Apothecaries' Systems, 1848
Nomogram for Estimating Surface Area of Infants and Young Children, 1849

Nomogram for Estimating Surface Area of Older Children and Adults, 1850

Table B-1	Metric Units and Symbols		
QUANTITY	**UNIT**	**SYMBOL**	**EQUIVALENT**
Length	Millimeter	mm	1,000 mm = 1 m
	Centimeter	cm	100 cm = 1 m
	Decimeter	dm	10 dm = 1 m
	Meter	m	1,000 m = 1 km
Volume	Cubic centimeter	cc or cm^3	1,000 cc = 1 cm^3 or liter
	Milliliter	ml or mL	1,000 mL = 1 liter
	Cubic decimeter	dm^3	1,000 dm^3 = 1 m^3
	Liter	L	1,000 L = 1 m^3
Mass	Microgram	μg	1,000 μg = 1 mg
	Milligram	mg	1,000 mg = 1 g
	Gram	g	1,000 g = 1 kg
	Kilogram	kg	1,000 kg = 1 metric ton (t)

To convert from pounds to kilograms, divide by 2.2.
To convert from kilograms to pounds, multiply by 2.2.

Table B-2	Celsius (Centigrade) and Fahrenheit Temperatures
DEGREES CELSIUS (CENTIGRADE)	DEGREES FAHRENHEIT
36.0	96.8
36.5	97.7
37.0	98.6
37.5	99.5
38.0	100.4
38.5	101.3
39.0	102.2
39.5	103.1
40.0	104.0
40.5	104.9
41.0	105.8
41.5	106.7
42.0	107.6

To convert degrees F to degrees C: Subtract 32, then divide by 1.8.
To convert degrees C to degrees F: Multiply by 1.8, then add 32.

Table B-3	Metric and Apothecaries' Systems			

(Approved *approximate* dose equivalents are enclosed in parentheses. Use exact equivalents in calculations.)

METRIC	APOTHECARIES	METRIC	APOTHECARIES
1 milligram (mg)	1/64 grain	3.888 cubic centimeters or grams	1 dram (4 cc or grams)
64.79 milligrams	1 grain (65 mg)	31.103 cubic centimeters or grams	1 ounce (30 cc or grams)
1 gram	15.43 grains (15 grains)	473.167 cubic centimeters	1 pint (500 cc)
1 cubic centimeter (cc)*	16 minims		

A cubic centimeter (cc) is the approximate equivalent of a milliliter (mL). The terms are used interchangeably in general medicine.

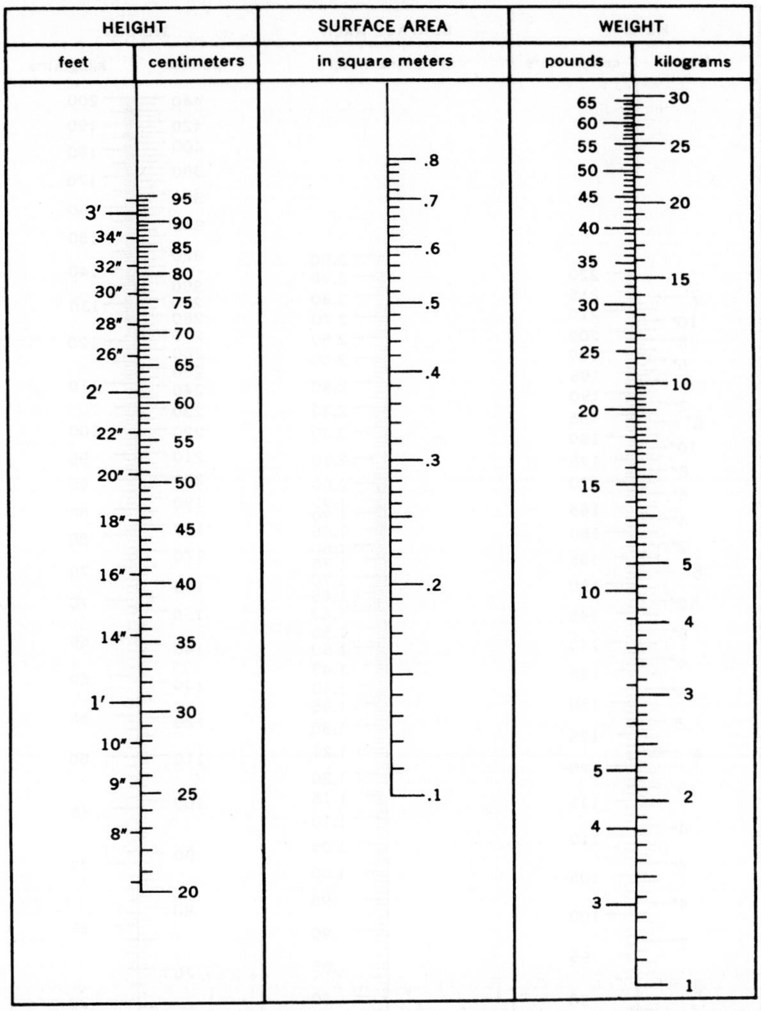

To determine the surface area of the patient, draw a straight line between the point representing the patient's height on the left vertical scale to the point representing the patient's weight on the right vertical scale. The point at which this line intersects the middle vertical scale represents the surface area in square meters. (Courtesy of Abbott Laboratories.)

Figure B-1. Nomogram for Estimating Surface Area of Infants and Young Children.

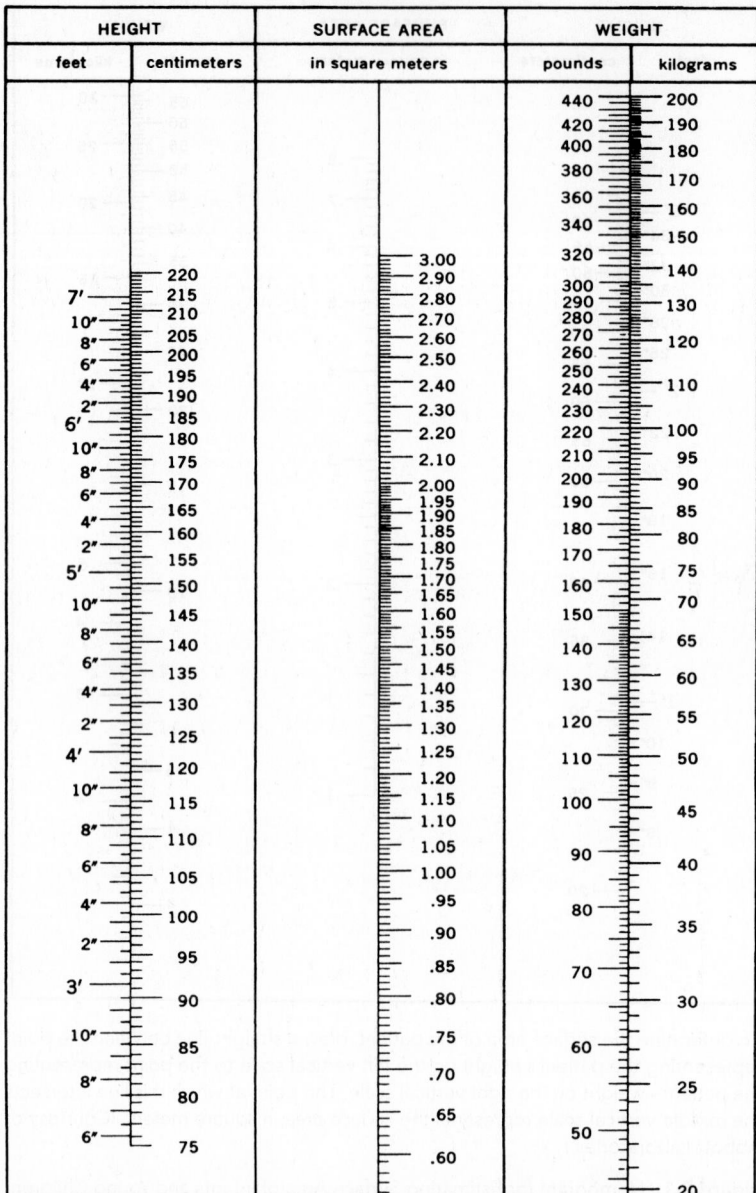

To determine the surface area of the patient, draw a straight line between the point representing the patient's height on the left vertical scale to the point representing the patient's weight on the right vertical scale. The point at which this line intersects the middle vertical scale represents the surface area in square meters. (Courtesy of Abbott Laboratories.)

Figure B-2. Nomogram for Estimating Surface Area of Older Children and Adults.

APPENDIX C
Pediatric Laboratory Values

Blood Chemistries, 1851
Normal Values—Hematology, 1852

Sample Conversions of Pounds
and Ounces to Grams, 1852

Table C-1	Blood Chemistries		
LABORATORY TEST	**QUALIFICATION**	**CONVENTIONAL UNITS**	**SI UNITS**
Carbon Dioxide (CO_2) Content	Cord blood	14–22 mmol/L	14–22 mmol/L
	Child	20–24 mmol/L	20–24 mmol/L
	Adult	24–30 mmol/L	24–30 mmol/L
Chloride	—	99–111 mEq/L	99–111 mmol/L
Creatinine (Serum)	**Age (years)**	**Upper Limits, mg/dL (μmol/L)**	
		Males	**Females**
	1	0.6 (53)	0.5 (44)
	2–3	0.7 (62)	0.6 (53)
	4–7	0.8 (71)	0.7 (62)
	8–10	0.9 (80)	0.8 (71)
	11–12	1.0 (88)	0.9 (80)
	13–17	1.2 (106)	1.1 (97)
	18–20	1.3 (115)	1.1 (97)
	Adult	1.2 (106)	1.4 (124)
Potassium	<age 10 days	4–6 mEq/L	4–6 mmol/L
	>age 10 days	3.5–5 mEq/L	3.5–5 mmol/L
Sodium	Premature	130–140 mEq/L	130–140 mmol/L
	Older	135–148 mEq/L	135–148 mmol/L
Urea Nitrogen	—	7–22 mg/dL	2.5–7.9 mmol/L

Table C-2   Normal Values—Hematology

AGE	HEMOGLOBIN (G %)	HEMATOCRIT (%)	MEAN CORPUSCULAR VOLUME (FL)	MEAN CELL HEMOGLOBIN CONCENTRATION (G/% RBC)
	Mean (–22 SD)	Mean (–22 SD)	Mean (–22 SD)	Mean (–22 SD)
26–30 Weeks' Gestation*	13.4 (11)	41.5 (34.9)	118.2 (106.7)	37.9 (30.6)
28 Weeks' Gestation	14.5	45	120	31
32 Weeks' Gestation	15	47	118	32
Term† (Cord)	16.5 (13.5)	51 (42)	108 (96)	33 (30)
1–3 Days	18.5 (14.5)	56 (45)	108 (95)	33 (29)
2 Weeks	16.6 (13.4)	53 (41)	105 (88)	31.4 (28.1)
1 Month	13.9 (10.7)	44 (33)	101 (91)	31.8 (28.1)
2 Months	11.2 (9.4)	35 (28)	95 (84)	31.8 (28.3)
6 Months	12.6 (11.1)	36 (31)	76 (68)	35 (32.7)
6 Months–2 Years	12 (10.5)	36 (33)	78 (70)	33 (30)
2–6 Years	12.5 (11.5)	37 (34)	81 (75)	34 (31)
6–12 Years	13.5 (11.5)	40 (35)	86 (77)	34 (31)
12–18 Years				
Male	14.5 (13)	43 (36)	88 (78)	34 (31)
Female	14 (12)	41 (37)	90 (78)	34 (31)

*Values are from fetal samplings.
†Younger than age 1 month, capillary Hb exceeds venous: age 1 hour, 3.6 g difference; age 5 days, 2.2 g difference; age 3 weeks, 1.1 g difference.
‡Mean (95% confidence limits).
Used with permission from Robertson, J., & Shilkofski, N. (Eds.). (2005). The Harriet Lane handbook (17th ed.). Philadelphia: Elsevier/Mosby.

Table C-3   Sample Conversions of Pounds and Ounces to Grams*

POUNDS	OUNCES									
	0	1	2	3	4	5	6	7	8	9
0	—	28	57	85	113	142	170	198	227	255
1	454	482	510	539	567	595	624	652	680	709
2	907	936	964	992	1,021	1,049	1,077	1,106	1,134	1,162
3	1,361	1,389	1,417	1,446	1,474	1,503	1,531	1,559	1,588	1,616
4	1,814	1,843	1,871	1,899	1,928	1,956	1,984	2,013	2,041	2,070
5	2,268	2,296	2,325	2,353	2,381	2,410	2,438	2,466	2,495	2,532
6	2,722	2,750	2,778	2,807	2,835	2,863	2,892	2,920	2,948	2,977

*1 ounce = approximately 30 g.

RETIC (%)	WHITE BLOOD CELL/MM³ × 100		PITS (10³/MM³)
	Mean (−2 SD)		Mean (±2 SD)
—	4.4 (2.7)		254
(5–10)	—		(180–327)
(3–10)	—		275
(3–7)	18.1 (9–30)*		290
(1.8–4.6)	18.9 (9.4–34)		290
—	11.5 (5–20)		192
(0.1–1.7)	10.8 (5–19.5)		252
—	—		—
(0.7–2.3)	11.9 (6–17.5)		—
—	10.6 (6–17)		(150–350)
(0.5–1.0)	8.5 (5–15.5)		(150–350)
(0.5–1.0)	8.1 (4.5–13.5)		(150–350)
(0.5–1.0)	7.8 (4.5–13.5)		(150–350)
(0.5–1.0)	7.8 (4.5–13.5)		(150–350)

10	11	12	13	14	15
283	312	340	369	397	425
737	765	794	822	850	879
1,191	1,219	1,247	1,276	1,304	1,332
1,644	1,673	1,701	1,729	1,758	1,786
2,098	2,126	2,155	2,183	2,211	2,240
2,551	2,580	2,608	2,637	2,665	2,693
3,005	3,033	3,062	3,090	3,118	3,147

APPENDIX D
Sources of Additional Information

Arthritis and Musculoskeletal Problems

American College of Rheumatology
2200 Lake Boulevard NE
Atlanta, GA 30319
(404) 633-3777
www.rheumatology.org

Arthritis Foundation
P.O. Box 7669
Atlanta, GA 30357
1-800-283-7800
www.arthritis.org

Lupus Foundation of America
2000 L. Street NW, Suite 410
Washington, DC 20036
(202) 349-1155
www.lupus.org

National Institute of Arthritis and Musculoskeletal and Skin Diseases
1 AMS Circle
Bethesda, MD 20892
(877) 22-NIAMS
www.niams.nih.gov

National Osteoporosis Foundation
1150 17th Street NW, Suite 850
Washington, DC 20036
(202) 223-2226
www.nof.org

United Scleroderma Foundation
300 Rosewood Drive, Suite 105
Danvers, MA 01923
(800) 722-HOPE
www.scleroderma.org

Asthma and Allergy and Respiratory Disease

American Academy of Allergy, Asthma, and Immunology
555 E. Wells Street, Suite 1100
Milwaukee, WI 53202
(414) 272-6071
www.aaaai.org

American College of Allergy, Asthma, and Immunology
85 West Algonquin Road, Suite 550
Arlington Heights, IL 60005
(847) 427-1200
www.acaai.org

American Latex Allergy Association
P.O. Box 198
Slinger, WI 53086
(888) 972-5378
www.latexallergyresources.org

American Lung Association
1301 Pennsylvania Avenue NW, Suite 800
Washington, DC 20004
(800) 548-8252
www.lungusa.org

National Institute of Allergy and Infectious Diseases
6610 Rockledge Drive, MSC 6612
Bethesda, MD 20892
(866) 284-4107
www.niaid.nih.gov

Birth Defects and Genetics

Cleft Palate Foundation
1504 E. Franklin Street, Suite 102
Chapel Hill, NC 27514
(919) 933-9044
www.cleftline.org

Esophageal Atresia/Tracheoesophageal Fistula (EA/TEF) Family and Child Support Connection
www.eatef.org

March of Dimes Birth Defects Foundation
1275 Mamaroneck Avenue
White Plains, NY 10605
(914) 997-4488
www.modimes.org

Cancer

American Cancer Society (ACS)
(800) ACS-2345
www.cancer.org

American Childhood Cancer Organization
P.O. Box 498
Kensington, MD 20895
(885) 858-2226
www.acco.org

Leukemia and Lymphoma Society
1311 Mamaroneck Avenue, Suite 310
White Plains, NY 10605
(914) 949-5213 or (800) 955-4572
www.leukemia-lymphoma.org

National Cancer Institute
(800) 4-CANCER

NCI Public Inquiries
6116 Executive Boulevard, Suite 300
Bethesda, MD 20892
(800) 422-6237
www.cancer.gov

National Coalition of Cancer Survivorship
1010 Wayne Avenue, Suite 770
Silver Spring, MD 20910
(301) 650-9127
www.canceradvocacy.org

National Marrow Donor Program
3001 Broadway Street NE, Suite 100
Minneapolis, MN 55413
(800) 627-7692
www.marrow.org

Diabetes and Endocrinology

American Diabetes Association
1701 N. Beauregard Street
Arlington, VA 22311
(800) 342-2383
www.diabetes.org

American Thyroid Association
6066 Leesburg Pike, Suite 550
Falls Church, VA 22041
(703) 998-8893
www.thyroid.org

Cushing's Support and Research Foundation
60 Robbins Road, #12
Plymouth, MA 02360
www.csrf.net

Juvenile Diabetes Foundation International
26 Broadway
New York, NY 10004
(800) JDF-CURE
www.jdf.org

National Adrenal Diseases Foundation
505 Northern Boulevard
Great Neck, NY 11021
(516) 487-4992
www.nadf.us

Gastrointestinal and Genitourinary Disease

American Association of Kidney Patients
2701 N. Rocky Point Drive, Suite 150
Tampa, FL 33607
(800) 749-AAKP
www.aakp.org

Association of Bladder Exstrophy Community
6737 W. Washington Street, Suite 3265
West Allis, WI 53214
(414) 918-9002
www.bladderexstrophy.com

Canadian Celiac Association
5025 Orbitor Drive, Building 1, Suite 400
Mississauga, ON, Canada L4W 4Y5
(905) 507-6208
www.celiac.ca

Celiac Disease Foundation
20350 Ventura Boulevard, Suite 240
Woodland Hills, CA 91364
(818) 716-1513
www.celiac.org

Celiac Sprue Association
P.O. Box 31700
Omaha, NE 68131
(877) CSA-4CSA
www.csaceliacs.org

Crohn's & Colitis Foundation of America, Inc.
386 Park Avenue South
New York, NY 10016
(800) 932-2423
www.ccfa.org

Cystic Fibrosis Foundation
6931 Arlington Road
Bethesda, MD 20814
(800) FIGHT CF
www.cff.org

National Institute of Diabetes, Digestive and Kidney Diseases
NIH Bldg. 31, Room 9A06
31 Center Drive MSC 2560
Bethesda, MD 20892
www.niddk.nih.gov

National Kidney Foundation
30 E. 33rd Street
New York, NY 10016
(800) 622-9010
www.kidney.org

United Ostomy Association of America
P.O. Box 512
Northfield, MN 55057
(800) 826-0826
www.uoaa.org

US TOO International (prostate cancer support)
5003 Fairview Avenue
Downers Grove, IL 60513
(630) 795-1002
www.ustoo.com

Heart and Blood

American Heart Association
772 Greenville Avenue
Dallas, TX 75231
(800) 242-8721
www.americanheart.org

American Sickle Cell Anemia Association
10900 Carnegie Avenue
Cleveland, OH 44106
(216) 229-8600
www.ascaa.org

Aplastic Anemia Foundation of America
100 Park Avenue, Suite 108
Rockville, MD 20850
(800) 747-2820
www.aamds.org

Children's Heart Society—Canada
Box 52088
Garneau Postal Outlet
Edmonton, AB, Canada T6G 2T5
(780) 454-7665
www.childrensheart.org

Congenital Heart Information Network
101 N. Washington Avenue, Suite 1A
Margate City, NJ 08402
(609) 822-1572
www.tchin.org

Cooley's Anemia Foundation
330 Seventh Avenue, #200
New York, NY 10001
(800) 522-7222
www.thalassemia.org

National Hemophilia Foundation
116 W. 32nd Street, 11th floor
New York, NY 10001
(212) 328-3700
www.hemophilia.org

Mental Health

Anxiety Disorders Association of America
8701 Georgia Avenue
Silver Spring, MD 20910
(240) 485-1001
www.adaa.org

National Alliance for Research on Schizophrenia and Depression
60 Cutter Mill Road, Suite 404
Great Neck, NY 11021
(516) 829-8289
www.narsad.org

National Alliance for Mental Illness
3803 N. Fairfax Dr., Suite 100
Arlington, VA 22203
(800) 950-NAMI
www.nami.org

International Foundation for Research and Education on Depression
P.O. Box 17598
Baltimore, MD 21297
www.ifred.org

Neurology and Neurosurgery

Alzheimer's Association
225 N. Michigan Avenue, 17th Floor
Chicago, IL 60601
(800) 272-3900
www.alz.org

American Brain Tumor Association
8550 W. Bryn Mawr Avenue, Suite 550
Chicago, IL 60631
(800) 886-2282
www.abta.org

Amyotrophic Lateral Sclerosis Association
27001 Agoura Road, Suite 250
Calabasas Hills, CA 91301
(800) 782-4747
www.alsa.org

The ARC (formerly Association for Retarded Citizens)
1825 K Street NW, Suite 1200
Washington, DC 20006
(800) 433-5255
www.thearc.org

Brain Injury Association of America
1608 Spring Hill Road, Suite 110
Vienna, VA 22182
(703) 761-0750
www.biausa.org

Children and Adults with Attention Deficit Disorders (CHADD)
8181 Professional Place, Suite 150
Landover, MD 20785
(301) 306-7070
www.chadd.org

Council for Learning Disabilities
P.O. Box 405
11184 Antioch Road
Overland Park, KS 66210
(913) 491-1011
www.cldinternational.org

Down Syndrome Parent Network
www.downsyndrome.com

Epilepsy Foundation of America
8301 Professional Place
Landover, MD 20785
(800) 332-1000
www.epilepsyfoundation.org

Guillain-Barré Syndrome Foundation International
104½ Forrest Avenue
Narberth, PA P1072
(610) 667-0131
www.gbs-cidp.org

Hydrocephalus Association
4340 East West Highway, Suite 905
Bethesda, MD 20814
(888) 598-3789
www.hydroassoc.org

Joseph P. Kennedy, Jr. Foundation (mental retardation)
1133 19th Street, N.W.
Washington, DC 20036
(202) 393-1250
www.jpkf.org

Learning Disability Association of America
4156 Library Road
Pittsburgh, PA 15234
(412) 341-1515
www.ldanatl.org

Muscular Dystrophy Association
3300 E. Sunrise Drive
Tucson, AZ 85718
www.mda.org

Myasthenia Gravis Foundation, Inc.
355 Lexington Avenue
New York, NY 10017
(800) 541-5454
www.myasthenia.org

National Down Syndrome Society
666 Broadway
New York, NY 10012
(800) 221-4602
www.ndss.org

National Fragile X Foundation
1615 Bonanza Street, Suite 202
Walnut Creek, CA 94596
(800) 688-8765
www.nfxf.org

NIH, Institute on Aging Alzheimer's Disease Education and Referral Center
31 Center Drive, MSC 2292
Bethesda, MD 20892
(800) 438-4380
www.alzheimers.org

National Multiple Sclerosis Society
733 Third Avenue
New York, NY 10017
(800) 344-4867
www.nmss.org

National Parkinson's Foundation
1501 NW 9th Avenue/Bob Hope Road
Miami, FL 33136
(305) 243-6666
www.parkinson.org

National Stroke Association
9709 E. Easter Lane
Centennial, CO 80112
(800) STROKES
www.stroke.org

Spina Bifida Association of America
4590 MacArthur Boulevard NW, Suite 250
Washington, DC 20007
(800) 621-3141
www.sbaa.org

United Cerebral Palsy Association
1825 K Street NW, Suite 600
Washington, DC 20006
(800) 872-5827
www.ucp.org

Prevention and Promotion of Health

American Dietetic Association
120 S. Riverside Street, Suite 2000
Chicago, IL 60606
(800) 877-1600
www.eatright.org

Take Off Pounds Sensibly (TOPS)
4575 S. Fifth Street
P.O. Box 070360
Milwaukee, WI 53207
(414) 482-4620
www.tops.org

Child Welfare Information Gateway
1250 Maryland Avenue SW
Washington, DC 20024
(800) 394-3366
www.childwelfare.gov

National Prevention Information Network (information on STD, TB, and AIDS prevention)
P.O. Box 6003
Rockville, MD 20849
(800) 232-4636
www.cdcnpin.org/scripts/index.asp

Overeaters Anonymous
P.O. Box 44020
Rio Rancho, NM 87174
(505) 891-2664
www.oa.org

Prevent Child Abuse America
228 S, Wabash Avenue
Chicago, IL 60604
(800) CHILDREN
www.preventchildabuse.org

Centers for Disease Control and Prevention
1600 Clifton Rd.
Atlanta, GA 30333
(800) 232-4636
www.cdc.gov

Sexually Transmitted Diseases

American Social Health Association
P.O. Box 13827
Research Triangle Park, NC 27709
(919) 361-8400
www.ashastd.org

CDC Sexually Transmitted Disease
1600 Clifton Road
Atlanta, GA 30333
(800) CDC-INFO
www.cdc.gov/STD

Centers for Disease Control and Prevention National STD and AIDS Hotline
(800) 227-8922

National Herpes Hotline
(919) 361-8488

Vision/Hearing

American Council for the Blind
2200 Wilson Boulevard, Suite 650
Arlington, VA 22201
(800) 424-8666
www.acb.org

American Foundation for the Blind
2 Penn Plaza, Suite 1102
New York, NY 10121
(800) 232-5463
www.afb.org

American Speech-Language-Hearing Association
2200 Research Boulevard
Rockville, MD 20850
(800) 638-8255
www.asha.org

Prevent Blindness America
211 W. Wacker Drive, Suite 1700
Chicago, IL 60606
(800) 331-2020
www.preventblindness.org

Women's Health

Endometriosis Association
8585 N. 76th Place
Milwaukee, WI 53223
(414) 355-2200
www.endometriosisassn.org

National Women's Health Information Center
200 Independence Avenue SW
Washington, DC 20201
(202) 690-7650
www.womenshealth.gov

North American Menopause Society
5900 Landerbrook Drive, Suite 390
Mayfield Heights, OH 44124
(440) 442-7550
www.menopause.org

Other

American Academy of Family Physicians Health Information
www.familydoctor.org

American Academy of Medical Acupuncture
1970 E. Grand Avenue, Suite 330
El Segundo, CA 90245
(310) 364-0193
www.medicalacupuncture.org

Baby Center (new and expectant parents)
163 Freelon Street
San Francisco, CA 94107
(866) 241-2229
www.babycenter.com

Caring Connections (National Hospice and Palliative Care Organizations)
(800) 658-8898
www.caringinfo.org

First Candle (miscarriage, stillbirth, and SIDS)
1314 Bedford Avenue, Suite 210
Baltimore, MD 21208
(800) 221-7437
www.firstcandle.org

MedicAlert Foundation
2323 Colorado Avenue
Turlock, CA 95382
(888) 633-4298
www.medicalert.org

National Information Center for Children and Youth with Disabilities (NICHCY)
1825 Connecticut Avenue NW, Suite 700
Washington, DC 20009
(800) 695-0285
www.nichcy.org

National Organization of Mothers of Twins Clubs, Inc.
2000 Mallory Lane, Suite 130-600
Franklin, TN 37067
(248) 231-4480
www.nomotc.org

National Organization for Rare Diseases
55 Kenosia Avenue
Danbury, CT 06810
(203) 744-0100
www.rarediseases.org

ART CREDITS

These illustrations were borrowed from Lippincott Williams & Wilkins sources.

CHAPTER 5

In Adult Physical Assessment: Figures 1, 8, 9, 10, 12, 14, 15, 33, 34, 35, 45, 46: Weber, J., and Kelley, J. (2003). *Health assessment in nursing* (2nd ed.). Philadelphia: Lippincott Williams & Wilkins. Photographs by Barbara Proud.

Figures 5-2, 5-5, 5-11,5-41: Craven, R., and Hirnle, C. (2000). *Fundamentals of nursing: Human health and function* (3rd ed.). Philadelphia: Lippincott Williams & Wilkins.

Figures 5-3, 5-19, 5-20, 5-28, 5-32, 5-36, 5-38, 5-39, 5-40: Bickley, L. (2003). *Bates' guide to physical examination and history taking* (8th ed.). Philadelphia: Lippincott Williams & Wilkins.

Figures 5-6, 5-7, 5-29: Smeltzer, S., and Bare, B. (2000). *Brunner and Suddarth's textbook of medical-surgical nursing* (9th ed.). Philadelphia: Lippincott Williams & Wilkins.

CHAPTER 6

Figure 6-2: Smeltzer, S., and Bare, B. (2000). *Brunner and Suddarth's textbook of medical-surgical nursing* (9th ed.). Philadelphia: Lippincott Williams & Wilkins.

CHAPTER 7

Figure 7-5: Smeltzer, S., and Bare, B. (2000). *Brunner and Suddarth's textbook of medical-surgical nursing* (9th ed.). Philadelphia: Lippincott Williams & Wilkins.

CHAPTER 8

Figure 8-1: Anatomical Chart Company.

CHAPTER 9

Box 9-2 (photographs): Weber, J., and Kelley, J. (2003). *Health assessment in nursing* (2nd ed.). Philadelphia: Lippincott Williams & Wilkins. Photographs by Barbara Proud.

Figure 9-2: Smeltzer, S., and Bare, B. (2000). *Brunner and Suddarth's textbook of medical-surgical nursing* (9th ed.). Philadelphia: Lippincott Williams & Wilkins.

Figure 9-4: Anatomical Chart Company.

CHAPTER 10

Figure 10-2A: Craven, R., and Hirnle, C. (2000). *Fundamentals of nursing: Human health and function* (3rd ed.). Philadelphia: Lippincott Williams & Wilkins.

Figure 10-4: Smeltzer, S., and Bare, B. (2000). *Brunner and Suddarth's textbook of medical-surgical nursing* (9th ed.). Philadelphia: Lippincott Williams & Wilkins.

Figure 10-5: Burton, G.C., and Hodgkin, J.E. (Eds.). (1984). *Respiratory care: A guide to practice* (2nd ed.). Philadelphia: J.B. Lippincott.

CHAPTER 12

Figure 12-7: Redrawn after Purcell, J.A., and Giffin, P.A. "Percutaneous transluminal coronary angioplasty." *American Journal of Nursing* 9:1620-1626, 1981.

In Procedure Guidelines 12-5: Smeltzer, S., and Bare, B. (2000). *Brunner and Suddarth's textbook of medical-surgical nursing* (9th ed.). Philadelphia: Lippincott Williams & Wilkins.

CHAPTER 13

Figure 13-1: Anatomical Chart Company.

Figure 13-3: Chaffee, E.E., and Greisheimer, E.M. *Basic physiology and anatomy* (3rd ed.). Philadelphia: J.B. Lippincott.

Figure 13-6: Porth, C.M. (2005). *Pathophysiology: Concepts of altered health states* (7th ed.). Philadelphia: Lippincott Williams & Wilkins.

CHAPTER 14

Figure 14-4: Smeltzer, S., and Bare, B. (2000). *Brunner and Suddarth's textbook of medical-surgical nursing* (9th ed.). Philadelphia: Lippincott Williams & Wilkins.

CHAPTER 15

Figure 15-1: Redrawn after Diepenbrock, N.H. (2004). *Quick reference to critical care* (2nd ed.). Philadelphia: Lippincott Williams & Wilkins.

Figures 15-3, 15-9: Porth, C.M. (1998). *Pathophysiology: Concepts of altered health states* (5th ed.). Philadelphia: Lippincott Williams & Wilkins.

Figure 15-6: LifeART image. (2004).

Figure 15-7: Anatomical Chart Company.

Figures 15-8, 15-10: Smeltzer, S., and Bare, B. (2000). *Brunner and Suddarth's textbook of medical-surgical nursing* (9th ed.). Philadelphia: Lippincott Williams & Wilkins.

Figure 15-12: Chaffee, E.E., and Greisheimer, E.M. *Basic physiology and anatomy* (3rd ed.). Philadelphia: J.B. Lippincott.

CHAPTER 16
Figure 16-2; in Procedure Guidelines 16-1: Smeltzer, S., and Bare, B. (2000). *Brunner and Suddarth's textbook of medical-surgical nursing* (9th ed.). Philadelphia: Lippincott Williams & Wilkins.

CHAPTER 17
Figure 17-2, 17-7: Smeltzer, S., and Bare, B. (2000). *Brunner and Suddarth's textbook of medical-surgical nursing* (9th ed.). Philadelphia: Lippincott Williams & Wilkins.

Figure 17-3: Galen, B. (1997). "Chronic recurrent sinusitis: Recognition and treatment." *Lippincott's Primary Care Practice,* 1(2), 183–197.

Figure 17-4: Bickley, L. (2003). *Bates' guide to physical examination and history taking* (8th ed.). Philadelphia: Lippincott Williams & Wilkins.

CHAPTER 18
Figure 18-3: Anatomical Chart Company.

Figure 18-6: Bickley, L. (2003). *Bates' guide to physical examination and history taking* (8th ed.). Philadelphia: Lippincott Williams & Wilkins.

Figures 18-10, 18-12: Rubin, E., and Farber, J.L. (1999). *Pathology* (3rd ed.). Philadelphia: Lippincott Williams & Wilkins.

Figures 18-11, 18-13: Smeltzer, S., and Bare, B. (2000). *Brunner and Suddarth's textbook of medical-surgical nursing* (9th ed.). Philadelphia: Lippincott Williams & Wilkins.

CHAPTER 19
Figure 19-1: Perrillo, R.P., & Regenstein, F.G. (1996). Viral and immune hepatitis. In Kelley, W.N. (Ed.). Textbook of internal medicine (3rd ed.). Philadelphia: J.B. Lippincott.

Figures 19-2, 19-4: Anatomical Chart Company asset.

In Procedure Guidelines 19-2: Smeltzer, S., and Bare, B. (2000). *Brunner and Suddarth's textbook of medical-surgical nursing* (9th ed.). Philadelphia: Lippincott Williams & Wilkins.

CHAPTER 21
Figure 21-1: Porth, C. (1998). *Pathophysiology: Concepts of altered health states* (5th ed.). Philadelphia: Lippincott-Raven Publishers.

Figures 21-2, 21-3, 21-4, 21-8, 21-9: Smeltzer, S., and Bare, B. (2000). *Brunner and Suddarth's textbook of medical-surgical nursing* (9th ed.). Philadelphia: Lippincott Williams & Wilkins.

Figure 21-5: Anatomical Chart Company.

Figure 21-6: Rubin, E., and Farber, J.L. (1999). *Pathology* (3rd ed.). Philadelphia: Lippincott Williams & Wilkins.

Figure 21-7: LifeART image.

CHAPTER 22
Figure 22-1: Premkumar, K. *The Massage Connection Anatomy and Physiology.* Baltimore: Lippincott Williams and Wilkins.

Figures 22-3, 22-5; in Procedure Guidelines 22-1: Smeltzer, S., and Bare, B. (2000). *Brunner and Suddarth's textbook of medical-surgical nursing* (9th ed.). Philadelphia: Lippincott Williams & Wilkins.

Figure 22-6: Reeder, S., Martin, L., and Koniak-Griffin, D. (1997). *Maternity nursing: Family, newborn, and women's health care* (18th ed.). Philadelphia: Lippincott-Raven Publishers.

Figures 22-8, 22-9: Anatomical Chart Company.

CHAPTER 24
Figure 24-3: Anatomical Chart Company.

Figure 24-4: Smeltzer, S., and Bare, B. (2000). *Brunner and Suddarth's textbook of medical-surgical nursing* (9th ed.). Philadelphia: Lippincott Williams & Wilkins.

Figure 24-5: Rubin, E., and Farber, J.L. (1999). *Pathology* (3rd ed.). Philadelphia: Lippincott Williams & Wilkins.

CHAPTER 25
Figure 25-2: Cameron, B.L. (2002). "Making diabetes management routine." *American Journal of Nursing*, 102(2), 27.

In Procedure Guidelines 25-2: Smeltzer, S., and Bare, B. (2000). *Brunner and Suddarth's textbook of medical-surgical nursing* (9th ed.). Philadelphia: Lippincott Williams & Wilkins.

CHAPTER 28
Figure 28-1: Anatomical Chart Company.

In Patient Education Guidelines: Nettina, S.M. (1997). "Patient education: Using an inhaler and a spacer." *Lippincott's Primary Care Practice*, 1(2), 231-232.

CHAPTER 32
Figure 32-1: Smeltzer, S., and Bare, B. (2000). *Brunner and Suddarth's textbook of medical-surgical nursing* (9th ed.). Philadelphia: Lippincott Williams & Wilkins. Photo by Barbara Proud.

Figures 32-2, 32-5, 32-6, 32-7, 32-8, 32-9, 32-10, 32-11, 32-12: Smeltzer, S., and Bare, B. (2000). *Brunner and Suddarth's textbook of medical-surgical nursing* (9th ed.). Philadelphia: Lippincott Williams & Wilkins.

CHAPTER 33
Figures 33-1, 33-3, 33-4, 33-5, 33-6A, 33-6B: Smeltzer, S., and Bare, B. (2000). *Brunner and Suddarth's textbook of medical-surgical nursing* (9th ed.). Philadelphia: Lippincott Williams & Wilkins.

Figure 33-6C: Porth, C.M. (1998). *Pathophysiology: Concepts of altered health states* (5th ed.). Philadelphia: Lippincott Williams & Wilkins.

CHAPTER 35

Figure 35-1: Smeltzer, S., and Bare, B. (2000). *Brunner and Suddarth's textbook of medical-surgical nursing* (9th ed.). Philadelphia: Lippincott Williams & Wilkins.

CHAPTER 36

Figures 36-6, 36-8: Pillitteri, A. (1999). *Maternal and child health nursing: Care of the childbearing and childrearing family* (3rd ed.). Philadelphia: Lippincott-Raven.

CHAPTER 37

Figures 37-4, 37-6: Pillitteri, A. (1999). *Maternal and child health nursing: care of the childbearing and childrearing family* (3rd ed.). Philadelphia: Lippincott-Raven.

Figure 37-10: Pillitteri, A. (2003). *Maternal and child health nursing: Care of the childbearing and childrearing family* (4th ed.). Philadelphia: Lippincott-Raven.

Figure 37-11: LifeART image.

CHAPTER 38

Figures 38-1, 38-3, 38-4: Reeder, S., Martin, L., and Koniak-Griffin, D. (1997). *Maternity nursing: Family newborn, and women's health care* (18th ed.). Philadelphia: Lippincott-Raven Publishers.

CHAPTER 39

Figures 39-1, 39-2, 39-3, 39-4, 39-7, 39-8; in Procedure Guidelines 39-1: Pillitteri, A. (1999). *Maternal and child health nursing: Care of the childbearing and childrearing family* (3rd ed.). Philadelphia: Lippincott-Raven.

Figure 39-6: Reeder, S., Martin, L., and Koniak-Griffin, D. (1997). *Maternity nursing: Family newborn, and women's health care* (18th ed.). Philadelphia: Lippincott-Raven Publishers.

CHAPTER 41

In pediatric physical assessment (first photograph): Pillitteri, A. (1999). *Maternal and child health nursing: Care of the childbearing and childrearing family* (3rd ed.). Philadelphia: Lippincott-Raven.

CHAPTER 42

Figure 42-3A, B, C: Pillitteri, A. (1999). *Maternal and child health nursing: Care of the childbearing and childrearing family* (3rd ed.). Philadelphia: Lippincott-Raven.

CHAPTER 43

In Procedure Guidelines 43-1 (photograph) and 43-2: Pillitteri, A. (1999). *Maternal and child health nursing: Care of the childbearing and childrearing family* (3rd ed.). Philadelphia: Lippincott-Raven. Photograph by Barbara Proud.

CHAPTER 44

Figure 44-2: Pillitteri, A. (1999). *Maternal and child health nursing: Care of the childbearing and childrearing family* (3rd ed.). Philadelphia: Lippincott-Raven.

CHAPTER 46

Figures 46-1, 46-2, 46-3: Pillitteri, A. (1999). *Maternal and child health nursing: Care of the childbearing and childrearing family* (3rd ed.). Philadelphia: Lippincott-Raven.

CHAPTER 47

Figure 47-1: Dershewitz, R.A. (1988). *Ambulatory pediatric care.* Philadelphia: J.B. Lippincott.

Figure 47-2: Pillitteri, A. (1999). *Maternal and child health nursing: Care of the childbearing and childrearing family* (3rd ed.). Philadelphia: Lippincott-Raven.

CHAPTER 48

Figure 48-1: Moore, K.L., & Dalley, A.F. (1999). *Clinically oriented anatomy* (4th ed.). Philadelphia: Lippincott Williams & Wilkins.

Figure 48-5: Rubin, E., & Farber, J.L. (1999). *Pathology* (3rd ed.). Philadelphia: Lippincott Williams & Wilkins.

Figure 48-6: Anatomical Chart Company.

Figure 48-7: LifeArt image.

CHAPTER 49

Figure 49-1: Smeltzer, S., and Bare, B. (2000). *Brunner and Suddarth's textbook of medical-surgical nursing* (9th ed.). Philadelphia: Lippincott Williams & Wilkins.

Figure 49-2B: Sadler, T. (2003). *Langman's medical embryology* (9th ed.). Philadelphia: Lippincott Williams & Wilkins.

Figure 49-3: Pillitteri, A. (1999). Maternal and child health nursing: Care of the childbearing and childrearing family, 3rd edition. Philadelphia: Lippincott-Raven.

CHAPTER 50

Figure 50-1: Anatomical Chart Company.

CHAPTER 52

Figure 52-1: Pillitteri, A. (1999). *Maternal and child health nursing: Care of the childbearing and childrearing family* (3rd ed.). Philadelphia: Lippincott-Raven.

CHAPTER 53

Figure 53-1: Pillitteri, A. (1999). *Maternal and child health nursing: Care of the childbearing and childrearing family* (3rd ed.). Philadelphia: Lippincott-Raven.

CHAPTER 54

Figure 54-3: Anatomical Chart Company.

Figure 54-4: Jackson, D.B., & Saunders, R.B. (1993). *Child health nursing.* Philadelphia: Lippincott Williams & Wilkins.

Figure 54-6; in Procedure Guidelines 54-2 (Buck's extension, Balanced suspension): Pillitteri, A. (1999). *Maternal and child health nursing: Care of the childbearing and childrearing family* (3rd ed.). Philadelphia: Lippincott-Raven.

INDEX

Note: Page numbers with b indicate boxes; those with f indicate figures; and those with t indicate tables.